Cancer Medicine

Cancer Medicine

Third Edition

VOLUME 1

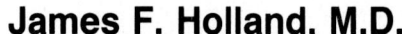

James F. Holland, M.D.
Jane B. and Jack R. Aron Professor of
    Neoplastic Diseases
Chairman, Department of Neoplastic Diseases;
    Professor of Medicine
Director, Derald H. Ruttenberg Cancer Center
Mt. Sinai Medical Center
New York, New York

Emil Frei III, M.D.
Director and Physician-in-Chief, Emeritus; Chief,
    Division of Cancer Pharmacology,
Dana-Farber Cancer Institute
Richard and Susan Smith Professor of Medicine
Harvard Medical School
Boston, Massachusetts

Robert C. Bast, Jr., M.D.
Wellcome Clinical Professor of Medicine in Honor of
    R. Wayne Rundles;
Director, Duke Comprehensive Cancer Center
Duke University Medical Center
Durham, North Carolina

Donald W. Kufe, M.D.
Chief, Laboratory of Clinical Pharmacology
Dana-Farber Cancer Institute
Professor of Medicine
Harvard Medical School
Boston, Massachusetts

Donald L. Morton, M.D.
Medical Director and Surgeon-In-Chief
John Wayne Cancer Institute at St. John's Hospital
    and Health Center
Santa Monica, California
Professor Emeritus, Department of Surgery/Oncology
UCLA School of Medicine
Los Angeles, California

Ralph R. Weichselbaum, M.D.
Harold H. Hines Jr. Professor and Chairman
Department of Radiation and Cellular Oncology,
    University of Chicago Hospital
Director, Chicago Tumor Institute
University of Chicago
Chicago, Illinois

Lea & Febiger • Philadelphia • London • 1993

Lea & Febiger
Box 3024
200 Chester Field Parkway
Malvern, Pennsylvania   19355-9725
U.S.A.
(215) 251-2230

Executive Editor—John Spahr, Jr.
Production Manager—Samuel A. Rondinelli
Project Editor—Dorothy A. DiRienzi

First Edition, 1973
   Reprinted, 1974
Second Edition, 1982
   Reprinted, 1982
Third Edition, 1993

NOTE: Although the author(s) and the publisher have taken reasonable steps to ensure the accuracy of the drug information included in this text before publication, drug information may change without notice and readers are advised to consult the manufacturer's packaging inserts before prescribing medications.

Library of Congress Cataloging-in-Publication Data

Cancer medicine / [edited by] James F. Holland . . . [et al.].—3rd ed.
      p.   cm.
   Includes bibliographical references and index.
   ISBN 0-8121-1422-1
   1. Cancer.   I. Holland, James F., 1925–
   [DNLM: 1. Neoplasms.   QZ 200 C21536]
RC261.C2735   1992
616.99′4—dc20
DNLM/DLC
for Library of Congress   91-25591
                                                                      CIP

Print number: 5   4   3   2   1

Reprints of chapters may be purchased from Lea & Febiger in quantities of 100 or more.
Contact Sally Grande in the Sales Department.

Preface

When the first edition of Cancer Medicine appeared in 1973, contemporaneously with the creation of medical oncology as a specialized discipline, it dealt in a comprehensive manner with accumulated and emerging knowledge that comprised the field. The second edition extended that enterprise.

This third edition is entirely new. The editorship has been triply expanded, the better to cover the much broader scientific and clinical aspects of modern oncology. The multidisciplinary nature of modern oncologic care has led to consideration of each clinical topic from the broader perspective of surgical and radiation oncology together with classic medical oncology. The authors, almost entirely new, were invited to participate because of their preeminence and special competence in their specific areas. The book is intended to provide the scientific foundations from which cancer medicine is derived. The new information about the cancer cell, the molecular mechanisms of the cancer process, and the impact of neoplasia on host systems form bedrock on which to build clinical understanding. The principles that underlie the diagnosis and treatment of patients with cancer are presented in several subsequent sections that are essential for a balanced and complete approach. The organ systems that are affected by cancer are then addressed in terms of their specific tumors, with multidisciplinary consideration of each neoplasm throughout its course. Complications of cancer and its treatment are presented by organ system, as are oncologic emergencies. Lastly, the relationship of the oncologist to government, to ethical standards, and to the information revolution are included.

Pediatric oncology has become a separate and distinct discipline. An extended consideration of pediatric oncology is nonetheless included so that the reader can understand the unique features of cancer in children, many of whom will now reach adulthood, and not as a reminescence of earlier times when medical oncologists were also expected to care for children. We thank Dr. G. Denman Hammond for his help with this.

This treatise aspires to serve as the premier single source on cancer that a reader can obtain. From it, a conscientious physician can learn in depth about cancer in general and about a specific disease in particular. With it, a student can embark on a wondrous journey of great intellectual challenge. In its pages, cancer scientists can locate their highly focused area of research with relationship to other endeavors and to its implications for human cancer. As a background source, oncology nurses can better understand the diseases that afflict the patients for whom they care. Cancer Medicine, 3rd edition, is also available as an electronic book, with its many advantages for immediate cross referencing, updating, and accessibility.

The editors are grateful to the authors whose scholarship defines the quality of the book. We are grateful to John Spahr, Jr., whose publishing instincts and commitments have been impeccable. We express our appreciation to Patricia Byron-Katzoff for her expert editorial assistance.

The editors are individually indebted to their patients, students, and colleagues for providing them with ongoing oncologic education, stimulus, and purpose. They are also mindful, with love, of the tolerance and support of their families despite the diversion of much personal time and energy to this undertaking.

James F. Holland
Emil Frei III
Robert C. Bast, Jr.
Donald W. Kufe
Donald L. Morton
Ralph R. Weichselbaum

Contributors

Stuart A. Aaronson, M.D.
Chief, Laboratory of Cellular and Molecular Biology, National Cancer Institute, Bethesda, Maryland

George Acs, M.D., Ph.D.
Professor of Biochemistry and Neoplastic Diseases, Mount Sinai School of Medicine, New York, New York

Edward P. Ambinder, M.D.
Associate Clinical Professor of Neoplastic Diseases and Medicine, Divisions of Hematology and Medical Oncology, Mount Sinai School of Medicine, New York, New York

Kenneth Anderson, M.D.
Associate Professor of Medicine, Harvard Medical School; Medical Director, Blood Component Laboratory, Dana-Farber Cancer Institute, Boston, Massachusetts

Karen H. Antman, M.D.
Associate Professor of Medicine, Division of Medicine, Harvard Medical School; Dana-Farber Cancer Institute, Boston, Massachusetts

Steven D. Averbuch, M.D.
Associate Director, Clinical Research, Merck Research Laboratories, Rahway, New Jersey; Assistant Clinical Professor, Department of Neoplastic Diseases, Mount Sinai School of Medicine, New York, New York

K. D. Bagshawe, M.D., F.R.S.
Professor Emeritus in Medical Oncology, Charing Cross and Westminster Medical School, London, England

John Baillie, M.B., Ch.B., F.R.C.P.
Assistant Professor of Medicine; Associate Director of Endoscopy, Duke University Medical Center, Durham, North Carolina

R. W. Baldwin, Ph.D., F.R.C. Path.
Professor, Director of Cancer Research Campaign Laboratories, University of Nottingham, Nottingham, England

Erik Barquist, M.D.
Department of Surgery, UCLA School of Medicine, Los Angeles, California

Lawrence W. Bassett, M.D.
Professor of Radiological Sciences, UCLA School of Medicine and Jonsson Comprehensive Cancer Center at UCLA; Director, Iris Cantor Center for Breast Imaging, UCLA Medical Center, Los Angeles, California

Robert C. Bast, Jr., M.D.
Wellcome Clinical Professor of Medicine in Honor of R. Wayne Rundles; Director, Duke Comprehensive Cancer Center, Duke University Medical Center, Durham, North Carolina

Poonam Batra, M.D., F.C.C.P.
Associate Clinical Professor, Department of Radiological Sciences, UCLA School of Medicine, Los Angeles, California

Kenneth A. Bauer, M.D.
Assistant Professor of Medicine, Department of Medicine, Harvard Medical School; Clinical Research Fellow, Department of Medicine, Beth Israel Hospital, Boston, Massachusetts

Stephen B. Baylin, M.D.
Professor of Oncology; Professor of Medicine, The Johns Hopkins Oncology Center, Baltimore, Maryland

William T. Beck, Ph.D.
Member, Department of Biochemical and Clinical Pharmacology, St. Jude Children's Research Hospital; Professor of Pharmacology, Department of Pharmacology, University of Tennessee, College of Medicine, Memphis, Tennessee

Robert M. Bell, Ph.D.
James B. Duke Professor of Biochemistry, Deputy Director, Duke Comprehensive Cancer Center; Head, Section of Cell Growth, Regulation and Oncogenesis, Duke University Medical Center, Durham, North Carolina

Robert S. Benjamin, M.D.
Professor of Medicine, Internist, and Chief, Melanoma/Sarcoma Section, Department of Medical Oncology, The University of Texas M. D. Anderson Cancer Center, Houston, Texas

Jonathan S. Berek, M.D.
Professor and Director, Division of GYN Oncology, UCLA School of Medicine, Los Angeles, California

Leslie Bernstein, Ph.D.
Associate Professor of Preventive Medicine, University of Southern California School of Medicine, Los Angeles, California

Steven H. Bernstein, M.D.
Instructor in Medicine, Harvard Medical School; Clinical Associate, Dana-Farber Cancer Institute, Boston, Massachusetts

Joseph R. Bertino, M.D.
Chairman and Member, Program of Molecular Pharmacology and Therapeutics; American Cancer Society Professor of Pharmacology and Medicine, Memorial Sloan-Kettering Cancer Center, New York, New York

William Bloomer, M.D.
Claude Worthington Benedum Professor of Radiation Oncology, University of Pittsburgh School of Medicine; Chairman, Department of Radiation Oncology, Joint Radiation Oncology Center, Pittsburgh Cancer Institute, Pittsburgh, Pennsylvania

Gerald P. Bodey, M.D.
Professor of Medicine and Chairman, Department of Medical Specialties; Chief, Section of Infectious Diseases, The University of Texas M. D. Anderson Cancer Center, Houston, Texas

Ernest C. Borden, M.D.
American Cancer Society Professor of Medicine and Microbiology; Director, Cancer Center of the Medical College of Wisconsin, Milwaukee, Wisconsin

Cynthia Boxrud, M.D.
Fellow, Ophthalmic Oncology and Orbital Disease, Cornell University Medical Center, New York Hospital, New York, New York

Cinda M. Boyer, Ph.D.
Assistant Medical Research Professor, Division of Hematology/Oncology, Duke University Medical Center, Durham, North Carolina

Edward C. Bradley, M.D.
Vice President, Research and Development, Sterling Oncology, Great Valley, Pennsylvania

Edward Bresnick, Ph.D.
James C. Chilcott Professor and Chairman, Department of Pharmacology and Toxicology; Deputy Director, Norris Cotton Cancer Center, Dartmouth Medical School, Hanover, New Hampshire

Nicholas Bruchovsky, M.D., Ph.D., F.R.C.P.(C)
Head, Department of Cancer Endocrinology, British Columbia Cancer Agency; Professor of Medicine, Department of Medicine, University of British Columbia, Vancouver, Canada

Howard W. Bruckner, M.D.
Professor of Neoplastic Diseases; Attending Physician, Mount Sinai Medical Center, New York, New York

Nancy Bunin, M.D.
Assistant Professor of Pediatrics, Division of Oncology and Children's Cancer Research Center, Children's Hospital of Philadelphia, Department of Pediatrics, The University of Pennsylvania, Philadelphia, Pennsylvania

Patrick A. Burch, M.D.
Instructor in Oncology, Mayo Medical School, Rochester, Minnesota

Ellyn Rackoff Bushkin, R.N., M.S., O.C.N.
Director, Clinical Nursing, Mount Sinai Medical Center, New York, New York; Chairman, The Board of Trustees, Oncology Nursing Foundation, Pittsburgh, Pennsylvania

V. S. Byers, M.D., Ph.D.
Associate Professor, Department of Dermatology, University of California, San Francisco; Special Lecturer, Cancer Research Campaign Laboratories, University of Nottingham, England

Blake Cady, M.D.
Associate Professor of Surgery, Harvard Medical School; Chief, Surgical Oncology, New England Deaconess Hospital, Boston, Massachusetts

M. Caggana, B.S., Sc.D.
Wadsworth Fellow, Wadsworth Center for Laboratories and Research, Albany, New York

Judith Campisi, M.D.
Senior Scientist, Lawrence Berkeley Laboratory, University of California, Division of Cell and Molecular Biology, Berkeley, California

George Canellos, M.D.
William Rosenberg Professor of Medicine, Harvard Medical School; Chief, Division of Clinical Oncology, Dana-Farber Cancer Institute; Physician, Brigham and Women's Hospital, Boston, Massachusetts

Robert L. Capizzi, M.D.
Executive Vice President, Worldwide Research and Development, U.S. Bioscience, Inc., West Conshohocken, Pennsylvania; Adjunct Professor of Medicine, Bowman Gray School of Medicine, Wake Forest University, Winston-Salem, North Carolina

R. W. Carlson, M.D.
Assistant Professor of Medicine, Division of Oncology, Stanford University, Stanford, California

C. Humberto Carrasco, M.D.
Professor of Radiology, The University of Texas, M. D. Anderson Cancer Center, Houston, Texas

Carol E. Cass, Ph.D.
Professor of Biochemistry and Senior Research Scientist, National Cancer Institute of Canada, Department of Biochemistry, University of Alberta, Edmonton, Alberta, Canada

A. Philippe Chahinian, M.D.
Professor of Neoplastic Diseases, Professor of Medicine, Mount Sinai Medical Center, New York, New York

Chusilp Charnsangavej, M.D.
Professor and Deputy Department Chairman for Academic Affairs, Department of Diagnostic Radiology, The University of Texas, M. D. Anderson Cancer Center, Houston, Texas

George T. Y. Chen, Ph.D.
Professor and Director, Medical Physics Section, Department of Radiation and Cellular Oncology, University of Chicago Hospital, Chicago, Illinois

Yung Chi Cheng, M.D.
Henry Bronson Professor of Pharmacology, Yale University School of Medicine, New Haven, Connecticut

George P. Chrousos, M.D.
Chief, Pediatric Endocrinology Section, National Institute of Child Health and Human Development, National Institutes of Health, Bethesda, Maryland

Kenneth C. Chu, Ph.D.
Health Scientist Administrator, Early Detection Branch, Division of Cancer Prevention and Control, National Cancer Institute, Bethesda, Maryland

John A. Cidlowski, Ph.D.
Professor, Departments of Physiology and Biochemistry and Biophysics, Lineberger Comprehensive Cancer Center, Cell Biology Program, University of North Carolina-Chapel Hill, Chapel Hill, North Carolina

James E. Cleaver, Ph.D.
Professor of Radiology (Radiobiology), Laboratory of Radiobiology and Environmental Health, University of California, San Francisco, California

Steven K. Clinton, M.D., Ph.D.
Instructor in Medicine, Harvard Medical School; Dana-Farber Cancer Institute, Boston, Massachusetts

Jeffrey I. Cohen, M.D.
Senior Staff Fellow, Laboratory of Clinical Investigation, National Institute of Allergy and Infectious Diseases, National Institutes of Health, Bethesda, Maryland

C. N. Coleman, M.D.
Professor and Chairman, Joint Center for Radiation Therapy, Harvard Medical School, Boston, Massachusetts

Michael Colvin, M.D.
Professor of Oncology and Medicine; Chief, Division of Pharmacology and Experimental Therapeutics, The Johns Hopkins University School of Medicine, Baltimore, Maryland

Ana Maria Comaru-Schally, Ph.D.
Professor of Clinical Medicine, Tulane University School of Medicine, New Orleans, Louisiana

Veronica L. Conley, Ph.D.
Health Scientist Administrator, Early Detection Branch, Division of Cancer Prevention and Control, National Cancer Institute, Bethesda, Maryland

James L. Connolly, M.D.
Associate Professor of Pathology, Harvard Medical School; Consultant in Breast Pathology, Dana-Farber Cancer Institute; Associate Pathologist and Associate Director of Surgical Pathology; Director of the Immunopathology Laboratory, Beth Israel Hospital, Boston, Massachusetts

Michael Cooper, M.D.
Senior Investigator, Clinical Pharmacology Branch, Clinical Oncology Program, Division of Cancer Treatment, National Cancer Institute, Bethesda, Maryland

Patricia H. Cotanch, R.N., Ph.D.
Professor, School of Nursing, Georgia State University; Assistant Professor, Emory University School of Medicine, Atlanta, Georgia

Peter B. Cotton, M.D., F.R.C.P.
Professor of Medicine; Chief of Endoscopy, Duke University Medical Center, Durham, North Carolina

Kenneth H. Cowan, M.D., Ph.D.
Head, Medical Breast Cancer Section, Medicine Branch, Clinical Oncology Branch, National Cancer Institute, Bethesda, Maryland

Kevin A. Craig, B.A.
Director, Medical and Scientific Communications, Roswell Park Cancer Institute, Buffalo, New York

William T. Creasman, M.D.
Sims-Hester Professor and Chairman, Department of Obstetrics and Gynecology, Medical University of South Carolina, Charleston, South Carolina

Christopher P. Crum, M.D.
Associate Professor of Pathology, Harvard Medical School; Director, Women's and Perinatal Pathology Division, Department of Pathology, Brigham and Women's Hospital, Boston, Massachusetts

Gregory A. Curt, M.D.
Associate Director of Clinical Oncology Program; Clinical Director, Division of Cancer Treatment, National Cancer Institute, Bethesda, Maryland

Giulio J. D'Angio, M.D.
Professor of Radiation Oncology; Professor of Pediatric Oncology; Professor of Radiology, University of Pennsylvania School of Medicine; Vice Chairman and Clinical Director, Department of Radiation Oncology, Hospital of the University of Pennsylvania, Philadelphia, Pennsylvania

Leslie J. DeGroot, M.D.
Professor of Medicine, Thyroid Study Unit, Department of Medicine, The University of Chicago Medical Center, Chicago, Illinois

Jean B. deKernion, M.D.
Professor of Surgery/Urology; Chief, Division of Urology, UCLA School of Medicine, Los Angeles, California

Thomas F. DeLaney, M.D.
Senior Investigator, Radiation Oncology Branch, Clinical Oncology Program, Division of Cancer Treatment, National Cancer Institute, Bethesda, Maryland

Alon Dembo, M.B., F.R.C.P.(C)*
Head, Division of Radiation Oncology; Professor, Departments of Radiology and Obstetrics and Gynecology, University of Toronto, Toronto-Bayview Regional Cancer Center, North York, Ontario, Canada

Eugene R. DeSombre, Ph.D.
Professor, Ben May Institute, University of Chicago, Chicago, Illinois

Marguerite Donoghue, R.N., M.N.
Vice President, Research and Regulatory Affairs, Capitol Associates, Inc.; Oncology Clinical Nurse Specialist, Washington, D.C.

Harold O. Douglass, Jr., M.D.
Associate Professor, Department of Research Surgery, State University of New York at Buffalo; Chief, Gastrointestinal Oncology and Associate Chief, Surgical Oncology, Roswell Park Cancer Institute, Buffalo, New York

Barbara S. Ducatman, M.D.
Assistant Professor of Pathology, Harvard Medical School; Associate Pathologist and Director of Cytopathology, Department of Pathology, Beth Israel Hospital, Boston, Massachusetts

Ann M. Dvorak, M.D.
Associate Professor of Pathology, Harvard Medical School; Senior Pathologist and Director, Electron Microscopy Unit, Department of Pathology, Beth Israel Hospital, Boston, Massachusetts

Harold F. Dvorak, M.D.
Mallinckrodt Professor of Pathology, Harvard Medical School, Pathologist-in-Chief, Department of Pathology, Beth Israel Hospital, Boston, Massachusetts

James S. Economou, M.D., Ph.D., F.A.C.S.
Assistant Professor of Surgery, Division of Surgical Oncology, UCLA School of Medicine, Los Angeles, California

Gary L. Eddy, M.D.
Associate Professor, Department of Obstetrics and Gynecology, Medical University of South Carolina, Charleston, South Carolina

Lawrence H. Einhorn, M.D.
Distinguished Professor of Medicine, Division of Hematology/Oncology, Indiana University, Department of Medicine, Indianapolis, Indiana

Robert M. Ellsworth, M.D.
Professor of Ophthalmology and Head, Ophthalmic Oncology Center, Cornell University, New York Hospital, New York, New York

Ezekiel J. Emanuel, M.D., Ph.D.
Fellow in Clinical Oncology, Division of Cancer Epidemiology and Control, Dana-Farber Cancer Institute; Fellow in Medicine, Harvard Medical School, Boston, Massachusetts

---

* Deceased

Paul F. Engstrom, M.D.
Vice-President, Population Science, Fox Chase Cancer Center; Professor of Medicine, Temple University School of Medicine, Philadelphia, Pennsylvania

William D. Ensminger, M.D., Ph.D.
Professor of Internal Medicine and Pharmacology and Director, Upjohn Center for Clinical Pharmacology, University of Michigan Medical School, Ann Arbor, Michigan

Michael S. Ewer, M.D., M.P.H.
Associate Professor of Medicine, Internist, and Director, Medical Intensive Care Unit, Department of Medical Specialties, The University of Texas M. D. Anderson Cancer Center, Houston, Texas

Jeffrey C. Faig, M.D.
Fellow in Endocrinology, Department of Medicine, Stanford University School of Medicine, Stanford, California

Louis D. Falo, Jr., M.D., Ph.D.
Clinical Fellow, Department of Dermatology, Massachusetts General Hospital; Research Fellow, Dana-Farber Cancer Institute, Boston, Massachusetts

Christopher H. Fanta, M.D.
Associate Professor of Medicine, Harvard Medical School; Clinical Director, Pulmonary Division, Brigham & Women's Hospital, Boston, Massachusetts

Eric R. Fearon, M.D., Ph.D.
Assistant Professor of Pathology, Yale University School of Medicine, New Haven, Connecticut

Robert A. Figlin, M.D.
Associate Professor of Medicine; Director, Bowyer Multidisciplinary Oncology Center, Department of Medicine, Division of Hematology-Oncology, UCLA School of Medicine, Los Angeles, California

Howard A. Fine, M.D.
Clinical Instructor in Medicine, Division of Clinical Oncology and Division of Human Retrovirology, Dana-Farber Cancer Institute, Boston, Massachusetts

Robert L. Fine, M.D.
Assistant Professor of Medicine and Pharmacology, Division of Hematology/Oncology, Duke University Medical Center; Durham Veterans' Administration Hospital, Durham, North Carolina

Howard J. Fingert, M.D.
Assistant Professor, Tufts University School of Medicine; St. Elizabeth's Hospital, Departments of Medicine and Biomedical Research, Division of Hematology/Oncology, Boston, Massachusetts

Bernard Fisher, M.D.
Distinguished Service Professor, Department of Surgery and Chairman, National Surgical Adjuvant Breast and Bowel Project (NSABP), University of Pittsburgh; Senior Scientific Advisor for Clinical Affairs, Pittsburgh Cancer Institute, Pittsburgh, Pennsylvania

T. B. Fitzpatrick, M.D., Ph.D.
Wigglesworth Professor of Dermatology, Emeritus, Harvard Medical School, Massachusetts General Hospital, Boston, Massachusetts

Mary R. Flack, M.D.
Senior Staff Fellow, National Institute of Child Health and Human Development, National Institute of Health, Bethesda, Maryland

Kathleen M. Foley, M.D.
Professor of Neurology and Neuroscience, and Professor of Clinical Pharmacology, Cornell University Medical College, New York, New York; Chief; Pain Service, Department of Neurology, Memorial-Sloan Kettering Cancer Center, New York, New York

Judah Folkman, M.D.
Julia Dyckman Andrus Professor of Pediatric Surgery and Professor of Anatomy and Cellular Biology, Harvard Medical School, Children's Hospital, Boston, Massachusetts

Arthur E. Frankel, M.D.
Adjunct Professor of Medicine, University of Florida, Gainesville, Florida

Arnold S. Freedman, M.D.
Assistant Professor of Medicine, Division of Tumor Immunology, Dana-Farber Cancer Institute, Harvard Medical School, Boston, Massachusetts

Emil Frei III, M.D.
Physician-in-Chief Emeritus; Chief, Division of Cancer Pharmacology, Dana-Farber Cancer Institute; Richard and Susan Smith Professor of Medicine, Harvard Medical School, Boston, Massachusetts

Christopher Fryer, F.R.C.P.(C)
Clinical Professor of Pediatrics, University of British Columbia; Head, Section of Pediatric Oncology, British Columbia Cancer Agency, Vancouver, British Columbia, Canada

William J. Fulkerson, Jr., M.D.
Associate Professor of Medicine; Director of Critical Care Medicine, Duke University Medical Center, Durham, North Carolina

Janice Lynn Gabrilove, M.D.
Assistant Attending Physician, Memorial Sloan-Kettering Cancer Center; Assistant Member, Sloan-Kettering Institute; Assistant Professor of Medicine, Cornell University Medical College, New York, New York

John F. Gaeta, M.D.
Professor of Pathology, State University of New York at Buffalo; Attending Pathologist, Buffalo General Hospital, Buffalo, New York

George T. Gallagher, D.M.D., D.M.Sc.
Assistant Professor of Oral Pathology, Department of Oral Pathology, Harvard School of Dental Medicine, Boston, Massachusetts

Marc B. Garnick, M.D.
Associate Clinical Professor of Medicine, Dana-Farber Cancer Institute, Harvard Medical School, Boston, Massachusetts; Vice President, Clinical Development, Genetics Institute, Inc., Cambridge, Massachusetts

Eli Glatstein, M.D
Professor and Chairman, Radiation Oncology Department, University of Texas Southwestern Medical School at Dallas, Dallas, Texas

L. Michael Glode, M.D.
Associate Professor of Medicine, University of Colorado Health Sciences Center; Staff Internist, Denver Veterans Administration Medical Center, Denver, Colorado

Harvey M. Golomb, M.D.
Professor, Department of Medicine and Director, Section of Hematology/Oncology, University of Chicago Medical Center, Chicago, Illinois

Edward G. Grant, M.D.
Professor of Radiological Sciences, UCLA School of Medicine; Chief, Department of Ultrasound, UCLA Medical Center, Los Angeles, California

F. Anthony Greco, M.D.
Professor of Medicine; Director, Department of Medical Oncology, Vanderbilt University Medical Center, Nashville, Tennessee

Daniel M. Green, M.D.
Professor of Pediatrics, State University of New York at Buffalo; Department of Pediatrics, Roswell Park Cancer Institute, Buffalo, New York

Warner C. Greene, M.D., Ph.D.
Professor of Medicine; Investigator, Howard Hughes Medical Institute, Duke University Medical Center, Durham, North Carolina

Michael R. Grever, M.D.
Acting Associate Director, Developmental Therapeutics Program, Division of Cancer Treatment, National Cancer Institute, Bethesda, Maryland

Charles K. Grieshaber, Ph.D.
Acting Director, Division of Research and Testing, Office of Research Resources, Center for Drug Evaluation and Research, Food anf Drug Administration, Rockville, Maryland

Elizabeth Grimm, Ph.D.
Associate Professor, Department of Tumor Biology, University of Texas M.D. Anderson Cancer Center, Houston, Texas

Astrid Gruber, M.D.
Department of Internal Medicine, Division of Hematology and Immunology, Karolinska Hospital, Stockholm, Sweden

Gerald M. Haase, M.D.
Associate Professor of Surgery, University of Colorado School of Medicine; Co-Chairman, Department of Pediatric Surgery, The Children's Hospital, Denver, Colorado

G. M. Hahn, Ph.D.
Professor of Radiation Oncology, Division of Radiation Biology, Department of Radiation Oncology, Stanford University School of Medicine, Stanford, California

John D. Hainsworth, M.D.
Associate Professor of Medicine, Division of Medical Oncology, Vanderbilt University Medical Center, Nashville, Tennessee

Dennis E. Hallahan, M.D.
Assistant Professor, Department of Radiation and Cellular Oncology, University of Chicago Hospital, Chicago, Illinois

Robert A. Halvorsen, Jr., M.D.
Professor and Vice-Chairman, Department of Radiology, University of California, San Francisco; Chief, Department of Radiology, San Francisco General Hospital, San Francisco, California

G. Denman Hammond, M.D.
Professor of Pediatrics, Associate Vice President of Health Affairs, University of Southern California, Los Angeles, California; Chairman, Children's Cancer Study Group; President, Orion Medical Sciences Institute, Arcadia, California

A.-R. Hanauske, M.D.
Deputy Chief, Division of Hematology and Oncology, Department of Medicine, Technical University, Munich, Federal Republic of Germany

Robert E. Handschumacher, Ph.D.
Professor of Pharmacology, Yale University School of Medicine, New Haven, Connecticut

Yusuf A. Hannun, M.D.
Assistant Professor, Division of Hematology/Oncology, Department of Medicine; Assistant Professor, Department of Cell Biology, Duke University Medical Center, Durham, North Carolina

Curtis C. Harris, M.D.
Chief, Laboratory of Human Carcinogenesis, National Cancer Institute, Bethesda, Maryland

William A. Haseltine, M.D.
Chief, Division of Human Retrovirology, Dana-Farber Cancer Institute; Professor in Pathology, Harvard Medical School, Boston, Massachusetts

Harley A. Haynes, M.D.
Director, Dermatology Division, Brigham and Women's Hospital; Associate Professor of Dermatology, Harvard Medical School, Boston, Massachusetts

Ronald E. Hempling, M.D.
Clinical Instuctor, Gynecology/Obstetrics, State University of New York at Buffalo; Associate Program Director, Department of Gynecologic Oncology, Roswell Park Cancer Institute, Buffalo, New York

Brian E. Henderson, M.D.
Professor of Preventive Medicine and Director, Kenneth Norris Jr. Comprehensive Cancer Center, University of Southern California School of Medicine, Los Angeles, California

Donald E. Henson, M.D.
Health Scientist Administrator, Early Detection Branch, Division of Cancer Prevention and Control, National Cancer Institute, Bethesda, Maryland

John W. Henson, M.D.
Instructor in Neurology, Massachusetts General Hospital and Harvard Medical School, Boston, Massachusetts

Arthur L. Herbst, M.D.
Joseph Bolivar DeLee Distinguished Service Professor and Chairman, Department of Obstetrics and Gynecology, University of Chicago, Chicago, Illinois

Andrew R. Hoffman, M.D.
Associate Professor of Medicine and Molecular and Cellular Physiology; Chief, Medical Service, Department of Veterans Affairs Medical Center, Palo Alto, California; Department of Medicine, Stanford University School of Medicine, Stanford, California

John Stanley Holcenberg, M.D.
Vice-President and Director of Clinical Affairs, Immunex Research and Development Corporation, Seattle, Washington

James F. Holland, M.D.
Jane B. and Jack R. Aron Professor of Neoplastic Diseases; Chairman, Department of Neoplastic Diseases; Director, Derald H. Ruttenberg Cancer Center, Mount Sinai School of Medicine, New York, New York

Jimmie C. Holland, M.D.
Chief of Psychiatry Service, Wayne E. Chapman Chair in Psychiatric Oncology, Memorial Sloan-Kettering Cancer Center; Professor of Psychiatry, Cornell University Medical College, New York, New York

Vincent Hollander, M.D., Ph.D.
Director, Endocrine Laboratory, Derald H. Ruttenberg Cancer Center, Mount Sinai Medical Center, New York, New York

E. Carmack Holmes, M.D.
Professor of Surgery and Executive Vice Chair, Division of Surgical Oncology, UCLA School of Medicine, Los Angeles, California

Waun Ki Hong, M.D.
Charles LeMaistre Chair in Thoracic Medicine, Professor of Medicine, Chief, Section of Head, Neck and Thoracic Medical Oncology, University of Texas M. D. Anderson Cancer Center, Houston, Texas

Antoinette F. Hood, M.D.
Associate Professor of Dermatology, The Johns Hopkins University School of Medicine, The Johns Hopkins Hospital, Baltimore, Maryland

Richard T. Hoppe, M.D.
Professor, Department of Radiation Oncology, Stanford University, Stanford, California

Peter J. Houghton, Ph.D.
Member, Department of Biochemical and Clinical Pharmacology, St. Jude Children's Research Hospital, Memphis, Tennessee

Stephen B. Howell, M.D.
Professor of Medicine and Director, Laboratory of Pharmacology, Cancer Center, University of California, San Diego, La Jolla, California

Andrew A. Jennis, M.D.
Fellow in Medicine, Harvard Medical School; Clinical Research Fellow, Department of Medicine, Beth Israel Hospital, Boston, Massachusetts

Elwood V. Jensen, Ph.D.
Professor Emeritus, Ben May Institute and Department of Biochemistry and Molecular Biology, University of Chicago, Chicago, Illinois; Scholar-in-Residence, Cornell University Medical College, New York, New York

V. Craig Jordan, Ph.D., D.Sc.
Professor of Human Oncology and Pharmacology and Director, Breast Cancer Program, University of Wisconsin Clinical Cancer Center, Madison, Wisconsin

A. Robert Kagan, M.D.
Chief, Department of Radiation Oncology, Southern California Kaiser Permanente Medical Group; Clinical Professor of Radiation Oncology, UCLA School of Medicine, Los Angeles, California

Shalom Kalnicki, M.D.
Associate Professor of Radiation Oncology, University of Pittsburgh School of Medicine, Joint Radiation Oncology Center, Pittsburgh Cancer Institute, Pittsburgh, Pennsylvania

Philip W. Kantoff, M.D.
Assistant Professor of Medicine, Harvard Medical School; Director of Genitourinary Oncology Program, Dana-Farber Cancer Institute, Boston, Massachusetts

Arlene F. Kantor, Dr.P.H.
Epidemiology and Biostatistics Program, National Cancer Institute, Bethesda, Maryland; Dana-Farber Cancer Institute, Department of Epidemiology and Biostatistics, Boston, Massachusetts

Lawrence D. Kaplan, M.D.
Assistant Clinical Professor of Medicine, University of California, San Francisco; AIDS Program and Clinical Oncology, San Francisco General Hospital, San Francisco, California

D. S. Kapp, Ph.D., M.D.
Professor of Radiation Oncology and Director, Clinical Hyperthermia, Department of Radiation Oncology, Stanford University School of Medicine, Stanford, California

Frederic Kass, M.D.
Clinical Assistant Professor of Medicine, University of Southern California School of Medicine, Los Angeles; Director of Clinical Research, Cancer Foundation of Santa Barbara, Santa Barbara, California

Peter A. Kaufman, M.D.
Assistant Professor of Medicine, Section of Hematology/Oncology, Department of Medicine, Dartmouth-Hitchcock Medical Center, Lebanon, New Hampshire

K. Kelsey, M.D.
Associate Professor of Occupational Medicine and Radiobiology, Department of Environmental Health; Department of Cancer Biology, Harvard School of Public Health, Boston, Massachusetts

B. J. Kennedy, M.D.
Regents Professor of Medicine, Masonic Professor of Oncology, Division of Medical Oncology, University of Minnesota Medical School, Minneapolis, Minnesota

Samir N. Khleif, M.D.
Medical Staff Fellow, Division of Cancer Treatment, National Cancer Institute, Bethesda, Maryland

Elliott Kieff, M.D.
Harriet Ryan Albee Professor, Department of Medicine and Microbiology and Molecular Genetics, Harvard University; Director, Infectious Disease Division, Brigham and Women's Hospital, Boston, Massachusetts

John M. Kirkwood, M.D.
Professor and Chief, Division of Medical Oncology, University of Pittsburgh School of Medicine; Associate Director, Pittsburgh Cancer Institute, Pittsburgh, Pennsylvania

Catherine Klein, M.D.
Associate Professor of Medicine, University of Colorado Health Sciences Center; Staff Internist, Denver Veterans Administration Medical Center, Denver, Colorado

George Klein, M.D., Ph.D.
Professor and Head, Department of Tumor Biology, Karolinska Institute, Stockholm, Sweden

James A. Knol, M.D.
Associate Professor of Surgery, University of Michigan Medical School, Ann Arbor, Michigan

Tatsuhei Kondo, M.D.
Professor Emeritus of Surgery, Nagoya University, Nagoya, Japan

Donald W. Kufe, M.D.
Chief, Laboratory of Clinical Pharmacology, Dana-Farber Cancer Institute; Professor of Medicine, Harvard Medical School, Boston, Massachusetts

Beatrice C. Lampkin, M.D.
Jacob G. Schmidlapp Professor of Pediatrics; Director, Hematology/Oncology Division, Children's Hospital Medical Center, Cincinnati, Ohio

George E. Laramore, M.D., Ph.D.
Professor of Radiation Oncology, and Clinical Director, Fast-Neutron Radiotherapy Project, University of Washington, Seattle, Washington

John Laszlo, M.D.
Senior Vice President for Research, American Cancer Society, Atlanta, Georgia

Lawrence Leichman, M.D.
Associate Professor of Medicine, University of Southern California School of Medicine, Los Angeles, California

Bernard Levin, M.D.
Professor of Medicine, Internist, and Chief, Section of Gastrointestinal Oncology and Digestive Diseases, Department of Medical Oncology, Division of Medicine, The University of Texas M. D. Anderson Cancer Center, Houston, Texas

Frederick P. Li, M.D.
Professor of Epidemiology, Harvard School of Public Health, Boston, Massachusetts; Head, Department of Epidemiology and Cancer Control, Dana-Farber Cancer Institute, Boston, Massachusetts

Terry L. Lierman, B.A., M.A.
President, Capitol Associates, Inc.; Executive Director, National Coalition for Cancer Research, Washington, D.C.

Lance A. Liotta, M.D., Ph.D.
Chief, Laboratory of Pathology, National Cancer Institute, National Institutes of Health, Bethesda, Maryland

Scott M. Lippman, M.D.
Associate Professor of Medicine, Section of Head, Neck and Thoracic Medical Oncology, University of Texas M. D. Anderson Cancer Center, Houston, Texas

John B. Little, M.D.
James Stevens Simmons Professor of Radiobiology, Department of Cancer Biology, Harvard School of Public Health; Lecturer on Radiation Therapy, Harvard Medical School, Boston, Massachusetts

Robert Livingston, M.D.
Professor of Medicine, Head, Division of Oncology, University of Washington Medical Center, Seattle, Washington

Robert Lufkin, M.D.
Associate Professor, Department of Radiological Sciences, UCLA School of Medicine, Los Angeles, California

Enrico Macchia, M.D.
Instituto di Endocrinologia, University of Pisa, Pisa, Italy

Michael T. Macfarlane, M.D.
Assistant Professor of Surgery/Urology, UCLA School of Medicine, Los Angeles; Chief of Urology, Sepulveda Veterans Administration Medical Center, Sepulveda, California

George D. Malkasian, M.D.
Professor, Department of Obstetrics and Gynecology, Mayo Clinic, Rochester, Minnesota

Cesare Maltoni, M.D.
Director, Bologna Institute of Oncology "F. Addarii," Bologna, Italy

V. A. Marcial, M.D., F.A.C.R.
Professor and Chairman, Division of Radiation Oncology, University of Puerto Rico, School of Medicine, San Juan, Puerto Rico

V. A. Marcial-Vega, M.D.
Assistant Professor, Department of Radiation Oncology, University of Miami School of Medicine, Miami, Florida

Richard Margolese, M.D., F.R.C.S.
Director of Oncology, Department of Surgery, Jewish General Hospital; Herbert Black Professor of Surgery, McGill University, Montreal, Canada

Harold M. Maurer, M.D.
Jessie Ball duPont Professor and Chairman, Department of Pediatrics, Children's Medical Center, Medical College of Virginia, Virginia Commonwealth University, Richmond, Virginia

Kenneth S. McCarty, Jr., M.D., Ph.D.
Associate Professor of Pathology, Assistant Professor of Medicine, Consultant Endocrinologist Durham Clinic, Director, Endocrine Oncology Laboratory and Co-Director Multidisciplinary Breast Clinic, Duke University Medical Center, Durham, North Carolina

Kenneth S. McCarty, Sr., Ph.D.
Professor of Biochemistry and Co-Director, Endocrine Oncology Laboratory, Duke University Medical Center, Durham, North Carolina

Katherine McGlynn, Ph.D.
Associate Member, Division of Population Science, Fox Chase Cancer Center; Adjunct Assistant Professor of Epidemiology in Medicine, University of Pennsylvania, Philadelphia, Pennsylvania

Anna T. Meadows, M.D.
Professor of Pediatrics and Director, Division of Oncology and Children's Cancer Research Center, Children's Hospital of Philadelphia, Department of Pediatrics, The University of Pennsylvania, Philadelphia, Pennsylvania

Franco Minardi, M.D.
Assistant, Institute of Oncology "F. Addarii," Bologna, Italy

David L. Mitchell, Ph.D.
Assistant Professor of Carcinogenesis, The University of Texas M. D. Anderson Cancer Center, Science Park Research Division, Smithville, Texas

John C. Morris, M.D.
Assistant Professor of Neoplastic Diseases, Assistant Professor of Medicine, Mount Sinai School of Medicine, New York, New York

Charles S. Morrow, M.D., Ph.D.
Fellow, Medicine Branch; Attending Physician, Pediatric Branch, National Cancer Institute, Bethesda, Maryland

Donald L. Morton, M.D.
Medical Director and Surgeon-in-Chief, John Wayne Cancer Institute at St. John's Hospital and Health Center, Santa Monica; Professor Emeritus, Department of Surgery/Oncology, UCLA, Los Angeles, California

Bina T. Motwani, M.D.
Instructor, Department of Neoplastic Diseases and Derald H. Ruttenberg Cancer Center, Mount Sinai School of Medicine, New York, New York

Piero Mustacchi, M.D.
Clinical Professor of Medicine and Epidemiology, University of California, San Francisco, School of Medicine; Attending Physician, University of California Hospitals, San Francisco; Attending Physician, Children's Hospital, San Francisco, California

Charles Myers, M.D.
Chief, Clinical Pharmacology Branch, Clinical Oncology Program, Division of Cancer Treatment, National Cancer Institute, Bethesda, Maryland

Lee M. Nadler, M.D.
Associate Professor of Medicine, Division of Tumor Immunology, Dana-Farber Cancer Institute; Department of Medicine, Harvard Medical School, Boston, Massachusetts

Craig R. Nichols, M.D.
Assistant Professor of Medicine, Division of Hematology/Oncology, Indiana University Department of Medicine, Indianapolis, Indiana

Larry Norton, M.D.
Chief, Breast and Gynecologic Cancer Medical Service, Department of Medicine, Memorial Sloan-Kettering Cancer Center, New York, New York; Associate Professor, Cornell University Medical Center, New York, New York

William D. Odell, M.D., Ph.D., M.A.C.P.
Professor and Chairman, Department of Internal Medicine, University of Utah Medical Center, Salt Lake City, Utah

Takao Ohnuma, M.D., Ph.D.
Professor of Neoplastic Diseases, The Derald H. Ruttenberg Cancer Center, Mount Sinai School of Medicine; Attending Physician, The Mount Sinai Hospital, New York, New York

Olufunmilayo I. Olopade, M.B., B.S.
Assistant Professor of Medicine, Section of Hematology/Oncology, University of Chicago, Chicago, Illinois

Richard J. O'Reilly, M.D.
Professor of Pediatrics, Cornell University Medical College; Chairman, Department of Pediatrics and Chief, Marrow Transplantation Service, Memorial Sloan-Kettering Cancer Center, New York, New York

C. Kent Osborne, M.D.
Professor of Medicine, Director, Medical Oncology Clinical Services, Head, Section of Clinical Medical Oncology, University of Texas Health Science Center, San Antonio, Texas

Robert F. Ozols, M.D., Ph.D
Chairman, Department of Medical Oncology, Fox Chase Cancer Center, Philadelphia, Pennsylvania

Esperanza B. Papadopoulos, M.D.
Clinical Assistant, Bone Marrow Transplantation Service, Memorial Sloan-Kettering Cancer Center, New York

Arthur B. Pardee, Ph.D.
Professor of Biological Chemistry and Molecular Pharmacology, Harvard Medical School; Chief, Division of Cell Growth and Regulation, Dana-Farber Cancer Institute, Boston, Massachusetts

Robert G. Parker, M.D.
Professor and Chair, Department of Radiation Oncology, UCLA School of Medicine, Los Angeles, California

William P. Peters, M.D., Ph.D.
Director, Bone Marrow Transplant Program; Associate Professor of Medicine, Duke University Medical Center, Durham, North Carolina

Herbert F. Pierson, Ph.D.
Toxicologist, Diet and Cancer Branch, National Cancer Institute, Rockville, Maryland

M. Steven Piver, M.D.
Chief, Department of Gynecologic Oncology, Roswell Park Cancer Institute; Clinical Professor and Chief, Division of Gynecologic Oncology, State University of New York at Buffalo, Buffalo, New York

Forrest Pommerenke, M.D.
Health Scientist Administrator, Early Detection Branch, Division of Cancer Prevention and Control, National Cancer Institute, Bethesda, Maryland

B. A. J. Ponder, M.A., M.B., B.Chir., Ph.D., F.R.C.P.
Director, Cancer Research Campaign Human Cancer Genetics Research Group, Department of Pathology, University of Cambridge, Cambridge, England; Honorary Consultant Physician, Addenbrooke's Hospital, Cambridge and Royal Marsden Hospital, London, England

Jerome B. Posner, M.D.
Professor of Neurology, Cornell University Medical College; Chairman, Department of Neurology, Memorial Sloan-Kettering Cancer Center, New York, New York

Milan Potmesil, M.D., Ph.D.
Professor of Radiology and Director, Laboratory of Experimental Therapy, New York University School of Medicine, New York, New York

Michael D. Prados, M.D.
Assistant Clinical Professor, Department of Neurological Surgery and Head, Division of Neuro-Oncology, School of Medicine, University of California, San Francisco, San Francisco, California

Douglas J. Pritchard, M.D.
Professor of Orthopedic Surgery, Professor of Oncology; Head, Subsection of Orthopedic Oncology, Mayo Clinic/Mayo Foundation, Rochester, Minnesota

A. Puras, M.D.
Associate Professor of Surgery; Chief, Urology Service, University of Puerto Rico School of Medicine, San Juan, Puerto Rico

Susan N. Rabinowe, M.D.
Instructor in Medicine, Harvard Medical School; Division of Tumor Immunology, Dana-Farber Cancer Institute, Boston, Massachusetts

Efraim Racker, M.D.
Albert Einstein Professor of Biochemistry, Section of Biochemistry, Molecular and Cell Biology, Cornell University, Ithaca, New York

Kristjan T. Ragnarsson, M.D.
Dr. Lucy G. Moses Professor and Chairman, Department of Rehabilitation Medicine, Mount Sinai School of Medicine; Director, Department of Rehabilitation Medicine, Mount Sinai Hospital, New York, New York

Kanti R. Rai, M.B., B.S.
Professor of Medicine, Albert Einstein College of Medicine; Chief, Division of Hematology/Oncology, Long Island Jewish Medical Center, New Hyde Park, New York

Malcolm Ranson, M.D., Ph.D.
EORTC/NCI Exchange Fellow, Clinical Pharmacology Branch, Clinical Oncology Program, Division of Cancer Treatment, National Cancer Institute, Bethesda, Maryland

Mark J. Ratain, M.D.
Associate Professor of Medicine and Clinical Pharmacology, Section of Hematology/Oncology, Department of Medicine, University of Chicago Pritzker School of Medicine, Chicago, Illinois

Mepur H. Ravindranath, Ph.D.
Assistant Research Oncologist, Division of Surgical Oncology, UCLA School of Medicine, Los Angeles, California

Peter Reizenstein, M.D., Ph.D.
Professor and Chairman, Hematology Collaborating Group; Head, Medical Division, National Institute of Radiation Protection, Karolinska Hospital, Stockholm, Sweden

C. Patrick Reynolds, M.D., Ph.D.
Associate Professor, Division of Hematology/Oncology, Department of Pediatrics, University of Southern California School of Medicine, Children's Hospital Los Angeles, Los Angeles, California

Jerome P. Richie, M.D.
Elliot Carr Cutler Professor of Urological Surgery, Harvard Medical School; Chief Surgeon, Division of Urological Surgery; Director, Harvard Program in Urology (Longwood Area), Brigham and Women's Hospital, Boston, Massachusetts

Barbara K. Rimer, M.P.H., Dr. P.H.
Director, Cancer Control Program, Duke Comprehensive Cancer Center, Durham, North Carolina

Cary N. Robertson, M.D.
Assistant Professor, Division of Urology, Department of Surgery, Duke University Medical Center, Durham, North Carolina

Barrett J. Rollins, M.D., Ph.D.
Assistant Professor, Department of Medicine, Harvard Medical School, Dana-Farber Cancer Institute, Boston, Massachusetts

Kenneth V. I. Rolston, M.D.
Associate Professor of Medicine, Section of Infectious Diseases, The University of Texas M. D. Anderson Cancer Center, Houston, Texas

Antonella Romanini, M.D.
Assistant Professor, Department of Clinical Pharmacology, Instituto Nazionale per la Ricerca sul Cancor, Genoa, Italy

Gerald Rosen, M.D.
Medical Director, The Cedars-Sinai Comprehensive Cancer Center; Attending Physician and Member of the Division of Oncology, The Cedars-Sinai Medical Center; Associate Professor and Member, The Jonsson Comprehensive Cancer Center, UCLA Center for the Health Sciences, Los Angeles, California

Ronald K. Ross, M.D.
Professor of Preventive Medicine; Associate Director, Cancer Cause and Prevention, Kenneth Norris Jr. Comprehensive Cancer Center, University of Southern California School of Medicine, Los Angeles, California

Warren E. Ross, M.D.
Executive Associate Dean, College of Medicine; Professor of Medicine, University of Florida, Gainesville, Florida

Bruce J. Roth, M.D.
Assistant Professor of Medicine, Division of Hematology/Oncology, Indiana University Department of Medicine, Indianapolis, Indiana

Jacob Rotmensch, M.D.
Associate Professor of Obstetrics and Gynecology, Division of Gynecologic Oncology, University of Chicago Pritzker School of Medicine, Chicago, Illinois

Leor D. Roubein, M.D.
Assistant Professor of Medicine, Assistant Internist; Medical Director of the Medical/Surgical Endoscopy Unit, Section of Gastrointestinal Oncology and Digestive Diseases, Department of Medical Oncology, Division of Medicine, The University of Texas M. D. Anderson Cancer Center, Houston, Texas

Janet D. Rowley, M.D.
Blum-Riese Distinguished Service Professor, Departments of Medicine and Molecular Genetics and Cell Biology, University of Chicago, Chicago, Illinois

E. Clifton Russell, M.D.
Associate Professor and Chairman, Division of Pediatric Hematology and Oncology, Department of Pediatrics, Children's Medical Center, Medical College of Virginia, Virginia Commonwealth University, Richmond, Virginia

Richard J. Santen, M.D.
Evan Pugh Professor of Medicine; Chief, Division of Endocrinology, The Milton S. Hershey Medical Center, The Pennsylvania State University, Hershey, Pennyslvania

Oliver Sartor, M.D.
Senior Investigator, Clinical Pharmacology Branch, Clinical Oncology Program, Division of Cancer Treatment, National Cancer Institute, Bethesda, Maryland

Edward Sausville, M.D., Ph.D.
Deputy Chief, Clinical Pharmacology Branch, Clinical Oncology Program, Division of Cancer Treatment, National Cancer Institute, Bethesda, Maryland

Andrew V. Schally, Ph.D., D.Sci., M.D.h.c.
Professor of Medicine; Head, Section of Experimental Medicine, Tulane University School of Medicine; Chief, Endocrine, Polypeptide and Cancer Institute, Veterans Affairs Medical Center, New Orleans, Louisiana; Senior Medical Investigator, The Veterans Administration, Nobel Prize in Medicine 1977

Charles A. Schiffer, M.D.
Professor of Medicine and Oncology; Chief, Division of Hematologic Malignancies, University of Maryland Cancer Center; Chief, Division of Hematology, Department of Medicine, University of Maryland School of Medicine, Baltimore, Maryland

Richard L. Schilsky, M.D.
Professor of Medicine and Director, Cancer Research Center, University of Chicago Pritzker School of Medicine, Chicago, Illinois

Julie A. Schneider, M.S.
Clinical Epidemiologist, Clinical Epidemiology Branch, National Cancer Institute, Bethesda, Maryland; Dana-Farber Cancer Institute, Department of Epidemiology and Biostatistics, Boston, Massachusetts

Stuart J. Schnitt, M.D.
Assistant Professor of Pathology, Harvard Medical School; Consultant in Breast Pathology, Dana-Farber Cancer Institute; Associate Pathologist, Associate Director of Surgical Pathology and Director of the Immunopathology Laboratory, Beth Israel Hospital, Boston, Massachusetts

Robert A. Schwartzman, B.S.
Department of Pharmacology, University of North Carolina at Chapel Hill, Chapel Hill, North Carolina

Leanne L. Seeger, M.D.
Assistant Professor, Department of Radiological Sciences, UCLA School of Medicine; Section Head, Musculoskeletal Radiology, UCLA School of Medicine, Los Angeles, California

Robert C. Seeger, M.D.
Professor, Division of Hematology/Oncology, Department of Pediatrics, University of Southern California School of Medicine, Children's Hospital Los Angeles, Los Angeles, California

Brenda Shank, M.D., Ph.D
Chairman and Professor of Radiation Oncology, Mount Sinai School of Medicine; Director and Attending, Radiation Oncology Department, Mount Sinai Hospital, New York, New York

Gerald Shklar, D.D.S., M.S.
Charles A. Brackett Professor of Oral Pathology; Head, Department of Oral Medicine and Oral Pathology, Harvard School of Dental Medicine; Lecturer in Oral Pathology, Tufts University School of Dental Medicine; Consultant in Oral Pathology, Brigham and Women's Hospital, Children's Hospital Medical Center, and Massachusetts General Hospital, Boston, Massachusetts

Robert Silber, M.D.
Professor of Medicine; Director, Division of Hematology, New York University Medical Center, Tisch Hospital, New York, New York

Richard T. Silver, M.D.
Clinical Professor of Medicine, Cornell University Medical College; Director, Section of Clinical Oncology Chemotherapy Research; Attending Physician, New York Hospital-Cornell Medical Center, New York, New York

Lewis R. Silverman, M.D.
Assistant Professor of Neoplastic Diseases, Mount Sinai School of Medicine; Clinical Assistant Attending, Mount Sinai Hospital; Chief of Oncology, Elmhurst Hospital Center, New York, New York

Murray Silverstein, M.D., Ph.D.
Professor of Medicine, Mayo Clinic, Rochester, Minnesota

David B. Skinner, M.D.
Professor of Surgery, Cornell University Medical College; Attending Surgeon and President/CEO, The New York Hospital, New York, New York

Kristin A. Skinner, M.D.
Surgical Oncology Fellow, UCLA School of Medicine, Department of Surgery, Division of Surgical Oncology, Los Angeles, California

Charles R. Smart, M.D.
Chief, Early Detection Branch, Division of Cancer Prevention and Control, National Cancer Institute, Bethesda, Maryland

Stephen T. Sonis, D.M.D., D.M.Sc.
Professor of Oral Medicine and Oral Pathology, Harvard School of Dental Medicine; Chief, Division of Dentistry, Brigham and Women's Hospital; Active Staff Member in Surgical Oncology, Dana-Farber Cancer Institute, Boston, Massachusetts

Sudhir Srivastava, Ph.D.
Health Scientist Administrator, Early Detection Branch, Division of Cancer Prevention and Control, National Cancer Institute, Bethesda, Maryland

Richard J. Steckel, M.D.
Director, Jonsson Comprehensive Cancer Center; Professor of Radiological Sciences and Radiation Oncology, University of California, Los Angeles, California

Patricia S. Steeg, Ph.D.
Senior Investigator, Laboratory of Pathology, National Cancer Institute, National Institutes of Health, Bethesda, Maryland

Glenn Steele, Jr., M.D., Ph.D.
William V. McDermott Professor of Surgery, Harvard Medical School; Chairman, Department of Surgery, New England, Deaconess Hospital, Boston, Massachusetts

William G. Stetler-Stevenson, M.D., Ph.D.
Senior Investigator, Laboratory of Pathology, National Cancer Institute, National Institutes of Health, Bethesda, Maryland

Charles D. Stiles, Ph.D.
Professor of Microbiology and Molecular Genetics, Departments of Microbiology and Molecular Genetics, Harvard Medical School and Dana-Farber Cancer Institute, Boston, Massachusetts

Richard M. Stone, M.D.
Instructor in Medicine, Harvard Medical School and Dana-Farber Cancer Institute, Boston, Massachusetts

Max W. Sung, M.D.
Assistant Professor, Department of Neoplastic Diseases and Derald H. Ruttenberg Cancer Center, Mount Sinai School of Medicine; Assistant Attending Physician, Mount Sinai Medical Center, New York, New York

Antonella Surbone, M.D.
Special Fellow in Breast and Gynecologic Oncology, Memorial Sloan-Kettering Cancer Center, New York, New York

Mario Sznol, M.D.
Senior Investigator, Cancer Therapy Evaluation Program, Division of Cancer Treatment, National Cancer Institute, Bethesda, Maryland

Tak Takvorian, M.D.
Assistant Professor of Medicine, Harvard Medical School and Dana-Farber Cancer Institute, Boston, Massachusetts

Victor F. Tapson, M.D.
Assistant Professor of Medicine, Department of Allergy, Pulmonary and Critical Care, Duke University School of Medicine, Durham, North Carolina

Joel Tepper, M.D.
Professor and Chair, Department of Radiation Oncology, University of North Carolina School of Medicine, Chapel Hill, North Carolina

Norman W. Thompson, M.D.
Henry King Ransom Professor of Surgery; Chief, Division of Endocrine Surgery, University of Michigan, Ann Arbor, Michigan

William M. Thompson, M.D.
Professor and Chairman, Department of Radiology, University Hospital, University of Minnesota, Minneapolis, Minnesota

A. K. F. Tong, M.D., B.S. (Lond)
Harvard University Health Service, Cambridge, Massachusetts

Timothy J. Triche, M.D., Ph.D.
Professor and Vice Chairman, Department of Pathology, University of Southern California School of Medicine; Pathologist-in-Chief and Chairman, Department of Pathology and Laboratory Medicine, Children's Hospital, Los Angeles, California

Michael E. Trigg, M.D.
Professor of Pediatrics and Director, Pediatric Bone Marrow Transplantation, Department of Pediatrics, The University of Iowa Hospitals and Clinics, Iowa City, Iowa

Bruce Trock, Ph.D.
Cancer Epidemiologist, Division of Population Science, Fox Chase Cancer Center; Adjunct Assistant Professor of Dermatology, University of Pennsylvania School of Medicine; Lecturer in Statistics and Epidemiology, Thomas Jefferson University School of Allied Health Sciences, Philadelphia, Pennsylvania

Steven R. Tronick, Ph.D.
Chief, Gene Structure Section, Laboratory of Cellular and Molecular Biology, National Cancer Institute, Bethesda, Maryland

Donald L. Trump, M.D.
Deputy Director, The Pittsburgh Cancer Institute; Professor of Medicine and Surgery, University of Pittsburgh, Pittsburgh, Pennsylvania

M. A. Tucker, M.D.
Chief, Family Studies Section, Environmental Epidemiology Branch, Public Health Service, National Cancer Institute, National Institutes of Health, Bethesda, Maryland

Andrew Turrisi III, M.D.
Associate Chairman and Director of Clinical Programs, Department of Radiation Oncology, University of Michigan Medical School, Ann Arbor, Michigan

John E. Ultmann, M.D.
Professor of Medicine, Division of Biological Sciences, The Pritzker School of Medicine; Director Emeritus, Cancer Research Center, University of Chicago, Chicago, Illinois

James Vardiman, M.D.
Associate Professor of Pathology; Director, Clinical Hematology Laboratory, University of Chicago Medical Center, Chicago, Illinois

Aaron I. Vinik, M.B.Bch., F.C.P., F.A.C.P., Ph.D.
Professor of Internal Medicine, Anatomy and Neurobiology; Director, Diabetes Research Institutes, Eastern Virginia Medical School, Norfolk, Virginia

Bert Vogelstein, M.D.
Professor of Oncology, Director, Molecular Genetics Laboratory, The Johns Hopkins Oncology Center, Baltimore, Maryland

Paul A. Volberding, M.D.
Professor of Medicine, University of California, San Francisco; Director, Center for AIDS Research; Chief, AIDS Program and Clinical Oncology, San Francisco General Hospital, San Francisco, California

D. D. Von Hoff, M.D., F.A.C.P.
Professor of Medicine, Head Section of Drug Development, Division of Oncology, Department of Medicine, University of Texas Health Science Center; Research Director, Cancer Therapy and Research Center, San Antonio, Texas

Sidney Wallace, M.D.
Professor and Chairman, Department of Diagnostic Radiology, Deputy Head, Division of Diagnostic Imaging, The University of Texas M.D. Anderson Cancer Center, Houston, Texas

Alan D. Waxman, M.D.
Clinical Professor of Radiology, University of Southern California; Director, Department of Nuclear Medicine, Cedars-Sinai Medical Center, Los Angeles, California

James L. Weese, M.D., F.A.C.S.
Director, Presbyterian Cancer Center; Chief, Surgical Oncology, Presbyterian Medical Center of Philadelphia, Philadelphia, Pennsylvania

Ralph R. Weichselbaum, M.D.
Harold H. Hines Jr. Professor and Chairman, Department of Radiation and Cellular Oncology; Director, Chicago Tumor Institute, University of Chicago, Chicago; Director, LaGrange Treatment Pavilion, LaGrange, Illinois

Ainsley Weston, Ph.D.
Visiting Scientist, Biochemical Epidemiology Section, Laboratory of Human Carcinogenesis, National Cancer Institute, National Institutes of Health, Bethesda, Maryland

Charles B. Wilson, M.D.
Tong-Po Kan Professor and Chairman, Department of Neurological Surgery, School of Medicine, University of California, San Francisco, California

Gregory T. Wolf, M.D.
Professor and Director, Head and Neck Surgery Division, Department of Otolaryngology, University of Michigan, Ann Arbor, Michigan

Jan H. Wong, M.D.
Associate Professor, Division of Surgical Oncology, UCLA School of Medicine, Los Angeles, California

Antoinette Wozniak, M.D.
Assistant Professor of Medicine, Wayne State University, Detroit, Michigan

Michael R. Zalutsky, Ph.D.
Professor of Radiology; Head, Laboratory of Radiopharmaceutical Chemistry, Duke University Medical Center, Durham, North Carolina

Marvin Zelen, Ph.D.
Professor of Statistical Science, Harvard School of Public Health; Chief, Division of Biostatistics and Epidemiology, Dana-Farber Cancer Institute, Boston, Massachusetts

Michael Zinner, M.D.
Professor and Chairman, Department of Surgery, UCLA School of Medicine, Los Angeles, California

Contents

Color Plates appear in Volume 1 following page 360.

I

Cancer Biology

I-1

Cell Proliferation and Differentiation

Howard J. Fingert
Judith Campisi
Arthur B. Pardee

Introduction

The biology of cell division and differentiation is exceedingly similar in normal and cancer cells. The cancer cell differs from its normal counterpart in that it is aberrantly regulated. Cancer cells generally contain the full complement of biomolecules necessary for survival, proliferation, differentiation, and expression of many cell-type-specific functions. However, failure to regulate these functions properly results in an altered phenotype and cancer.

Three cellular functions tend to be inappropriately regulated in a neoplasm. First, the normal constraints on cellular proliferation are relaxed. This is a necessary but often insufficient requirement for tumor formation. Second, differentiation can be distorted. The tumor cells may be blocked at a particular stage of differentiation, or they may differentiate into an inappropriate or abnormal cell type. Third, chromosomal and genetic organization may be destabilized such that variant cells arise with high frequency (see I-8). Some variants may have an increased growth advantage; others may be resistant to killing by chemotherapeutic drugs or radiation; and others may have increased motility or production of enzymes that permit invasion and metastases (see I-10).

To comprehend the biology of cancer, it is necessary to understand how these three functions, growth, differentiation, and chromosome stability, are controlled in normal cells, and how they become uncontrolled in cancer cells. This chapter will focus on the biology of cell proliferation and differentiation, and how these functions are linked in the development of neoplasia.

Proliferation

Tumor Growth and Cell Proliferation In Vivo

In terms of population kinetics, the growth of any tissue depends on three parameters: 1) rate of individual cell division (Tc); 2) growth fraction of the cell population; and 3) cell loss from the growing population through differentiation, cell death, or other means (Figure I-1-1). Normal cells reach a steady state of growth that provides a balanced economy for the body as a whole. Each organ maintains tight controls over the growth rate, growth fraction, and cell loss. Physiologic stimuli can alter these parameters in normal tissues, leading to increased tissue growth, but this growth will cease when the stimulus is withdrawn or a new steady state is achieved. Some normal tissues grow faster than cancers under physiologic conditions, so it is not simply rapid growth at a single time and place that distinguishes neoplasia. Biopsy samples from normal, inflammatory, and neoplastic lesions of the lung, cervix, vocal cord, or pharynx have been analyzed for the rate of cell proliferation. These studies showed that benign inflammatory lesions can grow over 20 times faster than cancer in a discrete time and place.[30,31,88] Similarly, rapid proliferation of human lymphoid cells is induced by immunostimulants; growth kinetics of these cells is similar to that observed in high-grade lymphomas.[12] Noncancerous tissues cease rapid growth when healing is complete, unlike neoplastic tissues, which continue to grow over time. In many ways, cancer can be thought of as a "wound that does not heal".[4]

In the early phases of tumor cell growth, it is generally believed that neoplastic cells multiply exponentially, for example, 1 cell becomes 2, 2 become 4, then 8, 16, etc. (see XV-1).[83] As the tumor mass increases, however, the rate of growth declines. Measuring tumor growth over time describes a curve with an exponential increase in the early period, and then a flattening out of the growth rate over time (Gompertzian curve).[87] Several mechanisms have been invoked to explain this change in growth rate with larger tumors: 1) decrease in the growth fraction; 2) increase in cell loss, i.e., exfoliation, necrosis; 3) nutritional depletion of tumor cells due to outgrowth of available blood supply (see I-11); or 4) lengthening of cell cycle time. Experimental tumor models suggest that cell cycle time changes only slightly

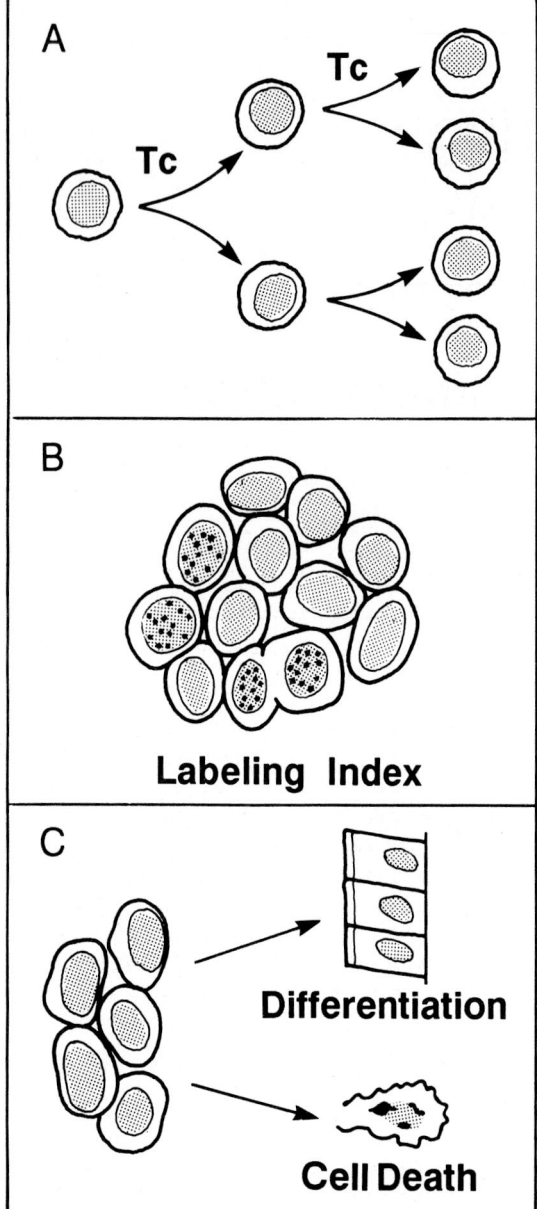

Figure I-1-1. Cell proliferation and cell loss. **A.** Tc is the average time required for one cell to divide into two daughter cells. Human cancer cells exhibit a broad range, many with Tc that is longer than rapidly-dividing normal tissues such as bone marrow and intestinal mucosa (Table I-1-1). **B.** Labeling index (LI) is a measure of the fraction of cells that are in DNA synthetic phase. This is commonly measured by uptake of radioactive substrate (thymidine) for DNA synthesis. After incubation with tritiated thymidine and then application of photographic emulsion, cells that incorporate thymidine are seen by development of black dots in the photographic emulsion that overlies the nucleus. This diagram shows 4/12 = 33% labeling. LI also correlates with growth fraction (GF), the proliferating fraction of the entire cell population under study. If four other cells were demonstrated to be proliferating, but in other phases of the cell cycle, then the GF would be 8/12 = 66%. **C.** Cell loss can occur by various means, including cell death and exfoliation or differentiation into nondividing cells. This diagram depicts stem cells of the gastrointestinal tract, differentiating into columnar cells that line the gastrointestinal mucosa.

Cell Proliferation

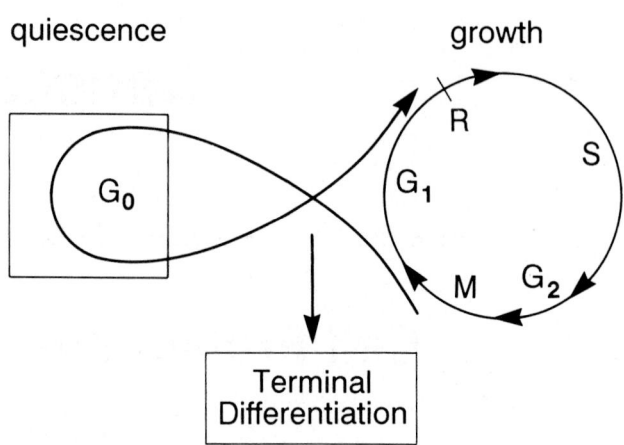

Figure I-1-2. Diagram of the cell cycle. When a cell is not synthesizing DNA (S phase), nor completing mitosis (M phase), it is commonly termed to be in a G (gap) phase. Normal cells are capable of resting in a nondividing state, called G_0. They can begin one or more cycles of cell division when there is a need to maintain or replace tissue, and they stop dividing when the necessary growth is complete. In G_1, protein and RNA synthesis are active. If conditions are permissive for subsequent cell division, cells pass through the R (restriction) point and quickly move into the S (synthetic) period when new DNA is synthesized. Another gap (G_2) follows when the newly duplicated chromosomes condense. In the M (mitosis) period, the chromosomes divide into two sets, and the cell forms two nuclei and then divides into two daughter cells. When normal cells differentiate, typically with gain in properties required for organ or tissue functions, they usually lose the capacity to continue cell division.

when tumor growth decreases.[34] Under adverse conditions, tumor cells often leave the growth fraction and enter a nongrowing state (G_0 or prolonged G_1; Figure I-1-2), although these same cells can reenter the division cycle when conditions improve or when stimulated by growth factors.

Analysis of Cell Proliferation

Autoradiography has been a useful tool for measuring growth rates of cell populations in vitro and in vivo.[63] This technique identifies growing cells by their uptake of radioactive precursors for DNA synthesis, such as tritiated thymidine. Samples of these tissues are then treated with photographic emulsion and developing agents. Black granules form over the nuclei of cells that have utilized the radioactive precursor and gone through DNA replication and cell division (Figure I-1-1B).[18,33] A similar technique exposes cells to bromodeoxyuridine (BrdU), a pyrimidine analog of thymidine selectively utilized by cells in DNA synthesis. Subsequently, the cell population is stained with an identifiable antibody that binds only BrdU-containing cells. This is a sensitive assay for the number of cells that are cycling through DNA synthesis (S phase).

The labeling index (LI) is a measure of cells synthesizing DNA, typically using thymidine incorporation to label S-phase cells by autoradiography. This technique provides a relatively simple method for estimating proliferative rates and growth fractions of cancerous or normal cells.[5] The average time for cell division within the growing population (Tc) can be estimated by taking multiple samples over time and counting the percentage of cells that are labeled at mitosis. Timed exposure to radioactive thymidine also provides a method for estimating the length of the cell cycle and the duration of cell cycle phases, for example, G_1, S, G_2, and M.

More recent studies to analyze cell proliferation employ staining with the Ki67 mouse monoclonal antibody, or quantification of DNA content by flow cytometry.[62] These latter techniques can be performed with small surgical tumor samples. Moreover, they do not require incubation of tissues in radioactive materials nor prior administration of drugs. The exact nature of the antigen bound by the antibody Ki67 is not known, but it is not appreciably expressed in quiescent (G_0) cells. Expression begins in cells that have entered the cell cycle (mid-G_1), and cells going through division (G_2-M) are heavily positive. Thus, the ratio of Ki67-positive cells to total cells represents the percent of cells cycling at any one time, a measure of the growth fraction.[73] Monoclonal antibodies to other proliferation-related antigens are currently under study. For example, monoclonal antibodies to "proliferation cell nuclear antigen", or PCNA, have been developed along with methods to measure this S-phase antigen in fixed, paraffin-embedded tissues. This technique may have practical advantages in terms of clinical studies.[36]

Flow cytometry, an automated technique to measure cell cycle distribution, is one of the most common methods to quantify the relative number of cells in $G_0 + G_1$, S, or $G_2 + M$ phases. Tissue samples are disaggregated, suspended as single cells, and stained with a fluorescent DNA dye. This sample then flows past a light source and a sensitive fluorescence detector that records the relative DNA content (measured by the amount of fluorescent signal per cell). These data are translated by computer to a histogram (Figure I-1-3), and computer programs are utilized to measure the relative number of cells with G_0-G_1, S, or G_2-M DNA content. This same technique provides a rapid method to quantify tumor ploidy, for example, cell populations with altered chromosome number. Tumor cells with normal chromosome content (2n) are diploid and the G_0-G_1 peak appears on the histogram at the same location as the G_0-G_1 peak from nontumor cells. However, the G_0-G_1 peak from tumor cells with abnormal (aneuploid) chromosome content appears at a different position in the histogram. For example, if the aneuploid

cells have more DNA in all phases of the cell cycle due to increased chromosome number, then the histogram is shifted to the right (Figure I-1-3).

Flow cytometry of DNA content has gained increasing use to measure proliferative activity of clinical tumor samples, due to its speed, relative simplicity with automated computer technology, and requirement of only small tumor samples. Many investigators use the S index or S-phase fraction (SPF), computed by the relative number of cells that do not have G_0-G_1 or G_2-M DNA content, to study proliferation of tumor cell populations. In patients with breast or ovarian cancer, a high S index was found to be an independent predictor of prognosis in patients with diploid tumors (see XXXII).[17,52] Similarly, the relative number of aneuploid tumor cells can have prognostic value, although such data are often linked to higher S-phase.[17,62] Other investigators measure the G_1 phase fraction (G_1PF) to represent cells that are not in other proliferative phases, and correlate a relative decrease in the G_1PF with higher proliferation.[54] However, this latter technique can be difficult if the tissue sample has variable concentrations of normal cells with G_0-G_1 DNA content.

These techniques to measure cell proliferation parameters provide useful information to understand the biology of tumor growth, and they may supplement routine histology to determine diagnosis and prognosis for many cancers.[73] Estimated mean values of LI and Tc for several neoplasms, and some of the most rapidly proliferating normal tissues, are listed in Table I-1-1. These data illustrate a wide range of Tc (1–10 days) and LI (3–40%), similar to the wide range of growth rates observed in clinical studies of human cancers.

The LI and growth fraction (GF) are the kinetic parameters that commonly distinguish cancer from normal tissues. In contrast, the actual rate of cell division, or Tc, is not a major determinant of abnormal growth of neoplasms. Many cancer cells grow at a slower Tc than normal tissues, especially

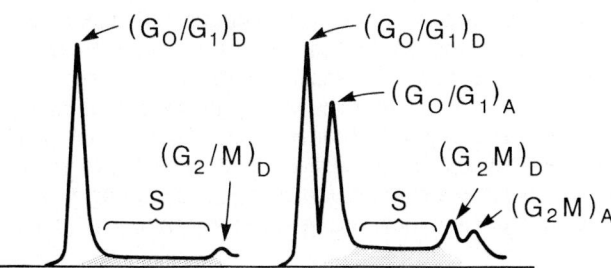

Figure I-1-3. Histograms of DNA content in normal and tumor cells. Using flow cytometry, areas under the curves are measured by computer, indicating the relative number of cells in G_0/G_1, S, or G_2/M phases of the cell cycle. L: Histogram of normal cells with 2N = diploid chromosomes. Shaded area represents cells in S phase. R: Histogram of a clinical breast cancer removed during surgery. In this tumor are both diploid (D) cells and aneuploid (A) cells, and it contains a larger number of cells in S phase (shaded area).

Table I-1-1. Growth Parameters of Human Neoplasms and Normal Tissues

Cell type	Labeling index (LI = %)	Estimated cell doubling time (Tc = days)
Normal bone marrow— myeloblasts	32–75	0.7–1.1
Acute myeloid leukemia	8–25	0.5–8
Normal B-cell lymphocytes	0–1	14–21 +
High-grade lymphoma	19–29	2–3
Normal intestinal crypts	12–18	1–2
Colon adenocarcinoma	3–35	1.6–5
Normal epithelium—pharynx	2–3	—
Squamous cell carcinoma of nasopharynx	5–16	2–4
Normal epithelium— bronchus	—	9–10
Epidermoid carcinoma of lung	5–8	8–10
Normal epithelium—cervix	4–8	—
Squamous cell carcinoma of cervix	13–40	—
Ovarian carcinoma	3–20	5–6
Benign mole of skin	0.3	—
Malignant melanoma of skin	12.8	—

those of the intestinal mucosa and bone marrow.[48,55] When comparisons have been possible between neoplastic and normal cells of the same histologic type (e.g., leukemia and normal bone marrow), it is also apparent that the Tc of cancer cells is the same as, or longer than, normal cells (Table I-1-1). Decreased cell loss is an important parameter in many neoplasms. Cancerous tissues increase in size faster than bone marrow or intestinal mucosa, even though the Tc and GFs predict slower growth of the tumors compared with the normal tissues.[19] However, the normal tissues balance high proliferative rates with cell loss through exfoliation or differentiation into nondividing cells.

Growth rates of individual tumors in vivo also demonstrate the importance of LI and the GF (Table I-1-2). Analysis of these data requires a clear distinction between the rate of cell division (Tc) and the doubling time of the tumor mass (Td). Tc refers to the time of cell division, i.e., the time required for an average cell to go through one complete cell division and return to the same phase of the cell cycle. Since autoradiography can identify radioactive thymidine-labeled cells as they pass through the DNA-replicative (S) phase of the cell cycle and into mitosis, Tc is often measured by the "intermitotic time" between two consecutive mitoses. In contrast, Td is the estimated time needed to double the size of an entire tumor mass using, for example, calipers or x-ray measurements. Td is usually much longer than Tc due to cell loss, change in growth rates over time, and a less than 100% growth fraction. For example, a Tc of about 2 to 3 days was measured in one tumor of the head and neck, and this tumor had a Td of 2l days during the same period of measurement.[11] Similarly, other human tumors have a Tc of 2 to 6 days, while the Td for the same tumor types has been in the range of 50 to 100 days. If all proliferating cells were to continue division with no cell loss, mathematical models can be employed to predict the "potential doubling time" of tumors. For example, squamous cell lung cancers may have an observed LI of about 7%, predicting a potential Td of 9 days; however, the observed Td is typically 1 to 2 months for these tumors, and this difference illustrates the high level of cell loss and variable growth that occurs with these and other solid neoplasms.[85]

The GF appears to correlate inversely with overall Td of solid tumors, i.e., an increased GF corresponds to a shorter Td and a faster growth of tumor masses. This was first dem-

Table I-1-2. Correlation Between Mass Doubling Time and Growth Fraction

Tumor	Growth fraction (%)	Doubling time (days)
Experimental tumors		
L1210 (mouse)	86	0.5
B 16 (mouse)	55	1.9
LL (mouse)	38	2.9
DMBA (rat)	10	7.4
Human tumors		
Embryonal carcinoma	90	27
Lymphoma—high grade	90	29
Squamous cell carcinoma	25	58
Adenocarcinoma	6	83

onstrated in animal tumors, which can be measured more frequently than most human cancers (Table I-1-2). A close correlation between increased LI and decreased Td has also been observed in studies of human cancers;[88] however, methodologic differences among various laboratories present many problems for such comparisons.[63,73] A correlation between histologic grade and LI has been observed in many cancers, including lymphoma, bladder, and breast carcinomas, and soft tissue sarcomas. In addition to grade or other traditional histologic criteria, several studies demonstrate that LI or S index can be an independent determinant of prognosis, especially in breast, colon, non-small cell lung, ovary, and primary brain neoplasms, chronic lymphocytic leukemia, and myeloma.[17,61,62]

Understanding the kinetics of tumor cell growth in vivo has provided direction for more basic investigations into the mechanisms of neoplasia at the cellular, subcellular, and molecular levels. The increased GF of cancer cells is a key property distinguishing most neoplasms from normal tissues. At the level of a single cell, the process that best determines the GF of a cell population is the initiation of cell division from a nongrowing state, i.e., the process of entering G_1-S phases from a quiescent state in which DNA replication is inactive. The events leading to cell division include a complex array of biochemical and genetic signals, and many of these have been clarified using cells in culture. In addition, tumor cell proliferation in vivo is influenced by a variety of local and systemic factors, and these will be reviewed in later chapters.

Cells in Culture

The importance of the individual cell in cancer is clear, since a single cancer cell injected into an appropriate animal is sufficient to give rise to a tumor. Many studies have therefore been performed with isolated normal and tumor cells in culture. Both normal and tumor-derived mammalian cells can be grown and compared in culture, although many are not readily established in culture initially.[3,70,71,90] Most studies have been done on fibroblasts since this cell type is easily cultured and is most likely to grow out of a tissue explant. Much has also been learned from hematopoetic cells.[22] Moreover, the culture of epithelial cells has advanced considerably.[75]

Cells are generally grown in a medium containing salts, amino acids, glucose, vitamins, and serum or growth factors. Normal cells, plated on a plastic surface to which they may attach, can grow until they have formed a confluent monolayer, whereupon growth ceases. Growth also ceases when cells have exhausted a nutrient or a factor provided by serum, or when such substances are removed by changing to a deficient medium. Thus, growth can be manipulated in culture.

Quiescence Versus Growth. Cells that have stopped growing are said to be in a G_0 state, or "quiescent". Most of the cells in adults are in G_0. They can be very active functionally and metabolically. Growth of G_0 cells can be initiated by appropriately changing the cell density or the supply of nutrients. These cells then enter the cell cycle (Figure I-1-2), beginning a sequence of events that culminates in cell division. For the 3T3 murine fibroblast line the durations of

G_1, S, G_2, and M are approximately 6, 8, 2, and 0.5 hours, respectively. The duration of a cycle is relatively constant. Thus, the fraction of time that a cell spends in quiescence as compared with its time in cycle determines its average growth rate. The switching of cells back and forth between quiescence and cycling depends on extracellular conditions, and is regulated differently in normal and tumor cells.

Molecular Events in Cell Proliferation. When a quiescent cell in culture is stimulated, for example by the addition of serum, the activated chain of events leads eventually to formation of two cells. This requires duplication of a multitude of molecules in the original cell.[9] At least three growth factors, provided in serum, have been found to act sequentially following resumption of proliferation of fibroblasts: platelet-derived growth factor (PDGF), epidermal growth factor (EGF), and insulin-like growth factor (IGF-1). These small polypeptides activate cells by binding to specific receptors on the cell surface (see I-3).[41,79]

Growth factor receptors are complex large proteins that span the plasma membrane. On the outside of the cell they have a specific domain that recognizes the growth factor, and their cytoplasmic portion may have an enzymatic function, such as a protein tyrosine kinase. Binding of a growth factor or ligand to its receptor can induce transmission of a signal to the cytoplasm through activation of the kinase.[26] The next step is a transduction of the cytoplasmic signal to the cell nucleus (see I-4). This is accomplished by a heterogeneous group of molecules known as second messengers. They include various proteins that are phosphorylated by kinases, small molecules such as inositol phosphates and cyclic AMP, and also ions, including Ca^{2+}, H^+, and Zn^{2+}. Within the nucleus, genes are then activated in response to these second messengers. The second messengers probably modify proteins that bind to regulatory DNA sequences located near specific functional genes. "Immediate-early" genes are activated quickly and include well known proto-oncogenes such as *fos* and *myc*. Production of new mRNAs, transcribed from these genes, does not require new protein synthesis, since production is not prevented by protein synthesis inhibitors. Other genes, including the *ras* and *raf* proto-oncogenes, are activated later.[26]

Protein and RNA synthesis are required for cells to enter S phase during which DNA is synthesized, since drugs that inhibit protein or RNA synthesis also block cell passage through G_1 to S (Figure I-1-4).[29,98] Cell proliferation, particularly progression through G_1, depends on factors present in growing cells that activate quiescent cells.[102] Experimental models have been developed to fuse growing and quiescent cells, and these fusions lead to rapid induction of cell division in the quiescent cells.[69] These positive factors are very likely proteins induced during the latter part of G_1.

A variety of proteins are produced during G_1 after cells leave quiescence. Some are enzymes that may expand metabolic functions lost by G_0 cells, such as those providing energy and more ribosomes for rapid protein synthesis. Others have so-called housekeeping functions that keep both quiescent and growing cells in metabolic balance. Only a few proteins appear to be key regulatory molecules. For example, enzymes are required for synthesis of isoprenoids, which are necessary for activity of the *ras* oncogene, and

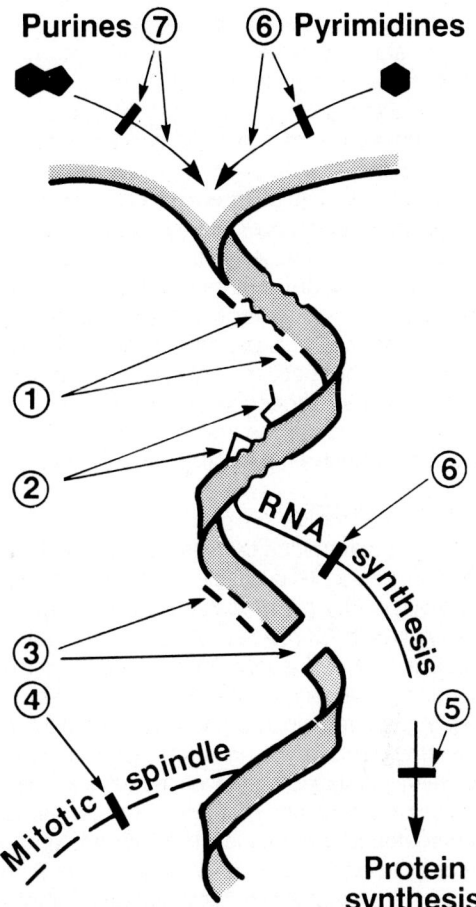

Figure I-1-4. Anticancer drugs and their effects on cell proliferation. Group 1. Antitumor, antibiotics and anthracyclines (doxorubicin, mitomycin, daunorubicin, mithramycin, idarubicin, dactinomycin, epirubicin, mitoxantrone). Effect: bind and disorganize DNA, prevent DNA replication and RNA synthesis. Group 2. Alkylating agents (mechlorethamine, cisplatin, cyclophosphamide, carboplatin, ifosfamide, nitrosoureas, thiotepa, dacarbazine). Effect: Crosslink DNA, prevent DNA replication and RNA synthesis. Group 3. Cleaving agents (bleomycin, etoposide). Effect: Cleave DNA after interaction with cellular components. Group 4. Tubulin binding agents (vincristine, taxol, vinblastine). Effect: Bind or disrupt mitotic spindles. Group 5. Protein synthesis inhibitor (L-asparaginase). Effect: Depletes extracellular asparagine, used for protein synthesis. Group 6. Antimetabolites (methotrexate, 5-fluorouracil, cytarabine, hydroxyurea, fludarabine). Effect: Block pyrimidine or purine conversion to nucleotide, misincorporate into DNA or RNA, terminate DNA synthesis. Group 7. Purine analogues (6-thioguanine, 6-mercaptopurine). Effect: Prevent purine ring biosynethesis, misincorporate into DNA or RNA (see XVI).

for the synthesis of polyamines, which have many functions including ionic binding to nucleic acids.

IGF appears to be the only factor necessary for progression through the end of the G_1 period. Enzymes involved in the synthesis of DNA, such as thymidine kinase and DNA polymerase, as well as histones, are synthesized just prior to S. These enzyme molecules relocate at the beginning of DNA synthesis, moving from the cytoplasm into the nucleus. A variety of experiments show that DNA is made by a high molecular weight multienzyme complex.[71,91] This complex contains many enzymes known to be involved in the process of DNA replication, but its size and other features are still a matter of debate. The onset of DNA replication has been investigated recently with in vitro systems. These studies reveal that the synthesis of helicase enzymes, which possess DNA unwinding ability, may provide the final factor for initiating S phase.[14]

After DNA synthesis has commenced, cell growth becomes relatively independent of external controls. After completing DNA duplication, the S phase cell then goes through G_2 and mitosis, and finally divides to form two daughter cells. Information is rapidly accumulating regarding molecular events related to mitosis.[27,57] The daughter cells, now in the G_1 phase, will then either pass through another cycle or arrest in a quiescent G_0 state, depending once more upon external conditions. If these conditions are not adequate, the cell will become arrested before it reinitiates DNA synthesis.

Proliferation Controls

Cell growth is determined by extracellular conditions that act prior to onset of DNA synthesis. The proliferation rate is initially determined by the probability of switching from the quiescent G_0 state to G_1 phase of the cell cycle. Cells in vivo and in culture may both spend long periods of time in the G_0 state, depending upon the cell type. Differentiated nerve and muscle cells remain quiescent permanently. Normal fibroblasts emerge to grow only when conditions are favorable and when stimulated by growth factors such as PDGF.

Two major control points exist (for 3T3 cells) between G_0 and S, competence and restriction (R). These are located approximately 12 and 2 hours prior to the start of S, respectively. PDGF permits sensitive cells, such as fibroblasts, to leave G_0, enter G_1, and reach competence. EGF and probably insulin allow passage through mid-G_1, while rapid protein synthesis and IGF-1 allow completion of G_1. The cycle, once initiated, thus is not free-running; rather it is highly regulated during the transition from G_1 to S phase.[23,71] All growth factors are dispensable a few hours prior to the onset of actual DNA synthesis, as is the requirement for a rapid rate of protein synthesis. This step of final regulation in G_1 is the R point.[71]

Relatively little is known about the kinds of molecules that regulate passage through these control points. Proto-oncogenes and tumor suppressor genes are of great interest in this regard (see I-5 and I-6). Some of these genes code for DNA binding proteins, such as *fos* and *jun*, which form a complex and bind to specific gene-regulatory DNA sequences during the competence process. Other proto-oncogenes code for growth factors; for example, c-*sis* codes for PDGF-B chain. Others code for growth factor receptors, such as the c-*erb* B gene which encodes the EGF receptor. And yet others, such as c-*raf*, appear to have other functions, for example, coding for protein kinases that act on substrates in the cascade involved in second messenger metabolism. Another set of gene products disappears when cells start to proliferate.[81] The proteins encoded by oncogenes similarly display diverse locations, some being on the plasma membrane, others in the nucleus, and still others inside the cytoplasm (see I-7).[7] Tumor suppressor genes produce proteins that are of increasing interest for their ability to regulate cell growth negatively.[80] Extracellular transforming growth factor beta (TGF-β) inhibits the growth of various epithelial cells by intracellular mechanisms still being investigated.[78] Several studies suggest that TGF-β inhibits cell growth by blocking expression of the c-*myc* gene, possibly through interaction with the retinoblastoma (RB) protein.[67] Paracrine production of TGF-β could limit growth of both normal and cancer cells, and experimental models suggest it may play a role in the regression of breast cancers in response to hormonal or drug therapies.[104]

Along with a general increase in metabolic activity during G_1, changes are observed in cell structural elements. For example, the cytoskeleton, composed of various filaments and microtubules, is modified. Actin, the major structural component of microfilaments, is produced more rapidly by stimulated cells. It is not clear at present which of these changes have regulatory consequences and which are simply reorganizations of the cell to provide greater metabolic activity.

Kinetic experiments show that normal cells must synthesize proteins rapidly in order to reach the restriction point and to proceed into division. The cell must make a sufficient amount of some special protein during late G_1 phase; this protein is unstable in normal cells, having a half-life of only about 2.5 hours in 3T3 cells. Therefore, the synthesis of this protein must be quite rapid; otherwise degradation prevents its sufficient accumulation. A protein with such properties has been identified.[71]

Cyclins are a family of proteins that accumulate in the G_1 phase of many eukaryotic cells, just before the transition into S phase (G_1 cyclins), and again during late S–G_2 phases before mitosis (mitotic cyclins).[57] After they reach a peak concentration, cyclin proteins are rapidly degraded. In several experimental systems, the cyclic levels of these proteins are necessary for transition through the cell cycle. These proteins bind to one of several enzymes with potent kinase activity, coded by a group of "cell division cycle" (cdc) genes. This cyclin-kinase complex becomes active to phosphorylate a variety of substrates. The identity and function of these substrates are not yet clear, but they appear to trigger initiation of DNA synthesis (S phase), or the mitotic apparatus needed for the final stage of cell division (M phase). First discovered in yeast and sea urchin eggs, similar protein-kinase complexes have been found in various eukaryotic species, and recent studies have focused on their possible role in regulation of neoplastic cell proliferation.

Relaxed Control in Tumor Cells

The biochemistry of growth appears to be qualitatively very similar in tumor and normal cells.[98] In spite of numerous efforts, universal differences in biochemical markers have not yet been discovered between normal and tumor cells.[1] The fundamental difference probably lies in a relaxation of regulatory machinery for cell growth.[71] Whereas normal cells generally are quiescent at physiologic levels of growth factors, the related tumor cells are able to proliferate at these levels. In some experimental models, tumor cells proliferate in the absence of growth factors or in very low levels. What biochemical reactions bring about this changed requirement? Several general mechanisms have been proposed. One is that the limiting growth factors are not needed because the tumor cells produce their own such as PDGF or TGF-α (Figure I-1-5) that activate their receptors (an autocrine mechanism). Alternatively, the receptors may be produced in excess, as is the case for EGF receptors in numerous clinical tumors, leading to adequate stimulation at the low growth factor concentrations found in vivo. Moreover, mutations that alter intracellular signaling mechanisms may bypass growth factor dependence. Mutated forms of proto-oncogenes, and inactivated tumor suppressor genes, can activate growth in these ways.

Growth control may be lost as a result of transformation by a DNA virus such as simian virus 40 (SV40) or papilloma viruses. These transformed cells are incapable of entering the G_0 state; rather, they proliferate very slowly and eventually die in vitro under conditions that cause normal cells to become quiescent, and they seem to bypass the normal G_1 phase controls.

Properties of Tumor Cells in Culture

Tumor and normal cells can be distinguished in culture by several tests. Tumorigenic cells are less sensitive to the presence of other cells in their immediate vicinity than are normal cells. Normal cells typically cease proliferation as the culture density increases, but tumor cells can reach several-fold higher densities in culture. If they are plated on a dense layer of nonproliferating, homogeneous normal cells, tumor cells can continue to grow and form foci of clustered cell colonies. Such colonies show altered interactions by the tumor cells, which grow randomly, criss-crossing one another and forming clusters of viable and necrotic cells. When these cultures are fixed and stained, the number of tumor colonies are easily quantitated against the background population of normal cells. This is the basis of the commonly used "focus forming assay" for detecting transformation, e.g., the capacity of mutagens or oncogenes to produce neoplastic transformation within a population of nontumor cells.

Cells of normal solid tissue lie on a secreted extracellular matrix (ECM), composed of various proteins that stimulate cell growth.[46] Transformed cells are often partly or completely independent of ECM for optimal growth, and they may secrete little matrix material.[59] In addition, the cytoskeleton within tumor cells tends to be less well organized, and its actin filaments are less highly polymerized. Tumor cells often can be grown in the absence of a substratum, as within a semisolid medium containing agar. This formation of colonies in suspension is also used as a test of neoplastic transformation.

These properties of tumor versus normal cells are used to detect cells that have been transformed in culture (see below). Each property provides the basis for an assay of neoplastic transformation. However, no one test is absolutely diagnostic for the ability of cells to form a tumor after implantation into a suitable animal such as an athymic mouse. Conditions in vivo differ sufficiently from those in culture that a correlation between the two methods is essential before one can conclude that a given property of the cultured cell is typical of cancer (see III-2).

Genetic Aspects of Cells in Culture

Nontumorigenic cells in culture can be transformed by a variety of agents so as to exhibit properties commonly seen in cells derived from in vivo tumors. Transformed cells can form foci on a normal cell monolayer, or colonies in a semisolid medium. The transformants can often, but not always, form tumors in experimental animals, whereas the original cells cannot.

The common thread in all these modes of transformation is that they cause changes in the DNA of the cells. The means by which this occurs differ widely. Transformation can occur spontaneously while cells continue to be cultured, although this is more commonly seen in certain rodent cells and almost never seen in human cells. Thus, murine embryo fibroblasts spontaneously give rise to cells with altered growth control properties and changes in their karyotypes. A cause–effect relationship between the chromosome rearrangements and the transformed properties is in accord with similar changes seen in cancer cells. Radiation, which creates reactive radicals, and certain chemicals, including many of the drugs used in cancer chemotherapy, are well known to have carcinogenic activities. These agents cause defects in DNA structure through chemical reactions, creating strand breaks and producing cross-links.[29] Transformation frequency has been correlated with degree of mutations, suggesting a mutational origin of carcinogenesis. However, the initiator–

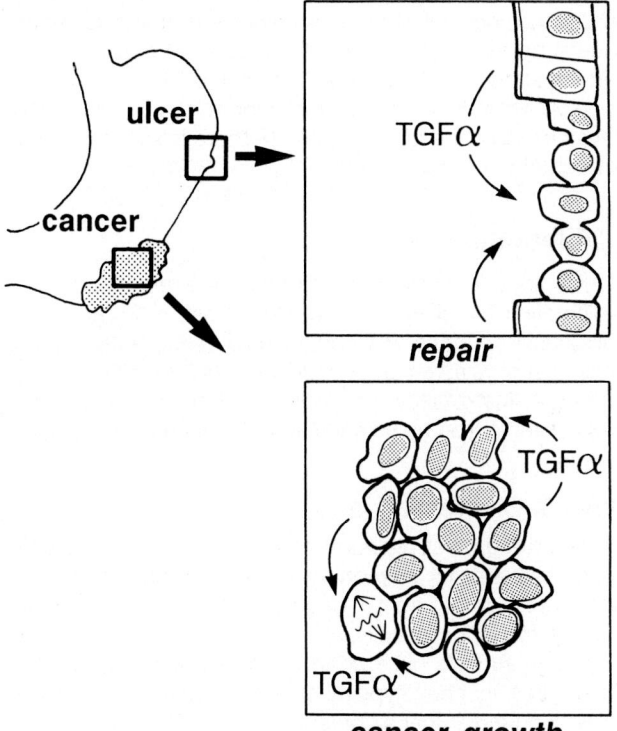

Figure I-1-5. Altered regulation of growth factors. **Top right:** As stem cells of the normal gastric mucosa differentiate, they gain the capacity to produce TGF-α and its surface receptor [the epidermal growth factor (EGF) receptor], both presumed to help regulate normal cell growth and repair. This figure depicts a hypothetical model with release of TGF-α (arrows) in response to a gastric ulcer, stimulating new cell growth and repair. When the ulcer is healed, the stimulation ceases. **Bottom right:** In gastric neoplasms, abnormal regulation of TGF-α and/or its receptor is hypothesized to contribute to the continued growth of cancer cells.[4]

promoter, multistep model of carcinogenesis in vivo suggests that mutation alone is insufficient for tumorigenesis. A few compounds have been reported to be antitumorigenic, acting to alter DNA repair after cells have been damaged, probably converting transforming reactions into lethal ones.[8]

Many carcinogens induce chemical changes in DNA.[35] For example, ultraviolet light creates thymine dimers, whereas X-rays produce chemical radicals within the cell that break DNA strands. Alkylating agents react with DNA bases at several sites, either on one strand or bifunctionally to cross-link DNA chains. In another mechanism, nonmethylated cytosine residues are produced by 5-azacytidine, and this change in DNA is commonly associated with transformation. Effects are sometimes more subtle as some carcinogens are not reactive until they have been activated by metabolism. Oxidative enzymes of the P450 system are found in the microsomal cell fraction of liver. They activate carcinogens such as benzo-[a]-pyrene and other aryl hydrocarbons. These changes are only the beginning of carcinogenesis. Most of the damage is eliminated by repair mechanisms that replace the damage with normal DNA components, so there is no permanent harm to the cell.[45] But when the chromosomes are altered by rearrangements or deletions, or a different base is substituted as a result of faulty repair, the resulting mutation can be either lethal, mutagenic, or even transforming. The repair mechanisms are of several types.[35] For example, in excision repair an endonuclease cleaves the DNA strand near the site of damage, other enzymes excise the damaged region, then DNA polymerases synthesize a replacement strand, and finally DNA ligase and topoisomerase(s) connect new and old segments. These enzymes have been identified as targets for cancer therapy (see XVI-7).[29]

Both RNA and DNA viruses can cause tumors by introducing new genetic information into cells. Retroviruses are small RNA viruses that form tumors in animals. They fall into two classes: 1) those that cause tumors with low efficiency; and 2) rare, highly oncogenic, and acutely transforming retroviruses. These latter viruses have acquired mutated sequences from mammalian cells. Such sequences have been designated oncogenes and, when reintroduced into normal cells by the virus, are responsible for transformation. Some of their functions have been mentioned above. An enormous amount of work has been performed on these oncogenes. Viral transformation appears to convert a normal cell into a tumor cell in a single step, as opposed to the multistep carcinogenesis observed with other agents. However, it is now evident that more than one oncogene is required for transformation. Furthermore, retroviral oncogenes may destabilize other genes in the chromosomes, owing to their flanking sequences, which are called long terminal repeats. These repeats can activate adjacent functional genes to cause further changes that eventually give rise to transformed phenotypes.

Tumor suppressor genes have more recently been proposed and identified (see I-6).[80] Two main lines of evidence support the existence of genes that suppress tumorigenicity in normal cells. First, the loss of certain genes is seen in tumors, as in retinoblastoma. Transfection of the normal RB gene has been reported to suppress the unregulated growth of these tumor cells.[51] Another suppressing protein is p53, whose mutated form (or loss) can be transforming. Mutations of p53 gene have been found in conjunction with chromosome 17p allelic deletions in tumors of the colon, brain, lung, breast, and bone.[2,86] Similar to the transfection experiments with the retinoblastoma gene, reintroduction of normal (not mutated) p53 genes into colon cancer cells inhibited tumor cell growth in vitro.[2] In normal cells the RB protein is produced throughout the cell cycle, but its phosphorylation increases at the G^1/S boundary, and this inactivates the RB protein and its negative effect on cell division.[60] Some studies suggest that the G_1 cyclin-kinase complex may phosphorylate the RB protein, releasing cells from G_1 arrest. Similarly, the p53 protein is likely phosphorylated by G_1 cyclin-kinase enzymes, leading to release from G_1 arrest, in addition to phosphorylation of other substrates required for initiation of S phase.[6]

A widely studied DNA virus is SV40.[60] The SV40 gene coding the T antigen is responsible for transformation of normal cells into tumor cells. Tumorigenic activity of the SV40 virus is probably related to inactivation of these tumor suppressor genes. Both the RB and p53 proteins are bound by the T-antigen, and by the E6 and E7 papilloma virus gene products. Tumor cell growth is suppressed by fusion with a normal cell, suggesting that the normal cell contains tumor suppressor genes.[80] Attempts have been made to isolate such suppressor genes using the (negative) assay of inhibited tumor cell proliferation by transfected DNA. A few have been obtained, including one that suppresses growth of cells transformed by the *ras* oncogene.[69] There is still much to be learned about these genes.

Differentiation

All tumor cells show abnormalities in the regulation of cell proliferation (neoplasia). In addition, most, if not all, tumor cells show abnormalities in differentiation (anaplasia). The anaplasia of tumors can provide insights into their etiology, degree of malignancy, prognosis, and sensitivity to therapeutic intervention by differentiation- or maturation-inducing agents.

What is Differentiation?

It is obvious that although somatic cells are genetically equal they are not phenotypically equal. Thus, skin fibroblasts are different from T lymphocytes, muscle cells differ from gastric mucosal cells, and so forth. However, within an organism, all cells have an identical complement of DNA. Differences in phenotype arise from differences in gene expression, not in gene content.

Differentiation and Gene Expression

The genes expressed by a particular cell comprise only about 10–20% of the coding capacity of the genome. In humans, there are roughly 100,000 genes that code for proteins; however, an individual cell generally expresses only 10,000–20,000 genes.

The genes expressed by a particular cell depend on its embryonic lineage, the developmental stage of the organism, the tissue and cellular environment, and the functions that the cell must fulfill. Differential gene expression (differentiation) occurs extensively during embryogenesis, but some cell types differentiate throughout life. The mechanisms that regulate differential gene expression are incompletely understood. They probably entail cascades or programs of nuclear factors, which repress or activate cell-type-specific genes. These programs of gene expression are generally instituted early in embryogenesis.[43]

Some genes are expressed by many, if not all, cell types. These "housekeeping" genes generally encode proteins that participate in basic or universal cellular functions (i.e., respiration or protein synthesis). Other genes, expressed only in specific cell types and/or stages of development, are said to be cell-type- or differentiation-specific genes. For example, keratinocytes, lymphocytes, and many other cells express the genes for the ribosomal proteins (housekeeping genes). Lymphocytes, but not keratinocytes, express genes for immunoglobulins. However, keratinocytes, but not lymphocytes, express cytokeratins (intermediate filament proteins whose expression is confined to cells of epithelial origin).[66] In addition, keratinocytes express particular cytokeratins, depending on the stage of differentiation (position in the epidermis). Finally, genes that encode the cornified envelope proteins are expressed only by keratinocytes that have undergone extensive differentiation and inhabit the uppermost epidermal layers.[76] Thus, the expression of specific gene products marks both the cell lineage and the stage of differentiation.

Differentiation and Cell Proliferation

Differentiation begins shortly after the first few cell divisions that follow fertilization. Throughout development, and in adult organisms, a cell's ability to proliferate is intimately connected to its state of differentiation.

In early embryos, cell proliferation is the primary means by which the cell mass increases. As the organism develops, proliferation becomes restricted. Some differentiated cells continue to proliferate; others irreversibly lose their ability to proliferate. Embryonic cells often display traits that confer on them a selective growth advantage over that of an adult cell. They proliferate vigorously, are capable of extensive migration, secrete factors that increase the local supply of blood (and, therefore, of nutrients), and produce enzymes capable of degrading basement membranes. In adult organisms, mutations or conditions that activate portions of embryonic programs of gene expression, or inactivate portions of the adult program, can produce cells having many properties of malignant tumor cells.[65]

Stem Cells

Stem cells have the capacity for both self-renewal (proliferation without a change in phenotype) and differentiation (changing into a new phenotype). Some stem cells have already undergone considerable differentiation so that further differentiation is restricted to a single cell type or lineage (for example, the basal keratinocytes of the epidermis, or stem cells of the intestinal crypts). Other stem cells are multipotent and differentiate into a variety of cell types, i.e., hematopoietic stem cells. It has been difficult to demonstrate

cells in adults that are totipotent, or capable of differentiating into many or all cell types.

In general, stem cell differentiation results in two types of changes: the expression of specialized, differentiation-specific gene products, and a partial or complete restriction of the cell's capacity for further proliferation. It follows, then, that another mechanism by which tumor cells might arise is by mutations that render a stem cell partly or wholly unable to differentiate.

Terminal Differentiation

Some cells, particularly in adults, are terminally differentiated. Terminally differentiated cells are irreversibly blocked in their ability to proliferate, although they may perform specialized functions for a long period of time. Some terminally differentiated cells, such as mature muscle and nerve cells, persist throughout much of the organism's lifespan. Others, such as keratinocytes in the outer epidermal layer, die soon after terminal differentiation. Terminal differentiation is an end state, the result of a stem cell that has gone through several successive stages of differentiation.

Tumors of terminally differentiated cells are rarely if ever found. Thus, tumors of mature muscle or nerve cells do not occur, although tumors of less differentiated myoblastic or neuronal stem cells do occur. Cell proliferation appears to be incompatible with the expression of a terminally differentiated program of gene expression. For example, cultured myoblasts or preadipocytes can be induced to differentiate terminally by modifying the culture conditions. When cells that are capable of terminal differentiation are forced to proliferate, i.e., by transfecting an oncogene into the cells or by providing a potent mitogen, terminal differentiation cannot be induced. Not only do the cells continue to proliferate, but they fail to express the gene products characteristic of the terminally differentiated state, i.e., muscle myosin or fat-metabolizing enzymes. Thus, the irreversible arrest of cell division and expression of the terminally differentiated phenotype are interdependent.

In healthy tissue, whether embryonic or adult, there is always a balance between cell proliferation and cell loss through death or terminal differentiation. In many tissues, proliferation is restricted to a subpopulation of cells, the stem cells, which undergo self-renewal as well as differentiation into less proliferative cell types. It follows, then, that mutations or conditions that interfere with the differentiation of stem cells will result in unbalanced proliferation and, thus, uncontrolled growth of the tissue. Mutations that drive proliferation are associated with an accumulation and overgrowth of less differentiated cells in the tissue. A common feature of tumor cells is their failure to differentiate terminally under appropriate conditions in vivo or in culture.[75,99,103]

Cellular Senescence

All normal, differentiated cells have only a limited capacity for cell division in vitro. Under suitable culture conditions, cells that can proliferate will go through an initial proliferative phase, but this is invariably followed by a gradual decline in growth of the culture. This progressive decline in proliferation is termed the finite lifespan phenotype or cellular senescence, and it is usually about 50 population doublings for human cells in culture.

In cell cultures derived from several rodent species, immortal cells (cells having an infinite lifespan in culture) arise spontaneously at a low frequency. These new cells can be propagated indefinitely in culture, and are called cell lines. Senescence is much more complete and irreversible with human cells cultured from normal tissues; establishment of immortal human cell lines rarely, if ever, occurs. Immortal cells, typically derived from embryonic rodent tissues, are much more susceptible to tumorigenic transformation than are cells that have a finite lifespan. Because many (but not all) human tumor cells are immortal, given appropriate culture conditions, it is thought that the acquisition of immortality is an important step in tumor progression.[80]

Once human cells senesce, it is virtually impossible to induce them to proliferate again.[72] In addition, senescent cells often show an altered pattern of gene expression.[82] Thus, in some ways, cellular senescence resembles terminal differentiation. One possibility is that the genes responsible for the loss of proliferation during terminal differentiation and senescence are either the same, or have common structural or functional features.

The "finite lifespan" phenotype and the nontumorigenic phenotype are generally dominant. When immortal cells are fused to normal cells, the hybrid cells undergo senescence and are not immortal. Similarly, when normal and tumor cells are fused, the hybrids are generally not tumorigenic. These findings support the idea that normal cells express one or more genes that ordinarily act to restrain growth. In cell hybrids, the suppressor genes, expressed by the normal cell, repress the immortal and transformed phenotypes. An important step in tumorigenesis may be the loss (by mutational inactivation or deletion due to chromosomal instability) of both alleles of a tumor suppressor gene (see I-6).[80] An intriguing hypothesis is that such tumor suppressor genes also function in pathways leading to cellular senescence and terminal differentiation.

Several types of normal tissues undergo involution in response to environmental stimuli. This property has been termed "programmed cell death" or "apoptosis". It has been studied in experimental models with cells or tissues from various mammalian species. One of these models is organ cultures of müllerian ducts from developing male embryos. These cultures undergo regression and cell death when exposed to the hormone called müllerian inhibiting substance (MIS).[25,95] This is similar to the growth and subsequent rapid degeneration of müllerian ducts within developing male embryos. MIS has structural similarity to TGF-β, and some studies suggest it causes tissue regression by inhibition of EGF-induced tyrosine phosphorylation.[16,21] Since embryonic cells that have not differentiated into müllerian ducts are not sensitive to MIS, programmed death is acquired as part of normal tissue differentiation. Prolonged viability and growth of tumor cells may be related to inhibition of usual apoptosis reactions. The protein coded by the bcl-2 oncogene, found in many human lymphoid neoplasms, may interfere with apoptosis through interaction with mitochondrial metabolism.[47]

The molecular events leading to apoptosis are not well defined; several studies implicate activation of endonucleases, new protein synthesis, soluble factors, and ion fluxes.[101] Future studies may provide new approaches to cancer therapy by selective enhancement of apoptosis in neoplastic tissues.[20] For example, MIS has been proposed as a potential therapeutic agent for gynecologic neoplasms, which have a müllerian duct origin and express appropriate receptors or depend on continued EGF-induced tyrosine phosphorylation.[95]

Extracellular Factors That Control Differentiation

During embryogenesis and in a number of adult tissues, differentiation depends upon external factors. These include insoluble factors such as the extracellular matrix (ECM) and the proximity and type of neighboring cells, as well as a growing list of soluble factors. In model systems, differentiation can be induced by a variety of biologic agents and drugs (Table I-1-3). The ECM and the differentiation-promoting soluble factors may be produced by the same cells that respond to these signals (autocrine regulation). They also may be produced by adjacent or distal cells (paracrine regulation).

Cell–cell and cell–ECM interactions are important for both the induction and maintenance of differentiation in several cell lineages. Unfortunately, relatively little is known at a molecular level about how insoluble factors act. In the case of the ECM, there are specific cell surface receptors that bind to particular components of the ECM.[28] One likely possibility is that the binding of an ECM component to its cellular receptor activates an intracellular signal transduction pathway, analogous to the signalling pathways that have been identified for polypeptide growth factors.

The soluble factors that regulate differentiation can be broadly classified into those that bind to cell surface receptors, and those that freely cross the plasma membrane and bind to cytoplasmic or nuclear receptors.

The first class includes molecules such as the fibroblast growth factors (FGF's), transforming growth factors alpha and beta (TGF-α and TGF-β), and hematopoietic factors such as colony-stimulating factor-1 (CSF-1), granulocyte colony-stimulating factor (G-CSF), granulocyte-macrophage colony-stimulating factor (GM-CSF), and the interleukins. These are all polypeptides, many of which were first identified as growth factors or inhibitors. The action of these polypeptides depends on production of cell-surface receptors, specific to certain cell types. For example, mononuclear phagocytes and their precursors express high-affinity CSF-1 receptors, coded by the c-fms gene. This receptor belongs to a family of protein–tyrosine kinases. The receptor for PDGF is structurally similar to the CSF-1 receptor, but activation of these receptors induces different intracellular responses, such as activation of specific phosphatidylinositol kinases and changes in intracellular calcium levels.[93]

FGF was identified as a fibroblast mitogen in brain and pituitary extracts, but recent data suggest that FGF induces mesodermal differentiation in early embryos.[56,77] FGF also inhibits the differentiation of some cells; terminal differentiation into mature myotubes cannot occur unless it is withdrawn from proliferating myoblasts. Similarly, TGF-β was first identified as a stimulator of anchorage-independent growth

Table I-1-3. Induction of Differentiation in Culture

Stem cell	Differentiation markers	Inducers
Preadipocyte	Adipocyte	Insulin, cort, cell density
Basal keratinocyte	Cornified envelope	RA—deficiency, cell density
Myoblast	Myotube	GF—deficiency, cell density
Squamous cell carcinoma	Cornified envelope	GF—deficiency, cort
Embryonal carcinoma	Endoderm, mesoderm, ectoderm	RA, ara-C, mito, HMBA, co-culture with blastocysts
Neuroblastoma	Neuron, neurotransmitter, action potential	PI, 6TG, ara-C, MTX, dox, bleo, RA, GF—deficiency
Melanoma	Dendrite, melanin, tyrosinase	PI, dox, DMSO, TPA, RA, MSH
Colon adenocarcinoma	Mucus, dome formation, CEA, columnar cell	NMF, DMSO, butyrate, low glucose, IFN, HMBA, cell density
Breast adenocarcinoma	Casein, dome formation	RA, PGE, DMSO
Bladder transitional cell carcinoma	Keratin filament, loss of surface antigen	HMBA
Erythroleukemia	Mature erythroid cell, hemoglobin	Dox, ara-C, 6TG, mito, dact, aza, hemin, DMSO, HMBA, CSF, RA, IFN
Promyelocytic	Granulocyte, macrophage	IFN, CSF, vitD, TPA, DMSO, NMF, dact, HMBA, aza, ara-C, RA
Myelocytic leukemia	Granulocyte, macrophage	CSF, RA, vitD, ara-C, dact, DMSO, TPA, cort, dox

Abbreviations: ara-C, cytarabine; aza, 5-azacytidine; bleo, bleomycin; CSF (G- or GM-), colony stimulating factor; cort, glucocorticoids; DMSO, dimethylsulfoxide; dact, dactinomycin; dox, doxorubicin; GF, growth factor; HMBA, hexamethylbisacetamide; IFN, alpha or gamma interferon; MSH, melanocyte stimulating hormone; MTX, methotrexate; mito, mitomycin C; NMF, N, N dimethylformamide; PGE, prostaglandin E; PI, phosphodiesterase inhibitor; RA, retinoic acid; TPA, 12-0-tetradecanoylphorbol-13-acetate; 6TG, 6-thioguanine; vitD, 1,25-dihydroxy vitamin D.
Modified from Cheson,[15] Reiss,[74] and Waxman.[97]

in mesenchymal cells, and later as an inhibitor of epithelial cell proliferation.[78,89] Like FGF, TGF-β stimulates the differentiation of some cells, i.e., keratinocytes or intestinal epithelial cells, but inhibits differentiation in others, i.e., myoblasts or preadipocytes. In some human tumor cells cultured in vitro or in athymic mice, TGF-β has been shown both to inhibit tumor growth and to promote a more differentiated phenotype in the remaining cells.[92]

The membrane-permeable regulators of differentiation include retinoic acid (vitamin A) and its derivatives (RA).[84] There is strong evidence that concentration gradients of RA are critical for the morphogenesis of some tissues in the early embryo.[24] RA can stimulate or inhibit growth and differentiation depending on the cell type. In general, RA is required for the differentiation of many epithelial cells. It diffuses freely into cells whereupon it binds to specific nuclear protein receptors (the retinoic acid receptors or RARs). At least three classes of RARs have been identified. Cell types vary in both the quality and quantity of RARs they express. In addition, other nuclear proteins, called RAR coregulators, have been found that interact with RARs and modulate their actions in various cell types.[38] These differences may explain why specific cells and tissues differ in their responses to RA. Some differentiation-specific genes that are regulated by RA contain 5′ sequences to which RA–RAR complexes bind, thereby activating transcription.[24,94] The sex steroids estrogen and testosterone may regulate differentiation by similar mechanisms. Like RA, the sex steroids freely cross the plasma membrane and bind to specific nuclear receptors. Steroid receptor complexes then activate or repress the transcription of differentiation-specific genes. Whether or not a cell can respond to RA, or a particular steroid, depends upon whether it expresses the gene for the appropriate nuclear receptor.

Tumor cells often produce factors that affect both growth and differentiation. These factors often change the growth and differentiated properties of the tumor cells themselves, as well as the surrounding normal tissue. For example, at least one type of FGF has been identified as an oncogene. FGF can itself confer neoplastic properties when expressed in an inappropriate cell type (e.g., a fibroblast). In addition, inappropriate expression of FGF by one cell may stimulate the growth and affect the differentiation of neighboring cell types.[77]

Intracellular Regulators

Cellular differentiation is controlled by external factors and by intrinsic programs of gene expression. In either case, the expression of differentiation-specific genes is generally under the control of a small number of master regulatory genes. A small number of genes have recently been identified that are potential "master regulators" of developmental stages and differentiation-specific gene expression. The most globally acting, master regulatory genes are known as homeotic genes. Homeotic genes were first identified as genetic loci that determined the developmental and spatial fates of cells in embryos of the fruit fly Drosophila. Similar genes have been identified in the genomes of higher organisms, including humans. Individual homeotic genes are expressed at different times during development and are also expressed in different adult tissues. Some homeotic genes code for extracellular factors while others code for nuclear proteins that are probably transcriptional regulatory factors. Homeotic genes regulate programs of differentiation, as opposed to individual differentiation-specific genes. Presumably they initiate a cascade of gene expression that involves regulatory genes having a more restricted range of actions.[37,49]

Some "master regulatory" genes appear to function only in cells of a restricted lineage. The best studied are those that regulate muscle differentiation.[58] The myoD and myd genes control the differentiation of mesenchymal stem cells into myoblasts, and the myogenin gene controls the differentiation of myoblasts into mature skeletal muscle. These genes all code for nuclear proteins that regulate the transcription of muscle-specific genes.[100] Mutations that interfere with the induction or function of myoD, myd, or myogenin select cells that cannot terminally differentiate and, therefore, have the potential to form a tumor.

DNA Methylation

In many cases, cells must go through one or more rounds of DNA replication before they can differentiate. This may be because there is often a need to modify the pattern of DNA methylation before differentiation can occur. Changes in DNA methylation are commonly introduced during DNA replication. The methylation of DNA on specific cytosine residues is believed to contribute to the changes in gene expression that occur during development. Presumably, DNA methylation affects gene expression because the transcriptional regulatory proteins that bind to methylated DNA differ from those that bind to unmethylated DNA. Many neoplastic tissues are hypomethylated relative to their normal counterparts.[32,39] Indeed, pharmacological agents that alter the pattern of DNA methylation induce differentiation in a number of cultured cell lines. However, DNA methylation is probably not a universal mechanism for differentiation, and some cells can be induced to differentiate with minimal or no change in cell cycle progression.[12]

Differentiation and Cancer Therapy

Analysis of differentiation by tumor cells often provides valuable information for both the diagnosis and therapy of human cancers. As tumor cells grow and die, they can release glycoproteins and other products similar to those of fetal tissues, and these oncofetal products can be detected in serum, or other body fluids, to assist in diagnosis, follow-up, and selection of therapies. Since these markers are usually antigenic, they are typically quantified with sensitive immunologic assays. Diagnosis of male testicular carcinomas and female gestational neoplasms is greatly assisted by measuring serum levels of human chorionic gonadotropin (hCG) or alpha feto-protein (AFP). Similarly, immunologic techniques can be used to assist the pathologist to identify the original tissue source for metastatic neoplasms that have no obvious origin by routine studies (see XXXVIII). Examples include estrogen receptors and alpha-lactalbumin in breast cancer, prostate-specific antigen and prostate acid phosphatase in prostate cancers, and myoglobin and desmin in sarcomas.[40]

Elevations of these markers in the serum often predict relapse of the neoplasm before any sign by routine examination or radiographic tests. In general, the specificity of such markers for a given neoplasm is poor, since minor elevations also occur with inflammatory and other benign conditions, or with several types of neoplasms. Clinical studies are ongoing to investigate serum or tissue markers of differentiation, aiming to "fine tune" either the timing or type of cancer therapy.[96] In carcinoma of unknown primary site, tissue markers for neuroendocrine differentiation select for a subgroup of patients with improved response to chemotherapy.[44] Similarly, neuroendocrine markers in non-small cell lung cancer may be associated with improved response rate to chemotherapy.[42]

Some tumor cells can be induced to differentiate terminally. This has been shown most extensively in cultured cell lines (Table I-1-3), but it has also been demonstrated in experimental animals.[74,92,97] After tumor cells have been induced to undergo terminal differentiation, their ability to grow as a tumor is often stably suppressed. In contrast to most anticancer drugs, which have nonspecific toxicity to both normal and cancer cells, drug-induced differentiation can be demonstrated with agents (or drug levels) that exert minimal effects on normal cells.[74] These observations have stimulated increased interest in clinical applications of differentiating agents to provide therapeutic gain with minimal toxicity.[97]

A number of agents known to induce differentiation in various model systems have been used clinically (Table I-1-3). Some of them are useful in only a particular type of tumor. For example, estrogens and androgens have been useful in treating some breast, prostate, and gynecologic tumors, providing, of course, that the tumor cells express the appropriate nuclear receptor. Other differentiation-inducing drugs have been more widely studied. For example, high doses of retinoic acid, hexamethylene bisacetamide, or 5-azacytidine, an inhibitor of DNA methylation, can induce differentiation and inhibit the growth of several types of tumors in laboratory models.[97]

In fresh cultures of human promyelocytic leukemia, retinoid-induced differentiation has been observed, similar to the effects seen in passaged leukemia cell lines.[10] All-trans retinoic acid has been used in clinical therapy of promyelocytic leukemia with promising initial results.[13,96A] Differentiation has been observed in cultured leukemia cells exposed to mithramycin and hydroxyurea, and some investigators have proposed this mechanism to explain remissions induced in patients with the accelerated phase of chronic myelogenous leukemia.[53] Since these and other proposed differentiating agents may also inhibit tumor cell growth by multiple mechanisms, it is difficult to prove specific differentiating actions of these agents when they are used in patients.[15,96A]

Retinoids and other differentiating agents are also used in clinical trials to prevent cancer in patients with premalignant lesions or with a high risk for developing cancer of the breast, cervix, colon, skin, lung, or oral cavity. Early results are encouraging, including the reversal of oral leukoplakia, and prevention of second neoplasms in patients with treated squamous cell carcinoma of the head and neck.[15,50] At present, it is difficult to predict whether or not the cells of a particular tumor (or precancerous lesion) can be induced to undergo terminal differentiation. In addition, retinoids can promote effects of carcinogens to induce new tumors in some experimental models, although other investigators using similar models found no such promoting effect.[68] Thus, the ultimate action of these drugs may be related to the target tissue, environmental factors, experimental methods, or other unknown events. However, greater knowledge about the molecular basis for the control of differentiation should lead to more accurate predictions, and to rational design of therapies for controlling tumor growth by manipulating the state of differentiation.[64,97]

References

1. Ashmun, R. A., Look, A. T., Roberts, W. M., Roussel, M. F., Seremetis, S., Ohtsuka, M., and Sherr, C. J.: Monoclonal antibodies to the human CSF-1 receptor detect epitopes on normal mononuclear phagocytes and on human myeloid leukemia blast cells. Blood, 73:827, 1989.
2. Baker, S. J., Markowitz, S., Fearon, E. R., Willson, J. K. V., and Vogelstein, B.: Suppression of human colorectal carcinoma cell growth by wild-type p53. Science, 249:912, 1990.
3. Baserga, R.: The Biology of Cell Reproduction. Cambridge, Harvard University Press, 1985.
4. Beauchamp, R. D., Barnard, J. D., McCutchen, C. M., Cherner, J. A., and Coffey, R. J., Jr.: Localization of transforming growth factor alpha and its receptor in gastric mucosal cells. J. Clin. Invest., 84:1017, 1989.
5. Bennington, J. L.: Cellular kinetics of invasive squamous carcinoma of the human cervix. Cancer Res., 29:1082, 1969.
6. Bischoff, J. R., Friedman, P. N., Marshak, D. R., Prives, C., and Beach, D.: Human p53 is phosphorylated by p60-cdc2 and cyclin B-cdc2. Proc. Natl. Acad. Sci., USA, 87:4766, 1990.
7. Bishop, J. M.: The molecular genetics of cancer. Science, 235:305, 1987.
8. Boothman, D. A., Schlegel, R., and Pardee, A. B.: Anticarcinogenic potential of DNA-repair modulators. Mutat. Res., 202:393, 1988.
9. Bourne, H. R.: Signals past, present, and future. Cold Spring Harbor Symp. Quant. Biol., LIII:1019, 1988.
10. Breitman, T. R., Collins, S. J., and Keene, B. R.: Terminal differentiation of human promyelocytic leukemic cells in primary culture in response to retinoic acid. Blood, 57:1000, 1981.
11. Bresciani, F., Pauluzi, R., Benassi, M., Nervi, C., Casale, C., and Ziparo, E.: Cell kinetics and growth of squamous cell carcinomas in man. Cancer Res., 34:2405, 1974.
12. Carlsson, M., Totterman, T. H., Matsson, P., and Nilsson, K.: Cell cycle progression of B-chronic lymphocytic leukemia cells induced to differentiate by TPA. Blood, 71:415, 1988.
13. Castaigne, S., Chomienne, C., Daniel, M. T., Ballerini, P., Berger, R., Fenaux, P., and Degos, L.: All-trans retinoic acid as a differentiation therapy for acute promyelocytic leukemia. I. Clinical Results. Blood, 76:1704, 1990.
14. Challberg, M. D., and Kelly, T. J.: Animal virus DNA replication. Annu. Rev. Biochem., 58:671, 1989.
15. Cheson, B. D., Jasperse, D. M., Chun, H. G., and Friedman, M. A.: Differentiating agents in the treatment of human malignancies. Cancer Treat. Rev. 13:129, 1986.
16. Cigarroa, F. G., Coughlin, J. P., Donahoe, P. K., White, M. F., Uitvlugt, N., and MacLaughlin, D. T.: Recombinant human müllerian inhibiting substance inhibits epidermal growth factor receptor tyrosine kinase. Growth Factors, 1:179, 1989.
17. Clark, G. M., Dressler, L. G., Owens, M.A., Pounds, G., Oldaker, T., and McGuire, W. L.: Prediction of relapse or survival in patients with node-negative breast cancer by DNA flow cytometry. N. Engl. J. Med., 320:627, 1989.
18. Clarkson, B., Ota, K., Ohkita, T., and O'Connor, A.: Kinetics of proliferation of cancer cells in neoplastic effusions in man. Cancer, 18:1189, 1965.
19. Coffey, D. S., and Isaacs, J. T.: Prostate tumor biology and cell kinetics–theory. Urology (Suppl. 3), 17:40, 1981.
20. Coffey, D. S., and Pienta, K. J.: New concepts in studying the control of normal and cancer growth of the prostate. Prog. Clin. Biol. Res., 239:1, 1987.
21. Coughlin, J. P., Donahoe, P. K., Budzik, G. P., and MacLaughlin, D. T.: Mullerian inhibiting substance blocks autophosphorylation of the EGF receptor by inhibiting tyrosine kinase. Mol. Cell. Endocrinol., 49:75, 1987.
22. Crabtree, G. R.: Contingent genetic regulatory events in T lymphocyte activation. Science, 243:355, 1989.
23. Cross, F., Weintraub, H., and Roberts, J.: Simple and complex cell cycle. Annu. Rev. Cell Biol., 5:341, 1989.
24. Dolle, P., Ruberte. E., Kastner, P., Petkovich, M., Stoner, C. M., Gudas, L. J., and Chambon, P.: Differential expression of genes encoding alpha, beta and gamma retinoic acid receptors and CRABP in the developing limbs of the mouse. Nature, 342:702, 1989.
25. Donahoe, P. K., Cate, R., MacLaughlin, D. T., Epstein, J., Fuller, A. F., Takahashi, M., Coughlin, J. P., Ninfa, E. G., and Taylor, L. A.: Müllerian inhibiting substance: Gene structure and mechanism of action of a fetal regressor. *In* Recent Progress in Hormone Research, Vol. 43. New York, Academic Press, 1987, pp. 431–467.
26. Druker, B. J., Mamon, H. J., and Roberts, T. M.: Oncogenes, growth factors, and signal transduction. N. Engl. J. Med., 321:1383, 1989.
27. Dunphy, W. G., and Newport, J. W.: Unraveling of mitotic control mechanisms. Cell, 55:925, 1988.
28. Ekblom, P., Vestweber, D., and Kemler, R.: Cell and extracellular matrix: Their organization and mutual dependence. Annu. Rev. Cell Biol., 2:27, 1986.
29. Epstein, R. J.: Drug-induced DNA damage and tumor chemosensitivity. J. Clin. Oncol., 8:2062, 1990.
30. Fabrikant, J. I., and Cherry, J.: The kinetics of cellular proliferation in normal and malignant tissues. J. Surg. Oncol., 1:23, 1969.
31. Fakuda, K., Iwasaka, T., Hachisuga, T.D, Sugimori, H.K., Tsugitomi, H., and Mutoh, F.: Immunocytochemical detection of S-phase cells in normal and neoplastic cervical epithelium by anti-BrdU monoclonal antibody. Anal. Quant. Cytol. Histol., 12:135, 1990.
32. Feinberg, A. P., and Vogelstein, B.: Hypomethylation distinguishes genes of some human cancers from their normal counterparts. Nature, 301:89, 1983.
33. Fettig, O., and Sievers, R.: 3H-index und mittlere Generationszeit des menschlichen Portiokarzinoms und seiner Vorstufen. Beitr. Pathol., 133:83, 1966.
34. Fingert, H. J., Campisi, J., Pardee, A. B.: Molecular Biology and Biochemistry of Cancer. *In* Gynecologic Oncology, 2nd edition. Edited by R. Knapp, and R. Berkowitz. New York, Macmillan Press, 1991, p. 30.
35. Friedberg, E. C.: DNA repair. New York, Freeman Press, 1987.
36. Garcia, R. L., Coltrera, M. D., and Gown, A. M.: Analysis of proliferative grade using anti-PCNA/cyclin monoclonal antibodies in fixed, embedded tissues. Am. J. Pathol., 134:733, 1989.
37. Gehring, W. J.: Homeoboxes in the study of development. Science 236:1245, 1987.
38. Glass, C. K., Devary, O. V., and Rosenfeld, M. G.: Multiple cell type-specific proteins differentially regulate target sequence recognition by the alpha retinoic acid receptor. Cell, 63:729, 1990.
39. Goelz, S. E., Vogelstein, B., Hamilton, S. R., and Feinberg, A. P.: Hypomethylation of DNA from benign and malignant human colon neoplasms. Science, 228:187, 1985.
40. Gorstein, F., and Thor, A.: Tumor Markers in Diagnostic Pathology, Vol. 10 in Clinics in Laboratory Medicine. Philadelphia, W.B. Saunders, 1990.
41. Goustin, A. S., Leof, E. B., Shipley, G. D., and Moses, H. L.: Growth factors and cancer. Cancer Res., 46:1015, 1986.
42. Graziano, S. L., Mazid, R., Newman, N., Tatum, A., Oler, A., Mortimer, J. A., Gullo, J. J., DiFino, S. M., and Scalzo, A. J.: The use of neuroendocrine immunoperoxidase markers to predict chemotherapy response in patients with non-small-cell lung cancer. J. Clin. Oncol., 7:1398, 1989.
43. Gurdon, J. B.: Embryonic induction–molecular prospects. Development 99:285, 1987.
44. Hainsworth, J. D., Johnson, D. H., and Greco, F. A.: Poorly differentiated neuroendocrine carcinoma of unknown primary site. Ann. Intern. Med., 109:364, 1988.
45. Hanawalt, P. C., Cooper, P. K., Ganesan, A. K., and Smith, C. A.: DNA repair in bacteria and mammalian cells. Annu. Rev. Biochem., 48: 783, 1979.
46. Hawkes, S., and Wang, J. L.: Extracellular Matrix. New York, Academic Press, 1982.
47. Hockenbery, D., Nunez, G., Milliman, C., Schreiber, R. D., and Korsmeyer, S. J.: Bcl-2 is an inner mitochondrial membrane protein that blocks programmed cell death. Nature, 348:334, 1990.
48. Hoffman, R. M., Connors, K. M., Meerson-Monosov, A. Z., Herrera, H., and Price, J. H.: A general native-state method for determination of proliferation capacity of human normal and tumor tissues in vitro. Proc. Natl. Acad. Sci. USA, 86:2013, 1989.
49. Holland P. W. H., and Hogan B. L. M.: Expression of homeobox genes during mouse development: A review. Genes Devel. 2:773, 1988.
50. Hong, W. K., Lippman, S. M., Itri, L. M., Karp, D. D., Lee, J. S., Byers, R. M., Schantz, S. P., Kramer, A. M. , Lotan, R., Peters, L. J., Dimery, I. W., Brown, B. W., and Goepfert, H.: Prevention of second primary tumors with isotretinoin in squamous-cell carcinoma of the head and neck. N. Engl. J. Med., 323:795, 1990.
51. Huang, H. J. S., Yee, J. K., Shew, J. Y., Chen, P. L., Bookstein, R., Friedmann, T., Lee, E. Y., and Lee, W. H.: Suppression of the neoplastic phenotype by replacement of the RB gene in human cancer cells. Science, 242:1563, 1989.
52. Kallioniemi, O., Punnonen, R., Mattila, J., Lehtinen, M., and Koivula, T.: Prognostic significance of DNA index, multiploidy, and S-phase fraction in ovarian cancer. Cancer, 61:334, 1988.
53. Koller, C. A., and Miller, D. M.: Preliminary observations on the therapy of the myeloid blast phase of chronic granulocytic leukemia with plicamycin and hydroxyurea. N. Engl. J. Med., 315:1433, 1986.
54. Kroese, M. C., Rutgers, D. H., Wils, I. S., Van Unnik, J. A., and Roholl, P. J.: The relevance of the DNA index and proliferation rate in the grading of benign and malignant soft tissue tumors. Cancer, 65:1782, 1990.
55. Lampkin, B. C.: Cell kinetics as related to treatment of patients with acute nonlymphoid leukemia. Am. J. Pediatr. Hematol. Oncol., 7:358, 1985.
56. Lemmon, S. K., Riley, M. C., Thomas, K. A., Hoover, G. A., Maciag, T., and Bradshaw, R. A.: Bovine fibroblast growth factor: Comparison of brain and pituitary preparations. J. Cell Biol., 95:162, 1982.
57. Lewin, B.: Driving the cell cycle: M phase kinase, its partners, and substrates. Cell, 61:743, 1990.
58. Linkhart, T. A., Clegg, C. H., and Hauschka, S. D.: Control of mouse myoblast commitment to terminal differentiation by mitogens. J. Supramol. Struct., 14:483, 1980.
59. Liotta, L. A.: Tumor invasion and metastases–role of the extracellular matrix. Cancer Res., 46:1, 1986.
60. Ludlow, J. W., De Caprio, J. A., Huang, C. M., Lee, W. H., Paucha, E., and Livingston, D. M.: SV40 large T antigen binds preferentially to an underphosphorylated member of the retinoblastoma susceptibility gene product family. Cell, 56:57, 1989.
61. McKeever, P. E., Feldenzer, J. A., McCoy, J. P., Laug, M., Gebarski, S., Chandler, W. F., Greenberg, H. S., Junck, L., D'Amato, C. J., and Varani, J.: Nuclear parameters as prognostic indicators in glioblastoma patients. J. Neuropathol. Exp. Neurol., 49:71, 1990.
62. Merkel, D. E., and McGuire, W. L.: Ploidy, proliferative activity and prognosis. Cancer, 65:1194, 1990.
63. Meyer, J. S.: Growth and cell kinetic measurements in human tumors. Pathol. Ann., 16:53, 1981.
64. Meyskens, F. L., Jr.: Coming of age–the chemoprevention of cancer. N. Engl. J. Med., 323:825, 1990.
65. Mintz, B., and Fleischman, R. A.: Teratocarcinomas and other neoplasms as developmental defects in gene expression. Adv. Cancer Res., 34:211, 1981.
66. Moll R., Francke W. W., Schiller D. L., Geiger B., and Krepler R.: The catalogue of human cytokeratins: Patterns of expression in normal epithelia, tumors and cultured cells. Cell 31:11, 1982.
67. Moses, H. L., Yang, E. Y., and Pientenpol, J. A.: TGF-beta stimulation and inhibition of cell proliferation: New mechanistic insights. Cell, 63:245, 1990.
68. Nauss, K. M., Bueche, D., and Newberne, P. M.: Effect of vitamin A nutriture on experimental esophageal carcinogenesis. J. Natl. Cancer Inst., 79:145, 1987.
69. Noda, M., Kitayama, H., Matsuzaki, T., Sugimoto, Y., Okayama, H., Bassin, R. H., and Ikawa, Y.: Detection of genes with a potential for suppressing the transformed phenotype associated with activated ras genes. Proc. Natl. Acad. Sci. USA, 86:162, 1989.
70. Pardee, A. B.: Molecules involved in proliferation of normal and cancer cells. Cancer Res., 47:1488, 1987.
71. Pardee, A. B.: G_1 events and regulation of cell proliferation. Science, 246:603, 1989.
72. Phillips P. D., and Cristofalo V. J.: A review of cellular aging research: Regulation of cell proliferation. Rev. Biol. Aging Res., 2:339, 1985.
73. Quinn, C. M., and Wright, N. A.: The clinical assessment of proliferation and growth in human tumours: evaluation of methods and applications as prognostic variables. J. Pathol., 160:93, 1990.
74. Reiss, M., Gamba-Vitalo, C., and Sartorelli, A.C.: Induction of tumor cell differentation as a therapeutic approach: preclinical models for hematopoietic and solid neoplasms. Cancer Treat. Rep., 70:201, 1986.
75. Rheinwald, J. G., and Beckett, M. A.: Defective terminal differentiation in culture as a consistent and selectable character of malignant human keratinocytes. Cell, 22:629, 1980.
76. Rice R. H., and Thacher S. M.: Involucrin: A constituent of cross-linked evelopes and

marker of squamous maturation. *In* Biology of the Integument 2. Edited by J. Bereiter-Hahn, A. G. Motolsky, and K. S. Richard. New York, Springer Verlag, 1986. pp. 752-761.

77. Rifkin D. B., and Moscatelli D.: Recent developments in the cell biology of basic fibroblasts growth factor. J. Cell Biol., 109:1, 1989.
78. Rizzino, A.: Transforming growth factor-beta: Multiple effects on cell differentiation and extracellular matrices. Dev. Biol., 130:411, 1988.
79. Rozengurt, E.: Early signals in the mitogenic response. Science, 234:161, 1986.
80. Sager, R.: Tumor suppressor genes: The puzzle and the promise. Science 246:1406, 1989.
81. Schneider, C., King, R. M., and Phillipson, L.: Genes specifically expressed at growth arrest of mammalian cells. Cell, 54:787, 1988.
82. Seshadri T., and Campisi J.: Repression of c-fos transcription and an altered genetic program in senescent human fibroblasts. Science, 247:205, 1990.
83. Skipper, H. E., and Schabel, F. M., Jr.: Quantitative and cytokinetic studies in experimental tumor systems. *In* Cancer Medicine, 2nd Edition. Edited by J. F. Holland, and E. Frei, III. Philadelphia, Lea and Febiger, 1982, pp. 663-684.
84. Sporn, M. B., Roberts, A. B., and Goodman, D. S.: The Retinoids, Vol. 2. New York, Academic Press, 9:56, 1984.
85. Steel, G. G.: Cytokinetics of Neoplasia. *In* Cancer Medicine, 2nd Edition. Edited by J. F. Holland, and E. Frei, III. Philadelphia, Lea and Febiger, 1982, pp. 177-189.
86. Takahashi, T., Nau, M. M., Chiba, I., Birrer, M. J., Rosenberg, R. K., Vinocour, M., Levitt, M., Pass, H., Gazdar, A. F., and Minna, J. D.: p53: A frequent target for genetic abnormalities in lung cancer. Science, 246:491, 1989.
87. Tannock, I.: Cell kinetics and chemotherapy: A critical review. Cancer Treat. Rep., 62:1117, 1978.
88. Teodori, L., Trinca, M. L., Goehdek, W., Hemmer, J., Salvatt, F., Storniello, G., and Mauro, F.: Cytokinetic investigation of lung tumors using the anti-bromodeoxyuridine (BUdR) monoclonal antibody method: comparison with DNA flow cytometric data. Int. J. Cancer, 45:995, 1990.
89. Todaro, G. J., DeLarco, J. E., Fryling, C., Johnson, P. A., and Sporn, M. B.: Tranforming growth factors: properties and possible mechanisms of action. J. Supramol. Struct. Cell Biochem., 15:287, 1981.
90. Todaro, G. J., and Green, H.: Quantitative studies of the growth of mouse embryo cells in culture and their development into established lines. J. Cell Biol., 17:299, 1963.
91. Tubo, R. A., and Berezney, R.: Pre-replicative association of multiple replicative enzyme activities with the nuclear matrix during rat liver regeneration. J. Biol. Chem., 262:1148, 1987.
92. Twardzik, D. R., Ranchalis, J. E., McPherson, J. M., Ogawa, Y., Gentry, L., Purchio, A., Plata, E., Todaro, G. J.: Inhibition and promotion of differentiation-like phenotype of a human lung carcinoma in athymic nude mice by natural and recombinant forms of transforming growth factor-beta. J. Natl. Cancer Inst., 81:1182, 1989.
93. Varticovski, L., Druker, B., Morrison, D., Cantley, L., and Roberts, T.: The colony stimulating factor-1 receptor associates with and activates phophatidylinositol-3 kinase. Nature, 342:699, 1989.
94. Vasios G. W., Gold J. D., Petkovich M., Chambon P., and Gudas L. J.: A retinoic acid-responsive element is present in the 5' flanking region of the laminin B1 gene. Proc. Natl. Acad. Sci. USA, 86:9099, 1989.
95. Wallen, J. W., Cate, R. L., Kiefer, D. M., Rieman, M. W., Martinez, D., Hoffman, R. M., Donohoe, P. K., Von Hoff, D. D., Pepinsky, B., and Oliff, A.: Minimal antiproliferative effect of recombinant müllerian inhibiting substance on gynecological tumor cell lines and tumor explants. Cancer Res., 49:2005, 1989.
96. Ward, A. M.: The value of markers in fine tuning of chemotherapy. Cancer Treat. Rev., 14:401, 1987.
96A.Warrell, R. P., Frankel, S. R., Miller, W. H., Scheinberg, D. A., Itri, L. M., Hittleman, W. N., Vyas, R., Andreef, M., Tafuri, A., Jakubowski, A., Gabrilove, J., Gordon, M. S., and Dmitrovsky, E.: Differentiation therapy of acute promyelocytic leukemia with tretinoin (all-trans-retinoic acid). N. Engl. J. Med., 324:1385, 1991.
97. Waxman, S., Rossi, G. B., and Takaku, F.: The Status of Differentiation Therapy of Cancer. New York, Raven Press, 1988.
98. Weber, G.: Biochemical strategy of cancer cells and the design of chemotherapy: G.H.A. Clowes Memorial Lecture. Cancer Res., 43:3466, 1983.
99. Wille, J. J., Maercklein, P. B., and Scott, R. E.: Neoplastic tranformation and defective control of cell proliferation and differentiation. Cancer Res., 42:5139, 1982.
100. Wright, W. E., Sasoon, D., and Lin, V. K.: Myogenin, a factor regulating myogenesis, has a homologous domain to Myo D. Cell, 56:607, 1989.
101. Wyllie, A. H.: Apoptosis: Cell death in tissue regulation. J. Pathol., 153:313, 1987.
102. Yanishevsky, R. M., and Stein, G. H.: Regulation of the cell cycle in eucaryotic cells. Int. Rev. Cytol., 69:223, 1981.
103. Yuspa, S. H., Lichti, U., Strickland, J., Jaken, S., Lowy, D., Harper, J., Roop, D., and Hennngs, H.: Aberrant regulation of differentiation in epidermal carcinogenesis. *In* Growth Factors, Tumor Promoters and Cancer Genes. Edited by N. H. Colburn, H. L. Moses, and E. J. Stanbridge. New York, Alan R. Liss, 1988; pp. 183-189.
104. Zugmaier, G., and Lippman, M. E.: Effects of TGF beta on normal and malignant mammary epithelium. Ann. N.Y. Acad. Sci., 593:272, 1990.

I-2

Molecular Biology

Barrett J. Rollins
Charles D. Stiles

Introduction

From the clinical perspective, cancer is a cellular disease. Abnormal cells are the fundamental unit of pathology in cancer, and most therapies are designed to attack the altered characteristics of the malignant cell. However, to gain the initiative in cancer detection and treatment, oncologists must begin to understand the molecular roots of the disease: genes, their messenger RNA's, and the proteins they produce. In short, oncologists should be conversant with the tools of molecular biology.

This chapter is a basic survey of molecular biology and is directed toward the clinician or trainee who wants a fundamental understanding of this discipline. It is "methods oriented" and will serve as a frame of reference for the other chapters in this section. It describes the principles that underlie procedures used most commonly by molecular biologists and provides examples of clinically relevant situations that draw upon particular techniques. It will become apparent that molecular biology already plays an important role in clinical cancer medicine, from the analysis of tumors for prognostic or pathogenetic information to the production of pharmacologic agents such as the colony stimulating factors and interleukins.

We will begin with an overview of genes, gene expression, and gene cloning. Our discussion of techniques will follow the flow of genetic information as we explain procedures used to analyze gene expression at the levels of DNA, RNA, and protein.

Overview–Gene Structure
Genes and Gene Expression

The gene is the fundamental unit of inheritance and the ultimate determinant of all phenotypes. The DNA of a normal human cell contains an estimated 30,000–40,000 genes, but only a fraction of these are used (or "expressed") in any particular cell at any given time.[38,39] For example, genes specific for erythroid cells, such as the hemoglobin genes, are not expressed in brain cells.

According to the "central dogma" of molecular biology, a gene exerts its effects by having its DNA "transcribed" into a messenger RNA (mRNA), which is in turn "translated" into a protein, the final effector of the gene's action. Thus molecular biologists often investigate gene "expression" or "activation", by which is meant the process of transcribing DNA into RNA, or translating RNA into protein. The process of transcription involves creating a perfect RNA copy of the gene using the DNA of the gene as a "template". Translation of mRNA into protein is a somewhat more complex process, since the structure of the gene's protein is "encoded" in the mRNA, and that structural message must be decoded during translation.

Functional Components of the Gene

Every gene consists of several functional components, each involved in a different facet of the process of gene expression (Figure I-2-1). Broadly speaking, however, there are two main functional units: the "promoter" region and the "coding" region.

The promoter region controls when and in what tissue a gene is expressed. For example, the promoter of the hemoglobin gene is responsible for its expression in erythroid cells and not in brain cells. How is this tissue specific expression achieved? In the DNA of the gene's promoter region, there are specific structural elements, "nucleotide sequences" (see Structural Considerations, below), that permit the gene to be expressed only in an appropriate cell. These are the elements in the hemoglobin gene that instruct an erythroid cell to transcribe hemoglobin mRNA from that gene. These structures are often referred to as "cis"-acting elements because they reside on the same molecule of DNA as the gene. In

some cases, other "cis"-acting elements, called "enhancers", reside on the same DNA molecule, but at great distances from the coding region of the gene.[1,45] In the appropriate cell, the "cis"-acting elements bind protein factors that are physically responsible for transcribing the gene. These proteins are often called "trans"-acting factors because they reside in the cell's nucleus separate from the DNA molecule bearing the gene. For example, brain cells would not have the right "trans"-acting factors that bind to the hemoglobin promoter, and therefore brain cells would not express hemoglobin. They would, however, have "trans"-acting factors that bind to neuron-specific gene promoters.

The structure of the protein that corresponds to a gene is specified by the gene's "coding" region. The coding region contains the information that directs an erythroid cell to assemble amino acids in the proper order to make the hemoglobin protein. How is this order of amino acids specified? As will be described below, DNA is a linear polymer consisting of four distinguishable subunits called nucleotides. In the coding region of a gene, the linear sequence of nucleotides "encodes" the amino acid sequence of the protein. This genetic code is in triplet form, so that every group of three nucleotides encodes a single amino acid. The number of triplets that can be formed by four nucleotides (64) exceeds the number of amino acids used to make proteins (20). This makes the code redundant and allows some amino acids to be encoded by several different triplets.[51] The nucleotide sequence of any gene can now be determined (see below). By translating the code, one can derive a predicted amino acid sequence for the protein encoded by a gene.

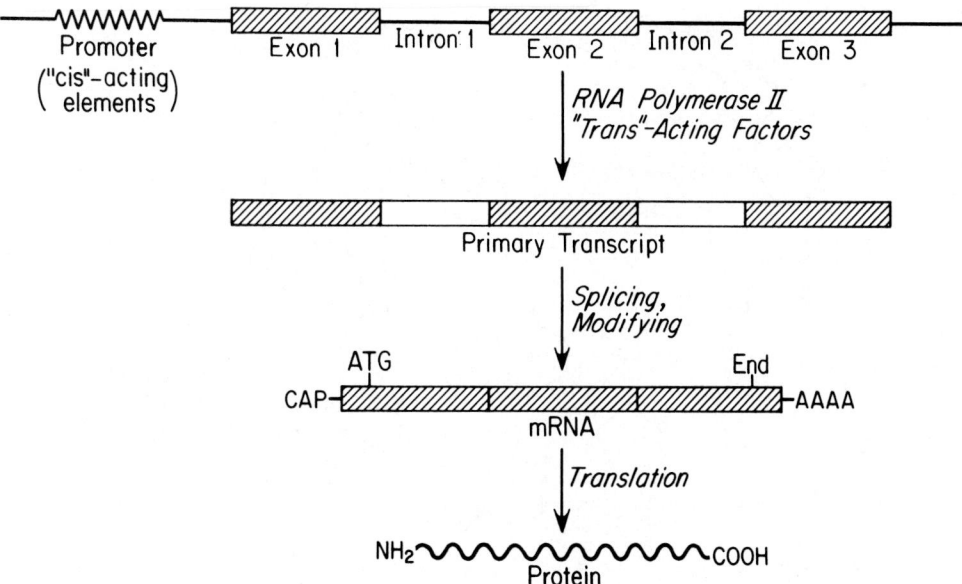

Figure I-2-1. Gene expression. A gene's DNA is transcribed into mRNA, which in turn is translated into protein. The functional components of a gene are schematically diagrammed here. Areas of the gene destined to be represented in mature mRNA are called exons, and intervening areas of DNA between exons are called introns. The portion of the gene that controls transcription, and therefore expression, is the promoter which is "upstream" (toward the 5' end). This control is exerted by specific nucleotide sequences in the promoter region (so-called "cis"-acting factors) and by proteins (so-called "trans"-acting factors) that must interact with promoter DNA and/or RNA polymerase II for transcription to occur.

The primary transcript is the RNA molecule made by RNA polymerase II that is complementary to the entire stretch of DNA containing the gene. Before leaving the nucleus, the primary transcript is modified by splicing together exons (thus removing intron sequences), adding a cap to the 5' end, and adding a poly-A tail to the 3' end. Once in the cytoplasm, mature mRNA undergoes translation to yield a protein.

Structural Considerations

Fine Structure. The basic repeating units of the DNA polymer are nucleotides (Figure I-2-2). Nucleotides consist of an invariant portion, a five-carbon deoxyribose sugar with a phosphate group, and a variable portion, the "base". Of the four bases that appear in the nucleotides of DNA, two are purines, adenine (A) and guanine (G), and two are pyrimidines, cytosine (C) and thymine (T). Nucleotides are connected to each other in the polymer through their phosphate groups, leaving the bases free to interact with each other through hydrogen bonding. This "base pairing" is specific, so that A interacts with T, and C interacts with G. DNA is ordinarily double-stranded, i.e., two linear polymers of DNA are aligned so that the bases of the two strands face each other. Base pairing makes this alignment specific, so that one DNA strand is a perfectly complementary copy of the other.

In every strand of a DNA polymer, the phosphate substitutions on the ribose molecules alternate between the 5' and 3' carbons. Thus there is a directionality to DNA: the genetic code reads in the 5' to 3' direction. In double-stranded DNA, the strand that carries the translatable code in the 5' to 3' direction is called the "sense" strand, while its complementary partner is the "antisense" strand.

Gross Structure. In eukaryotes, the coding regions of most genes are not continuous. Rather they consist of areas that are transcribed into mRNA, the "exons", which are interrupted by stretches of DNA that do not appear in mature mRNA, the "introns" (Figure I-2-1). The functions of introns are not known with certainty. A purpose of some sort is implied by their conservation in evolution. However, their overall physical structure might be more important than their specific nucleotide sequences, since the nucleotide sequences of introns diverge more rapidly in evolution than the sequences of exons. Overall, DNA that contains genes comprises a minority of total DNA. Between genes, there are vast stretches of untranscribed DNA that are assumed to play an important structural role.

In the nucleus, DNA is not present as naked nucleic acid. Rather DNA is found in close association with a number of accessory proteins, such as the histones, and in this form is called chromatin.[34] Although many of DNA's accessory proteins have no known specific function, they generally appear to be involved in the correct packaging of DNA. For example, DNA's double helix is ordinarily twisted on itself to form a super-coiled structure.[6] This structure must unwind

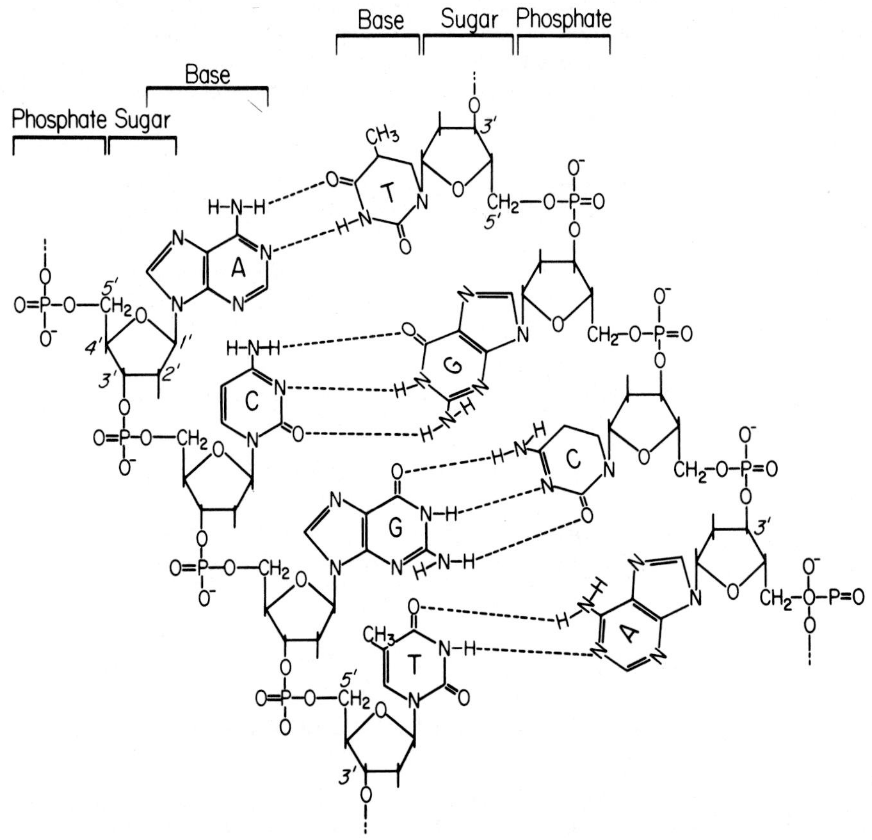

Figure I-2-2. Structure of base-paired, double-stranded DNA. Each strand of DNA consists of a backbone of five-carbon 2'-deoxyribose sugars connected to each other through phosphate bonds. Note that as one follows the sequence down the left-hand strand (A to C to G to T), one is also following the carbons of the deoxyribose ring, going from the 5' carbon to the 3' carbon. This is the basis for the 5' to 3' directionality of DNA. The 1' carbon of each 2'-deoxyribose is substituted with a purine or pyrimidine base. In double stranded DNA, bases face each other in the center of the molecule and base-pair via hydrogen bonds (dotted lines). Base-pairing is specific, so that adenine pairs with thymine, and guanine pairs with cytosine.

partially during DNA replication and transcription.[76] Some of the accessory proteins are involved in regulating this process.

Summary. Genes specify the structure of proteins that are responsible for the phenotype associated with a particular gene. While the nucleus of every human cell contains 30,000–40,000 genes, only a fraction of them are expressed in any given cell at any given time. The "promoter" (with or without an "enhancer") is the part of the gene that determines when and where it will be expressed. The "coding region" is the part of the gene that dictates the amino acid sequence of the protein encoded by the gene. DNA is a linear polymer of nucleotides. Ordinarily, the nucleotide bases of one strand of DNA interact with those of another strand (A with T, C with G) to make double-stranded DNA. In the cell's nucleus, DNA is associated with accessory proteins to make the structure called chromatin.

General Techniques

Restriction Endonucleases and Recombinant DNA

In eukaryotic chromosomes, individual molecules of DNA are several million base pairs long. Because these molecules are far too large to analyze directly, scientists are usually interested in cutting DNA into fragments of manageable size. Fortunately for molecular biologists, bacteria have evolved a highly diverse set of enzymes, the "restriction endonucleases", that cleave DNA internally within the polymer.[67]

In nature, these enzymes have evolved to protect bacteria from invasion by foreign DNA molecules, e.g., viruses. In order to discriminate between "domestic" and "foreign" DNA, these enzymes recognize specific nucleotide sequences. DNA without such specific sequences is left undisturbed by the enzymes. However, when a restriction endonuclease spots a "recognition site", it binds to the site and cleaves both strands of the DNA to which it has bound. Individual restriction endonucleases recognize specific sequences, usually on the order of four to six bases in length, and these sequences are often palindromes, i.e., the 5' to 3' sequence in the upper strand is identical to the 5' to 3' sequence in the lower strand (Figure I-2-3).[53]

While restriction endonucleases cut DNA into smaller fragments, there is a lower limit to the size of useful fragments. One would not want to cut DNA into such small pieces that

the informational content of each piece is negligible. Statistically, the longer a restriction endonuclease's recognition sequence, the less frequently this sequence will occur in a stretch of DNA. Therefore, the enzymes most commonly used to cut DNA into usefully large fragments are those that recognize a six nucleotide recognition site (so-called "six-base cutters"). For example, an endonuclease isolated from *E. coli*, called EcoRI, recognizes the sequence GAATTC, and wherever this occurs in double-stranded DNA, it will cleave between the G and A (Figure I-2-3). (Note that the anti-sense strand, which reads CTTAAG in the 3' to 5' direction, will also read GAATTC in the 5' to 3' direction. This is what is meant by a palindromic sequence.)

Gene Cloning

Mechanics The most powerful technique available for gene analysis, and the one technique that is the cornerstone for all others, is gene cloning (Figure I-2-4). In the gene cloning process, a discrete piece of DNA is faithfully replicated in the laboratory. Cloning provides quantities of specific DNA sufficient for biochemical analysis or for any other manipulation, including joining to a foreign piece of DNA. In the early 1970's, Cohen and Boyer drew upon two fundamental properties of bacteria and their viruses (phage) that made this innovation possible: plasmids and DNA ligases.[17]

Plasmids are circular molecules of DNA that replicate in the cytoplasm of bacterial cells, separate from the bacteria's own DNA. In nature, plasmids often carry genetic information useful to the host bacterium, such as genes that confer resistance to antibiotics. For the purposes of gene cloning, plasmids are important because they contain all the information necessary for directing bacterial enzymes to replicate the plasmid DNA, in some cases to many thousands of copies per bacterium.

DNA ligases are enzymes produced by bacteria (and some phage when they infect bacteria) that can link or ligate together separate pieces of DNA. The nucleotide sequence in a piece of DNA does not influence the activity of a DNA ligase, so that a DNA ligase can join two pieces of DNA that are not ordinarily connected to each other in nature.

In gene cloning, one uses a restriction endonuclease to cut open the circular plasmid DNA in a region of the plasmid not necessary for replication (Figure I-2-4). Suppose, for example, that the enzyme EcoRI cuts open the plasmid in such a non-essential area. EcoRI recognizes the sequence

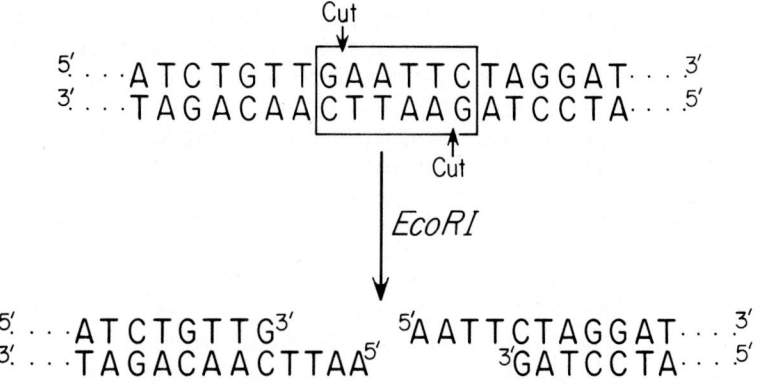

Figure I-2-3. Digestion of DNA with the restriction endonuclease EcoRI. The nucleotide sequence of this stretch of DNA contains the recognition sequence for EcoRI, GAATTC (boxed). EcoRI cuts the DNA in both strands between the indicated nucleotides, resulting in fragments with 5' single-stranded tails.

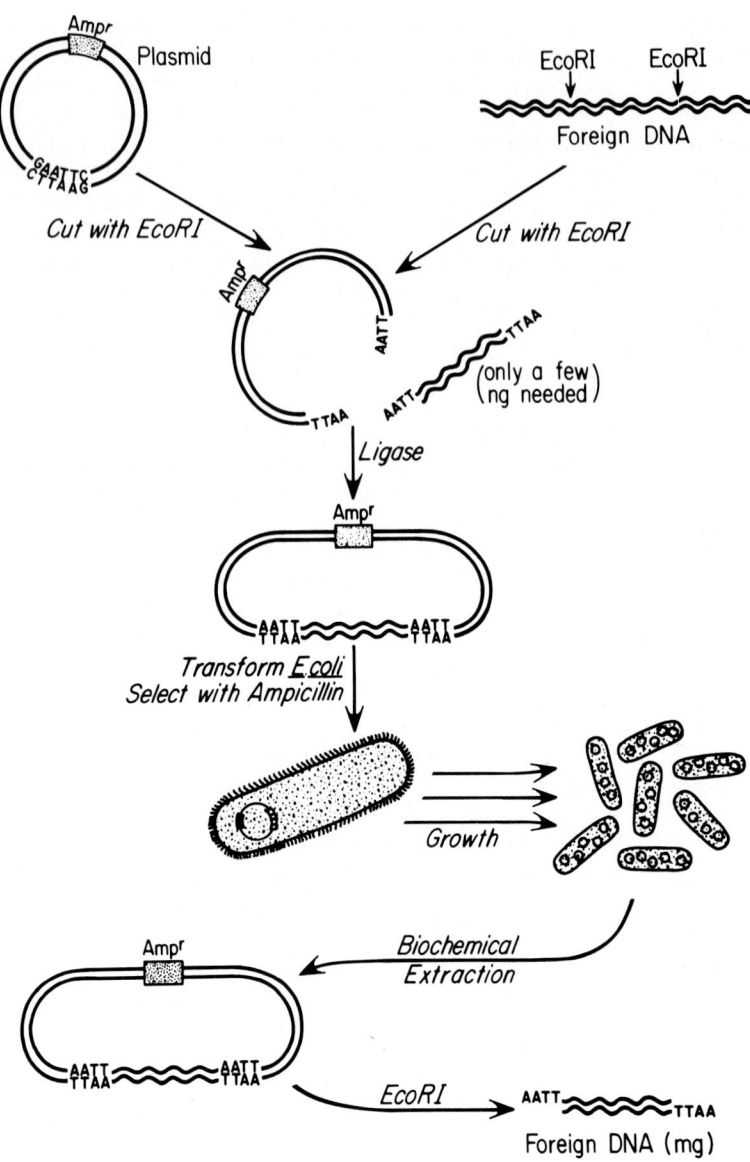

Figure I-2-4. Gene cloning. In this example, a small amount of foreign DNA (a few nanograms) is digested with EcoRI. This foreign DNA can come from any source, the only requirement being that it contain the same restriction endonuclease recognition sites as the vector. Plasmid vector is also digested with EcoRI to create a linear DNA molecule. The "sticky" single-stranded ends of the foreign DNA can align and base pair with the complementary "sticky ends" of the plasmid, after which DNA ligase covalently bonds foreign DNA to plasmid DNA. This recombinant DNA is introduced into *E. coli* by a process called transformation. Since the bacteria themselves are not resistant to ampicillin, growth in ampicillin will select only those bacteria that have taken up the plasmid DNA (which carries an ampicillin resistance gene). The plasmid is characterized by being able to originate synthesis in a bacterial system, so that as the bacterial culture grows, plasmids replicate resulting in several copies in each bacterium. When the culture has grown to sufficient size, plasmid DNA can be isolated biochemically, foreign DNA can be cut from the plasmid using EcoRI, and the resulting yield will often be milligrams of DNA, i.e., greater than a 10^6-fold amplification.

GAATTC, and cuts both DNA strands between the G and the A nucleotides. Protruding from the cut ends will be single-stranded DNA "tails" having the sequences AATT. (Note that the tail's sequence in the sense strand is the same as the sequence in the antisense strand when the nucleotides are read in the 5' to 3' direction). Any other piece of DNA that has been cut with EcoRI will also have single-stranded AATT tails, and the AATT tails on this foreign piece of DNA can base-pair with the complementary TTAA tails (reading 3' to 5') on the cut plasmid. When this happens, the foreign DNA piece physically closes the gap in the plasmid, forming a closed circular plasmid again (which is necessary for plasmid propagation).

Although the nucleotides at the ends of the plasmid and foreign DNA now abut each other, they are not covalently connected. This is an unstable situation which can be rectified by DNA ligase. When DNA ligase covalently joins the plasmid and foreign DNA, one has created a "recombinant" plasmid which still has all the information needed to be rep-

licated in a bacterium, but which also contains a foreign DNA "insert". Obviously, the EcoRI-cut ends of the plasmid can also base-pair with themselves again to re-form the native plasmid, but molecular biologists have developed a number of tricks to suppress this phenomenon. It should be pointed out that single-stranded tails are not always necessary for making recombinant DNA. Under certain conditions, DNA ligase can join together two fragments of "blunt-ended" DNA without these tails.

When a recombinant plasmid is re-introduced into a host bacterium (by a process called "transformation"), the plasmid will replicate as it usually does. Now, however, its foreign DNA insert is replicated along with the plasmid into which it was inserted. The transformed bacteria can then be grown to large numbers in liquid culture. With each bacterial cell division, the progeny bacteria contain plasmid molecules that continue to replicate. When the bacterial culture contains the desired quantity of this plasmid (this may be milligrams of plasmid DNA in a one liter culture), it can be re-isolated as pure DNA. The cloned foreign piece of DNA can then be cut out (with EcoRI in our example) for further analysis or manipulation. One can also use bacterial viruses (or phage) in the same manner by infecting host bacteria with recombinant phage bearing foreign DNA sequences. In all of these experiments, the plasmid or phage that houses the foreign DNA is called a "vector", because it is the vehicle that directs the foreign DNA into the host bacterium.

These extraordinarily powerful techniques, which are now standard practice in all molecular biology laboratories, have been responsible for the development of nearly all the analytical techniques described below. Several excellent manuals have been published that describe these techniques in detail.[2,8,57]

Gene Libraries. One exceptional application of these techniques has been the construction of gene libraries (Figure I-2-5).[15,41] A gene library contains the entire complement of DNA (and therefore genes) from an organism in the form of DNA inserts in recombinant plasmids or phage. DNA containing an organism's genes (i.e., genomic DNA) can be isolated from a cell or tissue of interest, including human tissue, and cut into pieces of manageable size using a restriction endonuclease. These DNA fragments, several million of them all of different lengths, can be cloned into bacterial plasmids or phage as described above so that each vector carries exactly one genomic DNA fragment. The recombinant vectors can then be re-introduced into bacteria, which can be plated onto agar plates and grown into individual bacterial colonies or phage plaques (areas of bacteria infected with phage). Now each bacterial colony, or each phage plaque, houses a recombinant plasmid bearing a different inserted fragment of DNA derived from the genomic DNA of the original cell or tissue. Each colony or plaque represents a different DNA "clone". Specific clones containing specific genes can be identified on the basis of their nucleotide sequences (see below), expanded into large-scale cultures, and their recombinant DNA isolated. In this way, new genes are cloned.[7,26]

Gene Probes and Hybridization

We shall see in the following sections that what lies at the heart of gene analysis is the ability to identify the presence of a specific gene (or mRNA) in a complex mixture of all the DNA (or RNA) in a cell or tissue. This can only be done when one already has a cloned fragment of DNA from the gene of interest. Such fragments are usually obtained from gene libraries constructed from genomic DNA (described above) or cDNA (to be described below). These DNA fragments can be almost any size, from a fraction of the size of the gene (a few hundred nucleotides) to the size of an entire gene (several thousand nucleotides). These cloned gene fragments are called "probes", because they are used to probe native DNA or RNA for the gene of interest.

In order to be useful, a gene probe must contain enough nucleotide sequences so that it will recognize the sequences of its corresponding gene. Recognition occurs by a process called "nucleic acid hybridization" in which two pieces of DNA can align themselves (or "anneal") by base pairing. One can tag the probe DNA (e.g., using ^{32}P-labeled nucleotides), split apart its two strands by heating ("denaturing")

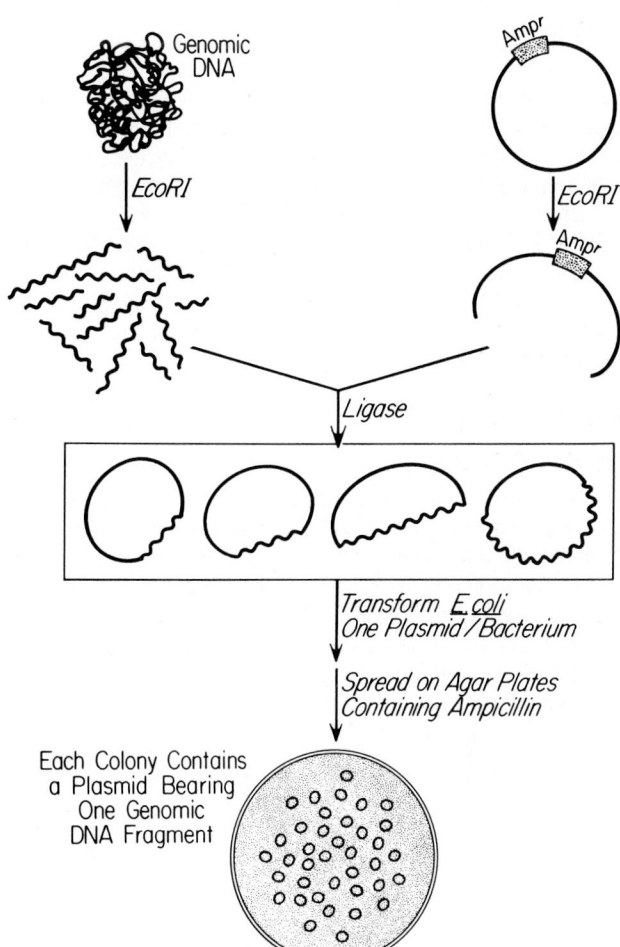

Figure I-2-5. Constructing a genomic library. Genomic DNA and plasmid DNA are cut with EcoRI in preparation for cloning, as in Figure I-2-4. (The vector DNA could also be bacteriophage DNA rather than plasmid DNA). In this case, all of the variously sized EcoRI-produced genomic DNA fragments are cloned individually into the EcoRI site of the plasmid, and the recombinant DNA is introduced into E. coli by transformation. Transformed bacteria are selected by growth in the presence of ampicillin, as in Figure I-2-4. Since each bacterium can be transformed by only one recombinant plasmid, and since each colony on the agar plate arose from a single transformed bacterium, each colony (or clone) contains amplified plasmid bearing a single genomic EcoRI fragment. Taken together, all the bacterial colonies represent the entire genetic complement of the organism from which the original genomic DNA was isolated. All of the clones on all of the plates can be thought of as a genomic library with each individual clone representing one volume.

and add it to the DNA mixture being studied, which has usually been immobilized by sticking it to an inert flat sheet. Under appropriate re-annealing conditions, wherever the probe DNA finds a complementary sequence, it will base pair with that sequence. All probe that has not specifically bound to its complementary DNA target can be washed away, and by exposing the flat sheet to X-ray film, the presence of the target DNA sequences can be revealed (see Southern Blotting, below).

Summary

Genes can be cut from total "genomic" DNA using restriction endonucleases that recognize specific nucleotide sequences. Individual genes can be captured and replicated in bulk for detailed analysis. This process is called "cloning" and employs bacterial plasmids and viruses (phage) as carriers for the cloned genes. Enzymes called DNA ligases join foreign DNA to plasmid or phage vectors which can then replicate within bacterial cells to create gene "libraries". Using nucleic acid hybridization, cloned genes act as probes to detect the presence of their native counterparts in complex mixtures of DNA or RNA.

Gene Analysis–DNA

Southern Blotting

One of the most useful techniques for analyzing a gene at the level of genomic DNA is Southern blotting, named for its originator, E.M. Southern.[68] In general, this technique allows one to determine whether specific nucleotide sequences in a cloned probe are present in a sample of genomic DNA. The presence of these sequences usually means that the gene itself is present in the genomic DNA. Figure I-2-6 diagrams the technique. Purified genomic DNA is digested with a specific restriction endonuclease which, as described above, will produce an array of differently sized DNA fragments. These fragments are then separated by size using electrophoresis through an agarose gel. (Since the phosphate groups in DNA make the molecules negatively charged, they will migrate toward the anode in an electric field. The semi-porous agarose will allow molecules of DNA to pass with varying degrees of ease, at a rate inversely proportional to their size. At any time after electrophoresis begins, small molecules will be closer to the anode than large molecules.) The agarose gel is usually cast in the form of a flat rectangle a few millimeters thick.

The final goal of Southern blotting is to identify specific fragments of cut DNA using nucleic acid hybridization. Because the agarose gel used in electrophoresis is thick and the DNA fragments can move within it, DNA in the gel is not in a suitable form for further analysis. The DNA fragments must be transferred to a solid support to which they can remain irreversibly bound in order to carry out nucleic acid hybridization studies. Thus, after electrophoresis, a paper-thin membrane microfilter (made of nitrocellulose or nylon) is placed over the flat portion of the gel. Liquid is then forced through the agarose gel in a direction perpendicular to the direction the DNA moved during electrophoresis. As the liq-

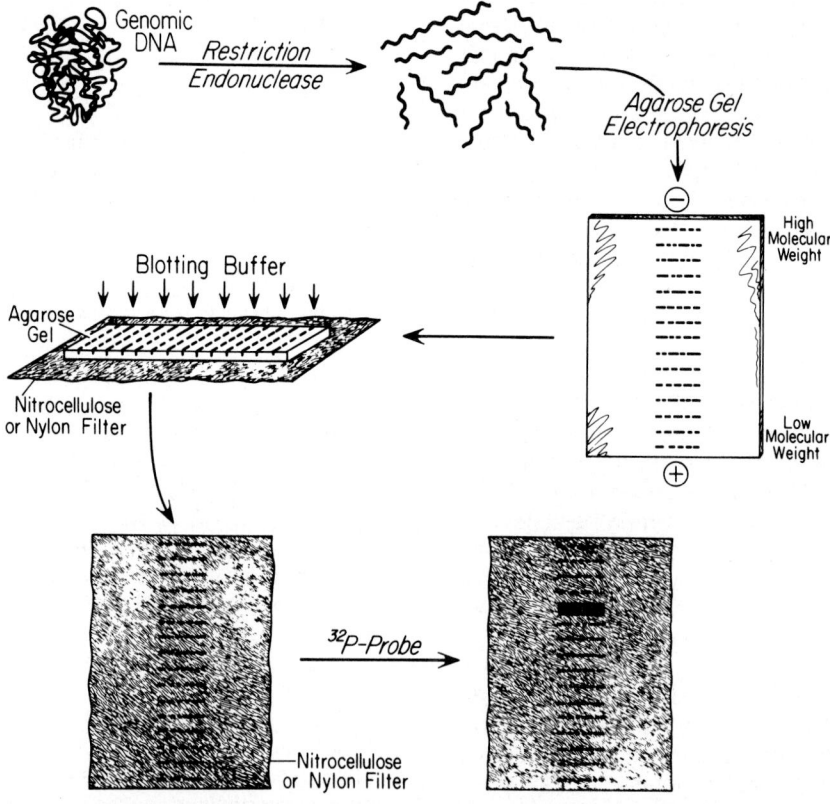

Figure I-2-6. Genomic Southern blotting. Genomic DNA is digested with a single restriction endonuclease resulting in a complex mixture of DNA fragments of different sizes, i.e., molecular weights. Digested DNA is arrayed by size using electrophoresis through a semi-solid agarose gel. Because DNA is negatively charged, fragments will migrate toward the anode, but their progress is variably impeded by interactions with the agarose gel. Small fragments interact less and migrate farther; large fragments interact more and migrate less. The arrayed fragments are then transferred to a sheet of nitrocellulose or nylon-backed filter paper by forcing buffer through the gel as shown. The DNA fragments are carried by capillary action and can be made to bind irreversibly to the filter. Now the DNA fragments, still arrayed by size on the filter, can be probed for specific nucleotide sequences using a ^{32}P-radiolabeled nucleic acid probe. The probe will hybridize to complementary sequences in the DNA, and the position of the fragment that contains these sequences can be revealed by exposing the filter to X-ray film.

uid perfuses through the gel, it carries the DNA fragments with it, depositing them on the membrane filter, to which the DNA sticks. After transfer, the DNA fragments are arrayed by size on the solid support.

At this point, a fragment of cloned DNA (the probe) is radiolabeled by using any of a variety of techniques. The membrane containing the transferred DNA is then soaked in a buffer containing the radiolabeled probe. If there are any sequences in the genomic DNA that are complementary to those in the probe, the probe will hybridize to those sequences on the filter, as described above. Unbound probe can be washed away, and the remaining specifically hybridized probe can be visualized by exposing the filter to X-ray film.

What results from these studies is a pattern of one or more radiolabeled bands on X-ray film. Each band corresponds to a restriction endonuclease-generated DNA fragment containing nucleotide sequences complementary to those in the radioactive probe. For any particular gene probe, the size (i.e., length) of the band it identifies will be the same from individual to individual within a species (see below for a discussion of RFLPs, an important exception). Therefore, if a gene has undergone a structural rearrangement, as, for example, when the c-abl oncogene is translocated from chromosome 9 to 22, the pattern may change. Suppose, for example, that the c-abl probe ordinarily recognizes a 2,000 base EcoRI fragment in normal genomic DNA. If the translocation breakpoint in a CML patient occurs within that fragment, part of the c-abl gene and one of its EcoRI sites will move to chromosome 22. Southern blot analysis of the patient's DNA may now detect either: A larger fragment than normal if the recipient chromosome has an EcoRI site farther away than the old EcoRI site; or a smaller fragment if it has an EcoRI site closer than the old one. Southern blotting is thus a sensitive technique for detecting large structural rearrangements in the genome, such as those that are occasionally associated with malignancy.

Since the amount of radiolabeled probe that hybridizes to a Southern blot is proportional to the number of copies of the specific gene present in the target DNA, this technique can be used quantitatively. For example, in an analysis of primary breast cancer tissue, Southern blotting was used to determine that 30% of these samples contained multiple copies of c-neu oncogene DNA, i.e., the gene was amplified.[64]

Restriction Fragment Length Polymorphisms (RFLPs)

Southern blots of the genomic DNA from two individuals may occasionally reveal a different pattern of bands when probed with a single cloned DNA. Such differences are considered polymorphic when they occur in a significant fraction of the population (usually greater than 1%). These "restriction fragment length polymorphisms" (RFLPs) are caused by stably inherited alterations in the nucleotide sequence of the genomic DNA to which the probe hybridizes.

There are two mechanisms whereby DNA polymorphisms become detectable by Southern blotting. First, a single nucleotide change (i.e., a mutation) can create a new restriction endonuclease site or destroy an old one. This would cause an alteration in the Southern blot pattern of that gene when the DNA is digested with a particular restriction endonuclease. For example, if a stretch of DNA with the sequence . . . AGGATTTCGA . . . underwent a mutation that changed the first T in that sequence to an A, the recognition site for EcoRI (GAATTC) would be created (Figure I-2-3). Digesting this individual's DNA with EcoRI would generate 2 new restriction fragments and remove 1 old one when compared to a "non-mutated" individual's DNA.

The second mechanism involves one of the more mysterious aspects of genomic DNA in eukaryotes, namely that it is replete with repeated sequences of unknown function. The sequences often repeat themselves along the DNA polymer, one repeat after the other, in so-called "tandem repeats". In humans, the best known repetitive sequence is called "alu", and its nucleotide sequence is so specific that it can be used to identify human DNA in a mixture of DNAs from many species. There are several examples of tandemly repeated sequences in which the number of tandem repeats varies among individuals.[49] One may have a DNA probe that recognizes a restriction fragment containing some tandem repeats. If the number of repeated sequences varies from one individual to the next, the size of the restriction fragment to which the probe hybridizes will vary between the individuals. This will appear as an RFLP.

By either mechanism, inherited genetic differences are often detected as RFLPs. One important use for RFLPs is in gene mapping. RFLPs occur at specific positions ("loci") in genomic DNA. If all the patients with a particular genetic disease have exactly the same RFLP, which is present in only 1% of the normal population, this is presumptive evidence that the gene for the disease is close (or "linked") to the RFLP locus. This analysis has been used to map the loci for the genes that, when mutated, give rise to Huntington's disease or cystic fibrosis.[27,72,75,80] These are the tools of "reverse genetics" which may some day lead to the identification of the multiple genes responsible for malignant transformation.

Another powerful application for RFLPs has been the demonstration of gene loss in cancer (Figure I-2-7). This relies on an individual being heterozygous for an RFLP, i.e., having one polymorphism on one chromosome and another polymorphism on the other. If an individual with cancer is heterozygous for a particular RFLP (termed an "informative" individual) his or her tumor can be analyzed by Southern blotting using the probe that recognizes the polymorphism, and compared to normal tissue analyzed the same way. If one of the RFLPs present in the heterozygous individual's normal DNA is missing from the tumor cell DNA, the tumor is said to have undergone a reduction to homozygosity. This implies a loss of genetic material from the tumor, specifically the DNA that includes the missing RFLP. This is the hallmark of a tumor suppressor gene.[32] It was in this way that the involvement of the suppressor gene p53 was found in human colon cancers.[4,74]

Nucleotide Sequencing

The nucleotide sequence of a gene's coding region encodes the amino acid sequence of its protein. This means that even in the absence of any knowledge about a gene's protein, we

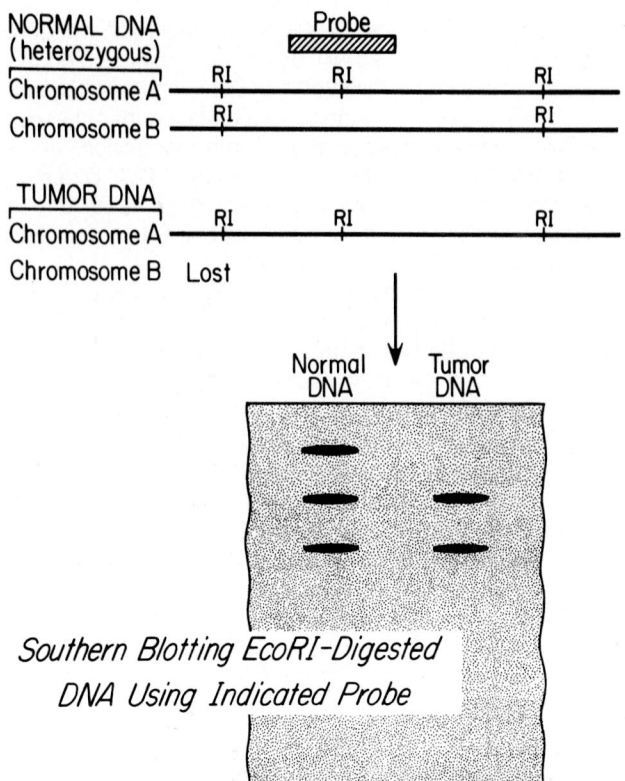

NORMAL DNA
(heterozygous)

Chromosome A

Chromosome B

TUMOR DNA

Chromosome A

Chromosome B Lost

Normal DNA   Tumor DNA

Southern Blotting EcoRI-Digested DNA Using Indicated Probe

Figure I-2-7. Using RFLPs and Southern blotting to detect loss of heterozygosity in tumor tissue. In this example, an individual is heterozygous for an EcoRI recognition site: The second EcoRI site on chromosome A is absent on its diploid partner chromosome B. The individual's tumor is assumed to be clonal and to have arisen from a cell that lost the region of chromosome B displayed in the figure. Southern blotting can then be performed using genomic DNA from the individual's normal DNA and tumor DNA in separate lanes of the agarose gel. Probing the DNA with the probe indicated at the top of the figure reveals a heterozygous banding pattern in normal DNA (reflecting the presence of both polymorphisms, one on each chromosome), and a loss of that pattern in the tumor DNA. This is one of the hallmarks of a tumor suppressor gene.

Figure I-2-8. DNA polymerase. In this schematic, the enzyme DNA polymerase is creating a new DNA chain (upper strand) using a template (lower strand). Specific nucleotides are added from the 5′ to the 3′ direction as determined by the next nucleotide in the template.

can predict the structure of that protein given the nucleotide sequence of the gene. How can the nucleotide sequence of a gene be determined? There are two methods used for sequencing DNA, the "chemical modification" method devised by Maxam and Gilbert, and the "enzymatic chain termination" method devised by Sanger and his colleagues.[44,58] Because of its ease and wider use, the chain termination method will be described here.

The chain termination method relies on properties of enzymes called DNA polymerases (Figure I-2-8). These are enzymes that create new DNA polymers starting from individual nucleotides. However, in order for a DNA polymerase to work, it needs a "template" of single stranded DNA on which to create the new polymer. DNA polymerase adds a new nucleotide to the 3′ end of a growing DNA chain, but the base of the new nucleotide must be able to base pair (i.e., be complementary) to the base on the template over which the polymerase is positioned. After the addition of that nucleotide, the polymerase moves to the next nucleotide on the template, and adds a new nucleotide to the 3′ end of

the growing chain. Again, the new nucleotide must be complementary to the next base in the template. When the process is completed, DNA polymerase will have made a new DNA chain whose nucleotide sequence is completely complementary to the template DNA.

Nucleotide sequencing is based on the observation that when DNA polymerase adds a synthetic abnormal nucleotide to a growing chain, the polymerization stops. The synthetic "terminating" nucleotides used most commonly are dideoxynucleotides that have lost oxygen from the 3′ carbon of their ribose groups. In the presence of the dideoxynucleotide, dideoxy-ATP (ddATP), chain termination will occur wherever an A appears in the new DNA sequence (a T in the template) (Figure I-2-9). These reactions are performed in vitro in a test-tube where millions of new DNA molecules are being made at once. If normal deoxy-ATP is mixed in the proper proportion with dideoxy-ATP, only a few of these molecules will terminate at each T in the template. This will generate a series of new DNA polymers, each one stretching from the beginning of the chain to the position of an A (i.e., a T in the template). If the newly formed DNA is radiolabeled, and the products of this reaction are separated electrophoretically in a polyacrylamide gel (see below), a ladder of radioactive bands will be generated. Each step of the ladder is a fragment of DNA that stretches from the start of the new polymer to the position of an A. Four separate reactions are performed using each of the four dideoxynucleotides. Each

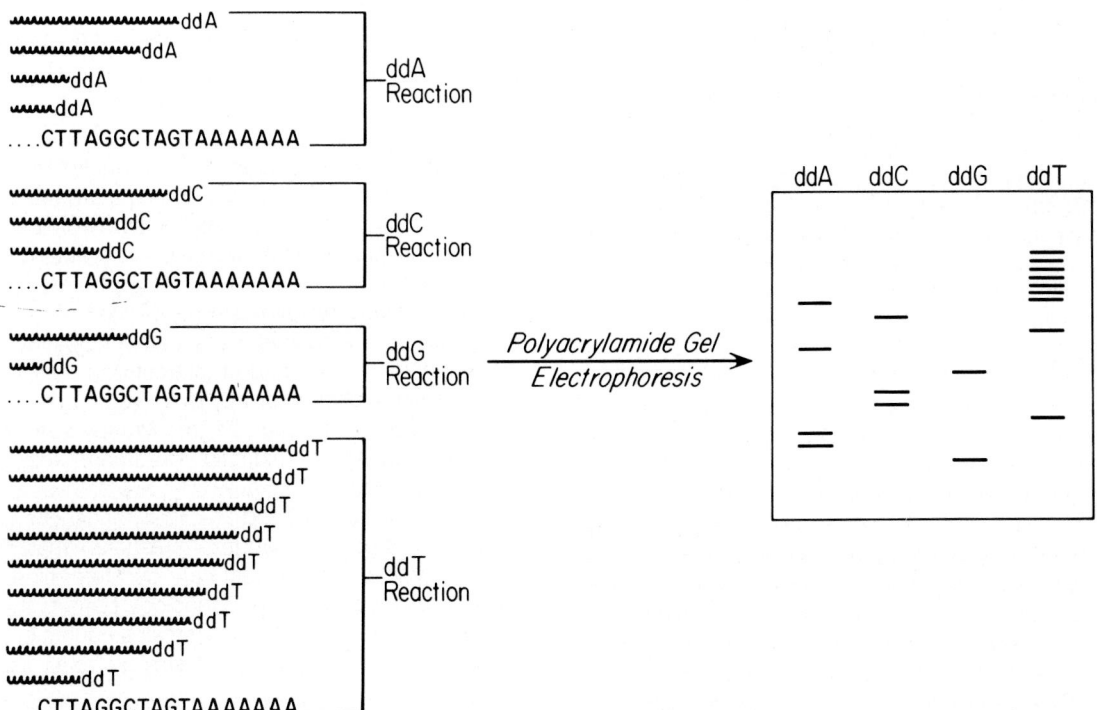

Figure I-2-9. DNA sequencing using the chain termination method. In this example, DNA ending with the sequence. . .CTTAGGCTAGTAAAAAAA is being analyzed. Four reactions are performed, each using this DNA as a template for a DNA polymerase reaction, and each containing one of the four dideoxynucleotides (dideoxyadenosine triphosphate [ddA], dideoxycytidine triphosphate [ddC], dideoxyguanosine triphosphate [ddG], and dideoxythymidine triphosphate [ddT]). In each reaction, chain elongation will terminate when the dideoxynucleotide is incorporated at the position of its complementary nucleotide in the template. This will result in a family of chains of differing lengths that correspond to the position at which polymerization terminated. These chains can be resolved by electrophoresis through a urea-containing polyacrylamide gel in which longer chains run near the top of the gel, and shorter chains near the bottom. Each new chain is radioactively labelled, and after autoradiography the pattern of bands can be read from X-ray film. By noting the order in which bands appear, starting at the bottom of the gel, one can read the sequence of the template by substituting the complement of each dideoxynucleotide at every position. Reading from the bottom yields GAATCCGATCATTTTTTT, and substituting the complementary base at each position yields CTTAGGCTAGTAAAAAAA, the sequence of the template.

reaction is run in an adjacent lane on a polyacrylamide gel so that the nucleotide sequence of a given piece of DNA can be read directly from the gel by reading up the steps of each ladder.

A specific application of DNA sequencing in cancer research has been the analysis of mutated sequences in the tumor suppressor gene *p53*. The hallmark of tumor suppressor gene involvement in cancer is loss of function of these genes. While loss of function can occur by wholesale loss of the gene, the same result can be achieved if the gene undergoes a mutation that inactivates its protein. Thus in many types of cancers that have retained a *p53* allele as determined by Southern blotting, DNA sequencing has shown that the remaining allele has often undergone a single nucleotide, or "point", mutation.[50,69]

Pulsed Field Gel Electrophoresis

One theoretical application for Southern blotting is the demonstration of gene linkage. If two different gene probes were to hybridize to the same restriction fragment in a Southern blot, this would prove that the loci of the two genes were closely linked. Unfortunately, eukaryotic genetic linkages ordinarily extend over millions of bases (megabases) of DNA, and the largest DNA fragments that can be resolved by conventional agarose gel electrophoresis are less than 100

thousand bases (100 kilobases). The reason for this limitation is the tendency for all DNA molecules above a certain size to become oriented with their long axes parallel to the electric field. This prevents any appreciable interaction between the DNA molecules and the agarose gel. In the absence of such interaction, the DNA molecules are not retarded during electrophoresis, and will migrate at the same rate regardless of size. If the long axes of these large molecules are periodically reoriented perpendicular to the direction of migration, they once again interact with the agarose. Such interactions force the DNA molecules to migrate at rates inversely proportional to their lengths, and resolution by size is achieved again.

A number of ingenious techniques have been designed to accomplish this purpose: pulsed-field gel electrophoresis in which two electrical fields are oriented perpendicularly and are alternately pulsed;[59] field inversion gel electrophoresis in which a single field is periodically inverted;[11] and contour-clamped homogeneous gel electrophoresis (CHEF) in which multiple fields of various orientations can be alternately applied.[14] These techniques now allow the separation of DNA fragments from 2–5 megabases in length.

Pulsed field gel electrophoresis has been used in the analysis of gene linkage on the long arm of chromosome 5. Genetic losses and alterations involving 5q have been associated with a variety of hematologic malignancies. The mapping of many of the genes encoding growth factors and growth factor receptors for hematologic cells on 5q has led to the suggestion that alterations in these genes are etiologic in these diseases.[36] By digesting DNA with restriction endonucleases that have rarely occurring recognition sites, and performing Southern blotting experiments after pulsed field gel electrophoresis, the genes for IL-3 and GM-CSF could be shown to lie on the same 436 kb fragment of DNA.[84] Ultimately, it was demonstrated that these genes are separated by only 9 kb of DNA.

Polymerase Chain Reaction

To detect gene sequences by Southern blotting, at least 1–2 μg of genomic DNA is required. This translates into milligram quantities of tissue that must be used fresh or freshly frozen. By amplifying specific fragments of DNA, the polymerase chain reaction (PCR) lowers the theoretical limit of detectable DNA sequences in a sample to a single molecule of DNA. With some advance knowledge of the nucleotide sequences in the DNA to be detected, microscopically small amounts of tissue, even a single cell, contain enough DNA to be amplified, and the amplified DNA can be easily analyzed. Fixed tissue in paraffin blocks or on slides can yield sufficient DNA for analysis using PCR.[82]

The concepts underlying PCR are diagrammed in Figure I-2-10. Two short single-stranded DNA fragments, called primers, bear sequences complementary to those that flank the stretch of DNA to be amplified. They are added to the target DNA, the mixture is heated to dissociate the paired double strands of target DNA, then the temperature is lowered to permit hybridization, or annealing, of the primers to their complementary sequences on the target DNA. A DNA polymerase enzyme is added to the mixture which will add nucleotides to the 3′ end of the primers using the target DNA as a sequence template. This step generates one copy of each of the strands of one target DNA molecule. The mixture is heated again to dissociate the strands, then cooled to allow more primers to anneal to the target sequences on both the original and new pieces of DNA. DNA polymerase is added again and now generates four copies of the target sequences. These steps are repeated, resulting in a geometrically increasing amount of target DNA, i.e., a chain reaction.

When it was first devised, this technique used a DNA polymerase from *E. coli*, which is inactivated by heating, so that fresh enzyme had to be added at every step.[47,56] With the discovery and cloning of the DNA polymerase from the thermophilic bacterium, *T. aquaticus* (the Taq polymerase), which retains activity after being heated to 95°C, heating and cooling steps could be carried out on the same mixture without adding new enzyme.[12,35,55] This allowed the procedure to be automated. There are now automated thermal cyclers in every molecular biology laboratory, and in many clinical laboratories, that will take PCR mixtures through 20–50 cycles, producing large amounts of synthetic DNA for subsequent analysis.

One recent application of this technique was the demonstration of HIV-1 DNA in high risk individuals who were seronegative.[28] The relative ease and reliability of PCR are certain to make it a commonly used technique in this type of viral diagnostics.

Summary

Genomic DNA is too large to be analyzed easily in the laboratory, but it can be cut into manageable fragments using restriction endonucleases isolated from bacteria. Electrophoresis through an agarose gel can separate these fragments by size. Pulsed field gel electrophoresis is a variation of this technique that allows the separation of extremely large DNA molecules. Fragments that carry nucleotide sequences corresponding to a gene of interest can then be detected by Southern blotting. For any given region of DNA, the size and number of restriction fragments may vary among individuals, leading to restriction fragment length polymorphisms (RFLPs). RFLPs are exploited both by basic scientists (in gene mapping) and clinicians (for cancer diagnostics). Specific nucleotide changes (mutations) that give rise to stable genetic differences can be determined by DNA sequencing. Finally, PCR technology permits the detection of specific genes in extremely small amounts of tissue or in tissue that has been fixed for histologic analysis.

Gene Expression–mRNA Transcript Analysis

Structural Considerations

The first step in gene expression is transcription of the genetic information in DNA into RNA. The individual building blocks of RNA, ribonucleotides, have the same structure as the deoxyribonucleotides in DNA, except that: 1) the 2′ carbon of the ribose sugar is substituted with an OH group instead of H; and 2) there are no thymine bases in RNA, only uracil (demethylated thymine) which also base pairs with adenine by hydrogen bonding. Just like the DNA polymerases described above, the enzyme RNA polymerase II uses the nucleotide sequence of the gene's DNA as a template to form a polymer of ribonucleotides with a sequence complementary to the DNA template.

In order for transcription to be "correct", RNA polymerase II must: 1) use the antisense strand of DNA as a template; 2) begin transcription at the start of the gene; and 3) end transcription at the end of the gene. The signals that assure correct transcription are provided to RNA polymerase II by the DNA in the form of specific nucleotide sequences in the promoter of the gene. After reading and interpreting these signals, RNA polymerase generates a primary RNA transcript that extends from the initiation site to the termination site in a perfect complementary match to the DNA sequence used as a template. However, not all transcribed RNA is destined to arrive in the cytoplasm as mRNA. Rather, by an incompletely understood process, sequences complementary to introns (see above) are excised from the primary transcript, and the ends of exon sequences are joined together in a process termed "splicing".[42,60]

In addition to splicing, the primary transcript is further modified by the addition of a methylated GTP "cap" at the 5′ end, and the addition of a stretch of anywhere from 20–40 A bases at the 3′ end.[10,61] These modifications appear to promote the "translatability" and relative stability of mRNA's,

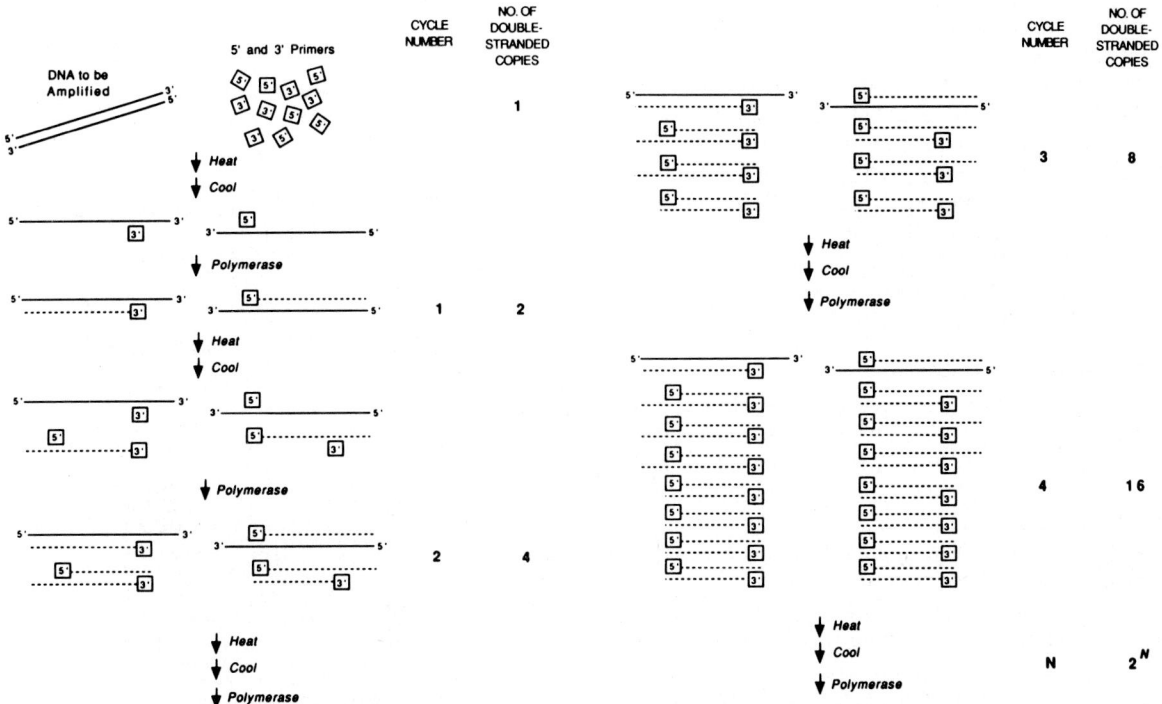

Figure I-2-10. Polymerase chain reaction (PCR). DNA is mixed with short (10–20 base) single-stranded oligonucleotide primers that are complementary to the 5′ and 3′ ends of the sequence to be amplified. The mixture is heated to dissociate or "melt" all double stranded DNA, and then cooled to permit the primers to anneal to their complementary sequences on the DNA to be amplified. Note that the 5′ primer will anneal to the "lower" strand, and the 3′ primer will anneal to the "upper" strand. A heat resistant (thermostable) DNA polymerase (*Taq* polymerase, see text) was added to the original mixture, and it now synthesizes DNA by starting at the primers using the strands to which the primers are annealed as a template. This results in the formation of two double-stranded DNA copies for every molecule of double-stranded DNA in the original mixture. The reaction is then heated to melt double-stranded DNA, cooled to allow reannealing, and the polymerase makes new double-stranded DNA again. There are now four double-stranded DNA copies for each original DNA molecule. This process can be repeated *n* times (usually 20 to 50) to result in 2^n copies of double-stranded DNA. Note that from the third cycle onward, short double-stranded DNA fragments (those that begin and end at the primer sites) will be amplified to great excess. These amplified fragments will dilute the original DNA template (and the DNA with 3′ and 5′ overhangs synthesized in cycle 2) to insignificant amounts.

and help direct the subcellular localization of mRNA's destined for translation.[24,62]

Northern Blotting

The fundamental question in the analysis of gene expression at the RNA level is whether RNA sequences derived from a gene of interest are present in cells or tissues. Detecting specific RNA sequences can be accomplished by Northern blotting, the whimsically named analog of Southern blotting applied to RNA analysis. RNA can be isolated from cells in its intact form, free from significant amounts of DNA.[13] Native RNA is much smaller than genomic DNA, so that it can be analyzed by agarose gel electrophoresis without the enzymatic digestion steps that are necessary for the analysis of high molecular weight DNA.

RNA is single stranded and has a tendency to fold back on itself. This allows complementary bases on the same stretch of RNA to base pair with each other and form what is termed "secondary structure". Because secondary structure can lead to aberrant electrophoretic behavior, RNA is electrophoretically separated by size in the presence of a denaturing agent such as formaldehyde or glyoxal/DMSO.[37,46] After electrophoresis through a denaturing agarose gel, the RNA is transferred to a nitrocellulose or nylon-based membrane in the same manner as DNA for Southern blotting

(Figure I-2-6). Hybridization schemes and blot washing are essentially the same for Northern blotting as for Southern blotting. In this manner, specific RNA sequences corresponding to those in cloned DNA probes can easily be identified.

There is a lower limit to the sensitivity of Northern blotting, so that only moderately abundant mRNA's can be detected using this technique. One way to increase the sensitivity of Northern blotting is to enrich the RNA preparation for messenger RNA. Ordinarily, mRNA makes up less than 10% of the total RNA content of a cell or tissue. When RNA is isolated from these sources, all RNA species are being isolated, i.e., ribosomal and transfer RNA as well as mRNA. As noted above, most mRNA's destined for the cytoplasm and translation are modified by the addition of a 3′ poly(A) tract. An RNA preparation can therefore be greatly enriched for mRNA species by removing all RNA molecules that lack the 3′ poly(A) tail.[3] This can be done by exposing the RNA preparation to a tract of poly(U) or poly(T) bound to an immobilized support, such as a plastic bead. The poly(A) portion of mRNA will bind to the poly(U) or poly(T) material, and non-poly(A)-containing RNA can be washed away. After washing, the poly(A)-containing mRNA can be recovered from the solid support and used in Northern blot analysis. This procedure improves the sensitivity of Northern blotting by nearly two orders of magnitude.

A dramatic use of Northern blotting in cancer research has been the demonstration of oncogene expression in some human tumors. RNA was isolated from human tumor samples and analyzed by Northern blotting using cloned DNA probes derived from various oncogenes. The earliest observations included expression of c-*abl* and c-*myc* in human tumor cell lines and leukemic blasts.[23,79] Since then, however, a large number of proto-oncogenes have been shown to be transcribed in primary human tumor tissue.[65]

Nuclease Protection Assays

Another technique used in the analysis of mRNA is the nuclease protection assay. This assay differs from Northern blotting in two general respects: it is more sensitive than Northern blotting, and is therefore used for the detection of rare mRNA species; and it provides detailed structural information about the mRNA being analyzed, and is thus often referred to as "transcript mapping".

Nuclease protection assays (diagrammed in Figure I-2-11) use a single-stranded radioactive DNA or RNA probe. The nucleotide sequence of the probe contains at least some nucleotides that are complementary to the mRNA being analyzed. The probe is annealed to the target mRNA by base pairing, and the regions of the probe that are complementary to the target mRNA now become double-stranded, while the non-complementary regions of the probe remain single-stranded. The annealed mixture is then subjected to digestion with an enzyme specific for single stranded DNA (usually S1 nuclease) when using a DNA probe, or RNA (usually a mixture of RNase A and RNase T1) when using an RNA probe.[9,40,87] The double-stranded annealed areas resist digestion, while all the single-stranded non-complementary parts of the probe are digested away. In essence, areas in the probe that anneal to the mRNA are "protected" from digestion by the nucleases. The surviving, undigested parts of the probe can then be analyzed by electrophoresis through an agarose or polyacrylamide gel. The amount of radiolabeled probe resistant to digestion is proportional to the amount of target mRNA in the sample.

Nuclease protection assays can also provide structural information about target mRNA sequences. If there are any mismatches in the sequence of the target mRNA compared to the probe, the areas corresponding to the mismatches will generate small single-stranded loops (Figure I-2-11). Since the nucleases used to digest the annealed probe/mRNA hybrid are specific for single stranded nucleotides, any mismatches between the probe and the target are susceptible to digestion. Thus a mismatch can be detected if the nuclease-digested radiolabeled probe is smaller than would have been expected, or when the probe has been digested into multiple fragments. In fact, by careful measurement of the length of the digested probe, one can determine exactly where the mismatch has occurred in the target mRNA.

This technique has been used to detect single base mutations or small deletions in cellular mRNA's. For example, the proposed pathogenetic role of tumor suppressor genes, such as *p53*, in cancer depends on the inactivation of these genes. One way to inactivate a gene is by a mutation that renders

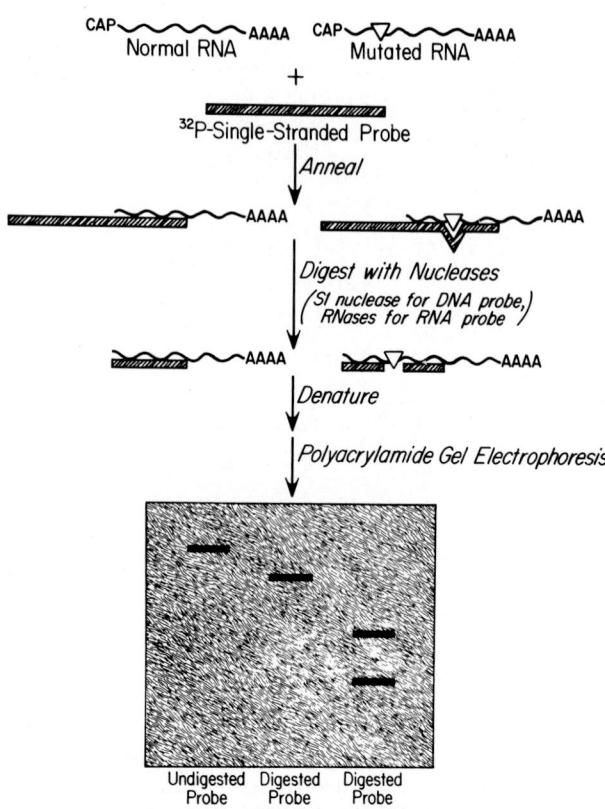

Figure I-2-11. Nuclease protection assay. In this example, an mRNA containing a point mutation (indicated by the inverted triangle in the mRNA on the right) is distinguished from its normal, nonmutated counterpart (mRNA on the left). The mRNA is mixed with a single-stranded ^{32}P-labeled DNA or RNA probe that has sequences perfectly complementary to the nonmutated region of interest in the mRNA, and extends for some length beyond the mRNA. The mixture is heated and then cooled to allow the probe to anneal to its complementary sequences in the mRNA. The annealed mixture is then treated with single-strand specific nucleases (S1 nuclease for a DNA probe, or RNases for an RNA probe). This results in digestion of the probe at all single-stranded areas: the extension beyond the mRNA sequences, and the single base-pair mismatch overlying the mutation (right). The radioactive digestion products are then separated by electrophoresis through a urea-containing polyacrylamide gel. The probe that annealed to normal, nonmutated mRNA is smaller than the undigested probe (by the length of the extended region not complementary to the mRNA) and will therefore migrate farther than undigested probe. The probe that annealed to the mutated mRNA will have been digested into two fragments whose summed length will equal that of the digested probe that annealed to non-mutated mRNA.

the protein product inactive. A recent study used a nuclease protection assay to demonstrate the presence of point mutations in the mRNA for *p53* in several primary human lung cancer samples.[69]

cDNA

The flow of genetic information usually runs from DNA to RNA to protein, following the so-called "central dogma" of molecular biology. There are, however, exceptions to this rule, the most prominent of which involves the life cycle of retroviruses. These viruses encode their genetic information in RNA rather than DNA. When they invade a susceptible host cell, they direct the synthesis of a DNA intermediate that is a complementary copy of their genomic RNA. The enzyme that accomplishes this task, reverse transcriptase, is a DNA polymerase (see above) that uses RNA, rather than DNA, as a template to form a complementary DNA (cDNA) copy of the RNA.[5,70] The enzyme has been purified and can be used in vitro to make cDNA copies of any available RNA.

One important application of cDNA synthesis has been the construction of cDNA libraries, analogs to the genomic libraries described above (Figure I-2-5).[21,54] A valuable tool for the analysis of gene expression would be a gene library that consisted only of the genes that were expressed in a cell or tissue of interest. Most of the time, one is really not concerned with all the information in the genome, e.g., intron sequences, promoters, and vast regions of "uninformative" DNA that lie between genes. For example, if one were interested in analyzing the genes expressed in a brain cell, why bother making a library that contained sequences for the hemoglobin gene? One way to construct a library comprised only of tissue-specific expressed genes would be to clone all the mRNA in a specific cell or tissue of interest. Unfortunately, there is no way to ligate single stranded RNA to a double stranded DNA cloning vector. However, one can use all the mRNA in a cell as a template for making double stranded cDNA, which can then be inserted into a cloning vector.

To make a cDNA library, one isolates all the mRNA from a cell or tissue. Then, using this mRNA as a template, reverse transcriptase makes cDNA copies of each mRNA molecule in the mixture. The cDNA is ligated into a plasmid or phage vector as described above for genomic libraries, and the recombinant vectors are introduced into bacteria. After growing the bacteria on agar plates, each bacterial colony or phage plaque of a cDNA library will house a unique recombinant vector containing the cDNA copy of a single mRNA. Desired clones can be detected by nucleic acid hybridization to the plaques or colonies using a radiolabeled gene probe.[7,26] Alternatively, if the vector containing the cDNA molecules can direct transcription of mRNA by host bacterial cells, mRNA will be synthesized and that mRNA will be translated. In this case, each bacterial colony or plaque will produce a different protein, and each protein will have been encoded by an mRNA from the original cell or tissue being investigated. If an antibody directed against a protein of interest is available, the cDNA clone corresponding to the mRNA that encodes that protein can be identified by binding the antibody to the colonies or plaques of the cDNA library.[85] This technique, called "expression cloning", often employs the bacteriophage λgt11 as the cloning vector.

cDNA libraries can be used to clone a cDNA for a known gene to discover the sequence of the mRNA it encodes. Alternatively, these libraries can be used to identify previously unknown genes. In a process called "differential screening", cDNA's can be discovered that owe their existence to a particular differentiation or activation state in the cell of origin. For example, this technique has been used to identify genes whose expression is turned on by hormones or by growth factors, such as platelet-derived growth factor (PDGF).[16]

PCR

Another important use of cDNA technology has allowed PCR (see above) to be applied to RNA. Since the *Taq* polymerase is a DNA polymerase (see above), it cannot use RNA as a template. Simply adding primers and *Taq* polymerase to an RNA preparation will not result in amplification. However, if an RNA of interest could be made into DNA, then PCR would proceed as usual.

The first step in this analysis is generating a cDNA copy of the mRNA of interest using reverse transcriptase. This can be done using a primer consisting of T's (complementary to the poly(A) tail) or of a sequence complementary to some portion of the 3' region of the mRNA. The 5' primer can then be added along with *Taq* polymerase, and the single-stranded cDNA made in the first step will be amplified as described above (Figure I-2-10). In one of the first applications of this technique, Ph' positive leukemias were diagnosed by identifying chimeric BCR-ABL mRNA species in clinical material using PCR. (BCR-ABL is the novel fused gene resulting from the translocation between chromosomes 9 and 22.) Since then, so-called "indirect transcript amplification" has come into widespread use.[31]

One inherent problem in using PCR to monitor mRNA expression is quantitation of the amplified PCR products. In Northern blotting or nuclease protection analysis, the intensity of the hybridization signal is directly proportional to the amount of target RNA in the sample. Thus one can compare the number of RNA molecules in one sample to another. With PCR, a slight change in the efficiency of polymerization in an early cycle in one sample will lead to a geometrically increasing discrepancy between the amount of amplified product in that sample compared to another sample. Fortunately, a number of techniques have been described for normalizing the products of PCR reactions to allow quantitative comparisons.[29] In general, they involve amplifying an easily distinguishable control RNA template in the same reaction as the RNA of interest. Normalization of the amplified experimental PCR products to the control products then allows comparisons to be made.

Ribozymes

One of the more surprising discoveries of the past decade was that some RNA molecules have enzymatic activity. These RNA's, called "ribozymes", can cleave RNA at sequence-specific sites.[86] They were originally discovered in *Tetrahymena* when it appeared that some of the primary RNA molecules in this species were capable of splicing out their introns without the aid of any protein enzymes. Ribozymes have also recently been described in higher organisms, and it is likely that they will be found to play a universal and important role in RNA processing. Their application to molecular biology and cancer research is only just beginning, but they will most likely be used to characterize RNA in much the same way that restriction endonucleases are used to characterize DNA. They may also eventually be used to sequence RNA directly.

Summary

The genetic information in DNA is copied, or "transcribed", into mRNA by the enzyme RNA polymerase II. Before being transported to the cytoplasm, primary transcripts in the nucleus are modified by splicing out introns, adding a 5' cap, and adding a 3' poly(A) tract. Cytoplasmic mRNA can be detected by Northern blotting, nuclease protection assays, or by modified PCR. Although nuclease protection assays are somewhat more technically demanding than Northern blotting, they are more sensitive assays and can also provide structural information about mRNA transcripts. A retroviral enzyme called reverse transcriptase can make cDNA copies of mRNA transcripts. These cDNA's can be cloned into cDNA libraries which are useful for isolating and analyzing expressed genes. In the future, ribozymes may be useful for RNA analysis by serving as the functional counterparts of the restriction endonucleases used to analyze DNA.

Gene Expression—Protein Analysis

Structural Considerations

Proteins are polymeric molecules consisting of amino acids linked by peptide bonds. The sequence of amino acids in a protein is dictated by the sequence of nucleic acids in the mRNA that encodes the protein. Since amino acids are joined to each other in a linear polymer, there is a directionality to proteins, just as there is to DNA and RNA. The 5' end of the mRNA corresponds to the amino end of its cognate protein and the 3' end corresponds to the carboxy end (Figure I-2-1).

For many proteins, the linear polymer of amino acids must undergo a number of alterations in order to be functional. These alterations are referred to as "post-translational modifications". For example, proteins destined to be secreted from a cell initially exist as propeptides with a 20 to 30 amino acid sequence at their amino ends. This highly hydrophobic tail, called a "leader sequence", remains embedded in the membranes of the endoplasmic reticulum and secretory granule until the protein is to be secreted, at which point the leader sequence is cleaved. There are many examples of propeptides that undergo cleavage of specific amino acids before they become mature, functional proteins.

Other post-translational modifications include the addition of various non-peptide substituents to the side chains of amino acids. These include simple and complex carbohydrate chains, sulfate groups, and phosphate groups. Phosphorylation of intracellular proteins, usually on serine, threonine, or tyrosine residues, plays an important regulatory role in protein function. For example, many of the cell surface receptors for growth factors, such as the PDGF receptor and the receptor for M-CSF, are themselves tyrosine protein kinases.[22,52,63] When this type of receptor binds its ligand, the receptor undergoes a conformational change that activates its kinase activity. The activated receptor then adds phosphate groups to some of its own tyrosine residues as well as to tyrosines in other proteins. It is presumed that the phosphorylation of these other proteins is part of the signal transduction process whereby a message is sent from the cell surface receptor to the nucleus. The importance of tyrosine phosphorylation in cell growth may be reflected in the fact that tyrosine kinases form the largest functional subset of oncogenes.

SDS-PAGE

As with nucleic acids, the most common analytical technique applied to proteins is separation by size using electrophoresis. However, unlike nucleic acids, not all proteins are anionic and they do not have a uniform charge-to-mass ratio. In the presence of an electric field, a mixture of unmodified and uncharacterized proteins would migrate in an unpredictable way, providing little or no information about their structures. This problem has been overcome by performing protein electrophoresis in the presence of the anionic detergent sodium dodecyl sulfate (SDS). SDS binds to proteins in a uniform way, approximately one molecule of SDS for every two amino acids. Thus all proteins become polyanions in the presence of SDS and the number of negative charges (supplied by the sulfate group in SDS) is directly proportional to the size, or molecular weight, of the protein.

Since proteins are generally smaller than the most commonly analyzed nucleic acids, electrophoresis is performed through a solid support made of polyacrylamide which provides better resolution than agarose at these sizes. In the presence of an electric field, proteins in SDS will migrate toward the anode at a rate inversely proportional to the log of their molecular weights.[33,78] Proteins can be analyzed by SDS-polyacrylamide gel electrophoresis (SDS-PAGE) in the presence or absence of β-mercaptoethanol (β-ME) which reduces sulfhydryl groups that can bind two protein chains together. Electrophoresis in the presence of β-ME permits the analysis of protein subunits, while electrophoresis in the absence of β-ME can reveal multimeric protein associations. SDS-PAGE is routinely employed to test the purity of a protein preparation. It is also an integral component of the techniques of immune precipitation and Western blotting.

Immune Precipitation

A primary goal of molecular biology is to use gene probes to detect the presence of a particular gene in a complex mixture of DNA's or RNA's. In a similar way, a specific antibody can be used as a probe to detect the presence of a particular protein in a complex mixture of proteins. An antibody directed against a protein of interest can be added to a mixture of proteins under conditions that allow the antibody to bind to its target protein (Figure I-2-12). One can then collect all the immunoglobulins (Ig's) in that mixture by adding a protein that binds to Ig's, such as anti-immunoglobulin antibodies or Staphylococcal protein A. These proteins are often bound to a solid support, e.g., polystyrene beads, that can be removed from solution by gentle centrifugation. As the beads collect at the bottom of the centrifuge tube, their attached Ig and target proteins collect there as well. When boiled in SDS and β-mercaptoethanol, the protein complexes dissociate, and they can be electrophoretically separated by SDS-PAGE. This process is called immune precipitation. To document the specificity of the antibody, a second immune precipitation is usually performed with a control antibody that does not bind the protein of interest. The two precipitations can be run side-by-side on SDS-PAGE, and the protein of interest identified by its presence in the experimental lane and its absence from the control lane. The proteins can be identified by staining reactions or, if the protein preparation is radiolabeled, by autoradiography.

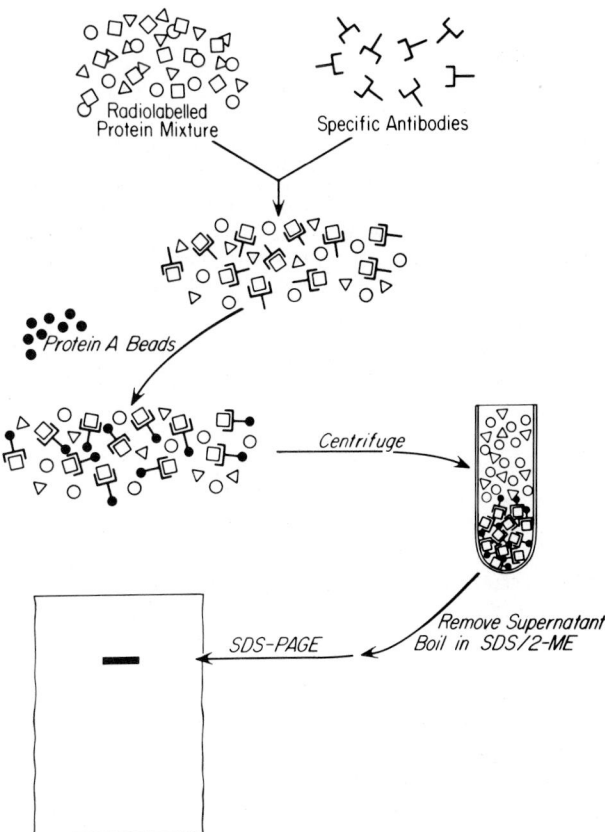

Figure I-2-12. Immune precipitation. A complex mixture of radio-labeled proteins (indicated by different geometric shapes) is incubated with antibodies specific for one of those proteins (in this case, the squares). After the antibodies have bound to their protein, small polystyrene or agarose beads containing staphylococcal protein A are added to the mixture. Protein A binds to the antibodies, and when centrifuged, the beads to which the protein A is bound will sediment to the bottom of the centrifuge tube, taking along the antibodies and the specific protein to which they have bound. The unbound proteins remain in the supernatant and can be removed. After boiling to dissociate the protein A/antibody/protein complex, specifically precipitated radiolabeled protein can be visualized by electrophoresis (SDS-PAGE) and autoradiography.

A recent application of this technique was the demonstration that the protein product of the retinoblastoma susceptibility gene (RB) binds to proteins encoded by DNA tumor viruses. Antibodies directed against adenovirus proteins were used in an immune precipitation of proteins from cells transformed or infected by adenovirus. In addition to the adenovirus proteins, the precipitated proteins contained another protein that was proven to be the protein encoded by retinoblastoma susceptibility gene.[81] Similar experiments using antibodies directed against the large T antigen of SV40 revealed an interaction between T antigen protein and the RB protein.[18] In both cases, these interactions may be central to the mechanisms whereby these viruses oncogenically transform susceptible host cells.

Western Blotting

Another valuable immunological identification technique is Western blotting (Figure I-2-13).[71] A mixture of proteins can be electrophoretically separated by SDS-PAGE, and the separated proteins can be transferred to a nitrocellulose or nylon-based filter by electrophoresis in a direction perpendicular to that of the first electrophoresis. The proteins will remain bound to the membrane support. By analogy to Southern blotting for DNA and Northern blotting for RNA, this technique for protein transfer has been called Western blotting.

The protein blot can be soaked in a solution that contains a specific antibody that binds to the protein of interest. The presence of the bound antibody on the blot can then be detected if the antibody is labelled. The label can be an enzyme that reveals its presence by catalyzing a color reaction, or it can be a radionuclide such as ^{125}I that can be detected by autoradiography. Alternatively, an unlabeled antibody can be detected by washing the blot in a solution that contains a labeled anti-immunoglobulin antibody.

This technique has been used to demonstrate overexpression of the HER-2/*neu* protein in some breast cancers in which Southern blotting revealed no gene amplification.[66] Since the protein is the effector of gene function and the determinant of phenotype, overexpression of the protein can be highly significant, and is often considered to be the "gold standard" of overexpression.

Sequencing

The ultimate in protein identification is direct determination of amino acid sequence. Automated sequenators are now available that have considerably simplified this technically demanding analysis. In addition, recent advances in protein chemistry have permitted sequencing to be performed on mere picomoles of protein. In fact, Western blotting can be used to purify small amounts of protein, and the fragment of the blot containing the stained protein of interest can be used directly in the automated sequenator.[43]

Direct protein sequencing was responsible for ushering in the modern era of molecular oncology. The empirically determined amino acid sequence of the B-chain of human platelet-derived growth factor (PDGF) was found to be nearly identical to the protein encoded by the oncogene v-*sis*, the transforming gene of the simian sarcoma virus.[20,77] This was the first demonstration of a connection between oncogenes and the components involved in normal cellular proliferation.

Engineered Protein Expression

The final goal of many experiments in molecular biology is the use of biological systems to synthesize the protein encoded by the gene being studied. This process, called engineered protein expression, can be an experimental end in itself. When the expressed protein synthesized by recombinant DNA methods can be shown to have all the properties of the natural protein, this is considered to be proof that the proper gene has been cloned. Alternatively, expression can be an end in itself when one wants to produce large amounts of a particular protein that might be difficult to obtain from natural sources.

In Vitro Translation. One very simple expression method is in vitro translation, in which translation occurs entirely in a test tube. All of the components necessary for translating mRNA can be obtained in a functional form from cells that are highly efficient in protein synthesis, such as reticulocytes

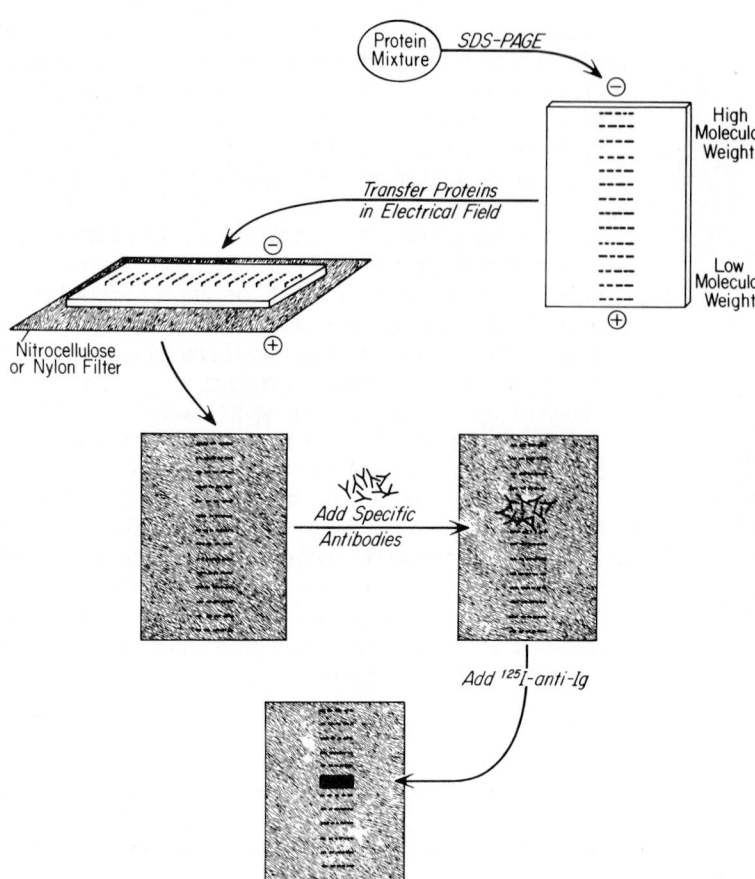

Figure I-2-13. Western blotting. A complex mixture of proteins can be separated by size using electrophoresis (SDS-PAGE). The separated proteins are then transferred to a nitrocellulose or nylon filter in an electric field, maintaining their size-specific spatial orientation on the filter. Antibodies directed against one specific protein in the original mixture are added to the filter and bind to the specific protein. Bound antibodies can be radiolabeled or enzymatically labeled themselves, or they can be visualized by incubating the filter with labeled anti-immunoglobulin antibodies.

(usually from rabbits) or wheat germ. Under the appropriate conditions, and in the presence of all 20 amino acids, a synthetic or purified RNA added to such a system will be efficiently translated into protein. If a radioactive amino acid, such as [^{35}S]methionine, is included in the mix, the reaction products can be analyzed by SDS-PAGE and autoradiography. Demonstrating an appropriately sized protein, or one that is recognized by a specific antibody, constitutes good evidence that the mRNA in hand is the one the investigator desires.

Large-Scale Production of Recombinant Proteins In vitro translation can only be applied at a small-scale analytical level. To produce large amounts of protein, one must turn to in vivo expression systems. One of the simplest involves cloning the cDNA for the desired protein into a bacterial plasmid or phage that contains a transcriptional promoter active in bacteria. When introduced into the appropriate bacterial host, large amounts of mRNA will be transcribed that, in turn, will be translated into protein. The recombinant protein can then be purified away from all the bacterial proteins. This is the way that many clinically available interferons have been produced.[19,25,48]

Many eukaryotic proteins require post-translational modifications for maximal activity. Bacteria do not have the machinery required to accomplish complex modifications, such as the addition of specific carbohydrate groups. Moreover, the interior milieu of a bacterial cell is a reducing environment, so that disulfide bonds essential to the structure

and function of many eukaryotic proteins cannot form. When these modifications are required, mammalian cells can be used for expression. The basic concept is the same as in bacterial systems: a cDNA is cloned into a vector having a eukaryotic transcriptional promoter and the resulting recombinant DNA is introduced into mammalian cells.

Expression systems have been modified to increase the levels of protein synthesis in number of ways. We present one particularly clever technique (diagrammed in Figure I-2-14) as an example of how observations in disparate areas of research oncology can be combined to great advantage. Here, a cDNA of interest is inserted in a plasmid downstream from a promoter sequence (in this case, one borrowed from adenovirus) and upstream from a cDNA for mouse dihydrofolate reductase (DHFR).[30] When mRNA is transcribed from this plasmid, the mRNA will be "dicistronic", i.e., it will contain the message sequences for two separate proteins on the same mRNA. Upstream, at the 5' end, will be the cDNA of interest, and downstream, at the 3' end, will be the DHFR cDNA. When the mRNA is translated, two separate proteins (not a fusion protein) will be made since the upstream cDNA has a termination codon at the end of its coding sequences.

This recombinant plasmid is then introduced, by means of a process called "transfection", into a cell line that has no endogenous DHFR gene.[73] Not all the cells in the transfection experiment take up the recombinant DNA, but by growing the cells in the absence of nucleosides in the growth medium, the only cells that will survive will be those that

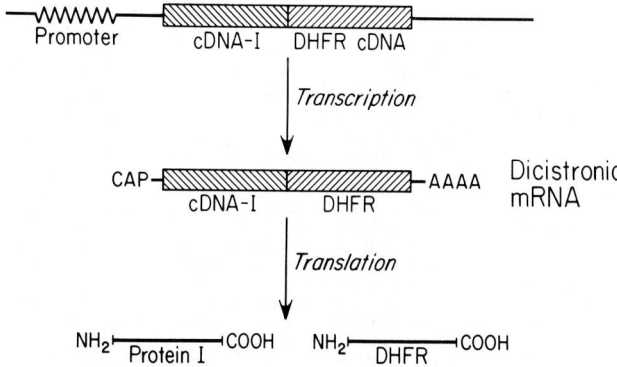

Figure I-2-14. Mammalian engineered protein expression system. A cDNA encoding the protein to be produced ("I") is cloned downstream (3′) of a promoter and upstream (5′) of a cDNA for dihydrofolate reductase (DHFR). After transfection into a mammalian cell the promoter directs transcription of a "dicistronic" mRNA, one that contains two independent coding regions. The cDNA for "I" is 5′ to the cDNA for DHFR. When the mRNA is translated, two separate proteins result, the "I" protein and DHFR. As described in the text, the cDNA for DHFR can be amplified by methotrexate selection. This process will also result in amplification of the closely linked DNA for cDNA-I, and will ultimately lead to large amounts of dicistronic mRNA and large amounts of "I" protein and DHFR.

have: 1) taken up the DNA; 2) have transcribed the DHFR cDNA into mRNA; and 3) have translated that mRNA into DHFR protein. These surviving cells will also necessarily be expressing the protein of interest, since its cDNA was upstream from the DHFR sequences.

One can now take advantage of the fact that the major mechanism of methotrexate (MTX) resistance in mammalian cells is amplification of the DNA encoding DHFR. The expressing cells can be exposed to gradually increasing concentrations of MTX in vitro to generate resistant lines. At each level of resistance, the transfected DHFR cDNA has undergone amplification, but so has the cDNA cloned immediately upstream from DHFR. Thus as DHFR protein expression reaches higher levels, so does the expression of the protein of interest. In this way, very high levels of several of the colony-stimulating factors have been produced for clinical use.[83]

There are still significant disadvantages to the use of mammalian cells for large-scale recombinant protein production. Mammalian cells are expensive to grow in vitro because they require a medium rich in nutrients and growth factors. Yeast cells, insect cells, and even plant cells are being exploited as an attractive compromise between mammalian cell culture and bacterial culture for protein expression. These eukaryotic cells can execute most of the post-translational modifications required by mammalian proteins, including disulfide bonding. At the same time, these cells are easier and more economical to grow in vitro. A number of expression vectors analogous to those described here for bacteria and animal cells have been developed for these alternative eukaryotic hosts.

Summary

The genetic information in DNA is transcribed into RNA, and the information in RNA is ultimately translated into protein. Like DNA and RNA, proteins are directional. The amino

and carboxy termini of proteins are specified by the 5′ and 3′ ends, respectively, of their cognate mRNA's. After translation, proteins may require further modification in order to be fully functional.

Proteins can be fractionated by size using electrophoresis through polyacrylamide gels in the presence of the anionic detergent, SDS (SDS-PAGE). SDS-PAGE is an integral component of the analytical techniques of immune precipitation and Western blotting. Automated analyzers are now available that can directly determine the amino acid sequence of a protein using vanishingly small amounts of material.

The mRNA that encodes a protein can be translated in vitro using cellular extracts of rabbit reticulocytes or wheat germ. The DNA that encodes a protein can be transcribed and the RNA translated in vivo by using appropriate vector and host cell combinations in culture. Bacterial cells are simple and economical vehicles for expressing foreign genes, but they cannot perform many of the post-translational modifications required by mammalian proteins. Vectors have been designed that permit mammalian cells to express foreign proteins with great efficiency and fidelity. However, mammalian expression systems are expensive. Simpler eukaryotic expression systems using yeast cells, insect cells, or plant cells have been developed as an acceptable middle ground.

References

1. Atchison, M. L.: Enhancers: mechanisms of action and cell specificity. Annu. Rev. Cell Biol., 4:127, 1988.
2. Ausubel, F. M., Brent, R., Kingston, R. E., Moore, D. D., Seidman, J. G., Smith, J. A., and Struhl, K.: Current Protocols in Molecular Biology. New York, John Wiley & Sons, 1989.
3. Aviv, H., and Leder, P.: Purification of biologically active globin messenger RNA by chromatography on oligothymidylic acid-cellulose. Proc. Natl. Acad. Sci. USA, 69:1408, 1972.
4. Baker, S. J., Fearon, E. R., Nigro, J. M., Hamilton, S. R., Preisinger, A. C., Jessup, J. M., vanTuinen, P., Ledbetter, D. H., Barker, D. F., Nakamura, Y., White, R., and Vogelstein, B.: Chromosome 17 deletions and p53 gene mutations in colorectal carcinomas. Science, 244:217, 1989.
5. Baltimore, D.: RNA-dependent DNA polymerase in virions of RNA tumor viruses. Nature, 226:1209, 1970.
6. Bauer, W. R., Crick, F. H. C., and White, J. H.: Supercoiled DNA. Sci. Am., 243:118, 1980.
7. Benton, W. D., and Davis, R. W.: Screening λgt recombinant clones by hybridization to single plaques in situ. Science, 196:180, 1977.
8. Berger, S. L., and Kimmel, A. R.: Guide to Molecular Cloning Techniques. In Methods in Enzymology. Edited by J. N. Abelson and M. I. Simon. San Diego, CA, Academic Press, 1987.
9. Berk, A. J., and Sharp, P. A.: Sizing and mapping of early adenovirus mRNAs by gel electrophoresis of S1 endonuclease-digested hybrids. Cell, 12:721, 1977.
10. Birnstiel, M. L., Busslinger, M., and Strub, K.: Transcription termination and 3′ processing: The end is in site! Cell, 41:349, 1985.
11. Carle, G. F., Frank, M., and Olson, M. V.: Electrophoretic separations of large DNA molecules by periodic inversion of the electric field. Science, 232:65, 1986.
12. Chien, A., Edgar, D. B., and Trela, J. M.: Deoxyribonucleic acid polymerase from the extreme thermophile Thermus aquaticus. J. Bacteriol., 127:1550, 1976.
13. Chirgwin, J. M., Przybyla, A. E., MacDonald, R. J., and Rutter, W. J.: Isolation of biologically active ribonucleic acid from sources enriched in ribonuclease. Biochemistry, 18:5294, 1979.
14. Chu, G., Vollrath, D., and Davis, R. W.: Separation of large DNA molecules by contour-clamped homogeneous electric fields. Science, 234:1582, 1986.
15. Clarke, L., and Carbon, J.: A colony bank containing synthetic Col E1 hybrid plasmids representative of the entire E. coli genome. Cell, 9:91, 1976.
16. Cochran, B. H., Reffel, A. C., and Stiles, C. D.: Molecular cloning of gene sequences regulated by platelet-derived growth factor. Cell, 33:939, 1983.
17. Cohen, S. N., Chang, A. C. Y., Boyer, H. W., and Helling, R. B.: Construction of biologically functional bacterial plasmids in vitro. Proc. Natl. Acad. Sci. USA, 70:3240, 1973.
18. DeCaprio, J. A., Ludlow, J. W., Figge, J., Shew, J. Y., Huang, C. M., Lee, W. H., Marsilio, E., Paucha, E., and Livingston, D. M.: SV40 large tumor antigen forms a specific complex with the product of the retinoblastoma susceptibility gene. Cell, 54:275, 1988.
19. Derynck, R., Remaut, E., Saman, E., Stanssens, P., DeClercq, E., Content, J., and Fiers, W.: Expression of human fibroblast interferon gene in Escherichia coli. Nature, 287:193, 1980.
20. Doolittle, R. F., Hunkapiller, M. W., Hood, L. E., Devare, S. G., Robbins, K. C., Aaronson, S. A., and Antoniades, H. A.: Simian sarcoma virus onc gene, v-sis, is derived from the gene (or genes) encoding a platelet-derived growth factor. Science, 221:275, 1983.
21. Efstradiatis, A., Kafatos, F. C., and Maniatis, T.: The primary structure of rabbit b-globin mRNA as determined from cloned cDNA. Cell, 10:571, 1977.

22. Ek, B., Westermark, B., Wasteson, A., and Heldin, C. H.: Stimulation of tyrosine-specific phosphorylation by platelet-derived growth factor. Nature, 295:419, 1982.
23. Eva, A., Robbins, K. C., Andersen, P. R., Srinivasan, A., Tronick, S. R., Reddy, E. P., Ellmore, N. W., Galen, A. T., Lautenberger, J. A., Papas, T. S., Westin, E. H., Wong-Staal, F., Gallo, R. C., and Aaronson, S. A.: Cellular genes analogous to retroviral *onc* genes are transcribed in human tumour cells. Nature, 295:116, 1982.
24. Filipowicz, W.: Functions of the 5′-terminal m7G cap in eukaryotic mRNA. FEBS Lett., 96:1, 1978.
25. Goeddel, D. V., Yelverton, E., Ullrich, A., Heyneker, H. L., Miozzari, K., Holmes, W., Seeburg, P. H., Dull, T., May, L., Stebbing, N., Crea, R., Maeda, S., McCandliss, R., Sloma, A., Tabor, J. M., Gross, M., Familletti, P. C., and Pestka, S.: Human leukocyte interferon produced by *E. coli* is biologically active. Nature, 287:411, 1980.
26. Grunstein, M., and Hogness, D. S.: Colony hybridization: a method for the isolation of cloned DNAs that contain a specific gene. Proc. Natl. Acad. Sci. USA, 72:3961, 1975.
27. Gusella, J. F., Wexler, N. S., Conneally, P. M., Naylor, S. L., Anderson, M. A., Tanzi, R. E., Watkins, P. C., Ottina, K., Wallace, M. R., and Sakaguchi, A. Y.: A polymorphic DNA marker genetically linked to Huntington's disease. Nature, 306:234, 1983.
28. Imagawa, D. T., Lee, M. H., Wolinsky, S. M., Sano, K., Morales, F., Kwok, S., Sninsky, J. J., Nishanian, P. G., Giorgi, J., Fahey, J. L., Dudley, J., Visscher, B. R., and Detels, R.: Long latency of human immunodeficiency virus-1 in seronegative high risk homosexual men determined by prospective virus isolation and DNA amplification studies. N. Engl. J. Med., 320:1428, 1989.
29. Innis, M. A., Gelfand, D. H., Sninsky, J. J., and White, T. J.: PCR Protocols. San Diego, CA, Academic Press, 1990.
30. Kaufman, R. J., Murtha, P., and Davies, M.: Translational efficiency of polycistronic mRNAs and their utilization to express heterologous genes in mammalian cells. EMBO J., 6:187, 1987.
31. Kawasaki, E. S., Clark, S. S., Coyne, M. Y., Smith, S. D., Champlin, R., Witte, O. N., and McCormick, F. P.: Diagnosis of chronic myeloid and acute lymphocytic leukemias by detection of leukemia-specific mRNA sequences amplified *in vitro*. Proc. Natl. Acad. Sci. USA, 85:5698, 1988.
32. Knudson, A. G.: Hereditary cancer, oncogenes, and antioncogenes. Cancer Res., 45:1437, 1985.
33. Laemmli, U. K.: Cleavage of structural proteins during the assembly of the head of bacteriophage T4. Nature, 227:680, 1970.
34. Laskey, R. A., and Earnshaw, W. C.: Nucleosome assembly. Nature, 286:763, 1980.
35. Lawyer, F. C., Stoffel, S., Saiki, R. K., Myambo, R., Drummond, R., and Gelfand, D. H.: Isolation, characterization, and expression in *Escherichia coli* of the DNA polymerase gene from *Thermus aquaticus*. J. Biol. Chem., 264:6427, 1989.
36. Le Beau, M. M., Pettenati, M. J., Lemons, R. S., Diaz, M. O., Westbrook, C. A., Larson, R. A., Sherr, C. J., and Rowley, J. D.: Assignment of the GM-CSF, CSF-1, and FMS genes to human chromosome 5 provides evidence for linkage of a family of genes regulating hematopoiesis and for their involvement in the deletion (5q) in myeloid disorders. Cold Spring Harbor Symp. Quant. Biol., 51:899, 1986.
37. Lehrach, H., Diamond, D., Wozney, J. M., and Boedtker, H.: RNA molecular weight determinations by gel electrophoresis under denaturing conditions, a critical reexamination. Biochem., 16:4743, 1977.
38. Lewin, B.: Gene Expression, 2nd Edition. New York, John Wiley & Sons, 1980.
39. Lewin, N.: Genes IV, 4th Edition. Oxford, UK, Oxford University Press, 1990.
40. Lynn, D. A., Angerer, L. M., Bruskin, A. M., Klein, W. H., and Angerer, R. C.: Localization of a family of mRNAs in a single cell type and its precursors in sea urchin embryos. Proc. Natl. Acad. Sci. USA, 80:2656, 1983.
41. Maniatis, T., Hardison, R. C., Lacy, E., Lauer, J., O'Connell, C., Quon, D., Sim, G. K., and Efstratiadis, A.: The isolation of structural genes from libraries of eukaryotic DNA. Cell, 15:687, 1978.
42. Maniatis, T., and Reed, R.: The role of small nuclear ribonucleoprotein particles in pre-mRNA splicing. Nature, 325:673, 1987.
43. Matsudaira, P.: Sequence from picomole quantities of proteins electroblotted onto polyvinylidene difluoride membranes. J. Biol. Chem., 262:10035, 1987.
44. Maxam, A. M., and Gilbert, W.: A new method for sequencing DNA. Proc. Natl. Acad. Sci. USA, 74:560, 1977.
45. McKnight, S., and Tjian, R.: Transcriptional selectivity of viral genes in mammalian cells. Cell, 46:795, 1986.
46. McMaster, G. K., and Carmichael, G. G.: Analysis of single- and double-stranded nucleic acids on polyacrylamide and agarose gels by using glyoxal and acridine orange. Proc. Natl. Acad. Sci. USA, 74:4835, 1977.
47. Mullis, K. B., and Faloona, F. A.: Specific synthesis of DNA *in vitro* via a polymerase-catalyzed chain reaction. Methods Enzymol., 155:335, 1987.
48. Nagata, S., Taira, H., Hall, A., Johnsrud, L., Streuli, M., Escodi, J., Boll, W., Cantell, K., and Weissman, C.: Synthesis in *E. coli* of a polypeptide with human leukocyte interferon activity. Nature, 284:316, 1980.
49. Nakamura, Y., Leppert, M., O'Connell, P., Wolff, R., Holm, T., Culver, M., Martin, C., Fujimoto, E., Hoff, M., Kumlin, E., and White, R.: Variable number of tandem repeat (VNTR) markers for human gene mapping. Science, 235:1616, 1987.
50. Nigro, J. M., Baker, S. J., Preisinger, A. C., Jessup, J. M., Hostetter, R., Cleary, K., Bigner, S. H., Davidson, N., Baylin, S., Devilee, P., Glover, T., Collins, F. S., Weston, A., Modali, R., Harris, C. C., and Vogelstein, B.: Mutations in the *p53* gene occur in diverse human tumor types. Nature, 342:705, 1989.
51. Nirenberg, M. W., and Leder, P.: RNA codewords and protein synthesis. Science, 145:1399, 1964.
52. Rettenmier, C. W., Chen, J. H., Roussel, M. F., and Sherr, C. J.: The product of the c-*fms* proto-oncogene: a glycoprotein with associated tyrosine kinase activity. Science, 228:320, 1985.
53. Roberts, R.: Restriction and modification enzymes and their recognition sequences. Nucl. Acids Res., 10:117, 1982.
54. Rougeon, F., and Mach, B.: Stepwise biosynthesis in vitro of globin genes from globin mRNA by DNA polymerase of avian myeloblastosis virus. Proc. Natl. Acad. Sci. USA, 73:3418, 1976.
55. Saiki, R. K., Gelfand, D. H., Stoffel, S., Scharf, S. J., Higuchi, R., Horn, G. T., Mullis, K. B., and Erlich, H. A.: Primer-directed enzymatic amplification of DNA with a thermostable DNA polymerase. Science, 239:487, 1988.
56. Saiki, R. K., Scharf, S., Faloona, F., Mullis, K. B., Horn, G. T., Erlich, H. A., and Arnheim, N.: Enzymatic amplification of β-globin genomic sequences and restriction site analysis for diagnosis of sickle cell anemia. Science, 230:1350, 1985.
57. Sambrook, J., Fritsch, E. F., and Maniatis, T.: Molecular Cloning, A Laboratory Manual, 2nd Edition. Cold Spring Harbor, NY, Cold Spring Harbor Laboratory Press, 1989.
58. Sanger, F., Nicklen, S., and Coulson, A. R.: DNA sequencing with chain-terminating inhibitors. Proc. Natl. Acad. Sci. USA, 74:5463, 1977.
59. Schwartz, D. C., and Cantor, C. R.: Separation of yeast chromosome-sized DNAs by pulsed field gradient gel electrophoresis. Cell, 37:67, 1984.
60. Sharp, P. A.: Splicing of messenger RNA precursors. Science, 235:766, 1987.
61. Shatkin, A. J.: Capping of eukaryotic mRNAs. Cell, 9:645, 1976.
62. Shatkin, A. J.: mRNA cap binding proteins: essential factors for initiating translation. Cell, 40:223, 1985.
63. Sherr, C. J., Rettenmier, C. W., Sacca, R., Roussel, M. F., Look, A. T., and Stanley, E. R.: The c-*fms* proto-oncogene product is related to the receptor for the mononuclear phagocyte growth factor, CSF-1. Cell, 41:665, 1985.
64. Slamon, D. J., Clark, G. M., Wong, S. G., Levin, W. J., Ullrich, A., and McGuire, W. L.: Human breast cancer: Correlation of relapse and survival with amplification of the HER-2/*neu* oncogene. Science, 235:177, 1987.
65. Slamon, D. J., deKernion, J. B., Verma, I. M., and Cline, M. J.: Expression of cellular oncogenes in human malignancies. Science, 224:256, 1984.
66. Slamon, D. J., Godolphin, W., Jones, L. A., Holt, J. A., Wong, S. G., Keith, D. E., Levin, W. J., Stuart, S. G., Udove, J., Ullrich, A., and Press, M. F.: Studies of the HER-2/*neu* proto-oncogene in human breast and ovarian cancers. Science, 244:707, 1989.
67. Smith, H. O.: Nucleotide sequence specificity of restriction endonucleases. Science, 205:455, 1979.
68. Southern, E. M.: Detection of specific sequences among DNA fragments separated by gel electrophoresis. J. Mol. Biol., 98:503, 1975.
69. Takahashi, T., Nau, M. M., Chiba, I., Birrer, M. J., Rosenberg, R. K., Vinocour, M., Levitt, M., Pass, H., Gazdar, A., and Minna, J. D.: p53: a frequent target for genetic abnormalities in lung cancer. Science, 246:491, 1989.
70. Temin, H. M., and Mizutani, S.: RNA-dependent DNA polymerase in virions of Rous sarcoma virus. Nature, 226:1211, 1970.
71. Towbin, H., Staehelin, T., and Gordon, J.: Electrophoretic transfer of proteins from polyacrylamide gels to nitrocellulose sheets: Procedure and some applications. Proc. Natl. Acad. Sci. USA, 76:4350, 1979.
72. Tsui, L. C., Buchwald, M., Barker, D., Braman, J. C., Knowlton, R., Schumm, J. W., Eiberg, H., Mohr, J., Kennedy, D., and Plavsic, N.: Cystic fibrosis locus defined by a genetically linked polymorphic DNA marker. Science, 230:1054, 1985.
73. Urlaub, G., and Chasin, L. A.: Isolation of Chinese hamster cell mutants deficient in dihydrofolate reductase activity. Proc. Natl. Acad. Sci. USA, 77:4216, 1980.
74. Vogelstein, B., Fearon, E. R., Kern, S. E., Hamilton, S. R., Preisinger, A. C., Nakamura, Y., and White, R.: Allelotype of colorectal carcinomas. Science, 244:207, 1989.
75. Wainwright, B. J., Scambler, P. J., Schmidtke, J., Watson, E. A., Law, H. Y., Farrall, M., Cooke, H. J., Eiberg, H., and Williamson, R.: Localization of cystic fibrosis locus to human chromosome 7cen-q22. Nature, 318:384, 1985.
76. Wang, J. C.: DNA topoisomerases. Annu. Rev. Biochem., 54:665, 1985.
77. Waterfield, M. D., Scrace, G. T., Whittle, N., Stroobant, P., Johnsson, A., Wasteson, A., Westermark, B., Heldin, C. H., Huang, J. S., and Deuel, T. F.: Platelet-derived growth factor is structurally related to the putative transforming protein p28*sis* of simian sarcoma virus. Nature, 304:35, 1983.
78. Weber, K., and Osborn, M.: The reliability of molecular weight determinations by dodecyl sulfate-polyacrylamide gel electrophoresis. J. Biol. Chem., 244:4406, 1969.
79. Westin, E. H., Wong-Staal, F., Gelmann, E. P., Dalla Favera, R., Papas, T. S., Lautenberger, J. A., Eva, A., Reddy, E. P., Tronick, S. R., Aaronson, S. A., and Gallo, R. C.: Expression of cellular homologues of retroviral *onc* genes in human hematopoietic cells. Proc. Natl. Acad. Sci. USA, 79:2490, 1982.
80. White, R., Woodward, S., Leppert, M., OConnell, P., Hoff, M., Herbst, J., Lalouel, J. M., Dean, M., and Vande Woude, G.: A closely linked genetic marker for cystic fibrosis. Nature, 318:382, 1985.
81. Whyte, P., Buchkovich, K. J., Horowitz, J. M., Friend, S. H., Raybuck, M., Weinberg, R. A., and Harlow, E.: Association between an oncogene and an anti-oncogene: the adenovirus E1A proteins bind to the retinoblastoma gene product. Nature, 334:124, 1988.
82. Wright, D. K., and Manos, M. M.: Sample Preparation From Paraffin-Embedded Tissues. *In* PCR Protocols: A Guide to Methods and Applications. Edited by M. A. Innis, D. H. Gelfand, J. J. Sninsky, and T. J. White. San Diego, CA, Academic Press, 1989, p. 153.
83. Yang, Y.-C., Ciarletta, A. B., Temple, P. A., Chung, M. P., Kovacic, S., Witek-Giannotti, J. S., Leary, A. C. , Kriz, R., Donahue, R. E., Wong, G. G., and Clark, S. C.: Human IL-3 (multi-CSF): identification by expression cloning of a novel hematopoietic growth factor related to murine IL-3. Cell, 47:3, 1986.
84. Yang, Y. C., Kovacic, S., Kriz, R., Wolf, S., Clark, S. C., Wellems, T. E., Nienhuis, A., and Epstein, N.: The human genes for GM-CSF and IL 3 are closely linked in tandem on chromosome 5. Blood, 71:958, 1988.
85. Young, R. A., and Davis, R. W.: Efficient isolation of genes using antibody probes. Proc. Natl. Acad. Sci. USA, 80:1194, 1983.
86. Zaug, A. J., Been, M. D., and Cech, T. R.: The Tetrahymena ribozyme acts like an RNA restriction endonuclease. Nature, 324:429, 1986.
87. Zinn, K., DiMaio, D., and Maniatis, T.: Identification of two distinct regulatory regions adjacent to the human β-interferon gene. Cell, 34:865, 1983.

Growth Factors

Stuart A. Aaronson
Steven R. Tronick

Introduction

The evolution of multicellular organisms has involved the development of intercellular communication required for such processes as embryonic development, tissue differentiation, as well as systemic responses to wounds and infections. These complex signalling networks are in large part mediated by growth factors, cytokines and hormones. Such factors can influence cell proliferation in positive or negative ways as well as inducing a series of differentiated responses in appropriate target cells. The interaction of a growth factor with its receptor by specific binding in turn activates a cascade of intracellular biochemical events that is ultimately responsible for the biological responses observed. Cytoplasmic molecules that mediate these responses have been termed second messengers. The eventual transmission of biochemical signals to the nucleus leads to effects on the expression of cassettes of genes involved in mitogenic and differentiation responses.

Over the past few years it has become increasingly evident that the pathogenic expression of critical genes in growth factor signalling pathways can contribute to altered cell growth associated with malignancy. The v-sis oncogene of simian sarcoma virus, which encodes a growth factor homologous to the B chain of human platelet derived growth factor (PDGF-B), is the paradigm for such genes.[34,185] The normal homologs of other oncogenes have been shown to encode membrane spanning growth factor receptors.[35,163] Other genes that act early in intracellular pathways of growth factor signal transduction have been implicated as oncogenes as well. Present knowledge indicates that the constitutive activation of growth factor signalling pathways through genetic alterations affecting these genes contributes to the development and progression of most if not all human cancers.

This chapter focuses on normal aspects of growth factor signalling, particularly those mediated by growth factor receptors possessing intrinsic protein tyrosine kinase activity. A discussion of G-protein mediated signalling pathways is presented as well. In addition, examples are provided where abnormalities in early steps in these pathways involving alterations in growth factor expression and/or receptor signalling have been implicated in the etiology of human malignancies. Finally, we will discuss how this knowledge may be useful in efforts to design new approaches towards therapeutic intervention with the malignant process.

History

Hormones which act at great distances from the cells producing them have been known for many years. Hormones as signalling molecules were isolated from tissue fluids and readily characterized by their in vivo effects. In contrast, knowledge of growth factors is relatively recent. Growth factor activity capable of stimulating the growth of chicken embryonic nerve cells was found to be released by mouse sarcoma cells.[102] During purification of this nerve growth factor (NGF), a second activity that promoted eyelid opening and incisor eruption in newborn mice and rats was discovered.[23] Because of recognition of its effects on epithelial cells, this factor was designated epidermal growth factor (EGF). Since the early days of tissue culture, it was recognized that serum was important for growth of cell cultures. A major mitogenic activity found in serum was shown to be derived from platelets and was, therefore, designated platelet derived growth factor (PDGF).[68,151] Subsequent studies by a number of laboratories have led to detection of a series of growth factors which were often given names based on the tissue or cell of origin or the target cell initially found to be stimulated.

An important discovery concerning growth factors came from the demonstration of a unique enzymologic activity associated with binding of EGF to its receptor.[15,23] Studies of the product of the viral oncogene, v-src, had led to the demonstration of its ability to act as a protein kinase.[11,24,73,103] Many protein kinases had been previously identified, but these had the capacity to phosphorylate serine and/or threonine residues. Moreover, it was well established that phosphorylations and dephosphorylations affected the activities of a variety of proteins. However, the src product was subsequently shown to have a unique specificity as a protein kinase in that it was capable of phosphorylating tyrosine residues.[24,73,103] Cohen then showed that addition of EGF led to phosphorylation of purified receptor on tyrosine residues.[15,23] Subsequent studies have demonstrated that the ability to perform this enzymatic function is central to the functions of a large number of mitogenic signalling molecules.

Since hormones act at long distances from their source and are produced by glandular tissues, their mode of action has been characterized as endocrine. Sporn and Todaro termed the modes of action of growth factors as paracrine or autocrine.[169] The former refers to the site of growth factor action on nearby or adjacent cells, whereas autocrine refers to the ability to activate mitogenic signalling pathways in the cell releasing the factor. In general, normal growth factors are thought to act by a paracrine mode, influencing and fine tuning the development and differentiation of cells nearby.

However, there are examples of growth factors that act in an endocrine-like manner as well as by autocrine routes.

Classification of Growth Factors that Act on Cells of Solid Tissues

A summary of some of the properties of the growth factors described below is presented in Table I-3-1.

Platelet-Derived Growth Factor Family

Platelet-derived growth factor is the major protein growth factor in human serum and is a markedly heat stable, cationic protein that consists of two related but non-identical (36.7% amino acid sequence identity) polypeptide chains designated A and B (also called PDGF-1 and PDGF-2).[34,185] PDGF molecules exist as AA and BB homodimers as well as an AB heterodimer.[68,151] PDGF-AB is the major PDGF form found in platelets and is released into serum upon blood clotting. However, there is evidence for the natural occurrence of each of the other forms. Connective tissue and glial cells in culture are highly sensitive to the mitogenic effects of PDGF,[66,151] and it is these cells that express PDGF receptors. The α and β PDGF receptors are encoded by distinct genes,[19,20,114,194] and there is evidence that they exist as receptor subunits that differentially interact with the three dimeric PDGF ligands.[61,64,68,114,115] Thus, PDGF-AA can bind only the αα receptor dimer while PDGF-BB can interact with αα, αβ, and ββ receptor dimers. The PDGF-AB heterodimer preferentially interacts with and triggers αα and αβ receptors and would bind the ββ receptor without, however, inducing its dimerization. This is an example of the fine degree of regulation that can evolve in the interactions of ligands with their receptors (Figure I-3-1). Presumably in the case of PDGF, this relates to quantitative regulation of responses based upon differential availability in tissues of ligands and receptors, since there is evidence that the two PDGF receptors, themselves, are each capable of mediating the major known PDGF responses including mitogenic signalling and chemotaxis.[115,188]

As noted earlier, the gene for the PDGF-B chain is the human homolog of the v-*sis* oncogene of simian sarcoma virus (SSV).[34,185] The transforming protein expressed by SSV shares close structural similarities with PDGF-B chain homodimers.[148,149] PDGF-B has been detected in human tumor cells that also possess PDGF receptors.[21,44,51,74] These findings taken together with the demonstration that the normal PDGF-B gene can act as an oncogene when expressed at high levels[51] suggest that PDGF-B plays a role in the development of certain human cancers. The PDGF-A chain is

Table I-3-1.   Growth Factors That Signal Through Protein Tyrosine Kinase Receptors

	Size Predicted from Sequence[1]		Size of Native Forms	
	Amino Acids	MW	MW	Source
PDGF Family				
PDGF-A	211	24,043	28,000–35,000	Platelets (α-granules)
PDGF-B	241	27,283	(Homo- and Hetero-	
			dimers of -A and -B)	
VEGF/VPF	192		45,000	Pituitary cells, Tumor cell lines
	(148/216)*		(Homodimers)	
EGF Family				
EGF	1207	13,945	6,200	Urine
				Submaxillary gland
TGF-α	160	17,007	5,500	Transformed cell lines, embryos
Amphiregulin	84	9,759	14,000	Tumor cell line
	(78)*			
Fibroblast Growth Factor Family				
A-FGF (FGF1/HBGF1)	155	17,254	17,000	Brain, pituitary
B-FGF (FGF2/HBGF2)	155	17,460	17,000	Brain, pituitary
int-2 (FGF3/HBGF3)	239	26,886	—	Mammary tumor cells
hst/KS3 (FGF4/HBGF4)	206	22,047	—	Tumor cell line (DNA transfection)
FGF5 (HBGF5)	267	29,370	—	Tumor cell line (DNA transfection)
FGF6[2]	—	—	—	Genomic library
KGF (FGF7)	194	22,512	28,000	Embryonic fibroblast cell line
Insulin Family				
Insulin	110	11,981	5,800	Pancreas
IGF-1	153	17,026	7,600	Plasma
	(195)*	(21,841)*		
Others				
HGF	728	83,132	70,000–90,000	Plasma

[1]Amino acid residues and molecular weight (unmodified polypeptide) of open reading frame of complete cDNA except where noted (includes signal sequence when present)
[2]Only partial sequence available
*Alternate forms of cDNA

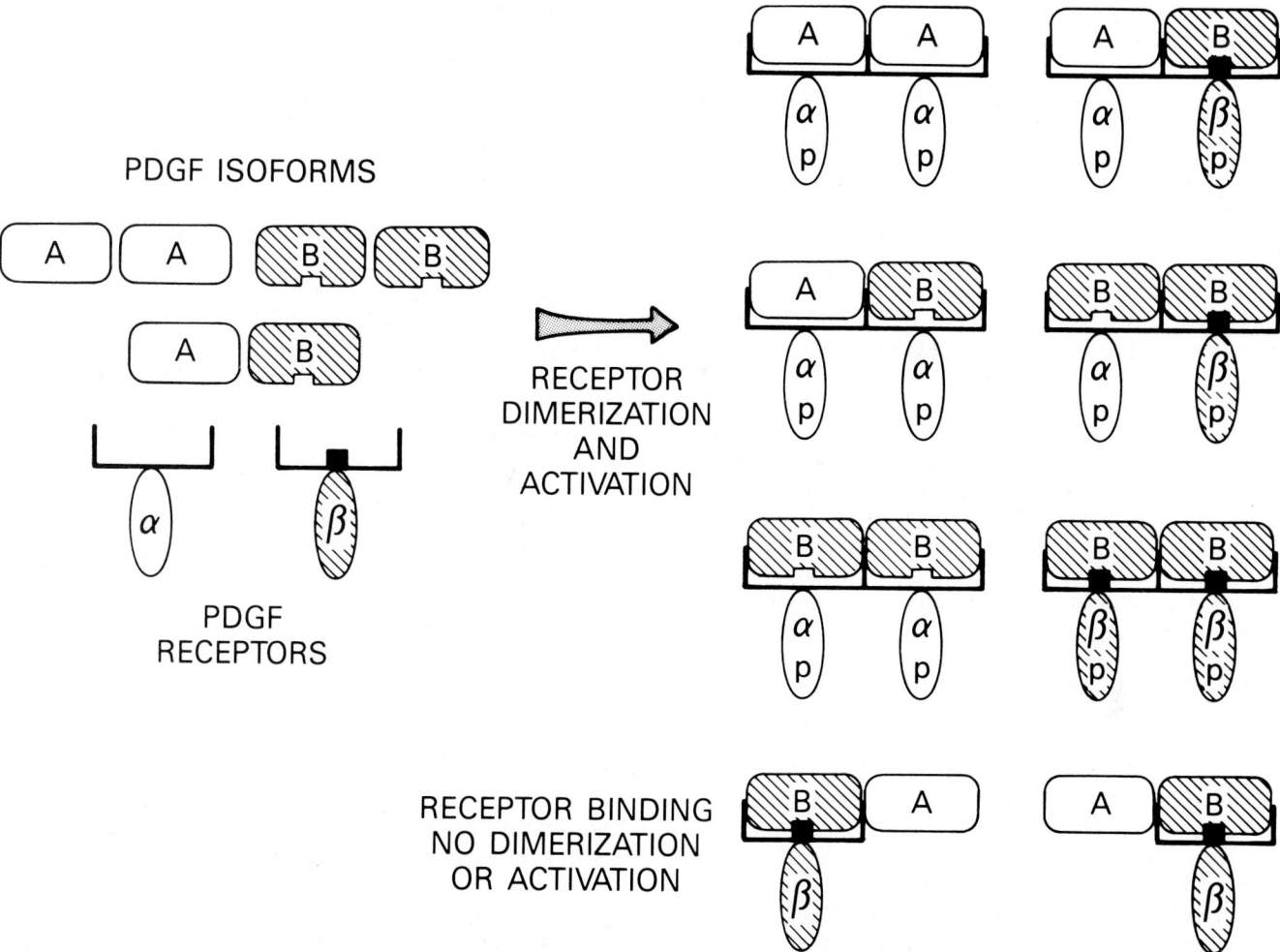

PDGF ISOFORMS

PDGF RECEPTORS

RECEPTOR DIMERIZATION AND ACTIVATION

RECEPTOR BINDING NO DIMERIZATION OR ACTIVATION

Figure I-3-1. Interactions between PDGF isoforms and PDGF receptors. Possible complexes that can form between the three dimeric PDGF isoforms and the α- and β-PDGF receptors are shown. The presence of the ligand-receptor complexes depicted would depend upon the relative levels of receptors in a particular cell as well as on the abundance of the various PDGF dimers. The lower part of the figure depicts a situation in which triggering of the β-receptor would be prevented when the PDGF-AB heterodimer is present in excess. The small letter "p" indicates ligand-triggered receptor autophosphorylation.

frequently expressed by human tumor cells, and AA homodimers are produced by osteosarcoma,[67] melanoma,[186] and glioblastoma cells.[135]

Efforts to identify factors that control angiogenesis recently led to the identification of a new growth factor that is a potent mitogen for vascular endothelial cells of small and large vessels, but has no effect on fibroblasts, lens epithelial cells, corneal endothelial cells, keratinocytes, or adrenal cortex cells. Vascular endothelial growth factor (VEGF) was isolated from the media of cultures of bovine pituitary follicular or folliculostellate cells and consists of two identical polypeptide chains of 23,000 daltons.[101] At the same time another group reported the cloning of a transcript encoding a protein termed vascular permeability factor (VPF) which also promotes endothelial cell growth and angiogenesis.[84] VPF was first identified in rodent tumor cell lines, but its purification and cDNA cloning was achieved by using the human histiocytic lymphoma cell line U937. Sequence comparisons revealed that VEGF and VPF are products of the same gene.

VEGF/VPF share sequence similarity with the PDGF-A and PDGF-B chains (18% identify). The eight cysteine residues in the PDGF-A and B chains are all conserved, but VEGF/VPF possesses an additional eight cysteines within its carboxy-terminal domain. Like PDGF, VEGF/VPF is heat (boiling) and acid stable and shows heterogeneity in size and charge upon electrophoretic analysis. The receptor for VEGF/VPF has not been identified, nor is it known whether growth factor triggering leads to tyrosine phosphorylation of target proteins. However, its structural similarity to PDGF suggests this possibility.

Epidermal Growth Factor Family

EGF purified from mouse submaxillary glands was found to promote precocious eyelid separation by enhancing epidermal growth and keratinization while it induced early incisor eruption by enhancing the differentiation of the lips of treated animals.[23] The proliferative effects of EGF on epidermal cells in organ and tissue cultures derived from avian and mammalian species were subsequently established.

Some years later, the discovery was made that urogastrone (URO), a hormone with gastric antisecretory activity was identical to EGF.[23,58] The role of EGF/URO in inhibiting gastric secretion long remained a mystery until Wright and colleagues reported the induction of novel EGF/URO secreting cells by mucosal ulceration.[191] Although EGF/URO was known to be a potent mitogen for cells of the intestine when administered parenterally, EGF/URO is not absorbed from the adult gut nor does it have an effect when given through the gut lumen when the mucosa is intact. The new cells that form following ulceration of the human gastrointestinal tract eventually form a small gland that secretes EGF/URO whose proliferative effects stimulate ulcer healing. This is likely to be a major in vivo role of EGF/URO.

The EGF chain consists of 53 amino acids constrained by three internal disulfide bonds and is generated from a 1200 residue precursor with a remarkable structure.[57,160] That is, the sequence of the precursor includes eight units similar to EGF and a hydrophobic stretch near its carboxy terminus such as those found in integral membrane proteins. The precursor has been detected as a glycosylated membrane protein in cells transfected with a prepro-EGF precursor and retains biological activity similar to that of EGF.[126]

Other members of the EGF family including tumor growth factor-α (TGF-α), amphiregulin (AR) and poxvirus growth factors share sequence similarities, high binding affinity to the EGF receptor and mitogenic effects on EGF-responsive cells.[150] Amphiregulin, like EGF and TGF-α, is generated by cleavage of a transmembrane precursor 252 amino acids in length but has, in contrast, a highly basic amino terminal 43 residue extension.[143] There is a distinct sequence motif $(X_nCX_7CX_{2-3}GXCX_{10-13}CXCX_3YXGXRCX_4LX_n)$ in each of these molecules that is also present in diverse proteins found on the cell surface or extracellularly but which are not, however, ligands for the EGF receptor.

Whereas EGF is normally expressed in kidney and submaxillary glands and is produced in response to GI tract injury as well,[23,150,191] TGFα appears to be normally expressed by a variety of epithelial cells.[30,150] AR transcripts have been detected in human placenta, ovarian and breast tissue as well as in cells derived from squamous carcinomas and mammary adenocarcinomas.[143]

Fibroblast Growth Factor Family

There are seven known members of the fibroblast growth factor (FGF) family, whose targets include cells derived from mesoderm and neuroectoderm. The best characterized, acidic and basic FGF are angiogenic in vivo and are thought to act during embryogenesis. Because heparin can bind to and modulate the biological activity of these proteins, they have also been termed heparin-binding growth factors (HBGFs).[14,17] The members include acidic FGF (aFGF, FGF-1), basic FGF (bFGF, FGF-2), int-2 (FGF-3), hst/KS3 (FGF-4), FGF-5, FGF-6, and keratinocyte growth factor (FGF-7).[14,17,47,110,154,174] The first to be isolated, bFGF, was recognized in certain hormone preparations by its mitogenicity for mouse 3T3 cells and chondrocytes and was later purified from bovine pituitary. aFGF was purified independently from acidic extracts of bovine brain.[14,17] Both aFGF and bFGF are single chain polypep-

tides of about 17,000 daltons and share 55% amino acid sequence identity. A striking feature of each of their structures, in contrast to those of other family members, is the lack of a consensus secretory signal peptide. This has generated a great deal of speculation regarding their mode of release from cells. Hypotheses have been proposed that argue for liberation of aFGF and bFGF from cells by lysis or escort out of intact cells by other proteins. Alternatively, the presence of a nuclear translocation signal and detection of aFGF and bFGF in the nuclei of endothelial and mesenchymal cells, respectively, indicate that they may act internally without requiring a secretory signal sequence.[10,75,156]

Analysis of DNA of mammary tumors induced by mouse mammary tumor virus (MMTV) revealed that the viral genome frequently integrates within a genetic locus termed int-2 and thereby induces the expression of this gene by insertional mutagenesis.[168] The protein encoded by int-2 is predicted to be 245 amino acids long and highly similar to aFGF and bFGF. The normal expression of int-2 is apparently limited to embryonic tissues and there is evidence from in vitro translation studies that it is a weak mitogen for mammary epithelial cells.[33] Recent transgenic mouse experiments have shown that int-2 expression leads to mammary gland hyperplasia in female mice and benign epithelial hyperplasia in the prostate of males.[128]

FGF-4 and FGF-5 were uncovered during searches for oncogenes in human tumor cells.[14,17,174] FGF-4 was isolated from both a human stomach tumor (hst)[172] and a Kaposi's sarcoma (KS3)[29] and is a mitogen for vascular endothelial cells, human melanocytes and mouse NIH/3T3 fibroblasts.[14] The FGF-5 gene was also isolated by DNA transfection but by using a culture system in which cell growth is dependent upon the presence of PDGF and FGF.[198] Thus, DNA from a human bladder carcinoma cell line induced morphological transformation in the absence of FGF. FGF-5 was found to be activated by a DNA rearrangement that juxtaposed a retrovirus transcriptional enhancer upstream of its natural promoter. Partially purified FGF-5 preparations were found to be mitogenic for mouse fibroblasts and bovine heart endothelial cells.[198]

Isolation of additional members of gene families is sometimes possible by low stringency molecular hybridization employing probes derived from the most highly conserved sequences among each gene. FGF-6 was isolated by this approach from a cosmid library prepared from a human lymphoblastoid cell line and was shown to act as a transforming gene for NIH/3T3 cells by transfection assays.[110] Other biological activities of FGF-6 have yet to be demonstrated.

KGF (FGF-7) was isolated from media conditioned by a human embryonic lung fibroblast cell line and was found to be a potent mitogen for epithelial cells (mouse keratinocytes) but lacked activity on fibroblasts or endothelial cells.[154] Thus, KGF is distinct in this regard not only from other members of the FGF family but from all other polypeptide growth factors as well. Molecular cloning and sequence analysis established it as a member of the FGF family whose predicted amino acid sequence is about 38% identical to those of aFGF and bFGF.[47] The functional role of KGF is perhaps better understood than those of any of the other FGF family members. Thus, KGF transcripts were found to be present in stromal fibroblast lines derived from epithelial tissues of embryonic, neonatal and adult sources but not in normal glial cells or a variety of epithelial cell lines. RNA of normal adult kidney and organs of the GI tract were positive but not from lung or brain. KGF mRNA was present in the dermis but not in the epidermal layer of mouse skin. Such striking specificity of expression in stromal cells from epithelial tissues supports the concept that this factor is important in the normal mesenchymal stimulation of epithelial cell growth.

The Insulin Family

The diversity of metabolic effects of insulin have been studied intensively for decades.[42] Its primary in vivo functions involve the regulation of rapid anabolic responses such as glucose uptake, lipogenesis and amino acid and ion transport. Besides its effects on metabolism, insulin stimulates DNA synthesis and cell growth. The activities of insulin-like growth factors (IGF-I and IGF-II) were first recognized as serum factors, antigenically distinct from insulin, that interacted with growth hormone in stimulating growth of skeletal tissues and were, as a result, termed somatomedins.[22] Subsequently it was determined that somatomedin C is identical to IGF-I, while a polypeptide known as multiplication stimulating factor (MSA) is homologous to IGF-II.

The IGFs contribute to the insulin-like effects of serum on muscle and adipose tissue, but there are major differences between insulin and the IGFs. For example, while insulin levels fluctuate widely according to carbohydrate level the IGFs are bound to carrier proteins and are maintained at steady concentrations in the blood stream. In contrast to the multiplicity of processes influenced by insulin the major biological effect of IGFs is to stimulate cell replication. The receptors for insulin and IGF-I are structurally related (see below) and possess tyrosine kinase activity, in contrast the IGF-II receptor which lacks this activity, is a single polypeptide chain and possesses only a very short cytoplasmic domain. At the structural level, IGF-I and insulin share 48% of their amino acid sequences, and their homology to IGF-II is 50%.[37,177] Insulin is synthesized as a 109 amino acid precursor (preproinsulin) which is processed to a 6 kilodalton protein consisting of two chains (A and B) linked by two disulfide bonds. The structures of IGF-I and IGF-II are analogous to proinsulin in that they consist of a single polypeptide chain.

In vivo studies indicate that IGF-I acts in an autocrine or paracrine mode, since infusion of IGF-I does not give rise to its growth promoting actions.[22] Although it is not known whether overexpression of insulin family members can lead to transformation, a recent report indicated that addition of exogenous IGF-I or supraphysiologic levels of insulin to mouse NIH/3T3 cells overexpressing IGF-I receptors introduced by transfection induced morphological transformation and enabled the cells to grow in soft agar and form tumors in nude mice.[81]

Hepatocyte Growth Factor

A growth factor (HGF) apparently specific for hepatocytes was isolated from plasma[55] or platelets.[130] HGF levels increase dramatically following acute liver injury and thus, may play an important role in liver regeneration. The biochemical and biological properties of HGF were found to differ from those of other known growth factors.[55,130] The molecular weight of native HGF was reported to be 70,000–90,000 daltons and consists of two polypeptide chains of about 70,000 and 34,000 daltons linked by disulfide bonds.[55,130] Cloning of HGF cDNA showed that the growth factor is encoded by a single transcript, whose 728 amino acid-long product is processed by proteolytic cleavage into heavy and light chains.[121,131] Unexpectedly, the predicted amino acid sequence of HGF was found to be related to plasminogen.[131] In addition to 38% sequence identity to plasminogen, including its serine protease domain, HGF was shown to possess disulfide bond-linked intrachain structures known as "kringles" which are typical of prothrombin, tissue plasminogen activator, urokinase and coagulation factor XII. Neither plasminogen nor plasmin have HGF-like activity, and HGF is not likely to be a protease since the histidine and serine residues in the region corresponding to the catalytic site are replaced by other amino acids. The receptor for HGF has been recently shown to be encoded by the MET proto-oncogene.[9A,131A]

Growth Factor Receptors with Tyrosine Kinase Activity

Membrane spanning tyrosine kinase receptors contain several discrete domains including their extracellular ligand binding, transmembrane, juxtamembrane, protein tyrosine kinase and carboxy-terminal tail domains (Figure I-3-1).[179,196] Interaction of a growth factor with its receptor at the cell surface leads to a tight association, so that growth factors are capable of mediating their activities at low nM concentrations. Following ligand binding, the growth factor-receptor complex is internalized leading to increased turnover of the receptor. In principle, the growth factor signal might be mediated by its internalization. However, there is substantial evidence that activation of the receptor tyrosine kinase is the trigger for the biochemical cascade of events that follows. It is possible that conformational changes induced by ligand binding to the receptor's external domain are somehow transmitted through the transmembrane domain to induce the conformational alterations of the receptor kinase resulting in its activation. In an alternative model, ligand binding induces receptor dimer or oligomer formation.[179] By this latter mechanism, molecular interactions between adjacent cytoplasmic domains leads to activation of kinase function. In the case of growth factors such as EGF, a single growth factor interacts with a single receptor.[179] There is evidence for dimerization of EGF receptors but activation by an intramolecular reaction has not been ruled out.[15] Dimeric ligands such as PDGF appear to be bivalent, as pointed out earlier, such that a single growth factor molecule initiates dimerization of two receptors (Figure I-3-1). There are other examples of growth factor receptor dimerization in response to ligand binding, and this property has been localized to the extracellular domains of at least some receptors.[179] However, it is not yet established whether dimerization precedes or follows receptor activation.

Most evidence indicates that the transmembrane domain

does not directly influence signal transduction and is instead a passive anchor of the receptor to the membrane. It is important to note, however, that point mutations in the transmembrane domain of one receptor-like protein, the neu/erbB-2 protein, enhances its transforming properties.[5] The juxtamembrane sequence that separates the transmembrane and cytoplasmic domains is not well-conserved between different families of receptors. However, juxtamembrane sequences are highly similar among members of the same family, and studies indicate that this stretch plays a role in modulation of receptor function. For example, addition of PDGF to many types of cells causes a rapid decrease in high affinity binding of EGF to its receptor. This has been shown to be a downstream effect of PDGF receptor activation in which protein kinase C, itself a serine protein kinase, is activated and, in turn, phosphorylates a site in the juxtamembrane domain of the EGF receptor.[196]

The tyrosine kinase domain is the most conserved among tyrosine kinase receptors and an intact protein tyrosine kinase domain is absolutely required for receptor signalling. For example, mutation of a single lysine in the ATP binding site, which blocks the ability of the receptor to phosphorylate tyrosine residues, completely inactivates receptor biological function. Yet, such kinase mutants retain the ability to bind ligand with high affinity and exhibit normal internalization and downregulation as well.[196]

The carboxy terminal domain of the receptor is thought to play an important role in regulation of kinase activity. This region typically contains several tyrosine residues, which are phosphorylated by the activated kinase. In fact, the receptor, itself, is often the major tyrosine phosphorylated species observed following ligand stimulation. Tyrosine phosphorylation of the carboxy terminal domain has been postulated to modulate kinase catalytic activity, and/or the ability of the kinase to interact with substrates. Thus, mutations which alter individual tyrosine sites or deletions of the carboxy terminal domain have the effect of attenuating kinase function in those receptors so far analyzed.[52,196]

The ability to molecularly clone related genes based upon the conserved nature of their kinase domains has led to the identification of structurally related members of different receptor families, but ligands for this increasing array of receptor-like proteins remain to be identified. Different families are schematically illustrated in Figure I-3-2. One includes the α and β PDGF receptors; the CSF-1 receptor; c-kit, a receptor for a newly identified hematopoietic growth factor that has a broad range of activities[189]; and a recently described gene, designated flt.[164] The external domains of each member of the PDGF receptor family show the same spacing of cysteine residues, consistent with the organization of five immunoglobulin-like domains.[18] A similar organization is present in other surface receptors including Thy 1, IgA, the T cell receptor, as well as IL-1 and IL-6 receptors.[184] Another feature of the PDGF receptor family is the presence of an insert (with respect to other tyrosine kinases) within the tyrosine kinase domain. These 80–100 amino acid stretches are highly divergent among different family members. There are reports that the kinase insert is required for interaction with certain substrates,[82] and deletions in this domain impair receptor mitogenic signalling.[41]

Another family of receptors, whose prototype is the EGF receptor, includes erbB-2,[86] also designated as c-neu,[6] or HER-2[161] and erbB-3.[93,144] In addition to their more conserved tyrosine kinases, the hallmark of these molecules is the presence in their external domains of two regions enriched in cysteine residues (Figure I-3-2). EGF and TGF-α do not bind the erbB-2 product, p185^{erbB-2}, but a distinct 30-kilodalton factor (gp30) secreted by human breast cancer cells was shown to compete with an antibody to p185^{erbB-2} for binding p185^{erbB-2} [106] suggesting that it is the erbB-2 ligand. The erbB-3 ligand remains to be identified.

A third family of receptor proteins includes the FGF receptor as its prototype.[14] This family most closely resembles the PDGF receptor family, but contains extracellular domain variants with two or three immunoglobulin-like motifs instead of five.[99] Moreover, the kinase insert within the tyrosine kinase domains of receptors of this family is shorter than in members of the PDGF receptor family (Figure I-3-2). A number of cDNAs structurally related to the FGF receptor have been isolated recently. One FGF receptor gene is likely represented by cek 1 (chicken),[140] flg,[155] and N-sam[65] (both human). The bek,[92] cek 3,[139] and K-sam genes,[65] from mouse, chicken and human, respectively, represent another, while cek 2 (chicken) represents a different gene.[139] Adding to this complexity are findings of alternatively spliced forms of FGF receptors expressed in different cell types.[78,147] The interaction of these gene products for different FGF family members awaits their further characterization.

A fourth family of receptors includes the insulin and IGF-1 receptors,[38,176,178] and a related gene, termed IR, of rodent origin.[165] The c-ros proto-oncogene product is most closely related to the IR family.[116] These receptors are encoded as a single chain, which is cleaved and processed to a disulfide linked heterodimer ($\alpha\beta$), and finally to a heterotetradimer ($\alpha_2\beta_2$). They each contain a single cysteine rich cluster in their extracellular domain.

Several other human protein tyrosine kinase receptor-like genes are distinct from these families and from one another. In each case, their ligands have not been identified. The eph gene was isolated by using a tyrosine kinase probe to screen a human genomic library.[69] It is not closely related to any other documented receptor by sequence similarity, has a single cysteine cluster in its extracellular domain, and lacks a prorecptor cleavage site (as in the insulin receptors) or kinase insert. Eph transcripts have been detected at high levels in human carcinomas. Closely related genes, designated eck and elk,[100] are apparently specifically expressed by epithelial cells and in brain, respectively. The met, ret, and trk genes were first isolated from human cells as oncogenes by transfection experiments.[43] The predicted structure of the met product is readily distinguishable from other receptors while its tyrosine kinase domain is highly similar to the corresponding region of the v-sea avian retroviral oncogene.[167] The degree of similarity outside this stretch is low, indicating that c-sea is unlikely to be the avian met homologue but it is not known if c-sea encodes a receptor. The met protein possesses a single small cysteine cluster in its extracellular domain and its kinase domain is not interrupted. Sequence analysis of its mouse homologue indicated that the met protein may be cleaved so as to generate

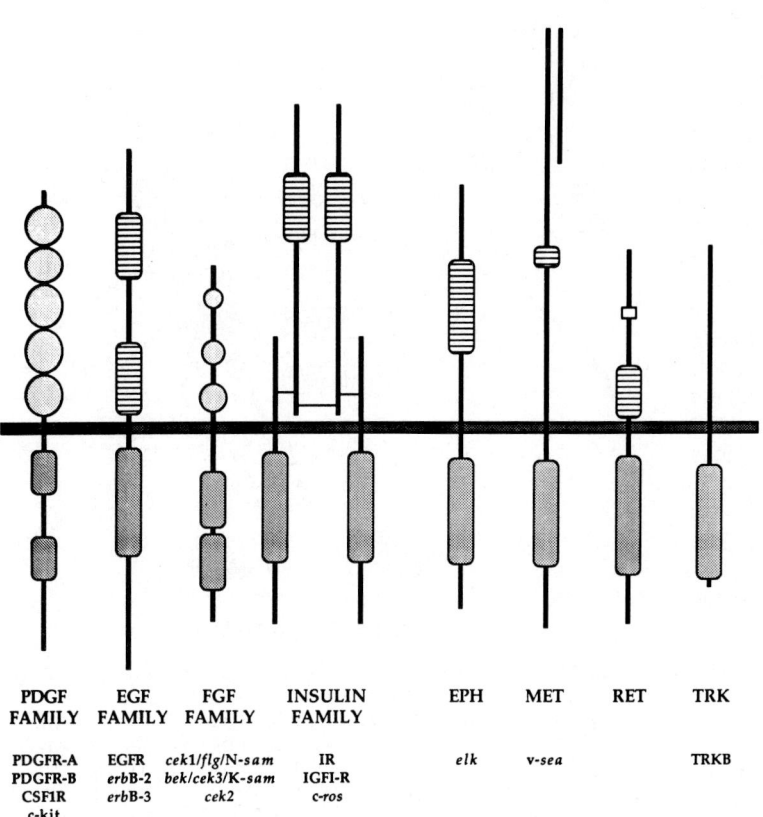

Figure I-3-2. Protein tyrosine kinase receptors. The thick horizontal line represents the cell membrane with the extracellular and intracellular environments above and below, respectively. Immunoglobulin-like domains = filled circles; cysteine-rich clusters = polygons with horizontal stripes; second transmembrane domain of RET = open box; tyrosine kinase domains = filled polygons.

PDGF FAMILY	EGF FAMILY	FGF FAMILY	INSULIN FAMILY	EPH	MET	RET	TRK
PDGFR-A	EGFR	cek1/flg/N-sam	IR	elk	v-sea		TRKB
PDGFR-B	erbB-2	bek/cek3/K-sam	IGFI-R				
CSF1R	erbB-3	cek2	c-ros				
c-kit							
flt							

an α,β heterodimer, and there is recent evidence for the existence of such a molecule.[16,54] Unlike *eph* and *met*, which are about equidistant in their sequence similarity from other receptors, *ret* is more closely (although still distantly) related to the FGF receptors (approximately 45% identity).[139] *Ret* is unique in that it possesses an additional predicted transmembrane domain near the amino terminal portion of its extracellular sequence.[173] The *trk* proto-oncogene product shows slightly higher similarity to the insulin receptor family compared to other receptors, lacks cysteine clusters and an interkinase region and has an unusually short C terminal domain.[111] A related gene, *trk*B, was isolated from mouse tissues, and its pattern of expression indicates that it may play a role in neural development.[88]

Growth Factor Signalling Pathways

The wide array of biochemical and biological responses to a particular growth factor has suggested that interaction with its cognate receptor initiates a cascade of biochemical events. Some of these are well documented and include alterations in phospholipid metabolism leading to the generation of two important second messengers, inositol 1, 4, 5 triphosphate (IP3) which causes release of calcium from intracellular compartments[8] and diacylglycerol (DAG), the natural activator of protein kinase C (PKC).[85] Recently, a direct biochemical link between the receptor kinase and this important second messenger pathway has been made with the discovery that phospholipase Cγ, one of several isoforms of phospholipase C responsible for IP3 and DAG release, is

rapidly tyrosine phosphorylated in response to EGF or PDGF triggering.[109,119,125,182,183] Moreover, there is evidence that tyrosine phosphorylation of PLCγ increases its enzymatic activity in vitro (G. Carpenter, personal communication). PLCγ appears to be a direct target of some,[13] but not all receptor tyrosine kinases.[183]

A second substrate of some receptor kinases is another enzyme involved in phospholipid metabolism, a phosphatidol inositol-3 kinase. This enzymatic activity has been shown to coimmunoprecipitate with activated PDGF or CSF-1 receptor kinases.[26,181] However, the role of this enzyme in mitogenic signal transduction remains to be determined.

A third potentially important target molecule is the GTPase activating protein (GAP),[72,175,187] intimately involved in the function of the *ras* proteins.[4,96] *Ras* encodes a 21,000 dalton guanine nucleotide binding protein (p21), which is active in the GTP bound form. There is substantial evidence that *ras* is a critical component of intracellular mitogenic signalling pathways since oncogenically activated *ras* p21 induces DNA synthesis upon microinjection[170] and antibodies to *ras* p21 can block mitogen induced DNA synthesis of normal cells.[127] Mutations which cause its oncogenic activation lead to accumulation of *ras* p21 GTP. GAP enhances the GTPase activity inherent in *ras* p21, but oncogenic mutations in *ras* block the ability of GAP to downregulate the *ras* p21 molecule to its GDP bound form.[72,175,187] There is evidence that GAP may also serve in a complex with *ras* p21 as an effector of its downstream signalling functions.[118,187] Thus, mutations which impair *ras* p21 interaction with GAP also block *ras* biological function.

Interactions between tyrosine kinase receptors and GAP have been uncovered recently. PDGF stimulation of fibroblasts leads to the rapid and sustained tyrosine phosphorylation of GAP with kinetics similar to those associated with activation of the receptor kinase.[122] Normally GAP is found as a cytosolic protein.[175] Yet in order for it to function, *ras* p21 must be membrane-associated.[4,96] Concomitant with activation of the receptor kinase, GAP appears to become more tightly associated with the membrane fraction, and the membrane-associated form of GAP undergoes tyrosine phosphorylation.[122] There is evidence that not all growth factor receptors with tyrosine kinase activity induce phosphorylation of the GAP protein. For example, the FGFs, which are highly potent mitogens for fibroblasts, do not induce GAP phosphorylation under conditions in which PDGF induces readily detectable tyrosine phosphorylation of the molecule. In addition to certain receptor kinases, many oncogenes which encode cytoplasmic tyrosine kinases induce GAP phosphorylation.[40]

The link between PDGF in mitogenic signalling and the *ras*-GAP complex was strengthened by findings that PDGF triggering of fibroblasts leads to an increase in the proportion of GTP bound *ras* p21 molecules.[157] Thus, it is possible that tyrosine phosphorylation of GAP transiently impairs its negative regulatory function. There is also evidence that tyrosine phosphorylated GAP coimmunoprecipitates in a complex not only with the receptor, but with proteins of 62,000 and 190,000 daltons. These proteins are tyrosine phosphorylated as well.[40] Thus, tyrosine phosphorylation may cause these proteins to form a complex required for *ras* effector function. In any case, tyrosine phosphorylation of GAP provides a direct biochemical link between growth factor triggered mitogenic pathways and the important *ras* p21 signalling molecules.

The *raf* proto-oncogene product, which is a serine/threonine kinase, has been reported to be tyrosine phosphorylated in response to PDGF triggering. However, its phosphorylation has been difficult to detect and does not represent stochiometrically significant levels.[124] There is evidence that the insulin[145] and EGF receptors[152] may regulate another serine/threonine kinase designated MAP kinase by tyrosine phosphorylation. MAP kinase in turn is known to phosphorylate and enhance the activity of S6 kinase whose substrate is the ribosomal protein S6.[171] The relevance of this kinase cascade to the mitogenic effects of EGF and insulin are unknown. Several other potential substrates for growth factor receptor kinases have been tentatively identified by their sizes on a gel without identification of any biochemical activity. Differences have been observed in the patterns of activities of distinct receptors, and further studies will be needed to identify the various second messengers whose activities are altered as a direct result of tyrosine phosphorylation by such receptors. Figure I-3-3 summarizes some of the putative substrates of different receptor kinases.

Neurotransmitters as Growth Factors

The transmission of signals generated by the reception of chemical and physical stimuli from the external and internal environments is mediated by a large variety of small molecules known as neurotransmitters. These molecules include

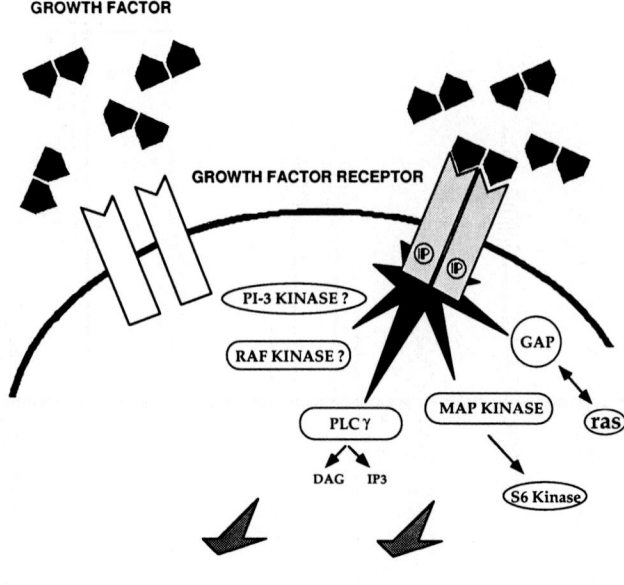

CELL GROWTH

Figure I-3-3.   Growth factor-mediated signalling pathways. The figure summarizes available experimental evidence for events that follow binding of growth factors to protein tyrosine kinase receptors. In this example the ligand is dimeric and bivalent and causes the receptor to dimerize. PLC-γ, GAP, MAP kinase, RAF kinase, and PI-kinase are primary targets of the receptor protein tyrosine kinase activity. GAP and MAP kinase are known to interact with *ras* and S6 kinase, respectively. Also shown are the second messengers (DAG and IP3) produced by the activity of PLC-γ. Question marks indicate uncertainties about the role of PI-3 kinase in mitogenesis and controversial findings regarding RAF phosphorylation by the PDGF receptor.

acetylcholine, amino acid derivatives such as epinephrine, norepinephrine, serotonin, dopamine and peptides, such as the angiotensins, β-endorphin, enkephalins and somatostatin. Although neurotransmitters are known to be involved in controlling an enormous array of bodily functions, their role in stimulating cell proliferation is just beginning to be appreciated. A recent example is the work of Ashkenazi and colleagues who found that a stable acetylcholine analog, carbachol was mitogenic, via muscarinic acetylcholine receptors (mACHR), in perinatal rat brain astrocytes and in brain-derived astrocytoma and neuroblastoma cell lines.[3] When Chinese hamster ovary (CHO) cells were transfected with human muscarinic acetylcholine receptor genes, carbachol stimulated DNA synthesis in those cells expressing mACHR subtypes which are known to activate PI hydrolysis most efficiently. These data are consistent with the observations that acetylcholine stimulates phosphoinositide hydrolysis at peak levels in the brain during the perinatal period when certain glial cells proliferate and differentiate. Besides these proliferative effects, it has been pointed out that neurotransmitter/receptor systems could act in other growth processes such as stimulating hypertrophy of, or inducing process extension in non-dividing neurons.[62]

Studies published in the mid-1970s demonstrated that angiotensin was mitogenic for adrenocortical cells,[53] but it was not until the era of tumor DNA-transfection experiments that the implications of these early observations with respect to growth control and cancer became more apparent. Thus, by using a cotransfection-tumorigenicity assay,[9,46] DNA isolated from a human epidermoid carcinoma was found to induce tumors in nude mice. The oncogene responsible, designated *mas,* was found to encode a protein that possesses seven membrane spanning regions characteristic of the G-protein linked receptors, visual rhodopsin and the α-subunit of the acetylcholine receptor.[197]

At about this same time, the sequences of additional neurotransmitter receptor genes were determined. Their structures were found to be closely related to *mas,* although overall amino acid sequence similarities were limited. These genes included the α_1,[25,159] α_2-,[91,105,146] β_1-,[50,108,195] and β_2-[89,90] adrenergic receptors, the muscarinic acetylcholine receptors (mACHR),[2,95,142] the serotonin receptors,[1,45] the substance K receptor[113] and dopamine receptors.[12,28,56,190,199]

Serotonin (5-hydroxytryptamine, 5-HT) was shown to be mitogenic for smooth muscle cells[133] and subsequently for fibroblasts.[162] There are several receptor subtypes for serotonin including those that couple either to signalling systems involving phospholipase C (PLC) activation ($5\text{-}HT_{1c}$ and $5\text{-}HT_2$ receptors) or adenylate cyclase ($5\text{-}HT_{1a}$ and $5\text{-}HT_{1b}$ receptors). Introduction of the $5\text{-}HT_{1c}$ gene into mouse NIH/3T3 fibroblasts induced morphological transformation which was dependent upon receptor activation by serotonin.[80] In such cells, serotonin was shown to mobilize intracellular Ca^{2+} probably via PLC activation and production of inositol triphosphate. Since diacyl glycerol is also released by the catalytic action of PLC, protein kinase C activation may also play a role in the induction of the transformed phenotype. In Figure I-3-4 the signalling pathways that are activated by the neurotransmitters and neuropeptides that have been found to be mitogenic are shown.[190]

Based on these studies and on the well known oncogenic effects of mutated *ras* p21 proteins, a reasonable prediction could be made that perturbations of signalling pathways downstream of the transmitter-receptor interaction could lead

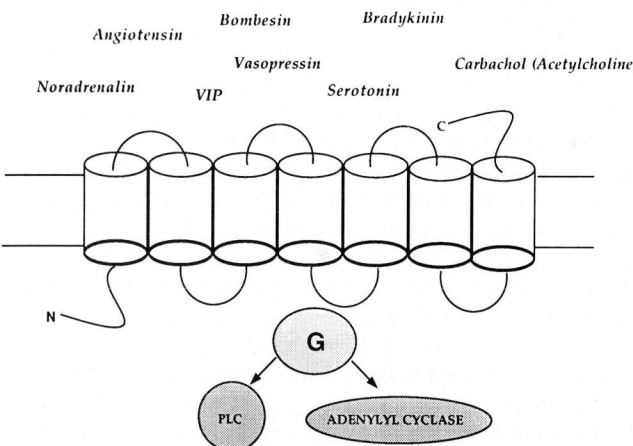

Figure I-3-4. Mitogenic neurotransmitters and neuropeptides. The signalling molecules shown interact with receptors possessing seven transmembrane domains. These receptors are linked to G proteins that affect either adenylyl cyclase or PLC activity resulting in the production of the second messengers cyclic AMP and DAG/IP3, respectively.

to malignant transformation. Signal transmission through the β-adrenergic receptor to adenylyl cyclase is mediated by the $G_{\alpha s}$ subunit of the G protein G_s. A link between alterations of this signalling system and oncogenesis was uncovered by studies on two distinct groups within a subset of growth hormone-secreting human pituitary tumors.[98] In one group, G_s was constitutively active resulting in elevated adenylyl cyclase activity and growth hormone levels. The $G_{\alpha s}$ component was found to be activated by point mutations in either a site at which cholera toxin inactivates G_s ($Arg^{201} \rightarrow$ Cys/His) or at a residue equivalent to a GTPase-inhibiting mutation that causes malignant activation of *ras* p21 ($Gln^{227} \rightarrow$ Arg). Since both mutations have the effect of destroying GTPase activity, $G_{\alpha s}$ (designated *gsp*) becomes constitutively activated in a manner analogous to the oncogenic activity of *ras* p21.

The two mutations are located in regions that are highly conserved among G_α proteins isolated from diverse eukaryotic species. With this knowledge, and under the assumption that all α chains of G proteins are proto-oncogenes, a search was conducted for tumors harboring GTPase-inhibiting mutations in genes for α chains and in other G proteins.[107] In this survey, 3/11 tumors of the adrenal cortex and 3/10 ovarian endocrine tumors, mutations of Arg^{179} (the cognate of Arg^{201} in G_α) to Cys or His were found in the α chain of G_{i2}. It was suggested that the mutant α_{i2} gene be considered as a putative oncogene designated *gip2*. Additional *gsp* mutations were found in 18/42 growth hormone-secreting pituitary tumors. In order to substantiate the hypothesis that these mutations are oncogenic, it will be necessary to show that the *gsp* and *gip2* proteins lack GTPase activity and are able to induce the malignant phenotype when introduced into the appropriate cell type.

Abnormalities Associated with Growth Factors in Cancer Cells

Following the demonstration that the v-*sis* oncogene encodes a protein closely related to human PDGF-B, substantial evidence has accumulated that the expression of PDGF-B in a cell possessing PDGF receptors is sufficient to act as one step in the neoplastic process. For example, when a retrovirus vector containing human PDGF-B is introduced either into cells in culture or in vivo, one observes growth alterations specific to cells that express PDGF receptors.[141] Other cell types in culture appear to be unaffected by expression of the same growth factor. Similarly, the PDGF-B retrovirus induces sarcomas and glial tumors in mice but does not cause tumors of other cell types. Thus, inappropriate expression of PDGF can be the initiating event in the formation of a malignant tumor. In some cases, such tumors can be shown to be comprised of clonally derived cells, indicating that additional steps are required to select for the fully malignant phenotype.[141]

In human tumors, at least one PDGF chain, and one of its receptors, have been detected in a high fraction of sarcomas as well as in glially derived neoplasms.[68,114,117,136] In tissue culture, such tumor cells exhibit evidence of a functional autocrine loop, in which chronic PDGF receptor activation can be demonstrated by the detection of tyrosine phosphorylated receptors and/or downregulation of the receptor protein. Thus, it appears that inappropriate expression of PDGF often plays an important role in such tumors.

By extrapolation, it follows that the expression of any growth factor and its specific receptor by the same cell could establish an autocrine loop that contributes to tumor progression. For example, TGFα is often detected in carcinomas that express high levels of EGF receptors.[30,32] The role of acidic or basic FGF in tumors is less well established. Because neither of these molecules possesses a secretory signal peptide sequence, their normal route of release by cells is not through the classical secretory route by which growth factor receptors are processed.[14,17] However, recent studies have demonstrated the expression of bFGF by human melanoma cell lines but not by normal melanocytes.[59] Moreover, only the former require bFGF for proliferation in culture.[60] Evidence that antagonists of FGF can inhibit growth of melanoma cells argues for a role of bFGF in the uncontrolled growth of these cells.[59] Since many more tyrosine kinase receptors have been identified than there are available ligands, the contribution of autocrine loops to malignancies is probably much more extensive than is presently documented.

Small cell lung carcinomas are thought to be of neuroectodermal origin. Cuttitta and colleagues reported that secretion by such tumors of bombesin-like peptides was growth stimulating.[27,123] The receptor has been recently identified and is a G-protein coupled membrane spanning receptor.[112] Antibodies to bombesin have been reported to inhibit proliferation of the small cell carcinoma cell lines both in vitro and in vivo.[129] Thus, bombesin appears to play a role as an autocrine growth factor in such tumors.

While several growth factors have been shown to induce transformation by an autocrine mode, it is also worth considering the possible role that growth factors might have in predisposing to cancer. It can be hypothesized that overexpression of growth factors by a paracrine mode might increase the proliferation of a polyclonal target cell population. This conceivably could increase the frequency of spontaneous genetic changes in the population, eventually selecting for a cancer cell. By such a model, increased production of a growth factor might act in a manner analogous to that of a tumor promoter. At the present time, this model is purely speculative and awaits experimental test.

Aberrations Affecting Growth Factor Receptors in Tumor Cells

While growth factor receptors can be constitutively activated by autocrine mechanisms, genetic alterations affecting receptor genes can also cause their activation as oncogenes (Figure I-3-5). The paradigm for such alterations is v-erbB, the oncogenic counterpart of the EGF receptor, transduced as the viral oncogene of avian erythroblastosis virus.[35,193] The mechanism of v-erbB activation involved deletion of its ligand binding domain. More subtle mutational changes are responsible for oncogenic activation of v-fms, whose normal homologue is the CSF-1 receptor.[163] Here, a small genetic alteration affecting the external domain of the molecule was responsible for constitutive activation of this receptor as an oncogene.[153]

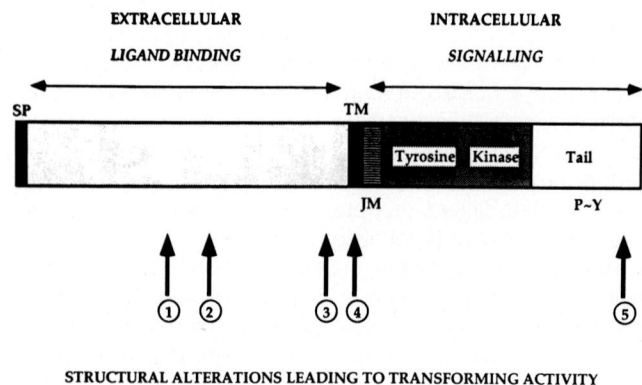

Figure I-3-5. Genetic alterations leading to malignant activation of protein tyrosine kinase receptors. The structure of a prototypical receptor is shown. The arrows indicate approximately where changes in receptor structure have been documented. SP = signal peptide; TM = transmembrane domain; JM = juxtamembrane domain; P ~ Y = major site of receptor autophosphorylation on tyrosine.

A member of the EGF receptor subfamily, designated neu, was initially identified as an oncogene by NIH/3T3 transfection analysis.[158] Thus, DNA from ethylnitroso urea-induced rat neuroblastomas was shown to reproducibly induce transformed foci in NIH/3T3 cells. The transforming gene was subsequently identified as having a specific mutation in its transmembrane domain responsible for its oncogenic activation.[5] Thus, subtle mutational changes in their transmembrane domains as well as in their external domains can in some cases activate the oncogenic potential of growth factor receptor genes.

By a completely independent approach, a new member of the EGF receptor family was initially identified as an amplified gene in a primary human mammary carcinoma[86] and a salivary gland tumor.[161] Designated erbB-2, this gene was cloned and the sequence of its predicted product revealed to be structurally related to the EGF receptor. Sequence analysis of rat neu later demonstrated that it was the rat homolog of human erbB-2.[6] Because erbB-2 was found to be commonly amplified and overexpressed in human breast carcinomas,[97,132,138,166] efforts were undertaken to determine the transforming potential of the normal overexpressed erbB-2 gene in model systems. It was found that erbB-2 overexpression beyond some critical threshold level in NIH/3T3 fibroblasts was sufficient to induce the malignant phenotype.[31] Since a putative ligand for the erbB-2 product has been identified,[106] it should be possible to determine whether overexpression of the erbB-2 proto-oncogene product leads to constitutive activation of its tyrosine kinase by an autocrine transforming mode or whether erbB-2 encodes an atypical receptor-like protein with constitutive kinase activity.

As indicated above, clinical studies have indicated that the normal erbB-2 gene is frequently amplified and/or over-expressed in human breast carcinomas as well as in ovarian carcinomas.[94,132,138,180] Moreover, there is evidence that detection in breast carcinomas of high levels of the erbB-2 protein may be a prognostic indicator of poor survival.[97,166] Thus, erbB-2 appears to be most commonly altered in human malignancies by mechanisms leading to its overexpression. Whereas erbB-2 overexpression has been observed primarily in adenocarcinomas, overexpression of an apparently normal EGF receptor has been reported frequently in squamous cell carcinomas[87] and glioblastomas.[104] A third member of the EGF receptor family, designated the erbB-3 has recently been isolated.[93] While knowledge of its role in malignancy is still at a very early stage, there is evidence that it may also be overexpressed in some human malignancies. The structures of the EGF receptor family members and a summary of their alterations detected in human tumors are presented in Figure I-3-6.

Implications for Cancer Therapy

Intervention with the pathologic expression of the subset of genes that can be activated as oncogenes might be most readily envisioned in the case of growth factors and receptors, whose products achieve a cell surface location. In the case of growth factors, this would only be advantageous if functional activation of the receptor target cell were confined to the tumor cell surface. Since both growth factor and receptor are processed through the same secretory pathway, it is also possible that receptor activation and functional coupling

with intercellular mitogenic signalling pathways occurs entirely within the cell. This has led to a so-called "internal autocrine" model. Efforts to establish whether autocrine growth stimulation can be blocked by surface-specific antagonists of ligand receptor interactions have intensified with evidence for the involvement of autocrine mechanisms in an increasing array of naturally occurring tumors.

Efforts to localize the site of v-sis action have led to conflicting findings and conclusions. Antibody to PDGF has been reported to inhibit growth of v-sis/PDGF transformants to various extents, consistent with at least some surface component to activity to the v-sis product.[49,70,79] Moreover, it has been reported that a v-sis mutant product that failed to achieve a cell surface location lacked transforming activity.[63] In contrast, others have reported evidence that internal forms of the PDGF receptors are tyrosine phosphorylated and exhibit greatly increased turnover in the absence of detectable mature PDGF receptor species.[71,83] These findings as well as evidence that PDGF mutants with anchor sequences that apparently lock them within the secretory pathway are transforming supported the internal autocrine model.[7]

It has been demonstrated that exogenous addition of PDGF to fibroblasts can transiently mimic the v-sis transformed state.[70,79] Such cells grow densely in a manner indistinguishable from that of v-sis transformants and form colonies in soft agar at an efficiency comparable to that of v-sis transformants. These findings have established that PDGF receptor activation at the cell surface would be sufficient to induce transformation, despite receptor downregulation that accompanies chronic exogenous growth factor stimulation. By use of chemically defined medium in which autocrine stimulation

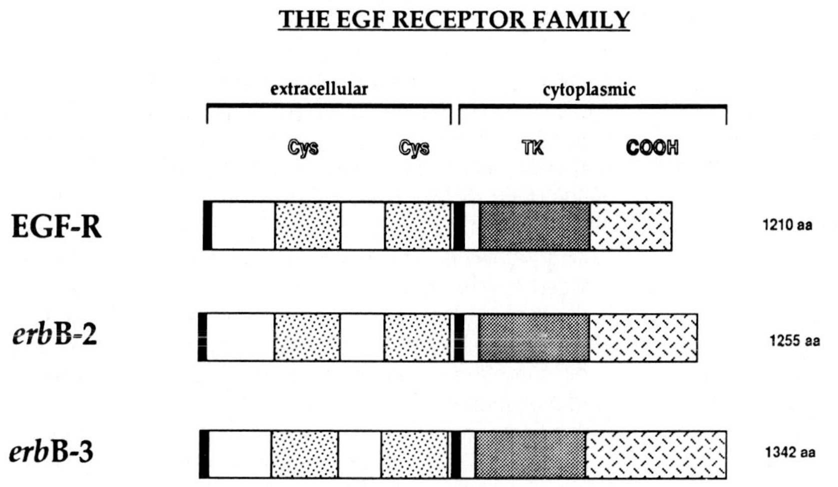

THE EGF RECEPTOR FAMILY

Figure I-3-6. Alterations in expression and structure of EGF receptor family members in human cancer.

ALTERATIONS OF EGF RECEPTOR FAMILY MEMBERS IN HUMAN CANCERS

	EGFR	erbB-2	erbB-3
Overexpression	squamous cell carcinoma adenocarcinoma glioblastoma	adenocarcionoma (breast, stomach, ovary, colon, salivary gland)	adenocarcinoma (breast)
Structural alteration	glioblastoma squamous cell carcinoma	intestinal adenocarcinoma	?

MECHANISM OF TRANSFORMATION	POTENTIAL INTERVENTION STRATEGIES		
	Antagonists of Ligand-Receptor Interaction	Inhibitors of Protein Tyrosine Kinase Activity	Receptor-Targeted Toxins
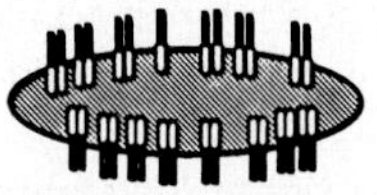 Receptor Overexpression	+	+	+
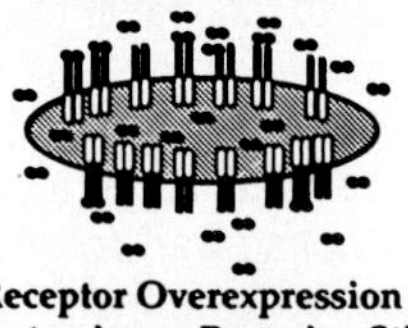 Receptor Overexpression with Autocrine or Paracrine Stimulation	+	+	+
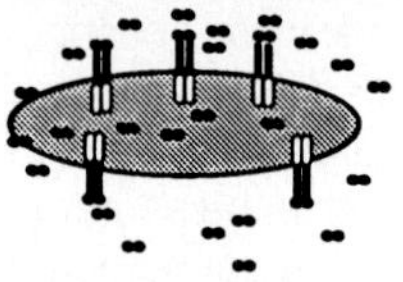 Normal Receptor Levels with Autocrine or Paracrine Stimulation	+	+ / −	+ / −
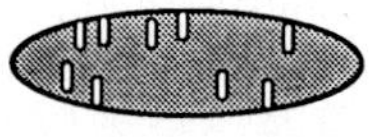 Alteration of Receptor Structure	−	+	−

Figure I-3-7. Therapeutic approaches for intervening in malignant activation of growth factor-mediated proliferative pathways. Intervention strategies that might be successful are indicated by "+." Treatments that could possibly affect normal cells as well as tumor cells are indicated by "+/−."

by the v-*sis* product was required to drive cell proliferation in the absence of added PDGF, it was possible to demonstrate partial growth inhibition by PDGF neutralizing antibody.[49] In contrast, there was essentially complete inhibition of v-*sis* directed proliferation in the presence of suramin, a highly anionic naphthalene sulfonic acid derivative,[39] which is known to interfere with ligand receptor interactions (see XVI-10). This action of suramin was specific, in that it did not alter the growth of cells transformed by other oncogenes. It was possible to further establish that immature forms of PDGF receptors that do not achieve a cell surface location are tyrosine phosphorylated in v-*sis* transformed cells, establishing that ligand binding and receptor activation do indeed occur within secretory pathway. However, mature PDGF receptors localized to the cell surface were tyrosine phosphorylated as well.

There is evidence that suramin may act within the cell as well as externally.[49] To determine its site of intervention with autocrine PDGF stimulation, v-*sis* transformed cells were exposed to suramin under conditions that led to profound growth inhibition. Under these conditions, tyrosine phosphorylation of surface forms of the receptor was markedly inhibited, while there was no inhibition of tyrosine phosphorylation of immature forms of the receptor.[49] Thus, it appears that suramin not only efficiently blocks new ligand-receptor interactions at the cell surface but is able to strip ligand

already bound to internally activated receptors as they achieve a cell surface location. Inhibitors of glycosylation that block maturation of the v-*fms* product have also been reported to induce reversion of v-*fms* transformed cells.[134,137] Thus, activation of this receptor may also require a cell surface location in order to couple efficiently with intracellular mitogenic signalling pathways. Whether such a mechanism can be generalized to other growth factors remains to be determined. If so, then surface acting molecules that can specifically interfere with ligand-receptor interactions may have applicability in efforts to intervene clinically in autocrine associated malignancies.

Such antagonists might be envisioned as a new generation of suramin-like compounds. They might also represent altered forms of a ligand with the capacity to bind more avidly to the receptor but be incapable of triggering receptor kinase activity. In the case of bivalent ligands like PDGF, which may interact with two receptors to induce dimer formation and receptor activation, a heterodimer composed of one active and one inactive PDGF chain could provide a model for a specific PDGF antagonist.

Therapeutic intervention may be possible in tumors that overexpress cell surface receptors. It is not uncommon for tumors that overexpress either the EGF receptor or *erb*B-2 to produce these proteins at levels as much as 100-fold higher than those associated with normal cells. In the case of *erb*B-2, antibodies which recognize its ligand binding domain have been shown in some cases to induce down-regulation of the receptor protein with associated growth inhibition in vitro and in vivo.[36] New approaches aimed at targeting toxins specifically to tumor cells by linkage of such toxins to antibodies or to the ligands themselves are presently underway.[48] Should the difficult problems associated with achieving necessary access to the tumor through systemic administration of such receptor targeted toxins be overcome, overexpressed growth factor receptors may prove to be important targets for such a strategy.

Another approach toward intervention with constitutively activated receptor kinases in cancer cells could conceivably involve highly specific inhibitors of tyrosine kinase activity. Imoto and colleagues reported the isolation of a microbial compound termed erbstatin which was found to inhibit the autokinase activity of the EGF receptor in a human epidermoid carcinoma cell line (A431) as well as that of the v-*src* oncogene product p60^{src}.[76] Yaish and colleagues designed a series of compounds based on the structure of erbstatin with the hopes of fulfilling the following criteria: The inhibitor would compete only with EGF receptor kinase and not with ATP, (since compounds that compete with ATP have been found to be highly toxic); other tyrosine kinase receptors would not be affected; and the solubility properties of the drug should enable it to traverse the membrane but still be water soluble.[192] The most potent compounds were more active by 3 logs against the EGF receptor compared to the insulin receptor kinase using exogenous substrates. EGF-dependent autophosphorylation of purified EGF receptor preparations was effectively inhibited. The proliferative response of A431 cells to EGF could also be inhibited, whereas growth in the absence of EGF was not affected. These drugs are referred to as "tyrphostins." Intervention strategies that could be used when malignant transformation is induced by the mechanisms described above are illustrated in Figure I-3-7. Thus, as evidence mounts that genetic alterations in growth factor signalling pathways underlies a major component of the malignant process, it is hoped that this knowledge will lead to new approaches towards therapeutic intervention with the cancer cell.

Note

The ligand for the *trk* proto-oncogene product has been recently identified as nerve growth factor (NGF),[200–202] and the ligands for the trkB product have been shown to be brain-derived neurotrophic factor and neutrotrophin-3.[203]

Acknowledgments

We thank M. Kraus, J. Rubin and W. LaRochelle for helpful discussions and contributing figures, and N. Lichtenberg for typing the manuscript.

References

1. Albert, P. R., Zhou, Q. Y., Van Tol, H. H., Bunzow, J. R., and Civelli, O.: Cloning, functional expression, and mRNA tissue distribution of the rat 5-hydroxytryptamine 1A receptor gene. J. Biol. Chem., 265:5825, 1990.
2. Allard, W. J., Sigal, I. S., and Dixon, R. A.: Sequence of the gene encoding the human M1 muscarinic acetylcholine receptor. Nucleic Acids Res., 15:10604, 1987.
3. Ashkenazi, A., Ramachandran, J., and Capon, D. J.: Acetylcholine analogue stimulates DNA synthesis in brain-derived cells via specific muscarinic receptor subtypes. Nature, 340:146, 1989.
4. Barbacid, M.: *ras* genes. Annu. Rev. Biochem., 56:779, 1987.
5. Bargmann, C. I., Hung, M. C., and Weinberg, R. A.: Multiple independent activations of the *neu* oncogene by a point mutation altering the transmembrane domain of p185, Cell, 45:649, 1986.
6. Bargmann, C. I., Hung, M. C., and Weinberg, R. A.: The *neu* oncogene encodes an epidermal growth factor receptor-related protein. Nature, 319:226, 1986.
7. Bejcek, B. E., Li, D. Y., and Deuel, T. F.: Transformation by v-*sis* occurs by an internal autoactivation mechanism. Science, 245:1496, 1989.
8. Berridge, M. J., and Irvine, R. F.: Inositol phosphates and cell signalling. Nature, 341:197, 1989.
9. Blair, D. G., Cooper, C. S., Oskarsson, M. K., Eader, L. A., and Vande Woude, G. F.: New method for detecting cellular transforming genes. Science, 218:1122, 1982.
9A. Bottaro, D. P., Rubin, J. S., Faletto, D. L., Chan, A. M., Kmiecik, T. E., Vande Woude, G. F., and Aaronson, S. A.: Identification of the hepatocyte growth factor receptor as the c-met proto-oncogene product. Science, *251*:802, 1991.
10. Bouche, G., Gas, N., Prats, H., Baldin, V., Tauber, J. P., Teissie, J., and Amalric, F.: Basic fibroblast growth factor enters the nucleolus and stimulates the transcription of ribosomal genes in ABAE cells undergoing G0----G1 transition. Proc. Natl. Acad. Sci. U.S.A., 84:6770, 1987.
11. Brugge, J. S., and Erikson, R. L.: Identification of a transformation-specific antigen induced by an avian sarcoma virus. Nature, 269:346, 1977.
12. Bunzow, J. R., Van Tol, H. H., Grandy, D. K., Albert, P., Salon, J., Christie, M., Machida, C. A., Neve, K. A., and Civelli, O.: Cloning and expression of a rat D2 dopamine receptor cDNA. Nature, 336:783, 1988.
13. Burgess, W. H., Dionne, C. A., Kaplow, J., Mudd, R., Friesel, R., Zilberstein, A., Schlessinger, J., and Jaye, M.: Characterization and cDNA cloning of phospholipase C-gamma, a major substrate for heparin-binding growth factor 1 (acidic fibroblast growth factor)-activated tyrosine kinase. Mol. Cell Biol., 10:4770, 1990.
14. Burgess, W. H., and Maciag, T.: The heparin-binding (fibroblast) growth factor family of proteins. Annu. Rev. Biochem., 58:575, 1989.
15. Carpenter, G., and Cohen, S.: Epidermal growth factor. J. Biol. Chem., 265:7709, 1990.
16. Chan, A. M., King, H. W., Deakin, E. A., Tempest, P. R., Hilkens, J., Kroezen, V., Edwards, D. R., Wills, A. J., Brookes, P., and Cooper, C. S.: Characterization of the mouse met proto-oncogene. Oncogene, 2:593, 1988.
17. Chiu, I. M.: Growth factor genes as oncogenes. Mol. Chem. Neuropathol., 10:37, 1989.
18. Claesson-Welsh, L., Eriksson, A., Moren, A., Severinsson, L., Ek, B., Ostman, A., Betsholtz, C., and Heldin, C. H.: cDNA cloning and expression of a human platelet-derived growth factor (PDGF) receptor specific for B-chain-containing PDGF molecules. Mol. Cell. Biol., 8:3476, 1988.
19. Claesson-Welsh, L., Eriksson, A., Westermark, B., and Heldin, C. H.: cDNA cloning and expression of the human A-type platelet-derived growth factor (PDGF) receptor establishes structural similarity to the B-type PDGF receptor. Proc. Natl. Acad. Sci. U.S.A., 86:4917, 1989.
20. Claesson-Welsh, L., Hammacher, A., Westermark, B., Heldin, C. H., and Nister, M.: Identification and structural analysis of the A type receptor for platelet-derived growth factor. Similarities with the B type receptor. J. Biol. Chem., 264:1742, 1989.
21. Clarke, M.F., Westin, E., Schmidt, D., Josephs, S. F., Ratner, L., Wong-Staal, F., Gallo, R. C., and Reitz, M. S., Jr.: Transformation of NIH/3T3 cells by a human c-sis cDNA clone. Nature, 308:464, 1984.
22. Clemmons, D. R.: Structural and functional analysis of insulin-like growth factors. Br. Med. Bull., 45:465, 1989.
23. Cohen, S.: Epidermal growth factor. Biosci. Rep., 6:1017, 1986.
24. Collett, M. S., and Erikson, R. L.: Protein kinase activity associated with the avian sarcoma virus src gene product. Proc. Natl. Acad. Sci. U.S.A., 75:2021, 1978.
25. Cotecchia, S., Schwinn, D. A., Randall, R. R., Lefkowitz, R. J., Caron, M. G., and Kobilka, B. K.: Molecular cloning and expression of the cDNA for the hamster alpha 1-adrenergic receptor. Proc. Natl. Acad. Sci. U.S.A., 85:7159, 1988.
26. Coughlin, S. R., Escobedo, J. A., and Williams, L. T.: Role of phosphatidylinositol kinase in PDGF receptor signal transduction. Science, 243:1191, 1989.
27. Cuttitta, F., Carney, D. N., Mulshine, J., Moody, T. W., Fedorko, J., Fischler, A., and Minna, J. D.: Bombesin-like peptides can function as autocrine growth factors in human small-cell lung cancer. Nature, 316:823, 1985.
28. Dearry, A., Gingrich, J. A., Falardeau, P., Fremeau, R. T., Jr., Bates, M. D., and Caron, M. G.: Molecular cloning and expression of the gene for a human D1 dopamine receptor. Nature, 347:72, 1990.
29. Delli Bovi, P., Curatola, A. M., Kern, F. G., Greco, A., Ittmann, M., and Basilico, C.: An oncogene isolated by transfection of Kaposi's sarcoma DNA encodes a growth factor that is a member of the FGF family. Cell, 50:729, 1987.
30. Derynck, R.: Transforming growth factor alpha. Cell, 54:593, 1988.
31. Di Fiore, P. P., Pierce, J. H., Kraus, M. H., Segatto, O., King, C. R., and Aaronson, S. A.: erbB-2 is a potent oncogene when overexpressed in NIH/3T3 cells. Science, 237:178, 1987.
32. Di Marco, E., Pierce, J. H., Fleming, T. P., Kraus, M. H., Molloy, C. J., Aaronson, S. A., and Di Fiore, P. P.: Autocrine interaction between TGF alpha and the EGF-receptor: quantitative requirements for induction of the malignant phenotype. Oncogene, 4:831, 1989.
33. Dixon, M., Deed, R., Acland, P., Moore, R., Whyte, A., Peters, G., and Dickson, C.: Detection and characterization of the fibroblast growth factor-related oncoprotein INT-2. Mol. Cell. Biol., 9:4896, 1989.
34. Doolittle, R. F., Hunkapiller, M. W., Hood, L. E., Devare, S. G., Robbins, K. C., Aaronson, S. A., and Antoniades, H. N.: Simian sarcoma virus onc gene, v-sis, is derived from the gene (or genes) encoding a platelet-derived growth factor. Science, 221:275, 1983.
35. Downward, J., Yarden, Y., Mayes, E., Scrace, G., Totty, N., Stockwell, P., Ullrich, A., Schlessinger, J., and Waterfield, M.D.: Close similarity of epidermal growth factor receptor and v-erbB oncogene protein sequences. Nature, 307:521, 1984.
36. Drebin, J. A., Link, V. C., Weinberg, R. A., and Greene, M. I.: Inhibition of tumor growth by a monoclonal antibody reactive with an oncogene-encoded tumor antigen. Proc. Natl. Acad. Sci. U.S.A., 83:9129, 1986.
37. Dull, T. J., Gray, A., Hayflick, J. S., and Ullrich, A.: Insulin-like growth factor II precursor gene organization in relation to insulin gene family. Nature, 310:777, 1984.
38. Ebina, Y., Ellis, L., Jarnagin, K., Edery, M., Graf, L., Clauser, E., Ou, J. H., Masiarz, F., Kan, Y. W., Goldfine, I. D., Roth, R. A., and Rutter, W. J.: The human insulin receptor

cDNA: the structural basis for hormone-activated transmembrane signalling. Cell, 40:747, 1985.
39. Ehrlich, P., and Shiga, K.: Berl. Klin. Wochenschr., 41:329, 1904.
40. Ellis, C., Moran, M., McCormick, F., and Pawson, T.: Phosphorylation of GAP and GAP-associated proteins by transforming and mitogenic tyrosine kinases. Nature, 343:377, 1990.
41. Escobedo, J. A., and Williams, L. T.: A PDGF receptor domain essential for mitogenesis but not for many other responses to PDGF. Nature, 335:85, 1988.
42. Espinal, J.: Mechanism of insulin action. Nature, 328:574, 1987.
43. Eva, A.: New human oncogenes. *In* The Oncogene Handbook. Edited by E. P. Reddy, A. M. Skalka, and T. Curran. Amsterdam, Elsevier, 1988, pp. 515–526.
44. Eva, A., Robbins, K. C., Andersen, P. R., Srinivasan, A., Tronick, S. R., Reddy, E. P., Ellmore, N. W., Galen, A. T., Lautenberger, J. A., Papas, T. S., Westin, E. H., Wong-Staal, F., Gallo, R. C., and Aaronson, S. A.: Cellular genes analogous to retroviral *onc* genes are transcribed in human tumour cells. Nature, 295:116, 1982.
45. Fargin, A., Raymond, J. R., Lohse, M. J., Kobilka, B. K., Caron, M. G., and Lefkowitz, R. J.: The genomic clone G-21 which resembles a beta-adrenergic receptor sequence encodes the 5-HT1A receptor. Nature, 335:358, 1988.
46. Fasano, O., Birnbaum, D., Edlund, L., Fogh, J., and Wigler, M.: New human transforming genes detected by a tumorigenicity assay. Mol. Cell. Biol., 4:1695, 1984.
47. Finch, P. W., Rubin, J. S., Miki, T., Ron, D., and Aaronson, S. A.: Human KGF is FGF-related with properties of a paracrine effector of epithelial cell growth. Science, 245:752, 1989.
48. FitzGerald, D., and Pastan, I.: Targeted toxin therapy for the treatment of cancer. J. Natl. Cancer Inst., 81:1455, 1989.
49. Fleming, T. P., Matsui, T., Molloy, C. J., Robbins, K. C., and Aaronson, S. A.: Autocrine mechanism for v-*sis* transformation requires cell surface localization of internally activated growth factor receptors. Proc. Natl. Acad. Sci. U.S.A., 86:8063, 1989.
50. Frielle, T., Collins, S., Daniel, K. W., Caron, M. G., Lefkowitz, R. J., and Kobilka, B. K.: Cloning of the cDNA for the human beta 1-adrenergic receptor. Proc. Natl. Acad. Sci. U.S.A., 84:7920, 1987.
51. Gazit, A., Igarashi, H., Chiu, I. M., Srinivasan, A., Yaniv, A., Tronick, S. R., Robbins, K. C., and Aaronson, S. A.: Expression of the normal human *sis*/PDGF-2 coding sequence induces cellular transformation. Cell, 39:89, 1984.
52. Gill, G. N., Rosenfeld, M. G., Chen, W. S., Bertics, P. J., and Lazar, C. S.: Analysis of functional domains in the epidermal growth factor receptor using site-directed mutagenesis. Adv. Exp. Med. Biol., 234:91, 1988.
53. Gill, G. N., Ill, C. R., and Simonian, M. H.: Angiotensin stimulation of bovine adrenocortical cell growth. Proc. Natl. Acad. Sci. U.S.A., 74:5569, 1977.
54. Giordano, S., Ponzetto, C., Di Renzo, M. F., Cooper, C. S., and Comoglio, P. M.: Tyrosine kinase receptor indistinguishable from the c-*met* protein. Nature, 339:155, 1989.
55. Gohda, E., Tsubouchi, H., Nakayama, H., Hirono, S., Sakiyama, O., Takahashi, K., Miyazaki, H., Hashimoto, S., and Daikuhara, Y.: Purification and partial characterization of hepatocyte growth factor from plasma of a patient with fulminant hepatic failure. J. Clin. Invest., 81:414, 1988.
56. Grandy, D. K., Marchionni, M. A., Makam, H., Stofko, R. E., Alfano, M., Frothingham, L., Fischer, J. B., Burke-Howie, K. J., Bunzow, J. R., Server, A. C., and Civelli, O.: Cloning of the cDNA and gene for a human D2 dopamine receptor. Proc. Natl. Acad. Sci. U.S.A., 86:9762, 1989.
57. Gray, A., Dull, T. J., and Ullrich, A.: Nucleotide sequence of epidermal growth factor cDNA predicts a 128,000-molecular weight protein precursor. Nature, 303:722, 1983.
58. Gregory, H.: Isolation and structure of urogastrone and its relationship to epidermal growth factor. Nature, 257:325, 1975.
59. Halaban, R., Kwon, B. S., Ghosh, S., Delli Bovi, P., and Baird, A.: bFGF as an autocrine growth factor for human melanomas. Oncogene Res., 3:177, 1988.
60. Halaban, R., Langdon, R., Birchall, N., Cuono, C., Baird, A., Scott, G., Moellmann, G., and McGuire, J.: Basic fibroblast growth factor from human keratinocytes is a natural mitogen for melanocytes. J. Cell Biol., 107:1611, 1988.
61. Hammacher, A., Mellstrom, K., Heldin, C. H., and Westermark, B.: Isoform-specific induction of actin reorganization by platelet-derived growth factor suggests that the functionally active receptor is a dimer. EMBO J., 8:2489, 1989.
62. Hanley, M. R.: Mitogenic neurotransmitters [news]. Nature, 340:97, 1989.
63. Hannink, M., and Donoghue, D. J.: Autocrine stimulation by the v-*sis* gene product requires a ligand-receptor interaction at the cell surface. J. Cell Biol., 107:287, 1988.
64. Hart, C. E., Forstrom, J. W., Kelly, J. D., Seifert, R. A., Smith, R. A., Ross, R., Murray, M. J., and Bowen-Pope, D. F.: Two classes of PDGF receptor recognize different isoforms of PDGF. Science, 240:1529, 1988.
65. Hattori, Y., Odagiri, H., Nakatani, H., Miyagawa, K., Naito, K., Sakamoto, H., Katoh, O., Yoshida, T., Sugimura, T., and Terada, M.: K-sam, an amplified gene in stomach cancer, is a member of the heparin-binding growth factor receptor genes. Proc. Natl. Sci. U.S.A., 87:5983, 1990.
66. Heldin, C. H., Hammacher, A., Nister, M., and Westermark, B.: Structural and functional aspects of platelet-derived growth factor. Br. J. Cancer, 57:591, 1988.
67. Heldin, C. H., Johnsson, A., Wennergren, S., Wernstedt, C., Betsholtz, C., and Westermark, B.: A human osteosarcoma cell line secretes a growth factor structurally related to a homodimer of PDGF A-chains. Nature, 319:511, 1986.
68. Heldin, C. H., and Westermark, B.: Platelet-derived growth factors: a family of isoforms that bind to two distinct receptors. Br. Med. Bull., 45:453, 1989.
69. Hirai, H., Maru, Y., Hagiwara, K., Nishida, J., and Takaku, F.: A novel putative tyrosine kinase receptor encoded by the *eph* gene. Science, 238:1717, 1987.
70. Huang, J. S., Huang, S. S., and Deuel, T. F.: Transforming protein of simian sarcoma virus stimulates autocrine growth of SSV-transformed cells through PDGF cell-surface receptors. Cell, 39:79, 1984.
71. Huang, S. S., and Huang, J. S.: Rapid turnover of the platelet-derived growth factor receptor in *sis*-transformed cells and and reversal by suramin. Implications for the mechanism of autocrine transformation. J. Biol. Chem., 263:12608, 1988.
72. Hunter, T., Angel, P., Boyle, W. J., Chiu, R., Freed, E., Gould, K. L., Isacke, C. M., Karin, M., Lindberg, R. A., and van der Geer P.: Targets for signal-transducing protein kinases. Cold Spring Harb. Symp. Quant. Biol., 53:131, 1988.
73. Hunter, T., and Sefton, B. M.: Transforming gene product of Rous sarcoma virus phosphorylates tyrosine. Proc. Natl. Acad. Sci. U.S.A., 77:1311, 1980.
74. Igarashi, H., Rao, C. D., Siroff, M., Leal, F., Robbins, K. C., and Aaronson, S. A.: Detection of PDGF-2 homodimers in human tumor cells. Oncogene, 1:79, 1987.
75. Imamura, T., Engleka, K., Zhan, X., Tokita, Y., Forough, R., Roeder, D., Jackson, A., Maier, J. A. M., Hla, T., and Maciag, T.: Recovery of mitogenic activity of a growth factor mutant with a nuclear translocation sequence. Science, 249:1567, 1990.
76. Imoto, M., Umezawa, K., Komuro, K., Sawa, T., Takeuchi, T., and Umezawa, H.: Antitumor activity of erbstatin, a tyrosine protein kinase inhibitor. Jpn. J. Cancer Res., 78:329, 1987.
77. Reference not used.
78. Johnson, D. E., Lee, P. L., Lu, J., and Willilams, L. T.: Diverse forms of a receptor for acidic and basic fibroblast growth factors. Mol. Cell. Biol., 10:4728, 1990.
79. Johnsson, A., Betsholtz, C., Heldin, C. H., and Westermark, B.: Antibodies against platelet-derived growth factor inhibit acute transformation by simian sarcoma virus. Nature, 317:438, 1985.
80. Julius, D., Livelli, T. J., Jessell, T. M., and Axel, R.: Ectopic expression of the serotonin 1c receptor and the triggering of malignant transformation. Science, 244:1057, 1989.
81. Kaleko, M., Rutter, W. J., and Miller, A. D.: Overexpression of the human insulinlike growth factor I receptor promotes ligand-dependent neoplastic transformation. Mol. Cell. Biol., 10:464, 1990.
82. Kazlauskas, A., and Cooper, J. A.: Autophosphorylation of the PDGF receptor in the kinase insert region regulates interactions with cell proteins. Cell, 58:1121, 1989.
83. Keating, M. T., and Williams, L. T.: Autocrine stimulation of intracellular PDGF receptors in v-*sis*-transformed cells. Science, 239:914, 1988.
84. Keck, P. J., Hauser, S. D., Krivi, G., Sanzo, K., Warren, T., Feder, J., and Connolly, D. T.: Vascular permeability factor, an endothelial cell mitogen related to PDGF. Science, 246:1309, 1989.
85. Kikkawa, U., and Nishizuka, Y.: The role of protein kinase C in transmembrane signalling. Annu. Rev. Cell Biol., 2:149, 1986.
86. King, C. R., Kraus, M. H., and Aaronson, S. A.: Amplification of a novel v-*erb*B-related gene in a human mammary carcinoma. Science, 229:974, 1985.
87. King, C. R., Kraus, M. H., Williams, L. T., Merlino, G. T., Pastan, I. H., and Aaronson, S. A.: Human tumor cell lines with EGF receptor gene amplification in the absence of aberrant sized mRNAs. Nucleic Acids Res., 13:8477, 1985.
88. Klein, R., Parada, L. F., Coulier, F., and Barbacid, M.: *trk*B, a novel tyrosine protein kinase receptor expressed during mouse neural development. EMBO J., 8:3701, 1989.
89. Kobilka, B. K., Dixon, R. A., Frielle, T., Dohlman, H. G., Bolanowski, M. A., Sigal, I. S., Yang-Feng, T. L., Francke, U., Caron, M. G., and Lefkowitz, R. J.: cDNA for the human beta 2-adrenergic receptor: a protein with multiple membrane-spanning domains and encoded by a gene whose chromosomal location is shared with that of the receptor for platelet-derived growth factor. Proc. Natl. Acad. Sci. U.S.A., 84:46, 1987.
90. Kobilka, B. K., Frielle, T., Dohlman, H. G., Bolanowski, M. A., Dixon, R. A., Keller, P., Caron, M. G., and Lefkowitz, R. J.: Delineation of the intronless nature of the genes for the human and hamster beta 2-adrenergic receptor and their putative promoter regions. J. Biol. Chem., 262:7321, 1987.
91. Kobilka, B. K., Matsui, H., Kobilka, T. S., Yang-Feng, T. L., Francke, U., Caron, M. G., Lefkowitz, R. J., and Regan, J. W.: Cloning, sequencing, and expression of the gene coding for the human platelet alpha 2-adrenergic receptor. Science, 238:650, 1987.
92. Kornbluth, S., Paulson, K. E., and Hanafusa, H.: Novel tyrosine kinase identified by phosphotyrosine antibody screening of cDNA libraries. Mol. Cell Biol., 8:5541, 1988.
93. Kraus, M. H., Issing, W., Miki, T., Popescu, N. C., and Aaronson, S. A.: Isolation and characterization of *erb*B-3, a third member of the *erb*B-epidermal growth factor receptor family: evidence for overexpression in a subset of human mammary tumors. Proc. Natl. Acad. Sci. U.S.A., 86:9193, 1989.
94. Kraus, M. H., Popescu, N. C., Amsbaugh, S. C., and King, C. R.: Overexpression of the EGF receptor-related proto-oncogene *erb*B-2 in human mammary tumor cell lines by different molecular mechanisms. EMBO J., 6:605, 1987.
95. Kubo, T., Fukuda, K., Mikami, A., Maeda, A., Takahashi, H., Mishina, M., Haga, T., Haga, K., Ichiyama, A., Kangawa, K., Kojima, M., Matsuo, H., Hirose, T., and Numa, S.: Cloning, sequencing and expression of complementary DNA encoding the muscarinic acetylcholine receptor. Nature, 323:411, 1986.
96. Lacal, J. C., and Tronick, S. R.: The *ras* oncogene. *In* The Oncogene Handbook. Edited by E. P. Reddy, A. M. Skalka, and T. Curran. Amsterdam, Elsevier, 1988, p. 255.
97. Lacroix, H., Iglehart, J. D., Skinner, M. A., and Kraus, M. H.: Overexpression of *erb*B-2 or EGF receptor proteins present in early stage mammary carcinoma is detected simultaneously in matched primary tumors and regional metastases. Oncogene, 4:145, 1989.
98. Landis, C. A., Masters, S. B., Spada, A., Pace, A. M., Bourne, H. R., and Vallar, L.: GTPase inhibiting mutations activate the alpha chain of Gs and stimulate adenylyl cyclase in human pituitary tumours. Nature, 340:692, 1989.
99. Lee, P. L., Johnson, D. E., Cousens, L. S., Fried, V. A., and Williams, L. T.: Purification and complementary DNA cloning of a receptor for basic fibroblast growth factor. Science, 245:57, 1989.
100. Letwin, K., Yee, S-P., and Pawson, T.: Novel protein-tyrosine kinase cDNAs related to *fps*/*fes* and *eph* cloned using anti-phosphotyrosine antibody. Oncogene, 3:621, 1988.
101. Leung, D. W., Cachianes, G., Kuang, W. J., Goeddel, D. V., and Ferrara, N.: Vascular endothelial growth factor is a secreted angiogenic mitogen. Science, 246:1306, 1989.
102. Levi-Montalcini, R.: The nerve growth factor 35 years later. Science, 237:1154, 1987.
103. Levinson, A. D., Oppermann, H., Levintow, L., Varmus, H. E., and Bishop, J. M.: Evidence that the transforming gene of avian sarcoma virus encodes a protein kinase associated with a phosphoprotein. Cell, 15:561, 1978.
104. Libermann, T. A., Razon, N., Bartal, A. D., Yarden, Y., Schlessinger, J., and Soreq, H.: Expression of epidermal growth factor receptors in human brain tumors. Cancer Res., 44:753, 1984.
105. Lomasney, J. W., Lorenz, W., Allen, L. F., King, K., Regan, J. W., Yang-Feng, T. L., Caron, M. G., and Lefkowitz, R. J.: Expansion of the alpha 2-adrenergic receptor family: cloning and characterization of a human alpha 2-adrenergic receptor subtype, the gene for which is located on chromosome 2. Proc. Natl. Acad. Sci. U.S.A., 87:5094, 1990.
106. Lupu, R., Colomer, R., Zugmaier, G., Sarup, J., Shepard, M., Slamon, D., and Lippman, M. E.: Direct interaction of a ligand for the *erb*B2 oncogene product with the EGF receptor and p185*erb*B2. Science, 249:1552, 1990.
107. Lyons, J., Landis, C. A., Harsh, G., Vallar, L., Grunewald, K., Feichtinger, H., Duh,

Q. Y., Clark, O. H., Kawasaki, E., Bourne, H. R., and McCormick, F.: Two G protein oncogenes in human endocrine tumors. Science, 249:655, 1990.
108. Machida, C. A., Bunzow, J. R., Searles, R. P., Van Tol, H., Tester, B., Neve, K. A., Teal, P., Nipper, V., and Civelli, O.: Molecular cloning and expression of the rat beta 1-adrenergic receptor gene. J. Biol. Chem., 265:12960, 1990.
109. Margolis, B., Rhee, S. G., Felder, S., Mervic, M., Lyall, R., Levitzki, A., Ullrich, A., Zilberstein, A., and Schlessinger, J.: EGF induces tyrosine phosphorylation of phospholipase C-II: a potential mechanism for EGF receptor signaling. Cell, 57:1101, 1989.
110. Marics, I., Adelaide, J., Raybaud, F., Mattei, M. G., Coulier, F., Planche, J., de Lapeyriere, O., and Birnbaum, D.: Characterization of the HST-related FGF.6 gene, a new member of the fibroblast growth factor gene family. Oncogene, 4:335, 1989.
111. Martin-Zanca, D., Oskam, R., Mitra, G., Copeland, T., and Barbacid, M.: Molecular and biochemical characterization of the human *trk* proto-oncogene. Mol. Cell. Biol., 9:24, 1989.
112. Marx, J.: Bombesin receptor gene cloned. Science, 249:1377, 1990.
113. Masu, Y., Nakayama, K., Tamaki, H., Harada, Y., Kuno, M., and Nakanishi, S.: cDNA cloning of bovine substance-K receptor through oocyte expression system. Nature, 329:836, 1987.
114. Matsui, T., Heidaran, M., Miki, T., Popescu, N., La Rochelle, W., Kraus, M., Pierce, J., and Aaronson, S. A.: Isolation of a novel receptor cDNA establishes the existence of two PDGF receptor genes. Science, 243:800, 1989.
115. Matsui, T., Pierce, J. H., Fleming, T. P., Greenberger, J. S., LaRochelle, W. J., Euggiero, M., and Aaronson, S. A.: Independent expression of human alpha or beta platelet-derived growth factor receptor cDNAs in a naive hematopoietic cell leads to functional coupling with mitogenic and chemotactic signaling pathways. Proc. Natl. Acad. Sci. U.S.A., 86:8314, 1989.
116. Matsushime, H., Wang, L. H., and Shibuya, M.: Human c-*ros*-1 gene homologous to the v-*ros* sequence of UR2 sarcoma virus encodes for a transmembrane receptorlike molecule. Mol. Cell. Biol., 6:3000, 1986.
117. Maxwell, M., Naber, S. P., Wolfe, H. J., Galanopoulos, T., Hedley-Whyte, E. T., Black, P. M., and Antoniades, H. N.: Coexpression of platelet-derived growth factor (PDGF) and PDGF-receptor genes by primary human astrocytomas may contribute to their development and maintenance. J. Clin. Invest., 86:131, 1990.
118. McCormick, F., Adari, H., Trahey, M., Halenbeck, R., Koths, K., Martin, G. A., Crosier, W. J., Watt, K., Rubinfeld, B., and Wong, G.: Interaction of *ras* p21 proteins with GTPase activating protein. Cold Spring Harb. Symp. Quant. Biol., 53:849, 1988.
119. Meisenhelder, J., Suh, P. G., Rhee, S. G., and Hunter, T.: Phospholipase C-gamma is a substrate for the PDGF and EGF receptor protein-tyrosine kinases *in vivo* and *in vitro*. Cell, 57:1109, 1989.
120. Reference not used.
121. Miyazawa, K., Tsubouchi, H., Naka, D., Takahashi, K., Okigaki, M., Arakaki, N., Nakayama, H., Hirono, S., Sakiyama, O., et al.: Molecular cloning and sequence analysis of cDNA for human hepatocyte growth factor. Biochem. Biophys. Res. Commun., 163:967, 1989.
122. Molloy, C. J., Bottaro, D. P., Fleming, T. P., Marshall, M. S., Gibbs, J. B., and Aaronson, S. A.: PDGF induction of tyrosine phosphorylation of GTPase activating protein. Nature, 342:711, 1989.
123. Moody, T. W., Pert, C. B., Gazdar, A. F., Carney, D. N., and Minna, J. D.: High levels of intracellular bombesin characterize human small-cell lung carcinoma. Science, 214:1246, 1981.
124. Morrison, D. K., Kaplan, D. R., Escobedo, J. A., Rapp, U. R., Roberts, T. M., and Williams, L. T.: Direct activation of the serine/threonine kinase activity of Raf-1 through tyrosine phosphorylation by the PDGF beta-receptor. Cell, 58:649, 1989.
125. Morrison, D. K., Kaplan, D. R., Rhee, S. G., and Williams, L. T.: Platelet-derived growth factor (PDGF)-dependent association of phospholipase C-gamma with the PDGF receptor signaling complex. Mol. Cell. Biol., 10:2359, 1990.
126. Mroczkowski, B., Reich, M., Chen, K., Bell, G. I., and Cohen, S.: Recombinant human epidermal growth factor precursor is a glycosylated membrane protein with biological activity. Mol. Cell. Biol., 9:2771, 1989.
127. Mulcahy, L. S., Smith, M. R., and Stacey, D. W.: Requirement for *ras* proto-oncogene function during serum-stimulated growth of NIH 3T3 cells. Nature, 313:241, 1985.
128. Muller, W. J., Lee, F. S., Dickson, C., Peters, G., Pattengale, P., and Leder, P.: The *int*-2 gene product acts as an epithelial growth factor in transgenic mice. EMBO J., 9:907, 1990.
129. Mulshine, J. L., Avis, I., Treston, A. M., Mobley, C., Kaspryzyk, P., Carrasquillo, J. A., Larson, S. M., Nakanishi, Y., Merchant, B., Minna, J. D., et al.: Clinical use of a monoclonal antibody to bombesin-like peptide in patients with lung cancer. Ann. N.Y. Acad. Sci., 547:360, 1988.
130. Nakamura, T., Nawa, K., Ichihara, A., Kaise, N., and Nishino, T.: Purification and subunit structure of hepatocyte growth factor from rat platelets. FEBS. Lett., 224:311, 1987.
131. Nakamura, T., Nishizawa, T., Hagiya, M., Seki, T., Shimonishi, M., Sugimura, A., Tashiro, K., and Shimizu, S.: Molecular cloning and expression of human hepatocyte growth factor. Nature, 342:440, 1989.
131A. Naldini, L., Vigna, E., Narsimhan, R. P., Gaudino, G., Zarnegar, R., Michalopoulos, G. K., and Comoglio, P. M.: Hepatocyte growth factor (HGF) stimulates the tyrosine kinase activity of the receptor encoded by the proto-oncogene c-MET. Oncogene, 6:501, 1991.
132. Natali, P. G., Nicotra, M. R., Bigotti, A., Venturo, I., Slamon, D. J., and Fendly, B. M.: Expression of the p185 encoded by HER2 oncogene in normal and transformed human tissues. Int. J. Cancer, 45:457, 1990.
133. Nemecek, G. M., Coughlin, S. R., Handley, D. A., and Moskowitz, M. A.: Stimulation of aortic smooth muscle cell mitogenesis by serotonin. Proc. Natl. Acad. Sci. U.S.A., 83:674, 1986.
134. Nichols, E. J., Manger, R., Hakomori, S. I., and Rohrschneider, L. R.: Transformation by the oncogene v-*fms*: the effects of castanospermine on transformation-related parameters. Exp. Cell Res., 173:486, 1987.
135. Nister, M., Hammacher, A., Mellstrom, K., Siegbahn, A., Ronnstrand, L., Westermark, B., and Heldin, C. H.: A glioma-derived PDGF A chain homodimer has different functional activities from a PDGF AB heterodimer purified from human platelets. Cell, 52:791, 1988.
136. Nister, M., Libermann, T. A., Betsholtz, C., Pettersson, M., Claesson-Welsh, L., Heldin, C. H., Schlessinger, J., and Westermark, B.: Expression of messenger RNAs for platelet-derived growth factor and transforming growth factor-alpha and their receptors in human malignant glioma cell lines. Cancer Res., 48:3910, 1988.
137. Ostrander, G. K., Scribner, N. K., and Rohrschneider, L. R.: Inhibition of v-*fms*-induced tumor growth in nude mice by castanospermine. Cancer Res., 48:1091, 1988.
138. Parkes, H. C., Lillycrop, K., Howell, A., and Craig, R. K.: C-*erb*B-2 mRNA expression in human breast tumours: comparison with c-*erb*B-2 DNA amplification and correlation with prognosis. Br. J. Cancer, 61:39, 1990.
139. Pasquale, E. B.: A distinctive family of embryonic protein-tyrosine kinase receptors. Proc. Natl. Acad. Sci. U.S.A., 87:5812, 1990.
140. Pasquale, E. B., and Singer, S. J.: Identification of a developmentally regulated protein-tyrosine kinase by using anti-phosphotyrosine antibodies to screen a cDNA expression library. Proc. Natl. Acad. Sci. U.S.A., 86:5449, 1989.
141. Pech, M., Gazit, A., Arnstein, P., and Aaronson, S. A.: Generation of fibrosarcomas *in vivo* by a retrovirus that expresses the normal B chain of platelet-derived growth factor and mimics the alternative splice pattern of the v-*sis* oncogene. Proc. Natl. Acad. Sci. U.S.A., 86:2693, 1989.
142. Peralta, E. G., Winslow, J. W., Peterson, G. L., Smith, D. H., Ashkenazi, A., Ramachandran, J., Schimerlik, M. I., and Capon, D. J.: Primary structure and biochemical properties of an M2 muscarinic receptor. Science, 236:600, 1987.
143. Plowman, G. D., Green, J. M., McDonald, V. L., Neubauer, M. G., Disteche, C. M., Todaro, G. J., and Shoyab, M.: The amphiregulin gene encodes a novel epidermal growth factor-related protein with tumor-inhibitory activity. Mol. Cell. Biol., 10:1969, 1990.
144. Plowman, G. D., Whitney, G. S., Neubauer, M. G., Green, J. M., McDonald, V. L., Todaro, G. J., and Shoyab, M.: Molecular cloning and expression of an additional epidermal growth factor receptor-related gene. Proc. Natl. Acad. Sci. U.S.A., 87:4905, 1990.
145. Ray, L. B., and Sturgill, T. W.: Insulin-stimulated microtubule-associated protein kinase is phosphorylated on tyrosine and threonine *in vivo*. Proc. Natl. Acad. Sci. U.S.A., 85:3753, 1988.
146. Regan, J. W., Kobilka, T. S., Yang-Feng, T. L., Caron, M. G., Lefkowitz, R. J., and Kobilka, B. K.: Cloning and expression of a human kidney cDNA for an alpha 2-adrenergic receptor subtype. Proc. Natl. Acad. Sci. U.S.A., 85:6301, 1988.
147. Reid, H. H., Wilks, A. F., and Bernard, O.: Two forms of the basic fibroblast growth factor receptor-like mRNA are expressed in the developing mouse brain. Proc. Natl. Acad. Sci. U.S.A., 87:1596, 1990.
148. Robbins, K. C., Antoniades, H. N., Devare, S. G., Hunkapiller, M. W., and Aaronson, S. A.: Structural and immunological similarities between simian sarcoma virus gene product(s) and human platelet-derived growth factor. Nature, 305:605, 1983.
149. Robbins, K. C., Leal, F., Pierce, J. H., and Aaronson, S. A.: The v-*sis*/PDGF-2 transforming gene product localizes to cell membranes but is not a secretory protein. EMBO J., 4:1783, 1985.
150. Roberts, A. B., and Sporn, M. B.: Principles of molecular cell biology of cancer: growth factors related to transformation. *In* Cancer Principles & Practice of Oncology. Edited by V. T. DeVita, Jr., S. Hellman and S. A. Rosenberg, Philadelphia, J. B. Lippincott Company, 1989, pp. 67–80.
151. Ross, R., Raines, E. W., and Bowen-Pope, D. F.: The biology of platelet-derived growth factor. Cell, 46:155, 1986.
152. Rossomando, A. J., Payne, D. M., Weber, M. J., and Sturgill, T. W.: Evidence that pp42, a major tyrosine kinase target protein, is a mitogen-activated serine/threonine protein kinase. Proc. Natl. Acad. Sci. U.S.A., 86:6940, 1989.
153. Roussel, M. F., Downing, J. R., Rettenmier, C. W., and Sherr, C. J.: A point mutation in the extracellular domain of the human CSF-1 receptor (c-*fms* proto-oncogene product) activates its transforming potential. Cell, 55:979, 1988.
154. Rubin, J. S., Osada, H., Finch, P. W., Taylor, W. G., Rudikoff, S., and Aaronson, S. A.: Purification and characterization of a newly identified growth factor specific for epithelial cells. Proc. Natl. Acad. Sci. U.S.A., 86:802, 1989.
155. Ruta, M., Howk, R., Ricca, G., Drohan, W., Zabelshansky, M., Laureys, G., Barton, D. E., Francke, U., Schlessinger, J., and Givol, D.: A novel protein tyrosine kinase gene whose expression is modulated during endothelial cell differentiation. Oncogene, 3:9, 1988.
156. Sano, H., Forough, R., Maier, J. A., Case, J. P., Jackson, A., Engleka, K., Maciag, T., and Wilder, R. L.: Detection of high levels of heparin binding growth factor-1 (acidic fibroblast growth factor) in inflammatory arthritic joints. J. Cell Biol., 110:1417, 1990.
157. Satoh, T., Endo, M., Nakafuku, M., Nakamur, S., and Kaziro, Y.: Platelet-derived growth factor stimulates formation of active p21*ras*-GTP complex in Swiss mouse 3T3 cells. Proc. Natl. Acad. Sci. U.S.A., 87:5993, 1990.
158. Schechter, A. L., Stern, D. F., Vaidyanathan, L., Decker, S. J., Drebin, J. A., Greene, M. I., and Weinberg, R. A.: The *neu* oncogene: an *erb*B-related gene encoding a 185,000-Mr tumour antigen. Nature, 312:513, 1984.
159. Schwinn, D. A., Lomasney, J. W., Lorenz, W., Szklut, P. J., Fremeau, R. T., Jr., Yang-Feng, T. L., Caron, M. G., Lefkowitz, R. J., and Cotecchia, S.: Molecular cloning and expression of the cDNA for a novel alpha 1-adrenergic receptor subtype. J. Biol. Chem., 265:8183, 1990.
160. Scott, J., Urdea, M., Quiroga, M., Sanchez-Pescador, R., Fong, N., Selby, M., Rutter, W. J., and Bell, G. I.: Structure of a mouse submaxillary messenger RNA encoding epidermal growth factor and seven related proteins. Science, 221:236, 1983.
161. Semba, K., Kamata, N., Toyoshima, K., and Yamamoto, T.: A v-*erb*B-related protooncogene, c-*erb*B-2, is distinct from the c-*erb*B-1/epidermal growth factor-receptor gene and is amplified in a human salivary gland adenocarcinoma. Proc. Natl. Acad. Sci. U.S.A., 82:6497, 1985.
162. Seuwen, K., Magnaldo, I., and Pouyssegur, J.: Serotonin stimulates DNA synthesis in fibroblasts acting through 5-HT1B receptors coupled to a Gi-protein. Nature, 335:254, 1988.
163. Sherr, C. J., Rettenmier, C. W., Sacca, R., Roussel, M. F., Look, A. T., and Stanley, E. R.: The c-*fms* proto-oncogene product is related to the receptor for the mononuclear phagocyte growth factor, CSF-1. Cell, 41:665, 1985.
164. Shibuya, M., Yamaguchi, S., Yamane, A., Ikeda, T., Tojo, A., Matsushime, H., and Sato, M.: Nucleotide sequence and expression of a novel human receptor-type tyrosine kinase gene (*flt*) closely related to the *fms* family. Oncogene, 5:519, 1990.
165. Shier, P., and Watt, V. M.: Primary structure of a putative receptor for a ligand of the insulin family. J. Biol. Chem., 264:14605, 1989.
166. Slamon, D. J., Godolphin, W., Jones, L.A., Holt, J. A., Wong, S. G., Keith, D. E., Levin,

W. J., Stuart, S. G., Udove, J., Ullrich, A., and Press, M. F.: Studies of the HER-2/*neu* proto-oncogene in human breast and ovarian cancer. Science, 244:707, 1989.

167. Smith, D. R., Vogt, P. K., and Hayman, M. J.: The v-*sea* oncogene of avian erythroblastosis retrovirus S13: another member of the protein-tyrosine kinase gene family. Proc. Natl. Acad. Sci. U.S.A., 86:5291, 1989.

168. Smith, R., Peters, G., and Dickson, C.: Multiple RNAs expressed from the *int*-2 gene in mouse embryonal carcinoma cell lines encode a protein with homology to fibroblast growth factors. EMBO J., 7:1013, 1988.

169. Sporn, M. B., and Todaro, G. J.: Autocrine secretion and malignant transformation of cells. N. Engl. J. Med., 303:878, 1980.

170. Stacey, D. W., and Kung, H. F.: Transformation of NIH/3T3 cells by microinjection of Ha-*ras* p21 protein. Nature, 310:508, 1984.

171. Sturgill, T. W., Ray, L. B., Erikson, E., and Maller, J. L.: Insulin-stimulated MAP-2 kinase phosphorylates and activates ribosomal protein S6 kinase II. Nature, 334:715, 1990.

172. Taira, M., Yoshida, T., Miyagawa, K., Sakamoto, H., Terada, M., and Sugimura, T.: cDNA sequence of human transforming gene *hst* and identification of the coding sequence required for transforming activity. Proc. Natl. Acad. Sci. U.S.A., 84:2980, 1987.

173. Takahashi, M., Buma, Y., Iwamoto, T., Inaguma, Y., Ikeda, H., and Hiai, H.: Cloning and expression of the *ret* proto-oncogene encoding a tyrosine kinase with two potential transmembrane domains. Oncogene, 3:571, 1988.

174. Thomas, K. A.: Transforming potential of fibroblast growth factor genes. Trends Biochem. Sci., 13:327, 1988.

175. Trahey, M., and McCormick, F.: A cytoplasmic protein stimulates normal N-*ras* p21 GTPase, but does not affect oncogenic mutants. Science, 238:542, 1987.

176. Ullrich, A., Bell, J. R., Chen, E. Y., Herrera, R., Petruzzelli, L. M., Dull, T. J., Gray, A., Coussens, L., Liao, Y. C., Tsubokawa, M., Mason, A., Seeburg, P. H., Grunfeld, C., Rosen, O. M., and Ramachandran, J.: Human insulin receptor and its relationship to the tyrosine kinase family of oncogenes. Nature, 313:756, 1985.

177. Ullrich, A., Berman, C. H., Dull, T. J., Gray, A., and Lee, J. M.: Isolation of the human insulin-like growth factor I gene using a single synthetic DNA probe. EMBO J., 3:361, 1984.

178. Ullrich, A., Gray, A., Tam, A. W., Yang-Feng, T., Tsubokawa, M., Collins, C., Henzel, W., Le Bon, T., Kathuria, S., Chen, E. et al.: Insulin-like growth factor I receptor primary structure: comparison with insulin receptor suggests structural determinants that define functional specificity. EMBO J., 5:2503, 1986.

179. Ullrich, A., and Schlessinger, J.: Signal transduction by receptors with tyrosine kinase activity. Cell, 61:203, 1990.

180. Van De Vijver M., Van De Bersselaar R., Devilee, P., Cornelisse, C., Peterse, J., and Nusse, R.: Amplification of the neu (c-*erb*B-2) oncogene in human mammary tumors is relatively frequent and is often accompanied by amplification of the linked c-*erb*A oncogene. Mol. Cell. Biol., 7:2019, 1987.

181. Varticovski, L., Druker, B., Morrison, D., Cantley, L., and Roberts, T.: The colony stimulating factor-1 receptor associates with and activates phosphatidylinositol-3 kinase. Nature, 342:699, 1989.

182. Wahl, M. I., Daniel, T. O., and Carpenter, G.: Antiphosphotyrosine recovery of phospholipase C activity after EGF treatment of A-431 cells. Science, 241:968, 1988.

183. Wahl, M. I., Nishibe, S., and Carpenter, G.: Growth factor signaling pathways: phosphoinositide metabolism and phosphorylation of phospholipase C. Cancer Cells, 1:101, 1989.

184. Waterfield, M. D.: Growth factor receptors. Br. Med. Bull., 45:541, 1989.

185. Waterfield, M. D., Scrace, G. T., Whittle, N., Stroobant, P., Johnsson, A., Wasteson, A., Westermark, B., Heldin, C. H., Huang, J. S., and Deuel, T. F.: Platelet-derived growth factor is structurally related to the putative transforming protein p28*sis* of simian sarcoma virus. Nature, 304:35, 1983.

186. Westermark, B., Johnsson, A., Paulsson, Y., Betsholtz, C., Heldin, C. H., Herlyn, M., Rodeck, U., and Koprowski, H.: Human melanoma cell lines of primary and metastatic orgin express the genes encoding the chains of platelet-derived growth factor (PDGF) and produce a PDGF-like growth factor. Proc. Natl. Acad. Sci. U.S.A., 83:7197, 1986.

187. Wigler, M. H.: GAPS in understanding *Ras*. Nature, 346:696, 1990.

188. Williams, L. T.: Signal transduction by the platelet-derived growth factor receptor. Science, 243:1564, 1989.

189. Witte, O. N.: Steel locus defines new multipotent growth factor. Cell, 63:5, 1990.

190. Woll, P. J., and Rozengurt, E.: Neuropeptides as growth regulators. Br. Med. Bull., 45:492, 1989.

191. Wright, N. A., Pike, C., and Elia, G.: Induction of a novel epidermal growth factor-secreting cell lineage by mucosal ulceration in human gastrointestinal stem cells. Nature, 343:82, 1990.

192. Yaish, P., Gazit, A., Gilon, C., and Levitzki, A.: Blocking of EGF-dependent cell proliferation by EGF receptor kinase inhibitors. Science, 242:933, 1988.

193. Yamamoto, T., Nishida, T., Miyajima, N., Kawai, S., Ooi, T., and Toyoshima, K.: The *erb*B gene of avian erythroblastosis virus is a member of the *src* gene family. Cell, 35:71, 1983.

194. Yarden, Y., Escobedo, J. A., Kuang, W. J., Yang-Feng, T. L., Daniel, T. O., Tremble, P. M., Chen, E. Y., Ando, M. E., Harkins, R. N., Francke, U., Fried, V. A., Ullrich, A., and Williams, L. T.: Structure of the receptor for platelet-derived growth factor helps define a family of closely related growth factor receptors. Nature, 323:226, 1986.

195. Yarden, Y., Rodriguez, H., Wong, S. K., Brandt, D. R., May, D. C., Burnier, J., Harkins, R. N., Chen, E. Y., Ramachandran, J., Ullrich, A., and Ross, E. M.: The avian beta-adrenergic receptor: primary structure and membrane topology. Proc. Natl. Acad. Sci. U.S.A., 83:6795, 1986.

196. Yarden, Y., and Ullrich, A.: Growth factor receptor tyrosine kinases. Annu. Rev. Biochem., 57:443, 1988.

197. Young, D., Waitches, G., Birchmeier, C., Fasano, O., and Wigler, M.: Isolation and characterization of a new cellular oncogene encoding a receptor with multiple potential transmembrane domains. Cell, 45:711, 1986.

198. Zhan, X., Bates, B., Hu, X. G., and Goldfarb, M.: The human FGF-5 oncogene encodes a novel protein related to fibroblast growth factors. Mol. Cell. Biol., 8:3487, 1988.

199. Zhou, Q-Y., Grandy, D. K., Thambi, L., Kushner, J. A., Van Tol, H. H. M., Cone, R., Pribnow, D., Salon, J., Bunzow, J. R., and Civelli, O.: Cloning and expression of human and rat D1 dopamine receptors. Nature, 347:76, 1990.

200. Hempstead, B. L., Martin-Zanca, D., Kaplan, D. R., Parada, L. F., and Chao, M. V.: High-affinity NGF binding requires coexpression of the trk proto-oncogene and the low-affinity NGF receptor. Nature, 350:678, 1991.

201. Klein, R., Jing, S. Q., Nanduri, V., O'Rourke, E., and Barbacid, M.: The trk proto-oncogene encodes a receptor for nerve growth factor. Cell, 65:189, 1991.

202. Nebreda, A. R., Martin-Zanca, D., Kaplan, D. R., Parada, L. F., and Santos, E.: Induction by NGF of meiotic maturation of Xenopus oocytes expressing the trk proto-oncogene product. Science, 252:558, 1991.

203. Soppet, D., Escandon, E., Maragos, J., Middlemas, D. S., Reid, S. W., Blair, J., Burton, L. E., Stanton, B. R., Kaplan, D. R., Hunter, T., Nikolics, K., and Parada, L. F.: The neurotrophic factors brain-derived neurotrophic factor and neurotrophin-3 are ligands for the trkB tyrosine kinase receptor. Cell, 65:895, 1991.

I-4

Signal Transduction in Cancer

Yusuf A. Hannun
Robert M. Bell

Introduction

The last decade has witnessed significant and exciting advances in understanding the mechanisms of cell regulation. This has been most notable in the area of cancer biology. The genetic and biochemical mechanisms underlying the pathogenesis of the cancerous phenotype have been yielding to the increasing sophistication and intensity of basic science approaches. In fact, it is now evident that cancer biology is amenable to investigation at a molecular level. While the complete and detailed understanding of the complex molecular pathways of cell regulation is not yet fully developed, many of the key elements responsible for control of cell growth and cell function in normal and malignant cells have been discovered and their mechanisms of action studied.

In normal cellular physiology, individual cells function in large part by responding to appropriate stimuli from their environment and by interacting with other cells. The healthy maintenance of normal physiology, therefore, demands that cells possess the ability to sense a multitude of external and internal stimuli, integrate those messages, and execute the appropriate responses (Figure I-4-1). For example, in the case of neutrophilic leukocytes, normal homeostasis requires

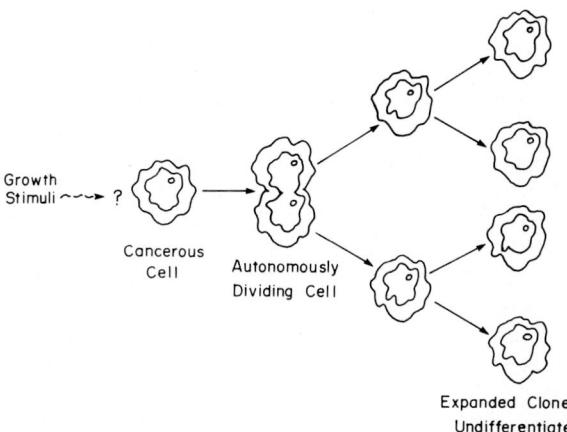

Figure I-4-1. Differentiation/proliferation in normal and cancerous cells. The specialized functions of most tissues (e.g., epithelial or hematopoietic) are carried out by fully differentiated cells with little or no capacity to divide and proliferate. Therefore, normal stem cells have to divide and proliferate in order to maintain an active pool of stem cells as well as to replenish lost differentiated cells. These processes of cell proliferation and differentiation are under strict control. Cells respond to environmental signals (such as growth factors and cytokines) and execute the appropriate responses. The intra- and intercellular pathways of signal transduction and cell regulation, therefore, play essential roles in ensuring normal cell function. Breakdown of these cell regulatory processes and signal transduction mechanisms may then result in autonomously dividing cells, hyperproliferation, and an expanded clone of undifferentiated cells with poor normal function.

these white blood cells to maintain an active pool of differentiated cells capable of responding to infectious agents. Similarly, the maintenance of normal epithelial tissues requires precursor cells to differentiate so as to regenerate epithelial surfaces while at the same time maintaining the precursor (stem cell) pool (Figure I-4-1). These examples illustrate the delicate balance that must be maintained between cellular proliferation and cell differentiation in different body tissues.

Cancer cells on the other hand, which are derived from normal counterparts, are characterized by their autonomous behavior and their unchecked proliferation. Cancer cells are afflicted by viruses, carcinogens, and/or endogenous muta-

tions so that they no longer respond to their environment (Figure I-4-1). This transformation is passed on to the progeny of a cancer cell, causing an expansion of this malignant clone. Such clonal expansion results in increased susceptibility to additional mutations and consequently greater loss of growth control, increasing the potential for metastasis and growth in otherwise unfavorable environments. The pathophysiology of cancer derives from these defects which accumulate in cancer cells (whether caused by exogenous agents or spontaneous mutations).

A major hypothesis of molecular cancer biology is that these defects modify the networks that control cell proliferation and/or differentiation. These networks are primarily composed of signal transduction and cell regulatory pathways that normally operate to tightly regulate cellular responses to the environment. Fundamental support for this hypothesis derives from the following: 1) oncogenes (cancer-causing genes) encode for essential components of signal transduction and cell regulatory pathways; 2) transforming viruses modulate the expression and/or function of endogenous cell regulatory molecules; 3) spontaneous oncogenic mutations are increasingly found to result in deranged behavior of cell regulatory molecules, and 4) various classes of tumor promoters, which are agents that enhance cell transformation, act by interacting with basic elements of signal transduction pathways. These and other observations have begun to unify heretofore disparate fields of cancer biology. In turn, cancer biology has unified different fields of physiology, biochemistry, and genetic research.

It is now clear that to understand cancer at a molecular level we must understand the pathways of cell regulation and signal transduction. The study of signal transduction has traditionally involved the dissection of biochemical pathways involved in the proximal events leading from external stimuli to cellular responses. As such, signal transduction is a major component of cell regulation. Advances in the study of cell regulation have merged areas of signal transduction (proximal events) with more distal events, thus blurring the demarcation of signal transduction events. The emphasis in this chapter will be predominantly on proximal events of cell regulation, i.e., signal transduction.

It is the aim of this chapter to review briefly the current state of knowledge regarding components of signal transduction, their regulation and normal operation, and their implicated roles in cancer pathogenesis. Not only is this knowledge beginning to unify our understanding of cancer biology, but it potentially identifies discrete biochemical targets for cancer therapeutics. The first section will describe the general components of signaling mechanisms while the second provides a more detailed description of individual signal transduction pathways. The third section provides a general overview of the interrelationships between different signaling pathways and describes their complexity and organization. The fourth section describes aberrations in signal transduction and their role in oncogenesis and tumor promotion while the fifth section outlines the therapeutic potential afforded by this increasing understanding of how cellular signaling impacts on cancer biology.

How Do Cells Transduce Signals?

Each cell type is capable of sensing numerous extracellular signals. While there are extracellular agents which penetrate the plasma membrane and interact with intracellular receptors (e.g., steroids and nitric oxide), the vast majority of these agents interact with receptors in the plasma membrane (Figure I-4-2). These cell surface receptors play a pivotal role by specifically recognizing and interacting with a unique extracellular agent (or with a closely related set of agents). They then communicate to intracellular macromolecules the status of their receptor occupancy. This initiates flow of information through a series of signaling components and ultimately results in modulation of cell function.

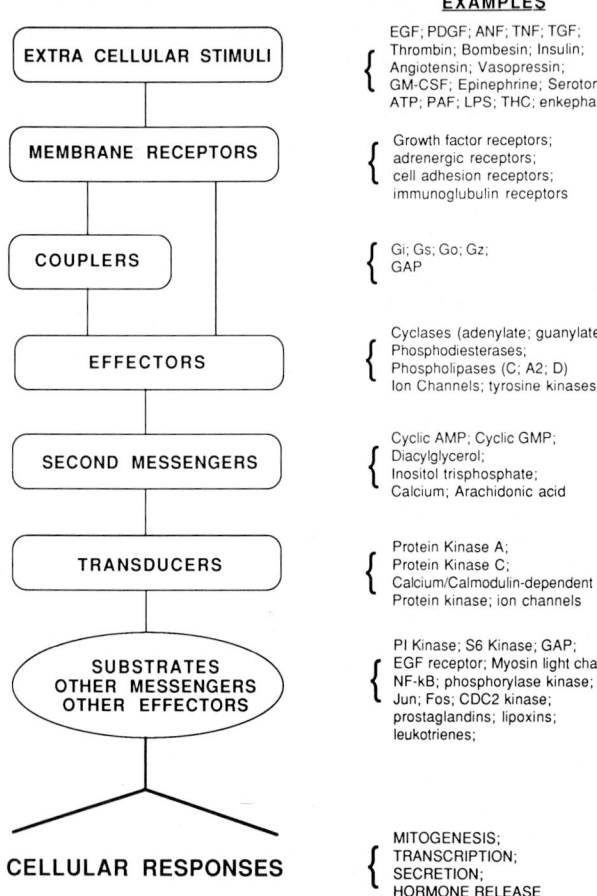

EXAMPLES

EXTRA CELLULAR STIMULI { EGF; PDGF; ANF; TNF; TGF; Thrombin; Bombesin; Insulin; Angiotensin; Vasopressin; GM-CSF; Epinephrine; Serotonin; ATP; PAF; LPS; THC; enkephalin

MEMBRANE RECEPTORS { Growth factor receptors; adrenergic receptors; cell adhesion receptors; immunoglobulin receptors

COUPLERS { Gi; Gs; Go; Gz; GAP

EFFECTORS { Cyclases (adenylate; guanylate); Phosphodiesterases; Phospholipases (C; A2; D) Ion Channels; tyrosine kinases

SECOND MESSENGERS { Cyclic AMP; Cyclic GMP; Diacylglycerol; Inositol trisphosphate; Calcium; Arachidonic acid

TRANSDUCERS { Protein Kinase A; Protein Kinase C; Calcium/Calmodulin-dependent Protein kinase; ion channels

SUBSTRATES OTHER MESSENGERS OTHER EFFECTORS { PI Kinase; S6 Kinase; GAP; EGF receptor; Myosin light chain; NF-kB; phosphorylase kinase; Jun; Fos; CDC2 kinase; prostaglandins; lipoxins; leukotrienes;

CELLULAR RESPONSES { MITOGENESIS; TRANSCRIPTION; SECRETION; HORMONE RELEASE

Figure I-4-2. Components of signal transduction pathways. Stimuli interact with membrane receptors that then couple effectors either directly or through couplers. Effectors usually act by generating second messengers which act on target transducers. These are usually protein kinases that modulate substrate phosphorylation. In other cases, initial signaling events lead to the activation of subsequent effectors and the generation of additional messengers. Examples of molecules belonging to each of these components are given to the right. EGF, epidermal growth factor; PDGF, platelet derived growth factor; ANF, atrial natriuretic factor; TNF, tumor necrosis factor; TGF, transforming growth factor; GM-CSF, granulocyte/macrophage-colony stimulating factor; PAF, platelet activating factor; LPS, lipopolysaccharide; THC, tetrahydrocannabinol; GAP, GTPase activating protein; Gi,Gs,Go,Gz, different G proteins; PI, phosphatidylinositol; NFκB, nuclear factor κB.

Extracellular Stimuli

The chemical composition of extracellular agents is quite diverse and includes proteins, small peptides, nucleotides, amino acid derivatives, carbohydrates, lipids, and other miscellaneous chemicals including neurotransmitters and many xenobiotics (Figure I-4-2). With very few exceptions, each of these extracellular agents has unique structural features that are recognized by its specific cell membrane receptor. This allows cells to recognize different stimuli accurately and initiate the appropriate response.

Growth factors form an important subset of extracellular stimuli (see below). They play essential roles in regulating cell proliferation and growth. Most known growth factors are polypeptides or glycoproteins; these include the transforming growth factors (TGF-α and TGF-β), interleukins, hematopoietic growth factors, epidermal growth factor (EGF), and platelet derived growth factor (PDGF). These growth factors are mitogenic (i.e., induce cell division) and, therefore, induce cell growth.[25] However, a few growth factors, such as transforming growth factor β (TGF-β), can also inhibit growth of many cell types.[47] An important feature of growth factors is that they possess multiple functions depending on the cell type.[68] For example, TGF-β can stimulate the growth of fibroblasts but inhibits the growth of many other cell types. Thrombin is a mitogen for fibroblasts and endothelial cells[76] but also functions as a critical component of blood coagulation and platelet activation.[66] Also, the action of growth factors may be dramatically influenced by the presence of other growth factors. TGF-β in the presence of PDGF stimulates the growth of fibroblasts, while the combination of TGF-β and EGF inhibits growth of these same cells.[61]

Membrane Receptors

Currently identified membrane receptors belong to a few large subfamilies. These include growth factor receptors[50] that are predominantly membrane spanning proteins (most receptors that have been studied are located at the plasma membrane; a few receptors have been suggested to also exist in the nuclear membrane). Receptors for growth factors are either single-chain proteins or multimers (usually homo or hetero dimers) (Figure I-4-3, Schemes I and VI). Many of the receptors in this group possess enzymatic activity in that they can phosphorylate other proteins and peptides on tyrosine residues (Figure I-4-3, Scheme I); i.e., they are tyrosine kinases (e.g., receptors for EGF, PDGF). Other receptors, however, do not possess tyrosine kinase activity (Figure I-4-3, Scheme V) such as those for TNF, interferon and interleukins.[1] Another major family of receptors is composed of protein molecules that appear to have seven transmembrane spanning regions.[30] These receptors (as well as some of those belonging to the first group) are able to specifically interact with intracellular proteins that function to couple bound-receptors to intracellular effector systems (Figure I-4-3, Schemes II and III). A third class of receptors is represented by the atrial natriuretic factor receptor which has an intracytoplasmic guanylate cyclase activity[36] (Figure I-4-3, Scheme IV). A major class of receptors, the immunoglobulin-receptor superfamily,[35] comprises receptors for immunoglobulins, T-cell antigens, and many cell-adhesion molecules. These and related receptors for cell adhesion molecules may play

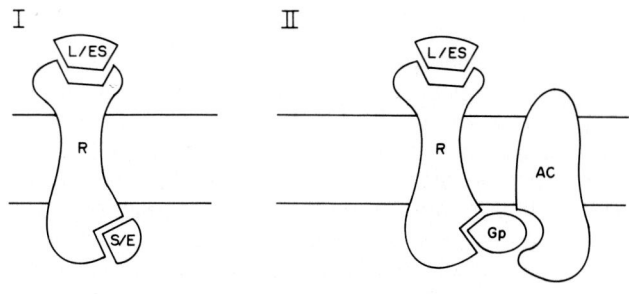

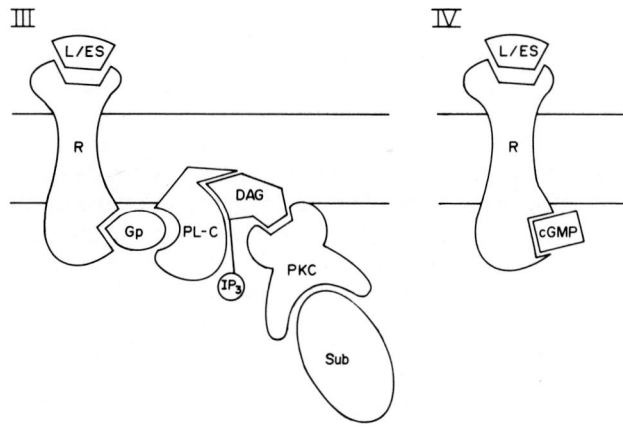

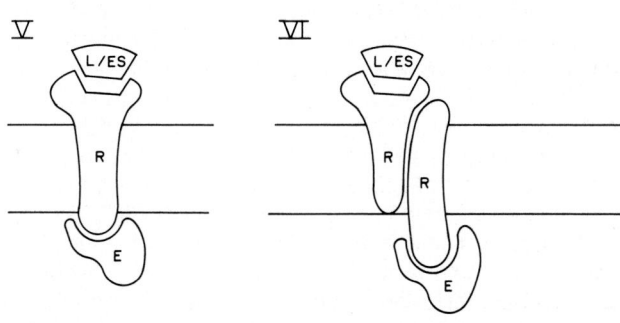

important roles in cell-cell interaction, cell adhesion, and mitogenesis. However, their coupling mechanisms are poorly understood. For all these receptor classes, a major question in the study of transmembrane signaling relates to the mechanism by which the binding of an extracellular agent to its membrane receptor initiates the biologic response. These are critical events that launch a series of sequential and parallel reactions in the cell. it is thought that significant changes in receptor conformation are imparted by receptor occupancy; however, the precise nature and mechanism of these changes are unknown.

G Proteins (Couplers)

The action of many membrane receptors is transduced by a distinct class of GTP-binding proteins known as G proteins.[14,17] These proteins appear to function primarily by coupling receptors to intracellular effectors (Figure I-4-2). They, therefore, play critical regulatory functions in directing intra-

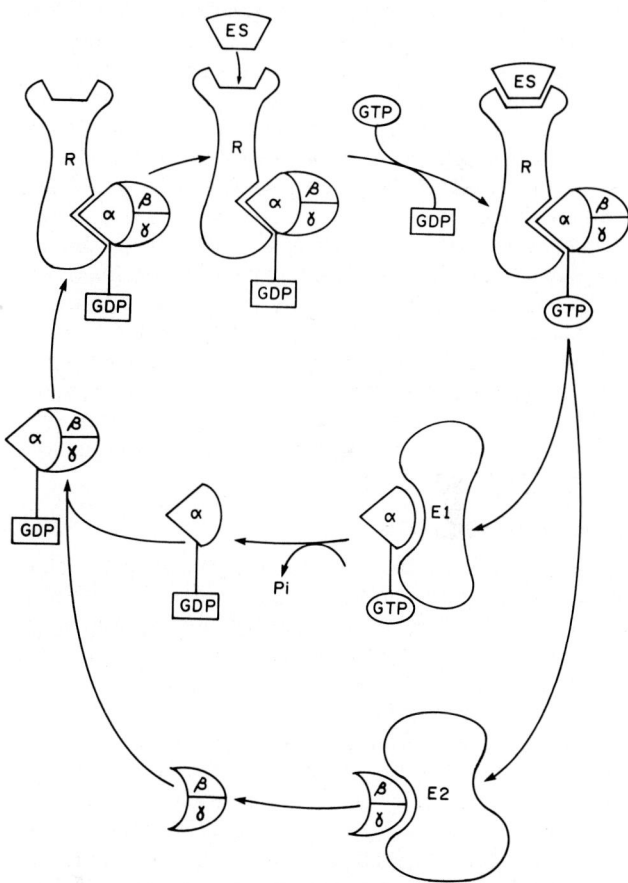

Figure I-4-3. Schematic of receptor classes. Most protein receptors are transmembrane proteins with an extracellular domain that contains the ligand binding site, an intramembranous domain, and an intracytoplasmic domain that usually harbors the site for interaction with couplers, effectors, or substrates. Many growth factor receptors are single or homodimer polypeptides with a single transmembrane domain (Scheme I and Scheme V) and an intracytoplasmic domain that has tyrosine kinase activity (Scheme I) or a short intracytoplasmic domain with no known effector function (Scheme V). A special case with the ANF receptor is the presence of guanylate cyclase activity in its intracytoplasmic domain (Scheme IV). Other receptors may exist as heterodimers with one or both components having ligand-binding sites (Scheme VI). Adrenergic and related receptors are characterized by seven transmembrane domains and an intracytoplasmic domain that couples to G proteins which in turn couple receptors to adenylate cyclase (Scheme II) or to phospholipase C (Scheme III). Growth factor receptors may also couple to phospholipase C and the PI cycle through G proteins (Scheme III). L/ES, ligand/extracellular stimulus; R, receptors; S/E substrate/effector; Gp, G protein; PL-C, phospholipase C; DAG, diacylglycerol; IP$_3$, inositol trisphosphate; PKC, protein kinase C; Sub, substrate.

Figure I-4-4. G protein cycle. Many membrane receptors may interact with G proteins which are trimers of α, β, and γ subunits with GDP bound to the α subunit. Upon receptor occupancy, the coupling of receptors to G proteins results in exchange of GDP for GTP. The GTP-bound α subunit then dissociates from the β γ subunit and regulates either directly or indirectly effector molecules such as adenylate cyclase. The β γ subunit may interact with other effector molecules such as ion channels and phospholipase A2. The α subunit possesses GTPase activity resulting in the release of phosphate from GTP and the generation of GDP. The GDP-bound α subunit then reassociates with the β γ subunit resulting in the formation of a resting complex.

cellular signaling traffic. Significant information has been amassed in the last decade regarding the nature, complexity, function, and roles of certain G-proteins in human disease. They are known to exist as two major families. The first is a family of large G-proteins which are heterotrimers composed of α, β, and γ subunits. There are multiple isoforms of these subunits that can associate in various combinations, resulting in distinct G proteins. In the resting state, the G protein exists with GDP tightly bound to the α chain (Figure I-4-4). Upon receptor occupancy, an appropriate conformational change in the receptor is triggered which results in modulation of the interaction of receptors with G proteins, causing replacement of bound GPD with GTP. GTP binding is accompanied by dissociation of the α chain from the β γ chains.[17] The released GTP-liganded α chain may then interact with certain effector molecules such as adenylate cyclase and phospholipase C[17] (Figure I-4-4), while the β γ chains may have function on their own (such as interaction with phospholipase A$_2$).[14] Signal termination results from the ability of G proteins to hydrolyze the bound GTP, thus regenerating GDP and reassociating the α with the β γ subunits.

Another family of G-proteins consists of small molecular weight G proteins (Smgs) that share homology with the α subunit of large molecular weight G proteins. These include the protooncogene ras, and other related molecules such as rev, rab, and rap. Smgs are also able to bind GTP and cause its hydrolysis, i.e., they possess GTPase activity.[38] GTPase activating proteins (GAPs), which potentiate the enzymatic activity of many Smgs, have been described. The GAPs serve as substrates of tyrosine kinases and may couple receptors to Smgs and possibly serve as down stream effectors. Although the role of small molecular weight G proteins in signal transduction is not clear, mutations in some of these molecules are oncogenic (see below). They also appear to be important for other cell function such as trafficking of macromolecules.

Effector Molecules

Effector molecules play a key role in transducing the action of extracellular agents following their interaction with their cell surface receptors. As noted above, many growth factor receptors possess intrinsic tyrosine kinase activity which is activated upon receptor occupancy.[50] This enzymatic activity then serves as an effector function for this class of receptors. For receptors that are coupled to G proteins,[17] however, it is these G proteins that regulate the activity of key effector enzymes (Figure I-4-2). The most notable such enzymes are adenylate cyclase and phospholipase C. Phospholipases C[46] serve to catalyze the hydrolysis of membrane phospholipids thereby generating diacylglycerol and inositol trisphosphates. Adenylate cyclase catalyzes the formation of cyclic AMP from ATP.[41] Diacylglycerol, inositol trisphosphates, and cyclic AMP then serve as important and potent second messengers.

While the effector function of either phospholipase C or adenylate cyclase appears to be utilized by many receptors, the extent and diversity of effector molecules is rapidly expanding (Figure I-4-2). Phospholipases C exist as a super family of enzymes that catalyze the hydrolysis of various membrane phospholipids (see below). Other signaling effectors include guanylate cyclase, which may either occur as an intrinsic element within certain membrane receptors[36] or as a separate soluble enzyme.[23] Another major effector is phospholipase A2, which hydrolyzes membrane phospholipids such as phosphatidylcholine. The main product of phospholipase A2 action is arachidonic acid from which many active metabolites are derived.[26,71] Other important effectors include ion channels[15] which may be directly or indirectly regulated by transducers such as G proteins and phosphodiesterases which hydrolyze and inactivate cyclic GMP.

Second Messengers and Mediators

The main function of effector molecules is the generation of second messengers that transduce the information generated by receptor occupancy into functional events. This function is achieved by altering the activity of key regulatory enzymes. Second messengers identified so far appear to be small molecules which are able to regulate target function specifically (Figure I-4-2). Most second messengers appear to derive from membrane lipids or intracellular nucleotides. The best studied and most ubiquitous second messengers are diacylglycerol, inositol trisphosphates, cyclic AMP, cyclic GMP, and calcium (Figures I-4-5 and I-4-6). Other emerging second messengers include arachidonic acid and its metabolites, phosphatidic acid, and sphingolipid-derived molecules. Many second messengers act by activating protein kinases either directly or indirectly (see below).

The formation of second messengers is under strict control. Their intracellular levels appear to be low in the resting state and increase, usually abruptly (Figure I-4-7), following receptor occupancy and activation of effectors such as phospholipase C or adenylate cyclase. The signal is then maintained for variable (Figure I-4-7), often short, durations (usually measured in seconds or minutes), and is terminated by metabolism of the second messenger into inactive metabolites. During this brief interval when the intracellular signal is generated, it is able to dramatically modulate the function of key target elements such as protein kinases. Obviously, deranged generation or metabolism of these second messengers could have profound effects on cell function (see I-7). The magnitude of the signal is also important in determining the extent of the cellular response. In turn, this is modulated by the potency of the extracellular stimulus, the degree of receptor occupancy, the nature of the coupling mechanisms, the effectiveness of cellular enzymes in metabolizing and extinguishing the signal, and a variety of positive and negative feedback mechanisms.

Immediate Targets for Second Messengers (Transducers)

The targets of action of second messengers play a key role in regulating diverse cellular activities ranging from short term effects such as hormone release and blood cell activation, to long term effects such as cell differentiation, tumor promotion, and oncogenesis. The best studied and most universal of these targets are protein kinases[21,28] that enzymatically transfer a phosphate from cellular ATP (or GTP) to serine, threonine, or tyrosine residues on various cellular proteins (see I-7). This phosphorylation event results in conformational changes in target substrates with significant

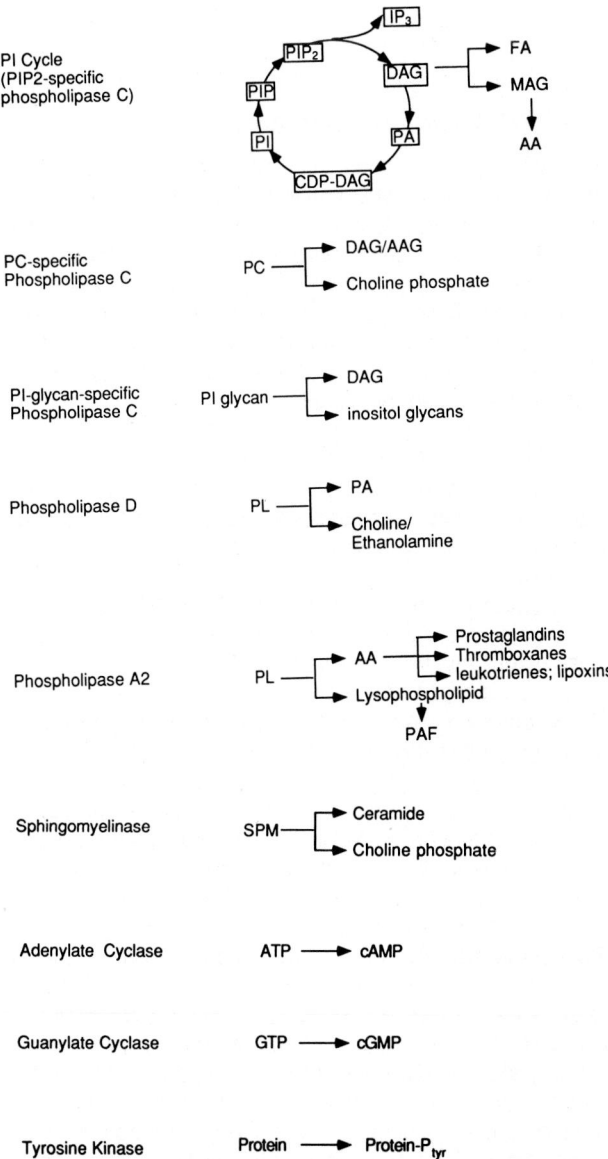

Figure I-4-5. Effector/second messenger systems. The different effector systems are shown. Enzyme activities are indicated on the left side, and schematic reactions showing precursors and second messengers are indicated on the right side of the figure. For structures and explanation of abbreviations see Figure I-4-6.

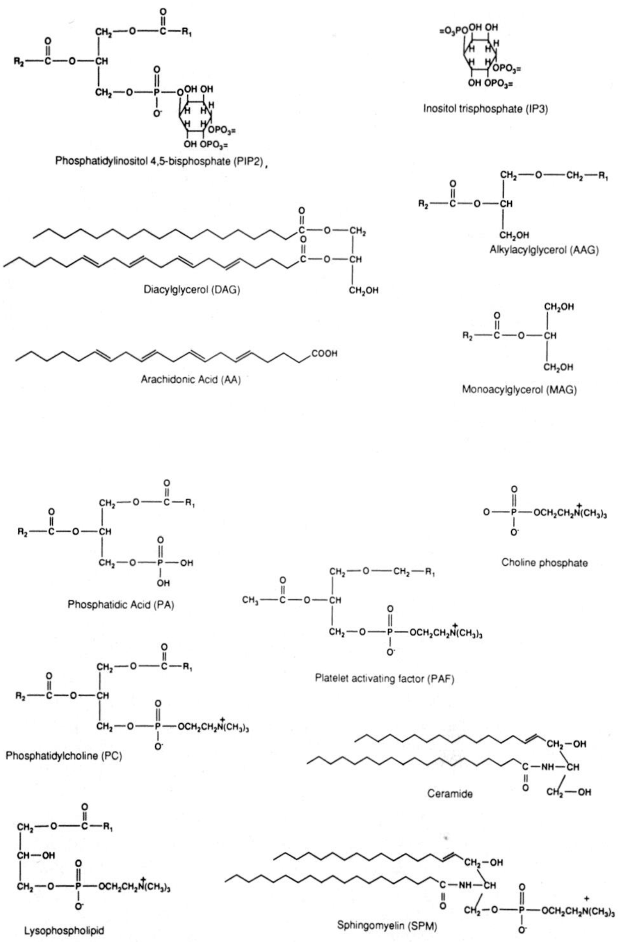

functional effects such as activation/inhibition of other kinases, metabolic enzymes, and/or transcriptional factors. Other known transducers of second messenger effects include protein phosphatases, proteases, and ion channels.

Major questions in molecular cell biology relate to the identification of physiologic targets for the action of transducers of second messenger action, and linking initial events of signal transduction to the functional outcome at a molecular level. At present, these remain largely elusive goals since not all components of the diverse signaling pathways have been defined and since the more distal mediators of cellular events have not yet been linked to proximal components of signaling pathways.

Figure I-4-6. Structures of second messengers and precursors.

Subsequent Messengers and Effectors

While many second messengers go on to directly interact with enzymes that mediate their effects, a number of second messengers operate by liberating a third stage of messenger molecules. For example, inositol trisphosphate activates intracellular calcium channels resulting in liberation of calcium from intracellular stores.[9] The generating of an intracellular calcium signal activates a number of calcium binding proteins, such as calmodulin, and leads to the modulation of the activity of a number of key regulatory enzymes and targets. In other cases, a second messenger may be metabolized to yield other messengers with distinct effects. This is best studied in the case of arachidonic acid which is further metabolized into active metabolites (Figures I-4-5 and I-4-6) with various biologic functions.[10] Diacylglycerol may be further metabolized to yield monoacylglycerol, which may have mitogenic activity,[69] and arachidonic acid (Figure I-4-5). Also, cascades of protein kinases exist whereby the activation of one kinase leads to phosphorylation and activation of a subsequent kinase (Figure I-4-2).[21]

Distal Components/Substrates of Protein Kinases

It appears that protein kinases play an essential role in signal transduction mechanisms. A major difficulty in under-

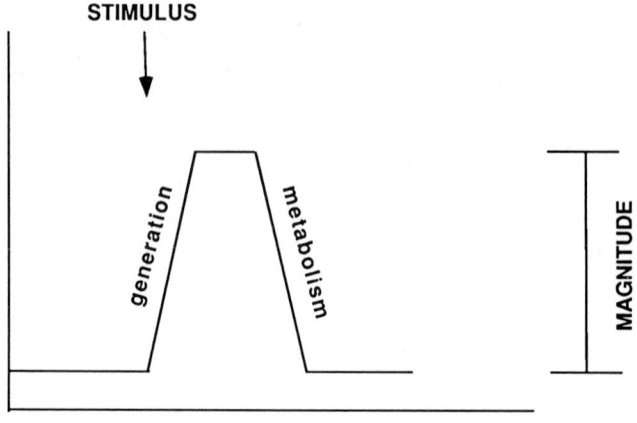

Figure I-4-7. The second messenger response. The interaction of extracellular stimuli with cells leads to the activation of effector molecules with the generation of second messengers such as diacylglycerol, cyclic AMP, cyclic GMP, inositol trisphosphate, and arachidonic acid. This results in a build up of levels of those second messengers from usually very low resting levels. The magnitude of peak intracellular levels of second messengers are determined primarily by the strength of the extracellular stimulus as well as by a variety of feedback mechanisms. In most cases, the duration of the second messenger response is limited by active metabolism of second messengers to either inactive metabolites or metabolites with different spectra of activities. The duration of the response is determined by the balance between generation and metabolism and is therefore modulated by the strength of the extracellular stimulus, the presence of multiple extracellular stimuli, feedback mechanisms, and degradation.

standing the mechanisms by which extracellular signals modulate discrete cellular functions relates to the identification of substrates whose phosphorylation by protein kinases results in modification of cellular responses. While many such substrates have been identified in vitro, correlating in vitro phosphorylation to an in vivo cellular response continues to be one of the most resistant problems facing investigators in this area of research.

As noted above, many of the substrates for protein kinases are protein kinases themselves. This results in signal amplification through a cascade of different protein kinases. Many of the ultimate substrates of protein kinases are rate limiting enzymes in metabolic cascades, a classic example being glycogen phosphorylase in the pathway of glycogen metabolism.

The pathways from protein kinases to more long term effects (Figure I-4-2) such as cell proliferation/differentiation appear to be particularly quite complex. At present, this trail appears to be lost in the cytoplasm but can be picked up again in the nucleus (see above). A number of transcription regulators appear to be phosphoproteins whose activities may be significantly regulated by phosphorylation/dephosphorylation. The best studied of these factors are Myc, Myb, Jun, Fos and NFκB, all of which have oncogenic counterparts (see below).

Signal Transduction Systems

Although signal transduction mechanisms are closely interrelated, a number of signal transduction pathways may, at a first level of approximation, be considered as discrete entities. The complexities generated by cross talk, feedback, divergence, and convergence of signal tranduction mechanisms are discussed below. A brief overview of the major known signal transduction pathways with special emphasis on their role in cell regulation, mitogenesis, and possible involvement in oncogenesis follows.

The Phosphatidylinositol Cycle

It has been almost four decades since investigators first observed changes in phospholipid levels following stimulation of pancreatic cells with acetylcholine.[32] The changes in phospholipids were rapid and involved the incorporation of labeled phosphate into phosphatidylinositol (PI) and phosphatidic acid. This was associated with acetylcholine-induced release of amylase from pancreatic acinar cells. Since these initial observations, it has become evident that the activation of many receptors leads to degradation of inositol phospholipids followed by resynthesis through the formation of phosphatidic acid as an intermediate (Figure I-4-5). This has come to be termed the phosphatidylinositol cycle of cell regulation (PI cycle). The enzymes involved in PI hydrolysis, the second messengers generated from the breakdown of inositol phospholipids, and the role of this important cycle in various cellular processes are being increasingly clarified.

Phospholipase C. The first regulated enzyme in the PI cycle is a phospholipase C which has specificity towards inositol phospholipids.[46] Coupling of surface receptors to phospholipase C appears to occur either through the intermediatory action of G proteins (e.g., receptors for thrombin, bombesin, and others) or through direct tyrosine phosphorylation of phospholipase C by activated receptors (e.g., receptors for epidermal growth factor or platelet derived growth factor) (Figure I-4-3). Phospholipase C is known to exist as a family of isoenzymes with variable tissue distribution, substrate specificity, and different requirements for calcium.[60] These phospholipases share an ability to hydrolyze inositol phospholipids, especially phosphatidylinositol bisphosphate. This results in the formation of two ubiquitous and important second messengers; inositol trisphosphate and diacylglycerol (Figures I-4-5 and I-4-6).

Inositol Trisphosphate. Inositol 1,4,5 trisphosphate, the released hydrophilic head group of phosphatidylinositol bisphosphate, mobilizes calcium from intracellular stores (thought to be the endoplasmic reticulum).[9] The resulting elevation in cytoplasmic calcium levels activates calcium-regulated enzymes. A critical result of calcium elevation is its binding to calmodulin, a major intracellular calcium binding protein. The calcium/calmodulin complex then interacts with a number of enzymes[18] including calcium/calmodulin dependent protein kinases, phosphatases and phosphodiesterases. Calcium/calmodulin dependent protein kinases consist of a family of related isoenzymes with wide tissue distribution.[21]

They include myosin light chain kinases, which play important roles in muscle function, as well neuron-specific isoenzymes with presumed functions in neural development, neurotransmission, and memory.

There are multiple species of inositol phosphates interconnected by complex metabolic pathways.[9,46] Only inositol 1,4,5-trisphosphate has a well-defined function in endogenous release of calcium. Another close relative, inositol tetrakisphosphate, may play a role in calcium entry into the cell.[49] The function of other inositol phosphates remains undetermined.

Diacylglycerol/Protein Kinase C. Diacylglycerol, the other product of phosphatidylinositol bisphosphate hydrolysis, is a neutral lipid second messenger[6] that specifically activates protein kinase C[55] (Figure I-4-3, Scheme III). This central event in signal transduction has not only linked protein kinase C to the PI cycle but also has linked PI turnover to the field of tumor promoters[55] (see below). Protein kinase C is a calcium- and phospholipid-dependent protein kinase that is specifically activated by diacylglycerols. It is also activated by phorbol ester-type tumor promoters. Protein kinase C is now known to consist of a family of closely related isoenzymes with different tissue distribution. Activation of protein kinase C occurs whenever the PI cycle is turned on in response to various extracellular stimuli. Protein kinase C appears to have multiple roles in hormone secretion, neurotransmission, cell proliferation, and cell differentiation.[55]

Protein kinase C phosphorylates a number of substrates that mediate the various physiologic responses associated with its activation. Although both the nature of these substrates and the signaling pathways leading to cellular responses remain poorly defined, certain pathways have received special attention as possible mediators of the effects of protein kinase C on mitogenesis and gene regulation (Figure I-4-8). The first involves the activation of the transcription factor NFκB. Activation of protein kinase C in lymphoid cells results in phosphorylation of IκB in cytosol, which is an inhibitor of NFκB.[24] This results in liberation of NFκB and its translocation to the nucleus where it acts by modulating the transcription of a number of genes including those for TNF and IL-2 receptor (Figure I-4-8).

Another transcription pathway, activated by protein kinase C, is that involving c-fos and c-jun protein products. The phosphorylation of as yet undetermined substrates results in dimerization of these two proteins to form the AP-1 transcription factor which modulates gene transcription (Figure I-4-8).[3] AP-1 function appears to be associated with sensitivity to tumor promotion.[7] A third pathway involves the phosphorylation of the transcription factor CREB-ATF by protein kinase C. This leads to dimerization and activation of CREB/ATF which then acts to modulate the transcription of a number of genes.[64] Because of the involvement of NFκB, CREB/ATF, Jun, and Fos in mitogenesis and oncogenesis, these studies implicate protein kinase C as an important regulator of these cell responses.

The discovery that protein kinase C is the predominant intracellular receptor for phorbol esters and that phorbol esters activate protein kinase C by substituting for endogenous diacylglycerol implicated protein kinase C in the process of tumor promotion and oncogenesis.[55] This has been further

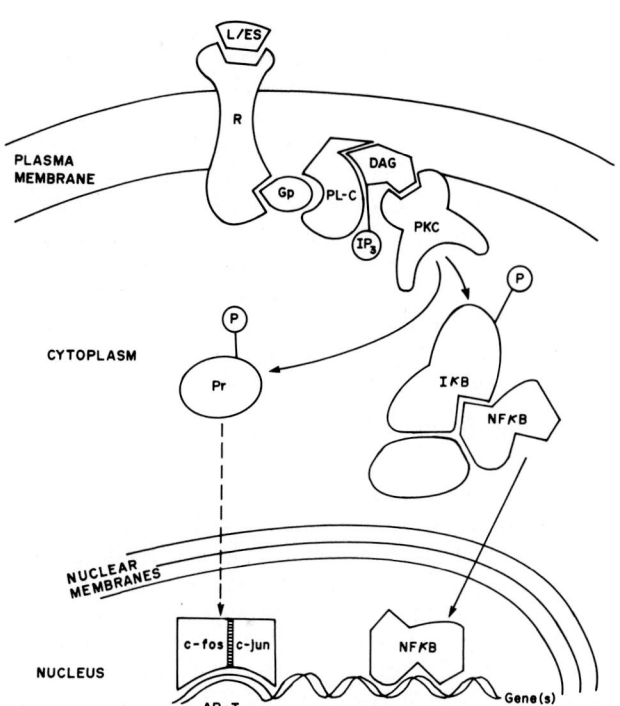

Figure I-4-8. Signaling pathways and gene regulation. This scheme illustrates two potential pathways relating signal transduction to gene regulation. The generation of diacylglycerol second messengers through the operation of the PI cycle (as shown above) or from other sources (see Figure I-4-5) leads to activation of protein kinase C which in turn phosphorylates a number of proteins. Phosphorylation of IκB results in dissociation of NFκB from this inhibitory cytoplasmic complex and translocation of NFκB to the nucleus where it is able to modulate transcription of nuclear genes as a homodimer, heterodimer, or tetramer. In another pathway, protein kinase C phosphorylation of, as yet unknown substrates, results in activation of AP-1 transcription factor, which is composed of a heterodimer of c-fos and c-jun that interacts with AP-1 sites on a number of genes thus modulating gene transcription. Other pathways (not shown) involve activation of CREB nuclear factors by protein kinase C and by cAMP-dependent protein kinase.

substantiated by multiple lines of evidence. First, many nonphorbol ester tumor promoters directly activate protein kinase C. Second, overexpression of protein kinase C in fibroblasts results in altered cell growth and acquisition of a transformed phenotype.[57] Third, fibroblasts containing overexpressed protein kinase C cause the formation of tumors in nude mice, a model for testing the oncogenic potential of various transformed cells.[57] Fourth, a mutated protein kinase C has been discovered in ultraviolet-transformed fibroblast cells; expression of the mutant PKC in normal fibroblasts resulted in cell transformation.[48] Finally, overproduction of protein kinase C increases the transforming potential of activated ras oncogenes.[34] These studies suggest that protein kinase C can act as an oncogene, a predictable result given its important role in cell regulation and mitogenesis.

Increasing evidence also implicates the phospholipase C/protein kinase C pathway as a potential target for a number of oncogenes. According to this hypothesis, the increased activity of oncogene products (due to overexpression or to expression of abnormal forms), observed in many cancers and transformed cell lines may primarily result in overdriving normal signal transduction pathways, especially the protein kinase C pathway. Support for this hypothesis has been forthcoming from a number of investigations. These studies have shown that overexpression of ras or sis oncogenes results in increased levels of diacylglycerol with consequent abnormal regulation of protein kinase C.[58] Prolonged elevation in intracellular diacylglycerol levels may mimic the action of tumor promoters. Thus, abnormal diacylglycerol metabolism may have oncogenic potential, and diacylglycerol may function as an endogenous tumor promoter. The exact mechanisms by which these effects are mediated and their overall contribution to the oncogenic potentials of these transforming oncogenes is yet to be determined.

Other Lipid-Derived Signal Transduction Pathways

Other Phospholipase Cs. Recent investigations have demonstrated the existence of phospholipases C with specificity towards phospholipids other than inositol phospholipids.[22] These appear to primarily act on phosphatidylcholine with the resulting generation of diacylglycerol and choline phosphate (Figures I-4-5 and I-4-6). Because plasma membrane content of phosphatidylcholine far exceeds that of inositol phospholipids (by a ratio of at least five or ten to one), induction of phosphatidylcholine hydrolysis may result in production of significantly larger quantities of diacylglycerol than observed with PI hydrolysis. This would result in prolonged elevation in diacylglycerol levels and sustained activation of protein kinase C. Therefore, the phosphatidylcholine pathway of signal transduction may be particularly relevant for mediation of mitogenic effects of cell surface receptors through the protein kinase C pathway. This has been suggested for the action of platelet-derived growth factor, interleukin-1, vasopressin, and phorbol esters. Although this pathway duplicates the ability of the PI cycle to generate diacylglycerol, a major distinguishing feature is the lack of concomitant generation of inositol trisphosphate with consequent elevation of intracellular calcium levels. Therefore, activation of phosphatidylcholine hydrolysis may lead to specific activation of protein kinase C independent of calcium mediated events. It has been suggested that oncogenic ras activates this pathway of signaling.[42]

Other phospholipases appear to have specificity towards complex inositol phospholipids termed PI glycans.[44] Hydrolysis of these lipids by a phospholipase C reaction results in the generation of diacylglycerol and inositol glycans (Figures I-4-5 and I-4-6). The latter may play important roles in mediating some of the actions of insulin and nerve growth factor. The structure of these putative second messengers is complex and appears to consist of inositol linked to complex carbohydrates composed of galactose, mannose, as well as ethanolamine. Again, the extent and significance of this signaling pathway is unclear.

Phospholipase D/Phosphatidic Acid Pathway. Hormone interaction with cell membrane receptor has recently been demonstrated to result in the activation of phospholipase D.[11] These stimuli include epinephrine, vasopressin, epidermal growth factor, platelet-derived growth factor, and others. The action of phospholipase D on membrane phospholipids results in a different chemical cleavage from that induced by phos-

pholipase C. When the substrate is phosphatidylcholine, the action of phospholipase D results in the formation of choline and phosphatidic acid (Figures I-4-5 and I-4-6). Phosphatidic acid may have its own cellular actions including mitogenesis. It may also serve as a precursor for the generation of diacylglycerol which would then activate protein kinase C.

The Phospholipase A$_2$/Arachidonic Acid Pathway. A major effect of the action of many extracellular stimuli is the activation of phospholipase A$_2$.[26,71] This enzyme liberates fatty acids from the 2 position of membrane phospholipids, where arachidonic acid is primarily located. The mechanisms responsible for activation of phospholipase A$_2$ remain poorly understood. Evidence appears to implicate either a role for calcium or the β and γ subunits of the heterotrimeric G proteins[14] (Figure I-4-4). Lysophospholipids (Figures I-4-5 and I-4-6), generated from the action of phospholipase A$_2$, may have their own effects on cells although these are not well defined. Lyso (alkyl) phosphatidylcholine may also serve as a precursor for platelet activating factor which has important mitogenic and cell-activating functions. Arachidonic acid, on the other hand, is known to exert effects of its own including interaction with membrane channels, protein kinase C, and other enzymes. More importantly, arachidonic acid appears to serve as a precursor for major cell regulatory molecules (Figures I-4-5 and I-4-6). These belong to different classes depending on the metabolic pathways involved in their synthesis. Metabolism through the cyclooxygenase pathway results in the formation of a number of prostaglandins, prostacyclins, and thromboxanes. Alternatively, arachidonic acid may be metabolized through the lipoxygenase pathway resulting in the formation of lipoxins and leukotrienes.[63] Many of these metabolites act as intercellular stimuli/messengers. These appear to have specific cell surface receptors[72] that transduce their action by activating adenylate cyclase, phospholipase C, or other signaling mechanisms. These metabolites have pleiotropic activities including effects on smooth muscle contractility, platelet aggregation, and mitogenesis.

Sphingolipids. Sphingolipids are important membrane lipids that show structural diversity and complexity that far exceeds that seen with glycerophospholipids. Investigations over many decades have established important roles for sphingolipids in different biologic processes, especially in cell contact, cell proliferation, and cell differentiation.[27,29] They have served as important tumor and differentiation markers. For example, the progression of human melanoma to more aggressive phenotypes is associated with the acquisition of novel sphingolipids. Their mechanisms of action, however, remain poorly understood.

Recent studies have begun exploring potential roles for sphingolipids and sphingolipid-derived molecules in signal transduction and as second messengers.[29] Sphingosine and related lysosphingolipids are potent inhibitors of protein kinase C. They also inhibit calcium/calmodulin dependent kinases and other biochemical targets although at somewhat higher concentrations. These molecules also appear to modulate the activity of tyrosine kinases such as the EGF receptor. Another sphingolipid, ceramide, appears to play important roles in cell differentiation. Ceramide is derived from membrane sphingomyelin upon the activation of a neutral sphingomyelinase in response to the action of a number of extracellular stimuli including vitamin D_3 and tumor necrosis factor (Figures I-4-5 and I-4-6). The existence of a sphingomyelin cycle analogous to the PI cycle of cell regulation has been proposed.[56] The diversity, regulation, and functional roles of these sphingolipid-derived molecules is under active investigation. These sphingolipids with negative effects on mitogenesis may provide the endogenous brakes and checks on signaling mechanisms involved in mediating the mitogenic action of various extracellular agents. As such, they may represent important targets for the action of oncogenes and anti-oncogenes.

Cyclases/Cyclic Nucleotide Signal Transduction Pathways

Adenylate Cyclase and Cyclic AMP. The first signaling mechanism to be dissected involved cyclic AMP as the second messenger. The interaction of many extracellular stimuli (e.g., adrenergic compounds, acetylcholine, serotonin) with their cell surface receptors is coupled to adenylate cyclase through the action of G proteins.[17,41] G protein-linked pathways exist for both the activation and inhibition of adenylate cyclase. This critical transmembrane enzyme catalyzes the formation of cyclic AMP from ATP (Figure I-4-5). Cyclic AMP acts as a second messenger to activate protein kinase A[21] (also known as cyclic AMP dependent protein kinase). Activation of protein kinase A results from interaction of cyclic AMP with a regulatory component of this enzyme, leading to dissociation of the catalytic subunit of the enzyme. The liberated catalytic subunit is then able to phosphorylate a number of protein substrates on serine and threonine residues, thereby modulating their activities.[21] Numerous substrates for protein kinase A have been identified in vitro and in vivo including the transcription factor(s) CREB/ATF.

Activation of the protein kinase A pathway of signaling has been implicated in a number of cellular processes including neurotransmission, hormone release, as well as in mitogenesis and cell differentiation.

Guanylate Cyclases and Cyclic GMP. Signaling mechanisms involving cyclic GMP as their second messenger have come under increasing investigation as a result of two, initially divergent, areas of cell biology. Cell biologists had identified the existence of factors termed EDRF (for endothelium derived relaxing factor) that act to cause smooth muscle relaxation. Recent evidence strongly suggests that this factor is in fact nitric oxide or a closely related molecule.[52] Nitric oxide (NO) appears to be not only the putative EDRF but also to be the mediator of action of a number of nitroso compounds such as nitrites and nitroprusside, agents of great importance in cardiovascular pharmacology. NO also appears to mediate tumor cell killing by macrophages. A major proximal target of NO appears to be a soluble form of guanylate cyclase. NO interacts with guanylate cyclase and liberates a heme moiety. This results in activation of the enzyme[23,52] and rapid intracellular formation of cyclic GMP. In turn, cyclic GMP is then able to activate cyclic GMP dependent protein kinase (protein kinase G).

Recent investigations have identified atrial natruretic peptide (or factor) as an important regulator of circulating fluid volume. Studies on the structure of the cellular receptor for atrial natruretic factor yielded the unexpected result that the intracellular domain of this receptor is a guanylate cyclase[36] (Figure I-4-3, Scheme IV). It is now established that the action of atrial natruretic factor on its receptor results in guanylate cyclase activation and the formation of cyclic GMP as a messenger. Atrial natruretic factor also has important mitogenic activities. These studies implicate cyclic GMP as a potentially important second messenger in the mitogenic response.

Receptor-Regulated Tyrosine Kinases

The receptors for many extracellular ligands possess a tyrosine kinase activity that is regulated by the status of receptor occupancy;[50] ligand interaction leads to activation of the tyrosine kinase activity of the receptor. It appears that this tyrosine kinase activity plays an essential role in receptor function. Mutant receptors biochemically engineered to lack the kinase activity lose their function. Major advances in understanding signaling through receptor tyrosine kinases came with the identification of a number of regulatory and effector molecules that are substrates for these receptors. These include a form of phospholipase C which is directly phosphorylated on tyrosine by receptors for epidermal growth factor and platelet-derived growth factor.[39] This phosphorylation may result in activation of the phospholipase C and initiation of signaling through that pathway (see above). Another emerging target for receptor tyrosine kinases is PI kinase.[75] This enzyme phosphorylates inositol phospholipids at the 3 position leading to the formation of a special class of inositol phospholipids. The role of this lipid in signaling, however, is poorly understood. GTPase activating protein (GAP) also appears to be a substrate for receptor tyrosine kinases,[51] and its phosphorylation may modulate its interaction with ras-like effector molecules. A number of other cellular substrates are known to be phosphorylated on tyrosine residues although it is not known whether this phosphorylation is due to receptor tyrosine kinases or other non-receptor tyrosine kinases. These substrates include the serine kinase encoded by the CDC2 gene which plays an important role in regulation of cell cycle.[53]

Other Components of Signal Transduction Mechanisms

A number of enzymes and molecules appear to play important roles in cell regulation and signal transduction. However, unlike the above described signaling pathways, their placement on a specific pathway has so far eluded investigators. These molecules include a number of serine-threonine protein kinases[21] such as S6 kinase and casein kinases, non-receptor tyrosine kinases[28] such as src kinase, and small molecular weight G-proteins such as ras.[59] It is generally accepted that these play essential roles in cell regulation. This is best attested to by the oncogenic potential of overexpression or mutation of these components, such as occurs with the oncogenic ras and src proteins. The direct activators of these molecules have not been determined nor have their substrates or targets of action. Many hypotheses have been generated as to what are important substrates for non-receptor tyrosine kinases and what are the effector mechanisms for ras and ras-like small molecular weight G-proteins. At this point, however, the position of these molecules in signaling pathways remains undetermined.

Complexity of Signal Transduction Pathways

Signaling pathways operate to transduce external stimuli to specific cellular responses. The basic structural and biochemical organization of signal transduction pathways as outlined in the previous section may, at a first level of approximation, be considered to consist of components that act in series to transduce the effect of extracellular signals. For example, growth factor interaction with cell receptors may lead to activation of phospholipase C through the coupling action of a G protein. This in turn generates a second messenger such as diacylglycerol, which activates a protein kinase. The consequent phosphorylation of key proteins would then modify cell function and lead to the desired response.

If a strict 1:1 correspondence between each two consecutive components of signal transduction pathways exists, then the action of any one extracellular agent would operate through a unique signal transduction pathway resulting in a distinct cellular response. While such a scenario would be conceptually easy to understand and would be more amenable to experimental study, it does not appear to approximate reality. In fact, had cells required each unique receptor to have its own unique coupling protein and unique effector mechanisms, cells would have required an enormous number of unique signaling pathways (probably measured in the hundreds). Apparently cells do not require a unique signaling mechanism for each response. This is understandable since each unique cell type is capable of carrying only a limited repertoire of functional activities even in response to diverse extracellular agents. Also, different cells may use similar signal transduction pathways to couple unique responses to various stimuli. For example, leukocytes and blood platelets may utilize the same or similar mechanisms to couple a "killing" response to foreign organisms on the one hand, and an aggregation response to thrombotic agents on the other. Similar pathways may couple the mitogenic response of epithelial cells to growth factors. These features allow significant simplification of signal transduction mechanisms. Paradoxically, this introduces substantial complexity in our understanding of signaling pathways. In the following section an overview of how signaling components may interact and how complexity is generated in signaling systems is presented.

Convergence of Signaling Pathways

A one to one correspondence of signaling components requires that each extracellular stimulus (S) binds to a unique receptor (R) which interacts with a unique coupler (C) allowing it to transmit information to a unique effector (E) which then generates one second messenger (SM) that in turn activates a unique transducer (T) which in the case of a protein kinase (PK) would phosphorylate a unique substrate (Sub) (Figure I-4-9, Scheme I). Examples of deviation occur at almost each and every level, so that it is the exception where unique consecutive targets interact in series coupling an extracellular stimulus to a cellular response. These different scenarios are illustrated in Figure I-4-9.

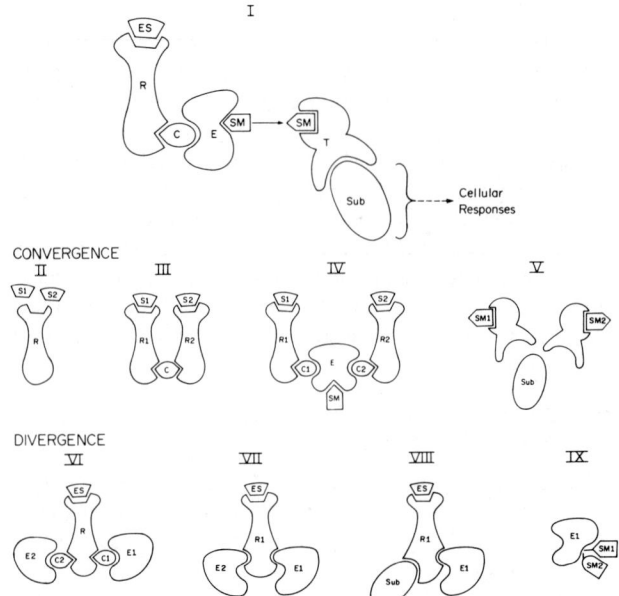

Figure I-4-9. Variations of signal transduction pathways. I: Schematic representation of a generic signal transduction pathway involving an extracellular stimulus, receptor, G protein, effector, second messenger, and transducer; the latter usually being a protein kinase phosphorylating a substrate. Phosphorylation of one or more substrates is then translated into a cellular response. II: More than one extracellular substrate may interact with the same receptor, such as occurs with TGFα and EGF. III: Two unique receptors may interact with the same G protein. IV: Two different G proteins may interact with the same effector, such as occurs with Gs and Gi acting on adenylate cyclase to stimulate and inhibit it, respectively. V: More distally in the signaling pathways, two protein kinases may act to phosphorylate the same substrate. VI: The same receptor may couple two distinct effectors via two distinct G proteins. VII: One receptor (such as tyrosine kinase receptors for growth factors) may phosphorylate two different effector molecules. VIII: A single receptor may phosphorylate one substrate and activate another effector. IX: A single effector may result in the generation of two distinct second messengers.

The one to one correspondence is best preserved in the interaction of unique extracellular stimuli with unique cell surface molecules. There are a few isolated exceptions whereby distinct, but closely related, extracellular stimuli interact with the same cellular receptor. This is best illustrated in the case of transforming growth factor α and epidermal growth factor, which appear to interact with the same cellular receptor,[73] the epidermal growth factor receptor (Figure I-4-9, Scheme II).

Many distinct receptors appear to utilize similar coupling mechanisms. For example, many distinct receptors couple to adenylate cyclase through identical G proteins[17] (Figure I-4-9, Scheme III). Similarly, different receptors may interact with different coupling proteins that would then interact with the same effector. This is also illustrated in the adenylate cyclase effector system whereby stimulatory and inhibitory adrenergic receptors couple to stimulatory and inhibitory G proteins, respectively.[17] This results in stimulation or inhibition of adenylate cyclase (Figure I-4-9, Scheme IV). As noted above, a number of growth factor receptors possess intrinsic tyrosine kinase activity. Therefore, the effector mechanism in this signaling pathway apparently resides in the receptor itself, obviating the need for a coupling mechanism.

Distinct signaling mechanisms may also converge at more distal components. For example, different protein kinases may phosphorylate the same substrates resulting in similar cellular responses (Figure I-4-9, Scheme V).

Divergence of Signaling

While the organization of many signaling events results in convergence of signaling pathways and induction of similar responses, signaling mechanisms also display significant divergence. A unique receptor may couple to more than one type of effector molecule (Figure I-4-9, Scheme VI). For example, certain cholinergic receptors may couple through G proteins to both adenylate cyclase and phospholipase C, thus launching these two important second messenger pathways.[4] Certain tyrosine-kinase receptors may directly activate other phospholipase Cs as well as other signaling effectors (such as GTPase activating proteins and PI kinase) which could then initiate alternate signaling mechanisms (Figure I-4-9, Scheme VII). In another variation (that is not welll-documented), these receptors may couple through G proteins to one effector set and by direct phosphorylation to another signaling pathway (Figure I-4-9, Scheme VIII).

Further divergence of signaling pathways occurs when certain effectors result in the generation of more than one second messenger molecule. The primary example for this event is the formation of both diacylglycerol and inositol trisphosphate upon the activation of phospholipase C (Figure I-4-9, Scheme IX). Similarly, activation of phospholipase A_2 generates arachidonic acid and lysophospholipids.

Redundancy

Further complexity in the organization of signal transduction mechanisms is introduced by the ability of distinct signaling pathways to mediate the same or closely related cellular responses. This is best studied in the events leading to the mitogenic response in various cell systems. It appears that activation of either the phospholipase C/protein kinase C pathway, cyclic AMP/protein kinase A pathway, tyrosine kinase pathway, or calcium mediated signaling may result in mitogensis. The level at which these pathways ultimately converge to induce a mitogenic response is not well delineated but may involve upregulation of distinct or similar transcription factors and cell cycle regulators.

This redundancy and overlap in the action of different growth factors allows individual cells to integrate their responses. This is of paramount importance under physiologic conditions where cells receive an ever-changing input from a multitude of positive and negative growth factors and regulators.

Cascades/Amplification

The earliest studies on biochemical pathways of signaling established the importance of the role of cascades and signal amplification. In those studies, it was established that activation of protein kinase A by cyclic AMP results in activation of phosphorylase kinase which in turn activates glycogen phosphorylase.[21] The interpolation of additional kinases and regulatory elements insures multiple steps of control of

signaling events. It also allows for amplification of intracellular signaling in which each kinase phosphorylates many copies of its substrate kinase, which in turn amplifies the signal by phosphorylating a larger amount of the next level of substrates.

The mediation of the mitogenic response, which plays an essential role in regulating the cell cycle, also appears to follow the same principles of a cascade of sequential signaling events resulting in signal amplification. Many of the involved messengers and kinases have been identified such as protein kinase C, protein kinase A, casein kinase 2, S6 kinase, and other kinases. The exact interaction, however, between these different kinases and the full identification of all components of this pathway have yet to be determined.

Feedback Control

Important regulation of the propagation of signaling events is achieved by feedback mechanisms. These are of two general varieties. Positive feedback mechanisms insure propagation and amplification of signals and second messengers. For example, inositol trisphosphate may release calcium from intracellular stores and, through yet unidentified mechanisms, may result in influx of extracellular calcium.[8] This serves to maintain a longer-lasting calcium signal. Similarly, activation of protein kinase C may result in further generation of diacylglycerol from membrane phospholipids with more prolonged activation of protein kinase C itself.

On the other hand, negative feedback mechanisms operate to attenuate ongoing signals. For example, activation of protein kinase C in certain cells may result in negative feedback effects on G proteins and phospholipase C,[55] thus insuring termination of further diacylglycerol generation. More sophisticated feedback mechanisms occur when protein kinases undergo autophosphorylation and modulate their own activity. This is best illustrated with calcium/calmodulin dependent protein kinases which, upon autophosphorylation, become intrinsically active and independent of further calcium/calmodulin regulation.[21]

Feedback regulation also operates at the intercellular level whereby the action of some growth factors leads to the generation and secretion of additional growth factors that proceed to act on the same or proximal cells.

While the operation of both positive and negative feedback mechanisms may appear contradictory, they play important roles in regulating the duration and intensity of signaling events. In situations where prolonged signaling is required, such as during mitogenesis, positive feedback may predominate, while in other situations negative feedback may insure prompt termination of signaling in response to subthreshold levels of extracellular stimuli.

Cross Talk Between Different Signaling Mechanisms

When different signaling mechanisms are launched independently by the action of the same or distinct extracellular stimuli, multiple interactions between those pathways insure that they do not operate totally independently of each other. This may serve important functions in integrating cellular responses to different stimuli and in tightly regulating unique responses to the same stimulus. For example, activation of adrenergic type receptors may lead to activation of endogenous kinases that serve to desensitize the cells to further action of the same or other stimuli.[30]

Spatial Organization of Signal Transduction

The initial events of signal transduction for most classes of extracellular agents appear to localize at the plasma membrane. The propagation of signals through effectors, second messengers, and transducing targets leads to interactions in different cellular compartments. Many events occur at the plasma membrane itself, and these usually involve positive and negative feedback effects. Many other events occur in the cytosolic compartment where protein kinases may phosphorylate soluble substrates. Other events, however, may occur in specialized cellular compartments. Inositol trisphosphates may release calcium from endoplasmic reticulum, protein kinases may associate with cytoskeletal or nuclear membrane compartments, phosphorylated substrates may migrate from cytosolic compartments to the nucleus where they may act to modulate transcriptional events.

It is also conceivable that further complexity may be introduced by compartmentalization of signaling events. This is a particularly difficult area of research. However, the complexity of intracellular organization may impose significant limitations as to the sites of generation of second messengers, sites of their action, and the topological pathways of propagation of signaling.

Temporal Regulation of Signal Transduction

The temporal aspects of signal transduction play critical roles in modifying cellular responses to the action of extracellular stimuli. The duration of exposure to extracellular stimuli may affect the degree and even the nature of the cellular response. Transient encounters between cells and extracellular stimuli may lead to suboptimal or aborted responses while more prolonged or intense encounters may lead to significant changes in cell function.

The generation of internal second messengers is also subject to tight temporal control. This is achieved by the regulation of both the generation and the metabolism of these second messengers. In many situations, the formation of the second messenger is transitory, leading to immediate and specific responses. This occurs, for example, when neutrophilic leukocytes encounter extracellular organisms and mount a chemotactic and bactericidal response.

For many cellular responses such as mitogenesis, a prolonged elevation of second messenger may be required for the response. The action of a number of growth factors on cell surface receptors leads to repetitive and oscillatory elevations in intracellular calcium that serve to maintain elevated calcium levels over a prolonged duration. Similarly, prolonged elevations in diacylglycerol levels may result in persistent activation of protein kinase C which would then result in a significant mitogenic response.

Additional temporal regulation of signal propagation is achieved by the cascade of sequential effector molecules and second messengers. While this allows for signal amplification, it may also play an important role in regulating the duration of signaling events.

These complexities of signaling mechanisms with redundancy, convergence, divergence, feedback, and cross talk between different signaling pathways provide individual cells with sophisticated control mechanisms that insure fidelity in signaling as well as allow fine tuning of cellular responses depending on the nature, intensity, and duration of extracellular stimuli. For the experimentalist, this lack of one to one correspondence between signaling components presents enormous problems for the dissection of physiologic pathways of signaling which mediate the effects of any one particular extracellular stimulus. Had signaling operated on a one to one correspondence, it would have been sufficient to demonstrate the effects of any one component on subsequent events to allow investigators to conclude that this component is vital for that particular cellular response. For example, demonstrating that an extracellular stimulus leads to the generation of diacylglycerol second messenger and demonstrating that diacylglycerol can cause mitogenesis would have been sufficient to conclude that the mitogenic effect in response to that extracellular stimulus is mediated through phospholipase C/diacylglycerol/protein kinase C. However, the redundancy, cross talk, and divergence of signaling mechanisms preclude such simple conclusions. Therefore, while many of the components of various signaling mechanisms are being assembled and studied, the exact relevance and contribution of each component to the overall cellular response has yet to be convincingly determined in any one situation. Clearly, this is an area of active investigation with profound implications for the understanding of cell regulation and carcinogenesis.

Oncogenesis and Signal Transduction

Disturbances in signal transduction mechanisms and cell regulatory processes provide the molecular basis to explain the induction and maintenance of the cancerous phenotype. In many cases, it appears that acquisition of an overactive or poorly regulated component of a signal transduction pathway is sufficient to drive cells into unchecked proliferation. In fact, disturbances in signal transduction and cell regulatory mechanisms appear to provide a unifying basis for the molecular analysis of traditionally distinct fields of carcinogenesis (genetic, viral, and acquired). A brief overview of the role of signal transduction during various processes and stages of carcinogenesis follows.

Oncogenes and Signal Transduction

Oncogenes were initially identified as transforming genes carried by carcinogenic retroviruses.[12] It became quickly evident, however, that these retroviral genes have cellular homologues, and that the retroviral oncogenes arose from their cellular counterparts, the proto-oncogenes. At this point, there is ample evidence supporting the involvement of proto-oncogenes in the generation and/or the maintenance of cancer (see I-5). For example, transfection (insertion of foreign DNA into cells) of cells in tissue culture with either high levels of proto-oncogenes or abnormally regulated proto-oncogenes results in cell transformation. Also, genes in retroviruses responsible for cell transformation are the viral counterparts of proto-oncogenes. When investigators searched for genes in cancer cells responsible for maintenance of the cancerous phenotype, mutated proto-oncogenes were often obtained.[12] Thus, a mutation in a proto-oncogene may lead to oncogenic activation by disrupting the control and function of its protein product. Alternatively, overexpression of a proto-oncogene, as may occur following chromosomal translocation, viral insertion, or deranged activity of an essential regulator, may also result in oncogenic transformation.[67]

The study of oncogenes has led to the classification of most proto-oncogene protein products as localizing to either the cytoplasm or the nucleus.[12] A tantalizing realization came with the repeated finding that cytoplasmic oncogenes (oncogenes whose protein product resides in the cytoplasm) are either actual components of signal transduction pathways or closely associated proteins. On the other hand, nuclear oncoproteins play important and critical roles in cell regulation and gene transcription although their precise function is less well defined than those of the cytoplasmic oncoproteins. Therefore most, if not all, proto-oncogenes encode normal cellular proteins which function to regulate cell growth.

While the study of signal transduction has generally been applied to transmembrane and cytoplasmic events, an ultimate and important target of many signal transduction pathways is modulation of the function of nuclear proteins. Many of the nuclear oncoproteins are phosphoproteins and appear to be substrates for different protein kinases, thus linking them to more general signal transduction pathways. Therefore, the products of most oncogenes appear to be integral members of signal transduction pathways. An understanding of their mechanism of action must by necessity involve dissection of their impact on signal transduction during normal cell function and determining how oncogenesis is related to disruption of these processes. In the simplest formulation, it appears that when any essential component of a signal transduction pathway is rendered hyperactive or autonomous, it may acquire the ability to drive the cell into unchecked proliferation. An active area of research is aimed at determining the mechanism of action of normal proto-oncogenes and their oncogenic variants.

The intimate relationship between oncogenes and components of signal transduction pathways has been established at almost every level (Figure I-4-10). For example, the earliest observation on a proto-oncogene with effects on cell growth came from the demonstration that the c-sis oncogene encodes for a platelet-derived growth factor (PDGF).[19] Cell transformation by an overexpressed c-sis oncogene then results in a mitogenic response by providing an overactive extracellular growth factor. V-erbB was then identified as a truncated form of the epidermal growth factor (EGF) receptor[20] with endogenous unchecked protein-tyrosine kinase activity. C-fms,[65] on the other hand, encodes the homologue of the receptor for the macrophage colony-stimulating factor (M-CSF), while c-mas may encode an angiotensin receptor.[37]

Mutated ras oncogenes are, so far, the most frequently detected mutated oncogenes in human cancer.[74] The ras oncogenes belong to the family of small molecular weight GTP-binding proteins, which are presumed to play essential roles in stimulus response coupling in analogy with the larger heterotrimeric GTP-binding proteins involved in the regulation of phospholipase C, adenylate cyclase, and cyclic GMP phosphodiesterase.

Many of the other extranuclear oncoproteins (protein products of oncogenes) appear to possess intrinsic protein-tyrosine kinase activity. These include Src, Abl, Fes, Fgr, Yes, Ros, and others.[12] By analogy with receptor tyrosine kinases, these cytoplasmic or membrane-associated tyrosine kinase oncoproteins are thought to play essential roles in signal transduction mechanisms although these remain poorly defined. Another category of extranuclear oncoproteins appears to possess protein-serine/threonine kinase activity, and these include Raf and Mos.[12] Mutated G proteins have been found in pituitary and other endocrine tumors,[45] while a mutated protein with homology to GAP may underlie the pathogenesis of neurofibromatosis.[77] Mutations in protein kinase C, an important serine/threonine kinase, have transforming potential.

Anti-Oncogenes and Cell Regulation

Just as increased and unchecked activity of essential components of promitogenic signaling pathways may contribute to carcinogenesis, it is equally conceivable that elimination of activity essential for inhibition of mitogenesis may also lead to increased proliferation. In fact, the existence of such suppressor oncogenes (also termed recessive oncogenes, or anti-oncogenes) has been postulated for many years. A number of such anti-oncogenes have recently been identified and these include the retinoblastoma gene, the elimination of whose activity results in retinoblastoma and a number of bladder and bone cancers.[33] The cellular localization of the protein product of the retinoblastoma gene appears to be nuclear, and its function appears to be related to inhibition of activity of positive transcriptional factors. The neurofibromatosis gene (NF) has been cloned and found to have homology to GAP. It is hypothesized that NF acts as a tumor suppressor gene that ordinarily functions to regulate the activity of ras or ras-like proteins.[77] P53, a 53 kD protein with as yet unidentified function, appears to be another anti-oncogene, especially in colon cancer.[54]

The study of anti-oncogenes has also led to identifying the K-rev (smg 21) gene as an anti-oncogene with homology to small molecular weight G proteins.[40] Its function appears to be to antagonize the role of the activity of ras oncogenes.

Tumor Promoters and Signal Transduction

Experimental models of carcinogenesis in the mouse are consistent with a two step carcinogenesis scheme consisting of an initiating event (step 1) followed by a tumor promoting event (step 2). These models have allowed the identification of a number of tumor promoters over the last three decades with pleiotropic biologic effects far exceeding their role as cancer promoting agents.[13] Studies in the past decade, however, have generated important insight into the mechanism of action of tumor promoters, and have led to unification of the field of study of tumor promotion with signal transduction (Figure I-4-11).

The best studied class of tumor promoters consists of phorbol esters and related molecules. Phorbol esters were known to exert profound effects on cellular functions including hormone release, blood cell activation, cell differentia-

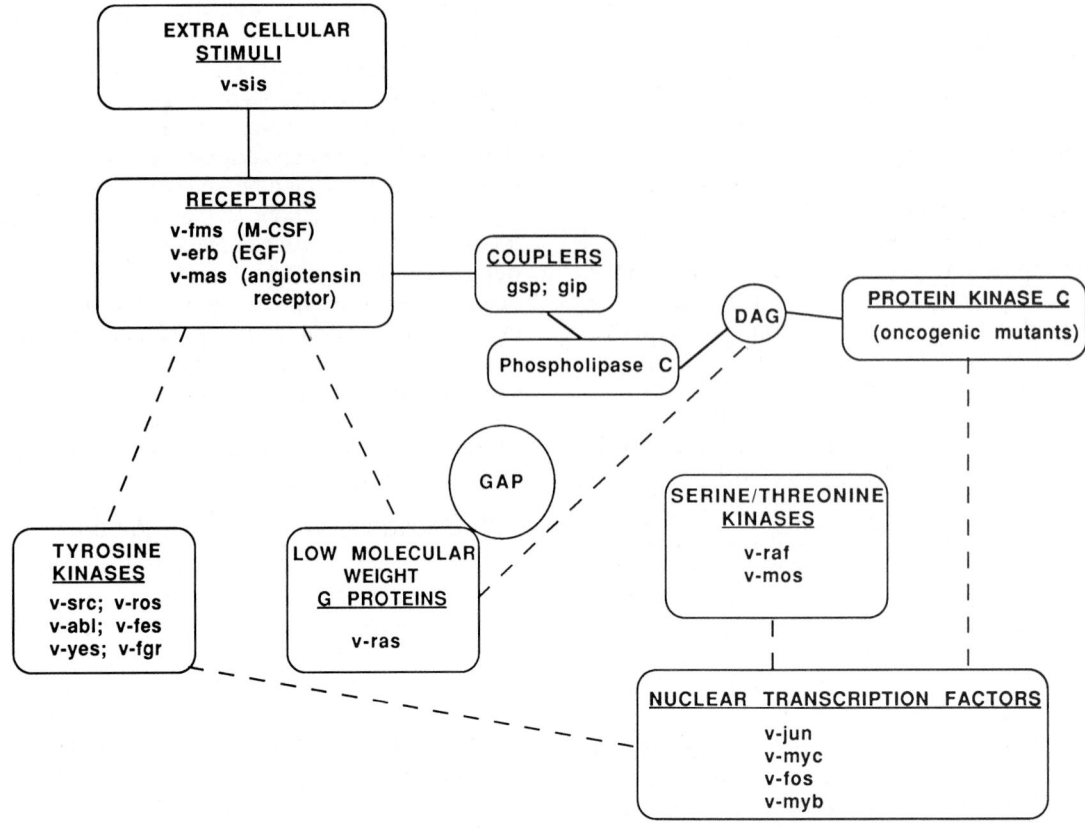

Figure I-4-10. Involvement of oncogene products in signal transduction pathways. This scheme illustrates components of signal transduction pathways and the role of products of oncogenes in signal transduction. v-Sis encodes an oncogenic counterpart of platelet-derived growth factor; c-fms, c-erb, and c-mas encode for receptors for M-CSF, EGF, and angiotensin, respectively; oncogenic counterparts of G proteins have been described (gsp and gip); while other oncogenes encode for tyrosine kinases, serine-threonine kinases, and nuclear transcription factors as indicated. GAP (GTPase activating proteins) may represent a family of proteins with possible oncogenic counterparts. Although the function of ras oncogenes in signal transduction is not well delineated, pathologically these molecules result in elevation of diacylglycerol (DAG) levels. Solid lines indicate established pathways of signaling while dashed lines indicate potential or poorly defined pathways.

tion, mitogenesis, and tumor promotion. Insight into their mechanism of action came with the identification of protein kinase C as the main intracellular receptor for these agents.[55] The interaction of phorbol esters with protein kinase C results in prolonged and unattenuated activation of this enzyme followed by its proteolytic inactivation. This interaction appears to explain most, if not all, the effects of phorbol esters on cell function. By extension, protein kinase C has been implicated as a main mediator of tumor promotion; this hypothesis and the mechanisms explaining these effects are yet to be demonstrated. Protein kinase C also appears to be the target of action of other nonphorbol ester tumor promoters. These include mezerein, aplysiatoxin, and lyngbyatoxin.

Arachidonic acid and its prostanoid metabolites also appear to exert tumor promoting activity. The mechanism of action, which may or may not involve protein kinase C, remains poorly understood.

More recently, two important additional links between tumor promotion and signal transduction have been established. First, it has been shown that thapsigargin, a potent tumor promoter, acts by primarily releasing calcium from intracellular stores[70] (Figure I-4-11). Okadaic acid, another tumor promoter, appears to inhibit serine/threonine protein

phosphatases[31] and thus results in increased phosphorylation of protein substrates (Figure I-4-11).

It appears that activation of either protein kinase C or calcium-dependent protein kinases (and other calcium-dependent events) or inhibition of protein phosphatases results in tumor promotion. Activation of kinases or inhibition of phosphatases results in increased phosphorylation of protein substrates. In the case of tumor promoters, it appears that a common final effect is to increase phosphorylation of critical substrates on serine and threonine residues (Figure I-4-11). The nature of these substrates has not been determined, but the convergence of the action of disparate tumor promoters on specific phosphorylation of proteins on serine and threonine residues strongly implicates signal transduction processes in tumor promotion and carcinogenesis.

Viruses and Oncogenesis

HTLV1 and Hepatitis B are major transforming human viruses (see III-9, III-11, and XXXVI-6). In this context, it is sufficient to point to the role of virally-encoded proteins in modifying essential components of signal transduction elements. This is especially true in the case of HTLV1 where the tax protein drives the expression of interleukin 2 and interleukin 2 receptor, two essential components of T lymphocyte growth and

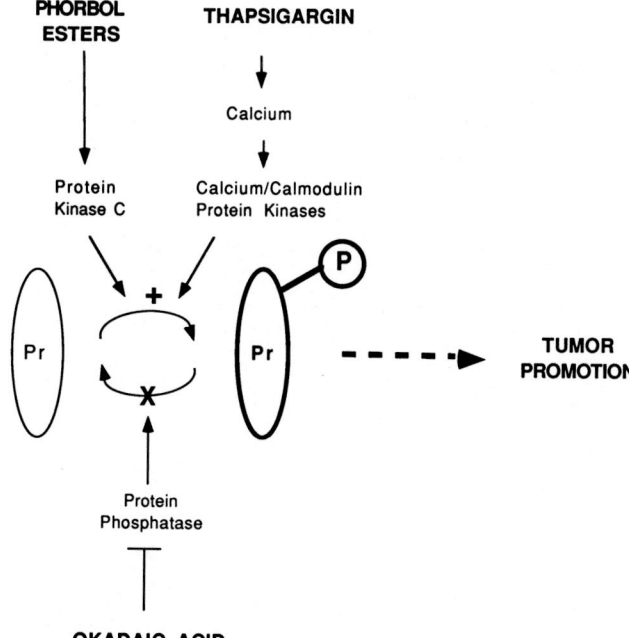

Figure I-4-11. Tumor promoters and protein phosphorylation. Three classes of tumor promoters are indicated. These are phorbol esters and non-phorbol ester tumor promoters that act by activating protein kinase C, thapsigargin which releases calcium from intracellular stores, and okadaic acid which inhibits protein phosphatases. Phorbol esters and thapsigargin activate protein kinases that increase endogenous substrate phosphorylation while okadaic acid inhibits protein phosphatases thus also enhancing substrate phosphorylation. The exact nature of the phosphorylated substrates and their roles in tumor promotion are not well delineated.

mitogenesis.[5] Hepatitis B may activate the N-myc proto-oncogene.

Metastasis and Signal Transduction

A crucial event in the progression of cancer is the acquisition by tumor cells of the ability to metastasize to new sites in the body. Recent evidence has begun to elucidate the mechanisms involved in metastasis. A gene has been isolated with the unique ability to suppress the ability of cancer cells to metastasize.[62] Loss of its function may be one mechanism allowing tumor cells to metastasize. Therefore this gene may function as an anti-oncogene.

An important link between metastasis and signal transduction came with the realization that this metastasis-suppressor gene may function as a nucleoside diphosphate kinase and that it may associate with G proteins.[43]

Implications for Treatment

The detailed mapping of signaling pathways and their precise roles in cell regulation and cell transformation offers a unique advantage in the development of specific preventative and therapeutic modalities for malignant disorders. These treatments may aim at any level of the signal transduction pathways; it is expected that detailed biochemical and molecular analysis of biopsy material from individual tumors will generate insight into the cause and pathogenesis

of individual tumors. This would then allow the development of specific therapeutic intervention. It is conceivable that modulation of receptors, coupling mechanisms, effectors, second messengers, protein kinases, and important substrates may also have profound therapeutic effects.

At present, a number of growth factors and hormones have found significant use in cancer therapy and prevention. Some, such as tumor necrosis factor, have been used for their direct toxic effect. Others, such as interleukins and interferons, have been used for their ability to modulate the body's immune response towards cancer, i.e., they are biologic response modifiers. Growth factors are playing increasingly important roles as adjunctive therapy to limit the toxicity and complications of chemotherapy. For example, erythropoietin may be used to stimulate red cell production. G-CSF and GM-CSF enhance the recovery of white blood cell counts, thus allowing the use of more effective chemotherapy and curtailing the morbidity and mortality associated with prolonged decreases in white blood cell counts (Section XVIII, Chapter 6).

One important area of research centers on the role of signal transduction in modulating the function of the proteins (e.g., gp 170) implicated in multiple drug resistance.[2] The ability to modulate the presumed pump activity of this protein may have significant therapeutic implications.

Another treatment potential arises from the observations that various tumor promoters appear to act, by different mechanisms, to increase protein phosphorylation through elements of signal transduction pathways. Therefore, it is possible that chemopreventive treatment aimed at preventing or reversing tumor promotion may make use of agents that counteract or preempt the effects of tumor promoters on signal transduction. Such agents may include protein kinase inhibitors, protein phosphatase activators, and modulators of calcium release.

Another area of cancer prevention relating to modulation of signal transduction may make use of dietary manipulation of signaling pathways. Diet contains carcinogens and tumor promoters, as well as inhibitors of carcinogenesis and tumor promotion, although the identity of the latter remains elusive.[16] Also, it is known that dietary habits may be associated with different composition of membrane lipids. Associations have been made between dietary fatty acid intake and risk of colon and breast cancer. It appears plausible that these dietary changes modulate the function of signaling pathways. For example, omega-3 fatty acids may substitute for arachidonic acids. When they are released in response to phospholipase A2 activation, they lead to the formation of inactive metabolites instead of the powerful thromboxanes and leukotrienes. Clearly, the understanding of normal signaling mechanisms and the impact of dietary manipulation on these pathways may open up an area of chemoprevention through dietary manipulation.

Conclusions

Signal transduction and cell regulatory mechanisms appear to offer a unifying molecular mechanism for the pathogenesis of cancer. Rapid advances in current knowledge of the components of signaling mechanisms, their regulation, and their interrelationships have provided a major breakthrough in our understanding on how normal cell function is regulated. This has been an essential step in applying this data base towards the understanding of how abnormalities in these pathways can impact on cancer pathogenesis and progression. Further studies to define all components of signaling and regulatory pathways and their precise roles in cell regulation are clearly indicated.

Such sophisticated understanding of signaling and regulatory mechanisms is no longer an unattainable task. The achievement of this goal should open multiple avenues for novel and innovative modalities for cancer prevention and treatment including dietary manipulation, biologic response modification, and treatments aimed at specific rectification of cancer cell behavior.

References

1. Akira, S., Hirono, T., Taga, T., and Kishimoto, T.: Biology of multifunctional cytokines: IL 6 and related molecules (IL 1 and TNF). FASEB J., 4:2860, 1990.
2. Ames, G.: The basis of multidrug resistance in mammalian cells: Homology with bacterial transport. Cell, 47:323, 1986.
3. Angel, P., Imagawa, M., Chiu, R., Stein, B., Imbra, R. J., Rahmsdorf, H. J., Jonat, C., Herrlich, P., and Karin, M.: Phorbol ester-inducible genes contain a common cis element recognized by TPA-modulated trans-acting factor. Cell, 49:729, 1987.
4. Ashkenazi, A., Winslow, J. W., Peralta, E. G., Peterson, G. L., Schimerlik, M. I., Capon, D. J., and Ramachandran, J.: An M2 muscarinic receptor subtype coupled to both adenylyl cyclase and phosphoinositide turnover. Science, 238:672, 1987.
5. Ballard, D. W., Bohnlein, E., Lowenthal, J. W., Wano, Y., Franza, B. R., and Greene, W. C.: HTLV-1 Tax induces proteins that activate the kB element in the IL-2 receptor a receptor gene. Science, 241:1652, 1988.
6. Bell, R. M.: Protein kinase C activation by diacylglycerol second messengers. Cell, 45:631, 1986.
7. Bernstein, L. R., and Colburn, N. H.: AP1/jun function is differentially induced in promotion-sensitive and resistant JB6 cells. Science, 244:566, 1989.
8. Berridge, M. J.: Calcium oscillations. J. Biol. Chem., 265:9583, 1990.
9. Berridge, M. J., and Irvine, R. F.: Inositol phosphates and cell signalling. Nature, 341:197, 1989.
10. Bevan, S., and Wood, J. N.: Arachidonic-acid metabolites as second messengers. Nature, 328:20, 1987.
11. Billah, M. M., Pai, J.-K., Mullmann, T. J., Egan, R. W., and Siegel, M. I.: Regulation of phospholipase D in HL-60 granulocytes. Activation by phorbol esters, diglyceride, and calcium ionophore via protein kinase C-independent mechanisms. J. Biol. Chem., 264:9069, 1989.
12. Bishop, J. M.: Viral oncogenes. Cell, 42:23, 1985.
13. Blumberg, P. M.: In vitro studies on the mode of action of the phorbol esters, potent tumor promoters. Crit. Rev. Toxicol., 8:153, 1980.
14. Bourne, H. R.: G-protein subunits: Who carries what message? Nature, 337:504, 1989.
15. Brown, A., and Birnbaumer, L.: Ion channels and G proteins. Hospital Practice, 124:139, 1989.
16. Carr, B. I.: Chemical carcinogens and inhibitors of carcinogenesis in the human diet. Cancer, 55:218, 1985.
17. Casey, P. J., and Gilman, A. G.: G protein involvement in receptor-effector coupling. J. Biol. Chem., 263:2577, 1988.
18. Cheung, W. Y.: Calmodulin—An Introduction. *In*: Calcium and Cell Function. Edited by W. Y. Cheung. New York, Academic Press, 1980, pp. 2–9.
19. Doolittle, R. F., Hunkapiller, M. W., Hood, L. E., De Vare, S. G., Robbins, K. C., Aaronson, S. A., and Antoniades, H. N.: Simian sarcoma virus onc gene, v-sis, is derived from the gene (or genes) encoding a platelet-derived growth factor. Science, 221:275, 1983.
20. Downward, J., Yarden, Y., Mayes, E., Scrace, G., Totty, N., Stockwell, P., Ullrich, A., Schlessinger, J., and Waterfield, M.D.: Close similarity of epidermal growth factor receptor and v-erb-B oncogene protein sequence. Nature, 307:521, 1984.
21. Edelman, A. M., Blumenthal, D. K., and Krebs, E. G.: Protein serine/threonine kinases. Annu. Rev. Biochem., 56:567, 1987.
22. Exton, J. H.: Signaling through phosphatidylcholine breakdown. J. Biol. Chem., 265:1, 1990.
23. Gerzer, R., Hofmann, F., and Schultz, G.: Purification of a soluble sodium-nitroprusside-stimulated guanylate cyclase from bovine lung. Eur. J. Biochem., 116:479, 1981.
24. Ghosh, S., and Baltimore, D.: Activation in vitro of NF-KB by phosphorylation of its inhibitor IKB. Nature, 344:678, 1990.
25. Green, A. R.: Peptide regulatory factors: Multifunctional mediators of cellular growth and differentiation. Lancet, 1:705, 1989.
26. Gronich, J. H., Bonventre, J. V., and Nemenoff, R. A.: Identification and characterization of a hormonally regulated form of phospholipase A2 in rat renal mesangial cells. J. Biol. Chem., 263:16645, 1988.
27. Hakomori, S.: Glycosphingolipids in cellular interaction, differentiation, and oncogenesis. Annu. Rev. Biochem., 50:733, 1981.
28. Hanks, S. K., Quinn, A. M., and Hunter, T.: The protein kinase family: Conserved features and deduced phylogeny of the catalytic domains. Science, 241:42, 1988.
29. Hannun, Y. A., and Bell, R. M.: Functions of sphingolipids and sphingolipid breakdown products in cellular regulation. Science, 243:500, 1989.
30. Hausdorf, W. P., Caron, M. G., and Lefkowitz, R. J.: Turning off the signal: Desensitization of β-adrenergic receptor function. FASEB J., 4:2881, 1990.
31. Haystead, T. A., Sim, A. T., Carling, D., Honnor, R. C., Tsukitani, Y., Cohen, P., and Hardie, D. G.: Effects of the tumour promoter okadaic acid on intracellular protein phosphorylation and metabolism. Nature, 337:78, 1989.
32. Hokin, M. R., and Hokin, L. E.: Enzyme secretion and the incorporation of ^{32}P into phospholipids of pancreas slices. J. Biol. Chem., 203:967, 1953.
33. Horowitz, J. M., Park, S.-H., Bogenmann, E., Cheng, J.-C., Yandell, D. W., Kaye, F. J., Minna, J. D., Dryja, T. P., and Weinberg, R. A.: Frequent inactivation of the retinoblastoma anti-oncogene is restricted to a subset of human tumor cells. Proc. Natl. Acad. Sci. USA, 87:2775, 1990.
34. Hsiao, W.-L. W., Housey, G. M., Johnson, M. D., and Weinstein, I. B.: Cells that overproduce protein kinase C are more susceptible to transformation by an activated H-*ras* oncogene. Mol. Cell. Biol., 9:2641, 1989.
35. Hunkapillar, T., and Hood, L.: Diversity of the immunoglobulin gene superfamily. Adv. Immunol., 4:1, 1989.
36. Inagami, T.: Atrial natriuretic factor. J. Biol. Chem., 264:3043, 1989.
37. Jackson, T. R., Blair, L. A., Marshall, J., Goedert, M., and Hanley, M. R.: The mas oncogene encodes an angiotensin receptor. Nature, 335:437, 1988.
38. Kawata, M., Matsui, Y., Kondo, J., Hishida, T., Teranishi, Y., and Takai, Y.: A novel small molecular weight GTP-binding protein with the same putative effector domain as the ras proteins in bovine brain membranes. J. Biol. Chem., 263:18965, 1988.
39. Kim, J. W., Sim, S. S., Kim, U.-H., Nishibe, S., Wahl, M. I., Carpenter, G., and Rhee, S. G.: Tyrosine residues in bovine phospholipase C-gamma phosphorylated by the epidermal growth factor receptor *in vitro*. J. Biol. Chem., 265:3940, 1990.
40. Kitayama, H., Sugimoto, Y., Matsuzaki, T., Ikawa, Y., and Noda, M.: A ras-related gene with transformation suppressor activity. Cell, 56:77, 1989.
41. Krupinski, J., Coussen, F., Bakalyar, H. A., Tang, W. J., Feinstein, P. G., Orth, K., Slaughter, C., Reed, R. R., and Gilman, A. G.: Adenylyl cyclase amino acid sequence: Possible channel- or transport-like structure. Science, 244:1558, 1989.
42. Lacal, J. C., Moscat, J., Aaronson, S. A.: Novel source of 1,2-diacylglycerol elevated in cells transformed by Ha-ras oncogene. Nature, 330:269, 1987.
43. Lacombe, M. L., Wallet, V., Troll, H., and Veron, M.: Functional cloning of a nucleoside diphosphate kinase from dictyostelium discoideum. J. Biol. Chem., 265:10012, 1990.
44. Low, M. G., and Saltiel, A. R.: Structural and functional roles of glycosyl-phosphatidylinositol in membranes. Science, 239:268, 1988.
45. Lyons, J., Landis, C. A., Harsh, G., Vallar, L., Grunewald, K., Feichtinger, H., Duh, Q. Y., Clark, O. H., Kawasaki, E., Bourne, H. R., and McCormick, F.: Two G protein oncogenes in human endocrine tumors. Science, 249:655, 1990.
46. Majerus, P. W., Connolly, T. M., Deckmyn, H., Ross, T. S., Bross, T. E., Ishii, H., Bansal, V., and Wilson, D.: The metabolism of phosphoinositide-derived messenger molecules. Science, 234:1519, 1986.
47. Massague, J.: The TGF-β family of growth and differentiation factors. Cell, 49:437, 1987.
48. Megidish, T., and Mazurek, N.: A mutant protein kinase C that can transform fibroblasts. Nature, 342:807, 1989.
49. Michell, B.: A second messenger function for inositol tetrakisphosphate. Nature, 324:613, 1986.
50. Michell, R. H.: Post-receptor signalling pathways. Lancet, 1:765, 1989.
51. Molloy, C. J., Bottaro, D. P., Fleming, T. P., Marshall, M. S., Gibbs, J. B., and Aaronson, S. A.: PDGF induction of tyrosine phosphorylation of GTPase activating protein. Nature, 343:711, 1989.
52. Moncada, S., Palmer, R. M. J., and Higgs, E. A.: Biosynthesis of nitric oxide from L-arginine. A pathway for the regulation of cell function and communication. Biochem. Pharmacol., 38:1709, 1989.
53. Morla, A. O., Draetta, G., Beach, D., and Wang, J. Y. J.: Reversible tyrosine phosphorylation of cdc2: Dephosphorylation accompanies activation during entry into mitosis. Cell, 58:193, 1989.
54. Nigro, J. M., Baker, S. J., Preisinger, A. C., Jessup, J. M., Hostetter, R., Cleary, K., Bigner, S. H., Davidson, N., Baylin, S., Devilee, P., Glover, T., Collins, F. S., Weston, A., Modali, R., Harris, C. C., and Vogelstein, B.: Mutations in the *p53* gene occur in diverse human tumour types. Nature, 343:705, 1989.
55. Nishizuka, Y.: Studies and prospectives of the protein kinase C family for cellular regulation. Cancer, 63:1892, 1989.
56. Okazaki, T., Bell, R. M., and Hannun, Y. A.: Sphingomyelin turnover induced by vitamin D_3 in HL-60 cells. Role in cell differentiation. J. Biol. Chem., 264:19076, 1989.
57. Persons, D. A., Wilkison, W. O., Bell, R. M., and Finn, O. J.: Altered growth regulation and enhanced tumorigenicity of NIH 3T3 fibroblasts transfected with protein kinase C-1 cDNA. Cell, 52:447, 1988.
58. Preiss, J., Loomis, C. R., Bishop, W. R., Stein, R., Niedel, J. E., and Bell, R. M.: Quantitative measurement of sn-1,2-diacylglycerols present in platelets, hepatocytes, and ras- and sis-transformed normal rat kidney cells. J. Biol. Chem., 261:8597, 1986.
59. Price, B. D., Morris, J. D. H., Marshall, C. J., and Hall, A.: Stimulation of phosphatidylcholine hydrolysis, diacylglycerol release, and arachidonic acid production by oncogenic ras is a consequence of protein kinase C activation. J. Biol. Chem., 264:16638, 1989.
60. Rhee, S. G., Suh, P. G., Ryu, S. H., and Lee, S. Y.: Studies of inositol phospholipid-specific phospholipase C. Science, 244:546, 1989.
61. Roberts, A. B., Anzano, M. A., Wakefield, L. M., Roche, N. S., Stern, D. F., and Sporn, M. B.: Type β transforming growth factor: A bifunctional regulator of cellular growth. Proc. Natl. Acad. Sci. USA, 82:119, 1985.
62. Rosengard, A. M., Krutzsch, H. C., Shearn, A., Biggs, J. R., Barker, E., Margulies, M. K., King, C. R., Liotta, L. A., and Steeg, P. S.: Reduced Mm23/Awd protein in tumour metastasis and aberrant Drosophila development. Nature, 342:177, 1989.
63. Samuelsson, B., Dahlen, S. E., Lindgren, J. A., Rouzer, C. A., and Serhan, C. N.: Leukotrienes and lipoxins: structures, biosynthesis, and biological effects. Science, 237:1171, 1987.
64. Sassone-Corsi, P., Ransone, L. J., and Verma, I. M.: Cross-talk in signal transduction: TPA-inducible factor jun/AP-1 activates cAMP-responsive enhancer elements. Oncogene, 5:427, 1990.
65. Sherr, C. J., Rettenmier, C. W., Sacca, R., Roussel, M. F., Look, A. T., and Stanley, E. R.: The c-fms proto-oncogene product is related to the receptor for the mononuclear phagocyte growth factor, CSF-1. Cell, 41:665, 1985.
66. Shuman, M. A., and Greenberg, C. S.: Platelet regulation of thrombus formation. *In*: Biochemistry of Platelets. Edited by D. R. Philips and M. A. Shuman. Orlando, Academic Press, 1986, pp 319–346.
67. Slamon, D. J.: Proto-oncogenes and human cancers. N. Engl. J. Med., 317:955, 1987.
68. Sporn, M. B., and Roberts, A. B.: Peptide growth factors are multifunctional. Nature, 332:217, 1988.

69. Takuwa, N., Takuwa, Y., and Rasmussen, H.: Stimulation of mitogenesis and glucose transport by 1-monooleoylglycerol in Swiss 3T3 fibroblasts. J. Biol. Chem., 263:9738, 1988.
70. Thastrup, O., Cullen, P. J., Drobak, B. K., Hanley, M. R., and Dawson, A. P.: Thapsigargin, a tumor promoter, discharges intracellular Ca^{2+} stores by specific inhibition of the endoplasmic reticulum Ca^{2+}-ATPase. Proc. Natl. Acad. Sci. USA, 87:2466, 1990.
71. Ulevitch, R. J., Watanabe, Y., Sano, M., Lister, M. D., Deems, R. A., and Dennis, E. A.: Solubilization, purification, and characterization of a membrane-bound phospholipase A2 from the P388D1 macrophage-like cell line. J. Biol. Chem., 263:3079, 1988.
72. Ushikubi, F., Nakajima, M., Hirata, M., Okuma, M., Fujiwara, M., and Narumiya, S.: Purification of the thromboxane A_2-prostaglandin H_2 receptor from human blood platelets. J. Biol. Chem., 264:16496, 1989.
73. Waterfield, M. D.: Epidermal growth factor and related molecules. Lancet, 1:1243, 1989.
74. Weinberg, R. A.: ras oncogenes and the molecular mechanisms of carcinogenesis. Blood, 64:1143, 1984.
75. Williams, L. T.: Signal transduction by the platelet-derived growth factor receptor. Science, 243:1564, 1989.
76. Wright, T. M., Rangan, L. A., Shin, H. S., and Raben, D. M.: Kinetic analysis of 1,2-diacylglycerol mass levels in cultured fibroblasts. J. Biol. Chem., 263:9374, 1988.
77. Xu, G., O'Connell, P., Viskochil, D., Cawthon, R., Robertson, M., Culver, M., Dunn, D., Stevens, J., Gesteland, R., White, R., and Weiss, R.: The neurofibromatosis type 1 gene encodes a protein related to GAP. Cell, 62:599, 1990.

I-5

Oncogenes

George Klein

Introduction

The word "oncogene" is a generally accepted misnomer; it is used as a collective term for a multiple set of growth regulatory genes that can contribute to the development of cancer after various types of pathological activation. Their discovery was an unexpected gift of viral oncology to cellular and cancer biology. The early work was based on the largely mistaken notion that oncogenic viruses owe their tumorigenic effect to indigenous viral sequences. This notion is only true for the DNA tumor viruses, but not for the RNA tumor viruses or retroviruses. The discovery of the oncogenes came from the RNA tumor virus field.

The RNA tumor viruses are a subclass of the retroviruses. They fall into two categories. Class I or acute viruses can cause tumors at the site of inoculation after short latency periods. They can also transform in vitro. The oncogenic effect of the Class II or chronic RNA tumor viruses is usually restricted to genetically susceptible hosts that are highly permissive for viral replication. Tumors appear only after relatively long latency periods and in remote and usually quite specific tissues, irrespective of the site of inoculation.

The development of the oncogene field started when it was discovered that Class I viruses carried modified host-cell derived sequences. They, rather than any indigenous viral sequences, were responsible for the transforming effect. They played no role in viral replication. On the contrary, they could be a burden to the virus. More often than not, they have actually impaired the replicative ability of their viral carrier and made it dependent on a "helper" virus that did not contain any cell-derived sequences.

The frequent "kidnapping" of cell derived genes can be seen in relation to the normal life cycle of the retroviruses. They carry their genetic information in RNA, but transcribe it in infected cells into DNA. The derived DNA provirus integrates with the host cell genome and replicates in synchrony with genes of the host cell. When the viral cycle is activated, the proviral DNA is again transcribed into RNA. This back-and-forth copying of the viral information between RNA and DNA favors the accidental pickup of host-cell derived sequences by illegitimate recombination.

The isolation of the Class I RNA tumor viruses must be regarded as a byproduct of experimentation. There is no evidence that such viruses ever induce tumors under natural conditions. Their survival has been favored under laboratory conditions by the horizontal passage by the investigator, under continuous selection for high tumorigenicity. This has not only preserved accidentally incorporated cellular sequences that could contribute to an oncogenic effect, but favored additional structural changes that increased the transforming ability of the incorporated sequences. The most striking examples of additional oncogenic modifications are provided by the Class I viruses that have picked up two different, unrelated but functionally complementary transforming genes in the course of this selection.

In spite of their artificial origin, the chimeric Class I viruses have provided an unexpectedly rich source of new information. The cell derived but virally carried, oncogenes (abbreviated as the v-onc genes), provided probes that have led to the discovery of previously unknown gene families that play important roles in the regulation of normal cell growth and division. Some of the corresponding normal cellular genes, also referred to as protooncogenes or c-onc genes, were found capable of contributing to natural tumor development, after they had been "activated" by specific mutations, chromosomal translocations, gene amplification, or the insertion of a viral enhancer in their vicinity.

The following section will briefly recapitulate some of the major features of this development, insofar as they are relevant for our present understanding. This is followed by a survey of the major known oncogene families. The chapter is concluded by considering the role of oncogene activation in natural tumor development and progression.

Discovery of the Oncogenes

The transforming gene of the Rous sarcoma virus (RSV), designated as v-src, was the first virally carried oncogene that has been discovered. RSV had been isolated from a spontaneously arising fowl sarcoma by Peyton Rous in 1911.[61] This was based on the successful transmission of the tumor by the inoculation of cell free filtrates to newly hatched chickens. It has been subsequently propagated by animal passage and concurrent selection for high tumorigenicity over several decades. The field of viral oncology remained relatively inactive until the 1950s, however, due to the lack of appropriate mammalian models. The discovery of the murine leukemia viruses by Gross and the polyoma virus by Gross, Stewart and Eddy in the 1950s has changed the climate of opinion and the pendulum has actually swung to the opposite extreme.[29,30,70] After having lingered on the shelf of unimportant curiosa, tumor viruses were suddenly brought into the center of attention. Major figures of the rapidly expanding field like Ludwik Gross who discovered the first mouse leukemia virus, Robert Huebner and George Todaro, who first coined the word "oncogene," but with a viral rather than cellular connotation, and Sol Spiegelman, one of the pioneers of modern molecular biology, argued forcefully that most if not all tumors may be caused by viruses.[34,68] They have emphasized that several of the class II RNA tumor viruses, such as the Gross leukemia virus and the mouse mammary tumor virus, were transmitted vertically from parents to offspring and remained latent for long periods of time.[9] Many other vertically transmitted retroviruses were discovered by this time that expressed little or no viral products during their prolonged latency, as judged by the technology of the period, and caused no apparent disease. Some of them were activated in tumors induced by other agents like chemical carcinogens, radiation or DNA tumor viruses. The proponents of the "panvirological" view of tumor origin argued that even these unrelated agents may induce tumors through the activation of latent retroviruses. They have quite overlooked the fact that most vertebrates carry endogenous, non-pathogenic retroviruses and that the oncogenic effect of the Class II RNA tumor viruses was restricted to a few subtypes. These were usually selected in the laboratory and were more often than not only pathogenic for specific inbred strains of mice, selected for high tumor incidence and/or high permissiveness for viral replication.

The "pan-virological" concept was not open to experimental verification or falsification. It was nevertheless highly productive, particularly at the interface between the scientists and their supporting bodies. The Virus Cancer Program became a major part of the concerted "war on cancer," initiated by the Cancer Act during the Nixon Administration. The large scale support of viral oncology failed to prove that most human tumors are caused by viruses, but it had several major spin-off effects. The rapid development of retrovirology was perhaps the most important among them. It has led to the discovery of the true, cell-derived oncogenes. In addition it has built up a technology that became crucially important when the unforeseen HIV pandemic struck two decades later.

The first oncogene theory of Huebner and Todaro did not distinguish conceptually between Class I and II RNA tumor viruses.[34] It has postulated that part of the *viral* genetic information acts as an "oncogene," i.e., transforms normal into malignant cells, whereas another part, the "virogene," is needed for viral replication. It is easy now to see the fallacy

of this reasoning. Small viruses can hardly afford to use a major part of their limited genetic information to no other purpose than to cause a lethal disease in their host.

The road that has led to the discovery of the cell-derived oncogenes was opened by the electron microscopic study of viral RNA and by genetic experiments with viral mutants. RSV was found to contain an approximately 16% larger RNA molecule than its most closely related but non-transforming relatives indicating the presence of some "extra" genetic information.[22] This was also suggested by experiments with a temperature sensitive (ts) RSV mutant that could only transform fibroblasts in vitro at a relatively low temperature.[46] Exposure of the tsRSV transformed cells to a non-permissive temperature induced reversion of the cells to a normal phenotype and they could shift back again at the permissive temperature. These modulations of the cellular phenotype had no effect on the *replication* of the mutant virus, however. This was interpreted to mean that the transforming gene played no essential part in viral replication. The development of molecular techniques has permitted the identification of closely homologous cellular sequences in all normal cells.[69] The virally carried oncogene was designated as *v-src,* its cellular homologue *c-src.* The latter was highly conserved in all vertebrates, indicating that it had some important "household" function. Similar cell-derived transforming sequences and corresponding, highly conserved cellular sequences could be subsequently identified in numerous other Class I RNA tumor viruses that had been isolated from various avian and mammalian species. More than 20 different oncogenes were detected in approximately 40 different viral isolates.[7] They are described in the next section.

Oncogene Families

Table I-5-1 shows an alphabetic list of the major retrovirally carried oncogenes, their pathogenicity, localization and, if known, the function of their product. The latter serves as the basis for the classification of the oncogenes, also indicated. The last column lists the involvement of the corresponding cellular protooncogene in the genesis or progression of some human tumors.

All known protooncogene functions are involved in the control of cell division. They can be classified under the following headings:

Growth factors;
Receptors;
Non-receptor kinases;
Signal transducers;
Transcription factors;
Nuclear proteins.

Growth Factors. This is a conceptually important group that contains only one presently known oncogene, v-*sis*, originally isolated from a simian sarcoma virus. Its cellular counterpart codes for one of two polypeptide chains that together constitute PDGF, platelet-derived growth factor.[80] PDGF is normally released by disintegrating thrombocytes and stimulates the division of fibroblasts, as part of the normal wound healing process. Fibroblasts respond to PDGF, but do not produce it. The accidental pickup of this gene by a simian retrovirus has turned it into a potent oncogene for fibroblasts,

Table I-5-1. Major Retrovirally Carried Oncogenes

Oncogene	Pathogenicity	Localization and Function*	Group†	Involvement of Cellular Counterpart in Human Tumors
v-abl	B cell tumors and fibrosarcomas	Membrane, tyrosine kinase	3	bcr/abl translocation in CGL, ALL
v-erbA	Supplemental	Nuclear receptor for thyroid hormone	2	
v-erbB	Erythroleukemia and fibrosarcomas	Membrane receptor for epidermal growth factor (EGF)	2	Amplified in squamous cell cancer and glioblastoma
v-ets	Supplemental		?	Occasional amplification in lymphoma; translocation in some leukemias
v-fes/fps	Sarcomas	Cytoplasmic tyrosine kinase	3	
v-fgr	Sarcomas	Membrane/cytoplasmic tyrosine kinase	3	
v-fms	Sarcomas	CSF-1 receptor	2	
v-fos	Sarcomas	DNA-binding nuclear regulatory protein	6	
v-jun	Sarcomas	Transcription factor, binds to proteins (incl fos) and DNA	5	
v-kit	Sarcomas	Related to protein kinase receptor family	2	
v-mil/raf	Sarcomas and supplemental	Cytosolic serine/threonine kinase	3	Rearrangement in primary stomach cancer
v-mos	Sarcomas	Cytoplasmic ser/thr kinase	3	
v-myb	Myeloblastosis	DNA binding nuclear regulatory protein	6	Occasional amplification in colon carcinomas, AML
v-myc	Carcinomas, leukemias, sarcomas	DNA binding nuclear regulatory protein	6	Translocation to an Ig locus in Burkitt lymphoma (c-myc), amplification in carcinomas (c-, N- or L-myc), neuroblastomas (N-myc), plasma cell leukemia (c-myc)
v-ras	Sarcomas	Membrane inner surface associated, signal transducing G-protein	4	Mutational activation in many carcinomas and leukemias; occasional amplification in carcinomas
v-rel	B-cell tumors	Nuclear DNA binding protein; transcriptional transactivator	5, 6	
v-ros	Sarcomas	Related to tyrosine kinase receptor family	2	
v-sea	Sarcomas, leukemias	Related to tyrosine kinase family	3	
v-sis	Sarcomas	Platelet derived growth factor (PDGF)	1	
v-ski	Carcinomas	Nuclear protein	6	
v-src	Sarcomas	Membrane inner surface associated tyrosine kinase	3	
v-yes	Sarcomas	Non-receptor type tyrosine kinase	3	

*Function may apply to both the virally carried oncogene and the cellular protooncogene, or to only one of them
†Group assignment: 1. growth factors; 2. receptors; 3. non-receptor kinases; 4. signal transducers; 5. transcription factors; 6. nuclear proteins

because the infected cells produce their own stimulatory factor. This stems from the fact that the retroviral genes are activated by a powerful enhancer/promoter complex, carried by the long terminal repeat (LTR) boxes at both ends of the viral RNA molecule. An attached cellular gene becomes constitutively activated, just like the viral genes. When the composite virus enters a fibroblast, the target cells produce PDGF that is normally produced by other cells, under physiologically regulated circumstances, never by the target cell itself. The illegitimate activation of the gene leads to an "autocrine,"

self stimulating cycle, manifested by the transformation of normal fibroblasts into sarcoma cells.[80]

The correctness of this explanation was proven by facsimile experiments. The normal cellular (c-sis) gene could be converted into a transforming oncogene by linking it to a retroviral LTR.[80]

It has yet not been proven that activated sis-genes contribute to natural tumor development. Numerous human sarcoma and glioma lines produce PDGF chains. Since these tumors originate from PDGF responsive tissues, this is consistent with a possible autocrine mechanism but the coexpression of the growth factor and its cognate receptor has not yet been documented, nor has it been shown that specific antibodies directed against the growth factor or its receptor can interrupt the autocrine circuit and thereby inhibit tumor growth.[21]

Receptors. Three virally transduced oncogenes have been identified as structurally altered versions of cellular genes that code for growth factor or hormone receptors. The cellular counterpart of the v-erbB oncogene that has been originally isolated from chicken erythroleukemia, codes for *epidermal growth factor (EGF) receptor*, while c-fms, the normal homolog of a feline sarcoma virus derived oncogene, codes for the CSF1 receptor.[21,66] The latter is the binding site for *macrophage* colony stimulating factor, an important regulator of the hemopoietic system. The product of the c-erbA gene has been recently identified as a thyroid hormone receptor.[79] Several other oncogenes encode proteins with a receptor like structure, although their ligands have not yet been identified. They include v-kit, v-ros and the *neu* or c-erb-B2 gene that has been detected by DNA transfection (see below). The latter technique has also detected receptor-like genes that encode tyrosine kinases (see left column of Table I-5-2). They all consist of an extracellular ligand-binding domain, a transmembrane domain and an intracellular domain. In addition to the tyrosine kinase receptor oncogenes, listed in italics, Table I-5-2 also includes, in regular print, some normal receptor genes that have a corresponding structure but no known involvement in oncogenic activity. The normally phosphorylated substrates of these kinases are unknown, but it may be surmised that they represent important regulatory proteins that can be activated or inactivated by phosphorylation. The functional control of each kinase must be tightly and differentially regulated in each cell type. Both the extracellular and the intracellular domains of kinase-receptor proteins are known to participate in this regulation. It is therefore not surprising that normal receptor genes may turn into activated oncogenes by several types of structural changes (Table I-5-3). Experimentally documented mechanisms include truncation of the extracellular, ligand binding part, mutations in the transmembrane domain, or viral insertions in the neighborhood of the gene. The best known member of this oncogene category v-erbB, is a truncated EGF receptor.[21] It lacks

Table I-5-2. Receptor Genes and Oncogenes with Protein Tyrosine Kinase Activity

Genes Encoding Protein Tyrosine Kinases with Transmembrane Domain	Genes Encoding Protein Tyrosine Kinases without Transmembrane Domain
EGF receptor gene/erbB	src
CSF-1 receptor gene/fms	yes
PDGF receptor gene	fgr
insulin receptor gene	hck
IGF-1 receptor gene	lyn
neu	fyn
trk	lck
met	abl
ros	fes/fps
ret	

From Westermark and Heldin[80]

Table I-5-3. Mechanism of Activation of Growth Factor Receptor-like Oncogenes

Mechanisms	Examples
Truncation	erbB, fms
Point mutation	neu
Chimeric molecule	trk, ret
Amplification	erbB, neu, met
Insertional mutagenesis	erbB

From Westermark and Heldin[80]

most of the extracellular ligand-binding domain, but contains the remaining part of the normal molecule, except for 32 C-terminal amino acids. This leads to a deregulation of the normal tyrosine kinase activity. A similar truncation of the c-erbB gene by retroviral insertion upstreams of the gene may lead to erythroleukemia, as discussed in the chapter on the Class II retroviruses below. Other documented cases of receptor gene activation include truncation of c-fms, point mutation of neu, also called c-erbB2, and rearrangement of trk and ret.

A recent study indicates that c-erbA, a normal thyroid hormone receptor, plays an important role in erythrocyte differentiation.[19] The v-erbA form has lost this function, due to the truncation of the gene. It can interfere with the action of the normal gene, acting as a dominant negative. It inhibits differentiation and favours progressive growth. This also shows how competition between a structurally changed gene and its normal counterpart can make the former into an oncogene and the latter into a tumor supressor gene, a frequently recurring new theme in oncogenetics.

Non-receptor Kinases. The right column of Table I-5-2 lists the tyrosine kinase oncogenes, discovered by retroviral transduction and/or by DNA transfection that do not have a receptor like transmembrane domain. Both the Rous sarcoma virus derived v-src and the Abelson mouse leukemia virus derived v-abl are in this category. Their protein products are at least partly associated with the inner surface of the plasma membrane. The normal c-src gene is mainly found in non-proliferating cells and its function may be more related to cell differentiation than to proliferation. Although c-src does not transform by itself, not even if linked to a retroviral enhancer, mutations that increase the kinase activity of the product can turn it into a transforming gene. Varmus has recently shown that a further mutant of activated c-src that has lost its kinase activity can serve as a dominant negative antagonist of the tumorigenic form and suppress its phenotypic effect in transformed cells.[33] This is an interesting competition model between transforming and suppressing variants of the same oncogene.

Several other oncogenes such as v-fes, v-fgr, v-ros, v-sea and v-yes belong to the non-receptor tyrosine kinase category, while others like v-raf and v-mos are serine/threonine kinases.[35] The mos-gene is noted for the extraordinary specificity of its expression, restricted to germ cells and early embryos.[65]

Similarly to the receptor group, the protooncogenes of the non-receptor kinase category can turn into oncogenes by structural changes that increase their kinase activity. Their natural phosphorylation targets are not known and their transforming mechanism is not understood. Current discussions are based on the assumption that the increased kinase activity changes the function of a membrane receptor or of signal transducer proteins.

Signal Transducers. Three *ras* genes, have been identified in the mammalian genome, designated H-, K-, and N-ras.[4] They resemble G-proteins that are known to participate in signal transduction from membrane receptors to the cell interior. It has been suggested, therefore, that the p21 protein product of the *ras* genes may be involved in signal transduction.[36] It is believed that most *ras* molecules exist in an inactive state in the resting cell where they bind GDP. Normal ras-proteins remain in this state until they receive a physiological stimulus from another protein, such as a transmembrane receptor. This stimulus leads to the synthesis of GTP from GDP, causing a conformational change of the ras protein. The activated protein may then interact with its as yet unknown effector molecule to continue the pathway of signal transduction. Subsequent to this interaction, the activated ras is deactivated immediately.

Numerous efforts have been made to identify the signal transduction pathways that include the ras proteins. It is very likely that the phosphatidylinositol (PI) pathway may be involved.

The ras genes can acquire transforming properties by qualitative (mutational) or quantitative (regulatory) changes. The vast majority of the known ras oncogenes owe their transforming properties, detected by the DNA transformation technique, to single point mutations at specific sites.[60,72] A 10 to 100-fold increase in the expression of *normal* ras can also transform susceptible cells, however.[4] Mutated ras is much more effective and induces more extensive changes. The mutated protein has a decreased ability to hydrolyze GTP or to bind to guanine nucleotides, compared to the normal protein. Since ras proteins exist in an equilibrium between an inactive and an active form, as already mentioned, the mutations may act by stabilizing the ras proteins in their active state. This may cause a continuous flow of signal transduction, leading to malignant transformation. Major overexpression of the normal ras protein can also create the necessary concentration of active proteins and thereby cause malignant transformation.

Transcription Factors. Originally isolated from a chicken sarcoma, the v-jun oncogene is closely homologous to AP-1, a known transcription factor.[10,45] Transcription factors play important roles in controlling gene expression. The role of the jun protein is also interesting because it can bind tightly to another nuclear oncoprotein, fos (see next section). The growth factors and oncogenes that can induce jun are components of mitotic signal chains.[76] They may be ordered in tentative sequences, such as: external growth factor-receptor-src-ras-mos....-fos-....-jun.

It may be surmised that the pathologically activated form of jun may no longer fulfill its physiological regulating function but acts as a carcinogen. Activation may occur by structural or by regulatory changes. Importantly, the transcriptional activator domain of jun is necessary for transformation, suggesting that jun induces cancer through its role as transcriptional regulator.

Most recently, the cellular counterpart of v-rel, the trans-

forming gene of a chicken reticuloendotheliosis and lymphoma virus, was also identified as a transcriptional transactivator.[75] The c-rel protooncogene is homologous to a Drosophila gene, involved in the regulation of dorsal-ventral polarity. It may be also homologous to NF kappa B, a well known transcription factor.

Nuclear Oncogenes. *Myc, myb, fos, rel* and *ski* code for DNA binding nuclear phosphoproteins that can transactivate other genes and can stimulate DNA replication, directly or indirectly. They may contribute to tumor development and/ or progression, after having been activated by structural and/ or by regulatory changes.[23] The best known gene of this category, *c-myc*,[53] is also most widely implicated in spontaneous tumor development in vivo. It is the cellular counterpart of v-myc that has been isolated from 4 different acute avian leukemia viruses. They can induce a broad spectrum of tumors, such as myelocytomatosis, endotheliomas, liver and kidney carcinomas, and erythroblastosis. One strain can also transform fibroblasts.

The cellular myc protooncogene encodes a short-lived nuclear phosphoprotein that is well conserved in vertebrates. It is a member of a family of structurally and functionally closely related genes. Next to c-myc, *N-myc* and *L-myc* are the best known members of the family. The c-myc gene can be constitutively activated by retroviral insertion on either side, or by translocation to a highly active chromosome region, such as an immunoglobulin locus in B-cells. It can also contribute to tumor progression by amplification, as will be discussed below. The extraordinary frequency of c-myc activation by these mechanisms in different tumors, and in the apparent absence of any structural changes in the protein, indicates that c-myc can turn into an oncogene by purely regulatory changes that lead to the constitutive expression of the gene and make it refractory to normal regulatory factors.

The role of the pathologically activated, constitutively expressed myc gene in the oncogenic process may be seen in relation to the normal expression of the gene.[40] Resting fibroblasts and lymphocytes do not express any detectable myc message but activated cells do. Growth factor or mitogen stimulation induces c-fos and c-myc. The induction of the "competence genes," involved in preparing the entry of resting cells into the mitotic cycle, is among the earliest activation asssociated changes.

A high constitutive myc expression can abrogate the growth factor requirements of normal cells. IL3 or IL2 dependent hemopoietic cell lines infected with v-myc-carrying retroviruses acquired the ability to grow in the absence of the stimulatory interleukin and became tumorigenic in mice.[59] This was not accompanied by constitutive IL3 or IL2 production and was therefore not due to an autocrine mechanism. It would appear that the uninterrupted expression of myc obviates the need of the cell for an external growth stimulatory signal.

When continuously proliferating leukemia, teratocarcinoma, neuroblastoma, or histiocytoma cells are induced to differentiate into a quiescent (Go) cell, myc expression is downregulated.[53] This can be prevented by the introduction of a constitutively expressed myc construct that fails to respond to normal regulatory signals. As long as myc expression is maintained, differentiation is inhibited.[18,57] Contrariwise, inhibition of c-myc expression by anti-sense RNA can lead to accelerated differentiation.[28,58] These experiments are consistent with the postulate that the pathological activation of myc expression by retroviral insertion or chromosomal translocation can prevent the cell from leaving the cycling compartment in accordance with its normal program. Such cells have an increased self renewal potential in vivo, and can readily grow as immortalized lines in vitro.

The v-fos oncogene has been originally detected in two different mouse osteosarcoma viruses. The normal c-fos protein is highly expressed in certain terminally differentiated cells and it has been therefore proposed that it plays a role in differentiation.[48] But c-fos is also believed to play a role in the activation of quiescent fibroblasts. Abrogation of fos-protein induction by antisense RNA prevented the cells from entering the cell cycle upon growth factor stimulation.[50] It is believed that the fos protein plays a multiple transregulatory function in modulating the expression of different sets of genes.

The molecular mechanisms involved in the activation of the non-tumorigenic c-fos gene into a powerful oncogene have been analyzed extensively. Considerable structural changes are required, but they do not involve the coding regions of the c-fos gene. The presence of a retroviral enhancer (LTR) region is necessary but not sufficient. In addition, a 67 bp element in the 3' non coding region must be deleted.[47] Other, C-terminal coding sequence deletions may have the same effect. This can be interpreted to mean that two changes are essential for the transforming effect: deregulation of transcription by the insertion of a constitutively active promoter/enhancer, and the elimination of a recognition signal for RNA degradation.[49]

The oncogene v-myb has been isolated from a defective avian leukemia virus. Its oncogenicity is restricted to myeloid cells. Activation of the normal c-myb proto-oncogene is dependent on the truncation of the coding region at both ends. Two independent viral isolates and several murine tumors with activated myb-genes showed similar deletions. The expression of c-myb decreases when immature cells are induced to differentiate. Therefore, c-myb is believed to play a role in the proliferation of hemopoietic cells.

Metabolic instability seems to be a common feature of several nuclear oncoproteins, such as myb, myc and fos, suggesting that they may be involved in the regulation of the cell cycle.

Sequence comparisons between v-onc genes and their normal cellular protooncogene counterparts have revealed considerable differences. Some of them may simply reflect random mutations and genetic drift during the prolonged passage of the virus, while others are responsible for an increased kinase or other relevant activity that contributes to transforming potential of the oncogene. Normal cellular protooncogene sequences, linked to viral enhancers, differ in their transforming or tumorigenic properties. Several of them are non- or less tumorigenic than the corresponding oncogenes but some are equally tumorigenic as the corresponding v-onc gene.

Convincing demonstration that a structurally or functionally activated normal oncogene may contribute to spontaneous tumor development came from the study of chromosomal translocations and the detection of oncogene amplification, as discussed below.

Oncogene Activation by Retroviral Insertion

The chronic or Class II RNA tumor viruses do not carry any oncogenes, but they often act through the activation of cellular protooncogenes.[15] Hayward et al have first raised the question whether avian leukosis virus (ALV) may cause tumors when a proviral DNA copy integrates in the neighbourhood of a protooncogene. If so, one of the two powerful enhancers located at each end of the viral genome could be expected to activate the juxtaposed cellular gene. Viral enhancers have evolved to compete with normal gene regulation. They may therefore switch on a nearby gene in a permanent, constitutive fashion. This was first verified by Hayward's detection of fused messages in the ALV-induced B-cell lymphomas of the chicken.[32] These messages originated from the viral promoter, and extended into the adjacent c-myc gene. Since retroviruses integrate at random with the cellular DNA, insertion in the neighborhood of c-myc in the correct orientation must be a very rare event. Many random integration events must take place prior to the "correct" hit. This explains some of the characteristic features of Class II retroviral oncogenesis such as the long latency period, the lack of a direct transforming effect and the need for long maintained virus production at a high level.

Table I-5-4 lists some of the better known oncogenic retroviral insertion systems. The protooncogene c-myc is activated by retroviral insertion upstream or downstream of the gene that does not disrupt the gene itself. In contrast, the insertional activation of c-erbB and c-myb is invariably associated with the truncation of the gene.

These experiments have not only explained the action of the Class II RNA tumor viruses, but they have also proven that the constitutive activation of *cellular* oncogenes may be an essential step in the tumorigenic process. Doubts about the significance of cellular oncogene activation in the natural history of spontaneously occurring tumors continued to prevail, however, because most of the Class II RNA tumor viruses had been selected for high tumorigenicity by prolonged passage in highly susceptible and usually inbred animal hosts. These doubts have only disappeared after it had been shown that cellular protooncogenes may be activated by non-viral mechanisms, such as mutation, translocation and amplification, and that they can contribute to tumor development. These mechanisms will be summarized in subsequent sections below.

The insertion of retroviral DNA into certain preferred integration sites has also identified some new, previously unknown protooncogenes that had been activated by the retrovirus. Several interesting integration domains like pim-1, MLVI-1, MLVI-4, evi-1, evi-2 and others have been detected with the help of the murine leukemia viruses.[51] The insertion preferences of the mouse mammary tumor agent (MMTV), has led to the identification of four new genes int-1, int-2, int-3, and int-4. At least one of them, int-1, had detectable transforming activity after insertion into a retrovirus.[14] It encodes a secretory protein, homologous to the product of the *wingless* gene

Table I-5-4. Cellular Protooncogenes Activated by Retroviral Insertion

Oncogene	Retrovirus	Tumor	Species	Note
c-myc	ALV or REV	B-cell lymphomas	Chicken	Fused cellular-viral messages
c-myc	REV	T-cell lymphomas	Chicken	The same
c-myc	MuLV	T-cell lymphomas	Mouse	Viral insertion into common high frequency integration sites
c-myc	FeLV	T-cell lymphomas	Cat	Generates myc-transducing virus
c-erbB	ALV	Erythroblastosis	Chicken	Chimeric viral-c-erbB messages, characteristic truncation
c-myb	Abelson MuLV	Early myeloid tumors, monocytic leukemias	Mouse	c-myb truncated at both ends. Viral insertions resemble changes in v-myb
c-myb	EU-8 avian leukosis virus	B-cell lymphomas with widespread metastasis	Chicken	Viral integration within c-myb. Abnormal transcripts
c-fms	Friend MuLV	Myeloid leukemias	Mouse	Overexpression and deregulation

From Cluman and Hayward[15]

in Drosophila, known to be involved in pattern formation. The function of int-2 is less known, but its virtually exclusive expression in early embryonic development has attracted wide attention from developmental biologists. Its activation generates a premalignant state in the mammary gland. Occasionally, MMTV insertion is found in the neighborhood of more than one gene, e.g., both int-1 and int-2, in the same tumor.[54] This may be regarded as a Class II counterpart of the double oncogene carrying Class I RNA tumor viruses.

Transformation with Tumor Derived DNA

The notion that activated *cellular* oncogenes can contribute to the development and/or progression of human tumors was stimulated by the discovery that DNA from a human bladder carcinoma and later from many other human and animal tumors could transform established strains of rodent fibroblasts in vitro and render them tumorigenic in vivo.[52] Serial passage of transforming DNA from transfected mouse fibroblasts permitted the isolation of the transforming human genes. Irrelevant human DNA is rapidly lost during such passage. The active human gene can be picked up by hybridization with the human species specific repetitive (Alu) sequences. The first bladder carcinoma study has led to the isolation of an activated *ras* gene.[52] This was followed by similar findings in many other tumors. The tumor derived transforming or "activated" forms of *ras* were found to carry point mutations in the same "hot spot" codons as the original, virally transduced *ras* genes.[4]

Transformation of rodent fibroblast lines with human tumor DNA has also identified other cellular oncogenes. Some of them had been previously known as virally transduced genes or were the close relatives of such genes, while others were first detected by the DNA technique (Table I-5-5). Repeated isolation of the same activated oncogene from the same tumor type was taken to indicate that its activation may contribute to the development and/or progression of the tumor.

Among the oncogenes detected by DNA transfection studies, *c-erbB2* or *neu* is of considerable interest.[5] Its product

Table I-5-5. Oncogenes Found in Tumor Cells by the DNA-mediated Transformation Technique

Oncogene	Localization and Function	Changes in Human Tumors
neu(c-erbB2)	Membrane receptor	Progression related amplification in breast carcinomas, glioblastomas
met	Tyrosine kinase	
trk	Tyrosine kinase	Activated in colon carcinoma
p53	Nuclear DNA binding protein	Activated in many carcinomas, sarcomas and leukemias

is highly homologous to, but distinct from c-erbB, the EGF receptor. The oncogenic mutation of neu was found to affect the transmembrane part of the protein. This implies that the transmembrane region has a critical role in the transduction of the mitogenic signal from the ligand binding external domain to the intracellular effector domain.

The *neu* gene can undergo amplification in breast carcinomas in a progression related fashion.[67] Amplification was also found in a salivary gland adenocarcinoma.

The *met* oncogene was identified in human osteosarcoma cells after in vitro treatment with the carcinogen methylnitrosourea (MNU).[17] The structural features of *met* indicate that it may encode a growth factor receptor for an unknown ligand. Oncogene activation is associated with rearrangement.

Oncogene Complementation

Following the discovery that established strains of rodent fibroblasts can be transformed by DNA from human tumors, Land, Parada and Weinberg have shown that even normal diploid rodent fibroblasts can be transformed, but only if two activated oncogenes are combined.[42] The first successful combination was myc and ras. Constitutively activated but otherwise normal myc genes immortalized the diploid fibroblasts, without any sign of morphological transformation. Mutationally activated ras genes changed the social relationships between the cells. The normal flat, two-dimensional monolayer transformed into disorderly and partly three dimensional growth. This was due to the lack of contact inhibition between the cells and was correlated with increased agarose clonability.

The oncogene complementation system was also helpful for the classification of other oncogenes as immortalizing or "myc related" and transforming or "ras related."[78] The former category includes, in addition to the other members of the *myc* family, also jun, myb, p53, ski and fos. This category also includes several DNA virus encoded transforming proteins, such as SV40 and polyoma large T, adenoviral E1A, and the human papillomavirus encoded E7 proteins. It is noteworthy that all immortalizing gene products in this group are nuclear proteins. In contrast, oncogenes of the ras-like group encode membrane associated proteins. In addition to other members of the ras family, the group includes polyoma middle T, a membrane associated, virally encoded transforming protein, and the cell-derived oncogenes src, erb B, ros, fms, fos, mil, mos and abl.

Weinberg has suggested that the nuclear proteins of the myc group may immortalize diploid fibroblasts by emancipating them from their requirement for exogenous signals.[78] Cells with constitutively expressed nuclear oncogenes can divide in the absence of growth factors secreted by other cells. Membrane proteins of the activated ras type liberate the cells from their own programmed, inner growth limitations. They can achieve this either by faulty signal transmission as in the case of ras, or by permanent damage to a membrane receptor, as in the case of v-erbB and v-fms, or by increased kinase activity that changes the normal membrane structure, as in the case of src and abl.

The activities of the nuclear and the cytoplasmic oncogenes are complementary rather than additive. Certain cancer traits are more effectively induced by nuclear proteins while others are more readily achieved by gene products that act in the cytoplasm, depending on the cell type and its actual position in the chain of tumor progression.[77]

Oncogene Activation by Chromosomal Translocation

A "natural" mode of cellular oncogene activation was discovered by the analysis of tumor associated chromosomal translocations.[38] Burkitt's lymphoma, a B-cell derived, immunoglobulin producing tumor, carries one of three alternative translocations in virtually 100% of the cases. The high endemic, largely EBV-carrying and the sporadic, mainly EBV-negative form contain the same translocations. They arise by a break in chromosome 8 at band q24, the location of the c-myc gene, and a break of one of the three immunoglobulin gene carrying chromosomes, followed by a reciprocal exchange of the terminal segments. In the most frequent or *typical* translocation, chromosome 14 breaks at the site of the IgH locus. In the two alternative *variant* translocations, 2;8 and 8;22, resp. chr 2 breaks at the site of the kappa and chr 22 at the site of the lambda gene. This juxtaposition of c-myc to the immunoglobulin (Ig) sequences subordinates them to the control of the constitutively active Ig-loci. The latter are not programmed to switch off at any time during the con-

tinued lifespan of the B-cell. The c-myc gene is regularly expressed in proliferating but not in resting cells.[53] The Ig-juxtaposed myc gene is constitutively expressed like an Ig-locus. In contrast to the normal, non-translocated myc gene, it does not obey the normal down regulation program of myc at the time when activated B-cells turn into long lived resting cells in G0. This happens on at least two different occasions during the life cycle of the B-cell: following the normal Ig-gene rearrangement when a pre-B turns into a virgin B-cell, and on the cessation of antigen induced B-cell proliferation when a stimulated blast turns into a memory cell.

Myc was first discovered as the transforming sequence of an avian leukemia virus.[53] The v-myc gene can transform a wide range of cells, including hemopoietic, mesenchymal and epithelial targets. Activation of its cellular (c-myc) counterpart can participate in the development and/or progression of many different tumors. Its activation by retroviral insertion is a regular event in the initiation of chicken bursal lymphoma. It is activated by chromosomal translocation to an Ig-locus, not only in Burkitt's lymphoma, but also in mouse and rat plasmacytoma. Moreover, the progression of several human tumors to more malignant forms can be favored by the amplification of c-myc or its close relatives, N- or L-myc, as discussed in the section on oncogene amplification below. This extraordinary frequency of myc activation by these three different mechanisms, and in so many different tumors probably reflects the fact that the normal protooncogene can turn into an oncogene by purely regulatory changes that lead to higher or more constitutive expression, without necessarily requiring any structural changes.

The dysregulation of c-myc by its juxtaposition to an Ig-locus is the clearest known example of tissue specific oncogene activation by a purely cellular mechanism. The molecular anatomy of the translocation is closely similar in the corresponding human, murine and rat tumors.[41] The breakpoints in and around the c-myc gene vary widely in different tumors, suggesting that the breakage is a random accident of cell division. The coding sequences always retain their integrity, indicating that the constitutively expressed myc protein needs to be intact in order to provide the translocation carrying cells with a selective advantage. The regular occurrence of the translocations indicates that they represent an essential rate limiting step in the tumorigenic process. This conclusion could be confirmed by "facsimile" experiments. Transgenic mice that carry a myc gene under the control of an immunoglobulin enhancer develop pre-B and B-cell derived lymphomas in 90% or more.[2] Mice infected with a retrovirally activated v-myc gene developed pristane oil induced plasmacytomas much faster and in a higher frequency than uninfected, pristane treated controls.[56] The plasmacytomas that expressed the experimentally introduced v-myc gene do not have any Ig/myc translocations, in contrast to those that did not express v-myc had either a typical or a variant translocation. These experiments confirmed that activated myc genes were tumorigenic for B-cells and supported the conclusion that the Ig/myc translocations trigger the development of the tumor by the constitutive activation of myc. They also showed that additional changes were required for the development of fully autonomous neoplasia, however, since all facsimile tumors were mono- or oligoclonal. Activation of additional oncogene(s) and/or loss of tumor suppressor genes may be required in addition. This is in line with our current knowledge concerning the multi-step development of most cancers.[39]

The CML- and ALL-associated Philadelphia (Ph$_1$) chromosome is another important case in point.[20] It also acts by the activation of a translocated oncogene, but in a different way. The typical form of the Ph$_1$ translocation arises by a reciprocal exchange between chromosomes 9 and 22. The apical breakpoint region of chr 9 contains the c-abl proto-oncogene. The corresponding v-abl oncogene was originally identified as the transforming sequence of the Abelson murine leukemia virus. This virus can transform pre-B cells and fibroblasts and is also a powerful accelerator of mineral oil induced murine plasmacytoma development. The retrovirally carried transforming gene is truncated at its 5' end. This lesion is associated with an increased enzymatic (tyrosine kinase) activity. In the typical 9;22 translocation, c-abl is truncated in an analogous way, due to its fusion with a cellular sequence, designated *bcr*, and has a similarly increased kinase activity. An abnormal 210 kD bcr/abl fusion protein is created that leads to the preleukemic condition known as CML. The Ph$_1$ translocation associated with a highly malignant variant of ALL in children and adults is cytogenetically identical but differs from the CML translocation at the molecular level. Only a minor part of the *bcr* sequences are involved. The fusion protein is smaller (185 kD) but it has a higher tyrosine kinase activity and has a greater transforming activity.

A comparison between the Ig/myc and the bcr/abl translocation provides some interesting parallels and contrasts. The Ig-sequences activate the myc-gene by a purely regulatory change, as mentioned, while the bcr/abl fusion protein is a structurally abnormal product. Moreover, while the constitutive expression of the translocated myc gene is accompanied by the down-regulation of the normal, untranslocated allele, the bcr/abl fusion protein is expressed together with the normal 160 kD c-abl protein.

The activation of the myc and abl oncogenes by purely cellular mechanisms has corroborated the notion that abnormally activated c-onc genes can contribute to tumor development under natural conditions. The subsequent study of other tumor associated translocations has generated important new information in its own right. Similarly to the DNA transfection approach, the translocation studies that have not only identified already known oncogenes, such as myc or abl, but revealed the existence of previously unknown oncogenes.

The study of the numerous translocations found in B- and T-cell lymphomas was particularly rewarding, since they involved the normally rearranging immunoglobulin or T-cell receptor sequences, respectively. The attached sequence that has become translocated from another chromosome could be identified by departing from the breakpoint.[31] The discovery of the bcl-2 oncogene, the chromosome 18-derived, IgH juxtaposed sequence in the follicular lymphoma associated 14;18 translocation was particularly important. Facsimile experiments with transgenic mice have shown that constitutive activation of the bcl-2 gene by a linked IgH enhancer (Emu) increase the life span of resting B-cells and prevent their programmed death by apoptosis. The corre-

sponding Emu-*myc* transgenics have gone one step farther. They had no resting B-cells at all. All their B-cells had transformed into proliferating immunoblasts.[1]

The myc/Ig translocation does not involve any specific sequences in or around the myc locus. In contrast, the IgH/bcl-2 (14;18) translocation takes place by recombination between J (joining) sequences of the IgH locus on chr 14 and corresponding homologous sequences in the neighborhood of the bcl-2 locus. The 14;18 translocation leads to the activation of the normal bcl-2 protein, lending further support to the notion that the major mode of oncogene activation in lymphoid malignancies is due to the action of juxtaposed (*cis*) regulatory sequences. It must be noted, however, that the oncogenic effect of different displaced oncogenes can be quite different. This can be best seen in the contrast between myc and bcl-2. The myc/Ig translocation leads to highly malignant lymphomas whereas the bcl-2/IgH translocation causes low grade malignancy.[31] This can be seen in relation to the different effects of the two genes in the transgenic mice, mentioned above. Occasionally a bcl-2/IgH carrying low grade lymphoma may progress to high malignancy by a second Ig/myc translocation. This is a good example of tumor progression by the sequential activation of different oncogenes. Progression of Ph$_1$ positive CML to acute leukemia provides another example.[20] Blast crisis can proceed through one of several alternative pathways. Duplication of the Ph$_1$ chromosome, appearance of an extra chromosome 8 and morphological change of chromosome 17 are the most common "major routes."

Myc and other oncogene translocations have also been identified in T-cell leukemias and lymphomas.[31] Instead of the Ig loci, the T-cell translocations involve one of the T-cell receptor (TCR) genes. The architecture of T-cell translocations resembles the variant (light chain), rather than the typical (heavy chain) translocations in the B-cells. The most common translocation disrupts J-segments of the TCR alpha locus on chromosome 14q11. The TCR beta locus on chromosome 7 is frequently involved.

Oncogene amplification in spontaneous human and animal tumors is an additional mechanism that has proven the role of pathologically active c-onc genes in tumor progression. Gene amplification is a well known phenomenon in the field of drug resistance.[64] Chronic exposure of bacteria or leukemic cells to methotrexate, a folic acid antagonist, leads to the amplification of the dihydrofolate reductase (DHFR) gene. Its enzyme product can detoxify the drug. The number of amplified gene copies increase with increasing levels of the drug. The amplified genes can be often visualized at the microscopic level. They can appear in two alternative forms. They may assemble into new chromosome domains that appear as homogeneously staining regions (HSR), because they lack the normal banding pattern. Alternatively, they can appear as multiple small chromosome-like elements, called double minutes (dms). HSR and dms are mutually exclusive. Gene amplification can also occur in the absence of cytogenetically visible changes, as detected by molecular hybridization with the appropriate gene probe.

Methotrexate resistant cells tend to lose their amplified DHFR gene sequences rapidly after the removal of the drug. Superficially, the amplification of resistance genes in drug treated cells and its reversal on the cessation of treatment look as induced adaptive responses, but they are not. A large variety of genes can be amplified in cells exposed to many different toxic agents, including chemical carcinogens, as part of a cellular stress reaction.[43] Following exposure to certain toxic agents that inhibit DNA synthesis, cells may respond with a random amplification of many actively transcribed sequences. Those cells that happen to contain extra copies of a gene that provides them with a selective advantage under the actual circumstances acquire a selective value and overgrow the rest. When selection is relaxed, the "extra gene burden" is usually not maintained—it is probably a handicap.

A wide variety of solid and hemopoietic tumors have been found to harbor amplified oncogenes.[3,16,67,71] Genes of the myc family were amplified most frequently. In small cell lung carcinoma (SCLC), myc-amplification was correlated with a "variant tumor cell phenotype",[44] characterized by shorter doubling time, higher cloning efficiency, increased radioresistance, increased invasiveness, increased tumorigenicity in nude mice, high metastatic ability and morphological and enzymatic changes associated with poor prognosis. Interestingly, the three known myc-genes, C-, N- and L-myc were alternatively amplified, suggesting a close functional relationship. N-myc has been originally discovered due to its prognostically unfavourable amplification in neuroblastoma[13] and L-myc through its amplification in some SCLC variants.[44] Their postulated functional relationship is consistent with the similar transforming potential of c- and N-myc, when cotransfected with activated ras genes into rat embryo fibroblasts.[65] This does not exclude minor functional differences, as suggested by the finding that SCLC variants with an N-myc amplification were less aggressive than their c-myc amplified counterparts.

Apparently, myc amplification conveys a growth advantage on the lung carcinoma cell, particularly after it had been displaced to a foreign tissue environment. In the neuroblastomas, Brodeur et al found a significant correlation between N-myc amplification and the more aggressive stage III-IV forms of the disease. There was a close correlation between patient survival and the N-myc copy number in the tumors.[13] In human B plasmacytomas, we have found a relationship between c-myc amplification, and the appearance of plasma cell leukemia,[71] the most malignant form of the disease.

Amplification of the *neu* oncogene in about 30% of breast carcinomas was correlated with poor prognosis and particularly in patients with extensive axillary lymph node involvement.[11,67] For node-positive patients, *neu* amplification was a significant predictor of early relapse and death.

It is not known how amplified oncogenes contribute to tumor progression, but their persistence during tumor growth and after metastasis suggests that the presence of the amplified copies is needed for the maintenance of highly malignant growth.

Amplified oncogenes may act by increasing the concentration of the relevant oncoprotein. An increased level of myc protein in the more invasive and metastatic forms of SCLC could act by increasing the proliferative drive of the cells, so that they become more apt to overcome local growth restricting forces in distant tissue compartments. Alterna-tively, gene amplification may not be accompanied by a parallel increase of the corresponding oncoprotein, but could act by titrating out regulatory factors that would normally inhibit the gene. A delicate balance may exist between the transcription of regulatory factors and their target DNA sequences in or near the gene. Amplification of the target sequences may tilt the balance in favor of cell division, at the expense of differentiation.[53] It may be noted that strong differentiation inducing signals elicited by TPA or DMSO, could down-regulate the 40-60 fold amplified, highly expressed myc genes in HL60, a promyelocytic leukemia line, concomitantly with terminal differentiation. Similarly, the highly expressed N-myc was downregulated when neuroblastoma cells were induced to differentiate by retinoic acid exposure.[74]

The Role of Oncogenes in the Multistep Evolution of Tumors

Few would contest the statement that the division and differentiation of somatic cells in higher organisms are regulated by multiple controls. Since cancer develops by the emancipation of a single cell from these controls, most, if not all cancers must arise through a series of sequential changes. Each step can be expected to provide the new mutant with a growth advantage, leading to the enrichment of the derived subclone. Cancer development can be viewed as a microevolutionary process that progresses toward increasing independence of the evolving subclonal series from host regulation.

The validity of this concept has been confirmed repeatedly. Statistical analysis of age incidence curves have shown that most solid tumors appear as a function of the fifth or sixth power of time.[24,55] This was taken to suggest that the tumors have arisen by five or six rate limiting mutational steps. Three to four changes appear to be involved in the origin of the leukemias.

The multistage concept of tumor development was also confirmed by the histological, cytogenetic and biological study of spontaneously occurring human and animal cancers.[26,27] The only known exceptions were found among the directly transforming class I retroviruses, mentioned in the beginning of this chapter. There is no doubt that v-src can transform cells and cause tumors in a single step for example. Serial laboratory passage of the oncogene carrying viruses, accompanied by continuous selection for high tumorigenicity by the investigator, tends to fix multiple genetic changes in the same transforming sequence, however, that contribute to high transforming capacity in a mutually complementary way. The most striking example of the same principle is demonstrated by the retroviruses that had picked up two unlinked oncogenes with complementary transforming effects.[78]

The natural process of spontaneous tumor development is quite different. Selection acts on cell clones, not on virally carried sequences. This favors single changes in multiple genes.[73] The resulting process whereby tumors go "from bad to worse" was called "progression" by Peyton Rous.[62] Foulds has described the natural history of tumor progression and formulated some of its basic rules.[26] He saw the neoplastic phenotype as being composed of several "unit characteristics," that could reassort independently. The same end stage, the relatively autonomous tumor phenotype, could be reached through several alternative pathways.

Foulds' progression rules tied in well with the important work of his contemporary, Jacob Furth. In a classical review on conditioned and autonomous neoplasms, Furth defined distinct stages in the development and progression of hormone dependent tumors.[27] His choice of the endocrine organs and their hormone dependent target tissues was based on the insight that they provided the only available system at the time that would permit an analysis of the relationship between growth regulatory host factors and their targets. He was convinced that the same principles must apply to tumor development in other tissues. This concept was fully vindicated by the modern development. One only needs to substitute growth factors and their receptors, instead of hormones and hormone receptors and the same general rules will emerge.

Furth has shown that a proliferative lesion can be induced in a hormone dependent tissue by the chronic overproduction of stimulating hormone or by the prolonged deficiency of an inhibitory hormone. This is consistent with the modern picture. The autocrine model of oncogene action is the clearest example of overstimulation. Faulty signaling from structurally changed receptors or from mutated signal transducers also belong to this category. The loss of an inhibitory factor is most clearly manifested in the inactivation of tumor suppressor genes such as Rb or p53 (see I-6). Immune defects that may permit the outgrowth of potentially highly antigenic, EBV and papilloma virus transformed cells are the only currently known examples at the host level.

In Furth's experiments, tumors induced by a certain hormonal imbalance were at least initially dependent on the persistence of the same imbalance. They ceased to grow or even regressed completely when the anomaly was corrected. This was referred to as the *conditioned* or *responsive* phase. Mutations that occurred at unpredictable intervals gave rise to *autonomous* subclones that could grow in normal, hormonally balanced hosts. They were often responsive, since they grew better in hosts with the original hormonal imbalance. Further changes could render them totally unresponsive.

The modern development has shown that activation of the growth factor-receptor circuits by autocrine mechanisms or by qualitative or quantitative changes in a receptor protein may first lead to a hyperplastic response of phenotypically normal cells.[37] This may be a necessary but not sufficient event in tumorigenesis. In terminally differentiating systems, such an event must be complemented by a differentiation block, in order to cause malignant growth.[80] A resulting subclone may be molded by further oncogene activation or suppressor loss events.

Both Furth and Foulds have viewed the growth momentum of the tumor cell population as the composite derivative of "intrinsic" and "responsive" growth. Most normal cells have a low intrinsic and a high responsive potential. Tumor progression is based on the stepwise increase of intrinsic growth, concurrent with the decrease of responsiveness. In Furth's view, "dependence and autonomy are relative and qualitative terms. Autonomy is never certain."[27]

There is still no better phenomenological description of tumor progression than the formulations of Foulds and Furth. Molecular biology has opened the way toward the precise identification of the underlying genetic changes. At least three functionally distinct gene groups can influence progression. Activation of the *oncogenes* by regulatory or structural changes can contribute to the intrinsic growth momentum of the cells. *Tumor suppressor* genes can facilitate tumor growth by their loss. The third group consists of miscellaneous genes that can *modulate* the growth of already established tumors, e.g. by influencing their invasive or metastatic behavior, or their sensitivity to immune rejection.

Activation of a single oncogene may play a unique, dominating role in the development of a given tumor, as illustrated by the chromosomal translocations in Burkitt's lymphoma and in chronic myelogenous leukemia. In the latter, the bcr/abl translocation is an essential, rate limiting event, while progression to highly malignant leukemia, referred to as the blast crisis, can occur through one of several alternative pathways. Multiple changes that may involve several alternative pathways have been also identified in T-cell leukemias, brain tumors and colorectal carcinomas. They are usually composed of both oncogene activation and suppressor loss events.

The prevalent mechanism of activation differs among the oncogenes and between different cell types. The preneoplastic history of the tumor, including events of initiation, promotion or chronic proliferation of the neoplastic precursor cell, can favor the probability of a given activation mechanism at the expense of another. In spite of all this diversity, there are a number of recurrent trends that are more striking than the variations. Oncogenes of the *ras* family are activated by the same point mutations in spontaneous and chemically induced human and animal tumors and in their virally transduced counterparts. The molecular anatomy of the corresponding virally transduced *versus* in situ activated cellular oncogene, shows close similarities in the case of *myb*, *abl*, *fos* and *erbB*. The range of transformation susceptible tissues can be similar or different for the corresponding v- and c-onc gene, depending on the host cell range of the carrier virus on the one hand, and the impact of the carcinogenic noxa, on the other.

The activation of cellular oncogenes in the course of tumor development and progression can be seen as experiments of nature. Their ability to contribute to the carcinogenic process *in humans* has been established beyond doubt. The cellular counterparts of at least nine retrovirally transduced oncogenes (see Table I-5-1), namely *abl*, *erbB*, *ets*, *mos*, *myb*, *myc*, *H-ras* and *sis* have been incriminated in the spontaneous, natural tumorigenic process.[8] Activated *ras*-oncogenes have been found in carcinomas of the bladder, breast, colon, kidney, liver, lung, ovary, pancreas, stomach, hematopoietic tumors of lymphoid and myeloid origin, fibrosarcomas, rhabdomyosarcomas, melanomas, neuroblastomas, gliomas and teratocarcinomas.[4] Approximately 10–25% of all human cancers have activated Ki-ras genes, although in certain tumors, such as colon carcinomas, the frequency may be as high as 40–50%. Activated k-ras can be often found in benign adenomas.[2626]

No single type of tumor has consistently harbored a mutated

taneous mammary tumor formation among inbred strains of mice led to the proposal by Haaland that tumorigenesis behaved in a formal sense as a mendelian genetic trait.[43] Similarly, analysis of the pedigrees of cancer patients at the University of Michigan Hospital between 1895 and 1913 identified four multigenerational families with susceptibilities to several specific cancer types that appeared to be transmitted as autosomal dominant mendelian traits (Figure I-6-1).[123] Although these studies suggested that in some cases a genetic basis for cancer might exist, other explanations for familial clustering were possible, and furthermore, it was argued that most cancers occurred as sporadic, isolated cases.

The notion that cancer might arise from a somatic alteration in the genetic material of the cell was first proposed by Boveri who noted that in sea urchin eggs fertilized by two sperm, abnormal mitotic divisions leading to the loss of chromosomes occurred in daughter cells, and atypical tissue masses could be seen in the resulting gastrula. He believed that these abnormal tissues appeared physically similar to the poorly differentiated tissue masses seen in tumors, and hypothesized that cancer arose from a cellular aberration that produced abnormal mitotic figures.[11] This hypothesis apparently did not gain favor at the time, initially because of the lack of direct experimental support from studies of the karyotypes of animal and human tumors, and later because of uncertainty about whether the changes in chromosome number in tumors were a cause or an effect of the neoplastic phenotype.

A landmark observation in the identification of a genetic

FAMILY G.

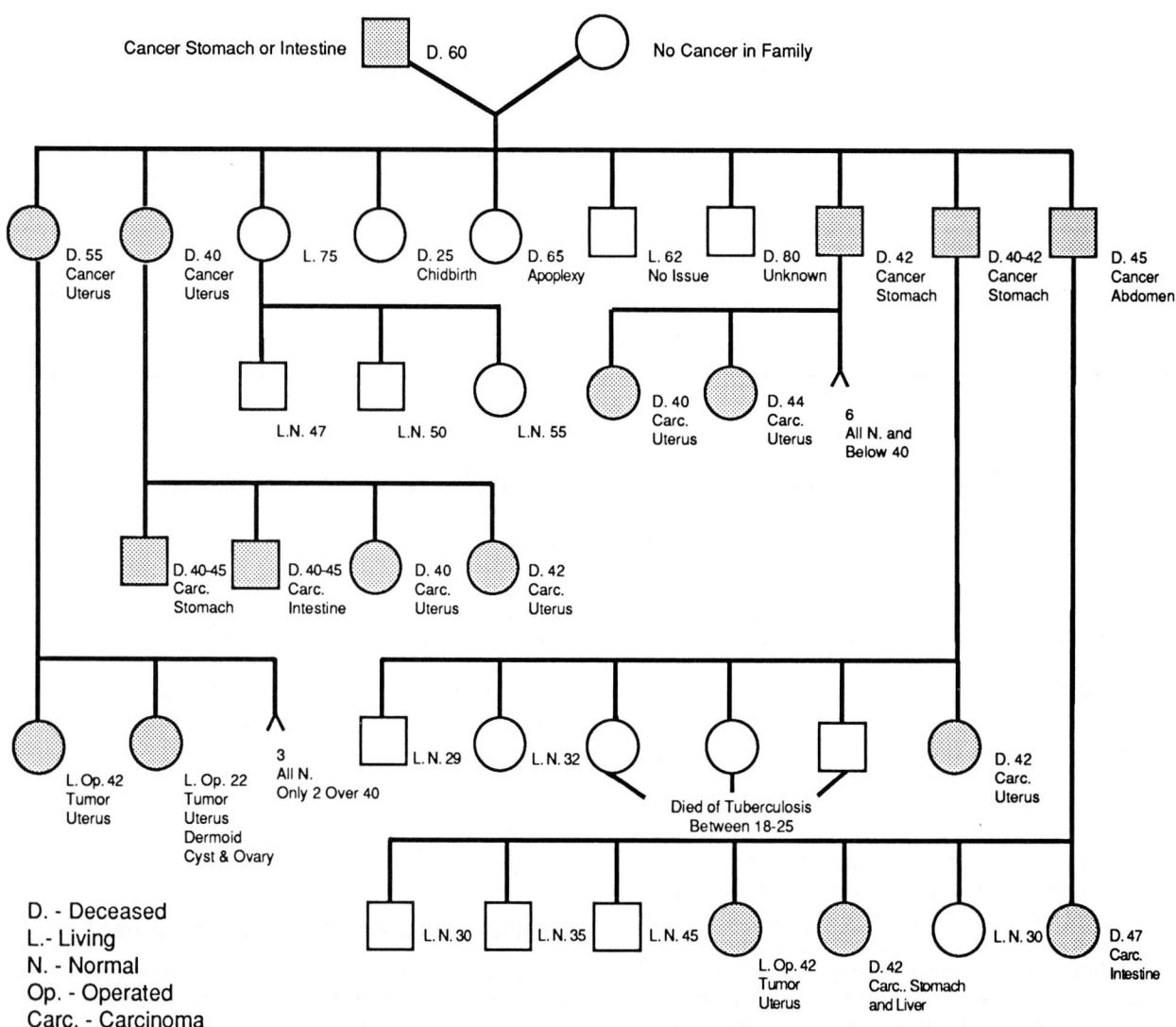

Figure I-6-1. The inheritance of cancer in a family (family G). The affected members with cancer are indicated by shaded figures, as well as the type of cancer in each case. The family demonstrates a dominant inheritance pattern for the development of cancer, either of the stomach, intestine, or uterus. (From A. S. Warthin.[123])

basis for cancer was reported by Rous in 1911, when he showed that sarcomas could be induced in chickens by cell-free filtrates of a sarcoma that arose spontaneously in a chicken.[99] Although this observation was interpreted as evidence that neoplasms could be virally-induced, the observation also was consistent with the idea that cancer could be attributed to discrete genetic elements. Sixty years after Rous' initial report, the oncogenic region of the Rous sarcoma virus was identified,[75] and further characterization and cloning of this region demonstrated that the oncogenicity of the virus resulted from the v-src gene, a transduced cellular gene.[114] Subsequently, it has been found that all oncogenes of acutely-transforming RNA tumor viruses are, in fact, transduced cellular genes.[7] The biochemical mechanisms by which viral oncogenes cause neoplastic transformation are still not precisely defined at present, but many of the cellular homologues of the viral oncogenes have been found to encode proteins that are intimately involved in the pathways of growth control in the normal cell. The viral oncogenes appear to cause transformation because they are mutated versions of the cellular genes and/or are expressed aberrantly; their effect is to alter cell growth in a positive fashion.[7]

It was thus hypothesized that human cancer might result, not from acutely-transforming tumor viruses per se, but from somatic mutations that might activate the cellular homologues of the oncogenes.[8,119] Although this was an attractive hypothesis, and oncogenes have been shown to play a significant role in many human tumors, they form only part of the story of the genetic bases for tumorigenesis.[44,125] For example, oncogenes have not been demonstrated to underlie the inherited predisposition to any human cancer. Furthermore, oncogenes appear to act in a positive fashion in neoplastic transformation. Many of the properties of neoplastic cells, however, including immortality and tumorigenicity, appear to result from the inactivation or loss of function of normal cellular genes. These cellular genes, hypothesized to regulate cellular proliferation and growth in a negative fashion, have been termed tumor suppressor genes.[59,100,112] Although the concept of tumor suppressor genes has proven useful for unifying a number of the diverse, and often seemingly unrelated observations on the genetic basis of cancer, the term itself provides little insight into the normal cellular functions of this class of genes.

Somatic Cell Genetic Studies of Tumorigenesis

While oncogenes were directly identified by their positive role in altering the growth properties of appropriate recipient cells, virtually all of the initial evidence supporting the existence of tumor suppressor genes was derived without direct identification of these genes. One of the essential difficulties in identifying tumor suppressor genes by direct selection methods is that these genes would be expected to suppress properties of tumor cells, such as their uncontrolled proliferation, unlimited life span, and tumorigenicity. The successful transfer of genes suppressing these properties would alter the properties of the tumor cells toward those of normal cells. Selection methods, however, for directly identifying suppressed cells in a background of transformed cells have

thus far proven elusive. Nevertheless, a number of somatic cell genetic studies of tumorigenesis using both rodent and human tumor cells have provided indirect evidence that at least two functional classes of tumor suppressor genes must exist.

The studies of Harris and colleagues provided the basis for the concept that the ability of cells to form a tumor is a recessive trait.[47,48,112] They observed that the growth of murine tumor cells in syngeneic animals could be suppressed when the malignant cells were fused to non-malignant cells, although reversion to tumorigenicity often occurred when the hybrids were propagated for extended periods in culture. The reappearance of malignancy was found to be associated with chromosome losses. Their interpretation–that malignancy can be suppressed in somatic cell hybrids–was subsequently supported by additional studies of mouse, rat, and hamster intraspecies somatic cell hybrids, as well as interspecies hybrids between rodent tumor cells and normal human cells.[57,101] The karyotypic instability of the rodent-human hybrids, however, greatly complicated the analysis of the human chromosomes involved in the suppression process. Stanbridge and his colleagues overcame this problem by studying hybrids made by fusing human tumor cell lines to normal, diploid human fibroblasts. Their analysis confirmed that hybrids retaining both sets of parental chromosomes were suppressed, with tumorigenic segregants arising only rarely after chromosome losses in the hybrids.[113] Moreover, it was demonstrated that the loss of specific human chromosomes, and not simply chromosome loss in general, correlated with the reversion to tumorigenicity.[57,113] Tumorigenicity could be suppressed even if activated oncogenes, such as mutated RAS genes, were expressed in the hybrids.[39]

The observation that the loss of specific chromosomes was associated with the reversion to malignancy suggested that a single chromosome (and perhaps even a single gene) might be sufficient to suppress tumorigenicity. To directly test this hypothesis, single chromosomes were transferred from normal cells to tumor cells, using the technique of micro-cell-mediated chromosome transfer. It was found that the transfer of a single chromosome 11 into the HeLa cervical carcinoma cell line suppressed the tumorigenic phenotype of the cells.[103] Similarly, transfer of chromosome 11 into a Wilms' tumor cell line was found to suppress tumorigenicity, while the transfer of several other chromosomes had no effect.[126] As shown in Table I-6-1, the tumorigenic phenotype of many different tumors can be suppressed by the transfer of a single chromosome.

Although the tumorigenic phenotype can often be suppressed in the hybrids resulting from fusion between malignant and normal cells (tumor X normal), many other traits characteristic of the parental tumor cells (such as immortality and anchorage-independent growth) are retained in the hybrids. This observation is consistent with the hypothesis that malignant tumors arise as a result of multiple genetic alterations. Suppression of tumorigenicity following cell fusion or microcell chromosome transfer might thus represent correction of only one of the alterations. Recent studies using microcell-mediated chromosome transfer have demonstrated that human chromosome 1 will cause an immortal, but non-tumorigenic, hamster cell line to undergo a process

Table I-6-1. Tumor Suppression by Single Chromosome Transfer.

| | Chromosome transferred | | |
Tumor cell line	Suppressive Effect	No Suppressive Effect	Reference
Cervical (Hela)	11	X	103
Wilms' (G401)	11	X, 13	126
Melanoma (UACC-903)(UACC-091)	6	NR	118
Cervical (SiHa)	11	12	87
Neuroblastoma (SK-N-MC)	1	11	87
Fibrosarcoma (HT1080)	1, 11	2, 7, 12	87
Endometrial (HHUA)	1, 6, 9, 11	19	87
Renal cell (YCR)	3	1, 11, X	106
Choriocarcinoma (CC1)	7	1, 2, 6, 9, 11	87
Rhabdomyosarcoma (A204)	11	NR	87

termed cellular senescence that results in cell death.[115] These data suggest that the genes that influence the life span of normal cells may be distinct from the genes that suppress the tumorigenic phenotype. However, because each of these classes of genes can suppress at least some of the phenotypic properties of tumor cells (i.e., tumorigenicity or immortality), the two classes of genes are not usually distinguished one from another and both types are referred to as tumor suppressor genes.

In summary, although the somatic cell genetic studies of tumorigenesis reviewed above did not directly identify tumor suppressor genes, they provided persuasive evidence for the existence of critical growth-regulating genes in normal cells that can suppress the phenotypic traits of immortal or even fully cancerous cells.

Retinoblastoma–A Paradigm for Suppressor Gene Function in Human Cancer

Concurrent with the initial cell fusion experiments of Harris and colleagues, Knudson's analysis of the age-specific incidence of retinoblastoma led him to propose that two hits or mutagenic events were necessary for the development of retinoblastoma.[58] Retinoblastoma is a childhood retinal tumor that occurs sporadically in most cases, but occurs in some families in a pattern consistent with autosomal dominant inheritance. In an individual with the inherited form of the disease, Knudson proposed that the first hit is present in the germline and thus in all cells of the body. The second hit was proposed to occur somatically and to result in tumor formation. In the non-hereditary form of retinoblastoma, both mutations were hypothesized to arise within the same somatic cell. The presence of a mutation at the susceptibility locus was proposed to be insufficient for tumor formation. However, given a high likelihood of a somatic mutation occurring in at least one retinal cell during development, the dominant inheritance pattern of the disease seen in some families could be explained. Although each of the two hits could have been in different genes, subsequent studies (see below) led to the conclusion that both hits were at the same genetic locus, with the first hit affecting the allele at the retinoblastoma susceptibility locus inherited from one parent and the second hit affecting the allele inherited from the other parent. Knudson's hypothesis served not only to illustrate the mechanisms through which inherited and somatic genetic changes might

interact to contribute to tumorigenesis, but it also linked the notion of recessive genetic determinants for human cancer to the observations of somatic cell genetic studies demonstrating the recessive nature of tumorigenesis.

The first clue to the location of the putative locus responsible for inherited retinoblastoma was obtained from the study of karyotypes of peripheral blood cells from patients with retinoblastoma. Deletions of chromosome 13 were observed in some cases.[34,86] Subsequent studies of a large number of patients with retinoblastoma revealed that in about 5% of the patients the deletion could be detected cytogenetically.[34] However, in cases where chromosome 13 deletions were observed, the common region of deletion was found to be centered around chromosome band q14. Levels of esterase D, an enzyme of unknown physiological function, were found to be reduced in patients with deletions of 13q14, as compared to karyotypically normal family members.[110] This finding suggested that the gene for esterase D might be contained within chromosome band 13q14. Indeed, analysis of the segregation patterns of esterase D isozymes and the retinoblastoma predisposition (RB1) locus in families established that the esterase D and RB1 loci were very closely genetically linked.[109] Furthermore, one child with inherited retinoblastoma was found to have no observed deletion of chromosome 13 in his blood cells and skin fibroblasts, and had approximately one-half the esterase D levels as those of normals. Interestingly, tumor cells from this patient had a complete absence of esterase D activity, but had one copy of chromosome 13 by karyotypic analysis. From these findings, it was proposed that the chromosome 13 remaining in the tumor carried a submicroscopic deletion that removed both the esterase D and RB1 loci.[6] The authors also hypothesized that the initial mutation in the child was recessive at the cellular level, i.e., cells with only the initial lesion had a normal phenotype. The effect of the predisposing mutation, however, could be unmasked in the tumor cells by a second event, such as the loss of the chromosome 13 carrying the wild-type allele. This proposal was entirely consistent with Knudson's two-hit hypothesis.

In an attempt to establish the generality of these observations, Cavenee, Whyte, and their colleagues undertook studies of retinoblastomas, both inherited and sporadic in nature, using DNA probes from chromosome 13.[15] They chose to perform the analysis with probes that detected restriction fragment length polymorphisms (RFLPs), so that the two parental chromosomes in the cells of the patient's normal and tumor tissues could be distinguished from one another. Using such molecular markers to compare paired normal and tumor samples from each patient, they were able to determine that loss of heterozygosity (i.e., the loss of one parental set of markers) for chromosome 13 markers had occurred during tumorigenesis in over 60% of the cases studied. The losses of heterozygosity for chromosome 13, and specifically the region of chromosome 13 containing the RB1 locus, occurred by a number of different chromosomal mechanisms (Figure I-6-2). In addition, through the study of inherited cases, it was shown that the chromosome 13 homologue retained in the tumor cells was derived from the affected parent and the chromosome carrying the wild-type RB1 allele had been lost.[16] The unmasking of initial predisposing mutations at the RB1 locus, whether the predisposing mutation

had been inherited or had arisen somatically, occurred by the same chromosomal mechanisms.

It had been noted previously that patients with the inherited form of retinoblastoma are at an increased risk for the development of second primary tumors, in particular osteosarcomas. A common pathogenic mechanism formed the basis for this clinical association, as shown by comparison of the RFLP patterns of chromosome 13 markers in osteosarcoma and normal tissues from such cases. It was observed that loss of heterozygosity for the chromosome region containing the RB1 locus had occurred during the development of the osteosarcomas in patients with the inherited form of the disease.[45] Similar losses of heterozygosity for chromosome 13 alleles were also observed in sporadic osteosarcomas.

The molecular studies of retinoblastomas and osteosarcomas using RFLPs to mark parental alleles in normal and

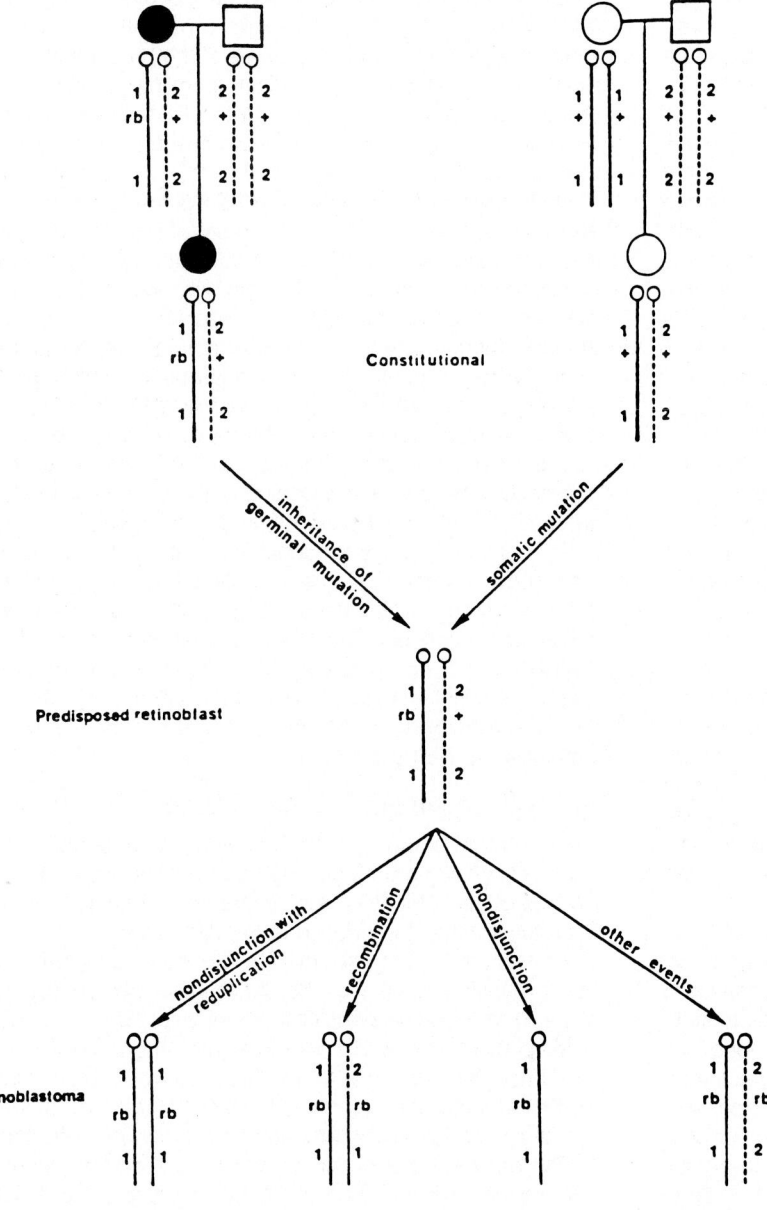

Figure I-6-2. Chromosomal mechanisms which result in loss of heterozygosity for alleles at the retinoblastoma locus at chromosome band 13q14. In the inherited form of the disease, the child inherits a chromosome 13 from her affected mother which carries a recessive mutation at the RB1 locus (this allele is designated rb) and a chromosome 13 from her father with no mutation at the locus (designated +). Thus, each of the cells of this girl contains one mutated and one wild-type RB1 allele (the genotype of the cells is rb/+). A retinoblastoma can arise after the loss or inactivation of the remaining wild-type retinoblastoma allele by one of the chromosomal mechanisms shown. In the non-inherited (sporadic) form of the disease, a recessive mutation arises somatically at one retinoblastoma allele in a developing retinal cell. Subsequently, a retinoblastoma will develop if the remaining RB1 allele in this predisposed retinoblast is inactivated by one of the chromosomal mechanisms shown. The two parental copies of chromosome 13 present in each cell of an individual can be distinguished by study of restriction fragment length polymorphisms (RFLPs) at loci flanking the RB1 locus on chromosome 13q (the polymorphic alleles are designated "1" and "2"). (Modified with the permission of Elsevier Press from W. Cavenee, A. Koufos, and M. Hansen, Mutat. Res., 168:3, 1986.)

tumor cells were of great significance. First, they provided strong support for Knudson's two-hit hypothesis, and illustrated the chromosomal mechanisms that might unmask recessive mutations at a tumor suppressor locus. Second, both the inherited and sporadic forms of a tumor appeared to arise by similar genetic alterations. Finally, osteosarcoma, a common second primary neoplasm in patients with inherited retinoblastoma, was found to have pathogenetic mechanisms in common with retinoblastoma.

Cloning and Analysis of the RB1 Gene

The isolation of the RB1 gene was facilitated by the identification of an anonymous DNA marker from the chromosome 13q14 region which detected DNA rearrangements in retinoblastomas.[34] Through the analysis of the DNA sequences flanking this DNA marker, a gene with the properties expected of the RB1 gene was identified.[35,37,67] This gene has been found to have a complex organization with 27 exons, spanning greater than 200 kilobases (kb) of DNA, spliced together to produce a messenger RNA transcript of about 4.7 kb. Interestingly, the RB1 gene appears to be almost ubiquitous in its expression pattern, rather than being restricted in its expression to retinoblasts and osteoblasts.[35,36,67,124]

The cloning of the RB1 gene allowed study of the mutations which inactivate the gene. Gross deletions of the DNA sequences containing the RB1 gene have been observed in several retinoblastomas and also in other tumors.[35–37,46,66,67,124] However, many retinoblastomas appear to express a full-length RB1 transcript and do not have detectable gene rearrangements when analyzed by Southern blots.[41] The detection of inherited and somatic mutations in most cases, therefore, has required detailed characterization of the sequence of the retinoblastoma gene.[23,132] Mutant alleles from both constitutional cells of individuals with the inherited form of the disease and from retinoblastomas of both inherited and sporadic type have now been sequenced. This analysis has provided molecular evidence supporting Knudson's two-hit model. As predicted by the model, patients with inherited retinoblastoma were found to have one mutated and one normal allele in their constitutional (blood) cells. In retinoblastomas of such individuals, the remaining RB1 allele was found to be inactivated by somatic mutation, usually by loss of the normal allele through a gross chromosomal event (Figure I-6-2), but in some cases by point mutation. Multiple tumors arising in an individual patient with inherited retinoblastoma all were found to contain the same germline (initial) mutation, but had different somatic mutations of the remaining RB1 allele. Finally, patients with single, sporadic retinoblastomas had two somatic mutations in their tumors, and two normal alleles in their blood cells.

While the identification of mutations in the RB1 gene in retinoblastomas provides strong support for the proposal that the cloned gene is indeed the gene whose inactivation is a crucial step in the formation of a retinoblastoma, a direct proof would be provided by evidence that the gene can function to suppress some aspects of retinoblastoma tumorigenesis. Indeed, the transfer of a cloned copy of the wild-type gene to retinoblastoma and osteosarcoma tumor cells in culture has been shown to affect a number of properties of the cells, including cell morphology, growth rate in culture,

and the ability of the cells to form colonies in soft agar and tumors in nude mice.[52]

The observation that the RB1 gene is almost ubiquitous in its expression pattern is puzzling with regard to the spectrum of tumors developing in patients with constitutional RB1 mutations and also the spectrum of tumors bearing somatic mutations of the gene. First, patients with constitutional mutations of the RB1 gene are at elevated risk for the development of only a rather limited number of rare tumor types, including a very high risk of retinoblastoma in childhood, and a high risk of osteosarcomas, soft tissue sarcomas, and melanomas later in life. Second, in addition to the identification of somatic mutations in the RB1 gene in sporadic retinoblastomas, somatic mutations have been observed in breast cancers, small cell cancers of the lung and other tissues, bladder cancer, and prostate cancer.[10,46,51,66] The reasons why somatic inactivation of the RB1 gene occurs during the development of these common cancers, but not in cancers of other cell types which also express the gene, are not clear. In addition, given that mutations of the RB1 gene apparently are involved in the development of some cancers of the breast, lung, and prostate in individuals with no RB1 germline mutations, the reasons why germline mutation of the RB1 gene does not predispose to an elevated risk for these common cancers also are not clear.

The cloning and analysis of the RB1 gene has ushered in an new era in the clinical management of patients and families with retinoblastoma. The identification of polymorphic DNA markers immediately flanking and within the retinoblastoma gene has provided a means with which to trace the inheritance of the predisposing mutant allele in families with inherited retinoblastoma. By determining which RFLPs are co-inherited with the predisposition to retinoblastoma development in a given family with the disease, it is possible to predict accurately whether a subsequent child or fetus in the family is at risk for developing retinoblastoma or osteosarcoma.[17] Furthermore, the cloning of the gene has given investigators the ability to identify specific mutations in the retinoblastoma gene in tumors of patients who do not have a family history of the disease. Blood cells from this group of affected individuals can then be studied to determine if the RB1 mutation(s) present in the tumor were inherited or arose somatically. Appropriate genetic counseling and further clinical follow-up can then be provided to those patients with inherited RB1 gene mutations.

Function of the RB1 Gene Product

The protein product of the RB1 gene is a nuclear phosphoprotein that has DNA-binding activity.[68] The protein (p105-Rb) has a few regions of very limited amino acid homology to proteins with known functions.[35,67] A discovery which suggested how the oncogenes of DNA tumor viruses might function to transform cells was the observation that the product of the E1A oncogene of the DNA tumor virus adenovirus type 5 complexed with the Rb protein in vitro and in vivo.[128] The E1A oncogene previously had been found to have many functions, including cell immortalization, induction of DNA synthesis, cooperation with other oncogenes in transformation, and regulation of transcription of viral and host genes.[79] The functional inactivation of Rb by its complexing to E1A may be responsible for some of these functions. Support for the proposal that complex formation between the E1A and Rb proteins is physiologically relevant in neoplastic transformation has been provided by the observation that mutations that inactivate the ability of E1A to bind to RB also inactivate the transforming ability of E1A.[129]

In addition to p105-Rb:E1A complexes, Rb has been found to form complexes with oncoproteins of two other DNA tumor viruses; i.e., the SV40 large T antigen and the human papillomavirus type 16 E7 protein (Figure I-6-3).[21,24] Genetic alterations that inactivate the transforming capability of these proteins also alter the ability of these oncoproteins to bind to the Rb protein. This observation argues that the associ-

Polyomaviruses

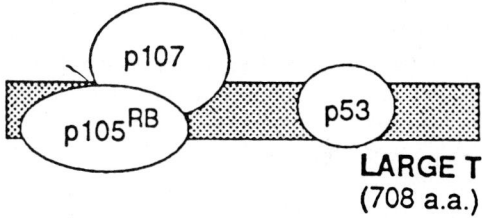

Adenoviruses

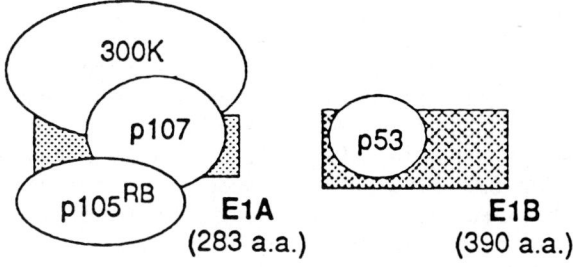

Papillomaviruses

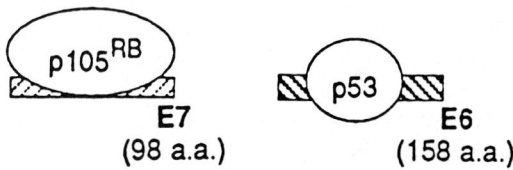

Figure I-6-3. A schematic representation of the interactions between the proteins of DNA tumor viruses and tumor suppressor gene products. Large T antigen, a product of SV40 polyomavirus, interacts with both p105-rb and p53 proteins, and an as yet unidentified 107 kilodalton phosphoprotein. In contrast, both p105-rb and p53 bind to different adenovirus and papillomavirus transforming proteins. It has been hypothesized that the interaction of tumor suppressor proteins of the host cell with transforming proteins of the DNA tumor viruses results in the inactivation of the normal suppressor function. (Reprinted with permission from Werness, B. A., Levine, A. J., Howley, P. M.: Association of human papillomavirus types 16 and 18 E6 proteins with p53. Science, 248:76, 1990.)

ation of oncoproteins with Rb is necessary for their ability to transform cells. It has been found that these oncoproteins appear to have a preferential affinity for the non-phosphorylated or underphosphorylated forms of Rb.[71] In addition, as the phosphorylation state of Rb appears to increase progressively through the cell division cycle from an unphosphorylated state in early G1 to a maximally phosphorylated state in late G2,[13,19] the binding of the E1A, T antigen, and E7 oncoproteins to p105-RB may functionally inactivate the RB protein's ability to regulate cell growth. The inactivation of p105-Rb function by oncoproteins of DNA tumor viruses would thus be analogous to inactivation of the RB1 gene, and thus p105-Rb, by mutational events.

Recently, support for the hypothesis that Rb functions to regulate gene expression has been provided. Expression of the c-Myc protein, a nuclear oncoprotein that is differentially expressed in proliferating compared to non-proliferating cells, has been found to be rapidly downregulated in a skin cell culture model system by treatment of the cells with the growth inhibitory factor TGF-beta (transforming growth factor beta). The downregulation of c-Myc expression occurs at the transcriptional level and is apparently dependent on function of the wild-type Rb protein.[89] Similarly, Rb appears to participate in the regulation of c-fos, another nuclear oncoprotein that is highly expressed in proliferating cells compared to non-proliferating cells.[97] It is tempting to speculate that Rb is a component of a growth inhibitory pathway(s) and regulates cell proliferation through the transcriptional down-regulation of genes whose function is to stimulate growth.

The Genetics of Wilms' Tumor

Wilms' tumor is the most common renal neoplasm of children, accounting for about 6% of all pediatric cancers. It is similar to retinoblastoma in a number of ways, as both tumors occur bilaterally or unilaterally, with single or multiple foci, and in a sporadic or inherited fashion. Hereditary cases, however, are not as common for Wilms' tumors as for retinoblastomas, and while almost all patients inheriting a mutation at the RB1 locus develop a retinoblastoma, only about 50% of individuals inheriting the predisposition to Wilms' tumor develop the disease.[59] Nevertheless, a statistical analysis of Wilms' tumor cases led Knudson and Strong to conclude in 1972 that the two-mutation model originally proposed for retinoblastoma was also likely to be valid for Wilms' tumor.[60] Specifically, Wilms' tumor was proposed to develop from two mutational events; the first of which could arise either in the germline or in somatic cells, and the second of which always arose somatically. The inheritance of one mutation at the Wilms' tumor predisposition locus was predicted to be associated with multiple tumors and an earlier onset, whereas sporadic tumors would occur singularly and would usually be diagnosed later.

The first finding suggesting a genetic basis for Wilms' tumor came from a report in 1964 describing six patients with Wilms' tumor and sporadic aniridia.[78] The likelihood, however, of this occurring simply by coincidence was extremely low. It was proposed, therefore, that the simultaneous occurrence of these two conditions might be a result of a chromosomal aberration involving more than one locus;

one locus leading to aniridia and the other to Wilms' tumor.[60] This hypothesis was subsequently supported by the discovery of interstitial deletions of chromosome 11p, involving band 11p13 in peripheral blood samples from children with the WAGR syndrome of Wilms' tumor, aniridia, genito-urinary abnormalities, and mental retardation.[96] In addition, a few cases of sporadic type Wilms' tumors and cytogenetic studies of the tumor tissues revealed deletions or translocations of chromosome band 11p13.[56,108] Subsequent studies of paired samples of Wilms' tumor and normal cells from patients, using probes which detect RFLPs on chromosome 11p, revealed that loss of heterozygosity for 11p markers occurred frequently in Wilms' tumors of both inherited and sporadic type.[28,62,85,94] These observations were consistent with the notion that the chromosomal events producing the loss of heterozygosity were unmasking recessive (inactivating) mutations at a tumor suppressor locus on chromsome 11p in Wilms' tumors. Further evidence that the loss or inactivation of a gene or genes on chromosome 11 is intimately involved in Wilms' tumorigenesis has been provided by somatic cell genetic studies. The introduction of a chromosome 11 from normal cells to a Wilms' tumor line by microcell-mediated chromosome transfer was found to suppress the ability of the tumor cells to form tumors in athymic mice (Table I-6-1).[126]

As described above, the 11p13 region had been implicated initially in Wilms' tumor development because of the constitutional deletions of this region in WAGR patients. Further analyses of this region using a variety of molecular techniques, including isolation of additional DNA clones from this region, mapping of these clones by pulsed-field gel electrophoresis, and chromosome walking and jumping studies, led to the identification of a gene which was inactivated in at least a subset of Wilms' tumor cases.[14,40] This gene, denoted WT1, appears to be a likely candidate for the Wilms' tumor gene located in chromosome band 11p13. The WT1 gene is expressed in the developing kidney and also in the genital ridge and fetal gonad of the embryo.[14,40,93] The predicted amino acid sequence specifies a protein with four tandem zinc-finger motifs, similar to those present in some proteins that control transcription. This finding, and the relative specificity of the gene's expression in developing kidney and urogenital tissues, have led to the hypothesis that inactivation of the gene may result in aberrant growth and differentiation of urogenital tissues.[14,40,93] At present, few mutations have been localized to the WT1 gene, and it is not known whether the gene is altered in the majority of Wilms' tumor cases.

Other findings suggest that Wilms' tumors may arise through mutations in genes besides the WT1 gene. First, the loss of heterozygosity of chromosome 11p markers in Wilms' tumors has been localized and often involves band 11p15, not 11p13 (and the WT1 gene), in many cases.[74,95] Second, the 11p15 region, but not the 11p13 region, has been found to be duplicated or rearranged in some patients with the Beckwith-Wiedmann syndrome, a congenital syndrome of hyperplasia of the kidneys, endocrine pancreas, and other internal organs, macroglossia, hemihypertrophy, and predisposition to embryonic tumors such as hepatoblastoma and Wilms' tumor.[2,90] Finally, linkage studies of three families with dominant inheritance of Wilms' tumor have excluded linkage of the susceptibility locus in these families to any part of chromosome 11p.[42,53] The data suggest that there are perhaps three different genes that, when mutated, can participate in Wilms' tumorigenesis. Whether a combination of inherited and somatic mutations in more than one of these genes (or even all three) are required for the development of Wilms' tumor, or whether alterative genetic pathways for the development of Wilms' tumor exist, is not yet resolved. Nevertheless, the genetic heterogeneity seen in Wilms' tumorigenesis provides an important contrast to the apparently less complex genetic pathway of retinoblastoma development. The genetics of Wilms' tumor may be, therefore, more akin to the genetics of common adult cancers, such as those of the colon, lung, and breast.

The p53 Gene—Oncogene or Tumor Suppressor Gene?

As noted above, genes that function to regulate cell proliferation and growth, and that are inactivated during tumor development, have been identified by a variety of different techniques. The isolation and molecular characterization of this presumably large and diverse family of genes has been, and will continue to be a difficult process to prove. In fact, even when cloned copies of a tumor suppressor gene are in hand, their functional identity can be confusing, as was the case for the p53 gene. The p53 gene was initially thought to be an oncogene, but recently it has been identified as a tumor suppressor gene by a number of converging lines of evidence.

The p53 protein was first identified because it formed a tight complex in cells with the SV40 large T antigen (SV40 LT) in virally infected cells.[64,65,70] Subsequently, it was found that the p53 protein formed complexes with other polyomavirus large T antigens, with the E1B oncoprotein of adenovirus type 5,[102] and with the E6 oncoprotein of papillomaviruses (Figure I-6-3).[127] Furthermore, the p53 protein of normal cells was found to be metabolically labile, and to be present only at low levels; however, high levels of the protein were found in many tumors and tumor cell lines.[20,65] These observations were interpreted initially as evidence that the p53 protein functioned in a positive fashion to participate in cellular transformation. Additional support for this interpretation was provided by experiments in which a cloned copy of a murine p53 gene acted as an oncogene when expressed at high levels. It was found that these p53 plasmid constructs could immortalize some cell types, and the p53 gene, in collaboration with a mutated ras oncogene, could fully transform rat fibroblasts to immortal, tumorigenic cells.[25,55,88]

Other observations, however, suggested that the p53 gene might be inactivated in some tumors. In Friend virus-induced mouse erythroleukemias, the gene was found to be a frequent target for mutation by viral integration events.[80] Although the functional effect of these mutations often was not clear, the identification of several tumors with deletions of much of the coding sequence established that the p53 gene was inactivated in at least some cases. Similarly, rearrangements and deletions of the p53 gene were observed in a human leukemic cell line and several human osteosarcomas.[76,131] These alterations also appeared to result in inactivation of the gene. A further line of evidence implicating the p53 gene as a tumor suppressor was obtained through the study of loss of heterozygosity in a number of human tumors, particularly colorectal cancers.[29] Loss of heterozygosity for alleles on the short arm of chromosome 17 was observed in greater than 75% of colorectal carcinomas. This observation was interpreted in accord with Knudson's hypothesis; the loss of chromosome 17p sequences was proposed to result in the unmasking of inactivating mutations at a tumor suppressor gene. In an attempt to identify such a tumor suppressor gene, the common region of loss on chromosome 17p was identified in colorectal tumors, and was found to contain the p53 gene.[3] No alterations of the remaining p53 allele in the colorectal tumors could be identified by Southern or Northern analyses. However, sequencing of the remaining p53 allele in colorectal tumors with 17p losses identified point mutations in the great majority of cases, resulting in amino acid substitutions at sites throughout the gene.[3,83] In addition to p53 mutations in colorectal tumors, a variety of other tumor types that frequently show loss of heterozygosity on 17p, including breast, lung, and brain tumors, have been observed to have mutations in the remaining p53 allele.[83,116] The common feature of the mutations identified was that they had occurred within highly conserved regions of the protein. Other tumor types, such as osteosarcomas, pediatric embryonal tumors, and blast cells of patients with chronic myelogenous leukemia in blast crisis, frequently have rearrangements and deletions of the p53 gene, in addition to point mutations.[1,81] The p53 gene is the most frequently altered gene in human cancer identified to date.

These findings suggesting that the wild-type p53 gene is a tumor suppressor gene were difficult to reconcile with the data establishing that the p53 gene could function in an apparently positive fashion to transform cells. Re-examination of the transformation studies provided an explanation for the apparent paradox. It was initially assumed that the conversion of p53 to an oncogene was due solely to its high expression levels in the plasmid constructs. However, a more complete analysis revealed that the cloned murine p53 genes that would cooperate in the cotransformation assay were not wild-type, but contained point mutations in their coding sequences.[25,50] Both the wild-type murine and human p53 genes have been shown to be incapable of mediating transformation in conjunction with mutated ras oncogenes; and furthermore, the wild-type genes have been found to inhibit the transforming ability of mutant p53 genes and other oncogenes.[26,32] Recently, it has been shown that the wild-type p53 gene functions to suppress the growth of human colorectal carcinoma cells with p53 mutations, and that mutations in the p53 gene abrogate its suppressor function.[4] The growth suppressive effect of the wild-type p53 gene was observed even though the cells had many other genetic alterations. The observation highlights the role of the wild-type p53 gene in the normal regulation of cell growth.

In order to reconcile the recent findings that the wild-type p53 gene is a suppressor gene with the earlier observations that mutant p53 can function as an oncogene, it has been postulated that many of the mutant p53 proteins function as dominant negative mutants in the cell.[3,49,64] The mutant p53 proteins may function in a dominant fashion (i.e., in the pres-

ence of the host cell wild-type p53 protein) in the co-transformation assay by binding to and inhibiting the function of the wild-type gene product. Alternatively, mutant p53 may compete with wild-type p53 for the normal substrate. Support for the first proposal has been provided by studies that show oligomerization between mutant and wild-type p53 proteins.[25,32] Mutant p53 would thus function in a manner analogous to T antigen by binding to and inactivating the wild-type p53.

In addition to the somatic mutations that are frequently detected in the p53 gene in different tumor types, recent studies have demonstrated that inherited mutations in the p53 gene are present in individuals with the dominantly inherited Li-Fraumeni syndrome (LFS).[73,111] Individuals affected with this syndrome are at a very elevated risk for the development of childhood soft tissue sarcomas, breast cancers, brain tumors, osteosarcomas, and a number of other neoplasms. The affected individuals in LFS families have one mutant and one normal p53 gene in each of their cells. The remaining wild-type p53 gene has been found to be inactivated during tumor development in tumors from individuals with LFS.[73] The identification of germline p53 mutations, although absent in the vast majority of individuals who develop cancer, provides additional support for the notion that wild-type p53 functions to regulate cell growth. Furthermore, similar to the RB1 gene, either somatic or inherited mutations in the p53 gene can inactivate its tumor suppressor function.

The Identification of Other Tumor Suppressor Gene Loci

The successful identification of the RB1 and p53 genes as tumor suppressor genes that are frequently inactivated during the development of human tumors, the identification of the WT1 gene, and the somatic cell genetic studies suggesting that the inactivation of normal cellular genes might be a general property of tumors have all served to spark a great deal of interest in the identification of additional tumor suppressor loci. The two leading approaches to the identification of novel tumor suppressor genes in human cancer are: linkage analysis to identify the genes predisposing to particular tumor susceptibility syndromes; and loss of heterozygosity (LOH) studies using paired normal and tumor specimens to identify chromosomal regions for which loss of parental alleles can be observed in the tumor material.

Identification by Linkage Analysis

The localization of genes involved in the predisposition to some inherited tumor syndromes has been carried out using linkage analysis (Table I-6-2). For example, the gene predisposing to familial adenomatous polyposis of the colon (FAP) has been mapped to chromosome 5q,[9,69] the neurofibromatosis type 1 (NF-1) gene to chromosome 17q,[5,104] and the multiple endocrine neoplasia type 2 (MEN-2) gene to chromosome 10.[77,107] In these 3 syndromes, allelic losses of the chromosome region linked to the inherited predisposition have been found to occur infrequently in the tumors of patients with the inherited forms of each of the diseases.[63,82,121] These observations contrast with the results seen in inherited retinoblastoma, and are not readily consistent with the idea that

Table I-6-2.   Evidence for Tumor Suppressor Gene Alterations in Selected Human Tumor Types or Tumor Syndromes from Linkage Analysis (LA), LOH Analysis, or the Detection of Specific Mutations.

Tumor Type or Tumor Syndrome	Chromosomal Region	Evidence
Retinoblastoma	13q14	LA, LOH, RB1 mutation
Osteosarcoma	13q14	LOH, RB1 mutation
	17p13	LOH, p53 mutation
Wilms'	11p13	WT-1 mutation
	11p15	LOH
	other	LA
Rhabdomyosarcoma	11p15	LOH
	17p13	LOH, p53 mutation
Hepatoblastoma	11p	LOH
Bladder (transitional cell)	9, 11p	LOH
	17p13	LOH, p53 mutation
Renal cell	3p	LA, LOH
Lung (small cell)	3p	LOH
	13q14	LOH, RB1 mutation
	17p13	LOH, p53 mutation
	others	LOH
Lung (non-small cell)	3p	LA, LOH
	13q14	LOH, RB1 mutation
	17p13	LOH, p53 mutation
	others	LOH
Colorectal	5q	LA, LOH
	17p13	LOH, p53 mutation
	18q	LOH, DCC mutation
	others	LOH
Breast	11p	LOH
	13q14	LOH, RB1 mutation
	17p13	LOH, p53 mutation
	others	LOH
Glioblastoma	10q	LOH
	17p13	LOH, p53 mutation
Neuroblastoma	1p	LOH
Neurofibromatosis type 1	17p13	p53 mutation
	17q	LA, NF-1 mutation
Neurofibromatosis type 2	22q	LA, LOH
Multiple endocrine neoplasia type 1	11q	LA, LOH
Multiple endocrine neoplasia type 2	10	LA
	1	LOH

both maternal and paternal copies of the predisposition genes must be inactivated in the cell for the growth-suppressive function to be eliminated. Rather, tumors in patients with some inherited predisposition syndromes may arise as a result of decreased levels of the wild-type suppressor gene product, in conjunction with alterations in other genes, even though one wild-type copy of the suppressor gene remains in the tumor cell.

As a result of linkage analyses, the gene predisposing to NF-1 has been identified. The NF-1 gene was mapped to the peri-centromeric region of chromosome 17 by linkage analysis of several large kindreds with von Recklinghausen neurofibromatosis (i.e., NF-1).[5,104] Subsequently, two neurofibromatosis patients with germline chromosomal translocations involving band 17q11 were identified, and found to have detectable alterations of the DNA sequences in this region.[33,84] Additional DNA markers were obtained from the chromosome regions flanking the breakpoints on chromosome 17q, and several additional patients were identified with DNA rearrangements and deletions in this region of

17q.[120] A cDNA for a large gene from this region was identified.[18,92,122] Mutations of this gene, both gross rearrangements and point mutations, have been identified in a number of NF-1 patients, and inactivation of this gene (the candidate NF-1 gene) appears to result in the predisposition to the development of peripheral neurofibromas and other tumors seen in NF-1 patients. The gene encodes a protein with homology to the family of molecules known as GTPase activating proteins (GAPs).[38] This class of molecules is of great interest to tumor biology, as one member (ras-GAP) has been shown to stimulate the GTPase activity of the ras oncoproteins, and many of the mutations that activate the ras protein alter its ability to interact with GAP.[117,130] Recent studies suggest that a domain of the NF-1 gene can function to stimulate the GTPase activity of both yeast and mammalian ras proteins. The mechanisms by which mutations alter/inactivate the normal function of the NF-1 protein and alter cell growth are not yet understood; however, it is likely that the NF-1 protein may function in signal transduction pathways involving cellular G proteins.

Identification by LOH

The study of LOH events in a wide variety of tumor types has led to the identification of many different chromosome regions which may contain novel tumor suppressor genes (Table I-6-2).[91,112] As can be seen from the table, LOH events for some of the chromosome regions have been identified in many different tumor types, and other LOH events appear to be restricted to either one or only a few tumor types. As noted previously, the study of mutations in the RB1 and p53 genes has provided support for the notion that mutations of a tumor suppressor gene that is expressed in many different tissues will not be restricted to a single tumor type. In contrast, alterations in other tumor suppressor genes that have more restricted expression patterns, such as the WT1 gene at 11p13, may be present only in a few, specific tumor types.

In general, LOH studies have been used to identify genes that may play a critical role in tumorigenesis by virtue of their somatic inactivation. However, the study of LOH events in tumors from patients with some of the inherited syndromes predisposing to cancer has also led to the mapping of the genes involved in multiple endocrine neoplasia type 1 (MEN-1) to chromosome 11q,[91] von Hippel-Lindau syndrome (VHL) to chromosome 3p,[105] and neurofibromatosis type 2 (NF-2) to chromosome 22q.[98]

The identification of allelic losses of chromosome 18q in more than 75% of colorectal cancers led to the proposal that the region contained a tumor suppressor gene. In an attempt to identify a candidate suppressor gene in the region, a contiguous stretch of DNA comprising 370 kb was isolated from a region of chromosome 18q suspected to reside near the gene. cDNA clones from a candidate tumor suppressor gene in this region were isolated.[28] This gene, termed DCC (for deleted in colorectal cancers), was found to be very large, extending more than 500 kb, and was found to encode a protein with significant homology to the immunoglobulin supergene family of cell adhesion molecules. The DCC gene was found to be expressed in many normal tissues, including colonic mucosa; however, its expression was greatly reduced or absent in most colorectal carcinomas studied. Somatic mutations of the DCC gene were identified in a number of colorectal tumors, using fragments of the cDNA clones. Thus, it has been suggested that the DCC gene may play a role in the pathogenesis of human colorectal neoplasia, perhaps through alteration of the normal cell-cell interactions controlling growth. Interestingly, an autosomal dominantly-inherited syndrome predisposing to carcinomas of the colon and other organs has been linked to chromosome 18q.[72] Whether the DCC gene is involved in this predisposition syndrome or other syndromes not yet mapped to a particular chromosomal region, remains to be determined.

Multiple Tumor Suppressor Genes Affected During Tumor Progression

Tumorigenesis has long been thought to be a multistep process in both man and experimental animal models. Measurements of age-dependent cancer incidence in man have shown that the rate of incidence for most epithelial cancers is proportional to the fifth to sixth power of elapsed time, suggesting that six to seven independent steps may determine the rate.[2] Thus, it can be predicted that several genetic alterations in both oncogenes and tumor suppressor genes are likely to be necessary for the development of most common cancers in man. Studies of a number of different types of human cancers have begun to provide molecular genetic evidence supporting this prediction.

In terms of the genetic alterations underlying tumor development, colorectal tumors are one of the best understood tumor types.[30] Abundant clinical and histopathological data suggest that the malignant form of the disease (carcinoma) arises from pre-existing benign tumors (adenomas). Tumors of various stages of development, from very small benign adenomas to large metastatic carcinomas can be obtained for study. The study of LOH events in such tumors has provided evidence for the inactivation of multiple tumor suppressor genes during colorectal tumorigenesis. The chromosomal regions affected by LOH events, the presumed target gene of each event, and the relative time of occurrence of the genetic alterations with respect to the different stages of colorectal tumorigenesis are outlined in Figure I-6-4. Although the alterations appear to occur in a preferred order, the order of the alterations is not invariant and the accumulation of the changes, rather than their order with respect to one another, seems most important in promoting tumor progression. In addition to the LOH events noted on chromosomes 5q, 17p, and 18q, other allelic losses can be observed in colorectal carcinomas. The median frequency of allelic losses in an individual colorectal carcinoma has been found to involve four to five chromosomal arms, and thus it is possible that inactivation of 4–5 tumor suppressor genes may be necessary to develop the fully malignant phenotype in some colorectal tumors. It has been shown that patients whose primary tumors have a high frequency of allelic losses have a higher risk of developing distant metastases and dying from their cancer than patients with a lower frequency of allelic losses in their tumors. Analysis of individual tumors for the extent of LOH events may, in the future, help to formulate prognosis more accurately.

Significant progress also has been made toward an understanding of the multiple genetic alterations arising in tumor suppressor genes in other human tumor types. Studies have demonstrated that LOH events can be observed for a number of chromosomal regions in each of these types of tumors (Table I-6-2). Studies of somatic alterations in gliomas of various stages have suggested that the progressive accumulation of alterations in tumor suppressor genes and oncogenes accompanies tumor progression in brain tumors,[54] as such alterations do in colorectal tumors.

Summary

An increasing body of evidence suggests that the inactivation of tumor suppressor genes is likely to play a critical role in the development of many types of human tumors. Only 20 years ago, it was proposed that tumorigenesis might result from the inactivation of normal cellular genes regulating growth in a negative fashion. Evidence for the existence of tumor suppressor genes and their importance in tumorigenesis has emerged gradually from somatic cell genetic

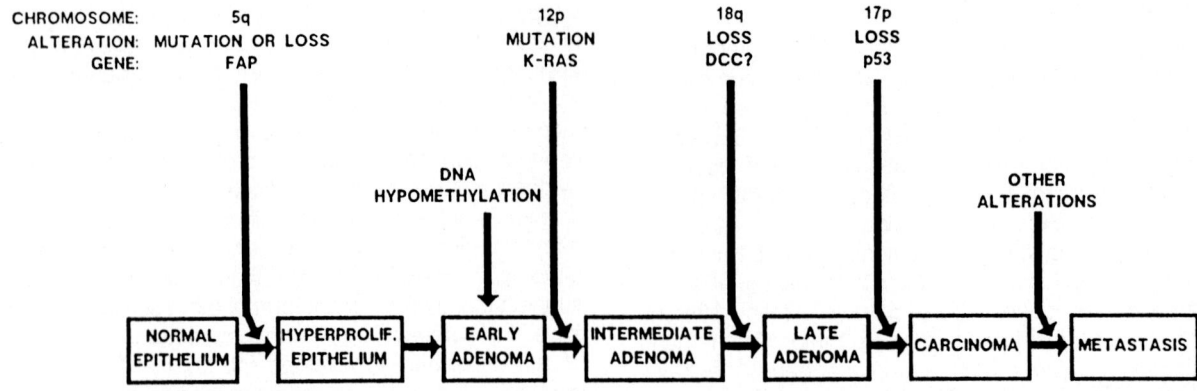

Figure I-6-4. A genetic model for colorectal tumorigenesis. Colorectal tumor arises and progresses through a series of genetic alterations involving oncogenes (ras) and tumor suppressor genes (particularly those on chromosomes 5q, 17p, and 18q). In the scheme shown, three stages of adenoma formation are represented and the progression from early to late adenoma stages is characterized by increasing size, dysplasia, and villous content of the tumors. In patients with familial adenomatous polyposis (FAP), a mutation on chromosome 5q is inherited. This alteration may be responsible for the hyperproliferative epithelium seen in these patients. In tumors arising in patients without polyposis, the same gene may inactivated by somatic mutation or LOH events on chromosome 5q. Hypomethylation is present in very small adenomas in patients with or without polyposis, and this alteration may lead to aneuploidy, resulting in the loss of suppressor gene alleles. Mutation in ras genes (usually K-ras) appears to occur in one cell of a pre-existing small adenoma and through clonal expansion produces a larger and more dysplastic tumor. The chromosomes most frequently affected by LOH events include 5q, 18q, and 17p; the putative target of the loss (i.e., the tumor suppressor gene) on each chromosome is indicated, as well as the relative timing of the loss with respect to the different stages of colorectal tumorigenesis. Although a preferred order for the series of genetic alterations exists, the order of the changes is not invariant. At present, it seems most likely that the accumulation of these genetic alterations is most important, rather than their order with respect to one another. (From Fearon and Vogelstein.[30])

studies, epidemiological studies, and studies of chromosome losses in tumor cells using cytogenetic and molecular genetic techniques. In the last few years, several tumor suppressor genes have been isolated by molecular cloning techniques. In some cases, these genes are lost or inactivated in the germline, and their inactivation may predispose to susceptibility to tumor formation. More often, tumor suppressor genes are functionally inactivated by somatic mutation.

While the normal cellular function of any of the tumor suppressor genes identified to date is not yet understood, it seems likely that they function in some manner to regulate the normal growth and differentiation of cells. Some of the products of tumor suppressor genes could be themselves capable of generating negative growth regulatory signals, in other cases, the gene products may function as transducers of normal growth-inhibitory signals. Just as the oncogenes are involved in many different levels of the growth regulatory circuits of the cell, the tumor suppressor genes can be predicted to function in a variety of pathways of cell growth control. The products of some tumor suppressor genes may act directly to oppose the function of oncogenes, while others may interact only indirectly with oncogenes in pathways of growth and differentiation. In the case of the retinoblastoma and p53 genes, the interaction between tumor suppressor genes and the oncogenes of DNA tumor viruses appears to be direct.

A more complete description of tumorigenesis will undoubtedly emerge with the identification of additional tumor suppressor genes and the characterization of their normal cellular function. In addition, these findings are likely to have great clinical importance for several reasons. The predisposition to the development of many human cancers, including rare tumor syndromes such as retinoblastoma, neurofi-

bromatosis, and multiple endocrine neoplasia, and common human cancers such as colon and breast tumors, can be inherited. It has been proposed that all of the predisposition syndromes may result from the germline inactivation of tumor suppressor genes (perhaps a unique gene in each case). Continued identification of the tumor suppressor genes involved in these predisposition syndromes should lead to more effective methods for the identification and clinical management of individuals who are at an increased risk of developing tumors. In addition, the further identification of the alterations in both oncogenes and tumor suppressor genes that underlie tumor development, in effect, a description of the molecular basis of cancer should provide clues to develop new methods to prevent disease, to detect disease at earlier and more curable stages, and to develop new chemotherapeutic agents that might selectively inactivate mutated oncogene products or that might mimic or restore the normal biological action of suppressor genes.

References

1. Ahua, H., Bar-Eli, M., Advani, S. H., Benchimol, S., and Cline, M. J.: Alterations of the p53 gene and the clonal evolution of the blast crises of chronic myelogenous leukemia. Proc. Natl. Acad. Sci. U.S.A., 86:6783, 1989.
2. Armitage, P., and Doll, R.: The age distribution of cancer and a multi-stage theory of carcinogenesis. Brit. J. Cancer, 8:1, 1954.
3. Baker, S. J., Fearon, E. R., Nigro, J. M., Hamilton, S. R., Preisinger, A. C., Jessup, J. M., van Tuinen, P., Ledbetter, D. H., Barker, D. F., Nakamura, Y., White, R., and Vogelstein, B.: Chromosome 17 deletions and p53 gene mutations in colorectal carcinomas. Science, 244:217, 1989.
4. Baker, S. J., Markowitz, S., Fearon, E. R., Willson, J. K. V., and Vogelstein, B.: Suppression of human colorectal carcinoma cell growth by wild-type p53. Science, 249:912, 1990.
5. Barker, D., Wright, E., Nguyen, K., Cannon, L., Fain, P., Goldgar, D., Bishop, D. T., Carey, J., Baty, B., Kivlin, J., Williard, H., Waye, J. S., Greig, G., Leinwand, L., Nakamura, Y., O'Connell, P., Leppert, M., Lalouel, J.-M., White, R., and Skolnick, M.: Gene for von Recklinghausen neurofibromatosis is in the pericentric region of chromosome 17. Science, 236:1100, 1987.
6. Benedict, W. F., Murphree, A. L., Banerjee, A., Spina, C. A., Sparkes, M. C., and Sparkes, R. S.: Patient with chromosome 13 deletion: Evidence that the retinoblastoma gene is a recessive cancer gene. Science, 219:973, 1983.
7. Bishop, J. M.: Viral oncogenes. Cell, 42:23, 1985.
8. Bishop, J. M.: The molecular genetics of cancer. Science, 235:305, 1987.

9. Bodmer, W. F., Bailey, C. J., Bodmer, J., Bussey, H. J. R., Ellis, A., Gorman, P., Lucibello, F. C., Murray, V. A., Rider, S. H., Scambler, P., Sheer, D., Solomon, E., and Spurr, N. K.: Localization of the gene for familial adenomatous polyposis on chromosome 5. Nature, 328:614, 1987.
10. Bookstein, R., Shew, J.-Y., Chen, P.-L., Scully, P., and Lee, W.-H.: Suppression of tumorigenicity of human prostate carcinoma cells by replacing a mutant RB gene. Science, 247:712, 1990.
11. Boveri, T.: The Origin of Malignant Tumors. Baltimore, Williams and Wilkins, 1929.
12. Broca, P. P.: Traite des Tumeurs. Paris, Asselin, 1986.
13. Buchkovich, K., Duffy, L. A., and Harlow, E.: The retinoblastoma protein is phosphorylated during specific phases of the cell cycle. Cell, 58:1099, 1989.
14. Call, K. M., Glaser, T., Ito, C. Y., Buckler, A. J., Pelletier, J., Haber, D. A., Rose, E. A., Kral, A., Yager, H., Lewis, W. H., Jones, C., and Housman, D. E.: Isolation and characterization of a zinc finger polypeptide gene at the human chromosome 11 Wilms' tumor locus. Cell, 60:509, 1990.
15. Cavenee, W. K., Dryja, T. P., Phillips, R. A., Benedict, W. F., Godbout, R., Gallie, B. L., Murphree, A. L., Strong, L. C., and White, R.: Expression of recessive alleles by chromosomal mechanisms in retinoblastoma. Science, 228:501, 19.
16. Cavenee, W. K., Hansen, M. F., Koch, E., Nordenskjold, M., Maumenee, I., Squire, J. A., Phillips, R. A., and Gallie, B. L.: Genetic origins of mutations predisposing to retinoblastoma. Science, 228:501, 1985.
17. Cavenee, W. K., Murphree, A. L., Shull, M. M., Benedict, W. F., Sparkes, R. S., Kock, E., and Nordenskjold, M.: Prediction of familial predisposition to retinoblastoma. N. Engl. J. Med., 314:1201, 1985.
18. Cawthon, R. M., Weiss, R., Xu, G., Viskochil, D., Culver, M., Stevens, J., Robertson, M., Dunn, D., Gesteland, R., O'Connell, P., and White, R.: A major segment of the neurofibromatosis type 1 gene: cDNA sequence, genomic structure, and point mutations. Cell, 62:193, 1990.
19. Chen, P.-L., Scully, P., Shew, J.-Y., Wang, J. Y. J., and Lee, W.-H.: Phosphorylation of the retinoblastoma gene product is modulated during the cell cycle and cellular differentiation. Cell, 58:1193, 1989.
20. Crawford, L. V., Pim, D. C., and Lamb, P.: The cellular protein p53 in human tumors. Mol. Bio. and Med., 2:261, 1984.
21. DeCaprio, J. A., Ludlow, J. W., Figge, J., Shew, J.-Y., Huang, C.-M., Lee, W.-H., Marsilio, E., Paucha, E., and Livingston, D. M.: SV40 large tumor antigen forms a specific complex with the product of the retinoblastoma susceptibility gene. Cell, 54:275, 1988.
22. Dryja, T. P., Rapaport, J. M., Joyce, J. M., and Petersen, R. A.: Molecular detection of deletions involving band q14 of chromosome 13 in retinoblastomas. Proc. Natl. Acad. Sci. U.S.A., 83:7391, 1986.
23. Dunn, J. M., Phillips, R. A., Zhu, X., Becker, A., and Gallie, B. L.: Mutations in the RB1 gene and their effects on transcription. Mol. Cel. Biol., 9:4596, 1989.
24. Dyson, N., Howley, P. M., Munger, K., and Harlow, E.: The human papilloma virus 16 E7 oncoprotein is able to bind to retinoblastoma gene product. Science, 243:934, 1989.
25. Eliyahu, D., Goldfinger, N., Pinhasi-Kimhi, O., Shaulsky, G., Shurnik, Y., Arai, N., Rotter, V., and Oren, M.: Meth A fibrosarcoma cells express two transforming mutant p53 species. Oncogene, 3:13, 1988.
26. Eliyahu, D., Michalovitz, D., Eliyahu, S., Pinhasi-Kimhi, O., and Oren, M.: Wild-type p53 can inhibit oncogene-mediated focus formation. Proc. Natl. Acad. Sci. U.S.A., 86:8763, 1989.
27. Eliyahu, D., Raz, A., Gruss, P., Givol, D., and Oren, M.: Participation of p53 cellular tumor antigen in transformation of normal embryonic cells. Nature, 312:651, 1984.
28. Fearon, E. R., Cho, K. R., Nigro, J. M., Kern, S. E., Simons, J. W., Ruppert, J. M., Hamilton, S. R., Preisinger, A. C., Thomas, G., Kinzler, K. W., and Vogelstein, B.: Identification of a chromosome 18q gene that is altered in colorectal cancers. Science, 247:49, 1990.
29. Fearon, E. R., Hamilton, S. R., and Vogelstein, B.: Clonal analysis of human colorectal tumors. Science, 238:193, 1987.
30. Fearon, E. R., and Vogelstein, B.: A genetic model for colorectal tumorigenesis. Cell, 61:759, 1990.
31. Fearon, E. R., Vogelstein, B., and Feinberg, A. P.: Somatic deletion and duplication of genes on chromosome 11 in Wilms' tumor. Nature, 309:176, 1984.
32. Finlay, C. A., Hinds, P. W., and Levine, A. J.: The p53 protooncogene can act as a suppressor of transformation. Cell, 57:1083, 1989.
33. Fountain, J. W., Wallace, M. R., Bruce, M. J., Seizinger, B. R., Menon, A. G., Gusella, J. F., Michels, V. V., Schmidt, M. A., Dewald, G. W., and Collins, F. S.: Physical mapping of a translocation breakpoint in neurofibromatosis. Science, 244:1085, 1989.
34. Francke, U.: Retinoblastoma and chromosome 13. Cytogenet. Cell Genet., 16:131, 1976.
35. Friend, S. H., Bernards, R., Rogel, S., Weinberg, R. A., Rapaport, J. M., Albert, D. M., and Dryja, T. P.: A human DNA segment with the properties of a gene that predisposes to retinoblastoma and osteosarcoma. Nature, 323:643, 1986.
36. Friend, S. H., Horowitz, J. M., Gerber, M. R., Wang, X. F., Bogenmann, E., Li, F. P., and Weinberg, R. A.: Deletions of a DNA sequence in retinoblastomas and mesenchymal tumors: organization of the sequence and its encoded protein. Proc. Natl. Acad. Sci. U.S.A., 84:9059, 1987.
37. Fung, Y.-K. T., Murphree, A. L., T'Ang, A., Qian, J., Hinrichs, S. H., and Benedict, W. F.: Structural evidence for the authenticity of the human retinoblastoma gene. Science, 236:1657, 1987.
38. Gangfeng, X., O'Connell, P., Viskochil, D., Cawthon, R., Robertson, M., Culver, M., Dunn D., Stevens, J., Gesteland, R., White, R., and Weiss, R.: The neurofibromatosis type 1 gene encodes a protein related to GAP. Cell, 62:599, 1990.
39. Geiser, A., Der, C. J., Marshall, C. J., and Stanbridge, E. J.: Suppression of tumorigenicity with continued expression of the c-Ha-ras oncogene in EJ bladder carcinoma X human fibroblast hybrid cells. Proc. Natl. Acad. Sci. U.S.A., 83:5029, 1986.
40. Gessler, M., Poustka, A., Cavenee, W. K., Neve, R. L., Orkin, S. H., and Bruns, G. A. P.: Homozygous deletion in Wilms' tumors of a zinc-finger gene identified by chromosome jumping. Nature, 343:774, 1990.
41. Goddard, A. D., Balakier, H., Canton, M., Dunn, J., Squire, J., Reyes, E., Becker, A., Phillips, R. A., and Gallie, B. L.: Infrequent genomic rearrangement and normal expression of the putative RB1 gene in retinoblastoma tumors. Mol. Cell. Biol., 8:2082, 1988.
42. Grundy, P., Koufos, A., Morgan, K., Li, F. P., Meadows, A. T., and Cavenee, W. K.: Familial predisposition to Wilms' tumor does not map to the short arm of chromosome 11. Nature, 336:374, 1988.
43. Haaland, M.: Spontaneous tumors in mice. Sci. Rep. Invest. Imp. Cancer Res. Fund, 4:1, 1911.
44. Hansen, M. F., and Cavenee, W. K.: Genetics of cancer predisposition. Cancer Res., 47:5518, 1987.
45. Hansen, M. F., Koufos, A., Gallie, B. L., Phillips, R. A., Fodstad, O., Grogger, A., Gedde-Dahl, T., and Cavenee, W. K.: Osteosarcoma and retinoblastoma: a shared chromosomal mechanism revealing recessive predisposition. Proc. Natl. Acad. Sci. U.S.A., 82:6216, 1985.
46. Harbour, J. W., Lai, S. L, Whang, P. J., Gazdar, A. F., Minna, J. D., and Kaye, F. J.: Abnormalities in structure and expression of the retinoblastoma gene in SCLC. Science, 241:353, 1988.
47. Harris, H.: The analysis of malignancy by cell fusion: the position in 1988. Cancer Res., 48:3302, 1988.
48. Harris, H., and Klein, G.: Malignancy of somatic cell hybrids. Nature, 224:1314, 1969.
49. Hershowitz, I.: Functional inactivation of genes by dominant negative mutations. Nature, 329:219, 1987.
50. Hinds, P., Finlay, C., and Levine, A. J.: Mutation is required to activate the p53 gene for cooperation with the ras oncogene and transformation. J. Virol., 63:739, 1989.
51. Horowitz, J., Yandell, D. W., Park, S.-H., Canning, S., Whyte, P., Buchkovich, K., Harlow, E., Weinberg, R. A., and Dryja, T. P.: Point mutational inactivation of the retinoblastoma antioncogene. Science, 243:937, 1989.
52. Huang, H.-J. S., Yee, J.-K., Shew, J.-Y., Chen, P.-L., Bookstein, R., Friedmann, T., Lee, E. Y.-H. P., and Lee, W.-H.: Suppression of the neoplastic phenotype by replacement of the RB gene in human cancer cells. Science, 242:1563, 1988.
53. Huff, V., Compton, D. A., Chao, L.-Y., Strong, L. C., Geiser, C. F., and Saunders, G. F.: Lack of linkage of familial Wilms' tumor to chromosomal band 11p13. Nature, 336:377, 1988.
54. James, C. D., Carlbom, E., Dumanski, J. P, Hansen, M., Nordenskjold, M., Collins, V. P., and Cavenee, W. K.: Clonal genomic alterations in glioma malignancy stages. Cancer Res., 48:5546, 1988.
55. Jenkins, J. R., Rudge, K., and Currie, G. A.: Cellular immortalization by a cDNA clone encoding the transformation associated phosphoprotein p53. Nature, 312:651, 1984.
56. Kaneko, Y., Egues, M. C., and Rowley, J. D.: Interstitial deletion of short arm of chromosome 11 limited to Wilms' tumor cells in a patient without aniridia. Cancer Res., 41:4577, 1981.
57. Klinger, H. P.: Suppression of tumorigenicity. Cytogenet. Cell Genet., 32:68, 1982.
58. Knudson, A. G., Jr.: Mutation and cancer: statistical study of retinoblastoma. Proc. Natl. Acad. Sci. U.S.A., 68:820, 1971.
59. Knudson, A. G., Jr.: Hereditary cancer, oncogenes, and anti-oncogenes. Cancer Res., 45:1437, 1985.
60. Knudson, A. G., Jr., and Strong, L. C.: Mutation and cancer: a model for Wilm's tumor of the kidney. J. Nat. Cancer Inst., 48:313, 1972.
61. Koufos, A., Grundy, P., Morgan, K., Aleck, K. A., Hadus, T., Lampkin, B. C., Kalbakji, A., and Cavenee, W. K.: Familial Wiedman-Beckwith syndrome and a second Wilms tumor locus both map to 11p15.5. Am J. Hum. Genet., 44:711, 1989.
62. Koufos, A., Hansen, M. F., Lampkin, B. C., Workman, M. L., Copeland, N. G., Jenkins, N. A., and Cavenee, W. K.: Loss of alleles at loci on human chromosome 11 during genesis of Wilms' tumor. Nature, 309:170, 1984.
63. Landsvater, R. M., Mathew, C. G. P., Smith, B. A., Marcu, E. M., Te Meerman, G. J., Lips, C. J. M., Geerdink, R. A., Nakamura, Y., Ponder, B. A. J., and Buys, C. H. C.: Development of multiple endocrine neoplasia type 2A does not involve substantial deletions of chromosome 10. Genomics, 4:246, 1989.
64. Lane, D. P., and Benchimol, S.: p53: oncogene or anti-oncogene? Genes Devel., 4:1, 1990.
65. Lane, D. P., and Crawford, L. V.: T-antigen is bound to host protein in SV40-transformed cells. Nature, 278:261, 1979.
66. Lee, E. Y.-H. P., To, H., Shew, J.-Y., Bookstein, R., Scully, P., and Lee, W.-H.: Inactivation of the retinoblastoma susceptibility gene in human breast cancer. Science, 241:218, 1988.
67. Lee, W.-H., Bookstein, R., Hong, F., Young, L.-H., Shew, J.-Y., and Lee, E. Y.-H. P.: Human retinoblastoma susceptibility gene: cloning, identification and sequence. Science, 235:1394, 1987.
68. Lee, W.-H., Shew, J. Y., Hong, F. D., Sery, T. W., Donoso, L. A., Young, L.-J., Bookstein, R., and Lee, E. Y.-H. P.: The retinoblastoma susceptibility gene encodes a nuclear phosphoprotein associated with DNA binding activity. Nature, 329:642, 1987.
69. Leppert, M., Dobbs, M., Scambler, P., O'Connell, P., Nakamura, Y., Stauffer, D., Woodward, S., Burt, R., Hughes, J., Gardner, E., Lathrop, M., Wasmuth, J., Lalouel, J.-M., and White, R.: The gene for familial polyposis coli maps to the long arm of chromosome 5. Science, 238:1411, 1987.
70. Linzer, D. I. H., and Levine, A. J.: Characterization of a 54K dalton cellular SV40 tumor antigen present in SV40 transformed cells and uninfected embryonal carcinoma cells. Cell, 17:43, 1979.
71. Ludlow, J. W., Decaprio, J. A., Huang, C.-M., Lee, W.-H., Paucha, E., and Livingston, D. M.: SV40 large T antigen binds preferentially to an underphosphorylated member of the retinoblastoma gene product family. Cell, 56:57, 1989.
72. Lynch, H. T., Schuelke, G. S., Kimberling, W. J., Albans, W. A., Lynch, J. F., Biscone, K. A., Lipkin, M. L., Deschner, E. E., Mikol, Y. B., Sandberg, A. A., Elston, R. C., Bailey-Wilson, J. E., and Danes, B. S.: Hereditary nonpolyposis colorectal cancer (Lynch syndromes I and II). II. Biomarker studies. Cancer, 56:939, 1985.
73. Malkin, D., Li, F. P., Strong, L. C., Fraumeni, J. F., Nelson, C. E., Kim, D. H., Gryka, M. A., Bischoff, F. Z., Tainsky, M. A., and Friend, S. H.: Germline p53 mutations in a familial syndrome of breast cancer, sarcomas, and other neoplasms. Science, 250:1233, 1990.
74. Mannens, M., Slater, R. M., Heytig, C., Blick, J., De Kraker, J., Coad, N., DePagter-Holthuizen, P., and Pearson, P. L.: Molecular nature of genetic changes resulting in loss of heterozygosity of chromosome 11 in Wilms' tumors. Hum. Genet., 81:41, 1988.
75. Martin, G. S.: Rous sarcoma virus: a function required for the maintenance of the transformed state. Nature, 227:1021, 1970.
76. Masuda, H. C., Miller, C., Koeffler, H. P., Battifora, H., and Kline, M. J.: Rearrangement of the p53 gene in human osteogenic sarcomas. Proc. Natl. Acad. Sci. U.S.A., 84:7716, 1987.
77. Mathew, C. G. P.,Chin, K. S., Easton, D. F., Thorpe, K., Carter, C., Liou, G. I., Fong,

S.-L., Bridges, C. D. B., Haak, H., Nieuwenhuijzen-Kruseman, A., Schifterr, S., Hansen, H. A., Telenius, H., Telenius-Berg, M., Ponder, B. A. J.: A linked genetic marker for multiple endocrine neoplasia type 2A on chromosome 10. Nature, 328:527, 1987.

78. Miller, R. W., Fraumeni, J. F., Jr., and Manning, M. D.: Association of Wilms tumor with aniridia, hemihypertrophy, and other congenital malformations. N. Engl. J. Med., 270:922, 1964.

79. Moran, E., and Matthews, M. B.: Multiple functional domains in the adenovirus E1A gene. Cell, 48:177, 1987.

80. Mowat, M., Cheng, A., Kicumca, N., Bernstein, A., and Benchimol, S.: The arrangements of the cellular p53 gene in erythroleukemic cells transformed by Friend virus. Nature, 314:633, 1985.

81. Mulligan, L. M., Matlashewski, G. J., Scrable, H. J., and Cavenee, W. K.: Mechanism of p53 loss in human sarcomas. Proc. Natl. Acad. Sci. U.S.A., 87:5863, 1990.

82. Nelkin, B. D., Nakumura, Y., White, R. W., deBustros, A. C., Herman, J., Wells, S. A., Jr., and Baylin, S. B.: Low incidence of loss of chromosome 10 in sporadic and hereditary human medullary thyroid carcinoma. Cancer Res., 49:4114, 1989.

83. Nigro, J. M., Baker, S. J., Preisinger, A. C., Jessup, J. M., Hostetter, R., Cleary, K., Bigner, S. H., Davidson, N., Baylin, S., Devilee, P., Glover, T., Collins, F. S., Wesxton, A., Modali, R., Harris, C. C., and Vogelstein, B.: Mutations in the p53 gene occur in diverse tumor types. Nature, 342:705, 1989.

84. O'Connell, P., Leach, R., Cawthon, R., Culver, M., Stevens, J., Viskochil, D., Fournier, R. E. K., Rich, D., Ledbetter, D., and White, R.: Two von Recklinghausen neurofibromatosis translocations map within a 600 kb segment of 17q11.2. Science, 244:1087, 1989.

85. Orkin, S. H., Goldman, D. S., and Sallan, S. E.: Development of homozygosity for chromosome 11p markers in Wilms' tumor. Nature, 309:172, 1984.

86. Orye, E., Delbek, M. J., and Vandenabeele, B.: Retinoblastoma and long arm deletion at chromosome 13: attempts to define the deleted segment. Clin. Genet., 5:457, 1974.

87. Oshimura, M., Kugoh, H., Koi, M., Shimizu, M., Yamada, H., Satoh, H., and Barrett, J. C.: Transfer of human chromosome 11 suppresses tumorigenicity of some but not all tumor cell lines. J. Cell. Biochem., 42:135, 1990.

88. Parada, L. F., Land, H., Weinberg, R. A., Wolf, D., and Rotter, V.: Cooperation between gene encoding p53 tumor antigen and ras in cellular transformation. Nature, 312:649, 1984.

89. Pientenpol, J., Stein, R. W., Moran, E., Yaciuk, P., Schlegel, R., Lyons, R. M., Pittelkow, M. R., Munger, K., Howley, P. M., and Moses, H. L.: TGF-beta 1 inhibition of c-myc transcription and growth in keratinocytes is abrogated by viral transforming proteins with pRB binding domains. Cell, 61:777, 1990.

90. Ping, A. J., Reeve, A. E., Law, D. J., Young, M. R., Boehuke, M., and Feinberg, A. P.: Genetic linkage of Beckwith-Wiedman syndrome to 11p15. Am. J. Hum. Genet., 44:720, 1989.

91. Ponder, B.: Gene losses in human tumors. Nature, 335:400, 1988.

92. Ponder, B.: Neurofibromatosis gene cloned. Nature, 346:703, 1990.

93. Pritchard-Jones, K., Fleming, S., Davidson, D., Bickmore, W., Porteous, D., Gosden, C., Bard, J., Buckler, A., Pelletier, J., Housman, D., van Heyningen, V., and Hastie, N.: The candidate Wilms tumor gene is involved in genitourinary development. Nature, 346:194, 1990.

94. Reeve, A. E., Housiaux, P. J., Gardner, R. J. M., Chewings, W. E., Grindley, R. M., and Millow, L. J.: Loss of a Harvey ras allele in sporadic Wilms' tumor. Nature, 309:174 1984.

95. Reeve, A. E., Sih, S. A., Raizis, A. M, and Feinberg, A. P.: Loss of allelic heterozygosity at a second locus on chromosome 11 in sporadic Wilms' tumor cells. Mol. Cell. Biol., 9:1799, 1989.

96. Riccardi, V. M., Hittner, H. M., Francke, U., Yunis, J. J., Ledbetter, D., and Borges, W.: The aniridia-Wilms' tumor association: the clinical role of chromosome band 11p13. Cancer Genet. Cytogenet., 2:131, 1980.

97. Robbins, P. D., Horowitz, J. M., and Mulligan, R. C.: Negative regulation of human c-fos expression by the retinoblastoma gene product. Nature, 346:668, 1990.

98. Rouleau, G. A., Wertelecki, W., Haines J. L., Hobbs, W. J., Trofatter, J. A., Seizinger, B. R., Martuza, R. L., Superneau, D. W., Conneally, P. M., and Gussela, J. F.: Genetic linkage of bilateral acoustic neurofibromatosis to a DNA marker on chromosome 22. Nature, 329:246, 1987.

99. Rous, P.: A sarcoma of the fowl transmissible by an agent separable from the tumor cells. J. Exp. Med., 13:397, 1911.

100. Sager, R.: Genetic suppression of tumor formation: a new frontier in cancer research. Cancer Res., 46:1573, 1986.

101. Sager, R.: Tumor suppressor genes: the puzzle and the promise. Science, 246:1406, 1989.

102. Sarnow, P., Ho, Y. S., Williams, J., and Levine, A. J.: Adenovirus E1b-58 Kd tumor antigen and SV40 large tumor antigen are physically associated with the same 54 Kd cellular protein in transformed cells. Cell, 28:387, 1982.

103. Saxon, P. J., Srivastan, E. S., and Stanbridge, E. J.: Introduction of human chromosome 11 via microcell transfer controls tumorigenic expression of HeLa cells. EMBO J., 5:3461, 1986.

104. Seizinger, B. R., Rouleau, G. A., Ozelius, L. J., et al.: Genetic linkage of von Recklinghausen neurofibromatosis to the nerve growth factor receptor gene. Cell, 49:589, 1987.

105. Seizinger, B. R., Rouleau, G. A., Ozelius, L. J., et al.: Von Hippel-Lindau disease

maps to the region of chromosome 3 associated with renal cell carcinoma. Nature, 332:268, 1988.

106. Shimizu, M., Yokota, J., Mori, N., Shuin, T., Shinoda, M., Terada, M., and Oshimura, M.: Introduction of normal chromosome 3p modulates the tumorigenicity of a human renal cell carcinoma cell line YCR. Oncogene, 5:185, 1990.

107. Simpson, N. E., Kidd, K. K., Goodfellow, P. J., McDermid, H., Myers, S., Kidd, J. R., Jackson, C. E., Duncan, A. M. V., Farrer, L. A., Brasch, K., Castiglione, C., Genel, M., Gertner, J., Greenberg, C. R., Gusella, J. F., Holden, J. J. A., and White, B. N.: Assignment of multiple endocrine neoplasia type 2A to chromosome 10 by linkage. Nature, 328:528, 1987.

108. Slater, R. M., and de Kraker, J.: Chromosome number 11 and Wilms' tumor. Cancer Genet. Cytogenet., 5:237, 1982.

109. Sparkes, R. S., Sparkes, M. C., Wilson, M. G., Towner, J. W., Benedict, W. F., Murphree, A. L., and Yunis, J. J.: Regional assignment of genes for human esterase D and retinoblastoma to chromosome 13q14. Science, 208:1042, 1980.

110. Sparkes, R. S., Murphree, A. L., Lingus, R. W., Sparkes, M. C., Field, L. L., Funderburk, S. J., and Benedict, W. F.: Gene for hereditary retinoblastoma assigned to human chromosome 13 by linkage to esterase D. Science, 219:971, 1983.

111. Srivastava, S., Zou, Z., Pirollo, K., Blattner, W., and Chang, E. H.: Germ-line transmission of a mutated p53 gene in cancer-prone family with Li-Fraumeni syndrome. Nature, 348:747, 1990.

112. Stanbridge, E. J., and Cavenee, W. K.: Heritable Cancer and Tumor Suppressor Genes: A Tentative Connection. In Oncogenes and the Molecular Origins of Cancer. Edited by R. A. Weinberg. Cold Spring Harbor, NY, Cold Spring Harbor Press, 1989.

113. Stanbridge, E. J., Der, C. J., Doerson, C. J., Nighimi, R. Y., Peehl, D. M., Weissman, B. E., and Wilkinson, J.: Human cell hybrids: Analysis of transformation and tumorigenicity. Science, 215:252, 1982.

114. Stehlin, D., Varmus, H. E., Bishop, J. M., and Vogt, P. K.: DNA related to the transforming gene(s) of avian sarcoma viruses is present in normal avian DNA. Nature, 260:170, 1976.

115. Sugawara, O., Oshimura, M., Koi, M., Annab, L.A., and Barrett, J. C.: Induction of cellular senescence in immortalized cells by human chromosome 1. Science, 247:707, 1990.

116. Takahashi, T., Nau, M. M., Chibu, I., Birrer, M. J., Rosenberg, R. K., Vinocour, M., Levitt, M., Pass, H., Gazdar, A. F., and Minna, J. D.: p53: A frequent target for genetic abnormalities in lung cancer. Science, 246:491, 1989.

117. Trahey, M., and McCormick F.: A cytoplasmic protein stimulates normal N-ras p21 GTPase, but does not affect oncogenic mutants. Science, 238:542, 1987.

118. Trent, J. M., Stanbridge, E. J., McBride, H. L., Meese, E. V., Casey, G., Araujo, D. E., Witkowski, C. M., and Nagle, R. B.: Tumorigenicity in human melanoma lines controlled by introduction of human chromosome 6. Science, 247:568, 1990.

119. Varmus, H. E.: The molecular genetics of cellular oncogenes. Annu. Rev. Genet., 18:553, 1984.

120. Viskochil, D., Buchberg, A. M., Xu, G., Cawthon, R. M., Stevens, J., Wolff, R. K., Culver, M., Carey, J. C., Copeland, N. G., Jenkins, N. A., White, R., and O'Connell, P.: Deletions and a translocation interrupt a cloned gene at the neurofibromatosis type 1 locus. Cell, 62:187, 1990.

121. Vogelstein, B., Fearon, E. R., Hamilton, S. R., Kern, S. E., Preisinger, A. C., Leppert, M., Nakumura, Y., White, R., Smits, A. M. M., and Bos, J. L.: Genetic alterations during colorectal-tumor development. N. Engl. J. Med., 319:525, 1988.

122. Wallace, M. R., Marchuk, D. A., Andersen, L. B., Letcher, R., Odeh, H. M., Saulino, A. M., Fountain, J. W., Bereton, A., Nicholson, J., Mitchell, A. L., Brownstein, B. H., and Collins, F. S.: Type 1 neurofibromatosis gene: identification of a large transcript disrupted in three NF1 patients. Science, 249:181, 1990.

123. Warthin, A. S.: Heredity with reference to carcinoma. Arch. Intern. Med., 12:546, 1913.

124. Weichselbaum, R. R., Beckett, M., and Diamond, A.: Some retinoblastomas, osteosarcomas, and soft tissue sarcomas may share a common etiology. Proc. Natl. Acad. Sci. U.S.A., 85:2106, 1988.

125. Weinberg, R. A.: Oncogenes, antioncogenes, and the molecular bases of multistep carcinogenesis. Cancer Res., 49:3713, 1989

126. Weissman, B. E., Saxon, P. J. Pasquale, S. R., Jones, G. R., Geiser, A. G., and Stanbridge, E. J.: Introduction of a normal human chromosome 11 into a Wilms' tumor cell line controls its tumorigenic expression. Science, 236:175, 1987.

127. Werness, B. A., Levine, A. J., and Howley, P. M.: Association of human papillomavirus types 16 and 18 E6 proteins with p53. Science, 248:76, 1990.

128. Whyte, P., Buchkovich, K. J., Horowitz, J. M., Friend, S. H., Raybuck, J., Weinberg, R. A., and Harlow, E.: Association between an oncogene and an anti-oncogene: the adenovirus E1A proteins bind to the retinoblastoma gene product. Nature, 334:124, 1988.

129. Whyte, P., Williamson, N. M., and Harlow, E.: Cellular targets for transformation by the adenovirus E1A proteins. Cell, 56:67, 1989.

130. Wigler, M. H.: GAPs in understanding Ras. Nature, 346:696, 1990.

131. Wolf, D., Admon, S., Oren, M., and Rotter, V.: Major deletions in the gene encoding the p53 tumor antigen cause lack of p53 expression in HL-60 cells. Proc. Natl. Acad. Sci. U.S.A., 82:790, 1984.

132. Yandell, D., Campbell, T. A., Dayton, S. H., Petersen, R., Walton, D., Little, J. B., McConkie-Rosell, A., Buckley, E. G., and Dryja, T. P.: Oncogenic point mutations in the human retinoblastoma gene: their application to genetic counseling. N. Engl. J. Med., 321:1689, 1989.

Products and Targets of Oncogenes

Efraim Racker

To be or not to be phosphorylated—that is not the question.

All cancer roads lead to phosphoproteins.

Historical Background and Overview

In 1984 Lewis Thomas wrote "cancer research has turned into something like a running hunt. The fox is not yet within sight, but it is at least known that there is indeed a fox, and this is a great change from the sense of things twenty years ago".[46] Today there are several foxes within sight (Table I-7-1) and there are many more somewhere out there. The hunt is on, more fierce in competition than ever. Let us make sure we shoot the foxes and not the hunters.

In 1911 Peyton Rous discovered that a sarcoma of chicken can be transmitted by a filtrable virus.[39] A tumor was formed without transfer of intact cells and abstract oncology was born. It then became possible to transform normal cells into cancer cells in tissue cultures.[18,48] They look like cancer cells, they grow in soft agar (anchorage independent) and, when injected into Balb/c mice, produce large tumors. The gene (v-src) responsible for this remarkable feat, was sequenced and shown to generate a protein tyrosine kinase.[8,19,27] Phosphorylation of proteins at serine or threonine residues is an important and well-known mechanism to regulate metabolism, but the src kinase was the first enzyme shown to phosphorylate tyrosine residues, an exciting discovery of great potential. Then came the surprising discovery that normal cells contain a closely related cellular gene (c-src) that also generates a protein tyrosine kinase.[5] In contrast to the v-src kinase the c-src kinase is under metabolic control and shows only little enzymatic activity in intact cells.

Here we are; it looked so simple! One gene—one protein kinase—one cancer. The end of the road seemed in sight. Yet over 12 years have passed since these monumental discoveries were made and fog has settled over the road. No relevant target for the protein tyrosine kinase of oncogenic src has been established. Based on differences in phosphorylation patterns between normal and v-src transformed cells many suspects were arrested but had to be released without bail after a short period of incarceration. I shall return to the reasons for the failure to identify relevant targets for src and other oncogene products with protein tyrosine kinases activity. Hopes were raised that an inhibitor of this protein tyrosine kinase would slow the growth of tumors, but new complications arose. Many normal proteins, such as the epidermal growth factor and insulin receptors, were also shown to catalyze phosphorylation of tyrosine residues of proteins. Obviously to find an anticancer agent we have to search for an inhibitor specific for the oncogenic tyrosine kinases. The prospects for this are not very good, but we

Table I-7-1. Partial List of Oncogenes, Anti-oncogenes (Growth Suppressor Genes) and Promoters Involving Phosphorylation

1. Oncogene products with protein tyrosine kinase activity (30 +)*
   a) src family (8)
   b) fps family (2)
   c) abl family (2)
   d) growth factor receptor mutants (3)
   e) constitutive receptor ligands (3)

2. Oncogene products and cell cycle regulators with protein serine (threonine) kinase activity
   a) raf (3)
   b) mos
   c) p34^{cdc2}
   d) MAP 2 (2)

3. Ras family
   Some oncogenes, some anti-oncogenes (50 +)

4. Promoter induced kinases
   PK-C (7)

5. Growth suppressor gene products (4 +)

*The numbers in parentheses indicate the currently identified members of the families

must continue to look and learn about differences between normal and oncogenic tyrosine kinases We are beginning to unravel some of these differences particularly with respect to their ability to communicate with other protein kinases and to transmit signals.

There are over 40 oncoproteins that catalyze or influence tyrosine phosphorylation.[11,35] Some are not protein tyrosine kinases, but stimulate phosphorylation of tyrosine residues of protein indirectly. The sis oncogene produces an oncoprotein that is a very close relative of the platelet-derived growth factor (PDGF) which activates the protein tyrosine kinase activity of the PDGF receptor in the plasma membrane. PDGF is a normal constituent of platelets released to aid the process of wound healing. Another oncogene product activates the tyrosine kinase of the fibroblast growth factor receptor. Indirect activation of protein tyrosine kinase activity is achieved by the ras and other oncoproteins (v-mos, v-fos, v-abl) that induce the secretion of transforming growth factor α, which stimulates the tyrosine kinase of the EGF receptor. Oncoproteins like mos and raf are protein serine (threonine) kinases. There are several important serine (threonine) kinases (p34^{cdc2}, MAP 2) in mammalian cells that are involved in cell cycle control. These protein serine kinases are members of signal transduction pathways that also involve protein tyrosine kinases that have not been identified as yet. Distortion of the cell cycle is a hallmark of cancer cells.

There are important families of GTP-binding and phosphorylated nuclear oncoproteins that are dealt with in other chapters of this book. They are intrinsic to the development of cancer in animals and are contributors to human cancers. Most of them have, like v-src, normal cousins that are present in cells without causing cancer. These normal genes are called protooncogenes, which is not a good name. Proto implies that they were here first, which is probably true, but why "oncogenes"? They have not been created to be mutated and to serve as punishment for cigarette smokers! These genes (c-src, c-ras, c-myc, etc.) have important functions of their own involving growth and differentiation. The name "protooncogene" will probably stay with us, like other misnomers such as "oxygen" (believed to be an acid former).

In addition to oncogenes which are c-genes that are either mutated, amplified or translocated, or are v-genes imported by viruses, there are other contributors to cancer. Tumor promoters are environmental toxins that contribute to malignancy. In animals they enhance formation of skin cancers. The best studied ones are phorbol esters that activate protein kinase C, a protein serine (threonine) kinase.

An important new family of genes that control growth of cancer has emerged recently. They are called growth or oncogene suppressor genes.[11] Their protein products which control growth and differentiation are regulated by phosphorylation and dephosphorylation. Their loss or mutation serves as another nail in the cancer coffin.

Cancer in man is clearly not a story of one gene-one enzyme-one tumor. There are multiple oncogenes involved, promoters and loss of growth suppressor genes and genes that facilitate metastasis. A large number of these cancer agents have one thing in common—they involve directly or indirectly phosphorylation-dephosphorylation reactions. But each acts differently. Like the British and Americans, they are separated by a common language. Their accents emphasize different phosphorylated amino acid residues and different target proteins. The question that we need to answer is not which proteins they phosphorylate, but which proteins are altered in function when phosphorylated. But this is not sufficient information; many proteins change function when they become phosphorylated. Such changes may or may not be relevant depending on the impact they make on the network of signal transductions. Stimulation of enzymes that are present in excess within a pathway (e.g., some of the glycolytic enzymes), is probably unimportant. For an evaluation of the relevance of protein phosphorylation modern genetic methods are available both in cells and in transgenic animals. I shall return to this problem in the discussion of specific protein kinases that participate in signal transduction pathways. Somewhat neglected until recently, protein phosphatases are becoming recognized as equally important players in the control of the network of communications. Finally, I want to contradict myself by pointing out that phosphorylation-dephosphorylation of proteins may be important even without changes in function. There is ample evidence that phosphorylation of proteins can alter their susceptibility to proteolysis.[25] Such regulations participate in oscillatory events

during the cell cycle, known to be controlled by phosphorylation-dephosphorylation and by proteolysis. Understanding of these complex control mechanisms of the cell cycle and their distortions in cancer cells, is likely to be the key task in the next decade of cancer research.

The huge network of phosphorylation-dephosphorylation reactions that control normal metabolism is very complex. There are interactions, "cross-talks" between kinases, one kinase phosphorylating a second kinase, thereby either stimulating or inhibiting its activity. There is "cross-talk" at the substrate level, one kinase phosphorylating a substrate and thereby changing its susceptibility to another kinase. I shall discuss later intracellular stress or heat-shock proteins, chaperones and match-makers that interact with substrates and either impair or facilitate phosphorylation processes.[38] Phosphorylations are orchestrated by counterpoint, one melody combining with another, as beautiful as an opera by Mozart and as bewildering as a symphony by Karl Husa. We need to know how this network is changed by cancer causing agents. In cancer there are distortions in the fine tuning of phosphorylation-dephosphorylation reactions that alter the cell cycle and lead to uncontrolled and metastatic growth. This chapter focuses on the phosphorylation of proteins describing the slow but steady progress we are making in solving this jigsaw puzzle.

Protein Tyrosine Kinases in Normal and Cancer Cells

In addition to the many oncogene products, several growth factor receptors are protein tyrosine kinases phosphorylating some of the same substrates phosphorylated by oncogenic tyrosine kinases. When specific ligands (e.g., EGF, CSF or insulin) bind to the extracellular domain of these receptors, which traverse the plasma membrane, the intracellular tyrosine kinase is activated. Why are these normal tyrosine kinases not tumorigenic? Is it because they don't phosphorylate tumor-relevant proteins or because they are only temporarily activated when the ligands combine with them? The fact that the erb B oncogene product is a truncated EGF receptor that lacks the EGF binding domain and is permanently activated, speaks for the second possibility. On the other hand different receptor kinases have different physiological functions and therefore must show different patterns of protein phosphorylation. For example, some of these specific phosphorylated targets may be critical for the action of insulin, but may not contribute to tumorigenicity.

In the past, the approach to identify relevant targets for protein tyrosine kinases was to compare the phosphorylation pattern, e.g., in a cell transformed by v-src with its untransformed parent cell line following exposure to inorganic radioactive phosphate; or to compare the tyrosine phosphorylation pattern between cells activated by different ligands such as insulin, PDGF, EGF, CSF, etc. The sensitivity of this approach has been greatly enhanced recently by using antibodies that recognize phosphotyrosine residues of proteins and by increasing the sensitivity and resolution of SDS-PAGE analysis. Between 20 to 50 proteins phosphorylated by tyrosine kinases of various oncoproteins and receptors have been discovered and more are emerging. As mentioned in the introduction none of these phosphoproteins have thus far been identified as relevant targets for growth. Protein kinases, and particularly protein tyrosine kinases, are promiscuous. We have shown several years ago that a synthetic random amino acid polymer of about 40,000 molecular weight that contains only glutamic acid and tyrosine (in a 4:1 ratio), is phosphorylated by every protein tyrosine kinase that we have tested thus far.[7] Yet insulin receptor and EGF receptor kinases phosphorylate different residues in this random polymer, apparently depending on the charge distribution in the vicinity of the tyrosine residue.[23] No wonder many innocent proteins that could not care less whether they are phosphorylated or not, become victims of these hungry protein tyrosine kinases. They act like criminals covering their tracks by phosphorylating proteins that are not relevant to their pathway of signal transduction. Therefore, to be or not to be phosphorylated—that is not the question.[37] The more important question is whether phosphorylation of a protein changes its function. But as pointed out earlier, even a change in function induced by the change in protein conformation caused by phosphorylation may be gratuitous. How can we design a rational search for relevant targets of protein kinases of oncoproteins instead of going on fishing expeditions without knowing which kind of fish we are looking for? This is where the extraordinary advances in molecular genetics and methods of analysis of signal transduction pathways come to the rescue as I shall discuss later.

Protein Serine (Threonine) Kinases in Normal and Cancer Cells

Protein serine (threonine) kinases can be divided into two main groups. Group A contains protein kinases that phosphorylate serine or threonine residues located at the proper distance from acidic residues such as glutamic or aspartic acid. They include casein kinase 1 and several members of the large family of casein kinase 2, including the membrane-associated protein kinase-P (PK-P). Several PKs in this group phosphorylate under appropriate conditions a large random polypeptide (ca 40,000 MW) containing only glutamic acid and threonine. Enzymes in group B phosphorylate serine (threonine) residues that are located at the proper distance from basic residues such as lysine or arginine. They include PK-A, cGMP-dependent PK, PK-C, calmodulin-dependent PK and p34 kinase. They phosphorylate synthetic random polypeptides of 15,000–60,000 molecular weight which contain only arginine and serine or arginine, proline and threonine.

PKs also phosphorylate synthetic peptides containing 7–15 amino acids that are custom-tailored according to the consensus sequence that surrounds the phosphorylation site of native target proteins. Their major advantage is greater specificity when compared to the large, random polypeptide substrates; their disadvanages are that they often have very high Km values and are more difficult to analyze. Many of these peptides are not commercially available and if available very expensive. The large random polypeptides are available and inexpensive. They are particularly useful for exploration of signal transduction between tyrosine and serine (threonine)

kinases and between serine kinases of group A and group B as will be described later.

The number of protein serine (threonine) kinases is staggering, but which ones are relevant to the cancer problem? In most instances we do not know their role in the life of the cell. In a few cases it was possible to elucidate their role because they are activated by external ligands. The stimulation of cAMP formation and of PK-A by epinephrine, and of PK-C by phorbol esters, are invaluable tools for the exploration of the biological role of these kinases. There is an abundance of other kinases that phosphorylate intracellular proteins at serine residues, apparently with no external ligand strings attached. I say apparently, because no external ligands for these protein-serine kinases have as yet been found. However, there are several protein serine kinases that are stimulated by ligand-activated tyrosine kinases. EGF receptor, insulin and PDGF receptors activate serine and threonine kinases. On the other hand, several serine (threonine) kinases influence ligand-activated protein tyrosine kinases.[2] PK-C inhibits EGF receptor kinase, PK-P stimulates EGF receptor kinase and inhibits insulin receptor kinase. Src kinase stimulates both PK-C and PK-P activity (casein kinase 2) which phosphorylate transcription factors.

These and many other observations point to a role of protein-serine (threonine) kinase in tumor growth. Phorbol esters that activate PK-C are mitogenic and over-expression of PK-C by transfection renders cells more susceptible to transformation by an activated ras oncogene.[20] Ras somehow stimulates PK-C activity. There are multiple forms of PK-C; at least one of them is present in the nucleus. C-raf is a cytoplasmic protein serine (threonine) kinase which contains a negative regulatory domain at its N-terminus. Truncation of this domain results in kinase activation.[13] Cells containing v-src or those that are activated by ligands of protein tyrosine kinases show increased raf kinase activity. PK-C also activates c-raf. There is suggestive evidence that activated raf goes to the nucleus and (perhaps indirectly) stimulates transcription. Three other important protein serine (threonine) kinases p34[cdc2], mos and MAP 2, play a role in the control of the cell cycle and are interlinked with protein tyrosine kinases.

Protein kinases of both groups A and B are ubiquitous enzymes that phosphorylate basic, neutral and acidic proteins. It should be stressed that proteins are complex in their charge distribution. An acidic protein such as casein contains appropriate basic sequences that serve as substrate for PK-A (group B) and some neutral or basic protein may be phosphorylated by group A kinases. Indeed, some proteins such as glycogen synthase were shown to serve as substrate for 10 different protein kinases of both groups A and B.

Signal Transduction Pathways from the Plasma Membrane to the Nucleus

A great deal of information has been obtained about signals emerging from the plasma membrane or from oncogene products that may or may not be associated with the plasma membrane. Many involve tyrosine protein kinases. Some involve protein serine (threonine) kinases. Rapid progress has also been made in identifying proteins and elucidating events at the receiving end of signals in the nucleus that influence DNA transcription. Many of these transcription factors have been shown to be controlled by phosphorylation-dephosphorylation. On the other hand, the interconnecting pathways from the plasma membrane to the nucleus are still mostly obscure. They are so complex and bewildering that it is easier to get lost in the crossroads of these kinase activities than in Tokyo, Boston or even in Brooklyn.

Among the new appoaches to this black box are the expression of oncogenic DNA sequences by transfection of normal (or quasi normal) cell lines. This has been the revolutionary method leading to the identification of human oncogenes. Over-expression of PK-C or suppression by down regulation of PK-C activity has led to an abundance (or over-abundance) of clues.[20] We can control expression of some transfected genes by using a promoter that can be activated e.g., by dexamethasone. Another important method is to inject individual cells with antibodies against an oncoprotein. For example, it was shown that injection of an antibody against c-ras prevents the transformation of 3T3 mouse fibroblasts by several oncogenes including v-src, but not by others (e.g., raf and mos).[44] It therefore looks as though c-ras is downstream from v-src. Does v-src phosphorylate ras? We have evidence that it does under certain conditions, but we need to obtain evidence that phosphorylated c-ras is oncogenic.[1] A more fashionable explanation is that another protein called GAP is involved. This GTPase activating protein greatly accelerates the conversion of c-ras-GTP into c-ras GDP, thereby rendering it inactive.[29] Significantly, GAP does not accelerate the GTPase activity of v-ras that is already low compared to that of c-ras. Several investigators are actively engaged in finding out whether GAP phosphorylated by a tyrosine kinase becomes inactivated thereby allowing a high steady-state concentration of c-ras-GTP. They have found that addition of ligands such as PDGF or EGF result in the phosphorylation of GAP and enhance the ratio of c-ras GTP/ c-ras GDP.[18,21,30] But more direct evidence is still needed: Is phosphorylated GAP inactive as GTPase activator? Some claim it is; others say it isn't. Several laboratories, including ours, are trying to obtain an unambiguous answer to this question. It is particularly important because oncogenic ras is found in several forms of human cancer (see I-5).

Instead of just looking for proteins phosphorylated by oncogene products at tyrosine residues, we have started a search for signal transduction in reconstituted systems. Since I have always considered that our reconstitution studies are relevant to mechanisms but may not represent physiological conditions, we do not hesitate to use a yeast system to aid us in studies of ras. In yeast, ras proteins are required for the production of c-AMP by adenylyl cyclase.[6] It so happens that mammalian GAP also accelerates the GTPase activity of a yeast ras protein. We therefore use a reconstituted system consisting of yeast adenylyl cyclase and yeast or mouse ras proteins and have demonstrated that GAP indeed inhibits cAMP formation. Now we are exploring the effect of phosphorylation on the activity of GAP. We find that several protein kinases, including c-src, v-src, PK-A and PK-C, phosphorylate GAP. Which ones are relevant, which ones gratuitous? We hope to find out. Some investigators believe that GAP

may have a second function, by interacting with growth factor receptors or even with ion channels.[18,29] If this is the case, these interactions may be influenced by phosphorylation of GAP by kinases that may not influence its GTPase activity.

Signal transduction in reconstituted systems may reveal features that are difficult to establish by other methods. For example, it is known that PK-C phosphorylates src kinase but a change in activity has not been demonstrated. We have preliminary data that show that src kinases enhance the activity of some protein serine kinases that are present in rate-limiting amounts with a random polymer as final phosphate acceptor. Other examples were reviewed previously.[37] It was shown recently that in vitro PDGF receptor phosphorylates raf resulting in a marked stimulation of its serine (threonine) kinase activity.[13]

I have emphasized signal tranductions from one protein kinase to another, but there are other actors in these pathways involving phosphorylations. We have observed that transfection with K-ras inhibits the autophosphorylation of the PDGF receptor and its signal transduction to the phosphoinositide cycle.[36] In some cells transfection with ras stimulates the PI cycle. The production of IP_3 that takes place on activation of the PI cycle, results in an increase of intracellular Ca^{2+} which stimulates PK-C. It is of interest, therefore, that thapsigargin, another tumor promoter which does not activate PK-C directly, increases intracellular Ca^{2+} by inhibiting a Ca^{2+} transport ATPase.[45] There is abundant evidence that Ca^{2+} is a growth regulator at several points of the cell cycle, which I shall discuss next. Okadaic acid, another tumor promoter, inhibits a protein phosphatase involved in the cell cycle.[15] Thus, three chemically unrelated promoters with different mechanisms of action influence phosphorylation-dephosphorylation reactions and are involved in signal transduction.

The Cell Cycle and Protein Kinases

The growth of normal cells is controlled at specific restriction points in the cell cycle.[34] As shown in Figure I-7-1, p34^{cdc2}, a protein serine (threonine) kinase, plays a critical role at the entry into mitosis as well as at a restriction point at G_1.[28,31,32] Cyclins, a family of proteins that oscillate during the cell cycle, interact with the p34 kinase to form the M-phase promoting factor complex (MPF). When p34 in this complex is phosphorylated at tyrosine and threonine residues, the enzyme is inactive. It is activated at the entry into the M phase by dephosphorylation. The role of cyclins in this process appears to resemble that of chaperones that influence phosphorylation reactions.[1,38] Like heat shock and stress proteins the cyclins are transient; they disappear at the exit from mitosis. It is not clear whether they disappear because of an activated protease or because their susceptibility to proteases is altered by phosphorylation-dephosphorylations. There may also be a change in the rate of their synthesis. Ca^{2+} which activates a protease and activates or inhibits various protein kinases, is probably a major actor in the cell cycle drama.

What is the role of protooncogenes and oncogenes in the control of the cell cycle? C-src kinase becomes transiently phosphorylated at both serine and threonine residues by p34 kinase during mitosis, resulting in an increase of its tyrosine

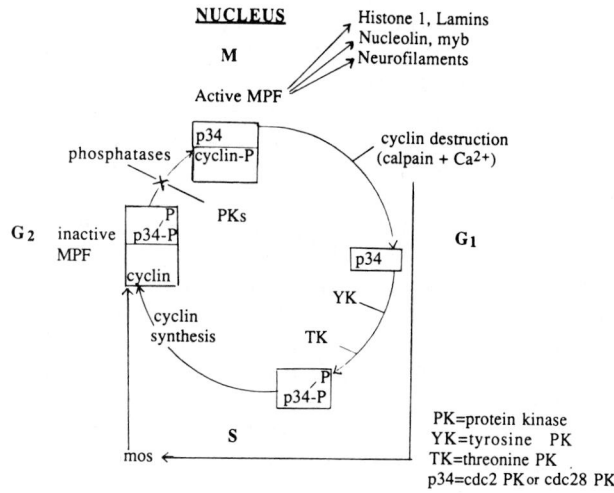

Figure I-7-1. This figure shows the current, tentative view of cyclic signal transduction pathways involving the cell cycle. Active maturation or mitosis factor (MPF) consists of two components, a cyclin and p34. The latter contains the active site of the protein kinase. In *S. cerevisiae* the p34 is the product of the cdc28 gene, in *S. pombe* the product of the cdc2 gene. An unidentified protein tyrosine kinase (YK) and an unidentified protein threonine (serine) kinase (TK) phosphorylate p34 and render it inactive. Prior to entry into mitosis p34 combines with a cyclin, and phosphatases activate the kinase by dephosphorylation. On exit from mitosis, cyclin is destroyed by a Ca^{2+} activated protease (calpain). Then p34 again becomes phosphorylated and inactive. There is a second role of p34 in the G_1 phase which has not as yet been clearly defined. Events in the plasma membrane that are triggered by hormones and growth factors also influence the cell cycle, but little is known about the pathways. EGF and PDGF are well-known mitogens. The raf proto oncogene has been proposed to transmit their signals to the nucleus. As described in the text, the ras pathway is controlled by GAP, oncogenic src requires c-ras for transformation. Protein kinase C is the signal transducer for phorbol esters that act as tumor promoters. Some of the arrows indicated in the figure suggest connections that have not been firmly established and are based on circumstantial evidence.

kinase activity.[43] These events have been lucidly discussed in an excellent review.[42] As mentioned earlier the kinase activity of c-src is very low. It has a domain at the c-terminus that is truncated in v-src. This segment contains a phosphotyrosine (at residue 527) that inhibits c-src kinase activity. Analogous control domains are found in other tyrosine kinases of protooncogenes such as fyn, yes and lck, as well as in PK-C and PK-A. It is possible that release from inhibitory domains also operates when receptors (EGF, insulin, PDGF) are activated by ligands. In any case, the stimulation of c-src during mitosis appears to be linked to its control domain, because site-directed mutagenesis of tyr 527 prevents the increase of c-src kinase activity during mitosis.[42] The question which enzyme(s) phosphorylates tyr 527 of c-src is still not settled.

There is evidence that c-src kinase itself may catalyze the phosphorylation of tyr 527; there is also evidence for a different kinase that phosphorylates this site. We reviewed these findings and proposed that both enzymes could participate,[1] but that c-src is not likely to catalyze the tyr 527 phosphorylation unless a chaperone is present. A variation of the c-src theme was observed with c-abl (p150) tyrosine kinase. Deletion of a regulatory region at the N-terminal, accompanied by a movement of the protein from the nucleus to the cytoplasm, gives rise to transformation.[48] As with c-src kinase there is a mitosis-linked phosphorylation of the c-abl protein probably catalyzed by p34 kinase, but no tyrosine kinase activation has been observed in the case of c-abl.[22]

As stressed earlier, no physiologically relevant target for any of the protein tyrosine kinases of receptors or oncogenes has been identified. However, there are many attractive candidates. Some of the biochemical (glycolysis, amino acid transport, etc.) and morphological changes observed in transformed cells are caricatures of transient changes seen in phases of the cell cycle. Several members of the cytoskeleton, of gap junction, of adhesion plaques and metabolic pathways are substrates for protein tyrosine kinases. Their phosphorylation could contribute to the morphological and metabolic changes that accompany transformation as well as certain phases of the cell cycle. The excitement that was first generated by these discoveries has been replaced by disillusions caused by many experiments negating the significance of these findings. Perhaps some of these phosphorylations should be re-investigated with a new perspective involving a second set of actors. Stress and heat-shock proteins were shown to affect phosphorylations and we have a new ballgame to watch.[1] Specific heat-shock proteins are present in transformed cells and interact with growth suppressor proteins. After all, isn't transformation of a cell a form of stress? Can we look at cytoskeletal associated proteins such as MAPs and tau as examples of chaperones that facilitate the formation of microtubules? After exposure of cells to mitogens, MAP2 kinase becomes phosphorylated at tyrosine and threonine residues, and in contrast to $p34^{cdc2}$, its kinase activity is increased by phosphorylation. Both threonine and tyrosine phosphorylation appear to be required for the activation of MAP2 kinase.[3] Such multiple requirements are possibly explained by the phenomenon of activation at the substrate level, mentioned earlier, in which the phosphorylation of a substrate by one kinase is required for the phosphorylation by a second kinase.[37] In line with this interpretation is the observation that a protein tyrosine phosphatase, injected into oocytes, activates p34. However, there are alternative explanations, e.g., both phosphorylations are required to block activity.

The c-mos gene product is also a protein serine (threonine) kinase and was the first protooncogene shown to be tumorigenic when over-expressed.[47] It participates in the cell cycle and oscillates probably because of destruction by calpain, a Ca^{2+} activated protease.[40,49] In the last few years there has been an explosion of new information about the numerous protein kinases and protein phosphatases that regulate the cell cycle.

I show some of these signal transduction connections in Figure I-7-1. In defense of the many interconnecting arrows in this figure, I can state with confidence that they represent an incomplete list of those we know today, and only a small fraction of those we shall know by the end of this century.[31] Clearly, anyone who is not thoroughly confused just does not understand the situation. Although the dust hasn't settled yet, it is becoming clear that several protooncogenes participate in the cell cycle and that their mutations to oncogenes are likely to distort the normal events in growth control.

Growth Supressor-, Heat Shock-, Stress Proteins, and Chaperones

Evidence for the existence of growth suppressor genes has been in the literature for many years. Only recently have specific proteins and their loss or mutations in human cancer been identified. These exciting discoveries are dealt with in another chapter (I-6). What is the role of phosphorylation-dephosphorylation in the activity of these growth suppressor proteins? The best documented example for such a role is the Rb protein which is missing or altered in retinoblastomas and other human tumors.[50] Although the exact mode of action of Rb is still subject to speculation, there is one important clue. Rb is a phosphoprotein and is phosphorylated by p34^{cdc2}. When it is dephosphorylated it interacts with oncoproteins such as large T of SV40, E1A of adenovirus and E7 of papilloma virus that are known to facilitate growth and immortalization of cells in tissue culture. This interaction with Rb prevents the oncogenic potential of these virus proteins. But what is the role of the Rb protein in normal growth? In the S and M phases of the cell cycle most Rb is found in the nucleus mainly in the phosphorylated (inactive) form. In the G0 and G1 phases some non-phosphorylated Rb is present.[9,10,12] Thus, there is a correlation between the state of Rb phosphorylation and cell cycle control, but there are gaps in our knowledge with respect to the identity of proteins that Rb interacts with in the absence of an oncogene. A candidate is c-myc. But what happens to its oncogenic potential if Rb leaves it to interact with an authentic oncogene like SV40? In any case, growth suppressor proteins appear to act as policemen who step in when a cell that is supposed to rest is trying to step out of G0.

We need to know more about the steady-state of growth suppressor proteins and how their levels are controlled during transcription and translation. A case in point is K$_{rev}$ 1 or Rap 1, representative of a class of small molecular GTP-binding proteins that have sequence homology with ras proteins and act as anti-oncogenes. An over-expression of K$_{rev}$ 1 induces resistance to oncogenic ras as well as to some other oncogenes, but not to all. A different pattern of resistance and susceptibility is observed with other growth suppressor genes and the list of growth suppressor genes with different specificities is steadily growing.[16] One growth suppressor protein is a 53,000 dalton protein which was shown to be phosphorylated by p34 kinase.[4,26] The observation that p53 interacts with a heat-shock protein, and the previously mentioned presence of stress proteins in transformed cells and their ability to modulate phosphorylation reactions, appear to justify a brief discussion of this class of proteins.[26]

"Heat-shock protein" is not a good name because a) other forms of stress (toxins, starvation, transformation) induce the appearance of the same or similar proteins, and b) there are heat-shock proteins that are constitutive and not induced by heat. They are still called heat-shock proteins because they are cursed by sequence homologies. These are often of obvious relevance with respect to function and evolution, but sometimes represent a trick of nature to confuse some over-enthusiastic evolutionist (as if this was necessary). The key point is that some "heat-shock proteins" are constitutively expressed without stress and have important physiological roles. There are families of the 70 kDa and of the 60 kDa protein. The 70 and 78 kDa chaperones function mainly in the cytosol facilitating the transport of proteins into mitochondria and into the endoplasmic reticulum. The family of 60 kDa proteins called "chaperonins"[14] are present in mitochondria, bacteria and chloroplasts and are related by sequence homology and immune cross-reactivity. In mitochondria 60 kDa protein assists in proper protein folding in cooperation with other chaperones.[33]

The name "molecular chaperone" was coined by Laskey[24] describing the action of nucleoplasmin which prevents the random interaction between histones and DNA and the formation of inactive aggregates. However, it has become apparent that some other "chaperones" actually facilitate protein folding and the formation of enzymatically active dimers and should therefore be called "match makers."[38] It was shown in elegant experiments[17] how two chaperonins, groEL and groES, participate in the formation of the photosynthetic enzyme called Rubisco. GroEL functions as a chaperone keeping the unfolded inactive enzyme in the extended form, while groES, acting as a matchmaker with the help of ATP and Mg, facilitates the formation of the enzymatically active dimer of Rubisco. Relevance to the cancer problem is suggested by the observations that groEL facilitates the phosphorylation of some substrates by the protein tyrosine kinase of the src gene product,[1] and other chaperones facilitate the phosphorylation of c-ras by src kinase. As said earlier the significance of these observations needs exploration, but in view of the massive evidence for the role of phosphorylation-dephosphorylation in the cell cycle and oncogenic transformation, it seems likely that chaperones participate.

Oncogenes, Growth Suppressor Genes and Protein Kinases in Human Cancer

Our knowledge of the events that lead to human cancer is very limited and speculations often exceed the speed limits dictated by our slow advances. Speculations based on experiments with animals and (to the horror of some clinicians) on work with cells grown in the ghetto of plastic dishes are viewed with justified suspicion. The onslaught of abstract oncology, using broken pieces of DNA, forced into pseudo normal 3T3 mouse fibroblasts by injury induced by Ca phosphate or even by guns, has not always been warmly greeted by men of medicine.

As a young M.D. I was impressed by the medical evidence in favor of environmental carcinogens and tumor promoters, irrespective of whether they were self inflicted via man-made products such as tar, cigarettes and atom bombs, or by uninsurable "acts of god" such as sunshine or cosmic radiation. Now I am convinced that the keys to cancer are the reactions catalyzed by protein kinases that control the cell cycle and are distorted by oncogene products. Moreover, I see no contradiction between these two points of view. The main obstacle to their integration is the complexity of cancer in humans. Each person is an individual and so is his cancer. The concept of individuality is acknowledged by all and ignored by most. A rose may be a rose, may be a rose, but a cancer is not a cancer, is not a cancer. The variations of the theme of cancer are staggering. The food I eat, the water I drink, the house I live in, the city I have chosen, the work I do, the people I associate with all contribute to the less important edges of the jig-saw puzzle we call cancer. I doubt that in any form of cancer we will ever see the whole picture. But in the center of the picture where the action is, the pieces are coming together. Human cancer is multigenic and the injuries to the genes are random processes that may not even have an order. Although there are hot spots in our DNA, the injuries are too varied for an ordered sequence of events in the progression from a normal tissue to a benign tumor, to a malignant growth that may or may not be metastatic.

The specific oncogenes that appear, the specific growth suppressor genes that disappear, the order of their appearance and disappearances, determines the character of the cancer. The response of the host with antibodies, immune cells, and stress proteins will modify its progression or even eliminate it, but will not likely change its basic character which is a function of the aquisitions of oncogenes and losses of suppressor genes.

Our new knowledge of the function of oncogenes as protein kinases and the control of the cell cycle by phosphorylation-dephosphorylations has opened up new approaches to cancer therapy. We do not know as yet whether the disruption of a phosphorylating cascade induced by a single oncogene will impede the growth of a human cancer. It does so in animals which are not ideal models, but the best we have. In contrast to normal cells that are only transiently exposed to ligands, such as EGF or PDGF, some tumors secrete TGFα and PDGF which by an autocrine mechanism constitutively activate protein tyrosine kinases. These transforming growth factors are obvious targets for therapeutic intervention and are being explored in animals and humans. We need to know more about the specificity of oncogenic protein kinases before we can design a drug that will not be toxic for other protein kinases that fulfill essential functions in normal cells. We can be very selective in our approach. We know several oncogenes associated with human cancer, with H-ras on the top of the list (Table I-7-2). We need to know whether TGFα, an activator of a protein tyrosine kinase in the plasma membrane, is secreted by ras-containing human cancers as it is by ras tumors in tissue cultures. The bcr-abl oncoprotein is a protein tyrosine kinase activated by chromosomal translocation and is present in most patients with chronic myelogenous leukemia. Would it make any difference to a patient with a ras containing colon cancer if we could stop the effect of TGFα, or if we could inhibit the abl kinase in a patient with chronic myelogenous leukemia? We do not know and need to find out. Which among the oncogenes present in a cancer cell dictates the distortion of the cell cycle? Do all of them contribute equally to malignancy? Or is one required for the function of a second one as observed

Table I-7-2. Proto-oncogenes and Human Tumors

Proto-oncogene	Neoplasm
H-ras	Carcinoma of colon, lung and pancreas; melanoma
K-ras	Acute myelogenous and lymphoblastic leukemia; carcinoma of thyroid; melanoma
N-ras	Carcinoma of genitourinary tract and thyroid; melanoma
Abl	Chronic myelogenous leukemia
Erbb-1	Squamous cell carcinoma; glioblastoma
Erbb-2 (neu)	Adenocarcinoma of breast and ovary
Myc	Burkitt's lymphoma Carcinoma of lung, breast and cervix
L-myc	Carcinoma of lung
N-myc	Neuroblastoma Small cell carcinoma of lung
Ret	Carcinoma of thyroid
Ros	Glioblastoma
Sis	Glioblastoma
Src	Carcinoma of colon
Trk	Carcinoma of thyroid

in protein kinase cascades? Could some of them contribute to malignancy yet be beneficial to the host by reducing metastatic potentials or by contributing to immune surveillance?

We need to match our ignorance by our determination to find out. It would be frustrating and tragic if we could not, because of lack of funds, explore all the exciting approaches that have become possible by the advances made in the past few years. The doors are wide open.

Acknowledgment

This investigation was supported by PHS grant CA08964, awarded by the National Cancer Institute, DHHS, and (in part) by a grant from the Cornell Biotechnology Program which is sponsored by the New York State Science and Technology Foundation, a consortium of industries, the U.S. Army Research Office and the National Science Foundation.

Abbreviations

PK: protein kinase; PK-A: catalytic subunit of cAMP-dependent PK; PK-C: Ca^{2+} and phospholipid-dependent PK; PK-P: polypeptide-dependent PK; p34: a product of the cdc2 gene and a serine (threonine) PK; MPF: maturation (M phase) promoting factor consisting of p34 and a cylcin; Tau: protein that facilitates the formation of microtubules; MAP: microtubule-associated proteins; MAP 2 kinase: a serine (threonine) PK which (among other substrates) phosphorylates some cytoskeleton proteins; EGF: epidermal growth factor; PDGF: platelet-derived growth factor; CSF: colony stimulating factor; SDS-PAGE: sodium dodecyl sulfate-polyacrylamide gel electrophoresis; c-src, c-ras, c-mos, c-raf, etc.: protooncogenes; GAP: GTPase activating protein, stimulates the GTPase activity of c-ras.

References

1. Abdel-Ghany, M., El-Gendy, K., Zhang, S., and Racker, E.: Control of src kinase activity by activators, inhibitors, and substrate chaperones. Proc. Natl. Acad. Sci. U.S.A., In press, 1990.
2. Abdel-Ghany, M., El-Gendy, K., Zhang, S., Raden, D., and Racker, E.: Brain protein kinase C phosphorylating poly(arginine, serine) or lamin B is stimulated by anions and by an activator purified from bovine serum albumin preparations. Proc. Natl. Acad. Sci. U.S.A., 86:1761, 1989.
3. Anderson, N. G., Maller, J. L., Tonks, N. K., and Sturgill, T. W.: Requirement for integration of signals from two distinct phosphorylation pathways for activation of MAP kinase. Nature (London), 343:651, 1990.
4. Bischoff, J. R., Friedman, P. N., Marshak, D. R., Prives, C., and Beach, D.: Human p53 is phosphorylated by p60-cdc2 and cyclin B-cdc2. Proc. Natl. Acad. Sci. U.S.A., 87:4766, 1990.
5. Bishop, J. M.: The molecular genetics of cancer. Science, 235:305, 1987.
6. Broek, D., Samiy, N., Fasano, O., Fujiyama, A., Tamanoi, F., Northup, J., and Wigler, M.: Differential activation of yeast adenylate cyclase by wild-type and mutant ras proteins. Cell, 41:763, 1985.
7. Braun, S., Raymond, W. E., and Racker, E.: Synthetic tyrosine polymers as substrates and inhibitors of tyrosine-specific protein kinases. J. Biol. Chem., 259:2051, 1984.
8. Brugge, J. S., and Erikson, R. L.: Identification of a transformation-specific antigen induced by an avian sarcoma virus. Nature, 269:346, 1977.
9. Buchkovich, K., Duffy, L. A., and Harlow, E.: The retinoblastoma protein is phosphorylated during specific phases of the cell cycle. Cell, 58:1097, 1989.
10. Chen, P.-L., Scully, P., Shew, J.-Y., Wang, J. Y. J., and Lee, W.-H.: Phosphorylation of the retinoblastoma gene product is modulated during the cell cycle and cellular differentiation. Cell, 58:1193, 1989.
11. Cooper, J. A.: Oncogenes and anti-oncogenes. Current Opinion in Cell Biology, 2:285, 1990.
12. DeCaprio, J. A., Ludlow, J. W., Lynch, D., Furukawa, Y., Griffin, J., Piwnica-Worms, J., Huang, C-M., and Livingston, D. M.: Gene product of the retinoblastoma susceptibility gene has properties of a cell cycle regulatory element. Cell, 58:1085, 1989.
13. Druker, B. J., Mamon, H. J., and Roberts T. M.: Oncogenes, growth factors, and signal transduction. N. Engl. J. Med., 321:1383, 1989.
14. Ellis, R. J., and Hemmingsen, S. M.: Molecular chaperones: proteins essential for the biogenesis of some macromolecular structures. TIBS, 14:339, 1989.
15. Felix, M.-A., Cohen, P., and Karsenti, E.: Cdc2 H1 kinase is negatively regulated by a type 2A phosphatase in the Xenopus early embryonic cell cycle: Evidence from the effects of okadaic acid. EMBO J., 9:675, 1990.
16. Function and Evolution of Ras Proteins, Symposium, May 9–13, 1990, Cold Spring Harbor, N.Y.
17. Goloubinoff, P., Christeller, J. T., Gatenby, A. A., and Lorimer, G. H.: Reconstitution of active dimeric ribulose bisphosphate carboxylase from an unfolded state depends on two chaperonin proteins and Mg-ATP. Nature, 342:884, 1989.
18. Hanafusa, H.: Cell transformation by RNA tumor viruses. In Comprehensive Virology, Volume 10. Edited by H. Fraenkel-Conrat, and R. R. Wagner. New York, Plenum Press, 1977, pp. 401-483.
19. Hunter, T., and Sefton, B. M.: Transforming gene product of Rous sarcoma virus phosphorylates tyrosine. Proc. Natl. Acad. Sci. U.S.A., 77:1311, 1980.
20. Jaken, S.: Protein kinase C and tumor promoters. Current Opinion in Cell Biology, 2:192, 1990.
21. Kaplan, D. R., Morrison, D. K., Wong, G., McCormick, F., and Williams, L. T.: PDGF β-receptor stimulates tyrosine phosphorylation of GAP and association of GAP with a signaling complex. Cell, 61:125, 1990.
22. Kipreos, E. T., and Wang, J. Y. J.: Differential phosphorylation of c-abl in cell cycle determined by cdc2 kinase and phosphatase activity. Science, 248:217, 1990.
23. Kole, H. K., Abdel-Ghany, M., and Racker, E.: Specific dephosphorylation of phosphoproteins by protein-serine and -tyrosine kinases. Proc. Natl. Acad. Sci. U.S.A., 85:5849, 1988.
24. Lasky, R. A., Honda, B. M., Mills, A. D., and Finch, J. T.: Nucleosomes are assembled by an acidic protein which binds histones and transfers them to DNA. Nature, 275:416, 1978.
25. Laumas, S., Abdel-Ghany, M., Leister, K., Resnick, R., Kandrach, A., and Racker, E.: Decreased susceptibility of a 70-kDA protein to cathepsin L after phosphorylation by protein kinase C. Proc. Natl. Acad. Sci. U.S.A., 86:3021, 1989.
26. Levine, A. J., Finlay, C. A., and Hinds, P. W.: The p53 proto-oncogene and its product. In Common Mechanisms of Transformation by Small DNA Tumor Viruses. Edited by L. P. Villarreal. American Society for Microbiology, Washington, DC, 1989, pp. 21-37.
27. Levinson, A. D., Oppermann, H., Levintow, L., Varmus, H. E., and Bishop, J. M.: Evidence that the transforming gene of avian sarcoma virus encodes a protein kinase associated with a phosphoprotein. Cell, 15:561, 1978.
28. Lewin, B.: Driving the cell cycle: M phase kinase, its partners, and substrates. Cell, 61:743, 1990.
29. McCormick, F.: ras GTPase activating protein: Signal transmitter and signal terminator. Cell, 56:5, 1989.
30. Molloy, C. J., Bottaro, D. P., Fleming, T. P., Marshall, M. S., Gibbs, J. B., and Aaronson, S. A.: PDGF induction of tyrosine phosphorylation of GTPase activating protein. Nature, 342:711, 1989.
31. Murray, A. W.: The cell cycle as a cdc2 cycle. Nature, 342:14, 1989.
32. Nurse, P.: Universal control mechanism regulating onset of M-phase. Nature, 344:503, 1990.
33. Ostermann, J., Horwich, A. L., Neupert, W., and Hartl, F.-U.: Protein folding in mitochondria requires complex formation with sp60 and ATP hydrolysis. Nature, 341:125, 1989.
34. Pardee, A. B.: G₁ events and regulation of cell proliferation. Science, 246:603, 1989.
35. Park, M., and Vande Woude, G. F.: Oncogenes: Genes associated with neoplastic disease. In The Metabolic Basis of Inherited Disease. Edited by C. R. Scriver, A. L. Baudet, W. S. Sly and D. Valle. New York, McGraw-Hill Inc., 1989, p. 251.
36. Parries, G., Hoebel, R., and Racker, E.: Oppposing effects of a ras oncogene on growth factor-stimulated phosphoinositide hydrolysis: Desensitization to platelet-derived growth factor and enhanced sensitivity to bradykinin. Proc. Natl. Acad. Sci. U.S.A., 84:2648, 1987.
37. Racker, E.: The search for oncogene targets. J. Natl. Cancer Inst., 81:247, 1989.
38. Racker, E.: Effect of chaperones and matchmakers on protein phosphorylations in membranes. In Current Topics of Cellular Regulation. Edited by G. R. Welch. New York, Academic Press, In press, 1990.
39. Rous, P.: A sarcoma of the fowl transmissible by an agent separable from the tumor cells. J. Exp. Med., 13:397, 1911.
40. Roy, L. M., Singh, B., Gautier, J., Arlinghaus, R. B., Nordeen, S. K., and Maller, J. L.: The cyclin B2 component of MPF is a substrate for the c-mosx proto-oncogene product. Cell, 61:825, 1990.
41. Rubin, H.: The behavior of cells before and after virus-induced malignant transformation. In The Harvey Lectures (The Harvey Society of New York 1965, 1966). New York, Academic Press, Series 61, 1967, p. 117.
42. Shalloway, D., and Shenoy, S.: Oncoprotein kinases in mitosis. In Advances in Cancer Research, Volume 52. Edited by G. Klein, and G. F. VandeWoude. Orlando, Academic Press, 1990, In press.
43. Shenoy, S., Choi, J-K., Bagrodia, S., Copeland, T. D., Maller, J. L., and Shalloway, D.: Purified maturation promoting factor phosphorylates pp60$^{c\text{-src}}$ at the sites phosphorylated during fibroblast mitosis. Cell, 57:763, 1989.
44. Smith, M. R., DeGudicibus, S. J., and Stacey, D. W.: Requirement for c-ras proteins during viral oncogene transformation. Nature, 320:540, 1986.
45. Thastrup, O., Cullen, P. J., Drobak, B. K., Hanley, M. R., and Dawson, A. P.: Thapsigargin, a tumor promoter, discharges intracellular Ca²⁺ stores by specific inhibition of the endoplasmic reticulum Ca²⁺-ATPase. Proc. Natl. Acad. Sci. U.S.A., 87:2466, 1990.
46. Thomas, L.: Cancer research, yesterday and today. In Cancer Today: Origins, Prevention, and Treatment. Edited by L. Roberts. Washington, D.C., National Academy Press, 1984.
47. Vande Woude, G. F., Gonzatti-Haces, M., Iyer, A., Park, M., Testa, J. R., Oskarsson, M., Paules, R. S., Propst, F., and Sagata, N.: The mos and met oncogenes: Transformation and reverse genetics. In The Regulation of Proliferation and Differentiation in Normal and Neoplastic Cells. New York, Academic Press, 1989, pp. 143-164.
48. Van Etten, R. A., Jackson, P., and Baltimore, D.: The mouse type IV c-abl gene product is a nuclear protein, and activation of transforming ability is associated with cytoplasmic localization. Cell, 58:669, 1989.
49. Watanabe, N., Vande Woude, G. F., Ikawa, Y., and Sagata, N.: Specific proteolysis of the c-mos proto-oncogene product by calpain on fertilization of Xenopus eggs. Nature, 342:505, 1989.
50. Weinberg, R. A.: The retinoblastoma gene and cell growth control. Trends Biochem. Sci., 15:199, 1990.

Recurring Chromosome Rearrangements in Human Cancer

Olufunmilayo I. Olopade
Janet D. Rowley

Introduction

Over the past several years, it has become clear that acquired clonal chromosomal abnormalities are found in the malignant cells of many patients with leukemia, lymphoma and solid tumors. A few of the genes involved in consistent chromosome rearrangements, notably translocations, have already been identified, and it is likely that the identity of most of the genes affected by these aberrations will be determined within the next decade. Moreover, for several of the rearrangements, some of the changes in gene structure and function have been defined. Therefore, some general principles that may be applicable to all chromosome rearrangements in human malignant disease are beginning to emerge. In this review we shall present the most current data on primary chromosomal rearrangements in hematologic malignancies as well as in solid tumors.

Much of the detailed information regarding the relevant chromosome rearrangements is contained in a number of recent reviews, and only a general summary will be presented here.[66,106A,128,133,152,173] Mitelman has published four editions of his Catalog of Chromosome Aberrations in Cancer.[104–106] A comparison of the number of abnormal karyotypes in the catalogues according to the type of neoplasia is summarized in Figure I-8-1. Although carcinomas account for the greatest proportion of malignant disease, they represent only about 20% of the karyotypic data, whereas most information is available for leukemia and lymphoma. It has been clear from the beginning of the cytogenetic analysis

of human malignant disease, that virtually all solid tumors, including the non-Hodgkin's lymphomas, had an abnormal karyotype and that some of these abnormalities were limited to a given tumor.[66,104,128,152,173] With regard to the leukemias, it appeared from studies in the 1960's and early 1970's, that only about 50% had an abnormal karyotype.[128,133,152] With improved culture techniques and with the development of processing methods that resulted in longer chromosomes with a larger number of more clearly defined bands, Yunis and associates have provided evidence that a karyotypic abnormality can be detected in virtually all leukemias as well.[173] Some malignant diseases, such as Hodgkin's disease or multiple myeloma, continue to show a high frequency of normal karyotypes, probably because of their low mitotic index.

Different chromosome changes have been observed in neoplastic cells, and these often occur in combination. This leads to great difficulty in trying to identify precisely the unique abnormalities in a particular cancer. A number of international meetings over the last 25 years have led to the establishment of a universally accepted system for chromosome nomenclature. The most authoritative document, An International System for Human Cytogenetic Nomenclature (1985) will be used here.[72] The simplest change is either a gain or a loss of a whole chromosome. Common structural alterations are translocations, which involve the exchange of material between two or more chromosomes, and deletions, which involve loss of DNA from a chromosome and thus from the affected cell (Figure I-8-2). Chromosome inversions have

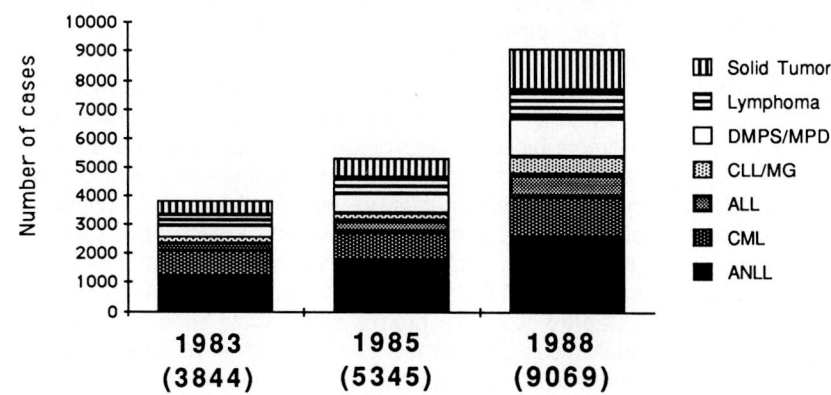

Number of Abnormal Karyotypes Mitelman's Catalog

Figure I-8-1. Graph showing the proportion of abnormal karotypes in the four Catalogs by disease type. The number in parenthesis below the date is the total number of abnormal karyotypes in each addition. CML patients with only a t(9;22) are not included.

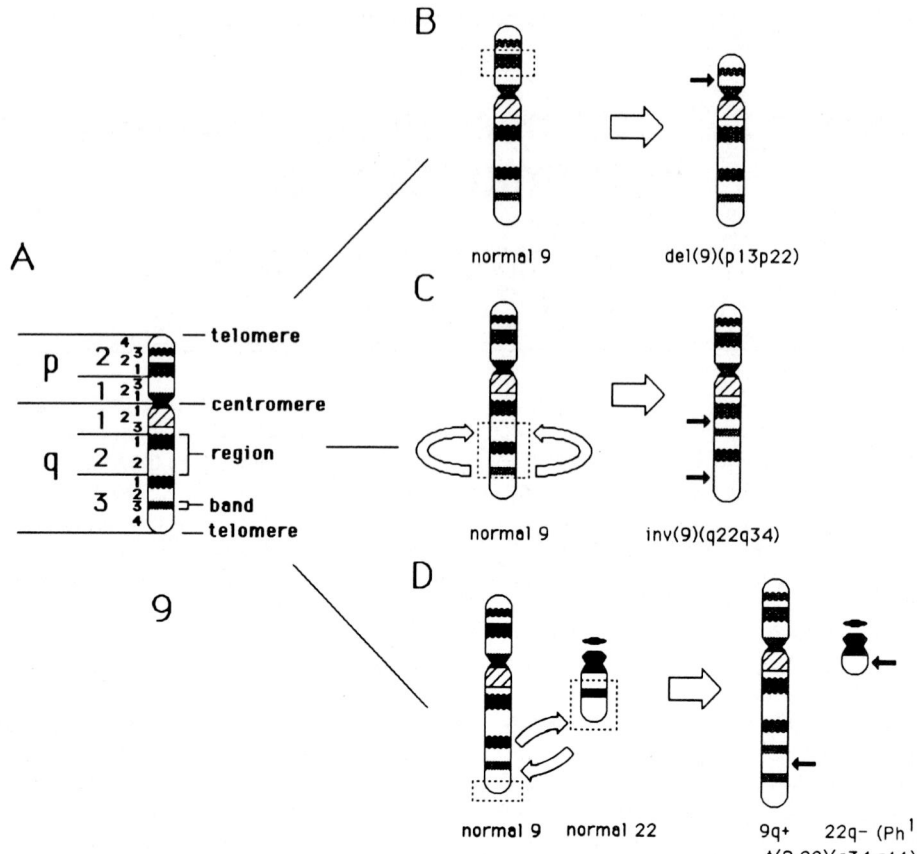

Figure I-8-2. Schematic diagram illustrating a normal chromosome and three chromosomal abnormalities observed in human neoplasms. *A*, Diagram of the banding pattern of a normal chromosome 9. The chromosome arms (p, short arm; q, long arm), regions, and band numbers are indicated on the left of the chromosome; specific chromosome structures are indicated on the right of the chromosome. *B*, Diagram of the mechanism of an interstitial deletion of the short arm of chromosome 9, a common abnormality in acute lymphoblastic leukemia. Chromosome breaks occur in bands 9p13 and 9p22, and the intervening chromosomal segment (band 9p21 and parts of bands 9p13 and 9p22) is lost [del(9)(p13p22)]. *C*, Diagram of the mechanism of a paracentric inversion. Chromosome breaks occur in two bands within a single chromosome arm, in this case, within 9p22 and 9q34; the intervening segment is inverted and the chromosome breaks are repaired [inv(9)(q22q34)]. *D*, Diagram of the mechanism of the reciprocal translocation involving chromosomes 9 and 22, t(9;22)(q34;q11), which gives rise to the Philadelphia (Ph[1]) chromosome in the malignant cells of patients with chronic myelogenous leukemia. Breaks occur in bands q34 and q11 of chromosomes 9 and 22, respectively, followed by a reciprocal exchange of chromosomal material. This rearrangement results in the translocation of the *ABL* oncogene, normally located at 9q34, adjacent to the *BCR* gene on chromosome 22, giving rise to a chimeric *BCR-ABL* gene, whose protein product plays a role in the transformation of myeloid cells. Source: Modified from Le Beau and Rowley: Cytogenetics. *In* Hematology. 4th Ed. Edited by W. J. Williams, E. Beutler, A. J. Ersler, and M. A. Lichtman. New York, McGraw Hill, 1990.

been observed; in this rearrangement, a single chromosome is broken in two places, and the central portion is inverted and rejoined to the ends of the chromosome. Each chromosome band is numbered.[72] The total chromosome number is followed by the sex chromosomes, and gains and losses of whole chromosomes are identified by a + or − before the chromosome number. A gain or loss of part of a chromosome is identified by a + or − after the chromosome arm involved; p and q represent the short and long arm, respectively. Translocations are indicated by t; the chromosomes involved are noted in the first set of brackets, and the breakpoints in the second set of brackets (see Table I-8-1). Other abnormalities will be defined when they are first described. The discussion will be restricted to clonal abnormalities which are defined as at least two cells with the same extra chromosome or structural rearrangement (identified with banding) or three cells with the same missing chromosome. Banding of chromosomes is essential to cytoge-

netic investigations because it allows identification of individual chromosomes. A band is defined as a chromosome area that is distinguished from adjacent segments by appearing darker or lighter by one or more banding techniques. Various banding methods are currently utilized which include quinacrine-mustard (Q bands), Giemsa stain (G bands), etc.

A new technique that will revolutionize chromosome analysis is the use of nonradiolabeled DNA probes (for example biotin labeled probes) that are detected by fluorescence microscopy. A large number of chromosome-specific centromere probes are now available which unequivocally mark a pair of chromosomes. Using these probes, gain or losses of chromosomes can be detected not only in metaphase cells but also in interphase cells (see I-8-Plate 2). Large size DNA probes that contain specific genes or anonymous DNA sequences, e.g., yeast artificial chromosomes or cosmids can be used to screen for recurring trans-

Table I-8-1A.   Glossary of Cytogenetic Terminology

Centromere	The constriction along the length of the chromosome that is the site of the spindle fiber attachment. The position of the centromere determines whether chromosomes are metacentric (X-shaped, e.g., chromosomes 1, 3, 16, 19, 20) or acrocentric (inverted V-shaped, e.g., chromosomes 13-15, 21, 22, Y). During mitosis the two exact copies of the DNA in each chromosome are separated by shortening of the spindle fibers attached to opposite sides of the dividing cell
Karyotype	Arrangement of chromosomes from a particular cell according to a well-established system such that the largest chromosomes are first and the smallest ones are last. See Figure I-8-3. Normal female karyotype is 46,XX; normal male karyotype is 46,XY
Translocation	A break in at least two chromosomes with exchange of material; in a reciprocal translocation, there is no obvious loss of chromosomal material. See Figure I-8-4
Deletion	A segment of a chromosome is missing as the result of two breaks and loss of the intervening piece. See Figure I-8-2
Inversion	Two breaks occur in the same chromosome with rotation of the intervening segment. If both the breaks are on the same side of the centromere, it is called a paracentric inversion. If they are on opposite sides it is called a pericentric inversion
Isochromosome	A chromosome that consists of identical copies of one chromosome arm with loss of the other arm. Thus an isochromosome for the long arm of No. 17 [i(17q)] contains two copies of the long arm (separated by the centromere) with loss of the short arm of the chromosome
Clone	In the cytogenetic sense, this is defined as two cells with the same additional or structurally rearranged chromosome or three cells with loss of the same chromosome
Diploid	Normal chromosome number and composition of chromosomes
Hyperdiploid	Additional chromosomes; therefore the modal number is 47 or greater
Hypodiploid	Loss of chromosomes with modal number 45 or less
Haploid	Only one-half the normal complement, i.e., 23 chromosomes

Table I-8-1B.   Karyotype Symbols

p	Short arm
q	Long arm
+	If before the chromosome, indicates a gain of a whole chromosome (e.g., +8) and if after the chromosome, indicates gain of part of the chromosome (e.g., 14q+, added material at the end of the long arm of No. 14)
−	If before the chromosome indicates a loss of a whole chromosome (e.g., −7) and if after the chromosome indicates loss of part of the chromosome (e.g., 5q−, loss of part of the long arm of No. 5)
?	Indicates uncertainty about the identity of the chromosome or band listed just after the ?
t	Translocation
del	Deletion
inv	Inversion
i	Isochromosome

a short period of time. The cells are exposed to a hypotonic solution, fixed, and stained according to a variety of protocols.[50] The use of amethopterin or fluorode-oxyuridine to synchronize cells combined with a brief exposure to mitotic inhibitors such as colchicine or the use of DNA-binding agents to elongate chromosomes have resulted in longer chromosomes that have an increased number of bands as well as improved morphology. The use of conditioned medium containing growth factors, the addition of PHA-stimulated conditioned medium or recombinant colony-stimulating factors to the culture medium have also contributed to the increased rate of successful cytogenetic analysis of different tumors. Cytogenetic analysis requires specimens that contain viable dividing cells, therefore specimens for analysis should be transported in suitable culture medium at room temperature to the cytogenetics laboratory without delay.

Myelo-Proliferative Disorders
Chronic Myeloid Leukemia

The first consistent chromosome abnormality in any malignant disease was the Philadelphia or Ph[1] chromosome identified in chronic myeloid leukemia (CML).[115] The abnormality was thought to be a deletion of chromosome No. 22 (22q−). The correct defect was later shown to be a translocation involving chromosome Nos. 9 and 22; [t(9;22)(q34;q11)] (Figure I-8-2).[135]

The Philadelphia chromosome occurs in a pluripotential stem cell that gives rise to cells of both lymphoid and myeloid lineage. The karyotypes of many Ph[1]+ patients with CML have been examined with banding techniques by a number of investigators. In a review of 1129 Ph[1]+ patients, the 9;22 translocation was identified in 1036 (92%).[133] The remaining patients had variant translocations; one appeared to be a simple translocation involving No. 22 and some chromosome other than No. 9 (about 4%), and the other was a complex translocation involving at least three or more different chromosomes, including chromosomes No. 9 and No. 22 (about 4%). Recent data clearly demonstrate that No. 9 is affected in the simple as well as the complex translocations, and that its involvement in the simple translocations initially had been overlooked.[39] Virtually all chromosomes have been involved in these variant translocations, but No. 17 is affected more often than any other chromosome. Other studies with fluor-

locations and to identify those that are split by the translocation breakpoints. This technique is currently being used by several groups in their search for genes involved in different translocations.[127]

To be relevant to the malignant disease, chromosomes for analysis must be obtained from the tumor cells. Thus for leukemia, bone marrow cells or peripheral blood cells processed directly or after 24–72 hr culture are used;[145] lymph nodes or solid tumors are minced to yield a single cell suspension that can be harvested immediately or cultured for escent markers or chromosome polymorphisms have shown that, in a particular patient, the same No. 9 and No. 22 are involved in each cell.[135]

The reciprocal nature of the translocation was established only recently, when the Abelson protooncogene, ABL, normally on No. 9, was identified on the Ph[1] chromosome. The ABL gene is the homolog of a viral oncogene isolated from a mouse pre B cell leukemia. The initial localization of ABL to chromosome 9 prompted de Klein and colleagues to investigate the involvement of this gene in the t(9;22), and they found that ABL is translocated to the Philadelphia chromosome.[40] This finding led Heisterkamp et al to screen samples from patients with CML, until one was identified which had an apparent DNA rearrangement in the vicinity of the v-abl homologous sequences. This led to cloning of the breakpoint involved in the t(9;22).[67] The site on the Ph[1] was called bcr, for breakpoint cluster region which in the majority of breaks, cluster in a small 5.8 kilobase (kb) region. In contrast the breaks on No. 9 occur over an incredible distance of more than 200 kb. The genetic consequences of the standard t(9;22) or the complex translocation involving at least 3 chromosomes is to move the ABL protooncogene on No. 9 next to a gene on No. 22, called BCR, whose function has recently been elucidated (Figure I-8-3).

The appearance of new abnormalities in the karyotype of a patient with CML often signals a change in the pace of the disease, usually to a more aggressive disorder. When patients with CML enter the terminal acute phase, about 10–20% appear to retain the 46, Ph[1] + cell line unchanged. However most patients show additional chromosome abnormalities which result in cells with modal chromosome numbers of

47–50.[133] During the acute phase of CML, different chromosomal abnormalities occur singly or in combination in a distinctly non-random pattern. In patients who have only a single new chromosome change, this most commonly involves a second Ph[1], an isochromosome for the long arm of chromosome No. 17 [i(17q)], or a +8, in descending order of frequency. Chromosome loss is rare but when it does occur a −7 is seen, which occurs in 3% of patients.[133]

Chronic myelogenous leukemia is a clonal stem cell disorder; the Ph[1] chromosome is present in granulocytic, erythroid, and megakaryocytic cells, in some B cells, and probably in a few T cells. In blast crisis, some blasts have intracytoplasmic IgM, which is characteristic of pre-B cells, and these cells have an immunoglobulin gene rearrangement.[7]

Marrow cells from some patients who appear to have CML on clinical and morphologic grounds lack a Ph[1] chromosome. The majority of these patients had a normal karyotype. Somewhat surprisingly, the survival of these patients was substantially shorter than those whose cells were Ph[1] +.[166] In two reviews of patients who were diagnosed as having Ph[1] negative CML, most of the patients were shown not to have CML, but rather have some type of myelodysplasia, most commonly chronic myelomonocytic leukemia or refractory anemia with excess blasts, leading to their shorter survival.[123,149] However, the situation has become more complex because it has recently been shown by molecular analysis that some patients with clinically typical CML who lack a Ph[1] chromosome cytogenetically,[9,110] have evidence of the insertion of ABL sequences into the BCR gene. Thus it can be proposed that the sine qua non of CML is the juxtaposition

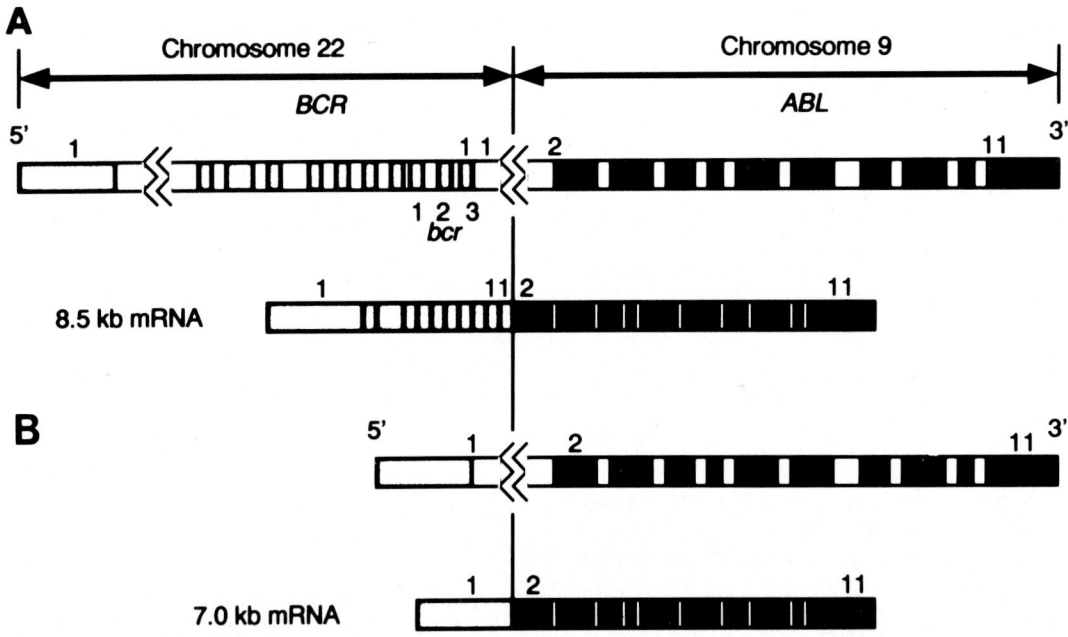

Figure I-8-3.   A, Map of the BCR-ABL fusion gene in CML and in some adult ALL patients. In this example, the breakpoint has occurred between the third and fourth exons included in the bcr region, which are equivalent to exons 11 and 121 in the BCR gene. The chimeric mRNA is diagrammed below the gene. B, Map of the fusion gene in some ALL patients showing the breakpoint in the first intron of BCR. The breakpoint in ABL is identical with that in CML in this example. Only one BCR exon is included so that the mRNA is much smaller than in CML.

of *BCR* and *ABL.* Several investigators are now trying to unravel the genetic consequences of the Ph[1] chromosome.

Acute Myeloid Leukemia De Novo

With initial banding analyses clonal chromosome abnormalities were detected in about 50% of patients with AML. This percentage has increased with improved banding and culture techniques; many laboratories are currently finding that at least 80% of patients have an abnormal karyotype. The most frequent abnormalities are a gain of No. 8 or a loss of No. 7 which are seen in most subtypes of AML.[51,133,152,173] Specific rearrangements are closely associated with particular subtypes of AML as defined by the French-American-British Cooperative Group (FAB classification) (Figure I-8-4)[10](I-8-Plate 1). The chromosome abnormalities associated and their frequency with each subtype are summarized in Table I-8-2.

A translocation between chromosomes 8 and 21 [t(8;21)(q22;q22)] was first identified in 1973 (Figure I-8-4).[130] The frequency with which this translocation is detected varies from one laboratory to another; it accounted for 10% (25/249) of the abnormal cases reviewed by Rowley and Testa,[133] and 12% of the patients with an abnormal karyotype reviewed at the Fourth IWCL.[51] However at the Sixth IWCL, only 44/656 or 7% of the patients had this abnormality.[56] The t(8;21) is the most frequent abnormality in children with AML, being reported in 17% (10 of 60) of karyotypically abnormal cases.[133] The 8;21 translocation is of interest for three other

reasons. First, chromosomes 8 and 21 can participate in three-way rearrangements similar to those involving chromosomes 9 and 22 in CML. Second, the t(8;21) is often accompanied by the loss of a sex chromosome; among the cases reviewed at the Fourth IWCL, 28 of 33 (85%) males were −Y and 8 of 12 (67%) females were −X.[51] This association is particularly noteworthy because sex chromosome abnormalities are otherwise rarely observed in AML. It has recently been shown that the gene for the receptor for *CSF2* (formerly *GMCSF*) is located in the pseudoautosomal region of the short arm of the X chromosome.[60] It is possible that loss of this receptor is an important factor leading to loss of X or Y chromosome in this subtype of leukemia. Third, this translocation has never been reported as a constitutional abnormality or observed in other malignant diseases (Rowley, unpublished observation). The molecular consequences of this translocation have been intensely investigated, and the translocation breakpoint has recently been cloned. A novel gene *AML* 1 was found to be rearranged in leukemic cells of patients with t(8;21).[109A]

A structural rearrangement involving chromosomes 15 and 17 in acute promyelocytic leukemia (APL) was first recognized in 1977 [t(15;17) (q22;q11–12)] (Figure I-8-4).[132] This rearrangement is unique to APL or the hypogranular variant. In our recent review, all 60 APL patients had a t(15;17).[133] The gene at the breakpoint on chromosome 17 has recently been identified as the alpha chain of the retinoic acid receptor *(RARA).*[24,43,95] Rearrangements of this gene

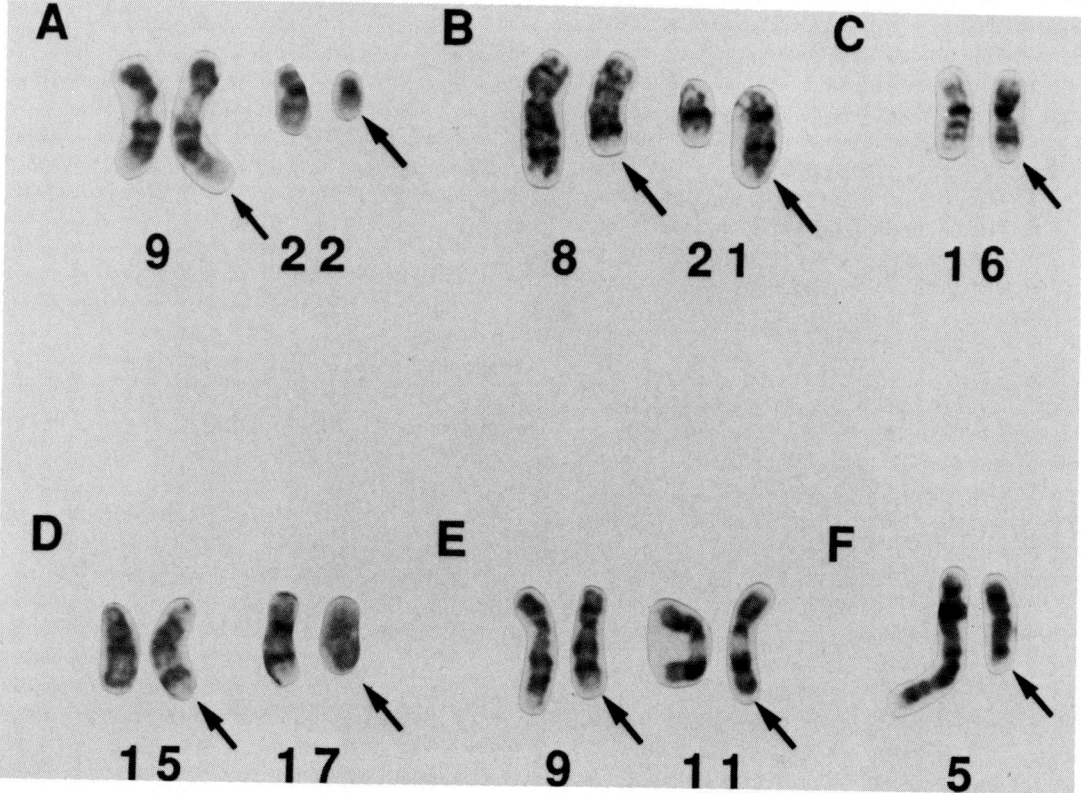

Figure I-8-4. Partial karyotypes from trypsin-Giemsa-banded metaphase cells depicting nonrandom chromosomal rearrangements observed in myeloid malignant diseases. *A,* t(9;22)(q34;q11), CML. *B,* t(8;21)(q22;q22), AML-M2. *C,* inv(16)(p13q22), AMMoL-M4Eo. *D,* t(15;17)(q22;q11–12), APL. *E,* t(9;11)(p22;q23). *F,* del(5)(q13q33) in t-ANLL. The rearranged chromosomes are identified with arrowheads.

on Southern blot analysis have been identified in the great majority of APL patients whose cells have been analyzed. The breakpoint in ten APL cases examined by Borrow and colleagues were shown to cluster in a 12-Kb region of chromosome 17, containing two Cp G-rich islands. The region is the first intron of the RARA gene.[24] Preliminary evidence suggests that the translocation results in a fusion mRNA which gives aberrant RARA transcripts in 100% of APL patients.[43]

A translocation involving chromosomes 6 and 9 [t(6;9) (p23;q34)] was first described in two patients in 1976, but no common features were detected. As a group, patients who have a t(6;9) have responded poorly to intensive therapy.[134] Slides from 9 patients with this translocation were recently reviewed and 8 of these 9 patients had an increase in basophils in the bone marrow ranging from 1.5–12% (the normal value is 0.2%); similar increases were noted in only 3% of other de novo AML patients.[120] Because the marrow in all biopsy specimens was hypercellular, this represents a marked increase in the total basophil count. The basophils appeared to be morphologically normal. This translocation has also been cloned recently.[161] The breakpoint on chromosome 9 is about 330 kb telomeric to ABL and has been called Cain (CAN). The gene on chromosome 6 has also been cloned.[161] As in CML, the translocation results in a fusion gene with an abnormally large mRNA.

The close association of translocations, or less often deletions, of the long arm of No. 11 (11q) and acute monoblastic leukemia (M5) was first observed by Berger and colleagues.[11] Abnormalities of 11q occurred most frequently in children with monoblastic leukemia (type a) (6 of 8); and less often in adults with monoblastic leukemia (5 of 16). Many of these children were less than 1 year of age. Aberrations of 11q differ from the t(8;22) and t(15;17) in two ways. First, the break point in 11q involves band 11q23–24, in about two-thirds of patients, but it can also occur in 11q13–14. Second, although translocations are more common, a terminal deletion of 11q occurs in about one-third of cases. Although the other chromosome involved in the translocation is variable, a t(9;11)(p22;q23) is most common.[63] Molecular analysis using a yeast artificial chromosome containing CD3 delta shows that the breakpoint in 11q23 is within 200 kb upstream of this gene.[127]

Another clinical-cytogenetic association that has been identified involves myelomonocytic leukemia with eosinophils that have unique morphologic changes (M4EO). Arthur and Bloomfield first reported on 5 patients with del(16)(q22) and an excess of eosinophils (8–54%).[4] Our group reported on 18 patients and then on a larger series of 33 patients.[84] Most of these patients had M4 leukemia with eosinophils that showed unique morphologic changes, including large and irregular basophilic granules; one-third lacked increased eosinophils because the marrow had fewer than 5% eosinophils. Twenty-seven patients had an inversion of No. 16, inv(16)(p13q22), and 6 had a t(16;16)(p13;q22). The strong correlation between abnormal eosinophils and structural rearrangements of No. 16 was confirmed at the Fourth IWCL.[51] In fact, the morphologic features of the eosinophils are so specific that our pathologists can accurately predict which patients will have either an inv(16) or a t(16;16) by examining the bone marrow aspirate. It appears that this relatively common (25% of our AMMoL patients have this aberration) but subtle chromosome aberration was undetected in the past, in part, because of poor morphology. This chromosome abnormality has clinical implications as well. Among 32 treated patients, 78% achieved a complete remission, compared with 36% of 58 other AMMoL patients. The median survival time was more than 65 weeks for patients with abnormal 16's compared with 29 weeks for those with a normal 16.[84]

A unique feature of abnormalities involving the long arm of chromosome 3 [inv(3)(q21;q26)] or t(3;3)(q21;q26) is the high frequency of platelet counts above 100×10^9/liter (100,000), sometimes over $1,000 \times 10^9$/liter. A consistent marrow finding is an increase in the number of megakaryocytes, essentially micromegakaryocytes.[18]

Gains and losses of part of or whole chromosomes occur frequently in AML, both as solitary changes usually found at diagnosis or as additional observations in later disease stages. Most of these structural rearrangements occur in younger patients with a median age in the thirties, whereas some of the numerical abnormalities such as −5 or loss of the long arm [del(5q)] or −7 or del(7q) occur in patients with a median age of over 50. Many of the latter patients have a history of working in environments that might have exposed them to mutagenic agents such as chemicals that include solvents, petroleum products or pesticides.[107] Secondary chromosome changes such as del(20q), del(9q) and i(17q) occur in AML and are also associated with other diseases; these changes are sometimes found as the sole aberrations in occasional AML patients.[66] Most patients with del 9q as a secondary abnormality had a t(8;21) initially. At the Fourth IWCL it was clearly shown that the type rather than the presence of a chromosome abnormality had prognostic importance. Thus although the projected median survival for all patients was 8 months, those with a t(8;21) had the longest median survival (13 months) while those with abnormalities of chromosomes 5 and 7, t(15;17) or hyperdiploidy, had the shortest survivals (3–4 mo.).[51]

Other Myeloproliferative Diseases

In P. Vera, an abnormal clone is present in 14% of untreated patients. This number increases to 39% of treated patients.[133] The malignant marrow cells frequently contain additional chromosomes, +8, or +9; the two abnormalities may also occur together. Del(20) and duplication of the long arm of chromosome 1 are also seen in 20% and 30% of patients, respectively. The presence of chromosomal abnormalities at diagnosis is not predictive of clinical outcome but a change in karyotype as with CML is an ominous sign.[145] In the terminal leukemic phase of P. Vera, −7 (20%) and del (5q) (40%) have been observed. It is not clear whether this abnormality is related to the therapy that these patients may have received. The presence of a (21q) marker was previously reported as a characteristic anomaly in essential thrombocythemia. However, in the largest series of 170 patients reviewed at the Third IWCL, 141 (95%) had a normal karyotype, and no consistent chromosome abnormality are associated with this disease.[148] About one-third of patients with agnogenic myeloid metaplasia have clonal abnormalities, commonly −7, +8, del(11q) or del(20q).[66,89]

Acute Myeloid Leukemia and Myelodysplastic Syndrome Associated with Prior Cytotoxic Therapy (t-AML/t-MDS)

A distinctive disorder of bone marrow morphology and function that terminates in myelodysplastic syndrome (MDS) or in AML has been recognized as a late complication of cytotoxic therapy used in the treatment of both malignant and non-malignant diseases.[86] Characteristic non-random chromosome abnormalities are commonly observed in bone marrow cells of patients with t-MDS/t-AML. These abnormalities differ in their type and frequency from those noted in de novo AML (Table I-8-2). We reported previously that part or all of chromosome Nos. 5 and/or 7 was lost in cells from 23 of 26 (88%) t-MDS/t-AML patients.[131] More recently 61 of 63 patients had an abnormal karyotype and 55 of these had an abnormality of one or both chromosomes 5 and 7.[86] These observations have been confirmed by others.[3,121] In contrast, only about 16% of patients with de novo AML have a similar abnormality of chromosome No. 5 or No. 7 or both.[85] Moreover, the latter patients frequently have had significant occupational exposure to potential environmental carcinogens, such as chemicals, solvents, or pesticides.[59,107] Of 17 patients with a del(5q), bands 5q23 and 5q31 were consistently missing in every patient. A number of genes encoding growth factors or growth factor receptors have been mapped to the region 5q23-32 that is consistently deleted in these patients. These include the granulocyte-macrophage colony-stimulating factor (CSF2), Interleukin-3,-4,-5 (IL-3,-4,-5), CD14, early growth response-1 (EGR-1), B₁-adrenergic receptor (B2AR), platelet-derived growth factor receptor (PDGFR), glucocorticoid receptor (GRL), and endothelial cell growth factor (ECGF) genes.[91] Whether any of them play a role in mutagen-associated leukemia is unknown.

Primary Myelodysplastic Syndrome

Clonal chromosome abnormalities have now been reported in more than 700 MDS patients; 40–79% of whom have clonal abnormalities at diagnosis.[66] The common chromosomal abnormalities, +8, −5/del(5q), 7/del(7q) and del (20q) are similar to those seen in AML de novo. However in a review of 247 patients at the Sixth IWCL, none had t(8;21), t(15;17), t(9;22), t(9;11); or inv (16).[56] This suggests that patients with the specific types of AML associated with these abnormalities only rarely exhibit a preleukemic phase of their disease. In general, unlike AML, chromosome changes show no close association with the specific subtypes of myelodysplastic syndrome but patients with complex karyotypes and abnormalities of chromosome 5 and/or 7 have a poor prognosis. The exception is the "5q-" syndrome in which there is an interstitial deletion of the long arm of 5. The syndrome occurs in a subset of older patients, frequently women, with refrac-

Table I-8-2. Non-random Chromosome Abnormalities in Malignant Myeloid Diseases

Disease*	Chromosome Abnormality	Percent of Patients
CML	t(9;22)(q34;q11)	~100%
CML blast phase	t(9;22)(q34;q11) with +8, +Ph¹, +19, or i(17q)	~70%
AML-M2	t(8;21)(q22;q22)	~20%
APL-M3, M3V	t(15;17)(q22;q11-12)	60-100%
AMMoL-M4Eo	inv(16)(p13q22) or t(16;16)(p13;q22)	100% (25% of M4)
AMMoL-M4 or M5	t(1;11)(q21;q23)	
	t(2;11)(p21;q23)	
	t(6;11)(q27;q23)	
	t(10;11)(p11-p15;q23)	−35%
	ins(10;11)(p11;q23q24)	
	t(11;17)(q23;q25)	
	t(11;19)(q23;p13)	
	t(11q13 or q23), del(11)(q23)	
AMoL-M5,	t(9;11)(p22;q23), t(11q13 or q23)	~30%
AML	+8	13%
	−7 or del(7q)	9%
	−5 or del(5q)	6%
	t(6;9)(p23;q34)	2%
	t(3;3)(q21;q26) or inv(3)(q21q26)	2%
	del(20q)	5%
	t(12p) or del(12p)	2%
	t(3;21)(q26;q22)	1%
Therapy-related AML	−7 or del(7q) and/or −5 or del(5q)	90%
	der(1)t(1;7)(p11;p11)	2%
	der(5)t(5;7)(q11;p11)	<1%
	t(9;11)(p22;q23)	<1%

*CML, chronic myelogenous leukemia; AML, acute myeloblastic leukemia; AML-M2, AML with maturation; AMMoL, acute myelomonocytic leukemia; AMMoL-M4Eo, acute myelomonocytic leukemia with abnormal eosinophils; AMoL, acute monoblastic leukemia; APL-M3, M3V, hypergranular (M3) and microgranular (M3V) acute promyelocytic leukemia

tory macrocytic anemia, generally low blast counts and normal or elevated platelet counts.[89,159]

Malignant Lymphoproliferative Diseases

The chromosome abnormalities in lymphoid disorders especially in the non-Hodgkin's lymphomas have been reviewed in considerable detail.[20,49,79,128,174] A high proportion of cases of lymphoma (79%) are characterized by recurring clonal chromosomal abnormalities; many of these abnormalities correlate with histologic and immunophenotypic subtypes (Table I-8-3). Chromosome band 14q32, is frequently involved in B-cell lymphoma, while T-cell lymphomas are characterized by rearrangements that involve 14q11, 7q35–36, or 7p15, the bands containing the genes for the T-cell receptor alpha/delta, beta, or gamma chain, respectively. This section will review the consistent translocations seen in Burkitt's lymphoma, follicular lymphoma, CLL, B-cell ALL, and in some T-cell disorders.

Lymphoma

In 1972, Manolov and Manolova discovered that the malignant cells of patients with Burkitt's lymphoma had an additional band at the end of the long arm of one chromosome No. 14 (14q+).[98] Zech and coworkers in 1976 first observed that the end of one chromosome No. 8 was consistently absent, and they suggested that the missing part of No. 8 was translocated to No. 14 [t(8;14)(q24;q32)].[177] The t(8;14) has also been observed in non-endemic Burkitt's tumors from America, Europe, and Japan. Thus, it is a highly characteristic chromosome anomaly in Burkitt's lymphoma. This translocation has also been observed in other lymphomas, particularly those of the diffuse large cell type. Two other, related translocations were later identified in Burkitt's tumors. All three translocations involve chromosome No. 8 with a break in the same band, 8q24. One variant translocation involved chromosome No. 2 with a break in the short arm [t(2;8)(p12;q24)], and the other involved No. 22 with a break in the long arm in band (22q11). All three translocations have also been identified in patients with B-cell ALL.

Other recurring abnormalities in B-cell lymphoma include the t(14;18)(q32;q21) and the t(11;14)(q13;q32). The t(14;18)(q32;q21), is, in fact, the most common translocation in lymphoma (Figure I-8-5). This was first identified by Fukuhara and coworkers in 6 of 9 patients with poorly differentiated lymphocytic lymphoma,[54] now called "malignant lymphoma, follicular, predominantly small cleaved cell" (FSC) in the International Classification System.[170] The correlation between karyotype and histology in 260 patients reviewed at the Fifth International Workshop on Chromosomes in Leukemia and Lymphoma is summarized in Figure I-8-6.[49] Among the 260 Workshop patients, 15% had a normal karyotype. The karyotypic pattern varies greatly among the different subgroups. The t(14;18) is common in follicular low grade lymphomas, whereas the t(8;14) is common in high grade small noncleaved cell lymphomas. Occasionally, the t(14;18) is seen in lymphomas with a more aggressive, high grade histology. Recent data suggest that patients with diffuse large

cell lymphoma who have a t(14;18) are likely to be older and to have a poorer prognosis than those who lack this translocation. Of 102 patients with large cell lymphoma, 19 had a t(14;18) and a rearrangement of BCL2 located on chromosome 18; their median disease-free survival was 33 months while the rate was not yet reached for the other patients without this rearrangement.[116] Recently Thangavelu and colleagues also reported on 6 patients whose malignant cells had t(14;18) in addition to either a t(8;14) or t(8;22) or t(2;8); all the patients had very poor prognosis (Figure I-8-7).[147] Analysis of the karyotypic pattern in low grade lymphomas also shows that certain additional chromosome changes, especially a gain of No. 7 or a deletion of the long arm of No. 6 [(del)6q] appear to correlate with a more aggressive phenotype.[79,174]

Another recurrent abnormality that has recently been described is the t(2;5)(p23;q35) in Ki-1 positive anaplastic large cell lymphoma.[17,88] Patients with this abnormality have unique clinico-morphologic characteristics and a more favorable prognosis when compared to other patients with large cell lymphoma.

The B-cell lymphoma/leukemia 1 gene (BCL1) has been identified as the gene in the breakpoint on chromosome 11 in the translocation t(11;14) while the BCL2 is the gene on chromosome 18 in the t(14;18).[16,33,153] Since the t(14;18) is the most common translocation in lymphomas, availability of DNA probes for the BCL2 gene has provided the basis for the molecular analysis of lymphomas in adults.[128] Molecular analysis of these translocations has resulted in the identification of genes involved in the translocations. The MYC protooncogene is located on chromosome 8 band q24 while the immunoglobulin genes (heavy chain, k and lambda light chains) are located on chromosome 14 (band q32), 2 (band p12), and 22 (band q11), respectively. Thus in Burkitt's lymphoma MYC sequences are juxtaposed to immunoglobulin gene sequences. The consequence of these translocations is deregulation of the MYC gene, and uncontrolled proliferation of the cells.[16,153]

Chronic Lymphocytic Leukemia

The early studies of the cytogenetic pattern in CLL showed a normal karyotype in most samples. As better culture and banding methods have been applied to these studies, nonrandom clonal abnormalities have been detected. These include translocations involving 14q32 such as the t(14;19)(q32;q13) and trisomy for chromosome 12.[15,55,64,104,126] The gene involved in the translocation t(14;19) has been cloned and identified as the BCL3 gene.[117] This protooncogene is related to genes implicated in cell lineage determination and cell cycle control. In two reports, translocations of 14q were observed in 17 of 87 patients or in 5 of 16 patients with abnormal karyotypes.[15,126] Trisomy 12 was even more common and was seen in 33 and 7 patients in the same two reports, respectively. These two abnormalities may occur together in the same leukemic cell. There are somewhat conflicting reports about the prognostic significance of these abnormalities.[15,64,126] However, the largest series of patients with CLL was recently published.[74] Clonal chromosomal changes were observed in 218 of 321 patients who could be examined cytogenetically. The most common abnormal-

Table I-8-3. Cytogenetic-Immunophenotypic-Genomic Correlations in Malignant Lymphoid Diseases

Phenotype	Rearrangement	Involved Genes	
Acute lymphoblastic leukemia			
Pre-B	t(1;19)(q23;p13)	PBX1	E2A
B(SIg+)	t(8;14)(q24;q32)	MYC	IGH
	t(2;8)(p11-12;q24)	IGK	MYC
	t(8;22)(q24;q11)	MYC	IGL
	t(5;14)(q31;q32)	IL3	IGH
	dic(9;12)(p11;p12)		
B or B-myeloid	t(9;22)(q34;q11)	ABL	BCR
	t(4;11)(q21;q23)		MLL1
Other hyperdiploidy (50–60 chromosomes)			
	del(9p),t(9p)	IFNA/B	BCL3*
	del(12p),t(12p)		
	t(8;17)(q24;q22)	MYC	
T	t(11;14)(p15;q11)	RBTN1	TCRD
	t(11;14)(p13;q11)	RBTN2	TCRD
	t(8;14)(q24;q11)	MYC	TCRA
	inv(14)(q11q32.3)	IGH	TCRA
	inv(14)(q11q32.1)/t(14;14)(q11;q32)	TCL1	TCRA
	t(10;14)(q24;q11)	HOX11	TCRD
	t(1;14)(p32;q11)	TCL5	TCRD
	t(7;9)(q35;q32)	TCRB	SUP-T3^
	t(7;9)(q35;q34)	TCRB	TCL3*
	t(7;7)(p15;q11)	TCRG	
	t(7;14)(p15;q11)	TCRG	
	t(7;14)(q35;q11)		
	t(7;19)(q35;p13)	TCRB	LYL1
	t(1;7)(p34;q34)	LCK	TCRD
Non-Hodgkin's lymphoma			
B	t(8;14)(q24;q32)	MYC	IGH
	t(2;8)(p11-12;q24)	IGK	MYC
	t(8;22)(q24;q11)	MYC	IGL
	t(14;18)(q32;q21)	IGH	BCL2
	t(11;14)(q13;q32)	BCL1#	IGH
	t(14;15)(q32;q15)	IGH	LTK
T	see T-cell ALL		
Chronic lymphocytic leukemia			
B	t(11;14)(q13;q32)	BCL1#	IGH
	t(14;19)(q32;q13)	IGH	BCL3
	t(2;14)(p13;q32)	IGH	
	t(18;22)(q21;q11)	BCL2	IGL
	t(14q32)		
	+12		
T	t(8;14)(q24;q11)	MYC	TCRA
	inv(14)(q11q32)	TCRA	TCL1
Multiple myeloma			
B	t(11;14)(q13;q32)	BCL1	IGH
	t(14q32)	IGH	
Adult T-cell leukemia			
	t(14;14)(q11;q32)		
	inv(14)(q11q32)		
	+3		

*Same name used for different translocation breakpoints
#No expressed gene identified at present
^Breakpoint not named; source of translocation for cloning listed

ities were trisomy 12 (67 patients), structural abnormalities of chromosome 13q14 (57 patients) and of chromosome 14 (41 patients). This study showed that patients with normal karyotypes had a median overall survival of more than 15 years in contrast to 7.7 years for patients with clonal changes. Patients with aberrations involving chromosome 14q also had a poorer prognosis.[74]

Acute Lymphocytic Leukemia

Whereas the correlation of cytogenetic changes with morphology in AML led to the identification of the specific associations described in a previous section, this correlation was not useful in ALL, except for the t(8;14) and its variants in L3, B-cell ALL. However with the widespread use of precise

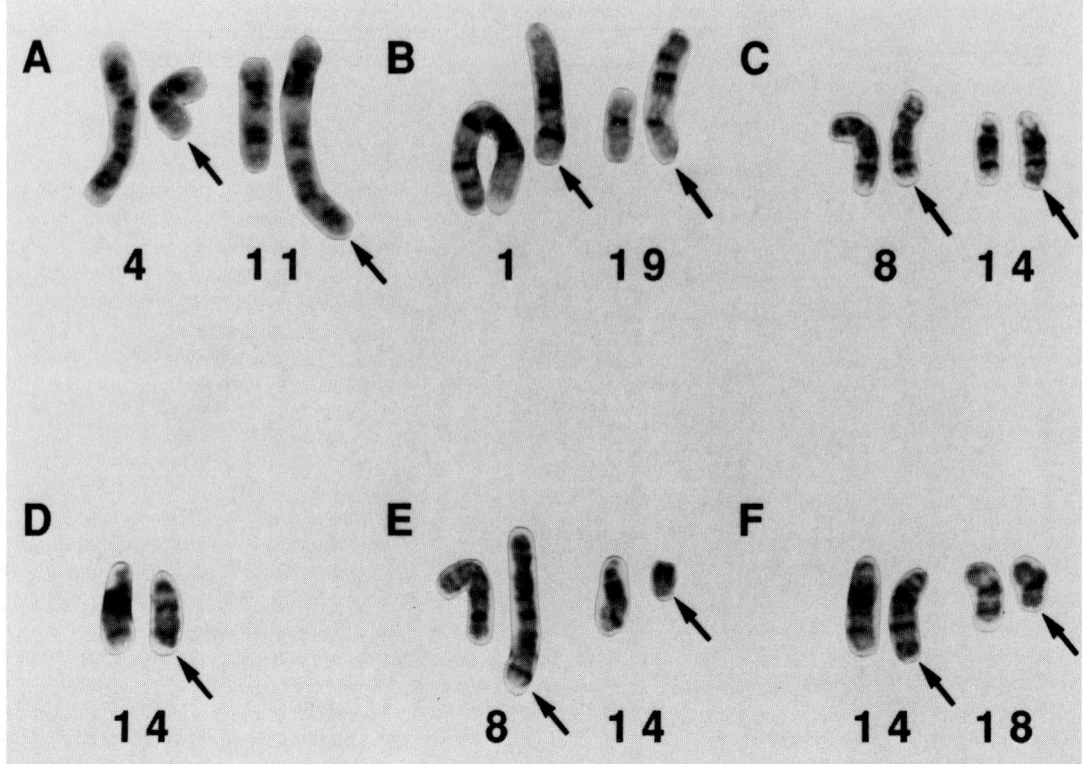

Figure I-8-5. Partial karyotypes of trypsin-Giemsa-banded metaphase cells depicting nonrandom chromosomal rearrangements observed in lymphoid malignant diseases. *A*, t(4;11)(q21;q23) in ALL; *B*, t(1;19)(q21;p13) in pre-B cell ALL; *C*, t(8;14)(q24;q32) in B cell ALL and Burkitt's lymphoma; *D*, inv(14)(9q11q32) in T cell leukemia/lymphoma; *E*, t(8;14)(q24;q11) in T cell leukemia/lymphoma; *F*, t(14;18)(q32;q21) in B cell NHL. The rearranged chromosomes are identified with arrowheads. (Modified from Le Beau and Rowley.[87])

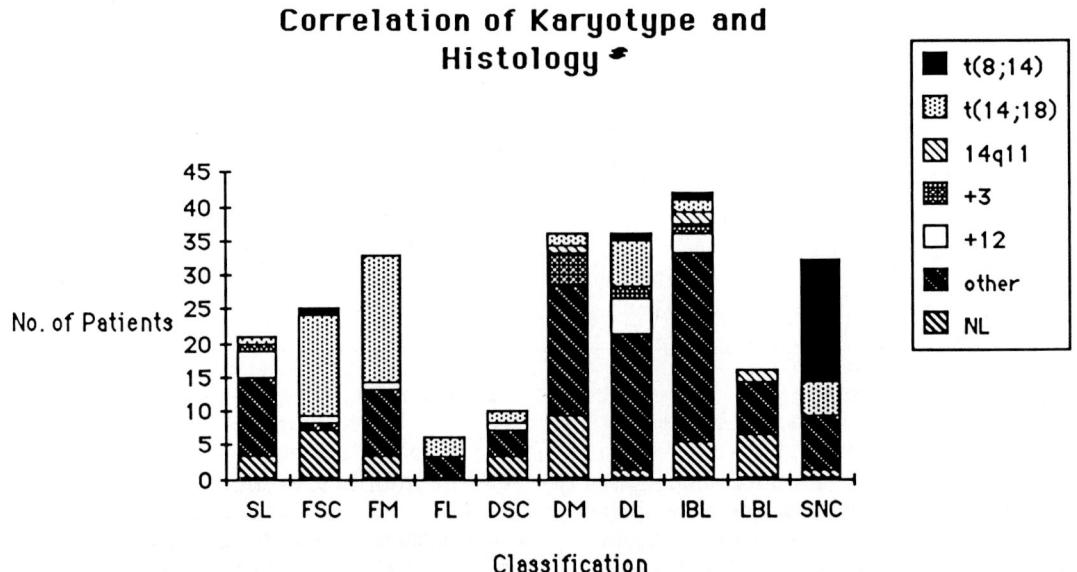

Figure I-8-6. Histogram showing the most common chromosome changes that were identified in 260 lymphomas studied prior to treatment and reviewed at the Fifth International Workshop on Chromosomes in Leukemia/Lymphoma; each tumor was classified according to the working formulation. (Modified from Rowley.[128A])

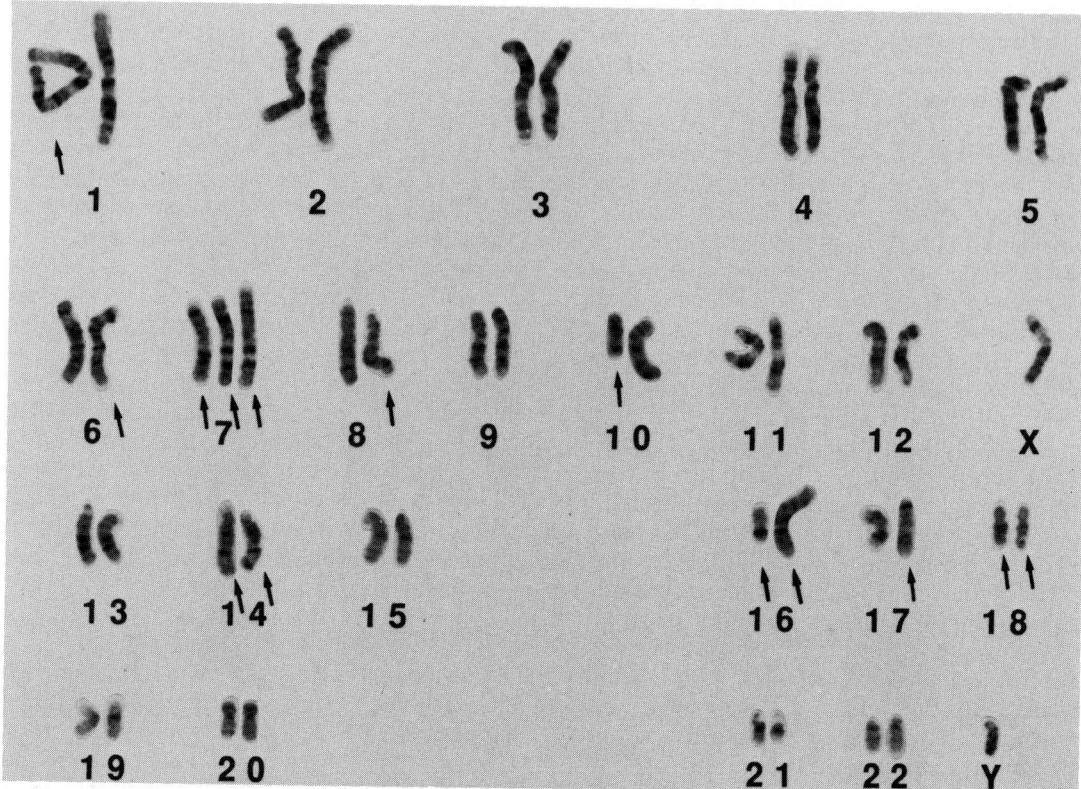

Figure I-8-7. Karyotype of a trypsin-Giemsa banded metaphase cell obtained from a bone marrow aspirate of a patient with malignant lymphoma. Chromosomal abnormalities are identified with arrows. Karotype: 47,XY,-18,t(1;?)(p36;?), dirdup(1)(q21q26),del(10)(q21q26),t(16;?)(p12;?),t(17;?)(p11;?),t(6;7)(p12;p15),t(7;16)(p22;p12),t(8;14)(q24;q32),t(14:18)(q32;q21),+der(7)(7;13)(q11;q14), +der(18)t(14;18)(q32;21). In pair 14, the first 14 is involved in the 8;14 translocation and the second in the 14;18 translocation.

immunophenotyping, the correlation of certain chromosome rearrangements with specific immunologic subsets of ALL has been established (Table I-8-3).

ALL is the most frequent leukemia in children. Patients who are between 3 and 7 years of age, with a WBC count of less than 10,000/mm³, and whose leukemic cells express the common acute lymphoblastic leukemic antigen (CALLA+ or CD10+), have the best prognosis. For many years metaphase chromosomes from ALL patients had poor morphology with indistinct bands making an accurate analysis difficult. Thus, there have been fewer reports of chromosome patterns in ALL than in AML. Recent improvements permit the correlation of the karyotype with other recognized prognostic factors.[20,148] It was rigorously demonstrated for the first time at the Third IWCL that the karyotype is an important independent prognostic factor in ALL.[148] Of 330 patients reviewed at the Third IWCL, 112 appeared to have a normal karyotype; the largest group (39 pts) with a well defined abnormality had a Ph¹ chromosome. Eighteen patients had a t(4;11), 16 had a t(8;14), and 15 had an abnormality of chromosome 14 not involving chromosome 8. Other patients with abnormalities were classified by the modal chromosome number. These patients were reviewed again at the Sixth IWCL; the data confirm that karyotype group is an independent prognostic factor for disease-free survival in children and that karyotype in combination with presenting WBC and FAB classification can identify groups of children and adults with a markedly different prognosis.[56]

At the Sixth IWCL, 29 of 172 (17%) adults and 9 of 157 (.06%) children had the Ph¹ chromosome. The Ph¹ chromosome is the most frequent rearrangement in adult ALL.[19,56] At the cytogenetic level, the breakpoints appear identical to those in CML; recent molecular analysis however indicates that the breakpoint in the BCR gene on No. 22 may be different in some patients with PH¹+ ALL than in those with CML.[41,68,128] Thus, in ALL, there are two subtypes of the Ph¹ chromosomes. The first subtype is identical to that seen in CML. The translocation breakpoints are within ABL and bcr and the same 8.5 kb fusion mRNA and chimeric p210 protein are produced. In the second subtype, the translocation breakpoint is also in ABL, but not within bcr; the chromosome 22 breakpoint falls upstream of the bcr, within the first intron of the BCR gene.[69] The transcript is a 7.0 kb fusion mRNA and the chimeric protein is known as the p185[bcr-abl].[31,32] Recent data suggest that sequences within the first exon of BCR bind to the ABL SH2 domain. This binding is needed for the activation of the ABL tyrosine kinase and the transforming potential of the chimeric BCR-ABL oncogene.[109A,122A] In ALL, where cytogenetic analysis may be more difficult than CML, pulse field gel electrophoresis or Southern blot analysis can be used to detect the Ph¹ chromosome by identification of a bcr rearrangement.[68,69] More recently the polymerase chain reaction (PCR) technique has been applied to the diagnosis of CML and ALL. This technique is very sensitive and can detect the presence of the abnormal BCR-ABL message in a dilution of 1:100,000 cells. This is useful in determining whether a patient with ALL has minimal residual disease after therapy. In the Sixth IWCL, the children with a Ph^1 chromosome had the second highest median leukocyte count (75,000/mm^3), all were non-B, non-T ALL, and they had a poor median survival of only 15 months. The Ph^1 + ALL in adults also carried a poor prognosis. Thus, by identifying this chromosomal abnormality, or its molecular equivalent, one can detect individuals who have a poor prognosis.

Of 216 Third IWCL patients with chromosomal abnormalities, 18 (8.3%) had a t(4;11)(q21;q23) rearrangement. One-half of the patients were children, most of whom were less than 1 year old. The association of the t(4;11) with neonatal or early-childhood ALL is particularly interesting in view of the low incidence of ALL in this age group; acute leukemias in this age group are usually of the myeloid type. Children with a t(4;11) had very high leukocyte counts (median WBC, 214,000/mm^3), which is a poor prognostic factor. Both children and adults with this abnormality had a short median survival of 9 and 7 months, respectively. Only patients with abnormalities involving 8q24 or 14q32 had shorter survivals. Although the morphology of some cells often appears lymphoid (L$_1$ and L$_2$), other features are more suggestive of a monocytic leukemia (biphenotypic leukemia). A t(4;11) cell line showed rearranged heavy and light chain (K) genes, although cells lacked cytoplasmic immunoglobulin and thus were probably in a very early stage of B cell differentiation.[142] However, when cultured with the phorbol ester, TPA, a monocytic-like phenotype was induced. Thus, these cells appear to be very early precursor cells that have dual lineage capabilities.

Another recurring chromosome abnormality is the t(1;19)(q21;p13) which has been identified in about 25% of patients with a pre B phenotype (cytoplasmic Ig+ and CALLA+).[29,103] This breakpoint has recently been cloned using the probe for a transcription factor (E2A) located on chromosome 19.[102] The translocation involves two genes that bind to DNA; the gene on chromosome 1 is called PBX. A fusion gene is formed and thus as in Ph^1 + CML and ALL, it is possible to use PCR technique to detect abnormal cells. This technique can also be used to detect minimal residual disease following completion of therapy in patients with this translocation.

Deletions of the long arm of chromosome 6 are relatively common changes in ALL, occurring in 5–10% of cases with clonal abnormalities.[66] The leukemic cells of some patients with ALL are characterized by a gain of many chromosomes and fewer structural abnormalities.[139,169] Chromosome numbers usually range from 50–60, and a few patients have up to 65 chromosomes (hyperdiploidy). Although identical karyotypes are unusual, certain additional chromosomes are commonly seen. Among 31 hyperdiploid patients at the Third IWCL (14% of patients with abnormalities), +21, +6, +18, +14, +4, and +10 in decreasing frequency were seen in 10–33% of patients.[148] It is interesting that some of these chromosomes, particularly Nos. 10, 18 and 21 are also seen as additional chromosomes in patients with near-haploidy, with chromosome numbers of 26–36 (median, 28). The median age of the 22 children with a hyperdiploid karyotype was 3 years, while the median age of all 31 patients (5 years) was less than that of patients with other abnormalities. The WBC

count was low (median of 6,000/mm^3). Thus, these patients have all of the previously recognized good prognostic factors, including age between 3 and 7 years, low WBC count, and CALLA+. In a follow-up study of these patients, the complete remission rate for children was 95% with a median remission duration that will be greater than 5 years. The median survival of the children with hyperdiploidy is longer than those of children with a normal karyotype; for adults, the median survival for the two groups is comparable. Chromosome losses were less frequent and involved No. 9, 7, 13, 20, or 8 in that order. The 3 translocations described for Burkitt's lymphoma are also seen in B-cell ALL. With regard to karyotype and age, patients with a deletion of 6q and a modal chromosome number greater than 50 were younger, and those with a Ph^1 chromosome or a 14q+ were older than patients with other abnormalities. In summary, the highest remission rates were in patients with a normal karyotype and a modal number greater than 50; the lowest were seen in patients with a Ph^1 chromosome, a 14q+ chromosome, a t(8;14), and a t(4;11).[19]

T-Cell Disorders

Although fewer leukemias of T-cell origin have been studied, a distinct pattern of nonrandom karyotypic abnormalities is emerging. Rearrangements involving the proximal bands of chromosome 14 (14q11-q13) are relatively common and those involving two regions of chromosome 7 (7q35–q36 and 7p15) also occur in T-cell malignancies, but have been observed in non-malignant T-cell disorders as well; breaks involving these regions are very rare in other malignant diseases (Table I-8-3). One recurring rearrangement in T-cell neoplasia, particularly CLL, is a paracentric inversion of chromosome 14 with a proximal breakpoint at q11 and a distal breakpoint at q32 [inv(14)(q11q32).[158,176] A closely related rearrangement, t(14;14)(q11;q32), is seen in T-cell neoplasia.[75,158] A number of reports from Japan have described the frequent occurrence of 14q11 breaks in adult T-cell leukemia-lymphoma patients.[109,137] Williams and her associates have described a t(11;14)(p13;q13) in the leukemic cells of 4 of 16 patients with T-cell acute lymphoblastic leukemia.[168] Thus, in some of these T-cell diseases, breaks occur in either 14q11 or 14q32, or in both bands in the same patient; in B-cell disorders, however, breaks occur essentially only in 14q32, and they rarely involve 14q11.[15] The data confirm the observation made some time ago that the proximal region of chromosome 14 was important in T-cell neoplasia.[75] In a manner similar to that observed in B-cell neoplasms, in which rearrangements frequently involve the chromosomal bands containing the immunoglobulin gene loci, T-cell neoplasms often have rearrangements involving band q11 of chromosome 14, the site of the T-cell receptor alpha-chain (TCRA) gene. Less often, one of two regions of chromosome 7 (7q35-36 and 7p15) to which the T-cell receptor beta-chain (TCRB) and gamma-chain (TCRG) genes have been localized, respectively, may be involved.[124]

Solid Tumors

Although solid tumors, in particular carcinomas, play a much larger part in human neoplasia than hematologic malignancies, much less is known about the cytogenetic abnormalities that characterize them. Among the reasons for this discrepancy is the difficulty of obtaining successful chromosome preparations from solid tumors because of extensive fibrosis or necrosis frequently associated with these tumors. Second, until recently, many investigators questioned the relevance of the chromosome changes in malignant cells, and therefore this difficult area of research was not pursued. Third, the karyotypes of the tumor cells frequently show high modal numbers, often 60–90 chromosomes with many bizarre marker chromosomes. It is therefore difficult to distinguish the primary change from those related to secondary evolution with progression of the malignant phenotype, since most of the studies have been made on highly advanced, often metastatic lesions. With newer culturing and banding techniques, patterns of relevant and consistent chromosomal rearrangements are emerging. To date, the cytogenetic abnormalities in solid tumors, unlike the case with hematologic malignancies, are merely associations and very few specific chromosome abnormalities have been described with specific types of cancers. For the purposes of this review of karyotypes in solid tumors, two broad groups of benign and malignant neoplasms are identified. Each group is then divided into six categories. These are: 1) epithelial, 2) mesenchymal, 3) neurogenic, 4) germ cell, 5) embryonal tumors, and 6) tumors of unknown histogenesis. Those changes that appear to be consistent are summarized in Table I-8-4.

Benign Tumors

Although much of the discussion in this chapter implies that chromosome aberrations are equivalent to a malignant phenotype, there are a number of exceptions. In the myeloproliferative disorders, patients with clonal chromosome abnormalities in marrow cells have been observed for up to 12 to 15 years without undergoing leukemic transformation.[133] Several benign tumors have clonal abnormalities of which the meningiomas described by Mark and colleagues and by Zankl and Zang have been studied most extensively.[100,175] However, there are now several reports of clonal cytogenetic abnormalities in benign solid tumors. Some examples are discussed below.

Epithelial Tumors

Salivary Gland Tumors. Mark and his associates have examined 100 parotid gland tumors and have noted clonal chromosome abnormalities in about 47%.[66,99] Of 47 adenomas with abnormal karyotypes, 34 had involvement of one of three particular chromosome regions; 8q12, 12q13–15, and 3p21. A translocation t(3;8)(p21;q12) was the most common abnormality. These abnormalities have not been reported in the few cases of malignant salivary gland tumors studied so far. The molecular consequences of these abnormalities are unknown.

Colonic Adenomas. Trisomies for chromosomes 7, 8, 13 and 14 have been identified in a few cases reported thus far.[66,108] Most attempts to study these tumors have failed because of insufficient mitotic cells from direct preparations or short term cultures. By using DNA probes, loss of heterozygosity for markers on chromosome 5q has been reported

Table I-8-4. Non-Random Chromosomal Abnormalities in Solid Tumors

Disease	Chromosomal Abnormalities
A. Benign Tumors	
Pleomorphic adenomas of the salivary glands	t(3;8)(p21;q12)
Meningioma and acoustic neuroma	Monosomy 22 or del(22q)
Lipoma	t(3;12)(q27-q28;q13-q14) ring chromosome
Ovarian tumors	Trisomy 12
Leiomyoma	t(12;14)(q14-q15;q23-q24)
B. Adult Cancers	
Breast	del(1p), del(11q)
Colon	del(17p), −18
Small cell lung carcinoma	del(3)(p14-p23)
Non small cell lung cancer	del(9p)
Renal carcinoma	del(3)(p11-p22)
Bladder cancer	i(5p), monosomy 9, del(19q)
Prostate	del(10)(q26)
Liposarcoma	t(12;16)(q13;p11)
Synovial sarcoma	t(X;18)(p11.2;q11.2)
Rhabdomyosarcoma (alveolar)	t(2;13)(q37;q14)
Malignant melanoma	del(1)(p11-p22), del(6)(q11q27), i(6p)
Testicular tumors	i(12p)
Glioma	−10, del(9p)
C. Involving Embryonic Cells	
Neuroblastoma	Del(1)(p32 to p36)
Ewing's sarcoma/peripheral neuroepithelioma	t(11;22)(q24;q12)
Wilms' tumor	Del(11)(p13) # Trisomy 1q
Retinoblastoma	Del(13)(q14)# Trisomy 1q

#Observed as a constitutional abnormality as well as in some tumors

in 20–50% of colorectal carcinoma and about 30% of patients with sporadic colonic adenomas.[47] The gene responsible for familial adenomatous polyposis has been mapped to chromosome 5q, but allelic losses of chromosome 5q are rare in adenomas from patients with familial adenomatous polyposis.[21,47]

Benign Ovarian Tumors. Trisomy 12 has been reported as the sole abnormality in five benign ovarian tumors, two other tumors have trisomy 12 in addition to other abnormalities. Thus, 7 out of 9 cytogenetically abnormal benign ovarian neoplasms are characterized by this trisomy.[122] The high frequency of trisomy 12 in benign ovarian tumors, often as the sole abnormality suggest that it may be a primary karyotypic event in the initiation of these tumors.

Mesenchymal Tumors

Leiomyomas. More than 100 leiomyomas with karyotypic abnormalities have been reported. It appears that breaks in 14q22–24 and in 12q14–15 are most common.[65,113,155] An identical translocation, t(12;14)(q14–15;q23–24) was found as the only abnormality in 4 of 34 leiomyomas.[61] Other abnormalities seen in leiomyomas include rearrangements of 6p, del (7)(q21 2q31,2) and t 12.[113]

Lipoma. Another benign mesenchymal neoplasm of special interest is lipoma. Of 26 lipomas karyotyped, 70% had consistent chromosome rearrangements; 13 of them had a reciprocal translocation involving 12q13–14.[66] This breakpoint has also been observed in liposarcomas. Analysis of 91 other cases of lipomas allowed a classification of lipomas into four cytogenetic subgroups; those with normal karyotypes, those with hyperdiploidy with ring chromosomes, those with pseudodiploidy with rearrangement of 12q(13–14) and those with hypodiploid or pseudodiploid karyotypes with other aberrations.[97] This region of chromosome No. 12 band q13–14 has now been observed to be involved in lipomas, liposarcomas, leiomyomas, and mixed salivary gland tumors. The molecular mechanism involved in abnormalities of this region is yet to be determined.

Neurogenic Tumors

Meningioma. This is the best characterized benign solid tumor. Mark and colleagues first described a loss of one chromosome 22 in meningioma. Monosomy 22 has now been reported in about 70% of cases or 95% of tumors with abnormal karyotypes.[100,175]

Malignant Tumors

Epithelial Tumors

Lung Cancer. Whang-Peng and coworkers reported a specific chromosome abnormality in small cell lung cancer (SCLC).[167] Specimens of 25 patients were successfully studied including 1 tumor specimen, 2 pleural effusions, 8 metastatic bone marrow cells, and 16 long-term SCLC cell lines. At least one chromosome 3 in all the metaphases examined had a deletion of the short arm. The shortest region of overlap in all the deletions was band 3p a14p23. In their study, this abnormality was not detected in any of the non-small cell lung cancer (NSCL) cancer cell lines. Other investigators have since confirmed this observation, but have failed to see del(3p) in every small cell lung cancer. Moreover Zech and associates have also reported this abnormality in all four subtypes of lung cancer.[178] Molecular analysis of lung cancer cells has also shown that loss of heterozygosity for markers on chromosome arm 3p occurs consistently in small cell lung carcinoma and occasionally in non-small cell lung carcinoma.[80,112]

Lukeis and colleagues have also reported chromosome 9p abnormalities in 9 of 10 lung cancers examined.[96] These included 5 adenocarcinomas, 3 squamous, and 2 large cell carcinomas. Non-reciprocal translocations, deletions or chromosome loss resulting in loss of material from the short arm of chromosome 9 with breakpoints in the region 9p11–p14 were observed. Thus, loss of genetic material from chromosome arm 9p may also contribute to the malignant process in these tumors.

Renal Cell Carcinoma. A translocation between chromosomes No. 3 and No. 11 confined to tumor cells was first reported in a patient with hereditary renal cell carcinoma, while a translocation between chromosome No. 3 and No. 8 was observed in the lymphocytes of 10 affected members of a family among whom bilateral renal carcinoma segregated in an apparently autosomal dominant fashion.[34,119,144] Deletions or structural rearrangements of the short arm of

chromosome 3 with breakpoints in bands 3p11–p21 are the changes most consistently seen in renal cell carcinoma. 3p deletion has also been found as the sole abnormality in some cases, or has been seen in 100% of cells showing clonal abnormalities.[144,162] These observations suggest that del (3p) may be a primary event in the development of these tumors.

Breast Cancer. There are no consistent changes in breast cancer but abnormalities of 1q seem to be most common, with breakpoints mapped to 1q12–23. Rearrangements of 1p with deletions or translocations affecting bands 1p11–1p21 also occur in about 25% of cases with cytogenetic abnormalities. Several laboratories have reported on the loss of heterozygosity at specific loci on chromosome regions 1p, 1q, 3p, 11p, 13q, 17p, 17q, and 18q in breast tumor.[66,150,152]

Colorectal Carcinomas. A considerable number of these tumors have been studied but the results are not easy to interpret. The most common changes include structural rearrangements of chromosomes 1 and 17 as well as trisomy 7 and trisomy 12.[104] Loss of chromosome 5 allele was reported by Solomon and colleagues. Reports of loss of material from the short arm of chromosome 17 and long arm of chromosome 18, prompted molecular geneticists to look at these chromosomes using DNA probes (as was the case with lung cancer and del(3p), as well as del(13q14) and retinoblastoma).[47] The most detailed molecular study of colorectal carcinomas has been provided by Vogelstein and coworkers who have demonstrated that the progressive accumulation of genetic changes parallels the clinical progression of colorectal tumors from normal epithelium to benign tumors and further to the malignant stage of the disease. By molecular analysis, loss of heterozygosity for DNA sequences from chromosome regions 5q, 17p, and 18q were found to occur in a great percentage of colorectal carcinomas.[47,160] Vogelstein proposes that colorectal tumorigenesis proceeds through a series of genetic alterations involving oncogenes (ras) and tumor suppressor genes (particularly those on chromosomes 5q, 17p, and 18q). Allelic deletions of chromosome 17p and 18q usually occur at a later stage of tumorigenesis than do deletions of chromosome 5q or *RAS* gene mutations. The accumulation of these genetic alterations rather than the order in which they occur appears to be most important in colorectal tumorigenesis. Most recently the *DCC* gene was identified from a segment of chromosome 18q and has been shown to be mutated in a few colorectal carcinomas.[47]

Bladder Carcinoma. Several studies of chromosome abnormalities in bladder cancer have reported abnormalities involving several chromosomes. Structural rearrangements of chromosomes 1, 5, and 11, as well as numerical aberrations involving chromosomes 7 and 9, appear to be the most frequent.[58,66] Monosomy 9 has been reported in 8 of 19 bladder tumors, one of which had monosomy 9 as the sole abnormality.[58] Isochromosome 5p (i[5p]) has been reported in 20% of all bladder tumors, while several copies of a chromosome 5 were deleted in a few cases. This may have the same effect as an isochromosome of 5p. Thus isochromosome 5p or del 5q may be important in this tumor.[58]

Malignant Mesenchymal Tumors

Sarcomas. Mesenchymal tumors are relatively rare, accounting for less than 1% of all human neoplasms. They are very heterogeneous, and may present diagnostic problems.[66,104] Recently, cytogenetic and molecular analysis of these tumors in their malignant (sarcoma) and benign forms have yielded some very important clues regarding the heretofore unsuspected relationship of some of these rare neoplasms, as well as providing help in classifying some of the undifferentiated forms of these tumors. Moreover, the fact that the benign and malignant forms have related karyotypic changes provides an important resource for identifying the additional genetic changes that occur in the malignant compared with the benign form.

Recurring translocations have recently been described in both liposarcoma and synovial sarcoma.[37,66,154,157] A t(12;16)(q13;p11) has been described, only in the myxoid subgroup of liposarcomas whereas other abnormalities including ring chromosomes appeared to be more frequent in well differentiated sarcomas. As previously discussed, a breakpoint cluster region on chromosome 12q13–14 is shared by both lipomas and myxoid liposarcomas.[154] The chromosome abnormality in synovial sarcoma [t(X;18) (p11.2;q11.2)] is also of interest because it is the first one involving a sex chromosome. This abnormality does not appear to be restricted to a particular histologic pattern.[157]

Neurogenic Tumors

Gliomas. There have been several reports on the cytogenetic abnormalities of these malignant brain tumors. The reports cover all the histologic subtypes of gliomas including astrocytomas, oligodendroglioma and glioblastoma multiforme. One of the largest series so far was that published in 1971 by Mark and colleagues who demonstrated that 37 of 50 gliomas had near diploid stem lines and that 26% contained double minutes (dmin).[101] This study was done prior to availability of banding techniques. With banding techniques several more gliomas have been studied. Jenkins and colleagues have also reported on 53 gliomas.[73] No specific abnormalities have been detected, but the most frequent findings have been dmin, structural abnormality of chromosome 9 (del 9p or translocation), trisomy 7 and loss of chromosomes 10, 18, and 22.[13,14,73] In a report by Bigner and colleagues, 8 of 22 tumors contained marker chromosomes derived from chromosome 9; in 3 tumors, both chromosome Nos. 9 participated in marker formation with different breakpoints, so that there were a total of 11 structural rearrangements of this chromosome.[14] In this series, the most prevalent finding was abnormalities of chromosome 9 with breakpoints at the centromere or in 9p. By molecular analysis we have found that hemizygous and homozygous deletions of the interferon genes (localized on chromosome 9p) occur in about 30% of gliomas (Olopade—unpublished). The potential role of these genes in the malignant transformation of gliomas is currently under investigation.

Neuroepitheliomas. Whang-Peng and colleagues in 1984 described a t(11;22)(q24;q12) in two cases of neuroepithelioma, the same translocation that has been reported in more than 90% of Ewing's sarcoma tumors.[6,165] Further, a comparison of Ewing's sarcoma and neuroepithelioma suggests that the two tumors are histogenetically related. It has recently been shown that the neuronal phenotype of Ewing's sarcoma and neuroepithelioma is the same. The similarity has been further substantiated by molecular analysis in which identical levels of protooncogene expression were found in Ewing's sarcoma and neuroepithelioma.[71] The discovery of the same identical translocation in neuroepithelioma and Ewing's sarcoma has changed the treatment modality in neuroepithelioma. Use of therapy similar to that used in Ewing's sarcoma has resulted in marked improvement in response of these tumors.

Embryonic Tumors

These tumors are of particular interest to the cytogeneticist because some of them occur in patients who have specific constitutional chromosome abnormalities. In all preceding sections, the karyotypic changes were somatic mutations in malignant cells and they were not present in other unaffected cells except in the few cases of familial renal cell carcinoma. In contrast, some patients at risk of developing retinoblastoma have a variable deletion of chromosome 13 that always includes 13q14, whereas other patients with a deletion of No. 11 (band 11p13) are at risk of developing Wilms' tumor. In general, these deletions are also associated with various phenotypic abnormalities.[52,66] Furthermore, analysis of tumor cells from patients with normal constitutional karyotypes indicated that about 5% of cases had tumor specific deletions of chromosome 13, each of which included deletions of chromosome 13, band q14. Relatively few tumors have been analyzed and monosomy 13 or del(13q) are observed in less than 20% of tumor cells from some patients with retinoblastoma. These deletion cases were useful in defining the region of the genome likely to contain a locus involved in the genesis of retinoblastoma. Further analysis of this locus using methods of molecular cloning led to the identification of the *RB1* gene.[30,45] The most common change that we have observed in Wilms' tumors is trisomy for the long arm of No. 1 (+1q), while deletions of 11p13 or unbalanced translocations occur in about 25% of cases.[81] Recent studies suggest that three genetic loci are implicated in the development of Wilms' tumor. One locus which is associated with the WAGR (Wilms' tumor, aniridia, genitourinary dysplasia, and mental retardation syndrome) maps to 11p13; another locus which is associated with the Beckwith-Wiedmann syndrome maps to 11p15; the third locus which may be involved in familial predisposition to Wilms' tumor was not genetically linked to any of the markers on 11p and may be on another chromosome.[62,82,125] Two groups have independently isolated a candidate gene *(WT1)* for Wilms' tumor at 11p13; the characterisation of mutations in tumor DNA suggests that the gene product contributes to the malignant process.[28,57] Complementary DNA (cDNA) clones representing transcripts of 2.5 (*WIT*-1) and 3.5 kb (*WIT*-2) mapping to a region which was homozygously deleted in a Wilms' (also representing candidate genes) tumor were also recently isolated from a kidney cDNA library; 11 of 12 tumors classified as histopathologically heterogenous exhibited absent or reduced expression of *WIT*-2.[22,70]

Recurring chromosome abnormalities, limited to the malignant cells, have also been observed in other childhood tumors, for example, a deletion of much of the long arm of chromosome 1 [del(1p)] has been noted in neuroblastomas.[26]

Neuroblastomas are also of interest because of their proclivity to undergo gene amplification which is manifested chromosomally as hundreds or thousands of small discrete pieces of chromosomes called double minutes, or long unbanded regions on chromosomes called homogeneously staining regions or HSR.[12] In some cell lines, these have been shown to represent amplification of MYCN.[138] MYCN amplification has also been identified in tumor samples; it is highly correlated with advanced stage (III and IV) and with a poor survival of these patients.[25]

Germ Cell Tumors

Atkin and Baker described an isochromosome for the short arm of chromosome No. 12 in four seminomas in 1983 [i(12p)].[5] The presence of this marker in various histologic types of germ cell tumors including seminomas, teratomas and embryonal cell carcinomas has subsequently been confirmed in several studies.[66,152] Thus, i(12p) appears to be a highly consistent and specific cytogenetic abnormality associated with testicular germ cell tumors.

Tumors of Uncertain Histogenesis

Ewing's Sarcoma. Aurias and colleagues as well as Turc-Carel and colleagues independently described a t(11;22)(q24;q12) in the malignant cells of patients with Ewing's sarcoma.[6,156] This translocation has now been detected in more than 90% of these tumors. The identification of the genes involved in this translocation is under investigation. As previously discussed the same chromosomal translocation has been described for neuroepithelioma and Ewing's sarcoma. The current thinking is that Ewing's sarcoma arises from cells of the neural crest. Both Ewing's sarcoma and neuroepithelioma are now treated the same way.

Malignant Melanoma. Chromosome changes involving chromosomes 1, 6, and 7 have often been reported in the malignant cells of patients with melanoma.[8] Most tumors studied have often been metastatic and there are few studies of early melanocytic lesions. Recent data from Parmiter and colleagues confirm that the predominant non-random abnormality in metastatic melanoma continues to be deletions and rearrangements of 1p, abnormalities of 6p and 6q, extra copies of chromosome 7 and losses of chromosome 10.[118] A translocation involving the terminal region 10q (q24–26) was also seen in some premalignant lesions. The abnormalities of chromosome 10 were seen in both early and late lesions suggesting that this may be a primary event in the malignant process.[118] Cowan and colleagues also described loss of one copy of chromosome 9 in 2 of 4 dysplastic nevi, and 4 of 11 melanomas.[35] Isochromosome 1q [i(1q)] or del(1p) occur in about 60% of all tumors while chromosome 6 is rearranged in more than 80% of all tumors.[66] Trent and colleagues recently presented evidence that the insertion of a normal chromosome 6 could revert some of the malignant phenotype in malignant melanoma.[151]

Molecular Analysis of Recurring Chromosome Abnormalities, Particularly Translocations

How and When Consistent Translocations Occur

We do not know how consistent structural rearrangements occur, but there are at least two possibilities.[129] The rearrangements may be random, but selection may act to eliminate the vast majority that do not provide the cell with a proliferative advantage. Alternatively, certain changes may occur preferentially and thus may be the ones we see. Some tantalizing data show an association of chromosome rearrangements in tumor cells from patients with fragile sites affecting one of the chromosome bands broken in the tumor cells.[90,143,172] However, much more research is required to clarify the role of fragile sites as a predisposing factor to malignant transformation.

Croce has proposed that many of the chromosome rearrangements in B and T cell tumors involve sequences used in the normal recombination of the V-D-J segments of the immunoglobulin and T cell receptor genes.[36] The presence of heptamer and nonamer sequences in the non-immunoglobulin gene at the site of the translocation, namely MYC and BCL2, has been reported. We have no indication at present that the genes involved in the translocations in myeloid leukemias undergo similar DNA rearrangements.

An equally important question is, when in the multistage process of malignant transformation of a particular cell do translocations or other chromosome aberrations occur? Some chromosome changes occur as part of the further evolution of the malignant phenotype, e.g., blast crisis of CML, and they are, therefore, relatively late events. But what about the occurrence of the t(9;22) in CML, for example? Does the Ph[1] occur in a single normal cell which becomes the progenitor of the leukemic clone, or is there expansion of a clone, possibly a leukemic one, in which a translocation occurs in one of these already abnormal cells? Fialkow and his colleagues have presented detailed evidence supporting the latter proposal.[48]

More recently, Adams and colleagues have constructed transgenic mice whose cells all have a vector containing the myc/IgH junction from a murine plasmacytoma.[1] All cells contain this construct; however the B cell tumors that occurred in every animal were clonal indicating that one or more additional changes occurred in one cell resulting in clonality.

Chromosome Location of Protooncogenes

One of the most surprising revelations in the recent past has involved the cellular oncogenes and their chromosome location. Much of the excitement derives from the observation that many protooncogenes are located in the bands that are involved in consistent translocations (Figure I-8-8).[1,16,46,77,92] The evidence in Burkitt's lymphoma and in CML clearly point the way for future research in this area. The gene for the protooncogene MYC (the cellular homolog of the avian myelocytomatosis virus) is on chromosome 8(q24). The immunoglobulin genes (heavy chain, and kappa and lambda light chain genes) are located at the breakpoints on the three chromosomes, other than No. 8, that are involved in the translocations in Burkitt's lymphoma, 14q32, 2p12, and 22q11 respectively. These translocations result in the aberrant juxtaposition of *MYC* and one of the immunoglobulin genes; this in turn leads to abnormal regulation of *MYC* expression, although the precise nature of the derangement is not presently understood.[77,92] Comparable chromosome translocations and gene rearrangements have been observed in mouse plasmacytomas.[76]

Investigators are now in the process of unraveling the mystery of the Ph[1] translocation in CML and ALL. In the t(9;22) in CML and ALL, the Abelson protooncogene *(ABL)* is translocated to the Ph[1] chromosome.[41] This was an important observation because *ABL* was the first gene known to be on No. 9 that was shown to translocate to No. 22, thus establishing the fact that the translocation was reciprocal.

With regard to Ph[1]-positive ALL, it has always been an enigma why the typical Ph[1] translocation is seen in ALL and in fact is the most common translocation in adults with ALL.[148] One relatively trivial explanation would be that the patients really had CML in lymphoid blast crisis with an undiagnosed chronic phase, and this may occur in some patients. However, analysis of DNA from some Ph[1]-positive ALL cells indicates that the breakpoint in the bcr region on No. 22 differs from that in CML.[41] In a recent report by the Cancer and Leukemia Group B (CALGB), 11 of 35 (32%) patients were molecularly positive for the Ph[1] chromosome by pulse field gel electrophoresis and Southern analysis. However only 2 of the 11 (7%) had the bcr rearrangement that is seen in CML, showing that these Ph[1] ALL patients did not have CML in lymphoid blast crisis.[69] Thus, the genetic analysis of what appeared to be a simple chromosome change, namely the 9;22 translocation, has revealed unexpected complexity. As previously described, it has been shown that the head to tail juxtaposition of the 5'-end of *ABL* with the truncated 3'-end of the *BCR* gene on chromosome 22 results in a new transcriptional unit producing a novel *BCR-ABL* fusion mRNA transcript.[136,140] The translation product of this hybrid 8.5 kb mRNA is a 210 KD protein with tyrosine kinase activity.[31,140] Daley and coworkers have now shown that this P210[bcr-abl] product is able to induce a CML-like disease when murine bone marrow was infected with a retrovirus encoding P210[bcr-abl] and transplanted into irradiated syngeneic recipients.[38] Thus it is likely that expression of this protein by bone marrow cells can induce chronic myelogenous leukemia.

Chromosome Location of Tumor Suppressor Genes

Chromosomal deletions in human tumors have been regarded as evidence that the deleted regions contain tumor suppressor genes (Table I-8-5). The tumor suppressor genes have been postulated to encode proteins that regulate normal growth and thus indirectly suppress neoplastic proliferation. In cells, these genes may act recessively, so that both maternal and paternal copies of the gene product must be inactivated in order for the tumor suppressor function to be eliminated. This model for tumor suppressor genes was originally postulated by Knudson[78] and has gained support from the study and molecular cloning of the retinoblastoma gene on chromosome band 13q14.

Patients with retinoblastoma have two patterns of inheritance, one as an autosomal dominant and one as a sporadic mutation. The age of the patient when the tumor was detected as well as other observations led Knudson to propose the "two-hit" hypothesis.[78] According to this hypothesis, in patients who inherited the predisposing gene, only one other change was needed for transformation of retinal cells to tumor cells and in these individuals, multiple tumors were diagnosed at a very early age. In sporadic cases, two independent mutations had to affect the same cell for transformation to occur; since this event was relatively uncommon, the tumors were unifocal and developed at an older age. Based on the consistent loss of chromosome band, 13q14, this band was thought to be the locus for the retinoblastoma or *RB1* gene. Studies confirming that No. 13 was the critical chromosome included the discovery that tumor cells frequently had loss of heterozygosity for DNA markers on chromosome 13q14. A gene from this region was molecularly cloned which had properties consistent with the *RB1* gene.[53,94] A 4.7 kb mRNA transcript of this gene was present in all normal tissues examined but was absent or altered in retinoblastoma cells and deletions within the gene have been detected in many retinoblastoma tissues. The protein product of the *RB1* gene is a nuclear phospho-protein of about 110 KD that has DNA binding activity.[93] This protein was recently shown to associate with large T antigen and EIA, the transforming proteins of DNA tumor viruses SV40 and adenovirus respectively.[93] These studies indirectly suggest that the RB protein has a role in regulating expression of other cellular genes, and may also mediate the oncogenic effects of some viral-transforming proteins. The protein product of the *RB1* gene has been implicated in the regulation of the cell cycle.[42] Bookstein has demonstrated suppression of tumorigenicity of human prostate carcinoma cells by replacing a mutated *RB1* gene.[23] Inactivation of the *RB1* gene has also been observed in different tumor types including osteosarcoma, synovial sarcoma and other soft tissue sarcomas, small-cell lung carcinoma, and breast carcinoma.

In this chapter, we have presented reports showing that several regions of different chromosomes are deleted in some malignant tumors. Extrapolating from the retinoblastoma experience, it is felt that these regions of the chromosome contain putative tumor suppressor genes. The somatic loss of both maternal and paternal copies of a gene have now been observed at a locus on 9p which includes the interferon genes, the *Tp53* locus on chromosome 17 and the *DCC* gene locus on chromosome 18 in malignant hematopoietic tissues, lung and colon cancers respectively.[44,47] Other tumors such as small cell lung cancer, colorectal carcinoma and gliomas are associated with chromosomal deletions, and similar mechanisms may be responsible for initiation and progression of disease in these tumors as well (Table I-8-5).

Specificity of Chromosome Rearrangements

The evidence presented in this chapter clearly demonstrates the remarkable specificity of certain chromosome rearrangements for particular subtypes of tumors especially leukemia or lymphoma. The mechanism or mechanisms by which this specificity is achieved are unknown, however a number of investigators have shown that certain proteins required for promotion of gene expression are synthesized

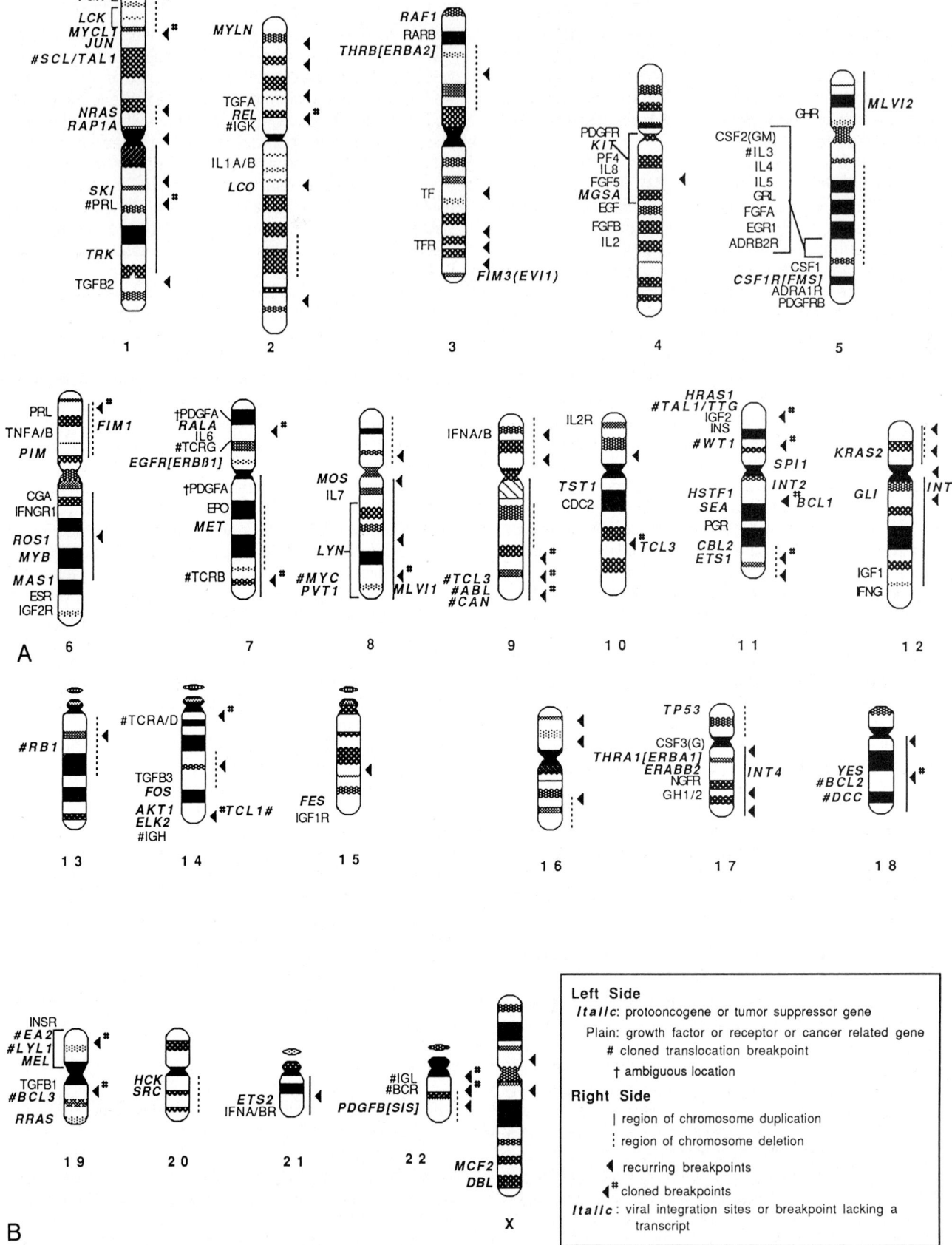

Figure I-8-8.   (Legend appears on facing page)

Table I-8-5. Neoplastic Diseases Associated with Putative Tumor Suppressor Genes

Malignant Diseases	Gene Locus
Neuroblastoma	1p32-ter
Renal cell carcinoma	3p
Small cell lung cancer	3p14-21
Familial adenomatous polyposis	5q21-22
Colorectal carcinoma	5q21-22
ALL, NHL	9p22
Glioblastoma	9p13-ter
Wilms' tumor	11p13
Embryonal rhabdomyosarcoma	11p15-ter
Transitional cell bladder carcinoma	11p
Retinoblastoma	13q14.1
Osteosarcoma	13q14.1
Ductal breast carcinoma	13q14.1
Meningioma	22q
Therapy-related AML	5q23-31

in a very cell-type specific manner.[114] These proteins are only present in the appropriate cell type and therefore the particular gene is activated only in that cell type. The chromosome rearrangements affecting *MYC* in B cell and T cell tumors strongly support the interpretation that the specificity resides in the gene that is uniquely active in a particular cell type. Thus the immunoglobulin genes are highly regulated in B cells and they can therefore serve as the switch or activator mechanism for *MYC* in B cells; on the other hand *TCRA* is an active gene in T cells with a strong enhancer/promotor and it clearly is an activator for *MYC* in T cells. A reasonable paradigm is that translocations bring together in an inappropriate manner a growth factor or growth factor receptor gene (the protooncogene in the examples defined to date) adjacent to an active cell specific gene.

As has been described in this chapter, the analysis of various tumors for alterations in protooncogenes or tumor suppressor genes has revealed that a number are abnormal as a result of translations, amplification, deletions or mutations. In some situations the relationship of the change in the protooncogene to the multistage process of malignant transformation is unclear.[46] Such ambiguity is not a problem with chromosome translocations; the evidence is overwhelming that the t(8;14) in Burkitt's lymphoma and the t(9;22) in CML are an integral component of the cascade of events leading to the transformation of a normal to a malignant cell. The ever-increasing number of translocations reviewed in this chapter provide a potential goldmine for identifying new genes that are unequivocally related to the malignant phenotype of the affected cell. The challenge is to isolate these translocation breakpoint junctions, to identify the genes that are located at these breakpoints, and then to determine the change in gene function that occurs as a consequence of the translocation. The ultimate measure of success, however, will be in the application of these new insights in the development of new, more effective treatments for cancer. In the future, each particular subtype of tumor will be treated in a uniquely defined way that is most appropriate for the specific genetic defect present in that tumor. This should lead to a new era of cancer therapy that is both more effective and less toxic.

REFERENCES

1. Adams, J. M. , Harris, A. W., Pinkert, C. A., Corcoran, L. M., Alexander, W. S., Cory, S., Palmiter, R. D., and Brinster, R. L.: The c-myc oncogene driven by immunoglobulin enhancers induces lymphoid malignancy in transgenic mice. Nature, 318:533, 1985.
2. ar-Rushdi, A., Nishikura, K., Erickson, J., Watt, R., Rovera, G., and Croce, C. M.: Differential expression of the translocated and the untranslocated c-myc oncogene in Burkitt lymphoma. Science, 222:390, 1983.
3. Arthur, D. C., and Bloomfield, C. D.: Banded chromosome analysis in patients with treatment-associated acute non-lymphocytic leukemia. Cancer Genet. Cytogenet., 12:189, 1984.
4. Arthur, D. C., and Bloomfield, C. D.: Partial deletion of the long arm of chromosome 16 and bone marrow eosinophilia in acute non-lymphocytic leukemia: A new association. Blood, 61:994, 1983.
5. Atkin, N. B., and Baker, M. C.: i(12p): Specific chromosome marker in seminoma and malignant teratoma of the testis? Cancer Genet. Cytogenet., 10:199, 1983.
6. Aurias, A., Rimbaut, C., Buffe, D., Dubousset, J., and Mazabraud, A.: Chromosomal translocations in Ewing's sarcoma. N. Engl. J. Med., 309:496, 1983.
7. Bakhshi, A., Minowada, J., Arnold, A., Cossman, J., Jensen, J. P., Whang-Peng, J., Waldmann, T. A, and Korsmeyer, S. J.: Lymphoid blast crises of chronic myelogenous leukemia represent stages in the development of B-cell precursors. N. Engl. J. Med., 309:826, 1983.
8. Balaban, G., Herlyn, M., Guerry, D., III, Bartolo, R., Koprowski, H., Clark, W. H., and Nowell, P. C.: Cytogenetics of human malignant melanoma and pre-malignant lesions. Cancer Genet. Cytogenet., 11:429, 1984.
9. Bartram, C. R.: Rearrangement of the c-abl and bcr genes in ph-negative CML and ph-positive acute leukemias. Leukemia, 2:63, 1988.
10. Bennett, J. M., Catovsky, D., Daniel, M. T., Flandrin, G., Galton, D. A. G., Gralnick, H. R., and Sultan, C.: Proposals for the classification of the acute leukemias: French-American-British (FAB) Co-operative Group. Br. J. Haematol., 51:189, 1985.
11. Berger, R., Bernheim, A., Sigaux, F., Daniel, M.-T., Valensi, F., and Flandrin, G.: Acute monocytic leukemia chromosome studies. Leuk. Res., 6:17, 1982.
12. Biedler, J. L., and Spengler, B. A.: Metaphase chromosome anomaly: Association with drug resistance and cell-specific products. Science, 191:185, 1976.
13. Bigner, S. H., Mark, J., Burger, P. C., Mahaley, M. S., Jr., Bullard, D. E., Muhlbaier, L. H., and Bigner, D. D.: Specific chromosomal abnormalities in malignant human gliomas. Cancer Res., 48:405, 1988.
14. Bigner, S. H., Mark, J., Bullard, D. E., Mahaley, M. S., Jr., and Bigner, D. D.: Chromosomal evolution in malignant glioma starts with specific and usually numerical deviations. Cancer Genet. Cytogenet., 22:121, 1986.
15. Bird, M. L., Ueshima, Y., Rowley, J. D., Haren, J. M., and Vardiman, J. W.: Chromosome abnormalities in B-cell chronic lymphocytic leukaemia and their clinical correlations. Leukemia, 3:182, 1989.
16. Bishop, J. M.: The molecular genetics of cancer. Leukemia, 2:199, 1988.
17. Bitter, M. A., Franklin, W. A., Larson, R. A., McKeithan, T. W., Rubin, L. M., LeBeau, M. M., Stephen, J. K., and Vardiman, J. W.: Morphology in Ki-1 (CD30)-positive non-Hodgkin's lymphoma is correlated with clinical features and the presence of a unique chromosomal abnormality, t(2;5)(p23;q35). Am. J. Surg. Pathol., 14:305, 1990.
18. Bitter, M. A., Neilly, M. E., LeBeau, M. M., Pearson, M. G., and Rowley, J. D.: Rearrangement of chromosome 3 involving bands 3q21 and 3q26 are associated with normal or elevated platelet counts in acute nonlymphocytic leukemia. Blood, 66:1362, 1985.
19. Bloomfield, C. D., Goldman, A. I., Alimena, G., Berger, R., Borgstrom, G. H., Brandt, L., Catovsky, D., de la Chapelle, A., Dewald, G. W., Garson, O. M., Garwicz, S., Golomb, M. H., Hossfeld, D. K., Lawler, S. D., Mitelman, F., Nilsson, P., Pierre, R. V., Philp, P., Prigogina, E., Rowley, J. D., Sakurai, M., Sandberg, M. A. P., Secker-Walker, L. M., Tricot, G., Vanden Berghe, H., Van Orshoven, A., Vupio, P., and Whang-Peng, J.: Chromosomal abnormalities identify high-risk and low-risk patients with acute lymphoblastic leukemia. Blood, 67:415, 1986.

Figure I-8-8. Map of the chromosome location of protooncogenes or of genes that appear to be important in malignant transformation and the breakpoints observed in recurring chromosome abnormalities in human leukemia, lymphoma, and solid tumors. Known protooncogenes are indicated in bold italics and other cancer related genes are listed in standard type. The protooncogenes and their locations are placed to the left of the appropriate chromosome band or region (indicated by a bracket). The breakpoints in recurring translocations, inversions, etc., are indicated with an arrow head to the right of the affected chromosome band. The solid vertical lines on the right indicate regions frequently present in triplicate; the dashed lines indicate recurring deletions. Recurring viral integration sites and cloned translocation breakpoints with no identified transcripts are indicated to the right of the appropriate band. Genes or recurring breakpoints that have been cloned are identified by #. The locations of the cancer-specific breakpoints are based on the Report of the Committee on Structural Chromosome Changes in Neoplasia, Human Gene Mapping 10.5.[70A] [Author's note. Any map of this sort involves selection as to the genes that should or should not be included; we have been relatively conservative. Also for recurring breakpoints and deletions, we have included only those listed as Status I or II in HGM10.5.]

20. Bloomfield, C. D., Arthur, D. C., Frizzera, G., Levine, E. G., Peterson, B. A., and Gajl-Peczalska, K. J.: Nonrandom chromosome abnormalities in lymphoma. Cancer Res., 43:2975, 1983.
21. Bodmer, W. F., Bailey, C. J., Bodmer, J., Bussey, H. J. R., Ellis, A., Gorman, P., Lucibello, F. C., Murday, V. A., Rider, S. H., Scambler, P., Sheer, D., Solomon, E., and Spurr, N. K.: Localization of the gene for familial adenomatous polyposis on chromosome 5. Nature, 328:614, 1987.
22. Bonetta, L., Kuehn, S. E., Huang, A., Law, D. J., Kalikin, L. M., Koi, M., Reeve, A. E., Brownstein, B. H., Herman, Y., Williams, B. R. G., and Feinberg, A. P.: Wilms' tumor locus on 11p13 defined by multiple CpG island-associated transcripts. Science, 250:994, 1990.
23. Bookstein, R., Shew, J. Y., Chen, R. L., Scully, P., and Lee, W. H.: Suppression of tumorigenicity of human prostate carcinoma cells by replacing a mutated RB gene. Science, 247:712, 1990.
24. Borrow, J., Goddard, A. D., Sheer, D., and Solomon, E.: Molecular analysis of acute promyelocytic leukemia breakpoint cluster region on chromosome 17. Science, 249:1577, 1990.
25. Brodeur, G. M., Seeger, R. L., Schwab, M., Vermus, H. E., and Bishop, J. M.: Amplification of N-myc in untreated neuroblastoma correlates with advanced disease stage. Science, 224:1121, 1984.
26. Brodeur, G. M., Green, A. A., Hayes, F. A., Williams, K. J., Williams, D. L., and Tsiatis, A. A.: Cytogenetic features of human neuroblastomas and cell lines. Cancer Res., 41:4678, 1981.
27. Caccia, N., Bruns, G. A., Kirsch, I. R., Hollis, G. F., Bertness, V., and Mak, T. W.: T cell receptor α-chain genes are located on chromosome 14 at 14q11–14q12 in humans. J. Exp. Med., 161:1255, 1985.
28. Call, K. M., Glaser, T., Ito, C. Y., Buckler, A. J., Pelletier, J., Hasen, D. A., Rose, E. A., Kral, A., Yeger, H., and Lewis, W. H.: Isolation and characterization of a zinc finger polypeptide gene at the human chromosome 11 Wilms' tumor locus. Cell, 60:509, 1990.
29. Carroll, A. J., Crist, W. M., Parmley, R. T., Roper, M., Cooper, M. D., and Finley, W. H.: Pre-B cell leukemia associated with chromosome translocation 1;19. Blood, 63:721, 1984.
30. Cavenee, W. K., Dryja, T. P., Phillips, R. A., Benedict, W. F., Godbout, R., Gallie, B. L., Murphree, A. L., Strong, L. C., and White, R. L.: Expression of recessive alleles by chromosomal mechanisms in retinoblastoma. Nature, 305:779, 1983.
31. Chan, L. C., Karhi, K. K., Rayter, S. I., Heisterkamp, N., Eridani, S., Powles, R., Lawler, S. D., Groffen, J., Foulkes, J. G., Greaves, M. F., and Wiedemann, L. M.: A novel *abl* protein expressed in Philadelphia chromosome positive acute lymphoblastic leukaemia. Nature, 325:635, 1987.
32. Clark, S. S., McLaughlin, J., Crist, W. M., Champlin, R., and Witte, O. N.: Unique forms of the abl tyrosine kinase distinguish Ph^1-positive CML from Ph^1-positive ALL. Science, 235:85, 1987.
33. Cleary, M. L., Smith, D. S., and Sklar, J.: Cloning and structural analysis of cDNA's for *bcl-2* and a hybrid bcl-2/immunoglobulin transcript resulting from the t(14;18) translocation. Cell, 47:19, 1986.
34. Cohen, A. J., Li, F. B., Berg, S., Marchetto, D. J., Tsai, S., Jacobs, S. C., and Brown, R. S.: Hereditary renal cell carcinoma associated with a chromosomal translocation. N. Engl. J. Med., 301:592, 1979.
35. Cowan, J. M., Halaban, R., and Francke, U.: Cytogenetic analysis of melanocytes from premalignant nevi and melanoma. J. Natl. Cancer Inst., 80:1159, 1988.
36. Croce, C. M., Isobe, M., Palumbo, A., Puck, J., Ming, J., Tweardy, D., Erikson, J., Davis, M., and Rovera, G.: Gene for α-chain of human T-cell receptor: Location on chromosome 14 region involved in T-cell neoplasms. Science, 227:1044, 1985.
37. Dal Cin, P., and Sandberg, A. A.: Chromosome changes in soft tissue tumors: Benign and malignant. Cancer Invest., 7:63, 1989.
38. Daley, G. Q., Van Etter, R. A., and Baltimore, D.: Induction of chronic myelogenous leukemia in mice by p210 bcr/abl gene of the Philadelphia chromosome. Science, 247:824, 1990.
39. de Klein, A., and Hagemeijer, A.: Cytogenetic and molecular analysis of the Ph^1 translocation in chronic myeloid leukemia. *In* Cancer Surveys 3. Edited by J. D. Rowley. Oxford, Oxford University Press, 1984, pp. 515–529.
40. de Klein, A., van Kessel, A. G., Grosveld, G., Bartram, C. R., Hagemeijer, A., Bootsma, D., Spurr, N. K., Heisterkamp, N., Groffen, J., Stephenson, J. R.: A cellular oncogene is translocated to the Philadelphia chromosome in chronic myelocytic leukemia. Nature, 300:765, 1982.
41. de Klein, A., Hagemeijer, A., Bartram, C. R., Houwen, R., Hoefsloot, L., Carbonell, F., Chan, L., Barnett, M., Greaves, M., Kleihamer, E., Heisterkamp, N., Groffen, J., and Grosveld, G.: BCR rearrangement and translocation of the c-*abl* oncogene in Philadelphia positive acute lymphoblastic leukemia. Blood, 68:1369, 1986.
42. De Caprio, J. A., Ludlow, J. W., Lynch, D., et al.: The product of the retinoblastoma gene has properties of a cell cycle regulatory element. Cell, 58:1085, 1989.
43. De The, H., Chomienne, C., Lanotte, M., Degos, L., and De Jean A.: The t(15;17) translocation of acute promyelocytic leukemia fuses the retinoic acid receptor alpha gene to a novel transcribed locus. Nature, 347:558, 1990.
44. Diaz, M. O., Ziemin, S., LeBeau, M. M., Pitha, P., Smith, S. D., Chilcote, R. R., Rowley, J. D.: Homozygous deletions of the α- and β1.-interferon genes in human leukemia and derived cell lines. Proc. Nat. Acad. Sci. USA, 85:5259, 1988.
45. Dryja, T. P., Cavenee, W. K., White, R., Rapaport, J. M., Petersen, R., Albert, D. M., Brins, G. A.: Homozygosity of chromosome 13 in retinoblastoma. N. Engl. J. Med., 310:550, 1984.
46. Duesberg, P. H.: Retroviruses as carcinogens and pathogens: Expectations and reality. Cancer Res., 47:1199, 1987.
47. Fearon, E. R., Cho, K. R., Nigro, J. M, Kearn, S. E., Simons, J. W., Ruppert, J. M., Hamilton, S. R., Presinger, A. L., Thomas, G., Kinzler, K. W., and Vogelstein, B: Identification of a chromosome 18q gene that is altered in colorectal cancers. Science, 247:49, 1990.
48. Fialkow, P. J., Singer, J. W., Raskind, W. H., Adamson, J. W., Jacobson, R. J., Bernstein, I. D., Dow, L. W., Najfeld, V., and Veith, R.: Clonal development, differentiation, and clinical remissions in acute nonlymphocytic leukemia. N. Engl. J. Med., 317:468, 1987.
49. Fifth International Workshop on Chromosomes in Leukemia-Lymphoma. Correlation of chromosome abnormalities with histologic and immunologic characteristics in non-Hodgkin's lymphoma and adult T-cell leukemia-lymphoma. Blood, 70:1554, 1987.
50. First International Workshop in Solid Tumors. Tucson, Arizona. March 3–5, 1985. Cancer Genet. Cytogenet., 19:3, 1986.
51. Fourth International Workshop on Chromosomes in Leukemia. Cancer Genet. Cytogenet., 11:249, 1984.
52. Francke, U.: Specific chromosome changes in the human heritable tumors retinoblastoma and nephroblastoma. *In* Chromosomes and Cancer. Edited by J. D. Rowley, and J. E. Ultmann. Bristol-Myers Symposia Series Vol. 5. New York, Academic Press, 1983, p. 99.
53. Friend, S. H., Bernards, R., Rogelj, S., Weinberg, R. A., Rapaport, J. M., Albert, D. M., and Dryja, T. P.: A human DNA segment with properties of the gene that predisposes to retinoblastoma. Nature, 323:643, 1986.
54. Fukuhara, S., Rowley, J. D., Variakojis, D., and Golomb, H. M.: Chromosome abnormalities in poorly differentiated lymphocytic lymphoma. Cancer Res., 39:3119, 1979.
55. Gahrton, G., and Robert, K.-H.: Chromosomal aberrations in chronic β-cell lymphocytic leukemia. Cancer Genet. Cytogenet., 6:171, 1982.
56. General report of the Sixth International Workshop on Chromosomes in Leukemia. Cancer Genet. Cytogenet., 40:149, 1989.
57. Gessler, M., Poustka, A., Cavene, W., Neve, R. L., Orkin, S. H., and Bruns, G. A.: Homozygous deletion in Wilms' tumor of a zinc finger gene identified by chromosome jumping. Nature, 343:774, 1990.
58. Gibas, Z., Prout, G., Connoly, J., Pontes, J. E., and Sandberg, A. A.: Nonrandom chromosomal changes in transitional cell carcinoma of the bladder. Cancer Res., 44:1257, 1984.
58A. Gishizky, M. L., McLaughlin, J., Pendergast, A. M., and Witte, O. N.: The 5′ noncoding region of the BCR/ABL oncogene augments its ability to stimulate the growth of immature lymphoid cells. Oncogene, 6:1299, 1991.
59. Golomb, H. M., Alimena, G., Rowley, J. D., Vardiman, J. W., Testa, J. R., and Sovik, C.: Correlation of occupation and karyotype in adults with acute nonlymphocytic leukemia. Blood, 60:404, 1982.
60. Gough, N. M., Geanig, D. P., Nicola, N. A., Baker, E., Pritchard, M., Callen, D. F., and Sutherland, G. R.: Localization of the human GM-GSF receptor gene to the X-Y pseudo-autosomal region. Nature, 345:734, 1990.
61. Groffen, J., Stephenson, J. R., Heisterkamp, N., deKlein, A., Bartram, C. R., and Grosveld, G.: Philadelphia chromosomal breakpoints are clustered within a limited region, bcr, on chromosome 22. Cell, 36:93, 1984.
62. Grundy, P., Cavenee, W. K., Koufos, A., Li, F. P., Meadows, A. T., and Morgan, K.: Familial predisposition to Wilms' tumor does not map to the short arm of chromosome 11. Nature, 336:374, 1988.
63. Hagemeijer, A., Hahlen, K., Sizoo, W., and Abels, J.: Translocation (9;11)(p21;q23) in three cases of acute monoblastic leukemia. Cancer Genet. Cytogenet., 5:95, 1982.
64. Han, T., Ozer, H., Sadamori, N., Emrich, L., Gomez, G. A., Henderson, E. S., Bloom, M. L., and Sandberg, A. A.: Prognostic importance of cytogenetic abnormalities in patients with chronic lymphocytic leukemia. N. Engl. J. Med., 310:288, 1984.
65. Heim, S., Nilbert, M., Vanni, R., Floderus, U. M., Mandahl, N., Liedgren, S., Lecca, U., Mitelman, F.: A specific translocation, t(12;14)(q14–15;q23–24) characterizes a subgroup of uterine leiomyomas. Cancer Gent. Cytogenet., 32:13, 1988.
66. Heim, S., and Mitelman, F.: Cancer Cytogenetics. New York, Alan R. Liss, Inc., 1987.
67. Heisterkamp, W., Stephenson, J. R., Groffen, J., Hansen, P. F., deKlein, A., Bertram, C. R., and Grosveld, G.: Localization of the C-abl oncogene adjacent to a translocation in chronic myelogenic leukemia. Nature, 306:239, 1983.
68. Hooberman, A. L., Rubin, C. M., Barton, K. P., and Westbrook, C. A.: Detection of the Philadelphia chromosome in acute lymphoblastic leukemia by pulsed-field gel electrophoresis. Blood, 74:1101, 1989.
69. Hooberman, A. L., Westbrook, C. A., Davey, F., Schiffer, C., Spiro, C., and Bloomfield, C. D.: Molecular detection of the Philadelphia chromosome (Ph^1) in adult acute lymphoblastic leukemia (ALL): Clinical, cytogenetic and immunophenotypic correlations in a CALGB study. Blood, 74:52a, 1989.
70. Huang, A., Campbell, C. E., Bonetta, L., McAndrews-Hill, M. S., Chilton-MacNeill, S., Coppes, M. J., Law, D. J., Feinberg, A. P., Yeger, H., and Williams, B. R. G.: Tissue, developmental, and tumor-specific expression of divergent transcripts in Wilms' tumor. Science, 250:991, 1990.
70A. Human Gene Mapping 10.5: Cytogenet. Cell Genet., 55:1, 1990.
71. Israel, M. A., Helman, L. J., and Miser, J.: Patterns of proto-oncogene expression: A novel approach to the development of tumor markers. Imp't. Adv. in Oncology, 1987.
72. ISCN (1985): An International System for Human Cytogenetic Nomenclature. Edited by D. G. Harnden, and H. P. Klinger. Published in collaboration with Cytogenet. Cell Genet., Basel, Karger, 1985.
73. Jenkins, R. B., Kimmel, D. W., Moertel, C. A., Schultz, C. G., Scheithamer, B. W., Kelly, P. J., and Dewald, G. W.: A cytogenetic study of 53 human gliomas. Cancer Genet. Cytogenet., 39:253, 1989.
74. Juliusson, G., Oscier, D. G., Fitchett, M., Ross, R. M., Stockdill, G., Mackie, M. J., Parker, A. C., Castoldi, G. L., Guneo, A, Kauutila, S., et al.: Prognostic subgroups in B-cell chronic lymphocytic leukemia defined by specific chromosomal abnormalities. N. Engl. J. Med., 323:720, 1990.
75. Kaiser-McCaw, B., Hecht, F., Harnden, D. G., and Teplitz, R. L.: Somatic rearrangement of chromosome 14 in human lymphocytes. Proc. Natl. Acad. Sci., 72:2071, 1975.
76. Klein, G.: Specific chromosomal translocations and the genesis of B-cell derived tumors in mice and men. Cell, 32:311, 1983.
77. Klein, G., and Klein, E.: Conditioned tumorigenicity of activated oncogenes. Cancer Res., 46:3211, 1986.
78. Knudson, A. G.: Mutation and cancer: Statistical study of retinoblastoma. Proc. Natl. Acad. Sci. U.S.A., 68:820, 1971.
79. Koduru, P. R. K., Filippa, D. A., Richardson, M. E., Jhanwar, S. C., Chaganti, S. R., Koziner, B., Clarkson, B. D., Lieberman, P. H., and Chaganti, R. S. K.: Cytogenetic and histologic correlations in malignant lymphomas. Blood, 69:97, 1987.
80. Kok, K., Osinga, J., Carritt, B., Davis, M. B., Van der Hout, A. H., Van der Veen, A. Y., deLeij, L. F., Berendsen, H. H., Postmus, P. E., Poppena, S., and Brys, C. H. C. M.: Deletion of a DNA sequence at the chromosomal region 3p21 in all major types of lung cancer. Nature, 330:578, 1987.
81. Kondo, K., Chilcote, R. R., Maurer, H. S., and Rowley, J. D.: Chromosome abnormalities in tumor cells from patients with sporadic Wilms' tumor. Cancer Res., 44:5376, 1984.

82. Koufos, A., Aleck, K. A., Cavenee, W. K., Grundy, P., Hadro, T., Kalbakji, A., Lampkin, B. C., and Morgan, K.: Familial Wiedemann-Beckwith syndrome and a second Wilms' tumor locus both map to 11p15.5. Am. J. Hum. Genet., 44:711, 1989.
83. Lang, R. A., Metcalf, D., Gough, N. M., Dunn, A. R., and Gonda, T. J.: Expression of a hemopoietic growth factor cDNA in a factor-dependent cell line results in autonomous growth and tumorigenicity. Cell, 43:531, 1985.
84. Larson, R. A., Williams, S. F., LeBeau, M. M., Bitter, M. A., Vardiman, J. W., and Rowley, J. D.: Acute myelomonocytic leukemia with abnormal eosinophils and inv(16) or t(16;16) has a favorable prognosis. Blood, 68:1242, 1986.
85. Larson, R. A., LeBeau, M. M., Vardiman, J. W., Testa, J. R., Golomb, H. M., Rowley, J. D.: The predictive value of initial cytogenetic studies in 148 adults with acute nonlymphocytic leukemia a 12 year study (1970–1982). Cancer Genet. Cytogenet., 10:219, 1983.
86. LeBeau, M. M., Albain, K. S., Larson, R. A., Vardiman, J. W., Davis, E. M., Blough, R. R., Golomb, H. M., and Rowley, J. D.: Clinical and cytogenetic correlations in 63 patients with therapy-related myelodysplastic syndromes and acute nonlymphocytic leukemia: Further evidence for characteristic abnormalities of chromosomes No. 5 and 7. J. Clin. Oncol., 4:325, 1986.
87. LeBeau, M. M., and Rowley, J. D.: Cytogenetics. *In* Hematology Ed. 4. Edited by W. J. Williams, C. Beutler, A. J. Erslow, and M. A. Lichtman. New York, McGraw Hill, 1989, pp. 78–89.
88. LeBeau, M. M., Bitter, M. A., and Larson, R. A.: The t(2;5)(p23;q35): A recurring chromosomal abnormality in Ki-1 positive anaplastic large cell lymphoma. Leukemia, 3:866, 1989.
89. LeBeau, M. M., and Larson, R. A.: Hematologic Malignancies in the Genetic Basis of Common Diseases. Edited by R. A. King, J. I. Rotter, and A. G. Motulsky. New York, Oxford Press, 1989.
90. LeBeau, M. M.: Chromosomal fragile sites and cancer-specific rearrangements. Blood, 67:849, 1986.
91. Le Beau, M. M., Pettenati, M. J., Lemons, R. S., Diaz, M. O., Westbrook, C. A., Larson, R. A., Sherr, C. J., and Rowley, J. D.: Assignment of the *GM-CSF, CSF-1,* and *FMS* genes to human chromosome 5 provides evidence for linkage of a family of genes regulating hematopoiesis and for their involvement in the deletion (5q) in myeloid disorders. Molecular Biology of Homo Sapiens, Cold Spring Harbor Symposium, 51:899, 1986.
92. Leder, P., Battey, J., Lenoir, G., Moulding, C., Murphy, W., Potter, H., Stewart, T., and Taub, R.: Translocations among antibody genes in human cancer. Science, 222:765, 1983.
93. Lee, W. H., Slew, J. Y., Hong, F. D., Sery, T. W., Donoso, L. A., Young, L. J., Bookstein, R., and Lee, E. Y. H.-P.: The retinoblastoma susceptibility gene encodes a nuclear phosphoprotein associated with DNA binding activity. Nature, 329:642, 1987.
94. Lee, W.-H., Bookstein, R., Hong, F., Young, L. T., Shew, J. Y., and Lee, E. Y.-H.P.: Human retinoblastoma susceptibility gene: Cloning, identification, and sequence. Science, 235:1394, 1987.
95. Longo, L., Pandolfi, P. P., Biondi, A., Rambaldi, A., Mancarelli, A., Lo-Coco, F., Diverio, D., Pegoraro, L., Avanzi, G., and Tabilio, A.: Rearrangements and aberrant expression of the retinoic acid receptor alpha gene in acute promyelocytic leukemias. J. Exp. Med., 172:1571, 1990.
96. Lukeis, R., Irving, L., Garson, M., and Hasthorpe, S.: Cytogenetics of non small cell lung cancer. Analysis of consistent non-random abnormalities. Genes, Chromosomes Cancer 3:116, 1991.
97. Mandahl, N., Heim, S., Arheden, K., Rydhom, A., Willen, H., and Mitelman, F.: Three major cytogenetic subgroups can be identified among chromosomally abnormal solitary lipomas. Hum. Genet., 70:203, 1988.
98. Manolov, G., and Manolova, Y.: Marker band in one chromosome 14 from Burkitt lymphomas. Nature, 237:33, 1972.
99. Mark, J., Dahlenfors, R., and Ekedahl, C.: Cytogenetics of the human mixed salivary gland tumor. Hereditas, 99:115, 1983.
100. Mark, J., Levan, G., and Mitelman, F.: Identification by fluorescence of the G chromosome lost in human meningiomas. Hereditas, 71:163, 1972.
101. Mark, J.: Chromosomal characteristic of neurogenic tumors in adults. Hereditas, 68:61, 1971.
102. Mellentin, J. D., Murre, C., Donlon, T., McCaw, P. S., Smith, S. D., Carroll, A. J., McDonald, M. E., Baltimore, D., and Cleary, M. L.: The gene for enhanced binding proteins E12/E47 lies at the t(1;19) breakpoint in acute leukemias. Science, 246:379, 1989.
103. Michael, P. M., Levin, M. D., and Garson, O. M.: Translocation 1;19—a new cytogenetic abnormality in acute lymphocytic leukemia. Cancer Genet. Cytogenet., 12:333, 1984.
104. Mitelman, F.: Catalog of Chromosome Aberrations in Cancer. New York, Alan R. Liss, Inc., 1988.
105. Mitelman, F.: Catalogue of chromosome aberrations in cancer. Cytogenet. Cell. Genet., 36:1, 1983.
106. Mitelman, F.: Catalog of chromosome aberrations in cancer. Progress and Topics in Cytogenetics Vol. 5. Edited by A. A. Sandberg. New York, Alan R. Liss, Inc., 1985.
106A. Mitelman, F.: Catalog of chromosome aberrations in cancer. 4th Edition. Edited by F. Mitelman. New York, Wiley-Liss, 1991.
107. Mitelman, F., Nilsson, P. G., Brandt, C., Alimena, G., Gastaldi, R., and Dallaicola, B.: Chromosome pattern, occupation and clinical features in patients with acute nonlymphocytic leukemia. Cancer Genet. Cytogenet., 4:187, 1981.
108. Mitelman, F., Mark, J., Nilsson, P. L., Dencker, H., Norryd., C., and Tranberg, K. G.: Chromosome banding pattern in colonic polyps. Hereditas, 78:63, 1974.
109. Miyamoto, K., Tomita, N., Ishii, A., Miyamoto, N., Nonaka, H., Kondo, T., Tanaka, T., Tsubota, T., and Kitajima, K.: Chromosome abnormalities of leukemia cells in adult patients with T-cell leukemia. J. Natl. Cancer Inst., 73:353, 1984.
109A. Miyoshi, H., Shimizu, K., Kozu, T., Maseki, N., Kaneko, Y., and Ohki, M: The t(8;21) breakpoints on chromosome 21 in acute myeloid leukemia are clustered within a limited region of a single gene, AML1. Proc. Natl. Acad. Sci. USA, 88:10431, 1991.
110. Morris, C. M., Reeve, A. E., Fitzgerald, P. H., Hollings, P. E., Beard, M. E. J., and Heaton, D. C.: Genomic diversity correlates with clinical variation in Ph^1-negative chronic myeloid leukemia. Nature, 320:281, 1986.
111. Murphree, A. L., and Benedict, W. F.: Retinoblastoma: Clues to human oncogenesis. Science, 219:1028, 1984.
112. Naylor, S. L., Johnson, B. E., Minna, J. D., and Sagakuchi, A. Y.: Loss of heterozygosity of chromosome 3p markers in small cell lung cancer. Nature, 329:451, 1987.
113. Nilbert, M., and Heim, S.: Uterine leiomyoma cytogenetics. Genes, Chromosomes and Cancer, 2:3, 1990.
114. Nomiyama, H., Fromental, C., and Xiao, J. H.: Cell-specific activity of the constituent elements of the simian virus 40 enhancer. Proc. Natl. Acad. Sci. U.S.A., 84:7881, 1987.
115. Nowell, P. C., and Hungerford, D. A.: A minute chromosome in human granulocytic leukemia. Science, 132:1497, 1960.
116. Offit, K., Hollis, R., Kodurn, P. R. K., Fillipa, D., Jhanwar, S. C., Clarkson, B. C., and Chaganti, R. S. K.: 18q21 rearrangement in diffuse large cell lymphoma. Incidence and clinical significance. Br. J. Haematol., 72:178, 1989.
117. Ohno, H., Takimoto, G., and McKeithan, T. W.: The candidate proto-oncogene bcl-3 is related to genes implicated in cell lineage determination and cell cycle control. Cell, 60:991, 1990.
118. Parmiter, A. H., Balaban, G., Clark, W. H., Jr., and Nowell, P. C.: Possible involvement of the chromosome region 10q24–26 in early stages of melanocytic neoplasia. Cancer, Genetics, Cytogenetics, 30:313, 1989.
119. Pathak, S., Strong, L. C., Ferrell, R. E., and Trindale, A.: Familial renal cell carcinoma with a 3:11 chromosome translocation united to tumor cells. Science, 217:939, 1982.
120. Pearson, M. G., Vardiman, J. W., LeBeau, M. M., Rowley, J. D., Schwartz, S., Kerman, S. L., Cohen, M. M., Fleishman, E. W., and Progogina, E. L.: increased numbers of marrow basophils may be associated with a t(6;9) in ANLL. Amer. J. Hemat., 18:393, 1985.
121. Pedersen-Bjergaard, J., and Philip, P.: Cytogenetic characteristics of therapy-related acute nonlymphocytic leukemia, preleukemia, and acute myeloproliferative syndrome: Correlation with clinical data for 61 consecutive cases. Br. J. Haematol., 66:199, 1987.
122. Pejovic, T., Heim, S., Mandahl, N., Elmfors, B., Floderus, U. M., Furgyik, S., Heim, G., Willen, H., and Mitelman, F.: Trisomy 12 is a consistent chromosome aberration in benign ovarian tumors. Genes, Chromosomes and Cancer, 2:48, 1990.
122A. Pendergast, A. M., Muller, A. J., Havlik, M. H., Maru, Y., and Witte, O. N.: BCR sequences essential for transformation by the BCR-ABL oncogene bind to the ABL SH2 regulatory domain in a non-phosphotyrosine-dependent manner. Cell, 66:161, 1991.
123. Pugh, W. C., Pearson, M., Vardiman, J. W., and Rowley, J. D.: Philadelphia chromosome-negative chronic myelogenous leukaemia: A morphologic reassessment. Br. J. Haematol., 60:457, 1985.
124. Raimondi, S. D., Pui, C.-H., Behm, F. G., and Williams, D. L.: 7q32–q36 translocations in childhood T cell leukemia: Cytogenetic evidence for involvement of the T cell receptor chain gene. Blood, 69:131, 1987.
125. Reeve, A. E., Sih, S. A., Raizis, A. M., and Feinberg, A. P.: Loss of allelic heterozygosity at a second locus in chromosome 11 in sporadic Wilms' tumor cells. Mol. Cell. Biol., 9:1799, 1989.
126. Robert, K.-H., Gahrton, G., Friberg, K., Zech, L., and Nilson, B.: Extra chromosome 12 and prognosis in chronic lymphocytic leukemia. Scand. J. Haematol., 28:163, 1982.
127. Rowley, J. D., Diaz, M. O., Espinosa, R., III, Patel, Y. D., Van Melle, E., Ziemin, S., Taillon-Miller, P., Lichter, P., Evans, G. A., and Kersey, J. H.: Mapping chromosome band 11q23 in human acute leukemia with biotingrated probes: Identification of 11q23 translocation breakpoints with yeast artificial chromosome. Proc. Natl. Acad. Sci. U.S.A., 87:9358, 1990.
128. Rowley, J. D.: Chromosome abnormalities in leukemia and lymphoma. Semin. Hematol., 27:122, 1990.
128A. Rowley, J. D.: Chromosomal abnormalities. *In* Cancer Principles and Practice of Oncology. 2nd Edition. Edited by V. T. DeVita, S. Hellman, and S. A. Rosenberg. Philadelphia, J. B. Lippincott, 1985, Vol. 1, p. 67.
129. Rowley, J. D.: Molecular cytogenetics: Rosetta stone for understanding cancer. Twenty-ninth GHA Clowes Memorial Award Lecture. Cancer Res., 50:3816, 1990.
130. Rowley, J. D.: Identification of translocation with quinacrine fluorescence in a patient with acute leukemia. Annal de Genet., 16:109, 1973.
131. Rowley, J. D., Golomb, H. M., and Vardiman, J. W.: Nonrandom chromosome abnormalities in acute leukemia and dysmyelopoietic syndromes in patients with previously treated malignant disease. Blood, 58:759, 1981.
132. Rowley, J. D., Golomb, H. M., and Daugherty, C.: 15/17 translocation, a consistent chromosomal change in acute promyelocytic leukemia. Lancet, 1:549, 1977.
133. Rowley, J. D., and Testa, J. R.: Chromosome abnormalities in malignant hematologic diseases. *In* Advances in Cancer Research. New York, Academic Press Inc., 1983, pp. 103–148.
134. Rowley, J. D., and Potter, D.: Chromosomal banding patterns in acute nonlymphocytic leukemia. Blood, 47:705, 1976.
135. Rowley, J. D.: A new consistent chromosomal abnormality in chronic myelogenous leukemia. Nature, 243:290, 1973.
136. Rubin, C. M., Carrino, J. J., Dickler, M. N., Leibowitz, D., Smith, S. D., and Westbrook, C. A.: Heterogeneity of genomic fusion of *BCR* and *ABL* in Philadelphia chromosome-positive acute lymphoblastic leukemia. Proc. Natl. Acad. Sci. U.S.A., 85:2795, 1988.
137. Sadamori, N., Nishino, K., Kusano, M., Tomonega, Y., Tagawa, M., Yao, E., Sasagawa, I., Nakamura, H., and Ichimaru, M.: Significance of chromosome 14 anomaly at band q11 in Japanese patients with adult T-cell leukemia. Cancer, 58:2244, 1986.
138. Schwab, M., Alitalo, K., Klempnauer, K.-H., Varmuss, H. E., Bishop, J. M., Gilbert, F., Brodeur, G., Goldstein, M., and Trent, J.: Amplified DNA with limited homology to myc cellular oncogene is shared by human neuroblastoma cell lines and a neuroblastoma tumour. Nature, 305:245, 1983.
139. Secker-Walker, L. M., Swansbury, G. J., Hardisty, R. M., Sallan, S. E., Garson, D. M., Sakamura, M., and Lawler, S. D.: Cytogenetics of acute lymphoblastic leukemia in children as a factor in the prediction of long-survival. Br. J. Haematol., 52:389, 1982.
140. Shtivelman, E., Lifshitz, B., Robert, P., Gale, R. P., and Canaani, E.: Fused transcript of abl and bcr genes in chronic myelogenous leukaemia. Nature, 315:550, 1985.
141. Solomon, E., Voss, R., Hall, V., Bodner, W. F., Jass, J. R., Jeffreys, A. J., Lucibello, F. C., Patel, I., and Rider, S. H.: Chromosome 5 allele loss in human colorectal carcinoma. Nature, 328:616, 1987.
142. Stong, R. C., Korsmeyer, S. J., Parkin, J. L., Arthur, D. C., and Kersey, J. H.: Human acute leukemia cell line with the t(4;11) chromosomal rearrangement exhibits B-lineage and monocytic characteristics. Blood, 67:391, 1986.

143. Sutherland, G. R., and Hecht, F.: Fragile Sites on Human Chromosomes. New York, Oxford University Press, 1985.
144. Szucs, S., Muller-Brechlin, R., De Riese, W., and Kovacs, G.: Deletion 3p: The only chromosome loss in a primary renal cell carcinoma. Cancer Genet. Cytogenet., 26:369, 1987.
145. Testa, J. R., and Rowley, J. D.: Chromosomes in leukemia and lymphoma with special emphasis on methodology. In The Leukemic Cell. Edited by D. Catovsky. Edinburgh, Churchill-Livingstone, 1981, p. 184.
146. Testa, J. R., Karnofsky, J. R., Rowley, J. D., Baron, J. M., and Vardiman, J. W.: Karyotypic patterns and their clinical significance in polycythemia vera. Am. J. Hematol., 11:29, 1981.
147. Thangavelu, M., Olopade, O. I., Beckman, E., Vardiman, J. W., Larson, R. A., McKeithan, T. W., LeBeau, M. M., and Rowley, J. D.: Clinical morphologic and cytogenetic characteristics of patients with lymphoid malignancies characterised by both t(14;8)(q32;q21) and t(8;14)(q23;q32) or t(8;22)(q24;q11). Genes, Chromosom. Cancer, 2:147, 1990.
148. The Third International Workshop on Chromosomes in Leukemia. Cancer Genet. Cytogenet., 4:95, 1981.
149. Travis, L. B., Pierre R. V., and DeWald, G. W.: Ph¹-negative chronic granulocytic leukemia: A nonentity. Am. J. Clin. Pathol., 85:186, 1986.
150. Trent, J. M.: The Third International Workshop on Chromosomes in Solid Tumors (IWCST). Tucson, Arizona. Cancer Genet. Cytogenet., 41:207, 1990.
151. Trent, J. M., Stanbridge, E. J., and McBride, H. L.: Tumorgenicity in human melanoma cell lines controlled by introduction of human chromosome 6. Science, 247:568, 1990.
152. Trent, J. M., Kaneko, Y., and Mitelman, F.: Report of the committee on structural chromosome changes in neoplasia. Human gene mapping 10. Cytogenet. Cell. Genet., 51:533, 1989.
153. Tsujimoto, Y., Finger, L. R., Yunis, J. J., Nowell, P. C., and Croce, C. J.: Cloning of the chromosome breakpoint of neoplastic B cells with the t(14;18) chromosome translocation. Science, 226:1098, 1984.
154. Turc-Carel C., Limon, J., Dal Cin, P., Rao, U., Karakousis, C., and Sandberg, A. A.: Cytogenetic studies of adipose tissue tumors. II Recurrent reciprocal translocation t(12;8)(q13;p11) in myxoid liposarcomas. Cancer Genet. Cytogenet., 23:291, 1986.
155. Turc-Carel, C., Dal Cin, P., Boghosian, L., Terk-Zakarian, J., and Sandberg, A. A.: Consistent breakpoints in region 14q22–q24 in uterine leiomyoma. Cancer Genet. Cytogenet., 32:25, 1988.
156. Turc-Carel, C., Philip, I., Berger, M. P., Philip, T., and Lenoir, G. M.: Chromosomal translocation (11;22) in cell lines of Ewing's sarcoma. C. R. Seances Acad. Sci. III, 296:1101, 1983.
157. Turc-Carel, C., Dal Cin, P., Limon, J., Rao, U., Li, F. P., Corson, J. M., Zimmerman, R., Parry, D. M., Cowan, J. M., and Sandberg, A. A.: Involvement of chromosome X in primary cytogenetic changes in human neoplasia: Nonrandom translocation in synovial sarcoma. Proc. Natl. Acad. Sci. U.S.A., 84:1981, 1987.
158. Ueshima, Y., Rowley, J. D., Variakojis, D., Winter, J., Gordon, L.: Cytogenetic studies on patients with chronic T cell leukemia/lymphoma. Blood, 63:1028, 1984.
159. Van den Berghe, H., Vermaelen, K., Mecucci, C., Barbieri, C., and Tricot, G.: The 5q-anomaly. Cancer Genet. Cytogenet., 17:189, 1985.
160. Vogelstein, B., Fearon, E. R., Hamilton, S. R., Kern, S. E., Aeisinger, A. C., Leppert, M., Nakamura, Y., White, R., Smits, A. M., and Bos, J. L.: Genetic alterations during colorectal-tumor development. N. Engl. J. Med., 319:525, 1988.
161. Von Lindern, M., Poustka, A., Lerach, H., and Grosveld, G.: The t(6;9) chromosome translocation associated with a specific subtype of acute nonlymphocytic leukemia. Mol. Cell. Biol., 10:4016, 1990.
162. Wang, N., and Perkins, K. L.: Involvement of band 3p14 in t(3;8) hereditary renal cancer. Cancer Genet. Cytogenet., 11:479, 1984.
163. Westbrook, C. A., Rubin, C. M., Carrino, J. J., LeBeau, M. M., Bernards, A., and Rowley, J. D.: Long-range mapping of the Philadelphia chromosome by pulsed-field gel electrophoresis. Blood, 71:697, 1988.
164. Westbrook, C. A., LeBeau, M. M., Diaz, M. O., Groffen, J., and Rowley, J. D.: Chromosomal localization and characterization of c-abl in the t(6;9) of acute nonlymphocytic leukemia. Proc. Natl. Acad. Sci. U.S.A., 82:8742, 1985.
165. Whang-Peng, J., Triche, T. J., Knutsen, T., Miser, J., Douglass, E. C., Israel, M. A.: Chromosome translocation in peripheral neuroepithelioma. N. Engl. J. Med., 311:584, 1984.
166. Whang-Peng, J., Canellos, G. P., Carbone, P. P., and Tjio, J. H.: Clinical implications of cytogenetic variants in chronic myelocytic leukemia (CML). Blood, 32:755, 1968.
167. Whang-Peng, J., Bunn, Jr., P.A., Kao-Shan, C. S., Lee, E. C., Carney, D. N., Gazdar, A., and Minna, J. D.: A nonrandom chromosomal abnormality, del 3p(14–23), in human small cell lung cancer (SCLC). Cancer Genet. Cytogenet., 6:119, 1982.
168. Williams, D. L., Look, A. T., Melvin, S. L., Roberson, P. K., Dahl, G., Flake, T., and Stass, S.: New chromosomal translocations correlate with specific immunophenotypes of childhood acute lymphoblastic leukemia. Cell, 36:101, 1984.
169. Williams, D. L., Tsiatis, A., Brodeur, G. M. G., Look, A. T., Melvin, S. L., Bowman, W. P., Kalwinsky, D. K., Rivera, G., and Dahl, G. V.: Prognostic importance of chromosome number in 136 untreated children with acute lymphoblastic leukemia. Blood, 60:864, 1982.
170. Working Formulation for Clinical Usage: National Cancer Institute sponsored study of classification of non-Hodgkin's lymphomas. Cancer, 49:2112, 1982.
171. Yoshida, M. A., Ohyashiki, K., Ochi, K., Gibas, A., Prout, G. R., Jr., Pontes, J. E., Huben, R., and Sandberg, A. A.: Rearrangement of chromosome 3 in renal cell carcinoma. Cancer Genet. Cytogenet., 19:351, 1986.
172. Yunis, J. J., and Soreng, A. L.: Constitutive fragile sites and cancer. Science, 226:1199, 1984.
173. Yunis, J. J.: The chromosomal basis of human neoplasia. Science, 221:227, 1983.
174. Yunis J. J., Frizzera, G., Oken, M. M., McKenna, J., Theologicdes, A., and Arnesen, M.: Multiple recurrent genomic defects in follicular lymphoma; a possible model for cancer. N. Engl. J. Med., 316:79, 1987.
175. Zankl, H., and Zang, K. D.: Cytological and cytogenetical studies on brain tumors. 4. Identification of the missing G chromosome in human meningiomas as no 22 by fluorescence technique. Human Genetik, 14:167, 1970.
176. Zech, L., Gahrton, G., Hammarstrom, L., Juliusson, G., Mallstedt, H., Robert, K. H., and Smith, C. I.: Inversion of chromosome 14 marks human T-cell chronic lymphocytic leukemia. Nature, 308:858, 1984.
177. Zech, L., Haglund, U., Nilsson, K., and Klein, G.: Characteristic chromosomal abnormalities in biopsies and lymphoid-cell lines from patients with Burkitt and non-Burkitt lymphomas. Int. J. Cancer, 17:47, 1976.
178. Zech, L., Bergh, J., and Nilsson, K.: Karyotypic characterization of established cell lines and short term cultures of human lung cancer. Cancer Genet. Cytogenet., 15:335, 1985.

Biochemistry of Cancer

Edward Bresnick

On Progress in Understanding the Biochemistry of the Cancer Cell

Phenomenal progress has occurred in the last 10 years, first in understanding the intricacies of communication within and between normal cells, and secondly in defining the biochemical differences between normal and cancer cells. Much of this progress is attributable to the discovery of oncogenes, their normal counterparts, protooncogenes, of the mechanisms of signal transduction, and of some of the details of the biochemistry of the cell cycle. Most of these topics will be covered in other chapters in this section.

Within this chapter, a brief historical perspective of the biochemistry of the cancer cell will be presented with concentration on the contributions of intermediary metabolism to the development of testable hypotheses relative to cancer etiology. In addition, some of the unique aspects of the biochemistry of the cancer cell will be discussed with the view of providing clues to early diagnosis of the disease in humans, of depicting potential targets for therapy, and of providing some beacon as to the causes for the aberrancies we understand as constituting the cancer cell.

In this discussion, information will be drawn from experiments with animal model systems, with cell cultures, and with humans, using both intact and *in vitro* systems. The central hypothesis is the universality of the mechanisms of cancer etiology and the applicability of data derived from these model systems to a discussion of the problem within the human population.

Early History of Research in Cancer Biochemistry

Energetics. The biochemistry of cancer received its real beginning with the work of Otto Warburg during the 1920's–1930's.[162] Warburg represented a dominant force in cancer research until 1940. Using predominantly the tissue slice technique, Warburg measured the utilization of glucose, the production of lactic acid and of carbon dioxide, and the utilization of oxygen by various tumors and normal tissues. He noted a high production of lactate by tumor slices in the presence of oxygen. In contrast, in rapidly-dividing normal systems, e.g., fetal tissue, the observed high rate of lactate production was completely abolished by oxygen.

The phenotype of elevated production of lactate in presence of oxygen was believed by him to represent a fundamental property of cancer cells which was not found in normal tissue. Consequently to Warburg, cancer represented a problem in intermediary metabolism. More specifically, a damage to some component of the respiratory chain was the underlying culprit.

Despite the claim by Warburg for a defect in respiration of tumor tissue, cogent arguments refuting this hypothesis were formulated and these have been summarized by Weinhouse.[164] The prevailing view currently accepts Weinhouse's analysis of the operation of both respiration and glycolysis within tumors. An excellent historical perspective of this problem is afforded in the review by Shapot.[135] Weinhouse pointed out that oxygen, which was consumed by neoplastic cells as effectively as by some normal cells, resulted in an inhibition of the formation of glycolytic end products. In fact, in a series of well-differentiated hepatomas, low rates of aerobic glycolysis were observed of the same magnitude as seen in normal liver with comparable rates of respiration .

The inhibition of glycolysis by oxidative phosphorylation has been called the *Pasteur Effect*. Respiration is markedly dependent upon the availabilities of intermediates such as ADP and inorganic phosphate, i.e., respiratory control. Competition for ADP and inorganic phosphate occurs in respiration and glycolysis, resulting in an apparent inhibition of glucose utilization by oxygen due in part to a reduced availability of these cofactors for phosphorylation under aerobic conditions.

Whether or not cancers can take full advantage of energetics which are potentially derivable from both respiration and glycolysis has been a question of major concern, although the current evidence would suggest not. For example, Urbach has reported a marked reduction in the partial pressure of oxygen in skin cancers as determined by inserting an oxygen electrode into the tumors as well as into the surrounding normal tissue.[153] A very interesting confirmation and extension of these results has been provided by the experiments of Malmgren and Flanigan in an animal model system.[88] Spores of *Clostridium tetani* were implanted in normal mice as well as in several murine tumors. The normal mice survived unaffected by these spores, while the tumor-bearing mice died because the spores were able to germinate in the low pO_2 environment of the tumors. Busch and colleagues have demonstrated the barely detectable level of citrate production by a tumor under *in vivo* conditions.[25] Yet, slices of the same tumor, when incubated in the presence of an appropriate amount of oxygen, produced citrate at a level which approximated that seen with normal liver.

All these studies strongly suggested local hypoxia as the underlying cause for the apparent deficiency in respiration of tumors; an inherent defect in respiration was not the problem. The problem of the utilization of glucose under rather unfavorable conditions by tumors, which confounded Warburg, is most probably due to the presence within tumor plasma membranes of a low K_m hexokinase which afforded a "trap" mechanism for the capture of this nutrient, even when present at low concentrations in the surrounding medium.[135] Indeed, a substantial body of literature has shown a hypoglycemic effect of large tumors as a result of this "trap"; this effect was not the result of ectopic hormone production.[133] The hypoglycemic effect may in part contribute to the problems associated with cachexia in the tumor-bearing host (see later section).

Other Examples from Intermediary Metabolism. Following the Warburg period, a number of technological advances resulted which enhanced the analytical capabilities of researchers by allowing for the better quantification of cofactors, enzymes and metabolic pathways in a large number of transplantable animal tumors. Based upon such measurements in a series of transplantable animal tumor models, Greenstein formulated a Convergence Hypothesis to explain a number of interesting aspects of neoplasia.[56] The Convergence Hypothesis was more of a descriptive formulation rather than a mechanistic discussion of tumor etiology. He noted that cancers tended to discard certain enzymes or pathways that were not required for growth processes. This observation was particularly true for transplanted tumors upon successive rounds of transplantation. For example, the latency times tended to decrease, i.e., a tumor of a certain size was reached within a shorter period of time after serial transplantations. Concomitant with this decrease in latency (and enhanced growth rate), the enzymatic profiles of the tumors tended to converge to a common pattern. In fact, the adoption of a similar enzymatic matrix by these tumors was really a reflection of the increase in growth rate and not an inherent feature of all cancers, slow- or fast-growing.

Chemically-induced hepatocarcinogenesis in rodents provided a number of models that could be analyzed for a number of different parameters. The Millers made several interesting observations relative to chemical hepatocarcinogenesis induced by the administration to rats of an azo dye, p-dimethylaminoazobenzene.[90] The azo dye tended to interact with certain proteins present in the livers of normal rats, i.e., a correlation existed between the formation of protein bound azo dye and hepatocarcinogenesis. The Millers believed that as a result of this interaction, a crucial protein(s) in the liver could have been altered in terms of function, or completely deleted. This protein purportedly would be involved in the regulation of a key event in growth but would not be essential for the survival of the target cells destined for cancer. Thus was born the Protein Deletion Theory of Carcinogenesis. Although the key protein or proteins have never been fully characterized, this hypothesis stimulated much research in the comparison of patterns in normal and neoplastic tissues and drove the field for a number of years.

In 1950, Van Potter modified the Protein Deletion Hypothesis after consideration of the results of a number of measurements of enzymatic content of neoplastic and normal liver.[113] Potter recognized the existence of alternate pathways involving common intermediates; some of these pathways favored anabolism and therefore growth, and some, catabolism. Furthermore, he noted that competition often existed in regard to the relative amounts of the component that was subjected to either anabolism or catabolism. Based upon his observations, he proposed the loss of systems of catabolism as a central feature of tumorigenesis, the Catabolic Deletion Hypothesis. The beauty of this hypothesis, and in fact of much of Potter's work, was the formulation of readily-testable questions. Although not providing any profound insight into the key event(s) underlying tumorigenesis, the Catabolic Deletion Hypothesis offered additional correlations between the rate of tumor growth and their enzymatic composition, i.e., the more rapidly proliferating tumors were associated with the greater loss of enzymes of catabolism.

A significant blow to the Catabolic Deletion Hypothesis as an explanation for cancer development came with the analysis of rapidly-proliferating normal systems, e.g., regenerating and fetal liver. As pointed out by Potter in the previous edition of this volume, a number of important enzymes that function in anabolism, e.g., DNA polymerase, were present in regenerating or fetal livers but not detectable in adult liver.[116] Conversely, catabolic enzymes, e.g., thymine reductase, were markedly diminished in these rapidly proliferating but normal systems when compared to adult liver. Consequently, the deletion or loss of catabolic enzymes could occur in *normal* albeit rapidly proliferating systems, as well as in tumors. Anabolic enzymes appeared in normal rapidly-proliferating systems as well as in tumors as a reflection of the rapidity of growth and were absent in adult liver.

Whether or not a *specific* protein regulator, but not an enzyme, is deleted prior to oncogenesis remains to be established. Such a protein, which has been postulated by Pitot and Heidelberger, could function as a key in triggering a panoply of regulatory steps.[110]

A further modification was proffered by Potter in his Minimal Deviation Hypothesis in which cancer cells were noted to deviate from normal cells with regard to a number of nonessential as well as some vitally important components.[114] Of great importance to this hypothesis, and subsequently to cancer research, was the development of the Morris hepatoma models. Accordingly, a brief digression on these hepatomas is germane to this discussion.

Through the selective use of a hepatocarcinogen, N-(2-fluorenyl)-phthalamic acid, Morris was able to develop a series of rat hepatomas that varied in growth rate, resulting in a transition from well differentiated tumors to poorly differentiated.[92] These were referred to as minimal deviation hepatomas. Subsequently, a number of these hepatomas were recruited into cell culture which added a further dimension to the quality of the questions that could be posed.

Potter believed that he and other investigators were now in position to reduce the differences between liver and hepatomas to only a few measurable effects. The analysis of the enzymatic composition of the slow, intermediate and fast growing varieties of the Morris hepatomas could clearly show what enzymes (either by appearance or deletion) would be inextricably linked to cancer, and which ones to growth rate. Although as viewed today, the Minimal Deviation Hypothesis would appear rather simplistic, it was responsible for several important findings, a) tumors of varying growth rates were analyzed as to enzyme content and the relationship between activity and proliferation rate was further corroborated, and b) the hypothesis forced the realization of the lack of importance of a number of documented enzymological changes in regard to the process of cancer development. An example of the remarkable correlation between the activity of a key enzyme in nucleotide metabolism, ribonucleotide reductase, and cell proliferation is afforded by the work of Elford et al. which is reproduced in Figure I-9-1.[38]

Refinement of Potter's hypothesis came with the development of the Molecular Correlation Concept by Weber who noted the quantitative and qualitative variations in the degree of neoplasia as related to the concentrations of certain enzymes that acted as regulators of key metabolic pathways.[163] The key enzymes were defined as a) regulating the rates and directions of competing (or opposing) metabolic pathways, e.g., glucokinase and glucose-6-phosphatase, b) overcoming thermodynamic barriers, e.g., phosphofructokinase, c) providing a common step in two or more metabolic pathways, e.g., citrate synthase, d) representing the first or last step in a reaction sequence, e.g., glutamine-dependent carbamyl phosphate synthetase, e) providing a target for feedback regulation of the allosteric variety, e.g., thymidine kinase, and f) exhibiting isoenzymic patterns, e.g., the hexokinases.

Those metabolic pathways that contained enzymes which fulfilled one or more of these criteria are indicated in Table I-9-1 along with the alteration that was observed in cancer.

One of the virtues of the Molecular Correlation Concept is the direction of attention to control of metabolic pathways at multiple steps as probably mediated by a single regulator.

Table I-9-1. Molecular Correlation Concept and Affected Processes*

Biochemical Process	Alteration in Cancer Cells
Pyrimidine and Purine Synthesis	Increased
Pyrimidine and Purine Catabolism	Decreased
RNA and DNA Syntheses	Increased
Glucose Catabolism	Increased
Glucose Synthesis	Decreased
Amino Acid Catabolism (for Gluconeogenesis)	Decreased
Urea Cycle	Decreased

*Adapted from Weber[161]

Table I-9-2. Expression of Oncofetal Proteins in Neoplasia

Fetal enzymes, e.g., hexokinase type I
Fetal antigens, e.g., α-fetoprotein
Plasminogen activator
Growth factors, e.g., PDGF
Polypeptide hormones, e.g., thyrocalcitonin
Cellular oncogene products, e.g., AP-1
Angiogenesis factors

This concept of a master regulator had previously been espoused as the Pleiotypic Response Hypothesis by Tomkins and his colleagues in which it was proposed that under normal conditions, a constant group of metabolically-unrelated steps would coordinately react in response to environmental modulation and as a result, affect the rate of growth.[65,148] As stated by Herschko and colleagues.[65]

"....the transformed phenotype itself may be the result of constant pleiotypic activation which, if true, could render transformed cells independent of growth stimulants normally required."

Therefore, a mutation in a *single* gene could affect a whole series of events which characterizes the malignant phenotype. This postulate predated and predicted the whole concept of signal transduction which is discussed in Chapter I-4.

Oncofetal Protein Expression in Cancer Cells

As indicated above, a number of the enzymatic changes that are observed in neoplastic tissues resemble those that are found in fetal systems. This observation has been responsible for the belief that neoplasia may in fact represent a dedifferentiation or retrodifferentiation of mature cells, as stated by Potter– "oncogeny is blocked ontogeny".[115] The fetal proteins that disappear as a result of maturation and are no longer expressed in adult tissues but reappear in cancerous tissues are referred to as oncofetal proteins. A representative list of such proteins is provided in Table I-9-2.

One of the first examples of oncofetal proteins was provided by the report of Schapira et al. who noted an unusual form of aldolase in primary liver cancer.[131] Aldolase occurs in multimolecular forms of tetrameric structure with aldolase A representing the predominant form in muscle; aldolase A is absent from normal adult liver. In fetal liver, aldolase A occurs associated with the liver-specific aldolase B. In primary hepatocellular carcinoma, only aldolase A is present.

A number of key enzymes occur as isoenzymes with the proportions of the different forms varying as a function of

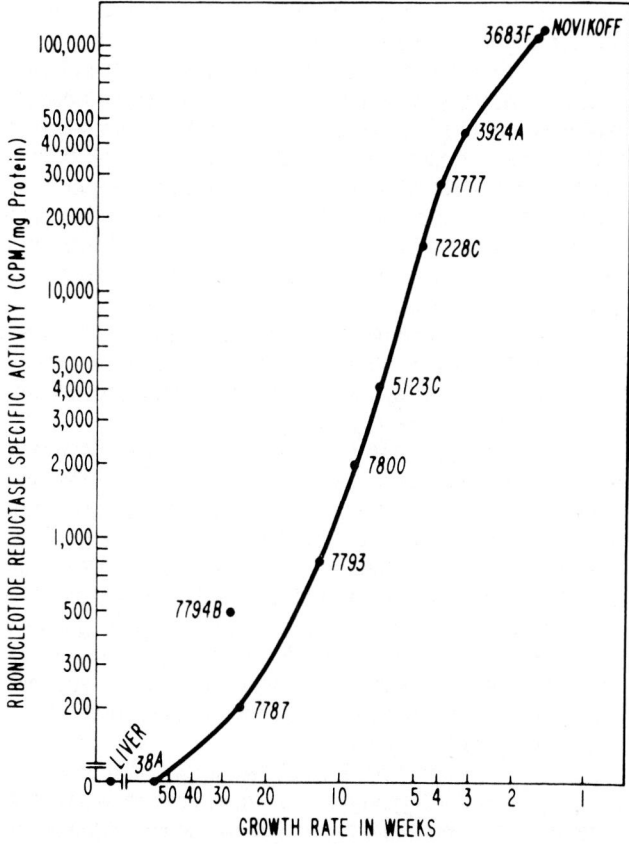

Figure I-9-1. Specific Activity of Ribonucleotide Reductase in Hepatomas of Varying Growth Rates. Rat hepatomas, indicated within the figure, were assayed for ribonucleotide reductase and the specific activity is plotted as a function of growth rate. The growth rate is expressed as the time required to reach a size that is normal for transplantation. (Data from Elfords et al.[38])

ontogeny. One of the prime examples in this regard are the hexokinases, i.e., glucose-ATP phosphotransferases. This family of enzymes, which plays a vital role in the utilization of glucose, occurs in 4 molecular forms, Types I through IV. Types I through III are referred to as hexokinases with all possessing a low K_m for glucose. Type IV phosphotransferase is glucokinase which is distinguished from the other hexokinases by its high K_m for glucose. The predominant forms in adult liver are Types I and IV. In fetal liver, Type IV glucokinase is barely detectable while Type I hexokinase is the major isoenzyme present. In hepatocarcinogenesis, a progressive reduction in the activity (and amount) of glucokinase is noted with a concomitant rise in Type I hexokinase.[160]

Phosphofructokinase, a key regulatory enzyme in glycolysis, also occurs in at least 4 molecular forms in eukaryotic systems with Isozyme I found predominantly in muscle, while Isozyme IV is noted mostly in liver. In the normal rapidly-proliferating systems, regenerating and fetal liver, as well as in a series of hepatomas, Type IV phosphofructokinase was also found but in much higher amount than in normal liver.[141] Pyruvate kinase, another key regulator of glycolysis, exists in isoenzymic forms with Type I pyruvate kinase occurring as the major type in adult liver, while representing only a minor type in fetal liver. In the latter, Type III pyruvate kinase is the major form. In transplanted hepatomas, the ratio of Type III/I increases as a reflection of decreasing differentiation.[141]

A considerable amount of research has been performed with the isoenzymes of alkaline phosphatase by Fishman and his colleagues.[45,46] The placental type of alkaline phosphatase, i.e., the Regan isoenzyme, was discovered in a patient with metastatic bronchogenic carcinoma. It is membrane-associated, heat-stable, L-phenylalanine-sensitive, and neuraminidase-cleavable. The Regan isoenzyme is found in the serum of one of seven cancer patients with the highest incidence in ovarian and other gynecological cancers.

Terminal Deoxynucleotidyltransferase (TdT) in Normal and Leukemic Cells. TdT has had a major impact upon the biotechnology industry because of its involvement in a number of cloning protocols. TdT catalyzes the linear polymerization of nucleotides onto a suitable template. The substrates for this enzyme are the deoxyribonucleoside-5'-triphosphates with a polydeoxynucleotide or DNA serving as the initiator. The product is the initiator covalently-linked to a polymer of deoxynucleoside monophosphates, the number of which depends upon the ratio of monomer to initiator.[17]

Chang was first to describe the ontogeny of TdT in the calf thymus gland where activity appeared late during fetal development and increased during the early postnatal period.[29] Subsequently, TdT was demonstrated in human and rodent bone marrow.[31,156] In normal humans, the TdT+ cells appear exclusively in the thymus cortex and bone marrow lymphocytes. As demonstrated by Bodger, TdT+ cells first appear in the lymphoid cells of the embryonic liver at the 12th–13th week, then in fetal thymus and bone marrow at 19–21 and 15–16 wk, respectively.[14] Within the fetal thymus, TdT+ cells constitute only 5–10% of the thymocytes; by 1–40 months of age postpartum, this number had increased to 60–85%. In children and young adults, less than 0.02%

of Ficoll-Hypaque-separated circulating lymphocytes are TdT+.[21]

The utility of the TdT+ phenotype as a marker of certain leukemias arose from the observation by McCaffrey of large amounts in circulating blast cells obtained from a patient with T-cell acute lymphocytic leukemia.[87] Subsequently, TdT+ cells were found in most forms of acute lymphocytic leukemia.[17] Consequently, this phenotype has provided another assist in the diagnosis of the specific type of leukemia where the affected cell is of the immature lymphoid variety.

Other Oncofetal Proteins. Oncofetal proteins of nonenzyme function are also found in a variety of neoplasms. These nonenzymatic proteins are often referred to as 'tumor-specific antigens.' A few examples will serve to illustrate this group, namely, a-fetoprotein (AFP) and carcinoembryonic antigen (CEA).

AFP is a serum protein that was first identified in human fetal cord blood but is not present in adult blood.[12] AFP is produced by fetal liver and to a lesser extent, by the yolk sac during prenatal development. It is the dominant serum protein in early extrauterine development. In many of its structural characteristics, AFP resembles albumin. However, the role of AFP has not been defined although it does bind estrogen to some extent.

Abelev and colleagues first observed the occurrence of what later turned out to be AFP in adult mice that were bearing a transplantable hepatoma.[1] Soon thereafter, elevated serum AFP levels were demonstrated in humans with hepatocellular carcinoma.[145] Using the rat Morris hepatomas, Sell and Morris have determined the concentration of AFP in the serum as a function of their growth rate.[134] Rats bearing poorly differentiated, rapidly-growing hepatomas exhibited levels of serum AFP as high as 18×10^6 ng/ml compared to 60 in the serum from normal rats. The serum AFP level in slow-growing, well-differentiated hepatoma-bearing rats was close to the normal value.

That elevations in serum AFP are not restricted to tumor-bearing hosts was demonstrated in the case of toxic injury to the liver. Partial hepatectomy or acute liver toxicity resulted in a transient increase in serum AFP.[154]

A second non-enzyme oncofetal protein of some import in cancer research and diagnosis is CEA, which was first reported by Gold and Freeman.[54] CEA is a serum glycoprotein of molecular weight of 200,000 Daltons that is present in adenocarcinoma of human digestive tract as well as in fetal tissues and is shed into the blood. CEA levels are also elevated in patients with cancers of the lung and genitourinary tract. Elevated serum CEA may be observed in noncancerous patients with colitis, liver cirrhosis or alcoholic pancreatitis. CEA is one of the most thoroughly characterized tumor-associated antigens.

With the cloning of the CEA cDNA, it has been possible to define different regions of the protein molecule.[100] CEA contains a 34 amino acid N-terminal sequence, followed by an 107 amino acid N-terminal domain, 3 highly homologous repeated domains of 178 amino acids, and a 26 residue hydrophobic C-terminal domain. The 3 homologous regions share extensive sequence homology with the immunoglobulin gene superfamily, supporting some type of evolutionary relationship.[104] The hydrophobic C-terminal region has suggested a membrane-anchoring function which has been pursued by Hefta et al.[64] The latter investigators have demonstrated the anchoring of CEA to plasma membranes by the covalent attachment to a ethanolamine-glycosyl phosphatidylinositol moiety which is added to the protein posttranslationally. Furthermore, it has been suggested that the increased levels of CEA in the serum of patients with certain cancers may be the result of its release from the membrane by some phospholipase or of the existence of some defect in the phosphatidylinositol complex.[64]

The function of CEA has been studied by a number of investigators. Benchimol has demonstrated the CEA-dependent, calcium-independent homotypic aggregation of cultured human colon adenocarcinoma cells and rodent cells that had been transfected with CEA cDNA.[10] CEA can facilitate the homotypic cell sorting of aggregating cells. It represents a new addition to the family of intercellular adhesion molecules and is structurally related to Thy-1 and neural cell adhesion molecule.[106] CEA has also been demonstrated in normal tissues to be localized to epithelial cell membranes facing the lumen.[10] In embryonic intestine and colonic tumors, CEA is found on the adjacent cell membranes. It has been postulated that the overproduction of CEA in colonic tumors may disrupt the normally-operating intercellular adhesion forces, resulting in more cell movement, less-ordered architecture, and more dedifferentiation.[10] These would constitute early steps in tumorigenesis.

Although neither AFP nor CEA is specific for tumors, they do increase the diagnostic capability and more importantly, allow for assessment of the efficacy of therapy or reappearance of cancer in the treated patient.

Ectopic Hormone Production by Cancer Cells

Tumors in experimental animal systems as well as in humans often exhibit 'bizarre' phenotypic expressions which can have very profound effects upon the host. These topics are covered in detail in Chapter XVI-10. In 1928, Brown reported an unusual Cushing's syndrome in a patient who presented with small cell lung carcinoma.[22] Her symptoms included diabetes, hirsutism, hypertension and adrenal hyperplasia. Subsequently, additional instances of this lung cancer-related syndrome were observed.

In 1965, Liddle and coworkers coined the phrase, *Ectopic ACTH Syndrome*, to describe such instances where the lung cancer was elaborating an ACTH-like substance (or ACTH itself) which was responsible for the hypercorticosteroidism.[82] It is now known that as many as 40% of patients with small cell lung carcinoma may elaborate such a polypeptide although in a large number of these individuals, the polypeptide is either nonfunctional or only possesses a small portion of biological activity. In the latter case, a precursor molecule, "big" ACTH (propiomelanocortin) is often present; this substance possesses only 4% of the biological activity of ACTH.

As indicated above, small cell lung carcinomas often display unusual phenotypic responses. They exhibit some characteristics of neuroendocrine cells in their uptake and decarboxylation of neuroactive amines.[107] In this regard, very elevated levels of serotonin, anti-diuretic hormone, calcitonin, as well as ACTH may be observed in small cell lung

cancer patients. These substances are responsible to varying degrees for the biologic syndromes seen.

Further evidence of the complications imposed upon the management of these cancer patients by ectopic production of a hormone by a nonendocrine tumor is afforded by the occurrence of hypercalcemia which often could be of life-threatening proportions. It was Gutman who in 1936 first reported an individual with hypercalcemia and hypophosphatemia as a result of a nonendocrine tumor which did not involve any osseous sites.[57] Subsequently, Tashjian demonstrated that extracts from nonparathyroid tumors contained a substance that was immunologically similar to parathyroid hormone (PTH).[143] The ectopic secretion of PTH (or PTH-like substances) occurs in a number of nonendocrine tumors, particularly in those originating in the lung and kidney. This elevated serum PTH leads to increased calcium resorption from bone and the occurrence of hypercalcemia. Hypercalcemia is relatively common in patients with disseminated cancer, occurring in approximately 10–20% of this population.[76]

Substances in addition to hormones have been demonstrated as ectopic secretions in various human cancers. Prostaglandins, particularly of the PGE family, have been reported as ectopic substances in cancers in both experimental animal systems and in humans.[122,144] In addition, the ectopic formation of a colony stimulating factor (CSF) has been noted in squamous cell carcinomas resulting in hypercalcemia.[78] In the latter instance, confirmation of the causative role of the carcinomas in generating hypercalcemia was provided by using the nude mouse model. The squamous cell carcinomas from two patients were removed, transplanted into nude mice, and a resultant hypercalcemia was noted. Upon resection of these tumors, the hypercalcemia in the nude mice resolved.

Finally, osteolytic substances have been reported in other types of cancers, e.g., Burkitt's lymphoma.[94] These substances were not PTH, PGE, or CSF and appeared to exert their action by directly resorbing bone independently of osteoclasts.

In summary, a number of nonendocrine cancer cells are able to manufacture and secrete ectopic substances including hormones and growth factors that enhance bone resorption and lead to increased levels of serum calcium. The mechanisms underlying the elaboration of these substances by the cancers is not understood although enhanced gene expression is involved.

Cancer, Cachexia, and Cachectic Factors

The growth of tumors in experimental animal systems and in humans is often accompanied by a very striking loss of weight, anorexia, asthenia and anemia, i.e., cachexia. In several instances, the cachectic response to the cancer is not directly related to the total cancer burden of the animal or patient but appears to depend more upon some inherent property. Cachexia oftentimes can be the primary cause of death of the patient with as many as 30% of the patients succumbing to its effect rather than from the tumor burden.[97,155] It certainly is a major confounder in the chemotherapy of cancer. Progress in the treatment of cachectic cancer patients has been poor; wasting is predictive of a poorer survival and lower rate of response to chemotherapy. Consequently, much interest has been generated in trying to understand the mechanisms underlying the tumor-induced cachectic response so that appropriate countering measures could be instituted.

Early on, several investigators had suggested that substances released from the tumors might be directly involved in eliciting the cachectic response.[97] Nakahara showed a marked depression in liver catalase activity in cancer patients and in tumor-bearing mice that had been treated with a water-soluble, ethanol-precipitable and heat-stable fraction extracted from human gastric or rectal carcinomas.[95] This polypeptide material was referred to as *Toxohormone*. Toxohormone also caused a reduction in the concentration of iron in plasma and in the amount of liver ferritin and NAD + NADH. Toxohormone administration involuted the thymus, produced hepato- and splenomegaly, and increased hepatic protoporphyrin. The exact mechanisms underlying these actions have never been established. However, it was clear that toxohormone played only a minor role in eliciting cachexia in the cancer patient.

A clearer picture of the cachectic response was afforded by a more detailed study of what happens in the tumor-bearing animal. In the sarcoma-bearing, non-cachectic rat, an increased gluconeogenesis, and an enhanced direction of glucose from peripheral tissues to the tumor are observed.[24,146] Plasma glucose levels in these rats were quite depressed and blood lactate was elevated. None of these changes were caused by alterations in insulin or glucagon levels.

Tumor-bearing rats or mice progressively lose weight and go into a negative nitrogen balance as the tumor weight increases.[93] Even force-feeding the host will not sustain an appropriate weight gain although growth of the tumor is enhanced by this treatment.[146] Thorough studies by Cameron and Ord and by Tanaka using several of the Morris hepatomas and a transplantable colon adenocarcinoma model, respectively, confirmed the utilization of the mechanisms of gluconeogenesis and the enhanced liver glycogenolysis to sustain glucose levels for the tumor.[26,142] The concept of a tumor as a "nitrogen trap" was espoused as early as 1948 by Mider who noted that rat tumors exhibited a positive nitrogen balance at the expense of the host's tissues.[89]

The effects of tumors upon the lipid status of the host were also consistent with an energy trap. Lindmark using a mouse sarcoma model system demonstrated increased fat oxidation, a decrease in body lipids and a greater expenditure of energy with regard to food consumption.[81]

In regard to cachexia and its effects, cancer patients behave very similarly to the experimental animal models. For example, Heber placed noncachectic lung cancer patients under conditions of constant calorie and nitrogen intake and then infused labeled lysine.[61] They noted an increased turnover rate of total body protein and an elevation in the catabolism of muscle protein as indicated by an enhanced 3-methyl-histidine/creatinine excretion rate. Although a profound increase in the rate of glucose production was observed, no changes were noted in serum ACTH, insulin, or glucagon; glucocorticoids were also normal as indicated by a 24 hour urinary cortisol level. In the blood of a number of patients with advanced cancer, an increased concentration of alanine is apparent. This alanine, which is present as a result of increased proteolysis, participates in the Cori cycle in liver and through lactic acid is converted to glucose for utilization by the malignancy.[34,42]

The above-cited representative examples in both experimental animals and in humans dramatically demonstrate the profound effects of the tumor upon intermediary metabolism in the host. The end result is to stimulate tumor growth at the expense of the host's tissue components. Furthermore, this result is accomplished by invoking very inefficient energy - producing mechanisms, i.e., glycolysis. The central question revolves about the nature of the component(s) present in tumors that is (or are) capable of directing the flow of energy from peripheral tissues to the tumor. Extensive research has shown that no shortage of willing candidates exists who are waiting to take their bows for this activity. Although IL-1 has been cast as one of the mediators of cachexia a greater role falls on the shoulders of a unique polypeptide, *cachectin or tumor necrosis factor (TNF)*.[136]

Tumor Necrosis Factor or Cachectin. The discovery of the role of TNF as a mediator in cachexia in the cancer patient draws upon two independent lines of research. A group of investigators at Rockefeller University were interested in the the process of cachexia that was observed in trypanosome-infected rabbits.[13,77,124] In these rabbits, an increase in circulating triglycerides was demonstrated which was caused by a systemic suppression of lipoprotein lipase (LPL). A bacterial lipopolysaccharide-inducible serum factor was isolated from these rabbits that could suppress LPL in mice as well as the activities of other lipogenic enzymes in an adipocyte cell line. This factor was called *Cachectin*. Chronic exposure of rabbits to cachectin led to all the signs and symptoms of cachexia seen in tumor-bearing rodents and in human cancer patients.[151]

More recent work by this group has demonstrated the suppression of the expression of several mRNA's that encode essential lipogenic enzymes (e.g., glycerol-3-phosphate dehydrogenase in adipocytes).[149] That the action of cachectin is not limited to lipid metabolism was apparent with the observations of a reduction in the resting transmembrane potential, a depletion in intracellular glycogen, an increase in efflux of lactate and an increased activity of the hexose transporters.[150]

The flip side of this story began nearly a century ago with the attempts of William Coley in the late 1800's to treat cancer by administering certain bacterial toxins to cancer patients. This strategy was based upon his observations of regression of some tumors in patients after a systemic bacterial infection.[101] Coley administered a mixture of killed bacteria directly into the tumor and noted some positive responses. However, with the improvement in surgical procedures, the advent of chemotherapy and of radiotherapy, the Coley treatment was abandoned.

Later, it was found that extracts of gram-negative bacteria could induce extensive hemorrhagic necrosis in mouse tumors. The active ingredient was demonstrated to contain *endotoxin*, a lipopolysaccharide. Indeed, the action of endotoxin appeared to be mediated through the stimulation of the production of a serum factor called *TNF*.[102] Human TNF has a molecular weight of 45,000 Daltons and is dissociable into components of molecular weight of 17,000.

TNF was soon demonstrated to be identical to cachectin.[13] The gene has been cloned by Wang.[161] The role of recombinant human cachectin/TNF was determined by Oliff who demonstrated the severe weight loss and increased mortality of mice that bore transgenic tumors which secreted this protein.[102]

Before completing this section of the chapter, a brief word about futile metabolic cycles would be in order. Futile cycles can operate in carbohydrate and lipid metabolism at a number of enzymatic steps. A futile cycle may occur in a portion of a metabolic pathway where antagonistic reactions operate simultaneously. Under these conditions, no net flux of metabolites occurs although a wasteful hydrolysis of ATP is observed resulting in the generation of excess heat. For this reason, futile cycles have been implicated in thermogenesis.[71,96] A major futile cycle occurs at the level of phosphofructokinase (PFK) and fructose-1,6-diphosphatase (FDP) as indicated below:

The formation of spermidine from putrescine and spermine from spermidine requires the addition of aminopropyl groups that are derived from decarboxylated S-adenosylmethionine. The enzymes catalyzing these steps are constitutive but are regulated by the availability of the decarboxylated substrate. S-Adenosylmethionine decarboxylase, which catalyzes the formation of the latter, is under both positive and negative feedback control with putrescine serving as an activator and spermidine as a repressor. The net result of this control mechanism is to regulate the supply of decarboxylated S-adenosylmethionine by the need for spermidine and the availability of putrescine.[66]

The synthesis of polyamines is required for the formation of the nucleolus and for appropriate embryonic development in certain worms; for oocyte maturation; and for rodent embryogenesis.[47,62,139] Some tissue hypertrophy and hyperplasia, e.g., renal and cardiac hypertrophy and regenerating liver, require polyamine synthesis.[87,108] Agents that induce terminal differentiation of the human HL60 promyelocytic cells increase putrescine and spermidine levels suggesting a role of the polyamines in this process.[70] An interesting but par-

$$\text{Inorganic PO}_4 \nwarrow \swarrow \begin{array}{c} \text{Fructose-6-phosphate} \\ \text{FDP} \qquad \text{PFK} \\ \text{Fructose-1,6-diphosphate} \end{array} \begin{array}{c} \text{ATP} \\ \\ \nearrow \searrow \text{ADP} + \text{Inorganic PO}_4 + \text{Heat} \end{array}$$

In the tumor-bearing patient, the fructose-6-phosphate/fructose-1,6-diphosphate cycle could be significantly enhanced, perhaps through the effect of TNF, with the resultant dephosphorylation of ATP and the production of heat instead of usable chemical energy. Indeed, the increased heat production may contribute to the appearance of fever in a number of advanced cancer patients. The major source of ATP under these circumstances becomes the oxidation of fatty acids with gluconeogenesis providing glucose for use by tissues that require this carbohydrate.

In brief, TNF/cachectin is elaborated by tumors or other cells within them, it binds to high affinity receptors present in a variety of tissues, e.g., adipose tissue, the resultant complex causes the suppression of specific mRNA synthesis, which then results in major changes in intermediary metabolism, as outlined above. The end result is the feeding of the tumor at the expense of the host, i.e., cachexia.

Polyamines and Cancer

The naturally-occurring polyamines, putrescine, spermidine and spermine, are ubiquitously distributed throughout the eukaryotes. Although their role has not been definitively established, cell proliferation and differentiation appear to require their biosynthesis and furthermore, their generation is tightly regulated.[73,109,140] The metabolic reactions leading to the formation of the polyamines and their biotransformation are indicated in Figure I-9-2. The parent substance from which putrescine (and hence, the other polyamines) is produced is ornithine in a reaction which is catalyzed by *ornithine decarboxylase* (ODC), the rate-limiting enzyme of this pathway.[127] We will return to ODC shortly.

adoxical requirement for polyamine synthesis in the cell cycle of normal and transformed cells has been reported. Inhibition of polyamine synthesis in Ehrlich ascites cells resulted in an accumulation of these cells in S and G_2 phases while normal cells under similar conditions of blockade arrested in the G_{z_1} phase.[63,126]

Animal tumor models require polyamine synthesis. High polyamine levels were present in Ehrlich ascites carcinoma cells; the rate of tumor cell proliferation correlated with the increases in polyamines.[73] Suppression of tumor growth has also been observed when inhibitors of polyamine synthesis were administered.[84] The impact of polyamines upon the growth of tumor systems included human neoplasms. Small cell lung carcinoma cell lines were very sensitive to inhibitors of polyamine synthesis both when added in culture or administered to nude mice bearing xenografts. Other sensitive human tumors included melanoma, prostatic carcinoma, and pancreatic carcinoma cells.[85]

Ornithine Decarboxylase As indicated above, ODC is a key regulatory enzyme in the biosynthesis of polyamines. Under normal conditions, the activity of ODC is very low in cells although the enzyme undergoes rapid induction upon exposure of cells to a variety of stimuli including growth factors, hormones and tumor promoters. These induced levels are quite ephemeral however as a result of the very short half-life of the protein.[99,132] ODC activity is markedly elevated in human skin tumors.[130] In a mouse model system, O'Brien and colleagues have demonstrated the occurrence of a functionally-altered ODC in skin tumors as compared to normal tissue; the tumor form of ODC is activated by GTP.[98] In a recent study from this laboratory, ODC was examined in

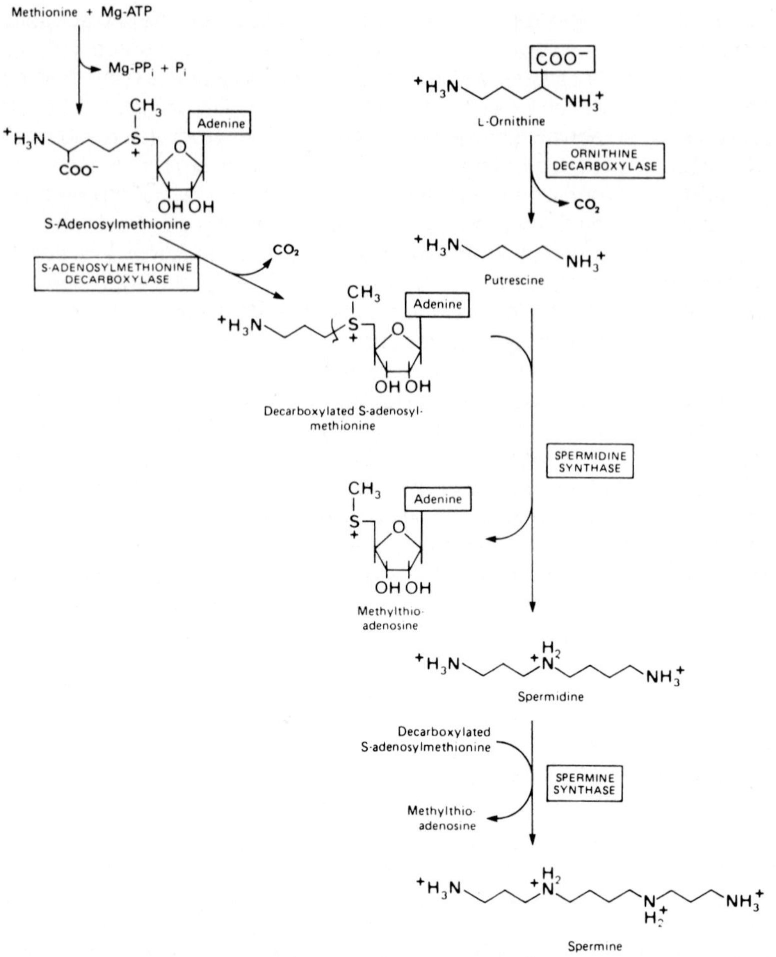

Figure I-9-2. Biosynthesis of Polyamines.

human skin and squamous cell carcinomas and a similar altered enzyme was observed in the human skin cancers which was activated by GTP.[67] These investigators have postulated that the altered protein allows for the escape of the polyamine biosynthetic pathway in these tumors from normal cellular regulation.

An interesting series of experiments has been reported from the Verma laboratory relating to the localization of at least one of the human ODC genes to chromosome 2 and to further defining the role of ODC and of polyamines in tumor cell biology.[35] In the normal ODC-deficient Chinese hamster ovary (CHO) cells, exogenous putrescine is required for cell growth. In CHO cells that have been transfected with the human ODC gene, the enzyme is overexpressed and the addition of putrescine is no longer required. Furthermore, in the transfected cells, considerably more $G_2 + M$ cells are noted when compared to the ODC-deficient parental cell line. These studies suggest that the polyamines, and putrescine in particular, may be required for the transition from S to $G_2 + M$; the studies reinforce the rate-limiting nature, and hence the importance, of ODC in this pathway.

Elevated ODC activity has been reported in certain premalignant conditions in humans. Increased ODC was observed in colon biopsy samples from familial polyposis patients, a condition in which increased proliferation of the colonic mucosa is present with a high risk for the develop-

ment of cancer.[84] Similarly, increased ODC activity has been reported in the epithelial dysplasia associated with Barrett's esophagus, another high risk situation for cancer development.[52]

Although the exact mechanism underlying the elevation of ODC in tumor tissue is not yet understood, considerable evidence based upon the induction of this regulatory enzyme in mouse skin and in cultured keratinocytes by phorbol ester has suggested a phosphorylation-mediated mechanism of gene activation. Phorbol ester is known to interact with and activate protein kinase C (see Chapter I-4). The action of protein kinase C should lead to the production of certain phosphorylated transacting proteins. These activators may be directly responsible for enhancing transcription of appropriate genes which contain phorbol ester responsive elements, including ODC.

The mechanisms underlying the elevation in ODC activity in malignant and premalignant tissues are important. ODC is a protein with a very rapid turnover, i.e., minutes. Some evidence indicates that the enhanced ODC activity in these tissues may be caused in part by a post-transcriptional effect, i.e., stabilization of existing ODC molecules. The manner by which intracellular protein degradation is accomplished is just being uncovered with at least three such mechanisms operative in mammalian cells, a) ubiquitin-dependent, ATP-requiring proteolysis where ubiquitin forms an isopeptide linkage with the ε-lysine of the protein to be degraded and the targeted molecule is subjected to proteolysis by a multisubunit protease, b) calcium-dependent proteases (calpains) although the role of this extralysosomal proteolytic mechanism is still unclear, and c) lysosomal degradation which is responsible for the proteolysis of many of the membranal proteins and of the long-lived cytosolic proteins.[35]

In addition to these mechanisms, some element of structure within the amino acid sequence of the ephemeral proteins has been suggested as contributing to the identification of molecules for degradation. In this regard, the PEST hypothesis is worthy of note. Rogers examined the amino acid sequence of a number of short-lived and long-lived proteins and noted an unusual richness of proline (P), glutamic acid (E), serine (S), and threonine (T) stretches within the primary structure of the proteins with the rapid turnover rates.[123] ODC is a protein with PEST sequences. It is interesting to speculate that in tumor tissues, perhaps some alteration in the PEST sequences has occurred which then stabilizes the existing ODC protein without compromising catalytic function. Indeed, Ghoda noted that the removal of 37 residues from the carboxyl-terminal end of ODC results in a marked stabilization of the molecule; the PEST sequences are contained within this region.[53] Whether or not alteration of the ODC gene occurs within tumors such that the PEST sequences are deleted or rendered nonfunctional, thus contributing to the increased activity of ODC, remains to be determined.

Cyclic Nucleotides as Regulators of Growth

Cyclic AMP (cAMP) may play an important role in the differentiation of certain cells. cAMP is formed from the catalytic action of adenyl cyclase, a membrane-bound enzyme which utilizes ATP as substrate (see Figure I-9-3). The intracellular level of cAMP is not only dependent upon the activity of adenyl cyclase but also upon a specific phosphodiesterase. As indicated in Figure I-9-3, the phosphodiesterase causes the hydrolytic cleavage of cAMP with the production of the relatively inert 5′-AMP. Although the details relative to biological role of cAMP are discussed in some detail in Chapter I-4, a brief summary of this involvement is presented below.

cAMP is involved in a number of phosphorylation reactions through the action of cAMP-dependent protein kinases, called A-kinases. Their dependency upon cAMP is based upon the existence of the A-kinases in an inactive form as a tetramer consisting of 2 regulatory and 2 catalytic subunits. cAMP

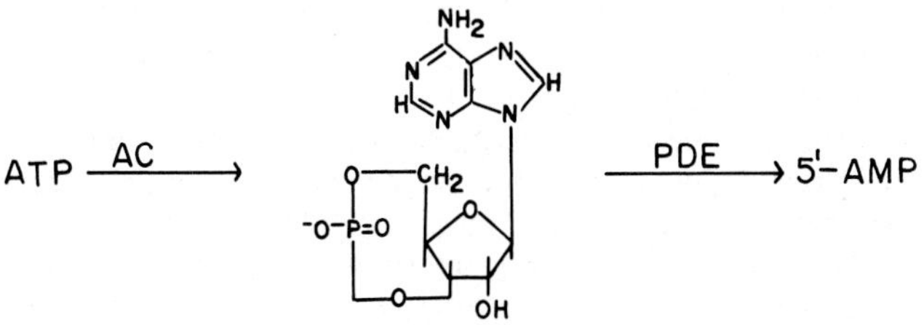

$$ATP \xrightarrow{\text{AC}} \text{cAMP} \xrightarrow{\text{PDE}} 5'-AMP$$

Figure I-9-3. The Biosynthesis and Catabolism of Cyclic AMP (cAMP). AC = adenyl cyclase; PDE = phosphodiesterase.

interacts with the regulatory subunits releasing the catalytic oligomer for enzymatic action. The active A-kinase then catalyzes the phosphorylation of appropriate protein substrates with ATP as the phosphorylating agent. The phosphorylated protein is responsible for eliciting a specific response relative to growth and proliferation of the cells.

cAMP levels are modulated by such external stimuli as growth factors and prostaglandins. This effect is mediated by the tight coupling that exists between the receptor for the external stimulus and the adenyl cyclase system. An excellent review of the interplay between growth factors, oncogene products, etc. and adenyl cyclase is offered by Bourne and DeFranco.[20]

The level of cAMP has been measured in a number of transformed cells and tumors.[117] In many cases, a decrease in cAMP was observed while in others, an increase. The addition of cAMP to cultured tumor cells led to a partial reversion to differentiated phenotype, i.e., more nearly normal. For example, neuroblastoma cells upon exposure to cAMP altered their morphology with the appearance of more normal long neurites and the concomitant appearance enzyme profiles that were closer to normal. A similar picture has been obtained with certain glioma cells. The effect of cAMP on these cells was reversible; with its removal, the cells reverted to their previous neoplastic phenotype.

The work of Burk is also worthy of note.[23] He showed that agents which inhibit phosphodiesterase activity and therefore increase intracellular cAMP levels significantly depressed the growth of both normal and virally-transformed baby hamster kidney cells. Furthermore, the cAMP levels increased concomitantly with the cessation of growth of nontransformed fibroblasts upon approaching confluence.[128] These observations formed the basis for the belief that cAMP levels may regulate the rate of cell proliferation. It is quite clear, however, that cAMP does not play a consistent role in neoplasia, although the enzymes which are phosphorylated through the action of the A-kinases are very important determinants of proliferation.

Poly(ADP-Ribose) Polymerase and Cell Death

Poly(ADP-ribose) polymerase or synthetase is a chromatin-bound enzyme that catalyzes the formation of poly(ADP-ribose) at the expense of NAD.[11,59] Poly(ADP-ribose) is capable of poly(ADP-ribosylation) of a number of proteins, thus altering their activity, e.g., DNA ligase, histones, the polymerase itself. The polymerase is involved in cell transformation, cell differentiation, and DNA repair, although the exact mechanisms in this regard have not been clearly defined. Borek and colleagues reported the inhibition of x-ray-, ultraviolet light- and chemical carcinogen-induced malignant transformation of hamster embryo cells and mouse C3H 10T1/2 cells by administration of inhibitors of poly(ADP-ribose) polymerase, thus implicating this enzyme in that process.[19]

Poly(ADP-ribosylation) is activated by DNA strand breaks, with successive transfer to nuclear proteins of the ADP-ribose moieties originating from NAD. This reaction in some manner facilitates the DNA repair process. Berger has proposed an interesting suicide response of cells with extensive DNA strand breaks which involves the poly(ADP-ribose) polymerase.[11] When the damage to DNA is severe, activation of the polymerase persists, leading to a depletion of the intracellular pools of both NAD and ATP. This depletion may result in rapid cell death before the DNA repair is consumated. However, some problems exist with this explanation for DNA damage-induced cell death. The depletion of NAD levels can be prevented by the administration of inhibitors of the poly (ADP-ribose) polymerase, e.g., 3-aminobenzamide. Yet, these polymerase inhibitors often *potentiate* the cell toxicity of the DNA damaging substance.[27]

The above discussion has raised the issue of damage-induced cell death. The rapid rate of DNA replication that is often seen in a number of cancer cells represents the chink in the armor that has stimulated a number of approaches to cancer therapy. Many of the useful drugs in cancer chemotherapy are alkylating agents that interact with DNA. The binding of these agents to DNA is however, not sufficient to explain the subsequent process of cell death. Some evidence exists that indicates that some cell cycle event(s) is or are associated with the toxicity of alkylating agents. For example, it is known that cis-platin, a useful cancer chemotherapeutic agent, is much more toxic to dividing cells although this drug is not a cell-cycle specific substance.[48] It is also known that the subsequent cell death is not related to a reduction in DNA synthesis mediated by cis-platin.[137] The latter investigators have postulated some critical event in G_2 that determines the fate of treated cells.

It was Wyllie and coworkers who first described the morphological events associated with *apoptosis*, or programmed cell death, a process which is observed in normal embryonic development, metamorphosis, differentiation, and general cell turnover.[166] Subsequently, it has been found that apoptosis is an active process which requires protein synthesis. Although lysosomes remain intact, the first step in apoptosis appears to be the degradation of DNA. Consequently, a specific endonuclease, the expression of which is turned on, has been postulated as the key protein in causing the programmed cell death.[37]

The purpose of this discussion is to provide the reader with a framework for understanding the use of *an already-existing* mechanism within normal and cancer cells to respond to the toxic action of a therapeutic agent. Furthermore, it is necessary to conceptualize some aberrancy in this mechanism occurring in some cancers. Thus, neoplastic cells, although exposed to an agent which can alkylate cellular DNA, may not trigger the apoptotic response, and the "resistant" cell will survive.

DNA Methylation in Cancer

There is a substantial amount of evidence that suggests a role for the methylation of DNA in the control of the expression of genes in eukaryotes. This methylation occurs exclusively in the 5-position of cytosine and more specifically, when this cytosine is part of the CpG dinucleotide. The first indications of this role came from the reports of Holliday and Pugh and Riggs in 1975.[68,121] A recent review by Jones and Buckley outlines the experimental details underlying the inverse relationship between the amount of 5-methylcytosine in DNA and the extent of gene expression.[75] The conclusion from many of these studies is that hypomethylation was necessary but not sufficient for enhanced gene activity.

The dinucleotide, CpG, is underrepresented in vertebrates and is generally clustered in so-called CpG islands. These islands are generally defined as GC-rich regions that are hypomethylated and that do not occur with any frequency in highly tissue-specific genes. Methylation of these CpG islands appears associated with transcriptional inactivity. Excellent examples of this type of regulation occur with genes associated with the inactive X-chromosome, e.g., hypoxanthine phosphoribosyltransferase and glucose-6-phosphate dehydrogenase. Although methylation of CpG islands within these genes is not the initial step in the inactivation, the 5-methylcytosine does stabilize the transcriptionally-inactive state.

Several investigators have examined the role of DNA methylation, e.g., at CpG islands, in the production of cancer and the maintenance of the cancerous state. This question has generally been addressed through the use of two techniques, a) the select sensitivity of certain restriction endonucleases to a methyl group, e.g., Msp I will cut CCGG independent of whether the second C (from the left) is methylated, while Hpa II will digest the DNA at this tetramer only when the middle CpG is unmethylated, and b) the utilization of 5-azacytidine, an inhibitor of DNA methyltransferase the enzyme which catalyzes the methylation of the CpG islands.

Kuo and colleagues have reported less methylation of the CpG sequences in the α-fetoprotein gene in hepatoma DNA when compared to normal liver DNA.[79] On the other hand, Baylin and colleagues[9,33] have noted hypermethylation of specific regions of human chromosomes in tumor cells, particularly through the use of chromosome 11 probes.[9,33] The latter studies raise the interesting possibility of increased methylation associated with the silencing of tumor suppressor genes. These studies suffer the disadvantage in their use of tumor cells that were maintained in culture. Under these conditions, it is not known if the effects on methylation were in fact imposed by the culture *per se*. However, many of these types of experiments have been repeated using primary tumor samples. Gama-Sosa has reported a reduced level of DNA methylation in a large number of human tumors.[51] Furthermore, the metastases exhibited a lower 5-methylcytosine content in their DNA when compared to that present in benign tumors or in nomal tissue. Feinberg has examined human colonic cells obtained from adenomas, adenocarcinomas and normal tissue.[41] He reported a hypomethylation of the DNA in the tumor with a reduction of approximately 10% in DNA 5-methylcytosine. No difference was noted in the levels of this parameter in benign versus malignant tumors. On the other hand, a hypermethylation of the calcitonin gene has been observed in over 90% of non-Hodgkin's type lymphoma and in 95% of the tumor cell DNA obtained from patients with acute myeloid leukemia.[8]

Several groups of investigators have examined the extent of DNA methylation as a function of tumor progression. Frost and his colleagues were first to report an alteration in the tumorigenicity by changing their immunogenicity after exposure to 5-azacytidine.[49,50] A reduction in DNA methylation after treatment with 5-azacytidine of clones of murine Lewis lung carcinoma cells that had been selected for their non-metastatic potential resulted in their conversion to a metastatic phenotype.[103,104,105] Therefore, treatment with this inhibitor of DNA methylation could result in either a loss or gain in metastatic potency depending upon the initial biological starting material.

The methylation of DNA, principally at the CpG islands, plays a role in the tumorigenesis process and in tumor progression. However, that role is not a simple one and may be unique for each individual tumor.

Proteases and Cancer Cells

The production and secretion of proteolytic enzymes by tumors represent very old observations. In 1925, Fischer reported that explants of virally-induced chicken tumors were able to lyse plasma clots while explants from normal connective tissue were inactive in this regard.[44] Subsequently, a number of investigators observed fibrinolytic activity released by a wide variety of transformed cells.[125]

Largely through the efforts of the Reich laboratory, it is clear that the fibrinolysis is the result of the secretion of plasminogen activator, which can convert the serum proteolytic zymogen, plasminogen, to an active enzyme.[119,152] Plasminogen activator is a serine protease that converts plasminogen to plasmin by cleavage of an arginine-valine bond that is present in the carboxyl-portion of the zymogen. It is plasmin that subsequently dissolves the fibrin clot noted by Fischer in 1925.

Two types of plasminogen activator have been described, tissue-type (t-PA) and urokinase (u-PA). They represent different gene products and possess different enzymatic characteristics. Furthermore, at least two specific inhibitors of plasminogen activator have been reported.

The plasminogen activators are involved in fibrinolysis, in tissue remodeling and in some stages of malignancy. In particular, the plasminogen activators are participants in a number of steps of metastasis; in the initial breakdown of the basement membrane allowing the detachment of tumor cells from the primary neoplasm; in the formation of the fibrin coat on circulating tumor cells facilitating evasion of the immune response; in the proteolysis of the extracellular matrix at the site of invasion; and in angiogenesis.[158]

Not only do the plasminogen activators play these roles in the malignant process, but urokinase also represents an excellent marker of malignancy. It is overexpressed in lung, colonic, breast and prostatic tumors.[74]

Hyperplastic Nodules, Foci, and Biological Markers

Hepatic preneoplastic foci can be induced in rodent liver by many different carcinogens.[40,133] These nodules are characterized both histologically and biochemically and are identified long before the appearance of the hepatocellular carcinoma, i.e., they are putative precursor lesions. In these foci, alterations in specific enzymes are observed.[111] The alterations in enzyme activity occurring within the liver preneoplastic foci or nodules are summarized in Table I-9-3. The changes in activity represent either increases in certain enzymes or decreases. In a number of instances, the enzymatic change is the result of a reversion to a fetal-type isozyme, representing an oncofetal protein, as presented earlier above.

Of the changes in enzyme activity occurring in hepatic

Table I-9-3. Marker Enzymes Found in Hepatic Preneoplastic Nodules*

Enzymes with Decreased Activity
  Specific isozymes of glucokinase, aldolase B, pyruvate kinase L
  Glucose-6-phosphatase and other gluconeogenic enzymes
  Liver-type glycogen phosphorylase
  Tryptophan 2,3-dioxygenase
  Serine dehydratase
  Various cytochrome P450's and P450-dependent monooxygenases
  NADPH-dependent cytochrome P450 reductase
  Selenium-dependent glutathione peroxidase
  Ca^{2+}, Mg^{2+}-dependent ATPase

Enzymes with Increased Activity
  Glucose-6-phosphate dehydrogenase
  Fetal-type isozymes of glycolysis
  Fetal-type (Type 1) UDP-glucuronosyltransferase
  Epoxide hydrolase
  Quinone reductase
  NADP-dependent aldehyde dehydrogenase
  Butyryl esterase
  Glutathione transferases
  γ-Glutamyltransferase
  Selenium-independent glutathione peroxidase
  Glutathione reductase

*Modified from Russel[127]

preneoplastic foci, three will be discussed in greater detail, γ-glutamyltranspeptidase (GGT), epoxide hydrolase and glutathione S-transferase-P (GST-P). These represent increases in enzyme activity and in several instances, the occurrence of a more fetal-type isozyme.

GGT. GGT has provided one of the most useful markers for preneoplasia of liver. The enzyme catalyzes the following reaction:

$$R{-}S{-}\underset{\underset{Glu}{|}}{\overset{\overset{Gly}{|}}{Cys}} \longrightarrow R{-}S{-}\underset{\underset{NH_2}{|}}{\overset{\overset{Gly}{|}}{Cys}} + Glu$$

(where R = H, as in glutathione itself or an adduct)

Fiala and coworkers were first to describe the appearance of GGT in experimental hepatomas and in preneoplastic liver.[43] GGT is apparently turned on rapidly in preneoplastic nodules. Histochemistry has revealed the GGT activity within proliferating ductular cells such as bile duct and hepatic oval cells as well as in the hepatic foci. The enzyme activity shows up in both the smooth endoplasmic reticulum and the bile canaliculus (the greater activity).

Epoxide Hydrolase. Farber and his colleagues had described the exclusive occurrence within the endoplasmic reticulum of hepatic hyperplastic nodules of an antigenic component which they tentatively termed *PN antigen*.[40] The PN antigen was purified and subsequently identified by Levin as a microsomal form of epoxide hydrolase.[80] This represented one of the first reports identifying an increased molecular form of an enzyme of biotransformation in preneoplastic nodules. The enzyme catalyzes the reaction shown below:

$$R—CH—CH—R_1 + H_2O \longrightarrow R—CH—CH—R_1$$

GST-P. The glutathione S-transferases represent a family of isozymes that were first identified in rat liver by Booth in 1961.[16] In the rat, approximately 12 molecular forms of the cytosolic enzyme involving 8 different subunits have been identified; these are divided into basic, neutral and acidic varieties.[124] The generic reaction catalyzed by this family of isozymes is indicated below:

$$Acceptor + GSH \longrightarrow Acceptor\text{-}SG$$

The glutathione S-transferases in the human also fall into basic, neutral and acidic categories.[129] For the present discussion, the isoenzyme of interest is the acidic GT-π which occurs in human fetal tissues as well as in adult lung, brain and spleen. GT-π corresponds to the rat GT 7-7.

A number of laboratories have studied the changes in isoenzymic pattern for the transferases during rat liver carcinogenesis.[129] Sato and coworkers first identified a form of this enzyme in rat placenta which was later established as occurring in hepatomas but not in any appreciable amounts in normal liver.[129] GT 7-7 turned out to be a good marker for preneoplastic liver foci and in fact may represent an accurate indicator of the "early" initiated cells after administration of carcinogens to rats.

Antibody to GT-π has been used in the detection of neoplasia and early preneoplastic states in a number of human organs. As reviewed by Sato, normal uterine cervical tissue was negative in response to this antibody while a positive reaction was observed in cases of mild dysplasia, e.g., koilocytosis.[129] Intense staining was seen in severe dysplasia and squamous cell carcinoma of the cervix. Similar positive reactions were apparent in esophageal dysplasia and carcinoma, in breast adenocarcinomas, in colon and hepatic tumors.

In summary, GT-π may prove to be an excellent marker of certain human cancers, particularly defining the early stages of tumorigenesis.

Cell Surface and Neoplasia

Substantial alterations to the plasma membrane of cells occurs in neoplastic transformation. In 1954, Abercrombie and Heaysman reported that cultured normal cells inhibited each other by mutual contact while many malignant cells did not cease growing under similar conditions.[2,3] This phenomenon of inhibition of the growth of normal cells was referred to as *contact inhibition.* For a variety of reasons, this repression of growth by contact was renamed *density-dependent inhibition of growth* by Stoker and Rubin in 1967.[138]

In culture, normal cells require a suitable surface for attachment, spreading and proliferation, a process that is referred to as *anchorage-dependent growth.* A number of transformed cells or malignant cells can grow in suspension or in semi-solid media and therefore are capable of anchorage-independent growth. The latter property has been useful in uncovering and subsequently growing malignant cells in a mixed population. Anchorage-independent growth has been closely associated with tumorigenicity.[91] It is germane to mention that anchorage-independent growth, although a property of transformed rodent cells, may not be characteristic of human tumor cells.

The lack of density-dependent inhibition of growth and the presence of anchorage-independence have suggested that neoplastic cells may have altered membranes as well as altered factor-mediated cell communication. Since the plasma membrane plays an important role in controlling movement and migration, adherence to supports and to other cells, in controlling the entry of nutrients and in the recognition of "nonself" in evoking an immune response, these alterations were pursued with some vigor.

Confirmation of a neoplasia-induced change(s) in cell membrane came with the use of a variety of lectins, each of which is capable of binding to a specific carbohydrate.[55] Aub was first to report the agglutination of several transformed cells by wheat germ agglutinin (WGA) while the normal counterparts were not so affected.[6] Several possibilities for this phenomenon would pertain, a) transformed cells might have more plasma membrane binding sites for lectins, b) surface binding sites for lectins might be more mobile resulting in a greater concentration of these receptors by lateral movement.

The latter possibility appears to be the correct one. The increased lateral mobility is undoubtedly the result of an increase in plasma membrane fluidity.

Attention was then focused on the chemistry of the cell surface and in particular on the glycoproteins and glycolipids. An excellent review of the aberrant glycosylation in malignancy has been written by Hakomori who has played a major role in this research area.[58] A more general review on alterations in neoplastic cell membrane components may be found in Ruddon.[125]

In the early literature, changes in membranal sialic acid had been reported to occur in neoplasia. Later, the affected culprits were identified as glycosphingolipids and glycolipids as well as glycoproteins. The alterations were the result of a) incomplete synthesis and/or processing of carbohydrate chains resulting in marked elevations in precursor forms, b) activation of glycosyltransferases that were normally absent or low in amount in normal cells, and c) rearrangements in the glycolipid components of the tumor cells.

With the development and the subsequent utilization of monoclonal antibodies, it was soon recognized that these oligosaccharides were tumor-associated antigens, some of which belonged to the class of oncofetal proteins.

Among the earliest evidence that indicated aberrant glycosylation in human cancer was the observation of the incompatible expression of A antigen or the reduction of A or B determinants. A large quantity of a number of fucose-containing glycolipids were found in various adenocarcinomas.[58]

Cell transformation was shown to alter the gangliosides and neutral glycolipids with a number of tumor systems expressing gangliotriosylceramide (Gg3), which had not been observed in normal cells.[58] The unique gangliosides found in tumors are shown in Tables I-9-4 to I-9-7.

Table I-9-4. Fucose-Containing Lipids and Gangliosides in Cancer

Name	Structure
Le^x	Galβ1$\rightarrow$4GlcNAcβ1$\rightarrow$3Galβ1$\rightarrow$R 3 $\uparrow$ Fucα1
Le^y	Galβ1$\rightarrow$4GlcNAcβ1$\rightarrow$3Galβ1$\rightarrow$R 2 3 $\uparrow$ $\uparrow$ Fucα1 Fucα1
Sialyl Le^x	Galβ1$\rightarrow$4GlcNAcβ1$\rightarrow$3Galβ1$\rightarrow$R 3 3 $\uparrow$ $\uparrow$ SA2 Fucα1
Trifucosyl Le^y	Galβ1$\rightarrow$4GlcNAcβ1$\rightarrow$3Galβ1$\rightarrow$4GlcNAc 2 3 3 $\uparrow$ $\uparrow$ $\uparrow$ Fucα1 Fucα1 Fucα1
ACFH18 Antigen	Galβ1$\rightarrow$[4GlcNAcβ1$\rightarrow$3Galβ1]$_n$$\rightarrow$3Gal$\beta$1$\rightarrow$4GlcNAc 6 3 $\uparrow$ $\uparrow$ SA2 Fucα1

Gal = galactose; β1$\rightarrow$4 = β—galactoside between 1-hydroxyl of one sugar to 4-hydroxyl of adjacent sugar; GlcNAcβ1-3Gal, 1-hydroxy group of N-acetyl-glucosamine bound by β-linkage to the 3-hydroxyl moiety of galactose; R = residue; Fucα1 = 1-hydroxy moiety of fucose linked to a group of an adjacent sugar (represented by the head of the arrow); SA2 = 2-position of sialic acid covalently linked to a group in the adjacent sugar (head of the arrow).

Table I-9-5. Ganglioside-Series of Antigens in Cancer Cells

Name	Structure
Gγ_3	GalNAc$\rightarrow$Gal$\rightarrow$Glc$\rightarrow$Cer
GM$_{1b}$	Gal$\rightarrow$GalNAc$\rightarrow$Gal$\rightarrow$Glc$\rightarrow$Cer $\uparrow$ SA
GM$_3$	Gal$\rightarrow$Glc$\rightarrow$Cer $\uparrow$ SA
GM$_2$	GalNAc$\rightarrow$Gal$\rightarrow$Glc$\rightarrow$Cer $\uparrow$ SA
GD$_2$	GalNAc$\rightarrow$Gal$\rightarrow$Glc$\rightarrow$Cer $\uparrow$ SA $\uparrow$ SA
GT$_2$	GalNAc$\rightarrow$Gal$\rightarrow$Glc$\rightarrow$Cer $\uparrow$ SA $\uparrow$ SA $\uparrow$ SA

Cer = ceramide. The other acronyms are indicated in Table I-9-4.

Table I-9-6. Globoside-Series of Antigens in Cancer Cells

Name	Structure
Forssman Antigen	GalNAcα1$\rightarrow$3GalNAcβ1$\rightarrow$3Galα1$\rightarrow$4Galβ1$\rightarrow$4Glcβ1$\rightarrow$Cer
SSEA-3	Galβ1$\rightarrow$3GalNAcβ1$\rightarrow$3Galα1$\rightarrow$4Galβ1$\rightarrow$4Glcβ1$\rightarrow$Cer
SSEA-4	NeuAcα2$\rightarrow$3Galβ1$\rightarrow$3GalNAcβ1$\rightarrow$3Galα1$\rightarrow$4Galβ1$\rightarrow$4Glcβ1$\rightarrow$Cer

GalNAcα1 = 1-hydroxyl group of N-acetylgalactosamine linked by α-configuration to an adjacent group of the sugar indicated at the head of the arrow; NeuAc = N-acetylneuraminic acid.

Table I-9-7. Tumor-Associated Glycoproteins in Cancer

Name	Structure
Tn	GalNAcα1-O-Ser/Thr
Sialyl Tn	NeuAcα2 $\downarrow$ 6 GalNAcα1-O-Ser/Thr

O-Ser/Thr = an ester between the hydroxyl of either serine (Ser) or threonine (Thr) and a sugar.

The tumor-associated carbohydrate antigens fell into 5 classes, a) epitope structures that were expressed in both glycosphingolipids and glycoproteins, b) epitopes expressed only in glycosphingolipids, c) epitopes expressed only in glycoproteins, d) polypeptide epitopes with antigenicity expressed when single or multiple threonine or serine moieties were glycosylated, and e) poorly defined epitopes.

The class a) antigens which were of the lacto series with Type 1 or 2 chains, were highly expressed in tumor cells, but not in progenitor cells, although a limited number were seen in some normal cells, e.g., di-or trimeric Le^x. Class b) antigens were significant components of tumor cells and only weakly expressed in normal counterparts, e.g., GM$_3$. Classes c, d, and e were of the mucin-type glycoproteins with Class c exclusively located in tumor cells, e.g., incompatible blood group antigens. Examples of the unusual antigenic components are indicated in Tables I-9-4 to I-9-7.

Aberrant glycosylation has also been reported in preneoplastic cells.[144] In rat liver preneoplastic nodules found in aryl amine-fed animals, fucosyl-containing carbohydrates that are absent in normal liver but highly expressed in hepatomas, are also observed. These result from the significant increase in fucosyltransferase that is specific for GM$_1$. In humans, Le^y presence correlated with the preneoplastic state that is seen in colonic polyps. Juvenile polyps of the non-malignant variety did not express this aberrant material.[58]

A very aberrant architecture is present in hepatocellular carcinoma, which may reflect changes in the ability of the neoplastic liver to adhere to their neighbors and/or to support the biomatrix. These interactions are important for tissue organization and for maintenance of differentiated function in normal liver cells. The aberrant architecture of hepatoma cells has been associated with a number of biochemical changes in the cell membranes. In this regard, Walborg et al. have reported the presence of a glycoprotein, dipeptidyl peptidase IV, which is related to a cell surface antigen, that is modulated as a function of the stage of malignancy.[157]

This protein, which cleaves X-proline dipeptides from the N-terminus, may be involved in the processing or binding of collagen, a major component of the biomatrix.

Extracellular Matrix

The extracellular matrix (ECM) is a complex medium which is formed from substances that are secreted by cells that make up the tissue in question. For epithelial tissues, cells from the epithelium and stroma or mesenchyme which form the base for the tissue produce the ECM components.

The ECM is important in the regulation of cell proliferation and differentiation as well as in determining the metastatic potential of malignant cells (Chapter I-10). In the latter context, the ECM represents the first barrier that must be traversed by cancer cells in order to invade through the lymphatic or vascular system. Consequently, it is not surprising that many cancer cells secrete proteases, glycosidases, heparanases and type IV collagenase since they are cells known to be able to compromise the integrity of the ECM.

The ECM is composed of: collagen types I-V depending upon the specific tissue; proteoglycans, such as chondroitin sulfate, heparan sulfate, dermatan sulfate; anchorage proteins such as fibronectin and laminin that serve as attachment sites to the matrix; and sometimes, elastin and entactin. The supporting structures of epithelial tissues such as in the gastrointestinal tract, mammary gland, or endocrine organs contain laminin, heparan sulfate-glycoproteins, and type IV collagen.

Fibronectin. This ECM material is a glycoprotein of MW = 450,000 which has the responsibility to anchor cells to the matrix. It consists of a disulfide-linked dimer that contains 5 N-linked oligosaccharides. Fibronectin occurs both as a cell-associated molecule and as a circulating form in the plasma.[167] Fibronectin binds to a number of macromolecules such as collagen, proteoglycans, the cell membrane itself, and participates, through the interaction with a fibronectin receptor, in cell spreading, movement and proliferation. In virally-transformed cells, the cell surface fibronectin is lost as a result of increased turnover and reduced binding.

As indicated, fibronectin binds to specific receptors present on cells. The major receptor consists of a noncovalent complex of two transmembrane glycoprotein subunits. This receptor is a member of the integrin family of cell surface heterodimers. The fibronectin receptor is also referred to as VLA-5. The latter has been examined in a number of normal and transformed human cells by Yamada and colleagues.[167] The fibronectin receptor in transformed cells underwent a more rapid intracellular processing mechanism, resulting in a reduction in the amount of this receptor and a more diffuse localization in the cell surface material. These events may contribute to the abnormal adhesion properties and invasiveness of the transformed human cells.

Laminin. This basement membrane protein is a glycoprotein of MW = 900,000 which contains multiple attachment points.[147] It consists of 2 chains with attachment sites for heparan sulfate and collagenase Type IV. Laminin is the first ECM protein to occur in embryonic development. It is lost from the cell surface of certain virally-transformed cells.[60]

Tenascin. This ECM component is a large oligomeric glycoprotein that is synthesized during embryonic development and is found prominently in a number of tumors.[61] In electron micrographs, the molecule has 6 long thin arms with a terminal knob on each arm, thick distal segment, thin proximal segment, a T-junction where 3 arms are joined to form a trimer, and a central knob where 2 trimers are united into a hexamer. The connections at the T-joint and at the central knob are disulfide bonds. Tenascin is secreted by fibroblasts and glial cells in culture, with various glioma cell lines representing some of the best sources for the human protein. Tenascin binds to chondroitin sulfate-containing proteoglycans.[30,156] In contrast to fibronectin or laminin, the interaction of tenascin with the cell surface is not associated with any flattening or spreading. The cells maintain their rounded to spindle or branching morphology.

Tenascin is not seen in mammary carcinoma or squamous carcinoma cells but is prominent in the surrounding connective tissue.[72,86] The synthesis of this ECM protein occurs in the mesenchyme that surrounds a transplantable breast cancer but not in the cancer cells *per se*. Transformed cells increase the ability of fibroblasts of underlying connective tissue to elaborate tenascin probably as a result of a soluble growth factor.

Tenascin is expressed in both mesenchymal tumors and carcinomas, but mostly in anaplastic tumors, e.g., in glioblastoma multiforme but not in the more differentiated astrocytomas. The presence of this substance may serve as a means for differential diagnosis of the gliomas.

Cytoskeletal Actin. Actin is one of the major components of the cytoskeleton and is ubiquitously present in eukaryotic cells.[112,165] Actin is necessary for regulation of cell shape, motility of the cell, secretion, intracellular transport, endocytosis and exocytosis, and cell division. Actin occurs in the cytoplasm as monomers, or G-actin or as microfilaments, F-actin.

Most transformed cells exhibit marked changes in patterns of actin filaments.[5,7,157] Cellular F-actin has been studied as a quantitative marker for transformation in relation to cell differentiation using human HL-60 cells.[160] The concentration of F-actin in untransformed cells was highest during the G_1 phase of the cycle. In transformed cells, on the other hand, a major increase occurred in the G2 + M phase. Phorbol ester which was able to differentiate the HL-60 cells caused a large decrease in the content of F-actin. Alterations in actin may be due to point mutations in the actin gene, altered regulation of F-actin assembly and/or changes in the actin polymerization process.

A number of actin-binding proteins occur in cells and these may play an important role in actin skeleton rearrangements in cell motility, division and differentiation. Among these proteins may be found: gelsolin which can bind to G-actin, cause aggregation to F-actin, and is important in the dynamic rearrangement of actin that occurs during spreading and locomotion of cells; villin, which is related to gelsolin but is able to bundle F-actin. During the differentiation of the cytoskeleton, a 50-fold increase occurs in gelsolin synthesis.[36] Villin is a component of brush border cells and is needed for the formation of microfilament bundles. It is the first actin-binding protein to appear at the site of microvilli assembly. The human colon carcinoma cell line, HT 29, can be induced to differentiate into a well-ordered brush border epithelium. Under these conditions, a marked increase in villin mRNA occurs up to levels that are found in normal intestinal mucosa.[118]

Conclusions

In the previous paragraphs, a small glimpse of the world of the neoplastic cell has been presented. It is apparent that many changes are noted in the biochemistry of this cell but a number of these changes appear to be related more to the rapid proliferation associated with some but not all human cancers. Growth-related alterations in enzyme activity or in secreted factors are adaptive mechanisms that make the cancer cell a better 'machine' in regard to cell division, invasion, and ability to avoid the negative influences of its neighbors. In this context, the cancer cell is truly a magnificent creature which proves its tremendous adaptability to adversity. The cancer cell is also quite remarkable in utilizing features that are already present in the normal cell but for reasons of ontogeny, may no longer be of value to the normal mature cell. The cancer cell however has resurrected these biochemical processes to be put to good advantage. Nevertheless, these phenotypic expressions provide the Achilles heel of the cancer cell by allowing for more definitive and early diagnosis, by providing targets for potential attack with some degree of specificity, and ultimately, perhaps, for reprogramming back to normalcy. It is a challenge to the molecular and biochemical oncologist to put these phenotypic expressions to better advantage so as to rid us of this remarkable but destructive cell.

Editors' Note: The structure of proteins and polypeptides will assume increasing importance in oncologic practice as receptor sites are characterized, mutations in gene products are described, and their role in oncogenesis and tumor progression is elucidated. Oncologists will surely be reading more about protein structure. An alphabetic nomenclature for amino acids has replaced the standard abbreviations and is presented here for convenience.

SYMBOLS FOR AMINO ACIDS

A	Ala	Alanine
B	Asx	Asparagine or aspartic acid
C	Cys	Cysteine
D	Asp	Aspartic acid
E	Glu	Glutamic acid
F	Phe	Phenylalanine
G	Gly	Glycine
H	His	Histidine
I	Ile	Isoleucine
K	Lys	Lysine
L	Leu	Leucine
M	Met	Methionine
N	Asn	Asparagine
P	Pro	Proline
Q	Gln	Glutamine
R	Arg	Arginine
S	Ser	Serine
T	Thr	Threonine
V	Val	Valine
W	Trp	Tryptophan
Y	Tyr	Tyrosine
Z	Glx	Glutamine or glutamic acid

References

1. Abelev, G. I., Perova, S. D., Khamkova, N. I., Postnikova, Z. A., and Irlin, I. S.: Production of embryonal a-globulin by transplantable mouse hepatomas. Transplantation 1:174, 1963.
2. Abercrombie, M., and Ambrose, E. J.: The surface properties of cancer cells: a review. Cancer Res. 22:525, 1962.
3. Abercrombie, M., and Heaysman, J. E. M.: Social behavior of cells in tissue culture II. Monolayering of fibroblasts. Exp. Cell Res. 6:293, 1954.
4. Akiyama, S. K., Larjava, H., and Yamada, K. M.: Differences in the biosynthesis and localization of the fibronectin receptor in normal and transformed cultured human cells. Cancer Res. 50:1602, 1990.
5. Antecol, M. H.: Ontogenic potential in fibroblasts from individuals genetically predisposed to cancer. Mutation Res. 199:293, 1988.
6. Aub, J. C., Sanford, B. H., and Cote. M. N.: Studies on reactivity of tumor and normal cells to a wheat germ agglutinin. Proc. Natl. Acad. Sci. 54:396, 1965.
7. Babiss, L. E., Liaw, W. S., Zimmer, S. G., Godman, G. C., Ginsberg, H. S., and Fisher, P. B.: Mutations in the E1a gene of adenovirus type 5 alter the tumorigenic properties of transformed cloned rat fibroblast cells. Proc. Natl. Acad. Sci. 83:2167, 1986.
8. Baylin, S. B., Fearon, E. R., Vogelstein, B., deBustros, A., Sharkis, S. J., Burke, P. J., Staal, S. D., and Nelkin, B. D.: Hypermethylation of the 5' region of the calcitonin gene is a property of human lymphoid and acute myeloid leukemia. Blood 70:412, 1987.
9. Baylin, S. B., Hoppener, J. W. M., deBustros, A., Steenbergh, P. H., Lips, C. J. M., and Nelkin, B. D.: DNA methylation patterns of the calcitonin gene in human lung cancers and lymphomas. Cancer Res. 46:2917, 1986.
10. Benchimol, S., Fuks, A., Jothy, S., Beauchemin, N., Shirota, K., and Stanners, C. P.: Carcinoembryonic antigen, a human tumor marker, functions as an intercellular adhesion molecule. Cell 57:327, 1989.
11. Berger, N. A.: Poly(ADP-ribose) in the cellular response to DNA damage. Radiation Res. 101:4, 1985.
12. Bergstrand, C. G., and Czar, B.: Demonstration of a new protein fraction in serum from the human fetus. Scand. J. Clin. Lab. Invest. 8:174, 1956.
13. Beutler, B., and Cerami, A.: Cachectin and tumor necrosis factor as two sites of the same biological coin. Nature 320:584, 1986.
14. Beutler, B., Mahoney, J., LeTrang, N., Pekala, P., and Cerami, A.: Purification of cachectin, a lipoprotein lipase-suppressing hormone secreted by endotoxin-induced RAW 264.7 cells. J. Exp. Med. 161:984, 1985.
15. Bird, A. P.: CpG-rich islands and the function of DNA methylation. Nature 321:209, 1986.
16. Bodger, M. P., Janossy, G., Bollum, F. J., Burford, G. D., and Hoffbrand, A. V.: The ontogeny of terminal deoxynucleotidyl transferase positive cells in the human fetus. Blood 61:1125, 1983.
17. Bollum, F. J., and Chang, L. M. S.: Terminal transferase in normal and leukemic cells. Adv. Cancer Res. 47:37, 1986.
18. Booth, J., Boyland, E., and Sims, P.: An enzyme from rat liver catalysing conjugations with glutathione. Biochem. J. 79:516, 1961.
19. Borek, C., Morgan, W. F., Ong, A., and Cleaver, J. E.: Inhibition of malignant transformation in vitro by inhibitors of poly(ADP-ribose) synthesis. Proc. Natl. Acad. Sci. 81:243, 1984.
20. Bourne, H. R., and DeFranco, A. L: Signal transduction and intracellular messengers. In Oncogenes and the Molecular Origins of Cancer. New York, Cold Spring Harbor Laboratory Press, p 79, 1989.
21. Bradstock, K. F., Kerr, A., and Bollum, F. J.: Antigenic phenotype of TdT-positive cells in human peripheral blood. Cell. Immunol. 90:590, 1985.
22. Brown, N. H.: A case of pluriglandular syndrome-diabetes of bearded women. Lancet 2:1022, 1928.
23. Burk, R. R.: Reduced adenyl cyclase activity in polyoma virus transformed cell line. Nature 219:1272, 1968.
24. Burt, M. E., Lowry, S. F., Gorshbath, C., and Brennan, M. E.: Metabolic alterations in a noncachetic animal tumor system. Cancer 47:2138, 1981.
25. Busch, H., Davis, J. R., and Olle, E.: Citrate accumulation in slices of transplantable tumors of the rat. Cancer Res. 17:711, 1957.
26. Cameron, I. L., and Ord, V. A.: Parenteral level of glucose intake on glucose homeostasis, tumor growth, gluconeogenesis, and body consumption in normal and tumor-bearing rats. Cancer Res. 43:5228, 1983.
27. Carson, D. A., Seto, S., Wasson, D. B., and Carrera, C. J.: DNA strand breaks, NAD metabolism, and programmed cell death. Exp. Cell Res. 164:273, 1986.
28. Carswell, E. A., Gold, L., Kassel, R. L., Green, S., Fiore, N., and Williamson, B.: An endotoxin-induced serum factor that causes necrosis of tumors. Proc. Natl. Acad. Sci. 72:3666, 1975.
29. Chang, L. M: Development of terminal deoxynucleotidyl transferase activity in embryonic calf thymus gland. Biochem. Biophys. Res. Commun. 44:124, 1971.
30. Chiquet, M., and Fambrough, D. M.: Chick myotendinous antigen II. A novel extracellular glycoprotein complex consisting of large disulfide-linked subunits. J. Cell Biol. 98:1937, 1984.
31. Coleman, M. S., Hutton, J. J., DeSimone, P., and Bollum, F. J.: Terminal deoxyribonucleotidyl transferase in human leukemia. Proc. Natl. Acad. Sci. 71:4404, 1974.
32. Dano, K., Andreasen, P. A., Grondahl-Hansen, J., Kristensen, P., Nielsen, L. S., and Skriver, L.: Plasminogen activators, tissue degradation and cancer. Adv. Cancer Res. 44:139, 1985.
33. deBustros, A., Nelkin, B. D., Silverman, A., Ehrlich, G., Poiesz, B., and Baylin, S. B.: The short arm of chromosome 11 is a "hot spot" for hypermethylation in human neoplasa. Proc. Natl. Acad. Sci. 85:5693, 1988.
34. DeWys, W.: Working conference on anorexia and cachexia of neoplastic disease. Cancer Res. 30:2816, 1970.
35. Dice, J. F.: Molecular determinants of protein half-lives in eukaryotic cells. FASEB. J. 1:349, 1987.
36. Dieffenbach, C. W., SenGupta, D. N., Krause, D., Sawzak, D., and Silverman, R. H.:

Invasion and Metastasis

Lance A. Liotta
William G. Stetler-Stevenson
Patricia S. Steeg

Invasion and metastasis is the most insidious and life threatening aspect of cancer.[9,32,63,74,126,142] It is well accepted that most invasive epithelial cancers are derived from pre-existing carcinoma in situ lesions, adenomas, or disorders of epithelial proliferation. Once the neoplasm becomes invasive, it has the capacity to disseminate via lymphatics and vascular channels. Local invasion can compromise the function of involved tissues. The most significant turning point in the disease, however, is the establishment of metastasis. At this stage the patient can no longer be cured by local therapy alone.

The patient with metastatic disease succumbs to direct anatomic compromise caused by the metastasis or to complications associated with metastasis therapy. Approximately 30% of patients with newly diagnosed cancers have clinically detectable metastases. At least 30–40% of the remaining patients clinically free of metastases actually harbor occult metastases. Thus, only a third of newly diagnosed patients can potentially be cured by local therapeutic modalities alone, a number which may be optimistic. Unfortunately, most patients suffer from multiple sites of metastatic disease, not all of which may present at any one time. The formation of metastatic colonies is a continuous process commencing early in the growth of the primary tumor and increasing with time. Metastases have the potential to metastasize: the presence of large identifiable metastases in a given organ are frequently accompanied by a greater number of micrometastases that may have been more recently disseminated from the primary tumor or the metastasis. The size and age variation in metastases, their dispersed anatomic locations, and their heterogeneous composition hinder complete surgical extirpation of disease and limit the effective concentration of anti-cancer drugs that can be delivered to tumor cells in metastatic colonies.

Tumors of comparable size and histology can have widely divergent metastatic potential depending upon their intrinsic aggressiveness. Thus, there is a great clinical need to a) predict the aggressiveness of a patient's individual tumor, b) identify clinically occult metastatic colonies, and c) eradicate established metastasis. New strategies to address these clinical goals have been provided by recent advances in our understanding of molecular mechanisms of metastasis. We now know that the malignant phenotype is the culmination of a series of genetic changes that involves both positive and negative regulatory elements (Figure I-10-1). Investigation of the activation, regulation, mutation, or somatic dele-

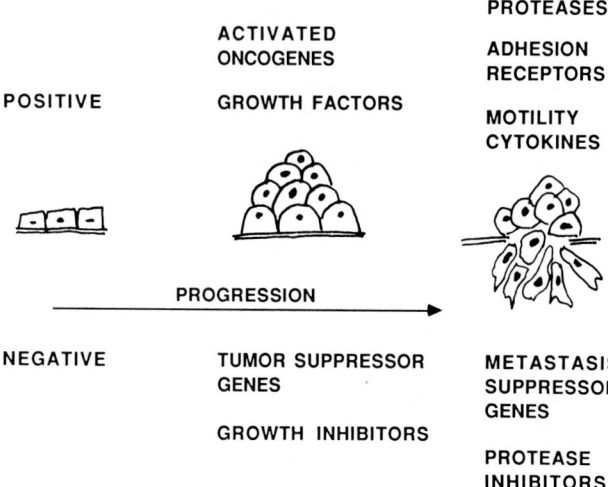

Figure I-10-1. Positive and negative regulation of proliferation, invasion and metastasis during multistep tumor progression.

tion of genes which encode these regulatory elements is a new frontier for metastasis research.

Tumor-Host Interactions in the Metastatic Cascade

The process of metastasis is a cascade of linked sequential steps involving multiple host-tumor interactions (Table I-10-1). To successfully create a metastatic deposit, a cell or group of cells must be able to leave the primary tumor, invade the local host tissue, and survive to proliferate (Figure I-10-2). This complex process requires the cells to enter into the circulation, arrest at the distant vascular bed, extravasate into the organ interstitium and parenchyma, and proliferate as a secondary colony. A large foundation of experimental work suggests that during each stage of the process, only the fittest tumor cells survive.[32,74,126] A very small percentage (<0.01%) of circulating tumor cells ultimately initiate successful metastatic colonies. Thus, metastasis is a highly selective competition favoring the survival of a minor subpopulation of metastatic tumor cells that preexist within the primary tumor.

The distribution of metastases varies widely depending on the histologic type and anatomic location of the primary tumor. The most frequent organ location of distant metastases in many types of cancers appears to be the first capillary bed

Table I-10-1.   Tumor-Host Interactions During the Metastatic Cascade

Metastatic Cascade Event	Potential Mechanisms
1. Tumor initiation	Carcinogenic insult, oncogene activation or derepression, chromosome rearrangement
2. Promotion and progression	Karyotypic, genetic, and epigenetic instability, gene amplification; promotion associated genes and growth factors; mutation or loss of suppressor gene products
3. Uncontrolled proliferation	Autocrine growth factors or their receptors, receptors for host hormones such as estrogen
4. Angiogenesis	Multiple angiogenesis factors including known growth factors
5. Invasion of local tissues, blood and lymphatic vessels	Serum chemoattractants, autocrine motility factors, attachment receptors, degradative enzymes, loss of expression of proteinase inhibitors
6. Circulating tumor cell arrest and extravasation	Tumor cell homotypic or heterotypic aggregation
a. adherence to endothelium	Tumor cell interaction with fibrin, platelets, and clotting factors, adhesions to RGD type receptors
b. retraction of endothelium	Platelet factors, tumor cell factors
c. adhesion to basement membrane	Receptors for laminin, thrombospondin and type IV collagen
d. dissolution of basement membrane	Metalloproteinases, serine proteinases, heparanase, cathepsins
e. locomotion	Autocrine motility factors, chemotaxis factors
7. Colony formation at secondary site	Receptors for local tissue growth factors, angiogenesis factors, mutation or loss of metastasis suppressor genes
8. Evasion of host defenses and resistance to therapy	Resistance to killing by host macrophages, natural killer cells and activated T cells, failure to express, or blocking of tumor specific antigens, amplification of drug resistance genes

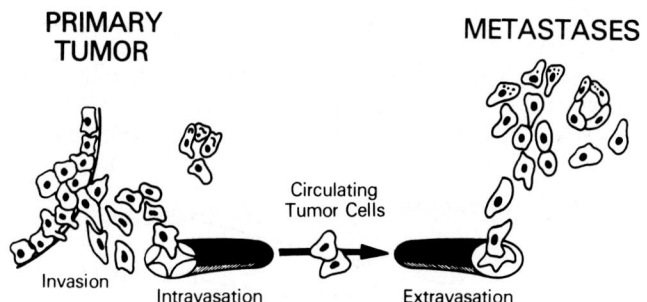

PRIMARY TUMOR   **METASTASES**

Circulating Tumor Cells

Invasion   Intravasation   Extravasation

Figure I-10-2.   Multistep cascade of metastasis.

encountered by the circulating cells. Examples of this are lung metastases from sarcoma, brain metastases from primary lung carcinoma, and colorectal cancer dissemination to liver. In the gynecologic tumors, distant metastases are seen in two forms; the first is serosal dissemination, e.g., liver capsule metastases from ovarian cancer, and the second is capillary-associated dissemination such as liver and lung parenchymal disease.

On the other hand there are many metastatic sites that cannot be predicted on the basis of anatomical considerations alone, and can be considered examples of organ tropism. Clear cell carcinoma of the kidney often metastasizes to thyroid, breast cancers to ovary, ovary rarely to breast, and ocular melanoma frequently metastasizes to liver. The predilection of breast and prostate cancer for bone may also reflect a degree of organ tropism. The molecular mechanisms mediating the organ distribution of metastasis has been the subject of study of a number of investigators.[101] Hamilton and coworkers developed a mouse xenograft model of human ovarian cancer using the NIH:OVCAR3 cell line developed from the ascites of a patient who had progressed on primary combination chemotherapy.[46] After intraperito-

neal inoculation, animals develop malignant ascites, tumor masses involving ovaries and bowel serosa, and may develop liver capsule metastases and very late lung metastases. This pattern accurately models what is seen in women with stage III and IV ovarian cancer. Another method for studying organ tropism involves the use of organs grafted into ectopic sites. Fidler and Hart observed that the intravenously injected B16-F10 melanoma cells colonized the native lung as well as subcutaneous lung grafts.[32] In order to find the ectopic site, the tumor cells must have either left the first capillary arrest site in the lungs and travelled to the ectopically implanted lung grafts, or entered the general circulation and then recognized signals from the ectopic lung to exit at that location. In control mice, ectopic kidney grafts were not colonized by the circulating tumor cells indicating a clear organ selectivity for lung but not kidney.

There are several theoretical mechanisms for organ tropism.[102] First, tumor cells disseminate equally in all organs, but preferentially grow only in specific organs. Preferential growth may be induced by local growth factors or hormones present in the target organ. For example, the insulin-like growth factors are present in liver and lung and have been shown to be important growth factors for breast cancer, lung cancer, and rhabdomyosarcoma. Second, circulating tumor cells may adhere preferentially to the endothelial luminal surface only in the targeted organ. This requires that there be special recognition signals on the endothelial cells which determine the organ specificity. Last, circulating tumor cells may respond to soluble factors diffusing locally out of the target organs.[62] Such factors could act in a chemotactic fashion to attract the tumor cells to extravasate. They could also cause the circulating tumor cells to aggregate and therefore embolize in the target organ. Kohn and colleagues have shown that the OVCAR3 human ovarian cancer cell line migrates in response to insulin and insulin-like growth factors, that are known to be present in many normal tissues and secreted by several tissues that are known metastatic target sites.[62] Nicolson and colleagues have identified endothelial surface antigens that may mediate preferential adhesion of circulating tumor cells to endothelium of particular organs.[101,102] Attempts at characterizing these antigens are underway.

Interaction of Metastatic Tumor Cells With the Extracellular Matrix

The mammalian organism is divided into a series of tissue compartments separated by the extracellular matrix. The basement membrane and its underlying interstitial stroma is the major connective tissue unit separating organ parenchymal compartments. During the transition from in situ to invasive carcinoma, tumor cells penetrate the epithelial basement membrane and enter the underlying interstitial stroma.[8,72] The continuous basement membrane is a dense meshwork of collagen, glycoproteins and proteoglycans which normally does not contain any pores large enough for tumor cell traversal without destructive enlargement. Therefore, invasion of the basement membrane must be an active process. In order to invade, cervical and endometrial carcinomas must penetrate the epithelial basement membrane separating the endometrial or cervical epithelium from the underlying submucosa and muscularis layers. Epithelial ovarian cancer cells must penetrate basement membranes and also the ovarian capsule in order to metastasize. Once the tumor cells enter the underlying stroma, they gain access to lymphatics and blood vessels for further dissemination. Fibrosarcomas and angiosarcomas, developing from stromal cells, invade surrounding muscle basement membrane and interstitium. Tumor cells must cross basement membranes to invade nerves and most types of organ parenchyma. During intravasation or extravasation, the tumor cells of any histologic origin must penetrate the subendothelial basement membrane. In the distant organ where metastatic colonies are established, extravasated tumor cells must migrate through the perivascular interstitial stroma before tumor colony growth occurs in the organ parenchyma.

General and widespread changes occur in the organization, distribution, and quantity of the epithelial basement membrane during the transition from benign to invasive carcinoma.[8] Benign proliferative disorders of the breast such as fibrocystic disease, sclerosing adenosis, intraductal hyperplasia, fibroadenoma, and intraductal papilloma are all characterized by disorganization of the normal epithelial stromal architecture. Extreme forms can mimic the appearance of invasive carcinoma. But regardless of the extensive nature of the architectural disorganization, these benign disorders are always characterized by a continuous basement membrane separating the epithelium from the stroma. In contrast, invasive ductal carcinoma,and invasive lobular carcinoma consistently possess a defective extracellular basement membrane with zones of basement membrane loss around the invading tumor cells in the stroma. The basement membrane is also markedly defective adjacent to tumor cells in lymph node and organ metastases. In some focal regions of well-differentiated carcinoma, partial basement mem-

brane formation by differentiated structures can be identified. These findings have direct application to diagnostic problems in surgical pathology, such as the differentiation of tangential sections of in situ lesions from true invasion or the differentiation of severe adenosis from invasive carcinoma. Loss of basement membranes in human carcinomas significantly correlates with increased incidence of metastases and poor five year survivals.

The general observation of defective basement membranes associated with cancer invasion and progression indicates that aggressive tumor cells may interact with basement membranes in a manner fundamentally different from normal cells. This provides the foundation for investigation of molecular mechanisms of tumor cell invasion. In this regard, the interactions of the tumor cell with the basement membrane can be separated into three steps (Figure I-10-3).[64,72,76] For the case of a circulating tumor cell, the basement membrane is exposed by retraction of the endothelium induced by the tumor cell. The tumor cell then attaches to the basement membrane surface. This is mediated by tumor cell surface proteins binding to glycoproteins such as laminin, type IV collagen, and fibronectin in the basement membrane. Following attachment, the tumor cells must create a rent in the basement membrane. Tumor cells both secrete degradative enzymes and induce the host to secrete proteinases to degrade the matrix and its component adhesion molecules. Matrix lysis takes place in a highly localized region close to the tumor cell surface where the amount of active enzyme outbalances the natural proteinase inhibitors pres-

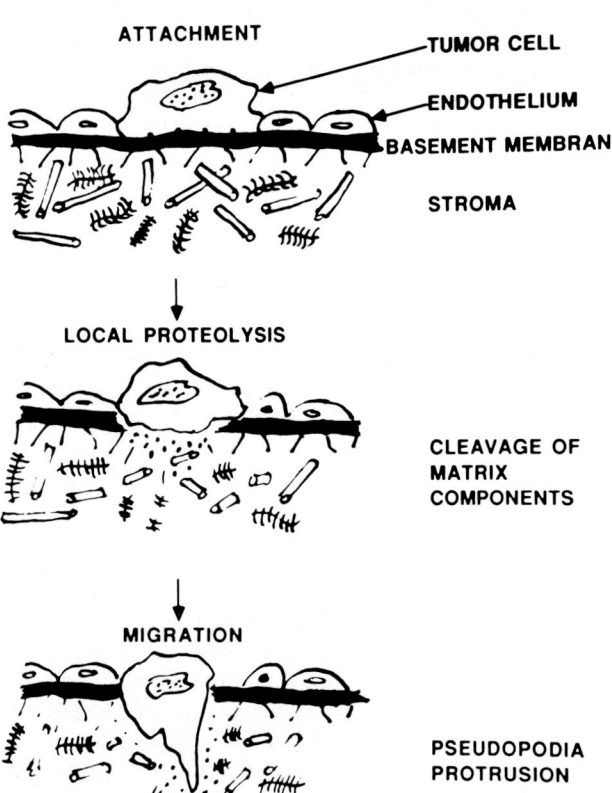

Figure I-10-3. Three step hypothesis for invasion of the extracellular matrix unit.

ent in the serum, in the matrix, or that secreted by normal cells in the vicinity. The third step of invasion is translocation of the tumor cell across the basement membrane via the hole created by the local proteolysis. The direction and site of the tumor cell locomotion may by influenced by host-derived chemoattractants or tumor cell-secreted motility factors. The invasive process is a dynamic one involving cyclic repetition of these steps.

Adhesion. The first step of basement membrane invasion requires tumor cell attachment. A major attachment protein found exclusively in the basement membrane is laminin. Laminin is a large complex cruciform glycoprotein with the ability to bind to multiple membrane components including type IV collagen, heparan sulfate, proteoglycan, and entactin.[77,115] Laminin plays a role in cell attachment, cell spreading, mitogenesis, neurite outgrowth, morphogenesis, and cell movement. Cell surface receptors for laminin mediate these varied functions of tumor cells. A nanomolar affinity cell surface laminin receptor of 67 kDa has been cloned from normal and neoplastic cells.[7,81,86,144] Laminin receptors may be altered in number or degree of occupancy in human carcinomas. This may be the indirect result of defective basement membrane organization in the carcinomas.[162] Breast carcinoma and colon carcinoma tissues contain a higher number of exposed, unoccupied laminin receptors compared to benign lesions. These receptors may be amplified and distributed over the surface of the cell in contrast to the architecture of the normal cell, in which the laminin receptors are polarized at the basal surface and are occupied by the laminin in the basement membrane.

There is experimental evidence to demonstrate that tumor cells exposed to the whole laminin molecule more avidly form metastases in animals. If, however, cells are treated with a fragment of laminin which cannot link the tumor cell to the basement membrane, metastases cannot be initiated. In other studies, linking an anti-laminin receptor monoclonal antibody onto adriamycin-containing liposomes markedly increased the cell kill of breast adenocarcinoma cells over normal control breast epithelial cells in vitro.[113] Further studies are necessary to determine the clinical applicability of these observations. Castronovo and colleagues showed that hormone dependent breast adenocarcinoma cells increased their laminin receptor mRNA 3-fold after treatment with estrogens and progestins; however, these effects were not seen in the hormone-independent cell line MDA-MB-231 cell line, suggesting that various cell-laminin interactions are mediated by steroid hormones.[18]

A second class of matrix receptors important in tumor cell attachment to the extracellular matrix is the "integrins." This family of cell surface glycoproteins bind a broad array of adhesion proteins with micromolar affinity.[55] The adhesion proteins which bind to integrins include fibronectin, vitronectin, fibrin, type I collagen, laminin, thrombospondin, and von Willebrand factor.[47] The integrin receptor consists of a heterodimer of alpha and beta chains which, in part, confer ligand specificity. Peptides of the Arg-Gly-Asp (RGD) group inhibit the functions of many of the integrins, a property for which the family was originally named. RGD sequences in a wide variety of proteins may serve as the recognition site for binding to the integrins. Preferential recognition of spe-

cific adhesion molecules may be conferred by ligand sequences flanking the RGD sites.[121] The integrin proteins are thought to align adhesion proteins such as fibronectin on the cell surface with cytoskeletal components such as talin and actin, thus altering cell shape.[52] In addition, these receptors may play an adhesive role in platelet-tumor interactions, binding of lymphoid cells to the endothelium, and the interaction of circulating tumor cells with endothelial surfaces, fibrin, von Willibrand factor, or thrombospondin. These adhesion ligands are important in the metastatic cascade. Co-injection of tumor cells with large quantities of RGD peptides inhibited metastasis formation in animal models.[54] Thus, the interaction of cells and adhesion molecules of low and high affinity receptors is important in metastasis development.

Proteolysis

The process of invasion is not a passive one due to pressure from excessive cellular proliferation alone, but is an active, dynamic process which requires protein synthesis and degradation.[42,145,146] Inhibitors of metalloproteinases or of protein synthesis, but not of DNA synthesis, block tumor cell invasion into the matrix. Tumor cells must traverse the extracellular matrix in the process of invasion and must be able to either secrete or activate enzymes which can degrade the major components of the matrix such as collagens types I, IV, and V, fibronectin, and proteoglycans.

Metalloproteinases

A critical proteolytic event early in the metastatic cascade appears to be the degradation of basement membrane collagen.[71] Basement membranes contain a distinct type of collagen, type IV collagen, as well as laminin and heparan sulfate proteoglycan. Type IV collagen may form the basement membrane architectural scaffolding on which laminin, heparan sulfate proteoglycan and minor components of the basement membrane are assembled. Much attention has focused on the ability of metastatic tumor cells to degrade type IV collagen.

Type IV collagenases are named for their selective ability to degrade type IV basement membrane collagen in a pepsin resistant triple helical domain generating characteristic ¼ amino terminal, and ¾ carboxyl terminal fragments.[31,73] They are members of the metalloproteinase gene family (Figure I-10-4). Other proteases, such as transin/stromelysin, may degrade type IV collagen in the pepsin sensitive non-helical domains in a less specific fashion.[163]

Recent work has demonstrated that there are at least two type IV collagenase enzymes . A 72 kDa and a 92 kDa type IV procollagenase exist.[20,164] Both are members of the matrix metalloproteinase gene family, and share structural homologies with other members of this family (Figure I-10-4). These type IV collagenases are distinguishable by immunologic, molecular and biochemical criteria, but not by substrate specificity. Both are secreted as latent proenzymes, are activated by organomercurial compounds with the concomitant autoproteolytic removal of an amino terminal fragment, are inhibited by members of the tissue inhibitor of metalloproteinase (TIMP) family, and form specific latent proenzyme-

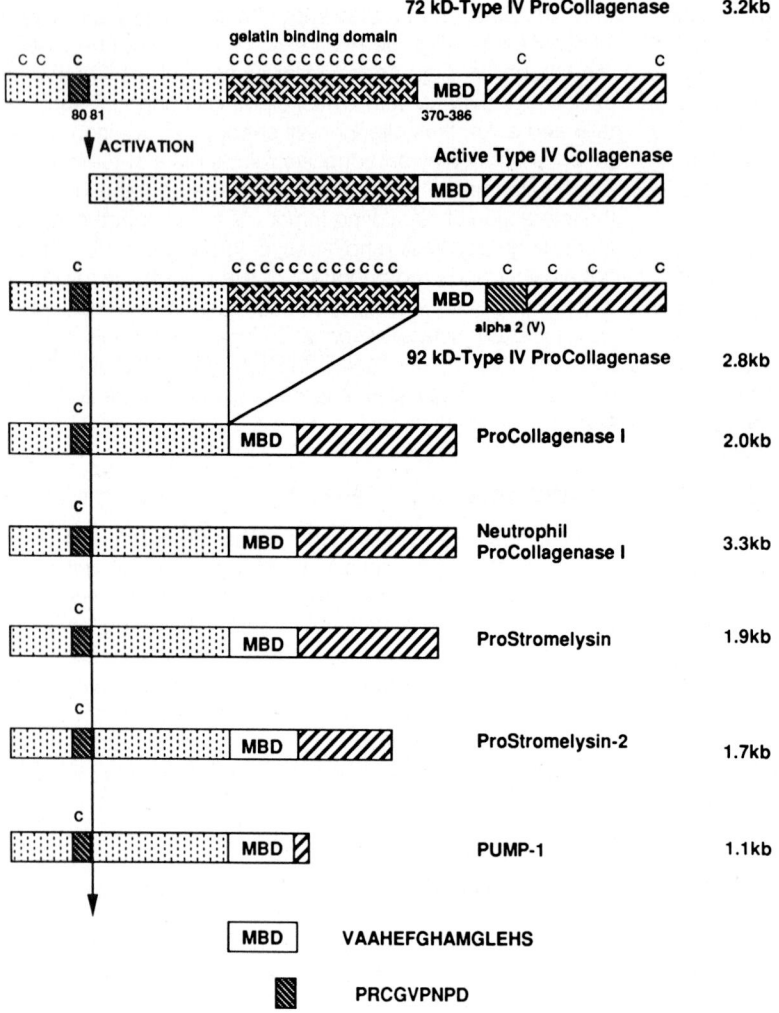

72 kD-Type IV ProCollagenase   3.2kb

gelatin binding domain

80 81   370-386

ACTIVATION

Active Type IV Collagenase

alpha 2 (V)

92 kD-Type IV ProCollagenase   2.8kb

ProCollagenase I   2.0kb

Neutrophil ProCollagenase I   3.3kb

ProStromelysin   1.9kb

ProStromelysin-2   1.7kb

PUMP-1   1.1kb

MBD   VAAHEFGHAMGLEHS

PRCGVPNPD

Figure I-10-4.   Metalloproteinase gene family. The proenzyme form of each proteinase member is shown. Activation involves cleavage of an amino terminal peptide 1-80 containing an unpaired cysteine residue. In the latent enzyme, the unpaired cysteine residue folds over and blocks the active site (MBD, metal binding domain) of the enzyme by forming a noncovalent interaction with the zinc metal atom. The type IV collagenases are distinguished by a cysteine repeat gelatin binding domain which mediates adhesion to type IV collagen. V = Val; A = Ala; H = His; E = Glu; F = Phe; G = Gly; M = Met; L = Lys; S = Ser; P = Pro; R = Arg; C = Cys; N = Asn; D = Asp; PUMP-I = putative metalloproteinase.

TIMP complexes with one or the other member of the TIMP family. Both enzymes also possess potent gelatinolytic activities and degrade native type V and VII collagens.

There is a substantial body of evidence which supports a positive correlation between type IV collagenase activity and tumor cell invasion.[37,79,90,98,117,150] Metastatic potential has been shown to correlate in a positive fashion with type IV collagenolytic activity in murine tumor models.[37,79,98,150] Highly aggressive human tumors such as carcinomas, melanomas, hepatomas, fibrosarcomas, and invasive lymphomas, all showed elevated levels of type IV collagenase activity when compared with benign controls. Studies have also shown a positive correlation between augmented type IV collagenase activity and the genetic induction of a metastatic phenotype.[37,150] Furthermore, use of agents which specifically inhibited type IV collagenase activity blocked invasion by tumor cells.[90,91,117]

Many earlier studies did not discriminate between the 72 kDa type IV collagenase which was originally identified and purified from a metastatic murine cell line, and the 92 kDa type IV collagenase which was originally characterized as a gelatinolytic activity from human polymorphonuclear leukocytes. However, recent studies using well characterized biochemical and molecular probes have demonstrated that in human tumor cells there is an excellent correlation between the 72 kDa type IV collagenase and enhanced metastatic potential. Immunohistochemical studies using affinity purified anti-72 kDa type IV collagenase antibodies have demonstrated that low levels of this enzyme are produced by normal, non-tumorigenic, non-metastatic cells such as the myoepithelial cells of the human breast.[92] Benign proliferative lesions of the breast were associated with some increase in 72 kDa type IV collagenase immunoreactivity that was again restricted to the myoepithelial cells. With progressive severity of breast lesions from atypical hyperplasia through carcinoma in situ to frankly invasive carcinoma, there was an increase in the immunohistochemical staining for the 72 kDa type IV collagenase that was specifically associated with the neoplastic breast epithelial cells (Figure I-10-5A).[92] Moreover, benign polyps of the colon, normal colorectal and gastric mucosa all show negligible immunoreactivity for 72 kDa type IV collagenase (Figure I-10-5B).[36] In contrast, almost all invasive colonic and gastric (Figure I-10-5C) adenocarcinomas were positive for this antigen.

Measurement of 72 kDa type IV collagenase mRNA levels and enzyme activity have shown a close correlation with the invasive and metastatic properties of c-Ha-ras transformed bronchial epithelial cells.[150] Down regulation of type IV col-

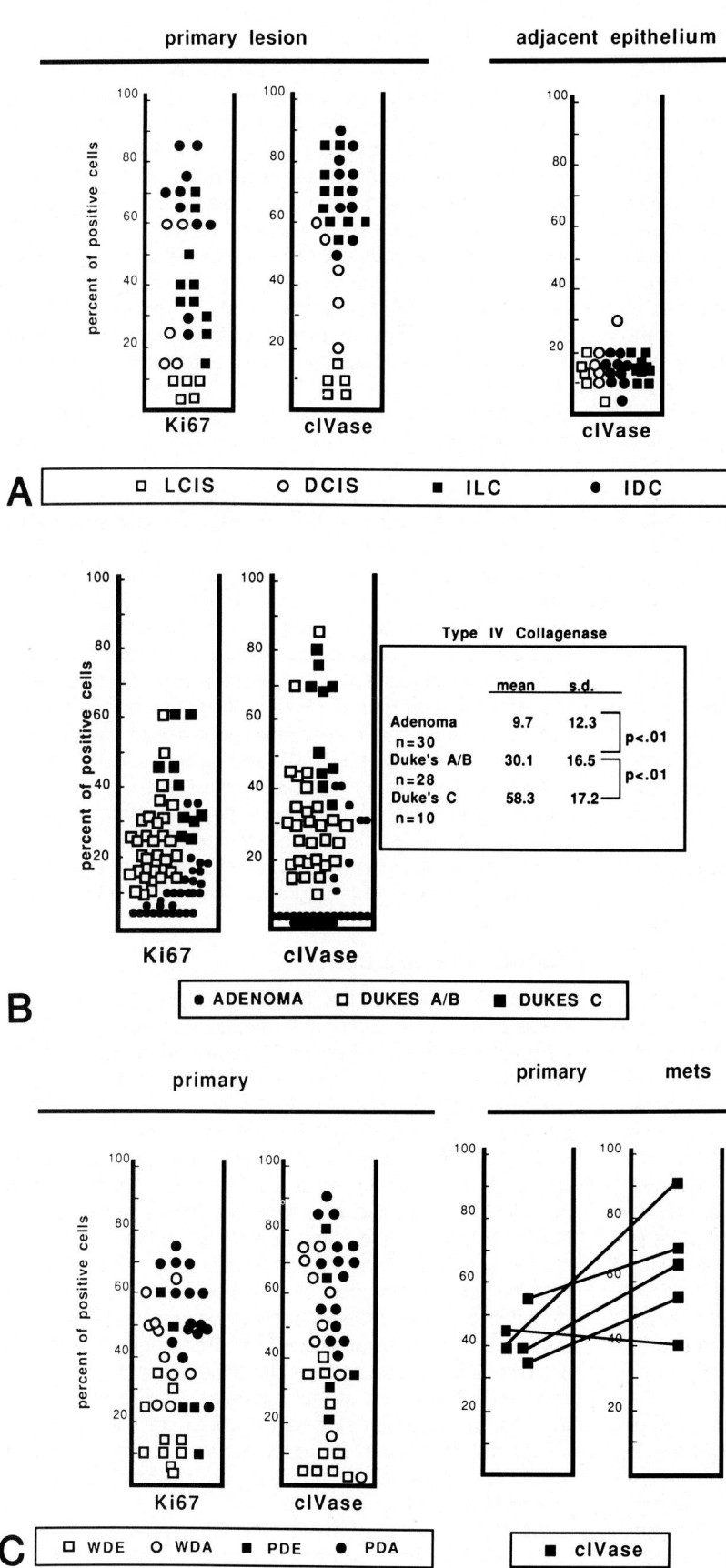

Figure I-10-5. Type IV collagenase augmentation during human carcinoma progression. Affinity purified anti-synthetic peptide antibodies were used in an immunohistochemical study of formalin fixed paraffin embedded human neoplasms. The Ki67 proliferation associated marker was used as a control. Each symbol represents an individual patient's primary tumor. In each tumor, 1,000 cells were scored by three independent pathologists. **A.** Breast Carcinoma. LCIS: Lobular Carcinoma in situ. DCIS: Ductal Carcinoma in situ. ILC: Infiltrating lobular carcinoma. IDC: Infiltrating ductal carcinoma. All invasive lesions had augmented levels of type IV collagenase (clVase) compared to adjacent non-cancerous epithelium. **B.** Colorectal Neoplasia. Duke's C cases had the highest proportion of cells positive for type IV collagenase (clVase). Duke's A/B tumors exhibited intermediate levels, and the majority of adenomas exhibited very low type IV collagenase content. The same pattern was found when the type IV collagenase mRNA levels were compared. **C.** Gastric Carcinoma. WDE: Well differentiated early (superficial). WDA: Well differentiated advanced (invading through the full thickness of the gastric wall). PDE: Poorly differentiated early. PDA: Poorly differentiated advanced. The advanced tumors contained the highest level of type IV collagenase.

lagenolytic activity by retinoic acid treatment of human melanoma cells has been correlated with a loss of the invasive phenotype. Studies of the mechanism of this effect have revealed that retinoic acid treatment of human melanoma cells results in a reduction of the steady state level of the 72 kDa type IV collagenase mRNA and loss of the invasive capacity.[48] Measurement of the steady state transcript levels for this enzyme in human colonic adenocarcinoma tissues have demonstrated a statistically significant increase over those of adjacent normal tissues which showed consistently low levels of expression. These studies suggest that the 72 kDa type IV collagenase enzyme is a normal cell component that is dramatically over-expressed in many invasive and metastatic human cancers. Endothelial cells in culture secrete a readily detectable level of type IV collagenase activity. Antisera against the 72 kDa type IV collagenase can inhibit basic fibroblast growth factor induced endothelial cell invasion of human amnion membrane in vitro.[91] These observations suggest that the 72 kDa type IV collagenase may also function in normal physiologic processes such as basement membrane turnover by myoepithelial cells and angiogenesis by endothelial cells.

Serine Proteinases

Malignant cells have been documented to have increased amounts of plasminogen activators.[21,41,82] In addition, oncogenic transformation of cells has been associated with increases in the extracellular release of plasminogen activators. The plasminogen activators, urokinase and tissue plasminogen activator, are independent gene products which are secreted as proenzymes. The only well-characterized physiologic substrate that is known for the plasminogen activators is plasminogen. Investigators from a number of laboratories have shown that plasminogen activator activity can be extracted from a number of human and animal tumors, and is predominantly urokinase.[16,83] Laboratory studies have indicated that matrix glycoproteins are susceptible to plasmin-mediated proteolytic degradation.[56,90,117] Direct evidence for the role of these enzymes in invasion has been reported using an in vitro invasion assay.[56] A positive correlation between plasminogen activator activity and metastatic potential has been established for the B16 murine melanoma line.[157] Highly metastatic cells of the F10 generation showed high levels in the primary tumors and even higher levels in the pulmonary metastases. A recent report demonstrated a significant (6-fold) elevation of urokinase mRNA in human primary lung and breast carcinomas when compared with nonmalignant tissues.[124] At present, urokinase levels are not considered sufficiently diagnostic of tumor aggressiveness to allow development as a tumor marker.

Cysteine Proteinases

Evidence for the role of the cysteine proteinases, cathepsins B, L, and D, in cancer progression and metastasis is growing.[84,116,131,132] Cathepsin B is a lysosomal acid hydrolase with a broad range of endopeptidase activity against substrates including myosin, actin, proteoglycans, fibronectin, laminin, and the nonhelical portions of type IV collagen. Cathepsin B activity has been found in association with the plasma membrane fraction of tumor cells, and in the conditioned media from tumor cell cultures.[131,132] The tumor cell-derived cathepsin B appears to be a different enzyme than that which is found in the lysosomes of normal cells. Studies using the B16 murine melanoma line have shown a correlation between cathepsin B activity and metastatic potential. Pietras and coworkers measured cathepsin B1 activity in the serum of patients with gynecologic malignancies and found a significant increase in cathepsin B1 activity in patients with stage III and IV squamous cell carcinoma of the uterine cervix. Minimal elevations were observed in women with lower stage disease, dysplasia, and controls.[107] They also showed that advanced stage adenocarcinomas of the ovary and endometrium were associated with markedly elevated levels of enzyme activity up to 2–3 fold higher than seen in early stage patients. A similarly positive correlation has been shown between cathepsin B levels in other human tumors and the malignant behavior of these tumors.

Cathepsin D is also a lysosomal acid proteinase.[118] It has documented mitogenic activity on estrogen-depleted MCF-7 human breast adenocarcinoma cells in culture, and its secretion is constitutive in hormone-independent breast cancer cell lines.[118] This proteinase has the ability to degrade extracellular matrix components such as proteoglycans, and is present in high levels in proliferative breast diseases both benign and malignant, but is present in very low amounts in resting mammary glands.[116] Two clinical studies of breast cancer patients have correlated high levels of cathepsin D with poor disease-free survival and overall survival, as an independent variable.[135,143] Cathepsin D was of most significant prognostic value in node-negative breast cancer patients. Hence, as markers of cancer invasion, cathepsin D and type IV collagenase are potential new diagnostic and prognostic markers of the aggressiveness of malignancy.

Tumor Cell Migration

An important step in the dynamic process of invasion and metastasis involves tumor cell translocation across biologic barriers. Tumor cell migration is necessary at the initiation of the metastatic cascade at which time the tumor cells leave the primary and gain access to the circulation, as well as at the end of invasion when the tumor cell is entering the secondary site. The movement of the cells through such biologic barriers may be driven by a number of factors.[43,85] These include tumor-derived chemotactic factors, host-derived chemoattractants, and combinations of the two. Laboratory studies of tumor cell locomotion have shown that tumor cells may respond chemotactically to growth factors, collagen peptides, adhesion proteins such as laminin and fibronectin, and tumor derived attractants.[5,44,85,86] These agents may both stimulate the initiation and maintenance of tumor cell motility and the directedness of that migration. The reliance upon the host for migration stimulation would not favor the sustained migration seen in highly metastatic populations of tumor cells, thus emphasizing the importance of tumor-derived chemoattractants.

Investigators have demonstrated the importance of autocrine growth factors for transformed cells, leading into the hypothesis that tumor cells also secrete autocrine motility-stimulating factors (AMF): For example, a 55 kDa protein which is secreted by the A2058 human melanoma cell line into its conditioned media.[44] The A2058 melanoma cells, as well as a broad array of other human carcinoma cell lines including MDA-231 human breast cancer, OVCAR3 human ovarian cancer, and lines of prostate cancer, colon cancer, and bladder cancer origin, respond to AMF with directed or chemotactic motility as well as random stimulated or chemokinetic migration. Several of these cell lines are under study to characterize their respective AMFs. AMF stimulates the initiation of pseudopodial extensions by cells prior to whole cell translocation.[44] Pseudopodia have clustering of laminin receptors, and have been found to have actin filament elongation at their core. The protruding pseudopodia may serve multiple functions including acting as sense organs for the migrating cell to locate directional clues, to secrete AMF for the body of the cell to sense, to provide propulsive traction for locomotion, and to induce matrix proteolysis to assist in the penetration of the matrix. The clinical importance of AMF has been demonstrated for bladder carcinoma patients. A blinded study was done in which urine from patients with benign genitourinary processes or transitional cell carcinoma of the bladder were studied for urinary motility-stimulating activity. A statistically significant correlation between the amount of AMF activity in the urine and the tumor stage and grade was demonstrated.[45] These observations suggest the potential diagnostic importance of markers of tumor cell locomotion.

The complexity of tumor cell migration requires that more than one agent be involved in the direction, location, and magnitude of the migratory response. During the course of invasion, the tumor cell must interact with the extracellular matrix components, and be exposed to host-derived factors. Tumor cells have receptors for many of these potential attractants. Growth factors produced by normal and malignant tissues, such as the insulin-like growth factors may also be important in the migration of tumor cells.[62] These factors primarily stimulate chemotactic, or directed motility and may play a role in tumor cell homing to certain secondary sites. Therefore, the response of the tumor cell to autocrine stimulation by AMFs and endocrine or paracrine stimulation by matrix components and host-derived growth factors is important in the initiation of tumor cell locomotion, its directedness, and potentially the determination of the location of the metastatic focus.

Genetic Regulation of Invasion and Metastasis

Invasion and metastasis is a very complicated multi-step process. Consequently one gene product is not sufficient for metastasis. Furthermore, it is now understood that negative factors may be just as important as the positive factors discussed in the preceding sections (Figure I-10-1). In order to manifest the metastatic phenotype, individual tumor cells must have either a deficiency in the negative factors or an augmentation in the positive factors. This is analogous to the positive and negative factors involved in tumorigenicity. Some genetic changes result in an imbalance of growth regulation, leading to uncontrolled proliferation. In terms of positive regulation, this can be due to mutational activation of oncogenes, increased production of growth factors, or a continuous activation of a growth factor signal pathway.[66,133,159]

Uncontrolled growth can also be caused by the loss of production of growth inhibitor cytokines such as TGFβ which have their action at the cell surface, or the loss of growth suppressor gene products such as Rb or P53 which operate inside the cell.[33,123,134] However unrestrained growth does not, by itself, cause invasion and metastasis. The latter phenotype may require additional genetic changes over and above those resulting in uncontrolled proliferation. Invasion and metastasis can be facilitated by proteins which stimulate tumor cell attachment to host cellular or extracellular matrix elements, tumor cell proteolysis of host barriers to invasion, such as the basement membrane, tumor cell locomotion, and tumor cell colony formation in the target organ for metastasis.[42,57,77,165] These positive elements are counterbalanced, however, by factors which can block their production, regulation or action. Two classes of metastasis suppressor gene products can be identified: a) those that act outside the cell to block key aspects of metastasis such as proteolysis,[1,4,13,17,26,40,49,58,80,93-95,127,138,139,151,152,160,161] and b) those that have their action inside the cell[10,22,67,96,100,110,114,120,125,128,136,137,147,149] in a regulatory pathway.[10,22-24,32-34,53,59-61,67-70,78,88,96,99,100,103-106,110,111,114,119,120,125,128-130,136-137,141,147,149,155,158]

Metastasis Suppressor Genes

Several lines of evidence have pointed to the existence of metastasis suppressor genes. Fusion of normal cells with metastatic tumor cells have yielded hybrids which were fully tumorigenic but no longer metastatic.[67,114,128,149] These results indicated that the normal cell contributed genes which suppressed some key aspect of the metastatic process which did not regulate tumorigenicity. The ras oncogene, which is capable of inducing the metastatic phenotype, fails to do so in all tumor cells.[110,147] C127 cells transfected with ras express high levels of p21 and are tumorigenic, but nonmetastatic.[97] This second line of evidence indicates that the cells resistant to the induction of metastasis by ras may express a suppressor gene. As an extension of this finding, injection of rats with N-Nitrosomethylurea induced specific activating mutations in ras, resulting in mammary tumor development;[96,136] however, only 10% of the resulting tumors were metastatic during observation periods of up to one year. The lack of metastatic behavior in 90% of NMU-induced tumors despite the presence of a metastasis-inducing gene suggested active suppression. It is therefore logical to postulate that highly invasive and metastatic tumor cells could be deficient in specific gene products which suppress metastasis in normal cells or in benign tumors. Given the complicated array of biological functions involved in the metastatic process (i.e., motility, adhesiveness, proteolysis, angiogenesis, avoidance of immune recognition), any gene product that effectively stops one component of the process may block metastatic behavior, and therefore have suppressor activity. In addition, regulatory genes may be identified that suppress a cascade of downstream metastasis-associated genes, or suppress some aspect of cellular communication or signal transduction. Suppressor genes may also include genes which promote the stability of tumor cells, thereby reducing the genetic instability thought to fuel progression to the metastatic phenotype.

The first non-immunologically related metastasis suppressor gene was described by Pozzatti and colleagues.[110] Rat embryo fibroblasts transfected with c-Ha-ras were highly metastatic upon intravenous injection, but cotransfection of rat embryo fibroblasts with c-Ha-ras and Adenovirus 2 Ela resulted in transformed but virtually nonmetastatic cells. The Ela gene therefore suppressed the metastasis-inducing activity of the ras gene. One component of the mechanism of action of Ela is the suppression of metalloproteinase production by the tumor cells.[37] Ela is a viral gene and cannot play a role in the fusion experiments in which genes from normal cells suppressed the metastatic phenotype. Other investigators therefore attempted to identify cellular genes capable of metastasis suppression.

TIMPs (Tissue Inhibitors of Metalloproteinases) Can Suppress Invasion

The first major approach to the indentification of metastasis suppressor genes employed a functional analysis. A key biochemical step required for invasion and metastasis was identified and used as a target for the isolation of a cellular factor which blocked the key step. In this manner the TIMP (tissue inhibitor of metalloproteinases) family has recently been proposed as a major natural inhibitor of cancer invasion.

The secretion and activation of metalloproteinases is not enough to insure that they will degrade the target matrix substrate. This is because natural inhibitor proteins, produced either by the host, or by the tumor cell itself can block the latent or the active metalloproteinases.[140,151,152] Natural inhibitor proteins, such as TIMPs, may therefore function as metastasis suppressor proteins which act to inhibit tumor cell invasion of the extracellular matrix.[94,161] TIMP-1, the first member of the TIMP family, is a glycoprotein with an apparent molecular size of 28.5 kDa which forms a complex of 1:1 stoichiometry with activated interstitial collagenase, activated stromelysin, and the 92 kDa type IV collagenase.[17,26,49,58,80,95,139,160] The gene coding for TIMP-1 has been cloned, sequenced and mapped to the X-chromosome.[17,80] The secreted protein has 184 amino acids and six intramolecular disulfide bonds. The same cells which produce interstitial collagenase are capable of synthesizing and secreting TIMP-1.[49] Thus, the net collagenolytic activity for these cell types is the result of the balance between activated enzyme levels and TIMP-1 levels. Studies have shown an inverse correlation between TIMP-1 levels and the invasive potential of murine and human tumor cells. Furthermore, it has been reported that transfection of antisense RNA which blocks TIMP-1 expression increases the malignant phenotype.[58] One explanation for this result is that the antisense RNA blocked the production of TIMP-1 which normally prevented the malignant phenotype.

Recently Stetler-Stevenson and colleagues have isolated, purified, determined the complete primary structure, and cloned a second member of the TIMP family, TIMP-2.[138,139] TIMP-2—from human AL058 melanoma cells—is a 21 kDa protein which selectively forms a complex with the latent proenzyme form of the 72 kDa type IV collagenase (Figure I-10-6). The secreted protein has 194 amino acid residues and is not glycosylated. TIMP-2 shows 37% identity and

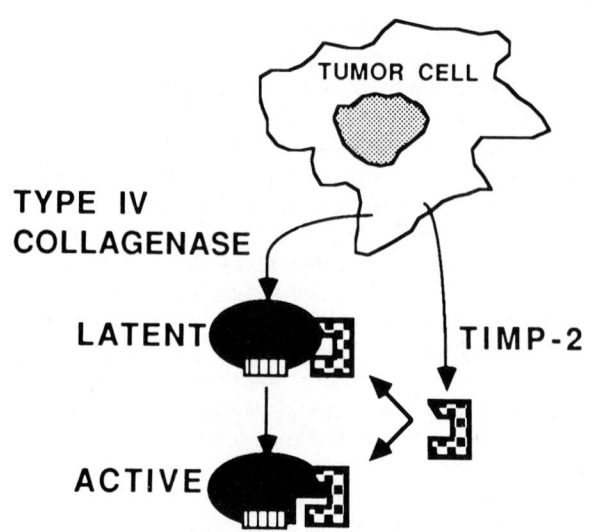

Figure I-10-6. Suppressor role for TIMP-2. Tumor cells can produce both metalloproteinases and TIMPs. TIMP-2 binds in a one to one molar ratio with latent 72 kDa type IV collagenase and blocks activation. It also binds to the activated form of the enzyme and to the activated form of all other members of the metalloproteinase family. Proteolysis via the 72 kDa type IV collagenase will occur only if the local levels of the activated enzyme molecules outnumber the local number of TIMP-2 molecules. Therapeutic administration of TIMP-2 can block enzyme activation as well as abolishing the activity of the activated enzyme species.

overall 65.6% homology to TIMP-1 at the deduced amino acid sequence level. The position of the twelve cysteine residues are conserved with respect to those present in TIMP-1, as are three of the four tryptophan residues. TIMP-2 has also been identified as a product of bovine endothelial cells. TIMP-2 inhibits the type IV collagenolytic activity and the gelatinolytic activity associated with the 72 kDa enzyme. Inhibition studies demonstrated that complete enzyme inhibition occurred at 1:1 molar ratio of TIMP-2 to activated 72 kDa type IV collagenase enzyme. Thus, unlike TIMP-1, TIMP-2 is capable of binding to both the latent and activated forms of the 72 kDa type IV collagenase. Cell culture studies using cell lines that produce a variety of collagenase family enzymes, as well as both TIMP-1 and TIMP-2, suggest that TIMP-2 preferentially interacts with the 72 kDa type IV collagenase. Thus, like interstitial collagenase activity which is the balance of activated enzyme and TIMP-1, the net 72 kDa type IV collagenase activity may depend upon the balance between the levels of activated enzyme and TIMP-2 (Figure I-10-6).

Northern blot analysis using *timp-2* cDNA clones reveals two mRNA transcript sizes of 3.5 and 1.0 kB.[138] These *timp-2* transcripts are clearly distinguished from the 0.9 kB *timp-1* mRNA. TGFβ1 treatment of human tumor cell lines and fetal lung fibroblasts resulted in a readily detectable decrease in both *timp-2* transcripts in all cell lines tested. These results are in contrast with the effect of TGF-β1 on *timp-1* mRNA levels. TGF-β1 induced a 1.5- to 6-fold increase in *timp-1* transcripts, depending on the cell line. Thus *timp-2* and *timp-1* are differentially regulated. Northern blot analyses of human colorectal tumor and adjacent normal tissues again demonstrated two mRNA transcripts when probed with the *timp-2* cDNA clone. *timp-2* transcript levels were present in both the normal mucosa and adenocarcinoma tissues. These results indicate that it is not the absolute level of 72kDa type IV collagenase or the absolute levels of TIMP-2 which is the determining factor. Rather, it is the balance between the local levels of TIMP-2 and the local concentration of the metalloproteinase.[40,138,139] TIMP-2 will form a 1:1 complex with both the latent or the activated enzyme. Further, binding of TIMP-2 to the latent form of type IV collagenase may block activation by serine proteinases such as plasmin. Binding of TIMP-2 to the active enzyme also abolishes its activity. The binding kd is in the picomolar range. In view of this stoichiometry, active proteolysis will only take place if the local number of type IV collagenase molecules is greater than the number of TIMP-2 molecules (Figure I-10-6).

The function of TIMP-1 and TIMP-2 may not be limited to metalloproteinase blockade. These proteins may also act as cytokines and recognize specific receptors. TIMP-2 and TIMP-1 have been cloned and sequenced from bovine endothelial cells and human fetal aorta cDNA libraries.[13] TIMP-1 stimulates the proliferation of human erythroleukemia cell line K562 in vitro.[4] Recently, the cartilage-derived angiogenesis inhibitor was shown to be identical to TIMP-1.[93] Furthermore, it was demonstrated that TIMP inhibited angiogenesis in vivo and both capillary endothelial cell proliferation and migration in vitro.[93] These results suggest that the TIMPs may have profound biologic effects that extend well beyond their role as inhibitors of the collagenase enzymes. Natural and recombinant TIMP-1 has been shown to prevent tumor cell invasion of human amnion in vitro, and to block metastasis formation in animal models.[1,127] TIMP-2 is also a potent inhibitor of tumor cell invasion in vitro, and animal studies of its efficacy in vivo are in progress.

Thus experimental evidence supports the concept that TIMPs may function as tumor suppressor proteins which inhibit matrix proteolysis and angiogenesis, phenomena which are necessary for tumor invasion and metastatic colony growth. It is conceivable that recombinant TIMP-2 could be considered for its therapeutic potential. TIMP-2 is not glycosylated, and is only 21 kDa in size. It should readily cross the capillary wall to enter the extracellular space. The attractiveness of this type of therapy relates to the potential low level of toxicity. The goal of the therapy would be to reverse the local deficiency of TIMP-2 at the tumor invasion front. Reversing this deficiency by systemic administration of TIMP-2 may not be harmful to normal epithelial cells, which require an intact basement membrane for anchorage and differentiation. TIMP-1 or TIMP-2 could potentially inhibit tumor growth by blocking angiogenesis. As a pure anti-invasion protein, TIMPs will still have important therapeutic potential. An anti-invasion compound could be used to prevent the transition from noninvasive neoplasms to invasive cancers, and to prevent disease progression due to local invasion. Applications involving long-term therapy could therefore be envisioned for carcinoma in situ of the breast or lung, adenomas of the colon, superficial transitional cell carcinomas of the bladder, intraperitoneal ovarian carcinoma, glioblastomas of the brain and basal cell carcinoma of the skin. In each of these diseases, the goal would be to limit or prevent invasion and therefore arrest cancer progression.

Other Metastasis Suppressor Genes

A second major method of identifying candidate metastasis suppressor genes has been the study of differentially expressed genes, i.e., genes whose expression decreased as tumor cells progress from low to high metastatic potential. Using either subtractive or differential colony hybridizations three such genes have been identified: WDNM1, fibronectin and nm23.

The WDNM1 gene was identified by subtractive hybridizations between nonmetastatic and metastatic clones of the rat mammary adenocarcinoma line DMBA-8 by Dear and colleagues WDNM1 RNA levels were quantitatively higher in low metastatic DMBA-8 clones than high metastatic counterparts, but were not detectable in normal tissue.[22] WDNM1 RNA levels did not vary with the growth state of the tumor cells. The DNA sequence of a WDNM1 cDNA clone was novel compared to Genebank sequences.

Schalken et al. performed differential hybridizations on low and high metastatic potential rat Dunning R-3327 prostatic tumor lines.[125] Six differentially expressed cDNA clones were identified, one of which was four- to eight-fold down-regulated in high metastatic ras transfected Dunning sublines. This differentially expressed gene was found to be homologous to the DNA sequence of the extracellular matrix component fibronectin.

The nm23 gene, the most extensively characterized metastasis associated gene, was identified on the basis of its reduced expression at the mRNA level in a series of seven cell lines, all derived from a single K-1735 murine melanoma. Nm23 mRNA levels were ten-fold reduced in five high metastatic potential K-1735 melanoma lines as compared to two related, low metastatic potential K-1735 melanoma lines. Quantitative reductions in expression of nm23 mRNA levels were observed in thirteen different cell lines in two rodent metastasis model systems, (Figure I-10-7) indicating its applicability to the metastasis of other tumor types. Nonmetastatic N-Nitrosomethylurea induced mammary tumors contained an average of two-fold greater nm23 RNA than did metastatic primary NMU tumors, and three-fold greater nm23 RNA than did pulmonary metastases.[136,137] Low metastatic potential tumors induced by the RIII strain of mouse mammary tumor virus (MMTV) contained three-fold greater nm23 RNA than did high metastatic potential tumors induced by the C3H strain of MMTV.[137] Low metastatic potential rat embryo fibroblasts transfected with c-Ha-ras + Adenovirus 2 E1a contained two- to eight-fold greater nm23 RNA than did high metastatic potential ras transfected rat embryo fibroblasts.[137] The latter model system identified the nm23 gene as the first cellular gene associated with E1a suppression of metastasis. Nm23 RNA and protein levels were also examined in a small scale prospective study of human infiltrating ductal breast carcinomas using in situ hybridization (Figure I-10-8) and immunoperoxidase staining.[10,120] At the mRNA level, all tumors from patients with evidence of metastasis to the lymph nodes at surgery contained low nm23 RNA levels. Among the patients without evidence of metastasis at surgery, nm23 RNA levels varied: Approximately 75% of these tumors contained significantly greater nm23 RNA levels, in agreement with a prediction of low metastatic poten-

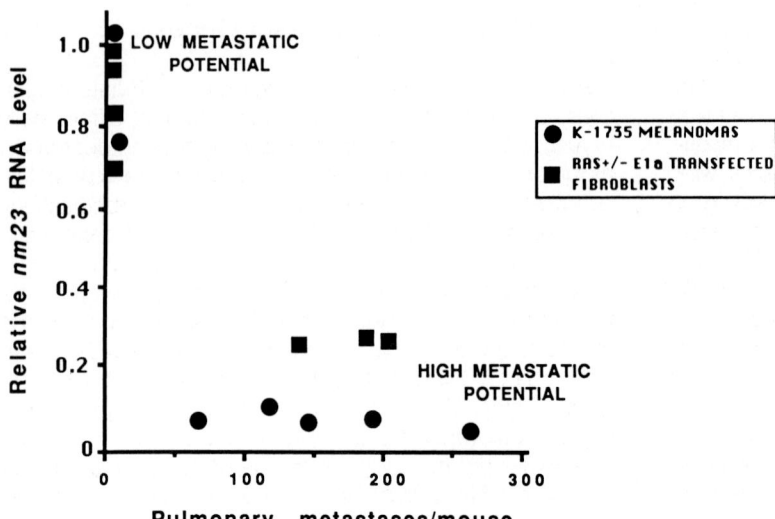

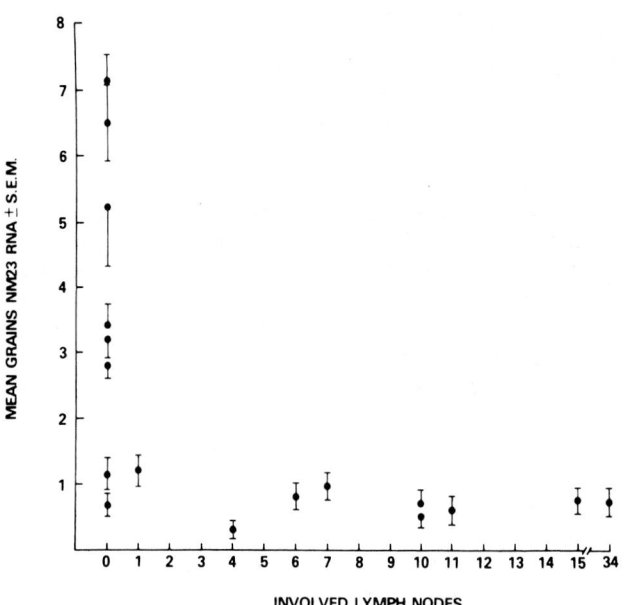

Figure I-10-7. Negative correlation of nm23 mRNA levels with the metastatic behavior in 13 different murine tumor cell lines from 2 different rodent model systems. The relative tumor cell mRNA is compared to the number of pulmonary metastases produced following intravenous injection of 2×10^5 tumor cells.[18,86]

Figure I-10-8. Negative correlation of nm23 mRNA levels with axillary lymph node metastasis in patients with infiltrating ductal breast carcinoma. The tumor cell nm23 mRNA levels were determined by quantitative in situ hybridization using a nm23 riboprobe. The horizontal axis shows the number of lymph nodes positive for metastasis. All metastatic tumors exhibited a profound loss of nm23 expression.

showing that nm23 RNA expression was reduced in high metastatic potential human breast tumors. This was associated with a reduction in survival which was highly statistically significant. Thus, nm23 expression may be of prognostic use for breast cancer. Large scale retrospective clinical studies will determine the prognostic significance of nm23 expression in breast cancer. Of particular interest is the prognostic significance of nm23 expression in lymph node-negative breast cancer, where statistics state that approximately 30% of patients will develop metastatic disease.[120] Decreased nm23 expression has also been found to prognosticate short disease-free intervals in patients with carcinoma of the colon.[18A]

The tumor metastatic process is known for its heterogeneity and complexity.[32] Tumor cells must invade the tumor border, host stroma and the circulatory system, avoid host immune defenses in the bloodstream, arrest and extravasate, establish angiogenic connections at the new location and grow in a new environment. This complexity is compounded by the observation that tumor cells can accomplish each required step by multiple mechanisms, i.e., tumor cells can degrade basement membranes using a host of different proteinases. This simple description of the metastatic process predicts that all tumor cells will not utilize the same mechanisms to metastasize. It is therefore unlikely that any one gene product will be predictive of metastatic potential in all cases. For example, proteins such as Cathepsin D and genetic events such as erb-b-2 or int-2 amplification have also been proposed to have prognostic use in breast cancer.[70,89,129,130] It is therefore expected that a comprehensive panel of genetic and expression data will ultimately provide the best means of cancer prognosis.

Suppressor genes have been identified for the tumorigenesis phase of cancer, including Rb, p53 and K-rev.[33,34,53,61,103] For Rb and p53, one line of evidence supporting their designation as a suppressor gene has been the somatic deletion of one chromosomal allele in tumor tissue. Paired normal lymphocyte and breast tumor DNAs have been examined for possible nm23-HI allelic deletion. A Bgl II restriction digest of human chromosomal DNA identified two allelic nm23 restriction fragment length polymorphisms

tial, but 25% of the tumors contained low nm23 RNA levels. Analysis of estrogen receptor expression and histologic degree of differentiation suggested that the 25% of tumors with low nm23 RNA levels were actually of increased metastatic potential: These tumors were estrogen receptor negative and of poorly differentiated histology. Short term (16 month) clinical followup data indicated that 12% of the low nm23 mRNA level patients, including one without evidence of lymph node metastases at surgery, developed disease progression, while none of the high nm23 RNA level patients did so.[10]

Although limited in size, the data from this study have recently been confirmed in a separate larger study, again

(RFLPs), at 3 and 7 kb, on Southern blots.[69] In 64% of the informative (heterozygous) pairs of normal lymphocyte-breast tumor DNAs studied, deletion of one nm23 allele was observed in the tumor tissue. Thus, one mechanism of nm23 down-regulation may be its deletion from one chromosome. This characteristic stands as genetic evidence that nm23 may be a metastasic suppressor gene in breast cancer. Final proof of this function awaits the results of transfection experiments.[119]

Mechanism of Action of nm23

What is known of the normal function of nm23?[23,24,69,78,156] The first clue to nm23 function(s) came from its high degree of identity with the Drosophila awd gene product.[120] Mutations which result in reduced awd expression or the production of a mutated protein do not significantly alter embryonic development, but do alter the development of multiple tissues post-metamorphosis, when presumptive adult tissue in the wing discs begins to divide and differentiate.[23,24] These abnormalities include altered morphology of the wing discs, larval brain and proventriculus, aberrant differentiation of the wing, leg and eye-antennae imaginal discs and ovaries, and cell necrosis, predominantly in the wing discs. Most striking is the heterogeneity in these abnormalities, where the pattern of cell death, for example, varies between the two imaginal discs of the same larva. Nm23/awd may contribute to the normal development of tissues, which may include cell division, cell-cell communication, and signal transduction. Loss of nm23/awd expression may lead to a disordered state, favoring aberrant development or tumor progression to the metastatic state.

The second clue to nm23 function came from the study of Wallet et al. who reported the identification of two developmentally regulated genes in Dictyostelium which encode NDP kinases.[78,156] These proteins are remarkably homologous to nm23 and awd. Gip 17 was identified by screening a Dictyostelium expressing cDNA library with ^{35}S-GTPgS. Guk 11.2 was identified in the same library by screening with an antibody to a Dictyostelium protein kinase. Compared to nm23/awd, the predicted amino acid sequences of gip 17 and guk 11.2 were 57 and 50% identical, respectively, and 70–75% homologous. The 17 kDa size of the Dictyostelium proteins is the same as nm23/awd. Considering that Dictyostelium represents one of the lowest branches of eukaryotic evolution, this degree of amino acid identity predicts functional similarity between the Dictyostelium proteins and nm23/awd.

NDP kinases comprise a ubiquitous class of enzymes which catalyze the transfer of the terminal phosphate group of 5'-trisphosphate nucleotides to 5'-diphosphate nucleotides (excluding ATP) through the formation of enzyme-bound high-energy phosphate intermediates.[60,99,106] The cellular NDP kinase is an oligomer of individual NDP kinase subunits, ranging from 3–6 subunits depending on the cell type. Each subunit has a size of 17–18 kDa. NDP kinases exhibit heterogeneity in their molecular sizes and amino acid sequences, membrane versus cytoplasmic localization, the number of NDP kinase subunits that are oligomerized into a functional enzyme, and percentage of enzyme that is phosphorylated. It is therefore expected that multiple NDP kinases exist, pos-

sibly each with separate functions. This heterogeneity is supported by the Wallet and colleagues data on the gip 17 and guk 11.2 mRNA expression in Dictyostelium differentiation, in that the expression of the two mRNAs varied at the end of serum starvation-induced development.[156] The two gene products may therefore have different functions.

NDP kinases are known to participate in at least two major functions which could play a role in cancer and development: Microtubule assembly/disassembly, and signal transduction through G-proteins.[59,60,87,99,104,105,141,158] Microtubule assembly requires the exchange, or transphosphorylation without exchange, of GDP to GTP. Nickerson and Wells have isolated a microtubule-associated NDP kinase which may catalyze such transphosphorylation.[99] In this fashion, nm23-like NDP kinases could regulate cellular functions utilizing microtubule machinery, including mitotic spindle formation and cell locomotion. One interesting possibility is that the high degree of aneuploidy observed in metastatic tumor cells may result, in part, from aberrant mitosis on a compromised spindle due to nm23-like NDP kinase down regulation or mutation.

Multiple lines of investigation support the role for nm23-like NDP kinases in the regulation of G protein activation through direct G-protein binding and high energy phospho-transfer reactions.[60,99,106] Nm23-like NDP kinases could function both as dominant oncogenes or as suppressor genes depending on whether they are normal or defective and which signal transduction pathway is involved. For metastasis, a likely signal pathway for nm23-like NDP kinase regulation is TGFβ. It is possible that nm23 NDP kinases could positively regulate the signal pathway resulting from TGFβ binding to its receptor. A defect in nm23 could therefore block the TGFβ induced suppression of metastatic colonies.

Replacement of deficient or defective nm23 protein in cancer cells constitutes a new approach to metastasis therapy. Transfection of nm23 cDNA into tumor cells may abrogate the metastatic phenotype. Transfection of the normal awd gene in Drosophila can prevent the abnormal organ development from the mutant awd. Advances in gene therapy could make it possible to consider epithelial organ specific gene targeting. Delivery of recombinant nm23 protein to breast cancer cells may require less technological advances prior to implementation, compared to gene therapy. Initial in vitro experiments will employ antibody coated or untreated liposomes to deliver the nm23 protein into human cancer cells. It may be possible to prepare a functionally active fragment of nm23 and deliver only this fragment, alone or coupled to an agent which stimulates internalization.

Changes in nm23 expression at the mRNA or protein level may be useful as a screening system for the identification of new hormones, cytokines, or synthetic compounds which may have anti-metastatic activity.

Oncogene Induction of Metastasis

A long list of oncogenes has been described which, either singly or in combinations, confer anchorage independent colony growth in soft agar, and in many cases, tumorgenicity in animal hosts.[50] Since cancer cells must be tumorigenic in order to grow as a metastatic colony, oncogenes must play a basic role, at least, in the growth phase of cancer metastasis. A growing body of evidence, however, indicates that some oncogenes may also directly induce the phenotype of invasion and metastasis. The mechanism of this induction involves pathways separate from those which regulate growth.

The most well studied oncogene capable of inducing the metastatic phenotype is H-ras. Each mammalian cell contains at least three functional ras genes: c-Ha ras, c-Ki-ras and N-ras.[11] Mutated forms of the ras protein product p21 have been identified in both human and carcinogen-induced animal tumors.[6] Thorgeirsson et al. were the first to report that acute myelogenous leukemia or bladder cancer tumor DNA containing activated (mutated) ras oncogene sequences, when transfected into mouse embryo derived fibroblasts (NIH-3T3 cells), produced numerous metastases upon intravenous injection.[147] These data were confirmed by direct transfection of the cloned activated ras oncogene. The resultant highly metastatic cells were not more resistant to host macrophage or NK lysis than conrol cells, indicating that the ras oncogene had augmented the intrinsic aggressiveness of the NIH-3T3 cells.

NIH-3T3 cells have been successfully transfected by multiple members of the ras gene family to induce the metastatic phenotype. This includes c-H-ras, N-ras, v-Ha-ras, T24 H-ras and yeast ras.[12,14,19,28,147,153] With regard to the normal ras proto-oncogenes, cells transformed with elevated levels of the ras proto-oncogene produced tumors at a rate comparable to cells transformed with activated ras.[97] However, when the same cells were tested for metastatic propensity, the cells transformed by the activated ras were much more efficient in the production of metastases compared to the proto-oncogene.[96] Nevertheless, very high levels of normal p21 could lead to metastasis production.[14,27,96]

A wide variety of other cell types were also also susceptible to ras induction of the metastatic phenotype.[19,153,154] These include the nonsenescing murine l0T1/2 fibroblast line, nonmetastatic murine BW51478 lymphoma cells, and two nonmetastatic murine mammary carcinoma lines, MTI Cl.5/7 and SP1.[19,28,153,154] In addition, Pozzatti et al. examined a series of diploid rat embryo fibroblasts transformed by ras alone or ras linked to an SV40 enhancer and a dominant selectable marker, pRSVneo.[109] These clones were all highly metastatic following intravenous, subcutaneous or intramuscular injection into nude mice. Muschel et al. found that differentiated diploid cells such as rat skin cells, rat muscle cells and Chinese hamster lung fibroblasts were induced by ras to become metastatic.[97] Thus, the ability of ras to induce the metastaic phenotype is not dependent on growth or karyotypic instability inherent in NIH-3T3 cells and tumor cells. Ras is not the only oncogene which can induce metastatic potential. The serine-threonine kinases v-mos, v-raf and A-raf, tyrosine kinases v-src, v-fes and v-fms and phosphoproteins myc and p53 have all been demonstrated to induce the metastatic phenotype.[30,35,108,122]

The mechanism of ras induction of the metastatic phenotype is under investigation. Egan et al. used a steroid responsive promoter to demonstrate the importance of ras oncogene transcript dose on metastasis production.[29] The p21 protein is associated with the inner plasma membrane, binds GTP and GDP with high affinity and has weak GTPase activity.[38,39,65,88,112,148] Based on these structural and functional properties, the ras p21 protein has been compared to classical G proteins, suggesting that p21 participates in the transduction of signals across the cell membrane.[38,88] The transforming activity of the ras gene is thought to result from mutations or overexpression which cause an increase in the relative level of the p21-GTP complex.[65] With regard to metastasis, Egan et al. examined the ability of two ras mutations on their ability to induce the metastatic phenotype: The substitution of leucine for glutamine at codon 61, which decreases GTPase activity and increases p21-GDP dissociation, resulting in a net inceade in p21-GTP, and mutation in the nucleotide binding region codons 116– 119, which also increase net p21-GTP due to the relative concentration difference of GTP and GDP pools in the cytoplasm.[27–30] Both mutations in ras were capable of inducing transformation and metastasis formation. Thus, the transforming and metastasis inducing activities of p21 may involve its association with guanine nucleotides in signal transduction. Neither the signals that activate the p21 protein in the cell membrane nor its downstream targets are well understood. Two observations, however, indicate that the signals used in ras induction of transformation and metastasis are dissimilar: (1) The Adenovirus 2 E1a gene has been demonstrated to suppress ras induction of metastatic potential without a similar effect on transformation; (2) C127 cells are capable of being transformed by ras, but do not metastasize.[97,109,110] For metastasis, several genes have been associated with ras activity, including type IV collagenase, cathepsin L, and extracellular matrix components.[37,84,125,150] In addition, a ras-responsive transcription element (RRE) has been identified which will regulate the transcription of linked genes in the presence of the ras signal, and shows sequence similarity to DNA sequences in the collagenase promoter[61] Thus, it is likely that a metastasis-specific set of genes are activated by ras, possibly in coordinated manner, to induce metastasis formation.

References

1. Alvarez, O. A., Carmichael, D. F., and DeClerck, Y. A.: Inhibition of collagenolytic activity and metastasis of tumor cells by a recombinant human tissue inhibitor of metalloproteinases. J. Natl. Cancer Inst., 82:589, 1990.
2. Amstad, P., Reddel, R. R., Pfeifer, A., Malan-Shibley, L., Mark, G. E., and Harris, C. C.: Neoplastic transformation of a human bronchial epithelial cell line by a recombinant retrovirus encoding viral Harvey ras. Mol. Carc., 1:151, 1988.
3. Ananthaswamy, H. A., Price, J. E., Tainsky, M. A., Goldberg, L. H., and Bales, E. S.: Correlation between Ha-ras gene amplification and spontaneous metastasis in NIH 3T3 cells transfected with genomic DNA from human skin cancers. Clin. Exp. Metastasis, 7:301, 1989.
4. Avalos, B., Kaufman, S., Tomonage, M., Williams, R., Golde, D., and Gasson, J.: K562 cells produce and respond to human erythroid potentiating activity. Blood, 71:1720, 1988.
5. Aznavoorian, S., Stracke, M. L., Krutzsch, H., Schiffmann, E., and Liotta, L. A.: Signal transduction for chemotaxis and haptotaxis by matrix molecules in tumor cells. J. Cell Biol., 110:1427, 1990.
6. Barbacid, M.: Ras genes. Annu. Rev. Biochem., 56:779, 1987.
7. Barsky, S. H., Rao, C. N., Williams, J. E., and Liotta, L. A.: Laminin molecular domains which alter metastasis in a murine model. J. Clin. Invest., 74:843, 1984.
8. Barsky, S. H., Siegal, G. P., Jannotta, F., and Liotta, L. A.: Loss of basement membrane components by invasive tumors but not by their benign counterparts. Lab. Invest., 49:140, 1983.
9. Bauer, W., Igot, J.-P., and Le Gal, Y.: Chronologie du cancer mammaire utilisant un modele de croissance Gompertz. Ann. Anat. Pathol. (Paris), 25:39, 1980.
10. Bevilacqua, G., Sobel, M. E., Liotta, L. A., and Steeg, P. S.: Association of low nm23 RNA levels in human primary infiltrating ductal breast carcinomas with lymph node involvement and other histopathological indicators of high metastatic potential. Cancer Res., 49:5185, 1989.
11. Bishop, J. M.: The molecular genetics of cancer. Science, 235:305, 1987.
12. Bondy, G. P., Wilson, S., and Chambers, A. F.: Experimental metastatic ability of H-ras-transformed NIH-3T3 cells. Cancer Res. 45:6005, 1985.
13. Boone, T., Johnson, M., DeClerck, Y., and Langley, K.: CDNA cloning and expression of a metalloproteinase inhibitor related to tissue inhibitor of metalloproteinases. Proc. Natl. Acad. Sci. U.S.A., 87:2800, 1990.
14. Bradley, M. O., Kraynak, A. R., Storer, R. D., and Gibbs, J. B.: Experimental metastasis

in nude mice of NIH-3T3 cells containing various ras genes. Proc. Natl. Acad. Sci. U.S.A., 83:5277, 1986.
15. Brown, P. D., Levy, A. T., Margulies, I. M. K., Liotta, L. A., and Stetler-Stevenson, W. G.: Independent expression and cellular processing of the 72-kDa type IV collagenase and interstitial collagenase in human tumorigenic cell lines. Cancer Res., 50:6184, 1990.
16. Cajot, J.-F., Sordat, B., Druithof, E. K. O., and Bachman, F.: Human primary colon carcinomas xenografted into nude mice. I. Characterization of plasminogen activators expressed by primary tumors and their xenografts. J. Natl. Cancer Inst., 77:703, 1986.
17. Carmichael, D. F., Sommer, A., Thomson, R., Anderson, D. C., Smith, C. G., Welgus, H. G., and Stricklin, G. P.: Primary structure and cDNA cloning of human fibroblast collagenase inhibitor. Proc. Natl. Acad. Sci. U.S.A., 83:2407, 1986.
18. Castronovo, V., Taraboletti, G., Liotta, L. A., and Sobel, M. E.: Modulation of laminin-receptor expression by estrogen and progestins in human breast cancer cell lines. J. Natl. Cancer Inst., 81:781, 1989.
18A. Cohn, K. H., Wang, F. S., DeSoto-LaPaix, F., Solomon, W. B., Patterson, L. G., Arnold, M. R., Weimar, J., Feldman, J. G., Levy, A. T., Leone, A., and Steeg, P. S.: Association of nm23-H1 allelic deletions with distant metastases in colorectal carcinoma. Lancet, 338:722, 1991.
19. Collard, J. G., Schijven, J. F., and Roos, E.: Invasive and metastatic potential induced by ras-transfection into mouse BW5147 T-lymphoma cells. Cancer Res., 47:754, 1987.
20. Collier, I. E., Wilhelm, S. M., Eisen, A. Z., Marmer, B. L., Grant, G. A., Seltzer, J. L., Kronberger, A., He, C., Bauer, E. A., and Goldberg, G. I.: H-ras oncogene transformed human bronchial epithelial cells (TBE-1) secrete a single metalloproteinase capable of degrading basement membrane collagen. J. Biol. Chem., 263:6579, 1988.
21. Dano, K., Andreasen, P. A., and Grondahl-Hansen, J.: Plasminogen activators, tissue degradation and cancer. Adv. Cancer Res., 44:139, 1985.
22. Dear, T. N., Ramshaw, I. R., and Keffard, R. F.: Differential expression of a novel gene in nonmetastatic rat mammary adenocarcinoma cells. Cancer Res., 48:5203, 1988.
23. Dearolf, C., Hersperger, E., and Shearn, A.: Developmental consequences of awd, a cell-autonomous lethal mutation of Drosophilia induced by hybrid dysgenesis. Develop. Biol., 129:159, 1988.
24. Dearolf, C., Tripoulas, N., Biggs, J., and Shearn, A.: Molecular consequences of awd, a cell-autonomous lethal mutation of Drosophila induced by hybrid dysgenesis. Develop. Biol., 129:169, 1988.
25. Denhardt, D. T., Greenberg, A. H., Egan, S. E., Hamilton, R. T., and Wright J. A.: Cysteine proteinase cathepsin L expression correlates closely with the metastatic potential of H-ras-transformed murine fibroblasts. Oncogene 2:55, 1987.
26. Docherty, A. J. P., Lyons, A., Smith, B. J., Wright, E. M., Stephens, P. E., Harris, T. J. R., Murphy, G., and Reynolds, J. J.: Sequence of human tissue inhibitor of metalloproteinases and its identity to erythroid potentiating activity. Nature, 318:66, 1985.
27. Egan, S. E., Broere, J. J., Jarolim, L., Wright, J. A., and Greenberg, A. H.: Coregulation of metastatic and transforming activity of normal and mutant ras genes. Int. J. Cancer, 43:443, 1989.
28. Egan S. E., McClarty, G. A., Jarolim, L., Wright, J. A., Spiro, I., Hager, G., and Greenberg, A. H.: Expression of H-ras correlates with metastatic potential: Evidence for direct regulation of the metastatic phenotype in IOT 1/2 and NIH-3T3 cells. Mol. Cell Biol., 7:830, 1987.
29. Egan, S. E., Spearman, M. A., Broere, J. J., Levy, A. B., Wright, J. A., and Greenberg, A. H.: myc/ras cooperation is insufficient for metastatic transformation (abstract). J. Cell Biochem., 13B(suppl):62, 1989.
30. Egan, S. E., Wright, J. A., Jarolim, L., Yanagihara, K., Bassin, R. H., and Greenberg, A. H.: Transformation by oncogenes encoding protein kinases induces the metastatic phenotype. Science, 238:202, 1987.
31. Fessler, L., Duncan, K., and Tryggvason, K.: Identification of the procollagen IV cleavage products produced by a specific tumor collagenase. J. Biol. Chem., 259:9783, 1984.
32. Fidler, I. J., and Hart, I. R.: Biologic diversity in metastatic neoplasms: Origins and implications. Science, 217:998, 1982.
33. Finlay, C. A., Hinds, P. W., and Levine, A. J.: The p53 proto-oncogene can act as a suppressor of transformation. Cell, 57:1083, 1989.
34. Friend, S. H., Bernards, R., Rojelj, S., Weinberg, R. A., Rapaport, J. M., Albert, D. M., and Dryja, T. P.: A human DNA segment with properties of the gene that predisposes to retinoblastoma and osteosarcoma. Nature, 323:643, 1986.
35. Gao, C., Wang, L.-C., Vass, W. C., Seth, A., and Chang, K. S. S.: The role of v-mos in transformation, oncogenicity and metastatic potential of mink lung cells. Oncogene, 3:267, 1988.
36. Garbisa, S., D'Errico, A., Grigioni, W. F., Biagini, G., Caenazzo, C., Fastelli, G., Stetler-Stevenson, W. G., and Liotta, L. A.: Type IV collagenase augmentation associated with colorectal and gastric cancer progression. *In* Genetic Mechanisms in Carcinogenesis and Tumor Progression. Edited by C. C. Harris and L. A. Liotta. UCLA Symposia on Molecular and Cellular Biology, New Series, Vol. 114. New York, Wiley-Liss, 1990, pp. 203-212.
37. Garbisa, S., Pozzatti, R., Muschel, R. J., Saffiotti, U., Ballin, M., Goldfarb, R. H., Khoury, G., and Liotta, L. A.: Secretion of type IV collagenolytic protease and metastatic phenotype: Induction by transfection with c-Ha-ras but not C-Ha-ras plus Ad2-Ela. Cancer Res., 47:1523, 1987.
38. Gibbs, J. B., Sigal, I.S., Poe, M., and Scolnick, E.M.: Intrinsic GTPase activity distinguishes normal and oncogenic ras p21 molecules. Proc. Natl. Acad. Sci. U.S.A., 81:5704, 1984.
39. Gilman A. G.: G proteins and dual control of adenylate cyclase. Cell, 36:577, 1984.
40. Goldberg, G. I., Marmer, B. L., Grant, G. A., Eisen, A. Z., Wilhelm, S., and He, C.: Human 72-kDa type IV collagenase forms a complex with a tissue inhibitor of metalloproteinase inhibitor. Proc. Natl. Acad. Sci. U.S.A., 86:8207, 1989.
41. Goldfarb, R. H., and Liotta, L. A.: Proteolytic enzymes in cancer invasion and metastasis. Semin. Thromb. Hemost., 12:294, 1986.
42. Gottesman, M.: The role of proteases in cancer. Sem. Cancer Biol., 1:97, 1990.
43. Grotendorst, G.R.: Alteration of the chemotactic response of NIH/3T3 cells to PDGF by growth factors, transformation, and tumor promoters. Cell, 36:279, 1984.
44. Guirguis, R., Margulies, I. M. K., Taraboletti, G., Schiffmann, E., and Liotta, L.A.: Cytokine-induced pseudopodial protrusion is coupled to tumor cell migration. Nature, 329:261, 1987.
45. Guirguis, R., Schiffmann, E., Liu, B., Birkbeck, D., Engel, J., and Liotta, L.: Detection of autocrine motility factor(s) in urine as markers of bladder cancer. J. Natl. Cancer Inst., 80:1203, 1988.
46. Hamilton, T.C., Young, R.C., Louie, K.G., Behrens, B.C., McKoy, W.M., Grotzinger, K.R., and Ozols, R.F.: Characterization of a xenograft model of human ovarian carcinoma which produces ascites and intra-abdominal carcinomatosis in mice. Cancer Res., 44:5286, 1984.
47. Heino, J., and Massague, J.: Transforming growth factor beta switches the pattern of integrins expressed in MG-63 human osteosarcoma cells and causes a selective loss of adhesion to laminin. J. Biol. Chem., 264:21806, 1989.
48. Hendrix, M. J. C, Wood, W. R., Seftor, E. A., Lotan, D., Nakajima, M., Misiorowsi, R. L., Seftor, R. E. B., Stetler-Stevenson, W. G., Bevacqua, S. J., Liotta, L. A., Sobel, M. E., Raz, A., and Lotan, R.: Retinoic acid inhibition of human melanoma cell invasion through a reconstituted basement membrane and its relation to decreases in the expression of proteolytic enzymes and motility factor receptor. Cancer Res., 50:4121, 1990.
49. Herron, G. S., Banda, M. J., Clark, E. J., Gavrilovic, J., and Werb, Z.: Secretion of metalloproteinases by stimulated capillary endothelial cells. II. Expression of collagenase and stromelysin activities is regulated by endogenous inhibitors. J. Biol. Chem., 261:2814, 1986.
50. Hill, R. P., Chambers, A. F., Ling, V., and Harris, J. F.: Dynamic heterogeneity: Rapid generation of metastatic variants in mouse B16 melanoma cells. Science, 224:998, 1984.
51. Hill, S. A., Wilson, S., and Chambers, A. F.: Clonal heterogeneity, experimental metastatic ability, and p21 expression in H-ras-transformed NIH-3T3 cells. J. Natl. Cancer Inst., 80:484, 1988.
52. Horwitz, A., Duggan, K., Buck, C., Beckerle, M. C., and Burridge, K.: Interaction of plasma membrane fibronectin receptor with talin–a transmembrane linkage. Nature, 320:531, 1986.
53. Huang, H.-J., Yee, J.-K., Shew, J.-Y., Chen, P.-L., Bookstein, R., Friedmann, T., Lee, E. Y.-H.P., and Lee, W.-H.: Suppression of the neoplastic phenotype by replacement of the RB gene in human cancer cells. Science, 242:1563, 1988.
54. Humphries, M. J., Olden, K., and Yamada, K. M.: A synthetic peptide from fibronectin inhibits experimental metastasis of murine melanoma cells. Science, 233:467, 1986.
55. Hynes, R. O.: Integrins: A family of cell surface receptors. Cell, 48:549, 1987.
56. Jones, P. A., and DeClerck, Y.A.: Extracellular matrix destruction by invasive tumor cells. Cancer Metast. Rev., 1:289, 1982.
57. Kerbel, R. S., Waghorne, C., Korczak, B., Lagarde, A., and Breitman M.L.: Clonal dominance of primary tumors by metastatic cells: genetic analysis and biological implications. Cancer Surveys, 7:597, 1988.
58. Khokha, R., Waterhouse, P., Yagel, S., Lala, P. K., Overall, C. M., Norton, G., and Denhardt, D. T.: Antisense RNA-induced reduction in metalloproteinase inhibitor causes mouse 3T3 cells to become tumorigenic. Science, 243:947, 1989.
59. Kimura, N., and Johnson, G.: Increased membrane associated nucleotide diphosphate kinase activity as a possible basis for enhanced guanine nucleotide dependent adenylate cyclase activity induced by picolinic acid treatment of simian virus 40-transformed normal rat kidney cells. J. Biol. Chem., 258:12609, 1983.
60. Kimura, N., and Shimada, N.: Membrane-associated nucleoside diphosphate kinase from rat liver. J. Biol. Chem., 263:4647, 1988.
61. Kitayama, H., Sugimoto, Y., Matsuzati, T., Ikawa, Y., and Noda, M.: A ras-related gene with transformation suppressor activity. Cell, 56:77, 1989.
62. Kohn, E.C., Francis, E.A., Liotta, L.A., and Schiffmann, E.: Heterogeneity of the motility responses in malignant tumor cells: A biological basis for the diversity and homing of metastatic cells. Int. J. Cancer, 1990, in press.
63. Koscielny, S., Tubiana, M., and Valleron, A.-J.: A simulation model of the natural history of human breast cancer. Br. J. Cancer, 52:515, 1985.
64. Kramer, R.H., Bensch, K.G., and Wong, J.: Invasion of reconstituted basement membrane matrix by metastatic human tumor cells. Cancer Res., 46:1980, 1986.
65. Lacal, J. S., and Aaronson, S. A.: Activation of ras p21 transforming properties associated with an increase in the release rate of bound guanine nucleotide. Mol. Cell Biol., 6:4214, 1986.
66. Landis, C., Masters, S., Spada, A., Pace, A., Bourne, H., and Vallar, L.: GTPase inhibiting mutations activate the alpha chain of Gs and stimulate adenylyl cyclase in human pituitary tumors. Nature, 340:692, 1989.
67. Layton, M. G., and Franks, L. M.: Selective suppression of metastasis but not tumorigenicity of a mouse lung carcinoma by cell hybridization. Int. J. Cancer, 37:723, 1986.
68. Leone, A., Flatow, U., King, C. R., Sandeen, M. A., Liotta, L. A., Steeg, P. S.: Nm23 suppression of murine melanoma metastasis. Submitted for publication.
69. Leone, A., McBride, O. W., Westin, A., Wang, M., Anglard, P., Cropp, C., Linehan, M. W., Rees, R., Callahan, R., Harris, C., Liotta, L. A., and Steeg, P. S.: Allelic deletion of nm23 in cancer. Submitted for publication.
70. Lidereau, R., Callahan, R., Dickson, C., Peters, G., Escot, C., and Ali, I. U.: Amplification of the *int-2* gene in primary human breast tumors. Oncogene Res., 2:285, 1988.
71. Liotta, L. A.: Tumor invasion and metastasis–role of the basement membrane. Am. J. Pathol., 117:339, 1984.
72. Liotta, L. A.: Tumor invasion and metastases–role of the extracellular matrix. Cancer Res., 46:1, 1986.
73. Liotta, L. A., Abe, S., Robey, P., and Martin, G.: Preferential digestion of basement membrane collagen by an enzyme derived from a metastatic murine tumor. Proc. Natl. Acad. Sci. U.S.A., 76:2268, 1979.
74. Liotta, L. A, Kleinerman, J., and Saidel, G. M.: Quantitative relationships of intravascular tumor cells, tumor vessels, and pulmonary metastases following tumor implantation. Cancer Res., 34:997, 1974.
75. Liotta, L. A., Mandler, R., Murano, G., Katz, D. A., Gordon, R. K., Chiang, P. K., and Schiffmann, E.: Tumor autocrine motility factor. Proc. Natl. Acad. Sci. U.S.A., 83:3302, 1986.
76. Liotta, L. A., Rao, C. N., and Barsky, S. H.: Tumor invasion and the extracellular matrix. Lab. Invest., 49:636, 1983.
77. Liotta, L. A., Rao, C. N., and Wewer, U. M.: Biochemical interactions with the basement membranes. Ann. Rev. Biochem., 55:1037, 1986.

78. Liotta, L., and Steeg, P.: Clues to the function of nm23 and Awd proteins in development, signal transduction, and tumor metastasis provided by studies of *Dictyostelium discoideum*. J. Natl. Cancer Inst., 82:1170, 1990.

79. Liotta, L. A., Tryggvason, K., Garbisa, S., Hart, I., Foltz, C.M., and Shafie, S.: Metastatic potential correlates with enzymatic degradation of basement membrane collagen. Nature, 284:67, 1980.

80. Mahtani, M. M., and Willard, H. F.: A primary genetic map of the pericentromeric region of the human X chromosome. Genomics 2:294, 1988.

81. Malinoff, H. L., and Wicha, M. S.: Isolation of a cell surface receptor protein for laminin from murine fibrosarcoma cells. J. Cell Biol., 96:1475, 1983.

82. Markus, G.: Plasminogen activators in malignant growth. *In* Progress in Fibrinolysis. Edited by J. F. Davidson. Edinburgh, Churchill Livingstone, 1983, p. 587.

83. Markus, G., Camiolo, S. M., Kohga, S., Madeja, J. M., and Mittelman, A. Plasminogen activator secretion of human tumors in short-term organ culture, including a comparison of primary and metabolic tumors. Cancer Res., 43:5517, 1983.

84. Mason, R. W., Gal, S., and Gottesman, M. M.: The identification of the major extracted protein (MEP) from a transformed mouse fibroblast cell line as a catalytically active precursor form of cathepsin L. Biochem. J., 248:449, 1987.

85. McCarthy, J. B., Basara, M. L., Palm, S. L., Sas, D. F., and Furcht, L. T.: The role of cell adhesion proteins–laminin and fibronectin–in the movement of malignant and metastatic cells. Cancer. Metast. Rev., 4:125, 1985.

86. McCarthy, J. B., Skubitz, A. P. N., Palm, S. L., and Furcht, L. T.: Metastasis inhibition of different tumor types by purified laminin fragments and a heparin-binding fragment of fibronectin. J. Natl. Cancer Inst., 80:108, 1988.

87. McCormick, F.: Gasp: Not just another oncogene. Nature, 340:678, 1989.

88. McCormick, F.: ras GTPase activating protein: Signal transmitter and signal terminator. Cell, 56:5, 1989.

89. McGuire, W. L., Tandon, A. K., Allred, D. C., Chamness, G. C., and Clark, G. M.: How to use prognostic factors in axillary node-negative breast cancer patients. J. Natl. Cancer Inst., 82:1006, 1990.

90. Mignatti, P., Robbins, E., and Rifkin, D.: Tumor invasion through the human amniotic membrane: Requirement for a proteinase cascade. Cell, 47:487, 1986.

91. Mignatti, P., Tsuboi, R., Robbins, E., and Rifkin, D.: In vitro angiogenesis on the human amniotic membrane: Requirement for basic fibroblast growth factor-induced proteinases. J. Cell Biol., 108:671, 1989.

92. Monteagudo, C., Merino, M., San-Juan, J., Liotta, L., and Stetler-Stevenson, W.: Immunohistologic distribution of type IV collagenase in normal, benign and malignant breast tissue. Am. J. Pathol., 136:585, 1990.

93. Moses, M. A., Sudhalter, J., and Langer, R.: Identification of an inhibitor of neovascularization from cartilage. Science, 248:1408, 1990.

94. Murphy, G., Cawston, T., and Reynolds, J.: An inhibitor of collagenase from human amniotic fluid. Purification, characterization and action on metalloproteinases. Biochem. J., 195:167, 1981.

95. Murphy, G., Reynolds, J. J., and Werb, Z.: Biosynthesis of tissue inhibitor of metalloproteinases by human fibroblasts in culture: stimulation by 12-0-tetradecanoyl-phorbol 13-acetate and interleukin-I in parallel with collagenase. J. Biol. Chem., 260:3079, 1985.

96. Muschel, R., and Liotta, L. A.: Role of oncogenes in metastasis. Carcinogenesis, 9:705, 1988.

97. Muschel, R. J., Williams, J. E., Lowy, D. R., and Liotta, L. A.: Harvey ras induction of metastatic potential depends upon oncogene activation and the type of recipient cell. Am. J. Pathol., 121:1, 1985.

98. Nakajima, M., Welch, D., Belloni, P. N., and Nicolson, G.L.: Degradation of basement membrane type IV collagen and lung subendothelial matrix by rat mammary adenocarcinoma cell clones of differing metastatic potentials. Cancer Res., 47:4869, 1987.

99. Nickerson, J., and Wells, W.: The microtubule-associated nucleoside diphosphate kinase. J. Biol. Chem., 259:11297, 1988.

100. Nicolson, G. L.: Tumor cell instability, diversification and progression to the metastatic phenotype: From oncogene to oncofetal expression. Cancer Res., 47:1473, 1987.

101. Nicolson, G. L.: Differential organ tissue adhesion, invasion and growth properties of metastatic rat mammary adenocarcinoma cells. Breast Cancer Res. Treat., 12:167, 1988.

102. Nicolson, G. L., Dulski, K., Basson, C., and Welch, D. R.: Preferential organ attachment and invasion in vitro by B16 melanoma cells selected for differing metastatic colonization and invasive properties. Invas. Metast., 5:144, 1985.

103. Nigro, J. M., Baker, S. J., Preisinger, A. C., Jessup, J. M., Hostetter, R., Cleary, K., Bigner, S. H., Davidson, N., Baylin, S., Devilee, P., Glover, T., Collins, F. S., Weston, A., Modali, R., Harris, C. C., and Vogelstein, B.: Mutations in the p53 gene occur in diverse human tumour types. Nature, 342:705, 1989.

104. Ohtsuki, K., Ikeuchi, T., and Yokoyama, M.: Characterization of nucleoside diphosphate kinase associated guanine nucleotide binding proteins from HeLa S3 cells. Biochem. Biophys. Acta, 882:322, 1986.

105. Ohtsuki, K., and Yokoyama, M.: Direct activation of guanine nucleotide binding proteins through a high-energy phosphate-transfer by nucleoside diphosphate-kinase. Biochem. Biophys. Res. Commun., 148:300, 1987.

106. Parks, R., and Agarwal, R.: Nucleoside diphosphokinases. *In* The Enzymes, Vol. VIII. Edited by P. Boyer. New York, Academic Press, 1973, pp. 307-334.

107. Pietras, R. J., Szego, C. M., Mangan, C. E., Seeler, B. J., and Burtnett, M. M.: Elevated serum cathepsin B1-like activity in women with neoplastic disease. Gynecol. Onc., 7:1, 1979.

108. Pohl, J., Goldfinger, N., Radler-Pohl, A., Rotter, V., and Schirrmacher, V.: p-53 increases experimental metastatic capacity of murine carcinoma cells. Mol. Cell Biol., 8:2078, 1988.

109. Pozzatti, R., McCormick, M., Thompson, M. A., and Khoury, G.: The EIA gene of adenovirus type 2 reduces the metastatic potential of ras transformed rat embryo cells. Mol. Cell Biol., 8:2984, 1988.

110. Pozzatti, R., Muschel, R., Williams, J., Padmanabhan, R., Howard, B., Liotta, L., and Khoury, G.: Primary rat embryo cells transformed by one or two oncogenes show different metastatic potential. Science, 232:223, 1986.

111. Price, J. E., Polyzos, A., Zhang, R. D., and Daniels, L.M.: Tumorigenicity and metastasis of human breast carcinoma cell lines in nude mice. Cancer Res., 50:717, 1990.

112. Pulciani, S., Santos, E., Long, L. K., Sorrentino, V., and Barbacid, M.: ras gene amplification and malignant transformation. Mol. Cell Biol., 5:2836, 1985.

113. Rahman, A., Pannerselvam, M., Guirguis, R., Castronovo, V., Sobel, M. E., Daddona, P. E., and Liotta, L. A.: Anti-laminin receptor antibody targeting of adriamycin encapsulated liposomes to human breast cancer cells in vitro. J. Natl. Cancer Inst., 81:1794, 1989.

114. Ramshaw, I. A., Carlsen, S., Wang, H. C., and Badenoch-Jones, P.: The use of cell fusion to analyze factors involved in tumor cell metastasis. Int. J. Cancer, 32:471, 1983.

115. Rao, C. N., Margulies, I. M. K., Tralka, S., Terranova, V. P., Madri, J. A. and Liotta, L. A.: Isolation of a subunit of laminin and its role in molecular structure and tumor cell attachment. J. Biol. Chem., 257:9740, 1982.

116. Recklies, A. D., Poole, A. R., and Mort, J. S.: A cysteine proteinase secreted from human breast tumours is immunologically related to cathepsin B. Biochem. J., 207:633, 1982.

117. Reich, R., Thompson, E., Iwamoto, Y., Martin, G. R., Deason, J. R., Fuller, G. C., and Miskin, R.: Effects of inhibitors of plasminogen activator, serine proteinases, and collagenase IV on the invasion of basement membranes by metastatic cells. Cancer Res., 48:3307, 1988.

118. Rochefort, H., Capony, F., Garcia, M., Cavailles, V., Freiss, G., Chambon, M., Morisset, M., and Vignon, F.: Estrogen-induced lysosomal proteases secreted by breast cancer cells: a role in carcinogenesis? J. Cell Biochem., 35:17, 1987.

119. Rosengard, A. M., Brown, P., Liotta, L. A., and Steeg, P. S.: Modulation of human breast carcinoma nm23 expression in vitro by transforming growth factor-beta. Manuscript in preparation

120. Rosengard, A. M., Krutzsch, H. C., Shearn, A., Biggs, J. R., Barker, E., Margulies, I. M. K., King, C. R., Liotta, L. A., and Steeg, P. S.: Reduced nm23/awd protein in tumor metastasis and aberrant Drosophila development. Nature, 342:177, 1989.

121. Ruoslahti, E., and Pierschbacher, M.D.: Arg-Gly-Asp: a versatile cell recognition signal. Cell, 44:517, 1986.

122. Sadowski, I., Pawson, T., and Lagarde, A.: v-fps protein-tyrosine kinase coordinately enhances the malignancy and growth factor responsiveness of pre-neoplastic lung fibroblasts. Oncogene, 2:241, 1988.

123. Sager, R.: Tumor suppressor genes: The puzzle and the promise. Science, 246:1406, 1989.

124. Sappino, A.-P., Busso, N., Belin, D., and Vassali, J.-D.: Increase of urokinase type plasminogen activator gene expression in human lung and breast carcinomas. Cancer Res., 47:4043, 1987.

125. Schalken, J. A., Ebeling, S. B., Issacs, J. T., Treiger, B., Bussemakers, M., de Jong, M., and Van de Ven, W.: Down modulation of fibronectin messenger RNA in metastasizing rat prostatic cancer cells revealed by differential hybridization analysis. Cancer Res., 48:2042, 1988.

126. Schirrmacher, V.: Experimental approaches, theoretical concepts, and impacts for treatment strategies. Adv. Cancer Res., 43:1, 1985.

127. Schultz, R. M., Silberman, S., Persky, B., Bajowski, A. S., Carmichael, D. F.: Inhibition by recombinant tissue inhibitor of metalloproteinases of human amnion invasion and lung colonization by murine B16-F10 melanoma cells. Cancer Res., 48:5539, 1988.

128. Sidebottom, E., and Clark, S. R.: Cell fusion segregates progressive growth from metastasis. Br. J. Cancer, 47:399, 1983.

129. Slamon, D. J., Clark, G. M., Wong, S. G., Levin, W. J., Ullrich, A., and McGuire, W. L.: Human breast cancer: Correlation of relapse and survival with amplification of the HER-2/neu oncogene. Science, 235:177, 1987.

130. Slamon, D. J., Godolphin, W., Jones, L. A., Holt, J. A., Wong, S. G., Keith, D. E., Levin, W. E., Stuart, S. G., Udove, J., Ullrich, A., and Press, M. F.: Studies of the HER-2/neu proto-oncogene in human breast and ovarian cancer. Science, 244:707, 1989.

131. Sloane, B. R., and Honn, K. V.: Cysteine proteinases and metastasis. Cancer Metast. Rev., 3:249, 1984.

132. Sloane, B. F., Rozhin, J., Johnson, K., Taylor, H., Crissman, J. D., and Honn, K. V.: Cathepsin B: association with plasma membrane in metastatic tumors. Proc. Natl. Acad. Sci. U.S.A., 83:2483, 1986.

133. Sporn, M., and Roberts, A.: Peptide growth factors: Current status and therapeutic opportunities. *In* Important Advances in Oncology. Edited by V. T. DeVita, Jr., S. Hellman, S. A. Rosenberg. Philadelphia, JB Lippincott Co., 1987, pp. 75-86.

134. Sporn, M., and Roberts, A.: Peptide Growth Ractors and their Receptors. Springer Verlag, 1990.

135. Spyratos, F., Maudelonde, T., Brouillet, J. P., Brunet, M., Defrenne, A., Andrieu, C., Hacene, K., Desplaces, A., Rouess, J., and Rockefort, H.: Cathepsin D: An independent prognostic factor for metastasis of breast cancer. Lancet, 2:1115, 1989.

136. Steeg, P. S., Bevilacqua, G., Kopper, L., Thorgeirsson, U. P., Talmadge, J. E., Liotta, L. A., and Sobel, M. E.: Evidence for a novel gene associated with low tumor metastatic potential. J. Natl. Cancer Inst., 80:200, 1988.

137. Steeg, P. S., Bevilacqua, G., Rosengard, A. M., Cioce, V., and Liotta, L. A.: Altered gene expression in tumor metastasis: The nm23 gene. *In* Cancer Metastasis, Molecular and Cellular Biology. Host Immune Responses and Perspectives for Treatment. Edited by V. Schirrmacher and Schwartz-Albiez. 1989, p. 44.

138. Stetler-Stevenson, W., Brown, P., Onisto, M., Levy, A., and Liotta, L.: Tissue inhibitor of metalloproteinase-2 (TIMP-2) mRNA expression in tumor cell lines and human tumor tissues. J. Biol. Chem., 265:13933, 1990.

139. Stetler-Stevenson, W. G., Krutzsch, H. C., and Liotta, L. A.: Tissue Inhibitor of Metalloproteinase-2 (TIMP-2), a new member of the metalloproteinase inhibitor family. J. Biol. Chem., 264:17374, 1989.

140. Stetler-Stevenson, W. G., Krutzsch, H. C., Wacher, M. P., Margulies, I. M. K., and Liotta, L. A.: The activation of human type IV collagenase proenzyme. Sequence identification of the major conversion product following organomercurial activation. J. Biol. Chem., 264:1353, 1989.

141. Stryer, L., and Bourne, H.: G-proteins: A family of signal transducers. Ann. Rev. Cell Biol., 2:391, 1986.

142. Sugarbaker, E. V.: Patterns of metastasis in human malignancies. Cancer Biol. Rev., 2:235, 1981.

143. Tandon, A. K., Clark, G. M., Chamness, G. C., Chirgwin, I., and McGuire, W. L.: Cathepsin D and prognosis in breast cancer. New Engl. J. Med., 322:297, 1990.

144. Terranova, V. P., Liotta, L. A., Russo, R. G., and Martin, G. R.: Role of laminin in the attachment and metastasis of murine tumor cells. Cancer Res., 42:2265, 1982.

145. Thorgeirsson, U. P., Liotta, L. A., Kalebic, T., Margulies, I. M. K., Thomas, K., Rios-

Candelore, M., and Russo, R. G.: Effect of natural protease inhibitors and a chemoattractant on tumor cell invasion in vitro. J. Natl. Cancer Inst., 69:1049, 1982 .

146. Thorgeirsson, U. P., Turpeenniemi-Hujanen, T., Neckers, L. M., Johnson, D. W., and Liotta, L. A.: Protein synthesis but not DNA synthesis is required for tumor cell invasion in vitro . Invas. Metast., 4:73, 1984 .

147. Thorgeirsson U. P., Turpeenniemi-Hujanen, T., Williams, J. E., Westin, E., Heilman, C. A., Talmadge, J. E., and Liotta, L. A.: NIH 3T3 cells transfected with human tumor DNA containing activated ras oncogenes express the metastatic phenotype in nude mice. Mol. Cell. Biol., 5:259, 1985.

148. Trahey, M., and McCormick, F.: A cytoplasmic protein stimulates normal N-ras p21 GTPase, but does not affect oncogene mutations. Science, 238:542, 1987.

149. Turpeenniemi-Hujanen, T., Thorgeirsson, U. P., Hart, I. R., Grant, S. S., and Liotta, L. A: Expression of collagenase IV (basement membrane collagenase) activity in murine tumor cell hybrids that differ in metastatic potential. J. Natl. Cancer Inst., 75:99, 1985.

150. Ura, H., Bonfil, R. D., Reich, R., Reddel, R., Pfeifer, A., Harris, C. C., and Klein, A. J. P.: Expression of type IV collagenase and procollagen genes and its correlation with the tumorigenic, invasive, and metastatic abilities of oncogene-transformed human bronchial epithelial cells. Cancer Res., 49:4615, 1989.

151. Vallee, B. L., and Auld, D. S.: Zinc coordination, function and structure of zinc enzymes and other proteins. Biochemistry, 29:5647, 1990.

152. Van Wart, H. E., and Birkedal-Hansen, H.: The cysteine switch: A principle of regulation of metalloproteinase activity with potential applicability to the entire matrix metalloproteinase gene family. Proc. Natl. Acad. Sci. U.S.A., 87:5578, 1990.

153. Vousden, K. H., Eccles, S. A., Purvies, H., and Marshall, C. J.: Enhanced spontaneous metastasis of mouse carcinoma cells transfected with an activated c-Ha-ras 1 gene. Int. J. Cancer, 37:425, 1986.

154. Waghorne, C., Kerbel, R. S., and Breitman, M.L.: Metastatic potential of SPI mouse mammary adenocarcinoma cells is differentially induced by activated and normal forms of c-H-ras. Oncogene, 1:149, 1987.

155. Wakefield, L. M., Thompson, N. L., Flanders, K. C., O'Conner-McCourt, K. C., and Sporn, M. B.: Transforming growth factor-beta: multifunctional regulator of cell growth and phenotype. Ann. N.Y. Acad. Sci., 551:290, 1989.

156. Wallet, V., Mutzel, R., Troll, H., Barzu, O., Wurster, B., Vernon, M., and Lacombe, M. A.: Dictyostelium nucleoside diphosphate kinase highly homologous to nm23 and awd proteins involved in mammalian tumor metastasis and Drosophila development. J. Natl. Cancer Inst., 18:1199, 1990.

157. Wang, B. S., McLoughlin, G. A., Richie, J. P., and Mannick, J.A.: Correlation of the production of plasminogen activator with tumor metastasis in B16 mouse melanoma cell lines. Cancer Res., 40:288, 1980.

158. Wieland, T., and Jakobs, K.: Receptor-regulated formation of GTP[gS] with subsequent persistent Gs-protein activation in membranes of human platelets. FEBS Lett, 245:189-193, 1989.

159. Weinberg, R. A.: Oncogenes, antioncogenes and the molecular basis of multistep carcinogenesis. Cancer Res., 49:3713, 1989.

160. Welgus, H. G., Jeffery, J. J., Eisen, A. Z., Roswit, W. T., and Stricklin, G. P.: Human skin fibroblast collagenase: Interaction with collagen and collagenase inhibitor. Collagen Rel. Res., 5:167, 1985.

161. Welgus, H. G., and Stricklin, G. P.: Human skin fibroblast collagenase inhibitor: Comparative studies in human connective tissues, serum, and amniotic fluid. J. Biol. Chem., 258:12259, 1983.

162. Wewer, U. M., Liotta, L. A., Jaye, M., Ricca, G. A., Drohan, W. N., Claysmith, A. P., Rao, C. N., Wirth, P., Coligan, J. E., Albrechtsen, R., Mudryj, M., and Sobel, M. E.: Altered levels of laminin receptor mRNA in various human carcinoma cells that have different abilities to bind laminin. Proc. Natl. Acad. Sci. U.S.A., 83:7137, 1986.

163. Wilhelm, S., Collier, I., Kronberg, A., Eisen, A., Marmer, B., Grant, G., Bauer, E. A., and Goldberg, G. I.: Human skin fibroblast stromelysin: structure, glycosylation, substrate specificity, and differential expression in normal and tumorigenic cells. Proc. Natl. Acad. Sci. U.S.A., 84:6725, 1987.

164. Wilhelm, S. M., Collier, I. E., Marmer, B. L., Eisen, A. Z., Grant, G. A., and Goldberg, G. I.: SV40-transformed human lung fibroblasts secrete a 92-kDa type-IV collagenase which is identical to that secreted by normal human macrophages. J. Biol. Chem., 264:17213, 1989.

165. Yamada, K. M., Akiyama, T., Hasegawa, T., Hasegawa, E., Humphries, M., Kennedy, D., Nagata, K., Urushihara, H., Olden, K., and Chen, W.-T.: Recent advances in research on fibronectin and other cell attachment proteins. J. Cell. Biochem., 28:79, 1985.

I-11

Tumor Angiogenesis

Judah Folkman

Historical Background: Confusion about the Cause of Tumor Hyperemia

It has been observed for over one hundred years that tumors appear to have an increased vascularity compared to normal tissues.[285] It was long believed that simple dilation of existing host blood vessels accounted for this tumor hyperemia.[42] Vasodilation was generally thought to be a "side-effect" of tumor metabolites of necrotic tumor products escaping from the tumor. Two reports suggested that tumor hyperemia could be related to *new* blood vessel growth, i.e., *neo*vascularization and not to dilation. Although these observations were largely overlooked, a 1939 paper showed that while neovascularization of a wound in a transparent chamber in a rabbit ear regressed completely after the wound had healed,[129] a tumor implant in the chamber was associated with accelerated growth of capillary blood vessels. The other report in 1945 revealed that new vessels in the neighborhood of a tumor implant arose from host vessels and not from the tumor itself.[3] These papers notwithstanding, a debate continued in the literature for two more decades about whether tumors were supplied by existing vessels or by neovascularization.[49] Even among a few investigators who accepted the notion of tumor-induced neovascularization, it was generally assumed that this vascular response was an inflammatory reaction, and was not necessary for tumor growth.[72]

Tumor Growth is Restricted in the Absence of the Vascular Response

A new view of the role of blood vessels in tumor growth was developed in the 1960s. Experiments with isolated perfused organs revealed that tumor growth was severely restricted in these organs because of the absence of neovascularization.[67,76,86,91] A series of experiments over the following decade showed that tumors implanted into animals consistently induced the growth of new capillary blood vessels.[77] This process was called "angiogenesis," a term coined in 1935 by Hertig to describe the proliferation of new vessels in the placenta.[123] Viable tumor cells released diffusible angiogenic factors which stimulated new capillary growth and endothelial mitosis in vivo,[70,87,152] even when tumor cell proliferation had been arrested by irradiation.[6] Necrotic tumor products were not angiogenic.

Hypothesis That Tumor Growth Is Angiogenesis-Dependent

From these observations a hypothesis was proposed that "once tumor take occurs, every further increase in tumor cell population must be preceded by an increase in new capillaries which converge upon the tumor."[70] According to this concept, a small focus of tumor cells (containing less than 10^6 cells in a volume of a few mm³) could not increase indefinitely without the induction of angiogenesis. The idea was based at first upon the difference in growth of immortalized tumor cell populations in flat tissue culture compared to spheroidal colonies in suspension culture (soft agar).[92] In two-dimensional flat cultures, a population of immortalized cells will expand indefinitely as long as fresh media is added and unlimited cell-free surface is provided. These conditions are satisfied by passage of the cells to new flasks. However, three-dimensional spheroids of the same cells, suspended in soft agar or methylcellulose, reach a diameter of a few mm, beyond which there is no further expansion of the population, despite repeated passage of the spheroids to fresh media. In such a spheroid, cell proliferation attains a steady state. The center of the spheroid contains dying cells, proliferating cells at the periphery and a middle layer of viable but non-dividing cells.[265,266] The spheroid stops enlarging when its external surface area can no longer provide sufficient diffusion of nutrients and wastes to and from the center of the cell population.[2] (Hollow fiber culture systems overcome this limitation and in a sense represent in vitro analogues of capillary blood vessels.)

Experimental Evidence That Tumor Growth Is Angiogenesis-Dependent

Further support for the hypothesis that tumor growth is angiogenesis-dependent was derived from the following experimental evidence: 1) Tumors implanted in subcutaneous transparent chambers grow very slowly before vascularization and tumor volume increases linearly. After vascularization, tumor growth is rapid and tumor volume may increase exponentially.[3] 2) Tumor growth in the avascular rabbit cornea proceeds slowly and at a linear rate, but switches to exponential growth after vascularization.[102] 3) Tumors suspended in the aqueous fluid of the anterior chamber of the rabbit eye remain viable, avascular and limited in size (< 1 mm³). These tumors induce neovascularization of iris vessels, but are too remote from these vessels to be invaded by them. Once a tumor spheroid is implanted contiguous to the proliferating iris vessels, the tumors may enlarge up to 16,000 times their original volume within 2 weeks.[104] 4) Human retinoblastomas which have metastasized to the vitreous are viable, avascular, and growth-restricted. 5) Within a solid tumor the ³H-thymidine labelling index of tumor cells decreases with increasing distance from the nearest open capillary. The mean labeling index for a given tumor is a function of the labeling index of the vascular endothelial cells in that tumor.[269] 6) Tumors implanted on the chorioallantoic membrane of the chick embryo are restricted in growth during the avascular phase but enlarge rapidly once they are vascularized.[154] 7) Tumors implanted on the chorioallantoic membrane in suc-

cessively older embryos grow at slower rates corresponding to the reduced rates of endothelial turnover with age.[154] 8) Vascular casts of metastases in the rabbit liver reveal that tumors up to a diameter of 1 mm are usually avascular, but beyond that size are vascularized.[171] 9) Carcinoma of the human ovary metastasizes to the peritoneal membrane as tiny avascular seeds. These implants rarely grow beyond a limited diameter of a few millimeters, until after vascularization. 10) Inhibitors of angiogenesis which are not cytostatic to tumor cells in vitro, inhibit tumor growth in vivo.[71] 11) In transgenic mice that develop carcinomas of the beta cells in the pancreatic islets, large tumors arise from a subset of preneoplastic hyperplastic islets that have become vascularized.[89] 12) In another experiment, neoplastic cells injected subcutaneously develop into tumors which become vascularized at about 0.4 mm³. As tumor size increases, blood vessels continue to proliferate and are enveloped by encroaching tumor. The vessels eventually occupy up to 1.5% of the tumor volume. This is a 400% increase in vascular density over normal subcutaneous tissue.[277] 13) In rat colon tumors arising spontaneously after administration of a carcinogen, the vascular phase can be further divided into two distinct stages.[257] In the early stage (<3.5 mm diameter) the tumor is supplied by pre-existing host microvessels which are dilated and widened. Some of this dilation may result from lateral proliferation of endothelial cells in post-capillary venules. In a later stage (>5.7 mm diameter) there is proliferation of new vessels with a greater microvessel density than normal.

These experiments[75] provide mainly correlative or indirect evidence that tumor growth is angiogenesis-dependent. Two recent experiments provide direct evidence. Basic fibroblast growth factor (bFGF) is mitogenic for vascular endothelial cells (and for other cell types), and is strongly angiogenic (see below). It is produced by endothelial cells and they also have receptors for it. A human colon carcinoma that lacks high-affinity receptors for bFGF and for which bFGF is not mitogenic in vitro was grown in nude mice.[116] Systemic injection of bFGF stimulated an increase in the density and branching of blood vessels in the tumor as well as a two-fold increase in tumor size. Receptor autoradiography of histologic tumor sections demonstrated the presence of bFGF receptors on the vascular endothelium. When the tumor-bearing mice received neutralizing monoclonal antisera against bFGF, tumor growth was significantly retarded. This study shows that changes in growth rate of tumor blood vessels directly govern tumor growth.

In another experiment, the cDNA for bFGF containing a signal sequence was transfected into normal mouse fibroblasts.[126A] The transfected fibroblasts became tumorigenic, secreted bFGF, and were also highly angiogenic. They formed large lethal tumors when implanted into mice, but administration of bFGF-specific antibodies inhibited tumor growth.

The hypothesis that tumor growth is angiogenesis-dependent is consistent with the observation that angiogenesis is necessary but not sufficient for continued tumor growth. While the absence of angiogenesis will severely limit tumor growth, the onset of angiogenic activity in a tumor permits, but does not guarantee, continued expansion of the tumor population. For example, adrenal adenomas are benign tumors which are highly neovascularized. Their tumor cells, however, lack the growth potential to take advantage of the new blood vessels they have induced. Thus, angiogenesis does not always correlate with malignancy.[227] Furthermore, leukemic cells and tumor cells that grow in ascites are not dependent upon angiogenesis, because they do not form a solid tumor or grow in a 3-dimensional tightly packed cell population. Angiogenesis may not be necessary for certain tumor cells capable of growth as a flat sheet between membranes, i.e., gliomatosis in the meninges.

Tumor Angiogenesis Permits Metastasis

Recent evidence suggests that metastasis is also angiogenesis-dependent. For a tumor cell to metastasize successfully it must breach several barriers and be able to respond to specific growth factors (see I-10).[19,66,207,288] Briefly, tumor cells must gain access to the vasculature in the primary tumor, survive the circulation, arrest in the microvasculature of the target organ,[206,208] exit from this vasculature,[24] grow in the target organ, and induce angiogenesis.[297] Angiogenesis is necessary at the beginning as well as at the end of this cascade of events (Figure I-11-1). Because of the clonal origin of metastasis,[147] it is possible that a primary tumor containing a high proportion of angiogenic cells will generate metastases which are already angiogenic when they arrive at the target tissue. Tumor cells rarely shed into the circulation before the primary tumor is vascularized.[173] Tumor cells can enter the circulation by penetrating through proliferating capillaries. Growing capillaries have fragmented basement membranes and are leaky (see VIII).[61,204] Mature capillaries have a thickened basement membrane. Furthermore, the migratory invasive endothelial cells at the tip of a new capillary vessel secrete increased collagenases and plasminogen activator.[197] When endothelial cell chemotaxis is stimulated in vitro by an angiogenic factor, there is a significant increase in cell-associated enzymatic activity capable of degrading both type IV and type V collagen.[145] These degradative enzymes may facilitate the entry of tumor cells into the circulation. An interesting experiment which supports this concept is the observation that India ink injected into

the rabbit cornea will remain at the injection site indefinitely as a tattoo, unless neovascularization is induced in the cornea. As new capillaries approach the ink spot, it fragments. Ink particles then appear in the cervical lymph nodes.[258]

Two clinical observations also point to a role for angiogenesis in metastasis. It has been recognized since 1970 that cutaneous melanomas less than 0.76 mm thick rarely metastasize and are rarely lethal.[30] Melanomas with a thickness of 1.0 mm or greater have an increasing metastatic and lethal potential. With few exceptions, this correlation has remained valid for more than 20 years.[190] However, a probable explanation for this high correlation has been suggested only recently.[262,263] Cutaneous melanomas less than 0.70 mm thick usually reside above the basement membrane which separates epithelium from dermis. They are rarely vascularized. Thicker melanomas are usually associated with angiogenesis in the dermis[259] and eventually with encroachment of tumor around new capillary blood vessels. It is likely that the increased tumor thickness and the increased metastatic potential both result from neovascularization.[73] In invasive breast cancer there is a significant direct correlation between the highest density of microvessels in a histological section and the occurrence of metastases (Fig. I-11-2).[286] It is now possible to quantitate neovascularization in a breast biopsy by staining the microsection with antibody to Factor VIII-related antigen, a specific marker for vascular endothelial cells.[286] Again, it must be emphasized that neovascularization permits, but does not guarantee metastasis, because a successful metastatic cell must overcome many other obstacles.

Capillary Proliferation Occurs in Sequential Steps

The complexity of the angiogenic process resembles blood clotting. Many sequential events are involved in the generation of a new capillary blood vessel. The morphological events of capillary growth include: endothelial cell induced-

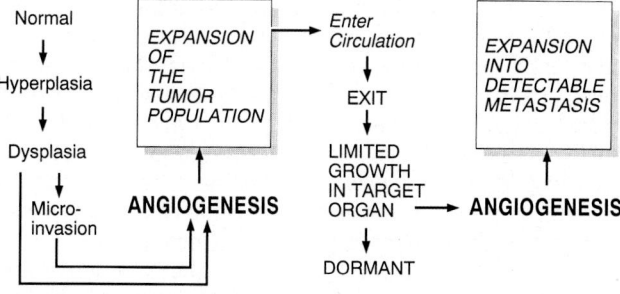

Figure I-11-1. Role of angiogenesis in metastasis. In this diagram, angiogenesis occurs at the beginning of the metastatic cascade. It permits expansion of the tumor population and it permits tumor cells to enter the circulation. Angiogenesis may also occur at the end of the metastatic cascade where it permits expansion of the metastatic implant. A metastatic implant that is not angiogenic may remain as an undetectable micrometastasis. Lack of angiogenic activity may be one cause of tumor dormancy.

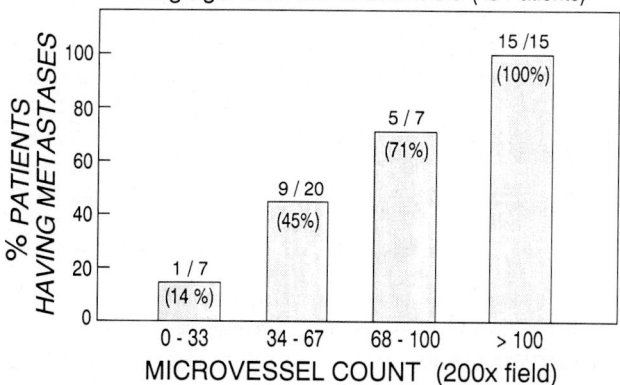

Figure I-11-2. Metastatic disease among 49 patients in relation to microvessel count in progressive increments. The incidence of metastatic disease increases as vessel counts in the primary tumor increases, reaching 100% among patients with counts above 100 per 200× field. (From Weidner et al.[286] with permission of the publisher.)

degradation of the basement membrane of the parent venule, directional locomotion in tandem with other endothelial cells, endothelial mitosis, lumen formation, development of sprouts and loops, generation of new basement membrane, and recruitment of pericytes.[10,194] This sequence is similar to the morphological steps of angiogenesis in a healing wound or in a developing embryo. However, many tumors impose modifications on a new capillary bed which differ from angiogenesis induced by non-neoplastic cells. For example, a histological cross-section of a capillary blood vessel in the normal brain reveals one or two endothelial cells per lumen. In a brain tumor however, such as a glioblastoma, 5–10 endothelial cells may occupy one lumen.[26] Tumor-induced vessels are often dilated and saccular and may even contain tumor cells within the endothelial lining.[139] Tumor microvasculature does not conform to the vasculature of normal tissues (e.g., artery to arteriole to capillary to post-capillary venule to venule to vein).[139] Tumors may contain giant capillaries, and arteriovenous shunts without intervening capillaries. Blood may even flow from one venule to another. Furthermore, organization of vessels may be different from one intratumoral location to the next.[139] Capillary growth rates (i.e., the velocity of neovascularization) range from 0.23–0.8 mm/day, depending on the experimental system used and the type of tumor.[69,291,292]

While actively growing capillaries are usually pericyte-poor, and do not regain their normal density of pericytes until after capillary growth has ceased, the capillaries in some tumors contain excessive numbers of pericytes.[242,282] Thus, some human tumors are pericyte-rich and others are pericyte-poor. It is not clear why these differences exist, nor whether they are clinically significant.

Many biochemical events also occur sequentially during the formation of a capillary blood vessel; however, these have not yet been elucidated in vivo at the level of detail of the morphological events. In the presence of an angiogenic molecule such as bFGF, there is a dramatic rise in production of plasminogen activator and collagenase by endothelial cells.[115] There are changes in basement membrane components. In new capillaries growing in the chick embryo: 1) sulfated glycosaminoglycan synthesis is decreased (e.g., heparan sulfate) but gradually increases as the vessel matures;[8] and 2) fibronectin is one of the earliest of the basement membrane components to appear, followed (within 2 days) by laminin, and finally by collagen type IV as the vessels mature.[9,94] Fibrin presumed to leak from the new vessels undergoes local degradation.[204] Little is known about what happens to endothelial production of plasminogen activator inhibitor (PAI-1), bFGF, PDGF, IGF-1 or other products of endothelial cells and pericytes during capillary proliferation.

In Vitro Bioassays for Components of Angiogenesis

Because angiogenesis *per se* is difficult to quantitate in vivo, the sequential events of capillary growth have been individually characterized by quantifiable in vitro bioassays. Capillary,[79] aortic,[110] and human umbilical vein endothelial cells,[103,138] are used in these systems. Locomotion in vitro is measured by chemokinetic assays which employ colloidal gold.[295] Endothelial chemotaxis is quantitated in Boyden chambers.[19] Mitosis and DNA synthesis are quantitated in subconfluent cultures of endothelial cells. Confluent endothelial cells, unlike fibroblasts, are generally refractory to mitogens.[119] Lumen formation is studied with endothelial cells that are cultured on collagen, fibronectin, or laminin substrata.[78,112,133,135,146,176,179,194,210,211] These in vitro bioassays have been successfully employed to discover and purify new angiogenic molecules,[254] as well as novel angiogenesis inhibitors.[131] However, whenever in vitro assays are used to guide purification of an angiogenic, or an angiostatic molecule, results must be confirmed in vivo. It is possible for a factor to be angiogenic in vivo but not mitogenic for endothelial cells in vitro (e.g., angiogenin, see below). Conversely, an endothelial mitogen in vitro may not be angiogenic in vivo (e.g., certain low density lipoproteins).[82]

In Vivo Bioassays for Angiogenesis

The currently available in vivo bioassays for angiogenesis are semi-quantitative and have many drawbacks. Nevertheless, they have served for the identification, purification and characterization of almost all of the known angiogenic molecules and the inhibitors of angiogenesis (see below). These bioassays have been extensively described and reviewed.[7,33,71,82] In brief, the chick embryo chorioallantoic membrane displays growth of new vessels toward an angiogenic factor implanted on the membrane in a pellet of methylcellulose or some other non-irritating vehicle. Embryos of 6–10 days are commonly used and examined 2–3 days later by stereomicroscopy. However, false-positive angiogenesis may be induced by any test material with abnormal osmolarity or pH which leads to cell damage. Furthermore, angiogenesis secondary to inflammation (where infiltrating macrophages or leukocytes are the source of angiogenic activity) cannot easily be distinguished from direct angiogenic activity without detailed histologic study.[233] Also, angiogenesis may be induced by fibrin degradation products which leak from embryonic vessels in response to injurious substances.[60,276] Several improvements have recently been made in the chick embryo assay.[260,268]

The cornea micropocket overcomes some of the disadvantages of the chick embryo assay. The putative angiogenic factor is implanted in the cornea of the rabbit,[102] mouse,[203] or rat,[95] usually in a polymeric sustained release vehicle.[164] The length and number of new capillaries which enter the avascular cornea can be quantitated with a slit-lamp microscope or by image analysis of specimens injected with India ink.[224] Vascularization of the cornea provides the most compelling evidence that new capillaries have been induced.[32] The major drawback of this method is the time and expense and the fewer substances that can be tested.

Other systems include the hamster cheek pouch[243] and the subcutaneous fascia in mice.[5] Recently, biodegradable[275] and non-biodegradable sponges[48] have been implanted in animals to study neovascularization induced by an angiogenic molecule within the sponge. These techniques facilitate histological and immuno-cytochemical studies of new vessels, but neovascularization is more difficult to quantitate than with other methods.

A simple, quantitative bioassay for angiogenesis would be

a major improvement for the field of angiogenesis research. The discovery of new angiogenic molecules in tumors and in body fluids, as well as the identification of new angiostatic molecules for therapeutic use, would be greatly facilitated by such an improved angiogenesis bioassay.

Human Tumors Usually Progress from a Pre-Vascular Phase to a Vascular Phase

The Prevascular Phase

Our current view is that tumors at their earliest origin may lack the capacity to induce neovascularization. Many observations of neoplasms arising in the epithelial compartment (e.g., carcinomas, melanomas), contribute to this concept. During the prevascular phase when angiogenic activity is absent or inadequate, in situ carcinomas in the cervix[256] or bladder,[124] for example, overlie an intact basement membrane beneath which normal capillary blood vessels are mature and non-proliferating. The prevascular phase of cutaneous melanoma presents a similar histologic picture.[262,263] These lesions are thin or flat, slowly growing, able to exist for years, and rarely metastatic. Most prevascular lesions are difficult to detect unless they are visible on an external surface, such as skin, oral cavity, or cervix. However, the prevascular phase is more readily observed microscopically, for example in breast cancer, where the multifocal origin of malignancy gives rise to ducts containing prevascular carcinoma in situ residing in the same neighborhood as normal ducts and ducts with highly neovascular carcinomas (Figure I-11-3).[286] The human breast contains between 6,000 and 10,000 ducts.[143] In a patient with a large vascularized invasive breast cancer, the same breast may harbor multiple areas of carcinoma in situ, with or without neovascularization or with or without microinvasion.[286] When such histological sections are stained with antibody to Factor VIII-related antigen, a specific marker for vascular endothelium, vessel density can be accurately counted and the prevascular and vascular phases of tumor growth are dramatically highlighted by the Factor VIII stain.

The Vascular Phase

Human tumors that have undergone neovascularization may enter a phase of rapid growth, increased metastatic potential, and accumulating symptoms.[286]

Neovascularization permits rapid tumor growth mainly because it temporarily solves the problem of exchange of nutrients, oxygen and wastes by a crowded three-dimensional cell population for which simple diffusion of these molecules across its outer surface would be inadequate. Furthermore, blood vessels themselves may stimulate tumor growth. When angiogenesis is generated in vitro in fibrin clot cultures, tumor cells added to the culture prefer to grow along capillary blood vessels despite the absence of blood flow.[209] Endothelial cells which line the myriads of new vessels induced by a tumor may also contribute growth factors such as bFGF, PDGF, IGF-1,[245,259] and cytokines such as IL-1, IL-6 and GM-CSF[200,220] which may augment tumor growth.

Neovascularization increases the probability of metastasis in part because it facilitates shedding of tumor cells into the circulation. In animals it was found that malignant cells appeared in the effluent circulation of the tumor, but only

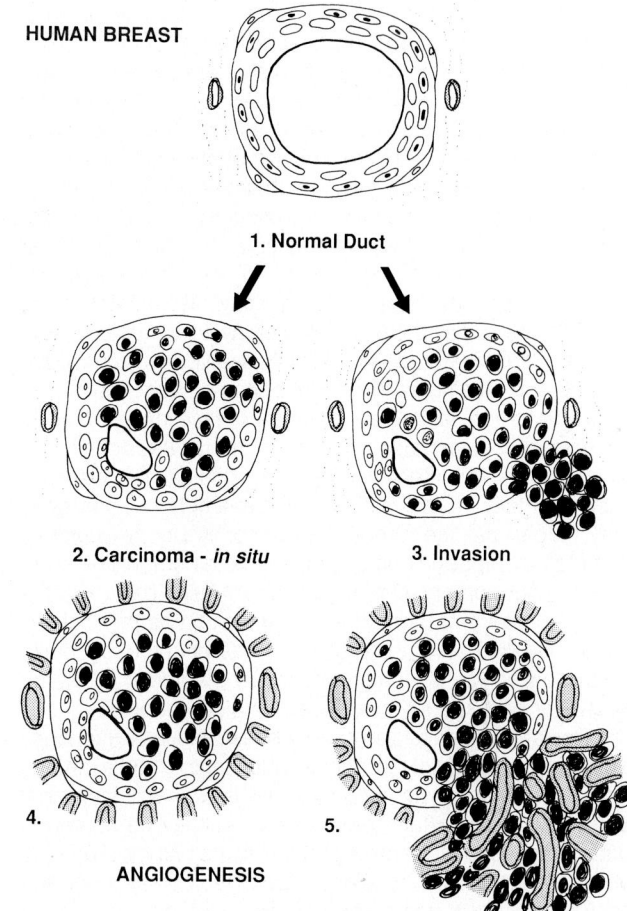

HUMAN BREAST

1. Normal Duct

2. Carcinoma - *in situ*

3. Invasion

4.

5.

ANGIOGENESIS

Figure I-11-3. Diagram of ducts in human breast. Each normal duct is lined by approximately two layers of epithelium. Proliferation occurs in the basal layer. Carcinoma in situ begins to fill the duct with abnormally proliferating cells. In the surgical specimen from a breast it is possible to find carcinoma in situ before and after the onset of angiogenesis. Also, one can see microinvasion before and after angiogenesis. Despite the presence of invasion, large tumor masses are usually not present until after neovascularization has taken place.

after neovascularization of the tumor had occurred.[173] In fact, the number of cells shed from the primary tumor correlated with the density of tumor blood vessels and also with the number of lung metastases observed later.

Neovascularization *per se* is responsible for some of the new symptoms which appear after a tumor has switched to the angiogenic phenotype. Blood in the urine, in the sputum or between menstrual periods, may signify the presence of a vascularized tumor in the bladder, bronchus or cervix. When ovarian carcinoma has metastasized to the peritoneal lining or to the omentum, tiny implants of a few millimeters diameter may remain white, avascular and nearly uniform in size. When some of these lesions become neovascularized, the ascites fluid in the peritoneum becomes bloody. Another cause of symptoms related to the onset of angiogenesis is local edema, especially in primary and metastatic brain tumors where highly permeable new capillary blood vessels contribute to protein leakage.[40,61,175] Of the known angiogenic molecules,[82] vascular endothelial growth factor (VEGF)[64] (also called VPF or FSdGF, see below) was identified because of its ability to increase vascular permeability.[247] Furthermore, while most solid tumors contain a vast network of new capillaries, they lack functioning lymphatics.[117,141] None of the angiogenic molecules discovered so far (see below) are known to stimulate proliferation of lymphatic endothelium. A novel form of cancer therapy which takes advantage of the hyperpermeability of new tumor vasculature and the hypoplasia of lymphatics within a tumor employs macromolecular drugs for prolonged tumor retention.[181] The paucity or absence of new lymphatics within a tumor may also contribute to elevated interstitial pressure as well as to increased local edema. Central necrosis is seldom observed in prevascular tumors or in carcinoma in situ but becomes common in vascularized tumors, especially as they increase in size. Vessels are compressed and occluded in the central areas of a tumor as a result of high interstitial pressure. This can be observed experimentally[106] and clinically. For example, angiography may reveal that the center of a tumor is poorly perfused because radiopaque dye cannot enter the compressed vessels. Vessel compression may also act as a barrier to the optimal delivery of therapeutic agents such as monoclonal antibodies.[140] These compressed areas become ischemic. Necrosis follows. It is inaccurate to say that these areas are avascular or that a tumor outgrew its blood supply.

Vascularized tumors also cause certain unique clinical signs which are related to the neovascularization. For example, retinoblastomas are accompanied by iris neovascularization. Bone pain in metastatic prostate cancer may be related in part to neovascularization. A problem in the biopsy of primary bone tumors is that if the biopsy specimen contains only the neovascular response at the periphery of the tumor, it may be mistaken for simple chronic granulation tissue or inflammation. The angiogenesis induced by cervical cancer may be observed by colposcopy,[256] a vascularized bladder carcinoma is detected by cystoscopy, and mammography often reveals the vascularized rim of a breast tumor. The appearance of telangiectasia or vascular spiders in a mastectomy scar may herald recurrence of tumor within the incision. Certain brain tumors induce angiogenesis in remote areas of the brain.

Angiogenic Molecules

At least eight polypeptide molecules have been demonstrated to be angiogenic in vivo. Some of these peptides are candidates for the mediators of tumor-induced angiogenesis. For 7 of them the complete amino acid sequence is known and their genes have been cloned (Table I-II-1). Two non-peptide low molecular weight compounds are also angiogenic.[56,160]

While much has been learned about the biochemistry and structure of the various angiogenic molecules since the first one was completely purified in 1984,[254] very little is understood about how these factors mediate angiogenesis in vivo or how they are regulated in normal and neoplastic tissue. Therefore, only a brief summary of the salient properties of each angiogenic molecule will be presented here.

Table I-11-1. Angiogenic Factors

Factor & In Vitro Activity	Molecular Weight		Reference
Mitogenic for Endothelial Cells and Other Cell Types			
Acidic FGF	16,500		82, 167, 278, 273, 274, 275
Basic FGF	18,000		82, 150, 253, 254
Transforming growth factor-alpha (TGFα)	5,500		53, 187, 243
Mitogenic for Endothelial Cells			
Platelet-derived endothelial cell growth factor (PD-ECGF)*	45,000		137, 193
*Vascular endothelial growth factor (VEGF)**	45,000	(23,000)	64, 169, 279
Vascular permeability factor (VPF)	40,000		38
Folliculostellate-derived growth factor (FSdGF)	23,000		108
Chemotactic* for Endothelial Cells**			
Angiotropin	4,500		125, 126
Effect on Endothelial Cells is Indirect or Unknown			
Angiogenin	14,100		65, 161, 228, 249, 264
Inhibit Endothelial Proliferation and Stimulate Tube Formation			
Transforming growth factor-beta (TGFβ)	25,000		148, 229, 230, 261
Tumor necrosis factor-alpha (TNFα)	17,000		98, 170, 215, 252

*PD-ECGF induces DNA synthesis, but not proliferation
**The amino acid sequences of VEGF, VPF, and FSdGF are nearly identical
***Chemotaxis is the only effect of angiotropin on endothelial cells reported to date. Other factors which are mitogenic for endothelial cells, are also chemotactic for them (e.g., aFGF, bFGF, and PD-ECGF)

Fibroblast Growth Factors

The fibroblast growth factors (FGFs) are among the most potent endothelial mitogens and are also highly angiogenic. FGF was first used to describe a polypeptide isolated from pituitary and brain that was mitogenic for 3T3 fibroblasts.[107] The first complete purification of an FGF was achieved by heparin-affinity chromatography of a factor isolated from rat chondrosarcoma.[254] This was determined to be basic fibroblast growth factor (bFGF) with a molecular weight of 17,000–18,000 and a pI of 9.6.[20] Acidic FGF (aFGF) was also found in brain[167,273] and when it was purified, had a molecular weight of 16–17 kD and a pI of 5.[274] Higher molecular weight forms of bFGF (up to 25 kD) have recently been found in normal tissues,[198] as well as in animal,[128] and human tumor cells.[153,223] In fact, bFGF is widely distributed in normal and malignant tissues,[121] while aFGF is localized mainly in neural tissues (e.g., brain, retina), and in bone.[82]

Three oncogenes encode for proteins that have a 40–50% homology for aFGF and bFGF. Int-2 is a product of integration of mammary tumor virus into the host genome.[55] The hst oncogene was isolated from a human gastric cancer.[236] A similar oncogene was later isolated from Kaposi's sarcoma and called K-FGF.[51] *FGF-5* is an oncogene isolated from a human bladder cancer.[299]

Both aFGF and bFGF are mitogenic[39,272] and chemotactic[39,223] for vascular endothelial cells as well as for fibroblasts and smooth muscle cells. Both FGFs are also potent angiogenic factors in the chick embryo and in the rabbit cornea at 10–100 ng.[1,82,253,271] A complex of aFGF and gelatin acts as a sustained-release depot that induces angiogenesis in the abdominal cavity of rats.[275] Angiogenesis can also be induced in vitro by FGF.[195]

A curious property of the fibroblast growth factors is their ability to bind to heparin.[177,254] This affinity for heparin was discovered by serendipity and was immediately employed to purify acidic and basic fibroblast growth factor. Purification of the FGFs by heparin-affinity chromatography was for a while thought to be the only application of this interesting property. It is now recognized, however, that many of the biological activities of the FGFs are mediated by interactions with heparin or heparin-like molecules (for review see 150). Heparin protects aFGF and bFGF from denaturation as well as from proteolytic degradation.[109,231,248] The mitogenic activity of aFGF is potentiated by heparin.[278] bFGF is stored in the subendothelial extracellular matrix in vitro[283] and in basement membrane in vivo,[84] where it is bound to heparan sulfate and can be mobilized by heparin, heparin fragments, heparinase or collagenase. It is also found in the basement membrane of all sizes of blood vessels.[41] The physiological role of sequestered FGF in the extracellular matrix is not clear, but it could be a mechanism for maintaining a biologically active supply of the growth factor in readiness for injury. We have used the term "stormone" to convey this unique characteristic.[84] The term may apply to other heparin-binding peptides which are stored in basement membrane, such as thrombospondin. When carcinoma in situ invades extracellular matrix, bFGF could be released as an early event in the induction of angiogenesis. However, this mechanism may also mediate pathological angiogenesis. For example, rapidly growing hemangiomas in newborn babies reveal large quantities of bFGF by immuno-staining (unpublished data). These hemangiomas are infiltrated with 20–30 times more mast cells than normal skin,[105] and the hemangiomas themselves are heparin-rich (unpublished data). It is possible that mast cell heparin mobilizes active bFGF and that a combination of heparin and FGF induces angiogenesis.

Both aFGF and bFGF are cell-associated, lack a consensus signal peptide and are normally not secreted.[153] In contrast, other growth factors such as PDGF, TGF-alpha, TGF-beta and TNF-alpha, are secreted. It is not clear how bFGF is delivered into the extracellular matrix. However, several alternative pathways of secretion have been proposed which do not involve the classic route of translocation through the rough endoplasmic reticulum.[201] It has been suggested instead, that bFGF may be secreted by exocytosis of vesicles. Nevertheless, the sequestration of FGFs within cells and in extracellular matrix may prevent this potent endothelial mitogen from acting under normal conditions. This could be one explanation for why normal vascular endothelial cells have such a low level of proliferation.[52] In tumors for which

FGF is a mediator of angiogenesis, there may be novel mechanisms of FGF secretion, release or amplification. For example, K-FGF from Kaposi's sarcoma is a secreted protein.[50]

bFGF-like activity has not been found in normal plasma.[10] However, significantly increased levels of a factor nearly identical to bFGF have been found in the plasma of patients with the familial multiple endocrine neoplasia type I syndrome (MEN-1) (see XXV-4). This syndrome is characterized by hyperplasia of parathyroid glands, pancreatic islets, and anterior pituitary glands.[301] Tumors also develop in these tissues. At this writing, sensitive immunoassays for FGF levels in plasma are under development to determine whether plasma levels of FGF are increased in the presence of other tumors. Increased levels of bFGF-like activity have been identified in the urine of patients with bladder and kidney cancer.[36]

Angiogenin

Angiogenin is a single chain cationic polypeptide containing 123 amino acids with a molecular weight of 14,123 and a pI of 9.5.[65,161,228,264] It contains a signal peptide, and is a secreted protein. It was first isolated from a line of human colon carcinoma cells, and was also found in lung carcinoma and hepatoma cells. Angiogenin is present in normal cells such as lymphocytes and circulates in human plasma at 60–50 μg/liter.[249] Angiogenin appears to be produced mainly in the liver,[287] and its gene was cloned from a human liver cDNA library.[161] Angiogenin has homology to pancreatic ribonuclease and exhibits ribonucleolytic activity, mainly hydrolysing 18S and 28S ribosomal RNA.[21,234,248] Pancreatic ribonuclease is not angiogenic. Angiogenin stimulates angiogenesis in the chick embryo at 0.5 ng and in the rabbit cornea at 50 ng.[65] This angiogenesis activity depends in part on angiogenin's ribonuclease activity because angiogenesis can be blocked by a human placental ribonuclease inhibitor.[250] Angiogenin does not appear to be mitogenic or chemotactic for endothelial cells. However, it does activate inositol-specific phospholipase C in vascular endothelial cells, thus leading to activation of protein kinase C.[18] It is not clear how these biochemical effects of angiogenin on endothelial cells relate to its angiogenic activity. Because angiogenin is secreted by both normal and tumor cells, its role in tumor angiogenesis is not yet understood, although it probably acts by a different mechanism than FGF.

Transforming Growth Factor-Alpha

TGF-alpha is a single chain polypeptide of 50 amino acids with a molecular weight of 5,500 which has a 40% homology to epidermal growth factor (EGF) and binds to the EGF receptor.[53,187] It is secreted by normal cells such as macrophages[180] and by some human tumor cells such as sarcomas.[280] TGF-alpha is mitogenic for fibroblasts, epithelial cells, and vascular endothelial cells.[243] It stimulates angiogenesis when injected subcutaneously or into the hamster cheek pouch at 0.3–1 μg. An evaluation of the role of TGF-alpha in tumor angiogenesis awaits further study.

Transforming Growth Factor-Beta

TGF-beta is a homodimeric polypeptide with a molecular weight of 25,000.[261] It is a completely different protein from

TGF-alpha. While the TGF-beta family contains several related molecules, and while TGF-beta 1 and TGF-beta 2 are highly homologous, they have different molecular weights and may have different receptors. TGF-beta was originally found in platelets, placenta, and kidney, but is also present in many other tissues including cartilage, bone, and tumor cells.[229] TGF-beta is secreted, but in a biologically inactive form. The latent form can be activated by heat, acid, and proteases.[148,166] Proteolytic activation of TGF-beta, for example by plasmin, could be a regulating mechanism for the functional activity of TGF-beta.

TGF-beta inhibits growth of many cell types in vitro such as fibroblasts, epithelial cells and endothelial cells,[11,97,120,202,281] and it induces production of extracellular matrix.[130] TGF-beta in vivo appears to mediate wound healing, inflammation, and possibly, differentiation of mesenchymal tissues.

TGF-beta induces angiogenesis in vivo,[230] despite its ability to inhibit endothelial cell proliferation in vitro. Subcutaneous injection of 1 μg into mice induces neovascular granulation tissue. TGF-beta is highly chemotactic to macrophages and fibroblasts.[284] Macrophages themselves induce angiogenesis.[127,155,221] They also release fibroblast growth factor[12] and produce other angiogenic factors such as tumor necrosis factor-alpha,[98,170] transforming growth factor-alpha[225,243] and angiotropin.[125] Thus, it is possible that the angiogenic activity of TGF-beta is mediated by macrophages.[261] After macrophage infiltration subsides, any residual TGF-beta might inhibit proliferation of vascular endothelial cells. TGF-beta could have a bifunctional effect on angiogenesis, depending on the local tissue density of macrophages. Unlike angiogenesis induced by FGF, there are conflicting data on the angiogenic activity of TGF-beta in other assay systems. For example, in the chick chorioallantoic membrane, TGF-beta is reported to stimulate[293] and to inhibit angiogenesis.[58]

Tumor Necrosis Factor-Alpha

TNF-alpha, also called cachectin, is an anionic polypeptide of up to 157 amino acids with a molecular weight of 17,000.[215,252] TNF-alpha is synthesized and secreted by tumor cells as well as by macrophages that have been activated by endotoxin or by fibrin degradation products. TNF-alpha has a wide range of activities. It induces cachexia. It stimulates the synthesis of interleukin-1, granulocyte-macrophage colony stimulating factor, and ELAM-1 by endothelial cells.[17,219] It inhibits endothelial cell proliferation in vitro but is chemotactic for endothelial cells.[98,170] TNF-alpha is also angiogenic in vivo, and is thought to be one of the major angiogenic molecules of macrophages.[170] Angiogenesis is induced in the chick chorioallantoic membrane at 1 ng and in the cornea at 3.5 ng without apparent inflammation. TNF-alpha is similar to TGF-beta, because both molecules promote angiogenesis in vivo and capillary tube formation in vitro, but inhibit endothelial cell proliferation in vitro. Thus, the in vivo and in vitro actions of these molecules seem to be paradoxical.[83] Another puzzle is, how can TNF-alpha be both angiogenic and tumor necrosing in vivo? One possible explanation is that TNF-alpha may have different effects upon vascular endothelium depending on whether the molecule is administered inside or outside of the vascular system.[83]

Vascular endothelial cells are bipolar with a luminal side and a basement-membrane side. When TNF-alpha is implanted in an extravascular location (basement-membrane side), capillary sprouts grow out from existing vessels. In contrast, the intravascular injection of TNF-alpha (luminal side), may stimulate procoagulant activity by endothelial cells,[16,205] but not capillary growth. Meth A sarcoma, for example, regresses when the host animal is injected with TNF-alpha in a sufficient dose to enter the vascular system.[215] The tumor vasculature undergoes thrombosis, disruption of small vessels, and hemorrhage. An early event is probably the procoagulant effect of TNF-alpha acting on the luminal side of proliferating endothelium. Other angiogenic factors (e.g., FGF, TGF-beta) may also have a differential effect on vascular endothelium in vivo depending upon the route of administration.

Platelet-Derived Endothelial Cell Growth Factor

PD-ECGF is a single chain polypeptide of 45,000 molecular weight[193] whose gene has recently been cloned.[137] It differs from platelet-derived growth factor (PDGF), because it is heat and acid labile, and because it is mitogenic for endothelial cells but not fibroblasts. Unlike FGF, it does not bind to heparin nor does heparin potentiate its activity. PD-ECGF is also angiogenic,[137] and it could act physiologically as a maintenance factor for vascular endothelium.[45]

Angiotropin

This copper-containing polyribonucleotide with a molecular weight of 4,500 has been isolated from peripheral porcine monocytes activated by concanavalin A.[125,126] No amino acid sequence or cDNA data are available at present. Angiotropin stimulates endothelial cell chemotaxis, but not proliferation and it has no effect on 3T3 fibroblasts. Angiotropin induces angiogenesis in the chick chorioallantoic membrane and in the rabbit cornea at a dose of 2,500 pg. Subcutaneous injections of angiotropin in the rabbit induce vasodilation followed by neovascularization, as well as epidermal and stromal proliferation and hair growth. The mechanism of angiotropin-mediated angiogenesis is not clear.

Vascular Endothelial Growth Factor

VEGF, a recently discovered angiogenic factor,[64] also known as VPF (vascular permeability factor)[38] and FSdGF (folliculo stellate-derived growth factor),[108] is a heparin-binding dimeric polypeptide of approximately 45,000–46,000 molecular weight which can be reduced to peptides of approximately 23,000 molecular weight. Its amino acid sequence deduced from a cDNA clone suggests partial homology to platelet-derived growth factor.[279] This factor has been isolated from the folliculo-stellate cells of the anterior pituitary gland, as well as from neuroblastoma cells,[169] a human colon adenocarcinoma cell line,[174] rat,[37] and human brain tumor cells,[37,191] and other tumor cell lines.[232,246] VEGF is an endothelial cell mitogen and also increases vascular permeability. It is angiogenic in the chick chorioallantoic membrane[168] and may be an important angiogenic mediator for brain tumors.

Low Molecular Weight Non-Peptide Angiogenic Factors

Several low molecular weight compounds are reported to be angiogenic. 1-butyryl glycerol is secreted by adipocytes that have differentiated from 3T3 fibroblasts.[56] It is angiogenic on the chick chorioallantoic membrane and is chemotactic to endothelial cells, but is not an endothelial mitogen. The prostaglandins PGE_1 and PGE_2 are angiogenic on the chorioallantoic membrane from 20 ng to 1 μg and in the rabbit cornea.[14,56,93,111] Prostaglandins are elevated in tumors, wounds and inflammatory exudates. Nicotinamide isolated from tumors is angiogenic.[160] Its mechanism of action is unclear. Related compounds such as adenosine are angiogenic in the chorioallantoic membrane and cornea.[59,96] Adenosine is a vasodilator that accumulates in response to hypoxia. It is not clear how adenosine induces vasoproliferation. Certain degradation products of hyaluronic acid are angiogenic[289] and these fragments could play a role in the mediation of angiogenesis by those tumors which produce hyaluronidase.

Several angiogenic factors have been isolated from tumors, wound fluid and from other tissues, but they have not yet been completely purified or characterized.[13,212]

Different Mechanisms of Switching to the Angiogenic Phenotype

Our current knowledge about the structure and biological activity of angiogenic molecules has not yet been translated to an understanding of how these factors are regulated in normal and neoplastic tissue. It is unclear how angiogenic activity is switched on either in normal tissues such as the ovary or in tumors. Furthermore, it is difficult to determine the precise time of onset of angiogenic activity in human or animal tumors, even though separable stages of tumor growth *before* and *after* neovascularization can be clearly distinguished in these tumors.[27,35,101,143,144,256,262,263,286]

These difficulties notwithstanding, the mechanism of switching to the angiogenic phenotype during tumorigenesis or tumor progression is currently a central question in cancer research. Several in vivo and in vitro experimental models have recently been developed and novel mechanisms of switching angiogenesis activity on, or of amplifying it, have been elucidated. Presumably, a given tumor may utilize more than one such mechanism. Some mechanisms are described here (with the caveat that many of these studies are still in progress).

Expression of a New Angiogenic Molecule

The switch to the angiogenic phenotype can be observed and quantitated in a recently reported transgenic mouse system.[89] In this system the large T antigen of the SV40 viral genome is hybridized to the rat insulin promoter.[118] This oncogene is then injected into the ova of pseudopregnant mice. When the mice are mated, half of their offspring express the oncogene only in the insulin-producing beta cells in the islets of the pancreas. Carcinomas develop in these islets at an age-dependent rate. The islets undergo hyperplasia at about 4 weeks, and at 6–7 weeks a few islets become angiogenic. Large vascularized tumors develop from these angiogenic islets. In this system, the induction of angiogenesis is mediated by a novel endothelial mitogen secreted by the angiogenic tumor cells but not by the pre-angiogenic cells (unpublished data). The expression of the oncogene

appears to induce proliferation in beta cells so that by 10–12 weeks more than 70% of the islets have become hyperplastic. The onset of angiogenic activity occurs in a subset of the hyperplastic islets and appears to arise from a secondary or later event. It is not clear whether this event requires the loss of a suppressor gene or the activation of a gene which codes for an angiogenic factor, or both. Nor, do we know what governs the timing of the onset of angiogenic activity and whether a critical number of cell divisions must occur before cells become angiogenic. We do know that not all of the cells in a vascularized tumor are angiogenic. It appears that once a threshold number of cells have switched to the angiogenic phenotype, sufficient neovascularization occurs so that the whole tumor population can expand. The volume of vascularized tumors is more than 1,000 times larger than the volume of non-angiogenic hyperplastic islets.

Secretion of bFGF

When cDNA for human bFGF containing a leader sequence is transfected into normal mouse fibroblasts they become angiogenic and tumorigenic.[126a] bFGF is the sole mediator of angiogenesis of the transfected cells and is secreted by them but not by the parental cells. Furthermore, a specific monoclonal antibody against the secreted bFGF, injected into mice intravenously, inhibits angiogenesis and suppresses growth of this tumor.

In a different system, fibromas of the skin arise in transgenic mice carrying the bovine papilloma virus genome.[162,172] The fibromas are flat, white, non-angiogenic lesions which grow slowly and do not metastasize. After several months a few fibromas develop into fibrosarcomas which are highly vascular, grow rapidly and kill the mice. The fibromas contain cell-associated bFGF but do not secrete it, while the fibrosarcomas secrete 95% of the bFGF they synthesize.[145A] In these systems, the angiogenic switch appears to depend on *secretion* of an angiogenic molecule that is normally cell-associated and not secreted.

Loss of Suppressor Gene Activity

In a hamster fibroblast cell line, "the inactivation of a suppressor gene during carcinogenesis results in a gain of angiogenic activity that parallels a gain in tumorigenicity."[22,23] The shift in angiogenic activity on suppressor gene loss can be attributed to a 10-fold decrease in the secretion of a 140-kD glycoprotein that acts as an inhibitor of angiogenesis.[226] The angiogenesis inhibitor, whose production is dependent on the expression of the suppressor gene, is a fragment of the matrix protein, thrombospondin. This model system may be a paradigm for other tumors where suppressor gene loss is associated with increased tumorigenicity.

Amplified Production of bFGF by Endothelial Cells

bFGF is produced by all vascular endothelial cells that have been examined so far. In certain human tumors such as colon carcinoma, neuroblastoma and adrenal carcinoma, vascular endothelial cells within the tumor stain intensely with antibody to bFGF compared to normal endothelial cells, or to the tumor cells.[244] This finding suggests that these tumors are releasing an unknown mediator which stimulates excessive production by bFGF by local endothelial cells. For comparison, basal cell carcinoma, squamous cell carcinoma, and hemangioma contain high levels of bFGF in their tumor cells, but not their endothelial cells. bFGF is not detected in either tumor cells or endothelial cells of Kaposi's sarcoma, ovarian carcinoma and hemangiosarcoma.

Recruitment of Macrophages

Certain tumors recruit macrophages[222] which themselves can release angiogenic activity.[157,196] The relative hypoxia in central areas of tumors may be conducive to increased production of angiogenic activity by macrophages, because high tissue lactate levels appear to stimulate maximal production of angiogenic activity by macrophages.[155] Thus, intratumoral activated macrophages may amplify tumor-induced angiogenesis.

Recruitment of Mast Cells

During tumor-induced angiogenesis in the chick embryo, there is a significant increase in mast cells prior to neovascularization.[149] Also, some human tumors are heavily infiltrated with mast cells. This has been quantitated in human hemangiomas where mast cells are significantly increased above normal.[105] When tumors are implanted in mast cell-deficient mice (W/W^v), angiogenesis and subsequent tumor growth are retarded.[54] Tumor growth is <60% of that observed in mice which have normal mast cell numbers. A significant increase in both neovascularization and tumor growth rate is observed when mast cell-deficient mice are injected with exogenous mast cells along with the original inoculation of tumor cells.[54] Mast cells are heparin-rich and heparin can mobilize bFGF from extracellular matrix and protect it from degradation. Furthermore, heparin can potentiate the mitogenic effect of FGF on endothelial cells.[278]

Mobilization of bFGF from Extracellular Matrix

As described in the section on bFGF, this angiogenic molecule is stored in extracellular matrix where it appears to be bound to heparan sulfate proteoglycan.[84] It can be released in a biologically active form by heparin, heparanases and collagenases,[84] or by plasminogen activator-mediated proteolytic activity.[241] All of these factors may be produced by tumor cells directly, or by cells which tumors recruit (e.g., macrophages and mast cells). Thus, for certain tumors such as carcinoma of the cervix or melanoma, mobilization of active FGF from the basement membrane may be an early event in the mechanism of switching to the angiogenic phenotype. FGF mobilization may occur as the tumor begins to invade from the epithelial compartment into the underlying stroma.

Suppression of Pericyte Inhibition of Endothelial Proliferation

Pericytes in the microvasculature appear to inhibit endothelial proliferation under physiological conditions.[46,47,217] This inhibitory action is offered as one of the possible mechanisms which normally maintain vascular endothelial cells in a quiescent, non-proliferating state.[151] The onset of neovascularization in the retina is often associated with pericyte loss. Both pericytes and capillary endothelial cells in vitro

release a latent form of TGF-beta which is activated when these cells contact each other during co-culture. Activated TGF-beta strongly inhibits endothelial cell proliferation.[4] However, it has been shown by immunostaining that pericytes may be significantly increased in tumor vasculature.[242] Therefore, tumors may employ unknown mechanisms to overcome the inhibitory effect of pericytes on endothelial cells.

Angiogenesis Inhibitors

In the early 1970s I proposed that inhibition of angiogenesis could be a potential anti-cancer therapy.[68] Demonstration of such anti-angiogenic therapy would require the administration of a specific angiogenesis inhibitor to tumor-bearing animals, and if successful, would strengthen the hypothesis that tumor growth is angiogenesis-dependent. No angiogenesis inhibitors were known in 1971 when this idea was put forward. Nevertheless, the concept of angiogenesis inhibitors has stimulated the search for them.[71,80] There are at least three strategies for anti-angiogenic therapy. One strategy would be to block tumor cells from expressing or producing angiogenic molecules. A second strategy would neutralize the activity of these angiogenic molecules after they are released from a tumor. A third strategy would be to block the cells which participate in blood vessel growth from responding to any angiogenic molecules. With but one exception, the angiogenesis inhibitors which have been discovered so far appear to operate by blocking the proliferation of capillary blood vessels in response to angiogenic molecules.

Collagenase Inhibitors

The first angiogenesis inhibitor was found in cartilage in 1973.[25,62,158,159,163] One form of this inhibitor has recently been completely purified from bovine cartilage and partially sequenced.[199] It has a molecular weight of 27,650. It inhibits angiogenesis in vivo and proliferation and migration of capillary endothelial cells in vitro. The protein is also an inhibitor of mammalian collagenase.[199] Of interest is the recent discovery of an angiogenesis inhibitor in the conditioned medium of a clonal human chondrosarcoma cell line.[267] The factor has not yet been completely purified and it is not known if it is a collagenase inhibitor.

Minocycline is a semisynthetic tetracycline antimicrobial that inhibits collagenase activity in the synovial fluid of patients with rheumatoid arthritis.[113] When implanted in a sustained release-pellet in the rabbit cornea, minocycline brought about a 4-fold reduction in neovascularization that had been induced by a tumor implant.[267A] In the cornea, minocycline inhibited angiogenesis as effectively as a cortisone-heparin pellet. Its effect in tumor-bearing mice has not been reported.

Medroxyprogesterone is a synthetic steroid that inhibits collagenolysis and tumor-induced angiogenesis in the rabbit cornea when the steroid is implanted in the cornea.[114] Medroxyprogesterone also inhibits plasminogen activator produced by endothelial cells. Plasminogen activator-mediated proteolytic activity can release basic fibroblast growth factor from endothelial cells.[241] Both of these properties may play a role in the anti-tumor effect of medroxyprogesterone acetate when it is used to treat patients with advanced or recurrent endometrial cancer.[99]

Chitin is a homogenous polysaccharide composed of N-acetyl-glucosamine residues. Chemically modified chitin derivatives into which 6-0-sulfate and 6-0-carboxymethyl groups are introduced (SCM-chitin) inhibit type IV collagenase and heparanase.[235] SCM-chitin inhibited tumor-induced angiogenesis and tumor growth in mice, when the polysaccharide was injected into the tumor.[235] It also prevented the invasion of endothelial cells through reconstituted basement membrane.

Angiostatic Steroids

While cortisone or hydrocortisone have little or no anti-angiogenic activity, they are converted to potent angiogenesis inhibitors by administration with heparin.[44,85,237] Neither the glucocorticoid nor the mineralocorticoid function of these steroids is necessary for anti-angiogenic activity,[43,238] but specific structure-activity relationships are critical.[81] Thus, pregnenolone, progesterone, and estrone have no anti-angiogenic activity, while tetrahydrocortisol and other angiostatic steroids have high anti-angiogenic activity (with heparin). The anticoagulant function of heparin is not necessary for its anti-angiogenic activity with steroids. Angiostatic steroids administered with heparin fragments which lack anticoagulant activity also inhibit angiogenesis. These steroid-heparin combinations also inhibit tumor growth[85] and metastasis[57,238] in tumor-bearing mice. While some tumors are potently inhibited or regress when treated with cortisone-heparin mixtures (but not with cortisone alone), others are refractory.[15,85] The explanation for this difference is unknown, but may lie in differences in output of angiogenic activity or differences in degradation of steroids or of heparin by different types of tumors. Furthermore, if exogenous heparin is omitted, angiostatic steroids can be equally well potentiated by a synthetic arylsulfatase inhibitor which protects endogenous heparin-like molecules from desulfation.[34] Synthetic sulfated cyclodextrins can also substitute for heparin.[90] Beta-cyclodextrin tetradecasulfate is 100–1,000 times more potent than heparin as a potentiator of angiostatic steroids. A critical ratio of cyclodextrin to steroid is necessary for optimum angiostatic activity. This observation taken together with other experimental results[90] suggests that the steroid enters the hydrophobic cavity of cyclodextrin to form a complex. In fact, the complex inhibits chemokinesis of capillary endothelial cells,[218] whereas either the steroid or the polysaccharide alone are ineffective.

The mechanism of action of angiostatic steroids is not completely understood.[239] However, in the presence of steroid-heparin combinations, the basement membranes of growing capillaries undergo rapid dissolution.[134] Endothelial cells round up and new capillary blood vessels retract. Basement membrane of nongrowing capillaries or of larger vessels is not degraded. Other studies suggest that the components of basement membrane such as fibronectin, collagen type IV and laminin may be undergoing rapid turnover in growing capillaries. Therefore, compounds which interfere with synthesis of these components, or increase their degradation rate, would act to increase the dissolution of basement membrane and to inhibit angiogenesis.[132,183]

Angiostatic steroids have not yet been used clinically, but their first application may be the treatment of corneal neovascularization which has failed conventional therapy.

Platelet Factor 4

Protamine was shown to be an angiogenesis inhibitor,[270] but cumulative toxicity from prolonged administration and a narrow window of angiostatic efficacy prevented its consideration for clinical use or further animal study. Platelet factor 4 was first tested for anti-angiogenic activity because it could bind and neutralize heparin similar to protamine.[88,270] It inhibited angiogenesis in the chick embryo, but there was insufficient material for testing in other systems because it could be obtained only by extraction and purification from platelets. Recently, recombinant human platelet factor-4 (rHuPF4) has been produced.[182] It specifically inhibits endothelial proliferation and migration in vitro.[251] Inhibition is associated with the carboxy-terminal, heparin-binding region of the molecule. A peptide as small as 12 amino acids retains full angiostatic activity. These inhibitory activities can be abrogated by heparin. The growth of human colon carcinoma in athymic mice, and the growth of murine melanoma are markedly inhibited by intralesional injections, while the tumor cells are insensitive to rHuPF4 in vitro at levels that inhibit normal endothelial cell proliferation. Thus, the anti-tumor effects of rHuPF4 are most likely due to inhibition of angiogenesis. Systemic administration of low dose rHuPF4 (μgs/mouse) is ineffective against tumor growth, perhaps because of rapid inactivation or efficient clearance of the peptide. However, higher doses await testing.

Bacterial-Derived Angiogenesis Inhibitors

A sulfated polysaccharide-peptidoglycan complex derived from the bacterial wall of an *Arthobacter* species inhibited angiogenesis in the chorioallantoic membrane and also inhibited the growth of sarcoma 180 tumor in mice.[136] The effect was greatly potentiated by corticosteroids. Other sulfated polysaccharides including dextran sulfates were relatively ineffective.

Fungal-Derived Angiogenesis Inhibitors

The synthesis of a family of novel angiogenesis inhibitors that are analogues of fumagillin, a naturally secreted antibiotic of Aspergillus fumigatus *fresenius,* has recently been reported (Figure I-11-4).[131] One of these angioinhibins, AGM-1470 (Figure I-11-5), inhibits proliferation and migration of capillary endothelial cells and inhibits angiogenesis in the chick embryo. It also suppresses growth of a wide variety of mouse tumors with little or no toxicity to the host. For example, treatment was not initiated until mice had palpable vascularized tumors of 100–200 mm^3. They received the inhibitor at 30 mgm/kg s.c. every other day for >100 days (e.g., about one-sixth the life of a mouse). They had little or no weight loss or hair loss. Survival time of treated mice was increased up to 260% over untreated controls. Tumor cell proliferation in vitro was refractory to AGM-1470. Animals bearing intraperitoneal leukemia P388 were unaffected by this compound. This tumor grows in an ascites form and is less dependent upon neovascularization. These findings

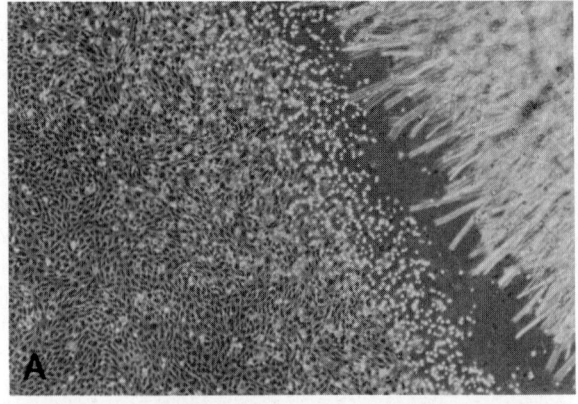

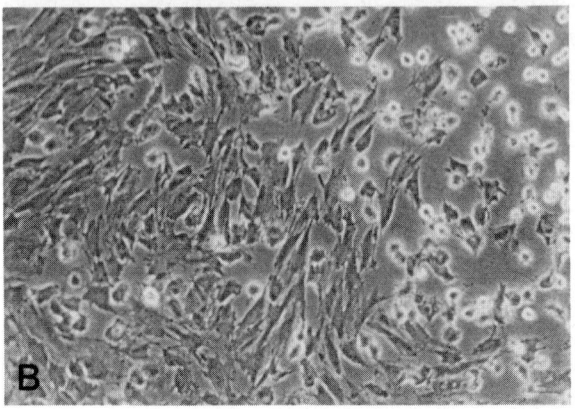

Figure I-11-4. Origin of angioinhibins. *A*, A contaminated culture of bovine capillary endothelial cells showing fungal hyphae at the right. *B*, Higher magnification showing an apparent diffusion gradient resulting in cell detachment and rounding nearest the edge of the fungal colony; cells only a few cell diameters away reveal normal morphology.

suggest that the angioinhibins exert their anti-tumor effect primarily by acting on the tumor vasculature.

Another fungal-derived angiogenesis inhibitor, herbimycin A, inhibits angiogenesis in the chick embryo.[214] However, it is relatively cytotoxic compared to other angiostatic antibiotics and its anti-tumor effect has not been determined.

Drugs Which Interfere with Basement Membrane Turnover

Basement membrane synthesis and degradation are essential steps in the process of angiogenesis.[184] After it was learned that dissolution of basement membrane of growing capillaries is one mechanism by which angiostatic steroids inhibit angiogenesis,[132,134,186] other specific modulators of matrix metabolism were examined.[132,185,192] Regression of growing capillaries in the chick embryo was induced by proline analogues such as l-azetidine-2-carboxylic acid, cis-hydroxyproline, dL-3,4,dihydroxyproline and thioproline. These compounds and a,a-dipyridyl, an inhibitor of prolylhydroxylase, all interfere with triple helix formation and prevent collagen deposition. Beta-aminoproprionitrile, an inhibitor of collagen cross-linking is also anti-angiogenic, although betamethyl d-xyloside, an inhibitor of glycosaminoglycan deposition is not. Co-administration of suboptimal doses of collagen modulators with angiostatic steroids and/or heparin

Figure I-11-5. Upper panel. Structure of fumagillin, the parent compound isolated from the culture contaminant [Aspergillus fumigatus *fresenius*] described in Figure I-11-4. Lower panel. The synthetic analogue AGM-1470, a related angioinhibin, which is a potent, nontoxic angiogenesis inhibitor. (From Ingber et al.[131] with permission of the publisher.)

potentiates inhibition of angiogenesis. These general inhibitors of collagen formation also inhibit tumor growth in mice, but are too toxic for long-term safe administration (up to 15% weight loss). Nevertheless, recent reports suggest that it may be possible to design collagen modulators that are more specific inhibitors of type IV collagen deposition, but are less toxic. Of interest is that tricyclodecan-9-yl xanthate (D609), an inhibitor of basement membrane collagen biosynthesis which has no effect on interstitial collagen synthesis, inhibits angiogenesis, tumor growth and metastasis, and prolongs survival in rats bearing Walker 256 carcinoma.[183] Taken together, these studies suggest that involution of growing capillaries may be induced by alterations in collagen metabolism that lead to loss of the structural integrity of basement membrane.

D-Penicillamine and Gold Thiomalate

Two drugs used to treat arthritis inhibit angiogenesis. D-penicillamine, a copper chelator, inhibits endothelial cell proliferation in vitro.[188] It also inhibits angiogenesis in the rabbit cornea at serum concentrations which are similar to the serum levels of this drug in treated patients. It has been proposed that D-penicillamine may play an important role in suppressing neovascularization in the joints of patients with rheumatoid arthritis. It is not clear whether the mechanism of anti-angiogenesis depends on the ability of D-penicillamine to act as a copper chelator. However, it is interesting that copper depletion in rats and rabbits that were treated with penicillamine and fed a copper-deficient diet markedly suppressed tumor-induced angiogenesis and tumor growth in the brain.[29]

Gold thiomalate and other gold derivatives have been effectively used to ameliorate the symptoms of arthritis. These gold compounds are now known to inhibit endothelial cell proliferation in vitro[189] and to block the release of angiogenic activity by activated macrophages.[156] The mechanism of action of gold compounds remains to be elucidated, but other macrophage functions do not appear to be suppressed when angiogenic activity is blocked.

Thrombospondin

Normal hamster cells were found to constituitively secrete a protein nearly identical to thrombospondin which inhibited endothelial cell proliferation and also inhibited angiogenesis in the cornea.[226] During malignant transformation of these hamster cells, expression of the inhibitor, which appears to be under the control of a cancer-suppressor gene, is down-regulated. Of interest is that thrombospondin is a heparin-binding protein which is also stored in extracellular matrix. Its effect as an anti-tumor agent has not been tested.

Vitamin D_3 Analogues

Two analogues of vitamin D_3 inhibited angiogenesis in the chick embryo chorioallantoic membrane in a dose-dependent manner and in the picomolar range.[213] The active metabolite of vitamin D_3, 1-alpha,25-dihydroxyvitamin D_3 and a synthetic analogue 22-oxa-1alpha,25-dihydroxyvitamin D_3 (which has no effect on calcium metabolism), are both able to inhibit angiogenesis, whereas vitamin D_3 is not effective.

Interferon

Interferons were previously reported to inhibit the migration of capillary endothelial cells in vitro[31] and to inhibit lymphocyte-induced angiogenesis in vivo.[255] Recently, interferon alpha (IFN-alpha) was used to successfully treat a child with pulmonary capillary hemangiomatosis.[290] This is a rare disease in which excessive growth of capillary blood vessels in the lung has usually led to a fatal outcome. The cause of this neovascularization is unknown. Nevertheless, long-term administration (months) of IFN-alpha at 3 million units/meter^2/day subcutaneously, caused regression of the pulmonary hemangiomas. The child returned to full activity, an unprecedented outcome for this disease.[74]

As a result of this report, several centers have begun during the past year to use IFN-alpha to treat life-threatening systemic hemangiomatosis in infants whose lesions have failed to respond to steroid therapy.[216] In this angiogenic disease, large hemangiomas consisting of rapidly proliferating capillary blood vessels suddenly appear after birth on the skin, in the orbits, in the airway and in abdominal organs.[63] Approximately 70% of patients fail to respond to steroid therapy. Mortality rates approach 60% or higher, especially if the liver is involved. Death is often due to unremitting platelet trapping and bleeding (Kassabach-Merritt syndrome). Prolonged treatment with IFN-alpha is required for 6 months or more, but newborns and infants tolerate this drug well with little toxicity. While it is too soon to say whether this therapy will stand the test of time, our early experience is that gradual regression of hemangiomas has occurred in 18 of 20 cases, there being two failures.

Now that several types of angiogenesis inhibitors are being studied experimentally, they are beginning to provide some insight as to how anti-angiogenic therapy may be used against tumors in the future. Whether anti-angiogenic therapy is used alone or in conjunction with conventional chemotherapy, it is becoming clear that angiogenesis inhibitors directed against growing capillary blood vessels may need to be administered for prolonged periods, i.e., months or years. Such long-term therapy will require systemic administration of compounds of relatively low toxicity, analogous to the treatment of malaria. An animal model of prophylactic anti-angiogenic tumor therapy has been reported.[178] The successful use of IFN-alpha to treat a patient suffering from pulmonary capillary hemangiomatosis[290] provides a glimpse of what anti-angiogenic therapy might be like in the future when more potent angiogenesis inhibitors[131] become available for clinical trial in cancer patients.

Interferon-alpha, however, has not proved to be a potent agent against a variety of solid tumors. This illustrates a second point, namely, that the effectiveness of certain angiogenesis inhibitors may be limited to specific capillary beds or to types of neovascularization induced by specific stimuli. For example, penicillamine may inhibit neovascularization in rheumatoid arthritis. But because penicillamine is destroyed by catalase, it would not be expected to inhibit the growth of catalase-rich tumors. Furthermore, some tumors are more highly angiogenic than others.[26] Angiogenesis inhibitors that are very potent (e.g., angioinhibins[131]), or combinations of different angiogenesis inhibitors may be required to successfully treat such tumors.

Summary and Future Directions

The field of angiogenesis research which began as an inquiry into the mechanisms by which tumors induce a new blood supply, has now broadened to include a diverse group of scientists who are addressing central questions. For example, the development of the vascular system itself is being explored. Genes which turn angiogenesis on or suppress angiogenic activity are being elucidated. Furthermore, angiogenic molecules are being employed to accelerate the healing of surgical wounds and peptic ulcers. Angiogenesis inhibitors intended for eventual anti-cancer therapy are also being studied for their potential use in ocular angiogenesis, arthritis and other non-neoplastic diseases.

These developments in fields parallel to oncology may bring new information to bear on the problem of tumor angiogenesis. We need to understand how tumors become angiogenic and what angiogenic molecules they employ. It will be important to know how these molecules are released, whether specific angiogenic molecules are produced by certain type of tumors, and how angiogenesis suppressor activity is down-regulated during tumor progression. It is still not clear what percent of tumor-induced angiogenesis must be blocked before tumor growth is inhibited, nor is it known if endothelial cells can become "resistant" to angiogenesis inhibitors.

Beyond these considerations lie questions for the more distant future. Can the onset of angiogenic activity be detected in the blood or other body fluids for use in diagnosis? Can the process of angiogenesis itself be manipulated by genetic therapies, for example by administration of anti-sense DNA? These questions and others provide the basis for continuing excitement in the field of angiogenesis research.

References

1. Abraham, J. A., Mergia, A., Whang, J. L., Tumolo, A., Friedman, J., Hjerrild, K. S. A., Gospodarowicz, D., and Fiddes, J. C.: Nucleotide sequence of a bovine clone encoding the angiogenic protein, basic fibroblast growth factor. Science, 233:545, 1986.
2. Adam, J. A., and Maggelakis, A. A.: Diffusion of regulated growth characteristics of a spherical prevascular carcinoma. Bulletin of Mathematical Biology, 52:549, 1990.
3. Algire, G. H., Chalkley, H. W., Legallais, F. Y., and Park, H. D.: Vascular reactions of normal and malignant tumors in vivo. I. Vascular reactions of mice to wounds and to normal and neoplastic transplants. J. Natl. Cancer Inst., 6:73, 1945.
4. Antonelli-Orlidge, A., Saunders, K. B., Smith, S. R., and D'Amore, P. A.: An activated form of transforming growth factor-beta is produced by co-cultures of endothelial cells and pericytes. Proc. Natl. Acad. Sci. U.S.A., 86:4544, 1989.
5. Auerbach, R.: Angiogenesis-inducing factors: A review. *In* Lymphokines. Edited by E. Pick. London, Academic Press, 1981, pp. 69–88.
6. Auerbach, R., Arensman, R., Kubai, L., and Folkman, J.: Tumor-induced angiogenesis: Lack of inhibition by irradiation. Intl. J. Cancer, 15:241, 1975.
7. Auerbach, R., Kubai, L., Knighton, D., and Folkman, J.: A simple procedure for the long-term cultivation of chicken embryos. Dev. Biol., 41:391, 1974.
8. Ausprunk, D. H.: Distribution of hyaluronic acid and sulfated glycosaminoglycans during blood vessel development in the chick chorioallantoic membrane. Amer. J. Anat., 177:313, 1986.
9. Ausprunk, D. H., Dethlefsen, S. M., and Higgins, E. R.: Distribution of fibronectin, laminin and type IV collagen during development of blood vessels in the chick chorioallantoic membrane. *In* The Development of the Vascular System. Edited by R. N. Feinberg, G. K. Sherer, and R. Auerbach. Basel, Switzerland, Karger, 1990, pp. 93–108.
10. Ausprunk, D. H., and Folkman, J.: Migration and proliferation of endothelial cells in preformed and newly formed blood vessels during tumor angiogenesis. Microvasc. Res., 14:53, 1977.
11. Baird, A., and Durkin, T.: Inhibition of endothelial cell proliferation by type-beta transforming growth factor: Interactions with acidic and basic fibroblast growth factors. Biochem. Biophys. Res. Commun., 138:476, 1986.
12. Baird, A., Mormede, P., and Bohlen, P.: Immunoreactive fibroblast growth factor in cells of peritoneal exudate suggests its identity with macrophage-derived growth factor. Biochem. Biophys. Res. Commun., 126:358, 1985.
13. Banda, M. J., Knighton, D. R., Hunt, T. K., and Werb, Z.: Isolation of a nonmitogenic angiogenesis factor from wound fluid. Proc. Natl. Acad. Sci. U.S.A., 79:7773, 1982.
14. Ben Ezra, D.: Neovasculogenic ability of prostaglandins, growth factors and synthetic chemoattractants. Am. J. Ophthalmol., 86:455, 1978.
15. Benrezzak, O., Madarnas, P., Pageau, R., Nigam, V., and Elhilali, M. M.: Evaluation of cortisone-heparin and cortisone-maltose tetrapalmitate therapies against rodent tumors. Anticancer Research, 9:1883, 1989.
16. Bevilacqua, M. P., Pober, J. S., Majeau, G. R., Fiers, W., Cotran, R. S., and Gimbrone, M. A., Jr.: Recombinant tumor necrosis factor induces procoagulant activity in cultured human vascular endothelium: Characterization and comparison with the actions of interleukin-1. Proc. Natl. Acad. Sci. U.S.A., 83:4533, 1986.
17. Bevilacqua, M. P., Pober, J. S., Wheeler, M. E., Cotran, R. S., and Gimbrone, M. A., Jr.: Interleukin 1 acts on cultured human vascular endothelium to increase the adhesion of polymorphonuclear leukocytes, monocytes and related leukocyte cell lines. J. Clin. Invest.: 76:2003, 1985.
18. Bicknell, R., and Vallee, B. L.: Angiogenin activates endothelial cell phospholipase C. Proc. Natl. Acad. Sci. U.S.A., 85:5961, 1988.
19. Blood, C. H., and Zetter, B. R.: Tumor interactions with the vasculature: angiogenesis and tumor metastasis. Biochemicia et Biophysica Acta, 1032:89, 1990.
20. Bohlen, P., Baird, A., Esch, F., Ling, N., and Gospodarowicz, D.: Isolation and partial molecular characterization of pituitary fibroblast growth factor. Proc. Natl. Acad. Sci. U.S.A., 81:5364, 1984.
21. Bond, M. D., and Vallee, B. L.: Replacement of residues 8–22 of angiogenin with 7–21 of RNASE-A selectively affects protein-synthesis inhibition and angiogenesis. Biochemistry, 29:3341, 1990.
22. Bouck, N.: Tumor Angiogenesis: The Role of Oncogenes and Tumor Suppressor Genes. Cancer Cells, 2:179, 1990.
23. Bouck, N., Stoler, A., and Polverini, P. J.: Coordinate control of anchorage independence, actin cytoskeleton and angiogenesis by human chromosome 1 in hamster-human hybrids. Cancer Res., 46:5101, 1986.
24. Boxberger, H. J., Paweletz, N., Spiess, E., and Kriehuber, R.: An in vitro model study of BSp73 rat tumour cell invasion into endothelial monolayer. Anticancer Research, 9:1777, 1989.
25. Brem, H., and Folkman, J.: Inhibition of tumor angiogenesis mediated by cartilage. J. Exp. Med., 141:427, 1975.
26. Brem, S., Cotran, R., and Folkman, J.: Tumor Angiogenesis: A Quantitative Method for Histologic Grading. J. Natl. Cancer Inst., 48:347, 1972.
27. Brem, S., Gullino, P., and Medina, D.: Angiogenesis: A marker for neoplastic transformation of mammary papillary hyperplasia. Science, 195:880, 1977.
28. Brem, S. S., Jensen, H. M., and Gullino, P. M.: Angiogenesis as a marker of preneoplastic lesions of the human breast. Cancer, 41:239, 1978.
29. Brem, S. S., Zagzag, D., Tsanaclis, A. M. C., Gately, S., Elkouby, M. P., and Brien, S. E.: Inhibition of angiogenesis and tumor growth in the brain. Am. J. Pathol., 137:1121, 1990.
30. Breslow, A.: Thickness, cross-sectional areas and depth of invasion in the prognosis of cutaneous melanoma. Ann. Surg., 172:902, 1970.
31. Brouty-Boye, D., and Zetter, B. R.: Inhibition of cell motility by interferon. Science, 208:516, 1980.
32. Burger, P. C., Chandler, D. B., and Klintworth, G. K.: Corneal neovascularization as studied by scanning electron microscopy. Lab. Invest., 48:169, 1983.
33. Castellot, J., Karnovsky, M., and Spiegelman, B.: Differentiation-dependent stimulation of neovascularization and endothelial cell chemotaxis by 3T3 adipocytes. Proc. Natl. Acad. Sci. U.S.A., 79:5597, 1982.
34. Chen, N. T., Corey, E. J., and Folkman, J.: Potentiation of angiostatic steroids by a synthetic inhibitor of arylsulfatase. Lab. Invest., 59:453, 1988.
35. Chodak, G. W., Haundeschild, C., Gittes, R. F., and Folkman, J.: Angiogenic activity as a marker of neoplastic and preneoplastic lesions of the human bladder. Ann. Surg., 192:762, 1980.
36. Chodak, G. W., Hospelhorn, Y., Judge, S. M., Mayforth, R., Koeppen, H., and Sasse, S. J.: Increased levels of fibroblast growth factor-like activity in urine from patients with bladder or kidney cancer. Cancer Research, 48:2083, 1988.
37. Conn, G., Soderman, D. D., Schaeffer, M. T., Wile, M., Hatcher, V. B., and Thomas, K. A.: Purification of a glycoprotein vascular endothelial mitogen from a rat glioma-derived cell line. Proc. Natl. Acad. Sci. U.S.A., 87:1323, 1990.
38. Connolly, D. T., Heuvelman, D. M., Nelson, R., Olander, J. V., Eppley, B. L., Delfino, J. J., Siegel, N. R., Leimgruber, R. M., and Feder, J.: Tumor vascular permeability factor stimulates endothelial cell growth and angiogenesis. J. Clin. Invest., 84:1470, 1989.
39. Connolly, D. T., Stoddard, B. L, Harakas, N. K., and Feder, J.: Human fibroblast-derived growth factor is a mitogen and chemoattractant for endothelial cells. Biochem. Biophys. Res. Commun., 144:705, 1987.
40. Coomber, B. L., Stewart, P. A., Hayakawa, E. M., Farrell, C. L., and Del Maestro, R. F.: A quantitative assessment of microvessel ultrastructure in C6 astrocytoma spheroids transplanted to brain and to muscle. Journal of Neuropathology and Experimental Neurology, 47:29, 1988.
41. Cordon-Cardo, C., Vlodavsky, I., Haimovitz-Friedman, A., Hicklin, D., and Fuks, Z.: Expression of basic fibroblast growth factor in normal human tissues. Lab. Invest., 63:832, 1990.
42. Coman, D. R., Sheldon, W. F.: The significance of hyperemia around tumor implants. Am. J. Pathol., 22:821, 1946.
43. Crum, R., and Folkman, J.: Anti-angiogenesis by steroids without glucocorticoid or mineralocorticoid activity in the presence of heparin. J. Cell Biol., 99:409a, 1984.
44. Crum, R., Szabo, S., and Folkman, J.: A new class of steroids inhibits angiogenesis in the presence of heparin or a heparin fragment. Science, 230:1375, 1985.
45. D'Amore, P.: Platelet-endothelial interaction and the maintenance of the microvasculature. Microvascular Research, 15:137, 1978.
46. D'Amore, P. A., and Orlidge, A.: Growth factors and pericytes in microangiopathy. Diabetes and Metabolism, 14:495, 1988.
47. D'Amore, P. A.: Modes of FGF release in vivo and in vitro. Cancer and Metastasis Reviews, 9:227, 1990.
48. Davidson, J. M., Klagsbrun, M., Hill, K. E., Buckley, A., Sullivan, R., Brewer, S., and Woodward, S. C.: Accelerated wound repair, cell proliferation, and collagen accumulation are produced by cartilage-derived growth factor. J. Cell Biol., 100:1219, 1985.
49. Day, E. D.: Vascular relationships of tumor and host. Prog. Exp. Tumor Res., 4:57, 1964.
50. Delli Bovi, P., Curatola, A. M., Newman, K. M., Sato, Y., Moscatelli, D., Hewick, R. M., Rifkin, D., and Basilico, C.: Processing, secretion and biological properties of a novel growth factor of the fibroblast growth family with oncogenic potential. Mol. Cell. Biol., 8:2933, 1988.
51. Delli Bovi, P. D., and Basilico, C.: Homology between fibroblast growth factor and a transforming gene from Kaposi's sarcoma. Proc. Natl. Acad. Sci. U.S.A., 84:5660, 1987.
52. Denekamp, J.: Vasculature as a target for tumour therapy. *In* Progress in Applied Microcirculation. Edited by F. Hammersen and O. Hudlicka. Basel, Karger, 1984, pp. 28–38.
53. Derynck, R., Roberts, A. B., Eaton, D. H., Winkler, M. E., and Goeddel, D. V.: Human transforming growth factor-alpha: precursor sequence, gene structure and heterologous expression. *In* Cancer Cells, Growth Factors and Transformation. Edited by Feramisco, J., Ozanne, B., and Stiles, C.: Cold Spring Harbor, New York, Cold Spring Harbor Laboratory, 1985, pp. 79–86.
54. Dethlefsen, S. M., Matsuura, N., and Zetter, B. R.: Tumor growth and angiogenesis in wild type and mast cell deficient mice. FASEB J., 4:A623 (Abstract #2070), 1990.
55. Dickson, C., and Peters, G.: Potential oncogene product related to growth factors. Nature, 326:833, 1987.
56. Dobson, D. E., Kambe, A., Block, E., Dion, T., Lu, H., Castellot, J. J., and Spiegelman, B. M.: 1-Butyryl-Glycerol: A Novel Angiogenesis Factor Secreted by Differentiating Adipocytes. Cell, 61:223, 1990.
57. Drago, J.: The evaluation of inhibitors of angiogenesis, platelet function and polyamine synthesis on metastasis in the NB rat prostatic carcinoma model. J. Urology, 135:337a, 1986.
58. Dugan, J. D. J., Roberts, A. B., Sporn, M. B., and Glaser, B. M.: Transforming growth factor beta (TGF-beta) inhibits neovascularization in vivo. J. Cell Biol., 107:579a, 1988.
59. Dusseau, J. W., Hutchins, P. M., and Malbasa, D. S.: Stimulation of angiogenesis by adenosine on the chick chorioallantoic membrane. Circ. Res., 59:163, 1986.
60. Dvorak, H. F.: Tumors: wounds that do not heal. Similarities between tumor stroma generation and wound healing. N. Engl. J. Med., 315:1650, 1986.
61. Dvorak, H. F., Nagy, J. A., Dvorak, J. T., and Dvorak, A. M.: Identification and characterization of the blood vessels of solid tumors that are leaky to circulating macromolecules. Amer. J. Pathol., 133:95, 1988.
62. Eisenstein, R., Sorgente, N., Soble, L., Miller, A., and Kuettner, K.: The resistance of certain tissues to invasion: penetrability of explanted tissues by vascularized mesenchyme. Am. J. Pathol., 73:765, 1973.
63. Enjolras, O., Riche, M. C., Merland, J. J., and Escande, J. P.: Management of alarming hemangiomas in infancy: A review of 25 cases. Pediatrics, 85:491, 1990.
64. Ferrara, N., Henzel, W. J.: Pituitary follicular cells secrete a novel heparin-binding growth factor specific for vascular endothelial cells. Biochem. Biophys. Res. Commun., 161:851, 1989.
65. Fett, J. W., Strydom, D. J., Lobb, R. F., Alderman, W. M., Bethune, J. L., Riordan, J. F., and Vallee, B. L.: Isolation and characterization of angiogenin, an angiogenic protein from human carcinoma cells. Biochemistry, 24:5480, 1985.
66. Fidler, I. J., Gersten, D. M., and Hart, I. R.: The biology of cancer invasion and metastasis. Advances in Cancer Research, 28:149, 1978.
67. Folkman, J.: The intestine as an organ culture. *In* Carcinoma of the Colon and Antecedent Epithelium. Edited by J. Burdette. Springfield, Illinois, Charles C Thomas, 1970, pp. 113–127.
68. Folkman, J.: Tumor angiogenesis: therapeutic implications. New England Journal of Medicine, 285:1182, 1971.
69. Folkman, J.: Tumor angiogenesis. *In* Cancer Biology, Vol. 3: Biology of Tumors. Edited by F. F. Becker. New York, Plenum Press, 1975, pp. 355–388.

70. Folkman, J.: Angiogenesis. *In* Biology of Endothelial Cells. Edited by Eric A. Jaffe. Boston, Martinus Nijhoff Publishers, 1984, pp. 412–428.
71. Folkman, J.: Angiogenesis and its inhibitors. *In* Important Advances in Oncology 1985. Edited by V. T. DeVita, Jr., S. Hellman, and S. A. Rosenberg. Philadelphia, J. B. Lippincott Co., 1985, pp. 42–62.
72. Folkman, J.: Toward an understanding of angiogenesis: search and discovery. *In* Perspectives of Biology and Medicine. 29(1):10-36, 1985.
73. Folkman, J.: What is the role of angiogenesis in metastasis from cutaneous melanoma? Eur. J. Cancer Clin. Oncol., 23:361, 1987.
74. Folkman, J.: Successful treatment of an angiogenic disease. New England Journal of Medicine, 320:1211, 1989.
75. Folkman, J.: What is the evidence that tumors are angiogenesis dependent? J. Natl. Canc. Inst., 82:4, 1990.
76. Folkman, J., Cole, P., and Zimmerman, S.: Tumor behavior in isolated perfused organs: In vitro growth and metastasis of biopsy material in rabbit thyroid and canine intestinal segment. Annals of Surgery, 164:491, 1966.
77. Folkman, J., and Cotran, R.: Relation of Vascular Proliferation to Tumor Growth. Internat. Rev. Exp. Pathol., 16:207, 1976.
78. Folkman, J., and Haudenschild, C. C.: Angiogenesis in vitro. Nature, 228:551, 1980.
79. Folkman, J., Haudenschild, C. D., and Zetter, B. R.: Long-term culture of capillary endothelial cells. Proc. Natl. Acad. Sci. U.S.A., 76:5217, 1979.
80. Folkman, J., and Ingber, D. E.: Angiostatic steroids: Method of discovery and mechanism of action. Annals of Surgery, 206:374, 1987.
81. Folkman, J., and Ingber, D. E.: Angiostatic steroids. *In* Anti-inflammatory Steroid Action—Basic and Clinical Aspects. Edited by R. P. Schleimer, H. N. Claman, and A. L. Oronsky. New York, Academic Press, 1989, pp. 330–350.
82. Folkman, J., and Klagsbrun, M.: Angiogenic factors. Science, 235:442, 1987.
83. Folkman, J., and Klagsbrun, M.: A family of angiogenic peptides. Nature, 329:671, 1987.
84. Folkman, J., Klagsbrun, M., Sasse, J., Wadzinski, M., Ingber, D., and Vlodavsky, I.: Heparin-binding angiogenic protein—basic fibroblast growth factor—is stored within basement membrane. Am. J. Pathol., 130:393, 1988.
85. Folkman, J., Langer, R., Linhardt, R., Haudenschild, C., and Taylor, S.: Angiogenesis inhibition and tumor regression caused by heparin or a heparin fragment in the presence of cortisone. Science, 221:719, 1983.
86. Folkman, J., Long, D., and Becker, F.: Growth and metastasis of tumor in organ culture. Cancer, 16:453-467, 1963.
87. Folkman, J., Merler, E., Abernathy, C., and Williams, G.: Isolation of a tumor factor responsible for angiogenesis. J. Exp. Med., 133:275, 1971.
88. Folkman, J., Taylor, S., and Spillberg, C.: The role of heparin in angiogenesis. Ciba Symposium, 100:132, 1983.
89. Folkman, J., Watson, K., Ingber, D., and Hanahan, D.: Induction of angiogenesis during the transition from hyperplasia to neoplasia. Nature, 339:58, 1989.
90. Folkman, J., Weisz, P. B., Joullie, M. M., Li, W. W., and Ewing, W. R.: Control of angiogenesis with synthetic heparin substitutes. Science, 243:1490, 1989.
91. Folkman, J., and Gimbrone, M.: Perfusion of the thyroid. *In* Karolinska Symposia on Research Methods in Reproduction Endocrinology. 4th Symposium: Perfusion Techniques (Acta Endocrinology). Edited by E. Dicsfalusy. 1971, pp. 237–248.
92. Folkman, J., and Hochberg, M.: Self-regulation of growth in three dimensions. J. Exp. Med., 138:745, 1973.
93. Form, D. M., and Auerbach, R.: PGE2 and angiogenesis. Proc. Soc. Exp. Biol. Med., 172:214, 1983.
94. Form, D. M., Pratt, B. M., and Madri, J. A.: Endothelial cell proliferation during angiogenesis. In vitro modulation by basement membrane components. Lab. Invest., 55:521, 1986.
95. Fournier, G. A., Lutty, G. A., Watt, S., Fenselau, A., and Patz, A.: A corneal micropocket assay for angiogenesis in the rat eye. Invest. Ophthalmol. Vis. Sci., 21:351, 1981.
96. Fraser, R. A., Ellis, M., and Stalker, A. L.: Experimental angiogenesis in the chorioallantoic membrane. *In* Current Advances in Basic and Clinical Microcirculatory Research. Basel, Karger, 1979, p. 25.
97. Frater-Schroder, M., Muller, G., Birchmeier, W., and Bohlen, P.: Transforming growth factor-beta inhibits endothelial cell proliferation. Biochem. Biophys. Res. Commun., 137:295, 1986.
98. Frater-Schroder, M., Risau, W., Hallmann, R., Gautschi, P., and Bohlen, P.: Tumor necrosis factor type a, a potent inhibitor of endothelial cell growth in vitro, is angiogenic in vivo. PNAS, 84:5277, 1987.
99. Fujimoto, J., Hosoda, S., Fujita, H., and Okada, H.: Inhibition of tumor angiogenesis activity by medroxyprogesterone acetate in gynecologic malignant tumors. Invasion and Metastasis, 9:269, 1989.
100. Gauthier, T., Maftouh, M., and Picard, C.: Rapid enzymatic degradation of I-125 (Tyr10) FGF(1-10) by serum in vitro and involvement in the determination of circulating FGF by RIA. Biochem. Biophys. Res. Commun., 145:775, 1987.
101. Gimbrone, M. A., and Gullino, P. M.: Angiogenic capacity of preneoplastic lesions of the murine mammary gland as a marker of neoplastic transformation. Cancer Res., 36:2611, 1976.
102. Gimbrone, M. A., Jr., Cotran, R., Leapman, S., and Folkman, J.: Tumor growth neovascularization: An experimental model using rabbit cornea. J. Natl. Canc. Inst., 52:413, 1974.
103. Gimbrone, M. A., Jr., Cotran, R. S., and Folkman, J.: Endothelial regeneration and turnover. Studies with human endothelial cell cultures. Ser. Haematol., 6:453, 1973.
104. Gimbrone, M. A., Jr., Leapman, S., Cotran, R. S., and Folkman, J.: Tumor dormancy in vivo by prevention of neovascularization. J. Exp. Med., 136:261, 1972.
105. Glowacki, J., and Mulliken, J.: Mast cells in hemangiomas and vascular malformations. Pediatrics, 70:48, 1982.
106. Goldacre, R., and Sylven, B.: On the access of blood-borne dyes to various tumour regions. Brit. J. Cancer, 16:306, 1962.
107. Gospodarowicz, D.: Localization of fibroblast growth factor and its effect alone and with hydrocortisone on 3T3 cell growth. Nature, 249:123, 1974.
108. Gospodarowicz, D., Abraham, J. A., and Schilling, J.: Isolation and characterization of a vascular endothelial cell mitogen produced by pituitary-derived folliculo stellate cells. Proc. Natl. Acad. Sci. U.S.A., 86:7311, 1989.
109. Gospodarowicz, D., and Cheng, J.: Heparin protects basic and acidic FGF from inactivation. J. Cell Physiology, 128:475, 1986.
110. Gospodarowicz, D., Moran, J., Braun, D., and Birdwell, C. R.: Clonal growth of bovine endothelial cells in culture: fibroblast growth factor as a survival factor. Proc. Natl. Acad. Sci. U.S.A., 73:4120, 1976.
111. Graeber, J. E., Glaser, B. M., Setty, B. N. Y., Jerdan, J. A., Walega, R. W., and Stuart, M. J.: 15-hydroxyeicosatetraenoic acid stimulates migration of human retinal microvessel endothelium in vitro and neovascularization in vivo. Prostaglandins, 39:665, 1990.
112. Grant, D. S., Tashiro, K. I., Sequi-Real, B., Yamada, Y., Martin, G. R., and Kleinman, H. K.: Two different laminin domains mediate the differentiation of human endothelial cells into capillary-like structures in vitro. Cell, 58:933, 1989.
113. Greenwald, R. A., Golub, L. M., Lavietes, B., Ramamurthy, N. S., Gruber, B., Laskin, R. S., and McNamara, T. F.: Tetracyclines inhibit human synovial collagenase in vivo and in vitro. J. Rheumatol., 14:28, 1987.
114. Gross, J., Azizkhan, R. S., Biswas, C., Bruns, R., Hseih, D., and Folkman, J.: Inhibition of tumor growth, vascularization, and collagenolysis in the rabbit cornea by medroxyprogesterone. Proc. Natl. Acad. Sci. U.S.A., 78:1176, 1981.
115. Gross, J. L., Moscatelli, D., and Rifkin, D. B.: Increased capillary endothelial cell protease activity in response to angiogenic stimuli in vitro. Proc. Natl. Acad. Sci. U.S.A., 80:2623, 1983.
116. Gross, J. L., Herblin, W. F., Dusak, B. A., Czerniak, P., Diamond, M., and Dexter, D. L.: Modulation of solid tumor growth in vivo by bFGF. Proc. Am. Assoc. Cancer Res., 31:79 (Abstract #469), 1990.
117. Gullino, P. M.: Extracellular compartments of solid tumors. *In* Cancer. Edited by F. F. Becker, New York, Plenum, 1975, pp. 327–354.
118. Hanahan, D.: Heritable formation of pancreatic beta-cell tumors in transgenic mice expressing recombinant insulin/simian virus 40 oncogenes. Nature, 315:115, 1985.
119. Haudenschild, C. C., Zahniser, D., Folkman, J., and Klagsbrun, M.: Human endothelial cells in culture. Lack of response to serum growth factors. Exp. Cell Res., 98:175, 1976.
120. Heimark, R. L., Twardzik, D. R., and Schwartz, S. M.: Inhibition of endothelial regeneration by type-beta transforming growth factor from platelets. Science, 233:1078, 1986.
121. Herlyn, M., Clark, W. H., Rodeck, U., Mancianti, M. L., Jambrosic, J., and Koprowski, H.: Biology of tumor progression in human melanocytes. Lab. Invest., 56:461, 1987.
122. Herman, I. M., and D'Amore, P. A.: Microvascular pericytes contain muscle and nonmuscle actin. J. Cell Biol., 101:43, 1985.
123. Hertig, A.: Angiogenesis in the early human chorio and in the primary placenta of the Macaque monkey. Contributions to Embryology, 25:37, 1935.
124. Hicks, R. M, and Chowaniec, J.: Experimental induction, histology, and ultrastructure of hyperplasia and neoplasia of the urinary bladder epithelium. Int. Rev. Exper. Pathol., 18:199, 1978.
125. Hockel, M., Jung, W., Vaupel, P., Rabes, H., Khaledpour, C., and Wissler, J. H.: Purified monocyte-derived angiogenic substance (angiotropin) induces controlled angiogenesis associated with regulated tissue proliferation in rabbit skin. J. Clin. Invest., 82:1075, 1988.
126. Hockel, M., Sasse, J., and Wissler, J. H.: Purified monocyte-derived angiogenic substance (angiotropin) stimulates migration, phenotypic changes and "tube formation" but not proliferation of capillary endothelial cells in vitro. J. Cell Physiol., 133:1, 1987.
126A. Hori, A., Sasada, R., Matsutani, E., Naito, K., Sakura, Y., Fujita, T., and Kozai, Y.: Suppression of solid tumor growth by immunoneutralizing monoclonal antibody against human basic fibroblast growth factor. Cancer Research, 51:6180, 1991.
127. Hunt, T., Knighton, D., Thakral, K., Goodson, W., and Andrews, W.: Studies on inflammation and wound-healing angiogenesis and collagen synthesis stimulated in vivo by resident and activated wound macrophages. Surgery, 96:48, 1984.
128. Iberg, N., Rogel, S., Fanning, P., and Klagsbrun, M.: Purification of 18- and 22 kDa forms of basic fibroblast growth factor from rat cells transformed by the *ras* oncogene. J. Biol. Chem., 264:19951, 1989.
129. Ide, A. G., Baker, N. H., and Warren, S. L.: Vascularization of the Brown-Pearce rabbit epithelioma transplant as seen in the transparent ear chamber. Am. J. Roentgenol., 42:881, 1939.
130. Ignotz, R., and Massague, J.: Transforming growth factor-beta stimulates the expression of fibronectin and collagen and their incorporation into the extracellular matrix. J. Biol. Chem., 261:4337, 1986.
131. Ingber, D., Fujita, T., Kishimoto, S., Sudo, K., Kanamaru, T., Brem, H., and Folkman, J.: Synthetic analogues of fumagillin that inhibit angiogenesis and suppress tumor growth. Nature, 348:555, 1990.
132. Ingber, D. E., and Folkman, J.: Inhibition of angiogenesis through modulation of collagen metabolism. Lab. Invest., 59:44, 1988.
133. Ingber, D. E., and Folkman, J.: Mechanochemical switching between growth and differentiation during fibroblast growth factor-stimulated angiogenesis in vitro: role of extracellular matrix. J. Cell Biol., 109:317, 1989.
134. Ingber, D. E., Madri, J. A., and Folkman, J.: A possible mechanism for inhibition of angiogenesis by angiostatic steroids: induction of capillary basement membrane dissolution. Endocrinology, 119:1768, 1986.
135. Ingber, D. E., Madri, J. A., and Folkman, J: Endothelial growth factors and extracellular matrix regulate DNA synthesis through modulation of cell and nuclear expansion. In Vitro Cell Dev. Biol., 23:387, 1987.
136. Inoue, K., Korenaga, H., Tanaka, N., Sakamoto, N., and Kadoya, S.: The sulfated polysaccharide-peptidoglycan complex potently inhibits embryonic angiogenesis and tumor growth in the presence of cortisone acetate. Carbohydrate Research, 181:135, 1988.
137. Ishikawa, F., Miyazono, K., Hellman, U., Wernstedt, C., Hagiwara, K., Usuki, K., Takaku, F., and Heldin, C. H.: Identification of angiogenic activity and the cloning and expression of platelet-derived endothelial cell growth factor. Nature, 338:557, 1989.
138. Jaffe, E. A., Nachman, R. L., Becker, C. G., and Minick, C. R.: Culture of human endothelial cells derived from umbilical veins: identification by morphologic and immunologic criteria. J. Clin. Invest., 52:2745, 1972.
139. Jain, R. K.: Determinants of Tumor Blood Flow. Cancer Research, 48:2641, 1988.
140. Jain, R. K.: Delivery of novel therapeutic agents in tumors: Physiological barriers and strategies. J. Natl. Cancer Inst., 81:570, 1989.
141. Jain, R. K., and Baxter, L. T.: Mechanisms of heterogenous distribution of monoclonal antibodies and other macromolecules in tumors: Significance of elevated interstitial pressure. Cancer Res., 48:7022, 1988.

142. Jakobsson, A., Sorbo, J., and Norrby, K.: Protamine and mast-cell-mediated angiogenesis in the rat. J. Exp. Pathol., 71:209, 1990.

143. Jensen, H. M.: Angiogenesis induced by normal human breast tissue. In Current Communications in Molecular Biology (Angiogenesis—Mechanisms and Pathobiology). Edited by D. B. Rifkin and M. Klagsbrun. Cold Spring Harbor, N.Y., Cold Spring Harbor Press, 1987, pp. 199–839.

144. Jensen, H. M., Chen, I., DeVault, M. R., and Lewis, A. E.: Angiogenesis induced by "normal" human breast tissue: A probable marker for precancer. Science, 218:293, 1982.

145. Kalebic, T., Garbisa, S., Glaser, B., and Liotta, L.: Basement membrane collagen degradation by migrating endothelial cells. Science, 221:281, 1983.

145A.Kandel, J., Bossy-Wetzel, E., Radvanyi, F., Klagsbrun, M., Folkman, J., and Hanahan, D.: Neovascularization is associated with a switch to the export of bFGF in the multistep development of fibrosarcoma. Cell, 66:1095, 1991.

146. Kawasaki, S, Mori, M., and Awai, M.: Capillary growth of rat aortic segments cultured in collagen gel without serum. Acta Pathologica Japonica, 39:712, 1989.

147. Kerbel, R. S., Waghorne, C., Korczak, B, Lagarde, A., and Breitman, M. L.: Clonal dominance of primary tumours by metastatic cells: genetic analysis and biological implications. Cancer. Surv., 7:597, 1988.

148. Keski-Oja, J., Lyons, R. M., and Moses, H. L.: Inactive secreted form(s) of transforming growth factor-beta: activation by proteolysis. J. Cell. Biochem., 11a (Suppl.):60, 1987.

149. Kessler, D., Langer, R., Pless, N., and Folkman, J.: Mast cells and tumor angiogenesis. International Journal of Cancer, 18:703, 1976.

150. Klagsbrun, M.: The affinity of fibroblast growth factors (FGFs) for heparan; FGF-heparan sulfate interactions in cells and extracellular matrix. Current Opinion in Cell Biology, 2:857, 1990.

151. Klagsbrun, M., and D'Amore, P. A.: Regulators of Angiogenesis. Annu. Rev. Physiol., 53:217, 1991.

152. Klagsbrun, M., Knighton, D., and Folkman, J.: Tumor angiogenesis activity in cells grown in tissue culture. Cancer Res., 36:110, 1976.

153. Klagsbrun, M., Sasse, J., Sullivan, R., and Smith, J. A.: Human tumor cells synthesize an endothelial cell growth factor that is structurally related to basic fibroblast growth factor. Proc. Natl. Acad. Sci. U.S.A., 83:2448, 1986.

154. Knighton, D., Ausprunk, D., Tapper, D., and Folkman, J.: Avascular and vascular phases of tumour growth in the chick embryo. Brit. J. Canc., 35:347, 1977.

155. Knighton, D., Hunt, T., Scheuenstuhl, H., Halliday, B. J., Werb, Z., and Banda, M. J.: Oxygen tension regulates the expression of angiogenesis factor by macrophages. Science, 221:1283, 1983.

156. Koch, A. E., Cho, M., Burrows, S., Leibovich, S. J., and Polverini, P. J.: Inhibition of production of macrophage-derived angiogenic activity by the anti-rheumatic agents gold sodium thiomalate and auranofin. Biochem. Biophys. Res. Commun., 154:205, 1988.

157. Koch, A. E., Polverini, P. J., and Leibovich, S. J.: Induction of neovascularization by activated human monocytes. J. Leukoc. Biol., 39:233, 1986.

158. Kuettner, K., and Pauli, B: Vascularity of cartilage. In Cartilage: Structure, Function and Biochemistry. Edited by B. Hall. New York, Academic Press, 1983, pp. 281–312.

159. Kuettner, K., Soble, L., Croxen, R., Marczynska, B., Hiti, J., and Harper, E.: Tumor cell collagenase and its inhibition by a cartilage-derived inhibitor. Science, 196:653, 1977.

160. Kull, F. C., Brent, D. A., Parikh, I., and Cuatrecasas, P.: Chemical identification of a tumor-derived angiogenic factor. Science, 236:843, 1987.

161. Kurachi, K., Davie, E. W., Strydom, D. J., Riordan, J. F., and Vallee, B. L.: Sequence of the cDNA and gene for angiogenin, a human angiogenesis factor. Biochemistry, 24:5494, 1985.

162. Lacey, M., Albert, S., and Hanahan, D.: Bovine papilloma virus genome elicits skin tumours in transgenic mice. Nature, 322:609, 1986.

163. Langer, R., Brem, H., Falterman, K., Klein, M., and Folkman, J.: Isolation of a cartilage factor that inhibits tumor neovascularization. Science, 193:70, 1976.

164. Langer, R., and Folkman, J.: Polymers for the sustained release of proteins and other macromolecules. Nature, 263:797, 1976.

165. Langer, R. S., Conn, H., Vacanti, J., Haudenschild, C., and Folkman, J.: Control of tumor growth in animals by infusion of an angiogenesis inhibitor. Proc. Natl. Acad. Sci. U.S.A., 77:4331, 1980.

166. Lawrence, D. A., Pircher, R., Kryceve-Martinerie, C, and Jullien, P.: Normal embryo fibroblasts release transforming growth factors in a latent form. J. Cell Physiol., 121:184, 1984.

167. Lemmon, S. K., and R. Bradshaw: Purification and partial characterization of bovine pituitary fibroblast growth factor. J. Cell. Biochem., 21:195, 1983.

168. Leung, D. W., Cachianes, G., Kuang, W. J., Goeddel, D. V., and Ferrara, N.: Vascular endothelial growth factor is a secreted angiogenic mitogen. Science, 246:1306, 1989.

169. Levy, A. P., Tamargo, R., Brem, H., and Nathans, D.: An endothelial cell growth factor from the mouse neuroblastoma cell line. Growth Factors, 2:9, 1989.

170. Liebovich, S. J., Polverini, P. J., Shepard, H. M., Wiseman, D. M., and Nusseir, S. V. N.: Macrophage-induced angiogenesis is mediated by tumour necrosis factor-a. Nature, 329:630, 1987.

171. Lien, W., and Ackerman, N.: The blood supply of experimental liver metastases. II. A microcirculatory study of normal and tumor vessels of the liver with the use of perfused silicone rubber. Surgery, 68:334, 1970.

172. Lindgren, V., Sippola-Thiele, M., Skowronski, J., Wetzel, E., Howley, P. M., and Hanahan, D.: Specific chromosomal abnormalities characterize fibrosarcomas of bovine virus papilloma type 1 transgenic mice. Proc. Natl. Acad. Sci. U.S.A., 86:5025, 1989.

173. Liotta, L., Saidel, G., and Kleinerman, J.: The significance of hematogenous tumor cell clumps in the metastatic process. Cancer Research, 36:889, 1976.

174. Lobb, R. R., Key, M. E., Alderman, E. M., and Fett, J. W.: Partial purification and characterization of a vascular permeability factor secreted by a human colon adenocarcinoma cell line. Int. J. Cancer, 36:473, 1985.

175. Long, D. M.: Capillary ultrastructure in human metastatic brain tumors. Neurosurgery, 51:53, 1979.

176. Maciag, T., Kadish, J., Wilkins, L., Stemerman, M. B., and Weinstein, R.: Organization behavior of human umbilical vein endothelial cells. J. Cell Biol., 94:511, 1982.

177. Maciag, T., Mehlman, T., Friesel, R., and Schreiber, A. B.: Heparin binds endothelial cell growth factor, the principal cell mitogen in bovine brain. Science, 225:932, 1984.

178. Madarnas, P., Benrezzak, O., and Nigam, V.: Prophylactic antiangiogenic tumor treatment. Anticancer Research, 9:897, 1989.

179. Madri, J., and Williams, S. K.: Capillary endothelial cell cultures: phenotypic modulation by matrix components. J. Cell Biol., 97:153, 1983.

180. Madtes, D. K., Raines, E. W., Sakariassen, K. S., Assoian, R. K., Sporn, M. B., Bell, G. I., and Ross, R.: Induction of transforming growth factor-alpha in activated human alveolar macrophages. Cell, 53:285, 1988.

181. Maeda, H., and Matsumura, Y.: Tumoritropic and lymphotropic principles of macromolecular drugs. Critical Reviews in Therapeutic Drug Carrier Systems, 6:193, 1989.

182. Maione, T. E., Gray, G. S., Petro, J., Hunt, A. J., Donner, A. L., Bauer, S. I., Carson, H. F., and Sharpe, R. J.: Inhibition of angiogenesis by recombinant human platelet factor-4 and related peptides. Science, 247:77, 1990.

183. Maragoudakis, M. E., Missirlis, E., Sarmonika, M., Panoutsacopoulou, M., and Karakiulakis, G.: Basement membrane biosynthesis as a target to tumor therapy. Journal of Pharmacology and Experimental Therapeutics, 252:753, 1990.

184. Maragoudakis, M. E., Panoutsacopoulou, M., and Sarmonika, M.: Rate of basement membrane biosynthesis as an index to angiogenesis. Tissue Cell, 20:531, 1988.

185. Maragoudakis, M. E., Sarmonika, M., and Panoutsacopoulou, M.: Inhibition of basement membrane synthesis prevents angiogenesis. J. Pharmacol. Exp. Ther., 244:729, 1988.

186. Maragoudakis, M. E., Sarmonika, M., and Panoutsacopoulou, M.: Antiangiogenic action of heparin plus cortisone is associated with decreased collagenous protein synthesis in the CAM system. J. Pharmacol. Exp. Ther., 251:679, 1989.

187. Marquardt, H., Hunkapiller, M. W., Hood, L. E., and Todaro, G. J.: Rat transforming growth factor type I: structure and relationship to epidermal growth factor. Science, 223:1079, 1984.

188. Matsubara, T., Saura, R., Hirohata, K., and Ziff, M.: Inhibition of human endothelial cell proliferation in vitro and neovascularization in vivo by D-Penicillamine. J. Clin. Invest., 83:158, 1989.

189. Matsubara, T., and Ziff, M.: Inhibition of human endothelial cell proliferation by gold compounds. J. Clin. Invest., 79:1440, 1987.

190. McGovern, V. J., and Murad, T. M: Pathology of Melanoma: An Overview. In Cutaneous Melanoma Clinical Management and Treatment Results Worldwide. Philadelphia, J. B. Lippincott, 1985, pp. 29-53.

191. Megyesi, J. F., Rosenthal, R. A., and Folkman, J.: Conditioned medium from a glioblastoma line contains a protein that reacts with an antibody to vascular permeability factor. J. Cell Biol., 111:227a (Abst. #1267), 1990.

192. Missirlis, E., Karakiulakis, G., and Maragoudakis, M. E.: Antitumor effect of GPA1734 in rat Walker 256 carcinoma. Invest. New Drugs, 8:145, 1990.

193. Miyazono, K., Okabe, T., Urabe, A., Takahu, F., and Heldin, C. H.: Purification and properties of an endothelial cell growth factor from human platelets. J. Biol. Chem., 262:4098, 1987.

194. Montesano, R., Orci, L., and Vassali, P.: In vitro rapid organization of endothelial cells into capillary-like networks is promoted by collagen matrices. J. Cell Biol., 97:1648, 1983.

195. Montesano, R., Vassali, J. D., Baird, A., Guillemin, R., and Orci, L.: Basic fibroblast growth factor induces angiogenesis in vitro. Proc. Natl. Acad. Sci. U.S.A., 83:7297, 1986.

196. Moore, J. W., III, and Sholley, M. M.: Comparison of the neovascular effects of stimulated macrophages and neutrophils in autologous rabbit corneas. Am. J. Pathol., 120:87, 1985.

197. Moscatelli, D., Gross, J., and Rifkin, D.: Angiogenic factors stimulate plasminogen activator and collagenase production by capillary endothelial cells. J. Cell Biol., 91:201a, 1981.

198. Moscatelli, D., Silverstein, J., Manejias, R., and Rifkin, D. B.: M 25,000 heparin binding protein from guinea pig brain is a high molecular weight form of basic fibroblast growth factor. Proc. Natl. Acad. Sci. U.S.A., 84:5778, 1987.

199. Moses, M. A., Sudhalter, J., and Langer, R.: Identification of an inhibitor of neovascularization from cartilage. Science, 248:1408, 1990.

200. Motro, B., Itin, A., Sachs, L., and Keshet, E: Pattern of interleukin 6 gene expression in vivo suggests a role for this cytokine in angiogenesis. Proc. Natl. Acad. Sci. U.S.A., 87:3092, 1990.

201. Muesch, A., Hartmann, E., Rohde, K., and Rapoport, T. A.: A novel pathway for secretory proteins? Trends Biochem. Sci., 15:86, 1990.

202. Muller, G., Behrens, J., Nussbaumer, U., Bohlen, P., and Birchmeier, W.: Inhibitory action of transforming growth factor-beta on endothelial cells. Proc. Natl. Acad. Sci. U.S.A., 84:5600, 1987.

203. Muthukkarauppan, V. R., and Auerbach, R.: Angiogenesis in the mouse cornea. Science, 205:1416, 1979.

204. Nagy, J. A., Brown, L. F., Senger, D. R., Lanir, N., Van de Water, L., Dvorak, A. M., and Dvorak, H. F.: Pathogenesis of tumor stroma generation: a critical role for leaky blood vessels and fibrin deposition. Biochim. Biophys. Acta, 948:305, 1989.

205. Nawroth, P., Handley, D., Matsueda, G., DeWaal, R., Gerlach, H., Blohm, D., and Stern, D.: Tumor necrosis factor/cachectin-induced intravascular fibrin formation in meth A fibrosarcomas. J. Exp. Med., 168:637, 1988.

206. Netland, P., and Zetter, B.: Organ-specific adhesion of metastatic tumor cells in vitro. Science, 224:113, 1984.

207. Nicolson, G.: Cancer metastasis. Scientific American, 240:66, 1979.

208. Nicolson, G. L.: Organ specificity of tumor metastasis: role of preferential adhesion, invasion and growth of malignant cells at specific secondary sites. Cancer and Metastasis Reviews, 7:143, 1988.

209. Nicosia, R., Tchao, R., and Leighton, J.: Angiogenesis-dependent tumor spread in reinforced fibrin clot culture. Cancer Res., 43:2159, 1983.

210. Nicosia, R. F., and Ottinett, A.: Growth of microvessels in serum-free matrix culture of rat aorta—a quantitative assay of angiogenesis in vitro. Lab. Invest., 63:115, 1990.

211. Nicosia, R. F., Tchao, R., and Leighton, J.: Histiotypic angiogenesis in vitro: light microscopic, ultrastructural and radiographic studies. In Vitro, 18:538, 1982.

212. Odedra, R., and Weiss, J. B.: A synergistic effect on microvessel cell proliferation between basic fibroblast growth factor (bFGF) and endothelial cell stimulating angiogenesis factor (ESAF). Biochem. Biophys. Res. Commun., 143:947, 1987.

213. Oikawa, T., Hirotani, K., Ogasawara, H., Katayama, T., Nakamura, O., Iwaguchi, T., and Hiragun, A.: Inhibition of angiogenesis by Vitamin D3 Analogues. Eur. J. Pharm., 178:247, 1990.

214. Oikawa, T, Hirotani, K., Shimamura, M., Ashino-Fuse, H., and Iwaguchi, T.: Powerful

antiangiogenic activity of herbimycin A (Named angiostatic antibiotic). Journal of Antibiotics, 42:1202, 1989.
215. Old, L. J.: Tumor necrosis factor (TNF). Science, 230:630, 1985.
216. Orchard, P., Smith, C., Woods, W., Dehner, L. P., Day, D. L., and Shapiro, R. S.: Treatment of hemangioendothiomas with alpha interferon. Lancet, 2:565, 1989.
217. Orlidge, A., and D'Amore, P. A.: Inhibition of capillary endothelial cell growth by pericytes and smooth muscle cells. J. Cell Biol., 105:1455, 1987.
218. Perles, T., Ingber, D. E., and Folkman, J.: Inhibition of Capillary Endothelial Cell Outgrowth: The role of complex formation between angiostatic steroids and beta-cyclodextrin tetradecasulfate. J. Cell Biol., 109:311a, 1989.
219. Pober, J. S., LaPierre, L. A., Stophen, A. H., Brock, T. A., Springer, T. A., Fiers, W., Bevilacqua, M. P., Mendrick, D. L., and Gimbrone, M. A. J.: Activation of cultured human endothelial cells by recombinant lymphotoxin: comparison with tumor necrosis factor and interleukin 1 species. J. Immunol., 138:3319, 1987.
220. Podor, T. J., Jirik, F. R., Loskutoff, D. J., Carson, D. A., and Lotz, M.: Human endothelial cells produce IL-6. Lack of responses to exogenous IL-6. Ann. N.Y. Acad. Sci., 557:374, 1989.
221. Polverini, P., Cotran, R., Gimbrone, M., Jr., and Unanue, E.: Activated macrophages induce vascular proliferation. Nature, 269:804, 1977.
222. Polverini, P. J., and Leibovich, J. S.: Induction of neovascularization in vivo and endothelial proliferation in vitro by tumor-associated macrophages. Lab. Invest., 51:635, 1984.
223. Presta, M., Moscatelli, D., Silverstein, J. J., and Rifkin, D. B.: Purification from a human hepatoma cell line of a basic FGF-like molecule that stimulates capillary endothelial cell plasminogen activator production, DNA synthesis and migration. Mol. Cell. Biology, 6:4060, 1986.
224. Proia, A. D., Chandler, M. B., Haynes, W. L., Smith, C. S., Suvarnamani, C., Erkel, F., and Klintworth, G. K.: Quantitation of corneal neovascularization using computerized image analysis. Lab. Invest., 58:473, 1988.
225. Rappolee, D. A., Mark, D., Banda, M. J., and Werb, Z.: Wound macrophages express TGF-alpha and other growth factors in vivo: analysis by mRNA phenotyping. Science, 241:708, 1988.
226. Rastinejad, F., Polverini, P. F., and Bouck, N. P.: Regulation of the activity of a new inhibitor of angiogenesis by a cancer suppressor gene. Cell, 56:345, 1989.
227. Ribatti, D., Vacca, A., Bertossi, M., De-Benedictis, G., Roncali, L., and Dammacco, F.: Angiogenesis induced by B-cell non-Hodgkins lymphomas—Lack of correlation with tumor malignancy and immunological phenotype. Anticancer Research, 10:401, 1990.
228. Riordan, J. F., and Vallee, B. L.: Human angiogenin, an organogenic protein. Br. J. Cancer, 57:587, 1988.
229. Roberts, A. B., Anzano, M. A., Lamb, L. C., Smith, J. M., and Sporn, M. B.: New class of transforming growth factors potentiated by epidermal growth factor: isolation from non-neoplastic tissues. Proc. Natl. Acad. Sci. U.S.A., 78:5339, 1981.
230. Roberts, A. B., Sporn, M. B., Assoian, R. K., Smith, J. M., Roche, N. S., Wakefield, L. M., Heine, U. I., Liotta, L. A., Falanga, V., Kehrl, J. H., and Fauci, A. S.: Transforming growth factor type-beta: rapid induction of fibrosis and angiogenesis in vivo and stimulation of collagen formation in vitro. Proc. Natl. Acad. Sci. U.S.A., 83:4167, 1986.
231. Rosengart, T. K., Johnson, W. V., Friesel, R., Clark, R., and Maciag, T.: Heparin protects heparin-binding growth factor-I from proteolytic inactivation in vitro. Biochem. Biophys. Res. Commun., 152:432, 1988.
232. Rosenthal, R. A., Megyesi, J. F., Henzel, W. J., Ferrara, N., and Folkman, J.: Conditioned medium from mouse sarcoma 180 cells contains vascular endothelial growth factor. FASEB J., 4:A1992 (Abstract #1737), 1990.
233. Ryan, T. J., and Stockley, A. T.: Mechanical versus biochemical factors in angiogenesis. Microvasc. Res., 20:258, 1980.
234. Rybak, S. M., and Vallee, B. L.: Base cleavage specificity of angiogenin with Saccharomyces cerevisiae and Escherichia coli 5S RNAs. Biochemistry, 27:2288, 1988.
235. Saiki, I., Murata, J., Nakajima, M., Tokura, S., and Azuma, I.: Inhibition by sulfated chitin derivatives of invasion through extracellular matrix and enzymatic degradation by metastatic melanoma cells. Cancer Res., 50:3631, 1990.
236. Sakamoto, H., Mori, M., Taira, M., Yoshida, T., Matsukawa, S., Shimizu, K., Sekiguchi, M., Terada, M., and Sugimura, T.: Transforming gene from human stomach cancers and a non-cancerous portion of stomach mucosa. Proc. Natl. Acad. Sci. U.S.A., 83:3997, 1986.
237. Sakamoto, N., Tanaka, N., Tohgo, A., and Ogawa, H.: Heparin plus cortisone acetate inhibit tumor growth by blocking endothelial cell proliferation. Cancer Journal, 1:55, 1986.
238. Sakamoto, N., and Tanaka, N. G.: Effect of angiostatic steroid with or without glucocorticoid activity on metastasis. Invasion and Metastasis, 7:208, 1987.
239. Sakamoto, N., and Tanaka, N. G.: Mechanism of synergistic effect of heparin and cortisone against angiogenesis and tumor growth. Cancer Journal, 2:9, 1988.
240. Saksela, O., Moscatelli, D., Sommer, A., and Rifkin, D. B.: Endothelial cell-derived heparin sulfate binds basic fibroblast growth factor and protects it from proteolytic degradation. J. Cell Biol., 107:743, 1988.
241. Saksela, O., and Rifkin, D. B.: Release of basic fibroblast growth factor-heparan sulfate complexes from endothelial cells by plasminogen activator-mediated proteolytic activity. J. Cell Biol., 110:767, 1990.
242. Schlingemann, R. O., Rietveld, F. J. R., de Waal, R. M. W., Ferrone, S., and Ruiter, D. J.: Expression of the high molecular weight melanoma-associated antigen by pericytes during angiogenesis in tumors and in healing wounds. Amer. J. Pathol., 136:1393, 1990.
243. Schreiber, A. B., Winkler, M. E., and Derynck, R.: Transforming growth factor-alpha: a more potent angiogenic mediator than epidermal growth factor. Science, 232:1250, 1986.
244. Schulze-Osthoff, K., Risau, W., Vollmer, E., and Sorg, C.: In Situ Detection of Basic Fibroblast Growth Factor by Highly Specific Antibodies. AJP, 137:85, 1990.
245. Schweigerer, L., Neufeld, G., Friedman, J., Abraham, J. A., Fiddes, J. A., and Gospodarowicz, D.: Capillary endothelial cells express basic fibroblast growth factor. Nature, 325:257, 1987.
246. Senger, D. R., Connolly, D. T., Van De Water, L., Feder, J., and Dvorak, H. F.: Purification and NH2-terminal amino acid sequence of guinea pig tumor-secreted vascular permeability factor. Cancer Research, 50:1774, 1990.
247. Senger, D. R., Galli, S. J., Dvorak, A. M., Perruzzi, C. A., and Harvey, V. S.: Tumor cells secrete a vascular permeability factor that promotes accumulation of ascites fluid. Science, 219:983, 1983.
248. Shapiro, R., Riordan, J. F., and Vallee, B. L.: Characteristic ribonucleolytic activity of human angiogenin. Biochemistry, 25:3527, 1986.
249. Shapiro, R., Strydom, D. J., Olson, K. A., and Vallee, B. L.: Isolation of angiogenin from normal human plasma. Biochemistry, 26:5141, 1987.
250. Shapiro, R., and Vallee, B. L.: Human placental ribonuclease inhibitor abolishes both angiogenic and ribonucleolytic activities of angiogenin. Proc. Natl. Acad. Sci. U.S.A., 84:2238, 1987.
251. Sharpe, R. J., Byers, H. R., Scott, C. F., Bauer, S. I., and Maione, T. E.: Growth inhibition of murine melanoma and human colon carcinoma by recombinant human platelet factor 4. J. Natl. Cancer. Inst., 82:848, 1990.
252. Sherry, B., and Cerami, A.: Cachectin/tumor necrosis factor exerts endocrine, paracrine, and autocrine control of inflammatory responses. J. Cell Biol., 107:1269, 1988.
253. Shing, Y., Folkman, J., Haudenschild, C., Lund, D., Crum, R., and Klagsbrun, M.: Angiogenesis is stimulated by a tumor-derived endothelial cell growth factor. J. Cell. Biochem., 29:275, 1985.
254. Shing, Y., Folkman, J., Sullivan, R., Butterfield, C., Murray, J., and Klagsbrun, M.: Heparin-affinity: purification of a tumor-derived capillary endothelial cell growth factor. Science, 223:1296, 1984.
255. Sidky, Y. A., and Borden, E. C.: Inhibition of angiogenesis by interferons: Effects on tumor- and lymphocyte-induced vascular responses. Cancer Research, 47:5155, 1987.
256. Sillman, F., Boyce, J., and Fruchter, R.: The significance of atypical vessels and neovascularization in cervical neoplasia. American Journal of Pathology, 139:154, 1981.
257. Skinner, S. A., Tutton, P. J. M., and O'Brien, P. E.: Microvascular architecture of experimental colon tumors in the rat. Cancer Res., 50:2411, 1990.
258. Smith, S. S., and Basu, P. K.: Mast cells in corneal immune reaction. Can. J. Ophthalmol., 5:175, 1970.
259. Smolle, J., Soyer, H. P., Hofmann-Wellenhof, R, Smolle-Juettner, F. M., and Kerl, H.: Vascular architecture of melanocytic skin tumors. Path. Res. Pract., 185:740, 1989.
260. Splawinski, J., Michna, M., Palczak, R., Konturek, S., and Splawinski, B.: Angiogenesis: quantitative assessment by the chick chorioallantoic membrane assay. Methods and Findings in Experimental Clinical Pharmacology, 10:221, 1988.
261. Sporn, M. B., Roberts, A. B., Wakefield, L. M., and deCrombrugghe, B.: Some recent advances in the chemistry and biology of transforming growth factor-beta. J. Cell Biol., 105:1039, 1987.
262. Srivastava, A., Laidler, P., Davies, R., and Horgan, K.: The prognostic significance of tumor vascularity in intermediate-thickness (0.76–4.0 mm thick) skin melanoma. Amer. Jour. Pathol., 133:419, 1988.
263. Srivastava, A., Laidler, P., Hughes, L. E., Woodcock, J., and Shedden, E. J.: Neovascularization in human cutaneous melanoma: A quantitative morphological and Doppler ultrasound study. Eur. J. Cancer Clin. Oncol., 22:1205, 1986.
264. Strydom, D. J., Fett, J. W., Lobb, R. R., Alderman, E. M., Bethune, J. L., Riordan, J. F., and Vallee, B. L.: Amino acid sequence of human-derived angiogenin. Biochemistry, 24:5486, 1985.
265. Sutherland, R. M.: Cell and environmental interactions in tumor microregions: the multicell spheroid model. Science, 240:177, 1988.
266. Sutherland, R. M., McCredie, J. A., and Inch, W. R.: Growth of multicell spheroids in tissue culture as a model of nodular carcinomas. J. Natl. Cancer Inst., 46:113, 1971.
267. Takigawa, M., Pan, H. O., Enomoto, M., Kinoshita, A., Nishida, Y., Suzuki, F., and Tajima, K.: A clonal human chondrosarcoma cell line produces an anti-angiogenic antitumor factor. Anticancer Research, 10:311, 1990.
267A.Tamargo, R., Bok, R. A., Brem, H.: Angiogenesis inhibition by minocycline. Cancer Research, 51:672, 1991.
268. Tanaka, N. G., Sakamoto, N., Tohgo, A., Nishiyama, Y., and Ogawa, H.: Inhibitory effects of anti-angiogenic agents on neovascularization and growth of the chorioallantoic membrane (CAM). The possibility of a new CAM assay for angiogenesis inhibition. Experimental Pathology, 30:143, 1986.
269. Tannock, I.: Population kinetics of carcinoma cells, capillary endothelial cells, and fibroblasts in a transplanted mouse mammary tumor. Cancer Res., 30:2470, 1970.
270. Taylor, S., and Folkman, J.: Protamine is an inhibitor of angiogenesis. Nature, 297:307, 1982.
271. Thomas, K., and Gimemez-Gallego, G.: Fibroblast growth factors: broad spectrum mitogens with potent angiogenic activity. Trends Biochem. Sci., 11:81, 1986.
272. Thomas, K. A.: Fibroblast growth factors. FASEB J., 1:4343, 1987.
273. Thomas, K. A., Riley, M. C., Lemmon, S. K., Baglan, N. C., and Bradshaw, R. A.: Brain fibroblast growth factor. J. Biol. Chem., 255:5517, 1980.
274. Thomas, K. A., Rios-Candelore, M., and Fitzpatrick, S.: Purification and characterization of acidic fibroblast growth factor from bovine brain. Proc. Natl. Acad. of Sci. U.S.A., 81:357, 1984.
275. Thompson, J. A., Anderson, K. D., DiPietro, J. M., Zweibel, J. A., Zametta, M., and Anderson, W. F.: Site-directed neovessel formation in vivo. Science, 241:1349, 1988.
276. Thompson, W. D., Campbell, R., and Evans, T.: Fibrin degradation response in the chick chorioallantoic membrane. J. Pathol. 145:27, 1985.
277. Thompson, W. D., Shiach, K. J., Fraser, R. A., McIntosh, L. C., and Simpson, J. G.: Tumours acquire their vasculature by vessel incorporation, not vessel ingrowth. Journal of Pathology, 151:323, 1987.
278. Thornton, S., Mueller, S., and Levine, E.: Human endothelial cells: Use of heparin in cloning and long-term serial cultivation. Science, 222:623, 1983.
279. Tischer, E., Gospodarowicz, D., Mitchell, R., Silva, M., Schilling, J., Lau, K., Crips, T., Fiddes, J. C., and Abraham, J. A.: Vascular endothelial growth factor: a new member of the platelet-derived growth factor gene family. Biochem. Biophys. Res. Commun., 165:1198, 1989.
280. Todaro, G. J., Fryling, C., and DeLarco, J. E.: Transforming growth factors produced by certain human tumor cells: polypeptides that interact with epidermal growth factor receptors. Proc. Natl. Acad. Sci. U.S.A., 77:5258, 1980.
281. Tucker, R. F., Shipley, G. D., Moses, H. L., and Holley, R. W.: Growth inhibitor from BSC-1 cells closely related to platelet type beta transforming growth factor. Science, 226:705, 1984.
282. Verhoeven, D., and Buyssens, N.: Desmin-positive stellate cells associated with angiogenesis in a tumour and non-tumour system. Arch. B Cell. Pathol., 54:263, 1988.
283. Vlodavsky, I., Folkman, J., Sullivan, R., Fridman, R., Ishai-Michaeli, R., Sasse, J., and

Klagsbrun, M.: Endothelial cell-derived basic fibroblast growth factor: synthesis and deposition into subendothelial extracellular matrix. Proc. Natl. Acad. Sci. U.S.A., 84:2292, 1987.

284. Wahl, S. M., Hunt, D. A., Wakefield, L. M., McCartney-Francis, N., Wahl, L. M., Roberts, A. B., and Sporn, M. B.: Transforming growth-factor beta (TGF-beta) induces monocyte chemotaxis and growth factor production. Proc. Natl. Acad. Sci. U.S.A., 84:5788, 1987.

285. Warren, B. A.: The Vascular Morphology of Tumors. In Tumor Blood Circulation: Angiogenesis, Vascular Morphology and Blood Flow of Experimental Human Tumors. Edited by Hans-Inge Peterson. Boca Raton, Florida, CRC Press, 1979, pp. 1–47.

286. Weidner, N., Semple, J. P., Welch, W. R., and Folkman, J.: Tumor angiogenesis and metastasis—correlation in invasive breast carcinoma. New England Journal of Medicine, 324:1, 1991.

287. Weiner, H. L., Weiner, L. H., and Swain, J. L.: Tissue distribution and developmental expression of the messenger RNA encoding angiogenin. Science, 237:280, 1987.

288. Weiss, L.: Biophysical aspects of the metastatic cascade. In Fundamental Aspects of Metastasis. Edited by Weiss L. 1976, pp. 51–70.

289. West, D. C., Hampson, I. N., Arnold, F., and Kumar, S.: Angiogenesis induced by degradation products of hyaluronic acid. Science, 228:1324, 1985.

290. White, C. W., Sondheimer, H. M., Crouch, E. C., Wilson, H., and Fan, L. F.: Treatment of pulmonary hemangiomatosis with recombinant interferon alfa-2a. NEJM, 320:1197, 1989.

291. Wurschmidt, F., Beck-Bornholdt, H. P., and Vogler, H.: Radiobiology of the rhabdomyosarcoma R1H of the rat: Influence of the size of irradiation field on tumor response, tumor bed effect, and neovascularization kinetics. Int. J. Radiation Oncology Biol. Phys., 18:879, 1990.

292. Yamaura, H., Yamada, K., and Matsuzawa, T.: Radiation effect on the proliferating capillaries in rat transparent chamber. Int. J. Radiat. Biol., 30:179, 1976.

293. Yang, E. Y., and Moses, H. L.: Transforming growth factor B1-induced changes in cell migration, proliferation, and angiogenesis in the chicken chorioallantoic membrane. 111:731, 1990.

294. Zetter, B. R.: Migration of capillary endothelial cells is stimulated by tumor-derived factors. Nature, 285:41, 1980.

295. Zetter, B. R.: Endothelial heterogeneity: influence of vessel size, organ localization, and species specificity on the properties of cultured endothelial cells. In Endothelial Cells. Edited by U. Ryan. Boca Raton, CRC Press, 1988, pp. 63–80.

296. Zetter, B. R.: Assay for capillary endothelial cell migration. Methods in Enzymology, 147:135, 1987.

297. Zetter, B. R.: Cellular mechanisms of site-specific tumor metastasis. N. Engl. J. Med., 322:605, 1990.

298. Zetter, B. R., Rasmussen, N., and Brown, L.: An in vivo assay for chemoattraction. Lab. Invest., 53:362, 1985.

299. Zhan, X., Bates, B., Hu, X., and Goldfarb, M.: The human FGF-5 oncogene encodes a novel protein related to fibroblast growth factors. Mol. Cell Biology, 8:3487, 1988.

300. Ziche, M., and Gullino, P. M.: Angiogenesis and neoplastic progression in vitro. J. Natl. Cancer Inst., 69:483, 1982.

301. Zimering, M. B., Brandi, M. L., DeGrange, D. A., Marx, S. J., Streeten, E., Katsumata, N., Murphy, P. R., Sato, Y., Friesen, H. G., and Aurbach, G. D.: Circulating Fibroblast Growth Factor-Like Substance in Familial Multiple Endocrine Neoplasia Type 1. J. Clin. Endocrinol. and Metab., 70:149, 1990.

II

Tumor Immunology

Robert C. Bast, Jr.
Cinda M. Boyer

Human Immune Response

The human immune response has evolved to distinguish "self" from "non-self" permitting the detection and elimination of foreign substances and organisms. This response is mediated by different lymphoreticular cells and their products (Table II-1-1). Bone marrow is the ultimate source of both B lymphocytes that produce antibodies and T lymphocytes that mediate cellular immunity.[201] B cells and T cells are small lymphocytes that cannot be distinguished morphologically before interaction with antigen, but that bear distinct cell surface receptors and that undergo distinctive programs of differentiation.

B-Cells

Mature B cells synthesize and express immunoglobulin on their cell surface.[138] After interaction with antigen and T cell products, different clones of B cells differentiate into one or more plasma cells that produce a single antibody which binds noncovalently to a particular antigen. Binding depends upon a precise complementarity between the antigen and the antibody's combining sites. The tertiary structure of the antibody combining site is determined by the primary amino acid sequence of each immunoglobulin. Immunoglobulin molecules consist of light (L) and heavy (H) polypeptide chains (Figure II-1-1). Each L and H chain can be divided into an amino-terminal variable (V) region and a carboxy-terminal constant (C) region. The V region of each H and L chain includes three complementarity determining regions (CDRs) which contribute to the antigen binding site and which determine the specificity of the antibody (Figures II-1-2 and II-1-3). Each H chain C region (C_H) determines the function and isotype of the antibody. These include IgG1, IgG2, IgG3, IgG4, IgA1, IgA2, IgM, IgD and IgE (Table II-1-2). The C_H region permits fixation of complement components, antibody dependent cell mediated cytotoxicity, immunoglobulin mediated phagocytosis and transport across the placenta. The effector functions of immunoglobulins are particularly important for controlling viremia, bacteremia and infection by gram positive and encapsulated bacteria.

Antibody diversity is generated by several mechanisms, including somatic recombination of immunoglobulin gene segments, association of different H and L chains as well as somatic mutation within the CDRs. Within the variable region of H chain genes there is recombination of segments from a library of more than 100 variable (V_H), 6 joining (J_H), and 30 diversity (D_H) segments.[233] To produce mature L chains, there is recombination of V_L and J_L gene segments with the L chain genes. Some imprecision in gene segment recombination is permitted and additional nucleotides are added to the H and L chain genes (N region) by terminal deoxynucleotidyl transferase (TDT) producing sequences of $V_H ND_H NJ_H C_H$ and $V_L NJ_L NC_L$. Heavy chain rearrangement precedes light chain rearrangement. Within a single B cell, only a single heavy and light chain associate. Following this association, hypermutable regions within the rearranged light and heavy chains undergo somatic mutation. Through these several mechanisms, more than 100,000 antibody specificities can be produced.

Development of the monoclonal antibody technology by Kohler and Milstein in 1975 has resulted in reagents that have permitted precise characterization of B cell differentiation and the interaction of B cells with T cells and their products.[145] Murine monoclonal antibodies are produced by somatic cell hybridization of murine plasmacytoma cells with B cells from immune donors. Hybridomas produce essentially unlimited amounts of antibody with defined specificity. Different monoclonal antibodies prepared against human leukocytes and tumor cells have defined "clusters of differentiation" or CD groups. Such CD groups (Table II-1-3) have defined different lineages, stages of differentiation and states of activation among normal lymphoid and hematopoietic cells. In addition, CD groups have permitted classification of lymphoreticular tumors based upon their similarity to normal lymphocytes of different lineages. Correlation between the phenotypes of benign and malignant cells is not always precise. A given CD determinant can be expressed by normal cells from different lineages. Individual tumor cells can express CD determinants characteristic of different lineages. In defining the phenotype of tumor cells, combinations of CD epitopes are often more helpful than single determinants.

Table II-1-1.   Phenotype and Functions of Human Lymphoreticular Cells

	Cell Type			
	T	B	Non-T Non-B	Monocyte/ Macrophage
Phenotype				
Surface membrane immunoglobulin	−	+	−	−
Fc Receptors (FCR)	+/−	+	+	+
C3 Receptors	−	+	−	+
Class II MHC	+/−*	+	+/−	+
TCR, CD3	+	−	−**	−
Function				
Antibody formation	−	+	−	−
Tumor cell killing	+	−	+	+
Induction	+	−	−	−
Suppression	+	−	−	+
Proliferation to:				
Mitogens	+	+	−	−
Alloantigens	+	−	−	−
Soluble proteins	+	−	−	−
Mediator production				
Interleukin 1	+/−	+/−	+/−	+
Interleukin 2	+	−	+/−	−
Interleukin 3	+	−	−	−
Interleukin 4	+	−	−	−
Interleukin 5	+	−	−	−
Interleukin 6	+	−	−	+
Antibody Dependent Cell Mediated Cytotoxicity (ADCC)	+/−*	−	+	+
Natural killing (NK)	−	−	+	−
Lymphocyte Activated Killing (LAK)	+	−	+	−
Tumor Infiltrating Lymphocytes (TIL)	+	−	+/−	−

*Present when activated
**CD3-zeta subunit is expressed on NK cells
Adapted from Bast et al.[18]

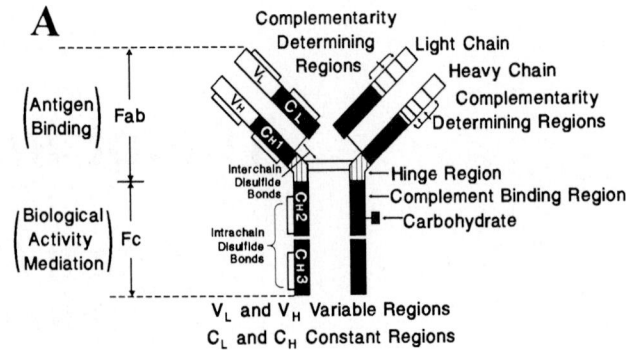

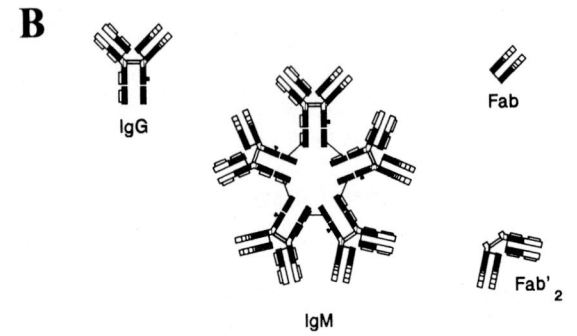

Figure II-1-1.   A. Structure of an immunoglobulin monomer. $V_{L, H}$, variable light and heavy chain regions; C_H1,2,3, constant heavy chain regions. (With permission from Wasserman[280] and Capra and Edmundson.[44]) B. Structure of IgG and IgM isotypes and immunoglobulin fragments. IgG consists of one immunoglobulin monomer. IgM is a pentamer consisting of five immunoglobulin monomers linked by interchain disulfide bonds. Fab fragments are generated by enzymatic cleavage with papain. Fab′$_2$ fragments are generated by enzymatic cleavage with pepsin.

Using murine monoclonal antibodies against human B lymphocytes, several stages in differentiation have been identified (Figure II-1-4). Initial B cell differentiation is independent of antigen, but subsequent differentiation requires antigen and proceeds optimally in the presence of T cell derived factors (such as IL-2, IL-4, IL-5 and IL-6). Pre-B cells are marked initially with CD19 followed by CD10 and CD20. In pre-B cells, the H chain rearranges, followed by the L chain producing cytoplasmic IgM. In immature B cells, monomeric IgM of a single specificity is displayed on the cell surface with class II MHC components (see below); CD10 is subsequently lost. IgD may be coexpressed with IgM. Activation of mature B cells, in contrast to that of T cells, can be triggered by antigen in the fluid phase. When antigen binds to cell membrane IgM in the presence of IL-1 and T cell factors such as IL-4, IL-5 and IL-6, mature virgin B cells proliferate, differentiate and switch isotypes to IgG, IgA or IgE. Signals are transduced with the aid of accessory molecules.[213] Both memory B cells and secretory plasma cells are produced. The latter lose cell surface immunoglobulin and CD19, but secrete IgG at rates up to 10^3 molecules/second.

B cells are organized in follicular aggregates within lymph nodes, spleen and gut associated lymphoid tissue, in proximity to T cells and antigen presenting cells. Antibody production can be augmented by T cell help and can be down regulated by T cell or macrophage mediated "suppression."

T-Cells

T-lymphocytes arise in bone marrow and differentiate within the thymus.[116] A significant fraction of T cells that recognize "self" determinants are eliminated during thymic differentiation. Mature T cells then traffic through the peripheral circulation and return to lymph through the venous and postcapillary venules of the skin and lymph nodes. T cells mediate the cellular response including delayed hypersensitivity, graft rejection and regulation of other T cells, B cells, monocytes and marrow progenitors. T cells are particularly important for resistance to viruses and to microbial pathogens that are destroyed by macrophages, including certain fungi, mycobacteria, *Salmonella* species and *Listeria monocytogenes*.

The specificity of interactions with different antigens is mediated by a large family of 90 Kd cell surface T cell recep-

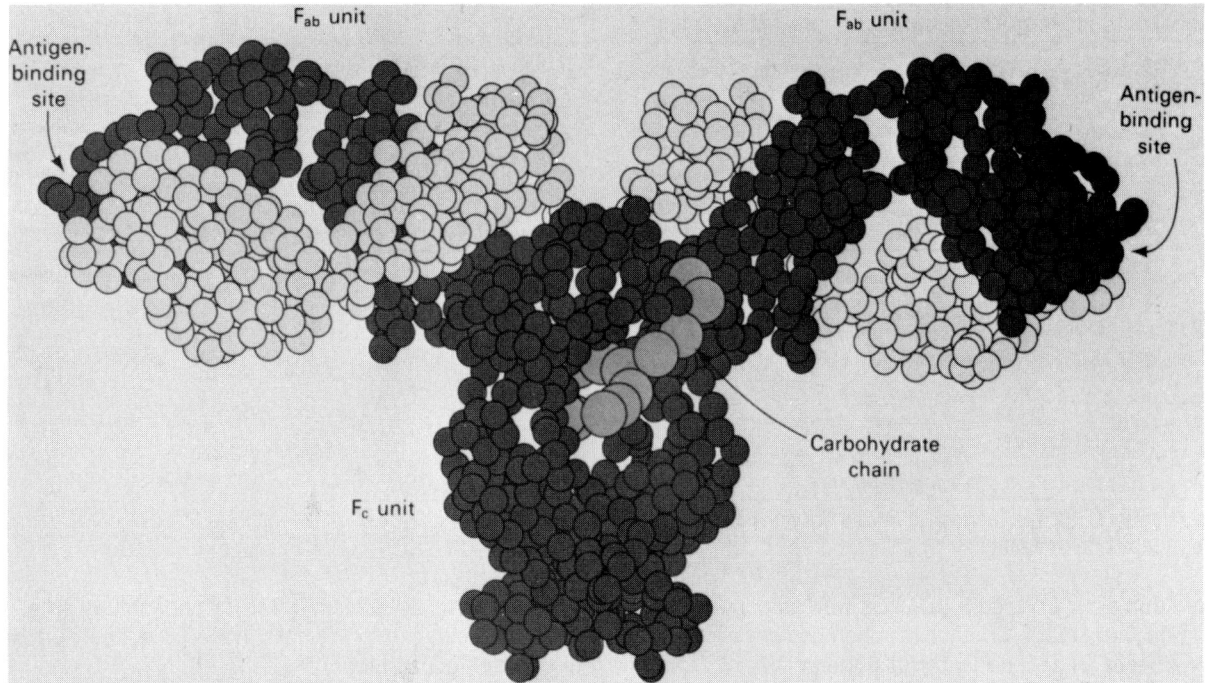

Figure II-1-2. Model of antibody molecule derived from x-ray crystallographic analysis. (With permission from Silverton et al.[239])

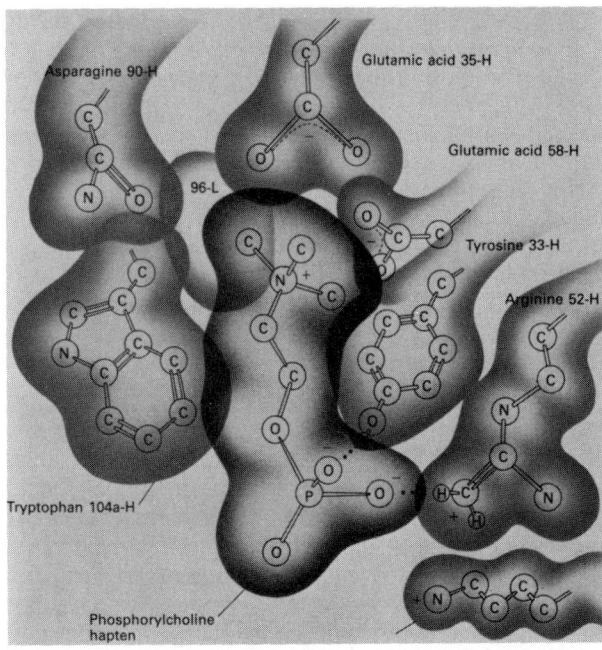

Figure II-1-3. Amino acids in the CDR regions forming the antigen binding site of an antibody molecule. Shown are those amino acids that contact the antigen, in this case the hapten phosphorylcholine. 96-L is the ninety-sixth residue of the light chain. (With permission from Capra and Edmundson.[44])

tors (TCR).[108,282] Different clones of T cells bearing distinctive TCR recognize different antigenic peptides. Diversity of TCR arises through somatic recombination of V, D, J and C gene segments analogous to that observed during generation of Ig diversity. In contrast to the process observed in B cells, somatic mutation is thought not to occur during T cell differentiation. Each TCR is an integral membrane heterodimer composed of either alpha/beta (95%) or gamma/delta (2–5%) chains. Additional diversity is probably generated by combinations of different α and β or γ and δ chains. Although uncommon in peripheral blood, γ/δ T cells are associated with the skin, lung and intestine. TCR of either type are found in close proximity to the 5 peptide chain complex of CD3 (Figure II-1-5). Antigen presenting cells (APC) including dendritic cells, macrophages and B cells digest exogenous proteins and display antigenic peptides at their surface in the context of Class II MHC antigens (HLA-DR, DQ and DP). Antigenic peptides from endogenous viral and cellular proteins become associated with Class I MHC antigens (HLA-A, B and C) during their synthesis and expression on the cell surface. In contrast to B cells that can recognize antigen in the fluid phase, T cells are thought to recognize antigen only on the surface of antigen presenting cells. CD8+ T cells interact with antigen bound to Class I MHC determinants, whereas CD4+ T cells recognize antigen bound to Class II MHC antigens. In either case the TCR binds to antigenic peptides that have bound to MHC molecules on the cell surface. Binding of TCR to antigen generates a signal that is transduced through CD3, releasing intracellular calcium and activating the phosphatidyl inositol or tyrosine kinase pathways.[231] In addition to the primary signal provided by antigen presented in an appropriate context, secondary signals are required to activate T cells fully, including soluble

Table II-1-2. Properties of Different Human Immunoglobulins

| Antibody | Heavy Chain | Serum Concentration (MG/ML) | Weight (Daltons) ($\times 10^3$) | Binding to Complement Activation | | Mediation of ADCC | Molecular Receptors on Mast Cells and Basophils |
				Classical Pathway	Alternate Pathway		
IgG1	γ1	9	150	+ +	– *	–	–
IgG2	γ2	3	150	+ / –	–	–	–
IgG3	γ3	1	150	+ + +	–	+	–
IgG4	γ4	0.5	150	–	+	+ / –	+
IgA1	α1	3	160	–	+	–	–
IgA2	α2	0.5	160	–	+	–	–
IgM	μ	1.5	950	+ + +	–	–	–
IgD	δ	0.03	175	–	+	–	–
IgE	ε	0.00005	190	–	–	?	+ +

*Aggregated IgG, IgA, IgM and IgE can also activate the alternate complement pathway.
Source: Adapted from Bast et al.[19]

factors such as interleukin-2 (IL-2) as well as contact with ligands on the surface of other lymphoreticular cells.[161,199] In the absence of secondary signals, the activity of T cells may be down regulated, producing tolerance to an otherwise foreign antigen. Activation of mature T cells by both primary and secondary signals can trigger morphologic change, proliferation, release of cytokines and acquisition of cytotoxic function.

T cells mature under the influence of thymic epithelium (Figure II-1-4). Early thymocytes, found in the outer cortex, express CD2 and CD7. Common thymocytes, found in the inner cortex, acquire CD1, CD4 and CD8. Mature thymocytes, found in the medulla, have lost CD1 but gained TCR, CD3 and CD5. Either CD4 or CD8 is expressed, but not both determinants. During maturation many clones that recognize "self" are eliminated and clones that recognize foreign antigens expanded. Mature T cells constitute 70–89% of normal peripheral blood lymphocytes, 30–40% of lymph node cells and 20–30% of splenic lymphocytes. T cells that contact appropriately presented and relevant antigens in the presence of stimulatory secondary signals are expanded into clones with the development of memory T cells.

Although there is not always a precise correlation, CD4+ T cells often exert helper/inducer function, whereas CD8+ T cells often mediate cytotoxicity and suppression. T inducer cells can "help" B cells, stimulate other cytotoxic T cells and activate monocytes. Suppressor T cells can affect B cells, T cells and hematopoietic precursors. Antigen specific and nonspecific suppression by T cells have been documented in different systems. Nonspecific suppression of immune function can also be mediated by macrophages. Both CD8+ and CD4+ T cells can be cytotoxic for targets which bear foreign class I and class II determinants respectively.

Non-T, Non-B Cells

A small population of lymphocytes lacks the markers associated with mature B cells or T cells. This third population of lymphocytes contains prominent intracytoplasmic granules and can bind the Fc region of IgG through specific receptors (FcR). Non-T, non-B cells can exert both antibody dependent cell mediated cytotoxicity (ADCC) and natural killer (NK) activity, destroying tumor cells in the presence or absence of specific IgG antibody.

Mononuclear Phagocytes

Monocytes, macrophages and dendritic cells can present antigen to lymphocytes and secrete cytokines such as Interleukin-1 (IL1), IL-6, tumor necrosis factor-alpha (TNF-α), interferons, prostaglandins and other monokines that can affect the function of both T cells and B cells. Mononuclear phagocytes (macrophages) are ultimately derived from promonocytes in the bone marrow that mature into monocytes which migrate to the liver, spleen, lymph nodes and lung. Tissue macrophages can phagocytize and digest microorganisms. Phagocytosis is enhanced by specific receptors for certain carbohydrates, complement and immunoglobulin. Human monocytes bear three distinct receptors for IgG (FcRI, FcRII, FcRIII) and are capable of mediating ADCC. After appropriate activation monocytes and macrophages can inhibit tumor growth in the absence of antibody.

Cytokines

T cells and monocytes produce a large number of factors which mediate intercellular communication. These include the interleukins and cytokines (Table II-1-4). A number of hematopoietic growth factors have been defined, many of which are expressed by lymphocytes and monocytes (Table II-1-5).[93] In addition, some tumors can produce one or more of these factors. Cytokines can interact synergistically and can stimulate the release of a cascade of secondary factors. Macrophages, for example, in addition to presenting antigen can secrete IL-1. In the presence of IL-1 and antigen, T inducer cell production of IL-2 is augmented and can further activate T cells, B cells, NK cells and monocytes. Activated T cells can, in turn, secrete IL-4, IL-5 and IL-6 that can stimulate the proliferation and differentiation of B lymphocytes. Activated T cells can also produce gamma-interferon that activates adjacent monocytes and modulates the proliferation of B cells and other T cells. Activation of monocytes and macrophages by T cells is essential for combating infec-

Table II-1-3. CD Designations

Group	Mr	Expression in Normal Leukocytes	Expression in Malignancies
CD 1	a gp49 b gp45 c gp43	80% of thymocytes; dendritic cells; B cell subset	Acute T lymphoblastic leukemia (<35%) and T lymphoblastic lymphoma (<35%)
CD 2	gp50	All T cells which form rosettes with sheep erythrocytes (E-rosette (CD58, LFA-3) receptor); 70–95% thymocytes; 100% T cells, and a variable percentage of LGLs	T cell malignancies (>70%)
2R		Activated T cells	
CD 3	complex (5 chns) gp/p 28, 26, 20, 16	Associated with the T cell antigen receptor (T1); 20–90% thymocytes; 100% T cells.	Chronic T lymphocytic leukemia (>70%) and cutaneous T cell lymphoma (>70%), Acute T lymphoblastic leukemia (<35%) and lymphoma (<35%)
CD 4	gp59	75–80% thymocytes; 60–70% T cells ("helper/inducer" subset); MHC Class II/HIV receptor	Acute T lymphoblastic leukemia (<35%), Chronic T lymphocytic leukemia (40–70%), Cutaneous T cell lymphoma (100%)
CD 5	gp67	10% thymocytes, most T cells and a subset of B cells	T cell malignancies (>70%) Chronic B lymphocytic leukemia (40–70%)
CD 6	gp100	Mature T cells; subset of B-cells	Acute T lymphoblastic leukemia (<35%), Chronic T lymphocytic leukemia (>70%) and cutaneous T cell lymphoma (>70%). Chronic B lymphocytic leukemia (40–70%)
CD 7	gp40	Thymocytes; 100% T cells; some LGLs	Acute T lymphocytic leukemia (40–70%), Cutaneous T cell lymphoma (<35%)
CD 8	gp33/33 gp33/31	50–80% thymocytes; 30% 35% T cells (cytotoxic/suppressor subset); MHC Class I receptor; some LGLs (low density)	Acute T-lymphoblastic leukemia (<35%) and chronic T-lymphocytic leukemia (<35%)
CD 9	p24	Pre-B cells; monocytes; platelets; granulocytes	Acute non-T non-B lymphoblastic leukemia (>70%), chronic B-lymphoblastic leukemia (<35%), multiple myeloma, acute myeloid leukemia
CD10	gp100 endopeptidase 24.11	Common acute lymphoblastic leukemia antigen; (CALLA); Pre-B cells; granulocytes	Acute non-T non-B lymphoblastic leukemia (>70%)
CD11a	gp180/95	Leucocytes (LFA-1)	
CD11b	gp165/95	C3Bi receptor (CR3); monocytes; granulocytes; LGLs	M4 (40–70%) and M5 (>70%) acute nonlymphocytic leukemia; acute lymphoblastic leukemia
CD11c	gp150/95	Monocytes; granulocytes; B cell subset	
CDw12	p90–120	Monocytes; granulocytes; platelets	M4 and M5 (<35%) stages of ANLL
CD13	gp 150 aminopeptidase N	Monocytes; granulocytes; early myeloid cells	M1 (>70%) and M4 or M5 (<35%) stages of ANLL, chronic myelogenous leukemia (40–70%)
CD14	gp55	70–93% monocytes; granulocytes; Langerhans cells	M4 (<35%) and M5 (40–70%) stages of acute nonlymphatic leukemia
CD15	Le^x determinant	100% monocytes; >95% mature granulocytes	Most ANLL; rare ALL; carcinoma
CD16	gp50–65	Fc receptor (FCRIII) LGLs (NK); granulocytes, monocytes, platelets	
CDw17	Lactosylceramide	Granulocytes, monocytes, platelets	ANLL
CD18	gp180, 95 Kd	β chain to CD11a,b,c; T cells; B cells; LGLs; monocytes; granulocytes	ANLL
CD19	gp95	100% of pre-B cells	All non-T ALL; some ANLL; B-CLL; B cell lymphoma
CD20	P37/32	B cells, ? ion channel	Some non-T ALL; B-CLL; B cell lymphoma
CD21	p140	Mature B cell subset; C3d/EBV-receptor (CR2)	Some non-T ALL; B-CLL; B cell lymphoma; hairy cell leukemia

Table II-1-3. CD Designations *Continued*

Group	Mr	Expression in Normal Leukocytes	Expression in Malignancies
CD22	gp135	B cell cytoplasm and surface in a subset	
CD23	gp45–50	B cell subset, activated macrophages; eosinophils; IgE receptor	B and T cell lymphomas; B-CLL; Hodgkin's disease
CD24	gp41/38	B cells; granulocytes	Non-T ALL; some ANLL; neuroblastoma
CD25	gp55	IL-2 receptor; activated T cells; B cells; monocytes; LGLs	T ALL
CD26	gp120 Dipeptidyl-peptidase IV	Activated T and B cells; macrophages	
CD27	p55 (dimer)	Thymocytes; T cell subset	T-CLL; Sezary cells
CD28	gp44	T cell subset	
CD29	gp120–130	VLAβ-chain; integrin β1-chain, platelet GPIIa; leukocytes, platelets	ALL (T and non-T), T-CLL
CD30	gp105	Activated T cells and B cells	Reed-Sternberg cells in Hodgkin's Disease
CD31	gp140	Platelets, monocytes, granulocytes, B cells	
CDw32	gp40	Monocytes, granulocytes, B cells	
CD33	gp67	Monocytes, marrow progenitors	ANLL
CD34	gp105–120	Marrow progenitors	ANLL
CD35	CR1	C3b receptor (CR1), granulocytes, B cells, monocytes, some T cells	ANLL
CD36	gp90	Monocytes, platelet GPIV, B cells	ANLL
CD37	gp40–52	B cells, T cells, monocytes	B lymphomas
CD38	p45	LGLs, B cells, activated T cells, monocytes, thymocytes, lymphoid progenitors	T-ALL, myeloma, some AML
CD39	gp70–100	B cell subset, monocytes	Burkitt's lymphoma cells
CD40	gp44/48	B cells	B lymphomas, B-CLL, Burkitt's lymphoma; some B-ALL; carcinomas
CD41	gp120/23	Platelet GPIIb-IIIa complex and GPIIb	
CD42a	gp23	Platelet GPIX	
CD42b	gp135/25	Platelet GPIB	
CD43	gp95	T cells, granulocytes, monocytes, brain	
CD44	gp80–95	Leukocytes, brain, erythrocytes (cellular adhesion molecule; T cell activation antigen)	
CD45	LCA, T200 tyrosine phosphatase	>95% of lymphocytes; monocytes and granulocytes	
CD45RA	gp220	T cell subset (appears to identify suppressor/inducers); B cells, monocytes	
CD45RB	gp220/205/190	B cells, T cell subset, monocytes, granulocytes	
CD45RO	gp180	T cells, B cell subset, monocytes	
CD46	gp66/56	Leukocytes	
CD47	gp47–52	Broad	
CD48	gp41	Leukocytes	
CDw49b	gp170 VLA-α chain, platelet GP1a	Platelets, cultured T cells	
CDw49d	gp150 VLA-α4 chain	Monocytes, T cells, B cells, Langerhans cells, thymocytes	
CDw49f	pg120/31/30 VLA-α6 chain, Plt GPIc	Platelets, T cells	
CDw50	gp148/108	Leukocytes	
CD51	gp125/25 VNR-α chain	Platelets	
CDw52	gp21–28	Leukocytes	
CD53	gp32–40	Leukocytes	
CD54	pg90 ICAM-1	Broad	
CD55	gp70 DAF	Broad	
CD56	gp220/135 L185	LGLs (NK); activated lymphocytes	LGL leukemias
CD57	gp110	LGLs (NK); T cells; B cell subset; brain	LGL leukemias
CD58	gp40–65	LFA-3; leukocytes, epithelial cell	

Table II-1-3. CD Designations *Continued*

Group	Mr	Expression in Normal Leukocytes	Expression in Malignancies
CD59	gp18–20	Broad	
CDw60	NeuAc- NeuAc- Gal-	T subset	
CD61	gp110 Integrin β3-, VNR- βchain, Plt GPIIIa	Platelets	
CD62	gp140	Platelets	
CD63	gp53 gran/12	Platelets, monocytes, granulocytes, T cells, B cells	
CD64	gp75	Monocytes	
CDw65	Ceramide dodecasaccharide 4c	Granulocytes, monocytes	
CD66	gp180–200	Granulocytes	
CD67	p100	Granulocytes	
CD68	gp110	Macrophages	
CD69	gp32/28	activated B cells and T cells	
CDw70	Ki-24	activated B cells and T cells	Reed-Sternberg cells
CD71	gp95 Transferrin receptor	Proliferating thymocytes, monocytes; activated T cells and B cells	
CD72	gp43/39	B cells	
CD73	p69	B cell subset, T cell subset	
CD74	gp41/35/33	B cells, monocytes	
CDw75	p53?	mature B cells, T cell subset	
CD76	gp85/67	mature B cells, T cell subset	
CD77	Gb3	resting B cells	
CDw78	?	B cells, monocytes	

Adapted from Knapp et al.,[144] Rosenberg et al.,[226] Reading,[211] and Zola.[294]

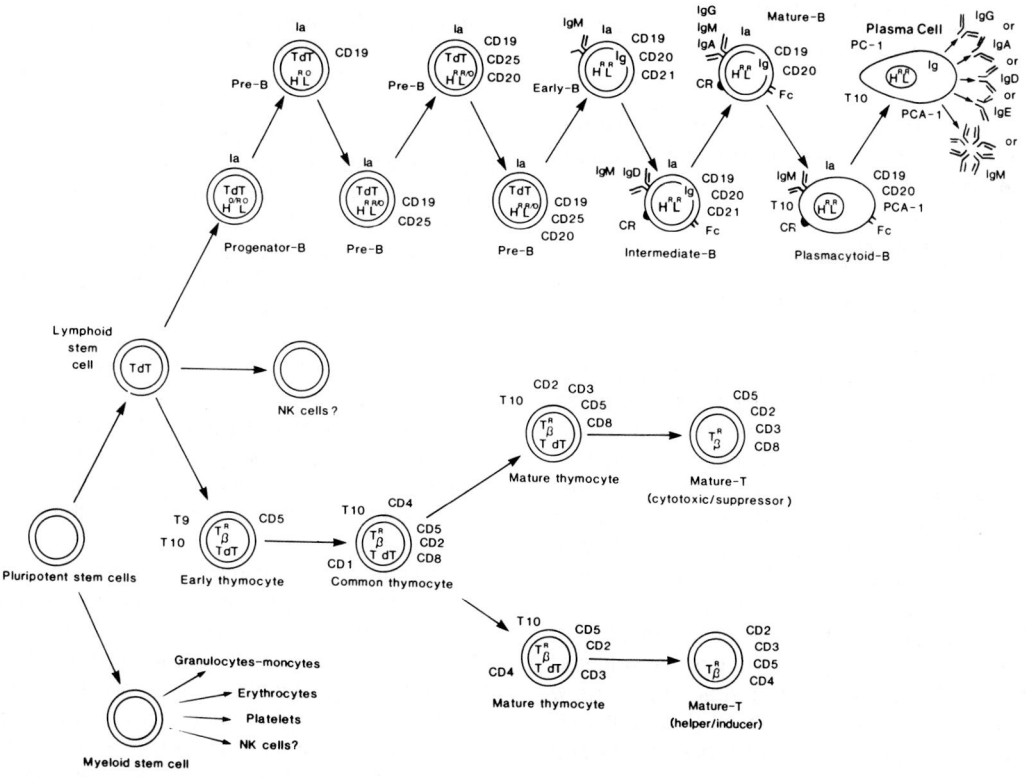

Figure II-1-4. Differentiation of lymphoreticular cells from pluripotent hematopoietic stem cells. TdT, terminal deoxynucleotidyl transferase; Ia, Class II MHC; H, heavy chain; L, light chain; O, germline configuration; R, rearranged gene; μ, cytoplasmic μ heavy chain; T^R_β, clonal rearrangement of the Tβ receptor; CR, complement receptor. (With permission from Foon and Todd.[81])

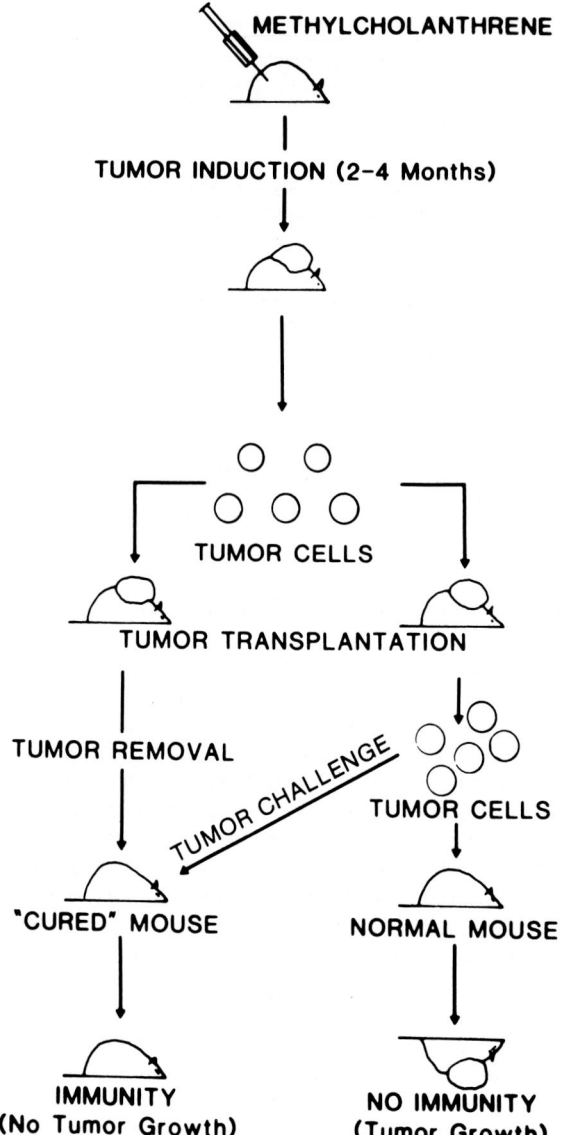

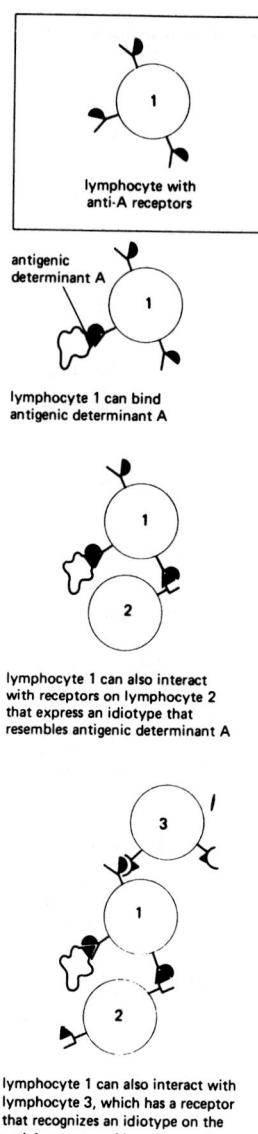

Figure II-1-7.   Demonstration of tumor-specific transplantation resistance. Tumors induced by an oncogenic DNA virus or a chemical carcinogen such as methylcholanthrene can be dissociated mechanically or enzymatically and transplanted to syngeneic recipients where the tumor will grow progressively. If the blood supply of the tumor is ligated to produce necrosis or if the tumor is excised before it can metastasize, the recipient will reject a second transplant of viable tumor cells that would grow progressively in a nonimmune recipient. The immune recipient would accept a graft of normal skin from the tumor donor, suggesting that the donor and recipient are indeed syngeneic and that rejection of the tumor transplant did not result from histoincompatibility of the donor and the recipient. (With permission from Bast.[18])

Figure II-1-8.   Idiotype-anti-idiotype network may play a role in the regulation of immune responses. (With permission from Alberts et al.[3])

cers have been induced by the injection of murine monoclonal antibodies directed against the same tumor associated antigens suggesting that anti-anti-idiotypic antibody had been formed.[53,112,156]

Cellular immunity to human cancers has also been demonstrated. T cells are the most prevalent leukocyte infiltrating tumors of several different histologic types. Delayed cutaneous reactivity has been evoked in patients with melanoma

using autologous tumor extracts, purified proteins and glycolipids. Lymphocyte proliferation has been produced by antigens associated with autologous tumor cells in up to 70% of patients, whereas lymphocyte mediated cytotoxicity has been produced against autologous tumor in up to 35% of patients.[199,272,277] Individually specific cytotoxic T cell clones have been isolated from melanoma, sarcoma, breast and ovarian carcinoma patients in the presence of IL-2. Studies with tumor infiltrating lymphocytes suggest that only a limited number of antigens are recognized. Cytotoxic effectors are most frequently CD3+CD8+CD4−, but CD3+CD8−CD4+ clones have been isolated from some patients. In some melanoma patients, cytotoxic reactivity has been MHC restricted,[192] particularly by HLA-A2 determinants.[54,58] MHC nonrestricted inhibition of clonogenic tumor cell growth has been produced against tumors of the same histologic type as that of the lymphocyte donor.[158] MHC nonrestricted cytotoxic T cells that preferentially kill pancreatic carcinoma cell lines have been grown from the lymph nodes of pancreatic cancer patients in the presence of IL-2 and allogeneic pancreatic cancer cells.[10] These T cells appear to recognize multiple antigenic determinants formed by the repeating 20 amino acid subunits of the core peptide of mucins that have been abnormally glycosylated within tumors. Similar observations have been obtained in breast cancer.[127]

Major Histocompatibility Complex (MHC) Antigens

Human histocompatibility antigens are encoded on chromosome 6 and are divided into two major classes.[219] Class I antigens (HLA-A, B and C) are cell surface proteins that contain a polymorphic 42 Kd peptide chain linked noncovalently to a 12 Kd β-2 microglobulin. Class I antigens are expressed by almost all body cells. Class II MHC antigens (HLA-DR, DP, DQ) are also integral membrane proteins. Each is a heterodimer with an α-chain and a β-chain, ranging in molecular weight up to 33 and 29 Kd, respectively. Class II MHC antigens are expressed primarily by lymphoreticular and endothelial cells. They can also be detected in epithelial cells after inflammation or treatment with gamma interferon.

MHC antigens can be expressed in tumor tissue.[71] Class I antigens can be down regulated in some tumors with a poor prognosis. Class II MHC antigens can be expressed ectopically. In normal epithelium, for example, Class II antigens cannot be detected, but are expressed by approximately 40% of epithelial ovarian cancers.[134] Class II antigens can also be expressed in some melanoma metastases,[55] but there is no consistent prognostic significance. In gestational trophoblastic neoplasia, paternal MHC antigens can be found in maternal circulating immune complexes following tumor regression.[148,210] Histoincompatibility of patients and their partners does not, however, correlate with prognosis.[28] Interestingly, interferons produce a highly selective induction of MHC antigens.[35] To the extent that these antigens are important for the recognition of tumor associated antigens, this might affect immunologic recognition of tumor cells.

Studies of MHC antigen expression on human tumors have most often examined monomorphic MHC determinants which are present on all Class I or Class II MHC molecules. It is possible that noncoordinate expression of MHC genes on one haplotype or that expression of certain MHC genes at a particular locus may be important.[54] These differences would be detectable only with antibodies reactive with subregion or polymorphic MHC determinants.

Studies of MHC in animal models have provided contradictory results.[71,96,257] Induction of MHC antigen expression by gene transfer or interferon attenuated the tumor growth of certain animal tumors, but did not affect other animal models.[71] A role for MHC antigens in tumor recognition was most often demonstrated in virally induced tumors susceptible to MHC-restricted cytotoxic T cells. Low levels of Class I MHC antigens on both animal and human cells correlated with increased susceptibility to NK cells.[251,252] A high level of MHC Class I expression on target cells is, however, important for recognition by cytotoxic T cells. Human peripheral blood lymphocytes transformed by Epstein Barr Virus (EBV) were killed by EBV specific MHC restricted cytotoxic T cells. EBV-positive Burkitt's lymphoma cells from the same individual expressed lower levels of MHC Class I antigens and were not killed.[164,221] The importance of MHC antigen expression for immune recognition of human tumors in vivo remains to be determined. Coexpression of class I MHC antigens with CD54 intercellular adhesion molecules appears to be important for generating a specific reaction against tumor cells in vitro.[273]

Oncofetal Antigens

Oncofetal antigens are expressed during fetal development. They are generally not expressed in adult tissues but may be re-expressed within neoplasms and in regenerating or inflamed tissues. A number of oncofetal antigens recognized by monoclonal or polyclonal reagents have provided useful serum markers for monitoring the course of different neoplasms. Ideally, tumor markers are sensitive, specific and correlate with changes in tumor burden. To impact on clinical practice, it is often important that alternative therapies that are more effective or less toxic could be utilized based upon changes in marker levels.

Human Chorionic Gonadotrophin (HCG). HCG is a glycoprotein heterodimer of 36.7 Kd synthesized by the syncytio-trophoblast during fetal development. The alpha subunit is encoded on chromosome 18 and the beta subunit on chromosome 19. Peak levels occur at 8–12 weeks of gestation during normal pregnancy. The half-life of the antigen in serum is 36 hours, assuring a rapid return of HCG to normal levels once the source of the antigen has been removed.

The major application of HCG has been in monitoring gestational trophoblastic neoplasia.[38] If there is no metastatic disease apparent at diagnosis, the HCG level can determine the need for chemotherapy. Failure of HCG to fall following chemotherapy reliably indicates drug resistance. Persistent normalization of HCG indicates cure of the disease. HCG can also be utilized as a marker in non-gestational choriocarcinoma of the ovary. These tumors are rare although most tumors secrete HCG. This is less reliable as a marker than in gestational trophoblastic disease. HCG has also been used in combination with alpha fetoprotein to follow patients with testicular carcinoma.

Alpha Fetoprotein (AFP). AFP is a glycoprotein of 70 Kd. The gene encoding AFP is linked to the serum albumin gene on chromosome 4. Peak levels during fetal development are observed at 13 weeks of gestation. The antigen is synthesized by fetal yolk sac, liver, and the upper gastrointestinal tract. AFP is immunosuppressive in high concentrations and may constitute one of several mechanisms that protect the fetus against a maternal immune response to fetal antigens. The half-life of AFP in serum is 4–6 days.

AFP can be a useful serum marker in hepatoma and in germ cell tumors of the ovaries and testes.[274] A small subset of gastric cancer patients also benefit from monitoring AFP concentration in that they have elevated serum levels of this marker despite normal levels of carcino-embryonic antigen. Occasional patients with other cancers have elevated AFP. AFP can be elevated in benign hepatocellular disease, ataxia telangiectasia, Wiscott-Aldrich Syndrome, and during pregnancy, particularly in the presence of fetal neural tube defects.

In monitoring testicular germ cell tumors with HCG and AFP both markers should be obtained preoperatively in all patients. Serial determinations have generally been obtained monthly for the first year and every two months for the second year. Persistently rising levels should prompt additional work-up and consideration of salvage therapy. Cross reaction between LH and HCG can sometimes produce false-positive elevations of HCG that decline after administration of androgens.

In monitoring ovarian germ cell tumors, AFP is particularly useful for a majority of endodermal sinus tumors (EST) and embryonal carcinomas. By contrast HCG is of greater value than AFP for nongestational choriocarcinomas. Failure to normalize is associated with persistent disease. Normal serum AFP can be associated with persistence of neoplastic elements other than endodermal sinus tumor and embryonal carcinoma. AFP is not expressed in pure dysgerminomas but should be measured in patients with this neoplasm in that chemotherapy is indicated for EST and embryonal carcinoma elements.

Carcinoembryonic Antigen (CEA). CEA is a glycoprotein of 200 Kd with greater than 50% carbohydrate. Anlaysis of its peptide core indicates that CEA is a member of the immunoglobulin supergene family.[202] The marker is associated with gastrointestinal, lung, breast, gynecological and genitourinary tumors as well as medullary carcinomas of the thyroid.[293] Recent studies point to the possible role of CEA in promoting metastasis.[128] Circulating levels of CEA have proven most useful in monitoring colon, pancreatic, stomach and lung cancer, particularly when tumor has metastasized to the liver. Changes in CEA levels reflect both tumor burden and the ability of the liver to clear CEA.[293]

Antigen levels in serum can be elevated (greater than 2.5 ng/ml) in inflammatory bowel disease, chronic obstructive pulmonary disease, cigarette smoking, cirrhosis and hepatobiliary disease. Consequently, CEA has not proven useful in screening for occult cancer.

The primary clinical application of CEA has been in monitoring colorectal carcinoma (see XXVIII-10). Preoperative CEA should be obtained in all patients with colorectal cancer. To detect persistent disease, CEA has been repeated one month postoperatively in Duke's B, C and resected Duke's D patients. The half life of CEA is approximately 10 days.[21] If CEA remains elevated (greater than 5 ng/ml) values can be repeated at 2–4 week intervals until it is clear whether values are rising or have normalized. If CEA is not elevated, values can be repeated every two months for two years and then every three months for three additional years. CEA levels have increased 4–6 months prior to disease recurrence in two thirds of patients.[21] Persistently rising CEA should prompt a non-invasive work-up and, in the absence of extraabdominal disease, second look laparotomy. Even with a negative CT scan, less than 5% of second look operations have been negative. In one large study of 400 patients, 63% of lesions could be resected when CEA was less than 11 ng/ml and 44% of these patients survived disease free for 5 years. With greater than 11 ng/ml of CEA 5 year survival is less than 25%.[169] In more than 100 patients who had undergone resection of 1–14 liver lesions, survival at 1 and 6 years was 91% and 50%.[168]

Differentiation and Lineage Associated Determinants

B and T Cell Antigens. Antigenic determinants are expressed in normal lymphoid cells that reflect distinct stages during differentiation.[81] Malignant cells can express combinations of the same antigens which may or may not correspond to the phenotypes of normal B and T cell precursors (see XXV-4 and XXXV-5).[6,66] The common acute lymphoblastic leukemia antigen (CALLA; CD10), for example, is a 100 Kd glycoprotein neutral endopeptidase found in 2–3% of normal bone marrow precursors and in approximately 50% of acute lymphoblastic leukemias, where expression of the antigen indicates a good prognosis. Acute lymphoblastic leukemias that express cell surface immunoglobulin (5%) or T cell antigens (25–30%) have a relatively worse prognosis, although differences are narrowing with improvements in therapy. Approximately 30% of ALLs lack CALLA, immunoglobulin or T cell markers. These "null cell" leukemias bear other B-cell determinants such as CD19 and also have a relatively poor prognosis compared to CALLA positive disease.

Chronic lymphocytic leukemia is more frequently of B cell (98%) than of T cell (2%) origin. Cutaneous T cell leukemia and mycosis fungoides display inducer phenotypes and express CD4. Hairy cell leukemia expresses CD11 and the IL-2 receptor (CD25). Large granular lymphocytic (LGL) leukemias express CD3, CD16, CD56, and CD57.

All nodular (follicular) lymphomas and a majority of all lymphomas express B cell antigens. A minority express T cell antigens.

Myeloid Antigens. A number of myeloid antigens have been defined which aid in distinguishing acute myelogenous leukemia from acute lymphoblastic leukemia (see XXXV-1).[6,120] In addition, certain phenotypes may have prognostic significance within the myeloid leukemias. MY7- MY4- AML may, for example, have a more favorable prognosis than leukemias that express these markers. Leukemias of mixed myeloid and lymphoid lineage that express CD7 have a poor prognosis.

Prostate Specific Antigen (PSA). Lineage or tissue specific markers have also proven useful in monitoring solid neoplasms. PSA is a glycoprotein of 33 Kd that contains 7% carbohydrate.[50] PSA is a serine protease that normally cleaves proteins in seminal fluid. The marker is elevated in serum more frequently than is prostatic acid phosphatase, particularly in early stages of the disease. Antigen is found in normal serum and can be elevated in benign prostatic hypertrophy, following prostatic examination and after prostatic surgery. After total prostatectomy, values should fall to 0. Rising levels can sometimes accompany localized disease that has recurred following prostatectomy and that can be treated with radiation therapy. For monitoring patients with prostate cancer both PSA and prostatic acid phosphatase have proven valuable. Immunocytochemical detection of PSA offers a highly specific test for tumors of prostatic origin.[61]

Mucins. Murine monoclonal antibodies have permitted detection of a number of epitopes on the high molecular weight mucins that are associated with normal epithelium and with carcinomas of the lung, breast, ovary and gastrointestinal tract. Mucin subunits are linked by sulfhydryl bonds and circulate in serum as random coiled moieties of >500 Kd. Mucins generally contain >50% carbohydrate and exhibit O-linked glycosylation. The protein core of each mucin contains repeating subunits of 20–30 amino acids, permitting each molecule to express multiple identical peptide as well as carbohydrate epitopes. The presence of multiple identical epitopes on each molecule has facilitated the development of double determinant "sandwich" immunoassays in which an antibody can be used to trap antigen on a solid phase immunoabsorbant. Radiolabeled or enzyme-conjugated antibody of exactly the same specificity can be used to detect additional free epitopes on the trapped antigen.

CA 19-9 is a sialylated Lewis blood group carbohydrate determinant associated both with a high molecular weight mucin and with cell membrane glycolipids.[160] A double determinant assay has been developed to detect CA 19-9 in serum.[64] Elevated levels of CA 19-9 (>37 units/ml) are found in serum from patients with pancreatic, gastric and colorectal carcinomas.[215] Early reports suggested that CA 19-9 might supplement CEA in monitoring patients with colorectal carcinoma. Among 220 patients with colorectal cancer, however, only 7 individuals had elevations of CA 19-9 in the absence of an elevated CEA. In the diagnostic workup of suspected pancreatic carcinoma an elevated CA 19-9 has a sensitivity of 70% and a specificity of 91%. Other mucin epitopes such as those recognized by DUPAN-2 have been used to monitor pancreatic cancer patients.[83,167]

A number of monoclonal and polyclonal antibodies have been prepared against mucins associated with breast cancers and normal human milk fat globule membranes including HMFG1,[42] HMFG2,[42] HME-Ags,[45] CA M26,[40] CA M29,[40] 115D8,[115] and DF3.[147] CA 15-3 is a heterodeterminant sandwich immunoassay that utilizes the 115D8 antibody as an immunoabsorbant and the DF 3 antibody as a probe.[107] Elevated levels of CA 15-3 (>30 units/ml) were found in sera from patients with breast, ovarian, lung and prostate cancers. Some 98.7% of healthy individuals have less than 30 units/ml CA 15-3, but elevated values have been found in normal pregnancy, during lactation and in the presence of hepatitis, endometriosis, benign gynecologic tumors and chronic pelvic inflammatory disease. CA 15-3 is more sensitive than CEA in detecting primary and metastatic breast cancer.[107] Approximately 20% of patients with primary breast cancer have elevated CA 15-3 levels. Some 38% of patients with locally recurrent disease have elevated CA 15-3 levels as do 70% of patients with bone and liver metastases. CA 15-3 levels have correlated with disease course in up to 74% of instances studied. A combination of CEA and CA 15-3 is not superior to CA 15-3 alone. Other assays for breast cancer mucin, including the IMx-BCM, may exhibit slightly greater sensitivity and specificity than CA 15-3,[57] but the utility of any of the mucin markers for managing breast cancer still remains to be defined.

CA 125. The CA 125 epitope is expressed on a high molecular weight glycoprotein whose smallest subunit is 220 Kd.[13,59] Each antigen molecule expresses multiple CA 125 epitopes, contains less than 50% carbohydrate and exhibits a buoyant density that sets CA 125 apart from the mucins. CA 125 is present in coelomic epithelium during embryonic development and can be detected in the fetal pleura, pericardium and peritoneum, as well as in most adult tissues derived from the coelomic epithelium.[133] Although CA 125 is rarely found in normal ovary, the antigen is detected in >80% of epithelial ovarian cancers.

A double determinant radioimmunoassay has been developed for CA 125 and can be used to monitor >80% of patients with ovarian cancer.[15] If elevated, serum CA 125 levels have correlated with disease course in 80–93% of instances studied.[123] Persistently rising CA 125 values are consistently associated with progressive disease. Elevation of CA 125 (>35 units/ml) at the time of a surgical surveillance procedure predicts persistence of disease with 96% accuracy.[123] CA 125 in a patient with primarily treated ovarian cancer can, however, return to less than 35 units/ml in response to surgery and chemotherapy prior to second look surgery and residual disease can be found in up to 60% of cases. The serum half-life of CA 125 is approximately 4.8 days and an apparent half-life of >20 days during initial chemotherapy is associated with an increased number of positive second look surgical surveillance procedures and a decreased survival.[119,271]

Although CA 125 can be elevated by adenocarcinomas that arise from a number of different sites, the marker is of some value in distinguishing malignant from benign pelvic masses.[68,162,243] In a postmenopausal patient with an adnexal mass, an elevated CA 125 (>95 units/ml) indicates some form of malignancy with a 96% positive predictive value. Thus, preoperative determination of CA 125 in patients with an adnexal mass could prompt referral for exploration to institutions with formal gynecologic oncology programs.

CA 125 is currently being evaluated as a marker for early detection of ovarian cancer.[142] Elevated levels of CA 125 can precede clinical presentation of cancer by 10–60 months.[17,295] CA 125 is elevated at the time of conventional diagnosis in 60% of ovarian cancer patients with early stage disease, whereas 2% of apparently healthy postmenopausal patients have comparable levels of CA 125. False positive values are more frequent in premenopausal patients, where CA 125 is elevated in pregnancy, endometriosis, pelvic inflammatory disease, pancreatitis, hepatic disease, renal disease and in any condition that can inflame the peritoneum, pleura or pericardium. In prospective studies, patients with early stage ovarian cancer have been detected using CA 125 to trigger pelvic examination and transabdominal sonography.[70,124,296] Current trials are evaluating CA 125 in combination with transvaginal sonography.[33]

Immunologic Mechanisms of Tumor Cell Killing

T-Cell Mediated Cytotoxicity

Tumor-specific transplantation resistance in murine systems is mediated by specific clones of T cells bearing unique receptors which are complementary to distinctive antigens associated with the tumor cell surface. Direct contact is required for specific killing, but soluble factors can also be produced. The precise mechanism of T cell mediated cytotoxicity is not known, but perforins, phospholipase, lymphotoxins, direct membrane interactions, and induction of apoptosis have all been proposed.[27,262,291,292] T cells are the most prevalent lymphoreticular cells to infiltrate many solid tumors. In the case of intraocular melanoma, the T cell receptor segment $V_{\alpha 7}$ was found in 7 of 8 tumors, consistent with the targeting of specific antigens by a limited repertoire of T cell receptors.[185] Both CD4+ and CD8+ T cells have been observed. CD4+ T cells are found at the implantation site of invasive moles and gestational trophoblastic neoplasia. Human melanomas, sarcomas and HTLV-1 induced leukemias are lysed in vitro by T-cells which recognize tumor-associated antigens in the context of the patient's MHC antigens. These have been CD3+, CD4-, CD8+ more often than CD3+, CD4+, CD8-.[91,260] Non-MHC restricted tumor cell killing by CD8+ T-cell clones has been observed in pancreatic and breast cancers. Mucin-like molecules may be the target insofar as killing can be blocked with monoclonal antibodies against the core protein of mucin.

Natural Killer Cells

Natural killer (NK) cells have the distinctive morphology of large granular lymphocytes.[261] Granules contain a cytotoxin that is transferred to tumor targets following adhesion of the natural killer. NK cells are CD56+, CD16+ (FcRIII+) and CD3-.[217,286,287] Direct contact with tumor cells is required for cytotoxicity, but previous immunization is not. The cytotoxic activity of NK cells is not MHC restricted and is not mediated through TCR. Recently, candidate molecules have been identified that may be the receptors which permit NK cells to recognize and to kill selectively both tumor cells and virus infected cells.[92,220] Some, but not all autologous, allogeneic and xenogeneic tumor cells are more sensitive than normal cells to NK activity. Tumor cells that are deficient in Class I MHC molecules are relatively more sensitive to natural killing, compatible with the possibility that MHC molecules inactivate NK or that they obscure a putative NK target structure.[126] Cytotoxicity can be augmented with interferons or IL-2 and can be inhibited by cyclic nucleotides, prostaglandins, phorbol esters, cyclophosphamide and corticosteroids. NK cells can produce IL-1, IL-2, interferons, colony-stimulating factors and cell growth factors in addition to cytotoxic factors.

Lymphokine Activated Killer Cells

LAK cells are produced from peripheral blood mononuclear cells by treatment with IL-2, lectins or alloantigens. Continued contact with IL-2 is required for optimal cytotoxicity. Both activated NK cells and T cells can be found in LAK populations that have been generated with high concentrations of IL-2.[111] LAK and cytolytic T cells contain both perforin and serine esterases.[191] In the case of LAK mediated by T cells that are CD3+ and TCR+, it is not clear whether tumor cell recognition depends upon the TCR or some other receptor. LAK cells are selectively cytotoxic for tumor cells and recognition is not MHC restricted. LAK can lyse some tumor cells which are resistant to NK cells. Direct contact is required between LAK cells and their targets.

Tumor infiltrating lymphocytes (TIL) have been obtained from several different human cancers. After growth in relatively low concentrations of IL-2, TIL have exhibited specific cytotoxicity for autologous tumor in many, but not all cases.

Cytotoxic effects have been mediated more frequently by CD3+CD8+ cells than by CD3+CD4+ lymphocytes.

Macrophage Mediated Cytotoxicity

Activated macrophages bind selectively to transformed cells and are selectively cytotoxic for them. In determining susceptibility to activated macrophages, studies with papillomavirus suggest that full transformation of cells by intact E7 protein is more important than the loss of suppressor gene function produced by mutant E7.[9] Direct contact between transformed tumor cells and macrophages is required. Tumor necrosis factor (TNF), a neutral protease, lysosomal hydrolases and reactive oxygen intermediates may all contribute to macrophage mediated cytotoxicity. Destruction of different tumor cell populations may proceed by different mechanisms.

Activation of macrophages can occur in distinct stages and requires at least two signals.[129] Gamma interferon and bacterial lipopolysaccharide (endotoxin) have been studied most intensively. Three different signaling pathways have been identified. Complex bacterial preparations including BCG and *Corynebacterium parvum* can activate macrophages.[1,166,182] Chemically defined mediators such as trehalose dimycolate and muramyl dipeptide can also activate macrophages. Activated macrophages produce prostaglandins which down regulate macrophages, neighboring lymphocytes and NK cells.

The number of macrophages found in human tumors is highly variable. Tumor cells have been shown to produce chemotactic factors as well as factors that inhibit chemotaxis. T cells associated with tumors can produce factors chemotactic for macrophages. IL-1, IL-6 and TNF produced by macrophages can stimulate the growth of a fraction of tumors. Breast and ovarian cancers can produce macrophage colony stimulating factor that is a potent chemotactic factor for monocytes. Consequently, monocytes and macrophages may participate in the paracrine growth stimulation of some tumors.

Neutrophil Mediated Cytotoxicity

After activation with phorbol myristate, granulocytes can lyse tumor cells.[152] Lysis by granulocytes is more protracted than lysis by T cells which generally requires less than 8 hours.

Complement Dependent Cytotoxicity

At least nine serum complement components can participate in the lysis of tumor cells.[230] Both conventional and alternative pathways for complement lysis have been described. The conventional pathway is initiated by binding of antibody to antigen. In the conventional pathway IgM is more potent than IgG. Nine serum proteins (C1–C9) interact sequentially to produce a "leaky patch" in the cell membrane destroying its osmotic integrity. Many nucleated tumor cells are relatively resistant to complement dependent cytotoxicity.[190] Fixed complement components have, however, been found at the site of rejection of tumors produced by monoclonal antibodies against glycolipid antigens.

Antibody Dependent Cell Mediated Cytotoxicity

In antibody dependent cell mediated cytotoxicity (ADCC), antibody acts as a bridge between tumor target cells and effector cells. Direct contact is required. Certain isotypes of IgG are effective, whereas IgM is not (Table II-1-2). Activated macrophages, lymphocytes, granulocytes and platelets can all serve as "effectors." All of these effector cells bear FcR. Antibody may bind first to the target and then to the effector. Alternatively, under certain conditions effectors can be armed before binding to the target. Effector cells can be activated by interaction with antibody and with tumor targets.

Relevance of Different Mechanisms In Vivo

The relative importance in vivo of different mechanisms for tumor cell killing has been difficult to assess.[237] In many studies with animal models, immune serum or lymphoid cells have been transferred locally with tumor cells or injected systemically into tumor bearing hosts. To prevent a contribution from host cells, the immune function of the recipient has often been suppressed by irradiation or through the use of congenitally immunodeficient nude or scid mice. In other studies, attempts have been made to ablate T cells, NK cells or macrophages using thymectomy and irradiation, antisera against lymphoid antigens or agents such as silica that are selectively toxic for phagocytic cells. In still other reports, tumor cells that have evaded host defenses in vivo have been tested for their susceptibility to different effector mechanisms in vitro.

In studies of tumor specific transplantation resistance, passive transfer of immunity has generally been achieved with lymphoid cells rather than with serum. T cells have been critical components of specific immunity to tumor associated antigens. In several murine models CD4+ T cells appear to be most important, whereas in others CD8+ T cells are required as well. Antibodies against glycolipid asialo-GM1 that is expressed on NK cells can potentiate pulmonary metastases after intravenous injection of murine tumor cells, arguing for a role of NK in controlling the growth of at least some tumors. UV-induced tumor cells that have evaded host defences are resistant to killing by T cells and macrophages, but are, however, susceptible to lysis by NK cells.[266] Tumor cells selected for resistance to macrophage mediated cytotoxicity in vitro were rejected by immunocompetent hosts. By contrast, tumor cells chosen for a loss of antigens recognized by T cells grew progressively in vivo.[267] Effective treatment with different immunotherapeutic agents might, of course, depend upon different effector mechanisms.

Mechanisms by Which Tumor Cells Escape Destruction

Lack of Antigen Expression

There are a number of mechanisms by which tumor cells may evade an established immune response. Not all tumor cells may express novel antigens; antigens may not appear at the cell surface or may not be presented in an appropriate context. Even if most cells within a tumor express potentially immunogenic antigens, a subpopulation of tumor cells may lack these antigens. Substantial heterogeneity has been observed in antigen expression within human tumors. Using a panel of 16 murine monoclonal antibodies, distinct antigenic phenotypes were found in 16 of 18 breast cancers and in each of 16 ovarian cancers.[34] Similar heterogeneity

has been demonstrated with polyclonal antisera and cell-mediated immunity. In some cases, heterogeneity in antigen expression relates to different phases of the cell cycle. In others, lack of antigen expression can be a stable phenotypic trait. Alternatively, cells which express a certain antigen can be grown from precursors that lack expression of that antigen, suggesting that loss of antigenic expression is not a stable phenotypic trait.

Antigenic Modulation and Circulating Antigen

Some antibodies are capable of inducing modulation of antigens from the cell surface. Antigenic modulation has been observed both in murine and in human leukemias.[193,216] Not all tumor-associated antigens modulate. Substantial amounts of antigen can be shed into serum. This can either be in soluble form or associated with cell membrane vesicles. Circulating antigen can suppress cytolytic T cell effector function and can induce suppressor cells that block generation of specific cytolytic T cells in murine melanoma models.[256] For those antigens that are immunogenic in the autologous host, antigen-antibody (immune) complexes can be formed. Circulating immune complexes have been found in a number of different cancers and in some cases tumor associated antigens have been detected within these complexes.[148,250,258,276] Prognostic correlations have been reported. To date, however, circulating immune complexes have not provided reliable markers for disease state.

Whether or not tumor associated antigens are shed or modulate, immunoglobulin might mask epitopes on "emergence-associated tumor immunogens," blocking cytolytic effectors.[163A] IgM antibodies have apparently exerted this effect in some murine systems.

Lack of Immunologic Recognition

Potentially immunogenic tumor associated antigens may be unable to bind to Class I or Class II MHC determinants from a given individual. Since many inducer T cells are of the CD4 phenotype and recognize antigens in the context of Class II determinants, whereas many cytotoxic T cells are of the CD8 phenotype and recognize antigens in the context of Class I MHC antigens, relevant epitopes from the same tumor may need to bind to both types of antigen to provide an effective cytolytic response. When T cell clones that recognize "self" are eliminated in the thymus, whole groups of rearranged variables β chain genes ($V_β$) are removed from the immunologic repertoire. Consequently, clones that would recognize potentially immunogenic tumor associated antigens may be deleted in some individuals depending upon their particular complement of "self" antigens.

Suppressor Cells and Factors

To the extent that tumor growth is affected by cytotoxic T lymphocytes, natural killer cells and activated macrophages, suppressor cells and soluble factors may be important. In recent years, the existence of antigen specific suppression has been questioned related to difficulties in obtaining T cell clones with specific suppressor activity and in characterizing relevant suppressor factors.[20] Substantial evidence has, however, accumulated documenting the importance of an idiotype-anti-idiotype network in regulating tumor immunity,[235] as well as the role of CD4+ and CD8+ T suppressor cells in well studied animal models.[65,186,187] Murine tumor specific transplantation resistance antigens can induce TS1 suppressor T cells that secrete a soluble suppressor factor which bears a receptor for antigen. The TSF1 suppressor factor can, in turn, induce TS2 suppressor cells that bear receptors which recognize the unique idiotope expressed on TSF1. The TS2 suppressor cells may induce yet another generation of suppressor cells (Figure II-1-9).[90] In the case of human melanoma, CD4+ T cells have also been isolated that suppress specific autologous cytotoxic responses.[46,176–180] These suppressor cells appear to interfere with the generation of high affinity IL-2 receptors on cytotoxic T lymphocytes.

Both humoral factors and lymphoreticular cells have been implicated in the nonspecific immunosuppression observed in cancer patients that affects their T cell, B cell or NK function. Cellular suppressors have included T lymphocytes, NK cells, monocytes and macrophages in different studies. Activation of macrophages can augment their immunosuppressive activity, related in part to secretion of prostaglandins. Prostaglandin E2 levels have been increased in bronchial lavage fluid from squamous cell lung cancer patients.[150] Humoral suppressor factors may be derived from tumor cells or host inflammatory cells.[14] Human tumor cells produce a variety of cytokines that can affect immune effectors including TGF-β and GM-CSF. The latter has been linked to immunosuppression in vivo in a murine mammary carcinoma model.[157]

Immunologic Surveillance

The theory of immunologic surveillance suggests that the cellular immune response has evolved to eliminate nascent clones of tumor cells before they can become clinically important.[4,12,43] In early studies T cells were considered the most likely effector for surveillance, but in more recent formulations NK cells, natural cytotoxic cells and activated macrophages have all been proposed as candidates for maintaining surveillance.[131] Evidence for immunologic surveillance has been obtained from animal models and clinical observations. Immunosuppression of mice with anti-thymocyte sera or thymectomy has increased their susceptibility to oncogenic DNA viruses. Greater numbers of tumors have arisen with shortened latent periods. In the case of RNA virus-induced tumors, thymectomy can have a paradoxical effect particularly in the case of viruses that affect T lymphocytes. With chemically-induced tumors, immunosuppression has increased oncogenesis in some studies, but not in others. Finally, tumors do not appear to arise more frequently in nude mice.

In patients with congenital immunodeficiency syndromes, an increased incidence of leukemias and lymphomas has been observed.[203] Similarly, in patients who are immunosuppressed after transplantation of organ allografts, large cell lymphomas of the CNS have been observed. In addition squamous cell carcinomas of the skin and cervix have also been seen more frequently. Interestingly, the incidence of other solid neoplams has not been substantially increased. In patients with AIDS, lymphomas, Kaposi's sarcoma, and anal carcinomas have been observed in excess (see XXXVII).[121,203] Whether this reflects the impact of multiple viral infections, cytokine secretion, abnormal proliferation of lymphocytes permitting promotion of tumor growth [206] or lack of immune surveillance is impossible to dissect from the current clinical data.

Immunocompetence of Cancer Patients

Immunocompetence varies inversely with tumor burden and directly with nutritional status. Protein calorie malnutrition may have a greater effect on cell-mediated immunity than upon a humoral response. Phagocytic function is also impaired.

Immunocompetence and Tumor Type

The underlying cancer can also affect immunocompetence (Table II-1-6). B cell defects have been observed in

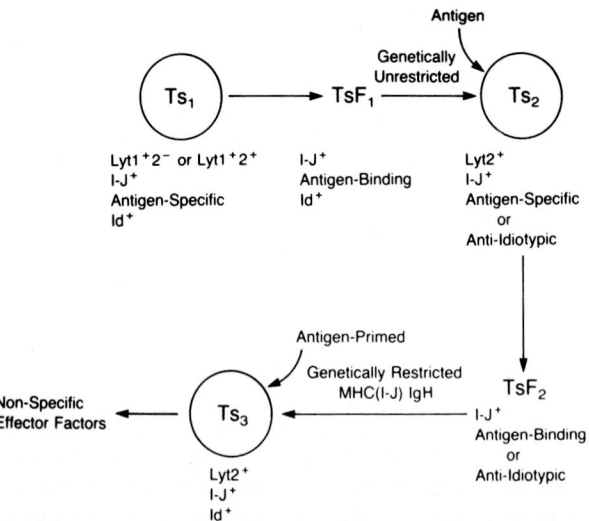

Figure II-1-9. A consensus pathway of T-cell mediated suppression. Ts, T suppressor cell; TsF, T suppressor factor; Lyt1, the murine T cell differentiation antigen analogous to CD4; Lyt2, the murine T cell differentiation antigen analogous to CD8; I-J, a marker for murine suppressor factors; Id, idiotype. (With permission from Hodes.[116])

Table II-1-6. Immunocompetence in Different Cancers

B-Cell Defects
Chronic lymphocytic leukemia
Multiple myeloma
Ovarian carcinoma
T-Cell Defects
Hodgkin's disease
Disseminated carcinomas
Kaposi's sarcoma/AIDS
Monocyte Defects
Carcinomas and sarcomas
Hodgkin's disease
Granulocyte Defects
Acute lymphoblastic leukemia
Acute myeloid leukemia
Chronic myelogenous leukemia
Multiple myeloma

chronic lymphocytic leukemia,[49,75,104,204] multiple myeloma,[39,143,205] and ovarian carcinoma.[78,163] T cell defects are observed in advanced disseminated carcinomas,[109,196,214] Hodgkin's disease,[2,79,84,85,95,264] and Kaposi's sarcoma.[203] In Hodgkin's disease both cellular and humoral suppressors have been identified. Monocyte defects are found in carcinomas and sarcomas as well as Hodgkin's disease. In addition to the reduced levels of granulocytes, functional defects have been identified in acute lymphocytic leukemia, acute myelogenous leukemia, chronic myelogenous leukemia and multiple myeloma. Exaggerated delayed hypersensitivity to mosquito bites has been observed in chronic lymphocytic leukemia,[281] and increased IgE has been observed in Hodgkin's disease,[279] possibly related to a loss of T suppressor cells.

Immunocompetence and Cancer Treatment

Surgical intervention produces a transient depression of T and B cell levels postoperatively.[26,130,240] T cell function generally recovers within 1 month. Splenectomy may predispose to a fulminant sepsis caused by *S. pneumoniae, H. influenza* or *N. meningitidis*.[67,73,218] This may relate both to loss of the spleen's phagocytic function and to decreased production of opsonizing antibodies.

Radiotherapy can depress levels of both T and B cells. B cell function recovers over a period of months, whereas certain T cell functions can be depressed for many years.[5,94] Total nodal irradiation prior to antigen injection facilitates the induction of immunologic tolerance mediated by T suppressor cells.[241] Small doses of total body irradiation can, however, eliminate precursors of suppressor cells.

Intermittent chemotherapy is generally less immunosuppressive than daily treatment.[114] T and B cell function generally rebounds between courses although persistent defects are observed after prolonged therapy when chemotherapy and radiotherapy are combined. Most cytotoxic drugs are immunosuppressive with the possible exception of vincristine and bleomycin. When given in conventional doses, steroids affect the recirculation of lymphocytes as well as their function. T cells are more markedly affected than B cells. By contrast cyclophosphamide has a much greater effect on B cells than on T cells.[263] When given in relatively small doses, cyclophosphamide can deplete suppressor T cells.[16] At higher doses, alkylating agents affect both B and T cells.[245]

Anaphylactoid reactions can occur following administration of a variety of chemotherapeutic agents including l-asparaginase, cyclophosphamide, cytosine arabinoside, bleomycin, doxorubicin, methotrexate, cisplatin, dacarbazine, and L-phenylalanine mustard.[283] Reactions to tartrazine dye have occurred following ingestion of hydroxyurea. Angioedema has been associated with administration of doxorubicin.

Approaches to Immunotherapy of Cancer

Over the years, two approaches have been utilized for immunotherapy of cancer. In active immunotherapy, attempts have been made to stimulate endogenous anti-tumor immunity within the host through the administration of bacterial products, chemically defined immunomodulators, cytokines and vaccines. In passive immunotherapy, antibodies, or lymphoreticular cells (adoptive immunotherapy) have been given to the host, providing exogenous immunity. Early attempts to treat cancers with immunotherapy were based upon empirical observations. Further development of these approaches has required a more fundamental understanding of the elements and regulation of the immune response, as well as the availability of new reagents. During the last two decades, somatic cell hybridization has facilitated the production of large amounts of monoclonal antibodies and recombinant DNA technology has provided novel cytokines and vaccines.

Active Immunotherapy

Bacterial Immunostimulants and Contact Allergens (See XVII-1). At the turn of the last century, William B. Coley had observed tumor regression in a patient who had developed a wound infection. Subsequently Coley treated cancer patients with supernatants from cultures of *Streptococcus pyogenes* and *Serratia marcescens*, observing a number of responses in different types of cancer.[183] More recent research has suggested that the efficacy of Coley's toxins may relate to their ability to evoke the release of TNF. In recent years, at least one randomized trial has tested the ability of Coley's toxins to augment chemotherapy for non-Hodgkin's lymphoma. Although early results suggested that patients who received chemotherapy plus toxins had a longer duration of response and survival than patients who received chemotherapy alone, differences between groups were not maintained over time.[136,137]

Active immunotherapy with contact allergens has produced regression of cutaneous squamous and basal cell carcinomas as well as cutaneous metastases from malignant melanoma.[52,139] Cancer cells appear to be destroyed as bystanders at the site of delayed cutaneous reactions to the chemical allergens.

Cutaneous metastases of malignant melanoma have also regressed in up to 60% of patients following direct intralesional injection of viable Bacillus Calmette Guerin (BCG), an attenuated strain of *Mycobacterium bovis* long used as a tuberculosis vaccine.[11,174] In 10–15% of patients, noninjected lesions have also regressed. Most attempts to utilize BCG alone for systemic therapy have failed to demonstrate an improvement in survival. The regional activity of BCG has been used to advantage in the treatment of recurrent papillomas and carcinomas of the bladder. Intravesical administration of BCG has delayed tumor recurrence and inhibited the development of new neoplasms. In randomized studies, BCG has proven superior to cytotoxic drugs such as thiotepa, mitomycin and doxorubicin.[113]

Other bacterial immunostimulants, including heat killed *Corynebacterium parvum (Propionobacter acnes),* have also failed to inhibit tumor growth consistently following systemic administration.[188] Intraperitoneal injection of *C. parvum* has, however, produced regression of small ovarian cancer metastases in 30% of patients.[25] Studies in animal systems have generally proven consistent with clinical experience, indicating that immunostimulants are most effective in immunocompetent hosts against small volumes of potentially immunogenic tumors growing in settings where direct contact can be achieved between cancer cells and the immunostimulant. Direct contact of immunostimulants with tumor cells optimizes not only the bystander killing by inflammatory cells, but also the development of specific immunity to tumor specific transplantation resistance antigens. Activated macrophages, T cells, NK cells and granulocytes have all been implicated as effectors of bystander killing in different systems. Cytokines including gamma interferon, TNF and IL-2 may also be important, but the precise mechanism(s) by which immunostimulants affect tumor growth have not yet been defined.

Chemically Defined Immunomodulators. Bacterial immunostimulants contain complex mixtures of immunomodulators. Chemically defined agents such as muramyl dipeptide and trehalose dimycolate have been utilized to activate macrophages and potentiate specific immunity in animal systems and in phase I clinical trials.[22,77,149] Despite their well defined structure and purity, these agents exert complex effects upon immuno-regulation that do not consistently induce tumor regression.

Immunorestorative agents can partially correct the lack of immunocompetence produced by tumor growth, malnutrition and therapy. Levamisole is a low molecular weight anti-helminthic drug that can affect macrophage and T cell function. Two recent randomized trials suggest that a combination of levamisole and 5-fluorouracil (5-FU) is significantly more effective than 5-FU alone in prolonging the survival of Dukes C colon cancer patients treated in an adjuvant setting.[103] Whether the additional activity provided by levamisole relates to immunomodulation or to some other effect of the drug remains to be determined.

Cytokines. Since nonspecific immunostimulants are now known to induce the release of different cytokines, purified or recombinantly derived preparations of cytokines have been evaluated individually for antitumor activity (see XVIII-3, XVIII-4, and XVIII-5). In general, clinical protocols to evaluate cytokines have mimicked the design of trials to evaluate cytotoxic drugs, in that a maximally tolerated dose has been sought and utilized to detect antitumor activity. Optimal effects upon particular immune responses may require relatively low concentrations of cytokines. Consequently the maximally tolerated dose may not coincide with the optimal dose.

Interferon-alpha has been most thoroughly examined with regard to efficacy and toxicity (see XVIII-3).[253] Lymphoreticular neoplasms have proven more susceptible to alpha interferon than have epithelial tumors. Particularly impressive responses have been observed in hairy cell leukemia (85%), chronic myelogenous leukemia (75%), and nodular non-Hodgkin's lymphoma (45%). A smaller fraction of patients with chronic lymphocytic leukemia and multiple myeloma have responded, and unlike most cytotoxic agents interferon-alpha has prolonged the duration of remissions in multiple myeloma. Among the solid neoplasms that respond to interferon-alpha are Kaposi's sarcoma (33%), glioblastoma (40%), mid-gut carcinoids (20%), melanoma (15%) and renal cell carcinoma (15%). Intralesional or regional administration of interferon has produced objective tumor regression in basal cell (75%), bladder (40%) and ovarian carcinomas (45%). When all trials are considered, systemic administration of interferon has produced objective responses in only

9% of 87 ovarian cancer patients, whereas intraperitoneal administration produced responses in 45% of 11 patients.[31] Life-threatening complications are rarely observed with recombinant interferons, but the patient's quality of life may not be improved given the side effects observed with optimally therapeutic doses which include fever, chills, malaise, myalgias, headache, anorexia, nausea, weight loss, reversible neutropenia and, on occasion, abnormalities in liver function and confusion.

Interferons exert a dual effect, inhibiting tumor growth directly through interaction with tumor cells and indirectly through modulation of the immune response. Among the immunologic effects of different interferons that may be relevant are increased expression of MHC antigens, increased NK activity, potentiation of cytotoxic T cells and activation of macrophages.[32]

Tumor necrosis factor is a cytokine now known to be one of the mediators released by macrophages after exposure to endotoxin (see XVIII-4). In animal models endotoxin produces hemorrhagic necrosis of established tumors. Serum from endotoxin treated animals mediates the same effects. The isolated activity was named tumor necrosis factor and was shown to be cytotoxic or cytostatic for tumor cells in vitro.[105] Administration of recombinant TNFα to cancer patients has been disappointing, however, with little direct antitumor activity at dose levels with manageable toxicity.[29,47,125,238]

Current studies are evaluating combinations of different cytokines as well as the use of cytokines with cytotoxic drugs. One of the most promising preliminary studies has combined 5-FU and interferon-alpha-2a to treat patients with colorectal carcinoma.[278] The administration of cytokines in combination may obviate the need for very high doses of a given cytokine that can produce untoward toxicity or exert undesirable pleiotropic effects upon the immune respone. Combination therapy with interferon gamma and TNFα has produced additive effects in animal models which may have been facilitated by the ability of interferon gamma to upregulate cellular receptors for TNF alpha.[232] Cytokines which stimulate the hematopoietic system such as IL-3, M-CSF, G-CSF and GM-CSF can not only reduce the duration and degree of leukopenia but can also activate immune effectors and affect the function of normal and malignant epithelial cells (see XVIII-6). GM-CSF, for example, can inhibit clonogenic ovarian tumor cell growth in anchorage independent assays.

Vaccines. In animal models, tumor specific transplantation resistance can sometimes be augmented by vaccines that present tumor associated antigens in an immunogenic form (see XVIII-2). Different vaccines have included tumor cells from autologous or allogeneic donors, virus infected tumor cells, purified tumor associated antigens and bacterial immunostimulants. Vaccines have generally been most effective against microscopic tumor burdens in immunocompetent hosts. There are few precedents for regression of palpable tumor nodules following vaccine treatment. In clinical studies, vaccines prepared from melanoma associated antigens and BCG or its components have evoked specific immune reactivity[154] and produced regression of clinically evident melanoma metastases in 8–16% of patients.[23,170]

Application of recombinant DNA technology has permitted isolation of genes that encode certain tumor associated peptides. Several of these genes have been incorporated into vaccinia virus and other potentially immunogenic viruses.[74] Whether the local response to viral antigens will potentiate antitumor immunity remains to be tested in the clinic. Genes for different cytokines including IL-2, IL-4, and gamma interferon have also been introduced into tumor cells, potentiating specific antitumor immunity in animal models.[76,88,89,94a] The efficacy of tumor cell vaccines is likely to depend upon the further definition of human tumor specific transplantation resistance antigens, as well as a more fundamental understanding of the peptides that are actually presented to inducer and effector T cells.

Even if tumor antigens are recognized, however, stimulation of the immune response may activate suppressor rather than cytotoxic effector mechanisms. Consequently, vaccines may form only one component of a program for immunoregulation that involves the inhibition of suppressor mechanisms and the stimulation of local or systemic inducer function. Some suppressor cells are unusually sensitive to low concentrations of cyclophosphamide.[16,24] To the extent that suppressor T cells exhibit a phenotype that is distinct from inducer T cells, monoclonal reagents might also be utilized. Cytokines such as IL-2 also need to be evaluated for their ability to augment responses to vaccines that contain tumor associated antigens.

Passive Immunotherapy

Serotherapy. (See XVII-7.) The use of antibodies as "magic bullets" was advocated by Paul Ehrlich in the early years of this century. Evaluation of polyclonal antisera for cancer treatment was hampered by difficulties in producing large quantities of high titered reagents that reacted selectively with tumor associated antigens. Clinical evaluation of serotherapy has been facilitated dramatically by the availability of monoclonal antibodies with defined specificity and high purity that can be produced in essentially unlimited amounts.[145]

Monoclonal and polyclonal antibodies prepared in different species have defined a large number of human tumor associated differentiation antigens.[6,37] Even with monoclonal reagents, however, few, if any, tumor-specific antigens have been identified. Tumor associated antigens are generally expressed in one or more normal cell types. Distribution of some tumor associated antigens may be restricted to a small population of normal host cells that are not required for survival. Most lymphomas are monoclonal and thought to be derived from single B or T lymphocytes that bear unique cell surface immunoglobulins or T cell receptors. Antibodies raised against the distinctive idiotopes expressed by the monoclonal immunoglobulins characteristic of each human B cell lymphoma, react with only a very small fraction of the patient's nonmalignant B cells. Similar specificity should be observed with antibodies against distinctive determinants on T cell receptors. Other tumor associated antigens may be expressed by a larger number of host cells, but quantitative differences in antigen expression might still permit effective therapy. In the case of those human cancers that are known to be induced by oncogenic viruses, specific viral antigens may be recognized in transformed cells. Not all of these components are, however, accessible for antibody binding at the cell surface. The human immune response may be capable of distinguishing tumor specific determinants. Human antibodies have been described which recognize antigens found only on autologous melanoma cells[188] and on tumor cells with differentially glycosylated blood group antigens.[132] Production of human monoclonal antibodies recognizing tumor-associated or tumor-specific antigens has, however, proven technically difficult.

Binding of antibodies to antigens on the surface of tumor cells is generally necessary, but not sufficient, to inhibit tumor growth. Antibodies reactive with certain growth factor receptors constitute an important exception to this generalization. Inhibition of anchorage dependent or anchorage independent growth can be observed with some, but not all antibodies that bind to the transferrin receptor, epidermal growth factor receptor, c-*erb* B-2 (HER-2/*neu*) gene product and the IL-2 receptor.[165,255] Antibodies with appropriate isotypes can trigger complement dependent cytotoxicity or participate in antibody dependent cell mediated cytotoxicity after binding to antigen. Many human tumor cells are, however, relatively resistant to lysis by human complement components. Effectors for antibody dependent cell mediated cytotoxicity may not be plentiful within the tumor compartment and their function may be impaired by several factors including the presence of endogenous antigen-antibody complexes. To compensate for deficiencies in host effector mechanisms, antibodies may be conjugated to cytotoxic drugs, isotopes or toxins, permitting the targeted delivery of these agents.

In addition to the potency of effector mechanisms, several other factors may impede the efficacy of monoclonal antibodies including complexing with shed antigen, failure to penetrate tissue, antigenic modulation, heterogeneity of antigen expression and the development of human anti-mouse antibodies (HAMA). Fortunately, not all cell surface antigens are shed and not all shed antigens impede reactivity of monoclonal antibodies with tumor cells. Saturation of antigenic sites on solid tumor nodules has proven difficult to achieve, although a significant fraction of sites can be occupied by monoclonal antibodies after intravenous injection. Even when antibody can gain access to a tumor nodule, a fraction of tumor cells may fail to express any given antigen. Use of multiple antibodies in combination can compensate for this heterogeneity.[34] Radionuclide conjugates may, in addition, have the ability to kill adjacent antigen negative tumor cells as bystanders. Although few allergic reactions have been related to HAMA, murine monoclonal antibodies are cleared more rapidly from the circulation in the presence of anti-murine immunoglobulins. Human monoclonal antibodies should be less immunogenic, but have been difficult to generate.[106] Using recombinant technology murine monoclonal antibodies have been "humanized" by inserting their complementarity determining regions into the framework of human immunoglobulins.[117,173] An immune response might still be generated to idiotypic determinants in the antigen combining region of human or chimeric antibodies.

Given the many potential limitations of serotherapy, it is remarkable that an objective response rate of 57% with two complete remissions lasting 29 and 72 months were observed when 14 patients with B cell lymphomas were treated with unconjugated anti-idiotypic antibodies.[151] Regression of melanoma metastases has also been produced with the systemic administration of antibodies against GD3[118,270] and the local injection of antibodies against GD2.[122] In addition, anti-idiotypic antibodies, at least in theory, can bear the internal image of tumor associated antigens and might be used as a vaccine.[112,171,184,285] Administration of unconjugated antibodies has generally been well tolerated.

Conjugates containing monoclonal antibodies and radionuclides have produced regression of lymphomas after intravenous injection.[63] Intraperitoneal administration of ^{131}I linked to antibodies against human milk fat globule protein has induced regression of small (<2 cm) ovarian cancer nodules in 36% of 24 patients treated.[72] Myelotoxicity has proven to be dose limiting in most phase I studies of radionuclide conjugates.

Several phase I trials of immunotoxins have been associated with unanticipated neurotoxicity, apparently related to the specificity of the antibody rather than to the direct effect of ricin A chain or *Pseudomonas* exotoxin.[30,82,200] Occasional responses have been observed in patients with melanoma[197,244] and lymphoma.[181] Thus, monoclonal antibodies have demonstrated some antitumor activity in the phase I and phase II studies performed to date (Table II-1-7). Based upon results in animal models, however, serotherapy is likely to have its greatest impact on microscopic disease and critical adjuvant trials have not yet been undertaken.

Adoptive Immunotherapy. From studies in animal tumor models, adoptive immunotherapy has been most effective when large numbers of lymphoid cells from intensely immune donors have been transferred to recipients with small tumor burdens.[242] In general, micrometastatic disease has been eradicated, whereas large or established tumors have been relatively more resistant to treatment. Immunogenic tumors have been better targets for adoptive immunotherapy than tumors with little or no demonstrable immunogenicity. Recruitment of specific or non-specific host effector cells may be important.[199]

With the production of IL-2 and other cytokines by recombinant DNA technology, clinical evaluation of adoptive immunotherapy has become feasible (see XVIII-5). Most clinical trials have, however, been performed in the setting of clinically evident metastatic disease. The immunogenicity of most human tumors has been difficult to define and the immune response of the patients has often been compromised. LAK cells have been generated from the patient's own peripheral blood lymphocytes by incubation ex vivo with high concentrations of IL-2.

When all of the available studies are considered, administration of autologous LAK cells with IL-2 has produced objective responses in 29% of patients with renal cancer, 20% with melanoma, and 16% with colorectal carcinoma.[223,225] Complete responses have sometimes been of long duration, but occur in less than 10% of patients treated. In different trials IL-2 alone has produced objective responses in approximately 20% of patients with renal cell carcinoma and melanoma. Consequently, the precise contribution of LAK cells requires further definition. Treatment with LAK and high doses of IL-2 has been associated with fever, nausea, vomiting, diarrhea, cutaneous erythema, fluid shifts, weight gain, oliguria, increased serum creatinine, hyperbilirubinemia, hypotension, supraventricular arrhythmias, and pulmonary edema. Although intensive support has been required, toxicity is generally reversible and few fatalities have been observed. Administration of IL-2 by continuous infusion may reduce toxicity to some extent.[284] Given the relatively modest rates of complete response and the substantial morbidity observed in clinical trials, it would be useful to be able to predict which patients might respond to combination therapy with LAK cells and IL-2.[208] At present there are no reliable prognostic markers for response.

Tumor infiltrating lymphocytes (TIL) can be isolated directly from tumors and cultured with IL-2 to expand the cell number.[227,290] In animal models TIL with specific anti-tumor reactivity have been grown in the presence of relatively low concentrations of IL-2 and have been shown to be 50–100 times more potent than LAK cells.[228] In contrast to LAK cells, TIL isolated from human tumors exhibit MHC-restricted cytotoxicity for the autologous tumor target. Treatment with TIL produced regression in 11 of 20 patients with metastatic melanoma.[227] In addition to specific anti-tumor reactivity, TIL may localize to tumor sites more effectively than LAK cells. In the future it may be possible to utilize gene transfer to track transferred lymphocytes and to produce lymphocytes with specificities and functional properties optimal for effective adoptive transfer of tumor rejection immunity.[224] Once again, critical adjuvant trials will be required to test the efficacy of adoptive immunotherapy.

Reference

1. Adams, D. O., Lewis, J. G., and Johnson, W. J.: Multiple modes of cellular injury by macrophages: Requirement for different forms of effector activation. *In* Progress in Immunology V. Edited by Y. Yamamura and T. Tada. Tokyo, Academic Press, Inc., 1983, p. 1009.
2. Aisenberg, A. C.: Lymphoma, leukemia and Hodgkin's disease. *In* Immunological Diseases. Edited by M. Samter. Boston, Little, Brown and Co., 1978, p. 530.
3. Alberts, B., Bray, D., Lewis, J., Raff, M., Roberts, R., and Watson, J. D.: Molecular Biology of the Cell. New York, Garland Publishing, Inc., 1983, p. 988.
4. Allison, A. C.: Immunological surveillance against tumor cells. *In* Cancer a Comprehensive Treatise. Biology of Tumors: Surfaces, Immunology, and Comparative Pathology. Edited by F. F. Becker. New York, Plenum Press, Vol. 4, 1975, p. 237.
5. Anderson, R. E., and Warner, N. L.: Ionizing radiation and the immune response. Adv. Immunol., 24:215, 1976.
6. Atwater, S. K., and Borowitz, M. J.: Immunophenotyping of Blood Cells. *In* Practical Laboratory Hematology. Second edition. Edited by J. Koepke. New York, Churchill Livingstone, 1991, p. 193.
7. Baldwin, R. W.: Specific antitumor immunity and its role in host resistance to tumors. *In* Basic and Clinical Tumor Immunology. Edited by R. B. Herberman. Boston, Martinus Nijhoff Publishers, 1983, p. 107.
8. Baldwin, R. W., and Price, M. R.: Neoantigen expression in chemical carcinogenesis. *In* Cancer a Comprehensive Treatise Etiology: Chemical and Physical Carcinogenesis. Edited by F. F. Becker. New York, Plenum Press, Vol. 1, 1975, p. 353.
9. Banks, L., Moreau, F., Vousden, K., Pim, D., and Matlashewski, G.: Expression of the human papillomavirus E7 oncogene during cell transformation is sufficient to induce susceptibility to lysis by activated macrophages. J. Immunol., 146:2037, 1991.

Table II-1-7. Trials of Unconjugated Monoclonal Antibodies to Treat Different Malignancies

Acute lymphocytic leukemia
Acute myeloid leukemia
Chronic lymphocytic leukemia
B-cell lymphoma
T-cell lymphoma
Gastrointestinal malignancies
Lung cancer
Prostate cancer
Breast cancer
Neuroblastoma
Renal cell carcinoma

Adapted from Bast[18]

10. Barnd, D. L., Lan, M. S., Metzgar, R. S., and Finn, O. J.: Specific major histocompatibility complex-unrestricted recognition of tumor-associated mucins by human cytotoxic T cells. Proc. Natl. Acad. Sci. USA, 86:7159, 1989.
11. Bast, R. C., Zbar, B., Borsos, T., and Rapp, H. J.: BCG and cancer. N. Engl. J. Med., 290:1413; 1458, 1974.
12. Bast, R. C., and Rapp, H. J.: The immunology of animal tumors. *In* Immunological Diseases. Third edition. Edited by M. Samter, D. W. Talmage, B. Rose, K. F. Austen, and J. H. Vaughan. Boston, Little, Brown and Co., 1978, p. 359.
13. Bast, R. C., Feeney, M., Lazarus, H., Nadler, L. M., Calvin, R. B., and Knapp, R. C.: Reactivity of a monoclonal antibody with human ovarian carcinoma. J. Clin. Invest., 68:1331, 1981.
14. Bast, R. C., Jr.: Effects of cancers and their treatment on host immunity. *In* Cancer Medicine. Second edition. Edited by J. F. Holland, E. and Frei, III. Philadelphia, Lea & Febiger, 1982, p. 1134.
15. Bast, R. C., Jr., Klug, T. L., St. John, E., Jenison, E., Niloff, J. M., Lazarus, H., Berkowitz, R. S., Leavitt, T., Griffiths, C. T., Parker, L., Zurawski, V. R., Jr., and Knapp, R. C.: A radioimmunoassay using a monoclonal antibody to monitor the course of epithelial ovarian cancer. N. Engl. J. Med., 309:883, 1983a.
16. Bast, R. C., Jr., Reinherz, E. L., Maver, C., Lavin, P., and Schlossman, S. F.: Contrasting effects of cyclophosphamide and prednisolone on the phenotype of human peripheral blood leukocytes. Clin. Immunol. Immunopathol., 28:101, 1983b.
17. Bast, R. C., Jr., Siegal, F. P., Runowicz, C., Klug, T. L., Zurawski, V. R., Jr., Schonholz, D., Cohen, C. J., and Knapp, R. C.: Elevation of serum CA125 prior to diagnosis of an epithelial ovarian carcinoma. Gynecol. Oncol., 22:115, 1985.
18. Bast, R. C., Jr.: Principles of Cancer Biology: Tumor immunology. *In* Cancer: Principles and Practice of Oncology. Second edition. Edited by V. T. DeVita, Jr., S. Hellman, and S. A. Rosenberg. New York. J. B. Lippincott, 1985, p. 125.
19. Bast, R. C., Jr., Bookman, M. A., and Knapp, R. C.: Concepts of gynecologic tumor immunology. *In* Gynecologic Oncology. Second edition. Edited by R. C. Knapp, and R. Berkowitz. New York, Macmillan, In press.
20. Batchelor, J. R., Lombardi, G., and Lechler, R. I.: Speculations on the specificity of suppression. Immunol. Today, 10:37, 1989.
21. Begent, R., and Rustin, G. J. S.: Tumour markers: From carcinoembryonic antigen to products of hybridoma technology. Cancer Surv., 8:107, 1989.
22. Bekierkunst, A., Levij, I. S., Yarkoni, E., Vilkas, E., and Lederer, E.: Suppression of urethan-induced lung adenomas in mice treated with trehalose-6, 6-dimycolate (cord factor) and living Bacillus Calmette-Guerin. Science, 174:1240, 1971.
23. Berd, D., Maguire, H. C., Jr., McCue, P., and Mastrangelo, M. J.: Treatment of metastatic melanoma with an autologous tumor-cell vaccine: Clinical and immunologic results in 64 patients. J. Clin. Oncol., 8:1858, 1990.
24. Berd, D., and Mastrangelo, M. J.: Active immunotherapy of human melanoma exploiting the immunopotentiating effects of cyclophosphamide. Cancer Invest., 6:337, 1988.
25. Berek, J. S., Knapp, R. C., Hacker, N. F., Lichtenstein, A., Jung, T., Spina, C., Obrist, R., Griffiths, C. T., Berkowitz, R. S., Parker, L., Zighelboim, J., and Bast, R. C., Jr.: Intraperitoneal immunotherapy of epithelial ovarian carcinoma with Cornebacterium parvum. Am. J. Obstet. Gynecol., 152:1003, 1985.
26. Berenbaum, M. C., Fluck, P. A., and Hurst, N. P.: Depression of lymphocyte responses after surgical trauma. Br. J. Exp. Pathol., 54:597, 1973.
27. Berke, G.: Functions and mechanisms of lysis induced by cytotoxic T lymphocytes and natural killer cells. *In* Fundamental Immunology. Second edition. Edited by W. E. Paul. New York, Raven Press, 1989, p. 735.
28. Berkowitz, R. S., Hornig-Rohan, J., Martin-Alosco, S., Klein, S., Goldstein, D. P., Bast, R. C., Jr., and DeWolf, W. C.: HL-A antigen frequency distribution in patients with gestational choriocarcinoma and their husbands. Placenta, 3 Suppl.:263, 1981.
29. Blick, M., Sherwin, S. A., Rosenblum, M., and Gutterman, J.: Phase I study of recombinant tumor necrosis factor in cancer patients. Cancer Res., 47:2986, 1987.
30. Bookman, M. A., Griffin, T., Godfrey, S., Padavic, K., Corda, J. P., Hamilton, T., Ozols, R. F., and Groves, E. S.: Anti-transferrin receptor immunotoxin (IT): Intraperitoneal (i.p.) phase-I trial. *In* Biology and Therapy of Ovarian Cancer. Marble Island Resort, Vermont, 1990.
31. Bookman, M. A., and Bast, R. C., Jr.: The immunobiology and immunotherapy of ovarian cancer. Semin. Oncol., 18:270, 1991.
32. Borden, E. C.: Interferons and cancer: How the promise is being kept. Interferon, 5:43, 1983.
33. Bourne, T., Campbell, S., Steer, C., Whitehead, M. I., and Collins, W. P.: Transvaginal colour flow imaging: A possible new screening technique for ovarian cancer. Br. Med. J., 299:1367, 1989.
34. Boyer, C. M., Borowitz, M. J., McCarty, K. S., Jr., Kinney, R. B., Everitt, L., Dawson, D. V., Ring, D., and Bast, R. C., Jr.: Heterogeneity of antigen expression in benign and malignant breast and ovarian epithelial cells. Int. J. Cancer, 43:55, 1989a.
35. Boyer, C. M., Dawson, D. V., Neal, S. E., Winchell, L. F., Leslie, D. S., Ring, D., and Bast, R. C., Jr.: Differential induction by interferons of major histocompatibility complex-encoded and non-major histocompatibility complex-encoded antigens in human breast and ovarian carcinoma cell lines. Cancer Res., 49:2928, 1989b.
36. Boyer, C. M., Knapp, R. C., and Bast, R. C., Jr.: Immunology and Immunotherapy. *In* Practical Gynecologic Oncology. Edited by J. S. Berek, and N. F. Hacker. Baltimore, Williams and Wilkins, 1989, p. 73.
37. Boyer, C. M., Lidor, Y., Lottich, S. C., and Bast, R. C., Jr.: Antigenic cell surface markers in human solid tumors. Antibody, Immunocon. Radiopharm., 1:105, 1988.
38. Braunstein, G. D.: Placental proteins as tumor markers. *In* Immunodiagnosis of Cancer, Second edition. Edited by R. B. Herberman, and D. W. Mercer. New York, Marcel Dekker, Inc., 1990, p. 673.
39. Broder, S., Humphrey, R., Durm, M., Blackman, M., Meade, B., Goldman, C., Strober, W., and Waldmann, T.: Impaired synthesis of polyclonal (non-paraprotein) immunoglobulins by circulating lymphocytes from patients with multiple myeloma: Role of suppressor cells. N. Engl. J. Med., 293:887, 1975.
40. Brown, J. P., Linsley, P. S., and Horn, D.: Breast carcinoma-associated mucins as tumor markers. *In* Immunodiagnosis of Cancer, Second edition. Edited by R. B. Herberman, and D. W. Mercer. New York, Marcel Dekker, Inc., 1990, p. 69.
41. Bugis, S. P., Lotzova, E., Savage, H. E., Hester, J. P., Racz, T., Sacks, P. G., and Schantz, S. P.: Inhibition of lymphokine-activated killer cell generation by blocking factors in sera of patients with head and neck cancer. Cancer Immunol. Immunother., 31:176, 1990.
42. Burchell, J., Wang, D., and Taylor-Papadimitriou, J.: Detection of the tumour-associated antigens recognized by the monoclonal antibodies HMFG-1 and 2 in serum from patients with breast cancer. Int. J. Cancer, 34:763, 1984.
43. Burnet, F. M.: The concept of immunological surveillance. Prog. Exp. Tumor Res., 13:1, 1970.
44. Capra, J. D., and Edmundson, A. B.: The antibody combining site. Sci. Am., 236:50, 1977.
45. Ceriani, R. L., and Rosenbaum, E. H.: Breast epithelial antigens in the circulation of breast cancer patients. *In* Immunodiagnosis of Cancer, Second edition. Edited by R. B. Herberman, and D. W. Mercer. New York, Marcel Dekker, Inc., 1990, p. 223.
46. Chakraborty, N. G., Twardzik, D. R., Sivanandham, M. T., Ergin, M. T., Hellstrom, K. E., and Mukherji, B.: Autologous melanoma-induced activation of regulatory T cells that suppress cytotoxic response. J. Immunol., 145:2359, 1990.
47. Chapman, P. B., Lester, T. J., Casper, E. S., Gabrilove, J. L., Wong, G. Y., Kempin, S. J., Gold, P. J., Welt, S., Warren, R. S., Starnes, H. F., Sherwin, S. A., Old, L. J., and Oettgen, H. F.: Clinical pharmacology of recombinant human tumor necrosis factor in patients with advanced cancer. J. Clin. Oncol., 5:1942, 1987.
48. Chieco-Bianchi, L., Collavo, D., and Biasi, G.: Immunologic unresponsiveness to murine leukemia virus antigens: Mechanisms and role in tumor development. Adv. Cancer Res., 51:277, 1988.
49. Chiorazzi, N., Fu, S. M., Montazeri, G., Kunkel, H. G., Rai, K., and Gee, T.: T cell helper defect in patients with chronic lymphocytic leukemia. J. Immunol., 122:1087, 1979.
50. Chu, T. M.: Prostate cancer-associated markers. *In* Immunodiagnosis of Cancer, Second edition. Edited by R. B. Herberman, and D. W. Mercer. New York, Marcel Dekker, Inc., 1990, p. 339.
51. Clark, S. C., and Kamen, R.: The human hematopoietic colony-stimulating factors. Science, 236:1229, 1987.
52. Cohen, M., Felix, E., Jessup, J., and Rosenberg, S.: Treatment of metastatic melanoma by intralesional injection of BCG, organic chemicals, and C. parvum. *In* Neoplasm Immunity: Mechanisms. Edited by R. G. Crispen. Chicago, ITR, 1976, p. 121.
53. Courtenay-Luck, N. S., Epenetos, A. A., Sivolapenko, G. B., Larche, M., Barkans, J. R., and Ritter, M. A.: Development of anti-idiotypic antibodies against tumour antigens and autoantigens in ovarian cancer patients treated intraperitoneally with mouse monoclonal antibodies. Lancet, 2:894, 1988.
54. Crowley, N. J., Darrow, T. L., Quinn-Allen, M. A., and Seigler, H. F.: MHC-restricted recognition of autologous melanoma by tumor-specific cytotoxic T cells. Evidence for restriction by a dominant HLA-A allele. J. Immunol., 146:1692, 1991.
55. Daar, A. S., Fuggle, S. V., Ting, A., and Fabre, J. W.: Anomolous expression of HLA-DR antigens on human colorectal cancer cells. J. Immunol., 129:447, 1982.
56. Dalianis, T.: Studies on the polyoma virus tumor-specific transplantation antigen (TSTA). Adv. Cancer Res., 55:57, 1990.
57. Daly, L., Ferguson, J., Cram, G., Haas, V., Beam, C., George, S., McCarty, K., Jr., and Bast, R.: Comparison of a new breast cancer serum marker, IM_xBCM to CA15-3 and CEA. Am. Soc. Clin. Oncol., 10:36, 1991.
58. Darrow, T. L., Slingluff, C. L., Jr., and Seigler, H. F.: The role of HLA class I antigens in recognition of melanoma cells by tumor-specific cytotoxic T lymphocytes. Evidence for shared tumor antigens. J. Immunol., 142:3329, 1989.
59. Davis, H. M., Zurawski, V. R., Jr., Bast, R. C., Jr., and Klug, T. L.: Characterization of the CA125 antigen associated with human epithelial ovarian carcinomas. Cancer Res., 46:6143, 1986.
60. Davis, M. M.: Molecular genetics of T cell antigen receptors. Hosp. Pract., 23:157; 169, 1988.
61. DeLellis, R. A., and Dayal, Y.: The role of immunohistochemistry in the diagnosis of poorly differentiated malignant neoplasms. Semin. Oncol., 14:173, 1987.
62. DeLeo, A. B.: Tumor rejection inducing antigens of mouse sarcomas: Biochemical and immunological characterization with monoclonal antibodies and CTL lines. *In* Tumor Immunol: Basic Mechanisms and Prospects for Therapy. Edited by R. H. Goldfarb, J., Heisler, and T. L. Whiteside. In press.
63. DeNardo, S. J., DeNardo, G. L., O'Grady, L. F., Levy, N. B., Mills, S. L., Macey, D. J., McGrahan, J. P., Miller, C. H., and Epstein, A. L.: Pilot studies of radiotherapy of B-cell lymphoma and leukemia using I-131 Lym-1 monoclonal antibody. Antibody, Immunocon. Radiopharm., 1:17, 1988.
64. Del Villano, B. C., Brennan, S., Brock, P., Bucher, C., Liu, V., McClure, M., Rake, B., Space, S., Westrick, B., Schoemaker, H., and Zurawski, V. R.: Radioimmunometric assay for a monoclonal antibody-defined tumor marker, CA 19-9. Clin. Chem., 29:549, 1983.
65. DiGiacomo, A., and North, R. J.: T cell suppressors of antitumor immunity. The production of Ly-1^-, 2^+ suppressors of delayed sensitivity precedes the production of suppressors of protective immunity. J. Exp. Med., 164:1179, 1986.
66. Drexler, H. G., and Minowada, J.: Lymphocytic leukemia and lymphomas. *In* Immunodiagnosis of Cancer. Second edition. Edited by R. B. Herberman, and D. W. Mercer. New York, Marcel Dekker, Inc., 1990, p. 243.
67. Editorial: Infective hazards of splenectomy. Lancet, 1:1167, 1976.
68. Einhorn, N., Bast, R. C., Jr., Knapp, R. C., Tjernberg, B., and Zurawski, V. R., Jr.: Preoperative evaluation of serum CA 125 levels in patients with primary epithelial ovarian cancer. Obstet. Gynecol., 67:414, 1986.
69. Einhorn, N., Knapp, R. C., Bast, R. C., and Zurawski, V. R., Jr.: The CA125 assay used in conjunction with CA 15-3 and TAG-72 assays for discrimination between malignant and non-malignant diseases of the ovary. Acta Oncol., 28:655, 1989.
70. Einhorn, N., Sjovall, K., Schoenfeld, D. A., Eklund, G., Knapp, R. C., Bast, R. C., Jr., and Zurawski, V. R., Jr.: Early detection of ovarian cancer using the CA 125 radioimmunoassay (RIA). Proc. Annu. Meet. Am. Soc. Clin. Oncol., 9:A607, 1990.
71. Elliott, B. E., Carlow, D. A., Rodricks, A. M., and Wade, A.: Perspectives on the role of MHC antigens in normal and malignant cell development. Adv. Cancer Res., 53:181, 1989.
72. Epenetos, A. A., Munro, A. J., Stewart, S., Rampling, R., Lambert, H. E., McKenzie, C. G., Soutter, P., Rahemtulla, A., Hooker, G., Sivolapenko, G. B., Snook, D., Courtenay-Luck, N., Dhokia, B., Krausz, T., Taylor-Papadimitriou, J., Durbin, H., and Bodmer, W. F.: Antibody-guided irradiation of advanced ovarian cancer with intraperitoneally administered radiolabeled monoclonal antibodies. J. Clin. Oncol., 5:1890, 1987.
73. Eraklis, A. J., Kevy, S. V., Diamond, L. K., and Gross, R. E.: Hazard of overwhelming infection after splenectomy in childhood. N. Engl. J. Med., 276:1225, 1967.

74. Estin, C. D., Stevenson, U. S., Plowman, G. D., Hu, S-L, Sridhar, P., Hellström, I., Brown, J. P., and Hellström, K. E.: Recombinant vaccinia virus vaccine against the human melanoma antigen p97 for use in immunotherapy. Proc. Natl. Acad. Sci. USA, 85:1052, 1988.
75. Faguet, G. B.: Mechanisms of lymphocyte activation: The role of suppressor cells in the proliferative responses of chronic lymphatic leukemia lymphocytes. J. Clin. Invest., 63:67, 1979.
76. Fearon, E. R., Pardoll, D. M., Itaya, T., Golumbek, P., Levitsky, H. I., Simons, J. W., Karasuyama, H., Vogelstein, B., and Frost, P.: Interleukin-2 production by tumor cells bypasses T helper function in the generation of a antitumor response. Cell, 60:397, 1990.
77. Fidler, I. J., Murray, J. L., and Kleinerman, E. S.: Systemic activation of macrophages in liposomes containing immunomodulators. *In* Biologic Therapy of Cancer. Edited by V. T. DeVita, Jr., S. Hellman, and S. A. Rosenberg. Philadelphia, J. B. Lippincott Co., 1991, p. 730.
78. Fisher, R. I., DeVita, V. T., Jr., Bostick, F., Vanhaelen, C., Howser, D. M., Hubbard, S. M., and Young, R. C.: Persistent immunologic abnormalities in long-term survivors of advanced Hodgkin's disease. Ann. Intern. Med., 92:595, 1980.
79. Fisher, R. I., and Young, R. C.: Immunologic aspects of Hodgkin's disease. *In* The Handbook of Cancer Immunology. Immune Status in Cancer Treatment and Prognosis. Part B, Vol. 4. Edited by H. Waters. New York, Garland STPM Press, 1978, p. 1.
80. Foley, E. J.: Antigenic properties of methylcholanthrene-induced tumors in mice of the strain of origin. Cancer Res., 13:835, 1953.
81. Foon, K. A., and Todd, R. F., III: Immunologic classification of leukemia and lymphoma. Blood, 68:1, 1986.
82. Frankel, A., Borowitz, M., Carter, P., Hertler, A., Moore, J. O., Brenckman, W., Groves, E. S., and Marafino, B.: A phase I study of continuous infusion immunotoxin for refractory metastatic breast cancer. Proc. Annu. Meet. Am. Soc. Clin. Oncol., 7:A121, 1988.
83. Fritsche, H. A., Jr., and Gelder, F. B.: Serum tumor markers for pancreatic cancer. *In* Immunodiagnosis of Cancer, 2nd edition. Edited by R. B. Herberman and D. W. Mercer. New York, Marcel Dekker, Inc., 1990, p. 289.
84. Fuks, Z., Strober, S., Bobrove, A. M., Sasazuki, T., McMichael, A., and Kaplan, H. S.: Longterm effects of radiation on T and B lymphocytes in peripheral blood of patients with Hodgkin's disease. J. Clin. Invest., 58:803, 1976.
85. Fuks, Z., Strober, S., King, D. P., and Kaplan, H. S.: Reversal of cell surface abnormalities of T lymphocytes in Hodgkin's disease after in vitro incubation in fetal sera. J. Immunol., 117:1331, 1976.
86. Furukawa, K. S., Furukawa, K., Real, F. X., Old, L. J., and Lloyd, K. O.: A unique antigenic epitope of human melanoma is carried on the common melanoma glycoprotein gp95/p97. J. Exp. Med., 169:585, 1989.
87. Furukawa, K., Yamaguchi, H., Oettgen, H. F., Old, L. J., and Lloyd, K. O.: Two human monoclonal antibodies reacting with the major gangliosides of human melanomas and comparison with corresponding mouse monoclonal antibodies. Cancer Res., 49:191, 1989.
88. Gansbacher, B., Bannerji, R., Daniels, B., Zier, K., Cronin, K., and Gilboa, E.: Retroviral vector-mediated τ-interferon gene transfer into tumor cells generates potent and long lasting antitumor immunity. Cancer Res., 50:7820, 1990.
89. Gansbacher, B., Zier, K., Daniels, B., Cronin, K., Bannerji, R., and Gilboa, E.: Interleukin 2 gene transfer into tumor cells abrogates tumorigenicity and induces protective immunity. J. Exp. Med., 172:1217, 1990.
90. Germain, R. N., and Benacerraf, B.: A single major pathway of T-lymphocyte interactions in antigen-specific immune suppression. Scand. J. Immunol., 13:1, 1981.
91. Gervois, N., Heuze, F., Diez, E., and Jotereau, F.: Selective expansion of a specific anti-tumor $CD8^+$ cytotoxic T lymphocyte clone in the bulk culture of tumor-infiltrating lymphocytes from a melanoma patient: Cytotoxic activity and T cell receptor gene rearrangements. Eur. J. Immunol., 20:825, 1990.
92. Giorda, R., Rudert, W. A., Vavassori, C., Chambers, W. H., Hiserodt, J. C., and Trucco, M.: NKR-P1, a signal transduction molecule on natural killer cells. Science, 249:1298, 1990.
93. Glaspy, J. A., and Golde, D. W.: The colony-stimulating factors: Biology and clinical use. Oncology, 4:25, 1990.
94. Goh, K.: Radiation, cell-mediated immunity, and cancer. *In* The Handbook of Cancer Immunology. Basic Cancer-Related Immunology. Vol. 1. Edited by H. Waters. New York, Garland STPM Press, 1978, p. 307.
94a. Golumbek, P. T., Lazenby, A. J., Levitsky, H. I., Jaffee, L. M., Karasuyama, H., Baker, M., and Pardoll, D. M.: Treatment of established renal cancer by tumor cells engineered to secrete interleukin-4. Science, 254:713, 1991.
95. Goodwin, J. S., Husby, G., and Williams, R. C.: Prostaglandin E and cancer growth. Cancer Immunol. Immunother., 8:3, 1980.
96. Gopas, J., Rager-Zisman, B., Bar-Eli, M., Hämmerling, G. J., and Segal, S.: The relationship between MHC antigen expression and metastasis. Adv. Cancer Res., 53:89, 1989.
97. Greenberg, P. D., Cheever, M. A., and Fefer, A.: Therapy of established tumors by adoptive transfer to T lymphocytes. *In* Basic and Clinical Tumor Immunology. Edited by R. B. Herberman. Boston, Martinus Nijhoff Publishers, 1983, p. 301.
98. Gregory, C. D., Murray, R. J., Edwards, C. F., and Rickinson, A. B.: Downregulation of cell adhesion molecules LFA-3 and ICAM-1 in Epstein-Barr virus-positive Burkitt's lymphoma underlies tumor cell escape from virus-specific T cell surveillance. J. Exp. Med., 167:1811, 1988.
99. Gross, L.: Intradermal immunization of C3H mice against a sarcoma that originated in an animal of the same line. Cancer Res., 3:326, 1943.
100. Habel, K.: Resistance of polyoma virus immune animals to transplanted polyoma tumors. Proc. Soc. Exp. Biol. Med., 106:722, 1961.
101. Hakomori, S.: Aberrant glycosylation in tumors and tumor-associated carbohydrate antigens. Adv. Cancer Res., 52:257, 1989.
102. Hamaoka, T., and Fujiwara, H.: Phenotypically and functionally distinct T-cell subsets in anti-tumor responses. Immunol. Today, 8:267, 1987.
103. Hamilton, J. M., Sznol, M., and Friedman, M. A.: 5-Fluorouracil plus levamisole: Effective adjuvant treatment for colon cancer. *In* Important Advances in Oncology 1990. Edited by V. T. DeVita, Jr., S. Hellman, and S. A. Rosenberg. Philadelphia, J. B. Lippincott Co., 1990, p. 115.
104. Han, T., and Dadey, B.: In vitro functional studies of mononuclear cells in patients with CLL: Evidence for functionally normal T lymphocytes and monocytes and abnormal B lymphocytes. Cancer, 43:109, 1979.
105. Haranaka, K., and Satomi, N.: Cytotoxic activity of tumor necrosis factor (TNF) on human cancer cells in vitro. Jpn. J. Exp. Med., 51:191, 1981.
106. Haspel, M. V., McCabe, R. P., Pomato, N., Janesch, N. J., Knowlton, J. V., Peters, L. C., Hoover, H. C., Jr., and Hanna, M. G., Jr.: Generation of tumor cell reactive human mononclonal antibodies using peripheral blood lymphocytes from actively immunized colorectal carcinoma patients. Cancer Res., 45:3951, 1985.
107. Hayes, D. F., Zurawski, V. R., Jr., and Kufe, D. W.: Comparison of circulating CA 15-3 and carcinoembryonic antigen levels in patients with breast cancer. J. Clin. Oncol., 4:1542, 1986.
108. Hedrick, S. M.: T lymphocyte receptors. *In* Fundamental Immunology, 2nd edition. Edited by W. E. Paul. New York, Raven Press, 1989, p. 291.
109. Heidenreich, W., Jagla, K., Schussler, J., Borner, P., Dehnhard, F., Kalden, J. R., Liebold, W., Peter, H. H., and Deicher, H.: Immunological characterization of mononuclear cells in peripheral blood and regional lymph nodes of breast cancer patients. Cancer, 43:1308, 1979.
110. Herberman, R. B.: Immunogenicity of tumor antigens. Biochim. Biophys. Acta., 473:93, 1977.
111. Herberman, R. B., Hiserodt, J., Vujanovic, N., Balch, C., Lotzova, E., Bolhuis, R., Golub, S., Lanier, L. L., Phillips, J. H., Riccardi, C., Ritz, J., Santoni, A., Schmidt, R. E., and Uchida, A.: Lymphokine-activated killer cell activity: Characteristics of effector cells and their progenitors in blood and spleen. Immunol. Today, 8:178, 1987.
112. Herlyn, D., Ross, A. H., and Koprowski, H.: Anti-idiotypic antibodies bear the internal image of a human tumor antigen. Science, 232:100, 1986.
113. Herr, H. W., Laudone, V. P., Badalament, R. A., Oettgen, H. F., Sogani, P. C., Freedman, B. D., Melamed, M. R., and Whitmore, W. F., Jr.: Bacillus Calmette-Guerin therapy alters the progression of superficial bladder cancer. J. Clin. Oncol., 6:1450, 1988.
114. Hersh, E. M., Gutterman, J. U., Mavligit, G., McCredie, K. B., Bodey, G. P., and Freireich, E. J.: Host defense, chemical immunosuppression, and the transplant recipient. Relative effects of intermittent versus continuous immunosuppressive therapy with reference to the objectives of treatment. Transplant. Proc. 5:1191, 1973.
115. Hilkens, J. F., Buijs, J., Hilgers, J., Hageman, Ph., Calafat, J., Sonnenberg, A., and van der Valk, M.: Monoclonal antibodies against human milk-fat globule membranes detecting differentiation antigens of the mammary gland and its tumors. Int. J. Cancer, 34:197, 1984.
116. Hodes, R. J.: T-cell-mediated regulation: Help and suppression. *In* Fundamental Immunology. 2nd Edition. Edited by W. E. Paul. New York, Raven Press, 1989, p. 587.
117. Houghton, A. N.: Building a better monoclonal antibody. Immunol. Today, 9:265, 1988.
118. Houghton, A. N., Mintzer, D., Cordon-Cardo, C., Welt, S., Fliegel, B., Vadhan, S., Carswell, E., Melamed, M. R., Oettgen, H. F., and Old, L. J.: Mouse monoclonal IgG3 antibody detecting G_{D3} ganglioside: A phase I trial in patients with malignant melanoma. Proc. Natl. Acad. Sci. USA, 82:1242, 1985.
119. Hunter, V. J., Daly, L., Helms, M., Soper, J. T., Berchuck, A., Clarke-Pearson, D. L., and Bast, R. C., Jr.: The prognostic significance of CA125 half-life patients with ovarian cancer who have received primary chemotherapy after surgical cytoreduction. Am. J. Obstet. Gynecol., 163:1164, 1990.
120. Hurwitz, C. A., Strauss, L. C., and Civin, C. I.: Immunodiagnosis of acute nonlymphocytic leukemia. *In* Immunodiagnosis of Cancer. Second edition. Edited by R. B. Herberman and D. W. Mercer. New York, Marcel Dekker, Inc., 1990, p. 265.
121. Ioachim, H. L.: The opportunistic tumors of immune deficiency. Adv. Cancer Res., 54:301, 1990.
122. Irie, R. F., and Morton, D. L.: Regression of cutaneous metastatic melanoma by intralesional injection with human monoclonal antibody to ganglioside GD2. Proc. Natl. Acad. Sci. USA, 83:8694, 1986.
123. Jacobs, I., and Bast, R. C., Jr.: The CA125 tumour-associated antigen: A review of the literature. Hum. Reprod., 4:1, 1989.
124. Jacobs, I., Stabile, I., Bridges, J., Kemsley, P., Reynolds, C., Grudzinskas, J., and Oram, D.: Multimodal approach to screening for ovarian cancer. Lancet, 1:268, 1988.
125. Jakubowski, A. A., Casper, E. S., Gabrilove, J. L., Templeton, M. A., Sherwin, S. A., and Oettgen, H. F.: Phase I trial of intramuscularly administered tumor necrosis factor in patients with advanced cancer. J. Clin. Oncol., 7:298, 1989.
126. Janeway, C. A., Jr.: Immune response: To thine own self be true . . . Curr. Biol., 1:239, 1991.
127. Jerome, K. R., Barnd, D. L., Boyer, C. M., Taylor-Papadimitriou, J., McKenzie, I. F. C., Bast, R. C., Jr., and Finn, O. J.: Adenocarcinoma reactive cytotoxic T lymphocytes recognize an epitope present on the protein core of epithelial mucin molecules. *In* Cellular Immunity and the Immunotherapy of Cancer. Edited by M. T. Lotze, and O. J. Finn. New York, Wiley-Liss Inc., 1990, p. 321.
128. Jessup, J. M., Wagner, H., Toth, C. A., Ford, R., and Thomas, P.: Carcinoembryonic antigen may promote metastasis by cell adhesion. Proc. Am. Assoc. Cancer Res., 31:A388, 1990.
129. Johnson, W. J., Somers, S. D., and Adams, D. O.: Expression and development of macrophage activation for tumor cytotoxicity. Contemp. Top. Immunobiol., 13:127, 1984.
130. Jubert, A. V., Lee, E. T., Hersh, E. M., and McBride, C. M.: Effects of surgery, anesthesia and intraoperative blood loss on immunocompetence. J. Surg. Res., 15:399, 1973.
131. Kärre, K., Ljunggren, H. G., Piontek, G., and Kiessling, R.: Selective rejection of H-2-deficient lymphoma variants suggests alternative immune defence strategy. Nature, 319:675, 1986.
132. Kabat, E. A., Liao, J., Shyong, J., and Osserman, E. F.: A monoclonal IgM lambda macroglobulin with specificity for lacto-N-tetraose in a patient with bronchogenic carcinoma. J. Immunol., 128:540, 1982.
133. Kabawat, S. E., Bast, R. C., Jr., Bhan, A. K., Welch, W. R., Knapp, R. C., and Colvin, R. B.: Tissue distribution of a coelomic-epithelium-related antigen recognized by the monoclonal antibody OC125. Int. J. Gynecol. Pathol., 2:275, 1983a.
134. Kabawat, S. E., Bast, R. C., Jr., Welch, W. R., Knapp, R. C., and Bhan, A. K.: Expression of major histocompatibility antigens and nature of inflammatory cellular infiltrate in ovarian neoplasms. Int. J. Cancer, 32:547, 1983b.

135. Kearney, J. F.: Idiotypic networks. *In* Fundamental Immunology, 2nd edition. Edited by W. E. Paul. New York, Raven Press, 1989, p. 663.
136. Kempin, S., Cirrincione C., Straus, D. S., Gee, T. S., Arlin, Z., Koziner, B., Pinsky, L., Nisce, L., Myers, J., Lee, B. J., III, Clarkson, B. D., Old, L. J., and Oettgen, H. F.: Improved remission rate and duration in nodular non-Hodgkin lymphoma (NNHL) with the use of mixed bacterial vaccine (MBV). Proc. Am. Soc. Clin. Oncol., 514, 1981.
137. Kempin, S., Cirrincione, C., Meyers, J., Lee, B., III, Straus, D., Koziner, B., Arlin, Z., Gee, T., Mertelsmann, R., Pinsky, C., Comacho, E., Nisce, L., Old, L., Clarkson, B., and Oettgen, H.: Combined modality therapy of advanced nodular lymphomas (NL): The role of nonspecific immunotherapy (MBV) as an important determinant of response and survival. Proc. Am. Soc. Clin. Oncol., 2:56, 1983.
138. Kincade, P. W., and Gimble, J. M.: B lymphocyets. *In* Fundamental Immunology. Second edition. Edited by W. E. Paul. New York, Raven Press, 1989, p. 41.
139. Klein, E.: Introduction: Immunotherapy of cancer in man, a reality. *In* Conference on the Use of BCG in Therapy of Cancer. National Cancer Institute Monograph 39. Edited by T. Borsos and H. J. Rapp. Washington, D. C., 1973, p. 139.
140. Klein, G., Sjogren, H. O., Klein, E., and Hellström, K. E.: Demonstration of resistance against methylcholanthrene-induced sarcomas in the primary autochthonous host. Cancer Res., 20:1561, 1960.
141. Klein, G.: Recent trends in tumor immunology. Isr. J. Med. Sci., 2:135, 1966.
142. Knapp, R. C., Berkowitz, R. S., Leavitt, T., Jr., and Bast, R. C., Jr.: Natural history and detection of ovarian cancer. *In* Gynecology and Obstetrics. Edited by J. W. Sciarra. Philadelphia, Harper & Row Publishers, 1988, p. 1.
143. Knapp, W., and Baumgartner, G.: Monocyte-mediated suppression of human B lymphocyte differentiation in vitro. J. Immunol., 121:1177, 1978.
144. Knapp, W., Dörken, B., Gilks, W. R., Rieber, E. P., Schmidt, R. E., Stein, H., and von dem Borne, A. E. G. Kr.: Leukocyte Typing IV White Cell Differentiation Antigens. Edited by W. Knapp, Oxford, Oxford University Press, 1989.
145. Kohler, G., and Milstein, C.: Continuous cultures of fused cells secreting antibody of predefined specificity. Nature, 256:495, 1975.
146. Kripke, M. L.: Immunology of murine skin cancers. Carcinog. Compr. Surv., 11:273, 1989.
147. Kufe, D., Inghirami, G., Abe, M., Hayes, D., Justi-Wheeler, H., and Schlom, J.: Differential reactivity of a novel monoclonal antibody (DF3) with human malignant versus benign breast tumors. Hydridoma. 3:223, 1984.
148. Lahey, S. J., Steele, G., Jr., Berkowitz, R., Rodrick, M. L., Ross, D. S., Goldstein, D. P., Zamcheck, N., Wilson, R. E., and Deasy, J. M.: Identification of material with paternal HLA antigen immunoreactivity from purported circulating immune complexes in patients with gestational trophoblastic neoplasia. J. Natl. Cancer Inst., 72:983, 1984.
149. Lederer, E., and Chedid, L.: Immunomodulation by synthetic muramyl peptides and trehalose diesters. *In* Immunological Aspects of Cancer Therapeutics. Edited by E. Mihich. New York, John Wiley & Sons, 1982, p. 107.
150. LeFever, A., and Funahashi, A.: Elevated prostaglandin E_2 levels in bronchoalveolar lavage fluid of patients with bronchogenic carcinoma. Chest, 98:1397, 1990.
151. Levy, R., and Miller, R. A.: Therapy of lymphoma directed at idiotypes. Monogr. Natl. Cancer Inst., 10:61, 1990.
152. Lichtenstein, A., Seelig, M., Berek, J., and Zighelboim, J.: Human neutrophil-mediated lysis of ovarian cancer cells. Blood, 74:805, 1989.
153. Livingston, D. M., and Bradley, M. K.: The simian virus 40 large T antigen. A lot packed into a little. Mol. Biol. Med., 4:63, 1987.
154. Livingston, P. O., Natoli, E. J., Calves, M. J., Stockert, E., Oettgen, H. F., and Old, L. J.: Vaccines containing purified GM2 ganglioside elicit GM2 antibodies in melanoma patients. Proc. Natl. Acad. Sci. USA, 84:2911, 1987.
155. Lloyd, K. O., and Old, L. J.: Human monoclonal antibodies to glycolipids and other carbohydrate antigens: Dissection of the humroal immune response in cancer patients. Cancer Res., 49:3445, 1989.
156. Loibner, H., Plot, R., Rot, A., Werner, G., Wrann, M., Samonigg, H., Schmid, M., Stoger, H., Truschnig, M., Herlyn, D. and Koprowski, H.: Immunoreactivity of patient with colorectal cancer metastasis after immunisation with anti-idiotypes. Lancet, 335:171, 1990.
157. Lopez, D. M., Fu, Y-X, and Watson, G. A.: Modulation of immune responses by tumor derived factors. Proc. Am. Assoc. Cancer Res., 31:236, 1990.
158. Lotze, M. T., and Finn, O. J.: Recent advances in cellular immunology: Implications for immunity to cancer. Immunol. Today, 11:190, 1990.
159. Lurquin, C., Van Pel, A., Mariame, B., De Plaen, E., Szikora, J. P., Janssens, C., Reddehase, M. J., Lejeune, J., and Boon, T.: Structure of the gene of tum-transplantation antigen P91A: The mutated exon encodes a peptide recognized with Ld by cytolytic T cells. Cell, 58:293, 1989.
160. Magnani, J. L., Steplewski, Z., Koprowski, H., and Ginsburg, V.: Identification of the gastrointestinal and pancreatic cancer-associated antigen detected by monoclonal antibody CA 19-9 in the sera of patients as a mucin. Cancer Res., 43:5489, 1983.
161. Makgoba, M. W., Sanders, M. E., and Shaw, S.: The CD2-LFA-3 and LFA-1-ICAM pathways: Relevance to T-cell recognition. Immunol. Today, 10:417, 1989.
162. Malkasian, G. D. Jr., Knapp, R. C., Lavin, P. T., Zurawski, V. R., Jr., Podratz, K. C., Stanhope, C. R., Mortel, R., Berek, J. S., Bast, R. C., Jr., and Ritts, R. E.: Preoperative evaluation of serum CA125 levels in premenopausal and postmenopausal patients with pelvic masses: Discrimination of benign from malignant disease. Am. J. Obstet. Gynecol., 159:341, 1988.
163. Mandell, G. L., Fisher, R. I., Bostick, F., and Young, R. C.: Ovarian cancer: A solid tumor with evidence of normal cellular immune function but abnormal B cell function. Am. J. Med., 66:621, 1979.
163A. Manson, L. A.: Does antibody-dependent epitope masking permit progressive tumor growth in the face of cell-mediated cytotoxicity? Immunol. Today, 12:352, 1991.
164. Masucci, M. G., Torsteindottir, S., Colombani, J., Brautbar, C., Klein, E., and Klein, G.: Down-regulation of class I HLA antigens of the Epstein-Barr virus-encoded latent membrane protein in Burkitt lymphoma lines. Proc. Natl. Acad. Sci. USA, 84:4567, 1987.
165. Masui, H., Moroyama, T., and Mendelsohn, J.: Mechanism of antitumor activity in mice for anti-epidermal growth factor receptor monoclonal antibodies with different isotypes. Cancer Res., 46:5592, 1986.
166. Meltzer, M. S., and Nacy, C. A.: Delayed-type hypersensitivity and the induction of activated, cytotoxic macrophages. *In* Fundamental Immunology. Second edition. Edited by W. E. Paul. New York, Raven Press, 1989, p. 765.
167. Metzgar, R. S., Rodriguez, N., Finn, O. J., Lan, M. S., Daasch, V. N., Fernsten, P. D., Meyers, W. C., Sindelar, W. F., Sandler, R. S. and Seigler, H. F.: Detection of a pancreatic cancer-associated antigen (DU-PAN-2 antigen) in serum and ascites of patients with adenocarcinoma. Proc. Natl. Acad. Sci. USA, 81:5242, 1984.
168. Minton, J. P.: Surgical management of recurrent colon and rectal cancers: Management of recurrent colorectal carcinoma. ASCO, Proc. Am. Soc. Clin. Oncol., Educational Booklet. 24th Annu. Meet., 1988, p. 143.
169. Minton, J. P., Hoehn, J. L., Gerber, D. M., Horsley, J. S., Connolly, D. P., Salwan, F., Fletcher, W. S., Cruz, A. B. Jr., Gatchell, F. G., Oviedo, M., Meyer, K. K., Leffall, L. D., Jr., Berk, R. S., Stewart, P. A., and Kurucz, S. E.: Results of a 400-patient carcinoembryonic antigen second-look colorectal cancer study. Cancer, 55:1284, 1985.
170. Mitchell, M. S., Harel, W., Kempf, R. A., Hu, E., Kan-Mitchell, J., Boswell, W. D., Dean, G., and Stevenson, L.: Active-specific immunotherapy for melanoma. J. Clin. Oncol., 8:856, 1990.
171. Mittelman, A., Chen, Z. J., Kageshita, T., Yang, T., Yamada, M., Baskind, P., Goldberg, N., Puccio, C., Ahmed, T., Arlin, Z., and Ferrone, S.: Active specific immunotherapy in patients with melanoma. A clinical trial with mouse antiidiotypic monoclonal antibodies elicited with syngeneic anti-high-molecular-weight-melanoma-associated antigen monoclonal antibodies. J. Clin. Invest., 86:2136, 1990; erratum appears: J. Clin. Invest. 87:757, 1991.
172. Moore, S. K., Kozak, C., Robinson, E. A., Ullrich, S. J., and Appella, E.: Cloning and nucleotide sequence of the murine hsp 84 CDNA and chromosome assignment of related sequences. Gene 56:29, 1987.
173. Morrison, S. L., and Ol, V. T.: Genetically engineered antibody molecules. Adv. Immunol., 44:65, 1989.
174. Morton, D. L., Eilber, F. R., Malmgren, R. A., and Wood, W. C.: Immunological factors which influence response to immunotherapy in malignant melanoma. Surgery, 68:158, 1970.
175. Morton, D. L., Miller, G. F., and Wood, D. A.: Demonstration of tumor-specific immunity against antigens unrelated to the mammary tumor virus in spontaneous mammary adenocarcinomas. J. Natl. Cancer Inst., 42:289, 1969.
176. Mukherji, B., Chakraborty, N. G., and Sivanandham, M.: T-cell clones that react against autologous human tumors. Immunol. Rev., 116:33, 1990.
177. Mukherji, B., Guha, A., Chakraborty, N. G., Sivanandham, M., Nashed, A. L., Sporn, J. R., and Ergin, M. T.: Clonal analysis of cytotoxic and regulatory T cell responses against human melanoma. J. Exp. Med., 169:1961, 1989.
178. Mukherji, B., Guha, A., Loomis, R., and Ergin, M. T.: Cell-mediated amplification and down regulation of cytotoxic immune response against autologous human cancer. J. Immunol., 138:1987, 1987.
179. Mukherji, B., Nashed, A. L., Guha, A., and Ergin, M. T.: Regulation of cellular immune response against autologous human melanoma. II. Mechanism of induction and specificity of suppression. J. Immunol., 136:1893, 1986.
180. Mukherji, B., Wilhelm, S. A., Guha, A., and Ergin, M. T.: Regulation of cellular immune response against autologous human melanoma. I. Evidence for cell-mediated suppression of in vitro cytotoxic immune response. J. Immunol., 136:1888, 1986.
181. Nadler, L. M., Breitmeyer, J., Coral, F., Spector, N., and Schlossman, S.: Anti-B4 blocked ricin immunotherapy for patients with B cell malignancies: Results of bolus and constant infusion phase I trials. Proceedings of the Second International Symposium on Immunotoxins, Orlando, 1990, p. 58.
182. Nathan, C. F., Murray, H. W., and Cohn, Z. A.: The macrophage as an effector cell. N. Engl. J. Med., 303:622, 1980.
183. Nauts, H. C.: Beneficial effects of acute concurrent infection, inflammation, fever or immunotherapy (bacterial toxins) on ovarian and uterine cancer. Cancer Res. Inst. Monog., 17:3, 1977.
184. Nepom, G. T., and Hellström, K. E.: Anti-idiotypic antibodies and the induction of specific tumor immunity. Cancer Metastatis Rev. 6:489, 1987.
185. Nitta, T., Oksenberg, J. R., Rao, N. A., and Steinmam, L.: Predominant expression of T cell receptor $V_\alpha 7$ in tumor-infiltrating lymphocytes of uveal melanoma. Science, 249:672, 1990.
186. North, R. J.: Down-regulation of the antitumor immune response. Adv. Cancer Res., 45:1, 1985.
187. North, R. J., DiGiacomo, A., and Dye, E. S.: Suppression of antitumor immunity. *In* Tumor Immunology—Mechanisms, Diagnosis, Therapy. Edited by W. den Otter, and E. J. Ruitenberg. New York, Elsevier Science Publishers, 1987, p. 125.
188. Oettgen, H. F., and Old, L. J.: The history of cancer immunotherapy. *In* Biologic Therapy of Cancer. Edited by V. T. DeVita, Jr., S. Hellman, and S. A. Rosenberg. Philadelphia, J. B. Lippincott Co., 1991, p. 87.
189. O'Garra, A., Umland, S., de France, T., and Christiansen, J.: 'B-cell factors' are pleiotropic. Immunol. Today, 9:45, 1988.
190. Ohanian, S. H., and Schlager, S. I.: Humoral immune killing of nucleated cells: Mechanisms of complement-mediated attack and target defense. Crit. Rev. Immunol., 1:165, 1981.
191. Ojcius, D. M., Zheng, L. M., Sphicas, E. C., Zychlinsky, A., and Young, J. D.: Subcellular localization of perforin and serin esterase in lymphokine-activated killer cells and cytotoxic T cells by immunogold labeling. J. Immunol., 146:4427, 1991.
192. Okubo, M., Sato, N., Wada, Y., Takahashi, S., Torimoto, K., Takahashi, N., Sato, T., Okazaki, M., Asaishi, K., and Kikuchi, K.: Identification by monoclonal antibody of the tumor antigen of a human autologous breast cancer cell that is involved in cytotoxicity by a cytotoxic T-cell clone. Cancer Res., 49:3950, 1989.
193. Old, L. J., Stockert, E., Boyse, E. A., and Kim, J. H.: Antigenic modulation. Loss of TL antigen from cells exposed to TL antibody. Study of the phenomenon in vitro. J. Exp. Med., 127:523, 1968.
194. Old, L. J.: Cancer immunology: The search for specificity—G. H. A. Clowes Memorial Lecture. Cancer Res., 41:361, 1981.
195. Old, L. J., and Boyse, E. A.: Immunology of experimental tumors. Annu. Rev. Med., 15:167, 1964.
196. Oldham, R. K., Wesse, J. L., Herberman, R. B., Perlin, E., Mills, M., Heims, W., Blom, J., Green, D., Reid, J., Bellinger, S., Law, I., McCoy, J. L., Dean, J. H., Cannon, G. B., and Djeu, J.: Immunological monitoring and immunotherapy in carcinoma of the lung. Int. J. Cancer, 18:739, 1976.
197. Oratz, R., Speyer, J. L., Wernz, J. C., Hochster, H., Meyers, M., Mischak, R., and Spitler, L. E.: Antimelanoma monoclonal antibody-ricin a chain immunoconjugate

(XMMME-001-RTA) plus cyclosphamide in the treatment of metastatic malignant melanoma: Results of a phase II trial. J. Biol. Response Mod., 9:345, 1990.
198. Paglieroni, T., and Mackenzie, M. R.: Multiple myeloma: An immunologic profile III: Cytotoxic and suppressive effects of the EA rosette-forming cell. J. Immunol., 124:2563, 1980.
199. Parmiani, G.: An explanation of the variable clinical response to interleukin 2 and LAK cells. Immunol. Today, 11:113, 1990.
200. Pastan, I., Pai, L., Bookman, M., Smith, J., Longo, D., Frankel, A., Willingham, M., and FitzGerald, D. J.: OVB3-PE clinical trial. *In* Biology and Therapy of Ovarian Cancer. Marble Island Resort, Vermont, 1990.
201. Paul, W. E.: The immune system: An introduction. *In* Fundamental Immunology. Second edition. Edited by W. E. Paul. New York, Raven Press, 1989, p. 3.
202. Paxton, R. J., Mooser, G., Pande, H., Lee, T. D., and Shively, J. E.: Sequence analysis of carcinoembryonic antigen: Identification of glycosylation sites and homology with the immunoglobulin supergene family. Proc. Natl. Acad. Sci. USA, 84:920, 1987.
203. Penn, I.: Principles of tumor immunity: Immunocompetence and cancer. *In* Biologic Therapy of Cancer. Edited by V. T. DeVita, Jr., S. Hellman, and S. A. Rosenberg. Philadelphia, J. B. Lippincott Co., 1991, p. 53.
204. Platsoucas, C. D., Galinski, M., Kempin, S., Reich, L., Clarkson, B., and Good, R. A.: Abnormal T lymphocyte subpopulations in patients with chronic B cell lymphocytic leukemia: An analysis by monoclonal antibodies. J. Immunol., 129:2305, 1982.
205. Platsoucas, C. D., Hansen, H. J., Redman, J. R., Berenson, S., Lee, B. J., and Clarkson, B. D.: T-cell imbalances in patients with multiple myeloma: An analysis of monoclonal antibodies. J. Clin. Immunol., 3:227, 1983.
206. Prehn, R. T.: The immune reaction as a stimulator of tumor growth. Science, 176:170, 1972.
207. Prehn, R. T., and Main, J. M.: Immunity to methylcholanthrene-induced sarcomas. J. Natl. Cancer Inst., 18:769, 1957.
208. Quirt, I. C., and Tannock, I. F.: Interleukin-2 for metastatic melanoma: Treating polyuria with insulin? J. Clin. Oncol., 8:1125, 1990.
209. Rapp, F.: Herpes simplex virus type 2 and cervical cancer. *In* Current Problems in Cancer. Vol. 6, No. 4. Edited by R. C. Hickey. Chicago, Year Book Medical Publishers, Inc., 1981, p. 3.
210. Rayner, A. A., Steele, G., Rodrick, M. L., Harte, P. J., Munroe, A. E., Zamcheck, N., and Wilson, R. E.: Application of polyethylene glycol turbidity assay to detection of circulating immune complexes in cancer patients. Am. J. Surg., 141:460, 1981.
211. Reading, C. L.: Elimination of residual tumor cells from autologous bone marrow grafts using monoclonal antibodies. *In* Principles of Cancer Biotherapy. Edited by R. K. Oldham. New York, Raven Press Ltd., 1987, p. 355.
212. Real, F. X., Mattes, M. J., Houghton, A. N., Oettgen, H. F., Lloyd, K. O., and Old, L. J.: Class I (unique) tumor antigens of human melanoma. Identification of a 90,000 dalton cell surface glycoprotein by autologous antibody. J. Exp. Med., 160:1219, 1984.
213. Reth, M., Hombach, J., Wienands, J., Campbell, K. S., Chien, N., Justement, L. B., and Cambier, J. C.: The B-cell antigen receptor complex. Immunol. Today, 12:196, 1991.
214. Ritts, R. E., Jr.: Immune status and role of immunotherapy: Overview. *In* Lung Cancer: Progress in Therapeutic Research and Therapy. Vol. 22. Edited by F. Muggia and M. Rozencweig. New York, Raven Press, 1979, p. 457.
215. Ritts, R. E., Jr., Del Villano, B. C., Go, V. L., Herberman, R. B., Klug, T. L., and Zurawski, V. R., Jr.: Initial clinical evaluation of an immunoradiometric assay for CA-19-9 using the NCI serum bank. Int. J. Cancer, 33:339, 1984.
216. Ritz, J., Pesando, J. M., Notis-McConarty, J., and Schlossman, S. F.: Modulation of human acute lymphoblastic leukemia antigen induced by monoclonal antibody in vitro. J. Immunol., 125:1506, 1980.
217. Robertson, M. J., and Ritz, J.: Biology and clinical relevance of human natural killer cells. Blood, 76:2421, 1990.
218. Robinette, C. D., and Fraumeni, J. F.: Splenectomy and subsequent mortality in veterans of the 1939-45 war. Lancet, 2:127, 1977.
219. Robinson, M. A., and Kindt, T. J.: Major histo-compatibility complex antigens and genes. *In* Fundamental Immunology, Second edition. Edited by W. E. Paul. New York, Raven Press, 1989. p. 489.
220. Roder, J.: Immune response: Killing comes naturally. Curr. Biol., 1:242, 1991.
221. Rooney, C. M., Rowe, M., Wallace, L. E., and Rickinson, A. B.: Epstein-Barr virus-positive Burkitt's lymphoma cells not recognized by virus-specific T-cell surveillance. Nature, 317:629, 1985.
222. Rosenberg, S. A.: Adoptive immunotherapy of cancer: Accomplishments and prospects. Cancer Treat. Rep., 68:233, 1984.
223. Rosenberg, S. A.: Adoptive cellular therapy: Clinical applications. *In* Biologic Therapy of Cancer. Edited by V. T. DeVita, Jr., S. Hellman, and S. A. Rosenberg. Philadelphia, J. B. Lippincott Co., 1991, p. 214.
224. Rosenberg, S. A., Aebersold, P., Cornetta, K., Kasid, A., Morgan, R. A., Moen, R., Karson, E. M., Lotze, M. T., Yang, J. C., Topalian, S. L., Merino, M. J., Culver, K., Miller, A. D., Blaese, R. M., and Anderson, W. F.: Gene transfer into humans-immunotherapy of patients with advanced melanoma, using tumor-infiltrating lymphocytes modified by retroviral gene transduction. N. Engl. J. Med., 323:570, 1990.
225. Rosenberg, S. A., Lotze, M. T., Muul, L. M., Chang, A. E., Avis, F. P., Leitman, S., Linehan, W. M., Robertson, C. N., Lee, R. E., Rubin, J. T., Seipp, C. A., Simpson, C. G., and White, D. E.: A progress report on the treatment of 157 patients with advanced cancer using lymphokine-activated killer cells and interleukin-2 or high-dose interleukin-2 alone. N. Engl. J. Med., 316:889, 1987.
226. Rosenberg, S. A., Longo, D. L., and Lotze, M. T.: Principles and applications of biologic therapy. *In* Cancer Principles and Practice of Oncology. Edited by V. T. DeVita, Jr., S. Hellman and S. A. Rosenberg. Philadelphia, J. B. Lippincott Company, 1989, p. 301.
227. Rosenberg, S. A., Packard, B. S., Aebersold, P. M., Solomon, D., Topalian, S. L., Toy, S. T., Simon, P., Lotze, M. T., Yang, J. C., Seipp, C. A., Simpson, C., Carter, C., Bock, S., Schwartzentruber, D., Wei, J. P., and White, D. E.: Use of tumor-infiltrating lymphocytes and interleukin-2 in the immunotherapy of patients with metastatic melanoma. A preliminary report. N. Engl. J. Med., 319:1676, 1988.
228. Rosenberg, S. A., Spiess, P., and Lafreniere, R.: A new approach to the adoptive immunotherapy of cancer with tumor-infiltrating lymphocytes. Science, 233:1318, 1986.
229. Rosenstein, M., Eberlein, T. J., and Rosenberg, S. A.: Adoptive immunotherapy of established syngeneic sold tumors: Role of T lymphoid subpopulations. J. Immunol., 132:2117, 1984.
230. Rosse, W. F.: Mechanisms of immune destruction: Complement and complement-dependent mechanisms. *In* Clinical Immunohematology: Basic Concepts and Clinical Applications. Boston, Blackwell Scientific Publications, 1990, p. 43.
231. Rudd, C. E.: CD4, CD8 and the TCR-CD3 complex: A novel class of protein-tyrosine kinase receptor. Immunol. Today, 11:400, 1990.
232. Ruddle, N. H.: Tumor necrosis factor and related cytoxins. Immunol. Today, 8:129, 1987.
233. Rudikoff, S.: Principles of tumor immunity: Biology of antibody-mediated response. *In* Biologic Therapy of Cancer. Edited by V. T. DeVita, Jr., S. Hellman and S. A. Rosenberg. Philadelphia, J. B. Lippincott Co., 1991, p. 22.
234. Sawada, Y., Urbanelli, D., Raskova, J., Shenk, T. E., and Raska, K., Jr.: Adenovirus tumor-specific transplantation antigen is a function of the E1A early region. J. Exp. Med., 163:563, 1986.
235. Schreiber, H.: Idiotype network interactions in tumor immunity. Adv. Cancer Res., 41:291, 1984.
236. Schreiber, H., Ward, P. L., Rowley, D. A. and Stauss, H. J.: Unique tumor-specific antigens. Annu. Rev. Immunol., 6:465, 1988.
237. Schreiber, H.: Tumor immunology. *In* Fundamental Immunology. Second edition. Edited by W. E. Paul. New York, Raven Press, 1989, p. 923.
238. Sherman, M. L., Spriggs, D. R., Arthur, K. A., Imamura, K., Frei, E., and Kufe, D. W.: Recombinant human tumor necrosis factor administered as a five-day continuous infusion in cancer patients: Phase I toxicity and effects on lipid metabolism. J. Clin. Oncol., 6:344, 1988.
239. Silverton, E. W., Navia, M. A., and Davies, D. R.: Three-dimensional structure of an intact human immunoglobulin. Proc. Natl. Acad. Sci. USA, 74:5140, 1977.
240. Slade, M. S., Simmons, R. L., Yunis, E., and Greenberg, L. J.: Immunodepression after major surgery in normal patients. Surgery, 78:363, 1975.
241. Slavin, S., and Strober, S.: Induction of allograft tolerance after total lymphoid irradiation (TLI): Development of suppressor cells of the mixed leukocyte reaction (MLR). J. Immunol., 123:942, 1979.
242. Sondel, P. M., Hank, J. A., Kohler, P. C., Sosman, J. A., Weil-Hillman, G., and Fisch, P.: The cellular immunotherapy of cancer: Current and potential uses of interleukin-2. Crit. Rev. Oncol/Hematol., 9:125, 1989.
243. Soper, J. T., Hunter, V. J., Daly, L., Tanner, M., Creasman, W. T., and Bast, R. C., Jr.: Preoperative serum tumor-associated antigen levels in women with pelvic masses. Obstet. Gynecol., 75:249, 1990.
244. Spitler, L. E., del Rio, M., Khentigan, A., Wedel, N. I., Brophy, N. A., Miller, L. L., Harkonen, W. S., Rosendorf, L. L., Lee, H. M., Mischak, R. P., Kawahata, R. T., Stoudemire, J. B., Fradkin, L. B., Bautista, E. E., and Scannon, P. J.: Therapy of patients with malignant melanoma using a monoclonal antimelanoma antibody-ricin A chain immunotoxin. Cancer Res., 47:1717, 1987.
245. Spreafico, F., and Anaclerio, A.: Immunosuppressive agents. *In* Immunopharmacology. Edited by J. W. Hadden, R. G. Coffey, and F. Spreafico. New York, Plenum Medical Book Co., 1977, p. 245.
246. Srivastava, P. K., DeLeo, A. B., and Old, L. J.: Tumor rejection antigens of chemically induced sarcomas of inbred mice. Proc. Natl. Acad. Sci. USA, 83:3407, 1986.
247. Srivastava, P. K., Chen, Y. T., and Old, L. J.: 5'-Structural analysis of genes encoding polymorphic antigens of chemically induced tumors. Proc. Natl. Acad. Sci. USA, 84:3807, 1987.
248. Srivastava, P. K., and Old, L. J.: Individually distinct transplantation antigens of chemically induced mouse tumors. Immunol. Today, 9:78, 1988.
249. Srivastava, P. K., and Old, L. J.: Identification of a human homologue of the murine tumor rejection antigen GP96. Cancer Res., 49:1341, 1989.
250. Stolbach, L., Pitt, A., Gandbhir, L., Dorsett, B., Barber, H., and Ioachim, H.: Ovarian cancer patient antibodies and their relationship to ovarian cancer associated markers. *In* Compendium of Assays for Immunodiagnosis of Human Cancer. Edited by R. B. Herberman. New York, Elsevier North Holland, Inc., 1979, p. 553.
251. Storkus, W. J., Alexander, J., Payne, J. A., Dawson, J. R., and Cresswell, P.: Reversal of natural killing susceptibility in target cells expressing transfected class I HLA genes. Proc. Natl. Acad. Sci. USA, 86:2361, 1989.
252. Storkus, W. J., Howell, D. N., Salter, R. D., Dawson, J. R., and Cresswell, P.: NK susceptibility varies inversely with target cell class I HLA antigen expression. J. Immunol., 138:1657, 1987.
253. Strander, H.: Interferons (IFNs). Adv. Cancer Res., 46:1, 1986.
254. Tada, T., Asano, Y., and Sano, K.: Present understanding of suppressor T-cells. Res. Immunol., 140:291, 1989.
255. Taetle, R., Castagnola, J., Mendelsohn, J.: Mechanisms of growth inhibition by anti-transferrin receptor monoclonal antibodies. Cancer Res., 46:1759, 1986.
256. Takahashi, K., Ono, K., Hirabayashi, Y., and Taniguchi, M.: Escape mechanisms of melanoma from immune system by soluble melanoma antigen. J. Immunol., 140:3244, 1988.
257. Tanaka, K., Yoshioka, T., Bieberich, C., and Jay, G.: Role of the major histocompatibility complex class I antigens in tumor growth and metastasis. Annu. Rev. Immunol., 6:359, 1988.
258. Theofilopoulos, A. N.: Immune complexes in cancer. N. Engl. J. Med., 307:1208, 1982.
259. Thurin, J.: Characterization and molecular biology of tumor-associated antigens. Curr. Opin. Immunol., 2:702, 1990.
260. Topalian, S. L., Solomon, D., and Rosenberg, S. A.: Tumor-specific cytolysis by lymphocytes infiltrating human melanomas. J. Immunol., 142:3714, 1989.
261. Trinchieri, G.: Biology of natural killer cells. Adv. Immunol., 47:187, 1989.
262. Tschopp, J., and Nabholz, M.: Perforin-mediated target cell lysis by cytolytic T lymphocytes. Annu. Rev. Immunol., 8:279, 1990.
263. Turk, J. L., and Parker, D.: The effect of cyclophosphamide on the immune response. J. Immunopharmacol., 1:127, 1979.
264. Twomey, J. J., and Rice, L.: Impact of Hodgkin's disease upon the immune system. Semin. Oncol., 7:114, 1980.
265. Ullrich, S. J., Robinson, E. A., Law, L. W., Willingham, M., and Appella, E.: A mouse tumor-specific transplantation antigen is a heat shock-related protein. Proc. Natl. Acad. Sci. USA, 83:3121, 1986.
266. Urban, J. L., Burton, R. C., Holland, J. M., Kripke, M. L., and Schreiber, H.: Mech-

anisms of syngeneic tumor rejection. Susceptibility of the host-selected progressor variants to various immunological effector cells. J. Exp. Med., 155:557, 1982.

267. Urban, J. L., Kripke, M. L., and Schreiber, H.: Stepwise immunologic selection of antigenic variants during tumor growth. J. Immunol., 137:3036, 1986.

268. Urbanelli, D., Sawada, Y., Raskova, J., Jones, N. C., Shenk, T., and Raska, K., Jr.: C-terminal domain of the adenovirus E1A oncogene product is required for induction of cytotoxic T lymphocytes and tumor-specific transplantation immunity. Virology, 173:607, 1989.

269. Vaage, J.: Nonvirus-associated antigens in virus-induced mouse mammary tumors. Cancer Res., 28:2477, 1968.

270. Vadhan-Raj, S., Cordon-Cardo, C., Carswell, E., Mintzer, D., Dantis, L., Duteau, C., Templeton, M. A., Oettgen, H. F., Old, L. J., and Houghton, A. N.: Phase I trial of a mouse monoclonal antibody against G$_{D3}$ ganglioside in patients with melanoma: Induction of inflammatory responses at tumor sites. J. Clin. Oncol., 6:1636, 1988.

271. van der Burg, M. E., Lammes, F. B., van Putten, W. L., and Stoter, G.: Ovarian cancer: The prognostic value of serum half-life of CA125 during induction chemotherapy. Gynecol. Oncol., 30:307, 1988.

272. Vanky, F., Masucci, M. G., Bejarano, M. T., and Klein, E.: Lysis of tumor biopsy cells by blood lymphocyte subsets of various densities. Autologous and allogeneic studies. Int. J. Cancer, 33:185, 1984.

273. Vanky, F., Wang, P., Patarroyo, M., and Klein, E.: Expression of the adhesion molecule ICAM-1 and major histocompatibility complex class I antigens on human tumor cells is required for their interaction with autologous lymphocytes in vitro. Cancer Immunol. Immunother., 31:19, 1990.

274. Vessella, R. L., and Lange, P. H.: Monitoring of patients with testicular cancer by assays for alpha-fetoprotein and human chorionic gonadotropin. In Manual of Clinical Laboratory Immunology. Third edition. Edited by N. R. Rose, H. Friedman, and J. L. Fahey. Washington, D. C., American Society for Microbiology, 1986, p. 810.

275. Vijayasaradhi, S., and Houghton, A. N.: Purification of an autoantigenic 75-kDa human melanosomal glycoprotein. Int. J. Cancer, 47:298, 1991.

276. Vlock, D. R.: Immune complexes and malignancy. In Immunodiagnosis of Cancer, 2nd edition. Edited by R. B. Herberman, and D. W. Mercer. New York, Marcel Dekker, Inc., 1990, p. 555.

277. Vose, B. M., and Howell, A.: Cultured human antitumour T cells and their potential for therapy. In Basic and Clinical Tumor Immunology. Edited by R. B. Herberman. Boston, Martinus Nijhoff Publishers, 1983, p. 129.

278. Wadler, S., Schwartz, E. L., Goldman, M., Lyver, A., Rader, M., Zimmerman, M., Itri, L., Weinberg, V., and Wiernik, P. H.: Flurouracil and recombinant alfa-2a-interferon: An active regimen against advanced colorectal carcinoma. Comment in: J. Clin. Oncol., 7:1764, 1989.; J. Clin. Oncol., 7:1769, 1989.

279. Waldmann, T. A., Bull, J. M., Bruce, R. M., Broder, S., Jost, M. C., Balestra, S. T., and Suer, M. E.: Serum immunoglobulin E levels in patients with neoplastic disease. J. Immunol., 113:379, 1974.

280. Wasserman, R. L., and Capra, J. D.: Immunoglobulins. In The Glycoconjugates.

Mammalian Glycoproteins and Glycolipids. Edited by M. I. Horowitz and W. Pigman. New York, Academic Press, 1977, p. 323.

281. Weed, R. I.: Exaggerated delayed hypersensitivity to mosquito bites in chronic lymphocytic leukemia. Blood, 26:257, 1965.

282. Weiss, A.: Structure and function of the T cell antigen receptor. J. Clin. Invest., 86:1015, 1990.

283. Weiss, R. B.: Hypersensitivity reactions to cancer chemotherapy. Semin. Oncol., 9:5, 1982.

284. West, W. H., Tauer, K. W., Yannelli, J. R., Marshall, G. D., Orr, D. W., Thurman, G. B., and Oldham, R. K.: Constant-infusion recombinant interleukin-2 in adoptive immunotherapy of advanced cancer. N. Engl. J. Med., 316:898, 1987.

285. Wettendorff, M., Iliopoulos, D., Tempero, M., Kay, D., DeFreitas, E., Koprowski, H., and Herlyn, D.: Idiotypic cascades in cancer patients treated with monoclonal antibody CO17-1A. Proc. Natl. Acad. Sci. USA, 86:3787, 1989.

286. Whiteside, T. L., and Herberman, R. B.: Short analytical review: The role of natural killer cells in human disease. Clin. Immunol. Immunopathol., 53:1, 1989.

287. Wunderlich, J. R., and Hodes, R. J.: Principles of tumor immunity: Biology of cellular immune response. In Biologic Therapy of Cancer. Edited by V. T. DeVita, Jr., S. Hellman and S. A. Rosenberg. Philadelphia, J. B. Lippincott Co., 1991, p. 3.

288. Yajima, H., Noda, T., de Villiers, E. M., Yajima, A., Yamamoto, K., Noda, K., and Ito, Y.: Isolation of a new type of human papillomavirus (HPV52B) with a transforming activity from cervical cancer tissue. Cancer Res., 48:7164, 1988.

289. Yamaguchi, H., Furukawa, K., Fortunato, S. R., Livingston, P. O., Lloyd, K. O., Oettgen, H. F., and Old, L. J.: Cell-surface antigens of melanoma recognized by human monoclonal antibodies. Proc. Natl. Acad. Sci. USA, 84:2416, 1987.

290. Yang, J. C. and Rosenberg, S. A.: Adoptive cellular therapy: Preclinical studies. In Biologic Therapy of Cancer. Edited by V. T. DeVita, Jr., S. Hellman, and S. A. Rosenberg. Philadelphia, J. B. Lippincott Co., 1991, p. 197.

291. Young, J. D.-E., and Liu, C.-C.: Multiple mechanisms of lymphocyte-mediated killing. Immunol. Today, 9:140, 1988.

292. Young, L. H. Y., Lui, C.-C., Joag, S., Rafii, S., and Young, J. D.-E.: How lymphocytes kill. Annu. Rev. Med., 41:45, 1990.

293. Zamcheck, N., Steele, G., Thomas, P., and Mayer, R. J.: Use of carcinoembryonic antigen in monitoring of patients. In Manual of Clinical Laboratory Immunology, 3rd edition. Edited by N. R. Rose, H. Friedman, and J. L. Fahey. Washington, D. C., American Society for Microbiology, 1986, p. 802.

294. Zola, H.: The surface antigens of human B lymphocytes. Immunol. Today, 8:308, 1987.

295. Zurawski, V. R., Jr., Orjaseter, H., Andersen, A., and Jellum E.: Elevated serum CA 125 levels prior to diagnosis of ovarian neoplasia: Relevance for early detection of ovarian cancer. Int. J. Cancer, 42:677, 1988.

296. Zurawski, V. R., Jr., Sjovall, K., Schoenfeld, D. A., Broderick, S. F., Hall, P., Bast, R. C., Jr., Eklund, G., Mattsson, B., Connor, R. J., Eng, D., Prorok, P. C., Knapp, R. C., and Einhorn, N.: Prospective evaluation of serum CA 125 levels in a normal population, Phase I: The specificities of single and serial determinations in testing for ovarian cancer. Gynecol. Oncol., 36:299, 1990.

III

Cancer Etiology

III-1

Genetic Predisposition to Cancer

B. A. J. Ponder

Introduction

Cancer as a Genetic Disease

Several steps are needed to turn a normal cell into a cancer cell. Most, if not all, of these involve mutational change. Cancer is, therefore, a genetic disease at the level of the somatic cell. Cancer may also be in some cases a genetic disease at the level of the germline. This chapter will consider the inherited contribution to cancer incidence, its importance and its investigation.

Inherited predisposition to cancer is potentially important for three reasons: 1) Individuals who are predisposed are a high-risk population who may benefit from efforts at prevention, or from early diagnosis and treatment. 2) The existence of genetic predisposition may provide a means to study the genetic steps of carcinogenesis. Most, if not all, cancers that result from inherited predisposition have a similar non-heritable counterpart; and in the cases so far studied, heritable and non-heritable cases are genetically similar. Study of the uncommon familial cases may therefore improve our understanding of the steps in development of cancers in general. 3) In some cases, genetic predisposition to cancer is accompanied by abnormalities in development and in growth control, both in the tissue from which the cancer will arise, and elsewhere. Many of the genes which, when mutated, are "cancer genes," may have important normal functions in growth and development. Cancer families are a way in which these genes are revealed and can be identified.

How Much of Cancer Is Due To Inherited Predisposition?

There is no clear answer to this question. In each case, inherited predisposition, environmental exposure and (since we are dealing with the accumulation of a series of stochastic events) chance will interact in different degrees. The question can be rephrased to ask in which cancers there is sufficiently strong inherited predisposition to be of practical significance for prevention or treatment.[1] The answer to this is also still unclear. Perhaps less than 1% of cancers occur in the "inherited cancer syndromes," described below; and a further 5–10% in recognizable familial clusters of the common cancers that probably have a genetic basis: but it will be argued below that important inherited predisposition may be much more extensive than this.

The Recognition of Inherited Predisposition

Because each heritable cancer has a histologically similar non-heritable counterpart, it can be difficult or impossible in an individual case to know whether a cancer is due to inherited predisposition or not.[54] Until the predisposing mutations themselves can be identified, the clues to inherited predisposition are: 1) in a few rare syndromes, a "marker phenotype"—for example, the multiple intestinal polyps characteristic of the inherited cancer syndrome familial polyposis (FAP) (Figure III-1-1); and 2) the clinical and family history[17]— if the cancer is rare, the occurrence of several cases in the family, or multiple primaries in the individual, is noticeable and probably significant. However, if the cancer is common—like breast cancer—the significance of several cases in a family may be much more difficult to determine. This point will be discussed further below in relation to breast and ovarian cancer (see Familial Cancers).

A classification of inherited predisposition to cancer for practical use can be based, not on biological mechanisms (which are still obscure) but on the ease of recognition, using marker phenotype and family clustering. Such a classification is given in Table III-1-1. The features of each group will be described in the following sections.

Inherited Cancer Syndromes

General Description

The inherited cancer syndromes[25,31,47] include all those cancers where a genetic effect is clearly apparent. Together they probably account for less than 1% of cancer incidence. The principal features of several of the syndromes are listed in Table III-1-2.

Recognition. Most cases of one of the inherited cancer syndromes can be recognized by a characteristic marker phenotype (Table III-1-2, Figure III-1-1A). Of course, a striking family history (Figure III-1-1B) may be the first clue: but it is important to realize that in many cases such a history is

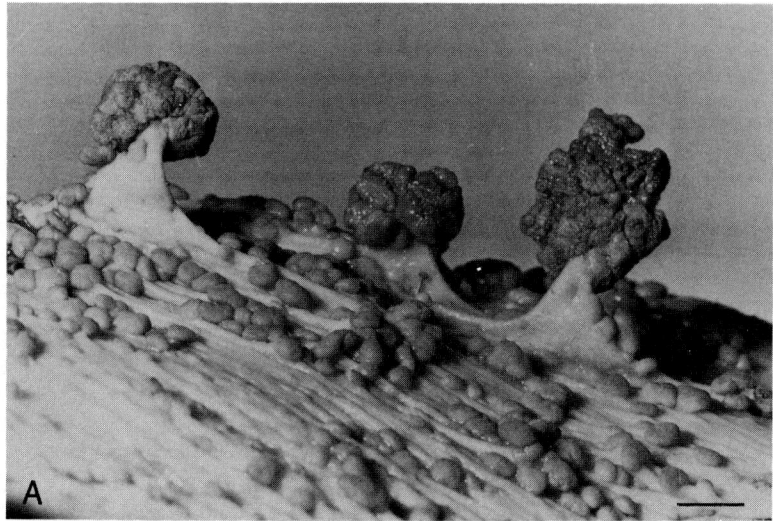

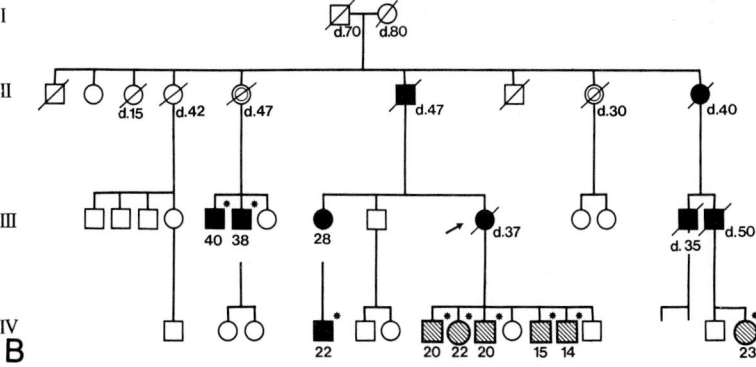

Figure III-1-1. A) Polyps in colon of an individual with familial polyposis. Two large polyps and a smaller one are shown arising from the surface of the colonic epithelium. Bar = 5 mm. (Photograph provided by the ICRF Colorectal Cancer Unit, St. Mark's Hospital). B) Pedigree of a family with familial polyposis of the colon (FAP).[8] The family was recognized when the individual in generation III (arrowed) presented with colonic cancer and was found to have multiple colonic polyps. Subsequently, other members of the family (indicated by asterisk) have been screened by sigmoidoscopy. Three were found to already have cancer; five siblings and a cousin in generation IV had polyps and were treated by prophylactic colectomy.

■ ● = colonic cancer
⚫ d37 = died age 37;
   ● = cancer diagnosed age 28
28
◎ = colonic cancer by history
▨ ⬨ = polyps, no cancer, with age
20 22   at diagnosis

Table III-1-1. Classification of Genetic Predisposition to Cancer by Strength of Familial Clustering

Class	Examples
Inherited cancer syndromes	Familial polyposis
	Multiple endocrine neoplasia types 1 and 2
	von Hippel-Lindau syndrome.
Familial clusters of cancer	Breast cancer
	Ovarian cancer
	Non-polyposis colorectal cancer
Genetic predisposition without evident familial clustering (still hypothetical)	Metabolic polymorphisms determining response to exogenous or endogenous carcinogens.

lacking, either because it has not been carefully sought, or because the patient is a new mutation, or the gene was not expressed in the parents ("incomplete penetrance").

In some cases (e.g., the polyps in FAP, C-cell hyperplasia in MEN 2) the marker phenotype is the result of a growth abnormality in the target tissue from which the cancer will arise, and can be regarded as a pre-neoplastic lesion. In other cases (e.g., the multiple cysts of abdominal organs in Von Hippel-Lindau syndrome, the ganglioneuromatosis of the intestine in MEN 2B, the osteomas in FAP), the phenotype results from developmental defects in tissues remote from

the cancer, and presumably reflects a pleiotropic effect of the inherited mutation. The diversity of tissues and effects (Table III-1-2) is puzzling because in most cases it does not conform to current ideas of lineage or physiological relationships.

In a few cases, for example retinoblastoma, there is no characteristic marker phenotype. In the case of retinoblastoma, the heritable form is usually easily recognized because the tumor is rare. Two cases in close relatives, or bilateral tumors in one individual, are therefore strong evidence of genetic predisposition. Difficulty arises when an individual has one tumor, and no family history: the majority of these are truly non-heritable, but a small number will be heritable cases who have by chance developed only one tumor, and who are new mutation cases—that is, the start of a new family. Because the retinoblastoma gene has been cloned, it is possible to detect the germline mutation in some of these cases and so prove that they are of the heritable type:[73] but in other syndromes where the gene has not been cloned, distinction between a truly non-heritable case and an isolated new mutation case in the absence of a marker phenotype is impossible.

Characteristic Features of the Inherited Cancer Syndromes

These will be illustrated mainly by reference to familial adenomatous polyposis (FAP).[6–8,29] The similar features of

Table III-1-2. Examples of Inherited Cancer Syndromes

Syndrome	Tissues Involved by Tumor[a]	Associated phenotype[b]	
		Associated with Tumor	In Other Tissues
Familial adenomatous polyposis (FAP)[8]	Colon, small intestine, thyroid, liver	Colonic polyps	Osteomas of jaw, hypertrophy of retinal pigment epithelium,[12] fibroblast proliferation of body wall (desmoid tumors), extra dentition.
Multiple endocrine neoplasia type 1 (MEN 1)[3]	Pituitary, parathyroid, pancreatic islets, adrenal cortex	Hyperplasia of target cells	—
Multiple endocrine neoplasia type 2 (MEN 2)[70]	Thyroid C-cells, adrenal medulla, parathyroid	Hyperplasia	(MEN type 2B only)[16] neuromas of lips, disordered autonomic ganglion plexus in viscera, skeletal abnormalities.
von Hippel-Lindau syndrome[27]	Kidney, haemangioblastoma of cerebellum, adrenal medulla	—	Angiomas of retina, multiple cysts of internal organs.
Basal cell nevus syndrome[25,66]	Skin, brain, (medulloblastoma)	—	Radiation sensitivity, skeletal abnormalities, plantar and palmar skin pits, jaw cysts, hamartoma of viscera.
Retinoblastoma	Retina, bone, (osteosarcoma), several epithelia, melanocytes[60]	—	
Neurofibromatosis type 1 (NF-1)[28,43]	Schwann cell, glia, adrenal medulla	Plexiform neurofibroma	Multiple, including: cafe au lait spots, axillary freckling, cutaneous neurofibroma, scoliosis, learning difficulties, short stature.
Neurofibromatosis type 2 (NF-2)[43]	Schwann cells of VIII cranial n. meninges	—	Occasional cutaneous neurofibroma, cafe au lait spots.

[a]Principal tumors underlined
[b]Note that while the range of abnormalities shown may reflect the effects of mutation of a single gene, it is not excluded that in some cases several genes may be involved in causing the phenotype

other inherited cancer syndromes are summarized in Table III-1-2.

The Pattern of Inheritance Is Autosomal Dominant. In FAP, as in all of the inherited cancer syndromes so far recognized, the pattern of cancers in the family is that expected of an autosomal dominant predisposing gene (Figure III-1-1b). In a few special cases, e.g., glomus tumors[71] and Beckwith-Wiedemann syndrome,[49] the pattern is modified according to the sex of the parent who transmitted the gene (see Genomic Imprinting below).

Predisposition Is Site-Specific. Predisposition is not to cancers in general, but to cancers of specific sites (Table III-1-2). In FAP, for example, the cancers are, in addition to colorectal carcinoma, carcinoma of the ampulla of Vater, hepatoblastoma and thyroid tumors. It is likely that many associations are still unrecognized; and others that are claimed are disputed. For example, very large studies of retinoblastoma families have recently revealed the previously unsuspected association of several common epithelial cancers with this tumor.[62]

There May Be Large Variations in Expression of the Syndrome

Variation may be in the spectrum of tumors and other phenotypic abnormalities ("expressivity"), or in the probability that each will be manifest by a certain age ("penetrance"). Two possibilities can be distinguished: clinically distinct syndromes which "breed true" in families and so are presumably due to different predisposing mutations (either at different loci, or different mutant alleles at the same locus);

and variation within a family, which cannot usually be due to differences in the predisposing mutation but must be due to some combination of modifying genes, environment, and chance.

Clinical Variation of Familial Colorectal Cancer. Several distinct syndromes are recognized (Table III-1-3).[1,20,48] In the group associated with adenomatous polyps, the traditional distinction between "polyposis" and "non-polyposis" syndromes is misleading, because the difference is in numbers of polyps rather than their absence in the non-polyposis group. The extent to which the different clinical syndromes are reflected in genetic differences is still unclear. Thus, FAP is defined genetically by linkage of the predisposing gene to a locus on chromosome 5q21.[6] Linkage to the Kidd blood group on chromosome 18 has been suggested for "non-polyposis" colorectal cancer families[38]—although this requires confirmation. Recently, however, a family with a pattern of dominantly inherited colonic cancer associated, on average, with numbers of polyps intermediate between those typically seen in FAP and in "cancer family syndrome" was reported also to show linkage to the FAP locus on 5q.[34] There may therefore be a spectrum of familial colorectal cancers associated with adenomatous polyps,[21] and with risk of other cancers to varying degree, that are due to different mutant alleles at the FAP locus. Further linkage studies in large colorectal cancer families, and characterization of mutant alleles at the FAP locus, will be needed to resolve this. A similar situation is seen in the multiple endocrine neoplasia type 2 (MEN 2) syndrome[70] where three clinically distinct

Table III-1-3. Some Syndromes Associated with Inherited Risk of Colonic Cancer

Associated with Adenomatous Polyps		Hamartomatous
Polyposis	Familial adenomatous polyposis (FAP) Turcot syndrome (Colorectal cancer, brain tumors, skin lesions).	Peutz-Jeghers Juvenile polyposis Cowden Gorlin
Non-polyposis	Cancer family syndrome (Lynch type II: colorectal plus cancer of endometrium, breast and ovary). Site specific colonic cancer Muir-Torre syndrome (cancer at multiple sites plus keratoacanthomas and sebaceous adenomas of face).	

For reviews see references 1, 20, 48

varieties breed true, but map to the same region of chromosome 10, suggesting they may be allelic.

Variation in Expression Within Single Families. Some families with typical FAP (colorectal carcinoma, multiple intestinal polyps) show the additional features of pancreatic ampullary tumors, desmoid tumors, and mandibular osteomas (Table III-1-2). This was originally delineated as a separate clinical variety, Gardner's syndrome.[21] Gardner's syndrome families map to the FAP locus on chromosome 5, so it seemed that FAP and Gardner's syndrome might be allelic; but now it is clear that the so-called Gardner's phenotype occurs to a greater or lesser degree in most FAP families.[38,48] This suggests that Gardner's syndrome is not a genetically distinct variant, but that the range of expression is the result of modifying influences (as yet undefined) acting on the expression of the same FAP mutation within a single family.

Variation in Penetrance Within and Between Families. The proportion of FAP gene carriers who manifest colorectal polyps increases with age.[48] Even by age 25, about 10% of carriers do not have detectable polyps (Figure III-1-2). Similarly, 10% of MEN 2A gene carriers are still not detected by a sensitive biochemical screening test at age 25, and 40% will not have developed clinically significant disease by age 70.[18] This variation may also be due to modifying genes, environmental, or chance effects; and to dissect these will be difficult. From a clinical standpoint, data about the age-related expression of marker phenotypes (or cancers) is important in family screening, because it is needed to estimate the probability that a family member with a negative screen or with apparently unaffected parents at a given age may still be a gene carrier[55] (see below).

If it were possible to predict the penetrance or expression of the predisposing gene in an individual family member, this would also have obvious application in clinical management. Unfortunately, this will not be possible until the causes of the variation are better understood.

Familial Cancers[17,30,31,54,67]

General Description

Of more general importance than the uncommon inherited cancer syndromes, this group comprises families that are at very high risk of a common cancer, such as breast, colon, or ovary. The coincidence of several cases in a single family has been reported at some time for cancers at almost all sites. There are two questions: is the clustering significant,

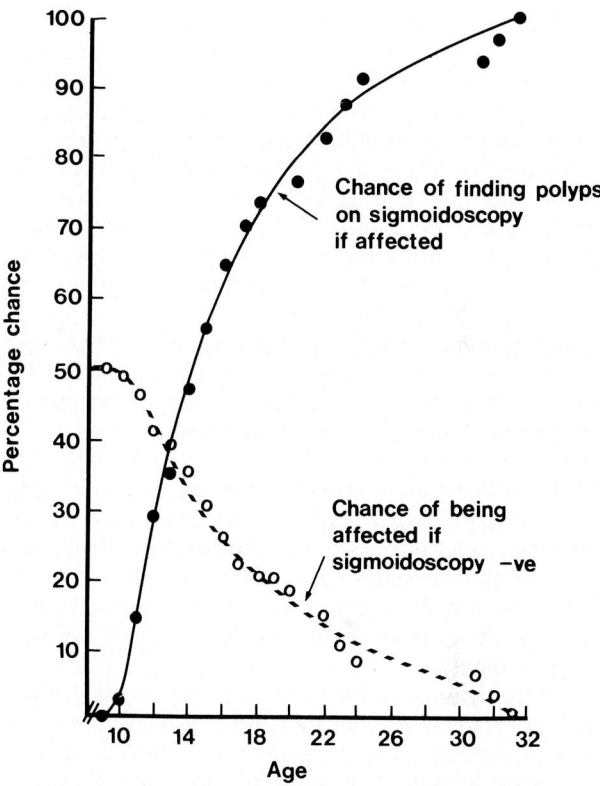

Figure III-1-2. Age at detection of polyps in a family member at risk of familial adenomatous polyposis (FAP). The chance of being affected is 50% at birth because FAP is dominantly inherited. (From Murday and Slack.[48])

and if so, is the pattern of occurrence of the cancers in the families best explained on a genetic or other basis? Final proof of genetic predisposition will come from demonstration of genetic linkage or of the inheritance of the germline mutation in affected families. Meanwhile, because in cancer families there are no marker phenotypes comparable to those in the inherited cancer syndromes, estimates of the probability of inherited predisposition in each family must be based on the strength and pattern of the familial association in each case.

Evidence that Familial Clustering of Cancers Is Significant

Most case reports of familial clusters are clinical anecdotes. Although some are very striking, there is always the question of a chance association. Solid evidence for significant familial clustering must come from truly population-based studies—that is, studies in which cases are initially ascertained in an unselected manner and without regard to their family history.[17]

The usual measure of familial clustering is the relative risk of cancer in the family members (either all first-degree relatives, or specified relatives, usually siblings) of an individual with cancer, compared to the risk in the population in general. The analysis may be stratified to look at groups who might be expected to be at higher risk, for example, the relatives of cases diagnosed before the age of 50, or relatives in a family where there are already two individuals affected.

For most common cancers, relative risks to siblings are of the order of 2 to 3 (Table III-1-4). Familial clustering of cancers is therefore real, but this does not tell us whether the clustering is of genetic origin. Nor does it tell us how the risk is distributed between individuals, because the relative risk is estimated as an average over the whole population. The same overall risk might in principle result either from a common gene which confers a slight increase in risk to many people, or from a rare gene with a very strong effect in a few. These questions can be tackled by segregation analysis.

Segregation Analysis. Segregation analysis[19,74] attempts to find the most likely explanation for an observed familial clustering of cancer by analysis of the pattern of occurrence of the cancer in the families of a large series of cases, ascertained without knowledge of family history. Typically, the analysis will give the relative likelihood of dominant, recessive or polygenic genetic predisposition, environmental predisposition, or mixed models incorporating genetic and environmental components. In the case of a genetic model, an estimate will be made of the gene frequency in the population, the penetrance, and the risk to gene carriers versus non-gene carriers.

Almost all analyses of the common cancers (breast, ovary, and colon) agree that the most likely explanation for the observed familial clustering is dominant predisposition by an uncommon gene of strong effect which affects a small number of families.[10,13,56,74] This conclusion is probably broadly correct, although segregation analysis alone can seldom provide conclusive evidence. Moreover, the detailed results of segregation analysis, especially on small data sets, depend

so much on the assumptions that are made that they should be treated with some caution. In particular, an additional contribution of a common gene of weaker effect may be difficult to resolve. Mathematical accounts of segregation analysis can be found in standard texts.[19]

Characteristic Features of Familial Cancers

The familial cancers resemble the inherited cancer syndromes in many of their features.

Predisposition Is Site-Specific, But There Is Variation Between and Within Families. Clinical observation of pedigrees, as well as population-based estimates of relative risks to siblings, indicate that specific cancers are associated in familial clusters. Some of these form well-known syndromes, for example, site-specific colonic cancer (Lynch type I) and "family cancer syndrome" (Lynch type II): colorectal, uterine, ovarian, gastric and breast.[38,39] Neither the boundaries between different syndromes nor the cancers which belong to each one are, however, always clear. For example, breast and ovarian cancer are often associated, but the clinical spectrum runs from "site specific" breast cancer, through "breast-ovarian" families with each cancer in different proportions, to "site specific" ovarian cancer (Figure III-1-3a,b,c).[40,64] There may be genetically determined differences in age at onset of breast cancer in different families. The Li-Fraumeni (or SBLA—sarcoma, breast, lung, adrenal) syndrome[35] is easy to recognize in its most florid form, which is quite uncommon, but there are many more families in which a woman with young-onset breast cancer has a single relative with a sarcoma or a brain tumor—do they fit? Recently, some typical Li-Fraumeni families have been shown to have germline mutations at the p53 locus,[42] and predisposition in some extensive families with young onset breast cancer has been shown to be linked to a locus on chromosome 17q.[23a] Findings such as this will be the key to genetic classification of these families. Genetic markers will also resolve the question of which cancers should be regarded as part of a syndrome, because it will be possible to compare their incidence in known gene carriers with that in the general population; and within a single family, markers will indicate which cancers can be attributed to inherited predisposition, and which are merely phenocopies (Figure III-1-4).

Inherited Predisposition Without Obvious Family Clustering

General Features

So far, we have considered only cases in which inherited predisposition is strong enough to cause obvious family clustering of cancer. However, it can easily be shown that with a slight reduction in the penetrance of the predisposing gene—that is, if only a few gene carriers actually develop cancer—there can still be very significant predisposition even though there are seldom enough close relatives actually affected to cause an obvious family cluster.[53] Thus a dominent gene that results in cancer at a specific site in only 1 in 10 of gene carriers will hardly cause any extended family clustering, because the risk is only $\frac{1}{2}$ times $\frac{1}{10} = \frac{1}{20}$ in each of the close relatives, and (on average) less in more distant relatives who are less likely to have the gene. Even so, over a

Table III-1-4. Summary of Estimates of Relative Risks of the Same Cancer in First Degree Relatives of Individuals Affected by Various Common Cancers

Site	Relative risk
Breast[13]	2.2
Ovary[56,63]	3
Endometrium[64]	2.7
Melanoma[51]	2.5
Lung[50]	2.7
Colon[37]	3.4
Stomach[41]	2.6

Adapted from Easton and Peto.[17] The references given are mostly to the most recent substantial study: others are given in reference 17

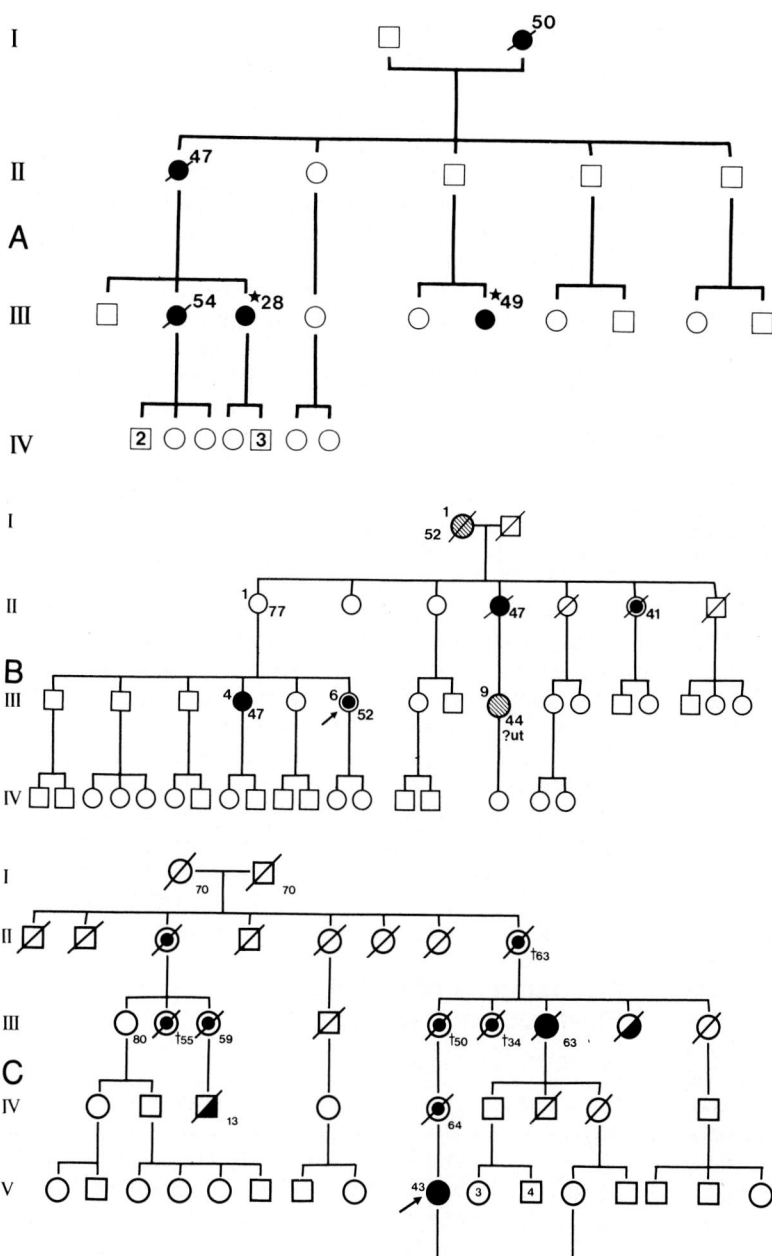

Figure III-1-3. Pedigrees to illustrate different types of "breast-ovarian cancer family." Each was seen within the past 5 years in the author's familial cancer clinic.

a) Site-specific breast cancer. Five family members have breast cancer, two of them (asterisked) have bilateral primary cancers.
●⁴⁹ = breast cancer, with age at diagnosis
③ = 3 sons.

b) 'Breast-ovarian' family. There are 2 cases of breast cancer and 2 of ovarian cancer, all at a fairly young age. Note that II-1 (now aged 77) is an obligatory gene carrier. III-9 has probable endometrial cancer: it is difficult to know whether this is significant and what is the risk of this cancer to other family members. I-1 had probable ovarian cancer and died age 52.
● = breast cancer
◉ = ovarian cancer, with ages at diagnosis.

c) Ovarian predominant family. There are 7 cases of ovarian cancer, and 2 (at ages 43 and 63) of breast cancer. Note the 13 year old boy in generation IV who had a brain tumor: it is impossible to know whether this was related to the presumed predisposing gene.
◎ = ovarian cancer
● = breast cancer; with ages at diagnosis (where known) or death (†)
◪◕ = other cancer.

range of plausible assumptions about gene frequency and relative risk in gene carriers, such a gene can lead to a remarkable concentration of risk in a predisposed minority of the population.[53] For example, if the gene confers a 100-fold increase in risk, from 1 in 1000 to 1 in 10, and it has a frequency in the population of 0.1, it will result in an overall incidence of the cancer of 1 in 50. Of the cases, however, 95% will be concentrated in the 19% of the population who have the predisposing gene. (The frequency distribution of alleles is given by the Hardy-Weinberg equilibrium p^2; $2pq$; q^2. If the frequency of the predisposing allele $q = 0.1$, then the wild-type gene frequency $p = 0.9$; 81% of the population

will be homozygous pp, 18% heterozygous, and 1% homozygous qq). The relative risk of cancer to siblings of a patient with the cancer (the usual measure of familial clustering) will be about 2.9-fold—roughly the value which is, in fact, found for many of the common cancers (Table III-1-4). In ovarian cancer the relative risk to siblings is around 3-fold, but much of this risk is probably accounted for by a minority of families at very high risk—and many of them are recognizable as multiple case families. In lung cancer, where by contrast family clusters are rare or absent, a similar relative risk to siblings is presumably the result of a more even distribution of risk among the population by a more common gene of

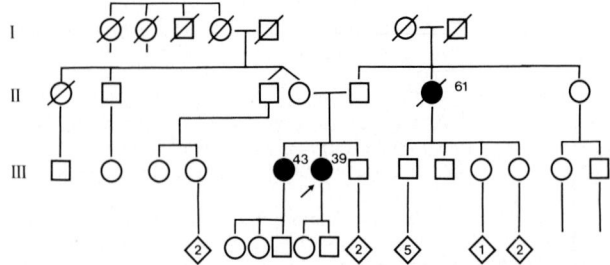

Figure III-1-4. The problems of incomplete penetrance and of phenocopies. There are 3 cases of breast cancer in the family, diagnosed at ages 39, 43 and 61. Two sisters affected at ages 39 and 43 are unlikely to be a coincidence: but if they are affected because of a dominant predisposing gene (see text), why is the family history not more extensive? A possible answer is incomplete penetrance of the gene, which would imply that other family members do carry the gene, but have not expressed it. A possible gene carrier is the aunt in generation II who developed breast cancer 61. If so, this would imply that inheritance is through the paternal side of the family, with implications for the risk to her daughters and other family members. But it is also possible that this individual is a phenocopy—that is, she developed breast cancer independently of the predisposing gene (● = breast cancer; ⬦̇ = 5 children, sex unspecified.)

less effect. Similar effects, in terms of concentration of cancer risk in a minority of the population, are predicted for recessive models.[53]

The Problem: How Can Such Predisposition Be Recognized?

These calculations suggest that familial cancers may be only the tip of the iceberg of inherited predisposition. In public health terms, the effects of common genes of weaker effect may be much more significant. The problem is to recognize the effects and to find the genes. In the inherited cancer syndromes and the familial cancers, recognition is provided by familial clusters and by marker phenotypes. The genes can be sought empirically, with no previous knowledge of what they are, by the methods of genetic linkage which exploit the occurrence of several cases in a family (see below). In the absence of family clustering or of obvious marker phenotypes, one has to start with candidate genes—that is, by guessing which genes may be involved, and testing them. If a sufficient number of pairs of affected siblings can be found, a modified form of genetic linkage may possibly be used;[5] but more often, the approach must be by case-control studies of a genetic variant of the candidate gene or its associated phenotype in subjects with and without cancer.

Possible Candidate Genes. In principle, almost any type of mechanism might be associated with a predisposing gene of low penetrance (see Mechanisms below); but in practice that which has attracted most interest is genetic polymorphisms which might affect interaction with potential environmental carcinogens.[2,4,22,23,45,68,75]

It is well known that individuals differ in metabolism of exogenous chemicals used as drugs, and there seems no reason to expect it will be any different for chemical carcinogens. Attention has therefore focused on the genes of the cytochrome P450 system,[2,4,22,23,45,75,76] which is involved in

metabolism of a variety of compounds, including polycyclic hydrocarbons and endogenous and exogenous steroid hormones; and on other enzymes involved in conjugation and detoxification and which are known to exhibit genetic variation, such as acetylating enzymes.[4] There is recent evidence, not yet conclusive, that variation at the locus for cytochrome P450 CYP1A1 may determine lung cancer risk in cigarette smokers;[23] and that acetylator status is associated with bladder cancer risk.[4]

Heterozygotes for the gene defects of the recessive DNA repair syndromes may be another group in this category. Although still controversial, there is increasing evidence from studies of the relatives of cases that heterozygotes for the recessive disorder AT (ataxia-telangiectasia) may be at substantially increased risk of several of the common cancers.[68] Depending on the frequency of the AT gene in the population, this might account for a significant minority of the incidence of these cancers at young ages.

Prospects

Precise definition of the contribution of this type of genetic variation to cancer incidence may never be possible because there will be a continuum of effects from the imperceptible to the highly significant. It is likely, however, that identification of gene-environment interactions in a minority of highly predisposed individuals will have significant impact on approaches to prevention and screening.[4] Starting with the genes and working through them to the chemicals with which they interact, a process of "reverse epidemiology" may lead to the identification of important environmental carcinogens, most of which are still unknown. The limiting factor at present is our ability to guess the relevant candidate genes.

Mechanisms of Genetic Predisposition to Cancer

General Description

In principle, predisposition could occur in one of three ways. The inherited mutation might: 1) provide one of the steps in carcinogenesis ready-made in the germ line; 2) make one of these steps more likely to happen; or 3) affect the consequences of one of the steps so as to make the subsequent steps more likely. Most of the inherited cancer syndromes seem to belong to the first category. An example of the second category is Xeroderma pigmentosum, in which an inherited defect in DNA repair makes somatic mutation more likely. The variations in carcinogen metabolism described in the last section potentially fall in this group. The third group might include, for example, altered endocrine or immune effects on the nascent cancer, but as yet there are no clear examples.

Inherited Cancer Syndromes

The paradigm for the mechanism of predisposition in the inherited cancer syndromes is retinoblastoma.[24] Since the germline mutation is present in every cell of the body, and not every cell becomes a tumor, it is clear that at least one further step is required. The second step might in principle entail either the loss of the remaining wild-type allele at the same locus as the inherited mutation, or mutation at another locus altogether. Either way, in non-hereditary cases both mutations have to occur by chance in the same somatic cell, whereas in hereditary cases the inheritance of one mutation in the germline will greatly increase the probability that at least one cell will acquire the second mutation and a cancer would result.[14,32] The model of mutations in both alleles at the same locus was confirmed in retinoblastoma, when it was shown that in a small proportion of familial cases the first mutation involved an inherited chromosomal deletion at the *Rb* locus, and that in the tumors the remaining (wild-type) allele inherited from the unaffected parent was also lost.[11] In non-familial cases, both alleles were inactivated by somatic mutation (Figure 111-1-5).

Tumor Suppressor Genes, Recessive Mutations and Dominant Pedigrees. The requirement for loss of the activity of both alleles of the *Rb* gene implies that the normal activity of the gene is to restrain or suppress tumorigenesis. This fits with the results from experiments in which hybrids between tumor cells and normal cells are found to be non-tumorigenic, again suggesting that, at the level of the cell, malignancy is the result of recessive mutations in a class of genes that have, therefore been called tumor suppressor genes (see I-6).[57] The apparent paradox that familial retinoblastoma has a dominant pattern of inheritance, but the mutation is reces-

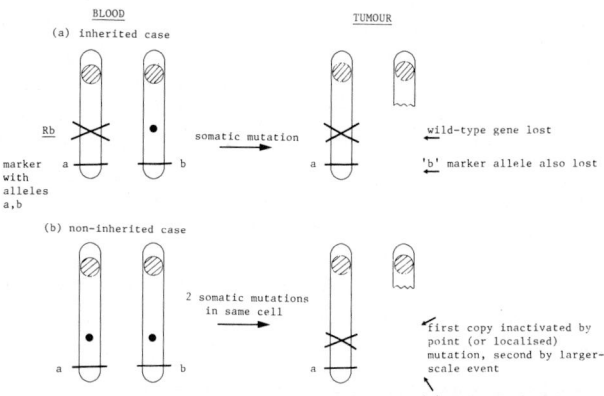

sive at the level of the cell, is explained because in cancer (unlike other diseases) only one cell need acquire the genetic lesion for the phenotype to be expressed. Thus, although the inherited mutation is recessive in terms of its effect in the cell, only one retinal cell need acquire the second, somatic mutation for a tumor to develop. The number of cells at risk is such that this is very probable, and almost everyone who inherits the mutation expresses the disease. The phenotype of tumor formation therefore appears to be dominant at the level of the family pedigree.

Are Other Inherited Cancers Like Retinoblastoma? This would imply that 1) the germline mutation results in loss of activity of the gene, and 2) that the wild-type allele is inactivated in tumors. Definitive proof is not available at the time of writing, because many of the genes are yet to be cloned; but in the syndromes in which the locus of inherited predisposition has been defined by genetic linkage, the evidence of germline deletions in some individuals or of loss of the corresponding region of the wild-type chromosome in tumors (Table III-1-5) suggests that it is likely. Multiple endocrine neoplasia type 2 (MEN 2) is a possible exception. Some caution is needed because only those syndromes can be discussed for which the chromosomal location of the gene is known. Because the syndromes associated with deletions are the easiest to map, a spurious impression may arise that all inherited cancers will be of this type.

Dosage Effects. The *Rb* mutation appears to be truly recessive in that there is no discernible phenotype associated with the first mutation. The widespread phenotypic abnormalities seen in other inherited cancer syndromes suggest that this is not always the case. In FAP, for example, some patients have probable germline deletions at the FAP locus, suggesting that the first mutation causes loss of activity of the gene. Yet already in childhood, FAP patients have a proliferative abnormality throughout their intestinal epithelium. Because every crypt is affected, this is presumably a direct expression of the germline mutation, without the need for a somatic mutation superimposed. This suggests a dosage effect—that is, an effect of copy number of the FAP

Figure III-1-5. Scheme of the genetic mechanism of development of retinoblastoma, and the concept of 'allele loss' in tumors. The figure shows a diagram of both copies of chromosome 13, which carries the retinoblastoma locus, in blood and in tumor cells from (1) an individual with the hereditary form of the cancer and (2) an individual with the non-hereditary form. ⬭ = the centromere of the chromosome, X = the germline mutation of one *Rb* allele in the hereditary case, and somatic mutation in the non-hereditary case, ● = wild type (normal) *Rb* allele. ____ a,b are marker alleles further down the chromosome, detectable by restriction fragment length polymorphisms.

Both alleles at the *Rb* locus must be inactivated for tumor to develop. In inherited cases, the loss of the first allele is inherited as a germline mutation. In non-inherited cases, both alleles must be inactivated in the same somatic cell. Usually (but not always) the first mutation is a point mutation or a small deletion within the *Rb* gene; but the second mutation may involve loss of part or all of the wild-type chromosome by a variety of genetic mechanisms which include non-disjunction, mitotic recombination, or chromosomal deletions.[11] It is possible to infer the occurrence of such events by comparison of DNA from tumor and blood in the same individual, with the finding loss of the appropriate marker allele (here, allele 'b'). A search for 'allele losses' in tumors using probes for different marker loci is now used to search for analogous genetic events in other tumors.[11,24,57]

Table III-1-5. Current Evidence of a Retinoblastoma-Like Genetic Mechanism in Other Inherited Cancer Syndromes.[a]

Syndrome	Chromosomal mapping by genetic linkage	Constitutional chromosomal abnormality[b]	Evidence of consistent allele loss in tumors
FAP	5q	deletion	(+)[c]
MEN 1	11q	not found	+
MEN 2	10	not found	not found
von Hippel-Lindau	3p	not found	+
NF-1	17q	translocation	(+)[d]
NF-2	22	not found	+

[a]Note that current lack of evidence does not necessarily imply it will not be found in future.

[b]In rare cases.

[c]Losses of the FAP region of 5q are rarely seen in FAP-associated colonic tumors until a late stage of cancer development.

[d]Awaiting confirmation.

See reference 57 for review.

gene on phenotype. It also raises the possibility that the focal lesions associated with many of the inherited cancer syndromes—the neurofibromas of NF1, the cysts of von Hippel-Lindau syndrome, the foci of C-cell hyperplasia in MEN 2 (Table III-1-2)—may be due to local threshold effects allowing expression of the inherited mutation, rather than necessarily due to second, somatic events, though this remains speculative.

Variable Expression. The concept of a dosage effect also implies that loss of activity of an allele may not be all or nothing. Different mutations in the gene may result in loss of activity to different extents, or in different functional domains of the gene; and in this way different germline mutations may cause different expressions of the same syndrome in different families—perhaps for example, predominance of breast or ovarian cancer in breast/ovarian families (Figure III-1-3). Variation *within* a family must have another cause; and here the concept of dosage may be broadened to include the idea of modification of expression of the germline mutation depending upon the genetic background, which, as it is probably composed of many unlinked genes, will differ from individual to individual in a family. Variation between families is open to investigation as soon as the predisposing genes are cloned; but to dissect the effects of modifying genes within a family has proved difficult even in Drosophila,[36] and so will probably remain an intractable problem in human cancers for some time to come.

Genomic Imprinting.[59,61] One particular type of variable expression within a family is easily identified, because it is specific to the sex of the parent from whom the gene has been inherited. In families with dominantly inherited susceptibility to glomus tumor, for example, the phenotype is only expressed when transmitted through the male germline.[71] After transmission through a female, the gene is almost silent until once more transmitted through a male. Similar effects are seen in families with rhabdomyosarcoma;[65] and in the expression of Beckwith-Wiedemann syndrome.

Until recently, it had been assumed that the paternally and maternally derived genomes were equivalent, but experiments in which mice with chromosomal translocations were bred to produce progeny in which both copies of one chromosome (or a part of a chromosome) were either of paternal or maternal origin, showed this not to be so. The mice develop differently. The phenomenon affects only a minority of chromosomal regions. Transgenic mice show similar parent-of-origin dependent expression of reporter genes such as β-galactosidase. This depends both upon the chromosomal localization of the transgene and, interestingly in view of the within-family variation of expression of human genetic disorders, on the genetic background of the mouse in which the transgene is expressed.

The molecular mechanism of imprinting is unclear, but it appears to result from diminished expression of one allele which may be related to differential methylation of genes in the male and female germline. Its physiological function is also unclear, but it may possibly provide a further level of control of expression of critical genes in embryogenesis. In the transgenic systems, imprinting effects diminish as the mice get older.

As inactivation of tumor suppressor genes is an important mechanism of carcinogenesis, the possibility of epigenetic inactivation by imprinting, which, moreover, may be subject to genetic background influences and changeable over time, has potentially exciting implications.[46] Only a very few cancers show imprinting, defined as parent of origin effects in expression. Unstable epigenetic modification independent of germline effects may be of much more general importance, but is also much harder to detect.

The Search for Inherited Predisposing Genes
General Principles

The gene for hemophilia could be found because sufficient was known about the mechanism of the disease—deficiency of clotting factor VIII—to work from the protein to the DNA sequence and hence the gene. Because there is no comparable understanding of the mechanisms of inherited predisposition to cancer, a different approach has been taken, starting with an empirical search for the gene by *genetic linkage*.

Genetic Linkage

The principle of genetic linkage is simple.[33,52] The pattern of inheritance of a specific cancer through a family is taken to indicate the inheritance of the predisposing gene or, in those who are unaffected, of the corresponding wild-type allele. The cancer gene can be located by testing in the same family the pattern of inheritance of the alleles at a "marker locus," whose chromosomal location is already known. If one allele of the marker is consistently coinherited with the cancer (and so, by inference, with the cancer gene), the marker and the cancer gene must be adjacent on the chromosome. Otherwise, they would tend to be separated by recombination at each meiosis, and their inheritance would be independent. As the human gene map expands, the number of markers and the power of linkage approaches will increase.

Problems with Linkage in Cancer Families

Phenocopies and Incomplete Penetrance. Unless there is a marker phenotype, as in some of the inherited cancer syndromes, the presence or absence of the cancer gene (rather than its wild-type allele) in each individual is inferred from the presence of the cancer. In the common cancers, such as breast cancer, this may be unsafe. Some individuals within a large family may have breast cancer by chance, rather than predisposition—they are phenocopies (see Figure III-1-4). Conversely, some individuals who do not have breast cancer, may still have inherited the cancer gene, but not expressed it. This will clearly be related to sex and age. With a marker phenotype, identification of gene carriers is potentially more accurate, provided good quality clinical data are available. Linkage is dependent, therefore, on accurate clinical data for affecteds and unaffecteds, which must include screening for the marker phenotype if one is available; and on the assumptions that are made about penetrance and numbers of phenocopies.

Heterogeneity. It is often necessary to combine data from several families to achieve significant evidence for linkage. Unless the families are predisposed at the same genetic locus, this is a potential disaster because positive scores from linked families will be cancelled by negatives from the unlinked. Although mathematical procedures exist to deal with the problem of heterogeneity, the power is much reduced and many more families must be analyzed—a problem, as availability of family material is usually a limiting factor. Every effort must therefore be made to start with large families, or failing that with families that are as homogenous as possible by clinical criteria, even though genetic homogeneity can still not be guaranteed. This problem is likely to be serious in common familial cancers such as breast cancer;[30] less so in the inherited cancer syndromes.

Specifying the Correct Genetic Model. Most linkage in familial cancers is run on the assumption of dominant inheritance because that is what segregation analyses and clinical observation suggest. If recessive inheritance is a possibility, that model should be run too; if the familial cancer is polygenic in origin, linkage may fail.

How To Start Looking

To scan the entire genome for linkage might take a small laboratory two or three years with today's resources. There are four possible clues to narrow the search: 1) Candidate genes. Try to guess the gene that is causing the syndrome. p53 in Li-Fraumeni syndrome is so far the only successful example.[42] 2) Constitutional chromosomal abnormalities. In rare cases the germline mutation may be associated with cytogenetically detectable deletions or translocations. Patients in whom young onset of cancer is associated with mental retardation or a developmental anomaly may be the best candidates, the additional features indicating the disruption of several genes in the chromosome region. Such cases have been crucial in the mapping of several cancer genes,[26] and a search for them may be well worth the effort. 10 ml heparinized blood should be taken for analysis by prophase banding. If positive, further blood should be taken to set up a lymphoblastoid cell line for detailed genetic mapping studies. 3) Allele losses. Assuming a retinoblastoma-like model, consistent regions of chromosomal loss in tumors, revealed by loss of marker alleles (see Figure III-1-5) may reflect loss of a critical suppressor gene and so the chromosome location of a gene, germline mutation of which will result in predisposition. Note however that by no means all suppressor gene loci defined in this way will correspond to loci for inherited predisposition.[57] 4) Exclusion mapping. Computer programs are available which will combine existing linkage data and generate an exclusion map, which indicates the residual probability that the gene is at any given location. This has proved useful in several of the inherited cancer syndromes, but if genetic heterogeneity is present it could be seriously misleading.

Problems with Incomplete or Small Families

Classical linkage as described above is applied to families in which there are several affected individuals in two or more generations. Often, however, real cancer families contain a small number of living distant relatives with all the intervening relatives dead. In other cases (i.e., lung cancer) extensive families are too rare for standard linkage approaches to be practical. Various modifications of linkage strategy have been

developed for such situations.[5,33] The reader contemplating such a study should seek expert advice at an early stage.

Investigation and Management of Cancer Families

General[58,67]

There is little doubt that in some types of familial cancer, especially the inherited cancer syndromes, screening and appropriate treatment of those at risk will reduce deaths and morbidity. Because the screened population is at very high risk, screening is likely to be highly cost-effective where curative treatment is available. Yet recognition and screening of such families is undoubtedly incomplete and often badly done. Even when effective screening or treatment is not available, families may benefit from information and advice. Most are well aware of their history, and worried by it. They often overestimate their risks, and can be reassured. The fear of many doctors, that they will provoke anxiety by discussing the issues, is usually unfounded.

When Is a Cancer Family Clinically Significant?

Putting to one side the syndromes with a clearly recognizable phenotype, this question reduces to: when is the family history so striking that it is unlikely to be due to chance? Clearly there can be no single answer. Two sisters at age 40 with breast cancer may be coincidence, but the figures for excess risk to sisters of cases of this age suggest about an 85% chance that such a pair is significant. Two sisters with breast cancer aged 70, by contrast, may be significant, but more likely are not.[17] The factors that suggest genetic predisposition are listed in Table III-1-6. In practice, one must take a thorough family history, evaluate these factors, and make an estimate for each new family. The decision will often depend critically on one or two diagnoses in family members now dead: if so, considerable effort may be needed to verify the information.

Familial Cancer Clinic

The purposes of a general familial cancer clinic are: to obtain as detailed a family history as possible, with confirmation of all important diagnoses; to estimate individual risks, discuss these with family members and their doctors, and advise on the options for management; and to maintain an overview of all the branches of the family (who may live at some distance from each other), to ensure that information from one branch that is relevant to the management of the other is passed on, and that continuity of follow up is maintained. This is difficult and time consuming, and usually beyond the resources of a busy medical or surgical clinic. The purpose of the familial cancer clinic is not, however, to take over clinical management; screening and treatment should remain

Table III-1-6. Features which Increase the Probability that a Familial Association of Cancer Is Due to Genetic Susceptibility

Association of specific (especially uncommon) tumors
Associated developmental or phenotypic abnormalities
Unusually early onset of cancer
Multiple primary cancers in one individual

the responsibility of local specialists, who will see the family regularly.

Experience in the UK suggests that a familial cancer clinic requires as a minimum a clinical geneticist with knowledge of cancer; one or more specially trained nurses who can obtain and confirm family information by telephone, home visits (often involving considerable travel); and seeking relevant records, and who can take and process blood samples; and a secretary/data manager. Close liaison with specialist clinicians in disciplines relevant to assessment of different syndromes (e.g., colonoscopy, ultrasound, mammography, ophthalmology) is essential, as well as with surgeons who will be responsible for prophylactic surgery—it is important to agree on management with the doctors who will carry it out, before advising the patient. Finally, close links with a molecular genetics laboratory are necessary as DNA-based diagnosis becomes possible for more familial cancers, and to foster research. To focus expertise, and to minimize the travelling required of families and of clinic nurses, a cooperative network of clinics has been set up throughout the UK, with clinicians in each region nominated to act as local sources of information and advice within their speciality.

Advising a Family

Risk Estimates. The first essential is to decide on the risk to the family member(s) concerned. The estimation may involve several steps (Figure III-1-6).[55] 1) What is the risk that the individual has inherited the predisposing gene, based on a given genetic model (usually autosomal dominant) and his relationship to known affected individuals? 2) Might DNA testing give a more precise answer? 3) How is this risk modified by the present age of the individual (the older without signs of the disease the lower the risk); by any suggestive marker phenotype (e.g., colonic polyps); by the present age (or age at death or prophylactic surgery) of any unaffected relative through whom the gene must have been inherited; and by uncertainty that this family, or branch of the family, does in fact carry a genetic predisposition (e.g., uncertainty whether the supposed gene carrier at the head of the branch might not be a phenocopy). 4) Is the risk of more than one type of cancer; if so, which; and are the risks different? 5) At what age does risk commence, and how is it distributed through life? 6) How is the risk affected by other known risk factors in this individual (e.g., age at menarche, parity, benign breast disease, and other factors).

Options for Management. In general, depending on the site, there will be three possibilities: do nothing, screening, and prophylactic surgery. Sensible advice about lifestyle may well be appropriate, but only in a few cases at present (e.g., familial melanoma—keep out of the sun) is specific advice on prevention likely to be a main option.

As a general rule, the patient or family should be helped to make their own decision, rather than have it imposed. The uncertainties of screening (e.g., for breast or ovarian cancer) and the benefits and drawbacks of surgery must be explained in detail appropriate to the individual. The implications for children, even though some years away, will probably be a major source of concern. It is often helpful to provide parents with a letter detailing the family tree, the discussions you have had, and your recommendations for the children, so

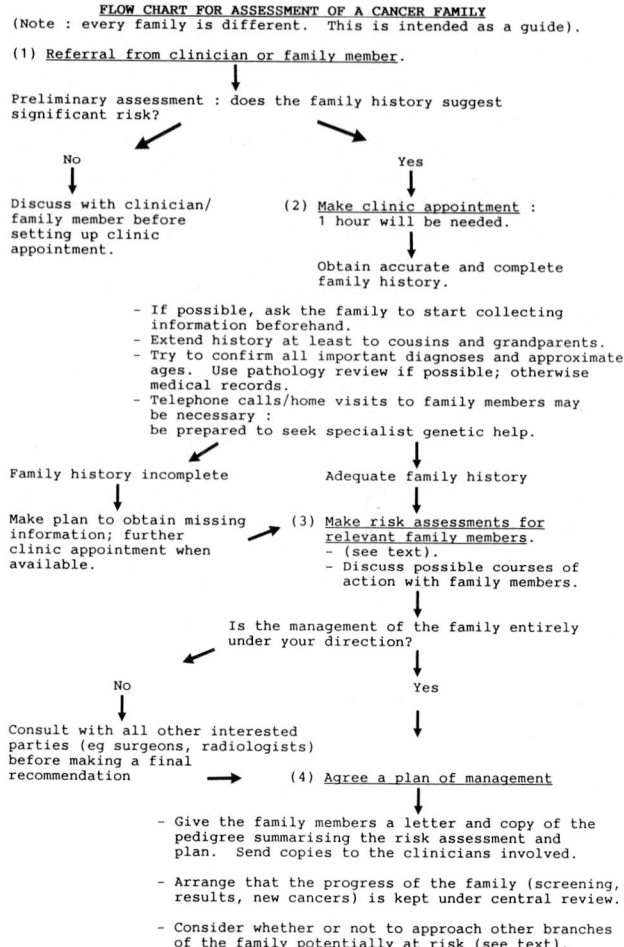

Figure III-1-6. Flow chart for clinical assessment of a cancer family.

that this can be passed on to the children for them to use at the appropriate time to seek advice.

Other branches of the family may also be at risk. The decision to approach them or not will depend primarily on whether they can expect to benefit. If they are not in contact with the branch who have sought advice, or are thought to be unaware of the problem, great caution is needed. Public records in the UK allow identification of the family doctor, who would be the recommended first contact in these circumstances.

Screening. A suggested outline of screening for some of the inherited cancer syndromes is given in Table III-1-7. Details must be sought elsewhere. For the common familial cancers, there is little general agreement and no present evidence of benefit. Some guidelines are suggested in Table III-1-8. Decisions to be made include the age to start, the interval, and the criteria for further investigation or surgery. Because of the generally small numbers, and the ethical difficulties of randomized studies in high risk families, there are few data on which to base these decisions or to prove that screening is beneficial.

DNA Diagnosis. Diagnosis using linked DNA markers[58] is currently possible with varying degrees of precision for FAP,[15] MEN 1,[9] MEN,[44] von Hippel Lindau syndrome,[72] NF-1,[72] and will soon be available for NF-2; others will be added

Table III-1-7.   A Summary of Current Screening Procedures for Individuals at Risk of Some Inherited Cancer Syndromes

Syndrome	Screening Procedure	Starting age
FAP	Examine for hypertrophy of retinal pigmented epithelium. Sigmoidoscopy for polyps.	Childhood Early teens
MEN 1	Plasma calcium.	Teens
MEN 2A	Measurement of stimulated plasma calcitonin; urinary catecholamines.	5 years
		Teens
von Hippel-Lindau	Examine for retinal angiomas urinary catecholamines.	5 years
	Renal ultrasound; cranial CT/MRI scan; CNS clinical exam.	Early 20s Baseline scans aged 20
NF-1	Diagnosis will usually be apparent in childhood (from CAL spots, iris nodules, other features). Once established, annual assessments for learning difficulties, visual impairment (optic glioma) and scoliosis.	
NF-2	MRI scan or brain stem auditory evoked responses for VIII n. tumor. Clinical exam for lens opacities.	Early teens

Table III-1-8.   A Guide to Possible Screening Policy for Individuals at High Risk in "Cancer Families"

Cancer	Screen	Start age (Usually controversial)
Breast	Mammography (possibly ultrasound if mammography unsatisfactory)	?35 years or 5 years earlier than earliest case in family
Ovary	Ultrasound; Doppler bloodflow scan of ovaries as 'second-line'; possibly serum CA-125	?25 years or 5 years earlier than earliest case in family
Colorectal (not FAP)	High-risk (>2 affected 1° relatives): colonoscopy: repeat every 3 years if polyps; 5 years if not Low risk: fecal occult blood	?30 years or 5 years before first case in family
Stomach	Gastroscopy	5 years before first case in family
Endometrium	Pelvic exam. ? Endometrial biopsy every 2 years	?35 years or 5 years before first case in family
Melanoma	Annual thorough skin exam by experienced doctor; patient/spouse education for change in nevus; excision biopsy of suspicious lesions	Childhood

Note: All screening should include a clinical examination directed to sites at risk. The procedures suggested here are not of proven effectiveness. Individual clinical judgement should always be used.

as the genes are mapped. Depending on the probes used and the family structure, however, many families may not be suitable for prediction.[69] Advice from a clinical geneticist should always be sought at an early stage. Diagnosis by direct identification of the inherited mutation is possible in most cases of retinoblastoma.[73]

Linkage-based prediction may be extremely useful in identifying non-gene carriers and excluding them from risk. For family members identified as gene carriers, the issue is potentially more complex. In many cases, the cancer will not develop for years, or at all, and one is reluctant to advise immediate prophylactic surgery. At present, in all the cancers for which DNA diagnosis is possible and where prophylactic surgery is an option, effective screening by marker phenotype is available. Individuals identified from DNA testing who are at risk are simply advised to continue in the screening program. When genetic prediction for breast cancer becomes possible, however, management of women shown to have inherited the gene will pose a much greater problem because of the uncertain penetrance of the gene, the lack of an effec-

tive screen for early disease, and the unacceptability of prophylactic surgery.

Future Prospects

The genes involved in predisposition to the inherited cancer syndromes and to many of the common cancers will probably be identified within the next few years. The challenges will then be to devise and evaluate effective means of screening for individuals at risk, and to use knowledge of the mechanisms of action of the genes to develop new approaches to prevention and treatment.

References

1. Alm, T., and Lieznerski, M.: The intestinal polyposes. Clinics in Gastroenterology, 2:577, 1973.
2. Ayesh, R., Idle, J. R., Ritchie, J. C., Crothers, M. J., and Hetzel, M. R.: Metabolic oxidation phenotypes as markers of susceptibility to lung cancer. Nature, 312:169, 1984.
3. Ballard, H. S., Frame, B., and Hartsock, R. J.: Familial multiple endocrine adenoma-peptic ulcer complex. Medicine, 43:481, 1964.
4. Banbury Report 16: Genetic Variability to Chemical Exposure. Edited by G. S. Omenn, and H. V. Gelboin. Cold Spring Harbor Laboratory, 1984.

5. Bishop, D. T., and Williamson, J A.: The power of identity by state methods for linkage analysis. Am. J. Hum. Genet., 46:254, 1990.
6. Bodmer, W. F., Bailey, C. J., Bodmer, J., Bussey, H. J. R., Ellis, A., Forman, P., Lucibello, F. L., Murday, V. A., Rider, S. H., Scambler, P., Sheer, D., Solomon, E., and Spurr, N. K.: Localisation of the gene for familial adenomatous polyposis on chromosome 5. Nature, 328:614, 1987.
7. Bulow, S.: Familial polyposis coli. A clinical and epidemiological study. Dan. Med. Bull., 34:1, 1987.
8. Bussey, H. J. R.: Familial polyposis coli. Family studies, histopathology, differential diagnosis and results of treatment. Baltimore, Johns Hopkins University Press, 1975.
9. Bystrom, C., Larsson, C., Blomberg, C., Sandelin, K., Falkner, U., Skogseid, B., Oberg, K., Werner, S., and Nordenskjold, M.: Localisation of the MEN 1 gene to a small region within chromosome band 11q13 by deletion mapping in tumours. Proc. Natl. Acad. Sci. USA, 87:1968, 1990.
10. Cannon-Albright, L. A., Skolnick, M. H., Bishop, D. T., Lee, R. G., and Burt, R. W.: Common inheritance of susceptibility to colonic adenomatous polyps and associated colorectal cancers. N. Engl. J. Med., 319:533, 1988.
11. Cavenee, W. K., Dryja, T. P., Phillips, R. A., Benedict, W. F., Godbout, R., Gallie, B. L., Murphree, A. L., Strong, L. C., and White, R. L.: Expression of recessive alleles by chromosomal mechanisms in retinoblastoma. Nature, 305:779, 1983.
12. Chapman, P. D., Church, W., Burn, J., and Gunn, A.: Congenital hypertrophy of retinal pigment epithelium: a sign of familial adenomatous polyposis. Br. Med. J., 298:353, 1989.
13. Claus, E. B., Risch, N. J., and Thompson, W. D.: Genetic analysis of breast cancer in the cancer and steroid hormone study. Am. J. Hum. Genet., 42:232, 1991.
14. De Mars, R.: In 23rd Annual Symposium on Fundamental Cancer Research, M. D. Anderson Hospital, 1969. Baltimore, Williams and Wilkins, 1970, p. 105.
15. Dunlop, M. G., Wyllie, A. H., Nakamura, Y., Steel, C. M., Evans, H. J., White, R. L., and Bird, C. C.: Genetic linkage map of six polymorphic DNA markers around the gene for familial adenomatous polyposis on chromosome 5. Am. J. Hum. Genet., 47:982, 1990.
16. Dyck, P. J., Carney, A., Sizemore, G. W., Okazaki, H., Brimijoin, W. S., and Lambert, E.: Multiple endocrine neoplasia type 2b:phenotype recognition. Ann. Neurology, 6:302, 1979.
17. Easton, D., and Peto, J.: The contribution of inherited predisposition to cancer incidence. In Cancer Surveys, Vol. 9. Genetic Predisposition to Cancer. Edited by W. Cavenee, B. A. J. Ponder, and E. Solomon. Oxford, Oxford University Press, 1991 (in press).
18. Easton, D. F., Ponder, M. A., Cummings, T., Gagel, R. F., Hansen, H. H., Reichlin, S., Tashjian, A. H., Telenius-Berg, M., and Ponder, B. A. J.: The clinical and screening age-at-onset distribution for the MEN 2 syndrome. Am. J. Hum. Genet., 44:208, 1989.
19. Elston, R. C.: Segregation Analysis. In Advances in Human Genetics II. Edited by H. Harris, and K. Hirschorn. Plenum, 1981, p. 63.
20. Erbe, R. W.: Inherited gastrointestinal syndromes. Ann. Intern. Med., 83:639, 1976.
21. Gardner, E. J.: Follow-up study of a family group exhibiting dominant inheritance for a syndrome including intestinal polyps and osteomatosis. Am. J. Hum. Genet., 14:376, 1962.
22. Gonzalez, F. J., Skoda, R. C., Kimura, S., Verno, M., Zanger, U. M., Nebert, D. W., Gelboin, H. V., Hardwick, J. P., and Meyer, U. A.: Characterisation of the common genetic defect in humans deficient in debrisoquin metabolism. Nature, 331:442, 1988.
23. Gough, A. C., Miles, J. S., Spurr, N. K., Moss, J. E., Gaedigk, A., Eichelbaum, M., and Wolf, C. R.: Identification of the primary gene defect at the cytochrome P450 CYP2D locus. Nature, 347:773, 1990.
23a. Hall, J. M., Lee, M. K., Newman, B., Morrow, J. E., Anderson, L. A., Huey, B., and King, M.-C.: Linkage of early-onset familial breast cancer to chromosome 17q21. Science, 250:1684, 1990.
24. Hansen, M. F., and Cavenee, W. K.: Retinoblastoma and the progression of tumour genetics. Trends in Genetics, 4:125, 1988.
25. Harnden, D., Morten, J., and Featherstone, T.: Dominant susceptibility to cancer in man. Adv. Cancer Res., 41:185, 1984.
26. Herrera, L., Kakati, S., Gibas, L., Pietrak, E., and Sandberg, A.: Gardner syndrome in a man with an interstitial deletion of 5q. Am. J. Med. Genet., 25:473, 1986.
27. Horton, W. A., Wong, V., and Eldridge, R.: Von Hippel-Lindau disease. Arch. Intern. Med., 136:769, 1976.
28. Huson, S. M., Harper, P. S., and Compston, D. A. S.: Von Recklinghausen neurofibromatosis: a clinical and population study in South-East Wales. Brain, 111:1355, 1988.
29. Jagelman, D. G.: Clinical management of familial adenomatous polyposis. Cancer Surveys, 8:159, 1989.
30. King, M.-C.: Genetic Analysis of Cancer in Families. In Cancer Surveys, Vol. 9. Genetic Predisposition to Cancer. Edited by W. Cavenee, B. A. J. Ponder, and E. Solomon. Oxford, Oxford University Press, 1991 (in press).
31. Knudsen, A. G.: Hereditary Cancers: Clues to mechanisms of carcinogenesis. Br. J. Cancer, 59:661, 1989.
32. Knudsen, A. G.: Mutation and cancer: Statistical study of retinoblastoma. Proc. Natl. Acad. Sci., USA, 68:820, 1971.
33. Lander, E. S.: Mapping complex genetic traits in humans. In Genome Analysis—A Practical Approach. Edited by K. E. Davies. Oxford, IRL Press, 1988, p. 171.
34. Leppert, M., Burt, R., Hughes, J. P., Samowitz, W., Nakamura, Y., Woodward, S., Gardner, E., Lalouel, J.-M., and White, R.: Genetic analysis of an inherited predisposition to colon cancer in a family with a variable number of adenomatous polyps. N. Engl. J. Med., 322:904, 1990.
35. Li, F. P., Fraumeni, J. F., Jr., Mulvihill, J. J., Blattner, W. A., Dreyfus, M. G., Tucker, M. A., and Miller, R. W.: A cancer family syndrome in twenty-four kindreds. Cancer Res., 48:5358, 1988.
36. Locke, J., Kotarski, M. A., and Tartof, K. D.: Dosage-dependent modifiers of positional effect variegation in Drosophila and a mass action model that explains their effect. Genetics, 120:181, 1988.
37. Lovett, E.: Family studies in cancer of the colon and rectum. Br. J. Surg., 63:13, 1976.
38. Lynch, H. T., Schuelke, G. S., Kimberling, W. J., Albano, W. A., Lynch, J. E., Biscone, K. A., Lipkin, M. L., Deschner, E. E., Mikol, Y. B., Sandberg, A. A., Elston, R. C., Bailey-Wilson, J. E., and Danes, B. S.: Hereditary nonpolyposis colorectal cancer (Lynch syndromes I and II). II. Biomarker studies. Cancer, 56:939, 1985.
39. Lynch, H. T., Kimberley, W., Albano, W. A., Lynch, J. F., Biscone, K., Schuelke, G. S., Sandberg, A. A., Lipkin, M., Deschner, E. E., Mikol, Y. B., Elston, R. C., Bailey-Wilson, J. E., and Shannon Danes, B.: Hereditary non polyposis colonic cancer (Lynch syndrome I and II). I. Clinical description of resource. Cancer, 56:934, 1988.
40. Lynch, H. T., and Lynch, J. F.: Breast Cancer Genetics: Clinical Nuances. In Cancer Genetics in Women, Vol. 1. Edited by Lynch, H. T., and Kullander, S. Boca Raton, CRC Press, 1987, p. 49.
41. Macklin, M. T.: Inheritance of cancer of the stomach and large intestine in man. J. Natl. Cancer Inst., 24:551, 1960.
42. Malkin, D., Li, F. P., Strong, L. C., Fraumeni, J. F., Nelson, C. E., Kim, D. H., Kassel, J., Gryka, M. A., Bischoff, F. Z., Tainsky, M. A., and Friend, S. H.: Germ line p. 53 mutations in a familial syndrome of breast cancer, sarcomas and other neoplasms. Science, 250:1233, 1990.
43. Martuza, R. L., and Eldridge, R.: Neurofibromatosis 2. N. Engl. J. Med., 318:684, 1988.
44. Mathew, C. G. P., Easton, D. F., Nakamura, Y., and Ponder, B. A. J.: Presymptomatic screening for multiple endocrine neoplasia type 2A using linked DNA markers. Lancet, 337:7, 1991.
45. McLenore, T. L., Adelberg, S., Liu, M., McMahon, N. A., Yu, S. J., Hubbard, W. C., Czerwincski, M., Wood, T. G., Stoneng, R., Lubet, R. A., Eggleston, J. C., Boyd, M. R. and Hines, R. N.: Expression of the CYP1A1 gene in patients with lung cancer. J. Natl. Cancer Inst., 82:1333, 1990.
46. Monk, M.: Variation in epigenetic inheritance. Trends in Genetics, 6:1, 1990.
47. Mulvihill, J. J., Miller, R. W., and Fraumeni, J. F.: Genetics of Human Cancer (Progress in Cancer Research and Therapy, Vol 3.) Raven Press, 1977.
48. Murday, V., and Slack, J.: Inherited disorders associated with colorectal cancer. Cancer Surveys, 8:137, 1989.
49. Nikawa, N., Ishikiriyama, S., Takahasi, S., Inagawa, A., Tonoki, H., Ohta, Y., Hase, N., Kamei, T., and Kajii, T.: The Wiedemann-Beckwith syndrome: pedigree studies on five families with evidence for autosomal dominent inheritance with variable expressivity. Am. J. Med. Genet., 211:41, 1986.
50. Ooi, W. L., Elston, R. C., Chen, V. W., Bailey-Wilson, J. E., and Rothschild, H.: Increased familial risk for lung cancer. J. Natl. Cancer Inst., 76:217, 1986.
51. Osterlind, A., Tucker, M. A., Hovi-Jensen, K., Stone, B. J., Engholm, G., and Jensen, O. M.: The Danish case-control study of cutaneous malignant melanoma. I. Importance of host factors. Int. J. Cancer, 42:200, 1988.
52. Ott, J.: A short guide to linkage analysis. In Human Genetic Diseases: A Practical Approach. Edited by K. E. Davies. Oxford, IRL Press, 1986.
53. Peto, J.: Genetic Predisposition to Cancer. In Cancer Incidence in Defined Populations, Banbury Report 4. Edited by J. Cairns, J. L. Lynch, and M. H. Skolnick. Cold Spring Harbor Laboratory, 1980, p. 203.
54. Ponder, B. A. J.: Inherited predisposition to cancer. Trends in Genetics, 6:213, 1990.
55. Ponder, B. A. J., Ponder, M. A., Coffey, R., Pembrey, M. E.: Gagel, R. F., Telenius-Berg, M., Semple, P., and Easton, D. F.: Risk estimation and screening in families of patients with medullary thyroid carcinoma. Lancet, 1:397, 1988.
56. Ponder, B. A. J., Easton, D., and Peto, J.: Risk of ovarian cancer associated with a family history. In Ovarian Cancer. Edited by F. Sharp, W. D. Mason, and R. E. Leake. London, Chapman and Hall, 1990, p. 3.
57. Ponder, B. A. J.: Gene losses in human tumours. Nature, 335:400, 1988.
58. Ponder, B. A. J.: Prospects for genetic diagnosis of inherited predisposition to cancer. Trends in Biotechnology, 8:98, 1990.
59. Reik, W.: Genomic imprinting and genetic disorders in man. Trends in Genetics, 5:331, 1989.
60. Riccardi, V. M., and Eichner, J. E.: Neurofibromatosis: Phenotype, Natural History and Pathogenesis. Baltimore, Johns Hopkins University Press, 1986.
61. Sapienza, C.: Genome imprinting, cellular mosaicism and carcinogenesis. Molecular Carcinogenesis, 3:118, 1990.
62. Saunders, B. M., Jay, M., Draper, G. J., and Roberts, G. M.: Non-ocular cancer in the relatives of retinoblastoma patients. Br. J. Cancer, 60:358, 1989.
63. Schildkraut, J. M., and Thompson, W. D.: Familial ovarian cancer: A population-based control study. Am. J. Epid., 128:456, 1988.
64. Schildkraut, J. M., Risch, N., and Thompson, W. D.: Evaluating genetic association among ovarian, breast and endometrial cancer: Evidence for a breast ovarian relationship. Am. J. Hum. Genet., 45:521, 1989.
65. Scrable, H., Cavenee, W. K., Ghevimi, F., Lovell, M., Morgan, K., and Sapienza, C.: A model for embryonal rhabdomyosarcoma tumorigenesis that involves genomic imprinting. Proc. Natl. Acad. Sci. USA, 86:7480, 1989.
66. Springate, J. E.: The nevoid basal cell carcinoma syndrome. J. Paed. Surg., 21:908, 1986.
67. Stoll, B. A.: Risk Factors and Multiple Cancer—New Horizons in Oncology, Vol. 3. Chichester, John Wiley, 1984.
68. Swift, M., Reitnauer, P. J., Morrell, D., and Chase, C. L.: Breast and other cancers in families with ataxia-telangiectasia. N. Engl. J. Med., 316:1289, 1988.
69. Telenius, H., Mathew, C. G. P., Nakamura, Y., Easton, D. F., Clark, J., Neumann, H. P. H., Ziegler, W. H., Schinzel, A., and Ponder, B. A. J.: Application of linked DNA markers to screening families with multiple endocrine neoplasia type 2A. Eur. J. Surg. Oncol., 16:134, 1990.
70. Thakker, R. V., and Ponder, B. A. J.: Multiple endocrine neoplasia. In Molecular Biology of Endocrinology (Bailliere's Clinical Endocrinology and Metabolism 2). Edited by M. C. Sheppard. London, Bailliere Tindall, 1988, p. 1031.
71. Van der Mey, A. G. L., Maaswinkel-Mooy, P. D., Cornelissa, C. J., Schmidt, P. H., and Van de Kamp, J. J. P.: Genomic imprinting in hereditary glomus tumours: Evidence of new genetic theory. Lancet, ii:1291, 1989.
72. Ward, K., O'Connell, P., Carey, J. C., Leppert, M., Jolley, S., Plaetke, R., Ogden,

B., and White, R.: Diagnosis of neurofibromatosis I by using tightly linked, flanking DNA markers. Am. J. Hum. Genet., 46:943, 1990.
73. Wiggs, J., Nordenskjöld, M., Yandell, D., Rapaport, J., Grondin, V., Janson, M., Werelius, B., Petersen, R., Craft, A., Riedel, K., Liberfarb, R., Walton, D., Wilson, W., and Dryja, T. P.: Prediction of the risk of hereditary retinoblastoma, using DNA polymorphisms within the retinoblastoma gene. N. Engl. J. Med., 318:151, 1988.
74. Williams, W. R., and Anderson, D. E.: Genetic epidemiology of breast cancer: segregation analysis of 200 Danish pedigrees. Genet. Epidemiol., 1:7, 1984.
75. Wolf, C. R.: Cytochrome P450's: a multigene family involved in carcinogen metabolism. Trends in Genetics, 2:209, 1986.
76. Wolf, C.R.: Metabolic factors in cancer susceptibility. In Cancer Surveys. Edited by Cavanee, W., Ponder, B. A. J., and Solomon, E. Oxford, Oxford University Press, 1991.

Acknowledgements

The author is a Gibb Fellow of the Cancer Research Campaign.

III-2

Chemical Carcinogenesis

Ainsley Weston
Curtis C. Harris

Introduction

A genetic basis for human carcinogenesis has been established through biochemical and molecular analyses of the disease.[25,107] Many different types of human cancer have been caused by occupational exposure, while others have been attributed to environmental exposure to chemical and/or viral agents (Table III-2-1).[58,95] The molecular mechanisms of human carcinogenesis are emerging through an increasing appreciation of the genetic and epigenetic changes that result from chemical-DNA interactions.

Chemical carcinogenesis is a multistage process that begins with exposure, usually to complex mixtures of chemicals found in the human environment. Once internalized, carcinogens are frequently subject to competing metabolic pathways of activation and detoxication, although some reactive environmental chemicals can act directly. Interindividual variations in metabolism together with differences in DNA-repair capacity and response to tumor promoters govern the relative risk of an individual.[43] The initial genetic change(s) that occurs as the result of the chemical-DNA interaction is termed tumor initiation. Initiated cells are irreversibly altered in such a way as to be at greater risk of malignant conversion than normal cells.[105] The epigenetic effects of tumor promoters facilitate the clonal expansion of the initiated cell.[116] This selective clonal growth advantage results in formation of a focus of preneoplastic cells. These cells are more vulnerable to progress towards tumorigenesis because they present a larger, more rapidly proliferating, target population for the further action of chemical carcinogens, oncogenic viruses or other cofactors. Additional genetic changes occur and consequently the accumulation of mutations, which may activate protooncogenes and inactivate tumor suppressor genes, leads to malignant conversion, tumor progression and metastasis. The underlying genetic mechanisms which regulate chemical carcinogenesis are becoming increasingly well understood, and the insights generated have assisted in the development of methodologies designed to assess human cancer risk and individual susceptibility factors. The results of these latter studies are further intended to mold strategies for cancer prevention.

Multistage Carcinogenesis

Carcinogenesis can be conceptually divided into four steps, tumor initiation, tumor promotion, malignant conversion and tumor progression (Figure III-2-1). The distinction between initiation and promotion was recognized through studies involving both viruses and chemical carcinogens.[92,93] This distinction was formally defined in a murine-skin carcinogenesis model where mice were treated topically with a single dose of a polycyclic aromatic hydrocarbon (initiator) followed by repeated topical doses of croton oil (promoter).[10] This mechanism has also been shown to operate in a range of other rodent tissues, including; bladder, colon, esophagus, liver, lung, mammary gland, stomach, and trachea.[116] During the last forty years the sequence of events comprising chemical carcinogenesis has been systematically dissected and the model has become increasingly refined. It is now recognized that carcinogenesis requires malignant conversion of hyperplastic cells from a benign or preneoplastic state and that invasion and metastasis are manifestations of further genetic and epigenetic changes.[20] Study of this process in humans is necessarily indirect. Measures of age-dependent cancer incidence have shown, however, that the rate of tumor development is proportional to the sixth power of time, suggesting that 4–6 independent steps are necessary.[84]

Tumor Initiation

Tumor initiation occurs as the result of irreversible genetic damage. For mutations to accumulate they must arise in cells that survive or give rise to descendants that survive the lifetime of the organism. A chemical carcinogen causes a mutation by modification of the molecular structure of the DNA. This is most often brought about by formation of an adduct between the chemical carcinogen or one of its functional

Table III-2-1. Examples of Tumors that are Considered to be Induced by Chemicals

Anatomical Site	Sub-category	Chemical or Mixture	Cofactor
External Epithelia (~56% human cancer)			
Lung		Arsenic	
		Asbestos	
		Bis (chloromethyl)ether	
		Chromium	
		Hematite	
		Nickel	
	Small cell & Squamous cell carcinomas	Tobacco smoke	Asbestos & Radon
		Diesel exhaust	
		Coke oven emission	
	Mesothelioma	Asbestos	
Esophagus	Squamous cell carcinoma	Tobacco smoke	Alcoholic beverages
Oral cavity	Squamous cell carcinoma	Betel nut	Calcium hydroxide
		Chewing tobacco	Alcoholic beverages
Skin	Basal cell carcinoma	Cutting oils	
		Soot	
		Coal tar	
Nasal sinuses		Nickel	
		Snuff (tobacco)	Glass powder
		Isopropyl alcohol	
Internal Epithelia (~8% human cancer)			
Liver	Hepatocellular carcinoma	Aflatoxin B1	Hepatitis virus B or C
			Alcoholic beverages
Bladder	Angioma	Vinyl chloride	
	Squamous cell carcinoma	Aromatic amines (Azo-dyes)	
Sarcoma/Leukemia (~8% human cancer)			
Hematologic	Acute lymphoblastic leukemia (ALL)	Benzene	

Information on carcinogenic risk of chemicals is found in reports by the International Agency on the Research of Cancer.[58]

MULTISTAGE CARCINOGENESIS

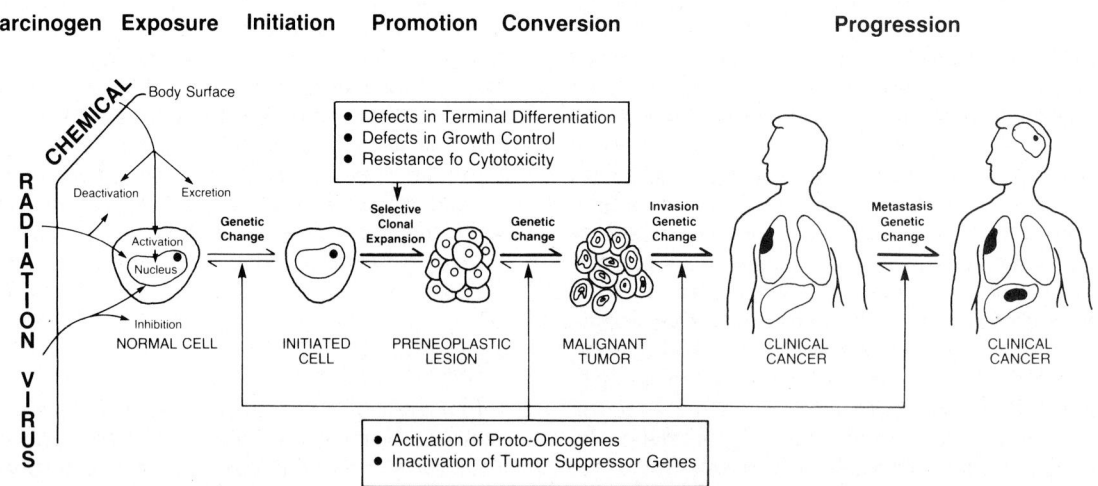

Figure III-2-1. Carcinogenesis can be conceptually divided into four steps: tumor initiation, tumor promotion, malignant conversion, and tumor progression. Activation of protooncogenes and loss of tumor suppressor genes are genetic changes that have been found in association with carcinogenesis. The accumulation of mutations and not necessarily the order in which they occur contributes to multistage carcinogenesis.

groups and a nucleotide in DNA (the process by which this occurs for the major classes of chemical carcinogens is discussed in detail under carcinogen metabolism). In general, a positive correlation is found between the amount of carcinogen-DNA adducts that can be detected in model systems and the resulting number of tumors that develop.[78,114] Thus tumors rarely develop in tissues that do not form carcinogen-DNA adducts. Carcinogen-DNA adduct formation is central to theories of chemical carcinogenesis, and can be considered to be a necessary, but not a sufficient, prerequisite for initiation. Some aspects of tumor initiation can also be accomplished by activation of protooncogenes; this topic will be discussed later (see tumor progression, oncogenes, and tumor suppressor genes below).

Tumor Promotion

Tumor promotion comprises the selective clonal expansion of initiated cells. Since the rate of accumulation of mutations is proportional to the rate of cell division, or at least the rate at which stem cells are replaced, it follows that clonal expansion of initiated cells produces a larger population of cells that are at risk of further genetic changes and malignant conversion.[20] Tumor promoters are generally non-mutagenic, not carcinogenic alone, and are often (but not always) able to mediate their biological effects without metabolic activation. These agents are characterized by their ability to reduce the latency period for tumor formation after exposure of a tissue to a tumor initiator, or increase the number of tumors formed in that tissue. In addition, they induce tumor formation in conjunction with a dose of an initiator too low to be carcinogenic alone. Chemicals or agents capable of both tumor initiation and promotion are known as complete carcinogens; examples of these are benzo[α]pyrene and 4-aminobiphenyl.

Croton oil (isolated from *Croton tiglium* seeds) has been used widely as a tumor promotor in murine skin carcinogenesis, and the mechanism of action of its most potent constituent, 12-O-tetradecanoylphorbol-13-acetate, via activation of protein kinase C is arguably the best understood among tumor promoters.[115] Protein kinase C is a calcium-phospholipid-dependent enzyme family that when activated causes phosphorylation of critical substrates and stimulates a cascade of epigenetic changes that can lead to cell growth.[3,11] The specific changes that have been observed to occur in cells treated with 12-O-tetradecanoylphorbol-13-acetate include; altered ion flux across the cell membrane, altered hormone binding and inhibition of cell-cell communication. Prostaglandin synthesis, that is also associated with tumor promotion, occurs as a result of stimulation of the arachidonic acid cascade that is mediated by protein kinase C. The cellular response to protein kinase C activation can result in modification of differentiation or cell proliferation, and is cell type dependent. The cell type dependent differential response may be explained by the fact that protein kinase C is a multigene family, the members of which are differentially expressed among animal species and tissue types.

The identification of new tumor promoters in animal models has accelerated with the increasingly sophisticated development of model systems designed to assay for tumor pro-

motion. Chemicals, complex mixtures of chemicals or other agents that have been shown to have tumor promoting properties include; dioxin (TCDD), benzoyl peroxide, bromomethylbenzanthracene, anthralin, phenol, saccharin, tryptophan, dichlorodiphenyltrichloroethane (DDT), phenobarbital, cigarette smoke condensate, polychlorinated biphenyls (PCBs), teleocidins, cyclamates, estrogens and other hormones, bile acids, ultraviolet light, wounding, abrasion and other chronic irritation (saline lavage).[116]

Okadaic acid is a powerful tumor promotor that is present in the marine sponge *Halichondria okadaii*. Okadaic acid, rather than acting through modulation of protein kinase C, is a specific inhibitor of protein phosphatase 1 (pp1) and 2A (pp2). Control of cellular processes occurs through reversible phosphorylation of pp1 and pp2.[26] Therefore, okadaic acid is actually capable of reversing cell transformation by some oncogenes (*c-raf*).

Malignant Conversion

Malignant conversion is the transformation of a preneoplastic cell into one that expresses the malignant phenotype. This process requires further genetic changes. It has been observed that the total dose of a tumor promoter is of less importance than frequently repeated administrations, and if the administration of a tumor promoter is discontinued before malignant conversion has occurred then premalignant or benign lesions may regress. The contribution of tumor promotion to the process of carcinogenesis is the expansion of a population of initiated cells which will then be at risk for malignant conversion. Conversion of a fraction of these to malignancy will be accelerated in proportion to the rate of cell division and the quantity of dividing cells in the benign tumor or preneoplastic lesion. In part these further genetic changes may be the result of infidelity of DNA synthesis.[71] The relatively low probability of malignant conversion can be substantially increased by exposure of preneoplastic cells to DNA damaging agents,[116] and it appears that this process may be mediated through the activation of protooncogenes and inactivation of tumor suppressor genes.

Tumor Progression

Tumor progression comprises the expression of the malignant phenotype and the tendency of already malignant cells to acquire more aggressive characteristics with time. Metastasis may also involve the ability of tumor cells to secrete proteases that allow invasion beyond the immediate location of the primary tumor. A prominent characteristic of the malignant phenotype is the propensity for genomic instability and uncontrolled growth. During this process further genetic changes can occur including the activation of protooncogenes and the functional loss of tumor suppressor genes. Protooncogenes are frequently activated by two major mechanisms: in the case of the *HRAS*-1 gene, point mutations are found in highly specific regions of the gene, (i.e., the 12th, 13th, 59th, or 61st codons), and members of the *myc, raf, neu,* and *jun* multigene families can be over-expressed, sometimes involving amplification of chromosome segments containing these genes. Loss of function of tumor suppressor genes usually occurs in a bimodal fashion involving deletion, point mutation, recombination, or chromosomal non-disjunction. These phenomena confer on the cells a growth advantage, and the capacity for regional invasion and ultimately distant metastatic spread. The accumulation of these mutations, and not the order or the stage in tumorigenesis in which they occur, appears to be an important determining factor that will be discussed below (see oncogenes and tumor suppressor genes).

Interindividual Variation

Polymorphisms arise through non-lethal mutations that occur during the course of evolution. The spectrum of polymorphisms among humans, for proteins that have a role in chemical carcinogenesis, includes; enzymes that metabolize (activate and detoxify) xenobiotic substances, enzymes that repair DNA damage and the cell surface receptors that activate the phosphorylation cascade. The cytochrome $P450$ multigene family is largely responsible for the metabolic activation and detoxication of many different chemical carcinogens that are present in the human environment.[37,40,75,77] However, acetylation (N-acetyltransferase) and formation of glutathione (glutathione-S-transferase) and glucuronide conjugates (β-glucuronidase) also contribute to xenobiotic metabolism.[28] The pathways of activation and detoxication are frequently in competition, so that an individual's propensity to convert a procarcinogen to an ultimate metabolite that can bind covalently with DNA varies considerably among the population.

Carcinogen Metabolism

The chemical etiology of occupationally-induced skin cancers was recognized as long ago as the eighteenth century.[86] In 1933, following a ten-year research program, the first chemically pure carcinogens were isolated from coal-tar pitch.[28,61] These chemicals were identified as polycyclic aromatic hydrocarbons, which are composed of variable numbers of fused benzene rings (Figure III-2-2). Polycyclic aromatic hydrocarbons are formed in the incomplete combustion of fossil fuels and vegetable matter (including cooked foods and tobacco), and are common environmental contaminants. The polycyclic aromatic hydrocarbons are chemically unreactive, and it was almost 20 years before it was shown that enzymic metabolites of these compounds could bind covalently to cellular macromolecules.[75]

Polycyclic aromatic hydrocarbons are activated in a multistep process involving initial epoxidation, hydration of the epoxide and subsequent epoxidation across the olefinic bond to form the ultimate carcinogenic metabolite, a diol-epoxide.[15,97] The first step in this process, the formation of the arene oxide is principally driven by cytochrome $P450_{IA1}$, the activity and inducibility of this enzyme (by exposure to polycyclic aromatic hydrocarbons) has been shown to vary among the human population.[43] The simple arene oxide is further metabolized to a dihydrodiol by epoxide hydrolase, the activity of which also varies among humans.[28,43] The second oxidation step at the site of the olefinic double bond is most extensively catalyzed by $P450_{IIIA4}$, which varies in activity among the population and is induced by steroids. Thus, for any individual there could be considerable day to day variation in enzyme activity.[40]

Metabolic activation of benzo[α]pyrene leads to the formation of the bay region benzo[α]pyrene-7,8-diol 9,10-oxide.[9,27] This vicinal diol-epoxide is asymmetrical and eight stereoisomers are possible. The reactivity of each isomer is variable and the isomers are formed in varying proportions by metabolism. Biological response to the different enantiomers in mammalian systems suggests that the (+)anti forms are the most active mutagens and carcinogens, and the (-)syn forms are the least active.

The arene ring of benzo[α]pyrene-7,8-diol 9,10-oxide opens spontaneously at the 10 position giving a highly reactive carbonium ion that can form a covalent addition product (adduct) with cellular macromolecules, including DNA. These adducts (an example of the structure of benzo[α]pyrene-7,8-diol 9,10-oxide bound to the exocyclic amino group [N2] of guanine is shown in III-2-Plate 1) cause the DNA to be damaged either by their persistence and consequent interference with replication or by aberrant DNA-repair. The same basic tenet holds true for carcinogen-DNA adducts of other chemical classes that may be activated by different metabolic pathways.

Another class of chemical carcinogens, aromatic amines, was first linked with increased bladder cancer among dye workers in 1895.[91] A principal aromatic amine thought to be responsible for bladder cancer incidence among workers in the rubber industry is 4-aminobiphenyl. This compound and many related compounds are components of cigarette smoke, diesel exhaust and the pyrolysis of certain foods. In addition nitrated polycyclic aromatic hydrocarbons are also environmental contaminants resulting from incomplete combustion of vegetable matter and diesel fuel, and are related to aromatic amines by nitroreduction.

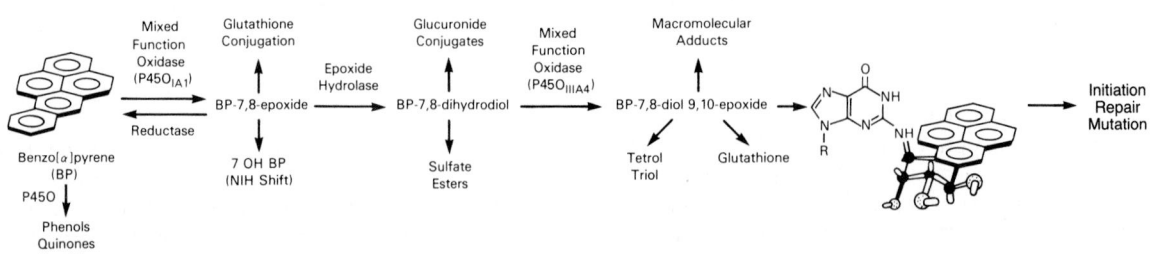

Figure III-2-2. Metabolism and activation of benzo[α]pyrene. The metabolic activation of benzo[α]pyrene (BP) proceeds by oxidation of the α-ring at the 7,8-position (cytochrome $P450_{IA1}$). Hydration of the arene oxide (epoxide hydratase) and further oxidation at the 9,10-position (cytochrome $P450_{IIIA4}$) produces a highly reactive vicinal diol-epoxide.

The metabolic activation of aromatic amines is complex.[9] They can be converted to an aromatic amide which is catalyzed by an acetyl coenzyme A dependent acetylation. The acetylation phenotype varies among the population and persons with the rapid acetylator phenotype are at higher risk of colon cancer,[57,68] whereas slow acetylators are at risk of bladder cancer.[23] This latter association may be due to the fact that activation of aromatic amines by N-oxidation is a competing pathway for aromatic amine metabolism, and the N-hydroxylation products when protonated (by the acid conditions in the urinary bladder) form reactive electrophiles that bind covalently with DNA or proteins to produce macromolecular damage.

An initial activation step for both aromatic amines and amides is N-oxidation by cytochrome $P450_{IA2}$. This $P450$ is inducible by phenobarbital, and since it is also responsible for the 3-demethylation of 1,3,7-trimethylxanthine (caffeine), the distribution of metabolic phenotypes in the population, and the disposition of an individual with respect to $P450_{IA2}$ metabolism, is relatively easy to determine.[19,40] The reaction of N-hydroxy-arylamines with DNA appears to be acid catalyzed, but they can be further activated by either an acetyl coenzyme A-dependent O-acetylase or a 3'-phosphoadenosine-5'phosphosulphate-dependent O-sulphotransferase. The N-arylhydroxamic acids, that arise as a result of the acetylation of N-hydroxy-arylamines or N-hydroxylation of aromatic amides, are not electrophilic and, therefore, require further activation. The predominant pathway for this seems to occur through acetyltransferase-catalyzed rearrangement to a reactive N-acetoxy-arylamine. Sulphotransferase catalysis results in the formation of N-sulphonyloxy arylamides. This complex pathway results in two major adduct types, amides (acetylated) and amines (non-acetylated).

The heterocyclic amines are formed during the preparation of cooked food, primarily from the pyrolysis (>150°C) of amino acids, creatinine and glucose. They have been recognized recently as food mutagens,[34,59,100] and have been shown to form adducts and cause liver tumors in primates.[1] In comparison to other carcinogens their metabolism is less well understood, but N-hydroxylation is considered to be a necessary step. Since they are similar in structure to the aromatic amines it is not surprising that they can be activated by cytochrome $P450_{IA2}$. The N-hydroxy metabolites of 3-amino-1-methyl-5H-pyrido[4,3-b]indole (Trp-P-1), 2-amino-6-methyldipyrido[1,2-a:3',2'-d]imidazole (Glu-P-1) and 2-amino-3-methyl-imidazo-[4,5-f]quinoline (IQ) can react directly with DNA. However, unlike the aromatic amines, this reaction is not facilitated by acid pH. Enzymic O-esterification of N-hydroxy metabolites is important in the activation of these food mutagens and the N-hydroxy metabolites are also good substrates for transacetylases. This suggests a possible etiological role for these chemicals in colorectal cancer, in combination with the rapid acetylator phenotype (mentioned above).

Aflatoxins (aflatoxin B_1, B_2, G_1, and G_2) are fungal mutagens that are formed primarily as metabolites of *Aspergillus flavus*, and they contaminate cereals, grain and nuts. A positive correlation exists between dietary aflatoxin exposure and liver cancer incidence in developing countries where grain spoilage is high. It should also be noted that a similar correlation exists between hepatitis B virus infection and incidence of hepatocellular carcinoma; chemical-viral interactive effects have been proposed.[45] Aflatoxins are activated by several cytochrome $P450s$ including $P450_{IIA3}$.[36] Aflatoxin B_1 and G_1 have an olefinic double bond at the 8,9-position and are more mutagenic and carcinogenic than aflatoxin B_2 and G_2 that are saturated and have an ethylenic bond at this position. This, and analysis of the DNA adducts, implies that the olefinic 8,9-bond is the site of activation.

Carcinogenic N-nitrosamines are ubiquitous environmental contaminants, and can be found in food, alcoholic beverages, cosmetics, cutting oils, hydraulic fluid, rubber, and tobacco.[7] Tobacco specific N-nitrosamines, for example 4-(methylnitrosoamino)-1-(3-pyridyl)-1-butanone, are carcinogenic in a wide range of animal species and may account for the carcinogenic nature of snuff and chewing tobacco.[51] Endogenous nitrosation can also occur as the result of the reaction of an amine with nitrate alone or nitrite in the presence of acid. Thus, nitrite (used in curing meats) and L-cysteine in the presence of acetaldehyde (a metabolite of alcohol) form N-nitrosothiazolidine-4-carboxylic acid. The N-nitrosamines are activated primarily by $P450_{IIE1}$. This isozyme is inducible by alcohol but it is not known whether $P450_{IIE1}$ is polymorphic.[40]

N-nitrosodimethylamine undergoes α-hydroxylation to form an unstable α-hydroxynitrosamine. The breakdown products are formaldehyde and methyl diazohydroxide. The alkyl groups of compounds like methyl diazohydroxide are good leaving groups and so methyl diazohydroxide is a powerful methylating agent that can add a small functional group (small alkyl-adduct, as opposed to the bulky aryl-adducts formed by the carcinogens discussed above) at more than ten different sites in DNA. The tobacco specific nitrosamines are not symmetrical and can also form bulky adducts, 4-(methylnitrosoamino)-1-(3-pyridyl)-1-butanone metabolism gives rise to either a positively charged pyridyl-oxobutyl ion or a positively charged methyl ion, both of which are able to alkylate DNA.[9,50,52]

DNA Damage and Repair

There are a number of ways in which the chemical structure of DNA can be altered by a carcinogen, these include: the formation of bulky aromatic type adducts, alkylation (generally small adducts), oxidation, dimerization and deamination. Chemical carcinogens can also cause epigenetic changes, for example, alteration in DNA methylation status.[112] Carcinogen-DNA adducts vary in their promutagenic potential, and this is exemplified for alkyl-adducts later in this section. Plate III-2-1 shows the binding of benzo[α]pyrene-7,8-diol 9,10-epoxide to the exocyclic (N2) amino group of deoxyguanosine. This is a bulky aromatic adduct that resides within the minor groove of the double helix, and is typical of polycyclic aromatic hydrocarbons. Although this adduct appears to be by far the most common form of DNA damage induced by benzo[α]pyrene in mammalian systems, others are possible, including covalent binding of metabolites to deoxyadenosine.[9,28]

Aromatic amine adducts are more complex, not only because they have both acetylated and non-acetylated (and deacetylated) metabolic intermediates but also because they form covalent bonds at the $C8$, $N2$, and sometimes $O6$ positions of deoxyguanosine as well as deoxyadenosine. However, the major adducts are $C8$-deoxyguanosine adducts, which reside predominantly in the major groove of DNA.[8]

Although the evidence for activation of aflatoxins B_1 and G_1 through hydroxylation of the olefinic 8,9-position is circumstantial, the structure of the adducts are known. They are formed at the $N7$-position of deoxyguanosine. These adducts are relatively unstable and have a half-life of about 50 hours at neutral pH, with resulting depurination. The aflatoxin B_1-N7-deoxyguanosine adduct can also undergo ring opening to yield two pyrimidine adducts, or alternately aflatoxin B_1-8,9-dihydrodiol could result. This latter possibility could restore the molecular structure of the DNA if hydrolysis of the original adduct occurs, but a potentially promutagenic lesion would result if formation of the 8,9-dihydrodiol is the result of degradation of ring-open adduct forms.[38,54]

Alkylation of DNA can occur at many sites either following the metabolic activation of certain N-nitrosamines or directly by the action of the N-alkylureas (N-methyl-N-nitrosourea) or the N-nitrosoguanidines. The protonated alkyl-functional groups that become available to form lesions in DNA generally attack the following nucleophilic centers: adenine ($N1$, $N3$, and $N7$); cytosine ($N3$); guanine ($N2$, $O6$ and $N7$); and thymine ($O2$, $N3$, and $O4$). Some of these lesions are known to be repaired ($O6$-methyldeoxyguanosine) while others are not ($N7$-methyldeoxyguanosine).[49] Furthermore, $O6$-methyldeoxyguanosine is a promutagenic lesion whereas $N7$-methyldeoxyguanosine is not.

Oxy-radical damage can result in the modification of DNA to form thymine glycol or 8-hydroxydeoxyguanosine adducts. Three major pathways have been identified. Exposure to organic peroxides (catechol, hydroquinone, and 4-nitroquinoline-N-oxide) leads to this type of oxy-radical damage. However, oxy-radicals and hydrogen peroxide can be generated in the catalytic cycling of some enzymes.[102] Cells can also be stimulated to produce peroxisomes by treatment with certain drugs and plasticizers.[90] Exposure to tumor promoters can indirectly increase oxy-radical formation; and perhaps the best known relationship is that between the phorbol esters and inflammatory cells. In this system, mediated through protein kinase C and the subsequent activation of a membrane localized pyridine nucleotide-dependent oxidase, oxy-radical formation is highly correlated with the relative potencies of the different phorbol esters.[35] Correspondingly, promoters that do not stimulate the protein kinase C signal transduction cascade do not effect oxy-radical production.

Another potentially mutagenic cause of DNA damage is deamination of methylated cytosine residues in DNA. In the case of methyl-cytosine at a CpG dinucleotide, deamination gives rise to a TpG mismatch. Repair of this lesion most often restores the CpG, however, a mutation may be fixed by repair to TpA.[101]

DNA repair enzymes act at sites of DNA damage caused by chemical carcinogens, and 4 major mechanisms are known; base excision repair, nucleotide excision repair, mismatch repair, and post-replication repair.[12,13,41] Discrimination between base excision repair and nucleotide excision repair is difficult, therefore it is appropriate to consider these processes together. Excision repair requires preincision recognition of the lesion and removal of the lesion by the action of a glycosylase. Repair of the damaged strand is then accomplished by the combined action of an exonuclease that degrades a portion of the damaged strand and a polymerase that synthesizes a "patch" containing the appropriate nucleotide sequence. The repair patch is synthesized in a 5' to 3' direction using the undamaged strand as a template and the patch is then ligated to the parental DNA at its 3' terminus. Some small alkyl-adducts, for example 3-methyladenine, as well as bulky aromatic adducts are repaired in this way. Larger adducts generally require removal of more than one or a few bases from the vicinity of the adduct, and nucleotide excision repair can remove up to 200 bases, including the adduct. DNA mismatches occur when conventional, but non-complementary, Watson-Crick bases lie opposite each other in the DNA helix. Transition mispairs (G-T or A-C) are repaired by the mismatch process more efficiently than transversion mispairs (G-G, A-A, G-A, C-C, C-T and T-T), probably due to differential recognition of the mispairings. Repair efficiency of mispairings is also dependent on their oligonucleotide environment for the same reason, mispairings in G-C rich regions are repaired more efficiently than those in A-T rich regions. The mechanism for correction of mispairings is essentially the same as that for excision-resynthesis repair described above, but generally involves the excision of large pieces of the DNA containing mispairings, obviously this process requires that the parental template strand is intact. Post-replication repair is the replication of DNA on a damaged template. When the DNA polymerase reaches a replication fork in the presence of damage to the parental strand, the polymerase can proceed past the lesion but a gap is left in the newly synthesized strand. The gap can be filled either by recombination of the daughter strand with the homologous parent strand that is mediated by the RecA protein, or in cases where single nucleotide gaps are left mammalian DNA polymerases can insert an adenine residue. These two possible mechanisms can therefore lead to recombinational events as well as base mispairing.

The rate but not the fidelity of DNA repair can be measured by adduct removal or unscheduled DNA synthesis. Substantial interindividual variations have been found in these rates.[43,81,94] Markedly reduced rates of excision repair are found in individuals with *Xeroderma pigmentosum*, and these individuals are at known risk of ultraviolet light induced skin cancer. However, among the general population approximately 5-fold variation in rates of excision repair are found in lymphocytes treated with carcinogens in vitro. An association has also been found between the reduced capacity of mononuclear leukocytes in vitro to repair aromatic amine adducts in individuals who have first degree relatives with cancer. Up to forty-fold variations among humans in the activity of o^6-alkylguanine-DNA alkyltransferase have also been reported. DNA repair rates are inhibited by aldehydes, alkylating agents and some chemotherapeutic drugs. Decreased DNA repair capacity has also been noted in the fibroblasts of lung cancer patients compared to those of melanoma patients or non-cancer controls. For benzo[α]pyrene-7,8-diol 9,10-epoxide-DNA adducts a unimodal distribution of repair rates has observed in lymphocytes, but interindividual variation has been found to be substantial.[94]

Response to Tumor Promoters

The tumor promoting effects of phorbol esters are reversible, and frequently repeated doses are necessary for promotion to occur.[115] This evidence suggests that tumor promotion occurs through an epigenetic mechanism based on selective clonal expansion. These effects are mediated primarily through protein kinase C activation. Resistance of initiated cells to phorbol ester mediated terminal differentiation may be related to alteration in the expression of protein kinase C (that may be related to the initiating event). Evidence to date supports this molecular model for the differential effects of tumor promoters between normal and initiated cells.

Phorbol esters produce different effects in different cell types. This may be explained by the expression of different classes of protein kinase C receptor among cell types. In addition, multiple protein kinase C genes and *m*RNA species have been identified in mammalian tissues,[29,64] and different rodent strains vary in their sensitivity to promoting agents.[16,83,98] Diversity in the elements that comprise the complex protein activation cascade, (including protein kinase C, its receptor and other protein kinase receptors) are likely to be differentially expressed among the population, either due to polymorphisms or differential exposures to environmental agents, and variation in individual response to tumor promoters could result.

Oncogenes and Tumor Suppressor Genes

Activation of protooncogenes and loss of tumor suppressor genes are genetic changes that have been found in association with carcinogenesis. The study of mechanisms by which chemical carcinogens cause these changes is an active area of interdisciplinary cancer research. It is clearly reasonable that chemical-DNA interactions and carcinogen-DNA adduct formation (either direct in the case of polycyclic aromatic hydrocarbons, or indirect in the case of oxy-radicals) lead to this type of genetic change in human cancer since these changes have been detected in tumors that have a recognized chemical etiology. Furthermore, recognition that carcinogen-DNA interaction was an important step in carcinogenesis and the results of short-term mutagenesis assays led to the conclusion that chemically induced DNA damage is an early step in the carcinogenic process.

The discovery of oncogenes, their role in cell transformation, and the realization that these genes arise from activation of normal cellular genes is dealt with elsewhere in this volume (see I-5). However, it should be emphasized that there are several possible mechanisms by which protooncogenes may be activated. These are: over-expression of the gene product leading to an increased concentration of the protein (dosage hypothesis); expression of the gene at an inappropriate time or context which could occur as a result of a mutation in the regulatory region of the gene (unscheduled gene expression); expression of a protooncogene in an inappropriate cell type; and structural alteration of the gene product. The primary mechanisms by which chemicals cause oncogene activation are discussed below. Activated *ras* genes predominate as the family of oncogenes to be isolated from solid tumors induced by chemicals in laboratory animals. Members of the *ras* gene family code for proteins of molecular weight 21,000 (*p*21), these proteins bind GTP, have GTPase activity and form complexes with other proteins, but the exact cellular function of *p*21 is the subject of ongoing research.[73] The first direct evidence of protooncogene activation by a chemical carcinogen was obtained from in vitro studies.[6,72] A wild-type recombinant clone of the human *HRAS*-1 gene (pEC) was modified with benzo[α]pyrene-diol-epoxide. The treated plasmid was then used to transfect NIH-3T3 cells with the result that the transformed cell foci produced contained the same specific point mutations (in either codon 12 or 61) that were known to exist in activated *ras* genes that were isolated from human tumors including the bladder (pEJ).

In animal model systems of chemical carcinogenesis and surveys of different types of human tumors that arise as a result of a variety of environmental-exposures (see Table III-2-1), *ras* mutations have been found.[6] In rodents, polycyclic aromatic hydrocarbons (3-methylcholanthrene, 7,12-dimethylbenz[α]anthracene and benzo[α]pyrene) have been used repeatedly to produce both benign tumors and malignant carcinomas. A large proportion of these premalignant and malignant lesions have been shown to have mutations in either the 12th or 61st codons. Similarly, treatment of rats with either 7,12-dimethylbenz[α]anthracene or *N*-methyl-*N*-nitrosourea resulted in the development of mammary carcinomas containing *ras* codon 12 or 61 mutations. These types of mutation have also been observed in mouse skin after initiation with 7,12-dimethylbenz[α]anthracene and tumor promotion with 12-*O*-tetradecanoylphorbol-13-acetate. Mutations in *ras* have been found in mouse liver after treatment with either vinyl carbamate, hydroxydehydroestragole or *N*-hydroxy-2-acetylaminofluorene. The same point-mutations have also been found in murine thymic lymphomas after treatment with *N*-methyl-*N*-nitrosourea or γ-radiation, and in other rodent skin models after treatment with either methylmethanesulphonate, β-propiolactone, dimethylcarbamyl chloride or *N*-methyl-*N'*-nitro-*N*-nitrosoguanidine.

These data suggest that chemical carcinogens may produce site specific mutations based in part on nucleoside selectivity of the ultimate carcinogen. However, persistence of a specific mutation is also dependent on the amino acid substitution in that the function of the mutant protein is altered to confer on the cell a clonal growth advantage. The types of mutations that are found in the chemically activated *ras* genes cause conformational changes that alter nucleotide binding to the *p*21 protein in such a way that the *p*21 GTPase activity is not reduced. There are data to support the hypothesis that *ras* activation is associated with malignant conversion as well as tumor initiation. Transfection of activated *ras* genes into benign papillomas that did not contain a constitutively activated *ras* gene caused malignant progression.[42]

Similarly normal human bronchial epithelial cells or those immortalized with SV40 T antigen have been shown to undergo malignant transformation when transfected with an activated *ras* gene.[2,87] In the immortalized cells, over-expression c-*raf*-1 and c-*myc* in combination but not in isolation also caused neoplastic transformation.[85] In addition Ki-*ras* gene mutations have been shown to be one of a number of changes that can arise either early or late in the development of colorectal carcinoma.[32] These findings suggest that the accumulation of mutations and not necessarily the order in which they occur contributes to multistage carcinogenesis. Furthermore, the stage of carcinogenesis in which each mutation occurs is not necessarily fixed. It appears that in the model for human colorectal carcinoma that *ras* mutations most often occur during malignant conversion, but they can be an early event (tumor initiation); whereas, in the rodent skin models *ras* mutations appear to be primarily a tumor initiating event. These differences may reflect the type of exposure both in terms of chemical class and chronic versus acute exposure or they may be a function of tissue type.

Loss of function of genes that may suppress the tumor phenotype was considered as a theoretical possibility in regard to retinoblastoma almost 20 years ago (see I-6). Firm experimental evidence for the existence of tumor suppressor genes has been provided by analysis of the molecular genetics of pediatric tumors (retinoblastoma, Wilms' tumor, rhabdomyosarcoma and bilateral acoustic neurofibromatosis). Examination of DNA-restriction fragment length polymorphisms by Southern hybridization shows loss of a restriction fragment from the tumor of a constitutive heterozygote if that genetic locus has been affected by certain mutational events (deletion, translocation, non-disjunction, mitotic recombination). This type of genetic analysis is termed loss of heterozygosity. In fact, in the case of the pediatric tumors' studies that showed loss of the normal allele and duplication of the inherited defective allele provided the first proof of mitotic recombination in humans.

Loss of a tumor suppressor gene is generally characterized by the presence of a mutation in one copy of the gene and loss of the homologous copy. Several genes that have these characteristics have been located on specific chromosomes: the retinoblastoma gene (13q); the Wilms' tumor gene (11p); the *p53* gene (17p); the deleted in colon carcinoma gene (DCC) (18q); the mutated colon cancer gene (MCC) (5q); the non-metastasis 23 gene (nm23) (17q); the protein tyrosine phosphatase gamma (PTP-γ) (3p) and the retinoic acid receptor gene (RAR).[5,24,30,63,65,67,70] The proof that these genes are tumor suppressor genes will come from experiments that test the tumor suppressive effects of a wild-type copy reintroduced into a tumor that has only a defective copy.

Other chromosomal loci have also been identified as candidates that contain tumor suppressor genes through loss of heterozygosity studies. Even though a model of carcinogenesis for retinoblastoma usually implies an inherited defect followed by a somatic mutation, spontaneous non-familial retinoblastoma is known. Therefore it is reasonable to suppose that chemical carcinogens may be responsible for causing genetic changes to tumor suppressor genes. This concept has been examined in the study of a growing number of adult tumors with etiologies of implied chemical exposure, i.e., the smoking related cancers. Frequent loss of heterozygosity has been observed in many of these tumor types.[46,74,111]

These studies have extended to DNA sequence analysis to determine if an associated mutation has occurred in a known tumor suppressor gene. Point mutations in the *p53*

gene, that give rise to amino acid changes or chain termination, are not only associated with loss of heterozygosity but can be frequently observed in lung cancer as well as colon cancer.[79,103] It has been implied above that some specificity with regard to DNA sequence may have a role in the determination of which site in the DNA may be altered by a particular chemical. Therefore, current efforts are directed toward the determination of the spectrum of mutations that are caused by a particular type of environmental exposure. A striking example of this type of analysis has recently implicated aflatoxin B_1 as the environmental agent responsible for specific *p53* mutations found in hepatocellular carcinomas of Chinese and southern African cancer patients.[17,56] These and other mutational spectra at the *p53* gene locus have been reviewed by Hollstein and colleagues.[55]

The general mechanism for loss of heterozygosity that occurs in tumors that have a familial origin may be different from that occurring in chemically induced cancer. Mitotic recombination is a common feature of pediatric neoplasms, however, the carcinogenic effects of the clastogens found in cigarette smoke appear in part to be mediated more typically through chromosomal deletions; these deletions are primarily terminal but are to a lesser extent interstitial.[111] Furthermore, given the complexity of tobacco smoke (a mixture of mutagens, carcinogens, and promoters) it is likely that these and other mutations are the result of both direct (adduct formation) and indirect (oxy-radical formation) damage to DNA. The determination of these types of disease-associated mutational spectra, that include both oncogenes and tumor suppressor genes, may eventually be useful in defining causal chemical exposure.

Clonal Evolution

The most extensively documented studies of sequential changes that address the question of clonality during human tumor evolution have used cytogenetic techniques in leukemia[80] (see I-8), and polymorphic gene loci in the molecular analysis of in colon cancer.[31,108] However, with the exception of a role for benzene in the etiology of acute myeloid leukemia, it is not certain whether either of these malignancies have a chemical etiology. Specifically, the clonal evolution of chemically induced mouse skin tumors has been studied in chimeric or mosaic animals.[88,89]

With reference to the case of chronic myelogenous leukemia, the early disease phase is characterized by a single reciprocal translocation, t(9;22) called the Philadelphia chromosome. This genetic change activates the *c-abl* protooncogene through the formation of a hybrid gene of *c-abl* with the break point cluster region (*bcr*). The resulting gene product has elevated tyrosine kinase activity. The later stages of chronic myelogenous leukemia are typified by overgrowth of one or more sub-clones that have additional karyotypic alterations.

In colorectal tumorigenesis a model has been developed in which accumulated alterations include at least one dominantly acting oncogene and several tumor suppressor genes.[31] These same studies provided evidence for the progressive nature of genetic changes in carcinogenesis. The fact that loss of heterozygosity in these and other types of tumors always results in loss of one of a pair of restriction fragments, that is the same allele (p53 for example) in all of the cells is evidence of clonality. The clonal origin of colorectal tumors in female cancer patients has been more convincingly demonstrated by differential methylation. Inactivation of the X chromosome (by methylation) during embryogenesis is random so that polyclonal female tissues develop with an approximately equal complement of inactivated maternal and paternal X chromosomes. If the tissues are monoclonal, the same inactive X chromosome should be present in all of the cells. Using a DNA-restriction fragment length polymorphism-based strategy all of the colorectal tumors were found to be monoclonal, and 95% of all human tumors so far studied, including leukemias, proved to be monoclonal.[31,108]

In chimeric or mosaic mice that differentially express isozymes of glucose phosphate isomerase or 3-phosphate kinase, a range of different carcinogens and initiation/promotion treatment regimes have been used to produce tumors that are monoclonal. Thus, the polyclonal tissues of the animals express more than one isotype and the tumor tissues express a single isotype indicating monoclonality. In a few rare cases polyclonal tumors were observed, probably due to the coalescence of two or more neighboring primary tumors. In experiments where the isozyme type was monitored at various stages in development, the malignant phenotype was always found to contain the same isotype as the benign papillomas. When human tumors have been examined in mosaic individuals evidence for monoclonality is most often found.

Chemical and Viral Interactions

A distinction between viral carcinogenesis and chemical carcinogenesis was made almost 50 years ago, and these seminal studies paved the way for the multistage theory of carcinogenesis.[10,92,93] Once inside a cell, certain viruses can integrate into the genome, and depending on their site of entry into the genome they can potentially activate protooncogenes and/or inactivate tumor suppressor genes. Since, in this way, viruses are able to act at every stage of carcinogenesis, it is reasonable that chemicals and viruses may have interactive effects in certain forms of carcinogenesis. There is now good evidence from experiments with in vivo experimental systems that viruses and chemicals can also interact in a synergistic manner.[48] The causation of cancer by purely chemical means has been discussed, and a number of studies have clearly demonstrated that certain forms of cancer have a viral etiology, these include; Burkitt's lymphoma and T-cell leukemia (see III-9, XXXVI-6 and XXXVI-10).

A number of human cancers are now considered to have both a viral component and chemical component to their etiology. Hepatitis B virus and aflatoxin B_1 or alcoholic beverages in hepatocellular carcinoma, Epstein-Barr virus and N-nitrosamines in nasopharyngeal carcinoma, and human papilloma virus and tobacco smoke components in cancers of the cervix, oral cavity, and larynx.[45,48] These studies have provided evidence of an association between environmental agents and carcinogenesis, but association does not imply causation. Therefore, experimental systems that provide evidence of chemical-viral interactive effects are discussed below.

In essence chemicals can act as tumor promoters following tumor initiation by viral agents, and viruses can act as promoters following chemical initiation. Cells pretreated with chemical carcinogens (benzo[α]pyrene, 4-nitroquinoline-N-oxide, 3-methylcholanthrene or thymidine analogues) have been shown to be more easily morphologically transformed by Simian virus 40 (SV40). Similarly enhanced transformation by other viruses (adenovirus SA7, mutant adenovirus type 5, or herpes simplex virus-2) has also been observed following pretreatment with several polycyclic aromatic hydrocarbons. In other cases alkylating agents have been used (methylmethane sulphate) prior to infection with wild type adenovirus 5, as a regime to morphologically transform rat embryo fibroblast cells in culture.

Human epithelial cells in vitro have proved more difficult for the study of chemical-viral interactions. Some reports exist where viruses (SV40 or Epstein-Barr) have been used to first immortalize the cells, however, and chemicals (3-methylcholanthrene or N-acetoxy-2-acetylaminofluorene, respectively) have been used to cause neoplastic transformation of the immortalized cells.[62] In Epstein-Barr immortalized B-lymphocytes, however, N-methyl-N-nitrosoguanidine treatment failed to cause neoplastic transformation. Taken together these studies may indicate that immortalization is required before malignant progression can occur, and that more than one gene is involved. However, it is difficult to assess the relevance of such an immortalization step to human carcinogenesis in vivo.

Implications for Molecular Epidemiology, Risk Assessment and Cancer Prevention

Increased understanding of mechanisms of carcinogenesis have led to the development of strategies for human cancer risk assessment.[47,110,113] These studies extend to the measurement of carcinogen-macromolecular adducts present in a target organ or surrogate, and the measurement of phenotypic determinants of disease disposition. The exposure of laboratory animals or cells in culture to chemical carcinogens has been shown to result in the formation of carcinogen-macromolecular adducts and suggest that it is reasonable to seek evidence for the presence of adducts in human tissues.

The biologically effective dose of a chemical carcinogen is governed by the amount of carcinogen that reaches a target tissue in a form that becomes activated in that tissue to a chemical species capable of causing lesions in DNA.[82] Because the chemical carcinogens in the human environment are not usually radioactive, and because humans are most commonly exposed to complex mixtures of chemicals, human carcinogen dosimetry at the molecular level requires sensitive and specific methods for carcinogen-macromolecular adduct quantitation. The low levels of adducts present in human DNA samples challenge the detection limits of conventional assay systems and complex mixtures of adducted materials confound simple assay systems.

A number of different methods have been developed for carcinogen-DNA dosimetry in humans. Specifically, the most commonly used techniques for human carcinogen-DNA adduct measurement are ^{32}P-nucleotide postlabeling, immunoassays, fluorescence spectroscopy, electrochemical conductance and gas chromatography/mass spectroscopy. Each of these techniques currently has its own advantages and limitations, and within the framework of epidemiological surveys multiple corroborative end-point analyses seem to provide the most useful information. These methodologies, their application and limitations are reviewed extensively elsewhere.[109,110,114]

Correlation of carcinogen-DNA adduct levels determined in humans with putative environmental exposure has rarely been shown in a convincing fashion. Probably the best example is the correlation of aflatoxin-DNA adducts that have been measured in urine samples from people in Africa. Aflatoxin-albumin adducts also correlated well with both exposure and 6-hydroxycortisol levels, indicating a role for $P450_{IIIA4}$ in aflatoxin activation.[39] Measurements of polycyclic aromatic hydrocarbon-DNA adducts in the peripheral white blood cells of occupationally exposed people have shown that this approach to human biomonitoring is feasible. Further research and development is required, however, to establish reliable methods.[96,109] With regard to measurement of 4-aminobiphenyl-hemoglobin adducts, however, a dose response relationship has been observed between the extent of smoking, type of tobacco used, and adduct levels.[18,106]

Assays for human cancer risk assessment that include the use of indicator drugs (an innocuous xenobiotic that shares the same pathway of metabolism as a known or suspect carcinogen; caffeine is an indicator of carcinogenic arylamine metabolism) are complementary to adduct studies, because of the implications for biologically effective dose following exposure.

Polymorphisms in xenobiotic metabolism may be determined by administration of an indicator drug and urinalysis to measure the metabolic ratio which characterizes the metabolic phenotype. Measures of metabolic ratio are the ratio between excretion of the unaltered drug to its metabolites, or a ratio of excreted metabolites. Caffeine is demethylated by the action of cytochrome $P450_{IA2}$.[19,40] The metabolites that are formed include theophylline (1,3-dimethylxanthine), paraxanthine (1,7-dimethylxanthine), theobromine (3,7-dimethylxanthine) and 1,3,7-trimethyluric acid. The formation of paraxanthine, demethylation of caffeine at the 3-position by $P450_{IA2}$, has been found to be highly correlated with metabolic N-oxidation of primary arylamines (e.g., the carcinogen, 4-aminobiphenyl, that is found in cigarette smoke and food items). N-acetyltransferase, which leads to the acetylation of primary arylamines, is an enzyme that competes with P450 demethylation. It is possible to discriminate between the slow and fast acetylator phenotypes by measuring other caffeine metabolites in urine. This is achieved by the determination of the ratio of 5-acetyl-6-formylamino-3-methyluracil (AFMU) to 1-methylxanthine. Therefore, determination of caffeine metabolic ratios in humans may be useful in assessing cancer risk of individuals with environmental exposures to aromatic amines in conjunction with genetic factors.

The extensive metabolizer phenotype of debrisoquine, an anti-hypertensive drug that is cleared through ring-hydroxylation by the hepatic cytochrome $P450_{IID6}$, is correlated with risk of lung cancer.[4,22,69] Extensive metabolizers of debrisoquine appear, therefore, to be at significantly greater risk of lung cancer than are poor metabolizers. There are two possible explanations for these findings; it has been hypothesized that $P450_{IID6}$ may activate a chemical carcinogen(s) found in tobacco smoke, and alternately, $P450_{IID6}$ may be in linkage disequilibrium with a lung cancer susceptibility gene. Even though the mechanistic basis for this association is obscure the debrisoquine polymorphism might still prove to be a valuable tool in risk assessment. Accordingly, research efforts in this area are continuing threefold: further epidemiological studies are in progress to firmly establish the association, carcinogen metabolism studies aimed at determination of a mechanistic basis for this association are being performed, and with the cloning of this gene molecular studies for the development of a genotyping test could also result in a better understanding of debrisoquine metabolizer disposition as a risk factor in lung carcinogenesis.[53]

Epidemiological and pharmacogenetic studies have postulated the existence of inherited predisposition for human lung cancer,[14] and certain genetic polymorphisms have been suggested to have an association with risk in human lung carcinogenesis. For DNA-restriction fragment length polymorphisms at the human HRAS-1 and L-myc loci, rare or minor restriction fragments (alleles) appear to either predispose to certain cancers[66] or are associated with poor prognosis.[60,76] A variable tandem repeat DNA sequence region tightly flanked by MspI restriction sites, which is located 3' with respect to the cellular HRAS-1 structural protooncogene (chromosome locus 11p15.5),[21,33] accounts for the DNA-restriction fragment length polymorphism. In the case of L-myc, the presence or absence of an EcoRI restriction site in the second intron of the gene defines a simple polymorphism. Both hypotheses have been tested in a formal case-control study.[99,104] Individuals with rare allelomorphs at the HRAS-1 protooncogene locus were found to be at greater risk of lung cancer.[99] No firm mechanistic basis is known for this association. The tandem repeat region may be sensitive to mitotic recombination and consequently a target for chemical carcinogens. No association was found with increased risk of metastasis and the L-myc protooncogene polymorphism.[104] Both the HRAS-1 and L-myc restriction fragment length polymorphisms were found to vary significantly with race.[99,104]

The goal of molecular epidemiology is to identify individuals at increased cancer risk by obtaining evidence of high exposure to carcinogens, leading to pathobiological lesions in target cells and/or increased susceptibility to cancer that are due to either inherited or acquired host factors. Interindividual variation among people in carcinogen biodistribution, metabolism, DNA adduct formation, DNA repair and potential response to tumor promoters have important implications in determination of cancer risk. An increased understanding of the molecular basis of these differences among humans and their connection with critical steps in carcinogenesis may assist the future potential to predict disease risk of the individual before clinical onset of disease.[44]

References

1. Adamson, R. H.: Induction of hepatocellular carcinoma in nonhuman primates by chemical carcinogens. Cancer Detect. Prev., 14:215, 1989.

2. Amstad, P., Reddel, R. R., Pfeifer, A., Malan-Shibley, L., Mark, G. E., and Harris, C. C.: Neoplastic transformation of a human bronchial epithelial cell line by a recombinant retrovirus encoding viral harvey *ras*. Mol. Carcinogenesis, 1:151, 1988.
3. Ashendel, C. L.: The phorbol ester receptor: A phospholipid-regulated protein kinase. Biochim. Biophys. Acta, 822:219, 1985.
4. Ayesh, R., Idle, J. R., Ritchie, J. C., Crothers, M. J., and Hetzel, M. R.: Metabolic oxidation phenotypes as markers for susceptibility to lung cancer. Nature, 312:169, 1984.
5. Baker, S. J., Fearon, E. R., Nigro, J. M., Hamilton, S. R., Preisinger, A. C., Jessup, J. M., van Tuinen, P., Ledbetter, D. H., Barker, D. F., and Nakamura, Y.: Chromosome 17 deletions and p53 gene mutations in colorectal carcinomas. Science, 244:217, 1989.
6. Barbacid, M.: Involvement of ras oncogenes in the initiation of carcinogen-induced tumors. Int. Symp. Princess Takamatsu Cancer Res. Fund, 17:43, 1986.
7. Bartsch, H., Ohshima, H., Shuker, D. E., Pignatelli, B., and Calmels, S.: Exposure of humans to endogenous N-nitroso compounds: Implications in cancer etiology. Mutat. Res., 238:255, 1990.
8. Beland, F. A. and Kadlubar, F. F.: Formation and persistence of arylamine DNA adducts in vivo. Environ. Health Perspect., 62:19, 1985.
9. Beland, F. A. and Poirier, M. C.: DNA adducts and carcinogenesis. *In* The Pathobiology of Neoplasia. Edited by A. E. Sirica. New York, Plenum Publishing Corp., 1989, p. 57.
10. Berenblum, I. and Shubik, P.: A new quantitative approach to the study of the stages of chemical carcinogenesis in the mouse skin. Br. J. Cancer, 1:383, 1947.
11. Blumberg, P. M.: In vitro studies on the mode of action of the phorbol esters, potent tumor promoters, part 2. CRC Crit. Rev. Toxicol., 8:199, 1981.
12. Bohr, V. A.: Gene specific DNA repair. Carcinogenesis, In press, 1991.
13. Bohr, V. A., Evans, M. K., and Fornace, A. J., Jr.: Biology of disease. DNA repair and its pathogenetic implications. Lab. Invest., 61:143, 1989.
14. Bonney, G. E.: Interactions of genes, environment, and life-style in lung cancer development. J. Natl. Cancer Inst., 82:1236, 1990.
15. Borgen, A., Darvey, H., Castagnoli, N., Crocker, T. T., Rasmussen, R. E., and Wang, I. Y.: Metabolic conversion of benzo(a)pyrene by Syrian hamster liver microsomes and binding of metabolites to deoxyribonucleic acid. J. Med. Chem., 16:502, 1973.
16. Boutwell, R. K.: Some biological aspects of skin carcinogenesis. Prog. Exp. Tumor Res., 4:207, 1964.
17. Bressac, B., Kew, M., Wands, J., and Ozturk, M.: Selective G to T mutations of p53 hepatocellular carcinoma from southern Africa. Nature, 350:429, 1991.
18. Bryant, M. S., Vineis, P., Skipper, P. L., and Tannenbaum, S. R.: Hemoglobin adducts of aromatic amines: Associations with smoking status and type of tobacco. Proc. Natl. Acad. Sci. USA, 85:9788, 1988.
19. Butler, M. A., Iwasaki, M., Guengerich, F. P., and Kadlubar, F. F.: Human cytochrome P-450_m PA (P-450IA2), the phenacetin O-deethylase, is primarily responsible for the hepatic 3-demethylation of caffeine and N-oxidation of carcinogenic arylamines. Proc. Natl. Acad. Sci. USA, 86:7696, 1989.
20. Cairns, J.: Mutation selection and the natural history of cancer. Nature, 255:197, 1975.
21. Capon, D. J., Chen, E. Y., Levinson, A. D., Seeburg, P. H., and Goeddel, D. V.: Complete nucleotide sequences of the T24 human bladder carcinoma oncogene and its normal homologue. Nature, 302:33, 1983.
22. Caporaso, N. E., Tucker, M. A., Hoover, R., Hayes, R. B., Pickle, L. W., Issaq, H., Muschik, G., Green-Gallo, L., Buivys, D., Aisner, S., Resau, J., Trump, B. F., Tollerud, D., Weston, A., and Harris, C. C.: Lung cancer and the debrisoquine metabolic phenotype. J. Natl. Cancer Inst., 85:1264, 1990.
23. Cartwright, R. A., Glashan, R. W., Rogers, H. J., Ahmad, R. A., Barham-Hall, D., Higgins, E., and Kahn, M. A.: Role of N-acetyltransferase phenotypes in bladder carcinogenesis: A pharmacogenetic epidemiological approach to bladder cancer. Lancet, 2:842, 1982.
24. Cavenee, W. K., Dryja, T. P., Phillips, R. A., Benedict, W. F., Godbout, R., Gallie, B. L., Murphree, A. L., Strong, L. C., and White, R. L.: Expression of recessive alleles by chromosomal mechanisms in retinoblastoma. Nature, 305:779, 1983.
25. Cavenee, W. K., Hansen, M. F., Nordenskjold, M., Kock, E., Maumenee, I., Squire, J. A., Phillips, R. A., and Gallie, B. L.: Genetic origin of mutations predisposing to retinoblastoma. Science, 228:501, 1985.
26. Cohen, P., Holmes, C. F., and Tsukitani, Y.: Okadaic acid: A new probe for the study of cellular regulation. Trends Biochem. Sci., 15:98, 1990.
27. Conney, A. H.: Induction of microsomal enzymes by foreign chemicals and carcinogenesis by polycyclic aromatic hydrocarbons: G. H. A. Clowes Memorial Lecture. Cancer Res., 42:4875, 1982.
28. Cooper, C. S., Grover, P. L., and Sims, P.: The metabolism and activation of benzo[α]pyrene. *In* Progress in Drug Metabolism. Edited by J. W. Bridges, and L. Chasseaud. England, Wiley and Sons, Ltd., 1983, p. 295.
29. Coussens, L., Parker, P. J., Rhee, L., Yang-Feng, T. L., Chen, E., Waterfield, M. D., Francke, U., and Ullrich, A.: Multiple, distinct forms of bovine and human protein kinase C suggest diversity in cellular signaling pathways. Science, 233:859, 1986.
30. Fearon, E. R., Cho, K. R., Nigro, J. M., Kern, S. E., Simons, J. W., Ruppert, J. M., Hamilton, S. R., Preisinger, A. C., Thomas, G., Kinzler, K. W., and Vogelstein, B.: Identification of a chromosome 18q gene that is altered in colorectal cancers. Science, 247:49, 1990.
31. Fearon, E. R., Hamilton, S. R., and Vogelstein, B.: Clonal analysis of human colorectal tumors. Science, 238:193, 1987.
32. Fearon, E. R. and Vogelstein, B.: A genetic model for colorectal tumorigenesis. Cell, 61:759, 1990.
33. Feinberg, A. P. and Vogelstein, B.: Hypomethylation of ras oncogenes in primary human cancers. Biochem. Biophys. Res. Commun., 111:47, 1983.
34. Felton, J. S., Knize, M. G., Shen, N. H., Wu, R., and Becher, G.: Mutagenic heterocyclic imidazoamines in cooked foods. *In* Carcinogenic and Mutagenic Responses to Aromatic Amines and Nitroarenes. Edited by C. M. King, L. J. Romano, and D. Schuetzle. New York, Elsevier Science Publishing Co., 1988, p. 73.
35. Floyd, R. A., Watson, J. J., Harris, J., West, M., and Wong, P. K.: Formation of 8-hydroxydeoxyguanosine, hydroxyl free radical adduct of DNA in granulocytes exposed to the tumor promoter, tetradecanoylphorbolacetate. Biochem. Biophys. Res. Commun., 137:841, 1986.
36. Gonzalez, F. J.: The molecular biology of cytochrome P450s. Pharmacol. Rev., 40:243, 1988.
37. Gonzalez, F. J.: Molecular genetics of the P-450 superfamily. Pharmacol. Ther., 45:1, 1990.
38. Groopman, J. D., Donahue, P. R., Zhu, J. Q., Chen, J. S., and Wogan, G. N.: Aflatoxin metabolism in humans: Detection of metabolites and nucleic acid adducts in urine by affinity chromatography. Proc. Natl. Acad. Sci. USA, 82:6492, 1985.
39. Groopman, J. D., Sabbioni, G., and Wild, C. P.: Molecular dosimetry of human aflatoxin exposures. *In* Molecular Dosimetry of Human Cancer: Epidemiological, Analytical, and Social Considerations. Edited by J. Groopman, and P. Skipper. New Jersey, Telford Press, 1991.
40. Guengerich, F. P.: Characterization of human microsomal cytochrome P-450 enzymes. Annu. Rev. Pharmacol. Toxicol., 29:241, 1989.
41. Hanawalt, P. C.: Preferential DNA repair in expressed genes. Environ. Health Perspect., 76:9, 1987.
42. Harper, J. R., Roop, D. R., and Yuspa, S. H.: Transfection of the EJ rasHa gene into keratinocytes derived from carcinogen-induced mouse papillomas causes malignant progression. Mol. Cell Biol., 6:3144, 1986.
43. Harris, C. C.: Interindividual variation among humans in carcinogen metabolism, DNA adduct formation and DNA repair. Carcinogenesis, 10:1563, 1989.
44. Harris, C. C.: Interindividual variation in human chemical carcinogenesis: Implications for risk assessment. *In* Scientific Issues in Quantitative Risk Assessment. Edited by S. H. Moolgavkar. Boston, Birkhauser, 1990, p. 235.
45. Harris, C. C.: Hepatocellular carcinogenesis: Recent advances and speculations. Cancer Cells, 2:146, 1990.
46. Harris, C. C., Reddel, R. R., Pfeifer, A., Amstad, P., Mark, G. E., Weston, A., Modali, R., Iman, D. S., McMenamin, M. G., Kaighn, M. E., Gabrielson, E. W., Jones, R., and Trump, B. F.: Oncogenes and tumor suppressor genes in human lung carcinogenesis. *In* Genetic Mechanisms in Carcinogenesis and Tumor Progression. Edited by C. C. Harris, and L. A. Liotta. New York, Wiley-Liss, 1990, p. 127.
47. Harris, C. C., Weston, A., Willey, J. C., Trivers, G. E., and Mann, D. L.: Biochemical and molecular epidemiology of human cancer: Indicators of carcinogen exposure, DNA damage, and genetic predisposition. Environ. Health Perspect., 75:109, 1987.
48. Haugen, A. and Harris, C. C.: Interactive effects between viruses and chemical carcinogens. *In* Carcinogenesis and Mutagenesis, Handbook of Experimental Pharmacology. Edited by C. S. Cooper, and P. L. Grover. London, Springer-Verlag, 1990, p. 249.
49. Hecht, S. S., Foiles, P. G., Carmella, S. G., Trushin, N., Rivenson, A., and Hoffmann, D.: Recent studies on the metabolic activation of tobacco-specific nitrosamines: Prospects for dosimetry in humans. *In* Banbury Report 23: Mechanisms in Tobacco Carcinogenesis. Edited by D. Hoffmann, and C. C. Harris. New York, Cold Spring Harbor Laboratory, 1986, p. 245.
50. Hecht, S. S. and Hoffmann, D.: Tobacco-specific nitrosamines, an important group of carcinogens in tobacco and tobacco smoke. Carcinogenesis, 9:875, 1988.
51. Hecht, S. S., and Hoffmann, D.: The relevance of tobacco-specific nitrosamines to human cancer. Cancer Surv., 8:273, 1989.
52. Hecht, S. S., Trushin, N., Castonguay, A., and Rivenson, A.: Comparative tumorigenicity and DNA methylation in F344 rats by 4-(methylnitrosamino)-1-(3-pyridyl)-1-butanone and *N*-nitrosodimethylamine. Cancer Res., 46:498, 1986.
53. Heim, M. and Meyer, U. A.: Genotyping of poor metabolizers of debrisoquine by allele-specific PCR amplification. Lancet, 336:529, 1990.
54. Hertzog, P. J., Smith, J. R., and Garner, R. C.: Characterisation of the imidazole ring-opened forms of trans-8,9-dihydro-8,9-dihydro-8-(7-guanyl)9-hydroxy aflatoxin B1. Carcinogenesis, 3:723, 1982.
55. Hollstein, M., Sidransky, D., Vogelstein, B., and Harris, C. C.: p53 mutations in human cancers. Science, 253:49, 1991.
56. Hsu, I. C., Metcalf, R. A., Sun, T., Welsh, J. A., Wang, N. J., and Harris, C. C.: Mutational hotspot in the p53 gene in human hepatocellular carcinomas. Nature, 350:427, 1991.
57. Ilett, K. F., David, B. M., Detchon, P., Castleden, W. M., and Kwa, R.: Acetylation phenotype in colorectal carcinoma. Cancer Res., 47:1466, 1987.
58. International Agency for Research on Cancer: IARC Monographs on the Evaluation of Carcinogenic Risks to Humans. Overall Evaluations of Carcinogenicity: An Updating of IARC Monographs Volumes 1 to 42. Lyon, IARC, 1987.
59. Kato, R.: Metabolic activation of mutagenic heterocyclic aromatic amines from protein pyrolysates. Crit. Rev. Toxicol., 16:307, 1986.
60. Kawashima, K., Shikama, H., Imoto, K., Izawa, M., Naruke, T., Okabayashi, K., and Nishimura, S.: Close correlation between restriction fragment length polymorphism of the L-MYC gene and metastasis of human lung cancer to the lymph nodes and other organs. Proc. Natl. Acad. Sci. USA, 85:2353, 1988.
61. Kennaway, E.: The identification of a carcinogenic compound in coal tar. Br. Med. J. Clin. Res., 2:749, 1955.
62. Kessler, D. J., Heilman, C. A., Cossman, J., Maguire, R. T., and Thorgeirsson, S. S.: Transformation of Epstein-Barr virus immortalized human B-cells by chemical carcinogens. Cancer Res., 47:527, 1987.
63. Kinzler, K. W., Nilbert, M. C., Vogelstein, B., Bryan, T. M., Levy, D. B., Kelly, J. S., Pressinger, A. C., Hamilton, S. R., Hedge, P., Markham, A., Carlson, M., Joslyn, G., Groden, J., White, R., Miki, Y., Miyoshi, Y., Nishisho, I., and Nakamura, Y.: Identification of a gene located at chromosome 5q21 that is mutated in colorectal cancers. Science, 251:1366, 1991.
64. Knopf, J. L., Lee, M. H., Sultzman, L. A., Kriz, R. W., Loomis, C. R., Hewick, R. M., and Bell, R. M.: Cloning and expression of multiple protein kinase C cDNAs. Cell, 46:491, 1986.
65. Koufos, A., Hansen, M. F., Lampkin, B. C., Workman, M. L., Copeland, N. G., Jenkins, N. A., and Cavenee, W. K.: Loss of alleles at loci on human chromosome 11 during genesis of Wilms' tumour. Nature, 309:170, 1984.
66. Krontiris, T. G., DiMartino, N. A., Colb, M., and Parkinson, D. R.: Unique allelic restriction fragments of the human Ha-ras locus in leukocyte and tumour DNAs of cancer patients. Nature, 313:369, 1985.
67. LaForgia, S., Morse, B., Cannizzaro, L. A., Li, F., Nowell, P. C., Boghosian-Sell, L., Glick, J., Weston, A., Harris, C. C., Drabkin, H., Patterson, D., Croce, C. M., Schlessinger, J., and Huebner, K.: Receptor-linker protein-tyrosine-phosphatase, PTPγ, is a candidate tumor suppressor at human chromosome region 3p21. Proc. Natl. Acad. Sci. U.S.A., 88:5036, 1991.
68. Lang, N. P., Chu, D. Z., Hunter, C. F., Kendall, D. C., Flammang, T. J., and Kadlubar,

F. F.: Role of aromatic amine acetyltransferase in human colorectal cancer. Arch. Surg., 121:1259, 1986.

69. Law, M. R., Hetzel, M. R., and Idle, J. R.: Debrisoquine metabolism and genetic predisposition to lung cancer. Br. J. Cancer, 59:686, 1989.

70. Leone, A. McBride, W. O., Weston, A., Wang, M., Anglard, P. Cropp, C. S., Goepel, J. R., Lidereau, R., Callahan, R., Linehan, W. M., Rees, R. C., Harris, C. C., Liotta, L. A., and Steeg, P. S.: Somatic allelic deletion of nm23 in human cancer. Cancer Res., 51:2490, 1991.

71. Loeb, L. A. and Cheng, K. C.: Errors in DNA synthesis: A source of spontaneous mutations. Mutat. Res., 238:297, 1990.

72. Marshall, C. J., Vousden, K. H., and Phillips, D. H.: Activation of c-Ha-ras-1 proto-oncogene by in vitro modification with a chemical carcinogen, benzo(a)pyrene diol-epoxide. Nature, 310:586, 1984.

73. McCormick, F.: ras GTPase activating protein: Signal transmitter and signal terminator. Cell, 56:5, 1989.

74. McGuire, W. L. and Naylor, S. L.: Loss of heterozygosity in breast cancer: cause or effect [editorial; comment]. J. Natl. Cancer Inst., 81:1764, 1989.

75. Miller, J. A.: Carcinogenesis by chemicals: an overview–G. H. A. Clowes memorial lecture. Cancer Res., 30:559, 1970.

76. Nau, M. M., Brooks, B. J., Jr., Battey, J. F., Sausville, E., Gazdar, A. F., Kirsch, I. R., McBride, O. W., Bertness, V., Hollis, G. F., and Minna, J. D.: L-myc, a new myc-related gene amplified and expressed in human small cell lung cancer. Nature, 318:69, 1985.

77. Nebert, D. W. and Negishi, M.: Multiple forms of cytochrome P-450 and the importance of molecular biology and evolution. Biochem. Pharmacol., 31:2311, 1982.

78. Neumann, H. G.: Role of extent and persistence of DNA modifications in chemical carcinogenesis by aromatic amines. Recent Results Cancer Res., 84:77, 1983.

79. Nigro, J. M., Baker, S. J., Preisinger, A. C., Jessup, J. M., Hostetter, R., Cleary, K., Bigner, S. H., Davidson, N., Baylin, S., Devilee, P., Glover, T., Collins, F. S., Weston, A., Modali, R., Harris, C. C., and Vogelstein, B.: Mutations in the p53 gene occur in diverse human tumor types. Nature, 342:705, 1989.

80. Nowell, P. C. and Croce, C. M.: Chromosomal approaches to oncogenes and oncogenesis. FASEB J, 2:3054, 1988.

81. Oesch, F., Aulmann, W., Platt, K. L., and Doerjer, G.: Individual differences in DNA repair capacities in man. Arch. Toxicol., 10(Suppl.):172, 1987.

82. Perera, F. P. and Weinstein, I. B.: Molecular epidemiology and carcinogen-DNA adduct detection: New approaches to studies of human cancer causation. J. Chronic. Dis., 35:581, 1982.

83. Peto, J.: Genetic predisposition to cancer. In Banbury Report No. 4. New York, Cold Spring Harbor Laboratory, 1980, p. 203.

84. Peto, R., Roe, F. J., Lee, P. N., Levy, L., and Clack, J.: Cancer and ageing in mice and men. Br. J. Cancer, 32:411, 1975.

85. Pfeifer, A., Mark, G. E., Malan-Shibley, L., Graziano, S. L., Amstad, P., and Harris, C. C.: Cooperation of c-raf-1 and c-myc protooncogenes in the neoplastic transformation of SV40 T-antigen immortalized human bronchial epithelial cells. Proc. Natl. Acad. Sci. USA, 86:10075, 1989.

86. Pott, P.: Chirurgical observations relative to the cancer of the scrotum. London, L. Hawes, W. Clark, and R. Collins, 1775.

87. Reddel, R. R., Ke, Y., Kaighn, M. E., Malan-Shibley, L., Lechner, J. F., Rhim, J. S., and Harris, C. C.: Human bronchial epithelial cells neoplastically transformed by v-Ki-ras: Altered response to inducers of terminal squamous differentiation. Oncogene Res., 3:401, 1988.

88. Reddy, A. L. and Fialkow, P. J.: Multicellular origin of fibrosarcomas in mice induced by the chemical carcinogen 3-methylcholanthrene. J. Exp. Med., 150:878, 1979.

89. Reddy, A. L. and Fialkow, P. J.: Papillomas induced by initiation-promotion differ from those induced by carcinogen alone. Nature, 304:69, 1983.

90. Reddy, J. K. and Lalwani, N. D.: Carcinogenesis by hepatic peroxisome proliferators: Evaluation of the risk of hypolipodemic drugs and industrial plasticizers to humans. CRC Crit. Rev. Toxicol., 12:1, 1984.

91. Rehn, C.: Blasengeschwulste bei Fuchsinarbeitern. Arch. Klin. Chir., 50:588, 1895.

92. Rous, P. and Friedwald, W. F.: The effect of chemical carcinogens on virus induced rabbit carcinomas. J. Exp. Med., 79:511, 1944.

93. Rous, P. and Kidd, J. G.: The carcinogenic effect of a papilloma virus on the tarred skin of rabbits. I. Description of the phenomenon. J. Exp. Med., 67:399, 1938.

94. Setlow, R. B.: Variations in DNA repair among humans. In Human Carcinogenesis. Edited by C. C. Harris, and H. Autrup. New York, Academic Press, 1983, p. 231.

95. Shields, P. G. and Harris, C. C.: Environmental causes of cancer. Med. Clin. North Am., 74:263, 1990.

96. Shields, P. G., Weston, A., Sugimura, H., Bowman, E. D., Caporaso, N. E., Manchester, D. K., Trivers, G. E., Tamai, S., Resau, J. H., Trump, B. F., and Harris, C. C.: Molecular Epidemiology: Dosimetry, Susceptibility and Cancer Risk. In Immunoassays for Monitoring Human Exposure to Toxic Chemicals in Foods and the Environment. Edited by M. Van der Laan. Washington, D.C., ACS Books, 1990, p. 186.

97. Sims, P., Grover, P. L., Swaisland, A., Pal, K., and Hewer, A. J.: Metabolic activation of benzo(a)pyrene proceeds by a diol-epoxide. Nature, 252:326, 1974.

98. Slaga, T. J., Fischer, S. M., Weeks, C. E., Klein-Szanto, A. J., and Reiners, J. J.: Studies of mechanisms involved in multistage carcinogenesis in mouse skin. In Mechanisms of Chemical Carcinogenesis. Edited by C. C. Harris, and P. A. Cerutti. New York, Alan R. Liss, Inc., 1982, p. 207.

99. Sugimura, H., Caporaso, N. E., Hoover, R. N., Modali, R., Resau, J., Trump, B. F., Lonergan, J. A., Krontiris, T. G., Mann, D. L., Weston, A., and Harris, C. C.: Association of rare alleles of the Harvey ras protooncogene locus with lung cancer. Cancer Res., 50:1857, 1990.

100. Sugimura, T., Sato, S., and Wakabayashi, T.: Mutagens: Carcinogens in pyrolysates of amino acids, proteins and cooked food; heterocyclic aromatic amines. In Chemical Induction of Cancer. Edited by Y. T. Woo, D. Y. Lai, J. T. Arcos, and M. F. Ardus. New York, Academic Press, 1988, p. 681.

101. Sved, J. and Bird, A.: The expected equilibrium of the CpG dinucleotide in vertebrate genomes under a mutation model. Proc. Natl. Acad. Sci. USA, 87:4692, 1990.

102. Taffe, B. G. and Kensler, T. W.: Free radicals and signal transduction in tumor promotion. In Genes and Signal Transduction in Multistage Carcinogenesis. Edited by N. H. Colburn. New York, Marcel Dekker, Inc., 1989, p. 391.

103. Takahashi, T., Nau, M. M., Chiba, I., Birrer, M. J., Rosenberg, R. K., Vinocour, M., Levitt, M., Pass, H., Gazdar, A. F., and Minna, J. D.: p53: A frequent target for genetic abnormalities in lung cancer. Science, 246:491, 1989.

104. Tamai, S., Sugimura, H., Caporaso, N. E., Resau, J. H., Trump, B. F., Weston, A., and Harris, C. C.: Restriction fragment length polymorphism analysis of the L-myc gene locus in a case-control study of lung cancer. Int. J. Cancer, 46:411, 1990.

105. Verma, A. K. and Boutwell, R. K.: Effects of dose and duration of treatment with the tumor-promoting agent, 12-O-tetradecanoylphorbol-13-acetate on mouse skin carcinogenesis. Carcinogenesis, 1:271, 1980.

106. Vineis, P., Caporaso, N., Tannenbaum, S. R., Skipper, P. L., Glogowski, J., Bartsch, H., Coda, M., Talaska, G., and Kadlubar, F.: Acetylation phenotype, carcinogen-hemoglobin adducts, and cigarette smoking. Cancer Res., 50:3002, 1990.

107. Vogelstein, B., Fearon, E. R., Hamilton, S. R., Kern, S. E., Preisinger, A. C., Leppert, M., Nakamura, Y., White, R., Smits, A. M., and Bos, J. L.: Genetic alterations during colorectal-tumor development. N. Engl. J. Med., 319:525, 1988.

108. Vogelstein, B., Fearon, E. R., Hamilton, S. R., Preisinger, A. C., Willard, H. F., Michelson, A. M., Riggs, A. D., and Orkin, S. H.: Clonal analysis using recombinant DNA probes from the X-chromosome. Cancer Res., 47:4806, 1987.

109. Weston, A., Manchester, D. K., Povey, A. C., and Harris, C. C.: Detection of carcinogen-macromolecular adducts in humans. J. Am. Coll. Toxicol., 8:913, 1989.

110. Weston, A., Willey, J. C., Manchester, D. K., Wilson, V. L., Brooks, B. R., Choi, J. S., Poirier, M. C., Trivers, G. E., Newman, M. J., Mann, D. L., and Harris, C. C.: Dosimeters of human exposure to carcinogens: Polycyclic aromatic hydrocarbon-macromolecular adducts. In Methods for Detecting DNA Damaging Agents in Humans: Applications in Cancer Epidemiology and Prevention. Edited by H. Bartsch, K. Hemminki, and I. K. O'Neill. Lyon, IARC, 1988, p. 181.

111. Weston, A., Willey, J. C., Modali, R., Sugimura, H., McDowell, E. M., Resau, J., Light, B., Haugen, A., Mann, D. L., Trump, B. F., and Harris, C. C.: Differential DNA sequence deletions from chromosomes 3, 11, 13 and 17 in squamous cell carcinoma, large cell carcinoma and adenocarcinoma of the human lung. Proc. Natl. Acad. Sci. USA, 86:5099, 1989.

112. Wilson, V. L., Smith, R. A., Longoria, J., Liotta, M. A., Harper, C. M., and Harris, C. C.: Chemical carcinogen-induced decreases in genomic 5-methyldeoxycytidine content of normal human bronchial epithelial cells. Proc. Natl. Acad. Sci. USA, 84:3298, 1987.

113. Wogan, G. N.: Markers of exposure to carcinogens. Environ. Health Perspect., 81:9, 1989.

114. Wogan, G. N. and Gorelick, N. J.: Chemical and biochemical dosimetry of exposure to genotoxic chemicals. Environ. Health Perspect., 62:5, 1985.

115. Yuspa, S. H.: Tumor promotion. In Accomplishments in Cancer Research. Edited by J. G. Fortner, and J. E. Rhoads. Philadelphia, Lippincott Co., 1986, p. 169.

116. Yuspa, S. H. and Poirier, M. C.: Chemical carcinogenesis: From animal models to molecular models in one decade. Adv. Cancer Res., 50:25, 1988.

Hormones and the Etiology of Cancer

Brian E. Henderson
Leslie Bernstein
Ronald K. Ross

Introduction

There is a substantial and convincing body of experimental, clinical and epidemiological evidence indicating that hormones play a major role in the etiology of several human cancers. The concept that hormones can increase the incidence of neoplasia was first proposed by Bittner, based on experimental studies of estrogens and mammary cancer in mice.[16] This concept has been refined into epidemiologic hypotheses related to cancers of the breast, endometrium, prostate, ovary, thyroid, bone, and testis.[49,53] A key element of these hypotheses is that neoplasia is the consequence of excessive hormonal stimulation of the particular target organ, the normal growth and function of which is under the control of one or more steroid or polypeptide hormones (Figure III-3-1). In this model, hormones exert an effect that may be independent of outside initiators such as chemicals or ionizing radiation.[95]

Neoplasia of tissues that are responsive to hormones currently account for more than 20 percent of all newly diagnosed male, and more than 40 percent of all newly diagnosed female, cancers in the United States. Because of the evidence that endogenous hormones affect the risk of these cancers and the importance of these cancers in absolute frequency, reason for concern exists about the effects on cancer risk if the same or closely related hormones are administered for therapeutic purposes; for example, as contraceptives, as hormone replacement therapy, or for the prevention of miscarriage.[49,53] This chapter reviews the epidemiological and endocrinological evidence for the role of hormones in the development of specific cancers and the current status of the relationship between exogenous hormones and cancer of the breast, endometrium and ovary.

Endometrial Cancer

Among the hormone-related cancers, etiologically the best understood is endometrial cancer. All the major demographic characteristics of the disease, as well as the major non-demographic risk factors, are explicable on the basis of cumulative exposure of the endometrium to that fraction of estrogen which is unopposed by the modifying influences of progesterone (Table III-3-1).[49]

Key and Pike have recently summarized the existing data on endometrial mitotic activity during normal menstrual cycles.[63] Mitotic rates are low during days 1–4 of the cycle,

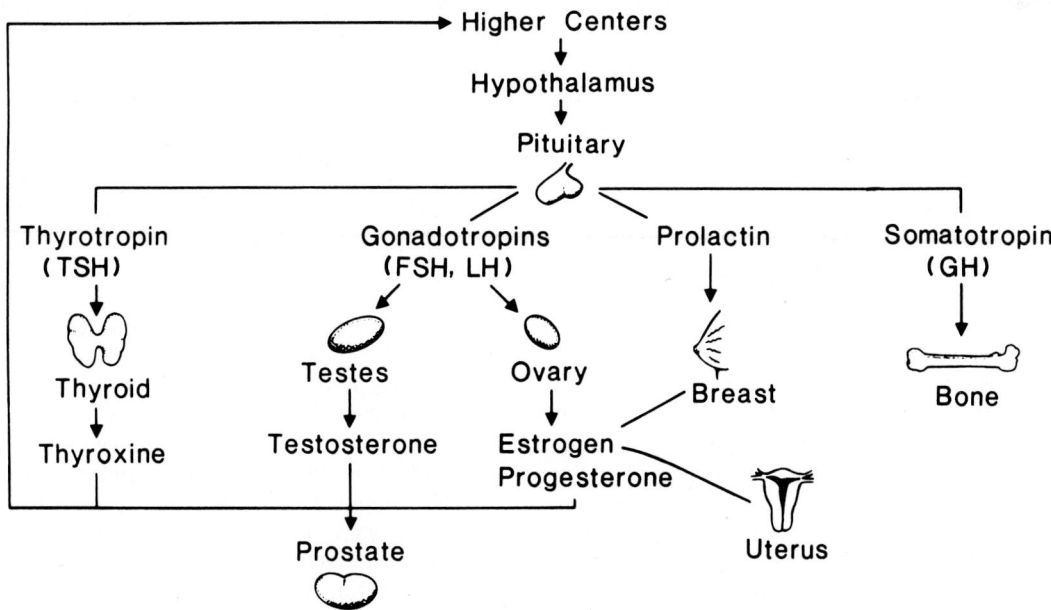

Figure III-3-1. Hypothesized relationships between steroid and polypeptide hormones and human cancer.

Table III-3-1. A Summary of Established Hormonal Risk and Protective Factors for Endometrial Cancer

Risk factors (increased exposure to "unopposed" estrogen)
 Estrogen replacement therapy
 Obesity
 Sequential oral contraceptives
 Late menopause

Protective factors (decreased exposure to unopposed estrogen)
 Pregnancy
 Oral contraceptives

then increase rapidly and remain stable thereafter until day 19, after which rates drop to essentially zero for the remainder of the cycle. There appears to be a lag period of about 4 days before the full stimulatory effects of unopposed estrogen, or the modifying influence of progesterone on endometrial mitotic activity, are fully apparent.

The cellular basis for the antiestrogenic activity of progestogens on the endometrium is well understood.[49] Progestogens reduce the concentration of estradiol receptors and increase the activity of the enzyme system that converts estradiol to estrone, a biologically less potent estrogen due to its lower affinity for cellular estrogen receptors. Luteal phase progesterone causes endometrial cells to differentiate to a secretory state and progestogen withdrawal leads to cyclic sloughing of endometrial tissue.

The age-incidence curve of endometrial cancer consists essentially of two straight lines of different slopes intersecting at the menopause.[63] During the premenopausal period the slope is steep and most likely determined by the accumulation of mitotic activity during the first half of the menstrual cycle, when estrogen is unopposed by progesterone. With cessation of ovarian function at the menopause, the slope of the age-incidence curve decreases dramatically, although endometrial cancer rates continue to increase in the postmenopausal period. The most likely explanation for the latter phenomenon is weight-related estrogen formation and use of estrogen replacement therapy.

Based on the concept that frequency of mitotic activity is the primary determinant of endometrial cancer risk and that such activity is controlled by cumulative exposure to unopposed estrogens, one can readily predict the most important risk factors for this disease. Pregnancies and oral contraceptives (OCs), which expose the endometrium to constant high levels of both estrogen and progestogen, should protect against endometrial cancer development. Estrogen replacement therapy and obesity should increase risk. All of these predicted effects have been well documented by a large series of epidemiologic studies.

Hormone replacement therapy in the form of unopposed estrogen therapy gained widespread popularity in the United States in the 1960's and into the 1970's. By 1974, there were nearly 30 million prescriptions of estrogen replacement being filled annually and the most popular brand, a type of conjugated equine estrogen, had become the fourth most frequently prescribed drug in the country.[62] Concomitant with this increasing usage, endometrial cancer incidence rates in postmenopausal women also increased rapidly, especially on the West Coast, where use of estrogen replacement ther-

apy (ERT) was particularly common.[6] By 1975, the results of epidemiologic case-control studies were being published, demonstrating a strong overall association between estrogen use and endometrial cancer risk.[69,123] Although the methodologic strengths and weaknesses of these early studies were the subject of intense scrunity and much debate, it soon became apparent that this association represented a cause and effect relationship. Literally dozens of studies have now documented a high relative risk of endometrial cancer following ERT.[12] Risk is strongly related to both dose and duration of use, but high risk follows even moderate doses taken for moderately long periods of time. Women who use ERT for 5 or more years have about a 6- to 8-fold increase in risk compared with women who never used such therapy.[119]

While the incidence of aggressive endometrial cancer is clearly increased by estrogen use, somewhat paradoxically the overall mortality among affected users is much lower than among non-users who develop endometrial cancer.[23] In fact, such women have little reduction in lifespan, compared with healthy women the same age.[23] The reasons for this are not completely known, but this phenomenon is likely to be explicable largely on the basis of increased medical surveillance among estrogen users. Women who use ERT tend to be closely followed since the drug is known to induce vaginal bleeding. Part of this favorable survival experience is probably also due to patients with estrogen-induced benign hyperplasia being mislabeled as endometrial cancer cases. While past users of ERT have a risk of endometrial cancer which is intermediate between that of current users of comparable duration and lifetime non-users, risk in such women remains substantially elevated over baseline even after many years of treatment.[86]

High weight leads to increased risk for endometrial cancer at all ages.[33,45,61,65] The three studies of postmenopausal women with the largest number of endometrial cancer cases and controls all show at least a doubling of risk between the thinnest and heaviest women.[31,61,65] The reason for this increase in risk with increasing weight is straightforward—obese postmenopausal women have increased plasma concentrations of estradiol.[124] Adipose tissue is rich in an aromatase enzyme system that converts androstenedione to estrone. Estrone, in turn, can be converted directly to estradiol. In addition, sex-hormone binding globulin (SHBG) levels are lower in obese women, so that the amount of bioavailable estradiol in obese women is higher than would be expected from the peripheral conversion of androstenedione to estrone alone.[124]

The explanation for the substantially increased risk of endometrial cancer with obesity in premenopausal women, as observed in the studies of Henderson and colleagues,[45] and LaVecchia and colleagues,[65] is less obvious. Although obesity does appear to be associated with slightly increased levels of bioavailable estradiol in premenopausal women, this alone appears insufficient to account for such a profound effect of obesity on risk. The more likely explanation is that obesity in premenopausal women is associated with amenorrhea and subnormal luteal phase progesterone levels, resulting in prolonged exposure of the endometrium to unopposed estrogen.[100]

The role of estrogens as the principal cause of endometrial cancer is further supported by the marked increase in risk after a relatively short duration of use of sequential OCs, which deliver an unopposed estrogen during most of the monthly cycle.[45] As potent as the effects are of ERT and sequential OCs in modifying risk of endometrial cancer, these effects can be mitigated by the simultaneous administration of progestogens. A series of case-control studies have consistently demonstrated that combination OCs, which deliver an estrogen and progestogen simultaneously during each day of use, decrease the risk of endometrial cancer by 50% or more.[12] Two prospective studies, the Walnut Creek Contraceptive Drug Study,[98] and the Royal College of General Practitioner's Oral Contraceptive Study,[9] have demonstrated similar decreases in risk. In most of these studies, endometrial cancer risk steadily decreased with increasing duration of use. In the largest case-control study, the protective effect of combination OC use persisted for women who discontinued using OCs 15 years prior to participation in the study.[21]

The newer regimens of hormone replacement therapy typically follow a pattern not unlike that of sequential OCs, with an unopposed estrogen given early in a monthly cycle followed by estrogen combined with a progestogen for the last 10–12 days. This regimen attempts to reproduce the hormonal pattern of the normal menstrual cycle, albeit at lower levels of both estrogen and progestogen. One might predict therefore that this method of hormone replacement therapy might only partially offset the increased risk of endometrial cancer associated with unopposed ERT. There has been only one study reported to date on the effects of combination hormone therapy on endometrial cancer risk, which meets acceptable methodologic standards. Although endometrial cancer risk in this prospective study was clearly reduced to a level below that of women using unopposed ERT, the study was not sufficiently large to determine with confidence whether risk was reduced to baseline.[87] A continuous combined regimen of hormone replacement therapy in which estrogen and progestogen are administered together each day, as with combination OCs, has been growing in popularity. This regimen presumably could totally obviate the risk of endometrial cancer, but could also reduce some of the benefit of unopposed estrogen on heart disease risk and may also adversely affect risk of breast cancer.[51]

The other major, established risk factor for endometrial cancer, low parity, is also readily explained by the unopposed estrogen hypothesis.[68] The highest risk of endometrial cancer occurs in either married or unmarried nulliparous women and decreases in risk occur with each increase in parity; nulliparous women have an endometrial cancer risk which is 3–5 times that of women of parity greater than 3.[68] This effect is expected since no endometrial mitotic activity occurs during pregnancy, due to the persistently high progesterone levels.

Breast Cancer

The available evidence regarding the hormonal etiology of breast cancer is most consistent with the hypothesis that estrogen is the primary stimulant for breast cell prolifera-tion.[49,53] The simultaneous presence of progesterone probably further increases the rate of proliferation.[63] This latter conclusion is based largely on the fact that breast mitotic activity peaks during the luteal phase of the menstrual cycle.[35]

Among non-demographic factors, the most consistently documented risk factors for breast cancer are: early age at menarche, late age at menopause, late age at first full-term pregnancy, and weight (Table III-3-2).[48] The age incidence curve for breast cancer emphasizes the importance of ovulation in determining risk. The initial cases occur in early adulthood and the rate of increase in incidence then rises sharply with age to the time of the menopause, when it slows dramatically. The rate of increase in the postmenopausal period is only about one-sixth the rate of increase in the premenopausal period. This age incidence curve appears, then, to be shaped in a major way by the effects of ovarian activity.

Early age at menarche has been demonstrated as a risk factor for breast cancer in most case-control studies.[48] In general, an approximately 20% decrease in breast cancer risk results from each year that menarche is delayed. In a study of young women, Henderson and colleagues recorded both age at onset of menstruation and age when "regular", i.e., predictable, menstruation was first established.[47] For a fixed age at menarche, the establishment of regular menstrual cycles within 1 year of the first menstrual period more than doubled the risk of breast cancer, when compared to women with a 5-year or longer delay for menses to regularize. Women with early menarche, age 12 or younger, and rapid establishment of regular cycles had an almost 4-fold increased risk of breast cancer when compared to women with late menarche, age 13 or older, and long duration of irregular cycles.

These observations suggest that regular ovulatory cycles increase a woman's risk of breast cancer and support results from an earlier study comparing circulating hormone levels in daughters of breast cancer cases and with those in age matched daughters of controls.[50] The daughters of the breast cancer cases, who as a group have at least twice the breast cancer risk of the general population, had higher levels of circulating estrogen and progesterone than did the controls.[46]

Other evidence supporting the concept that the cumulative number of ovulatory cycles, i.e., cumulative estrogen and progesterone exposure, is a major determinant of breast

Table III-3-2. A Summary of Established Hormonal Risk and Protective Factors for Breast Cancer

Risk factors (increased exposure to estrogen and/or progesterone)
    Early menarche
    Late menopause
    Obesity (postmenopausal women)
    Hormone replacement therapy
    Pregnancy ("early" effect)

Protective factors (reduced exposure to estrogen and/or progesterone)
    Lactation
    Pregnancy ("late" effect)
    Obesity (premenopausal women)

long-lasting, i.e., 10–15 years after discontinuing OC use the risk remains at a very low level.[22,120]

Casagrande and coworkers suggested that, since the protection afforded by pregnancies and by OC use appeared to act through a common mechanism, periods of pregnancy and OC use could be combined into a single measure of "protected time".[20] They demonstrated that the risk of ovarian cancer clearly decreased as protected time increased. Other epidemiological studies have confirmed this observation.[36,120]

As with breast and endometrial cancer, the age incidence curve for ovarian cancer emphasizes the importance of ovulation in determining risk. The age incidence curve of ovarian cancer can be brought into line with the familiar linear log-log plot of other nonhormone-dependent epithelial tumors if ovarian age is considered as starting at menarche and proceeding at a reduced rate (roughly 30% of normal) during periods of anovulation, including the postmenopausal period.[30,120]

Prostate Cancer

Prostate cancer has become the most frequently diagnosed cancer among men in the United States, exceeding lung cancer by a narrow margin. Approximately 106,000 cases will be diagnosed in 1990 alone, resulting in about 30,000 deaths.[2] The most important risk factor for prostate cancer is age. Prostate cancer is extremely rare prior to age 40, but thereafter the rate of increase, i.e., the slope of the age incidence curve, is greater than for any other cancer.[102] There is substantial international variation in prostate cancer incidence, with 50- to 100-fold differences in rates among countries with the highest and lowest reported incidence. Among countries with reasonably reliable cancer reporting, China and Japan have the lowest prostate cancer rates, whereas Black Americans have, by far, the highest prostate cancer rates in the world.[78]

Testosterone, through metabolism to dihydrotestosterone, controls mitotic activity in the prostate although the quantitative relationship between testosterone levels and rate of cell proliferation in the prostate is unstudied. Free testosterone, the small proportion (about 2%) of testosterone that is not bound to either serum albumin or SHBG, diffuses into prostate cells where it is rapidly and irreversibly converted to dihydrotestosterone through the action of the enzyme 5-α reductase. Dihydrotestosterone is bound to cytosol receptors which, in turn, are translocated to the nucleus of prostate cells.[24]

There exist several lines of evidence which contribute information helpful in understanding the relationship between hormones and prostate cancer.

Laboratory animals have a very low spontaneous incidence of adenocarcinomas of the prostate and few experimental strategies are known to increase tumor yield.[99] The first and most successful experimental model was that produced by Noble, who demonstrated that exogenous administration of subcutaneous testosterone propionate could, in a dose-related fashion, dramatically increase the incidence of adenocarcinoma of the prostate in Nb rats.[82] Pollard has similarly induced prostatic carcinoma in germ free Lobund

Wistar rats through hormonal manipulation.[92] Attempts to chemically induce prostatic adenocarcinomas other than by hormonal manipulation have been largely unsuccessful. In recent years, Bosland has been able to induce invasively growing metastasizing adenocarcinomas in the prostate of Wistar rats by a single intravenous injection of N-methyl-N-nitrosourea.[17] Hormonal priming with testosterone to induce maximal cell proliferation was required in this model for any tumor induction. All clearly established experimental models of prostatic adenocarcinomas have an androgen requirement for tumor induction.

A number of studies have compared circulating testosterone levels measured by radioimmunoassay in cases of prostate cancer with those in controls of similar age with no known prostatic disease. The largest and best designed of these studies tend to find higher levels of serum testosterone in cases.[102] For example, Ghanadian and colleagues showed that patients with prostatic cancer had higher testosterone levels than healthy controls of similar age.[38] Ahlawalia and co-workers also found levels of serum testosterone to be significantly higher in patients with prostatic cancer than in age-matched controls in United States, but not African blacks.[1] Drafta and colleagues similarly found higher circulating T levels among cases than in "normal ambulatory controls".[32] However, others have not found such differences, especially those studies which have utilized non-healthy controls for comparison.[58]

There have been three prospective studies of prostate cancer and circulating testosterone levels reported to date, with inconsistent results. One found higher levels in cases but the others did not.[42] In a case-control study nested within a large Hawaiian prospective study, Nomura and co-workers observed no difference in testosterone levels between 98 prostate cancer cases and age- and hour-of-sampling matched controls.[83] Barrett-Conner and colleagues recently reported results from an ongoing prospective study among a cohort of elderly residents of Rancho Bernardo, California.[8] They found no consistent relationship between circulatory testosterone levels and subsequent prostate cancer risk, but rather unexpectedly found that prostate cancer increased with increased estradiol levels, and with increased levels of the adrenal androgen androstenedione.

The hypothesis of a hormonal etiology for prostatic cancer would predict that healthy black males should have higher testosterone levels than healthy white males. Since differences in the ratio of prostate cancer incidence among racial-ethnic groups are maximal early in the age range in which prostate cancer occurs, hormonal patterns at young ages might be particularly important determinants of risk.[102] Ross and colleagues studied circulating steroid hormone levels in white and black college students in Los Angeles.[103] After adjustment for minor differences in age, alcohol use, smoking habits and time of sampling as well as weight, the mean testosterone level in blacks was 15% higher than that of whites, and the free testosterone level was 13% higher. Although this difference is not large, it is sufficient to explain the two-fold excess of this disease in blacks if such differences were persistent throughout adolescence and adult life.[103]

Endocrine manipulation has remained a mainstay of treatment of prostatic cancer for nearly half a century. Administration of estrogens, and more recently of luteinizing hormone releasing hormone (LHRH) agonists, to reduce pituitary luteinizing hormone (LH) production, and thereby greatly reduce testicular testosterone production, is a common strategy for treating advanced disease. Use of anti-androgens to block androgen activity at the cellular level is also growing in popularity.[79]

There does not currently exist an extensive or strong body of epidemiologic literature supporting an etiologic relationship between testosterone and prostate cancer. One important reason for this may be that there exist no definitive and reproducible markers of hormonal events in men, such as pregnancies or menstrual experiences in women. Nonetheless, there do exist data which lend credibility to this hypothesis and support the need for more definitive research in this area.

Castration leads to an approximately 80% reduction in prostatic size. Although there has been no systematic study of this association, there has never been a case report of prostatic cancer occurring in such patients.[102]

A number of investigators have found evidence that factors associated with increased sexual activity are associated with increased prostate cancer risk, e.g., early age at first intercourse,[57] frequency of intercourse,[106] number of sexual partners,[110] and venereal disease history,[57,106,110] although, with the exception of the latter observation, results are not entirely consistent across studies.[102] Findings such as these have suggested the possibility that prostate cancer may be caused by transmission of an infectious agent through sexual activity. However, in a cohort study of cancer mortality in Catholic priests in Los Angeles, Ross and colleagues found a small but statistically non-significant excess of prostate cancer deaths.[104] The absence of a marked deficit of prostate cancer mortality among such men is evidence against sexual transmission of the disease. An obvious alternate explanation is that these sexual activity measures are indices of underlying androgen production.

The other fairly well established risk factor for prostatic cancer that is of interest in terms of a hormonal etiology is dietary fat consumption. There is a strong correlation between per capita fat consumption and prostate cancer mortality on an international basis.[5] Moreover, the four largest epidemiologic case-control studies find that cases tend to consume more fat than controls.[39,55,64,106] These studies have involved diverse target populations including blacks, whites and Asians in the United States. Studies which have evaluated prostate cancer risk in association with intake of specific high fat content foods, e.g., beef and pork, milk, eggs, or cheese, rather than as a specific nutrient also support the notion that fat is a risk factor.[109,111] It has been hypothesized that dietary fat might affect prostate cancer occurrence through an alteration in the hormonal environment. In support of this hypothesis, Hill and Wynder a decade ago showed in a small study that switching from a Western diet (40% of calories from fat) to an isocaloric vegetarian low-fat diet (25% calories from fat) resulted in a substantial reduction in circulating testosterone levels.[56] There exist preliminary data, using the Lobund-Wistar rat model, suggesting that dietary fat may enhance the effects of testosterone in inducing prostatic cancer, but isocaloric diets have not yet been evaluated in this system.[91]

Adolescent and Young Adult Genital Cancer

The work of Herbst and colleagues describing the association between in utero diethylstilbestrol (DES) exposure and vaginal adenocarcinoma provided the initial suggestion that estrogen might induce anomalous development in utero which would later have neoplastic consequences in the postpubertal period.[53] They showed that there was a greatly limited age range during which these neoplasms developed (approximately ages 15–29) and the relevant exposure nearly always occurred during the first trimester of the index pregnancy. Vaginal adenocarcinomas appear to develop from Mullerian duct remnants that are induced by DES exposure to persist beyond early fetal life. These remain dormant during childhood and are activated at puberty.

The age-specific incidence rates of malignant germ cell tumors of the testis peak in early adult life, in a pattern that is similar to that of DES-induced vaginal adenocarcinoma.[105] This correspondence suggests that the etiology of testicular germ cell neoplasms may also involve in utero hormonal exposure. Risk factors for testis cancer include a history of cryptorchidism, caucasian race and in utero exogenous estrogen exposure, and may include maternal nausea and maternal obesity as well.

Men with a history of cryptorchid testis have been reported to have relative risks of testis cancer ranging from 3 to 14, compared to men who experienced normal testicular descent.[28,43,93] A persistently undescended testis is often accompanied by other structural abnormalities. The testis is smaller and tubule development and spermatogenesis are retarded. Sertoli cell development is delayed and there are abnormalities of the Leydig cells.[54] It is not the abdominal location of the undescended testis that increases the risk of cancer in the undescended testis. After descent is achieved by surgical treatment, previously undescended testes retain a higher than normal risk of cancer.[31,93] Furthermore, the contralateral, normally descended testis in patients with unilateral cryptorchidism is reported to have a 2-fold increased risk of cancer.[43,60,76]

Normal descent of the testis is under hormonal control. Animal experiments have shown that estrogen treatment of pregnant mice can lead to undescended and hypogenetic testes.[84] Similar abnormalities have been reported in the male offspring of women exposed to DES and to OCs during pregnancy.[84] Thus, it is likely that cryptorchidism is tied to estrogen levels early in pregnancy and represents another, sometimes intermediate, outcome of the pathway leading to germ cell testicular tumors.

Other potential risk factors for testis cancer may also be manifestations of excess estrogen during the critical gestation period. Excessive nausea during pregnancy of mothers of patients with testis cancer may be associated with an increased risk of testis cancer; the risk is greatest for nausea requiring medical treatment and most noticeable for sons who were the mother's first live birth.[28,43] Increased levels of bioavailable estradiol are found in the first trimester of pregnancy of women with hyperemesis gravidarum compared to controls and in the first trimester of a woman's first compared to her second pregnancy.[11,27] Since adipose tissue is a source of estrogen, and since obesity is associated with reduced levels of SHBG, the increasing risk of testis cancer observed with increased weight of the mother prior to the index pregnancy may also reflect an excess of bioavailable estrogen.[67]

Three of four studies of the relationship of exogenous sex steroid exposure in pregnancy and testis cancer have shown higher risk of testis cancer in sons who experienced in utero exposure to either DES, OCs, estrogen, or the estrogen-progestin combinations used in pregnancy tests, with reported relative risks ranging from 2.8–5.3.[28,43,77,107]

The rarity of testis cancer and, correspondingly, cryptorchidism, in black males, may represent a slight variation of this "estrogen excess" hypothesis.[105] The substantially higher plasma testosterone as well as estrogen levels in black women compared to white women early in gestation suggest the possibility that both hormones may be important factors in the development of the testis.[44] The absolute excess of testosterone in the early gestation blood of black women, by providing a "protected" environment for testicular development and descent, is one possible explanation for the subsequent lower incidence of testis cancer in black male offspring. In rats, estrogen-inhibited testicular descent can be reversed by treatment with androgens.[97]

There are similarities in the epidemiology of ovarian and testicular germ cell tumors even though the former are comparatively rare. The ovarian tumors tend to have a peak incidence rate in the young adult age range and, as for testis cancer, these rates have been increasing.[115] Furthermore, risk of these tumors is associated with maternal exposure to hormonal drugs during the index pregnancy.[114]

Thyroid Cancer

The pituitary hormone thyroid stimulating hormone (TSH) is the principal hormone regulating the growth and function of the thyroid gland and thus, excess TSH may be of etiologic importance in the development of thyroid cancer.[59] This hypothesis is supported by the observation that growth of some thyroid cancers depends on TSH secretion, so that suppression of TSH release by administration of thyroxin is often an effective treatment for thyroid carcinomas.[25] Experimental studies provide further support for this hypothesis. Sustained elevation of TSH induces thyroid tumors in rodents.[7,40] The actual mechanism by which elevated TSH levels have been achieved in these studies appears unimportant as thyroid tumors have been produced by iodine-deficient diets, by blocking thyroid hormone synthesis, by administering TSH directly, and by chemical goitrogens.[75]

In the United States, thyroid cancer is roughly 2.5 times more common in women than men. Incidence rates in women increase sharply from childhood to age 30 and then plateau, whereas in men, thyroid cancer incidence rates increase gradually over the lifespan. The ratio of female-to-male incidence rates is greatest between the ages of 20 and 35, during which women have 4–5 times the risk of men. This ratio remains above 3 until the menopause when it begins to level off around 1.5. This suggests that sex hormones may play an important role in the development of thyroid

cancer. A history of pregnancy has been associated with elevated risk of thyroid cancer in three case-control studies.[74,94,101] There is increased activity of the thyroid gland during pregnancy, as estrogen increases thyroxine-binding globulin (TBG) concentrations.[19] The level of TBG in normal females is 10–20% higher than in males, and in pregnancy, a 50% increase in the level of TBG globulin results in an increase in TSH of similar magnitude.[37,73,85] It therefore is also likely that TSH levels of nonpregnant normal females may vary and be elevated above the level of males at some point in the menstrual cycle, although not necessarily throughout the cycle.

Osteosarcoma

The age-specific incidence curve of osteosarcoma shows a distinct peak in the adolescent period.[49] Epidemiological findings strongly suggest that the adolescent peak in incidence is associated with the pattern of childhood skeletal growth. Osteosarcomas in adolescents occur most frequently in the epiphyses of long bones, sites of maximal bone growth, and often occur in conjunction with the adolescent growth spurt when skeletal growth is maximal.[96,116] Skeletal growth results from a combination of factors, but hormonal activity is a primary stimulus.

During the preadolescent period from about age 5 to 11, girls grow faster than boys, but their growth stops earlier so that, by the middle to late teenage years, males are considerably taller.[112] The age-specific incidence curves for osteosarcoma follow the same pattern. Osteosarcoma rates for girls up to about age 13 are roughly 30% higher than are the rates in boys. In the age group 15–24, the male rate exceeds the female rate by some 140%. Blacks are known to have proportionately longer legs and arms than do whites despite similar adult height and they have a higher rate of osteosarcoma under age 25 than do whites, all the excess being in long-bone tumors.[34]

Conclusion

As our understanding of the relationship between epidemiological risk factors and the circulatory levels of the rel-

Table III-3-4. Summary of the Established Effects of Combination Oral Contraceptives and Estrogen Replacement Therapy on Cancer Risk

	Exposure*	Relative Risk†
Oral Contraceptives		
Ovary	Ever	0.5–0.8
Endometrium	Ever	0.4–0.6
Breast	>8 years	1.7
Testis	In utero	2.8–5.3
Estrogen Replacement Therapy		
Endometrium	>5 years	6–8
Breast	>10 years	1.5–2.0

*Compared to non-use
†An estimate derived from a summary of effects observed in relevant studies; see reference 12 for comprehensive review.

evant hormones grows, avenues to primary prevention are becoming apparent. The control of obesity has obvious implications for endometrial cancer and postmenopausal breast cancer. More information on the relationship between childhood diet and physical activity and the onset of puberty should provide opportunities for prevention of breast and perhaps prostate cancer.[14] Hormonal chemoprevention trials for breast cancer are being seriously evaluated based on our current understanding of the hormonal etiology of that tumor.[26,90] Clearly the knowledge accumulated about the potential adverse impact of exogenous steroids in the form of contraceptives and hormone replacement therapy (Table III-3-4) has led to continuing improvements in these products.

References

1. Ahluwalia, B., Jackson, M. A., Jones, G. W., Williams, A. O., Rao, M. S., and Rajguru, S.: Blood hormone profiles in prostate cancer patients in high risk and low risk populations. Cancer, 48:2267, 1981.
2. American Cancer Society: Cancer Facts and Figures– 1990.
3. Apter, D., Reinila, M., and Vihko, R.: Some endocrine characteristics of early menarche, a risk factor for breast cancer, are preserved into adulthood. Int. J. Cancer, 44:783, 1989.
4. Apter, D., and Vihko, R.: Early menarche, a risk factor for breast cancer, indicates early onset of ovulatory cycles. J. Clin. Endocrinol. Metab., 57:82, 1983.
5. Armstrong, B. G., and Doll, R.: Environmental factors and cancer incidence and mortality in different countries, with special reference to dietary practices. Int. J. Cancer, 15:617, 1975.
6. Austin, D.F., and Roe, K.M.: Increase in cancer of the corpus uteri in the San Francisco–Oakland standard metropolitan statistical area 1960–1975. J.N.C.I., 62:13, 1979.
7. Axelrad, A. A., and Leblond, C. P.: Induction of thyroid tumors in rats by a low iodine diet. Cancer, 8:339, 1955.
8. Barrett-Conner, E., Garland, C., McPhillips, J. B., Khaw, K. T., and Wingard, D. L.: A prospective population-based study of androstenedione, estrogens, and prostatic cancer. Cancer Res., 50:169, 1990.
9. Beral, V., Hannaford, P., and Kay, C.: Oral contraceptive use and malignancies of the genital tract. Lancet, 2:1331, 1988.
10. Bergkvist, L., Adami, H.-O., Persson, I., Hoover, R., and Schairer, C.: The risk of breast cancer after estrogen and estrogen-progestin replacement. N. Engl. J. Med., 321:293, 1989.
11. Bernstein, L., Depue, R. H., Ross, R. K., Judd, H. L., Pike, M. C., and Henderson, B. E.: Higher maternal levels of free estradiol in first compared to second pregnancy: Early gestation differences. J. Natl. Cancer Inst., 76:1035, 1986.
12. Bernstein, L., and Henderson, B. E.: Exogenous hormones. In Cancer Epidemiology and Prevention. Edited by D. Schottenfeld and J. F. Fraumeni. New York, W.B. Saunders, Co., In press.
13. Bernstein, L., Pike, M. C., Ross, R. K., Judd, H. L., Brown, J. B., and Henderson, B. E.: Estrogen and sex hormone-binding globulin levels in nulliparous and parous women. J. Natl. Cancer Inst., 74:741,1985.
14. Bernstein, L., Ross, R. K., Lobo, R. A., Hanisch, R., Krailo, M. D., and Henderson, B. E.: The effects of moderate physical activity on menstrual cycle patterns in adolescence: Implication for breast cancer prevention. Br. J. Cancer, 55:681, 1987.
15. Bernstein, L., Yuan, J. M., Ross, R. K., Pike, M. C., Hanisch, K., Lobo, R., Stanczyk, F., Gao, Y.-T., and Henderson, B. E.: Serum hormone levels in premenopausal Chinese women in Shanghai and white women in Los Angeles: Results from two breast cancer case-control studies. Cancer Causes and Control, 1:51, 1990.
16. Bittner, J. J.: The causes and control of mammary cancer in mice. Harvey Lect., 42:221, 1947.
17. Bosland, M. C., Prinsen, M. K., and Kroes, R.: Adenocarcinomas of the prostate induced by N-nitroso-N-methylurea in rats pretreated with cyproterone acetate and testosterone. Cancer Lett., 18:69, 1983.
18. Bruzzi, P., Negri, E., La Vecchia, C., Decarli, A., Palli, D., Parazzini, F., and Del Turco, M. R.: Short term increase in risk of breast cancer after full term pregnancy. Br. Med. J., 297:1096, 1988.
19. Burrow, G. N.: Thyroid Function in Relation to Age and Pregnancy. In The Thyroid Gland. Edited by M. DeVisscher. New York, Raven Press, 1980, p. 215.
20. Casagrande, J. T., Louie, E. W., Pike, M. C., Roy, S., Ross, R. K., and Henderson, B. E.: "Incessant ovulation" and ovarian cancer. Lancet, 2:170, 1979.
21. Centers for Disease Control: Oral contraceptive use and the risk of endometrial cancer. JAMA, 249:1600, 1983.
22. Centers for Disease Control: The reduction in risk of ovarian cancer associated with oral contraceptive use. N. Engl. J. Med., 316:650, 1987.
23. Chu, J., Schweid, A. I., and Weiss, N. S.: Survival among women with endometrial cancer: A comparison of estrogen users and non-users. Am. J. Obstet. Gynecol., 143:569, 1982.
24. Coffey, D. S.: Physiology of Reproduction. In Androgen Excess and the Sex Accessory Tissue. Edited by E. Knoble, and J. Neill. Need Publishers, 1988, p. 1081 .
25. Crile, G.: Endocrine dependency of papillary carcinomas of the thyroid. J.A.M.A., 195:721, 1966.
26. Cuzick, J., Wang, D. Y., and Bulbrook, R. D.: The prevention of breast cancer. Lancet, 2:83, 1986.
27. Depue, R. H., Bernstein, L., Ross, R. K., Judd, H. L., and Henderson, B. E.: Hyperemesis gravidarum in relation to estradiol levels, pregnancy outcome, and other maternal factors: A seroepidemiologic study. Am. J. Obstet. Gynecol., 156:1137, 1987.
28. Depue, R. H., Pike, M. C., and Henderson, B. E.: Estrogen exposure during gestation and risk of testicular cancer. J. Natl. Cancer Inst., 71:1151, 1983.
29. DeWaard, F., and Baanders-van Halewijn, E. A.: A prospective study in general practice on breast cancer risk in postmenopausal women. Int. J. Cancer, 14:153, 1974.
30. Doll, R.: The age distribution of cancer. J. Royal Stat. So. A., 134:133, 1977.
31. Dow, J. A., and Mostofi, F. K.: Testicular tumors following orchiopexy. South. Med. J., 60:193, 1967.
32. Drafta, D., Proca, E., Zamfir, V., Schindler, A. E., Neacsu, E., and Stroe, E.: Plasma steroids in benign prostatic hypertrophy and carcinoma of the prostate. J. Steroid Biochem., 17:689, 1982.
33. Elwood, J. M., Cole, P., Rothman, K. J., and Kaplan, S. D.: Epidemiology of endometrial cancer. J. Natl. Cancer Inst., 59:1055, 1977.
34. Eveleth, P. B., and Tunner, J. M.: Worldwide Variation in Growth. Cambridge, England, Cambridge University Press, 1976.
35. Ferguson, D. J. P., and Anderson, T. J.: Morphological evaluation of cell turnover in relation to the menstrual cycle in the "resting" human breast. Br. J. Cancer, 44:177, 1981.
36. Franceschi, S., LaVecchia, C., Helmrich, S. P., Magnioni, C., and Toynoni, G.: Risk factors for epithelial ovarian cancer in Italy. Am. J. Epidemiol., 115:714, 1982.
37. Gershengorn, M. C., Glinoer, D., and Robbins, J.: Transport and Metabolism of Thyroid Hormones. In The Thyroid Gland. Edited by M. DeVisscher. New York, Raven Press, 1980, p. 81.
38. Ghanadian, R., Puah, C. M., and O'Donoghue, E. P .N.: Serum testosterone and dihydrotestosterone in carcinoma of the prostate. Br. J. Cancer, 39:696,1979.
39. Graham, S., Haughey, B., Marshall, J., Priore, R., Byers, T., Rzepka, T., Mettlin, C., and Pontes, J. E.: Diet in the epidemiology of carcinoma of the prostate gland. J.N.C.I., 70:687, 1983.
40. Griesback, W. E., Kennedy, T. H., and Purves, H. D.: Studies on experimental goitre III. The effect of goitrogenic diet of hypophysectomized rats. Br. J. Exp. Pathol., 22:249, 1941.
41. Hadjimichael, O. C., Boyle, C. A., and Meigs, J. W.: Abortion before first live birth and risk of breast cancer. Br. J. Cancer, 53:281, 1986.
42. Henderson, B. E.: Summary report of the sixth symposium on cancer registries in the Pacific Basin. J.N.C.I., 82:1186, 1990.
43. Henderson, B. E., Benton, B., Jing, J., Yu, M. C., and Pike, M. C.: Risk factors for cancer of the testis in young men. Int. J. Cancer, 23:598, 1979.
44. Henderson, B. E., Bernstein, L., Ross, R. K., Depue, R. H., and Judd, H. L.: The early in utero oestrogen and testosterone environment of blacks and whites: Potential effects on male offspring. Br. J . Cancer, 57:216, 1988.
45. Henderson, B. E., Casagrande, J. T., Pike, M. C., Mack, T., Rosario, I., and Duke, A.: The epidemiology of endometrial cancer in young women. Br. J. Cancer, 47:749, 1983.
46. Henderson, B. E., Gerkins, V., and Rosario, I.: Elevated serum levels of estrogen and prolactin in daughters of breast cancer patients. N. Engl. J. Med., 293:790, 1975.
47. Henderson, B. E., Pike, M. C., and Casagrande, J. T.: Breast cancer and the estrogen window hypothesis. Lancet, 2:363, 1981.
48. Henderson, B. E., Pike, M. C., and Ross, R. K.: Epidemiology and Risk Factors. In Breast Cancer: Diagnosis and Management. Edited by G. Bonadonna. New York, John Wiley and Sons, Ltd., 1984, p. 15.
49. Henderson, B. E., Ross, R. K., and Bernstein, L.: Estrogens as a cause of human cancer: The Richard and Hinda Rosenthal Foundation Award Lecture. Cancer Res., 48:246, 1988.
50. Henderson, B. E., Ross, R. K., Judd, H. L., Krailo, M. D., and Pike, M. C.: Do regulatory ovulatory cycles increase breast cancer risk? Cancer, 56:1206, 1985.
51. Henderson, B. E., Ross, R. K., Lobo, R. A., Pike, M. C., and Mack, T. M.: Reevaluating the role of progestogen therapy after the menopause. Fertility and Sterility, 49:98, 1988.
52. Henderson, B. E., Ross, R. K., and Pike, M. D.: Breast Neoplasia. In Menopause: Physiology and Pharmacology. Edited by D. R. Mischell. Chicago, Year Book Medical Publishers, 1987, p. 261.
53. Henderson, B. E., Ross, R. K., Pike, M. C., and Casagrande, J. T.: Endogenous hormones as a major risk factor in human cancer. Cancer Res., 43:3232, 1982.
54. Herbst, A. L., Cole, P., Norusis, M. J., Welch, W. R., and Scully, R. E.: Epidemiologic aspects and factors related to survival in 384 registry cases of clear cell adenocarcinoma of the vagina and cervix. Am. J. Obstet. Gynecol., 135:876, 1979.
55. Heshmat, M. Y., Kaul, L., Kovi, J., Jackson, M. A., Jackson, A. G., Jones, G. W., Edson, M., Enterline, J. P., Worrell, R. G., and Perry S. L.: Nutrition and prostate cancer. A case-control study. Prostate, 6:7, 1985.
56. Hill, P. B., and Wynder, E. L.: Effect of vegetarian diet and dexamethasone on plasma prolactin, testosterone and dehydroepiandrosterone in men and women. Cancer Lett., 7:273, 1979.
57. Honda, G. D., Bernstein, L., Ross, R. K., Greenland, S., Gerkins, V., and Henderson, B. E.: Vasectomy, cigarette smoking, and age at first sexual intercourse as risk factors for prostate cancer in middle-aged men. Br. J. Cancer, 57:326, 1988.
58. Hulka, B. S., Hammond, J. E., DiFerdinanado, G., Mickey, D. D., Fried, F. A., Checkoway, H., Strumpf, W. E., Beckman, W., and Clark, D. C.: Serum hormone levels among patients with prostatic carcinoma or benign prostatic hyperplasia and clinic controls. Prostate, 11:171, 1987.
59. Ingbar, S. H., and Woeber, K. A.: The Thyroid Gland. In Textbook of Endocrinology. Edited by R. H. Williams. Philadelphia, W.B. Saunders: Philadelphia, 1974, p. 95.
60. Johnson, D. E., Woodhead, D. M., Pohl, D. R., and Robison, J.: Cryptorchidism and testicular tumorigenesis. Surgery, 63:919, 1968.
61. Kelsey, J. L., LiVolsi, V. A., Holford, T. R., Fischer, D. A., Morton, E. D., Schwartz, P. E., O'Connor, T., and White, C.: A case-control study of cancer of the endometrium. Am. J. Epidemiol., 116:333,1982.
62. Kennedy, D. L., Baum, C., and Forbes, M. B.: Noncontraceptive estrogens and progestins: Use patterns over time. Obstetrics and Gynecology, 65:441, 1985.
63. Key, T. J. A., and Pike, M. C.: The role of oestrogens and progestagens in the epidemiology and prevention of breast cancer. Eur. J. Cancer Clin. Oncol., 24:29, 1988.

64. Kolonel, L. N., Yoshizawa, C. N., and Hankin, J. H.: Diet and prostatic cancer: A case-control study in Hawaii. Am. J. Epidemiol., 127:999, 1988.

65. LaVecchia, C., Franceschi, S., Decarli, A., Gallus, G., and Toynoni G.: Risk factors for endometrial cancer at 3 different ages. J. Natl. Cancer Inst., 73:667, 1984.

66. Lipschultz, L., Caminos-Torres, R., Greenspan, C. S., and Snyder, P. J.: Testicular function after orchiopexy for unilaterally undescended testis. N. Engl. J. Med., 295:15, 1976.

67. MacDonald, P. C., Edman, C. D., Hemsell, D. L., Porter, J. C., and Siiteri, P. K.: Effect of obesity on conversion of plasma androstenedione to estrone in postmenopausal women with and without endometrial cancer. Am. J. Obstet. Gynecol., 130:448, 1978.

68. Mack, T., Cozen, W., and Quinn, M.: Epidemiology of gynecological cancer II: endometrium, ovary, vulva, vagina. In press, 1990.

69. Mack, T. M., Pike, M. C., Henderson, B. E., Pfeffer, R. I., Gerkins, V. R., Arthur, M., and Brown S. E.: Estrogens and endometrial cancer in a retirement community. N. Engl. J. Med., 294:1262, 1976.

70. MacMahon, B., Cole, P., Brown, J. B., Aoki, K., Lin, T. M., Morgan, R. W., and Woo, N.-C.: Urine estrogen profiles of Asian and North American women. Int. J. Cancer, 14:161, 1974.

71. MacMahon, B., Cole, P., Lin, T. M., Lowe, C. R., Mirra, A. P., Ravnihar, B., Salber, E. J., Valaoras V. G., and Yuasa, S.: Age at first birth and cancer of the breast. A summary of an international study. Bull. WHO, 43:209,1970.

72. MacMahon, B., Trichopoulos, D., Brown, J., Andersen, A. P., Aoki, K., Cole, P., deWaard, F., Kauraniemi, T., Morgan, R. W., Purde, M., Ravihar, B., Stormby, N., Westlund, K., and Woo, N.-C.: Age at menarche, probability of ovulation and breast cancer risk. Int. J. Cancer, 29:13, 1982.

73. Malkasian, G. D., and Mayberry, W. E.: Serum total and free thyroxine and thyrotropin in normal and pregnant women, neonates, and women receiving progestogens. Am. J. Obstet. Gynecol., 108:1234, 1970.

74. McTiernan, A. M., Weiss, N. S., and Daling, J. R.: Incidence of thyroid cancer in women in relation to reproductive and hormonal factors. Am. J. Epidemiol., 120:423, 1984.

75. Morris, H. P.: Experimental thyroid tumors. Brookhaven Symposia in Biology, 7:192, 1954.

76. Morrison, A. S.: Cryptorchidism, hernia and cancer of the testis. J. Natl. Cancer Inst., 56:731, 1976.

77. Moss, A. R., Osmond, D., Bacchetti, P., Torti, F. M., and Gurgin, V.: Hormonal risk factors in testicular cancer: A case-control study. Am. J. Epidemiol., 124:39, 1986.

78. Muir, C., Waterhouse, J., Mack, T., Powell, J., and Whelan, S.: Cancer Incidence in Five Continents, Volume V, IARC, Lyon, 1987.

79. Murphy, G. P., Natarajan, N., Pontes, J. E., Schmitz, R. L., Smart, C. R., Schmidt, J. D., and Mettlin, C.: The national survey of prostate cancer in the United States by the American College of Surgeons. J. Urol., 127:928, 1982.

80. Musey, V. C., Collins, E. C., Musey, P. I., Martino-Saltzman, D., and Preedy, J. R.: Long-term effect of a first pregnancy on the secretion of prolactin. N. Engl. J. Med., 316:229, 1987.

81. Newhouse, M. L., Pearson, R. M., Fullerton, J. M., Boesen, E. A. M., and Shannon H. S.: A case-control study of carcinoma of the ovary. Br. J. Prev. Soc. Med., 31:148, 1979.

82. Noble, R. L.: The development of prostatic adenocarcinoma in Nb rats following prolonged sex hormone administration. Cancer Res., 37:1929, 1977.

83. Nomura, A., Heilbrun, Z. K., Stemmermann, G. N., and Judd, H. L.: Prediagnostic serum hormones and the risk of prostate cancer. Cancer Res., 48:3515, 1988.

84. Nomura, T., and Kanzaki, T.: Induction of urogenital anomalies and some tumors in the progeny of mice receiving diethylstilbestrol during pregnancy. Cancer Res., 37:1099, 1977.

85. Pacchiarotti, A., Martino, E., Bartalena, L., Buratti, L., Mammoli, C., Strigini, F., Fruzzetti, F., Melis, G. B., and Pinchera, A.: Serum thyrotropin by ultrasensitive immunoradiometric assay and serum free thyroid hormones in pregnancy. J. Endcrinol. Invest., 9:185, 1986.

86. Paganini-Hill, A., Ross, R. K., and Henderson, B. E.: Endometrial cancer and patterns of use of oestrogen replacement therapy: a cohort study. Br. J. Cancer, 59:445, 1989.

87. Persson, I, Adami, H. O., Bergkvist, K., Lundgren, A., Petterson, B. Hoover, R., and Schairer, C.: Risk of endometrial cancer after treatment with oestrogens alone or in conjunction with progestogens: Results of a prospective study. Br. Med. J., 298:147, 1989.

88. Pike, M. C., Henderson, B. E., Casagrande, J. T., Rosario, I., and Gray, G. E.: Oral contraceptive use and early abortion as risk factors for breast cancer in young women. Br. J. Cancer, 43:72, 1981.

89. Pike, M. C., Krailo, M. C., Henderson, B. E., Casagrande, J. T., and Hoel, D. G.: "Hormonal" risk factors, "breast tissue age" and the age-incidence of breast cancer. Nature, 303:767, 1983.

90. Pike, M. C., Ross, R. K., Lobo, R. A., Key, T. J. A., Potts, M., and Henderson B. E.: LHRH agonists and the prevention of breast and prostate cancer. Br. J. Cancer, 60:142, 1989.

91. Pollard, M., and Luckert, P. H.: Prostate cancer in a Sprague-Dawley rat. Prostate, 6:1, 1985.

92. Pollard, M., Luckert, P. H., and Schmidt, M. A.: Induction of prostate adenocarcinomas in Lobund Wistar rats by testosterone. Prostate, 4:563, 1982.

93. Pottern, L. M., Brown, L. M., Hoover, R. N., Javadpour, N., O'Connell, K. J., Stutzman, R. E., and Blattner, W. A.: Testicular cancer risk among young men: Role of cryptorchidism and inguinal hernia. J. Natl. Cancer Inst., 74:377,1985.

94. Preston-Martin, S., Bernstein, L., Pike, M. C., Maldonado, A. A., and Henderson, B. E.: Thryoid cancer among young women related to prior thyroid disease and pregnancy history. Br. J. Cancer, 55:191,1987.

95. Preston-Martin, S., Pike, M. C., Ross, R. K., Jones, P. A., and Henderson, B. E.: Increased cell division as a cause of human cancer. Cancer Res., 50:7415, 1990.

96. Price, C. H. G.: Primary bone-forming tumors and their relationship to skeletal growth. J. Bone Jt. Surg. Br., 40:574, 1958.

97. Rajfer, J., and Walsh, P. C.: Hormonal regulation of testicular descent: Experimental and clinical observations. J. Urol., 118:985, 1977.

98. Ramcharan, S., Pellegrin, F. A., Ray, R., and Hsu, J. P.: A prospective study of the side effects of oral contraceptive use. In: The Walnut Creek Contraceptive Drug Study, NIH Publ. 81-564, Vol. 3. Washington, D.C., USC Government Printing Office, 1981.

99. Rivenson, A., and Silverman, J.: Prostatic Cancer in Laboratory Animals. In Endocrinology of Cancer. Edited by D. P. Rose. Boca Raton, FL, CRC Press, 1979, p 2.

100. Rogers, J., and Mitchell, G. W.: The relation of obesity to menstrual disturbances. N. Engl. J. Med., 247:53, 1952.

101. Ron, E., Kleinerman, R. A., Boice, J. D., LiVolsi, V. A., Flannery, J. T., and Fraumeni, J. F.: A population-based case-control study of thyroid cancer. J. Natl. Cancer Inst., 79:1, 1987.

102. Ross, R. K.: Prostate Cancer. In Cancer Epidemiology and Prevention, 2nd Edition. Edited by D. Schottenfeld, and J. Fraumeni. Philadelphia, W.B. Saunders Co., In press.

103. Ross, R. K., Bernstein, L., Judd, H., Hanisch, R., Pike, M., and Henderson, B. E.: Serum testosterone levels in young black and white men. J.N.C.I., 76:45, 1986.

104. Ross, R. K., Deapen, D. M., Casagrande, J. T., Paganini-Hill, A., and Henderson, B. E.: A cohort study of mortality from cancer of the prostate in Catholic priests. Br. J. Cancer, 43:233, 1981.

105. Ross, R. K., McCurtis, J. W., Henderson, B. E., Menck, H. R., Mack, T. M., and Martin, S. P.: Descriptive epidemiology of testicular and prostatic cancer in Los Angeles. Br. J. Cancer, 39:284, 1979.

106. Ross, R. K., Shimizu, H., Paganini-Hill, A., Honda, G., and Henderson, B. E.: Case-control studies of prostate cancer in blacks and whites in Southern California. J.N.C.I., 78:869, 1987.

107. Schottenfeld, D., Warshauer, M. E., Sherlock, S., Zauber, A. G., Leder, M., and Payne, R.: The epidemiology of testicular cancer in young adults. Am. J. Epidemiol., 112:232, 1980.

108. Shimizu, H., Ross, R. K., Bernstein, L., Pike, M. C., and Henderson, B. E.: Serum estrogen levels in postmenopausal women: comparison of US whites and Japanese in Japan. Br. J. Cancer, 62:451, 1990.

109. Snowdon, D. A., Phillips, R. L., and Choi, W.: Diet, obesity, and risk of fatal prostate cancer. Am. J. Epidemiol., 120:244, 1984.

110. Steele, R., Lees, R. E. M., Kraus, A. S., and Rao, R.: Sexual factors in the epidemiology of cancer of the prostate. J. Chron. Dis., 24:29, 1971.

111. Talamini, R., LaVecchia, C., Decarli, A., Negri, E., and Franceschi, S.: Nutrition, social factors and prostatic cancer in a Northern Italian population. Br. J. Cancer, 53: 817, 1986.

112. Tanner, J. M.: Growth at Adolescence, 2nd Ed. Oxford, England, Blackwell Scientific Publication, 1962, p. 1.

113. Trichopoulos, D., MacMahon, B., and Cole, P.: The menopause and breast cancer. J. Natl. Cancer Inst. 48:605, 1972.

114. Walker, A. H., Ross, R. K., Haile, R. W. C., and Henderson, B. E.: Hormonal factors and risk of ovarian germ cell cancer in young women. Br. J. Cancer, 57:418, 1988.

115. Walker, A. H., Ross, R. K., Pike, M. C., and Henderson, B. E.: A possible rising incidence of malignant germ cell tumors in young women. Br. J. Cancer, 49:669, 1984.

116. Weinfeld, M. S., and Dudley, H. R.: Osteogenic sarcoma. J. Bone Jt. Surg. Am., 44:269, 1962.

117. Weiss, N.: Ovary. In Cancer Epidemiology and Prevention. Edited by D. Schottenfeld and J. F. Fraumeni. Philadelphia, W. B. Saunders, 1982, p. 871.

118. Willett, W. C., Browne, M. L., Bain, C., Lipnick, R. J., Stampfer, M. J., Rosner, B., Colditz, G. A., Hennekens, C. H., and Speizer, F. E.: Relative weight and risk of breast cancer among premenopausal women. Am. J. Epidemiol., 122:731, 1985.

119. World Health Organization: Research on the menopause. Geneva, World Health Organization Technical Report Series 670, 1981.

120. Wu, M. L., Whittemore, A. S., Paffenbarger, R. S., Sarles, D. L., Kampert, J. B., Grosser, S., Jung, D. L., Ballon, S., Hendrickson, M., and Mohle-Boetani, J.: Personal and environmental characteristics related to epithelial ovarian cancer. 1. Reproductive and menstrual events and oral contraceptive use. Am. J. Epidemiol., 128:1216, 1988.

121. Yu, M. C., Gerkins, V. R., Henderson, B. E., Brown, J. B., and Pike, M. C.: Elevated levels of prolactin in nulliparous women. Br. J. Cancer, 43:826, 1981.

122. Yuan, J.-M., Yu, M. C., Ross, R. K., Gao, Y. T., and Henderson, B. E.: Risk factors for breast cancer in Chinese women in Shanghai. Cancer Res., 48:1949, 1988.

123. Ziel H. K., and Finkle W. D.: Increased risk of endometrial carcinoma among users of conjugated estrogens. N. Engl. J. Med., 293:1167, 1975.

124. Zumoff, B.: Relationship of obesity to blood estrogens. Cancer Res., 42:3289S, 1982.

Ionizing Radiation

John B. Little

Introduction

The hazards of exposure to ionizing radiation were recognized shortly after Roentgen's discovery of the x-ray in 1895. Acute skin reactions were observed in many individuals working with early x-ray generators, and by 1902 the first radiation-induced cancer was reported arising in an ulcerated area of the skin. Within a few years, a large number of such skin cancers had been observed, and the first report of leukemia in 5 radiation workers appeared in 1911.[53] Indeed, Marie Curie and her daughter Irene are both thought to have died of radiation-induced leukemia. Since that time, many experimental and epidemiologic studies have confirmed the oncogenic effects of radiation in many tissues of many species.

There are a number of characteristics specific to ionizing radiation which differentiate it from chemical toxic agents or other physical carcinogens. Notably among these is its ability to penetrate cells and to deposit energy within them in a random fashion, unaffected by the usual cellular barriers presented to chemical agents. All cells in the body are thus susceptible to damage by ionizing radiation; the amount of damage incurred will be related to the physical parameters that determine the radiation dose received by the particular cells or tissue. Furthermore, the physical characteristics of ionizing radiation allow us to measure accurately very low levels of exposure, doses several orders of magnitude below those that produce measurable biologic effects in human cells.

This chapter will review briefly the principal cellular and tissue effects of radiation, as well as current knowledge concerning cellular and molecular mechanisms for radiation carcinogenesis. The term carcinogenesis is used in its broad sense to include the development of all types of malignant neoplasms. A more detailed description will then be presented of current knowledge concerning the induction of cancer by radiation in experimental animals and human beings. Human risk estimates are derived primarily from epidemiologic studies following relatively high dose radiation exposures. As ionizing radiation appears in reality to be a relatively weak carcinogen and mutagen compared to many chemical agents, few reliable human data are available on its oncogenic effects in the dose range below 50 cGy.

Development of Radiation Injury

A schematic representation of the interaction of ionizing radiation with biologic tissues and the subsequent development of radiation injury is shown in Figure III-4-1. Such radiation is of two major types, electromagnetic waves or ionizing particles. In either case, interaction with orbital elec-

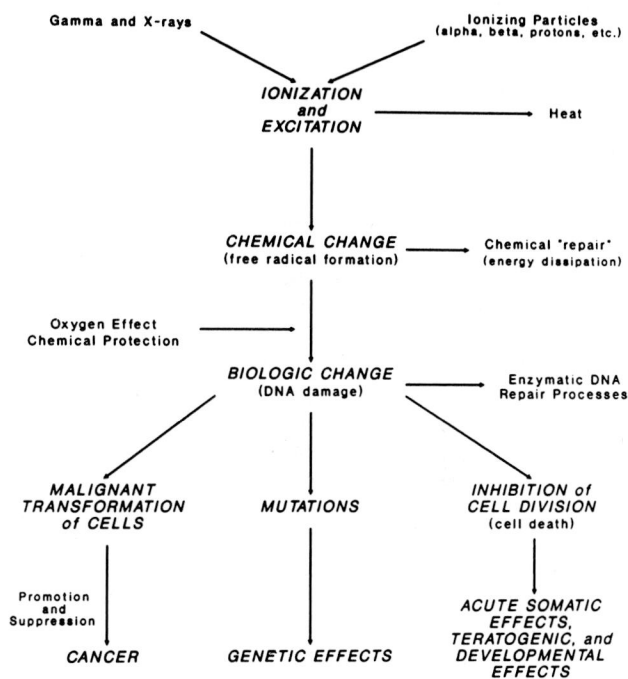

Figure III-4-1. Development of radiation injury.

trons results in ionizations and excitations. The initial deposition of energy in irradiated cells thus occurs in the form of ionized and excited atoms or molecules distributed at random throughout the cells. It is the ionizations that cause most of the chemical changes in the vicinity of the event; this energy may be subsequently transferred through a chain of chemical reactions finally producing irreversible damage to critical molecules of biologic importance to the cell. It appears that the energy that goes into producing excited molecules produces relatively few chemical reactions and is eventually dissipated in the form of heat.

The ionizing event involves the ejection of an orbital electron from a molecule, producing a positively charged or "ionized" molecule. These molecules are highly unstable and rapidly undergo chemical change. This change results in the production of "free radicals," which are atoms or molecules containing unpaired electrons. These free radicals are extremely reactive and may lead to permanent damage of the affected molecule, or the energy may be transferred to another molecule. Most of the energy deposited within a cell results in the production of aqueous free radicals, as approximately 80% of the cell is water. Chemical damage may be repaired before it is irreversible by the recombination of radicals and dissipation of the associated energy, or it may be modified by agents such as molecular oxygen or sulfhydryl radioprotective compounds.

The initial biologic change is thought to be damage to DNA molecules in the cell. The time required for the entire chain of physical and chemical events as shown in Figure III-4-1 from the initial interaction until the production of DNA damage is of the order of a microsecond or less. The subsequent development of biochemical and physiologic changes, however, may take hours to days, whereas the induction of cancer may take many years.

Principal Cellular and Tissue Effects of Radiation

Cell Killing

Radiation in sufficient doses can inhibit mitosis; that is, the cell's ability to divide and proliferate indefinitely. The inhibition of cell proliferation is the mechanism by which radiation kills most cells. The nature and kinetics of the cytotoxic effects of radiation in mammalian cells has been reviewed elsewhere.[27] They are discussed in detail in Section XIII, Chapter 1 of this text, particularly as they relate to tumor cells and radiation oncology. As radiation kills cells by inhibiting their ability to divide, its effects in human beings occur primarily in tissues with high cell turnover or renewal rates characterized by a large amount of proliferative activity. These include tissues such as the bone marrow and mucosal lining of the stomach and small intestine. Symptoms of acute exposure to whole-body irradiation in human beings are usually observed only following doses of 150 cGy or greater, whereas significant cell killing in vitro can be detected with doses as low as 50 cGy.

Another important somatic effect related to cell killing arises from irradiation of the developing embryo and fetus.[4,35] Irradiation of experimental animals with doses in the order of 200–400 cGy during the first trimester of pregnancy has led to a variety of congenital anomalies in the offspring. However, no such effects have been observed in human beings, or in large populations of mice exposed to doses below 25 cGy.[4] Recent epidemiologic studies in the atom bomb survivors of Hiroshima and Nagasaki have focused on mental retardation and other measures of intelligence such as test scores and school performance. These are presumably more sensitive indicators of radiation effects owing to cell depletion amongst the neuroblasts during development. Neuroblasts comprise by far the largest population of cells in the early fetus, and continue proliferating until the 5th or 6th month of pregnancy.

The number of children with such disorders in the atom bomb survivor study is small, and the mean values for all endpoints are not significantly different from controls for the dose groups below 50–100 cGy. The BEIR V Committee concluded that for mental retardation, the best documented of the developmental abnormalities, the prevalence appeared to increase with dose in a linear manner for individuals irradiated between 8 and 15 weeks, the most sensitive time period after conception.[19] However, the data do not exclude a threshold in the range of 20–40 cGy.[19] On the assumption of a linear, non-threshold relationship, the magnitude of the risk would be approximately a 4% chance of occurrence per

10 cGy for exposure at 8–15 weeks of gestational age, with less risk occurring for exposure at other ages.

Mutagenesis

The mutagenic effects of ionizing radiation were first described by Herman Muller in 1927 in his classic experiments with the fruit fly, drosophila. Subsequent experiments showed the dose-response relationship for such mutations to be a linear function of exposure over a wide range of radiation doses from as low as 10 to 1000 cGy. Studies of the induction of single gene mutations in human cells have been limited to several genetic loci. However, results of these studies also suggest that the induction of mutations in human cells is a linear function of dose with doses as low as 10 and perhaps 1 cGy.[18] There appears to be relatively little dose-rate effect for the induction of mutations in human cells.[18,47] DNA structural analyses have shown that the majority of radiation-induced mutations in human cells result from large-scale genetic events involving loss of the entire active gene and often extending to other loci on the same chromosome.[59]

The major potential consequence of radiation-induced mutations in human populations are heritable genetic effects resulting from mutations induced in germinal cells. Such effects have been examined in several different animal systems.[19] For high dose-rate exposure, the induced mutation rate per gamete per cell generally falls in the range of 10^{-4}–10^{-5} per cGy. The rates per locus are in the range of 10^{-7}–10^{-8} per cGy. Protraction of exposure appears to decrease the mutation rate in rodent systems by a factor of 5 or greater. When all of the experimental data for the various genetic endpoints are considered, the genetic doubling dose (radiation dose necessary to double the spontaneous mutation rate) for low dose-rate exposure appears to be in the range of 100 cGy. Although significant heritable genetic effects of radiation have not yet been demonstrated in human populations, a doubling dose of 100 cGy is not inconsistent with the absence of a statistically significant increase in hereditary disease amongst the children of atom bomb survivors.[1] Indeed, 100 cGy represents approximately the lower 95% confidence limit for the human doubling dose.[19]

Chromosomal Aberrations

Radiation can induce two types of chromosomal aberrations in mammalian cells. The first have been termed "unstable" aberrations, in that they are usually lethal to dividing cells. They include such changes as dicentrics, ring chromosomes, large deletions and fragments. These types of aberrations do not allow the equal distribution of genetic material into daughter cells; in many cases, the frequency of such aberrations correlates well with the cytotoxic effects of radiation.

The second type has been termed "stable" aberrations. These include changes such as small deletions, reciprocal translocations and aneuploidy which do not preclude the cell from dividing. A karyotype of a human cell showing a stable aberration is shown in Figure III-4-2. Radiation-induced reciprocal translocations such as have occurred in this cell may be passed on through many generations of cell replication and emerge in clonal cell populations.[21,22]

It is well known that such deletions and translocations can

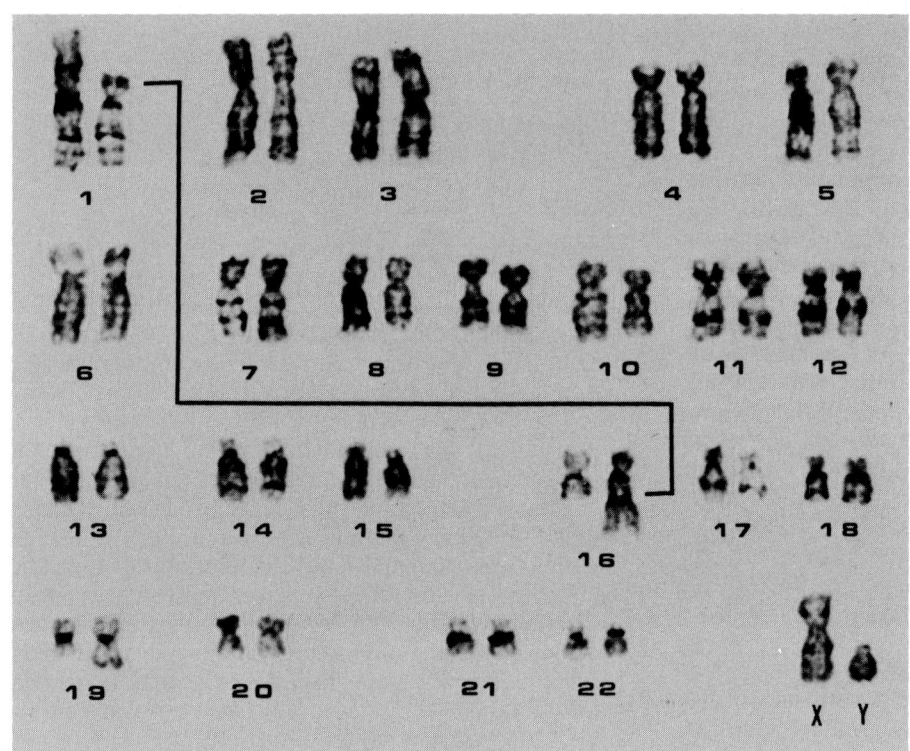

result in gene mutations. It is tempting to speculate that they may play a more fundamental role in the process of carci-nogenesis. Typically, cancer cells are aneuploid and contain multiple stable chromosomal aberrations. In a number of cases, specific chromosomal abnormalities have been asso-ciated with specific tumor types.[39] This phenomenon is dis-cussed in detail in I-8. In some instances, such as the chro-mosome 8:16 translocation in Burkitt's lymphoma, the chromosomal change results in the activation of a specific oncogene. In others, such as the chromosome 13 deletion found in retinoblastoma, tumor development has been ascribed to loss or inactivation of a suppressor gene. Further work is required, however, to define the role of such events in radiation-induced cancer.

Neoplastic Transformation

The final important cellular effect of radiation is neoplastic transformation, or the conversion of a normal cell to one with the phenotype of a cancer cell including the ability to form an invasive, malignant tumor upon reinjection into syngeneic hosts. Current knowledge concerning the transformation of cells in vitro by ionizing radiation is described in the following section.

Neoplastic Transformation In Vitro By Radiation

Most human cancers have been shown to be clonal in origin. That is, all of the cells within a tumor are descendants of a single cell that has undergone the process of neoplastic transformation. The transformation of one or more normal cells in a tissue in vivo is thought to represent the earliest step in the overall process of carcinogenesis.[28] Whether or not such a transformed cell can successfully give rise to an invasive, malignant tumor depends upon a number of tissue and systemic factors.

Although a number of different in vitro transformation sys-tems involving various species and cell types are under active investigation, those which generate reliable quantitative data have been restricted to rodent cells and in none of these is the entire process of malignant transformation measured.[5] Rather, surrogate features of transformation are assayed such as changes in colony morphology, focus formation or growth under anchorage independent conditions. Furthermore, no quantitative human cell system has as yet been developed.[34]

Stages In Neoplastic Transformation

Studies of transformation induced by radiation or chemical agents indicate that it is a progressive, multi-step process by which normal cells acquire the various phenotypic char-acteristics of cancer cells. There appear to be three major independent stages in the malignant transformation of cells in vitro: the development of morphological changes; cellular immortality; and tumorigenicity.[7] Morphologic changes are many and varied including the development of abnormalities in cytology, growth pattern and the control of cell prolifera-tion. Immortalization occurs frequently in rodent cells but extremely rarely in human cells, either spontaneously or as a result of treatment with radiation or chemical carcinogens. It may thus be an important rate-limiting step in human cell transformation and perhaps in human carcinogenesis in vivo.[7] Tumorigenicity also appears to be an independent pheno-type that generally occurs only in previously immortalized cells. Such immortal cells may gain a selective growth advantage over cells which become senescent during cultivation in vitro or are programmed for terminal differentiation in vivo.

Dose Response Relationships

The observed frequency of neoplastic transformation per viable cell increases with dose up to the range of 400–600 cGy, reaching a plateau at higher doses. As radiation is highly cytotoxic in this higher dose range, the yield of transformants per initial cell at risk actually declines. The latter parameter, the yield of transformed cells per initial cell at risk, would be the more relevant one for the induction of cancer in vivo. The in vitro results thus predict a most effective dose for transformation in the range of 400–600 cGy, a phenomenon that reflects a balance between transformation and cell killing. Ionizing radiation is not a potent inducer of transformation as compared with many chemical agents. Polycyclic hydrocarbons, for example, can induce much higher frequencies of transformation at doses which produce very little cell killing.[28]

Dose response curves for the induction of transformation in two very similar mouse cell systems are shown in Figure III-4-3. Although the transformation frequencies reached a similar plateau at doses above 600 rads, the shapes of the curves at lower doses differed significantly. Such findings, as well as the fact that transformation represents but an early event in the overall process of carcinogenesis, suggest that it is not relevant to predict the shape of the dose response curve for carcinogenesis in vivo at low radiation doses from the findings with transformation in vitro. For irradiation with densely-ionizing, high linear energy transfer (LET) radiation,

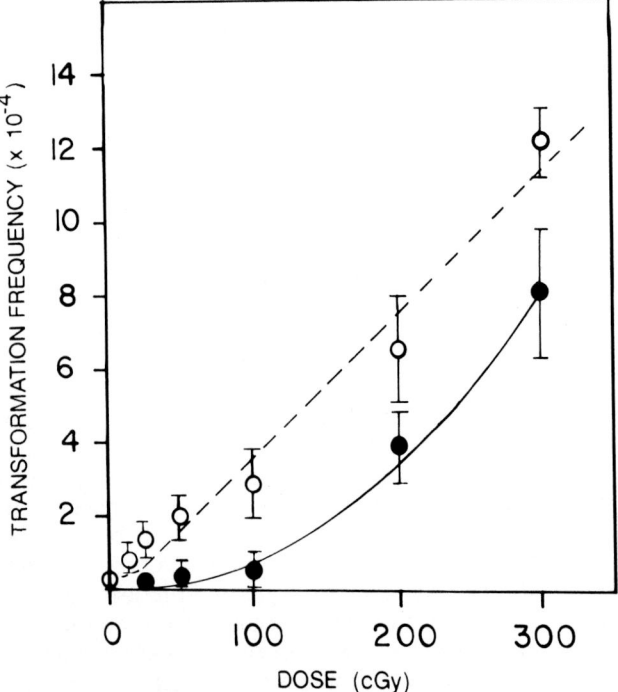

Figure III-4-3. Dose-response curves for the induction of neoplastic transformation in mouse cells by X-irradiation. The upper curve is for BALB/3T3 cells and the bottom curve for C3H/10T1/2 cells.

the frequency of transformation rises much more rapidly at low doses, reaching a roughly similar plateau. Relative Biological Effectiveness (RBE) factors in the range of 3 to 10 have been calculated for high LET radiations such as fast neutrons, alpha particles, and heavy charged ions.

Modifying Factors

Incubation of cells with various agents during the 4–6 week post-irradiation expression period can markedly modify the ultimate yield of transformed cells.[6,29] For example, the phorbol ester compound 12-0-tetradecanoyl-phorbol-13-acetate (TPA) acts as a potent promoter of x-ray transformation if applied repeatedly beginning either immediately after irradiation, or several weeks later. Indeed, these in vitro findings offered the first evidence that the initiation-promotion phenomenon was a general one and not simply limited to mouse skin. The promoting effect of TPA in vitro is shown graphically in Figure III-4-4A.

A number of different classes of agents applied by a similar experimental protocol can suppress transformation. These include protease inhibitors, selenium and certain vitamins, in particular analogs of vitamin A also known as retinoids. Transformation can also be modulated by certain hormones, growth factors and anti-inflammatory agents.[6] Notable among these is thyroid hormone, specifically T3.

Thus, it has become evident that a number of non-carcinogenic secondary factors can markedly modulate the frequency of radiation-induced transformation. As transformation can be markedly enhanced, suppressed or completely inhibited, such factors may become the controlling ones in the overall process of transformation of cells exposed to radiation. In most cases, effects of such agents in vitro have been predictive of those observed in experimental animal systems. It therefore seems likely that they may be of similar importance in human radiation carcinogenesis, though very little epidemiological data to support this contention are as yet available.

The effects of dose-rate on radiation transformation have proven somewhat complex. In general, protraction of exposure to low LET radiation leads to a lower frequency of transformation. However, protraction of exposure to fission spectrum neutrons at total doses up to 100 cGy has been reported to enhance the frequency of transformation.[20] The latter phenomenon has not been observed for other high LET radiations, and thus needs further investigation.

Two-Event Hypothesis of Radiation Transformation

Studies of the kinetics of radiation transformation in vitro indicate that it involves two distinct events.[23,24] The first is a frequent event which involves a large fraction of the irradiated cell population, whereas the second or transforming event is a low frequency one involving progeny of the original irradiated cells after many rounds of cell division. This second step occurs with a constant frequency per cell per generation and has the characteristics of a mutagenic event.[30]

This finding is in contradistinction to classical theories of carcinogenesis in which the initiating event is thought to be a rare one and likely mutagenic in nature. However, evidence

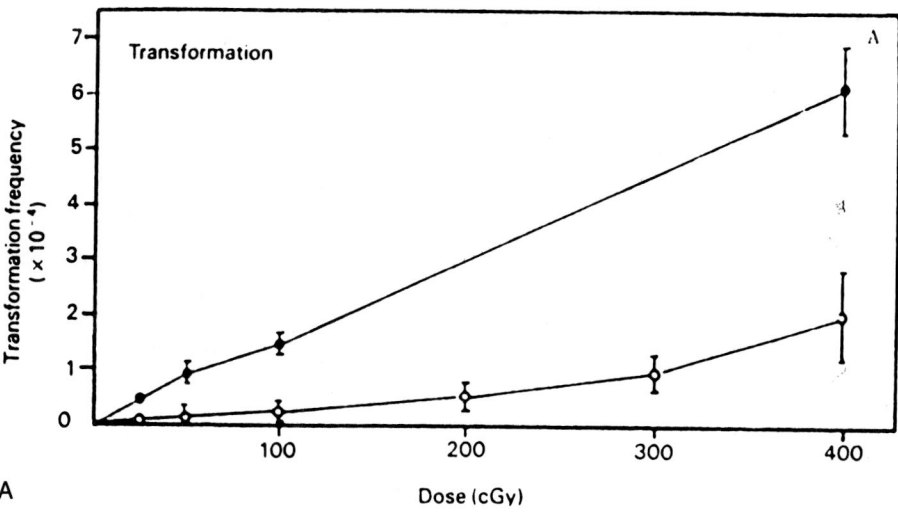

A

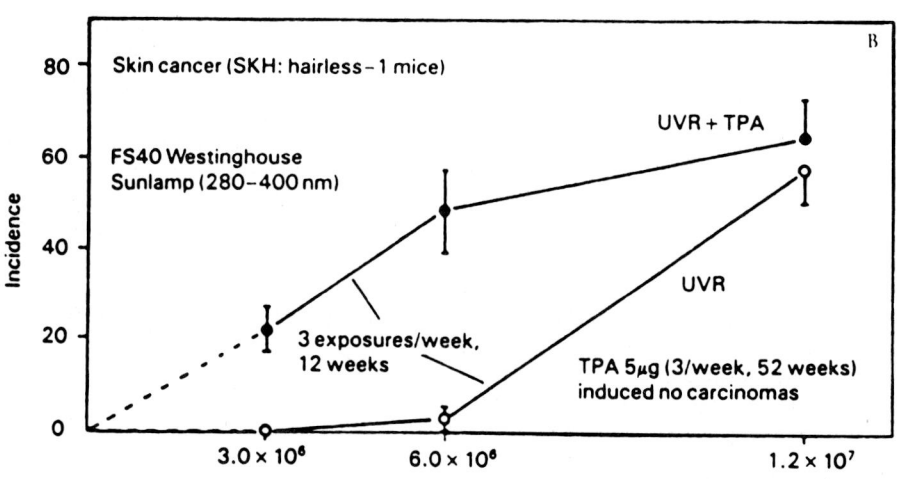

B

Figure III-4-4. Enhancement of radiation-induced transformation in vitro and carcinogenesis in vivo by post-irradiation exposure to the phorbol ester tumor promoting agent TPA. Panel A: Neoplastic transformation in mouse 10T1/2 cells; lower curve is for cells treated with x-rays alone whereas upper curve is for x-irradiated cells continuously incubated with TPA post-irradiation. Panel B: Skin tumors in mice treated with ultraviolet light irradiation; lower curve is for mice treated with radiation alone, whereas the upper curve is for irradiated mice receiving repeated applications of TPA post-irradiation. Reproduced from Little; the data in Panel B are from Fry and Ley.[13,28]

is now emerging from experimental animal systems indicating that the initiating event may indeed be a frequent one.[30] Moreover, it now appears that other cellular effects of radiation may also be delayed, appearing in the progeny of irradiated cells after many generations of replication. These include specific gene mutations, cell death, and the finding that intragenic recombinational activity persists in yeast cells for many generations of replication following exposure to ionizing radiation.[11,17,43]

These findings are all consistent with the hypothesis that radiation induces genetic instability in cells, as a cellular response to the non-specific DNA damage it produces. This genetic instability results in malignant transformation or other cellular effects in progeny cells, sometimes after many generations of replication. The various factors modulating transformation may act on this process. Interestingly, this concept is consistent with the emerging findings in human populations which suggest that radiation-induced cancer may follow a Relative Risk model (see below); that is, a given dose of radiation increases the spontaneous cancer rate at all follow-up times rather than inducing a specific cohort of new tumors.

Molecular Mechanisms

DNA Damage

It is well recognized that DNA damage is central to the initiation phase of carcinogenesis induced by ionizing or ultraviolet light radiation, as well as by many chemical carcinogens.[57] The cellular enzyme protein kinase C (PKC) plays a critical role in growth control, and may be central to the promotional phase of carcinogenesis. PKC, activated by phorbol ester tumor promoters such as TPA, can produce a cascade of events resulting in alterations in gene expression, membrane function and ultimately cellular differentiation and proliferation.[57] The role of these factors is described in more detail in Section I of this text. Given the complex multi-stage nature of carcinogenesis, it is reasonable to speculate that clonal evolution toward neoplasia involves a sequence of changes in gene expression driven by both genetic and epigenetic changes.

From studies of radiation-induced carcinogenesis in human populations and experimental systems, it appears that radiation acts primarily as an initiating agent by its ability to damage DNA. Radiation can induce both specific base damage and DNA strand breaks, and mammalian cells possess efficient enzymatic mechanisms for repairing these types of damage. Although it has long been assumed that unrejoined DNA double strand breaks are important in the lethal effects of radiation on cells, evidence is now emerging to suggest that incorrectly rejoined DNA double strand breaks may be important mutagenic and carcinogenic lesions.[32,48] This DNA misrepair appears to lead to DNA deletions and rearrangements; DNA structural analyses of radiation-induced mutants at specific gene loci in human cells indicate that most of them arise as a result of such large-scale genetic and chromosomal changes.[59]

It is now well established that certain chromosomal rearrangements including translocations and deletions are associated with a wide variety of human cancers.[39] These are described in Section I, Chapter 8. Though no consistent non-random chromosomal changes have as yet been associated with radiation carcinogenesis in vivo or in vitro, there is evidence to implicate specific chromosomal rearrangements in pre-leukemic clones in ataxia telangiectasia patients and in two types of radiation-induced murine leukemia.[7]

Oncogenes

The involvement of various oncogenes in experimental and human carcinogenesis is well established.[9,56] This area has been reviewed in detail in Section I of this text. The role of specific oncogene activation in radiation-induced cancer is less clear.[3,7] Activation of ras oncogenes occurs though in relatively low frequencies in mouse lymphomas induced by radiation, whereas activation of c-Ki-ras as well as amplification of c-myc has been reported in some radiation-induced rat skin tumors, but not in mouse skin tumors.[3,36,40] Recently, amplification and rearrangement of c-myc has been reported in a small fraction (6–30%) of radiation-induced murine osteosarcomas.[45]

If myc and ras oncogenes play a significant role in radiation carcinogenesis, activation or amplification of these genes should be found in vitro as well as in vivo. Although evidence of dominant transforming activity has been found in cells transformed by radiation in vitro, this activity has not been associated with a number of known oncogenes.[25,46] Specifically, no evidence has been found for activation or overexpression of ras genes, nor for increased expression or amplification of c-myc. Such findings along with those of in vivo studies have led to the conclusion that distinctive, as yet unidentified transforming genes may be involved in radiation carcinogenesis.

Finally, it is not clear from such studies whether oncogene activation arose as a consequence of a direct interaction of radiation with cellular DNA, or from a complex series of events initially triggered by DNA damage. The activation of ras oncogenes by chemical carcinogens may be either an early or a late event. In one study in which the timing of oncogene activation was studied during radiation transformation, it appeared to occur as a later event.[25] As discussed above, mutations arising as a result of exposure to ionizing radiation usually involve large-scale DNA structural changes and rearrangements. As ras activation usually occurs by point mutations, it may not be unexpected that activation of the ras proto-oncogene is not an important mechanism of radiation

transformation and carcinogenesis. Although the whole question of the association of oncogenes with radiation carcinogenesis needs further investigation, it is clear that the pattern of oncogene activation differs significantly for transformation and carcinogenesis induced by radiation as compared with chemical carcinogens.

Tumor Suppressor Genes

Evidence for the potential importance of tumor suppressor genes in human carcinogenesis has been derived largely from studies of the retinoblastoma gene. These studies and the characteristics of suppressor genes are described in Section I, Chapter 6. Mutations in the retinoblastoma gene are also associated with several other types of tumors including osteosarcomas, soft tissue sarcomas, small cell lung cancer and breast cancer.[55]

Interestingly, retinoblastoma patients appear to be at an unusually high risk for radiation-induced secondary osteosarcomas occurring in the treatment field. The fact that inactivation of a suppressor gene may result from large-scale genetic events including deletions and gene conversion or recombinational processes, suggests that tumors which arise as a result of the loss of suppressor gene activity may be particularly susceptible to induction by radiation. Although this is an intriguing hypothesis, there is at present insufficient data to establish suppressor gene inactivation as an important mechanism in radiation carcinogenesis.

Experimental Radiation Carcinogenesis

General Characteristics of Radiation Carcinogenesis

Ionizing radiation has been called a "universal carcinogen" in that it will induce cancer in most tissues of most species at all ages including the fetus. It is one of the few definitely established carcinogens in human beings, and perhaps the only one with firm dose-response data in human populations. It is, however, a relatively weak carcinogen and mutagen when compared to certain chemical agents. The cancers induced by radiation are of the same histological types as occur spontaneously, but the distribution of types may differ. For example: A higher percentage of small cell carcinomas of the lung occur as a result of exposure to alpha-radiation in uranium miners; radiation induces follicular and papillary carcinomas of the thyroid but not anaplastic and medullary carcinomas; chronic lymphocytic leukemia is apparently not induced by radiation whereas other common types of leukemia are. There is a distinct latent period between exposure to radiation and the clinical appearance of a tumor.

Dose-Response Relationships

It has been generally accepted that radiation carcinogenesis is a stochastic process. That is, the probability of the occurrence of the effect increases with dose with no threshold, but the severity of the effect is not influenced by dose. This is in contradistinction to a non-stochastic effect for which both the probability and the severity of the effect vary with dose. There is no clear experimental evidence to suggest that the grade of malignancy including its invasive or metastatic properties is a function of dose; radiation-induced cancer appears to be an all or none effect. Stochastic effects are those which may arise from damage to a few cells or even a single cell. If this is the case, any dose no matter how small carries with it the finite probability of producing the effect. Studies of radiation-induced carcinogenesis in experimental animals and human populations have been designed to test this hypothesis, as most environmental exposures are in the low dose range. Unfortunately, however, it is very difficult to obtain statistically significant data in either human or animal studies at doses below 50 cGy of low LET radiation.

Many earlier studies of the effects of radiation in small animals involved its life shortening properties. Although this effect was originally ascribed to "radiation-induced aging" in which the natural causes of death were accelerated by radiation, a critical examination of this phenomenon by use of techniques such as serial sacrifice experiments and life table analyses have shown that practically all of the life shortening effect of radiation in experimental animals can be accounted for by the induction of cancer, except perhaps in the high, sublethal dose range.[44,49] Thus, the dose response relationship for life shortening in animals should represent that for cancer deaths from all types of radiation-induced tumors in that species. Such a dose response curve is shown in Figure III-4-5. A generally linear response has been observed for life shortening in a number of different studies.

The dose response relationships for the induction of cancers in specific tissues vary with site, with sex and with species.[14,51,52] For low LET radiation, the frequency of induced cancers generally rises with dose in the range of 0–300 cGy. In some cases, tumor incidence levels off at higher doses and may even decline. This phenomenon is thought to reflect cell killing. The carcinogenic effect of low LET radiation in rodents is usually reduced with protraction of exposure. In the dose range up to 200–300 cGy, the dose response curves for individual tumor types vary but generally assume a linear-quadratic to near linear relationship.

For high LET radiation, the rise in cancer incidence with dose is much steeper. The dose response curves are approximately linear within the range of 0–20 cGy, though in some cases they bend over reaching a plateau at higher

doses.[14,50] In contradistinction to low LET radiation, significant increases in cancer and life-shortening can be observed after doses as low as 10 cGy of neutrons, alpha particles or heavy ions.[14,31,50] RBE values in the range of 3–15 have been estimated for the carcinogenic effects of these radiations at low doses. There is usually no dose-rate effect for high LET radiation exposure. However, an outstanding example is the induction of mouse mammary tumors by low doses of fast neutrons in which protraction of exposure appears to increase the carcinogenic effectiveness by a factor of 2–3 at doses of 2.5–10 cGy.[50]

Modifying Factors

As in the case of neoplastic transformation, radiation carcinogenesis in experimental animals can also be modulated by non-carcinogenic secondary factors. Data on the promotion by TPA of ultraviolet light induced skin cancer in mice are shown in Figure III-4-4B. This can be compared with the effect of this tumor promoter on neoplastic transformation in Figure III-4-4A. A similar phenomenon has been shown for the induction of malignant squamous cell carcinoma of the skin of mice by ionizing radiation, and evidence is accumulating that the two-stage model of initiation and promotion generally applies to tumor induction in epithelial tissues.[3,8]

As an illustration of the possible effects of innocuous seeming secondary factors, 8 weekly intratracheal instillations of 0.2 ml of isotonic saline given to hamsters 4 months after exposure to a relatively low dose of alpha radiation led to a ten-fold enhancement in the induction of lung cancer as compared to that occurring in animals receiving radiation alone.[29] It appeared that the saline instillations, which were non-carcinogenic in themselves, had induced a transient round of cell proliferation among the target cells in the lungs of these animals facilitating expression of the initial radiation-induced damage.

Post-irradiation treatment with agents such as the protease inhibitors which inhibit radiation transformation in vitro can also suppress the induction of carcinogenesis in vivo, as can the presence of certain thiol radioprotective compounds during irradiation. The hormonal environment is also important in certain radiation induced rodent cancers, particularly ovarian and mammary tumors. These and other observations again emphasize the importance of non-carcinogenic secondary factors in the induction and expression of experimental radiation carcinogenesis. However, the extent to which such factors are important in radiation-induced cancer in human populations is not clear.

Another factor which may modify the carcinogenic effects of radiation is genetic susceptibility. Should a fraction of the population be genetically predisposed to radiation-induced cancer, this fact could be of considerable importance in the setting of protection standards. Clearly, there are marked differences in the susceptibility to radiation-induced cancer among different strains of mice; in general, such susceptibility correlates with the spontaneous incidence of the particular tumor. On the other hand, there is little evidence to suggest that such genetic factors are involved in most human cancer, though they do appear to play a role in certain rare disorders. Patients with hereditary retinoblastoma are at increased risk for the development of radiation-induced bone

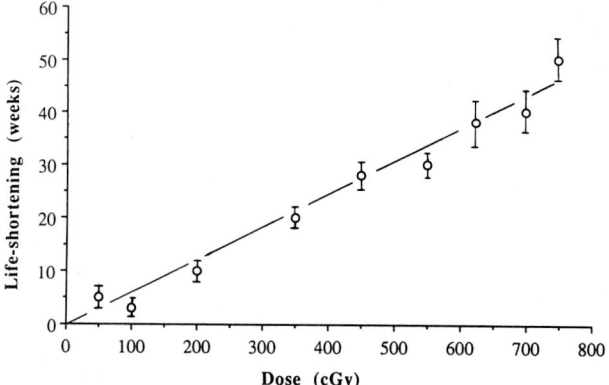

Figure III-4-5. Life shortening in mice as a function of dose of ionizing radiation. The shortening of lifespan is ascribed to early death owing to induced cancers. Reproduced from Lindop and Rotblat.[26]

cancers, whereas patients with the nevoid basal cell carcinoma syndrome are at high risk for the development of basal cell cancers in irradiated areas. Thus, models for genetic predisposition to radiation carcinogenesis do exist in human beings.

Human Epidemiologic Studies

There is now a large body of data derived from epidemiologic studies in irradiated human populations, and it is largely on the basis of these data that current risk estimates are derived. These data are reviewed in detail in the latest report from the National Research Council Committee on the Biological Effects of Radiation (BEIR V).[19] They are derived primarily from two sources: 1) the long-term follow-up of survivors of the atom bombings of Hiroshima and Nagasaki; and 2) populations exposed to medical x-rays.[2,41] Information is also available from certain occupational exposures, particularly from individuals with pulmonary and skeletal exposure to alpha radiation. The results of these studies have yielded significant dose response data for the induction of cancer in at least 5 tissue sites. Such dose response data are extremely important in ascribing radiation as the causal agent for the increased incidence of cancer, as well as for estimating the risks associated with a given exposure. Unfortunately, however, the epidemiologic studies yielding useful dose-response data all involve relatively high dose exposures (above 50 cGy). Thus, risk estimates in the low dose range must be derived from an extrapolation from the high dose data. The shape of the dose-response relationship becomes of critical importance in making such extrapolations. The observed dose-response curves from the human epidemiologic studies appear to be either linear or linear-quadratic in form (that is, a linear component at low doses with a quadratic component at higher doses). A linear curve implies a constant risk per cGy at all doses, whereas the linear-quadratic model implies a smaller risk per cGy in the low dose range. The assumption of a linear model simplifies the extrapolation from high to low doses and the corresponding estimation of risks. Furthermore, it is a conservative technique; that is, if anything it would overestimate rather than underestimate the potential risk. There is no evidence for a proportionally greater effect at low doses.

A final parameter of importance in determining the hazards of a given dose of radiation is the choice of risk models. For many years, risks were estimated on the basis of an Absolute Risk model. This model assumed that a given number of excess cancers were induced by a given radiation dose. Radiation-induced cancers occurred in addition to the natural incidence. Thus, the increased risk could be expressed as the number of excess cancer cases (or cancer deaths) per 10^6 exposed people per year per cGy (the rate per year), or as the total number of excess cancers per 10^6 exposed people per cGy (the total risk or yield of cancers to be expected from a given radiation dose). The Absolute Risk model generally assumes a linear dose-response relationship, though with certain corrections it can be applied to the linear-quadratic situation.

An analysis of the recent data from the atom bomb survivors suggests that radiation-induced cancer more likely follows a Relative Risk model.[19,41] This is also true for several different tumor types in mice.[44] The Relative Risk model implies that radiation increases the natural incidence of cancer in all ages by a dose-dependent factor. As the excess cancer risk is proportional to the natural incidence, radiation-induced cancers would occur primarily at the times when natural tumors arose, independent of the age at irradiation. Thus, the largest cohort of radiation-induced cancers would appear in older individuals. Indeed, this is proving to be the case amongst the atom bomb survivors and is one of the primary reasons why risk estimates based on this population have been revised upward within the last few years.

Leukemia

At one time, leukemia was thought to be the major radiation-induced cancer to arise from whole body exposure. We now know the two reasons for this assumption: 1) the spontaneous occurrence of leukemia is low, thus radiation-induced cases are more readily recognizable; and 2) the latent period in human beings is very short relative to other types of cancer, thus leukemias are recognized earlier. Excess leukemias begin appearing within 2 years after acute radiation exposure, reaching a peak incidence within 10 years then falling off steadily. This is in comparison to other cancers in which the minimum latent period is 10–15 years, and the rate of appearance of new radiation-induced tumors increases at least up to 30 years. The major sources of data for the induction of leukemia are from the 76,000 members of the life span study of the atom bomb survivors from whom DS86 (1986) dose estimates are available, and from a study of approximately 14,000 patients in Great Britain treated with radiation for ankylosing spondylitis of the spine.

The dose response relationship for the induction of leukemia in the atom bomb survivors, based on the DS86 dosimetry measurements of organ-absorbed dose, is shown in Figure III-4-6A. Various dose-response models fitted to the data are also shown on this graph. The data are best described by a linear quadratic model with a cell killing term (dashed line), although statistically speaking the linear quadratic fit is not significantly better than a straight linear fit.[41] Based on these data, the relative risk at 100 cGy is 6.21, and the attributable risk is estimated to be 2.94 excess cancer deaths/10^6/yr/cGy. This latter figure is approximately 5-fold higher than that estimated from the data for the British ankylosing spondylitis patients. This may be ascribed to the younger age of the atom bomb survivors at the time of irradiation, and the fact they received a single acute whole body exposure.[19] Children appear to be twice as sensitive as adults to the leukemogenic effects of radiation, whereas the unborn child may be about 10 times more sensitive following in utero irradiation.[33]

Radiation-induced leukemia in human populations differs in several characteristics from solid tumors. These include the unusually short latent period, high relative risk (Table III-4-1), and the fact that the epidemiologic data best fit a linear-quadratic dose response relationship. This may be related to the nature of the bone marrow and blood stream which contain no stroma as do most tissues. Therefore, there may be fewer constraints on cell proliferation, in essence allowing

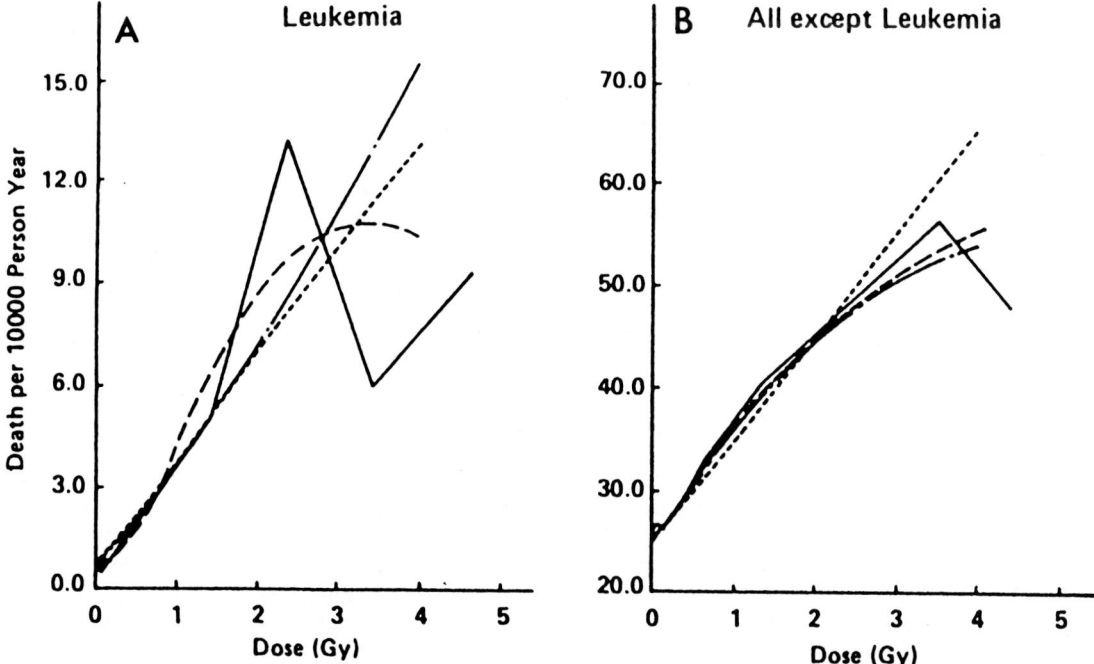

Figure III-4-6. Dose-response curves for induction of cancer in human populations receiving uniform whole body radiation exposure, derived from epidemiological data from the atom bomb survivors of Hiroshima and Nagasaki. Panel A: Leukemia. Panel B: All cancer except leukemia. The solid lines represent the actual data, whereas the others represent mathematically fitted dose response curves based on different models: (-----) linear; (–·–·–) linear-quadratic; (– – – –) with cell killing correction. Reproduced from Shimizu et al.[41]

Table III-4-1. Summary Measures of Radiation Dose-response for Mortality at Statistically Significant Tissue Sites in Atom Bomb Survivors of Hiroshima and Nagasaki[a]

Site of Cancer	Relative Risk at 100 cGy	Excess Deaths per 10⁶/yr/cGy	Attributable Risk (%)[b]
Leukemia	6.21	2.94	58.6
All Cancers (except leukemia)	1.41	10.13	8.1
Female Breast	2.19	1.20	22.1
Lung	1.63	1.68	12.3
Esophagus	1.58	0.45	13.0
Stomach	1.27	2.42	5.7
Colon	1.85	0.81	16.3
Ovary	2.33	0.71	22.3
Urinary Tract	2.27	0.68	21.5
Multiple Myeloma	3.29	0.26	31.8

[a]Includes both sexes, all ages at exposure, 1950–1985 data. Estimates based on organ-absorbed dose measurements and linear extrapolation model. Data from Shimizu et al.[41]

[b]Percent of all cancer observed that can be attributed to the radiation exposure.

a few transformed cells to grow rapidly and be detected earlier as a clinical cancer.

Other Tumors

The dose-response relationship for all cancers except leukemia is shown in Fig. III-4-6B; the data are best described by a linear model. The various risk estimates for all types of cancer in which mortality was significantly increased among the atom bomb survivors is shown in Table III-4-1. These data are based upon 42,000 subjects exposed to greater than 1 cGy. This group includes approximately 140 leukemia deaths of which 80 are ascribed to radiation exposure, and about 3300 other cancer deaths of which 260 are ascribed to radiation exposure. Approximately 8% of all cancer deaths in this population so far are associated with radiation, though the overall mortality rate is not significantly increased. As can be seen in Table III-4-1, the relative risk at 100 cGy is considerably lower for all other cancers than it is for leukemia. The excess cancer deaths/10⁶/yr/cGy is approximately 10 for all cancers, ranging from 0.26–2.4 in individual tissues.

In addition to breast, lung and leukemia, dose response data from human epidemiologic studies are available for two other sites not shown in the atom bomb survivor data in Table III-4-1; these are, thyroid and bone. The incidence of bone cancer was not significantly elevated in the atom bomb studies; the relative and absolute risks are low for the induction of this type of cancer by low LET radiation. The dose-response data have come from studies of persons with elevated body burdens of alpha-emitting radium isotopes as a result of occupational or medical exposures.

Thyroid cancer, on the other hand, is very efficiently induced by low LET radiation. Dose response relationships are derived from populations receiving therapeutic irradiation either for an enlarged thymus gland or tinea capitis. Relative risk estimates for the development of thyroid cancer have ranged from 7–69 among various age groups, ethnic origins and different studies.[19] However, cancer death rates are not significantly elevated in these populations, as radiation apparently induces only papillary and follicular type tumors which are readily curable.

In addition to the results from the atom bomb survivors, dose-response data are available for breast cancer from several medically exposed populations. The results of these studies are generally consistent in terms of risk estimates. Taken as a whole, however, several other interesting findings have arisen. Radiation-induced breast cancers are similar in histopathological types and age distribution to those arising spontaneously. Women under 20 years of age at exposure are at a higher relative risk than adults, similar to the observations for leukemia. As in the case of thyroid cancer, the development of breast cancer is profoundly dependent on hormonal status. Finally, protraction of exposure does not appear to reduce the risk of radiation-induced breast cancer.

Additional epidemiologic studies are also available for the induction of lung cancer.[19] Of particular interest among the underground uranium workers in the Colorado plateau has been an apparent multiplicative interaction with cigarette smoking. This observation is consistent with certain experimental findings on alpha-radiation induced lung cancer. However, statistically significant evidence for a more than additive effect between smoking and low LET radiation on lung cancer not been observed in other epidemiologic studies. This important question needs further investigation.

Radiation-Induced Second Tumors

An increase in secondary tumors in the treatment field has now been observed in patients treated for several different types of cancer by radiation therapy, often in conjunction with chemotherapy. This phenomenon is described in detail in Section XL, Chapter 17. In some cases the incidence of radiation associated second tumors appears to be proportional to dose at the treatment portal, though some epidemiologic data suggest that for leukemia in particular the tumor incidence may decline at high doses owing to killing of the target cells.[2] The significance of such an effect for most other cancers remains unclear.

Increased susceptibility to radiation-induced second tumors clearly occurs in certain rare genetic disorders. The extent to which genetic factors play a more general role in susceptibility to spontaneous or treatment-induced secondary tumors in cancer patients is unknown. It is certain, however, that the entire process is a complex one in which many factors may contribute including the type of primary cancer, exposure to other environmental mutagens, immune-surveillance mechanisms and hormonal factors.

Low-Dose Exposures

There have been a number of epidemiologic studies over the past decade that purport to show carcinogenic effect of environmental radiation exposures in the dose range below 10 cGy. The populations involved are varied but include military personnel exposed during nuclear bomb testing, workers in various nuclear and weapons facilities, and members of the general population living near nuclear facilities or exposed to fall-out. There has also been considerable recent concern about exposure to naturally occurring radon in the air of homes and the workplace; however, the biolog-

ical significance of these exposures remains unclear at the present time.[37]

There have been several recent reports analysing various of these low-dose epidemiologic studies.[16,33,37,54] Based on the relative and absolute risk estimates shown in Table III-4-1, a significant increase in radiation-associated cancer in populations of these sizes exposed to doses in the range of 10 cGy or less would imply a markedly enhanced sensitivity at low doses. That is, the dose response curve should be concave upward at low doses, with the excess cancer incidence rising rapidly at very low doses. There are no experimental data to support such a phenomenon.

In reality, a careful analysis of nearly all of these low-dose studies indicates no significant increase in the incidence of all cancers or of cancers at specific sites. Owing to small numbers, the confidence limits in some cases are large, such that a two or three fold effect cannot be excluded. For example, the observed over expected ratios for leukemia occurring in the population living in the vicinity of each of five different Canadian nuclear facilities were not significantly elevated, but ranged from 0.31–2.46.

A seeming exception has been the population surrounding the Selafield nuclear plant in West Cumbria, Great Britain, in which a small cluster of leukemias has been observed in young people.[15] The effect appears not to correlate with irradiation of the individuals who developed leukemia, but rather with paternal irradiation in fathers receiving doses greater than 10 cGy prior to conception. In this context, it is of interest to note that the purported increase in leukemia in the population living near the Pilgrim Power Plant in Massachusetts occurred in elderly people, rather than the 0–24 year age group as at Selafield.

There is no experimental or epidemiologic precedent for such an effect of paternal irradiation. No increase in leukemia was observed in children born to 7,300 fathers exposed to a mean of 49 cGy at the time of the atomic bombings in Hiroshima and Nagasaki.[60] Furthermore, no increase in other heritable diseases or abnormalities has been detected in the Selafield population. A wider study of nuclear facilities in England and Wales concluded that there was no general increase in cancer mortality near these nuclear facilities, a finding which is in agreement with similar investigations in other countries.[12] It seems quite likely that the apparent effect may be related to exposure to chemicals or other factors related to the nuclear industry.[10]

In summary, no consistent trend has emerged from a large variety of epidemiologic studies of low dose radiation exposures such as to suggest an unexpected increase in sensitivity in the range from 0 to 10–20 cGy. The data are in general consistent with a linear extrapolation from the high dose results. This conclusion is supported by the lack of correlation between cancer incidence and background radiation observed in several different studies. Low dose epidemiologic studies in populations of limited size must be very carefully controlled and are often prone to bias by confounding factors.

Risk Assessment

The lifetime excess cancer risk estimates as determined by the National Research Council Committee on the Biological Effects of Ionizing Radiation and presented in their 1990 Report (BEIR V) are shown in Table III-4-2.[19] These estimates were derived from a composite of the epidemiological data from the atom bomb survivors and various medical x-ray exposures. They were derived by use of the Relative Risk model, on the assumption of a linear-quadratic dose-response relationship for leukemia and a straight linear relationship for other tumors. In addition, characteristics such as the latent period, age at exposure, time after exposure and interaction effects were taken into consideration.

The risk estimates shown in Table III-4-2 are for the mean of all ages at exposure. For children under 20, excess cancer mortality per cGy is about 50% higher than the mean for all tumors, whereas it is much lower at ages over 65. The leukemia risk, on the other hand, rises quite steeply in middle and old age where the risk is nearly 4 times that of young adults and twice that of children.[19] It should be pointed out that the risk estimates in Table III-4-2 are probably maximal ones and might be reduced by a factor of 2 or 3 if different dose response and risk models and parameters were used.

The lifetime excess yield of death from all cancers including leukemia as shown in Table III-4-2 is approximately 800 per 10^6 exposed people per cGy. On an individual basis, this is approximately 1:1250 (0.8×10^{-3}) effect per cGy. For an example, a person receiving 10 cGy whole body exposure would have a 0.8% change of developing cancer as a result of this exposure, whereas his chances of dying of cancer unrelated to radiation exposure are approximately 20%. It should be pointed out, however, that these risks are for uniform whole body exposure to radiation. For localized radiation exposures, the risks will be much lower and related to the critical tissues including the bone marrow included within the radiation field. For localized exposures, estimates are based on data such as those shown in Table III-4-2 and the utilization of models developed for specific tissue sites as described by the BEIR Committee.[19]

It is often the perception of risk rather than the actual risk itself which is particularly important in the promotion and regulation of health and safety.[42] For example, members of the League of Women Voters and a group of college students were asked to order their perception of the risk of fatality for 30 activities and technologies. Both placed nuclear power in first position ahead of smoking, alcoholic beverages and motor vehicles. The risk experts ranked motor vehicle accidents first (there are about 60,000 motor vehicle deaths in the United States each year), whereas they ranked nuclear power 20th–in the same range as food coloring and home appliances.

Table III-4-2. Lifetime Excess Cancer Risk Estimates for Acute Radiation Exposure[a]

Type of Cancer	Cancer Deaths per 10^6 exposed per cGy	
	Males	Females
Leukemia	110	80
Non-Leukemias	660	730
All Cancers	770	810

[a]Estimates from BEIR V Report.[19] See text for discussion of these estimates.

It is thus of interest to compare the risk of death from various activities associated with everyday living.[58] Such a comparison is shown in Table III-4-3. In general, it turns out that the risk from radiation exposure is relatively small compared with other risks associated with everyday living. Similarly, a comparison of occupational hazards shows that the risks to radiation workers are much lower than those associated with many other occupations.[38] In this context, it is of interest to note the estimation that 300,000 excess deaths each year are currently associated with cigarette smoking in the United States. On the assumption that 50% of the population smokes, such an excess death rate would be comparable to that resulting from approximately 250 cGy of uniform whole-body radiation exposure

Of concern to the clinical oncologist, however, is the risk of inducing a second malignant tumor as a result of exposure to high doses of radiation often in conjunction with chemotherapy. This will of course depend upon the particular tissue sites included in the radiation field. One could then derive risk estimates based on the type of information shown in Table III-4-1. However, the information in Table III-4-1 was

Table III-4-3. Risk of Death from Various Environmental Sources (Risks of One in One Million).[a]

Source	Amount of Exposure	Risk
Ionizing radiation (uniform whole body)	12 uGy	Cancer
Cigarettes	1 cigarette	Cancer, heart disease
Living with Cigarette Smoker	2 months	Cancer, heart disease
Wine	0.5 liter	Cirrhosis of the liver
Peanut Butter	10 tablespoons	Liver cancer caused by aflatoxin
Miami drinking water	1 gallon	cancer caused by chloroform
Visit to Denver	1 week	cancer caused by cosmic rays
Jet flying	1500 miles	cancer caused by cosmic rays
Living near polyvinylchloride plant	20 years	cancer caused by vinyl chloride
In stone or brick building	1 week	cancer caused by radioactivity
In New York or Boston	1 day	air pollution
In coal mine	3 hours	accident
In coal mine	1 hour	black lung disease
Canoeing	6 minutes	drowning
Jet flying	2500 miles	accident
In automobile	50 miles	accident
On motorcycle	5 miles	accident

[a]Estimates derived from various sources on assumption of linear, nonthreshold response for all effects.

derived from presumably normal people in the general population exposed to tens to hundreds rather than thousands of cGy. As discussed earlier, there may be a number of factors which determine susceptibility to second tumors in cancer patients treated with high doses of radiation. One risk factor is the irradiation of large tissue volumes as in the treatment of disorders such as Hodgkins' disease. Genetic factors would be another important risk factor. It is well known, for example, that retinoblastoma patients are at very high risk for developing second tumors in the irradiated field. The extent to which genetic hypersusceptibility may be important in some of the more common cancers remains to be determined.

In most cases it would seem that a benefit/risk estimation would be positive; that is, the benefit of treatment would outweigh the risk of developing secondary tumors. However, we have very little information concerning the relative carcinogenicity of various combinations of radiation and chemotherapeutic agents. It is possible that certain combinations might be particularly carcinogenic whereas others may not. Clearly, additional knowledge is needed concerning treatment regimens which might minimize their carcinogenic effects, and thus the risk of developing secondary treatment-induced tumors, while producing an optimal therapeutic gain.

References

1. Abrahamson, S.: Risk estimates: Past, present, and future. Health Physics, 59:99, 1990.
2. Boice, J. D., Jr.: Carcinogenesis—A synopsis of human experience with external exposure in medicine. Health Physics, 55:621, 1988.
3. Bowden, G. T., Jaffe, D., and Andrews, K.: Biological and molecular aspects of radiation carcinogenesis in mouse skin. Radiation Res., 121:235, 1990.
4. Brent, R. L.: Radiation teratogenesis. Teratology, 21:281, 1980.
5. Chadwick, K. H., Seymour, C., and Barnhart, B.: Cell Transformation and Radiation-induced Cancer. New York, Adam Hilger, 1989.
6. Chan, G. L., and Little, J. B.: Neoplastic transformation in vitro. In Radiation Carcinogenesis. Edited by A. C. Upton, R. E. Albert, F. J. Burns and R. E. Shore. New York, Elsevier, 1986, p. 107.
7. Cox, R., and Little, J. B.: Oncogenic Cell Transformation In Vitro. In Advances in Radiation Biology, Vol. 15. Edited by O. F. Nygaard, W. K. Sinclair and J. T. Lett. New York, Academic Press, 1991.
8. Drinkwater, N. R.: Experimental models and biological mechanisms for tumor promotion. Cancer Cells, 2:8, 1990.
9. Druker, B. J., Mamon, H. J., and Roberts T. M.: Oncogenes, growth factors, and signal transduction. N. Engl. J. Med., 321:1383, 1989.
10. Evans, H. J.: Leukaemia and radiation. Nature, 345:16, 1990.
11. Fabre, F.: Mitotic transmission of induced recombinational ability in yeast. In Cellular Responses to DNA Damage. New York, Alan R. Liss, 1983, p. 379.
12. Forman, D., Cook-Mozaffari, P., Darby, S., Davey, G., Stratton, I., Doll, R., and Pike, M.: Cancer near nuclear installations. Nature, 329:499, 1987.
13. Fry, R. J. M., and Ley, R. D.: Ultraviolet radiation carcinogenesis. In Mechanisms of Tumor Promotion, Vol. II: Tumor Promotion and Skin Carcinogenesis. Edited by T. J. Slaga. Boca Raton, Fl, CRC Press, 1984, p. 73.
14. Fry, R. J. M., and Storer, J.B.: External Radiation Carcinogenesis. In Advances in Radiation Biology, Vol. 13. Edited by J.T. Lett. New York, Academic Press, 1987, p. 31.
15. Gardner, M. J., Snee, M. P., Hall, A. J., Powell, C. A., Downes, S., and Terrell, J. D.: Results of case-control study of leukaemia and lymphoma among young people near Sellafield nuclear plant in West Cumbria. British Med. J., 300:423, 1990.
16. Gilbert, E. S., Fry, S. A., Wiggs, L. D., Voelz, G. L., Cragle, D. L., and Petersen, G. R.: Analyses of combined mortality data on workers at the Hanford Site, Oak Ridge National Laboratory, and Rocky Flats Nuclear Weapons Plant. Radiation Res., 120:19, 1989.
17. Gorgojo, L., and Little, J. B.: Expression of lethal mutations in progeny of irradiated mammalian cells. Int. J.Radiat. Biol., 55:619, 1989.
18. Grosovsky, A. J., and Little, J. B.: Evidence for linear response for the induction of mutations in human cells by x-ray exposures below 10 rads. Proc. Natl. Acad. Sci., USA 82:2092, 1985.
19. Health Effects of Exposure to Low Levels of Ionizing Radiation: BEIR V. Committee on the Biological Effects of Ionizing Radiations, National Research Council, Washington, National Academy Press, 1990.
20. Hill, C. K., Buonaguro, F. M., Myers, C. P., Han, A., and Elkind, M. M.: Fission-spectrum neutrons at reduced dose rates enhance neoplastic transformation. Nature, 298:67, 1982.
21. Kano, Y., and Little, J. B.: Persistence of x-ray-induced chromosomal rearrangements in long-term cultures of human diploid fibroblasts. Cancer Res., 44:3706, 1984.
22. Kano, Y., and Little, J. B.: Mechanisms of human cell neoplastic transformation: X-ray-induced abnormal clone formation in long-term cultures of human diploid fibroblasts. Cancer Res., 45:2550, 1985.
23. Kennedy, A. R., Fox, M., Murphy, G., and Little, J. B.: Relationship between x-ray exposure and malignant transformation in C3H 10T1/2 cells. Proc. Nat. Acad. Sci. U.S.A., 77:7262, 1980.
24. Kennedy, A. R., and Little, J. B.: Evidence that a second event in x-ray induced oncogenic transformation in vitro occurs during cellular proliferation. Radiation Res., 99:228, 1984.
25. Krolewski, B., and Little, J. B.: Molecular analysis of DNA isolated from the different stages of x-ray-induced transformation in vitro. Molec. Carcinogenesis, 2:27, 1989.
26. Lindop, P., and Rotblat, J.: Long-term effects of a single whole-body exposure of mice to ionizing radiations. I. Life-shortening. Proc. R. Soc. Lond., B., 154:332, 1961.
27. Little, J.B.: Cellular effects of ionizing radiation. I & II. New Eng. J. Med. 273:308 & 369, 1968.
28. Little, J. B.: The relevance of cell transformation to carcinogenesis in vivo. In Low Dose Radiation–Biological Basis of Risk Assessment. Edited by K. F. Baverstock and J. W. Strather. London, Taylor and Francis, 1989, p. 396.
29. Little, J. B.: Low-Dose Radiation Effects: Interactions and Synergism. Health Physics, 59:49, 1990.
30. Little, J. B.: Characteristics of radiation-induced neoplastic transformation in vitro. Leukemia Res., 10:719, 1986.
31. Little, J. B., Kennedy, A. R., and McGandy, R. B.: Lung cancer induced in hamsters by low doses of alpha radiation from polonium-210. Science, 188:737, 1975.
32. Little, J. B., Whaley, J. M., and Liber, H. L.: Role of energy distribution in DNA on the mutagenic effects of internal emitters. In Mechanisms of Anti-Carcinogenesis and Radiation Protection. Edited by O. F. Nygaard and A. C. Upton. New York, Plenum Press, 1990.
33. MacMahon, B.: Some recent issues in low-exposure radiation epidemiology. Environ. Health Perspect., 81:131, 1989.
34. McCormick, J. J., and Maher, V. M.: Towards an understanding of the malignant transformation of diploid human fibroblasts. Mutation Res., 199:273, 1988.
35. Miller, R. W.: Effects of prenatal exposure to ionizing radiation. Health Phys., 59:57, 1990.
36. Newcomb, E. W., Steinberg, J. J., and Pellicer, A.: Ras oncogenes and phenotypic staging in N-methylnitrosourea- and gamma-irradiation-induced thymic lymphomas in C57BL/6J mice. Cancer Res., 48:5514, 1988.
37. Peto, J.: Radon and the risks of cancer. Nature, 345:389, 1990.
38. Pochin, E. E. Occupational and other fatality risks. Community Health Stud., 6:2, 1974.
39. Rowley, J. D.: Molecular cytogenetics: Rosetta Stone for understanding Cancer. Cancer Res., 50:3816, 1990.
40. Sawey, M. J., Hood, A. T., Burns, F. J., and Garte, S. J.: Activation of myc and ras oncogenes in primary rat tumors induced by ionizing radiation. Mol. Cell. Biol., 7:932, 1987.
41. Shimizu, Y., Kato, H., and Schull W. J.: Studies of the Mortality of A-Bomb Survivors. 9. Mortality, 1950-1985: Part 2. Cancer Mortality Based on the Recently Revised Doses (DS86). Radiation Res., 121:120, 1990.
42. Slovic, P.: Perception of Risk. Science, 236:280, 1987.
43. Stomato, T., Weinstein, R., Peters, B., Hu, J., Doherty, B., and Giaccia, A.: Delayed mutation in Chinese hamster cells. Som. Cell Molec. Genet., 13:57, 1987.
44. Storer, J. B., Mitchell, T. J., and Fry, R. J. M.: Extrapolation of the relative risk of radiogenic neoplasms across mouse strains and to man. Radiat. Res., 114: 331, 1988.
45. Sturm, S. A., Strauss, P. G., Adolph, S., Hameister, H., and Erfle, V.: Amplification and rearrangement of c-myc in radiation-induced murine osteosarcomas. Cancer Res., 50:4146, 1990.
46. Suzuki, K., Suzuki, F., Watanabe, M., and Nikaido, O.: Multistep nature of x-ray induced neoplastic transformation in golden hamster embryo cells: Expression of transformed phenotypes and stepwise changes in karyotypes. Cancer Res., 49:2134, 1989.
47. Tabocchini, M. A., Little, J. B., and Liber, H.L.: Mutation induction in human lymphoblasts after protracted exposure to low doses of tritiated water. In Low Dose Radiation–Biological Basis of Risk Assessment. Edited by K. F. Baverstock and J. W. Stather. London, Taylor and Francis, 1989, p. 439.
48. Thacker, J.: The use of recombinant DNA techniques to study radiation-induced damage, Int. J. Radiat. Biol., 50:1, 1986.
49. Thomson, J. F., and Grahn, D.: Life shortening in mice exposed to fission neutrons and gamma-rays VII. Effects of 60 once-weekly exposures. Radiat. Res., 115:347, 1988.
50. Ullrich, R. L.: Tumor induction in BALB/c mice after fractionated or protracted exposures to fission-spectrum neutrons. Radiation Res., 97:587, 1984.
51. Ullrich, R. L., and Storer, J. B.: Influence of gamma irradiation on the development of neoplastic disease in mice I. Reticular tissue tumors. Radiation Res., 80:303, 1979.
52. Ullrich, R. L., and Storer, J. B.: Influence of gamma irradiation on the development of neoplastic disease in mice II. Solid tumors. Radiation Res., 80: 317, 1979.
53. Upton, A. C. Historial perspectives on radiation carcinogenesis. In Radiation Carcinogenesis. Edited by A. C. Upton, R. E. Albert, F. J. Burns and R. E. Shore. New York, Elsevier, 1986, p. 1.
54. Webster, E. W.: On the question of cancer induction by small x-ray doses. Am. J. Roentgenol., 137:647, 1981.
55. Weichselbaum, R. R., Beckett, M. A., and Diamond, A. A.: Some retinoblastomas, osteosarcomas, and soft tissue sarcomas may share a common etiology. Proc. Natl. Acad. Sci. U.S.A., 85:2106, 1988.
56. Weinberg, R. A.: Oncogenes, antioncogenes, and the molecular bases of multistep carcinogenesis. Cancer Res., 49:3713, 1989.
57. Weinstein, I. B.: The origins of human cancer: Molecular mechanisms of carcinogenesis and their implications for cancer prevention and treatment. Cancer Res., 48:4135, 1988.
58. Wilson, R., and Crouch, E. A. C.: Risk Assessment and Comparisons: An Introduction. Science, 236:267, 1987.
59. Yandell, D. W., Dryja, T. P., and Little, J. B.: Molecular genetic analysis of recessive mutations at a heterozygous autosomal locus in human cells. Mutation Res., 229:89, 1990.
60. Yoshimoto, Y.: Cancer risk among children of atomic bomb survivors. J.A.M.A., 264: 596, 1990.

Ultraviolet Radiation Carcinogenesis

James E. Cleaver
David L. Mitchell

Mad dogs and Englishmen go out in the mid-day sun.

Noel Coward

Skin Tumor Induction

Skin cancers occur in uniquely accessible sites and are caused by well-defined environmental agents; consequently, their formation illustrates numerous salient features of carcinogenesis. Skin tumors in man account for about 30% of all new cancers reported annually.[63,64] Epidemiological and laboratory studies provide evidence for a direct causal role of sunlight exposure in the induction of cancer,[29] and the high rate of skin carcinogenesis is a direct result of the high dose rate from this causative agent. Both basal cell and squamous cell carcinomas are found on sun-exposed regions of the head and neck, and their incidence is correlated with cumulative sunlight exposure. Melanoma, although also likely to be associated with sunlight exposure, shows a weaker dependence on total exposure to sunlight and a distribution over the body that is not correlated to exposed areas.[4]

Evidence for the carcinogenic role of sunlight includes the following: basal and squamous cell carcinomas appear on parts of the body unprotected from the sun's rays (e.g., the face and trunk in men, face and legs in women); tumor incidence and mortality increase with decreasing latitude, corresponding to exposure; skin cancers are less frequent in dark-skinned populations than in lighter-skinned peoples; and tumor incidence increases with occupational exposure, such as in ranchers and fishermen.

Exposure to direct sunlight in the mid-United States latitudes results in the accumulation of a mean lethal dose to unprotected human cells within approximately 30 minutes.[70] The only other carcinogen to which we are exposed that even approaches these exposure levels would be cigarette smoke in very heavy smokers. Variations in individual susceptibility are also clearly observed in skin carcinogenesis. Human skin can be classified into types I–IV, ranging from individuals who always burn and never tan, to those who tan but never burn; skin cancer susceptibility varies accordingly.[85] But the most dramatic examples of variations in human susceptibility occur in the human genetic disorders that show increased responses to sunlight exposure.[22] These include xeroderma pigmentosum, Cockayne syndrome, basal cell nevus syndrome, dysplastic nevus syndrome, Bloom syndrome, Rothmund-Thompson syndrome, the porphyrias, and phenylketonuria. Some other disorders are associated with an acquired sun sensitivity, including polymorphous light eruption, actinic reticuloid, solar urticaria, lupus erythematosus, and Darier's disease. Less specific factors contributing to sun sensitivity include skin type, race, eye and hair color, and tendency for freckling; additional factors can include medication and immunological status. Sunlight exposure also has a major immunosuppressive effect leading to loss of antigen-presenting Langerhans cells and the appearance of dyskeratotic keratinocytes (sunburn cells) in the upper epidermis, together with the erythemal sunburn response associated with vasodilation caused by a release of prostaglandin.[43]

A major player in all of these responses is the absorption of sunlight quanta in cellular molecules in the skin. The importance of DNA as a chromophore for the shorter wavelengths is illustrated by the autosomal recessive disease xeroderma pigmentosum (XP). In this disease a failure in one cellular protective mechanism, DNA repair, is associated with a major increase in the rate of onset of squamous and basal cell carcinoma and melanoma.[22] Median onset for skin cancer in the general United States population occurs at 50–60 years of age; in XP patients carcinogenesis is accelerated and median onset is within the first decade (Figure III-5-1). This early onset is a direct consequence of sunlight-induced changes in DNA of skin cells. An appreciation of the significance of these changes requires describing the photochemical responses of DNA, mechanisms of DNA repair, and their mutagenic and carcinogenic consequences.

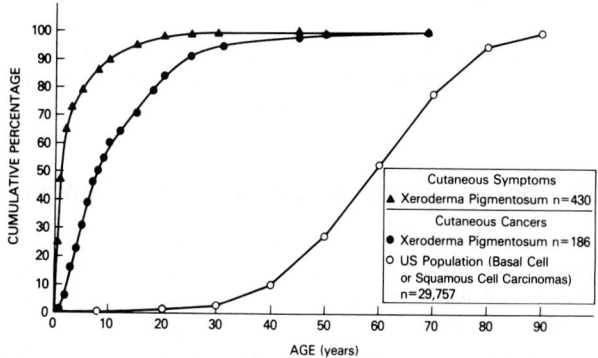

Figure III-5-1. Age at onset of XP symptoms. Age at onset of cutaneous symptoms (generally sun sensitivity or pigmentation) was reported for 430 patients. Age at first skin cancer was reported for 186 patients and is compared with age distribution for 29,757 patients with basal cell carcinoma or squamous cell carcinoma in the United States general population. (Reproduced from Kraemer et al.,[42] with permission.)

strand breaks. This suggests that during excision repair a dynamic balance is established between strand breakage and rejoining. The actual number of sites involved in excision repair at any one time is small, no more than about 1 in 2 × 10⁸ daltons of DNA. Only about 1% of the dimers produced in DNA by a dose of 10 J/m² are undergoing excision at any instant. Excision must therefore be rate-limited by the enzymes involved in the early steps of repair, which presumably move along the DNA repairing different sites in sequence.

There is considerable difference between cyclobutane dimers and (6-4) photoproducts in their rates of excision from the overall genome of rodent and human fibroblasts and skin (Figures III-5-5 and III-5-6).[54] (6-4) Photoproducts are the more rapidly excised, 50% being removed from human and rodent cells in 2–6 hours. Cyclobutane dimers are much more slowly removed; one-half are removed from human cell DNA in 12–24 hours,[18,30] but negligible amounts are removed from rodent DNA for even longer times. There are also large variations in dimer excision between human subjects.[30] The different rates of excision may reflect the fact that (6-4) photoproducts are preferentially located in internucleosomal regions of DNA, whereas dimers are more randomly located.[55] The linker regions are likely to be more accessible to excision enzymes. When excision is considered on an individual gene basis, additional variation exists according to transcriptional activity. Pyrimidine dimers are excised more rapidly from actively transcribed genes, especially the DNA strand used as the template for transcription.[48] An increased excision rate in active genes may also occur for (6-4) photoproducts, but this is less easily resolved against the greater overall rate of excision of these photoproducts in the genome as a whole.

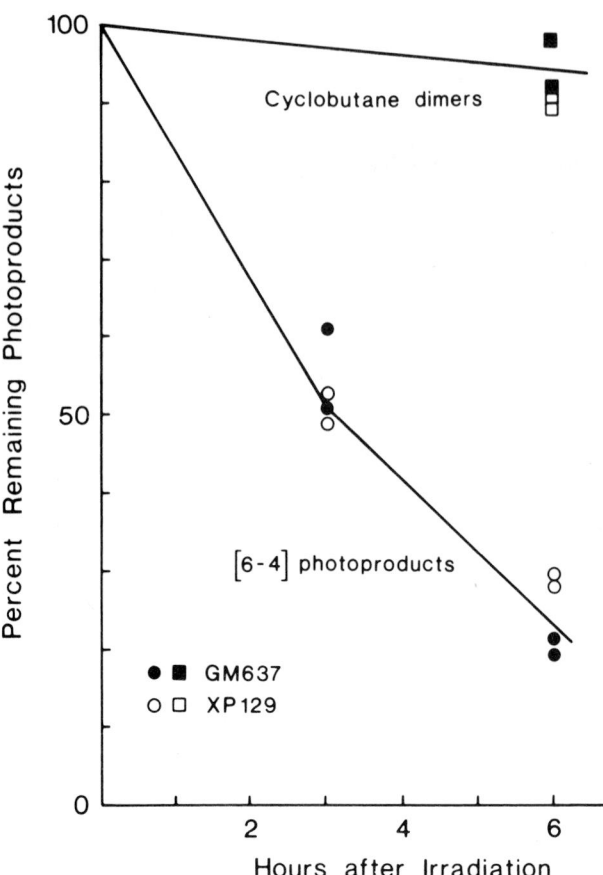

Figure III-5-6. Repair of (6-4) photoproducts and cyclobutane dimers in human fibroblasts in culture. Radioimmunoassays that specifically detect (6-4) photoproducts (circles) or cyclobutane dimers (squares) were used to monitor the removal of lesions from the DNA of normal (GM637) or XP revertant (XP129) cells. (Cleaver, unpublished data.)

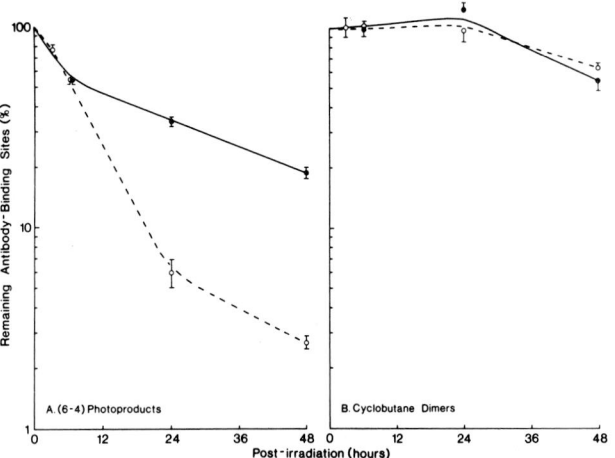

Figure III-5-5. Repair of (6-4) photoproducts and cyclobutane dimers in mouse skin and cultured cells. Radioimmunoassays that specifically detect (6-4) photoproducts (A) or cyclobutane dimers (B) were used to monitor the removal of these lesions from the DNA of irradiated mouse skin (○) and mouse cells in culture (●). Means and standard error bars are shown for 3, 6, 24, and 48 h after UVB irradiation of mouse skin (n = 10) and for 3, 4, and 24 h after UVC irradiation of 3T3 and 10T1/2 cels (n = 4). (Reproduced from Mitchell et al.,[56] with permission.)

Mutagenicity of UV Photoproducts

Two molecular mechanisms are currently considered important in the initiation of carcinogenesis: activation of proto-oncogenes, and inactivation of tumor-suppressor genes. Both sites of action are vulnerable to the lethal and mutagenic effects of UV light. A gene, such as the *ras* proto-oncogene, can be activated by a point mutation.

The lethality of a particular type of DNA damage (photoproduct) may ultimately influence its mutagenicity and tumorigenicity. This relationship has been considered in terms of a "pass/fail" rule:[7] lesions that block DNA polymerization are lethal but nonmutagenic. In other words, the more cytotoxic a lesion (assuming its lethality results from termination of DNA synthesis) the less likely it will be to allow continued synthesis and mutation induction at that site. In terms of this model, the mutagenicity of the major photoproducts in mammalian cells is inversely related to their cytotoxicity; their cytotoxicity is in turn modulated by repair.

Tumor progression can also be affected by UV damage in DNA. Cell death, due to the lethal effects of UV light, may enhance the clonal expansion of surviving cells that may have been mutated or initiated, increasing the probability of tumor progression. Thus, the interplay of UV lethality and mutagenesis in human skin cells may determine the onset and progression of UV carcinogenesis.

Site-specific determination of photoproduct induction in the *lacI* gene of *E. coli* suggested a correlation between UV mutation hotspots and hotspots of (6-4) photoproduct induction.[6] Analysis of sites of (6-4) photoproduct induction suggested that this lesion was responsible for the major fraction of cytosine-to-thymine transition mutations in *E. coli.* Consistent with this observation, it was shown that the exclusive induction of cyclobutane dimers by acetophenone and UVB light did not increase the induction of transition mutations in lambda phage.[91] A similar relationship was observed in a study of photoreactivation in *E. coli;* whereas cyclobutane dimers and (6-4) photoproducts were similarly cytotoxic, the latter were much more mutagenic.[69]

Recently, it has become possible to evaluate the role of specific photoproducts in UV mutagenesis in human cells with the use of shuttle vectors. In these systems UV-irradiated simian virus (SV)40-based plasmids are transfected into human cells, where they are replicated by the host. The plasmids are subsequently recovered, amplified in bacteria, and analyzed for mutation induction by DNA sequencing. Sites of mutations can then be compared with sites of photoproduct induction in the target sequence. Results of these studies are similar to those obtained in *E. coli:* sites of transition mutations correlate with sites of increased (6-4) photoproduct induction (Table III-5-1). In particular, sites and frequencies of mutation hotspots in the *lacI* gene transfected into human cells were identical to those determined in *E. coli.*[44] In a shuttle vector system in which photoproduct induction and sites of mutation were examined in the *supF* gene, transfection into SV40-transformed human fibroblasts and monkey kidney cells indicated a similar correlation.[36] In the *supF* gene inserted into the mouse L cell chromosome[34] and in the endogenous *APRT* gene of CHO cells,[24] most of the mutations consisted of cytosine-to-thymine transitions occurring at thymine-cytosine and cytosine-cytosine sequences.

Since the spectrum of damage induced by UVB radiation is different from that induced by UVC light, differences in the mutagenic action of these wavelengths are likely. After UVB irradiation of human cells, the ratio of ouabain-resistant mutants to thioguanine-resistant mutants is 10-fold higher than after UVC irradiation, suggesting that a unique type of premutagenic lesion is induced by the longer wavelengths.[75] Mutations induced by UVB radiation have been analyzed at the sequence level in simian cells and show significant differences when compared with those induced by UVC light.[41] Although GC to AT transition mutations still predominate from UVB, there are variations in the location of mutation hotspots, which are associated with regions of multiple base changes. In addition, UVB light induces more deletions and insertions than UVC light.

The predominance of cytosine-to-thymine transition mutations in both prokaryotic and eukaryotic cells has been explained in terms of the "A rule." This rule states that polymerases predominantly insert adenine opposite a site that lacks base coding information.[71] In terms of this model, thymine-thymine cyclobutane dimers, the predominant photoproduct, would not usually be mutagenic since adenine is

Table III-5-1. UVC-Induced Mutations Observed in Shuttle Vector pZ189 Replicated in XP or Normal Human Cells[a]

Mutations	Number of plasmids with base changes[b]	
	XP	Normal
Independent plasmids sequenced[c]	61 (100%)	89 (100%)
Point mutations		
Single base substitution	47[d] (77%)	48 (53%)
Tandem base substitutions[e]	12 (20%)	16 (18%)
Multiple base substitutions[f]	1[d] (2%)	24 (28%)
Base insertions and deletions		
Single base insertion	0	2
Single or tandem base deletions	1	3
Types of single or tandem base substitutions and number of changes		
Transitions	67[d] (94%)	61 (75%)
GC to AT	66[d] (93%)	59 (73%)
AT to GC	1 (1%)	2 (2%)
Transversions	4[d] (6%)	20 (25%)
GC to TA	0[d]	8 (10%)
GC to CG	1 (1%)	5 (6%)
AT to TA	3 (4%)	6 (8%)
AT to CG	0	1 (1%)

[a]Modified from Bredberg et al.,[8] and previously published by Cleaver and Kraemer[22]

[b]50 to 300 J/m² from XP cells, 100–5,000 J/m² for normal cells

[c]From separate transfections or different mutations in the same transfection including all experiments

[d]$p < 0.01$ versus normal

[e]Two base substitutions 0 to 2 bases apart, or 3 adjacent base substitutions

[f]At least 2 base substitutions more than 3 bases apart

often correctly inserted opposite thymine. However, incorporation of adenine opposite a cytosine in a dipyrimidine photoproduct would result in a cytosine-to-thymine transition mutation. Hence, cyclobutane dimers and (6-4) photoproducts containing noninstructive cytosine base(s) are considered mutagenic whereas thymine-thymine dimers are not.

Cyclobutane dimers and (6-4) photoproducts can both form at sequences shown to be mutation hotspots in shuttle vectors, and the identity of the mutagenic lesion has been tested by photoreactivation of the *supF* sequence in plasmids before transfection.[7,60] Enzymatic photoreversal of cyclobutane dimers reduced the mutation frequency in normal cells by 75% and in XP group A cells by 90%. Since cotransfection of monkey cells with a mixture of unirradiated *supF* plasmid and irradiated plasmid without the *supF* gene did not generate mutations, the role of an SOS-like system, as observed in *E. coli,* did not appear to be responsible for the results.[60] These results are not consistent with the model developed in *E. coli* and suggest that (6-4) photoproducts may be less mutagenic in human cells. A similar analysis with photoreactivation suggested that cyclobutane dimers occurring at thymine-cytosine, cytosine-thymine, and cytosine-cytosine dipyrimidine sites were the predominant mutagenic lesions induced in human cells and that (6-4) photoproducts at these sites accounted for only about 10% of the mutations.[7] However, this same study indicated that the frequencies of both cyclobutane dimers and (6-4) photoproducts at individual dipyrimidine sites did not correlate with mutation frequency, suggesting that, although UV-induced lesions are required for mutagenesis, mutation hotspots are determined by other factors.

Genetic Regulation of Repair of DNA Damage

Selection of UV-sensitive hamster and mouse cells in culture and the study of human sunlight-sensitive disorders have identified a large series of genetic loci that control the response of mammalian skin to damage (Table III-5-2). These loci are all characterized by significant increases in sensitivity to UVC or UVB radiation and include the following groups: excision repair cross complementing (ERCC) series (approximately nine complementation groups);[10,11] XP (approximately 8 complementation groups);[22] Cockayne syndrome (CS) (approximately three complementation groups);[45] trichothiodystrophy (TTD) (approximately three distinct phenotypic types);[9] and basal cell nevus syndrome (BCNS).[3]

With the exception of BCNS, all of these disorders represent increased sensitivity to UVB and UVC wavelengths

Table III-5-2. Complementation Groups in XP and UV-Sensitive Chinese Hamster Ovary (CHO) Cells

Group	Human chromosome location	Central nervous system disorders	Relative repair (%)
Xeroderma pigmentosum			
A	9	Yes	2–5
B (Cockayne and ERCC3)[a]	2	Yes	3–7
C		No	5–20
D (Cockayne)[a,b]	19	Yes	25–50
E		No	50
F	15[c]	No	18
G		Yes	<2
Variant		No	100
CHO (ERCC)[d]			
1	19		Low
2	19		Intermediate
3	2		Intermediate
4	16		Low
5	13		Intermediate

[a]Patients also exhibit symptoms commonly associated with Cockayne syndrome: dwarfism, cutaneous features, and mental retardation. Group B and ERCC3 represent the same complementation group, as do Group D and ERCC2.

[b]Some patients also have symptoms of trichothiodystrophy.

[c]Although this chromosome is the only one to demonstrate complementation of XP group F, the degree of correction is not complete. See Cleaver[19] for further discussion of this point.

[d]Genes in the ERCC series are found in human and rodent cells, and were first identified through selection of UV-sensitive hamster cells. ERCC1 does not correspond to any XP group, but ERCC3 and XP group B are identical. There are 8 or more CHO complementation groups, but the higher numbered groups are rare and still being characterized. Relative repair in the ERCC series is classified approximately on the basis of relative sensitivity to DNA damage.

due to recessive mutations. BCNS, however, exhibits a unique sensitivity to UVB wavelengths and is a dominant disorder. The recessive disorders can be thought of as subsets within a large family of genes that regulate human cell DNA repair (Figure III-5-7). These subsets are not mutually exclusive, because CS overlaps with XP groups B and D, and TTD overlaps with group D. The XP group B corresponds to ERCC3 as well as to a CS group. Chromosome locations are known, and the genes have been cloned for several of these loci (Table III-5-2). Thus, mutations in individual genes have pleiotropic effects on cellular sensitivity to UV light and DNA repair and are associated with a range of clinical syndromes involving skin, nervous system, and immunological changes.

ERCC Gene Family

These genes were identified by selection of UV-sensitive rodent cells in culture (Table III-5-2).[10,11,72] ERCC1 and ERCC2 have been cloned and exhibit DNA sequence similarity to bacterial and yeast genes. ERCC1 encodes a protein of 297 amino acids and shows sequence similarity to *UVR A* and *C* of *E. coli* and *rad10* of yeast.[79–81] ERCC2 encodes a protein of 760 amino acids and is similar to *rad3*, which is an essential gene, and exhibits properties of an ATP-dependent DNA helicase.[87,88] ERCC1 is located on human chromosome 19 but does not appear to be represented among human sunlight-sensitive disorders. ERCC3, on the other hand, corresponds to XP group B, a patient who also exhibited clinical symptoms of CS. This gene may code for a DNA helicase, and the complex phenotype appears due to homozygosity at a single locus from parents who were recessive for different mutations.[89]

All of the ERCC genes appear to regulate the excision of

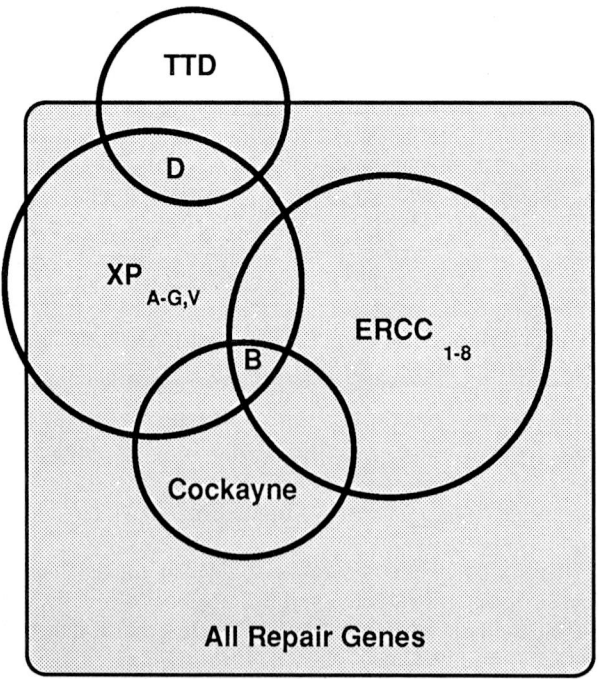

Figure III-5-7. Representation of the total set of mammalian repair genes, with XP, Cockayne syndrome, the ERCC series, and trichothiodystrophy (TTD) as subsets within the field.

DNA photoproducts, and *ERCC1* and *ERCC2* appear to correspond to important enzymatic functions of photoproduct recognition and removal.

Xeroderma Pigmentosum

XP is a rare autosomal recessive disease that occurs at a frequency of about 1:250,000 in the United States.[22] Affected patients (homozygotes) have sun sensitivity resulting in progressive degenerative changes of sun-exposed portions of the skin and eyes, often leading to neoplasia. Some XP patients have, in addition, progressive neurologic degeneration. Obligate heterozygotes (parents) are generally asymptomatic. The median age of onset is 1–2 years of age, with skin rapidly taking on the appearance of that seen in individuals with many years of sun exposure. Pigmentation is patchy, and skin shows atrophy and telangiectasia with development of basal and squamous cell carcinomas. The frequency of cancers is 2,000 times that seen in the general population under 20 years of age, with an approximate 30-year reduction in life span.

Cells from patients with XP excise pyrimidine dimers and (6-4) photoproducts at reduced rates of 0–90% of normal, except for the variant group, which has near-normal rates (Table III-5-3). Reduced excision is correlated with low levels of repair replication. The reductions are similar in all tissues thus far investigated, including skin in vivo, peripheral lymphocytes, fibroblasts, liver cell cultures, and tumor cells. Genetic heterogeneity in XP patients whose cells are defective in excision repair is suggested by the differing residual activities of dimer excision and repair replication and by the differing clinical patterns.[22] Somatic cell hybridization studies have demonstrated complementation in multinucleated cells with nuclei from each XP patient (heterokaryons). Heterokaryons from some combinations of XP patients exhibit complementation and increased repair, whereas other combinations remain repair deficient. Complementation is an indication that the cell types contain defects in different genes and that each supplies what the other is lacking. At least 7 complementation groups are known among patients who are deficient in excision repair, and an eighth, the XP variant, has a defect in replication of damaged DNA (Table III-5-2).

The existence of 8 complementation groups (group I was recently withdrawn and group H is under some dispute as a separate complementation group[19]) in XP probably indicates that the initial step of excision involves cooperative action between multiple proteins that bind to damaged sites and to each other, to unwind and modify the site before endonuclease cleavage, and are then displaced by helicase and polymerases.[19] These products therefore have a variety of DNA- and protein-binding activity with varied specificity. Considerable genetic diversity exists within these disorders, and the capacity for excision repair correlates in many cases with the ability to survive UV irradiation. Compared with normal cells, cells from XP groups A and D are very sensitive to the lethal effects of UV light and are unable to excise the two major types of UV damage, the cyclobutane dimer and the (6-4) photoproduct (Table III-5-3). XP group A cells also have a reduced capacity to repair the Dewar pyrimidinone, an important lesion induced with increased efficiency by UVB light.[50,53] Consistent with this pattern, XP group E cells display an intermediate phenotype, both in their UV sensitivity and their capacity to excise UV damage, and lack a damage-specific binding protein.[13,58]

Group C is one of the largest groups and is often referred to as the common or classic form of XP. The patients show only skin disorders, which vary considerably in severity, depending on the climate. Tumors of the tongue have been observed in several patients. Cells have low but heterogeneous levels of excision repair (10–20% of normal) and are less sensitive to killing by UV light and chemical carcinogens than cells in groups A and D. One characteristic of repair unique to group C is that in nonproliferating cells the reduced repair is not widespread in their genome, as in groups A, D, and others, but is confined to certain genomic regions.[17,39] These cells insert repair patches into small regions of their genome at normal rates, probably corresponding to (6-4) and cyclobutane dimer repair,[17,39] and excise thymine dimers preferentially from transcriptionally active regions.[84] This raises the dilemma that high rates of cell killing, somatic mutation, and cancer from UV light in XP group C are associated with repair deficiencies in the nontranscribed regions of the genome. This in turn suggests that activating rather than silencing mutations may be important, or that mutations arise from unrepaired lesions in the nontranscribed strand of active genes.

Group E is a rare group that exhibits mild symptoms and residual levels of repair that are as much as 50% of normal. Some of these cells lack an inducible DNA-binding protein

Table III-5-3.   DNA Repair Characteristics of Human Cells

Phenotype	Typical cell lines	(6-4) Photoproducts repaired at 6 h (% of normal)	Incision (% of normal)	Repair synthesis (% of normal)	Cyclobutane dimer repair (% of normal)	UV resistance (% of normal)
Normal	AG1518A	100	100	100	100	100
Normal	HeLa	100	100	100	100	100
XP-A	XP12RO, XP12BE	<10	<10	<5	<5	<15
XP-A revertant	XP129	80	>80	50–90	<5	100
XP-C	XPIBE	~25	~30	<15	<10	40
XP-D	XP6BE, XP102LO	<10	15–40	25	<20	10
XP-E	XP2RO	~75		40–60	~40	70
XP variant	XP4BE, XP13BE	100	>100	70	>90	65
XP-D-like	TTD1GL	100	100	100	100	100
XP-D-like	TTD1BI	75	~50	~50	100	100
XP-D-like	TTD2GL	<25	10–40	10–40	<20	10

that has many similarities to yeast photolyase, but its binding capacity is specific for (6-4) photoproducts and does not involve any functional photolyase activity.[13,58] The role of this binding protein may therefore be to increase the signal provided by DNA damage to other binding proteins and endonucleases.

The mechanism of UV cytotoxicity in XP variant cells does not seem to be associated with an obvious excision repair defect. These cells appear near normal in their ability to excise DNA damage (Table III-5-3), yet show a slight but significant sensitivity to UV light. Critical regions in DNA during the S phase, such as replication forks, may be under-repaired or abnormally replicated, resulting in reduced UV resistance. It is enigmatic that the genetic defect responsible for the slight reduction in UV resistance in XP variant cells is still capable of producing elevated levels of mutation and the severe clinical symptoms displayed by XP patients.[22]

Cockayne Syndrome

CS is an autosomal recessive disease characterized by cachectic dwarfism, retinal abnormalities, microcephaly, deafness, neural defects, and retardation of growth and development after birth. Carcinomas of the skin as a result of hyperphotosensitivity are not seen in patients with CS, setting this disease apart from XP.

CS patients are distributed unevenly within the complementation groups.[45] Of a total of 11 patients, two are assigned to group A, eight to group B, and one to group C. The one patient in group C is the patient classified as the sole representative of XP group B. An additional complementation group may be represented by the patient once assigned as the sole representative of XP group H,[25] but there is uncertainty about this assignment.[37,61] The UV sensitivity of most CS cells lies in a narrow range, with a D_{37} about half of normal, unlike XP cells, which exhibit a wide range of sensitivity.

Characteristic cellular changes in CS include a failure of DNA and RNA synthesis to recover to normal levels after UV irradiation.[16,47] The excision of DNA photoproducts from total genomic DNA of CS cells is normal, but repair of transcriptionally active genes may be reduced.[83]

Cockayne syndrome and XP group C therefore make an interesting contrast. CS cells repair only transcriptionally inactive genes, whereas XP group C cells repair only transcriptionally active genes. They show a similar increased sensitivity to cell killing, indicating that all regions of the genome must be repaired for normal survival. But only XP group C shows elevated mutagenesis and carcinogenesis, indicating that defective repair of transcriptionally inactive genes is more important for these endpoints.

Trichothiodystrophy

TTD is a rare autosomal recessive disorder characterized by sulfur-deficient brittle hair and ichthyosis. Hair shafts split longitudinally into small fibers, and this brittleness is associated with levels of cysteine/cystine in hair proteins that are 15–50% of those in normal individuals. The condition is also accompanied by physical and mental retardation of varying severity. The patients often have an unusual facial appearance, with protruding ears and a receding chin. Mental abil-

ities range from low normal to severe retardation.[46] Three categories of the disease can be recognized on the basis of cellular responses to UV damage: the most severe has repair deficiencies and complementation properties that place them in XP group D; intermediate cases show reduced DNA repair but normal UV sensitivity; and the third is indistinguishable in UV response from normal cells.[9]

Repair profiles of three fibroblast lines derived from patients with TTD have been characterized; each displays a unique phenotype.[9] One TTD cell line shows normal UV resistance and DNA repair properties; another shows an XP group D response to UV irradiation, with greatly reduced survival and repair; cells derived from a third patient show normal survival after UV irradiation, but the repair capacity, as evidenced by repair synthesis and repair incision, is significantly reduced. Although the excision rate of the (6-4) photoproduct in this third TTD class is slightly reduced, cyclobutane dimer repair appears normal, suggesting either that the (6-4) photoproduct is not lethal in these cells or that the observed defect in its repair is not sufficient to affect survival.

Basal Cell Nevus Syndrome

BCNS is an autosomal dominant disorder with high penetrance (>97%). The principal manifestations of this syndrome are multiple tumors (average, 50–100), primarily on sun-exposed skin, that usually appear at puberty, and during the second and third decade of life.[35] Other symptoms include palmar and plantar pitting and musculoskeletal abnormalities (i.e., scoliosis, bifurcated rib, spina bifida). The high incidence of developmental anomalies suggests that the normal allele of the BCNS gene may play a role in growth and development in addition to the acceleration of sunlight-induced carcinogenesis.

Development of other tumors in BCNS, including medulloblastoma and ovarian and uterine fibromas, suggests that BCNS fits Knudson's two-mutation model for carcinogenesis.[3,35] However, the number of such mutations required to induce cancers in individuals with BCNS is unknown and could be higher than two. Nevertheless, in BCNS, one of the mutations is inherited as an autosomal dominant gene in all somatic cells, whereas the remaining mutation(s) can be induced by UV or ionizing radiation. This hypothesis is supported by the observation that presymptomatic children with BCNS who were treated with radiation for medulloblastoma developed multiple basal cell carcinomas in the area that received radiation six months to three years later.

Fibroblasts from individuals with BCNS have not shown consistent increases in sensitivity to X rays or UVC (254 nm) radiation. They do, however, show characteristic sensitivity to UVB, with about a 5-fold reduction in the 50% survival dose.[3] Although cyclobutane dimer repair is normal in these cells, excision of (6-4) photoproducts may be reduced, resembling that shown for TTD group 3 patients.[61a] The reduced repair of the (6-4) photoproduct may not be sufficient to affect survival after UVC irradiation. The increased sensitivity of these cells to UVB light may thus reflect an inability to excise photodamage induced with greater frequency by these wavelengths (e.g., Dewar pyrimidinones).

The dominant genetics and lack of any sensitivity to UVC radiation make it unlikely that this disorder represents a primary deficiency in repair of the major UV photoproducts. Rather, there seems to be a specific change in some factors involved in gene expression subsequent to primary damage and repair events. In an analogy with retinoblastoma, BCNS may involve cell cycle factors and chromosome stability during progression. Alternatively, the specificity for UVB sensitivity may indicate a deficit in some products associated with melanin production or protection from UVB.[49]

Reversion of XP and Hamster Repair Deficiencies

UV cytotoxicity in human and other mammalian cells is evidently influenced by extremely complex mechanisms. In some cells, loss of a repair function correlates well with cell survival; in other systems there appears to be little correlation between DNA repair, cell survival, and an array of clinical symptoms. Reversion of UV-hypersensitive cells to normal resistance is a useful tool in understanding the fine structure of UV cytotoxicity and may shed some light on this complex problem. The repair phenotypes of two XP group A revertants have been characterized and suggest that of the two major types of photodamage, the (6-4) photoproduct may be intrinsically more lethal than the cyclobutane dimer (Table III-5-3).[18,20] These cell lines are as resistant to the killing effects of UV light as normal human cells, yet are incapable of removing cyclobutane dimers from bulk genomic DNA and from actively transcribing sequences.[21] Since (6-4) photoproduct excision is near normal in these cells, it is presumed that these lesions must play a primary role in cell killing. Support for this idea has recently been obtained from another mammalian revertant cell line isolated from a Chinese hamster UV-sensitive mutant.[52] This hamster revertant has recovered much of the normal capacity to survive UV light, yet cannot repair cyclobutane dimers in a transcribing gene. Oddly, the mutation rate at the transcribing locus where cyclobutane dimer repair was measured has recovered to normal levels. Since the kinetics of (6-4) photoproduct repair are normal in this revertant, this photoproduct may ultimately be an important premutagenic lesion in mammalian cells.

Carcinogenesis

Carcinogenesis often appears to proceed by a multi-step process, the first being an initiation event with subsequent promotional events that can often occur much later. One view of carcinogenesis would correlate initiation with the induction of somatic mutations, and promotion with alterations in the expression of these mutations.

Carcinogenesis appears to involve the activity of a large number of genes. These include genes for detoxifying carcinogenic chemicals, the DNA repair gene family, some 50 or more dominantly acting proto-oncogenes activated by mutation, deletion, translocation, or amplification, and tumor suppressor genes whose loss may contribute to the development of cancer.[62,66,86]

The sequence of events seen in colorectal cancer and retinoblastoma may provide a useful model for skin carcinogenesis.[66,86] Early events may correspond to activating mutations, and various stages of tumor development occur as a result of progressive chromosome loss or conversion of heterozygosity to homozygosity. On the basis of studies with XP, early events in the skin may correspond to UV-induced mutations. Not only are major genetic defects in repair related to cancer in XP, but variations in repair among individuals also show a correlation with basal cell carcinoma.[1] Here, however, recent studies on ras activation lead to a dilemma. Several investigations have led to identification of activating mutations in the Ha-ras and N-ras oncogenes at codon 61, from solar UV exposure.[2,40,68] However, although over 75% of UV-induced mutations are C to T transitions at TC or CC dimer photoproduct sites,[8] Ha-ras and N-ras activation occurred in tumors at a TT site and are transversions not previously identified in model culture systems.[8] Clearly, detailed investigation of oncogene activation in a number of mouse and human systems is needed to clarify the relationship between UV-induced mutations and ras activation.

Inactivation of tumor suppressor genes has been demonstrated in retinoblastoma,[31] Wilms' tumor,[12] and acoustic neuromas, and allelic loss resulting in conversion from heterozygosity to homozygosity appears to be a common consequence of tumor progression.[86] Interestingly, chromosome 6 appears to carry a melanoma suppressor gene.[73] The high levels of skin cancer in XP patients may result from increased levels of UV damage caused by defective repair, which lead to activating mutations and chromosome instability. Tumor suppressor genes could contribute to tumor advancement by incremental effects on cell growth and intercellular regulation. The observation that promotion involves alterations in cell–cell communication is consistent with this interpretation. Tumor promoters may be environmental factors that mimic the effect of regulatory genes. Analysis of the various stages of skin tumor development would seem to be especially promising at this time since so many stages are accessible and the environmental causative factors are so well known.

Note

Recent studies[92] have demonstrated that a large proportion of human skin tumors contain mutations in the p53 tumor suppressor gene that are caused by UV photoproducts. This demonstrates a direct causal role for UVB from sunlight in causing one of the mutagenic events in skin carcinogenesis.

References

1. Alcalay, J., Freeman, S. E., Goldberg, L. H., and Wolf, J. E., Jr.: Excision repair of pyrimidine dimers induced by simulated solar radiation in the skin of patients with basal cell carcinoma. J. Invest. Dermatol., in press.
2. Ananthaswamy, H. N., Price, J. E., Goldberg, L. H., and Bales, E. S.: Detection and identification of activated oncogenes in human skin cancers occurring on sun-exposed body sites. Cancer Res., 48:3341, 1988.
3. Applegate, L. A., Goldberg, L. H., Ley, R. D., and Ananthaswamy, H. N.: Hypersensitivity of skin fibroblasts from basal cell nevus syndrome patients to killing by ultraviolet B but not by ultraviolet C radiation. Cancer Res., 50:637, 1990.
4. Armstrong, B. K.: Epidemiology of malignant melanoma: Intermittent or total accumulated exposure to the sun? J. Dermatol. Surg. Oncol., 14:835, 1988.
5. Bose, S. N., Kumar, S., Davies, R. J. H., Sethi, S. K., and McCloskey, J. A.: The photochemistry of d(T-A) in aqueous solution and in ice. Nucl. Acids Res., 12:7929, 1984.
6. Brash, D. E., and Haseltine, W. A.: UV-induced hotspots occur at DNA damage hotspots. Nature, 298:189, 1982.
7. Brash, D. E., Seetharam, S., Kraemer, K. H., Seidman, M. M., and Bredberg, A.: Photoproduct frequency is not the major determinant of UV base substitution hot spots or cold spots in human cells. Proc. Natl. Acad. Sci. USA, 84:3782 1987.
8. Bredberg, A., Kraemer, K. H., and Seidman, M. M.: Restricted ultraviolet mutational spectrum in a shuttle vector propagated in xeroderma pigmentosum cells. Proc. Natl. Acad. Sci. USA, 83:8273, 1986.
9. Broughton, B. C., Lehmann, A. R., Harcourt, S. A., Arlett, C. F., Sarasin, A., Kleijer, W.

J., Beemer, F. A., Nairn, R., and Mitchell, D. L.: Relationship between pyrimidine dimers, 6-4 photoproducts, repair synthesis and cell survival: Studies using cells from patients with trichothiodystrophy. Mutat. Res., 235:33, 1990.

10. Busch, D. B., Cleaver, J. E., and Glaser, D. A.: Large-scale isolation of UV-sensitive clones of CHO cells. Somat. Cell Genet., 6:407, 1980.

11. Busch, D., Greiner, C., Lewis, K., Ford, R., Adair, G., and Thompson, L.: Summary of complemention groups of UV-sensitive CHO cell mutants isolated by large-scale screening. Mutagenesis, 4:349, 1989.

12. Call, K. M., Glaser, T., Ito, C. Y., Buckler, A. J., Pelletier, J., Haber, D. A., Rose, E. A., Kral, A., Yeger, H., Lewis, W. H., Jones, C., and Housman, D. E.: Isolation and characterization of a zinc finger polypeptide gene at the human chromosome 11 Wilms' tumor locus. Cell, 60:509, 1990.

13. Chu, G., and Chang, E.: Xeroderma pigmentosum group E cells lack a nuclear factor that binds to damaged DNA. Science, 242:564, 1988.

14. Cleaver, J. E.: Defective repair replication of DNA in xeroderma pigmentosum. Nature, 218:652, 1968.

15. Cleaver, J. E.: Xeroderma pigmentosum: A human disease in which an initial stage of DNA repair is defective. Proc. Natl. Acad. Sci. USA, 63:428, 1969.

16. Cleaver, J. E.: Normal reconstruction of DNA supercoiling and chromatin structure in Cockayne syndrome cells during repair of damage from ultraviolet light. Am. J. Hum. Genet., 34:566, 1982.

17. Cleaver, J. E.: DNA repair in human xeroderma pigmentosum group C cells involves a different distribution of damaged sites in confluent and growing cells. Nucleic Acids Res., 14:8155, 1986.

18. Cleaver, J. E.: DNA damage and repair in normal, xeroderma pigmentosum and XP revertant cells analyzed by gel electrophoresis: Excision of cyclobutane dimers from the whole genome is not necessary for cell survival. Carcinogenesis, 10:1691, 1989.

19. Cleaver, J. E.: Do we know the cause of xeroderma pigmentosum? Carcinogenesis, 11:875, 1990.

20. Cleaver, J. E., Cortes, F., Lutze, L. H., Morgan, W. F., Player, A. N., and Mitchell, D. L.: Unique DNA repair properties of xeroderma pigmentosum revertant. Mol. Cell. Biol., 7:3353, 1987.

21. Cleaver, J. E., Jen, J., Charles, W. C., and Mitchell, D. L.: Cyclobutane dimers and (6-4) photoproducts are mended in human cells with the same patch sizes. Photochem. Photobiol., 54:393, 1991.

22. Cleaver, J. E., and Kraemer, K. H.: Xeroderma pigmentosum. In The Metabolic Basis of Inherited Disease, 6th ed. Vol. II. Edited by C. R. Scriver, A. L. Beaudet, W. S. Sly, and D. Valle. New York, McGraw-Hill, 1989, pp. 2949-2971.

23. Demple, B., and Linn, S.: 5,6-Saturated thymine lesions in DNA: Production by ultraviolet light or hydrogen peroxide. Nucl. Acids Res., 10:3781, 1982.

24. Drobetsky, E. A., Grosovsky, A. J., and Glickman, B. W.: The specificity of UV-induced mutations at an endogenous locus in mammalian cells. Proc. Natl. Acad. Sci. USA, 84:9103, 1987.

25. Dupuy, J.-M., Moshell, A. N., Lutzner, M. A., and Robbins, J. H.: A new patient with both xeroderma pigmentosum and Cockayne syndrome is not in complementation group B. (Abstract) J. Invest. Dermatol., 78:356, 1982.

26. Elkind, M. M., Han, A., and Chiang-Liu, C.-M.: "Sunlight"-induced mammalian cell killing: A comparative study of ultraviolet and near-ultraviolet inactivation. Photochem. Photobiol., 27:709, 1978.

27. Ellison, M. J., and Childs, J. D.: Pyrimidine dimers induced in Escherichia coli DNA by ultraviolet radiation present in sunlight. Photochem. Photobiol., 34:465, 1981.

28. Epstein, J. H., Fukuyama, K., Reed, W. B., and Epstein, W. L.: Defect in DNA synthesis in skin of patients with xeroderma pigmentosum demonstrated in vivo. Science, 168:1477, 1970.

29. Fitzpatrick, T. B., and Sober, A. J.: Sunlight and skin cancer. N. Engl. J. Med., 313:818, 1985.

30. Freeman, S. E.: Variations in excision repair of UVB-induced pyrimidine dimers in DNA of human skin in situ. J. Invest. Dermatol., 90:814, 1988.

31. Friend, S. H., Horowitz, J. M., Gerber, M. R., Wang, X.-F., Bogenmann, E., Li, F. P., and Weinberg, R. A.: Deletions of a DNA sequence in retinoblastomas and mesenchymal tumors: Organization of the sequence and its encoded protein. Proc. Natl. Acad. Sci. USA, 84:9059, 1987. Published erratum appears in Proc. Natl. Acad. Sci. USA, 85:2234, 1988.

32. Gallagher, P. E., and Duker, N. J.: Detection of UV purine photoproducts in a defined sequence of human DNA. Mol. Cell. Biol., 6:707, 1986.

33. Gasparro, F. P., and Fresco, J. R.: Ultraviolet-induced 8,8-adenine dehydrodimers in oligo-and polynucleotides. Nucl. Acids Res., 14:4239, 1986.

34. Glazer, P. M., Sarkar, S. N., and Summers, W. C.: Detection and analysis of UV-induced mutations in mammalian cell DNA using a lambda phage shuttle vector. Proc. Natl. Acad. Sci. USA, 83:1041, 1986.

35. Gorlin, R. J., and Goltz, R. W.: Multiple nevoid basal-cell epithelioma, jaw cysts and bifid rib: A syndrome. N. Engl. J. Med., 262:908, 1960.

36. Hauser, J., Seidman, M. M., Sidur, K., and Dixon, K.: Sequence specificity of point mutations induced during passage of a UV-irradiated shuttle vector plasmid in monkey cells. Mol. Cell. Biol., 6:277, 1986.

37. Johnson, R. T.: Reply to letter by J. H. Robbins, Hum. Genet., 84:101, 1989.

38. Jones, C. A., Huberman, E., Cunningham, M. L., and Peak, M. J.: Mutagenesis and cytotoxicity in human epithelial cells by far-and near-ultraviolet radiations: Action spectra. Radiat. Res., 110:244, 1987.

39. Karentz, D., and Cleaver, J. E.: Excision repair in xeroderma pigmentosum group C but not group D is clustered in a small fraction of the total genome. Mutat. Res., 165:165, 1986.

40. Keijzer, W., Mulder, M. P., Langeveld, J. C., Smit, E. M., Bos, J. L., Bootsma, D., and Hoeijmakers, J. H.: Establishment and characterization of a melanoma cell line from a xeroderma pigmentosum patient: Activation of N-ras at a potential pyrimidine dimer site. Cancer Res., 49:1229, 1989.

41. Keyse, S. M., Amaudruz, F., and Tyrrell, R. M.: Determination of the spectrum of mutations induced by defined-wavelength solar UVB (313-nm) radiation in mammalian cells by use of a shuttle vector. Mol. Cell. Biol., 8:5425, 1988.

42. Kraemer, K. H., Lee, M. M., and Scotto, J.: Xeroderma pigmentosum. Cutaneous, ocular, and neurological abnormalities in 830 published cases. Arch. Dermatol., 123:241, 1987.

43. Kripke, M. L.: Immunological unresponsiveness induced by ultraviolet radiation. Immunol. Rev., 80:87, 1984.

44. Lebkowski, J. S., Clancy, S., Miller, J. H., and Calos, M. P.: The lac1 shuttle: Rapid analysis of the mutagenic specificity of ultraviolet light in human cells. Proc. Natl. Acad. Sci. USA, 82:8606, 1985.

45. Lehmann, A. R.: Three complementation groups in Cockayne syndrome. Mutat. Res., 106:347, 1982.

46. Lehmann, A. R., Arlett, C. F., Broughton, B. C., Harcourt, S. A., Steingrimsdottir, H., Stefanini, M., Taylor, A. M. R., Natarajan, A. T., Green, S., King, M. D., Mackie, R. M., Stephenson, J. B. P., and Tolmie, J. L.: Trichothiodystrophy, a human DNA repair disorder with heterogeneity in the cellular response to ultraviolet light. Cancer Res., 48:6090, 1988.

47. Lehmann, A. R., Kirk-Bell, S., and Mayne, L.: Abnormal kinetics of DNA synthesis in ultraviolet light-irradiated cells from patients with Cockayne's syndrome. Cancer Res., 39:4237, 1979.

48. Mellon, I., Bohr, V. A., Smith, C. A., and Hanawalt, P. C.: Preferential DNA repair of an active gene in human cells. Proc. Natl. Acad. Sci. USA, 83:8878, 1986.

49. Mentor, J. M., Willis, I., Tounsel, M. E., Williamson, G. D., and Moore, C L.: Melanin is a double-edged sword. In Photobiology, The Science and Its Applications. Edited by E. Riklis. Plenum Press, in press.

50. Mitchell, D. L.: The induction and repair of lesions produced by the photolysis of (6-4) photoproducts in normal and UV-hypersensitive human cells. Mutat. Res., 194:227, 1988.

51. Mitchell, D. L., and Cleaver, J. E.: Photochemical alterations of cytosine account for most biological effects after ultraviolet irradiation. In Trends in Photochemistry and Photobiology. Research Trends, Council of Scientific Research Integration, Sreekanteswaram, Trivandrum, India, pp. 107–119, 1990.

52. Mitchell, D. L., Cleaver, J. E., Jen, J., Mullenders, L. H., Venema, J., van Hoffen, A., Simons, J. W. I. M., and Zdzienicka, M.: The relative biological effectiveness of pyrimidine (6-4)pyrimidone photoproducts in mammalian cells. (Abstract) 18th Annual Meeting of the American Society for Photobiology, Vancouver, British Columbia, June 16–20, 1990.

53. Mitchell, D. L., and Nairn, R. S.: The (6-4) photoproduct and human skin cancer. Photo-Dermatology, 5:61, 1988.

54. Mitchell, D. L., and Nairn, R. S.: The biology of the (6-4) photoproduct. Photochem. Photobiol., 49:805, 1989.

55. Mitchell, D. L., Nguyen, T. D., and Cleaver, J. E.: Nonrandom induction of pyrimidine-pyrimidone (6-4) photoproducts in ultraviolet-irradiated human chromatin. J. Biol. Chem., 265:5353, 1990.

56. Mitchell, D. L., Cleaver, J. E., and Epstein, J. H.: Repair of pyrimidine(6-4)-pyrimidone photoproducts in mouse skin. J. Invest. Dermatol., 95:55, 1990.

57. Niggli, H. J., and Cerutti, P. A.: Cyclobutane-type pyrimidine photodimer formation and excision in human skin fibroblasts after irradiation with 313-nm ultraviolet light. Biochemistry, 22:1390, 1983.

58. Patterson, M., and Chu, G.: Evidence that xeroderma pigmentosum cells from complementation group E are deficient in a homolog of yeast photolyase. Mol. Cell. Biol., 9:5105, 1989.

59. Peak, M. J., and Peak, J. G.: Single-strand breaks induced in Bacillus subtilis DNA by ultraviolet light: Action spectrum and properties. Photochem. Photobiol., 35:675, 1982.

60. Protic-Sabljic, M., Tuteja, N., Munson, P. J., Hauser, J., Kraemer, K. H., and Dixon, K.: UV light-induced cyclobutane pyrimidine dimers are mutagenic in mammalian cells. Mol. Cell. Biol., 6:3349, 1986.

61. Robbins, J. H.: No lack of complementation for unscheduled DNA synthesis between xeroderma pigmentosum complementation groups D and H. (Letter) Hum. Genet., 84:99, 1989.

61a. Rosenstein, B., and Mitchell, D. L.: Unpublished observation.

62. Sager, R.: Tumor suppressor genes: The puzzle and the promise. Science, 246:1406, 1989.

63. Scotto, J., Fears, T. R., and Fraumeni, J. F.: Incidence of nonmelanoma skin cancer in the United States. U.S. Department of Health and Human Services, NIH Publication No. 83-2433, 1983.

64. Scotto, J., and Fraumeni, J. F., Jr.: Skin (other than melanoma). In Cancer Epidemiology and Prevention. Edited by D. Schottenfeld and J. R. Fraumeni, Jr. Philadelphia, W. B. Saunders, 1982, pp. 996-1011.

65. Smith, P. J., and Paterson, M. C.: Abnormal responses to mid-ultraviolet light of cultured fibroblasts from patients with disorders featuring sunlight sensitivity. Cancer Res., 41:511, 1981.

66. Stanbridge, E. J.: Identifying tumor suppressor genes in human colorectal cancer. Science, 247:12, 1990.

67. Sterenborg, H. J. C. M., and van der Leun, J. C.: Tumorigenesis by a long wavelength UV-A source. Photochem. Photobiol., 51:325, 1990.

68. Suarez, H. G., Daya-Grosjean, L., Schlaifer, D., Nardeux, P., Renault, G., Bos, J. L., and Sarasin, A.: Activated oncogenes in human skin tumors from a repair-deficient syndrome, xeroderma pigmentosum. Cancer Res., 49:1223, 1989.

69. Tang, M.-S., Hrncir, J., Mitchell, D., Ross, J., and Clarkson, J.: The relative cytotoxicity and mutagenicity of cyclobutane pyrimidine dimers and (6-4) photoproducts in Escherichia coli cells. Mutat. Res., 161:9, 1986.

70. Taylor, J. -S., and Cohrs, M. P.: DNA, light, and Dewar pyrimidinones: The structure and biological significance of TpT3. J. Am. Chem. Soc., 109:2834, 1987.

71. Tessman, I.: In Abstracts of the Bacteriophage Meeting. Edited by A. Bukhari, and E. Ljungquist. Cold Spring Harbor Laboratory, Cold Spring Harbor, New York, 1976, p. 87.

72. Thompson, L. H., Rubin, J. S., Cleaver, J. E., Whitmore, G. F., and Brookman, K.: A screening method for isolating DNA repair-deficient mutants of CHO cells. Somat. Cell Genet., 6:391, 1980.

73. Trent, J. M., Stanbridge, E. J., McBride, H. L., Meese, E. U., Casey, G., Araujo, D. E., Witkowski, C. M., and Nagle, R. B.: Tumorigenicity in human melanoma cell lines controlled by introduction of human chromosome 6. Science, 247:568, 1990.

74. Trosko, J. E., Krause, D., and Isoun, M.: Sunlight-induced pyrimidine dimers in human cells in vitro. Nature, 228:358, 1970.

75. Tyrrell, R. M.: Mutagenic action of monochromatic UV radiation in the solar range on human cells. Mutat. Res., 129:103, 1984.

76. Tyrrell, R. M., and Keyse, S. M.: New trends in photobiology: The interaction of UVA radiation with cultured cells. J. Photochem. Photobiol., B, 4:349, 1990.

77. Tyrrell, R. M., and Pidoux, M.: Endogenous glutathione protects human skin fibroblasts

against the cytotoxic action of UVB, UVA and near-visible radiations. Photochem. Photobiol., 44:561, 1986.

78. Tyrrell, R. M., and Pidoux, M.: Action spectra for human skin cells: Estimates of the relative cytotoxicity of the middle ultraviolet, near ultraviolet, and violet regions of sunlight on epidermal keratinocytes. Cancer Res., 47:1825, 1987.

79. Van Duin, M., de Wit, J., Odijk, H., Westerveld, A., Yasui, A., Koken, M. H. M., Hoeijmakers, J. H. J., and Bootsma, D.: Molecular characterization of the human excision repair gene ERCC-1: cDNA cloning and amino acid homology with the yeast DNA repair gene RAD10. Cell, 44:913, 1986.

80. Van Duin, M., Koken, M. H. M., van den Tol., J., ten Dijke, P., Odijk, H., Westerveld, A., Bootsma, D., and Hoeijmakers, J. H. J.: Genomic characterization of the human DNA excision repair gene ERCC-1. Nucleic Acids Res., 15:9195, 1987.

81. Van Diun, M., van den Tol, J., Warmerdam, P., Odijk, H., Meijer, D., Westerveld, A., Bootsma, D., and Hoeijmakers, J. H. J.: Evolution and mutagenesis of the mammalian excision repair gene ERCC-1. Nucleic Acids Res., 16:5305, 1988.

82. Van Houten, B.: Nucleotide excision repair in Escherichia coli. Microbiol. Rev., 54:18, 1990.

83. Venema, J., Mullenders, L. H. F., Natarajan, A. T., van Zeeland, A. A., and Mayne, L. V.: The genetic defect in Cockayne syndrome is associated with a defect in repair of UV-induced DNA damage in transcriptionally active DNA. Proc. Natl. Acad. Sci. USA, 87:4707, 1990.

84. Venema, J., Van Hoffen, A., Natarajan, A. T., van Zeeland, A. A., and Mullenders, L. H.: The residual repair capacity of xeroderma pigmentosum complementation group

C fibroblasts is highly specific for transcriptionally active DNA. Nucl. Acids Res., 18:443, 1990.

85. Vitaliano, P. P., and Urbach, F.: The relative importance of risk factors in nonmelanoma carcinoma. Arch. Dermatol., 116:454, 1980.

86. Vogelstein, B., Fearon, E. R., Kern, S. E., Hamilton, S. R., Preisinger, A. C., Nakamura, Y., and White, R.: Allelotype of colorectal carcinomas. Science, 244:207, 1989.

87. Weber, C. A., Salazar, E. P., Stewart, S. A., and Thompson, L. H.: Molecular cloning and biological characterization of a human gene, ERCC2, that corrects the nucleotide excision repair defect in CHO UV5 cells. Mol. Cell. Biol., 8:1137, 1988.

88. Weber, C. A., Salazar, E. P., Stewart, S. A., and Thompson, L. H.: ERCC2: cDNA cloning and molecular characterization of a human nucleotide excision repair gene with high homology to yeast RAD3. EMBO J., 9:1437, 1990.

89. Weeda, G., Reinier, C. A., van Ham, H., Vermeulen, W., Bootsma, D., van der Eb, A. J., and Hoeijmakers, J. H. J.: A presumed DNA helicase encoded by the excision repair gene ERCC-3 is involved in the human repair disorders xeroderma pigmentosum and Cockayne syndrome. Cell, in press.

90. Weiss, R. B., Gallagher, P. E., Brent, T. P., and Duker, N. J.: Cytosine photoproduct-DNA glycosylase in Escherichia coli and cultured human cells. Biochemistry, 28:1488, 1989.

91. Wood, R. D., Skopek, T. R., and Hutchinson, F.: Changes in DNA base sequence induced by targeted mutagenesis of lambda phage by ultraviolet light. J. Mol. Biol., 173:273, 1984.

92. Brash, D. E., Rudolph, J. A., Simon, J. A., Lin, A., McKenna, G. J., Baden, H. P., Halperin, A. J., and Ponten, J.: A role for sunlight in skin cancer: UV-induced p53 mutations in squamous cell carcinoma. Proc. Natl. Acad. Sci. USA, 88:10124, 1991.

III-6

Physical Carcinogens

Cesare Maltoni
Franco Minardi

Introduction

Broadly, the term "physical carcinogens" includes a wide range of agents: radiations of different kinds, low and high temperatures, mechanical traumas, and solid and gel materials. More restrictively, however, the term is currently used to define solid and gel materials, water-insoluble or only slightly soluble, which are capable of producing cancer. This meaning will be used in this chapter, although "solid and gel carcinogens" would be a more precise definition. Both "physical carcinogens" and "solid carcinogens" have been widely used in an oversimplified manner to identify agents that produce cancer mainly, if not exclusively, through their physical properties and physical effects, rather than through their chemical properties and actions, as opposed to "chemical carcinogens". Physical carcinogens include hard and soft materials, fibrous particles, non-fibrous particles, and gel materials.

The first scientific demonstration of the carcinogenic capacity of the physical agents was made by Turner, who found that Bakelite disks, implanted in rats, evoked fibrosarcomas.[26] Anecdotal cases of tumors that arose around foreign bodies (including bullets in wartime) were reported earlier.

The identification of physical carcinogens is based on epidemiological and/or experimental data. The extrapolation of experimental results to humans is improved by the use of experimental models as closely equivalent to human situations as possible. The following examples may serve to illustrate this concept. Intratissue inserts of metallic alloys or plastics may well reproduce the situations in which allogenic prostheses are implanted surgically in the human body; conversely, the inhalation of particulate materials may correctly reproduce the exposure of laborers working in a dusty occupational environment.

The Known Physical Carcinogens
Hard and Soft Materials

The category of hard and soft materials includes metals and metallic alloys, synthetic products, and other natural materials, in the form of disks, squares, films, and foams. The studies performed in this field are nearly exclusively experimental, and the majority have been made on rats by intratissue implantations, mainly in the subcutaneous tissues, and more infrequently in other sites. The experiments of Oppenheimer and colleagues, and of Nothdurft on squares and disks of metals and plastics are classical.[21–24]

The most relevant available experimental data on the carcinogenicity of these materials are presented in Table III-6-1. The observed tumors arise around implants and are sarcomas of different types: fibrosarcomas (Figure III-6-1), rhabdomyosarcomas (Figure III-6-2), and osteosarcomas.

Studies on the sequence of changes taking place at the site of implants for reconstructing the histogenesis of sarcomas have shown that the implanted material induces a fibrous reaction that remains apparently unchanged for several months and may even undergo hyalinization. After several months the cells in the more internal layer of the fibrous capsule, in direct contact with the implanted material, may

Table III-6-1.   Hard and Soft Materials, of Different Shape and Dimension, Found to Be Carcinogenic When Implanted in Rodents

Metals
  Gold
  Platinum
  Silver
  Steel
  Tantalum
Metallic alloys
  Vitallium (chromium, cobalt, molybdenum)
Water-insoluble polymers
  Hydrocarbon polymers (synthetic)
    Polyethylene (Polythene)
    Polymethylmetacrylate (Lucite)
    Polyvinylbenzol (Polystyrol)
    Cross linked polyvinyl alcohol (Ivalon)
    Polyester condensate of terephthalate and ethylene glycol
      (Dacron)
    Phenol-formaldehyde condensate (Bakelite)
  Halogenated-hydrocarbon polymers (synthetic)
    Polyvinylidene chloride (Saran)
    Polyvinyl chloride (PVC, Igelit, Vestolit, Vinnol)
    Polyfluor(chlor)-olefine (Teflon)
    Polymethylmetacrylate chloride (Pliofilm)
    Copolymer of vinyl chloride and acrylonitrile (Vinyon N,
      Dynel)
  Aminized hydrocarbons polymers (polyamides) (synthetic)
    Polyhexamethylene diamine adilpanide (nylon)
    Poly-e-caprolactam, polyurethane (Perlon)
  Hydrocarbon polymers (semisynthetic and natural)
    Processed latex gum (rubber)
    Processed polyglucose (cellulose) (cellophane)
    Processed cellulose (linen, parchment paper, silk, keratin,
      ivory)
  Silicon polymers (synthetic)
    Processed polydimethylsiloxane (silicon rubber) (Silastic)

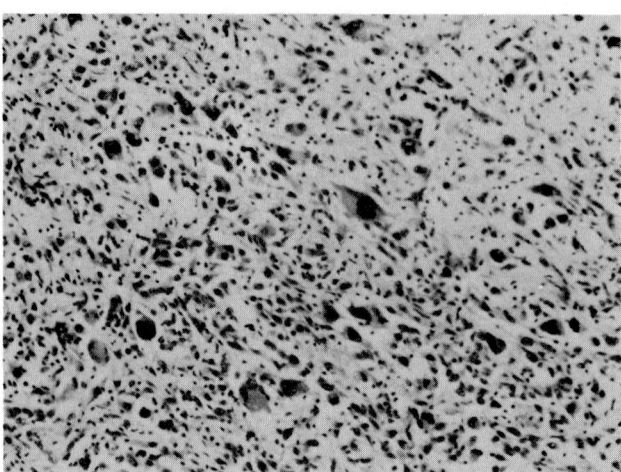

Figure III-6-2. Rhabdomyosarcoma that arose around an implant of an intact disk of vitallium in a female Sprague-Dawley rat.

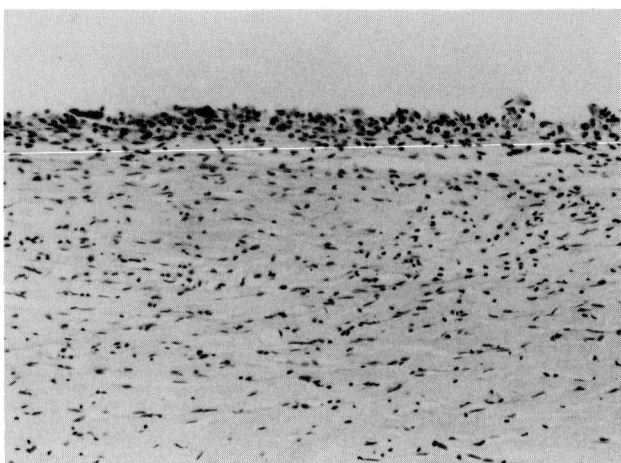

Figure III-6-3. Cellular proliferation in a fibrous capsule formed around an implant of an intact disk of vitallium at the edge of the cavity containing the implant, and therefore in direct contact with the implanted material, after 15 months from the implant in a male Sprague-Dawley rat.

start to proliferate (Figure III-6-3) and then evolve to the formation of sarcomas. These changes and their sequence take place independently from the nature of the implanted material.

Various investigators have shown that intact films of certain polymers have more potent carcinogenic effects than films of the same polymer carrying perforations and are considerably more potent than powdered films.[23] Other investigators, studying a different material, have been unable to confirm such a specific relationship between physical form and carcinogenesis.[19] Testing vitallium in the form of intact disks, holed disks of the same diameter and thickness, and fragments (in the amount equivalent to the weight of the intact disks), the fragmentation effect has been confirmed, but not that of holing: holed disks proved to be as carcinogenic as intact disks (Table III-6-2).

Surgical prostheses of metals, metallic alloys, and polymers are widely used nowadays. Only a few isolated cases

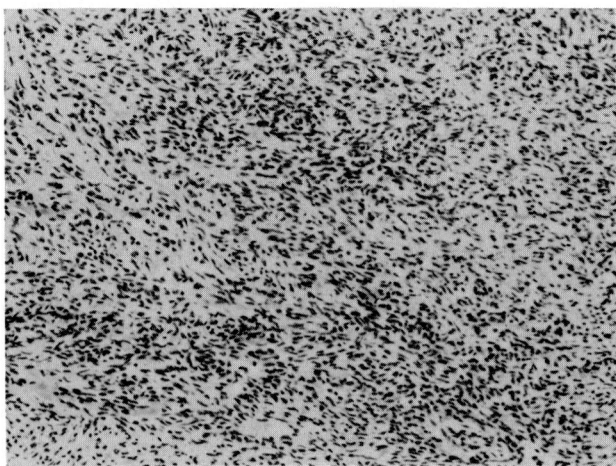

Figure III-6-1. Fibrosarcoma that arose around an implant of a holed disk of vitallium in a female Sprague-Dawley rat.

Table III-6-2.   Results of Long-term Carcinogenicity Bioassays of Vitallium, in Different Forms, Implanted in Subcutaneous Tissues of Sprague-Dawley Rats

Treatment	No.	Animals Developing Sarcomas at Site of Implantation
Intact disks	30	13
Holed disks	30	15
Fragments	30	2
None (controls)	30	0

Data extracted from Maltoni et al.[19]

of human sarcomas around surgical implants of metals and plastics have so far been reported in the literature.[18,19] More information on the potential carcinogenic risks of surgically implanted hard and soft materials could be provided by programmed long-term follow-up of implanted patients.

Fibers

The category of fibers includes natural mineral fibers and man-made mineral fibers. The carcinogenicity of these materials has been investigated by epidemiological and/or experimental studies.

Asbestos. Among the fibrous materials, asbestos has attracted the most attention because of its industrial and commercial relevance (about 3,000 uses) and its diffusion in the occupational and general environment, and because of the early detection of its pathogenicity and carcinogenicity. Six fibrous silicates are currently characterized as asbestos: the fibrous serpentine mineral chrysotile (white asbestos), and the amphyboles actinolite, amosite, anthophyllite, crocidolite (blue asbestos), and tremolite. The most commercially important minerals of asbestos are chrysotile, amosite, and crocidolite. Chrysotile is produced in the largest amounts and is the most widely used and diffused into the environment. In the last decades asbestos has been mined at the rate of 5–8 million tons per year worldwide. Asbestos is mainly used in buildings, pipes, the paper industry, maritime and railway carriers, and the clutch and brake industry. Its wide use for insulation is the major cause of environmental and occupational exposure.

Because of its great production and wide and numerous uses, asbestos may be considered ubiquitous. It is present in workplaces, the general environment, and the family environment, where it is brought by exposed workers on their clothes and in their hair. It is found in air, and traces of the mineral have been detected in water (including drinking water), in foods and drugs, and in a variety of consumer products. The following worker categories must be considered exposed: miners and millers of the mineral, manufacturers of asbestos products, laborers who repair, maintain, and clean structures and materials containing asbestos, and workers handling waste made of, or contaminated with asbestos.

The possible association between asbestos and cancer was suspected for the first time in 1935. In that year Lynch and Smith described a lung carcinoma in a patient with asbestosis (fibrosis of the lung due to the inhalation of asbestos dust).[12] The carcinogenic effect of asbestos fibers of different types on various tissues and organs, both in humans and in experimental animals, is now definitively established by a large number of clinical, epidemiological, and experimental studies. Several comprehensive reviews on asbestos carcinogenicity are available.[8,11,25]

The major route of exposure in humans is inhalation. In animals (mainly rats, but also mice and hamsters) asbestos has been tested by inhalation, by intraperitoneal, intrapleural, and subcutaneous injection, and by ingestion. The tumors observed following exposure to asbestos fibers in humans and in experimental animals are listed in Table III-6-3. Mesothelioma in its different sites (mainly pleura and peritoneum) is the tumor most specifically connected to asbestos, both in humans and in animals (Figures III-6-4 and III-6-5). Mesotheliomas in humans have been found after occupational, environmental, and family exposure.

The time of latency of asbestos-correlated tumors is long. In general, tumors start to appear 20 years after start of exposure. Lung carcinomas and mesotheliomas, in people exposed to asbestos, may be preceded by or associated with lung fibrosis and pleural plaques. These changes represent a marker of asbestos exposure, but a possible role in the natural history of the tumors has not been proved, and has been denied by several investigators. The number of occupational groups at risk of asbestos cancer has been growing, and the incidence of asbestos-correlated tumors in some occupational categories has also been increasing in recent years. A clear example is represented by the mortality due to mesothelioma among workers exposed to asbestos used in the railroads (Figure III-6-6).[17]

Table III-6-3.   Tumors Related to Asbestos Exposure in Humans and Experimental Animals

In Humans	In Experimental Animals
Lung cancer	Lung cancer
Pleural mesothelioma	Pleural mesothelioma
Peritoneal mesothelioma	Peritoneal mesothelioma
Other site mesothelioma	and possibly sarcoma
and possibly sarcoma	
Pharyngo-laryngeal cancer	
Gastrointestinal cancer	
Kidney cancer	

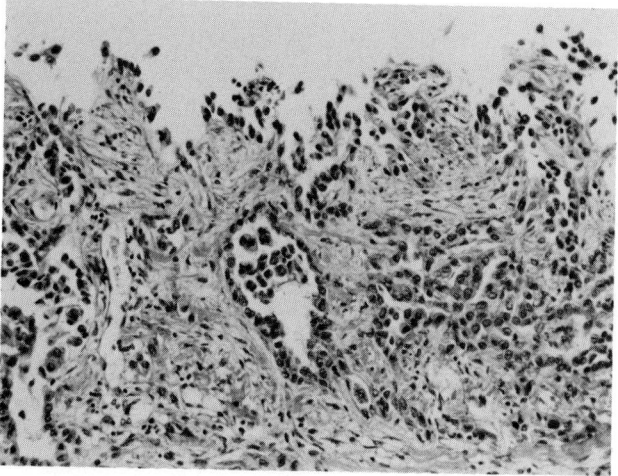

Figure III-6-4. Tubular epitheliomorphic mesothelioma of the pleura in an Italian railroad machinist.

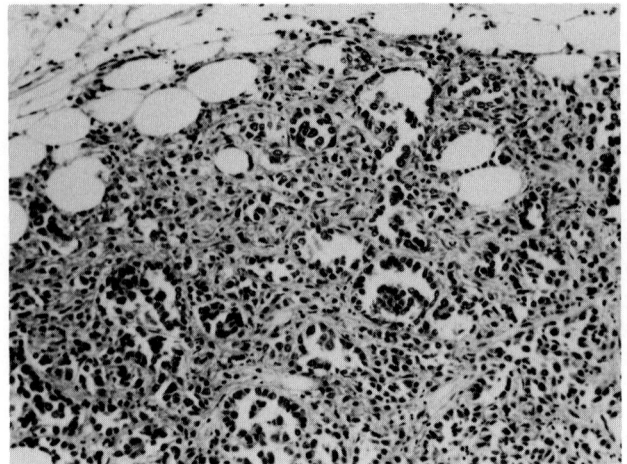

Figure III-6-5. Tubular epitheliomorphic mesothelioma of the peritoneum of a male Sprague-Dawley rat injected with 25 mg of Canadian chrysotile in 1 ml of H_2O.

In experimental systems, the various asbestos minerals show a similar carcinogenic potency (Table III-6-4). There is evidence that each of the major non-neoplastic and neoplastic diseases associated with asbestos in humans is produced by all the different forms of the mineral, the amphiboles as well as the serpentine (chrysotile).[3]

The diffusion of asbestos minerals in the environment, the number of people exposed, and the high degree of carcinogenicity of these materials make asbestos carcinogenicity a major worldwide problem of public health.

Erionite. Erionite is a fibrous zeolite, whose fibers are similar in dimension to asbestos fibers, though they are probably shorter in length on average. Zeolites are crystalline aluminosilicates, in which the primary "building blocks" are tetrahedra consisting of either silicon or aluminum atoms surrounded by four oxygen atoms. These tetrahedra combine, linked together by oxygen bridges and cations, to yield

an ordered three-dimensional framework. Although there are more than 30 known natural zeolites, only four are fibrous (chabazite, clinoptilolite, erionite, mordenite). Zeolite minerals are found as major constituents in numerous sedimentary volcanic tuffs, especially where these were deposited and have been altered by saline lake water. Many hundreds of occurrences have been recorded of zeolite deposits in over 40 countries.

Natural zeolites have many commercial uses, most of which are based on the ability of these minerals to adsorb molecules from air or liquid selectively. The exposure of humans can be occupational or environmental.

An excess of mortality due to pleural and peritoneal mesotheliomas, both in males and females, has been reported in three remote Anatolian villages in the same area where erionite occurs. In two of those villages, lung cancer appeared to be excessive. The high incidence of mesothelioma and lung cancer has been attributed to the presence of erionite in the soil, road dust, and building stones of those villages.[2,9] Asbestos is not more common in erionite villages than in control villages where the excess of mesothelioma was not found.

The hypothesis that erionite is the causative agent of the Turkish mesotheliomas and therefore that it is a human carcinogen has been supported by experimental evidence. Following inhalation exposure and intraperitoneal and intrapleural injection, erionite causes the onset of peritoneal and pleural mesotheliomas in rats and mice.[9,13–16] In rats erionite has been shown to be the most powerful mesotheliomatogenic agent for pleura (Table III-6-5).

The demonstration of the carcinogenic effect of erionite is also of particular relevance considering the large amount and diffusion of natural fibrous and non-fibrous zeolites, their widespread industrial uses (which are expected to increase), and the production of man-made zeolites for several industrial applications (as detergents and as catalysts in the petrochemical and refining industries). A systematic and integrated project of long-term carcinogenicity bioassays of natural

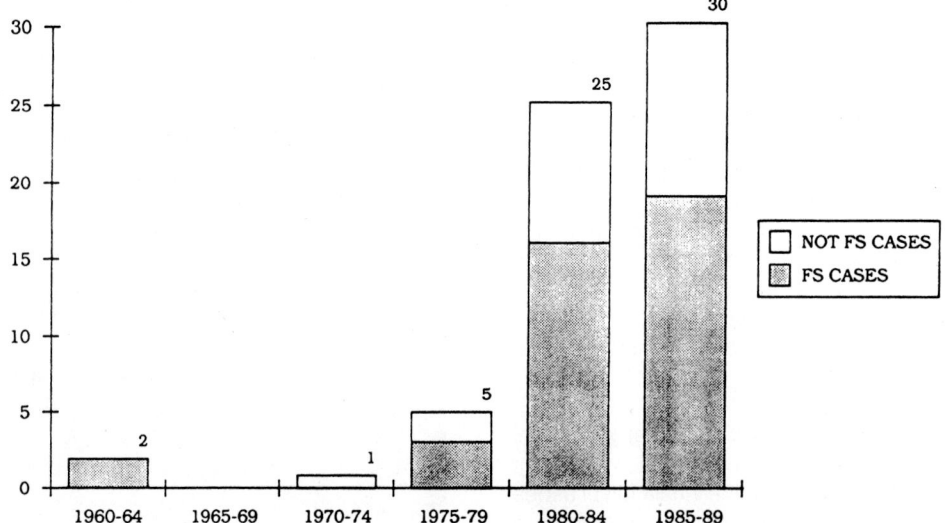

Figure III-6-6. Distribution, by 5-year periods, of the cases of mesothelioma among machinists (especially) and other workers of the Italian State Railroads (FS) and among rolling-stock machinists in workshops not belonging to the FS in Italy. Data from Maltoni et al.[17]

Table III-6-4. Results of Long-term Carcinogenicity Bioassays on Various Asbestos Minerals, Injected into Peritoneal Cavity[a] of Sprague-Dawley Rats

Test Material	No.	Animals Bearing Peritoneal Mesotheliomas
Amosite	40	36
Anthophyllite	40	33
Chrysotile (California)	40	29
Chrysotile (Canada)	40	32
Chrysotile (Rhodesia)	40	33
Crocidolite	40	39
H_2O (controls)	150	0

[a]A single injection of 25 mg in H_2O
Data extracted from Maltoni and Minardi[15]

Table III-6-5. Comparative Mesotheliomatogenic Effects on Rat Pleura of Erionite and Asbestos (Crocidolite and Chrysotile), Following Injection into Pleural Cavity[a]

Material	No.	Animals Bearing Peritoneal Mesotheliomas
Erionite	40	35
Crocidolite	40	18
Chrysotile (Canada)	40	26
H_2O (controls)	150	0

[a]A single injection of 25 mg in H_2O
Data extracted from Maltoni and Minardi[15]

and man-made fibrous and non-fibrous zeolites was begun several years ago at the Bologna Institute of Oncology, and is now ongoing.

Other Natural and Man-Made Fibers. Other fibers include: among the natural fibers, wollastonite (a fibrous silicate), attapulgite (a fibrous silicate), and the asbestiform fibers present in commercial talc; and among the man-made fibers, glasswool, rockwool and slagwool (produced by blowing, centrifuging, and drawing molten rock or slag), and ceramic fibers.

Data on the carcinogenicity of natural and man-made fibers is of great public interest, because of the various industrial uses (the large majority as asbestos substitutes). At present more than 5 million tons of man-made mineral fibers are produced annually in more than 100 factories located throughout the world. Glass fiber products comprise over 50% of the total.

Most of the carcinogenicity data comes from experimental studies, and only to a limited extent from epidemiological investigations. The experimental bioassays on carcinogenicity have been performed on rodents (mostly rats, but also mice and hamsters) in which the materials were administered by inhalation and/or intrapleural and intraperitoneal injection or implantation. The data on the carcinogenicity of these fibers have been extensively reviewed.[9–11]

Results of the epidemiological and experimental studies are shown in Table III-6-6.

Non-Fibrous Particulate Materials

Non-fibrous particulates include powdered metallic cobalt and nickel, and crystalline silica.

Particles of pure metallic cobalt (sizes ranging from 3.5 × 3.5 μm to 17 × 12 μm) with large numbers of long, narrow particles on the order of 10 × 4 μm and clumps of particles measuring up to 100 × 100 μm, when injected in the thigh muscles, cause the onset of sarcomas (mainly rhabdomyosarcomas) at the site of injection.[5]

After intrafemoral (marrow cavity) and subcutaneous introduction into rats, particles of pure metallic nickel ranging in diameter from 2–50 μm (mean, 10–30 μm) have been shown to produce sarcomas of different histotypes in about 28% of the implanted animals.

Various forms and preparations of crystalline silica (quartz, cristobalite, and tridymite) have been tested for carcinogenicity. Quartz, with particle sizes in the respirable range, administered by inhalation or by intratracheal instillation in rats, produced adenocarcinomas and squamous cell carcinomas of the lung in three of five experiments performed. When injected in the pleural and peritoneal cavities, quartz of several types, with particles in the respirable range, resulted in thoracic and abdominal malignant lymphomas, primarily of the histiocytic type. Cristobalite and tridymite, with particles in the respirable range, also resulted in malignant lymphomas, primarily of the histiocytic type, when injected in the pleural cavity.

Gel Materials

Two types of silicone gel used for breast prostheses have been tested by subcutaneous implantation in male and female Sprague-Dawley rats by Dow-Corning.[4] Tumors, the large majority of which are fibrosarcomas, developed at the site of implantation in 22–32% of the animals in the treated groups.

The relevance of this finding for public health may be large, considering that silicone implants are widely used for mammary prostheses. According to the U.S. Food and Drug Administration, 130,000 silicone gel breast prostheses are currently being implanted annually, and there are approximately 2 million implanted women to date. Of the breast prostheses implanted, 85% are for augmentation (cosmetic) purposes, and the remainder are for breast reconstruction following mastectomy. Other uses of silicone gel implants are for testicular prostheses. Though the silicone gel is encased in a silicone envelope when used in breast prostheses, there is good evidence that silicone gel "bleeds" through the envelope and can thus get into surrounding tissues and to other distant places in the body.[11] To our knowledge, no cases of mammary sarcomas have been reported in women following implants with breast silicone prostheses. However, widespread use of these prostheses in plastic surgery has only occurred since the 1970s, while the latency period of the majority of tumors, due to exogenous agents, is usually over 20 years. On the basis of the experimental results, clinical-epidemiological surveillance of women implanted with breast prostheses should be undertaken.

Mechanisms of Carcinogenesis

It has been hypothesized that physical carcinogens produce cancer by some physical mechanisms rather than by chemical reaction. Such physical mechanisms have been

Table III-6-6. Results of Long-Term Carcinogenicity Bioassays and Epidemiologic Investigations on Natural (Other Than Asbestos and Erionite) and Man-Made Mineral Fibers

Fibrous material	Tumors in experimental animals	Tumors in humans
Wollastonite	Pleural "sarcomas"	—
Attapulgite	Mesotheliomas	—
Talc containing asbestiform fibers	Mesotheliomas[a]	Lung cancer Mesotheliomas[b]
Glass wool	Lung tumors Mesotheliomas	Lung cancer[b]
Rockwool	Mesotheliomas	
Slagwool	(Equivocal findings)	
Rockwool + slagwool		Lung cancer[b]
Ceramic fibers	Lung tumors[b] Mesotheliomas	—

[a]Data extracted from Minardi et al.[20]
[b]The evidence is still limited[9,10]

regarded as a mere non-specific irritative effect of hypothetical surface factors on cells, which could cause cellular proliferation, selection of spontaneously occurring transformed clones, and, finally, neoplasms. In support of this view, it has also been hypothesized that the fibrous reaction observed around implanted disks, squares, and films would "immunologically protect" the transformed clones formed within the core of the capsule, in contact with implants, thereby favoring the formation of tumors. Such claims have been supported mainly by the experimental evidence of various investigators, which has shown that physical changes of the implanted materials such as perforation of polymeric disks and fragmentation of polymeric materials inhibited the carcinogenic effect. This physical hypothesis comes from the assumption that solid carcinogens are inert.

There are, however, other facts that oppose the physical hypothesis, and support a chemical mechanism. There are many observations, by several investigators and by ourselves, demonstrating that many plastic polymers (the most specific example of inert material), embedded in tissues, undergo progressive deterioration at varying rates, indicating some chemical interaction between the xenobiotic material and biological substrates. The perforation effect has not been confirmed by other investigators nor by us, in the course of vitallium disk carcinogenesis. The discrepancy between these experimental results may be explained by the different experimental conditions in various laboratories (for example, the duration of experiments), particularly when one is analyzing experiments performed many years ago, at a time when the standards of good laboratory procedures may not have been uniform. The fragmentation effect may be explained by the fact that fragments or powders, after insertion, usually form a compact mass in the body tissues, with a lesser surface of interaction with biological substrate than the surface area of a disk. Therefore the chemical mechanism cannot be discarded. The leaching of microquantities of soluble material from the physical carcinogens into the body might be sufficient to transform cells that are in intimate contact with the xenobiotic material.

For many years there was wide agreement that asbestos fibers (and by extension, all mineral fibers) acted simply by an irritative mechanism. The hypotheses on the pathogenetic mechanisms of asbestos carcinogenesis must now be reviewed on the basis of new findings. Recent data have shown that asbestos (crocidolite and chrysotile) is mutagenic per se.[6] Moreover, it has been demonstrated that chrysotile fibers have the ability to introduce plasmid DNA into cells, and that this DNA is able to function in both replication and gene expression. The introduction of exogenous DNA into eukaryotic cells could cause mutations in several ways and thus contribute to asbestos-induced carcinogenesis.[1]

The hypotheses on the mechanism of action of physical carcinogens are not only scientific puzzles, but have specific practical implications: a chemical mechanism would imply a possible mutagenic effect and therefore a non-threshold dose.

Conclusions

Physical carcinogenesis may be considered at present an important public health, economic, and social problem, because of the large diffusion of particulate non-fibrous and fibrous industrial materials in the general and domestic environment and in workplaces, and the wide and increasing use of xenobiotic implants, in plastic, orthopedic, vascular, dental, and other specialized surgery.

The dramatic carcinogenic effect of asbestos, the available data about other industrial mineral fibers, the expected introduction of new types of fibrous and non-fibrous materials in the environment, and the expanding use of alloplastic surgery, all call for more systematic studies of physical carcinogenesis. When such studies are positive, the consequent measures of control will be mainly preventive.

References

1. Appel, J. D., Fasy, T. M., Kohtz, D. S., Kohtz, J. D., and Johnson, E. M.: Asbestos fibers mediate transformation of monkey cells by exogenous plasmid DNA. Proc. Natl. Acad. Sci. U.S.A., 85:7670, 1988.
2. Baris, Y. I., Sahin, A. A., Oezesmi, M., Kerse, E., Oezen, E., Kolacan, B., Altinoers, M., and Goektepeli, A.: An outbreak of pleural mesothelioma and chronic fibrosing pleurisy in the village of Karain/Uerguep in Anatolia. Thorax, 33:181, 1978.
3. Cullen, M. R., Lopez-Carrillo, L., Alli, B., Pace, P. E., Shalat, S. L., and Baloyi, R. S.: Chrysotile asbestos and health in Zimbabwe. Am. J. Ind. Med., 19:161, 1991.
4. Food and Drug Administration: Analysis of Dow-Corning data regarding carcinogenicity of silicone gels. Washington, D.C., Federal Drug Administration, 1988.
5. Heath, J. C.: The production of malignant tumours by cobalt in the rat. Br. J. Cancer, 10:668, 1956.
6. Hei, T., and Waldren, C.: Personal communication.
7. Hueper, W. C.: Experimental studies in metal carcinogenesis. IV. Cancer produced by parenterally introduced metallic nickel. J. Natl. Cancer Inst., 16:55, 1955.

8. International Agency for Research on Cancer: Monographs on the Evaluation of Carcinogenic Risk of Chemicals to Man. Asbestos, Volume 14. Lyon, International Agency for Research on Cancer, 1977.

9. International Agency for Research on Cancer: Monographs on the Evaluation of the Carcinogenic Risk of Chemicals to humans. Silica and Some Silicates, Volume 42. Lyon, International Agency for Research on Cancer, 1987.

10. International Agency for Research on Cancer: Monographs on the Evaluation of the Carcinogenic Risk to humans. Man-made Mineral Fibres and Radon, Volume 43. Lyon, International Agency for Research on Cancer, 1988.

11. International Programme on Chemical Safety: Asbestos and Other Natural Mineral Fibres. Geneva, World Health Organization, 1986.

12. Lynch, K. M., and Smith, W. A.: Pulmonary asbestosis. III. Carcinoma of lung in asbestos–silicosis. Am. J. Cancer, 24: 56, 1935.

13. Maltoni, C., and Minardi, F.: The comparative potency of asbestos and erionite in producing mesothelioma, following intrapleural and intraperitoneal injection into Sprague-Dawley rats. Acta Oncol., 4:69, 1983.

14. Maltoni, C., and Minardi, F.: Unpublished data.

15. Maltoni, C., and Minardi, F.: Recent results of carcinogenicity bioassays of fibres and other particulate materials. In Nonoccupational Exposure to Mineral Fibres. Edited by E. Bignon, J. Peto, and R. Saracci. Lyon, International Agency for Research on Cancer, 1989, p. 46.

16. Maltoni, C., Minardi, F., and Morisi, L.: Pleural mesotheliomas in Sprague-Dawley rats by erionite: First experimental evidence. Environ. Res., 29:238, 1982.

17. Maltoni, C., Pinto, C., and Mobiglia, A.: Mesotheliomas following exposure to asbestos used in railroads: The Italian cases. Toxicol. Ind. Health, In press.

18. Maltoni, C., and Sinibaldi C.: Carcinogenicity of acrylic resins (polymethyl methacrylate) used in dentistry. Long-term bioassays on Sprague-Dawley rats by subcutaneous implantation. Acta Oncol., 3:13, 1982.

19. Maltoni, C., Sinibaldi, C., and Morisi, L.: Carcinogenicity of vitallium. Long-term bioassays on Sprague-Dawley rats and Swiss mice by subcutaneous implantation. Acta Oncol., 1:11, 1980.

20. Minardi, F., Belpoggi, F., Franch, A., and Maltoni, C.: La cancerogenesi da talco grezzo contaminato con amianto: Primi risultati dei saggi sperimentali dell'Istituto di Oncologia di Bologna. In Recenti Progressi nelle Conoscenze e nel Controllo dei Tumori. Edited by E. Triggiani, G. Sammarco, G. Liguori, D. Carretti, and C. Maltoni. Bologna, Monduzzi, 1990, p. 279.

21. Nothdurft, H.: Die experimentalle Erzeugung von Sarkomen bei Ratten und Mausen durch Implantation von Rundscheiben aus Gold, Silber, Platin oder Elfenbein. Naturwissenschaften, 42:75, 1955.

22. Oppenheimer, B. S., Oppenheimer, E. T., Danishefsky, I., and Stout, A. P.: Carcinogenic effect of metals in rodents. Cancer Res., 16:439, 1956.

23. Oppenheimer, B. S., Oppenheimer, E. T., Danishefsky, I., Stout, A. P., and Eirich, F. R.: Further studies of polymers as carcinogenic agents in animals. Cancer Res., 15:333, 1955.

24. Oppenheimer, B. S., Oppenheimer, E. T., Stout, A. P., and Danishefsky, I.: Malignant tumours resulting from embedding plastics in rodents. Science, 118:305, 1953.

25. Selikoff, I. J., and Lee, D. H. K.: Asbestos and Disease. New York, Academic Press, 1978.

26. Turner, F. C.: Sarcomas at sites of subcutaneous implanted Bakelite disks in rats. J. Natl. Cancer Inst., 2:81, 1941.

III-7

Trauma and Inflammation

John F. Gaeta

The normal wear and tear of life induces a multiplicity of traumas which are rarely noted or quickly forgotten until the time arises to make something out of them.

—Stewart, 1946

Introduction

The role of trauma in the causation of cancer is a subject fraught with gross exaggerations and contradictions. The literature abounds with points of view ranging from detailed descriptions of case reports of trauma followed by malignant neoplasms to others in which this relationship is minimized or flatly denied.[1,13,26,33,36,45,48,50]

This problem is further obscured when the medicolegal implications are brought into the picture. Compensation claims for development of a tumor ascribed to trauma are not infrequent, and although they rarely have a factual basis, some of them have been settled in favor of the injured party. Many of the causes found in the literature claiming a causal relationship between trauma and neoplasia try to fulfill a number of criteria postulated by different authors.[18,53]

Most of the conditions listed include: (1) Authenticity of trauma, (2) sufficient severity of the trauma, (3) reasonable evidence of prior integrity of the injured area, (4) tumor appearance at the site of trauma, and (5) time interval not too remote for reasonable association of trauma and tumor.[41]

Additional criteria to further authenticate this possible relationship are: (1) Trauma of such magnitude that reparative proliferation of cells occurs, and (2) tumor of a type that might reasonably develop as a result of the regeneration and repair of specific tissues damaged during injury.[53]

Unfortunately, the application of these criteria is not in itself a warranty to a scientific and objective approach to this problem. One of the main sources of disagreement between advocates and detractors of the role of trauma in the causation of cancer has been the length and significance of the time interval between the two. This factor appears to be somewhat flexible when compared to the appearance time of other neoplasms brought about by known carcinogens. The sequence of events leading to the development of leukemia following irradiation exposure is not well known, but in the case of radiation-related leukemia in Nagasaki and Hiroshima after atomic bomb exposure, we have good documentation to indicate a peak appearance time of 7.2 - 9.4 years between exposure and onset of leukemia.[6] A similar time interval (8.5 years) has been demonstrated in the case of thyroid neoplasms in children following neck irradiation.[55] Recent studies that correlate the appearance of some forms of vaginal adenocarcinoma in young women with mothers who received stilbestrol therapy during the gestation period indicate that the neoplasm may follow 14–22 years after the chemical traumatic event.[22]

Mechanisms of Possible Traumatic Causation

A wide variety of malignant neoplasms has been described in the literature in association with trauma. In many cases the association is purely coincidental, judging by the lack of scientific evidence, but it emphasizes the fact that mechanical trauma often serves to alert the patient to the presence of a pre-existing neoplasm in the affected parts. Accepting the definition of trauma as a mechanical force received by the body and followed by a local reaction characteristic of injury, we exclude ionizing irradiation, chemical insults, and ultraviolet radiation as different forms of injury to be discussed elsewhere in their respective relation to cancer.[41] Different forms of skin cancer have been known to result from mechanical injury.

Draining Sinuses

In 1828, Marjolin described the development of malignant neoplastic changes in an old skin ulcer, probably the site of a draining sinus.[34] In 1931, Benedict described 12 cases of cancer occurring in draining osteomyelitic sinuses and collected 52 similar cases from the literature.[4] He studied 2,400 cases of osteomyelitic sinuses and found 0.5% incidence of malignant change. The draining sinus in which cancer occurred had been present for an average of 30 years, and the subsequent neoplastic lesions were invariably slow growing. A review of all reports of cases in which metastases had occurred proved the presence of metastases in only four cases.[5] Emphasizing the rarity of spread, this study postulated that some of the cases reported could have been instances of pseudoepitheliomatous hyperplasia of the skin around the sinus, mistakenly diagnosed as carcinoma.

Thermal Injury

Since the description of Dupuytren in 1839 of a patient treated for cancer arising in the scar of a burn caused by sulfuric acid, many cases have been described in which heat has been the initial insult that allegedly triggered the development of cancer at the site of injury and subsequent scar.[16] Excellent reviews on this subject are available, concluding that the potentiality of a scar to undergo malignant neoplastic degeneration, and the type of epithelioma resulting, are related to the extent of the surface area involved and the depth of the burn.[27,47] The type of burn inflicted upon the tissue is also related to the nature of the agent (tar, flame, metal), to its temperature, to the tissue's capacity for heat absorption, and to the duration of contact.[1] Although most of the reported malignant lesions that follow burns correspond to epidermoid carcinomas, basal cell cancers can also originate by the same mechanism, usually when the burn is superficial and when the thermal injury results from hot solids. Based on a study of 2,465 cases of skin cancer, 2% of all epidermoid carcinomas and 0.3% of all basal cell carcinomas originate on skin subjected to thermal injury.[28,47]

Kangri Burn Cancer. The Indian kangri is an earthenware bowl heated by charcoal and worn against the skin of the thighs and abdomen. Owing to the constant application of heat, the skin in these areas becomes dry and horny and frequently shows a variable degree of chronic dermatitis. Scars resulting from previous kangri burns are frequent and apt to undergo malignant change. The average age of onset is 55 years and the average duration of life is 15 months from the recognized time of onset of the cancer. The gross lesion is variable in appearance, but microscopically it consistently shows an epidermoid type of carcinoma.[37]

Kairo Burn Cancer. The kairo burn cancer in Japan relates to another system for the maintenance of body warmth, the use of a light tin box that fits snugly against the contour of the abdomen. It is generally worn for a period of at least three hours at a time. The continued or prolonged use of this utensil produces erythematous burns or chronic dermatitis leading to malignant neoplastic changes.[47]

Lung Cancer

A relationship between lung cancer and pulmonary scars was first noted by Friedrich and Rossle, and their association has been the subject of numerous reports.[2,9,19,33,35,40,42,59] The exact frequency of this association is difficult to determine from previous reports. Luders and Themel found a frequency of 28% in their study of 2,032 autopsies, whereas others report only an incidence of 14%.[21,29] These findings led to the concept of "scar cancer" as a morphologic entity embracing any inflammatory or vascular pulmonary lesion leading to the formation of scar tissue followed by the development of a local carcinoma. In most instances, the tumor arises peripherally and histologically shows the characteristics of pulmonary adenocarcinoma or bronchiolar carcinoma.[9] Exact criteria have been postulated to differentiate true pulmonary scars from the dense connective tissue often encountered in lung cancer.[10] Still some believe that this association is probably much higher than suspected because of the common difficulty of convincingly demonstrating the presence of pre-existing scar tissue when examining large pulmonary lesions either in surgical or in autopsy material.[59]

Cancer of the Esophagus

This type of cancer is often related to previous injury. Studies of a substantial number of cases of stricture of the esophagus following lye ingestion indicate that at least 5.2% of the lye strictures are followed by squamous cell carcinoma.[25] A number of other irritants have been implicated, such as strong alcohol, tobacco smoking and ingestion of material, but thermal irritation has been quoted as the most constant factor predisposing to esophageal cancer.[49,54] Some authors have stressed the frequency of this form of cancer in geographic locations where ingestion of hot tea is a common habit.

Cancer of the Oral Cavity. The role of these irritants is apparently reversed in relation to cancer of the oral cavity. Observations of 659 cases of carcinoma of the oral cavity emphasize the role of tobacco and alcohol in the etiology of oral cancer and diminish the significance of local trauma and dental irritation.[57]

Moles and Malignant Melanoma

Although the exact cellular origin of malignant melanomas can still be debated, a significant number are related to pre-existing nevi (moles).[30] A low percentage of nevi undergo malignant changes, but the true nature of this transformation is not well known. The fact that most malignant melanomas occur on exposed surfaces of the body, and the reported higher incidence of the disease in the sunnier parts of some countries, suggested that trauma or injury plays a part in their causation.[11,31] Another evidence in favor of the same hypothesis is the higher incidence of malignant melanoma in patients affected by xeroderma pigmentosum, a congenital disease characterized by failure to repair injury to DNA manifested as hypersensitivity to sunlight.[27]

Evidence in favor of trauma playing a role in the development of malignant melanoma also includes reports of a significant incidence of this lesion in Sudanese patients.[23] However, some studies of malignant melanoma in Australia showed that the most frequent location is the skin of the back, at least in the male, but this failed to show any direct relation to the belt area of the trunk where the incidence of constant trauma is obviously higher.[11]

Trauma and Bone Tumors

The etiologic aspect of single trauma has been repeatedly mentioned, although never elucidated, in relation to bone tumors. The preponderant number of bone tumors occurs in the same young age group in which the incidence of trauma is especially high. Most of the reports in the literature deal with observations of single cases. A general review of this problem in 1967 includes six cases of osteogenic sarcomas following a history of trauma.[37] All of them, however, presented such a short time interval (eight days to four months) that their causal relationship seems highly improbable. The lack of any significant increase of the number of bone tumors following the two world wars also speaks against such a relationship.[14]

Other Types of Cancer

Other types that have been reported occasionally in association with trauma include: Mammary carcinoma, brain tumors, carcinoma of uterine cervix, meningioma, glioma, and testicular tumors, but the evidence of etiologic significance is not persuasive.[3,7,36,39,44,51]

Interactions of Trauma and Tissue Repair

There is no evidence to substantiate the production of experimental tumors by the direct action of trauma, but there are numerous studies indicating its significance as a "co-carcinogen." Since the studies of Rous and his co-workers, it became apparent that, although repeated application of tar can induce tumors in rabbits under certain circumstances, a trauma can precipitate the formation of a tumor when the cells have been conditioned with previous tar treatment or by local promoters.[20,43] However, if trauma is to be considered independently as a tumor-causative factor, this could only take place as a rare event during the process of regeneration and repair. Normal regenerative process implies the restoration of lost parts by structurally and often functionally similar cells. There are some who would evoke a variety of organ-specific wound hormones liberated from the site of injury which exert a stimulating effect on homologous tissue.[46] Such putative hormonal factors have been further studied more recently, and it was concluded that the hormones (chalones) liberated from the wound have a specific role as mitotic inhibitors.[8] According to this view, liberation of the chalone releases cells to divide. This might also explain the mitogenic capacity of estrogens, which provide an increase of mitotic activity, possibly through neutralization of chalone substances. It is conceivable that persistent cell damage by

trauma could trigger an excessive proliferative effect because of the absence of the inhibiting effect of local chalones.

Other authors have advanced the possibility of direct mutation from chronic inflammation or repair.[52] This concept was chiefly based upon the proposition that a sudden transformation of a gene could result from trauma leading to a change of the basic characteristics of a cell and its progeny. Because cell mutations can be brought about by different stimuli, some investigators have concluded that the effect of repeated trauma upon tissues can be analogous to chemical carcinogens in their ability to induce cellular mutation.[12]

Another hypothesis unrelated to a humoral factor and recently related to carcinogenesis suggests a regulatory mechanism between cytoplasmic and nuclear structures.[38] Since the endoplasmic reticulum modulates DNA biosynthesis in some way, any stimulus (trauma) capable of destroying critical cytoplasmic structures or proteins could lead to a loss of a feedback mechanism with the cell beginning actively to synthesize DNA, causing polyploidy or cell division. In this manner, the differentiation of the tissue would be lost and a large increase of immature, undifferentiated cell population would result from which a malignant neoplasm might emerge. Electron microscope studies corroborate the destruction of endoplasmic reticulum structures during cancerization of the liver by means of dimethylnitrosamine.[17]

References

1. Abbas, J. S., and Beecham, J. E.: Burn wound carcinoma: case report and review of the literature. Burns Incl. Therm. Inj., 14:222, 1988.
2. Balo, J., Juhasz, E, and Temes, J.: Pulmonary infarcts and pulmonary carcinoma. Cancer, 9:918, 1956.
3. Barnett, G. H., Chou, S. M., and Bay, J. W.: Post-traumatic intracranial meningioma: A case report and review of the literature. Neurosurgery 18:75, 1986.
4. Benedict, E. B.: Carcinoma in osteomyelitis. Surg. Gynecol. Obstet., 53:1, 1931.
5. Bereston, E. S., and Ney, C.: Squamous cell carcinoma arising in a chronic osteomyelitic sinus tract with metastasis. Arch. Surg., 43:257, 1941.
6. Bizzozero, O. J., Johnson, K. G., and Ciocco, A.: Radiation-related leukemia, Hiroshima and Nagasaki, 1946-1964. I. Distribution, incidence and appearance time. N. Engl. J. Med., 274:1095, 1966.
7. Boyd, J. T., and Doll, R.: A study of the etiology of carcinoma uteri. Br. J. Cancer, 18:419, 1964.
8. Bullough, W. S.: Mitotic and functional homeostasis: a speculative review. Cancer Res., 25:1683, 1965.
9. Carroll, R.: The significance of lung scars on primary lung cancer. J. Path. Bact., 83:293, 1962.
10. Castleman, B.: Healed pulmonary infarcts. Arch. Path., 30:130, 1940.
11. Davis, N. C., Herrow, J. J., and McLeod, G. R.: Malignant melanoma in Queensland. Analysis of 400 skin lesions. Lancet, II:407, 1966.
12. Demerec, M.: Mutations induced by carcinogens. Br. J. Cancer, 2:114, 1948.
13. DeNayer, P. P., Delloye, C., and Malghem, J.: Bone injury and late giant cell tumor occurrence: A possible relation—A case report. Orthopedics, 10:1279, 1983.
14. Dietrich, A.: Krebs Nach Kriegsverletzungen. Zschr. f. Krebsforsch, 52:91, 1942.
15. Dolberg, D. S., Hollingsworth, R., and Hertle, M.: Wounding and its role in RSV-mediated tumor formation. Science, 230: 676, 1985.
16. Dupuytren, G.: Leçons Orales de Clinique Chirurgicale. 2nd Edition, Paris, 1839.
17. Emmelot, E., and Benedetti, E. L.: Changes in the fine structure of rat liver brought about by dimethylnitrosamine. J. Biophys. Biochem. Cytol., 7:393, 1960.
18. Ewing, J.: Bulkley Lecture: Modern Attitude Toward Traumatic Cancer. Arch. Path., 10:690, 1935.
19. Friedrich, G.: Periphere Lungenkrebse auf dem bodem Pleuraher Narben. Virchon Arch. Path. Anat., 304: 230, 1939.
20. Friedwald, W. F., and Rous, P.: The pathogenesis of deferred cancer. J. Exp. Med., 91:459, 1950.
21. Gelzer, J.: Uber die peripheren Lungenkrebse in Bereich von Lungernarben. Virchon Arch. Path. Anat., p. 329, 1956.
22. Herbst, A. L., Ulfelder, H., and Poskanzer, D. C.: Adenocarcinoma of the vagina: Association of maternal stilbestrol therapy with tumor appearance in young women. N. Engl. J. Med., 284:878, 1971.
23. Hewer, T. F.: Malignant melanoma in colored races: role of trauma in its causation. J. Path. Bact., 41:473, 1935.
24. Johnson F. M.: The development of carcinoma in scar tissue following burns. Am. Surg., 83:165, 1926.
25. Joske, R. A., and Benedict, E. B.: The role of benign esophageal obstruction in the development of carcinoma of the esophagus. Gastroenterology, 36:749, 1959.
26. Langer, F., Pritzker, K. P., Gross, A. E., and Shapiro, I. L.: Giant cell tumor associated with trauma. Clin. Orthop., 164:245, 1982.

27. Lever, W. F.: Histopathology of the Skin. Philadelphia, J.B. Lippincott Co., 4th ed., 1967, p. 63.
28. Lifeso, R. M., Rooney, R. J., and Shaker, M.: Post-traumatic squamous cell carcinoma. J. Bone Joint Surg., 72:12, 1990.
29. Luders, C. J., and Themel, K. G.: Die Narbenkrebse der Lungen als Beitrag zur Pathogenese des peripheren Lungencarcinoms. Virchon Arch. Path. Anat., 325:499, 1954.
30. McGovern, J. J.: Malignant Melanoma: Clinical and Histological Diagnosis. New York, Wiley, 1976, pp. 47-54.
31. McKie, R. M., and Atchison, T.: Severe sunburn and subsequent risk of primary cutaneous malignant melanomas in Scotland. Br. J. Cancer, 46.955, 1982.
33. Madri, J. A, and Carter, D.: Scar cancers of the lung: Origin and significance. Hum. Pathol., 15 625, 1984.
34. Marjolin, J. N.: Ulcère. Dict. de méd., 2nd ed., 1846, XXX, 10. SCARS, p. 22.
35. Meyer, E., and Liebow, A.: Relationship of interstitial pneumonia, honeycombing and atypical epithelial proliferation to cancer of the lung. Cancer, 18:322, 1965.
36. Mosinger, M., Glaunes, J. P., Fiorentini, H., and Bandler, H.: Tumeurs et Cancers Post Traumatiques. Ann. Med. Leg., 41:472, 1961.
37. Neve, E. F.: Kangri Burn Cancer. Br. J. Med., 21:1255,1923.
38. Oehlert, W.: The mechanism of regeneration, hyperplasia and cancerization. Acta. Un. Int. Cancer, 19:605, 1963.
39. Perez-Diaz, C., Cabello, A., and Lobato, R. D.: Oligodendrogliomas arising in the scar of a brain contusion: Report of two surgically verified cases. Surg. Neurol., 24:581, 1985.
40. Raeburn, C., and Spencer, H.: Lung scar cancers. Brit. J. Tuberc., 51:237, 1957.
41. Rigdon, R. H.: Trauma and cancer: A relationship based upon cell mutation. South. Med. J., 55:341, 1962.
42. Rossle, R.: Die Narbenkrebse der Lungen. Schweiz. Med. Wschr., 73:1200, 1943.
43. Rous, P., and Kidd, J. G.: Conditional neoplasms and sub-threshold neoplastic states. J. Exp. Med., 73:365, 1941.
44. Stewart, F. W.: Occupational and post-traumatic cancer. Bull. N.Y. Acad. Med., 22:145, 1947.
45. Stoll, H. L., and Crissey, J. T.: Epithelioma from single trauma. N. Y. State J. Med., 62:496, 1962.
46. Tier, H., Kiljunen, A., and Putkonen, T.: Existence of growth promoting factor in the skin of the white rat. Ann. Chir. Gynaecol. Fenn., p. 40, 1951.
47. Treves, N., and Pack, G. T.: The development of cancer in burn scars. Surg. Gynec. Obstet., 51:749, 1930.
48. Troost, D., and Tulleken, C. A.: Malignant glioma after bombshell injury. J. Clin. Neuropathol., 3:139, 1984.
49. Victoria, C. G., Munoz, N., and Day, N. E.: Hot beverages and esophageal cancer in Southern Brazil: A case control study. Int. J. Cancer, 39:710, 1987.
50. Voutilainen, A., Teir, H., and Kivivouri, A.: Causal relationship between trauma and malignant tumors. Ann. Chir. Gynaecol. Fenn. Supp., 56(Suppl. 152):1, 1967.
51. Walshe, F.: Head injuries as a factor in the etiology of an intracranial meningioma. Lancet, 2:993, 1961.
52. Warren, S.: In Pathology. Edited by W. A. D. Anderson. St. Louis, The C.V. Mosby Co., 1961, p. 447.
53. Warren, S.: Minimal criteria to prove causation of traumatic or occupational neoplasms. Ann. Surg., 117:585, 1943.
54. Watson, W. L., and Goodner, J.: Carcinoma of esophagus. Am. J. Surg., 93:259, 1957.
55. Winship, T., and Rosvoll, R. V.: Childhood thyroid carcinoma. Cancer, 14:734, 1961.
56. Wojewski, A.: Reticulum cell sarcoma with primary manifestation in testis. J. Urol., 89:709, 1963.
57. Wynder, E. J., Bross, I. J., and Feldman, R. M.: A study of the etiological factors in cancer of the mouth. Cancer, 10:1300, 1957.
58. Yamamura, T., Aozasa, K., and Honda, T.: Malignant fibrous histiocytoma developing in a burn scar. Br. J. Dermatol., 110:725, 1984.
59. Yokoo, H., and Suckow, E.: Peripheral lung cancers arising in scars. Cancer, 14:1205, 1961.

RNA Tumor Viruses

Howard A. Fine
William A. Haseltine

Introduction

The retroviruses are small single-stranded RNA containing animal viruses. The life cycle of these intracellular parasites is unique. By converting their genomic RNA into DNA and inserting it into the chromosomes of their host cells, these viruses can mutate, capture, and even transfer vital genetic information from one cell to another. The resultant effect is often an alteration in cellular growth and differentiation, leading to a wide variety of neoplastic and immunodeficient disease states in a broad range of animal hosts. The study of these viruses has thus resulted in profound insights into factors regulating the growth of normal and neoplastic cells.

The first retrovirus was identified in 1911 by Peyton Rous when he found a transmissible agent able to cause sarcomas in chickens.[122] The implications of this discovery were not immediately appreciated, since most scientists believed that this phenomenon was a peculiarity specific to the avian system only. Over the next forty years, however, interest in retroviruses dramatically increased with the recognition that these agents could cause neoplasms in other animals including mammals.[14]

Although quantitative assays for these viruses were developed as early as the 1950s, our present understanding of the biology of retroviruses occurred only after discovery of the enzyme, reverse transcriptase, in 1970.[7,142,147] This finding significantly increased the general interest in retroviruses. However, they continued to be viewed as an enigma of nature, and their relevance to normal cellular growth and spontaneously occurring animal neoplasms remained obscure.

This all changed in 1976 when it was demonstrated that the apparent transforming genes (oncogenes) carried by these viruses were homologs of endogenous cellular genes (proto-oncogenes).[133] This discovery led to an explosion of interest in the field of retrovirology and to the identification of no less than 60 proto-oncogenes. The impact of these discoveries has changed the way science now views how cellular genes control normal as well as neoplastic cellular growth.

This contribution to our current knowledge has alone made the study of retroviruses vitally important. Additional discoveries in the 1980s, however, made the direct relevance of these viruses to humans frightfully clear.[164] These discoveries included the finding in 1980 of the first infectious human retrovirus, Human T Cell Leukemia virus (HTLV-1). This virus has been etiologically linked to a specific type of T cell lymphoma/leukemia and to several degenerative neurologic diseases (see XXXVI-6).[45,110,128,166] It soon became clear that HTLV was not to be the only human pathogenic virus, for in 1984, the human immunodeficiency virus (HIV) was found to be the etiologic cause of AIDS.[8,46,86]

With the increased understanding of how retroviruses can stably introduce and express their own genes in host cells, researchers have begun to manipulate these viruses to express heterologous genes of interest into target cells.[94,145] Thus in a real way the study of retroviruses has brought the futuristic idea of "gene therapy" to the modern day clinic.[121]

With this as a background to the history and relevance of retrovirology, this chapter will proceed to summarize some key features concerning the classification and life cycles of retroviruses. Next, there will be a discussion of the mechanisms by which these viruses cause neoplastic transformation and the demonstration how our study of the life cycle of retroviruses has contributed to our understanding of cell growth regulation. The chapter will conclude with a brief discussion of endogenous retroviruses and the potential for retroviral vectors to impact dramatically on the therapy of cancer and other diseases in the future.

Classification

The family of viruses known as retroviradae comprise a large group of animal viruses with roughly similar structures. The viral particles are composed of a nuclear capsid or core made up of several protein products of the *gag* gene (Figure III-8-1). This core is surrounded by a lipid membrane derived from the host plasma membrane and contains viral glycoprotein projections encoded by the *env* gene. In whole, the viral particle measures approximately 100 nm in diameter. Within the nuclear capsid resides several enzymatic proteins encoded by the *pol* gene. Also within the core resides the genome of the virus consisting of two single stranded RNA molecules.

The family of retroviruses has been subclassified using various schemas.[140] Historically, they have grouped based on their apparent effects on their host cells. These three subfamilies include the spumaviruses, lentiviruses, and the oncoviruses. These subfamilies have been further broken down into seven different groups based on genomic structures (Table III-8-1). Another somewhat dated classification groups retroviruses A through D based on their electron microscopic morphology (Table III-8-2). Finally, retroviruses are also described as being exogenous if they only infect somatic cells, or endogenous if they are integrated into the germ line of the organism.

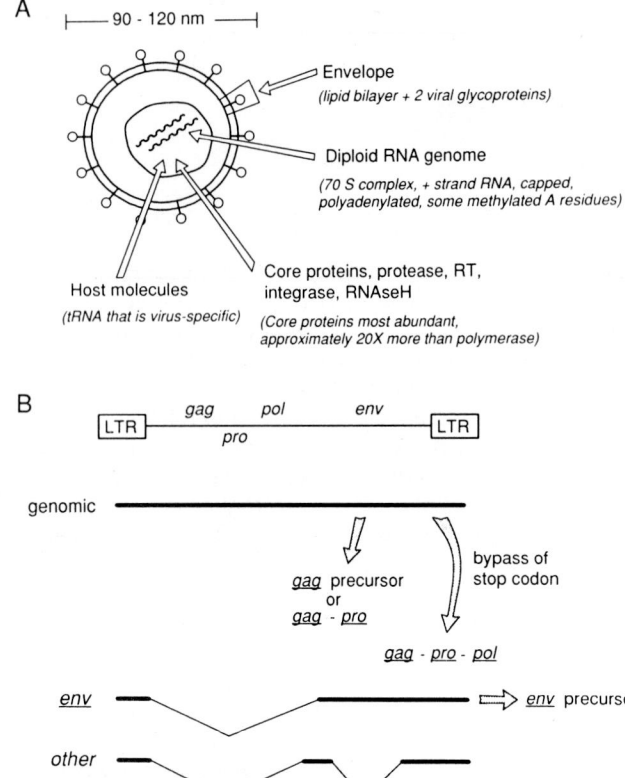

A

|— 90 - 120 nm —|

Envelope
(lipid bilayer + 2 viral glycoproteins)

Diploid RNA genome
(70 S complex, + strand RNA, capped, polyadenylated, some methylated A residues)

Core proteins, protease, RT, integrase, RNAseH
(Core proteins most abundant, approximately 20X more than polymerase)

Host molecules
(tRNA that is virus-specific)

B
LTR   gag   pol   env   LTR
pro

genomic

gag precursor
or
gag - pro

bypass of stop codon

gag - pro - pol

env   env precursor

other

Figure III-8-1. *A,* Structure of typical retrovirus virion. *B,* Structure of typical retroviral genome. All replication competent retroviruses generate a full-length genomic RNA that encodes the *gag* and *pol* products and a singly-spliced RNA that encodes the *env* product. Some retroviruses also generate smaller multiply-spliced messages. (*Pro* - protease; *pol* - polymerase; *env* - envelope; *gag* - core proteins.)

Table III-8-1.   Retrovirus Groups

Oncornaviruses
  Avian leukosis-sarcoma viruses (ALSV)
  Avian reticuloendotheliosis virus
  Mammalian leukemia and sarcoma viruses (mouse/cat type C viruses)
  Mouse mammary tumor virus
  Primate type D viruses (Mason-Pfizer monkey virus/SAIDS virus)
  Human T cell leukemia virus/bovine leukemia virus/simian T cell leukemia virus
Lentiviruses (including immunodeficiency viruses)
Spumaviruses

Structure

All replication competent retroviral genomes contain at least three major structural genes (*gag, pol,* and *env*) and 5′ and 3′ regulatory regions known as the long terminal repeats (LTR) (see Figure III-8-1). Replication defective retroviruses have the same general genomic structure, but contain large deletions of some of the structural genes. These deleted structural genes are often replaced by oncogenes (see below). This section will describe the genomic and protein components of a replication-competent retrovirus.

Table III-8-2.   Retrovirus Morphology

A-type particles
  Intracellular core formation *and* budding
  Intracisternal A-type particles are products of endogenous proviruses
  Non-infectious

B-type particles (MMTV)
  Core formation occurs in the cytoplasm
  After budding at the plasma membrane, maturation to an eccentric core occurs
  Prominent surface spikes

C-type particles
  Most oncornaviruses
  Initially form electron-dense patches at the plasma membrane
  Budding at plasma membrane
  Maturation of core to yield centrally located cores
  Spikes may or not be prominent

D-type particles
  Mason-Pfizer monkey virus, simian AIDS virus
  Intracellular nucleocapsid formation, budding at plasma membrane
  Eccentric core
  Less prominent spikes

Lentiviruses
  Visna-maidi, EIAV, CAEV, SIV, HIV, FIV, BIV
  Core formation and budding as for C-type particles
  Condensed mature core forms pyramidal shape

Spumaviruses
  IAP-like cores

LTR

The LTR plays a vital role in the life cycle of the retrovirus, not only responsible for viral gene expression, but also necessary for viral genomic integration into the host cell chromosomes. Relative to this latter function it is of interest that retroviral LTRs share structural homology with the eukaryotic transposible elements known as retrotransposons.[153] The LTRs contain many regulatory signals necessary for the efficient expression and replication of the retroviral genome. Structurally, it has generally been separated into three regions, U5, R and U3 (see Figure III-8-2). U5 is bounded by the primer binding site (see below). It is the first portion of the retroviral genome to be transcribed by the reverse transcriptase and thus becomes the 3′ LTR of the integrated provirus. This repeated structure is necessary for the reverse transcriptase process. U3 starts out adjacent to R at the 3′ end of the genomic RNA, but after reverse transcription becomes the 5′ end of the virus. This region, therefore, contains many of the regulatory elements necessary for efficient proviral transcription. It is important to keep in mind that all primary retroviral transcripts are initiated at the 5′ LTR and are terminated in the 3′ LTR.

At the 5′ end of U3 are a series of enhancer sequences that help regulate levels of proviral gene expression. These sequences are responsive to host cell transcriptional factors. Examples of such sequences are the NF-κβ consensus sequence in HIV-1, the cyclic AMP responsive elements in HTLV-1 and binding sites for the glucocorticoid receptor in the MMTV LTR.[10,50,107,165] It is precisely because of the

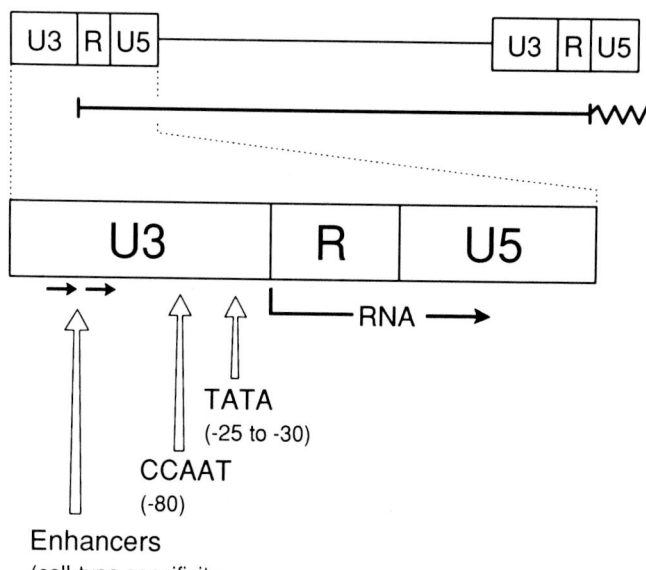

Enhancers

(cell-type specificity,

leukemogenic potential,

expression of endogenous proviruses)

Figure III-8-2. LTR structure. Replication competent retroviruses contain identical long terminal repeats (LTR) at the 5' and 3' ends. The U3 portion of the 5' LTR contains all the enhancer and promoter elements necessary for efficient initiation of transcription of either retroviral or cellular genes. (MuLV, murine leukemia virus; FeLV, feline leukemia virus; MMTV, Moloney mammary tumor virus; MA, matrix protein; CA, capsid; NC, nuclear capsid; PR, protease; RT, reverse transcriptase; IN, integrase.)

dependence on these host cellular factors for efficient proviral LTR directed transcription, that the LTR ultimately plays a major role in determining the host range of the virus.

There are several other important sequences within the LTR. They include "CAT" and "TATAAA" box which lie downstream of the enhancer sequences and function as the promoter for RNA transcription from the proviral DNA.[36,47] At the junctions of U3 and R lies the CAP site where RNA transcription is actually initiated.[18] In the 3' region of R exists the polyadenylation signal for the termination of transcription.

Leader Sequence

Between the 5' LTR and the initiation codon of the *gag* gene lies the leader sequence. Within this short stretch of nucleotides lies three extremely important sequences. One is the primer binding site (PBS). This is the area where a specific cellular tRNA specifically binds to its complementary sequence. The tRNA serves as the primer for the reverse transcriptase (see below).[139]

The second important structure within the leader sequences is the splice donor site for generation of subgenomic messages, usually the *env* transcript.

The third important function of the leader sequence is that it provides the so-called packaging sequences that allow full-length viral RNA to be recognized by *gag* proteins and to be incorporated into the virion particle for export out of the cell.[27,85]

gag

The most 5' structural gene in the genome of all retroviruses is *gag*. The mRNA that encodes for *gag* is the same size as the genomic RNA and is identical to the RNA species that encodes the *pro* (protease) and *pol* (polymerase) genes.[40,112,113,155] The *gag* protein is synthesized as a large precursor that is eventually cleaved into three to five smaller *gag* proteins by both cellular and virally encoded proteases. The viral protease is encoded as a carboxy extension to the *gag* precursor protein as is the *pol* gene product.

The three major *gag* proteins are the nucleic acid binding protein, the capsid protein, and the matrix protein. The nuclear binding proteins are small basic proteins located in the capsid core and are associated with the RNA molecules. Their positive charges are probably vital for effective RNA packaging by neutralizing the negative charges of the RNA phosphate moieties. Another structural motif within the nuclear binding protein that allows for efficient RNA packaging is the zinc finger. This is a peptide stretch containing cysteines and histidines placed in specific positions such that a zinc atom can be incorporated. This structure is known to bind avidly to nucleic acids and is clearly necessary for the packaging of the genomic RNA into the virion.[49,126] Whether a zinc atom is actually necessary, however, remains controversial.

The capsid protein is the major structural protein of the virus and by itself forms the shell of the capsid structure. The matrix protein lies on the outside of the capsid shell and interacts with the overlying membrane of the viral particle. This hydrophobic interaction occurs via the post-translational addition of a myristic acid to the matrix protein.[127]

pro/pol

It is somewhat imprecise to describe *pol* or *pro/pol* as a separate gene, since as mentioned above, these proteins are transcribed from the same RNA species as the *gag* proteins. In essence, they are merely carboxy terminal extensions of the *gag* gene. By necessity the level of production of *gag* protein, however, is usually greater than that of either *pro* or *pol*. How the virus regulates the level of *gag* production compared to the *pol* product varies with the specific types of virus (Figure III-8-3). In the murine leukemia virus (MuLV) there exists a stop codon at the end of the *gag* reading frame, thus ensuring that most transcripts only encode the *gag* protein. The virus, however, has the ability to periodically cause termination suppression by allowing the cellular transcription apparatus to insert a random amino acid at this codon, thus allowing for a read-through *gag-pro-pol* fusion precursor.[167] In contrast, The Rous sarcoma virus (RSV) maintains a greater level of *gag* production compared to *pol* by having the two genes in different but overlapping reading frames. The *pol* product is occasionally made as a *gag/pol* fusion protein by virtue of a short *gag* sequence and resultant downstream DNA secondary structure that allows the ribosome to frameshift into the *pol* reading frame.[67,68,98] In one retrovirus, ALV, the level of *gag* production is the same as *pol* because both genes are contained in one long open reading frame, and thus transcriptional regulation does not occur.

As complex as the creation of these *pro-pol* RNA products

A Suppressor Termination

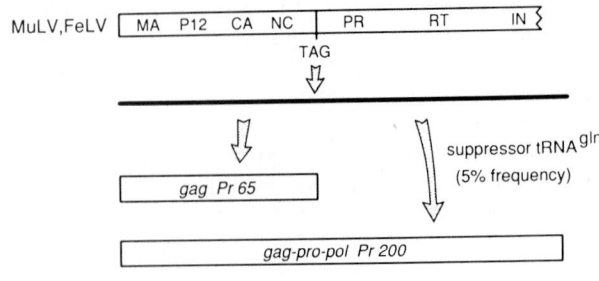

B Ribosomal Frameshifting

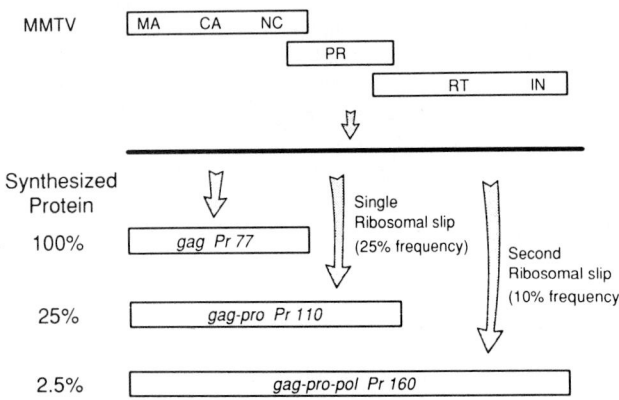

Figure III-8-3. Alternative methods different retroviruses utilize to bypass the *gag* stop codon in order to generate the *pro-pol* products from the full-length genomic transcripts.

is, the function of their protein products is even more complex. As described above, the basic function of the protease is to cleave the *gag* or *gag/pol* fusion precursor into their individual components.

The *pol* gene actually encodes three different enzymes, the reverse transcriptase, a ribonuclease, and the integrase. Although reverse transcriptase was originally discovered in retroviruses, it has recently become clear that reverse transcriptase can be found in many other types of viruses and in eukaryotic cells.[64,136] Nevertheless, retroviruses remain the only known group of viruses whose entire life cycle is fully dependent on the activity of this enzyme. This accounts for why reverse transcriptase is one of the most highly conserved parts of the retroviral genome, particularly at the amino acid level.[23,24] The major function of the reverse transcriptase is as an RNA dependent DNA polymerase. However, the reverse transcriptase enzyme also has significant RNase H activity located towards the carboxyl terminus of the protein.[70] This activity is essential for the removal of the RNA template from the reverse transcribed negative DNA strand, in order to allow synthesis of the positive DNA strand. Another unusual feature of this polymerase is its ability to utilize either RNA or DNA as a primer. As previously discussed, it is in fact a host cell tRNA that serves as the natural primer for retroviral reverse transcriptase.

Integrase is the second enzyme product of the *pol* gene. As its name implies, integrase is a vital component in the

process of proviral integration into the host genome (see below).

Envelope

The final gene that is consistently found in all replication competent retroviruses is the *env* gene. In contrast to the *gag* and *pol* genes which are transcribed from a full-length proviral mRNA, the *env* message is the result of a single splicing event.[95,158] The cellular RNA splicing machinery utilizes the splice donor sequence localized in the leader segment and the splice acceptor sequences invariably found slightly upstream of the envelope initiation codon. Like the *gag* gene, *env* encodes a large precursor protein ranging in size from 150 to 160 kDs in different viruses.[31,37,39] This precursor is then cleaved by cellular proteases to produce a larger and smaller envelope protein. The large envelope protein is seen in electron micrographs as the spike coming out of the virion particle. This larger envelope component is glycosylated and sits outside of the viral membrane.[89] Its major function is to specifically bind to a host cell surface protein that serves as the receptor for that virus.[30,78] It is for this reason that the large envelope protein is generally the immunodominant portion of the virus for host neutralizing antibodies.[104]

The smaller envelope component is the transmembrane protein. It is composed of three segments including the cytoplasmic, transmembrane, and external region. The external region of the transmembrane protein interacts with the larger envelope component effectively holding it onto the surface of the virion.[82] The transmembrane portion of the protein is composed of hydrophobic amino acids and essentially anchors the entire envelope complex onto the membrane of the virus. The function of the cytoplasmic portion of this protein remains obscure. Besides its role as an anchor of the larger envelope component, the transmembrane protein also plays a vital role in the fusion of the virion membrane with the infected cellular membrane following receptor binding.[82]

Variations in Genomic Structure

It should again be re-emphasized that the genomic composition of the retrovirus as outlined above is a generalization of the minimal amount of genetic information carried by replication-competent retroviruses. There are many retroviruses whose genomes encode other structural and/or regulatory proteins.

In particular, the lentiviruses carry many more than just the *gag, pol* and *env* genes. HIV-1, for example, encodes at least eight other regulatory or structural genes, many for which a function has not yet been ascribed.[55] The HTLV-1/ BLV family of retroviruses also encodes at least three additional proteins in a 1–2 kb stretch of genome located between the *env* gene and U3. This region, known as the X region, has many other potential reading frames that may encode proteins that have yet to be identified. Likewise, MMTV, and the spumaviruses have 3′ open reading frames that may encode proteins.

In contrast to the complicated genomic organization of the lentiviruses are some of the acutely transforming retroviruses (i.e., RSV, A-MuLV) which are defective for replication secondary to replacement of some or all of their structural genes with host cellular sequences (i.e., oncogenes, see below).

Life Cycle

The life cycle of a retrovirus is extraordinarily complex, and the details are beyond the scope of this chapter. Nevertheless, the uniqueness of the process, and the importance in understanding the general strategy the virus takes is vital to understanding the mechanism of transformation, and thus will be briefly outlined below (Figure III-8-4). Although retroviral virions may non-discriminantly attach to almost any cell membrane, actual infection is quite specific. The large exterior glycoprotein envelope functions as a specific ligand for cellular membrane-associated proteins. Thus these proteins are effectively receptors for retroviral infection. To date, only the receptors for the HIV family of viruses and the murine ecotropic retroviruses (MuLV) have been identified.[3,88] In 1984 CD4 became the first recognized retroviral receptor with the demonstration that the large HIV exterior glycoprotein (gp120) specifically bound to it. The MuLV receptor was identified by Albritton and co-workers as a multiple membrane-spanning protein.[3]

The frequency with which a particular retroviral receptor is found in different types of cells will play a major role in the host range of that virus. The two known human retroviruses, HIV and HTLV-1, provide a dramatic contrast to this idea of receptor-mediated host range. HTLV-1 has the ability to infect a broad range of cell types, including cells from non-primate mammals. HIV, on the other hand, has a very restricted host range limited to CD4-positive primate cells.

The frequency with which a particular retroviral receptor occurs is not, however, the only envelope property that determines retroviral host range. Following receptor binding, another envelope mediated event must occur. This is the fusion of the viral membrane with the cellular membrane. The transmembrane envelope component is thought to mediate this function.[82] This reaction has apparent specificity as demonstrated by the observation that mouse cells, transfected with and expressing human CD4 still cannot be infected with HIV. This demonstrates that infection requires more than just receptor binding.

When a retrovirus does bind to its appropriate receptor in a fusion-permissive cell, the virion particle is internalized. During the internalization process, the virion loses its membrane coat and the naked core begins to break down in the cytoplasm. At this point the process of proviral DNA generation directed by the reverse transcriptase is initiated (Figure III-8-5). This process can be summarized as follows. Using the tRNA hybridized to the primer binding sequence (located within the leader segment) as an RNA primer, the RT makes a DNA complementary template in the 5 to 3' direction, thereby creating a minus strand U5 R LTR. This

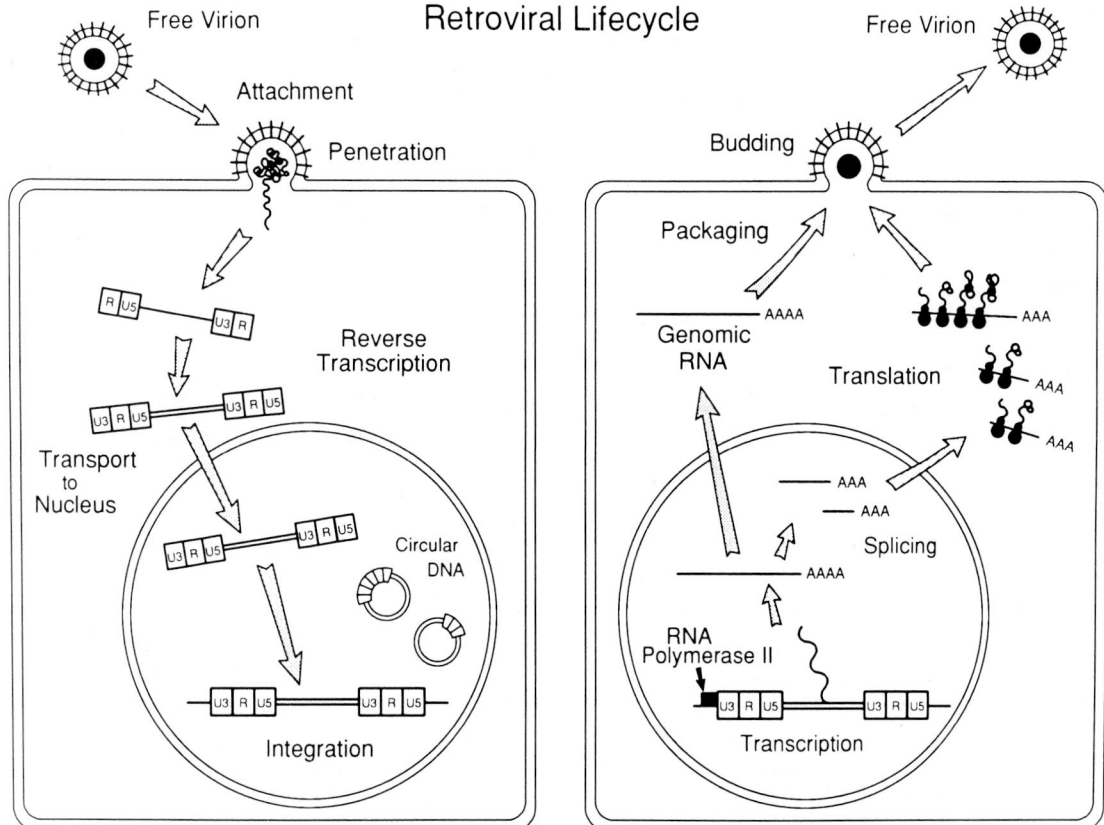

Figure III-8-4. Life cycle. Following the retroviral binding to its specific cell membrane receptor, the viral and cellular membranes fuse, and the core virion is internalized into the cell. Reverse transcriptase directed double-stranded retroviral genomic DNA is then generated, followed by integrase directed integration into host cell DNA. Retroviral transcripts using host transcriptional machinery then proceed with the eventual formation of new retroviral virions that bud from the cell surface allowing for a new round of infection to occur.

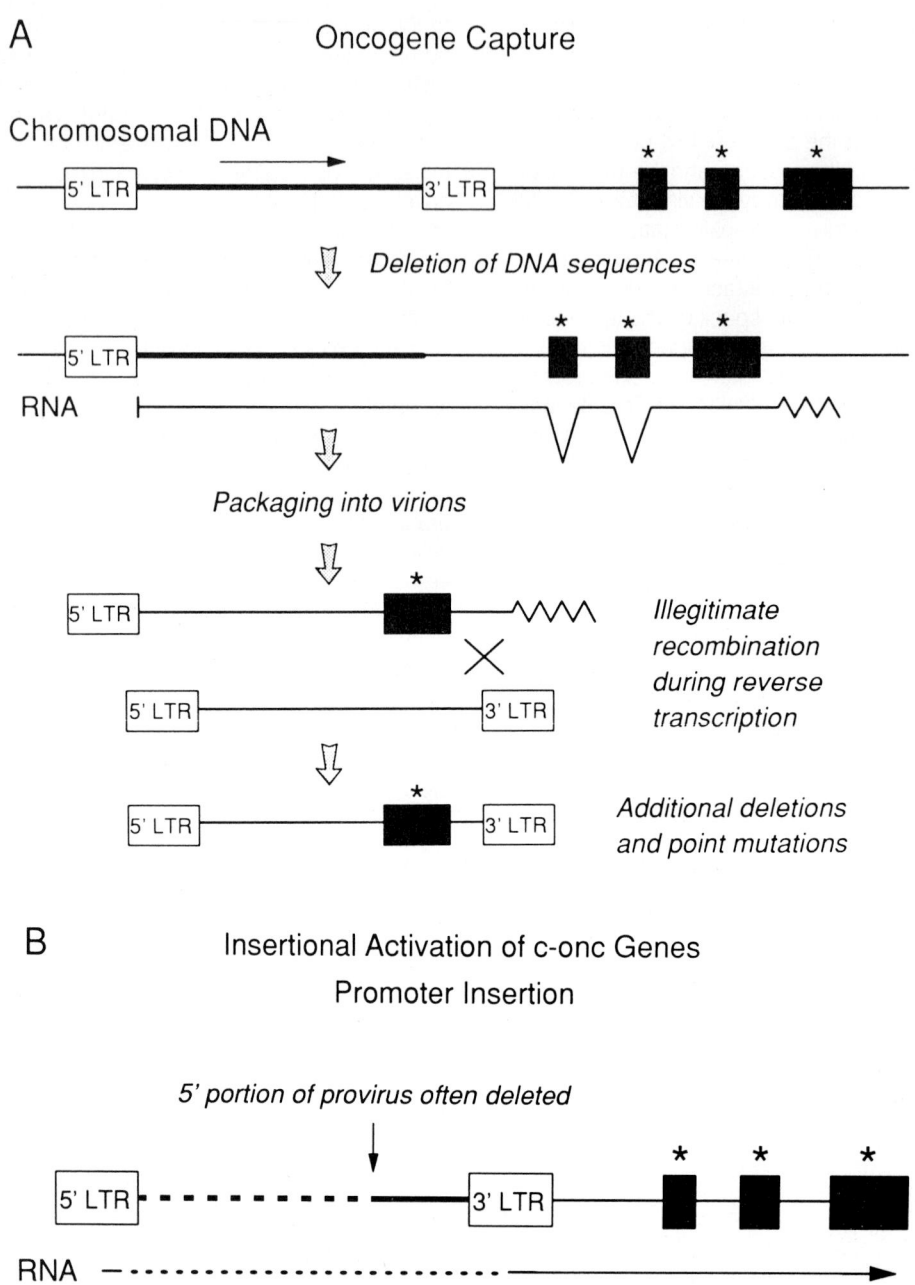

Figure III-8-5. Four mechanisms of retroviral induced oncogenesis. *A*, Oncogene capture. A mutated form of a cellular proto-oncogene (v-onc) is transferred (transduced) to a normal cell, thus inducing transformation. (* - c-oncogene.) *B*, Insertional activation. There is a significant increase in the rate of proto-oncogene expression secondary to LTR directed transcriptional enhancement. (* - c-oncogene.)

piece of DNA is known as "strong stop."[54] Utilizing the RNAse activity the RT digests the U5/R genomic RNA template. The strong stop DNA, along with the RT, thus makes the first of two "jumps" by hybridizing to the genomic RNA at the 3' end using the R genome as the homologous sequence. From here the remainder of the negative DNA strand is synthesized in the 5 to 3' direction. The RNAse activity now removes most of the remaining RNA genomic template except for a short stretch just 5' to U3. This remaining small RNA piece is now used as the primer to create the second strong stop DNA, now consisting of U3, R, and U5 sequences. The 3'

PBS on the negative DNA strand is now cleaved by RNAse activity which allows the positive strong stop DNA to make the second primer "jump" and hybridize at the 5' end of the minus DNA template using the 5' primer binding sequence as the homologous region. From here, the reverse transcriptase can complete the synthesis of the positive strand DNA. In all, the RT reaction has taken a single strand of RNA with unique ends and created a double-stranded DNA species with duplicated LTRs.

Once this double-stranded DNA is created, it must be inserted into the host genome for successful continuation of

C   Growth Stimulation and Two-step Oncogenesis

D   Transactivation (HTLV-1 *tax*)

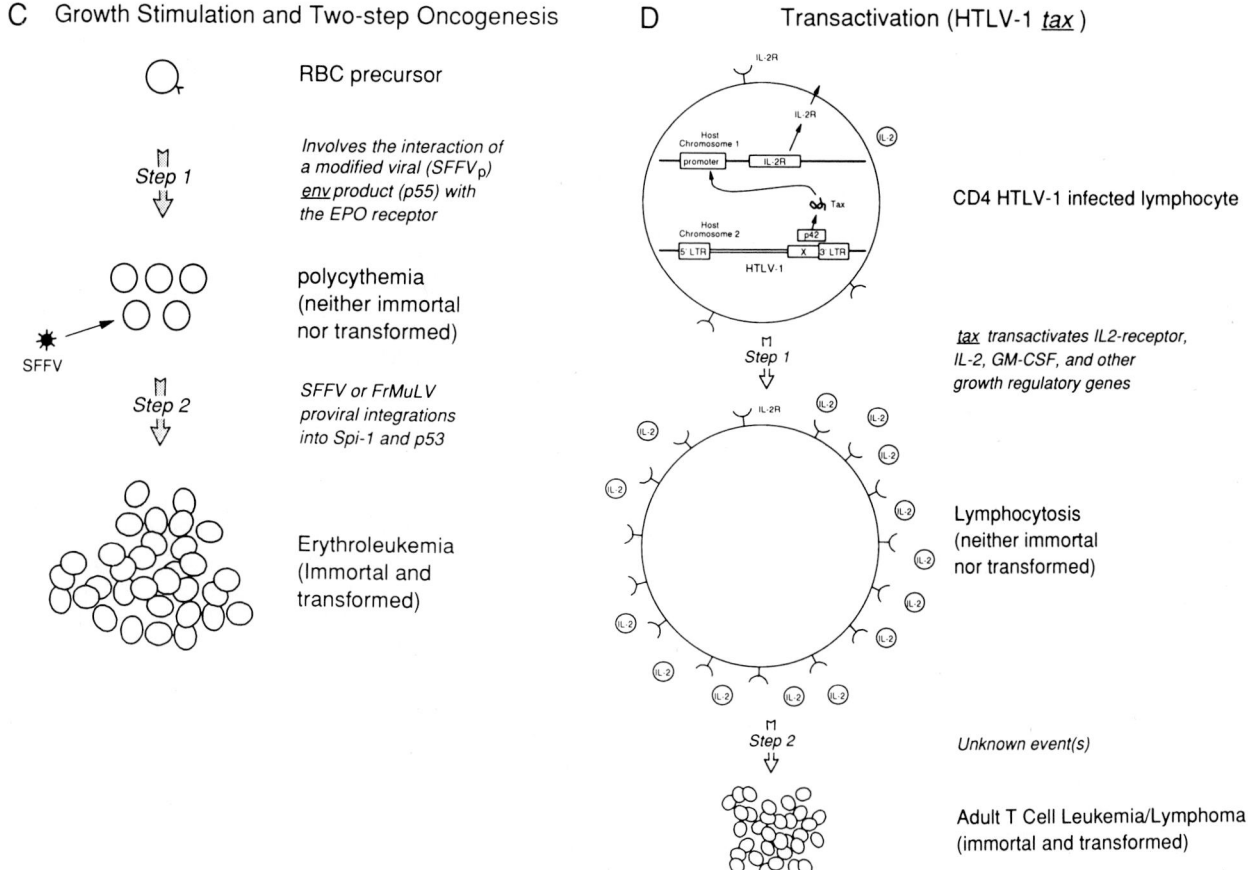

RBC precursor

Step 1

Involves the interaction of
a modified viral (SFFV$_p$)
env product (p55) with
the EPO receptor

polycythemia
(neither immortal
nor transformed)

SFFV

Step 2

SFFV or FrMuLV
proviral integrations
into Spi-1 and p53

Erythroleukemia
(Immortal and
transformed)

CD4 HTLV-1 infected lymphocyte

Step 1

tax transactivates IL2-receptor,
IL-2, GM-CSF, and other
growth regulatory genes

Lymphocytosis
(neither immortal
nor transformed)

Step 2

Unknown event(s)

Adult T Cell Leukemia/Lymphoma
(immortal and transformed)

Figure III-8-5 *Continued.*   *C*, Growth stimulation plus two-step oncogenesis. A mutated *env* protein from the defective SFFV binds to the erythropoietin (EPO) receptor causing an erythrocyte hyperplasia. This increases the susceptible target population to the actual transforming event, a retroviral insertional disruption of the Spi-I or p53 gene. SFFV, spleen focus forming virus; FrMuLV, Friend murine leukemia virus. *D*, Transactivation. The viral transactivating protein (*tax* in the case of HTLV-1) causes expansion of the potential target population through transactivation of growth regulatory genes. Some unknown second event then induces the actual transformation of a clone of these cells.

the viral life cycle. This insertion is dependent on the virally encoded integrase protein (Figure III-8-6). At this point the integrase directs both the viral DNA and a piece of the host DNA to undergo a specific cleavage that creates staggered ends on both pieces of DNA. This reaction is accompanied by deletion of two base pairs from each end of the viral DNA and by duplication of four to six base pairs at the site of the host DNA cleavage. Following this reaction, the DNA is inserted and ligated into the chromosomal DNA. Recent studies using purified integrase preparations have successfully demonstrated that the integrase protein is capable and sufficient for performing all these functions.[21]

Once integrated, viral transcription can proceed. As previously discussed, most retroviruses transcribe two species of mRNA. The full-length transcript can either be used as genomic RNA or as the message for the *gag* or *gag/pol* products. Factors determining how these two transcripts will be utilized have yet to be identified. The second mRNA species made by almost all retroviruses is a singly spliced message encoding the *env* gene. For most retroviruses the splicing reaction is fully dependent on host factors. Some retroviruses such as the HTLV/BLV group and the lentiviruses, however, encode regulatory proteins that influence

how the viral messages will be spliced.[33,58] The *gag* and the *gag/pol* messages are transcribed by free ribosomes and the precursor proteins localize to the cell membrane. This is directed by the fatty acid, myristic acid, which is added post-transcriptionally to the matrix protein.[57,127] At the cell surface it is the precursor *gag* protein that specifically interacts and binds to the genomic RNA.[163]

The envelope mRNA is transcribed by endoplasmic reticulum associated ribosomes for eventual export to the cell surface, following extensive glycosylation in the Golgi body.[119] How the *gag* precursor protein reverse transcriptase complex associates with the envelope protein is still not known. It does appear, however, that full processing of both the envelope and *gag* precursors only appear to occur at or soon after the budding of the nascent virion particle from the cell surface.[168] The retrovirus can now begin a new replication cycle.

Before leaving the subject of the retroviral life cycle, several key points should be re-emphasized. There is no other intracellular parasite that is so consistently efficient at integrating its entire genome into the host cell's DNA. The integration is stable and becomes a permanent genetic component of the cell and its progeny. Thus, not only are

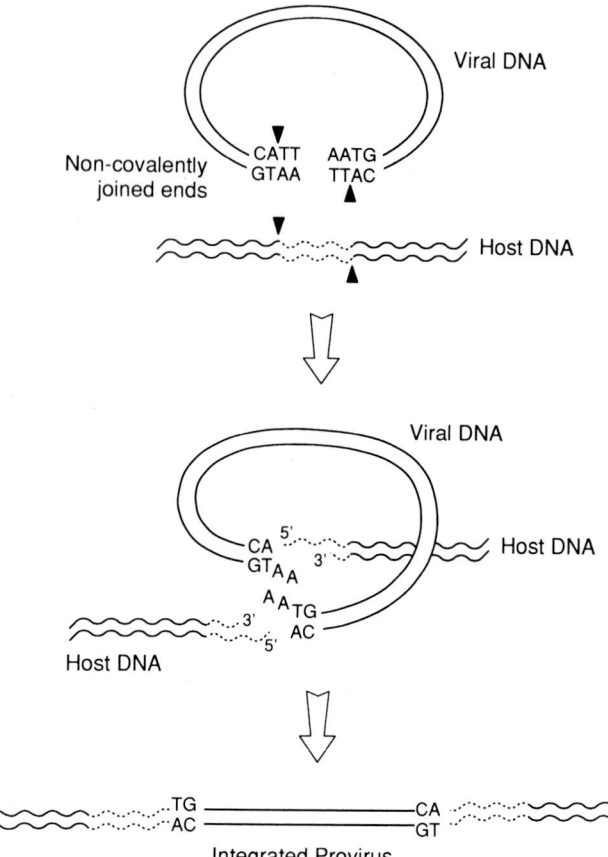

Figure III-8-6. Integration. The newly reversed transcribed double-stranded retroviral DNA genome and a piece of chromosomal DNA are specifically cleaved by the retroviral integrase protein. This is accompanied by a deletion of two base pairs from the retroviral genome and a duplication of four to six base pairs from the host DNA. Following retroviral genomic insertion into the cleaved host DNA, the DNA is relegated.

retroviruses passed down the lineage of a particular cell line, but when they infect germ cells, they become permanent genetic components of the organism. In humans, those proviruses constitute as much as 2–5% of the entire genome.[144] Although certain DNA viruses also have the ability to integrate into host cell DNA, their persistence over a cell lineage is limited by the fact that they usually cause cell death. Retroviruses, on the contrary, are generally not cytopathic and have even developed strategies that potentiate the growth of the infected host cell line. Through these mechanisms, retroviral infection has become ubiquitous in almost all higher organisms.

Another key point to remember is that once a retrovirus has become integrated within a host cell chromosome, its transcription and replication is almost totally dependent on host cell factors. Thus, when the host cell is inactive, so is the virus. Alternately, cellular activating signals (i.e., steroid hormones in mammary tissue) will similarly activate retroviral transcription. The retrovirus has, however, evolutionarily developed some control over this process by selectively incorporating specific cellular enhancer sequences within the LTR (as previously described). This retroviral-mediated control of transcription is taken to another level in the lentiviruses and in the HTLV/BLV group of retroviruses where transcription is directly affected by virally encoded regulatory proteins.

The final point to be made is that retroviral integration does not always proceed without problems. Sometimes only part of the retroviral genome is incorporated into the host cell chromosome. If the incorporated segment includes the LTR and the appropriate packaging signals, a fusion transcript including both viral and cellular sequences could conceivably be made and packaged into a virion. This is exactly what occurs with the oncogene transducing retroviruses as will be described below.

Mechanisms of Oncogenesis

The currently accepted idea that neoplastic growth is a result of genetic alterations stems directly from the study of retroviruses.[22,79,142] Rous was the first to show that sarcomas in chickens could be induced by a transmissible agent.[122] The concept that genetic changes were responsible for these tumors, however, was not appreciated until the isolation of mutant retroviruses that were conditionally defective (i.e., temperature sensitive) for transformation but not replication.[5,77,90] These viruses were uniformly found to have mutations in a 3′ extra open reading frame known as *src*.[154] Through a series of experiments using recombinant viruses it was demonstrated that this intact *src* gene could act as a dominant inducer of the transformed phenotype (oncogene). Thus, for the first time it could be shown that a genetic element was directly responsible for transformation. The significance of these observations was further enhanced when it was demonstrated that the *src* gene hybridized with an endogenous cellular gene found in non-infected host cell DNA.[133] The demonstration that normally occurring cellular genes could, in the correct context, lead to malignant transformation has shaped present day ideas of how neoplastic growth is initiated and how it is maintained.

Since these early discoveries the study of other retroviruses has led to the identification of no less than 50 oncogenes.[11,12] Oncogenes are defined as genetic elements that either alone, or in cooperation with other oncogenes, transform normal cells. They are derived from their normal cellular homologs, the proto-oncogenes. Although the functions of these proto-oncogenes are quite variable, they all share the common property of being important for normal cellular growth and differentiation. It is not surprising, therefore, that either abnormal expression or mutation of these genes could result in neoplastic transformation. In the last 10 years much has been learned about the biochemistry of these proto-oncogene protein products, and how they contribute to the malignant phenotype. This subject is dealt with in detail in I-5. The following section of this chapter will concentrate on describing several different mechanisms by which retroviruses transform cells, and discuss several representative retroviruses that utilize these mechanisms (Figure III-8-7).

Oncogene Transduction

As discussed above, the first oncogenic retrovirus to be described was the Rous sarcoma virus (RSV). It has become

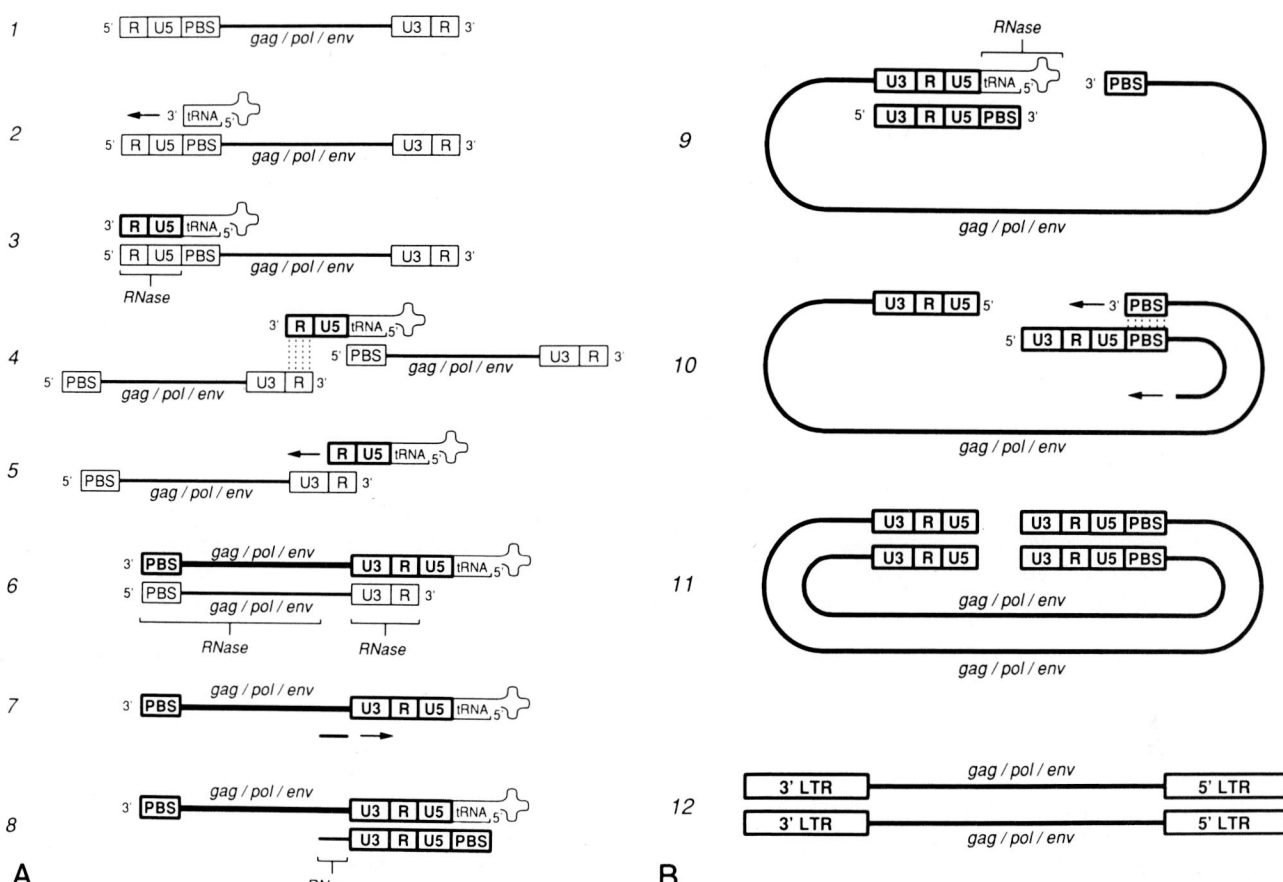

Figure III-8-7. Reverse transcription. From a single stranded RNA genomic precursor, the reverse transcriptase synthesizes a double stranded DNA provirus ready for integration into host cell DNA.

the prototypic virus representative of the group of retroviruses that transform cells by the delivery (transduction) of an oncogene (src in the case of RSV) from the host cell to a target cell. These oncogene transducing retroviruses have several common characteristics. First, these viruses are replication-defective secondary to some or all of their structural genes having been replaced by oncogenes.[13,62,66] Ironically, despite RSV being the prototype of this group, it is the only member of this group that is replication competent. This is because the transduced src oncogene is located 3' to the intact gag, pol and env genes.[27] Along with replication defectiveness, another common characteristic of this group of retroviruses is that they are acutely transforming. This means these viruses will produce tumors in vivo and in vitro within days to weeks of infection.[35] In fact, retrovirally transduced oncogenes are the most potent carcinogens known. The final common property of this diverse group of viruses is that they cause the formation of polyclonal tumors. This probably reflects their high efficiency of transformation and thus any given tumor is made up of many different clones of cells that are the result of multiple different transformation events.

The life cycle of RSV is like that of the typical retrovirus described in the last section. The difference, however, is that in the correct cell type, RSV induces malignant transformation. RSV induces fibrosarcomas and histiocytic sarco-

mas when injected into young chickens.[122] When these chicks (less than one month old) are infected, tumor formation is seen within two to three days. The tumors grow rapidly and in multiple locations (lungs, liver, spleen) and are eventually fatal. Similar tumors are seen when the same viral inoculum is used to infect adult chickens. These tumors, however, spontaneously regress if the bird's immune response is intact.[9,52]

RSV also has the capability of forming sarcomas in mammals, especially if young animals are inoculated. Tumors, however, only occasionally form, and usually only at the sites of inoculation. Furthermore, these tumors spontaneously regress as the animals grow older. This reduced oncogenic potential in mammals has been attributed to the inability of most RSV strains to replicate in mammalian cells in vivo.[4,16]

The virally encoded src gene (v-src) is expressed in all tumors and its central role in tumor induction is supported by the experimental observation that injection of the src DNA into young birds can induce the same tumors.[43] Interestingly, these DNA induced tumors generally regress as is seen when the virus infects adult birds. Such regression demonstrates the importance of continued viral replication and infection of other host cells for the development of the full malignant phenotype.

Another example of an oncogene transducing retrovirus

is the Abelson murine leukemia virus (A-MuLV). The life cycle of this virus is more typical of other transducing oncogenes, than is RSV, because A-MuLV is replication-defective. A-MuLV originally arose in nude mice treated with prednisolone and the Moloney murine leukemia virus (M-MuLV).[1,2] It was found that a transmissible agent from these animals induced lymphosarcomas in both adult and newborn nude mice.[129] Unlike the well-described T cell lymphomas induced by the M-MuLV, however, these nude mice developed B cell lymphomas. This discrepancy was finally explained by the work of Scher and co-workers who isolated a new retroviral strain from these mice, the A-MuLV.[125] A-MuLV induces a B cell lymphoma in most strains of young mice, although adult animals seem to be resistant to tumor induction.

Molecular analysis of A-MuLV revealed a provirus of almost 5700 basepairs long with two open reading frames.[120] The larger reading frame encodes a fusion protein consisting of the 5′ end of *gag* joined to the v-*abl* oncogene. One strain of A-MuLV utilizes the entire v-*abl* oncogene while another strain utilizes a v-*abl* that contains a 263 amino acid internal deletion.[84] These two A-MuLV strains, therefore, encode a p160 and a p120 *gag-abl* fusion oncogene respectively, both of which are transforming. Although the v-*abl* oncogene was clearly derived from the c-*abl* proto-oncogene, sequence analysis demonstrates that c-*abl* and v-*abl* differ substantially from each other.[109] This demonstrates a very important principle underlying retroviral oncogene transduction. Never does the mere addition of a retroviral sequence to a cellular gene allow for the creation of a transforming protein. Rather, all transduced oncogenes to date have been shown to have some (often extensive) changes within the proto-oncogene sequence itself. Specific examples of some of these changes are noted in Table III-8-3.

Another important principle highlighted by A-MuLV is that since it does not contain an intact *gag*, *pol*, or *env* gene it cannot replicate. A-MuLV does, however, infect and transform multiple target cells both in vivo and in vitro. This is

Table III-8-3.   Differences Between v-*onc* and c-*onc* Genes

Only a portion of the cellular oncogene is often present in v-*onc*
v-*onc* is derived from processed MRNA, devoid of introns and flanking sequences
Loss of cellular control elements (promoters/repressors as well as RNA destabilizers)   for some oncogenes (*myc* and *mos*), ↑ level of expression in itself may be transforming

Deletions/rearrangements may affect the structure of the protein itself
    loss of C-terminal Tyr-containing region of c-*src* causes loss of phosphorylation-mediated control by host cell kinases
    v-*erb* B differs from EGF receptor by deletion of the extracellular domain

v-onc genes are often fused to viral sequences important for transforming function
    gag-abl acquires a myrisitilation signal → membrane localization important for transforming activity
    v-*fms* is the CSF-1 receptor fused to *gag* gene product, the latter providing a signal sequence for placement into the cell membrane

achieved through coinfection with a "helper virus." A helper virus is defined as a replication competent virus that produces the structural components necessary for the packaging and infection of the defective transforming retroviral genome. In the case of A-MuLV, the helper virus is usually another murine leukemia virus like M-MuLV. In some transformed cell lines, only defective transforming retrovirus is present. These cell lines are appropriately called "non-producers," since no infectious virus can be made. These replication-defective transforming retroviruses can, however, be "rescued" and used to infect other target cells by the addition of a helper virus to the non-producer cell line. The ability of retroviruses to package heterogeneous RNA genomes is a vitally important property that can be exploited in the laboratory for the creation of retroviral vectors as will be discussed later.

Before leaving the subject of oncogene transduction, it is worth briefly reviewing several proposed mechanisms for how cellular sequences are incorporated into the retroviral genome. It is important to realize the process of retroviral gene transduction has never been reproduced in the laboratory, presumably because it is such a rare event. Nevertheless, there are two leading hypotheses on how this process may occur (Figure III-8-5A). In the most commonly cited hypothesis, a replication-competent retrovirus integrates into the host DNA 5′ to a particular proto-oncogene.[143,151] At some point a deletion occurs that removes the 3′ portion of the retrovirus and the 5′ portion of the proto-oncogene. This deletion leaves the remaining structural retroviral gene (usually the *gag* gene) in frame with the proto-oncogene. This allows for the *gag*/proto-oncogene fusion transcript to be generated. This transcript then undergoes processing, including intron splicing, and is packaged into a virion along with a wild type retroviral genome. Upon subsequent infection of another cell, these two RNA species undergo reverse transcriptase mediated recombination between their 3′ ends. This places a 3′ LTR onto the end of the transduced oncogene, thus allowing for this defective, but oncogene containing genome to be integrated into chromosomal DNA.

The alternative model of oncogene transduction suggests that an intact replication competent retrovirus integrates just upstream of a proto-oncogene (Figure III-8-5B). On occasion, the viral genomic transcript is not appropriately terminated at the 3′ LTR termination signal but instead the RNA polymerase continues to read through into the open reading frame of the downstream proto-oncogene. This creates a full retroviral genomic RNA/proto-oncogene fusion message. At this point either a splicing event or a homologous recombination deletes the viral 3′ and proto-oncogene 5′ sequences thus creating the fusion oncogene message. This latter mechanism necessitates that there exist areas of homology between proto-oncogene and viral sequences for recombination, or that there are appropriate splicing signals for the creation of the hybrid message. Of interest, is the observation that there are extensive homologous sequences between some retroviral structural genes and proto-oncogenes. One such example is the CMII strain of the acutely transforming avian retrovirus subgroup, MC29. In this virus there is a stretch of nucleotides in the *pol* gene that is nearly identical to a nucleotide stretch in c-*myc*. This area corresponds directly with the junction of the gag Δpol/v-myc fusion junction in the CMII virus.[157] This supports the possibility of a recombination event being responsible for the fusion protein. Alternately, Walther and co-workers have reported that the Δgag/v-myc junction in CMII corresponds to a splice acceptor site in c-myc.[157] This site may have been used in conjunction with a potential splice donor site present in some retroviral gag sequences, thus generating the fusion message entirely by a splicing mechanism. In many other retroviruses, however, neither splicing site nor homologous sequences can be found.[71,80] In summary then, it seems most likely that onco-genes have been transduced by various retroviruses using either of these two mechanisms described above, and in some cases, a combination of both.

Insertional Activation

The majority of transforming retroviruses are placed into the group called the leukemia viruses (this name is actually inaccurate since many of the acutely transforming oncogene transducing retroviruses also cause leukemias). In contrast to the oncogene transducing retroviruses, these viruses contain the entire set of structural genes and are replication competent. They are, however, much less efficient at inducing in vivo transformation than are the transducing viruses and generally cause tumors only after long latent periods. Furthermore, they do not induce transformation of cells in vitro. The tumors they do induce are usually monoclonal, again suggesting the rarity of the transforming event. In these virtually induced tumors, the provirus is generally found within the vicinity of the proto-oncogene. It is thought that through its proximity to this gene, the proviral LTR functions as a positive enhancer of increased proto-oncogene expression. This mechanism of transformation is, therefore, often termed insertional or cis oncogene activation. The prototypic retrovirus in this group is the strain of avian leukosis virus (ALV) known as the lymphoid leukosis virus (LLV). LLV is passed from bird-to-bird by both vertical and horizontal transmission. After infection, B cell lymphoblasts begin to accumulate in the bursa of Fabricius within one to two months.[29,102] Although most of the enlarged follicles regress with the natural involution of the bursa, some tumor nodules continue to grow. Within 6–8 months the chicken usually has developed a widespread metastatic lymphoma. Molecular analyses of these tumors have revealed several important points. First, although LLV appears to integrate randomly into host cell chromosomes, all tumor cells were found to have at least one provirus inserted in the vicinity of the c-myc gene.[44,56,101,147] Furthermore, the level of c-myc transcription in these tumor cells is significantly elevated compared to normal cells. Another important feature of this mechanism of transformation is that once the provirus is integrated adjacent to the proto-oncogene in question (i.e., c-myc in the LLV example), continued transcription of viral sequences is no longer necessary to induce or maintain the malignant phenotype.[101,115] That transcription of the proto-oncogene seems to be initiated by the U3 region of the LTR is also characteristic of this mechanism of transformation. For this reason most retroviruses that are acting as enhancers for proto-oncogene expression are found to be oriented with the 3' LTR upstream of the proto-onco-gene.[115]

The mouse mammary tumor virus (MMTV) represents another interesting example of a retrovirus that transforms cells via insertional activation of a proto-oncogene. MMTV was first detected over 50 years ago as a transmissible virus in the milk of a specific strain of inbred mice.[98] These mice were known to have a very high incidence of breast carci-noma, with 90% of animals developing tumors by the age of nine months. Animal breeding experiments showed that MMTV could be transferred horizontally or vertically as an endogenous provirus and that nearly 80% of mammary epi-thelium becomes infected. Although the MMTV proviral DNA has been shown to be randomly integrated in all tissue types, the breast tumor cells were found to consistently have one provirus integrated into a very discrete area of chromosome 15.[106] Although examination of multiple tumors revealed that the exact integration site was always slightly different, it uni-formly occurred around a discrete 30 kb sequence. In addition the provirus, although always adjacent to, never inter-rupted this sequence.[105,150] This DNA segment has now been identified as the proto-oncogene, int-1.[149] It has now been established that int-1 is normally expressed only in the neural tube in midgestational embryos and in the testicular post-meiotic cells.[69,128] However, expression of this gene in the mammary carcinoma cells induced by MMTV suggests a role in the development of the transformed phenotype.[106,116]

The role of int-1 in the induction of mouse breast carcinoma was further suggested by the work of Tsukamoto and co-workers when they demonstrated that transgenic mice carrying an MMTV/int-1 transgene developed breast carci-noma.[148] The specificity of int-1 expression for the devel-opment of breast tumors in transgenic mice must be ques-tioned, however, since it has now been shown that either v-Ha-ras, c-myc, c-neu, or TGF-α when driven by the MMTV promoter all induce the development of breast tumors in transgenic mice.[17,92,130,134] This ability of different genes to induce the same type of tumor suggests that the specificity of mammary tumor induction in these mice is a function of the viral LTR, and not the specific oncogene.

Growth Stimulation and Two-Step Oncogenesis

The defective spleen focus forming virus (SFFV) and its helper, the Friend murine leukemia virus (Fr-MuLV) represent retroviruses with a unique mechanism of tumor induction. Infection of mice with Fr-MuLV and SFFV induces a polyclonal erythrocytosis associated with splenomegaly and hep-atomegaly.[53,162] The cells, however, are neither immortal nor capable of forming tumors in nude mice. Maintenance of this erythrocytosis is dependent on continued viral replication. After a relative long latent period one (or a few) of these proliferating clones of erythroblasts will transform into a tumorigenic clone, and the animal will develop frank eryth-roid leukemia. Individually, the Fr-MuLV never induces the erythrocytosis stage of the disease and can only rarely induce the erythroid leukemia when injected into nude newborn mice after a very long latent period. The defective SFFV always induces the erythrocytosis stage of the disease but this usu-ally remits in time since no more infectious virus is being made. Only rarely can helper-free SFFV induce progression to a full-blown erythroid leukemia (Figure III-8-5C).

Over the last several years, molecular analysis of these

viruses has elucidated the mechanism of this two-stage oncogenic process. The erythroid hyperplasia occurs as a result of the synthesis of the one gene product of the defective SFFV, a mutant envelope protein known as gp55. Recent work has demonstrated that gp55 binds to and stimulates the erythropoietin receptor on erythroid precursors.[87] It is through this mechanism that SFFV can induce erythroid hyperplasia.[124] This represents a novel method by which a retrovirus stimulates cell growth. Although there are retroviruses known to transduce oncogenes which encode proteins that are homologs of normal cellular growth factors (i.e., v-sis and PDGF), this is the only known example where a structurally unique viral protein can mimic the function of a cellular protein.

The second component of the Fr-MuLV/SFFV transformation process can be explained by the observation that rearrangement of the cellular tumor suppressor gene, p53, occurs in a high percentage of Friend erythroleukemia cell lines.[25,99,123] In most of these cell lines, the p53 gene disruption is secondary to SFFV (or to a lesser extent Fr-MuLV) proviral integration. In these tumor cells, p53 protein is either entirely absent or mutated. This concept of insertional mutagenesis of a tumor suppressor gene is another novel retroviral mechanism of transformation. These two mechanisms can be used to explain the synergistic ability of both SFFV and Fr-MuLV to induce erythroid tumors. SFFV provides a proliferation signal to expand the pool of potential target cells for transformation. Fr-MuLV, on the other hand, supplies the needed helper function for the SFFV to continue to infect new target cells. Since proviral integration tends to be a random event, the more integration events that can occur in a larger number of target cells, the greater the likelihood of a specific disruption of the p53 locus and resultant cellular transformation.

Transactivation

The human T cell leukemia virus type 1 and 2 (HTLV-1 and 2) and bovine leukemia virus (BLV) transform cells by an unknown but apparently unique mechanism. Like the *cis*-activation group of transforming retroviruses, HTLV-1 is replication competent, carries no oncogene, and induces a monoclonal leukemia (adult T cell leukemia, ATL) after a long latent period.[15,45,110,137,166] Like the oncogene-transducing retroviruses, however, HTLV-1 can immortalize lymphocytes in vitro, and has no specific site of proviral integration in the transformed cell (Figure III-8-5D).

The transforming capability of these viruses resides in their unique 3' genomic structure called the X region. This area is a 1–2 kb stretch of DNA containing several potential open reading frames. The X region has been implicated in the transformation process from the time it was first identified. This was based largely on the observation that many HTLV-1 transformed cell lines contain defective proviral genomes that encode only the X region product. The X region of HTLV-1 is known to encode at least three proteins, *tax* (p42), *rex* (p27), and p21.[108,131,156] Although *rex* (a post-transcriptional regulator of viral RNA processing) and p21 (unknown function) may still be involved in the transformation process, most attention has focused on the *tax* protein. The role of *tax* in the viral life cycle is to transactivate the viral LTR, which

results in a 100 to 200 fold increase in the rate of proviral transcription.[131] Of even greater potential significance, however, is the ability of *tax* to transactivate endogenous cellular enhancers and promoters. These elements include the enhancer and promoters of the IL-2 receptor gene, the GM-CSF gene, the c-*fos* gene, the vimentin gene, and others.[42,65,96,108] It has been suggested that through transcriptional transactivation of some or all of these growth regulatory genes, *tax* plays a vital role in the transformation process. In recent years three sets of experiments have added support to the idea that the X region and in particular *tax* is involved in oncogenesis. In the first experiment *tax* was shown to induce fibrosarcomas in transgenic mice when incorporated as the transgene.[103] In the second set of experiments, *tax* was shown to induce soft agar colony formation when transfected into a partially transformed rat fibroblastic cell line, and to have the capability of cooperating with an activated *ras* oncogene to transform primary rat embryo cells.[118,138] These experiments clearly demonstrated the oncogenic potential of *tax*. The third experiment demonstrated the relevance of the X-region to ATL, the in vivo disease. In this experiment the X-region was inserted into a novel vector derived from the primate herpes virus, *Herpes saimiri*. Infection of human bone marrow and cord blood with the *H. saimiri*/X region vector resulted in the immortalization of CD4-positive T lymphocytes that had the exact immunophenotype of ATL cells in vivo. These results provide compelling evidence that the X region, and *tax* in particular, are involved in the transformation process. It is possible, however, that these genes do not directly cause the development of ATL in vivo, but rather serve mainly as a proliferative stimulus to increase the number of potential transformation target cells, in much the same way as the gp55 envelope mutant of the SFFV does in the Fr-MuLV system. If this is the case, a second transforming event would be necessary for the full development of ATL. The search for this second event remains an active area of research in the field of human retrovirology.

Immunodeficiency

Besides neoplastic and degenerative neurologic diseases, the other major disease category associated with retroviral infection are immune deficiencies. The prototypic virus in this category is the human immune deficiency virus, HIV, the etiologic agent of AIDS.[8,46] Patients with AIDS have an extraordinarily increased rate of developing high grade lymphomas and Kaposi's sarcoma (KS). Most investigators believe that the relationship between HIV and the development of these tumors is indirect.[41] Clinical experience with other types of both congenital and iatrogenically induced immune suppression has demonstrated the development of a high rate of secondary tumors in these patients. These tumors are generally high grade lymphomas, though other tumors, including KS, can be seen. The mechanism of tumor induction during immune deficiency is thought to be secondary to decreased immune surveillance resulting in inefficient destruction of early transformed cells. It has also been suggested that other viruses, particularly EBV, have a direct role in tumor induction in the immune deficient state. It is of interest that many of the high grade lymphomas in AIDS patients have been found to harbor EBV genomic DNA.[51]

Some investigators, however, have suggested a more direct role for HIV in tumor induction. This is based on several studies that have demonstrated that when the *tat* protein of HIV (the transactivating protein) is placed into transgenic mice, the animals develop KS-like lesions.[154] In other experiments, *tat* protein applied directly to in vitro human endothelial cells induced a pattern of growth that morphologically resembled KS.[38] The significance of these findings to KS induction in AIDS patients, however, remains unclear at this time.

Before leaving the subject of immune deficiency, it is noteworthy to mention another example where tumor induction appears to be intimately related to immune deficiency. It has been known for some time that the Duplan strain of MuLV causes a severe immune deficiency disease in mice. The manifestations of this disease include a polyclonal B cell proliferation resulting in lymphadenopathy, splenomegaly, hypergammaglobinemia, B- and T-lymphocyte functional abnormalities, increased susceptibility to infections, and malignant B cell lymphomas.[20,81,91,111] In 1989 it was demonstrated that the viral stocks of the Duplan MuLV actually consisted of both a helper MuLV and a novel 4.8 kb defective retrovirus. This defective virus was shown to be the actual disease inducing agent since helper-free defective virus could cause the immune deficiency disease in vivo.[34] Subsequent studies revealed that this defective retrovirus is oncogenic and contributes to the transformation of several B cell clones in vivo. This oligoclonal pattern of proliferation apparently then leads to an immune deficiency state as an epiphenomenon of the leukemia or as a paraneoplastic syndrome.[63] It is of interest to speculate whether other immune deficiency inducing retroviruses will be found to be oncogenic in the future.

Endogenous Retroviruses

An important aspect in the relationship of a retrovirus to its host is that proviral DNA can become an inheritable genetic element of that organism if the retrovirus infects a germ cell. Indeed, it has now been estimated that as much as 0.5–1% of the mammalian genome is composed of sequences identifiable as retroviral proviruses.[144] It is generally believed that these endogenous retroviruses have arisen rather late in evolution. This is based on the observation that there is a huge variance in the type and number of endogenous retroviruses between closely related species, thus suggesting the acquisition of these viruses after divergence of closely linked species.[26]

Endogenous retroviruses have several general properties. First, most of these viruses are defective, although a few endogenous retroviruses of mice and chickens can generate infectious virions. In principle, endogenous retroviruses are structurally similar to their exogenous counterparts in that they contain the *gag, pol,* and *env* gene, although they often have large deletions in their genomes sometimes leaving only the LTRs intact. There are some endogenous retroviruses, however, that have only subtle mutations such as frameshifts or point mutations in *gag* and *env* initiation codons. Whether defective or not, it would appear that all these endogenous retroviruses were integrated into the host chromosome by the usual integrase-mediated process as deduced from sequence analysis of their LTR-host DNA junctions.

A second property of these endogenous retroviruses is that not only are there significant differences in endogenous retroviral content between species, but also significant variations within a given species. This suggests that endogenous retroviruses are evolutionarily unstable, and thus not essential to their host. In vivo support of this hypothesis can be found by the existence of totally normal chickens and mice that were specifically bred not to contain endogenous retroviruses. It is still plausible, however, that some type of subtle evolutionary advantage is associated with the presence of specific endogenous retroviruses in a given organism (i.e., immunity against infection from certain pathogenic retroviruses).

Another interesting feature of endogenous retroviruses is their variable level of expression in the host cell. This can span the spectrum from complete lack of transcription to production of infectious virions. There are several potential explanations for this including different sites of integration within a given chromosome allowing for local chromatin structure to control general levels of transcription of genes within that region. Another probable mechanism of transcriptional variation is post-integration chemical modification of the provirus. The most well understood of these mechanisms is methylation of enhancer regions within the LTR which thereby inhibits RNA polymerase transcriptional initiation.[60] A final explanation for the variable expression of endogenous retroviruses probably relates to tissue tropism. Many endogenous retroviruses have been found to harbor glucocorticoid responsive elements in their LTRs, much like the MMTV LTR. It is of interest that retroviral particles have been most often reported in humans in steroid responsive tissues such as embryonic and reproductive organs. These particles have been seen in as many as 66% of all normal placentas and testicular tumors such as teratomas.[6,19,32] It is also reasonable to speculate that other endogenous retrovirus LTRs will be found to contain additional tissue-specific enhancer sequences, thus accounting for much of the variable levels of expression seen with endogenous retroviruses.

The final general principle of endogenous retroviruses is that they are generally not pathogenic. This is not surprising since any inherited genetic element that is deleterious to the host and serves no vital function will be strongly selected against. MMTV is at least one exception, however, where an endogenous retrovirus can be shown to be directly responsible for disease induction. Another example of a pathogenic endogenous retrovirus can be found in the AKR mouse, a strain of animals bred specifically to select for a high rate of leukemia/lymphoma.[141] It has now been demonstrated that through a complex multistage process of endogenous retroviral recombination, re-infection, and proto-oncogene *cis*-activation, most mice develop a fatal T cell lymphoma by the second year of life. Whether there will be other examples of pathogenic endogenous retroviruses, particularly in the human, has yet to be seen. Numerous reports of retroviral particles in human tumor specimens have not been verified. For now it appears that few, if any, replication competent human endogenous retroviruses capable of causing disease exist.

Whether or not infectious endogenous retroviral virions can be found in man, it is clear that endogenous retroviral RNA is produced in all human cells. One specific type of human endogenous retroviral RNA accounts for .05% of the total placental RNA.[76] The types of proteins encoded by these RNAs and their cellular functions remain speculative at this time. One particularly interesting endogenous retroviral transcriptional product is the RNA generated by ERV-3. The three RNA species known to be generated by this virus are 9, 7.3, and 3.5 kb in size. All three RNAs are initiated at the 5' LTR and utilize the same splice donor site within the upstream leader sequence. The smallest RNA species is the natural subgenomic spliced env-coding RNA that is terminated in the 3' LTR. The 9 and 7.3 kb RNA, however, extend through the 3' LTR and are spliced into a human sequence measuring 5.5 and 3.8 kb, respectively.[28,75] The cellular function, if any, of these RNAs remains unknown. Nevertheless, the observation that all normal tissues express at least the 9.0 and 3.5 RNA species, while several different choriocarcinoma cell lines do not, is intriguing.[75]

A final point about the potential ability of endogenous retroviruses to induce disease is notable. Up to this point we have described the potential for these viruses to encode gene products that would produce a dominant cellular phenotype. Endogenous retroviruses, however, through insertional mutagenesis, could result in recessive phenotypes. Two examples of this are well described in mice, namely the D (dilute brown) and Hr (hairless) mutations. Genetic linkage mapping has placed the position of a specific endogenous murine retrovirus at the loci of these genes. Spontaneous reversions of these mutations are almost always associated with deletion of the provirus.[72,135] It is possible that some (or possibly many) variable human phenotypes are secondary to endogenous retroviral insertional mutations of a specific allele. Furthermore, with our growing understanding of tumor suppressor genes, like retinoblastoma and p53, it is conceivable that insertional mutagenesis of one of these alleles may eventually be identified as the recessive defect underlying some of the familial cancer syndromes.

Retroviral Vectors

As investigators begin to understand more about specific genes and their functions, the concept of gene therapy moves closer to reality.[145] The problem of how to deliver a gene of interest to a target cell, however, remains a major obstacle. Traditional laboratory approaches to this problem have included inducing transient changes in the cellular membrane of a target cell, thus allowing passive influx of foreign DNA. These changes have been induced using either electrical current or chemicals.[159] These methods are quite inefficient, however, allowing less than 1 in 10^4–10^6 cells to take up the DNA. Direct microinjection of the DNA has also been used to introduce genes into target cells.[132] This technique is hampered, however, by the frequent acquisition by the target cells of multiple tandem repeats of the microinjected gene in the target cells. Furthermore, this is only useful for introducing foreign DNA into a few cells at a time.

Investigators have also used viruses such as the papilloma virus and herpes viruses as vectors to carry the foreign gene into target cells.[48,100,169] These vectors suffer from being large and difficult to manipulate genetically. In addition, they carry with them many of their own viral genes. Another problem with these vectors is that many of them are maintained episomally and therefore are not integrated into cellular DNA. Thus, the heterologous gene may not be subject to the same transcriptional controls active on endogenous genes.

Retroviral based vectors can potentially overcome all these problems. Retroviruses are efficient at infecting multiple cells simultaneously and integrating a single copy of genetic information into the target cell genome. In addition, the host range of these viruses can be targeted to a particular cell type by changing the type of envelope on the virion ("pseudotyping"). Although many different types of retroviral vectors have been created, the majority have been derived from the Moloney murine leukemia virus (Mo-MuLV). The general principle underlying retroviral-based vectors is that the structural components of the virion can be supplied to any given genomic RNA in trans, as long as the genomic RNA contains the appropriate packaging signals. As described previously, most of these signals are contained in the nucleotide sequences in the 5' leader segment and in the LTRs. Thus, at a minimum a retroviral vector must contain these elements. The gene of interest can then be inserted into the vector and be driven by the vector LTR or by a heterologous promoter (see Figure III-8-6).

Besides the vector itself, the other major components of this system are the genes encoding the structural proteins necessary for virion production. In most retroviral vector systems, these genes are stably introduced into cell lines ("packaging cell lines") such that these cells constitutively make viral proteins and virions. The structural genes, however, have been manipulated such that their RNAs do not contain the appropriate packaging signals, and thus the virions produced in these packaging cell lines do not contain RNA. When the vector, with the gene of interest, is introduced into these packaging cell lines, the vector RNA (which does possess the packaging signals) is incorporated into the virion. These virions then bud from the cell into the supernatant and can be collected and used to infect target cells.

The development of useful retroviral vectors has quickly progressed over the last five years. To date, Mo-MuLV based vectors have been shown to efficiently infect and express heterologous genes in various cell types including murine, canine, and human cells.[59,61,83] Despite these early successes, the development of clinically useful retroviral vectors will have to address several key problems. One such problem is the generation of helper or wild-type viruses. This occurs through recombination between homologous areas of the vector and the structural gene expressors, such that a replication-competent genome with sufficient packaging signals for virion incorporation is generated. This problem has been largely eliminated by placing the different structural genes on different expressors, thus requiring multiple recombination events to correctly occur for the generation of wild-type virus. A second strategy to reduce the yield of helper viruses has been to minimize areas of homology between the vector and the structural gene expressor. One common method for achieving this is by replacing the native retroviral

LTR of the structural gene expressor with a heterologous promoter or heterologous polyadenylation signal.

Another problem with many retroviral vectors is that in vivo gene expression does not always parallel in vitro expression. This is exemplified by a series of experiments utilizing a Mo-MuLV based vector carrying the human adenosine deaminase gene (ADA). These experiments demonstrated that cells infected with this vector produced high levels of ADA in vitro. When these same cells, however, were injected into an animal (mouse or monkey) the level of ADA production was significantly reduced.[73,74,93,160] The reason for this remains unexplained, but maintenance of a high level of expression of the transferred gene in vivo is a problem that must be overcome if retroviral vectors are to become clinically useful.

Another potential problem with the use of retroviral vectors is the possibility of insertional mutagenesis by the vector. With the use of Mo-MuLV based vectors in primates, this concern is highly theoretical and seems quite unlikely for the following reasons. First, even wild-type Mo-MuLV induced transformation has never been shown to occur in primate cells. Furthermore, persistent viremia with replication-competent Mo-MuLV is an important factor in tumor induction in the mouse. With the recent advancement in the development of helper-free Mo-MuLV vectors systems, it seems unlikely that the vector could induce tumors in a mouse, let alone a primate. Finally, tumor induction is usually associated with multiple viral genomic insertions into the target cells, while retroviral vectors generally insert a single copy. In summary then, it would appear that the likelihood of Mo-MuLV vector induced insertional mutagenesis of a primate cell leading to malignant transformation is highly improbable if not impossible. Nevertheless, this theoretical problem remains a concern for vectors based on other retroviruses.

A final major problem associated with the potential clinical usefulness of retroviral vectors relates to their ability to carry only one or a few genes. These vectors, therefore, hold immediate clinical promise only for diseases caused by loss of function by a single gene, such as ADA-deficiency, Lesch-Nyhan syndrome, Tay-Sachs disease, sickle cell cell anemia, and hemophilia. Unfortunately most diseases, like cancer, are the result of a pathogenic process involving multiple genetic perturbations. It is unlikely, even with the discovery of tumor suppressor genes, that the addition of a single gene will completely correct the neoplastic phenotype. Thus for cancer therapy, retroviral vectors hold most promise not for reversing the malignant phenotype but rather for the delivery of a gene that will inhibit the growth of or accelerate the destruction of the neoplastic cells. One example of how such a strategy might work can be found in the ongoing experiments at the National Cancer Institute, where a vector carrying the tumor necrosis gene has been used to infect tumor infiltrating lymphocytes ("TIL cells"). It is hoped that these cells will then target the specific tumor they were derived from and elicit tumor cell death secondary to very high local levels of TIL cell produced tumor necrosis factor.

Conclusion

The study of retroviruses has contributed much to our present day knowledge in many areas of biology. Retrovirologists were the first to show that cellular transformation was the result of genetic perturbations. Through the study of these genetic changes came the discovery of oncogenes, and with it the realization that abnormal expression or mutations of a cellular gene could result in malignant transformation.

The study of the retroviral life cycle has also given us new insights into other general concepts in molecular biology. Examples include new mechanisms of transcriptional regulation such as the glucocorticoid responsive element in the MMTV LTR. Retroviruses have also demonstrated much about the complicated mechanism of RNA splicing and factors that regulate it such as the rev protein in HIV. Scientists have also learned novel aspects of translational control from retroviruses such as the ribosomal frameshifting and termination suppression used to translate the polymerase protein from the gag/pol RNA. The study of gag and envelope processing and assembly has also taught us much about how macromolecules interact.

Outside of the advancements made in basic science knowledge, the study of retroviruses has had an even greater direct benefit. Secondary to the work in the late 1970s elucidating the basic biology underlying the life cycle of these viruses, it finally became possible to isolate two pathogenic human retroviruses, HIV and HTLV-1. In the short time period since their discovery, more has been learned about HIV than any other virus. This knowledge has already translated into the discovery of a clinically useful anti-viral drug (AZT), with other drugs and vaccines already in the clinical testing phase.

Finally, an important lesson learned from retrovirology has been the knowledge of how to utilize these viruses as vectors to carry heterologous genes to target cells. These vectors are uniquely equipped to deliver a single copy of the gene to multiple primary target cells, allowing for integration into the host cell genome, and for expression of that gene at high levels. Through the use of these vectors, the age of gene therapy is at hand. It is an irony of nature that the very agents that are responsible for so many types of disease states may eventually be exploited therapeutically to eradicate these same diseases.

References

1. Abelson, H. T., and Rabstein, L. S.: Influence of prednisone on Moloney leukemogenic virus in BALB/c mice. Cancer Res., 30:2208, 1970.
2. Abelson, H. T., and Rabstein, L. S.: Lymphosarcoma: Virus induced thymic-independent disease in mice. Cancer Res., 30:2213, 1970.
3. Albritton, L. M., Tseng, L., Scadden, D., and Cunningham, J. M.: A putative murine ecotropic retrovirus receptor gene encodes a multiple membrane-spanning protein and confers susceptibility to virus infection. Cell, 57:659, 1989.
4. Altaner, C., and Temin, H. M.: Carcinogenesis by Rous sarcoma virus XII. A qualitative study of infection of rat cells by avian sarcoma viruses. Virology, 40:118, 1970.
5. Bader, J. P.: Temperature-dependent transformation of cells infected with a mutant of Bryan Rous sarcoma virus. J. Virol., 10:267, 1972.
6. Baller, K., Frank, H., Lower, J., Lower, R., and Kurth, R: Structural organization of unique retrovirus-like particles budding from human terato-carcinoma cell lines. J. Gen. Virol., 64:2549, 1983.
7. Baltimore, D.: RNA–dependent DNA polymerase in virions of RNA tumor viruses. Nature, 226:1209, 1970.
8. Barré-Sinoussi, F., Chermann, J. C., Rey, F., Nugeyre, M. T., Chamaret, S., Gruest, J., Diouguet, G., Axler-Blin, C., Vezinet-Brun, F., Rouzioux, C., Rozenbaum, W., and Montagnier, L.: Isolation of a T-lymphotropic retrovirus from a patient at risk for acquired immune deficiency syndrome (AIDS). Science, 220:868, 1983.
9. Beard, J. W.: Biology of oncorna viruses. In Viral Oncology. Edited by G. Klein. New York, Raven Press, 1980, p. 55.
10. Bielinska, A., Krashow, B., and Nabel, G. J.: NF-kappa B-mediated activation of the human immunodeficiency virus enhancer: Site of transcription initiation is independent of the TATA box. J. Virol., 63:4097, 1989.
11. Bishop, J. M.: Viral oncogenes. Cell, 42:23, 1985.
12. Bishop, J. M.: The molecular genetics of cancer. Science, 235:305, 1987.

13. Bister, K., and Vogt, P. K.: Genetic analysis of the defectiveness in strain MC29 avian leukemia virus. Virology, 88:213, 1978.
14. Bittner, J. J.: Some possible effects of nursing on mammary gland tumor incidence. Science, 84:162, 1936.
15. Blattner, W. A., Kalyanaraman, V. S., Robert-Guroff, M., Lister, T. A., Galton, D. A., Sarin, P. S., Crawford, M. H., Catovsky, D., Greaves, M., and Gallo, R. C.: The human type-C retrovirus, HTLV, in Blacks from the Caribbean region, and relationship to adult T-cell leukemia/lymphoma. Int. J. Cancer, 30:257, 1982.
16. Boettiger, D., Love, D. M., and Weiss, R. A.: Virus envelope markers in mammalian tropism of avian RNA tumor viruses. J. Virol., 15:108, 1975.
17. Bouchard, L., Lamore, L., Tremblay, P. J., and Jolicoeur, P.: Stochastic appearance of mammary tumors in transgenic mice carrying MMTV/c-neu oncogene. Cell, 57:931, 1989.
18. Breathnach, R., and Chambon, P.: Organization and expression of eucaryotic split gene coding for proteins. Annu. Rev. Biochem., 50:349, 1981.
19. Bronson, D., Saxinger, W., Ritz, D., and Fraley, E.: Production of virions with retrovirus morphology by human embryonal carcinoma cells in vitro. J. Gen. Virol., 65:1043, 1984.
20. Buller, R. M. L., Yetter, R. A., Fredrickson, T. N., Morse, H. C., III: Abrogation of resistance to severe mousepox in C47BL/6 mice infected with LP-BM5 murine leukemia viruses. J. Virol., 61:383, 1987.
21. Bushman, F. D., Fujiwara, T., and Craigie, R.: Retroviral DNA integration directed by HIV integration protein in vitro. Science, 249:1555, 1990.
22. Cairns, J.: Mutation selection and the natural history of cancer. Nature, 255:197, 1975.
23. Chiu, I. M., Callahan, R., Tronick, S. R., Schlom, J., and Aaronson, S. A.: Major pol gene progenitors in the evolution of oncoviruses. Science, 223:364, 1984.
24. Chiu, I. M., Yasiv, A., Dahlberg, J. E., Gazit, A., Skuntz, S. F., Tronick, S. R., and Aaronson, S. A.: Nucleotide sequence evidence for relationship of AIDS retrovirus and lentiviruses. Nature, 387:364, 1985.
25. Chow, V., Ben-David, Y., Bernstein, A., Benchimol, S., and Mowat, M.: Multistage Friend erythroleukemia: Independent origin of tumor clones with normal or rearranged p53 cellular oncogenes. J. Virol., 61:3777, 1987.
26. Coffin, J.: Endogenous viruses. *In* RNA Tumor Viruses. Edited by R. Weiss, N. Teich, H. Varmus, and J. Coffin. Cold Spring Harbor, New York, Cold Spring Harbor Laboratory, 1984, p.1109.
27. Coffin, J. M.: Structure of the retroviral genome. *In* RNA Tumor Viruses. Edited by R. Weiss, N. Teich, H. Varmus, and J. Coffin. Cold Spring Harbor, New York, Cold Spring Harbor Laboratory, 1984, p. 261.
28. Cohen, M., Kato, N., and Larsson, E.: ERV3 human endogenous provirus mRNAs are expressed in normal and malignant tissues and cells, but not in choriocarcinoma tumor cells. J. Cell Biochem., 36:121, 1988.
29. Cooper, M. D., Payne, L. N., Dent, P. B., Burmester, B. R., and Good, R. A.: Pathogenesis of avian lymphoid leukosis. J. Natl. Cancer Inst., 41:373, 1968.
30. DeLarco, J., and Todaro, G. J.: Membrane receptors for murine leukemia viruses: Characterization using the purified viral envelope glycoprotein, gp71. Cell, 8:365, 1976.
31. Dickson, C., Puma, J. P., and Nandi, S.: Identification of a precursor protein to the major glycoproteins of mouse mammary tumor virus. J. Virol., 17:275, 1976.
32. Dirksen, E., and Levy, J.: Virus-like particles in placentas from normal individuals and patients with systemic lupus erythematosus. J. Natl. Cancer Inst., 59:1187, 1977.
33. Dokhelar, M. C., Pickford, H., Sodroski, J., and Haseltine, W. A.: HTLV–1 p27rex regulates gag and env protein expression. J. Acquir. Immune Defic. Syndr., 2:431, 1989.
34. Douglas, C. A., Hanna, Z., and Jolicoeur, P.: Severe immunodeficiency disease induced by a defective murine leukemia virus. Nature, 338:505, 1989.
35. Duesberg, P. H.: Retroviral transforming genes in normal cells? Nature, 304:219, 1983.
36. Efstratiadle, A., Posakony, J. W., Maniatle, T., Lawn, R. M., O'Connell, C., Spritz, R. A., DeRiel, J. R., Forget, B. G., Weissman, S. M., Slightom, J. L., Blachi, A. E., Smithiers, O., Baralle, F. E., Shouldere, C. C., and Proudfoot, N. J.: The structure and evolution of the human β-globin gene family. Cell, 21:653, 1980.
37. England, J. M., Bolognesi, D. P., Dietzschold, B., and Halpern, M. S.: Evidence that a precursor glycoprotein is cleaved to yield the major glycoprotein of avian tumor virus. J. Virol., 21:810, 1977.
38. Ensoli, B., Barillari, G., Salahuddin, S. Z., Gallo, R. C., and Wong-Staal, F.: Tat protein of HIV-1 stimulates growth of cells derived from Kaposi's sarcoma lesions of AIDS patients. Nature, 345:84, 1990.
39. Famulari, N. G., Buchhagen, D. L., Klenk, H. D., and Fleissner, E.: Presence of murine leukemia virus envelope proteins gp70 and p15 (E) in a common polyprotein of infected cells. J. Virol., 20:501, 1976.
40. Fan, H., and Verma, I. M.: Size analysis and relationship of murine leukemia virus-specific mRNAs: Evidence for transposition of sequences during synthesis and processing of subgenomic mRNA. J. Virol., 26:468, 1978.
41. Fauci, A. S.: The human immunodeficiency virus: Infectivity and mechanisms of pathogenesis. Science, 239:617, 1988.
42. Fujii, M., Sassone-Corsi, P., and Verma, I. M.: c-fos promoter trans-activation by the tax1 protein of human T cell leukemia virus type 1. Proc. Natl. Acad. Sci. U.S.A., 85:8526, 1988.
43. Fung, Y. K., Crittenden, L. B., Fadly, A. M., and Kung, H. J.: Tumor induction by direct injection of cloned v-src DNA into chickens. Proc. Natl. Acad. Sci. U.S.A., 80:353, 1983.
44. Fung, Y. K., Fadly, A. M., Crittenden, L. B., and Kung, H. J.: One of the mechanisms of retrovirus-induced avian lymphoid leukosis: Deletion and integration of the provirus. Proc. Natl. Acad. Sci. U.S.A., 78:3418, 1981.
45. Gallo, R. C., Blattner, W. A., Reitz, M. B., Jr., and Ito, Y: HTLV: The virus of adult T-cell leukemia in Japan and elsewhere (letter). Lancet, 1:683, 1982.
46. Gallo, R. C., Salahuddin, S. Z., Popovic, M., Shearer, G. M., Kaplan, M., Hayns, B. F., Palker, T. S., Redfield, R., Oleske, J., Safai, B., White, B., Fester, P., and Markham, P. D.: Frequent detection and isolation of cytopathic retroviruses (HTLV-III) from patients with AIDS and at risk for AIDS. Science, 224:500, 1984.
47. Gannon, F., O'Hare, K., Perrin, F., LePennec, J. P., Benoist, C., Cochet, M., Breathnach, R., Royal, A., Garapin, A., Cami, B., and Chambon, P.: Organization and sequences at the 5′ end of a cloned complete ovalbumin gene. Nature, 278:428, 1979.
48. Grassman, R., Dengler, C., Muller-Fleckenstein, I., Fleckenstein, B., McGuire, K., Dokhelar, M. C., Sodroski, J. G., and Haseltine, W. A.: Transformation to continuous growth of primary human T lymphocytes by human T-cell leukemia virus type I X-region genes transduced by a Herpesvirus saimiri vector. Proc. Natl. Acad. Sci. U.S.A., 86:3351, 1989.
49. Green, L. M., and Berg, J. M.: A retroviral Cys-Xaa_2-Cys-Xaa_4-His-Xaa_{-4}-Cys peptide binds metal ions: Spectroscopic studies and a proposed three-dimensional structure. Proc. Natl. Acad. Sci. U.S.A., 86:4047, 1989.
50. Griffin, G. E., Leung, K., Folks, T. M., Kunkel, S., and Nabel, G. J.: Activation of HIV gene expression during monocyte differentiation by induction of NF-kappa B. Nature, 339:70, 1989.
51. Groopman, J. E., Sullivan, J. L., Mulder, C., Ginsburg, D., Orkin, S. H., O'Hara, C. J., Falchuk, K., Wong-Staal, F., and Gallo, R.C.: Pathogenesis of B cell lymphoma in a patient with AIDS. Blood, 87:612, 1986.
52. Gross, L.: The Rouse chicken sarcoma. *In* Oncogenic Viruses. 2nd Ed. Oxford, Pergamon Press, 1970, pp. 99–157.
53. Hankins, W. D., Kost, T. A., Koury, M. J., and Krantz, S. B.: Erythroid bursts produced by Friend leukemia virus in vitro. Nature, 276:506, 1978.
54. Haseltine, W. A., Kleid, D. G., Panet, A., Rothenberg, E., and Baltimore, D.: Ordered transcription of RNA tumor virus genomes. J. Med. Biol., 106:109, 1976,
55. Haseltine, W. A., and Wong-Staal, F.: The molecular biology of the AIDS virus. Sci. Am., 259:52, 1988.
56. Hayward, W. S., Neel, B. G., and Astrin, S. M.: Activation of a cellular on gene by promoter insertion in ALV-induced lymphoid leukosis. Nature, 290:475, 1981.
57. Henderson, L. E., Krutzsch, H. C., and Oroszlan, S.: Myristyl amino-terminal acylation of murine retrovirus proteins: An unusual post-translational protein modification. Proc. Natl. Acad. Sci, U.S.A., 80:339, 1983.
58. Hidakka, M., Inoue, J., Yoshida, M., and Seiki, M.: Post-transcriptional regulator (rex) of HTLV–1 initiates expression of viral structural proteins but suppresses expression of regulatory proteins. EMBO J., 7:519, 1988.
59. Hock, R. A., and Miller, A. D.: Retrovirus-mediated transfer and expression of drug resistance genes in human haematopoietic progenitor cells. Nature, 320:275, 1986.
60. Hoffman, J. W., Steffer, D., Gusella, J., Tabin, C., Bird, S., Cowing, D., and Weinberg, R. W.: DNA methylation affecting the expression of murine leukemia proviruses. J. Virol., 44:144, 1982.
61. Hogge, D. E., and Humphries, R. K.: Gene transfer to primary normal and malignant human hemopoietic progenitors using recombinant retroviruses. Blood, 69:611, 1987.
62. Hu, S. S., Moscovici, C., and Vogt, P. K.: The defectiveness of Mill Hill 2, a carcinoma-inducing avian oncovirus. Virology, 89:162, 1978.
63. Huang, M., Simard, C., and Jolicoeur, P.: Immunodeficiency and clonal growth of target cells induced by helper-free defective retrovirus. Science, 246:1614, 1989.
64. Hull, R., and Covey, S. N.: Does the cauliflower moseric virus replicate by reverse transcription? Trends in Bioch. Sci., 8:119, 1983.
65. Inoue, J., Seiki, M., Taniguchi, T., Tsuru, S., and Yoshida, M.: Induction of interleukin 2 receptor gene expression by p40x encoded by human T cell leukemia virus type 1. EMBO J., 5:2883, 1986.
66. Ishizaki, R., Langlois, A. J., Chabot, J., and Beard, J. W.: Component of strain MC29 avian leukosis virus with the property of defectiveness. J. Virol., 8:821, 1971.
67. Jacks, T., and Varmus, H. E.: Expression of the Rous sarcoma virus pol gene by ribosomal frameshifting. Science, 320:1237, 1985.
68. Jacks, T., Townsley, K., Varmus, H. E., and Major, J.: Two efficient ribosomal frameshifting events are required for synthesis of mouse mammary tumor virus gag-related polyproteins. Proc. Natl. Acad. Sci. U.S.A., 84:4298, 1987.
69. Jakobovits, A., Shackleford, G. M., Varmus, H. E., and Martin, G. R.: Two proto-oncogenes implicated in mammary carcinogenesis, int-1 and int-2, are independently regulated during mouse development. Proc. Natl. Acad. Sci. U.S.A., 83:7806, 1986.
70. Janese, N., and Goff, S. P.: Domain structure of the Moloney murine leukemia virus reverse transcriptase: Mutational analysis and separate expression of the DNA polymerase and RNAse H activities. Proc. Natl. Acad. Sci. U.S.A., 85:1777, 1988.
71. Jansen, H. W., and Bister, K.: Nucleotide sequence analysis of the chicken gene c-mil, the progenitor of the retroviral oncogene v-mil. Virology, 143:359, 1985.
72. Jenkins, N. A., Copeland, N. G., Taylor, B. A., and Lee, B. K.: Dilute (d) coat color mutation of DBA/2j mice is associated with the site of integration of an ecotropic MuLV genome. Nature, 293:370, 1981.
73. Kantoff, P. W., Gillio, A. P., McLachlin, J. R., Bordignon, C., Eglitis, M. A., Kernan, N. A., Moen, R. C., Kohn, D. B., Yu, S. F., Karson, E., Karlsson, S., Zwiebel, J. A., Gilboa, E., Blaese, R. M., Nienhuis, A., O'Reilly, R. J., and Anderson, W. F.: Expression of human adenosine deaminase in nonhuman primates after retrovirus-mediated gene transfer. J. Exp. Med., 166:219, 1987.
74. Kantoff, P. W., Kohn, D. B., Mitsuya, H., Armentano, D., Sieberg, M., Zwiebel, J. A., Eglitis, M. A., McLachlin, J. R., Wiginton, D. A., Hutton, J. J., Horowitz, S. D., Gilboa, E., Blaese, R. M., and Anderson, W. F.: Correction of adenosine deaminase deficiency in cultured human T and B cells by retrovirus-mediated gene transfer. Proc. Natl. Acad. Sci. U.S.A., 83:6563, 1986.
75. Kato, N., Larsson, E., and Cohen, M.: Absence of expression of a human endogenous retrovirus is correlated with choriocarcinoma. Int. J. Cancer, 41:380, 1988.
76. Kato, N., Pfeifer-Ohlsson, S., Kato, M., Larsson, E., Rydnert, J., Ohlsson, R., and Cohen, M.: Tissue-specific expression of human provirus ERV3 mRNA in human placenta: Two of the three ERV3 mRNAs contain human cellular sequences. J. Virol., 61:2182, 1987.
77. Kawai, S., and Hanafusa, H.: The effects of reciprocal changes in the temperature on the transformed state of cells infected with a Rous sarcoma virus mutant. Virology, 46:470, 1971.
78. Kennel, S. J., Del Villano, B. C., Levy, R., and Lesner, R. A.: Properties of an oncornavirus glycoprotein: Evidence for its presence on the surface of virions and infected cells. Virology, 55:464, 1973.
79. Klein, G.: The role of gene dosage and genetic transpositions in carcinogenesis. Nature, 294:313, 1981.
80. Klempnauer, K. H., Gonda, T. J., and Bishop, J. M.: Nucleotide sequence of the retroviral leukemia gene v-myb and its cellular progenitor c-myb: The architecture of a transduced oncogene. Cell, 31:453, 1982.
81. Klinken, S. P., Fredrickson, T. N., Hartley, J. W., Yetter, R. A., and Morse, H. C., 3d.:

Evolution of B cell lineage lymphomas in mice with a retrovirus induced immunodeficiency syndrome, MAIDS. J. Immunol., 140:1123, 1988.
82. Kowalski, M., Potz, J., Basiripour, L., Dorfman, T., Goh, W. C., Terwilliger, E., Dayton, A., Rosen, C., Haseltine, W., and Sodroski, J.: Functional regions of the envelope glycoprotein of human immunodeficiency virus type 1. Science, 237:1351, 1987.
83. Laneuville, P., Chang, W., Kamel-Reid, B., Fauser, A. A., and Dick, J. E.: High efficiency gene transfer and expression in normal human hematopoietic cells with retrovirus vectors. Blood, 71:811, 1988.
84. Lee, R., Paskind, M., Wang, J. Y. J., and Baltimore, D.: Abelson (p160) murine leukemia virus (ab-MLV) abl gene. *In* RNA Tumor Viruses. Edited by R. Weiss, N. Teich, H. Varmus, and J. Coffin. New York, Cold Spring Harbor Laboratory, 1985, p. 861.
85. Lever, A., Gottlinger, H., Haseltine, W., and Sodroski, J.: Identification of a sequence required for efficient packaging of human immunodeficiency virus type 1 RNA into virions. J. Virol., 63:4085, 1989.
86. Levy, J. A., Hoffman, A. D., Kramer, S. N., Landis, J. A., and Shimabukura, J. M.: Isolation of lymphocytopathic retroviruses from San Francisco patients with AIDS. Science, 225:84, 1984.
87. Li, J. P., D'Andrea, A. D., Lodish, H. F., and Baltimore, D.: Activation of cell growth by binding of Friend spleen focus-forming virus gp55 glycoprotein to the erythropoietin receptor. Nature, 343:762, 1990.
88. Madden, P. J., Dalgleish, A. G., McDougal, J. S., Chapman, P. R., Weiss, R. A., and Axel, R.: The TH gene encodes the AIDS virus receptor and is expressed in the immune system and the brain. Cell, 47:333, 1986.
89. Marguardt, H., Gilden, R. V., and Oroszlan, S.: Envelope glycoproteins of Rauscher murine leukeima virus: Isolation and chemical characterization. Biochemistry, 16:710, 1977.
90. Martin, G. S.: Rous sarcoma virus: A function required for the maintenance of the transformed state. Nature, 227:1021, 1970.
91. Masier, D. E., Yetter, R. A., and Morse, H. C., III: Retroviral induction of acute lymphoproliferative disease and profound immunosuppression in adult C57BL/6 mice. J. Exp. Med., 161:766, 1985.
92. Matsui, Y., Halter, S. A., Holt, J. T., Hogan, B. L., and Coffey, R. J.: Development of mammary hyperplasia and neoplasia in MMTV-TFGα transgenic mice. Cell, 61:1147, 1990.
93. McLachlin, J. R., Bernstein, S. C., and Anderson, W. F.: Separation of human from mouse and monkey adenosine deaminase by ion-exchange chromatography following retroviral-mediated gene transfer. Anal. Biochem., 163:143, 1987.
94. McLachlin, J. R., Cornetta, K., Eglitis, M. A., and Anderson, W. F.: Retroviral-mediated gene transfer. Progress in Nucl. Acid Res. and Mol. Biol., 38:91, 1990.
95. Mellon, P., and Duesberg, P. H.: Subgenomic cellular Rous sarcoma virus RNAs contain oligonucleotides from the 3′ half and the 5′ terminus of virion RNA. Nature, 270:631, 1977.
96. Miyatake, S., Seiki, M., Yoshida, M., and Arai, K.: T-cell activation signals and human T-cell leukemia virus type 1–encoded p40x protein activate the mouse granulocyte-macrophage colony-stimulating factor gene through a common DNA element. Mol. Cell Biol., 8:5581, 1988.
97. Moore, D. H., Long, C. A., Vaidya, A. D., Sheffield, J. B., Dion, A. S., and Lasfargues, E. Y.: Mammary tumor viruses. Adv. Cancer Res., 29:347, 1979.
98. Moore, R., Dixon, M., Smith, R., Peters, G., and Dickson, C.: Complete nucleotide sequence of a milk-transmitted mouse mammary tumor virus: Two frameshift suppression events are required for translation of gag and pol. J. Virol., 61:480, 1987.
99. Mowat, M., Cheng, A., Kimura, N., Berstein, A., and Berchimel, S.: Rearrangements of the cellular p53 gene in erythroleukemia cells transformed by Friend virus. Nature, 314:633, 1985.
100. Mulligan, R. C., Howard, B. H., and Berg, P.: Synthesis of rabbit beta-globin in cultured monkey kidney cells following infection with a SV40 beta-globin recombinant gemome. Nature, 277:108, 1979.
101. Neel, B. G., Hayward, W. S., Robinson, H. L., Frang, J., and Astrin, S. M.: Avian leukosis virus-induced tumors have common proviral integration sites and synthetic discrete new RNAs: Oncogenesis by promoter insertion. Cell, 23:323, 1981.
102. Neiman, P. E., Jordan, L., Weiss, R. A., and Payne, L. N.: Malignant lymphoma of the bursa of Fabricius: Analysis of early transformation. Cold Spring Harbor Conf. Cell Proliferation, 7:519, 1980.
103. Nerenberg, M., Hinrichs, S. W., Reynolds, R. K., Khoury, G., and Jay, G.: The tat gene of human T-lymphotropic virus type 1 induce mesenchymal tumors in transgenic mice. Science, 237:1324, 1987.
104. Nowinski, R. C., Fleissner, E., Sarkar, N. H., and Aoki, T.: Chromatographic separation and antigenic analysis of proteins of the oncornaviruses. J. Virol., 9:359, 1972.
105. Nusse, R., and Varmus, H. E.: Many tumors induced by mouse mammary tumor virus contain a provirus integrated in the same region of the host genome. Cell, 31:99, 1982.
106. Nusse, R. A., von Ooyen, A., Cox, D., Fung, Y. K., and Varmus, H.: Mode of proviral activation of a putative mammary oncogene (int–1) on mouse chromosome 15. Nature, 307:131, 1984.
107. Ohtan, K., Nakamura, M., Saito, S., Nada, T., Yoshiaki, I., Sugamura, K., and Hinumia, Y.: Identification of two distinct elements in the long terminal repeat of HTLV–1 responsible for maximum gene expression. EMBO J., 6:389, 1987.
108. Okada, M., Maeda, M., Tagaya, Y., Taniguchi, Y., Tashigawara, K., Yoshiki, T., Diamantstein, T., Smith, K. A., Uchiyama, T., Honjo, T., and Yodoi, J. O.: TCGF (IL 2)-receptor inducing factor(s). II. Possible role of ATL-derived factor (ADF) on constitutive IL 2 receptor expression of HTLV–1(+) T cell lines. J. Immunol., 135:3995, 1985.
109. Opp, C., Shore, S. C., and Reddy, E. P.: Nucleotide sequence analysis of testis-derived c-abl cDNAs: Implications for testis-specific transcription and abl oncogene activation. Proc. Natl. Acad. Sci. U.S.A., 84:8200, 1987.
110. Pandolfi, F., Blattner, W. A., de Rossi, B., Semenzato, G., Strong, D. M., and Gallo, R. C.: T-cell leukemia-lymphoma virus and heterogeneity of chronic T-cell malignancies (letter). Lancet, 2:1273, 1982.
111. Pattengale, P. K., Taylor, C. R., Twomey, P., Hill, S., Jonasson, J., Beardsley, T., and Haas, M.: Immunopathology of B-cell lymphomas induced in C47BL/6 mice by dual tropic murine leukemia virus (MuLV). Am. J. Pathol., 107:362, 1982.
112. Pawson, T., Harvey, R., and Smith, A. E.: The size of Rous sarcoma virus mRNAs active in cell-free translation. Nature, 268:416, 1977.
113. Pawson, T., Martin, G. S., and Smith, A. E.: Cell-free translation of virion RNA from nondefective and transformation-defective Rous sarcoma viruses. J. Virol., 19:950, 1976.
114. Payne, G. S., Bishop, J. M., and Varmus, H. E.: Multiple arrangements of viral DNA and an activated host oncogene in bursal lymphomas. Nature, 295:209, 1982.
115. Payne, G. S., Courtneidge, S. A., Crittenden, L. B., Fadly, A. M., Bishop, J. M., and Varmus, H. E.: Analysis of avian leukosis virus DNA and RNA in bursal tumors: Virus gene expression is not required for maintenance of the tumor state. Cell, 33:311, 1981.
116. Peters, G., Lee, A., and Dickson, C.: Concerted activation of two potential proto-oncogenes in mouse mammary carcinomas. Nature, 320:628, 1986.
117. Poisz, B. J., Ruscetti, F. W., Gazdar, A. D., Bunn, F. A., Minna, J. D., and Gallo, R. C.: Detection and isolation of type C retrovirus particles from fresh and cultured lymphocytes of a patient with cutaneous T-cell lymphoma. Proc. Natl. Acad. Sci. U.S.A., 77:7415, 1980.
118. Pozzatti, P., Vogel, J., and Jay, G.: The human T-lymphotropic virus type I tax gene can cooperate with the ras oncogene to induce neoplastic transformation of cells. Mol. Cell Biol., 10:413, 1990.
119. Purchio, A. F., Jonanovich, S., and Erikson, R. L.: Sites of synthesis of viral proteins in avian sarcoma virus-infected chicken cells. J Virol., 35:629, 1986.
120. Reddy, E. P., Smith, M. J., and Srinivason, A.: Nucleotide sequence of Abelson murine leukemia virus genome. Structural similarity of its transforming gene product to other onc gene products with tyrosine-specific kinase activity. Proc. Natl. Acad. Sci. U.S.A., 80:3623, 1983.
121. Rosenberg, S. A., Asbersold, P., Gornetta, K., Kasid, A., Morgan, R. A., Moen, R., Karson, E. M., Lotze, M. T., Yang, J. C., Topalian, S. L., Merino, M. J., Culver, K., Miller, A. D., Blaese, R. M., and Anderson, W. F.: Gene transfer into humans. Immunotherapy of patients with advanced melanoma using tumor-infiltrating lymphocytes modified by retroviral gene transduction. N. Engl. J. Med., 323:570, 1990.
122. Rous, F. P.: Sarcoma of the fowl transmissible by an agent separable from the tumor cells. J. Exp. Med., 13:392, 1911.
123. Rovinski, B., Munroe, D., Peacock, J., Mowat, M., Bernstein, A., and Benchimol, S.: Deletion of 5′-coding sequences of the cellular p53 gene in mouse erythroleukemia: A novel mechanism of oncogene regulation. Mol. Cell Biol., 7:847, 1987.
124. Ruscetti, S. K., Janesch, N. J., Chakraborti, A., Sawyer, S. T., and Hankins, W. D.: Friend spleen focus-forming virus induces factor independence in an erythropoietin-dependent erythroleukemia cell line. J. Virol., 64:1057, 1990.
125. Scher, C. D., and Siegler, R.: Direct transformation of 3T3 cells by Abelson murine leukemia virus. Nature, 253:729, 1975.
126. Schiff, L. A., Nibert, M. L., and Fields, B. N.: Characterization of a zinc blotting technique: Evidence that a retroviral gag protein binds zinc. Proc. Natl. Acad. Sci. U.S.A., 85:4195, 1988.
127. Schultz, A. M., and Oroszlan, S.: In vivo modification of retroviral gag gene-encoded polyproteins by myristic acid. J. Virol., 46:355, 1983.
128. Shackleford, G. M., and Varmus, H. E.: Expression of the proto-oncogene int–1 is restricted to postmeiotic male germ cells and the neural tube of mid-gestational embryos. Cell, 50:89, 1987.
129. Siegler, R., Zajdel, S., and Lane, I.: Pathogenesis of Abelson virus-induced murine leukemia. J. Natl. Cancer Inst., 48:189, 1972.
130. Sinn, E., Muller, W., Pattengale, P., Tepler, I., Wallace, R., and Leder, P.: Co-expression of MMTV/v-Ha-ras and MMTV/c-myc genes in transgenic mice: Synergistic action of oncogenes in vivo. Cell, 49:465, 1987.
131. Sodroski, J., Rosen, C., Goh, W. C., and Haseltine, W.: A transcriptional activator protein encoded by the x-lor region of the human T-cell leukemia virus. Science, 228:1430, 1985.
132. Stacey, D. W., and Allfrey, V. G.: Microinjection studies of duck globin messenger RNA translation in human and avian cells. Cell, 9:725, 1976.
133. Stehelin, D., Varmus, H. E., Bishop, J. M., and Vogt, P. K.: DNA related to the transforming gene of avian sarcoma virus is present in normal avian DNA. Nature, 260:170, 1976.
134. Stewart, T. A., Pattengale, P. K., and Leder, P.: Spontaneous mammary adenocarcinomas in transgenic mice that carry and express MTV/c-myc fusion genes. Cell, 38:627, 1984.
135. Stoye, J. P., Fenner, S., Greenoak, G. E., Moran, C., and Coffin, J. M.: Role of endogenous retroviruses as mutations: The hairless mutation of mice. Cell, 54:383, 1988.
136. Summers, J., and Mason, W. S.: Replication of the genome of a hepatitic B-like virus by reverse transcription of an RNA intermediate. Cell, 29:403, 1982.
137. Tajima, K., Tominaga, S., Suchi, T., Kawagoe, T., Komoda, H., Hinuma, Y., Oda, T., and Fujita, K.: Epidemiological analysis of the distribution of antibody to adult T-cell leukemia-virus-associated antigens: Possible horizontal transmission of adult T-cell leukemia virus. Gann, 73:893, 1982.
138. Tanaka, A., Takahashi, C., Yamaoka, S., Nosaka, T., Maki, M., and Hatanaka, M.: Oncogenic transformation by the tax gene of human T cell leukemia virus type I in vitro. Proc. Natl. Acad. Sci. U.S.A., 87:1071, 1990.
139. Taylor, J. M., and Illmensee, R.: Site on the RNA of an avian sarcoma virus at which primer is bound. J. Virol., 16:653, 1975.
140. Teich, N.: Taxonomy of retrovirus. *In* RNA Tumor Viruses. Edited by R. Weiss, N. Teich, H. Varmus, and J. Coffin. Cold Spring Harbor, New York, Cold Spring Harbor Laboratory. 1984, p. 25:509
141. Teich, N., Wyke, J., Mak, T., Bernstein, A., and Hardy, W.: Pathogenesis of retrovirus-induced disease. *In* RNA Tumor Viruses. Edited by R. Weiss, N. Teich, H. Varmus, and J. Coffin. Cold Spring Harbor, New York, Cold Spring Harbor Laboratory, 1984, p. 785.
142. Temin, H. M.: On the origin of the genes for neoplasia: G.H.A. Clowes memorial lecture. Cancer Res., 34:2835, 1974.
143. Temin, H. M.: Do we understand the genetic mechanisms of oncogensis? Keynote address for Honey Harbor meeting on cellular and molecular biology of neoplasia. J. Cell Physiol. Supp., 3:1, 1984.
144. Temin, H. M.: Reverse transcription in the eukaryotic genome: Retroviruses, pararetroviruses, retrotransposons, and retro-transcripts. Mol. Biol. Eval., 6:455, 1985.
145. Temin, H. M.: Retrovirus Vectors: Promise and Reality. Science, 244:983, 1989.
146. Temin, H. M., and Mizutani, S.: RNA-dependent DNA polymerase in virions of Rous sarcoma virus. Nature, 226:1211, 1970.

147. Temin, H. M., and Rubin, H.: Characteristics of an assay for the Rous sarcoma virus and Rous sarcoma cells in tissue culture. Virology, 6:669, 1958.
148. Tsukamoto, A. S., Gross, C. R., Guzman, R. C., Parslow, T., and Varmus, H. E.: Expression of the int-1 gene in transgenic mice is associated with mammary gland hyperplasia and adenocarcinomas in male and female mice. Cell, 55:619, 1988.
149. Van Ooyen, A., Kwee, V., and Nusse, R.: The nucleotide sequence of the human int-1 mammary oncogene; Evolutionary conservation of codon and non-codon sequences. EMBO J., 4:2905, 1985.
150. Van Ooyen, A., and Nusse, R.: Structure and nucleotide sequence of the putative mammary oncogene int-1; proviral insertions leave the protein-encoding–domain intact. Cell, 39:233, 1984.
151. Varmus, H. E.: Form and function of retroviral proviruses. Science, 216:812, 1982.
152. Varmus, H. E.: In Mobile Genetic Elements. Edited by J. Shapiro. New York, Academic Press, 1983, p. 411.
153. Vogel, J., Hinrichs, S. H., Reynolds, R. K., Luciw, P. A., and Jay, G.: The HIV tat gene induces dermal lesions resembling Kaposi's sarcoma in transgenic mice. Nature, 334:636, 1989.
154. Vogt, P. K.: Spontaneous segregation of non-transforming viruses from cloned sarcoma viruses. Virology, 46:939, 1971.
155. von der Helm, K., and Duesberg, P. H.: Translation of Rous sarcoma virus RNA in a cell-free system from ascites Krebs II cells. Proc. Natl. Acad. Sci. U.S.A., 72:614, 1975.
156. Wachsman, W., Gold, D. W., Temple, P.A., Orr, E. C., Clark, B. C., and Chen, I. S.: HTLV X-gene product: Requirement for the env methionine initiation codon. Science, 228:1534, 1985.
157. Walther, N., Lurz, R., Patschinsky, T., Jansen, H. W., and Bister, K.: Molecular cloning of proviral DNA and structural analysis of the transduced myc oncogene of avian oncovirus CMII. J. Virol., 54:576, 1985.
158. Weiss, S. R., Varmus, H. E., and Bishop, J. M.: The size and genetic composition of virus-specific RNAs in the cytoplasm of cells producing avian sarcoma-leukemia viruses. Cell, 12:983, 1977.
159. Wigler, M., Pellicer, A., Silverstein, S., and Axel, R.: Biochemical transfer of single-copy eucaryotic genes using total cellular DNA as donor. Cell, 14:724, 1978.
160. Williams, D. A., Orkin, S. H., and Mulligan, R. C.: Retrovirus-mediated transfer of human adenosine deaminase gene sequences into cells in culture and into murine hematopoietic cells in vivo. Proc. Natl. Acad. Sci. U.S.A., 83:2566, 1986.
161. Wolff, J. A., Yae, J. K., Skelly, H. F., Moores, J. C., Respess, J. G., Friedmann, T., and Leffert, H.: Expression of retrovirally transduced genes in primary cultures of adult rat hepatocytes. Proc. Natl. Acad. Sci. U.S.A., 84:3344, 1987.
162. Wolff, L., and Ruscetti, S.: Malignant transformation of erythroid cells in vivo by introduction of a non-replicating retrovirus vector. Science, 228:1549, 1985.
163. Wong, T. C., Lewis, R. B., Bose, H. R., and Kang, C. Y.: Assembly of avian reticuloendotheliosis virus: Association of the core precursor, polypeptide with the intracellular ribonucleoprotein complex. J. Virol., 34:484, 1980.
164. Wong-Staal, F., and Gallo, R. C.: Human T-lymphotropic retroviruses. Nature, 317:395, 1985.
165. Yamamoto, K. R.: Steroid receptor regulated transcription of specific genes and gene networks. Am. Rev. Genet., 19:209, 1985.
166. Yoshida, M., Miyoshi, I., and Hinuma, Y.: Isolation and characterization of retrovirus from cell lines of human adult T-cell leukemia and its implication in the disease. Proc. Natl. Acad. Sci. U.S.A., 79:2031, 1982.
167. Yoshinaka, Y., Katoh, I., Copeland, J. D., and Ozoszlan, S.: Murine leukemia protease is encoded by the gag-pol gene and is synthesized through suppression of an amber termination codon. Proc. Natl. Acad. Sci. U.S.A., 82:1618, 1985.
168. Yoshinaka, Y., and Luftig, R. B.: Murine leukemia virus morphogenesis: Cleavage of p70 in vitro can be accompanied by a shift from a concentrically coiled internal strand ("immature") to a collapsed ("mature") form of the virus core. Proc. Natl. Acad. Sci. U.S.A., 74:3446, 1977.
169. Zinn, K., Mellon, P., Ptashne, M., and Maniatis, T.: Regulated expression of an extra-chromosomal human beta-interferon gene in mouse cells. Proc. Natl. Acad. Sci. U.S.A., 79:4897, 1982.

III-9

Herpesviruses

Jeffrey I. Cohen
Elliott Kieff

Virology

Properties of Herpesviruses

Herpesviruses are enveloped virions which contain a DNA core surrounded by an icosahedral nucleocapsid and a tegument. The viral genome consists of linear, double-stranded DNA varying in size from 120–230 kilobase pairs depending on the virus. Virions contain 30–35 structural proteins.

Seven herpesviruses have been isolated from humans. Herpes simplex 1, herpes simplex 2, and varicella-zoster virus are members of the alphaherpesvirus subfamily. Cytomegalovirus, human herpesvirus 6, and human herpesvirus 7 are betaherpesviruses. Epstein-Barr virus is a gammaherpesvirus. Herpesviruses are ubiquitous in nature and nearly every animal species is infected by at least one herpesvirus. The animal herpesviruses discussed below include herpesvirus saimiri which naturally infects squirrel monkeys, herpesvirus aeteles which infects spider monkeys, Marek's disease virus which infects birds, and Lucke herpesvirus which infects frogs.

Infection of cells with herpesviruses begins with adsorption and fusion of the virion envelope with the cell membrane. The envelope glycoproteins are important mediators of adsorption and fusion. The viral capsid is released into the cytoplasm and transported to the nucleus where the linear viral DNA circularizes. In lytic infection, immediate-early, early, and subsequently late viral genes are transcribed in the nucleus and their proteins are synthesized in the cytoplasm, while translation of host cell RNAs is inhibited. Immediate-early genes encode regulators of virus gene expression. Early genes encode proteins that are involved in viral DNA synthesis. Late genes encode structural proteins of the virus. Early lytic replication is associated with irreversible cytocidal inhibition of host DNA, RNA, and protein synthesis. Virion DNA is replicated and assembled into nucleocapsids in the nucleus. Nucleocapsids undergo initial envelopment by budding through the inner lamella of the nuclear membrane. Viral proteins and glycoproteins modify the host cell's cytoplasmic membranes. Virions are released by exocytosis or by cytoplasmic deenvelopment and reenvelopment at the plasma membrane.

Herpesviruses have the capacity to establish latent infection as well as lytic infection. Reactivation from latent infection is controlled by cellular factors, although virus immediate-early genes mediate the initial reactivation from latency. The capacity to establish latent infection in vivo and to reactivate from latency assures a source of virus to infect previously uninfected individuals. Herpesviruses are ubiquitous in most human populations. Almost all adults are latently infected with herpes simplex 1, varicella-zoster virus, human herpesvirus 6, and Epstein-Barr virus. Reactivation in adults results in transmission of virus to infants, children, or young adults, perpetuating nearly uniform adult infection and persistence of the virus over many generations.

Oncogenic Features of Herpesviruses

Several features of herpesvirus replication are important for maintenance of latency and for oncogenicity. In order to be oncogenic, herpesviruses must be able to maintain their viral genome in the cell, avoid killing the cell, avoid destruction of the cell by the immune system, and activate appropriate cellular growth control regulatory pathways. Since Epstein-Barr is the best studied of the human herpesviruses that latently infects cells and has a strong association with human neoplasia, this virus will be used to illustrate the principles of herpesvirus infection relevant to oncogenicity.

First, viral DNA must be maintained in the cell. Epstein-Barr virus establishes latent infection in B lymphocytes. B lymphocytes replicate so that the virus must have a way to assure transmission to cell progeny.[49] The Epstein-Barr virus genome is usually maintained either as a multicopy circular episome in the host cell or the viral DNA can integrate into the host genome. Episomes are formed by fusion of the terminal direct repeats which are present at both ends of the linear genome present in virions.[15] The Namalwa Burkitt tumor cell line contains a complete copy of the entire Epstein-Barr virus genome integrated into the host cell DNA and no additional episomal viral DNA. Analysis of the DNA sequence indicates that the viral genome is integrated into the host DNA at the terminal direct repeat sequence of the virus. There is no homology between the viral DNA and the cell DNA at the site of recombination.[53]

Second, a cell transformed by a virus may only express a limited number of viral genes so as to avoid killing the cell and to avoid inciting destruction of the cell by the immune system. Replication of herpesviruses in cells results in inhibition of host cell protein synthesis and lysis of the host cell. Analysis of the Epstein-Barr virus DNA sequence indicates nearly 100 possible gene products; however, infection of B cells with Epstein-Barr virus results in expression of only ten genes.[40] This limited repertoire of gene products prevents frequent viral replication with death of the infected cell and limits the ability of the immune system to recognize a cell latently infected with the virus. Epstein-Barr virus also encodes a viral protein (BCRF1) which is highly homologous to interleukin-10 and has interleukin-10 activity.[35] Recombinant BCRF1 inhibits interferon-gamma synthesis by activated human peripheral blood mononuclear cells; interferon-gamma has been shown to inhibit outgrowth of Epstein-Barr virus-infected B cells in vitro. While BCRF1 is transcribed in the late phase of the viral replication cycle, expression of this gene in the small number of latently infected cells that do enter the lytic cycle may prevent activation of the immune system with subsequent destruction of other latently infected cells.

Third, viral genes may interact with other cell proteins or directly transactivate other cell genes to provide additional functions necessary for immortalization. Proteins from several DNA tumor viruses, including SV40, adenovirus, and human papillomavirus, have been shown to interact with cell proteins such as the retinoblastoma gene product which appear to normally have tumor suppressor activity. In addition, proteins from these viruses also transactivate expression of cell genes which may be important to initiate or maintain neoplasia. While proteins from the Epstein-Barr virus have not yet been shown to interact with tumor suppressor gene products, at least one gene expressed during latent infection (EBNA-2) has been shown to transactivate expression of both viral and B cell genes (see below).

Oncogenic Animal Viruses

Marek's Disease Virus

Marek's disease virus induces fatal lymphoproliferation in its natural host, the chicken. Inoculation of the virus into these animals results in T-cell lymphomas four to six weeks later. Lymphoblastoid cell lines derived from the tumors contain episomal copies of the Marek's disease virus genome and generally do not produce infectious virus. RNAs are transcribed from multiple regions of the genome in cell lines obtained from Marek's disease virus induced tumors.[84] Loss of RNA transcripts from one region of the viral genome (BamHI-H) is correlated with loss of viral oncogenicity.[7] Serial passage of the virus in chicken embryo fibroblasts results in attenuation with loss of oncogenicity. Vaccination of animals with an attenuated strain of Marek's disease virus, or with a different avian herpesvirus (herpesvirus of turkeys) results in protection of animals from tumors.[66,72] T-cell immunity is thought to play a major role in protection against Marek's disease. Thus, Marek's disease is one of the first DNA tumor viruses in which disease can be prevented by vaccination.

Lucke Herpesvirus

Lucke herpesvirus induces renal adenocarcinomas in its natural host, the frog. Inoculation of the virus into frog embryos, during a specific stage in development of the kidney, reproducibly results in renal carcinoma; however, inoculation during a later period of development fails to induce tumor formation. The virus is maintained in the latent state in warm temperatures, while viral replication is induced by exposure to cold temperatures.[57]

Herpesvirus Saimiri

Herpesvirus saimiri is not oncogenic in its natural host, the squirrel monkey. However, inoculation of the virus into several other species of monkeys (e.g., tamarins, owl monkeys, and marmosets) or New Zealand white rabbits results in fatal lymphoproliferative disease with T cell leukemia, lymphoma, or lymphosarcoma. Three strains of herpesvirus saimiri have been identified. Strains A and C (but not B) can transform peripheral blood lymphocytes from marmosets. In contrast, strain C (but not strains A or B) is oncogenic in New Zealand white rabbits.[54] The herpesvirus saimiri genome is present in a latent state in tumor cells. A small region of the viral genome (2.3 kilobase pairs) is required for immortalization of primate T cells in vitro and for inducing lymphomas in owl monkeys.[18] It is not known whether this region is sufficient for cell transformation. The region is not necessary for viral replication.[18] The region contains an open reading frame that can encode a membrane-spanning protein with a potential zinc finger domain.[64] Inoculation of cotton-top marmosets with virus-free herpesvirus saimiri antigen preparations results in protection of the animals from tumors on challenge with virus.[67]

Herpesvirus Aeteles

Like herpesvirus saimiri, herpesvirus aeteles is not oncogenic in its natural host (the spider monkey), but it induces T cell lymphomas in other primates (including tamarins and owl monkeys). The virus also immortalizes T cells from tamarins in vitro.[24]

Epstein-Barr Virus: An Oncogenic Human Herpesvirus

Pathogenesis

Effect on B Cell Growth In Vitro.   Infection of primary B cells with Epstein-Barr virus in vitro results in transformation of the cells which can then proliferate indefinitely.[33] The resulting lymphoblastoid cell lines show several phenotypic changes which differentiate them from resting B cells. The lymphoblastoid cells are larger, grow in large dense clumps and secrete polyclonal immunoglobulin.[65,74] B cell activation antigens are also expressed on the surface of the lymphoblastoid cells including antigens defined by monoclonal antibodies AC2, Ki-1, Ki-24,[76] and the CD23 cell surface protein.[85,90] While CD23 (EBVCS) is expressed on the surface of Epstein-Barr virus-transformed B cells, it is not present on normal resting B cells.[41] The supernatant of Epstein-Barr virus-transformed B cells contains a 35 kDa protein thought to represent a soluble, cleaved form of CD23.[91] The soluble, cleaved form of CD23 may possess autocrine growth factor activity in Epstein-Barr virus-transformed B cells.[88] Subsequent attempts to duplicate these findings with recombinant CD23 have been unsuccessful.[93] Other evidence that antibodies to CD23 can block the uptake of B cell growth factor on the surface of the B cells, suggests that CD23 could be a receptor for B cell growth factor.[27]

Epstein-Barr Virus Gene Expression in Transformed Lymphocytes

Six different Epstein-Barr virus nuclear proteins, two membrane proteins, and two nontranslated RNAs are known to be expressed in latently infected B lymphocytes that have been growth transformed by Epstein-Barr virus in vitro. The Epstein-Barr virus nuclear proteins, EBNA-1, EBNA-2, EBNA-LP, EBNA-3A, EBNA-3B, and EBNA-3C make up the Epstein-Barr virus nuclear antigen complex. EBNA-1 binds to the oriP sequence of Epstein-Barr virus and allows maintenance of the Epstein-Barr virus genome as an episome in transformed B cells.[103] Binding of EBNA-1 to oriP also has a small effect on transactivation of oriP as a cis enhancer of transcription.[71] Mutational analysis of EBNA-1 indicates that the carboxy portion is required for the trans-activation function.[52]

EBNA-2 is required for B cell transformation by Epstein-Barr virus. Expression of EBNA-2 in rodent fibroblasts reduces serum requirements,[16] and in Epstein-Barr virus-negative Burkitt lymphoma cells causes growth in tight clumps and induces expression of two B cell activation antigens CD23 and CD21.[97,98] EBNA-2 also transactivates expression of the Epstein-Barr virus gene LMP-1 and c-fgr, a cellular gene which encodes a protein tyrosine kinase and is a member of the src gene family.[43,100]

Recombinant viruses with EBNA-2 deletion mutants fail to transform B cells.[14,30] Mutational analysis indicates that at least four separate EBNA-2 domains are necessary for lymphocyte transformation. Mutations in EBNA-2 that abolish transforming activity also abolish LMP-1 transactivation by EBNA-2. In addition, EBNA-2 is a major determinant of the type-specific transforming difference between the two naturally occurring types of Epstein-Barr virus.[14]

EBNA-LP is encoded by the leader sequence in EBNA-2 mRNAs (and possibly for EBNA-1 and EBNA-3).[80] EBNA-LP localizes to the nucleus in linear arrays of granules, suggesting a possible role in RNA processing.[99] EBNA-LP has DNA binding activity,[81] but has no discernable effects when expressed in rodent fibroblasts or B lymphoma cells.[97] A recent study showed that deletion of the carboxy portion of EBNA-LP does not abolish transformation.[30]

EBNA-3A, EBNA-3B, and EBNA-3C are encoded by three tandem open reading frames. These three proteins are distantly related.[68,69] EBNA-3C transactivates expression of CD21,[98] but not other B cell activation antigens; the function of EBNA-3A and EBNA-3B is unknown.

Two latent membrane proteins, LMP-1 and LMP-2, are also expressed in B cells that have been growth transformed by Epstein-Barr virus. LMP-1 functions as a transforming oncogene when transfected into established rodent cell lines.[3,94,95] Expression of LMP-1 in Epstein-Barr virus-negative Burkitt lymphoma cells results in a change in morphology and increased expression of the B cell activation antigen CD23, cellular adhesion molecules including ICAM-1, LFA-1, LFA-3 (96), and vimentin.[5] LMP-1 interacts with cellular proteins, including vimentin, to form a patch in the cytoplasmic membrane of the B cell.[47] Mutational analysis of LMP-1 indicates that the amino terminus and membrane spanning domains are required for transformation of rodent cells, while the carboxy portion is not essential.[4,95]

LMP-1 may play a role in epithelial cell neoplasia since LMP-1 is one of only two Epstein-Barr virus genes expressed in nasopharyngeal carcinoma (see below). Expression of LMP-1 in epithelial cells inhibits differentiation of the cells.[17] Expression of LMP-1 in the skin of transgenic mice induces epithelial hyperplasia with increased expression of keratin 6.[102]

LMP-2 has multiple transmembrane domains and colocalizes with LMP-1 in the cytoplasmic membrane of B cells.[51] The association of LMP-2 with LMP-1 may contribute to the transforming function of the latter.

The two Epstein-Barr virus encoded RNAs, EBER 1 and EBER 2, are the two most abundant Epstein-Barr virus RNAs in latently infected B cells; however, they have no role in latent or lytic Epstein-Barr virus infection or cell transformation in vitro.[87] These RNAs are not polyadenylated and form a complex with the nuclear antigen La.[46] Recombinant Epstein-Barr virus deleted for both EBER genes is able to transform B lymphocytes in vitro. The transformed B lymphocytes are indistinguishable from cells transformed by wild type virus and express the usual complement of EBNA and LMP proteins. The levels of spontaneous or induced lytic cycle Epstein-Barr virus gene expression are unaffected by the EBER deletions.[87]

Animal Models. Three types of animal models have been used to study Epstein-Barr virus oncogenesis. In the first model, Epstein-Barr virus-infected, growth transformed, lymphoblastoid cell lines produce B cell tumors when inoculated intracerebrally into nude mice.[26] Inoculation into subcutaneous tissue of nude mice usually is not tumorigenic. However, lymphoblastoid cell lines have induced tumors when inoculated into animals treated with antilymphocyte serum.[2] Furthermore, Rat-1 cells converted to Epstein-Barr virus LMP-1 expression by gene transfer are tumorigenic when inoculated subcutaneously into nude mice.[94]

In the second model, inoculation of peripheral blood leukocytes from Epstein-Barr virus-seropositive humans into mice with severe combined immunodeficiency results in development of B cell lymphomas in the animals. The tumor cells are human in origin and contain Epstein-Barr virus DNA. Inoculation of mice with peripheral blood leukocytes from Epstein-Barr virus-seronegative humans results in engraftment of a functional human immune system, but without development of lymphomas.[60] If these latter mice are subsequently inoculated with cell-free Epstein-Barr virus, the animals develop immunoblastic lymphomas. Inoculation of lymphoblastoid cell lines into mice with severe combined immunodeficiency also results in lymphomas. These B cell tumors contain Epstein-Barr virus genomes, and express the full complement of EBNA and LMP genes characteristic of latently infected, growth transformed cell lines.[78] The cells do not have chromosomal translocations.[11]

In the third model, cotton-top tamarins inoculated with a large dose of cell-free Epstein-Barr virus develop multifocal large cell lymphomas over the ensuing few weeks.[56] These tumors contain Epstein-Barr virus genomes, do not have chromosomal translocations,[12] and express EBNA-1, EBNA-2, EBNA-LP, and LMP-1.[106] Tumors at different sites within an animal arise from different B cell clones. At each site the tumors are monoclonal or oligoclonal in origin. This model has been useful in assessing efficacy of candidate Epstein-Barr virus vaccines. Inoculation of cotton-top tamarins with recombinant vaccinia virus expressing Epstein-Barr virus envelope glycoprotein 350,[59] or gp350 incorporated into iscoms (immune-stimulating complexes[58]) protects the animals from development of lymphoma when challenged with virus.

Clinical Aspects

Introduction

Two types of human malignancies have been associated with Epstein-Barr virus infection; those which occur shortly after Epstein-Barr virus infection and those which occur long after infection. To understand the distinction it is necessary to consider normal Epstein-Barr virus infection. Epstein-Barr virus infection is usually spread by saliva. Virus infection initiates in the oropharyngeal epithelium and spreads to subepithelial B lymphocytes. In the course of primary Epstein-Barr virus infection, up to several percent of the peripheral blood B lymphocytes are infected with Epstein-Barr virus and have the capacity to proliferate indefinitely in vitro.[55] The

pharyngeal tonsils may be infiltrated with Epstein-Barr virus infected B lymphocytes. NK cells,[6] suppressor T cells,[92] and rapidly evolving HLA and EBNA,[10,62] or LMP-1 restricted cytotoxic T cells control the latently infected B lymphocytes.[63] T and B cell interactions release lymphokines and cytokines giving rise to many of the clinical manifestations of acute infectious mononucleosis. After recovery, the fraction of B lymphocytes latently infected with Epstein-Barr virus in the peripheral blood remains at 1 in 10^5 to 1 in 10^6. These lymphocytes or their precursors are the primary site of Epstein-Barr virus persistence and a source of virus for persistent infection of epithelial surfaces.

B lymphocyte tumors which occur early after Epstein-Barr virus infection are usually lymphoproliferative processes in which latent virus infection in B lymphocytes is the principal cause of proliferation. Oral hairy leukoplakia may be the epithelial counterpart.[28] In contrast, Burkitt lymphoma and nasopharyngeal carcinoma occur long after primary Epstein-Barr virus infection; although etiologically related to Epstein-Barr virus, viral gene expression may not be important to the growth of the clinically evident malignant cells.

Lymphoproliferative Disease

Epstein-Barr virus is associated with B cell lymphoproliferative disease in patients with congenital immunodeficiency. The X-linked lymphoproliferative syndrome is an inherited immunodeficiency in which affected males experience morbidity and mortality with Epstein-Barr virus infection.[29] Before infection with the virus, the patients have apparently normal cellular and humoral immune responses.[86] With primary Epstein-Barr virus infection, most of the patients die of fulminant hepatitis or another complication of infectious mononucleosis, one-fourth develop malignant lymphoma, and one-fourth develop acquired hypogammaglobulinemia.[29] Epstein-Barr virus nuclear antigens and viral DNA has been detected in lesions from these patients. The mutation responsible for the X-linked lymphoproliferative syndrome has been linked to a restriction fragment length polymorphism which may now allow prenatal diagnosis and identification of female carriers.[82]

Epstein-Barr virus has also been associated with fatal infectious mononucleosis in individuals with no known underlying genetic predisposition,[73,83] or in patients with immunodeficiency states. These include congenital immunodeficiencies such as the Wiskott-Aldrich syndrome and severe combined immunodeficiency.[38,79] Epstein-Barr virus lymphoproliferative disease occurs in patients who are immunosuppressed due to bone marrow transplantation, solid organ transplantation, or the acquired immunodeficiency syndrome (AIDS).[13] Most patients present with symptoms within 3 years of transplantation. The most common symptoms are fever, lymphadenopathy or gastrointestinal symptoms. Lymphoproliferative lesions are most commonly seen in the lymph nodes, liver, lungs, kidney, bone marrow, or small intestine. Tumors in transplant patients are usually classified as lymphomas or immunoblastic sarcomas; some patients have hyperplastic lesions. The proliferating lymphocytes in these tumors generally do not have chromosomal translocations. Monoclonal, oligoclonal, and polyclonal B lymphocyte growth has been reported. Tumors in patients with AIDS are frequently Burkitt or Burkitt-type lymphomas and often have chromosomal translocations with c-myc rearrangements. The mortality rate in patients with acquired immunodeficiency and Epstein-Barr virus lymphoproliferative disease is about 70%. Tissue from organ or bone marrow transplant recipients or from patients with AIDS who have Epstein-Barr virus lymphoproliferative disease contains Epstein-Barr virus genomes and shows expression of EBNA-1, EBNA-2, LMP-1, CD23, and the intercellular adhesion molecules ICAM-1 and LFA-3.[89,104]

Burkitt's Lymphoma

Burkitt's lymphoma is the most common childhood tumor in equatorial Africa and New Guinea. In Africa and New Guinea, the tumor is associated with holoendemic malaria. Areas with malaria control programs have a lower incidence of Burkitt's lymphoma. Burkitt's lymphoma also occurs less frequently throughout the rest of the world. In Africa, most children (60%) present with tumors involving the face, while 30% have abdominal tumors; in the United States children present at a slightly later age and 75% have abdominal tumors. Even in Africa or New Guinea where the tumors occur at a younger age and are closely associated with Epstein-Barr virus infection, the tumors occur at least several months to years after primary infection.[19]

Burkitt's lymphoma is classified as a high-grade malignant lymphoma with small noncleaved cells. The cells are monoclonal B cells which usually contain chromosomal translocations. In contrast to many other childhood lymphomas, the peripheral blood and bone marrow are rarely involved with tumor.

Seroepidemiologic studies show a strong association between Burkitt's lymphoma and Epstein-Barr virus in Africa.[19] Over 90% of African Burkitt's lymphomas are associated with Epstein-Barr virus, while only about 20% of Burkitt's lymphomas in the United States are associated with Epstein-Barr virus. African patients with Burkitt's lymphoma often have high levels of antibody to Epstein-Barr virus antigens.[32] In fact, antibody titers correlate with the onset of tumors, compatible with the hypothesis that virus burden is pathophysiologically linked to tumor. Tumor tissue contains Epstein-Barr virus genomes and virus can be recovered from the tissue.[77] Burkitt's lymphoma tissues express EBNA-1, but frequently do not express EBNA-2 or LMP-1, two genes that are important in Epstein-Barr virus induced B cell proliferation. Similarly, cell lines derived from Burkitt's lymphoma that grow as individual cells express EBNA-1, but not EBNA-2, EBNA-3A, EBNA-3B, EBNA-3C, EBNA-LP, or LMP-1. These cell lines do not express the B cell activation antigen CD23, or the intercellular adhesion molecules ICAM-1 or LFA-3. However, when Burkitt lymphoma cell lines are maintained in culture they tend to grow in tight clumps, with a lymphoblastoid cell-like morphology, and express EBNA-1, EBNA-2, EBNA-3A, EBNA-3B, EBNA-3C, EBNA-LP, LMP-1, CD23 and intercellular adhesion molecules.[75]

Burkitt's lymphomas contain a chromosomal translocation which results in c-myc dysregulation. The most common chromosomal translocation is the 8/14 translocation which places a portion of the c-myc oncogene (chromosome 8) adjacent to the immunoglobulin heavy chain constant region (chromosome 14). The 8/22 translocation seen in other Burkitt's tumors places the c-myc oncogene (chromosome 8) at a distance from the lambda light chain constant region (chromosome 22). These latter translocations are often associated with mutations in the c-myc gene. These translocations result in deregulation and high constitutive c-myc expression. Transgenic animals that overexpress c-myc in breast epithelial or B lymphoid cells develop monoclonal tumors at a characteristic age.[1,45] Two conclusions emerge from these transgenic studies. First, c-myc is etiologically related to these experimental transgenic tumors. Second, dysregulated c-myc expression is not sufficient per se for malignancy.

Expression of c-myc (under a heterologous promoter) in Epstein-Barr virus immortalized lymphoblastoid cell lines results in transformation of the cells with anchorage-independent growth and tumors when injected into immunodeficient mice.[50] In addition, expression of c-myc in these cells results in down-regulation of LFA-1, an intercellular adhesion molecule, with loss of homotypic B cell adhesion in vitro. This reduction in LFA-1 may be important for the escape of Burkitt lymphoma cells from immunosurveillance and killing by cytotoxic T cells, since LFA-1 is known to be involved in B cell adhesion to natural killer cells and cytotoxic T cells.[36]

Epstein-Barr virus associated endemic Burkitt's lymphoma may develop in steps.[42] First, Epstein-Barr virus infection may expand the pool of differentiating and proliferating B lymphocytes. Second, chronic holoendemic malaria may cause T lymphocyte suppression and B lymphocyte proliferation. Third, enhanced proliferation of differentiating B cells may favor the chance occurrence of a reciprocal c-myc (8/14 or 8/22) translocation placing c-myc partially under the control of immunoglobulin related transcriptional enhancers with development of a monoclonal tumor.

Nasopharyngeal Carcinoma

Nasopharyngeal carcinoma is the second most common malignancy in Southern China or overseas Chinese who originated from Southern China. Some northern native American populations also have a high incidence of nasopharyngeal carcinoma. North African populations have an intermediate incidence and most caucasian or black populations have a low incidence.

The tumor may present with a metastatic lymph node in the jugular chain, with a bloody nasal discharge and nasal speech, or with unilateral secretory otitis media (secondary to compression of the eustachian tube). The third, fourth, fifth, and sixth cranial nerves may be destroyed by the tumor which may also invade the cavernous sinus. Nasopharyngeal carcinoma frequently shows a nonkeratinizing squamous cell histopathology.

The nonkeratinizing nasopharyngeal carcinomas are uniformly associated with Epstein-Barr virus. Seroepidemiologic studies indicate that patients with nasopharyngeal carcinoma have high levels of antibodies to Epstein-Barr virus antigens. Patients usually have elevated levels of IgA antibody to the viral capsid antigen (VCA) and early antigen (EA). Epstein-Barr virus antibody titers are useful in screening patients for early detection of nasopharyngeal carcinoma.[20] Nasopharyngeal carcinoma tissue contains Epstein-Barr virus genomes in every cell. Biopsy tissue shows expression of EBNA-1 with variable expression of LMP-1 (40–70% of biopsies show LMP-1). EBNA-2, EBNA-3, and EBNA-LP are not expressed.[23,105] These tumors are monoclonal with regard to Epstein-Barr virus infection, indicating that Epstein-Barr virus infection precedes malignant cell outgrowth at the cellular level. Unlike Burkitt's lymphoma, the association of Epstein-Barr virus with nasopharyngeal carcinoma is uniform and universal.

Other Tumors Associated With Epstein-Barr Virus

Epidemiological studies suggest an association of Epstein-Barr virus with Hodgkin's disease. Patients with a history of infectious mononucleosis have an increased risk of developing Hodgkin's disease.[44] Patients with Hodgkin's disease generally have higher titers of antibody to Epstein-Barr virus viral capsid antigen (VCA) than the general population;[22] some patients with Hodgkin's disease have elevated antibody titers to Epstein-Barr virus VCA and nuclear antigens before development of the disease.[61] Tissues from about 20% of patients with Hodgkin's disease have Epstein-Barr virus genomes. These lesions are usually monoclonal proliferations and the Epstein-Barr virus genome is present in the Reed-Sternberg cells in most of the patients.[101]

Epstein-Barr virus genomes have been detected in three patients with T cell lymphomas presenting with fever, pneumonia, and numerous hematologic abnormalities. All three patients had markedly elevated antibody titers to Epstein-Barr virus VCA and early antigen.[39] Epstein-Barr virus DNA has also been detected in a central nervous system lymphoma from a patient with no underlying immunodeficiency,[34] patients with carcinoma of the palatine tonsil,[9] or patients with supraglottic laryngeal carcinoma.[8] Epstein-Barr virus DNA and Epstein-Barr virus nuclear antigens have been detected in thymic carcinomas,[47] or T cell lymphomas in patients with lethal midline granuloma.[31]

Oncogenic Potential of Other Human Herpesviruses

Cytomegalovirus has not been shown to be oncogenic in humans. While viral antigens or viral DNA has been demonstrated in some tumors (e.g., Kaposi's sarcoma in AIDS patients, colon carcinomas, cervical carcinomas), a similar level of cytomegalovirus antigens or DNA indicative of latent infection in nontumor tissue from control patients favors the hypothesis that cytomegalovirus is not causally linked to these tumors. In fact, cytomegalovirus transforms animal cells in vitro with a very low efficiency;[70] thus, the virus does not encode for a highly efficient transforming protein. Three potential, low efficiency, transforming domains have been mapped in cytomegalovirus DNA. One DNA segment can transform both primary and continuous cell lines, while the other two DNA segments can transform immortalized cell lines.[37] These DNA segments probably exert their effects by low frequency integration into cell DNA.

While initial seroepidemiologic studies suggested a role for herpes simplex virus 2 in cervical carcinoma, there has been no convincing evidence for viral antigens or viral DNA in these tissues. More recent studies suggest that human papillomavirus may be a cause of cervical carcinoma and that herpes simplex virus 2 infections are seen in the same populations as that of human papillomavirus. Herpes simplex virus 2 infection could be an adjuvant to human papillomavirus mediated cell transformation.

Hamster embryo fibroblasts infected with either inactivated herpes simplex virus 2,[21] or live varicella-zoster virus yield transformed foci with a very low frequency.[25] Inoculation of the transformed cells into hamsters results in tumors. However, the transformed cells stop producing viral antigens and lose their herpesvirus DNA. This phenomenon has been referred to as the "hit-and-run" mechanism in which a viral DNA segment could activate a cell growth control regulatory pathway. The viral DNA might then no longer be necessary for transformation and would be lost from the cell with successive passage. The frequency of herpes simplex virus 2 or varicella-zoster virus transformation in vitro is so low that it has been difficult to rigorously establish the validity of the "hit-and-run" hypothesis using tumor formation in experimental animals as an endpoint.

References

1. Adams, J. M., Harris, A. W., Pinkert, C. A., Corcoran, L. M., Alexander, W. S., Cory, S., Palmiter, R. D., and Brinster, R. L.: The c-myc oncogene driven by immunoglobulin enhancers induces lymphoid malignancy in transgenic mice. Nature, 318:533, 1985.
2. Adams, R. A., Hellerstein, E. E., Pothier, L., Foley, G. F., Lazarus, H., and Stuart, A.: Malignant potential of a cell line isolated from the peripheral blood in infectious mononucleosis. Cancer, 27:651, 1971.
3. Baichwal, V. R., and Sugden, B.: Transformation of Balb 3T3 cells by the BNLF-1 gene of Epstein-Barr virus. Oncogene, 2:461, 1988.
4. Baichwal, V. R., and Sugden, B.: The multiple membrane-spanning segments of the BNLF-1 oncogene from Epstein-Barr virus are required for transformation. Oncogene, 4:67, 1989.
5. Birkenbach, M., Liebowitz, D., Wang, F., Sample, J., and Kieff, E.: Epstein-Barr virus latent infection membrane protein increases vimentin expression in human B-cell lines. J. Virol., 63:4079, 1989.
6. Blazer, B., Patarroyo, M., Klein, E., and Klein, G.: Increased sensitivity of human lymphoid lines to natural killer cells after induction of the Epstein-Barr viral cycle by superinfection or sodium butyrate. J. Exp. Med., 151:614, 1980.
7. Bradley, G., Lancz, G., Tanaka, A., and Nonoyama, M.: Loss of Marek's disease virus tumorigenicity is associated with truncation of RNAs transcribed within BamHI-H. J. Virol., 63:4129, 1989.
8. Brichacek, B., Hirsch, I., Sibl, O., Vilikusova, E., and Vonka, V.: Association of some supraglottic laryngeal carcinomas with EB virus. Int. J. Cancer, 32:193, 1983.
9. Brichacek, B., Hirsch, I., Sibl, O., Vilikusova, E., and Vonka, V.: Presence of Epstein-Barr virus DNA in carcinomas of the palatine tonsil. J. Natl. Cancer Inst., 72:809, 1984.
10. Burrows, S. R., Sculley, T. B., Misko, I. S., Schmidt, C., and Moss, D. J.: An Epstein-Barr virus-specific cytotoxic T cell epitope in EBNA 3. J. Exp. Med., 171:345, 1990.
11. Cannon, M. J., Pisa, P., Fox, R. I., and Cooper, N. R.: Epstein-Barr virus induces aggressive lymphoproliferative disorders of human B cell origin in SCID/hu chimeric mice. J. Clin. Invest., 85:1333, 1990.
12. Cleary, M. L., Epstein, M. A., Finerty, S., Dorfman, R. F., Bornkamm, G. W., Kirkwood, J. K., Morgan, A. J., and Sklar, J.: Individual tumors of multifocal EB virus-induced malignant lymphomas in tamarins arise from different B-cell clones. Science, 228:722, 1985.
13. Cohen, J. I.: Epstein-Barr virus lymphoproliferative disease associated with acquired immunodeficiency. Medicine, 70:137, 1991.
14. Cohen, J. I., Wang, F., Mannick, J., and Kieff, E.: Epstein-Barr virus nuclear protein 2 is a key determinant of lymphocyte transformation. Proc. Natl. Acad. Sci. U.S.A., 86:9558, 1989.
15. Dambaugh, T., Beisel, C., Hummel, M., King, W., Fennewald, S., Cheung, A., Heller, M., Raab-Traub, N., and Kieff, E.: Epstein-Barr virus (B95-8) DNA: Molecular cloning and detailed mapping. Proc. Natl. Acad. Sci. U.S.A., 77:2999, 1980.
16. Dambaugh, T., Wang, F., Hennessy, K., Woodland, E., Rickinson, A., and Kieff, E.: Expression of the Epstein-Barr virus nuclear protein 2 in rodent cells. J. Virol., 59:453, 1986.
17. Dawson, C. W., Rickinson, A. B., and Young, L. S.: Epstein-Barr virus latent membrane protein inhibits human epithelial cell differentiation. Nature, 344:777, 1990.
18. Desrosiers, R. C., Bakker, A., Kamine, J., Falk, L. A., Hunt, R. D., and King, N. W.: A region of the herpesvirus saimiri genome required for oncogenicity. Science, 228:184, 1985.
19. deThe, G., Geser, A., Day, N. E., Tukei, P. M., Williams, E. H., Beri, D. P., Smith, P. G., Dean, A. G., Bornkamm, G. W., Feorino, P., and Henle, W.: Epidemiological evidence for causal relationship between Epstein-Barr virus and Burkitt's lymphoma from Ugandan prospective study. Nature, 274:756, 1978.
20. deThe, G., and Zeng, Y.: Population Screening for EBV Markers: Toward Improvement of Nasopharyngeal Carcinoma Control. In The Epstein-Barr Virus: Recent Advances. Edited by M. A. Epstein, and B. G. Achong. New York: John Wiley & Sons, 1986, p. 237.
21. Duff, R., and Rapp, F.: Oncogenic transformation of hamster cells after exposure to herpes simplex virus type 2. Nature New Biology, 233:48, 1971.
22. Evans, A. S., and Gutensohn, N. M.: A population-based case-control study of EBV

and other viral antibodies among persons with Hodgkin's disease and their siblings. Int. J. Cancer, 34:149, 1984.
23. Fahraeus, R., Fu, H. L., Ernberg, I., Finke, J., Rowe, M., Klein, G., Falk, K., Nilsson, E., Yadav, M., Busson, P., Tursz, T., and Kallin, B.: Expression of Epstein-Barr virus-encoded proteins in nasopharyngeal carcinoma. Int. J. Cancer, 42:329, 1988.
24. Falk, L., Johnson, D., and Deinhardt, F.: Transformation of marmoset lymphocytes in vitro with Herpesvirus ateles. Int. J. Cancer., 21:652, 1978.
25. Gelb, L., and Dohner, D.: Varicella-zoster virus-induced transformation of mammalian cells in vitro. J. Invest. Dermatol., 83:77s, 1984.
26. Giovanella, B., Nilsson, K., Zech, L., Yim, O., Klein, G., and Stehlin, J. S.: Growth of diploid, Epstein-Barr virus-carrying human lymphoblastoid cell lines heterotransplanted into nude mice under immunologically privileged conditions. Int. J. Cancer, 24:103, 1979.
27. Gordon, J., Webb, A. J., Walker, L., Guy, G. R., and Rowe, M.: Evidence for an association between CD23 and the receptor for a low molecular weight B cell growth factor. Eur. J. Immunol., 16:1627, 1986.
28. Greenspan, J. S., Greenspan, D., Lennette, E. T., Abrams, D. I., Conant, M. A., Petersen, V., and Freese, U. K.: Replication of Epstein-Barr virus within the epithelial cells of oral "hairy" leukoplakia, an AIDS-associated lesion. N. Engl. J. Med., 313:1564, 1985.
29. Grierson, H., and Purtilo, D. T.: Epstein-Barr virus infections in males with the X-linked lymphoproliferative syndrome. Ann. Intern. Med., 106: 538, 1987.
30. Hammerschmidt, W., and Sugden, B.: Genetic analysis of immortalizing functions of Epstein-Barr virus in human B lymphocytes. Nature, 340:393, 1989.
31. Harabuchi, Y., Yamanaka, N., Kataura, A., Imai, S., Kinoshita, T., Mizuno, F., and Osata, T.: Epstein-Barr virus in nasal T-cell lymphomas in patients with lethal midline granuloma. Lancet, 1:128, 1990.
32. Henle, G., Henle, W., Clifford, P., Diehl, V., Kafuko, G. W., Kirya, B. G., Klein, G., Morrow, R. H., Munube, G. M., Pike, P., Tukei, P. M., and Ziegler, J. L.: Antibodies to Epstein-Barr virus in Burkitt's lymphoma and control groups. J. Natl. Cancer Inst., 43:1147, 1969.
33. Henle, W., Diehl, B., Kohn, G., zur Hausen, H., and Henle, G.: Herpes-type virus and chromosome marker in normal leukocytes after growth with irradiated Burkitt cells. Science, 157:1064, 1967.
34. Hochberg, F. H., Miller, G., Schooley, R. T., Hirsch, M. S., Feorino, P., and Henle, W.: Central-nervous-system lymphoma related to Epstein-Barr virus. N. Engl. J. Med., 309:745, 1983.
35. Hsu, D.-H., de Waal Malefyt, R., Fiorentino, D. F., Dang, M.-N., Vieira, P., deVries, J., Spits, H., Mosmann, T. R., Moore, K. W.: Expression of interleukin-10 activity by Epstein-Barr virus protein BCRF1. Science, 250:830, 1990.
36. Inghirami, G., Grignani, F., Sternas, L., Lombardi, L., Knowles, D. M., and Dalla-Favera, R.: Down-regulation of LFA-1 adhesion receptors by c-myc oncogene in human B lymphoblastoid cells. Science, 250:682, 1990.
37. Jariwalla, R. J., Razzaque, A., Lawson, S., and Rosenthal, L. J.: Tumor progression mediated by two cooperating DNA segments of human cytomegalovirus. J. Virol., 63:425, 1989.
38. Joncas, J. H., Russo, P., Brochu, P., Simard, P., Brisebois, J., Dube, J., Marton, D., Leclerc, J. M., Hume, H., Rivard, G. E.: Epstein-Barr virus polymorphic B-cell lymphoma associated with leukemia and with congenital immunodeficiencies. J. Clin. Oncol., 8:378, 1990.
39. Jones, J. F., Shurin, S., Abramowsky, C., Tubbs, R. R., Sciotto, C. G., Wahl, R., Sands, J., Gottman, D., Katz, B., and Sklar, J.: T-cell lymphomas containing Epstein-Barr viral DNA in patients with chronic Epstein-Barr virus infections. N. Engl. J. Med., 318:733, 1988.
40. Kieff, E., and Liebowitz, D.: Epstein-Barr Virus and Its Replication. *In* Virology. Edited by B. N. Fields, D. M. Knipe, R. M. Chanock, M. S. Hirsch, J. L. Melnick, T. P. Monath, and B. Roizman. New York, Raven Press, 1990, p.1889.
41. Kinter, C., and Sugden, B.: Identification of antigenic determinants unique to the surfaces of cells transformed by Epstein-Barr virus. Nature, 294:458, 1981.
42. Klein, G.: Lymphoma development in mice and humans: diversity of initiation is followed by convergent cytogenetic evolution. Proc. Natl. Acad. Sci. U.S.A., 76:2442, 1979.
43. Knutson, J. C.: The level of c-fgr RNA is increased by EBNA-2, an Epstein-Barr virus gene required for B-cell immortalization. J. Virol., 64:2530, 1990.
44. Kvale, G., Hoiby, E. A., and Pedersen, E.: Hodgkin's disease in patients with previous infectious mononucleosis. Int. J. Cancer, 23:593, 1979.
45. Leder, A., Pattengale, P. K., Kuo, A., Stewart, T. A., and Leder, P.: Consequences of widespread deregulation of the c-myc gene in transgenic mice: Multiple neoplasms and normal development. Cell, 45:485, 1986.
46. Lerner, M. R., Andrews, N. C., Miller, G., and Steitz, J. A.: Two small RNAs encoded by Epstein-Barr virus and complexed with protein are precipitated by antibodies from patients with systemic lupus erythematosus. Proc. Natl. Acad. Sci. U.S.A., 78:805, 1981.
47. Leyvraz, S., Henle, W., Chahinian, A. P., Perlmann, C., Klein, G., Gordon, R. E., Rosenblum, M., and Holland, J. F.: Association of Epstein-Barr virus with thymic carcinoma. N. Engl. J. Med., 312:1296, 1985.
48. Liebowitz, D., Kopan, R., Fuchs, E., Sample, J., and Kieff, E.: An Epstein-Barr virus transforming protein associates with vimentin in lymphocytes. Mol. Cell. Biol., 7:2299, 1987.
49. Lindahl, T., Adams, A., Bjursell, G., Bornkamm, G. W., Kaschka-Dierich, C., and Jehn, U.: Covalently closed circular duplex DNA of Epstein-Barr virus in a human lymphoid cell line. J. Mol. Biol., 102:511, 1976.
50. Lombardi, L., Newcomb, E. W., and Dalla-Favera, R.: Pathogenesis of Burkitt lymphoma: Expression of an activated c-myc oncogene causes the tumorigenic conversion of EBV-infected human B lymphocytes. Cell, 49:161, 1987.
51. Longnecker, R., and Kieff, E.: A second Epstein-Barr virus membrane protein (LMP2) is expressed in latent infection and colocalizes with LMP1. J. Virol., 64:2319, 1990.
52. Lupton, S., and Levine, A. J.: Mapping genetic elements of Epstein-Barr virus that facilitate extrachromosomal persistence of Epstein-Barr virus-derived plasmids in human cells. Mol. Cell. Biol., 5:2533, 1985.
53. Matsuo, T., Heller, M., Petti, L., O'Shiro, E., and Kieff, E.: Persistence of the entire Epstein-Barr virus genome integrated into human lymphocyte DNA. Science, 226:1322, 1984.
54. Medveczky, M. M., Szomolanyi, E., Hesselton, R., DeGrand, D., Geck, P., and Medveczky, P. G.: Herpesvirus saimiri strains from three DNA subgroups have different oncogenic potentials in New Zealand White rabbits. J. Virol., 63:3601, 1989.
55. Miller, G.: Epstein-Barr Virus. *In* Virology. Edited by B. N. Fields, D. M. Knipe, R. M. Chanock, M. S. Hirsch, J. L. Melnick, T. P. Monath, and B. Roizman. New York, Raven Press, 1990, p.1921.
56. Miller, G., Shope, T., Coope, D., Waters, L., Pagano, J., Bornkamm, G. W., and Henle, W.: Lymphoma in cotton-top marmosets after inoculation with Epstein-Barr virus: Tumor incidence, histologic spectrum, antibody responses, demonstration of viral DNA, and characterization of viruses. J. Exp. Med., 145:948, 1977.
57. Mizell, M.: Lucke frog carcinoma herpesvirus: Transmission and expression during early development. Adv. Viral. Oncol., 5:129, 1985.
58. Morgan, A. J., Finerty, S., Lovgren, K., Scullion, F. T., and Morein, B.: Prevention of Epstein-Barr (EB) virus-induced lymphoma in cottontop tamarins by vaccination with the EB virus envelope glycoprotein gp340 incorporated into immune-stimulating complexes. J. Gen. Virol., 69:2093, 1988.
59. Morgan, A. J., Mackett, M., Finerty, S., Arrand, J. R., Scullion, F. T., and Epstein, M. A.: Recombinant vaccinia virus expressing Epstein-Barr virus glycoprotein gp340 protects cottontop tamarins against EB virus-induced malignant lymphomas. J. Med. Virol., 25:189, 1988.
60. Mosier, D. E., Gulizia, R. J., Baird, S. M., and Wilson, D. B.: Transfer of a functional human immune system to mice with severe combined immunodeficiency. Nature, 335:256, 1988.
61. Mueller, N., Evans, A., Harris, N. L., Comstock, G., Jellum, E., Magnus, K., Orentreich, N., Polk, B. F., and Vogelman, J.: Hodgkin's disease and Epstein-Barr virus: Altered antibody pattern before diagnosis. N. Engl. J. Med., 320:689, 1989.
62. Murray, R. J., Kurilla, M. G., Griffin, H. M., Brooks, J. M., Mackett, M., Arrand, J. R., Rowe, M., Burrows, S. R., Moss, D. J., Kieff, E., and Rickinson, A. B.: Human cytotoxic T- cell responses against Epstein-Barr virus nuclear antigens demonstrated by using recombinant vaccinia viruses. Proc. Natl. Acad. Sci. U.S.A., 87:2906, 1990.
63. Murray, R. J., Wang, D., Young, L. S., Wang, F., Rowe, M., Kieff, E., and Rickinson, A. B.: Epstein-Barr virus-specific cytotoxic T-cell recognition of transfectants expressing the virus-coded latent membrane protein LMP. J. Virol., 62:3747, 1988.
64. Murthy, S. C. S., Trimble, J. J., and Desrosiers, R. C.: Deletion mutants of herpesvirus saimiri define an open reading frame necessary for transformation. J. Virol., 63:3307, 1989.
65. Nilsson, K., and Klein, G.: Phenotypic and cytogenetic characteristics of human B-lymphoid cell lines and their relevance for the etiology of Burkitt's lymphoma. Adv. Cancer Res., 37:319, 1982.
66. Okazaki, W., Purchase, H. G., and Burmester, B. R.: Protection against Marek's disease by vaccination with a herpesvirus of turkeys. Avian Dis., 14:413, 1970.
67. Pearson, G. R., and Scott, R.E.: Isolation of virus-free Herpesvirus saimiri antigen-positive plasma membrane vesicles. Proc. Natl. Acad. Sci. U.S.A., 74:2546, 1977.
68. Petti, L., and Kieff, E.: A sixth Epstein-Barr virus nuclear protein (EBNA3B) is expressed in latently infected growth-transformed lymphocytes. J. Virol., 62:2173, 1988.
69. Petti, L., Sample, J., Wang, F., and Kieff, E.: A fifth Epstein-Barr virus nuclear protein (EBNA3C) is expressed in latently infected growth-transformed lymphocytes. J. Virol., 62:1330, 1988.
70. Rapp, F., and Robbins, D.: Cytomegalovirus and Human Cancer. *In* CMV: Pathogenesis and Prevention of Human Infection. Birth Defects: Original Article Series, Vol. 20, No. 1. Edited by S. A. Plotkin, S. Michelson, J. S. Pagano, and F. Rapp. March of Dimes Birth Defects Foundation. New York: Alan R. Liss, p. 175, 1984.
71. Reisman, D., and Sugden, B.: Trans-activation of an Epstein-Barr viral transcriptional enhancer by the Epstein-Barr viral nuclear antigen 1. Mol. Cell. Biol., 6:3838, 1986.
72. Rispens, B., van Vloten, H., Mastenbroek, N., and Maas, H.: Control of Marek's disease in the Netherlands II. Field trials on vaccination with an avirulent strain (CVI 988) of Marek's disease virus. Avian Dis., 16:126, 1972.
73. Robinson, J. E., Brown, N., Andiman, W., Halliday, K., Francke, U., Robert, M. F., Andersson-Anvret, M., Horstmann, D., and Miller, G.: Diffuse polyclonal B-cell lymphoma during primary infection with Epstein-Barr virus. N. Engl. J. Med., 302:1293, 1980.
74. Rosen, A., Gergely, P., Jondal, M., Klein, G., and Britton, S.: Polyclonal Ig production after Epstein-Barr virus infection of human lymphocytes in vitro. Nature, 267:52, 1977.
75. Rowe, M., and Gregory, C.: Epstein-Barr virus and Burkitt's lymphoma. Adv. Viral. Oncology, 8:237, 1989.
76. Rowe, M., Rooney, C. M., Rickinson, A. B., Lenoir, G. M., Rupani, H., Moss, D. J., Stein, H., and Epstein, M. A.: Distinctions between endemic and sporadic forms of Epstein-Barr virus-positive Burkitt's lymphoma. Int. J. Cancer, 35:435, 1985.
77. Rowe, M., Rowe, D. T., Gregory, C. D., Young, L. S., Farrell, P. J., Rupani, H., Rickinson, A. B.: Differences in B cell growth phenotype reflect novel patterns of Epstein-Barr virus latent gene expression in Burkitt's lymphoma cells. EMBO J., 6:2743, 1987.
78. Rowe, M., Young, L. S., Crocker, J., Stokes, H., Henderson, S., Rickinson, A. B.: Epstein-Barr virus (EBV)-associated lymphoproliferative disease in the SCID mouse model: implications for the pathogenesis of EBV-positive lymphomas in man. J. Exp. Med., 173:147, 1991.
79. Saemundsen, A. K., Purtilo, D. T., Sakamoto, K., Sullivan, J. L., Synnerholm, A. C., Hanto, D., Simmons, R., Anvret, M., Collins, R., and Klein, G.: Documentation of Epstein-Barr virus infection in immunodeficient patients with life-threatening lymphoproliferative disease by Epstein-Barr virus complementary RNA/DNA and viral DNA/DNA hybridization. Cancer Res., 41:4237, 1981.
80. Sample, J., Hummel, M., Braun, D., Birkenbach, M., and Kieff, E.: Nucleotide sequences of mRNAs encoding Epstein-Barr virus nuclear proteins: A probable transcriptional initiation site. Proc. Natl. Acad. Sci. U.S.A., 83:5096, 1986.
81. Sauter, M., Boos, H., Hirsch, F., and Mueller-Lantzsch, N.: Characterization of a latent protein encoded by the large internal repeats and the BamH1 Y fragment of the Epstein-Barr virus (EBV) genome. Virology, 166:586, 1988.
82. Skare, J. C., Milunsky, A., Byron, K. S., and Sullivan, J. L.: Mapping of the X-linked lymphoproliferative syndrome. Proc. Natl. Acad. Sci. U.S.A., 84:2015, 1987.
83. Snydman, D. R., Rudders, R. A., Daoust, P., Sullivan, J. L., and Evan, A. S.: Infectious mononucleosis in an adult progressing to fatal immunoblastic lymphoma. Ann. Intern. Med., 96:737, 1982.
84. Sugaya, K., Bradley, G., Nonoyama, M., and Tanaka, A.: Latent transcripts of Marek's disease virus are clustered in the short and long repeat regions. J. Virol., 64:5773, 1990.

85. Sugden, B., and Metzenberg, S.: Characterization of an antigen whose cell surface expression is induced by infection with Epstein-Barr virus. J. Virol., 46:800, 1983.

86. Sullivan, J. L., Byron, K. S., Brewster, F. E., Baker, S. M., and Ochs, H. D.: X-linked lymphoproliferative syndrome: natural history of the immunodeficiency. J. Clin. Invest., 71:1765, 1983.

87. Swaminathan, S., Tomkinson, B., and Kieff, E.: Recombinant Epstein-Barr virus with small RNA (EBER) genes deleted transforms lymphocytes and replicates in vitro. Proc. Natl. Acad. Sci. U.S.A., 88:1546, 1991.

88. Swendeman, S., and Thorley-Lawson, D. A.: The activation antigen BLAST-2, when shed, is an autocrine BCGF for normal and transformed B cells. EMBO J., 6:1637, 1987.

89. Thomas, J. A., and Crawford, D. H.: Epstein-Barr virus associated B-cell lymphomas in AIDS and after organ transplantation. Lancet, Letter, 1:1075, 1989.

90. Thorley-Lawson, D. A., Nadler, L. M., Bhan, A. K., and Schooley, R. T.: BLAST-2 (EBVCS), an early cell surface marker of human B cell activation, is superinduced by Epstein-Barr virus. J. Immunol., 134:3007, 1985.

91. Thorley-Lawson, D. A., Swendeman, S. L., and Edson, C. M.: Biochemical analysis suggests distinct functional roles for the BLAST-1 and BLAST-2 antigens. J. Immunol., 136:1745, 1986.

92. Tosato, G., Magrath, I., Koski, I., Dooley, N., and Blase, R. M.: Activation of suppressor T cells during Epstein-Barr virus-induced infectious mononucleosis. N. Engl. J. Med., 301:1133, 1979.

93. Uchibayashi, N., Kikutani, H., Barsumian, E., Hauptmann, R., Schneider, F. J., Schwendenwein, R., Sommergruber, W., Spevak, W., Maurer-Fogy, I., Svemura, M., and Kishimoto, T.: Recombinant soluble Fc-epsilon receptor II (Fc$_E$RII/CD23) has IgE binding activity but no B cell growth promoting activity. J. Immunol., 142:3901, 1989.

94. Wang, D., Liebowitz, D., and Kieff, E.: An EBV membrane protein expressed in immortalized lymphocytes transforms established rodent cells. Cell, 43:831, 1985.

95. Wang, D., Liebowitz, D., and Kieff, E.: The truncated form of the Epstein-Barr virus latent-infection membrane protein expressed in virus replication does not transform rodent fibroblasts. J. Virol., 62:2337, 1988.

96. Wang, D., Liebowitz, D., Wang, F., Gregory, C., Rickinson, A., Larson, R., Springer, T., and Kieff, E.: Epstein-Barr virus latent membrane protein alters the human B-

97. lymphocyte phenotype: Deletion of the amino terminus abolishes activity. J. Virol., 62:4173, 1988.

97. Wang, F., Gregory, C. D., Rowe, M., Rickinson, A. B., Wang, D., Birkenbach, M., Kikutani, H., Kishimoto, T., and Kieff, E.: Epstein-Barr virus nuclear antigen 2 specifically induces expression of the B-cell activation antigen CD23. Proc. Natl. Acad. Sci. U.S.A., 84:3452, 1987.

98. Wang, F., Gregory, C., Sample, C., Rowe, M., Liebowitz, D., Murray, R., Rickinson, A., and Kieff, E.: Epstein-Barr virus latent membrane protein (LMP-1) and nuclear proteins 2 and 3C are effectors of phenotypic changes in B lymphocytes: EBNA-2 and LMP-1 cooperatively induce CD23. J. Virol., 64:2309, 1990.

99. Wang, F., Petti, L., Braun, D., Seung, S., and Kieff, E.: A bicistronic Epstein-Barr virus mRNA encodes two nuclear proteins in latently infected, growth-transformed lymphocytes. J. Virol., 61:945, 1987.

100. Wang, F., Tsang, S. F., Kurilla, M. G., Cohen, J. I., and Kieff, E.: Epstein-Barr virus nuclear antigen 2 transactivates latent membrane protein. J. Virol., 64:3407, 1990.

101. Weiss, L. M., Movahed, L. A., Warnke, R. A., and Sklar, J.: Detection of Epstein-Barr viral genomes in Reed-Sternberg cells of Hodgkin's disease. N. Engl. J. Med., 320:502, 1989.

102. Wilson, J. B., Weinberg, W., Johnson, R., Yuspa, S., and Levine, A. J.: Expression of the BNLF-1 oncogene of Epstein-Barr virus in the skin of transgenic mice induces hyperplasia and aberrant expression of keratin 6. Cell, 61:1315, 1990.

103. Yates, J., Warren, N., Reisman, D., and Sugden, B.: A cis-acting element from the Epstein-Barr viral genome that permits stable replication of recombinant plasmids in latently infected cells. Proc. Natl. Acad. Sci. U.S.A., 81:3806, 1984.

104. Young, L., Alfieri, C., Hennessy, K., Evans, H., O'Hara, C., Anderson, K. C., Ritz, J., Shapiro, R. S., Rickinson, A., Kieff, E., and Cohen, J. I.: Expression of Epstein-Barr virus transformation-associated genes in tissues of patients with EBV lymphoproliferative disease. N. Engl. J. Med., 321:1080, 1989.

105. Young, L. S., Dawson, C. W., Clark, D., Rupani, H., Busson, P., Tursz, T., Johnson, A., and Rickinson, A. B.: Epstein-Barr virus gene expression in nasopharyngeal carcinoma. J. Gen. Virol., 69:1051, 1988.

106. Young, L. S., Finerty, S., Brooks, L., Scullion, F., Rickinson, A. B., and Morgan, A. J.: Epstein-Barr virus gene expression in malignant lymphomas induced by experimental virus infection of cottontop tamarins. J. Virol., 63:1967, 1989.

III-10

Papillomaviruses and Cervical Neoplasia

Christopher P. Crum

Introduction

In recent years, human papillomaviruses (HPV) have become the principal focus of efforts to implicate a transmissible virus in the genesis of lower genital tract neoplasia. As would be expected, the explosion in technology has dictated both the tempo and direction of this research, which began with descriptive and experimental pathology, progressed to molecular biology, and finally, involved molecular immunology in efforts to both implicate the virus directly in producing neoplasia while unraveling the mechanisms of host response.

For example, elegant biochemical work by several laboratories has unraveled potential mechanisms by which HPV infection may produce neoplastic transformation. Putting this information in some morphological perspective has been made possible by studies with keratinocyte cultures, in which features of HPV-related neoplasia have been reproduced.[59,85] Further, direct analysis of HPV nucleic acids in clinical material has identified the nature of HPV expression, and provided morphological clues to why certain HPV nucleic acids may be associated with cancer. Clinical application of this information has been attempted, based principally upon the strong association between HPV and cancer. Unfortunately, the strict association between HPV nucleic acids and cervical cancer has been hampered by the discovery of

"latent" or occult virus infection, which in turn has complicated the picture of a diagnostic molecular test which would highlight women at risk for developing cancer. Finally, the advent of molecular immunology has produced sobering observations, balancing the hope for a serological test for HPV exposure with the reality that HPV infection (or exposure) is extremely common while cervical cancer is not. The goal of this chapter is to detail these different facets while putting them into perspective from the point of pathogenesis, diagnosis and clinical management of HPV-related diseases.

Definitions, Mechanisms and Pathobiology of Genital HPV Infection

Definition of Infection

Genital papillomavirus (HPV) "infections" are best defined by the presence of clinically or colposcopically identifiable "lesions" which contain infectious virus, the prototype of which is genital warts. In this instance, infectious virus is likely to be identified within the epithelium (Figure III-10-1A). More recently, the term infection has been expanded to include HPV-related precancerous lesions, or even cancers, infection being used loosely to identify the presence of viral DNA. However, virions are less likely to be identified in these processes (Figures III-10-1B and III-10-1C).[56] As will be detailed

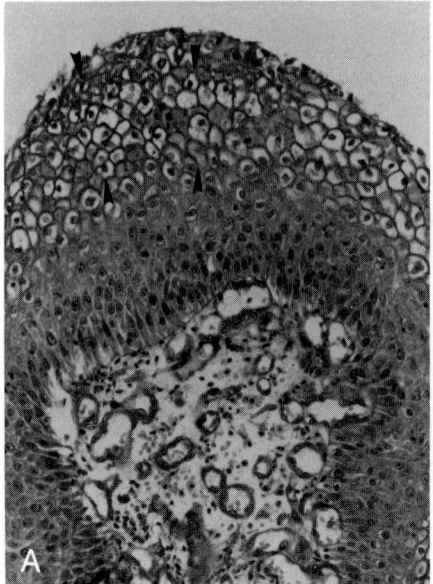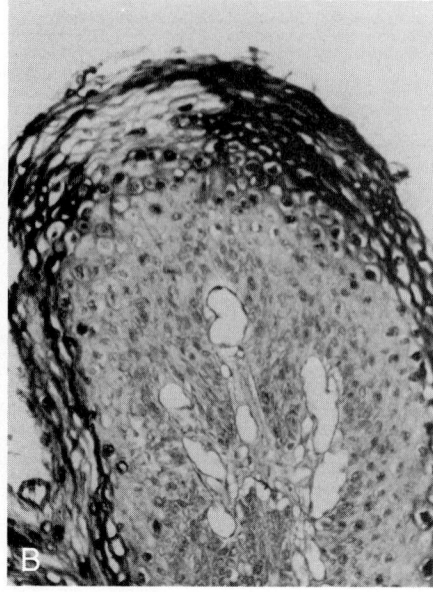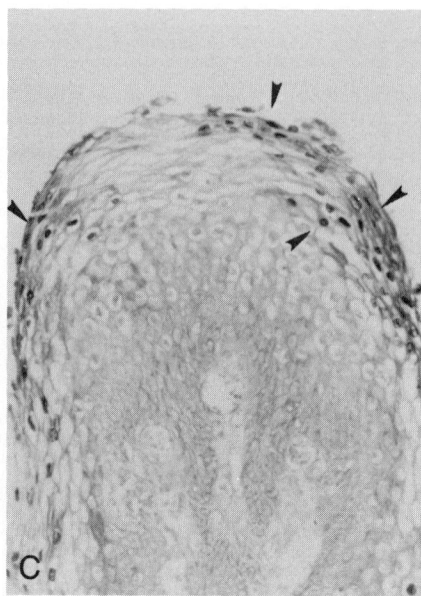

Figure III-10-1.   Histopathology of a classical papillomavirus (HPV) infection (condyloma) of the cervix associated with "low risk" HPV types (HPV types 6 or 11). A. Illustrates the morphological features which include nuclear atypia in the superficial epithelial cells with prominent cytoplasmic halos (arrows). The lower cell layers contain minimal cytological atypia. B. Following in situ hybridization with a biotin-labeled mixed DNA probe containing HPV types 6 and 11 (VIRATYPE, Life Technologies, Gaithersburg, MD). The dark staining in the superficial cell nuclei and cytoplasm represent viral DNA and RNA produced during viral replication. C. An immunoperoxidase stain for HPV capsid proteins, highlighting several darkly staining nuclei in the superficial epithelium (arrows).

subsequently, the presence of HPV DNA should not be held synonymous with infection, in that it may be recovered from individuals with no history (or future prospects) of genital warts, in which case the biological importance of HPV DNA remains unclear (Table III-10-1).

As alluded to above, the hallmark of HPV infection is a morphological "transformation" of the target tissue. This should not be confused with the term transformation as classically applied to changes in cultured cells produced after introduction of HPV nucleic acids. Rather, it defines the morphological alterations which can be most consistently associated with the presence of HPV nucleic acids. It may, depending upon the host response and HPV type involved in the infection, be defined as a genital wart or a genital precancer, either of which is distinct from normal epithelium (Figures III-10-1 and III-10-2).

Mechanism of Infection

Papillomaviruses are epitheliotropic circular double stranded DNA viruses which infect squamous epithelium, and the interval from exposure to the development of a lesion may vary, ranging from a few weeks to several months and perhaps longer.[52,62] It is presumed that the virus gains access to the cervix or lower female genital tract via defects in the epithelium which expose basal epithelial cells to virion particles. In support of this hypothesis is the demonstration of papillomavirus DNA and RNA in basal cells and the observation that experimental infection of squamous mucosa by HPV is enhanced by disturbing the epithelial surface (and hence exposing the basal cells) prior to exposure.[5,50] Of particular interest is the hypothesis that the viral DNA exists either in or in proximity to the epithelium for an extended interval without causing morphological changes.[93] This has

Table III-10-1.   Definitions

HPV	=	Human papillomavirus
HPV infection	=	Production of a lesion (condyloma) which contains HPV virions. Usually synonymous with condyloma or very low grade CIN (see Figure III-10-1).
CIN	=	Cervical intraepithelial neoplasia, synonymous with cancer precursor and distinct from condyloma. Low grade lesions (also called "flat condyloma") may contain HPV virions and be similar in appearance to condyloma (see Figure III-10-2).
HPV-related lesion	=	Includes HPV infection, but also any lesion associated with papillomaviruses, including high grade CIN and various invasive carcinomas.
Occult or Latent HPV infection	=	Defined as the presence of HPV DNA in the absence of demonstrable evidence of HPV infection (i.e., no lesion is present). Natural history is unclear.
High Risk HPV	=	HPV associated with CIN and/or carcinomas.
Low Risk HPV	=	HPV associated with condylomata.
Open reading frame	=	Interval of DNA capable of encoding a protein of sufficient length to functionally justify designation as a potential "gene."

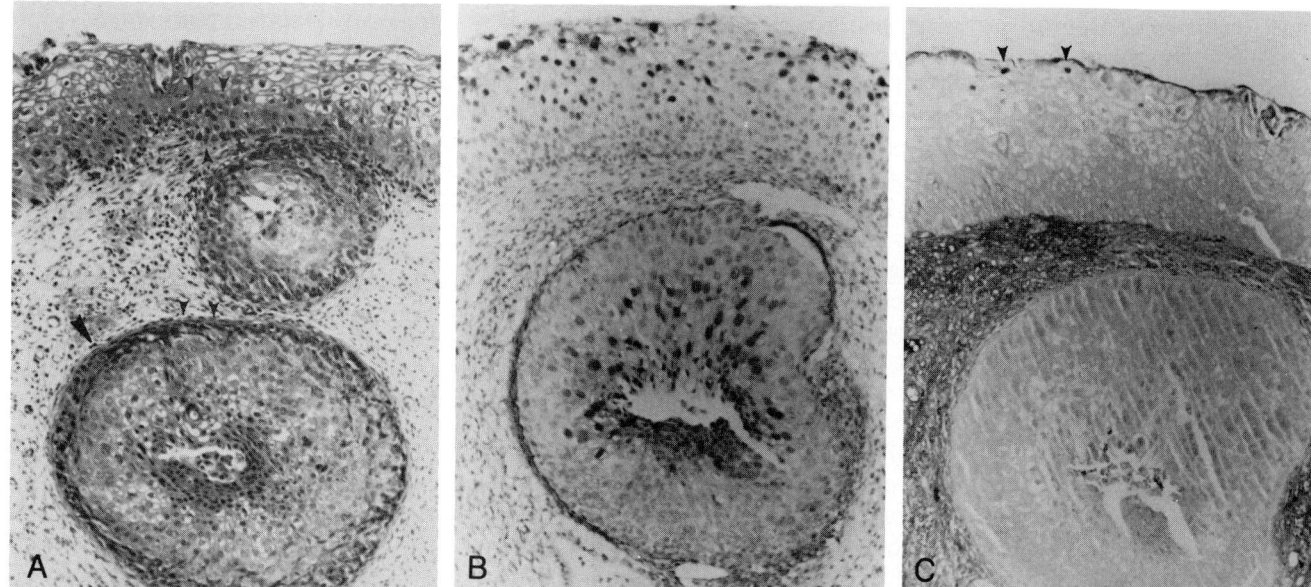

Figure III-10-2.   Histopathology of cervical intraepithelial neoplasm associated with "high risk" HPV types (ie., 16, 31, 33, 35 etc.). A. Illustrates a lesion involving the superficial and crypt (gland) epithelium (large arrow). Koilocytotic atypia is present (upper right), but in addition, nuclear atypia is conspicuous in the lower cell layers (small arrows). B. Following in situ hybridization with a mixed probe containing HPV types 31, 33 and 35. Note the similar distribution of staining as in Figure III-10-1B. In contrast to Figure III-10-1C, capsid proteins are infrequently identified by immunostaining, with rare positive nuclei observed (arrows).

been termed "latent" or occult infection; however, the precise definition of latency and the reservoir of latent infection remain unclear.[5]

As the cells containing the viral DNA approach the upper layers of the epithelium, the virus replicates and assembles into virions, which can be detected by electron microscopy or immunohistochemistry (Figure III-10-1).[97] A portion of the superficial cells in the infected epithelium characteristically display enlarged, hyperchromatic nuclei, with or without cytoplasmic halos (koilocytotic atypia), and the mature virus usually concentrates in this cell population (Figure III-10-1).[48,97] Whether koilocytosis per se is due exclusively to viral replication is controversial, principally because this cytological phenomenon may exist in the absence of abundant capsid proteins or virions. The implication is therefore that koilocytotic cells represent a cytopathic change which may be related to either viral replication, a more fundamental alteration in the morphologically transformed epithelium which is manifest in the superficial cells, or a combination of both processes.[48,97]

Although genital squamous epithelium appears to be the principal site for HPV infection, there is evidence that infection may occur in germinal or undifferentiated epithelial cells which give rise to both the squamous and glandular components of the cervical mucosa. HPV nucleic acids have been isolated from neoplasms not clearly derived from squamous-committed epithelial cells, most notably adenocarcinomas and undifferentiated carcinomas (small cell carcinoma).[90,95]

Site Specificity

Squamous epithelium is most susceptible to HPV infections. In particular, squamo-columnar junctions where the glandular portion is undergoing replacement or "transformation" by squamous epithelium (transformation zones) are most vulnerable to the genital papillomaviruses.[80] Infection with "genital types" has been demonstrated in other mucosal sites in which this process of epithelial transformation takes place, including: the larynx,[1] oro-pharyngeal mucosa,[16] anus,[2] esophagus,[101] subungual mucosa (nail bed),[66] and conjunctiva.[60] Kreider and colleagues demonstrated that some of the above sites were particularly vulnerable to experimental infection with genital viruses.[51] This indicates that genital HPV types require specific conditions provided by certain locales for infection to occur or characteristics facilitating morphological transformation once infection has taken place. Favoring the latter is the unusual predisposition of certain HPV types for the cervix over other genital HPVs.[79]

HPV and Human Genital Neoplasia

Evolution of the Concept

Although studies with animal papillomaviruses established their potential role in the genesis of neoplasia, the most significant link between HPV and human cervical neoplasia came in the form of observations that a common cytological feature of abnormal Papanicolaou smears—koilocytotic atypia—was a cellular marker for the presence of genital HPV infection.[48,61,77] By virtue of its high frequency, this cytological abnormality focused researchers on this virus and its association with not only genital warts, but cervical precancerous lesions (cervical intraepithelial neoplasia (CIN) or cervical dysplasia). Thus, the hypothesis that HPV was an oncogenic virus was derived almost entirely from morphological evidence via the association between genital papillomaviruses, abnormal Papanicolaou smears, and cervical precancers.[62]

The cloning of genital HPVs re-directed attention from the morphology of HPV infection to the molecular pathology of HPV-related diseases, in that molecular probes could identify HPV nucleic acids in the absence of viral particles or capsid proteins. Thus it became possible to identify HPV nucleic acids in not only condylomata, but also squamous precancers and carcinomas of the female genital tract.[3,5,24,33] As part of this progression, the discovery of a variety of different HPV types laid the foundation for establishing that specific HPV types are associated with certain types of genital lesions.[14] Currently over 60 distinct types of HPV have been identified, many of which are associated with specific clinical and pathological characteristics.[5] For example, genital warts and condylomata are associated with certain viral types (i.e., types 6, 11, and others) whereas precancerous lesions (CIN) and invasive cancer are frequently associated primarily with types 16, 18, 31, 33, 35, and others (Table III-10-2).[5] In essence, the "higher grade" precancers are more likely to harbor "high risk" HPV types, implying that, as a group, these lesions are more likely to progress to carcinoma if not treated (Figure III-10-2). The association of high risk HPV types with both high grade precursors and cancers has strengthened the hypothesis that infection by specific types produces specific kinds of precursor lesions which may evolve into carcinoma, depending upon host factors.[3,13,24]

One interesting departure from the above concept occurs with HPV type 18, which is associated infrequently with squamous precursors and more frequently with invasive squamous, glandular and undifferentiated cervical cancers.[54,90,94,95] In contrast to squamous disease, which may persist in a precursor stage for many years, infection and lesion development associated with certain HPV-18 infections may evolve more rapidly, producing cancer, often in young individuals, over a short period of time.

Table III-10-2.   Most Common Genital HPV Types

Low Risk HPVs		
HPV 6	=	Most common HPV type associated with exophytic warts; most common in vulvar condylomata, and uncommon cervical exophytic condylomata.
HPV 11	=	Second most commonly associated with exophytic warts. Uncommon in the cervix.
HPV 42	=	Associated with benign genital warts.
High Risk HPVs		
HPV 16	=	Most common cervical HPV, associated with a spectrum of squamous lesions, including cervical cancer.
HPV 18	=	Associated principally with squamous carcinoma, uncommonly (less than 3%) with squamous precursor lesions. Predominant type in adenocarcinomas and small cell carcinomas.
HPV 31, 33, 35, 51	=	Additional types associated with squamous precursors and invasive cancers, less common than HPV 16.

Molecular Basis for HPV-Related Neoplasia

Lesions associated with "high risk" HPV types frequently possess morphological and biological characteristics which distinguish them from infections by other HPV types, suggesting that molecular events occur during infection which are unique to these virus-host relationships.[13,14,29,30] For example, HPV-16 related precursors produce fewer virions, are associated with greater cytological atypia, and by inference, frequently contain aneuploid cell populations (Figure III-10-2).[29,30] The supposition is that some component of infection by this and similar viruses produces fundamental changes in the biology of the epithelium, which in turn increases the risk of persistence in morphological abnormalities and, in some cases, progression to cancer. Clues to what make HPV-16 infection unique vis-a-vis so-called low risk (HPV-6) infection have been forthcoming from several lines of investigation, all of which center on the viral genome itself (Figure III-10-3).[89] Mechanisms which have been studied and which may distinguish low from high risk viruses include: 1) differences in the expression of so-called transforming genes, such as the E6/E7 and E5 oncoproteins; 2) the process of genomic integration; and 3) mechanisms by which the upstream regulatory region is influenced by exogenous factors such as receptor complexes. These mechanisms are summarized in Figure III-10-4.[6,25,75,88,100]

Most of what is known about HPVs is derived from analogous studies with bovine papillomaviruses (BPV). Lowy and colleagues established that 69% of the BPV genome was capable of altering the growth characteristics of cells in culture (transformation).[57] Subsequent sequencing of this viral DNA and that of HPVs have established that both human and animal HPVs share similar genomic organization, in which the region corresponding to the transforming region of BPV is designated as the early ("E") region. In contrast the late ("L") region encodes capsid proteins and does not possess transforming potential.[5,88] Studies of cell transfection and in-vitro biochemical assays combined with mutational analysis have identified specific open reading frames (ORFs) which produce gene products (proteins) possessing different biological properties (Figure III-10-3).[5]

The E6/E7 region of HPV-16 appears to be critical to HPV-16 mediated transformation of human keratinocytes in culture.[75] The mechanisms of action may involve complexing with certain regulatory (anti-oncogene) proteins such as the Rb (retinoblastoma anti-oncogene) and P53 proteins.[25,100] In contrast to HPV-16, HPV-6 and HPV-11 do not possess the same binding capability, and this may be related to distinct amino acid sequences—termed cell division (CD) motifs—which are conserved among "high risk" viruses and which confer these binding properties.[34] The relationship between this potential binding of cellular regulatory proteins and subsequent events in neoplasia are unclear.

A second component of E6/E7 activity which is relatively unique to high risk HPVs is a spliced message (mRNA) from the E6 ORF. This produces a unique protein (called E6*) which is found in cancers associated with these viruses.[86] The precise role of this molecular phenomenon is unclear.

In addition to the functional properties of the E6/E7 region, host genomic integration by the viral DNA distinguishes high

Genomic Map of HPV-16

(Circular Genome)

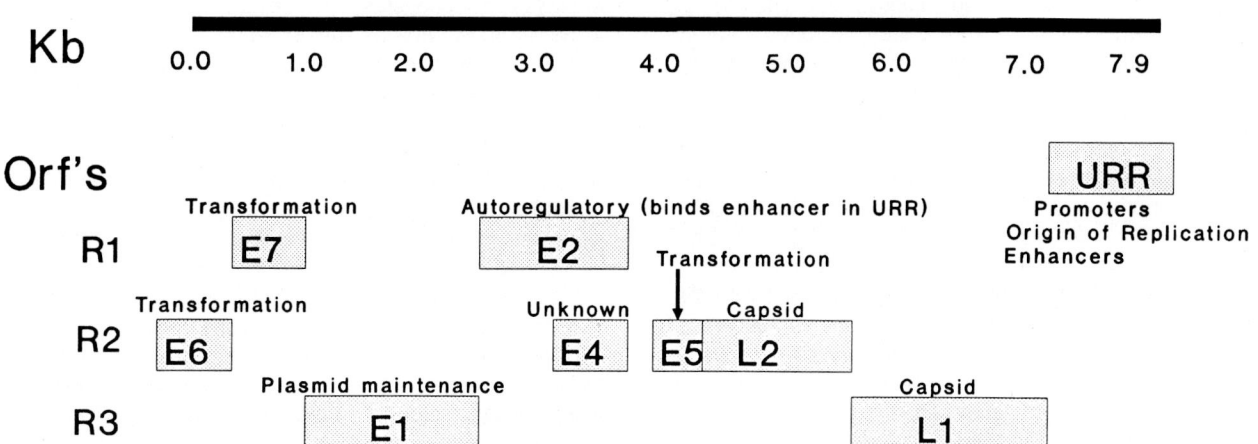

Figure III-10-3.   Schematic of the HPV-16 genome, outlining potential "genes" (open reading frames) and their possible functions.

Molecular Basis for HPV-Related Neoplasia Associated With "High Risk" Viruses

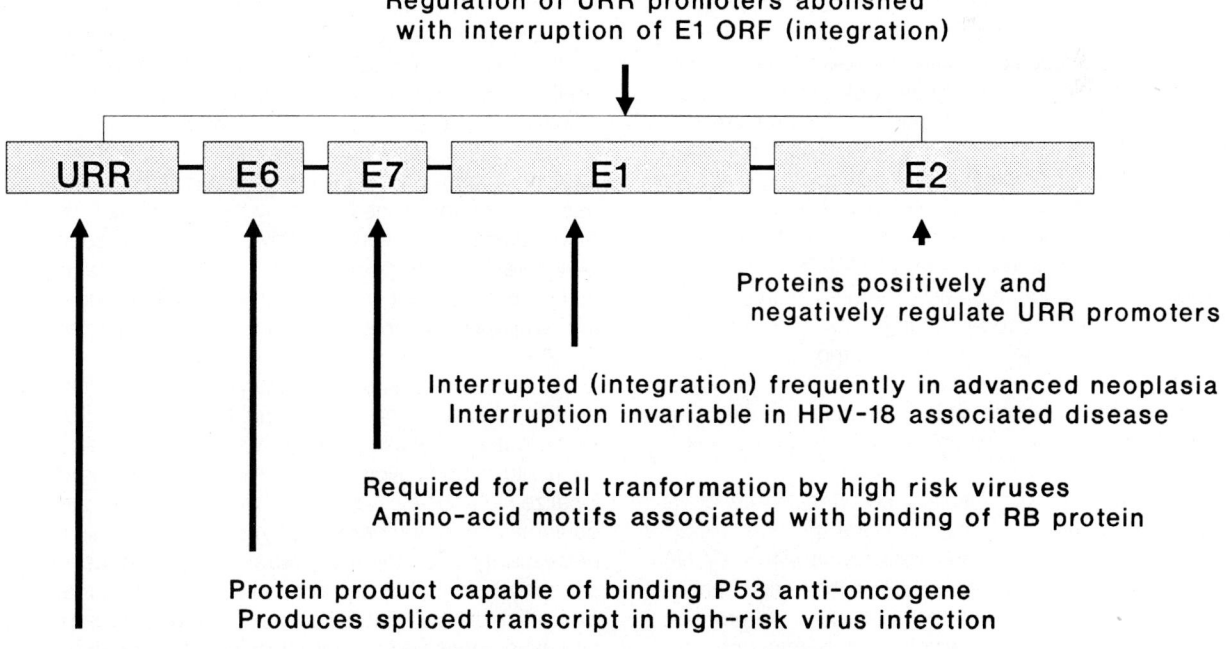

Figure III-10-4.   Schematic of potential mechanisms of HPV-related neoplastic transformation.

risk papillomaviruses. Although the site of integration in the host chromosome is variable, the portion of the HPV genome which is interrupted when integration occurs is relatively constant, occurring within the span of the E1 and E2 ORFs. Integration raises at least four questions. The first is whether it signifies progression to cancer, since integration is rarely found in conventional condylomata (HPV-6), found inconsistently in precursors, and frequently (but not invariably) in invasive cancers associated with HPV-16. The second question is whether integration changes the pattern of viral gene expression. Most compelling is the fact that integration interrupts the genome and silences expression of the E2 ORF. The latter encodes positive and negative autoregulatory proteins, the absence of which may lead to increased expression of the E6/E7 ORFs, which remain continuous with the upstream promoters (Figure III-10-4). This is certainly observed in cell cultures of cancer cell lines, wherein the only HPV DNA present is in integrated form. However, in many cancers and most precancers, integrated sequences, if present, often co-exist with episomal (free viral) DNA, which would theoretically produce the necessary autoregulatory proteins from intact HPV molecules. Finally, integration is most strongly associated with certain HPV types, such as type 18.[95] Lesions associated with this viral DNA almost always exhibit integration, suggesting that while integration is not essential to neoplasia, it may be a marker for more aggressive viral DNA types, or aid more directly in the neoplastic process.[86]

Another ORF with potential transforming ability is the E5 ORF, although the evidence in support of this is limited principally to the BPV system.[20] The relationship of this protein to human disease is unknown. A final region which may distinguish high from low risk HPV is the upstream regulatory region (URR), or long control region (LCR). This region contains sequences which bind nuclear proteins and which contain sequences which will enhance transcription in a variety of HPV types when exposed to glucocorticoids. Studies by Pater and colleagues demonstrated that dexamethasone was required for oncogenic transformation of cultured cells by HPV-16 DNA and *Ras* oncogene, and that this phenomenon was not reproduced with HPV-11.[74] This is of particular interest in light of epidemiological studies associating oral contraceptives with the risk of cervical cancer.[36]

Other ORFs include those encoding capsid proteins (L1,L2) of unknown function, such as the E4 ORF.[68] The latter is produced in abundance in some HPV infections.[4,13,15,23] In addition, the E2 ORF encodes an important product which both positively and negatively regulates the upstream regulating region.[92] Finally, the intact E1 ORF is required for maintenance of the plasmid state, perhaps explaining why it is the site of interruption when genomic integration takes place.[58]

In recent years, the experimental infection of cervical grafts with HPV-11 has produced genital warts in nude mice.[55] Moreover, transfection of human keratinocytes with HPV DNA has verified the necessity of the E7 ORF in the transformation process, and demonstrated that HPV-16 alone will produce an aneuploid cell population which exhibits many characteristics of a precursor lesion.[59] Co-transfection of HPV-16 DNA with oncogenes has likewise produced similar lesions and, in some studies, neoplasms with metastatic potential.[21]

What has not been accomplished has been the successful completion of the life cycle of the virus in tissue culture, or the production of infectious virus from cells into which DNA alone has been introduced. These remain the principle obstacles to successfully mimicking in vitro the in vivo state of the virus, as well as manipulating the viral genome to identify the critical components of infection.

Occult Infection

Considerable evidence has accumulated identifying HPV DNA in tissue or cell preparations which do not exhibit significant morphological abnormalities. The basis for the hypothesis that clinically occult HPV infection exists has been established previously, if simply from the observation that new disease may occur in sites where previously there had been no lesion. In the first molecular analysis of this phenomenon, Steinberg and colleagues reported finding HPV DNA sequences in normal appearing laryngeal mucosa from patients with a history of laryngeal papillomas, but who were at the time in apparent remission.[93] Ferenczy and colleagues linked occult infection to clinical disease in their study of patients with vulvar warts or precancers undergoing laser therapy. They found that grossly normal squamous epithelium adjacent to the treatment field often contained HPV DNA, and that patients with this clinically "occult" infection had a higher frequency of recurrences vis-a-vis those that did not.[27] This is reinforced by observations that warts may preferentially occur at sites of trauma, emphasizing the relationship between healing and viral activation.[73]

It must be emphasized that the studies described above addressed populations with documented HPV-associated lesions either concurrently or in the past. It is possible that despite appearing normal, tissue contained HPV DNA due to its proximity to tissue clinically infected by the virus or from shed cellular material (contamination) in adjacent lesions. Whatever the mechanism, the important questions to be addressed are whether it occurs in women with no history of HPV infection or abnormal Papanicolaou smears, and specifically, if it has prognostic importance.

Numerous studies have reported the detection of HPV DNA in women with no history of previous HPV-related disease.[49] Although some extremely high estimates have been made using either very sensitive techniques such as the polymerase chain reaction or relatively nonspecific techniques such as slot blot hybridization, most studies place the range of occult infection in non-pregnant women at from 5–12%.[32,44]

It is important to stress that the precise epithelial location of HPV DNA sequences in normal epithelium is not known. Numerous studies using relatively sensitive techniques such as in situ hybridization have (with rare exception) failed to localize HPV nucleic acids in normal epithelium, despite the confirmation on Southern blot hybridization.[70] This does not necessarily exclude the potential importance of these sequences, in that Nuovo and colleagues found that a large proportion of HPV-related lesions contain more than one HPV type when analyzed by polymerase chain reaction, despite the fact that only one HPV type could be detected by in-situ hybridization.[71] This would suggest that when a lesion develops from infection by a single virus type, other virus types in the vicinity are in some way inhibited from co-inflicting and also producing morphological changes. In fact, the frequency of histologically demonstrable double infection is less than 5%.[71] Nevertheless, Nuovo and colleagues demonstrated that recurrent lesions following ablation were frequently associated with HPV types other than the original.[72] While the role of occult infection in these recurrences is unknown, this and other findings suggest that occult infection may have clinical significance under certain circumstances.

The above issue again concerns patients with disease, not addressing the question of whether HPV DNA testing will provide information about the natural history of occult infection in women without a history of an abnormal Papanicolaou smear or clinical warts. Even with carefully planned prospective studies, there are two major methodological problems to be overcome. One is the need to identify a population of women who are clearly HPV DNA negative to serve as a control group, because the "control" group may vary as a function of the number of HPV DNA tests performed.[78] The second is confirming that a specific population of HPV-DNA-positive women are truly disease-free at the start of follow-up. Studies indicate that blind re-review of cytologically negative women who are HPV-DNA positive will uncover significant cytological abnormalities in 15–20% which were missed on the first analysis.[56,100] Thus, if careful quality control is not performed, there is the possibility that lesions missed (or not sampled cytologically) and then subsequently discovered will be misinterpreted as having "progressed". In one of the most carefully executed studies, Lorincz and colleagues found that 15 and 5% of HPV positive and negative cases, respectively, developed a significant cytological abnormality over a mean follow-up of two years.[55] However, they noted that the majority of lesions were discovered in women with a prior history of HPV-related disease and represented recurrence versus incidence cases. Only two of twenty-eight (7%) HPV positive women with no history of HPV-related disease developed a lesion over two years of follow-up.[55]

Host Response

The above studies have set the stage for evaluating the relationship between exposure, disease development and the host response. There is ample historical evidence to indicate that a host immune response exists to HPV-related genital disease.[31,63–65,84] The most fundamental is the data documenting spontaneous regression of warts without therapy.[9] Both humoral and cell mediated mechanisms have been implicated in this process. Studies using papillomavirions from cutaneous warts have described higher reactions to intradermal testing in patients with plantar warts (53–79%) than controls (6%).[9] In-vitro tests of leukocyte migration inhibition (LMI) have also complemented these observations. LMI has been reported positive in up to 16% and 79%, respectively, of patients before and after cure of cutaneous warts.[9]

In the cervix, as in other sites, some immune phenomena appear to operate in preventing recurrence following therapy.[26,81] Richart and colleagues demonstrated that the risk of developing new cervical HPV-related precursor lesions following ablative therapy was not greater than that for the population at risk, once short term recurrences were excluded.[81] Recent data by Nuovo and colleagues suggests further that even short term recurrences may not signify an immune defect, because they are frequently related HPV types other than those associated with the original lesion.[72]

Because of the unique problems associated with the study of HPV, in particular the lack of a system for propagating virus in culture, the technology has evolved for producing specific viral proteins selectively in-vitro.[76,91,98] This has made it possible to explore both expression of HPV proteins in tissues and acquire reagents to evaluate the human immune response. Typically used systems involve expression vectors in which a HPV DNA sequence corresponding to a particular ORF (or "gene") is cloned in tandem with a gene which encodes a protein which can be induced artificially in bacterial culture. Using sequence information from both the vector and the HPV DNA insert, the insert can be cloned in such a way to insure that the insert HPV portion is then expressed as part of the "fusion protein".

With the applications of fusion protein technology to express portions or all of ORFs of HPVs and the widespread availability of sequence data from which linear epitopes could be predicted, a multitude of studies have attempted to characterize the immune response to genital papillomaviruses. Several of these studies are summarized in Table III-10-3 (Figure III-10-5).[8,18,19,37–41]

A summary of the studies includes the following points: 1) There are relatively small differences in immunoreactivity to late proteins between cases and controls in studies using Western blot as the mode of detection. Whether this is due to exposure to these proteins early in life, or cross-reactivity with late proteins of other HPVs (such as cutaneous viruses) is unclear;[39,41] 2) Western blot analysis of early proteins such as E4 and particularly E7, point to a greater correlation with disease.[41] However, this depends upon the degree of seroreactivity in the control population. One study reported a 14 fold greater frequency of seroreactivity in cases (21%) which depended upon an extremely low (1.4%) rate in the controls;[41] 3) studies using enzyme-linked-immunoabsorbant assays (ELISA) and oligopeptides have identified "linear" epitopes in a high proportion of cases versus controls, using peptides from the L1 and E2 ORFs. These last studies have employed an exhaustive analysis of the entire coding region, and their completeness is only marred by the limitations inherent in analyzing linear molecules which may or may not represent the critical immunodeterminants present in the native folded protein (17–19); and 4) certain issues have not been resolved, including the following: Discrepancies between studies; the "type-specificity" of immunoreactivity; the status of HPV infection in the control population; route of exposure; the potential of serology to identify patients at risk for invasive cancer and the role of local immunity.[35,96]

Epidemiologic Discrepancies

From the above data it appears that a significant proportion of women who are HPV DNA positive do not exhibit clinical disease, questioning the epidemiological significance of the prevalence of HPV DNA in a population. Kjaer and colleagues reaffirmed the powerful relationship between sexual behavior and cervical cancer in their study of two similar populations in Greenland and Denmark.[47] However,

Table III-10-3.   Serological Reactivity to Genital Papillomaviruses

Reference	Population Studied	Antigen Used	Percent Cases	Percent Controls	Comment
48	STD Clinic	HPV 6b L1	66	57	(a)
		HPV 16 L2	47	30	
		HPV 18 L2	25	26	
		HPV 16 E7	13	12	
		HPV 18 E7	3	1	
41	Colposcopy Clinic	HPV 16 E4	32.6	11.4	p = .004
		HPV 16 E7	6.5	3.8	NS
	Cervical Cancer	HPV 16 E4	15.9	7.8	p = .053
		HPV 16 E7	20.5	1.4	p = .00001
17	CIN and Cancer	HPV 16 E2P (a)	78.0	21.0	
18	Cervical Cancer	HPV 16 L1P (a)	60	7	

(a) Controls are listed here as hospitalized children from this study
NS, Not stated

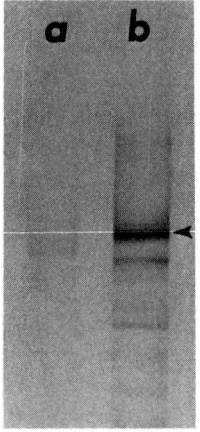

Figure III-10-5.   Immunoblot (western blot) with human serum demonstrating seroreactivity to an in-vitro synthesized pATH fusion protein containing HPV-16 L2 (capsid) protein. The sera reacts with the fusion protein (86 kilodaltons) in lane B (arrow). Lane A, containing a vector (pATH) protein alone as a control, is negative.

when a comparison of prevalence rates for HPV nucleic acids was completed, it appeared that the low risk population exhibited a higher rate of HPV-DNA positivity.[45] Their preliminary conclusion was that the risk of invasive cancer was not directly related to prevalence of HPV DNA, as detected by DNA detection methods. Corroborating evidence has surfaced in other studies as well. Kiviat and colleagues found equal prevalence rates in populations of women with different sexual histories.[44] The conclusion from these studies would be that perhaps only a subset of HPV-DNA positive women are at risk for cancer, and that the assay used to detect HPV DNA is detecting HPV which is not directly related to risk factors associated with cancer.[45] This therefore contrasts to the clear relationship between sexual factors such as sexual partners and herpes virus II infection and clinical cervical or genital HPV-related disease.[42,45,47,83] Nevertheless, a third study by Kjaer and colleagues unearthed a potential explanation for the lower index of HPV DNA positives in the high risk group, which was that factors in the high risk group (such as repeated early exposures and development of immunity) prevented a precise documentation of HPV exposure via DNA testing.[46] In other words, a

"high risk" individual with numerous previous exposures might be less likely to be HPV DNA positive than a "low risk" individual who has fewer exposures but was exposed in the more recent past. In support of this, Burkett and colleagues found that the detection of HPV DNA was unrelated to lifetime sexual partners, but was significantly related to the number of sexual partners in the past year.[7] Thus, a high number of sexual partners and number of years with an "unprotected" cervix (i.e., years in which sexual intercourse was not accompanied by barrier contraception) may identify a high risk group while paradoxically reducing the likelihood of recovering HPV DNA. In this context, the absence of correlation between prevalence of HPV DNA and cancer argues less against the importance of HPV infection as for the significance of other primary factors and co-factors in the genesis of genital neoplasia,[36,69] the most powerful appear to be cigarette smoking, age, immune status, and contraceptive use.[49]

Applications to Clinical Medicine

While HPV DNA positivity clearly identifies a group of women who are more likely to have a cervical lesion, the value of this technique for predicting a lesion in the future is limited, as is the specificity of the technique, particularly in the general population. Because of the way in which the screening protocols are structured (i.e., around the Papanicolaou smear), the potential value of widespread HPV testing is limited to complementing the Papanicolaou smear and reducing false negatives.[56,82,99] Assuming that more sophisticated approaches to Papanicolaou smear screening (i.e., with computerized image analysis) may accomplish the above, HPV DNA testing as currently used will have questionable value, particularly given the uncertain predictive value of HPV DNA positivity for incidence of disease.

Although HPV DNA testing is an imperfect alternative to the Papanicolaou smear for preventing cancer, a significant proportion of cancer cases do develop despite screening, in a addition to about one-third which develop in women who have never been screened.[68] The question is how this subset of women can be identified. More thorough health care delivery via Papanicolaou smear screening is the most effective alternative, essentially rendering the question moot if high risk populations are more thoroughly screened. However, women who do not have access to a gynecological exam will, by definition, benefit neither from a Papanicolaou smear or viral testing as conventionally applied.

At present, the importance of focusing on sexual transmission per se is unclear. Male sexual partners carry the viruses, and in general, manifest no clinical disease, or subtle infections on the penile shaft, scrotum, and urethral meatus. Efforts to detect and eradicate disease in this group have been encouraged, but, as implied above, the actual impact of this approach on the cancer incidence rates are unclear, as are the importance of benign genital warts on areas less susceptible to neoplastic change, such as the vulva and vagina. The failure of high technology (laser therapy, etc.) to eradicate these infections, much less latent virus infection, has encouraged a more conservative approach to generic HPV infection, and focused efforts on identifying subsets of women who are at greater risk. This group includes blacks, smokers, and individuals who have disease on the cervix as depicted by clear-cut Papanicolaou smear abnormalities.[49] The most perplexing component of HPV-related disease remains those cancers which develop rapidly and appear to comprise an aggressive subset associated in part with HPV-18. Unraveling the mechanisms of disease progression in this group and identifying susceptible individuals may be particularly critical to preventing cancer related deaths in this group, which is generally young and which frequently has a history of normal Papanicolaou smears. Ultimately the impetus will shift toward reducing morbidity and mortality by focusing upon methods by which immunology may be exploited to produce protective antibodies, which may eventually lead to successful vaccine development.[10,11]

References

1. Abramson, A. L., Steinberg, B. M., and Winkler, B.: Laryngeal papillomatosis: clinical histopathologic and molecular studies. Laryngoscope, 97:678, 1987.
2. Beckmann, A. M., Daling, J. R., Sherman, K. J., Miller, B. A., Coates, R. J., Kiviat, N. B., Myerson, D., Weiss, N. S., Hislop, T. G., Beagrie, M., and McDougall, J.K.: Human papillomavirus and anal cancer. Int. J. Cancer, 43:1042, 1989.
3. Boshart, M., Gissman, L., Ikenberg, H., Scheurlen, W., and zur Hausen, H.: A new type of papillomavirus DNA, its presence in genital cancer biopsies and in cell lines derived from cervical cancer. EMBO, 3:1151, 1984.
4. Breitburd, F., Croissant, O., and Orth, G.: Expression of human papillomavirus type-1 E4 gene products in warts. In Cancer Cells 5: Papillomaviruses. Edited by B. M. Steinberg, J. L. Brandsma, and L. B. Taichman. New York, Cold Spring Harbor Laboratory, 1987, p. 115.
5. Broker, T. R., and Botchan, M.: Papillomaviruses: Retrospectives and prospectives. In Cancer Cells 4: DNA Tumor Viruses. Edited by M. Botchan, T. Grodzicker, and P. A. Sharp. New York, Cold Spring Harbor Laboratory, 1986, p. 17.
6. Broker, T. R., Chow, L. T., Chin, M. T., Rhodes, C. R., Wolinsky, S. M., Whitbeck, A., and Stoler, M.: A molecular portrait of human papillomavirus carcinogenesis. In Cancer Cells 7: Molecular Diagnostics of Human Cancer. Edited by M. Furth, and M. Greaves. New York, Cold Spring Harbor Laboratory, 1989, p. 197.
7. Burkett, B., Peterson, C., Ward, B. E., Nuckols, M., Burch, L., Brennan, C., and Crum, C. P.: The relationship between contraceptives, sexual practices, and cervical human papillomavirus infection among a college population. J. Clin. Epidemiol., 1991. Submitted.
8. Cason, J., Patel, D., Naylor, J., Lunney, D., Shepherd, P. S., Best, J. M., and McCance, D. J.: Identification of immunogenic regions of the major coat protein of human papillomavirus type 16 that contain type-restricted epitopes. J. Gen. Virol., 70:2973, 1989.
9. Chardonnet, Y., Viac, J., Staquet, M. J., and Thivolet, J.: Cell mediated immunity to human papillomaviruses. Clin. Dermatol., 3:156, 1985.
10. Christensen, N. D., and Kreider, J. W.: Antibody mediated neutralization in vivo of infectious papillomaviruses. J. Virol., 64:3151, 1990.
11. Christensen, N. D., Kreider, J. W., Cladel, N. M., and Galloway, D. A.: Immunological cross-reactivity to laboratory-produced HPV-11 virions of polysera raised against bacterially derived fusion proteins and synthetic peptides of HPV-6b and HPV-16 capsid proteins. Virology, 175:1, 1990.
12. Crum, C. P., Barber, S. R., Symbula, M., Snyder, K., Saleh, A. M., and Roche, J. K.: Co-expression of the human papillomavirus type 16 E4 and L1 open reading frames in early cervical neoplasia. Virol., 178:238, 1990.
13. Crum, C. P., Ikenberg, H., Richart, R. M., and Gissman, L.: Human papillomavirus type 16 and early cervical neoplasia. N. Engl. J. Med., 310:380, 1984.
14. Crum, C. P., Mitao, M., Levine, R. U., and Silverstein, S.: Cervical papillomaviruses segregate within morphologically distinct precancerous lesions. J. Virol., 54:675,1985.

15. Crum, C. P., Nuovo, G., Friedman, D., and Silverstein, S. J.: Accumulation of RNA homologous to human papillomavirus type 16 open reading frames in genital precancers. J. Virol., 62:84, 1988.
16. de Villiers, E. M., Weidauer, H., Otto, H., and zur Hausen, H.: Papillomavirus DNA in human tongue carcinomas. Int. J. Cancer, 36:575, 1985.
17. Dillner, J., Dillner, L., Robb, J., Willems, J., Jones, I., Lancaster, W., Smith, R., and Lerner, R.: A synthetic peptide defines a serologic IgA response to a human papillomavirus-encoded nuclear antigen expressed in virus-carrying cervical neoplasia. Proc. Natl. Acad. Sci. U.S.A., 86:3838, 1989.
18. Dillner, J., Dillner, L., Utter, G., Eklund, C., Rotoloa, A., Costa, S., and Diluca, D.: Mapping of linear epitopes of human papillomavirus type 16: The L1 and L2 open reading frames. Int. J. Cancer, 45:529, 1990.
19. Dillner, J., Bekassy, Z., Jonsson, N., Moreno-Lopez, J., and Blomberg, J.: Detection of IgA antibodies against human papillomavirus in cervical secretions from patients with cervical intraepithelial neoplasia. Int. J. Cancer, 43:36, 1989.
20. DiMaio, D., Guralski, D., and Schiller, J. T.: Translation of open reading frame E5 of bovine papillomavirus is required for its transforming activity. Proc. Natl. Acad. Sci. U.S.A., 83:1797, 1986.
21. DiPaolo, J. A., Woodworth, C. D., Popescu, N. C., Notario, V., and Doniger, J.: Induction of human cervical squamous cell carcinoma by sequential infection with human papillomavirus 16 DNA and viral Harvey ras. Oncogene, 4:395, 1989.
22. Doorbar, J., Campbell, D., Grand, R. J. A., and Gallimore, P. H.: Identification of the human papillomavirus-1a E4 gene products. EMBO, 5:355, 1986.
23. Doorbar, J., Coneron, I., and Gallimore, P. H.: Sequence divergence yet conserved characteristics among the E4 proteins of cutaneous human papillomaviruses. Virology, 172:51, 1989.
24. Durst, M., Gissman, L., Ikenberg, H., and zur Hausen, H.: A papillomavirus DNA from a cervical carcinoma and its prevalence in cancer biopsy samples from different geographic regions. Proc. Natl. Acad. Sci. U.S.A., 80:3812, 1983.
25. Dyson, N., Howley, P. M., Munger, K., and Harlow, E.: The human papillomavirus-16 E7 oncoprotein is able to bind to the retinoblastoma gene product. Science, 243:934, 1989.
26. Erickson, K.: Treatment of the common wart by induced allergic inflammation. Dermatologica, 160:161, 1980.
27. Ferenczy, A., Mitao, M., Nagai, N., Silverstein, S. J., and Crum, C. P.: Latent papillomavirus and recurring genital warts. N. Engl. J. Med., 313:784, 1985.
28. Firzlaff, J. M., Kiviat, N. B., Beckmann, A. M., Jenison, S. A., and Galloway, D. A.: Detection of human papillomavirus capsid antigens in various squamous epithelial lesions using antibodies directed against the L1 and L2 open reading frames. Virology, 164:467, 1988.
29. Fu, Y. S., Huang, I., Beaudenon, S., Ionesco, M., Barrasso, R., de Brux, J., and Orth, G.: Correlative study of human papillomavirus DNA, histopathology, and morphometry in cervical condyloma and intraepithelial neoplasia. Int. J. Gynecol. Pathol., 7:297, 1988.
30. Fu, Y. S., Reagan, J. W., and Richart, R. M.: Definition of precursors. Gynecol. Oncol., 12(Suppl.):220, 1981.
31. Genner, J.: Verrucal vulgares: II. Demonstration of a complement fixation reaction. Acta. Derm. Venereol. (Stockh.), 51:365, 1971.
32. Gissman, L.: Personal Communication.
33. Gissman, L., De Villiers, E-M., and zur Hausen, H.: Analysis of human genital warts (condylomata acuminata) and other genital tumors for human papillomavirus type 6 DNA. Int. J. Cancer, 29:143, 1982.
34. Goldsborough, M. D., DiSilvestre, D., Temple, G. F., and Lorincz, A. T.: Nucleotide sequence of human papillomavirus type 31: A cervical neoplasia-associated virus. Virology, 171:306, 1989.
35. Head, J. R., and Billingham, R. E.: Concerning the immunology of the uterus. Am. J. Reprod. Immunology and Microbiol., 10:76, 1986.
36. Hildesheim, A., Reeves, W. C., Brinton, L. A., Lavery, C., Brenes, M., De La Guardia, M. E., Godoy, J., and Rawls, W. E.: Association of oral contraceptive use and human papillomavirus in invasive cervical cancers. Int. J. Cancer, 45:860, 1990.
37. Jenison, S. A., Firzlaff, J. M., Langenberg, A., and Galloway, D. A.: Identification of immunoreactive antigens of human papillomavirus type 6b using Escherichia coli-expressed fusion proteins. J. Virol., 62:2115, 1988.
38. Jenison, S. A., Yu, X-P., Valentine, J. M., and Galloway, D. A.: Human antibodies react with an epitope of the human papillomavirus type 6b L1 open reading frame which is distinct from the type-common epitope. J. Virol., 63:809, 1989.
39. Jenison, S. A., Yu, X-P., Valentine, J. M., Koutsky, L. A., Christiansen, A. E., Beckmann, A. M., and Galloway, D. A.: Evidence of prevalent genital-type human papillomavirus infections in adults and children. J. Inf. Dis., 1990. In press.
40. Jenson, A. B., Rosenthal, J. D., Oson, C., Pass, F., Lancaster, W. D., and Shah, K.: Immunologic relatedness of papillomaviruses from different species. J. Natl. Cancer Inst., 64:495, 1980.
41. Jochmus-Kudielka, I., Schneider, A., Braun, R., Kimmig, R., Koldovsky, U., Schneweis, K. E., Seedorf, K., and Gissmann, L.: Antibodies against the human papillomavirus type 16 early proteins in human sera: correlation of anti-E7 reactivity with cervical cancer. J. Natl. Cancer Inst., 81:1698, 1989.
42. Kessler, I.: Human cervical cancer as a venereal disease. Cancer Res., 36:783, 1976.
43. Kienzler, J. L.: Humoral immunity to human papillomaviruses. Clin. Derm., 4:144, 1985.
44. Kiviat, N. B., Koutsky, L. A., Paavonen, J. A., Galloway, D. A., Critchlow, C. W., Beckmann, A. M., McDougall, J. K., Peterson, M. L., Stevens, C. E., Lipinski, C. M., and Holmes, K. K.: Prevalence of genital papillomavirus infection among women attending a college student health clinic or a sexually transmitted disease clinic. J. Infect. Dis., 159:293, 1989.
45. Kjaer, S. K., de Villers, E. M., Haugaard, B. J., Christensen, R. B., Teisen, C., Moller, K. A., Poll, P., Jensen, H., Vestergaard, B. F., Lynge, E., and Jensen, O. M.: Human papillomaviruses, herpes simplex virus and cervical cancer incidence in Greenland and Denmark. A population-based cross-sectional study. Int. J. Cancer, 41:518, 1988.
46. Kjaer, S. K., Engholm, G., Teisen, C., Haugaard, B. J., Lynge, E., Poll, P., Vestergaard, B. F., deVilliers, E-M., and Jensen, O. M.: Risk factors for cervical human papillomavirus and herpes simplex virus infections in Greenland and Denmark: a population-based study. Am. J. Epidemiol., 131:669, 1990.
47. Kjaer, S. K., Teisen, C., Haugaard, B. J., Lynge, E., Christensen, R. B., Moller, K. A., Jensen, H., Poll, P., Vestergaard, B. F., de Villiers, E-M., and Mensen, O. M.: Risk

factors for cervical cancer in Greenland and Denmark: a population-based cross-sectional study. Int. J. Cancer, 44:40, 1989.

48. Koss, L. G., and Durfee, G. R.: Unusual patterns of squamous epithelium of the uterine cervix: cytologic and histologic study of koilocytotic atypia. Ann. N.Y. Acad. Sci., 63:1245, 1956.

49. Koutsky, L. A., Galloway, D. A., and Holmes, K. K.: Epidemiology of genital human papillomavirus infection. Epidemiol. Rev., 10:122, 1988.

50. Kreider, S.: Personal Communication.

51. Kreider, J. W., Howett, M. K., Stoler, M. H., Zaino, R. J., and Welsh, P.: Susceptibility of various human tissues to transformation in-vivo with human papillomavirus type 11. Int. J. Cancer, 39:459, 1987.

52. Kreider, J. W., Howett, M. K., Wolfe, S. A., Bartlett, G. L., Zaino, R. J., Sedlacek, T., and Mortel, R.: Morphological transformation in-vivo of human uterine cervix with papillomavirus from condylomata acuminata. Nature, 317:639, 1985.

53. Kurman, R. J., Shah, K. H., Lancaster, W. D., and Jenson, A. B.: Immunoperoxidase localization of papillomaviral antigens in cervical dysplasia and vulvar condyloma. Am. J. Obstet. Gynecol., 140:931, 1981.

54. Kurman, R. J., Shiffman, R. M., Lancaster, W. D., Reid, R., Jenson, A. B., Temple, G. F., and Lorincz, A. T.: Analysis of individual human papillomavirus types in cervical neoplasia: a possible role for type 18 in rapid progression. Am. J. Obstet. Gynecol., 159:1631, 1988.

55. Lorincz, A. T., Schiffman, M. H., Jaffurs, W. J., Marlow, J., Quinn, A. P., and Temple, G. F.: Temporal associations of human papillomavirus infection with cervical cytologic abnormalities. Am. J. Obstet. Gynecol., 162:645, 1990.

56. Lorincz, A. T., Temple, G. F., Patterson, J. A., Jenson, A. B., Kurman, R. J., and Lancaster, W. D.: Correlation of cellular atypia and human papillomavirus deoxyribonucleic acid sequences in exfoliated cells of the uterine cervix. Obstet. Gynecol., 68:508, 1986.

57. Lowy, D. R., Dvoretzky, I., Shober, R., Law, M.-F., Engel, L., and Howley, P.: In-vitro tumorigenic transformation by a defined sub-genomic fragment of bovine papillomavirus DNA. Nature, 287:72, 1980.

58. Lusky, M., and Botchan, M. R.: Genetic analysis of bovine papillomavirus type 1 trans-acting replication factors. J. Virol., 53:955, 1985.

59. McCance, D. J., Kopan, R., Fuchs, E., and Laimans, L. A.: Human papillomavirus type 16 alters human epithelial cell differentiation in-vitro. Proc. Natl. Acad. Sci. U.S.A., 85:7169, 1988.

60. McDonnell, J. M., Mayr, A. J., and Martin, W. J.: DNA of human papillomavirus type 16 in dysplastic and malignant lesions of the conjunctiva and cornea. N. Engl. J. Med., 320:1442, 1989.

61. Meisels, A., and Fortin, R.: Condylomatous lesions of the cervix and vagina I. Cytologic patterns. Acta. Cytol., 20:505, 1976.

62. Meisels, A., and Morin, C.: Human papillomavirus and cancer of the uterine cervix. Gynecol. Oncol., 12(Suppl.):111, 1981.

63. Morison, W. L.: Survey of viral warts, herpes zoster, and herpes simplex in patients with secondary immunodeficiency and neoplasms. Brit. J. Dermatol., 91:18, 1974.

64. Morison, W. L.: Cell-mediated immune responses in patients with warts. Brit. J. Dermatol., 93:553, 1975.

65. Morris, H. H., Gatter, K. C., Sykes, G., Casemore, V., and Mason, D. Y.: Langerhans' cells in human cervical epithelium: effects of wart virus infection and intraepithelial neoplasia. Brit. J. Obstet. Gynecol., 90:412, 1983.

66. Moy, R. L., Eliezri, Y. D., Nuovo, G. J., Zitelli, Z. A., Bennett, R. G., and Silverstein, S. J.: Squamous cell carcinoma of the finger is associated with human papillomavirus type 16 DNA. J.A.M.A., 261:2669, 1989.

67. National Cancer Institute: Cancer control objectives for the nation: 1985-2000. Bethesda, MD, U.S. Department of Health and Human Services, Public Health Service, 1986, NIH publication no. 86-2880 (NCI monographs, no. 2).

68. Neary, K., Horwitz, B. H., and DiMaio, D.: Mutational analysis of open reading frame E4 of bovine papillomavirus type 1. J. Virol., 61:1248, 1987.

69. Neill, S. M., Lessanaleibowitch, M., Pelisse, M., and Moyalbarracco, M.: Lichen sclerosis, invasive squamous cell carcinoma and human papillomavirus. Am. J. Obstet. Gynecol., 162:1633, 1990.

70. Nuovo, G. J.: Correlation of histology with human papillomavirus DNA detection in the female genital tract. Gynecol. Oncol., 31:176, 1988.

71. Nuovo, G. J.: Human papillomavirus (HPV) DNA in genital tract lesions histologically negative for condylomata: analysis by in situ, Southern blot hybridization and the polymerase chain reaction. Am. J. Surg. Pathol., 1990. In press.

72. Nuovo, G. J., and Pedemonte, B. M.: Human papillomavirus types and recurrent cervical warts. J.A.M.A., 263:1223, 1990.

73. Papay, F., Wood, B., and Coulson, M.: Squamous cell papilloma at the tracheoesophageal puncture stoma. Arch. Otolaryngol. Head Neck Surg., 114:564, 1988.

74. Pater, M. M., Hughes, G. A., Hyslop, D. E., Nakshatri, H., and Pater, A.: Glucocorticoid-dependent oncogenic transformation by type 16 but not type 11 human papillomavirus DNA. Nature, 335:832, 1988.

75. Phelps, W. C., Yee, C. L., Munger, K., and Howley, P. M.: The human papillomavirus

type 16 E7 gene encodes transactivation and transformation functions similar to those of adenovirus E1A. Cell, 53:539, 1988.

76. Pilacinsky, W. P., Glassman, D. L., Krzyzek, R. A., Sadowski, P. L., and Robbins, A. K.: Cloning and expression in Escherichia coli of the bovine papillomavirus L1 and L2 open reading frames. Biotechnology, 2:356, 1984.

77. Purola, E., and Savia, E.: Cytology of gynecologic condyloma acuminatum. Acta. Cytol., 21:26, 1977.

78. Reeves, W. C., Arosemena, J. R., Garcia, M., de Lao, S. L., Cuevas, M., Wuiroz, E., Caussy, D., and Rawls, W. E.: Genital human papillomavirus infection in Panama City prostitutes. J. Inf. Dis., 160:599, 1989.

79. Reid, R., Greenberg, M., Jenson, A. B., Husain, M., Willett, J., Daoud, Y., Temple, G., Stanhope, C. R., Sherman, A. I., Phibbs G. D., and Lorincz, A. T.: Sexually transmitted papillomaviral infections. I. The anatomic distribution and pathologic grade of neoplastic lesions associated with different viral types. Am. J. Obstet. Gynecol., 156:212, 1987.

80. Richart, R. M.: Cervical intraepithelial neoplasia. In Pathology Annual. Edited by S. C. Sommers. New York, Appleton-Century-Crofts, 1973, p. 301.

81. Richart, R. M., Townsend, D. E., Crisp, W., DePetrillo, A., Ferenczy, A., Johnson, G., Lickrish, G., Roy, M., and Villa Santa, U.: An analysis of "long term" follow-up results in patients with cervical intraepithelial neoplasia treated by cryotherapy. Am. J. Obstet. Gynecol., 137:823, 1980.

82. Ritter, D. B., Kadish, A. S., Vermund, S. H., Romney, S. L., Villari, D., and Burk, R. D.: Detection of human papillomavirus deoxyribonucleic acid in exfoliated cells as a predictor of cervical neoplasia in a high-risk population. Am. J. Obstet Gynecol., 159:1517, 1988.

83. Rotkin, I. D.: Epidemiology of cancer of the cervix. III. Sexual characteristics of a cervical cancer population. Am. J. Public Health, 57:815, 1967.

84. Samuel, M., Shirodaria, P. V., and McMillan, S. A.: Incidence of virus-specific antibodies and autoantibodies in sera of patients with warts. Clin. Exp. Dermataol., 1:269, 1976.

85. Schlegel, R., Phelps, W. C., Zhang, Y.-L., and Barbosa, M.: Quantitative keratinocyte assay detects two biological activities of human papillomavirus DNA and identifies viral types associated with cervical carcinoma. EMBO J., 7:3181, 1988.

86. Schwartz, E., Schneider-Gadicke, A., and zur Hausen, H.: Human papillomavirus type-18 transcription in cervical carcinoma cell lines and in human cell hybrids. In Cancer Cells 5: Papillomaviruses. Edited by B. M. Steinberg, J. L. Brandsma, and L. B. Taichman. New York, Cold Spring Harbor Laboratory, 1987, p. 47.

87. Seedorf, K., Krammer, G., Durst, M., Suhai, S., and Rowenkamp, W.: Human papillomavirus type 16 DNA sequence. Virology, 145:181, 1985.

88. Seedorf, K., Oltersdorf, T., Krammer, G., and Rowenkamp, W.: Identification of early proteins of the human papillomaviruses type 16 (HPV 16) and 18 (HPV 18) in cervical carcinoma cells. EMBO J., 6:139,1987.

89. Sekine, H., Fuse, A., Inaba, N., Takamizawa, H., and Simizu, B.: Detection of the human papillomavirus 6b E2 gene product in genital condyloma and laryngeal papilloma tissues. Virology, 170:92, 1989.

90. Smotkin, D., Berek, J. S., Fu, Y. S., Hacker, N. F., Major, F. G., and Wettstein, F. O.: Human papillomavirus deoxyribonucleic acid in adenocarcinoma and adenosquamous carcinoma of the uterine cervix. Obstet. Gynecol., 68:241, 1986.

91. Smotkin, D., and Wettstein, F. O.: Transcription of human papillomavirus type 16 early genes in a cervical cancer and a cancer-derived cell line and identification of the E7 protein. Proc. Natl. Acad. Sci. USA, 83:4680, 1986.

92. Spalholz, B. A., Wang, Y.-C., and Howley, P. M.: Transactivation of a bovine papillomavirus transcriptional regulatory element by the E2 gene product. Cell, 42:183, 1985.

93. Steinberg, B. M., Topp, W. C., Schneider, P. S., and Abramson, A. L.: Laryngeal papillomavirus infection during clinical remission. N. Engl. J. Med., 308:1261, 1985.

94. Stoler, M. H., Rhodes, C. R., Whitbeck, A., Chow, L. T., and Broker, T. R.: Gene expression of HPV type 16 and 18 in cervical neoplasia. In Papillomaviruses. Edited by P. Howley, T. Broker. UCLA Symposium Mol. Biol., 124:1, 1990.

95. Stoler, M. H., Walker, A. N., and Mills, S.E.: Small cell neuroendocrine carcinoma of the cervix: a human papillomavirus type 18 associated cervix cancer. Lab. Invest., 60:92A, 1989.

96. Syrjanen, K. J.: Immunocompetent cells in uterine cervical lesions of human papillomavirus origin. Gynecol. Obstet. Invest., 16:327, 1983.

97. Taichman, L. B., Reilly, S. S., and LaPorta, R. F.: The role of keratinocyte differentiation in the expression of epitheliotropic viruses. J. Invest. Dermatol., 1:137, 1983.

98. Tanese, N., Roth, M., and Goff, S. B.: Expression of enzymatically active reverse transcriptase in Escherichia coli. Proc. Natl. Acad. Sci. U.S.A., 82:4944, 1985.

99. Ward, B. E., Burkett, B. A., Peterson, C., Nuckols, M., Brennan, C., Birch, L., and Crum, C. P.: Cytological correlates of cervical papillomavirus infection. Int. J. Gynecol. Pathol., 1991. In press.

100. Werness, B. A., Levine, A. J., and Howley, P. M.: Association of human papillomavirus types 16 and 18 E6 proteins with p53. Science, 248:76, 1990.

101. Winkler, B. W., Capo, V., Reumann, W., LaPorta, R., Reilly, S., Green, P., Richart, R. M., and Crum, C. P.: Human papillomavirus infection of the esophagus: a clinicopathologic study with demonstration of papillomavirus antigen by the immunoperoxidase technique. Cancer, 55:149, 1985.

Hepatitis Viruses

Max W. Sung
George Acs

Introduction

Clinical hepatitis produced by viral infection has been documented for at least five specifically hepatotropic viruses. These include: 1) Hepatitis A virus (HAV), an RNA picornavirus that is transmitted fecal-orally and produces a self-limiting clinical course.[66] 2) Hepatitis B virus (HBV), a partially double stranded hepadnavirus that is transmitted parenterally and may produce a self-limiting clinical course with clearance of the virus, or persist with viral replication leading to chronic hepatitis, cirrhosis, and hepatocellular carcinoma (HCC).[155] 3) Hepatitis C virus (HCV), a single-stranded RNA virus related to the *Flaviviridae* that is transmitted parenterally and accounts for the majority of parenterally transmitted non-A, non-B hepatitis.[32] Similar to HBV, HCV infection may be self-limiting or persistent as chronic hepatitis, cirrhosis, and hepatocellular carcinoma. 4) Hepatitis D virus (HDV or delta virus), an RNA virus which requires the presence of HBV for infection, and which may affect the clinical course of HBV infection.[124] 5) Hepatitis E virus (HEV), an RNA virus that is transmitted fecal-orally and accounts for the majority of enterically transmitted non-A, non-B hepatitis.[4,153] HEV infection, like HAV, is self-limiting and has not been implicated in the development of hepatocellular carcinoma. Other viruses, not specifically hepatotropic, may also produce clinical hepatitis; these include cytomegalovirus, Epstein-Barr virus, human immunodeficiency virus, herpes simplex virus, yellow fever virus, rubella, and the Ebola, Lassa and Marburg viruses.[214] This discussion will concern those viruses associated with hepatocellular carcinoma, namely, hepatitis B, C, and D viruses.

Hepatitis B Virus (HBV)

Structure and Pathogenicity

The hepatitis B virus is a 42 nm particle with envelope proteins (HBsAg) enclosing a 27 nm core particle, which consists of a partially double stranded circular DNA genome, a core protein (HBcAg), and a DNA polymerase. The HBV genome contains four open reading frames which are transcribed and translated into proteins. These include the envelope proteins (large, middle, and major HBsAg), produced by the S-gene, pre-S1 and pre-S2 gene sequences; the core protein (HBcAg), produced by the C-gene and pre-C gene sequence, and which is also truncated and secreted as the e antigen (HBeAg); the DNA polymerase protein and X-protein, produced by the P- and X-genes, respectively.[119,151,176] Hepatitis B virus is transmitted parenterally from infected patients,[154] where concentrations in the blood may approach 10^{10} per ml (concentrations in body secretions such as semen and saliva are only 1/1000 that of blood).[73,91] Settings where HBV may be transmitted include parenteral exposure to infected blood products such as during transfusions,[2] contamination of needles used in intravenous drug administrations,[27] sexual intercourse,[180] from mother to infant perinatally or in utero.[11,64,161,162] Infants of HBeAg positive mothers have a 70% chance of infection, and following acute infection, a 90% chance of chronic infection.[63] Transmission has also been reported in institutions for the mentally retarded,[181] day care centers,[69] and family environments within close interpersonal contacts.[72,132,146] The virus has been shown to be quite stable at ambient temperatures, and contamination of surfaces in homes of chronically infected persons has been documented.[14,15] The mode of transmission in intra-family contacts may be through inapparent percutaneous exposure, although oral spread cannot be excluded, since accidental ingestion of HBsAg positive human serum has been reported to result in HBV infection.

Following entry into the bloodstream, the hepatitis B virus circulates to the liver, where it enters a hepatocyte, possibly via membrane receptors recognizing a sequence from the pre-S1 gene product.[136] Within the hepatocyte, the virus replicates via an RNA intermediate, encapsidates, and is released from the host cell.[204] The infected cells also secrete large amounts of HBsAg (major protein) in the form of 22 nm particles and tubules, and HBeAg, a truncated portion of the core protein.[51,139] HBV is generally not cytopathic; the viral gene products, HBcAg and HBeAg, become associated with the membranes of infected hepatocytes and elicit a Class I immune response from cytotoxic T-lymphocytes, which in turn produces hepatocellular necrosis.[121,122,123,186] Antibodies are also formed against viral proteins (anti-HBs, anti-HBc, anti-HBe) but these do not appear to produce hepatocellular damage, except in immune-complex mediated disease such as polyarteritis and polyarthritis occasionally seen during acute infection.[50,197] In the majority of adult patients following acute infection, viral replication ceases and HBeAg and HBsAg are cleared from the circulation in less than three and six months, respectively.[79] Viral replication persists however in up to 10% of adults and 90% of neonates following acute infection, with continued presence of HBsAg, HBeAg, and HBV DNA in blood.[117,159] The frequency of viral persistence following acute infection is related to age, sex and immune deficiency; 90% of infants less than one year of age, 30% of children ages one through five, 10% of adults;[117] men twice as likely as women;[179] immune deficient individuals such as those with HIV infection,[185] those with renal insufficiency requiring hemodialysis,[182] and those with Down's syndrome.[80] Patients exposed to large pools of potentially infected plasma such as hemophiliacs also are at risk for chronicity.[62] Clearance of the virus in chronic infections may occur spontaneously, with seroconversion to negativity for HBeAg and HBsAg in 10% and 1–2% of cases, respectively.[117] Chronically infected patients exhibit a wide range of pathology, from asymptomatic carriers, to a continuum of hepatic pathology from chronic persistent, chronic lobular, and chronic active hepatitis, to eventual cirrhosis and/or hepatocellular carcinoma.[145]

HBV and Hepatocellular Carcinoma

Epidemiological Considerations. Population surveys of markers of HBV infection (HBsAg, HBeAg, anti-HBs, anti-HBc, HBV DNA) have shown wide geographic variations.[170] In high endemic areas, such as sub-Saharan Africa, China, and Southeast Asia, the prevalence of HBsAg, a marker for chronic infection, is 5–15% and overall infection rates 70–90%.[99] In these areas, transmission is primarily vertical from mother to infant and horizontal in children less than five years of age. Low endemic areas include North America, Western Europe, Australia, temperate South America, where prevalence for HBsAg is less than 1% and overall infection rates 5–7%, with primarily horizontal transmission involving high risk groups such as recipients of contaminated blood products, intravenous drug users, sexual partners, and institutionalized mentally retarded individuals. The evidence for epidemiologic association between chronic HBV infection and hepatocellular carcinoma (HCC) is overwhelming. Close to 300 million people worldwide are chronic carriers of HBV and the risk of developing HCC in this population is more than 200-fold higher than in the non-infected population.[178] In low endemic areas, HCC found on autopsies is about 0.4%,[78,208] while in high endemic areas where HBV infection is 10-fold higher, 20–40% of all cancers are HCC.[97,113,150,177] In the best prospective study from Taiwan, 22,707 males were tested for hepatitis B surface antigen, of whom 3,454 were positive (15.2%).[10] At the seven-year follow-up, 116 cases of HCC were diagnosed, 113 of the cases in the patients who had previously tested positive for HBsAg; the other three cases had other serological markers indicating that infection with HBV had occurred. None of the HBsAg negative controls developed HCC. In another study, it was demonstrated that HVB can be passaged vertically and that HCC patients more frequently have HBsAg positive mothers than fathers.[8,107] These two studies indicate not only an association between HBV and HCC but also strongly suggest a causal relationship. It is generally accepted that carcinogenesis is a multistep process involving initiation, promotion, and progression.[202] The question arises, despite this overwhelming epidemiological evidence, whether HBV infection alone can be responsible for all these processes. There are several observations indicating that other agents alone or in combination with HBV play a role in the etiology of HCC. In industrialized countries 68% and in developing countries 11% of the HCC patients do not have serological markers of HBV infection. These data must be treated cautiously since they depend on the sensitivities of the assays for serological markers. The numbers may change substantially by using

the polymerase chain reaction which can detect minimal amounts of HBV DNA in serum or tissue.[20,95,140]

More compelling evidence for the contribution of other factors to hepatic carcinogenesis are the following: 1) within one region, the prevalence of HBV infection may be relatively uniform but HCC is not;[141,195,209,210] 2) HCC is more frequently found in males than in females;[187] and 3) in some endemic areas, variation in HCC rates have been reported by ethnic group or place of birth.[109] Besides HBV, other factors in the development of HCC may include genetic disposition, and the role of the immune system. In addition alcohol, cigarette smoking, oral contraceptives, and aflatoxin have been implicated as etiological agents, as have alpha-1-antitrypsin deficiency and schistosomiasis.

Aflatoxin exposure from ingestion of aflatoxin-contaminated foods has been implicated as a cause of HCC. Most of these correlation studies were done in high HBV endemic areas, did not take into account HBV status, and were plagued by inaccurate assessments of aflatoxin exposure.[24,142,143,165,195] A 1987 study in Swaziland addressed the relationship between aflatoxin exposure, HBV infection, and the incidence of HCC.[141] In this study, HBsAg prevalence varied little from region to region, while aflatoxin exposure varied by as much as five fold. Incidence of hepatocellular carcinoma also varied by up to five fold and correlated well with aflatoxin exposure, suggesting that aflatoxin may act as an independent risk factor. Alcohol consumption and cigarette smoking have also been implicated in the causation of HCC in case control and cohort studies.[77,105,189] However, when HBV status was taken into account, alcohol consumption remained a risk factor, while cigarette smoking did not.[5,138,189,211] The role of cirrhosis as the actual etiologic link was addressed in a cross sectional study from France which showed that the relative risk for hepatocellular carcinoma was about twice greater in HBV-associated cirrhosis as in alcoholic cirrhosis patients.[67] Of note is a study from Taiwan where up to 27% of HBV-associated hepatocellular carcinoma did not have cirrhosis.[10] Oral contraceptive use has also been recognized as a risk factor, but HBV status was not not taken into account in these studies.[58,75,133]

Mechanisms of Oncogenicity. Application of the technology of molecular biology to HBV infection gave several clues regarding the mechanisms by which HBV infection leads to HCC. A uniform mechanism, valid for every HCC, is still elusive however. In the following sections we will review the genetic organization of HBV during infection, and the possible mechanism(s) by which it can cause HCC.

The availability of cloned HBV DNA made it possible to detect HBV DNA in hepatocellular carcinomas. The epidemiological studies based on serological markers were confirmed, since all the HCCs induced by HBV infection contained chromosomally integrated HBV DNA in various forms. The long latency period which elapses between infection and the development of HCC makes it very unlikely that the HBV DNA codes for a dominantly acting classical oncogene. Furthermore during this latency period the HBV DNA gets fragmented and rearranged; thus neither the HBV DNA sequences inserted nor the chromosomal site of insertion are uniform in the various HCCs. The chromosomally integrated HBV DNA may release the growth control of hepatocytes by: coding for a factor like the X-protein which activates otherwise dormant genes, or activates proto-oncogenes or silences anti-oncogenes; insertion of HBV DNA sequences which can also activate and influence the transcription of cellular genes; and causing chronic inflammation with cell death and hepatocyte regeneration, fibrosis, and activating the immune system by liberating cytokines at the wrong time at the wrong place.

The Role of X Protein in HCC. The X-protein coded by the X-gene of HBV has a transactivating activity on a number of viral and cellular genes which may be involved in the development of HCC.[33,87,163,164,171,190,191,192,193] Its genomic localization is analogous to that of the human T cell lymphotropic viruses (HTLV-I, II and HIV) namely it is at the 3' end of the linearized genome.[120] Interestingly, other DNA viruses with oncogenic activity also code for a transactivating activity, for example the T antigen of SV40,[18,19] the MS-EA protein of Epstein-Barr virus,[112] the IE protein of herpes simplex,[54,60] and the tat protein of the human immunodeficiency virus,[39] which despite being an RNA virus shares some steps in its replicative cycle with HBV. The sequence coding for the X-protein is well conserved between the various subtypes of HBV and in the woodchuck and ground squirrel hepatitis viruses. Despite similar genetic organization of the hepadnaviruses, duck hepatitis virus does not contain the sequences coding for the X-protein and infection with this virus does not lead to HCC. In many HCCs the viral DNA is inserted near or within the coding sequences of the X-protein;[205] thus the possibility that expression of this protein, or of a fusion protein with cellularly coded genes, plays an important role in the development of HCC. That specific cellular proteins in concert with virally coded proteins are involved in HCC is suggested by the finding that chimpanzees infected with HBV display the classical symptoms and signs of hepatitis as judged morphologically in liver, and by the appearance of elevated serum enzymes together with viral antigens and the corresponding antibodies. In contrast to human disease, however, HBV infection in the chimpanzee does not lead to HCC.

Activation of Oncogenes, Growth Factors and Receptors in HCC. Although the woodchuck hepatitis virus DNA sequences are not adjacent to the coding sequences of the myc gene, rearrangements of the myc gene with a 5–50-fold higher expression was found in several HCCs. The rearrangements found in woodchuck HCCs are similar to those found in human B and T cell leukemias, Burkitt's lymphoma and mouse plasmacytoma.[127] Mutations and activation of the genes belonging to the ras family are associated with a wide variety of human cancers. Mutations in the ras gene(s) are not found in human HCCs, but activated H-ras and K-ras genes have been detected in some HCCs.[88,184] Since in other tissues, high expression of the ras genes, as well as mutated sequences, are associated with malignant transformation, the role of ras gene in HCCs cannot be overlooked. Among the growth factors analyzed in HCCs, insulin-like growth factor II (IGF II), originally called somatomedin A, seems to be involved in the development of HCCs. IGF II RNAs are differentially spliced; the most abundant species found in fetal woodchuck liver represents the predominant species in both precancerous liver nodules and HCCs in the woodchuck.

Furthermore, the pattern of IGF II RNAs in precancerous liver nodules is similar to that found in fully malignant HCCs. Thus the activation of IGF II transcripts may contribute to the growth of precancerous nodules.[199] Since the development of carcinomas can be viewed as a disturbance of the signal transducing system, it is intriguing that HBV DNA is sometimes integrated in frame next to a liver cell sequence which bears a striking homology not only to v-erb-A oncogene but also to the DNA binding domains of the human glucocorticoid receptor, estrogen receptor genes, and of the retinoic acid receptor. The inappropriate expression of these genes due to HBV DNA integration might be a contributory factor to the development of HCCs. HBV-DNA integration into chromosomal DNA was found to have relationships to oncogenes, receptors and growth factors, and, at least in one case to a normal protein, cyclin A.[40,41,44,86,200] Cyclin A and B are well conserved during evolution and play an important role in mitotic division. The finding that HBV DNA is inserted into the intron of cyclin A might influence the progression phase of HCCs. This brief and by no means complete summation of the insertion sites of HBV DNA leads unequivocally to the conclusion that the integration of HBV DNA can be viewed only as guilt by association; the "smoking gun" has not yet been identified.

Tumor Suppressor Genes in HCC. Several lines of evidence indicate that HBV DNA insertion into chromosomes may be associated with the inactivation of a tumor suppressor gene. First, the long latency period which elapses between infection and the development of HCC and the fact that not all infections lead to HCC is compatible with the notion, as in retinoblastoma, that one allele is altered genetically while the other allele is somatically mutated. Indeed, in children with the Beckwith-Wiedeman congenital malformation syndrome, 10% of the cases are associated with mutations on chromosome 11. This leads to tumor formation which includes hepatoblastoma, Wilms' tumor, rhabdomyosarcoma and adrenal carcinoma.[101] That chromosome 11 codes for a tumor suppressor gene was shown by Stanbridge, who found that the malignant phenotype was repressed when the normal chromosome 11 was present in somatic hybrids between tumorigenic and nontumorigenic cells.[172] The loss of this chromosome led to a reversion to the malignant phenotype. The suppressor gene in retinoblastoma was mapped to chromosome 13.[59,110] In 45% of HCC cases alleles from chromosome 11p are missing and in 50% of HCCs alleles from chromosome 13q are missing.[198] In addition, HBV DNA integration was mapped to chromosome 11 in many cases. It has also been shown that the p53 gene functions as a tumor suppressor, and in many human cancers including HCC, mutations occur in this gene, with the mutated gene subsequently acting as an oncogene.[21,85] Further, albeit circumstantial, evidence for the role of suppressor genes in HCC is furnished by transgenic mice carrying the SV40 gene coding for T antigen. The tumorigenic activity of the SV40 T antigen is associated with its ability to bind to suppressor gene product. In transgenic mice expressing SV40 T antigen, after a long period of hyperplasia, HCC develops.[74] Furthermore, mouse hepatocytes which were immortalized by T antigen were transfected with a selectable gene and

HBV DNA. All the cells in which HBV replicated displayed malignant growth characteristics and were tumorigenic.

HBV-Induced Hepatocytic Hyperplasia and Necrosis in HCC. As a consequence of HBV infection leading to HCC hepatocytic nodules, ground glass-appearing cells containing HBsAg, hyperplasia, necroinflammation, fibrosis, portal inflammation, and in many cases, cirrhosis, can be detected in the liver.[61,89] The causal relation between the infection and the liver cell injury is not yet elucidated. We have only circumstantial evidence that the immune system is involved.[52,125] The availability of vaccines and the production of viral antigens by recombinant DNA technology made it possible to determine that the production of antibodies against HBsAg is T cell dependent, while HBcAg is more immunogenic and elicits antibodies in T cell dependent and independent ways.[121,122] HBcAg specific, functionally competent CD4+ helper and CD8+ suppressor T cells were detected in chronic infection, wheres HBsAg specific T cells were not found.[57] The T cell clones which were HBcAg specific were HLA-DR restricted and secreted IL2, gamma-IFN, and tumor necrosis factor. For this involvement of the immune system it is obligatory that HBV enter the cells of the immune system in order to present the antigen, and there are indications that, albeit rarely, lymphocytes and monocytes are infected with HBV in vivo.[70,106] Although the involvement of the immune system could adequately explain the cascade of events which lead from infection through inflammation, necrosis, and regeneration, with subsequent genetic changes leading to HCC, the results obtained with transgenic mice indicate that HCC can develop without the contributions of the immune system. Transgenic mice carrying HBV DNA sequences have been produced in several laboratories.[29,30,56] The livers of these animals produce surface antigens and secrete virus into the serum but the immune system does not respond since they are tolerant. In one case a programmed response characterized by inflammation, regenerative hyperplasia, and aneuploidy led to the development of HCC. The incidence of HCC was influenced by sex and age and was directly related to liver cell injury and non-secreted HBsAg content of the liver cells.[30]

Thus, in summation several factors, directly or indirectly, alone or in combination, can lead to HCC, but the integration of HBV DNA in one form or another is obligatory.

Control of HBV Related Hepatocellular Carcinoma

In view of the strong association of hepatocellular carcinoma to chronic HBV infection and the poor response of advanced HCC to treatment, the strategic control of HCC most logically lies in the prevention and treatment of chronic HBV infection.

Treatment of Chronic HBV Infection. Patients with persistent viral replication following acute HBV infection are at the highest risk for developing chronic hepatitis, cirrhosis, and hepatocellular carcinoma.[178] Treatments to terminate viral replication in chronic HBV infection have generally not been satisfactory. Alpha-interferon, when given at doses of 5 million units subcutaneously daily for 16 weeks, produced HBeAg and HBsAg seroconversion, as well as decreases in, or loss of circulating HBV DNA in approximately one-third

of patients.[84] Antiviral therapy with Ara-A or Ara-AMP have in some reports produced decreases in HBV DNA levels and effected seroconversion of HBeAg, but not of HBsAg.[188] Follow-up controlled trials showed that the rate of HBeAg seroconversion following Ara-AMP was not higher than untreated controls.[82,203] Corticosteroids appear beneficial only in clinically severe cases of HBV-associated chronic active hepatitis.[130,131] In patients with only low to moderate aminotransferase elevations, corticosteroids may delay spontaneous recovery and increase morbidity and mortality.[104] Long term steroid administration may postpone spontaneous seroconversion of HBeAg to anti-HBe. Short courses, usually given with rapid withdrawal in order to precipitate seroconversion, may actually exacerbate clinical HBV infection.[81] Combination of alpha-interferon with other agents has been attempted. A controlled trial of prednisone for six weeks followed by subcutaneous interferon alpha-2b daily for six weeks produced HBeAg seroconversion rates indistinguishable from interferon alone (36 vs. 37%).[144] The combination of alpha interferon with gamma-interferon only increased adverse side effects, and did not produce additive or synergistic antiviral activity.[26,46]

Newer investigational agents include the Thymosin preparations fraction 5 and alpha-1, which in a pilot study produced clearance of HBV-DNA in 6 of 7 treated patients compared with no effect in 5 control patients.[129] Confirmation awaits completion of a multi-institutional phase III trial in progress. 2′,3′-Dideoxynucleotides have been used to inhibit HBV replication in vitro with limited success.[108] The carbocyclic analog of 2′-deoxyguanosine, 2′-CDG, however, has been shown to produce virtual cessation of viral replication in cell culture studies.[149] 2′-CDG was nontoxic at concentrations 200 times the minimum effective inhibitory concentration.

Prevention of Hepatitis B Infection: Pre-exposure Prophylaxis. Krugman in 1981 reported on the effectiveness of a crude vaccine prepared by inactivating human serum containing HBsAg, and demonstrated protection against subsequent hepatitis B infection in treated patients.[102] More sophisticated vaccines have been developed since that time, such as plasma-derived vaccines prepared from purification of HBsAg particles from seropositive patients,[76,183] and recombinant vaccines prepared from purification of the protein product of *Saccharomyces cerevisiae* (Baker's yeast) following transfection with viral vectors expressing the HBsAg genome.[13,115] Over 90% of patients developed adequate levels of anti-HBs (≥ 10 SRU) following a series of three injections at 0, 1, and 6 months, and, in these patients, protection from subsequent hepatitis B infection was essentially complete.[116,183] Side effects included mild pain at the site of injection, and mild temperature elevations. There have been no reported cases of HIV transmission with either the plasma-derived or recombinant vaccines.[201] However, 5% of the treated patients developed inadequate responses (between 2.1 to 9.9 SRU), while the remaining 5% produced no anti-HBs. Lack of response may be due to immune suppression, such as those with renal failure or HIV infection;[34,68,174] older age (more than 60 years),[43] or route of injection, since intramuscular is superior to subcutaneous or intradermal administration.[42,111,152,196,213] For nonresponders or inadequate responders, an additional dose produced adequate levels of anti-HBs in 25%; an additional series of three injections produced adequate anti-HBs in 50–60%.[92,93] For the remainder, co-administration of the vaccine with interferon-alpha, thymopentin, or interleukin-2 is being investigated for enhancement of response.[49,65,94,212]

Post-Exposure Prophylaxis. For prevention after HBV exposure, such as following delivery of a neonate from an infected mother, needle-stick puncture from an infected patient, or sexual intercourse with an infected partner, administration of Hepatitis B Immune Globulin (HBIG) followed by HBV vaccination was more than 90% effective.[175,206] Vaccination without HBIG produced only 70–80% anti-HBs responses.[9,148,207] Administration of the vaccines to patients with prior HBV infection (anti-HBs positive), or with chronic infection (HBsAg positive) produced no amelioration of the chronic HBV infection.[6,48]

Developments in New HBV Vaccines. A synthetic vaccine containing amino acid sequences analogous to the p25 HBsAg protein has been developed, which produced rapid antibody responses (1–2 weeks) following primary immunization in mice.[160] HBsAg vaccines incorporating the pre-S(2) polypeptide may induce responses in individuals who failed to respond with the conventional vaccine.[90,134,135] The use of live vaccines, incorporating the HBsAg genome to viral promoters such as the vaccinia and adenoviruses, are attractive because of the low cost of production and the ease of administration (multiple pressure or scratch techniques, or oral administration).[38,126,128,169] The use of baculovirus expression vectors in insects or worms may also decrease the cost of large scale HBsAg production.[118]

Hepatitis C Virus (HCV)

Hepatitis C virus RNA was first isolated from non-A, non-B infectious plasma in 1989, and assays for antibodies to this virus (anti-HCV, RIBA) produced.[3,31,103] HCV RNA in plasma can be detected by the polymerase chain reaction,[96,201] but a commercial assay has yet to be developed. HCV is a 30–60 nm spherical particle comprising the RNA genome in a lipid containing envelope; it is the major etiologic agent in parenterally transmitted non-A, non-B hepatitis.[32] HCV produces a picture clinically similar to hepatitis B.[47] Acute hepatitis C goes on to develop chronic infection in 54% of patients and of these, 10–25% progress to cirrhosis. Modes of transmission are also similar to HBV, via primarily parenteral exposure. Evidence for transmission via sexual intercourse, intrafamily contact, and maternal-neonatal transfer is controversial.[1,53,55,156,194]

The epidemiologic evidence for an association of HCV with hepatocellular carcinoma is compelling. Case control studies from Japan, Italy, Spain, South Africa, and Taiwan have shown that the prevalence of anti-HCV positivity in patients with HCC is substantially higher than in the control population.[22,28,35,71,98,100] In Central Japan, 73.5% (61/83) of HCC patients have anti-HCV, compared with 0.9–1.2% in the control population. Moreover, when HCC patients with positive HBsAg were excluded, 94% tested positive for anti-HCV. In Sicily, 76% (152/200) of HCC patients were positive for anti-HCV; when HBsAg positive patients were excluded, 79%

tested positive for anti-HCV.[166] Virtually 100% of HCC patients with only anti-HCV positivity also had cirrhosis. It is possible that the oncogenicity of HCV is due largely to cirrhosis resulting from chronic infection.

Preliminary randomized double blind controlled trials with alpha-interferon have shown it to be effective in diminishing the clinical severity of HCV associated hepatitis, both in level of aminotransferases and in the extent of necrosis in liver biopsies.[37,45]

Hepatitis D Virus (HDV)

Hepatitis D virus (delta virus), a 36 nm particle containing a closed circularized RNA genome encapsidated by HBsAg major protein, requires the presence of HBV for infection and replication.[7] Acute HDV infection may occur concurrently with acute HBV infection (HDV/HBV coinfection), producing clinical hepatitis with a self-limiting course. Acute HDV infection may also occur in the setting of chronic HBV infection (HDV superinfection), produce an exacerbation of clinical hepatitis, and persist with chronic viral replication leading to cirrhosis. In 15% of cases, HDV superinfection produces an accelerated course of chronic HBV infection.[16,17] Although chronic HDV infection in cirrhotic patients does not pose an increased risk for HCC, the increased risk for cirrhosis in chronic HDV infection may in itself increase the oncogenicity of chronic HBV infection.[23,137,147] HDV infection can be diagnosed by identification in serum of anti-HD, HDAg, or HDV RNA.[12,25,167,168] Treatment of chronic HDV infection with alpha interferon has been reported to produce virological and biochemical improvement in a small proportion of patients. These effects are only transient however, with return of virological and biochemical parameters to baseline soon after cessation of treatment.[83,114,157,158]

References

1. Alter, M. J., Coleman, P. J., Alexander, W. J., Kramer, E., Miller, J. K., Mandel, E., Hadler, S. C., and Margolis, H. S.: Importance of heterosexual activity in the transmission of hepatitis B and non-A, non-B hepatitis. J. Am. Med. Assoc., 262:1201, 1989.
2. Alter, H. J., Holland, P. V., and Purcell, R. H.: The emerging pattern of post-transfusion hepatitis. Am. J. Med. Sci., 270:329, 1975.
3. Alter, H. J., Tegtmeier, G. E., Jett, B. W., Quan, S., Shih, J. W., Bayer, W. L., and Polito, A.: The use of a recombinant immunoblot assay in the interpretation of anti-hepatitis C virus reactivity among prospectively followed patients, implicated donors, and random donors. Transfusion, 31:771, 1991.
4. Asher, L. V. S., Innis, B. L., Shrestha, M. P., Ticehurst, J., and Baxe, W. B.: Virus-like particles in the liver of a patient with fulminant hepatitis and antibody to hepatitis E virus. J. Med. Virol., 31:229, 1990.
5. Austin, H., Delzell, E., Grufferman, S., Levine, R., Morrison, A. S., Stolley, P. D., and Cole, P.: A case-control study of hepatocellular carcinoma and the hepatitis B virus, cigarette smoking, and alcohol consumption. Cancer Res., 46:962, 1986.
6. Barin, F., Yvonnet, B., Goudeau, A., Coursaget, P., Chiron, J. P., Denis, F., and Mar, I. D.: Hepatitis B vaccine: further studies in children with previously acquired hepatitis B surface antigenemia. Infect. Immun., 41:83, 1983.
7. Baroudy, B. M., Smedile, A., Korba, B. E., Bergmann, K. F., Pohl, C., Wells, F. V., and Gerin, J. L.: Transcription and replication of hepatitis delta virus. Prog. Clin. Biol. Res., 234:89, 1987.
8. Beasley, R. P.: Hepatitis B virus as the etiologic agent in hepatocellular carcinoma-epidemiologic considerations. Hepatology, 2:21S, 1982.
9. Beasley, R. P., Huang, L. Y., Stevens, C. E., Lin, C. C., Cahsieh, F. J., Wang, K. Y., Sung, T. S., and Szmuness, W.: Efficacy of hepatitis B immune globulin for prevention of perinatal transmission of the hepatitis B carrier state: final report of a randomized double-blind placebo-controlled trial. Hepatology, 3:135, 1983.
10 Beasley, R. P., Hwang, L. Y., Lin, C. C., and Chien, C. S. Hepatocellular carcinoma and hepatitis B virus: a prospective study of 22,707 men in Taiwan. Lancet, 2:1129, 1981.
11. Beasley, R. P., Trepo, C., Stevens, C. E., and Szmuness, W.: The e antigen in vertical transmission of hepatitis B surface antigen. Am. J. Epidemiol., 105:94, 1977.
12. Bergmann, K., and Gerin, J. L.: Antigens of hepatitis delta virus in the liver and serum of humans and animals. J. Infect. Dis., 154:945, 1986.

13. Bitter, G. A., Egan, K. M., Burnette, W. N., Samal, B., Fieschko, J. C., Peterson, D. L., Downing, M. R., Wypych, J., and Langley, K. E.: Hepatitis B vaccine produced in yeast. J. Med. Virol., 25:123, 1988.

14. Bond, W. W., Favero, M. S., Petersen, N. J., Gravelle, C. R., Ebert, J. W., and Maynard, J. E.: Survival and hepatitis B virus after drying and storage for one week. Lancet, 1:550, 1981.

15. Bond, W. W., Petersen, N. J., and Favero, M. S.: Viral hepatitis B: Aspects of environmental control. Health Lab. Sci., 14:235, 1977.

16. Bonino, F., Brunetto, M. R., and Negro, F.: Factors influencing the natural course of HDV hepatitis. In The Hepatitis Delta Virus. Edited by J. L. Gerin, R. H. Purcell, and M. Rizzetto. New York, Wiley-Liss, 1991, p. 137.

17. Bonino, F., Negro, F., Baldi, M., Brunetto, M. R., Chiaberge, E., Capalbo, M., Maran, E., Lavarini, C., Rocca, N., and Rocca, G.: The natural history of chronic delta hepatitis. In The Hepatitis Delta Virus and Its Infection. Edited by M. Rizzetto, J. L. Gerin, and R. H. Purcell. New York, Alan R. Liss, 1987, p. 145.

18. Brady, J., Bolen, J. B., Radonovich, M., Salzman, N., and Khoury, G.: Stimulation of simian virus 40 late gene expression by simian virus 40 tumor antigen. Proc. Natl. Acad. Sci. USA, 81:2040, 1984.

19. Brady, J. Loeken, M. R., and Khoury, G.: Interactions between two transcriptional control sequences required for tumor-antigen-mediated simian virus 40 late gene expression. Proc. Natl. Acad. Sci. USA, 82:7299, 1985.

20. Brechot, C.: Hepatitis B virus (HBV) and hepatocellular carcinoma. HBV DNA status and its implications. J. Hepatol., 4:269, 1987.

21. Bressac, B., Kew, M., Wands, J., and Ozturk, M.: Selective G to T mutations of p53 gene in hepatocellular carcinoma from southern Africa. Nature, 350:429, 1991.

22. Bruix, J., Barrera, J. M., Calvet, X., Ercilla, G., Costa, J., Sanchez-Tapias, J. M., Ventura, M., Vall, M., Bruguera, M., Bru, C., Castillo, R., and Rodes, J.: Prevalence of antibodies to hepatitis C virus in Spanish patients with hepatocellular carcinoma and hepatic cirrhosis. Lancet, 2:1004, 1989.

23. Brunetto, M. R., Oliveri, F., Baldi, M., Capalbo, M., Piantino, P., Smedile, A., Chiaberge, E., Verme, G., and Bonino, F.: Hepatocellular carcinoma and hepatitis delta virus infection. J. Hepatol. 9 (Suppl.):S123, 1989.

24. Bulatao-Jayme, J., Almero, E. M., Castro, C. A., Jardeleza, T. R., and Salamat, L. A.: A case-control dietary study of primary liver cancer risk from aflatoxin exposure. Int. J. Epidemiol., 11:112, 1982.

25. Buti, M., Esteban, R., Roggendorf, M., Fernandez, J., Jardi, R., Rashofer, R., Allende, H., Genesca, J., Esteban, J. I., and Guardia. J.: Hepatitis D virus RNA in acute delta infection: serological profile and correlation with other markers of hepatitis D virus infection. Hepatology, 8:1124, 1988.

26. Caselman, W. H., Eisenburg, J., Hofschneider, P. H., and Koshy, R.: Beta-and gamma-interferon in chronic active hepatitis B: A pilot trial of short-term combination therapy. Gastroenterol., 96:449, 1989.

27. Centers for Disease Control.: Changing patterns of groups at high risk for hepatitis B in the United States. MMWR, 37:429, 1988.

28. Chen, D. S., Kuo, G. C., Sung, J. L., Lai, M. Y., Shey, J. C., Chen, P. J., Yang, P. M., Hsu, H. M., Chang, M. H., Chen, C. J., Hahn, L. C., Choo, Q. L., Wang, T. H., and Houghton, M.: Hepatitis C virus infection in an area hyperendemic for hepatitis B and chronic liver disease: the Taiwan experience. J. Infect. Dis., 162:817, 1990.

29. Chisari, F. V., Filippi, P., Buras, J., McLachlan, A., Popper, H., Pinkert, C. A., Palmiter, R. D., and Brinster, R. L.: Structural and pathological effects of synthesis of hepatitis B virus large envelope polypeptide in transgenic mice. Proc. Natl. Acad. Sci. USA, 84:6909, 1987.

30. Chisari, F. V., Klopchin, K., Moriyama, T., Pasquinelli, C., Dunsford, H. A., Sell, S., Pinkert, C. A., Brinster, R. L., and Palmiter, R. D.: Molecular pathogenesis of hepatocellular carcinoma in hepatitis B virus transgenic mice. Cell, 59:1145, 1989.

31. Choo, Q. L., Kuo, G., Weiner, A. J., Overby, L. R., Bradley, D. W., and Houghton, M.: Isolation of cDNA cline derived from a blood-borne non-A, non-B viral hepatitis genome. Science, 244:359, 1989.

32. Choo, Q. L., Weiner, A. J., Overby, L. R., Kuo, G., Houghton, M., and Bradley, D. W.: Hepatitis C virus: The major causative agent of viral non-A, non-B hepatitis, Br. Med. Bull., 46:423, 1990.

33. Colgrove, R., Simon, G., and Ganem, D.: Transcriptional activation of homologous and heterologous genes by the hepatitis B virus X gene product in cells permissive for viral replication. J. Virol., 63:4019, 1989.

34. Collier, A. C., Corey, L., Murphy, V. L., and Handsfield, H. H.: Antibody to human immunodeficiency virus and suboptimal response to hepatitis B vaccination. Ann. Intern. Med., 109:101, 1988.

35. Colombo, M., Kuo, G., Choo, Q. L., Donato, M. F., Del Ninno, E., Tommasini, M. A., Dioguardi, N., and Houghton, M.: Prevalence of antibodies to hepatitis C virus in Italian patients with hepatocellular carcinoma. Lancet, 2:1006, 1989.

36. Reference deleted.

37. Davis, G. L., Balart, L. A., Schiff, E. R., Lindsay, K., Bodenheimer, H. C., Jr., Perrillo, R. P., Carey, W., Jacobson, I. M., Payne, J., Dienstag, J. L., Van Thiel, D. H., Tamburro, C., Lefkowitch, J., Albrecht, J., Meschievitz, C., Ortego, T. J., and Givas, A.: The Hepatitis Interventional Therapy Group: Treatment of chronic hepatitis C with recombinant interferon alfa. A multicenter randomized, controlled trial. N. Engl. J. Med., 321:1501, 1989.

38. Davis, A. R., Kostek, B., Mason, B., Hsiao, C. L., Morin, J., Dheer, S. K., and Hung, P. P.: Expression of hepatitis B surface antigen with a recombinant adenovirus. Proc. Natl. Acad. Sci. USA, 82:7560, 1985.

39. Dayton, A. I., Sodroski, J. G., Rosen, C. A., Goh, W. C., and Haseltine, W. A.: The trans-activator gene of the human T-cell lymphotropic virus type III is required for replication. Cell, 44:941, 1986.

40. Dejean, A., Bougueleret, L., Grzeschik, K. H., and Tiollais, P.: Hepatitis B virus DNA integration in a sequence homologous to v-erb-A and steroid receptor genes in a hepatocellular carcinoma. Nature, 332:70, 1986.

41. Dejean, A., Carloni, G., Brechot, C., Tiollais, P., and Wain-Hobson, S.: Organization and expression of hepatitis B sequences cloned from hepatocellular carcinoma tissue DNA. J. Cell. Biochem., 20:293, 1982.

42. DeLalla, F., Rinaldi, E., Santoro, D., and Pravettonic, G.: Immune response to hepatitis B vaccine given at different injection sites and by different routes: a controlled randomized study. Eur. J. Epidemiol., 4:256, 1988.

43. Denis, F., Mounier, M., Hessel, L., Michel, J. P., Gualde, N., Dubois, F., Barin, F., and Goudeau, A.: Hepatitis B vaccination in the elderly. J. Infect. Dis., 149:1019, 1984.

44. DeThe, H., Marchio, A., Tiollais, P., and Dejean, A.: A novel steroid thyroid hormone receptor-related gene inappropriately expressed in human hepatocellular carcinoma. Nature, 330:667, 1987.

45. Di Bisceglie, A. M., Martin, P., Kassianides, C., Lisker-Melman, M., Murray, L., Waggoner, J., Goodman, Z., Banks, S. M., and Hoofnagle, J. H.: Recombinant interferon alfa therapy for chronic hepatitis C. A randomized, double-blind, placebo-controlled trial. N. Engl. J. Med., 321:1506, 1989.

46. Di Bisceglie, A. M., Rustgi, V. K., Kassianides, C., Lisker-Melman, M., Park, Y., Waggoner, J. G., and Hoofnagle, J. H.: Therapy of chronic hepatitis B with recombinant human alpha and gamma interferon. Hepatology, 11:266, 1990.

47. Dienstag, J. L.: Non-A, non-B hepatitis. I. Recognition, epidemiology, and clinical features. Gastroenterol., 85:439, 1983.

48. Dienstag, J. L., Stevens, C. E., Bhan, A. K., and Szmuness, W.: Hepatitis B vaccine administered to chronic carriers of hepatitis B surface antigen. Ann. Intern. Med., 96:575, 1982.

49. Donati, D., and Gastaldi, L.: Controlled trial of thymopentin in hemodialysis patients who fail to respond to hepatitis B vaccination. Nephron, 50:133, 1988.

50. Duffy, J., Lidsky, M. D., Sharp, J. T., Davis, J. S., Person, D. A., Hollinger, F. B., and Min, K. W.: Polyarthritis, polyarteritis and hepatitis B. Medicine (Baltimore), 55:19, 1976.

51. Eble, B., Lingappa, V., and Ganem, D.: Hepatitis B surface antigen—an unusual secreted protein initially synthesized as a transmembrane polypeptide. Mol. Cell Biol., 6:1454, 1986.

52. Eggink, H. G., Houthoff, H. J., Huitema, S., Poppema, S., and Gips, C. H.: Cellular and humoral immune reactions in chronic active liver disease: lymphocyte subsets in liver biopsies of patients with untreated idiopathic autoimmune hepatitis, chronic active hepatitis B and primary biliary cirrhosis. C;in. Exp. Immunol., 50:17, 1982.

53. Esteban, J. I., Esteban, R., Viladomiu, L., Lopez-Talavera, J. C., Gonzalez, A., Hernandez, J. M., Roget, M., Vargas, V., Genesca, J., Buti, M., Guardia, J., Houghton, M., Choo, Q. L., and Kuo, G.: Hepatitis C virus antibodies among risk groups in Spain. Lancet, 2:294, 1989.

54. Everett, R. D.: Transactivation of transcription by herpes virus products: requirement for two HSV-1 immediate early polypeptdes for maximum activity. EMBO J., 3:3135, 1984.

55. Everhart, J. E., Di Besceg"ie, A. M., Murray, L. M., Alter, H. J., Melpolder, J. J., Kuo, G., and Hoofnagle, J. H.: Risk for non-A, non-B (type C) hepatitis through sexual or household contact with chronic carriers. Ann. Int. Med., 112:544, 1990.

56. Farza, H., Hadchouel, M., Scotto, J., Tiollais, P., Babinet, C., and Pourcel, C.: Replication and gene expression of hepatitis B virus in a transgenic mouse that contains the complete viral genome. J. Virol., 62:4144, 1988.

57. Ferrari, C., Penna, A., Giuberti, T., Tong, M. J., Ribera, E., Fiaccadori, F., and Chisari, F. V.: Intrahepatic nucleocapsid antigen-specific T cell in chronic active hepatitis B. J. Immunol., 139:2050, 1987.

58. Forman, D., Doll, R., and Peto, R.: Trends in mortality from carcinoma of the liver and the use of oral contraceptives. Br. J. Cancer, 48:349, 1983.

59. Fung, Y. K. T., Murphree, A. L., T'Ang, A., Qian, J., Hinrichs, S. H., and Benedict, W. F.: Structural evidence for the authenticity for the human retinoblastoma gene. Science, 236:1657, 1987.

60. Gelman, I. H., and Silverstein, S.: Identification of immediate early genes from herpes simplex virus that transactivate the virus thymidine kinase gene. Proc. Natl. Acad. Sci. USA, 82:5265, 1985.

61. Gerber, M. A., Hadziyannis, S., Vissoulis, C., Schattner, F., Paronetto, F., and Popper, H.: Hepatitis B antigen: nature and distribution of cytoplasmic antigen in hepatocytes of carriers. Proc. Soc. Exp. Biol. Med., 145:863, 1974.

62. Gerety, R. J., and Barker, L. F.: Viral antigens and antibodies in hemophiliacs. In Unresolved Therapeutic Problems in Hemophilia. NIH publication No. 77-1089. Washington, D. C., Government Printing Office, 1976, p. 51.

63. Gerety, R. J., Hoofnagle, J. H., Markenson, J. A., and Narker, L. F.: Exposure to hepatitis B virus and development of chronic HBsAg carrier state in children. J. Pediatr., 84:661, 1974.

64. Gerety, A. J., and Schweitzer, K.: Viral hepatitis type B during pregnancy, the neonatal period, and infancy. J. Pediatr., 90:368, 1977.

65. Grob, P. J., Joller-Jemelka, H. I., Binswanger, U., Zaruka, K., Descoeudres, C., and Fernex, M.: Interferon as an adjuvant for hepatitis B vaccination in non-and low-responder populations. Eur. J. Clin. Microbiol., 3:195, 1984.

66. Gust, I. D., and Feinstone, S. M.: Hepatitis A. Prog. Liver Diseases, 9:371, 1990.

67. Hadengue, A., N'Dri, N., and Benhamou, J. -P.: Relative risk of hepatocellular car-

cinoma in HBsAg positive vs. alcoholic cirrhosis. A cross-sectional study. Liver, 10:147, 1990.

68. Hadler, S. C.: Hepatitis B prevention and human immunodeficiency virus infection. Ann. Intern. Med., 109:92, 1988.

69. Hadler, S. C., and McFarland, L.: Hepatitis in day care centers: epidemiology and prevention. Rev. Infect. Dis., 8:548, 1986.

70. Harisson, T. J.: Hepatitis B virus DNA in peripheral blood leukocytes: a brief review. J. Med. Virol., 31:33, 1990.

71. Hasan, F., Jeffers, L. J., De Medina, M., Reddy, K. R., Parker, T., Schiff, E. R., Houghton, M., Choo, Q. L., and Kuo, G.: Hepatitis C-associated hepatocellular carcinoma. Hepatology, 12:589, 1990.

72. Heathcote, J., Gateau, P., and Sherlock, S.: Role of the hepatitis-B antigen carriers in non-parenteral transmission of the hepatitis-B virus. Lancet, 2:370, 1974.

73. Heathcote, J., Jenny, M. R. C. P., Cameron, C. H., Path, M. R. C., Dane, B. S., and Path, F. R. C.: Hepatitis B antigen in saliva and semen. Lancet, 1:71, 1974.

74. Held, W. A., Mullins, J. J., Kuhn, N. J., Gallagher, J. F., Gu, G. D., and Gross, K. W.: T antigen expression and tumorigenesis in transgenic mice containing a mouse major urinary protein/SV40 T antigen hybrid gene. EMBO J., 8:183, 1989.

75. Henderson, B. E., Preston-Martin, S., Edmondson, H. A., Peters, R. L., and Pike, M. C.: Hepatocellular carcinoma and oral contraceptives. Br. J. Cancer, 48:437, 1983.

76. Hilleman, M., Buynak, E. B., Roehm, R. R., Tytell, A. A., Bertland, A. U., and Lampson, G. P.: Purified and inactivated human hepatitis B Vaccine. Progress report. Am. J. Med. Sci., 270:401, 1975.

77. Hirayama, T.: A large-scale cohort study on the relationship between diet and selected cancers of digestive organs. In Gastrointestinal Cancer: Endogenous Factors. Edited by W. R. Bruce, P. Correa, M. Lipkin, S. Tanenbaum, and T. Wilkins. Cold Spring Harbor, CSH Press, 1981, p. 409.

78. Hollinger, F. B., and the North American Regional Study Group: Controlling hepatitis B virus transmission in North America. Vaccine, 8 Suppl: S122, 1990.

79. Hollinger, F. B., Dienstag, J. L.: Hepatitis Viruses. In Manual of Clinical Microbiology 4th ed. Edited by A. Lennette, A. Balows, W. H. Hausler, Jr., H. J. Shadomy. Washington, American Society of Microbiology, Washington, 1985, p. 813.

80. Hollinger, F. B., Goyal, R. K., Hersh, T., Powell, H. C., Schulmen, R. J., Melnick, J. L.: Immune response to hepatitis virus type B in Down's syndrome and other mentally retarded patients. Am. J. Epidemiol., 95:356, 1972.

81. Hoofnagle, J. H., Davis, G. L., Pappas, S. C., Hanson, R. G., Peters, M., Avigan, M. I., Waggoner, J. G., Jones, E. A., Seeff, L. B.: A short course of prednisolone in chronic type B hepatitis: report of a randomized, double-blind placebo-controlled trial. Ann. Int. Med., 104:12, 1986.

82. Hoofnagle, J. H., Hanson, R. G., Minuk, G. Y., Pappas, S. C., Schafer, D. F., Dusheiko, G. M., Strauss, S. E., Popper, H., Jones, E. A.: Randomized controlled trial of adenine arabinoside monophosphate for chronic type B hepatitis. Gastroenterology, 86:150, 1984.

83. Hoofnagle, J., Mullen, K., Peters, M., Avigan, M., Park, Y., Waggoner, J., Gerin, J. L., Hoyer, B., Smedile, A.: Treatment of chronic delta hepatitis with recombinant human alpha interferon. In The Hepatitis Delta Virus and Its Infection. Edited by M. Rizzetto, J. L. Gerin, R. H. Purcell. New York, Alan R. Liss, 1987, p. 291.

84. Hoofnagle, J. H., Peters, M., Mullen, K. D., Jones, D. B., Rustgi, V. D., DiBisceglie, A., Hallahan, C., Park, Y., Meschievitz, C., and Jones, E. A.: Randomized, controlled world trial of recombinant human alpha-interferon in patients with chronic hepatitis B. Gastroent., 95:1318, 1988.

85. Hsu, I. C., Metcalf, R. A., Sun, T., Welsh, J. A., Wang, N. J., Harris, C. C.: Mutational hotspot in the p53 gene in humam hepatocellular carcinomas. Nature, 350:427, 1991.

86. Hsu, T., Moroy, T., Etiemble, J., Louise, A., Trepo, C., Tiollais, P., and Buendia, M. A.: Activation of c-myc by woodchuck hepatitis virus insertion in hepatocellular carcinoma. Cell, 55:627, 1988.

87. Hu, K. Q., Vierling, J. M., and Siddiqui, A.: Trans-activation of HLA-DR gene by hepatitis B virus X gene product. Proc. Natl. Acad. Sci. USA, 87:7140, 1990.

88. Ichiyada, T., Fujiyama, A., Fukushige, S., Hatada, I., and Matsubara, K.: Molecular cloning of an oncogene from a human hepatocellular carcinoma. Proc. Natl. Acad. Sci. USA, 83:4993, 1986.

89. Ishak, K. G.: Light microscopic morphology of viral hepatitis. Am. J. Clin. Path., 65:787, 1976.

90. Itoh, Y., Takai, E., Ohnuma, H., Kitajima, K., Tsuda, F., Machida, A., Mishiro, S., Nakamura, T., Miyakawa, Y., and Mayumi, M.: A synthetic peptide vaccine involving the product of the pre-S(2) region of the hepatitis B virus DNA: protective efficacy in chimpanzees. Proc. Natl. Acad. Sci. USA, 83:9174, 1986.

91. Jenison, S. A., Lemon, S. M., Baker, L. N., and Newbold, J. E.: Quantitative analysis of hepatitis B virus DNA in saliva and semen of chronically infected homosexual men. J. Infect. Dis., 156:299, 1987.

92. Jilg, W., Schmidt, M., and Deinhardt, F.: Immune response to hepatitis B revaccination. J. Med. Virol., 24:377, 1988.

93. Jilg, W., Schmidt, M., and Deinhardt, F.: Prolonged immunity after late booster doses of hepatitis B vaccine. J. Infect. Dis., 157:1267, 1988.

94. Kakumu, S., Fuji, A., Tahara, H., Yoshioka, K., and Sakamoto, N.: Enhancement of antibody production of hepatitis B surface antigen by interleukin 2. J. Clin. Lab. Immunol., 26:25, 1988.

95. Kaneko, S., Miller, R. H., Feinstone, S. M., Unoura, M., Kobayashi, K., Hattori, N., and Purcell, R. H.: Detection of serum hepatitis B virus DNA in patients with chronic hepatitis using the polymerase chain reaction assay. Proc. Natl. Assoc. Sci. USA, 86:312, 1989.

96. Kaneko, S., Unoura, M., Kobayashi, K., Kuno, K., Murakami, S., and Hattori, N.: Detection of serum hepatitis C virus RNA. Lancet, 335:976, 1990.

97. Kew, M. C., Desmyter, J., Bradburne, A. F., and Macnab, G. M.: Hepatitis B virus infection in southern African blacks with hepatocellular cancer. J. Natl. Cancer Inst., 62:517, 1979.

98. Kew, M.C., Houghton, M., Choo, Q. L., and Kuo, G.: Hepatitis C virus antibodies in southern African blacks with hepatocellular carcinoma. Lancet, 2:873, 1990.

99. Kiire, C. F., and the African Regional Study Group: Hepatitis B infection in sub-Saharan Africa. Vaccine, 8(Suppl.):S107, 1990.

100. Kiyosawa, K., Sodeyama, T., Tanaka, E., Gibo, Y., Yoshizawa, K., Nakano, Y., Furuta, S., Akahane, Y., Nishioka, K., Purcell, R. H., and Alter, H. J.: Interrelationship of blood transfusion, non-A, non-B hepatitis and hepatocellular carcinoma: Analysis by detection of antibody to hepatitis C virus. Hepatology, 12:671, 1990.

101. Koufos, A., Hansen, M. F., Copeland, N. G., Jenkins, N. A., Lampkin, B. C., and Cavenee, W. K.: Loss of heterozygosity in three embryonic tumours suggests a common pathogenetic mechanism. Nature, 316:330, 1985.

102. Krugman, S., Giles, J. P., and Hammond, J.: Viral hepatitis type B (MS-2 strain): studies on active immunization. JAMA, 217:41, 1971.

103. Kuo, G., Choo, Q. L., Alter, H. J., Gitnick, G. L., Redeker, A. G., Purcell, R. H., Miyamura, T., Dienstag, J. L., Alter, M. J., Stevens, C. E., Tegtmeier, G. E., Bonino, F., Colombo, M., Lee, W.-S., Kuo, C., Berger, K., Shuster, J. R., Overby, L. R., Brandley, D. W., and Houghton, M.: An assay for circulating antibodies to a major etiologic virus of human non-A, non-B hepatitis. Science, 244:362, 1989.

104. Lam, K. C., Lai, C. L., Trepo, C., and Wu, P. C.: Deleterious effect of prednisolone in HBsAg-positive chronic active hepatitis. N. Engl. J. Med., 304:390, 1981.

105. Lam, K. C., Yu, M. C., Leung, J. W. C., and Henderson, B. E.: Hepatitis B virus and cigarette smoking: risk factors for hepatocellular carcinoma in Hong Kong. Cancer Res., 42:5246, 1982.

106. Lamelin, J. P., and Trepo, C.: The hepatitis B virus and the peripheral blood mononuclear cells: a brief review. J. Hepatol., 10:120, 1990.

107. Larouze, B., Saimot, G., Lustbader, E. D., London, W. T., Werner, B. G., and Payet, M.: Host responses to hepatitis-B infection in patients with primary hepatic carcinoma and their families: A case/control study in Senegal, West Africa. Lancet, 2:534, 1976.

108. Lee, B., Luo, W. X., Suzuki, S., Robbions, M. J., and Tyrrell, D. L.: In vitro and in vivo comparison of the abilities of purine and pyrimidine 2',3'-dideoxynucleotides to inhibit duck hepadna virus. Antimicrob. Agents Chemother., 33:336, 1989.

109. Lee, H. P., Day, N. E., and Shanmugaratnam, K.: Trends in Cancer Incidence in Singapore, 1968-1982. IARC Scientific Publications, No. 91. Lyon, France, International Agency for Research on Cancer, 1988.

110. Lee, W. H., Bookstein, R., Hong, F., Young, L. J., Shew, J. Y., Lee, E. Y. H. P.: Human retinoblastoma susceptibility gene: cloning, identification, and sequence. Science, 235:1394, 1987.

111. Lemon, S. M., and Weber, D. J.: Immunogenicity of plasma-derived hepatitis B vaccine: Relationship to site of injection and obesity. J. Gen. Intern. Med., 1:199, 1986.

112. Lieberman, P. M., O'Hare, P., Hayward, G. S., and Hayward, S. D.: Promiscuous trans-activation of gene expression by an Epstein-Barr virus-encoded early nuclear protein. J. Virol., 60:140, 1986.

113. Lingao, A. L., Domingo, E. O., and Nishioka, K.: Hepatitis B virus profile of hepatocellular carcinoma in the Philippines. Cancer, 48:1590, 1981.

114. Marinacci, G., Hassan, G., DiGiacomo, C., Barlattani, A., Costa, F., Rasshofer, R., and Roggendorf, M.: Long-term treatment of chronic delta hepatitis with alpha recombinant interferon. In The Hepatitis Delta Virus. Edited by J. L. Gerin, R. H. Purcell, and M. Rizzetto. New York, Wiley-Liss, 1991, p. 405.

115. McAleer, W. J., Buynak, E. B., Maigetter, R. Z., Wampler, D. E., Miller, W. J., and Hilleman, M. R.: Human hepatitis B vaccine from recombinant yeast. Nature, 307:178, 1984.

116. McLean, A. A., Hilleman, M. R., McAleer, W. J., and Buynak, E. B.: Summary of worldwide experience with HB-Vax (R) (B,MSD). J. Infect. Dis. 7(Suppl.):95, 1983.

117. McMahon, B. L., Alward, W. L. M., Hall, D. B., Heyward, W. L., Bender, T. R., Krantz, T. P., and Maynard, J. E.: Acute hepatitis B infection: Relation of age to the clinical expression of disease and subsequent development of the carrier state. J. Infect. Dis., 151:599, 1985.

118. Miller, L. K.: Baculoviruses as gene expression vectors. Am. Rev. Microbiol., 42:177, 1988.

119. Miller, R. H., Kaneko, S., Chung, C. T., Girones, R., and Purcell, R. H.: Compact organization of the hepatitis B virus genome. Hepatology, 9:322, 1989.

120. Miller, R. H., and Robinson, W. S.: Common evolutionary origin of hepatitis B virus and retrovirus. Proc. Natl. Acad. Sci. USA, 83:2531, 1986.

121. Milich, D. R.: Genetic and molecular basis for T-and B-cell recognition of hepatitis B viral antigen. Immunol. Rev., 99:71, 1987.

122. Milich, D. R., McLachlan, A., Moriarty, A., and Thornton, G. B.: Immune response to hepatitis B virus core antigen (HNcAg): localization of T cell recognition sites within HBcAg/HBeAg. J. Immunol., 139:1223, 1987.

123. Mondelli, M., Eddleston, A. L. W. F.: Mechanisms of liver cell injury in acute and chronic hepatitis B. Sem. Liver Dis., 4:47, 1984.

124. Monjardino, J. P., and Saldanha, J. A.: Delta hepatitis. The disease and the virus. Br. Med. Bull., 46:399, 1990.

125. Montano, L., Aranguibel, F., Boffill, M., Goodall, A. H., Janossy, G., and Thomas, H. C.: An analysis of the composition of the inflammatory infiltrate in autoimmune and hepatitis B virus-induced chronic liver disease. Hepatology, 3:292, 1983.

126. Morin, J. E., Lubeck, M. D., Barton, J. E., Conley, A. J., Davis, A. R., and Hung, P.

P.: Recombinant adenovirus induces antibody response to hepatitis B virus surface antigen in hamsters. Proc. Natl. Acad. Sci. USA, 84:4626, 1987.

127. Moroy, T., Marchio, A., Etiemble, J., Trepo, C., Tiollais, P., and Buendia, M. A.: Rearrangement and enhanced expression of c-myc in hepatocellular carcinoma of hepatitis virus infected woodchucks. Nature, 324:276, 1986.

128. Moss, B., Smith, G., Gerin, J. L., et al.: Use of vaccinia virus as a vector for the construction of live recombinant hepatitis B virus vaccines. In Viral Hepatitis and Liver Disease. Edited by G. N. Vyas, J. L. Dienstag, J. H. Hoofnagle. Orlando, FL, Grune & Stratton, 1984, p. 293.

129. Mutchnik, M. G., Appelman, H. D., Chung, H. T., Aragona, E., Gupta, T. P., Cummings, G. D., Waggoner, J. G., Hoofnagle, J. H., and Shafritz, D. A.: Thymosin treatment of chronic hepatitis B: a placebo-controlled pilot trial. Hepatology, 14:409, 1991.

130. Nair, P. V., Tong, M. J., Stevenson, D., Roskamp, D., and Boone, C.: Effect of short term, high-dose prednisone treatment of patients with HBsAg-positive chronic active hepatitis. Liver, 5:8, 1985.

131. Nair, P. V., Tong, M. J., Stevenson, D., Roskamp, D., and Boone, C.: A pilot study on the effects of prednisone withdrawal on serum hepatitis N virus DNA and HBeAg in chronic active hepatitis B. Hepatology, 6:1319, 1986.

132. Nernier, R. H., Sampliner, R., Gerety, R., Tabor, E., Hamilton, F., and Nathanson, N.: Hepatitis B infection in households of chronic carriers of hepatitis B surface antigen factors associated with prevalence of infection. Am. J. Epidemiol., 116:199, 1980.

133. Neuberger, J., Forman, D., Doll, R., and Williams, R.: Oral contraceptives and hepatocellular carcinoma. Br. Med. J., 292:1355, 1986.

134. Neurath, A. R., Kent, S. B. H., Strick, N., Taylor, P., and Stevens, C. E.: Hepatitis B virus contains pre-S gene-encoded domains. Nature, 315:154, 1985.

135. Neurath, A. R., Kent, S. B. H., Strick, N., Stark, D., and Sproul, P.: Genetic restriction of immune responsiveness to synthetic peptides corresponding to sequences in the pre-S region of the hepatitis B virus (HBV) envelope gene. J. Med. Virol., 17:119, 1985.

136. Neurath, A. R., Kent, S. B. H., Strick, N., and Parker, K.: Identification and chemical synthesis of a host cell receptor binding site on hepatitis B virus. Cell, 46:429, 1986.

137. Oliveri, F., Brunetto, M. R., Baldi, M., Piantino, P., Ponzetto, A., Forzani, B., Smedile, A., Verme, G., and Bonino, F.: Hepatitis delta virus and hepatocellular carcinoma. In The Hepatitis Delta Virus. Edited by J. L. Gerin, R. H. Purcell, and M. Rizzetto. New York, Wiley-Liss, 1991, p. 217.

138. Oshima, A., Tsukuma, H., Hiyama, T., Fujimoto, I., Yamano, H., and Tanaka, M.: Follow-up study of HBsAg positive blood donors with special reference to effect of drinking and smoking on development of liver cancer. Int. J. Cancer, 34:775, 1984.

139. Ou, J. H., Laub, O., and Rutter, W. J.: Hepatitis B virus gene function: the precore region targets the core antigen to cellular membranes and causes the secretion of the e antigen. Proc. Natl. Acad. Sci. USA, 83:1578, 1986.

140. Paterlini, P., Gerken, G., Nakajima, E., Terre, S., D'Errico, A., Grigiono, W., Halpas, B., Franco, D., Wands, J., Kew, M., Pisi, E., Tiollais, P., and Brechot, C.: Polymerase chain reaction to detect hepatitis B virus DNA and RNA sequences in primary liver cancers from patients negative for hepatitis B surface antigen. N. Engl. J. Med., 323:80, 1990.

141. Peers, F., Bosch, X., Kaldor, J., Linsell, A., and Pluijmen, M.: Aflatoxin exposure, hepatitis B virus infection and liver cancer in Swaziland. Int. J. Cancer, 39:545, 1987.

142. Peers, F. G., Gilman, G. A., and Linsell, C. A.: Dietary aflatoxins and human liver cancer. A study in Swaziland. Int. J. Cancer, 17:167, 1976.

143. Peers, F. G., and Linsell, C. A.: Dietary aflatoxins and liver cancer. A population based study in Kenya. Br. J. Cancer, 27:473, 1973.

144. Perrillo, R. P., Schiff, E. R., Davis, G. L., Bodenheimer, H. C., Jr., Lindsay, K., Payne, J., Dienstag, J. L., O'Brien, C., Tamburro, C., Jacobson, I. M., Sampliner, R., Feit, D., Lefkowictch, J., Kuhns, M., Meschievitz, C., Sanghvi, B., Albrecht, J., Gobas, A., and the Hepatitis Interventional Therapy Group. A randomized, controlled trial of interferon alfa-2b alone and after prednisone withdrawal for the treatment of chronic hepatitis B. N. Engl. J. Med., 323:295, 1990.

145. Peters, R. L.: Viral hepatitis: a pathologic spectrum. Am. J. Med. Sci., 270:17, 1975.

146. Peters, C. J., Purcell, R. H., Lander, J. J., and Johnson, K. M.: Radioimmunoassay for antibody to hepatitis B surface antigen shows transmission of hepatitis B virus among household contacts. J. Infect. Dis., 134:218, 1976.

147. Ponzetto, A., Hele, C., Forzani, B., Avanzini, L., and Rizzetto, M.: Hepatocellular carcinoma and hepatitis delta virus in the woodchuck animal model. Gastroenterology, 94:A583, 1988.

148. Poovorawan, Y., Sanpavat, S., Pongpunlert, W., Chomdermpadetsuk, S., Sentrakul, P., Chitinands, and Tannirundorn, Y.: Comparison of a recombinant DNA hepatitis B vaccine alone or in combination with hepatitis B immunoglobulin for the prevention of perinatal acquisition of hepatitis B carriage. Vaccine, 8(Suppl.):S56, 1990.

149. Price, P. M., Banerjee, R., and Acs, G.: Inhibition of the replication of hepatitis B virus by the carbocyclic analogue of 2'-deoxyguanosine. Proc. Natl. Acad. Sci. USA, 86:8541, 1989.

150. Prince, A. M., Szmuness, W., Michon, J., Desmaille, J., Diebolt, G., Linhard, J., Quenum, C., and Sankale, M.: A case-control study of the association between primary liver cancer and hepatitis B infection in Senegal. Int. J. Cancer, 16:376, 1975.

151. Pugh, J. C., and Bassendine, M. F.: Molecular biology of hepadnavirus replication. Br. Med. Bull., 46:329, 1990.

152. Redfield, R. R., Innis, B. L., Scott, R. M., Cannon, H. G., and Bancroft, W. H.: Clinical evaluation of low-dose intradermal administered hepatitis B vaccine, a cost-reduction strategy. JAMA, 254:32030, 1985.

153. Reyes, G. R., Purdy, M. A., Kim, K. P., Luk, K. C., Young, L. M., Fry, K. E., and

Bradley, D. W.: Isolation of a cDNA from the virus responsible for enterically transmitted non-A, non-B hepatitis. Science, 247:1335, 1990.

154. Robinson, W. S., and Lutwick, L. I.: The virus of hepatitis, type B (part 1). N. Engl. J. Med., 295:1169, 1976.

155. Robinson, W. S., and Marion, P. L.: Biological features of hepadna viruses. In Viral Hepatitis and Liver Disease. Edited by A. J. Zuckerman, New York, Alan R. Liss, 1988, p. 449.

156. Roggendorf, M., Deinhardt, F., Rasshofer, R., Eberle, J., Hopf, U., Moller, B., Zachoval, R., Pape, G., Schramm, W., and Rommel, F.: Antibodies to hepatitis C virus. Lancet, 2:324, 1989.

157. Rosina, F., Pintus, C., Meschievitz, C., and Rizzetto, M.: Long-term interferon treatment of chronic delta hepatitis: a multicenter Italian study. In The Hepatitis Delta Virus. Edited by J. L. Gerin, R. H. Purcell, and M. Rizzetto. New York, Wiley-Liss, 1991, p. 385.

158. Rosina, F., Saracco, G., Lattore, V., Quatrone, V., Rozzetto, M., Verme, G., Trinchero, P., Sansalvadore, F., and Smedile, A.: Alpha-2 recombinant interferon in the treatment of chronic hepatitis delta virus hepatitis. In The Hepatitis Delta Virus and Its Infection. Edited by M. Rizzetto, J. L. Gerin, and R. H. Purcell. New York, Alan R. Liss, 1987, p. 299.

159. Rumi, M. G., Colombo, M., Romeo, R., Colucci, G., Gringer, A., and Mannucci, P. M.: Serum hepatitis B virus DNA detects cryptic hepatitis B virus infections in multitransfused hemophilic patients. Blood, 75:1654, 1990.

160. Sanchez, Y., Ionescu-Matiu, I., Sparrow, J. T., Melnick, J. L., and Dreesman, G. R.: Immunogenicity of conjugates and micelles of synthetic hepatitis B surface antigen peptides. Intervirology, 18:209, 1982.

161. Schweitzer, K.: Vertical transmission of the hepatitis B surface antigens. Am. J. Med. Sci., 270:287, 1975.

162. Schweitzer, K., Dunn, A. E. G., Peters, R. L., and Spears, R. L.: Viral hepatitis B in neonates and infants. Am. J. Med., 55:762, 1973.

163. Seto, E., Mitchell, P. J., and Yen, T. S. B.: Transactivation by the hepatitis B virus X protein depends on AP-2 and other transcription factors. Nature, 344:72, 1990.

164. Seto, E., Yen, T. S. B., Peterlin, B. M., and Ou, J. H.: Trans-activation of the human immunodeficiency virus long terminal repeat by the hepatitis B virus X protein. Proc. Natl. Acad. Sci. USA, 85:8286, 1988.

165. Shank, R. C., Gordon, J. E., Wogan, G. N., Nondasuta, A., and Subhamani, B.: Dietary aflatoxins and human liver cancer: III. Field survey of rural Thai families for ingested aflatoxins. Fed. Cosmet. Toxicol., 10:71, 1972.

166. Simonetti, R. G., Cottone, M., Craxi, A., Pagliaro, L., Rapicetta, M., Chionne, P., and Costantino, A.: Prevalance of antibodies to hepatitis C virus in hepatocellular carcinoma. Lancet, 2:1338, 1989.

167. Smedile, A., Baroudy, B. M., Bergman, K. F., Rizzetto, M., Purcell, R. H., and Gerin, J. L.: Clinical significance of HDV-RNA in HDV disease. Prog. Clin. Biol. Res., 234:235, 1987.

168. Smedile, A., Rizzetto, M., Denniston, K., Bonino, F., Wells, F., Verme, G., Consolo, F., Hoyer, B., Purcell, R. H., and Gerin, J. L.: Type D hepatitis. The clinical significance of hepatitis D. virus RNA in serum as detected by hybridization-based assay. Hepatology, 6:1297, 1986.

169. Smith, G. L., Mackett, M., and Moss, B.: Infectious vaccinia virus recombinants that express hepatitis B virus surface antigen. Nature, 302:490, 1983.

170. Sobeslavsky, O.: Prevalence and markers of hepatitis B infection in various countries. A WHO collaborative study. Bull. WHO, 58:621, 1980.

171. Spandau, D. F., and Lee, C. H.: Trans-activation of viral enhancers by the hepatitis B virus X protein. J. Virol., 62:427, 1988.

172. Stanbridge, E. J., Flandermeyer, R. R., Daniels, D. W., and Nelson-Rees, W. A.: Specific chromosome loss associated with the expression in tumorigenicity in human cell hybrids. Somat. Cell Genet., 7:699, 1981.

173. Stevens, C. E.: No increased incidence of AIDS in recipients of hepatitis B vaccine. N. Engl. J. Med., 308:1163, 1983.

174. Stevens, C. E., Alter, H. J., Taylor, P. E., Zang, E. A., Harley, E. J., and Szmuness, W.: Hepatitis B vaccine in patients receiving hemodialysis. Immunogenicity and efficacy. N. Engl. J. Med., 311:496, 1984.

175. Stevens, C. E., Taylor, P. E., Tong, M. J., Toy, P. T., Vyas, G. N., Nair, E. V., Weissman, J. Y., and Krugman, S.: Yeast-recombinant hepatitis B vaccine. Efficacy with hepatitis immune globulin in prevention of perinatal hepatitis B virus transmission. JAMA, 257:2612, 1987.

176. Summers, J.: The replication cycle and hepatitis B viruses. Cancer, 61:1957, 1988.

177. Sung, J. L., and the Asian Regional Study Group: Hepatitis B virus eradication strategy for Asia. Vaccine, 8(Suppl.):S95, 1990.

178. Szmuness, W.: Hepatocellular carcinoma and the hepatitis B virus: evidence for a causal association. Prog. Med. Virol., 24:40, 1978.

179. Szmuness, W., Harley, E. J., Kram, H., and Stevens, C. E.: Sociodemographic aspects of the epidemiology of hepatitis B. In Viral Hepatitis. Edited by G. N. Vyas, S. N. Cohen, and R. Schmid. Philadelphia, PA, Franklin Institute Press, 1987, p. 297.

180. Szmuness, W., Much, M. I., Prince, A. M., Hoofnagle, J. H., Cherubin, C. E., Harley, E. J., and Block, G. H.: On the role of sexual behavior in the spread of hepatitis B infection. Ann. Intern. Med., 83:489, 1975.

181. Szmuness, W., Pick, K., and Prince, A. M.: The serum hepatitis virus specific antigens (SH): a preliminary report of epidemiologic studies in an institution for the mentally retarded. Am. J. Epidemiol., 92:51, 1970.

182. Szmuness, W., Prince, F. M., Grady, G. F., Mann, M. K., Levine, R. W., Friedman, E. A., Jacobs, M. J., Josephson, A., Ribot, S., Shapiro, F. L., Stenzel, K. H., Suki, W.

N., and Vyas, G.: Hepatitis B infection: a point prevalence study in 15 U. S. hemo-dialysis centers. JAMA, 227:901, 1974.

183. Szmuness, W., Stevens, C. E., Harley, E. J., Zang, E. A., Oleszko, W. R., William, D. C., Sadovsky, R., Morrison, J. M., and Kellner, A.: Hepatitis B vaccine. Demonstration of efficacy in a controlled clinical trial in a high-risk population in the United States. N. Engl. J. Med., 303:833, 1980.

184. Takada, S., and Koike, K.: Activated N-ras gene was found in human hepatoma tissue but only in a small fraction of the tumor cells. Oncogene, 4:189, 1989.

185. Taylor, P. Z., Stevens, C. E., De Cordoba, S. R., and Rubinstein, P.: Hepatitis B virus and human immunodeficiency virus: possible interactions. In Viral Hepatitis and Liver Disease. Edited by A. J. Zuckerman. New York, Alan R. Liss, 1988, p. 190.

186. Thomas, H. C., Pignatelli, M., Arodall, A., Waters, J., Karayiamis, P., and Brown, D.: Immunologic mechanisms of cell lysis in hepatitis B virus infection. In Viral Hepatitis and Liver Disease. Edited by G. N. Vyas, J. L. Dienstag, and J. H. Hoofnagle. Orlando, Florida, Grune and Stratton, 1984, p. 167.

187. Tong, M. J., Thursby, M. W., Lin, J. H., Weissman, J. V., and McPeak, C. M.: Studies on the maternal-infant transmission of the hepatitis B virus and HBV infection within families. Prog. Med. Virol., 27:137, 1981.

188. Trepo, C., Hantz, O., Ouzan, D., Chossegros, P., Chevallier, P., Berthillon, P., and Brette, R.: Therapeutic efficacy of ARA-AMP in symptomatic HBeAg positive CAH: A randomized placebo controlled study. Hepatology, 4:1055, 1984.

189. Trichopoulos, D., Day, N. E., Kaklamani, E., Tzonou, A., Munoz, N., Zavitsanos, X., Koumantaki, Y., and Trichopoulou, A.: Hepatitis B virus, tobacco smoking and ethanol consumption in the etiology of hepatocellular carcinoma. Int. J. Cancer, 29:45, 1987.

190. Twu, J. S., Chu, K., and Robinson, W. S.: Hepatitis B virus X gene activates KB-like enhancer sequences in the long terminal repeat of human immunodeficiency virus 1. Proc. Natl. Acad. Sci. USA, 86:5168, 1989.

191. Twu, J. S., and Robinson, J. S.: Hepatitis B virus X gene can transactivate heterolgous viral sequences. Proc. Natl. Acad. Sci. USA, 86:2046, 1989.

192. Twu, J. S., Rosen, C. A., Haseltine, W. A., and Robinson, W. S.: Identification of a region within the human immunodeficiency virus type 1 long terminal repeat that is essential for transactivation by the hepatitis B virus gene X. J. Virol., 63:2857, 1989.

193. Twu, J. S., and Schloemer, R. H.: Transcriptional trans-activating function of hepatitis B virus. J. Virol., 61:3448, 1987.

194. Van der Poel, C. L., Reesink, H. W., Lelie, P. N., Leentvaar-Kuypers, A., Choo, Q. L., Kuo, G., and Houghton, M.: Anti-hepatitis C antibodies and non-A, non-B post-transfusion hepatitis in the Netherlands. Lancet, 2:297, 1989.

195. Van Rensburg, S. J., Cook-Mozafarri, P., van Schalkwyk, D. J., van der Watt, J. J., Vincent, T. J., and Purchase, I. F.: Hepatocellular carcinoma and dietary aflatoxin in Mozambique and Transkei. Br. J. Cancer, 51:713, 1985.

196. Wahl, M., and Hermodsson, S.: Intradermal, subcutaneous or intramuscular administration of hepatitis B Vaccine: side effects and antibody response. Scand. J. Infect. Dis., 19:617, 1987.

197. Wands, J. R., Alpert, E., and Isselbacher, K. T.: Arthritis associated with chronic active hepatitis: complement activation and characterization of circulating immune complexes. Gastroenterol., 69:1286, 1975.

198. Wang, H. P., and Rogler, C. E.: Deletions in human chromosome arms 11p and 13q in primary hepatocellular carcinomas. Cytogenet. Cell Genet., 48:72, 1988.

199. Wang, H. P., and Rogler, C. E.: personal communication, 1990.

200. Wang, J., Chenivesse, X., Henglein, B., and Brechot, C.: Hepatitis B virus integration in a cyclin A gene in a hepatocellular carcinoma. Nature, 343:555, 1990.

201. Weiner, A. J., Kuo, G., Bradley, D. W., Bonino, F., Saracco, G., Lee, C., Rosenblatt, J., Choo, Q. L., and Houghton, M.: Detection of hepatitis C viral sequences in non-A, non-B hepatitis. Lancet, 335:1, 1990.

202. I. B. Weinstein: Synergistic interactions between chemical carcinogens, tumor promoters, and viruses and their relevance to human liver cancer. Cancer Detect. and Prev., 14:253, 1989.

203. Weller, I. V., Lok, A. S., Mindel, A., Karayiannis, P., Galpin, S., Monjardino, J., Sherlock, S., and Thomas, H. C.: Randomized controlled trial of adenine arabinoside 5'-monophosphate in chronic hepatitis virus infection. Gut, 26:745, 1985.

204. Will, H., Reiser, W., Weimer, T., Pfaff, E., Buscher, M., Sprengel, R., Cattaneo, R., and Schaller, H.: Replication strategy of human hepatitis B virus. J. Virol., 61:904, 1987.

205. Wollersheim, M., Debelka, U., and Hofscheider, P. H.: A transactivating function encoded in the hepatitis B virus X gene is conserved in the integrated state. Oncogene, 3:545, 1988.

206. Wong, V. C. W., Ip, H. M. H., Reesink, H. W., Lelie, P. N., Reerink-Brongers, E. E., Yeung, C. Y., and Ma, H. H.: Prevention of the HBsAg carrier in newborn infants of mothers who are chronic carriers of HBsAg and HBeAg by administration of hepatitis-B vaccine and hepatitis-B immunoglobulin. Double-blind randomized placebo-controlled study. Lancet, 1:921, 1984.

207. Xu, D. Z., Liu, C. B., Francis, D. P., Purcell, R. H., Gun, Z. I., Duan, S. C., Chen, R. J., Margolis, H. S., Huang, C. H., Maynard, J. E., and the United States-China Cooperative Study Group on Hepatitis B: Prevention of perinatal acquisition of hepatitis B carriage using vaccine: preliminary report of a randomized, double-blind placebo-controlled and comparative trial. Pediatrics, 76:713, 1985.

208. Yarrish, R. L., Werner, B. G., and Blumberg, B. S.: Association of hepatitis B virus infection with hepatocellular carcinoma in American patients. Int. J. Cancer, 26:711, 1980.

209. Yeh, F. S., Mo, C. C., Luo, S., Henderson, B. E., Tong, M. J., and Tu, M. C.: A serological case-control study of primary hepatocellular carcinoma in Guangxi, China. Cancer Res., 45:872, 1985.

210. Yeh, F. S., Mo, C. C., and Yen, R. C.: Risk factors for hepatocellular carcinoma in Guangxi, People's Republic of China. Natl. Cancer Inst. Monograph., 69:47, 1985.

211. Yu, M. C., Mack, T., Hanisch, R., Peters, R. L., Henderson, B. E., and Pike, M. C.: Hepatitis, alcohol consumption, cigarette smoking and hepatocellular carcinoma in Los Angeles. Cancer Res., 43:6077, 1983.

212. Zaruba, K., Grob, P. J., and Bolla, K.: Thymopentin as adjuvant therapy to hepatitis B vaccination in formerly non- or hyporesponding hemodialysis patients. Surv. Immunol. Res., 4(Suppl 1):102, 1985.

213. Zoulek, G., Lorbeer, B., Jilg, W., and Deinhardt, F.: Evaluation of a reduced dose of hepatitis B vaccine administered intradermally. J. Med. Virol., 14:27, 1984.

214. Zuckerman, A. J.: The history of viral hepatitis from antiquity to the present. In Viral Hepatitis: Laboratory and Clinical Science. Edited by F. Deinhardt, J. Deinhardt. New York, Marcel Dekker, 1983, p. 3.

Parasites

Piero Mustacchi

Introduction

When relatively uncommon neoplasms are noted with undue frequency in countries with high prevalence of parasitic diseases, the question of the role of the parasite arises. In this respect, the two most intriguing examples are probably the relationships of schistosomiasis to bladder cancer, and malaria to Burkitt's lymphoma.

Schistosomiasis and Cancer of the Bladder

Epidemiologic Aspects

The data associating schistosomiasis and neoplasia are overwhelming, but explanations for this association remain speculative.[11,28] Published data so far have been retrospective and therefore have yielded only relative frequencies with their well-known inherent limitations.

Geography. In Africa, squamous carcinoma of the bladder is greatly over-represented among the fellaheen of Egypt and the Africans of Mozambique and Rhodesia, all countries where Schistosoma hematobium is endemic. This has led to the hypothesis that infestation predisposes to malignant bladder neoplasms. Observations made in Ghana are only suggestive of an association, however, and none emerges from Tanzania, Uganda, and French-speaking West Africa, where schistosomiasis is endemic but bladder cancer is apparently rare.

No prospective study measuring the risk of developing bladder cancer in infested and noninfested persons is as yet available; thus conflicting conclusions derived from relative frequency data remain unresolved. Although differences in relative frequencies may reflect differences in risk, the interplay of other factors such as geopolitical variations in case finding, can result in spurious differences and erroneous associations. If the postulated association is correct, a certain condition must obtain: the worm produces a carcinogen, or carries a virus, or is cocarcinogenic to other exposures. In this case a number of unanswered questions arise to explain geographic differences in vesical cancer observed where schistosomiasis is endemic. These range from whether there is geographic uniformity in the host's reaction to infestation, to whether other environmental variables (such as the bright food coloring used in the candy so popular in the Nile Delta) are more directly responsible for vesical neoplasia.

Age and Sex. Bilharzial bladder cancer attacks men preferentially. In Egyptian hospital series their mean age is 41 years, or about 5 years less than the nonbilharzial type, and the sex ratio ranges from 5:1 to 9:1.[1,32] In Ghana, 5 of 13 males with bladder cancer came to autopsy before age 36.[56] In Mozambique, too, bilharzial bladder cancer occurs earlier

in life, but the sex ratio is nowhere as striking as in Egypt (M/F = 1.75:1).[60] The question whether this difference from Egypt reflects a greater susceptibility of females, a lesser risk of males, or simply a vagary resulting from under-reporting remains unresolved.

Urban/Rural Distribution. In Egypt, additional support for an association with bilharzial infestation can be found in the relative paucity of bladder cancer cases reported from hospitals serving the nonparasitized Italian and Greek residents of metropolitan Cairo, compared with the large number observed in hospitals attending Egyptian peasants.[1]

Similarly, a survey of consecutive Egyptian patients, 624 urban and 848 rural, yielded 107 malignant neoplasms. Of the 33 observed in urban patients, ten, or less than one third, occurred in the bladder. The fellaheen living in rural areas contributed 74 cancers, of which 45 (60%) were vesical.[56]

Frequency and Severity of Infestation. The association of bladder cancer with schistosomal infestation seems to become stronger with the duration and severity of the infestation.[27,56] In the Nile Delta, a progressively larger proportion of patients is found to have Schistosoma ova in the urine as the study progresses from bladders with cytologically benign epithelium to those with squamous metaplasia, benign tumors and, finally, cancer.

The severity of infestation tends to rise sharply with opportunities for exposure. In Egypt it is directly related to the extent of perennial irrigation through canals with constant risk of re-infestation. In Ghana, where different agricultural conditions prevail, schistosomiasis is essentially a prepubertal disease, and a small proportion of the population is infested compared to the extent found in Egypt. Comparative studies in these two countries indicate a rather good direct relationship between parasitic infestation and frequency of bladder cancer.[56] Thus, the peculiar agricultural setting of the Nile Valley singles this region for a dose-response relationship not encountered in other parts of Africa.

Variability in Diagnostic Criteria of Schistosomiasis. Many reports on schistosomal bladder cancer fail to define the diagnostic criteria for infestation; moreover, there is no assurance that uniform criteria were used throughout a study. For instance, negating a diagnosis of schistosomiasis because of the absence of ova in the centrifuged urinary specimen would be unrealistic in many cases of contracted bladder due to bilharzial fibrosis, in which the dense scar tissue precludes shedding of ova from the submucosa. Conversely, sound epidemiologic practices require that when evidence of infestation in ova-negative bilharzial patients is sought by rectal scrapings or x-ray studies, the same diagnostic refinements be used in every member of the group studied.

One such study conducted in the Nile Delta concluded

that only 11% of the men and 3% of the women could be considered infested, on the basis of presence of schistosomal ova in the initial urinalysis. Based on this diagnostic criterion, only a suggestive association of infestation and cancer of the bladder was demonstrated (p = 0.04). By expanding the criteria for diagnosis of schistosomiasis to include the presence of ova in any centrifuged urinary sample and other evidence of infestation obtained by endoscopic or radiologic procedures, the prevalence of infestation was increased threefold. In either instance, after correcting for age, sex, and residence, the relative risk of developing bladder cancer among the bilharzial patients was double that experienced by the comparison population group. By adopting the expanded definition of schistosomiasis, the association became much more probable (p = 0.002).[56]

A similar change in the force of the association emerges when the pathologist, who had established a diagnosis of schistosomiasis on a surgical specimen of limited dimensions, expands the anatomic substrate for infestation to a complete autopsy.[32] In this situation, the p value for the association changes from 0.05 to less than 0.001.

Geographic Variability in Schistosomal Virulence. Within East Africa, a coastal strain of *S. hematobium* is more virulent than that at Lake Victoria, where infested bladders do not show severe changes.

When *S. mansoni* is considered, the Brazilian and Puerto Rican strains are the most virulent when measured by the production of liver disease in infested mice. Under the same experimental conditions, the Egyptian strain caused the least liver damage and the Tanzanian strain produced the fewest eggs.[70] Variability in *S. mansoni* virulence has been invoked to explain the high frequency of liver cancer in Mozambique, but not in Egypt, even though schistosomal liver cirrhosis is common in both countries. This type of explanation is at best tentative, because other, and as yet undetected, environmental carcinogenic hazards can be at work.

Role of Urinary Infection. In Egypt, but not in Mozambique, bladder calculi and incrustations of vesical ulcers are frequent complications of schistosomal infestation. The experimental work linking some nitroso products of bacterial metabolism to carcinogenesis may perhaps refurbish the old carcinogenic hypothesis of the early Egyptian workers who incriminated "alkaline urine."

Pathology of Benign and Preneoplastic Schistosomal Bladder Lesions

An intense, delayed-sensitivity reaction is elicited by viable Schistosoma eggs plugged in the vesical venules. Depending on how severe and widespread the reaction, this results in tubercles, nodules, or polyps. Thus, in bilharzial cystitis, the papilloma is essentially a granuloma and not a precancerous lesion, covered as it is by one or two layers of flattened cells, which merge with the transitional epithelium at its base.[60]

With recurrent inflammation and fibrosis, some transitional epithelial cells become sequestered in the vesical submucosa and acquire a globular arrangement around a central cavity. By opening into the bladder cavity, the cystic formations become pseudoglands. These structures, as part of cystitis glandularis, are at times precancerous; an adenocarcinoma may arise from the columnar epithelium into which their lining has differentiated.

In patients with bilharzia, squamous metaplasia is frequently encountered, because it is a common concomitant of chronic inflammation.[14] This type of metaplasia is a nearly consistent precursor of bladder cancer and, for this reason, leukoplakia acquires clinical importance as a precancerous condition.

Site of Origin. In Western countries bladder cancer frequently arises in the trigone; in Egypt it develops in areas remote from the ureters, mostly in the anterior and posterior bladder walls. This peculiarity tends to strengthen its association with schistosomal infection, because the scanty or altogether absent submucosal tissue of the trigone discourages significant deposition of ova (Table III-12-1).

Histologic Classification. Table III-12-2 contrasts the overrepresentation of squamous cell carcinoma of the bladder in areas like Egypt, Mozambique, and South Africa (Bantu population), where the association with schistosomiasis is considered important, with the Uganda and white South African experience where the reverse applies.

Within the same country, squamous cell carcinoma of the bladder is markedly overrepresented only in areas where schistosomiasis is endemic.[41]

Experimental Data. Half a century ago, papillomatous hyperplasia of the vesical wall was observed in African Sooty monkeys within three months of infestation with *S. hematobium* and, more recently, a carcinoma of the bladder was diagnosed in a baboon killed 26 weeks after infestation.[30] In a number of nonhuman primates, infection with *S. hematobium* resulted in epithelial proliferation, squamous metaplasia, and transitional cell carcinoma of the urinary bladder.[44] The American opossum has been found a suitable experimental animal for infection with *S. hematobium*.[45] These experimental observations are important because neither eggs of *S. hematobium* nor lyophilized worms nor urine from bilharzial patients have been found to be carcinogenic to mice.[20,65] Furthermore, schistosoma ova, either dry or in the presence of 3-methycholanthrene, lacked urothelial topical carcinogenicity or co-carcinogenicity in mice.[4] However, 2-acetyl-amino-fluorene appears to promote malignant and benign bladder neoplasms of mice infested with bilharzia more often than does the schistosomiasis alone or the carcinogen alone.[31] Similarly, N-methyl-N-nitrosourea and *S. hematobium* caused bladder tumors in 5 of 16 hamsters, whereas given singly, no oncogenic effect was seen. Three *S. hematobium* infected baboons treated with N-butyl-N-butazolnitrosamine all developed extensive bladder cancer.[34]

Table III-12-1. Anatomical Distribution of Vesical Cancer in Egypt and United States

	Egypt %	USA %
Trigone	3	21
Lateral wall	34	47
Anterior wall	22	8
Posterior wall	30	18
Vault	11	6

Table III-12-2. Histologic Types of Bladder Cancer in Africa

	Egypt[1,14]	East African[30]	South Africa[35]		Uganda[15]
			Bantu	White	
Squamous	232	58	16	11	26
Transitional	134	28	2	0	31
Anaplastic	2	13	4	129	7
Adenocarcinoma	20	0	1	0	5
Total	389	100	23	140	69

Information from Aboul Naser,[1] Dimmette,[14] Dodge,[15] Gillman,[30] and Higginson.[35]

Cancer development was felt to have been accelerated by schistosomal infection, presumably acting as a late-stage or co-carcinogen by virtue of its direct proliferative effect on urothelium.[33]

Analogously, an increased incidence of hepatoma has been described after administration of carcinogen to mice infested with *S. mansoni*.[20] This occurs even though the toxic morphologic alterations occurring in liver are fewer than those observed in noninfested mice exposed to the same hepatocarcinogen.[48]

Helminthic Infestation and Viruses. No information seems to be available on the relationship between helminthic parasites and oncogenic viruses. One knows, however, that parasitic diseases exacerbate viral infection. In one of four capuchin monkeys C-type virus particles were found in a papillary carcinoma induced by *S. hematobium* which had not been present earlier in the normal bladder tissue. Mice inoculated subcutaneously with Japanese B virus are resistant to the development of encephalitis unless they are challenged with the canine roundworm *Toxocara canis*. Also, overt disease in adult rats inoculated with encephalomyocarditis virus is promoted by concurrent trichinosis. Finally, in mice infested with *S. mansoni,* the parasitic disease may enhance the acute effect of hepatitis virus, but no evidence has been found as yet that the chronic cirrhosis-like picture results therefrom.[71]

Metabolic Observations during Schistosomiasis

Increased urinary excretion of free 3-hydroxykynurenine, 3-hydroxyanthranilic acid, and 2-amino-3-hydroxyacetophenone has been documented in some patients with bladder cancer. These 0-aminophenol derivatives of tryptophan are generally excreted as conjugates of sulfuric acid or glucuronic acid. They are related to the carcinogenic metabolites of β-naphthylamine and are themselves carcinogenic to mice.

The relative resistance of the trigone to schistosomal bladder cancer would make less tenable an etiologic hypothesis predicated upon the topical action of an endogenous urinary carcinogen, were it not for the increased activity of urinary β-glucuronidase in vesical infections, including schistosomiasis. Under these circumstances the enzymatic release of the active carcinogen from its glucuronide could well become a significant biologic factor determining the anatomic localization of the neoplasm. Thus, in the study of bilharzial cancer, the metabolism of tryptophan along the formylkynurenine pathway leading to nicotinic acid has elicited considerable interest.[54] The basic justification for this interest originally stemmed from industrial oncology. However epidemiologic support is also derived from the high prevalence of classic pellagra in Egypt, but not in other parts of Africa where squamous bladder cancer seems to be infrequent despite endemic schistosomiasis. In pellagra, exaggeration of the pathway from tryptophan to nicotinic acid occurs, producing larger amounts of tryptophan intermediates along the formylkynurenine pathway.

Our understanding of the role played by schistosomal infestation in disturbed tryptophan metabolism is complicated by geographic variations of dietary habits. In fact, serotonin metabolites such as 5-hydroxyindoleacetic acid, which are excreted in large amounts by plantain-eating Africans, are low in Africans on other diets.[25,68] Similar differences attributable to dietary habits have been found between bilharzial patients in Mozambique and their"controls" in South Africa. Egyptian peasants are not plantain-eaters but subsist mostly on beans and lentils. Those with bilharzial cancer metabolize tryptophan in a manner reminiscent of the pattern seen in many patients with spontaneous bladder cancer, because they have increased excretion of 3-hydroxyanthranilic acid, anthranilic acid, 5-hydroxyindoleacetic acid, and kynurenine. The excretion of these metabolites is enhanced by a loading dose of tryptophan.

Schistosomiasis should not be considered the only causal factor in the associated excretion of abnormal tryptophan metabolites because, with or without cancer, vesical schistosomiasis is almost universally accompanied by urinary tract infection. The bacterial flora may thus contribute to a spurious accumulation of some metabolites of tryptophan. Moreover, untreated pellagra is associated with increased urinary excretion of anthranilic acid, acetylkynurenine, and 5-hydroxyindoleacetic acid.

Potentially carcinogenic metabolites of tryptophan, which may be the true oncogenic agent in the presence of bilharzial bladder inflammation, are principally determined by hepatic metabolic patterns. Factors that bear on this are coincident infestation of the liver by *S. mansoni,* pyridoxine deficiency, and chronic protein starvation. In the presence of advanced abnormalities in any of these factors, lesser amounts of potential carcinogenic metabolites are formed owing to lack of hepatic enzyme or co-factor, but no mutagens were detected by the Ames test in the urine of patients suffering from bilharzial bladder cancer.[22]

Similarly, a study on the frequency of active *ras* oncogenes in bilharzial bladder cancer concluded that the carcinogenic process involved in the endemic neoplasm is not associated with detectable point mutations within *ras* genes at a higher frequency than those in non-bilharzial cancer.[26]

In view of its isolation from direct exposure to putative

carcinogens present in the urine, a defunctioned bilharzial bladder may seem an unlikely site for the development of neoplastic changes. None the less this has been reported in a defunctioned bladder showing extensive metaplasia.[18] Quantitative estimates of infection with *S. haematobium* have shown that its overall severity is unlikely to be the sole factor in the pathogenesis of endemic vesical cancer.[19]

Schistosomiasis and Cancer of Other Sites

Large Intestine. While Egyptian data tend to discount any association of *S. mansoni* or *S. hematobium* with cancer of the large intestine, in Asia, intestinal infestation with *S. japonicum* is considered a significant contributory factor to the development of cancer of the colon and rectum.[32]

In one report from China, where, in endemic areas, the prevalence of schistosomiasis may reach 44 per 100,000, 48% of colectomy specimens for colorectal carcinoma obtained from 1951 to 1974 were associated with *Schistosoma japonicum* infestation. The mean age of the schistosomal group was 6.5 years less than for idiopathic colorectal carcinoma. Associated inflammatory changes, pseudopolyps, and transitional mucosal changes of schistosomal granulomatous disease progressing to mucosal atypia and to carcinoma were reminiscent of bowel carcinoma in patients with ulcerative colitis, save for the ova deposited in all layers of the bowel.[12] Nonetheless, 92% were well differentiated, compared to 69% in the nonschistosomal group.

In Shanghai, patients with intestinal schistosomiasis and cancer of the large intestine are on the average six years younger than patients with spontaneous intestinal cancer.[36,50]

However, Chinese patients whose history of schistosomiasis entailed an elevated relative risk of rectal cancer (RR = 8.3; CI = 3.1–22.6) did not show a parallel increase in their relative risk for cancer of the colon.[70]

Breast. In Egyptian hospital material, male breast cancer seems to be over-represented. If corroborated by incidence studies, this observation would be a valuable epidemiologic observation worthy of further investigation. Hyperestrogenism secondary to bilharzial liver fibrosis has been invoked as one possible cause.

Liver. Discordant observations on the association of schistosomiasis and hepatic cancer are difficult to reconcile without further data. In Egypt and Mozambique bilharzial liver cirrhosis is very common; however carcinoma of the liver is prevalent only in Mozambique, where it is the most common cancer among males.[32,60] Differences in chronic hepatitis from hepatitis B virus have been postulated. The association of cirrhosis from *S. japonicum* with hepatoma has been infrequently reported and appears invalid.

In Japan, liver cancer correlated highly with 3 factors: HBsAg (RR = 10.0), history of schistosomiasis (RR = 9.5), and daily intake of alcohol (RR = 3.2) with the combination of hazards acting multiplicatively or at least synergistically.[39,42]

Lymphoma. Eight cases of solitary follicular lymphoma of the spleen were found among 863 spleens removed from patients with hepatosplenic schistosomiasis. The rarity of an isolated tumor of this site and of this type suggests a causal link possibly mediated by cycles of follicular hyperplasia and involution occurring in the spleen in the course of advanced schistosomiasis.[5]

In a Nigerian series, lymphoreticular tumors were over-represented in infected individuals (16%) compared to uninfested ones.[17]

Miscellaneous Organs. Immunohistochemically-confirmed invasive squamous cell carcinoma of the prostate was diagnosed in two patients with prostatic schistosomiasis coming from a population where prostatic cancer is uncommon.[3]

On the other hand, Egyptian material indicates no relationship between bilharziasis and cancer of the lungs, pancreas, prostate, seminal vesicles, urethra, vulva, vagina, cervix uteri, body of the uterus, or ovaries.[32] As would be expected, surgical or autopsy material in countries with high schistosomal endemicity from time to time shows the presence of schistosoma ova in various tissues including cancers. The literature contains a number of isolated reports of such coincidences.

Moreover, in areas where infestation is endemic, schistosomal tissue reaction may be so intense and proliferative as to be mistaken clinically for cancer of the large intestine or the cervix.[55,64]

Oriental Distomiasis

Liver and Pancreas. *Clonorchis sinensis* is endemic in parts of Japan, Korea, China, and Hong Kong; a similar species, *Opisthorchis viverrini*, causes distomiasis in Thailand. Liver fluke infections have been associated with intrahepatic bile-duct carcinoma in those areas of Asia where distomiasis is endemic; in Indonesia, and in Taipei, Taiwan, where distomiasis is considered uncommon, cholangiocarcinoma is infrequent. Imported cases of distomiasis are seen in the United States.[29]

Human infection results from eating raw or undercooked parasitized freshwater fish. In man, the ingested parasites excyst in the duodenum and ascend the bile ducts and capillaries where they mature, causing biliary epithelial hyperplasia and fibrosis. An association of *C. sinensis* with multifocal hepatoma arising typically from second-order bile ducts has been reported in man and in the dog. Etiologic mechanisms that have been invoked include mechanical or chemical irritation produced by the worm, and the possible elaboration of carcinogens from a biliary substrate. In man, the presence of stones is apparently not necessary for the induction of intrahepatic cholangiocarcinoma, for stones are generally absent in human clonorchiasis.[29] Metaplasia, but not cancer, has been reported in ductal lesions associated with pancreatic clonorchiasis.

Amebiasis

The association of amebiasis with neoplasms of the large intestine remains speculative at best.

Malaria

The geographic distribution of Burkitt's lymphoma in the classic malarial belt suggested initially the possible role of an arthropod vector in oncogenesis.[8] The notion that drugs taken for malaria prophylaxis contribute to the development of Burkitt's lymphoma was unlikely because no increase, and a possible decrease, in endemic Burkitt's lymphoma (eBL) was observed in the Malagasy Republic and in Imesi, West Africa, where intensive antimalarial prophylaxis is practiced; moreover, cases occur in Africa, Israel, and elsewhere among individuals not receiving malaria prophylaxis.[2,7,38,49,61,62]

More significant are the epidemiologic observations that have linked eBL to the combined effect of malaria and infection with the Epstein-Barr virus (EBV).[23]

Regarding malaria, eBL is only found in areas where malaria is holoendemic or hyperendemic, and within these areas it is absent in pockets of no malaria such as urban centers or high altitudes. Within endemic areas, the peak incidence of eBL follows closely the one of severe *P. falciparum* malaria and malaria prophylaxis reduces the incidence of the lymphoma.

Also very plausible is the argument that the persistent reticuloendothelial stimulation experienced by malarial populations conditions the EBV-infected African patient to develop a neoplasm rather than a self-limited disease such as infectious mononucleosis.[58] This view finds support in the observation that each one of the erythrocytic, exo-erythrocytic, and sexual forms of the parasite is structurally differentiated and probably contains a multitude of biologically active antigenic constituents.[57] In this respect it is interesting to note that in endemic malarial areas, the distribution of hyper-reactive malarial splenomegaly parallels the distribution of eBL.[23]

One way of explaining the observation that the malarial patient harboring a multitude of parasite-derived antigens becomes a host greatly susceptible to eBL is the suggestion that malarial patients produce so many nonspecific and"useless" antibodies that they are unable to recognize and respond to the threat posed by a small clone of malignant lymphoid cells.[72] This view is supported by experimental data. In mice, antigenic stimulation and immunologic suppression often result in an increased incidence of lymphomas; mice repeatedly injected with *Plasmodium berghei* sometimes develop malignant lymphoma morphologically similar to Burkitt's lymphoma, and sometimes develop persistent antigenic stimulation without significant tumorigenesis.[21,43,67] Lymphomas are frequently induced by Moloney leukemogenic virus in mice infected with *P. berghei* but rarely occur in mice given either plasmodium or virus alone.[73]

Of considerable interest are studies on the frequency of sickle trait in eBL patients and controls. People with sickle trait are not protected from being bitten by mosquitoes or from malarial infection, but they are protected against the lethal effect of overwhelming *P. falciparum* malaria in early childhood and from the intense reticuloendothelial stimulation that sometimes progresses to hyper-reactive malarial splenomegaly ("big spleen" disease).[51] Sickle cells do not support the growth of parasites when exposed to low oxygen tension *in vitro,* and this may explain why children with the sickle-cell trait have a lower *P. falciparum* parasitemia. As a result, lower mortality rate, lower IgM levels, and reduced lymphoproliferation (as measured by spleen size) are found among individuals with hemoglobin AS genotype. However, most studies attempting to link eBL to that hemoglobinopathy

have failed to reach statistical significance.[23] Other hemoglobinopathies, e.g., hereditary ovalocytosis, also protect against malaria. If eBL turns out to be under-represented in populations where, as in Papua New Guinea, both ovalocytosis and malaria are prevalent such information would provide strong supporting evidence for malaria as a cofactor in the genesis of eBL.[9,23] In this event the observation that in Uganda malarial endemicity also correlates with non-Burkitt's, non-Hodgkin's lymphoma, would acquire added significance.[63]

The small differences in titers of malarial antibodies observed in BL patients and controls were attributed to the fact that many in the experimental group had received several courses of anti-malarial drugs, something likely to have lowered the level of malaria-specific antibodies.[23,52] A probable role of malaria emerges also from the following considerations. African children with eBL develop autoantibodies, the elevated titers of which show no linear correlation with EBV titers (VCA or EBNA),. suggesting that a factor independent of EBV causes an immunologic imbalance and autoantibody production.[69] The notion that this could be due to malaria is supported by the observation that Caucasians suffering from an acute *P. falciparum* malaria develop autoantibodies and that *in vitro* experiments demonstrated that normal human lymphocytes will produce autoantibodies as a response to malarial antigens.[13,40,53]

It has been pointed out that in the genesis of eBL, regardless of whether one considers malaria the initiator and EBV the promoter or vice versa, neither hypothesis accounts for the fact that *in vitro* infection of B cells with EBV and stimulation of EBV-genome-negative or -positive B cells with malaria antigens has yet to produce a cell carrying any one of the chromosomal tumorigenic translocations found in both sporadic and eBL.[23] Thus it seems likely that other unidentified factors, genetic, nutritional or environmental play a significant role in this type of tumorigenesis.

American Burkitt's Lymphoma. By the early seventies approximately 100 cases of Burkitt's lymphoma had been confirmed by the American Burkitt's lymphoma registry.[46] Space-time clustering is suggested by the American data.[47,59] Although malaria is associated with Burkitt's lymphoma in Africa, the relative rarity of the tumor in relation to the holoendemic nature of malaria indicates that a combination of genetic factors plus specific environmental factors may be operative. Host and environmental factors other than malaria are probably important in North American cases.[46]

Cancer in Animals

Observations made by Fibiger on gastric cancer in rats infested with a nematode are now all but discredited.[24] A question that remains to be evaluated is whether the nematode helped localize some unidentified carcinogens in the diet, similar to the induction of sarcomas at the site of subcutaneous injection of sodium chloride in rats being fed 3-methylcholanthrene.[37,66]

Sarcoma is an almost inevitable complication of infestation of the liver or the subcutaneous tissues of rats with *Cysticercus fasciolaris,* the larval form of the common tapeworm of the cat, *Taenia taeniaformis.* Washed, ground-up C. fas-

ciolaris produced peritoneal sarcomas in half the injected rats, the proportion reaching 91% if the animals were genetically related to the parasitized host. The active agent appears to be associated with the calcium carbonate corpuscles of the parasite, but the mechanism is not clear.[16] Although not directly implicated in vesical carcinogenesis, there is suggestive evidence that infestation with another nematode, *Trichosomoides crassicauda,* will increase the incidence of tumors in the bladders of rats receiving 2-acetyl-amino-fluorine.[10]

Another nematode, *Spirocerca lupi,* has been associated with the development of esophageal sarcoma in dogs. Here the reported association seems to be described only in the southern United States, thereby adding a possible geographic dimension to the problem.

Some neoplastic responses to parasitic infestation are a kind of cecidiosis, and may represent the end of an hypothesized evolutionary sequence by which parasite secretions stimulate the host to form protective structures (cecidia) that benefit the parasite.[6]

References

1. Aboul Nasr, A. L., Gazayerli, M. E., Fawzi, R. M., and El-Sibai, I.: Epidemiology and pathology of cancer of the bladder in Egypt. Acta Unio Internat. Contra Cancrum. 18:528, 1962.
2. Aghai, E., Hulu, N., Virag, I., Kende, G., and Ramot, B.: Childhood non-Hodgkin's lymphoma–a study of 17 cases in Israel. Cancer, 33:1411, 1974.
3. Al Adnani, M. S.: Schistosomiasis, metaplasia and squamous cell carcinoma of the prostate: histogenesis of the squamous cells determined by localization of specific markers. Neoplasma, 32:613, 1985.
4. Al-Hussaini, M., and McDonald, D.F.: Lack of urothelial topical tumorigenicity and cotumorigenicity of Schistosome ova in mice. Cancer Res., 27:228, 1967.
5. Andrade, Z. A., and Abreu, W. N.: Follicular lymphoma of the spleen with hepatosplenic schistosomiasis mansoni. Am. J. Trop. Med. Hyg., 20:237, 1971.
6. Audy, J. R.:"Hostology"–an alternative view. Trop. Med. Hyg. News, 19:15, 1970.
7. Bruce-Chwatt, L. J.: Antimalarial drugs and Burkitt's lymphoma. Lancet, 1:223, 1974.
8. Burchenal, J. H.: Geographic chemotherapy–Burkitt's tumor as a stalking horse for leukemia: Presidential address. Cancer Res., 26:2393, 1966.
9. Castelino, D., Saul, A., Myler, P., Kidson, C., Thomas, H., and Cooke, R.: Ovalocytosis in Papua New Guinea–Dominantly inherited resistance to malaria. Southeast Asian J. Trop. Med. Public Health, 12:549, 1981.
10. Chapman, W. H.: The incidence of a nematode, *Trichosomoides crassicauda*, in the bladder of laboratory rats: Treatment with nitrofurantoin and preliminary report of their influence on urinary calculi and experimental tumors. J. Invest. Urol., 2:52, 1964.
11. Cheever, A. W.: Schistosomiasis and neoplasia. J. Nat. Cancer Inst., 61:13, 1978.
12. Chen, M.-C., Chuang, C.-Y., Chang, P.Y., and Hu, T.-C.: Evolution of colorectal cancer in schistosomiasis. Cancer, 46:1661, 1980.
13. Daniel-Ribeiro, C. T., de Roquefeuil, S., Druilhe, P., Monjour, L., Homberg, J.-C., and Gentilini, M.: Abnormal anti-single stranded (ss) DNA activity in sera from Plasmodium falciparum infected individuals. Trans. R. Soc. Trop. Med. Hyg., 78:742, 1983.
14. Dimmette, R. M., Sproat, H. F., and Sayegh, E. S.: The classification of carcinoma of the urinary bladder associated with schistosomiasis and metaplasia. J. Urol., 75:680, 1956.
15. Dodge, O. G.: Tumours of the bladder in Uganda Africans. Acta Unio Internat. Contra Cancrum, 18:548, 1962.
16. Dunning, W. F., and Curtis, M. R.: Multiple peritoneal sarcoma in rats from intraperitoneal injection of washed ground Taenia larvae. Cancer Res., 6:668, 1946.
17. Edington, G. M., von Lichtenberg, F., Nwabuebo, I., Taylor, J. R., and Smith, J. H.: Pathologic effects of schistosomiasis in Ibadan, western state of Nigeria. I. Incidence and intensity of infection; distribution and severity of lesions. Am. J. Trop. Med., 19:982, 1970.
18. Elem, B., Alam, S. Z.: Total intestinal metaplasia with focal adenocarcinoma in a schistosoma-infested defunctioned urinary bladder. Brit. J. Urol., 56:331, 1984.
19. Elem, B., and Purohit, R.: Carcinoma of the urinary bladder in Zambia. A quantitative estimation of Schistosoma haematobium infection. Brit. J. Urol., 55:275, 1983.
20. El-Ghaffar, Y. A.: Failure to induce bladder cancer in mice. Bladder implantation with paraffin wax pellets of lyophilized urine from bilharzial patients. Cancer, 19:1225, 1966.
21. Evans, A. S.: Clinical syndromes associated with EB virus infection. Adv. Intern. Med., 18:77, 1972.
22. Everson, R. B., Gad-el-Mawla, N. M., Attia, M. A., Chevlen, E. M, Thorgeirsson, S. S., Alexander, L. A., Flack, P. M., Staiano, N., and Ziegler, J. L.: Analysis of human urine for mutagens associated with carcinoma of the bilharzial bladder by the Ames Salmonella plate assay. Interpretation employing quantitation of viable lawn bacteria. Cancer, 51:371, 1983.
23. Facer, C. A., and Playfair, J. H. L.: Malaria, Epstein-Barr virus and the genesis of lymphomas. Adv. Cancer Res., 53:33, 1989.
24. Fibiger, J.: Untersuchung fiber eine Nematode (Spiroptera sp. n.) und deren Fähigkeit, papillomatöse und karzinomatöse Geschwulstbildungen im Magen der Ratte hervorzurufen. Z. Krebsforsch, 13:217, 1913.
25. Fripp, P. H.: Bilharziasis and bladder cancer. Brit. J. Cancer, 19:292, 1965.
26. Fujita, J., Nakayama, H., Onoue, H., Rhim, J. S., El-Bolkainy, M. N., El-Aaser, A. A., and Kitamura, Y.: Frequency of active *ras* oncogenes in human bladder cancers associated with schistosomiasis. Jpn. J. Cancer Res. (Gann), 78:915, 1987.
27. Gelfand, M., Weinberg, R. W., and Castle, W. M.: Relation between carcinoma of the bladder and infestation with Schistosoma haematobium. Lancet, 1:1249, 1967.
28. Gentile, J. M.: Schistosome related cancers: A possible role for genotoxins. Exp. Mutagen., 7:775, 1985.
29. Gibson, J. B., and Chan, W. C.: Primary carcinomas of the liver in Hong Kong: Some possible actiologic factors. Recent Results in Cancer Res., *39*:107, 1971.
30. Gillman, J., and Prates, M. D.: Histologic types and histogenesis of bladder cancer in the Portuguese East African with special reference to bilharzial cystitis. Acta Unio Internat. contra Cancrum, 18:560, 1962.
31. Hashem, M., and Boutros, K.: The influence of bilharzial infection on the carcinogenesis of the mouse bladder. An experimental study. J. Egypt. Med. Assoc., 44:598, 1961.
32. Hashem, M., Zaki, S. A., and Hussein, M.: The bilharzial bladder cancer and its relation to schistosomiasis. A statistical study. J. Egypt. Med. Assoc., 44:579, 1961.
33. Hicks, R. M.: The canopic worm: Role of bilharziasis in the aetiology of human bladder cancer. J. R. Soc. Med. 76:16, 1983.
34. Hicks, R. M., James, C., Webbe, G., and Nelson, G. S.: Schistosoma haemotobium and bladder cancer. Trans. Roy. Soc. Trop. Med. Hyg., 71:288, 1977.
35. Higginson, J., and Oettie, A. G.: Cancer of the bladder in the South African Bantu. Acta Unio Internat. contra Cancrum, 18:580, 1962.
36. Huan-Wen, T., and Yueh-Ying, Y.: A pathologic study of intestinal schistosomiasis associated with cancer. Chinese Med. J., 77:244, 1958.
37. Huggins, C., and Grand, L. C.: Sarcoma induced remotely in rats fed 3-methyl-cholanthrene. Cancer Res., 23:477, 1963.
38. Hutt, M. S. R., and Burkitt, D. P.: Aetiology of Burkitt's lymphoma. Lancet, 1:439, 1973.
39. Inaba, Y., Maruchi, N., Matsuda, M., Yoshihara, N., and Yamamato, S.: A case-control study on liver cancer with special emphasis on the possible aetiological role of schistosomiasis. Int. J. Epid., 13:408, 1984.
40. Kataaha, P. K., Hacer, C. A., and Holborow, E. J.: Stimulation of autoantibodies production in normal blood lymphocytes by malaria culture supernatants. Parasite Immunol., 6:481, 1984.
41. Kitinya, J. N., Lauren, P. A., Eshleman, L. J., Paljarvi, L., and Tanaka, K.: The incidence of squamous and transitional cell carcinomas of the urinary bladder in northern Tanzania in areas of high and low levels of endemic *Schistosoma haematobium* infection. Trans. R. Soc. Trop. Med. Hyg., 80:935, 1986.
42. Kojiro, M., Kakizoe, S., Yano, H., Tsumagari, J., Kenmochi, K., and Nakashima, T.: Hepatocellular carcinoma and *Schistosomiasis japonica*. A clinicopathologic study of 59 autopsy cases of hepatocellular carcinoma associated with chronic *Schistosomiasis japonica*. Acta Path Jpn. 36:525, 1986.
43. Krüger, G., and O'Conor, G. T.: Epidemiologic and immunologic considerations on the pathogenesis of Burkitt's tumor. Recent Results Cancer Res., 39:211, 1972.
44. Kuntz, R. E., Cheever, A. W., and Meyers, B. J.: Proliferative epithelial lesions of the urinary bladder of nonhuman primates infested with *Schistosoma haematobium*. J. Natl. Cancer Inst., 48:223, 1972.
45. Kuntz, R. W., Myers, B. J., Moore, J. A., and Huang, T. C.: Parasitologic aspects of Schistosoma haematobium (Iran) infections in the American opossum (Didelphis marsupialis L.). Int. J. Parasitol., 5:21, 1975.
46. Levine, P. H., and Cho, B. R.: Burkitt's lymphoma: Clinical features of North American cases. Cancer Res., 34:1219, 1974.
47. Levine, P. H., Sandler, S. G., Komp, D. M., O'Conor, G. T., and O'Connor, D. M.: Simultaneous occurrence of"American Burkitt's lymphoma" in neighbors. N. Engl. J. Med., 288:562, 1973.
48. Liu, L. B., Domingo, E. O., Stenger, R. J., Warren, K. S., Confer, D. B., and Johnson, E. A.: An ultrastructural study of the toxic and carcinogenic effects of 2-amino-5-azotoluene on the livers of schistosome-infected and uninfected mice. Cancer Res., 29:837, 1969.
49. McGucken, R. B.: Antimalarial drugs and Burkitt's lymphoma. Lancet, 1:68, 1974.
50. Ming-Chai, C., and Shan-Chi, C. W.: Acute colonic obstruction in Schistosomiasis japonica. A clinical study of 40 cases–14 associated with carcinoma. Chinese Med. J., 75:517, 1957.
51. Morrow, R. H., Sever, J. L., and Henderson, B. E.: Antibody levels in infectious agents other than Epstein-Barr virus in Burkitt's lymphoma patients. Cancer Res., 34:1212, 1974.
52. Morrow, R. H.: Epidemiological Evidence for the Role of Falciparum Malaria. *In* Burkitt's Lymphoma: A Human Cancer Model. Edited by G. Lenoir, G. O'Connor, and C. Olweny. Lyons, IARC, Science Publication No. 60, 1985, pp. 177–185.
53. Mortazavi-Milani, S. M., Stierle, H. E., and Holborow, E. J.: Antibody to intermediate filaments of the cytoskeletons in the sera of patients with acute malaria. Clin. Exp. Immunol., 55:177, 1983.
54. Mousa, A. H., Abdel Wahab, A. F., Mousa, W., Abdel-Tawab, G. A., Saad, A. A., and Kelada, N. L.: Tryptophan metabolism in hepatosplenic bilharziasis. Trans. Roy. Soc. Trop. Med. Hvg., 61:640, 1967.
55. Mustacchi, P. O., and El-Sibai, I.: Advanced schistosomal proctitis simulating clinically cancer of the rectum. Gastroenterology, 19:137, 1951.
56. Mustacchi, P., and Shimkin, M. B.: Cancer of the bladder and infestation with Schistosoma hematobium. J. Natl. Cancer Inst., 20:825, 1958.
57. Neva, F. A., Sheagren, J. N., Shulman, N. R., and Canfield, C. J.: Malaria: Host-defense mechanisms and complications. Ann. Intern. Med., 73:295, 1970.
58. O'Conor, G. T.: Persistent immunologic stimulation as a factor in oncogenesis with special reference to Burkitt's tumor. Am. J. Med., 48:279, 1970.
59. Patton, L. L., McMillan, C. W., and Webster, W. P.: American Burkitt's lymphoma: A 10-year review and case study. Oral Surg. Oral Med. Oral Pathol., 69:307, 1990.
60. Prates, M. D., and Gillman, J.: Carcinoma of the urinary bladder in the Portuguese East African with special reference to bilharzial cystitis and preneoplastic reactions. S. Afr. J. Med. Sci., 24:13, 1959.
61. Sadoff, L.: Aetiology of Burkitt's lymphoma. Lancet, 2:1414, 1972.
62. Sadoff, L.: Antimalarial drugs and Burkitt's lymphoma. Lancet, 2:1262, 1973.
63. Schmauz, R., Mugerwa, J. W., and Wright, D. H.: The distribution of non-Burkitt, non-Hodgkin's lymphoma in Uganda in relation to malarial endemicity. Int. J. Cancer, 45:650, 1990.
64. Schwartz, D. A.: Carcinoma of the uterine cervix and schistosomiasis in West Africa. Gynec. Oncol., 19:365, 1984.

65. Shimkin, M. B., Mustacchi, P. O., Cram, E. B., and Wright, W. H.: Lack of carcinogenicity of lyophilized Schistosoma in mice. J. Natl. Cancer Inst., 16:471, 1955.
66. Shimkin, M. B., and Triolo, V. A.: History of chemical carcinogenesis: Some prospective remarks. International Symposium on Carcinogenesis and Carcinogen Testing, 1969, Boston, Mass. Progr. Exp. Tumor Res., 11:1, 1969.
67. Sizaret, P., O'Conor, G. T., Beaumont, R., and Laval, M.: Serum protein patterns in mice following primary and challenge infection with Plasmodium berghei. Z. Tropenmed. Parasitol., 22:260, 1971.
68. Trout, G. E., Gillman, J., and Prates, M. D.: Bilharzial cystitis and the urinary excretion of tryptophan metabolites in the Portuguese East African. Acta Unio Internat. contra Cancrum, 18:575, 1962.
69. Vainio, E., Lenoir, G. M., and Franklin, R. M.: Autoantibodies in three populations of Burkitt's lymphoma patients. Clin. Exp. Immunol., 54:387, 1983.
70. Warren, K. S.: A comparison of Puerto Rican, Brazilian, Egyptian, and Tanzanian strains of Schistosoma mansoni in mice: Penetration of cercarise, maturation of schistosomes and production of liver disease. Trans. Roy. Soc. Trop. Med. Hyg., 61:795, 1967.
71. Warren, K. S., Rosenthal, M. S., and Domingo, E. O.: Mouse hepatitis virus (MHV$_3$) infection in chronic murine Schistosomiasis mansoni. Bull. N.Y. Acad. Med., 45:211, 1969.
72. Warrens, A. E.: Burkitt's lymphoma and disordered immunoglobulin response. Lancet, 1:742, 1974.
73. Wedderburn, N.: Effect of concurrent malarial infection on development of virus-induced lymphoma in Balb/c mice. Lancet, 2:1114, 1970.
74. Xu, Z., and Su, D.-L.: Schistosoma japonicum and colorectal cancer: An epidemiologic study in the People's Republic of China. Int. J. Cancer, 34:315, 1984.

III-13

Immunological Aspects of Cancer Etiology

R. W. Baldwin
V. S. Byers

Antigenic Profiles on Tumor Cells

Experiments dating from the 1950's showing that immunity could be induced against tumors arising following exposure of animals to chemical carcinogens or oncogenic viruses provided the basis upon which contemporary tumor immunology has evolved. These early experiments demonstrated that immunity could be induced by various manipulations against experimental animal tumors transplanted into syngeneic (inbred) recipients, this manoeuvre being utilized so as to exclude immune responses to normal tissue transplantation antigens.[4,57] Surgical resection of a growing tumor, providing all tumor was removed, proved to be an effective method for inducing resistance to a subsequent challenge with cells of the same transplanted tumor. Other procedures which have subsequently formed the basis of trials of human cancer immunotherapy include implantation of tumor cells rendered incapable of continuous growth, e.g., by treatment with X or gamma-irradiation, often together with immunological adjuvants such as BCG.[61] Critical control experiments showing that grafting normal tissues, e.g., skin, did not induce immunity to transplanted tumors indicated that residual heterozygosity between tumor donor and recipient of tumor tissue was not responsible for eliciting the tumor rejection response. Investigations then went on to show that immunity could be induced against an autochthonous tumor. This is illustrated by the induction of immunity against mouse sarcomas produced by 3-methylcholanthrene (MCA) following complete resection of the primary tumor and then rechallenge of the cured mouse some time later with the same tumor maintained by transplantation into a secondary (syngeneic) mouse.

Chemically Induced Tumors

Tumor specific rejection antigens (TSRA) were originally identified with MCA induced sarcomas in mice and rats.[4]

This led to the now classical observation that MCA-induced sarcomas express individually distinct tumor rejection antigens. For example, induction of immunity to one tumor did not confer host resistance to another tumor induced by MCA, even where the two tumors arose in a single mouse. Many other types of chemical carcinogen-induced tumor have been investigated for TSRA expression (Table III-13-1). These include sarcomas and carcinomas induced with a range of polycyclic hydrocarbons such as benzo[a]pyrene (BP) and 7-12-dimethylbenz[a]anthracene (DMBA).

In addition neoplastic transformation in vitro by exposure of mouse fibroblasts to 3-methylcholonthrene leads to the expression of surface components which function in vivo to elicit specific immunity against in vivo growth of transformed cells.[20] Transformed cell lines derived from separate colonies each expressed individually distinct tumor rejection antigens reflecting the findings observed in animals treated with polycyclic hydrocarbon carcinogens.

Tumor rejection antigens are also expressed on aromatic amine-induced tumors of diverse histological types such as mammary carcinomas, hepatocellular carcinomas and ear duct carcinomas. Hepatocellular carcinomas induced by alkylnitrosamines (e.g., diethylnitrosamine) and aromatic aminoazobenzenes (e.g., 4-dimethylaminoazobenzene) also express tumor rejection antigens.

Radiation induced tumors express TSRA, this being exemplified by studies with ultraviolet light induced skin tumors.[36] These are so immunogenic that their growth on transplantation into syngeneic mice can only be effected if the recipient is immunosuppressed.

In all of these examples the tumor rejection response is directed specifically against the immunizing tumor indicating that the tumor rejection antigen is a unique component associated with the malignant cell.

It is notable that many of the experimentally-induced animal tumors shown to express tumor rejection antigens have

Table III-13-1. Expression of Tumor-Specific Rejection Antigens on Carcinogen-Induced Tumors

Carcinogen	Tumor Type	Species
Polycyclic Hydrocarbons		
3-methylcholanthrene (MCA)	Sarcoma	Mouse
		Rat
		Guinea pig
	Mammary carcinoma	Mouse
		Rat
	Lymphoma	Mouse
	Skin papilloma/carcinoma	Mouse
	Bladder papilloma/carcinoma	Mouse
		Rat
	In vitro transformed prostate cells	Mouse
	3T3 cells transformed in vitro, maintained in vivo	Mouse
Dibenz[a,h]anthracene	Sarcoma	Mouse
		Guinea pig
7,12-Dimethylbenz[a]anthracene (DMBA)	Sarcoma	Mouse
		Guinea pig
Benzo[a]pyrene	Sarcoma	Mouse
		Rat
Aminoazo Dyes		
4-Dimethylaminoazo-benzene (DAB)	Hepatocellular carcinoma	Rat
o-Aminoazotoluene	Hepatocellular carcinoma	Mouse
Aromatic Amines		
N-2-Fluorenyl-aceta-mide	Mammary carcinoma	Rat
	Hepatocellular carcinoma	Rat
	Zymbal gland carcinoma	Rat
Alkylnitrosamines		
Diethylnitrosamine	Hepatocellular carcinoma	Rat
		Guinea pig
Miscellaneous		
Urethan	Pulmonary adenoma	Mouse
Mineral oil	Plasmacytoma	Mouse
Plastic film	Sarcoma	Mouse
UV radiation	Skin carcinoma	Mouse

been induced by carcinogens identified or suspected to be human carcinogens.[1,63] Polycyclic hydrocarbons are associated with combustion products including tobacco smoke and other air pollutants. Alkylnitrosamines are associated with cooked food products and beverages and aromatic amines, such as benzidine and 2-naphthylamine produced in industrial processes, have long been associated with human cancer induction. Finally ionizing radiation is causally associated with leukaemia and lung tumors, while ultraviolet light-radiation is associated with skin tumors. The findings from extensive animal studies on the induction of immunity to carcinogen-induced tumors can be summarized as follows: 1) All chemical carcinogens tested induce tumors expressing tumor rejection antigens. 2) Tumor rejection antigens are specific for individual tumors. Evidence for cross-reactive

tumor rejection antigens is inconclusive. 3) Expression of tumor rejection antigens is not a necessary feature of carcinogen induced neoplastic transformation. Variability of tumor rejection antigen expression has been observed within populations of tumors induced with a particular carcinogen, e.g., MCA. The reasons for this variability of TSRA expression have not been explained, although the dose of carcinogen and latent period of tumor induction have been cited as related factors. This may reflect the degree of DNA damage leading to target gene mutation and directly or indirectly to TSRA expression. This is emphasized by an intriguing approach showing that highly immunogenic variants of tumor cells are obtained in very high frequency by treating mouse tumor cells in vitro with mutagens such as N-methyl-N' nitro-N-nitrosoguanidine.[8,10] These variants are termed tum+ cells since they do not produce tumors in syngeneic mice, whereas the original tumor (tum−) will produce progressive tumor growth. Rejection of tum+ cells is mediated by a T lymphocyte mediated response. 4) When expressed, tumor rejection antigens are stable components of the neoplastic cell and cannot be selected against even when tumors are passaged into immune recipients. 5) Cellular immunity to carcinogen-induced tumors has been defined by adoptive transfer assays showing that T lymphocytes from tumor-immune donors transfer immunity to the tumor into naive animals. This T cell mediated immunity is specific for the immunizing tumor reflecting the specific characteristics of the tumor rejection antigen.[24] Demonstration of specific T cell responses in vitro has not been satisfactory in the past because of the effects of lymphocytes non-specifically cytotoxic for tumor cells.[26] Identification of specific cytotoxic T cells has been resolved recently by culturing murine MCA sarcoma infiltrating lymphocytes in medium containing interleukin-2 (IL-2) and further stimulating cells with irradiated autologous tumor.[6] These cells were specifically cytotoxic for the tumor from which they were derived and were therapeutically effective in eliminating established micrometastases of the tumor. 6) Identification of antibody responses to tumor antigens on carcinogen-induced tumors has been inconsistent. Antibodies in sera from rats immunized against several types of tumor including MCA-induced sarcomas and aminoazo-dye induced hepatomas have been identified by membrane immunofluorescence staining of tumor cells and by antibody-mediated complement cytotoxicity tests.[4] These antibodies identified specific tumor antigens identical to those detected by tumor rejection methods. Serological assays have proved inconclusive in typing antigens on murine tumors since reactivities detected following tumor cell immunization have generally been directed to cross-reactive envelope and internal antigens of endogenous murine leukemia viruses (MULV) associated with these tumors.[57] These MULV cross reactions need to be appreciated since they prevent detection of antibodies to the individually distinct antigens on murine tumors induced by chemical carcinogens. There is little or no conclusive evidence therefore that murine tumor antigens arising from carcinogen induced neoplastic transformation initiate B lymphocyte responses leading to the production of tumor specific antibodies. 7) The characteristics of the TSRA associated with carcinogen-induced tumors which mediate tumor rejection are still not defined. Recent studies with MCA-induced sarcomas have led to the conclusion that the TSRA's associated with two examples belong to a new family of cell surface glycoproteins (gp96). It has been further proposed that the polymorphism of the gp96 molecule is due to modifications in the amino acid sequence possibly discrete and restricted to a particular region of the molecule.[57] 8) The molecular events leading to the expression of cell surface molecules recognized by the host as tumor rejection antigens following exposure to chemical carcinogens remain unknown. Early investigations correlated tumor antigen expression with interaction of carcinogen metabolites with cellular macromolecules such as protein and DNA.[4] This has led to the widely accepted, but unproven, view that the neoantigens are products of mutated genes. Progress in resolving this question is hampered by limited confidence of in vitro assays, particularly for antibody mediated responses, to tumor rejection antigens. This is illustrated by studies defining the individually distinct tumor rejection antigens on methylcholanthrene-induced sarcomas. Tumor immunity was elicited by a 96 kDa cell surface glycoprotein (gp96) the specificity being identical to that of intact tumor cells. From biochemical studies evidence indicates that the gp96 antigens are encoded by a single gene specifying a single mRNA species. Nucleotide and deduced amino acid sequences of DNA clones show no significant similarity with any known protein. The gene coding for this gp96 molecule has subsequently been mapped to mouse chromosome 10. From these studies Old and his colleagues have proposed that the polymorphism of the gp96 molecules is due to modifications in the amino acid sequences possibly restricted to a particular region of the molecule.[56,57] The relationship between the gp96 glycoproteins on 3-methylcholanthrene-induced tumors and specific tumor antigens on other experimental tumors is unknown. For example, murine sarcomas induced with UV-radiation express tumor rejection antigens related to class I major histocompatability determinants.[58,59] Immunogenic tumor cell variants have been obtained in high frequency by treating mouse tumor cells in vitro with mutagens.[8,9] Analysis of tumor responses and patterns of tumor cell lysis by cytolytic T cell lymphocytes have indicated that most of these so-called "tum⁻ variants" express new transplantation antigens specific for each variant. This has made possible the cloning of genes coding for tum⁻ antigens. They show no homology with any genes recorded in DNA data libraries and their expression has been reported to result from point mutations located in an exon causing a change in amino acid.

Virus Induced Tumors

DNA-Tumor Viruses

Animal tumors induced by oncogenic viruses express neoantigens which elicit cell mediated immune responses resulting in tumor rejection.[25,32,47] This was originally demonstrated in the early 1960's by showing that adult mice infected with the DNA polyoma virus or by implantation of polyoma-virus induced tumors rejected challenge with transplants of syngeneic polyoma tumors. Other tumors induced by DNA viruses include SV40-induced mouse and hamster tumors, human adenovirus induced mouse tumors, Rous chicken sarcoma virus induced tumors, and Shope papilloma virus rabbit tumors.

In these examples the tumor rejection antigens are common to tumors induced by a specific virus (common group-specific tumor rejection antigens). For instance, polyoma virus induced tumors in different species (mice, hamsters) express a common tumor rejection antigen. This antigen is not present on the mature virion and is present on cells whether or not they release virus. The DNA viruses encode proteins intracellularly, predominantly as nuclear proteins (T antigens) which are also expressed at the cell surface and these function as tumor rejection antigens. In this respect the tumor rejection antigens are tumor specific since they are not encoded by genes of the host, are not expressed on normal cells and are not present on virion particles.

RNA-Tumor Viruses

RNA tumor viruses such as murine leukemia viruses and mammary tumor virus induce the expression of neoantigens which function to induce rejection of tumors induced by each virus type.[7,42,47] All of these RNA oncogenic viruses induce the expression of virus encoded antigens on the surface of tumor cells. These represent virus encoded protein including virus envelope glycoprotein gp70. Differing from the proteins encoded by DNA tumor viruses which are not expressed on virus particles but only by infected/transformed cells, tumor antigens encoded by RNA viruses are associated with virus particles as well as the surface of virus-infected and transformed cells.

Human Cancer Viruses

Worldwide viruses, either directly or indirectly, have been estimated to account for around 20 percent of human cancers. These include hepatocellular carcinoma (HPC), Burkitt's lymphoma/nasopharyngeal carcinoma, cervical cancer, some skin cancers, and some leukemias/lymphomas. Viral and host factors involved in the pathogenesis of these tumors are still not well understood but immunocompetence is an important factor both in limiting virus infection of host cells and in growth of tumor cells.

Hepatitis B Virus. Primary liver cancer, hepatocellular carcinoma (HCC), is one of the ten most common human cancers, and around 80% of cases are associated etiologically with hepatitis B virus infection (HBV), often early in life.[18,72] For example, in Taiwan and South Africa, 66–80% of patients with HCC are hepatitis B surface antigen (HBsAg) positive compared to 8–15% of the normal population. In the light of this relationship between HBV infection and HCC development, vaccination procedures to eradicate HBV infection are being pursued.

Viral vaccines are prepared from intact virus or fractions. Another source of viral antigen for vaccination is HBsAg, the non-infectious surplus coat of the virus, isolated and purified from plasma of asymptomatic carriers. More recently recombinant DNA techniques have been employed for expressing hepatitis B surface antigen and core antigen in prokaryotic and eukaryotic cells. This has led to the development of a range of preparations for vaccine development including hepatitis B subunit vaccines, polypeptide vaccine hybrid vaccine virus/hepatitis B virus vaccines and chemically synthesized products.[72]

Papilloma Viruses. The human papilloma viruses (HPV) are a widespread family of viruses causing various proliferative diseases in infected epithelium. It is now thought that infection with specific types of HPV are necessary, but not sufficient, factors for the development of cervical, vulvar, penile and perianal cancers.[73] HPV16 is the most prevalent of the HPV viruses, reported to account for around 50% of all genital HPV infections. This raises the possibility of devising vaccination procedures for stimulating immune responses for suppressing HPV infection and so arresting the development of malignant disease.

Epstein-Barr Virus. Epstein-Barr virus (EBV) is one of the most common infective agents in humans with in excess of 90 percent of the world population being persistently infected. The virus is the causative agent of infectious mononucleosis and is associated with several human malignancies such as Burkitt's lymphoma nasopharyngeal carcinoma and polyclonal B cell lymphomas in immunosuppressed individuals.[16] Immunological studies have been cited as evidence that EBV might be at least one of the causative agents of Burkitt's lymphoma and nasopharyngeal carcinoma and a range of EBV antigens associated with these tumors have been identified.[48] These include viral capsid antigens, so-called early antigens, membrane antigens, EBV-induced nuclear antigens, and lymphocyte defined membrane antigens. EB virus vaccines are being developed using a range of types of EBV antigens such as envelope glycoproteins. Future clinical trials will establish whether this type of vaccination will restrict the spread of virus and control EBV-related disease such as nasopharyngeal cancer.

Human T Cell Lymphotropic Virus (HTLV-I). Human T cell lymphotropic virus type I (HTLV-I) isolated in 1980 is a retrovirus causing a unique T cell malignancy; adult T cell leukemia/lymphoma, a disease that is endemic in Southern Japan, Central Africa and the Carribbean basin.[54,71] This is the first authentic human cancer virus although HTLV-I causes less than 1 percent of all leukemias. However, blood donor surveys conducted by the American Red Cross indicate that approximately 20 per 100,000 of the population were seropositive for HTLV-I.[68] The viral and host factors involved in HTLV-I pathogenesis are being studied, one aim being to develop immunological measures to control viral infection.

Human Tumor Antigens

Human tumors express an array of intracellular and cell surface molecules identified as antigens through their reaction with murine monoclonal antibodies.[11] This approach is illustrated by the identification of glycoprotein, glycolipid and mucin-like antigens on colorectal cancer cells.[11] Monoclonal antibodies have also been used to identify mucin-like glycoproteins on breast cancer.[30] In this case the polypeptide epitope binding several monoclonal antibodies have been identified as a tandem repeat of a continuous sequence of amino acids.[12,51,55] Monoclonal antibodies have been particularly effective in defining melanoma associated antigens. There are well in excess of 20 monoclonal antibodies specifying protein and glycoprotein structures expressed upon melanoma cells.[11]

Tumor antigens identified by murine monoclonal antibodies cannot be classified as specific human tumor antigens since this is dependent upon showing that they are capable of inducing immune responses in patients. In some instances, however, murine monoclonal antibodies may recognize antigens that can evoke an immune response in cancer patients. This evidence is now being accrued through the manipulation of anti-idiotypic antibodies to stimulate anti-tumor immune responses. This approach is based upon the concept that an anti-idiotypic antibody (Ab$_2$) reacting with the binding site of an antibody (Ab$_1$) reacting with antigen (Ag) will itself be able to generate an immune response to the original antigen.[35] Anti-idiotypic antibody therapy of colorectal cancer is being explored using heterologous (goat) anti-idiotypic antibody reacting with monoclonal antibody CO17-1A,[27] and with a human anti-idiotypic monoclonal antibody reacting with monoclonal antibody 791T/36.[2] The original monoclonal antibodies recognise glycoproteins on colorectal cancer and the idiotypic immunotherapy approach suggests that under the right conditions immune responses can be initiated in patients.

Specific neoantigens associated with human tumors, especially malignant melanoma, have been identified by analysis of autologous tumor-cell lymphocyte interactions. Initially this approach produced inconclusive results since lymphocytes derived from various sources, e.g., peripheral blood, contain populations of cells such as natural killer cells showing broad cytotoxicity. Definition of tumor specific lymphocyte cytotoxicity has become possible with the development of methods for expanding T cells in vitro to produce T cell clones. For example, lymphocytes cultured from tumor-infiltrating cells (TIL) from melanoma patients are in some cases specifically cytotoxic for autologous melanoma cells, but not allogeneic melanomas.[64] These highly specific TIL's were identified as T cell by phenotyping (CD3+, CD8+, CD4-) and lack of binding with antibody (Leu 7) reacting with NK Cells. Several other groups have identified cytotoxic lymphocytes (CTL) derived from peripheral blood lymphocytes of melanoma patients.[65] The consensus of opinion is that the CTL's reacting only with autologous tumor cells are produced in response to recognition of melanoma specific antigen presented in association with major histocompatibility complex (MHC) molecules. Evidence for the production of autologous T cell responses to antigens on other types of human cancer cell is still equivocal.

Immunocompetence and Cancer

The concept of immunosurveillance in cancer gained popularity in the mid 1970's.[4,33,44] This proposed that "the phenomenon of homograft rejection represents a primary mechanism for the natural defence against neoplastic cells." From this it was argued firstly that most, if not all, neoplastic cells express antigens that are not present on normal cells. Secondly, cellular immune responses mediated by T lymphocytes that recognize these tumor antigens protect the host against neoplasia. Thirdly, aberration of the immune system (immunosuppression) allows neoplasms to develop.

Experimental studies cited in support of immunosurveillance include the finding of increased tumor incidences in immunosuppressed animals treated with oncogenic viruses.[70] For example, immunosuppression by neonatal thymectomy or treatment with anti-lymphocyte antibody so as to ablate T lymphocyte activity results in increased tumorigenic responses to oncogenic viruses. These include DNA viruses such as polyoma virus which induces a range of tumors in mice and Shope fibroma virus in rabbits. Tumors induced by RNA viruses (murine leukemia virus, mouse mammary tumor virus) are also subject to immunological control. Murine skin tumors induced by UV radiation are also under immunological control and can only be propogated in immunodeficient hosts.[37] In contrast no differences were found in the incidences of tumors induced by chemical carcinogens when immunocompetent or T cell deficient e.g., athymic mice were studied.[4] There was also no significant increase in the incidence of naturally arising tumors in T cell deficient hosts.[38,60] It is likely, therefore, that the enhanced oncogenic responses to viruses following immunosuppression reflects suppression of T cell immunity to viral antigens or virus encoded tumor antigens.

The observation of an association between immune deficiency and lymphoid malignancies in humans was also cited initially in support of cancer immunosurveillance, but further investigations indicated that the frequency of different types of tumors in immunodeficient patients was quite different from that in the general population.[49] In particular, there was a much higher incidence of non-Hodgkin's lymphomas which it has been suggested is related to Epstein-Barr virus infection. Malignant lymphomas occurring in x-linked lymphoproliferative syndrome and associated with HIV-I associated immunodeficiency show evidence of Epstein-Barr virus infection.[22,34]

The clinical impact of immunosuppression is most clearly seen in relation to infection with retroviruses known to be causative agents for a number of neoplastic diseases.[21] This includes HTLV-1 in adult T cell leukemia, HTLV-2 in some cases of hairy cell leukemia and T cell chronic lymphocytic leukemia, and probably most importantly, HIV-1 in acquired immunodeficiency syndrome associated with B cell lymphoma and Kaposi's sarcoma.[45] An important pathway of immunosuppression by retroviruses involves T lymphocyte infection leading to their destruction or loss of functional activity. Other indirect mechanisms of immunosuppression such as generation of suppressor T cells or soluble factors and abnormal lymphokine production have been postulated.[41]

The available evidence, therefore, suggests that where tumors express neoantigens which evoke T cell mediated immunity, then immunocompetence of the host is a significant factor in tumor development. This, in turn, raises the issue of whether common types of human cancer express tumor antigens as they evolve from the initial clone of transformed cells to primary tumors and then to metastatic disease.

The other related issue is the now widely accepted view that host resistance to human cancers is mediated by a broad spectrum of effector cells, driven by a range of cytokines.[5] Effectors include non-specific cytotoxic cells such as natural killer (NK) cells and lymphokine activated (LAK) cells in addition to antigen-restricted T lymphocytes.

Evidence for the effectiveness of both antigen-restricted and non-antigen restricted effector cells is being accrued from therapeutic trials with interleukin 2 (IL-2) activated lymphocytes derived from peripheral blood or tumor infiltrating cells.[52] For example, lymphocytes infiltrating human melanomas (TIL) are specifically cytotoxic for the autologous tumor providing evidence of MHC-restricted human tumor immune responses in the use of TIL for immunotherapy.[64] In addition, non-MHC restricted cytotoxic cells derived by IL-2 treatment of peripheral blood lymphocytes are being used for melanoma immunotherapy.[53]

Defects in MHC-restricted and non-MHC restricted cytotoxic cells has been observed in tumor bearing patients.[13,29] Factors responsible for this include suppressor cells,[62] and tumor derived factors.[39] Although the suppressor mechanisms observed in tumor bearing hosts are poorly defined, the view is gaining ground that the immunosuppression influences cancer development.[46] Immune deficiency may influence the survival of early transformed cells, their progression to tumor colonies and their metastatic spread. These findings have drawn attention to the need to consider the overall impact of immunocompetence on the initiation of cancer cells and their subsequent development.

Immunosuppressive Action of Environmental Agents

Xenobiotic agents introduced into the human environment have long been recognised by epidemiologists as a major cause of human cancer.[17] Health assessment of environmental agents, particularly in relation to their carcinogenic potential is being carefully scrutinized.[1,50] A selection of agents initially considered for their carcinogenic potential is listed in Table III-13-2. These represent only a small fraction of the chemical substances introduced into the environment, but

Table III-13-2. Chemical Agents Known or Suspected to be Carcinogenic and Immunotoxic

Air Pollutants	
Aromatic compounds	Benzene
Polycyclic Hydrocarbons	Benzo[a]pyrene
Dioxins	TCDD
Chlorinated Hydrocarbons	Trichloroethylene
Food/Beverage	
Fungal products	Aflatoxin
Alkylnitrosamines	Dimethylnitrosamine
Water Pollutants	
Polychlorinated Biphenyls	
Chlorinated Hydrocarbons	Tricholorethylene
Aromatic compounds	Benzene
Occupational Exposure	
Aromatic compounds	Benzene
Chlorinated Hydrocarbons	Trichloroethylene
Polycyclic Hydrocarbons	Benzo[a]pyrene
Metals	Nickel/Chromium compounds
Formaldehyde	
Aromatic amines	Benzidine
Mineral oils	

provide at least a starting point for considering their immunotoxic properties. For example, over 700 organic chemicals have been shown to be present in the U.S. drinking water supply.[23] There are numerous airborne pollutants arising from multiple sources such as cigarette smoke, automobile engine exhaust emissions and industrial emissions. These include combustion products such as dioxins and polycyclic hydrocarbons. Thirdly, there are many potential and proven immunotoxic substances introduced through the food chain including agricultural chemicals and agents used in various aspects of food processing. Only a small fraction of these chemical substances have been examined for their influence on immune functions.[43] Furthermore assessment of the effects of human exposure has not been defined in any precise fashion since this has usually been examined in environmental or workplace exposure and exposed subjects are rarely exposed to a single substance.

Polycyclic Aromatic Hydrocarbons

Polycyclic aromatic hydrocarbons are ubiquitous in the environment arising from numerous sources especially tobacco smoke, incomplete combustion of fossil fuels and as by-products of industrial processes. The immunosuppressive action of 7,12,-dimethylbenz[a]anthracene (DMBA) has been examined in some detail as one example of this class of compound. Significant and long-lasting suppression of numerous lymphocyte functions was observed in DMBA-treated mice. These include susceptibility to challenge with tumor cells and bacterial infection, reduced ability to generate cytotoxic T cells and reduced splenocyte IL-2 production.[28,66] Other polycyclic hydrocarbons shown to suppress lymphocyte function include benzo[a]pyrene,[15,19] and 3-methylcholanthrene.[69]

Benzene

Benzene is extensively used industrially and is a widespread environmental pollutant through its emission in automobile exhaust fumes and as a trace contaminant in ground water. Workplace exposure has been estimated at a daily average dose in the 70kg adult of 2.4mg and indoor air pollution ranging up to 1,000μg/day.[50] Benzene is metabolized to phenol and the principal secondary metabolites are hydroquinone, benzoquinone and catechol. Suppression of cell growth and function in bone marrow and lymphoid organs correlates with the concentration of these metabolites. These metabolites also affect immune function at exposure levels which are not cytotoxic. Metabolites of benzene can depress mitogen-induced proliferation of B and T lymphocytes, depress IL-2 production, and inhibit gamma-interferon synthesis.

The influence of non-cytotoxic levels of benzene exposure on hematopoiesis or lymphocyte function in human subjects is inadequately documented even from studies on workplace exposure.[31] Low level workplace exposure (15–20 ppm) did not result in overt reduction of WBC counts but immune function was not assessed. Waterborne exposure of human populations to benzene cannot be adequately assessed since ground water contains a multiplicity of contaminants. Experimental studies have reported depressed cell mediated immunity in mice exposed to benzene in drinking water.[14]

Dioxins

Dioxins represent a class of agents recognized as environmental pollutants.[1,50] The prototype of this class of compound is 2,3,7,8,-tetrachlorodibenzo-p-dioxin (TCDD). This compound produces a number of toxic manifestations including carcinogenesis, teratogenesis, and immunotoxicity. Administration of TCDD to several species of laboratory animals caused lymphoid atrophy, suppression of lymphoid function, and sustained immunosuppression. The specific effects of TCDD exposure on lymphoid function depends upon the age of the recipient. The primary effect after perinatal exposure is persistent suppression of T cell functions but this is less apparent in adults. Here the primary effect is on hematopoietic stem cells and B lymphocytes.

In a review of human health hazards of polychlorinated dibenzo-p-dioxins, it was concluded that TCDD is a toxic chemical that can have adverse effects upon the immune system. There is a wide variation in susceptibility between species with humans being among the least susceptible to the immunotoxic effects of TCDD. The possibility of perinatal exposure to TCDD in human milk was noted as a particular concern.

Chlorinated Hydrocarbons

The general population is exposed to very low levels of chlorinated hydrocarbons including trichloroethylene in air, water and food.[50] For example, the average daily dose/70kg adult of TCE is 14μg. For occupational exposure this rises to up to 4g/day. The OSHA time weighted average permissable exposure level (1989) was chosen as 50 parts/million in air. Animal studies have demonstrated immunotoxic effects of TCE.[67] The influence of human exposure has not been adequately evaluated but the increased incidence of childhood leukemia in regions of Woburn, Massachusetts related to contaminated well water was compared with immunological parameters of exposed families.[13,40]

Conclusions

Host immune responses to tumor associated antigens influence to varying degrees the oncogenic process and so will impact on the incidence of cancer or the extent of cancer metastatic spread. Tumors induced in animals by oncogenic viruses frequently are highly immunogenic and so are particularly susceptible to immunological control. Tumors induced by chemical carcinogens are generally less immunogenic and the frequency of TSRA expression on these tumors is less than with virus-induced tumors. This may reflect in some way, as yet unexplained, the degree of genetic damage induced following carcinogen exposure. For example, several studies have reported that tumor immunogenicity is related to the dose of carcinogen used in their induction. Also tumors arising early were frequently more immunogenic than those with longer latent induction times. This may be relevant to the observation that animal tumors arising naturally, i.e., without the deliberate exposure to chemical carcinogens are at best only weakly immunogenic.[33]

The concept of immunosurveillance as a component of the carcinogenic process has undergone modification from the original view on the role of MHC restricted T lymphocytes and now includes non-MHC restricted T cells as well as natural killer cells. The impact of immunosuppression is most clearly seen with highly immunogenic tumors, particularly virus-induced tumors. On the other hand there is substantial evidence that down-regulation of immune function occurs in cancer patients and many investigators feel that this influences the progression of disease. These findings raise the issue of immunosuppression by environmental agents in cancer development. This may arise because the carcinogenic agent itself, e.g., benzo[a]pyrene is immunosuppressive. Alternatively, immunosuppressive agents in the environment may act synergistically with carcinogens and thereby enhance the development of malignancy.

The essential problem in environmental exposure is to evaluate immunosuppressive agents present at low levels in the human environment. This has been approached by laboratory studies to define "chemical immunosuppressants" and will, in the future, be incorporated in legislation regarding human exposure to chemical agents.

References

1. Ames, B. N., Magraw, R., and Gold, L. S.: Ranking possible carcinogenic hazards. Science, 236:271, 1987.
2. Austin, E. B., Robins, R. A., Durrant, L. G., Price, M. R., and Baldwin, R. W.: Human monoclonal anti-idiotypic antibody to the tumour-associated antibody 791T/36. Immunology, 67:525, 1989
3. Balch, C. M., Tilden, A. B., Dougherty, P. A., Cloud, G. A., and Abo, T.: Heterogeneity of natural killer lymphocyte abnormalities in colon cancer patients. Surgery, 95:63, 1984.
4. Baldwin, R. W.: Immunological aspects of chemical carcinogenesis. Adv. Cancer Res., 18:1, 1973.
5. Balkwill, F. R., and Burke, F.: The cytokine network. Immunol. Today, 10:299, 1989.
6. Barth, R. J., Bock, S. N., Mule, J. J., and Rosenberg, S. A.: Unique murine tumor-associated antigens identified by tumor infiltrating lymphocytes. J. Immunol., 144:1531, 1990.
7. Bentvelzen, P., and Hilgers, J.: Murine mammary tumor virus. In Viral Oncology. Edited by G. Klein. New York, Raven Press, 1980, p. 311.
8. Boon, T.: Antigenic tumor cell variants obtained with mutagens. Adv. Cancer. Res., 39:121, 1983.
9. Boon, T. and Kellerman, O.: Rejection by syngeneic mice of all variants obtained by mutagenesis of a malignant teratocarcinoma cell line. Proc. Natl. Acad. Sci. U.S.A., 74:272, 1977.
10. Boon, T., Van Pel, A., Deplaen, E., Van Den Eynde, B., and Hainaut, P.: Genes Coding for TUM-Transplantation Antigens. A model for TSTA. In Progress in Immunology, VII. Edited by F. Melcheis, et al. New York, Springer-Verlag, 1989, p.1063.
11. Boyer, C. M., Lidor, Y., Lottich, C., and Bast, R .C.: Antigenic cell surface markers in human solid tumors. Antibody Immunoconjugates and Radiopharmaceuticals, 1:105, 1988.
12. Burchell, J., Taylor-Papadimitriou, J., Boshell, M., Gendler, S., and Duhig, T.: A short sequence within the amino acid tandem repeat of a cancer-associated mucin, contains immunodominant epitopes. Int. J. Cancer, 44:691, 1989.
13. Byers, V. S., Levin, A. S., Ozonoff, D. M., and Baldwin, R. W.: Association between clinical symptoms and lymphocyte abnormalities in a population with chronic domestic exposure to industrial solvent-contaminated domestic water supply and a high incidence of leukemia. Cancer Immunol. Immunother., 27:77, 1988.
14. Cheung, S. C., Nerland, D. E., and Sonnefeld, G.: Inhibition of interferon gamma production by benzene and benzene metabolites. J. Natl. Cancer Inst., 80:1069, 1988.
15. Dean, J. H., Luster, M. I., Boorman, G. A., Lauer, L. D., Leubke, R. W., and Lawson, L.: Selective immunosuppression resulting from exposure to the carcinogenic congener of benzopyrene in B6C3F1 mice. Clin. Exp. Immunol., 52:199, 1983.
16. De-The, G.: Role of Epstein-Barr Virus in Human Diseases: Infectious Mononucleosis, Burkitt's Lymphoma, and Nasopharyngeal Carcinoma. In Viral Oncology. Edited by G. Klein. New York, Raven Press, 1980, p.769.
17. Doll, R., and Peto, R.: The Causes of Cancer. Oxford, England, Oxford Univ. Press, 1981.
18. Dusheiko, G. M.: Hepatocellular carcinoma associated with chronic viral hepatitis. Aetiology, diagnosis and treatment. Br. Med Bull., 46:492, 1990.
19. Ehrlich, R., Efrati, M., Malatzky, E., Shochat, L., Bar Eyal, A., and Witz, I. P.: Natural host defence during oncogenesis. NK activity and dimethylbenzanthracene carcinogenesis. Int. J. Cancer, 31:67, 1983.
20. Embleton, M. J., and Heidelberger, C.: Antigenicity of clones of mouse prostate cells transformed in vitro. Int. J. Cancer, 9:8, 1972.
21. Essex, M.: Role of retroviruses in immune suppression that may result in cancer. In GMCRF Accomplishments in Cancer Research. Edited by J. G. Fortner and J. E. Rhoads. Philadelphia, J.B. Lippincott, 1987, p.183.
22. Harrington, D. S., Weisenburger, D. D., and Purtilo, D. T.: Malignant lymphoma in the X-linked lymphoproliferative syndrome. Cancer, 59:1419, 1987.
23. Harris, R. H., Page, T., and Reiches, N. A.: Carcinogenic Hazards of Organic Chemicals in Drinking Water. In Book A: Incidence of Cancer in Humans. Edited by H. H. Hiatt, J. D. Watson, and J. A. Winsten. Cold Spring Harbor, New York, Cold Spring Harbor Laboratory, 1977, p.309.
24. Hellstrom, I., and Hellstrom, K. E.: Cellular immunity against tumor specific antigens. Adv. Cancer Res., 12:167, 1969.
25. Hellstrom, K.E., and Hellstrom, I.: Oncogene-associated tumor antigens as targets for immunotherapy. FASEB J., 3:1715, 1989.
26. Hercend, T., and Schmidt, R. E.: Characteristics and uses of natural killer cells. Immunol. Today, 9:291, 1988.
27. Herlyn, D., Wettendorff, M., Schmoll, E., Iliopoulos, D., Schedel, I., Dreikhausen, F., Raab, R., Ross, A. H., Jaksche, M., Scriba, M., and Koprowski, H.: Anti-idiotype immunization of cancer patients: Modulation of the immune response. Proc. Natl. Acad. Sci. U.S.A., 84:8055, 1987.
28. House, R. V., Pallardy, M. J., and Dean, J. H.: Suppression of murine cytotoxic T lymphocyte induction following exposure to 7,12-dimethylbenz[a]anthracene: Dysfunction of antigen recognition. Int. J. Immunopharmacol., 11:207, 1989.
29. Itoh, K., Pellis, N. R., and Balch, C. M.: Monocyte dependent serum-borne suppressor of induction of lymphokine-activated killer cells in lymphocytes from melanoma patients. Cancer Immunol. Immunother., 29:57, 1989.
30. Kenemans, P., Bast, R. C., Yedema, C. A., Price, M. R., and Hilgers, J.: CA 125 and polymorphic epithelial mucin as serum tumor markers. Cancer Rev., 11-12:119, 1988.
31. Kipen, H. M., Cody, R. P., Crump, K. S., Allen, B. C., and Goldstein, B. D.: Hematological effects of benzene: A thirty five year longitudinal study of rubber works. Toxicol. Ind. Health., 4:411, 1988.
32. Klein, G.: Tumour antigens. Annu. Rev. Microbiol., 20:223, 1966.
33. Klein, G., and Klein, E.: Immunosurveillance against virus-induced tumors and non-rejectability of spontaneous tumors: Contrasting consequences of host versus tumor evolution. Proc. Nat. Acad. Sci. U.S.A., 74:2121, 1977.
34. Knowles, D. M., Chamulak, G. A., Subar, M., Burke, J. S., Dugan, M., Wernz, J., Slywotzky, C., Pelicci, G., Della-Favera, R., and Raphael, B.: Lymphoid neoplasia associated with the acquired immunodeficiency syndrome (AIDS). The New York University Medical Center experience with 105 patients (1981-1986). Ann. Intern. Med., 108:744, 1988.
35. Kohler, H., Kieber-Emmons, T., Rinivasan, S., Kaveri, S., Morrow, W. J. W., Muller, S., Kang, C.-Y., and Raychaudhuri, S.: Short Analytical Review. Revised Immune Network Concepts. Clin. Immunol. Immunopathol., 52:104, 1989.
36. Kripke, M. L.: Immunologic mechanisms in UV radiation carcinogenesis. Adv. Cancer. Res. 34:69, 1981.
37. Kripke, M. L.: Immunoregulation of carcinogenesis: past present and future. J. Natl. Cancer Inst., 80:722, 1988.
38. Kripke, M. L.: Effects of UV radiation on tumor immunity. J. Natl. Cancer Inst., 82:1392, 1990.
39. Kuppner, M. C., Hamou, M. F., Bodmer, S., Fontana, A., and De Tribolet, M.: The glioblastoma-derived T cell suppressor factor 1 transforming factor beta 2 inhibits the generation of lymphokine activated killer (LAK) cells. Int. J. Cancer, 42:562, 1988.
40. Lagakos, S. W., Wessen, B. J., and Zelen, M.: An analysis of contaminated well water and health effects in Woburn, Massachusetts. J. Amer. Stat. Assoc., 81:583, 1986.
41. Levy, J. A.: Mysteries of HIV; challenges for therapy and prevention. Nature, 333:519, 1988.
42. Lilly, F., and Mayer, A.: Genetic Aspects of Murine Type-C Viruses and Their Hosts in Oncogenesis. In Viral Oncology. Edited by G. Klein. New York, Raven Press, 1980, p.89.
43. Luster, M. I., and Blank, J. A.: Molecular and cellular basis of chemically induced immunotoxicity. Annu. Rev. Pharmacol. Toxicol., 27:23, 1987.
44. Milief, C. J. M., and Schwartz, R. S.: Immunocompetence and Malignancy. In Cancer: A Comprehensive Treatise. Edited by F. F. Becker. New York, Plenum, 1975, p. 121.
45. Nerurkar, L. S., and Gallo, R. C.: Human retroviruses: cancer and AIDS. Int. J. Cancer Suppl., 4:2, 1989.
46. North, R. J.: Down regulation of the anti-tumor immune response. Adv. Cancer Res. 45:1, 1985.
47. Old, L. J.: Cancer Immunology: The search for specificity–G.H.A. Clowes Memorial Lecture. Cancer Res. 41:361, 1981.
48. Pearson, G. R.: Epstein-Barr Virus: Immunology. In Viral Oncology. Edited by G. Klein. New York, Raven Press, 1980, p.739.
49. Penn, I.: Depressed immunity and the development of cancer. Clin. Exp. Immunol., 46:459, 1981.
50. Perera, F., and Boffetta, P.: Perspectives on comparing risks of environmental carcinogens. J. Natl. Cancer Inst., 80:1282, 1988.
51. Price, M. R., Hudecz, F., Baldwin, R. W., Edwards, P. M., and Tendler, S. J. B.: Immunological and structural features of the protein core of human breast carcinoma-associated epithelial mucin. Mol. Immunol., 27:795, 1990.
52. Rosenberg, S. A.: Immunotherapy of cancer using interleukin 2. Immunol. Today, 9:58, 1988.
53. Rosenberg, S. A., Lotze, M. T., Muul, L. M., Chang, A. E., Avis, F. P., Leitman, S., Linehan, W. M., Robertson, C. N., Lee, R. E., Rubin, J. T., et al.: A progress report on the treatment of 157 patients with advanced cancer using lymphokine-activated killer cells and interleukin-2 or high-dose interleukin-2 alone. N. Engl. J. Med., 316:889, 1987.
54. Sarma, P. S., and Gruber, J.: Human T-cell lymphotropic viruses in human diseases. J. Natl. Cancer Inst., 82:1100, 1990.
55. Siddiqui, J., Abe, M., Hayes, D., Shani, E., Yunis, E., and Kufe, D.: Isolation and sequencing of a cDNA coding for the human DF3 breast carcinoma associated antigen. Proc. Natl. Acad. Sci. U.S.A., 85:2320, 1988.
56. Srivastava, P. K., Deleo, A. B., and Old, L. J.: Tumour rejection antigens of chemically induced sarcomas of inbred mice. Proc. Natl. Acad. Sci. U.S.A., 83:3407, 1986.
57. Srivastava, P. K., and Old, L. J.: Individually distinct transplantation antigens of chemically induced mouse tumors. Immunol. Today, 9:78, 1988.
58. Strauss, H. J., and Schreiber, H.: Tumor Specific Antigens on Experimental Tumors. In Progress in Immunology VI. New York, Academic Press, 1986, p.706.
59. Stauss, H. J., Van Waes C. S., Fink, M. A., Starr, B., and Schreiber, H.: Identification of a unique tumor antigen as rejection antigen by molecular cloning and gene transfer J. Exp. Med. 164:1516, 1983.
60. Stutman, O.: Immunodepression and malignancy. Adv. Cancer Res., 22:261, 1975.
61. Terry, W., and Rosenberg, S. A.: Immunotherapy of Human Cancer. Edited by W. D. Terry and S. A. Rosenberg. 1982.
62. Toge, T., Kuroi, K., Kuninobu, H., Yamaguchi, Y., Kegoya, Y., Baba, N., and Hattori, T.: Role of the spleen in immunosuppression of gastric cancer: Predominance of

suppressor precursor and suppressor induced T cells in the recirculating spleen cells. Clin. Exp. Immunol. 74:409, 1988.

63. Tomatis, L., Atio, A., Wilbourn, J., and Shuber, L.: Human carcinogens so far identified. Jpn. J. Cancer. Res. (Gann), 80: 795, 1989.

64. Topalian, S. I., Solomon, D., and Rosenberg, S. A.: Tumor-specific cytolysis by lymphocytes infiltrating human melanomas. J. Immunol., 142:3714, 1989.

65. Van Den Eynde, B., Hainaut, P., Herin, M., Knuth, A., Lemoine, C., Weynants, P., Van Der Bruggen, P., Fauchet, R., and Boon, T.: Presence on a human melanoma of multiple antigens recognized by autologous CTL. Int. J. Cancer, 44:634, 1989.

66. Ward, E. C., Murray, M. J., Lauer, L. D., House, R. V., and Dean, J. H.: Persistent suppression of humoral and cell-mediated immunity in mice following exposure to the polycyclic aromatic hydrocarbon 7,12-dimethylbenz[a]anthracene. Int. J. Immunopharmacol., 8:13, 1986.

67. WHO: Trichloroethylene. Environmental Health Criteria 50, 1985.

68. Williams, A. E., Fang, C. T., Slamon, D. J., et al.: Seroprevalence and epidemiological correlates of HTLV-I infection in U.S. blood donors. Science, 240:643, 1988. (Erratum. Science, 244: 757, 1989)

69. Wojdani, A., and Alfred, L. J.: Alterations in cell-mediated immune functions induced in mouse splenic lymphocytes by polycyclic aromatic hydrocarbons. Cancer Res., 44:942, 1984.

70. Woodruff, M .F. A.: The Interaction of Cancer and Host: Its Therapeutic Significance. New York, Grune and Stratton, 1980, p. 467.

71. Yoshida, M., and Seiki, M.: Recent advances in the molecular biology of HTLV-1: Trans-activation of viral and cellular genes. Annu. Rev. Immunol., 5:541, 1987.

72. Zuckerman, A. J.: Prevention of primary liver cancer by immunization. Cancer Detection Prev., 14:309, 1989.

73. Zur Hausen, H.: Papillomaviruses in anogenital cancer as a model to understand the role of viruses in human cancers. Cancer Res., 49:4677, 1989.

IV
Cancer Epidemiology

Frederick P. Li
Julie A. Schneider
Arlene F. Kantor

Introduction

In 1992, newly diagnosed cancers in the United States are estimated to exceed 1.13 million, and cancer deaths will equal 520,000 for the first time.[19A] These figures highlight the steady rise in cancer occurrence and deaths among Americans throughout this century. Aging and numerical growth of the United States population are the major causes of these increases. Presently, one person in three will develop cancer within a lifetime and one in five will die of cancer. The human suffering due to cancer is enormous, and the cost of care for cancer patients contributes substantially to the rising expenditures for medical services in the U.S. In this era of medical cost containment, oncologists need to develop not only better treatments for cancer but also effective programs of cancer prevention.

The prevention of cancer requires knowledge of its causes. History shows that epidemiological studies have been key to the control of a wide range of infectious diseases, such as tuberculosis, smallpox, cholera, and plague.[83] In recent decades, epidemiological studies have also contributed to our understanding of the origins of chronic diseases, notably heart disease and cancer.[37,41,104,128] This chapter describes methods used to conduct epidemiological studies, and summarizes the current state of knowledge of causes of human cancer.

Cancer epidemiology can be defined as the study of the frequencies, patterns of distribution, and determinants of tumor occurrence in humans.[91] By examining who develops cancer, epidemiologists generate and test hypotheses regarding why certain individuals develop cancer. Characterizing cancer patients helps to identify host factors in the genesis of neoplasia. The impact of environmental carcinogens is examined by determining exposures to candidate agents, and correlating these exposures with disease incidence. For most human cancers, cancer risk increases with dose and duration of exposure to a carcinogen. The time interval from initial oncogenic exposure to disease development is often a decade or longer, and the search for cancer causation needs to explore both the present and past histories of patients.[42] In addition, the suspected carcinogen should have biological properties that are consistent with a role in the pathogenesis of cancer. These and other tests of causal association permit exclusion of factors that have a non-causal relationship to cancer development. Identification of etiological influences can lead to early cancer detection and prevention, particularly among populations at increased risk. Thus, scarce health care resources can be allocated to those most likely to benefit from appropriate interventions.

Design of Epidemiologic Studies

Descriptive Studies

Epidemiologic studies often begin with descriptions of the patients who develop cancer. These patients are examined to uncover demographic characteristics, medical histories, occupations, habits, and lifestyles that may predispose to cancer. The likelihood of a causal effect can be further evaluated in analytical studies.

The patterns of cancer in populations are described by several standard measures of frequency. Cancer occurrence can be expressed in terms of number of cases, a proportion, or a rate.[63] These measures can be applied to new occurrences of cancer (incidence) or cancer deaths (mortality) within a defined time interval, usually one year. The enumeration of cancer cases is useful, for example, in assessing levels of need for medical services. A proportion is often used to identify the fraction of total deaths that are due to cancer, or the fraction of all cancers that arise at an anatomic site. Rates (number of cancers per 100,000 persons) serve to standardize the measurement of disease frequency, allowing for ease of comparison among different populations. In epidemiological studies, rates are the most useful measure of cancer incidence and mortality. Crude rates measure cancer frequency in a population without regard for its composition. Cancer rates can be specific for age, race, and sex, or adjusted to account for the influence of these factors. An age-adjusted rate is a weighted summary of age-specific rates which removes differences in age composition among populations.

Prevalence measures the proportion of the population who have cancer at a specified point or during an interval of time. Cancer prevalence reflects both incidence and survival of cancer, and provides a measure of the cancer burden within a population.[48] However, the measure includes patients who are dying of cancer, under active treatment, in complete remission, and long-term survivors. This heterogeneity limits the utility of prevalence as a measure of cancer frequency. Cancer incidence and mortality are better indicators in most circumstances.[9]

Clinicians often need to measure the impact of therapy on survival of their patients. Absolute survival rates measure the proportion of cancer patients who survive for a specified period of time after diagnosis. However, survivorship from time of diagnosis can be diminished by diseases other than cancer, particularly among elderly patients. The relative survival rate is used to measure survival of cancer, after eliminating the effects of deaths from other causes.[22]

Sources of Data. Data on cancer incidence and mortality are obtained from several sources. Mortality data in the U.S. are derived primarily from death certificates. Population-based cancer registries have been established in a number of states to provide cancer incidence data. A consortium of these registries under the Surveillance, Epidemiology and End Results (SEER) Program has been the principal source of U.S. cancer rates since 1973. The SEER Program, administered through the National Cancer Institute, monitors cancer incidence, mortality, and survival in approximately 10% of the U.S. population. SEER data are not representative of this population but do encompass diverse geographic, ethnic, and racial groups. The quality of cancer frequency data available outside the U.S. is variable. Several European countries have established nationwide cancer incidence registries of high quality; registration of cancer incidence and mortality is more limited in developing nations. The available data are summarized and updated periodically in Cancer Incidence in Five Continents.[26]

The quality and completeness of data vary among cancer registries, which often employ different methods of case ascertainment. Diagnostic practice and classification of cancers differ between geographic areas, and change over time. Ascertainment is usually less complete among elderly patients and those with limited access to medical care. Treatable cancers (such as skin cancers) may not be identified by the surveillance mechanisms of cancer registries, whereas cancer deaths are more likely to be recorded. Comparability of data must be considered in analyses of incidence and mortality figures from different cancer registries.[63]

Cancer Incidence and Mortality. Table IV-1-1 shows the estimates of the annual numbers of new cancers and cancer deaths in 1990 in the U.S. Cancers of the breast, lung, colon and rectum account for nearly one-half of the one million incident cases. Cancers of the prostate, oral cavity, pancreas, endometrium, and bladder are also commonly diagnosed. Data for almost 500,000 cancer deaths show the same general patterns. Lung cancer is, by far, the leading

Table IV-1-1. Estimated Numbers of New Cancer Cases and Cancer Deaths in the United States, 1992*

Tumor Type	New Cases (Thousands)	Deaths (Thousands)
Oral cavity	30.3	8.0
Esophagus	11.1	10.0
Stomach	24.4	13.3
Colon and rectum	156.0	58.3
Liver	15.4	12.3
Pancreas	28.3	25.0
Larynx	12.5	3.7
Lung	168.0	146.0
Breast	181.0	46.3
Cervix	13.5	4.4
Endometrium	32.0	5.6
Ovary	21.0	13.0
Prostate	132.0	34.0
Melanoma	32.0	6.7
Bladder	51.6	9.5
Kidney	26.5	10.7
Thyroid	12.5	1.0
Leukemias	28.2	18.2
Lymphomas	48.4	20.9
Multiple myeloma	12.5	9.2
Brain	16.9	11.8
Other sites	75.9	52.1
All cancers	1130.0	520.0

Excluded are all in-situ cancers and carcinomas of the skin.
*Boring et al.[19A]

cause of cancer death, accounting for approximately 30% of the total. Mortality also approximates incidence for multiple myeloma, brain tumors, and cancers of the esophagus and pancreas. By comparison, survival is better for colorectal and breast cancers, with reported mortality equaling 30–40% of incidence.

Table IV-1-2 shows age-adjusted U.S. mortality and incidence rates, by sex, 1986–1987. The mortality rate in males for all sites combined is more than 50% higher than that in females. At present, lung cancer is the leading cause of cancer deaths in men and women in the United States. The lung cancer mortality rate in women recently surpassed that for breast cancer, but is much lower than the lung cancer rate in men. Mortality rates are also at least twice as high in men for cancers of the oral cavity, esophagus, stomach, liver, larynx, bladder, and kidney. Cancers of the male reproductive organs (prostate and testis) account for approximately 11% of all cancer deaths in men, whereas cancer of the breast and female reproductive organs account for 30% of cancer deaths in women. Cancer incidence data reiterate these patterns, and will be described in subsequent discussions only when noteworthy divergences from mortality data are found.

Cancer Patterns by Age. Cancer is rare in childhood, rises in frequency throughout adulthood, and occurs most often in the elderly. The high frequency of cancer in the elderly is consistent with the multistage nature of carcinogenesis which usually requires decades for cancer to develop following exposures to etiological agents.[42] Approximately 20% of the U.S. population is 55 years of age or older, but more than 80% of invasive cancers occur in this age group.

Table IV-1-2. Age-adjusted Incidence and Mortality Rates per 100,000 Population, United States, All Races, by Sex, 1986–87.*

Tumor Type	Incidence Rate		Mortality Rate	
	Males	Females	Males	Females
Oral cavity	17.0	6.2	4.7	1.7
Esophagus	6.4	2.0	5.8	1.5
Stomach	11.9	5.2	7.2	3.2
Colon and rectum	60.9	42.1	24.5	16.8
Liver	4.0	1.7	3.7	1.7
Pancreas	10.9	8.0	10.0	7.2
Larynx	8.2	1.6	2.6	0.5
Lung	83.2	37.3	74.5	27.6
Breast	0.8	108.9	0.2	27.2
Cervix	—	8.6	—	3.1
Uterus	—	21.3	—	3.6
Ovary	—	13.2	—	7.7
Prostate	95.1	—	24.2	—
Testis	4.3	—	0.3	—
Melanoma	12.3	9.3	3.0	1.5
Bladder	30.3	7.4	5.7	1.7
Kidney	11.6	5.6	4.8	2.3
Thyroid	2.5	6.2	0.3	0.4
Leukemias	12.6	7.3	8.3	4.9
Multiple myeloma	5.0	3.6	3.5	2.4
Brain	7.2	5.3	4.9	3.3
Hodgkin's disease	3.2	2.3	0.8	0.5
Non-Hodgkin's lymphoma	16.1	10.6	7.1	4.8
Other sites	32.8	22.2	23.0	15.9
All sites	436.3	335.9	219.1	139.5

Rates are age-adjusted to the 1970 U.S. standard population
*American Cancer Society[2]

At these ages, the leading causes of cancer mortality include lung, colon, and pancreas (Figure IV-1-1). Prostate cancer in men, and cancers of the breast and ovary in women, are also common in elderly patients.

Patterns of cancer differ between the elderly and persons ages 15–54. In young adults, the leading cause of cancer mortality is breast cancer in women and lung cancer in men. Brain tumors, leukemias, lymphomas, and melanoma also account for a substantial proportion of deaths in young adults. Mortality from cancers of the colon and ovary start to rise after age 35.

Childhood cancers comprise less than 1% of all incident cancers. However, cancer accounts for more than 10% of mortality from all causes in children under 15 years of age.[151] Cancer mortality rates in children have decreased almost 50% in the last few decades due to improved treatment of many childhood cancers.[150] Leukemia accounts for approximately one-third of all cancer mortality in children 0–14 and remains one of the most common causes of cancer death in young adults. From childhood onward, more males develop cancer than females, a trend that continues into adulthood.

Time Trends. Heart disease mortality, the leading cause of death in the U.S., has declined in frequency in recent years. More people live to die of cancer, which now accounts for more than 20% of deaths from all causes. Overall, age-adjusted cancer mortality rates have risen approximately 10% since 1950. Lung cancer mortality is a major contributor to this increase.[2]

Rates of certain cancers in the U.S. have changed substantially in recent decades, suggesting an effect of the introduction or disappearance of environmental oncogenic factors (Figure IV-1-2A). Lung cancer mortality has risen sharply over the past several decades due to the increase in tobacco use by men dating to World War I and by women during World War II.[42] The sex-specific mortality curves depicted in Figure IV-1-2B and -2C show sharper rises in lung cancer mortality after 1940 in men and after 1960 in women. The lag time between the start of habitual tobacco use and lung cancer development typifies the long latency of most carcinogens. Recently, tobacco consumption has declined, and lung cancer rates in men have plateaued, although rates in women continue to rise unabated. Reported mortality rates for cancers of the stomach have decreased dramatically since 1950. Among women, mortality rates for uterine cancers, particularly cancers of the uterine cervix, have declined steadily, primarily due to decreased incidence of invasive lesions. Breast cancer mortality has not changed in any apparent way since 1950, despite an increase in reported incidence. Colorectal cancer mortality has fallen slightly in recent decades, whereas prostate cancer mortality rates have increased slightly. These trends reflect changes in disease incidence, diagnostic practices, screening, and treatment effects.[142]

Racial, Ethnic, and International Variation. In the United States, overall cancer incidence is reportedly 6% higher in blacks than in whites, while cancer mortality for blacks is approximately 30% higher. Socioeconomic status and access to health care appear to account for part of this differential.[3,11,30,96] Compared with whites in the U.S., blacks currently have higher mortality rates for multiple myeloma and

MORTALITY FOR THE FIVE LEADING CANCER SITES FOR MALES BY AGE GROUP, UNITED STATES, 1986

All Ages	Under 15	15–34	35–54	55–74	75+
All Cancer 250,559	All Cancer 1,033	All Cancer 4,171	All Cancer 25,581	All Cancer 137,927	All Cancer 81,825
Lung 85,057	Leukemia 383	Leukemia 771	Lung 8,819	Lung 54,050	Lung 21,999
Colon & Rectum 27,469	Brain & CNS 244	Skin 483	Colon & Rectum 2,206	Colon & Rectum 14,532	Prostate 15,888
Prostate 27,262	Non-Hodgkin's Lymphomas 103	Non-Hodgkin's Lymphomas 477	Skin 1,308	Prostate 11,066	Colon & Rectum 10,530
Pancreas 11,403	Bone 46	Brain & CNS 459	Non-Hodgkin's Lymphomas 1,305	Pancreas 6,673	Pancreas 3,571
Leukemia 9,565	Connective Tissue 37	Hodgkin's Disease 300	Brain & CNS 1,251	Stomach 4,445	Bladder 3,376

Source: Vital Statistics of the United States, 1986.

MORTALITY FOR THE FIVE LEADING CANCER SITES FOR FEMALES BY AGE GROUP, UNITED STATES, 1986

All Ages	Under 15	15–34	35–54	55–74	75+
All Cancer 218,817	All Cancer 798	All Cancer 3,548	All Cancer 27,210	All Cancer 107,681	All Cancer 79,556
Breast 40,539	Leukemia 284	Breast 668	Breast 8,391	Lung 25,153	Colon & Rectum 14,231
Lung 40,465	Brain & CNS 198	Leukemia 472	Lung 4,967	Breast 20,166	Breast 11,308
Colon & Rectum 28,347	Connective Tissue 40	Uterus 368	Colon & Rectum 1,948	Colon & Rectum 11,993	Lung 10,230
Pancreas 12,055	Kidney 36	Brain & CNS 325	Uterus 1,798	Ovary 6,563	Pancreas 5,506
Ovary 11,903	Bone 34	Non-Hodgkin's Lymphomas 215	Ovary 1,688	Pancreas 5,784	Ovary 3,510

Source: Vital Statistics of the United States, 1986.

Figure IV-1-1. Cancer deaths for the five leading cancer sites, by sex and age, United States, 1986. Reproduced from American Cancer Society[1] with permission.

CANCER DEATH RATES* BY SITE, UNITED STATES, 1930-86

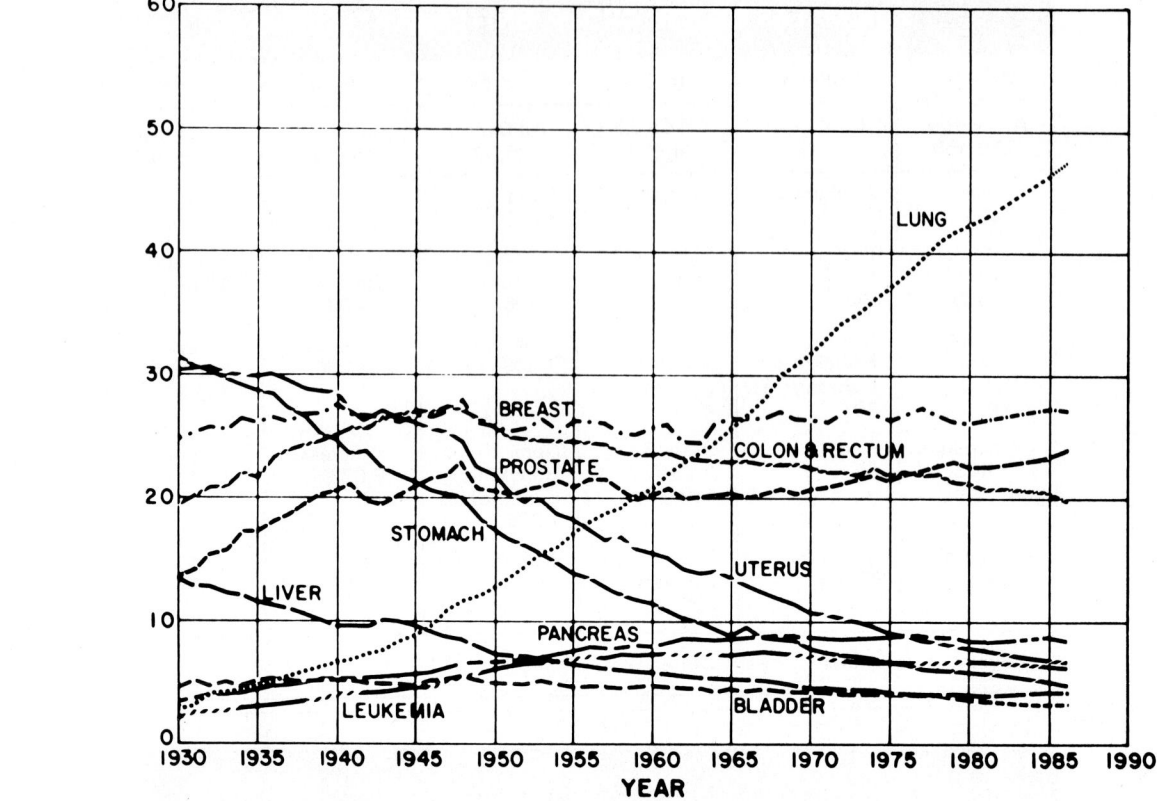

*Rate for the population standardized for age on the 1970 US population.
Sources of Data: National Center for Health Statistics and Bureau of the Census, United States.
Note: Rates are for both sexes combined except breast and uterus (female population only) and prostate (male population only).

A

Figure IV-1-2.   A, Trends in age-adjusted cancer mortality rates per 100,000 population, by site, both sexes, United States, 1930–1986. Reproduced from American Cancer Society[1] with permission.

cancers of the esophagus, cervix, prostate, larynx, stomach, oropharynx, liver, corpus uteri, pancreas, and lung. (Figure IV-1-3). Blacks tend to smoke more than other groups in the U.S., which likely accounts for their higher rates of cancers of the lung and several other sites.[54]

Other ethnic groups in the U.S. also differ from U.S. whites with regard to certain site-specific cancer rates.[26] Relative to whites, age-adjusted incidence and mortality rates among Mexican-Americans (Hispanics) are higher for gallbladder, stomach, and cervical cancers. In addition, increased rates have been reported for gallbladder, stomach, and cervical cancers among American Indians; stomach cancer among Japanese Americans; nasopharyngeal and liver cancers in Chinese Americans; lung, stomach, and cervical cancers among Hawaiians; and liver cancer among Filipino Americans.

Cancer incidence rates differ throughout the world, and migrant studies have helped elucidate environmental factors in cancer development. Migrants to the U.S. tend to acquire the patterns of cancer rates of whites in the U.S. For example, the low incidence rates of breast and colon cancers in Japan have increased in those who migrate to the U.S., while the high stomach cancer rates have fallen.[60]

Worldwide, developed countries generally have higher reported incidence rates for cancers of the breast (North America, Europe), lung (British Isles), and prostate (U.S. blacks, Scandinavia). Elevated rates have been reported for cancer of the stomach in Japan and China, nasopharyngeal cancer in Southern China, colon cancer in Denmark and New Zealand, cervical cancer in Brazil, liver cancer in parts of China and sub-Saharan Africa, and melanoma in Australia. Investigations of the exceptionally high rates of esophageal cancers in parts of China and the Caspian littoral have shown associations with vitamin and other dietary deficiencies.[77] Data for developing countries are more difficult to evaluate due to underreporting. In these countries, cancers of the cervix uteri, liver, stomach, and esophagus often occur more frequently.[26]

Analytical Studies

Case Control Studies. Descriptive epidemiological findings and observations at the bedside can be further assessed in analytical studies of suspected risk factors. A case-control method is usually employed, which can both test specific etiologic hypotheses and generate new hypotheses for further examination.[121] These studies compare a group of can-

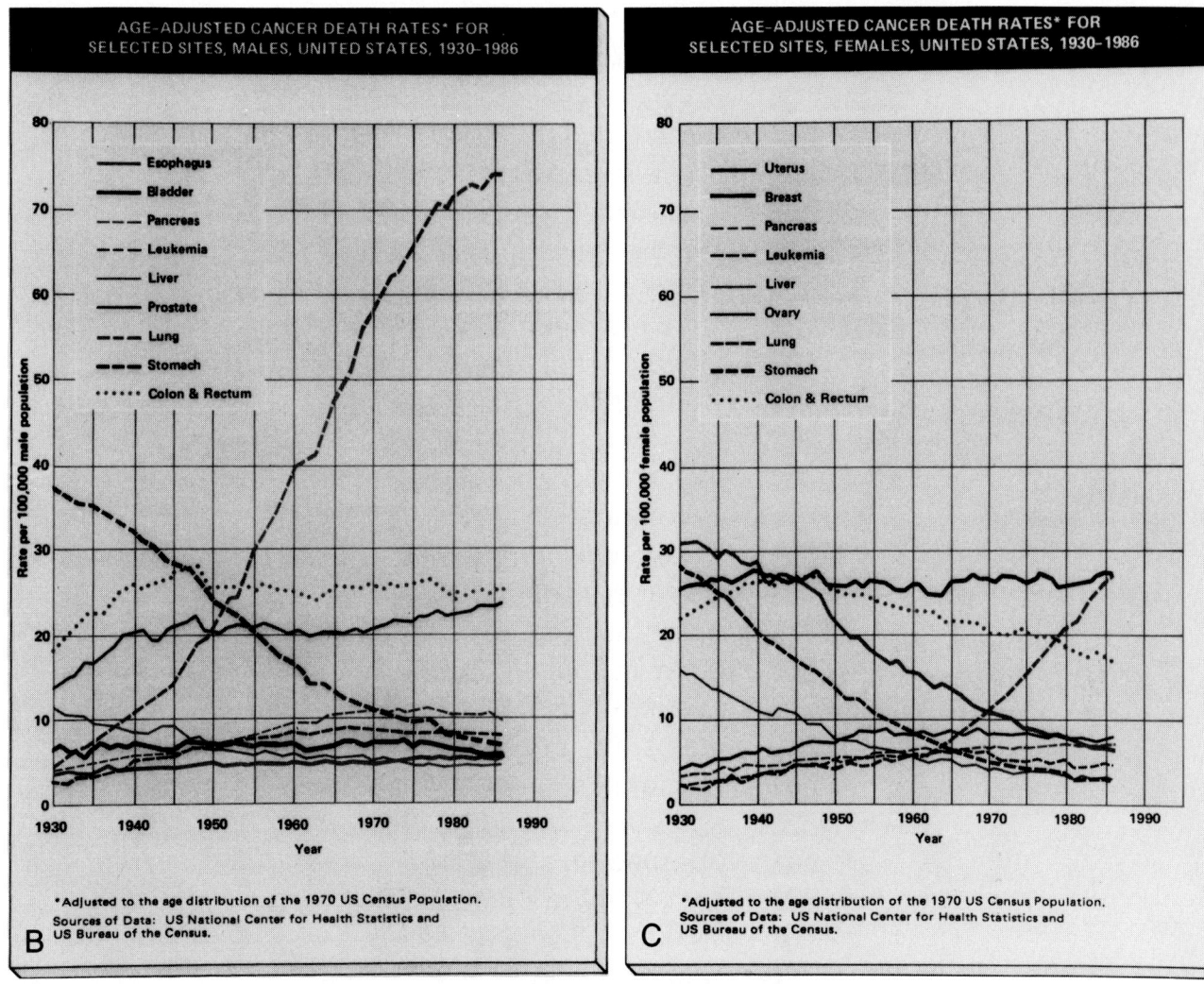

AGE-ADJUSTED CANCER DEATH RATES* FOR
SELECTED SITES, MALES, UNITED STATES, 1930–1986

AGE-ADJUSTED CANCER DEATH RATES* FOR
SELECTED SITES, FEMALES, UNITED STATES, 1930–1986

*Adjusted to the age distribution of the 1970 US Census Population.
Sources of Data: US National Center for Health Statistics and
US Bureau of the Census.

Figure IV-1-2 (cont.)   B, Trends in age-adjusted cancer mortality rates per 100,000 population, by site, males, United States, 1930–1986. C, Trends in age-adjusted cancer mortality rates per 100,000 population, by site, females, United States, 1930–1986. Reproduced from American Cancer Society[1] with permission.

cer patients (cases) to a group of individuals who are free of cancer (controls). Cases can be chosen, for example, from cancer patients diagnosed during a defined time period in a geographic area or hospital. Controls can be drawn from the same region or hospital as the cases, or from other appropriate sources. The case-control method has been useful, for example, in clarifying aspects of the relation between vaginal adenocarcinoma and in utero exposure to diethylstilbestrol.[65,66]

At the outset of a case-control study, the investigators may know of certain characteristics such as sex, race and age that are strongly related to the distribution of the cancer. To account for these influences, a decision is often made to individually match controls to cases on these variables, or to obtain the same frequency or proportion of subgroups in both series (frequency matching). Additionally, a control series which is larger than the case series has statistical advantages in certain situations.

Information for cases and controls on oncogenic exposures and risk factors can be obtained through various means.

Clinical data are usually obtained from medical records and pathology reports. In-person or telephone interviews of cases and controls are conducted in a similar manner. The data may be supplemented by employment records and other relevant documents. For deceased patients, interviews of next-of-kin may be conducted. Mail questionnaires are used less often than direct interviews because the quality of information and response rate tend to be inferior.

Case-control studies are well suited and practical for the evaluation of uncommon diseases such as cancer. The sizes of the case and control series are defined at the outset, and results from a case-control study are achieved relatively quickly. Ideally, the case series should be a representative sample of all cases in a population or demographic subgroup. A control series must also be carefully chosen. In a population-based case-control study, an unbiased sample of cases from a roster of all patients diagnosed in a geographic area is compared to a series of controls randomly selected from the general non-diseased population in the same area. If this is not practical, as with a hospital-based

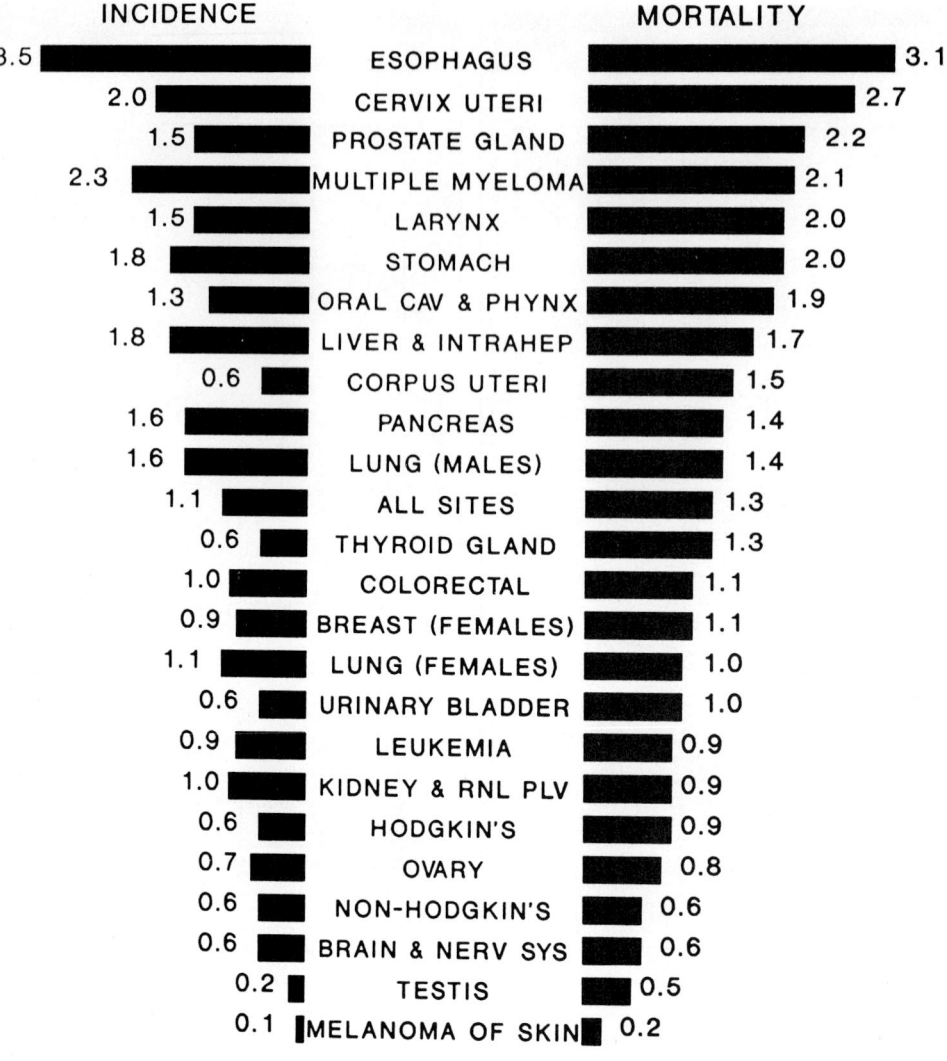

Figure IV-1-3. Ratios of cancer incidence and mortality rates for blacks and whites, by site, all ages, United States, 1983–1987. Reproduced from Field.[49]

case series, the use of more than one type of control group is helpful in searching for consistent findings across all comparisons.

The case-control design is vulnerable to bias. Information on past events obtained in records or by personal recall may be flawed or incomplete. Moreover, cases and controls may interpret and respond differently to questions. The choice of a control group can be the most vexing aspect of this type of study. The population-based case-control study theoretically avoids such selection bias, but it is not used in the majority of situations because of logistical problems and expense. Hospital- or practice-based studies are more common, but also more hazardous when controls are selected from the same patient population. Selection bias for admission may not be similar for different diagnoses, or the controls may suffer from a condition that is also related to the exposure under study. Health plan enrollees, relatives, friends and neighbors of the cases have also been used as controls.

Recently, random-digit dialing has been used to selected controls by telephone. Once a study is underway, an additional bias in an interview study is a suboptimal response rate, particularly among controls as compared to cases.

Cohort Studies. In contrast to the case-control method, a study can be conducted in which a group (cohort) of cancer-free individuals are observed for disease development over time. After adequate numbers of years or cancers have been accrued, tumor occurrence is examined in relation to level of exposure to the risk factor under investigation.[99] Thus, cohort studies compare the rate of cancer in exposed and non-exposed individuals. In a prospective cohort study, exposed and non-exposed persons will be followed over a period of years for the development of cancer. A retrospective cohort study analyzes exposure and cancer occurrence data for events that have already taken place. The cohort method has been useful, for example, in follow-up of atomic bomb survivors for carcinogenic effects of radiation.[33]

Cohort studies are useful in evaluating etiologic hypotheses and confirming leads from case-control studies. Prospective cohort studies accurately categorize exposure to the study factor at the start of follow-up, and the quality of this information is usually unaffected by subsequent disease status. Surrogates for exposure dose, such as DNA adducts in tissues of cancer patients, may facilitate the classification of exposure levels, and quantitation of risk estimates.[107,108] Cohort studies can also provide incidence rates associated with various levels of exposure to carcinogens. However, a large cohort study often involves thousands of subjects. A long period of time must elapse to yield a sufficient number of persons with cancer. For these reasons cohort studies are expensive. The retrospective cohort design is less costly, and more often used in cancer epidemiology. However, it poses some difficulties in categorizing exposure based on historic data. Both types suffer from losses to follow-up and changes over time in diagnostic criteria for the tumor under study.

A newer approach to examining causes of cancer is the intervention study. These are clinical trials in which the effect of an intervention, designed to reduce or eliminate exposure to a known or suspected carcinogen, is evaluated for its capacity to reduce or delay cancer development. A finding of no effect among the group receiving treatment might be due to insufficient study sample size (which should be addressed in the design phase of the study), poor compliance, losses to follow-up, or a period of observation that is too short to detect a beneficial effect. Random allocation of subjects in intervention trials reduces the likelihood of false-positive results. Harm from the intervention should not outweigh the potential benefits from the intervention.

Intervention trials in the area of cancer prevention are limited by the long latent period between initiation of an intervention (such as a vaccine, or a change in diet or lifestyle) and a resultant reduction in cancer occurrence. The role of hepatitis-B virus (HBV) in the etiology of hepatocellular carcinoma is being assessed in clinical trials of a HBV vaccine in areas where liver cancer is endemic.[17] The role of nutrients and micronutrients in cancer prevention and etiology is being explored, but there are few definitive data regarding beneficial effects. Recently, biological markers of intermediate endpoints are being sought that indicate retardation or reversal of the oncogenic process as a result of nutritional or other interventions. For example, recent biomarker studies have shown possible reduction of oral leukoplakia, the premalignant lesions of oral cancer, by 13-cis-retinoic acid. Additional uses of such biomarkers in epidemiologic studies and intervention studies are being developed.[88]

Analysis of Results. In assessing the degree of the association between a risk factor and a disease, a standard concept for comparison is the relative risk. Relative risk is defined as the ratio of the disease rate (usually incidence rate) among those exposed, to the disease rate among those not exposed. Thus, the relative risk can only be obtained from a cohort study. However, it can be estimated from a case-control study through a figure called the odds ratio (ratio of the odds of the factor among cases to the odds of the factor among controls). The odds ratio is easily calculated from a fourfold table, as shown in Table IV-1-3. The odds ratio would be (a/

Table IV-1-3. Odds Ratio Calculation Table

	Cases	Controls
Exposed	a	b
Not exposed	c	d

b)/(c/d), or ad/bc. The odds ratio is considered an adequate approximation of the relative risk when the disease is relatively uncommon (as is the case with cancer).

The validity of a study may be enhanced by controlling for confounding factors. These are extraneous independent factors that are associated with both the exposure factor of interest and the disease under study. Common confounding variables are sex, age, race and socioeconomic status. These can be handled through stratification in the analysis (or alternatively through matching during the study's design).[50] Analysis may also include multivariate techniques, in particular multiple regression.[23]

Since valid associations may suggest prevention strategies, it is important to evaluate causal plausibility versus spurious association. If an association is not statistically significant, it may be disregarded, or alternatively, pursued in a larger study group. However, in order to demonstrate causation, several additional criteria beyond statistical significance must be met. Evidence to support a causative role for the exposure includes the following: strength of association (i.e., larger relative risks, dose-response effects are more likely to indicate a causal relationship); consistency of the association across appropriate subgroups in the study as well as across studies of various populations and methods; temporality (a reasonable induction period has elapsed from time of exposure to disease); and biological plausibility.

Cancer epidemiology research has produced a number of conflicting reports of an association. In evaluating these reports, appropriate questions would include not only standard statistical considerations, but also the following: 1) did the conflicting studies use different designs, e.g., case-control versus cohort? 2) was the exposure rare, so that the number of cases is not sufficiently large to detect an association? 3) were so many "fishing expedition" (a posteriori) comparisons made that a few showed a statistically significant association by chance alone? 4) if a case-control interview design was used, was the response rate suboptimal, particularly among controls? and 5) if a cohort was used, was the follow-up rate sufficiently high?

Oncogenic Influences in Humans

The literature on cancer epidemiology is voluminous and often difficult for clinicians to evaluate.[152] Some reports have failed to distinguish unproven etiological hypotheses from established oncogenic effects by such agents as tobacco and ionizing radiation. The lay press have added to this confusion by touting preliminary reports of suspected environmental carcinogens as proven fact. Carcinogens that account for many thousands of deaths annually in the U.S. have on occasion received less attention than agents that are responsible for only rare cases of cancer, such as diethylstilbestrol.[65] In the following discussion, effort is made to distinguish commonly encountered carcinogens from exposures limited to small subgroups and suspected hazards (Table IV-1-4).

Commonly Encountered Human Carcinogens

Tobacco. Cigarette smoking is the most important cause of preventable morbidity and mortality in the U.S.[49] An estimated 350,000 excess deaths occur annually from cigarette smoking nationwide. The majority of these deaths are due to cardiac and pulmonary diseases, but one-third (130,000 deaths) are due to cancer. Cigarette smoking is the predominant cause of lung cancer and a major cause of cancers of the larynx, oral cavity, and bladder.[128] Smoking has also been linked to development of cancers of the esophagus, pancreas, and kidney.[128] The annual cost of smoking-related illness and lost productivity in the U.S. is many billions of dollars. Carcinomas of the lung, due largely to smoking, have been the leading cause of cancer death in the U.S. for more than 2 decades.[128] One cancer death in three among American men is the result of lung cancer, which has also surpassed breast cancer as the leading cause of neoplastic disease mortality among women. Smoking is associated primarily with squamous and small cell carcinomas of the lung, but also increases the risk of adenocarcinoma. Elimination of tobacco use is the major method of cancer prevention available.[71]

The oncogenic effect in humans of cigarette smoking is beyond doubt. Data show that increased tobacco consumption in the U.S. and elsewhere was followed several decades later by a rise in lung cancer rates. A series of reports of the U.S. Surgeon General has summarized the data from diverse epidemiologic studies.[128] At least 9 large prospective cohort studies of up to 1 million subjects each, and 50 case-control studies worldwide have consistently shown that cigarette smoking increases the risk of lung cancer. The cancer risk is correlated with the amount of smoke exposure as measured by years of tobacco use, number of cigarettes consumed daily, their tar and nicotine content, and depth of inhalation of the smoke. The risk declines with smoking cessation, but lapse of a decade is required for the lung cancer risk in former smokers to approximate the low risk of nonsmokers.[140] These findings indicate that early cessation is important among current smokers, and that adolescents need to be strongly discouraged from starting the habit.[138,139] (See Chapter VI-1.) Recent studies suggest that Mendelian traits may influence susceptibility to lung cancer carcinogens.[28,123]

Cigarette smoking and alternative methods of tobacco use also increase risk of cancer.[24,47] Pipe and cigar smokers develop relatively fewer lung cancers but are at particularly high risk of oral cancers, including lip cancer in pipe users, and buccal cancers in snuff dippers. Recent evidence suggests oncogenic effects in non-smokers who inhale the smoke of nearby cigarette smokers. Although the risk to individual "passive smokers" appears relatively small, the aggregate

Table IV-1-4. Established Environmental Causes of Human Cancer*

Carcinogen	Cancer Site
Industrial Chemicals and Fibers	
Arsenicals	Skin, lung
Asbestos	Lung, pleura, peritoneum, pericardium
Benzene	Acute myelocytic leukemia
Bis(chloromethyl) ether	Lung
Chromium	Lung
Isopropyl alcohol production	Nasal sinuses
Mustard gas	Lung, larynx, nasal sinuses
Nickel dust	Lung, nasal sinuses
Polycyclic hydrocarbons	Lung, scrotum, skin (squamous carcinoma)
Vinyl chloride	Liver (angiosarcoma)
Drugs	
Alkylating agents (melphalan, cyclophosphamide, chlorambucil, nitrosoureas)	Acute myelocytic leukemia (also bladder, osteosarcoma for cyclophosphamide)
Androgenic steroids	Liver
Diethylstilbestrol (prenatal exposure)	Vagina (adenocarcinoma)
Immunosuppressive drugs (azathioprine, cyclosporine)	Non-Hodgkin's lymphoma
Phenacetin	Renal pelvis, bladder
Synthetic estrogens	Endometrium
Radiation	
Ionizing radiation	Almost all organs
Sunlight (UV)	Skin, intraocular melanoma
Personal Habits	
Alcoholic beverages	Liver, esophagus, mouth, pharynx, larynx
Tobacco	Lung, mouth, pharynx, larynx, esophagus, pancreas, bladder, kidney, renal pelvis
Viruses	
Chronic hepatitis B infection	Liver
HTLV-I	Adult T cell leukemia

*Only well established carcinogens in humans are listed

oncogenic effect on the population appears to be substantial.[15,141] Pregnant women who smoke can harm the developing fetus, and young parents who smoke increase the frequency of respiratory diseases in their young children. The increased risk of oral cancer among users of snuff and chewing tobacco is of concern in view of their growing popularity among youth.[94,149]

Clinicians are familiar with the difficulties of convincing patients to cease smoking, but need to persevere. The resistance of patients is primarily due to the habituating effects of cigarette smoking, particularly among heavy smokers. Nevertheless, per capita cigarette sales for adults in the United States have declined steadily in recent years.[140] Historically, the decline in tobacco use appeared first in physicians and dentists who had knowledge of its hazards.[46] Lung cancer death rates among physicians in the U.S. and England have declined steadily as a consequence of smoking cessation. Other health-conscious segments of society have also reduced tobacco consumption. The poor and the under-educated in the U.S. and the peoples of the Third World may gradually become the remnant population who smoke with high frequency. Many smokers have quit on the advice of their physicians, who are well-situated to influence the lifestyles of their patients.[4] In addition, limitations on advertising of tobacco products as well as increasing tobacco prices through taxation have contributed to a reduction in smoking.[36] With time, reduction in smoking in the population will inevitably result in a decline in tobacco-induced cancers.[138] (See Chapter VI-1.)

Alcohol. Tobacco and alcohol consumption combine to multiply the risk of cancers of the upper aerodigestive tract, including the mouth, tongue, esophagus pharynx and larynx.[43,95] Epidemiological studies in humans strongly implicate alcohol as a causal factor in these neoplasms, though ethanol rarely induces cancers in laboratory animals. Cancer might be due to other ingredients in alcoholic beverages or oral mucosal injury by alcohol, which magnifies the oncogenic effects of tobacco products.[111] Heavy drinkers also tend to have poor oral hygiene and poor diet, which may contribute to cancer development.[92] Cancers of the esophagus and liver often occur among chronic alcoholics in the United States.[21] In addition, recent data have raised the possibility that moderate alcohol ingestion elevates the risk of breast cancer, although other studies have failed to find an association.[97,118,120,146] Excessive alcohol consumption often starts in adolescence under the same social and psychological influences that promote cigarette smoking. Prevention of addiction to drugs and alcohol is beginning to receive more attention from educational, social, and legal agencies.[45,87]

Ionizing Radiation. Oncogenic effects of ionizing radiation have been identified in studies of nuclear bomb survivors, occupationally irradiated workers, and patients treated for cancer and other diseases.[33] Data have been gathered on types of radiation-induced tumors, time from exposure to tumor development (latency), radiation dose effects, and the influence of sex and age at exposure.[51] Assessment of risk for humans is often hindered by incomplete radiation dose data, paucity of large study populations, and diversity of conditions of exposures. Nevertheless, the aggregate data show that under certain conditions, ionizing radiation induces many types of leukemia as well as cancers of the thyroid, breast, respiratory system, digestive system, skin, bone, soft tissues, and other sites.[18] An apparent exception is chronic lymphocytic leukemia, which has not developed excessively among large study populations, such as atomic bomb survivors and patients irradiated for ankylosing spondylitis.

Data on radiation carcinogenesis have been gleaned primarily from studies of persons exposed to doses of tens to hundreds of centigray (cGy; rem). The radiation was delivered as either whole body exposure, or partial-body radiotherapy for diverse diseases.[19,112] Among atom bomb survivors, excess leukemias developed within 3 years of exposure, with a peak rate at 5–8 years after irradiation.[112] Acute lymphocytic leukemia has been observed primarily in those who were children at the time of the bombing. The myelogenous leukemias developed in both exposed children and adults. Chronic myelogenous leukemia tended to develop sooner following radiation exposure than acute myelogenous leukemia, which continues to occur excessively 4 decades after the bombing. The time to diagnosis of solid tumors has been longer than a decade from radiation exposure. Brain tumors, carcinomas and sarcomas have occurred excessively among atom bomb survivors and patients irradiated for tinea capitis, thymic enlargement in infancy, metropathia hemorrhagica, postpartum mastitis, and follow-up of pneumothorax therapy for pulmonary tuberculosis.[18] In patients who received partial-body radiation, the excess cancers have developed in tissues within or adjacent to the radiation portal.

Malignant tumors have been induced by radiotherapy in doses of thousands of centigray for childhood cancers, Hodgkin's disease, and carcinoma of diverse sites. Second neoplasms after childhood cancer include a high proportion of sarcomas, but also leukemias, lymphomas, and carcinomas of the skin, breast and lung.[14,18] It has been difficult to separate the role of radiotherapy in these patients from the effects of host susceptibility. Among patients irradiated for carcinoma of the cervix, a small excess of leukemia and solid tumors has been observed in several large studies.[19] The failure to detect a continuing rise in cancer risk with higher doses of radiotherapy might be due to dominance of the cell-killing effects over the transforming effects of the exposure.

The oncogenic effects in humans of low dose radiation (less than 20 cGy) cannot be quantified with precision.[135] Estimates of risk have been based on extrapolation from effects detected at higher doses. Recently the BEIR (Biological Effects of Ionizing Radiation) Committee of the National Research Council issued its fifth report, Health Effects of Exposure to Low Levels of Ionizing Radiation (BEIR-V).[33] After reviewing relevant epidemiological and laboratory data on radiation carcinogenesis, the report concluded that children are more susceptible than adults to the oncogenic effects of ionizing radiation. For doses up to several hundred cGy, excess cancer mortality (excluding leukemia) increases in a direct linear relationship to dose (doubling the dose doubles the cancer risk). The slope of the line suggests no more than 1,000 excess cancer deaths over the lifetime of 100,000 persons exposed to 10 rem, a dose approximating the lifetime dose from background irradiation. The figure is a small fraction of the 23,000 cancer deaths from all causes expected in a U.S. population of 100,000. Nevertheless, the excess radiation-induced cancer mortality is higher than prior BEIR estimates by several fold.[51] The upward revision is due in part to accumulation of data favoring the relative risk model for radiation effects. According to this model, a given dose of radiation increases cancer frequency by a fraction of the underlying cancer risk, which rises sharply with age. This model is consistent with the finding, for example, that breast irradiation is much more hazardous to females who have higher underlying risk of the cancer. Radiogenic breast cancers also arise more frequently in older women, who have higher underlying breast cancer rates compared to younger women. However, considerable uncertainty exists in present dose-risk estimates for humans, particularly with regard to lifetime effects. Additionally, the issue of threshold dose for tumor induction is unresolved, and is not readily measured in human populations.[114] For purposes of protection of radiation workers and the public, it is assumed that oncogenic effects of ionizing radiation do not have a threshold. A minute radiation dose is presumed to have a small oncogenic potential.

Studies of the oncogenic effects of radionuclides have focused primarily on occupationally exposed workers such as uranium miners and radium dial painters, and on patients injected with thorotrast. However, recent concern has been raised about the development of lung cancer and perhaps acute myelogenous leukemias after inhalation of radon gases within dwellings.[16,64] Some studies have raised the possibility of thousands of lung cancers annually in the U.S. as a consequence of radon exposure, but additional studies are needed.[16]

Sunlight. Excessive sunlight exposure increases the risk of several forms of skin cancer in exposed surfaces. These include basal and squamous cell carcinomas, and to a lesser extent, melanoma.[80,134] The risk of cancer is higher among Caucasian populations residing in tropical areas as compared with more temperate climates. A particularly high risk of sun-induced skin cancer has been found among fair-skinned individuals of Celtic origin, and groups with ultraviolet light sensitivity such as patients with xeroderma pigmentosum and dysplastic nevus syndrome.[10,116] The increase in popularity of sunbathing and outdoor activities among adolescents and young adults has heightened exposure to ultraviolet radiation. Education regarding the protective effects of clothing and topical sunscreens can be effective methods of reducing sunlight exposure, particularly among sensitive individuals.

Asbestos Fibers. Asbestos is an important cause of cancers of the respiratory tract, notably lung cancer and mesothelioma of both pleura and peritoneum.[34] The oncogenic hazards of asbestos exposure were recognized after lung cancers were found in patients with asbestosis. In 1960, Wagner and coworkers reported 33 cases of mesothelioma in workers and residents near an asbestos mine in South Africa.[137] Subsequent studies have reported mesothelioma in other asbestos workers and exposed populations.

Asbestos is a useful thermal insulator that has been mined in large quantities over the last century. The material is a family of fibrous silicates that are widely distributed geographically.[34] Oncogenic asbestos fibers are the rod-like amphiboles (crocidolite, amosite, anthophyllite, tremolite, and actinolyte). The oncogenic effect of asbestos appears to be a consequence of its physical properties rather than its chemical structure. Linear fibers of narrow diameter are more likely to induce tumors in laboratory animals. The widespread presence of asbestos in urban industrialized environments is illustrated by the use of asbestos in fire retardant ceiling materials in nearly 10% of U.S. schools.[130] No cancers have yet been linked to attendance in these schools, but pleural and peritoneal mesotheliomas have been reported to develop after a single exposure to asbestos. In contrast, lung cancer develops chiefly among heavily exposed workers, such as pipe fitters and shipyard employees. Lung cancer risk in asbestos workers is multiplied several-fold by cigarette smoking, and the combination of these exposures is particularly hazardous.[100]

Asbestos is estimated to be a causal factor in thousands of cancers, primarily lung cancers, each year in the U.S. The number may increase in the future because the latency for asbestos-associated cancers is 3–4 decades. The incidence of asbestos-induced mesothelioma is difficult to assess.[129] The neoplasm is not easy to diagnose, and death certificate data are unreliable. A reasonable estimate is that 2,000 new cases of mesothelioma occur annually in the United States.[129] Projections of future incidence suggest that the number of mesothelioma cases will rise moderately early in the next century and then decline when the benefits of environmental protection regulations of the 1970's and beyond are realized.

Deterioration of asbestos-containing products over time can cause release of asbestos fibers into the environment.[34] Demolition and repair of structures with friable asbestos also pose health hazards. Proper handling of these materials can be difficult and costly. Removal of the asbestos is a permanent solution. However, removal is costly and requires installation of effective barrier systems to avoid asbestos dissemination during removal. Encapsulation of friable asbestos is another option, but the solution is not permanent because encapsulating materials can deteriorate over time. The cost of dealing with asbestos in schools alone is billions of dollars, and homes, factories, offices, and public buildings are also contaminated.[100]

Candidate Oncogenic Influences

A number of prevalent environmental influences have been examined as human carcinogens with inconsistent results. In general, evidence of an oncogenic role for these factors is less convincing than for agents described in the last section. The distinction is quite arbitrary, and made in part to help readers distinguish established carcinogens in humans from candidate carcinogens. If future studies confirm the oncogenic activity of these candidate carcinogens, the number of cancers attributable to these agents could be substantial.

Dietary Factors. Available experimental and epidemiological data implicate diet as a factor in the etiology of cancers of the digestive tract and other sites.[102] Diet alters risk of tumors in certain laboratory animals. In addition, migrant studies and international comparisons of cancer rates have provided evidence that dietary factors can modify risk of cancers of the esophagus, stomach, colon, rectum, breast, endometrium, and prostate.[145] However, epidemiologic investigations of dietary differences among subgroups within a population have often yielded inconsistent results.

Precise dietary causes of cancers in humans remain uncertain despite extensive investigations.[105] The lengthy list of suspected oncogenic influences include the basic nutritional components of foods (fats, total calories, and low fiber content), food additives (dyes), flavoring agents (saccharin), contaminants (aflatoxin), preservatives (salt curing, pickling), and cooking methods (smoking, charcoal broiling).[102,105,145,147] Animal and human studies of obesity and cancer are complicated by the difficulty of separating the effects of calories, fat, and body weight.[119,144] Moreover, some animal studies suggest that marked restriction in total caloric intake is needed to reduce cancer incidence. Epidemiological studies have noted a correlation between diets low in fiber and increased risk for colon cancer, but results are not fully consistent.[144] Work in progress is examining the effects of different types of fiber on cancer occurrence. Other reports raise the possibility of protective factors in the diet, such as calcium, selenium, and vitamins A, C, D, E, and beta-carotenes.[102] Lower risk of carcinomas of the oral cavity, bladder, stomach, ovary and lung have been reported with ingestion of higher levels of vitamin A, carotenoids, or fruits and vegetables.[98,102,126,150] However, the possibility exists that the protection originates from other constitutents in fruits and vegetables, or other differences in lifestyle. Dietary intervention studies are difficult to perform because of requirements for accurate reporting, large patient series, problems with long-term compliance and the lapse of years required to detect reductions in cancer occurrence.[98] Intermediate biochemical markers of effects of diet modification are being developed. In rare instances, discernible reduction in cancer occurrence has been reported in small series of patients.[102]

Controversy remains regarding the appropriate recommendations to the public regarding diet modification in cancer prevention.[102,105] Dietary studies of the Seventh-Day Adventists, who are often vegetarian and nonsmokers, show lower rates for cancers of the lung and digestive tract.[109] For the general American population, some have advocated cancer control through major public education programs that encourage consumption of a balanced diet adequate in protein and other needed nutrients, with energy content sufficient to maintain a stable and normal body weight. These measures include reducing caloric and alcohol intake, decreasing fats to less than 30% of total calories, and increasing consumption of fresh fruits and vegetables.[145] While research continues, these recommendations seem prudent. A recent study of over 88,000 nurses reveals increased risk of colon cancer among those who consumed more meat and animal fat.[148] Even if benefits in terms of prevention of breast, colon, prostate, and other cancers were small, these measures are likely to provide protection against cardiovascular diseases, the leading cause of death nationally. (See VI-2.)

Viruses. Viruses have long been invoked as causes of human cancers.[59] Both DNA and RNA viruses have been demonstrated to induce cancers in experimental animals.

With recent advances in molecular biology, the role of viruses in human cancer development is now under intensive study. Results to date show the presence of diverse viruses in cancer patients, but their contributions to the oncogenic process often remains uncertain.[62] Some viruses appear to be etiological agents; others might enhance the oncogenic process by stimulating cellular proliferation or suppressing immunity; and the remainder are found in association with cancer but have no apparent causal role. Better understanding of the molecular mechanisms of oncogenesis should help distinguish etiologic agents from secondary changes. Studies of the oncogenic RNA viruses have unexpectedly shown that transforming virogenes originate from cellular genes acquired during the intracellular phase of the viral life cycle. These cellular genes (proto-oncogenes) gain tumorigenic potential when incorporated into the viral genome. Additional studies have shown that proto-oncogenes have been strictly conserved through evolution, suggesting that they produce proteins vital to the function and survival of the organism. Some proto-oncogenes have now been shown to encode proteins that are growth factors or growth factor receptors. Qualitative or quantitive changes (activation) of these genes can confer certain behavioral characteristics of neoplasia. Oncogenes that are involved in the development of many human cancers are usually activated by mechanisms unrelated to viral infection.

Squamous cell carcinoma of the uterine cervix is associated with viral infections which may be acquired through sexual intercourse.[136] The incidence of the neoplasm is increased in prostitutes and in women who have had multiple sexual partners, early age at first coitus, and history of venereal diseases.[62,136] Cervical carcinoma has also been reported to occur excessively in women whose partners have carcinoma of the penis.[127] Other studies show that these male partners tend to have a history of multiple sexual partners, suggesting that an infectious oncogenic agent is transmitted by males.[125] Genital infections, particularly with papillomavirus types 16 and 18, are suspected as etiologic factors.[136,153] (See III-10.) Temporal trends show that mortality rates for cervix cancer have declined substantially over the last several decades in the United States.[40] The decline may be due to both screening for cervix cancer with the Papanicolaou smear and lower disease incidence attributable to reduced exposure to risk factors. A worrisome exception is a recently reported increase in cervical cancer in young women.[6]

Human T-cell leukemia/lymphoma virus I (HTLV-I) has recently been linked to the development of a rare aggressive form of leukemia in young adults.[13] The disease has an unusual geographic distribution, with clusters in parts of Japan and the Caribbean. Human immunodeficiency disease virus (HIV; HTLV-III), the cause of AIDS, is associated with markedly increased risk of Kaposi's sarcoma, non-Hodgkin's lymphoma, and perhaps other cancers in early adulthood.[75] (See XXXVII-1.) HIV might not be the etiologic agent for these neoplasms; co-infection with an unidentified second virus has been suggested as the cause of Kaposi's sarcoma.[35] Non-Hodgkin's lymphoma in AIDS patients might be in part the consequence of the profound immunosuppression that accompanies the infection.

Other viruses have been implicated in human oncogenesis. Epstein-Barr (EB) virus is a suspected oncogenic virus that is associated with development of non-Hodgkin's lymphoma, Burkitt's lymphoma, and nasopharyngeal carcinoma.[58] (See III-9.) A recent study of EB virus antibody titers in Hodgkin's disease patients revealed that elevations of certain titers often preceded the neoplasm by several years. The finding suggests that enhanced activation of EB virus might be involved in the pathogenesis of Hodgkin's disease, or serve as a marker of altered immune control of the infection.[101]

Cancer of the liver is a relatively rare disease in the United States and occurs largely among patients with alcoholic cirrhosis.[20,76] Worldwide, primary liver cancer is a leading cause of cancer death in developing nations, particularly in Africa and Asia. The major risk factor in these patients is chronic hepatitis-B infection acquired initially in infancy.[8] (See III-11 and XXIX-3.) Risk of primary liver cancer is increased up to 200-fold among carriers of hepatitis-B virus. Hepatitis-B vaccination decreases the risk of infection and holds the promise of reducing the incidence of liver cancer; trials are in progress in several endemic areas. In areas endemic for liver cancer, the contamination of food by aflatoxins and other mycotoxins might be an additional etiologic factor.[7] Evidence for an oncogenic role of non-B hepatitis viruses is much more tenuous.[73]

Cancer Clusters. In recent decades, much public attention has focused on reports of localized temporal-geographical clusters of cancer which may indicate the action of a point exposure to carcinogens.[25] Many clusters have involved childhood cancers, notably leukemia, occurring within a short period of time in a small geographic area. Investigations of most suspected clusters have failed to identify an etiologic agent. Moreover, application of appropriate statistical methods to analyze such aggregates have shown that these "clusters" were probably explainable on the basis of chance.[53] An exception is a study of Woburn, Massachusetts, showing that childhood leukemia rates were double the expected frequency between 1969 and 1979.[81,82] Prospective observation of the community has revealed that childhood leukemias have continued to develop excessively. The explanation is unknown, and extensive efforts are in progress to identify the cause. Many other reports of cancer clusters have involved residents near chemical dumps such as in Love Canal, New York.[72] In most instances, no excess cancers have been shown to be caused by ambient pollutants.[38] However, the latent period for carcinogenesis is long, and clean-up of these toxic sites needs to proceed.

Another pattern of clustering is based on linking cancer patients who have a history of personal contact with each other, despite dissimilar times and geographic locations at diagnosis of cancer.[59] This model postulates person-to-person transmission of a hypothetical infectious agent, perhaps an oncogenic virus. Clustering of cancer by personal contact has been most often examined in connection with Hodgkin's disease in young adults, but the results are inconsistent.[59]

Carcinogens in Population Subgroups

This section discusses the oncogenic effects of high-dose carcinogen exposures that are limited to subgroups in the population. Since oncogenic effects generally increase with dose, resultant cancers are most readily discerned in these subgroups. The question remains of the risk of exposure to minute doses of these agents among the general population.

Chemical Exposures in the Workplace. Among hundreds of chemicals examined in some detail for oncogenic effects, approximately 20 have been determined to be oncogenic in humans (Table IV-1-4).[114] These compounds are shown along with the cancers that occur as a result of exposure. Most chemical carcinogens induce carcinomas of the lung and upper airway; others cause acute leukemia and carcinomas of the bladder, liver, skin, and other organs. Additional chemicals have been found to induce cancer in laboratory animals, but the relevant data for humans are insufficient or inconsistent and additional research is needed. Oncogenic chemical exposures often occur in the workplace, and these are estimated to account for approximately 5 percent of all cancers in the U.S.[42] Lung cancer has developed excessively among workers exposed to chromium, arsenic, mustard gas, polycyclic hydrocarbons, and bis(chloro-methyl)ether. Bladder cancer develops excessively after exposure to certain aromatic amines in dye workers, rubber workers, tanners and organic chemical workers. Liver damage by vinyl chloride predisposes to angiosarcomas of the liver. Acute myelogenous leukemia occurs excessively in benzene workers. There is uncertainty whether atmospheric pollution resulting from the release of industrial chemicals causes a small portion of lung and other cancers.[42] However, other ill effects of these pollutants are well documented, and control measures should be instituted.

Preliminary data suggest that dioxins might increase risk of soft tissue sarcomas among forestry workers but additional data are needed. Dioxins are an ingredient in the defoliant Agent Orange, and its effects on exposed Vietnam War veterans remains the subject of intense scientific and political debate. Studies of Vietnam-era veterans are reported to show no overall excess of cancers, but non-Hodgkin's lymphoma rates are elevated. It has been difficult to relate cancer occurrence in these veterans to their exposure to defoliants. Recently, herbicides have been linked to non-Hodgkin's lymphoma in several groups of farmers in the U.S., Canada and elsewhere.[67] The oncogenic herbicide has not been identified with certainty although phenoxyacetic acids, particularly 2,4-D, are suspected to be causal agents.[12,67,143]

Medications. Drugs are routinely tested for oncogenic activity in animals prior to approval for clinical use in humans.[122] The few medications strongly implicated as carcinogens in humans are listed in Table IV-1-4.[122] The risk of cancer associated with most of these drugs is small, and for some diseases, better treatment alternatives are not available. Alkylating agents, alone or in combination with other therapies, are the treatment of choice for certain cancers and immunological diseases, even though a few patients may subsequently develop acute myelogenous leukemia.[29,55,79,113] All alkylating agents appear to have leukemogenic potential, including cyclophosphamide, melphalan, mechlorethamine, procarbazine, and nitrosoureas.[29] Recent data raise concern about the possible role of etoposide in the development of secondary acute myelogenous leukemia in children treated for acute lymphocytic leukemia.[113] Bladder cancers have also been reported after cyclophosphamide-associated cystitis.[132] Bladder cancer after administration of chlornaphazine, an alkylating agent that is no longer in use, may be the result of its biotransformation to the bladder carcinogen, beta-naphthylamine. Recently, secondary osteosarcoma has been reported to occur in association with alkylating agent therapy among a series of survivors of childhood cancer, but confirmation is needed.[133] Drugs and diagnostic agents used for non-neoplastic diseases, such as hormones, radionuclides and immunosuppressants have also been linked to the development of malignant tumors.[31,110,122] Some of these drugs, such as inorganic arsenicals and thorium dioxide (Thorotrast), are no longer in use but continue to produce cancers because their latency period extends for decades.

Organ transplant recipients are at high risk of non-Hodgkin's lymphoma, Kaposi's sarcoma, and skin cancer.[68] The lymphomas may appear within several weeks after renal or cardiac transplantation, and differ from most environmental cancers which arise many years after exposure to carcinogens. Molecular analyses reveal the lymphoproliferative diseases in transplant recipients to be monoclonal, oligoclonal or polyclonal.[32] The transplant-associated lymphomas have a predilection for the central nervous system. Immunosuppressive therapy with azathioprine and cyclosporin has been implicated as a risk factor in transplant recipients, although the transplanted organ may also have an oncogenic influence. Among leukemic patients who received bone marrow transplantation, leukemia was found to recur occasionally in the transplanted donor cells.

Hormonal factors, both endogenous and exogenous, have been implicated in the development of cancers of the breast, ovary, endometrium, and other sites.[70,104,124] The evidence appears strongest for the proliferative effects of conjugated estrogens on the endometrium, which produces a form of endometrial carcinoma with an excellent prognosis. Data are less consistent regarding increased risk of breast cancer after prolonged use of oral contraceptives starting in early adulthood.[31]

Host Susceptibility Factors

Inherited susceptibility to cancer is often manifest by occurrence of the same neoplasm among multiple blood relatives. These neoplasms tend to occur at earlier ages than usual, bilaterally in paired organs, and in multiple primary foci within the predisposed organ. Familial aggregation has been reported for virtually every form of cancer in humans. In general, close relatives of a cancer patient appear to have a 2–3-fold increase in risk of that tumor. Among cancer families, however, the level of excess risk is heterogeneous and ranges up to 10,000-fold, as in carriers of the retinoblastoma gene.[78] Survivors of hereditary retinoblastoma are prone to second cancers, particularly osteosarcoma and soft tissue sarcomas. Clinicians are often asked by patients about the clinical implications of a family history of cancer. To provide an informative response, data are needed on the sex of affected family member(s), the relationship to the patient, age(s) at diagnosis, primary site and histology of each tumor, and disease outcome. A pedigree can be used as a concise record of cancer occurrence in multiple members of a family. In families of particular interest, confirmation of the medical history of family members should be sought through examinations of pathology reports, medical records, and death certificates. If indicated, available family members should be examined for physical evidence of inherited disorders that predispose to cancer.[106] It is noteworthy that cancer is a common disease over a lifetime in the United States, occurring in 1 of every 3 persons.[106] Therefore, a family history of cancer is the rule, and not the exception. Seemingly striking family aggregates of cancer can occur solely on the basis of chance. However, cancers in childhood are rare, and their occurrence in families are much less likely to be due to chance association.[106] Estimates vary on the proportion of human cancers that are due to hereditary influences. A substantial proportion of cancers of the colon, breast and other common sites of involvement demonstrate a familial tendency.[84] On the other hand, few cancers consistently follow a strictly Mendelian (autosomal dominant, autosomal recessive or X-linked) pattern, or occur excessively in association with an underlying single-gene disorder such as hereditary retinoblastoma. When the retinoblastoma gene was cloned, however, it was found to be altered in a wide spectrum of cancers, including sarcomas and carcinomas of the lung, breast, and other sites. In addition, genetic factors can play a role in the development of cancers triggered by environmental factors, through inherited mechanisms that influence the metabolism of carcinogens.[74]

An inherited susceptibility to certain cancers can be recognized by the presence of a predisposing syndrome (Table IV-1-5). More than 200 single gene traits are known to be associated with the development of neoplasia.[78] The frequency of tumors differs markedly among these inherited disorders. Benign and malignant tumors are the sole manifestation of some disorders, but are rarely featured in others. Hereditary cancers can present as multiple primary tumors in organs that share the same embryological origins, as in the multiple endocrine neoplasia (MEN) syndromes.[78] In addition, neoplasia occurs as a feature of diverse inherited diseases, such as neurofibromatosis, types 1 and 2, which predispose to tumors of peripheral nerves and brain.[69] A list of the most important of these predisposing conditions is shown in Table IV-1-5. In addition, families have been reported with cancer syndromes that affect diverse anatomic sites and tissues. These families generally have no characteristic clinical features, and they are identified primarily on the basis of statistical association. A syndrome of multiple primary adenocarcinomas of the colon, endometrium, breast and other sites has been described, but remains difficult to diagnose.[89,90] Another syndrome of breast cancer in young women, childhood sarcomas, and other neoplasms (the Li-Fraumeni Syndrome) has been extensively studied.[86] Prospective study of these families has shown a marked excess of the component neoplasms during follow-up observation. The syndrome of breast cancer and childhood neoplasms has also been identified in population-based series of children with sarcomas and in segregation analysis of families with a case of childhood sarcoma.[61,131] A tumor suppressor gene, p53, has been implicated in tumor development in sporadic and familial cases of diverse tumors, including those of the Li-Fraumeni Syndrome.[103] The recent finding of a germ-line mutant p53 in the affected members of five Li-Fraumeni fam-

Table IV-1-5. Single-Gene Traits Associated with Cancers of Internal Organs*

Organ System	Predisposing Genetic Disorder (Inheritance†)	Type of Cancer
Digestive and respiratory	Polyposis coli (AD), and Gardner's syndrome (AD)	Carcinoma of colon and rectum
	Hereditary hemochromatosis (AD), and Tyrosinemia (AR)	Primary liver cancer
	Palmar-plantar hyperkeratosis (tylosis) (AD)	Esophageal carcinoma
	Hereditary pancreatitis (AD)	Pancreatic carcinoma
	Fibrocystic pulmonary dysplasia (AD)	Carcinoma of lung
Genitourinary organs	Gonadal dysgenesis (AR)	Dysgerminoma of ovary
	von Hippel-Lindau syndrome (AD)	Renal carcinoma (also retinal tumor)
Brain and endocrine	Neurofibromatosis (AD), and tuberous sclerosis (AD)	Tumors of brain and peripheral nerves
	Multiple endocrine neoplasia Type I (AD)	Parathyroid, pituitary, pancreatic islet tumors
	Nevoid basal cell carcinoma syndrome (AD)	Medulloblastoma (and other tumors)
	Multiple endocrine neoplasia types II, III (AD)	Medullary thyroid carcinoma, pheochromocytoma
	Multiple hamartoma syndrome (Cowden's disease) (AD)	Thyroid and breast cancer (also colon and other)
Hematologic system	Agammaglobulinemia (XL, AR), Wiskott-Aldrich syndrome (XL), ataxia-telangiectasia (AR), and X-linked lymphoproliferative syndrome (XL)	Lymphoma
	Bloom's syndrome (AR), and Fanconi's anemia (AR)	Leukemia
Musculoskeletal system	Multiple exostosis (AD), Paget's disease (AD), and multiple enchondromatosis (AD)	Osteogenic sarcoma
	Werner's syndrome (adult progeria) (AR)	Soft-tissue sarcoma

*Excluding familial site-specific cancers and cancer syndromes
†AD = autosomal dominant, AR = autosomal recessive, XL = X-linked

ilies indicates that p53 mutants can confer a heritable susceptibility to certain cancers.[93]

Family aggregation of cancer can be due to both hereditary influences and shared exposure to environmental carcinogens.[85] Dietary factors may modify the frequency of colonic tumors in patients with familial adenomatous polyposis. A recent study showed that reduction in dietary fat intake and grain fiber supplementation inhibit development of new rectal polyps in a small series of patients.[39] Carcinomas of the skin and malignant melanomas are, for example, often considered neoplasms induced by environmental factors, particularly sunlight and other sources of ultraviolet radiation. However, skin cancers differ markedly in frequency among the races. They are commonest among fair-skinned Caucasians but rare among blacks. The finding indicates that genetically determined skin pigmentation is also an important etiological factor. Furthermore, in several rare hereditary disorders of DNA repair, such as xeroderma pigmentosum (XP), exceptionally high risk of skin cancers has been found.[115] In-vitro studies of cells of XP patients show reduced repair of ultraviolet radiation damage, which normally involves a multistep process of incision near the damaged strand, excision of the dimer, repair of the DNA and rejoining.[44] At least 9 distinct mutations (complementation groups) along this enzymatic pathway have been identified. A second disease featuring increased sensitivity to ionizing radiation is ataxia telangiectasia (AT).[52] Patients with AT are at very high risk of lymphoid neoplasms that, when treated with standard doses of radiotherapy, can produce fatal toxicity.

Knowledge that a family history of cancer is a consistent risk factor for neoplasia can be used to enhance primary and secondary prevention of cancer.[106] In families with a known predisposing gene, the risk of cancer can often be estimated and used in genetic counseling. Inherited precursor lesions of cancer can be useful in early diagnosis and surveillance, as illustrated in families with dysplastic nevus syndrome and susceptibility to melanoma.[10,56] These kindreds can be identified by obtaining a complete family history and performing a thorough skin examination of all blood relatives. Suspicious pigmented lesions should be excised and submitted for histopathological examination.[57] High risk individuals should be taught to recognize changes in size, color and shape of lesions that might indicate early melanoma. Since ultraviolet radiation is an etiologic factor in melanoma, avoidance of exposure is particularly important in predisposed families. In addition, early cancer detection can be undertaken in susceptible families that have no discernible precursor lesions and biomarkers of a carrier state. In breast cancer, early detection has been demonstrated to reduce breast cancer mortality rates and a family history of breast cancer is known to elevate a woman's risk of the neoplasm. The magnitude of the effect of a family history of breast cancer is determined by the number of affected relatives.[117] Breast cancer in these families tends to occur in younger women, and studies in progress should help quantify benefits of directed screening of women in high risk families.[5] A similar rationale argues for early detection of colorectal carcinomas in predisposed families, particularly in light of new evidence that inherited factors contribute to the development of a high proportion of colonic adenomas and carcinomas.[27]

References

1. American Cancer Society: Ca-A Cancer Journal for Clinicians. Edited by A. I. Holleb. New York, H&W Publishing, Volume 40, No.1, 1990.
2. American Cancer Society: Cancer Facts and Figures–1990.
3. American Cancer Society: Special report on cancer in the socioeconomically disadvantaged. American Cancer Society Subcommittee on cancer in the economically disadvantaged, 1986.
4. Anda, R. F., Remington, P. L., Sienko, D. G., and Davis R. M.: Are physicians advising smokers to quit? The patient's perspective. J.A.M.A., 257:1916, 1987.
5. Anderson, D. E., and Badzioch, M. D.: Risk of familial breast cancer. Cancer, 56:383,1985.
6. Anello, C., and Lao, C.: U.S. trends in mortality from carcinoma of cervix. Lancet, I:1038, 1979.
7. Ayoola, E. A.: Synergism between hepatitis B virus and aflatoxin in hepatocellular carcinoma. IARC Science Publishers, 63:167, 1984.
8. Arthur, M. J. P., Hall, A. J., and Wright, R.: Hepatitis B, hepatocellular carcinoma, and strategies for prevention. Lancet, 1:607, 1984.
9. Bailar, J. C., and Smith, E. M.: Progress against cancer? N. Engl. J. Med., 314:1226, 1986.
10. Bale, S. J., Dracopoli, N. C., Tucker, M. A., Clark, W. H., Fraser, M. C., Stanger, B. Z., Green, P., Donis-Keller, H., Housman, D. E., and Greene, M. H.: Mapping the gene for hereditary cutaneous malignant melanoma-dysplastic nevus to chromosome 1p. N. Engl. J. Med., 320:1367, 1989.
11. Baquet, C. R., and Ringen, K.: Cancer among blacks and other minorities. Publication #86-2785. U.S. Department of Health and Human Services, Public Health Service, National Institutes of Health, March 1986.
12. Blair, A.: Herbicides and non-Hodgkin's lymphoma: New evidence from a study of Saskatchewan farmers. J. Natl. Cancer Inst., 82:544, 1990.
13. Blattner, W. A., Nomura, A., Clark, J. W., Ho, G. Y., Nakao, Y., Gallo, R., and Robert-Guroff, M.: Modes of transmission and evidence for viral latency from studies of human T-cell lymphotrophic virus type I in Japanese migrant populations in Hawaii. Proc. Natl. Acad. Sci. U.S.A., 83:4895, 1986.
14. Blayney, D. W., Longo, D. L., Young, R. C., Greene, M. H., Hubbard, S. M., Postal, M. G., Duffey, P. L., and DeVita, V. T., Jr.,: Decreasing risk of leukemia with prolonged follow-up after chemotherapy and radiotherapy for Hodgkin's disease. N. Engl. J. Med., 316:710, 1987.
15. Blot, W. J., and Fraumeni, J.F., Jr: Passive smoking and lung cancer (editorial). J. Natl. Cancer Inst., 77:993, 1986.
16. Blot, W. J., Xu, Z. Y., Boice, J. D., Jr., Zhao, D. Z., Stone, B. J., Sun, J., Jing, L. B., and Fraumeni, J.F., Jr.: Indoor radon and lung cancer in China. J. Natl. Cancer Inst., 82:1025, 1990.
17. Blumberg, B. S., and London, W. T.: Hepatitis B virus and the prevention of primary cancer of the liver. J. Natl. Cancer Inst., 74:267, 1985.
18. Boice, J. D., Jr., and Fraumeni, J. F., Jr.: Radiation Carcinogenesis. Epidemiology and Biological Significance. *In* Progress in Cancer Research and Therapy, Volume 26. New York, Raven Press, 1984.
19. Boice, J. D., Jr., Blettner, M., Kleinerman, R. A., Stovall, M., Moloney, W. C., Engholm, G., Austin, D. F., Bosch A., Cookfair, D. L., Krementz, E. T., Latourette, H. B., Peters, L. J., Schulz, M. D., Lundell, M., Pettersson, F., Storm, H. H., Bell, C. M. J., Coleman, M. P., Fraser, P., Palmer, M., Prior, P., Choi, N. W., Hislop, T. G., Koch, M., Robb, D., Robson, D., Spengler, R. F., vonFournier, D., Frischkorn, R., Lochmüller, H., Pompe-Kirn, V., Rimpela, A., Kjørstad, K., Pejovic, M. H., Sigurdsson, K., Pisani, P., Kucera, H., and Hutchison, G. B.: Radiation dose and leukemia risk in patients treated for cancer of the cervix. J. Natl. Cancer Inst., 79:1295, 1987.

19A. Boring, C. C., Squires, T. S., and Tong, T.: Cancer Statistics 1992. Ca. A cancer journal for clinicians, 42:19, 1992.

20. Boutron, M. C., Faivre, J., Milan, C., Bedenne, L., Hillon, P., and Klepping, C.: Primary liver cancer in Cote D'Or (France). Int. J. Epidemiol., 17:21, 1988.
21. Brechot, C., Nalpas, B., Courouce, A., Duhamel, G.,, Callard, P., Carnot, F., Tiollais, P., and Berthelot, P.: Evidence that hepatitis B virus has a role in liver-cell carcinoma in alcoholic liver disease. N. Engl. J. Med., 306:1384, 1982.
22. Breslow, L., Bailar, J. C., III, Brown, B. W., Jr., Brown, H. G., Darity, W. A., Defendi, V., Fisher, B., Goodman, R. L., Mosteller, F., and Shapiro, S.: Measurement of progress against cancer. J. Natl. Cancer Inst., 82:825, 1990.
23. Breslow, N. E., and Day, N. E.: Statistical Methods in Cancer Research, Volume I. The Analysis of Case-Control Studies. Lyon, IARC Scientific Publications, 1981.
24. Brinton, L. A., Schairer, C., Haenszel, W., Stolley, R., Lehman, H. F., Levine, R., and Savitz, D. A.: Cigarette smoking and invasive cervical cancer. J.A.M.A., 255:3265, 1986.
25. Caldwell, G. C., and Heath, C. W.: Case clustering in cancer. South. Med. J., 69:1598, 1976.
26. Cancer Incidence in Five Continents, Volume V. Edited by C. Muir, J. Waterhouse, T. Mack, et al. Lyon, France, IARC Scientific Publications, 1987.
27. Cannon-Albright, L. A., Skolnick, M. H., Bishop, D. T., Lee, R. G., and Burt, R. W.: Common inheritance of susceptibility to colonic adenomatous polyps and associated colorectal cancers. N. Engl. J. Med., 319:533,1988.
28. Caporaso, N. E., Tucker, M. A., Hoover, R. N., Hayes, R. B., Pickle, L. W., Issaq, H. J., Muschik, G. M., Green-Gallo, L., Buivys, D., Aisner, S., Resau, J. H., Trump, B. F., Tollerud, D., Weston, A., and Harris, C. C.: Lung cancer and the debrisoquine metabolic phenotype. J. Natl. Cancer Inst., 82:1264, 1990.
29. Casciato, D. A., and Scott, J. L.: Acute leukemia following prolonged cytotoxic agent therapy. Medicine, 58:32, 1979.
30. Centers for Disease Control. Black-white differences in cervical cancer mortality–United States, 1980–1987. Morbidity and Mortality Weekly Reports, 39:245, 1990.
31. Chilvers, C., McPherson, K., Peto, J., Pike, M. C.; and Vessey, M.P.: Oral contraceptive use and breast cancer risk in young women. Lancet, 1:973, 1989.
32. Cleary, M. L., and Sklar, J.: Lymphoproliferative disorders in cardiac transplant recipients are multiclonal lymphomas. Lancet, II:489, 1984.
33. Committee on the Biological Effects of Ionizing Radiations: Health Effects of Exposure to Low Levels of Ionizing Radiation. Beir V. Washington, DC, National Academy Press, 1990.
34. Craighead, J. E., and Mossman, B. T.: The pathogenesis of asbestos-associated diseases. N. Engl. J. Med., 306:1446, 1982.
35. Cremer, K. J., Spring, S. B., and Gruber, J.: Role of human immunodeficiency virus type 1 and other viruses in malignancies associated with acquired immunodeficiency disease syndrome. J. Natl. Cancer Inst., 82:1016, 1990.
36. Davis, R. M.: Current trends in cigarette advertising and marketing. N. Engl. J. Med., 316:725, 1987.
37. Dawber, T. R.: The Framingham Study: The Epidemiology of Atherosclerotic Disease. Cambridge, MA, Harvard University Press, 1980.
38. Day, R., Ware J. H., Wartenberg, D., and Zelen, M.: An investigation of a reported cancer cluster in Randolph, Massachusetts. J. Clin. Epidemiol., 42:137, 1989.
39. DeCosse, J. J., Miller, H. H., and Lesser, M. L.: Effect of wheat fiber and vitamins C and E on rectal polyps in patients with familial adenomatous polyposis. J. Natl. Cancer Inst. 81:1291, 1989.
40. Devesa S. S.: Descriptive epidemiology of cancer of the uterine cervix. J. Am. College of Obstet. Gynecol., 63:605, 1984.
41. Doll, R., and Hill, A. B.: Lung cancer and other causes of death in relation to smoking: A second report on the mortality of British doctors. Brit. Med. J., 10:1071, 1965.
42. Doll, R., and Peto, R.: The causes of cancer: Quantitative estimates of avoidable risks of cancer in the United States today. J. Natl. Cancer Inst., 66:1193, 1981.
43. Editorial: Alcohol and Cancer. Lancet 335:634, 1990.
44. Editorial: Sunlight, DNA repair, and skin cancer. Lancet I:1362, 1989.
45. Ellickson, P. L., and Bell, R. M.: Drug prevention in junior high: A multi-site longitudinal test. Science, 247:1299, 1990.
46. Enstrom, J. E.: Trends in mortality among California physicians after giving up smoking: 1950–79. Br. Med. J., 286:1101, 1983.
47. Ernster, V. L., Grady, D. G., Greene, J. C., Walsh, M., Robertson, P., Daniels, T. E., Benowitz, N., Siegel, D., Gerbert, B., and Hauck, W. W.: Smokeless tobacco use and health effects among baseball players. J.A.M.A., 264:218, 1990.
48. Feldman, A. R., Kessler, L., Myers, M. H., and Naughton, M. D.: The prevalence of cancer: Estimates based on the Connecticut Tumor Registry. N. Engl. J. Med., 315:1394, 1986.
49. Fielding, J. E.: Smoking: Health effects and control. N. Engl. J. Med., 313:491, 1985.
50. Fleiss, J. L.: Statistical Methods for Rates and Proportions. New York, John Wiley and Sons, 1981.
51. Fry, R. J., and Sinclair, W. K.: New dosimetry of atomic bomb radiations. Lancet, 2:845, 1987.
52. Gatti, R. A., Berkel, I., Boder, E., Braedt, G., Charmley, P., Concannon, P., Ersoy, F., Foroud, T., Jaspers, N.G., Lange, K., et al.: Localization of an ataxia-telangiectasia gene to chromosome 11q22-23. Nature, 336:577,1988.
53. Glass, A. G., and Mantel, N.: Lack of time-space clustering of childhood leukemia in Los Angeles County, 1960–1964. Cancer Res., 29:1995, 1969.
54. Gloeckler Ries, L. A., Hankey, B. F., and Edwards, B. K.: Cancer Statistics Review 1973–1987. Department of Health and Human Services, NIH Publication No. 90-2789, 1989.
55. Greene, M. H., Boice, J. D., Greer, B. E., Blessing, J. A., and Dembo, A. J.: Acute nonlymphocytic leukemia after therapy with alkylating agents for ovarian cancer. N. Engl. J. Med., 307:1416, 1982.
56. Greene, M. H., Clark, W. H., Jr., Tucker, M. A., Kraemer, K. H., Elder, D. E., and Fraser, M. C.: High risk of malignant melanoma in melanoma-prone families with dysplastic nevi. Ann. Intern. Med., 102:458, 1985.
57. Greene, M. H., Clark, W. H., Jr., Tucker, M. A., Elder, D. E., Kraemer, K. H., Guerry, D., IV, Witmer, W. K., Thompson, J., Matozzo, I., and Fraser, M.C.: Acquired precursors of cutaneous malignant melanoma. N. Engl. J. Med., 312:91, 1985.
58. Grufferman, S., Raab-Traub, N., Marvin, K., Borowitz, M. J., and Pagano, J. S.: Burkitt's and other non-Hodgkin's lymphomas in adults exposed to a visitor from Africa. N. Engl. J. Med., 313:1525, 1985.
59. Gutensohn, N., and Cole P.: Childhood social environment and Hodgkin's disease. N. Engl. J. Med., 304:135, 1981.
60. Haenszel, W.: Migrant Studies. *In* Cancer Epidemiology and Prevention. Edited by D. Schottenfeld, and J. F. Fraumeni. Philadelphia, W.B. Saunders Company, 1982, p. 194.
61. Hartley, A. L., Birch, J. M., Marsden, H. B., and Harris, M.: Breast cancer risk in mothers of children with osteosarcoma and chondrosarcoma. Br. J. Cancer, 54:819, 1986.
62. Henderson, B. E.: Establishment of an association between a virus and a human cancer. J. Natl. Cancer Inst., 81:320, 1989.
63. Hennekens, C. H., and Buring, J. E.: Epidemiology in Medicine. Edited by S. L. Mayrent. Boston, Little, Brown, and Co., 1987.
64. Henshaw, D. L., Eatough, J. P., and Richardson, R. B.: Radon as a causative factor induction of myeloid leukemia and other cancers. Lancet, 335:1008, 1990.
65. Herbst, A. L., Ulfelder, J., and Poskanzer, D. C.: Adenocarcinoma of the vagina: Association of maternal stilbestrol therapy with tumor appearance in young women. N. Engl. J. Med., 284:878, 1971.
66. Herbst, A. L., Anderson, S., Hubby, M. M., Haenszel, W. M., Kaufman, R. H., and Noller, K. L.: Risk factors for the development of diethylstilbestrol-associated clear-cell adenocarcinoma: a case-control study. Am. J. Obstet. Gynecol., 154:814, 1986.
67. Hoar, S. K., Blair, A., Holmes, F. F., Boysen, C. D., Robel, R. J., Hoover, R., Fraumeni, J. F., Jr.: Agricultural herbicide use and risk of lymphoma and soft-tissue sarcoma. J.A.M.A., 256:1141, 1986.
68. Hoover, R., and Fraumeni, J. F., Jr.: Risk of cancer in renal-transplant recipients. Lancet, 2:55, 1973.
69. Hope, D. G., and Mulvihill, J. J.: Malignancy in neurofibromatosis. *In* Neurofibromatosis: Genetics, Cell Biology, and Biochemistry. Edited by V. M. Riccardi, and J. J. Mulvihill. New York, Raven Press, 1981, p. 33.
70. Hulka, B. S., Chambless, L. E., Kaufman, D. G., Fowler, W. C., and Greenberg, B. G.: Protection against endometrial carcinoma by combination-product oral contraceptives. J.A.M.A., 247:475, 1982.
71. Iglehart, J. K.: The campaign against smoking gains momentum. N. Engl. J. Med., 314:1059, 1986.
72. Janerich, D. T., Burnett, W. S., Feck, G., Hoff, M., Nasca, P., Polednak, A. P., Greenwald., P., and Vianna, N.: Cancer incidence in the Love Canal area. Science, 212:1404, 1981.
73. Johnson, P. J., and Williams, R.: Hepatitis C antibodies and hepato-cellular carcinoma: New clues or a false trail? J. Natl. Cancer Inst., 82:986, 1990.
74. Kaisary, A., Smith, P., Jacqz, E., McAllister, C.B., Wilkinson, G.R., Ray, W..A., and

Branch, R. A.: Genetic predisposition to bladder cancer: Ability to hydroxylate debrisoquine and mephenytoin as risk factors. Cancer Res., 47:5488, 1987.

75. Kaplan, M. H., Susin, M., Pahwa, S. G., Fetten, J., Allen, S. L., Lichtman, S., Sarngadharon, M. G., and Gallo, R. C.: Neoplastic complications of HTLVIII infection: Lymphomas and solid tumors. Am. J. Med., 82:389, 1987.

76. Keller, A. Z.: Alcohol, tobacco and age factors in the relative frequency of cancer among males with and without liver cirrhosis. Am. J. Epidemiol. 106:194, 1977.

77. Kmet, J., and Mahboubi, E.: Esophageal cancer in the Caspian littoral of Iran: Initial studies. Science 175:846, 1972.

78. Knudson, A. G., Jr.: Hereditary cancers disclose a class of cancer genes. Cancer, 63:1888, 1989.

79. Kraemer, K. H., DiGiovanna, J. J., Moshell, A. N., Tarone, R. E., and Peck, G. L.: Prevention of skin cancer in xeroderma pigmentosum with the use of oral isotretinoin. N. Engl. J. Med., 318:1633, 1988.

80. Kripke, M. L., and Sass, E. R.: International Conference on Ultraviolet Carcinogenesis. Department of Health, Education and Welfare Publication No. (NIH) 78-1532. Washington, D.C., U.S. Government Printing Office, 1977.

81. Lagakos, S. W., Wessen, B., et al.: The Woburn Health Study. (unpublished data).

82. Lagakos, S. W., Wessen, B. J., et al.: An analysis of contaminated well water and health effects in Woburn, Massachusetts. J. Am. Stat. Assoc., 81:583, 1986.

83. Langmuir, A. D.: The surveillance of communicable diseases of national importance. N. Engl. J. Med., 268:182, 1963.

84. Leppert, M., Burt, R., Hughes, J. P., Samowitz, W., Nakamura, Y., Woodward, S., Gardner, E., Lalouel, J. M., and White, R.: Genetic analysis of an inherited predisposition to colon cancer in a family with a variable number of adenomatous polyps. N. Engl. J. Med., 322:904, 1990.

85. Li, F. P.: Cancer epidemiology and prevention. Scientific American, 10:12, 1978.

86. Li, F. P., Fraumeni, J. F., Jr., Mulvihill, J. J., Blattner, W. A., Dreyfus, M. G., Tucker, M. A., and Miller, R.W.: A cancer family syndrome in twenty-four kindreds. Cancer Res., 48:5358, 1988.

87. Li, F. P., and Mulvihill, J. J.: Preventative Pediatric Oncology: The Childhood Origins of Adult Cancer. In Principles and Practices of Pediatric Oncology. Edited by P. A. Pizzo, and D. G. Poplack. Philadelphia, JB Lippincott Company, 1988, p. 1075.

88. Lippman, S. M., Lee, J. S., Lotan, R., Hittelman, W., Wargovich, M. J., and Hong, W. K.: Biomarkers as intermediate end points in chemoprevention trials. J. Natl. Cancer Inst., 82:555, 1990.

89. Lynch, H. T., and Krush, A. J.: Cancer family "G" revisited: 1895–1970. Cancer, 27:1505, 1971.

90. Lynch, H. T., and Lynch, P. M.: Hereditary and gastrointestinal tract cancer. In Gastrointestinal Tract Cancer. Edited by M. Lipkin, and R. A. Good. New York, Plenum Medical Book Company, 1980, p. 259.

91. MacMahon, B., and Pugh, T. F.: Epidemiology: Principles and Methods. Boston, Little, Brown, and Co., 1970.

92. Mahboubi, E., and Sayed, G. M.: Oral Cavity and Pharynx. In Cancer Epidemiology and Prevention. Edited by D. Schottenfeld, and J. F. Fraumeni. Philadelphia, W.B. Saunders Company, 1982, p. 583.

93. Malkin, D., Li, F. P., Strong, L. C., Fraumeni, J. F., Jr., Nelson, C. E., Kim, D. H., Kassel, J., Gryka, M. A., Bischoff, F. Z., Tainsky, M. A., and Friend, S. H.: Germ line p53 mutations in a familial syndrome of breast cancer, sarcomas, and other neoplasms. Science 250:1233, 1990.

94. Mattson, M. E., and Winn, D. M.: Smokeless tobacco: association with increased cancer risk. NCI Monograph, 8:13, 1989.

95. McMichael, A. J.: Increases in laryngeal cancer in Britain and Australia in relation to alcohol and tobacco consumption trends. Lancet, 2:1244, 1978.

96. McWhorter, W. P., Schatzkin, A. G., Horm, J. W., and Brown, C. C.: Contribution of socioeconomic status to black/white differences in cancer incidence. Cancer, 63:982, 1989.

97. Meara, J., McPherson, K., Roberts, M., Jones, L., and Vessey, M.: Alcohol, cigarette smoking, and breast cancer. Br. J. Cancer, 60:70, 1989.

98. Menkes, M. S., Comstock, G. W., Vuilleumier, J. P., Helsing, K. J., Rider, A. A., and Brookmeyer, R.: Serum beta-carotene, vitamins A and E, selenium, and the risk of lung cancer. N. Engl. J. Med., 315:1250, 1986.

99. Monson, R. R.: Occupational Epidemiology. Boca Raton, CRC Press, 1980.

100. Mossman, B. T., and Gee, J. B. L.: Asbestos-related diseases. N. Engl. J. Med., 320:1721, 1989.

101. Mueller, N., Evans, A., Harris, N. L., Comstock, G. W., Jellum, E., Magnus, K., Orentreich, N., Polk, B. F., and Vogelman, J.: Hodgkin's disease and Epstein-Barr virus. N. Engl. J. Med., 320:689, 1989.

102. Nestle, M., and Bailar, J.: The Surgeon General's Report on Nutrition and Health. U.S. Government Printing Office, Washington, DC DHHS Publication No. 88-50210, 1988.

103. Nigro, J. M., Baker, S. J., Preisinger, A. C., Jessup, J. M., Hostetter, R., Cleary, K., Bignerm, S. H., Davidson, N., Baylin, S., Devilee, P., Glover, T., Collins, F. S., Weston, A., Modali, R., Harris, C. C., and Vogelstein, B.: A tumor suppressor gene, p53, has been implicated in tumor development in sporadic and familial cases of diverse tumors, including those of the Li-Fraumeni Syndrome. Nature, 342:705, 1989.

104. Oral-contraceptive use and the risk of breast cancer. The Cancer and Steroid Hormone Study of the Centers for Disease Control and the National Institute of Child Health and Human Development. N. Engl. J. Med., 315:405, 1986.

105. Pariza, M. W.: A perspective on diet, nutrition, and cancer. J.A.M.A., 251:455, 1984.

106. Parry, D. M., Mulvihill, J. J., Miller, R. W., Berg, K., and Carter, C. L.: Strategies for controlling cancer through genetics. Cancer Res., 47:6814, 1987.

107. Perera, F., Mayer, J., Jaretzki, A., Hearne, S., Brenner, D., Young, T. L., Fischman, H. K., Grimes, M., Grantham, S., Tang, M. X., Tsai, W.-Y., and Santella, R. M.: Comparison of DNA adducts and sister chromatid exchange in lung cancer cases and controls. Cancer Res. 49:4446, 1989.

108. Perera, F. P., and Weinstein, I. B.: Molecular epidemiology and carcinogen-DNA adduct detection: new approaches to studies of human cancer causation. J. Chron. Dis., 35:581, 1982.

109. Phillips, R. L.: Role of life-style and dietary habits in risk of cancer among Seventh-Day Adventists. Cancer Res., 35:3513, 1975.

110. Piper, J. M., Tonascia, J., and Matanoski, G. M.: Heavy phenacetin use and bladder cancer in women aged 20 to 49 years. N. Engl. J. Med., 313:292, 1985.

111. Pollack, E. S., Nomura, A. M. Y., Heilbrun, L. K., Stemmerman, G. N., and Green, S.

B.: Prospective study of alcohol consumption and cancer. N. Engl. J. Med., 310:617, 1984.

112. Preston, D. L., Kato, H., Kopecky, K. J., and Fujita, S.: Studies of the mortality of A-bomb survivors. Radiat. Res., 111:151, 1987.

113. Pui, C. H., Behm, F. G., Raimondi, S. C., Dodge, R. K., George, S. L., Rivera, G. K., Mirro, J., Jr., Kalwinsky, D. K., Dahl, G. V., and Murphy, S. B.: Secondary acute myeloid leukemia in children treated for acute lymphoid leukemia. N. Engl. J. Med., 321:136, 1989.

114. Report of an IARC Working Group: An evaluation of chemicals and industrial processes associated with cancer in humans based on human and animal data. IARC monographs volumes 1 - 20. Cancer Res., 40:12, 1980.

115. Robbins, J. H.: Xeroderma pigmentosum. Defective DNA repair causes skin cancer and neurodegeneration. J.A.M.A., 260:384, 1988.

116. Rosen, S.: Xeroderma pigmentosum. Defective DNA repair causes skin cancer and neurodegeneration. J.A.M.A., 260:384, 1988.

117. Sattin, R. W., Rubin, G. L., Webster, L. A., Huezo, C. M., Wingo, P. A., Ory, H. W., and Layde, P. M.: Family history and the risk of breast cancer. J.A.M.A., 253:1908, 1985.

118. Schatzkin, A., Carter, C. L., Green, S. B., Kreger, B. E., Splansky G. L., Anderson, K. M., Helsel, W. E., and Kannel, W. B.: Is alcohol consumption related to breast cancer? Results from the Framingham heart study. J. Natl. Cancer Inst., 81:31, 1989.

119. Schatzkin, A., Greenwald, P., Byar, D. P., and Clifford, C. K.: The dietary fat-breast cancer hypothesis is alive. J.A.M.A., 261:3284, 1989.

120. Schatzkin, A., Jones, D. Y., Hoover, R. N., Taylor, P. R., Brinton, L. A., Ziegler, R. G., Harvey, E. B., Carter, C. L., Licitra, L. N., Dufour, M. C., and Larson, D. B.: Alcohol consumption and breast cancer in the epidemiologic follow-up study of the first National Health and Nutrition Examination Survey. N. Engl. J. Med., 316:1169, 1987.

121. Schlesselman, J. J.: Case-Control Studies: Design, Conduct, Analysis. New York, Oxford University Press, 1982.

122. Schmahl, D., Thomas, C., and Auer, R.: Iatrongenic Carcinogenesis. Berlin, Springer-Verlag, 1977.

123. Sellers, T. A., Bailey-Wilson, J. E., Elston, R. C., Wilson, A. F., Elston, G. Z., Ooi, W. L., and Rothschild, H.: Evidence for Mendelian inheritance in the pathogenesis of lung cancer. J. Natl. Cancer Inst., 82:1272, 1990.

124. Shapiro, S., Kelly, J. P., Rosenberg, L., Kaufman, D. W., Helmrich, S. P., Rosenshein, N. B., Lewis, J.L., Jr., Knapp, R. C., Stolley, P. D., and Schottenfeld, D.: Risk of localized and widespread endometrial cancer in relation to recent and discontinued use of conjugated estrogens. N. Engl. J. Med., 313:969, 1985.

125. Skegg, D. C., Corwin, P. A., Paul, C., and Doll, R.: Importance of the male factor in cancer of the cervix. Lancet, II:581, 1982.

126. Slattery, M. L., Schuman, K. L., West, D. W., French, T. K., and Robison, L. M.: Nutrient intake and ovarian cancer. Am. J. Epidemiol., 130:497, 1989.

127. Smith, P. G., Kinlen, L. J., White, G. C., Adelstein, A. M., and Fox, A. J.: Mortality of wives of men dying with cancer of the penis. Br. J. Cancer, 41:422, 1980.

128. Smoking and Health: A report of the surgeon general. US Dept of Health, Education, and Welfare, DHEW Publication No (PHS) 79-50066. Government Printing Office, Washington, DC, 1979.

129. Spirtas, R., Beebe, G. W., Connelly, R. R., Wright, W. E., Peters, J. M., Sherwin, R. P., Henderson, B. E., Stark A., Kovasznay, B. M., and Davies, J. N.: Recent trends in mesothelioma incidence in the United States. Am. J. Med., 9:397, 1986.

130. Sponner, C. M.: Asbestos in schools: A public health problem. N. Engl. J. Med., 301:782, 1979.

131. Strong, L. C., Stine, M., and Norsted, T. L.: Cancer in survivors of childhood soft tissue sarcoma and their relatives. J. Natl. Cancer Inst., 79:1213, 1987.

132. Travis, L. B., Curtis, R. E., Boice, J. D., Jr., and Fraumeni, J. F., Jr.: Bladder cancer after chemotherapy for non-Hodgkin's lymphoma. N. Engl. J. Med., 321:544, 1989.

133. Tucker, M. A., D'Angio, G. J., Boice, J. D., Jr., Strong, L. C., Li, F. P., Stovall, M., Stone, B. J., Green, D. M., Lombardi, F., and Newton, W.: Bone sarcomas linked to radiotherapy and chemotherapy in children. N. Engl. J. Med., 312:588, 1987.

134. Tucker, M. A., Shields, J. A., Hartge, P., Augsburger, J., Hoover, R. N., and Fraumeni, J. F., Jr.: Sunlight exposure as risk factor for intraocular malignant melanoma. N. Engl. J. Med., 313:789, 1985.

135. Upton, A. C.: oncogenic effects of low-level ionizing radiation. J. Natl. Cancer Inst., 82:448, 1990.

136. Villa, L. L., and Franco, E. L.: Epidemiologic correlates of cervical neoplasia and risk of human papillomavirus infection in asymptomatic women in Brazil. J. Natl. Cancer Inst., 81:332, 1989.

137. Wagner, J. C., Sleggs, C. A., and Marchang, P.: Diffuse pleural mesothelioma and asbestos exposure in the North Western Cape Province. Br. J. Ind. Med., 17:260, 1960.

138. Walker, W. J., and Brin, B. N.: U.S. lung cancer mortality and declining cigarette tobacco consumption. J. Clin. Epidemiol., 41:179, 1988.

139. Walter, H. J., Vaughan, R. D., and Wynder, E. L.: Primary prevention of cancer among children: Changes in cigarette smoking and diet after six years of intervention. J. Natl. Cancer Inst., 81:995, 1989.

140. Warner, K. E.: Cigarette smoking in the 1970's: The impact of the antismoking campaign on consumption. Science, 211:729, 1981.

141. White, J. R., and Froeb, H. F.: Small-airways dysfunction in nonsmokers chronically exposed to tobacco smoke. N. Engl. J. Med., 302:720, 1980.

142. White, E., Lee, C. Y., and Kristal, A. R.: Evaluation of the increase in breast cancer incidence in relation to mammography use. J. Natl. Cancer Inst., 82:1546, 1990.

143. Wigle, D. T., Semenciw, R. M., Wilkins, K., Riedel, D., Ritter, L., Morrison, H. I., and Mao, Y.: Mortality study of Canadian male farm operators: Non-Hodgkin's lymphoma mortality and agricultural practices in Saskatchewan. J. Natl. Cancer Inst., 82:575, 1990.

144. Willett, W.: The search for the causes of breast and colon cancer. Nature, 338:389, 1989.

145. Willett, W. C., and MacMahon, B.: Diet and cancer–an overview (pt1). N. Engl. J. Med., 310:633, 1984.

146. Willett, W. C., Stampfer, M. J., Colditz, G. A., Rosner, B. A., Hennekens C. H., and Speizer, F. E.: Moderate alcohol consumption and the risk of breast cancer. N. Engl. J. Med., 316:1174, 1987.

147. Willett, W. C., Stampfer, M. J., Colditz, G. A., Rosner, B. A., Hennekens, C. H., and

Speizer, F. E.: Dietary fat and the risk of breast cancer. N. Engl. J. Med., 316:22, 1987.

148. Willett, W. C., Stampfer, M. J., Colditz, G. A., Rosner, B. A., and Speizer, F. E.: Relation of meat, fat, and fiber intake to the risk of colon cancer in a propective study among women. N. Engl. J. Med., 323:1664, 1990.

149. Winn, D. M., Blot, W. J., Shy, C. M., Pickle, L. W., Toledo, A., and Fraumeni, J. F., Jr.: Snuff dipping and oral cancer among women in the southern United States. N. Engl. J. Med., 304:745, 1981.

150. You, W. C., Blot, W. J., Chang, Y. S., Ershow, A. G., Yang, Z. T., An, Q., Henderson, B., Xu, G. W., Fraumeni, J. F., Jr., and Wang, T. G.: Diet and high risk of stomach cancer in Shandong, China. Cancer Res., 48:3518, 1988.

151. Young, J. L., Gloekler Ries, L., Silverberg, E., Horm, J. W., and Miller, R. W.: Cancer incidence, survival, and mortality for children younger than age 15 years. Cancer, 58:598, 1986.

152. Zeckhauser, R. J., and Viscusi, W. K.: Risk within reason. Science, 248:559, 1990.

153. Zur Hausen, H.: Papillomaviruses in anogenital cancer as a model to understand the role of viruses in human cancers. Cancer Res., 49:4677, 1989.

V

Theory and Practice of Clinical Trials

Marvin Zelen

Introduction

The modern era of therapeutics in cancer is dominated by clinical data arising from cancer clinical trials. The reliance on clinical trial methodology to generate scientific data on the value of therapies has not only been adopted by the oncology community, but is true for all chronic diseases. The United States' effort to find AIDS therapies is relying solely on clinical trials. Applications for drug approval to the U.S. Food and Drug Administration (FDA) can only be made on the basis of scientific evidence generated by clinical trials. The development and widespread acceptance of clinical trials is one of the major conceptual advances in experimental therapeutics made in the latter half of the twentieth century. Sir Bradford Hill was one of the key biostatistical scientists who recognized the importance of clinical trials in medicine and formulated many of the present-day foundations.[6]

A clinical trial is defined as an experiment on humans being carried out in order to evaluate one or more potentially beneficial therapies. The clinical investigator is assumed to have control of both the therapies that are to be evaluated and the patient population to which these therapies will be administered.

The basic ideas associated with clinical trials have been discussed for at least 150 years. An important intellectual landmark is the treatise *Essays in Clinical Instruction,* written by French physician, P.C.A. Louis in 1834.[8] His book advocated the use of the "numerical method" to study the benefits of therapy. His view was that only with "counting" is it possible to learn about the scientific basis of medicine. However, counting is not easy. It is necessary to take into account the different circumstances of age, sex, temperament, physical condition, natural history of the disease, and errors in giving therapy. He wrote, "The only reproach which can be made to the Numerical Method is that it offers real difficulties in its execution. . . . this method requires much more labor and time than the most distinguished members of our profession can dedicate to it." Dr. Louis's comments are just as appropriate today as when he wrote them.

Types of Clinical Trials

Ordinary clinical trials are characterized by three phases, which are referred to as Phase I, II, or III trials. The characterization of these trials has arisen from drug trials, but the language has been used for radiotherapy and surgery trials as well.

A Phase I trial refers to a new treatment (usually a drug) that is to be tried on humans for the first time. The aim is to find an acceptable dose and schedule with respect to toxicity. The use of the term "acceptable" is particularly important. Therapies for life-threatening illnesses will generally allow for greater risks of serious side effects than those therapies that are targeted at less serious illnesses. In cancer, patients who are refractory to therapies believed to be beneficial are usually the patients who are entered on Phase I trials. As a result, the evaluation of side effects on this very advanced disease population may not necessarily be the same for patients who ultimately will receive the therapy for an evaluation of benefit.

Phase II cancer trials are initiated after the completion of Phase I trials. The goal is to determine if the therapy has any beneficial effect. Sometimes the patient population in Phase II trials is composed of newly diagnosed patients with advanced cancer. Entering newly diagnosed patients may be justified in non-small cell lung cancer trials, but may not be appropriate for cancer sites for which therapies with proven benefit do exist. As a result, most patients entering Phase II trials are those who are no longer benefiting from therapies believed to be beneficial. The dilemma of Phase II trials is that the trial may not be a satisfactory test of an experimental therapy if a patient population is used that has failed or has been found to be unresponsive to therapies with proven benefit. Another criticism of Phase II trials is that some trials are designed to investigate a single dose and schedule while others are testing combinations of drugs. The particular dose-schedule combination(s) of a drug(s) may be far from optimal. Scientific considerations dictate that tests of drugs in Phase II trials should be over a spectrum of doses and schedules that still have acceptable toxicity. In some circumstances it may be appropriate to combine Phase I and II trials into a single Phase I–II trial.

Phase III studies are always comparative trials: one or more experimental therapies are compared with the best standard therapy or competitive therapies. They tend to have many more patients than Phase II trials and often require patients from many cooperating hospitals.

Randomized vs. Nonrandomized Clinical Trials

The fundamental scientific principle underlying the comparison of patient groups receiving different therapies is that the groups must be alike in all important aspects and only differ in the treatment that each group receives. Otherwise, differences between the groups may not be due to the treatments under study, but may be attributed to the particular characteristics of the group. In clinical experimentation, the patients may vary widely in their ability to respond to therapy. Furthermore, the therapies cannot be exactly reproduced from occasion to occasion, in contrast to the physical sciences, in which the treatments applied to the experimental units are exactly reproducible and the experimental units are homogeneous. Variability in clinical experimentation arises from the heterogeneity of the patient populations and the lack of exact reproducibility of the treatment, whereas in the physical sciences variability is often a secondary factor and arises from slight changes in the ambient environment and the variability of the measuring instrument.

The use of randomization refers to the process used to generate comparable patient groups. The term randomization refers to allocating the treatments to the patients using a chance mechanism. It is equivalent to tossing a coin to assign therapies when only two treatments are under investigation. Classical randomized clinical trials require that neither the physician nor the patient know in advance the treatment to be given prior to entering a trial. The device of randomization makes the treatment groups "alike on the average" with respect to all factors that are likely to affect the principal end-points of a trial. Randomization ensures that each patient in a study has the same opportunity of being assigned to any of the therapies in the trial. In actual practice a randomization schedule is chosen from a table of random numbers.[13] These are tables in which every number has the same chance of occurring in every part of the table.

Randomized clinical trials (often designated as RCTs) are regarded by many investigators as the "ideal" scientific standard for comparing therapies. The device of randomization creates balanced patient subgroups that have the same average baseline characteristics. This "balance" not only applies to known prognostic factors, but to unknown prognostic factors as well. Randomization eliminates both physician and patient selection biases. The former refers to the physician creating a bias by only putting a special class of patients on one of the treatments, e.g., assigning the patients in poorest physical condition to the least toxic treatment. The patient selection bias refers to a comparable bias, but is induced by the patient.

Another implicit advantage of an RCT is that the experimental therapy is compared with a concurrent control group. Hence every group in the trial will have the same criteria for diagnosing and staging of the disease, patient management, and supportive care and the same data quality and methods of evaluation.

Despite the widespread acceptance of the scientific merits of randomization, many physicians are reluctant to participate in RCTs.[12] The principal reason for non-participation is that physicians feel that the patient–physician relationship is compromised if the physician has to explain to the patient that the treatment for their cancer would be chosen by a "toss of a coin" or by a "computer." The U.S. Code of Federal Regulations governing human experimentation has been interpreted to imply that a physician must tell the patient about the use of randomization. As a result of the non-participation by elements of the population with disease, the results of an RCT may not necessarily apply to the entire patient population. Caution must be exercised when extrapolating the inference from a clinical trial to the entire population with disease.

An interesting example of biases which arise in physician and patient selection is illustrated in the trial reported by Antman et al.[2] An RCT was carried out jointly by the Dana Farber Cancer Institute and the Massachusetts General Hospital for the treatment of sarcoma (intermediate, high grade). The trial compared Adriamycin against observation (no active treatment). Over a period of time, there were 84 eligible patients seen in both institutions of whom only 36 were entered on the RCT. Among the 48 patients who did not go on trial, half was due each to patient or physician refusal. Of the 48 patients, 29 did not receive any active treatment and for all practical purposes received the same treatment as the control treatment of the RCT. Thus, the control arm of the RCT and a portion of the patient population (non-randomized) can be compared. The 20-month disease-free survival for the control patients in the RCT was 64% compared with 16% for the non-randomized patients receiving no treatment; the 30-month survival was 68% for the RCT controls compared with 29% of the non-randomized controls. Even after adjustment for differences in prognostic factors, the differences still persisted. This example illustrates the need for concurrent control groups.

As a consequence of the unpopularity of RCTs with many physicians, there are many non-randomized trials aimed at making conclusions about the value of an experimental treatment. Generally, data on an experimental treatment is generated prospectively and compared with an historical "control" group of patients. Of course, if the value of treatment is overwhelmingly beneficial no comparison may be necessary. For example, if patients with pancreatic cancer are living long periods of time (say, 5 years) without evidence of disease, no formal comparison is necessary since we know the prognosis of this disease is uniformly dismal. Unfortunately, the available therapies for cancer are not likely to result in dramatic benefits. Consequently, the benefit of an active therapy is likely to be of moderate magnitude, requiring care in the evaluation. Moderate benefits are of real clinical importance, e.g., increasing the cure rate of breast cancer by 10–20%, will result in the savings of thousands of lives.

The use of historical controls for evaluating the benefits of an experimental therapy is fraught with many problems. There are ample opportunities for serious biases to distort the conclusions. Even when known biases are considered, there may be other unknown biases that can distort the conclusions of a clinical trial.

Nevertheless, non-randomized trials may be important as part of the overall scientific process in evaluating an experimental treatment. They have a role in pilot and exploratory studies as well as Phase II trials. Consider a Phase II study to identify an active drug or drug combination. Good scientific strategy would dictate that the study be carried out in the most desirable conditions possible to identify an active therapy, e.g., selection of patient population. However, the comparison of the magnitude of the effect with other available therapies is best done with an RCT.

The reporting of a non-randomized trial requires special care—especially when claims are made about efficacy. The reporting should address the potential biases that could affect the conclusions. Below are six sources of biases that arise in all non-randomized trials that employ a comparison with an historical control group.

Physician Selection Bias. Selection of patients for the experimental treatment may be biased. This is not true in RCTs.

Patient Selection Bias. Patients self-select themselves for the experimental treatment. There is no self-selection in the historical control group. This leads to potential biases in comparing outcome with an historical control group. RCTs have patient self-selection only for those who enter the trial. However, since the assignment to treatment is randomized, the self-selection does not bias comparisons between therapies within the same trial.

Diagnosis and Staging. Methods of diagnosis and staging must be the same for the experimental therapy and the historical groups. If methods have improved during recent years this may not be reflected in the historical control group. For example, a significant number of newly diagnosed breast cancer cases are found by mammography. This precludes using an historical group for comparisons of adjuvant treatment unless one takes account of the method of diagnosis. The problem does not exist with a concurrent control group.

Patient Management and Supportive Care. This must be the same for both groups.

Evaluation Methods. This factor reflects on the quality of the data. If the historical control group has significant missing or unknown data for important variables, then unbiased comparisons may be impossible.

Prognostic Factors. The key prognostic factors must be the same for both groups. Statistical adjustments can often be used to make the groups comparable when the prognostic factors are known. It is not possible to adjust when data are missing or if there are unknown prognostic factors.

E. Frei III has suggested that complex staging is a strong argument against the use of historical controls. He cites the time when metastatic colon cancer was considered incurable. Early stages had variable prognoses, with a high death rate. When adjuvant therapy became available, through clinical trials, staging was pursued much more vigorously. As a result, more lymph nodes are examined, multiple step sections are made, and liver biopsies are carried out. Consequently, a higher proportion of more recent patients may be in a better prognostic state than controls, even though they

may both be classified in the same stage. Since they have better prognoses, their survival will be greater than the historical controls.

Use of consecutive patients for generating data on the new treatment and use of "matched" controls are two common methods for investigating new treatments without resorting to randomization. Both have their drawbacks. Entering consecutive patients on a study eliminates the opportunity for physician bias associated with the selection of patients. However, if patient consent is necessary, a patient selection bias will still be present. If the mix of patients has not changed over time, the prognostic variables associated with each group may be comparable. However, issues such as patient bias, diagnosis and staging, patient management and supportive care, and different methods of evaluation must still be considered. The consecutive patient experimental design is targeted mainly at eliminating the bias arising from physician selection of patients.

Employment of matched controls is another method often used to compare a new treatment with an historical control. This involves forming a group of one or more control patients for each patient receiving the new treatment. Patients are selected from the historical group so that they are comparable to the new treatment group on a patient-by-patient basis for known prognostic variables. This method is limited in that only a few key variables can be matched on any practical basis. For example, in matching one would perhaps aim to have patients who are comparable with respect to anatomic staging, pathology, performance status, and extradisease characteristics such as demographic factors, prior treatment history, and so forth.

Statistical modeling is a generalization of matching that enables one to adjust for several factors simultaneously. However, this method also has limitations, as the statistical adjustment for bias introduces additional variability in the analysis due to the "uncertainty" of the adjustment. Such adjustments can be made only for known prognostic factors. Patient and physician self-selection cannot be factored into the adjustments. Neither can questions about different criteria for diagnosis and staging, different methods of patient support and management, and different methods of evaluation.

In summary, the non-randomized methods for evaluation of new therapies are useful for exploratory and pilot studies. They are not to be relied on for generating credible conclusions, unless the issues of potential biases are carefully discussed, or the therapy outcome is so dramatic that it could not be credited to the aggregate effect of the potential biases.

Another type of non-randomized study which is likely to gain more popularity in the future is the study that attempts to correlate disease markers with survival. The simplest example is to relate tumor response for measurable disease with eventual survival. The logic is that patients enter a trial with a positive disease marker (e.g., tumor), receive treatment and the tumor becomes smaller or disappears. Survival comparisons are made between patient groups with positive marker versus negative marker (tumor has significant reduction in volume or disappears). A straightforward comparison as described is *invalid*;[1] the reason being that the longer a patient lives, the greater the opportunity to observe a change in disease marker status. This means that even if change of marker status is *not* related to increased survival, a direct comparison of survival data negative vs. positive disease markers will show a positive relationship. This relationship is spurious. However, new statistical techniques of analysis are now being developed that can overcome this problem.[7] It is expected that the new techniques will strengthen Phase II studies in that they will enable inferences to be made relating change in marker status to survival (or any other appropriate time metric). However, inference will only be able to answer the question, "Is a change in disease marker positively related to survival for the patients under study?"

Multicenter vs. Single-Center Trials

The available experimental therapies for cancer are likely to have only moderate therapeutic benefit. Nevertheless, a moderate benefit can be important. For example, the number of new female breast cancer cases diagnosed in a year is estimated to be more than 85,000. Approximately half of these new cases have positive axillary nodal involvement. If the cure rate were increased by 10%, then at least 4,000 more women would be cured every year.

The end-points for nearly all definitive Phase III studies are survival or the disease-free period. Furthermore, the clinical course of the disease is complicated and highly variable. As a consequence of both the need for making an inference on survival and the variability of the data, it is necessary to have a relatively long follow-up time on a large number of patients. Since few hospitals have enough patients to meet this need, it is necessary to carry out these Phase III trials using many cooperating hospitals. Consequently, nearly all Phase III trials are multicenter trials in which patients are pooled into a common study. Carrying out a multicenter trial results in increased administrative difficulties and quality assurance problems. It is one of the most difficult and complicated experiments in science.

Multicenter studies are used not only in Phase III clinical trials, but in Phase II trials as well. The use of multicenters enables patient accrual goals to be achieved much more rapidly. Table V-1-1 is a summary of current practice with regard to multicenter studies and their use in Phases I, II, and III trials.

Planning Clinical Trials

Overall Considerations in Planning Clinical Trials

The overall planning for a clinical trial depends critically on whether the trial is an "exploratory" or "management" trial. A management trial seeks to determine whether a therapy is beneficial under conditions as close to clinical circumstances as possible. Sometimes the term "demonstra-

tion trial" is used to describe a management trial. A management trial should be carried out by a large number of hospitals. In this way it will be possible to determine if a therapy is beneficial when the trial is collecting data from a large group of representative hospitals. An exploratory trial seeks to determine whether a therapy is efficacious under ideal or restricted circumstances, which may not necessarily correspond to a practical clinical situation.

Objectives in clinical trials may greatly vary. Possible objectives are: 1) to find the best treatment; 2) to find the best treatment by prognostic subgroup; 3) to determine the relationship between the natural history of disease and treatment; 4) to identify an active treatment; and 5) to evaluate the effects of augmenting a beneficial therapy.

The choice of the eligible patient population in a trial is crucial to reaching accrual goals in a reasonable time. It is necessary to decide whether to have narrow eligibility requirements so that patients are relatively homogeneous with regard to baseline prognostic variables or to have broad eligibility requirements that will accelerate accrual. The pros and cons about the choice of the population depend on whether the trial is a management or exploratory trial. If the trial is an exploratory trial, then having a relatively homogeneous patient population will result in less variability in the end-points of the trial and will make the trial more sensitive in showing differences among the treatments. Alternatively, if the trial is a management trial, there is some advantage in having broad eligibility criteria as one will be able to explore how therapy benefit varies among subgroups of patients. Using post-hoc stratification and statistical modeling in the analysis of the trial will reduce the statistical fluctuations generated from having heterogeneous patient groups. An operational problem with defining narrow eligibility criteria is that accrual may take a long time.

Another basic decision in the choice of population is to determine whether the patient population should be newly diagnosed or should include patients who have been shown to be refractory to beneficial therapies. A newly diagnosed patient represents the most promising patient material for study. On the other hand, it is necessary to consider the ethics of withholding therapies of proven benefit in favor of an experimental treatment having unknown benefit. If one chooses to use a patient population that is refractory to beneficial therapies, then it may not be possible to evaluate the experimental therapy suitably. The decision on choice of patient population in a trial must strike a balance between the ethics of denying a patient a beneficial (but still noncurative) therapy compared with the opportunity of a patient's receiving an experimental therapy with the potential of significantly better benefit relative to the withheld treatment.

Another consideration in planning a study is to determine the treatment plan if the patient has failed or does not appear

Table V-1-1. Characterization of Clinical Trials

| Phase | Single Center | | Multicenter | |
	Randomized	Non-Randomized	Non-Randomized	Randomized
I	Never	Yes	Never	Rare
II	Rare	Yes	Yes	Yes
III	Yes	Use of historical controls	Yes	Use of historical controls

to be benefitting from the treatment. Does one not change the treatment or should a new therapy plan be prescribed? If the end-point is survival, then introducing a new therapy may complicate the interpretation of the survival data. On the other hand, if the protocol does not specify what to do after failure, the attending physicians may introduce a large number of new therapies, which will even further complicate the interpretation of the survival information.

It is generally accepted that Phase III trials should be randomized. However, should Phase II trials be randomized? Since the object of a Phase II trial is to determine if there is any activity against the disease rather than to make comparisons with other therapies, most Phase II trials are non-randomized. One reason for evaluating several therapies in the same Phase II trial, though, is to try to evaluate them simultaneously with the same clinical trial process and for the same patient population. Another strategy is to include as one of the therapies a treatment that has proven benefit, but which has not yet been used on the Phase II patient population. If the therapy with prior proven benefit cannot demonstrate benefit, then the Phase II trial may not have a suitable patient population to permit the evaluation of the experimental therapies. Thus, if several therapies are to be evaluated in the same Phase II trial, randomization should be used for the treatment assignment.

What end-points should be chosen to evaluate the therapies? There is widespread agreement that adjuvant trials should use survival as an end-point. However, patients who have recurrent disease will receive additional or alternate therapies. This will certainly be true for placebo or no treatment control patients. Those on therapy will also receive alternate therapies on recurrence. Thus the survival data may not be clear-cut. Other end-points could be the disease-free period, and time to "progression" (progression must be carefully defined). Phase II trials often use tumor response or other disease markers. In practice, there will be a number of end-points in any trial.

During the past few years, there has been an increase in the use of surrogate markers as the major end-point of Phase III studies. Some disease markers have a high correlation with survival. The idea is that conclusions about treatment benefit can be made in a shorter time frame. For example, many Phase III trials in AIDS use the CD4 + counts as the major end-point. In cancer, complete responses may have high correlation with survival. A problem with using a gross measurement like complete response in cancer, versus a survival end-point, is that in many cancers the anticipated frequency of complete responses is still too low to provide meaningful comparisons.

Quality of life issues are being widely recognized as important end-points in cancer. (See XX.) A patient cured of leukemia by bone marrow transplantation who has chronic graft versus host disease has a severely compromised quality of life. The paper by Goldhirsch et al.[5] discusses new methods for objectively evaluating quality of life. It represents an important advance. They call their method Q-TWiST (Quality-adjusted Time Without Symptoms and Toxicity of treatment).

Statistical Tests and Probabilities of Reaching Incorrect Conclusions

Almost all clinical trials are analyzed using statistical procedures that are based on the frequency theory of proba-

bility. This simply means that if, for example, an outcome has a probability of happening of 10% in an experiment, then in an infinite number of repetitions of the experiment, one would observe the outcome 10% of the time. It will be assumed in all that follows that probability statements refer to the relative frequency notion of probability.

Consider a trial in which two treatments are being evaluated. After the trial is completed and an analysis is made, the two main conclusions are that: 1) the treatments are equivalent; or 2) the treatments differ. These two conclusions are referred to as the null and alternate hypothesis, respectively. The statistical procedures (called tests) chosen for analysis enable the specification of the error probabilities (α, β), i.e.,

$\alpha = $ probability of concluding treatments are different when they are actually the same

$\beta = $ probability of concluding treatments are the same when they are actually different

The two probabilities are often referred to as type I and II errors, respectively. These error probabilities are the false-positive and false-negative rates, respectively, i.e., calling a result positive when it should be negative and calling a result negative when it should be positive.

The practical application of these tests is that using the observed data from the trial one calculates a probability or significance level. This is the probability of observing the same or more extreme differences among therapies than those observed if in actuality the two treatments are equivalent. The reasoning behind the probability calculations is that if the investigator is willing to accept the differences observed in the trial as being scientific evidence in favor of a difference between the two treatments, then the scientific evidence would be stronger if the differences were larger than those observed. This probability is called a tail area, significance level, or simply the P value. If the P value is less than .05, then the practice is to accept the hypothesis that the treatments do differ. Thus, if the treatments are truly equivalent, the probability would be less than 5% that the observed differences among the treatments could have arisen from statistical fluctuations in the data.

The power or sensitivity of a test is equal to $1 - \beta$ and denotes the probability that the clinical trial will be able to detect differences among the treatments when in fact the differences are real. The power is fundamental in planning all clinical trials. It depends on: the significance level chosen, the number of patients in the trial, and the magnitude of the difference between the treatments. Large numbers of patients and large differences between treatments increase the power. In studies in which survival is an end-point, longer follow-up time also increases the power.

When a trial comes to the conclusion that there is "no difference between the treatments" or the result is not "statistically significant," it may be because: 1) either there is no difference between the treatments; or 2) the power of the trial was so low that the trial was unable to detect a difference.

We will illustrate the concept of power and its relation to sample size in a Phase I trial. Suppose a Phase I trial is being conducted to determine the probability of life-threatening toxicity from an experimental drug. Suppose that if no life-threatening toxicity is observed the drug will be declared to be "free of life-threatening toxicity." Table V-1-2 shows the relationship between true toxicity rate, number of patients, and the power (probability of observing at least one life-threatening toxic event). For example, if only five patients are in the trial and the true toxicity rate is 10%, there is only a 41% probability of observing one or more toxic reactions. As the sample size increases this probability goes to unity. Similarly, if the true toxic rate is high, it is easy to show that the power is increased, e.g., if the toxic rate is 40% and only five patients are in the trial, the power is 0.92. This same table can also be used to determine the probability of observing one or more responses or solutions to any problem in which events are being observed.

As another example of the use of power in a clinical trial, consider a trial in which the proportion of recurrences is the principal end-point of interest. Suppose one desires to calculate the sample size necessary to detect a difference between two groups when one group has a recurrence rate of 60% and another group may have a possible recurrence rate within the range 30 to 55%. Table V-1-3 shows the number of patients per treatment for different levels of power comparing the two recurrence rates. For example, one needs more than 2,000 patients for each treatment group in order to have a power of .9 to detect a difference between 55% vs. 60%. However, the sample size is reduced to 130 patients per group to test 40% vs. 60% for the same power (.9). It is clear that increasing the number of patients results in an increase in power. Also, as the differences between groups become large, a high level of power can be attained for the same sample size.

In practice one does not know the recurrence rates to compare. A range of comparisons is chosen, based on past data that are of clinical interest, and a sample size is then chosen that will give high power. Generally, a power less than 80% for clinically important differences is unacceptable in planning a clinical trial.

Data Collection and Forms Design

There is a great deal of misunderstanding of the amount of data required to evaluate a clinical trial properly. Ordinarily clinical trials carried on by the pharmaceutical industry with the intent of submitting the trial to the FDA for drug approval collect very large amounts of data. A great deal of this data may be unnecessary. It is not uncommon to have data forms exceeding 100 pages for each patient. One reason motivating the large collection of data items is the "antagonistic" relationship between FDA and industry. Essentially, industry-sponsored data collection plans have the theme "to leave no stone unturned." Another motivating factor is that many trials are planned to show that two treatments are equivalent ("me too trials"). Usually a new drug is compared with a competitor's drug that has already received FDA approval. Large amounts of data are collected in these trials in order to be able to answer unanticipated questions that might be raised by the FDA.

Disregarding the special problems between the FDA and industry, the data chosen for collection in a clinical trial must supply information to determine: 1) eligibility of patient; 2) whether the protocol was followed; and 3) objective measures of the study end-points. In general, the more data collected the greater the opportunity for data degradation. A non-randomized study attempting to make treatment comparisons would ordinarily require a greater amount of data to check for biases than a randomized study. A randomized study, by definition, has comparable patient groups that differ only in the treatment assigned to the groups.

In general a cancer clinical trial is likely to have six different types of forms for collecting data as well as special forms. The data forms and types of information collected are outlined in Table V-1-4.

The data forms should be designed so that they are self-

Table V-1-2. Probability of Observing at Least One Toxic Event as a Function of True Rate and Number of Patients in Trial[a]

True Toxicity (%)	Number of Patients			
	5	10	20	30
10	.41	.65	.88	.96
20	.67	.89	.99	.999
30	.89	.97	.999	1.0
40	.92	.994	1.0	1.0
50	.97	.999	1.0	1.0

[a]Example: If true toxicity is 10% and observations are made on 10 patients, there is a probability of 0.65 that at least one of the patients will show toxicity.

Table V-1-3. Number of Patients Per Treatment Required to Detect Differences Between Proportions for Different Values of Power[a]

Proportion Comparisons	Power				
	0.3	0.5	0.7	0.8	0.9
55% vs. 60%	406	752	1,202	1,530	2,050
50% vs. 60%	103	190	304	390	520
40% vs. 60%	27	48	77	97	130
30% vs. 60%	12	22	34	44	56

[a]The test assumes a two-sided false-positive rate of 5%.

Table V-1-4. Characteristics of Data Collection Forms in Cancer Clinical Trials

Form Identification	Data Items
On Study	Identification, demographic characters, disease presentation, prior treatment history, special tests, protocol treatment
Flow Sheet(s)	Record of each visit, treatment given, tests, disease assessment, intercurrent medications, toxicity, psychologic assessment, other events
Evaluation (at end of every step in study)	Summary of outcome, toxicity, medications received, confounding events
Follow-up (periodic)	Patient status
Death Form	Cause of death, autopsy results if available
Final Evaluation	Summary of relevant patient information
Special Forms	Surgery, pathology, radiation therapy, psychological assessments (self or observer), special diagnostic tests

coding. As much as possible, boxes need only be checked to supply information. Care should be taken to prevent the person filling in the form from making interpretive decisions, e.g., calling a toxicity life-threatening. Space should be provided to allow the physician to note or comment on special features of the patient that were not collected by the data form or that require further comment.

Experimental Design

In this section we briefly discuss experimental design for randomized studies. Generally Phase III cancer clinical trials have two to four treatment groups. The reason for keeping the number of treatments small is that the patient consent process requires the physician to discuss all treatment options with the patient. Having more than four different treatment programs is likely to be too confusing to the patient. The logistics of having a large number of treatments in a multicenter trial may also be overwhelming.

Clinical trials utilizing randomization are ordinarily designed using stratified randomization.[13] After a patient is found eligible for a trial, he/she may be classified into two or more subgroups or strata that are defined by data available at the time of registering a patient in the trial. The subgroup should be defined so that patients in the same strata have a more common prognosis than patients from different strata. For example, a study for advanced breast cancer may have eight strata defined by: 1) performance status (0, 1 vs. 2, 3); 2) number of recurrent sites (two or less vs. more than two); and 3) disease-free interval (1 year vs. greater than 1 year). All possible combinations of these three factors result in eight distinct strata. Within each stratum, the treatments are assigned at random. Stratification tends to balance the treatment assignments so that the treatment groups are equally balanced among the different strata. This is especially important in the early stages of a study in which only a small number of patients have been registered. If unexpected events are observed (e.g., unusual toxicities) within a treatment group, one would be able to analyze whether the event arose due to an aggregate of prognostic factors in one treatment group that was not present in other groups. As the number of patients becomes large, the patient groups tend to be comparable on the average and the need for stratification diminishes or even disappears. Relatively small clinical trials should always be stratified however.

There are obvious practical limits to the number of strata that can be utilized. If there is a large number of strata relative to the number of patients, then many of the strata will not have any patients. Having empty strata does not cause a loss of efficiency. If the number of patients in a single stratum is less than the number of treatments, however, there will be a loss of efficiency. For example, if there are two treatments, then all strata containing only one patient will not contribute to the analysis, unless additional modeling assumptions are made. In practice, the maximum number of patient/disease variables in a trial is about 12–15 for trials involving several hundred patients. A rough "rule of thumb" is that the (number of patients per treatment)/(number of strata) ≥ 4.

Table V-1-5 shows a variety of experimental designs that have been found to be useful in Phase III trials. It is assumed in all of these experimental designs that the only patients who are randomized are those who have given patient consent. As the designs become more complicated, the statistical methods for analysis also become more complex.

Another kind of experimental design that should be used more often is the factorial experiment. Suppose the class of therapies can be characterized by two factors, which will be designated A and B, e.g., A might refer to drug A and B to drug B. Suppose that drugs A and B are given at two doses A_0, A_1 for drug A and B_0, B_1 for drug B. Then there will be four drug combinations given by A_0B_0, A_0B_1, A_1B_0, and A_1B_1. If the clinical trial is carried out with these four groups then one can determine: 1) if a low dose is different from a higher dose of A or B; and 2) if there is an interaction (synergy) between A and B. In general, the factors may refer to different modalities of treatment, or dose or schedule. The advantage of a factorial design is that it enables two questions to be answered for the same patient. Factorial experiments need not be restricted to two factors, and the number of conditions for each factor need not be two. However, due to the need to keep the number of treatment groups small, the factorial design with two factors each under two different conditions appears to be the most practical in clinical trials.

In some instances it may be possible to investigate three factors, each at two conditions, simultaneously by having only four treatments. Consider the case where an investigation is planned to explore three drugs (denoted by A, B, C) each at two different doses. All possible combinations result in eight distinct treatments. However, by choosing a special set of four treatments it is possible to investigate the contribution to outcome for each drug by changing the dose. There are two sets of four treatments that can be chosen for this purpose. If the dose levels are designated by (A_0, A_1), (B_0, B_1), and (C_0, C_1), then any treatment combinations will be made up of three letters where the subscript 0 or 1 denotes the dose. The two sets of four treatment combinations, each of which is suitable for a trial, are:

$$\text{Set I: } A_0B_0C_0, \ A_0B_1C_1, \ A_1B_0C_1, \ A_1B_1C_0$$

$$\text{Set II: } A_0B_0C_1, \ A_0B_1C_0, \ A_1B_0C_0, \ A_1B_1C_1$$

Note that the two sets together comprise the eight possible treatment combinations. This experimental design is called a Latin square or equivalently a "1/2 replicate of a 2^3 factorial design."

The Role of Compliance

One of the key problems in interpreting the results of a clinical trial is the effect of compliance on the conclusions. If the conclusions of a trial result in no difference between the therapies under investigation, it may be due to lack of compliance. The effect of non-compliance is to lower the sensitivity of a trial to find differences as well as to create possible biases.

As an example of the potential for bias consider a randomized clinical trial comparing two treatment programs for the treatment of head and neck cancer. One therapy is radiation followed by surgery; the other is surgery followed by radiation. Patients in whom the disease has disappeared after radiation may refuse surgery whereas patients doing poorly after surgery may refuse radiation. For the first treat-

Table V-1-5. Experimental Designs for Phase III Randomized Trials[a]

Name	Design	Comment
Simple Two Treatment	R — A / — B	Compare A vs. B
Adjuvant Treatment	R — A / — A + B	Does addition of B to A result in greater benefit?
Combination	R — A / — B / — A + B	Is A + B superior to each alone?
New Treatment after Event (Event may be failure, response, or a fixed period of time)	R — A / — B → E — C	Compare treatment programs A or B followed by C
Common Initial Treatment	A — E — R — B / — C	Compare treatment program A followed by B or C
Cross-Over	R — A — E — B / — B — E — A	Compare A vs. B both before and after event
Two Randomizations	R — A / — B → E — R — C / — D	Compare A vs. B; Compare C vs. D after event

[a]R, randomize; E, event

ment program the better prognosis patients do not comply, while in the other program, the poorer prognosis patients do not comply.

In order to understand more fully the role of bias and loss of efficiency we will use a simple mathematical model. Consider a trial comparing two treatments A and B. Let the proportion of non-compliers be P_a and P_b for the two treatments, respectively. Also let the outcome for each treatment be m_a and m_b for compliers and m'_a and m'_b for non-compliers. (The outcome could be the proportion of responders, the median survival, or whatever is appropriate.) Then the average outcome for each treatment group will consist of a mixture of outcomes of compliers and non-compliers. Define M_a and M_b as the aggregate outcome for each group. We can write M_a and M_b as

$$M_a = (1-P_a)\, m_a + P_a m'_a$$
$$M_b = (1-P_b)\, m_b + P_b m'_b.$$

Note that the effect of non-compliance is to dilute the outcomes for each group. The comparison $(M_a - M_b)$ which compares treatment A with treatment B is

$$M_a - M_b = (m_a - m_b) + P_a(m'_a - m_a) - P_b(m'_b - m_b). \quad (1)$$

Let us consider a case in which there is no difference between treatments for compliers $(m_a = m_b = m)$ and non-

compliers $(m'_a = m'_b = m')$. Then the value of $(M_a - M_b)$ is

$$M_a - M_b = (P_a - P_b)\,(m' - m)$$

which will result in a bias if the non-compliance rates P_a, P_b are different and if $m \neq m'$. As a result the analysis could show a difference between treatments when in truth there is none.

As another example, suppose that treatment A is an observation group having complete compliance $(P_a = 0)$. Suppose that treatment B is an experimental therapy and non-compliance is simply not taking the medication. Then the non-compliers on the intervention arm are likely to have the same outcome as the compliers on the observation treatment arm $(m'_b = m_a)$. Hence substituting $P_a = 0$ and $m'_b = m_a$ in Equation 1 gives

$$M_a - M_b = (1 - P_b)\,(m_a - m_b).$$

Thus the effect of non-compliance is to make the treatment difference smaller. (The multiplier $(1 - P_b)$ is always less than 1 unless $P_b = 0$, in which case it is unity.) The net effect of noncompliance for patients assigned to B is to lower the statistical efficiency. The statistical efficiency is $(1 - P_b)^2$. Table V-1-6 is an instructive table of statistical efficiencies for various values of P_b. The statistical efficiency means that if, for example, the proportion not complying is 10%, it is equivalent to utilizing effectively only 81% of the accrual. In

Table V-1-6.   Proportion Not Complying vs. Statistical Efficiency (One Treatment Group is an Observational Group)

Proportion Not Complying	Statistical Efficiency
0.0	1.0
0.10	0.81
0.25	0.56
0.50	0.25

Table V-1-7.   Average Compliance vs. Statistical Efficiency Trials (Non-compliance Refers to Receiving Intervention Treatment of Other Group)

$P = (P_a + P_b)/2$	Statistical Efficiency
0.0	1.0
0.10	0.64
0.25	0.25
0.40	0.04

other words, 100 patients having a 10% non-compliance rate is equivalent to having 81 patients who completely comply.

Compliance issues are of fundamental importance in cancer prevention trials. Consider a clinical trial in which A is an observation arm and B is an intervention aimed at preventing cancer. Contemplated interventions may be to reduce smoking, reduce intake of dietary fats, or similar activity. However, it is quite possible that individuals in the control group will not comply because they eliminated smoking or changed their diet. In this case $m'_a = m_b$ and $m'_b = m_a$. (Those in the control group who adopt the intervention are noncompliers, but will have the same expected outcome as compliers in the intervention group; similarly those in the intervention group who do not comply will have the same outcome as the compliers in the control groups). Substituting $m'_a = m_b$ and $m'_b = m_a$ in Equation 1 results in

$$M_a - M_b = (1 - P_a - P_b)(m_a - m_b).$$

Note that it is necessary for the sum of the two non-compliance rates to be less than unity ($P_a + P_b < 1$), otherwise the multiplier will be negative, and even though ($m_a - m_b$) may be positive, $M_a - M_b$ will be negative. Thus trials with very large noncompliance rates will be worthless. The statistical efficiency in this case is $(1 - P_a - P_b)^2$. Table V-1-7 shows how the statistical efficiency changes with the average compliance rate $P = (P_a + P_b)/2$. Thus a trial with a 10% noncompliance rate is only 64% efficient and is losing approximately one-third of its effective number of patients.

As an example of the reality of noncompliance, one can use the experience of the Multiple Risk Factor Intervention Trial, often referred to as the MR FIT Trial.[9] The intervention consisted of an educational program to change the lifestyle habits thought to be risk factors for coronary heart disease. Smoking was the most important risk factor. It is interesting to note that 30% of the control group gave up smoking compared with 46% of the intervention group. Thus $P_a = 0.30$ and $P_b = 0.54$. Hence, the statistical efficiency of this trial is $(1 - 0.30 - 0.54)^2 = 0.0256$. The study enrolled 12,866 men. Therefore, with a statistical efficiency of 2.56%, this trial was equivalent to having $(0.0256) \times (12,866) = 320$ men who complied 100%.

Interim Analyses, Multiple Looks at the Data, and Early Stopping

Nearly all ongoing clinical trials are monitored at periodic intervals both in the accrual and follow-up phases of the study. A common time period for such monitoring is every 6 months. At these times, an interim analysis is carried out for the purposes of reviewing the toxicity and endpoint data. If the toxicity is unexpectedly high, the trial is likely to be modified. Also if one treatment appears to be significantly superior or inferior to the other therapies under investigation, ethical considerations would dictate that the trial be terminated or modified. The results of these interim analyses are reviewed by the principals responsible for carrying out the trial (Study Chair, Study Statistician, Key Investigators). In some instances, there may be a disinterested formal monitoring committee charged with the responsibility of reviewing interim analyses. Ordinarily, in a multicenter trial, detailed interim analyses are not made available to all trial participants unless the outcome information is blinded with respect to treatment identification. The reason for masking treatment identification with respect to endpoint data is to avoid accrual to a study being influenced by statistical fluctuations in the endpoint data. Toxicity information is usually identified, but even this can influence the subsequent conduct of a trial.

The decision to terminate a trial early because of the apparent inferiority or superiority of one or more therapies is a difficult problem. The difficulty arises because the false positive rate (probability of concluding a therapy is beneficial when it is not) increases as the number of interim analyses increases. For example, if a clinical trial is planned to have a false positive rate of 5%, then the false positive rate would be changed to 14% if there were five interim analyses. The false positive rate is changed because the more occasions the data are reviewed the greater the opportunity to have a large statistical fluctuation that may be mistaken for a real effect. Table V-1-8 shows how the false positive rate changes with a varying number of multiple looks at the data.

In recent years, new statistical techniques have been developed to aid decision on the early stopping of clinical trials. The idea behind these methods is that one specifies not only the overall false positive and false negative rates as in conventional clinical trials, but also the number of "looks" at the data and the maximal sample size of the trial. This results in objective early stopping rules. These methods are

Table V-1-8.   Multiple "Looks" at Data vs. False Positive Rate[a]

Number of "Looks"	False Positive Rate
1	.05
2	.08
3	.11
4	.13
5	.14
10	.19

[a]The larger the number of interim analyses ("looks"), the greater the chance of finding false positive effects. This same table can be used to determine the overall false positive rate of an experiment when the analysis "looks" at several subgroups separately. For example, if there are five subgroups in a study, where each is analyzed separately with a 5% false positive rate, then the overall false positive rate is 14%.

called "sequential methods" and are modifications of concepts from the era of World War II when sequential methods were developed for the acceptance sampling of equipment. Essentially, these sequential methods are derived so that at each interim analysis the trial may be stopped if the significance level of the statistical tests comparing the treatments is very low. For example, an early stopping rule for a trial having five interim analyses may stop the trial if the first analysis was significant at the $P = .00001$ level; stopping at the second analysis would be done if the results were significant at the $P = .001$ level, with subsequent stopping rules if the significance levels were $P = .008$, $P = .023$, and $P = .041$ for the third, fourth, and fifth interim analyses, respectively. This set of rules preserves an overall 5% false positive rate for the trial. In essence the trial results would have to be very dramatic to result in early stopping of the trial.

In practice these early stopping rules should only serve as a guide to aid investigators. It is especially important in using these rules that the data are current, recently reviewed, and that prognostic subgroups are comparable between the various treatments being compared.

If sequential method trials continue to the last interim analysis, it generally results in about a 5–20% increase in sample size compared with a study design with a pre-assigned fixed number of patients. The potential gain in using sequential methods is to have the option of terminating the trial in the accrual phase of the study. This option may be realizable for trials in which the end-point is the proportion of responders, but is not likely to happen when the end-point is survival. An experiment carried out by Rosner and Tsiatis is particularly instructive.[10] They obtained 72 recently completed studies from the Eastern Cooperative Oncology Group (ECOG) in which survival or some other time metric was an end-point. Various sequential experimental plans were superimposed on the studies to determine what would have happened if the studies had originally been designed to have early stopping. They found that among the 72 studies, 66 (92%) would have terminated earlier utilizing the best sequential plan. (They simulated four different sequential plans.) Among these, 26 (36%) would have been terminated while in the accrual phase. It is particularly important to note that all conclusions made from the sequential analysis simulation agreed with those made by the clinical investigators using the full data set. This study shows that the use of sequential methods in clinical trials can result in a positive gain.[10] A fuller discussion of sequential methods in the context of cancer trials can be found in Geller.[4]

Strategy of Experimentation

There are a very large number of cancer clinical trials being carried on throughout the world. A positive outcome is likely to affect clinical practice. One question that arises is: what proportion of these trials reporting beneficial results is true? The answer to this question is important in deciding when a practicing physician should adopt a new therapy.

In order to discuss this problem, it is necessary to understand how conclusions from a trial are made. All analyses of clinical trials utilize statistical methods that are based on the concepts of probabilities of making incorrect decisions.

The previous section discussed statistical tests and the role of false positive and false negative rates, i.e., the false positive rate refers to the probability of concluding positive benefit when there is no benefit; the false negative rate is the probability of concluding there is no benefit when a treatment is beneficial. In addition to these two concepts, we need another concept, which is the "prior probability of success." It depends on the level of clinical innovation and basic science that motivates the trial. The prior probability of success is subjective and cannot be measured objectively. However, it increases with knowledge of successful exploratory or pilot studies. Phase III studies should only be initiated on the basis of successful exploratory and Phase II studies. If a trial tests a drug combination in which each individual drug is without benefit, the prior probability of success will be low. What values of the prior probability of success should one adapt for cancer trials? Since the concept is subjective, it is difficult to be precise, but prior probabilities in the range of 5–15% seem reasonable for most cancer trials.

Define α, β, and θ to be:

$$\alpha = \text{false positive rate}$$
$$\beta = \text{false negative rate}$$
$$\theta = \text{prior probability of success}$$

Let us adopt the values $\alpha = .05$, $\beta = .7$, and $\theta = .10$. The value of $\alpha = .05$ is commonly chosen as a false positive rate in most studies; a false negative rate of $\beta = .7$ arises if one has 50 patients in each of two groups and is attempting to determine if there is a 50% difference in the median survivals of two groups. Figure V-1-1 illustrates this process if we have 1,000 trials. Since the false positive rate is $\beta = .7$, the true positive rate is $1 - \beta = 0.30$. With the value of $\theta = .10$, one can expect 100 true positive trials. However, only 30% of these will be reported as positive. In addition, among the true negative trials, 5% or 45 trials will be reported as false positives. Thus there will be a total of 75 reported positive trials from among the 1,000 trials. The true positive trials are indistinguishable from the false positive trials. Thus the proportion of true positives among the reported 75 positives is 30/75 = .40. Hence, with these parameters, among every 10 reported positive therapies, we would expect (on the average) 4 to be true positive.

If the trials had very large patient numbers, the false negative rate β would be close to zero. If $\beta = 0$, then all 100 true positive trials will be reported to be positive and the proportion of true positives would be 100/145 = 0.69, i.e., approximately 7 of 10 reported positive trials are true positives. Thus we have shown that with a prior probability of success of 0.10, the probability that a treatment reported to be beneficial is in truth beneficial may range from .40 to .69.

If $P(+)$ denotes the probability that a reported positive trial is a true positive, then we can write

$$P(+) = 1/[1 + \frac{1 - \theta}{\theta} \frac{\alpha}{1 - \beta}]$$

which shows that $P(+)$ depends on θ, α, and β. If θ is close to unity, then $P(+)$ is close to unity.

Table V-1-9 is a summary of $P(+)$ for a variety of values of θ and β with $\alpha = .05$. Note that as θ goes toward unity,

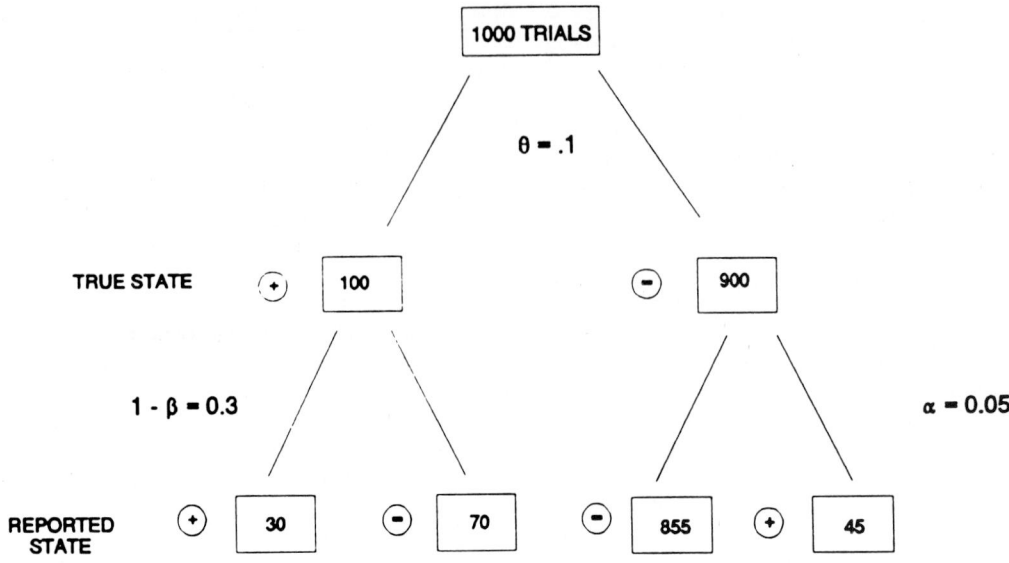

$$P(+) - PROBABILITY\ REPORTED + TREATMENT\ IS\ EFFECTIVE - \frac{30}{75} - .40$$

Figure V-1-1. The clinical trial process is shown. θ, prior probability of success; α, false-positive probability; β, false-negative probability.

Table V-1-9. Probability that a Reported Positive Treatment is a True Positive (False Positive Probability is Fixed at 5%)[a]

θ	β		
	.7	.4	.1
.1	.40	.57	.67
.2	.60	.75	.82
.4	.80	.89	.92
.6	.90	.95	.96

[a]θ, prior probability of success; β, false-negative probability.

$P(+)$ will approach unity. These considerations indicate that in assessing the conclusions of a trial reported to be positive, it is necessary to review the prior scientific evidence that led up to the trial. Also one should avoid initiating Phase III trials that are not preceded by positive pilot and Phase II studies.

Reporting of Clinical Trials

The practicing oncologist must rely heavily on the published literature to help make therapy decisions. There are too many cancer sites and the current views on the systemic treatment of disease may appear to be moving too quickly for most oncologists to have personal experience with the "latest treatments." In this section, we outline guidelines for assessing the quality of the reporting of a clinical trial. These guidelines should be useful both to readers of the literature and authors of clinical trial manuscripts.[13]

General Guidelines

Population Under Study. There should be clear statements describing the population under study. Major sub-

groups of patients who are excluded should be mentioned, e.g., "patients over age 65 were not eligible for the study."

Therapy. The reporting of the protocol therapy (especially chemotherapy) should be outlined in sufficient detail so that the therapy can be duplicated by another physician. Not only the contents of the written protocol, but also the therapy actually received by patients. This is especially important for chemotherapy, for which full doses as written in a protocol may not have been given often to patients. Summary measures such as average dose per course, proportion of patients receiving incomplete courses, proportion of patients receiving full doses, and average number of courses should be provided. Their effect on outcome should be analyzed. If the written protocol provided for a de-escalation or escalation of dose(s) as a function of toxicity, details should be given. Information should be given on the extent to which dose changes followed protocol criteria.

Study Design. The study design should be outlined. A schema, which is a pictorial display of the study design, is helpful to the reader. If the study is randomized, it is not sufficient to state simply that it was a randomized study. A statement should indicate how the randomization was carried out, e.g., central randomization, closed envelope, or other methods. The actual randomization scheme should be described. Occasionally a randomization schedule or procedure may be changed during the course of the study. If this was done, details should be given regarding the reasons for the change. If there is institutional balancing or other kinds of stratification, it should be so stated.

Patient Accounting. There should be a detailed accounting of all patients registered for the study. Registration should be carefully defined. How is a patient officially registered? Are all patients officially registered prior to first day of treatment, or after treatment has begun? It is disappointing to learn that in many single-institution non-randomized studies, registration may take place months after the first day of treatment. This leaves open the possibility that not all patients on a protocol are registered. In a randomized study, patients are registered from the moment of randomization. Non-randomized studies should have similarly precise rules for registration.

The number of patients who are classified as "canceled" or "evaluable" should be given by treatment. A canceled patient is defined as a registered patient who withdrew from the study before the first day of treatment. An unevaluable patient may be one who has incomplete information. Some studies classify an unevaluable patient as one who has major deviations from the protocol. If the reasons for patients being classified as canceled or unevaluable are related to the treatment assignment, then it is mandatory that all patients be included in the treatment comparisons. Otherwise the selective inclusion of patients may result in wrong conclusions being drawn from the study.

Follow-Up. The follow-up period for patients should be given separately for each treatment. Statistics should be included on the average follow-up time, the number followed for each time period (1 year, 2 years), and maximum and minimum follow-up times. The number of patients lost to follow-up and the reasons should be reported for each treatment. If a relatively large number of patients is lost to follow-up (say 10%), then statements about long-term effects may not be correct.

Data Quality. There should be a discussion of the quality control methods used for the data. Was there "Second-Party Review?" A Second-Party Review is defined as a patient data review by individuals other than the investigator generating the patient record. This could be carried out by the study chairman or a special committee. If there was central data management, it should be mentioned. The review should be centered on answering three major questions for each patient: 1) was the patient eligible? 2) was the protocol followed? 3) was there objective documentation of the major end-points? There should be statements about the quality control of radiotherapy and surgery if these treatment modalities were involved in the study. Similar remarks hold for pathology quality control.

End-points and Censored Data. Trials in which the end-point for evaluating therapy is a time metric, such as survival or disease-free survival, may often have patients with incomplete data. This happens if patients are still alive or in the disease-free state at the time of analysis. Such observations are called censored observations. Several situations arise in defining censored observations that could seriously skew the results. We mention only two, which are in widespread use and could lead to incorrect conclusions. The first of these occurs when a patient dies from a cause other than cancer, e.g., cardiovascular disease, suicide, etc. When there are appreciable numbers of patients dying from competing causes of death, it could seriously alter the conclusions of the study if these patients were treated as censored observations. The cancer may have been an important contributing factor in

their death. The other reporting problem arises when a patient is taken off the protocol treatment, due to lack of response or progression of disease, and receives some other therapy that may be more beneficial. If the survival time is classified as censored (still alive) at the time the patient ceased to be on protocol therapy, then the statistical analysis will be biased (being purged of an imminent death) and it will bias a poor therapy to make it appear better. It is unfortunate that such practices are widespread. It is for this reason that the report of a clinical trial should indicate the reasons for classifying patients as censored when the classification arises, other than the usual situation where not enough follow-up time has elapsed to have a complete observation.

Statistical Analysis. The report on therapeutic benefit should be presented so that there is no ambiguity if a treatment difference refers to the entire patient population or to special subgroups of patients. It is necessary that the analysis consider all known major prognostic factors that can affect the outcome. Otherwise there may be disappointment when the therapy is applied in practice. The comparison of response proportions, and disease-free and survival curves, must be made using objective statistical procedures. If a complicated statistical model is used, it should be described in the paper or in an appendix. The description of the statistical methods must be adequate for another statistician to reproduce the analysis if the source data were available.

The outcome of statistical tests depends on both the existence of a true difference and the number of patients in the study. If the number of patients is small, then the study will have low sensitivity (power) to detect small or moderate treatment differences. Failure to find statistical significance may be due to small numbers, rather than to lack of benefit. It is for this reason that every paper reporting a null effect should have a discussion of statistical power and how it can influence the conclusions of the paper.

The analysis should also contain a discussion relating to ending patient entry to the study. For example, was the trial (or part of the trial) stopped because of an unusual outcome associated with a treatment—a very good or poor result? Was patient accrual terminated after a predetermined number of patients entered the trial? Was an early stopping rule used? All of these affect the reader's interpretation of the study conclusions.

Statistical Techniques

The most common end-points in cancer clinical trials are: "success" (defined in the context of the trial), response (complete, partial, or both), toxicity (lethal, life-threatening, severe, moderate or mild), survival, disease-free survival, and duration of response. These end-points fall into two general classes, which are often called categorical data (success, response, toxicity) and time metric or survival data (survival, disease-free survival, and duration of response). Categorical data are characterized by having outcomes that belong in a category and can be counted, e.g., number of successes or failures, or other events. The survival data (this is the term most often used to describe time metric data, even though the data may not actually refer to survival) are characterized by two events (beginning and end); the time between these two events is the time measurement.

Categorical Data

Suppose a trial evaluating objective tumor response observed 20 complete or partial responses from 100 patients. The reported response rate is 20%. The statistical model for this study envisions a true or theoretical response rate that could only be calculated if the experiment enrolled the entire population of patients with the particular disease characteristics. Theoretically this number would be very large. The clinical trial enrolling 100 patients is a sample from this population. The proportion 20% is only an estimate of the true proportion as it is based on a sample of patients. How close is the reported value to the true value? In order to judge how close the reported or sample value is to the true value one utilizes a statistical technique called a confidence interval. The formula for the confidence interval is

$$\hat{p} \pm 2\sqrt{\hat{p}(1-\hat{p})/n} \qquad (2)$$

where n is the sample size and $\hat{p}$ = (number of successes)/(sample size). The caret (ˆ) is often used to remind one that the proportion is based on a sample of observations; the true value would be designated by p. More correctly, the formula given by Equation 2 is an approximate 95% confidence limit. The confidence interval for our example is calculated to be $0.20 \pm .08$. The operational interpretation of the confidence interval is that the true value of response is within the interval (12%, 28%). The reason it is referred to as a 95% confidence interval is that on the average 95% of such confidence intervals will be correct, i.e., the true value of response will be within the interval. It is possible to raise the "confidence" to 99% or even higher at the expense of widening the interval. In practice most scientists use 95%.

Another common statistical problem arising in the analysis of a clinical trial is to compare two proportions. The comparison can be made by calculating a confidence interval between two proportions or carrying out a statistical test of significance. To illustrate the problem suppose that outcome is measured by success and failure and the proportion of successes for two treatments, designated as A and B, are $\hat{p}_a = 50/90 = .56$ and $\hat{p}_b = 40/100 = .40$, respectively. The formula for calculating an approximate 95% confidence interval for the (true) difference ($p_a - p_b$) is

$$(\hat{p}_a - \hat{p}_b) \pm 2\sqrt{\frac{\hat{p}_a(1-\hat{p}_a)}{n_a} + \frac{\hat{p}_b(1-\hat{p}_b)}{n_b}} \qquad (3)$$

where n_a and n_b are the respective sample sizes. Carrying out the calculations results in $0.16 \pm .14$. The interpretation is that the true value of the difference can be as low as 0.02 or as high as 0.30. The interval (0.02, 0.30) is referred to as a 95% confidence interval for the difference between two proportions. The formula in Equation 3 is only an approximation for the 95% confidence interval but is accurate enough for sample sizes above 20. The interpretation of the 95% confidence intervals is that out of every 100 intervals so

calculated, on the average 95 of them will have the true difference within the interval. In the particular example, we conclude that there is a real difference between the success proportions, as a difference of 0 is not a possible value of the true difference.

Another common way to compare proportions is to carry out a statistical test of significance. Usually the data are put in the form of a 2 × 2 table, as shown in Table V-1-10.

The statistical test calculates the probability of obtaining a result that was observed as well as outcomes more extreme if actually there is no difference between the treatments. The calculation is based on the following reasoning: If the outcome is regarded as scientific evidence in favor of a treatment difference, then outcomes having a greater difference would constitute even stronger evidence of a real difference between the treatments. Essentially the probabilities of all the more extreme tables are calculated where the totals in the margins are kept constant. The probabilities are then summed to form a P value. For example, a more extreme table is depicted in Table V-1-11, and the data would be even stronger evidence in favor of a difference.

If the P value is small then the probability of the observed table or more extreme tables arising by chance (no difference between treatments) is unlikely. Hence we would conclude that the premise on which the calculation is made (no treatment difference) is incorrect and the treatments do differ. Usually a P value less than 0.05 is declared "significant," resulting in a conclusion that treatments differ.

The statistical test is based on a hypothesis, called the "null hypothesis," in which the true values are equal. This is usually designated as $H_0: p_a = p_b$. The alternative hypothesis is that the true proportions are different, e.g., usually specified by $H_1: p_a \neq p_b$. This alternative hypothesis is called a two-sided alternative, as it refers to either $p_a < p_b$, or $p_a > p_b$. Occasionally the alternative hypothesis would be a one-sided hypothesis, e.g., $H_1: p_a > p_b$. As a working rule, one should routinely use two-sided alternative hypotheses. A one-sided hypothesis is used when one treatment can never have a less beneficial effect than the other treatment. In some instances, investigators have reasoned that in comparing a potentially beneficial treatment against a control or observation group, a one-sided test would be suitable, i.e., the therapy will be no different from having no treatment or will be better. This excludes the possibility that the active treatment may result in adversely affecting the patient. There have been instances when one-sided tests have been used to

Table V-1-10. Statistical Test of Significance (2 × 2 Table)

Group	Success	Failure	Total
A	50	40	90
B	40	60	100
Total	90	100	190

Table V-1-11. Statistical Test of Significance (More Extreme 2 × 2 Table)

Group	Success	Failure	Total
A	51	39	90
B	39	61	100
Total	90	100	190

evaluate the outcome of clinical trials in which, on further follow-up, the active treatment was found to be detrimental.

The statistical test for calculating the test of significance is often referred to as Fisher's exact test after R. A. Fisher the statistician who derived it. The numerical procedure for the test is complicated. However, it is available in almost all computer software programs for statistical analyses. The statistical test for computing Fisher's exact test comparing the two proportions

$$\hat{p}_a = \frac{50}{90} = 0.56 \text{ vs } \hat{p}_b = \frac{20}{100} = 0.20$$

resulted in a P value of $P = .0415$.

Since any value less than 0.05 is significant, we would conclude that the proportions do differ. An approximate test for comparing the two proportions can be carried out by calculating the chi-square test for comparing two proportions. The formula is

$$X^2 = (\hat{p}_a - \hat{p}_b)^2 / \left[\frac{\hat{p}_a(1 - \hat{p}_a)}{n_a} + \frac{\hat{p}_b(1 - \hat{p}_b)}{n_b} \right] \qquad (4)$$

and then comparing the calculated values from a table of the chi-square distribution. Large values of X^2 reflect evidence of a treatment difference. Table V-1-12 is a short table of the chi-square distribution. Note that if $X^2 > 3.8$, the P value is certainly less than 0.05. Using the same data from which Fisher's exact test was carried out results in a value of $X^2 = 4.97$. This gives a P value of .03. If the sample sizes are of moderate size (say at least 20 for each group) the chi-square test will give an answer that is quite close to Fisher's exact test.

The difference between the confidence interval approach and the test of significance is that the significance test does not indicate the magnitude of the difference between the two proportions. The significance test refers to the probability of observing the given difference or larger differences between the two observed proportions if actually the two theoretical proportions are the same. In other words, it calculates the probability of these differences arising from chance fluctuations.

Survival Data

A characteristic of survival data is that, at the time of analysis, some of the patients may still be alive. The observations are called "censored observations" and represent incomplete data. However, they do contain important information by providing a lower bound on survival. Both complete and censored observations must be included in any analysis of survival-type data. Censored data arise from a variety of different circumstances. The two chief reasons for observing a censored observation are: 1) the period of follow-up is short, and 2) the patient may have been lost to follow-up. The first reason for censoring is referred to as "non-informative censoring" as, apart from providing a lower bound on survival, the fact that the patient is censored conveys no further information about the treatment. Lost to follow-up patients may have arisen because the patient has moved leaving no trace, or may have died without the investigator being aware of the death. In some cases, the loss of contact may have arisen because the treatment was unsuccessful or too toxic. Alternatively, the loss to follow-up may be unrelated to the patient's progress. The latter represents non-informative censoring; however, the other reasons contain information about the treatment and may be informative. Since information on the reasons for patients being lost to follow-up is not generally available, clinical trials with a significant number of patients who are lost to follow-up could be seriously biased. A rule of thumb is that if there are more than 10% of the patients who are lost to follow-up, then care must be taken in the interpretation of the data. One way to assess the importance of the lost to follow-up patients is to carry out the analysis in two separate ways: 1) regarding all the lost to follow-up patients as censored; and 2) assuming the observations on the lost to follow-up patients are complete and represent the survival time. If the general conclusions of both analyses are the same, then the lost to follow-up patients do not constitute a source of bias.

A theoretical survival distribution exists for any defined population of patients. It may be altered by treatment. The theoretical survival distribution is the probability distribution of the different survival times if a (conceptually) infinite number of patients has received the same therapy. Figure V-1-2 is a plot of a theoretical survival function. It is a plot of a probability versus time. Denoting the survival function by $S(t)$ it represents the proportion of patients who will have a longer survival than time t. For example, if t_m is the time for which the survival time is exceeded by half of the patients, then $S(t_m) = \frac{1}{2}$. The quantity t_m is called the *median survival*. The median survival in Figure V-1-2 is $t_m = 2$ years. In general, one can define the survival time t_p such that $S(t_p) = p$. The survival time t_p represents that point on the theoretical survival curve such that a proportion p of patients will have longer survival time. For example, if $p = .25$, then 25% of the patients are expected to have longer survival times than $t_{.25}$. The value t_p is called the pth percentile or upper pth percentile.

The theoretical survival distribution is never really known. Instead, in any real life situation, we have a limited amount of data. One aspect of the statistical analysis is to use these data to *estimate* the theoretical survival distribution. The estimate of the theoretical survival distribution can be considered as a summary or condensation of the data.

There are two principal ways of estimating the survival curve from actual data. These are called the life-table method and the Kaplan-Meier or maximum likelihood method. The life table method is generally used with a large number of

Table V-1-12.   Key Values of the Chi-Square Distribution and Their Associated Probabilities (One Degree of Freedom)

P	X^2	P	X^2
.50	0.46	.04	4.20
.40	0.71	.03	4.71
.30	1.08	.02	5.43
.20	1.64	.01	6.56
.10	2.69	.001	10.82
.05	3.84		

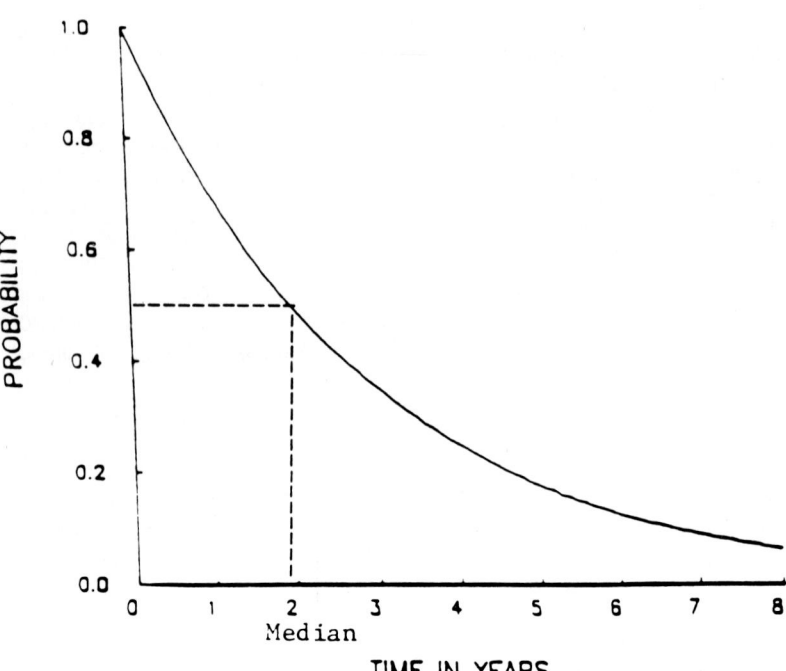

Figure V-1-2. Plot of theoretical survival distribution. The median is 2 years and corresponds to the time for which half of the patients survive a longer time.

observations, whereas the maximum likelihood method is used when there is a small number of observations. There is a large number of different computer programs that will automatically calculate these estimates. We shall illustrate the calculations for the life table method as this is the more common method encountered. The calculations for data on $n = 118$ patients with advanced adenocarcinoma of the lung are outlined in Table V-1-13. The starting point for the calculations is to select a time interval in order to summarize the survival times. In Table V-1-13, the time interval is 1 month. A summary of the data is given in columns 2–4. The calculations in this table are self-explanatory. Figure V-1-3 is a plot of the survival function. Note that it is plotted as a

step function. The last column of Table V-1-13 refers to the survival probability. For example, the probability is .897 of surviving 1 month and .809 of surviving two months. The number at risk within any interval is the number of patients who are "candidates" for dying within the interval. For example, for the first interval, 118 patients were alive at the beginning of the interval, but 3 were censored within the interval. The number at risk is calculated by assuming that three censored patients are equivalent to half of that number who would be available for a potential death. Hence the number at risk is calculated as $118 - \frac{3}{2} = 116.5$. The larger the number of patients at risk, the greater the reliability of the survival probability. As a result, the survival probabilities in

Table V-1-13. Estimating the Survival Function for Patient with Advanced Carcinoma of the Lung (n = 118)

Interval No.	Interval (month)	No. Censored (a)	No. Deaths (b)	No. Alive at Beginning of Interval* (c)	No. at Risk (d = c − a/2)	Probability of Surviving (e = 1 − b/d)	Survival**
1	0–1	3	12	118	116.5	.897	.897
2	1–2	3	10	103	101.5	.901	.809
3	2–3	5	13	90	88	.852	.689
4	3–4	9	8	72	67.5	.881	.607
5	4–5	6	6	55	52	.885	.537
6	5–6	2	5	43	42	.881	.473
7	6–7	6	5	36	33	.848	.402
8	7–8	1	5	25	24.5	.796	.320
9	8–9	1	3	19	18.5	.838	.268
10	9–10	3	2	15	13.5	.852	.228
11	10–11	3	1	10	8.5	.882	.201
12	11–12	1	2	6	5.5	.636	.128
13	12+	3	0	3	3		

*The number of patients alive at the beginning of each interval is calculated by setting $c_1 = 118$ (the sample size of the study) for interval 1. The calculation for c_2, c_3, etc. proceeds by using the formula $c_i = c_{i-1} - (a_{i-1} + b_{i-1})$. For example, $c_2 = c_1 - (a_1 + b_1) = 118 - (3 + 12) = 103$.

**The last column gives the survival probabilities. The formulas for these entries are $f_1 = e_1$, $f_2 = e_2 f_1$, $f_3 = e_3 f_2$, . . . $f_i = e_i f_{i-1}$. For example, $f_2 = (.901)(.897) = .809$.

SURVIVAL FOR PATIENTS WITH ADENOCARCINOMA OF LUNG (N=118)

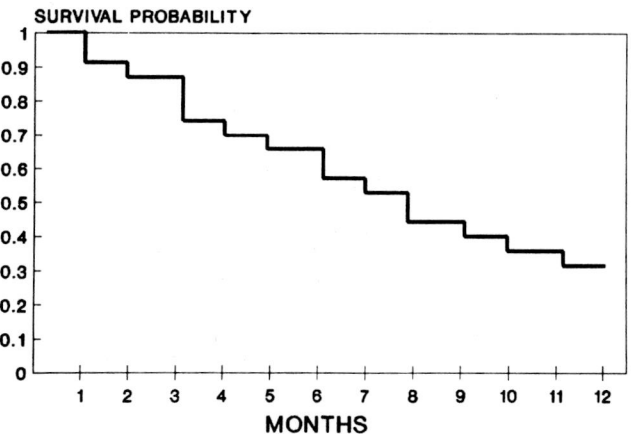

Figure V-1-3. Survival for patients with adenocarcinoma of the lung ($N = 118$), plotted as a step function.

the "tails" of the distribution do not have the same reliability as those in the beginning of the distribution.

Test of Significance for Comparing Two Survival Distributions. There are several ways of carrying out a statistical test of significance for comparing two survival distributions. The most widely used test is called the "log rank test." The calculation of the test is relatively complicated; however, it is widely available on computer systems. The key assumption in using the log rank test is that if the two survival distributions are denoted by $S_1(t)$ and $S_2(t)$, then the ratio of their logarithms is always a constant, i.e. log $S_1(t)$ / log $S_2(t)$ = β (constant independent of time). The log rank procedure tests the null hypothesis that $\beta = 0$. If the assumption is that the ratio of the logarithms of the survival function is not constant, then the log rank test would be inappropriate to use for comparing two survival distributions. The assumption described above is sometimes referred to as the "proportional hazard" assumption. (See section on Statistical Models for a discussion of hazard functions.) One situation in which this assumption does not hold is when the two survival distributions are observed to cross or intersect. This corresponds to the case in which one therapy appears to be better during the early follow-up, but as time progresses a higher proportion of patients on the other therapy live longer periods of time.

Statistical Models

The evaluation of any therapy in a clinical trial should take into consideration all factors that influence outcome. In addition to the potential for the therapy under investigation to influence outcome, features associated with the natural history of the disease also influence the outcome. For example, it is well known that the probability of observing a response for advanced lung cancer depends both on performance status and weight loss. Another example is that the survival of women participating in adjuvant breast cancer trials is affected by: menopausal status, nodal involvement, tumor

size, and ER status. The incorporation of these baseline variables in the statistical analysis ordinarily results in a more precise analysis.

The way in which these covariates are incorporated into a statistical analysis is to use statistical models. General statistical models have been developed for both categorical and survival data. The models commonly used for these two kinds of end-points are referred to as logistic and proportional hazards models, respectively. Very often the proportional hazards models are called "Cox models" in honor of D. R. Cox, who first proposed them. The computations for utilizing these models are extensive and ordinarily would be impossible to carry out on a hand calculator. However, the calculations for both types of models are widely available in many statistical software analysis packages. In this chapter, it is only appropriate to give the basic concepts.

The basic idea of models will be presented as if one had two therapies that are being compared, and a single covariant. The generalization of these ideas to many covariants is straightforward.

Logistic Models

Suppose we have two therapies (labeled A and B) having theoretical response probabilities p_a and p_b, which are unknown. The odds of response for each therapy is defined as the ratio of the probability of a response to the probability of no response, i.e., p_a/q_a and p_b/q_b where $q_a = 1 - p_a$ and $q_b = 1 - q_b$. The model for comparing two therapies would be to write the logarithm of the odds ratio as

$$\log (p_a / q_a) = \alpha, \qquad \log (p_b / q_b) = \alpha + \beta.$$

The quantities α and β are unknown parameters in the model. If $\beta = 0$, then the two treatments are the same. This formulation of the modeling is equivalent to writing

$$p_a = e^{\alpha}/1 + e^{\alpha}, \ q_a = 1/1 + e^{\alpha}$$

$$p_b = e^{\alpha+\beta}/1 + e^{\alpha+\beta}, \ q_b = 1/1 + e^{\alpha+\beta}$$

The quantities p_a and p_b are expressed in terms of parameters α and (α, β) respectively. The functional form is the logistic function; hence the name logistic models. Often the logarithms of the odds ratios $\log(p_a/q_a)$ and $\log(p_b/q_b)$ are called logits.

Now suppose that the response is affected by gender. This is incorporated into the model by writing the logit for response as

Treatment A:	$\log (p_a/q_a) = \alpha + \gamma$	for males
	$\log (p_a/q_a) = \alpha$	for females
Treatment B:	$\log (p_b/q_b) = \alpha + \beta + \gamma$	for males
	$\log (p_b/q_b) = \alpha + \beta$	for females

where the parameters (α, β, γ) are unknown. The above model assumes that the effect of gender is additive and is independent of treatment. A more complex model would be to allow the effect of treatment to depend on gender. This can be done by defining a new parameter δ and writing the model for males receiving treatment B as $\log(p_b/q_b) = \alpha + \beta + \gamma + \delta$. The quantity δ is called an interaction term. The parameters for the logit model with interaction can be summarized in Table V-1-14.

Statistical methods exist for finding the numerical values

Table V-1-14. Summary of Logit Model

	Female	Male
Treatment A	α	$\alpha + \gamma$
Treatment B	$\alpha + \beta$	$\alpha + \beta + \gamma + \delta$
Difference in logits	β	$\beta + \delta$

Table V-1-15. Model Interpretation

Parameter values	Interpretation
$\delta = 0$	Gender does not affect response differently for each treatment
$\delta \neq 0$	Treatments do differ but difference depends on gender
$\delta = 0, \beta = 0$	No difference between treatments
$\delta \neq 0, \beta = 0$	No difference in treatment for females, but difference in treatment for males
$\beta = -\delta \neq 0$	No difference in treatment for males, but difference in treatment for females
$\delta = 0, \gamma = 0$	Gender does not influence outcome
$\delta \neq 0, \gamma = 0$	Gender only influences outcome for treatment B

of the parameters and for making tests of significance. The numerical calculations are readily carried out on computers. The model is very flexible and gives an organized way to interpret the data. Table V-1-15 summarizes the various possibilities for drawing conclusions from this data set. The extension to many more covariates can be made.

In using a statistical model to analyze data, there are many opportunities to draw incorrect conclusions because the model was incorrect. For example, if the interaction term (δ) was omitted in the model and the effect of treatment depended on gender, then conclusions from the analysis might be wrong. Unfortunately details of the goodness of fit of mathematical models are often omitted from scientific papers so that it is difficult for even the most experienced reader to verify the adequacy of a model.

Proportional Hazard Models for Survival (Cox Survival Models)

Modeling of survival data to take account of other factors that influence survival is carried out by modeling the "hazard function" or "failure rate." To illustrate these ideas, consider the survival (years) of ten patients: .2+, .5+, .5, 1.2+, 1.2, 1.8, 2.0, 2.1, 3.5, 5.0+, where + denotes a censored observation. Out of 10 observations there are 6 deaths. Hence, the proportion of deaths is $p = \frac{6}{10} = 0.6$. However, the proportion of deaths depends on the length of the follow-up time. The longer the follow-up time the greater the proportion of deaths. (The total follow-up time is the sum of all of the observations. In this example, it is 18 years.) A more useful summary of the data is provided by the ratio of the proportion of deaths to the average follow-up time. This results in an expression that has units of "deaths per unit follow-up time" or, equivalently, "proportion of failures per average follow-

up time." This quantity is called the "failure rate" (FR) and is calculated by

$$FR = \begin{array}{c} \text{observed proportion} \\ \text{of deaths/average} \\ \text{follow-up time} \end{array} = \frac{6/10}{18/10} = \frac{1}{3} \begin{array}{c} \text{deaths per patient} \\ \text{per year.} \end{array}$$

Sometimes it is convenient to report the deaths as per 100 patients or per 1,000 patients. In our example, the failure rate could be reported as 1 death per 3 patients per year, or 33 deaths per 100 patients per year, or 333 deaths per 1,000 patients per year. Alternatively, the time units may be changed to be deaths per month, in which case the death rate would be 2.75 deaths per 100 patients per month. The FR = 0.333 represents an average failure rate over the entire set of data. One could have calculated separate failure rates for the first year, second year, etc. These calculations are shown in Table V-1-16.

It is clear that the failure rate keeps dropping with time and that the FR = 0.33 is an average failure rate. With a very large number of patients the failure rate can be calculated for smaller and smaller time intervals, e.g., monthly, weekly, daily. One can envision an interval of time that gets progressively smaller as the interval shrinks to a point. With each of these smaller and smaller intervals a failure rate can be calculated, provided the number of patients is very large (theoretically infinite). This limiting process defines the "instantaneous failure rate" or the "hazard function." The hazard function is directly related to the survival function. If one knows the hazard function, then the survival function is completely defined and vice versa. Letting $S(t)$ define the survival function and $h(t)$ the hazard function, the relationship between the two is given by

$$h(t) = -\frac{d}{dt} \log S(t)$$

or

$$S(t) = \exp\left[-\int_0^t h(x)dx\right]$$

Suppose a clinical trial is comparing two treatments denoted by A and B. The proportional hazards model for making the comparison is to specify that $h_B(t) = e^\beta h_A(t)$ where $h_A(t)$, $h_B(t)$ are the hazard functions for the two treatments and β is an unknown constant. Clearly, if $\beta = 0$, the two treatments have the same hazard function and consequently the same survival functions. A more formal way of writing this model is

$$h_A(t) = h_0(t)$$
$$h_B(t) = h_0(t)e^\beta$$

Thus, the hazard function of treatment B is proportional to the hazard function of treatment A. This model leads to the log rank test, which has been discussed earlier. Note that

$$S_A(t) = \exp\left[-\int_0^t h_0(x)dx\right]$$

and

$$S_B(t) = \exp\left[-e^\beta\int_0^t h_0(x)dx.\right]$$

Table V-1-16. Calculation of Interval Failure Rates

Time Interval	Proportions of Failure	Average Follow-up Time	FR
First year	1/3	1.2/3 = 0.4	0.82
Second year	2/3	4.2/3 = 1.4	0.48
Third year and beyond	3/4	12.6/4 = 3.15	0.24

Therefore $\log S_B(t)/\log S_A(t) = \beta$, which is the assumption for the log rank test discussed earlier.

Now suppose that survival not only depends on the treatment, but on gender. The hazard function can then be modeled in a similar way as the logistic function. Explicitly, we can model the hazard function for each treatment by

$$\log h_A(t) = \log h_0(t) \qquad \text{for treatment A, females}$$
$$\log h_B(t) = \log h_0(t) + \beta \qquad \text{for treatment B, females}$$
$$\log h_A(t) = \log h_0(t) + \delta \qquad \text{for treatment A, males}$$
$$\log h_B(t) = \log h_0(t) + \beta + \delta \qquad \text{for treatment B, males}$$

The quantities β, γ, δ can be estimated from the data. Statistical tests are available for making inferences on these parameters. Note that this is a parallel model to the logistic regression model. The only difference is that $h_0(t)$, which is the baseline hazard rate, replaces α in the logistic model. The inferences from this proportional hazard model with respect to the parameters are the same as in the logistic model (see Table V-1-15).

Many applications of this type of model fail to verify whether the proportional hazards assumption is correct. Furthermore, it is rare that an interaction term is included in the model. Investigators should be wary of the presentation of a statistical analysis that does not address the issues of the inclusion of interaction terms to determine if the treatment effect depends on one or more prognostic or other baseline factors as well as the correctness of the proportional hazard assumption. In order to illustrate further how modeling for proportional hazard models is carried out, a detailed example is presented.

Example. The Eastern Cooperative Oncology Group carried out a randomized clinical trial on recurrent head and neck cancer with three treatment groups: low-dose (40 mg/M^2) methotrexate (M), high-dose (240 mg/M^2) methotrexate plus leucovorin rescue (ML), high-dose (240 mg/M^2) methotrexate plus leucovorin rescue plus cyclophosphamide (500 mg/M^2) plus cytosine arabinoside (300 mg/M^2) (MLCC). It is known that survival depends on performance status, time since first symptoms, disease site, and weight loss. The trial registered 237 patients. Table V-1-17 summarizes the median survivals by treatment and various subgroups.

It is clear that this trial is complex and is a candidate for statistical modeling. The particular variables chosen for modeling and their associated levels are summarized in Table V-1-18.

Table V-1-18 represents a condensation of the data since performance status is measured on a 5-point scale (0, 1, 2, 3, 4). An ambulatory patient is someone with a performance status of 2 or less. Similarly, the time from first symptoms has been condensed to three levels. Even with this condensation, the number of possible combinations is $3 \times 2 \times 3$

Table V-1-17. Summary of Median Survival by Treatment and Prognostic Factors: Head and Neck Trial ECOG

	Sample Size	Median Survival (weeks)
Treatment		
M	81	22
ML	80	19
MLCC	76	14
Total	237	
Performance Status		
Ambulatory	144	24
Nonambulatory	93	10
Weight Loss		
None	93	24
< 5%	61	14
5–10%	39	14
> 10%	44	16
Disease Site		
Tongue	45	21
Larynx	42	21
Hypopharynx	19	17
Oral mesopharynx	33	14
Floor of mouth	30	16
Other (mouth)	16	9
Other	34	22

Table V-1-18. Factors for Modeling

Variable	Levels	No. of Levels
Treatment	M, ML, MLCC	3
Performance Status	Ambulatory, nonambulatory	2
Time Since First Symptoms	< 1 year, 1–2 years, > 2 years	3
Site	Other, tongue, hypopharynx, larynx	4
Weight Loss	None, < 5%, 5–10%, > 10%	4

$\times 4 \times 4 = 288$. The entire trial only registered 237 patients. There are more experimental combinations than patients.

In setting up the statistical model, each variable will generate parameters in the model. Ordinarily, the number of parameters is one less than the number of levels. For example, treatment will have two parameters because it has three groups. This can be modeled by using the parameters β_1 and β_2, i.e., $h(M) = h_0(t)$, $h(ML) = h_0(t)e^{\beta_1}$, $h(MLCC) = h_0(t)e^{\beta_2}$. Since $h(ML)/h(M) = e^\beta$, positive values of β_1 imply that treatment ML has a higher failure rate than M. A similar interpretation holds for $h(MLCC)/h(M) = e^{\beta_2}$. The comparisons of ML to MLCC results in $h(MLCC)/h(ML) = e^{\beta_2 - \beta_1}$. Hence if $\beta_2 > \beta_1$, then MLCC has a higher failure rate than ML. The same scheme is set up for the other variables.

Table V-1-19 summarizes the elements of the model. Note that weight loss is only one parameter (δ) even though there are four levels. This variable has been modeled as a continuous variable where a new variable x is introduced that takes on values (0, 2, 3, 4) corresponding to increasing levels of weight loss. The estimates β_1 and β_2 are significantly greater than zero. Hence M (low-dose methotrexate) has better survival (smaller hazard function) than the other two treatments. In order to compare the hazard ratios of h(ML) to h(MLCC) we have $h(ML)/h(MLCC) = e^{\beta_1 - \beta_2}$. Making the comparison, we have $(\hat{\beta}_1 - \hat{\beta}_2) = -0.13 \pm .25$. Since zero is a possible value of $(\hat{\beta}_1 - \hat{\beta}_2)$, we would conclude that the two high-dose methotrexate arms have the same survival. Reviewing the other parameters, we note that performance status, time since first symptoms, weight loss, and disease sites are all significant.

This model is an example of an additive model. There are no interaction terms with treatment. It concludes that low-dose methotrexate is superior, but does not explore (for example) how this superiority is related to ambulatory status, i.e., does the superiority hold in the same way for both ambulatory and nonambulatory patients? Similar remarks can be made about the other prognostic factors. Another potential criticism is that the way the weight loss is modeled requires further documentation.

Meta-Analysis

In the last decade there has been increasing use of the statistical technique termed "meta-analysis." This term refers to the use of formal statistical techniques to sum up a collection of separate studies that are attempting to investigate the same hypothesis. Its purpose is the same as the scientific review of independent studies all aimed at studying the same hypothesis. The difference between meta-analysis and an ordinary scientific review is that a scientific review of the literature tends to be somewhat personal, reflecting the views of the reviewer. On the other hand, the meta-analysis attempts to synthesize the data in a quantitative way. The end product is a numerical estimate of a quantity that usually reflects the advantage of a treatment or a method.

The impetus for carrying out meta-analyses of cancer clinical trials is that the trials may be too small to be able to find small, but important therapeutic effects. For example, there are approximately 40,000 annual deaths from breast cancer every year in the United States. If the cure rate was increased by 10%, then one would expect 4,000 fewer deaths. A clinical trial to compare a treatment with a very low cure rate, in the neighborhood of 10–20%, with one that caused a 10% increase would require approximately 10,000–25,000 patients in a clinical trial. No breast cancer trials have ever been designed with this large a sample size.

Meta-analytic methods have been utilized in a wide variety of fields with different subject matters. They have been applied to observational as well as randomized studies. The initial applications were made in the field of education research, but now these ideas are being applied to a large number of scientific fields. Although carrying out a meta-analysis is relatively straightforward, carrying out a good analysis is difficult.

The principal difficulties in applying meta-analysis to clinical trials are: the therapies may be different, the patient populations may be different, the follow-up times may vary, and the quality of the studies may vary. To illustrate these ideas, suppose a meta-analysis is to be performed to determine if adjuvant chemotherapy prolongs survival for breast cancer patients. A recent meta-analysis of this kind has been carried out (the Early Breast Cancer Trialists' Collaborative Group).[3] Which trials should be included in this analysis? Trials exist that are both randomized and non-randomized. To include non-randomized studies would introduce all of the well-known biases associated with non-randomized trials. Hence, the meta-analysis should be restricted to randomized studies only. Among the randomized trials, some exist comparing chemotherapy vs. placebo or observation group, whereas others may be comparing chemotherapy plus post-operative radiation vs. post-operative radiation. Should the latter trials be included in a meta-analysis? Hypothetically, if the radiation therapy is of no benefit, then such trials should be included. Alternatively, if the radiation therapy does improve survival, then it will ameliorate the effect of chemotherapy to improve survival. Among the randomized chemotherapy trials, there are a variety of treatment regimens. Some have utilized tamoxifen, cyclophosphamide, combination therapy [cyclophosphamide-methotrexate-5-fluorouracil (CMF)], CMF with prednisone, or melphalan. The schedules have ranged from short intensive courses to long courses of therapy. Doses may have differed among the studies. Some studies have been made on node-negative patients only, and some have been on node-positive patients. Still other have included both. The eligibility requirements for the trials may differ in substantial ways.

Should the meta-analysis be restricted to published studies only, or should it include both published and unpublished studies? Published studies tend to be positive, whereas

Table V-1-19.   Elements of Proportional Hazard Model

Variable	Level	Model	Estimates of Parameters*
Performance Status	Ambulatory	1	
	Nonambulatory	e^{α}	$\hat{\alpha} = .66 \pm 16$
Treatment			
	M	1	
	ML	e^{β_1}	$\hat{\beta}_1 = .36 \pm .17$
	MLCC	e^{β_2}	$\hat{\beta}_2 = .49 \pm .18$
Site			
	Other	1	
	Tongue	e^{γ_1}	$\hat{\gamma}_1 = .26 \pm .26$
	Hypopharynx	e^{γ_2}	$\hat{\gamma}_2 = .18 \pm .32$
	Larynx	e^{γ_3}	$\hat{\gamma}_3 = .45 \pm .26$
Weight Loss			
	None ($x = 0$)	1	
	< 5% ($x = 2$)	$e^{2\delta}$	
		$e^{\delta x}$	$\hat{\delta} = .14 \pm .05$
	5–10% ($x = 3$)	$e^{3\delta}$	
	> 10% ($x = 4$)	$e^{4\delta}$	

*± figures represent 95% confidence intervals.

unpublished studies tend to be negative. However, the data quality of unpublished studies may not be the same as for published studies. How does one find unpublished studies? Finally, the methods used to carry out the meta-analysis give more weight to studies with larger sample sizes and do not give any weight to the quality of a study. Nevertheless, the proponents of meta-analysis believe that despite all of these problems, a meta-analysis is worthwhile.

To discuss the basic issues, the meta-analysis carried out by the Early Breast Cancer Trialists' Collaborative Group of cytotoxic therapy for early breast cancer patients will be reviewed.[3] The meta-analysis includes almost all randomized clinical trials (published and unpublished) that were made available for analysis. The only exclusions were trials in Japan and the USSR. The number of trials in the analysis totalled 35, which were divided into four major subgroups: 1) trials of CMF or [CMF–prednisone (CMFP)]; 2) trials of CMF + extra cytotoxic agents; 3) trials of combination therapy that include some C, M, or F; 4) trials of single agents. The analysis was divided into two sets corresponding to women less than 50 years of age at time of entry to trial and those 50 or greater. We shall only consider the analysis for the younger women. The essential summary of the analysis has been put in graphical form by the authors and appears as Figure V-1-4. The columns are self-explanatory except for the last two. The authors have calculated the difference between the observed number of deaths (O) and the expected number of deaths (E) for the treatment, assuming there is no difference between treatment and control. This difference is written as O − E and the results are given for each trial. A negative value reflects that the treatment group had less deaths than expected. The value of O − E is given for each trial. The graphical portion of the figure plots the ratio of treatment to control mortality rates with a 99% confidence interval for each trial. A value less than unity indicates that mortality is less for the treatment than control. The diamond symbol is centered on the average ratio of mortality rates. Its length represents a 95% confidence interval. The figure contains the average mortality ratios for each of the four subgroups of trials as well as an overall ratio, which appears at the bottom. The overall conclusions are that: 1) trials including CMF (group a) have a significant reduction in the annual mortality rate (37% ± 9%); 2) none of the other three clinical trial groups indicate a significant reduction in mortality; and 3) all four groups combined together share a 22% ± 6% reduction in overall mortality. This last conclusion mainly reflects the inclusion of the CMF trials in the overall average.

If we examine the CMF (group a) trials, among the 11 trials listed, 3 have less than 5 patients per treatment group and did not warrant inclusion. Of the remaining 8 trials, all had a no treatment control group except Glasgow, which had a control group receiving radiotherapy. Both the ECOG (6177) and the Ludwig III trials added prednisone to the CMF, with the Ludwig trial also adding tamoxifen. With the exception of the Leiden and UK/Asia trials, all had a 12-month course of therapy, with the former having a 24-month course of therapy. Thus, the trials were not all comparable, but reasonably close with respect to therapy. It is questionable whether the Glasgow study should be included because it does not have a no treatment control group. In any event,

excluding trials with small numbers, of the remaining 8 trials, all produced a negative O − E, which indicates an excess of deaths in the control group. The chance of this happening, if treatment is not beneficial, is the same as tossing a fair coin eight times and observing all heads or all tails. This probability is $P = .016$ and is unlikely to have happened by chance. Hence one could have readily concluded that the aggregate of trials having CMF as their therapy reduces mortality. Among the eight mature trials, five are individually significant at the .05 level, i.e., INT Milan 7205, Glasgow, Leiden, Guys/Manch II, INT Milan 8004. Thus, it is no surprise that the meta-analysis reached a similar conclusion. The use of a 99% confidence interval for the individual trials obscures those trials significant at the conventional 5% level. It is not clear why this was done.

The overall value of O − E essentially gives more weight to trials having the larger number of patients. There is no attempt to weight or judge the quality of these studies. However, one clue to the quality of these studies is that there should be equal numbers of patients in each treatment group for every trial except for chance fluctuations. Note that the total number of patients in the treatment and control groups are 635 and 554, respectively, in the group a analysis. The probability that such a split could arise by chance is $P = .02$. In other words, the split is not random and probably reflects differential quality among these trials. The major contributors to this imbalance are: INT Milan 7205, Glasgow, and UK/Asia. These trials represent 40% of the total number of patients in group a. Additional trials have been analyzed in a recent report of the Early Breast Cancer Trialists.[3A]

It is not at all certain that many poor trials considered as a constellation in a meta-analysis will shed more light than two good trials which reach similar conclusions. The strength of meta-analysis is numbers, but the weakness is failure to consider the inherent quality of the research design and execution by better investigators. Babe Ruth and Hank Aaron could doubtless teach more about home run hitting than their 16 additional teammates combined.

References

1. Anderson, J. R., Cain K. C., and Gelber, R. D.: Analysis of survival by tumor response. J. Clin. Oncol., 1:710, 1983.
2. Antman, K., Amato, D., Wood, W., et al: Selection bias in clinical trials. J. Clin. Oncol., 3:1142, 1985.
3. Early Breast Cancer Trialists' Collaborative Group: Effects of adjuvant tamoxifen and of cytotoxic therapy on mortality in early breast cancer. N. Engl. J. Med., 319:1687, 1988.
3A.Early Breast Cancer Trialists' Collaborative Group: Systemic Treatment of Early Breast Cancer by Hormonal, Cytotoxic, or Immune Therapy. One hundred thirty-three randomized trials involving 31,000 recurrences and 24,000 deaths among 75,000 women. Lancet, 339:1(Part 1), 85(Part 2), 1992.
4. Geller, N. L.: Planned interim analysis and its role in cancer clinical trials. J. Clin. Oncol., 5:1485, 1987.
5. Goldhirsch, A., Gelber, R. D., Simes, R. J., et al: Costs and benefits of adjuvant therapy in breast cancer: A quality adjusted survival analysis. J. Clin. Oncol., 7:36, 1989.
6. Hill, A. B.: Principles of Medical Statistics (5th Edition). London, The Lancet Limited, 1956.
7. Lefkopoulou, M., and Zelen, M.: Unpublished data, 1992.
8. Louis, P. C. A.: Essays in Clinical Instruction (translated). London, P. Martin, 1834.
9. Neaton, J. D., Brose, S., Fishman, E. L., et al: The Multiple Risk Factor Interventions Trial (MRFIT) VII. A comparison of risk factor changes between two study groups. Prev. Med., 10:519, 1981.
10. Rosner, G. L., and Tsiatis, A. A.: The impact that group sequential tests would have made on ECOG clinical trials. Stat. Med., 8:505, 1989.
11. Simes, R. J., and Zelen, M.: Exploratory data analysis and the use of the hazard function for interpreting survival data: An investigator's primer. J. Clin. Oncol., 3:1418, 1985.
12. Taylor, K. M., Margolese, R. G., and Saskolne, C. L.: Physicians' reasons for not entering eligible patients in a randomized clinical trial of surgery for breast cancer. N. Engl. J. Med., 310:1363, 1984.

(A) Women aged < 50 years at entry

Study Name	Treatment	Basic Data (Deaths/Patients) Treatment Group	Control Group	Deaths in Treatment Group Observed - Expected	Variance of O-E	Ratio of Treatment to Control Mortality Rates (Result, Confidence Interval & % improvement)
(a) Trials of CMF (N.B: includes CMFPr, but not CMF + other cytotoxics)						
INT Milan 7205	CMF	41/95	46/75	-8.3	15.4	
Manchester I *	CMF	8/21	9/24	-0.2	3.8	
Glasgow	CMF	16/47	18/34	-4.8	6.9	
Leiden Mamma	CMF	15/96	23/90	-5.2	8.6	
Danish BCG 77b *	CMF	46/149	44/130	-2.3	20.5	
ECOG EST6177	CMFPr	0/1	1/8	-0.1	0.1	
UK/Asia Collab.	CMF	21/131	20/99	-2.7	9.1	
Ludwig III *	CMF	1/2	4/4	-0.4	0.5	
Guy's/Manch. II	CMF	9/63	19/60	-7.0	6.3	
INT Milan 8004	CMF	0/26	5/29	-2.2	1.2	
Danish BCG 82c	CMF	0/4	0/1			
Subtotal (a): CMF		157/635	189/554	-33.3	72.4	37% ± 9
(b) Trials of CMF with extra cytotoxics						
West Midlands	CMFVALeu	48/119	59/119	-6.9	23.0	
Vienna	CMFV	9/32	9/27	-0.8	4.1	
SWOG 7827 A	CMFVPr	-/14	-/13	blind	0.2	
Case Western B	CMFVPr	2/19	0/20	1.0	0.5	
GROCTA Italy	CMF then E	1/38	1/39	0.0	0.5	
Subtotal (b): CMF plus		61/222	69/218	-6.3	28.3	20% ± 17
(c) Trials of regimes without some or all of C, M, F						
Mayo Clinic	CFPr	3/5	1/3	0.8	0.7	
East Berlin	various	22/59	16/28	-1.0	6.9	
DFCI 74063	AC	1/2	1/1	-0.3	0.2	
UK MCCG 003	CVF/CVM	32/61	25/47	2.1	11.4	
Northwick Park	MefV	7/21	8/24	0.0	3.4	
King's CRC I	MeIM	35/85	29/62	-1.8	13.6	
West Midlands	LeuMF	19/122	20/131	-0.3	9.2	
Oxford *	MeIMF	13/45	19/48	-2.4	7.3	
MD Anderson8026	MV	1/51	6/63	-2.1	1.7	
N Sweden BCG	AC	1/16	7/22	-2.1	1.8	
SE Sweden BCG	BAC	0/0	1/1			
Subtotal (c): other polychem		134/467	133/430	-7.2	56.2	12% ± 13
Total (a + b + c): any polychem		352/1324	391/1202	-46.7	156.9	26% ± 7
(d) Trials of single agents						
Birmingham & WM	C/F	38/77	13/28	1.7	8.7	
NSABP B-05	Mel	24/68	38/61	-7.2	11.8	
Edinburgh II	F	39/59	42/56	-4.3	15.2	
Guy's/Manch. I *	Mel	26/69	34/74	-2.6	13.2	
Dublin	F	5/8	5/10	0.9	2.0	
Danish BCG 77b *	C	39/128	44/130	-2.1	19.0	
Oxford *	Mel	17/44	19/48	-0.3	7.8	
S Swedish BCG	C	17/98	10/90	3.7	6.5	
Subtotal (d): single agents		205/551	205/497	-10.3	84.2	11% ± 10
Total (a + b + c + d): any chem		557/1875	524/1497	-54.6	219.8	22% ± 6

```
          0.0      0.5      1.0      1.5      2.0
             Treated better  |  Treated worse
```

Figure V-1-4. Results of meta-analysis of clinical trials evaluating cytotoxic drugs as adjuvant treatment for breast cancer: Woman aged < 50 years at entry. (From Early Breast Cancer Trialists' Collaborative Group.[3])

13. Zelen, M.: The randomization and stratification of patients to clinical trials. J Chron. Dis., 27:365, 1974.
14. Zelen, M.: Guidelines for publishing papers on cancer clinical trials: Responsibilities of editors and authors. J. Clin. Oncol., 1:1614, 1983.

Additional Readings

A good overall book on general features of clinical trials is Pocock, S. J.: *Clinical Trials: A Practical Approach,* Chichester, John Wiley & Sons, 1983. There are a number of books devoted to clinical trials in which individual authors have written chapters on specialized topics. Among those that contain expository chapters on statistical methods are: Miké, V., and Stanley, K. E. (eds.): *Statistics in Medical Research,* New York, John Wiley & Sons, 1982; and Shapiro, S. H., and Louis, T. A. (eds.), *Clinical Trials,* New York, Marcel Dekker, 1983. A more general compilation that stresses the practical problems in carrying out cancer clinical trials is: Buyse, M. E., Staquet, M. J., and Sylvester, R. J. (eds.), *Cancer Clinical Trials,* Oxford, Oxford University Press, 1984. A compilation of chapters targeted at early breast cancer trials is found in Baum, M., Kay, R., and Scheurlen, H. (eds.): *Clinical Trials In Early Breast Cancer: Second Heidelberg Symposium.* Basel, Birkhaeuser Verlag, 1982.

There are a number of papers that provide charts or extensive tables for making sample size calculations. Among these are: Feigl, P.: A graphical aid for determining sample size when comparing two independent proportions. *Biometrics,* 34:111, 1978; Freedman, L. S.: Tables of the number of patients required in clinical trials using the logrank test. *Statistics in Medicine,* 1:121, 1982; Schoenfeld, D. A., and Richter, J. R.: Nomograms for calculating the number of patients needed for a clinical trial with survival as an endpoint. *Biometrics,* 38:163, 1982.

Meta-analysis of clinical trials will continue to be a source of debate in medical research. A popular, but not dispassionate account of this topic, is Mann, C.: Meta-analysis in the breech. *Science,* 249:476, 1990. Another overview of breast cancer adjuvant trials that uses hazard functions is Zelen, M., and Gelman, R.: Assessment of adjuvant trials in breast cancer. NCI Monograph. *Adjuvant Chemotherapy and Endocrine Therapy for Breast Cancer.* Washington, D.C., U.S. Government Printing Office, 1986.

The planning of sequential trials requires complex calculations and specialized software that is not widely available. A software package, suitable for personal computers, that is easy to use is expected to be available at the end of 1991 from Cytel, Inc., Cambridge, MA.

COLOR
PLATES

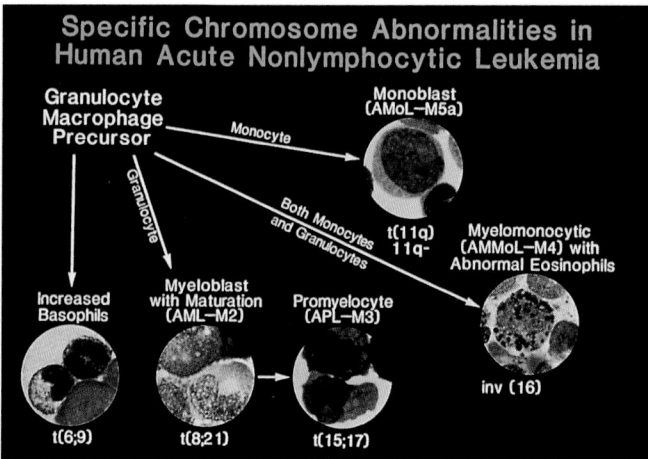

I–8–PLATE 1. Specific chromosome abnormalities associated with specific types of human acute nonlymphocytic leukemia.

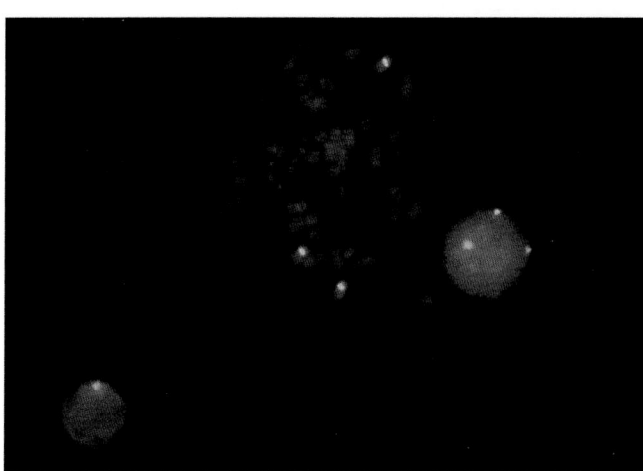

I–8–PLATE 2. In situ hybridization with biotinylated DNA probe to chromosome 8 centromere demonstrates three copies of chromosome 8 in a metaphase and in an interphase cell. The probe was detected with fluoresceinated avidin (yellow) and the cells were counterstained with propidium iodide (red). Magnification: X1,000.

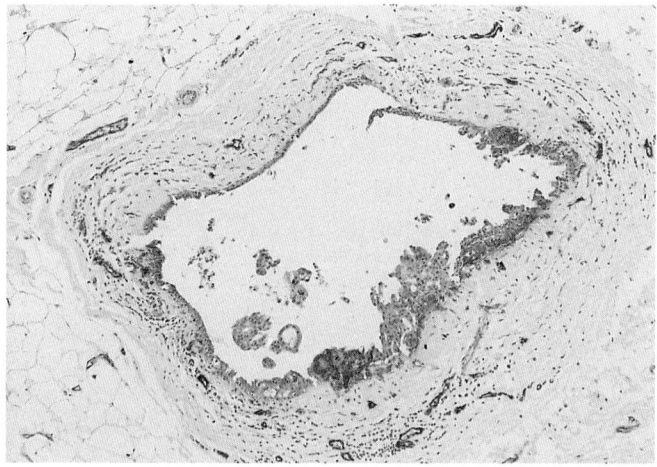

I–11–PLATE 1. Hematoxylin and eosin stained section with immunoperoxidase staining for Factor VIII shows cluster of endothelial cells (brown) immediately adjacent to segment of human breast duct with early carcinoma in situ. This represents earliest switch to angiogenic state. Angiogenesis is absent near remaining normal epithelium of the duct.

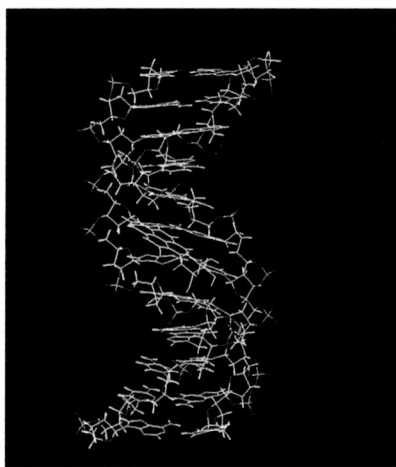

III–2–PLATE 1. Computer modeled image of the anti-benzo {alpha} pyrene-diol-epoxide deoxyguanosine adduct formed in the minor groove of a 12-base pair DNA sequence (5'-ATCGGCGCGGTA-3'). The structure is a half-bond color stick model. C=grey, N=blue, O=red, P=green, H=white. All atoms of the polycyclic hydrocarbon moiety are yellow.

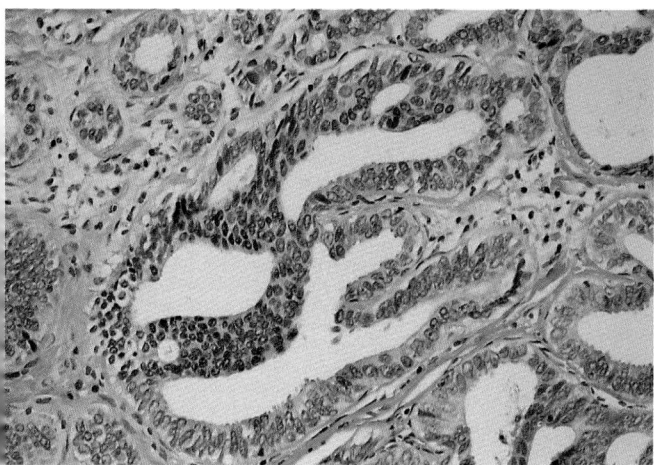

VIII–1–PLATE 1. Adenocarcinoma of the breast. The tumor is arranged in the form of fairly well differentiated glands separated by a fibrous connective tissue stroma. Moderate numbers of inflammatory cells, mostly lymphocytes, are present in the stroma. H&E, X65.

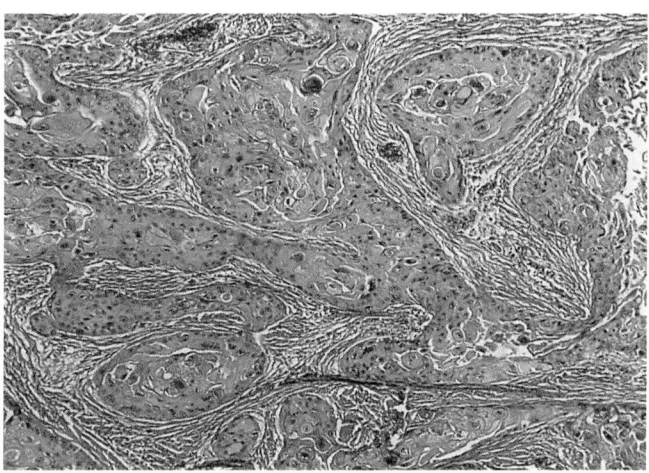

VIII–1–PLATE 2. Squamous cell carcinoma of the skin of the face. The tumor consists of islands of well differentiated squamous epithelium separated by fibrous connective tissue stroma. Note that epithelium forms "keratin pearls." H&E, X60.

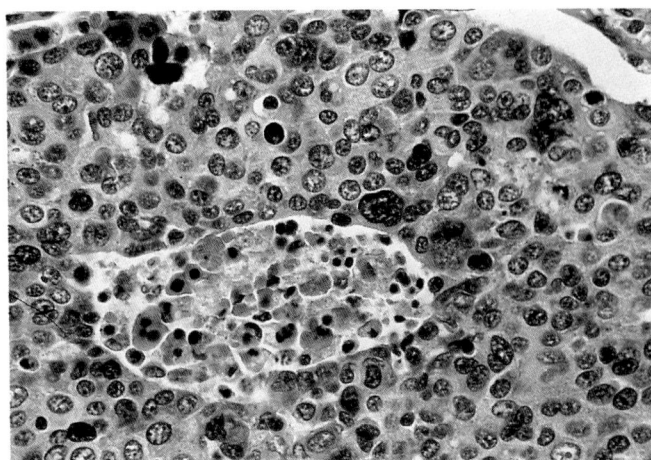

VIII–1–PLATE 3. Undifferentiated carcinoma of the lung. The tumor is comprised of irregularly arranged pleomorphic tumor cells with large nuclei and prominent nucleoli. A central necrotic zone, typical of this type of tumor, is present. There is little stroma. H&E, X100.

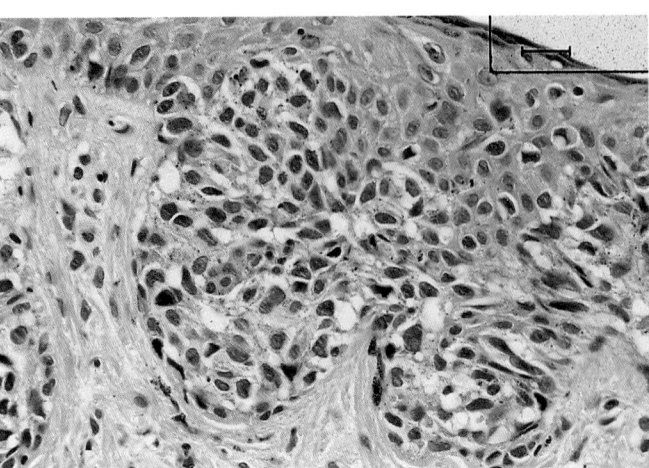

VIII–1–PLATE 4. Malignant melanoma arising in the skin. Tumor is comprised of large, irregular cells with large nuclei, prominent nucleoli, and abundant, clear cytoplasm, peppered with dots and larger accumulations of melanin pigment. H&E, X100.

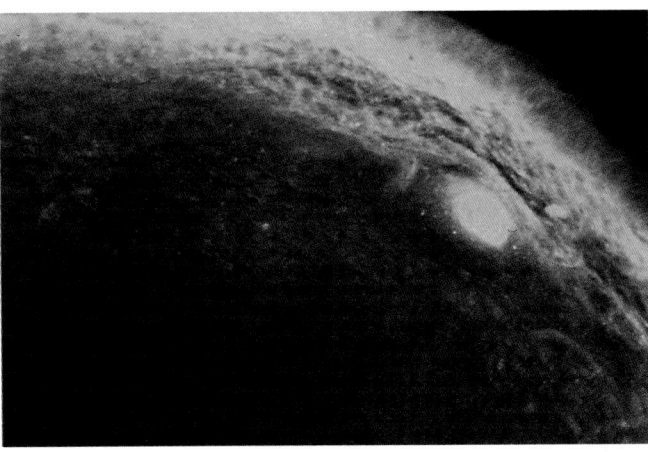

VIII–1–PLATE 5. Lewis lung carcinoma growing in the flank of a syngeneic C57Bl/6 mouse that had received a macromolecular tracer, 70kDa fluoresceinated dextran, 15 minutes previously. Bright-staining apple green fluorescence forming a rim around the tumor represents extensive extravasation of tracer into the surrounding normal connective tissue from leaky blood vessels at the tumor-host interface. The tumor itself is virtually unstained, appearing as a "black hole," because tracer at its periphery diffuses poorly into the tumor. Fluorescence microscopy, X15.

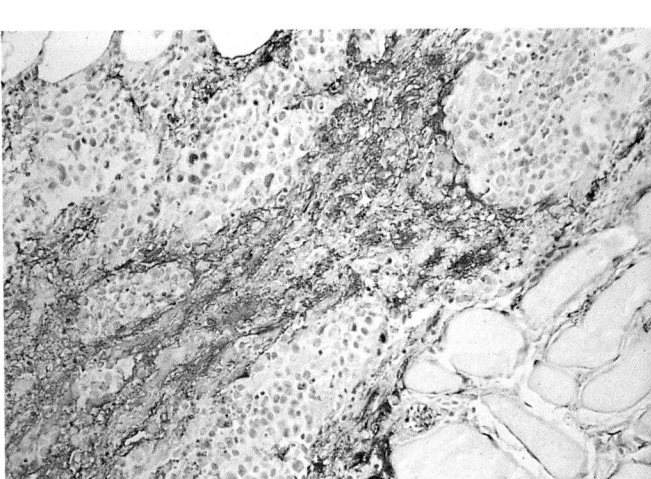

VIII–1–PLATE 6. Immunoperoxidase staining reaction of the line 10 guinea pig undifferentiated bile duct carcinoma exposed to a monoclonal antibody specific for fibrin (kindly supplied by Dr. Gary Matsueda). Tumor is comprised of nests of malignant cells interspersed in a stroma that stains heavily for fibrin. Immunoperoxidase, X50.

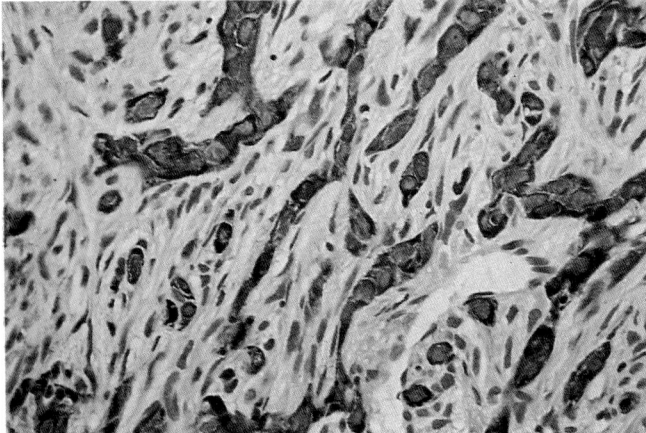

VIII–1–PLATE 7. Immunoperoxidase staining of a monoclonal antibody specific for keratin in a poorly differentiated squamous cell carcinoma of the skin. This "spindle cell" form of the tumor mimics tumors of connective tissue origin and its true nature can often be determined only by immunohistochemistry. Immunoperoxidase, X100.

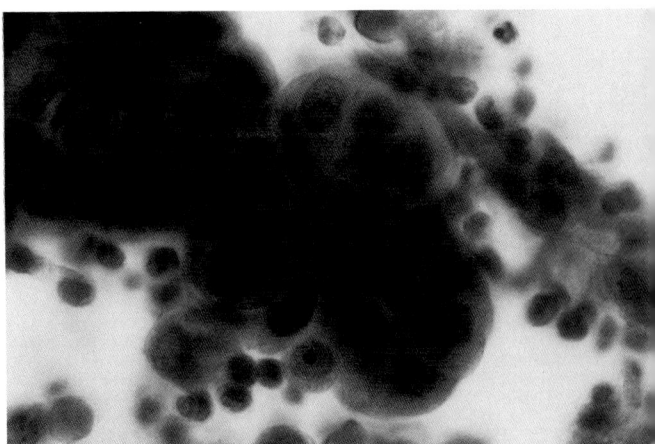

VIII–1–PLATE 8. Ovarian papillary serous adenocarcinoma in ascitic fluid. The cells are present in three-dimensional clusters with nuclear molding and irregular hyperchromatic nuclei. Papanicolaou, X250.

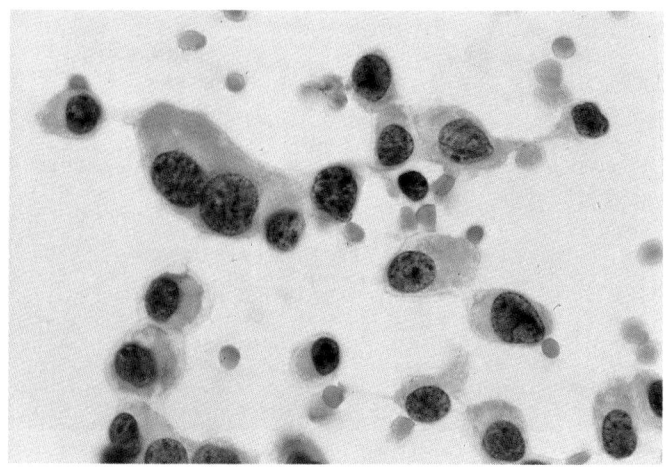

VIII–1–PLATE 9. Metastatic neuroendocrine tumor as seen in a fine needle aspiration of liver. Note the eccentric nuclei with "salt and pepper" chromatin and abundant granular cytoplasm. Immunocytochemical stains confirmed the diagnosis. Papanicolaou, X250.

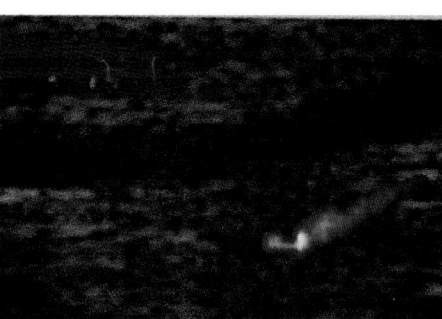

IX–1–PLATE 1. Fifty-five-year-old woman following a left mastectomy and subsequent irradiation presented with acute onset of severe left arm swelling. Color Doppler imaging revealed extensive thrombosis of left subclavian/brachial venous system. Note arterial flow (red) adjacent to vein (uncolored), which shows no flow and is filled with low level echoes representing blood clot.

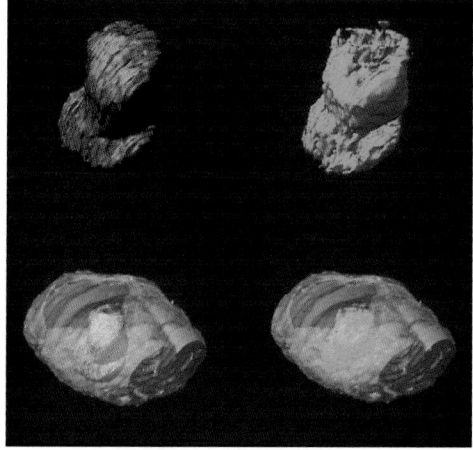

IX–1–PLATE 2. Brown three-dimensional model of a rat brain tumor (upper left) was constructed of thionine-stained histologic sections and corresponds almost exactly with green three-dimensional tumor model (upper right) constructed from autoradiograms. Autoradiograms were made using tritiated ligand, which binds to peripheral benzodiazepine receptors on tumor. Both tumor models are depicted within transparent rat brain in the lower panels.

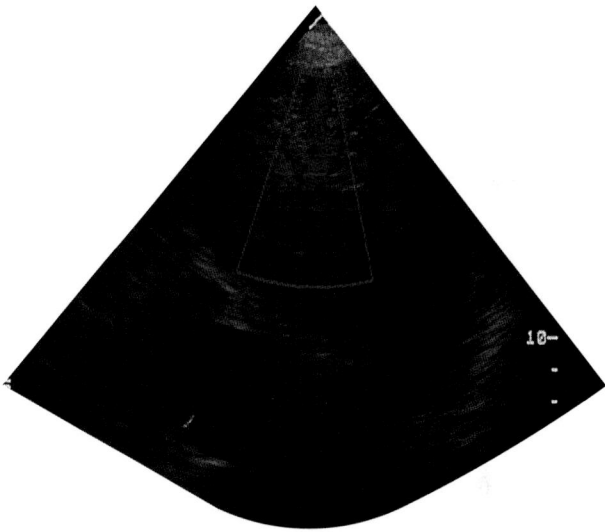

IX–1–PLATE 3. Color flow Doppler reveals normally directed flow in one hepatic vein branch (blue, lower left) and reversed flow in an adjacent branch (red). This finding is diagnostic of Budd-Chiari syndrome.

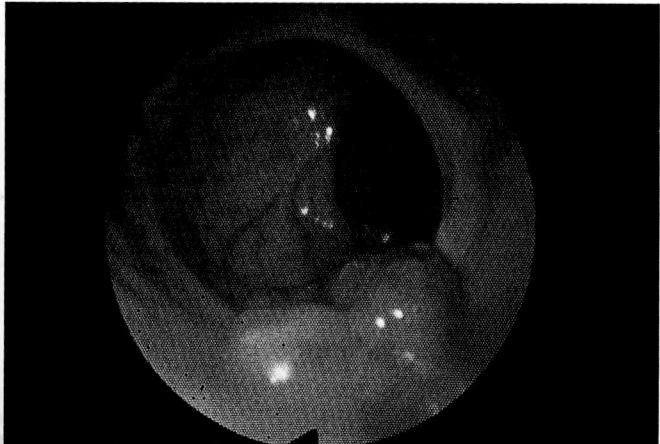

XI–1–PLATE 1. Sessile adenocarcinoma of the rectum discovered during screening colonoscopy in an asymptomatic 50-year-old male. First-degree relatives of patient had had colon cancer.

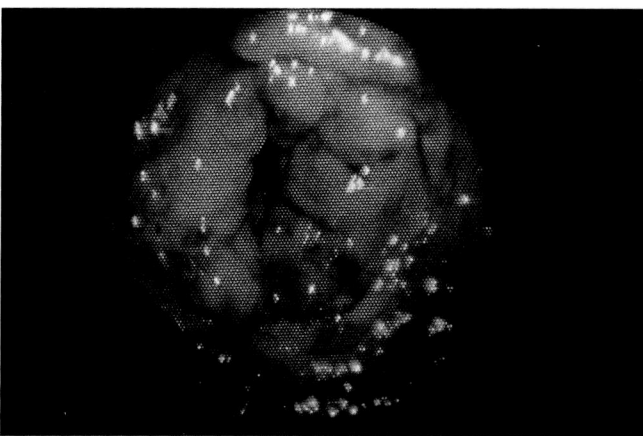

XI–1–PLATE 2. Nearly complete rectal obstruction in an elderly male unfit for surgery. Nd-YAG laser photo ablation provided effective palliation by widening the lumen and reducing the friability of the tumor.

5

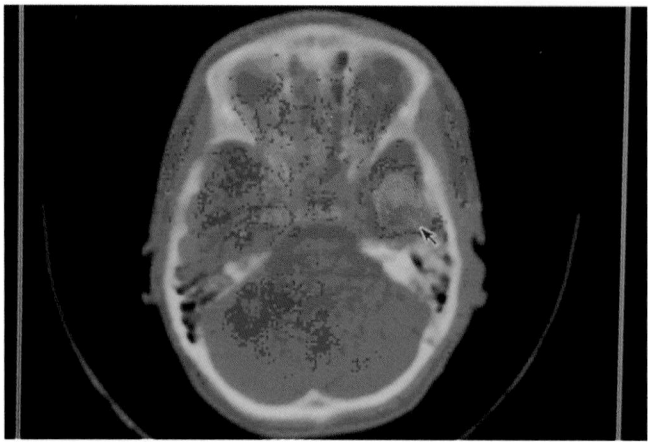

XIII–1–PLATE 1. Image correlation of two complementary imaging modalities, here magnetic resonance imaging (MRI) of tumor and computerized tomography (CT) of skull. Positron emission tomography (PET scanning) or single photon emission computerized tomography (SPECT) can also be correlated in similar fashion.

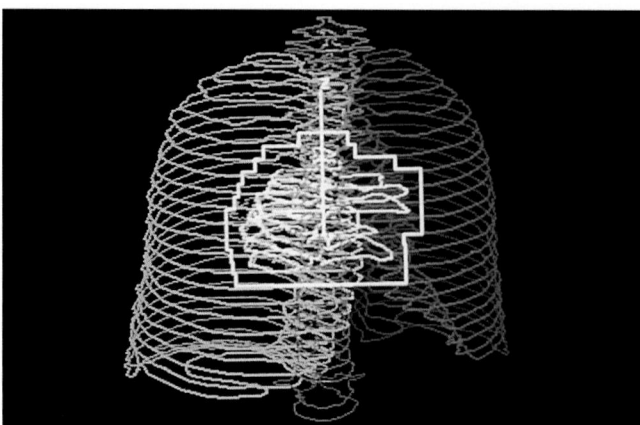

XIII–1–PLATE 2. A beam's eye view graphic of a three-dimensional tumor volume contoured on sequential axial CT scans (white), depicting its location relative to the right lung (yellow), left lung (blue), verebral column (green) and spinal canal (red). A margin of 1 cm defines a suitable aperture to fully encompass the target volume (white border). Rotating the viewing perspectives to oblique angles yields a range of angles that encompass the target yet avoid the spinal cord.

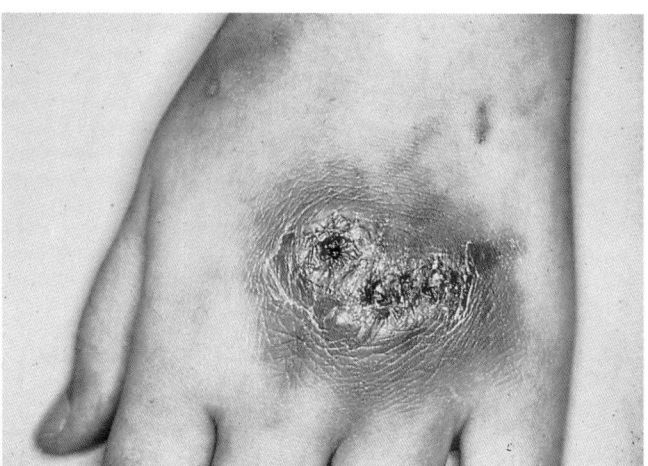

XVI–5–PLATE 1. Necrosis and inflammation from extravasation of doxorubicin.

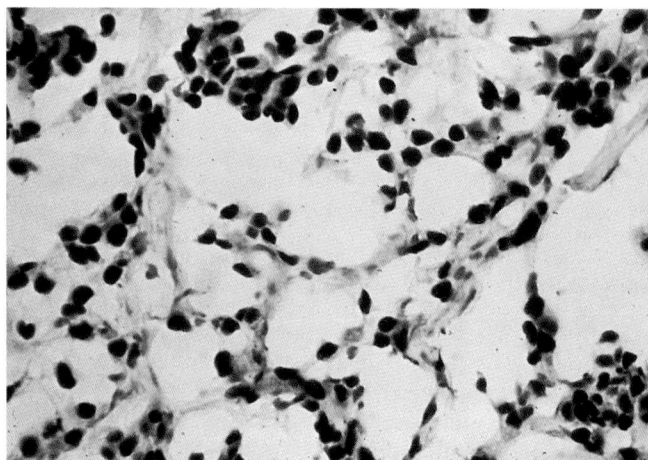

XVII–1–PLATE 1. Immunochemical identification of estrogen receptors in individual cells of 8 μm frozen section of human breast cancer using monoclonal antibody H222 to MCF-7 cell receptor and methods described by King et al. Picric acid-formalin fixation, diaminobenzidine stain, hematoxylin counterstain. X250.

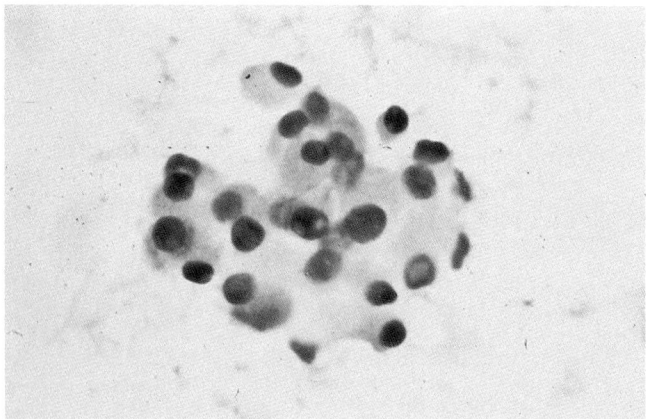

XVII–1–PLATE 2. Same as XVII–1–1; fine needle aspiration.

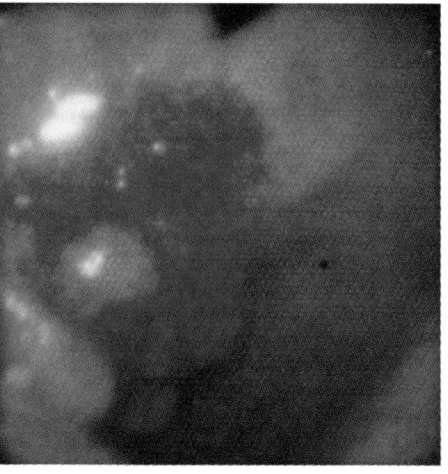

XXVIII–1–PLATE 1. Fiberoptic bronchoscopic picture of carcinoma at interbronchial carina.

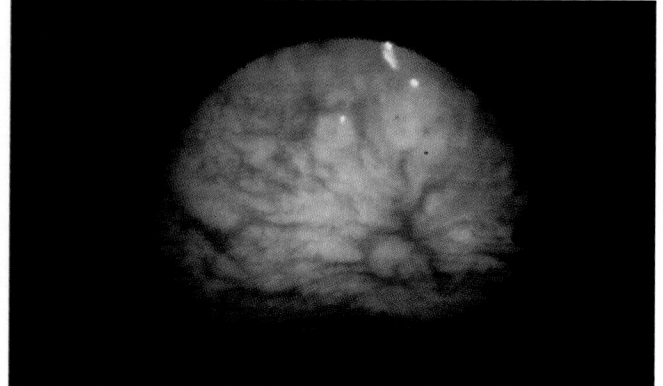

XXIX–1–PLATE 1. Fiberoptic gastroscopic picture of carcinoma of the stomach.

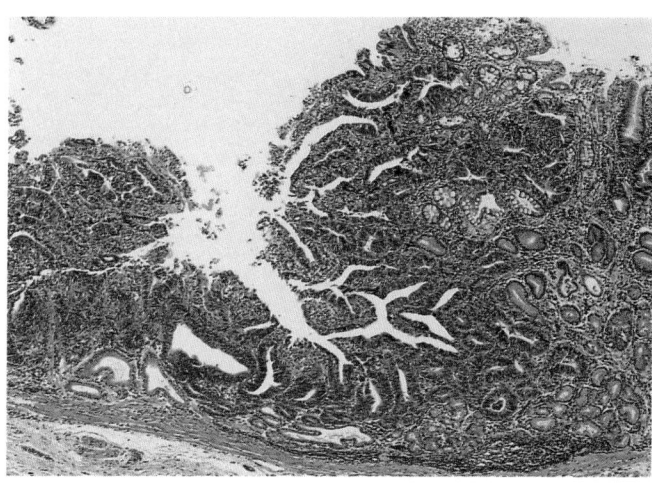

XXIX–2–PLATE 2. Adenocarcinoma of the stomach.

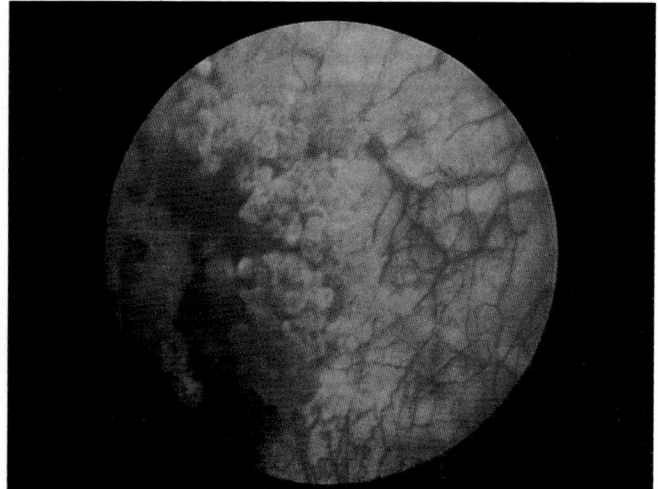

XXX–3–PLATE 1. Cystoscopic view of multiple papillary carcinomas of bladder.

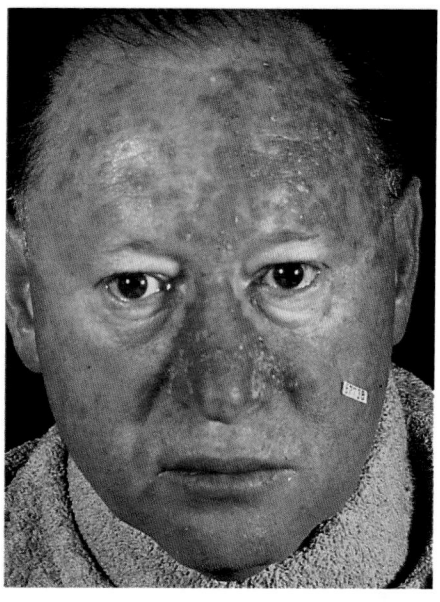

XXXIII–1–PLATE 1. Actinic keratosis. Extensive actinic keratosis on the face. Note that the right half has been used as a control and the left half of the forehead and the nose was treated with 5% 5-fluorouracil for 14 days. One month later the entire face had been treated and had healed, much improved.

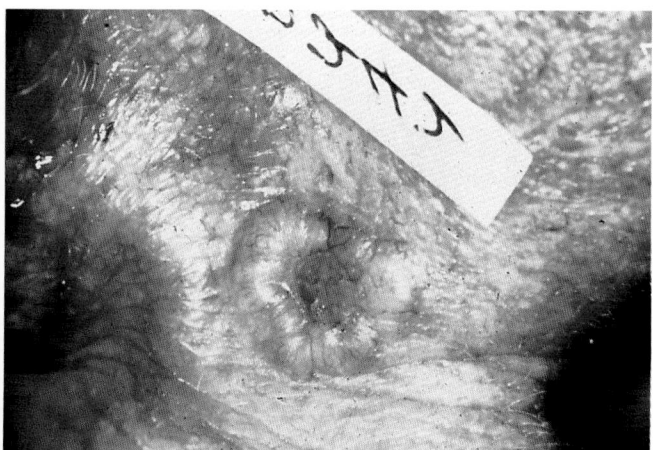

XXXIII–1–PLATE 2. Basal cell carcinoma. The lesion is quite limited clinically.

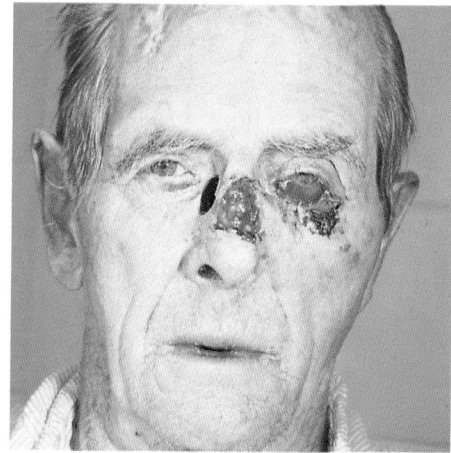

XXXIII–1–PLATE 3. Basal cell carcinoma. Note the erosive nature of longstanding lesions.

7

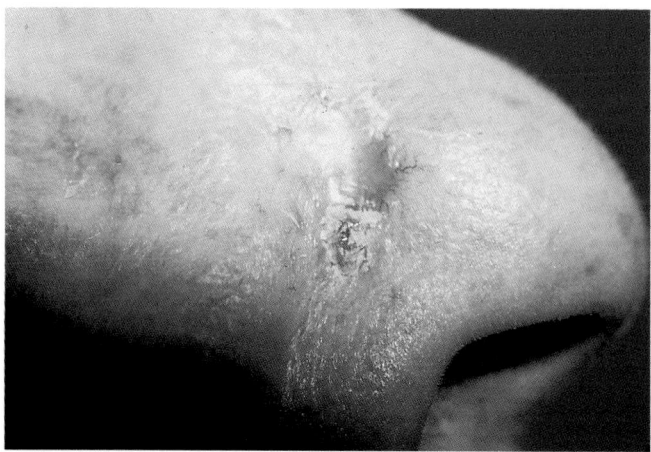

XXXIII–1–PLATE 4. Basal cell carcinoma. A pearly nodule with an umbilicated, ulcerated center and telangiectasia.

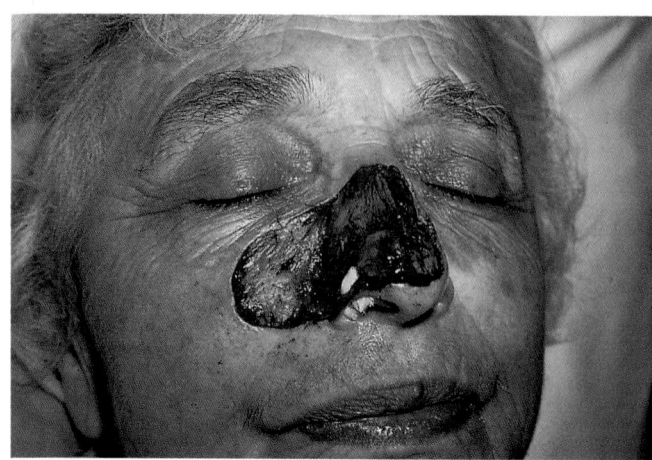

XXXIII–1–PLATE 5. Same patient as XXXIII-1-Plate 4 after treatment with Mohs' surgery, illustrating the cryptic extension far beyond the clinically evident border.

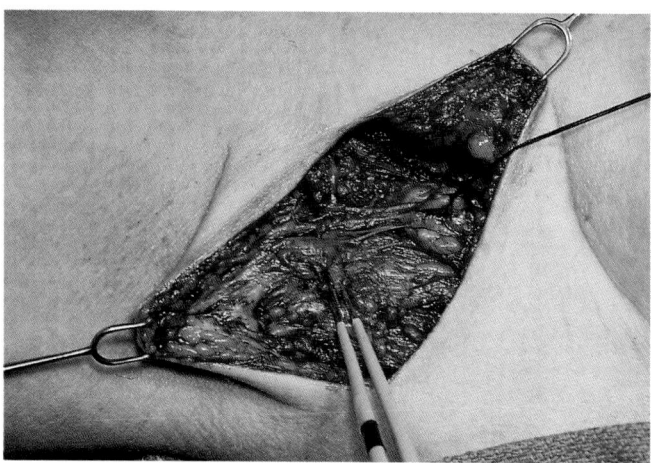

XXXIV–1–PLATE 1. Malignant melanoma. Intraoperative mapping of regional lymphatics for selective lymphadenectomy. Blue lymphatic channel drains into "sentinel" lymph node, which is also stained.

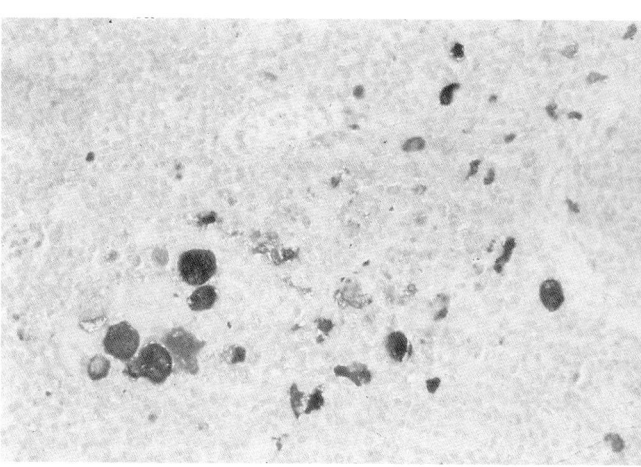

XXXIV–1–PLATE 2. Occult melanoma cells metastatic to lymph node detected by immunohistologic chemical technique using monoclonal antibody to S-100 protein.

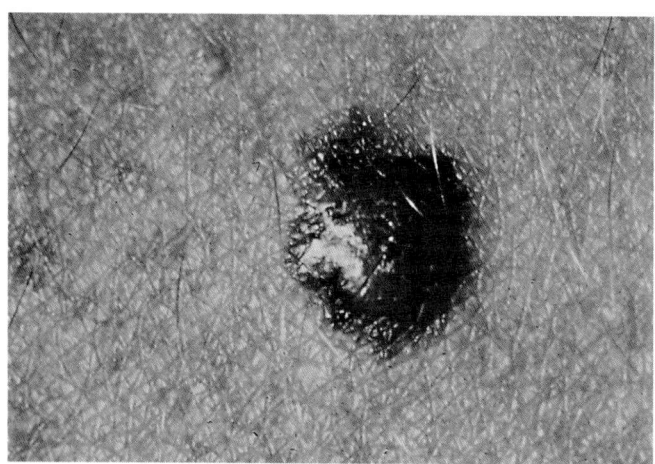

XXXIV–1–PLATE 3. Nodular melanoma.

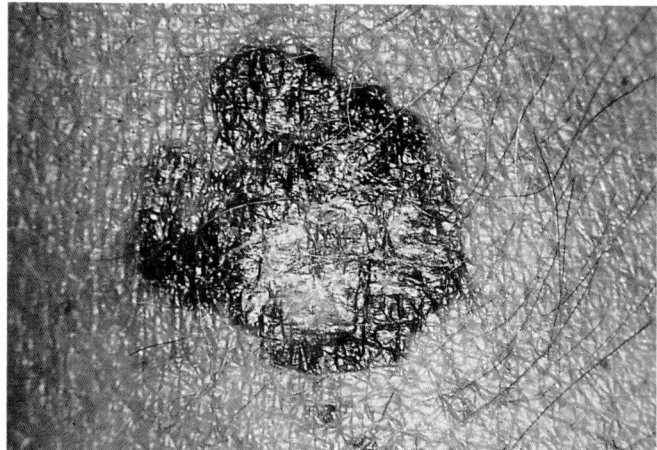

XXXIV–1–PLATE 4. Superficial spreading melanoma. Note irregular border, variations in color and area of partial regression.

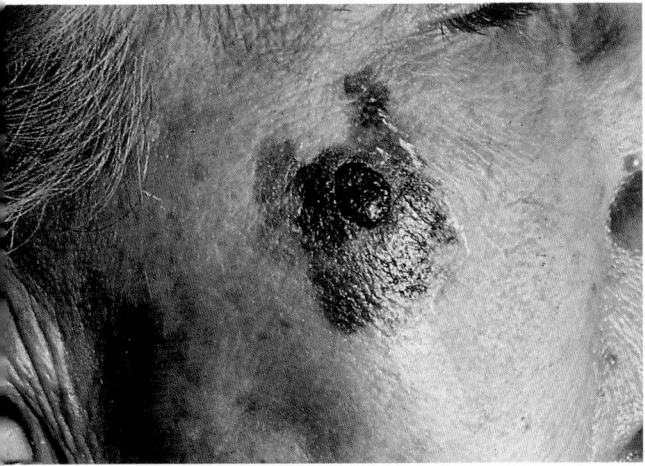

XXXIV–1–PLATE 5. Lentigo maligna melanoma with a nodular area of accelerated growth.

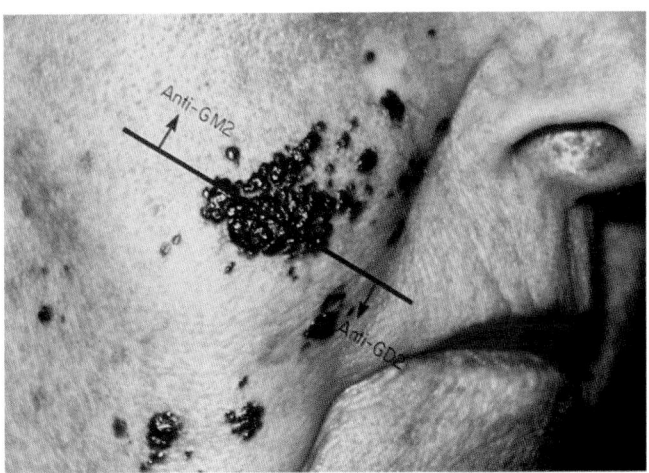

XXXIV–1–PLATE 6. Recurrent melanoma, unresponsive to radiotherapy, prior to immunotherapy with intralesional injections of human monoclonal antibody to GM_2 or GD_2.

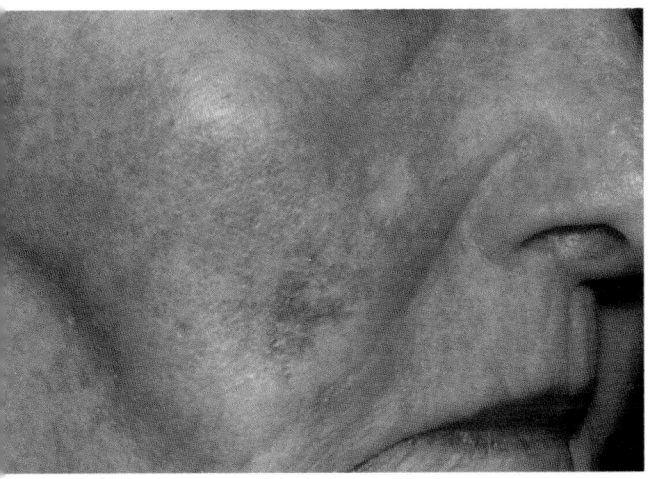

XXXIV–1–PLATE 7. The same patient 2 ½ years later following complete regression of all disease.

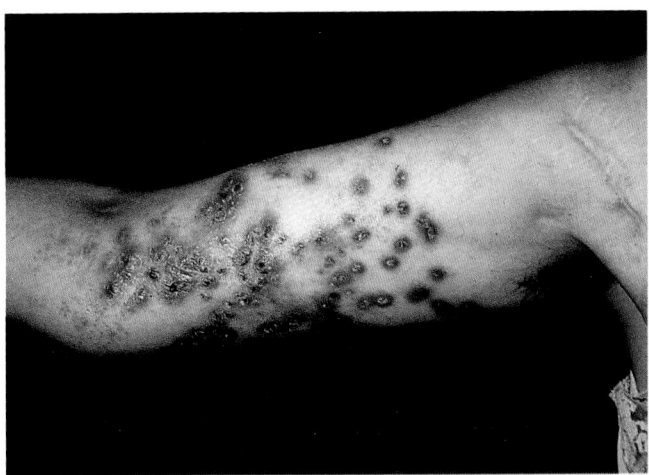

XXXIV–1–PLATE 8. Recurrent melanoma treated with intralesional BCG injections.

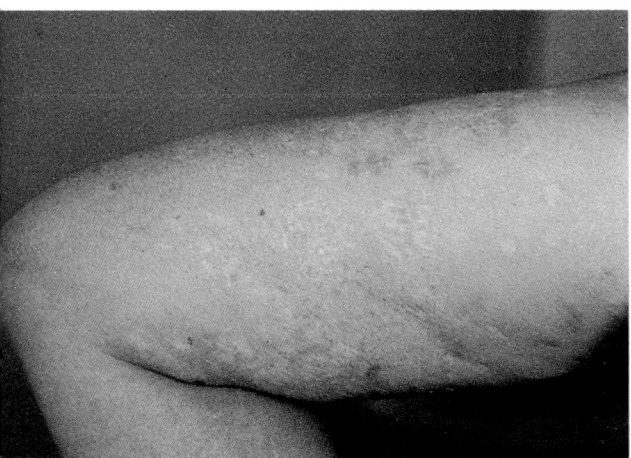

XXXIV–1–PLATE 9. Complete regression of patient in XXXIV-1-Plate 8 five years later. Patient free of disease at last follow-up ten years later.

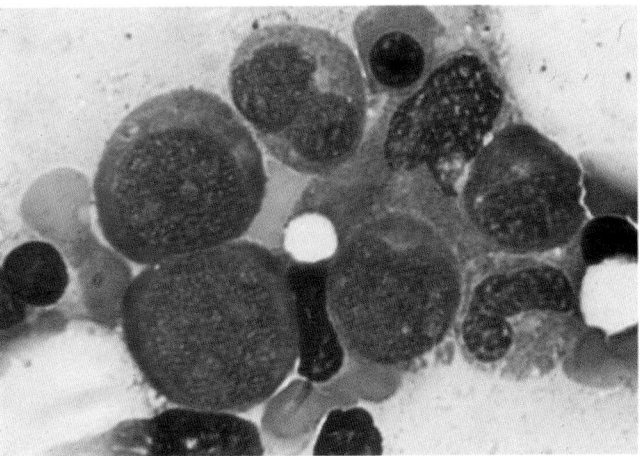

XXXVI–1–PLATE 1. Myelodysplastic syndrome. Left shifted myeloid series in bone marrow with immature blasts containing prominent nucleoli, a giant metamyelocyte with hypogranulation and megaloblastoid erythropoiesis. These are characteristic features of disordered maturation and differentiation.

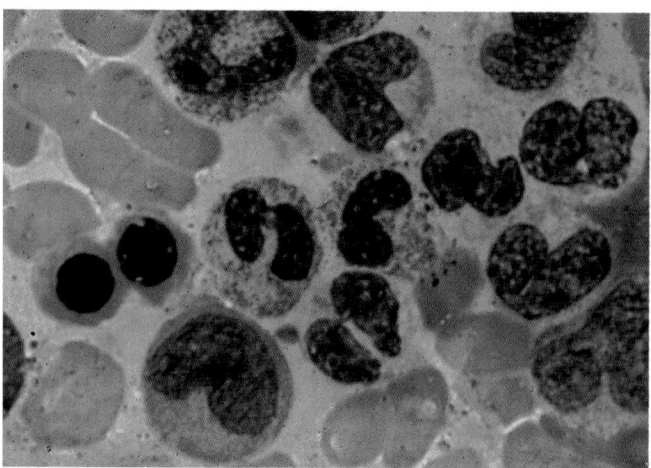

XXXVI–1–PLATE 2. Myelodysplastic syndrome. Bone marrow of a different patient shows maturing bilobed granulocytes with acquired psuedo-Pelger-Huet anomaly, metamyelocytes, promonocyte, and megaloblastoid erythropoiesis.

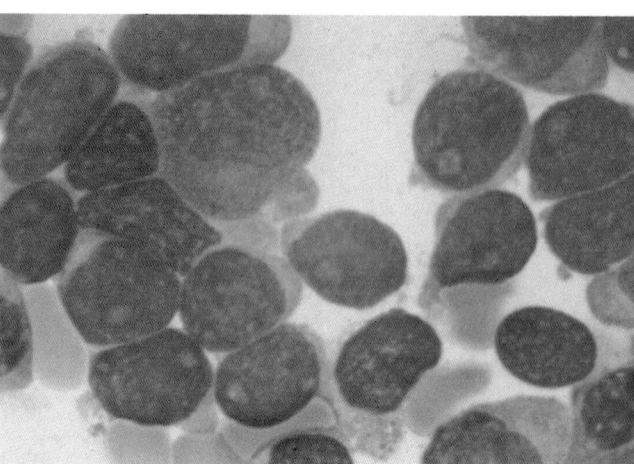

XXXVI–2–PLATE 1. FAB MO. Marrow blasts from patient with this undifferentiated type of acute myelogenous leukemia can have variable amounts of agranular cytoplasm without Auer rods. The cells are peroxidase and Sudan black negative and can be confused with FAB M7 or FAB L2. The myeloid commitment of these blasts can be confirmed by immunophenotyping with antibodies against myeloid antigens and/or demonstration of ultrastructural peroxidase positive granules using transmission electron microscopy.

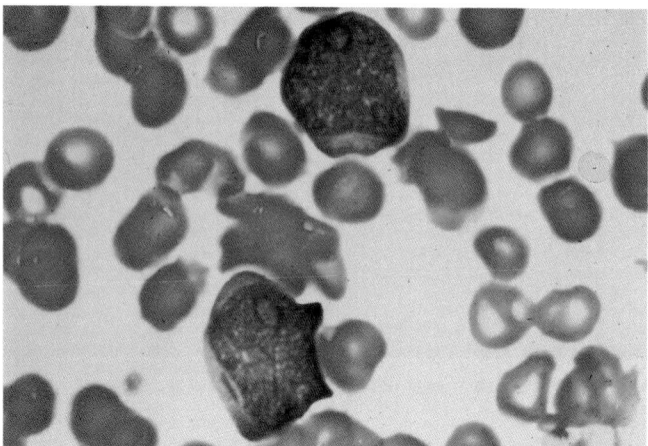

XXXVI–2–PLATE 2. FAB M1. Typical appearance of blasts in this category. A prominent Auer rod is seen.

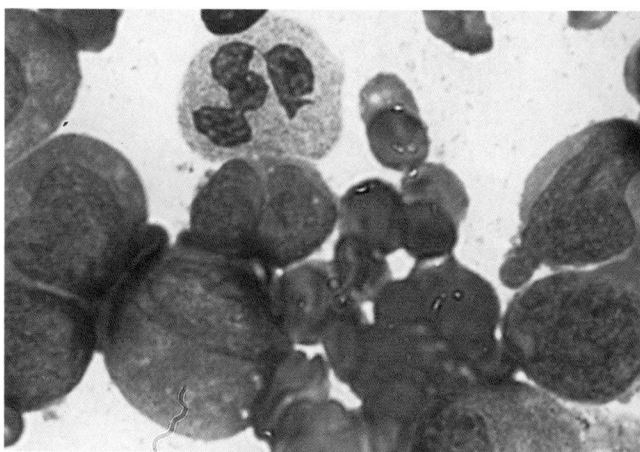

XXXVI–2–PLATE 3. FAB M2. Leukemia is characterized by evidence of continued myeloid differentiation with myelocytes and more mature myeloid elements present.

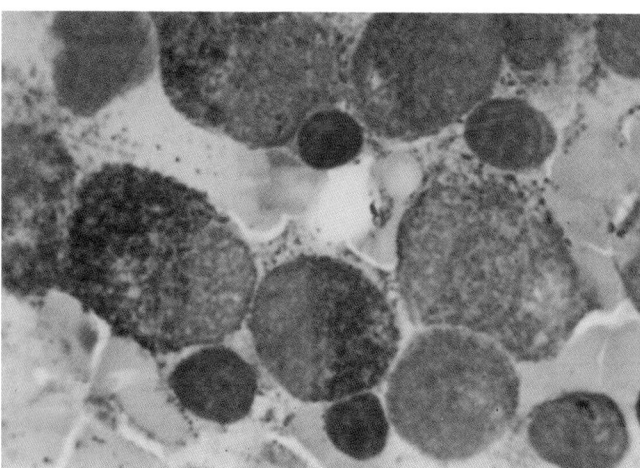

XXXVI–2–PLATE 4. FAB M3. Progranulocytic leukemic cells usually have round nuclei with heavily granulated cytoplasm. Extracellular granules from disrupted cells are often noted, and blasts with multiple Auer rods (not shown) are common. This leukemia has typical 15, 17 translocation, and a characteristic clinical picture of disseminated intravascular coagulation.

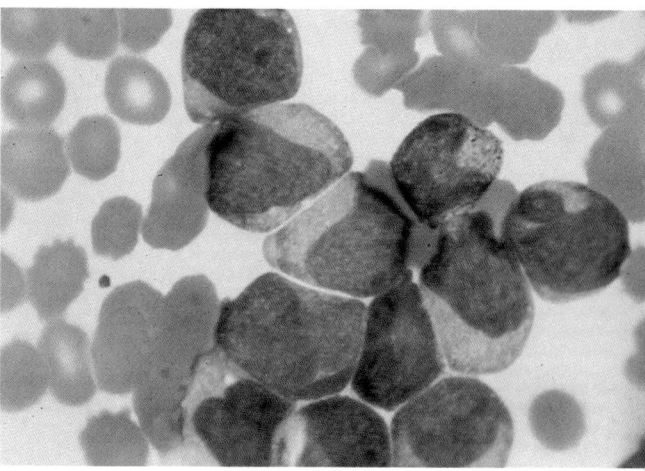

XXXVI–2–PLATE 5. FAB M4. Myelomonocytic leukemia has blasts with both myeloid and monocytoid appearance.

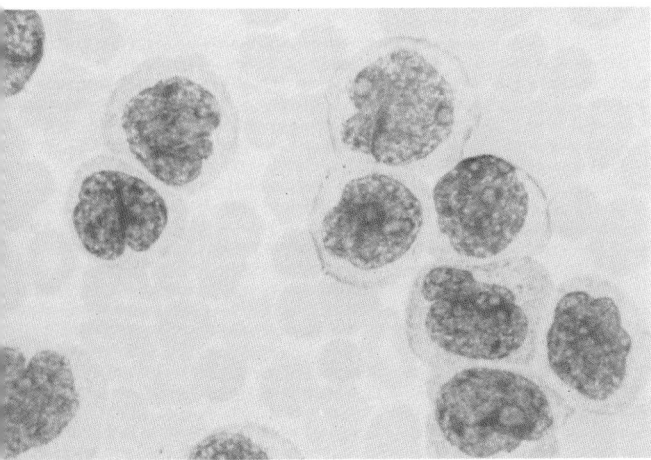

XXXVI–2–PLATE 6. FAB M5. Monocytic leukemia. Prominent nuclei filled with nucleoli in some cells, light granulation and large amount of lightly basophilic cytoplasm give these cells the appearance of promonocytes.

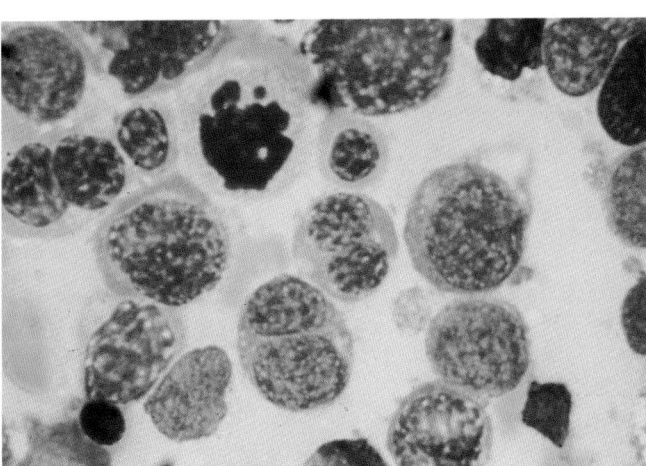

XXXVI–2–PLATE 7. FAB M6. Erythroleukemia is characterized by the presence of bizarre megaloblastic and often multinucleated erythroid precursors. Karyorrhexis is seen in some cells. The somewhat arbitrary distinction between FAB M6 and myelodysplastic syndrome with excess blasts in transformation is made by quantification of the fraction of myeloid blasts.

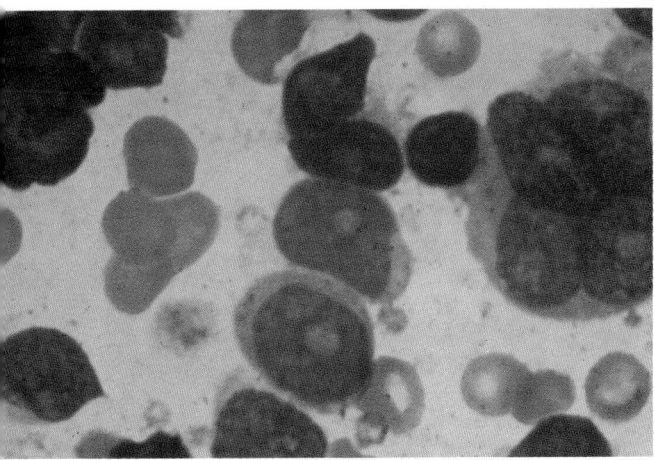

XXXVI–2–PLATE 8. FAB M7. Megakaryocytic leukemia. Blasts in this category are often morphologically undifferentiated. The presence of multinucleated cells, dysplastic micromegakaryocytes and cytoplasmic budding can be helpful diagnostic clues. The diagnosis is confirmed by immunophenotyping or ultrastructural studies.

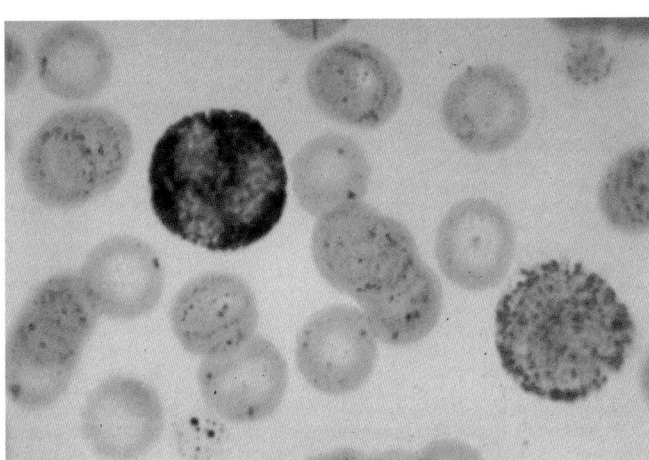

XXXVI–2–PLATE 9. Typical granular staining with Sudan black B of a blast and a neutrophil from a patient with FAB M1 AML.

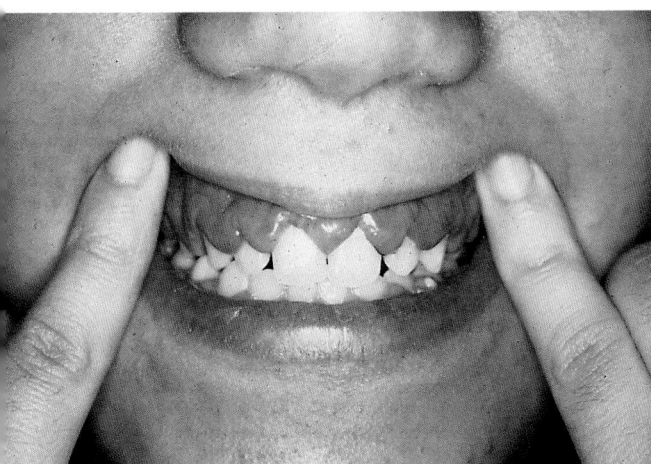

XXXVI–2–PLATE 10. FAB M5. Gingival hypertrophy due to infiltration by leukemic cells in acute monocytic leukemia.

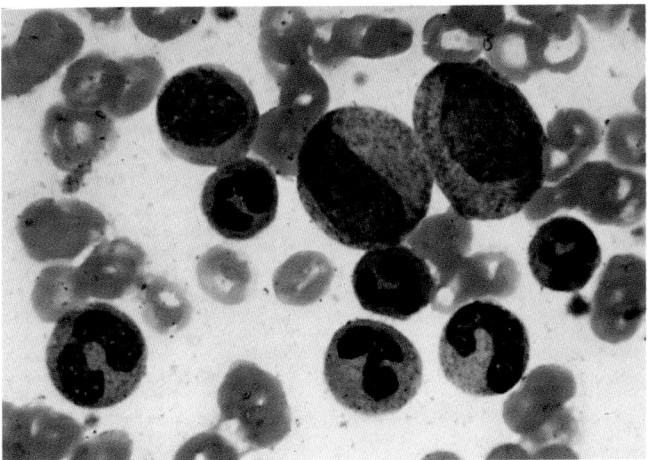

XXXVI–3–PLATE 1. Chronic myelocytic leukemia. Leukocytosis with myelocytes, metamyelocytes, band cells and polymorphonuclear leukocytes are characteristic of the peripheral blood in the chronic phase of this disease.

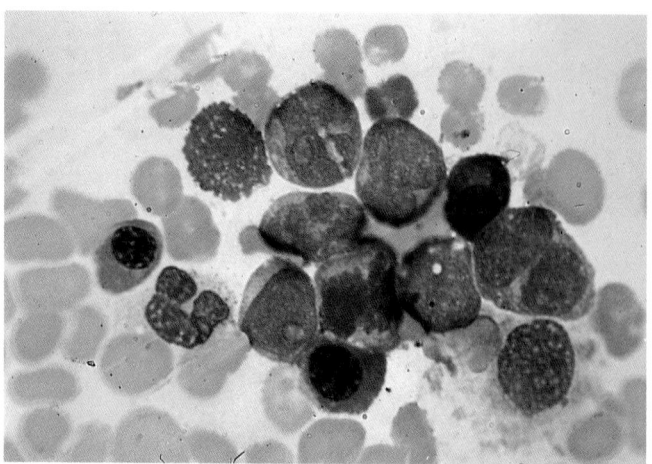

XXXVI–3–PLATE 2. Chronic myelocytic leukemia, blastic crisis. Marrow aspiration shows predominance of blastic forms, which may have myeloid or lymphoid appearance.

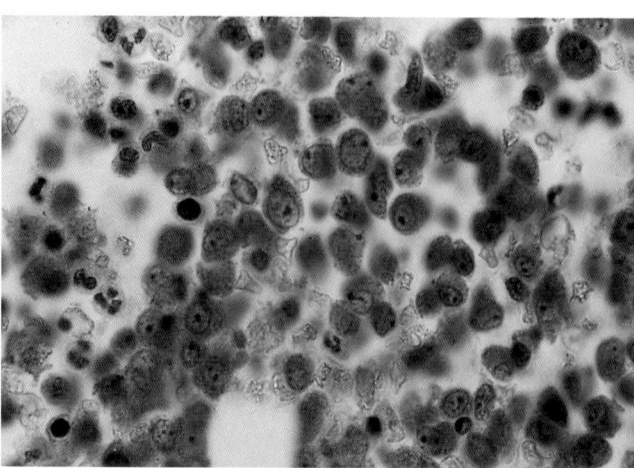

XXXVI–3–PLATE 3. Chronic myelocytic leukemia, blastic crisis. This bone marrow biopsy shows that blasts with prominent nucleoli comprise about 75% of the marrow cells.

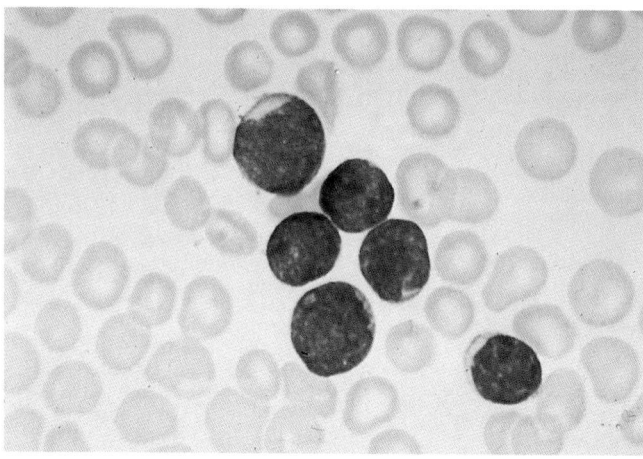

XXXVI–5–PLATE 1. FAB L1 characterized by blasts that are relatively homogeneous in size and appearance with sparse agranular cytoplasm. The nuclei are round and nucleoli are usually small and not prominent. Occasionally it is difficult to distinguish FAB L1 morphology from other more differentiated lymphoproliferative disorders: immunophenotyping is of critical value in such circumstances.

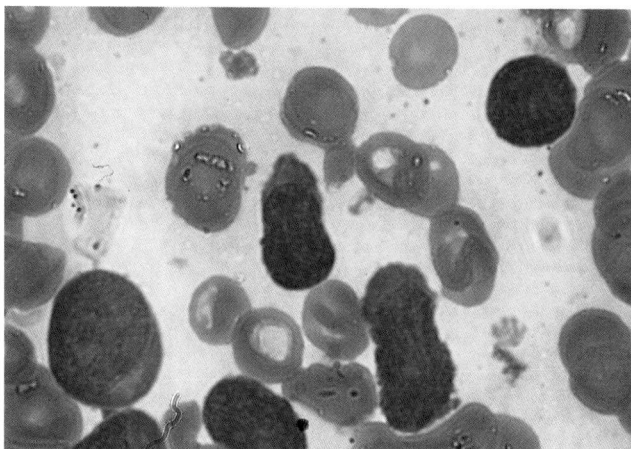

XXXVI–5–PLATE 2. FAB L2 blasts are generally larger and more heterogeneous in size and shape than FAB L1. The nucleoli are more numerous and prominent. Variable amounts of lightly basophilic agranular cytoplasm are seen. Diagnostic confusion may occur with poorly differentiated myeloid leukemias or megakaryocytic leukemia, which can be resolved with histochemical stains, Tdt assay or immunophenotyping.

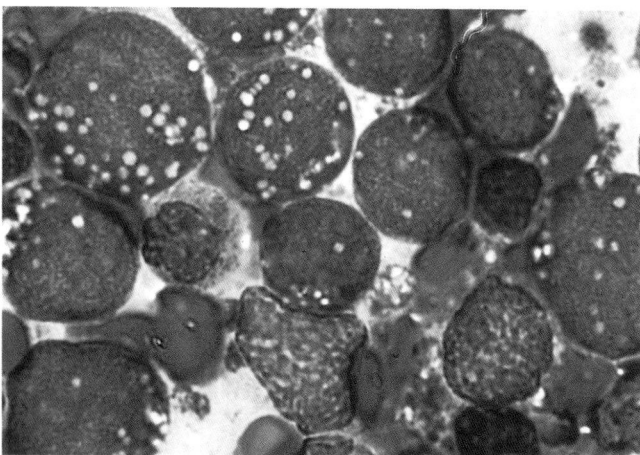

XXXVI–5–PLATE 3. FAB L3. Burkitt-type blasts are larger and have nuclei with less condensed chromatin and prominent nucleoli. The cytoplasm is deeply basophilic and usually heavily vacuolated; the vacuole will stain with oil Red O. Surface immunoglobulin is present in a monoclonal pattern.

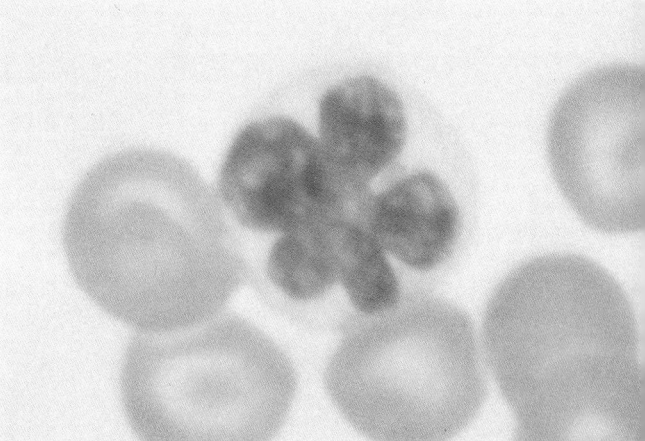

XXXVI–6–PLATE 1. HTLV-1 associated adult T cell leukemia (ATLL). Typical medium sized ATLL cell with characteristic flower-petal-shaped lobulated nucleus and moderately well condensed nuclear chromatin.

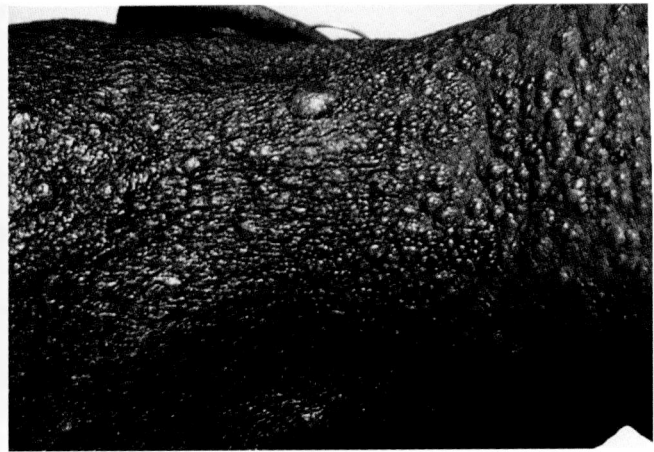

XXXVI–6–PLATE 2. Characteristic generalized non-exfoliative nodular cutaneous eruption in a patient with HTLV-1 associated adult T cell leukemia.

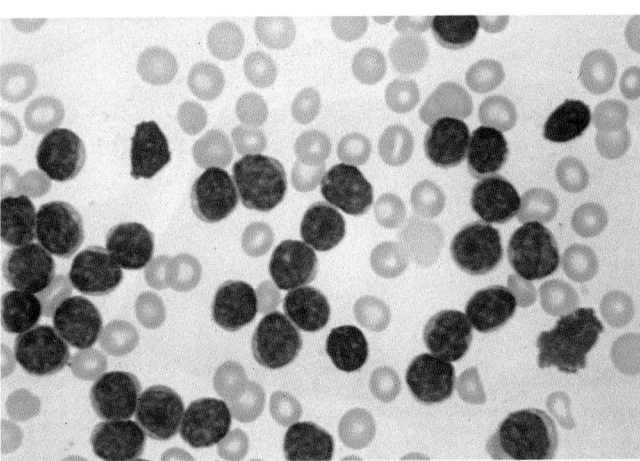

XXXVI–7–PLATE 1. Chronic lymphocytic leukemia. Lymphocyte morphology in peripheral blood smear. Leukocyte count 100,000/μl. The majority of lymphocytes are mature appearing. One smudge cell is present. Platelets are absent in this thrombocytopenic patient. Wright-Giemsa.

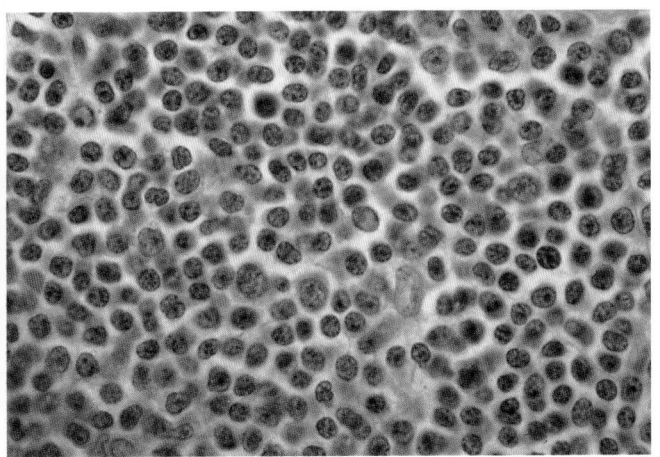

XXXVI–7–PLATE 2. Chronic lymphocytic leukemia. Marrow biopsy with diffuse infiltration with CLL cells. H&E.

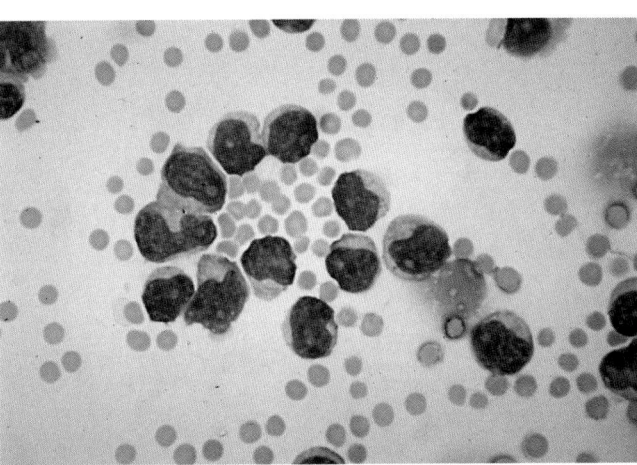

XXXVI–7–PLATE 3. Prolymphocytic leukemia. Peripheral blood smear shows cells with prominent nucleoli and abundant cytoplasm. Wright-Giemsa.

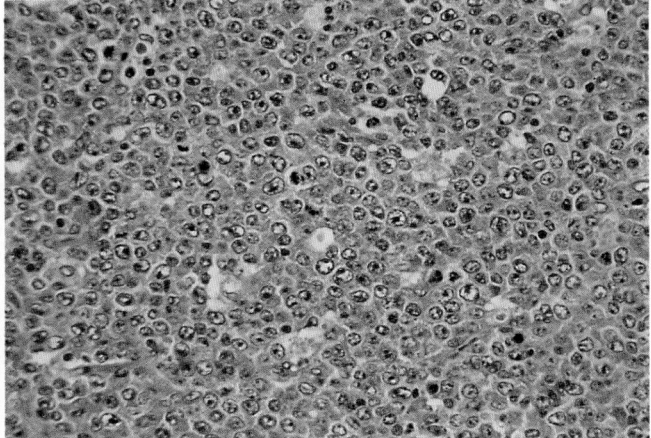

XXXVI–7–PLATE 4. Chronic lymphocytic leukemia, Richter's syndrome. Section of lymph node with immunoblastic proliferation consisting of large cells with prominent nucleoli. H&E.

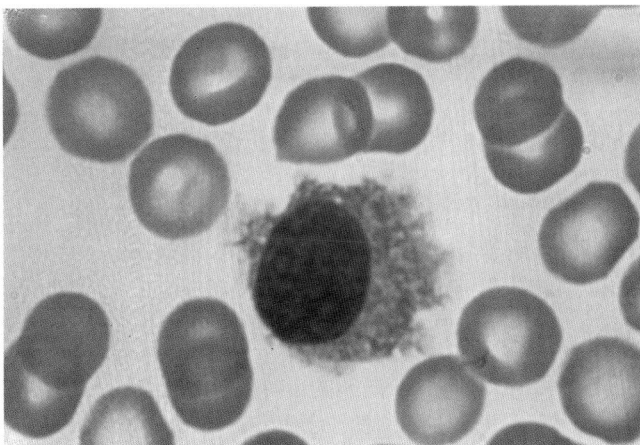

XXXVI–8–PLATE 1. Hairy cell leukemia. The cell is characterized by an eccentrically located nucleus with fine chromatin, indistinct nucleoli, and an abundant amount of gray-blue cytoplasm with shaggy margins. Wright's stain, X1,000.

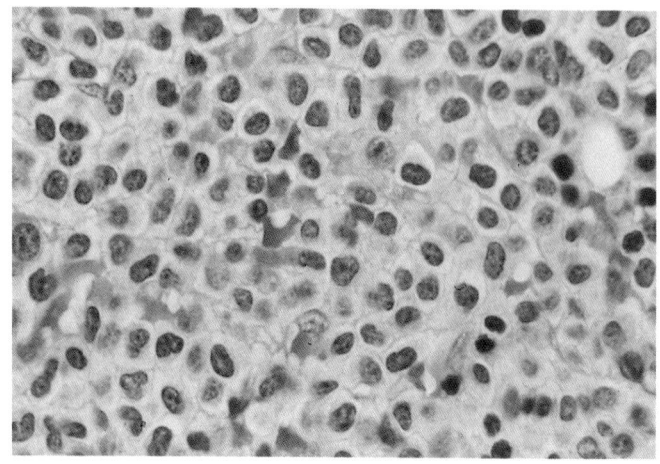

XXXVI–8–PLATE 2. Hairy cell leukemia. The marrow biopsy shows leukemic cells with abundant clear cytoplasm, oval or slightly indented nuclei, and the appearance of a "water-clear" rim separating each nucleus. H&E, X400.

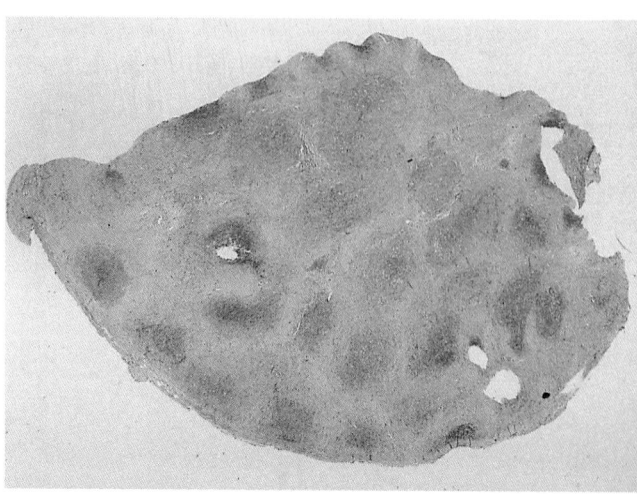

XXXVI–9–PLATE 1. Hodgkin's disease. Nodular sclerosis.

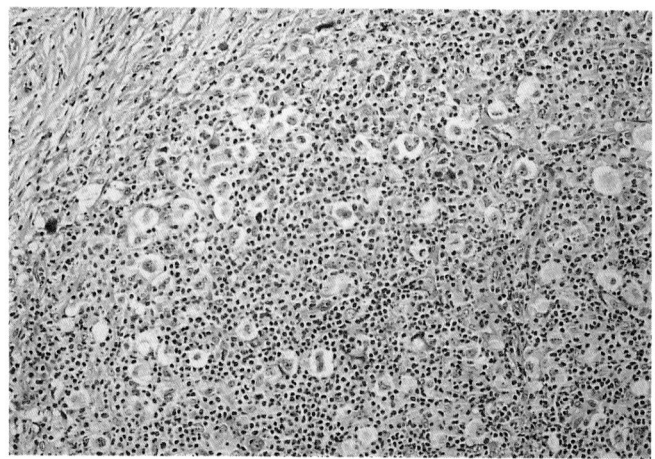

XXXVI–9–PLATE 2. Hodgkin's disease. Lacunar cells in nodular sclerosis.

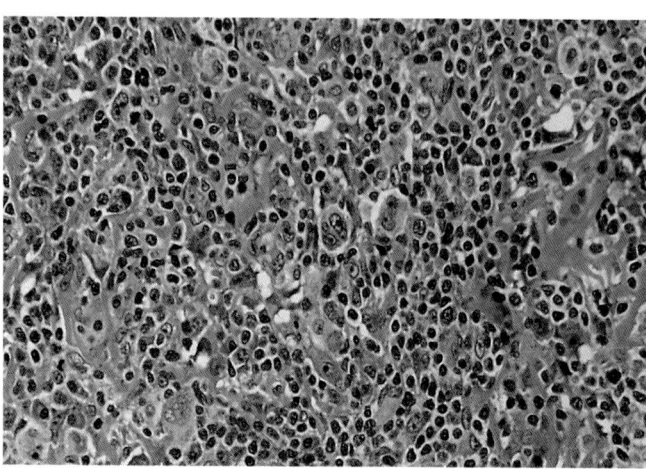

XXXVI–9–PLATE 3. Hodgkin's disease. Mixed cellularity. Several Reed Sternberg cells are seen.

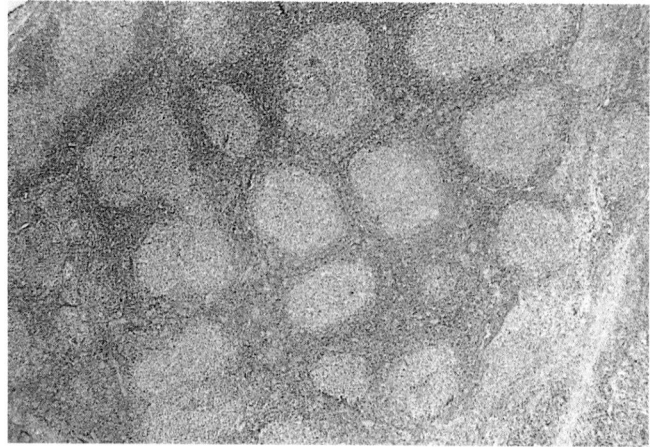

XXXVI–10–PLATE 1. Nodular poorly differentiated lymphoma.

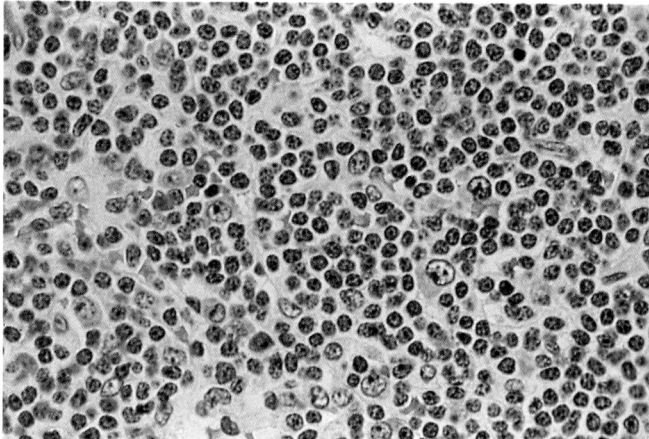

XXXVI–10–PLATE 2. Diffuse well differentiated lymphoma.

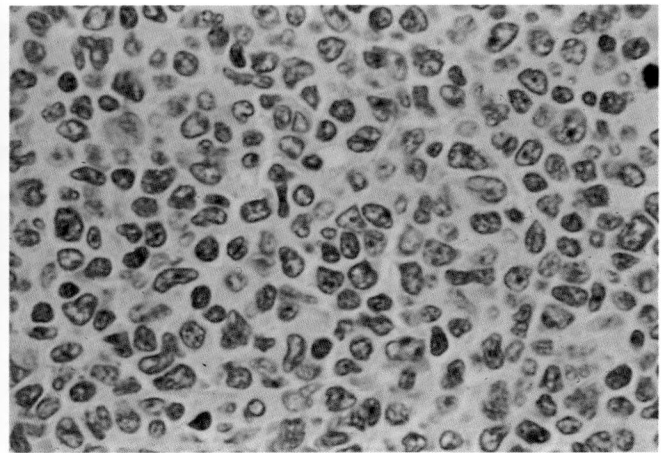

XXXVI–10–PLATE 3. Diffuse poorly differentiated lymphoma.

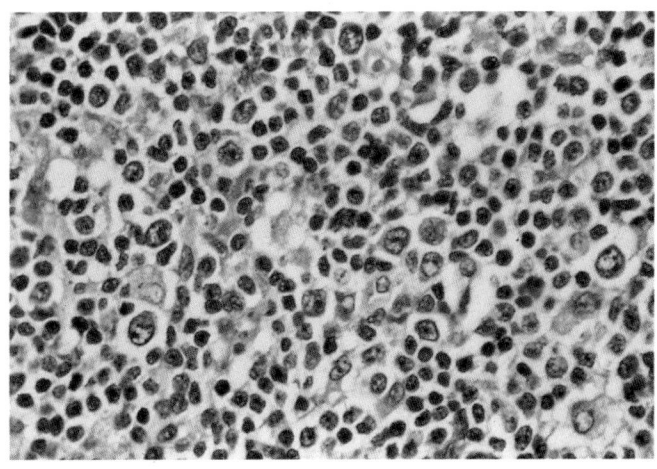

XXXVI–10–PLATE 4. Diffuse mixed lymphoma.

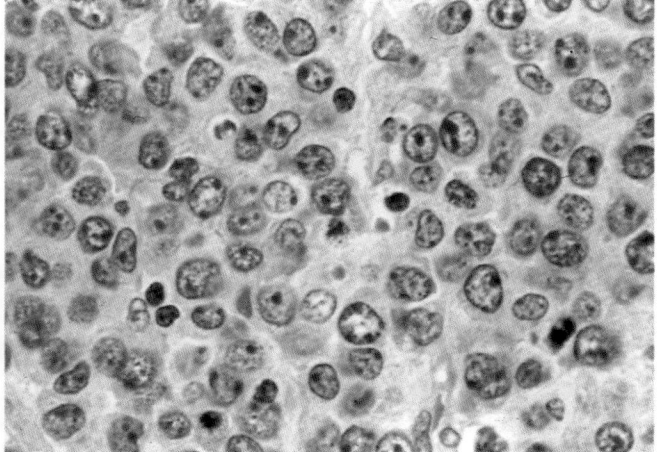

XXXVI–10–PLATE 5. B cell immunoblastic lymphoma.

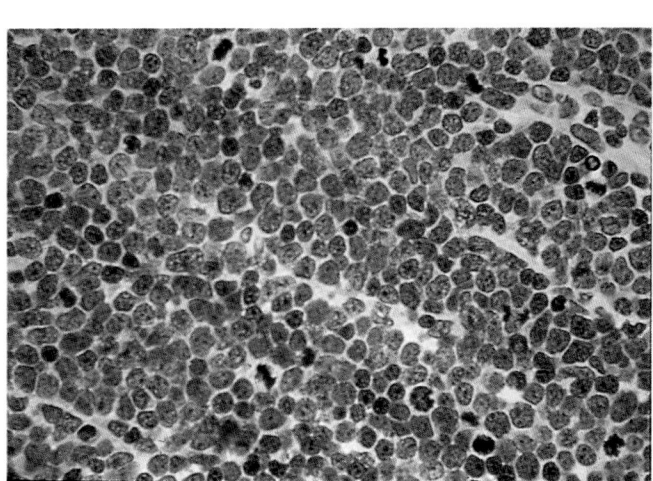

XXXVI–10–PLATE 6. T cell lymphoblastic lymphoma.

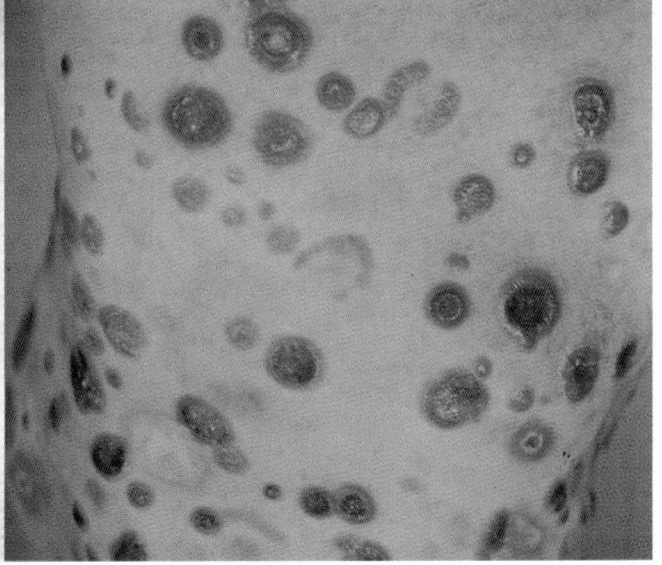

XXXVI–11–PLATE 1. The flank of a patient with typical plaques of mycosis fungoides, many of which have evolved into tumors with central ulceration.

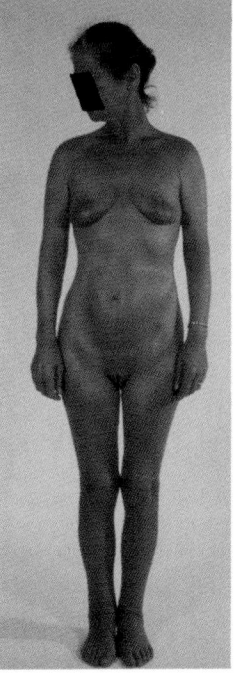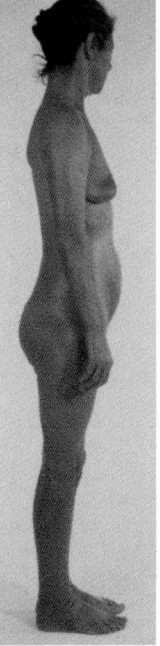

XXXVI–11–PLATE 2. Generalized erythroderma (or "l'homme rouge"), often with very atrophic skin, is typical of patients with the Sézary syndrome.

15

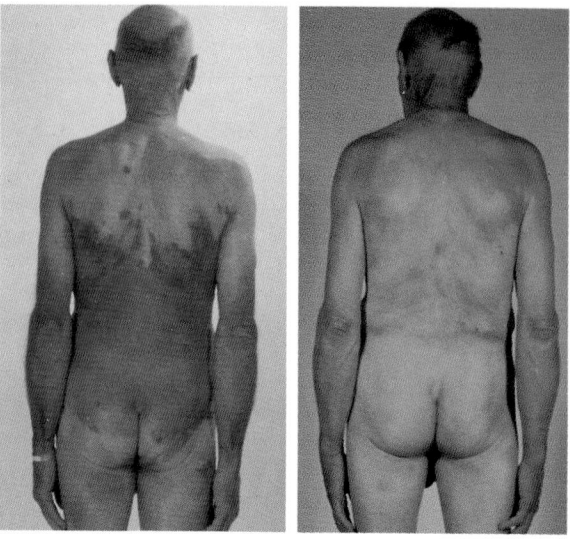

XXXVI–11–PLATE 3. A typical patient with extensive plaque disease at the time of presentation (A, left) and three years after a course of total skin electron beam therapy (B, right).

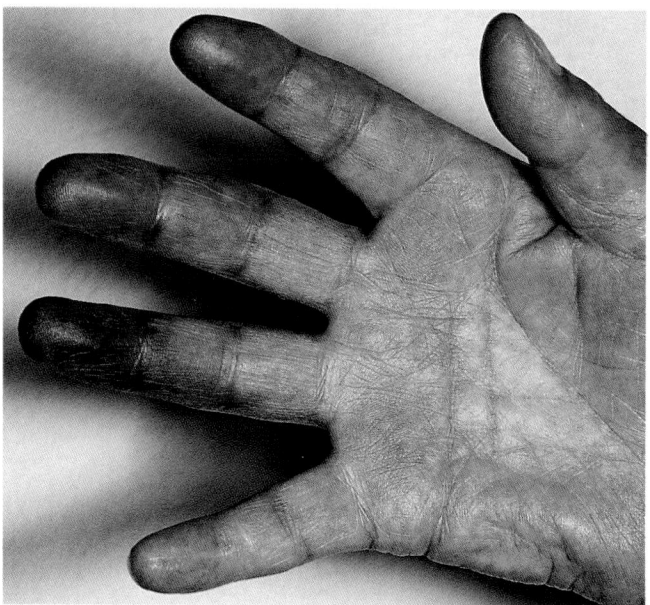

XXXVI–14–PLATE 2. Raynaud's phenomenon in polycythemia vera with cyanotic fingertips.

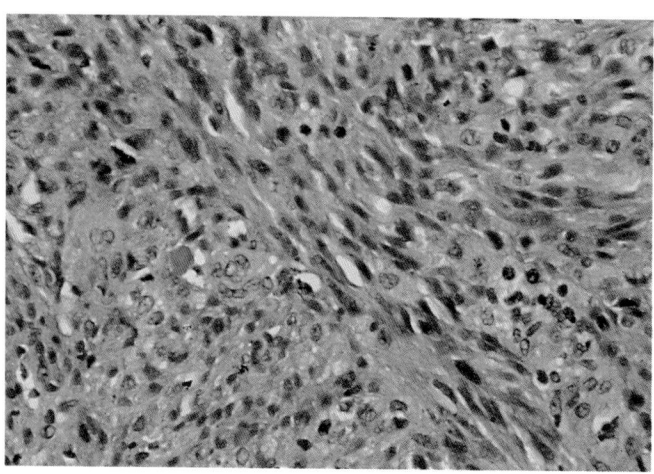

XXXVII–1–PLATE 2. Kaposi's sarcoma. Typical microscopic appearance showing spindle cells, slit-like vascular spaces and extravasated red blood cells.

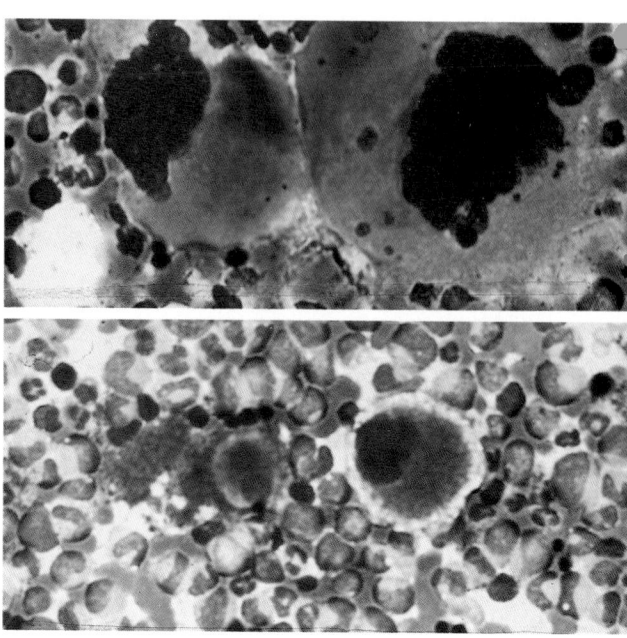

XXXVI–14–PLATE 1. Large polynucleated megakaryocytes in po[l] cythemia vera contrast sharply with small mononuclear megakaryocyt[e] in chronic myelocytic leukemia.

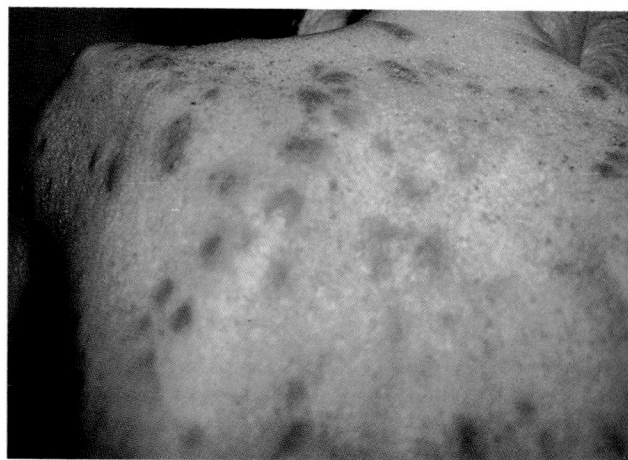

XXXVII–1–PLATE 1. Kaposi's sarcoma of the back in a patient w[ith] AIDS.

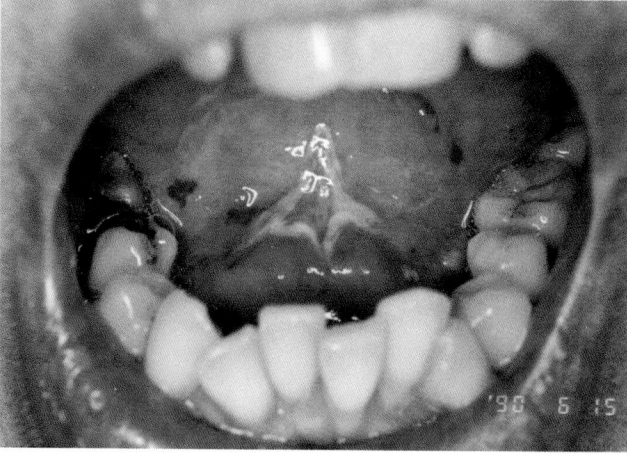

XL–14–PLATE 1. Stomatitis from chemotherapy. Sublingual wh[ite] thickened mucosa due to necrosis and edema. Focal hemorrhages a[re] seen. These changes may occur throughout the oral pharyngeal cavit[y]

VI

Cancer Prevention

VI-1

Prevention of Tobacco-Related Cancers

Paul F. Engstrom
Bruce Trock
Barbara K. Rimer

Introduction

In the United States, over 59 million people smoke, and each year nearly 400,000 people die prematurely from tobacco-related diseases. This includes 136,000 deaths from cancer, 115,000 from coronary heart disease, 60,000 from chronic obstructive pulmonary disease, 27,000 from stroke, and another 50,000 deaths from other causes, including peptic ulcer disease, stillbirths and low birthweight. Cigarette smoking remains the greatest cause of preventable mortality in the United States.

Americans have dramatically altered their smoking behavior since the first Surgeon General's report on tobacco was released in 1964. At that time, about 40% of the United States population smoked; in 1987, it was 29%. Smoking is higher among men (32% smoke) than among women (27%); it is also higher among African Americans (34%) than among whites (29%). Smoking is inversely related to level of education: 36% of those with less than a high school education smoke compared to 33% with a high school education, 26% with some college and 16% who graduated from college.[116] There also is a similar pattern of higher smoking rates among blue-collar and service workers compared to white-collar workers. Tobacco use is influenced heavily by the tobacco industry's $2 billion annual advertising and marketing campaigns. Women, minorities, blue-collar workers, adolescents, and even children are bombarded by clever, often insidious, marketing and advertising gimmicks.

In this chapter, we review the pathogenesis and epidemiology of smoking-related cancer and discuss addiction, prevention and cessation of tobacco use.

Physicochemical Composition of Tobacco Smoke

More than 4,000 known compounds are estimated to be present in tobacco smoke. These occur as volatile constituents forming a vapor phase, and in particulate form suspended in the vapor phase. The majority of carcinogens and mutagens are found in the particulate phase. Currently, 43 carcinogens have been identified in tobacco smoke, including polynuclear aromatic hydrocarbons (PAH), nitrosamines, heterocyclic hydrocarbons, benzene, and radioactive polonium-210.[116] Tobacco-specific nitrosamines (TSNA) are the carcinogens present in the highest concentration (they occur in even higher concentrations in smokeless tobacco). For purposes of risk assessment, tobacco smoke is classified as mainstream smoke (MS) and sidestream smoke (SS). The former represents smoke which is directly inhaled through the butt end of the cigarette, while the latter is continuously emitted from the burning end into the environment. Although most of the components that have been identified in tobacco smoke occur in both MS and SS, the concentrations of many toxic and tumorigenic agents are higher in SS (e.g., nitrosamines).[51]

Nicotine is the pharmacologic agent responsible for the addictive properties of tobacco, and is also a major source of TSNA through N-nitrosation reactions.[51] It is present in both MS and SS, and is rapidly absorbed from the small airways and alveoli of the lung. Nicotine from smokeless tobacco is absorbed through the oral mucous membranes. Once in the blood, nicotine is transported to specific receptor sites on the brain. Interaction with these receptor sites is believed to be the basis for producing a chemical dependence on tobacco. The liver is the primary site of nicotine metabolism, with cotinine as the major metabolite.[117]

Carcinogenesis Bioassays and Markers of Genotoxicity

Tobacco smoke and smokeless tobacco contain compounds which function as tumor initiators, promoters, or cocarcinogens. Tumor initiators are mutagens which bond covalently to cellular DNA; their effects are generally irreversible and may require only a single exposure. Promoters are compounds which stimulate excessive proliferation of initiated cells; they produce reversible effects which result in cancer after prolonged application. Cocarcinogens enhance the effects of carcinogens, but are not essential to the carcinogenic process and may have little or no direct carcinogenic activity.[6]

Experimental simulation of human smoking was conducted on beagle dogs by Auerbach and colleagues. Cigarettes were held in a Teflon tube that was inserted in a tracheostoma, and smoke was delivered by deep voluntary inhalation of the dog. After a maximum of 14 months of exposure, no tumors developed in 10 exposed dogs, but sections of bronchial epithelium exhibited atypical nuclei, loss of ciliated columnar cells with squamous replacement, and hyperplasia. These histologic changes, which were similar to those seen in tissue from lung cancer patients, were almost entirely absent in sections from unexposed dogs.[3]

Only limited success has been achieved in inducing respiratory cancers in animals in response to tobacco smoke inhalation, due both to acute toxic effects and animals' resistance to deep inhalation of tobacco smoke. In these studies, animals are placed in exposure chambers and exposed to alternating short periods of tobacco smoke diluted with air, followed by air alone. Excess incidence of respiratory tumors has been demonstrated in mice, rats, dogs, and hamsters (the latter develop laryngeal tumors only) compared to unexposed controls. However, overall incidence has been low, and dominated by adenomas and alveologenic adenocarcinomas.[51,118]

The majority of carcinogenesis bioassays in animals have used direct application of tobacco smoke condensates ("tars"), or subfractions of the particulate phase. Tumor initiation and cocarcinogenesis have primarily been associated with the neutral subfractions that are rich in polynuclear aromatic hydrocarbons (PAH), while promoters are found in the weakly acidic subfractions.[51] Intrapulmonary administration of tobacco smoke condensates or fractions have produced lung carcinomas and adenomas in rats and hamsters, respectively.[51,118] Tumors of the nasal cavity, lung, liver, and esophagus have been produced in rats by intraperitoneal administration of tobacco-specific nitrosamines (TNSA).[48] The most extensive assays have examined tumorigenesis of tars on mouse skin. Skin-painting of cigarette smoke condensates has consistently produced papillomas and carcinomas in over 40% of mice, compared to near-zero incidence in control animals. Condensates from pipes and cigars have also produced high tumor incidence in animal bioassays.

A large number of in vitro studies have been conducted with tobacco smoke (both MS and SS) as well as condensates. Mutagenicity has been demonstrated for smoke and condensates in Salmonella typhimurium (the Ames test).[2] Urine from smokers has also been shown to be mutagenic in this system, with some evidence of a dose-response. In mammalian tissue culture systems, condensates, fresh tobacco smoke, and the gas phase of smoke have induced sister chromatid exchange and other mutations, cell transformation, and inhibition of both DNA repair and intercellular communication.[51]

A number of markers of genetic damage occur with significantly greater frequency in smokers than non-smokers. Excess prevalence of sister chromatid exchanges and micronuclei has been observed in peripheral blood lymphocytes and bone marrow of smokers compared to non-smokers. Many of these studies have demonstrated dose-response trends with number of cigarettes or duration of smoking.[51]

DNA adducts (addition products) represent covalent bonding of carcinogen with DNA, and serve as a marker of initiation. These adducts have been found in the lung, bronchus, larynx, esophagus, bladder, kidney, blood, and heart of smokers; adduct levels correlate with dose and duration of smoking. The adducts probably arise from exposure to PAH and other aromatic compounds, since adducts are not seen in association with smokeless tobacco, and polycyclic aromatics are generated by burning tobacco.[84,87] Detectable DNA adduct levels are observed in less than 20% of smokers, presumably representing heterogeneity in ability to metabolize PAH or repair adducts. This is in good agreement with the 10–20% of heavy smokers who develop lung cancer.[39]

The predictive value of DNA adducts and sister chromatid exchange (SCE) as markers of cancer risk has not yet been determined, although a number of studies are currently underway. A recent small case-control study of lung cancer found that, among current smokers, PAH-adduct levels were higher in peripheral blood leukocytes of cases than controls. However, adduct levels did not differ significantly between smokers and non-smokers for cases and controls combined. Sister chromatid exchange was more frequent in smokers than non-smokers, but did not differ between cases and controls.[82] Other small studies have also observed no correlation between cigarette smoking and PAH-adducts in peripheral blood leukocytes, and lung tissue.[83,84] Interpretation of these results must be tempered by the small numbers of subjects, potential confounding factors, significant interindividual variation in DNA binding, and the fact that the assay is relatively crude, i.e., it does not discern between different but structurally related PAHs.[82] At present, adducts and SCEs should be considered important chiefly as markers of carcinogen-induced genetic damage. The significance of this initiating step with respect to cancer risk or susceptibility is modified by environmental and host factors (metabolic activation, detoxification, DNA repair mechanisms).

Genetic Variation in Susceptibility

Susceptibility to the carcinogenic effects of tobacco smoke appears to be genetically determined. A number of epidemiologic studies have observed an apparent familial aggregation of lung cancer risk; with one study demonstrating possible synergism between familial risk and cigarette smoking.[30,74,114] A recent segregation analysis has provided evidence that such familial clustering is strongly consistent with mendelian codominant inheritance of a two-allele autosomal gene, with age of onset dependent on genotype. In other words, if A and B are the two alleles, with greater susceptibility associated with A, then mean age of onset (for a given smoking level) increases with genotype in the order AA, AB, BB.[101] The analysis suggested that the joint effect of the gene and cigarette smoking could be responsible for 42% of lung cancer cases at age 50, 34% at age 60, and 13% at age 70. In contrast, the corresponding percentages attributable to smoking alone were 27% at age 50, 49% at age 60, and 72% at age 70.[101]

Several enzyme systems involved in the metabolism of xenobiotics exhibit distinct genetic polymorphisms that may be associated with differential susceptibility. This raises the possibility that certain phenotypes could serve as markers to identify individuals at increased risk. The enzymes that have received the most study include the P450 enzymes involved in debrisoquine metabolism, the N-acetyltransferases which acetylate aryl amines in the liver, and aryl hydrocarbon hydroxylase (AHH) which catalyses monooxygenation of aromatic hydrocarbons.

The cytochrome P450 superfamily of genes encodes a system of enzymes responsible for oxidative metabolism of endogenous compounds (e.g., fatty acids, prostaglandins), as well as drugs and other xenobiotics. Because enzymatic oxidation produces highly reactive intermediates, it is thought that metabolism by P450 enzymes activates carcinogens such as PAH. Genetic variation in P450 enzymes may alter the capacity to metabolically activate certain carcinogens, thus influencing cancer risk. The metabolism of debrisoquine (a beta-blocker used as an antihypertensive agent) involves a P450 enzyme encoded by the gene CYP2D6. It is hypothesized that the CYP2D6 enzyme may also be involved in metabolism of carcinogenic compounds in cigarette smoke. Polymorphisms of this gene are manifested by variation in extent of metabolism, with phenotypes categorized as extensive, intermediate, or poor metabolizers. Individuals who exhibit the "extensive" metabolizer phenotype (as determined by the ratio of unchanged debrisoquine to 4-hydroxydebrisoquine in the urine) have an increased risk of lung cancer, compared to intermediate or poor metabolizers.[9,10,68] A recent well-designed case-control study found that the risk associated with the extensive metabolizer phenotype was higher in whites (odds ratio = 10.2) than in blacks (odds ratio = 4.5), after controlling for age, sex, and smoking.[10] Risk for individuals occupationally exposed to asbestos may be increased 18-fold. Risk is greatest for squamous and small cell carcinomas, but not significantly elevated for adenocarcinoma. The latter histologic type is not strongly associated with smoking, which provides indirect evidence for a role of the CYP2D6 gene in tobacco carcinogenesis. The extensive and poor metabolizer phenotypes occur in 20–30% and 5–10% of Caucasians respectively; the former is an autosomal dominant trait.[9,68]

Acetylation rates are under genetic control at a single locus, with two different phenotypes categorized as "rapid" and "slow." The latter is autosomal recessive and occurs in approximately 50–60% of Western populations, compared to 10% among Asian populations.[72] Slow acetylators are less efficient at detoxifying aryl amines, which are potent bladder carcinogens. A number of studies have shown excesses of slow acetylators among occupationally exposed bladder cancer cases compared to controls, but no difference in acetylation status when comparing cases unrelated to occupational exposure to controls.[11,63] Although aryl amines are present in tobacco smoke, studies have either found no difference in acetylation status between smoking and nonsmoking bladder cancer cases, or nonsignificant excesses of slow acetylators among smoking cases.[11,43,69] Thus, there is little evidence to date for a role of acetylator status in smoking-induced bladder cancer.

Aryl hydrocarbon hydroxylase (AHH) is a P450-dependent monooxygenase which can be induced to a variable degree by exposure to aromatic compounds such as benzpyrene. Considerable disagreement exists as to whether this trait is associated with variation in lung cancer susceptibility.[81] Kouri and colleagues found significantly higher AHH-inducibility

in lymphocytes from lung cancer cases compared to controls with other pulmonary disease, matched for age, sex, and cigarette smoking.[58] They claimed that inconsistent results seen in other studies were due to poor control of experimental conditions, and failure to make comparisons at the time of peak activity (which can vary from 48–120 hours in culture). However, another study that examined inducibility in lung tissue from lung cancer patients, and lymphocytes from smoking and nonsmoking controls as well as cases found no evidence of excess risk associated with high inducibility. These authors concluded that AHH inducibility exhibits wide variation between individuals, but is not systematically associated with lung cancer risk.[54] In a more recent study, the P450 gene CYP1A1, which is associated with AHH activity, was shown to correlate with smoking status in normal tissue from lung cancer patients. In this study, CYP1A1 messenger RNA (mRNA) levels were higher in current smokers than in non-smokers or patients who had quit smoking for more than 6 weeks, suggesting that gene expression is induced by active smoking. The association was somewhat less consistent for tumor tissue, although an abnormal CYP1A1 mRNA that was absent in normal tissue was observed in 5 of 10 tumors that did express the CYP1A1 gene.[67] However, because a control series was not included, it is not possible to determine whether CYP1A1 expression (and thus, AHH activity) is a marker of increased risk of lung cancer, or only a marker of smoking status. At present, no firm conclusions can be drawn about the usefulness of AHH as a marker of increased susceptibility.

In addition to the enzyme systems described above, a number of oncogenes have been identified in tobacco-related cancers. However, the association between oncogene activation and exposure to tobacco in these cancers has not been studied. Activation of the *ras* and/or *myc* oncogenes has been observed in several tobacco-related cancers including lung,[59,105] head and neck,[24,31] bladder,[113] and kidney.[105] Most studies have examined human tumor cell lines or tumor and non-tumor tissue from small numbers of cancer patients. However, a recent study utilizing a case-control design found significantly higher frequency of rare alleles of the *Ha-ras* locus in lung cancer cases in blacks than in controls, and a suggestive but non-significant trend toward higher frequencies in lung cancer in whites.[112] Cases and controls were matched for age, race, and smoking habit. Stronger trends were observed when adenocarcinoma cases were excluded, suggesting that the gene may influence susceptibility to carcinogens in tobacco.

Cancers Associated with Tobacco Use

The 1989 Surgeon General's report on smoking and health characterized specific cancers as to whether tobacco smoke plays a causal role, acts as a contributory factor, or is merely associated with the cancer. Cancers in each of these categories are listed in Table VI-1-1, which also summarizes data on mortality and attributable risk from the 1989 report.[116]

All of the cancer sites shown in Table VI-1-1 exhibit a dose response with level of cigarette smoking (e.g., cigarettes per day). Lung, larynx, oral, esophageal, and bladder cancers also exhibit a dose response with duration of smoking; duration effects have been less widely studied for other cancer sites.[118] Pipe and cigar smoking are also associated with

Table VI-1-1. Tobacco Smoke and Risks of Specific Cancers in Western Countries[a]

Cancer Site	Mortality Ratios[b]	Attributable Risk (%)[e]
A. Causal role of tobacco		
Lung and bronchus	7.0–15.9	90 (M), 79 (F)
Larynx	6.1–13.1	81 (M), 87 (F)
Oral cavity[c]	1.0–12.5	92 (M), 61 (F)
Esophagus	1.7–6.6	78 (M), 75 (F)
B. Contributory role of tobacco		
Bladder	0.7–3.0	47 (M), 37 (F)
Kidney	1.1–1.6	48 (M), 12 (F)
Pancreas	1.6–6.0	29 (M), 34 (F)
C. Association with tobacco		
Stomach	0.9–2.3	NA
Cervix (invasive)	0.7–2.9[d]	NA

[a]Data taken from 1989 Surgeon General's report on smoking and health,[116] except for cervix.[51]
[b]Males only
[c]Buccal cavity and pharynx
[d]Estimated relative risks
[e]% risk attributable to tobacco
M, males, F, females, NA, data not available

increased risk of cancers of the lung, oral cavity, larynx, and esophagus; for all but the former the excess risk is similar to that for cigarettes. Cessation of smoking is associated with a gradual decline in risk relative to nonsmokers.[116] In addition, patients with oral cancer who quit smoking have approximately one-half the risk of second primaries as do patients who continue to smoke.[104]

Smoking cessation has had the largest effect on lung cancer mortality rates among white males. From 1973–74 to 1985–86, cancer mortality increased 15.9% in white males (from 62.4 to 72.3 per 100,000), compared to 28.7% in black males (76.3 to 98.2 per 100,000). The corresponding figures for females were a 96.2% increase among whites (13.8 to 27.1 per 100,000), and 87.4% among blacks (13.8 to 25.9 per 100,000). Black males also exhibit higher mortality rates and less favorable mortality trends for cancers of the larynx, esophagus, oral cavity, and pancreas.[119]

Sidestream Smoking and Cancer

A large number of investigations of the risk associated with sidestream smoking (passive smoking, involuntary smoking) have been conducted since the early 1970's. The most extensive area of investigation has been the risk of lung cancer in non-smokers in relation to spouses' smoking habits. Although some studies have not found an association with passive smoking, the majority have found small increases in risk.[21,32,53,108] Exposure to passive smoke in the workplace has also been linked to excess lung cancer risk among non-smokers. Case-control studies have estimated relative risks ranging from 1.3–2.2 for workplace exposure.[55,108,130] Both the 1986 Surgeon General's report, and the National Research Council have estimated an increase in risk of approximately 30% associated with exposure to sidestream smoke, and consider such exposure to be a cause of lung cancer in non-smokers.[70,120] Because many studies were too small to estimate such a modest increase in risk with precision, a meta-

analysis was conducted by Wald. This analysis was based on 13 studies from 1982–1986 and concluded that environmental tobacco smoke was associated with a 35–50% increase in lung cancer risk.[125]

Limited reports of associations with cancers of other sites have been reported, but for the most part they have been sites which are not associated with mainstream smoking (e.g., brain, nasal sinus). However, a recent study found that cervical cancer risk in non-smokers increased with the number of hours per day exposed to passive smoke; risk remained elevated after adjustment for sexual practices and other potential confounding factors. The magnitude of the effect was similar to that associated with mainstream smoking.[106] Because of the correlation between smoke exposure and sexual practices associated with high cervical cancer risk, and the difficulty of adequately controlling for confounding by sexual practice, this intriguing finding requires confirmation.

Studies of childhood cancer in relation to parents' smoking habits have generally found no evidence of increased risk.[51] However, a recent report demonstrated a doubling of adult lung cancer risk among non-smokers and ex-smokers associated with heavy exposure to passive smoke during childhood and adolescence.[52] Unlike most other studies, there was no excess risk associated with exposure from spousal smoking, all passive smoke exposure in adulthood, or lifetime passive smoke exposure. Although the lack of association with these other sources of exposure raises the question of undetected bias or confounding, the study was carefully designed and showed no change in risk when controlling for potential known sources of error. Furthermore, these results are consistent with the increased prevalence of respiratory problems in children exposed to passive smoke, and the presence of tobacco-related carcinogens in the blood of adults with passive smoke exposure.

Factors Modifying Tobacco-Related Cancer Risk

Several factors strongly potentiate the carcinogenic effects of tobacco smoke. The strongest synergistic effects have been seen for asbestos and radon. Several studies have found evidence suggesting that the effects of asbestos and cigarette smoking are multiplicative, particularly in insulation workers who are exposed to high levels of asbestos dust.[40,46,51,95] In one very large cohort of insulation workers, the mortality ratio for the combined exposure was 53.2 compared to unexposed non-smokers.[40] Most of the data concerning radon exposure are based on studies of uranium miners. Studies have produced widely varying estimates of the combined risk, and some studies have been based on small numbers. Nevertheless, it is likely that the combined effect is more than additive and may be multiplicative; relative risks exceeding 10 have been observed for the combined exposure in several studies.[51,93] Currently there are few data on the combined effects of smoking and indoor radon. Recent results from the largest case-control study to date did not have sufficient numbers of subjects with high radon exposure to generate separate risks for smokers and non-smokers.[98] Only women were included in this study to minimize bias from non-residential radon exposure or other occupational carcinogens.

Synergistic effects of alcohol have been observed in a large number of studies of oral, laryngeal and esophageal cancers, with relative risks as high as 10–20 for heavy smoking and drinking.[19,45,73] In most studies, the combined effect of alcohol and tobacco appeared to be multiplicative, that is, the risk associated with the combined exposure was approximately equal to the product of the risks associated with the individual exposures.[51] In animals, alcohol increases the carcinogenicity of PAH, and potentiates the activity of microsomal enzyme systems.[118] Further evidence for synergism comes from a study that observed significantly elevated levels of micronucleated cells in buccal mucosa from persons with heavy smoking and drinking habits, but no elevation in subjects with exposure to only alcohol or tobacco.[109]

Organic solvents have been associated with increased lung cancer risk.[99] Blue-collar occupations which involve significant exposure to these compounds are also characterized by a high prevalence of cigarette smoking. It is thought that the potential for synergism exists in a manner similar to that hypothesized for alcohol and tobacco, that is, volatilization facilitating exposure to carcinogens in tobacco smoke. However, studies of the interaction between smoking and solvent exposure on lung cancer risk have not been conducted.

In contrast to the agents described above, a large number of studies suggest that high intake of dietary beta-carotene reduces the risk of lung cancer among smokers.[8,41,47,60] In most studies, reductions in risk on the order of 30–60% have been observed. Effects have been strongest for squamous cell and small cell cancers, suggesting inhibition of tobacco-related carcinogenesis. Studies of serum retinol levels have produced inconsistent results.[124,127] This may reflect the fact that serum vitamin A levels tend to remain fairly constant among individuals with good nutritional status. Protective effects of beta-carotene have also been observed for other squamous cell cancers associated with smoking, such as oral cavity,[66,128] larynx,[64] esophagus,[7] bladder and cervix.[36] The magnitude of protective effects has been similar to those seen for lung cancer.

Several recent studies of the synthetic retinoid isotretinoin (13-cis retinoic acid) have demonstrated significant response rates in advanced head and neck and larynx cancers, although numbers have been small.[62] Isotretinoin has also been effective in preventing second malignant tumors in squamous cell head and neck tumors rendered disease-free by surgery and/or radiation.[49] Treatment of premalignant oral lesions (i.e., oral leukoplakia) with isotretinoin and beta-carotene has also been successful.[102,110] A number of trials to investigate the therapeutic effects of retinoids in head and neck cancers are currently in progress.

The effects of vitamins C and E on tobacco-associated cancers have also been studied, although not as extensively as vitamin A. Increased risk of cancers of the esophagus, lung, larynx, oral cavity, stomach, cervix and bladder have been associated with low intake of dietary vitamin C.[4,5,65] However, there is much less epidemiologic data on these vitamins than for vitamin A; at present these associations must be considered tentative.[116]

Tobacco Addiction

In the 1964 Surgeon General's Report, smoking was described as an habituation.[122] In 1988, for the first time, the United States Department of Health and Human Services (USDHHS) identified tobacco use as nicotine addiction, concluding that ". . . cigarettes and other forms of tobacco are addictive."[117] Nicotine is the drug in tobacco that causes addiction. Moreover, the processes that determine tobacco addiction are similar to those that determine addiction to drugs such as heroin and cocaine."[117] Drug dependence involves the repeated administration of a substance which contains a psychoactive chemical. Like other drug dependencies, nicotine dependence is a progressive, chronic, relapsing disorder characterized by: stereotypic patterns of use, use despite harmful effects, relapse following abstinence and recurrent drug cravings. Dependence-producing drugs often produce tolerance, physical dependence and pleasant effects.[117]

The intensity of nicotine's effects is related to the dose given, time since last dose and the level of preexisting or acquired tolerance.[117] There is an interplay between the addictive nature of cigarettes and their behaviorally-reinforcing properties. Over time, smoking becomes associated with a number of cues which reinforce the behavior.[25] It is this combination of physiologic and psychological dependence that makes cessation such a challenge.

Prevention of Tobacco Use

Clearly, the best strategy is to prevent smoking. This means early intervention through school and family health education as well as environmental and policy changes, such as bans on tobacco advertising and promotion and restrictions on sales.[22] A recent review of smoking initiation showed that among all race-ethnic groups, smoking initiation occurred as young as age nine, increased rapidly from 11–17 years-of-age and then declined after age 19.[22] Educational attainment was the greatest predictor of smoking initiation. The targets of prevention programs have shifted from junior high and high school students to younger children. The most successful prevention programs provide accurate information on smoking, increase the social skills of adolescents to resist peer pressures to smoke, correct normative expectations about smoking, inoculate students against mass media messages, use opinion leaders, involve parents and provide information about the consequences of use.[12,18,42,85,96] A recent meta-analysis of 47 school-based smoking and alcohol intervention programs showed impressive improvements in knowledge and modest attitude changes and behavior changes for the intervened students.[91]

Strategies For Cessation

To be effective, smoking cessation programs should include most of the following techniques: stimulus control, methods for dealing with withdrawal, social support, coping skills training, relaxation training, encouragement of exercise and other positive coping behaviors and relapse prevention. Programs also should be tailored to the patient's stage in the smoking cessation process–precontemplation, contemplation, action or maintenance.[86] Here, we will summarize several smoking cessation strategies that have proven utility, can be cost-effective and have minimal side effects. These include: self-help methods, smoking cessation clinics, physician interventions and pharmacologic adjuncts. Quit rates refer to point prevalence where abstinence rates are noted at a specific time during the follow-up period. For example, at 6 months post treatment, smokers are asked if they have smoked during the past 7 days. Although self-reports of quitting appear reasonably accurate, smoking status can be measured through cotinine assays, saliva thiocyanate or carbon monoxide monitoring.[94]

Self-Help Methods. The majority of smokers quit on their own without outside help. It has been estimated that 90% of the smokers who quit do so on their own, without entering formal treatment programs.[116] In fact, as Cohen and colleagues concluded, the apparent success of self-quitting is in contrast to what appears to be the disappointing performance of formal treatment programs.[13] This does not mean smokers quit in a void or without the use of strategies and techniques.[26] Among smokers quitting on their own, the most powerful predictor of outcome in one study was the number of coping mechanisms used by the smoker. Such techniques may include: avoiding situations where people are smoking, taking up exercise, monitoring one's smoking, using cognitive strategies like positive self-talk, substituting other behaviors for smoking (such as chewing gum) or calling upon others for support.[103]

Self-help programs, including quitting guides, have been developed by a number of organizations, including the USDHHS (*Clearing the Air*), American Cancer Society (*Fresh Start, Smart Move*), American Lung Association (*Freedom From Smoking® For You and Your Family*) and by other organizations seeking to develop more targeted programs for special audiences (e.g., Fox Chase Cancer Center's Clear Horizons Program for smokers aged 50 and older). One of the first evaluations of self help, the assessment of *Freedom From Smoking,* found gradually increasing quit rates over time with one year quit rates of 18%.[16] In an analysis of data from ten NCI-funded self-help trials, twelve-month point prevalence rates ranged from 5.1–26.9% with a median of 13.9%. As in most self-help studies, heavy smoking self-quitters were less likely to quit than light smokers; the latter were 2.2 times more likely to report continuous abstinence at 12 months.[13]

Smoking Cessation Clinics. Smoking cessation clinics are sponsored by voluntary organizations (e.g., American Cancer Society, American Lung Association), proprietary organizations (e.g., Smokenders), hospitals, health plans, health departments and other organizations. The most effective group programs and clinics help smokers to prepare for quitting and continue through maintenance. Like exemplary self-help programs, they teach smokers to understand why they smoke and to develop appropriate coping strategies to use after cessation. Schwartz examined the quit rates of 46 group trials, the majority of which had at least one year follow-up: Success rates ranged from 0–71% success with a median

quit rate of 27%.[100] Group cessation methods appeal to only a small subset of smokers, such as those who cannot quit on their own or who lack supportive quitting environments. Physicians should maintain a list of reliable group programs for referral. In selecting group programs for patient referral, it is important to know whether purported success rates are based on all enrollees or only on those completing the program.

Physician-Based Interventions. Glynn and Manley estimate that as many as 4.5 million smokers in the United States might be motivated to quit each year through brief physician counseling if 150,000 office-based physicians participated.[100] Only 25% of smokers report that their physicians ever talked to them about smoking.[28] Even brief physician interventions can have an important, cost-effective impact on patients' smoking cessation.[15,25,35,37,57,76] The role of physicians in smoking cessation counseling may range from brief physician advice to more intensive counseling, physician-initiated contracting for cessation, and referral to community services for assistance.[28]

The NCI has developed a four-step smoking cessation protocol to assist physicians in providing cessation counseling.[35] These steps include: 1) *ask* about smoking at every opportunity; 2) *advise* patients to stop; 3) *assist* the patient in stopping; and 4) *arrange* follow-up visits. Thus, within the context of a smoke-free office, physicians should take a smoking history on all patients and label the charts of smokers. All smokers should be given a strong message to quit, encouraged to set a quit date, and informed that the physician will monitor their progress on subsequent visits with progress notes entered into the patient's chart.[14,77] Minimal contact interventions, such as brief counseling with a plan for cessation plus self-help guides, should be offered to all patients who express an interest in quitting. Finally, intensive treatments in the practice or from outside referral generally offer help beyond that available in do-it-yourself programs and tend to attract smokers seeking extra help.[76]

Clinical trials have shown that physicians trained to provide "behavioral cessation counseling" are even more successful at helping patients to quit smoking than physicians who provide advice only (8.45 quit rate vs. 3.6%).[61,129] Clinical trials show that intensive physician interventions can produce quit rates of 20–25%.[34] In a meta-analysis of physician intervention trials, Kottke and colleagues found the best results when face-to-face counseling or advice were used, compared to programs using nicotine gum alone.[57]

Pharmacologic Treatments. Recognition of the addictive properties of nicotine has led to pharmacologic treatments to aid smokers in coping with the physiological aspects of withdrawal. Such treatments include Clonidine, an antihypertensive medication that reduces opiate and alcohol withdrawal.[27] While early reports of Clonidine were promising, more recent trials have not shown significant differences between placebo and Clonidine.[17,33]

To date, nicotine polacrilix (Nicorette®) remains the most effective pharmacologic intervention and the only FDA-approved drug for treating nicotine dependence. Nicorette® is a prescription drug in the form of a sugar-free chewing gum containing nicotine, obtained from the tobacco plant, which is bound to an ion exchange resin to allow slow release of nicotine when chewed.[100] Nicotine polacrilix can reduce symptoms of tobacco withdrawal, such as anxiety, weight gain, decreased mental concentration and diminished task performance.[44] A number of randomized controlled trials now show its efficacy when used with behavioral interventions, such as counseling.[29,38,56,88,115] Without such intervention, Nicorette® may be little better than a placebo. Fagerstrom found quit rates of 68% at one year when Nicorette® was supplemented with psychotherapy.[23] However, not all studies show significant findings.[50]

Unfortunately, Nicorette® often is used incorrectly, and this may account for some of the inconsistent results. In fact, it is a sustained release medication and should not be chewed like a gum.[94] The patient must stop smoking entirely and use the medication for at least several months.[97] Russell and colleagues show that quit rates are related to the amount of drug used; at least three boxes appears essential.[92] Success rates also are higher for patients who have more follow-up visits.[129] Finally, patients must wean off Nicorette®.

The transdermal nicotine patch shows promising results in trials and might have greater acceptability for both patients and their physicians.[1] Other pharmacological adjuncts under development include doxapin, ACTH and nasal nicotine solution.

Smokers at Special Risk

The profile of smokers is changing. Today, smokers are more likely to come from minority groups and from women. They are likely to have at most a high school education and to be blue-collar workers.[111,121] Older smokers with long smoking histories are at special risk. Cancer patients represent another group that has received too little attention. Here, we briefly highlight some of the smoking characteristics of these groups.

Women. Tobacco is the greatest preventable cause of death in American women, and is responsible for 125,000 deaths per year.[116] Women began smoking during World War II and have been more resistant to quitting than men. Lung cancer now has overtaken breast cancer as the number one cancer killer of women.[116]

Overall, 26.8% of women smoke, but that disguises considerable subgroup differences. As education rises, women are more likely to be never smokers or former smokers than current smokers. Smoking among college graduates has dropped by half since 1966, while smoking among those with less than high school education has hardly changed.[15]

Women seem to have special problems quitting (although this is not well-documented). This may be due to lack of social support for quitting, fear of weight gain and greater reliance on cigarettes for stress control. It is not yet known to what extent this reflects gender differences in the physiologic mechanism of addiction, social or behavioral factors or a combination thereof. Except for adolescent females, since 1979, smoking cessation trends among women have approached those of men.[75] It is essential that women patients be assessed for smoking and then encouraged to quit using the NCI protocol described earlier.

Minorities. African Americans represent the nation's largest minority group. They have the highest smoking rates and lowest quit rates of any ethnic/racial group: 35% of African Americans smoke.[79] African Americans also suffer the highest rates of morbidity and mortality in the United States from smoking-related diseases, including lung cancer and cardiovascular disease.[80] Although African Americans smoke fewer cigarettes, they are more likely to smoke brands with higher tar/nicotine yields. The higher smoking prevalence among African Americans probably can be explained by the fact that they are more likely than white smokers to be low income and low education. It appears that African Americans and whites are equally likely to have ever smoked, but African Americans are less likely to have quit, regardless of socio-demographic factors.[71,80] To be appropriate for use with minorities, educational materials must be matched to the smoker's cultural background and reading level. Medical advice to quit is essential, because it appears that fewer African American smokers are being advised to quit by physicians.[80] Self-help interventions combined with medical advice should be offered in public health and hospital clinics and emergency rooms as well as in more traditional medical settings.[76] All of these recommendations are especially important in view of the fact that African American smokers attempt to quit as often as white smokers but succeed less often.[79,80] Similar recommendations should be followed for other minority groups with high smoking rates, for example, Hispanic, American Indian and Asian men.

Older Smokers. Until recently, older smokers were all but ignored. Yet, there are thirteen million smokers aged 50 and over and eight million smokers aged 60 and over.[116] A nationwide survey of American Association of Retired Persons (AARP) members showed that 26% of the older respondents had never tried to quit smoking, and, only 39% reported that their physicians had told them to stop smoking. A significantly higher proportion of older smokers than non-smokers reported the presence of smoking-related symptoms, including frequent coughing, trouble breathing, tiring easily and other respiratory conditions.[89] Older smokers are most likely to quit for health reasons, so physician interventions are likely to be especially effective. As Fisher and Hill advised, "Remembering not to underestimate the benefits of quitting among older smokers, even the busiest specialist should view such interventions as worth the small time they consume."[27]

Cancer Patients. Cancer patients also were not considered as a target for smoking cessation until recently. This may explain why smoking rates for cancer patients parallel the general United States population.[107] Continued smoking among cancer patients may not only impair patients' quality of life; it may predispose some patients, especially those with head and neck cancers, to a second primary malignancy. The evidence suggests that smoking cessation has a therapeutic benefit for many cancer patients, especially those with early-stage, tobacco-related malignancies, such as lung cancer and head and neck cancers.[20] Patients with life-threatening illnesses may stop smoking spontaneously or on the basis of medical advice. Eriksen and Kondo concluded that 39–75% of cancer patients stop smoking following intervention, although many return to smoking once the immediate illness crisis has passed.[20] Preliminary data from Orleans and colleagues suggest that cancer patients want to stop smoking and desire help in doing so.[78] In a survey of 688 cancer patients who were smokers, over two-thirds expressed a strong desire to quit, and over three-fourths were interested in self-help materials.

It is important that cancer patients be advised to stop smoking and be given concrete quitting assistance following the protocol recommended by Glynn and Manley.[35] Cancer patients, especially those with early-stage cancers and those with tobacco-related malignancies, may not realize that their health can benefit following smoking cessation. Referral to individual or group counseling and/or nicotine replacement therapy may be appropriate for some cancer patients who are unable to stop smoking without additional assistance.

Conclusion

Given the immensity of the health problem, the number of Americans who now smoke or begin to smoke each year, and the addiction associated with using tobacco, the issue of how to achieve a reduction in smoking must be a national priority. There is no one way to reduce smoking in our society. Smoking control requires multi-faceted, concurrent and complementary interventions that include targeted health education programs, mass media campaigns, legislative and policy strategies and changes in taxation and export policies. Legislative efforts such as tax increases, advertising restrictions, labeling requirements, and regulatory actions to prevent smoking in a variety of public places or prohibit cigarette sales to minors are associated with reduced tobacco use.[90] For instance, a 10% increase in the price of cigarettes produces about a 4% decrease in adult consumption and a 14% decrease in teenage consumption.[126]

Trends toward restricting smoking in public places already have made smoking a socially unacceptable activity in many places. In 1990, over 42 states and more than 320 communities restrict smoking in public; an estimated one-half of large businesses have a smoking policy for their employees.[116] Such policies are vital in creating non-smoking social norms and are likely to continue. However, unless similar strategies are adopted around the world, total deaths from tobacco-related causes will continue to rise especially in Asia, Africa, and South America where cigarettes are heavily advertised and marketed. For example, in Thailand, 65% of men over the age of 20 now smoke, and one out of every five male cancer patients is afflicted with lung cancer.[123] In China, 61% of males over age 15 are smokers; it is estimated that by 2025, two million Chinese will die annually from smoking.[131]

In 1984, the Director of the National Cancer Institute commissioned a plan to reduce the nations's cancer mortality by 50% by the end of this century. This plan included an objective to reduce smoking prevalence for adolescents and adults to below 15%. Similarly, in 1989 the Surgeon General called for a smoke-free society by the year 2000. Physicians can play a pivotal role in facilitating a smoke-free society. They can make their offices and hospitals smoke-free, assess all patients for smoking status and intervene with smokers. They also can serve as leaders in community coalitions aimed at bringing about a smoke-free United States by the year 2000. In addition, physicians, as individuals, or as part of the powerful organizations to which they belong, can express their opposition to United States and other governmental policies which sanction the growth of the international tobacco trade. For example, they can oppose United States enforcement of trade sanctions under Section 301 of the United States Trade Act.[123] Physicians and other health professionals must continue to be leaders in the quest for a smoke-free world.

References

1. Abelin, T., Buehler, A., Muller, P., Vesanen, K., and Imhof, P. R.: Controlled trial of transdermal nicotine patch in tobacco withdrawal. Lancet, 1:7, 1989.
2. Ames, B. N., Durston, W. E., Yamasaki, E., and Lee, F. D.: Carcinogens are mutagens: A simple test system combining liver homogenates for activation and bacteria for detection. Proc. Natl. Acad. Sci. USA, 70:2281, 1973.
3. Auerbach, O., Hammond, E. C., Kirman, D., Garfinkel, L., and Stout, A. P.: Histologic changes in bronchial tubes of cigarette-smoking dogs. Cancer, 20:2055, 1967.
4. Bertram, J. S., Kolonel, L. N., and Meyskens, F. L.: Rationale and strategies for chemoprevention of cancer in humans. Cancer Res., 47:3012, 1987.
5. Boone, C. W., Kelloff, G. J., and Malone, W. E.: Identification of candidate cancer chemopreventive agents and their evaluation in animal models and human clinical trials: A review. Cancer Res., 50:2, 1990.
6. Boutwell, R. K.: On the Role of Tumor Promotion in Chemical Carcinogenesis. In Models, Mechanisms, and Etiology of Tumour Promotion. Edited by M. Borzsonyi, and N. E. Day. Lyon, IARC, 1984, p. 3.
7. Brown, L. M., Blot, W. J., Schuman, S. H., Smith, V. M., Ershow, A. G., Marks, R. D., and Fraumeni, J. F.: Environmental factors and high risk of esophageal cancer among men in coastal South Carolina. J.N.C.I., 80:1620, 1988.
8. Byers, T., Vena, J., Mettlin, C., Swanson, M., and Graham, S.: Dietary vitamin A and lung cancer risk: An analysis by histologic subtypes. Am. J. Epidemiol., 120:769, 1984.
9. Caporaso, N., Hayes, R., Dosemeci, M., Hoover, R., Ayesh, R., Hetzel, M., and Idle, J.: Lung cancer risk, occupational exposure, and the debrisoquine metabolic phenotype. Cancer Res., 49:3675,1989.
10. Caporaso, N. E., Tucker, M. A., Hoover, R. N., Hayes, R. B., Pickle, L. W., Issaq, H. J., Muschik, G. M., Green-Gallo, L., Buivys, D., Aisner, S., Resau, J. H., Trump, B. F., Tollerud, D., Weston, A., and Harris, C. C.: Lung cancer and the debrisoquine metabolic phenotype. J.N.C.I., 82:1264, 1990.
11. Cartwright, R. A., Glashan, R. W., Rogers, H. J., Ahmad, R. A., Barham-Hall, D., Higgins, E., and Kahn, M. A.: Role of n-acetyltransferase phenotypes in bladder carcinogenesis: A pharmacogenetic epidemiological approach to bladder cancer. Lancet, October 16:842, 1982.
12. Christenson, G. M., Gold, R. S., Katz, M., and Kreuter, M. W.: Preface. J. Sch. Health, 55:295, 1985.
13. Cohen, S., Lichtenstein, E., Prochaska, J. O., Rossi, J. S., Gritz, E. R., Carr, C. R., Orleans, C. T., Schoenbach, V. J., Biener, L., Abrams, D., DiClemente, C., Curry, S., Marlatt, G. A., Cummings, K. M., Emont, S. L., Giovino, G., and Ossip-Klein, D.: Debunking myths about self-quitting. Am. Psychol., 44:1355, 1989.
14. Cohen, S. J., Christen, A. G., Katz, B. P., Drook, C. A., Davis, B. J., Smith, D. M., and Stookey, G. K.: Counseling medical and dental patients about cigarette smoking: The impact of nicotine gum and chart reminders. Am. J. Public Health, 77:313, 1987.
15. Cummings, S. R., Rubin, S. M., and Oster, G.: The cost-effectiveness of counseling smokers to quit. J.A.M.A., 261:75, 1989.
16. Davis, M. F., Rosenberg, K., Iverson, D. C., Vernon, T. M., and Bauer, J.: Worksite health promotion in Colorado. Public Health Rep., 99:538, 1984.
17. Davison, R., Kaplan, K., Fintel, D., Parker, M., Anderson, L., and Haring, O.: The effect of clonidine on the cessation of cigarette smoking. Clin. Pharmacol. Ther., 44:265, 1988.
18. Ellickson, P. L., and Bell, R. M.: Drug prevention in junior high: A multi-site longitudinal test. Science, 247:1299, 1990.
19. Elwood, J. M., Pearson, J. C. G., Skippen, D. H., and Jackson, S. M.: Alcohol, smoking, social, and occupational factors in the aetiology of cancer of the oral cavity, pharynx and larynx. Int. J. Cancer, 34:603, 1984.
20. Eriksen, M. P., and Kondo, A. T.: Smoking cessation for cancer patients: Rationale and approaches. Health Education Research, 4:489, 1989.
21. Eriksen, M. P., Lemaistre, C. A., and Newell, G. R.: Health hazards of passive smoking. Ann. Rev. Public Health, 9:47, 1988.
22. Escobedo, L. G., Anda, R. F., Smith, P. F., Remington, P. L., and Mast, E. E.: Sociodemographic characteristics of cigarette smoking initiation in the United States. J.A.M.A., 264:1550, 1990.
23. Fagerstrom, K. O.: A comparison of psychological and pharmacological treatment in smoking cessation. J. Behav. Med., 5:343, 1982.
24. Field, J. K., and Spandidos D. A.: Expression of oncogenes in human tumours with special reference to the head and neck region. Oral Pathol., 16:97, 1987.
25. Fisher, E. B., Bishop, D. B., Goldmuntz, J., and Jacobs, A.: Implications for the practicing physician of the psychosocial dimensions of smoking. Chest, 93:69S, 1988.
26. Fisher, E. B., Harie-Joshu, D., Morgan, G. D., Rehberg, H., and Rost, K.: State of the art: Smoking and smoking cessation. Am. Rev. Respir. Dis., In review.
27. Fisher, E. B., and Hill, R. D.: Perspectives on older smokers. (Editorial) Chest, 97:517, 1990.
28. Fisher, E. B., and Rost, K.: Smoking cessation: A practical guide for the physician. Clin. Chest Med., 7:551, 1986.
29. Fortmann, S., Killen, J., Telch, M., and Newman, B.: Minimal contact treatment for smoking cessation. J.A.M.A., 260:1575, 1988.
30. Fraumeni, J. F., Jr., Wertelecki, W., Blattner, W. A., Jensen, R. D., and Leventhal, B. G.: Varied manifestations of a familial lymphoproliferative disorder. Am. J. Med., 59:145, 1975.
31. Gallick, G. E., Sacks, P. G., Maxwell, S. A., Steck, P. A., and Gutterman, J. U.: Head and neck squamous cell carcinoma lines as a model system for the study of oncogene

expression during tumor progression and metastasis. Prog. Clin. Biol. Res., 212:97, 1986.
32. Garfinkel, L.: Time trends in lung cancer mortality among nonsmokers and a note on passive smoking. J.N.C.I., 66:1061, 1981.
33. Glassman, A. H., Jackson, W. K., Walsh, B. T., Roose, S. P., and Rosenfeld, B.: Cigarette craving, smoking withdrawal, and clonidine. Science, 226:864, 1984.
34. Glynn, T. J.: Relative effectiveness of physician-initiated smoking cessation programs. The Cancer Bulletin, 40:359, 1988.
35. Glynn, T. J., and Manley, M. W.: Physicians, cancer control and the treatment of nicotine dependence: Defining success. Health Education Research, 4:479, 1989.
36. Graham, S.: Epidemiology of retinoids and cancer. J.N.C.I., 73:1423, 1984.
37. Gritz, E. R.: Cigarette smoking: The need for action by health professionals. CA, 38:194, 1988.
38. Hall, S. M., Tunstall, C. D., Ginsberg, D., Benowitz, N. L., and Jones, R. T.: Nicotine gum and behavioral treatment: A placebo controlled trial. J. Consult. Clin. Psychol., 55:603, 1987.
39. Hammond, E. C., Garfinkel, L., and Lew, E. A.: Longevity, selective mortality, and competitive risks in relation to chemical carcinogenesis. Environ. Res., 16:153, 1978.
40. Hammond, E. C., Selikoff, I. J., and Seidman, H.: Asbestos exposure, cigarette smoking and death rates. Ann. N.Y. Acad. Sci., 330:473, 1979.
41. Hankin, J. H., Kolonel, L. N., and Hinds, M. W.: Dietary history methods for epidemiologic studies: Application in a case-control study of vitamin A and lung cancer. J.N.C.I., 73:1417, 1984.
42. Hansen, W. B., Malotte, C. K., and Fielding, J. E.: Evaluation of a tobacco and alcohol abuse prevention curriculum for adolescents. Health Educ. Q., 15:93, 1988.
43. Hanssen, H. P., Agarwal, D. P., Goedde, H. W., Bucher, H., Huland, H., Brachmann, W., and Ovenbeck, R.: Association of n-acetyltransferase polymorphism and environmental factors with bladder carcinogenesis. Study in a North German population. Eur. Urol., 11:263, 1985.
44. Henningfield, J. E.: Understanding nicotine addiction and physical withdrawal process. J. Am. Dent. Assoc., (Suppl.)2S, 1990.
45. Herity, B., Moriarty, M., Daly, L., Dunn, J., and Bourke, G. J.: The role of tobacco and alcohol in the aetiology of lung and larynx cancer. Br. J. Cancer, 46:961, 1982.
46. Hilt, B., Langard, S., Andersen, A., and Rosenberg, J.: Asbestos exposure, smoking habits, and cancer incidence among production and maintenance workers in an electrochemical plant. Am. J. Ind. Med., 8:565, 1985.
47. Hirayama, T.: Diet and cancer. Nutr. Cancer, 1:67, 1979.
48. Hoffman, D., Melikian, A., Adams, J. D., Brunnemann, K. D., and Haley, N. J.: New aspects of tobacco carcinogenesis. Carcinogenesis, 8:239, 1985.
49. Hong, W. K., Lippman, S. M., Itri, L. M., Karp, D. D., Lee, J. S., Byers, R. M., Schantz, S. P., Kramer, A. M., Lotan, R., Peters, L. J., Dimery, I. W., Brown, B. W., and Goepfert, H.: Prevention of second primary tumors with isotretinoin in squamous-cell carcinoma of the head and neck. N. Engl. J. Med., 323:795, 1990.
50. Hughes, J., Gust, S., Keehan, R., Fenwick, J., and Healey, M.: Nicotine vs placebo gum in general medical practice. J.A.M.A., 261:1300, 1989.
51. IARC: IARC Monographs on the Evaluation of the Carcinogenic Risk of Chemicals to Humans: Vol. 38–Tobacco Smoking. Lyon, IARC, 1986.
52. Janerich, D. T., Thompson, W. Douglas, Varela, L. R., Greenwald, P., Chorost, S., Tucci, C., Zaman, M. B., Melamed, M. R., Kiely, M., and McKneally, M. F.: Lung cancer and exposure to tobacco smoke in the household. N. Engl. J. Med., 323:632, 1990.
53. Kabat, G. C., and Wynder, E. L.: Lung cancer in nonsmokers. Cancer 53:1214, 1984.
54. Karki, N. T., Pokela, R., Nuutinen, L., and Pelkonen, O.: Aryl hydrocarbon hydroxylase in lymphocytes and lung tissue from lung cancer patients and controls. Int. J. Cancer, 39:565, 1987.
55. Kawachi, I., Pearce, N. E., and Jackson, R. T.: Deaths from lung cancer and ischaemic heart disease due to passive smoking in New Zealand. N. Z. Med. J., 102:337, 1989.
56. Killen, J. D., Maccoby, N., and Taylor, C. B.: Nicotine gum and self-regulation training in smoking relapse prevention. Behavior Therapy, 15:234, 1984.
57. Kottke, T. E., Battista, R. N., DeFriese, G. H., and Brekke, M. L.: Attributes of successful smoking cessation interventions in medical practice. J.A.M.A., 259:2883, 1988.
58. Kouri, R. E., McKinney, C. E., Slomiany, D. J., Snodgrass, D. R., Wray, N. P., and McLemore, T. L.: Positive correlation between high aryl hydrocarbon hydroxylase activity and primary lung cancer as analyzed in cryopreserved lymphocytes. Cancer Res., 42:5030, 1982.
59. Krontiris, T. G., DiMartino, N. A., Mitcheson, H. D., Lonergan, J. A., Begg, C., and Parkinson, D. R.: Human hypervariable sequences in risk assessment: Rare Ha-ras alleles in cancer patients. Environ. Health Perspect., 76:147, 1987.
60. Kvale, G., Bjelke, E., and Gart, J. J.: Dietary habits and lung cancer risk. Int. J. Cancer, 31:397, 1983.
61. Li, V. C., Coates, T. J., Ewart, C. K., and Young, J. K.: The effectiveness of smoking cessation advice given during routine medical care: Physicians can make a difference. Am. J. Prev. Med., 3:81, 1987.
62. Lippman, S. M., Garewal, H. S., and Meyskens, F. L.: Retinoids as potential chemopreventive agents in squamous cell carcinoma of the head and neck. Prev. Med., 18:740, 1989.
63. Lower, G. M., Nilsson, T., Nelson, C. E., Wolf, H., Gamsky, T. E., and Bryan, G. T.: N-acetyltransferase phenotype and risk in urinary bladder cancer: Approaches in molecular epidemiology. Preliminary results in Sweden and Denmark. Environ. Health Perspect., 29:71, 1979.
64. Mackerras, D., Buffler, P. A., Randall, D. E., Nichaman, M. Z., Pickle, L. W., and Mason, T. J.: Carotene intake and the risk of laryngeal cancer in coastal Texas. Am. J. Epidemiol., 128:980, 1988.
65. Malone, W. F., Kelloff, G. J., Pierson, H., and Greenwald, P.: Chemoprevention of bladder cancer. Cancer, 60(Suppl.):650, 1987.
66. Marshall, J., Graham, S., Mettlin, C., Sheed, D., and Swanson, M.: Diet in the epidemiology of oral cancer. Nutr. Cancer, 3:145, 1982.
67. McLemore, T. L., Adelberg, S., Liu, M. C., McMahon, N. A., Yu, S. J., Hubbard, W. C., Czerwinski, M., Wood, T. G., Storeng, R., Lubet, R. A., Eggleston, J. C., Boyd, M. R., and Hines, R. N.: Expression of CYP1A1 gene in patients with lung cancer: Evidence for cigarette smoke-induced gene expression in normal lung tissue and for altered gene regulation in primary pulmonary carcinomas. J.N.C.I., 82:1333, 1990.
68. McManus, M. E., Boobis, A. R., Minchin, R. F., Schwartz, D. M., Murray, S., Davies, D. S., and Thorgeirsson, S. S.: Relationship between oxidative metabolism of 2-acetylaminofluorene, debrisoquine, bufuralol, and aldrin in human liver microsomes. Cancer Res., 44:5692, 1984.
69. Mommsen, S., and Agaard, J.: Susceptibility in urinary bladder cancer: Acetyltransferase phenotypes and related risk factors. Cancer Letter, 32:199, 1986.
70. National Research Council: Environmental Tobacco Smoke. Measuring Exposures and Assessing Health Effects. Washington, National Academy Press, 1986.
71. Novotny, T., Warner, K. E., Kendrick, J. E., and Remington, P. L.: Socioeconomic factors and racial smoking differences in the United States. Am. J. Public Health, 78:1187, 1988.
72. Office of Technology Assessment: The Role of Genetic Testing in the Prevention of Occupational Disease. Washington, Office of Technology Assessment, 1983, p. 95.
73. Olsen, J., Sabroe, S., and Fasting, U.: Interaction of alcohol and tobacco as risk factors in cancer of the laryngeal region. J. Epidemiol. Community Health, 39:165, 1985.
74. Ooi, W. L., Elston, R. C., Chen, V. W., Bailey-Wilson, J. E., and Rothschild, H: Increased familial risk for lung cancer. J.N.C.I., 76:217, 1986.
75. Orlandi, M. A.: Gender differences in smoking cessation. Women Health, 11:237, 1986.
76. Orleans, C. T.: Smoking cessation in primary care settings. N.J. Med., 85:116, 1988.
77. Orleans, C. T.: Understanding and promoting smoking cessation: Overview and guidelines for physician intervention. Annu. Rev. Med., 36:51, 1985.
78. Orleans, C. T., Lindblad, A., Davis, S., Rose, M., James, J., Engstrom, P., Robinson, R., Brody, D., Angel, I., and Gritz, E.: The need for brief physician-initiated quit smoking strategies in CCOP settings. Presented at the 14th Annual Meeting of the American Society of Preventive Oncology, Bethesda, MD, March 19-20, 1990.
79. Orleans, C. T., Schoenbach, V. J., Salmon, M. A., Strecher, V. J., Kalsbeek, W., Quade, D., Brooks, E. F., Konrad, T. R., Blackmon, C., and Watts, C. D.: A survey of smoking and quitting patterns among Black Americans. Am. J. Public Health, 79:176, 1989.
80. Orleans, C. T., Strecher, V. J., Schoenbach, V. J., Salmon, M. A., and Blackmon, C.: Smoking cessation initiatives for Black Americans: Recommendations for research and intervention. Health Education Research, 4:13, 1989.
81. Pelkonen, O., Karki, N. T., and Sotaniemi, E. A.: Determination of carcinogen-activating enzymes in the monitoring of high-risk groups. In Human Cancer. Its Characterization and Treatment. Edited by W. Davis, K. R. Harrap, and G. Stathopoulos. Amsterdam, Excerpta Medica, 1980, pps. 48-57.
82. Perera, F., Mayer, J., Jaretzki, A., Hearne, S., Brenner, D., Young, T. L., Fischman, H. K., Grimes, M., Grantham, S., Tang, M. X., Tsai, W. Y., and Santella, R. M.: Comparison of DNA adducts and sister chromatid exchange in lung cancer cases and controls. Cancer Res., 49:4446, 1989.
83. Perera, F. P., Poirier, M. C., Yuspa, S. H., Nakayama, J., Jaretzki, A., Curnen, M. M., Knowles, D. M., and Weinstein, I. B.: A pilot project in molecular cancer epidemiology: Determination of benzo(a)pyrene-DNA adducts in animal and human tissues by immunoassays. Carcinogenesis, 3:1405, 1982.
84. Perera, F. P., Santella, R. M., Brenner, D., Poirier, M. C., Munshi, A. A., Fischman, H. K., and Van Ryzin, J.: DNA adducts, protein adducts, and sister chromatid exchange in cigarette smokers and nonsmokers. J.N.C.I., 79:449, 1987.
85. Perry, C. L., Baranowski, T., and Parcel, G. S.: How individuals, environments, and health behavior interact: Social learning theory. In Health Behavior and Health Education Theory, Research, and Practice. Edited by K. Glanz, F. M. Lewis, and B. K. Rimer. San Francisco, Jossey-Bass Inc., 1990, pp. 161-186.
86. Prochaska, J. O., and DiClemente, C. C.: Common Processes of Self-Change in Smoking, Weight Control, and Psychological Distress. *In* Coping and Substance Use. Edited by S. Shiffman and T. Wills. New York, Academic Press, 1985, pp. 345-364.
87. Randerath, E., Miller, R. H., Mittal, D., Avitts, T. A., Dunsford, H. A., and Randerath, K.: Covalent DNA damage in tissues of cigarette smokers as determined by 32P-postlabeling assay. J.N.C.I., 81:341, 1989.
88. Raw, M., Jarvis, M. J., Feyerabend, C., and Russell, M. A. H.: Comparison of nicotine chewing-gum and psychological treatments for dependent smokers. Br. Med. J., 281:481, 1980.
89. Rimer, B. K., Orleans, C. T., Keintz, M. K., Cristinzio, S., and Fleisher, L.: The older smoker: Status, challenges and opportunities for intervention. Chest, 97:547, 1990.
90. Roemer, R.: Recent Developments in Legislation to Combat the World's Smoking Epidemic. Geneva, World Health Organization, 1986.
91. Rundall, T. G., and Bruvold, W. H.: A meta-analysis of school-based smoking and alcohol use prevention programs. Health Educ. Q., 15:317, 1988.
92. Russell, M. A., Merriman, R., Stapleton, J., and Taylor, W.: Effect of nicotine chewing gum as an adjunct to general practitioners' advice against smoking. Br. Med. J., 287:1782, 1983.
93. Saccomanno, G.: The contribution of uranium miners to lung cancer histogenesis. Recent Results. Cancer Res., 82:43, 1982.
94. Sachs, D. P. L.: Smoking cessation strategies: What works, what doesn't. J. Am. Dent. Assoc., (Suppl.):13S, 1990.
95. Saracci, R.: Asbestos and lung cancer: An analysis of the epidemiological evidence on the asbestos-smoking interaction. Int. J. Cancer, 20:323,1977.
96. Schinke, S. P., Gilchrist, L. D., Snow, W. H., and Schilling, R. F.: Skills-building methods to prevent smoking by adolescents. J. Adolesc. Health Care, 6:439, 1985.
97. Schneider, N. G.: Psychopharmacologic treatment of cigarette smoking. J. Am. Dent. Assoc., (Suppl.):7S, 1990.
98. Schoenberg, J. B., Klotz, J. B., Wilcox, H. B., Gil-del-Real, M., Stemhagen, A., and Nicholls, G. P.: Lung cancer and exposure to radon in women–New Jersey. M.M.W.R., 38:715, 1989.
99. Schottenfeld, D., and Fraumeni, J. F.: Cancer Epidemiology and Prevention. Philadelphia, W. B. Saunders Co., 1982, p. 572.
100. Schwartz, J. L.: Review and Evaluation of Smoking Cessation Methods: The United States and Canada, 1978–1985. Washington, Division of Cancer Prevention and Control, National Cancer Institute, U. S. Department of Health and Human Services, Public Health Service, National Institutes of Health (NIH Pub. No. 87-2940), 1987.
101. Sellers, T. A., Bailey-Wilson, J. E., Elston, R. C., Wilson, A. F., Elston, G. Z., Ooi, W. L., and Rothschild, H.: Evidence for Mendelian inheritance in the pathogenesis of lung cancer. J.N.C.I., 82:1272, 1990.
102. Shah, J. P., Strong, E. W., and DeCosse, J. J.: Effect of retinoids on oral leukoplakia. Am. J. Surg., 146:466, 1983.

103. Shiffman, S.: Relapse following smoking cessation: A situational analysis. J. Consult. Clin. Psychol., 50:71, 1982.

104. Silverman, S., Gorsky, M., and Greenspan, D.: Tobacco usage in patients with head and neck carcinomas: A follow-up study on habit changes and second primary oral/oropharyngeal cancers. J. Am. Dent. Assoc., 106:33, 1983.

105. Slamon D. J., deKernion, J. B., Verma, I. M., and Cline, M. J.: Expression of cellular oncogenes in human malignancies. Science, 224:256, 1984.

106. Slattery, M. L., Robison, L. M., Schuman, K. L., French, T. K., Abbott, T. M., Overall, J. C., Jr., and Gardner, J. W.: Cigarette smoking and exposure to passive smoke are risk factors for cervical cancer. J.A.M.A., 261:1593, 1989.

107. Spitz, M. R., Fueger, J. J., Eriksen, M. P., and Newell, G. R.: Profiles of cigarette smoking among patients in a cancer center. Journal of Cancer Education, 3:265, 1988.

108. Spitzer, W. O., Lawrence, V., Dales, R., Hill, G., Archer, M. C., Clark, P., Abenhaim, L., Hardy, J., Sampalis, J., and Pinfold, S. P.: Links between passive smoking and disease: A best evidence synthesis. A report of the Working Group on Passive Smoking. Clin. Invest. Med., 13:17, 1990.

109. Stich, H. F., and Rosin, M. P.: Quantitating the synergistic effect of smoking and alcohol consumption with the micronucleus test on human buccal mucosa cells. Int. J. Cancer, 31:305, 1983.

110. Stich, H. F., Rosin, M. P., and Hornby, A. P.: Remission of oral leukoplakias and micronuclei in tobacco/betel quid chewers treated with beta-carotene and with beta-carotene plus vitamin A. Int. J. Cancer, 42:195, 1988.

111. Strecher, V. J., Rimer, B. K., and Monaco, K. D.: Development of a new self-help guide–Freedom From Smoking® For You and Your Family. Health Educ. Q., 16:101, 1989.

112. Sugimura, H., Caporaso, N. E., Modali, R. V., Hoover, R. N., Resau, J. H., Trump, B. F., Lonergan, J. A., Krontiris, T. G., Mann, D. L., and Weston, A.: Association of rare alleles of the Harvey ras protooncogene locus with lung cancer. Cancer Res., 50:1857, 1990.

113. Tabin, C. J., Bradley, S. M., Bargmann, C. I., Weinberg, R. A., Papageorge, A. G., Scolnick, E. M., Dhar, R., Lowy, D. R., and Chang, E. H.: Mechanism of activation of a human oncogene. Nature, 300:143, 1982.

114. Tokuhata, G. K., and Lilienfeld, A. M.: Familial aggregation of lung cancer in humans. J.N.C.I., 30:289, 1963.

115. Tonnesen, P., Fryd, V., Hansen, M., Helsted, J., Gunnesen, A. B., Forchammer, H., and Stockner, M.: Effect of nicotine chewing gum in combination with group counseling on the cessation of smoking. N. Engl. J. Med., 381:15, 1988.

116. United States Department of Health and Human Services: Reducing the Health Consequences of Smoking: 25 Years of Progress. A Report of the Surgeon General. Washington, U.S. Department of Health and Human Services, Public Health Service, Centers for Disease Control, Center for Chronic Disease Prevention and Health Promotion, Office on Smoking and Health (DHHS Publication No. (CDC) 89-8411), 1989.

117. United States Department of Health and Human Services: The Health Consequences

118. of Smoking: Nicotine Addiction. A Report of the Surgeon General 1988. Washington, U.S. Department of Health and Human Services, Public Health Service, Centers for Disease Control, Center for Health Promotion and Education, Office on Smoking and Health (DHHS Publication No. (CDC) 88-8406), 1988.

118. United States Department of Health and Human Services: The Health Consequences of Smoking: Cancer. A Report of the Surgeon General. Washington, U.S. Department of Health and Human Services, Public Health Service, Office on Smoking and Health (DHHS Publication No. (PHS) 82-50179), 1982.

119. United States Department of Health and Human Services: Cancer Statistics Review 1973-1986. Bethesda, U.S. Department of Health and Human Services, Public Health Service, National Cancer Institute (NIH Publication No. 89-2789),1989.

120. United States Department of Health and Human Services: The Health Consequences of Involuntary Smoking. A Report of the Surgeon General. Washington, U.S. Department of Health and Human Services, Public Health Service, Centers for Disease Control, (DHHS Publication No. (CDC) 87-8398), 1986.

121. United States Department of Health and Human Services: Smoking Tobacco and Health A Fact Book. Washington, U.S. Department of Health and Human Services, Public Health Service, Centers for Disease Control, Center for Chronic Disease Prevention and Health Promotion, Office on Smoking and Health (DHHS Publication No. (CDC) 87-8397), Revised October,1989.

122. United States Public Health Service: Smoking and Health. Report of the Advisory Committee to the Surgeon General of the Public Health Service. Washington, U. S. Department of Health, Education, and Welfare, Public Health Service, Center for Disease Control (PHS Publication No. 1103), 1964.

123. Vateesatokit, P.: The latest victim of tobacco trade sanctions. J.A.M.A., 264:1522, 1990.

124. Wald, N., Idle, M., and Boreham, J.: Low serum vitamin-A and subsequent risk of cancer. Lancet, 2:813, 1980.

125. Wald, N. J., Nanchahal, K., Thompson, S. G., and Cuckle, H.S.: Does breathing other people's tobacco smoke cause lung cancer? Br. Med. J., 293:1217, 1986.

126. Warner, K. E.: Cigarette taxation: Doing good by doing well. J. Public Health Policy, September:312, 1984.

127. Willett, W. C., Polk, B. F., Underwood, B. A., Stampfer, M. J., Pressel, S., Rosner, B., Taylor, J. O., Schneider, K., and Hames, C. G.: Relation of serum vitamins A and E and carotenoids to the risk of cancer. N. Engl. J. Med., 310:430, 1984.

128. Winn, D. M., Ziegler, K. G., and Pickle, L. W.: Diet in the etiology of oral and pharyngeal cancer among women from the southern United States. Cancer Res., 44:1216, 1984.

129. Wilson, D. M. C., Taylor, D. W., Gilbert, J. R., Best, J. A., Lindsay, E. A., Willms, D. G., and Singer, J.: A randomized trial of a family physician intervention for smoking cessation. J.A.M.A., 260:1570, 1988.

130. Wu, A. H., Henderson, B. E., Pike, M. C., and Yu, M. C.: Smoking and other risk factors for lung cancer in women. J.N.C.I., 74:747, 1985.

131. Yu, J. J., Mattson, M. E., Boyd, G. M., Mueller, M. D., Shopland, D. R., Pechacek, T. F., and Cullen, J. W.: A comparison of smoking patterns in the People's Republic of China with the United States. J.A.M.A., 264:1575, 1990.

VI-2

Nutrition in the Etiology and Prevention of Cancer

Steven K. Clinton

Introduction

Throughout the course of human evolution, the often precarious food supply, was typically low in fat and high in complex carbohydrates and fiber. Over the last two centuries, improvements in food production, processing, storage, and distribution have led to major changes in diet composition within the industrialized nations. During this period, life expectancy dramatically increased in economically developed countries due to a combination of factors including public health measures, improved occupational safety, and major reductions in nutrient deficiency syndromes. As the population has aged, we have seen a shift in the major causes of morbidity and mortality towards chronic diseases such as cancer and cardiovascular disease. These changes have been associated with an increasingly overweight and sedentary population. Although nutritional deficiencies still plague subpopulations in industrial nations such as the poor, aged, alcoholics, and chronically ill, we now recognize the "afflu-

ent" diet as a contributor to the pathogenesis of chronic diseases which afflict the vast majority of the population. Efforts to understand the etiologies of the cancers have led to epidemiologic and laboratory studies that have strongly implicated certain dietary patterns and specific nutrients.

The diet is not only a source of nutrients, but serves as a vehicle for many other substances that may participate in promoting or inhibiting carcinogenesis. Although frequently implicated by the popular press and public, it appears that food additives, such as dyes, artificial sweeteners, and flavoring agents contribute very little to the overall cancer burden.[204,206] The potential risks of man-made contaminants such as pesticides, herbicides, and industrial wastes which enter the food chain have not yet been clearly defined. Many natural carcinogens produced by plants or fungi, such as aflatoxins in moldy grains, probably play a role in the etiology of some human cancers. Increasing evidence implicates food processing or cooking methods, for example salt-pickling and charcoal-broiling, as sources of carcinogens or tumor promoting substances.[204,206] A rapidly expanding area of research focuses upon the identification of natural substances in foods, such as phytochemicals, which are not nutrients but have anti-carcinogenic properties that may ultimately be utilized in chemoprevention programs.[16,86,204,206] The role of non-nutritive components of the diet in cancer cause and prevention is the focus of chapter VI-3.

This review is devoted to the role of nutrients in the etiology of cancer. Although nutrients are not carcinogenic *per se*, laboratory studies have proven that nutritional status has a major influence upon host susceptibility to oncogenic events. The nutrients may be classified into six main categories: protein, carbohydrate, fat, vitamins, minerals, and water. The only components providing energy are protein, carbohydrates, and fat at approximately 4, 4, and 9 kilocalories per gram, respectively. The vitamins and minerals provide no energy but function as structural components or as cofactors in numerous vital metabolic processes. Dietary fiber has not been considered as an essential nutrient category, although considerable efforts have recently been devoted to understanding the complexities of dietary fiber and its role in human health and disease. Alcohol has been a component of the human diet throughout recorded history and has numerous metabolic and physiologic effects in addition to its contribution to energy intake (7 kcal/gm). The potential complex interactions among the dozens of established nutrients and the genetic and environmental factors participating in human carcinogenesis has precluded precise quantification of the risks and benefits associated with any single nutrient. Recent publications have provided comprehensive overviews of the nutrition and cancer field.[3,31,104,206,240,246] Rather than detailing the complex, often incomplete, and occasionally contradictory literature concerning the role of nutrients in the etiology of human cancer, this chapter is intended to be a general guide to a rapidly expanding discipline with an emphasis upon the major emerging concepts in the area.

Historical Perspectives on Nutrition and Cancer

The preventative or curative properties of foods have been a part of the folklore and religion of all ancient cultures. The teachings of Hippocrates formed the basis for the understanding of cancer from approximately 450 B.C. through the middle ages.[271,272] Not only did he define the word cancer based upon the crab-like spread of the disease, but he formulated a concept that diseases, including cancer, resulted from an imbalance of the four humors which composed the body. The four humors where referred to as blood, phlegm, yellow bile, and black bile. Cancer was the result of an excess of black bile, also known as melencole. Health was the result of maintaining the four humors in proper and harmonious proportion. Hippocrates appreciated the importance of diet in the maintenance of health. As quoted by Byers and Graham,[31] Hippocrates wrote:

". . . this I know, moreover, that to the human body it makes a great difference whether the bread be fine or coarse; with or without the hull, whether mixed with much or little water, strongly wrought or scarcely at all, baked or raw . . . Whoever pays no attention to these things, or, paying attention, does not comprehend them, how can he understand the diseases which befall man? For, by everyone of these things, man is affected and changed this way or that, and the whole of his life is subjected to them, whether in health, convalescence, or disease. Nothing else, then, can be more important or more necessary to know than these things."

Galen, about 200 A.D., accepted and extended the teachings of Hippocrates concerning diet and cancer.[110] He recommended special diets, avoiding foods which were the sources of excess black bile associated with cancer such as wine, vinegar, cabbage, aged cheese, nuts, and pickled meats. Foods which were thought to restore the appropriate balance of black bile were vegetables, milk, young goat's flesh, veal, fowl, oysters, and light wine. He also recommended fasting from time to time, showing remarkable foresight into current research concerning the inhibition of tumorigenesis by diet restriction.

For over 1,500 years following the birth of Christ the humoral theory, heavily overladen with mysticism and religious beliefs, dominated European concepts of cancer and became more elaborate with the introduction of abnormal as well as normal humors. By the Renaissance, the holistic humoral approach to cancer was being replaced by newer concepts. Paracelsus discarded and ridiculed the doctrine of the four humors and introduced the iatrochemical theory that cancer was a result of an imbalance of chemicals, such as an excess of arsenic derived from the diet.[272] However, observations by medical practitioners soon implicated a number of lifestyle and occupational factors in the etiology of cancer and directed the scientific inquiry into the origins of cancer away from the unsubstantiated dietary beliefs which have always remained popular among the public. Bernardino Rammazzini, in the early 1700s, implicated lifestyle in the etiology of breast cancer when he observed that breast cancer was more common among nuns than other women.[326] Percivall Pott's description in 1775 of scrotal cancer in the chimney sweeps of London was the first clear example of occupational cancer.[225] In the same era, tobacco products were implicated in cancer causation based upon the association between cancer of the lip and pipe smoking, and between nasal cancer and snuff.[272]

From the 18th through the early 20th centuries the emerging scientific disciplines of nutrition and carcinogenesis evolved independently. During the 1800s, efforts to define the origins of cancer focused primarily upon environmental exposures associated with the industrial revolution. Skin cancer in petrochemical workers, lung cancer in miners, and bladder cancer among workers in the aniline dye industry were recorded. During the early decades of the 20th century many chemicals were purified from substances associated with human cancers and rodent models for cancer were developed.[271,272]

Lavoisier is considered the originator of modern nutrition based upon his discovery of the chemical basis of respiration and metabolism during the late 1700s. Advances in chemistry during the 19th century led to efforts directed at defining the chemical composition of food and the roles of different chemical fractions in animal growth and health. The first half of the 20th century was the golden era in nutritional science when the essential vitamins, minerals, and amino acids were isolated, characterized, synthesized, and their deficiency syndromes defined and treated.

Important interactions between the disciplines of carcinogenesis and nutrition developed in the years surrounding World War II. During this period the nutrient requirements of rodents were defined and purified components of foods were available for the preparation of carefully controlled experimental diets. The effects of nutrients upon tumorigenesis could be investigated in the expanding list of rodent cancer models utilizing carcinogens found in the diet or workplace. For example, a number of nutrients were found to modify liver carcinogenesis induced by p-dimethylaminoazobenzene, more well known at that time as the food dye called "butter yellow."[194a] The meticulous studies of Tannenbaum and coworkers during the 1940s delineated the important roles of fat and energy intake, as well as many other nutrients, in the genesis of experimental cancers.[287] Although the relevance of the laboratory data to human cancer was frequently discussed, the epidemiologic methodology needed to investigate nutrition and cancer hypotheses in humans had not been adequately developed in the years immediately following World War II.

During the 1950's, the possibility that nutrients indirectly modify human cancer incidence was overshadowed by the perceived hazard of additives and environmental contaminants in the food supply. These concerns were the focus of attention by the United States Congress and led to the passage in 1958 of the Delaney Amendment which stated that no additive is to be permitted in any amount in the food supply if it has been shown to produce cancer in animal studies or in other appropriate tests. The requirement that food additives and contaminants from food production and processing be extensively tested for carcinogenicity or mutagenesis directed research efforts away from the role of nutrients as modifiers of carcinogenesis. However, after intensive investigations, the National Academy of Sciences concluded in a series of reports that food preservatives, antioxidants, food colors and other intentionally added substances probably did not account for a significant proportion of human cancers.[202,204–206] In contrast, the contribution of indirect additives, contaminants, and by-products of food processing and cooking to cancer risk remains an area of uncertainty and the focus of continuing research.

Advances in nutrition and cancer epidemiology during the 1960s and 1970s refocused attention upon the indirect effects that nutrients may have on carcinogenesis. The observations that human cancers exhibit several hundred-fold variations in incidence among different geographic and cultural areas and that migrants from low risk areas to high risk areas frequently showed dramatic increases in cancer incidence suggested that lifestyle plays a major role. Variations in diet and nutrient intake were among the factors most frequently found to change in concert with risk for many human cancers, especially those of the gastrointestinal tract, breast, and prostate.[10,34,65] The major advances in recent decades in understanding the relationship of diet to cardiovascular disease further emphasized the plausibility of modulating cancer risk by nutrient modification.

By the 1980s, interest in cancer prevention increased in political and lay circles due to the perceived failure of the medical and scientific community to develop cures for major cancers despite huge financial expenditures. The National Academy of Sciences summarized the literature in nutrition and cancer and issued a report in 1982, which included controversial recommendations.[204] The expert committee concluded that most major cancers were influenced by dietary patterns but that data were insufficient to quantify accurately the contribution of diet to cancer risk and the benefits that could be achieved by dietary modifications. However, specific recommendations for changes in the American diet were made by the National Academy of Sciences[204] and subsequently by the National Cancer Institute[207] and the American Cancer Society.[4,5] The approach was to define dietary goals which would be readily achievable by the American population, even though the limited research data suggest that even more extensive changes in the diet may be necessary to reduce cancer risk significantly. The World Health Organization has also completed a report addressing the role of diet in the protection against chronic diseases, including cancer.[325] This report documents the shift towards an "affluent" diet associated with modest increases in prosperity in developing countries. A series of population nutrient goals, similar to those proposed by the National Academy of Sciences in 1982, have been established to serve as a guide for nutrient intakes necessary to minimize diet-related diseases in all countries throughout the world.

As we move towards the 21st century the current research strategies in the area of nutrition and cancer can be divided into two major philosophical approaches, best described as proscriptive and prescriptive. Proscriptive efforts are focused primarily upon the identification and elimination of dietary components that are associated with increased cancer risk. Major alterations in the American diet, such as a reduction in fat intake, would require significant changes in consumer behavior, farming practice, government subsidies to the agricultural community, and the food processing industry. The obstacles to proscriptive change to prevent cancer are readily apparent after years of efforts to reduce the use of tobacco products. The scientific basis for limiting tobacco use has been firmly established yet political, economic, and social considerations prevent implementation of educational, medical and agricultural programs that could have significant benefits in public health. Interest in the prescriptive or pharmacologic approach to cancer prevention is gaining momentum. This concept circumvents the problems of the "affluent" diet by trying to define substances that can be utilized as supplements or in the fortification of foods to counteract the components of the current diet that increase risk for cancer and other chronic diseases. This strategy, referred to as chemoprevention, focuses upon the identification of specific micronutrients, natural compounds in foods, and synthetic agents which can be integrated into the diet of specific high risk individuals or the entire population to reduce cancer incidence. Judgment concerning the scientific validity or effectiveness of these divergent philosophies will be reserved for future historians.

Methodological Issues in Diet and Cancer Studies

The obstacles to precisely defining the role of specific nutrients in human cancer are numerous.[49,115,127] The unbiased detection and quantification of risks associated with variations in nutrient intake would ideally be achieved through randomized prospective trials. Unfortunately the large costs of long term nutrition studies and scientific difficulties in controlling or measuring nutrient intake limit feasibility. Current nutritional guidelines for disease prevention and future refinements will be based upon the integration of information derived from a variety of different epidemiologic approaches and laboratory investigations. The etiologies of most chronic diseases, including cancer, are multifactorial. Human cancers show striking variations based upon such factors as age, sex, race, time, socioeconomic status, and many occupational and lifestyle factors. The potential for complex interactions between these factors and nutrients is enormous and emphasizes the difficulties in demonstrating causal associations with the same clarity as demonstrable for high-risk environmental exposures such as cigarette smoking.

Assessment of the Human Diet

The critical limiting feature of most human studies designed to address the role of nutrients in cancer is the imprecision of quantifying nutrient intake. An accurate estimate of human nutrient intake is derived from a two step process. First, the amounts and types of foods consumed must be determined by interviews, questionnaires, or food diaries. This information can then be utilized to calculate nutrient intake if an accurate data base has been established that quantifies the amount of each nutrient contained in the foods consumed by the population under investigation. Each of these steps can be associated with significant error which often makes nutrient-cancer associations difficult to detect.

A very active and critical area of research involves the design and validation of dietary questionnaires and interview techniques to measure long and short term dietary intake.[49] A number of issues must be addressed by investigators in this field. The human diet is a complex array of foods which exhibits significant day-to-day and seasonal variation. The complexity of the diet differs widely among populations, cultures, and geographic areas. This often requires the development of different assessment methods for each population. For example, food variety in specific counties within the People's Republic of China is very homogeneous and may be limited to less than 25 items produced locally.[128] In contrast, 90% by weight of the American diet is derived from over 500 different food items.[223] Within a geographic area, food selections among individuals also shows significant variation with age, gender, and social and economic status. Among individuals evaluated in studies, the perceived and actual food selections and their quantities may differ significantly. Most human cancers have a long latency, and the methodological difficulties associated with estimating the intake of foods or nutrients consumed many years prior to the diagnosis of cancer are a major concern for retrospective studies.[334]

Accurate quantification of nutrient intake depends upon a data base which defines the nutrient composition of the chosen foods. The United States Department of Agriculture Handbooks provide an accurate estimate of the nutrient composition of most foods consumed in North America.[313] However, the nutrient content of foods found in many under-

developed nations has not been as precisely defined. The content of some nutrients in a food may be relatively constant and even regulated by law in some nations, such as the amount of fat in whole milk. However, the contents of other nutrients in food items may be highly variable. For example, the selenium concentration in grains and vegetables will vary greatly depending upon the soil selenium content. In nations where foods are shipped large distances, an estimate of selenium intake may require direct measurement of its content in food samples from the study population.

In many studies, the consumption of certain foods which account for the greatest variance for the nutrient of interest serve as a surrogate indicator of nutrient intake. For example, many investigators present an analysis of meat intake relative to the risk of certain cancers as a surrogate indicator of saturated fat intake. Similarly, the consumption of certain vegetables and citrus fruits is often used as an estimate of vitamin C intake. Studies using surrogate measures for nutrient intake can greatly underestimate or fail to detect a real association between a nutrient and cancer due to the imperfect exposure data. In addition, most foods are a source of more than one potentially active nutrient. For example, many fruits and vegetables are not only a source of vitamin C but contribute significantly to carotenoid, vitamin A, and fiber intake. Caution should be used when making assumptions concerning the role of specific nutrients when investigators use food items or groups as the primary focus of the analysis.

Biochemical Assessment of Nutrient Intake

Future progress will depend, in part, upon innovative epidemiologic strategies employing accurate biochemical indicators for the intake of many nutrients.[49,217] Markers for nutrient intake will provide important corroborative data for information derived from questionnaires and interviews. An additional application will be in the measurement of compliance with dietary regimens during prospective intervention trials. For some nutritional factors such as total fat intake, we have no useful screening test that can be applied to a large population. For others, such as cholesterol consumption, the measurement of serum cholesterol provides only a crude indictor of intake and is modulated by many other genetic and dietary factors. Serum retinol as a measure of vitamin A status is buffered by tissue stores and reflects nutrient status only at the extremes of deficiency or excess.[318] In contrast, measuring selenium content of hair or toenail clippings provides an integrated measure of selenium intake over an extended period of time and can be utilized in epidemiologic studies.[198] Since the presence of a disease may alter dietary intake and the metabolism of specific nutrients, the biochemical measurements of nutrient intake will be less useful in retrospective and case-control studies. They will be most informative in prospective and cohort studies, geographic correlational investigations, and studies of migrant populations.

Correlation and Ecologic Studies

International studies have observed large variations in the incidence of many cancers between nations and geographic areas. The age-adjusted rates for specific cancers have been found to be strongly associated with the estimated *per capita* intakes of certain foods or nutrients. For example, Armstrong and Doll reported a correlation of 0.89 between the estimated average fat intakes and breast cancer mortality rates in nations around the world.[10] Researchers must be particularly careful not to draw premature or inappropriate conclusions based upon correlations between cancer rates and single nutrients. Nations showing large variations in cancer incidence often exhibit dietary patterns so dramatically different that conclusions concerning the contribution of individual dietary components or nutrients are impossible. For example, the Chinese exhibit an overall age-adjusted breast cancer mortality that is approximately 10% of that found in the United States and consume a diet which is lower in total fat, animal protein, refined carbohydrates, vitamin A, and calcium but higher in carotenoids, starches, and fiber (Table VI-2-1).[128] In addition to the differences in nutrient content, human diets also exhibit significant differences in food processing and preparation associated with the shift from an agrarian to an industrial society. Although the contribution of a single dietary component, such as dietary fat, cannot be precisely defined by these studies, one can derive information concerning the potential impact of the overall dietary background. Despite the inherent difficulties in interpretation, the ecologic studies will continue to provide a very important resource for the generation of nutrition and cancer hypotheses. Improvements in the epidemiologic and biochemical methodology for the measurement of nutrient exposure will allow future researchers to maximize the value of data obtained by these studies.

Case-Control Studies

Most case-control studies in the area of nutrition and cancer have been disappointing. The inaccuracies in quantifying previous nutrient intake over the long period of tumor development prior to diagnosis and the changes in diet associated with the disease itself, are among the many limitations of these studies.[334] In addition, national or geographic areas may be very homogeneous relative to the intake of certain nutrients and differences between cancer cases and matched controls may not be demonstrable. For example, within a population of American women nurses, the mean proportions of total calories derived from fat for the lowest and highest quintiles are 32 and 44%, respectively, based upon data derived from a food frequency questionnaire.[319] The mean fat intake for the lowest quintile exceeds the current popu-

Table VI-2-1. Estimated Average Intake of Several Dietary and Nutritional Factors in The Peoples Republic of China and United States

Dietary Intake	China	United States
Plant protein (% of total)	89	30
Starch (g/day)	371	120
Fat (% of calories)	14	39
Vitamin A (retinol equivalents/day)	28	990
Total carotinoids (retinol equivalents/day)	836	429
Vitamin C (mg/day)	140	73
Total fiber (gms/day)	33	11

From Junshi et al.[128]

lation target recommendation of 30% of calories for dietary fat.[4,5,204–207] Few Americans consume diets similar to populations exhibiting low-risk of colon, breast, or prostate cancer, such as the Chinese, where fat intake averages 14.5% of calories.[128] It would be unlikely that case control studies using current assessment methods would consistently detect an effect of fat on cancer risk within the American population. Case-control studies may prove to be most useful in migrant populations moving to areas exhibiting dramatic differences in dietary content. For example, migrants from countries exhibiting a low-risk of colon cancer, such as China, moving to high-risk areas such as the United States.[317] Cases and controls can then be evaluated according to the degree of adaptation to the high-risk American diet.

Prospective and Cohort Studies

The prospective approach defines a study population and monitors the incidence of disease over time as well as exposure to potential risk factors. A well known example of a cohort study is the Nurses' Health study, composed of approximately 100,000 American women nurses responding to an initial food-frequency questionnaire designed to evaluate various dietary and life-style factors in 1976.[49] A six-year follow-up identified 150 cases of colon cancer, and risk could then be correlated with estimates of nutrient intake or specific foods based upon the previously obtained data.[322] These studies avoid some of the inaccuracies of estimating dietary intake retrospectively and the recall bias typically found in case-control studies since a description of dietary exposures can be obtained prior to the development of the disease. Unfortunately, the number of prospective studies is limited by the high costs associated with the large numbers of subjects and the long follow-up periods required for the evaluation of diseases such as cancer. An additional consideration for some cancers, such as breast cancer, is that nutrients acting during childhood and adolescence may be crucial and a prospective study initiated in middle-aged women may not accurately identify critical dietary risk factors.

Prospective studies are especially useful when evaluating biochemical markers for nutrient intake utilizing samples of blood, urine, feces, or tissue, that may ultimately be correlated with cancer risk. One approach, referred to as a nested case-control study, requires that biological specimens have been collected from all members of the cohort. Since it may not be cost effective to measure nutrient markers in samples from all individuals, the experiment can be limited to those developing a specific cancer and matched controls from the cohort. For example, several studies utilized this technique to examine the relationship between serum beta-carotene and lung cancer risk.[187,214] Prospectively collected sera from those developing lung cancer were analyzed and compared to controls matched by age, sex, time of serum collection, and smoking history. In each study, serum beta-carotene was observed to be lower among individuals subsequently developing lung cancer compared to controls.

Randomized Trials and Intervention Studies

Oncologists routinely utilize the randomized trial to assess the utility of therapeutic interventions in the treatment of cancer or the prevention of relapse. Despite the scientific advantages, this method is difficult to implement for the evaluation of many nutrition and cancer hypotheses. Experiments in otherwise healthy individuals can only be justified when considerable observational data has been collected and supported by studies from the laboratory. It is critical that the potential benefits be well defined and that adverse outcomes be unlikely. For some nutritional variables, such as a low fat diet, it may be difficult to insure that a large population would adhere to a strict diet over a long period of time. The biochemical methodology to assess compliance with a low-fat diet does not currently exist. In addition, the intake of fat in the control group may change over time based upon societal adaptation to current recommendations. Randomized trials will be most useful in the testing of potential cancer inhibitors, such as certain vitamins, minerals, and other chemopreventive agents that can be incorporated into pills or capsules and provided in a double-bind fashion over a period of years. Several randomized trials evaluating nutrition and cancer hypotheses are underway in the area of chemoprevention.[85,86] For example, the Physicians Health Study has randomized 22,000 American male physicians to either 30 mg beta-carotene or placebo treatment on alternate days.[96] This population will be followed for a variety of end points including cancer incidence.

Even when scientifically and ethically feasible, the large costs of randomized trials limit their implementation. Since the time interval between changing a dietary factor and a change in cancer incidence may be many years or decades, trials must be of long duration to eliminate the possibility that a negative result is not secondary to an insufficient period of follow-up. For this reason, many studies focus upon nutrients which have been shown to modulate later events in carcinogenesis rather than initiation. It is critical that surrogate markers associated with cancer risk be identified that can also be utilized in short term studies to investigate nutritional hypotheses. For example, studies have demonstrated the ability of supplemental wheat bran to decrease colon mucosal cell proliferative rates[2] and reduce polyp formation[58] in patients at high risk for colon cancer. Efforts to define intermediate markers for common cancers, which can be utilized in prospective studies is of major importance to the nutrition and cancer field.

Laboratory Animal Models

The effects of nutrients, and their interactions, on carcinogenesis can be rigorously tested in animal models. Although the information derived from animal models must be extrapolated to humans with caution, it does provide important evidence for the biologic plausibility of relationships suggested by epidemiologic studies. The nutrient requirements of most laboratory animals have been precisely defined and purified ingredients can be utilized to formulate diets for cancer studies.[6,7,203,211] Unfortunately, numerous published studies have failed to provide useful information due to a failure to appreciate two critical observations derived from decades of experimentation.[246] The first is the strong positive correlation between energy intake and the incidence or growth of tumors in virtually every animal model system.[1,8,71,204,206,246,255,287] The second issue is the frequent observation that animals fed nutritionally complete diets

composed of unrefined foods, usually referred to as chow, often exhibit a reduction in tumorigenesis compared to those fed a complete diet derived from purified nutrients.[204,246,314]

Since energy intake has a major influence upon tumorigenesis (Figure VI-2-1), the recording of food consumption and body weight is an essential aspect of all rodent studies.[286] Unfortunately, the failure to document the effects of the dietary treatments upon feed (energy) intake frequently limits the interpretation of published experiments. Nutritional deficiencies, imbalances, or excesses can significantly alter energy intake. For example, vitamin A deficiency, or the supplementation of the diet with selenium at high concentrations, can inhibit carcinogenesis through an indirect effect upon energy intake. Readers of nutrition and carcinogenesis literature must carefully evaluate dietary treatments, identify the variables present, and determine if energy intake has confounded the interpretation of the data. In some cases, pair-feeding and other methods of compensating for treatment induced differences in energy intake can be utilized.

Another problem, frequently found in the literature is the inappropriate use of cereal-based commercial laboratory chows. Some investigators use these products as the control or "normal" diet for comparison against synthetic diets with a different concentration of a specific nutrient. Although commercial laboratory chows provide excellent nutrition, they vary over time and between companies in the sources of natural ingredients. Chow diets are composed of varying concentrations of cereals, vegetables, legumes, fish meal, and milk products which are a function of local market availability and cost. Although the nutrient content of these diets satisfy the established minimum requirements for mice and rats, the concentrations of individual nutrients may vary substantially. For example, the vitamin A and beta-carotene content of different batches of the NIH-07 chow diet varied over 6- and 20-fold respectively.[237] In addition, detectable levels

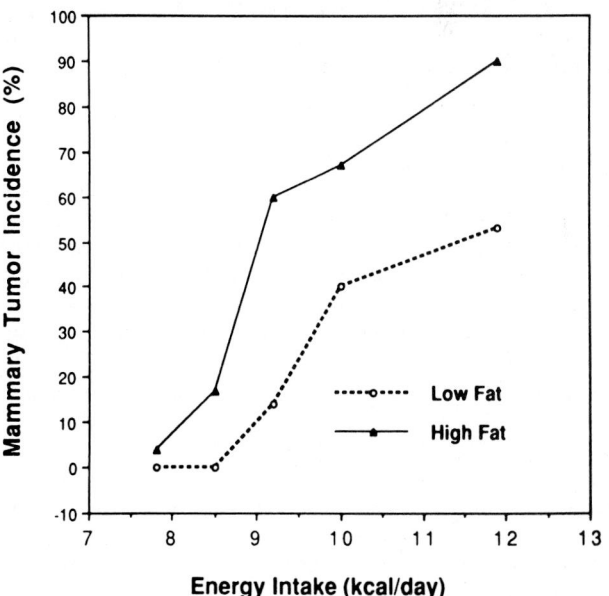

Figure VI-2-1. The effects of low- and high-fat diets at different levels of caloric intake on spontaneous mammary tumorigenesis in C3H female mice.[286]

of aflatoxins, nitrosamines, antioxidants, pesticides, herbicides and heavy metals are observed.[237] Many undefined substances found in grains and vegetables are thought to have anti-carcinogenic activity and contribute to the tumor preventive properties associated with chow diets. In general, natural ingredient diets are inconsistent and therefore inadequate for use in experiments designed to quantify the subtle effects of specific nutrients on carcinogenesis. Diets need to be defined in publications and confounding variables eliminated whenever possible.

Nutrition and the Etiology of Common Cancers

It is unlikely that any nutrient will influence all cancers uniformly. In reviewing the relationships between nutrition and cancer it is convenient to examine the data for each tissue or organ separately. However, this approach will ultimately prove to be inadequate. A key feature of human cancer is heterogeneity in biological characteristics and response to treatment. It is clear that cancer of the breast, colon, or any tissue represents a family of diseases. As laboratory methodology improves, we will be able to subclassify cancers according to molecular, biochemical, and biologic characteristics. The more precise classification of human cancers, coupled with future improvements in nutritional assessment, will allow a more accurate quantification of the relationship between nutrients and specific neoplasms. Parallels can be drawn from our experience in cancer therapy. Alpha-interferon has been found to be an excellent therapy for a very rare type of leukemia, hairy cell leukemia. However, if all leukemias are grouped together and treated with alpha interferon, the overall effectiveness of the drug would be nonsignificant. In the same manner we may find that a particular nutrient may prove to inhibit the growth of cancers having specific oncogene mutations, or to promote tumors exhibiting other mutations. In the following section, the major hypotheses are reviewed concerning the role of nutrients in the pathogenesis of the human cancers most frequently linked to diet and nutrition.

Lung

In affluent nations, lung cancer is the leading cause of cancer related death.[25] Cigarette smoking accounts for the vast majority of cases.[62] Certain occupational exposures, such as asbestos or irradiation, may act synergistically with cigarette smoking to increase risk.[62] Potential interactions between smoking and nutritional status have not been adequately assessed. An accumulating body of evidence suggests a role for vitamin A, carotenoids, or other undefined constituents in fruits and vegetables in modulating risk.[16,48,204,206] A series of studies from Norway,[22,143] Japan,[106] England,[87] and the United States[90] have reported inverse associations between estimated intakes of vitamin A and lung cancer risk. Bjelke's prospective study involved over 8,000 Norwegian men responding to a mailed food frequency questionnaire designed to assess dietary vitamin A intake.[32] The relative risk for lung cancer was increased by 2.5 for smokers in the low vitamin A group compared to those in the high intake group. It is difficult to conclude from these studies alone if the critical component is vitamin A, beta-carotene, or other undefined dietary components derived from foods which are coincidentally rich in vitamin A.[32,102,106,169,257,270,336] Prospective studies have compared serum beta-carotene levels in individuals subsequently developing lung cancer to matched controls and found them to be inversely correlated with risk.[187,214] Similar inverse correlations with serum vitamin A have not been consistently observed.[72,187,222,256,308,309] This is not surprising since serum levels are a poor reflection of vitamin A status except at the extremes of intake. Studies in rodent models have occasionally observed protective effects of vitamin A or analogues against respiratory tract carcinogenesis induced by a variety of polycyclic aromatic hydrocarbons, which are found in cigarette smoke, or nitrosamines.[8] Overall, the evidence suggests that vitamin A and carotenoids should be further studied relative to the risk of the lung cancer in smokers. However, most of the plant foods rich in vitamin A and carotenoids may contain other dietary constituents, not yet characterized, which may also modulate cancer risk.

A number of other nutrients, such as vitamin C,[32,102,143] total fat,[32,331] total protein,[310] and cholesterol[101] have been investigated relative to modulating risk of lung cancer in human or rodent studies.[204,206,246] However, their roles remain obscure. Overall, elimination of cigarette smoking and occupational risk factors will have the greatest impact upon decreasing the incidence of lung cancer. Among high-risk individuals, the frequent consumption of green and yellow vegetables, leading to the higher intake of vitamin A, carotenoids and other associated constituents, may provide some degree of protection against lung cancer.

Oral Cavity, Larynx, and Oropharynx

Cancers of the oral cavity and the larynx, like lung cancer, are strongly related to the use of tobacco prod-

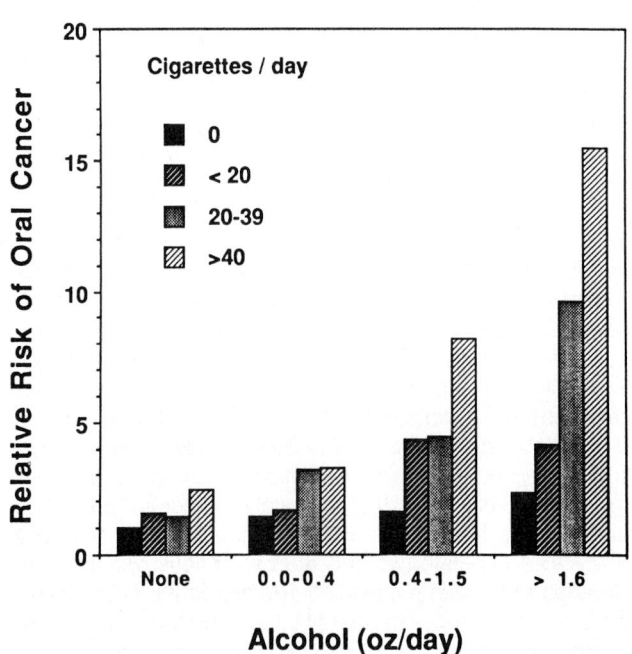

Figure VI-2-2. The interactions between alcohol intake and cigarette smoking on the relative risk of oral cancer.[282]

ucts.[11,173,179,247,296] Case-control studies, completed over several decades, have also documented associations between alcohol and cancers of these tissues.[78,131,134,178,269,321,328] A dose-response relationship of alcohol and oral cancer, independent of tobacco usage has been observed in a number of studies (Figure VI-2-2).[29,68,97,216,252,327] Additional evidence is derived from studies of populations, such as alcoholics that exhibit increased risk and Seventh-Day Adventists and Mormons in the United States that abstain from alcohol and have lower risk.[61,162] It is of interest that the feeding of pure alcohol as part of a nutritionally sound diet does not produce oral cancers in experimental animals.[247] The extent that this represents biochemical differences between man and rodents, the lack of a direct carcinogenic effect of ethanol, the presence of carcinogens in alcoholic beverages consumed by man, the passive inhalation of ambient tobacco smoke in the places where ethanol is consumed, or the importance of other interacting carcinogens and nutritional deficits needs to be further evaluated.

Vitamin A deficiency leads to squamous metaplasia which is corrected by treatment with vitamin A and a number of related retinoids. The metaplasia associated with vitamin A deficiency is similar histologically to the premalignant changes observed following exposure of the oral mucosa to chemical carcinogens. Several animal studies have suggested that vitamin A, carotenoids, or synthetic retinoids may retard carcinogenesis of the oral cavity. Case-control studies have occasionally reported increased risk associated with lower estimated vitamin A intake.[177] A number of chemoprevention trials have been undertaken utilizing leukoplakia, a premalignant condition of the oral mucosa, as the end-point. In a randomized trial, Stich and colleagues treated patients having leukoplakia with beta-carotene, beta-carotene plus vitamin A, or placebo for six months.[282] Upon re-evaluation, the complete remission rates were 15%, 28%, and 3%, respectively. A subsequent study reported a 57% complete remission rate in a group treated with vitamin A at 200,000 IU/week compared to only 3% in the placebo group.[282] A number of non-randomized studies using synthetic retinoids have also suggested dramatic reversals in oral leukoplakia. Subsequent randomized studies using 13-cis-retinoic acid also showed significantly lower relapse rates in the treated groups.[111]

The beneficial effects of vitamin A and synthetic retinoids in preventing premalignant changes of the oral mucosa, led to a trial designed to determine its effectiveness in preventing second primary tumors of the areodigestive tract.[112] Second cancers occur at a rate of 3–4% per year in patients that have received potentially curative treatment of their initial early stage cancer. Patients rendered disease-free after primary treatment of their head and neck cancer were randomized to placebo or 13-cis-retinoic acid. There were no significant differences in the local, regional, or distant recurrences of the primary cancers (Table VI-2-2). However, the treated group had significantly fewer second primary tumors compared to placebo controls, at 4 vs. 24% respectively after 32 months (see XXVII-1).[112] This study suggests that vitamin A or retinoids influence early stages in carcinogenesis and that these compounds probably have little utility for the treatment of established cancers of the oral pharynx. These clin-

Table VI-2-2. The Effects of 13-Cis Retinoic Acid on the Incidence of Primary-Treatment Failure and the Incidence of Second Primary Tumors in Squamous-Cell Carcinoma of the Head and Neck

Type of Failure	13-cis retinoic acid (N=49)	Placebo (N=51)	P value
Disease			
progression	31%	33%	0.772
Local	8%	14%	0.373
Regional	16%	14%	0.719
Distant	14%	10%	0.490
Second primary			
tumor	4%	24%	0.005

Retinoid treatment had no effect upon the progression of the primary tumor but significantly reduced the incidence of second primary cancers (see XXVII-1)
From Hong et al.[112]

ical studies support the hypothesis that increased risk may be associated with infrequent consumption of fruits and vegetables, the main source of dietary vitamin A and its precursors.[177,204,206]

Esophagus

Cancer of the esophagus varies several hundred-fold between countries and between regions within nations.[25] The incidence is particularly high in an area extending from the southern border of the Caspian Sea in Iran across central Asia to China. Within nations, such as China or Iran, there are frequently large differences in risk between different locations and population groups.[172] For example, age-adjusted annual mortality in the Caspian region of Iran is 165 and 195 per 100,000 for males and females, respectively, but is 10- and 20-fold lower in other areas of the country.[172] The incidence of esophageal cancer in the United States is relatively low at less than 7 per 100,000.[25]

In most affluent nations, correlational analyses and case-control studies indicate that the major risk factors are ethanol and cigarette smoking.[204,206,247] The risk increases in proportion to the amount of alcohol consumed.[178,294,295,296,327] A number of studies have shown a dose-response relationship after controlling for cigarette smoking although the two factors may show a significant additive effect.[132,178,295] In the United States, mortality from esophageal cancer in the white population has decreased gradually over recent decades whereas the mortality has doubled for black men in the last 25 years.[266,267] It has been postulated that the three-fold greater risk in African Americans compared to whites may be due to differences in alcohol intake, tobacco smoking, and undefined dietary or nutritional factors.[227,267,335] Increasing consumption of alcohol is generally associated with the marginal intake of many nutrients which is thought to predispose individuals to greater risk.[335] A case-control study in the U.S. observed an inverse relationship between esophageal cancer and the consumption of fresh fruits and vegetables and the estimated intake of vitamins A and C.[83,191]

Alcohol consumption does not explain the high-risk for esophageal cancer in certain parts of Asia.[204] Populations in these areas frequently consume diets which are marginal or deficient in a number of nutrients.[52,113,302,332] Low intakes of fresh fruits, vegetables, and animal products are noted and the estimated intakes of vitamin A, vitamin C, riboflavin, zinc, and several trace elements, such as molybdenum, are frequently cited as being low.[50–52,113,332] It has been postulated that dietary deficiencies may alter susceptibility to carcinogens indigenous to these populations. Although not firmly established, a role for N-nitroso compounds in pickled foods and mycotoxins from moldy grains, has been postulated.[52,113,176,332] In some areas, associations have been found with the intake of foods which are at high temperatures when consumed.[52,59,332]

Several nutrient hypotheses have been evaluated in animal models using nitrosamine-induced esophageal cancer.[8] Overall, vitamin A and several synthetic analogues have shown little effect upon risk in these models.[209,304] Some, but not all, studies with supplemental selenium,[208,304] or molybdenum[161,304] have reduced tumorigenesis. A role for zinc has been proposed based upon the prevalence of zinc deficiency in many of the high risk areas of the world.[200,204,206] Some animal studies have observed increased risk with zinc deficiency and a reduction in carcinogenesis with supplementation, although a number of experiments found no significant effect.[13,69,70,74,301,303,304]

In summary, cigarette smoking and alcohol consumption are the most important etiologic factors in affluent nations. The possibility that marginal intakes of one or more nutrients, secondary to the infrequent consumption of fruits and vegetables, may contribute to risk in affluent populations has been suggested, but not firmly established. In some areas of the world, such as the high-risk area between Iran and China, micronutrient deficiencies coupled with the exposure to carcinogenic substances associated with intake of salt-pickled vegetables or mouldy foods may be contributing factors.

Stomach

The incidence of gastric carcinoma varies widely among countries and is highest in parts of Asia, such as Japan, and South America (Figure VI-2-3).[25] In addition, subpopulations within a nation can show risks several fold greater than other groups.[55] A dramatic decrease in the incidence of stomach cancer in many affluent nations, especially the U.S., has been observed over the last 50 years. In the U.S., the current rates are among the lowest in the world, whereas in 1930, gastric cancer was the most frequently diagnosed cancer in Americans.[118] Studies of Japanese migrants to Hawaii or North America show that risk is significantly reduced in the second- and third-generation after migration.[90,91,135] This may indicate that critical risk factors are active early in life or that life-style factors, such as diet and nutrition, change gradually over succeeding generations.

Although there is general agreement that diet plays a role in gastric carcinogenesis, the mechanisms which underlay the geographic and temporal incidence patterns have not been firmly established.[55,204,206] Efforts to define the causes of stomach cancer have proceeded in several directions: 1) the identification of natural carcinogens or precursors found in the food; 2) the production of carcinogens during food processing or cooking; 3) the synthesis of carcinogens from dietary precursors in the stomach; 4) the identification of

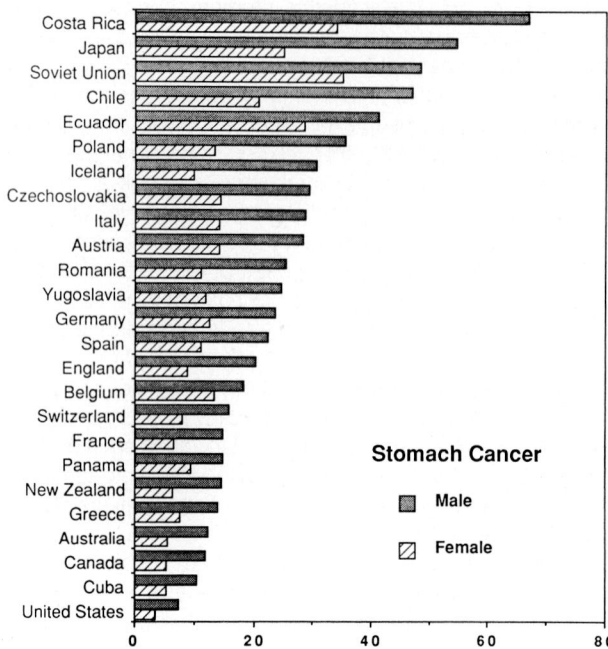

Figure VI-2-3. Age-adjusted death rates per 100,000 population from gastric cancer in selected countries.[25]

dietary protective factors which may be consumed in inadequate quantities by high risk groups; 5) the identification of nutrients which increase risk for initiation by carcinogens or act directly as promoters; and 6) the role of infectious agents.

The polycyclic aromatic hydrocarbons are a heterogeneous class of lipophilic compounds, many of which are carcinogenic and mutagenic. When administered orally, several of these compounds have been reported to produce forestomach tumors in mice and hamsters.[39,242] These compounds are produced during the heating of foods to high temperatures or incorporated into foods cooked over a flame or smoked. They are found in high quantities in grilled, charbroiled, and smoke-cured meats.[114,149,151] For example, the quantity of polycyclic aromatic hydrocarbons in a large, well done charcoal broiled steak is equivalent to that found in the smoke of 600 cigarettes.[147] Hot air drying and roasting of grains and coffee also produces polycyclic aromatic hydrocarbons.[73] Subpopulations at high risk for gastric cancer in Iceland, Hungary, and Latvia were found to have greater exposure to polycyclic aromatic hydrocarbons in smoked meats.[38,66,280,307] Overall, dietary exposure to polycyclic aromatic hydrocarbons has not been fully evaluated in large populations differing in gastric cancer risk.[204]

It has been postulated that nitrosamines found in food or produced in the stomach from precursors may play a role in gastric carcinogenesis.[55,196,204,265] Many nitrosamines are potent mutagens and stomach carcinogens in experimental animals. Several studies have suggested an association between increased levels of nitrate in the diet or drinking water and gastric cancer risk.[55,204] Nitrate itself is not carcinogenic, however. Dietary nitrate must first undergo reduction to nitrite which in turn nitrosates other compounds in the stomach contents producing nitrosamines.[218,258] Factors which modulate the conversion of dietary nitrate to nitrite are probably more important than the amount of nitrate in the diet.[55] One hypothesis suggests that the disruption of the gastric mucosa by surgery, dietary irritants, or nutritional deficits produces focal areas of gastritis or atrophy leading to colonization by bacteria known to produce nitrate reductases.[93] These changes are thought to promote increased formation of nitrosamines and initiate the malignant cascade. For example, pernicious anemia is a well known metabolic disease of nutrient metabolism which leads to atrophic gastritis and increased risk of carcinoma.[254] A number of food items and drugs have been found to yield mutagens after nitrosation. For example, nitrosation of a substance in fish consumed in Japan yields a carcinogen for the stomach of rats.[316] A compound found in fava beans, consumed by high-risk populations in Colombia, also yields a potent mutagen after nitrosation.[224] Bile acids can be nitrosated and may contribute to carcinoma at the anastomotic site following partial gastrectomy.[144,272] Laboratory studies suggest that vitamins C or E and other antioxidants may protect against the formation of nitrosamines.[129,158]

Continuing efforts are directed toward the identification of dietary factors which may accentuate the endogenous production of mutagens, alter mucosal cell susceptibility to transformation, or act as promoters. Epidemiologic studies have consistently identified increased risk associated with the intake of excessive salt, used in many cultures as a preservative of dried meats and pickled vegetables.[54,91,92,104,126,201,243,297] Salt cured foods induce gastric irritation in man and rodents.[167,259,260] Although salt alone will not induce tumors in experimental models, increased intake potentiates tumorigenesis induced by other agents.[264,283]

The populations consuming abundant quantities of fresh fruits and vegetables generally have a low risk of stomach cancer.[55,77,89,91,99,103,221,243] Efforts to identify components of these foods which have protective properties are underway. Several possibilities have been proposed, including vitamin A, carotenoids, tocopherols, and vitamin C.[55,129,158] Other studies have suggested a protective effect of dairy products, better refrigeration and sanitation, and the increased use of antioxidants by the food industry.[55,104]

Infection of the gastric mucosa with *Helicobacter pylori* (previously known as *Campylobacter pylori*) has been strongly associated with chronic atrophic gastritis and gastric carcinoma.[214,220] However, the vast majority of infected individuals do not develop gastric cancer. The dietary and environmental factors, which interact with *Helicobacter pylori* infection to modulate risk have not been defined.

Although gastric cancer has been associated with several dietary variables, it is not possible at this time to quantitate the contribution of these components or their mechanisms of action. In general the diet of high risk populations is low in animal products, high in complex carbohydrates derived from grains, high in salt-preserved and pickled foods, and low in fresh fruits and leafy green vegetables.[55,204,206] In some populations additional risk may be derived from diets high in smoked foods or nitrates.

Liver

Primary hepatocellular carcinoma is very rare in the United States and Northern Europe.[25] In contrast, it is one of the most frequent types of cancer in sub-Saharan Africa, China, and southeast Asia.[25] Hepatitis B infection appears to be the major etiologic factor in many high-risk areas where the carrier state imparts a relative risk of approximately 200-fold.[14] Contamination of foods with carcinogenic fungal products, such as certain aflatoxins, may also contribute to risk in some populations.[9,148,204,206,323] Aflatoxins are found in geographic areas where food processing and storage are not optimal. Some aflatoxins induce hepatocellular carcinoma in rodent models at concentrations found in the diet of high-risk populations.[324] The ability to precisely quantify the contribution of aflatoxins to hepatocellular carcinoma incidence in many high-risk developing nations is limited by the difficulties of accurately assessing aflatoxin intake and the actual incidence of cancer in these populations. In addition, groups with high aflatoxin exposure often have high rates of hepatitis B infection, parasitic infections, and nutritional deficiencies which may interact to determine risk.

In low-risk nations, it has been proposed that alcohol intake may be an important dietary factor in the pathogenesis of liver cancer.[10,12,236,247,294] The data are inconsistent,[100,164,165,291] however, and other cofactors may act in an additive or synergistic fashion.[26,333] It has been hypothesized that liver cancer occurs primarily in those whose cumulative experience with ethanol, viral hepatitis, and toxin exposure leads to cirrhosis. The cellular and molecular events associated with cirrhosis and regenerative nodules which may participate in the initiation and progression to cancer are under investigation. Additional evidence suggests that vinyl chloride, oral contraceptives and androgenic-anabolic steroids may also participate in liver carcinogenesis in susceptible individuals.

Animal studies have shown that a number of dietary factors modulate experimental liver carcinogenesis utilizing various carcinogens including aflatoxin. Diets high in protein, energy or lipid or deficient in lipotropes generally enhance hepatocarcinogenesis.[8,204,206,246] The role of these and other nutrients in modulating hepatocellular carcinoma in humans has not been defined.

Pancreas

The important roles for nutrients in regulating normal pancreatic growth and function suggests that diet and nutrition may contribute to the pathogenesis of pancreatic cancer.[156] The exocrine pancreas, which is the origin for 90% of the pancreatic cancers, readily alters the pattern of digestive enzyme secretion in response to the nutrient content of the diet.[279] Dietary restriction produces acinar cell atrophy, reduces DNA synthesis,[210] and inhibits experimental pancreatic carcinogenesis.[244] Pancreatic cell replication and differentiation are modulated by a number of gastrointestinal hormones, such as cholecystokinin and gastrin, and many dietary factors are potent mediators of gastrointestinal hormone secretion.[156] Non-nutritive components, such as trypsin inhibitors, frequently found in certain vegetables and legumes, have dramatic stimulatory effects on pancreatic cell DNA synthesis, induce hyperplasia and hypertrophy, and enhance pancreatic carcinogenesis in laboratory studies.[156]

The strong evidence supporting a role for dietary and nutritional factors in modulating pancreatic cell replication and differentiation suggests that diet may be important in pancreatic carcinogenesis.

The descriptive epidemiology of pancreatic cancer is complicated by the fact that estimates of incidence are dependent upon conventions of medical care which vary in different geographic areas and socioeconomic conditions.[168] The symptoms of pancreatic cancer are often vague, and significant cost and risk is associated with obtaining tissue for histologic diagnosis in many nations. Errors in clinical impressions and the difficulty of accurately reporting clinical diagnoses from medical records by cancer registries suggests that extreme caution should be used in comparing rates from populations having different standards of medical care or living in different times and places. Meaningful clues from epidemiologic studies concerning diet and nutrition in the pathogenesis of pancreatic cancer are likely to be obscured by inconsistencies in diagnosis among different geographic and socioeconomic population groups. Overall, reports have suggested a higher incidence in affluent populations of North America and Northern Europe.[25] Descriptive studies have suggested associations between risk for pancreatic cancer and a number of components characteristic of the affluent diet, such as meat, fat, protein, eggs, milk and alcohol.[10,156,168,170,204,206,330]

Several animal models for pancreatic cancer have been characterized and utilized to examine the roles of dietary and nutritional components in modulating carcinogenesis under precisely controlled conditions.[8,152,229] Diet and energy restriction dramatically reduces the number of pancreatic cancers in rodent models[8,244] consistent with many studies showing a strong inhibitory effect of diet or energy restriction on carcinogenesis in other tissues.[8,255] High fat diets, in the range of those consumed in affluent nations, enhance azaserine- and N-nitrosobis(2-oxopropyl)amine-induced pancreatic carcinogenesis.[8,18,19,21,245] The effects of protein quantity and quality on pancreatic carcinogenesis have not yet been clearly defined. Protein or amino acid deficiency and lower protein quality leads to pancreatic atrophy which is reversible upon improvement of the diet.[274,275,315] Roebuck and colleagues observed no effect of increasing protein on azaserine-induced cancer in rats,[244] whereas others[19,230,232] have reported reduced N-nitrosobis(2-oxopropyl)amine-induced pancreatic carcinoma incidence in hamsters with a severe protein deficiency. A potential interaction between fat and protein has been reported in the hamster model.[19] Those fed diets high in both fat and protein develop more pancreatic neoplasms than those fed diets low in both components.

Among the vitamins, studies suggest that vitamin A and synthetic retinoids may modulate experimental pancreatic carcinogenesis.[8,156] Several of the retinoids have been found to inhibit azaserine-induced pancreatic cancer in rats,[153–155] but results using the hamster model have been less conclusive.[17,20,154,155] Other studies have observed stimulatory effects of vitamin A and retinoids.[8] The effects of retinoid supplementation appear to depend upon the dose, the baseline vitamin A status, and a number of host factors. Additional efforts to define synthetic retinoids which can be utilized as chemopreventative or therapeutic agents should be encour-

aged, although findings based upon pharmacologic doses of compounds not naturally found in foods may have little relevance to the role of dietary vitamin A status and pancreatic cancer risk.

Laboratory studies suggest that the pancreas is sensitive to dietary selenium intake. Selenium-deficiency has been observed to produce pancreatic atrophy and fibrosis which is reversed with selenium supplementation.[156,215] However, supplemental selenium has not significantly altered experimental pancreatic carcinogenesis in several studies.[8]

Trypsin inhibitors found in many legumes and vegetables may contribute to the pathogenesis of pancreatic cancer.[156] The heat labile trypsin inhibitors are thought to be the factors responsible for pancreatic acinar hyperplasia and the spontaneous carcinomas observed in rats fed diets containing raw soy flour.[181,182,183] Diets containing trypsin inhibitors also enhance the progression of pancreatic carcinomas induced by carcinogens, such as azaserine.[152,182,197] The ability of trypsin inhibitors to enhance pancreatic carcinogenesis is probably closely related to an increased production of trophic hormones and growth factors which contribute to acinar cell hyperplasia. However, it is unlikely that the average cooked human diet characteristic of high-risk nations contains significant concentrations of active trypsin inhibitors. Additional information concerning the risk associated with various amounts and durations of exposure to the wide variety of different trypsin inhibitors is necessary.

A role for alcohol intake remains speculative.[156] Ethanol does produce toxic injury to pancreatic cells and the recurrent injury and regeneration may enhance risk in a fashion similar to partial pancreatectomy[61] and other chemical injuries.[184] Laboratory[232,300] and epidemiologic studies[156,168,170] remain inconclusive, however.

In summary, laboratory studies clearly indicate that pancreatic carcinogenesis is sensitive to a number of dietary and nutritional components. In some cases, the experimental data and very limited epidemiologic data are in agreement. However, additional studies designed to define more clearly the associations identified and the mechanisms involved must be completed in order to identify dietary changes which will significantly decrease the risk of this devastating cancer.

Colon and Rectum

Colorectal cancer is a major public health problem in affluent westernized cultures.[25] In the U.S. and western Europe, up to 5% of the population may develop cancer of the large bowel by the age of 75.[312] The international variation in large bowel cancer is large (Figure VI-2-4). Although diagnostic differences may account for some of the international variation, it is unlikely to account for the greater than 10-fold variations observed between many nations.[25] The lower rates in Japan suggest that cultural and lifestyle factors rather than industrialization are the critical factors.[25] The geographic incidence patterns for colon and rectal cancer generally vary in concert suggesting that some similarity in etiology exists.[124,312] Studies in migrant populations, such as Chinese migrants to the United States,[317] clearly indicate that international variations are primarily due to environmental influences rather than genetic background.[90,124,185] Japanese migrants to the U.S. also show a definite shift towards the

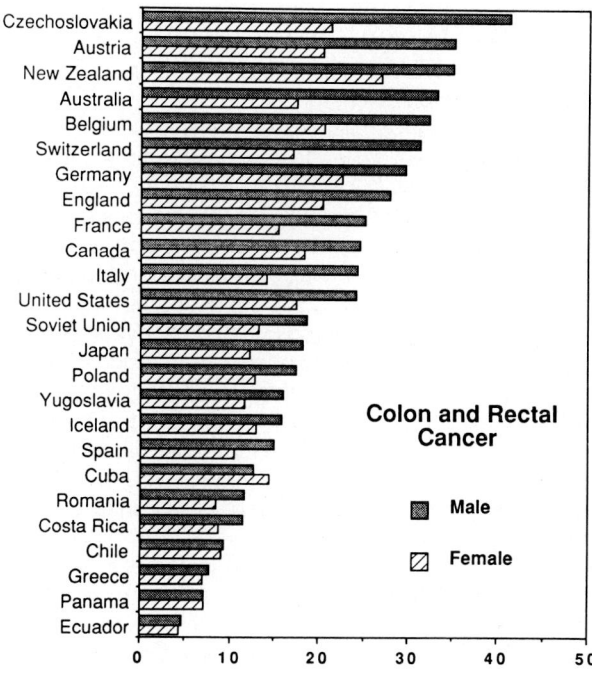

Figure VI-2-4. Age-adjusted death rates per 100,000 population from colon cancer in selected countries.[25]

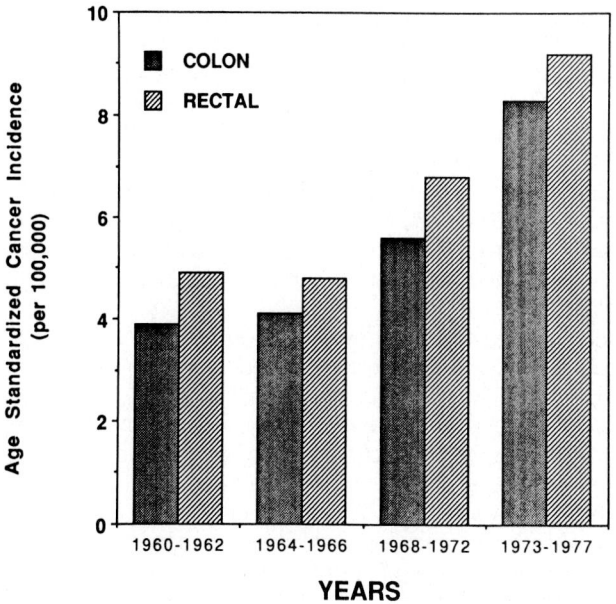

Figure VI-2-5. Age-standardized colon and rectal cancer incidence per 100,000 men in Japan from 1960 through 1977.[125]

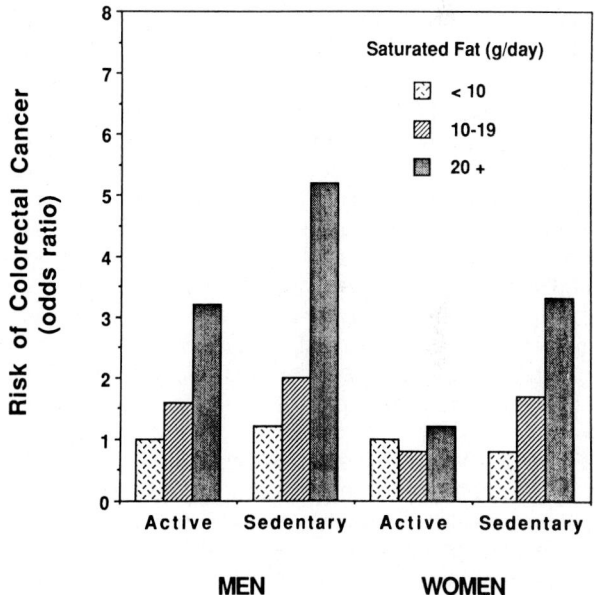

Figure VI-2-6. The risk of colorectal cancer in Chinese migrants to the United States according to dietary fat intake and level of physical activity.[317]

colorectal cancer rates of the adopted country within the first generation.[90] Examination of time trends in colorectal cancer incidence also suggests major contributions for environmental and lifestyle factors.[124] Increases in large bowel cancer have been particularly striking within Japan in recent decades (Figure VI-2-5).[124,142,321] The desire to understand these variations in incidence and to institute preventive measures has prompted efforts to identify specific substances which are initiators or promoters of colon cancer. The role of diet and nutrition in the production of initiators and promoters or in modulating the sensitivity of the host to these agents has led to the generation of a number of hypotheses.

Diets most frequently associated with increased colorectal cancer risk have several characteristics: high in total fat, high in total protein, frequent meat intake, a high proportion of saturated fats, low in fruits and vegetables, and low in fiber.[124,204,206,239] In addition, excess caloric intake and obesity have been implicated in some but not all studies.[146,317] The relative contribution of each variable alone and the potential interactions among them are currently under investigation in human and laboratory studies.

Fat. Among the nutritional variables, dietary fat has been most extensively studied. Food consumption data from geographically defined populations has shown striking correlations between estimated fat intake, especially saturated fat, and colorectal cancer incidence[10,34,249] which has been supported by many,[82,122,140,141,166,226,276,317] but not all,[124,180,246,281,299] case-control investigations. A recent population based case-control study suggests that dietary fat may account for 60% of colorectal cancer risk among Chi-

nese migrants to the United States (Figure VI-2-6).[317] A recent prospective study in a cohort of 88,000 American nurses supports a role for animal fat in colon cancer.[322] An increased relative risk of 1.89 (95% confidence interval, 1.13 to 3.15) was observed for the highest quintile (over 65 g/day) compared with the lowest quintile (less than 39 g/day) of animal fat intake.

The majority of studies in carcinogen-induced rodent models for colon cancer have observed increased tumor incidence and multiplicity in rats fed diets containing fat concentrations similar to those observed in the high-risk human diet.[8,138,239] A promotional effect has been observed for both saturated and unsaturated fats.[8] However, several well controlled rodent studies have failed to document increased tumor incidence with greater dietary fat suggesting that the effect of fat may not be a simple direct relationship and may depend upon other variables which have yet to be clearly defined such as timing of carcinogen exposure relative to dietary intervention, type of carcinogen and its mechanism of action, and the consumption of other interacting nutrients.[212]

Potential mechanisms whereby fat may enhance colon cancer have been postulated, based upon both human and rodent studies. A popular hypothesis suggests that dietary fat increases the concentration of bile acids in the colon which alters the metabolic activity of the gut microflora in a manner that favors the production of bile acid metabolites. These metabolites may be weak carcinogens, increase susceptibility of the mucosa to other carcinogens, or act directly as promoters.[239] Low risk populations in Asia and Africa have lower concentrations of bile acids and their metabolites in the stool compared to high risk populations of North America.[239] Similar results have been observed in rats fed diets varying in fat content.[239] The intrarectal administration of bile acid metabolites has also been reported to increase carcinogen-induced colon cancer in some studies[239] but not in others.[45]

Protein. A role for dietary protein in colorectal cancer has been postulated.[204,206,290,306] The international variation in total protein intake is much less than for fat. However, the source of protein does vary significantly and is primarily derived from vegetable sources in low-risk populations and from meat and dairy products in those exhibiting high-risk.[204,206] Few rodent studies have investigated the role of protein in colon carcinogenesis. Increasing protein intake enhanced 1,2-dimethylhydrazine induced colon intestinal carcinogenesis in rats whereas no effect of protein source was observed.[41,290] It has been proposed that protein may modulate colon carcinogenesis via increasing colonic ammonia concentrations.[45]

Fiber. Burkitt and Trowell popularized the hypothesis that low dietary fiber intake may be a critical variable enhancing colon cancer risk.[30] Trowell provided a useful definition of fiber as components of plant cells that resist digestion by secretions of the human gastrointestinal tract.[293] However, the precise definition continues to be debated and refined among nutritional scientists.[204,206] In general, dietary fiber is a complex collection of substances, including cellulose, hemicelluloses, pectin, lignin, gums, some polysaccharides, and mucilages. It is possible to expand the definition to include indigestible substances which are not derived from plant sources, such as chitins from fungi and crustaceans, aminopolysaccharides from animals, or nonenzymatic browning products formed during food processing. The chemistry of dietary fiber is exceptionally complex and the standardization of analytical techniques is a dynamic and evolving field of nutritional science. The different fiber components have widely varying physical and chemical properties, such as water holding capacity or ion-exhange properties. At the present time our limited understanding of the physical and chemical characteristics has not allowed adequate insight into the biologic properties of high fiber foods, which makes it particularly difficult to understand their roles in diseases, such as colon cancer.[204,206]

Studies of several populations consuming diets similar in fat but differing in total fiber intake suggest a protective role for fiber.[123,174,238,292] Most international and intracountry studies have provided little insight.[10,15,150,163] This should not be surprising since there is a lack of complete analytical data concerning the content of fiber components in foods consumed by many populations. Superimposed upon the analytic difficulties, the epidemiologic methodology for estimating fiber intake exhibits tremendous imprecision. Several case-control studies have attempted to correlate colon cancer risk with total fiber intake, but have provided inconsistent results.[122,140,141,166,226,322] Case-control studies of dietary fiber are complicated by the small variation in fiber intake frequently observed within a population of colon cancer patients and matched controls.

The chemical complexity of fiber suggests that an estimate of total fiber intake may not be an adequate measure for epidemiologic studies attempting to determine its role in colon cancer, emphasizing the need for standardized analytic techniques in fiber chemistry. A number of case-control studies have not attempted to calculate fiber intake per se, but utilize the frequency of consumption of high-fiber foods as an indirect indicator. In general, these studies suggest a protective effect of fiber-rich diets and especially vegetable consumption.[23,57,79,171,175,195,292] Intervention trials with dietary fiber are now beginning to yield results relative to the colon cancer risk. A recent double-blind, placebo-controlled study showed that a daily supplement of 22.5 g of wheat bran significantly reduced the number of adenomatous polyps in the sigmoid colon and rectum of familial polyposis patients.[58] A subsequent single arm study reported a reduction in rectal mucosal cell DNA synthesis rates in patients with a history of resected colon or rectal cancer fed wheat bran fiber.[2] Future randomized studies will determine if supplements of wheat bran fiber prevent the development of colon cancer in a high-risk population. Studies to determine the validity of colon cell proliferative rates as a marker of carcinogenic risk are also needed. An intermediate marker will be especially useful for the rapid assessment of the chemopreventative effects of various types of dietary fiber.

Animal studies have reinforced the concept that fiber nutrition may play a role in colon carcinogenesis, but that the relationship is not simple.[119,120,137,204,206] Studies have observed no effect, increased, or decreased tumorigenesis depending upon the amount, type, and source of fiber, its particle size, the amount of other nutrients, the type of carcinogen, the timing of fiber feeding relative to carcinogen administration, and the strain and species of animal. The results of rodent studies reflect the complexities of fiber nutrition and emphasize the importance of avoiding strong conclusions based upon single studies. Among the fiber sources evaluated, wheat bran has shown a relatively consistent ability to inhibit experimental colon carcinogenesis.[137,204,206]

A number of mechanisms may contribute to the protective effect of dietary fiber against colon cancer.[137,204,206] Fiber may increase fecal bulk and reduce the concentration of colon mutagens or promoters. Many high fiber diets decrease transit time, providing another mechanism to reduce exposure of the colon to genotoxic agents or tumor promoters in the fecal stream. Many fibers may also bind carcinogens found in the diet further limiting exposure.[47] Most fibers are metabolized to varying degrees by the bacterial flora which may lead to the production of metabolites that can increase or decrease risk. In summary, each fiber type has unique properties which may modulate carcinogenesis by different mechanisms. Evidence suggests that diets containing foods that have varying amounts and sources of fiber probably influence colon cancer risk, although the details of this relationship remain to be defined.

Colon Carcinogens. The recent characterization of a series of very specific mutational events in human colon cancer must ultimately be linked with etiologic agents which induce these genotoxic events. At the present time, there are no definitive data implicating specific ingested carcinogens for human large bowel cancer. However, the potential for the production of initiators or promoters during cooking and food processing has not been thoroughly investigated.[27] Food preparation varies among different cultures and could be a critical factor contributing to the large geographic differences in cancer incidence. For example, in China many foods are prepared with steam whereas similar foods are more frequently fried by Chinese migrants to the U.S. These differences in food preparation may lead to a different pattern or concentration of pyrolysis products in food. A number of mutagenic pyrolysis products are produced during cooking and several have been found to be carcinogenic in laboratory animals although very few have been found to be specific for the colon.[27,262,263] Short term studies, which examine nuclear aberrations and microadenoma formation in the colonic mucosa have been utilized as an indirect measure of carcinogenic potential.[27] Rodents fed diets containing cooked food items, such as fried bacon or hamburger, show a higher frequency of nuclear aberrations in the colon mucosa than do controls.[27,53]

Other investigations have focused upon the production of mutagens within the digestive tract as a result of bacterial metabolism.[27] Human feces contain substances which are mutagenic in bacterial test systems.[27] Correlational studies have indicated that fecal mutagenicity is greater in populations at high risk for colorectal cancer.[67,199] For example, the concentration of stool mutagens in rural black South Africans at low risk of colon cancer was lower than in urban blacks and whites who experience greater risk.[67] Human subjects fed a high risk diet rich in protein, fat, energy, and animal products showed greater concentrations of fecal mutagens than those fed a low risk diet.[139]

One class of mutagenic compounds, known as fecapentaenes, was characterized and found to be produced by the colonic bacteria.[64,88,305] However, fecapentaenes have not yet been proven to be carcinogenic for the colon.[311] The concentrations of these compounds have been reported to decrease in individuals whose diet is supplemented with ascorbic acid and α-tocopherol,[63] or dietary fiber.[241] However, a randomized study on polyp recurrence found no beneficial effect of these supplements.[27] Another large study found no significant differences between 68 colon cancer

patients and 114 controls in the content of stool fecapentaenes.[262,263] Although fecapentaenes may have some role in colon cancer, it does not appear that they are the major or only initiator. Metabolites, such as the ketosteroids, produced by bacteria or during food processing from cholesterol or bile acids also have genotoxic and cytotoxic properties.[27] The concentration of these compounds in the fecal contents varies widely and the dietary factors which modulate their formation remain to be defined.

In summary, increased colorectal cancer risk is strongly associated with an affluent diet, which is rich in high fat foods, especially from animal products, and low in fruits, grains, and vegetables. The individual contributions of fat, protein, energy intake, numerous vitamins and minerals, and specific fiber components have not been clearly defined. The potential interactions among these components are numerous. At the present time, it is prudent to consider the impact of the total diet when making recommendations rather than focusing upon a single nutrient.

Breast

Cancer of the breast is frequent in the affluent nations of North America and Western Europe and relatively rare in many parts of Asia and Africa.[25] Migrants from low risk nations show increasing risk after moving to a high risk nation.[28,90,204,206,246] The increase in breast cancer risk among Japanese immigrants to the U.S. is most noticeable over several generations, in contrast to colon cancer risk which increases significantly over the lifespan of the original migrant population.[321] This observation suggests that nutritional or other environmental factors active during youth and adolescence may have a long term and major impact upon subsequent breast cancer risk. These findings are consistent with the hypothesis that some dietary patterns established early in life are associated with increased height and weight, leading to a hormonal environment contributing to an earlier age of menarche, which is in turn associated with increased risk of breast cancer.[84]

A number of dietary and nutritional factors have been proposed to enhance or protect against breast cancer. Ecologic studies have defined associations between national breast cancer rates and diets high in fat, protein, milk, eggs, refined sugar, animal products, and beef in particular.[10,34,76,194,204,206] All of these components are characteristic of the Western diet and the individual contribution of each factor to breast cancer risk cannot be determined by correlational studies alone. Case-control studies have frequently supported associations between breast cancer and components of the affluent diet.[108,109,115,159,192,284,289] but results have not been uniform.[80,107] Since a large number of studies have focused upon nutrition and breast cancer, several nutrients will be examined separately.

Fat. The controversy concerning the contribution of dietary fat to breast cancer risk can best be appreciated through the examination of representative data presented in Figure VI-2-7 and Tables VI-2-3 and VI-2-4. Geographic studies show strong correlations between national rates of breast cancer and the estimated per capita fat consumption.[34,36,233] There are wide international variations in breast cancer rates as well as per capita fat consumption or the percentage of

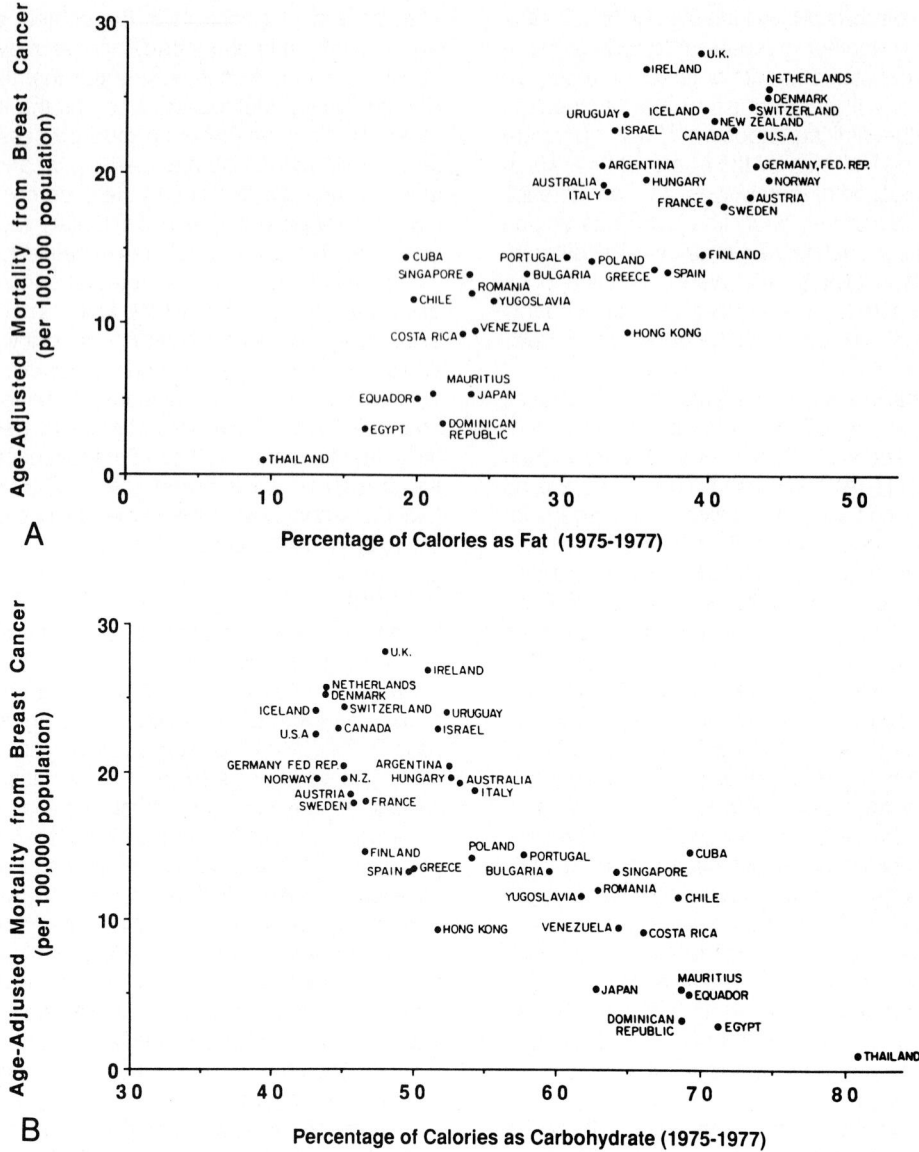

Figure VI-2-7. International correlation of (A) estimated dietary fat intake (percentage of calories as fat) or (B) estimated carbohydrate intake (percentage of calories as carbohydrate) and age-adjusted breast cancer mortality.[36]

calories derived from fat. In general the relationship between dietary fat and breast cancer appears to be linear and correlation coefficients range between 0.75 and 0.90.[34,36,233] Breast cancer rates have also been observed to increase significantly in populations migrating from low risk areas, such as Japan, where diets are low in fat to high risk areas, such as the United States, where populations consume diets high in fat.[28,90,204,206,246] Time trend studies also support the fat-breast cancer association. Within Japan, estimates of per capita daily fat intake rose from 23 g/day to 52 g/day over the 15 year period prior to 1973.[105] During this period, breast cancer mortality increased in Japan by over 30%.[142] Ecologic studies are frequently criticized since they utilize grouped data and the estimates of fat intake are crude. However, a major advantage is the very wide range of fat intake observed when countries are the experimental unit. Correlation does not prove cause and effect and many investigators argue

that fat intake may be an indictor of some other unidentified environmental component that is the critical risk factor. The strong correlations observed may be indicative of the overall effect of many nutrients which change simultaneously.

In contrast to the ecologic studies, most case control or prospective investigations have failed to detect a significant relationship between breast cancer risk and estimates of fat intake.[76,204,206,246,248] For example, Willet and colleagues examined breast cancer risk in a cohort of American nurses evaluated at intervals with a food frequency questionnaire designed to estimate the intake of a number of nutrients, including fat.[319] No significant relationships between the estimates of total fat, saturated fat, or cholesterol intake and breast cancer risk were observed (Table VI-2-3). In general, the case control and prospective studies have examined populations showing very homogeneous fat intake.[234,261] For example, the quintile means for total fat intake among par-

Table VI-2-3. Dietary Fat and the Risk of Breast Cancer in a Cohort of 89,538 American Nurses Aged 34 to 59 at the Time of Initial Evaluation in 1980

Measurement	Quintile				
	1	2	3	4	5
Total fat					
Mean calorie-adjusted (gms/day)	56	64	69	72	78
Mean % of calories	32	36	39	41	44
Multivariate relative risk	1.00	0.80	0.88	0.80	0.82
Saturated fat					
Mean calorie-adjusted (gms/day)	19	22	24	26	30
Mean % of calories	11	13	14	15	17
Multivariate relative risk	1.00	0.80	0.91	0.77	0.84
Cholesterol					
Mean calorie-adjusted (mg/day)	216	268	301	337	423
Multivariate relative risk	1.00	1.06	1.02	1.07	0.91

During four years of follow-up, there were 601 cases of breast cancer diagnosed among participants. The multivariate age-adjusted relative risk of breast cancer is expressed according to the quintile estimates of calorie-adjusted total fat, saturated fat, and cholesterol intake
From Willett et al.[319]

Table VI-2-4. The Effects of Dietary Fat Intake (12, 24, 48% of Calories) on 7,12-dimethylbenz(a)anthracene (DMBA)-induced Mammary Carcinogenesis in Female Rats

Dietary Fat (% kcal)	Number of Rats	Daily Energy Intake (kcal/day)	Final Body Weight (grams)	Adeno-carcinoma Incidence (%)	Number of Cancers
12	120	46	263	19	34
24	120	47	262	35	53
48	120	47	260	62	125

Rats were fed diets with corn oil providing 12, 24, or 48% of total energy from 4 weeks of age for a period of 30 weeks. DMBA was given as a single dose (2.0 mg/100 g body weight) after 4 weeks of feeding. Each doubling of energy intake from fat multiplied the odds of developing an adenocarcinoma by 2.7 (P < 0.001)
From Clinton et al.[42]

ticipants in the Nurses' Health Study cohort were very narrow at 32, 36, 39, 41, and 44% of calories.[319] The lowest quintile was still significantly higher than the populations around the world exhibiting lower breast cancer risk and consuming diets containing dietary fat at 20–30% of calories.

Although the epidemiologic data has not provided definitive results concerning dietary fat and breast cancer, accumulated evidence from over 100 animals studies using chemical carcinogens, hormones, irradiation, or viruses to induce breast cancer indicate that fat as a single variable enhances mammary carcinogenesis.[71] For example, a large study in rats utilizing diets containing dietary fat concentrations ranging from 12–48% of calories clearly indicates a strong enhancement of mammary carcinogenesis over the range of fat intake observed in human populations.[42–44] Well

controlled rodent studies have also shown that dietary fat enhances breast cancer risk independently of caloric intake (Figure VI-2-1).[42,43,286] In addition, both saturated or polyunsaturated fats will similarly enhance mammary carcinogenesis once a minimal amount of essential fatty acids has been provided.[35]

Overall, the large body of data from animal investigations and human geographic epidemiologic studies supports the hypothesis that dietary fat may be one component of an affluent diet contributing to increased breast cancer risk. However, the negative findings from recent analytic epidemiologic studies have led many to believe that the hypothesis has been proven false. Many investigators have expressed the opinion that most of the recent analytic epidemiologic studies are severely compromised by several major limitations: 1) the substantial measurement error in the assessment of dietary fat intake; 2) the very narrow range of fat intake in studies; and 3) the important effects of fat may have occurred earlier in life.[234,261] These studies therefore lack the sensitivity required to detect a relationship between fat and cancer risk. Ultimately, an intervention trial may provide the only possible scientific approach to determining whether a reduction in dietary fat can have a significant impact upon the risk of cancers of the breast, colon, or prostate.

Protein. Dietary protein has a major impact upon early growth and development of humans and laboratory animals. Marginal intakes of protein and energy may be factors contributing to the later onset of menarche in many populations exhibiting lower risk of breast cancer. In general, geographic correlational and case-control studies have not shown strong or consistent associations. Laboratory studies show no major influence on breast cancer when protein is varied over a wide range after rats have reached sexual maturity.[42,44] In contrast, a stimulatory effect of protein has been observed in a two-generation model.[94] High protein diets fed to dams throughout mating and lactation, and then fed to female offspring, accelerated sexual maturation and increased the incidence of chemically induced mammary cancer. The role of protein nutrition during childhood and adolescence as a risk factor for breast cancer later in life has not been carefully examined.

Alcohol. The issue of alcohol and breast cancer is controversial.[95] A significant increase in risk with greater alcohol intake was suggested by a recent review of the accumulated case-control and cohort studies.[157] Overall, it was estimated that 13–14% of all breast cancer in the U.S. may be attributed to alcohol alone.[157,320] The relative risk from the consumption of one typical serving of beer, wine, or liquor (approximately 12 gms of ethanol) per day was estimated to be 1.4 whereas three drinks per day would approximately double the risk. However, much more effort will be required to eliminate the controversy surrounding this issue.[95,288]

Vitamins. Some human epidemiologic studies suggest an inverse correlation between breast cancer risk and estimated intakes of vitamin A.[188,204,206,246] The majority of rodent experimentation also supports a protective effect of vitamin A and related compounds.[8] Vitamins E and C have frequently been investigated relative to breast cancer risk but no major role for these or other vitamins has been firmly established.

Minerals. Among the minerals, selenium has been most

extensively studied relative to breast cancer risk, primarily in animal models.[8,204,206] It is difficult to assess human selenium intake by dietary questionnaires, since plants are very sensitive to the soil selenium content, leading to tremendous variation in selenium content of foods. Although questionnaires are of little utility, tissue samples can be used to estimate recent intake, but this approach will be useful only if evaluated prospectively since the presence of a cancer may alter the results obtained.[198,206] Due to the difficulties in assessment, human studies have not provided strong evidence for increased risk with low intakes. Animal studies have suggested that elevated selenium intake may inhibit mammary carcinogenesis under some conditions.[8,40,206] However, it is apparent that the protective effect of selenium is dependent upon other nutritional factors such as the amount and source of fat and protein in the diet and possibly vitamin E and antioxidants. Since the role of selenium in human cancer is uncertain and it has potential for significant toxicity, individuals should be discouraged from consuming selenium as a supplement.[8,204,206]

In summary, geographic epidemiologic data, studies of migrant populations, and rodent experiments strongly suggest that diet may have a significant impact upon breast cancer risk. However, the contribution of individual components of the diet and the time period during a women's life when they may be most active are not well understood. In addition to the possible risk associated with the affluent diet, particularly fat intake, alcohol consumption may play a role in mammary cancer and warrants further study.

Prostate

Cancer of the prostate has become one of the most frequent cancers in the United States, and is especially high among the African-American population.[37,251] Prostate cancer is a disease of aging men and is rare under the age of 45. The international distribution of prostate cancer is similar to that of colon and breast cancer and is, therefore, correlated with Western culture and affluent diets.[25] The role of nutrition in prostate cancer has not been widely investigated.

International and intracountry correlational studies have suggested associations between prostate cancer mortality and the per-capita intake of total fat.[10,24,117,249] Similarly, several analytical epidemiologic studies have reported associations between total fat or the consumption of high-fat foods and prostate cancer.[81,98,136,253,268,278] Few rodent models of prostate cancer have been characterized and utilized to investigate nutritional hypotheses derived from epidemiologic studies. Essential fatty acid deficiency was found to inhibit the growth rate of a transplantable prostate adenocarcinoma, whereas dietary fat concentrations over the wide range of intake observed in human populations had no significant effect.[46] This observation does not preclude the possibility of significant effects of dietary fat on earlier stages in the carcinogenic process, which cannot be evaluated in a transplantable tumor model.

Increasing evidence supports a role for vitamin A, carotenoids, or synthetic retinoids in prostate carcinogenesis. However, the relationship of these substances to prostate cancer may be very complex. In a series of studies, estimates of Vitamin A intake have been reported to have no relationship, or to be associated with increased or decreased risk of prostate cancer.[81,98,136,249,251,270] It is clear that the relationship between vitamin A status, ranging from deficiency to excess, and prostate cancer has not been defined. The high intake of foods rich in carotenoids, which have biological characteristics in addition to their contribution to vitamin A status, have been associated with decreased risk.[250,268] Increased body weight or obesity has been associated with prostate cancer risk in some,[146,278,285] but not all, studies.[136]

In summary, a role for diet in prostate cancer has been suggested by epidemiologic studies and a limited number of laboratory investigations. Prostate cancer is higher in nations consuming an affluent diet, although the contribution of specific components such as fat and energy intake have not been well defined. The biological plausibility is further enhanced by the knowledge that many nutrients modulate the secretion of, or tissue sensitivity to hormones, such as testosterone, which are thought to participate in prostate carcinogenesis. The possible relationship of vitamin A and related compounds needs further clarification.

Endometrium

In general, endometrial cancer shows an international distribution similar to other cancers of affluence, such as breast, colon, and prostate.[25] An association between endometrial cancer and excess weight has often been reported.[204,206,246] One established risk factor is the use of exogenous estrogens at high-dosages.[204,206] It has been postulated, although evidence is minimal, that dietary factors contributing to obesity may influence risk though changes in the hormonal environment. The potential interactions between dietary components and supplemental estrogens should be investigated (see XXXI-3).

Ovary

There are considerable international and geographic variations in the incidence and mortality rates of ovarian cancer. The disease is more common in nations exhibiting Western culture, especially among those in the higher socioeconomic groups.[25,145,204,206,246] Although some of the geographic variation may be due to reproductive variables, there are also suggestive relationships to dietary components.[204,206,246] Several studies have implicated fat, particularly from animal sources.[56,145] In contrast, the consumption of vegetables and grain products was associated with lower risk.[145] At the present time no conclusive role for dietary components in the pathogenesis of ovarian cancer has been established, but additional studies are needed.

Bladder

Bladder cancer is more frequent in industrialized nations, especially among those in urban areas and of lower socioeconomic status.[25] Bladder cancer is associated with cigarette smoking, occupational exposures to certain industrial chemicals, and parasitic bladder infections. There is very limited evidence to suggest an important role for nutrients or other dietary factors in bladder cancer.[10,204,206,246] Laboratory studies have found that the non-nutritive sweeteners, cyclamates and saccharine, may be weak initiators or promoters of bladder carcinogenesis in rodents,[235] but their contribution to human cancer is probably very small.[204,205,206] Although some studies have suggested an association between coffee consumption and bladder cancer,[189,277] the majority of studies do not support a significant relationship.[121,125,206]

Summary of Research Efforts Concerning Nutrients and Cancer

Energy. Due to the inaccuracies associated with the methodology used in studies to assess the balance between energy intake and energy expenditures in human populations we have very little direct information relative to its contribution to the pathogenesis of human cancers. In contrast, striking and consistent inhibitory effects of reduced energy intake on most types of cancer have been observed in rodent studies.[8,71,204,206,246,255] An understanding of the diverse mechanisms underlying these observations should have relevance to human cancer prevention. Experimental evidence suggests that energy intake modulates a range of metabolic, endocrinologic, and immunologic processes which influence cellular proliferative rates, proto-oncogene expression, and DNA repair capabilities.[255] Many questions concerning cancer risk and the interactions between energy intake, energy expenditure, metabolic rate, and relative body weight or obesity, remain to be answered.

Protein. Dietary protein, like energy intake, has dramatic effects upon many physiologic and biochemical processes that may participate in carcinogenesis.[306] The Western diet is associated with a number of humans cancers and is typically in excess of the recommended protein requirement. The major change in protein intake as nations develop economically is a shift from plant products to animal products as the major source of protein. It has not been possible to delineate the specific contribution of protein quantity or source in human cancer since its consumption is closely related to the intake of other dietary factors such as energy and fat. Laboratory studies have generally found minimal effects of dietary protein content except at the extremes of feeding.[204,246,306] Experimental studies of the breast,[94] colon,[45,290] and liver[204,206] have provided some evidence for increased risk with greater protein intake.

Lipids. Defining the contribution of dietary fat in the etiology of many cancers, especially those of the breast, colon, pancreas, endometrium, and prostate, is an active area of investigation.[138,204,206,246] Improved epidemiologic and biochemical methods are needed to assess accurately past and current lipid intake in humans. Many previous studies lack the sensitivity and specificity necessary to quantify risk associated with high fat diets. Although the human studies at this time are not totally consistent, precisely controlled laboratory studies in rodent models support a contribution of dietary fat concentration and source in the pathogenesis of several malignant neoplasms, such as breast and colon cancer. Dietary fat modulates many metabolic and endocrine processes which may alter tissue susceptibility to transformation and progression. In addition, dietary lipids influence the lipid composition of cell membranes and may thereby modulate the cellular response of many growth stimulating and inhibitory pathways by altering ligand-receptor binding and signal transduction.

Cholesterol. Dietary cholesterol is derived from meat and dairy products and is therefore correlated with cancers which are frequent in affluent nations. The close association of cholesterol with other nutrients, such as fat, has made it difficult to establish a contribution to breast, colon, or prostate cancer risk.[108,130,180,204,206,226,246] Several long term prospective studies originally designed to evaluate cardiovascular disease have reported an inverse relationship between overall cancer risk and serum cholesterol levels at the start of the study.[186] These observations, have created a potentially difficult problem for those concerned with public health and dietary guidelines. However, at the present time it is not clear if the information relative to a preexisting low serum cholesterol level can be extrapolated to a population that has deliberately lowered serum levels in order to reduce risk of cardiovascular disease. Overall, the relationship between dietary cholesterol, serum cholesterol, and cancer risk in humans is far from clear.

Carbohydrates. Very few studies have examined the relationship between carbohydrates and cancer.[36] The limited number of laboratory studies have suggested that carcinogenesis in some models can be modulated to a limited degree by the source of carbohydrate, although the mechanisms remain obscure.

Fiber. The complexities of dietary fiber chemistry and in vivo physiologic effects have made it impossible to define the overall contribution of total fiber intake or specific fractions to cancer risk.[137,204,206] However, the recent data concerning the inhibition of colon polyp formation by specific fiber supplements suggests potential benefits for high risk individuals. This is a rapidly expanding area of nutrition research and significant improvements in our understanding of dietary fiber in health and disease should be forthcoming.

Vitamins. The public perceives vitamin supplements as an important form of self-therapy for the prevention and treatment of many ailments, including cancer.[188] Vitamin supplements are inexpensive, easy to consume, relatively free of side effects when consumed at recommended dosages, and can be obtained without a prescription. A particularly attractive aspect of vitamin supplementation is the belief that these nutrients may counteract the adverse effects of diet or lifestyle that are much more difficult to change. These issues emphasize the importance of scientifically sound studies to define the risks and benefits of vitamin nutrition in the origins of human cancer. It is important to stress that major organizations providing dietary guidelines emphasize the importance of obtaining proper vitamin nutrition through the consumption of foods rich in vitamins rather than through the use of supplements. Caution is advisable since vitamin supplementation may not be uniformly beneficial and enhanced tumor promotion may occur in some situations.

The role of vitamin A in the normal growth and development of epithelial tissues has been known for decades. Vitamin A is provided in the diet as retinol and its esters, primarily from milk and organ meats, and as β-carotene in yellow and leafy green vegetables. Interest in vitamin A and related compounds in the etiology, prevention, and treatment of cancer is rapidly expanding. Epidemiologic studies evaluated a role for vitamin A in cancers of the lung, breast, oropharynx, stomach, bladder, prostate and colon.[188] In some cases a protective effect of consuming foods rich in retinoids has been suggested with prostate cancer being the exception, where both protective and inhibitory associations have been reported.[188,204,206,246] Improvements in estimating vitamin A intake through questionnaires and by biochemical testing are needed to improve the quality of data obtained from future studies. The majority of studies in laboratory models indicate that vitamin A deficiency increases the susceptibility of many tissues to chemical carcinogenesis. The role of vitamin A excess has not been frequently assessed. The use of vitamin A and synthetic retinoids in chemoprevention trials to determine their effectiveness as supplements should be encouraged.

There are very few studies investigating the role of vitamin D in human cancer.[188,206] Several studies have suggested a relationship between lower vitamin D intake and colon cancer.[188,206] Cancer cells derived from many human tumors have been shown to express the receptor for 1,25-dihydroxyvitamin D3 and respond to this agent in vitro, but the pathophysiologic significance to human cancer remains to be determined.[188]

Vitamin E is a family of eight compounds collectively referred to as tocopherols. Vegetable oil, eggs, and whole grains are the major sources of dietary vitamin E. The antioxidant and free radical scavenger properties of vitamin E have suggested a possible role as an antineoplastic vitamin.[188] However, too few in vivo experimental or epidemiologic studies have been completed to provide evidence to support or refute this hypothesis. The limited knowledge concerning potential risks of large doses of this fat soluble vitamin should discourage excessive supplementation.

Vitamin C, which includes ascorbic acid and dehydroascorbic acid, functions as a general antioxidant and as a component of several enzymatic reactions in intermediary metabolism.[188] Citrus fruits, leafy vegetables, tomatoes, and potatoes are rich sources of vitamin C. Despite the large volume of publications in the last decade, there is a very little evidence to support a critical role of vitamin C in the etiology of most human cancers.[188,204,206] The strongest evidence concerns the ability of vitamin C to inhibit the formation of carcinogenic nitrosamines, which may ultimately reduce the incidence of cancers that are thought to be associated with nitrosamines, such as gastric cancer. At the present time there is no evidence to suggest that the consumption of vitamin C supplements at levels higher than can be achieved in a well-balanced diet, containing ample fresh fruits and vegetables, is useful in the prevention or treatment of human cancer.

Minerals. A number of minerals are required for normal structural development of the skeleton and soft tissue and for numerous biochemical and physiologic reactions. Those required in large amounts such as calcium, phosphorus, and magnesium are considered macrominerals. The trace elements are needed in much smaller amounts and include zinc, selenium, fluoride, iron, copper, iodine, manganese, and molybdenum. The contributions of most minerals to carcinogenesis have not been clearly defined,[188,204,206,246] and specific recommendations concerning intake should be avoided. Among the minerals, roles for selenium and calcium in human cancer have been actively investigated.

Recent evidence suggests a role for calcium in colon carcinogenesis. A prospective cohort study in the United States found that those developing colon cancer had a significantly lower intake of calcium and vitamin D.[75] Case-control studies have been inconsistent.[206] Calcium supplementation of 1.2 g per day reduced the proliferative rate of colonic cells in patients considered to be at increased risk of colon cancer.[149] Laboratory studies have reported that calcium reduces the loss of superficial epithelial cells and the proliferation of basal crypt cells.[33] Clinical trials to determine the effects of calcium supplementation on polyp formation are currently underway.

Selenium is an essential constituent of glutathione peroxidase and participates in the destruction of hydrogen peroxide and organic hydroperoxides using reducing equivalent from glutathione. Selenium therefore participates in cellular and tissue defense against oxidative damage. Marginal selenium intake does not produce major physiologic changes, but does predispose to injury by other agents, such as chemical carcinogens. A major obstacle for epidemiologic studies is that estimates of dietary selenium intake are unreliable, especially in industrialized nations where foods are extensively processed and shipped large distances, since food content is very sensitive to soil concentrations. An inverse association between the selenium levels in forage crops and mortality rates from certain cancers in different geographic areas has been suggested.[40,206] Other studies have compared blood selenium levels in cancer patients and controls.[206] Although these studies are frequently small and do not control for other risk factors, many have observed lower selenium levels in cancer patients. Prospective studies, where serum has been obtained prior to the onset of disease, have provided inconsistent results.[206] Animal studies have also provided contradictory results concerning the effects of excess selenium or selenium deficiency and carcinogenesis.[206] Overall, conclusions concerning a role of selenium in human cancer cannot be justified, and supplementation of the diet with a mineral that has significant risk of toxicity cannot be supported. However, further studies are warranted in order to define the types of cancer which may be affected and the conditions under which adjustments of selenium intake may be beneficial.

Ethanol. The chronic consumption of alcohol is strongly associated with cancers of the oropharynx, larynx, and esophagus.[206,247] Tobacco smoking acts synergistically with alcohol in the pathogenesis of these cancers. Ethanol probably contributes to liver cancer and may have a role in gastric, pancreatic, colon, and breast cancer although additional studies are necessary in order to firmly establish and quantify risk for the latter tissues. The risks associated with moderate alcohol intake and cancer are not well established but have been suggested in some studies.[206,247] Ethanol itself is probably not a carcinogen and a number of mechanisms are under investigation whereby ethanol may modulate carcinogenesis.[247] Ethanol may have direct effects upon the target tissue altering cell turnover, permeability to carcinogens, or carcinogen metabolism. Ethanol may alter nutrient requirements of the target tissue, thereby disrupting normal structure and function and altering carcinogenic risk. Some alcoholic beverages may contain chemical substances which are carcinogens or tumor promoters. The systemic effects of alcohol upon hepatic carcinogen or hormone metabolism may indirectly alter risk of cancer in many tissues. Ethanol may contribute to malnutrition with regard to a number of nutrients by altering absorption and metabolism or through the poor dietary habits associated with excessive consumption of alcoholic beverages.

Dietary and Nutritional Recommendations

Considerable controversy exists within the lay public, scientific community, food industry, and government regulatory agencies concerning the establishment of dietary guidelines to prevent cancer. Some argue that dietary changes should not be recommended until scientific uncertainties have been resolved, whereas others believe that the associations observed justify institution of changes in the diet while more definitive data are obtained. Since cancer ranks as the second leading cause of death in affluent nations, there is a large public demand for nutritional remedies to prevent cancer. In the absence of sound guidelines, the public will indulge in the overinterpretation of inconclusive studies and will pursue dietary habits, including supplements which are useless and even harmful. Unfortunately, absolute proof for many of the diet and cancer hypotheses will be difficult to obtain due to the expense required to support long term studies in large numbers of subjects. The decisions to formulate recommendations must take into account several factors, including: strength of the evidence, potential benefits to society if the disease could be avoided, likelihood and severity of an adverse effect, and the feasibility of reducing exposure to the risk factor. In addition, economic issues relative to the food and agricultural industry are factors which may influence decisions of committees assembled to define nutritional guidelines. Although much remains to be learned before the impact of proposed recommendations on health can be precisely quantified, most experts in the field agree that a number of recommendations can be made with a reasonable degree of certainty, with the likelihood of minimal risk, and the potential for significant public health benefits.[206]

In general, there are two different, but complementary approaches to reducing dietary risk factors for cancer and other chronic diseases. One focuses upon the individuals or groups and is aimed at identifying those at high risk and providing dietary intervention. A second addresses the population as a whole and is the public health approach. For some cases, we can identify individuals, with a very high degree of certainty, who will develop a specific cancer and institute preventive measures. For example, those with familial polyposis have a very high incidence of colon cancer, and a prophylactic colectomy is frequently performed prior to the age at which tumor risk increases. However, most cancer patients cannot be identified with a similar degree of certainty prior to the onset of their disease. The future application of sophisticated individually based nutritional or chemopreventative interventions will be greatly facilitated by the identification of susceptible genotypes, and by identifying additional environmental risk factors.

The public health approach is a preventive strategy designed to decrease overall disease incidence by reducing adverse dietary habits of the entire population. Implementation of dietary recommendations requires cooperation among the media, food industry, nutritional scientists, public health personnel, medical practitioners, educators, and the government.[206] In order to achieve success, dietary recommendations must be simple and feasible to implement, have minimal risk, low cost to society, and the potential to benefit many people.[206] Past efforts have been successful in the area of nutrition. For example, iron fortification of cereals benefits a large number of children and adult women, while risk is limited to a small number of individuals with hemochromatosis.

Tables VI-2-5 and VI-2-6 present population based dietary recommendations published over the last decade by several organizations in order to lower risk from chronic diseases.[4,5,204,206] Most groups recommend reducing total fat intake to 30% or less of calories with saturated fats reduced to less than 10% of calories and cholesterol limited to less than 300 mg/day. Although the role(s) of fat level, saturation, and cholesterol in cancer have not been precisely quantified, a large body of evidence also supports a contribution of these dietary factors to cardiovascular diseases. These goals can be accomplished by substituting fish, poultry without skin, lean meats and low- or nonfat dairy products for fatty meats and whole-milk dairy products, and by selecting more fruits, vegetables, cereals, and legumes in conjunction with limiting fats and oils in cooking, spreads, and dressings.[206] With a decrease in lipid calories, carbohydrates should increase to approximately 55% of total energy through an increase in the consumption of green and yellow vegetables, citrus fruits, whole-grain cereals and breads, which are typically low in fat and rich in many vitamins, minerals, and fiber. Most groups suggest moderation in protein intake. Protein is an essential nutrient, but in many affluent nations, intake is in two fold excess of the established recommended daily allowance. The contribution of protein to risk of cancer and other major diseases is less clear than for lipid intake. The NAS has recommended protein intake at levels lower than twice the RDA for all age groups. The consumption of meat is frequently associated with certain cancers and cardiovascular disease. However, at this time it is not possible to implicate meat per se, other than through its contribution to high total or saturated fat and cholesterol intake. Lean meats can remain a component of a low fat diet.

Excess weight has been associated with increased morbidity and mortality from a number of diseases including diabetes, hypertension, cardiovascular disease, and some forms of cancer.[4,5,204,206] Laboratory studies indicate a strong relationship between energy intake and carcinogenesis, but the relevance of these studies, which frequently use severely restricted diets, to the human situation is unknown. The increasingly sedentary populations of many affluent nations exhibit higher average body weight or other indices of body mass even while total energy intake is slightly decreasing. It is recommended that food intake and physical activity be balanced to maintain appropriate body weight.

Most expert committees do not recommend alcohol consumption based upon its role in cancer, other diseases, acci-

Table VI-2-5. A Comparison of Dietary Recommendations to Lower Cancer Risk in the United States[4,204,206,207]

Organization	Maintain Appropriate Body Weight	Limit or Reduce Total Fat (%kcal)	Ratio of Saturated to Unsaturated Dietary Fats	Fruit and Vegetable Intake	Complex Carbohydrate Intake	Sodium Intake	Food Preparation and Processing	Food Additives and Contaminants	Alcohol	Other
National Research Council, National Academy of Sciences, 1982[204]	No Comment	<30%	Not defined	Increase citrus fruits, green and yellow and cruciferous vegetables	Increase whole grain products	Indirectly	Reduce cured, pickled, and smoked foods	Continue to monitor, test, and reduce exposure	Drink less, if at all	Monitor and test for mutagens
American Cancer Society, 1984[4]	Yes	<30%	Not defined	Especially those with vitamin A and C, cruciferous vegetables	Whole grain foods and high fiber foods	Not defined	Reduce cured, pickled, and smoked foods	No comment	Drink less, if at all	
National Cancer Institute, 1987[207]	Yes	<30%	Not defined	Citrus fruits, cruciferous vegetables, vitamin A rich green and yellow vegetables	Whole grain products, eat 20–30 g fiber per day	Not defined	Reduce cured, pickled, and smoked foods. Avoid frying and high temperature cooking	No comment	Drink less, if at all	Varied and balanced diet
National Research Council, National Academy of Sciences, 1989[206]	Yes	<30%	Reduce saturated fat to <10% of energy, reduce cholesterol intake to <300 mg/day	Eat 5 or more servings of green and yellow vegetables and citrus fruits per day	Eat 6 or more servings of breads, cereals, and legumes per day	Limit salt intake to 6 gms or less per day	Highly processed salty, salt-preserved, and salt-pickled foods should be consumed sparingly	No comment	Limit pure alcohol intake to <1 oz per day, if at all	Avoid taking dietary supplements in excess of the RDA in any one day

dents, and birth defects. The NAS has suggested limiting intake, for those who drink, to less than 1 ounce of alcohol per day which is equivalent to two cans of beer or small glasses of wine.[206] Salt intake should be limited to less than 6 grams per day, primarily by reducing its use in cooking and at the table.[206] The evidence linking salt intake to hypertension is strong. The consumption of salt-preserved or salt-pickled foods should be limited, based upon the frequent association with stomach cancer although the causative agents in these foods have not been identified. The NAS does not recommend calcium intake above the current recommended daily allowances.[206] Benefits of intake above these levels to prevent osteoporosis, hypertension, or colon cancer have not been adequately documented. It is recommended that fluoride intake be optimized especially during the years of tooth formation.[206] There is no substantial evidence linking fluoride intake to cancer risk.

An increasing proportion of the American population consumes some type of self-prescribed nutritional supplement on a daily basis. The benefits of nutrient supplements which are in great excess of the recommended daily allowances have not been proven, although significant risks are well known. The appropriate mechanism to obtain the recommended concentrations of nutrients is through a diverse and varied diet. It is important to view these guidelines as reflecting an overall dietary pattern rather than individual recommendations. Most of the evidence suggests that a major impact upon cancer incidence would require the combination of changes recommended in these guidelines.

References

1. Albanes, D.: Caloric intake, body weight and cancer. A Review. Nutr. Cancer, 9:199, 1987.
2. Alberts, D. S., Einspahr, J., Rees-McGee, S., Ramanujam, P., Buller, M. K., Clark, L., Ritenbaugh, C., Atwood, J., Pethigal, P., Earnest, D., Villar, H., Phelps, J., Lipkin, M., Wargovich, M., and Meyskens, F. L., Jr.: Effects of dietary wheat bran fiber on rectal epithelial cell proliferation in patients with resection for colorectal cancers. J. Natl. Cancer Inst., 82:1280, 1990.
3. Alfin-Slater, R. B., and Kritchevsky, D.: In Human Nutrition: A Comprehensive Treatise, Volume 7, Cancer and Nutrition. New York, Plenum Press, 1991.
4. American Cancer Society: Nutrition and cancer: Cause and prevention. American Cancer Society Special Report, N. Y., 1984.
5. American Cancer Society: Guidelines on diet, nutrition, and cancer, CA, 41:334, 1991.
6. American Institute of Nutrition: Report of the AIN ad hoc committee on standards for nutritional studies. J. Nutr., 110:1340, 1977.
7. American Institute of Nutrition. Second report of the AIN ad hoc committee on standards for nutritional studies. J. Nutr., 110:1726, 1980.
8. Angres, G., and Beth, M.: Effects of dietary constituents on carcinogenesis in different tumor models: an overview from 1975 to 1988. In Human Nutrition: A Comprehensive Treatise, Volume 7, Cancer and Nutrition. Edited by R. B. Alfin-Slater, and D. Kritchevsky. New York, Plenum Press, 1991, p. 51.
9. Anthony, P. P.: Cancer of the liver: Pathogenesis and recent aetiological factors. Trans. R. Soc. Trop. Med. Hyg., 71:466, 1977.
10. Armstrong, B., and Doll, R.: Environmental factors and cancer incidence and mortality in different countries, with special reference to dietary practices. Int. J. Cancer, 15:617, 1975.
11. Austin, D. F.: Larynx. In Cancer Epidemiology and Prevention. Edited by D. Schottenfeld, and J. F. Fraumeni, Jr. Philadelphia, Saunders, 1982, p. 554.
12. Austin, H., Delzell, E., Grufferman, S., Levine, R., Morrison, A., Stolley, P. D., and Cole, P.: A case control study of hepatocellular carcinoma and the hepatitis B virus, cigarette smoking, and alcohol consumption. Cancer Res., 46:962, 1986.
13. Barch, D. H., Kuemmerle, S. C., Hollenberg, P. F., and Iannaccone, P. M.: Esophageal microsomal metabolism of N-nitrosomethylbenzylamine in the zinc-deficient rat. Cancer Res., 44:5629, 1984.

Table VI-2-6. Population Nutrient Goals Established by the World Health Organization to Prevent Diet-Related Chronic Diseases

	Lower Limit	Upper Limit
Total fat	15% of energy	30% of energy*
Saturated fats	0% of energy	10% of energy
Polyunsaturated fats	3% of energy	7% of energy
Dietary cholesterol	0 mg per day	300 mg per day
Total carbohydrate	55% of energy	75% of energy
Complex carbohydrates†	50% of energy	70% of energy
Dietary fiber‡ as non starch polysaccharides	16 gm per day	24 gm per day
Total dietary fiber	27 gm per day	40 gm per day
Free sugars§	0% of energy	10% of energy
Protein	10% of energy	15% of energy
Salt	Not defined	6 gm per day
Total energy	Energy intake needs to be sufficient to allow for normal childhood growth, for the needs of pregnancy and lactation, and for work and desirable physical activities, and to maintain appropriate body reserves of energy in children and adults. Adult populations on average should have a body-mass index (BMI) of 20–22 (BMI = body mass in kg/[height in meters]^2	

*An interim goal for nations with high fat intakes: further benefits would be expected by reducing fat intake towards 15% of total energy

†A daily minimum intake of 400 gm of vegetables and fruits, including at least 30 g of pulses, nuts, and seeds, should contribute to this component

‡Dietary fiber includes the non-starch polysaccharides (NSP), the goals for which are based on NSP obtained from mixed food sources. Since the definition and measurement of dietary fiber remain uncertain, the goals for total dietary fiber have been estimated from the non-starch polysaccharide values

§These sugars include monosaccharides, disaccharides, and other short-chain sugars extracted from carbohydrates by refining. These refined or purified sugars do not include the natural sugars consumed when eating fruits and vegetables or drinking milk

14. Beasley, R. P., Lin, C. C., Hwan, L. Y., and Chien, C. S.: Hepatocellular carcinoma and hepatitis B virus: A prospective study of 22,707 men in Taiwan. Lancet, 2:1129, 1981.

15. Bingham, S. A., Williams, D. R. R., and Cummings, J. H.: Dietary fiber consumption in Britain: New estimates and their relation to large bowel cancer mortality. Br. J. Cancer, 52:399, 1985.

16. Birt, D. F., and Bresnick, E.: Chemoprevention by nonnutrient components of vegetables and fruits. In Human Nutrition: A Comprehensive Treatise, Volume 7, Cancer and Nutrition. Edited by R. B. Alfin-Slater, and D. Kritchevsky. New York, Plenum Press, 1991, p. 221.

17. Birt, D. F., Sayed, S., Davies, M. H., and Pour, P. M.: Sex differences in the effects of retinoids on carcinogenesis by N-nitrosobis(2-oxopropyl)amine in Syrian hamsters. Cancer Lett., 14:13, 1981.

18. Birt, D. F., Salmasi, S., and Pour, P. M.: Enhancement of experimental pancreatic cancer in Syrian golden hamsters by dietary fat. J. Natl. Cancer Inst., 67:1327, 1981.

19. Birt, D. F., Stepan, K. R., and Pour, P. M.: Interaction of dietary fat and protein on pancreatic carcinogenesis in Syrian golden hamsters. J. Natl. Cancer Inst., 71:355, 1983.

20. Birt, D. F., Davies, M. H., Pour, P. M., and Salmasi, S.: Lack of inhibition by retinoids of bis(2-oxopropyl)nitrosamine-induced carcinogenesis in Syrian hamsters. Carcinogenesis, 4:1216, 1983.

21. Birt, D., Julius, A., White, L., and Pour, P.: Enhancement of pancreatic carcinogenesis in hamsters fed a high-fat diet ad libitum and at a controlled calorie intake. Cancer Res., 49:5848, 1989.

22. Bjelke, E.: Dietary vitamin A and human lung cancer. Int. J. Cancer, 15:561, 1975.

23. Bjelke, E.: Dietary factors and the epidemiology of cancer of the stomach and large bowel. Aktuel. Ernaehrungsmed. Klin. Prax., Suppl. 2:10, 1978.

24. Blair, A., and Fraumeni, J. F., Jr.: Geographic patterns of prostate cancer in the United States. J. Natl. Cancer Inst., 61:1379, 1978.

25. Boring, C. C., Squires, T. S., and Tong, T.: Cancer Statistic, 1991. CA, 41:19, 1991.

26. Brechot, C., Nalpas, B., Courouce, A., Duhamel, G., Callard, P., Carnot, F., Tiollais, P., and Berthelot, P.: Evidence that hepatitis B virus has a role in liver-cell carcinoma in alcoholic liver disease. N. Engl. J. Med., 306:1384, 1982.

27. Bruce, W. R.: Recent hypotheses for the origin of colon cancer. Cancer Res., 47:4237, 1987.

28. Buell, P.: Changing incidence of breast cancer in Japanese-American women. J. Natl. Cancer Inst., 51:1479, 1973.

29. Burch, J. D., Howe, G. R., Miller, A. B., and Semenciw, R.: Tobacco, alcohol, asbestos, and nickel in the etiology of cancer of the larynx: A case-control study. J. Natl. Cancer Inst., 67:1219, 1981.

30. Burkitt, D. P., and Trowell, H. C.: Refined Carbohydrate Foods and Disease: Some Implications of Dietary Fibre. London, Academic Press, 1975.

31. Byers, T. E., and Graham, S.: The epidemiology of diet and cancer. Adv. Cancer Res., 41:1, 1984.

32. Byers, T. E., Graham, S., Haughey, B. P., Marshall, J. R., and Swanson, M. K.: Diet and lung cancer risk: Findings from the Western New York Diet Study. Am. J. Epidemiol., 125:351, 1987.

33. Caderni, G., Stuart, E. W., and Bruce, W. R.: Dietary factors affecting the proliferation of epithelial cells in the mouse colon. Nutr. Cancer, 11:147, 1988.

34. Carroll, K. K., and Khor, H. T.: Dietary fat in relation to tumorigenesis. Prog. Biochem. Pharmacol., 10:308, 1975.

35. Carroll, K. K., and Hopkins, G. J.: Dietary polyunsaturated fat versus saturated fat in relation to mammary carcinogenesis. Lipids, 14:155, 1979.

36. Carroll, K. K.: Carbohydrate and Cancer In Human Nutrition: A Comprehensive Treatise, Volume 7, Cancer and Nutrition. Edited by R. B. Alfin-Slater, and D. Kritchevsky. New York, Plenum Press, 1991, p. 97.

37. Chiarodo, A.: National Cancer Institute roundtable on prostate cancer: Future research directions. Cancer Res., 51:2498, 1991.

38. Choi, N. W., Entwistle, D. W., Michaluk, W., and Nelson, N.: Gastric cancer in Icelanders in Manitoba. Isr. J. Med. Sci., 7:1500, 1971.

39. Chu, E. W., and Malmgren, R. A.: An inhibitory effect of vitamin A on the induction of tumors for forestomach and cervix in the Syrian hamster by carcinogenic polycyclic hydrocarbons. Cancer Res., 25:884, 1965.

40. Clark, L. C.: The epidemiology of selenium and cancer. Fed. Proc., 44:2584, 1985.

41. Clinton, S. K., Destree, R., Anderson, D. B., Truex, C. R., Imrey, P. B., and Visek, W. J.: 1,2-dimethylhydrazine-induced colon cancer in rats fed beef or vegetable protein. Nutr. Repts. International, 20:335, 1979.

42. Clinton, S. K., Imrey, P. B., Alster, J. M., Simon, J., Truex, C. R., and Visek, W. J.: The combined effects of dietary protein and fat on 7,12-dimethylbenz(a)anthracene-induced breast cancer in rats. J. Nutr., 114:1213, 1984.

43. Clinton, S. K., Alster, J. M., Imrey, P. B., Nandkumar, S., Truex, C. R., and Visek, W. J.: Effects of dietary protein, fat and energy intake during an initiation phase study of 7,12-dimethylbenz[a]anthracene-induced breast cancer in rats. J. Nutr., 116:2290, 1986.

44. Clinton, S. K., Alster, J. M., Imrey, P. B., Simon, J., and Visek, W. J.: The combined effects of dietary protein and fat intake during the promotion phase of 7,12-dimethylbenz[a]anthracene-induced breast cancer in rats. J. Nutr., 118:1577, 1988.

45. Clinton, S. K., Bostwick, D. G., Olson, L. M., Mangian, H. J. H., and Visek, W. J.: Effects of ammonium acetate and sodium cholate on N-methyl-N-nitrosoguanidine-induced colon carcinogenesis on rats. Cancer Res., 48:3035, 1988.

46. Clinton, S. K., Palmer, S. S., Spriggs, C. E., and Visek, W. J.: The growth of Dunning transplantable prostate adenocarcinomas in rats fed diets varying in fat content. J. Nutr., 118:1577, 1988.

47. Clinton, S. K., and Visek, W. J.: Wheat bran and the induction of intestinal benzo(a)pyrene-hydroxylase by dietary benzo(a)pyrene. J. Nutr., 119:395, 1989.

48. Colditz, G. A., Stampfer, M. J., and Willett, W. C.: Diet and lung cancer. A review of the epidemiologic evidence in humans. Arch. Intern. Med., 147:157, 1987.

49. Colditz, G. A., and Willet, W. C.: Epidemiologic approaches to the study of diet and cancer. In Human Nutrition: A Comprehensive Treatise, Volume 7, Cancer and Nutrition. Edited by R. B. Alfin-Slater, and D. Kritchevsky. New York, Plenum Press, 1991, p. 51.

50. Cook-Mozaffari, P.: The epidemiology of cancer of the oesophagus. Nutr. Cancer, 1:51, 1979.

51. Cook-Mozaffari, P. J., Azordegan, F., Day, W. E., Ressicaud, A., Sabai, C., and Aramesh, B.: Oesophageal cancer studies in the Caspian littoral of Iran: Results of a case-control study. Br. J. Cancer, 39:293, 1979.

52. Coordinating Group for Research on Etiology of Esophageal Cancer in North China: The epidemiology and etiology of esophageal cancer in North China. A preliminary report. Chin. Med. J. (Peking, Engl. Ed.), 1:167, 1975.

53. Corpet, C. E., Stamp, D., Medline, A., Minkin, S., Archer, M., and Bruce, W.: Promotion of colonic microadenoma growth in mice and rats fed cooked sugar or cooked casein and fat. Cancer Res., 50:6955, 1990.
54. Correa, P., Cuello, C., Fajardo, L. F., Haenszel, W., Bolanos, O., and deRamirez, B.: Diet and gastric cancer: Nutrition survey of a high-risk area. J. Natl. Cancer Inst., 70:673, 1983.
55. Correa, P.: The new era of cancer epidemiology. Can. Epidemiol. Control, 1:5, 1991.
56. Cramer, D. W., Welch, W. R., Hutchinson, G. B., Willett, W., and Scully, R. E.: Dietary animal fat in relation to ovarian cancer risk. Obstet. Gynecol., 63:833, 1984.
57. Dales, L. G., Friedman, G. D., Ury, H. K., Grossman, S., and Williams, S. R.: A case-control study of relationships of diet and other traits to colorectal cancer in American blacks. Am. J. Epidemiol., 109:132, 1979.
58. DeCosse, J. J., Miller, H. H., and Lesser, M. L.: Effect of wheat fiber and vitamins C and E on rectal polyps in patients with familial adenomatous polyposis. J. Natl. Cancer Inst., 81:1290, 1989.
59. de Jong, U. W., Breslow, N., Hong, J. G. E., Sridharan, M., and Shanmugaratnam, K.: Aetiological factors in oesophageal cancer in Singapore Chinese. Int. J. Cancer, 13:291, 1974.
60. DeLint, J., and Levinson, T.: Mortality among patients treated for alcoholism: A 5-year follow-up. Can. Med. Assoc. J., 113:385, 1975.
61. Denda, A., Inui, S., Sunagawa, M., Takahashi, S., and Konishi, Y.: Enhancing effect of partial pancreatectomy and ethionine-induced pancreatic regeneration on the tumorigenesis of azaserine in rats. Gann, 69:633, 1978.
62. DHEW (Department of Health, Education, and Welfare): Smoking and Health: A Report of the Surgeon General. 1979. DHEW Publ. No. (PHS) 79-50066. Office on Smoking and Health, Office of the Assistant Secretary for Health, Public Health Service, U. S. Department of Health, Education and Welfare, Rockville, Md., pp. 1164.
63. Dion, P. W., Bright-See, E. B., Smith, C. C., and Bruce, W. R.: The effect of dietary ascorbic acid and alpha-tocoperhol on fecal mutagenicity. Mutation Res., 102:27, 1982.
64. Dion, P., and Bruce, W. R.: Mutagenicity of different fractions of extracts of human feces. Mutation. Res., 119:151, 1983.
65. Doll, R., and Peto, R.: Quantitative estimates of avoidable risks of cancer in the United States today. J. Natl. Cancer Inst., 66:1191, 1981.
66. Dungal, N.: The special problem of stomach cancer in Iceland. With particular reference to dietary factors. J.A.M.A., 176:789, 1961.
67. Ehrich, M., Aswell, J. E., Van Tassell, R. L., and Wilkins, T. D.: Mutagens in the feces of 3 South African populations at different levels of risk for colon cancer. Mutation Res., 64:231, 1979.
68. Flanders, W. D., and Rothman, K. J.: Occupational risk for laryngeal cancer. Am. J. Public Health, 72:369, 1982.
69. Fong, L. Y. Y., Sivak, A., and Newberne, P. M.: Zinc deficiency and methylbenzyl-nitrosamine-induced esophageal cancer in rats. J. Natl. Cancer Inst., 61:145, 1978.
70. Fong, L. Y. Y., Lee, J. S. K., Chan, W. C., and Newberne, P. M.: Zinc deficiency and the development of esophageal and forestomach tumors in Sprague-Dawley rats fed precursors of N-nitro-N-benzylmethylamine. J. Natl. Cancer Inst., 72:419, 1984.
71. Freedman, L. S., Clifford, C., and Messina, M.: Analysis of dietary fat, calories, body weight, and the development of mammary tumors in rats and mice: A review. Cancer Res., 50:5710, 1990.
72. Freidman, G. D., Blaner, W. S., Goodman, D. S., Vogelman, J. H., Brind, J. L., Hoover, R., Fireman, B. H., and Orentreich, N.: Serum retinol and retinol-binding protein levels do not predict subsequent lung cancer. Am. J. Epidemiol., 123:781, 1986.
73. Fritz, W.: Zum Losungsverhalten der Polyaromaten beim Kochen von Kaffee-Ersatzstoffen und Bohnenkaffee. Dtsh. Lebensm. Rundsch., 65:83, 1969.
74. Gabrial, G. N., Schrager, T. F., and Newberne, P. M.: Zinc deficiency, alcohol, and a retinoid: Association with esophageal cancer in rats. J. Natl. Cancer Inst., 68:785, 1982.
75. Garland, C., Shekelle, R. B., Barrett-Connor, E., Criqui, M. H., Rossof, A. H., and Paul, O.: Dietary vitamin D and calcium and risk of colorectal cancer: A 19-year prosective study in men. Lancet, 1:307, 1985.
76. Goodwin, P. J., and Boyd, N. F.: Critical appraisal of the evidence that dietary fat intake is related to breast cancer risk in humans. J. Natl. Cancer Inst., 79:473, 1987.
77. Graham, S., Schotz, W., and Martino, P.: Alimentary factors in the epidemiology of gastric cancer. Cancer, 30:927, 1972.
78. Graham, S., Dayal, H., Rohrer, T., Swanson, M., Sultz, H., Shedd, D., and Fischman, S.: Dentition, diet, tobacco, and alcohol in the epidemiology of oral cancer. J. Natl. Cancer Inst., 59:1611, 1977.
79. Graham, S., Dayal, H., Swanson, M., Mittelman, A., and Wilkinson, G.: Diet in the epidemiology of cancer of the colon and rectum. J. Natl. Cancer Inst., 61:709, 1978.
80. Graham, S., Marshall, J., Mettlin, C., Rzepka, T., Nemoto, T., and Byers, T.: Diet in the epidemiology of breast cancer. Am. J. Epidemiol., 116:68, 1982.
81. Graham, S., Haughey, B., Marshall, J., Priore, R., Byers, T., Rzepka, T., Mettlin, C., and Pontes, J. E.: Diet in the epidemiology of carcinoma of the prostate gland. J. Natl. Cancer Inst., 70:687, 1983.
82. Graham, S., Marshall, J., Haughey, B., Mittelman, A., Swanson, M., Zielezny, M., Byers, T., Wilkinson, G., and West, D.: Dietary epidemiology of cancer of the colon in western New York. Am. J. Epidemiol., 128:490, 1988.
83. Graham, S., Marshall, J., Haughey, B., Brasure, J., Freudenheim, J., Zielezny, M., Wilkinson, G., and Nolan, J.: Nutritional epidemiology of cancer of the esophagus. Am. J. Epidemiol., 131:454, 1990.
84. Gray, G. E., Pike, M. C., and Henderson, B. E.: Breast cancer incidence and mortality rates in different countries in relation to known risk factors and dietary practices. Br. J. Cancer, 39:1, 1979.
85. Greenwald, P., Sondik, E., and Lynch, B. S.: Diet and chemoprevention in NCI's research strategy to achieve national cancer control objectives. Ann. Prev. Public Health, 7:267, 1986.
86. Greenwald, P., Nixon, D. W., Malone, W. F., Kelloff, G. J., Stern, H. R., and Witkin, K. M.: Concepts in cancer chemoprevention research. Cancer, 65:1483, 1990.
87. Gregor, A., Lee, P. N., Roe, F. J. C., Wilson, M. J., and Melton, A.: Comparison of dietary histories in lung cancer cases and controls with special reference to vitamin A. Nutr. Cancer, 2:93, 1980.
88. Gupta, I., Suzuki, K., Bruce, W. R., Krepinsky, J. J., and Yates, P. A.: A model study of fecapentaenes: Mutagens of bacterial origin with alkylating properties. Science, 255:521, 1984.
89. Haenszel, W.: Variation in the incidence of and mortality from stomach cancer, with particular reference to the United States. J. Natl. Cancer Inst., 21:213, 1958.
90. Haenszel, W.: Cancer mortality among the foreign-born in the United States. J. Natl. Cancer Inst., 26:37, 1961.
91. Haenszel, W., Kurihara, M., Segi, M., and Lee, R. K. C.: Stomach cancer among Japanese in Hawaii. J. Natl. Cancer Inst., 49:969, 1972.
92. Haenszel, W., Kurihara, M., Locke, F. B., Shimuzu, K., and Segi, M.: Stomach cancer in Japan. J. Natl. Cancer Inst., 56:265, 1976.
93. Hawksworth, G., Hill, M. J., Gordillo, G., and Cuello, C.: Possible relationship between nitrates, nitrosamines and gastric cancer in southwest Colombia, in N-nitroso Compounds in the Environment. *In* IARC Scientific Publication, Lyon, France, No. 9, 1975, p. 229.
94. Hawrylewicz, E. J., Huang, H. H., Kissane, J. Q., and Drab, E. A.: Enhancement of 7,12-dimethylbenz(a)anthracene (DMBA) mammary tumorigenesis by high protein in rats. Nutr. Rept. Int., 26:793, 1982.
95. Henderson, I. C.: What can a woman do about her risk of dying of breast cancer? Curr. Probl. Cancer, 14:163, 1990.
96. Hennekens, C. H., Eberlein, K. A., and the Physicians' Health Study Research Group: A randomized trial of aspirin and beta-carotene among U. S. physicians. Prev. Med., 14:165, 1985.
97. Herity, B., Moriarty, M., Daly, L., Dunn, J., and Bourke, G. J.: The role of tobacco and alcohol in the aetiology of lung and larynx cancer. Br. J. Cancer, 46:961, 1982.
98. Heshmat, M. Y., Kaul, L., Kovi, J., Jackson, M. A., Jackson, A. G., Jones, G. W., Edson, M., Enterline, J. P., Worrell, R. G., and Perry, S. L.: Nutrition and prostate cancer: A case-control study. Prostate, 6:7, 1985.
99. Higginson, J.: Etiological factors in gastro-intestinal cancer in man. J. Natl. Cancer Inst., 37:527, 1966.
100. Hinds, M. W., Kolonel, L. N., Lee, J., and Hirohata, T.: Associations between cancer incidence and alcohol/cigarette consumption among five ethnic groups in Hawaii. Br. J. Cancer, 41:929, 1980.
101. Hinds, M. W., Kolonel, L. N., Hankin, J. H., and Lee, J.: Dietary cholesterol and lung cancer risk in a multiethnic population in Hawaii. Int. J. Cancer, 32:727, 1983.
102. Hinds, M. W., Kolonel, L. N., Hankin, J. H., and Lee, J.: Dietary vitamin A, carotene, vitamin C and risk of lung cancer in Hawaii. Am. J. Epidemiol., 119:227, 1984.
103. Hirayama, T.: A study of the epidemiology of stomach cancer, with special reference to the effect of diet factor. Bull. Inst. Publ. Health, 12:85, 1963.
104. Hirayama, T.: The epidemiology of cancer of the stomach in Japan, with special reference to the role of diet. Gann Monogr., 3:15, 1968.
105. Hirayama, T.: Epidemiology of breast cancer with special reference to the role of diet. Prev. Med., 7:173, 1978.
106. Hirayama, T.: Diet and cancer. Nutr. Cancer, 1:67, 1979.
107. Hirohata, T., Shigematsu, T., Nomura, A. M., Nomura, Y., Horie, A., and Hirohata, I.: Occurrence of breast cancer in relation to diet and reproductive history: A case-control study in Fukuoka, Japan. Natl. Cancer Inst. Monogr., 69:187, 1985.
108. Hirohata, T., Nomura, A. M., Hankin, J. H., Kolonel, L. N., and Lee, J.: An epidemiologic study on the association between diet and breast cancer. J. Natl. Cancer Inst., 78:595, 1987.
109. Hislop, T. G., Coldman, A. J., Elwood, J. M., Brauer, G., and Kan, L.: Childhood and recent eating patterns and risk of breast cancer. Cancer Detect. Prev., 9:47, 1986.
110. Hoffman, F. L.: Cancer and Diet. Baltimore, The Williams & Wilkins Co., 1937.
111. Hong, W. K., Endicott, J., Itri, L. M., Doos, W., Batsakis, J. G., Bell, R., Fofonoff, S., Byers, R., Atkinson, E. N., Vaughan, C., Toth, B., Kramer, A., Dimery, I., Skipper, P., and Strong, S.: 13 cis-retinoic acid in the treatment of oral leukoplakia. N. Engl. J. Med., 315:1501, 1986.
112. Hong, W. K., Lippman, S. M., Itri, L. M., Karp, D. D., Lee, J. S., Byers, R. M., Schantz, S. P., Kramer, A. M., Lotan, R., Peters, L. J., Dimery, I. W., Brown, B. W., and Goepfert, H.: Prevention of second primary tumors with isotretinoin in squamous-cell carcinoma of the head and neck. N. Engl. J. Med., 323:1278, 1990.
113. Hormozdiari, H., Day, N. E., Aramesh, B., and Mahboubi, E.: Dietary factors and esophageal cancer in the Caspian littoral of Iran. Cancer Res., 35:3493, 1975.
114. Howard, J. W., and Fazio, T.: Review of polycyclic aromatic hydrocarbons in foods. Analytical methodology and reported findings of polycyclic aromatic hydrocarbons in foods. J. Assoc. Off. Anal. Chem., 63:1077, 1980.
115. Howe, G. R.: The use of polytomous dual response data to increase power in case-control studies: An application to the association between dietary fat and breast cancer. J. Chronic Dis., 38:663, 1985.
116. Howe, G. R., Miller, A. B., and Jain, M.: Re: "Total energy intake: implications for epidemiologic analyses." Am. J. Epidemiol., 124:157, 1986.
117. Howell, M. A.: Factor analysis of international cancer mortality data and per capita food consumption. Br. J. Cancer, 29:328, 1974.
118. Howson, C. P., Hiryama, T., and Wynder, E. L.: The decline in gastric cancer: epidemiology of an unplanned triumph. Epidemiol. Rev., 8:1, 1986.
119. Jacobs, L. R.: Relationship between dietary fiber and cancer: metabolic, physiologic and cellular mechanisms. Proc. Soc. Exp. Biol. Med., 183:290, 1986.
120. Jacobs, L. R.: Dietary fiber and cancer. J. Nutr., 117:1319, 1987.
121. Jacobsen, B. K., Bjelke, E., Kvale, G., and Heuch, I.: Coffee drinking, mortality and cancer incidence: Results from a Norweigan prospective study. J. Natl. Cancer Inst., 76:823, 1986.
122. Jain, M., Cook, G. M., Davis, F. G., Grace, M. G., Howe, G. R., and Miller, A. B.: A case-control study of diet and colo-rectal cancer. Int. J. Cancer, 26:757, 1980.
123. Jensen, O. M., Maclennan, R., and Wahrendorf, J.: Diet, bowel function, fecal characteristics and large bowel cancer in Denmark and Finland. Nutr. Cancer, 4:5, 1982.
124. Jensen, O. M.: The epidemiology of large bowel cancer. *In* Diet, Nutrition, and Cancer: A Critical Evaluation, Vol. 1, Macronutrients and Cancer. Edited by B. S. Reddy and L. A. Cohen. Boca Raton, CRC Press, Inc., 1986, pp. 27–46.
125. Jensen, O. M., Wahrendorf, J., Knudsen, J. B., and Sorenson, B. L.: The Copenhagen case-control study of bladder cancer. II. The effect of coffee and other beverages. Int. J. Cancer, 37:651, 1986.
126. Joosens, J. V., and Geboers, J.: Dietary salt and risks to health. Am. J. Clin. Nutr., 45:1277, 1987.
127. Johansen, H. L., and Neutel, C. I.: Epidemiological studies in nutrition: Utility and limitations. J. Nutr., 118:137, 1988.
128. Junshi, C., Campbell, T. C., Junyao, L., and Peto, R.: Diet, Life-style, and Mortality in China. Oxford, Oxford University Press, 1990.

129. Kamiyama, S., Ohshima, H., Shimada, A., Saito, N., Bourgade, M., Ziegler, P., and Bartsch, H.: Urinary excretion of N-nitrosamino acids and nitrate by inhabitants in high- and low-risk areas for stomach cancer in northern Japan. IARC Scil. Publ., 84:497, 1987.
130. Katsouyanni, K., Willett, W., Trichopoulos, D., Boyle, P., Trichopoulou, A., Vasilaros, S., Papadiamanits, J., and MacMahon, B.: Risk of breast cancer among Greek women in relation to nutrient intake. Cancer, 61:181, 1988.
131. Keller, A. Z., and Terris, M.: The association of alcohol and tobacco with cancer of the mouth and pharynx. Am. J. Public Health, 55:1578, 1965.
132. Keller, A. Z.: The epidemiology of esophageal cancer in the west. Prev. Med., 9:607, 1980.
133. Kennaway, E. L., and Kennaway, N. M.: Further study of incidence of cancer of lung and larynx. Br. J. Cancer, 1:260, 1947.
134. Kirchner, J. A., and Malkin, J. S.: Cancer of larynx; 30-year survey at New Haven Hospital. Arch. Otolaryngol., 58:19, 1953.
135. Kolonel, L. N., Hinds, M. W., and Hankin, J. H.: Cancer patterns among migrant and native-born Japanese in Hawaii in relation to smoking, drinking, and dietary habits. *In* Genetic and Environmental Factors in Experimental and Human Cancer. Edited by H. V. Gelboin, M. MacMahon, T. Matsushima, T. Sugimura, S. Takayama, and H. Takebe. Tokyo, Japan Scientific Societies Press, 1980, pp. 327.
136. Kolonel, L. N., Yoshizawa, C. N., and Hankin, J. H.: Diet and prostatic cancer: A case-study control in Hawaii. Am. J. Epidemiol., 127:999, 1988.
137. Kritchevsky, D., and Klurfeld, D. M.: Dietary fiber and Cancer. *In* Human Nutrition: A Comprehensive Treatise, Volume 7, Cancer and Nutrition. Edited by R. B. Alfin-Slater and D. Kritchevsky. New York, Plenum Press, 1991, p. 211.
138. Kritchevsky, D., and Klurfeld, D. M.: Fat and Cancer. *In* Human Nutrition: A Comprehensive Treatise, Volume 7, Cancer and Nutrition. Edited by R. B. Alfin-Slater and D. Kritchevsky. New York, Plenum Press, 1991, p. 51.
139. Kuhnlein, H., Kuhnlein, U., and Bell, P. A.: The effect of short-term dietary modification on human fecal mutagenic activity. Mutation Res., 113:1, 1983.
140. Kune, G. A., and Kune, S.: The nutritional causes of colorectal cancer: an introduction to the Melbourene study. Nutr. Cancer, 9:1, 1987a.
141. Kune, S., Kune, G. A., and Watson, L. F.: Case-control study of dietary etiological factors: The Melbourne Colorectal Cancer Study. Nutr. Cancer, 9:21, 1987b.
142. Kurihara, M., Aoki, K., and Tominaga, S.: Cancer Mortality Statistics in the World. Nagoya, University of Nagoya Press, 1984.
143. Kvale, G., Bjelke, E., and Gart, J. J.: Dietary habits and lung cancer risk. Int. J. Cancer, 31:397, 1983.
144. Langhans, P., Heger, R. A., Hoberstein, J., and Bunte, H.: Operation-sequel carcinoma. An experimental study. Hepato-Gastroenterology, 28:34, 1981.
145. La Vecchia, C., Decarli, A., Negri, E., Parazzini, F., Gentile, A., Cecchetti, G., Fasoli, M., and Franceschi, S.: Dietary factors and the risk of epithelial ovarian cancer. J. Natl. Cancer Inst., 79:663, 1987.
146. Lew, E. A., and Garfinkel, L.: Variations in mortality by weight among 750,000 men and women. J. Chronic Dis., 32:563, 1979.
147. Lijinsky, W., and Shubik, P.: Benzo(a)pyrene and other polynuclear hydrocarbons in charcoal-broiled meat. Science, 145:53, 1964.
148. Linsell, C. A., and Peers, F. G.: Aflatoxin and liver cell cancer. Trans Roy. Soc. Trop. Med. Hyg., 71:471, 1977.
149. Lipkin, M.: Calcium modulation of intermediate biomarkers in the gastrointestinal tract. *In* Calcium, Vitamin D and Cancer. Edited by M. Lipkin, G. Kelloff, and H. Newmark. Boca Raton, CRC Press, 1991.
150. Liu, K., Stamler, J., Moss, D., Garside, D., Persky, V., and Soltero, I.: Dietary cholesterol, fat, and fibre, and colon-cancer mortality. Lancet, 2:782, 1979.
151. Lo, M.-T., and Sandi, E.: Polycyclic aromatic hydrocarbons (polynuclears) in foods. Residue Rev., 69:35, 1978.
152. Longnecker, D. S., Roebuck, B. D., Yager, J. D., Jr., Lilja, H. S., and Siegmund, B. T.: Pancreatic carcinoma in azaserine-treated rats: Induction, classification, and dietary modulation of incidence. Cancer, 47:1562, 1981.
153. Longnecker, D. S., Curphey, T. J., Kuhlmann, E. T., and Roebuck, B. D.: Inhibition of pancreatic carcinogenesis by retinoids in azaserine-treated rats. Cancer Res., 42:19, 1982.
154. Longnecker, D. S., Kuhlmann, E. T., and Curphey, T. J.: Divergent effects of retinoids on pancreatic and liver carcinogenesis in azaserine-treated rats. Cancer Res., 43:3219, 1983.
155. Longnecker, D. S., Kuhlmann, E. T., and Curphey, T. J.: Effects of four retinoids in N-nitrosobis(2-oxopropyl)amine-treated hamsters. Cancer Res., 43:3226, 1983.
156. Longnecker, D. S., and Morgan, R G. H.: Diet and cancer of the pancreas: epidemiological and experimental evidence: *In* Diet, Nutrition, and Cancer: A Critical Evaluation. Vol. 1. Macronutrients and Cancer. Edited by B. S. Reddy, and L. A. Cohen. Boca Raton, CRC Press, Inc., 1986, p. 11.
157. Longnecker, M. P., Berlin, J. A., Orza, M. J., and Chlmers, T. C.: A metaanalysis of alcohol consumption in relation to risk of breast cancer. J.A.M.A., 260:652, 1988.
158. Lu, S., Ohshima, H., Fu, H., Tian, Y., Li, F., Blettner, M., Wahrendorf, J., and Bartsch, H.: Urinary excretion of N-nitrosoamino acids and nitrate by inhabitants of high- and low-risk areas for esophageal cancer in northern China: Endogenous formation of nitrosoproline and its inhibition by vitamin C. Cancer Res., 46:1485, 1986.
159. Lubin, J. H., Burns, P. E., Blot, W. J., Ziegler, R. G., Lees, A. W., and Fraumeni, J. F., Jr.: Dietary factors and breast cancer risk. Int. J. Cancer, 28:685, 1981.
160. Lubin, F., Wax, Y., and Modan, B.: Role of fat, animal protein, and dietary fiber in breast cancer etiology: A case-control study. J. Natl. Cancer Inst., 77:605, 1986.
161. Luo, X. M., Wei, H. J., and Yang, S. P.: Inhibitory effect of molybdenum on esophageal and forestomach carcinogenesis in rats. J. Natl. Cancer Inst., 71:75, 1983.
162. Lyon, J. L., Klauber, M. R., Gardner, J. W., and Smart, C. R.: Cancer incidence in Mormons and non-Mormons in Utah, 1966–1970. N. Engl. J. Med., 294:129, 1976.
163. Lyon, J. L., and Sorenson, A. W.: Colon cancer in a low-risk population. Am. J. Clin. Nutr., 31:S227, 1978.
164. Lyon, J. L., Gardner, J. W., and West, D. W.: Cancer risk and lifestyle: Cancer among Mormons (1967–1975). *In* Genetic Environmental Factors in Experimental and Human Cancer. Edited by H. V. Gelboin, B. MacMahon, T. Matsushima, T. Sugimura, S. Takayama, and H. Takebe. Tokyo, Japan Scientific Societies Press, 1980a, pp. 273–290.
165. Lyon, J. L., Gardner, J. W., and West, D. W.: Cancer risk and lifestyle: Cancer among Mormons (1967–1975). *In* Cancer Incidence in Defined Populations. Banbury Report 4. Edited by J. Cairns, J. L. Lyon, and M. Skolnick. Cold Spring Harbor, NY, Cold Spring Harbor Laboratory, 1980b, p. 3.
166. Lyon, J. L., Mahoney, A. W., West, D. W., Gardner, J. W., Smith, K. R., Sorenson, A. W., and Stanish, W.: Energy intake: Its relationship to colon cancer risk. J. Natl. Cancer Inst., 78:853, 1987.
167. MacDonald, W. E., Anderson, F. H., and Hashimoto, S.: Histological effect of certain pickles on the human gastric mucosa. Can. Med. Assoc. J., 96:1521, 1967.
168. Mack, T. M.: Pancreas. *In* Cancer Epidemiology and Prevention. Edited by D. Schottenfeld and E. F. Fraumeni, Jr. Philadelphia, W. B. Saunders, 1982, p. 638.
169. MacLennan, R., DaCosta, J., Day, N. E., Law, C. H., Ng, Y. K., and Shanmugaratnam, K.: Risk factors for lung cancer in Singapore Chinese, a population with high female incidence rates. Int. J. Cancer, 20:854, 1977.
170. MacMahon, B.: Risk factors for cancer of the pancreas. Cancer, 50:2676, 1982.
171. Macquart-Moulin, G., Riboli, E., Cornee, J., Charnay, B., Berthezene, P., and Day, N.: Case-control study on colorectal cancer and diet in Marseilles. Int. J. Cancer, 38:183, 1986.
172. Mahboubi, E., Kmet, J., Cook, P. J., Day, N. E., Ghadirian, P., and Salmasizadeh, S.: Oesophageal cancer studies in the Caspian Littoral of Iran: the Caspian cancer registry. Br. J. Cancer, 28:197, 1973.
173. Mahboudi, E., and Sayed, G. M.: Oval Cavity and Pharynx. *In* Cancer Epidemiology and Prevention. Edited by D. Schottenfeld, and J. F. Fraumeni, Jr. Philadelphia, Saunders, 1982, p. 583.
174. Malhotra, S. L.: Dietary factors in a study of colon cancer from cancer registry, with special reference to the role of saliva, milk and fermented milk products and vegetable fibre. Med. Hypotheses, 3:122, 1977.
175. Manousos, O., Day, N. E., Trichopoulos, D., Gerovassilis, F., Tzonou, A., and Polychronopoulou, A.: Diet and colorectal cancer: A case-control study in Greece. Int. J. Cancer, 32:1, 1983.
176. Marasas, W. F. O., van Rensburg, S. J., and Mirocha, C. J.: Incidence of Fusarium species and the mycotoxins, deoxynivalenol and zearalenone, in corn produced in esophageal cancer areas in Transkei. J. Agric. Food Chem., 27:1108, 1979.
177. Marshall, J., Graham, S., and Mettlin, C.: Diet in the epidemiology of oral cancer. Nutr. Cancer, 3:145, 1982.
178. Martinez, I.: Factors associated with cancer of the esophagus, mouth and pharynx in Puerto Rico. J. Natl. Cancer Inst., 42:1069, 1969.
179. Mashberg, A., Garfinkel, L., and Harris, S.: Alcohol as a primary risk factor in oral squamous carcinoma. CA, 31:146, 1981.
180. McGee, D., Reed, D., Stemmermann, G., Rhoads, G., Yano, K., and Feinleib, M.: The relationship of dietary fat and cholesterol to mortality in 10 years: The Honolulu Heart Program. Int. J. Epidemiol., 14:97, 1985.
181. McGuinness, E. E., Morgan, R. G. H., Levison, D. A., Frape, D. L., Hopwood, D., and Wormsley, K. G.: The effects of long-term feeding of soya flour on the rat pancreas. Scand. J. Gastroenterol., 15:497, 1980.
182. McGuinness, E. E., Morgan, R. G. H., Levison, D. A., Hopwood, D., and Wormsley, K. G.: Interaction of azaserine and raw soya flour on the rat pancreas. Scand. J. Gastroenterol., 16:49, 1981.
183. McGuinness, E. E., Hopwood, D., and Wormsley, K. G.: Further studies of the effects of raw soya flour on the rat pancreas. Scand. J. Gastroenterol., 17:273, 1982.
184. McGuinness, E. E., Hopwood, D., and Wormsley, K. G.: Potentiation of pancreatic carcinogenesis in the rat by DL-ethionine-induced pancreatitis. Scand. J. Gastroenterol., 18:189, 1983.
185. McMichael, A. J., McCall, M. G., Hartshome, J. M., and Woodlings, T. L.: Patterns of intestinal cancer in European migrants to Australia: The role of dietary change. Int. J. Cancer, 25:431, 1980.
186. McMichael, A. J.: Serum cholesterol and human cancer. *In* Human Nutrition: A Comprehensive Treatise, Volume 7, Cancer and Nutrition. Edited by R. B. Alfin-Slater, and D. Kritchevsky. New York, Plenum Press, 1991, p. 141.
187. Menkes, M. S., Comstock, G. W., Vuilleumier, J. P., Helsing, K. J., Rider, A. A., and Brookmeyer, R.: Serum beta-carotene, vitamins A and E, selenium, and the risk of lung cancer. N. Engl. J. Med., 315:1250, 1986.
188. Merrill, A. H., Foltz, A. T., and McCormick, D. B.: Vitamins and Cancer. *In* Human Nutrition: A Comprehensive Treatise, Volume 7, Cancer and Nutrition. Edited by R. B. Alfin-Slater and D. Kritchevsky. New York, Plenum Press, 1991, p. 262.
189. Mettlin, C., and Graham, S.: Dietary risk factors in human bladder cancer. Am. J. Epidemiol., 110:255, 1979.
190. Mettlin, C., Graham, S., and Swanson, M.: Vitamin A and lung cancer. J. Natl. Cancer Inst., 62:1435, 1979.
191. Mettlin, C., Graham, S., Priore, R., Marshall, J., and Swanson, M.: Diet and cancer of the esophagus. Nutr. Cancer, 2:143, 1980.
192. Miller, A. B., Kelly, A., Choi, N. W., Matthews, V., Morgan, R. W., Munan, L., Burch, J. D., Feather, J., Howe, G. R., and Jain, M.: A study of diet and breast cancer. Am. J. Epidemiol., 107:499, 1978.
193. Miller, A. B., Howe, G. R., Jain, M., Craib, K. J. P., and Harrison, L.: Food items and food groups as risk factors in a case-control study of diet and colo-rectal cancer. Int. J. Cancer, 32:155, 1983.
194. Miller, A. B.: Nutrition and the Epidemiology of Breast Cancer. *In* Diet Nutrition, and Cancer: A Critical Evaluation, Vol. 1, Macronutrients and Cancer. Edited by B. S. Reddy and L. A. Cohen. Boca Raton, CRC Press, Inc., 1986.
194a. Miller, J. A., Carcinogenesis by chemicals: An overview—GHA Clowes Memorial Lecture. Cancer Res., 30:559, 1970.
195. Modan, B., Barell, V., Lubin, F., Modan, M., Greenberg, R. A., and Graham, S.: Low-fiber intake as an etiologic factor in cancer of the colon. J. Natl. Cancer Inst., 55:15, 1975.
196. Montes, G., Cuello, C., Gordillo, G., Pelon, W., Johnson, W., and Correa, P.: Mutagenic activity of gastric juice. Cancer Lett., 7:307, 1979.
197. Morgan, R. G. H., Levinson, D. A., Hopwood, D., Saunders, J. H. B., and Wormsley, K. G.: Potentiation of the action of azaserine on the rat pancreas by raw soya bean flour. Cancer Lett., 3:87, 1977.
198. Morris, J. S. I., Stampfer, J. J., and Willet, W. C.: Dietary selenium in humans. Toenails as an indicator. Biol. Trace Element Res., 5:529, 1983.
199. Mower, H. F., Ichinotsubo, D., Wang, L. W., Mandel, M., Stemmermann, G., Nomura, A., Heilbrun, L., Kamiyama, S., and Shimada, A.: Fecal mutagens in two Japanese populations with different colon cancer risks. Cancer Res., 42:1164, 1982.
200. Munoz, N., Wahrendorf, J., Lu, J. B., Crespi, M., Day, N. E., Thurnham, D. I., Zhang,

C. Y., Zheng, H. J., Li, B., Li, W. Y., Lin, G. L., Lan, X. Z., Correa, P., Grassi, A., O'Connor, G. T., and Bosch, F. X.: No effect of riboflavine, retinol, and zinc on precancerous lesions of the oesophagus: A randomized double-blind intervention study in a high-risk population in China. Lancet, 2:111, 1985.
201. Nagai, M., Hashimoto, T., Yanagawa, H., Yokoyama, H., and Minowa, M.: Relationship of diet to the incidence of esophageal and stomach cancer in Japan. Nutr. Cancer, 3:257, 1982.
202. National Academy of Sciences: Toward Healthful Diets. National Academy Press, Washington, DC, 1978.
203. National Academy of Sciences, National Research Council: Nutrient Requirements of Laboratory Animals, No. 10, Washington, DC, 1978.
204. National Academy of Sciences: Committee on Diet, Nutrition, and Cancer. *In* Diet, Nutrition, and Cancer, National Academy Press, Washington, DC, 1982.
205. National Academy of Sciences, National Research Council: Evaluation of cyclamate for carcinogenicity. Report of Committee on the Evaluation of Cyclamate for Carcinogenicity, Commission of Life sciences, National Academy Press, Washington, D. C., 1985.
206. National Academy of Sciences, Committee on Diet and Health, Food and Nutrition Board, Commission on Life sciences, National Research Council. *In* Diet and Health: Implications for Reducing Chronic Disease Risk. National Academy Press, Washington, DC, 1989.
207. National Cancer Institute. Diet, Nutrition, and Cancer Prevention: A Guide to Food Choices. NIH Pub. No. 87-28-78, National Institutes of Health, Public Health Service, U.S. Dept. Health and Human Services. U.S. Government Printing Office, Washington, DC, 1987.
208. Nauss, K. M., Bueche, D., Soule, N., Fu, P., Yew, K., and Newberne, P. M.: Effect of dietary selenium levels on methylbenzylnitrosamine-induced esophageal cancer in rats. Cancer Lett., 33:107, 1986.
209. Nauss, K. M., Bueche, D., and Newberne, P. M. Effect of vitamin A nutriture on experimental esophageal carcinogenesis. J. Natl. Cancer Inst., 79(1):145, 1987.
210. Nevalainen, T. J., and Janigan, D. T.: Degeneration of mouse pancreatic acinar cells during fasting. Virchows. Arch. B, 15:107, 1974.
211. Newberne, P. M., Bieri, J. G., Briggs, G. M., and Nesheim, M. C.: Control of diets in laboratory animal experimentation. ILAR News, 21:A3, 1978.
212. Newberne, P. M., and Nauss, K. M.: Dietary fat and colon cancer: Variable results in animal models. Prog. Clin. Biol. Res., 222:311, 1986.
213. Nomura, A. M., Stemmermann, G. N., Heilbrun, L. K., Salkeld, R. M., and Vuilleumier, J. P.: Serum vitamin levels and the risk of cancer of specific sites to men of Japanese ancestry in Hawaii. Cancer Res., 45:2369, 1985.
214. Nomura, A., Stemmermann, G., Chyou, P., Kato, I., Perez-Perez, G., and Blaser, M.: Helicobacter pylori infection and gastric carcinoma among Japanese Americans in Hawaii. N. Engl. J. Med., 325:1132, 1991.
215. O'Connor, T. P., Youngman, L. D., and Campbell, T. C.: Effect of selenium on development of L-azaserine induced preneoplastic abnormal acinar cell nodules in rat pancreas. Fed. Proc., 42:670, 1983.
216. Olsen, J., Sabreo, S., and Fasting, U.: Interaction of alcohol and tobacco risk factors in cancer of the laryngeal region. J. Epidemiol. Community Health, 39:165, 1985.
217. Olson, J. A.: Nutrition monitoring and nutrition status assessment: An overview. J. Nutr., 120:1431–1432, 1990.
218. Oshima, H., and Bartsch, H.: Quantitative estimation of endogenous nitrosation in humans by monitoring N-nitrosoproline excreted in the urine. Cancer Res., 41:3568, 1981.
219. Paganini-Hill, A., Chao, A., Ross, R. K., and Henderson, B. E.: Vitamin A, β-carotene, and the risk of cancer: a prospective study. J. Natl. Cancer Inst., 79:443, 1987.
220. Parsonnet, J., Friedman, G., Vandersteen, D., Chang, Y., Vogelman, J., Orentreich, N., and Sibley, R.: Helicobacter pylori infection and the risk of gastric carcinoma. N. Engl. J. Med., 325:1127, 1991.
221. Paymaster, J. C., Sanghvi, L. D., and Gangadharan, P.: Cancer in the gastrointestinal tract in Western India. Epidemiologic study. Cancer, 21:279, 1968.
222. Peleg, I., Heyden, A., Knowles, M., and Hames, C. G.: Serum retinol and risk of subsequent cancer: Extension of the Evans County, Georgia, study. J. Natl. Cancer Inst., 73:1455, 1984.
223. Pennington, J. A. T.: Revision of the total diet study food list and diets. J. Am. Dietetic Assoc., 82:166, 1983.
224. Piacek-Llanes, B., and Tannenbaum, S. R.: Formation of an activated N-nitroso compound in nitrite-treated fava beans (Vicia faba). Carcinogenesis, 3:1379, 1982.
225. Pott, P.: Cancer scroti, *In:* Chirurgical Observations Relative to the Cataract, the Polypus of the Nose, the Cancer of the Scrotum, the Different Kind of Ruptures, and the Mortification of the Toes and Feet, 1775.
226. Potter, J. D., and McMichael, A. J.: Diet and cancer of the colon and rectum: a case-control study. J. Natl. Cancer Inst., 76:557, 1986.
227. Pottern, L. M., Morris, L. E., Blot, W. J., Ziegler, R. G., and Fraumeni, J. F.: Esophageal cancer among black men in Washington, D.C. I. Alcohol, tobacco and other risk factors. J. Natl. Cancer Inst., 67:777, 1984.
228. Pottern, L. M., Morris, L. E., Blot, W. J., Ziegler, R. G., and Fraumeni, J. F.: Prospective study of alcohol consumption and cancer. N. Engl. J. Med., 310:617, 1984.
229. Pour, P. M., Runge, R. G., Birt, D., Gingell, R., Lawson, T., Nagel, D., Wallacave, L., and Salmasi, S. Z.: Current knowledge of pancreatic carcinogenesis in the hamster and its relevance to the human disease. Cancer, 47:1573 1981.
230. Pour, P. M., and Birt, D. F.: Modifying factors in pancreatic carcinogenesis in the hamster model. IV. Effects of dietary protein. J. Natl. Cancer Inst., 71:347, 1983.
231. Pour, P. M., Birt, D. F., Salmasi, S. Z., and Gotz, U.: Modifying factors in pancreatic carcinogenesis in the hamster model. I. Effect of protein-free diet fed during the early stages of carcinogenesis. J. Natl. Cancer Inst., 70:141, 1983.
232. Pour, P. M., Reber, H. A., and Stepan, K.: Modification of pancreatic carcinogenesis in the hamster model. XII. Dose-related effect of ethanol. J. Natl. Cancer Inst., 71:1085, 1983.
233. Prentice, R. L., Kakar, F., Hursting, S., Sheppard, L., Klein, R., and Kushi, L. H.: Aspects of the rationale for the Women's Health Trial. J. Natl. Cancer Inst., 80:802, 1988.
234. Prentice, R. L., Pepe, M., and Self, S. G.: Dietary fat and breast cancer: A quantitative assessment of the epidemiological literature and a discussion of methodological issues. Cancer Res., 49:3147, 1989.
235. Price, J. M., Biava, C. G., Oser, B. L., Vogin, E. E., Steinfeld, J., and Ley, H. L.: Bladder tumors in rats fed cyclohexamine or high doses of a mixture of cyclamate and saccharin. Science, 167:1131, 1970.
236. Purtilo, D. T., and Gottlieb, L. S.: Cirrhosis and hepatoma occurring at Boston City Hospital (1917–1968). Cancer, 32:458, 1973.
237. Rao, G. N., and Knapka, J. J.: Contaminant and nutrient concentrations of natural ingredient rat and mouse diet used in chemical toxicology studies. Fund. Appl. Toxicol., 9:329, 1987.
238. Reddy, B. S., Hedges, A. R., Laakso, K., and Wynder, E. L.: Metabolic epidemiology of large bowel cancer: Fecal bulk and constituents of high-risk North American and low-risk Finnish population. Cancer, 42:2832, 1978.
239. Reddy, B. S.: Diet and colon cancer: Evidence from human and animal model studies. *In* Diet, Nutrition, and Cancer: A Critical Evaluation. Vol. 1. Macronutrients and Cancer. Edited by B. S. Reddy and L. A. Cohen. Boca Raton, CRC Press, Inc., 1986, p. 47.
240. Reddy, B. S., and Cohen, L. A.: Diet, Nutrition and Cancer: A Critical Evaluation. Vol. 1. Macronutrients and Cancer. Boca Raton, CRC Press, Inc., 1986.
241. Reddy, B. S., Sharma, C., Simi, B., Engle, A., Laakso, K., Puska, P., and Korpela, R.: Metabolic epidemiology of colon cancer: effect of dietary fiber on fecal mutagens and bile acids in healthy subjects. Cancer Res., 47:644, 1987.
242. Rigdon, R. H., and Neal, J.: Relationship of leukemia to lung and stomach tumors in mice fed benzo(a)pyrene. Proc. Soc. Exp. Biol. Med., 130:146, 1969.
243. Risch, H. A., Jain, M., Choi, N. W., Fodor, J. G., Pfeiffer, C. J., Howe, G. R., Harrison, L. W., Craib, K. J., and Miller, A. B.: Dietary factors and the incidence of cancer of the stomach. Am. J. Epidemiol., 122:947, 1985.
244. Roebuck, B. D., Yager, J. D., Jr., and Longnecker, D. S.: Dietary modulation of azaserine-induced pancreatic carcinogenesis in the rat. Cancer Res., 41:888, 1981.
245. Roebuck, B. D., Yager, J. D., Jr., Longnecker, D. S., and Wilpone, S. A.: Promotion by unsaturated fat of azaserine-induced pancreatic carcinogenesis in the rat. Cancer Res., 41:3961, 1981.
246. Rogers, A. E., and Longnecker, M. P.: Biology of disease. Dietary and nutritional influences on cancer: A review of epidemiological and experimental data. Lab. Invest., 59:729, 1988.
247. Rogers, A. E., and Conner, M. W.: Interrelationships of alcohol and cancer. *In* Human Nutrition: A Comprehensive Treatise, Volume 7, Cancer and Nutrition. Edited by R. B. Alfin-Slater and D. Kritchevsky. New York, Plenum Press, 1991, pp. 51–68.
248. Rohan, T. E. I., and Bain, C. J.: Diet in the etiology of breast cancer. Epidemiol. Rev., 9:120, 1987.
249. Rose, D. P., Boyar, A. P., and Wynder, E. L.: International comparisons of mortality rates for cancer of the breast, ovary, prostate, and colon, and per capita food consumption. Cancer, 58:2363, 1986.
250. Ross, R. K., Paganini-Hill, A., and Henderson, B. E.: The etiology of prostate cancer: What does the epidemiology suggest? Prostate, 4:333, 1983.
251. Ross, R. K., Shimizu, H., Paganini-Hill, A., Honda, G., and Henderson, B. E.: Case-control studies of prostate cancer in blacks and whites in Southern California. J. Natl. Cancer Inst., 78:869, 1987.
252. Rothman, K., and Keller, A.: The effect of joint exposure to alcohol and tobacco on risk of cancer of the mouth and pharynx. J. Chronic Dis., 25:711, 1972.
253. Rotkin, I. D.: Studies in the epidemiology of prostatic cancer: Expanded sampling. Cancer Treat. Rep., 61:173, 1977.
254. Ruddell, W. S. J., Bone, E. S., Hill, M. J., and Walters, C. L.: Pathogenesis of gastric cancer in pernicious anaemia. Lancet, 1:521, 1978.
255. Ruggeri, B.: The effects of caloric restriction on neoplasia and age-related degenerative processes. *In* Human Nutrition: A Comprehensive Treatise, Volume 7, Cancer and Nutrition. Edited by R. B. Alfin-Slater, and D. Kritchevsky. New York, Plenum Press, 1991, p. 187.
256. Salonen, J. T., Salonen, R., Lappetelainen, R., Maenpaa, P. H., Alfthan, G., and Puska, P.: Risk of cancer in relation to serum concentrations of selenium and vitamins A and E: Matched case-control analysis of prospective data. Br. Med. J., 290:417, 1985.
257. Samet, J. M., Skipper, B. J., Humble, C. G., and Pathak, D. R.: Lung cancer risk and vitamin A consumption in New Mexico. Am. Rev. Respir. Dis., 131:198, 1985.
258. Sander, J., Burkle, G., and Schweinsberg, F.: Induktion malignen tumoren bei ratten durch gleichzeitge verfutterung von nitrit und sek underen aminen. Z. Krebsforsch., 73:54, 1969.
259. Sato, T., Fukuyama, T., Susuki, T., and Takayanagi, J.: The relationship between gastric cancer mortality rate and salted food intake in several places in Japan. Bull. Inst. Publ. Health, 8:187, 1959.
260. Sato, T., Fukuyama, T., Urata, G., and Suzuki, T.: Bleeding in the glandular stomach of mice by feeding highly salted foods and a comment on salted foods in Japan. Bull. Inst. Publ. Health, 8:10, 1959.
261. Schatzkin, A., Greenwald, P., Byer, D., and Clifford, C.: The dietary fat-breast cancer hypothesis is alive. J. Am. Med. Assoc., 261:3284, 1989.
262. Schiffman, M. H., Andrews, A. W., Van Tassell, R. L., Smith, L., Daniel, J., Robinson, A., Hoover, R. N., Rosenthal, J., Weil, R., Nair, P. P., Schwartz, S., Pettigrew, H., Batist, G., Shaw, R., and Wilkins, T. D.: Case control study of colorectal cancer and fecal mutagenicity. Cancer Res., 49:3420, 1989.
263. Schiffman, M. H., and Felton, J. S.: Re: "Fried foods and the risk of colon cancer." Am. J. Epidemiol., 131:376, 1990.
264. Schirai, T., Imaida, K., Fukushima, S., Hasegawa, R., Tatematsu, M., and Ito, N.: Effects of NaCl, Tween 60 and a low dose of N-ethyl-N′-nitro-N-nitrosoguanidine on gastric carcinogenesis of rats given a single dose of N-methyl-N′-nitro-N′-nitrosoguanidine. Carcinogenesis, 12:1419, 1982.
265. Schlag, P., Ulrich, H., Merkle, P., Bockler, R., Peter, M., and Herfarth, C.: Are nitrite and N-nitroso compounds in gastric juices risk factors for carcinoma of the operated stomach? Lancet, 1:727, 1980.
266. Schoenberg, B., Bailar, J. C., and Fraumeni, J. F.: Certain mortality patterns of esophageal cancer in the United States 1930–1967. J. Natl. Cancer Inst., 46:63, 1971.
267. Schottenfeld, D.: Epidemiology of cancer of the esophagus. Semin. Oncol., 11:92, 1984.
268. Schuman, L. M., Mandel, J. S., Radke, A., Seal, U., and Halberg, F.: Some selected features of the epidemiology of prostatic cancer: Minneapolis-St. Paul, Minnesota case-control study, 1976–1979. *In* Trends in Cancer Incidence: Causes and Practical Implications. Edited by K. Magnus. Washington, D. C., Hemisphere Publishing Corp., 1982, p. 345.

269. Schwartz, D., Lellouch, J., Flamant, R., and Denoix, P. F.: Alcohol and cancer. Results of a retrospective investigation. Rev. Fr. Etud. Clin. Biol., 7:590, 1962.

270. Shekelle, R. B., Lepper, M., Liu, S., Maliza, C., Raynor, W. J., Jr., Rossof, A. H., Paul, O., Shryock, A. M., and Stamler, J.: Dietary vitamin A and risk of cancer in the Western Electric study. Lancet, 2:1186, 1981.

271. Shimkin, M. B.: Contrary to Nature. U.S. Dept. of Health, Education, and Welfare, Public Health Service, National Institutes of Health, DHEW Publication No. (NIH) 76-720, 1977.

272. Shimkin, M. B.: Silvergirls's Medicine—Oncology. Austin, Silvergirl, Inc. 1986.

273. Shuker, D. E. G., Tannenbaum, S. R., and Wishnok, J. S.: N-nitroso bile acid conjugates. I. Synthesis, chemical reactivity and mutagenic activity. J. Org. Chem., 46:2092, 1981.

274. Sidransky, H.: Chemical pathology of nutritional deficiency induced by certain plant proteins. J. Nutr., 71:387, 1960.

275. Sidransky, H.: Chemical and cellular pathology of experimental acute amino acid deficiency. Methods Achiev. Exp. Pathol., 6:1, 1972.

276. Slattery, M. L., Schumacher, M. C., Smith, K. R., West, D. W., and Abd-Elghany, N.: Physical activity, diet, and risk of colon cancer in Utah. Am. J. Epidemiol., 128:989, 1988.

277. Snowdon, D. A., and Phillips, R. L.: Coffee consumption and risk of fatal cancers. Am. J. Public Health, 74:820, 1984.

278. Snowdon, D. A., Phillips, R. L., and Choi, W.: Diet, obesity and risk of fatal prostate cancer. Am. J. Epidemiol., 120:244, 1984.

279. Solomon, T. E.: Regulation of exocrine pancreatic cell proliferation and enzyme systhesis. In Physiology of the Gastrointestinal Tract, Vol 2. Edited by L. R. Johnson. New York, Raven Press, 1981, p. 873.

280. Soos, K.: The occurrence of carcinogenic polycyclic hydrocarbons in foodstuffs in Hungary. Arch. Toxicol., Suppl. 4:446, 1980.

281. Stemmermann, G. N., Nomura, A. M. Y., and Heilbrun, K. L.: Dietary fat and the risk of colorectal cancer. Cancer Res., 44:4633, 1984.

282. Stich, H. F., Rosin, M. P., Hornby, A. P., Mathew, B., Sankaranarayanan, R. and Nair, M. K.: Remission or oral leukoplakias and micronuclei in tobacco/betel quid chewers treated with beta-carotene and with beta-carotene plus vitamin A. Int. J. Cancer, 42:195, 1988.

283. Takahashi, M., Kokuho, T., Furukawa, F., Kurokawa, Y., Tatematsu, M., and Hayashi, Y.: Effect of high salt diet on rat gastric carcinogenesis induced by MNNG. Gann Monogr., 74:28, 1983.

284. Talamini, R., LaVecchia, C., Decarli, A., Francechi, S., Grattoni, E., Grigoletto, E., Liberati, A., and Tognoni, G.: Social factors, diet and breast cancer in northern Italian population. Br. J. Cancer, 49:723, 1984.

285. Talamini, R., LaVecchia, C., Decarli, A., Negri, E., and Francechi, S.: Nutrition, social factors and prostatic cancer in Northern Italian population. Br. J. Cancer, 53:817, 1986.

286. Tannenbaum, A.: The dependence of tumor formation on the composition of the calorie-restricted diet as well as on the degree of restriction. Cancer Res., 5:616, 1945.

287. Tannenbaum, A.: Nutrition and Cancer. In The Physiopathology of Cancer. Edited by F. Homburger. New York, Hoeber-Harper, 1959.

288. Toniolo, P., Riboli, E., Protta, F., Charrel, M., and Cappa, A. P. M.: Breast cancer and alcohol consumption: A case-control study in northern Italy. Cancer Res., 49:5203, 1989.

289. Toniolo, P., Riboli, E., Protta, F., Charrel, M., and Cappa, A. P. M.: Calorie-providing nutrients and risk of breast cancer. J. Natl. Cancer Inst., 81:278, 1989.

290. Topping, D. C., and Visek, W. J.: Nitrogen intake and tumorigenesis in rats injected with 1,2-dimethylhydrazine. J. Nutr., 106:1583, 1976.

291. Trichopoulos, D., Day, N. E., Kaklamani, E., Tzonou, A., Munoz, N., Zavitsanos, X., Koumantaki, Y., and Trichopoulou, A.: Hepatitis B virus, tobacco smoking, and ethanol consumption in the etiology of hepatocellular carcinoma. Int. J. Cancer, 39:45, 1987.

292. Trock, B., Ianza, E., and Greenwald, P.: Dietary fiber, vegetables, and colon cancer: critical review and meta-analysis of the epidemiologic evidence. J. Natl. Cancer Inst., 82:650, 1990.

293. Trowell, H.: Definition of dietary fiber and hypotheses that it is a protective factor in certain diseases. Am. J. Clin. Nutr., 29:417, 1976.

294. Tuyns, A.: Alcool et Cancer. International Agency for Research on Cancer, Lyon, 1978.

295. Tuyns, A. J., Pequignot, G., and Abbatucci, J. S.: Oesophageal cancer and alcohol consumption; Importance of type of beverage. Int. J. Cancer, 23:443, 1979.

296. Tuyns, A. J.: Alcohol. In Cancer Epidemiology and Prevention. Edited by D. Schottenfeld, and J. F. Fraumeni, Jr. Philadelphia, W. B. Saunders, 1982, pp. 293–303.

297. Tuyns, A. J.: Sodium chloride and cancer of the digestive tract. Nutr. Cancer, 4:198, 1983.

298. Tuyns, A. J.: Oesophageal cancer in non-smoking drinkers and in non-drinking smokers. Int. J. Cancer, 32:433, 1983.

299. Tuyns, A. J., Haelterman, M., and Kaaks, R.: Colorectal cancer and the intake of nutrients: oligosaccharides are a risk factor, fats are not: A case-control study in Belgium. Nutr. Cancer, 10:181, 1987.

300. Tweedie, J. H., Reber, H. A., Pour, P. M., and Pounder, D. M.: Protective effect of ethanol on the development of pancreatic cancer. Surg. Forum, 32:222, 1981.

301. van Rensburg, S. J., du Bruyn, D. B., and van Schalkwyk, D. J.: Promotion of methylbenzylnitosamine-induced esophageal cancer in rats by subclinical zinc deficiency. Nutr. Rep. Int., 22(6):891, 1980.

302. van Rensburg, S. J.: Epidemiologic and dietary evidence for a specific nutritional predisposition to esophageal cancer. J. Natl. Cancer Inst., 67:243, 1981.

303. van Rensburg, S. J., Hall, J. M., and du Bruyn, D. B.: Effects of various dietary staples on esophageal carcinogenesis induced in rats by subcutaneously administered N-nitrosomethylbenzylsamine. J. Natl. Cancer Inst., 75(3):561, 1985.

304. van Rensburg, S. J., Hall, J. M., and Gathercole, P. S.: Inhibition of esophageal carcinogenesis in corn-fed rats by riboflavin, nicotinic acid, selenium, molybdenum, zinc, and magnesium. Nutr. Cancer, 8:163, 1986.

305. Van Tassell, R. L., Schram, R. M., and Wilkins, T. D.: Microbial biosynthesis of fecapentaenes. In Genetic Toxicology of the Diet. Edited by I. Knudson. New York, Alan R. Liss, 1986, p. 199.

306. Visek, W. J., and Clinton, S. K.: Dietary Protein and Cancer. In Human Nutrition: A Comprehensive Treatise, Volume 7, Cancer and Nutrition. Edited by R. B. Alfin-Slater, and D. Kritchevsky. New York, Plenum Press, 1991, p. 103.

307. Voitalovich, E. A., Deekoon, P. P., Deemarsky, L. U., and Shabad, L. M.: Comparative study of malignant tumor frequency in Tookoom District of the Latvian SSR. Vopr. Onkol., 3:351, 1957.

308. Wald, N., Idle, M., Boreham, J., and Bailey, A.: Low serum-vitamin-A and subsequent risk of cancer. Preliminary results of a prospective study. Lancet, 2:813, 1980.

309. Wald, N., Boreham, J., and Bailey, A.: Serum retinol and subsequent risk of cancer. Br. J. Cancer, 54:957, 1986.

310. Walters, M. A., and Roe, F. J. C.: The effect of dietary casein on the induction of lung tumours by the injection of 9,10-dimethyl-1,2benzanthracene (DMBA) into newborn mice. Br. J. Cancer, 18:312, 1964.

311. Ward, J. M., Anjo, T., Ohannesian, L., Keefer, L. K., Devor, D. E., Donovan, P. J., Smith, G. T., Henneman, J. R., Streeter, A. J., Konishi, N., Rehm, S., Reist, E. J., Bradford, W. W., and Rice, J. M.: Inactivity of fecapentaene-12 as a rodent carcinogen or tumor initiator and guidelines for its use in biological studies. Cancer Lett., 42:49, 1988.

312. Waterhouse, J., Muir, C. S., Shanmugaratnam, K., and Powell, J.: Incidence in five Continents, Vol. 4, IARC Scientific Publ. No. 42, International Agency for research on Cancer, Lyon, 1982.

313. Watt, B. K., and Merrill, A. L.: Composition of Foods, Agriculture Handbook, No. 8, USDA, Washington, D. C. 1975.

314. Wattenberg, L. W.: Inhibitors of chemical carcinogens. In Cancer: Achievements, Challenges, and Prospects for the 1980's. Vol. 1. Edited by J. H. Burchenal, and H. F. Oettgen. New York, Grune and Stratton, 1981, p. 517.

315. Weisblum, B., Herman, L., and Fitzgerald, P. J.: Changes in pancreatic acinar cells during protein deprivation. J. Cell. Biol., 12:313, 1962.

316. Weisburger, J. H., Marquardt, H., Hirota, N., Mori, H., and Williams, G. M.: Induction of cancer of the glandular stomach in rats by extract of nitrite-treated fish. J. Natl. Cancer Inst., 64:163, 1980.

317. Whittemore, A. S., Wu-Williams, A. H., Lee, M., Shu, Z., Gallagher, R. P., Deng-as, J., Lun, Z., Xianghui, W., Kun, C., Jung, D., Teh, C.-Z., Chengde, L., Yao, X. J., Paffenbarger, R. S., Jr. and Henderson, B. E.: Diet, physical activity, and colorectal cancer among chinese in North America, and China. J. Natl. Cancer Inst., 82:915, 1990.

318. Willet, W. C., Stampfer, M. J., Underwood, B. A., Sampson, L. A., Hennekens, C. H., Wallingford, J. C., Cooper, L. C., Hsieh, C. C., and Speizer, F. E.: Vitamin A supplementation and plasma retinol levels: a randomized trial among women. J. Natl. Cancer Inst., 73:1445, 1984.

319. Willett, W. C., Stampfer, M. J., Colditz, G. A., Rosner, B. A., Hennekens, C. H., and Speizer, F. E.: Dietary fat and the risk of breast cancer. N. Engl. J. Med., 316:22, 1987a.

320. Willett, W. C., Stampfer, M. J., Colditz, G. A., Rosner, B. A., Hennekens, C. H., and Speizer, F. E.: Moderate alcohol consumption and the risk of breast cancer. N. Engl. J. Med., 316:1174, 1987b.

321. Willet, W.: The search for the causes of breast and colon cancer. Nature, 338:389, 1989.

322. Willet, W. C., Stampfer, M. J., Colditz, G. A., Rosner, B. A., and Speizer, F. E.: Relation of meat, fat, and fiber intake to the risk of colon cancer in a prospective study among women. N. Engl. J. Med., 323:1664, 1990.

323. Wogan, G. N.: Dietary factors and special epidemiological situations of liver cancer in Thailand and Africa. Cancer Res., 35:3499, 1975.

324. World Health Organization: Environmental Health Criteria 11. Mycotoxins. WHO, Geneva, 1979.

325. World Health Organization: Diet, Nutrition and the Prevention of Chronic Diseases. Technical Report Series, No. 797, WHO, Geneva, 1990.

326. Wright, W. C.: De Morbis Artificum by Bernardino Ramazzini. The Latin Text of 1713. University of Chicago Press, 1940.

327. Wynder, E. L., Bross, I. J., and Feldmann, R. M.: A study of the etiological factors in cancer of the mouth. Cancer, 10:1300, 1957.

328. Wynder, E. L., Hultberg, S., Jacobson, F., and Bross, I. J.: Environmental factors in cancer of the upper alimentary tract: A Swedish study with special reference to Plummer-Vinson (Paterson-Kelly) syndrome. Cancer, 10:470, 1957.

329. Wynder, E. L., and Bross, I. J.: A study of etiological factors in cancer of the esophagus. Cancer, 14:389, 1961.

330. Wynder, E. L.: An epidemiological evaluation of the causes of cancer of the pancreas. Cancer Res., 35:2228, 1975.

331. Wynder, E. L., Hebert, J. R., and Kabat, G. C.: Association of dietary fat and lung cancer. J. Natl. Cancer Inst., 79:631, 1987.

332. Yang, C. S.: Research on esophageal cancer in China: A review. Cancer Res., 40:2633, 1980.

333. Yu, M. C., Mack, T., Hanisch, R., Peters, R. L., Henderson, B. E., and Pike, M. C.: Hepatitis, alcohol consumption, cigarette smoking, and hepatocellular carcinoma in Los Angeles. Cancer Res., 43:6077, 1983.

334. Zaridze, D. G., Muir, C. S., and McMichael, A. J.: Diet and cancer: Value of different types of epidemiological studies. In Diet and Human Carcinogenesis. Edited by J. V. Joossens, M. J. Hill, and J. Geboers. New York, Excerpta Medica, 1985, pp. 221–233.

335. Ziegler, R. G., Morris, L. E., Blot, W. J., Pottern, L. M., Hoover, R., and Fraumeni, J. F., Jr.: Esophageal cancer among black men in Washington, D. C. II. Role of nutrition. J. Natl. Cancer Inst., 67:1199, 1981.

336. Ziegler, R. G., Mason, T. J., Stemhagen, A., Hoover, R., Schoenberg, J. B., Gridley, G., Virgo, P. W., Altman, R., and Fraumeni, J. F., Jr.: Dietary carotene and vitamin A and risk of lung cancer among white men in New Jersey. J. Natl. Cancer Inst., 73:1429, 1984.

Diet, Chemoprevention and Cancer

Herbert F. Pierson

Introduction

Biomedical scientists and clinical practitioners are becoming more aware of the importance of the relationship between diet and cancer. Every molecule in the human body originates from the diet, which is a complex mixture of chemical substances. The functions of the essential nutrients, whose absence from the body produces a characteristic deficiency syndrome often contributing to predisposition to disease, have been studied for decades. The preceding chapter has reviewed the role of nutrients in cancer cause and prevention. The human diet contains many additional man-made and natural substances, however, that may enhance or reduce the risk of cancer. Chemical constituents in the diet, especially those of plant origin not considered to be essential (i.e., dozens of classes of small organic molecules consumed daily in significant quantities), also may prove to modulate homeostatic balance, cellular and tissue integrity, and metabolism in directions potentially useful for chemoprevention of chronic diseases like cancer.[6,50,64,192,294,295] This chapter will focus primarily upon the role of these substances in human cancer and the potential to utilize this knowledge in cancer prevention. The relationship of diet to cancer chemoprevention is under intensive study and this field of research represents one of the most exciting and important subspecialties in cancer medicine.

Chemoprevention

Chemoprevention is a term used to indicate the inhibition or reversal of carcinogenesis, primarily in the preneoplastic stage, by specific chemical compounds. Ongoing research indicates that chemoprevention will become an important complement to other cancer-control approaches involving optimization of nutrient intake and reduction of exposure to carcinogenic agents. Agents useful for chemoprevention of cancer derive from a variety of sources. They include the pharmacologic intake of specific minerals or vitamins, and related synthetic analogs. Natural ingredients derived from plants or animals which are not nutrients, but have specific anticarcinogenic biologic properties are under investigation. Many pharmaceutical agents have been shown to inhibit carcinogenesis in experimental models and are undergoing further evaluation as chemopreventive agents.

The identification of high-risk individuals or groups forms the basis for chemoprevention research. In general, four risk groups may be targeted for chemoprevention: the general population, high-risk groups, patients with preneoplastic lesions, and previous cancer patients at risk for second primaries. Since the large majority of these subjects is relatively healthy compared to those with an active cancer, it is critical that the risks of toxicity from the chronic administration of chemopreventive agents be well defined. In general, the acceptable toxicity of chemopreventive agents varies in proportion to the spectrum of cancer risk in the target population. Those in higher risk groups may acceptably be exposed to a greater risk of side-effects. Laboratory and clinical studies must therefore carefully evaluate long term toxicity as well as efficacy of potential chemopreventive agents.

The Chemoprevention Branch of the National Cancer Institute is continuously identifying potential cancer chemopreventive agents and has over 1,000 compounds undergoing consideration for further development.[71B,136A] The agents are selected and prioritized using the criteria of high efficacy and low toxicity, consistency and magnitude of benefit in different animal models and multiple target sites, and specificity of the chemopreventive effect against specific classes of known human carcinogens. Table VI-3-1 provides a partial list of promising chemopreventive agents currently undergoing investigation, along with their source and putative mechanism of action.[171B,136A] Although a large number of agents may be screened in laboratory studies, the number that actually reach clinical evaluation will be small.

Intervention trials are ultimately needed to determine the effectiveness of an agent in reducing cancer incidence. In addition, the trials help to define which animal models are most applicable to human cancer, to evaluate toxicity and risk benefit relationships, and to determine the costs and feasibility of applying a specific chemopreventive agent to a larger population.[171A] A partial list of chemoprevention trials which are now underway is presented in Table VI-3-2.[171A]

Biomarkers and Intermediate Endpoints

An expanding area of research is the development of biologic markers for the early detection (screening) of high risk individuals and as intermediate end points for chemoprevention trials.[163A,163B] Intermediate end points may include cytology (dysplasia and atypia), genomic markers (micronuclei, DNA-adducts), biochemical indices (ornithine decarboxylase, prostaglandin synthetase), differentiation markers (surface antigens), growth regulatory or inhibitory factors (epidermal growth factor, transforming growth factors), and proliferation indices (polyamines, proliferating cell nuclear antigen). A major research focus in the future will be the development and validation of sensitive and specific markers of early events in the multistage process of carcinogenesis which are predictive for the future development of invasive cancer. Using these markers, high-risk individuals can be enrolled in chemoprevention trials to determine the reversal of early steps in the carcinogenesis process.[136A,171B]

Table VI-3-1.   Chemopreventive Agents Undergoing Laboratory or Clinical Investigation*

Agent	Source	Possible Mechanism of Action
β-Carotene	Green and yellow vegetables	Antioxidant, retinoid activity
4-Hydroxyphenyl retinamide	Synthetic retinoid	Stimulates differentiation
13-cis retinoic acid	Retinoid	Stimulates differentiation
Retinol	Green and yellow vegetables	Stimulates differentiation
Selenite, selenate selenomethionine	Grains, meat	Component of glutathione peroxidase, antioxidation
Tamoxifen	Pharmaceutical	Binds estrogen receptor
Vitamin E	Wheat, soybeans, synthetic pharmaceutical	Antioxidant, terminates free radical-mediated reactions
DHEA, DHEA analog(s) (dehydroepiandrosterone)	Natural metabolite and synthetic pharmaceutical	Glucose-6-phosphate dehydrogenase inhibitor
Piroxicam	Pharmaceutical	Prostaglandin synthesis inhibitor
Bromoergocryptine	Pharmaceutical	Anterior pituitary suppressant
Molybdate	Mineral, ubiquitous meats, vegetables	Cofactor for xanthine oxidase; maintains differentiation
Fluocinolone acetonide	Synthetic pharmaceutical	Glucocorticoid analog cyclic AMP modulator
Difluoromethylornithine	Synthetic pharmaceutical	Ornithine decarboxylase inhibitor; antiproliferative
Hexamethylene bisacetamide	Pharmaceutical	Differentiating agent
Dithiolthiones	Pharmaceutical	Induces hepatic carcinogen detoxification
Ellagic acid	Nuts, berries, fruits	Binds benzo(a)pyrene
Benzyl isothiocyanate	Cruciferous vegetables	Induces hepatic carcinogen detoxification
Indole-3-carbinol	Cruciferous vegetables	Induces carcinogen detoxification
Butylated hydroxyanisole	Synthetic food additive	Antioxidant and induces carcinogen detoxification
Sulfasalazine	Pharmaceutical	Prostaglandin synthesis inhibitor
b-glycyrrhetinic acid	Licorice	Antimutagen

*Adapted from Malone et al.[171B]

Metabolic Targets For Chemopreventive Agents

There are numerous mechanisms whereby dietary components may modulate the carcinogenic process. Some compounds exert their effect by blocking the cellular uptake of carcinogens or promoters and enhancing those cell membrane processes which eliminate harmful substances from cells.[81,293,296] Intracellular events, such as the activity of enzyme systems that enhance the detoxification of harmful substances, can be modulated by dietary components.[46] Dietary components can also directly induce the synthesis of enzyme systems, such as cytochrome P-450 dependent enzymes, that prevent carcinogenic damage to cellular components. In addition, the stimulation of enzymic repair of damage to critical intracellular sites is a critical target for modulation.[53]

Intracellular events also include the modulation of cyclic nucleotide ratios that govern mitotic rates.[7,73,88,190,328] Nucleotide triphosphates are metabolized to yield cyclic nucleotides which play a key regulatory role in cell division or serve as substrates for a variety of protein kinases many of which are related to critical proto-oncogenes.[27,108,173] New areas of intracellular research emphasize the importance of inhibition by dietary components of protooncogene and oncogene protein products.[23]

The reduction of molecular oxygen yielding active oxygen radicals (superoxide) may contribute to carcinogenesis and other chronic diseases. Oxygen free radicals are normally dismutated to superoxide and hydrogen peroxide, and then to water by zinc, iron, manganese, and copper-containing superoxide dismutases and iron-containing catalase, respectively. Conditions which imbalance hydrogen peroxide detoxification and favor accumulation, predispose to spontaneous formation of the hydroxyl free radical. This hydroxyl free radical is a potent oxidizing agent catalyzing lipid peroxidation and causing nucleic acid damage.[98,112,166] Natural and synthetic substances which are antioxidants or modulate the cellular response to free-radicals may be used in cancer prevention. Dietary antioxidants like vitamin E and carotenoids, and possibly others, are thought to exert their protective action by binding to and sequestering the free radicals which cause toxic oxidations.[156] Similarly, cellular damage which liberates metallic cations, (iron and copper) facilitates the conversion of hydrogen peroxide into damaging oxygen radicals.[130] Activated white blood cells may also contribute to oxygen radical damage to tissues.[285] Peroxides generated by the metabolism of superoxides are metabolized by catalase. Another enzyme which detoxifies peroxides is glutathione peroxidase. This selenium-containing enzyme system helps detoxify both hydrogen peroxide and lipid peroxides.[242]

Numerous dietary studies have linked the inhibition of glucose-6 phosphate dehydrogenase activity with prevention of tumor promotion in animals.[89,230] An endogenous steroidal metabolite, dehydroepiandrosterone (DHEA), specifically

Table VI-3-2.   Representative Chemoprevention Intervention Studies Currently Underway*

Target Site Organ	Target/Risk Group	Inhibitory Agents
Lung	Chronic smokers	Folic acid
		Vitamin B-12
Lung	Men, asbestosis	β-Carotene
		Retinol
Lung	Cigarette smokers	β-Carotene
		Retinol
Lung	Asbestos exposed men	β-Carotene
		Retinol
Lung	Chronic smokers	13-*cis* Retinoic acid
Oral cavity	Leukoplakia	13-*cis* Retinoic acid
Oral cavity	Leukoplakia	β-Carotene
		13-*cis* Retinoic acid
Breast	Women, previous breast cancer	4-Hydroxyphenyl retinamide
Breast	Women, high risk	Tamoxifen
Skin	Albinos in Tanzania	β-Carotene
Skin	Previous basal cell carcinoma of skin	β-Carotene
Skin	Actinic keratoses patients	Retinol
Skin	Previous non-melanoma skin cancer	Selenium
Skin	Previous basal cell carcinoma of skin	Retinol
		13-*cis* Retinoic acid
Cervix	Women, mild, moderate dysplasia	Retinyl acetate
Cervix	Women, cervical dysplasia	Folic acid
Colon	Familial polyposis	Vitamins C and E and fiber
Colon	Previous adenoma of colon	Calcium
Colon	Previous adenoma of colon	β-Carotene, vitamins C and E
Colon	Previous adenoma of colon	Piroxicam
Colon	Previous adenoma of colon	Fiber, calcium
All sites	Physicians	β-Carotene

*Adapted from Malone et al.[171A]

inhibits the generation of reduced nicotinamide adenine dinucleotide phosphate (NADPH) by glucose-6 phosphate dehydrogenase. Although partial or selective inhibition of NADPH appears to be beneficial for cancer prevention, complete inhibition of NADPH may be undesirable as this reductant is a required cofactor for glutathione reductase, a key enzyme which ensures that the cell has a sufficient supply of reduced glutathione for the glutathione transferase activity. This enzyme system covalently combines reduced glutathione with potential carcinogens often rendering the carcinogens biologically inert. Glutathione conjugation is a primary means of drug metabolism, excretion and detoxification.[138] NADPH is also required as a co-factor for assuring the proper oxidative status of prosthetic iron in cytochrome P_{450}, mixed-function oxidases utilizing riboflavin. This series of enzymes is largely responsible for transforming lipid soluble toxins in the body into water soluble oxidized metabolites; these are capable of being further conjugated with either sulfate, glucuronic acid, or glutathione prior to elimination in biological fluids such as urine, saliva, or bile.[208]

Evidence at the tissue and organism level suggests a variety of possible protective mechanisms linked to dietary components. Modulation of prostaglandin biosynthesis may prevent accumulation of procarcinogenic prostaglandin species,[55] accentuate the immune response,[77,215] and regulate circulating biochemical messages required for cell differentiation.[66] Modulation of physiologic and biochemical processes involved in drug metabolism by dietary components can alter the pharmacokinetic profiles of both endogenous and exogenous toxins and thereby enhance whole body detoxification and excretion.[210] Modulation of steroid hormone metabolism can result in less potent metabolites, which are consequently less capable of sustaining hormone-dependent processes known to be tumor promoting.[181] In addition, the modulation of chemical reactions in the gastrointestinal lumen by dietary components probably inhibits the action of food mutagens and tumor promoters by competing for receptors, sequestering toxins and mutagens before absorption, altering intraluminal pH to prevent reabsorption of toxins, and by changing transit time.[61,286]

Identification of Dietary Chemopreventive Compounds

Protease Inhibitors

Among the protective elements associated with the consumption of some plant proteins are the protease inhibitors.[163] Laboratory evidence for the cancer preventive actions of protease inhibitors includes preclinical observations of suppression of dimethyl hydrazine-induced colon carcinogenesis in mice,[246] modulation of mammary tumor development in rats,[278] reduction in cellular H-ras mRNA levels,[85] anticarcinogenic activity,[278] suppression of x-ray induced chromosomal aberrations,[137] and reduced increase in c-myc RNA in cell cultures.[45]

Garlic and Onion Family

Current research indicates that vegetable protein obtained from members of the *Allium* species (garlic and onion family) is rich in sulfur-containing amino acids and other sulfur containing compounds, which have strong nucleophilic binding activity for activated carcinogens. Notable in this area is a report associating the daily consumption of gram quantities of garlic with reduced stomach cancer incidence in populations at high risk.[323] Numerous laboratory studies designed to feed sulfur-rich constituents of garlic to animals exposed to potent chemical carcinogens indicated that diallyl sulfide and S-allylcysteine prevented the formation of the expected colon tumors.[20,120,199,299] One preventive mechanism proposed to explain this protection includes a direct chemical reaction between the electron-rich sulfur containing compound and the electron-deficient carcinogen, resulting in a covalently bonded detoxified product.[281] Another mechanism may involve enhancement of naturally occurring antioxidant defenses like the induction of glutathione transferase isozymes and modulation of cytochrome P_{450} isozymes that help detoxify electrophilic carcinogenic species.[37,228,243,287]

Research also indicates that the form of food processing used to prepare foods rich in sulfur compounds for human consumption dictates the pharmacological nature of the garlic activity. For example, heating garlic in oil during cooking causes molecular rearrangements of the sulfur compounds. Some of these are potent prostaglandin modulating species which act as non-steroidal anti-inflammatory analgesics and antithrombotics.[30] Other preparations of garlic formed from aqueous alcoholic extractions were studied in humans and found to reduce hypercholesterolemia.[158] Similar aqueous preparations of garlic were correlated with an enhancement of cell mediated immunity in humans.[131]

Cancer preventive activity of food forms of garlic in laboratory animal models is well documented[199,288,289] and the role of dietary garlic in the prevention of human cancer appears promising. Future research will elucidate which fractions of *Allium* vegetables are indicated for dietary cancer prevention.

Phytosterols

Steroidal compounds are also consumed in the diet, especially if the diet is rich in edible plant protein or protein extracts. Kaweol and caffestol palmitates, found in the protein of coffee beans, elevate glutathione-S-transferase activity in the liver and intestinal mucosa of mice and exhibit cancer preventive activity against chemical carcinogens.[155] The triterpenoid sterols like glycyrrhetinic acid isolated from licorice root modulate cellular metabolism in directions many scientists feel are potentially cancer preventive. This modulation includes inhibition of ornithine decarboxylase, the rate limiting biosynthetic enzyme for nucleic acid synthesis,[200,207] inhibition of cyclic nucleotide phosphodiesterase activity and thereby mitotic rates,[5] inhibition of metabolic cooperation between carcinogen-treated cells,[279] reversal of intercellular junctional communication known to occur after carcinogen exposure,[63] inhibition of biosynthesis of mitogenic prostaglandin species,[121,206] inhibition of the mutagenicity of tryptophan pyrrolysis products and furylacrylamides,[261] induction of differentiation of malignant cells in vitro,[1] inhibition of

protein kinase C activated by tumor promoters,[205] inhibition of oral cancer in hamster induced by DMBA,[22] and blockage of estrogen receptors on breast epithelium.[154] Licorice root extract, from the legume *Glycyrrhiza glabra,* used as a food flavoring and sweetener, contains isoflavones and triterpenoid sterols. The isoflavone antioxidant glabrene is also an antimutagenic factor in licorice root in in vitro tests.[180]

Legumes like alfalfa, and alfalfa sprouts, are a rich source of phytosterols. Major sterols include medicarcinogenic acid and soyasapogenol A and B.[99,117] As a class, these sterols are also called saponins since they impart a bitter taste and foaming property to water. Saponins in the diet affect mammalian physiology and metabolism, and the safety of large amounts is not known. For example, alfalfa meal as a sole protein source inhibited growth of rats, chickens, monkeys, and rabbits unless the diet was supplemented with cholesterol.[57]

Feeding plant sterols in the diet to laboratory animals significantly inhibited colon carcinogenesis.[219] Saponins are thought to induce binding of bile salts to polysaccharides in vegetable fiber via strong surface active properties.[203] Feeding saponins increased bile acid production and excretion of neutral sterols and bile acids in feces of rats and guinea pigs.[116,275] A 30% alfalfa diet significantly increased hepatic aminopyrine demethylase activity in rats.[84] Soybean saponins inhibit proteases like chymotrypsin and trypsin in the intestinal tract.[122] Saponins form insoluble complexes with zinc and iron and may cause a fecal loss of these minerals.[309]

One of the most important dietary sources of plant sterols is the *Curcurbitaceae* family, representing 114 genera of which 22 are cultivated and found in the human diet.[72] The *Cucurbitaceae* or the cucumber and squash family, are consumed worldwide as both fruits and vegetables. One species, the balsam pear *(Momordica charantia),* or bitter melon, has found use in both folk and recent medicine. The balsam pear has demonstrated both anti-tumor properties and cancer preventive activity. One laboratory characterized an acid-stable, heat-sensitive aqueous extract from the ripe fruit of *Momordica* with tumor growth inhibiting activities. The active preparation contained a compound with a molecular weight of less than 12,000.[82,282] Up to 40% of the seed oil can be a complex mixture of naturally occurring sterols.[141]

Against a transplanted prostate adenocarcinoma injected into rats, an intraperitoneal injection of an aqueous extract of bitter melon reduced tumor growth by 61%.[82] The growth inhibiting activity of the bitter melon extract was related to its ability to inhibit guanylate cyclase activity of tumor cells.[252] This finding is important because exposure to nitroso-containing carcinogens is associated with stimulation of cyclic GMP synthesis.[73,88,190,328] Inhibition of the carcinogen stimulation of cyclic GMP production by the extract of the bitter melon accounted for its cancer inhibitory activity.[51]

Protein extracts of the bitter melon also inhibited tumor growth in transplanted cell systems. The treatment of mice intraperitoneally with a bitter melon extract following injection with L1210 leukemia cells, produced a significant delay in both tumor onset and inhibition of tumor growth.[60] A heat labile protein characterized in the bitter melon extract was thought to account for the biological activity of this tumor system. This protein also inhibited guanylate cyclase activity and was found to be cytotoxic in vitro toward human leukemia cells.[129,259] Studies with preclinical tumor systems suggested anti-tumor activity of other bitter melon components.[82,129,259,282]

In other studies, the examination of crude pumpkin extracts yielded data suggesting potential cancer preventive activity. Boiled pumpkin juice injections suppressed DMBA-induced chromosomal aberrations in rat bone marrow assays.[124] In laboratory animals fed a diet supplemented with 10% pumpkin on a weight/weight basis, some hepatic enzymes, most notably glucose-6-phosphatase and NADPH-cytochrome C reductase, were enhanced while other enzyme activities, such as NADPH-cytochrome C reductase and aniline hydroxylase, were selectively inhibited.[204]

One series of steroid-like compounds found in the *Cucurbitaceae* are called cucurbitacins, which are tetracyclic triterpenoids that have been recognized for some time to demonstrate cytotoxic activity. Among the transformed mammalian cells found to be sensitive to these compounds are KB,[10] HeLa,[314] Ehrlich ascites, and sarcoma 180.[87] Inhibition of cell proliferation occurs upon exposure to several of the many known cucurbitacins. The mechanism of cytotoxic action is not well understood, but inhibition of macromolecular biosynthesis such as DNA, RNA, and protein is observed with cucurbitacin I in HeLa cells.[314] It is also postulated that such anti-proliferative effects may be mediated through a glucocorticoid receptor because cucurbitacin I binds specifically to such receptors on intact HeLa cells.[313]

Three cucurbitacins are reported to inhibit tumor growth in vivo: cucurbitacin E, elatericin A, and elatericin B. Against a transplanted tumor model system in mice, these three compounds inhibited the growth of transplanted Ehrlich ascites, and sarcoma 180 cells up to 57% of untreated controls when injected intraperitoneally 24 hours after tumor cell implantation.[87]

Virtually no information exists on the gastrointestinal absorption of biologically active peptides and sterols from squash, cucumbers, melons, pumpkins and gourds consumed as food. Hence the dietary role of these constituents in cancer prevention awaits clarification through clinical feeding studies.

Identification of Dietary Carcinogenic Agents

The identification of compounds in the diet which may be carcinogenic or enhance the activity of carcinogens should be vigorously pursued. In addition to instituting specific recommendations to avoid these substances the food science industry may develop and institute processing methods which eliminate or minimize their concentration in foods. Recommendations for alternative recipes can be made if procarcinogenic substances are the result of specific cooking methods. Identification of dietary carcinogenic agents for humans may allow scientists to define specific chemopreventive programs targeted at the populations experiencing high exposure. The following section is devoted to the identification of substances found in the food supply which may contribute to cancer risk that require additional investigation.

Cooking, Food Processing and Cancer

The characterization of carcinogenic substances in the diet is now an active area of investigation. Research indicates that the manner and temperatures used in food preparation influence the production of amino acid metabolites that may exert chronic adverse influences on sensitive tissue sites in the human body.[127,191,251,257] Research shows that high temperatures used for cooking can be linked with the production of toxic mutagenic amino acid pyrolysis products: Trp-P-1 and Trp-P-2 from tryptophan;[123,319] GLU-P-1 and GLU-P-2 from glutamic acid; PHE-P-1 from phenylalanine; LYS-P-1 from lysine; ORN-P-1 from ornithine;[322] as well as two mutagenic metabolites from soybean globulin.[254] Most of the heat-induced metabolites of amino acids are heterocyclic amines,[256] and have been shown to require bioactivation by microsomal cytochrome P_{450} mixed function oxidases to exert mutagenic activity in vitro.[123,202,254,319] Carcinogenicity tests conducted on TRP-P-1, TRP-P-2, GLU-P-1, GLU-P-2, and others, all prove to be positive in mice, with some specificity for females and some unusual tumor types.[253,255]

Two active mutagenic substances have been isolated from broiled, dried sardines, IQ and MeIQ.[134,135] The specific mutagenicity of MeIQ was found to be higher than that of aflatoxin-B1.[134] Another report indicates the presence of mutagenic activity from hamburger fried under normal cooking conditions and suggests a highly potent new mutagen, MeIQX.[133] These mutagens require metabolic activation in the in vitro bacterial mutagenicity screen.

Follow-up studies showed that cytochrome isozyme-P448, which is typically induced by 3-methylcholanthrene, is most effective in converting these heterocyclic amines to heterocyclic hydroxylamines.[252] The hydroxylamine derivative of TRP-P-2 reacts directly with DNA in vitro and acetylated forms of hydroxylamines are thought to be the ultimate carcinogens capable of rapidly reacting with DNA bases to produce tumors.[100,101]

The human risk for cancer from amino acid pyrolysates resulting from excessively cooking dietary protein has yet to be clarified in epidemiological studies, but most authorities agree that excessively cooking protein rich foods should be contraindicated in our lifestyle practices.

Cyanide Containing Food Substances

Another class of compounds consumed along with dietary protein of plant origin are cyanide-containing substances. Edible plants exhibiting 2,000 ppm of cyanide per fresh weight of edible plant material are acutely lethal.[86] The average lethal single oral dose of hydrogen cyanide for humans, sheep and cattle is about the same at 2 mg per kilogram of body weight.[247]

Protein derived from sorghum and legumes contains cyanogenic glycosides like the compound Dhurrin, (S)-p-hydroxymandelonitrile-beta-D-glycopyranoside.[56] This compound is hydrolyzed by β-glucosidases of microbial origin to form p-hydroxymandelonitrile and the corresponding glycoside in the intestinal tract of mammals.

The tropical root food cassava (manioc) is another source of dietary cyanide and constitutes a staple for millions of people in lowland, humid, tropical areas. Cassava root contains the cyanogenic glycosides linamarin (2-hydroxyiso-butyronitrile-β-D-glucopyranoside) and (R)-lotaustralin (methyl-linamarin), which are hydrolyzed by enzyme action when the plant material is crushed during preparation. Cyanide is largely eliminated by cooking. Both linamarin and lotaustralin also have been reported to occur together in various species of legumes and edible grains in approximately equivalent amounts.[39–41,178]

It is important to note that cyanide toxicity results when either hydrocyanic acid forms cyanomethemoglobin in red cells or cyanide anion inactivates the cytochrome P$_{450}$ mixed function oxidases required for conjugation, excretion, and detoxification of foreign materials in the body.[56] The chronic impairment of cytochrome P$_{450}$ detoxification is thought to be a factor contributing to the developmental process of preneoplastic lesions.[6,42,64,84,168,208,320,321]

Glucosinolates

Glucosinolates are a class of compounds whose metabolites, isothiocyanates, nitrites, and thiocyanates, can adversely affect growth and reproduction in animals.[80] In the mammalian intestinal tract a glucosinolate molecule may be hydrolyzed to form an isothiocyanate molecule, a substituted nitrile, and a thiocyanate molecule. When two nitriles and a sulfur atom react together they produce the ring compound 5-vinyl oxazolidine-2-thione, also called goitrin, which stimulates the secretion of thyrotropin by the pituitary.[65]

These compounds are abundantly common in protein of cruciferous vegetables like cabbage, swiss chard, brussels sprouts, mustard greens, cauliflower, turnip, broccoli, radish, Chinese cabbage, and in prepared mustard. As early as 1966 the chronic consumption of cruciferous plants was linked to the formation of goiters in animals and in humans who drank the milk of animals consuming kale or turnips.[311] Goiters produced in humans by chronic consumption of goitrin in milk or vegetables are unresponsive to dietary administration of iodine as potassium iodide.[148]

Laboratory studies indicate that some cruciferous glucosinolates in the diet break down and yield compounds which are potentially important for modulating carcinogenesis. Two classes of aromatic aglycones are formed after intestinal microbial hydrolysis. The first are phenyl- and benzyl-isothiocyanates. These are inhibitive of benzopyrene-induced forestomach cancer in mice,[298] nitrosamine-DNA adduct formation in rat lung in vivo,[297] DMBA-induced mammary cancer in rats,[299] DMH-induced colon cancer in rodents,[179] and inducive of glutathione-s-transferase activity in many rodent tissues.[245] Cabbage feeding modulated DMH-induced colon cancer in rodents.[179]

The second class of aromatic aglycones in cruciferous vegetables formed by microbial hydrolysis of glucosinolates are the indoles such as indole-3-acetonitrile, 3,3′-diindolyl-methane, and indole-3-carbinol. These substances are inhibitive of benzopyrene-induced and DMBA-induced forestomach and mammary cancer in rodents,[248,300] and inducive of both glutathione-s-transferase activity and microsomal cytochrome P$_{450}$ mixed function oxidase activity.[238] Indole-3-carbinol modulates the hepatic cytochrome P$_{450}$ mixed function oxidases and the biotransformation of estradiol favoring the production of 2-hydroxylated steroids which bioinactivate estrogen, and therefore may lower risk for the development of hormone-dependent breast cancer.[181,189,229]

Nitrates, Nitrites, and Nitrosamines

Among the potential toxicants present naturally, the most widely distributed in edible plant protein are nitrates and nitrites. Their concentrations in edible plant protein are increased by careless applications of inorganic nitrogenous fertilizers, which may be avoided by following present agricultural recommendations to harvest plants 60–70 days after nitrate fertilizing.[209,315] Nitrite can originate in the saliva, produced by enzymes of the oral microflora from ingested nitrates. Nitrite toxicity may act in two general directions. First, by reaction with hemoglobin to form methemoglobin, or secondly, with amines to form nitrosamines.[3,283] Amaranth, which is a leafy vegetable consumed in salads, may contain a nitrate content of up to 3.25% on a dry weight basis, which can cause fatal methemoglobinemia.[283]

In humans the potential formation of carcinogenic nitrosamines is a threat to health, since nitrosamines are extremely carcinogenic compounds. They are formed in food from available precursors such as nitriles, nitrates, amines, and amino acids. Nitrites can be formed by the bacterial reduction of nitrate.[3] Dietary amines can form during heating of proteinaceous foods since free amino acids are always present. N-nitroso compounds like nitrosamines may be formed from nitrites and amines during digestion in the stomach or by bacteria during transit through the intestines.[6,157,177,185,186,283]

Numerous hepatotoxic disorders and preneoplastic lesions in farm animals have been shown to be due to the presence of dimethylnitrosamine in fish meal diets,[145–147,233] and the carcinogenic activity of dimethylnitrosamine has been known since 1956.[170] This initial study indicated that even a small quantity fed to laboratory animals over a prolonged period resulted in the development of cancer of the liver, while larger acute doses produced renal tumors.

Studies have indicated a clear epidemiological relationship between the content of nitrosamines in foods and cancer of the digestive tract in humans.[59,110] Antioxidants like ascorbic acid, tocopherols, and plant phenolics have been used to prevent nitrosamine formation in foods and to inactivate toxic alkylating moieties of nitrosamines.[15,157,185]

Oxalates

Oxalates occur in some edible plant protein sources at relatively high levels, mainly as the soluble sodium and potassium salt, or as the insoluble calcium oxalate. Ingestion of some plant protein may be accompanied by ingestion of potentially toxic quantities of oxalate. High levels of oxalates generally occur in spinach and in some species of lamb's quarters. Potentially toxic levels also are found in a variety of *Amaranthus,* sunflower leaves, sugar beet tops, and various edible grasses.[194]

The exact association between the dietary consumption of oxalates in proteinaceous food and carcinogenesis in humans remains to be proved, although oxalates may be dietary factors contributing to susceptibility to carcinogenic substances and to chronic irritation and inflammation within the gastrointestinal tract.

It is important to note that oxalate-containing edible plants used as sources of protein by humans may also have high levels of nitrates or cyanogenic glycosides. These latter compounds may increase the severity of the toxic effect of met-hemoglobinemia, inducing degenerative changes in the kidney which can lead to impaired excretion of the oxalates and exacerbate renal toxicity.[35]

Animal studies indicate that the ingestion of large quantities of oxalate containing food plants may cause alkalosis, hypocalcemia, and acute uremia due to blockage of kidney tubules by calcium oxalate crystals. Ingestion of five grams or more of oxalic acid can be fatal to humans, causing corrosive gastroenteritis, shock, convulsions, and renal damage. Corrosive substances in the digestive tract can facilitate the permeability of epithelial cells to other toxic substances and their entry into the circulation.[227,260] Oxalate poisoning in humans is thoroughly described in cases of consumption of rhubarb leaves.[162]

Phytoestrogens

Research of phytoestrogens was originally stimulated by interest in alfalfa as a source of dietary protein. Forage plants such as alfalfa, clover, and legumes in general are a rich source of phytoestrogens, many of which have been linked since 1940 with serious reproductive disturbances in animals.[21]

In laboratory animal tests assessing the effect of estrogens on uterine weight gain and estrus cycling, the phytoestrogens as a class exhibit weak estrogenicity.[48] The primary phytoestrogens in edible proteinaceous legumes are a class of bioflavonoids called isoflavones. Representative isoflavones include genistein, formononetin, biochanin A, and daidzein.[218] Relative to milligram quantities of diethylstilbesterol, the potency of genistein was found to be 0.019 and that of biochanin A, was very similar. Diadzein was found to be the most active with a potency of 0.042, while formonetin had the lowest estrogenicity in this test which amounted to 0.009 diethylstilbesterol activity.[49] Coumesterol, found in edible legumes, has exhibited up to 35 times greater estrogenic activity than the other isoflavones.[24,36] The relationship between the consumption of phytoestrogens by humans and adverse health effects, including cancer, was reviewed by Setchell.[234]

Although the phytoestrogen content in the blood of humans consuming either legumes or meats from animals fed legumes has not been well quantified, research on food animals has indicated that isoflavones do enter into the plasma of grazing sheep. Evidence suggests that the phytoestrogens are metabolized by the intestinal flora by demethylation and reduction and that these processes modulate estrogenicity in a compound specific manner.[17]

Knowledge of the consumption of phytoestrogens in protein sources may prove to be useful in understanding cancer prevention, as well as causation, in humans. In vitro data suggest that certain legume isoflavones, like biochanin A, also inhibit carcinogenic activation in cells by inhibiting the binding of activated benzopyrene metabolites to DNA.[44] Other recent studies have suggested that isoflavones may be naturally occurring inhibitors of oncogene protein product expression.

The soybean isoflavone genistein is a highly specific inhibitor of tyrosine kinase activity.[4,174,292] If one accepts the hypothesis that tyrosine kinase activity is over-expressed in preneoplastic cells, and that dietary isoflavones enter into the systemic circulation and penetrate into cells in which tyrosine kinase activity has been amplified, the protective influences of the phytoestrogen might account in part for inhibition of cancer in some human populations, e.g., Asians who are heavy users of legume protein.[143] Of particular relevance to the development of human breast cancer is the important observation that tyrosine kinase activity is progressively elevated in breast epithelium as a function of the state of progression to frank carcinoma.[108]

It is conceivable that bathing preneoplastic lesions rich in over-expressed tyrosine kinase with phytoestrogens from dietary sources may retard the tumorigenic activity.[108] Future research is required to clarify the potential benefit of chronic legume isoflavone consumption on the modulation of over-expressed tyrosine kinase activity in preneoplastic breast lesions.

Amino Acid Derivatives

There are approximately 320 amino acids found in edible plants, but only 20 are incorporated into proteins. Some of the non-protein amino acids are toxic to humans because of their close similarity to the protein amino acids which allows them to antagonize basic functions by competing with normal amino acids at specific biosynthetic sites. Consumption of the seeds and leafy parts of *Lathyrus* species (sweet peas) as a major source of dietary protein caused severe toxic effects in humans.[2]

Protein from parts of the edible jack-bean plant *(Canavalia)* are rich in a compound called L-canavanine, 2-amino-4-(guanidinoxy) butyric acid, a naturally occurring toxic structural analogue of L-arginine.[270] The biological effects and mechanism of action of L-canavanine have been reviewed extensively.[224] The biosynthesis of canavanine-containing proteins in vivo disrupts important reactions of RNA and DNA metabolism, and affects arginine metabolism. Canavanine changes central biochemical reactions, becomes a potent anti-metabolite of L-arginine, and is teratogenic in laboratory animals. This and other compounds, such as beta-cyano-L-alanine, are also found in edible *Lathyrus* species. Studies in laboratory rats demonstrated their ability to induce severe neurotoxicity, and extensive degenerative damage in bones and connective tissues.[301] The ability of toxic amino acids to impair cell division, normal development of tissues, and subsequently alter cellular chemistry correlates closely with changes in cells formed during carcinogenic processes.[6] Little attention has been paid to the impact of inadvertent toxic amino acid consumption on human cancer incidence.

Edible plants used for dietary protein and for flavoring foods may be rich sources of sulfur-containing compounds.[78] Certain cruciferous vegetables such as cabbage, kale, rape, and brussels sprouts cause severe changes in the blood, jaundice, and cessation of milk production in ruminants and cattle feeding on them as a major dietary component for several weeks.[96] Studies further showed the anemia factor to be S-methylcysteine sulfoxide.[239,258] Other studies have also implicated dietary sulfur-containing compounds.[97,240] Depletion of reduced glutathione in erythrocytes accounted for the toxic effect of these sulfur-containing compounds,[6,46,102,112] and such a mechanism in major tissue systems is linked to carcinogen susceptibility.[23,107,236,242,245,299]

Conversely, reports exist that similar dietary sulfur compounds may contribute to an overall cancer preventive action, as noted above. For example, garlic is rich in sulfur-containing compounds exhibiting allylic moieties positioned close to the sulfur atom.[290] Such compounds in garlic are reactive and thought to contribute to the nucleophilic trapping activity rendering electrophilic carcinogens inactive.[29,302]

Other studies have suggested that garlic compounds, including those with allylic sulfur functional groups, elevate intracellular reduced glutathione levels and serve as a means for accentuating anti-oxidant defenses against the toxic effects of carcinogens on cells and tissues.[244,245] An epidemiological study in China examining populations at high risk for stomach cancer correlated the daily consumption of gram quantities of garlic with the inhibition of gastric cancer attributable to nitrosamine consumption.[177,323]

Simpler, volatile sulfhydryl compounds in allinaceous and cruciferous vegetables have the propensity for reacting with reduced glutathione and forming mixed disulfides that deplete glutathione stores and render cells susceptible to oxidative injury.[46] Consuming large quantities of fresh garlic or onions indicate that large doses of volatile sulfur compounds may be hemolytic and act acutely.[102] This knowledge may help differentiate toxic from potential beneficial sulfur compounds in the diet.

References

1. Abe, H., Ohya, N., Yamamoto, K. F., Shibuya, T., Arichi, S., and Odashima, S.: Effects of glycyrrhizin and glycyrrhetinic acid on growth and melanogenesis in cultured B16 melanoma cells. Eur. J. Cancer Clin. Oncol., 23:1549, 1987.
2. Adiga, P. R., Rao, S. L. N., and Sarma, P. S.: Some structural features and neurotoxic action of a compound from Lathyrus sativus seeds. Curr. Sci., 32:153, 1963.
3. Achtzehn, M. K., and Howat, H.: Nitrate content of vegetables. Nahrung, 13:667, 1969.
4. Akiyama, T., Ishida, J., Nakagawa, S., Ogawara, H., Watanabe, S., Itoh, N., Shibuya, M., and Fukami, Y.: Genistein, a specific inhibitor of tyrosine-specific protein kinases. J. Biol. Chem., 262:5592, 1987.
5. Amer, M. S., McKinney, G. R., and Akcasu, A.: Inhibition of cyclic nucleotide phosphodiesterase activity by glycyrrhizin in rat, guinea pig, and dog stomach. Biochem. Pharmacol., 23:3085, 1974.
6. Ames, B. N.: Dietary carcinogens and anticarcinogens (oxygen radicals and degenerative diseases). Science, 221:1256, 1983.
7. Anderson, W. B., Estival, A., Tapiovaara, H., and Gopalkrishna, R.: Altered subcellular distribution of protein kinase C (a phorbol ester receptor). Possible role in tumor promotion and the regulation of cell growth: relationship to changes in adenylate cyclase activity. Adv. Cyclic Nucleotide Protein Phosphorylation Res., 19:287, 1985.
8. Aoki, K.: Epidemiology of gastric cancer, with reference to etiology. Igan To Shudan Kenshin, 48:44, 1980.
9. Appleton, B. S., and Campbell, T. C.: Inhibition of aflatoxin-inititated preneoplastic liver lesions by low dietary protein. Nutr. Cancer, 3:200, 1982.
10. Arisawa, M., Pezzuto, J. M., Kinghorn, A. D., Cordell, G. A., and Farnsworth, N. R.: Plant anticancer agents XXX: Cucurbitacins from Ipomopsis aggregata (Polemoniaceae). J. Pharm. Sci., 73:411, 1984.
11. Armstrong, B., and Doll, R.: Environmental factors and cancer incidence and mortality in different countries with special reference to dietary practices. Int. J. Cancer, 15:617, 1975.
12. Ashida, H., Kanazowa, K., and Natake, M.: Decrease of NADPH level in rat liver on oral administration of secondary autoxidation products of linoleic acid. Agric. Biol. Chem., 51:2951, 1987.
13. Babbs, C. F.: Free radicals and the etiology of colon cancer. Free Radicals Biol. Med., 8:191, 1990.
14. Balducci, L., Wallace, C., Khansur, T., Vance, R. B., Thigpen, J. T., and Hardy, C.: Nutrition, cancer, and aging: An annotated review. I. Diet, carcinogenesis, and aging. J. Am. Geriatr. Soc., 34:127, 1986.
15. Barale, R., Zucconi, D., Bertani, R., and Loprieno, N.: Vegetables inhibit in vivo the mutagenicity of nitrite combined with nitrosable compounds. Mut. Res., 120:145, 1983.
16. Bas, J. L.: The ras gene family and human carcinogenesis. Mut. Res., 195:255, 1988.
17. Batterham, T. J., Shutt, D. A., Braden, A. W., and Tweedale, H. J.: Metabolism of intraluminally administered 14C-formonetin and 14C-biochanin A in sheep. Aust. J. Agric. Res., 22:131, 1971.
18. Baumann, C. A., Jacobi, H. P., and Rusch, H. P.: The effect of diet on experimental tumor production. Am. J. Hyg., 30:1, 1939.
19. Baumann, C. A., and Rusch, H. P.: Effect of diet on tumors induced by ultraviolet light. Am. J. Cancer, 35:213, 1939.
20. Belman, S., Solomon, J., Segal, A., Block, E., and Barany, G.: Inhibition of soybean lipoxygenase and mouse skin tumor promotion by onion and garlic components. J. Biochem. Toxicol., 4:151, 1989.
21. Bennetts, H. W.: Two sheep problems on subterranean clover dominant pastures. 1. Lambing trouble (Dystokia) in Merinos. 2. Prolapse of the womb (inversion of the uterus). West. Austr. Dep. Agric. J., 21:104, 1944.
22. Berry, C., and Vora, P.: Modulation of glycyrrhizin of DMBA-induced tumors in hamsters. Am. Assoc. Dental Res., March 7-11, Cincinnati, Ohio, 1990.
23. Bertram, J. S., Kolonel, L. N., and Meyskens, F. L., Jr.: Rationale and strategies for chemoprevention of cancer in humans. Cancer Res., 47:3012, 1987.
24. Bickhoff, E. M., Livingston, A. L., Hendrickson, A. P., and Booth, A. N.: Relative potencies of several estrogen-like compounds found in forages. J. Agric. Food. Chem., 10:410, 1962.
25. Birt, D. F.: Effects of the intake of selected vitamins and minerals on cancer prevention. Magnesium, 8:17, 1989.
26. Birt, D. F.: Update on the effects of Vitamins A, C, and E and selenium on carcinogenesis. Proc. Soc. Exp. Biol. Med., 183:311, 1986.
27. Bishop, J. M.: The molecular genetics of cancer. Science, 235:305, 1987.
28. Bjelke, E.: Epidemiology of colorectal cancer, with emphasis on diet. Int. Congr. Ser., 484:158, 1980.
29. Block, E.: The chemistry of garlic and onions. Sci. Am., 252:114, 1985.
30. Block, E., Ahmad, S., and Jain, M.: (E,Z)-ajoene: a potent antithrombotic agent from garlic. J. Am. Chem. Soc., 106:8295, 1984.
31. Boissonneault, G. A., Elson, C. E., and Pariza, M. W.: Net energy effects of dietary fat on chemically induced mammary carcinogenesis in F344 rats. J. Natl. Cancer Inst., 76:335, 1986.
32. Bongiorno, C. P.: Appropriate prevention and detection of gastrointestinal neoplasms in the elderly. Clin. Geriatr. Med., 41:222, 1988.
33. Boutwell, R. K., Brush, M. K., and Rusch, M. D.: The stimulating effect of dietary fat on carcinogenesis. Cancer Res., 9:741, 1949.
34. Boutwell, R. K., Brush, M. K., and Rusch, H. P.: Some physiological effects associated with chronic caloric restriction. Am. J. Physiol., 154:517, 1948.
35. Boyce, W. H., Garvey, F. K., and Strawcutter, H. E.: Incidence of urinary calculi among patients in general hospitals, 1948-1952. J. Am. Med. Assoc., 161:1437, 1956.
36. Braden, A. W. H., Hart, N. K., and Lamberton, J. A.: The estrogenic activity and metabolism of certain isoflavones in sheep. Austr. J. Agric. Res., 18:335, 1967.
37. Brody, J. F., Li, D. C., Ishizaki, H., and Yang, C. S.: Effect of diallyl sulfide on rat liver microsomal nitrosamine metabolism and other monooxygenase activities. Cancer Res., 48:5937, 1988.
38. Bruce, A.: Dietary recommendations in cancer prevention. Ann. Clin. Res., 19:313, 1987.
39. Butler, G. W.: The distribution of the cyanoglycosides linamarin and lotaustralin in higher plants. Phytochem., 4:127, 1965.
40. Butler, G. W., Bailey, R. W., and Kennedy, L. D.: Studies on the glucosidase "Linamarase." Phytochem., 4:369, 1965.
41. Butler, G. W., and Conn, E. E.: Biosynthesis of the cyanogenic glycosides: linamarin and isolinamarin. J. Biol. Chem., 239:1674, 1964.
42. Campbell, T. C., and Hayes, J. R.: Role of nutrition in the drug metabolizing enzyme system. Pharmacol. Rev., 26:171, 1974.
43. Carroll, K. K.: Experimental evidence of dietary factors and hormone-dependent cancers. Cancer Res., 35:3374, 1975.
44. Cassady, J. M., Zennie, T. M., Chae, Y. H., Ferin, M. A., Portuonda, N. E., and Baird, W. M.: Use of a mammalian cell culture benzo(a)pyrene metabolism assay for the detection of potential anticarcinogens from natural products: inhibition of metabolism by biochanin A, an isoflavone from Trifolium pratense L. Cancer Res., 48:6257, 1988.
45. Chang, J. D., and Kennedy, A. R.: Cell cycle progression of C3H/10T1/2 and 3T3 cells in the absence of an increase in c-myc RNA levels. Carcinogenesis, 9:17, 1988.
46. Chasseud, L. F.: The role of glutathione and glutathione-s-transferases in the metabolism of chemical carcinogens and other electrophilic agents. Adv. Cancer Res., 29:176, 1979.
47. Chen, L. H., Boissonneault, G. A., and Glauert, H. P.: Vitamin C, Vitamin E, and cancer (Review). Anticancer Res., 8:739, 1988.
48. Cheng, E., and Burroughs, W.: Estrogenic substances in forages. In Grasslands. Sprague, H. B. (ed.) Am. Assoc. Adv. Sci., 53:195, 1959.
49. Cheng, E., Yoder, L., Story, C. D., and Burroughs, W.: Estrogenic activity of some isoflavone derivatives. Science, 120:575, 1954.
50. Chen, M. C., and Meguid, M. M.: Postulated cancer prevention diets. A guide to food selections. Surg. Clin. North Am., 66:931, 1986.
51. Claflin, A. J., Vesely, D. L., Hudson, J. L., Bagwell, C. B., Lehotay, D. C., Lo, T. M., Fletcher, M. A., Block, N. L., and Levey, L. S.: Inhibition of growth and guanylate cyclase activity of an undifferentiated prostate adenocarcinoma by an extract of the balsam pear (Momordica charantia abbreviata). Proc. Natl. Acad. Sci., U. S. A., 75:989, 1978.
52. Clarke, B. A. C., and Clarke, M. L.: Garners Veterinarian Toxicology, 3rd edition, London, Tindall and Corsell, 1967.
53. Clarke, C., and Shankel, D. M.: Antimutagenesis in microbial systems. Bacteriol. Rev., 39:33, 1975.
54. Clinton, S. K., Truex, C. G., and Visek, W. J.: Dietary protein, aryl hydrocarbon hydroxylase and chemical carcinogenesis in rats. J. Nutr., 109:55, 1975.
55. Cohen, L. A., Thompson, D. O., Choi, K., Karmeli, R. A., and Rose, D. P.: Dietary fat and mammary cancer. II. Modulation of serum and tumor lipid composition and tumor prostaglandins by different dietary fats: association with tumor incidence patterns. J. Natl. Cancer Inst., 77:43, 1986.
56. Conn, E. E.: Cyanide and cyanogenic glycosides. In Herbivores, Their Interactions with Secondary Plant Metabolites. Edited by G. A. Rosenthal. Academic Press, New York, 1979.
57. Cookson, F. B., and Federoff, S.: Quantitative relationships between administered cholesterol and alfalfa required to prevent hypercholesterolemia in rabbits. Brit. J. Exp. Pathol., 49:348, 1968.

58. Cramer, D. W., Welch, W. R., Hutchinson, G. B., Willet, W., and Scully, R. E.: Dietary animal fat in relation to ovarian cancer risk. Obstet. Gynecol., 63:833, 1984.
59. Crosby, N. J.: Nitrosamines in foodstuffs. Residue Rev., 64:77, 1976.
60. Cunnick, J. E., and Takemoto, D. J.: Modulation of murine immune cells by the bitter melon *(Momordica charantia)*. Proc. Am. Assoc. Cancer Res., 26:277, 1985.
61. Cummings, J.: Dietary fiber, treatment time, faecal bacterias, steroids, and colon cancer in two Scandinavian populations. Lancet, 2:207, 1977.
62. Dales, L. G., Friedman, G. D., Ury, H. K., Grossman, S., and Williams, S. R.: A case-control study of relationships of diet and other traits to colorectal cancer in American blacks. Am. J. Epidemiol., 109:132, 1979.
63. Davidson, J. S., Baumgarten, I. M., and Harley, E. H.: Reversible inhibition of intercellular junctional communication by glycyrretinic acid. Biochem. Biophys. Res. Commun., 134:29, 1986.
64. Davis, D. L.: Natural anticarcinogens, carcinogens and changing patterns in cancer: some speculation. Environ. Res., 50:322, 1989.
65. Daxenbichler, M. E., van Etten, C. H., and Wolff, I. A.: Diastereomeric episulfides from epigoitrin upon autolysis of crambe seed meal. Phytochem., 7:989, 1968.
66. De Luca, L. M.: Essential function deficiency as the result of tumor promotion and establishment of biological autarchy. J. Natl. Cancer Inst., 70:405, 1983.
67. Diet and Health: Implications for reducing chronic disease risk. Washington, DC, National Academy of Sciences, 1989.
68. Diet, Nutrition and Cancer. Washington, DC, National Academy of Sciences, 1982.
69. Di Palma, J. R., and McMichael, R.: The interaction of vitamins with cancer chemotherapy. CA, 29:280, 1979.
70. Doll, R.: Prevention of cancer: Practical prospects. Ann. Acad. Med. Singapore, 13:194, 1984.
71. Drasar, B., and Irving, D.: Environmental factors and cancer of the colon and breast. Brit. J. Cancer, 27:167, 1973.
72. Dreker, M. L., Weber, C. W., Bemis, W. P., and Berry, J. W.: Cucurbit seed coat composition. J. Agric. Food Chem., 28:364, 1980.
73. Dumont, J. E., Jauniaux, J. C., and Roger, P. P.: The cyclic AMP-mediated stimulation of cell proliferation. Trends Biochem. Sci., 14:67, 1989.
74. Dunaif, G. E., and Campbell, J. C.: Dietary protein level and aflatoxin B_1-induced preneoplastic hepatic lesions in the rat. J. Nutr., 117:1298, 1987.
75. Dunaif, G. E., and Campbell, J. C.: Relative contribution of dietary protein level and aflatoxin B_1 dose in generation of presumptive preneoplastic foci in rat liver. J. Natl. Cancer Inst., 78:365, 1987.
76. Edenharder, R.: Nutrition and the etiology of colon cancer: From descriptive epidemiology to dietary prevention. Z. Ernahrungswiss, 26:143, 1987.
77. Erickson, K. L., Adams, D. A., and McNeill, C. J.: Dietary lipid modulation of immune responsiveness. Lipids, 18:468, 1983.
78. Etthinger, M. G., and Kjaer, A.: Sulfur compounds in plants. *In* Recent Advances in Phytochemistry, Vol. 1, Edited by T. J. Mabry, R. E. Alston, and V. C. Runeckless, New York, Appleton-Century-Crafts, 1968.
79. Fakunle, J. B.: Evaluation of garlic extracts on cancer growth in rats fed diets with varying levels of protein. Diss. Abstr. Int. (Sci); 44:116-B, 1983.
80. Fenwick, G. R., Heaney, R. N., and Mullin, W. J.: Glucosinolates and their breakdown products in food and food plants. CRC Crit. Rev. Food Sci. Nutr., 18:123, 1983.
81. Fiala, E. S., Reddy, B. S., and Weisburger, J. H.: Naturally occurring anticarcinogenic substances in foodstuffs. Ann. Rev. Nutr., 5:295, 1985.
82. Fletcher, M. A., Caldwell, K., Claflin, A. J., and Malinin, T.: Further characterization of a tumor cell growth inhibitor from the balsam pear. Fed. Proc., 3:414, 1980.
83. Freudenheim, J. L., and Marshall, J. R.: The problem of profound mismeasurement and the power of epidemiological studies of diet and cancer. Nutr. Cancer, 11:243, 1988.
84. Garrett, B. J., Cheake, P. R., Miranda, C. L., Goeger, D. E., and Buhler, D. R.: Consumption of poisonous plants *(Senecio jocobaes, Symphytum officinala, Pteridium aquilinum, Hypericum perforatum)* by rats: Chronic toxicity, mineral metabolism, and hepatic drug-metabolizing enzymes. Toxicol. Lett., 10:183, 1982.
85. Garte, S. J., Currie, D. D., and Troll, W.: Inhibition of H-ras oncogene transformation of NIH 3T3 cells by protease inhibitors. Cancer Res., 47:3159, 1987.
86. Garz, H. J., Haag, W. I., Specht, J. E., and Haskins, F. N.: Assay of p-hydroxybenzaldehyde as a measure of hydrocyanic acid potential in sorghums. Crop Sci., 17:578, 1977.
87. Gitter, S., Gallily, R., Shomat, B., and Lavie, D.: Studies on the antitumor effect of cucurbitacins. Cancer Res., 21:516, 1961.
88. Goldberg, W. D., and Haddox, M. K.: Cyclic GMP metabolism and involvement in biological regulation. Ann. Rev. Biochem., 46:823, 1977.
89. Gordon, G. B., Shantz, L. M., and Talalay, P.: Modulation of growth, differentiation, and carcinogenesis by dehydroepiandrosterone. Adv. Enzyme Regul., 26:355, 1987.
90. Gori, G. B.: Priorities in cancer prevention: A conference appraisal. Prev. Med., 9:305, 1990.
91. Graham, S.: Toward a dietary prevention of cancer. Epidemiol. Rev., 5:38, 1983.
92. Graham, S.: Diet and Cancer. Am. J. Epidemiol., 112:247, 1980.
93. Graham, S., Dayal, H., Swanson, M., Mittelman, A., and Wilkinson, G.: Diet in the epidemiology of cancer of the colon and rectum. J. Natl. Cancer Inst., 61:709, 1978.
94. Graham, S., Humphrey, B., Marshall, J., Priore, R., Byers, T., Rzepka, T., Mettlin, C., and Pontes, J. E.: Diet in epidemiology of carcinoma of the prostate gland. J. Natl. Cancer Inst., 70:687, 1983.
95. Gregor, O., Toman, R., and Prusova, F.: Gastrointestinal cancer and nutrition. Gut, 10:1031, 1969.
96. Greenholgh, J. F. D., Aitken, J. N., and Gunn, J. B.: Kale anemia III. A survey of kale feeding practices and anemia in cattle on dairy farms in England and Scotland. Res. Vet. Sci., 13:15, 1972.
97. Gruhzit, O. M.: The haemolytic principles of onion juice. Am. J. Med. Res., 181:815, 1931.
98. Haliwell, B.: How to characterize a biological antioxidant. Free Radical Res. Commun., 9:1, 1990.
99. Hanson, C. H., Pederson, M. W., Berrang, B., Wall, M. E., and Davis, K. H.: The saponins in alfalfa cultivars. *In* Antiquality component of Forages, Madison, WI, Crop Science Society of America, 1973.
100. Hashimoto, Y., Shirdo, K., and Okamoto, T.: Metabolic activation of a mutagen, 2-amino-6-methyldipyrido [1,2-A:3′,2′,-d] imidazole. Identification of 2-hydroxyamino-6-methyldipyrido [1,2-a:3′,2′,-d] imidazole and its reaction with DNA. Biochem. Biophys. Res. Commun., 92:971, 1980.
101. Hashimoto, Y., Shido, K., and Okamoto, T.: Activation of a mutagen, 3-amino-1-methyl-5H-pyrido [4,3-b] indole. Identification of 3-hydroxyamino-1-methyl-5H-pyrido [4,3-b] indole and its reaction with DNA. Biochem. Biophys. Res. Commun., 96:355, 1980.
102. Harvey, J. W., and Rachear, D.: Experimental onion-induced hemolytic anemia in dogs. Veterinary Pathol., 22:387, 1985.
103. Hayatsu, H., Arimoto, S., and Negishi, T.: Dietary inhibitors of mutagenesis and carcinogenesis. Mutat. Res., 202:429, 1988.
104. Hems, G.: Associations between breast-cancer mortality rates, childbearing and diet in the United Kingdom. Brit. J. Cancer, 41:429, 1980.
105. Hems, G.: The contributions of diet and childbearing to breast-cancer rates. Brit. J. Cancer, 37:974, 1978.
106. Henderson, B. E., Pike, M. C., and Ross, R. K.: Breast cancer: Epidemiology and risk factors. Cancer Invest. Manage., 1:15, 1984.
107. Hendrich, S., and Pitot, H. C.: Enzymes of gluthathione metabolism as biochemical markers during hepatocarcinogenesis. Cancer Metastasis Rev., 6:155, 1987.
108. Hennipnan, A., Van Oirschot, B. A., Smits, J., Rijhsen, G., and Staal, G. E. J.: Tyrosine kinase activity in breast cancer, benign breast disease, and normal breast tissue. Cancer Res., 49:519, 1989.
109. Heshmat, M. Y., Kaul, L., Korr, J., Jackson, M. N., Jackson, A. G., Jones, G. W., Edson, M., Enterline, J. P., Worrell, R. G., and Perry, S. L.: Nutrition and prostate cancer: A case-control study. Prostate, 6:7, 1985.
110. Hill, M. J.: Bacterial metabolism and human carcinogenesis. Brit. Med. Bull., 36:89, 1980.
111. Hirono, I.: Natural carcinogenic products of plant origin. CRC Crit. Rev. Toxicol., 8:235, 1981.
112. Hockstein, P., and Atallah, A. S.: The role of oxidants and antioxidants in the inhibition of mutation and cancer. Mut. Res., 202:363, 1988.
113. Hocman, G.: Prevention of cancer: Vegetables and plants. Comp. Biochem. Physiol., 93:201, 1989.
114. Hocman, G.: Prevention of cancer: Restriction of nutritional energy intake (Joules). Comp. Biochem. Physiol., 91:209, 1988.
115. Homburger, F., and Boger, E.: The carcinogenicity of essential oils, flavors, and spices: A review. Cancer Res., 28:2372, 1968.
116. Hood, R. L., Oakenfull, D. G., and Topping, D. L.: Dietary saponins and plasma cholesterol. Proc. Nutr. Soc., 38:78A, 1979.
117. Horber, E., Leath, K. T., Berrang, B., Marcarian, V., and Hanson, C. H.: Biological activities of saponin components from DuPritts and Lahortan alfalfa. Entomol. Exp. Appl., 17:410, 1974.
118. Howe, G. R.: The use of polytomas dual response data to increase power in case-control studies: an application to the association between dietary fat and breast cancer. J. Chronic Dis., 38:663, 1985.
119. Howe, G. R., Miller, A. B., and Jain, M.: Total energy intake: implications for epidemiologic analysis. Am. J. Epidemiol., 124:157, 1986.
120. Hussain, S. P., Janner, L. N., and Rao, N. R.: Chemopreventive action of garlic on methylcholanthrene-induced carcinogenesis in the uterine cervix of mice. Cancer Lett., 49:175, 1990.
121. Inoue, H., Saito, H., Koshihara, Y., and Murota, S.: Inhibitory effect of glycyrrhetinic acid derivatives on lipoxygenase and prostaglandin synthetase. Chem. Pharm. Bull., 34:897, 1986.
122. Ishaaya, I., and Birk, Y.: Soybean saponins. IV. The effects of protein on the inhibitory activity of soybean saponins on certain enzymes. J. Food Sci., 30:118, 1965.
123. Ishii, K., Ando, M., Kamataki, T., Kato, R., and Nagoo, M.: Metabolic activation of mutagenic tryptophan pyrolysis products (Trp-P-1 and Trp-P-2) by a purified cytochrome P-450 dependent monooxygenase system. Cancer Lett., 9:271, 1980.
124. Ito, Y., Maeda, S., and Sugiyama, T.: Suppression of 7, 12-dimethylbenz(a)anthracene-induced chromosome aberrations in rat bone marrow cells by vegetable juices. Mutat. Res., 172:55, 1986.
125. Jacobs, L. R.: Fiber and colon cancer. Gastroenterol. Clin. North Am., 17:747, 1988.
126. Jacobi, H. P., and Baumann, C. A.: The effect of fat on tumor formation. Am. J. Cancer, 39:338, 1940.
127. Jagerstad, M., Reutersward, A. L., Dahlqvist, A., Greves, S., Nyhammer, T., Olson, K., Westesson, A. K., and Oste, R.: Creatinine and Maillard reaction products as precursors of the mutagenic IQ-compounds (imidazo-quinolines and quinoxaline) formed in fried beef. Maillard Symposium in Las Vegas, AOC-Symposium Series, 1983.
128. Jain, M., Cook, G. M., Davis, F. G., Grace, M. G., Howe, G. R., and Miller, A. B.: A case-control study of diet and colorectal cancer. Int. J. Cancer, 26:757, 1980.
129. Jilka, C., Strifler, B., Fortner, G. W., Hayes, E. F., and Takemoto, D. J.: In vivo antitumor activity of the bitter melon *(Momordica charantia)*. Cancer Res., 43:5151, 1983.
130. Kabayashi, S., Veda, K., and Komano, T.: The effect of metal ions on the DNA damage induced by hydrogen peroxide. Agric. Biol. Chem., 54:69, 1990.
131. Kandil, O. M., Abdullah, T. H., and Elkadi, A.: Garlic and the immune system in humans: its effect on natural killer cells. Fed. Proc., 46:441, 1987.
132. Karmali, R. A.: Eicosanoids in neoplasia. Prevent. Med., 16:493, 1987.
133. Kasai, H., Yamaizumi, Z., Shiomi, T., Yokoyama, S., Miyezawa, T., Wakabayashi, K., Nagoo, M., Sugimura, T., and Nishimura, S.: Structure of a potent mutagen isolated from fried beef. Chem. Lett., 485, 1981.
134. Kasai, H., Yamagumi, Z., Wakabayashi, K., Nagoo, M., Sugimura, T., Yokoyama, S., Muyazawa, T., and Nishimura, S.: Structure and chemical synthesis of Me-IQ, a potent mutagen isolated from broiled fish. Chem. Lett., 1391, 1980.
135. Kasai, H., Yamaizumi, Z., Wakabayashi, K., Nagoo, M., Sugimura, T., Yokoyama, S., Miyazawa, T., Spingarn, N. E., Weisburger, J. H., and Nishimura, S.: Potent novel mutagens produced by broiling fish under normal conditions. Proc. Jap. Acad. Sci., 56B:278, 1980.
136. Katsouyami, K. D., Trichopoulos, D., Boyle, P., Xirouchaki, E., Trichopoula, A., Lisseos, B., Vasilaros, S., and MacMahon, B.: Diet and breast cancer: a case-control study in Greece. Int. J. Cancer, 38:815, 1986.
136a. Kelloff, G. J., Malone, W. F., Boone, C. W., Sigman, C. C., and Fay, J. R.: Progress in applied chemoprevention research. Semin. Oncol., 17:438, 1990.
137. Kennedy, A. R., and Little, J. B.: Effects of protease inhibitors on radiation transformation in vitro. Cancer Res., 41:2103, 1981.
138. Ketterer, B., Meyer, D. J., Coles, B., Taylor, J. B., and Pemble, S.: Glutathione trans-

ferases and carcinogenesis. *In* Antimutagenesis and Anticarcinogenesis Mechanisms, Edited by D. M. Shankel, P. E. Hartman, T. Kada, and A. Hollaender. New York, Plenum Press, 1986, p. 103.
139. Khojasteh, A., and Kraybill, W. G.: Cancer of the esophagus: The environmental connection. South. Med. J., 81:878, 1988.
140. Kinlen, L. J.: Meat and fat consumption and cancer mortality: a study of strict religious orders in Britain. Lancet, 1:946, 1982.
141. Kikuchi, M., Ishikawa, T., Iida, T., Seto, S., Tamura, T., and Matsumoto, T.: Triterpene alcohols in the seed oils of *Momordica charantia* L. Agric. Biol. Chem., 50:2921, 1986.
142. Klurfeld, D. M., Weber, M. M., and Kritchevsky, D.: Inhibition of chemically induced mammary and colon tumor promotion by caloric restriction in rats fed increased dietary fat. Cancer Res., 47:2759, 1987.
143. Kolonel, L. W., Hinds, M. W., and Hankin, J. H.: Cancer patterns among migrant and native-born Japanese in Hawaii in relation to smoking, drinking, and dietary habits. *In* Genetic and Environmental Factors in Experimental and Human Cancer. Edited by H. V. Gelboin, B. MacMahon, T. Matsushima, T. Sugimura, S. Taitayama, and H. Takebe. Tokyo, Japan Scientific Societies Press, 1980, p. 237.
144. Kolonel, L. N., Nomura, A. M., Hinds, M. W., Hirohata, T., Hankin, J. H., and Lee, J.: Role of diet in cancer incidence in Hawaii. Cancer Res., 43(Suppl.):2397S, 1983.
145. Koppang, N.: Dimethylnitrosamine. Formulation in fish meal and toxic effects in pigs. Am. J. Pathol., 74:95, 1974.
146. Koppang, N.: Toxic effect of dimethylnitrosamines in cows. J. Natl. Cancer Inst., 52:523, 1974.
147. Koppang, N.: Toxic effect of dimethylnitrosamines in sheep. Acta Vet. Scand., 15:533, 1974.
148. Kreula, M., and Kiisvaara, M.: Determination of 1-5-vinyl-2-thioxazolidone from plant material in milk. Acta Chem. Scard., 13:1375, 1959.
149. Kretz, J.: Cancer Prevention. Krebsarzt, 18(1/2):1, 1963.
150. Kritchevsky, D.: Fat, calories and fiber. Prog. Clin. Biol. Res., 222:495, 1986.
151. Kritchevsky, D., Weber, M. M., Buch, C. L., and Klurfeld, D. M.: Calories, fat and cancer. Lipids, 21:272, 1986.
152. Kritchevsky, D., Weber, M. M., and Klurfeld, D. M.: Dietary fat versus caloric content in initiation and promotion of 7,12-dimethylbenzanthracene-induced mammary tumorigenesis in rats. Cancer Res., 44:3174, 1984.
153. Kritchevsky, D., Tepper, S. A., and Story, J. A.: Isocaloric, isogravic diets in rats. III. Effects of nonnutritive fiber (alfalfa or cellulose) on cholesterol metabolism. Nutr. Reports Inter., 9:301, 1974.
154. Kumagi, A., Nishimo, K., Shimomura, A., Kin, T., and Yamamura, Y.: Effects of glycyrrhizin on estrogen action. Endocrinol., 14:34, 1967.
155. Lam, L. K. T., Sparins, V. L., and Wattenberg, L. W.: Isolation and identification of kaweol palmitate and cafestol palmitate as active constitutents of green coffee beans that enhance glutathione S-transferase activity in the mouse. Cancer Res., 42:1193, 1982.
156. Larson, R. A.: The antioxidants of higher plants. Phytochem., 27:969, 1988.
157. Lathia, D., and Blum, A.: Role of vitamin E as nitrite scavenger and N-nitrosamine inhibitor: A review. Inter. J. Vitamin Nutr. Res., 59:430, 1990.
158. Lau, B. H. S., Adetumbi, M. A., and Sanchez, A.: *Allium sativum* (garlic) and atherosclerosis: a review. Nutr. Res., 3:119, 1983.
159. Lavik, P. S., and Bauman, C. A.: Further studies on the tumor promoting action of fat. Cancer Res., 3:749, 1943.
160. Le, M. G., Moulton, L. H., Hill, C., and Kramer, A.: Consumption of dairy products and alcohol in a case-control study of breast cancer. J. Natl. Cancer Inst., 77:633, 1986.
161. Leonard, T. K., Mohs, M. E., Ho, E. E., and Watson, R. R.: Nutrient intakes: cancer causation and prevention. Prog. Food Nutr. Sci., 10:237, 1986.
162. Libert, B.: Breeding a low-oxalate rhubarb: A genetic approach to improve the nutritional quality of oxalate-accumulating crop plants. Upsaala, Sweden, Swedish University of Agricultural Sciences, p. 1, 1986.
163. Liener, I.: Significance for humans of biologically active factors in soybeans and other food legumes. J. Am. Oil Chem. Soc., 56:121, 1979.
163a. Lippman, S. M., Hittelman, W. N., Lotan, R., Pastorino, U., and Hong, W. K.: Recent advances in cancer chemoprevention. Cancer Cells, 2:59, 1991.
163b. Lippman, S. M., Lee, J. S., Lotan, R., Hittelman, W., Wargovich, M. J., and Hong, W. K.: Biomarkers as intermediate end ponts in chemoprevention trials. J. Natl. Cancer Inst., 82:555, 1990.
164. Lubin, F., Wax, Y., and Modan, B.: Role of fat, animal protein, and dietary fiber in breast cancer etiology: a case-control study. J. Natl. Cancer Inst., 77:605, 1986.
165. Lubin, J. H., Burns, P. E., Blot, W. J., Ziegler, R. G., Lees, A. W., and Fraumeni, J. F.: Dietary factors and breast cancer risk. Int. J. Cancer, 28:685, 1981.
166. Lutz, W. K.; Endogenous genotoxic agents and processes as a basis of spontaneous carcinogenesis. Mut. Res., 238:287, 1990.
167. Macquart-Moulin, G., Riboli, E., Cornee, J., Charny, B., Berthezene, P., and Day, N.: Case-control study on colo-rectal cancer and diet in Marseilles. Int. J. Cancer, 38:183, 1986.
168. Magbodile, M. U. K., and Campbell, T. C.: Effect of protein deprivation on male weanling rats on kinetics of hepatic microsomal enzyme activity. J. Nutr., 102:53, 1972.
169. Madhaven, T. V., and Gopalan, C.: The effect of dietary protein on carcinogenesis of aflatoxin. Arch. Pathol., 55:133, 1968.
170. Magee, P. N., and Barnes, J. M.: The production of malignant primary hepatic tumors in the rat by feeding dimethylnitrosamine. Brit. J. Cancer, 10:114, 1956.
171. Malinow, M. R., McLaughlin, P., Naits, H. K., Lewis, L. A., and McNutty, W. P.: Effect of alfalfa meal on shrinkage (regression) of atherosclerotic plagues during cholesterol feeding in monkeys. Atherosclerosis, 30:27, 1978.
171a. Malone, W. F.: Studies evaluating antioxidants and beta-carotene as chemopreventives. Am. J. Clin. Nutr., 53;305s, 1991.
171b. Malone, W. F., Kelloff, G. J., Boone, C., and Nixon, D. W.: Chemoprevention and modern cancer prevention. Prev. Med., 19:553-561, 1989.
172. Manousos, O., Day, N. E., Trichopoulos, D., Gerovassilis, F., Tzonou, A., and Polychronopoulou, A.: Diet and colorectal cancer: a case-control study in Greece. Int. J. Cancer, 32:1, 1983.
173. Markovits, J., Linassin, C., Fosse, P., Couprie, J., Pierre, J., Jacqrumin-Sablon, A., Saucier, J. M., Le Peca, J. B., and Larsen, A. K.: Inhibitory effects of the tyrosine kinase inhibitor genistein on mammalian DNA topoisomerose II. Cancer Res., 49:5111, 1989.
174. Markovits, J., Linassier, C., Fosse, P., Couprie, J., Pierre, J., Jacquemin-Sablon, A., Saucier, J. M., LePecau, J. B., and Larsen, A. K.: Inhibitory effects of the tyrosine kinase inhibitor genistein a mammalian DNA topoisoinerase II. Cancer Res., 49:517811, 1989.
175. McCarty, M. F.: Nutritional modulation of mineralocorticoid and postaglandin production: Potential role in the prevention and treatment of gastric pathology. Med. Hypoth., 11:381, 1983.
176. McKeown-Eyssen, G., Holloway, C., Jazmaji, V., Bright-See, E., Dion, P., and Bruce, W. R.: A randomized trial of vitamins C and E in the prevention of recurrence of colorectal polyps. Cancer Res., 48:4701, 1988.
177. Mei, X., Wang, M. C., Xu, H. X., Pan, X. P., Gao, C. Y., Han, N., and Fu, M. Y.: Garlic and gastric cancer—the effect of garlic on nitrite and nitrate in gastric juice. Acta Nutr. Sinica., 4:53, 1982.
178. Melville, J., and Doak, B. W.: Cyanogenesis of white clover. II. Isolation of the glucosidose constitutent. New Zealand Sci. Technol., Sect. B., 22:367, 1940.
179. Messina, M. J.: Experimental colon cancer: Effects of route of administration of 1,2-dimethylhydrazine (DMH) administration, cabbage consumption and prior exposure to DMH. Diss. Abstr. Inst. [E], 48:3534, 1988.
180. Metscher, L. A., Drake, S., Gollapudi, S. R., Hannis, J. A., and Shankel, D. M.: Isolation and identification of higher plant agents active in antimutagenic assay systems. *Glycyrrhiza glabra*. Basic Life Sciences, 39:153, 1986.
181. Michnovitz, J. J., and Bradlow, H. L.: Induction of estradiol metabolism by dietary indole-3-carbinol in humans. Science, 82:947, 1990.
182. Miller, A. B.: Diet and cancer, A review. Rev. Oncology, 3:87, 1990.
183. Miller, A. B., Howe, G. R., Jain, M., Craib, K. J., and Harrison, L.: Food items and food groups as risk factors in a case-control study of diet and colo-rectal cancer. Int. J. Cancer, 32:155, 1983.
184. Miller, A. B., Kelley, A., Choi, N. W., Matthews, R. W., Morgan, L., Manan, J. D., Burch, J., Howe, G. R., and Joen, M.: A study of diet and breast cancer. Am. J. Epidemiol., 107:499, 1978.
185. Mirvish, S. S., Wallacave, L., Eagen, M., and Shubik, P.: Ascorbate-nitrite reaction: Possible means of blocking the formation of carcinogenic-N-nitroso compounds. Science, 177:65, 1972.
186. Montesano, R., and Hall, J.: Nitrosamine metabolism and carcinogenesis. Environ. Sci. Res., 31:447, 1984.
187. Mulinos, M. G., and Pomerantz, L.: Pseudo-hypophysectomy; condition resembling hypophysectomy produced by malnutrition. J. Nutr., 19:493, 1940.
188. Murphy, G. P.: Urologic cancer. Cancer, 62:1800, 1988.
189. Musey, P. I., Collins, D. C., Bradlow, H. L., Gould, K. G., and Preedy, J. R. K.: Effect of diet on oxidation of 17-beta-estradiol in mice. J. Clin. Endocrinol. Metab., 65:792, 1987.
190. Murad, F., Arnold, W. P., Mittal, C. K., and Broughler, J. M.: Properties and regulation of guanylate cyclase and some proposed functions for cyclic GMP. Adv. Cyclic Nucleotide Res., 11:175, 1979.
191. Nageo, M., Honda, M., Seino, Y., Yahagi, T., and Surgimura, T.: Mutagenesis of smoke condensates and the charred surface of fish and meat. Cancer Letter, 2:221, 1977.
192. Natori, S.: Plant secondary metabolites as chemical carcinogens. Bioactive Mol., 2:217, 1987.
193. Newberne, P. M.: Chemical carcinogenesis: Mycotoxins and other chemicals to which humans are exposed. Semin. Liver Dis., 4:122, 1984.
194. Newberne, P. M., and Conner, M. W.: Dietary modifiers in cancer. Prog. Clin. Biol. Res., 259:105, 1988.
195. Newberne, P. M., and Rogers, A. E.: Labile methyl groups and the promotion of cancer. Ann. Rev. Nutr., 6:407, 1986.
196. Newmark, H. L., Lipkin, M., and Makehwari, N.: Colonic hyperplasia and hyperproliferation induced by a nutritional stress diet with four components of Western-style diet. J. Natl. Cancer Inst., 82:491, 1990.
197. Nigro, N. D., and Bull, A. W.: Prospects for the prevention of colorectal cancer. Dis. Colon Rectum, 30:751, 1987.
198. Nigro, N. D.: Animal studies implicating fat and fecal steroids in intestinal cancer. Cancer Res., 41:3769, 1981.
199. Nishima, H., Iwashima, A., Itakura, Y., Matsura, H., and Fuwa, T.: Anti-tumor promoting activity of garlic extracts. Oncology, 46:277, 1989.
200. Nishino, H., Nishino, A., Takayosu, J., Hasegawa, T., Iwashima, H., Hirabayaski, K., Iwata, S., and Shibata, S.: Inhibition of the tumor-promoting action of 12-0-Tetradecanoylphorbol-13-acetate by some oleanic-type triterpenoid compounds. Cancer Res., 48:5210, 1988.
201. Nomura, A., Henderson, B. E., and Lee, J.: Breast cancer and diet among the Japanese in Hawaii. Am. J. Clin. Nutr., 31:2020, 1978.
202. Nuva, T., Yamazoe, Y., and Kato, R.: Metabolic activation of 2-amino-9H-pyrido [2,3-b] indole by rat liver microsomes. Mut. Res., 95:159, 1982.
203. Oakenfull, D. G., and Fenwick, D. E.: Absorption of bile salts from aqueous solution by plant fiber and cholestyramine. Brit. J. Nutr., 40:299, 1978.
204. Obidoa, O., and Okoro, D. C.: Effect of short term ingestion of *Telforia occidentalis* (fluted pumpkin) on the liver. I. Microsomal interactions with aflatoxin B_1. Qual. Plant Foods Human Nutr., 37:77, 1987.
205. O'Brian, C. A., Ward, N. E., and Vogel, V. G.: Inhibition of protein kinase C by the 12-0-tetradecanoylphorbol-13-acetate antagonist glycyrrhetinic acid. Cancer Lett., 49:9, 1990.
206. Ohuchi, K., Kamada, Y., Levine, L., and Tsurufuji, S.: Glycyrrhizin inhibits prostaglandin E2 production by activated peritoneal macrophages from rats. Prostaglandin Medicine, 7:457, 1981.
207. Okamoto, H., Yoshida, D., Saito, Y., and Mizusaki, S.: Inhibition of 12-0-tetradecanoylphorpol 13-acetate-induced ornithine decarboxylase activity in mouse epidermis by sweetening agents and related compounds. Cancer Lett., 21:29, 1983.
208. Okay, A. B., Roberts, B. A., Harper, P. A., and Dennison, M. S.: Induction of drug-metabolizing enzymes: mechanisms and consequences. Clin. Biochem., 19:132, 1986.
209. Ostgard, O.: Fodder rape. The effect of sowing methods and nitrogen fertilization on yield and chemical composition at different times of harvesting. Forsk. Fors. Landbruket, 24:577, 1973.

210. Pantuch, E. J., Pantuch, C. B., Garland, W. A., Min, B. H., Wattenberg, L. W., Anderson, K. E., Kappas, A., and Conney, A. H.: Stimulating effect of brussels sprouts and cabbage on human drug metabolism. Clin. Pharmacol. Ther., 25:88, 1979.
211. Pariza, M. W.: Fat, calories, and mammary carcinogenesis: net energy effects. Am. J. Clin. Nutr., 45:261, 1987.
212. Pariza, M. W.: Calorie restriction, ad libium feeding, and cancer. Proc. Soc. Exp. Biol. Med., 183:293, 1986.
213. Phillips, R. L.: Role of life style and dietary habits in risk of cancer among Seventh-Day Adventists. Cancer Res., 35:3513, 1975.
214. Pinto, J., Raiczyk, G. B., Huang, Y. P., and Rivlin, R. S.: New approaches to the possible prevention of side effects of chemotherapy by nutrition. Cancer, 58:1911, 1986.
215. Plescid, O. J., Brown, J., Lombardi, D., Lenti, L., Racis, S., and Pontieri, G. M.: Tumor-mediated immunosubversion: role of dietary essential fatty acids. Prostagl. Leukotr. Cancer, 6:321, 1989.
216. Potter, J. D., and McMichael, A. J.: Diet and cancer of the colon and rectum: a case-control study. J. Natl. Cancer Inst., 76:557, 1986.
217. Prentice, R. L., Kakar, F., Hursting, S., Sheppard, L., Klein, R., and Kreski, L. H.: Aspects of the rationale for the women's health trial. J. Natl. Cancer Inst., 80:802, 1988.
218. Price, K. R., and Fenwick, G. R.: Naturally occurring estrogens in foods—A review. Food Additives Contam., 2:73, 1985.
219. Raicht, R. F., Cohen, B. I., Fazzini, E. P., Sarwal, A. N., and Takahashi, M.: Protective effect of plant sterols against chemically induced colon tumors in rats. Cancer Res., 40:403, 1980.
220. Reddy, B. S.: Etiology of colon cancer. Prostaglandins Leukotrienes Cancer, 6:153, 1989.
221. Reddy, B. S.: Dietary fat and colon cancer: Animal models. Prevent. Med., 16:460, 1987.
222. Reddy, B. S.: Influence of types and levels of dietary fat on colon cancer. ACS Symp. Ser., 277:119, 1985.
223. Rohan, T. E., McMichael, A. J., and Baghurst, P. A.: A population-based case-control study of diet and breast cancer in Australia. Amer. J. Epidemiol., 128:478, 1988.
224. Rosenthal, G. A.: The biological effects and mode of action of L-canavanine, a structural analogue of L-arginine. Q. Rev. Biol., 52:155, 1977.
225. Ross, M. H., and Bras, G.: Tumor incidence patterns and nutrition in the rat. J. Nutr., 87:245, 1965.
226. Ross, M. H., and Bras, G.: Influence of protein under- and over-nutrition on spontaneous tumor prevalence in the rat. J. Nutr., 103:944, 1973.
227. Rydout, C. L., Wharf, S. G., Prue, K. R., Johnson, I. T., and Fenwick, G. R.: UK mean daily intakes of saponins-intestine-permeabilyzing factors in legumes. Food Sciences and Nutrition, 42F:111, 1988.
228. Sadhana, A. S., Rao, A. R., Kucheria, K., and Bijani, V.: Inhibitory action of garlic oil on the initiation of benzo [a] pyrene-induced skin carcinogenesis in mice. Cancer Lett., 40:193, 1988.
229. Schneider, J., Kinne, D., Fracchia, A., Pierce, V., Anderson, K. E., Bradlow, H. L., and Fishman, J.: Abnormal oxidative metabolism of estradiol in women with breast cancer. Proc. Natl. Acad. Sci., 79:3047, 1982.
230. Schwartz, A. G., Paskko, L., and Witcomb, J. M.: Inhibition of tumor development by dihydroepiandrosterone and related steroids. Toxicol. Pathol., 14:357, 1986.
231. Schulsinger, D. A., Root, M. M., and Campbell, T. C.: Effect of dietary protein quality on development of aflatoxin B_{-1}-induced hepatic preneoplasic lesions. J. Natl. Cancer Inst., 81:1241, 1989.
232. Schuman, L. M., Mandell, J. S., Raddke, A., Seal, V., and Halberg, F.: Some selected cases of the epidemiology of prostate cancer 1976–1979. *In* Trends in Cancer Incidence, Edited by K. Magnus. New York, Hemisphere Corp., 1982, p. 345.
233. Sen, N. P., Schwinghamer, L. A., Donaldson, B. A., and Miles, W. F.: N-nitrosodimethylamine in fish meal. J. Agric. Food Chem., 20:1281, 1972.
234. Setchell, K. D. R., Borriella, S. P., Hulme, P., Kirk, D. W., and Axelson, M.: Nonsteroidal estrogens of dietary origin: possible roles in hormone-dependent disease. Am. J. Clin. Nutr., 40:569, 1984.
235. Shabad, L. M.: Some principles on the prevention of cancer due to chemical substances. Med. Hyg. (Geneve), 22:1063, 1964.
236. Shan, X., Aw, T. Y., and Jones, D. P.: Glutathione-dependent protection against oxidative injury. Pharmacol. Ther., 47:61, 1990.
237. Silverman, J.: Nutritional aspects of cancer prevention: an overview. J. Am. Vet. Med. Assoc., 179:1404, 1981.
238. Shirtzer, H. G.: Indole-3-carbinol and indole acetonitrile influence on hepatic microsomal metabolism. Toxicol. Appl. Pharmacol., 64:353, 1982.
239. Smith, R. H.: S-methylcysteine sulphoxide, the Brassica anemia factor (a valuable dietary factor for man?). Vet. Sci. Commun., 2:47, 1978.
240. Smith, R. H.: Kale poisoning. Rep. Rowett Inst., 30:112, 1974.
241. Snowden, D. A., Philips, R. L., and Choi, W.: Diet, obesity, and risk of fatal prostate cancer. Am. J. Epidemiol., 120:244, 1984.
242. Spallholz, J. E.: Selenium and glutathione peroxidase: essential nutrient and antioxidant component of the immune system. Adv. Exp. Med. Bid., 262:145, 1990.
243. Sparins, V. L., Barany, G., and Wattenberg, L. W.: Effects of organosulfur compounds from garlic and onions on benzo [a] pyrene-induced neoplasia and glutathione S-transferase activity in the mouse. Carcinogenesis, 9:131, 1988.
244. Sparins, V. L., Mott, A. W., Barany, G., and Wattenberg, L. W.: Effects of allyl methyl trisulfide on glutathione-S-transferase activity and benzopyrene induced neoplasia in the mouse. Nutr. Cancer, 8:211, 1986.
245. Sparins, V. L., and Wattenberg, L. W.: Enhancement of glutathione S-transferase activity of the mouse forestomach by inhibitors of benzo(a)pyrene-induced neoplasia of this anatomic site. J. Natl. Cancer Inst., 66:769, 1981.
246. St. Clair, W. H., Billings, P. C., Carew, J. A., Keller-McGandy, C., Newberne, P., and Kennedy, A. R.: Suppression of dimethylhydazine-induced carcinogenesis in mice by dietary addition of the Bowman-Birk protease inhibitor. Cancer Res., 50:580, 1990.
247. Steyn, D. G.: Modern trends in methods of food production, food processing and food preparation which constitute a potential hazard to human and animal health. Repub. South Africa Dept. Agric. (Pretoria) Tech. Serv. Tech. Commun., 136:13, 1977.
248. Stowesard, G. S., Anderson, J. L., and Munson, L.: Protective effect of dietary brussels sprouts against mammary carcinogenesis in Sprague-Dawley rats. Cancer Lett., 39:199, 1988.
249. Sugiura, K., and Rhoads, C. P.: Experimental liver cancer in rats and its inhibition by rice-bran extract, yeast and yeast extract. Cancer Res., 1:3, 1940.
250. Sugimura, T.: Complexity of human carcinogenesis and new causes. Proc. Annu. Meet. Am. Assoc. Cancer Res., 30:683, 1989.
251. Sugimura, T.: Mutagens, carcinogens, and tumor promoters in our daily food. Cancer, 49:1970.
252. Sugimura, T.: Mutagens in cooked food. *In* Genetic Toxicology: An Agricultural Perspective, Edited by R. A. Fleck and A. Hollaender. New York, Plenum Press, 1982, p. 243.
253. Sugimura, T.: The Ernest W. Bertner Memorial Award Lecture: Tumor inhibitors and promoters associated with ordinary foods. *In* Molecular Interventions of Nutrition and Cancer. Edited by M. A. Arnat, J. Van Eys, and Y. M. Wang. New York, Plenum Press, 1982, p. 3.
254. Sugimura, T., and Sato, S.: Mutagen-carcinogenesis in foods. Cancer Res., 43(Suppl.):2415S, 1983.
255. Sugimura, T., Kawachi, T., Nagoo, M., and Yakagi, T.: Mutagens in food as causes of cancer. Prog. Cancer Res. Ther., 17:59, 1981.
256. Sugimura, T., Nagoo, M., and Wakabayashi, K.: Mutagenic heterocyclic amines in cooked foods. *In* Carcinogens: Selected Methods of Analysis, Vol. 4. Edited by H. Egan, L. Fishbein, M. Castegnaro, I. K. O'Neill, H. Bartsch, and W. Davis. Lyon, IARC Scientific Publication No. 40, 1981, p. 251.
257. Sugimura, T., Nageo, M., Kawacki, T., Honda, M., Yahagi, T., Seino, Y., Sato, S., Matsukura, N., Matsushima, T., Shiva, A., Sawanura, M., and Matsumo, H.: Mutagens-carcinogens in food, with special reference to highly mutagenic pyrolytic products in broiled foods. *In* Origins of Human Cancer, Book C. Edited by H. H. Hiatt, J. D. Watson, and J. A. Winsten. New York, Cold Spring Harbor, 1977, p. 1561.
258. Synge, R. L. M., and Wood, J. C.: (+)-(S-methylcysteine-S-oxide) in cabbage. Biochem. J., 64:252, 1956.
259. Takemoto, D. J., Dunford, C., and McMurray, M. M.: The cytotoxic and cytostatic effects of the bitter melon *(Momordica charantia)* on human lymphocytes. Toxicon, 20:593, 1982.
260. Takeuchi, K., Okada, M., Niida, H., and Okabe, S.: Role of sulfhydryls in mucosal injury caused by ethanol: relation to microvascular permeability, gastric motility and cytoprotection. J. Pharmacol. Exper. Ther., 248:836, 1989.
261. Tanaka, M., Mano, N., Okazai, E., Narui, Y., and Koyama, Y.: Inhibition of mutagenicity by glycyrrhiza extract and glycyrrhizin. J. Pharmacobiodyn., 10:685, 1987.
262. Tannenbaum, A.: Nutrition and Cancer. *In* The Pathophysiology of Cancer, 2nd Edition. Edited by F. F. Homburger. New York, Harper, 1959, p. 517.
263. Tannenbaum, A.: The role of nutrition in the origin and growth of tumors. *In* Approaches to Tumor Chemotherapy. American Association for the Advancement of Science, Washington, D. C., 1947, p. 96.
264. Tannenbaum, A.: The dependence of tumor formation on the composition of the calorie restricted diet as well as on the degree of restriction. Cancer Res., 5:616, 1945.
265. Tannenbaum, A.: A dependence of tumor formation on the composition of the calorie restriction. Cancer Res., 5:609, 1945.
266. Tannenbaum, A.: The dependence of the genesis of induced skin tumors on the calorie intake during different states of carcinogenesis. Cancer Res., 4:673, 1944.
267. Tannenbaum, A.: The genesis and growth of tumors. II. Effects of caloric restriction per se. Cancer Res., 2:460, 1942.
268. Tannenbaum, A.: The genesis and growth of tumors. III. Effects of a high fat diet. Cancer Res., 2:468, 1942.
269. Tao, Z., Jiao, G. S., Zhang, W., Li, Z. J., Shi, K. X., Qiu, X. Y., Wang, Y. D., Huang, W. H., Shi, R., and Chen, L.: The application of conditional logistic regression model to A 1:2 case control study on 200 cases of gastric cancer in Shanghai. First Shanghai International Symposium on Gastrointestinal Cancers. 11/14–16/88. Shanghai, 1989, p. 210.
270. Telek, L. 1979. Preparation of leaf protein concentrates in low and humid tropics. *In* Tropical Foods, Chemistry and Nutrition, Vol. 2, Edited by G. E. Inglett, and G. Charalambous. New York, Academic Press, 1979.
271. Temcharoen, P., Anukarahanonta, T., and Bhamarapravati, N.: Influence of dietary protein and vitamin B12 on the toxicity and carcinogenicity of aflatoxins in rat liver. Cancer Res., 38:2185, 1978.
272. Thomas, D. B., and Chu, J.: Nutritional and endocrine factors in reproductive organ cancers: Opportunities for primary prevention. J. Chronic Dis., 39:1031, 1986.
273. Thompson, H. J., Mecker, L. D., Tagliaferro, A. R., and Roberts, J. S.: Effect of energy intake on the promotion of mammary carcinogenesis by dietary fat. Nutr. Cancer, 7:37, 1985.
274. Tomatis, L.: Diet, nutrition and cancer: Concluding remarks and future perspectives. Int. Symp. Princess Takamatsu Cancer Res. Fund, 16:325, 1985.
275. Topping, D. L., Hood, R. L., Illman, R. J., Storer, G. B., and Oakenfull, D. G.: Effects of dietary saponins on bile acid secretion and plasma cholesterol in the rat. Proc. Nutr. Soc. August 3, 1968, 1978.
276. Troll, W.: Plant protease inhibitors as anticarcinogens. Fed. Proc. 44(3):xiii, 1985.
277. Troll, W., Frenhal, K., and Wiesner, R.: Protease inhibitors as anticarcinogens. J. Natl. Cancer Inst., 73:1245, 1984.
278. Troll, W., Wiesner, R., Shellaberger, C. J., Holtzman, S., and Stone, J. P.: Soybean diet lowers breast tumor incidence in irradiated rats. Carcinogenesis, 1:469, 1980.
279. Tsuda, H., and Okam, O. H.: Elimination of metabolic cooperation by glycyrrhetinic acid, on anti-tumor promoter, in cultured Chinese hamster cells. Carcinogenesis, 7:1805, 1986.
280. Tuyns, A. J., Hoelterman, M., and Kaaks, R.: Colorectal cancer and the intake of nutrients: oligosaccharides are a risk factor, fats are not. A case control study in Belgium. Nutr. Cancer, 10:181, 1987.
281. Unnikrishnan, M. C., Soudamini, K. K., and Kutlan, R.: Chemoprevention of garlic extract toward cyclophosphamide toxicity in mice. Nutr. Cancer, 13:201, 1990.
282. Vesely, D. L., Graves, W. R., Lo, T. M., Fletcher, M. A., and Levey, G. S.: Isolation of a guanylate cyclase inhibitor from the balsam pear *(Momordica charantia abbreviata)*. Biochem. Biophys. Res. Commun., 77:1294, 1977.
283. Walker, R.: Naturally occurring nitrate/nitrite in foods. Review J. Sci. Food Agric., 26:1735, 1975.
284. Walters, M. A., and Roe, F. J. C.: The effect of dietary casein on the induction of lung tumors by the injection of 9,10-dimethyl-1,2-benzanthracene (DMBA) into newborn mice. Brit. J. Cancer, 18:312, 1964.

285. Ward, P. A., Warren, J. S., Till, G. O., Varani, J., and Johnson, K. J.: Modification of disease by preventing free radical formation: A new concept in pharmacological intervention. Bailliares Clin. Haematol., 2:391, 1989.

286. Wargovich, M. J.: New dietary anticarcinogens and prevention of gastrointestinal cancer. Dis. Colon Rectum, 31:72, 1988.

287. Wargovich, M. J.: Diallyl sulfide, a flavor component of garlic *(Allium sativum)*, inhibits dimethylhydrazene-induced colon cancer. Carcinogenesis, 8:487, 1987.

288. Wargovich, M. J., Woods, C., Eng. V. W., Stephens, L. C., and Gray, K.: Chemoprevention of N-nitrosomethylbenzylamin-induced esophageal cancer in rats by the naturally occurring thioether, diallyl sulfide. Cancer Res., 48:6872, 1988.

289. Wargovich, M. J., and Lointier, P. H.: Calcium and Vitamin D modulate mouse colon epithelial proliferation and growth characteristics of a human colon tumor cell line. Can. J. Physiol. Pharmacol., 65:472, 1987.

290. Wargovich, M. J., and Goldberg, M. T.: Diallyl sulfide: A naturally thioether that inhibits carcinogen-induced nuclear damage to colon epithelial cells *in vivo*. Mutation Res., 143:127, 1985.

291. Watanobe, J., Kawgiri, K., Yonekawa, H., Nagoo, M., and Togashira, Y.: Immunological analysis of the roles of two major types of cytochrome P-450 in mutagenesis of compounds isolated from pyrolysates. Biochem. Biophys. Res. Commun., 104:193, 1982.

292. Watanabe, T., Shiraiski, T., Sasaho, H., and Oiski, M.: Inhibitors for protein-tyrosine kinases, ST638 and genistein: induce differentiation of mouse erythroleukemia cells in a synergistic manner. Exp. Cell Res., 183:335, 1989.

293. Watson, R. R., and Leonard, T. K.: Selenium and vitamins A, E, and C.: Nutrients with cancer prevention properties. J. Am. Diet Assoc., 86:505, 1986.

294. Wattenberg, L. W.: Inhibition of carcinogenesis by naturally-occurring and synthetic compounds. Basic Life Sci., 52:155, 1990.

295. Wattenberg, L. W.: Chemoprevention of cancer. Cancer Res., 45:1, 1985.

296. Wattenberg, L. W.: Inhibition of neoplasia by minor dietary constitutents. Cancer Res., 43(Suppl.):2448S, 1983.

297. Wattenberg, L. W.: Inhibition of carcinogen-induced neoplasia by sodium cyanate, tert-butyl-isocyanate and benzyl isothiocyanate administered subsequent to the carcinogen exposure. Cancer Res., 41:2991, 1981.

298. Wattenberg, L. W.: Inhibition of carcinogenic effects of polycyclic hydrocarbon by benzyl isothiocyanate and related compounds. J. Natl. Cancer Inst., 58:195, 197.

299. Wattenberg, L. W., Sparins, V. L., and Barany, G.: Inhibition of N-nitrosodiethylamine carcinogenesis in mice by naturally occurring organosulphur compounds and monoterpenes. Cancer Res., 49:2689, 1989.

300. Wattenberg, L. W., and Loub, W. D.: Inhibition of polycyclic hydrocarbon-induced neoplasia by naturally occurring indoles. Cancer Res., 38:1410, 1978.

301. Wawzonek, S., Ponsetti, I. V., Shephard, R. S., and Wiedemann, L. G.: Epiphyseal plate lesions, degenerative arthritis and dissecting aneurism of the aorta predicted by amino nitriles. Science, 121:63, 1955.

302. Weisburger, A. S., and Pensky, J.: Tumor inhibition by a sulfhydryl-blocking agent related to an active principle of garlic. Cancer Res., 18:1301, 1958.

303. Weisburger, J. H., and Wynder, E. L.: Etiology of colorectal cancer with emphasis on mechanism of action and prevention. Important Adv. Oncol., 1987, p. 197.

304. Weisburger, J. H., and Horn, C. L.: Human and laboratory studies on the causes and prevention of gastrointestinal cancer. Scand. J. Gastroenterol., 104(Suppl.):15, 1984.

305. Weisburger, J. H., Wynder, E. L., and Horn, C. L.: Nutritional factors and etiologic mechanisms in the causation of gastrointestinal cancers. Cancer, 50:2541, 1982.

306. Weisburger, J. H., Hegsted, D. M., Gori, G. B., and Lewis, B.: Extending the prudent diet to cancer prevention. Prev. Med., 9:297, 1980.

307. Weisburger, J. H., Marquardt, H., Mower, H. F., Hirota, N., Mori, H., and Williams, G.: Inhibition of carcinogenesis: Vitamin C and the prevention of gastric cancer. Prev. Med., 9:352, 1980.

308. Wells, P., Alftergood, L., and Alfin-Slater, R. B.: Effect of varying levels of dietary protein on tumor development and lipid metabolism in rats exposed to aflatoxin. J. Am. Oil Chem. Soc., 53:559, 1976.

309. West, L. G., Greger, J. L., and Nonnamaker, B. J.: Saponin-mineral interactions. Fed. Proc. Am. Soc. Exp. Biol., 37:667, 1978.

310. Willet, W., and Stampfer, M. J.: Total energy intake: implications for epidemiologic analysis. Am. J. Epidemiol., 124:17, 1986.

311. Wills, J. R.: Goitrogens in foods. *In* Toxicants Occurring Naturally in Foods. Natl. Acad. Sci. Natl. Res. Council, Washington, D. C., Publ. 1354, 1966.

312. Wilpart, M.: Dietary lipids and experimental colonic carcinogenesis. Critical review of the literature. Acta Gastroenterol. Belg., 51:357, 1989.

313. Witkowski, A., and Konopa, J.: Binding of the cytoxic and antitumor triterpenes, cucurbitacins, to glucocorticoid receptors of HeLa cells. Biochim. Biophys. Acta, 674:246, 1981.

314. Witkowski, A., Woynarowska, B., and Konopa, J.: Inhibition of the biosynthesis of deoxyribonucleic acid, ribonucleic acid, and protein in HeLa S3 cells by cucurbitacins, glucocorticoid acid-like cytoxic triterpenes. Biochem. Pharmacol., 33:995, 1984.

315. Wojtych, B., Podusowska, I., and Strawinska, Z.: Effect of rate of nitrogen on the contents of nitrates and goitrogens (vinyl) thioxazolidone and isothiocyanates in kale *(Brassica oleracea* var. *acephala)* and winter rape *(Brassica napus)*. Acta Agrar. Silvestria Ser. Agrar., 13:87, 1973.

316. Wynder, E. L.: Dietary factors related to breast cancer. Cancer, 46:899, 1980.

317. Wynder, E. L.: The dietary environment and cancer. J. Am. Diet Assoc., 71:385, 1977.

318. Yamanaka, W. K.: Vitamins and cancer prevention. How much do we know? Postgrad. Med., 82:149, 1987.

319. Yamazoe, Y., Ishii, K., Kamatachi, T., Kato, R., and Sugimura, T.: Isolation and characterization of active metabolites of tryptophan pyrolystate mutagen, Trp-P-2, formed by rat liver microsomes. Chem. Biol. Inter., 30:125, 1980.

320. Yang, C. S.: Modification of carcinogenesis by dietary and nutritional factors. Environ. Sci. Res., 31:465, 1984.

321. Yang, C. S., and Newmark, H. L.: The role of micronutrient deficiency in carcinogenesis. CRC Crit. Rev. Oncol. Hematol., 7:267, 1987.

322. Yokota, M., Narita, K., Kosuye, T., Wakabayashi, K., Nagoo, M., Sugimura, T., Yamaguchi, K., Shudo, K., Iitaka, Y., and Akamoto, T.: A potent mutagen isolated from a pyrolate of L-ornithine. Chem. Pharm. Bull., 29:1473, 1981.

323. You, W. C., Blot, W. J., Chang, Y. S., Ershow, A., Yang, Z. T., An, Q., Henderson, B. E., Fraumeni, J. F., and Wang, T. G.: Allium vegetables and reduced risk of stomach cancer. J. Natl. Cancer Inst., 81:162, 1989.

324. Young, V. R., and Newberne, P. M.: Vitamins and cancer prevention: Issues and dilemmas. Cancer, 47:1226, 1981.

325. Young, V. R., and Pellett, P. L.: Protein intake and requirements with reference to diet and health. Am. J. Clin. Nutr., 45:1323, 1987.

326. Youngman, L. D., Houghton, L. A., Bell, R. C., and Campbell, T. C.: The modulation of aflatoxin B1 (AFB1)-induced tumors by dietary protein. FASEB J., 3:A473, 1989.

327. Yu, L. Y. 1988. Nutritional factors in gastric cancer in China. First Shanghai International Symposium on Gastrointestinal Cancers. 11/14–16/88, Shanghai, China, 1989, p. 52.

328. Zeilig, C. E., and Goldberg, N. D.: Cell-cycle-related changes of 3/5-cyclic GMP levels in Naukoff hepatoma cells. Proc. Natl. Acad. Sci., 74:1052, 1977.

329. Ziegler, R. G.: A review of epidemiologic evidence that carotenoids reduce the risk of cancer. J. Nutr., 119:116, 1989.

330. Willett, W. C., Stampfer, M. J., Colditz, G. A., Rosner, B. A., and Speizer, F. E.: Relation of meat, fat, and fiber intake to the risk of colon cancer in a prospective study among women. N. Engl. J. Med., 323:1664, 1990.

VII

Cancer Screening and Early Detection

Charles R. Smart
Kenneth C. Chu
Veronica L. Conley
Donald E. Henson
Forrest Pommerenke
Sudhir Srivastava

Introduction

In 1992, an estimated 1,130,000 people in the United States will be diagnosed as having cancer and 520,000 will die of these diseases.[2] How many of these deaths could be avoided through early detection? Estimates vary from 3% to 35% depending on the criteria. Early detection via screening for breast and cervical cancer alone is projected to result in a 3% reduction in cancer deaths.[77] Adding early detection recommendations for these and other cancers to ordinary medical practice in physicians' offices could reduce the number of cancer deaths by one-third.[1] In 1987, the National Cancer Institute, with consultation from professional medical organizations and from the American Cancer Society developed early cancer detection guidelines for cancers of skin, oral, breast, colon & rectum, cervix, prostate, and testis.

In developing these guidelines the following definitions were used: *screening* is looking for disease in asymptomatic populations; *early detection* is looking for disease in asymptomatic and symptomatic patients (case-finding) in the physician's office; *detection* examinations, tests or procedures used in early detection or screening are usually not diagnostic, but suspicious for the presence of disease; and *diagnosis* is made following a work-up, a biopsy or other tests in pursuing symptoms or positive detection procedures.

The NCI Guidelines for Early Cancer Detection refer to individual case-finding in the physician's office. The purpose of this chapter is to present the NCI Guidelines, their rationale and supporting evidences.

Guideline Development

In developing the Guidelines, NCI called upon the major professional medical organizations in the U.S. for assistance.

The organizations responded by sending consultants knowledgeable in the detection of cancer. They were from the following organizations: American Academy of Dermatology; American Academy of Family Practice; American Academy of Otolaryngology Surgery; American Cancer Society; American College of Obstetricians and Gynecologists; American College of Physicians; American College of Radiology; American College of Surgeons; American Gastroenterology Association; American Medical Association; American Society of Clinical Oncology; American Society of Colon and Rectal Surgeons; American Society of Internal Medicine; American Urological Association; and Society of Surgical Oncology.

The guidelines are based on the best statistical and clinical information currently available. Evidence of a mortality reduction from a randomized trial is present only for breast cancer. All experimental data as well as other scientific evidence, such as incidence, stage of disease, treatment, survival and mortality statistics are considered.

The term "guideline" is used rather than "recommendation," because a physician considering a particular patient's background, medical history, and circumstances, may properly choose to make a different recommendation. They are considered "working guidelines" being subject to modification as new evidence becomes available. These guidelines are intended to promote greater uniformity and compliance in cancer detection practices within the medical profession. Moreover, the guidelines should encourage patients to be responsible for their own health, to the extent practicable. Patients should be encouraged in good health principles, such as abstinence from smoking, avoidance of sunburning, avoidance of dietary and other factors that predispose to cancer. They should also be encouraged and instructed in self examination of the skin, the breasts in women, and the testes in men.

The Scientific Basis

Two requirements must be met for early detection to be useful: 1) there must be a test or procedure that will detect cancers earlier and, 2) there must be evidence that earlier treatment will result in an improved outcome.

Detection

The majority of all detectable cancers (this includes skin cancer) can be suspected on a routine physical examination.

Observation is the most widely available examination for the detection of early cancer. It is useful in identifying suspicious lesions on the skin, lip, oral, larynx, external genitalia, and cervix. In white individuals skin cancer alone equals all other cancers combined. Fortunately, most skin cancers are highly curable, including melanomas, if detected early.

The second most valuable detection procedure is palpation. It is particularly valuable in detecting lumps, nodules, or tumors in the breast, mouth, salivary glands, thyroid, and subcutaneous tissues; enlarged lymph nodes in the neck, axilla, and groin; in the anus, and rectum; in the prostate and testis; and of the ovaries and uterus.

Internal cancers require an extension of observation through scopes, x-rays and ultrasound. Laboratory tests such as the Pap smear, and occult blood testing of the feces or urine have also proven helpful for some of these cancers. However, concerns regarding effectiveness, yield and cost play an important role in decisions to detect these internal cancers in asymptomatic individuals. The performance of these tests are measured in terms of sensitivity, specificity and positive predictive values. These measurements are more easily applied to laboratory tests than to physical examination.

There are some cancers where early detection does not appear useful; those where no early detection tests exist, as in cancer of the pancreas; and in cancers with no apparent localized phase, as in leukemia.

Improved Outcomes

The relation of stage to survival and mortality is the basis of clinical cancer management. It is the major factor in prognosis, in the determination of treatment and in the evaluation of end results. In the 1940's, a generalized staging classification of localized, regional and distant (LRD) was developed to show long term trends, and it is still useful. In the more detailed TNM system the (T)umor size, the status of the lymph (N)odes and the status of distant (M)etastases is also categorized. These elements are then grouped into Stages 0–4 according to their survival characteristics. The science of cancer classification by prognostic factors has developed through the extensive study of thousands of cases followed for many years. As malignant tumors increase in size they have a greater propensity to metastasize to regional lymph nodes and to distant sites (Figures VII-1-1 and VII-2-2; Table VII-1). Stage has such a profound effect that all randomized treatment trials require the comparison of similar stages in

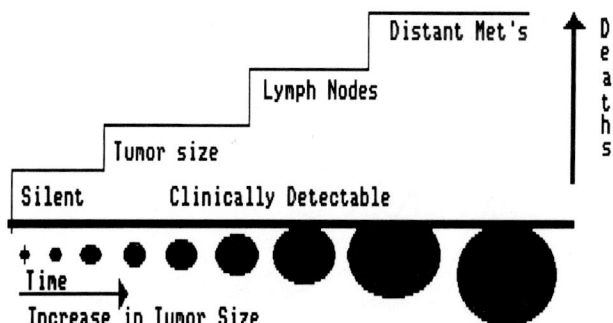

Figure VII-1-1. Dynamics of cancer spread.

evaluating differences in outcome. In the breast randomized screening trial, the reductions in mortality have been shown to be due to shifts in stage.[24,27] In other sites shifts in stage appear to herald improved survival and decreased mortality. Even in lung cancer where the randomized trial failed to show any difference in mortality between the study and the control arms it was because screening was occurring in both arms with nearly equal shifts to earlier stage disease (35.8% and 35.5%) compared to the usual 20% seen in clinical practice. There was a 30% over-all 5 year survival rate of all lung cancers in the trial.[13] Therefore even in lung cancer stage shift is an intermediate indicator of outcome.[23,98]

The Natural Experiment. The Surveillance, Epidemiology, and End Results (SEER) Program of the NCI, gathers data from 9 geographic areas, covering approximately 12% of the U.S. population. This data set, because of its total population coverage and long duration (1973–1987) is a unique and important resource in considering the potential for early cancer detection. Some cancers with a localized phase are shown in Table VII-1-2. Those with localized cancers have a better outcome than those with regional or distant spread. In considering over 1 million cancers (excluding in situ carcinomas and squamous and basal cell skin cancers) by stage the 5 year relative survival rate is 78% for localized cancer, 45% for regional cancer, and 12% for distant metastatic cancer.[78]

In geographic population based registries, studies of incidence, stage, treatment, survival and mortality that includes all cases, minimize selection, lead-time, length and healthy volunteer biases. When differences in over-all survival exist between two geographic areas, races, sexes, religious or socioeconomic groups, it is often due to stage differences reflecting detection practices.[100] An example is in oral cancers where the survival rate for black males is one-half that for white males (see section on oral cancer).

Where all patients with cancer within a geographic area have been followed for many years, case-fatality rates (1 – the survival rates) become a more accurate comparative measurement than mortality rates. Mortality rates are based upon information from death certificates, which is less accurate than the detailed information gathered in cancer registries from operative and pathology reports. In case fatality rates measurement begins at the time of diagnosis and is measured in months or years thereafter until death. It is generally reported as a percentage, number dying/100 with cancer at 1 year, 2 etc. A mortality rate (#/100,000 population/year),

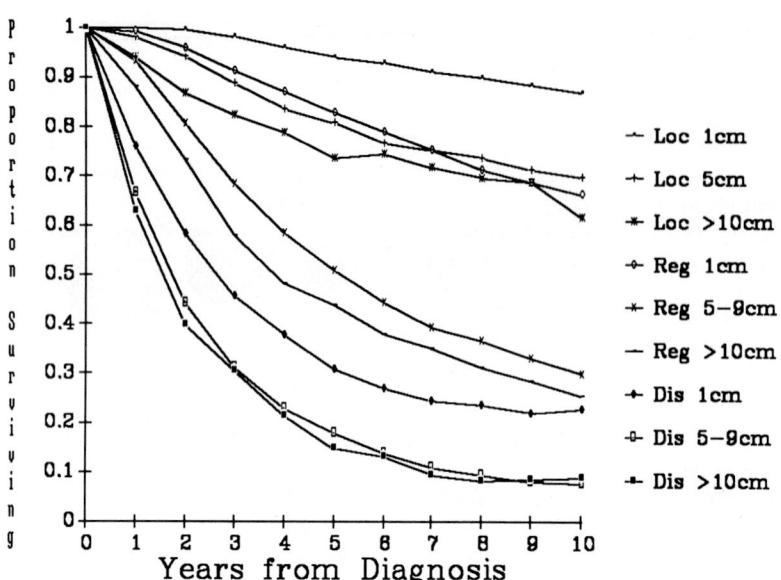

Figure VII-1-2.   Breast cancer relative survival by stage and tumor size.

Table VII-1-1.   Historical Stage Distribution & 5-Year Relative Survival Rate. SEER Program 1974–85

Site	Number	Distribution (%)				5-Year Survival (%)				
		Loc	Reg	Dist	Unk	Tot	Loc	Reg	Dist	Unk
Oral & Pharynx	24,937	38	40	12	9	52	76	41	18	45
Esophagus	7,929	28	20	27	25	6	12	4	1	5
Stomach	20,466	16	35	37	13	16	56	16	2	10
Colon	77,312	31	40	23	6	53	87	58	6	28
Rectum	33,810	39	34	18	9	50	79	46	4	33
Pancreas	21,410	11	20	52	16	3	6	4	1	4
Larynx	10,521	53	35	7	6	66	82	53	27	54
Lung	114,872	21	30	39	10	13	36	13	1	8
Bone	1,909	36	36	17	11	53	70	55	14	50
Soft Tissue	4,682	59	14	16	11	61	76	54	17	50
Melanoma	18,345	76	10	5	9	80	90	55	14	65
Breast	108,763	48	41	7	3	75	90	68	18	55
Cervix	13,222	45	31	9	14	67	88	51	14	67
Corpus	32,090	79	9	7	5	85	92	68	25	72
Ovary	16,656	24	12	60	5	38	85	45	18	30
Prostate	73,464	60	13	20	7	70	84	73	29	66
Testis	5,021	59	23	15	3	87	96	90	53	78
Bladder	36,374	72	20	3	5	75	87	43	9	60
Kidney	14,887	41	25	29	5	52	84	52	7	29
Brain	12,457	81	11	1	7	21	22	20	21	18
Thyroid	9,492	58	32	7	3	93	99	91	54	75

Table VII-1-2.   Median Survival Time in Years by Size of Tumor and Stage of Disease. SEER Program Data 1973–1986

	Breast Cancer 155,920			Colon Cancer 158,240			Lung Cancer 152,656		
	Loc	Reg	Dis	Loc	Reg	Dis	Loc	Reg	Dis
<1 cm	>13	12	1	>10	5	0.7	6	2	0.6
1 cm	>13	13	2	>10	4	0.8	6	2	0.7
2 cm	>13	11	2	>10	4	0.9	4	2	0.7
3 cm	12	8	2	9	4	0.9	3	2	0.6
4 cm	11	7	2	9	4	0.9	2	2	0.6
5-9 cm	10	6	2	8	4	0.8	1	1	0.6
>10	10	4	2	8	4	0.8	0.8	0.8	0.6

is concerned with the number dying within a specific year, but were diagnosed in that or previous years. Case fatality is looking from the time of diagnosis and thereafter, while mortality is looking from the time of death toward the diagnosis. The patterns are nearly identical mirror images (Figure VII-1-3). In oral cancer most deaths occur within the first 3 or 4 years following the diagnosis. Case fatality is an accurate measurement of death in a population based registry. In oropharyngeal cancer it gives evidence of an improved outcome in white males compared to black males from the earlier detection of oral cancers (as discussed later). Much can be learned regarding the value of early detection through the evaluation of these naturally occurring experiments.

There is a possibility through screening and early detection to discover some cancers that may never have surfaced in life.[39,85,92] This is particularly true in prostate cancer where autopsy series have shown a high percentage of occult carcinomas in elderly men.[46] The discovery of these cancers could increase the number of cases, give the appearance of stage shift and increased survival without necessarily reducing mortality. Therefore the strongest measures of an improved outcome are from greatest to least: a decrease in mortality, a stage shift in stage, an increase in survival, an increase in detection rates.

Designed Experimental Trials. Designed experimental trials are to correct for selection, lead-time, length, healthy volunteer and other biases when prospectively testing a detection procedure to determine its direct effect on outcome. The most direct evidence of benefit is mortality reduction in a randomized trial. Where such evidence is available, as with breast cancer,[97] it forms the basis for a guideline. For other sites, such evidence is not, and may never be available. Theoretically it is possible, but the sample size that is needed (Figure VII-1-4), the expense and the duration for such trials in other sites, such as melanoma, oral, or gastric cancers, is unrealistic. Therefore, evidence developed by other methods must be used.

Case Control and Cohort Studies. They provide indirect, but substantial evidence for the effectiveness of early detection. Such studies do not prove a mortality reduction effect, but they indicate the potential for mortality reduction through reduction of incidence of advanced disease and increased survival time. Such evidence is particularly compelling for the effectiveness of screening for cervical cancer.[105]

Descriptive Uncontrolled Studies. These studies based upon the experience of individual doctors, groups, hospitals, and non-population based registries yield important information for screening and early detection. The performance of various detection tests, such as sensitivity, specificity and positive predictive values, are generally first reported in descriptive studies. The first evidence that early detection is successful is an increase of early cancers with shifts in stage and increased survival rates. Later a reduction in deaths may occur. These are generally first reported in descriptive studies. Examples are the two sigmoidoscopy studies, which together include over 44,000 patients followed for 15–25 years, showing a 85–90% survival rate of those detected with rectal cancer.[44,51]

In addition to the organs in which cancers may be detected as part of screening, that are considered below, other sites are important for early diagnosis during screening examinations. The thyroid should be examined by inspection and palpation in every patient. Enlargement or nodularity requires additional inquiry which is detailed in chapter XXVI-2. Search for lymph nodes in the neck, axillae, groins and femoral areas should be performed in every physical examination. A node that is significantly enlarged without suitable explanation for more than 3 weeks deserves further diagnostic study. The contours of the body should be symmetrical and undistorted by masses in the cutaneous and subcutaneous tissues. Detection of such a mass by inspection and palpation requires differential diagnosis among many inflammatory, developmental and traumatic events. If the differential diagnosis includes a neoplasm, many lumps and bumps are benign tumors, such as lipomas and neurofibromas. The early diagnosis of soft tissue sarcomas requires detection of the mass

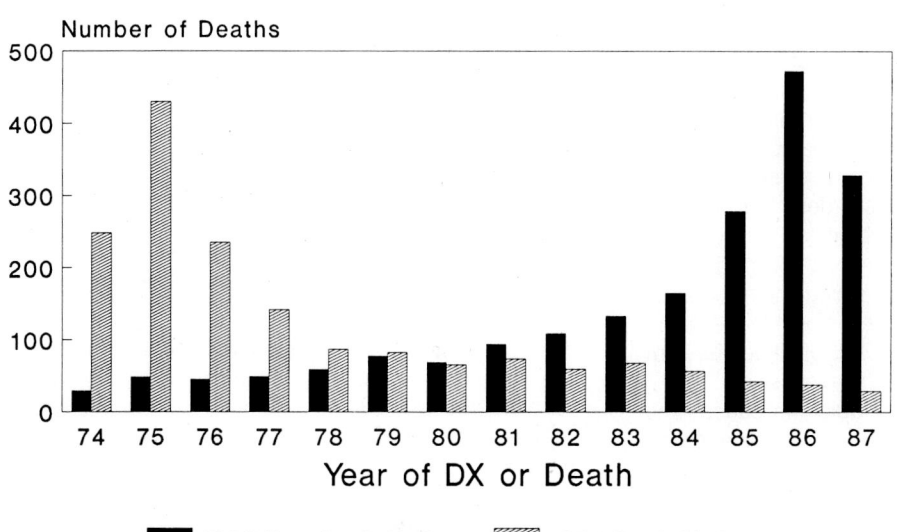

Figure VII-1-3. Oropharyngeal cancer, case fatality for 1974 vs. mortality 1987.

Number of Deaths

Year of DX or Death

■ 1987 Deaths & Yr Dx   ▨ 1974 Dx & Yr Death

SEER Data 1974-1987

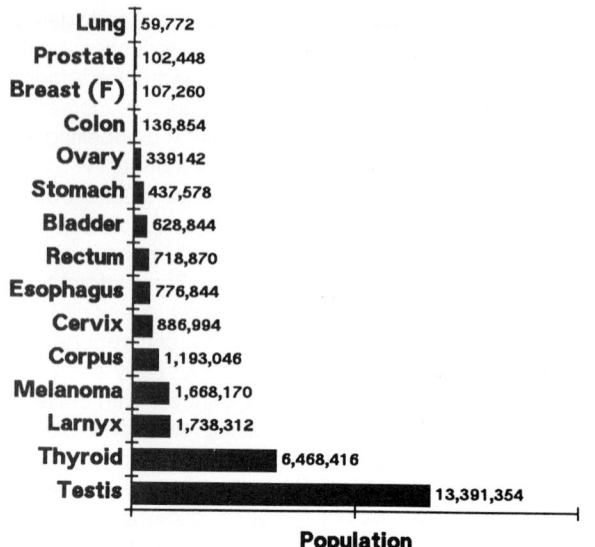

Figure VII-1-4. Sample size calculations, 90% power to decrease mortality 25%.

and the clinical judgment concerning those masses which require histologic evaluation.

Skin Cancer

Guideline

That primary care physicians be encouraged to examine the skin as part of the periodic health examination and in other patient encounters.

That all individuals should be encouraged to examine their skin thoroughly on a regular basis.

That special attention be given to pigmented nevi and also to high risk individuals with a personal or family history of skin cancer, melanoma or dysplastic nevi.

Significance

Skin cancer is the most common cancer in the U.S., affecting some 600,000 white Americans every year. It accounts for 1.7% of all cancer deaths.[2] Nearly all occur in fair skinned individuals who have been exposed to the sun, x-rays or ultra-violet light for prolonged periods. There are three main types—basal cell, the most prevalent; squamous cell; and malignant melanoma. Basal and squamous cell cancers have an excellent prognosis. They are easily detected clinically and are often cured by an excision biopsy. This does not mean that they are unimportant or should be neglected. When neglected they may be very deforming and may cause death. However, melanoma, the rarest but most virulent, (Figures VII-1-5, 6) is responsible for 75% of all deaths from skin cancer and will be the focus of this discussion.

The incidence of melanoma rises rapidly in caucasians after age 20 (Figure VII-1-7). Fair-skinned individuals exposed to the sun are at higher risk. The best defense against skin cancer is protection from the sun and ultra-violet light. Individuals with the familial or sporadic form of the dysplastic nevus syndrome are at high risk for melanoma.[78]

In recent years, the mortality from melanoma has increased rapidly especially in white males,[74] possibly as a result of

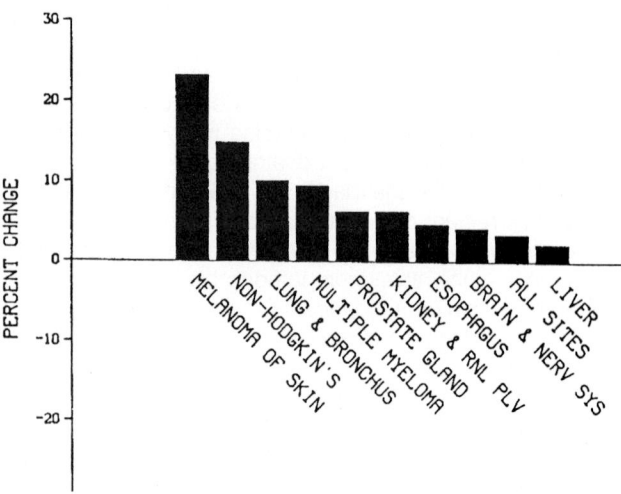

Figure VII-1-5. Increases in cancer mortality in the United States, 1975–1984 in white males.

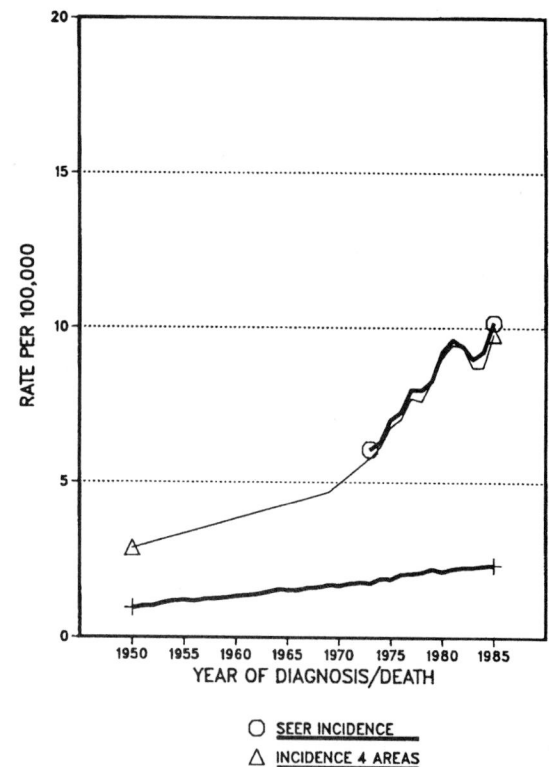

Figure VII-1-6. Melanoma of skin in white males and females.

increased recreational exposure to sunlight. In 1992, 32,000 individuals are expected to develop melanoma and 6,700 are expected to die.[2] There is an increase in mortality as well as in the incidence. Incidence has increased nearly 80% between 1973 and 1987, at nearly 10% per year.[78]

Evidence of Benefit

Progress can be measured in overall survival rates. The 5-year survival has continued to increase over time. In 1973, the overall 5-year survival was 71.9% whereas in 1986 it had

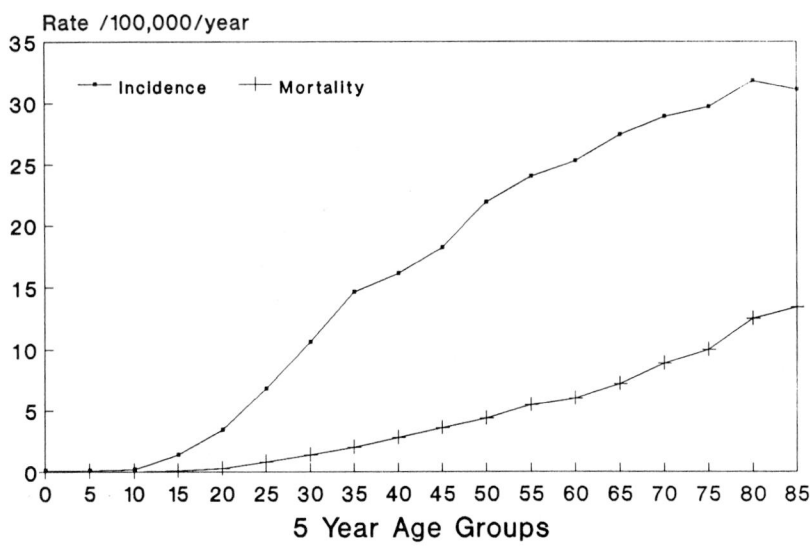

Rate /100,000/year

5 Year Age Groups

SEER Data 1983-1987

Figure VII-1-7.   Melanoma in white males and females, age specific incidence and mortality.

Figure VII-1-7.   Melanoma in white males and females, age specific incidence and mortality.

increased to 81.4%. The 5-year relative survival rate for localized stage is 90% (Figure VII-1-8).[78]

Over 90% of melanomas that arise in the skin can be recognized with the naked eye. Very often there is a prolonged horizontal growth phase during which time the tumor expands centrifugally beneath the epidermis but does not invade the underlying dermis. This horizontal growth phase provides lead time for early detection. Melanoma is 100% curable if treated prior to the onset of the vertical growth phase with its metastatic potential.[42] Two countries, Australia and Scotland, have had vigorous public and professional education programs resulting in a shift to earlier stage disease and improved survival.

In Queensland, Australia, which has the highest incidence of melanoma in the world, the overall survival rate for 1,187 patients was greater than 82%. No deaths were recorded for Stage I patients and Stage II patients had a 10-year survival of 90%. More importantly, Australia, with its rising incidence, has registered the first documented stabilization in population based mortality rates for melanoma associated with professional and public education.[52]

A similar program in Scotland also led to the detection of early disease.[32] Following a public education program in Scotland, the proportion of patients with primary melanomas categorized "thin, good prognosis" had risen from 38% to 62%. The proportion of tumors categorized as "thick, poor prognosis" had fallen from 34% to 15%.

The probability of tumor recurrence in 10 years is less than 10% with tumors less than 1.4 mm in thickness. For patients with tumors less than 0.76 mm in thickness, the likelihood of recurrence is less than 1% in 10 years.[11]

An important additional advantage of early detection is a reduction in the need for admission to the hospital and thus a decrease in hospital costs. A high proportion of patients with thin melanomas require only local excision which can be performed on an outpatient basis. The treatment of early lesions is less morbid than the treatment of advanced lesions.

Oral Cancer

Guideline

That starting at age 50 a complete oral examination be performed as part of the periodic health examination and other appropriate patient encounters.

That special attention be given those individuals at high risk due to tobacco and alcohol use and socioeconomic status.

That patients be counseled on smoking cessation and on alcohol moderation or abstention.

Significance

Cancers of the oral cavity and pharynx are a major cause of death from cancer in the U.S. An estimated 30,300 new cases of oral cancer will be diagnosed in the United States in 1991.[2] This disease will affect approximately 20,600 men and 9,700 women. In the same year, oral cancer is expected to cause 7,950 deaths. This form of cancer accounts for about 4% of cancers in men and 2% in women. It occurs

MELANOMA OF SKIN

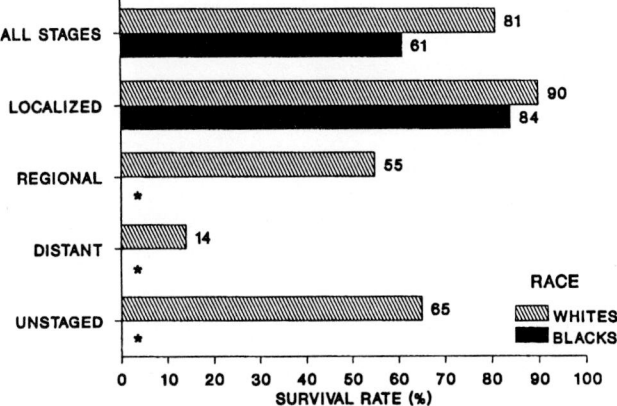

Figure VII-1-8.   Survival rates for 5 years, SEER program, 1981–1986.

more frequently in blacks than whites.[78] More than 90% of oral cancers occur in patients over the age of 45 (Figure VII-1-9). The incidence increases steadily with age until 65, when the rate levels off. Over the past 11 years there has been no change in incidence, but there has been a slight decrease in mortality rate (Figure VII-1-10).

Trends over the same years have shown little change in early stage disease varying from 2–27% in men of all races.

The primary risk factors for oral cancer in American men and women are tobacco and alcohol use; lower socioeconomic status, poor oral hygiene and decayed teeth have also been implicated.[37]

Oral cancer occurs in a region of the body that is generally accessible to physical examination by the patient, the dentist and the physician. Screening can be made more efficient by inspecting the high risk sites where 90% of all squamous cell cancers arise: the floor of the mouth, the ventrolateral aspect of the tongue and the soft palate complex.[67] It has been pointed out that high risk individuals visit their medical doctors more frequently than their dentists. An inspection of the oral cavity should be part of every physical examination in a dentist's or physician's office without additional costs.

Although easily detected and often cured in its early stages, most oral cancers are moderately advanced (regional stage) at the time of diagnosis. Unfortunately, this trend has not changed. An oral examination should also look for erythroplastic lesions, the earliest sign of squamous cell carcinoma.[20] The overall survival rate also has not changed over the past few years (Figure VII-1-11).

Evidence of Benefit

The routine examination of asymptomatic and symptomatic patients results in the detection of earlier stage cancers. In 1982, routine oral examinations were performed on 672,000 initial exam veteran patients with the detection of 814 oral squamous cell cancers. In high risk heavy smokers and drinkers over 40 years of age, the detection rate can be as high as one cancer in every 200–250 individuals examined.[67] In a regional oral cancer detection program in the

Boston area, early stage disease increased from 20% to 33% over a three year period by stressing the importance of the routine oral examination.[86] It did not require an intricate time consuming examination, just an examination. In Sri Lanka, primary health care workers were trained in the oral examination and they sent to a referral center 660 suspected cancers of which only 10% had no lesion, and 58% were confirmed as having oral cancer.[110]

When an entire population is monitored, white males have a higher percentage of oral cancer diagnosed and treated earlier than black males (Figure VII-1-12). White males with localized cancer have a better survival than black males. This indicates either more advanced localized disease in black males or a difference in treatment (Figure VII-1-13). Unfortunately most oral cancers are advanced in both races when detected and early detection does not result in a better outcome for them.

Breast Cancer
Guideline

That women should be encouraged to do monthly breast self examination.

That clinical examination of the breasts and mammography are the basic detection methods. The examinations are complementary and both are necessary to achieve maximum detection rates.

That the screening process should begin by age 40 and consist of annual clinical examination with screening mammography performed at 1–2 year intervals.

That beginning at age 50, both clinical examination and mammography should be performed on an annual basis.

That special surveillance be given women with a personal history of breast cancer or history of breast cancer in a mother or sister.

Significance

In 1992 in the United States breast cancer is the number one cancer in women with an estimated 181,000 new cases.[2]

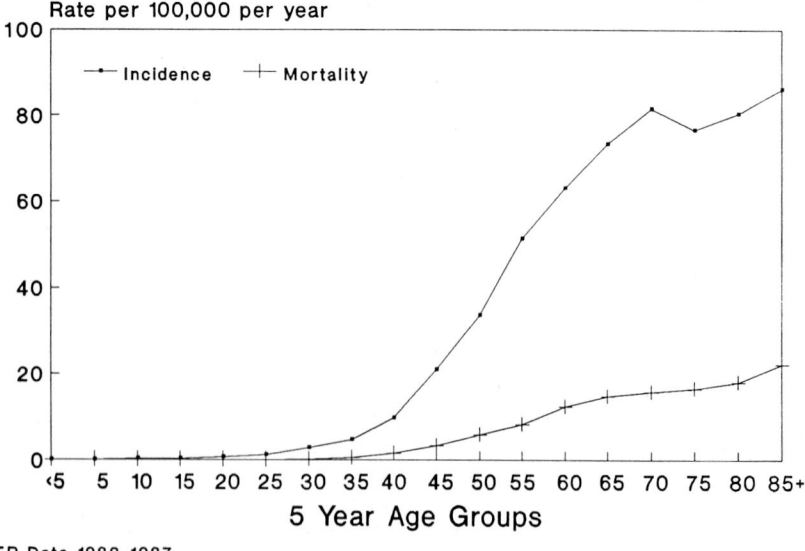

Rate per 100,000 per year

5 Year Age Groups

SEER Data 1983-1987

Figure VII-1-9. Cancer of the oral cavity and pharynx, age specific incidence and mortality rate.

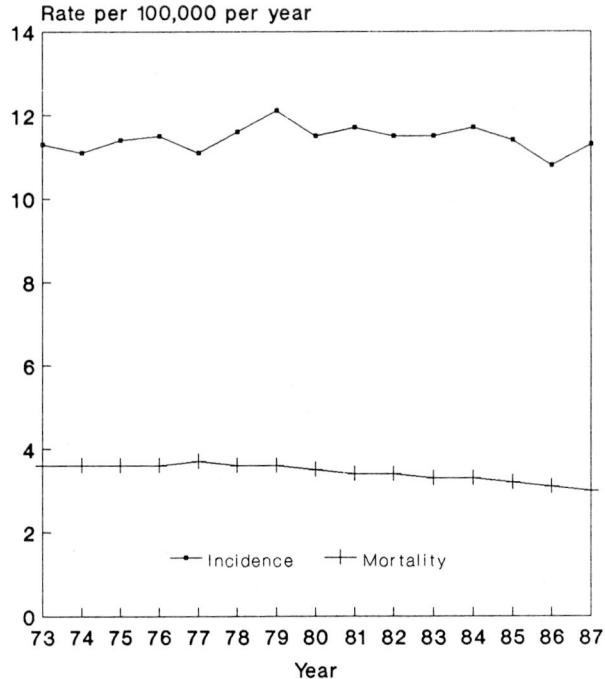

SEER Data 1973 - 1987 All Races & Sexes

Figure VII-1-10. Oral and pharyngeal cancer, trends in incidence and mortality.

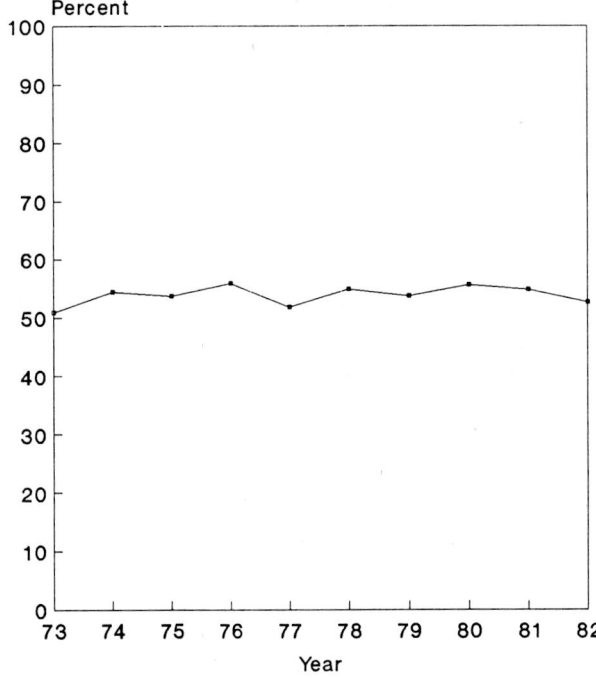

SEER Data 1973-1982 White Race

Figure VII-1-11. Oral and pharyngeal cancer, trends in relative 5-year survival rates.

The incidence has been increasing 1% per year over the past 50 years with only a slight increase in the mortality rate. A woman's lifetime risk is now 1:9 of developing breast cancer. In 1992, 46,300 breast cancer deaths are expected. It was the leading cause of death from cancer in women until 1987, when lung cancer took first place. The incidence has been increasing in an interesting way, to be discussed later, but the mortality rate is rather constant having increased only 1.5% since 1973 (Figure VII-1-14). Breast cancer in American males constitutes approximately 1% of the annual incidence of breast cancer. In African males it constitutes 5–15% of the annual incidence.

The risk of developing breast cancer is increased in women who have already had cancer in one breast or where there is a history of breast cancer in a mother or sister. However, for 85% of women the major risk factors are sex and age (Figure VII-1-15).[78]

Evidence of Benefit

In 1973–1974 there was a sharp increase in the incidence of breast cancer in the U.S. This rise in incidence was due to the sudden increase in early detection activity associated with the publicity given the President and Vice President's wives' diagnoses of breast cancer. Much of this was due to self-examination. There was not only an increase in the number of cancers but a shift toward earlier stage and earlier age. This demonstrated the potential of early detection to have an immediate effect.

In 1980, there began a second acute increase in breast cancer detection which followed the publishing of the American Cancer Society's breast cancer detection guidelines[3] and the initiation of a Breast Cancer Awareness Campaign. NCI and other organizations also joined in the effort. Between 1980 and 1987 there was a 32% increase in breast cancer incidence (Figure VII-1-14).[78]

This increase is due largely to mammographic detection, since it has been associated with a similar increase in the sale of new mammographic machines[12] and in the number of mammograms.[26] The percentage of women over 40 years of age who obtained at least one mammogram rose from 37% in 1987 to 64% in 1990, and the percentage of women who had more than one and who followed the guidelines rose from 17% to 31%.[107] The increase has been in smaller cancers and in early stage disease (Figures VII-1-16 and VII-1-17).

The 5 year survival rate for breast cancer remained at 75% until 1980 when it increased to 79% over a three-year period. (In situ cancers were excluded from both the incidence and survival rates). The staging system of localized, regional, and distant disease is useful in showing long term trends.

From 1981 to 1986 the 5-year relative survival rate for localized disease was 91% for white and 86% for black women, for regional disease 70% and 56%, and for distant disease it was 19% and 14% respectively (Figure VII-1-18).

Screening Trials

Randomized clinical trials have shown that early detection of breast cancer does reduce mortality. A study through the Health Insurance Plan of Greater New York (HIP) for early detection was conducted from 1963 through 1969. It involved

Stage

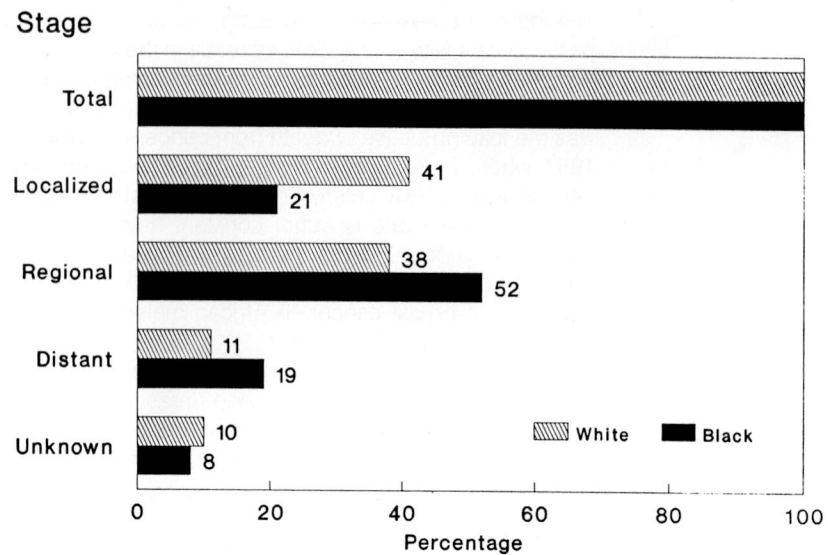

Figure VII-1-12. Oral and pharyngeal cancer in males, stage at diagnosis by race.

SEER Data 1974 - 1986, 1990 Report

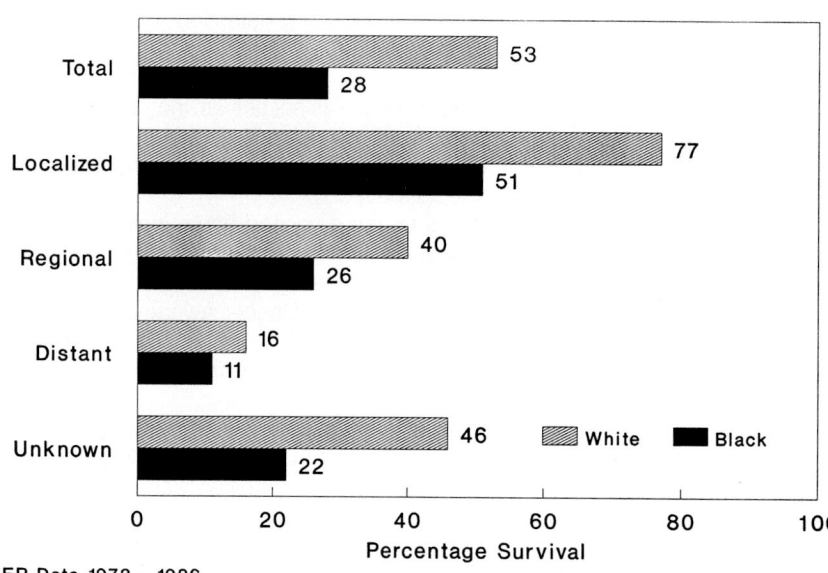

Figure VII-1-13. Oral and pharyngeal cancer in males, 5-year relative survival by race.

SEER Data 1973 - 1986

62,000 women 40–64 years of age who were randomized into a study group of 31,000. The study group of 31,000 were offered a clinical breast examination and mammography; 21,000 women (67%) accepted, and 10,000 (33%) refused. After the initial screen, three subsequent annual screens were offered with a 39.4% compliance rate for all four screens.[97]

The control group of 31,000 women received usual medical care but were followed closely to determine the number of breast cancers, their stage, survival and the number of ensuing deaths from breast cancer. Despite the large size of the HIP trial with 62,000 women, it was not designed to permit subgroup analysis by age groups. Thirty-one cancers were detected in the under 50 age group, 66 in the 50–59 category, and 35 in the over 60 group. Five women under 50 who were screen-detected died of breast cancer within the first five years, 9 women age 50–59 died, and 3 women 60 or older died. Even though the breast cancer deaths in

the interval and refused groups are added to the screen-detected to constitute the study group for comparison with the control group, the numbers still remain small: 39 vs. 63. The mortality difference between study and control groups was statistically significant by five years after entry for women age 50 and older (Figure VII-1-19). At ten years from entry there were 30% fewer breast cancer deaths in the study group than in the control group. In the subgroup of women 40–49 years of age, the mortality difference was not significant until the 9th year after entry, and continued through the 18 years of followup at which time it was 24% for the younger women and 23% for the older (Figure VII-1-20).[24] This decrease in mortality was in women who had their breast cancers diagnosed when they were under 50 years of age.

Improved Mammography and Detection

Using 1960's technology in the HIP Trial, and despite the fact that only 43% of the study group were detected through

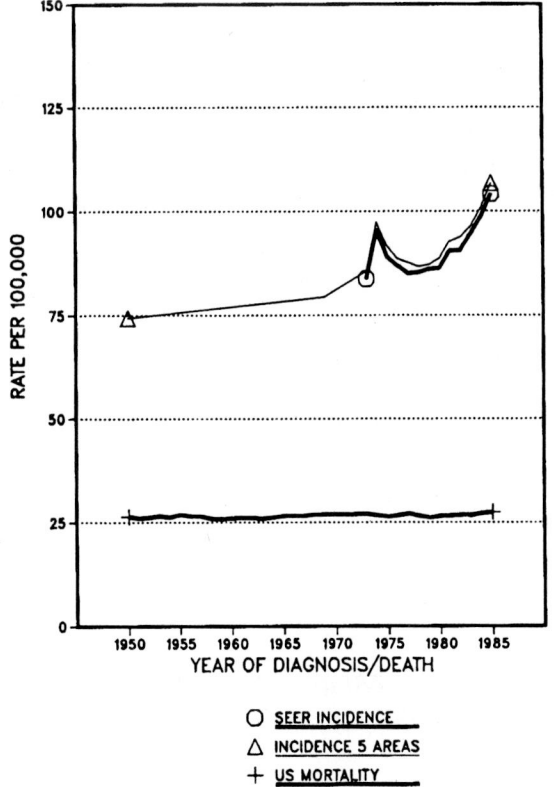

Figure VII-1-14.   Breast cancer—white females.

- ○ SEER INCIDENCE
- △ INCIDENCE 5 AREAS
- + US MORTALITY

This project was not a randomized trial, but a demonstration that large numbers of American women, (280,000, 35–74 years of age), could be recruited for five yearly clinical and mammographic breast examinations. It was also designed to determine whether breast cancers detected earlier would be more amenable to treatment than the usual cases seen in community practice. The women in the BCDDP had an incidence rate nearly double that of the Third National Cancer Survey (TNCS) that was conducted from 1969–1971 (Figure VII-1-21).[9]

The TNCS was a cancer incidence population-based survey covering 10 cities and 2 states. The women in the BCDDP were a self-selected volunteer high risk group. They were characterized by a higher than average income, more white, and more with a personal and family history of breast cancer than was seen in either the HIP Trial or in the general U.S. population. It is noteworthy, not only that the incidence rate was double the expected rate as compared to the TNCS, but the incidence of cancer in the age group 45–49 was the same as that in the 55–59 year age group. The data in Figure VII-1-21 were developed in 1977, in the middle of the BCDDP, considering only the first two screenings, while routine mammographic screening of women in their forties was still in force.[9]

Mammography techniques improved in the 1970's (Table VII-1-3). In the HIP Trial, mammography was only able to detect 40% of the cancers in women 40–49 and in 60% of women with cancer 50–59. In the BCDDP, mammography had improved and detected breast cancer at nearly the same rate: 91% in women 40–49 and 92.0% for women age 50–59.[5,9,95,99,102]

screening (mammography or physical examination), the trial resulted in a 30% decrease in mortality. In women over 50 years of age, shifts occurred from Stage III to Stage II, and from Stage II to Stage I. For women age 40–49 at the time of screening the delayed benefit was due to a shift to smaller sizes of cancers within Stage I in the screened group.[24,27] From 1973–1982, as a result of the proven benefits of screening in the HIP Trial, the ACS and NCI jointly funded the Breast Cancer Detection Demonstration Project (BCDDP).[5,9,99,102]

Trials in Other Countries

Many trials have been conducted in other countries as outlined in Table VII-1-4. The majority of trials have shown early detection from screening, however few have reached statistical significance.

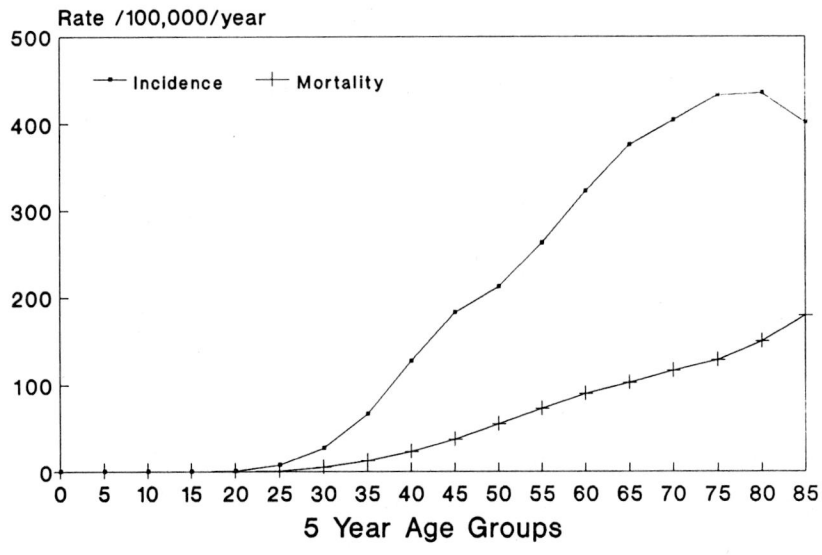

Figure VII-1-15.   Breast cancer in females, age specific incidence and mortality.

SEER Data 1983-1987

PERCENTAGE

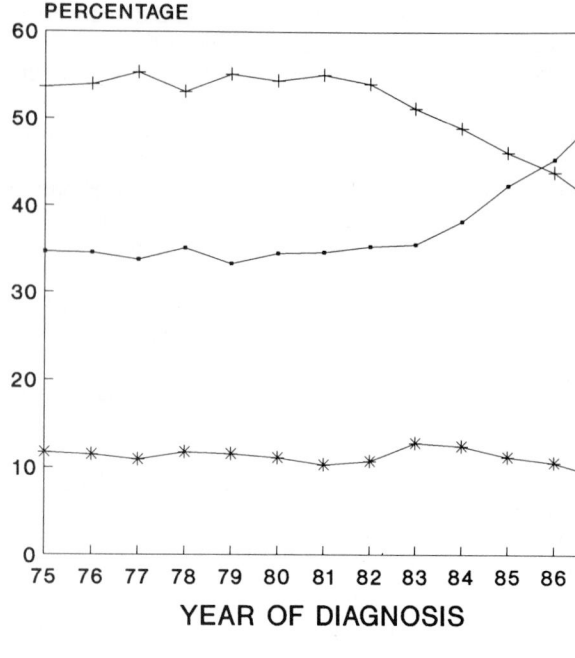

YEAR OF DIAGNOSIS

Figure VII-1-16. Breast cancer trends in size. SEER program 1975–1987.

RATE PER 100,000 /YEAR

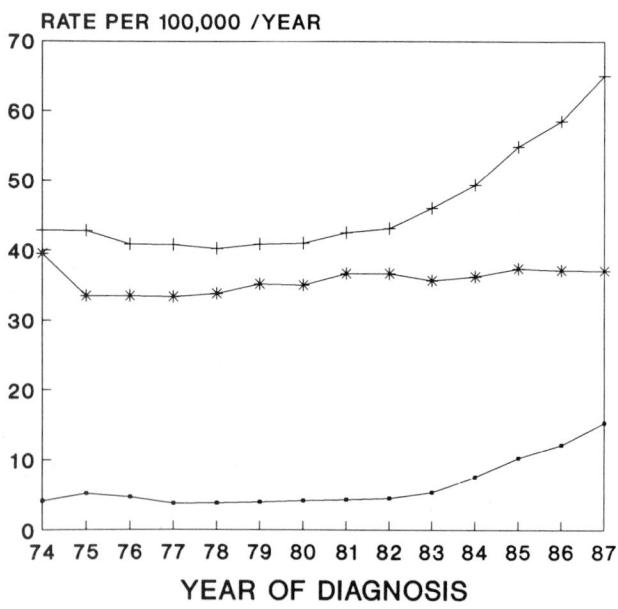

YEAR OF DIAGNOSIS

Figure VII-1-17. Breast cancer trends in stage. SEER program 1974–1987.

Benefits in Age 40–49

The segment of the guideline recommending that women age 40–49 have a mammogram every 1 or 2 years has been controversial. The reasons in support of it follow.

Twenty-four percent of all deaths from breast cancer occur in women who had the diagnosis made when they were

BREAST (FEMALES)

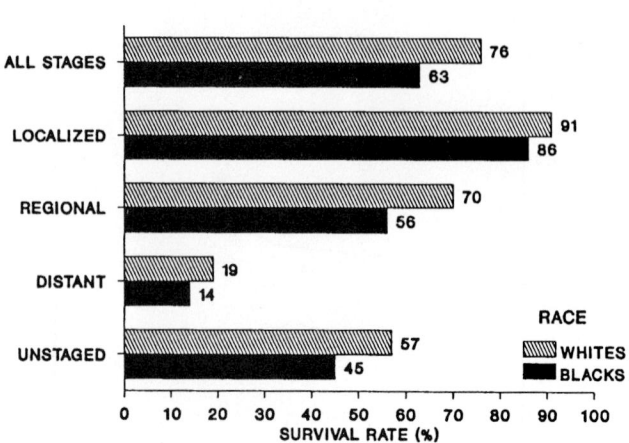

Figure VII-1-18. Survival rates for 5 years. SEER program, 1981–1986.

HIP Mortality Curves
50–64 Age-at-Entry

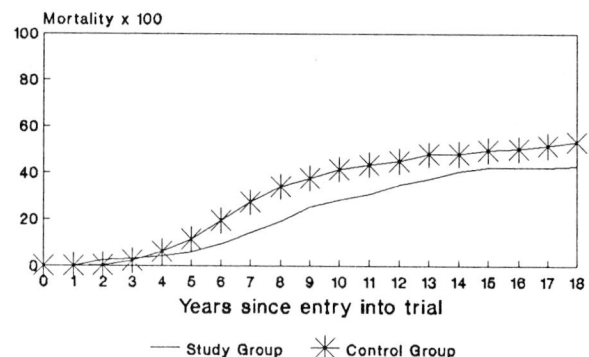

Figure VII-1-19. Mortality trends.

HIP Mortality Curves
40–49 Age-at-Entry

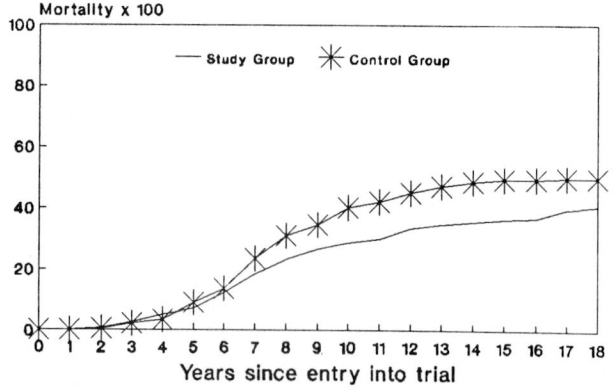

Figure VII-1-20. Trends in mortality for women 40–49.

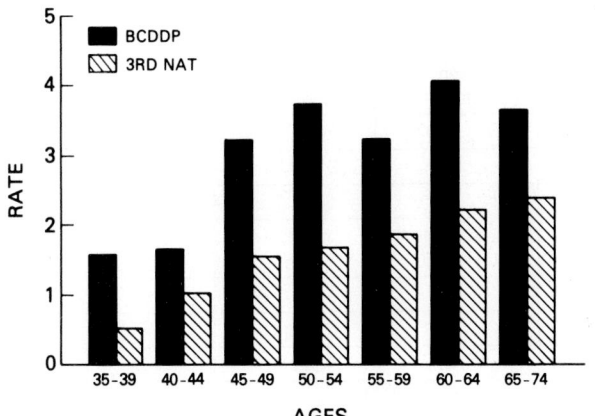

Figure VII-1-21.   Estimated incidence of breast cancer: BCDDP vs. 3rd National Cancer Survey.

Table VII-1-3.   Improvements in Mammographic Breast Cancer Detection

	1960's HIP	1970's BCDDP
Age 40-49	39%	91%
Age 50-59	60%	92%
Minimal Cancers	8%	35%
Radiation Dosage (1990 0.3-0.4 rads)	3.2 rads	1 rad

BCDDP Beahrs report

under 50 years of age.[78] Forty-one percent of all years of life lost from breast cancer in women under 80 years of age results from breast cancer diagnosed in women 35–49 years of age.[97]

In the HIP study a mortality reduction occurred in women 40–49 years of age as well as in those 50 and older.[24]

Mammography improved greatly between the time of the HIP study and the BCDDP. It improved to the point that breast cancer could be detected nearly as well in younger as in older women. This was also confirmed by in situ, tumor size and lymph node involvement. Mammography was better in the 1970's (BCDDP) and is even better in the 1990's.

Self-selection greatly increases the yield in screening for breast cancers. In the HIP study this was true in the comparison of those that accepted screening compared to those that refused. It was especially true in the BCDDP volunteer (self-selected) group of women with more than the usual number of risk factors, i.e., mother or sister with breast cancer, higher income, and higher education. While screening was still active in younger women in the BCDDP (up to 1977) the rate of cancer detection was virtually the same in women 45–49 as in women 55–59. This was also true in the national incidence rates during the years 1974, 1976, 1977 before the moratorium on screening younger women. Afterward the rate in younger women fell to nearly half of the previous rate.

Mammographic screening moves the diagnosis forward in time, such that women who would ordinarily have their cancer diagnosed without screening at ages 50–53 in 1973 would be detected through screening at ages 46–49 in 1986. This is due to lead-time and the prevalence effect which is

seen in comparing the SEER age specific incidence rates for 1973 with those for 1986 (Figure VII-1-22).

There has been a 11% mortality reduction in the SEER areas for women under the age of 50, even though the incidence has been increasing.[78] This reduction has not as yet occurred for older women. In the San Francisco Oakland area where there has been active breast cancer screening there has been a significant decrease in mortality for all age groups (Figure VII-1-23).[14]

In the light of present information, the guidelines of the National Cancer Institute seem reasonable with a mammogram every 1–2 years in asymptomatic 40–49 year old women and yearly in older women.

Breast Self-Examination

One cohort study examined mortality and 5-year survival among women with breast cancer who did not report performing BSE. It found fewer deaths due to breast cancer (14% vs. 26%) and improved estimated 5-year survival rates (75% vs. 59%) among women who reported performing BSE than among women who reported no BSE.[28,83]

In a non-randomized breast cancer screening controlled trial which included BSE, in England, the preliminary results suggest that following training in BSE, women found slightly smaller tumors. At one study site, the mean tumor size decreased from 2.8–2.0 cm after women were invited to a lecture on BSE.[104]

Since it is free, and can be practiced monthly for life, BSE should be taught, encouraged, and reinforced as part of every cancer screening and health awareness program. Heightened awareness about breast cancer will increase the use of mammography.

Colorectal Cancer
Guideline

That a rectal examination be included as a part of the periodic health examination.

That at the age of 50, annual fecal occult blood testing and a sigmoidoscopy every three to five years be done.

That the physician should identify for special surveillance high risk patients including those with a strong family history of colon cancer, or with a personal history of adenomas, colon cancer or inflammatory bowel disease.

Significance

Colorectal cancer is the second leading cause of death from cancer in the U.S. It is estimated that there will be 156,000 new cases and 58,300 deaths in the United States in 1992.[2] The incidence is increasing but the mortality rate is decreasing (Figure VII-1-24). The incidence is slightly higher in men than in women (60.4 vs. 40.9 per 100,000 per year). Age-specific incidence and mortality rates show that nearly all cases are diagnosed after 50 years of age (Figure VII-1-25).[78]

Most patients (65%) present with advanced disease. The case fatality rate is 50%. For localized disease the 5 year survival rate approaches 90% for cancer of the colon and 80% for cancer of the rectum. Although the colon and rectum are different segments of the same organ, their stage and

Table VII-1-4.   Controlled Studies of Breast Cancer Screening, 1963–1989, Determining Effect on Mortality

Study	Dates	Type	Age	Study #	Partici-pation %	Control #	Screening Interval	Modalities	Change in Mortality	Statistical Significance
U.S.									Decr.	
HIP	1963-1969	Rand	40-64	30,239	67-39	30,756	1 × 4	CBE + Mamm2	30%	Yes
Sweden										
W-E 2 county		Rand	40-74	78,085	89, 83	56,782	2 yr 40-49 3 yr > 50	Mamm1	31%	Yes
Malmo	1977-	Rand	45-69	21,088	74	21,195		Mamm 1 & 2		No
Stockholm	1981-		40-64	40,318	81	20,000	2 yrs	Mamm1		
Goteborg	1982-		40-59	22,000		30,000	1.5 yrs	Mamm2		
UK										
Edinborough	1979-		45-64	65,000			Mamm1 alt CBE	20		
8 Areas	1979-							2 Mamm1, BSE		
Netherlands										
Nijmegen	1975-	Case-Ct	35-65	23,205	85			Mamm1	53	
DOM	1974-	Case-Ct	50-64	20,555	72-30		1, 1.5, 2, 4	Mamm2		
Italy, Florence	1970	Case-Ct	40-70				2.5 yrs	Mamm2	76	
Canada	1080	Rand	40-49	50,000				Mammo2, CBE, BSE		
			50-59	40,000						

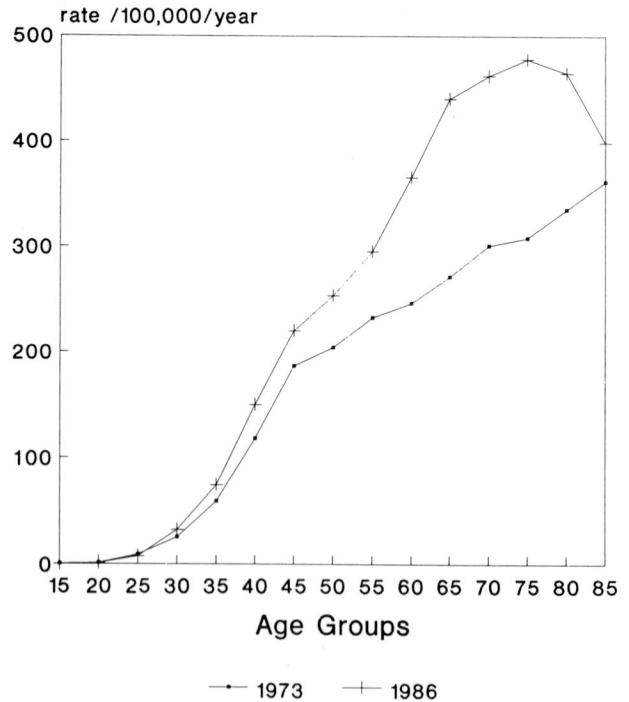

Figure VII-1-22. Carcinoma of the breast, age specific incidence 1973 vs. 1986.

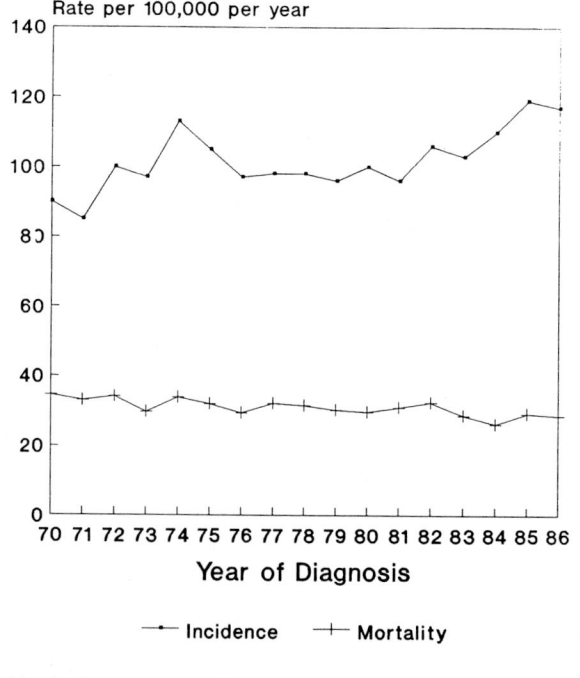

California Technical Report #5

Figure VII-1-23. San Francisco-Oakland breast cancer. Incidence and mortality 1970–1986.

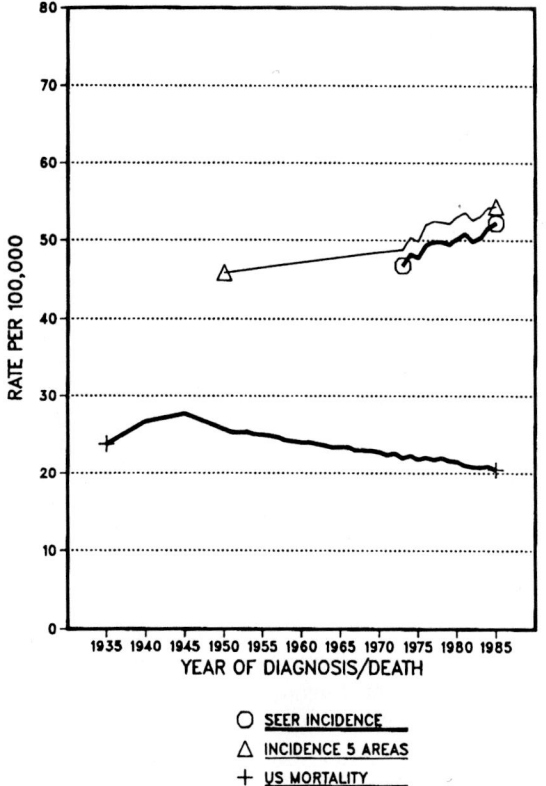

Figure VII-1-24. Cancer of colon/rectum in white males and females.

O SEER INCIDENCE
Δ INCIDENCE 5 AREAS
+ US MORTALITY

an increased risk include: a personal history of colorectal cancer or adenomas (1.5–3.0%), first degree family history of colorectal cancer or adenomas (7%) and a personal history of ovarian, endometrial or breast cancer (7%). These high risk groups account for only 23% of all colorectal cancers. Limiting screening or early cancer detection to only these high risk groups would miss the majority of colorectal cancers.[49]

Evidence of Benefit

A high percentage of early cancers can be detected by screening asymptomatic individuals over 50 years of age with a digital rectal examination, fecal occult blood testing and sigmoidoscopy. The flexible fiberoptic sigmoidoscopy was introduced in 1969. The 60 cm flexible sigmoidoscope became available in 1976 and then the 35 cm flexible sigmoidoscope.[38] The flexible sigmoidoscope permits a more complete examination of the distal colon with more acceptable patient tolerance. It is estimated that the rigid instrument can discover 25–35% of polyps, the 35 cm flexible scope around 50–55% and the 60 cm scope as many as 65–75%. The removal of premalignant polyps should decrease incidence and mortality. The discovery of polyps in the distal colon or rectum, or the presence of occult blood mandates an evaluation of the entire colon.

Virtually all screening studies using any of these modalities have demonstrated an increase in the proportion of early cases and a corresponding increase in survival compared to cases diagnosed in a non-screening environment.

The Memorial-Strang Clinic sigmoidoscopy study[44] was conducted between 1946 and 1954 in 26,124 patients. The survival rate in the 58 discovered patients with cancer was 90% after a followup period of 15 years.

The Gilbertsen study, over a 25 year period, which subjected 18,158 patients to periodic rigid sigmoidoscopy, showed a significant reduction in the incidence of cancer in the rectosigmoid colon when compared to statewide data.[51] There were 14 rectal cancers in the study group which was

survival characteristics are similar. Therefore, only the survival data by stage for colon cancer is shown (Figure VII-1-26).

There are groups that have a high incidence of colorectal cancer. These include hereditary conditions, such as familial polyposis, nonpolyposis syndromes, the cancer family syndrome (autosomal dominant), and hereditary site specific colon cancer, and ulcerative colitis. Together they account for 6% of colorectal cancers. More common conditions with

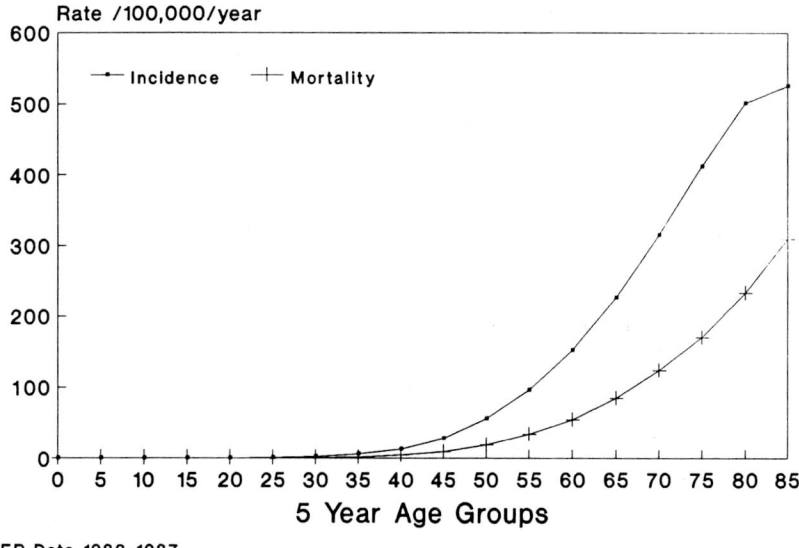

Figure VII-1-25. Colorectal cancer in males and females. Age specific incidence and mortality.

SEER Data 1983–1987

COLON

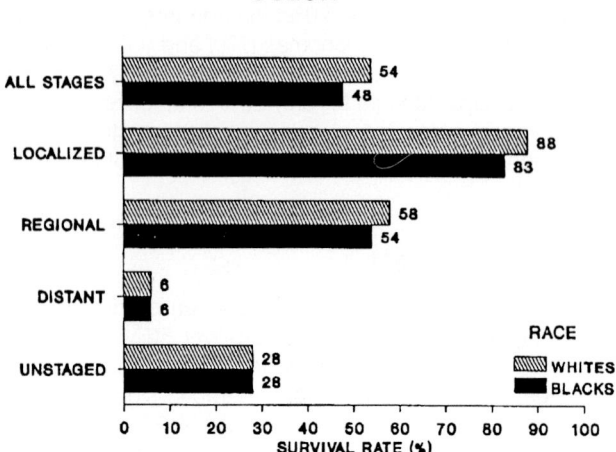

Figure VII-1-26. Survival rates for 5 years. SEER program, 1981–1986.

Table VII-1-5.   Colorectal Cancer Screening Trials

Trial	Population	Positivity	Predictive Value	Dukes' A&Bs(%) Screened	Dukes' A&Bs(%) Control
MSKCC	22,000	1.7%	30%	65	33
Sweden	27,000	1.9%	22%	65	33
England	20,000	2.1%	40%	90	40
Minnesota	48,000	2.4%	31%	78	—
Denmark	62,000	1.0%	17%	71	55

only 15% of expected in that state. However this study was not controlled and had minimal follow-up data provided.

The Kaiser-Permanente Multiphasic Health Checkup was a randomized study of 10,713 health plan members aged 35–54, after 16 years showed a more favorable stage distribution, survival rate and a reduction in mortality between the study and control groups (12 vs. 29 deaths) which was statistically significant. However, in a recent re-evaluation considering only those cancers within reach of the sigmoidoscope no statistical difference could be demonstrated.[41]

There are five controlled clinical trials that have been completed or that are in progress to evaluate the efficacy of screening utilizing the fecal occult blood test. The Memorial Sloan-Kettering Cancer Center–Strang Clinic (MSKCC) trial was completed in 1985.[112] This was a randomized trial. There was no preselection possible on the part of the patient or physician since the patient and control groups were selected by calendar periods. The Swedish trial is a targeted study for the 60–64 age group.[58] The English program selects candidates from lists of family practitioners.[49] The Minnesota program enrolls volunteers.[45] The Danish trial offers screening to a population age group between 45–75 years of age allocated at random to a control and a study group.[60]

The positivity and predictive value for neoplastic lesions (both cancers and adenomas) is as follows: All trials have shown a consistent improvement in the stage of disease in the screened population. Recent data from the Danish trial indicates a high percentage of Dukes' A and B lesions compared to the control groups (Table VII-1-5). Cancers diag-

nosed in the screened group were also smaller than in the control group.

In the MSKCC trial two different groups of patients were studied. The "annual" group had a history of periodic checkups at the Strang Clinic. The "initial" group were new patients at the Clinic. The "initial" group had different characteristics from the "annual" group. They reported more symptoms (8–9%), the rate of positivity was higher and more findings were present on the initial proctosigmoidoscopy than in the "annual" group. The preliminary analysis of survival indicates a highly significant difference between the "initial" study and control group. At this time the comparison of the "initial" groups also reveals a large difference in colorectal cancer mortality but of borderline significance because of the small number of colon cancer deaths. This correlates with the survival data. Final conclusions about mortality will require completion of patient follow up and final data analysis.

Mathematical models have been constructed to estimate outcome and costs of screening strategies for average risk and high risk groups. These models project a significant reduction in colorectal cancer mortality utilizing currently available screening methodology. For example, utilizing the most accurate available information, an annual fecal occult blood test might result in a mortality reduction of 30%. An annual fecal occult blood test and flexible sigmoidoscopy every 5 years might reduce mortality by 40%.[34,36]

National trends show an increase in earlier stage (in situ + localized) disease from 32% in 1973 to 43% in 1987 (Figure VII-1-27). In addition, there has been an increase in survival (Figure VII-1-28) and a decrease in mortality for colorectal cancer (Figure VII-1-24).

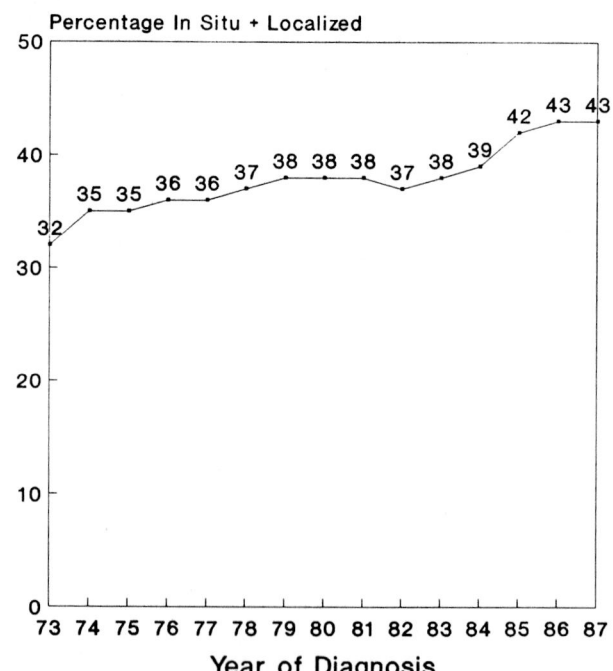

SEER Program

Figure VII-1-27. Colorectal cancer. Trends in stage, 1973–1987.

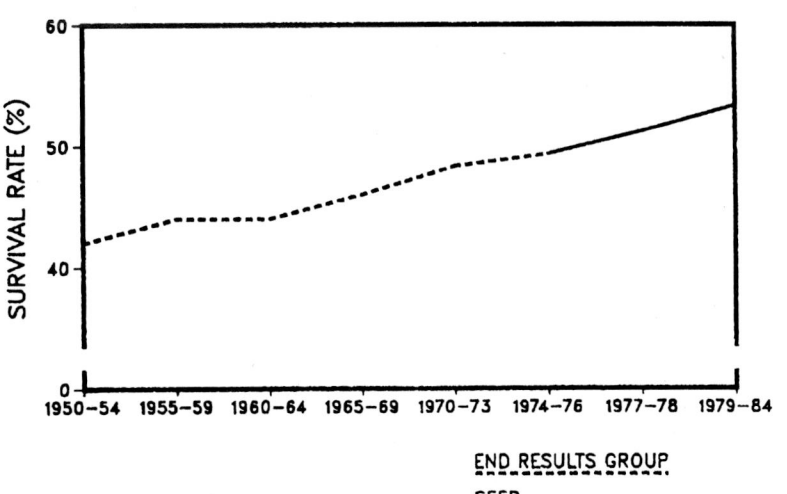

Figure VII-1-28. Five-year survival rate of colon/rectum cancer in white males and females.

Prostate Cancer

Guideline

That annual digital rectal examination of the prostate be performed on all males over 40 years of age.

Significance

Prostate cancer is the most common malignant cancer in American men (excluding skin). It is estimated that in 1991 approximately 132,000 new cases and 34,000 prostate cancer related deaths will occur in the U.S.A.[2] Prostate and colorectal cancer are tied for second leading cause of death from cancer in men being exceeded only by lung cancer. Prostate cancer amounts to 20% of all male cancers and 11% of male cancer related deaths. While incidence rates have increased significantly over the past 35 years, the mortality rates have increased only slightly (Figure VII-1-29).[78]

Prostate cancer is rarely seen in men under age 50 and then rises rapidly with each decade thereafter (Figure VII-1-30). The incidence is highest in black males (125.5/100,000) as compared to white males (83.4/100,000).

Although the incidence of prostate cancer found at autopsy steadily increases for each decade after age 50, many of these lesions are clinically silent. The tumor doubling time is long, in the range of months to years, and the ability of a given tumor to progress is highly variable.

The 1980 survey conducted by the American College of Surgeons and the 1990 cancer statistics report from the National Cancer Institute indicate that 50 to 65% of cases of prostate cancer are localized (clinical Stages A and B), 9–17% are regional (clinical Stage C), and 20–25% are metastatic (clinical Stage D) at time of diagnosis.

However, the inaccuracy and frequent clinical understaging of prostate cancer is recognized by urologists. From a review of the literature, the pathologic stage of prostate cancer at the time of diagnosis more likely is Stage A or B in 5–10% of cases, Stage C in 45%, and Stage D in 40–45% of cases.[33,68]

Progress has been made in predicting the biologic behavior of these tumors. The semiquantitative histopathologic grading scheme proposed by Gleason is reproducible among

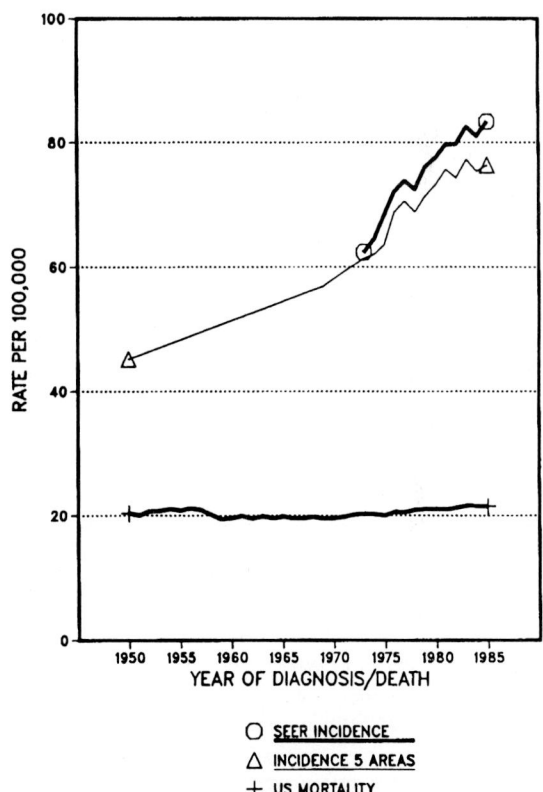

Figure VII-1-29. Prostate gland. White males.

pathologists and correlates with the incidence of nodal metastases and with patient survival in a number of reported studies.[90]

There has been a correlation of primary tumor volume to local extent of disease, progression and survival.[70] Recently, a review of a large number of prostate cancers in radical prostatectomy, cystectomy, and autopsy specimens showed that capsular penetration, seminal vesicle invasion, and lymph node metastases were virtually limited to tumors larger than 1.4 cm in volume.[70]

Five-year survival rates for prostate cancer have improved

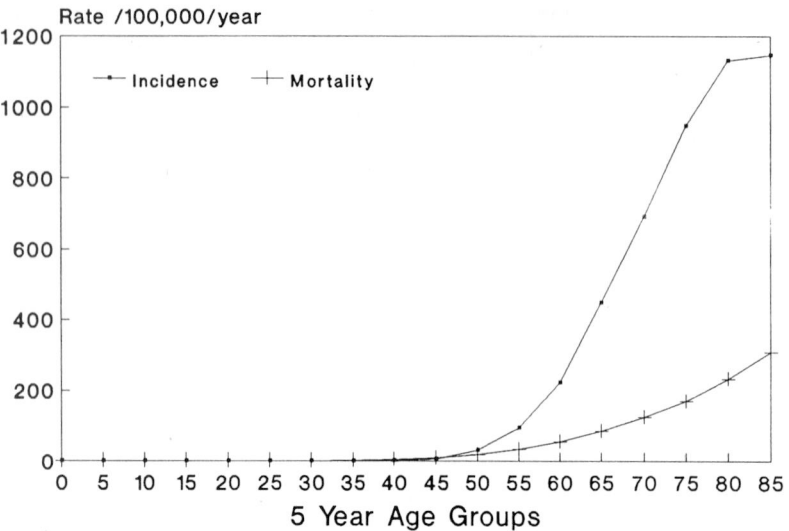

Figure VII-1-30. Prostate cancer. Age specific incidence and mortality.

SEER Data 1983-1987

for each of four consecutive periods from 1960 to 1983 (Figure VII-1-31). Survival remains lower for black patients than for white patients 62% vs. 72% relative 5-year survival. This is also true for survival by various stages of disease with 81% vs. 85% for those with localized cancer, 66% vs. 74% with regional cancer and 23% vs. 30% with distant metastatic disease (Figure VII-1-32).

Evidence of Benefit

One of the earliest studies on the rectal exam for the early detection of prostate cancer was in 1954 when 136 cases were diagnosed in military personnel at Walter Reed Army Hospital between 1940–1952.[106] These patients were subject to mandatory rectal examination as part of the annual physical examination of men over 40 years of age. Fifty-four percent of cases (74/136) had disease confined to the gland and were considered candidates for radical prostatectomy. The rectal exam was erroneous in only 10% of cases and the differential diagnosis of a palpable prostatic lesion was easy clinically.

In 1960, survival time was higher among men found to have prostate cancer on a subsequent rectal exam after negative initial exam than in patients with tumor on the initial

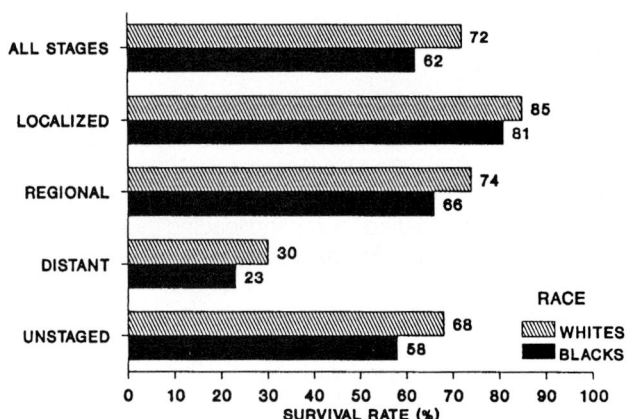

PROSTATE GLAND

Figure VII-1-32. Survival rates for 5 years. SEER program, 1981–1986.

exam. Survival rates for the two respective groups were 86% vs. 57%, with a mean followup of 32 months. The implication was that routine interval rectal exam was detecting new cases that were more likely localized.[54]

In 1971, a report on 5,856 men who underwent annual rectal examination for five years detected a 1.3% (75 cases) incidence of prostatic cancer. One-third of the cases were considered clinically localized and amenable to cure by radical prostatectomy.[43]

In 1980, a routine prostatic biopsy was performed on 71 men over 50 years of age. No cases of prostate cancer were detected in men with a palpably normal gland, however, 2–20% were positive in other series.[17] The rectal exam and nine other tests for prostate cancer were evaluated in 300 elderly men presenting with symptoms of urinary obstruction. The nine other tests were serum acid phosphatase by radioimmunoassay and counter-immune electrophoresis; aspiration urine cytology; prostatic secretion cytology after prostate massage; urine cytology before and after massage;

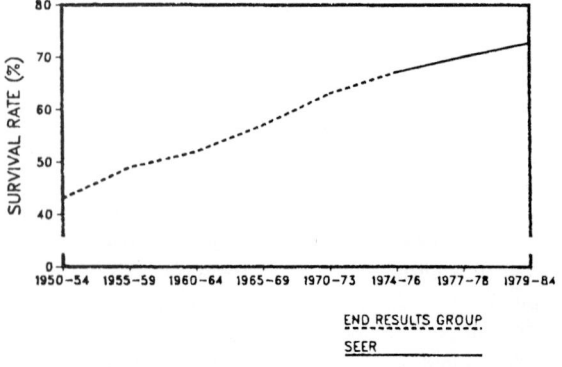

Figure VII-1-31. Five-year survival rate of prostate cancer in white males.

serum lactic dehydrogenase V/I enzyme ratio; and leukocyte adherence inhibition. Digital rectal examination had a sensitivity of 0.69 and specificity of 0.89, which was the highest of any of the 10 methods tested.[48]

In 1984, 811 unselected patients from 50–80 years of age who underwent rectal examination and followup were reported. Thirty-eight of 43 patients with a palpable abnormality in the prostate agreed to undergo biopsy. The positive predictive value of a palpable nodule, i.e., prostate cancer on biopsy, was 29% (11/38). Further evaluation revealed the stages were: B in 45%, C in 36%, and D in 18% of cases.[21] Some additional investigators also report a high proportion of localized disease when prostate cancer is detected by routine rectal examination.[33,43,103] In contrast, others have reported that even with annual rectal examination, only 20% of cases are localized at the time of diagnosis.[108]

A summary of the literature on the rectal examination for detection of prostate cancer is as follows: sensitivity 55–69%, specificity 89–97%, positive predictive value 11–26%, negative predictive value 85%–96%.[89] Digital rectal examination for prostate cancer could be easily taught to all physicians, is inexpensive, is noninvasive, nonmorbid, and is already part of the recommended physical examination for the early detection of colorectal cancer.

Prostatic imaging by transrectal ultrasound has the following characteristics: sensitivity 71%, specificity 86%; positive predictive value 31%; and negative predictive value 95%.[50] The relatively low specificity, the invasiveness and cost of the procedure, preclude the use of ultrasound or other current imaging techniques for the routine early detection of prostate cancer.

A long list of blood, tissue, and urine markers, including acid phosphatase, prostate specific antigen, creatine phosphokinase, alkaline phosphatase, and lactic dehydrogenase, to name only a few, have been carefully studied in prostate cancer.[89] The overall reported results for enzymatic prostatic acid phosphatase are as follows: sensitivity 70%, specificity 95%, positive predictive value 61%, and negative predictive value 97%. Despite these results, none of the available tumor markers has been found to have the overall efficiency to recommend its use as a early detection test. Prostatic specific antigen appears to be superior to other prior laboratory approaches, and is currently undergoing evaluation.

Given the imperfections of every available method, annual digital rectal examination for men beyond 40 years of age seems to be the most reasonable for the early detection of prostate cancer.

Cancer of the Cervix

Guideline

That all women who are, or have been sexually active, or have reached age 18 years, have an annual Pap test and pelvic examination.

That after a woman has had three or more consecutive satisfactory normal annual examinations, the Pap test may be performed less frequently at the discretion of her physician.

Significance

In 1992 more than 13,500 cases of invasive cervical cancer will be diagnosed and 4,400 women will die from this disease.[2] From 1950–1970, the incidence and mortality rates of invasive cervical cancer fell impressively by more than 70 percent (Figure VII-1-33).[78] Since the early 1980's, however, the rates for incidence and mortality appear to be decreasing more slowly. According to incidence and mortality rates, screening for cervical cancer should start in the late teens when these rates begin their upward trend. Rates for carcinoma in situ reach a peak for both black and white women between 20 and 30 years of age (Figures VII-1-34 and VII-1-35).

After the age of 25, however, the incidence of invasive cancer in black women increases dramatically with age while in white women the incidence rises more slowly. Mortality also increases with advancing age with dramatic differences between black and white women (Figure VII-1-36). Because of the continuously rising incidence and mortality rates with advancing age, screening should continue for most women, and particularly black women, with no upper age limit.

It is of interest to note that the survival rates of white and black women by stage of disease (Figure VII-1-37) are very similar, suggesting that equally early detection occurs at least in the pre-menopausal years as has been verified by a number of surveys. Extra effort is warranted to reach older women who have not been screened. Over 25% of the total number of invasive cervical cancers occur in women older than 65, and 40–50% of all women who die from cervical

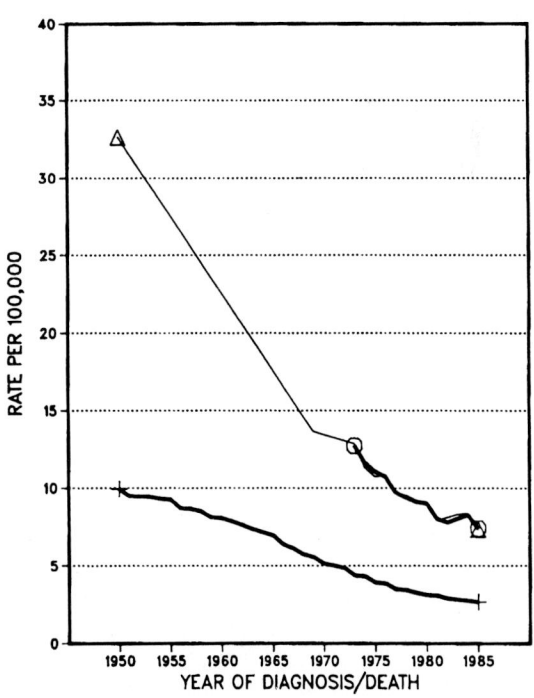

Figure VII-1-33. Cervix uteri in white females.

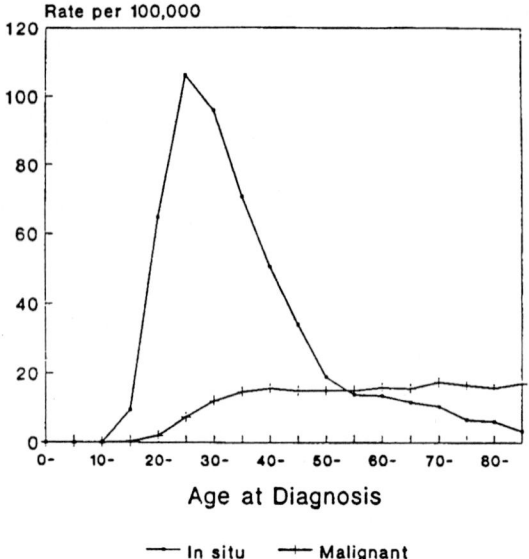

Source: NCI SEER Program

Figure VII-1-34. Age-specific cervical cancer incidence rates in white women, 1983–1987.

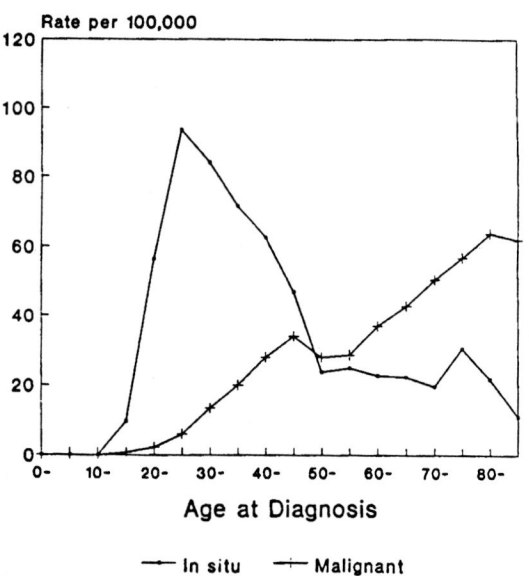

Source: NCI SEER Program

Figure VII-1-35. Age-specific cervical cancer incidence rates in black women, 1983–1987.

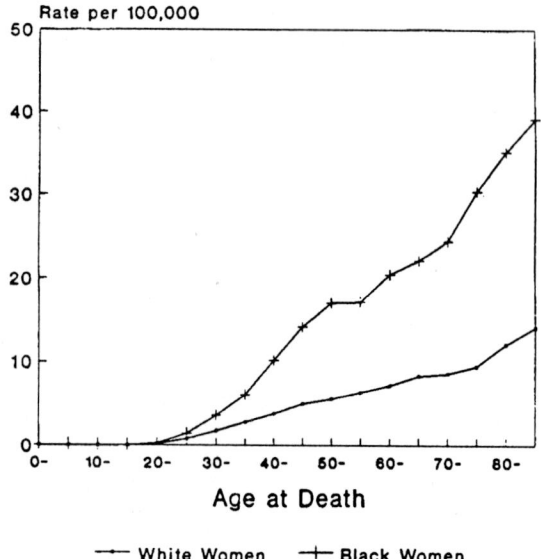

Source: NCHS Mortality Data

Figure VII-1-36. Age-specific cervical cancer mortality rates by race, 1983–1987.

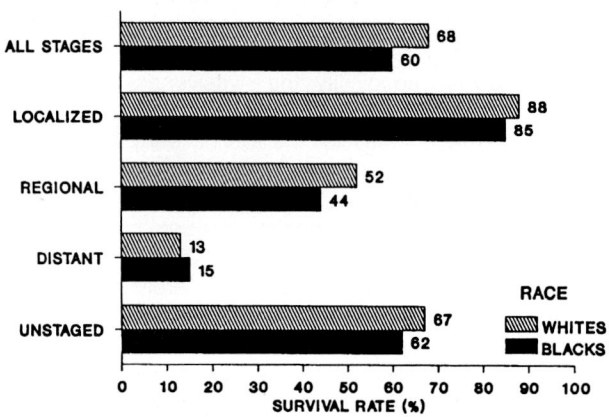

Figure VII-1-37. Cervix uteri.

cancer are over 65 years of age.[79,88] A large proportion of women, particularly elderly black women and middle aged poor women, have not had regular Pap smears.[65] In some areas, as many as 75% of women over 65 have not had a Pap smear within the previous five years.[66] These patterns underscore the importance of special screening efforts targeted to reach women who do not receive regular screening.

Evidence of Benefit

The widespread acceptance of the Pap smear makes the possibility of testing the efficacy of cervical cytology by ran-

domized trials remote. There is, nevertheless, substantial evidence from observational studies that mortality from cervical cancer can be reduced by screening.

Mortality from cervical cancer has decreased in several large populations following the introduction of well-run screening programs.[22,29,61,72] Data from several large Scandinavian studies show sharp reductions in incidence and mortality following the start of organized screening programs. Iceland reduced mortality rates by 80% over 20 years, and Finland and Sweden reduced their mortality 50% and 34% respectively.[61] Similar reductions have been found in large populations in the United States and Canada.[22,72]

Reductions in incidence and mortality seem to be proportional to the intensity of screening efforts. The Scandinavian countries with the highest rates of screening activity reported greater reductions in mortality than those countries with lower rates of screening.[61] Mortality in the Canadian provinces was reduced most remarkably in British Columbia which had screening rates 2–5 times those of the other provinces.[72]

Case control studies have found the risk of developing invasive cervical cancer is from 3–10 times greater in women who have not been screened for cervical cancer.[4,25,62] Risk also increases with longer duration following the last normal Pap smear, or similarly, with decreasing frequency of screening.[18,53] Screening every 2–3 years, however, has not been found significantly to increase the risk of finding invasive cervical cancer above the risk expected with annual screening.[53,59] The analysis of survival data shows that survival appears to be directly related to the stage of disease at diagnosis (Figure VII-1-38). The 5-year relative survival rate for cervical cancer is 88% for women with an initial diagnosis of localized disease. For those initially diagnosed with distant disease the survival is only 13%.[78] Early detection, using cervical cytology, is currently the only practical means of detecting cervical cancer in localized or pre-malignant stages.

Targeting High Risk Patients. Progress in mortality reduction will be accelerated most significantly by increasing the percentage of cervical neoplasms discovered in the precancerous or localized stages. This can be done most effectively by screening women at greatest risk for cervical cancer, i.e., those who have not had a Pap test or those who have not had one for several years. These women are often older, are often of lower socioeconomic status, may be members of minority groups, and are often seen by physicians for a variety of acute and chronic conditions unrelated to preventive medical care.[59,65,66,88] Other well-known risk factors, such as early age of first intercourse and multiple sexual partners, have less practical clinical significance due to the difficulty in obtaining adequate histories of these risk factors.

Testicular Cancer

Guideline

That periodic testicular self-examination be encouraged.

That routine palpation of the testicles continue to be encouraged as part of the physical examination.

That high risk individuals with a history of cryptorchidism,

gonadal dysgenesis and Kleinfelter's syndrome receive special attention.

Significance

It is estimated that 6,300 new cases of testicular cancer will be diagnosed and 350 men will die of the disease in 1991.[2] Testicular cancer accounts for only 1% of all cancers in men. Despite a slow apparent increase in incidence there has been a dramatic change in the mortality (Figure VII-1-39) as a result of recent new treatments.

Unlike most other cancers, this disease is generally found in young men.[78] It is the most common cancer in white men 20–34 years of age, the second most common from 35–39 years, and the third most common from 15–19 years (Figure VII-1-40).

This type of cancer is 4.5 times more common among white men than black, with intermediate incidence rates for Hispanics, American Indians, and Asians. High risk groups exist. Males with cryptorchidism have 3–17 times the average risk, meaning that for every 10 patients with the condition one will develop testicular cancer. There is also an increased risk in males with gonadal dysgenesis and in Kleinfelter's syndrome[50] as well as in the sons of women who took DES to minimize spontaneous abortion.

Most testicular cancers are discovered by patients themselves, by accident or by self-examination. Approximately 60% are localized, 24% regional, and 14% distant stage at diagnosis.

In 1974, cisplatin and multidrug combination chemotherapy, and radical retroperitoneal lymph node dissections were

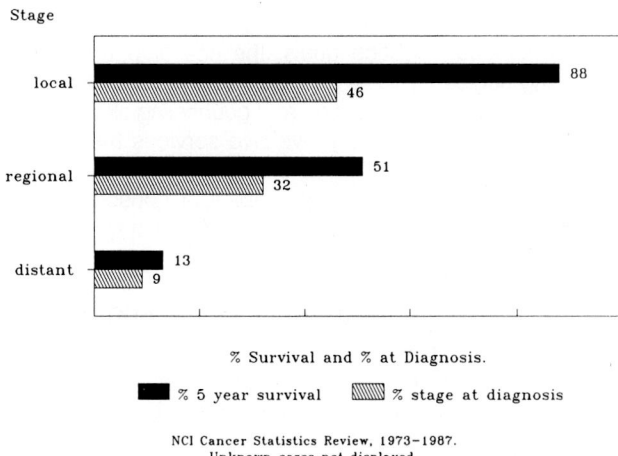

% Survival and % at Diagnosis.

■ % 5 year survival   ▨ % stage at diagnosis

NCI Cancer Statistics Review, 1973–1987.
Unknown cases not displayed.

Figure VII-1-38. Cervical cancer: Stage at diagnosis and 5-year survival.

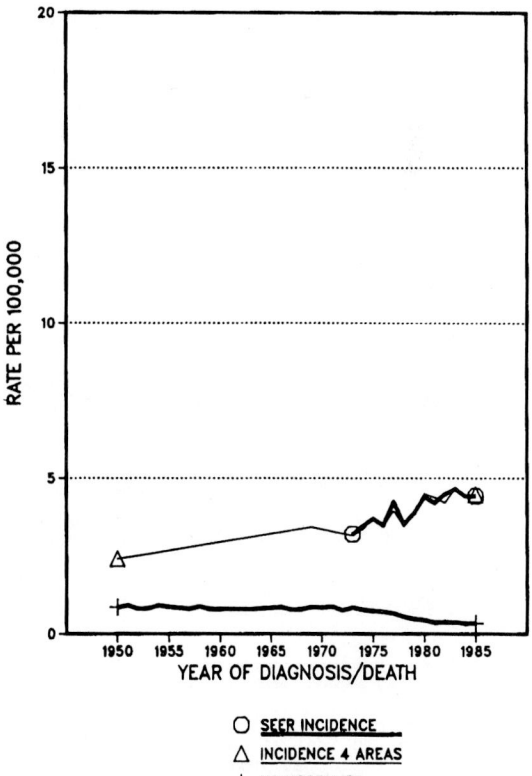

○ SEER INCIDENCE
△ INCIDENCE 4 AREAS
+ US MORTALITY

Figure VII-1-39. Cancer of the testis in white males.

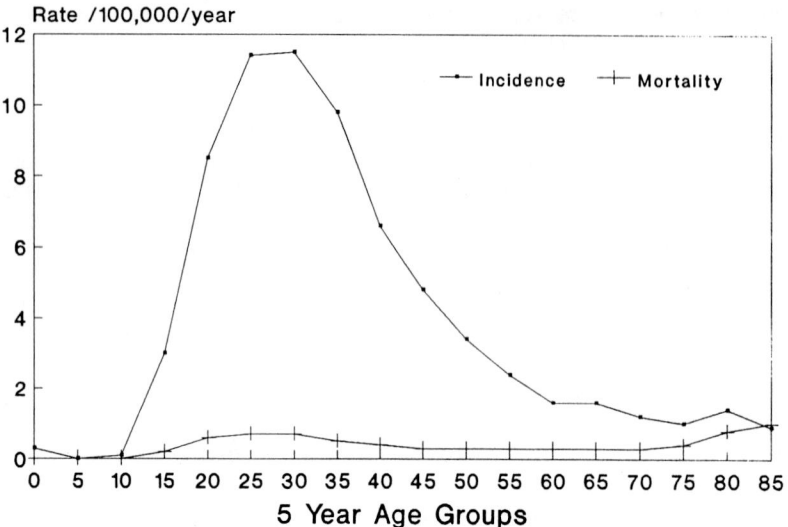

Rate /100,000/year

5 Year Age Groups

SEER Data 1983-1987

Figure VII-1-40. Cancer of the testis. Age specific incidence and mortality.

introduced for the treatment of advanced stage disease. Excellent results are now achieved in regional stage as well as in localized stage (Figure VII-1-41). There is, however, still a 30% case fatality rate in patients diagnosed with disseminated non-seminoma testicular cancer including a 5% death rate from the toxicity of chemotherapeutic regimens.[73] In Einhorn's initial experience with platinum-based multiagent chemotherapy, 93–96% of patients with minimal pulmonary or minimal pulmonary plus minimal abdominal disease, respectively, attained complete response following treatment. In contrast, only 65% of patients with advanced or bulky abdominal disease responded completely. Complete response usually means cure, while partial response is followed by relapse and death in a high percent of cases.

Nevertheless the majority of patients with regional and early advanced disease benefited by the new treatment resulting in a marked increase in over-all survival.

There has also been a 60% decrease in mortality, without any appreciable change in the stage distribution at diagnosis (Figure VII-1-42).

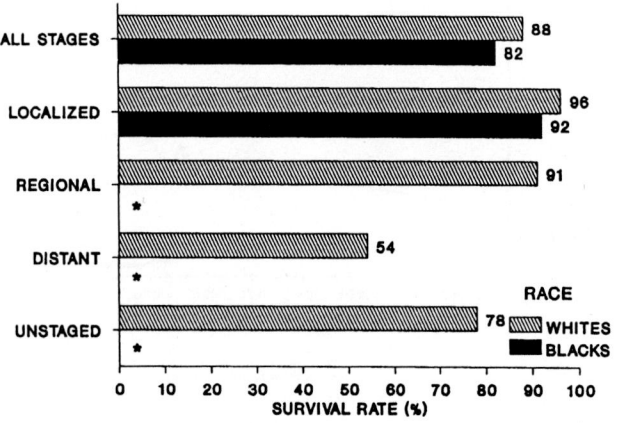

Figure VII-1-41. Cancer of the testis. *Valid survival rate could not be calculated.

Evidence of Benefit

Most testicular cancers are first detected by the patient by accident or by self examination. Some are discovered by routine physical examination. Both detection methods entail little cost or morbidity.

Delayed diagnosis leading to advanced disease has detrimental effects beyond a decrease in patient survival. The amount of treatment required in terms of courses of chemotherapy and extent of surgery is greater and carries higher morbidity and cost than for patients with early diagnosis and low tumor stage.[93]

Implementation of Guidelines

The National Cancer Institute and others have identified several major factors which consistently encourage early detection activity within physicians' offices. The factors most frequently associated with high levels of early detection activity include the use of reminder systems, the development of skills in early detection procedures, and careful attention to staff training. Other important attributes include the establishment of clear practice goals, the use of performance enhancing logistic and organizational systems, and the improvement of communication and counseling skills. Basic principles of implementing preventive services have been derived from these performance enhancing attributes. There is good evidence that these principles, if conscientiously applied, can enhance the performance of preventive activity in a variety of practice settings.

Identify Baseline Performance Rates and Set Measurable Practice Goals

A quantitative description of the current state of activity is fundamental for most managerial decisions. For physicians interested in providing preventive services this means establishing baseline levels of activity which can be used to develop realistic practice goals and to track progress in achieving these goals.[10,15,80,81]

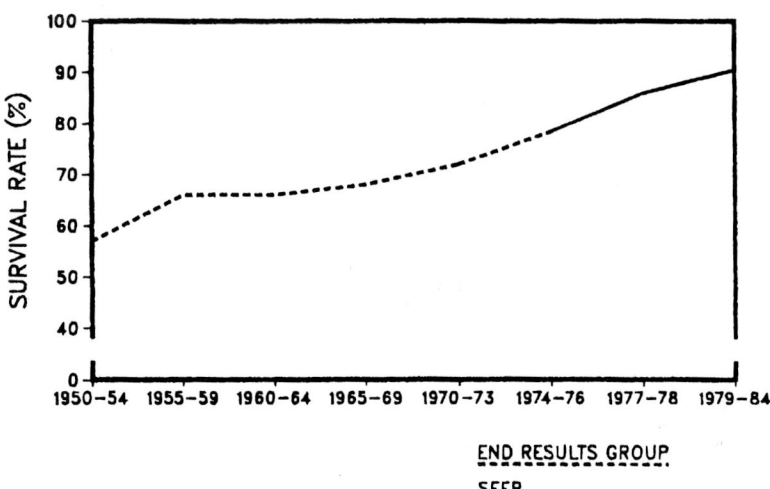

Figure VII-1-42. Five-year survival rate of cancer of the testis in white males.

Develop a Comprehensive Plan to Achieve and Maintain Practice Goals

Existing practice patterns are difficult to change and can impede efforts to increase preventive activity. Changing these institutionalized practice patterns requires careful planning. Otherwise, improvements in preventive activity may not last as old practice patterns re-emerge.[64,94]

Give a High Priority to Staff Training and Participation

A highly trained and motivated staff is a great asset for preventive activity. The opinions, input, and attitudes of office staff and the quality of their training are crucial to the success of changing the direction of a practice towards prevention. In addition, delegating certain tasks and procedures to trained staff will relieve the physician from being consciously responsible for every aspect of preventive care.[47,57]

Be Sure That Office Systems, Design, and Organization Facilitate Preventive Care

Improvements in practice performance are difficult to maintain unless the changes are institutionalized into organizational systems and behavior. Clear protocols for follow-up and referral, and provisions for patient comfort and modesty can encourage preventive activity. Other aids include attractive educational materials, a "smoke free" office, and a well trained and organized staff.[16,57]

Develop State of the Art Skills in Early Detection Procedures

Early detection activity requires certain procedural skills. Flexible sigmoidoscopy, obtaining an adequate Pap smear, and the clinical examination of the breast, prostate, and skin are skills found to vary widely between physicians. Continuing medical education efforts to develop and enhance important early detection skills should be encouraged.[40,91,111]

Develop State of the Art Counseling and Communication Skills

Communication skills are vital for educating patients about early detection procedures, smoking cessation, and diet modification. Physicians with special training and effective communication skills are more successful in counseling their patients on the need for preventive procedures and life style changes such as smoking cessation and diet modification. Continuing medical education efforts to develop and to improve communication skills should also be encouraged.[63,87,101,109,114]

Use Reminder Systems to Ensure That Patients at Risk Are Identified, Screened, and Followed

Such systems remind physicians, patients, and office staff of the need for early detection activities, particularly for patients who are at high risk for cancer. Flow charts, computerized reminders, chart stickers, and chart review by staff are examples of useful systems that cue physicians to the need for early detection activity in individual patients.[30,69,71,84]

Use Every Opportunity to Perform Unscheduled Preventive Procedures

Many patients do not schedule periodic preventive examinations. Most patients, however, are regularly seen by physicians for other reasons. Therefore, the organizational capability to integrate preventive activity into a variety of encounters should be considered in order to reach patients who do not schedule preventive care.[6,7,8,19,31,76]

When Possible, Minimize Cost Barriers for Patients and Optimize Reimbursement for Preventive Activity

Problems concerning reimbursement and costs are not completely beyond the ability of physicians to control. These barriers can be minimized by careful attention to insurance provisions, referral to low cost screening facilities, and special arrangements. Consideration may be given to lowering costs for screening tests and combining services into economical attractive packages.

References

1. American Cancer Society: Cancer Facts and Figures—1990. Atlanta, Ga, ACS publication, 1989.
2. Reference not used.
3. American Cancer Society: Guidelines for the cancer-related checkup: Recommendations and rationale. CA, 30(4):194, 1980.

4. Aristizaball, N., Cuello, C., Correa, P., Collazos, T., and Hainszel, W.: The impact of vaginal cytology on cervical cancer risks in Calli, Colombia. Int. J. Cancer, 34:5, 1984.

5. Baker, L. H.: Breast Cancer Detection Demonstration Project: Five-Year Summary Report, CA Vol. 32, No. 4, p. 4, 1982.

6. Battista, R. N.: Adult cancer prevention in primary care: Patterns of practice in Quebec. AJPH, 73:1036, 1983.

7. Battista, R. N., and Spitzer, W. O.: Adult cancer prevention in primary care: Contrasts among primary care practice settings in Quebec. AJPH, 73:1040, 1983.

8. Battista, R. N., Williams, I. J., and MacFarlane, L. A.: Determinates of primary medical practice in adult cancer prevention. Med. Care, 24:216, 1986.

9. Beahrs, O. H., Shapiro, S., Smart, C. R., and McDivitt, R. W.: Report of the working group to review the National Cancer Institute-American Cancer Society Breast Cancer Detection Demonstration Projects. J. NCI, 62(3):641, 1979.

10. Berwick, D. M., and Knapp, M. G.: Theory and practice for measuring health care quality. Health Care Financing Revew, Annual Supplement, 49-55, 1987.

11. Blois, M. S., Sagebiel, R. W., Abarbanel, R. M., Caldwell, T. M., and Tuttle, M. S.: I. Malignant melanoma of the skin. The association of tumor depth and type, and patient sex, age, and site with survival. Cancer, 52:1330, 1983.

11a.Boring, C.C., Squires, T.S., and Tong, T.: Cancer Statistics, 1992. Cancer J for Clinicians 42:19,1992.

12. Brown, M.: Is the supply of mammographic X-ray machines outstripping need and demand? An economic analysis. Ann. Int. Med., 113:547, 1990.

13. Buncher, C. R.: Final Report Central Statistical Group for Collaborative Study in Lung Cancer, Natl. Cancer Inst., contract no N01-CN-33937, unpublished, January 31, 1985.

14. California Tumor Registry, Trends in Female Breast Cancer Incidence, Mortality, Diagnosis and Treatment, 1970–1986, San Francisco–Oakland Metropolitan Statistical Area, Technical Report No. 5,Department of Health Services, State of California, p. 8, 1989.

15. Caper, P.: The epidemiologic surveillance of medical care. AJPH, 77:669, 1987.

16. Carter, W. B., Belcher, D. W., and Inui, T. S.: Implementing preventive care in clinical practice: II. Problems for managers, clinicians, and patients. Medical Care Review, 38:195, 1981.

17. Catalona, W. J.: Yield from routine prostatic needle biopsy in patients more than 50 years old referred for urologic evaluation; a preliminary report. J. Urol., 124:844, 1980.

18. Celantano, D. D., Klassen, A. C., Weisman, C. S., et al.: Cervical cancer screening practices among older women: results from the Maryland cervical cancer case-control study. J. Clin. Epidemiol., 41:531, 1989.

19. Celentano, D. D., Klassen, A. C., Weisman, C. S., and Rosenshein, N. B.: Duration of relative protection of screening for cervical cancer. Preventive Medicine, 18:411, 1989.

20. Chiodo, G. T., Eigner, T., and Rosenstein, D. I.: Oral cancer detection: the importance of routine screening for prolongation of survival. Postgrad. Med., 80:231, 1986.

21. Chodak, G. W., and Schoenberg, H. W.: Early detection of prostate cancer by routine early detection. JAMA, 252:3261, 1984.

22. Christopherson, W. M., Lundin, F. E., Mendez, W. M., and Farker, J. E.: Cervical cancer control: A study of morbidity and mortality trends over a twenty-one year period. Cancer, 38:1357, 1976.

23. Chu, K. C., Byar, D., and Smart, C. R.: Re-Analysis of Lung Screening Data, NCI unpublished, 1990.

24. Chu, K. C., Smart, C. R., and Tarone, R. E.: Analysis of breast cancer mortality and stage-distribution by age for the Health Insurance Plan Study: A randomized trial with breast cancer screening. J. Natl. Cancer Inst., 80:1125, 1988.

25. Clarke, E. A., and Anderson, T. W.: Does screening by "Pap" smears help prevent cervical cancer? A case-control study. Lancet, 2:1, 1979.

26. Commission on Cancer, American College of Surgeons, Personal Communication.

27. Connor, R. I., Chu, K. C., and Smart, C. R.: Stage-shift cancer screening model. J. Clin. Epidemiol., 42:1083, 1989.

28. Costanza, M. C., and Foster, R. S.: Relationship between breast self-examination and death from breast cancer by age groups. Cancer Detect. Prev., 7:103, 1984.

29. Cramer, D. W.: The role of cervical cytology in the declining morbidity and mortality of cervical cancer. Cancer, 34:2018, 1975.

30. Davidson, R. A., Fletcher, S. W., Retchin, S., and Duh, S.: A nurse-initiated reminder system for the periodic health examination: implementation and evaluation. Arch. Itern. Med., 144:2167, 1984.

31. Dietrich, A. J., and Goldberg, H.: Preventive content of adult primary care: do generalists and subspecialists differ? AJPH, 74:223, 1984.

32. Doherty, V., and Mackie, R. M.: Reasons for poor prognosis in British patients with cutaneous malignant melanoma. Brit. Med. J., 292:987, 1986.

33. Donohue, R. E., Fauver, H. E., Whitese, L., and Pfister, R. R: Staging prostatic cancer: a different distribution. J. Urol., 122:327, 1979.

34. Eddy, D. M.: Screening for colorectal cancer. Ann. Int. Med., Sept. 1990.

35. Eddy, D. M., Hasselblad, V., McGivney, W., and Hendee, W.: The value of mammography screening in women under age 50 years. JAMA, 259:1512, 1988.

36. Eddy, D. M., Nugent, W. F., Eddy, J. F., Coller, J., Gilbertsen, V., Gottlieb, R. R., Sherlock, P., and Winawer, S. J.: Screening for colorectal cancer in a high-risk population. Gastroenterology, 92:682, 1987.

37. Elwood, J. M., and Gallagher, R. P.: Factors influencing early diagnosis of cancer of the oral cavity. Can. Med. Assoc. J., 133:651, 1985.

38. Fath, R. B., and Winawer, S. J.: Endoscopic screening by flexible fiberoptic sigmoidoscopy. In Rosen, P., ed. Frontiers of Gastrointestinal Research. Switzerland, Karger and Basel, 1986; 10:102.

39. Feinleib, M., and Zelen, M.: Some pitfalls in the evaluation of screening programs. Arch. Environ. Health, 19:412, 1969.

40. Fletcher, S. W., O'Malley, M. S., and Bunce, L. A.: Physicians' ability to detect lumps in silicone breast models. JAMA, 253:2224, 1985.

41. Friedman, G. D., Collen, M. F., and Fireman, B. H.: Multiphasic health checkup evaluation: A 16-year follow-up. J. Chron. Dis., 39:453, 1986.

42. Friedman, R. J., Rigel, D. S., and Kopf, A. W.: Early detection of malignant melanoma: The role of physician examination and self-examination of the skin. CA, 35:130, 1985.

43. Gibertsen, V. A.: Cancer of the prostate gland. JAMA, 215:81, 1971.

44. Gilbertsen, V. A.: Proctosigmoidoscopy and polypectomy in reducing the incidence of rectal cancer. Cancer, 34:936, 1974.

45. Gilbertsen, V. A., McHugh, R., Schuman, L., and Williams, S. E.: The early detection of colorectal cancers: A preliminary report of the results of the occult blood study. Cancer, 45:2959, 1980.

46. Gittes, R. F., and Chu, T. M: Detection and diagnosis of prostate cancer. Semin. Oncol., 3:123, 1976.

47. Glynn, T. J., and Manley, M. W.: How to help your patients stop smoking: a National Cancer Institute manual for physicians. Bethesda, MD: National Institutes of Health, DHHS publications number (NIH)89-3064, 1989.

48. Guinan, P., Bush, I., and Ray, V.: The accuracy of the rectal examnation in the diagnosis of prostate carcinoma. NEJM, 303:499, 1980.

49. Hardcastle, J. D., Armitage, N. C., Chamberlain, J., Amar, S. S., James, P. D., and Balfour, T. W.: Fecal occult blood screening for colorectal cancer in the general population: Results of controlled trial. Cancer, 58:397, 1986.

50. Henderson, B. E., Benton, B, Jing, J., Yu, M. C., and Pike, M. C.: Risk factors for cancer of the testes in young men. Cancer, 23:598, 1979.

51. Hertz, R. E., Dedish, M. R., and Day, E.: Value of periodic examinations in detecting cancer of the rectum and colon. Postgrad. Med., 27:290, 1960.

52. Holman, C. D., James, I. R., Gattey, P. H., and Armstrong, B. K.: An analysis of trends in mortality from malignant melanoma of the skin in Australia. Int. J. Can., 26:703, 1980.

53. International Agency for Research on Cancer Working Group on Evaluation of Cervical Cancer Screening Programmes. Screening for squamous cervical cancer: duration of low risk after negative results of cervical cytology and its implication for screening policies. Br. Med. J., 293:659, 1986.

54. Jenson, C. B., Shahon, D. B., and Wangensteen, O. H.: Evaluation of annual examinations in the detection of cancer. JAMA, 174:1783, 1960.

55. Johannesson, G., Geirsson, G., and Day, N.: The effect of mass screening in Iceland, 1965–1974, on the incidence and mortality of cervical carcinoma. Int. J. Cancer, 21:418, 1978.

56. Kamerow, D. B., Mickalide, A. D., and Woolf, S. H.: Preventive services in the office. Help Newsletter 3(1). Kansas City, MO: American Academy of Family Physicians, 1989.

57. Kadmon, D.: Methods of detecting prostatic tumors. In: Ratliff, T. L., and Catalona, W. J., eds. Genitourinary Cancer. Boston: Martinus Nijhoff, 77, 1987.

58. Kewenter, J.: Progress report on a randomized controlled trial of screening for colorectal cancer in Göteborg, Sweden. UICC proceedings, 1986.

59. Kleinman, J. C., and Kopstein, A.: Who is being screened for cervical cancer? AJPH, 71:73, 1981.

60. Kronborg, O., Fenger, C., Sondergaard, O., Pedersen, K. M., and Olsen, J.: Initial mass screening for colorectal cancer with fecal occult blood test. A prospective randomized study at Funen in Denmark. Scand. J. Gastroenterol., 2:677, 1987.

61. Laara, E., Day, N. E., and Hakama, M.: Trends in mortality from cervical cancer in the Nordic countries: association with organized screening programmes. Lancet, 1:1247, 1987.

62. La Vecchia, C. L., Franceschi, S., Decarli, A., Fasoli, M., Gentile, A., and Tognoni, G.: "Pap" smear and the risk of cervical neoplasia: quantitative estimates from a case-control study. Lancet, 2:779, 1984.

63. Lipkin, M., Quill, T. E., and Napadano, R. J.: The medical interview: A core curriculum for residencies in internal medicine. Ann. Intern. Med., 100:177, 1984.

64. Love, R. R.: The physician's role in cancer prevention and screening. Cancer Bulletin, 40:380, 1988.

65. Makuc, D. M., Freid, V. M., and Kleinman, J. C.: National trends in the use of preventive health care by women. Am. J. Public Health, 79:21, 1989.

66. Mandelblatt, J., Gopaui, I., and Wistreich, M.: Gynecological care of elderly women: Another look at Papanicolaou smear testing. JAMA, 256:367, 1986.

67. Mashberg, A., and Barsa, P.: Screening for oral and oropharyngeal squamous carcinomas. CA, 34:262, 1984.

68. McCullough, D. L.: Diagnosis and staging of prostatic cancer. In Genitourinary Cancer, Skinner, D. G., and deKernion, J. B., eds. W. B. Saunders Co., Philadelphia, p. 295, 1978.

69. McDonald, C. J., Hui, S. L., Smith, D. M., Tierney, W. M., Cohen, S. J., Weinberger, M., and McCabe, G. P.: Reminders to physicians from an introspective computer medical record. Ann. Intern. Med., 100:130, 1984.

70. McNeal, J. E., Bostwick, D. G., Kidrachuk, R. A., Redwine, E. A., Freiha, F. S., and Stamey, T. A.: Patterns of progression in prostate cancer. Lancet, 1:60, 1986.

71. McPhee, S. J., Bird, J. A., Jenkins, C. N., and Fordham, D.: Promoting cancer screening: a randomized, controlled trial of three interventions. Arch. Intern. Med., 149:1866, 1989.

72. Miller, A. B., Lindsay, J., and Hill, G. B.: Mortality from cancer of the uterus in Canada and its relationship to screening for cancer of the cervix. Int. J. Cancer, 177:602, 1976.

73. Morse, M. J., and Whitmore, W. F.: Neoplasms of the testis. Campbell's Urology. W. B. Saunders Co., Philadelphia, p. 1535, 1986.

74. National Cancer Institute: 1986 Annual Cancer Statistics Review, p. III-B-2, NIH, Bethesda, MD, 1986.

75. National Cancer Institute: 1987 Annual Cancer Statistics Review. p. III-B-2, NIH, Bethesda, MD, 1987.

76. National Cancer Institute: Cancer Control Objectives for the Nation: 1985–2000. NCI Monograph No. 2, 1986, p. 9.

77. National Cancer Institute. Cancer Statistics Review 1973–1987, Bethesda, MD, NCI, publication No. (NIH) 90-2789, 1990.

78. National Cancer Institute, Division of Cancer Prevention and Control, Surveillance Program. Unpublished data. 1990.

79. NCI Breast Cancer Screening Consortium. Screening Mammography: A missed clinical opportunity? JAMA, 264:54, 1990.

80. Nutting, P. A.: Community-oriented primary care: researchable questions for family practice. Journal of Family Practice, 30:633, 1990.

81. Nutting, P. A.: Population-based family practice: the next challenge of primary care. Journal of Family Practice, 24:83, 1987.

82. Percy, C., Ries, L. G., and Holten, V. D.: The accuracy of liver cancer as the underlying cause of death on death certificates. Pub. Health Reports, 105:361, 1990.

83. Philip, J., Harris, W. G., Flaherty, C., Joslin, C. A., Rustage, J. H., and Wijesinghe,

D. P.: Breast self-examination: Clinical results from a population-based prospective study. Br. J. Cancer, 44:618, 1984.

84. Prislin, M. D., Vandenbark, M. S., and Clarkson, Q. D.: The impact of a health screening flow sheet on the performance and documentation of health screening procedures. Family Medicine, 18:290, 1986.

85. Prorok, P. C., and Miller, A. B.: Screening for Cancer, International Union Against Cancer Technical Report Series, Vol. 78, 1984.

86. Prout, M.: Follow-up studies on head and neck screening, NCI report 2 R18 CA40667-06, unpublished, 1990.

87. Quill, T. E.: Recognizing and adjusting to barriers in doctor-patient communication. Ann. Intern. Med., 111:51, 1989.

88. Remington, P., Lantz, P., and Phillips, J. L.: Cervical cancer deaths among older women: implications for prevention. Wis. Med. J., 89:30, 1990.

89. Resnick, M. I.: Background for early detection—epidemiology and cost effectiveness. Prog. Clin. Biol. Res., 269:131, 1988.

90. Resnick, M. I.: Editorial comment. In Genitourinary Cancer, Ratliff, T. L., and Catalona, W. J., eds. Martinus Nijhoff Publ. Boston, p. 94, 1987.

91. Rodney, W. M., Beaber, R. J., and Johnson, R.: Physician compliance with colorectal cancer screening (1978–1983): the impact of flexible sigmoidoscopy. Journal of Family Practice, 20:265, 1985.

92. Sackett, D. L.: Screening in family practice: Prevention, levels of evidence, and the pitfalls of common sense. J. Fam. Pract., 24:233, 1987.

93. Sagalowsky, A. I.: Expectant management of Stage A nonseminomatous testicular tumors. Genitourinary Cancer. Martinus Nijhoff, Boston, p. 225, 1987.

94. Segall, A., Barker, W. H., and Cobb, S.: Development of a competency-based approach to teaching preventive medicine. Prev. Med., 10:726, 1981.

95. Seidman, H., Geib, S. K., Silverberg, E., La Verda, N., and Lubera, J. A.: Survival Experience in the Breast Cancer Detection Demonstration Project; CA Vol 37, No. 5, pp. 258, 1987.

96. Shapiro, S.: The status of breast cancer screening: A quarter of a century of research. World J. Surg., 13:9, 1989.

97. Shapiro, S., Venet, W., Stax, P., and Venet, L.: Periodic Screening for Breast Cancer—The Health Insurance Plan Project and Its Sequelae, 1963–1986, Johns Hopkins Univ. Press, Baltimore, 1988, p. 1.

98. Shukla, R., Deddens, J. A., and Buncher, C. R.: Survival benefits of x-ray screening for lung cancer after bias adjustments, computers and mathematics with applications. 18:937, 1989.

99. Smart, C. R.: The role of mammography in the prevention of mortality from breast cancer. Cancer Prevention. Lippincott, Phila. Pa. 1–16, June 1990.

100. Smart, C. R., and Chu, K.: Stage as a measure of evaluating changing patterns in early cancer detection: A clinical perspective. Sem. Clin. Oncol. In Press.

101. Solberg, L. I., Maxwell, P. L., and Kottke, T. E.: A systematic primary care office-based smoking cessation program. Journal of Family Practice, 30:647, 1990.

102. Tabar, L., and Dean, P. B.: The present state of screening for breast cancer. Sem. Oncol., 5:94, 1989.

103. The US Preventive Services Task Force, Guide to Clinical Preventive Services: An Assessment of 169 Interventions. Baltimore, MD, Williams & Wilkins, 1989.

104. Thompson, I. M., Ernst, J. J., Gongai, M. P., and Spence, C. R.: Adenocarcinoma of the prostate: results of routine urological early detection. J. Urol., 132:690, 1984.

105. UK Trial of Early Detection of Breast Cancer Group: Trial of early detection of breast cancer: Description of method. Br. J. Cancer, 44:618, 1981.

106. Vanchiere, C.: New surveys show use of mammography rising. JNCI, 82:1451, 1990.

107. Van Buskirk, K. E., and Kimbrough, J. C.: Cancer of the prostate. J. Urol., 71:742, 1954.

108. Wajsman, Z., and Chu, T. M.: Detection and diagnosis of prostatic cancer. In Murphy, G. P., ed. Prostatic Cancer. Littleton, Mass.: PSG, p. 111, 1979.

109. Wallace, R. B., Wiese, W. H., and Lawrence, R. S.: Inventory of knowledge and skills relating to disease prevention and health promotion. American Journal of Prev. Med., 6:51, 1990.

110. Warnakulasuriya, S., and Pindborg, J. J.: Reliability of oral precancer screening by primary health care workers in Sri Lanka. Community Dent. Health 7:73, 1990.

111. Wigton, R. S., Nicolas, J. A., and Blanck, L. L.: Procedural skills of the general internist: a survey of 2500 physicians. Ann. Intern. Med., 111:1023, 1989.

112. Winawer, S. J.: Final Progress Report Grant No. CA 15429, 1985.

113. Winawer, S. J.: Screening for colorectal cancer. In De Vita, V. T., Hellman, S., and Rosenberg, S. A., eds. Cancer: Principles & Practice of Oncology Updates (1):1–16, 1987. J. B. Lippincott Co., Phila.

114. Zinn, W. M.: Transference phenomena in medical practice: being whom the patient needs. Ann. Intern. Med., 113:293, 1990.

VIII

Principles of Cancer Pathology

James L. Connolly
Barbara S. Ducatman
Stuart J. Schnitt
Ann M. Dvorak
Harold F. Dvorak

Introduction

Pathologists are physicians who are concerned primarily with the study of disease in all of its aspects, i.e., causation, diagnosis, pathogenesis, mechanisms, natural history, anatomic and biochemical features, progression, and prognosis. There is a great deal of truth in the old adage that pathologists are "doctors' doctors," consultants with specialized knowledge that can be helpful to the clinician who is caring directly for the patient. Nowhere in medicine is this adage more true than in the care of patients with cancer.

Pathologists engage in three major types of activity: anatomic pathology, which includes both surgical and autopsy pathology; clinical pathology, also known as laboratory medicine, i.e., the operation and direction of clinical laboratories; and experimental pathology, or basic investigations into the pathogenesis of disease. While oncologists are apt to interact most closely, most consistently, and on a more personal level with surgical pathologists in the course of their practice, they need to be aware of the roles played by pathologists of all three types if they are to provide optimal patient care. This is particularly true as the distinctions differentiating the several traditional types of pathologist have blurred as advances in technology (i.e., immunohistochemistry, flow cytometry, molecular biological approaches to cancer diagnosis) have moved from the research laboratory into the clinic.

This chapter will review some of the basic principles of pathology as they apply to neoplastic disease. Primary emphasis will be on solid tumors, though much of what will be said also applies to tumors of other types, e.g., lymphomas, leukemias. The goal will be to provide for oncologists a better feel for what pathologists do, how they arrive at diagnoses, what tools, and especially what modern tools, they have at their disposal, and how the oncologist can inter-act most productively with the pathologist to achieve the greatest benefit for the patient.

Solid Tumor Structure and Tumor Stroma Generation

The Structure of Solid Tumors

What is a tumor? Although physicians know very well what they mean when they use the term, the question is not a simple one to answer in a concise and comprehensive manner. The word "tumor" is of Latin origin and means "swelling." But not all swellings (e.g., the swellings of inflammation and repair) are tumors in the modern sense of the term. The distinguished pathologist, Sir Rupert Willis, has offered what is widely considered to be the best definition of a tumor: "A neoplasm (tumor) is an abnormal mass of tissue, the growth of which exceeds and is uncoordinated with that of the normal tissues and persists in the same excessive manner after cessation of the stimuli which evoked the change."[153] To this definition have been added three additional properties:[26] tumors are apparently purposeless, they prey on the host, and they are virtually autonomous. Even this definition is not perfectly satisfactory in that it fails to consider tumors that do not form discrete masses, e.g., leukemias, ascites tumors.

Solid tumors have a distinct structure.[26,38,107] At all but perhaps their earliest stage of development, they form a mass that is composed of two distinct but interdependent compartments: the parenchyma (neoplastic cells) and the stroma that the neoplastic cells induce and in which they are dispersed. In tumors of epithelial cell origin, a basal lamina generally separates clumps of tumor cells from stroma. However, the basal lamina is often incomplete, especially at points of tumor invasion.

Stroma is interposed between malignant cells and normal host tissues and is essential for tumor growth. Stroma is a product of the host that is induced by tumors. Thus, it is comprised of nonmalignant supporting tissue and includes connective tissue, blood vessels, and very often inflammatory cells. Stroma provides the vascular supply that tumors require for obtaining nutrients, gas exchange, and waste disposal. Most tumors, and certainly all solid tumors, regardless of their type or cellular origin, require stroma if they are to grow beyond a minimal size of 1–2 mm.[47] On the other hand, stroma may also limit the influx of inflammatory cells, or, alternatively, may limit the egress of tumor cells (invasion). Stroma, therefore, at once provides a lifeline that is necessary for tumor growth and imposes a barrier that inhibits and may regulate interchange of fluids, gases, and cells with the host.

The bulk of tumor stroma is comprised of interstitial connective tissue. For the most part, this connective tissue is formed by elements that are derived from the circulating blood and from adjacent host connective tissues. Plasma components include water and plasma proteins, together with various types and numbers of inflammatory cells. Almost any element found in the various normal connective tissues of the body may be represented in tumor stroma, even including bone and cartilage. Generally speaking, the major components of tumor stroma include structural proteins; interstitial fluid; proteoglycans and glycosaminoglycans; new blood vessels (angiogenesis); interstitial collagens (types I, III, and, to a lesser extent, V); fibrin (see VIII-1-Plate 6); fibronectin; and cells of two general types, fixed tissue cells such as fibroblasts that reside in normal connective tissue and inflammatory cells that are derived from the blood.

Although the same basic building blocks comprise all tumor stroma, pathologists have long recognized that tumors differ markedly from each other in stromal content. Sometimes these differences are primarily quantitative. At one extreme are desmoplastic tumors, such as many carcinomas of the breast, stomach, and pancreas, in which up to 90% or more of the total tumor mass consists of stroma. At the other extreme are tumors such as medullary carcinomas of the breast and many lymphomas in which only minimal stroma is deposited.

In other cases, differences in stromal content between different tumors are largely qualitative. For example, some carcinomas of the breast provoke the deposition of abundant elastic tissue along with collagen whereas others (e.g., medullary carcinoma of the breast) may induce an extensive lymphocytic infiltrate and little else in the way of stroma. Even within a single tumor there may be significant variations in stromal composition from one area to another.

Tumor Stroma Generation

Studies of transplantable tumors have revealed important information concerning the pathogenesis of tumor stroma generation (Figure VIII-1-1).[38,107] The initial event in this process, evident within an hour or less of tumor transplant, is locally increased vascular permeability. In general, the permeability increase cannot be accounted for by mast cell release of mediators, such as histamine, or by an immune or inflammatory response on the part of the host. Recently a tumor-secreted protein has been identified that apparently accounts for the vascular hyperpermeability found in many tumors. This protein, vascular permeability factor (VPF), is

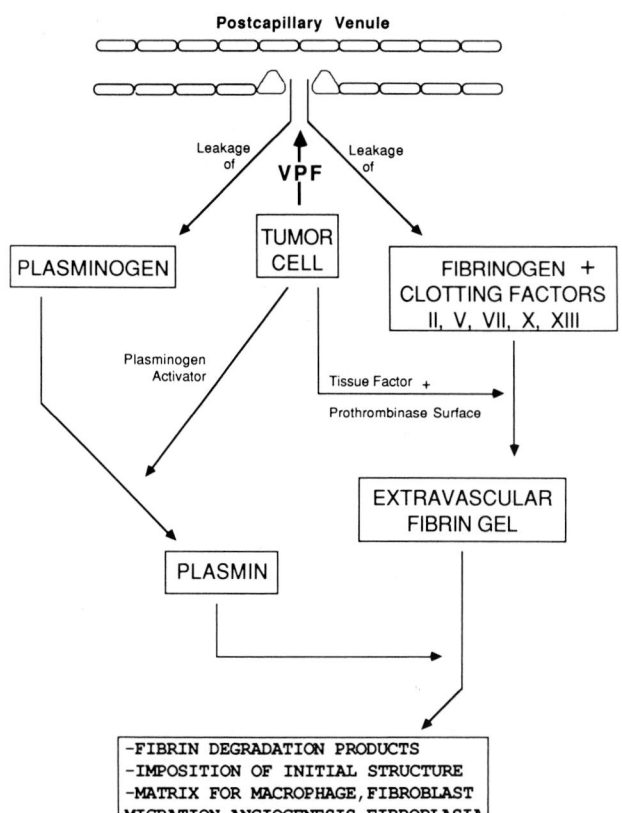

Figure VIII-1-1. Schematic diagram depicting the pathogenesis of tumor stroma generation. VPF, vascular permeability factor.

secreted by a wide variety of tumor cells of both epithelial and connective tissue cell origin and has the property of rendering the local microvasculature strikingly hyperpermeable to plasma and plasma proteins (see VIII-1-Plate 5).[19,129,130] VPF has recently been purified to homogeneity and cloned;[77,89,130] its structure is extensively conserved in species as diverse as mouse and humans. When injected into skin or other normal tissues, VPF, like mediators of inflammation such as histamine, provokes the extravasation of a protein-rich plasma exudate; like histamine, the primary target of VPF action is postcapillary venules and small veins.

An important and almost immediate consequence of vascular hyperpermeability is plasma protein leakage with coagulation and crosslinking of fibrinogen to form an extravascular fibrin gel.[38,107] Fibrinogen extravasates along with other plasma proteins from leaky blood vessels and is rapidly clotted by thrombin to form fibrin monomers that polymerize spontaneously and subsequently are covalently crosslinked by clotting factor XIII, a plasma protein transglutaminase that also extravasates from leaky vessels and is itself activated by thrombin. Thrombin is generated from prothrombin by activation of the extrinsic clotting pathway, primarily through the agency of tissue factor, a phospholipoprotein that is associated with tumor cells and also with various host inflammatory and connective tissue cells. In addition to tissue factor, several extravasated plasma clotting factors (i.e., clotting factors V and VII, in addition to prothrombin) and a suitable surface are required for prothrombinase assembly and thrombin generation. The overall result is that within a few hours of transplant tumor cells are surrounded by leaky host blood vessels and are enmeshed in a fibrin gel "cocoon" (Figure VIII-1-1).

Over the course of days and weeks, the fibrin gel cocoon is modulated by proteases (see VIII-1-Plate 6) and is gradually replaced by the ingrowth of fibroblasts and new blood vessels that give rise to loose connective tissue, similar to the "granulation tissue" of healing wounds. After an additional period of time, this granulation tissue is further transformed into the poorly vascularized, densely collagenous scar-like connective tissue characteristic of tumor desmoplasia. Simultaneously, of course, other tumor cells have broken away from the original tumor site and have begun to recapitulate at nearby sites and particularly at the tumor's growing edge the same sequence of events—increased vascular permeability and new fibrin deposition. Thus, at any one time, growing desmoplastic tumors consist of older, generally more centrally placed portions comprised of tumor cell units that are encased in poorly vascularized, dense collagenous stroma and a more active, newer, fibrin-rich peripheral zone that interfaces with the surrounding host tissue.

From this description it is apparent that the events of tumor stroma generation closely resemble those of wound healing. In both processes the initial event is a local increase in vascular permeability, followed, in turn, by extravascular clotting, fibrin deposition, fibrin proteolysis, and infiltration by inflammatory and connective tissue cells, leading to the development of granulation tissue and finally of dense fibrous connective tissue (termed "desmoplasia" in tumors and "scar" in healed wounds). There are also, however, at least two notable differences between these processes. In wounds, increased vascular permeability results from trauma of one sort or another and is accompanied by local tissue injury, extravasation of blood cells, and platelet degranulation with the release of clotting and growth factors that stimulate the wound-healing response. Platelets, which play several critical roles in wound healing, seem not to participate in tumor stroma generation; apparently platelet functions are subsumed by tumor cells that make similar or analogous products. Tumors differ from healing wounds in another important respect. At wound sites vascular hypermeability is self-limited and returns to normal within a few days; by contrast, vascular hyperpermeability persists indefinitely in tumors. Thus, tumors behave in some sense as wounds that do not heal.[38]

The analogy between wound healing and tumor stroma generation may be taken one step farther. Except in lower vertebrates, wound healing does not recapitulate ontogeny but, instead, replaces zones of injury with connective tissue whose functional capacities fall well short of the original normal tissue. In the same manner, tumor stroma, especially that of poorly differentiated malignant tumors, is generally a disorganized and poorly supportive parody of normal connective tissue. The vascular supply is particularly deficient. Tumor blood vessels are very often poorly differentiated, unevenly spaced, and, despite their increased numbers, unequal to the task of supporting the growth and even the life of rapidly metabolizing tumor cells.[144] The result is irregular blood flow, uneven perfusion, shifting zones of anoxia,

low pH, and, commonly, coagulative necrosis—a necrosis resulting from vascular insufficiency.[139] In fact, the presence of necrosis may be helpful to the pathologist in recognizing malignant tumors and distinguishing them from their benign counterparts and certain nonneoplastic processes.

The Role of the Surgical Pathologist in the Diagnosis and Management of the Cancer Patient

Surgical pathologists have the definitive role in tumor diagnosis. No matter how high the index of clinical suspicion, the diagnosis of cancer is not conclusively established nor safely assumed in the absence of a tissue diagnosis. With very few exceptions, definitive therapy for cancer should not be undertaken in the absence of a tissue diagnosis. Policies supporting this practice are written into the bylaws of most hospitals and are regularly monitored by hospital tissue committees and by accrediting agencies.

It is the task of the surgical pathologist to provide an accurate, specific and sufficiently comprehensive diagnosis to enable the clinician to develop an optimal plan of treatment and, to the extent possible, estimate prognosis. There was a time not many years ago when the simple designation "benign" or "malignant" provided the clinician with all of the information necessary to provide appropriate patient care. This is no longer the case. Cancer is not a single disease. There are more than 300 distinct varieties of tumors, each with a characteristic biology. Moreover, tumors have a course of historical development and progression; in an individual patient, they may be first recognized at any stage along that course. The tremendous advances in all fields of oncology require a great deal of additional information, and nearly every case, in fact, requires a fuller understanding of the patient's particular tumor to allow the most appropriate classification for research, for prognosis and for therapeutic intervention. Details of the type and origin of the tumor, its differentiation, level of invasion, the numbers of lymph nodes with and without metastatic tumor, lymph node architecture, the presence or absence of hormone receptors, the activity of specific enzymes, ploidy, and frequency of mitosis and cells in S phase may all be relevant in virtually every pathologic assessment of neoplasia. Molecular pathology, using DNA probes with or without amplification by the polymerase chain reaction to detect expression of specific genes in neoplasms, has not yet reached standard practice but promises a golden age for pathology in the 1990s.

Surgical pathologists deal primarily with structure. Careful gross examination of excised tissue, first with the naked eye or with the help of a dissecting microscope, is followed by a more detailed examination of tissue sections in the compound light microscope. Preliminary examination may make use of frozen tissue sections, but in most instances pathologists rely on the better preservation of structure afforded by permanent tissue sections stained with hematoxylin and eosin (H&E) and occasionally other dyes. Histochemistry, immunohistochemistry, and electron microscopy are helpful or necessary supplements for diagnosis in 10–15% of solid tumors. In addition, surgical pathologists collaborate closely with cytopathologists in diagnoses involving exfoliated cells or needle aspirates and with clinical pathologists who make use of other techniques such as culture for microorganisms, flow cytometry, and specialized laboratory tests of a biochemical, immunological, or molecular nature. In order to perform many of these supplementary studies, the specimen must be specially processed while it is still fresh, i.e., prior to routine fixation. It is a responsibility of the surgical pathologist to coordinate these various activities and to synthesize the information provided by each into a comprehensive diagnosis that is maximally informative to the clinician caring for the patient.

Methods for Obtaining Specimens

Tissue may be obtained in a number of ways, each with its appropriate place and uses depending on the clinical circumstances. Cytological examination of exfoliated, scraped, or brushed cells can be a rapid, efficient, and low-risk technique for establishing an accurate diagnosis. This approach, along with the related technique of fine needle aspiration is discussed in greater detail later; for obvious reasons, these approaches do not always reveal the primary tumor site or the extent of disease. Cutting needle biopsies or drill biopsies obtain tissue cores for histological examinations or special studies that permit evaluation of architectural structure but may result in tissue distortion and have a greater risk of bleeding and patient discomfort than use of fine needles. Incisional biopsy (along with fine needle aspiration) is often the method of choice for lesions that are inoperable or too large for ready excision, or when excision could lead to functional or cosmetic impairment. Care must be taken that incisional biopsies are performed in a fashion that will not comprise definitive therapy, i.e., the tissue excised should be confined to an area that will be encompassed by subsequent treatment. Excisional biopsy is often favored because it provides generous amounts of tissue for diagnosis and may itself afford sufficient surgical therapy for some tumors, e.g., small- to medium-sized breast cancers.

There are many potential pitfalls in biopsy interpretation. These include inadequate tissue sampling and artifacts induced by the procedure itself, such as thermal damage caused by an electrocautery or laser. Except for excisional biopsies, negative findings do not exclude the possibility that a tumor or other significant pathologic condition is present but was not included in the tissue submitted for examination. Thus, for procedures short of complete excision, the clinician must be prepared to perform a second, often more extensive procedure if the first does not yield sufficient diagnostic information.

Gross Handling of Specimens

The pathologist must regard, and therefore properly triage, biopsies, and particularly excisional biopsies, as the definitive surgical specimen. To do this well, the pathologist must be informed about the clinical history, differential diagnosis, and relevant laboratory results. These, together with the gross tissue examination and frozen section, if any, may individually or together dictate whether special studies are required. Specimens should be marked with clips or sutures to provide anatomic orientation, and these should be described in the pathology submission sheet. Often, tissue arrives in the pathology lab in formalin or other fixatives. At that stage it is already too late to perform many special studies (e.g., microbiological cultures, certain types of immunohistochemistry and electron microscopy) that may prove to be critical for diagnosis. This fact emphasizes the importance of consulting the pathologist in advance in order to avoid the need for rebiopsy. Frequently the goal of biopsy is to determine whether the lesion is benign or malignant with the expectation of performing additional surgery if the lesion proves malignant. In this case, supplementary tests may properly be deferred to subsequent, more definitive surgery at which time larger amounts of tissue become available.

The gross specimen should be described with regard to its appearance and characteristics, taking care to measure in three dimensions the size of the specimen and, if visible, the lesion itself along with the distances between the lesion edges and the excision (resection) margins. Excision margins should be identified and marked with ink prior to any dissection, thus permitting accurate measurement of these distances microscopically. Depending upon the type of specimen and the clinical circumstances, margins can be evaluated by analysis of frozen sections. All lymph nodes associated with the specimen need to be dissected out, described along with their location, and processed for histology.

A still more careful examination is required for radiographically directed biopsies and for breast biopsies where no lesion may be visible to the naked eye. Specimens with calcification often require specimen radiography. Ideally, a radiograph should be made of the intact specimen, following which the margins should be inked, the specimen "bread-loafed," and radiographs taken of each slice. Sections should then be coded, processed individually for histology and correlated with the corresponding radiographs.[25,113]

Preparation of Microscopic Sections

Microscopic examination requires that tissues be cut with a microtome into sections that can be stained with dyes that enhance contrast and thereby facilitate delineation of tissue and cell structure. Two types of sectioning methods are most commonly used: frozen sections (typically stained with toluidine blue or H&E) and paraffin embedded or permanent sections (typically stained with H&E). Frozen sections can be prepared rapidly (within minutes) during the course of surgery while the patient is still under anesthesia and therefore are of the greatest practical value in situations requiring an immediate answer to an important clinical question. At one time, frozen sections were commonly performed intraoperatively in patients with suspected breast cancer with the expectation that definitive radical surgery would follow immediately if cancer were found. With the less aggressive surgical therapy now common for treatment of breast cancer, this practice has precipituously declined.

However, frozen sections continue to have many important applications. First, they are useful for determining whether a lesion is a neoplasm, and, if so, whether it is benign or malignant. Second, they can provide information as to the extent of regional tumor metastases which may govern decisions concerning further surgery, e.g., mediastinal lymph node involvement in primary carcinoma of the lung, peripancreatic lymph node involvement by carcinoma of the pancreas. Third, they allow the pathologist to determine whether the resection margins are adequate following definitive cancer surgery, such as resection of skin, gut, or pulmonary lesions. If resection margins are inadequate, additional tissue can be removed immediately, without the need for a subsequent operation. For some tumors, however, such as those arising in soft tissues or breast, resection margins are best evaluated in permanent sections. Finally, perhaps the most common current use of frozen sections is to determine the appropriate additional workup necessary for a particular tissue specimen while it is still fresh, e.g, if the metastatic tumor found in a lymph node is recognized as a poorly differentiated carcinoma, electron microscopy and hormone receptor studies may be required for proper diagnosis. On the other hand, if the tumor is a lymphoma, an entirely different set of studies may be required, such as those for cell surface antigen markers and gene rearrangement.

In contrast to frozen sections, permanent sections are prepared from tissues that have been fixed, dehydrated, and embedded in paraffin wax as a supporting medium prior to sectioning. Though requiring more time for preparation (generally 12–24 hours), permanent sections offer a number of important advantages over frozen tissue sections. Sections are generally thinner (typically 5 μm) and, by avoiding freezing artifacts, are of better overall quality and therefore permit greater certainty of interpretation. A broader repertoire of stains is also available for permanent sections. Certain tissues, such as those containing fat or bone, cut poorly or cannot be cut as frozen sections but may be satisfactorily studied in permanent sections. As a general rule, if insufficient tissue is available for both frozen and permanent sections, only permanent sections should be prepared. While the opinions just expressed certainly represent a majority view, some excellent pathology departments routinely diagnose tumors on the basis of frozen sections and prepare permanent sections primarily for archival purposes.

Microscopic Interpretation of Tissue Sections

In cases of suspected cancer the first task of the surgical pathologist is to decide whether a neoplasm is present. As noted above, the word "tumor" is Latin for "swelling," and various types of "swelling" can masquerade as neoplasms. These include inflammatory lesions, repair, hypertrophy, hyperplasia (e.g., keloids), choristomas (ectopic rests), and hamartomas (masses of mature cells that are appropriate to a given site but are arranged in a disorganized fashion as the result of aberrant differentiation). This initial distinction is often made easily, e.g., hyperplastic polyps of the colon, nasal polyps, and skin tags are not likely to be confused with true neoplasms. Sometimes, however, the task is less straightforward. Tumors not infrequently generate an extensive inflammatory response, and it is not unusual, for example in endoscopic biopsies of gastric carcinomas, to find only after a prolonged search rare individual cancer cells "buried" in an extensive inflammatory cell infiltrate. Healing ulcerations of the gastrointestinal or cervical mucosae may sometimes closely resemble the carcinomas or premalignant lesions (e.g., cervical intraepithelial neoplasia I, II, or III) that arise in those tissues. Finally, atypical hyperplasia can be

very difficult to distinguish from in situ carcinoma, and, even when no evidence of tumor is found, may represent an important diagnostic finding. For example, patients whose biopsies show atypical hyperplasia and have a positive family history for breast cancer have a nine-fold increased risk for developing breast cancer at a later time.[32]

Having decided that a neoplasm is present on the basis of criteria such as cellular abnormalities or invasion (see below), the pathologist's next task is to classify it. A number of classification schemes are possible, but the most important of these is based on the tumor's histogenetic or cytogenetic origin. Histogenetic/cytogenetic classification is often supplemented by other useful descriptors such as those provided by the tumor's gross or microscopic appearance (e.g., polypoid, papillomatous), the degree of cellular differentiation (e.g., well- or poorly differentiated, see VIII-1-Plate 3), and, perhaps most importantly, by the expected biological behavior (benign versus malignant). Broadly speaking, tumors of epithelial cell origin are termed adenomas or papillomas when benign and carcinomas when malignant. Carcinomas account for ~80% of all malignant tumors. Their classification is often further qualified on the basis of the type of epithelium present, e.g., glandular (adenocarcinoma, see VIII-1-Plate 1), squamous (squamous cell carcinoma, see VIII-1-Plate 2), transitional cell (transitional cell carcinoma). Addition of the suffix -oma to the cell of origin also describes benign tumors of mesenchymal origin (e.g., lipomas, fibromas, leiomyomas). Malignant tumors of mesenchymal origin are designated sarcomas (e.g., liposarcomas, fibrosarcomas, leiomyosarcomas). Most tumors are comprised of a single type of neoplastic cell. However, a few tumors contain neoplastic cells of more than a single type. Adenoacanthomas contain both squamous cell carcinoma and adenocarcinoma elements. Carcinosarcomas are so called because some of the epithelial cells resemble sarcomatous elements. A few tumors contain neoplastic cells from more than one germ layer, such as Wilms' tumor and teratomas. Certain tumors have long been identified with trivial names that do not follow any well-ordered classification scheme. Examples include seminomas (for carcinomas of testicular epithelial cell origin), hypernephromas (for renal cell carcinomas), and melanomas (for melanocarcinomas) (see VIII-1-Plate 4). Other tumors, due to prolonged use, continue to bear eponyms (e.g., Hodgkin's disease, Ewing's sarcoma, Kaposi's sarcoma).

The pathologist must carry classification further still. Even within a single organ and within a single type of epithelium, several different types of tumors may arise, each with its own special characteristics, prognosis, and response to therapy. In the breast, for example, the two most common types of malignant tumor are infiltrating ductal carcinoma (sometimes designated as carcinoma "not otherwise specified" or N.O.S.), which accounts for ~78% of breast cancers, and infiltrating lobular carcinomas, which account for an additional ~9% of breast cancers. These two tumors, together accounting for nearly 90% of breast cancers, have similar prognoses that are less favorable than those of the other, less common types of breast carcinoma (i.e., tubular, mucinous or colloid, medullary, papillary, and adenoid cystic carcinomas).[95]

One of the most important distinctions the surgical pathologist can make is that between tumors that are benign or malignant. In general, benign tumors share certain properties. The neoplastic cells comprising the tumor are usually well differentiated, closely resembling the corresponding cells of normal tissue. Benign tumors tend to expand uniformly in all directions unless impeded from doing so by surrounding structures, e.g., compression by the bony skull often causes meningiomas to take on a flattened appearance. As expansile masses, benign tumors cause compression atrophy of surrounding normal tissues that results in the formation of a thin rim of fibrous connective tissue; this enveloping connective tissue rim may serve as a "capsule" that renders benign tumors discrete, readily palpable, and easily movable. Not all benign tumors have capsules, however, e.g., leiomyomas of the uterus, hemangiomas, and adenomatous polyps of the large intestine.

Malignant tumors, or cancers, are characterized primarily by the increased numbers and abnormality of their neoplastic cells. Cellular abnormalities are of two general types, those involving intercellular relationships and those affecting individual neoplastic cells. With regard to the former, malignant tumors commonly exhibit abnormal orientation of both neoplastic cells and stroma that may be best described as "helter-skelter" or disorganized. For example, carcinomas of the skin may be comprised of squamous cells that differentiate and mature fairly normally; however, the cells are organized into nests in which the least differentiated cells are situated peripherally, and the most differentiated cells are positioned centrally where they form keratin pearls. Further, these tumor cell nests are surrounded by disorganized stroma. Disturbed intercellular arrangements such as these are of great help to the pathologist reading a tissue section; much of tumor diagnosis depends on the pathologist's ability to recognize altered microscopic tissue patterns.

Abnormalities of individual neoplastic cells may also be helpful in diagnosis, particularly increased numbers of mitoses and cytological features relating to the state of tumor cell differentiation. Cytological features of malignancy include altered polarity, tumor cell enlargement, increased ratio of nuclear to cytoplasmic area (may approach 1:1 instead of the normal 1:4 or 1:6, though exceptions exist), pleomorphism (variation in size and shape) of tumor cells and their nuclei, clumping of nuclear chromatin and distribution of chromatin along the nuclear membrane, enlarged nucleoli, atypical or bizarre mitoses (e.g., tripolar), and tumor giant cells with one or more nuclei. Some malignant tumors, however, are well differentiated, so well differentiated, in fact, that their malignant cells cannot be distinguished from those of benign tumors, or even from normal cells by any available diagnostic method. In such instances the recognition of abnormal cellular relationships becomes especially important for correct diagnosis.

"Anaplasia" (Greek, "to form backwards") is the term pathologists commonly use to describe the degree of tumor differentiation, or, more correctly, the lack thereof. Though well-entrenched, the term is an unfortunate one. It implies that tumors arise from mature, differentiated cells by a process of dedifferentiation (i.e., differentiation in reverse). Few pathologists hold that view today. Mammalian cells, once differentiated, generally lack the capacity to reverse that

process. Also, there is strong and growing evidence for the alternate explanation, namely that tumors arise from populations of undifferentiated "stem" or "reserve" cells that are present in many, perhaps in all, organs.[118] Stem cells comprise a minority cell population that lacks differentiation markers, making them difficult to identify. However, positive recognition of stem cells has been achieved in several organs, e.g., bone marrow, epidermis, liver, and gastrointestinal tract mucosa.[122] Stem cells have a high capacity for cell proliferation, but, unless stimulated, may divide infrequently. Stem cells alone have the capacity to regenerate normal tissues and, by extension, tumor cell populations. Oncologists of course are well aware that stem cells are the critically important target of cancer therapy. Destruction of differentiated tumor cells, without simultaneous killing of tumor stem cells, will not lead to permanent tumor eradication.

Malignant tumors invariably lack a capsule. Instead, they extend crab-like projections into the surrounding host tissues without respect for normal anatomic boundaries. This behavior is referred to as invasion. Malignant tumor cells often invade lymphatics and veins and are transported by lymph or blood flow to distant sites, opening the possibility of metastasis (see I-10). Invasion is not a property confined to malignant tumor cells; many proliferations in fetal life, placental trophoblasts, and inflammatory cells also have the capacity to "invade" tissues. However, cancers need not be invasive at the time of removal, either because they have been "caught" before they had time to invade or because they have not yet progressed to the point where they have acquired the capacity to invade. Epithelial tumors with all other properties of malignancy that have not extended though the underlying basement membrane at the time of diagnosis are described as in situ carcinomas and can almost certainly be cured by complete excision.[128]

Ancillary Staining and Analytical Methods

Special stains are commonly employed to aid in tumor differential diagnosis and classification. Examples include van Gieson's stain or the Masson trichrome method for distinguishing collagen and muscle, Weigert's stain for elastic tissue, silver stains for reticulin fibers, and special stains for mucins, amyloid, lipids, myelin, and glycogen—all substances whose identification may aid in the diagnosis of one or another type of tumor. Other special stains are useful for recognizing and classifying bacteria, fungi, and certain types of virus that may complicate the course of cancer patients, especially following immunosuppressive therapies. Enzyme histochemistry may be essential for defining tumor cell lineage, as in certain types of leukemia, e.g., chloroacetate esterase or endogenous peroxidase staining for cells of myelomonocytic lineage, alpha naphthyl butyrate esterase (so-called nonspecific esterase) staining for cells of monocyte-macrophage origin.

Other techniques that may occasionally aid the surgical pathologist in tumor diagnosis are specimen x-ray (e.g., for localizing and analyzing crystalline materials, such as calcium, in breast biopsies) and morphometry.

Excision Margins

An important concern for the pathologist is the adequacy of tumor excision. Depending on the tissue, this decision can be made on either frozen or permanent sections. If the tumor forms a discrete mass and the margins of the specimen are clearly recognizable, determination of excision margins is usually straightforward. Examples of tumors whose excision is likely to give clearly defined margins include those arising in the gastrointestinal tract, lung, and skin. On the other hand, the margins of tumors arising in soft tissues (e.g., many sarcomas and breast carcinomas) and diffusely infiltrating tumors (e.g., infiltrating lobular carcinoma of the breast, signet ring tumors of the gastrointestinal tract, nerve-invading tumors such as adenoid cystic carcinomas of the salivary glands, gliomas, and glioblastomas) may be much more difficult to define. With at least certain histologic patterns of breast carcinoma, factors such as the extent of intraductal growth may be more reliable predictors of residual tumor than adequate excision margins.[71,127]

Tumor Staging, Progression, Grading, and Prognosis

Tumor staging (e.g., the well-known TNM system) has proved to be of great value in estimating prognosis. Staging attempts to measure the extent of spread of a cancer within a patient based on such parameters as the size of the primary tumor, the degree of lymph node involvement, and the presence of metastases. It is obvious that objective determinations made by the pathologist on resected tumor specimens have a critical impact on accurate tumor staging. With perhaps only one exception (papillary carcinoma of the thyroid), the presence of metastases to regional lymph nodes is the single most important risk factor in determining tumor prognosis. Therefore, the pathologist must search diligently to find, examine, and prepare histological sections from all lymph nodes included in resected tissue.

Before discussing tumor grading, it is necessary to recognize that tumors are not static entities; rather, they tend to progress from "bad to worse." Progression refers to a tumor's acquisition of increasingly malignant properties over time, e.g., faster growth rate, anaplasia, loss of hormonal responsiveness, invasiveness, chromosomal aberrations, drug resistance, and metastatic potential.[49,70] These individual properties develop stepwise, independently, and often in a preferred but not invariant order. None is inevitable. Some tumors do not progress beyond a certain point, e.g., basal cell carcinomas of the skin have the capacity to invade but seldom if ever develop the capacity to metastasize. Rarely, in fact, tumors regress spontaneously, e.g., neuroblastomas in children. In a given tumor, progression can never be regarded as complete and it may be remarkably incomplete by the time of the patient's death.

Progression is thought to depend on clonal evolution. Cancer is associated with genetic and epigenetic plasticity and perhaps an increased mutation rate, which together lead to variation and selection.[108] Selection is always in the direction of survival, which, in the case of cancer, favors those mutant clones that have the greatest capacity for proliferation, for metastasis, and for drug resistance. Implicit in the concept of tumor progression is tumor heterogeneity. Pathologists have recognized for many decades that the cells comprising a tumor are not morphologically homogeneous. In fact, morphological heterogeneity provides one criterion for grading

tumors (see below). More recently, it has been recognized that the individual cells that comprise tumors are often heterogeneous with regard to many other properties as well.

The multistage nature of carcinogenesis illustrates the concept of tumor progression. It is now clear that many tumors develop over time from individual clones of normal stem cell precursors in a series of distinct steps that include, at the least, dysplasia (sometimes accompanied by metaplasia), carcinoma in situ, and frank malignancy. Subsequent steps may include invasion of basement membrane and of local host tissues, induction of an independent vascular supply, extension into lymphatics and/or blood vessels, survival in the circulation, and colonization at discontinuous sites (metastasis). Carcinoma of the cervix clearly illustrates progression in that well-defined stages of dysplasia [cervical intraepithelial neoplasia (CIN)] and carcinoma in situ regularly precede the development of invasive carcinoma. A similar progression can be traced in the development of carcinoma of the colon.[145] Field carcinogenesis recognizes that the neoplastic process is ongoing at various stages of progression in a tissue that has been uniformly exposed to a carcinogen. Thus repeated instances of neoplasia of the bladder mucosa and oral mucosa are common. Semiserial sectioning of nearby regions in these and other organs usually reveals incipient changes chronologically younger or pathogenetically less advanced than the signal cancer.

Once they have become malignant, tumors vary considerably in their capacity for further progression. Tumors of bone marrow and lymphoid origin are most likely to undergo further morphological change, e.g., chronic myelogenous leukemia commonly progresses to blast crisis, and chronic lymphocytic leukemia, though less frequently, may proceed to a large-cell phase (Richter's syndrome). Solid tumors, on the other hand, are less apt to change morphologically. The fact that pathologists are able to make accurate diagnoses of solid tumor metastases and late recurrences depends on the morphological stability that most solid tumors maintain over a period of many years.

Tumor grading has traditionally referred to a pathologist's judgment as to a tumor's degree of differentiation and growth rate, often on a scale of I to III or IV, where III or IV represents the least differentiated, fastest dividing tumors (i.e., those tumors presumed to have the worst prognosis). Formal grading systems based on these criteria are less popular today than formerly because of their shortcomings. First, a different scale is required for each type of tumor, and scoring is subjective and not always reproducible. Second, tumors are typically heterogeneous and areas differing significantly in differentiation and mitotic activity may coexist, with the attendant risk of sampling error. Because prognosis is invariably linked to the most malignant portions of a tumor, it follows that, for accurate diagnosis and grading, sufficient tissue and microscopic sections must be sampled so that the most malignant areas are found. Finally, the correlation between histological appearance and biological behavior is seldom perfect. Because of these shortcomings, many pathologists have abandoned attempts to grade cancers and have instead adopted a descriptive terminology such as "well-differentiated mucin-secreting adenocarcinoma of the colon" or "poorly differentiated squamous cell carcinoma of the lung."

This is not to say, however, that pathologists are not still on the lookout for more useful tumor-specific features that may be important independent predictors of tumor prognosis. Recent attempts to identify such predictors have borne fruit in certain specific cancers. Thus, carcinomas of the prostate may be usefully graded on the basis of tissue architecture and neoplastic cell pattern.[60] A number of different criteria including nuclear differentiation, degree of gland or tubule formation, and mitotic activity have been usefully combined to grade breast carcinomas.[12,41,126] Two common and much studied solid tumors, cutaneous melanomas and carcinoma of the breast, illustrate other tumor-specific factors that affect prognosis in important ways. These will now be discussed in greater detail.

Histologic Grading and Prognosis of Cutaneous Melanomas. Cutaneous melanomas (see VIII-1-Plate 4) are subclassified clinically as being of the nodular (NM), superficial spreading (SSM), and lentigo maligna (LMM) types. LMM generally have the best prognosis and NM the worst.[23,24,56,75,86,96,98,99] In addition to clinical subtype, many additional factors affect the prognosis of patients bearing these tumors, including tumor ulceration, thickness, cell type (i.e., spindle, epithelioid, etc), mitotic activity, lymphocytic reaction, presence or absence of pigment, regression, vascular invasion and anatomic site of the primary tumor, sex of the patient, and histologic regression.[97]

Recently, a model incorporating 23 separate tumor characteristics was developed.[23] By multivariate analysis, six of these characteristics were found to be independent prognosticators: 1) mitotic rate, 2) presence of tumor-infiltrating lymphocytes, 3) tumor thickness, 4) anatomic site, 5) sex of the patient, and 6) evidence of histologic regression.[23] One of the most useful prognostic factors was the extent (i.e., the depth) of vertical invasion into the skin. Two widely regarded systems have been developed to classify melanomas using this criterion. Clark and colleagues[24] originally categorized melanoma invasion as follows: level 1, tumor confined to the epidermis (in situ): level 2, tumor invasion into the papillary dermis; level 3, tumor fills papillary dermis and abuts on, but does not involve, the reticular dermis; level 4, tumor invades the reticular dermis; and level 5, tumor invades the subcutaneous fat. Utilizing this system, level 1 tumors were found not to metastasize and level 2 tumors rarely did so. However, tumors scored as levels 3 to 5 commonly metastasized and yielded progressively worse survival rates[24] (see XXXIV).

One confounding limitation to the Clark system is that dermal anatomy varies significantly in different parts of the body. Breslow, therefore, developed an alternate scoring method, measuring with an ocular micrometer the vertical dimension of tumor invasion from the top of the granular cell layer of the epidermis.[18] Patients whose tumors measured ≤ 0.75 mm in vertical dimension rarely developed metastases, whereas patients with thicker lesions had an increasingly worse prognosis. The Breslow system of measurement also has its limitations, e.g., when pseudoepitheliomatous hyperplasia or tumor ulceration is present.

Using measurement schemes such as these, the supposed differences in prognosis between SSM and NM tend to blur because NM have generally extended deeper into the dermis at the time of diagnosis than have SSM.[43,97–99] LMM, however, continue to be an exception, maintaining their more favorable prognosis even when tumor thickness is taken into consideration.[87] For this reason, it is important to determine if a melanoma has arisen in the context of lentigo maligna.

Factors Important in Predicting Risk for Local Recurrence or Distant Metastases in Patients With Invasive Breast Cancer. Separate consideration must be given to the risks of *local recurrence* of cancer in the breast and *distant metastases;* the factors that affect each are not identical (see XXXII).

Local recurrence. In patients treated for infiltrating ductal carcinoma with breast-conserving surgery and radiation therapy, the factors predictive of local recurrence are not clearly related to known factors that predict for the development of distant metastasis. A recent large study on a total of 584 patients with clinical stage I or II infiltrating ductal carcinoma of the breast makes this point.[17] Treatment consisted of complete surgical excision of the primary tumor followed by radiation therapy totalling at least 60 Gy to the primary site. Of 34 separate tumor characteristics that were subjected to multivariate analysis, the only factor that was found to be associated with an increased risk of local breast recurrence was the presence of an extensive intraductal component (EIC-positive). EIC positivity was identified in two distinct groups of tumors: 1) tumors that were predominantly ductal carcinomas in situ with areas of focal invasion; and 2) primarily invasive tumors in which the ducts and lobules were not obliterated, virtually all preserved ducts were involved by ductal carcinoma in situ (this often corresponded to as much as 25% of the tumor volume), and tumors in which ductal carcinoma in situ was present adjacent to the invasive tumor.

Twenty-eight percent of all cases fell into the EIC-positive group and 26% of such patients developed local tumor recurrence as compared with only 7% of patients with EIC-negative tumors ($P = 0.001$).[17] A number of other investigators have now confirmed the finding that the presence of EIC is associated with a higher risk for breast recurrence after local excision and radiation therapy.[73,116] Still others disagree (see XXXII).

There seem to be two likely explanations for the increased risk of local recurrence in patients with EIC-positive tumors. One is that the residual tumor in this group of patients is less radiosensitive than in patients with EIC-negative tumors. The second is that the subclinical residual tumor burden following excision is consistently larger in EIC-positive than in EIC-negative patients and may be too large to have been eradicated by the cosmetically acceptable doses of radiation therapy that were delivered. While both of these explanations are possible, it has been found that the residual tumor burden is consistently larger in EIC-positive than in EIC-negative patients.[71]

Distant metastases. As with many other tumors, the single most important factor predictive of the systemic spread of breast cancer is involvement of the regional lymph nodes. Unless treated, most patients with involved axillary lymph nodes will ultimately die from metastatic spread of their disease. Since the natural history of breast cancer is often protracted, clinically evident metastases may not appear for many years, e.g., ≥10–20 years after the primary tumor and axillary lymph nodes have been removed. The greater the number of involved axillary lymph nodes, the greater is the likelihood that tumor cells have spread elsewhere in the body to indeterminate locations only to become clinically manifest at a later time. Thus, in one large series, 87% of the patients with ≥13 involved axillary lymph nodes developed metastatic spread within 10 years whereas only 20% of node-negative patients did so.[46]

Given the important prognostic significance of positive lymph nodes and recent evidence that patient survival improves with adjuvant therapy, criteria are now urgently needed to identify the 20–30% of lymph node-negative patients who will nonetheless develop metastatic disease after primary breast treatment. Factors worthy of consideration include the degree of tumor differentiation and the mitotic index. In addition, other, more specific factors may play a role. One likely candidate is the capacity of tumor cells to find their way into vascular spaces such as lymphatics or small blood vessels.[42,88,123,142]

Criteria for grading breast carcinomas. Several scoring systems have been used to grade breast cancers. Generally speaking, most include the degree of nuclear differentiation, the degree to which the tumor is able to form glands, and some attempt to estimate tumor growth rate by measuring mitotic activity. Using such criteria, the survival rates at 5 years in one series of node-negative patients with grade I through grade III tumors varied from 86% through 64%, and at 15 years from 49% through 25%.[11]

One newer approach for assessing tumor differentiation involves the use of flow cytometry. Tumors with normal diploid or tetraploid DNA content have been repeatedly shown to have a better prognosis than aneuploid tumors.[22,44,146] However, not all workers agree with this conclusion as it applies to node-negative patients.[105,121]

Tumor growth rate may be measured in a number of ways, including standard counts of mitotic figures per high power field, the percentage of cells in S-phase as determined by flow cytometry, [^{3}H] thymidine labeling index, and fraction of Ki-67-positive cells.[12,22,41,58,126,132] In a large study of DNA ploidy and S-phase fraction in lymph node-negative patients with breast cancer, no correlation was found between S-phase fraction and survival among patients with aneuploid tumors.[22] These aneuploid tumors constituted two-thirds of cases studied. Among diploid tumors, however, the S-phase fraction was highly predictive for the risk of recurrence.[22]

One of the most intensively studied and widely used measures for grading breast tumors is their expression of estrogen and progesterone hormone receptors (ERP). These are in fact the only measures for which standardized quality control is currently available. Most studies have shown that lymph node-negative patients with ERP-positive tumors have a significantly better disease-free survival, and, in some cases, better overall survival than patients whose tumors are ERP-negative.[45] The difference between the survival rates of patients with ERP-positive tumors and ERP-negative tumors decreases with time, and some studies have suggested that the survival curves will eventually merge.[64] Taken together, these observations suggest that tumors expressing estrogen and progesterone receptors tend to proliferate more slowly than tumors lacking such receptors. Thus, ERP measurements may not represent an independent prognostic factor per se but may instead provide yet another method of assessing tumor growth rate.

A large number of studies are now in progress attempting to identify other factors that may predict for risk in node-negative patients. These include evaluation of Ki-67 protein,[54] epidermal growth factor receptors,[13,114,125] insulin-like growth factors,[15,80] transforming growth factor-α,[4,149] cathepsin D,[138] and various oncogenes and their products. For a recent review of prognostic factors in breast cancer, see Harris et al.[68]

The Report Issued by the Surgical Pathologist

The gross and microscopic findings should be presented descriptively and comprehensively in terms that are understandable to both the pathologist and the clinicians caring for the patient. The report should provide enough information so that the clinician caring for the patient can follow the thought processes of the pathologist, much as if he or she were viewing the case with the pathologist at a double-headed microscope. The report should include the results of all specialized tests performed, their interpretation, and the synthesis and coordination of all clinically useful information available to the pathologist that may be of aid in diagnosis and management. Finally, reports should be issued in a timely manner so that they are available to the clinician within a few days of tissue submission. Failure to report results promptly may delay patient care (thus uselessly adding to the cost of medical care), lead to error and confusion, and at the very least prolong anxiety in patients who are often already distraught.

The Role of the Cytopathologist

Cytology is used for screening purposes and for the definitive diagnosis of suspicious lesions that may represent cancer or its precursors. Specific benefits include cost effectiveness, rapid turnaround time, and tissue diagnosis with minimal patient risk. Because diagnosis is usually made on only a small sample of cells or tissue, optimal technique is crucial both for specimen collection and preparation. Diagnosis should only be attempted by experienced personnel on well-fixed, appropriately stained specimens. Moreover, as in all areas of pathology, cytological diagnosis should never be made "in a vacuum"; pertinent clinical data on the requisition slip will facilitate rapid, accurate, and definitive cytologic diagnoses. Communication between the cytopathologist and clinician is therefore crucial.

A "positive" cytology report should indicate that the pathologist is sufficiently confident of the diagnosis that he or she is prepared to have the patient undergo definitive treatment such as surgical resection or chemotherapy based on that diagnosis alone. Where there is any doubt, the report should be less definitive, indicating by a term such as "atypia" that cellular abnormalities are present whose significance is not known. Often, a repeat cytology sample, biopsy, or other diagnostic test will be in order. Definitive therapy should never be initiated solely on the basis of "atypia." A "negative" cytology means that no abnormal cells were found in the sample examined. It is important for all to realize that this does not necessarily indicate absence of malignant disease in the patient. False-negative cytologies are often the result of sampling error.[55] However, laboratory error may result in both false-negative and false-positive results.

Exfoliative Cytology

Cells exfoliated from the respiratory and urinary tracts and from the female genital organs are studied principally to screen for cancer and its precursors. The use of the Pap smear has been instrumental in lowering the mortality rate from cervical cancer over the last four decades.[21,27,63,78,103,104] A problem inherent in all screening tests is the need to balance sensitivity and specificity. Lowering the threshold for diagnosis of atypia means that fewer cases of neoplasia will be missed. However, the statistically necessary price is that more patients without neoplastic disease will require additional, expensive studies such as colposcopy to rule out the presence of cancer.

The importance of sample collection and preparation needs to be emphasized. False-negative results are due most often to inadequate sampling or to poor sample preparation. Failure to fix samples immediately, thick smears, and the presence of significant amounts of blood may all result in specimens that are inadequate for diagnosis. Sensitivity can be increased by using a cytobrush because of its ability to sample a broad area.[16] In urinary and respiratory cytology, as with cervical cytology, larger and higher grade lesions are less likely to be missed because of problems related to either sampling or interpretation. In the case of smaller, lower grade lesions, multiple samples may be required to make a positive diagnosis. Cytopathologists generally feel that the economic and noninvasive advantages of cytology are lost after collection of three indeterminate specimens.

Endoscopic Cytology

In areas amenable to endoscopy, such as the bronchial tree and gastrointestinal tract, cytology may serve as a screening technique and may also provide a definitive diagnosis. Paired cytology and biopsy specimens give the greatest likelihood of diagnosing malignancy.[8] Because brush samples cover a wide surface area, they provide greater diagnostic sensitivity, particularly for the diagnosis of nonmalignant infectious diseases such as fungal infections. However, endoscopic biopsies generally provide more information, particularly in determining tumor type.

Cytology of Body Cavity and Cerebrospinal Fluids

Fluids are generally obtained from these sites for the purpose of diagnosing metastatic disease. Certain clues may allow the cytopathologist to pinpoint the site of primary tumor origin. For example, effusions obtained from female patients that exhibit three-dimensional clusters of adenocarcinoma cells are most often derived from tumors that arise in breast, ovary, or lung (see VIII-I-Plate 8). In men, metastatic adenocarcinomas diagnosed in effusions are most likely to be of pulmonary or gastrointestinal tract origin. If consistent with the clinical findings and results from other studies, a positive cytologic diagnosis can lead directly to treatment without the need for additional biopsies. As always, current cytology specimens should be compared to previous cytology or histology specimens, if available.

Reactive mesothelial cells share certain characteristics with malignant carcinoma cells including large nuclei with prominent nucleoli and even mitotic figures. Features such as cellular aggregates with smooth outlines, nuclear moulding and irregularity, and lack of intercellular spaces or "windows" help to distinguish carcinoma cells from reactive mesothelial cells. Panels of immunocytochemical stains may sometimes prove useful (see below). Unfortunately, there are at present no available antibodies that distinguish benign from malignant mesothelial cells and very few that reliably identify the site of origin of metastatic cancers.[31,94] Mesothelial cells survive and multiply when exfoliated into effusions. Therefore, although immediate fixation is not necessary, fluids do need to be refrigerated promptly and also require anticoagulation (heparin, 1 U/10 ml).

The chance of detecting malignancy in cerebrospinal fluid is lower than that in most other body fluids. This probably reflects the small number of malignant cells exfoliated into the cerebrospinal fluid (CSF) coupled with the small amounts of fluid normally available for study. In contrast, large volumes of fluid are typically collected from effusions into body cavities, and cells can be concentrated substantially from such fluids by centrifugation or filtration.

Aspiration Cytology

The earliest work on aspiration cytology was reported from the Memorial Hospital in New York in the 1930s.[93] Subsequently, the impetus for this technique shifted to Europe[90] and was not "rediscovered" in the United States until the 1970s. Prior to aspiration, the skin is prepared with alcohol; local anesthetic may be administered but often is not necessary. A 22–25-gauge needle is inserted into the center of palpable lesions, and 5–20 cc of suction is applied to the syringe. The needle may be moved rapidly from side to side within the lesion to sample as broadly as possible. Suction is then released, and the needle is withdrawn. The needle should always be withdrawn immediately if any blood enters its hub; however, cysts need to be drained completely with reaspiration if any mass remains. In highly vascular tissues, such as the thyroid, it is often advisable to start with a smaller gauge needle (e.g., 25-gauge) and to move to a larger size needle if tissue is not aspirated.

Considerable controversy exists over who is best qualified to perform fine needle aspirates (FNA). At present, cytopathologists, surgeons, and other clinicians successfully perform such aspirations.[51] In fact, the most critical and technically demanding step in aspiration cytology is generally not the aspiration itself but rather the preparation of adequate slides after the sample has been obtained.[50,91,111] Smears can be made directly, or the needle can be rinsed with a preservative solution, such as Saccomanno's, 50% ethanol, or a balanced electrolyte solution.[1,30] For preparation of smears, the needle is detached from the syringe, the syringe is filled with air and reattached, and the contents are expelled onto glass slides where they are spread in much the same manner as a blood smear, using a second slide or coverslip. Such preparations can be air dried for staining with Romanovsky's stains. Alternatively, smears can be alcohol-fixed and stained with Papanicolaou's or H&E stains. Fixation must be immediate and is generally performed with 95% ethanol or with commercially available spray fixatives.

In the case of lesions that are not directly palpable, aspiration is best performed by a radiologist under computed tomography (CT), ultrasound, or fluoroscopic guidance. Such deep aspiration procedures are expensive, time-consuming, and invasive. For these reasons it is desirable that a cytotechnologist or cytopathologist attend the procedure to ensure specimen adequacy and optimal slide preparation. A further advantage of this attendance is the ability of experienced personnel to triage material effectively for special studies, such as immunocytochemistry, electron microscopy, and flow cytometry.

Definitive aspiration cytology diagnoses, rendered by an experienced cytopathologist, can provide the basis for definitive therapy. However, such diagnoses need to be viewed in the context of all other laboratory studies and clinical findings. Specific problems and pitfalls that attend aspirations of various sites will now be briefly discussed.

Thyroid. FNA permits the accurate diagnosis of papillary, medullary, and anaplastic carcinomas but is less useful in the diagnosis of follicular nodules. There are cytologic features that help to distinguish among the various types of follicular disease,[79] but a definitive diagnosis may not always be possible by FNA, particularly the distinction between follicular adenomas and carcinoma. Thus, in some instances, FNA will serve only to distinguish patients needing immediate surgery for thyroid disease from those who may be safely followed with or without hormonal suppression.[50,65,66] However, even this limited information will eliminate much unnecessary surgery.

Breast. The specificity of breast aspiration is very high in the hands of an experienced cytopathologist, and a positive diagnosis may safely lead to mastectomy or other definitive treatment.[50,81,82] Of course, atypical and suspicious cases will require further workup. Aspiration cytology of the breast may also be performed on nonpalpable lesions under the guidance of conventional or stereotaxic mammography or ultrasound,[2,10,28,67,92] but the exact role for this new technique is not yet clear. Inherent problems for breast cytology include the inability to distinguish infiltrating from in situ ductal carcinoma and the limited accuracy in distinguishing correctly between premalignant and benign lesions (e.g., lobular carcinoma in situ, atypical ductal hyperplasia, ductal hyperplasia, intraductal papilloma).[39,134,148]

Lung. Aspiration cytology of the lung may lead to the diagnosis of both primary and metastatic tumors and nonneoplastic lesions such as tuberculosis and fungal infections.[50,111,140] As with histologic tissue sections, it is not always possible to distinguish primary from metastatic carcinomas.

Abdomen. Aspiration cytology is particularly useful in diagnosing cancers arising in the liver, pancreas, kidney, and retroperitoneum that would otherwise necessitate major surgery.[111] Poorly differentiated tumors may be difficult to type, but the use of adjunct techniques may aid in establishing a definitive diagnosis (see VIII-1-Plate 9).

Lymph Nodes. Many cytopathologists believe that aspiration cytology has only a limited role in the diagnosis of lymph node lesions. However, FNA can provide useful information such as obviating the need for surgery in cases of metastatic carcinoma to palpable lymph nodes with a known primary. Aspirates may also be useful for diagnosing lymphoproliferative diseases.[51,52]

There have been few diagnostic tests introduced into medicine that have actually lowered the cost of high-quality patient care. Cytopathology is such a test. It offers the advantages of low morbidity, rapid turnaround time, and outstanding cost effectiveness. The problems and pitfalls of cytology should not detract from its usefulness. All procedures have limitations, and the oncologist needs to be informed as to both the benefits and the pitfalls of this approach.

The Role of the Immunohistochemist

During the past decade, immunohistochemistry has become an important adjunct in the evaluation of human neoplasms. A detailed discussion of the technical aspects of immunohistochemistry is beyond the scope of this chapter, and the interested reader is referred to several review articles and monographs.[72,131,135,141] The commercial availability of a broad range of reagents (including prediluted reagents in kit form) has made it possible for high-quality immunohistochemistry to be performed in most pathology laboratories. The most commonly employed immunohistochemical techniques are those in which enzymes such as horseradish peroxidase or alkaline phosphatase are used in conjunction with specific antibodies. Methods such as the peroxidase–antiperoxidase (PAP) technique and the avidin–biotin complex (ABC) technique are the most widely utilized in current practice. In the PAP technique, antigen-containing tissue sections, cytospins, or smears are sequentially incubated with: 1) an unlabeled specific rabbit antibody directed against the antigen of interest (primary antibody); 2) a secondary (bridging) reagent consisting, for example, of swine antibodies directed against rabbit immunoglobulin if the primary antibody was prepared in rabbits; and 3) a tertiary reagent consisting of peroxidase–rabbit anti-peroxidase complexes. The second (swine) anti-rabbit immunoglobulin antibody serves as a bridge that links the primary rabbit antibody with rabbit peroxidase–anti-peroxidase complexes. The ABC procedure also requires three sequential steps: an unlabeled primary antibody, a biotin-labeled antiimmunoglobulin secondary antibody, and, finally, preformed avidin–biotin–peroxidase complexes. Although both the PAP and ABC methods provide satisfactory staining results, the latter is often somewhat more sensitive.[155] It should be noted that the sensitivity of any immunohistochemical procedure is, in large part, related to the reagents and detailed procedures employed. As a consequence it is difficult to compare the results of immunohistochemical studies from different institutions that employ different reagents and methods.

Virtually any type of pathologic specimen may be suitable for immunohistochemical staining including fresh-frozen tissue, fixed tissue, and cytologic preparations. Unfortunately, however, not all antigens are equally well preserved after these various treatments. Fixation masks or destroys many antigens, and the approach taken for immunohistochemical staining must depend upon the antigen(s) of interest. For example, while a large number of cytoplasmic antigens are detectable in fixed, paraffin-embedded tissue, many cell surface-associated antigens are demonstrable only in fresh-frozen tissue sections or in smears. Pretreatment with proteolytic enzymes such as trypsin or pepsin may permit the identification of certain otherwise undemonstrable antigens in fixed, paraffin-embedded tissue sections. Finally, not all fixatives are equivalent with regard to antigen preservation. While crosslinking fixatives such as formaldehyde are often suitable, they are suboptimal for detecting certain antigens of diagnostic importance such as those located on intermediate filaments, which are best demonstrated in fresh-frozen or alcohol-fixed tissue.[5,106,120]

Applications

Immunohistochemistry is widely useful in the evaluation of human tumors. Some more common applications are listed in Table VIII-1-1 and are discussed below.

Categorization of "Undifferentiated" Malignant Tumors. Not infrequently, a pathologist examining routine H&E-stained paraffin sections recognizes the presence of a malignant tumor but is unable to characterize the tumor further. This is understandable in that "undifferentiated" tumors often lack characteristics that permit more accurate classification. However, further classification is often important in making clinical decisions related to appropriate therapy and prognosis. Immunohistochemistry may be helpful in such situations (see VIII-1-Plate 7). Before performing immunohistochemistry, however, the pathologist must first develop a differential diagnosis, and this will depend on the tumor's histologic appearance, its anatomic location, and the clinical setting. Only then is he or she in a position to select a panel of antibodies that will permit a more definitive diagnosis.

One common problem in tumor diagnosis will serve as an example. Undifferentiated tumors composed of large cells with an epithelioid appearance may suggest undifferentiated carcinoma, lymphoma, or melanoma. The distinction among these tumor types can often be made using a panel of antibodies, as illustrated in Table VIII-1-2. Unfortunately, this table presents an ideal result that is not always achieved in practice. Some carcinomas show aberrant staining for vimentin[3,62] or S100 protein,[29] some lymphomas demonstrate

Table VIII-1-1. Common Applications of Immunohistochemistry in the Evaluation of Human Tumors

Categorization of "undifferentiated" malignant tumors
Determination of site of origin of metastatic tumors
Subclassification of tumors in various organ systems and tissue compartments (e.g., central nervous system tumors, germ cell tumors, sarcomas)
Distinction between carcinomas and malignant mesotheliomas
Categorization of leukemias and lymphomas
Detection of antigens of potential prognostic or therapeutic importance:
  Estrogen and progesterone receptors
  Oncogene products
  Markers of proliferative activity
  P-glycoprotein

Table VIII-1-2. Immunohistochemical Evaluation of the "Undifferentiated" Malignant Tumor in which the Differential Diagnosis Includes Carcinoma, Lymphoma, and Melanoma (see text)

Antigen	Carcinoma	Lymphoma	Melanoma
Keratin	+	−	−
Epithelial membrane antigen	+	−	−
Vimentin	−	+ or −	+
Leukocyte common antigen	−	+	−
S-100 protein	−	−	+
Melanoma-associated antigen	−	−	+

Table VIII-1-3. Antigens with Highly Restricted Specificity

Antigen	Tumor Specificity
Factor VIII-related antigen	Vascular tumors
Gross cystic disease fluid protein	Breast carcinomas; cutaneous tumors with apocrine differentiation
Melanoma-associated antigen	Melanoma
Muscle-specific actin	Smooth muscle and skeletal muscle tumors
Myoglobin	Skeletal muscle tumors
Prostate specific antigen	Prostatic carcinomas
Thyroglobulin	Thyroid follicular cell tumors

epithelial membrane antigen,[119] and some melanomas exhibit immunoreactivity for keratin.[154] Such results emphasize the need to use a panel of antibodies, rather than a single antibody, when evaluating tumors.

Determination of Site of Origin of Metastatic Tumors. Routine microscopic examination may permit general classification of a tumor (e.g., carcinoma) but not identification of its site of origin. Immunohistochemistry may sometimes be helpful in providing this additional information, and a number of useful antigens that may be identified are listed in Table VIII-1-3. Unfortunately, appropriate organ- or tissue-specific antibodies are not currently available for many important tumors, including such common carcinomas as those arising in the lung, colon, endometrium, and pancreas, thereby limiting the ability of immunohistochemistry to resolve such problems in every instance. Furthermore, some of the antigens listed in Table VIII-1-3 have now been found aberrantly in neoplasms other than those for which they were initially thought to be "specific." For example, the melanoma-associated antigen detected by one widely used antibody (HMB-45) has recently been found in some breast carcinomas.[14]

Subclassification of Tumors in Various Organ Systems. In some organs and tissue compartments, it may be difficult to subclassify certain tumors based on histological grounds because of overlapping features. Some of these distinctions are of academic interest only (e.g., determining whether a high-grade spindle cell sarcoma shows neural, myogenous, or fibrohistiocytic differentiation), but others have therapeutic and prognostic significance. For example, in some cases it may be difficult or impossible to distinguish with certainty an anaplastic seminoma from an embryonal carcinoma of the testis by routine microscopic examination, a distinction with both therapeutic and prognostic implications. However, immunostaining for the intermediate filament keratin is often useful in making this distinction, because seminomas are typically keratin negative, whereas embryonal carcinomas are usually keratin positive.[6,102] Similar situations may be encountered in other organ systems and tissue compartments.

Distinction Between Carcinomas and Malignant Mesotheliomas. A common problem encountered by the surgical pathologist is the distinction between metastatic adenocarcinoma and malignant mesothelioma involving the pleura or peritoneum.[110,112,152] Immunohistochemical staining using a panel of antibodies may be useful in assisting in this distinction (Table VIII-1-4).

Categorization of Leukemias and Lymphomas. One of the most common uses for immunohistochemistry is the correct diagnosis and classification of leukemias and lymphomas (see XXXVI-2). A detailed discussion of this subject is beyond the scope of this chapter, and the interested reader is referred to several recent articles and reviews.[9,83,110,117,152] In brief, immunohistochemistry, in conjunction with morphology and histochemistry, is a useful adjunct in making the distinction between acute leukemias of lymphoid and nonlymphoid types and in distinguishing hairy cell leukemia from other types of leukemic infiltrates in the bone marrow and at other sites. In addition, immunohistochemistry is useful for subclassifying non-Hodgkin's lymphomas and Hodgkin's disease and in distinguishing them from each other in problematic cases (see XXXVI-10).

Detection of Antigens of Potential Prognostic or Therapeutic Significance. A variety of antigens of possible prognostic and therapeutic importance can be detected using immunohistochemistry including estrogen and progesterone receptors in breast cancers,[115,134] protein products of oncogenes (such as HER-2/*neu* in breast cancers and c-myc in neuroblastomas[133,143]), antigens associated with tumor cell proliferation such as Ki-67 and PCNA/cyclin,[53,58] and the P-glycoprotein product of the multiple drug resistance (MDR) gene.[150] Ki-67 is of particular interest.[57] It is a nuclear antigen present in all proliferating cells, i.e., present in G_1, S, G_2, and M phases of the cell cycle but absent in G_0 cells. Therefore, by staining for this antigen, it is possible to measure the tumor growth fraction directly and in a simpler manner that is more readily applicable to clinical specimens than are radioactive labeling methods using [^{3}H]thymidine. Ki-67 staining also yields results that are more reproducible than those obtained by mitotic figure counting.

Table VIII-1-4. Immunohistochemical Distinction Between Metastatic Adenocarcinoma and Malignant Mesothelioma Involving the Pleura or Peritoneum

	Adenocarcinoma	Mesothelioma
Keratin	+	+
Vimentin	+ or −	+ or −
Carcinoembryonic antigen	+ or −	−
LeuM1	+ or −	−
B72.3	+ or −	−

Limitations

An appreciation of the limitations of immunohistochemistry in tumor diagnosis is as important as an understanding of its many useful applications. Potential limitations in the immunohistochemical evaluation of solid tumors can be broadly characterized as technical and interpretive.

Technical Limitations. Because demonstration of different types of antigens by immunostaining requires appropriate tissue preparation, advance planning for immunohistochemistry is essential so that the specimen is handled appropriately. For example, if on clinical grounds or at intraoperative examination (i.e., frozen section or tissue imprint) an excised lymph node has features that suggest a lymphoma, a portion of the specimen should be snap-frozen to permit reliable demonstration of lymphocyte surface markers, since these cannot be well demonstrated in fixed, paraffin-embedded tissue. In cases of suspected carcinoma, in which the demonstration of intermediate filament proteins is likely to be important, fixation of a portion of the tumor in an alcohol-based fixative is advisable.

As with any laboratory procedure, the use of appropriate positive and negative controls is mandatory in immunohistochemistry and serves as a check on the technical adequacy of the procedure. Results of immunostaining must always be viewed with caution if the appropriate controls are omitted or suboptimal.

Interpretive Limitations. The usefulness of immunohistochemical staining depends not only on the technical adequacy of the procedure but also upon proper selection of antibodies and correct interpretation of both positive and negative staining. In most situations, it is more useful to employ a panel of antibodies than a single antibody. The antibodies comprising the panel must be selected carefully, based on a thoughtful differential diagnosis. A "shotgun" approach to immunostaining is strongly discouraged and may only serve to compound diagnostic confusion.

Accurate interpretation of staining requires familiarity with the characteristics of "true-positive," "false-positive," "true-negative," and "false-negative" staining. Negative reactions are more difficult to interpret than are positive reactions. Even with the use of other controls, it is difficult to be certain that a reaction is a "true-negative" unless the section in question stains positively for a complementary antigen. For example, in the analysis of an undifferentiated malignant tumor in which the differential diagnosis includes lymphoma and carcinoma, a negative reaction for keratin (the intermediate filament characteristic of many carcinomas) does not by itself rule out the possibility of carcinoma. However, if a negative keratin stain is accompanied by positive staining for leukocyte common antigen (a marker present in most lymphomas), the likelihood of lymphoma is greatly enhanced.

Some antibodies are of great diagnostic value in terms of both sensitivity and specificity (e.g., antibodies to prostate-specific antigen), whereas others are of limited diagnostic value even when used as part of a panel (e.g., antibodies to the intermediate filament vimentin). Pathologists who use immunohistochemistry must be experienced and aware of the limitations of a methodology that is evolving at a rapid pace. An antigenic profile suitable today for diagnosing a particular type of tumor may tomorrow be shown to be suboptimal or less specific than was originally thought. Immunohistochemistry is a valuable tool for aiding in the diagnosis of difficult tumors. However, it is only an adjunct to diagnosis, and the results must be interpreted in the context of other findings, particularly routine histological sections and the clinical setting.

The Role of the Electron Microscopist

Though making use of radically different technology, electron microscopy (EM) seeks the same type of information as that gleaned from immunohistochemistry, i.e., detection of differentiation markers that permit more accurate tumor identification and classification. EM is generally not useful in determining whether individual cells are malignant or benign (but see ref. 100 for an exception). It is a powerful tool for recognizing subcellular structures that are not detectable by light microscopy but that, when present, allow confident identification of cells of epithelial or melanocyte origin, for example. Although advances in immunohistochemistry have somewhat reduced the need for EM in tumor diagnosis, they have by no means eliminated this need altogether, and EM remains at present an underutilized technique for tumor diagnosis.[59,69,74] Moreover, validation of new immunohistochemical reagents is often best accomplished by ultrastructural study of replicate tissue samples.

Technical Considerations

Appropriate tissue handling, fixation, and processing are of even greater importance in EM than they are for immunohistochemistry.[33] Advanced planning and consultation between the clinician, surgical pathologist, and electron microscopist are therefore imperative. In many cases, it is advantageous to have a pathologist or knowledgeable technician in the operating room or at the bedside at the time of biopsy in order that tissue may be fixed immediately and trimmed appropriately. Tissues must be cut into small pieces because chemical fixatives penetrate tissues slowly (over minutes to hours), and the electron microscope glaringly exposes artifacts in poorly fixed tissues that are not detectable at the lower resolution afforded by light microscopy. In at least one dimension, tissues must be no thicker than 1 mm, and to achieve this small size, further trimming may be necessary after brief preliminary fixation. Mixtures of glutaraldehyde and paraformaldehyde (e.g., Karnovsky's fixative) provide optimal fixation.[33] Although these reagents are best when freshly prepared, it is also possible to freeze vials of fixative beforehand that may be thawed immediately prior to use. Tissues fixed in formalin or in other "routine" fixatives designed for light microscopy give inadequate tissue preservation for electron microscopy. Once tissues are fixed inappropriately, they generally cannot be recovered for adequate electron microscopy, and rebiopsy becomes the best option. Peripheral blood, bone marrow, and cell-containing fluids (e.g., pleural effusions, spinal, or synovial fluids) are handled somewhat differently from samples of solid tissue and require that a member of the electron microscopy staff be present as the sample is obtained.[33]

Applications

The great strength of EM lies in its exquisite resolution, which permits the recognition of intracellular structures, organelles or products, that are undetectable by light microscopy. EM is often helpful in the diagnosis of "undifferentiated" malignant tumors and in determining the origin of metastatic tumors of unknown primary site (Figures VIII-1-2, VIII-1-3).[36] The recognition of cytoplasmic premelanosomes within tumor cells permits the distinction of amelanotic malignant melanomas from undifferentiated carcinomas and lymphomas with which they can be confused. Other ultrastructural features whose recognition may permit definitive diagnosis are the cytoplasmic granules characteristic of carcinoid tumors; the norepinephrine- and epinephrine-containing granules found in pheochromocytomas; terminal webs characteristic of primary gastrointestinal carcinomas arising from absorptive epithelial cells;[34] lamellar (surfactant) bodies found only in type II pneumocytes and therefore diagnostic of alveolar cell carcinomas of the lung;[37] tonofilaments and desmosomes found in mesothelial cells and squamous cells; and cyto-

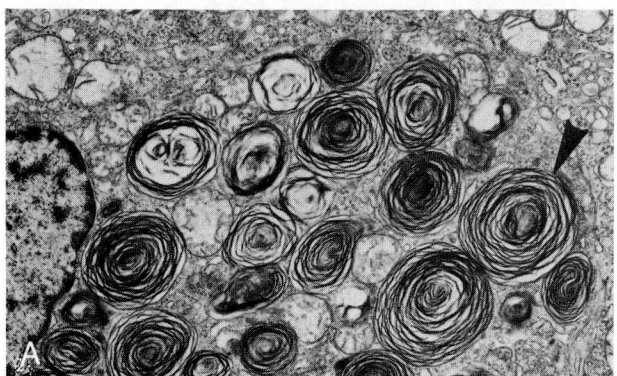

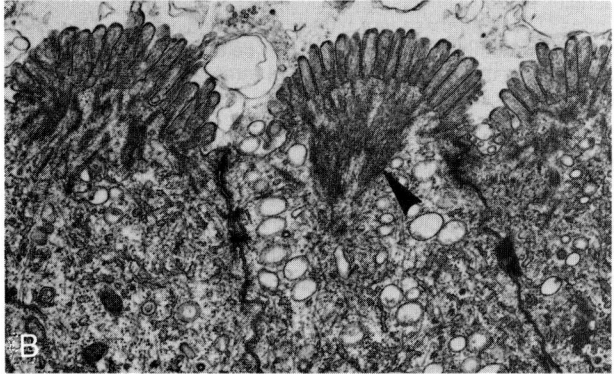

Figure VIII-1-2.   *A.* Electron micrograph from lung mass shows typical surfactant-containing lamellar bodies (surfactant bodies) (arrowhead) that fill the cytoplasm of a tumor cell, allowing the specific diagnosis of primary alveolar cell carcinoma of the lung to be made. *B.* Electron micrograph from lung mass shows apical cytoplasm of three tumor cells at high magnification. Note short, blunt surface microvilli and the dense terminal web (arrowhead) of cytoskeletal filaments that traverse the apical cytoplasm horizontally and run vertically within individual microvilli. Tumor cells are joined by epithelial junctions and contain numerous apical cytoplasmic vesicles. The identification of the differentiated organelle, the terminal web, allows the specific diagnosis of metastatic adenocarcinoma of gut absorptive epithelial cell origin to be made. *A,* ×12,500; *B,* ×19,000.

128. Schnitt, S. J., Silen, W., Sadowsky, N. L., Connolly, J. L., and Harris, J. R.: Ductal carcinoma in situ (intraductal carcinoma) of the breast. N. Engl. J. Med., 318:898, 1988.

129. Senger, D. R., Galli, S. J., Dvorak, A. M., Perruzzi, C. A., Harvey, V. S., and Dvorak, H. F.: Tumor cells secrete a vascular permeability factor that promotes accumulation of ascites fluid. Science, 219:983, 1983.

130. Senger, D. R., Connolly, D. T., Van De Water, L., Feder, J., and Dvorak, H. F.: Purification and NH_2-terminal amino acid sequence of guinea pig tumor-secreted vascular permeability factor. Cancer Res., 50:1774, 1990.

131. Sheibani, K., and Tubbs, R. R.: Enzyme immunohistochemistry: Technical aspects. Semin. Diagn. Pathol., 1:235, 1984.

132. Silvestrini, R., Daidone, M. G., Valagussa, P., Salvadori, B., Rovini, D., and Bonadonna, G.: Cell kinetics as a prognostic marker in locally advanced breast cancer. Cancer Treat. Rep., 71:375, 1987.

133. Slamon, D. J., Godolphin, W., Jones, L. A., Holt, J. A.: Wong, S. G., Keith, D. E., Levin, W. J., Stuart, S. G., Udove, J., Ullrich, A., and Press, M. F.: Studies of the HER-2/neu proto-oncogene in human breast and ovarian cancer. Science, 244:707, 1989.

134. Sneige, N., White, V. A., Katz, R. L., Troncoso, P., Libshitz, H. I., and Hortobagyi, G. N.: Ductal carcinoma-in-situ of the breast: Fine-needle aspiration cytology of 12 cases. Diagn. Cytopathol., 5:371, 1989.

135. Sternberger, L. A.: Immunocytochemistry, 3rd Edition. New York, John Wiley & Sons, 1986.

136. Symposium on Estrogen Receptor Determination with Monoclonal Antibodies. Cancer Res., 46:4231S, 1986.

137. Symposium on the Autopsy: A Professional Obligation Dissected. Hum. Pathol., 21:127, 1990.

138. Tandon, A. K. C., Chamness, G. C., Chirgwin, J. M., and McGuire, W. L.: Cathepsin D and prognosis in breast cancer. N. Engl. J. Med., 322:297, 1990.

139. Tannock, I. F., and Rotin, D.: Acid pH in tumors and its potential for therapeutic exploitation. Cancer Res., 49:4373, 1989.

140. Tao, L.-C.: Lung, pleura, and mediastinum. In Guides to Clinical Aspiration Biopsy. Series. Edited by T. S. Kline. New York/Tokyo, Igaku-Shoin, 1988, p. 1.

141. Taylor, C. R.: Immunomicroscopy: A Diagnostic Tool for the Surgical Pathologist. Philadelphia, W. B. Saunders, 1986.

142. Toikkanen, S., Joensuu, H., and Klemi, P.: Nuclear DNA content as a prognostic factor in $T_{1-2}N_0$ breast cancer. Am. J. Clin. Pathol., 93:471, 1990.

143. Van de Vijver, J. J., Peterse, J. L., Mooi, W. J., Wisman, P., Lomans, J., Dalesio, O., and Nusse, R.: Neu-protein overexpression in breast cancer. Association with comedo-type ductal carcinoma in situ and limited prognostic value in stage II breast cancer. N. Engl. J. Med., 319:1239, 1988.

144. Vaupel, P., Kallinowski, F., and Okunieff, P.: Blood flow, oxygen and nutrient supply, and metabolic microenvironment of human tumors: A review. Cancer Res., 49:6449, 1989.

145. Vogelstein, B., Fearon, E. R., Hamilton, S. R., Kern, S. E., Preisinger, A. C., Leppert, M., Nakamura, Y., White, R., Smits, A. M. M., and Bos, J. L.: Genetic alterations during colorectal-tumor development. N. Engl. J. Med., 319:525, 1988.

146. von Rosen, A., Rutqvist, L. E., Carstensen, J., Fallenius, A., Skoog, L., and Auer, G.: Prognostic value of nuclear DNA content in breast cancer in relation to tumor size, nodal status, and estrogen receptor content. Breast Cancer Res. Treat., 13:23, 1989.

147. Wainscoat, J. S., and Fey, M. F.: Assessment of clonality in human tumors: A review. Cancer Res., 50:1355, 1990.

148. Wang, H. H., Ducatman, B. S., and Eick, D.: Comparative features of ductal carcinoma in situ and infiltrating ductal carcinoma of the breast on fine needle aspiration biopsy. Am. J. Clin. Pathol., 92:736, 1989.

149. Watson, P., Barrett, J., Pantazis, C., and Guthrie, T.: Color video analysis of transforming growth factor alpha expression in female breast cancer. Proc. Am. Soc. Clin. Oncol., 7:36, 1988.

150. Weinstein, R. S., Kuszak, J. R., Kluskens, L. F., and Coon, J. S.: P-glycoproteins in pathology: The multidrug resistance gene family in humans. Hum. Pathol., 21:34, 1990.

151. Weiss, L. M., Hu, E., Wood, G. S., Moulds, C., Cleary, M. L., Warnke, R., and Sklar, J.: Clonal rearrangements of T-cell receptor genes in mycosis fungoides and dermatopathic lymphadenopathy. N. Engl. J. Med., 313:539, 1985.

152. Wick, M. R., Loy, T., Mills, S. E., Legier, J. F., and Manivel, J. C.: Malignant epithelioid pleural mesothelioma versus peripheral pulmonary adenocarcinoma: A histochemical, ultrastructural, and immunohistologic study of 103 cases. Hum. Pathol., 21:759, 1990.

153. Willis, R. A.: The Spread of Tumors in the Human Body. London, Butterworths & Co., 1952.

154. Zarbo, R. J., Gown, A. M., Nagle, R. B., Visscher, D. W., and Crissman, J. D.: Anomalous cytokeratin expression in malignant melanoma: One- and two-dimensional Western blot analysis and immunohistochemical survey of 100 melanomas. Mod. Pathol., 3:494, 1990.

155. Zuo-Rong, S., Itzkowitz, S. H., and Kim, Y. S.: A comparison of three immunoperoxidase techniques for antigen detection in colorectal carcinoma tissues. J. Histochem. Cytochem., 36:317, 1988.

Acknowledgements

This work was supported by US Public Health Service grants CA-28471, CA-28834, and CA-50453, by the Beth Israel Hospital Pathology Foundation, Inc., and under terms of a contract from the National Foundation for Cancer Research. The authors thank Mr. Peter K. Gardner for his expertise in compiling this manuscript.

IX

Principles of Imaging

IX-1

Introduction

Richard J. Steckel

The technologic revolution which is being fueled by the development of increasingly powerful computer hardware and software is currently affecting all branches of medicine. Nowhere has this revolution had a greater impact, however, than on the science and practice of diagnostic imaging. Malignant tumors frequently alter the normal spatial relationships of tissues and organs, and diagnostic imaging is critical not only for cancer diagnosis but also for staging tumors and following patients after they are treated. In the near future it is expected that technologic advances which are related to imaging (MR spectroscopy; PET scans with new metabolic agents; labelled monoclonal antibodies) will assist the clinician to evaluate better the *functional* aspects of tumors and their treatments.[2,3,6,8]

It may be appropriate to review briefly some of the technical similarities, as well as the differences, between the three most sophisticated cross-sectional or planar imaging techniques that are now available–computerized tomography (CT), magnetic resonance imaging (MRI) and positron emission tomography (PET) scanning. All three of these techniques require computerized image reconstructions of 2-dimensional "slices" through the body that are oriented in various planes. More recently, 3-dimensional volume or surface images have also become possible. With CT scans, an external radiation source and a radiation detector are required on opposite sides of the body, which is similar in concept to ordinary radiographic imaging techniques. On the other hand, MRI uses a powerful magnet and a source of radio-frequency waves to create images of the head or body, without the need for ionizing radiation (see below). PET scanning uses tracer amounts of short-lived radionuclides that have been produced in a medical cyclotron, injected intravenously into patients and concentrated in tumors or various organs within the body; the small amounts of radioactivity from these radionuclides can be picked up by external radiation detectors and then used to create planar or volume images. The radionuclides that are used for PET scanning actually emit subatomic particles called positrons, and each positron combines with an electron in the tissues to produce two x-ray photons that can then be detected outside the body. The radiation doses to tissues are less than those with ordinary radiographic studies.

With CT scanning, the recorded densities of tissues on the CT images have the same significance as the film densities on x-ray radiographs: The CT densities indicate the relative amounts of x-rays absorbed by each tissue depicted on the image, but CT is much more sensitive to minor differences in tissue absorption ("contrast") than ordinary radiographs. In addition, the cross-sectional or planar imaging capability of CT can "peel off" superimposed layers of tissue that are visible on ordinary radiographs of the chest, abdomen and other body structures, showing the radiographic anatomy of a single layer or "slice" of tissue in an axial plane. Since an external ionizing radiation source is required, the x-ray doses to tissues with CT studies are similar to those that are experienced with ordinary chest, abdomen, bone and skull radiographs.

In MRI a powerful unidirectional magnetic field is used to orient or polarize some of the body's hydrogen atoms in the direction of the magnetic field. Short pulses of radiowaves are then sent into the head or body at a specific frequency which is "resonant" with the polarized hydrogen atoms. The hydrogen atoms in the body that are already oriented in the direction of the magnetic field are momentarily deflected from their axes by these radiowave pulses. When they return to their original orientation in the magnetic field immediately after each radiowave pulse, the hydrogen atoms will emit radiowaves at the resonant frequency; these emissions can be picked up by an external radiowave detector. Using a computer, the radiowave emissions from hydrogen atoms within the body can then be used to synthesize a 3-dimensional volume image (or multiple adjacent planar images) of the region of the body that is under study. Therefore, the MR images actually represent a computer-generated map of hydrogen atom radiowave emitters in one body region. The radiowave emissions from hydrogen atoms within the body are referred to as "echoes," and the TE or "echo delay time" for a given MR image is the split-second time period that elapses between the excitation of hydrogen atoms in the tissues by pulsed radiowaves from the MR machine, and the detection or "sampling" of echoes from inside the body by the external radiowave detector (see above). The time delay between each successive radiowave pulse from the MRI machine (which, like the echo delay time, can be determined by the operator of the MRI unit) is called the TR or "repetition time." Depending upon the TE and TR settings (measured in milliseconds, or msec) that are chosen by the MRI operator for each clinical imaging examination, one can produce an image which is characterized as a "T1-weighted (T1W) image" or as a "T2-weighted (T2W) image." With the most commonly used MR imaging technique, known as "spin echo" imaging, the T1W images require relatively short TE and TR settings (a TE of 40 msec and a TR of 200 msec, for example), and T2W images require longer settings (e.g., a TE of 120 msec and a TR of 2,000 msec). Tumors appear relatively dark on T1-weighted MR images when compared to surrounding normal tissues, and they appear relatively bright on T2-weighted images. Anatomic detail is somewhat better on T1-weighted images, whereas tumors (and the edema and reactive tissue which surrounds them) often stand out in better contrast to surrounding normal tissues on T2-weighted studies.

It should also be noted that: (1) MR images can be obtained easily in any plane (not just the axial plane, as with CT images), (2) the contrast between different soft tissues is superior with MRI, and (3) one can discern vessels that contain flowing blood on MRI studies without the need to inject vascular contrast materials, because the vessel lumens often appear as "signal voids" (e.g., they appear black on the MR images). On the other hand, small amounts of calcium cannot be detected easily with MRI, as opposed to CT which is exquisitely sensitive to calcification in tissues. Unfortunately, standard MRI scans also take a relatively long time to obtain as compared to CT scans; they require several minutes rather than a few seconds to perform. Body motion therefore remains a potential problem with some MRI studies. The physical confines of the MRI machine are also quite restrictive, and up to 10% of patients experience severe claustrophobic reactions in the machine. For the same reason, very ill patients who are on life support systems are difficult to study with MRI equipment.

It is possible now to do semiquantitative "spectroscopic analyses" of metabolites in tissues with magnetic resonance, while producing images of tumors and normal tissues. There is some hope that the spectroscopic analyses might contribute to diagnostic specificity in the future and/or help to assess the responses of tumors to therapy. These assumptions are still being subjected to investigation, however.

PET scanning, like the spectroscopic analyses which are now possible with high magnetic field MR imaging, also may provide unique information about the metabolic activities of tumors, including metabolic changes that may occur with treatment. The short-lived positron emitting radionuclides that are required for PET scanning can be used to "tag" certain normal metabolites (e.g., radioactive fluorine-labelled glucose analogues) which are injected into the body prior to PET scanning. The rate and intensity of accumulation of a radioactive metabolite within a tumor and its surrounding normal tissues can then be analyzed with serial PET scans, leading to important inferences about tumor metabolism and metabolic changes that may occur with treatment. The ability to examine the metabolism of targeted volumes of tissue in situ is an important complement to the imaging ability of PET scans, and in this connection PET may offer a powerful new approach for studying tumors in the laboratory as well as in clinical situations.

The technologic advances which have generated transmission (CT) and positron emission (PET) computerized tomography and magnetic resonance imaging (MRI), as well as modern ultrasound (US) methods, have already led to fundamental improvements in our ability to visualize tumors and to assess their metabolic as well as physical effects on the body. Whereas the "traditional" radiologic imaging techniques which are still being used daily throughout the world (e.g., radiographs of the chest, bones and abdomen; gastrointestinal contrast studies; bone scans) may either visualize tumors "directly" (e.g., show tumor nodules in the lung) or "indirectly" (e.g., demonstrate widening of the duodenal loop on a G.I. series, from which one may infer the presence of a pancreatic mass), the newer cross-sectional imaging techniques can produce direct images of tumor masses anywhere in the body. In addition to showing the internal structure or texture of a tumor, these techniques can also delineate the tumor margins and demonstrate its effects upon surrounding anatomic structures. Some tumors may become more visible (enhance) when intravenous contrast materials are infused during CT or MRI scans, or when particular MRI sequences are used (e.g., T-2 images). This ability to visualize a tumor directly as well as to show its effects upon surrounding organs, and the corresponding ability of cross-sectional scans to "strip away" overlying structures which may otherwise obscure a tumor mass, constitute fundamental advances for evaluating and managing cancer which have come about with modern planar imaging.[7,9,12]

Even with these advances it is necessary to emphasize that the *radiologist still is not able to make a tissue diagnosis*, and that relevant clinical information is essential for a proper interpretation of diagnostic images using any radiologic technique. Furthermore, US, CT and MRI have not replaced most of the "standard" radiologic techniques that have been part of our diagnostic armamentarium for generations. Instead, they serve to complement the standard techniques. Planar imaging methods have also made cancer diagnosis, staging and patient followup more accurate (or at least more sensitive) and more rapid than ever before. In spite of their relatively high costs, particularly for CT and MRI studies, the total impact of these newer imaging techniques upon the economics of cancer care may be mixed. In fact, a good argument can be made that these techniques may contribute to a decrease in the overall costs of patient care and the non-medical costs of cancer in several ways.[5] First, planar imaging methods have greatly lessened or eliminated the demand for invasive diagnostic techniques such as angiography, pneumoencephalography, and standard myelography. They have also facilitated the differential diagnosis of cancer *versus* other (non-malignant) conditions, and they may obviate unnecessary surgery in individuals who have been shown to have metastatic or locally advanced disease. The newer imaging methods have also helped to guide deep needle aspirations or biopsies as well as to plan open biopsies and surgical resections, and they have lessened the requirements for hospitalization by facilitating diagnosis and staging on an outpatient basis. For these reasons and others, modern diagnostic imaging techniques have not only improved cancer care and lessened patient suffering, they may have reduced overall medical expenditures as well as losses of income to patients, by shortening and simplifying diagnostic procedures, lessening hospitalization requirements and helping to tailor therapeutic approaches more appropriately to individual patient needs.

As opposed to the major impact of new technologies on cancer diagnosis, staging and followup, only one imaging method has had a significant impact upon screening asymptomatic individuals for cancer, and that is low-dose mammography. Breast cancer mortality within a defined population of women can be reduced by approximately one-third through the regular use of screening mammography as recommended in nationally published guidelines.[1,4] It should also be cautioned that while cross-sectional or planar imaging techniques have greatly increased our sensitivity in detecting masses and delineating their extent, these techniques may not have succeeded in improving our specificity for diagnosing cancer to the same degree.[11] Stated differently, the clinician as well as the diagnostic radiologist should be cautious in interpreting "positive" findings on imaging examinations in patients who have recognized cancers, with specific reference to diagnosing metastatic disease or extensions of tumors into contiguous organs. There are numerous conditions besides metastases which can present as nodules in the lungs on a CT scan or as "hot" lesions in the bones on radionuclide scans. As always, careful correlation of abnormalities on imaging studies with clinical and laboratory findings is essential. Comparing serial images over time will also help to improve diagnostic specificity when certain abnormalities are noted: tumor masses in the lungs shouldn't double in size over a few days, and, conversely, metastatic lesions usually do not remain stable for months or years. Comparison with a "baseline" imaging study from a year earlier may sometimes be critical to reach the correct diagnosis when evaluating an abnormality on a current CT, MRI or chest radiographic examination. The correlation of findings from different kinds of imaging studies (e.g., comparing bone scan abnormalities with radiographs of the same body areas in patients with suspected breast cancer metastases) may be as important as the correlation of imaging abnormalities with symptoms and clinical findings.

It should be evident from this introductory chapter on imaging, as well as from other contributions to *Cancer Medicine*, that much research still remains to be done on the appropriate uses of diagnostic imaging in cancer management. In fact, one could surmise that some of the nonreproducible results which may emerge from therapeutic trials might be directly related to inaccurate stratification of cancer patients in these trials.[12] A heterogeneous group of patients who have been improperly stratified together prior to randomization may have different stages or different forms of the disease under study. The current applications of imaging techniques in clinical practice for diagnosing and staging cancer are still considerably less than optimal, and some

clinical cancer studies may in fact be "mixing apples and oranges." Controlled investigations to determine the appropriate uses of diagnostic imaging in cancer patients will help to establish new standards upon which better clinical practices must ultimately be based.

One area of continuing concern is the type and appropriate periodicity of imaging examinations for following cancer patients after they are treated. The clinical questions pertinent to this important area of concern must also be subjected to carefully controlled studies. The actual needs for post-treatment surveillance with imaging examinations should be conditioned on whether effective palliative or salvage methods ("second- or third-line" treatments) are currently available when patients experience tumor recurrences. Equally germane to the design of investigations on imaging examinations to follow treated cancer patients is whether or not a second- or third-line therapy is more effective when a recurrence is detected "early," as opposed to "late": Some treatments for recurrent disease may be just as effective (or as ineffective) when a recurrence becomes evident through the appearance of new symptoms or physical findings, rather than by regular surveillance with laboratory studies and imaging examinations. It is a virtual certainty that some diagnostic imaging techniques are now being used inappropriately to follow cancer patients at major cancer treatment centers as well as in community practices, in the absence of reliable data from controlled clinical trials to determine what the actual effects of periodic imaging studies are upon patient outcomes.

The principles of diagnostic imaging and their current applications to clinical cancer management, as described in this book, represent the most informed recommendations currently available from a number of contributing experts. While these recommendations must suffice for now, additional carefully designed studies and corroborative data are urgently needed if recent technical developments in diagnostic imaging are to be applied optimally to cancer patient care.

References

1. Cady, B.: New diagnostic, staging and therapeutic aspects of early breast cancer. Cancer, 65(3 Suppl.):634, 1990.
2. Carrasquillo, J. A., Bunn, P. A., Keenan, A. M., Reynolds, J. C., Schroff, R. W., Foon, K. A., Su, M. H., Gazdar, A. F., Mulshine, J. L., Oldham, R. K., Perentesis, P., Horowitz, M., Eddy, J., James, P., and Larson, S. M.: Radioimmunodetection of cutaneous T-cell lymphoma with ^{111}In-labelled T101 monoclonal antibody. N. Engl. J. M., 315:673, 1986.
3. Dodd, G. D.: Advances in cancer diagnosis. Cancer, 65 (3 Suppl.):595, 1990.
4. Henson, D. E., and Ries, L. A.: Progress in early breast cancer detection. Cancer, 65(9 Suppl.):2155, 1990.
5. Kuhns, L. R., Thornbury, J. R., and Tryback, D.: Decisionmaking in Imaging. Chicago, Year Book Publishers, 1989.
6. Larson, S. M.: Positron emission tomography in oncology and allied diseases. Principles and Practice of Oncology Updates, 3:1, 1989.
7. Platt, J. F., Glazer, G. M., Gross, B. H., Quint, L. E., Francis, I. R., and Orringer, M. B.: CT evaluation of mediastinal lymph nodes in lung cancer: Influence of lobar site of the primary neoplasm. AJR, 149:683, 1987.
8. Schlom, J.: Innovations in monoclonal antibody tumors targeting. Diagnostic and therapeutic implications. J.A.M.A., 261:744, 1989.
9. Siegelman, S. S., Khouri, N. F., Leo, F. P., Fishman, E. K., Braverman, R. M., and Zerhouni, E. A.: Solitary pulmonary nodules: CT assessment. Radiology, 160:307, 1986.
10. Simon, R.: The importance of prognostic factors in clinical trials. Cancer Treat. Rev., 68:185, 1984.
11. Steckel, R. J., and Kagan, A. R.: Pitfalls in the diagnosis of metastatic disease or local tumor extension with modern imaging techniques. Invest. Radiol., 25:818, 1990.
12. Zerhouni, G. A., Stitik, F. P., Siegelman, S. S., Naidich, D. P., Sagel, S. S., Proto, A. V., Muhm, J. R., Walsh, J. W., Martinez, C. R., and Heelan, R. T.: CT of the pulmonary nodule: A cooperative study. Radiology, 160:319, 1986.

Imaging Cancer of Unknown Primary Site

A. Robert Kagan
Richard J. Steckel

Oncologists may perceive that the more they know about an individual patient, the better they can treat the patient. Unfortunately, when this perception is applied uncritically to the use of imaging examinations in a patient with disseminated cancer and an unknown primary, errant clinical judgments may sometimes be made.

Unknown primary tumors are far from rare. We see about one new patient per week with metastatic disease and an unknown primary in a large radiation oncology referral practice. A group of 255 patients with unknown primary tumors have been reported in one study, and autopsy results were available in 34.[12] The primary site could be identified at autopsy in only 14 of the 34 patients, of which seven were in the lung (not small cell), two in the pancreas, one each in the kidney, bladder, biliary ducts, and mediastinum, and one visceral Kaposi's sarcoma. In none of the 14 tumors that were identified at autopsy would prior knowledge of the primary site have affected the patient's course. In patients presenting with metastatic disease and unknown primaries, the most common primary tumors identified later in the patient's course or at autopsy are in the lung or pancreas; these are incurable when they have spread beyond the primary site, and in most there is still no effective palliation available. On the other hand, palliation is attainable with some disseminated carcinomas of the breast, prostate, endometrium, thyroid and ovary, and identification of a primary could be helpful. Curative treatments might also be undertaken for certain disseminated cancers including lymphomas, testicular germ cell tumors, and gestational choriocarcinomas.[6] However, treatable conditions still represent only a small fraction (less than 10%) of disseminated cancers presenting with "unknown primaries."

Patients with unknown primaries that are metastatic to cervical lymph nodes are often referred to an otolaryngologist, but those with isolated axillary or inguinal lymph node metastases may be referred directly to a medical oncologist.[3,11] The differential diagnosis when a patient presents initially with metastatic cervical lymph nodes includes lymphoma, germ cell tumor, thyroid or an upper airway tumor, carcinoma from another site, or melanoma. A final diagnosis can often be made by biopsy using histochemical, immunohistologic or electron microscopic techniques (see Section XXXVIII), not by performing extensive imaging studies or laboratory tests. Isolated lymph node metastases that first present in the supraclavicular fossa usually originate from primary tumors below the clavicle.[2] However, many patients who present with masses that are confined to the supraclavicular area and a biopsy diagnosis of "undifferentiated carcinoma" are

Table IX-2-1. Diagnostic Imaging Recommendations for Patients with Metastatic Carcinoma and an Occult Primary*

Presenting Site of Metastatic Disease	Imaging Studies to Consider Initially (Chest Radiographs are Always Indicated)
Abdominal mass	Abdominal CT scan
Hepatomegaly	Abdominal CT scan
	Consider barium enema/UGI series
Biliary tract (painless jaundice)	Percutaneous and/or endoscopic cholangio-pancreatogram
	Abdominal CT scan
Malignant ascites	Abdominal CT scan
	Consider barium enema/UGI series
Malignant pleural effusion	Mammogram in women
	Consider chest CT scan
Upper cervical lymph nodes	MRI or CT of upper airways, if endoscopy is negative
	Consider thyroid scan
Lower cervical lymph nodes	CT chest/abdomen
	Consider mammogram in women
Axillary lymph nodes (undifferentiated CA)	Mammography in women
	Consider chest CT scan
Brain (diagnosed on CT or MRI)	Chest/abdominal CT scans (if chest radiographs are nondiagnostic)
Spinal epidural space (on myelogram, contrast CT, or MRI)	Chest CT (if radiographs are nondiagnostic)
Bone	Radionuclide bone scan survey with correlative radiographs
	CT of chest/abdomen (if chest radiographs are nondiagnostic)
	Consider ultrasound of prostate (men) or mammogram (women)
Lungs (multiple nodules)	CT abdomen/pelvis
	Consider BE/UGI series

*Adapted from *Investigative Radiology*[8]

still being referred for CT and/or MRI of the head and neck. Many are also subjected to triple endoscopy with "blind" biopsies of the nasopharynx, tonsil, base of tongue, pyriform sinus and/or esophagus, in a fruitless search for an upper aerodigestive tract lesion.

It has been suggested that patients presenting with a nonlymphomatous anterior mediastinal mass on chest radiographs and undifferentiated histology be managed as if they had a germ cell neoplasm, whether or not they have elevated serum levels of human chorionic gonadotropin and/or alpha fetoprotein.[4] A similar approach has been recommended for patients who present initially with infradiaphragmatic adenopathy and no identifiable primary. However, Abeloff was not able to corroborate these recommendations.[1]

With the exception of breast cancer, malignant ascites or malignant pleural effusions often arise from primary tumors that are within the cavity containing the fluid.[12] Only for cancer of the ovary, small cell carcinoma of the lung, or lymphoma are there effective palliative treatments potentially available, however. For the most part, these primary tumor types can be diagnosed by cytology or by a serosal biopsy and concurrent clinical findings, not by the extensive use of imaging.

The imaging examinations which can be justified in initial attempts to establish the site of origin of an unknown primary tumor are relatively few in number (Table IX-2-1). In one clinical series, 65 consecutive patients with a diagnosis of "unknown primary" were subjected to extensive imaging studies.[7] In only 18 of these 65 patients was a diagnostic imaging procedure later identified as having been helpful: A chest roentgenogram in nine, barium enema in four, transhepatic cholangiogram in three, and renal arteriogram and xeromammogram in one patient each.

Some clinicians may use the "shotgun approach" and perform multiple imaging examinations on patients with unknown primaries, in part to deflect peer criticism by covering all clinical possibilities and avoiding diagnostic pitfalls. However, clinicians are not the only ones who use this approach. After careful microscopic analysis of a solitary brain metastasis in a patient with an unknown primary and a negative chest roentgenogram, a pathologist may suggest the ovary, thyroid, breast, or gastrointestinal tract as possible primary sources for the patient's tumor. This diffuse opinion may lead, in turn, to a further exhaustive search for the primary tumor which is often fruitless.[9] Diagnostic radiologists may also contribute to the shotgun approach by suggesting that gastrointestinal imaging studies be repeated following optimal bowel preparation, that questionable CT findings be checked with an MRI or vice versa, or that angiography and/ or endoscopy be performed to confirm possible abnormalities that were suggested on other diagnostic studies.

In conclusion, extended diagnostic workups that are performed for metastatic disease with a persistently unknown primary site will frequently not identify the primary tumor.[5,10] Furthermore, even if the primary tumor is eventually found, exhaustive studies including multiple imaging examinations often do not provide information that contributes to the length and/or quality of the patient's life. Therefore, except in carefully defined clinical circumstances the use of multiple imaging examinations to evaluate patients who have a disseminated cancer, with the purpose of uncovering a stubbornly occult primary tumor, may yield little information of direct benefit to the afflicted patient.

References

1. Abeloff, M. D.: Adenocarcinoma of Unknown Primary. The John Hopkins Medical Grand Rounds, Vol. XII: Program 2, Presentation 4, 1985.
2. Batsakis, J. G.: The Pathology of Head and Neck Tumors: The Occult Primary and Metastases to the Head and Neck, Part 10. Head Neck Surg. (May/June):409, 1987.
3. Guarischi, A., Keane, T. J., and Elhakim, T.: Metastatic inguinal nodes from an unknown primary neoplasm. Cancer, 59:572, 1987.
4. Hainsworth, J. D., and Greco, F. A.: When the primary site is unknown: Issues in diagnosis and management. Advances in Oncology, 5:20, 1989.
5. Hamilton, C. S., and Langlands, A. O.: ACUPS (adenocarcinoma of unknown primary site): A clinical and cost benefit analysis. Int. J. Radiat. Oncol. Biol. Phys., 13:1497, 1987.
6. Horning, S. J., Carrier, E. K., Rouse, R. V., Warnke, R. A., and Michie, S. A.: Lymphomas presenting as histologically unclassified neoplasms: Characteristics and response to treatment. J. Clin. Oncol. 7:1281, 1989.
7. Kagan, A. R., and Steckel, R. J.: Diagnosis of metastatic cancer with an unknown primary site. In Cancer Diagnosis, New Concepts and Techniques. Edited by R. J. Steckel and A. R. Kagan. New York, Grune and Stratton, 1982, p. 289.
8. Kagan, A. R., and Steckel, R. J.: Diagnostic imaging in clinical cancer management of metastases from unknown primary tumors. Invest. Radiol., 23:545, 1988.
9. LeChevalier, T., Smith, F. P., Caille, P., Costans, J. P., and Rouesse, J. G.: Sites of primary malignancies in patients presenting with cerebral metastases. Cancer, 56:880, 1985.
10. Nystrom, J. S., VanEgmond, E. M., and Leonard, R. J.: Appropriate therapy for metastatic cancer of unknown primary origin. Advances in Oncology 5:27, 1989.
11. Patel, J., Nemoto, T. Rosner, D., Dao, T. L., and Pickren, J. W.: Axillary lymph node metastasis from an occult breast cancer. Cancer, 47:2923, 1981.
12. Ringenberg, Q. S., Doll, D. C., Loy, T. S., and Yarbro, J. W.: Malignant ascites of unknown origin. Cancer, 64:753, 1989.
13. Steckel, R. J., and Kagan, A. R.: Metastatic tumors of unknown origin. Cancer, Accepted for Publication, 1990.

IX-3

Imaging Neoplasms of the Head and Neck and Central Nervous System

Robert Lufkin

Magnetic resonance imaging (MRI) has come to dominate the diagnostic imaging of extracranial head and neck structures and the central nervous system in the few years since its introduction. In spite of its negative impact on the use of computerized tomography (CT) and myelography, as well as its lesser impact on angiographic studies, there are still situations where MRI does not provide sufficient diagnostic information and a more invasive study is indicated. In order to appreciate their relative roles in imaging cancer of the head and neck and central nervous system, it is particularly important to consider the strengths and weaknesses of MRI as compared to CT.

MRI–Advantages

Lack of Ionizing Radiation

The fact that the MR images use only magnetism and radiowaves is an advantage over other studies that require ionizing radiation. This is particularly important in individuals requiring many serial examinations, in the pediatric patient, or during pregnancy.

Sensitivity to Flow

The exquisite sensitivity of MRI to flow is based on the fact that any change in location of protons due to arterial, venous or CSF pulsations during MR imaging or spectroscopy results in a change in signal. This obviates the need for intravenous contrast materials (as with X-ray CT) to demonstrate vascular structures. In fact, most experts agree that in most clinical situations, MR without contrast is superior to x-ray CT with contrast for the definition of vascular anatomy. Intravenous contrast material may also be valuable with MR in the central nervous system to show blood-brain barrier disruption, but it is not necessary for the simple demonstration of flowing blood. The inherent sensitivity of MR to flow is being applied at some research centers to perform projection images of flowing blood in patients using a new technique referred to as "MR angiography."

Multiplanar Capabilities

With x-ray CT the scan plane is defined by the x-ray tube-detector axis through the gantry. In most patients this means that scanning is limited to the axial and, in some cases, the coronal plane. With MRI the scan plane is defined instead by the selection of RF frequencies and magnetic field gradients, which can be varied and are under electronic rather than physical control.

Iron Sensitivity

Because of the paramagnetic and ferromagnetic properties of many forms of iron with their unpaired electrons, these substances have special effects on MR images. Many types of iron result in subtle alterations in the local magnetic field environment of tissue protons, which in turn causes relaxation enhancement or shortening of T1 or T2 relaxation times. The type and amount of shortening reflect the form and quantity of the iron-containing compounds. As a result of the high sensitivity of MR to iron it has been said that "iron is to MR as calcium is to CT."

Accumulation of nonheme iron in the form of ferritin has been demonstrated in the brain by MR with normal aging.[2] Ferritin iron results in a loss of MR signal due to preferential T2 shortening. It is found most commonly in the globus pallidus, red nucleus, and substantia nigra.

Heme iron has a characteristic appearance on MR because of the changes it undergoes as hemoglobin passes through several breakdown stages. While the iron in normal oxyhemoglobin does not result in any significant relaxation enhancement, the reversible transformation to deoxyhemoglobin results in preferential T2 shortening on MR images. After 72–90 hours the deoxyhemoglobin in extravasated blood is irreversibly converted to methemoglobin which has a characteristic high signal on T1 weighted images because of its T1 shortening effect. Gradually, this breakdown product is converted to hemosiderin, which will show up as a low MR signal because of T2 shortening. While CT is sensitive to acute hemorrhage because of the protein content of blood within brain tissue, MR is far more sensitive to the later phases of a hematoma (>72 hours) after much of the protein has broken down.

High Soft Tissue Contrast Resolution

The high sensitivity of MRI to variations in tissue proton density and in T1 and T2 relaxation times is extremely valuable for imaging CNS pathology. All forms of cerebral edema are generally shown better with MRI than with CT. The lack of beam hardening artifact from bone, a common problem with CT, results in superior MR imaging of the vertex, posterior fossa, floor of the middle fossa, skull base and spinal contents.

MRI–Disadvantages

Low Calcium Sensitivity

MRI is inferior to CT for detecting calcification in masses and/or in association with hyperostosis. In some cases this lower sensitivity to calcium is more than offset by the superior soft tissue resolution of MRI. Newer types of pulse sequences, which have a higher T2 sensitivity, may improve the ability of MRI to detect calcium.

Acute Hemorrhage

While MRI is clearly superior to CT for the evaluation of subacute (>72 hours) and chronic hemorrhage (see above), the high sensitivity of CT to blood protein in acute CNS hemorrhage has made it the study of choice for patients with recent bleeding. Other pulse sequences with high T2 sensitivity are under investigation for the evaluation of acute hemorrhage with MRI.

MRI–Contraindications

Despite the noninvasive nature of MRI, exposures to magnetic fields and radiofrequencies (RF) may be contraindicated in certain patients. These patients are best studied with other techniques such as CT. The operation of cardiac and other forms of pacemakers may be adversely affected by MR scanning, so patients with these devices are generally excluded from examination. Newly-inserted clips for intracranial aneurysms may develop torque from changing magnetic fields and may actually twist off vessels, so these patients are also excluded from MR study. New nonferromagnetic clips which are unaffected by magnetic fields are now available for aneurysm clipping.[2] MRI studies of patients with skull plates, wires, surgical clips that have been in place for a long time, or even large metallic implants may contain some image artifacts but are safe to perform. These appliances are well fixed in the tissues and are resistant to magnetic field torques, and therefore do not represent contraindications to MRI.

Slow Image Acquisition

Conventional MR scanning is generally slower than a comparable CT study. This means that patients who are too ill to be placed within the MR magnet for scan times in excess of 10 minutes are best studied with techniques other than MRI. The problem of slow data acquisition with MR may be overcome in the near future as newer pulse sequence strategies are developed. These may allow scan times comparable to or shorter than CT, and several investigators are even considering MR fluoroscopy.

High Cost

MRI studies generally are more expensive than CT. This is a relative disadvantage for MRI in situations where CT and MRI can provide similar information. With the introduction of lower cost MR scanners, it is anticipated that the cost per MR examination will decrease in the near future. As a result the cancer imaging applications of MR will continue to increase.

Extracranial Head and Neck Cancer

Magnetic resonance imaging has replaced computed tomography as the study of choice for many lesions of the extracranial head and neck. The notable exceptions where CT is still essential are lesions in which subtle bone destruction or new bone formation (e.g., osteomas of the sinuses) are essential to recognize. Magnetic resonance easily surpasses CT in its ability to differentiate subtle differences in soft tissue boundaries and local extensions of tumors of the head and neck. The role of intravenous gadolinium-DTPA, gd-DTPA (Magnevist, Berlex, New York) in MRI examinations of the head and neck is currently under investigation.[24] Preliminary studies indicate that, while tumor enhancement occurs with contrast infusions, little clinically relevant information is added in many cases. When intracranial tumor extension is present, however, the gadolinium contrast can improve the detection of blood-brain barrier and leptomeningeal abnormalities (e.g., cerebral edema and tumor involvement).

Salivary Glands

MRI has replaced CT for the imaging evaluation of most masses in the major salivary glands.[3,19,21,23,28,29] Since MRI can rarely suggest the histology of tumors, its value in most cases (as with CT) is to define the tumor outline. While poor tumor margination may be a clue to malignancy, it is certainly not a pathognomonic finding in MRI or in CT studies. Deep parapharyngeal space involvement may be demonstrated with CT; however, MRI provides much better soft tissue contrast. The real advantage of magnetic resonance in evaluating masses in the parotid area is its ability to define more accurately the extent of a mass, to localize a tumor as extraparotid or intraparotid, and to determine whether an intraparotid tumor is in the superficial or deep lobes of the gland.

Paranasal Sinuses

While CT remains the study of choice for inflammatory sinus disease, MRI is extremely valuable for evaluating masses of the paranasal sinuses. It allows excellent delineation of soft tissue masses that are surrounded by secretions within the sinuses. Erosions of the bony walls can also be dem-

onstrated on MR by the absence of the signal void which is normally present with cortical bone. For tumor extensions outside the bony sinuses, MRI is clearly the study of choice because it can differentiate normal skeletal muscle from deep tumor extension, which can sometimes be difficult on CT studies. In cases where there is a question of extension into the anterior or middle cranial fossa, MRI with gadolinium enhancement is now the study of choice.

Nasopharynx

The relative lack of motion and the abundant fascial planes of the nasopharynx result in high quality MR imaging.[10,30] Retropharyngeal adenopathy, tumor infiltration beyond the pharyngobasilar fascia, and hypertrophic lymphoid tissue are all identified more easily with MRI than CT.[31] In particular, direct coronal and sagittal MR scans can be valuable to assess the craniocaudal extent of a tumor and possible intracranial involvement. While CT scanning is unquestionably more accurate in detecting small amounts of calcification or losses of bone, magnetic resonance examinations are quite adequate to evaluate skull base invasion. Abnormalities of the skull base are detected on MRI by replacement of the normal low signal cortical bone with the higher signal of a neoplasm. The capability of multiplanar imaging and the far superior soft tissue resolution of MRI therefore make it the imaging study of choice to evaluate the nasopharynx.

Tongue and Oropharynx

In general, MRI produces soft tissue detail that is superior to CT for evaluating the tongue and oropharynx (Figure IX-3-1). Therefore, MRI is also considered the study of choice for cancer in this area. Lack of artifacts from dental amalgam and beam hardening artifacts from the mandible on MRI also eliminates two major shortcomings of CT in examining the area. Finally, the ability of MRI to obtain direct coronal and sagittal scan planes is a distinct advantage in evaluating the intrinsic tongue musculature and assessing tumor volume for treatment planning.[18,32]

Larynx and Hypopharynx

Rarely does an imaging modality play a significant role in making the primary diagnosis of malignancy in the larynx or hypopharynx. These regions are so easily accessible to clinical examination that the combination of visual inspection and cytology/biopsy usually suffices to confirm a diagnosis of cancer. Therefore, the role of MRI is the same as CT for cancer in this area: to define the extent of disease. While laryngoscopy can show normal mucosal surfaces and masses involving the airway, deep tumor extensions are difficult to detect from clinical examination alone. In several areas these extensions may have profound implications for the management and control of disease. CT, and now MR to an even greater degree, can define this critically important deep anatomy.[2,7,8,13-15,20,26,27]

Compared with CT, MRI provides superior soft tissue definition. Direct coronal and sagittal scanning planes allow the visualization of intrinsic laryngeal musculature and will better

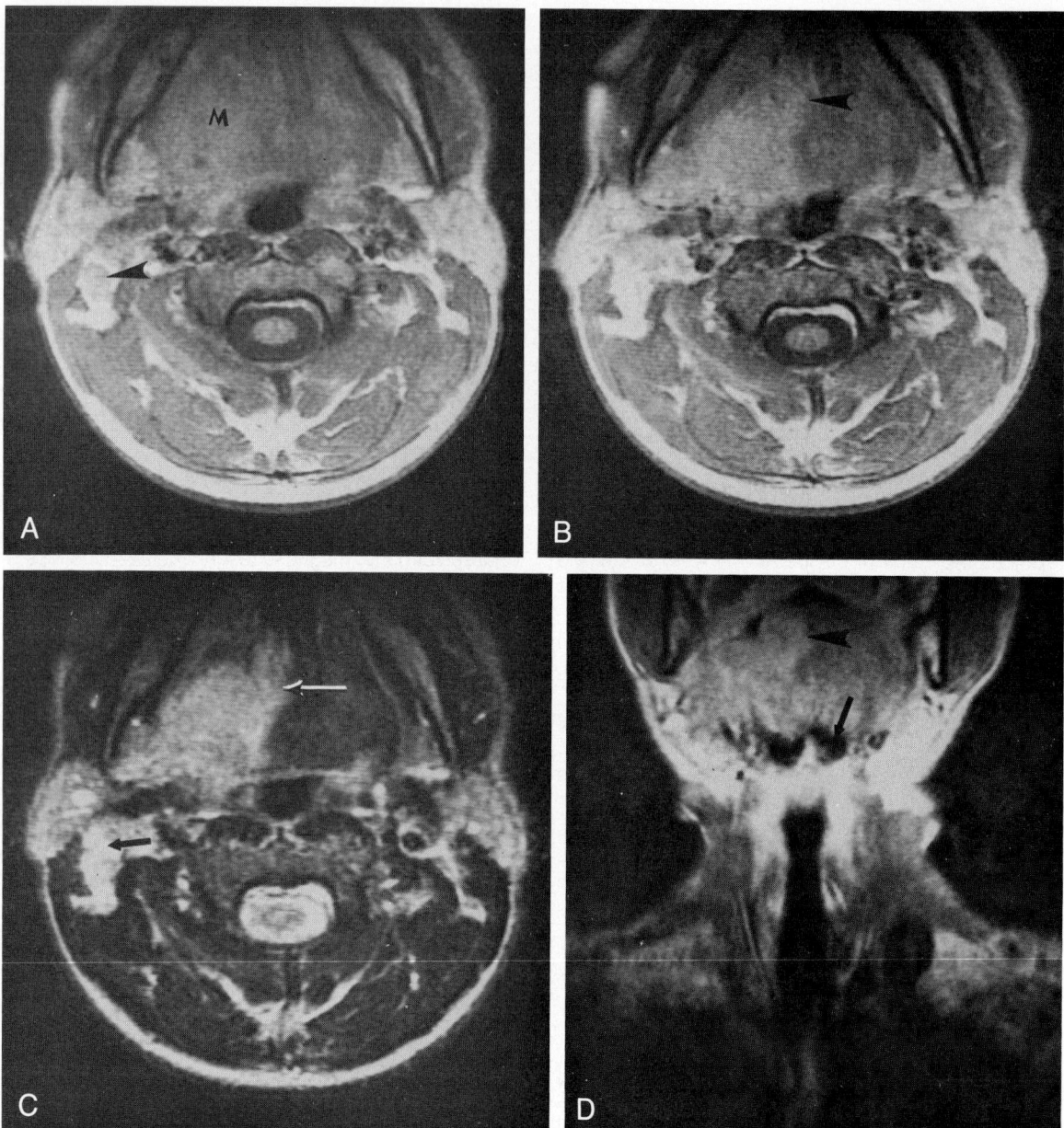

Figure IX-3-1. Squamous carcinoma of the tongue base. MR imaging, with and without gadolinium contrast. (A) Axial T1-weighted image (Se/800/30) through the tongue base reveals mass effect (M) on the left and associated adenopathy (arrowhead). The spinal cord is well demonstrated with this pulse sequence (note central gray matter and low-signal CSF surrounding the cord). Bone cortices in the mandible and vertebral bodies appear as areas of low signal (black). CT scanning is generally more sensitive than MRI for detecting small calcifications or subtle bone erosions. (B) MR image at similar level to (A), with same pulse sequence, following administration of gadolinium DTPA. Mild enhancement of the tongue mass is noted (arrowhead), with slight decrease in visibility of the abnormal lymph node. (C) T2-weighted image (SE/2000/85) without gadolinium reveals high signal in the tongue mass (white arrowhead) and increased signal in the area of adenopathy (arrow), somewhat similar to appearance with gadolinium on T1-weighted images (B). (D) Coronal T1-weighted image is useful for defining the extent of the mass (arrowhead) and showing that there is no extension to the supraglottic larynx. The vallecula is free of tumor (arrow).

define cranial-caudal tumor extensions. Thus, MRI is now the imaging study of choice to evaluate tumor stage within the larynx and hypopharynx.

Thyroid

Ultrasound and nuclear medicine techniques are generally more cost-effective than MRI for imaging malignancies of

the thyroid. However, the latter is valuable for demonstrating extensions of thyroid tumors into the mediastinum where ultrasound is a less effective modality.

Central Nervous System Cancer

It is difficult to generalize on the role of MRI in brain tumor imaging, because there is such variability in the results for

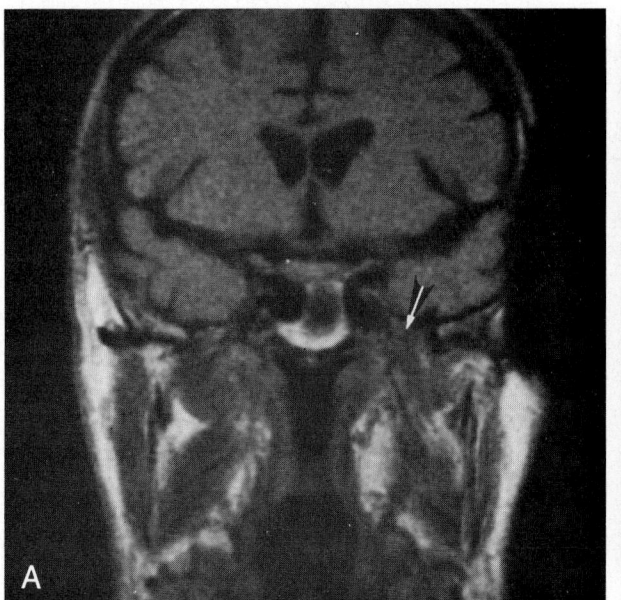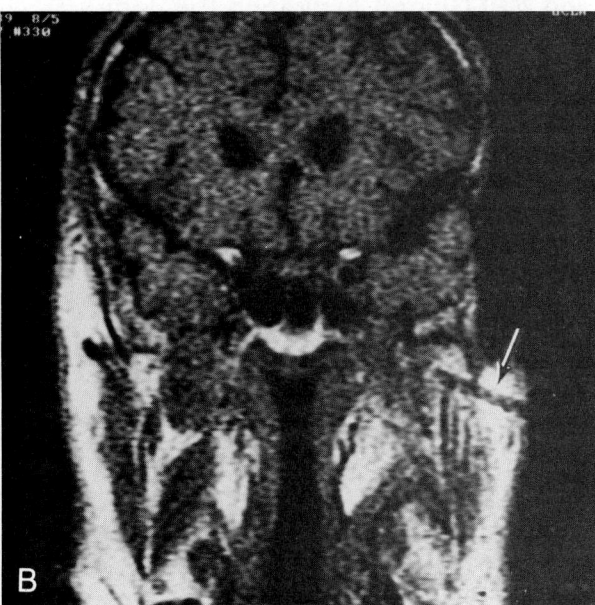

Figure IX-3-2. Diagnosis made by MRI-guided aspiration cytology, of recurrent squamous carcinoma in the parapharyngeal space extending to the skull base. (A) Coronal image (SE/700/30) shows mass high in the infratemporal fossa (arrow). (B) Gradient echo image after needle placement. Although image quality is less with newer rapid scanning techniques, the needle is well visualized (arrow) and scan time is reduced to 48 seconds (SE/480/30/60° flip angle).

different tumors and for different locations.[22,33] In general, MRI is effective for detecting intracranial tumors, because it is so sensitive to the cerebral edema which accompanies most tumors. Therefore MRI is particularly advantageous for detecting small lesions such as metastases which are found in greater numbers by MRI than by CT.[12]

Bleeding into a CNS tumor may also be appreciated better by MRI than by CT, both because the abnormal signal from blood persists longer on MRI and because there is no problem in distinguishing hemorrhage from calcification. Cysts associated with tumors are visible with MRI, as they are with CT, but considerable information may be available from MRI regarding the contents of the cysts since the signal intensity of fluid varies greatly with protein content.

MRI also has disadvantages for detecting and defining CNS tumors. Tumors may frequently be obscured by the high signal from surrounding brain edema. The use of a variety of MRI sequences may allow the tumor to be seen in such cases. MR imaging may also benefit from the use of intravenous paramagnetic contrast media that pass into CNS regions lacking an effective blood-brain barrier, thus highlighting some tumors. Gadolinium-DTPA therefore results in a clear MRI demonstration of most neoplasms.[6,9]

Initially, it was hoped that it might be possible to perform tissue characterization in brain tumors by determining T1 and T2 values. However, there appears to be such a wide overlap in these values that neither tumor type nor the degree of malignancy can be predicted.[10] The inability of MRI to demonstrate calcification is also a disadvantage in characterizing some brain intracranial tumors. MRI probably gives a better representation of the extent of a primary brain tumor than does CT. It is known that primary CNS tumors often extend beyond the apparent outlines of a mass as demonstrated by either CT or MRI, and it may be safer to consider

that a brain tumor has spread throughout the surrounding zone of visible edema which is better delineated by MRI.[25]

While it appears, at present, that both MRI and CT are quite effective in demonstrating brain tumors, MRI has the advantage of greater sensitivity for detecting edema as well as the potential for demonstrating lesions in several different planes or projections. With the use of intravenous gadolinium DTPA, MRI is better able to show meningiomas and can help to characterize brain neoplasms better. While tumor boundaries may be obscured with either CT or MRI by extensive brain edema, contrast enhancement may be valuable for delineating blood-brain barrier abnormalities and subarachnoid tumor spread.[11] Standard arteriography with contrast injections via catheters into the carotid or vertebro-basilar systems is required relatively rarely to characterize CNS neoplasms in the era of CT and MRI. Its remaining applications for studying space-occupying lesions lie principally in the realm of arteriovenous malformations and aneurysms.

A solitary brain metastasis may be difficult to differentiate from a glioma. However, multiplicity of lesions strongly suggests metastatic disease. MRI is particularly valuable for evaluating the common complication of bleeding into brain metastases which may be seen with melanoma, choriocarcinoma, and oat cell carcinoma of the lung.

CT scanning can better define tumoral calcifications and the associated hyperostosis of a meningioma. However, both CT and MRI can easily demonstrate meningeal lesions with intravenous contrast enhancement. MRI consistently demonstrates small acoustic angle tumors with greater detail than CT. This eliminates the need for injecting intrathecal air or other contrast materials. Acoustic neuromas show striking intravenous contrast enhancement with both CT and MRI, however.

CT and MRI-Guided Aspiration Cytology

The use of guided aspiration cytology for deep or impalpable lesions has contributed to the evaluation of many patients with extracranial head/neck and CNS tumors.[16,17] With this technique, aspiration of cells through fine needles allows a diagnosis by cytology rather than by histology which requires a larger specimen and a formal biopsy. While the aspiration technique has long been used with ultrasound and CT guidance, there are a number of areas such as the skull base where beam hardening artifacts limit the effectiveness of CT scanning to guide this procedure.

At UCLA, MRI has been the modality of choice for guiding aspiration cytology procedures in the head and neck over the last three years (Figure IX-3-2). In addition to the lack of beam hardening artifacts and the availability of high soft tissue contrast and flow sensitivity, the ability to do multiplanar imaging with MRI is particularly advantageous in complex cases.

References

1. Brothers, M., Fox, A. J., Lee, D. H., et al.: MR of postoperative cerebral aneurysm. A.J.N.R. (Abstract), Radiology, In press.
2. Castelijns, J. A., Gerritsen, G. J., Kaiser, M. C., Valk, J., Jansen, W., Meyer, C. J., and Snow, G. B.: MRI of normal or cancerous laryngeal cartilages: Histopathologic correlation. Laryngoscope, 97:1085, 1987.
3. Casselman, J. W., and Mancuso, A. A.: Major salivary gland masses: Comparison of MR imaging and CT. Radiology, 165:183, 1987.
4. Dillon, W. P., Mills, C. M., Kjos, B., Degroot, J., and Brant-Zawadzki, M.: Magnetic resonance imaging of the nasopharynx. Radiology, 152:731, 1984.
5. Drayer, B., Burger, P., Darwin, R., Riederer, S., Herfkens, R., and Johnson, G. A.: MRI of brain iron. AJR Am. J. Roentgenol.,147:103, 1986.
6. Felix, R., Schnorner, W., Laniado, M., Niendorf, H. P., Claussen, C., Flieger, W., and Speck, U.: Brain tumors: MR imaging with gadolinium-DTPA. Radiology, 156:681, 1985.
7. Glazer, H. S., Niemeyer, J. H., Balfe, D., Devieni, V. R., Emami, B., Hayden, R. E., Aronberg, D. J., Levitt, R. G., Ward, M. P., Sagel, S. S., and Lee, J. K: Neck neoplasms: MR imaging. Part I. Initial evaluation. Radiology, 160:343, 1986.
8. Glazer, H. S., Niemeyer, J. H., Balfe, D., Hayden, R. E., Emami, B., Devineni, V. R., Levitt, R. G., Aronberg, D. J., Ward, M. P., Lee, J. K., and Sagel, S. S.: Neck neoplasms: MR imaging. Part II. Post treatment evaluation. Radiology, 160:349, 1986.
9. Graif, M., Bydder, G., Steiner, R., Niendord, P., Thomas, D. G., and Young, I. R.: Contrast-enhanced MR imaging of malignant brain tumors. A.J.N.R., 6:855, 1985.
10. Komiyama, M. Yaguro, H., Baba, M., Yasui, T., Hakuba, A., Nishimura, S., and Inoue, Y.: MR imaging: possibility of tissue characterization of brain tumors using T1 and T2 values. A.J.N.R., 8:65, 1987.
11. Krol, G., Sze, G., Malkin, M., and Walker, R.: MR of cranial and spinal meningeal carcinomatosis; comparison with CT and myelography. AJR Am. J. Roentgenol., 151:583, 1988.
12. Lee, B., Kneeland, J., Cahill, P., and Deck, M.: MR recognition of supratentorial tumors. A.J.N.R., 6:871, 1985.
13. Lufkin, R. B., and Hanafee, W. N.: Application of surface coils to MR anatomy of the larynx. AJR Am. J. Roentgenol., 145:483, 1985.
14. Lufkin, R., Hanafee, W., Wortham, D., and Hoover, L.: MRI of the larynx and hypopharynx using surface coils. Radiology, 158:747, 1986.
15. Lufkin, R., Larsson, S., and Hanafee, W.: NMR anatomy of the larynx and tongue. Radiology, 148:173, 1983.
16. Lufkin, R., Teresi, L., Chiu, L., and Hanafee, W.: A technique for MR guided needle placement in the head and neck. AJR Am. J. Roentgenol., 151:193, 1988.
17. Lufkin, R., Teresi, L., and Hanafee, W.: New needle for MRI guided aspiration cytology. AJR Am. J. Roentgenol., 149:380, 1987.
18. Lufkin, R. B., Wortham, D. G., Dietrich, R. B., Hoover, L. A., Larsson, S. G., Kangarloo, H., and Hanafee, W. N.: Tongue and oropharynx: Findings on MR imaging. Radiology 161:69, 1986.
19. Mandelblatt, S. M., Braun, I. F., Davis, P. C., Fry, S. M., Jacobs, L. H., and Hoffman, J. C., Jr.: Parotid masses: MR Imaging. Radiology 163:411, 1987.
20. McArdle, C. B., Bailey, B. J., and Amparo, E. G.: Surface coil magnetic resonance imaging of the normal larynx. Arch. Otolaryngol. Head Neck Surg., 112:616, 1986.
21. Mirich, D. R., McArdle, C. B., and Kulkarni, M. V.: Benign pleomorphic adenomas of the salivary glands: Surface coil MR imaging versus CT. J. Comput. Assist. Tomogr., 11:620, 1987.
22. Muller-Forell, W., Schroth, G., and Egan, P. J.: MR imaging in tumors of the pineal region. Neuroradiology, 30:224, 1988.
23. Rice, D. H., and Becker, T.: Magnetic resonance imaging of the salivary glands. Arch. Otolaryngol. Head Neck Surg., 113:78, 1987.
24. Robinson, J. D., Crawford, S., Teresi, L., Schiller, V. L., Lufkin, R. B., Harnsberger, H. R., Dietrich, R. B., Crim, J. R., Duckwiler, G. R., Spickler, E., and Hanafee, W.: Gadolinium MR imaging in the head and neck. Radiology, In press.
25. Shuman, W., Griffin, B., Haynor, D., Jones, D. C., Johnson, D. S., Cromwell, L. D., and Laramore, G. E.: The utility of MR in planning the radiation therapy of oligodendroglioma. A.J.N.R., 151:583, 1988.
26. Stark, D. D., Moss, A. A., Gamsu, G., Glark, O. H., Gooding, G. W., and Webb, W. R.: Magnetic resonance imaging of the neck. Part 1. Normal anatomy. Radiology, 150:447, 1984.
27. Stark, D. D., Moss, A. A., Gamsu, G., Clark, O. H., Gooding, G. W., and Webb, W. R.: Magnetic resonance imaging of the neck. Part 2. Pathologic findings. Radiology, 150:455, 1984.
28. Teresi, L., Lufkin, R., Kolin, E., Hanafee, W., : MRI of the intraparotid facial nerve. American Journal of Neuroradiology, 8:253, 1987.
29. Teresi, L., Lufkin, R., Wortham, D., Abemayor, E., and Hanafee, W.: Parotid masses: magnetic resonance imaging. Radiology, 163:405, 1987.
30. Teresi, L. M., Lufkin, R. B., Vinuela, F., Dietrich, R. B., Wilson, G. H., Bentson, J. R., and Hanafee, W. N.: MR imaging of the nasopharynx and floor of the middle crania fossa. Part I. Normal anatomy. Radiology, 164:811, 1987.
31. Teresi, L. M., Lufkin, R. B., Vinuela, F., Dietrich, R. B., Wilson, G. H., Bentson, J. R., and Hanafee, W. N.: MR imaging of the nasopharynx and floor of the middle crania fossa. Part II. Malignant tumors. Radiology, 164:817, 1987.
32. Unger, J. M.: The oral cavity and tongue: magnetic resonance imaging. Radiology, 155:151, 1985.
33. Yuh, W. T., Barloon, T. J., Jacoby, C. G., and Schultz, D. H.: MR of fourth-ventricular epidermoid tumors. A.J.N.R., 9:794, 1988.

IX-4

Imaging Neoplasms of the Thorax

Poonam Batra

Lung Cancer

Conventional posteroanterior and lateral chest radiographs obtained with high kilovoltage (kVp) technique represent the most valuable and cost effective imaging examination for lung cancer. Oblique or overpenetrated views may be obtained in selected cases to evaluate equivocal findings on the chest radiographs, and fluoroscopy may be used to verify the presence or absence of a suspected lung lesion. In the case of a solitary pulmonary nodule, a radiograph obtained with low kVp technique or fluoroscopy may show a benign pattern of calcification and obviate further study. An obvious exception may be a "scar cancer," in which a calcific focus may be present in an eccentric location and the nodule spiculated or irregular in appearance. Fluoroscopy may also be used to guide a percutaneous biopsy of a lesion in the lung, mediastinum or pleura.

Computerized tomography (CT), by virtue of its cross-sectional display of anatomy and its superior contrast resolution, has become the principal radiographic technique to supplement chest radiographic findings. The morphology of a lung lesion, including its size, margins, and presence or absence of calcification, can be demonstrated well by CT. In general, a lung lesion less than 3 cm in size, with clearly defined margins and a high attenuation value suggesting that it might contain calcium (Hounsfield numbers greater than 164) can be considered as benign.[24] A lung lesion with an irregular spiculated border and a diameter greater than 3 cm may be regarded as particularly suspicious for cancer. CT can depict the segmental and subsegmental bronchial anatomy, and therefore it can help to determine the exact location of endobronchial cancers.[17] Furthermore, it can assess the extraluminal component of an endobronchial cancer, which is not visible to the bronchoscopist. Because of its relatively low signal-to-noise ratio and respiratory motion problems, MRI is not as useful as CT at this point for imaging lung cancer.[1] Difficulty in recognizing calcification is also a limitation in evaluating primary lung lesions with MRI. Coronal or sagittal MR images can be particularly useful for detecting the superior extent of tumors at the lung apex (Figure IX-4-1) or assessing involvement of the subclavian artery or brachial plexus.

Accurate preoperative staging of non-small cell lung cancer is essential to select patients with localized disease for curative surgery and those with widespread neoplasms for palliative therapy.[2] CT is clearly superior to conventional radiography in demonstrating the extent of the primary lesion, invasion of the hilum or mediastinum, and the presence of enlarged lymph nodes.[4,15] Most potential surgical candidates with non-small cell lung cancer should have a preoperative chest CT scan, but the role of CT when a small peripheral lesion is the only radiographic abnormality is controversial. Some investigators believe that a patient with a small peripheral nodule and a normal mediastinum on plain chest radiographs (presumed $T_1 N_0 M_0$) does not require a CT scan, since the likelihood of detecting mediastinal lymphadenopathy is low.[20] Others maintain that CT is indicated even with these patients, since occult mediastinal adenopathy, a contralateral lung lesion, or adrenal metastases may be detected in a minority of cases.[12] In patients with an enlarged hilum, it may be difficult on plain films to distinguish between hilar adenopathy and a dilated pulmonary artery.

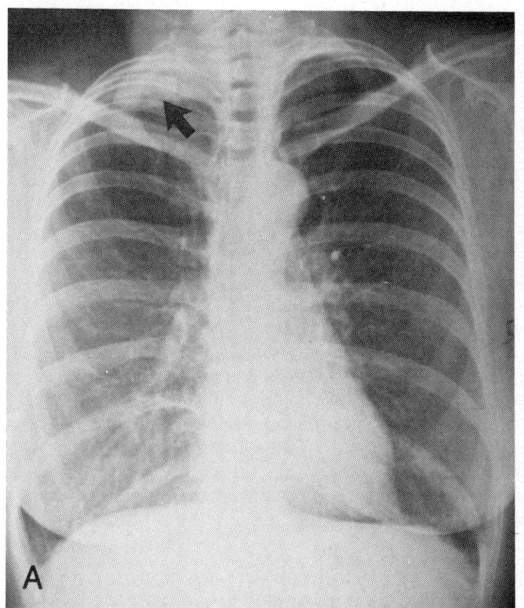

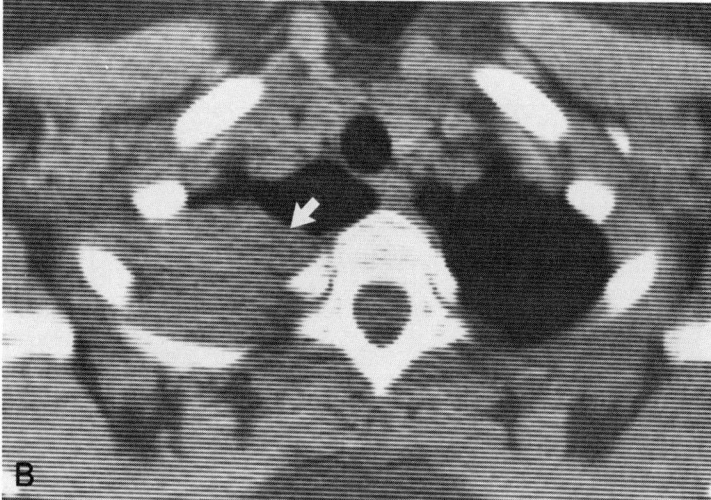

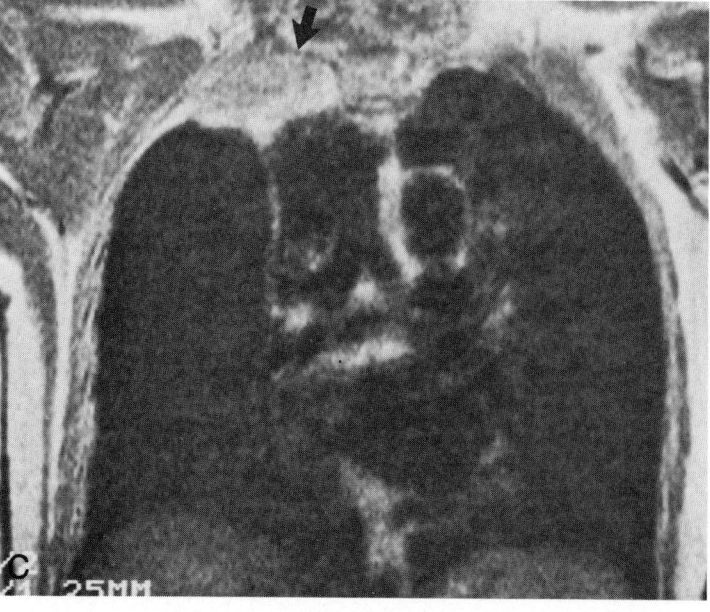

Figure IX-4-1. Superior sulcus lung cancer in a 46-year-old woman. (A) Posteroanterior chest radiograph reveals a soft-tissue density at the right lung apex (arrow). The ribs are intact. (B) CT scan shows lung mass at the right apex (arrow). (C) MRI coronal image (T1-weighted spin-echo image obtained with a TE of 28 msec, and TR gated to heart rate) clearly demonstrates the cephalad extent of tumor (arrow).

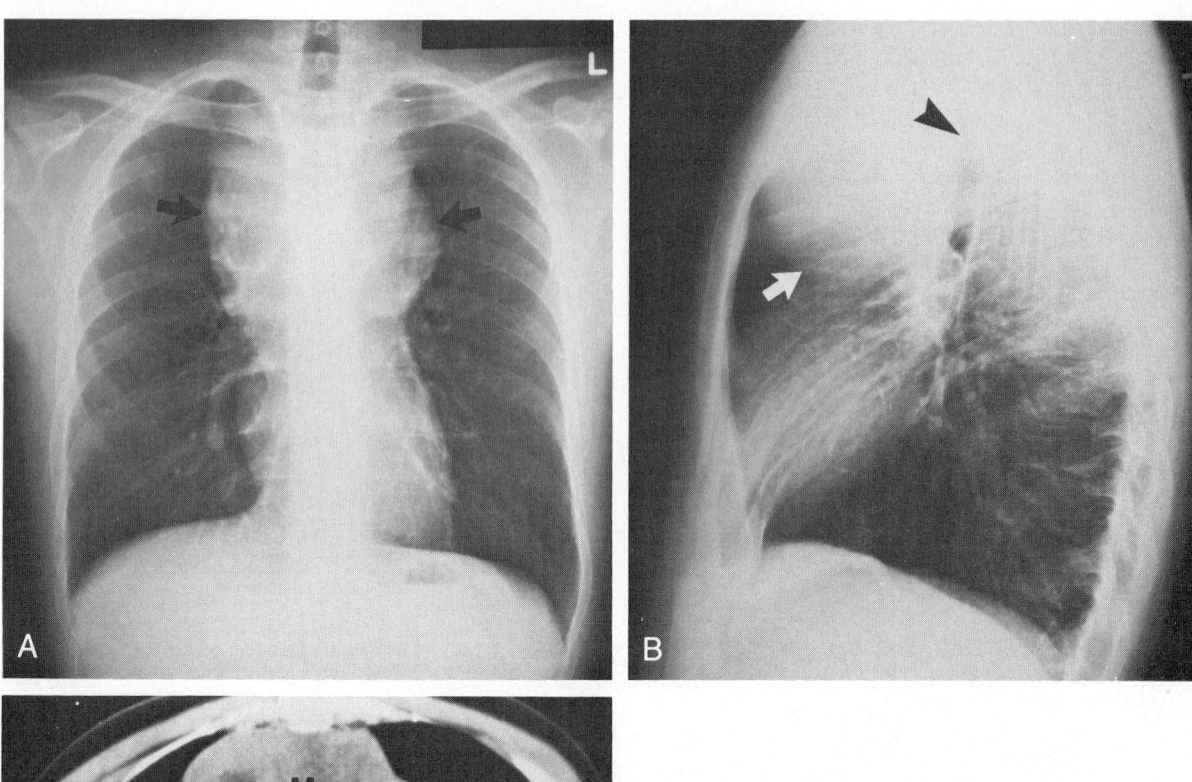

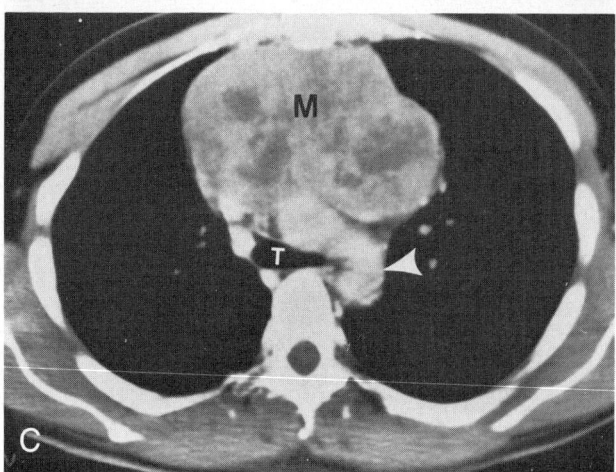

Figure IX-4-2. Non-seminoma germ cell tumor in a 25-year-old man. Posteroanterior (A) and lateral (B) chest radiographs reveal a large, well-defined mass in the anterior mediastinum (arrows). Note marked narrowing of the tracheal air column (arrowhead). CT scan (C) 1 cm above the level of carina shows a large anterior mediastinal mass (M) containing low density regions of fat or necrosis. The mass has displaced the aortic arch (arrowhead) posteriorly, which in turn has compressed the anterolateral aspect of the trachea (T).

Both CT and MRI can be used to make this distinction; however, it may be somewhat easier with MRI, particularly in those patients who cannot tolerate intravenous contrast agents during CT.[25] Either or both of these cross-sectional imaging techniques may also be used to diagnose or rule out hilar adenopathy in patients with equivocal enlargement of the hilum on plain chest radiographs.[5] CT is reported to have a sensitivity of 88 to 95% in diagnosing mediastinal adenopathy.[6,19] The specificity is low (50%), however, because some enlarged nodes may be tumor-free. Patients with enlarged mediastinal nodes that are demonstrated by CT must have the nodes biopsied. While it was originally hoped that MRI could differentiate benign from malignant nodes on the basis of their signal intensities on T_1 and T_2 weighted images, no significant difference in T_1 or T_2 values has been noted between inflammatory and malignant nodes.[8] MRI and CT have proved to be comparable for detecting abnormal mediastinal lymph nodes. While some normal-sized nodes may harbor microscopic metastases, the predictive value of

a negative CT scan is good. It has been stated that patients who have a completely normal mediastinum on a CT scan can proceed directly to thoracotomy without prior mediastinoscopy.[22] On the other hand, patients who have unequivocal mediastinal adenopathy on plain chest radiographs precluding resection usually do not require CT for staging purposes.[6] Nevertheless CT may be valuable in such cases for biopsy planning or for radiation therapy planning.

Conventional radiographic examinations and CT can detect chest wall invasion when rib destruction is seen. However, in the absence of rib destruction or a definite mass within the chest wall, CT may be inaccurate in assessing chest wall invasion by a peripheral lung cancer.[21] Recently, it has been shown that MR imaging can detect chest wall invasion in some patients with lung cancer when the CT findings are equivocal.[11]

Thoracic CT scanning should include the upper abdomen in patients with lung cancer, given the frequency of metastases to the adrenals, liver, and upper abdominal lymph

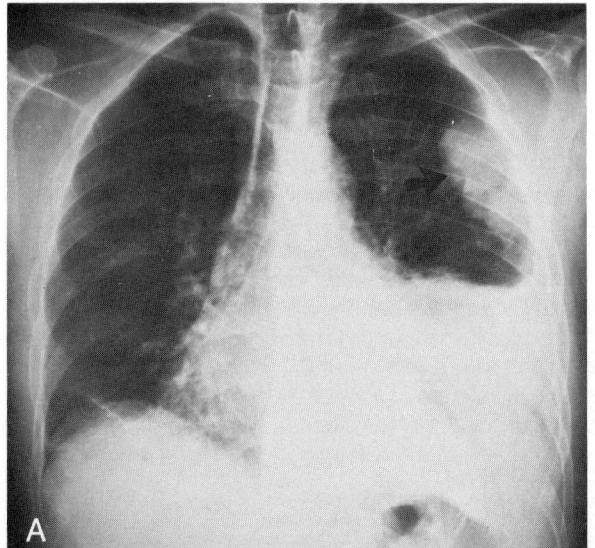

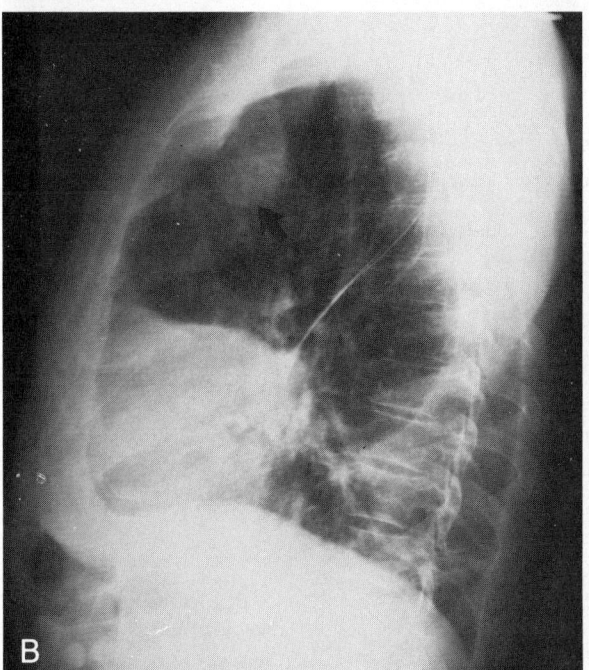

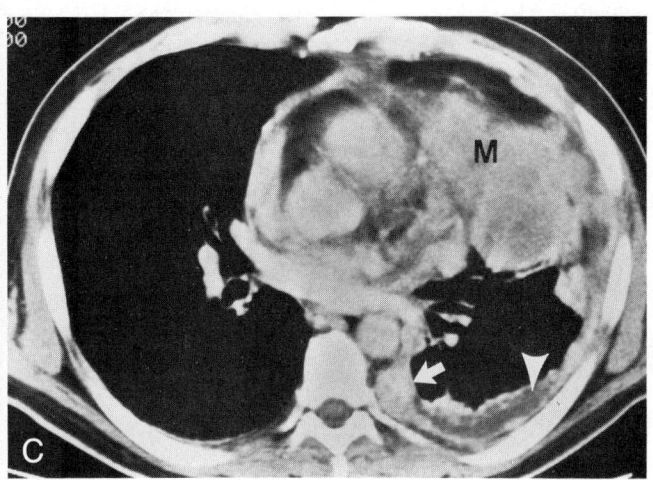

Figure IX-4-3. Malignant mesothelioma in a 55-year-old man. Postero-anterior (A) and lateral (B) chest radiographs show a pleural effusion associated with a lobulated mass in the lateral and anterior portion of the left hemithorax (arrows). CT scan with intravenous contrast (C) reveals enhanced pleural neoplasm (arrow) and nonenhanced pleural effusion (arrowhead). The inhomogenous mass (M) is seen to invade the anterior mediastinal fat. Circumferential involvement of the left hemithorax is well demonstrated.

nodes. A small adrenal nodule in a patient with lung cancer is still more likely to represent an adenoma than a metastasis, however, and needle biopsy is currently required to make an absolute diagnosis.[18] In the future, MR imaging may have a role in helping to distinguish adrenal metastases from incidental adenomas.[9]

Mediastinal Masses

Close to one-half of patients with mediastinal tumors are asymptomatic. Posteroanterior and lateral chest radiographs continue to be the most valuable imaging modality for detecting primary mediastinal tumors. Oblique views or fluoroscopy may assist in evaluating patients with equivocal chest radiographic abnormalities. In most institutions, CT has now replaced conventional tomography as the most useful tech-

nique for evaluating mediastinal abnormalities after they have been identified or suspected on plain chest radiographs, or when clinical findings suggest the possibility of disease in this region.[3] As an example, CT examination is indicated in patients with myasthenia gravis to search for an occult thymoma, even when the chest radiographs are normal. CT can also serve as an important adjunct to plain chest radiographs in planning radiotherapy, and it can direct the best approach for biopsy or resection of a mediastinal mass. The superior contrast of CT allows differentiation of mediastinal tumors from lymph nodes, vessels and airways. When required, intravenous contrast can help to distinguish between vascular and nonvascular abnormalities. CT delineates the morphology of a mass as well as its size, extent, and relationships to adjacent mediastinal structures (Figure IX-4-2). Calcifications, fat or fluid components within the mass can be demonstrated, but a reliable distinction between benign and malignant lesions is not always possible. Demonstration by CT of invasion into adjacent pleura, pericardium or lung with encasement or narrrowing of vessels and bronchi, will indicate the malignant nature of a mass, however.

More recently, MRI has been shown to be equivalent to CT in detecting enlarged mediastinal lymph nodes and masses.[5,14] While MRI is no more specific than CT in differentiating benign from malignant masses for purposes of primary diagnosis, there is evidence to suggest that it may be helpful in distinguishing post-radiation fibrosis from residual or recurrent mediastinal and lung tumor.[7] Invasion or encasement of vessels and cardiovascular structures by tumor may also be demonstrated better on MRI than CT, without the need for contrast injections.

Pleural Cancers

Extensive pleural involvement from a malignant mesothelioma is easily demonstrated on plain chest radiographs. While the distinction between some pleural masses and loculated pleural effusions may be difficult with chest radiographs alone, it can be accomplished easily with a CT examination (Figure IX-4-3). A malignant mesothelioma frequently appears to be more extensive on a CT scan than on plain chest radiographs.[10,16] Invasion of pleural tumor into the mediastinum or chest wall can also be suggested by CT.[23] The CT appearance of malignant mesothelioma is not specific, however, and a similar radiographic appearance may occur in metastatic disease to the pleura.[13] At present, MRI does not play a significant role in evaluating pleural cancers.

Metastatic Disease in the Thorax

While the focus of this section has been on primary malignancies occurring within the chest, a word is in order here on the use of imaging techniques to detect and evaluate thoracic metastases. Bone metastases are covered in Section IX on Radionuclide Imaging. Planar imaging techniques (MRI and/or CT) may be used to clarify abnormalities that have been detected by bone scans and/or by clinical symptoms, or by plain radiographs in the case of mediastinal or hilar enlargement. However, the largest amount of additional information has been made available by CT in detecting small lung metastases and pleural nodules. In some geographic areas, however, benign lung nodules (healed granulomas) are relatively common, and the clinical context of positive CT findings must be taken carefully into account. CT can also be used to guide percutaneous needle biopsies of suspected metastatic lesions.

Conclusion

Conventional PA and lateral chest radiographs continue to be the most useful study for the detection and initial evaluation of cancer in the chest. CT, by virtue of its cross-sectional imaging display which allows thoracic structures to be visualized without superimposition, is now the imaging modality of choice to supplement the chest radiographic findings. MR imaging, because of its inferior spatial resolution, its longer data acquisition times, and its inability to display calcifications, still has a limited role to play in evaluating intrathoracic cancers. Furthermore, MRI is not suitable for critically ill patients who require close monitoring or those with implanted pacemakers. Accordingly, MR imaging is currently used as a "problem solving" modality to clarify complex findings on other studies, by virtue of its direct coronal or sagittal imaging capability. MR imaging can also be used to define mediastinal or hilar masses which may be difficult to distinguish from vessels on CT, to confirm chest wall invasion, to evaluate the causes of adrenal nodules, or to distinguish recurrent tumor from postradiation fibrosis.

References

1. Batra, P., Brown, K., Collins, J. D., Ovenfors, C. O., and Steckel, R. J.: Evaluation of intrathoracic extent of lung cancer by plain chest radiography, computed tomography, and magnetic resonance imaging. Am. Rev. Respir. Dis., 137:1456, 1988.
2. Batra, P., Brown, K., and Steckel, R.: Diagnostic imaging techniques in lung carcinoma. Am. J. Surg., 153:517, 1987.
3. Batra, P., Brown, K., and Steckel, R.: Diagnostic imaging techniques in mediastinal malignancies. Am. J. Surg., 156:4, 1988.
4. Faling, L. J., Pugatch, R. D., Jung-Legg, Y., Daly, B. D., Jr., Hong, W. K., Robbins, A. H., and Snider, G. L.: Computed tomographic scanning of the mediastinum in the staging of bronchogenic carcinoma. Am. Rev. Respir. Dis., 124:690, 1981.
5. Gefter, W. B.: Chest applications of magnetic resonance imaging: an update. Radiol. Clin. North Am., 26:573, 1988.
6. Glazer, G. M., Gross, B. H., Quint, L. E., Francis, I. R., and Orringer, M. B.: Staging of non-small cell lung cancer. In Staging of Neoplasms. Edited by G. M. Glazer. New York, Churchhill Livingstone, 1986, p. 101.
7. Glazer, H. S., Levitt, R. G., Lee, J. K., Emami, B., Gronemeyer, S., and Murphy, W. A.: Differentiation of radiation fibrosis from recurrent pulmonary neoplasm by magnetic resonance imaging. AJR Am. J. Roentgenol., 143:729, 1984.
8. Glazer, G. M., Orringer, M. B., Chenevert, T. L., Borrello, J. A., Penner, M. W., Quint, L. E., Li, K. C., and Aisen, A. M.: Mediastinal lymph nodes: relaxation time/pathologic correlation and implications in staging of lung cancer with MR imaging. Radiology, 168:429, 1988.
9. Glazer, G. M., Woolsey, E. J., Borrello, J., Francis, I. R., Aisen, A. M., Bookstein, F., Amendola, M. A., Gross, M. D., Bree, R. L., and Martel, W.: Adrenal tissue characterization using MR imaging. Radiology, 158:73, 1986.
10. Grant, D. C., Seltzer, S. E., Antman, K. H., Finberg, H. J., and Koster, K.: Computed tomography of malignant pleural mesothelioma. J. Comput. Assist. Tomogr., 7:626, 1983.
11. Haggar, A. M., Pearlberg, J. L., Froelich, J. W., Hearshen, D. O., Beute, G. H., Lewis, J. W., Jr., Schkudor, G. W., Wood, C., and Gniewek, P.: Chest-wall invasion by carcinoma of the lung: detection by MR imaging. AJR Am. J. Roentgenol., 148:1075, 1987.
12. Heavey, L. R., Glazer, G. M., Gross, B. H., Francis, I. R., and Orringer, M. B.: The role of CT in staging radiographic $T_1 N_0 M_0$ lung cancer. AJR Am. J. Roentgenol., 146:285, 1986.
13. Leung, A. N., Muller, N. L., and Miller, R. R.: CT in differential diagnosis of diffuse pleural disease. AJR Am. J. Roentgenol., 154:487, 1990.
14. Levitt, R. G., Glazer, H. S., Roper, C. L., Lee, J. K., and Murphy, W. A.: Magnetic resonance imaging of mediastinal and hilar masses: comparison with CT. AJR Am. J. Roentgenol., 145:9, 1985.
15. Lipshitz, M. I.: Computed tomography in bronchogenic carcinoma. Semin. Roentgenol., 25:64, 1990.
16. Kawashima, A., and Lipshitz, M. I.: Malignant pleural mesothelioma: CT manifestations in 50 cases. A. J. R., 155:965, 1990.
17. Mayr, B., Heywang, S. H., Ingrisch, H., Huber, R. M., Haussinger, K., and Lissner, J.: Comparison of CT with MR imaging of endobronchial tumors. J. Comput. Assist. Tomogr., 11:43, 1987.
18. Oliver, T. W., Bernardino, M. E., Miller, J. I., Mansour, K., Greene, D., and Davis, W. A.: Isolated adrenal masses in nonsmall-cell bronchogenic carcinoma. Radiology, 153:217, 1984.
19. Osborne, D. R., Korobkin, M., Ravin, C. E., Putman, C. E., Wolfe, W. G., Sealy, W. C., Young, W. G., Breiman, R., Heaston, D., Ram, P., and Halber, M.: Comparison of plain radiography, conventional tomography, and computed tomography in detecting intrathoracic lymph node metastases from lung carcinoma. Radiology, 142:157, 1982.
20. Pearlberg, J. L., Sandler, M. A., Beute, G. H., and Madrazo, B. L.: $T_1 N_0 M_0$ bronchogenic carcinoma: assessment by CT. Radiology, 157:187, 1985.
21. Pennes, D. R., Glazer, G. M., Wimbish, K. J., Gross, B. H., Long, R. W., and Orringer, M. B.: Chest wall invasion by lung cancer: limitations of CT evaluation. AJR Am. J. Roentgenol., 144:507, 1985.
22. Rea, H. H., Shevland, J. E., and House, A. J. S.: Accuracy of computed tomographic scanning in assessment of the mediastinum in bronchial carcinoma. J. Thorac. Cardiovas. Surg., 81:825, 1981.
23. Sagel, S. S., and Glazer, H. S.: Lung, pleura, chest wall. In Computed Body Tomography with MRI Correlation. Edited by J. K. T. Lee, S. S. Sagel, and R. J. Stanley. New York, Raven Press, 1989, p. 295.
24. Siegelman, S. S., Khouri, N. F., Leo, F. P., Fishman, E. K., Braverman, R. M., and Zerhouni, E. A.: Solitary pulmonary nodules: CT assessment. Radiology, 160:307, 1986.
25. Webb, W. R., Gamsu, G., Stark, D. D., and Moore, E. H.: Magnetic resonance imaging of the normal and abnormal pulmonary hila. Radiology, 152:89, 1984.

Imaging Neoplasms of the Abdomen and Pelvis

Robert A. Halvorsen, Jr.
William M. Thompson

Introduction

With the introduction of computed tomography (CT) in the late 1970's and with the more recent development of magnetic resonance imaging (MRI), imaging techniques have been able to provide much more accurate delineation of tumors and adjacent structures in the abdomen and pelvis than was possible previously. The relative roles of the newer imaging modalities in comparison to "conventional" techniques such as barium studies or intravenous urograms vary not only with the organ system involved but with the point in the individual patient's management at which the study is performed.

The choice of whether to use CT or MRI to evaluate abdomino-pelvic abnormalities depends upon the organ system being studied and the individual patient's condition. CT has the advantages of lower cost, greater availability, and the ability to evaluate a number of organs with one diagnostic study (see below, and Table IX-5-1). Disadvantages of CT include ionizing radiation and potential allergic reactions to intravenous contrast media. Advantages of MRI include lack of ionizing radiation and its ability to obtain direct sagittal and coronal images, which can be especially helpful in the pelvis. Early studies have suggested that the use of intravenous Gd-DTPA may further increase the accuracy of MRI in the abdomen and pelvis. Disadvantages of MRI include the longer scanning times now required, which limit high quality studies to patients who are capable of remaining immobile for long periods. MRI studies also cover only a limited anatomical area. For example, a thorough MRI study of the liver may require several pulse sequences and will provide images only of the upper abdomen, taking up to one hour to complete. In order to evaluate the entire abdomen and pelvis with MRI, two or three additional scanning periods may be required. Since some patients with claus- trophobia, severe illnesses requiring continuous monitoring, intracerebral surgical clips, other metallic foreign bodies, or cardiac pacemakers are not candidates for MRI studies, CT is likely to remain the primary modality for staging and following cancers of the abdomen and pelvis in the immediate future.

Diagnosis

Visualization of the mucosal surfaces is essential to diagnose early lesions in the hollow organs of the gastrointestinal tract. The conventional upper gastrointestinal series (UGI), small bowel follow-through and barium enema (or endoscopic evaluation of the upper and lower tracts) are superior to either CT or MRI for detecting mucosal lesions (Table IX-5-2). On the other hand, both CT and MRI are superior to barium studies for evaluating the wall and extramural portions of the GI tract for tumor involvement, and both may be helpful also in detecting distant metastases.[1,3,15]

Both CT and MRI have also proved useful for detecting neoplasms of the solid organs in the abdomen and pelvis. For instance, prior to the development of CT, pancreatic cancer was usually diagnosed by indirect means such as an upper gastrointestinal study which demonstrated displacement of the stomach or duodenum. CT makes direct imaging of pancreatic masses possible, as well as CT-guided biopsies of primary and metastatic lesions (Figure IX-5-1). In conjunction with endoscopic retrograde cholangiopancreatography (ERCP), CT is now used in the evaluation of most patients with potential pancreatic neoplasms.

With current third and fourth generation CT scanners, scan times have been reduced to 1 to 2 seconds per CT image, thereby eliminating most motion artifacts. MRI technology is advancing rapidly, as well. The initial enthusiasm for MRI was due not only to the lack of ionizing radiation, but more importantly the potential for improved tissue characterization. When MRI was introduced, it was hoped that differences

Table IX-5-1. Imaging: CT vs MRI

	CT	MRI
Cost	$860.00[a]	$1,180.00[a]
Availability	Generally available	Limited in some areas
Detectability of tumor	Good	Superior
Spatial resolution	Excellent	Excellent (if pt cooperative)
Scan planes	axial only	Multiple planes
Ionizing radiation	Yes	No
IV contrast required	Yes	No (may change)
Body areas covered	Large	Smaller

[a]Cost at University of Minnesota; 1990

Table IX-5-2. Imaging Techniques for Diagnosis

	Barium	IVU	US	CT	MRI
GI Tract	+ +	− −	− −	− −	− −
Liver	− −	− −	+	+ +	+ +
Pancreas	− −	− −	+	+ +	− −
Kidneys		+	+	+ +	− −
Uterus/Ovaries	− −	− −	+ +	+	+ +
Prostate	− −	+	+ +	− −	− −

+ +, Superior; +, Helpful; −, Not useful; Barium, Intraluminal Contrast; IVU, Intravenous Urography; US, Ultrasonography; CT, Computed Tomography; MRI, Magnetic Resonance Imaging.

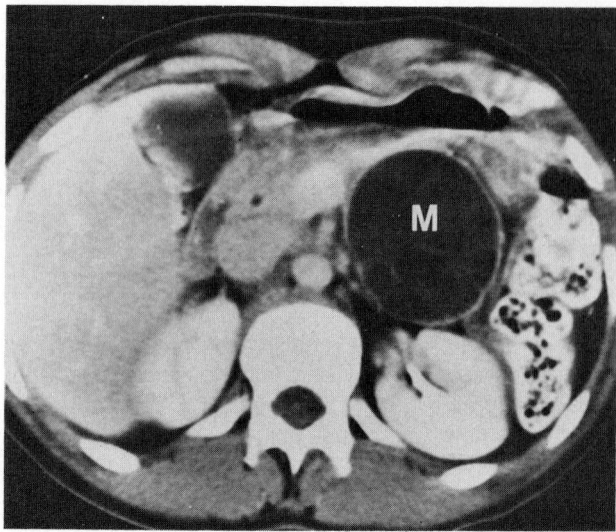

Figure IX-5-1. Cystic pancreatic mass. Contrast enhanced CT of upper abdomen demonstrates large cystic mass (M) in tail of pancreas anterior to left kidney and posterior to stomach. Operative specimen diagnosed as pancreatic cystadenoma.

in the signal intensities of abnormal tissues would enable differentiation of benign from malignant masses. Unfortunately, tissue characterization has not proved to be reliable, and in the abdomen and pelvis the only tumor that has a relatively "pathognomonic" appearance is adrenal pheochromocytoma. All other tumors overlap in signal characteristics with other types of neoplasms and inflammatory processes.

The standard pulse sequence used in MRI has been spin echo.[16] T1-weighted spin echo images have a higher spatial resolution than T2-weighted images and are therefore more helpful in providing anatomical information. T2-weighted images show the contrast differences more clearly between normal and abnormal tissues. In general, pathologic lesions will appear as relatively dark (low signal) areas on T1 and as bright (high signal) areas on T2-weighted images.

Unfortunately, many different pathologic processes, and not just tumors, may produce these "dark-bright" appearances.[9,17] For instance, edema adjacent to a tumor as well as the tumor itself may have similar appearances under some circumstances. A simple cyst may also be "dark-bright" on T_1 and T_2 images, as will abscesses and some benign tumors. Therefore, while MRI may be quite sensitive for detecting an abnormality, absolute characterization of the abnormality is usually not possible.

Recently, new pulse sequences have been developed that allow MRI imaging data to be acquired in 20 seconds or less, during one breath-hold. This eliminates respiratory motion artifacts.[4] The new rapid acquisition techniques currently do not match the contrast sensitivity of standard spin echo techniques in the abdomen and pelvis. Therefore, they are useful as problem solving tools but have not yet replaced standard MRI techniques for tumor detection and staging.

Intravenous contrast is used routinely with CT. Initially, no contrast injection was thought to be necessary with MRI, but gadolinium-DTPA (Gd-DTPA) has been approved recently

by the FDA for use with MRI in the central nervous system as an intravenous contrast agent (see IX-3). While still investigational, the use of Gd-DTPA during abdominal and pelvic MRI appears promising. Like conventional iodinated contrast agents, MRI contrast media diffuse rapidly from the blood into the interstitial space. Therefore, MRI scanning with Gd-DTPA should be performed during, and not following, the intravenous administration of this agent. Standard spin echo techniques will probably not be optimal, and fast scanning techniques may eventually be required to maximize the effectiveness of intravascular contrast materials with MRI. The combination of fast MRI scanning and intravenous contrast has great promise and may eventually replace CT with contrast as the standard imaging technique for solid organs in the abdomen and pelvis, but the technique still remains investigational.

Staging

After a malignant lesion has been diagnosed in the abdomen or pelvis, imaging techniques can be helpful for tumor staging (Table IX-5-3). With certain limitations, the cross-sectional imaging abilities of both CT and MRI are helpful in detecting extramural spread of tumor from the GI tract.[14] For instance, either CT or MRI can detect abnormal tissue infiltrating the fat that surrounds the rectum, but neither may be able to differentiate inflammatory strands from neoplastic invasion. Another limitation of both CT and MRI is their inability to detect tumor in normal-sized lymph nodes. CT can be helpful with cancers such as seminoma and lymphoma that may produce considerable lymph node enlargement, as opposed to GI tract carcinomas which often replace regional lymph nodes rather than enlarge them. Neither CT nor MRI can determine the depth of invasion of a mucosal or submucosal tumor within the wall of the GI tract. Therefore, the major role of CT and MRI in staging abdominopelvic malignancies is the detection of distant metastases.

Post-Treatment Surveillance

CT is now the standard imaging technique in most institutions for following patients with cancers of the abdomen and pelvis. It is also used routinely for detecting liver metastases. While MRI now approaches or equals CT in depicting liver metastases, it is relatively limited in its sensitivity for detecting extrahepatic metastatic disease in the abdomen. Therefore, a CT examination of the upper abdomen can potentially detect more metastatic lesions than an MRI study. The higher cost and limited availability of MRI have also

Table IX-5-3. Imaging Techniques for Staging/Follow-up

	Barium	IVU	US	CT	MRI
GI Tract	+	− −	+	+ +	+ +
Liver	− −	− −	+	+ +	+ +
Pancreas	− −	− −	− −	+ +	+
Kidneys	− −	− −	+	+ +	+ +
Uterus/Ovaries	− −	− −	+ +	+	+ +
Prostate	− −	− −	+ +	+	+

+ +, Superior; +, Helpful; −, Not useful; Barium, Intraluminal Contrast; IVU, Intravenous Urography; US, Ultrasonography; CT, Computed Tomography; MRI, Magnetic Resonance Imaging.

permitted CT to maintain its role as the primary abdominal imaging modality for post-treatment surveillance of cancer patients.

Gastrointestinal Tract: Hollow Organs

While evaluation of the mucosal surfaces with barium studies and endoscopy still plays a primary role in diagnosing cancers of the stomach, small bowel and colon, staging and followup of these tumors are generally done now with the assistance of CT scanning.[13,15] CT is somewhat limited in its ability to detect mesenteric pathology because of the difficulty in differentiating unopacified loops of bowel from tumor masses, but it may be useful for detecting metastases to solid organs and retroperitoneal lymph nodes (see above). MRI has achieved only limited use in the upper abdomen until now because of the lack of a suitable oral contrast medium, as well as the prolonged imaging times required. As described in IX-9, endoscopic ultrasound techniques, especially transrectal sonography, represent an evolving technology which has promise for evaluating wall invasion by tumors in the GI tract.[2,12] Endoscopic sonography is limited by its inability to depict lesions more than 5 cm from the GI lumen, however, and by problems of access to the ultrasound probe. Tumors that prevent passage of the probe because of obstruction or severe narrowing cannot be evaluated adequately by endosonography. The role of nuclear medicine in the diagnosis, staging and followup of GI tract cancers has declined with the introduction of newer imaging modalities. CT, MRI and ultrasound are all more sensitive and reliable techniques for demonstrating liver metastases than is radionuclide scanning.

Liver Metastases

The diagnosis, staging and followup of primary and metastatic liver lesions can now be attained with multiple imaging modalities. CT is the most widely used technique in the United States for ascertaining liver involvement by cancer. In Europe, many institutions use hepatic ultrasound first, and then employ CT or MRI only in problem cases. MRI has the potential for replacing CT and ultrasound as the primary diagnostic tool for liver pathology, but CT and MRI of the liver currently should be considered as complementary procedures (Figure IX-5-2).[4] Neither study is perfect, and not infrequently lesions that are missed by CT will be detected by MRI, or vice versa. Therefore, in patients in whom it is important to detect all metastatic lesions within the liver, both CT and MRI may be indicated.

Currently, the most widely-used technique for CT examination of the liver is dynamic bolus-enhanced CT (DBCT), which requires a continuous slow infusion of intravenous contrast media during the examination. Unenhanced CT is less sensitive than DBCT for liver lesions. CT scans obtained following, rather than during the administration of intravenous contrast are even less sensitive, since the contrast material may diffuse into a liver tumor and make it indistinguishable from the normal liver. Not only can DBCT detect more lesions than other CT techniques, but it can also help to characterize some masses. Cavernous hemangioma, the most frequent benign hepatic mass, may appear on DBCT as a liver mass with well-defined margins. It will demonstrate rim-enhance-

ment during the infusion of intravenous contrast material and then show progressive enhancement from the periphery to the center of the mass following completion of the contrast infusion. When the CT findings are suggestive but not characteristic of a hemangioma, MRI can also be useful. The characteristic MRI appearance of a liver hemangioma is that of a well-defined, low-signal-intensity mass on T1-weighted images and a "light-bulb" or high signal intensity mass on T2-weighted pulse sequences.[4,9,17] Unfortunately, this MRI appearance can sometimes be encountered also with necrotic neoplasms or with metastases from hypervascular primary tumors such as islet cell carcinomas.

A radionuclide scan procedure performed with technetium-99m labelled red blood cells (Tc-RBC) can also be used to make a specific diagnosis of hemangioma of the liver. The diagnosis is made when there is diminished radionuclide activity in a liver lesion during the early (vascular) phase of a labelled red cell infusion, and increased activity (a hot spot) on delayed or blood-pool scan images. While this "flip-flop" in the appearance of a liver mass on such a scan is diagnostic of a hemangioma, the Tc-RBC study is limited in its ability to detect hemangiomas that are less than two centimeters in diameter.

CT and sonography both play important roles in evaluating the jaundiced cancer patient. Sonographic studies are quite accurate in diagnosing bile duct dilatation and in helping to determine whether "medical" or "surgical" jaundice is present. CT can then be used to confirm the presence of ductal dilatation, and it is usually superior to sonography in determining the cause of obstruction. This is because of CT's ability to image the extrahepatic biliary tree and to diagnose the actual obstructing lesion such as a pancreatic mass.

Both CT and ultrasound can also be helpful in guiding fine-needle biopsies of liver lesions. While sonographically-guided biopsies require more technical expertise than biopsies monitored with CT, the ability to image the needle tip with sonography while advancing the needle into a lesion is a definite advantage over CT. The performance of a CT-guided biopsy can be considered as partially "blind," since the needle tip cannot be visualized while it is being advanced inside the liver. Sonographic biopsies are also less expensive than CT-directed ones in many institutions.

Pancreas

CT has also become the primary imaging modality to evaluate suspected pancreatic pathology. Pancreatic CT using a bolus of intravenous contrast material and thin collimation can detect a majority of pancreatic adenocarcinomas and islet cell tumors, and CT-guided biopsies can confirm the diagnosis (see Figure IX-5-1). Ultrasound has been used to evaluate the pancreas, but in general its application is limited by interposed bowel gas which makes evaluation of the entire pancreas difficult in most patients. MRI is still limited in evaluating the pancreas, because of the difficulty in differentiating pancreatic tissue from adjacent bowel. Once adequate oral contrast agents become available for use with MRI, the role of MRI in pancreatic imaging will increase. Angiography of the pancreas has declined in popularity following the advent of CT, but it still can be helpful as a complementary problem-solving tool in certain circumstances.

who subsequently underwent radical prostatectomy, CT staging had an accuracy of 65%; with MRI staging, accuracy increased to 83%.[6]

Conclusion

Conventional imaging techniques, including barium studies and intravenous urography, remain the primary diagnostic tools of the radiologist for evaluating the luminal portions of the GI and GU tracts. Diagnosis of tumors of the solid organs usually requires a cross-sectional imaging method such as CT, MRI or occasionally sonography, often followed by guided biopsy. CT and, potentially, MRI have replaced conventional radiologic imaging studies for staging and following abdominopelvic malignancies.

References

1. Butch, R. J., Stark, D. D., Wittenberg, J., Tepper, J. E., Saini, S., Simeone, J. F., Mueller, P. R., and Ferrucci, J. T., Jr.: Staging rectal cancer by MR and CT. AJR Am. J. Roentgenol., 146:1155, 1986.
2. Carroll, B. A.: US of the gastrointestinal tract. Radiology, 172:605, 1989.
3. De Lange, E. E., Fechner, R. E., and Wanebo, H. J.: Suspected recurrent rectosigmoid carcinoma after abdominoperineal resection: MR imaging and histopathologic findings. Radiology, 170:323, 1989.
4. Glazer, G. M.: MR imaging of the liver, kidneys, and adrenal glands. Radiology, 166:303, 1988.
5. Hricak, H., Demas, B. E., Williams, R. D., McNamara, M. T., Hedgcock, M. W., Amparo, E. G., and Tanagho, E. A.: Magnetic resonance imaging in the diagnosis and staging of renal and perirenal neoplasms. Radiology, 154:709, 1985.
6. Hricak, H., Dooms, G. C., Jeffrey, R. B., Avallone, A., Jacobs, D., Benton, W. K., Narayan, P., and Tanagho, E. A.: Prostatic carcinoma: staging by clinical assessment, CT, and MR imaging. Radiology, 162:331, 1987.
7. Hricak, H., Stern, J. L., Fisher, M. R., Shapeero, L. G., Winkler, M. L., and Lacey, C. G.: Endometrial carcinoma staging by MR imaging. Radiology, 162:297, 1987.
8. Johnson, C. D., Dunnick, N. R., Cohan, R. H., and Illescas, F. F.: Renal adenocarcinoma: CT staging of 100 tumors. AJR Am. J. Roentgenol., 148:59, 1987.
9. Li, K. C., Glazer, G. M., Quint, L. E., Francis, I. R., Aisen, A. M., Ensminger, W. D., and Bookstein, F. L.: Distinction of hepatic cavernous hamangioma from hepatic metastases with MR imaging. Radiology, 169:409, 1988.
10. Mitchell, D. G., Mintz, M. C., Spritzer, C. E., Gussman, D., Arger, P. H., Coleman, B. G., Axel, L., and Kressel, H. Y.: Adnexal masses: MR imaging observations at 1.5 T, with US and CT correlation. Radiology, 162:319, 1987.
11. Quint, L. E., Glazer, G. M., Chenevert, T. L., Fechner, K. P., Gikas, P. W., Shireman, P. K., Grossman, H. B., and Li, K. C.: In vivo and in vitro MR imaging of renal tumors: histopathologic correlation and pulse sequence optimization. Radiology, 169:359, 1988.
12. Rifkin, M. D., Ehrlich, S. M., and Marks, G.: Staging of rectal carcinoma: prospective comparison of endorectal US and CT. Radiology, 170:319, 1989.
13. Sussman, S. K., Halvorsen, R. A., Jr., Illescas, F. F., Cohan, R. H., Saeed, M., Liverman, P. M., Thompson, W. M., and Meyers, W. C.: Gastric adenocarcinoma: CT versus surgical staging. Radiology, 167:335, 1988.
14. Thompson, W. M., and Halvorsen, R. A., Jr.: Computed tomographic staging of gastrointestinal malignancies. Part II. The small bowel, colon and rectum. Invest. Radiol., 22:96, 1987.
15. Thompson, W. M., Halvorsen, R. A., Foster, W. L., Jr., Roberts, L., and Gibbons, R.: Preoperative and postoperative CT staging of rectosigmoid carcinoma. AJR Am. J. Roentgenol., 146:703, 1986.
16. Turnbull, L. W., and Kean, D. M.: Tumour identification using magnetic resonance imaging. Cancer Surv., 6:343, 1987.
17. Wittenberg, J., Stark, D. D., Forman, B. H., Hahn, P. F., Saini, S., Weissleder, R., Rummeny, E., and Ferrucci, J. T.: Differentiation of hepatic metastases from hepatic hamangiomas and cysts by using MR imaging. AJR Am. J. Roentgenol., 151:79, 1988.

IX-6

Imaging Musculoskeletal Neoplasms

Leanne L. Seeger

Since the advent of cross-sectional scanning techniques, the evaluation of the patient with a primary musculoskeletal cancer has changed dramatically. The choice of which imaging modality is best suited to a particular problem can be complex and will depend on several factors.

A diagnosis of a musculoskeletal tumor can often be suspected clinically and may be supported by the findings on plain radiographs. Radionuclide scans may be used to screen for additional lesions within or invading bone, and the tissue diagnosis is confirmed by biopsy. In this situation, the role of magnetic resonance imaging (MRI) and computerized tomography (CT) scanning is not to obtain a diagnosis, but rather to supply additional information about the location and extent of the tumor.[6]

If one is attempting initially to determine the presence or absence of a lesion (e.g., bone pain, with negative or equivocal radiographic findings), MR imaging is now generally considered to be the modality of choice. Because of its inherent high contrast between normal and abnormal marrow and soft tissues, MRI provides a highly sensitive means to document or exclude pathology. However, the findings on MR images are often nonspecific, and malignant and benign tumors, infection and trauma may have similar appearances.[5]

When a lesion is known to exist and additional information is needed for a differential diagnosis, CT is usually the favored imaging modality. This reflects not only the nonspecificity of MRI abnormalities, but also the fact that MRI may be relatively insensitive to tumor mineralization and to the presence of subtle cortical defects (see below).

When obtaining cross-sectional images in patients with a known primary neoplasm in the extremities, the information of greatest interest includes a determination of the extent of the tumor in the marrow and soft-tissues, a definition of the tumor's relationship to major neural and vascular structures, and evaluation of adjacent joints for intra-articular and/or synovial infiltration. If amputation or limb salvage is anticipated, MRI and CT can also be used to provide accurate measurements of tumor size and distance to adjacent joints. These measurements may be used to manufacture endoprostheses and/or for surgical planning. For primary pelvic tumors involving the ilium or sacrum, preoperative imaging must be capable of identifying infiltration into pelvic soft tissues or the epidural space, and defining the relationships of tumor to sacral and sciatic nerves, major vessels, and the hip and sacroiliac joints.

Either MRI or CT can answer many of these questions during the preoperative evaluation, and one of the two studies will usually suffice (Figure IX-6-1). However, there are some advantages to each modality, and the study that is chosen will depend largely on the experience of the referring physician and the radiologist. Several studies have compared MRI and CT for the evaluation of primary bone tumors.[1-4,7] Since these studies address many different facets in tumor evaluation, it is difficult to determine from the reports if one modality is superior overall. There is, however, fairly uniform agreement that MRI is superior to CT for delineating the margins of a tumor with respect to adjacent normal muscle, and that CT is superior in evaluating subtle cortical invasion. Under most circumstances, MRI and CT are comparable in their abilities to determine the extent of intramedullary tumor involvement to a level of accuracy that is clinically important. This is especially true if CT scans are acquired with the help of intravenous contrast, and if thin section images are obtained through the tumor margins.

Using conventional spin echo techniques for MR imaging, a determination of tumor extent and the relationships to major neurovascular structures and to adjacent joints is done by comparing T1- and T2-weighted images. With CT scanning, optimal visualization of the extraosseous (soft tissues) and intramedullary extent of a tumor usually requires the administration of intravenous contrast media. In the case of pelvic

tumors, when preliminary radiographs reveal little or no calcified tumor matrix in the soft tissues, ingested contrast material to opacify pelvic bowel loops may also be helpful for determining the presence or absence of intra-pelvic soft-tissue invasion. If an extra-osseous pelvic tumor mass is highly mineralized, however, it may be difficult to differentiate osteoblastic tumor from contrast-filled loops of bowel on a CT scan. All CT images should be evaluated with bone as well as soft-tissue window settings. Bone windows will best display calcified tumor matrix and cortical involvement. Soft-tissue window settings are needed to evaluate the marrow space for tumor invasion (which appears as loss of normal low-density fat in the marrow cavity), the soft tissue extent of the tumor, and the relationships of the tumor to major neurovascular structures (with the assistance of IV contrast material).

Either MRI or CT may be used for the postoperative evaluation of patients who have undergone amputation, hemipelvectomy, or local tumor excision. Cross-sectional studies may be useful for identifying recurrent tumor in patients who have undergone limb salvage with a custom endoprosthesis (Figure IX-6-2), especially if the region of concern lies proximal or distal to the endoprosthesis. With both MRI and CT, metal-induced artifacts may sometimes be a problem. The

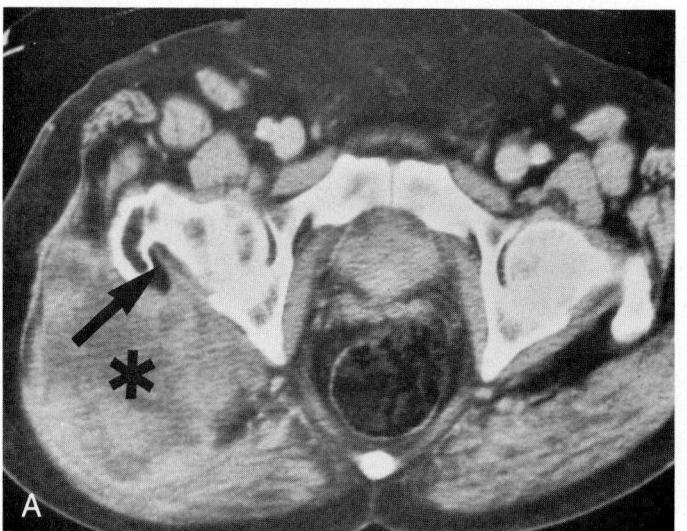

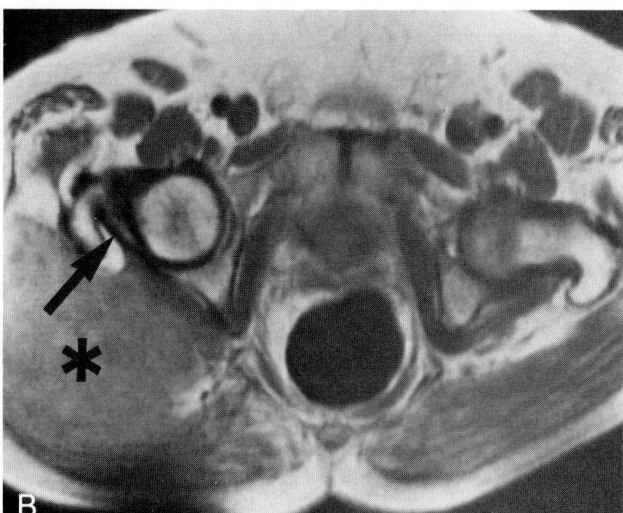

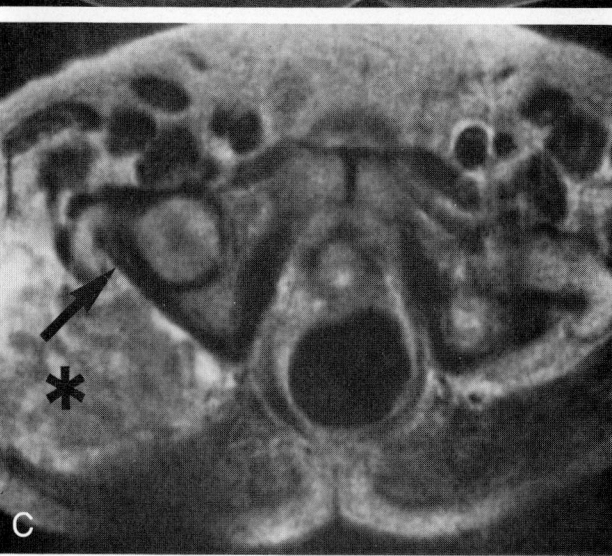

Figure IX-6-1. MRI vs. CT: 69-year-old male with liposarcoma of the right buttock (*). Both imaging modalities clearly show tumor extent. Tumor extends to the hip joint posteriorly, but the capsule is not invaded (arrow). (A) Contrast-enhanced CT scan, soft tissue window. (B) Axial T1-weighted MR scan (SE 22/700). (C) Axial T2-weighted MR scan (SE 85/2000).

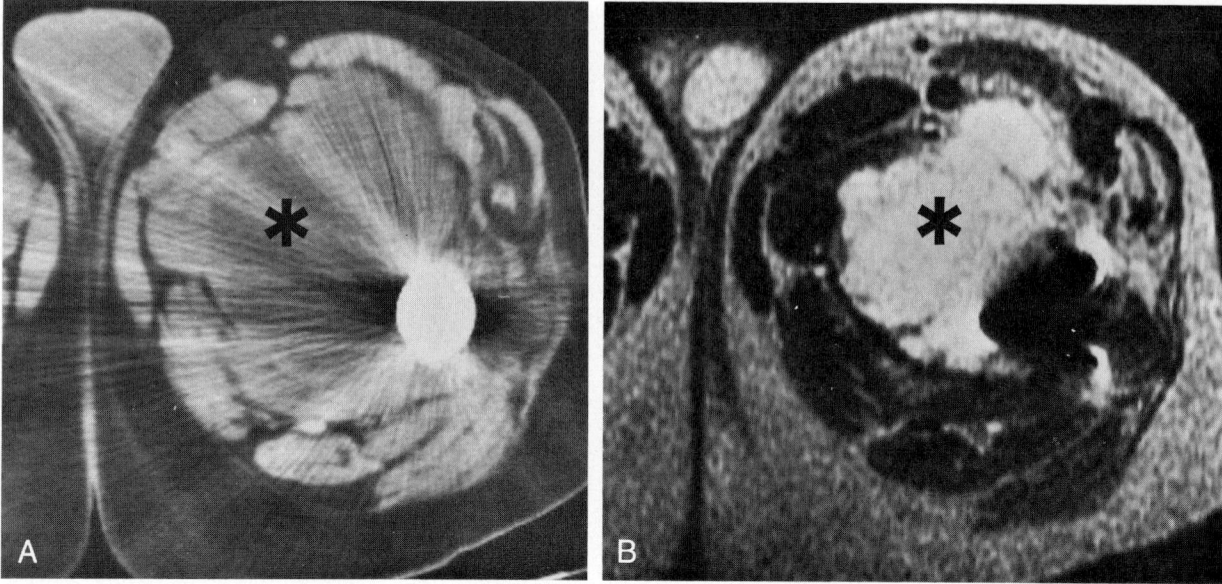

Figure IX-6-2.   MRI vs. CT: 71-year-old male with recurrent chondrosarcoma (*) following proximal femoral limb salvage with custom endoprosthesis (titanium alloy). (A) Contrast-enhanced CT scan (soft tissue window). Despite significant artifact, recurrent tumor is readily evident. (B) Axial T2-weighted MR scan (SE 85/2000) obtained on a 0.3 Tesla MR system. Titanium causes minimal artifact with low- to mid-field strength magnets. The recurrent tumor is evident as a high signal intensity mass surrounding the prosthesis.

severity of an artifact will, in part, be determined by the type of metal used for endoprosthesis manufacture (e.g., ferrous metals degrade MR images). For MRI, the field strength of the imaging system is also important, with low-field magnets inducing the least amount of artifact.

In the case of limb salvage, methylmethacrylate bone cement is frequently used to anchor the endoprosthesis. The cement will appear as a well-defined band of high density on CT images and as a signal void on MR images, and it should not be mistaken for residual or recurrent osteoblastic tumor. Confusion can be avoided by correlating the MR or CT images with radiographs.

References

1. Aisen, A. M., Martel, W., Braunstein, E. M., McMillan, K. I., Phillips, W. A., and Kling, T. F.: MRI and CT evaluation of primary bone and soft-tissue tumors. AJR Am. J. Roentgenol., 146:749, 1986.
2. Bloem, J. L., Taminiau, A. H. M., Eulderink, F., Hermans, J., and Pauwels, E. K.: Radiologic staging of primary bone sarcoma: MR imaging, scintigraphy, angiography, and CT correlated with pathologic examination. Radiology, 169:805, 1988.
3. Gillespy, III, T., Manfrini, M., Ruggieri, P., Spanier, S. S., Pettersson, H., and Springfield, D. S.: Staging of intraosseous extent of osteosarcoma: Correlation of preoperative CT and MR imaging with pathologic macroslides. Radiology, 167:765, 1988.
4. Pettersson, H., Gillespy, T., III, Hamlin, D. J., Enneking, W. F., Springfield, D. S., Andrew, E. R., Spanier, S., and Slone, R.: Primary musculoskeletal tumors: Examination with MR imaging compared with conventional modalities. Radiology, 164:237, 1987.
5. Seeger, L. L., Dungan, D. H., Eckardt, J. J., et al.: Nonspecific findings on MRI: The importance of correlative studies and clinical information. Clin. Orthop. Rel. Res., In press.
6. Seeger, L. L., Eckardt, J. J., and Bassett, L. W.: Cross-sectional imaging in the evaluation of osteogenic sarcoma: MRI and CT. Sem. Roentgenol., 24:174, 1989.
7. Zimmer, W. D., Berquist, T. H., McLeod, R. A., Sim, F. H., Pritchard, D. J., Shives, T. C., Wold, L. E., and May, G. R.: Bone tumors: Magnetic resonance imaging versus computed tomography. Radiology, 155:709, 1985.

Imaging the Breast

Lawrence W. Bassett

Introduction

An estimated 181,000 new cases of breast cancer will occur in the United States in 1992, and 46,300 women will die of the disease.[28] The greatest risk is for women over the age of 40 years, and the incidence increases with age. While some women are known to be at higher risk, 75 percent of women who develop breast cancer have no known risk factors other than age.[23] The best hope for improved survival is early detection, and the most successful method of breast cancer screening is mammography.[24,32]

Indications for Mammography

There are two types of mammography, (1) consultative or diagnostic mammography and (2) screening mammography. Consultative mammography, also called diagnostic or problem-solving mammography, is indicated whenever there are suspicious clinical findings. It should be performed even when a biopsy is being planned. The consultative mammographic examination involves a complete work-up which is tailored to the symptomatic patient. It often includes additional views of the abnormal breast using spot compression and magnification devices, and the correlation of mammographic findings with physical examination and breast sonography. The purpose of mammography prior to a possible biopsy is to help identify the nature of a mass and to find occult cancers, including multifocal carcinomas.

Screening mammography is performed on asymptomatic women to detect clinically occult breast cancer. On June 27, 1989, the American Cancer Society and ten other national research and medical associations put forward consensus screening guidelines recommending: (1) annual clinical breast examinations by a health professional for women 40 and older; (2) mammograms every 1–2 years for women age 40–49; and (3) mammograms annually for women 50 years and older.[9] In women at higher risk because of a history of breast cancer in a mother or sister occurring at a young age, screening mammography might be instituted earlier (several years before the age of clinical detection in the first degree relative may be a reasonable guideline).

Performing the Examinations

Today, breast radiography should only be performed with special film-screen mammography or xeromammography equipment. Clinical investigations have failed to reveal a significant difference in diagnostic accuracy between these two methods.[21,30] In the 1980s, a trend towards using low dose film-screen mammography began and continues up to today. As a result, in February 1989 the Xerox company announced that it would discontinue the production of xeromammography equipment.

Film-screen mammography employs three primary views: oblique, lateral and craniocaudal. The oblique is the most effective single view (Figure IX-7-1), because it depicts well the upper-outer quadrant and axillary tail, the most common locations for carcinomas.[4] Screening mammography should include two views–oblique and craniocaudal. In the past, some investigators have argued for screening with a single view to reduce radiation exposure, cost and examination time.[17] However, others have found that the rate of cancer detection is too low with single view screening, with up to 11 percent of lesions being missed.[19,27] With single view screening, greater numbers of patients also need to be called back for additional views; therefore, two view screening examinations may actually be more cost-effective.[3,27]

Film-screen mammography must be performed with special equipment dedicated to breast radiography. Dedicated units have an x-ray target suitable for soft-tissue imaging and a breast compression device. Adequate breast compression is essential for high-quality mammograms.[18] Exag-

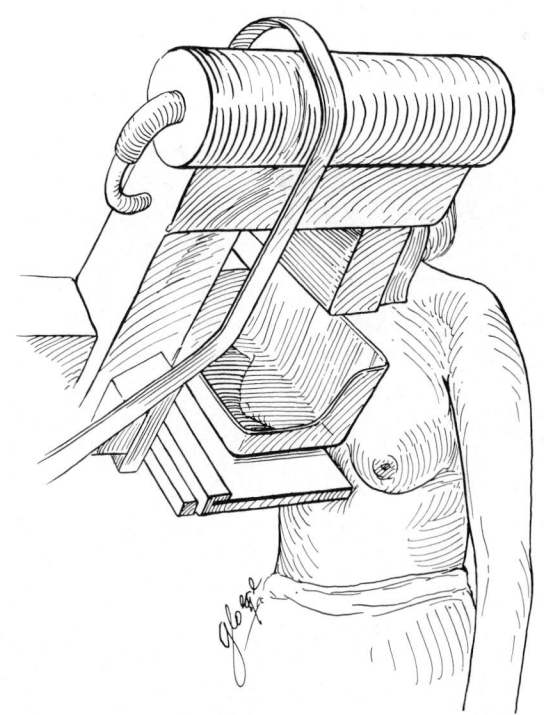

Figure IX-7-1. Positioning of the breast for the oblique projection. The film is placed under the breast, parallel to the pectoral muscle inferior border. The x-ray beam is directed from superomedial to inferolateral, perpendicular to the pectoral muscle border, which should be included in the upper half of the image. This view provides the most complete visualization of the upper-outer quadrant, including the axillary tail of breast tissue.

gerated positioning to optimize visualization of one portion of the breast, magnification, and spot compression restricted to a specific area of interest are used to better define or to verify a lesion once it is identified.

The Normal Mammogram

The breasts of younger women are often relatively radiopaque, because they are composed primarily of dense fibroglandular tissue. This significantly limits the accuracy of mammography. With increasing age and after childbearing, much of the dense glandular tissue is replaced by radiolucent fat, providing a background in which small cancers can be detected more readily (Figures IX-7-2 and IX-7-3). The breast tissue should be bilaterally symmetrical, and mammograms should be viewed so that the right and left breasts can be compared.

Features of Malignant and Benign Lesions

Mammographic features of malignancy can be divided into primary, secondary and indirect signs. Primary signs include a mass and/or microcalcifications (Figure IX-7-4). Secondary signs, such as skin thickening and retraction, are often obvious from clinical examinations. Subtle or indirect signs, which include distortion of the internal breast architecture and the appearance of a neodensity in the breast, have been reported to be the only findings in up to 20 percent of mammographically detected cancers.[25] To recognize these relatively subtle signs, it may be necessary to have previous mammograms for comparison. Furthermore, biopsies can often be avoided when findings have not changed from previous mammograms. Some commonly encountered mammographic findings are defined briefly here:

Malignant Masses. An irregular or spiculated margin is

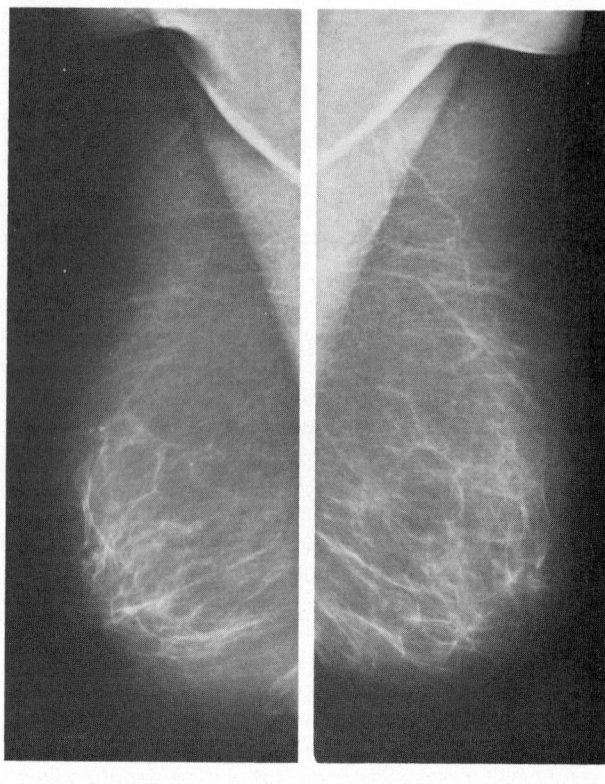

Figure IX-7-3.   Bilateral oblique views of a 65-year-old woman. Almost all of the parenchymal tissue has been replaced by radiolucent fat. Even the smallest tumor could be seen within this breast pattern.

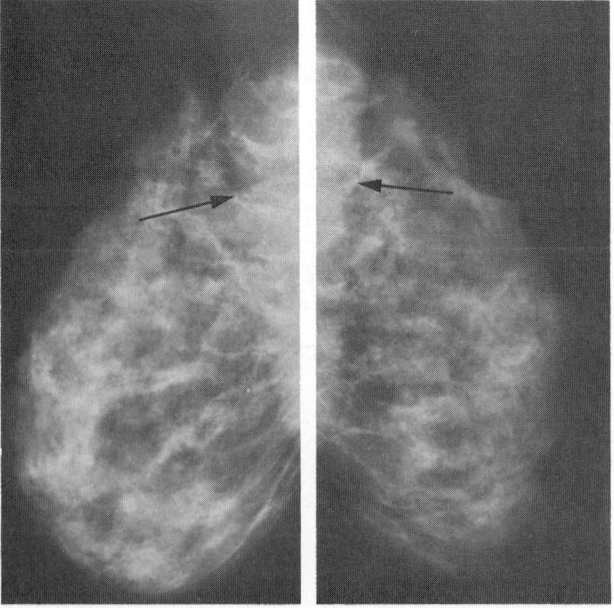

Figure IX-7-2.   Bilateral oblique views of a 45-year-old woman. The breasts are a mixture of radiodense (white) parenchymal tissue and radiolucent fat. The pectoral muscle (arrow) is seen at the posterior aspect of the breast. A small carcinoma could easily be obscured within one of the areas of dense parenchymal tissue.

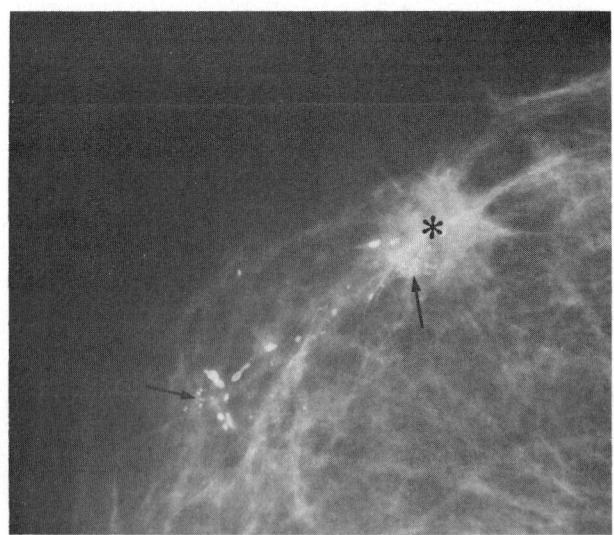

Figure IX-7-4.   Ductal carcinoma manifested by a spiculated mass (*) and clusters of fine malignant calcifications (arrows).

the most important feature indicating that a mass is malignant. The more highly infiltrative the lesion, the more spiculated the margin will appear in the mammogram (Figure IX-7-4).[8]

Malignant Calcifications. Malignant calcifications may occur with or without an apparent mass.[7] The microcalcifications typically are quite fine, numerous, clustered and variable in size and shape (Figure IX-7-4).

Benign Masses. The majority of benign masses, such as cysts, intramammary lymph nodes and fibroadenomas, have well-circumscribed margins (Figure IX-7-5).

Benign Calcifications. Benign calcifications are more likely to be round, uniform, coarse and scattered in distribution (Figure IX-7-5).

Pitfalls in Mammographic Interpretation

While masses with spiculated or ill-defined margins are usually malignant, a similar appearance may be seen in benign radial scars, sclerosing adenosis, post-traumatic fat necrosis, or biopsy scars (Figure IX-7-6). Less infiltrating cancers may have only slightly irregular, or even well-circumscribed, margins. Occasionally, a carcinoma is so well circumscribed that it is identical to a benign lesion (Figure IX-7-7). Papillary, medullary, and colloid carcinomas are particularly likely to be well circumscribed.

Calcifications associated with fibrocystic changes in the breast often mimic those seen in malignancy, leading to unavoidable false-positive mammograms. Therefore, clustered microcalcifications are a sensitive but not a specific sign of breast cancer.

Prebiopsy Needle Localization

Mammographically-guided needle localization prior to biopsy is indicated for any suspicious lesion that is seen in mammograms but not identified on clinical examination. The

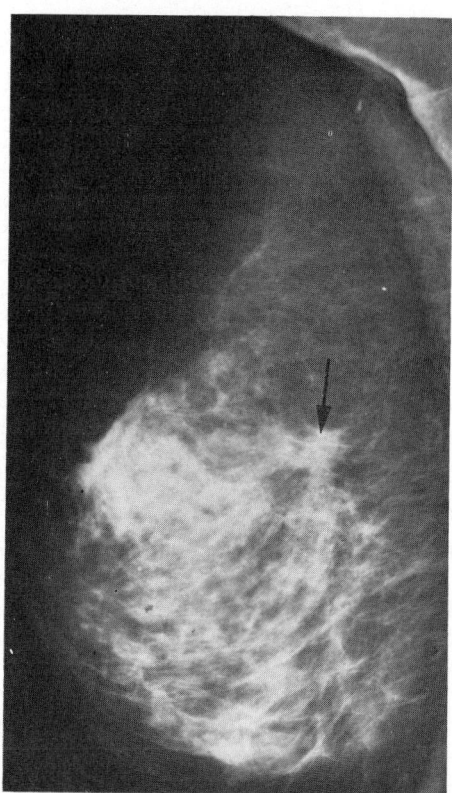

Figure IX-7-6. Biopsy scar mimicking malignancy. Routine mammogram six months after surgery shows architectural distortion (arrow) at the site where a fibroadenoma had been excised. The history of recent surgery at this location and the absence of a palpable mass are consistent with a postsurgical scar. Follow up mammograms six months later showed a decrease in the size of the scar.

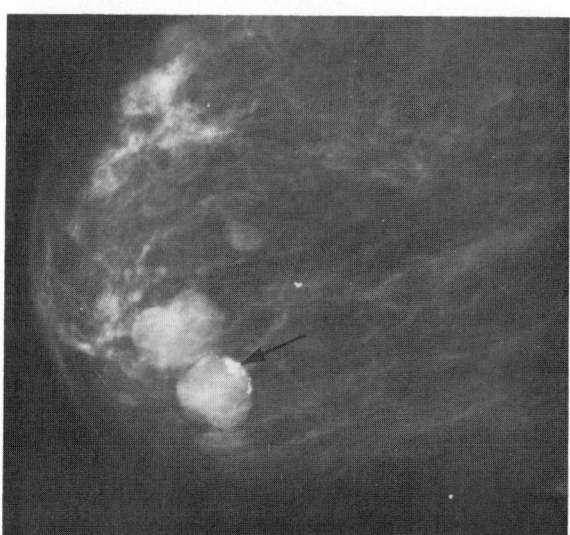

Figure IX-7-5. Benign masses in a 42-year-old woman. The well-circumscribed margins and the multiplicity and coarseness of calcifications (arrow) in the wall of one of the masses are all signs of benignity. Accordingly, biopsy was not done. The most likely diagnosis is multiple fibroadenomas.

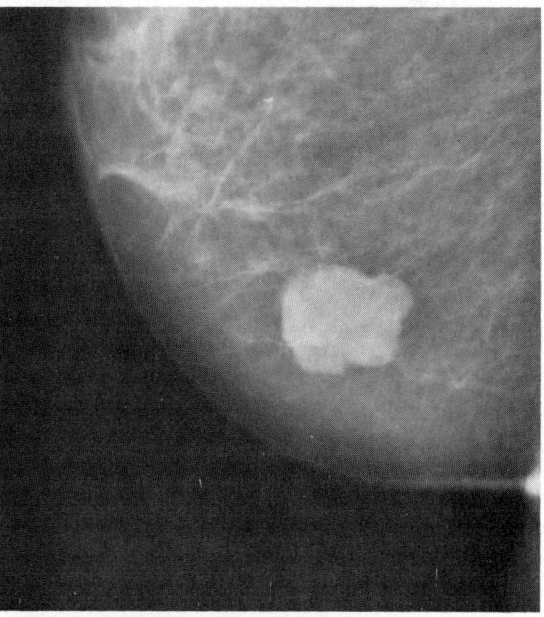

Figure IX-7-7. Well-circumscribed cancer in a 55-year-old woman. A solitary mass like this one, when shown to be solid by ultrasound, should be viewed with suspicion even when the margins of the mass are well-circumscribed. Biopsy revealed medullary carcinoma.

purpose of needle localization is to ensure removal of an occult lesion with the smallest possible breast deformity. Variations on the needle localization method include: (1) a direct needle approach where the tip of a hypodermic needle is inserted as close as possible to the mammographic abnormality and left in place when the patient goes to surgery; (2) a "spot" method which involves injecting methylene blue dye (0.1 cc) into the breast tissue through a needle positioned near the mammographic abnormality before the needle is removed; and (3) use of a needle to introduce a malleable wire with a barbed or round end which is placed at the site of the suspected tumor before biopsy.[13,16,33]

Specimen radiographs should be performed to verify that a nonpalpable lesion has been removed.[29] If the abnormality is not identified in the specimen radiograph, removal of more tissue is usually indicated.

The Postsurgical Breast

Postsurgical changes on mammograms include skin thickening or retraction, architectural distortion (Figure IX-7-6), asymmetry, calcification and fat necrosis.[22] Since some postsurgical changes may be mistaken for carcinomas, it is helpful to perform a baseline mammogram at 4–6 months after operation for comparison with later mammograms. When patients have undergone limited surgical resections for carcinomas, it is particularly useful to perform such baseline studies. Regular follow-up mammograms are then done at intervals of six months to one year. After limited surgical treatment for an extensive ductal carcinoma in situ, mammography can be useful prior to radiotherapy to identify residual tumor calcifications.[31]

Mammography for Staging

In addition to the clinical examination and diagnostic blood work, the pretreatment staging protocol for breast cancer should include chest radiography and bilateral mammography. Mammography prior to biopsy of a palpable abnormality is used to exclude bilateral and multifocal lesions. While normal-sized or enlarged axillary nodes can be visualized in a mediolateral oblique film-screen mammogram, there are no mammographic criteria which can exclude nodal involvement. Therefore, histologic assessment is essential for staging.[15]

The Underutilization of Screening Mammography

The 1987 National Health Interview Survey reported that only 40 percent of eligible American women had ever had a mammogram.[5] The underuse of mammography has stimulated investigators to identify the present barriers to mammographic screening in the U.S.: (1) lack of awareness by women and their physicians of breast cancer screening guidelines and benefits; (2) physician expectation of noncompliance by their patients; (3) concern about radiation; (4) concern about overdiagnosis; (5) women's fear of discovering cancer and losing a breast; (6) perception that mammography involves discomfort and inconvenience; and (7) physicians' perception of the examination as high in cost/low in yield.[14] Recent efforts by government agencies, professional societies and the mass media have resulted in increased use of screening mammography. As of January 1990, 64% of American women had had at least one mammogram, but only 31% followed the guidelines for annual screening.[34]

Overcoming the Barriers to Screening

Physicians are now more inclined to order mammograms than they were five years ago.[1] The major reasons for the increased acceptance of mammography as a screening technique include support by major medical societies, a realization that the examination has been technically improved and is safer and more effective, and a conviction that earlier detection can save lives. In response to concerns about overdiagnosis, radiologists are being encouraged to monitor their biopsy results and strive for an acceptable rate of true positive results in their practices.[20]

High cost has persisted as a barrier to breast cancer screening with mammography. Some health maintenance organizations now support screening, and public pressures for mandatory insurance coverage for mammography to screen normal women is increasing. A number of bills have been introduced for mandatory insurance coverage at both the federal and state levels, and many states now have legislation requiring reimbursement for screening mammography by insurance companies.

Quality Assurance

Concerns of radiologists, national medical organizations and the public about the variable quality of mammographic examinations have led the American College of Radiology (ACR) to develop a voluntary mammography accreditation program.[11] The ACR Mammography Accreditation Program offers radiologists an objective evaluation of their equipment, staff qualifications, image quality and radiation dosage. ACR accreditation in mammography is rapidly becoming the standard by which mammography facilities will be deemed acceptable by referring physicians, consumers, third party and government reimbursement sources, and local and national professional medical organizations. By March 1, 1991, over 4,274 of approximately 8,000 mammography facilities nationwide had applied for accreditation and over 2,170 had been accredited.[10]

Other Breast Imaging Methods

Breast ultrasound is a useful adjunct to mammography for well-circumscribed masses in order to discern cysts from solid tumors, especially when the masses are non-palpable.[12] On the other hand, clinical investigations have shown that modalities such as ultrasound, diaphanography (breast transillumination with light scanning), and thermography can not detect early breast cancers reliably and are not cost-effective for this purpose. Therefore, these methods should not be part of the basic screening process for breast cancer.[2]

Magnetic resonance imaging (MRI) of the breast has also been the subject of recent investigations. Thus far, considerable overlap in the MRI features of malignant and benign lesions has been observed.[22] The high cost of MRI and its inability to resolve smaller masses and microcalcifications make it impractical for breast imaging at this time.

References

1. American Cancer Society. 1989 Survey of Physicians' Attitudes and Practices in Early Cancer Detection. CA, 40:77, 1990.
2. American College of Radiology, Policy Statement on Breast Imaging Centers. A.C.R. Bulletin, 41:18, 1985.
3. Bassett, L. W., Bunnell, D. H., Jahanshahi, R., Gold, R. H., Arndt, R. D., and Linsman, J.: Breast cancer detection: One versus two views. Radiology, 165:95, 1987.
4. Bassett, L. W., and Gold, R. H.: Breast radiography using the oblique projection. Radiology, 149:585, 1983.
5. CDC. Provisional estimates from the National Health Interview Survey supplement on cancer control–United States, January–March 1987. M.M.W.R., 37:417, 1988.
6. Egan, J. F., Sayler, C. B., and Goodman, M. J.: A technique for localizing occult breast lesions. CA, 26:32, 1976.
7. Egan, R. L., McSweeney, M. B., and Sewell, C.: Intramammary calcifications without an associated mass in benign and malignant diseases. Radiology, 137:1, 1980.
8. Gold, R. H., Montgomery, C. K., and Rambo, O. N.: Significance of margination of benign and malignant infiltrative mammary lesions: roentgenographic-pathological correlation. AJR Am. J. Roentgenol., 118:881, 1973.
9. Gordillo, C: Breast cancer screening guidelines agreed on by AMA, other medically related organizations. J.A.M.A., 262:1165, 1989.
10. Hendrick, R. E.: Personal Communication.
11. Hendrick, R. E.: Standardization of image quality and radiation dose in mammography. Radiology, 174:648, 1990.
12. Hilton, S. V., Leopold, G. R., Olson, L. K., and Willson, S. A.: Real-time breast sonography: Application in 300 consecutive patients. AJR, 147:479, 1986.
13. Homer, M. J.: Nonpalpable breast lesion localization using a curved-end retractable wire. Radiology, 157:259, 1985.
14. Howard, J.: Using mammography for cancer control: An unrealized potential. CA, 37:33, 1987.
15. Kalisher, L., Chu, A. M., and Peyster, R. G.: Clinicopathological correlations of xeroradiography in determining involvement of metastatic axillary nodes in female breast cancer. Radiology, 121:333, 1976.
16. Kopans, D. B., and Meyer, J. E.: Versatile spring hookwire breast lesion localizer. AJR, 138:586, 1982.
17. Lundgren, B., and Jakobsson, S.: Single view mammography: A simple and efficient approach to breast cancer screening. Cancer, 38:1124, 1976.
18. Mammography-User's Guide Recommendations of the National Council On Radiation Protection And Measurements. N. C. R. P. Report No. 85, 1986.
19. Moskowitz, M., and Libshitz, H.: Mammographic screening for breast cancer by lateral view only: Is it practical? J. Can. Assoc. Radiol., 28:259, 1977.
20. Murphy, W. A., Destouet, J. M., and Monsees, B. S.: Professional quality assurance for mammography screening programs. Radiology, 175:319, 1990.
21. Pagani, J. J., Bassett, L. W., Gold, R. H., Benedetti, J., Arndt, R. D., Linsman, J., and Scanlan, R. L.: Efficacy of combined film-screen/xeromammography: Preliminary report. AJR, 135:141, 1980.
22. Ross, R. J., Thompson, J. S., Kim, K., and Bailey, R. A.: Nuclear magnetic resonance imaging and evaluation of human breast tissue: Preliminary clinical trials. Radiology, 143:195, 1982.
23. Seidman H., Stellman, S. D., and Mushinski, M. H.: A different perspective on breast cancer risk factors: some implications for the nonattributable risk. CA, 32:301, 1982.
24. Shapiro, S.: Evidence on screening for breast cancer from a randomized trial. Cancer, 39:2772, 1977.
25. Sickles, E. A.: Mammographic features of 300 consecutive nonpalpable breast cancers. A. J. R., 146:661, 1986.
26. Sickles, E. A., and Herzog, K. A.: Mammography of the postsurgical breast. AJR, 136:585, 1981.
27. Sickles, E. A., Weber, W. N., Galvin, H. B., Ominsky, S. H., and Sollitto, R. A.: Baseline screening mammography: One vs. two views per breast. AJR, 147:1149, 1986.
28. Silverberg, E., Boring, C. C., and Squires, T. S.: "Cancer statistics, 1990." CA, 40:9, 1990.
29. Snyder, R. E.: Specimen radiography and preoperative localization of nonpalpable breast cancer. Cancer, 46:950, 1980.
30. Snyder, R. E., and Kirch, R. L.: Comparison study of xeromammography and low-dose mammography. In Early breast cancer detection and treatment. Edited by H. S. Galagher. Wiley, New York, 1975, p. 199.
31. Stomper, P. C., Connelly, J. L., Meyer, J. E., and Harris, J. R.: Clinically occult ductal carcinoma in situ detected with mamography: Analysis of 100 cases with radiologic-pathologic correlation. Radiology, 172:235, 1989.
32. Tabar, L., Fagerberg, C. J., Gad, A., Baldetorp, L., Holmberg, L. H., Grontoft, O., Ljungquist, U., Lundstrom, B., Manson, J. C., Eklund, G., Day, N. E., and Pettersson, F.: Reduction in mortality from breast cancer after mass screening with mammography. Randomized trial from the Breast Cancer Screening Working Group of the Swedish National Board of Health and Welfare. Lancet, 1:829, 1985.
33. Threatt, B., Appelman, H., Dow, R., and O'Rourke, T.: Percutaneous needle localization of clustered mammary microcalcifications prior to biopsy. Am. J. Roentgenol. Radium Ther. Nucl. Med., 121:839, 1974.
34. Use of mammography—United States 1990. M.M.W.R., 38:321, 1990.

Ultrasound in Cancer Medicine
Edward G. Grant

Sonography has been used for over 30 years for the simple differentiation of cystic and solid lesions. While variations in this application continue to have great clinical value, advancements in technology now enable ultrasound to be used for an increasing number of applications that appear to be far removed from its original purpose. Technical breakthroughs in ultrasound equipment have led, in particular, to improvements in spatial resolution and tissue contrast. Ultrasound imaging can also be performed now in "real time" (like fluoroscopic imaging). The incorporation of Doppler (both duplex and color) also permits the noninvasive evaluation of vascular abnormalities, including some which may be associated with tumors.

In spite of these technologic advancements, some basic limitations of ultrasound imaging persist, particularly the inability of sound waves to penetrate bone or gas. Therefore, ultrasound is infrequently used in the evaluation of the central nervous system (CNS) or the parenchyma of the lung.

Central Nervous System Ultrasound

There is one notable exception in the CNS, however, which is the use of ultrasound during intracranial neurosurgery. In this procedure, a sheathed ultrasound transducer is placed directly on the exposed brain to facilitate the approach to a known lesion and minimize damage to surrounding normal brain (Figure IX-8-1).[11] In addition, ultrasound can be used to ensure that a resection has been complete. Intraoperative sonography can also be used to assist in the resection of spinal masses,[16] including tumors and arteriovenous malformations.[21]

Head and Neck Ultrasound

While the role of ultrasound imaging inside the skull is limited, the soft tissues of the head and neck are readily accessible to high-resolution ultrasound. Ultrasound has been used to differentiate cystic from solid thyroid nodules, and it can readily depict small thyroid masses. In this regard, ultrasound has better resolution than either nuclear scintigraphy or CT. The ability to identify small lesions can be of particular value in differentiating solitary from multiple nodules, and it makes sonography an excellent method to evaluate and follow patients with a history of thyroid irradiation early in life. In addition, the ability to identify small thyroid masses and to guide biopsies makes sonography the preferred method for finding an occult thyroid cancer in a patient who presents with metastatic disease that is compatible with a thyroid origin.[25] Sonography can also distinguish adenopathy involving anterior cervical nodes from thyroid masses. A recent study by Gooding and colleagues also shows that sonography is uniquely capable of determining whether or not there is carotid involvement by cervical adenopathy.[7]

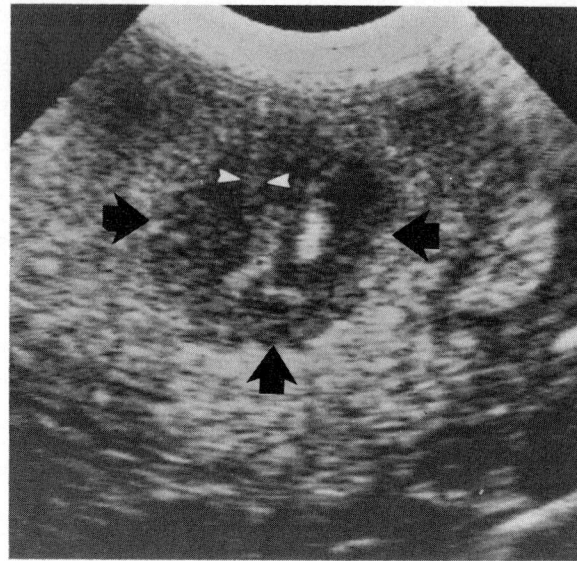

Figure IX-8-1. Intraoperative ultrasound: patient with history of melanoma who was found to have a small, superficial mass in right frontal lobe on CT scan. At surgery, lesion was not palpable, and ultrasound was used to guide biopsy and resection. Note well defined, hypoechoic mass (arrows) and biopsy needle within the metastasis (arrowheads).

While sonography is less commonly used in the United States for this purpose than in Europe, a number of studies also indicate that it may be useful for staging patients with cancer of the floor of the mouth.[6,10] The relative lack of enthusiasm in the United States for using ultrasound to evaluate oral neoplasms probably reflects the ready availability of CT and MRI. Ultrasound does have the advantage of being a real-time examination, however, and therefore may be of particular value in identifying fixation when a tumor invades the tongue, vocal cords or other normally mobile structures. Other uses for sonography in the head and neck include the identification of enlarged parathyroid glands in patients with hypercalcemia (Figure IX-8-2) and the evaluation of parotid masses.[18,28]

Thoracic Ultrasound

In the thorax, the use of sonography is usually limited to localizing or evaluating pleural opacities that have been identified previously on radiographs. Sonography should be capable of differentiating between free and loculated effusions, determining which are amenable to thoracentesis (an effusion with numerous internal septae or locules may require thoracotomy), and finding the optimum site for puncture. Tube insertion for pleural drainage or drug administration

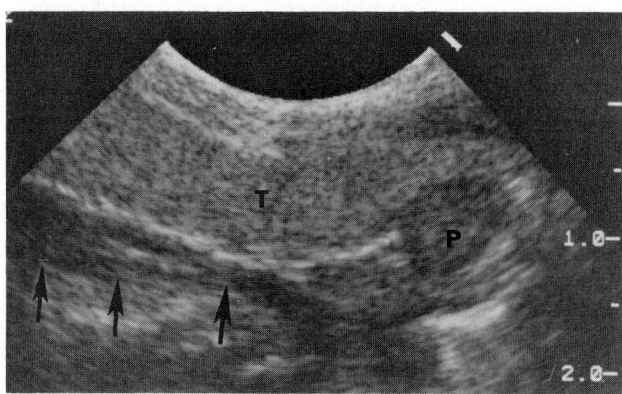

Figure IX-8-2. Parathyroid adenoma: ultrasound study on patient with metastatic breast carcinoma and elevated calcium levels. On a longitudinal (sagittal) section through left thyroid gland (T), note the well-defined, hypoechoic mass inferior to thyroid which is typical of parathyroid adenoma (P). Arrows point to longus colli muscle. Head of patient is to the left; foot is to the right; skin of anterior neck is at top.

and other interventional procedures can also be performed under ultrasound guidance.[15] Within the effusion itself, sonography can also identify collapsed lung and differentiate it from consolidation without atelectasis.

Breast Ultrasound

Outside the pleural cavity, the main application of thoracic ultrasound is in breast imaging. It is used typically to differentiate solid from cystic masses. Some investigators have attempted to use ultrasound Doppler analysis to differentiate benign from malignant breast masses, but the technique is not yet sufficiently developed to obviate the need for biopsy.[23] Another recent application of ultrasound in breast cancer has been to detect adenopathy in the internal mammary lymph node chain.[22] The addition of color Doppler imaging will facilitate identification of the internal mammary vessels as they course beneath the upper ribs, and therefore help to define adjacent adenopathy.

Vascular Ultrasound

Color Doppler can also be used to evaluate vessels in the neck, upper thorax and arms. Thrombosed vessels can be differentiated readily from normal ones or those compressed by extraluminal masses. The ability to depict venous flow may be of particular value in the cancer patient who presents with acute or chronic arm swelling, and color Doppler sonography should be highly accurate for evaluating thromboses in the jugular, subclavian, and axillary veins (Plate IX-1).[9,12] The proximal subclavian and innominate veins may be difficult to image with sonography, however, and may require MRI or contrast venography. The potential of color Doppler for evaluating patients with the superior vena cava syndrome remains to be investigated.

Endoscopic ultrasound is a relatively new adaptation of sonography. This technique requires the incorporation of a minute transducer into the tip of an endoscope and enables the operator to see tissues that are deep to mucosal surfaces. This technique is being used increasingly, and it is an excellent method for assessing the depth of penetration

of esophageal and gastric malignancies, identifying nodal involvement, and defining the internal characteristics of submucosal masses, both benign and malignant (Figure IX-8-3).[26] Endoscopic ultrasound may eventually prove to be an essential component in evaluating the mediastinum of patients who have potential nodal spread to that area, since neither CT nor MRI has proven to be as accurate as once hoped.

Abdominal Ultrasound

Sonography is often considered to be an adjunctive imaging technique for evaluating the abdomen in the cancer patient. Screening for metastatic liver disease, for example, is better done with CT. However, ultrasound can be of practical use in many situations, such as the differentiation of cystic and solid lesions in the liver. Hill and colleagues have recently found ultrasound to be of particular value when further characterization is necessary for small indeterminate lesions identified on a CT scan.[2] Sonography is also an excellent method for following measurable abdominal disease in patients who are on treatment protocols. The spatial resolution of ultrasound is currently comparable to CT, it is far less expensive (usually one third to one half the cost of CT), it requires no contrast injection, and it may be more readily available at some institutions.

While CT is generally preferred now for evaluating metastatic liver disease, sonography has been applied widely as the primary screening modality for asymptomatic patients who are at risk of hepatocellular carcinoma.[3] Yearly ultra-

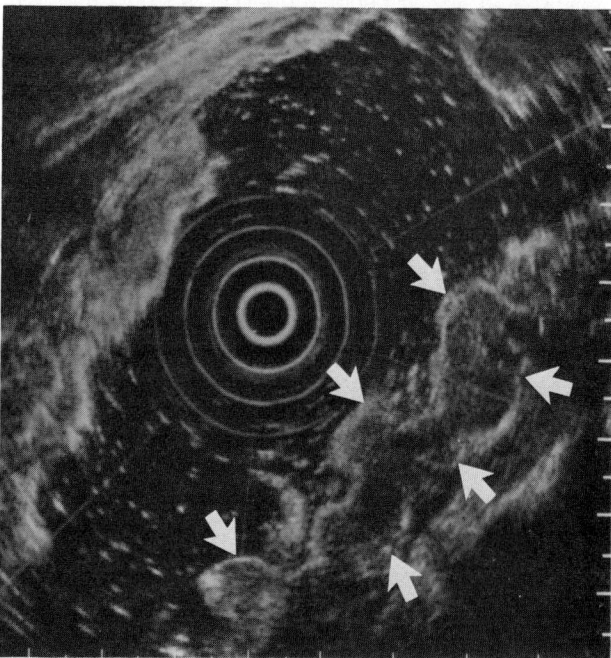

Figure IX-8-3. Endoscopic ultrasound: patient with weight loss. Thickened gastric folds were noted on upper GI study. Endoscopic ultrasound is suggestive of lymphoma. Note marked thickening of wall of stomach (arrows), with preservation of mucosa. Central ring-like structure is a combination of the endoscopic ultrasound scanner itself and reverberation artifact. Dark, speckled area is water (with small air bubbles) which has been instilled into the stomach for better imaging of the wall. No perigastric lymph nodes were identified.

sound studies are recommended in people with chronic active hepatitis and some forms of cirrhosis. In patients with hepatocellular carcinoma, ultrasound has also been used to monitor the placement of needles for percutaneous ethanol ablation.[14] Ultrasound remains an excellent and cost-efficient method for guiding percutaneous biopsy of any hepatic (Figure IX-8-4) or other abdominal mass, and it has also been used to guide the placement of radiation trocars in patients with metastatic liver disease.[4]

Sonography is the primary imaging modality in the initial evaluation of patients with jaundice and can define intrahepatic ductal dilation quite accurately. While the actual identification of an obstructing lesion may not always be possible (strictures and stones may be particularly difficult to image), pancreatic masses or adenopathy should be visualized in the majority of patients and can then be biopsied under ultrasound guidance.[13] Once biliary obstruction is identified, color Doppler can be used to differentiate dilated biliary radicals from adjacent portal veins. This can be of practical import when percutaneous biliary drainage is being considered, since ultrasound can be used to guide the needle into a nonvascular lumen.

While most of the uses for conventional sonography in the liver are now well established, color Doppler has opened up several new windows of opportunity. In particular, this technique provides a noninvasive method for evaluating the hepatic vasculature. Portal vein thrombosis or compression by external masses is readily depicted with color Doppler imaging. Color Doppler is also an excellent method for evaluating patients who are suspected of having a Budd-Chiari syndrome, and it is capable of differentiating those patients with venous compression by tumor from those with thrombosis (bland or neoplastic) of the hepatic veins or inferior vena cava (Plate IX-3).[8] A unique group of cancer patients at risk for hepatic veno-occlusive disease are those who have undergone certain regimens of intensive chemotherapy and bone marrow transplantation. Unlike most patients with Budd-Chiari syndrome who have gross thrombosis or tumor involvement of the major hepatic veins, patients with the syndrome who have undergone chemotherapy and bone marrow transplantation are obstructed at the level of the hepatic venules. The major hepatic veins remain patent, and contrast venography may be normal. However, Doppler may indicate the correct diagnosis by showing reversal of portal vein flow.[1] While Doppler can be of assistance in evaluating the hepatic veins and the portal vein, it has not led to increased specificity in characterizing hepatic masses. Color Doppler can determine if a mass is relatively vascular or nonvascular, but so far it seems incapable of distinguishing between primary cancers, metastatic and benign lesions (particularly hemangiomas).

In the retroperitoneum, the primary uses for sonography include assessments of kidney size, contour and internal echo characteristics, the detection of hydronephrosis, and the characterization of cystic or solid masses. While several authors have reported specific Doppler signal patterns in renal carcinomas, this is probably of little practical significance since surgery or biopsy must still be performed on all solid renal masses.[17] However, color Doppler can be used to identify renal vein thrombosis (with or without tumor) and the level of extension of a thrombus into the inferior vena cava. In fact, inferior vena caval obstruction of any type can be assessed using color Doppler, and ilio-femoral thromboses also should now be assessed using duplex or color Doppler. Color Doppler sonography has also become the primary examination for evaluating deep venous thromboses in the leg and should replace contrast venography in all but the most unusual cases.[5,22] A particular advantage of ultra-

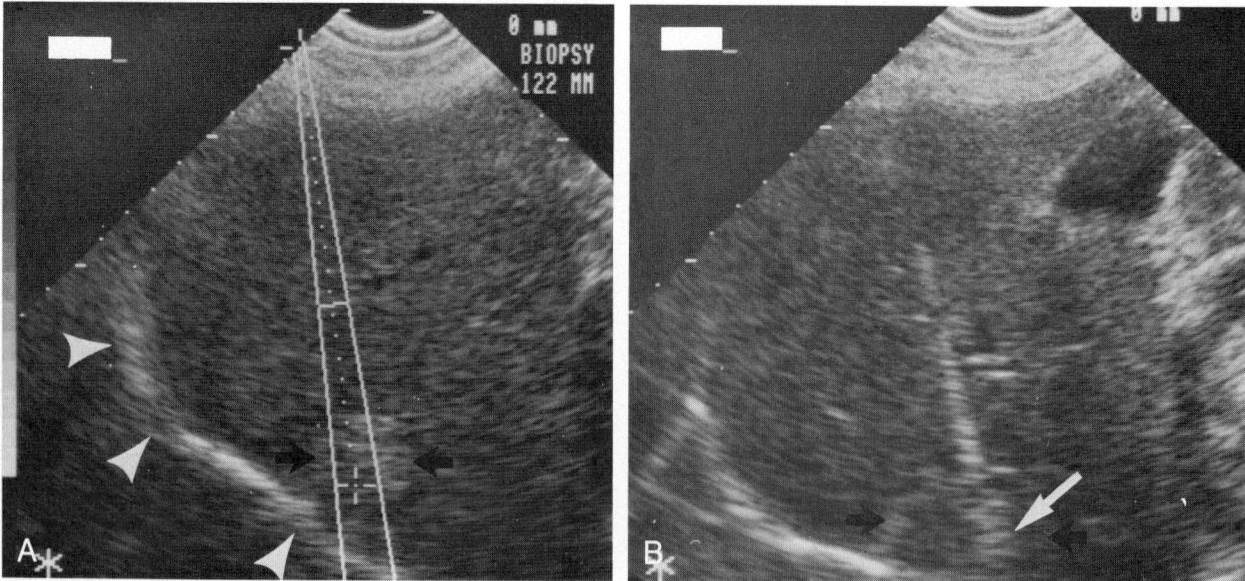

Figure IX-8-4.   Ultrasound-guided biopsy (sagittal scans): Echogenic mass identified in posterior right lobe of liver in patient with history of ovarian carcinoma. Arrows in (A) depict liver mass adjacent to diaphragm (arrowheads). Needle guide has been placed on ultrasound transducer, and expected path of biopsy needle through the liver is displayed electronically (white lines) on ultrasound monitor. Depth of lesion can also be determined. Repeat scan (B) during biopsy confirms proper position of needle (white arrow). Head of patient is toward left on both scans; foot is toward right. Anterior abdominal wall is at top.

sound over venography in the cancer patient is its ability to differentiate thromboses inside a vessel from a neoplasm compressing or invading the vessel.

While sonography can readily evaluate vessels in the retroperitoneum, the presence or absence of adenopathy is usually better determined by CT. A notable exception may be patients with testicular tumors.[24] However, the improved accuracy of sonography for identifying para-aortic adenopathy in this disease may be the result of the thinner body habitus of many young patients with testicular cancer, and it is probably not inherent in the pathology. In general, sonography may be an excellent alternative to CT for evaluating the retroperitoneum in thin patients.

Pelvic Ultrasound

In pelvic neoplastic diseases, current staging procedures now rely primarily on CT for definitive imaging information. However, the preliminary evaluation of most pelvic masses continues to be done with ultrasound. Sonography has been quite successful in separating lesions which are gynecologic from those which are not, and in helping to characterize lesions of the uterus and ovaries. A new variation in sonographic examination technique is endovaginal sonography. The proximity of the endovaginal transducer to the uterus and ovaries produces images which are far superior to those obtained with transabdominal scanning methods. The endovaginal technique is readily accepted by most women (including postmenopausal women) and does not require a full bladder.

In examining the uterus, thickening of the endometrial lining is exquisitely depicted by endovaginal ultrasound (Figure IX-8-5A), as are small submucosal leiomyomas. In particular, small leiomyomas which may be sources for vaginal bleeding are often not seen with conventional transabdominal scanning techniques. In a patient with a known or suspected adnexal mass, endovaginal sonography can define

the lesion's internal characteristics far better than a conventional ultrasound scan and provide a more definitive diagnosis in many cases (Figure IX-8-5B). The improved resolution of this technique also may facilitate differentiation of a large ovary from a true mass. A recent potential application of endovaginal sonography is to screen asymptomatic women for ovarian carcinoma, since the technique is capable of identifying ovarian lesions before they cause a palpable mass. Unfortunately, unlike mammographic screening, endovaginal sonography in its present form would probably not be cost-effective as a screening technique if it were applied to the general population. Selected patients who are at higher risk but not symptomatic (women who have a strong family history of ovarian cancer, a personal history of breast cancer, or middle-aged women who are nulliparous) may benefit from its application.[27]

Prostatic Ultrasound

Sonography is also used to evaluate tumors in the male pelvis. A minor adaptation of the endovaginal probe allows it to be inserted into the rectum, thereby affording excellent images of the prostate and seminal vesicles. Again, however, its utility as a screening procedure for prostate cancer remains in question. At this point we know relatively little about the natural history of small asymptomatic prostatic nodules, which are quite common. The transrectal technique is also nonspecific with regard to differentiating between benign and malignant nodules.[19] Transrectal sonography can be an excellent guidance method for biopsying a small prostate nodule, however.

Testicular Ultrasound

High-resolution sonography remains the primary imaging modality for testicular masses. Intratesticular masses may be differentiated from those which arise outside the gland (Figure IX-8-6) and lesions rendered impalpable by overlying

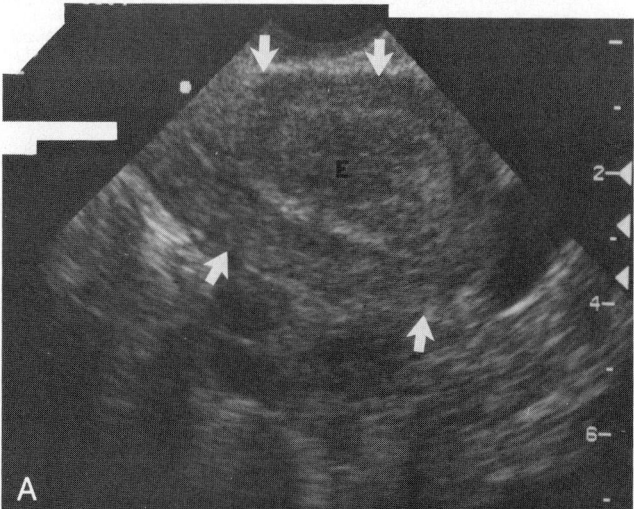
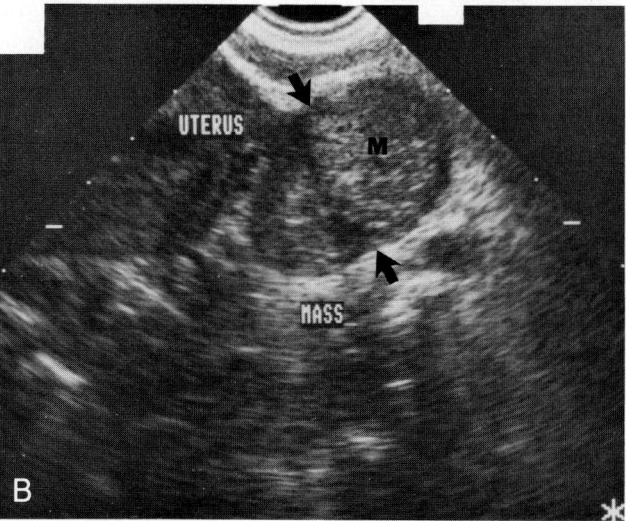

Figure IX-8-5.   Transvaginal sonography: (A) Longitudinal ultrasound scan through uterus of 66-year-old woman with vaginal bleeding. Uterus (arrows) is enlarged for a postmenopausal patient, measuring 4.2 cm. Endometrium (E) is markedly thickened, a finding suggestive of endometrial carcinoma. (B). Postmenopausal patient with vague pelvic pain. Endovaginal ultrasound scan through left adnexal area reveals a normal-size ovary containing 1-cm echogenic mass (M). Lesion proved to be a benign ovarian fibroma. Upper limit of both scans represents the ultrasound transducer within the vagina.

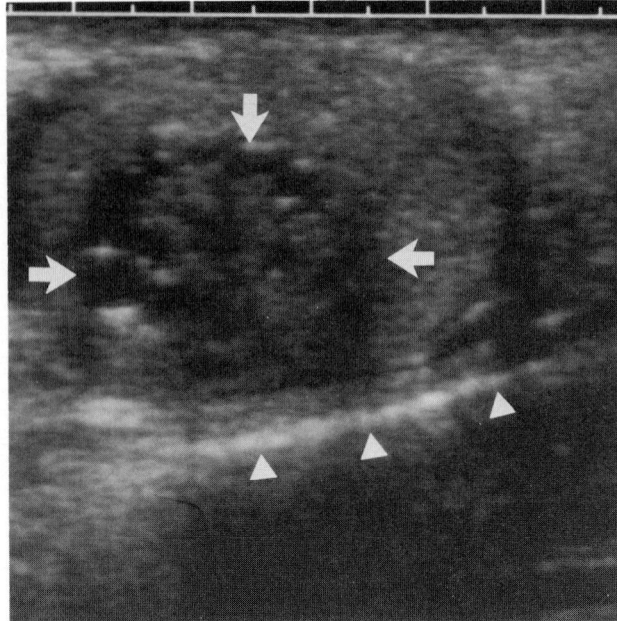

Figure IX-8-6. Testicular sonogram: Longitudinal section through right side of scrotum of 20-year-old man with painless enlargement of testis. A well defined, hypoechoic mass is identified posteriorly (arrows). Mass contained multiple cystic spaces; other scanning sections revealed internal calcifications. Although sonographic appearance is not usually specific for cell type, calcifications are typical of teratocarcinoma. Diagnosis was confirmed at surgery. Arrowheads outline anterior scrotal wall. Epididymis is not visible in this particular plane of section.

pathologic processes (e.g., a hydrocele or varicocele) should be easily identifiable. In this connection also, patients who present with metastatic nodes in the retroperitoneum or mediastinum and whose histology is compatible with a testicular origin should undergo testicular sonography to identify a possible occult primary. In patients with lymphoma or leukemia, sonography may also define residual disease in the testis which may not be palpable.

In summary, modern sonography is an extemely versatile tool with applications to cancer management in many areas of the body. The uses for conventional (B mode or real-time) techniques are well established and are known to most clinicians. The newer adaptations of ultrasound (color Doppler and endoluminal scanning, in particular) provide incremental advantages that support their inclusion in the imaging techniques available to modern cancer medicine.

References

1. Abu-Yousef, M. M., Brown, B. P., Gingrich, R. D., and LaBrecque, D. R.: Duplex doppler sonography in the diagnosis of veno-occlusive disease. (Scientific Presentation.) J. Ultrasound Med., 9:S1, 1990.
2. Brick, S. H., Hill, M. C., and Lande, I. M.: Mistaken or indeterminate CT diagnosis of hepatic metastases: The value of sonography. A.J.R., 148:723, 1987.
3. Choi, B. I., Kim, C. W., Han, M. C., Kim, C. Y., Lee, H. S., Kim, S. T., and Kim, Y. I.: Sonographic characteristics of small hepatocellular carcinoma. Gastrointest. Radiol., 14:255, 1989.
4. Dritschilo, A., Grant, E. G., Harter, K. W., Holt, R. W., Rustgi, S. N., and Rodgers, J. E.: Interstitial radiation therapy for hepatic metastases: Sonographic guidance for applicator placement. A.J.R., 147:275, 1986.
5. Foley, W. D., Middleton, W. D., Lawson, T. L., Erickson, S., Quiroz, F. A., and Macrander, S.: Color Doppler ultrasound imaging of lower-extremity venous disease. A.J.R., 152:371, 1989.
6. Fruehwald, F., Salomonowitz, E., Neuhold, A., Pavelka, R., and Mailath, G.: Tongue cancer: Sonographic assessment of tumor stage. J. Ultrasound. Med., 6:121, 1987.
7. Gooding, G. A. W., Langman, A. W., Dillon, W. P., and Kaplan, M. J.: Malignant carotid artery invasion: Sonographic detection. Radiology, 171:435, 1989.
8. Grant, E. G., Perrella, R. R., Tessler, F. N., Lois, J., and Busuttil, R.: Budd-Chiari syndrome: The results of duplex and color Doppler imaging. A.J.R., 152:377, 1989.
9. Grassi, C. J., and Polak, J. F.: Axillary and subclavian venous thrombosis: Follow-up evaluation with color Doppler flow US and venography. Radiology, 175:651, 1990.
10. Gritzmann, N., Traxler, M., Grasl, M., and Pavelka, R.: Advanced laryngeal cancer: Sonographic assessment. Radiology, 171:171, 1989.
11. Hatfield, M. K., Rubin, J. M., Gebarski, S. S., and Silbergleit, R.: Intraoperative sonography in low-grade gliomas. J. Ultrasound Med., 8:131, 1989.
12. Knudson, G. J., Wiedmeyer, D. A., Erickson, S. J., Foley, W. D., Lawson, T. L., Mewissen, M. W., and Lipchik, E. O.: Color Doppler sonographic imaging in the assessment of upper-extremity deep venous thrombosis. A. J. R., 154:399, ????.
13. Laing, F. C., Jeffrey, R. B., Jr., Wing, V. W., and Nyberg, D. A.: Biliary dilatation: defining the level and cause by real-time US. Radiology, 160:39, 1986.
14. Livraghi, T., Salmi, A., Bolondi, L., Marin, G., Arienti, V., Monti, F., and Vettori, C.: Small hepatocellular carcinoma: Percutaneous alcohol injection—results in 23 patients. Radiology, 168:313, 1988.
15. O'Moore, P. V., Mueller, P. R., Simeone, J. F., Saini, S., Butch, R. J., Hahn, P. F., Steiner, E., Stark, D. D., and Ferruchi, J. T., Jr.: Sonographic guidance in diagnostic and therapeutic interventions in the pleural space. A.J.R., 149:1, 1987.
16. Raghavendra, N., Epstein, F. J., and McCleary, L.: Intramedullary spinal cord tumors in children: Localization with intraoperative sonography. A.J.N.R., 5:395, 1984.
17. Ramos, I. M., Taylor, K. J. W., Kier, R., Burns, P. N., Snower, D. P., and Carter, D.: Tumor vascular signals in renal masses: Detection with Doppler US. Radiology, 168:633, 1988.
18. Reading, C. C., Charboneau, J. W., James, E. M., Karsell, P. R., Purnell, D. C., Grant, C. S., and Van Heerden, J. A.: High resolution parathyroid sonography. A.J.R., 139:539, 1982.
19. Rifkin, M. D.: Endorectal sonography of the prostate: Clinical implications. A.J.R., 148:1137, 1987.
20. Rose, S. C., Zwiebel, W. J., Nelson, B. D., Preist, D. L., Knighton, R. A., Brown, J. W., Lawrence, P. F., Stults, B. M., Reading, J. C., and Miller, F. J.: Symptomatic lower extremity deep venous thrombosis. Accuracy, limitations, and role of color duplex flow imaging in diagnosis. Radiology, 175:639, 1990.
21. Rubin, J. M., Hatfield, M. K., Chandler, W. F., Black, K. L., and Dipietro, M. A.: Intracerebral arteriovenous malformations: Intraoperative color Doppler flow imaging. Radiology, 170:219, 1989.
22. Scatarige, J. C., Hamper, U. M., Sheth, S., and Allen, III, H. A.: Parasternal sonography of the internal mammary vessels: Technique, normal anatomy, and lymphadenopathy. Radiology, 172:453, 1989.
23. Schoenberger, S. G., Sutherland, C. M., and Robinson, A. E.: Breast neoplasms: Duplex sonographic imaging as an adjunct in diagnosis. Radiology, 168:665, 1988.
24. Schwerk, W. B., Schwerk, W. N., and Rodeck, G.: Testicular tumors: Prospective analysis of real-time US patterns and abdominal staging. Radiology, 164:369, 1987.
25. Simeone, J. F., Daniels, G. H., and Mueller, P. R.: High-resolution real-time sonography of the parathyroid. Radiology, 145:431, 1982.
26. Tio, T. L., Coene, P. P. L. O., Schouwink, M. H., and Tytgat, G. N. J.: Esophagogastric carcinoma: Preoperative TNM classification with endosonography. Radiology, 173:411, 1989.
27. Van Nagell, J. R., Higgins, R. V., Donaldson, E. S., Gallion, H. H., Powell, D. E., Pavlik, E. J., Woods, C. H., and Thompson, E. A.: Transvaginal sonography as a screening method for ovarian cancer. Cancer, 65:573, 1990.
28. Whyte, A. M., and Byrne, J. V.: Comparison of computed tomography and ultrasound in the assessment of parotid masses. Clin. Radiol., 38:339, 1987.

Radionuclide Imaging in Cancer Medicine

Alan D. Waxman

Introduction

The use of radionuclides for evaluating cancer patients is of interest to all practicing oncologists. Several new applications using thallium-201 and gallium-67 have recently been reported, and they impact on the management of many tumor types. Positron emission tomography (PET) is an emerging technology which, while costly, appears to have great promise for detecting and staging tumors as well as determining the effects of therapy on tumor viability. Monoclonal antibodies labelled with isotopes are being proposed for therapeutic as well as diagnostic purposes. The development of new radiopharmaceuticals for diagnosis and therapy and the emergence of new instrumentation for detecting tumors have given further impetus recently to the field of Nuclear Oncology.

Bone Scan

The most common Nuclear Medicine procedure performed in oncology is the bone scan. This is an extremely sensitive and cost-effective test for detecting osseous metastases even before radiographs become abnormal.[22,25] In addition to its sensitivity, the bone scan is a total body screening procedure which can survey all body sites in less than one hour. Specificity has been a concern in the interpretation of bone scans, since many processes other than cancer can cause positive studies. However, given a careful history and correlation with other imaging modalities, the bone scan has a high degree of accuracy in predicting metastasis.

Specific carcinomas, particularly breast, lung, kidney and prostate are well suited for baseline bone scans, since the appearance of bone metastases as one manifestation of metastatic disease is relatively frequent.[19,22,32] The quality and reproducibility of bone scans is excellent using current detectors, and with multiple-headed cameras these studies can be completed in 20 minutes.

Single photon emission computed tomography (SPECT) is now being used in conjunction with other imaging modalities to better define and characterize osseous lesions. In particular, differentiation of vertebral body metastases from degenerative processes is considerably improved using SPECT.[5]

Metastases are often detected on bone scans before symptoms occur or objective findings can be appreciated on radiographs or CT scans. The radiation dose is extremely low, and repetitive studies on an annual or a more frequent basis pose no danger to the patient.

Gallium-67 Scintigraphy

Gallium-67 scintigraphy for tumor detection has been available for at least 20 years. In the last 7–8 years, however, there has been a significant decline in the use of gallium for tumor detection with the emergence of computed tomography and magnetic resonance imaging. With its limitations in spatial resolution, radionuclide imaging does not give the morphologic detail of CT or MRI. However, because of the physiologic nature of gallium scanning, it is capable of depicting tumor viability more accurately than other techniques.[11,12] For this reason, it is still widely used in determining tumor response to therapy. Kaplan and co-workers have shown that in diffuse large cell lymphomas the detection of gallium-67 within a tumor at the mid-course of chemotherapy is indicative of suboptimal tumor cell killing and is associated with an eventual mortality approaching 100%.[12] The presence of a true positive gallium finding in a lymphoma patient may be accompanied by a negative or equivocal CT or MRI. A number of groups have reported prognostically important results from the use of gallium in Hodgkin's disease as well as in diffuse large cell lymphoma.[2,11,37]

When gallium images are interpreted along with CT or MRI images, it is possible to determine more accurately the significance of a post-therapy fibrotic process or "scar." If the gallium study is positive, residual tumor exists within the fibrotic process. If the gallium scan becomes negative, the remaining tissue most likely represents only fibrosis with no tumor. Gallium scans can also be a valuable adjunct in other tumors (e.g., testicular and lung cancers) when the same logic is applied.

Thallium-201 in Oncology

Thallium-201 (Tl-201) is an isotope which is now used most commonly to assess myocardial perfusion. It is a safe, nontoxic radiopharmaceutical which gives a low radiation dose to the patient. However, there are also a large and growing number of reports in the literature regarding the clinical utility of thallium-201 in several areas of oncology.[1,6,13-15,20,24,28-30,33-36,38]

Thallium has proved useful in the detection and localization of parathyroid adenomas and carcinomas.[6,20,38] The current sensitivity of Tl-201, as reported in the literature for the detection and localization of parathyroid adenomas, ranges from 70–90%.[6,20,26,38] This figure generally exceeds the sensitivity of other imaging modalities, including ultrasound.

The use of thallium-201 to evaluate thyroid nodules has been reported by several groups; however, it is nonspecific and cannot differentiate malignant masses from benign adenomas.[33] Tl-201 has recently been shown to be useful for locating differentiated thyroid cancer tissue in thyroidectomized patients who have undergone prior I-131 therapy.[10,30] Its sensitivity in this clinical situation has been shown to be higher than scanning with diagnostic doses of I-131.[10,30]

The use of Tl-201 to detect bronchogenic carcinoma metastases in the hilar and mediastinal regions has also been described. While there is a potential use for thallium-201 in staging lung cancer, no definitive studies are available at this time to determine its absolute sensitivity or specificity.

Brain masses have been evaluated using thallium-201, and the successful detection and localization of primary brain tumors has been demonstrated.[1,14,15,24,28] Its application to clinical grading of astrocytomas has been proposed by several groups, who have demonstrated that the intensity of thallium activity within a tumor parallels the tumor grade. High-grade brain tumors demonstrate greater intensity than low-grade lesions, and some low-grade lesions can appear entirely normal on Tl-201 scans.[15,24] Tumor viability has also been evaluated using thallium-201. Successful treatment of brain tumors using chemotherapy or radiation has led to significant reductions or to complete resolution of positive findings on thallium-201 studies. It is not yet clear whether radiation necrosis can be separated from residual tumor using thallium-201 scintigraphy, but preliminary studies indicate promise in this area.

Thallium-201 has also been used to evaluate primary bone tumors. Tl-201 can determine the local extent of a bone tumor as well as the tumor's response to chemotherapy or radiation therapy.[29] There is an excellent correlation with the amount of thallium activity remaining in a bone tumor following therapy and the degree of tumor necrosis noted pathologically.

Staging lymph nodes above the diaphragm or in the inguinal region with Tl-201 scintigraphy appears to be equivalent to scans using gallium-67 in patients who have intermediate- and high-grade non-Hodgkin's lymphoma.[36] Thallium-201 is clearly superior to gallium with low-grade tumors (Figure IX-9-1).[13] Serial thallium scans can also be an excellent predictor of therapeutic response in patients with non-Hodgkin's lymphoma.

Preliminary studies indicate that there is significant uptake of Tl-201 in primary breast cancers, while benign lesions tend to have minimal or absent uptake. Thallium does not appear to be a good indicator of axillary node involvement in breast cancer, however, since the sensitivity for axillary adenopathy is approximately 50%.[34,35]

Patients with Kaposi's sarcoma often demonstrate strongly positive thallium-201 studies in areas involved by tumor, particularly inguinal and/or mediastinal nodes.[18] The corresponding gallium scans in these patients may be entirely negative. Thallium studies done in conjunction with gallium scans are, in fact, often able to detect the presence of Kaposi's sarcoma in immunocompromised patients, especially when the thallium scan is strongly positive and the gallium study is negative or equivocal in the same body areas.

Tumor uptake of thallium-201 appears to rely upon cell membrane transport functions which are related to two predominant mechanisms, an ATPase sodium-potassium pump as well as a co-transport mechanism within the cell membrane.[31] Assessments with Tl-201 of responses to chemotherapy or radiation therapy may be directly linked to their ability to disrupt these membrane transport functions.

Monoclonal Antibodies in Nuclear Medicine

Radiolabelled monoclonal antibodies directed toward a variety of antigens associated with specific tumor types, and using several different radionuclides, are currently under investigation in many institutions. Several different radionuclides are also being used to label the monoclonals. Bale and co-workers demonstrated the feasibility of irradiating tumors with I-131-labelled antibodies directed against fibrin approximately 30 years ago.[3] In 1980, Pressman demonstrated the use of radiolabelled antibodies for diagnostic purposes with external imaging techniques.[27] At the present time there are no radiolabelled monoclonal antibodies commercially available for tumor imaging, since clinical trials are still in progress to determine the safety and efficacy of these agents. Depending upon tumor type, as well as tumor location and size, the reported sensitivity of labelled monoclonal antibodies in recent clinical studies has varied from 40% to 95%.[7,8]

Several advances have occurred recently in tumor detection technology using monoclonals. These include the use of antibody fragments, labelling different sites on the antibody molecule or fragment, enhancement of in vivo antibody clearance, the use of more desirable labelling isotopes such as Tc-99m and I-123, improvements in protein chemistry which minimize damage to the antibody during labelling, and other improvements in antibody production techniques.

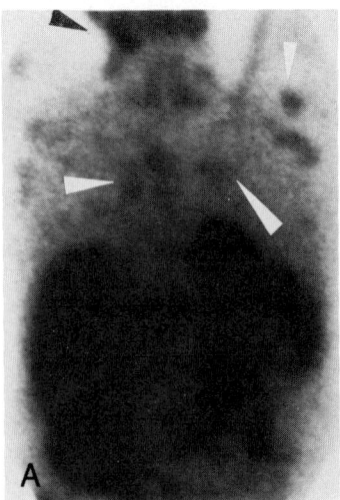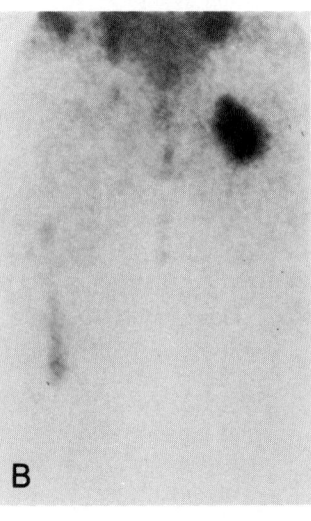

Figure IX-9-1. Tl-201 scan in patient with low-grade lymphoma. (A) Focal uptake of thallium in cervical (dark arrowhead), axillary, and hilar-mediastinal (white arrowheads) lymph nodes, indicating tumor involvement. Intense uptake in liver and spleen and excretion into bowel are nonspecific findings which limit the usefulness of this scanning technique in abdomen and retroperitoneum. (B) Anterior view of lower pelvis and thighs shows intense uptake in left inguinal nodes and in shaft of right femur, indicating lymphomatous involvement.

Widespread clinical use of monoclonal antibodies for tumor detection and staging may not occur for another 3–5 years. While progress has been slow, the results of the most recent clinical trials are extremely encouraging. Figure IX-9-2 depicts a patient with a large subperitoneal deposit from an adenocarcinoma of the colon who was studied 1, 3 and 9 days following injection of an Indium-111 labelled monoclonal antibody, B72.3 (IN-111-CYT-103).

Positron Emission Tomography

Positron emission tomography (PET) is an evolving technology in which positron emitting isotopes of fluorine, nitrogen, carbon or oxygen can be used to detect and characterize tumors. Deoxyglucose labelled with fluorine-18 has been shown to detect lymph node metastases on PET scans of patients with carcinoma of the lung.[17] Detection of metastases to the hilum and mediastinum as small as 1.0 cm have been reported with this method. Whole body techniques are currently being developed using positron detector devices which will permit a "total body screen" for metastases (see Figure IX-8-6). The labelling of many different compounds and biologicals is possible with positron emitters, which in turn creates a wide variety of clinical possibilities for detecting tumors and studying their metabolism.

Recently, fluorine-18 labelled estrogen was used successfully to image human breast cancer. In this study with PET scanning, there was an excellent correlation between tumor uptake and estrogen-receptor concentration, but correlation with progestin-receptor concentration was poor.[23]

As PET detectors are improved and resources for applying this technique increase, it is possible that PET may become a leading modality for noninvasive staging of patients with cancer. Currently, the technology is costly and the production of positron-emitting radiopharmaceuticals requires a cyclotron facility. Government reimbursement is still an issue. However, the applications of this technology within the field of oncology are expected to have a major impact in the near future.

Therapeutic Applications of Radionuclides

I-131 is a beta emitting isotope of iodine which has been used effectively in the treatment of differentiated thyroid cancers. Treatment with I-131 results in a high concentration of radiation delivered selectively to this tumor. Localized doses approaching 50,000 cGy to the tumor are possible. I-131 therapy has resulted in a significant reduction in recurrences and improvements in survival of patients who have differentiated thyroid cancers, when compared to controls in whom I-131 was not used.[4,21]

Radiolabelled monoclonal antibodies are also being used for the investigative treatment of specific tumors including cutaneous B cell lymphoma, Hodgkin's disease, non-Hodgkin's lymphoma, and ovarian cancer.[9] Current research efforts are being directed to improving tumor uptake of antibody as opposed to uptake by normal tissues, thus allowing higher doses of alpha or beta emitting compounds to be administered.

Phosphorus-32 has been used for the treatment of intracavitary tumors for many years. Peritoneal and mesenteric metastases from ovarian carcinoma may be treated with peritoneal infusions of P-32 if chemotherapy is unsuccessful. Intravenous administration of sodium phosphate labelled with P-32 has also been used to treat polycythemia vera.

Clinical trials are now in progress using strontium-89 and samarium-153 to treat painful skeletal metastases in patients with breast or prostate cancers. Preliminary results are encouraging, with bone pain responses approaching 80%.[16]

With specific biologic agents and new radionuclides becoming available, it is important to recognize the increasing potential for therapeutic application of Nuclear Medicine techniques in oncology, and to encourage the oncologist, radiation therapist, and Nuclear Medicine physician to work closely as a team to deliver optimum care for the cancer patient.

References

1. Ancri, D., Basset, J. Y., Lonchampt, M. F., and Etavard, C.: Diagnosis of cerebral lesions by thallium-201. Radiology, 128:417, 1978.
2. Armitage, J. O., Weisenburger, D. D., Hutchins, M., Moravec, D. F., Dowling, M., Sorensen, S., Mailliard, J., Okerbloom, J., Johnson, P. S., Howe, D., Bascome, G. K., Casey, J., Linder, J., and Purtilo, D. T.: Chemotherapy for diffuse large-cell lymphoma–Rapidly responding patients have more durable remissions. J. Clin. Oncol., 4:160, 1986.
3. Bale, W. F., Spar, I. L., Goodland, R. L.: Experimental radiation therapy of tumors with I-131-carrying antibodies to fibrin. Cancer Res., 20:1488, 1960.
4. Beierwaltes, W. H.: The treatment of thyroid carcinoma with radioactive iodine. Semin. Nucl. Med., 8:79, 1978.
5. Collier, B. D., Hellman, R. S., Jr., and Krasnow, A. Z.: Bone SPECT. Semin. Nucl. Med., 17:247, 1987.

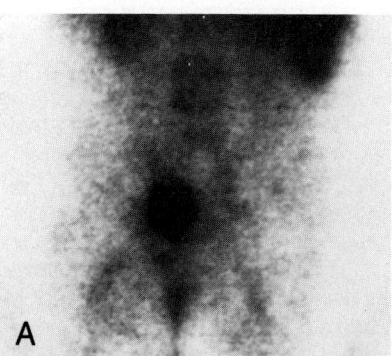 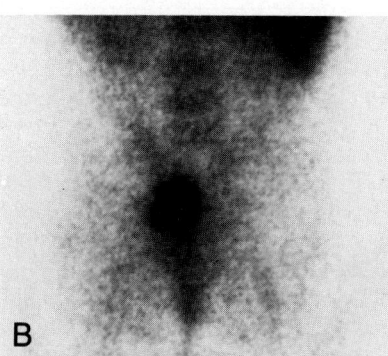 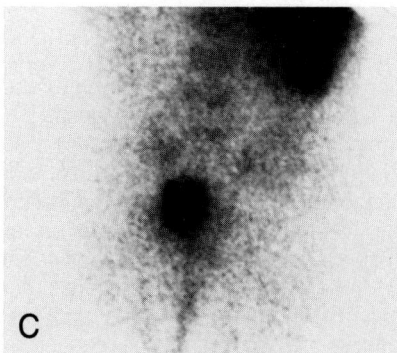

Figure IX-9-2. An indium-111 labelled monoclonal antibody (B72.3) scan targeted to a mucin antigen produced by tumor. Labelled antibody was supplied by the Cytogen Corporation. Adenocarcinoma of colon is located immediately anterior to sacrum, and it was nonresectable at surgery. Note the progressive improvement in target-to-nontarget ratio of antibody uptake on delayed images. Spleen (upper right) also retains the antibody. (A) Day 1; (B) Day 3; (C) Day 9.

6. Ferlin, G., Borsato, M., Camerani, M., Conte, N., and Zotti, D.: New perspectives in localizing enlarged parathyroids by technetium-thallium subtraction scan. J. Nucl. Med., 24:438, 1983.
7. Freeman, L. M., and Blaufox, M. D., editors. *In* Monoclonal Antibodies I. Semin. Nucl. Med., 19(4):157, 1989.
8. Freeman, L. M., Blaufox, M. D., editors. *In* Monoclonal Antibodies II. Semin. Nucl. Med., 19(4):251, 1989.
9. Goldenberg, D. M.: Future role of radiolabeled monoclonal antibodies in oncological diagnosis and therapy. *In* Monoclonal Antibodies II. Edited by L. M. Freeman, and M. D. Blaufox. Semin. Nucl. Med., 19:4, 1989.
10. Hoefnagel, C. A., Delprat, C. C., Marcuse, H. R., and de Vijlder, J. J.: Role of thallium-201 total-body scintigraphy in follow-up of thyroid carcinoma. J. Nucl. Med., 27:1854, 1986.
11. Israel, O., Front, D., Epelbaum, R., Ben-Haim, S., Jerushalmi, J., Kleinhaus, U., Even-Sapir, E., and Robinson, E.: Residual mass and negative gallium scintigraphy in treated lymphoma. J. Nucl. Med., 31:365, 1990.
12. Kaplan, W. D., Jochelson, M., Herman, T., et al.: Ga-67 imaging: A predictor of residual tumor viability in patient with diffuse large cell lymphoma (DLCL). (Abstract). J. Clin. Oncol., 6:230, 1988.
13. Kaplan, W. D., Southee, M. L., Annese, M. S., Jochelson, L. M., and Nadler, L. M.: Evaluating low and intermediate grade non-Hodgkin's lymphoma (NHL) with gallium-67 (Ga) and thallium-201 (Tl) imaging. (Abstract). J. Nucl. Med., 31:793, 1990.
14. Kaplan, W. D., Takvorian, T., Morris, J. H., Rumbaugh, C. L., Connolly, B. T., and Atkins, H. L.: Thallium-201 brain tumor imaging: A comparative study with pathological correlation. J. Nucl. Med., 28:47, 1987.
15. Kim, K. T., Black, K. L., Marciano, D., Mazziotta, J. C., Guze, B. H., Grafton, S., Hawkins, R. A., and Becker, D. P.: Thallium-201 SPECT imaging of brain tumors: Methods and results. J. Nucl. Med., 31:965, 1990.
16. Kloiber, R., Molnar, C. P., and Barnes, M.: Sr-89 therapy for metastatic bone disease: Scintigraphic and Radiographic follow-up. Radiology, 163:719, 1987.
17. Knopp, M. V., Strauss, L. G., Haberkorn, U., Dimitrakopoulou, A., Bischoff, H., Manke, H., Oberdorfer, F., Ostertag, H., and Lorenz, W. J.: Optimizing therapy management unresectable bronciogenic carcinoma by metabolic imaging with PET. (Abstract). J. Nucl. Med., 31:767, 1990.
18. Lee, V. W., Rosen, M. P., Baum, A., Cohen, S. E., Cooley, T. P., and Liebman, H. A.: AIDS-related Kaposi Sarcoma: Findings on thallium-201 scintigraphy. A. J. R., 151:1233, 1988.
19. Levenson, R. M., Sauerbrunn, B. J., Bates, H. R., Newman, R. D., Eddy, J. L., and Ihde, D. C.: Comparative value of bone scintigraphy and radiography in monitoring tumor response in systemically treated prostatic carcinoma. Radiology, 146:513, 1983.
20. MacFarlane, S. D., Hanelin, L. G., Taft, D. A., Ryan, J. A., Jr., and Fredlund, P. N.: Localization of abnormal parathyroid glands using thallium-201. Am. J. Surg., 148:7, 1984.
21. Mazzaferri, E. L., and Young, R. L.: Papillary thyroid carcinoma: A 10 year follow-up report of the impact of therapy in 576 patients. Am. J. Med., 7:511, 1981.
22. McNeil, B. J.: Value of bone scanning in neoplastic disease. Seminars in Nucl. Med., 14:277, 1984.
23. Mintun, M. A., Welch, M. J., Siegel, B. A., Mathias, C. J., Brodack, J. W., McGuire, A. H., and Katzenellenbogen, J. A.: Breast cancer: PET imaging of estrogen-receptors. Radiology, 169:45, 1988.
24. Mountz, J. M., Stafford-Schuck, K., McKeever, P., Liebert, M., Raymond, P., Taren, J. A., and Beierwaltes, W. H.: The tumor/cardiac ratio: A new method to estimate residual high grade astrocytoma using thallium-201. (Abstract). J. Nucl. Med., 707, 1987.
25. Paulson, D. F.: The impact of current staging procedures in assessing disease extent of prostatic adenocarcinoma. J. Urol., 121:300, 1979.
26. Picard, D., D'Amour, P., Carrier, L., Chartrand, R., and Poisson, R.: Localization of abnormal parathyroid gland(s) using thallium-201/iodine 123 subtraction scintigraphy in patients with primary hyperpara-thyroidism. Clin. Nucl. Med., 12:60, 1987.
27. Pressman, D.: The development and use of radiolabeled antitumor antibodies. Cancer Res., 40:2960, 1980.
28. Ramanna, L., Waxman, A. D., Binny, G., Waxman, S., Brachman, M. B., Tanasescu, D. E., Tourje, J. E., and Pressman, B. D.: Increasing specificity of brain scintigraphy using thallium-201. J. Nucl. Med., (Abstract) 28:658, 1987.
29. Ramanna, L., Waxman, A., Binney, G., Waxman, S., Mirra, J., and Rosen, G.: Thallium-201 scintigraphy in bone sarcoma: Comparison with gallium-67 and technetium-MDP in the evaluation of chemotherapeutic response. J. Nucl. Med., 31:567, 1990.
30. Ramanna, L., Waxman, A. D., Brachman, M. B., Tanasescu, D., and Braunstein, G.: T1-201 (T1) and I-131 discordance in pts with differentiated thyroid CA (DTC): Is there a rationale for T1 thyroglobin (Tg) screening? J. Nucl. Med., (Abstract) 29:753, 1988.
31. Sessler, M. J., Geck, P., Maul, F. D., Hop, G., and Munz, D. L.: New aspects of cellular T1-201 uptake: T^+-Na^+-2 Cl^--cotransport is the central mechanism of ION uptake. Nucl. Med., 25:24, 1986.
32. Strender, L. E., Lagergren, C., Wallgren, A., and Liljevall, S.: Role of bone scans in the initial assessment of operable patients with breast cancer. Acta Radiol. Oncol., 20:187, 1981.
33. Tonami, N., Bunko, H., Michigishi, T., Kuwajima, A., and Hisada, K.: Clinical application of thallium-201 scintigraphy in patients with cold thyroid nodules. Clin. Nucl. Med., 3:217, 1978.
34. Waxman, A. D., Ramanna, L., Brachman, M. B., Gleishman, S., and Brenner, J.: Thallium scintigraphy in primary carcinoma of the breast: Evaluations of primary and axillary metastasis. J. Nucl. Med., (Abstract) 30:844, 1989.
35. Waxman, A. D., Ramanna, L., Memsic, A., Silberman, A., and Brenner, J.: Thallium scintigraphy in the differentation of malignant from benign mass abnormalities of the breast. J. Nucl. Med., (Abstract) 31:767, 1990.
37. Wylie, B. R., Southee, A. E., Joshua, D. E., McLaughlin, A. F., Gibson, J., Hutton, B. F., Morris, J. G., and Kronenberg, H.: Gallium screening in the management of mediastinal Hodgkin's disease. Eur. J. Haematol., 42:344, 1989.
38. Young, A. E., Gaunt, J. L., Croft, D. N., Collins, R. E., Wells, C. P., and Coakley, A. J.: Location of parathyroid adenomas by thallium-201 and technetium-99m subtraction scanning. Br. Med. J., 286:1384, 1983.

IX-10

Perspectives in Imaging

Richard J. Steckel

A number of new, or imminent, developments in diagnostic imaging which have potential import for the detection, diagnosis, staging and followup of cancer patients have been described in the preceding chapters of this section. They include rapid MR imaging sequences which will mitigate the problem of motion during MRI examinations, new scanning agents, Doppler ultrasound, as well as endoluminal (e.g., endovaginal, endorectal, endoesophageal and endobronchial) ultrasound scanning techniques, and other improvements in existing modalities. New applications of PET (positron emission tomography) to cancer management also appear to be on the horizon. These include not only new compounds to evaluate tumor metabolism with PET scanning, but also new approaches to multiplanar imaging of the entire body using the PET principle to evaluate tumors (Fig-

ure IX-10-1). Also under development are scanning agents which have greater specificity for certain tumors, including "designer compounds" which attach to epitopes that are concentrated on the surfaces of tumor cells and not on surrounding normal cells (Plate IX-2, courtesy of K. L. Black, MD, Division of Neurosurgery, UCLA School of Medicine). In vivo imaging capability of the ligand for benzodiazepine receptors in Plate IX-2, using a radionuclide "tag" for external scanning, is currently being studied for possible application to clinical diagnosis and staging of brain tumors. Even more important perhaps than engineering and biotechnologic developments which can be anticipated over the next several years, is the need for a more concerted evaluation of existing diagnostic imaging methods and their appropriate applications to cancer management: We now have a plethora

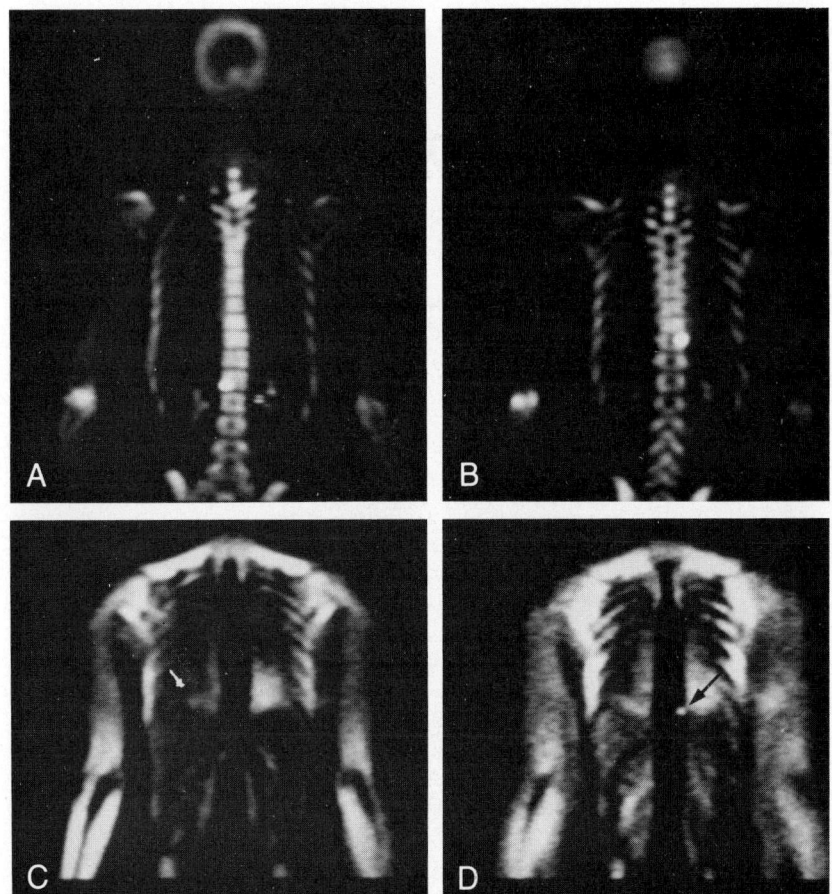

Figure IX-10-1. A and B: Anterior coronal images of a fluorine-18 PET bone scan in a patient with breast cancer demonstrating focal activity at several levels of the spine. In (A), focal osteoblastic activity is evident in metastatic lesions at T1 and T12 levels. In (B), at a slightly more posterior level, focal uptake is seen at T10 level. On both images, "hot" area is noted in right antecubital fossa at radionuclide injection site. C and D: Posterior coronal images of 18-fluoro-deoxy-glucose scan of the same patient. In (C), focal increase in metabolic activity is confirmed at site of metastatic lesion in pedicle and transverse process of T10 (white arrow). In (D), similar increase in metabolic activity is seen in T12 vertebra (black arrow).

of imaging techniques available to us, without sufficient data to use them in the most efficient manner to detect and diagnose cancer, to guide treatment and followup care, and to prevent morbidity. Accelerating medical costs will force us to take the difficult steps that are needed to evaluate our present imaging methodologies systematically for their contributions to clinical cancer management and to determine their appropriate places, relative to one another and to non-imaging studies in our diagnostic armamentarium. In this introductory presentation we have touched upon many unresolved issues concerning the appropriate use of diagnostic imaging techniques in cancer medicine that still call for careful investigation.

X

Interventional Radiology

Sidney Wallace
C. Humberto Carrasco
Chusilp Charnsangavej

Introduction

Utilizing imaging that best defines the target organ, the interventional radiologist applies percutaneous procedures for a more aggressive and invasive approach to the diagnosis and management of the patient with cancer.[79] Both percutaneous vascular and nonvascular interventional radiologic techniques, adapted from established surgical procedures, are done more rapidly and efficiently.[78] At the University of Texas M. D. Anderson Cancer Center (MDACC) more than 3,000 interventional radiologic procedures are performed each year which include biopsy and drainage; intra-arterial infusion, embolization and chemoembolization; reposition of central venous catheters; placement of metallic stents and inferior vena caval filters; and intravascular foreign body retrieval, among others.

Biopsy

Almost all tissues, including the myocardium, are accessible to percutaneous biopsy. Its success depends upon the expertise and interest of the radiologist and the cytologist. A variety of needles (14g to 25g) as well as biopsy forceps are efficient in obtaining representative specimens. Superficial palpable masses are biopsied by the cytologist while others requiring imaging techniques–fluoroscopy, ultrasonography (US), computed tomography (CT) and magnetic resonance imaging (MRI)–are sampled by the radiologist. Most biopsies of lesions in adults are scheduled electively on an outpatient basis. Prothrombin time, partial thromboplastin time and platelet counts are necessary and any correctable coagulopathies are remedied. Intravenous sedation and local analgesia are usually adequate while general anesthesia is reserved for children. After the biopsy, the patient is observed for approximately one hour before discharge from the radiology department.

Thoracic. Guidance by fluoroscopy or CT is usually adequate for biopsy of the lung or mediastinum. The reported accuracy (sensitivity) of percutaneous transthoracic needle biopsy of patients with lung cancer is 90–98%.[72,83] The results for pulmonary metastases are virtually the same as for a primary neoplasm. Lymphangitic carcinoma can be defined in approximately 50%.[83] The diagnostic yield by percutaneous biopsy for focal pulmonary infection in the immunocompromised patients was reported as 73%.[17] Positive cytology was disclosed in 72% of attempted biopsies of mediastinal masses with a 9% incidence of complications.[66] The major complication of lung biopsy is pneumothorax which occurs in 15–30% with 5% necessitating a thoracic tube which can be placed by the interventional radiologist.[83]

Breast. The combination of the clinical examination, mammography and cytology establishes a correct diagnosis of malignancy in 95–98% of breast lesions.[46] At MDACC, cytology, especially with ultrasonography for guidance, yields positive results in 75–80% of suspicious lesions.[29] Localization of small lesions, less than 1 cm in diameter, for surgical excision is frequently accomplished utilizing mammography.

Abdomen. Guided by fluoroscopy, US, CT and more recently MRI, 84–93% of patients biopsied yielded adequate diagnostic material for cytologic analysis. Using 20g–23g needle biopsies of the liver, pancreas, kidney, adrenal, spleen and ovary among others were accomplished with a sensitivity of 86.6%, a specificity of 98.6%, and an accuracy of 90%.[57] The overall complication rate in another study of 63,180 biopsies was 0.16%.[73] Seeding of malignant cells along the needle tract was 0.05%.

Lymph Nodes. Metastatic lymphadenopathy from carcinoma can be detected by fine needle aspiration (FNA) directed by fluoroscopy of lymph nodes opacified by lymphography, CT or US with a high degree of accuracy of 83–95%.[33,89] At MDACC the accuracy of needle biopsy of lymph nodes involved by lymphoma has improved from 54% to 80% with the help of immunocytochemical cell markers, DNA flow cytometry, cytogenetics, molecular studies, cytospin and cell block for cytology (Figure X-1-1).[15]

Musculoskeletal. The diagnostic accuracy of percutaneous skeletal biopsy is 80% with a range of 50–94%.[13] At MDACC an overall diagnostic accuracy of 78.6% was reported

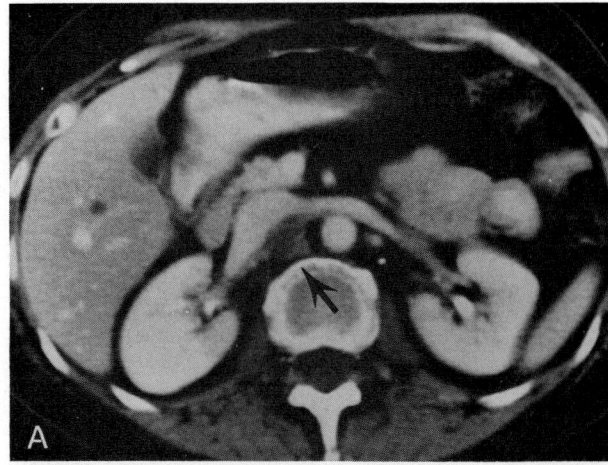

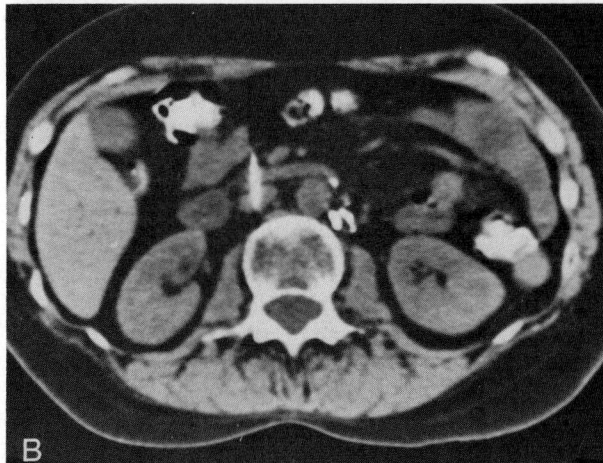

Figure X-1-1. Percutaneous lymph node biopsy, CT guidance. A. 2-cm mass (arrow) is noted behind the inferior vena cava and right renal vein in a patient with previously treated lymphoma. B. Percutaneous biopsy (note vertical biopsy needle) revealed recurrent lymphoma.

in a series of 178 patients with primary skeletal tumors who underwent percutaneous needle biopsy, more accurate in malignant neoplasms (83%) than in benign tumors (64.2%).[6] In unsuspected infectious diseases the frequency of positive bacterial cultures has been low.[13,75]

Drainage Procedures

Percutaneous catheter drainage of obstructed urinary, biliary and gastrointestinal tracts as well as abnormal fluid collections such as abscesses, bilomas, urinomas, and lymphocysts is accomplished under radiologic guidance utilizing the Seldinger technique with needle, wire and catheter.[14]

Nephrostomy. In cancer patients, urinary tract obstruction usually develops as the result of compression or direct extension of primary or metastatic neoplasms in the pelvis or retroperitoneum. Less frequently, obstruction in these patients is caused by calculi or benign strictures. Metastases to the urinary tract occur in only 2–5% of patients who die of malignant neoplasms.[48] Percutaneous nephrostomy is performed to improve renal function and decrease blood pressure, to treat sepsis in cases of pyonephrosis and to divert flow away

from a urinary fistula. It is particularly important in patients whose therapy will include agents that depend on renal excretion and are also potentially nephrotoxic. The decision to perform a nephrostomy takes into consideration the patient's expected survival and the available therapeutic options. The mortality rate for percutaneous nephrostomy is less than 0.2%.[38] The 0.7% incidence of complications immediately following the nephrostomy procedure consisted of hemorrhage, septicemia and endotoxic shock.[38] Although clinically detectable retroperitoneal hemorrhage is unusual, computed tomography detected its presence in 13% of patients.[27]

Ureteral stents, internal-external or indwelling, offer a more comfortable alternative to nephrostomy for long term urinary tract decompression. Permanent nephrostomy and ureteral stenting provide adequate palliation for ureteral obstructions by malignant neoplasms. In cancer patients, benign fibrotic ureteral strictures may occur after pelvic surgery, at ureteral anastomotic sites and, less frequently, after radiation therapy. In a series of 44 patients with benign ureteral strictures, immediately successful dilatation was accomplished in 48% of the patients.[8] The best results are achieved in patients with relatively recent strictures, whereas balloon dilatation of longstanding severely fibrotic strictures is more likely to fail. Other endourological methods of treating strictures include endoscopic incision and electrolysis.

Ureteral fistulas usually occur secondary to anastomotic leakage, inadvertent ligation or transection during surgery, ischemia, radiation therapy or neoplastic invasion of the ureter. A rare complication is a ureteroarterial fistula caused by erosion of the stent into the common iliac artery where it is crossed by the ureter.[1] Treating malignant distal ureteric and vesical fistulas with surgical urinary diversion is not usually justified. Percutaneous nephrostomy may offer some palliation to patients extremely incapacitated by urinary tract fistulas (cutaneous, vaginal or rectal) but only when performed in conjunction with complete ureteral occlusion will flow through the fistula cease. Ureteral occlusion with butyl-2-cyano-acrylate has been only temporary, but detachable balloons seem to provide a longer lasting occlusion.[34,35]

Biliary Drainage. Percutaneous drainage of an obstructed biliary system is achieved by inserting a catheter through the hepatic parenchyma into the bile duct. The endoscopic approach is employed with increasing frequency. Three types of biliary drainage are performed percutaneously—external, combined external-internal and drainage through indwelling stents. Percutaneous drainage is an important adjunct to palliative treatment of inoperable cancer patients in whom it is performed to improve the metabolic and nutritional status, provide relief of pruritus and allow the administration of chemotherapeutic agents which require unimpeded biliary excretion evidenced by low serum bilirubin levels. In addition, percutaneous drainage is used to treat acute suppurative cholangitis, in failed bilioenteric bypass and for diversion of bile flow in treating bile leaks and fistulas where it may be used in conjunction with percutaneous drainage of the extraductal bile collections.

In 131 patients at MDACC with cancer, the overall median survival from the time of percutaneous drainage until death was only 57 days.[16] The short survival time reflects the terminal nature of these patients with biliary obstruction who frequently undergo the procedure before starting chemotherapy for their neoplasms. Patients who underwent subsequent biliary bypass had a better median survival time (172 days) suggesting the better clinical status of the surgical candidates, most of whom had carcinoma of the pancreas, in which jaundice often occurs relatively early.

The acute complications of biliary drainage are those due to the procedure, whereas delayed complications are related to chronic catheter drainage. The incidence of acute complications is low; a review of 200 patients showed sepsis in 7, hemorrhage in 6 and death in 3. Fever and hemobilia occurred in 21 and 18 patients respectively.[50] Cholangitis, the most frequent complication in chronic drainage was experienced by 47% of 161 patients. This often happened during periods of myelosuppression. Dislodgement of the catheter was noted in 18% and in 14% the catheter became occluded.[16] Intrahepatic vascular lesions including pseudoaneurysms and arterioportal fistulas have been reported in 26–33% but are usually asymptomatic.[36,55] Pleural empyema, hemothorax, pneumothorax and bilious pleural effusion may occur in 1–2.5% of patients.[50,56] A cholerrhagic state with bile output of 7L per day was seen in 5% of our patients.[16] It is usually temporary but it creates severe fluid and electrolyte loss with hypotension and hyponatremia requiring aggressive replacement therapy.

The adequacy of catheter drainage depends on the physical properties of the catheter material, its luminal diameter, its length and the total area of its inflow and outflow side holes as well as the pressure gradient and the type of fluid being drained. Although stents larger than 8 to 10F are best for internal drainage, their transhepatic insertion is painful and requires a well-established tract. A combined peroral-transhepatic method and an endoscopic technique have been described for passage of larger endoprostheses.[40,71] Multiple endoprostheses can be placed adjacent to one another. More recently expandable metallic stents are being evaluated but thus far mucosal hypertrophy and tumor ingrowth through interstices limit their usefulness.

Percutaneous Gastrostomy. Percutaneous gastrostomy offers a useful route for nutritional support in patients who have esophageal and head and neck neoplasms that compromise swallowing function. Those patients who have chronic intestinal obstruction caused by unresectable neoplasms and those who have multiple enteric strictures secondary to irradiation need decompressive gastrostomies. Although previously considered exclusively a surgical procedure, endoscopic creation of a gastrostomy through a gastroscope perforating outward has been described in 1983. The patients with an obstructive lesion involving the pharynx and esophagus were excluded from that study.[62] In 1979, percutaneous placement of a gastrostomy through the skin and stomach penetrating inward was done in two patients with previously discontinued Stamm gastrostomies and in 1981 percutaneous gastrostomies without complications were reported in 17 patients with a Stamey percutaneous cystostomy catheter.[63,68]

Percutaneous gastrostomy was performed in 100 cancer patients at MDACC.[54] In 67 patients with bowel obstruction the procedure was done for gastric drainage with 24–28F Malecot catheters inserted in one sitting. The remaining 33 patients had supragastric obstructions or fistulas and required 10–14F pigtail catheters for feeding purposes. The average postgastrostomy hospitalization was 3.6 days. Drainage gastrostomies were ready for use immediately after the procedure, whereas the use of feeding gastrostomies started an average of two days after tube insertion. There were no major complications or deaths related to the procedure. Percutaneous gastrostomy is a simple safe technique even when large caliber catheters are used and it does not require gastric fixation to the abdominal wall to prevent spillage into the peritoneum.

Abscess Drainage. In patients with cancer, an intra-abdominal abscess is life-threatening, usually caused by perforation of a hollow viscus affected by a neoplasm or by a postoperative complication. A septic episode is often accompanied by renal, pulmonary or cardiovascular failure, and when untreated has a mortality rate of nearly 100%. Thirty-six percent of intra-abdominal abscesses are located intraperitoneally, 38% retroperitoneally, and 26% are visceral.[4]

Computed tomography, ultrasonography and radionuclide scintigraphy are used to diagnose and localize abscesses. The radiologic features are nonspecific and must be differentiated from biloma, urinoma, lymphocele, seroma, pancreatic pseudocyst, hematoma, neoplasm, and fluid-filled viscus. Cross-sectional scans are used to determine the depth, the cutaneous entry site and the angle through which the collection is best approached.[32,37]

A diagnostic fine needle (21–22g) puncture is made and a sample taken for gram stain and culture. If the gram stain is negative, the remaining fluid is aspirated for bacterial culture and cytologic assay and the needle is withdrawn. A catheter may be left in place until the results of the culture are known but no longer than 48 hours to avoid infecting a sterile collection. A drainage catheter is inserted if the presence of infection has been confirmed.

Selection of a safe route for diagnostic puncture and drainage is the most crucial aspect of the procedure. Nonviscous collections are drained adequately by 6–10F catheters which are also used to drain renal and hepatic parenchymal abscesses.[52] For viscous nonparenchymal collections 12–14F sump catheters are employed. Irrigating drainage catheters with saline, chemical or antibiotic solutions is usually not necessary and may disseminate the infection. If the exudate is viscous, gentle irrigation with 5–10 ml of physiologic solution may be necessary to maintain catheter patency. Drainage of simple abscesses usually ceases by the 5th to 10th day. With an associated fistula, drainage may persist for weeks.[70] Successful percutaneous drainage was accomplished in 83.6% of 250 abdominal abscesses and fluid collections with 21 failures and 20 recurrences.[77] Treatment failures occurred with multiloculated abscesses and with cellulitis associated with fistulas, viscous hematomas or organized collections. The overall complication rate was 10% (3% severe and 7% minor) which included septicemia, infection of a previously sterile cavity, bowel perforation and one death.

Intra-Arterial Therapy

Intra-arterial management of patients with neoplasms by the percutaneous transcatheter approach necessitates the participation of chemotherapist, surgeon, radiotherapist and the interventional radiologist in the infusion of chemotherapeutic agents, embolization and chemoembolization.

Infusion

Most cytotoxic agents have a steep dose-response curve; that is, the higher the concentration, the greater the tumor effect.[31] Intra-arterial infusion exposes the neoplasm to a higher local concentration of chemotherapy with no increase in systemic toxicity but frequently an increase in local side effects. The pharmacokinetics of regional chemotherapy will be discussed in detail in a later chapter (XV-4). Those agents most effective when delivered systemically should be the initial choice for intra-arterial therapy. Neoplasms refractory to intravenous chemotherapy may respond to the intra-arterial infusion of the same drugs at the same dose rate. Those drugs tolerated by the local tissues can be administered intra-arterially, while others can be delivered intravenously at the same time or sequentially. Doxorubicin and the vinca-alkaloids are local irritants which cause endarteritis and are better tolerated by the liver than the extremities. Intra-arterial delivery, however, can be accomplished even with these agents by decreasing the dose per unit of time and extending the infusion over a longer period.

Hypervascular neoplasms act as a sump to draw the blood and chemotherapy almost exclusively to the tumor. Intra-arterial delivery is even more essential for hypovascular neoplasms to increase the drug concentration to the neoplasm which may be associated with a higher incidence of local complications.

The delivery of chemotherapeutic agents requires selective arterial catheterization which is accomplished by tailoring the catheter configuration to the vascular anatomy.[21] A nonthrombogenic environment is created by systemic heparinization (15,000–25,000 units of aqueous heparin over each 24 hours) injected intra-arterially or intravenously maintaining the clotting parameters at 1.5 to 2 times normal.[82] Heparin and doxorubicin are incompatible and must be infused through different catheters; one intravenous while the other is intra-arterial.

Occlusion for Infusion. Temporary or permanent occlusion of branch vessels using Gelfoam segments and/or stainless steel coils can minimize the exposure of normal tissues and maximize the infusion of the tumor. This is especially helpful in the pelvis where the superior and inferior gluteal arteries are occluded to decrease the chemodermatitis in the buttocks and to increase the concentration to neoplasms of pelvic viscera.[84] Occlusion of the superficial temporal and middle meningeal arteries directs flow into the internal maxillary artery in treating neoplasms of the maxillary sinuses. The gastroduodenal artery may be occluded at its junction with the common hepatic artery to lessen gastric, duodenal and pancreatic complications.[25] Selective occlusion is not associated with ischemia because of adequate collateral circulation.

Alteration of the vascular supply by selective occlusion of most of the major vessels contributing to the neoplasm allows a single artery through collateral circulation to supply the entire organ and neoplasm. This is especially effective in converting multiple arteries supplying the liver to a single artery to be infused through a single catheter.[24]

Pulsatile Flow. The flow rate for intra-arterial infusion is 50–200 ml/hr delivered at constant pump pressure. This slow rate results in laminar flow or streaming and unequal distribution of the chemotherapeutic agent. A pulsatile pump (Pulser, Cook Inc., Bloomington, IN) devised by Gianturco can be attached to the constant infusion pump to create turbulence at the tip of the catheter dispersing the infusate.[86] The Pulser has been helpful in significantly improving distribution in 20% of patients treated by hepatic arterial infusion and controlling chemodermatitis in 90% of the children with osteosarcoma of the extremity treated by arterial infusion.

Flow Studies. Radionuclide flow studies are used routinely to evaluate distribution following catheter placement for intra-arterial chemotherapy infusion.[40] One to 5 mCi of Technetium 99^m macro-aggregated albumin (MAA) in a volume of 0.5–1 cc is delivered by a mechanical pump at a rate similar to that of the chemotherapy infusion. Scintigraphy of the area of interest is obtained; flow distribution is evaluated as to tumor uptake, normal adjacent organ uptake and systemic escape. This information assists the prediction of tumor response, the possibility of complications and dose adjustment.

Therapeutic Agents for Intra-Arterial Delivery. The cytotoxic agents delivered by the intra-arterial route include 5FU, floxuridine (FUDR), doxorubicin (Adriamycin), mitoxantrone, bleomycin, methotrexate, cisplatin, carboplatin, cyclophosphamide, ifosfamide (ifex), dacarbazine (DTIC), vincristine (VCR), vinblastine(VLB), vindesine, mitomycin C, etoposide (VP16-213), phenylalanine mustard (Melphalan), nitrogen mustard (mechlorethamine), actinomycin-D, aziridinyl-benzoquinone (AZQ), acridinylanisidide (AMSA), and streptozotocin. Immunomodifiers that have been administered intra-arterially include interferon, interleukin-2, tumor necrosis factor (TNF), Bacille Calmette Guerin (BCG) and corynebacterium parvum. Almost all water soluble antibiotics can be delivered intra-arterially. Corticosteroids have also been administered by this route. Before the use of a new agent intra-arterially, laboratory examination is necessary to determine the tolerated dose to the patient, the organ and the artery infused.

Embolization

Embolization is the occlusion of the arterial supply of the tumor to create ischemia, tumor necrosis and to arrest tumor growth by the intra-arterial delivery of particulate materials, sclerosing solutions and substances introduced in the liquid state that eventually solidify. Interruption of a vessel at its origin has an effect similar to that of a surgical ligation. Collateral circulation is available immediately; the more central the occlusion, the more abundant the collateral circulation. The closer the occlusion is to the tumor, the smaller is the opportunity for collateral circulation.

The materials available for embolization include autologous clot and tissue, clot modified by thrombin, epsilon aminocaproic acid (Amicar), and heat; absorbable gelatin sponge (Gelfoam); oxidized cellulose (Oxycel); polyvinyl alcohol foam (Ivalon); cyanoacrylates; silastic, resin and dextran microspheres (Dowex, Sephadex, and Spherex); Ethibloc; microfibrillar collagen hemostat (Avitene, Angiostat); sodium tetradecyl sulphate (Sotradecol); absolute alcohol; balloon catheters and detachable balloons; and metallic devices such as brushes and stainless steel coils.

In general, at MDACC, peripheral embolization is accomplished with absorbable gelatin sponge particles or powder (Gelfoam) or polyvinyl alcohol foam (Ivalon) granules, and central occlusion with absorbable gelatin sponge segments or stainless steel coils.

The indications for transcatheter embolization of neoplasms are: 1) to control hemorrhage; 2) preoperatively, to facilitate surgical resection by decreasing blood loss and operating time; 3) to inhibit tumor growth; and 4) to relieve pain by decreasing tumor bulk (Fig. X-1-2).

Chemoembolization

This technique as proposed by Kato et al is the combination of intra-arterial infusion of chemotherapeutic agents and arterial embolization of the vascular supply to the neoplasm.[41] In addition to the direct effect of ischemia on the neoplasm by occlusion, the emboli prolong the transit time

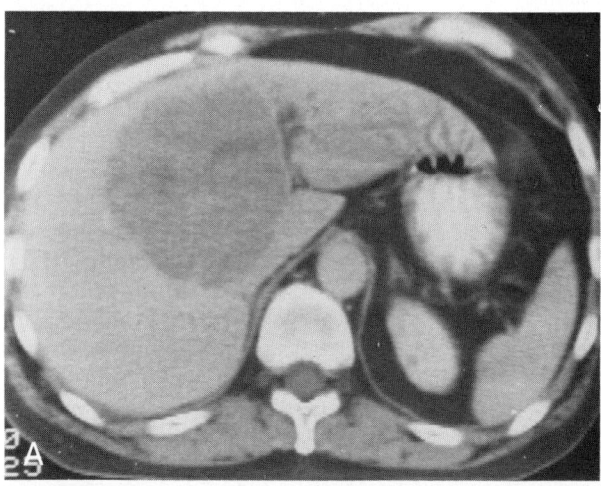

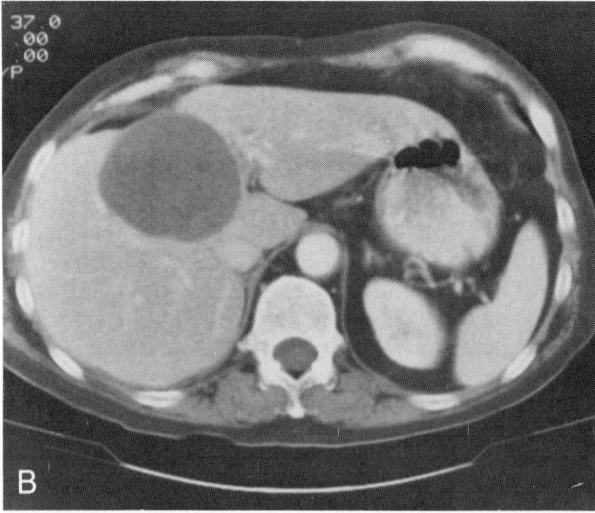

Figure X-1-2. Sequential embolization. A. This inoperable metastasis from an adrenal cortical carcinoma was treated by transcatheter embolization with Ivalon. B. The right and left lobes treated one month apart demonstrate an excellent response.

through the tumor vascular bed, theoretically increasing the contact time between the chemotherapeutic agent and the neoplastic cell. The increased local drug concentration is enhanced by the increased tissue permeability caused by anoxia. The overall effect is cytotoxic not only to the neoplasm but to the vessels embolized and infused, compounding the vasculitis and occlusion. The systemic toxic effect may be reduced by metabolism of the drug on its first passage through the infused organ, thereby confining the higher concentration to the target organ.

Mitomycin C has been incorporated in ethylcellulose microcapsules (225 μm in diameter) for gradual and sustained release.[41] Starch microspheres (40 μm in diameter), injected prior to the intra-arterial infusion of chemotherapy are gradually degraded by serum amylase to slow flow and increase contact time.[5,28] In Japan, management of hepatocellular carcinoma and to a lesser extent hepatic metastases includes the intra-arterial delivery of gelfoam, Lipiodol and chemotherapeutic agents, primarily mitomycin C but at times adriamycin, actinomycin D, neocarcinostatin or cisplatin.[53,88] Ethibloc, a solution of prolamine in alcohol has also been used in Europe in combination with pulverized lyophilized cytotoxic drugs, mitomycin C (10 mg), adriamycin (25 mg) and cisplatin (25 mg).[42]

At MDACC, Ivalon or Gelfoam has been vigorously combined with cisplatin, mitomycin C, floxuridine, adriamycin, actinomycin-D, streptozotocin, and Bacille Calmette-Guerin (BCG) for chemoembolization.[18] These combinations frequently increase tumor response but also increase local toxicity. In our laboratory, floxuridine (FUDR) and cisplatin have been encapsulated in 100 μm particles; cisplatin and iodine-containing contrast materials have been formulated into 1 μm degradable and nondegradable microcapsules for chemoembolization.[87]

Hemorrhage

The control of hemorrhage in patients with neoplastic diseases is often a life-saving procedure and may allow the opportunity for more specific antitumor therapy by surgery, irradiation or chemotherapy. Low grade chronic bleeding from a neoplasm may be managed by the intra-arterial infusion of chemotherapy directly to the tumor. Otherwise embolization may be necessary but this too has its limitations and may be temporary.

Gastrointestinal. The intravenous infusion of vasopressin (Pitressin), the preferred treatment for bleeding from esophageal varices, is at times effective in the management of diffuse gastrointestinal hemorrhage as seen in patients with leukemia and lymphoma. Intra-arterial vasopressin usually is ineffective in the control of gastrointestinal bleeding from malignant neoplasms but is used in the treatment of a hemorrhage of benign etiology in the cancer patient.[9]

Gastrointestinal bleeding from neoplasms of the liver, stomach, duodenum and rectosigmoid as well as from radiation change, especially in the rectum, is more readily controlled by embolization of the hepatic, left gastric, gastroduodenal, superior and inferior pancreaticoduodenal, inferior mesenteric or internal iliac arteries.[22,26] Rarely, extremely selective limited embolization of short segments of the superior and inferior mesenteric arteries may be possible but ischemia with infarction is a more frequent and catastrophic complication.[20,26,64]

Embolization may also be the preferred management of bleeding from a benign cause in a patient with cancer. Hemobilia as the result of catheter placement for biliary drainage may be controlled by embolization of the traumatized branch of the hepatic artery.[61]

Genitourinary. Hemorrhage from neoplasms of the genitourinary tract has been treated successfully by the intra-arterial infusion of chemotherapy if the bleeding is chronic or by intra-arterial embolization. This has been accomplished in patients with neoplasms of the bladder, uterine cervix and corpus. Bleeding caused by irradiation cystitis may be controlled by bilateral internal iliac artery embolization.[45,69]

A chronically indwelling ureterostomy catheter may erode the ureter into the adjacent common iliac artery creating a uretero-arterial fistula resulting in intermittent massive hematuria.[76] The interventional radiologist can occlude the artery and the fistula with coils after the vascular surgeon by-passes the vessel to be occluded.

Gastrointestinal Neoplasms

Hepatocellular Carcinoma. Our intra-arterial regimen consists of an infusion of FUDR ($100 \ mg/m^2/day \times 5$), adriamycin ($40 \ mg/m^2$) and mitomycin C ($10 \ mg/m^2$). The treatment is repeated every four weeks. A response rate of 62% was achieved; the median survival was 11.5 months. With associated hepatic artery occlusion, the median survival was 17 months.[50]

Yamada and colleagues reported 1, 2, and 3 year survival rates of 44%, 29% and 15% respectively in 120 patients with hepatocellular carcinoma treated by chemoembolization using gelfoam and mitomycin C or adriamycin.[7] Ohishi and colleagues used gelfoam with lipiodol and mitomycin C or adriamycin resulting in a one year survival rate of 69% among 97 patients treated. A significant decrease in serum alpha-fetoprotein was observed in 90% of patients.[60]

In patients with inoperable hepatocellular carcinoma, our current protocol is chemoembolization with Ivalon and floxuridine (400 mg), adriamycin (50 mg) and mitomycin (10 mg) or cisplatin (50–100 mg).

Metastatic Colorectal Carcinoma. Hepatic metastases from carcinoma of the colon have a 20% response rate when treated by intravenous 5FU. Intra-arterial therapy through surgically or radiologically placed catheters has response rates ranging from 44–88% based on varied criteria including clinical examination, carcinoembryonic antigen or scanning techniques (computed tomography, ultrasonography, radionuclide scintigraphy and/or magnetic resonance imaging). Despite effective control of hepatic metastases, extrahepatic disease is eventually the major cause of death.[7,50,51,60]

The chemotherapy regimen at MDACC consists of FUDR ($100 \ mg/m^2$ infused continuously over 24 hours each day for five days and mitomycin C (added at $10 \ mg/m^2$ infused over two hours on the first day). The treatment is repeated every four weeks for at least three cycles. In another regimen, mitomycin C is replaced by cisplatin ($100 \ mg/m^2$ over two hours on the first day).

For the FUDR and mitomycin C regimen, the response rate for intra-arterial therapy in those patients who had previously failed systemic 5FU was 45%; a 61% response rate was achieved in previously untreated patients.[50,60] The median survival time for responders was 16 months. A response rate of 52% was found in patients who were treated with FUDR and cisplatin.

More recently, there has been an increased interest in the use of chemoembolization for the treatment of metastases to the liver from colorectal carcinoma. In general, the protocols used for intra-arterial infusion combined with embolic material are our initial choices for chemoembolization. Thus far, FUDR (up to 800 mg) or cisplatin (150 mg) added to Ivalon and/or Gelfoam used sequentially each month for three months has produced less than dramatic results.

Patients with colorectal cancer whose pelvic disease has recurred following initial treatment with radiotherapy and intravenous chemotherapy (5FU) have been effectively managed by bilateral internal iliac artery infusion of 5FU ($500 \ mg/m^2/day$ for five days) and mitomycin C ($10 \ mg/m^2$ over two hours). Eleven of the 15 patients who complained of pelvic pain had significant relief of symptoms. Cisplatin ($100 \ mg/m^2$ over two hours) was substituted for mitomycin C with similar results.

Metastatic Anal Carcinoma. All three patients with hepatic metastases from carcinoma of the anus recently treated with FUDR ($100 \ mg/m^2/day$ for five days and cisplatin ($100 \ mg/m^2$ over two hours) intra-arterially have responded.[3]

Metastatic Breast Carcinoma. Several regimens have been used for hepatic artery infusion of chemotherapy in patients with hepatic metastases from carcinoma of the breast, but these are used mostly as second line treatment after the patients have failed systemic chemotherapy.

Hepatic arterial infusion of cisplatin ($120 \ mg/m^2$ over two hours at monthly intervals) yielded a 19% response rate among 26 patients with a median response period of slightly more than 15 weeks and a median survival period of 11 months. Using a combination of cisplatin ($100 \ mg/m^2$) and vinblastine sulfate ($1.7 \ mg/m^2$ daily for 3.5 days) a partial response rate of 33% was achieved. For the 33 patients who underwent this regimen, a similar median survival period of 11 months was observed.[30]

More recently, chemoembolization with cisplatin (150 mg), vinblastine (10 mg) and Ivalon delivered into one lobe of the liver at a time sequentially every four to six weeks for two to three cycles has been most promising in patients with hepatic metastases from breast cancer who have failed systemic chemotherapy with 5FU in combination.

Metastatic Ocular Melanoma. The median survival time of patients with hepatic metastases from melanoma of the eye is two to six months after diagnosis despite hepatic arterial infusion or embolization. For 30 patients, chemoembolization with cisplatin (150 mg) and Ivalon (150 mg) for one lobe of the liver treated sequentially at one month intervals for three treatments has been most effective resulting in a 46% response rate with a median survival time of 11 months. Further chemoembolization depended upon the response to the initial course. The longest survivor lived almost five years from the first chemoembolization.[49]

Metastatic Neuroendocrine Tumors. The best results of hepatic artery embolization with Ivalon and/or Gelfoam were observed in patients with metastatic neuroendocrine tumors to the liver with carcinoid syndrome. Twenty (87%) of the 23 patients responded to embolization with a median response duration of more than 11 months. The symptomatic responses correlated with a decrease in the extent of the hepatic metastases and a decrease in the urine 5-hydroxyindolacetic acid values to a mean of 41% of pretreatment levels.[12]

Of the 20 patients with symptoms from islet cell carcinoma metastatic to the liver, 16 (80%) achieved objective tumor regression after embolization. Sequential and periodic embolization is required for effective palliation.[2] Thus far, as many as 21 embolizations have been administered to a patient and the longest survivor with metastatic neuroendocrine tumor to the liver is now 10 years.

Newer Approaches. Chemoembolization combining particles of Ivalon and/or Gelfoam powder and segments with one or more chemotherapeutic agents are yielding interesting results in a variety of primary and secondary cancers of the liver. Chemoembolization with Ivalon and cisplatin followed by an intra-arterial infusion of vinblastine also has therapeutic potential. However, the intra-arterial infusion of immunomodifiers including interleukin II, interferon and tumor necrosis factor delivered into the hepatic or splenic artery has been disappointing.

Skeletal Neoplasms

Osteosarcoma. The rationale for preoperative intra-arterial infusion in osteogenic sarcoma is to control the local primary tumor, to facilitate local resection with limb salvage rather than amputation and to identify effective chemotherapeutic agents for adjuvant therapy based on the degree of tumor necrosis of the resected specimen.[65]

Patients younger than 16 years of age received seven courses of intra-arterial cisplatin (150 mg/m^2 over two hours) every two weeks. Patients over 16 years old received in addition, intravenous doxorubicin (90 mg over 96 hours) before each of three to six courses of intra-arterial cisplatin at a dose of 120–200 mg/m^2 diluted in 300 ml of 3% saline over 2–24 hours. Vigorous hydration with intravenous fluids and mannitol diureses was given in both groups.[10,39]

Most patients experienced pain relief within days of the initial administration of cisplatin. Limb salvage was possible in 24 of the first 40 patients, whereas, only six were considered candidates prior to preoperative chemotherapy. Currently approximately 80% of our skeletally mature patients undergo limb salvage.

The overall disease-free survival of 65% is superior to our historical controls of 20%.[74] The 28 patients treated since 1983 have a 75% disease-free survival at two years, compared to 62% for those treated between 1979 and 1982.

Giant Cell Tumors. Most tumors in this group of 21 patients were located in the sacrum, ilium and thoracolumbar spine and had not responded to chemotherapy, irradiation or surgery. Sequential embolization resulted in complete control of pain and radiographic healing of the tumors in 48% of the patients. Partial relief of symptoms was observed in an additional 19% of patients for a total response rate of 67%. After embolization, seven patients received chemotherapy or irradiation. One patient underwent subsequent surgery for an iliac tumor that responded to embolization.[23]

Ischemic neuropathy and a single instance of unexplained death were complications seen after extrinsic pelvic arterial embolization.

Metastatic Skeletal Neoplasms. Embolization of skeletal neoplasms was initially performed as an adjunct to surgical resection for hypervascular tumors to decrease operative blood loss. Subsequently, this technique was used for palliation of pain caused by skeletal metastases. Our efforts have been mostly concentrated on hypervascular metastases such as those from hypernephroma and thyroid carcinoma.[11]

Genito-Urinary

Renal Carcinoma. Renal artery embolization, usually performed with Ivalon, gelfoam and stainless steel coils, is reserved preoperatively for those neoplasms greater than 9 cm in diameter. In the presence of pulmonary metastases alone, renal artery embolization followed by a therapeutic delay of five to seven days or more, nephrectomy and Depo-Provera (400 mg IM twice weekly) resulted in a 28% response rate with a median survival of 18 months for the responders. This compares well with a median survival of six months for historical controls.[81]

More frequently, embolization of the renal carcinoma is done when the patients are not candidates for surgery because of their general medical status or the extent of their metastases. Sequential renal artery embolization, preserving as much renal parenchyma and function as possible, has been used in the management of congestive heart failure in association with arteriovenous shunting though the renal carcinoma, and for hypertension, hypercalcemia, polycythemia, and hemorrhage. Selective embolization is especially effective in patients with an elevated serum creatinine or a solitary kidney.[81] At times, embolization of the neoplasm itself can be done preserving at least 50% of the kidney. In patients with metastases, renal artery embolization debulks the tumor in preparation for subsequent systemic treatment with 5-FU, Mitomycin C and alpha Interferon. This regimen has a 38% response rate. Embolization is as effective in reducing tumor cell population as nephrectomy.[70]

The diagnostic studies and the embolization are done with a two day interval and hydration to prevent renal failure. Complications of renal artery embolization include the post-embolization syndrome of pain, fever, nausea and vomiting. A decrease in urine output in the immediate post-embolization period must be investigated as an emergency with a conventional radiograph of the abdomen to ascertain that coils have not been displaced to the normal renal artery. Patients with a recent history of pyuria and/or renal calculi are treated prophylactically prior to and following embolization with antibiotics to prevent an abscess.

Carcinoma of the Bladder. Patients with locally advanced bladder carcinoma with or without nodal metastases have been treated with combined intravenous and intra-arterial CISCA (cisplatin, cytoxan and adriamycin) chemotherapy. Cytoxan (650 mg/m^2) and adriamycin (50 mg/m^2) were delivered intravenously on the day the catheters were placed. The next day following adequate hydration, cisplatin (75–100 mg/m^2) was infused intra-arterially along with intravenous mannitol (40 gm) for diuresis. An overall complete remission rate of 50% and objective response rate of 18% for a total

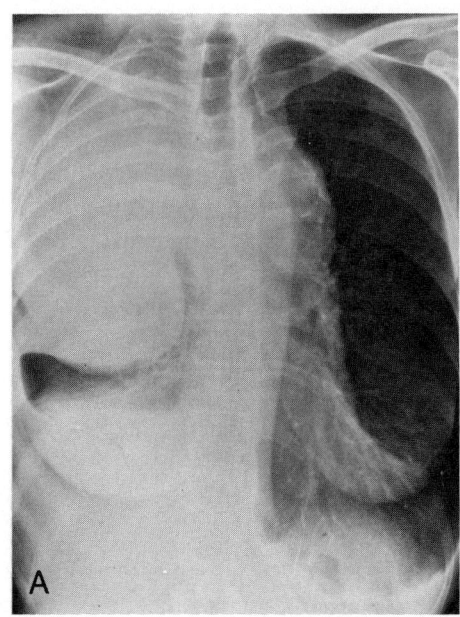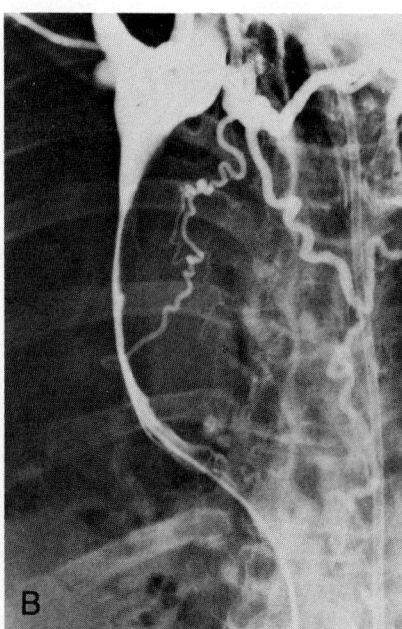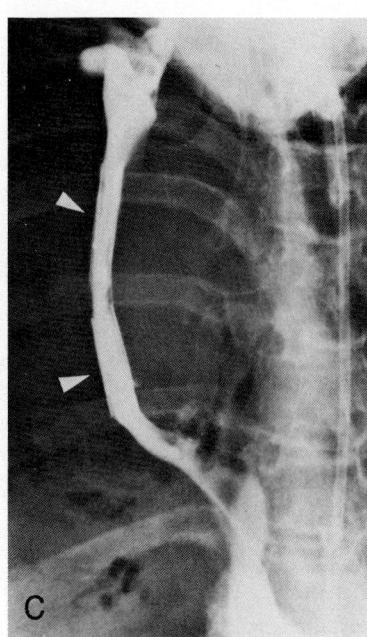

Figure X-1-3. Superior vena caval syndrome: management by expandable metallic stents. A. This carcinoma of the lung encircled the superior vena cava. B. Venacavography demonstrated a marked narrowing and collateral circulation. C. Expandable metallic stents adequately dilated the superior vena cava allowing improvement in flow. Collateral circulation was no longer opacified. The patient's symptoms were immediately relieved.

response rate of 68% was achieved.[80] This served as the basis for subsequent systemic chemotherapy.

Carcinoma of the Cervix. Patients with Stages III and IV cervical cancer were treated with intra-arterial infusion of mitomycin C (10 mg/m^2 over 24 hours every other course), bleomycin (20–40 mg/m^2 over 24 hours) and cisplatin (100 mg/m^2 over 2 hours). After three cycles spaced 3 to 4 weeks apart, the patients were evaluated for further definitive radiotherapy.

Of 47 patients treated, 42 were evaluated. Twenty-nine of the 42 patients (69%) had a partial response with a reduction of the tumor by more than 50%. Of the 42 patients, 21 remain disease free with a median duration of follow up of 18 months. Of the 29 patients who responded to chemotherapy, 20 (69%) remain disease-free.[43]

Carcinoma of the Genitalia. Intra-arterial infusion for cancers of the vagina, vulva and penis has been delivered through the internal pudendal branch of the internal iliac artery, the external pudendal branch of the internal iliac artery and external pudendal branch of the deep femoral artery. The chemotherapy regimen consisted of mitomycin C (10 mg/m^2 over 24 hours), bleomycin (20–40 mg/m^2 over 24 hours) and cisplatin (100 mg/m^2 over two hours). Although the number of patients treated under this regimen is too small for analysis, dramatic responses have been observed in several patients.

Head and Neck

Paranasal Sinuses. Patients with advanced paranasal sinus neoplasms have been treated with combined selective intra-arterial (cisplatin) and systemic (5FU) chemotherapy yielding an immediate and satisfactory tumor response rate of 91%. Repetitive uncomplicated catheterization of the pterygoid

segment of the internal maxillary artery using a coaxial system with a 2.7F catheter was essential to success. The effectiveness of intra-arterial chemotherapy seemed to be dependent on the tumor sensitivity and the ability to encompass the entire tumor within the anatomic territory of the infused artery.[47]

Metallic Stents

Self-Expandable Stents. The management of patients with stenosis of a tubular structure due to neoplasm or the result of treatment of a neoplasm led to the development of metallic endoprostheses to reestablish patency. The percutaneous placement of such devices allows the introduction through catheters of relatively small diameter with subsequent expansion once deployed. Metallic stents now available include self-expandable and balloon-assisted.[67,58,85]

At MDACC the Gianturco self-expandable "Z" stent is being investigated in the treatment of patients with stenoses of the vascular system, tracheobronchial tree and the biliary ducts.[19] The stents are constructed of stainless steel wire (0.010–0.022 inch in caliber) bent in zig-zag pattern and encircled to form a cylinder. The expansile force varies directly with the caliber of wire, diameter of the stent in its resting state, the number and angle of the bends and indirectly with the length. Lateral barbs minimize migration. The stents are covered by the lining of the tubular structure in one to three months.

These devices have been successful in the management of venous stenoses including patients with superior (Fig. X-1-3) or inferior vena cava syndrome. In the presence of thrombosis, thrombolysis through a catheter placed directly into the clot must precede dilatation. Venous stenosis as the result of radiation fibrosis can be treated effectively. Tracheobronchial narrowing secondary to primary and secondary tumors of the lung or mediastinum are successfully dilated by metallic stents. A myocutaneous graft following resection of a tracheal carcinoma has been supported by a stent; postoperative anastomotic stenoses have easily been expanded. Obstructive jaundice produced by malignant neoplasms, i.e., primary carcinomas of the biliary ducts, pancreas, gallbladder, and ampulla of Vater have been palliated with stents. Inoperable cholangiocarcinoma was best managed by a combination of stents and irradiation. Complications include obstruction, penetration, infection, hemorrhage and migration of the stents.

These results are still early and limited but are promising. Indications and contraindications are still to be defined. The current selection of patients is on the basis of little or no alternative therapy. The "Z" stent may provide relief of the immediate luminal obstruction so that definitive therapy can follow.

Summary

The percutaneous procedures described represent only a portion of the activities of the interventional radiologist in the diagnosis and management of neoplasms. These techniques, still in their infancy, expand our therapeutic potential. Tumor debulking is readily accomplished through this approach. Phase 2 studies initiated by the intra-arterial route may allow a better appreciation of effectiveness and toxicity. Targeted microparticles containing chemotherapy and/or immunomodifiers delivered intra-arterially should enhance the efficiency of these agents. Interventional radiology allows diagnosis and therapy with less morbidity and mortality, at a reduced emotional and financial burden, for cancer patients.

References

1. Adams, P. S., Jr.: Iliac artery-ureteral fistula developing after dilatation and stent placement. Radiology, 153:647, 1984.
2. Ajani, J., Carrasco, C. H., Charnsangavej, C., Samaan, N. A., Levin, B., and Wallace, S.: Islet cell tumors metastatic to the liver: Effective palliation by sequential hepatic artery embolization. Ann. Surg., 108:340, 1988.
3. Ajani, J. A., Carrasco, C. H., Jackson, D. E., and Wallace, S.: Combination of cisplatin plus fluoropyrimidine chemotherapy effective against liver metastases from carcinoma of the anal canal. Am. J. Med., 87:221, 1989.
4. Altemeier, W. A., Culbertson, W. R., Fullen, W. D., and Shook, C. D.: Intra-abdominal abscesses. Am. J. Surg., 125:70, 1973.
5. Aronsen, K. F., Hellekant, C., Holmberg, J., Rothman, U., and Teder, H.: Controlled blocking of hepatic artery flow with enzymatically degradable microspheres combined with oncolytic drugs. Eur. Surg. Res., 11:99, 1979.
6. Ayala, A. G., and Zornoza, J.: Primary bone tumors: Percutaneous needle biopsy: radiologic-pathologic study of 222 biopsies. Radiology, 149:675, 1983.
7. Balch, C. M., Urist, M. M., Soong, S.-J., and McGregor, M.: A prospective phase II clinical trial of continuous FUDR regional chemotherapy for colorectal metastases to the liver using a totally implantable drug infusion pump. Ann. Surg., 198:567, 1983.
8. Banner, M. P., and Pollack, H. M.: Dilatation of ureteral stenoses: techniques and experience in 44 patients. A.J.R., 143:789, 1984.
9. Baum, S., and Nusbaum, M.: The control of gastrointestinal hemorrhage by selective mesenteric arterial infusion of vasopressin. Radiology, 98:497, 1971.
10. Benjamin, R. S., Chuang, V. P., and Wallace, S.: Preoperative chemotherapy for osteosarcoma. ASCO, Abstract C-675, 1:174, 1982.
11. Bowers, T. A., Murray, J. A., Charnsangavej, C., Soo, C. S., Chuang, V. P., and Wallace, S.: Bone metastases from renal carcinoma. J. Bone Joint Surg., 64:749, 1982.
12. Carrasco, C. H., Charnsangavej, C., Ajani, J., Samaan, N., Richli, W., and Wallace, S.: The carcinoid syndrome: Palliation by hepatic artery embolization. Radiology, 149:79, 1983.
13. Carrasco, C. H., Charnsangavej, C., Richli, W. R., and Wallace, S.: Bone Biopsy. In Interventional Radiology. Edited by R. F. Dondelinger, P. Rossi, J. C. Kurdziel, and S. Wallace. New York, Thieme Medical Publishers, Inc., 1990, p. 58.
14. Carrasco, C. H., Charnsangavej, C., Richli, W. R., and Wallace, S.: Percutaneous Drainage. In Current Problems in Cancer, Vol. X, No. 12. Edited by R. C. Hickey. Chicago, Year Book Medical Publishers Inc., 1986, p. 596.
15. Carrasco, C. H., Richli, W. R., Lawrence, D., Katz, R. L., and Wallace, S.: Fine needle aspiration biopsy of lymphoma. Radiol. Clin. North Am., 28:879, 1990.
16. Carrasco, C. H., Zornoza, J., and Bechtel, W.: Malignant biliary obstruction: Complications of percutaneous biliary drainage. Radiology, 152:343, 1984.
17. Castellino, R., and Blank, N.: Etiologic diagnosis of focal pulmonary infection in immu-

18. Charnsangavej, C., Carrasco, C. H., Richli, W. R., and Wallace, S.: Liver Tumors. In Interventional Radiology. Edited by R. F. Dondelinger, P. Rossi, J. C. Kurdziel, and S. Wallace. New York, Thieme Medical Publishers, 1990, p. 448.
19. Charnsangavej, C., Carrasco, C. H., Wright, K. C., Wallace, S., and Gianturco, C.: Expandable Stents. In Interventional Radiology. Edited by R. F. Dondelinger, P. Rossi, J. C. Kurdziel, and S. Wallace. New York, Thieme Medical Publishers, 1990, p. 692.
20. Cho, K. J., Schmidt, R. W., and Lenz, J.: Effects of experimental embolization of superior mesenteric artery branch on the intestine. Invest. Radiol. 14:207, 1979.
21. Chuang, V. P., Soo, C. S., Carrasco, C. H., and Wallace, S.: Superselective catheterization technique in hepatic angiography. A.J.R., 141:803, 1983.
22. Chuang, V. P., Soo, C. S., and Wallace, S.: Ivalon embolization in abdominal neoplasms. A.J.R., 136:723, 1981.
23. Chuang, V. P., Soo, C. S., Wallace, S., and Benjamin, R. S.: Arterial occlusion: Management of giant cell tumor and aneurysmal bone cyst. A.J.R., 136:1127, 1981.
24. Chuang, V. P., and Wallace, S.: Hepatic arterial redistribution for intra-arterial infusion of hepatic neoplasms. Radiology, 135:295, 1980.
25. Chuang, V. P., Wallace, S., Stroehlein, J., Yap, H. Y., and Patt, Y. Z.: Hepatic artery infusion chemotherapy: Gastroduodenal complications. A.J.R., 137:347, 1981.
26. Chuang, V. P., Wallace, S., Zornoza, J., and Davis, L. J.: Transcatheter arterial occlusion in the management of rectosigmoidal bleeding. Radiology, 133:605, 1979.
27. Cronan, J. J., Dorfman, G. S., Amis, E. S., and Denny, J. F., Jr.: Retroperitoneal hemorrhage after percutaneous nephrostomy. A.J.R., 144:801, 1985.
28. Dakhil, S., Ensminger, W., Cho, K., Niederhuber, J., Doan, K., and Wheeler, R.: Improved regional selectivity of hepatic arterial BCNU with degradable microspheres. Cancer, 50:631, 1982.
29. Fornage, B., Faroux, M. J., and Simatos, A.: Breast masses: US guided fine-needle aspiration biopsy. Radiology, 147:409, 1987.
30. Fraschini, G., Yap, H. Y., Chuang, V. P., Hortobagyi, G. N., Blumenschien, G. R., and Wallace, S.: Remission consolidation in metastatic breast carcinoma to the liver with hepatic arterial infusion chemotherapy. Proc. Am. Soc. Clin. Oncol., 2:107, 1983.
31. Frei, E., III.: Effect of Dose and Schedule on Response. In Cancer Medicine, 2nd Edition. Edited by J. F. Holland, and E. Frei III. Philadelphia, Lea & Febiger, Inc., 1973, p. 717.
32. Gerzof, S. G.: Percutaneous Drainage Technique. In Interventional Radiology. Edited by R. F. Dondelinger, P. Rossi, J. C. Kurdziel, and S. Wallace. New York, Thieme Medical Publishers, Inc., 1990, p. 96.
33. Gothlin, J. H., and MacIntosh, P. K.: Interventional radiology in the assessment of the retroperitoneal lymph nodes. Radiol. Clin. North Am., 17:461, 1979.
34. Gunther, R., Klose, K., and Alken, P.: Transrenal ureteral occlusion with a detachable balloon. Radiology, 142:521, 1982.
35. Gunther, R., Marberger, M., and Klose, K.: Transrenal ureteral embolization. Radiology, 132:317, 1979.
36. Hoevels, J., and Nilsson, U.: Intrahepatic vascular lesions following nonsurgical percutaneous transhepatic bile duct intubation. Gastrointest Radiol., 5:127, 1980.
37. Holm, H. H., Kristensen, J. K., Rasmussen, S. N., Northeved, A., and Barlebo, H.: Ultrasound as a guide in percutaneous puncture technique. Ultrasonics, 10:83, 1972.
38. Hruby, W., and Marberger, M.: Late sequellae of percutaneous nephrostomy. Radiology, 152:383, 1984.
39. Jaffe, N., Knapp, J., Chuang, V. P., Wallace, S., Ayala, A., Murray, J., Cangir, A., Wang, A., and Benjamin, R. S.: Osteosarcoma: Intra-arterial treatment of the primary tumor with cis-diammine-dichloroplatinum II (CDP). Cancer, 51:402, 1983.
40. Kaplan, W. D., D'Orsi, C. J., Ensminger, W. D., Smith, E. H., and Levin, D. C.: Intra-arterial radionuclide infusion: A new technique to assess chemotherapy perfusion patterns. Cancer Treat. Rep., 62:699, 1978.
41. Kato, T., Nemoto, R., Mori, H., Takahashi, M., Tamakawa, Y., and Harada, M.: Arterial chemoembolization with microencapsulated anticancer drug. J.A.M.A., 245:1123, 1981.
42. Kauffmann, G. W., Rasweiler, J., Richter, G., Hanenstein, K. H., Rohrbach, R., and Friedburg, H.: Capillary embolization by EthiblOc: A new embolization concept tested in dog kidney. A.J.R., 137:1163, 1981.
43. Kavanaugh, J. J.: Regional chemotherapeutic approaches to the management of pelvic malignancies. Cancer Bull., 36:52, 1984.
44. Kerlan, R. K., Ring, E. J., Pogany, A. C., and Jeffrey, R. B.: Biliary endoprostheses: Insertion using a combined peroral-transhepatic method. Radiology, 150:828, 1984.
45. Kobayashi, I., Kusano, S., Matsubayashi, T., and Uchida, T.: Selective embolization of the vesical artery in the management of massive bladder hemorrhage. Radiology, 136:345, 1980.
46. Lamarque, J. L., and Rodiere, M. J.: Breast Biopsy. In Interventional Radiology. Edited by R. F. Dondelinger, P. Rossi, J. C. Kurdziel, and S. Wallace. New York, Thieme Medical Publishers, Inc., 1990, p 27.
47. Lee, Y. Y., Dimery, I. W., Van Tassel, P., De Pena, C., Blacklock J. B., and Goeepfert, H.: Superselective intra-arterial chemotherapy of advanced paranasal sinus tumors. Arch. Otolaryngol. Head Neck Surg., 115:503, 1989.
48. Linger, M. E.: Secondary tumors of the genitourinary tract. J. Urol., 65:144, 1951.
49. Mavligit, G. M., Charnsangavej, C., Carrasco, C. H., Patt, Y. Z., Benjamin, R. S., and Wallace, S.: Regression of ocular melanoma metastatic to the liver after hepatic artery chemoembolization with cisplatin and polyvinyl sponge. J.A.M.A. 260:974, 1988.
50. Mueller, P. R., van Sonnenberg, E., and Ferrucci, J. T.: Percutaneous biliary drainage: Technical and catheter related problems in 200 procedures. A.J.R., 138:17, 1982.
51. Niederhuber, J. E., Ensminger, W., Gyves, J., Thrall, J., Walker, S., and Cozzi, E.: Regional chemotherapy of colorectal cancer metastatic to the liver. Cancer, 53:1336, 1984.
52. Novy, S., Wallace, S., Goldman, A. M., and Ben-Menachem, Y.: Pyogenic liver abscess: Angiographic diagnosis and treatment by closed aspiration. A.J.R., 121:388, 1974.
53. Ohishi, H., Uchida, H., Yoshimura, H., Ohue, S., Ueda, J., Katsuragi, M., Matsuo, N., and Hosogi, Y.: Hepatocellular carcinoma detected by iodized oil. Radiology, 154:25, 1985.
54. O'Keeffe, F., Carrasco, C. H., Charnsangavej, C., Richli, W. R., Wallace, S., and Freedman, R. S.: Percutaneous drainage and feeding gastrostomies in 100 patients. Radiology, 172:341, 1989.
55. Okuda, K., Musha, H., Nakajima, Y., Takayasu, K., Suzuki, Y., Morita, M., and Yamasaki, T.: Frequency of intrahepatic arteriovenous fistula as a sequela to percutaneous needle puncture of the liver. Gastroenterology, 74:1204, 1978.

56. Oleaga, J. A., and Ring, E. J.: Interventional biliary radiology. Semin. Roentgenol., 16:116, 1981.
57. Otto, R. C., Dondelinger, R. F., and Kurdziel, J. C.: Abdominal Biopsy. In Interventional Radiology. Edited by R. F. Dondelinger, P. Rossi, J. C. Kurdziel, and S. Wallace. New York, Thieme Medical Publishers, Inc., 1990, p. 33.
58. Palmaz, J. C., Sibbitt, R. R., Reuter, S. R., Tio, F. O., and Rice, W. J.: Expandable intraluminal graft: A preliminary study. Radiology, 156:73, 1985.
59. Patt, Y. Z., Chuang, V. P., Wallace, S., Hersh, E. M., Freireich, E. J., and Mavligit, G. M.: The palliative role of hepatic arterial infusion and arterial occlusion in colorectal carcinoma metastatic to the liver. The Lancet, 1:349, 1981.
60. Patt, Y. Z., Peters, R. E., Chuang, V. P., Wallace, S., and Mavligit, G. M.: Effective retreatment of patients with colorectal cancer and liver metastases. Am. J. Med., 75:237, 1983.
61. Perlberger R.: Control of hemobilia by sequelae embolization. A.J.R., 128:672, 1977.
62. Ponsky, J. L., Gauderer, M. W. L., and Stellato, T. A.: Percutaneous endoscopic gastrostomy: Review of 150 cases. Arch. Surg., 118:913, 1983.
63. Prenshaw, R. M.: A percutaneous method for inserting a feeding gastrostomy tube. Surg. Gynecol. Obstet., 152:659, 1981.
64. Rosch, J.: Lower Gastrointestinal Bleeding. In Interventional Radiology. Edited R. F. Dondelinger, P. Rossi, J. C. Kurdziel, and S. Wallace. New York, Thieme Medical Publishers, Inc., 1990, p. 349.
65. Rosen, G., Marcove, R. C., Caparros, B., Nirenberg, A., Kosloff, C., and Huvos, A. S.: Primary osteogenic sarcoma: The rationale for preoperative chemotherapy and delay surgery. Cancer, 43:2163, 1979.
66. Rosenberger, A., and Adler, O. B.: Mediastinal Biopsy. In Interventional Radiology. Edited by R. F. Dondelinger, P. Rossi, J. C. Kurdziel, and S. Wallace. New York, Thieme Medical Publishers, Inc., 1990, p.18.
67. Rousseau, H., Puel, J., Joffre, F., Sigwant, U., Duboucher, C., Imbert, C., Knight, C., Kroft, L., and Wallsten, H.: A new type of self-expanding endovascular stent prosthesis: Experimental study. Radiology, 164:709, 1987.
68. Sacks, B. A., and Glotzer, D. J.: Percutaneous reestablishment of feeding gastrostomies. Surgery, 85:575, 1979.
69. Schwartz, P. E., Goldstein, H. M., Wallace, S., and Rutledge, F.: Control of arterial hemorrhage using percutaneous arterial catheter technique in patients with gynecologic malignancies. Gynecol. Oncol., 3:276, 1975.
70. Sella, A., Logothetis, C., Dexeus, F., Amato, R., Kilbourn, R., Fitz, K., Gutterman, J., and Wallace, S.: Increased response rate with the combination of chemotherapy 5-Fluorouracil (5-FU) and Mitomycin-C (MMC) [with interferon (Roferon)] in patients (Pts) with metastatic renal cell carcinoma (RCC). Preceedings of ASCO Annual Meeting, Abstract, 1990.
71. Siegel, J. H., and Daniel, S. J.: Endoscopic and fluoroscopic sequelae placement of a large caliber biliary endoprosthesis. Am. J. Gastroenterol., 79:461, 1984.
72. Skinner, W. N.: Transthoracic needle biopsy of small peripheral malignant lung lesions. Intervent. Radiol., 8:305, 1973.
73. Smith, E. H.: The hazards of fine needle aspiration biopsy. Ultrasound Med. Biol., 10:629, 1984.
74. Sutow, W. W., Sullivan, M. P., Wilbur, J. R., and Cangir, A.: A study of adjuvant chemotherapy in osteogenic sarcoma. J. Clin. Pharmacol., 7:530, 1975.
75. Tehranzadeh, J., Freiberger, R. H., and Ghelman, B.: Closed skeletal needle biopsy: Review of 120 cases. A.J.R., 140:113, 1983.
76. Toolin, E., Pollack, H. M., Mclean, G. K., Banner, M. R., and Wein, A. J.: Ureteroarterial fistula: A case report. J. Urol. 132:553, 1984.
77. von Sonnenberg, E., Mueller, P. R., and Ferrucci, J. T.: Percutaneous drainage of 250 abdominal abscesses and fluid collections. Radiology, 151:337, 1984.
78. Wallace, S., Carrasco, C. H., Charnsangavej, C., Lee, Y. Y., Wright, K. C., and Gianturco, C.: Percutaneous Transcatheter Infusion and Infarction in the Treatment of Human Cancer, Part II. In Current Problems in Cancer, Vol. No. 18. Edited by R. C. Hickey. Chicago, Year Book Medical Publishers, Inc., 1984, p.1.
79. Wallace, S., Charnsangavej, C., Carrasco, C. H., Bechtel, W., and Wright, K. C., Gianturco C.: Percutaneous Transcatheter Infusion and Infarction in the Treatment of Human Cancer: Part I. In Current Problems in Cancer, Vol. VI, No. 17. Edited by R. C. Hickey. Chicago, Year Book Medical Publishers, Inc., 1984, p. 1.
80. Wallace, S., Chuang, V. P., Samuels, M. L., and Johnson, D.: Transcatheter intraarterial infusion of chemotherapy in advance bladder cancer. Cancer, 42:640, 1982.
81. Wallace, S., Chuang, V. P., Swanson, D. A., Bracken, B., Hersh, E. M., Ayala, A., and Johnson, D.: Embolization of renal carcinoma: Experience with 100 patients. Radiology, 138:563, 1981.
82. Wallace, S., Medellin, H., de Jongh, D. S., and Gianturco, C.: Systemic heparinization for angiography. A.J.R., 116:204, 1972.
83. Westcott, J. L.: Lung Biopsy. In Interventional Radiology. Edited by R. F. Dondelinger, P. Rossi, J. C. Kurdziel, and S. Wallace. New York, Thieme Medical Publishers, Inc., 1990, p. 9.
84. Woods, D., Bechtel, W., Charnsangavej, C., Haynie, T. P., Kim, E. E., Carrasco, C. H., and Wallace, S.: Gluteal artery occlusion: Intra-arterial chemotherapy of pelvic neoplasms. Radiology, 155:341, 1985.
85. Wright, K. C., Wallace, S., Charnsangavej, C., Carrasco, C. H., and Gianturco, C.: Percutaneous endovascular stents: an experimental evaluation. Radiology, 156:69, 1985.
86. Wright, K. C., Wallace, S., Kim, E. E., Haynie, T. P., Charnsangavej, C., Chuang, V. P., and Gianturco, C.: Pulsed arterial infusions: chemotherapeutic implications. Cancer, 57:1952, 1986.
87. Wright, K. C., Wallace, S., Mosier, B., and Mosier, D.: Microcapsules for arterial embolization: appearance an in vitro drug release characteristics. J. Microencapsul., 5:13, 1988.
88. Yamada, R., Sato, M., Kawabata, M., Nakatsuka, H., Nakamura, K., and Takashima, S.: Hepatic artery embolization in 120 patients with unresectable hepatoma. Radiology, 148:397, 1983.
89. Zornoza, J., Jonsson, K., Wallace, S., and Lukeman, J. M.: Fine needle aspiration biopsy of retroperitoneal lymph nodes and abdominal masses: An updated report. Radiology, 125:87, 1977.

XI

Endoscopy

XI-1

Gastrointestinal Endoscopy

John Baillie
Peter B. Cotton

Introduction

The gastrointestinal tract is long and tortuous. For the first half of this century, detection and diagnosis of its diseases (and those of its associated organs such as the liver and pancreas) relied upon barium contrast radiology, and open surgery. Rigid esophagoscopes and proctoscopes provided only glimpses of the long tunnels beyond. Semiflexible lens gastroscopes were introduced in the 1930s and used by few enthusiasts; examinations were incomplete and uncomfortable, and biopsy facilities were inadequate. Subsequently, a miniaturized intragastric camera was used extensively in Japan for detection of early gastric cancer.

These techniques have all been sidelined by flexible endoscopy, which began in 1958 with the publication by Hirschowitz and colleagues of the first clinical application of a fiberoptic endoscope.[40] Commercial versions were introduced in the 1960's and widely applied for diagnostic purposes in the upper and lower GI tract in the 1970's. This wave was followed, predominantly in the 1980's, by development of numerous endoscopically-based therapeutic techniques.

Within the last five years, light sensitive transistors (charged coupled devices, or CCDs) have wrought a new revolution.[50] Video endoscopes employ these devices to create high resolution television images that can be analyzed and manipulated to provide information never before available to endoscopists. These electronic refinements—which include image enhancement,[70] reflectance spectrometry,[13] and mucosal blood flow mapping[25]—have greatly increased the potential of endoscopy for diagnosis and treatment of gastrointestinal cancer.

Diagnostic and therapeutic endoscopy has become a subspecialty of its own. Gastroenterologists and surgeons undertaking such procedures require appropriate supervised training and certification. As few medical oncologists have had formal endoscopic training, the oncologist and the endoscopist work as a team to investigate and treat GI cancer. Increasingly, GI endoscopy is being performed in the outpatient setting. It is unusual to require more than intra-venous sedation; some basic therapeutic procedures (e.g., dilatation of esophageal strictures, colonoscopic polypectomy) do not require hospitalization. However, the patients undergoing more aggressive endoscopy therapy (e.g., laser ablation, biliary stent placement) need to be observed in hospital after their procedures.

Diagnostic Endoscopy

The major advances in diagnostic endoscopy have followed refinement of endoscopes and their accessories. Modern endoscopes are much more flexible than their predecessors, allowing them to reach previously inaccessible or poorly visualized areas of the GI tract. However, the small intestine from the distal duodenum to the distal ileum remains relatively difficult to view endoscopically; a variety of research instruments have been developed but none are in routine use. Using standard endoscopes, we can directly visualize the esophagus, stomach, duodenum, the last 10 cm of the ileum and the entire colon. In addition, we can opacify the biliary tree and pancreatic ducts by retrograde injection of contrast agents. Finally, rigid laparoscopy allows us to view the peritoneum and peritoneal aspects of the liver and small intestine. Technical aspects of these procedures are well described elsewhere.[15]

A significant proportion of the work of the gastrointestinal endoscopist involves a search for, and characterization of, cancers. Sometimes a gut tumor can be diagnosed as malignant with a high degree of confidence solely from the macroscopic appearance at endoscopy. However, other adjuvant techniques such as vital staining and endoscopic ultrasound can provide additional diagnostic information, and histologic and/or cytologic confirmation of the diagnosis. It is almost always necessary to determine the cell type and degree of differentiation to plan the most effective therapy.

Biopsy and Cytology

Samples must be taken from all suspicious lesions. Standard endoscopic biopsies are rather small and usually do not penetrate beyond the mucosa. As a result, submucosally spreading and intramural tumors may be missed by the usual biopsy technique. For example, Kaposi's sarcoma[97] (a frequent accompaniment of AIDS), gastric lymphoma, and leiomyoma are rarely diagnosed by standard biopsy forceps. When there is evidence that the bowel wall is thickened, larger and deeper biopsies than normal can be taken using large particle (jumbo) forceps, or the submucosa can be accessed by so-called "tunneling"; repeated biopsies in the same site allow the endoscopist to tunnel down to the lesion of interest.[4] Endoscopic needle aspiration biopsy is an alternative that has yet to gain widespread acceptance.[28] It is essential for the endoscopist to ensure that the pathologist receives specimens in appropriate fixative. For example, biopsies destined for immuno-peroxidase staining (e.g., for lymphoma markers) and electron microscopy require special handling, and should not be fixed in standard formalin. As endoscopic biopsies are very small (frequently only a few millimeters in diameter), multiple specimens are taken to improve the diagnostic yield. It is rarely difficult to target malignant tissue in gross tumors, but more subtle lesions may resist diagnosis. Biopsies taken from the rim of a malignant ulcer are often positive, as this represents the growing edge of the tumor, whereas biopsies of the base may show only necrotic material.

Brush cytology, alone or in combination with biopsy, can increase the diagnostic yield in malignancy. So-called "salvage cytology" assures that no potentially diagnostic material is wasted;[29] in one method washings from the endoscope biopsy channel are centrifuged and the resulting solid pellet stained for cytologic examination.

Vital Staining

Vital staining with iodine (Lugol's solution), indigocarmine, India ink or methylene blue has been known for many years to highlight the mucosal pattern of the gut.[22,88] When used with a magnifying endoscope, dye staining can help identify areas of dysplasia or carcinoma in situ. With rapid advances being made in electronic image analysis, vital staining is likely to regain popularity. Recent work has shown that fluorescence of colonic mucosal cells exposed to monochromatic (laser) light may be highly specific for epithelial dysplasia.[13] This exciting development requires further evaluation but potentially offers a way to look for dysplasia and carcinoma without the need to take biopsies.

Endoscopic Ultrasound

Relatively recent innovations in ultrasound transducer design have made it possible to place a small ultrasound probe on the tip of a modified flexible endoscope.[9,80] This has the benefit of affording direct access to mucosal lesions, close proximity to submucosal ones, and a superior view of structures within and surrounding the bowel wall. By varying the frequency of the ultrasound signal (e.g., 7.5 MHz, 10 MHz, or 12 MHz) the depth of the image (i.e., millimeters into the bowel wall) can be altered. The resolution of endoscopic ultrasound is so good that individual layers of the bowel wall can be identified, which has immediate implications for tumor staging. The marriage of endoscopic ultrasound with tar-

geted biopsies—possibly using a modified Tru-Cut biopsy gun housed within the endoscope—is eagerly awaited.

Therapeutic Techniques

Gastrointestinal endoscopy during the 1960s focused almost exclusively on diagnosis. However, with the advent of more flexible endoscopes with large instrument channels in the early 1970s, therapy became a possibility. There is now a wide range of therapeutic techniques ranging from snare polypectomy to laser ablation of tumors. The adenoma-carcinoma sequence in the stomach and colon is well-established;[60] we know that the likelihood of malignant change in polyps increases with size, especially when the polyp head is over 2 cm in diameter. Using electrocautery, polyps can be removed and recovered for histologic examination. The search for adenomatous polyps and their removal has become a major focus of colon cancer screening. As yet, statistical evidence that endoscopic removal of adenomatous polyps reduces the risk of cancer is not available, but this will require a longitudinal study involving thousands of patients over twenty years or more. However, there is good evidence that aggressive screening of patients with rectal bleeding provides a worthwhile yield of polyps and cancers.[32] It has only recently been appreciated that very small, sessile polyps (e.g., 1 mm–2 mm), which we used to assume were benign, hyperplastic lesions, are not infrequently microadenomas.[73] It has now been recommended that all sessile polyps should be biopsied to look for adenomatous change. The histologic appearance of the polypectomy specimen determines whether or not the procedure has been curative. Even if the head of the polyp contains a malignant focus, polypectomy is regarded as curative if the stalk shows no evidence of invasion by tumor cells (i.e., carcinoma-in-situ). Extension of tumor into the stalk mandates surgical exploration for segmental bowel resection and local lymph node dissection.[12]

Malignant Structures and Tumor Ablation

There is interest also in using therapeutic endoscopy methods for palliation of patients unsuitable for definitive surgical management. These techniques include the placement of plastic prostheses to bypass obstruction[19,59] (e.g., in the esophagus, stomach, bile ducts, and pancreas), debulking of tumors by injection of sclerosing agents (e.g., absolute alcohol) and laser photocoagulation of obstructing tumors.[51] Potentiation of laser energy absorption by administering porphyrins (photodynamic therapy) has not yet proved superior to standard laser therapy for obstructing gut tumors. So-called "smart lasers" that can identify and specifically target abnormal tissue have been developed for laser coronary angioplasty. It is likely that this technology will soon be adapted to allow specific targeting of tumor tissue. This has obvious implications for treatment of small tumors in confined spaces, such as the biliary tree. Smart lasers may eventually offer the potential for cure of small malignant lesions, such as early gastric cancer.[87] Western doctors have lagged behind their Japanese colleagues in searching for these lesions, some even assuming that early gastric cancer is a Japanese disease. However, all cancers everywhere must start off small, wherein lies the greatest potential for cure. It is likely that new technology such as laser fluorescence analysis and endoscopic ultrasound will eventually be employed during routine endoscopic screening for cancer.

Diagnostic and Therapeutic Role in Specific Organs

Esophagus

Most patients with esophageal neoplasia eventually develop disturbance of swallowing caused by mechanical obstruction, upset motility or a combination of the two. The usual complaint is of dysphagia (food and/or liquid sticking) with or without regurgitation. Painful swallowing (odynophagia) is usually due to mucosal inflammation but can also accompany mechanical obstruction, especially at the gastric cardia.

Other patients may have non-specific signs and symptoms of cancer such as unexplained weight loss, lassitude and anemia. There is considerable debate regarding the relative merits of contrast radiology (barium swallow) and endoscopy; the choice of initial investigation is often dictated by local availability and expertise. Although endoscopy has the diagnostic edge as biopsies and cytology specimens can be obtained, contrast radiology provides valuable complementary information. It is the authors' preference that all patients presenting with progressive dysphagia have a contrast study prior to endoscopy. The endoscopic literature suggests that endoscopy alone will make a diagnosis of cancer in at least 73% of cases, with biopsy and/or cytology increasing the yield to around 95%.[36,68,71,92] False positive results from cytology occur in between 0.1% and 1% of cases, especially in the presence of active inflammation.[78,79] Multiple biopsies increase diagnostic accuracy considerably. If a tight esophageal stricture is present, this usually requires endoscopic dilatation for access before biopsies or cytology can be taken. Malignant tumors arising in the distal third of esophagus may be either squamous carcinoma or adenocarcinoma, the latter arising from ectopic columnar epithelium (Barrett's esophagus). It is vital to identify the cell type as this determines initial management, squamous tumors being relatively sensitive to irradiation and chemotherapy compared with adenocarcinoma.

Palliation of Dysphagia. Beyond initial diagnosis, the role of the gastrointestinal endoscopist in esophageal cancer is usually to provide palliation for progressive dysphagia. Surgical intervention provides the best palliation by tumor bypass.[39] Unfortunately, few patients are suitable candidates for surgery but it is important that all should undergo appropriate evaluation before the decision is made to pursue a non-surgical approach. The standard method for endoscopic palliation of malignant dysphagia has been to place a plastic prosthesis across the stricture, a procedure associated with significant morbidity and mortality.[26] This technique cannot be used in the presence of significant tracheal compression, as the act of placing the prosthesis in the esophagus can precipitate acute respiratory embarrassment. All patients being considered for esophageal prosthesis placement should have a lateral chest X-ray to assess tracheal patency. The standard esophageal prosthesis has

been modified to help manage the difficult problems of tracheo- and broncho-esophageal fistulae. These fistulae commonly follow radiotherapy, although they may also be spontaneous. Modified esophageal prostheses with a polyvinyl alcohol (foam) cuff can be inflated when the stent is appropriately positioned across the fistula.[57] Cuffed stents have proved highly effective in preventing the distressing sequelae of pulmonary aspiration through fistulae. However, they should be used only when there is sufficient narrowing of the esophagus (either from exophytic tumor or extrinsic compression) to hold the prosthesis in place. Increasingly, endoscopists are seeing patients with fistulae from a relatively normal looking esophagus, usually following irradiation or endobronchial laser therapy to primary lung tumors. These cases are unsuitable for endoscopic stenting. Other endoscopic means of palliation of malignant esophageal strictures are currently being evaluated. These include the injection of sclerosant agents to produce tumor necrosis,[64] laser photoablation,[7,8] the use of the bipolar tumor probe,[48] and endoluminal irradiation using endoscopically-placed catheters.[33]

Endoscopic assessment of post-surgical esophageal strictures requires particular care. When a patient who has had esophago-gastrectomy for esophageal cancer develops an anastomotic stricture, it can be very difficult to distinguish mediastinal fibrosis from local tumor recurrence, especially by CT scanning. Endoscopic brushings and biopsy may need to be performed repeatedly to yield malignant cells. Endoscopic ultrasound now offers a superior way to image the esophageal wall and adjacent structures, which will undoubtedly improve the accuracy of diagnosis and staging of esophageal malignancy including recurrence.

Benign Tumors. Benign tumors of the esophagus are rare and seldom of clinical significance. However, squamous papillomas associated with human papilloma virus (HPV) infection[11] may grow sufficiently large to become symptomatic. These can be removed by snare cautery. The natural history of this disease, which is increasingly common, is unknown. There is concern that prolonged exposure to HPV may be associated with increased risk of malignant change, as in the uterine cervix. Longterm follow-up of patients with esophageal papillomas will be needed to determine if this is indeed a risk factor for carcinoma. An unusual but interesting benign tumor which may cause symptoms is the fibro-lamellar polyp,[93] which can grow very large indeed. As fibro-lamellar polyps can have a very vascular stalk, large ones are more safely removed by surgery than by endoscopic polypectomy.

Stomach

Gastric Cancer

Gastric cancers often present insidiously with unexplained weight loss, anorexia and chronic iron-deficiency anemia. They may ulcerate, mimicking benign ulcers. Alternatively, they can be unequivocally malignant-looking exophytic masses or can spread submucosally, causing gross thickening and loss of distensibility of the stomach wall (linitis plastica). Adenocarcinoma of the stomach is a particular challenge to the gastrointestinal endoscopist; by the time it causes obvious symptoms such as esophageal or gastric outlet obstruction, bleeding, or marked anorexia and loss of weight, the tumor has almost always grown beyond the stage of curative resection. The challenge is to diagnose gastric cancer early. Barium studies have a low detection rate for early gastric cancer of between 1 and 2 per 1,000, and a high false positive rate.[45] Endoscopy in patients over 40 years of age in high risk areas yields five early gastric cancers per 1,000 patients but reportedly detects only 60% of these lesions at initial examination.[86] When early gastric cancer is suspected, the changes may be subtle. As there is a false negative rate of up to 15%,[14] suspicious lesions must be re-examined and re-biopsied when initial biopsies are negative for malignancy. It is desirable to confirm the benign nature of all gastric ulcers by endoscopy and biopsy, especially as small malignant ulcers may heal transiently. Follow-up endoscopy should be performed 4–8 weeks after the initial examination, and repeated at regular intervals until healing is confirmed. As dysplasia is difficult to interpret in gastric mucosa, only the most severe dysplasia should be considered as having malignant potential. The natural history of gastric dysplasia is unknown[63] and there is no consensus on how to manage early gastric cancer. Laser photoablation has been suggested as a conservative alternative to radical gastric surgery.[46]

Gastric adenomas larger than 20 mm in diameter carry a significant risk of malignancy and should be removed endoscopically. Below 20 mm the risk is small—possibly around 2%[49] but it is good practice to remove these lesions by snare cautery or "hot biopsy" technique. The screening of patients with putative high-risk associations for gastric adenocarcinoma is addressed below.

Gastric lymphoma is frequently difficult to diagnose, although large folds and/or decreased motility seen on barium studies or at endoscopy should raise suspicion of this lesion.[90] Superficial mucosal biopsies are inadequate for diagnosis; once thickening of the gastric wall has been confirmed by CT scanning or endoscopic ultrasound, multiple large biopsies should be taken from suspect areas. Sufficient biopsies should be taken to allow some material to be sent for immunohistochemical analysis for lymphoma markers. Occasionally, laparotomy is required to obtain full-thickness biopsies of the stomach wall before a diagnosis of lymphoma can be confirmed.

Tumor metastatic to the stomach is unusual but certain cancers appear to have a predisposition for this site, including adenocarcinoma of breast and malignant melanoma.[62] With the increasing prevalence of the acquired immunodeficiency syndrome (AIDS), endoscopists have become familiar with the esophageal, gastric and colonic lesions of Kaposi's sarcoma.[24] The typical histologic appearances are rarely seen in superficial biopsies; suspected Kaposi's sarcoma is another indication for multiple, large particle biopsies.

Benign Tumors. Excluding congenital abnormalities such as the pancreatic rest, the most common benign tumor of clinical significance seen in the stomach is the leiomyoma,[61] which has a characteristic cylindrical shape with an apical depression. Leiomyomas can grow very large; they frequently ulcerate and bleed. As leiomyomas may undergo malignant degeneration to form leiomyosarcoma, large lesions should be surgically excised. Small neuroendocrine tumors such as carcinoids are an occasional finding in gastric biopsies;[31] they are rarely functional. Pathologic gastric acid hypersecretion (the Zollinger-Ellison syndrome) may be caused by a primary gastric gastrinoma. Almost invariably, these lesions are too small to be identified radiologically or by endoscopy. The majority of benign gastric tumors are submucosal—other histologic types include fibroma, lipoma, eosinophilic granuloma and a variety of cysts—and are therefore difficult to diagnose by mucosal biopsy. Endoscopic ultrasound has proved useful in characterizing these lesions.[9]

Endoscopic Treatment. Therapeutic endoscopy has not been especially helpful in the management of gastric cancer. Endoscopically-placed prostheses are useful for palliating dysphagia in obstructing tumors of the gastric cardia but have proved less satisfactory for more distal lesions, mainly due to the technical difficulty of inserting them. Laser therapy can provide palliation in noncircumferential lesions of the gastric cardia.[58] However, the use of the neodymium-yttrium argon garnet (Nd-YAG) laser to debulk large, exophytic stomach tumors seldom provides clinical benefit since gastric emptying problems result as much from disordered or absent motility as from mechanical factors. Furthermore, laser therapy in the normally thin-walled stomach carries a significant risk of perforation. Microwave radiation may provide a safer alternative; probes suitable for endoscopic use are currently being evaluated.[53] Laser photocoagulation can occasionally be helpful in management of bleeding from ulcerating tumors.

Screening for Esophageal and Gastric Cancer

Endoscopic screening has been recommended for patients at risk of developing esophageal and gastric cancers. The risk of esophageal cancer is increased in patients who smoke, drink or who have nutritional deficiencies, and in those with, or who have had, corrosive strictures, tylosis, celiac disease, the Plummer-Vinson (Brown-Kelly-Patterson) syndrome, achalasia, head, neck and pulmonary neoplasms, radiation therapy and, especially, those with Barrett's esophagus.[20,41,42,72,83,89,99] For the majority of these conditions, no specific screening recommendations exist. Barrett's esophagus, heterotrophic columnar mucosa, is associated with the development of adenocarcinoma; the relative risk is calculated to be 40 times greater than that of the general population.[84] Surveillance in Barrett's esophagus remains controversial;[85] the pendulum of opinion swings back and forth between annual surveillance endoscopy with multiple biopsies and doing nothing until symptoms supervene. There is as yet no evidence that periodic surveillance alters outcome in Barrett's esophagus. However, the finding of severe dysplasia in Barrett's epithelium warrants early re-biopsy at the very least; surgical resection (esophago-gastrectomy) must be considered. Screening of patients at increased risk for gastric cancer is even more contentious. There is no established role for endoscopic surveillance in asymptomatic patients who have undergone gastric surgery, at least within the first 20 years.[10] In patients who develop symptoms, any abnormality seen at endoscopy should be biopsied; many invisible early lesions have been detected by routine biopsy close to the gastric stoma. There may be an increased risk of gastric cancer in young patients with pernicious anemia and atrophic gastritis with intestinal metaplasia.[81] Controlled studies are required to assess risk-benefit ratios before general screening recommendations can be made. Gastric adenomas greater than 2 cm in diameter carry a significant risk of malignancy, which makes endoscopic resection mandatory for large lesions. The risk of malignant transformation in multiple gastric adenomatosis of familial polyposis syndromes (e.g., Gardner's, Peutz-Jehger) has yet to be defined.

Duodenum and Small Intestine

Endoscopists tend to consider the duodenum as a separate entity from the remainder of the small intestine, as it is readily accessible with standard endoscopic equipment. Anatomically the duodenum can be divided into four parts, the first part (or bulb) beyond the pylorus leading to the second (D_2), third (D_3) and fourth (D_4). Standard gastroscopes routinely reach D_2. As the duodenal papilla is usually located on the medial wall of D_2, adequate inspection requires the use of a side-viewing instrument (duodenoscope). A pediatric colonoscope can frequently be advanced to D_4 but rarely further (unless this is done at surgery, when the surgeon can "feed" the endoscope through the loops of small bowel). Endoscopic evaluation of the jejunum and ileum using per-oral endoscopy has proved unsatisfactory, and remains largely a research tool. A variety of push, pull, and Sonde-type enteroscopes have been tried; their supporters claim to identify pathology with them in about one-third of cases of unexplained GI bleeding.[55] Enteroscopy is difficult, time-consuming and unpleasant for the patient however. The distal 10 cm or so of the ileum can be inspected by intubating the ileocecal value during colonoscopy. The remainder of the small intestine is best seen endoscopically in the operating room, when the surgeon can assist the endoscopist by manually advancing the instrument through the bowel. A carefully performed enteroclysis (small bowel enema) remains the investigation of first choice for identifying mass lesions within the small intestine.

Tumors of the duodenum are uncommon and the majority are benign. It is so rare to find malignancy in duodenal ulcers that they are not biopsied routinely at endoscopy. Occasionally a primary duodenal or pancreatic carcinoma will masquerade as a benign duodenal ulcer; it is usually not long before the true nature of the lesion declares itself. Tumors of the ampulla (duodenal papilla) are discussed in the section on pancreatic and biliary cancers. Metastases to the duodenum from distant cancers are rare.

A variety of benign tumors occur in the duodenum. There have been several case reports of duodenal gastrinoma causing Zollinger-Ellison syndrome.[94] Carcinoid tumors are rarely of clinical significance. One common benign tumor is Brunner's gland hyperplasia,[65] which has no pathologic significance. Lymphoid nodular hyperplasia[23] is associated with a relative deficiency of intestinal IgA, which encourages small bowel colonization by the protozoan parasite, Giardia lamblia. Pathologic dilatation of intestinal lymphoid channels, lymphangiectasia,[38] results in the formation of submucosal cysts filled with chylous fluid. Again, this is a benign condition. Duodenal adenomas may be solitary, or multiple in familial polyposis syndromes[82] (e.g., Peutz-Jehger syndrome, Gardner's syndrome). The malignant potential of small bowel adenomas in these syndromes is not zero, as was previously supposed, although it is considerably less than that of the corresponding colon polyps. It has been recommended that patients with multiple duodenal adenomas as part of a familial polyposis syndrome should have periodic screening endoscopy.[77]

Benign and malignant tumors of the small bowel present in the same way, with acute or chronic bleeding, or mechanical obstruction, including intussusception. Benign tumors such as leiomyoma bleed because they ulcerate. Intussusception tends to occur when tumors are large enough to cause mechanical irritation but are too small to completely obstruct the lumen of the bowel. Although the small bowel is rarely the target of distant metastases except for melanoma, it may be involved by direct extension from adjacent organs. Primary lymphoma of the small intestine occurs with increased frequency in patients with gluten enteropathy (Celiac sprue).[91] Endoscopy has little to offer in the diagnosis and treatment of small bowel tumors. However, percutaneous endoscopic gastrostomy (PEG) tube placement has reportedly been used with good results to palliate small intestinal obstruction in metastatic ovarian cancer. In this situation, the PEG tube is used for decompression and not for feeding. It spares terminally ill patients the added discomfort of a nasogastric tube.

Colon

It was estimated that in 1989, 161,000 new cases of adenocarcinoma of the colon would be diagnosed in the United States, and that over 60,000 would die from the disease.[37] Other primary neoplasms of the colon (e.g., lymphoma) are rare. The colon can be involved in metastatic tumor by direct extension from adjacent organs, or by hematogenous or lymphatic spread. The discrete nodular lesions of Kaposi's sarcoma may be seen at colonoscopy in patients with AIDS. Since >50% of colon cancers present clinically when the tumor is beyond curative resection, considerable effort is being directed towards identification and screening of patients at increased risk of developing colon cancer. (See Plate XI-1-1.) The risk of any individual increases after age 40. Patients with inflammatory bowel disease, a family history of colon cancer (first degree relatives), adenomas of the colon, previous colon cancer, and familial polyposis syndromes are at substantially increased risk.[44] As the progression of benign adenomatous polyps of the colon to adenocarcinoma is indisputable, the identification and endoscopic removal of polyps is one of the primary objectives of colon cancer screening. The American Cancer Society and the U.S. National Cancer Institute recommend annual digital rectal examinations with fecal occult blood testing for patients over 50. In addition, they advocate flexible sigmoidoscopy every 3–5 years.[3] Clearly, these examinations will identify a proportion of patients with colon polyps and cancer. However, flexible sigmoidoscopy, while 3–5 times more sensitive than rigid proctoscopy,[6] provides access to less than 50% of the colon. This is a particular worry, as proximal migration of colon cancer is well-documented in Western societies.[76] Double contrast barium enema can detect most cancers but several studies have shown that single and double contrast barium enemas are significantly less accurate than colonoscopy.[52] In one study, barium enemas missed 45% of adenomas, 28% of carcinomas in situ, and 26% of invasive carcinomas subsequently identified at colonoscopy.[98]

Screening Strategies. How should we screen for colon cancer? Consensus studies from the US and Britain suggest that routine screening of average risk patients cannot be justified at present.[47] For this reason, gastroenterologists are devoting their energies to surveillance of high risk groups. In patients suspected of having colon cancer, flexible sigmoidoscopy followed by double contrast barium enema is probably the minimum acceptable screening. However, colonoscopy is being adopted widely as a more sensitive single procedure alternative.[98] Epidemiological studies suggest that patients with multiple colon polyps, and those with previous colon cancer, should be followed up at least every 2 years, and those with single polyps at least every 4 years.[96] Carcinoma in patients with longstanding total ulcerative colitis occurs in approximately 8–10% of patients at 15 years. It is recommended that surveillance examinations should be performed every 2–3 years after 7–10 years of pancolitis, although even these studies may miss the development of a cancer.[54] The finding of epithelial dysplasia is significant, particularly when associated with any form of colonic mass.[5] The risk of GI tract malignancy is slightly increased in patients with Crohn's disease,[30] but not sufficiently to justify routine cancer screening. Siblings and offspring of patients with familial polyposis syndromes should be offered colon cancer screening in early adulthood. There is no evidence to justify the routine use of screening for relatives of patients with sporadic adenomatous polyps.

It is too early to identify any impact of surveillance on the incidence and mortality of colon cancer. However, if vigorous screening programs succeed in identifying and removing adenomatous polyps, and permit diagnosis of colon cancers at a stage where cure is possible (i.e., Dukes' A and B lesions), there should be measurable benefit. The public has been made aware of the association between cigarette smoking and lung cancer, as well as the benefits of screening for cancers of the breast, uterine cervix, testes, and skin. A major health education effort is needed to encourage those most likely to benefit from colon cancer screening to seek it.

Tumor Ablation. Therapeutic endoscopy can palliate bleeding and/or obstructing colon cancers in selected patients whose comorbid diseases make them unsuitable for conventional surgical management. (See Plate XI-1-2.) The surface of acutely or chronically bleeding tumors can be coagulated using an Nd-YAG laser. This laser can also be used at higher energy levels to vaporize tissue to restore a lumen through obstructing cancers.[21] Laser treatment is not without risk; colon perforation is a recognized complication of laser therapy. Photodynamic therapy of colon tumors—using a porphyrin derivative to selectively sensitize tumor cells to laser energy—and technical enhancements such as contact probes and water-guided laser delivery systems[74] remain experimental.

Biliary and Pancreatic Cancer

When managing a patient who presents with symptoms suggestive of pancreatic or biliary cancer, the first goal of the clinician is to define the nature and extent of the problem, as quickly as possible with minimal interference and cost. Twenty years ago most of these cases were diagnosed at laparotomy. Since then, developments in pancreatic and biliary imaging have been spectacular (see IX-5), so that diagnosis is often straightforward, allowing more attention to be focused where it is really needed—on treatment.

This section concentrates on the contribution which can be made by the gastrointestinal endoscopist, especially with endoscopic retrograde cholangiopancreatography (ERCP). This method for imaging the biliary tree and pancreas became available before ultrasound and computed tomographic scanning, and was the first modality to provide meaningful radiographs of the pancreas. Developments in scanning techniques have reduced somewhat the relevance of ERCP in pancreatic diagnosis, but its role in the bile duct has increased markedly, because of its therapeutic potential in patients with obstruction due to stones, strictures and cancer.

Technical Aspects of ERCP. ERCP[15] is performed with a lateral-viewing duodenoscope passed under light sedation in a patient lying prone on a standard radiographic table. The equipment and all ancillaries (e.g., catheters, guidewires) are fully disinfected before use. The tip of the endoscope is negotiated into the second part of the duodenum and the papilla of Vater brought into a direct face on position. A catheter is advanced through the working channel of the endoscope out into view in the duodenum, where it can be directed into the papilla by combined movements of the endoscope tip and the cannula elevator. Perpendicular insertion into the papilla usually provides a pancreatogram; a more upward path finds the biliary axis. Contrast is injected under fluoroscopy, and relevant radiographs taken in appropriate positions (Figure XI-1-1). Fine detail can be obtained by selective deep cannulation of the ducts and their branches. Obstructions (for example, in the bile duct) which appear to be complete radiographically can usually be negotiated with guidewires; these allow subsequent passage of a catheter and demonstration of the ductal systems "upstream" of the apparent obstruction (Figure XI-1-2).

The success rate for cannulating the desired duct or ducts varies with experience. Experts will fail in less than 5% of cases, but the success rate may be as low as 70% in the hands of endoscopists who have performed less than 100 procedures. Some problems of access to the papilla (e.g., surgical diversions and peripapillary diverticula) make ERCP more difficult, and duct entry may be inhibited by disease such as tumor or stone. The congenital anomaly of pancreas divisum (in which most of the pancreas drains through Santorini's duct and the accessory papilla) occurs in about 7% of the population; in these cases complete pancreatography necessitates cannulation also of the minor papilla, which is technically more demanding.

The main risk involved in diagnostic ERCP (apart from the rare risks of any gastrointestinal endoscopy procedure) is that of pancreatitis.[16] Injection of too much contrast under excessive pressure is the commonest cause, but many other factors are involved. The risk of pancreatitis should be less than 3% (depending on definition). Injection of contrast into an obstructed biliary tree can aggravate infection unless

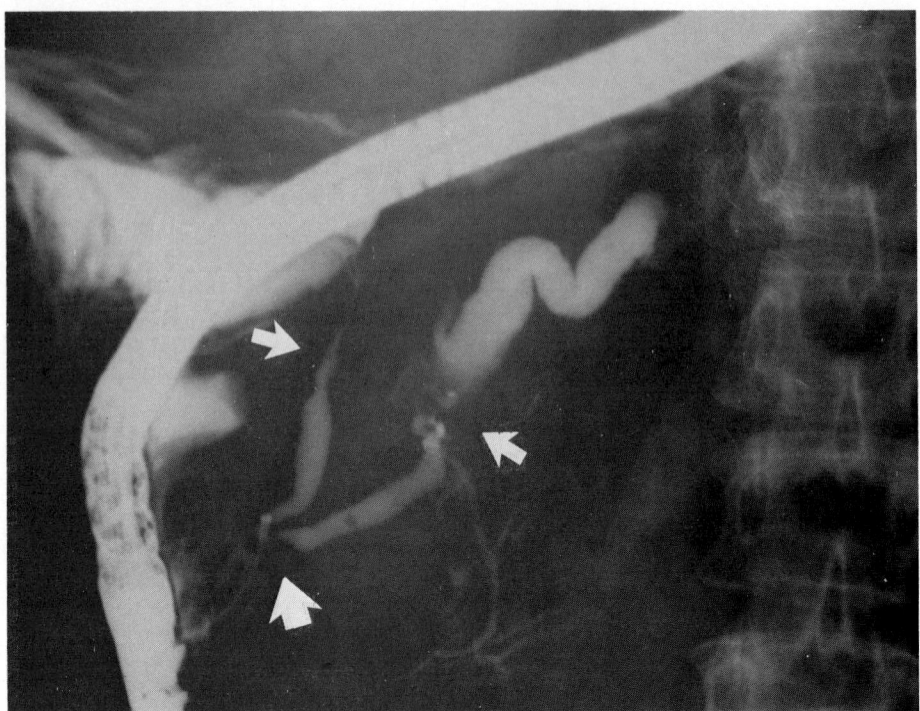

Figure XI-1-1. Endoscopic retrograde cholangiogram and pancreatogram. The metal tip of catheter can be seen in the orifice of the papilla. There is a tight stricture of the pancreatic duct in the head with some upstream dilatation. The bile duct is strictured in the same area; radiographic findings characteristic of pancreatic cancer. Large arrow indicates tip of ERCP cannula. Upper and lower small arrows indicate sites of common bile duct and pancreatic duct strictures, respectively.

appropriate drainage is provided promptly, preferably by endoscopic techniques. For this reason, training and practice in ERCP should be restricted to those who have ambition or skill to perform all of the therapeutic applications as well as diagnostic indications.

ERCP in Diagnosis. The sensitivity of pancreatography in detection of pancreatic cancer is often claimed to be in excess of 90%, by which is meant that an obstructed or strictured duct system is seen, consistent with a mass lesion. Unfortunately, the radiographic distiction between chronic pancreatitis and pancreatic cancer (especially when causing complete duct obstruction) is not absolute. Thus, pancreatography is more effective in detecting pancreatic pathology than in differential diagnosis. A good quality normal pancreatogram (including first and second order branches) makes pancreatic cancer very unlikely, but tumors arising in the uncinate process, and islet cell neoplasms, are rarely detected.

ERCP is now most widely used in the investigation and management of patients with biliary obstruction, usually after preliminary ultrasound and/or CT scanning. The double duct sign (contiguous strictures or obstruction of both pancreatic and bile ducts—Figure XI-1-1) is almost pathognomonic of pancreatic head cancer. Most strictures and obstructions to the bile duct are malignant (apart from those occurring as a result of operative trauma), but there are rare isolated benign strictures which cause diagnostic difficulty. Even more difficult is the detection of cholangiocarcinoma in the presence of multiple strictures in patients with sclerosing cholangitis. Tumors of the gallbladder, hilar nodes, and intrahepatic metastases give fairly characteristic cholangiographic appearances.

Duodenoscopy (with a side-viewing instrument) is the investigation of choice in patients suspected of having tumors in and around the papilla of Vater. Exquisite views are obtained, and the extent of the disease can be judged both by the endoscopic view and the depth of the strictures on ERCP cholangiography and pancreatography.

Tissue Diagnosis. Tumors of the papilla and deeper lesions invading the duodenum are accessible to standard endoscopic biopsy and cytology techniques. The same probes (or variations) can be passed up the pancreatic and biliary ductal systems (Figure XI-1-3). The sensitivity of brushing cytology is 70–80% when the lesion can be reached. Biopsy yield is lower unless the tumor is exophytic. Attempts are being made to develop new devices such as duct "scrapers" or endoscopic needle aspiration. Collection of bile and pancreatic juice for cytology has proven to be less worthwhile.

Enthusiasm for these ERCP techniques for establishing the diagnosis of cancer has increased recently because more and more patients are being treated without laparotomy, and because alternative tissue techniques (such as percutaneous fine needle aspiration biopsy under CT control) are not always successful.[1,35]

Endoscopic Techniques for Tumor Staging. Staging becomes the most important issue once a tumor has been detected. Unfortunately, most biliary and pancreatic cancers are unresectable at the time of diagnosis.[18] Since there are now effective non-operative methods for palliation, the ability to detect unresectability without laparotomy has become more important. The mere size of a tumor may predict unresectability, but other parameters, such as distant metastases and invasion of major vessels, are more specific. Standard ERCP has little contribution to make in this context, but its fledgling companion—endoscopic ultrasound—may provide a contribution over and above that available from standard ultrasound scanning, computed tomography, nuclear magnetic resonance and angiography. Laparoscopy also has a role.

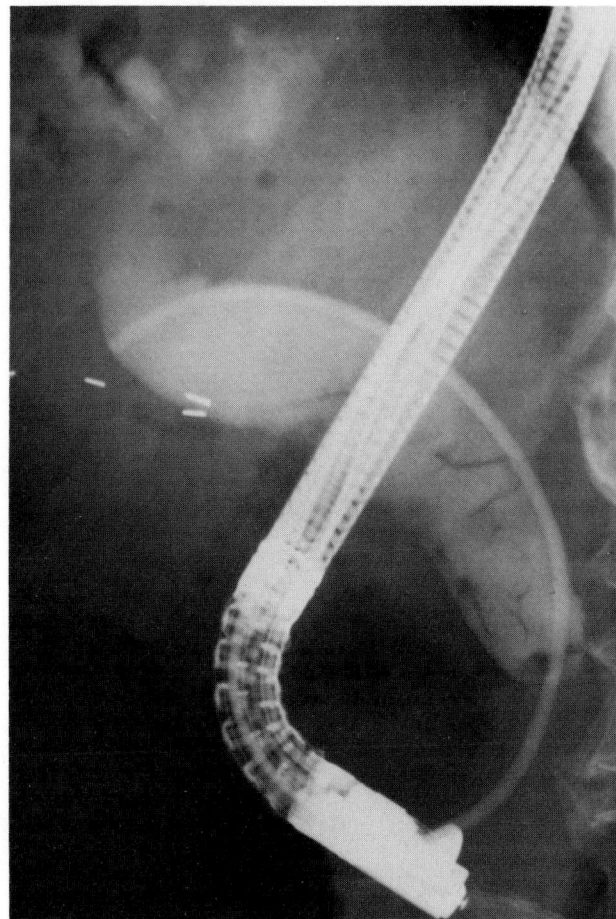

Figure XI-1-2. After a guidewire has been passed through the malignant bile duct stricture a catheter is slid over it for injection of contrast, demonstrating marked upstream dilatation.

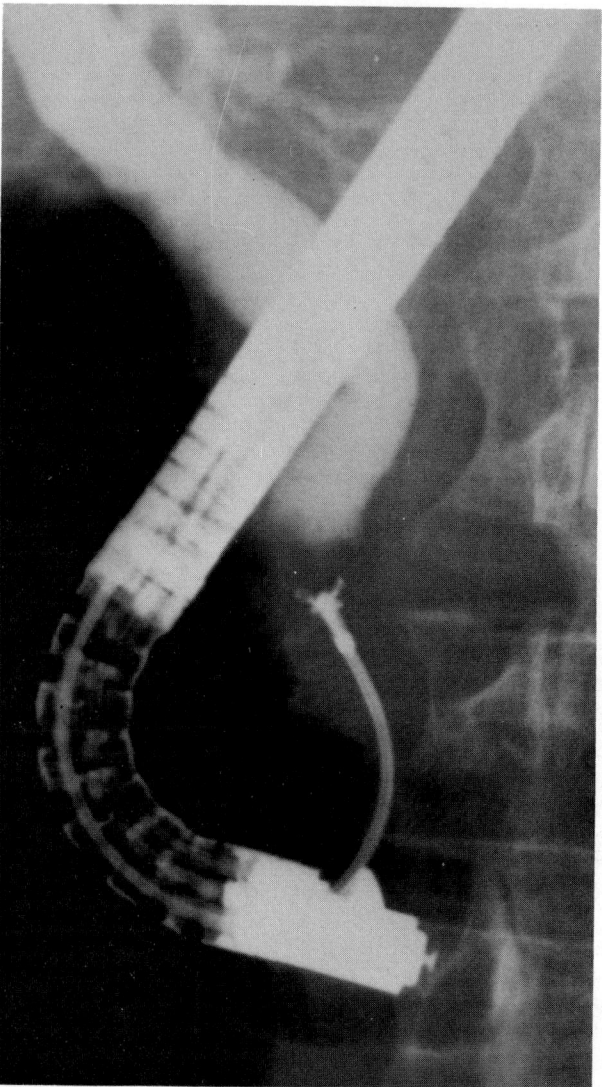

Figure XI-1-3. Biopsy forceps passed up the bile duct for tissue diagnosis of cholangiocarcinoma.

Endoscopic Treatment

So far the main therapeutic contribution of endoscopy has been in the palliation of malignant obstructive jaundice, using plastic stents.[18] Once a guidewire has been passed through a malignant biliary stricture, it is relatively simple to railroad a stent (Figures XI-1-4 and XI-1-5). This technique is now widely used in poor risk patients with unresectable disease; the success rate for relief of jaundice in patients with low obstruction is 85–90%, with minimal complications. The main problem with biliary stenting currently is that standard stents (10 or 11.5 French gauge) have a tendency to clog after about six months. This factor becomes more important as patients with less advanced disease are treated. Approximately 30% of patients with pancreatic cancer treated by endoscopic biliary stenting have required one or more stent changes.

Obstructive jaundice can also be relieved by surgical bypass, and by percutaneous transhepatic radiological stenting. The relative roles for these techniques are hotly debated.[18] Undoubtedly, results depend considerably on individual expertise so that each institution may develop its own bias. Randomized studies have shown that endoscopic stenting is safer and more effective than the percutaneous transhepatic approach, and has substantial short-term advantages over surgical bypass.[18] However, these conclusions apply only to the groups of patients in which the studies were performed, and should not be extrapolated to other patients—or other centers.

The problem of stent clogging is being addressed by exploring new materials, and the value of changing bile composition. Most encouraging at present is the development of expandable wire mesh stents. These can be placed through standard duodenoscopes (in a catheter of 8 French gauge), and expand in situ up to a maximum of 10 mm (30 French gauge). Preliminary experience has been encouraging.

Management of hilar tumors is more troublesome, both technically and conceptually; it is difficult to provide effective drainage to all obstructed segments.[67] Endoscopists approach these strictures from below, and interventional radiologists from above; increasingly endoscopists and radiologists combine to insert two or more stents, in an attempt to provide

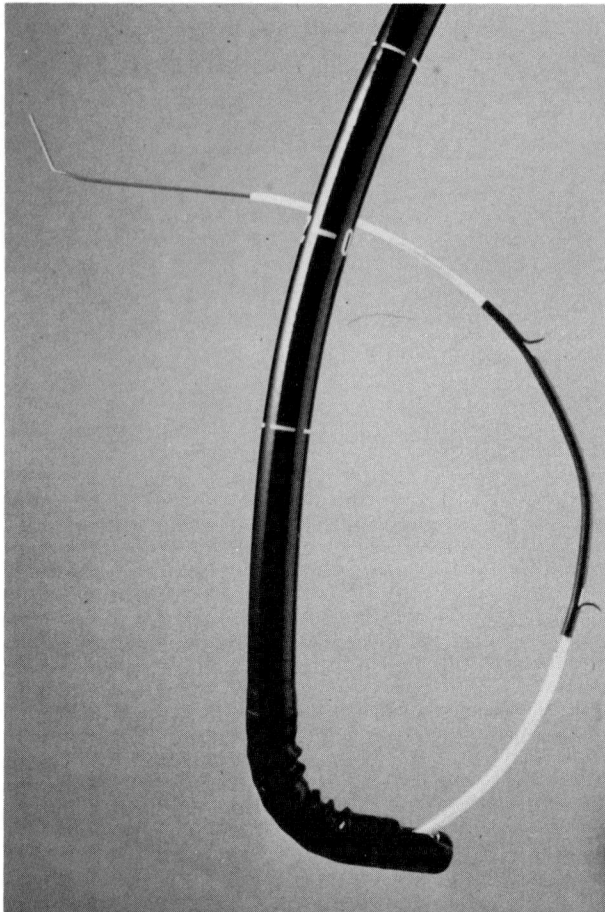

Figure XI-1-4. Endoscopic equipment for stent insertion: large channel duodenoscope with a three layer system comprising a guidewire, cathether and stent with anchoring flaps.

comprehensive drainage, thereby reducing the risk of sepsis in undrained segments.

Tumors of the papilla of Vater causing jaundice or pancreatitis can also be managed endoscopically when there are strong contraindications to surgical resection (e.g., advanced age or distant metastases). The tumor can be debulked by snare diathermy or laser, and the obstructed orifices opened by endoscopic diathermy sphincterotomy, with or without stenting. Some patients have been managed successfully for several years, but there is a need for repeated intervention, and some patients have problems with bleeding and eventual duodenal obstruction.[43]

Some endoscopists have advocated placing stents in malignant strictures of the pancreatic duct in the hope of relieving pain and improving digestion. The value of this treatment has not been proven.

Techniques for tumor destruction have been developed.[18] Iridium[192] wires can be placed in the bile duct through endoscopically inserted nasobiliary tubes or stents. Unfortunately, as with intraoperative or percutaneous iridium treatment, there are no randomized controlled data to prove benefit. Attempts to debulk intraluminal bile duct tumors by laser balloons or other tumor probes are in their infancy. Such techniques may eventually be linked to endoluminal ultrasound probes to

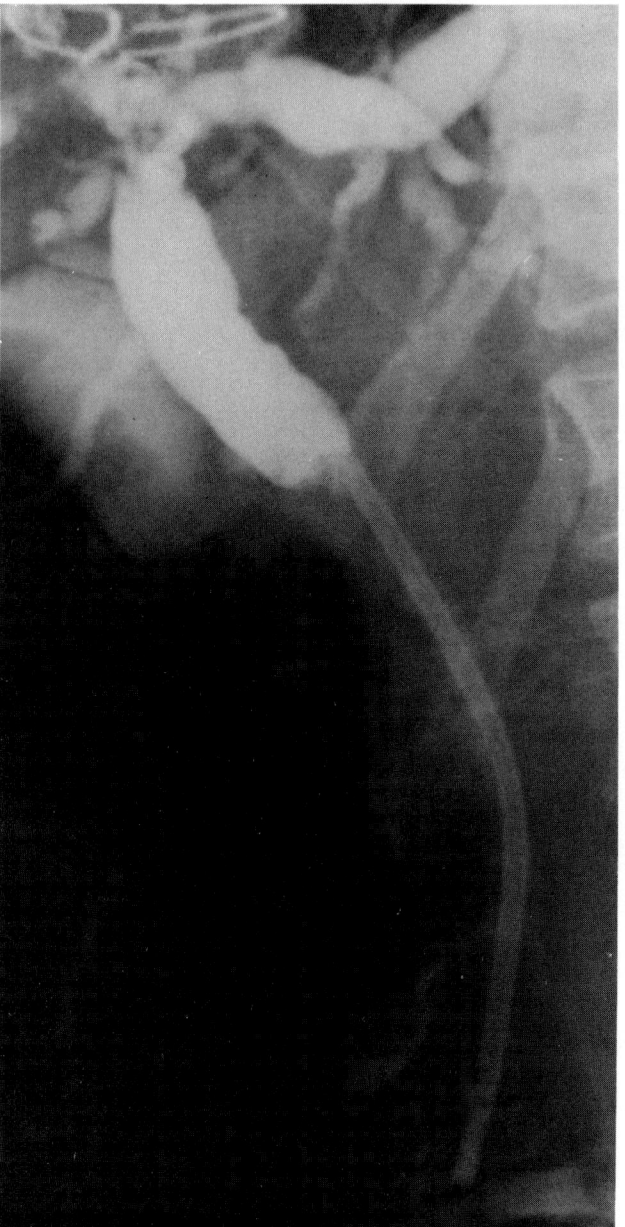

Figure XI-1-5. Stent in place through a mid duct cholangiocarcinoma with good drainage into the duodenum.

demonstrate the depth of tumor invasion and results of treatment.

Peroral Transpapillary Cholangioscopy and Pancreatoscopy

The development of "mother and baby" endoscope systems (Figure XI-1-6) now permit direct peroral visualization of the biliary and pancreatic ductal systems. The smallest "miniscopes" can be passed through the intact papilla, but are limited in their functions. Endoscopes large enough (4 mm) to have tip deflection and an operating channel require a sphincterotomy for insertion. Cholangioscopy and pancreatoscopy occasionally permit diagnosis of tumors which had previously escaped detection (especially small mucus

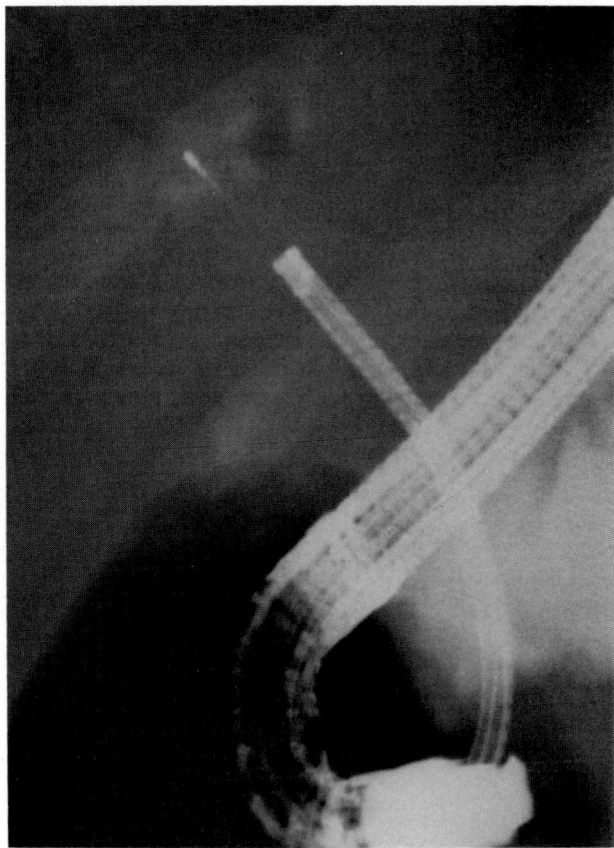

Figure XI-1-6. "Mother and baby" endoscope system. A small fiberscope is passed through the channel of a larger instrument, allowing direct examination of the bile duct, and tissue sampling under direct vision.

secreting lesions). Tumor destruction and manipulation under direct vision may be possible eventually. Similar instruments and techniques can be applied in the bile duct (and pancreas) in patients who have a suitable stoma formed at surgery or by percutaneous intervention.

Clinical Contexts

Patients with symptoms suggestive of pancreatic cancer (without jaundice) are normally investigated with ultrasound, CT scanning and upper GI endoscopy to rule out gastric or duodenal disease. Scans will detect most pancreatic cancers (because they are large at presentation), and the diagnosis can be confirmed by percutaneous biopsy. Patients in whom a suspicion of pancreatic disease persists despite negative or equivocal scanning should undergo ERCP. Pancreatography will detect tumors of duct origin (and pancreatitis) in some patients with negative scans, and a normal examination in this context provides considerable reassurance.

Endoscopic methods have their greatest contribution in patients with jaundice. Percutaneous transhepatic cholangiography is a very effective diagnostic technique, but the endoscopic approach has a greater diagnostic and therapeutic range. Where expertise is available, ERCP will be required in most jaundiced patients, whatever the scans demonstrate, unless there is a clear indication for immediate

surgery. Good quality ERCP will refine the diagnosis (perhaps with tissue confirmation) and start the treatment process. Stones are managed by sphincterotomy, and strictures by stenting.[17] We recommend stenting patients with malignant strictures even if there is a strong possibility of subsequent surgical resection. The risks of stent insertion are probably less than those of leaving instrumented ducts undrained, and it is likely that preoperative drainage may have some beneficial effect on surgical morbidity. Enthusiasm for preoperative external drainage has evaporated after several negative randomized trials,[66] but the endoscopic approach is different. Bile drains internally, there are none of the risks of transhepatic puncture, and the stent can remain in place for permanent palliation if the decision is eventually made not to attempt resection.

Management of patients with biliary and pancreatic malignancy is a multidisciplinary task. Endoscopists have powerful diagnostic and therapeutic skills, which are most effective if they work closely with colleagues in radiology, surgery and oncology. It is equally true that more prospective collaborative studies are needed to evaluate and improve our management.

Laparoscopy

Laparoscopy, direct visualization of the peritoneal cavity using a rigid teleoscope (laparoscope), has become an infrequently used tool in the hands of most gastroenterologists, largely because of significant advances in imaging by ultrasound, computerized tomography (CT), and magnetic resonance (MRI) techniques. In addition, ERCP has greatly improved visualization of the biliary tree and pancreas. However, a renaissance may be just around the corner: a spin-off of the current vogue for laparoscopic cholecystectomy[69] is likely to be a renewed appreciation of the diagnostic uses of laparoscopy (see XI-3).

Laparoscopy has been shown to provide a diagnosis in many patients with obscure abdominal pain.[27] Indeed, it has been suggested, albeit by supporters of the technique, that no patient should have his or her abdominal pain labeled as "psychogenic" unless laparoscopy has been performed. Although innovative Japanese workers have described a sophisticated technique for directly visualizing the pancreas,[95] the usual application of the laparoscope in pancreatic disease is to perform peritoneoscopy for staging.[56] Patients with adenocarcinoma of the pancreas can be spared major surgery for attempted curative resection if liver and/or peritoneal metastases are seen and biopsied at laparoscopy. Laparoscopic biopsy of tumor nodules can provide a histologic diagnosis in metastatic cancer when the primary is unknown.

Perhaps the unique diagnostic value of laparoscopy is in the evaluation of focal, superficial liver lesions. Not only can biopsy of nodules on the liver surface confirm the presence and type of tumor, but it may yield a diagnosis of chronic granulomatous disease such as tuberculosis[2] and brucellosis, or one of the systemic mycoses.[75] Peritoneoscopy and biopsy of peritoneal nodules can also provide valuable diagnostic information in ascites.[34] To date, there have been few therapeutic applications of laparoscopy in malignancy, but this is certain to change with the rapid development of laparoscopic surgery and the miniaturization of flexible endoscopes and accessories. With increasing endoscopic access to organs and body cavities previously only reached by surgical exploration, the possibilities for laser photoablation, cryosurgery, local irradiation, and surgical procedures through the laparoscope seem considerable.

Conclusion

Endoscopy clearly has the primary role in diagnosis of tumors arising in the esophagus, stomach and large bowel. Refinements in some techniques, and concentration on high risk groups, will eventually result in earlier diagnosis and more effective treatment. The relatively new technology of endoscopic intraluminal ultrasound provides an intriguing new perspective in staging, and enhances the possibility of tumor cure by endoscopic techniques, validated by submucosal scanning. Current crude techniques for palliation of malignant luminal strictures (esophagus and colon) will be refined.

Endoscopic access to the biliary tree and pancreas has equally dramatic diagnostic and therapeutic consequences, which, through lack of training, are not being exploited fully at the present time. The spread of these techniques and collaboration with other cancer specialists will provide an increasingly tight focus on specific problems and patients.

References

1. Aabakken, L., Karesen, R., Serck-Hanssen, A., and Osnes, M.: Transpapillary biopsies and brush cytology from the common bile duct. Endoscopy, 18:49, 1986.
2. Alvarez, S. Z., and Carpio, R.: Hepatobiliary tuberculosis. Dig. Dis. Sci., 28:193, 1983.
3. American Cancer Society: Guidelines for the cancer-related check-up. Recommendations and Rationale. CA, 30:4, 1980.
4. Bjork, J. T., Geenen, J. E., Soergel, K. H., Parker, H. W., Leinicke, J. A., and Komorowski, R. A.: Endoscopic evaluation of large gastric folds: A comparison of biopsy techniques. Gastrointest. Endosc., 24:22, 1977.
5. Blackstone, M., Riddell, R. H., Rogers, B. H. G., and Levin, B.: Dysplasia-associated lesions or mass (DALM) detected by colonoscopy in longstanding ulcerative colitis: An indication for colectomy. Gastroenterology, 80:366, 1981.
6. Bohlman, T., Katon, R., Lipshultz, G., McCool, M. F., Smith, F. W., and Melnyk, C. S.: Fiberoptic pansigmoidoscopy. An evaluation and comparison with rigid sigmoidoscopy. Gastroenterology, 72:644, 1977.
7. Bown, S. G., Hawes, R., Matthewson, K., Swain, C. P., Barr, H., Boulos, P. B., and Clark, C. G.: Endoscopic laser palliation for advanced malignant dysphagia. Gut, 28:799, 1987.
8. Buset, M., Des Mares, B., Baize, M., Bourgeois, N., de Boelpaepe, C., de Toeuf, J., and Cremer, M.: Palliative endoscopic management of obstructive esophagogastric cancer: Laser or Prosthesis? Gastrointest. Endosc., 33:357, 1987.
9. Caletti, G. C., Zani, L., Bolondi, L., Brocchi, E., Rollo, V., and Barbara, L.: Endoscopic ultrasonography in the diagnosis of gastric submucosal tumor. Gastrointest. Endosc., 35:413, 1989.
10. Caygill, C., Hill, M., Kirkham, J., and Northfield, T. C.: Mortality from gastric cancer following gastric surgery for peptic ulcer. Lancet, 1:929, 1986.
11. Colina, F., Solis, J. A., and Munoz, M. T.: Squamous papilloma of the esophagus. Am. J. Gastro., 74:410, 1980.
12. Conte, C. C., Welch, J. P., Tennant, R., Forouhar, F., Lundy, J., and Bloom, G. P.: Management of endoscopically removed malignant colon polyps. J. Surg. Oncol., 36:116, 1987.
13. Cothren, R. M., Richards-Kortum, R., Sivak, M. V., Fitzmaurice, M., Rava, R. P., Boyce, G. A., Doxtader, M., Blackman, R., Ivanc, T. B., Hayes, G. B., Feld, M. S. and Petras, R. E.: Gastrointestinal tissue diagnosis by laser-induced fluorescence spectroscopy at endoscopy. Gastrointest. Endosc., 36:105, 1990.
14. Cotton, P. B., and Shorvon, P. J.: Analysis of endoscopy and radiography in the diagnosis, followup, and treatment of peptic ulcer disease. Clin. Gastroenterol., 13:383, 1986.
15. Cotton, P. B., and Williams, C. B.: Practical Gastrointestinal Endoscopy. Third Edition, Boston, Blackwell Scientific Publications, 1990.
16. Cotton, P. B.: Complications of ERCP and Therapeutic Procedures. In Gastrointestinal Emergencies. Edited by M. B. Taylor. Baltimore, Williams & Wilkins, 1989.
17. Cotton, P. B.: Endoscopy can replace surgery for treatment of many patients with biliary obstruction. N. C. Med. J., 5:210, 1990.
18. Cotton, P. B.: Management of malignant bile duct obstruction. J. Gastroenterology Hepatology, 5:63, 1990.
19. Cox, J., and Bennett, J. R.: Light at the end of the tunnel? Palliation for oesophageal carcinoma. Gut, 28:781, 1987.
20. Day, N., Munoz, N., and Ghadrian, P.: Epidemiology of Esophageal Cancer: A Review. In Epidemiology of Cancer of the Digestive Tract. Edited by P. Correa and W. Haenszel. The Hague, Netherlands, Nijhoff, 1982, pp. 21–55.
21. Eckhauser, M. L., Imbembo, A. L., and Mansour, E. G.: The role of pre-resectional laser recanalization for obstructing adenocarcinoma of the rectum—comparison of costs and complications. Gastrointest. Endosc., 21:81, 1989.
22. Endo, M., Takeshita, K., and Yoshida, M.: How can we diagnose the early stage of esophageal cancer? Endoscopic diagnosis. Endoscopy, 18:1, 1986.
23. Feller, E. R., Weiser, M. M., and Schapiro, R. H.: Endoscopic visualization of nodular lymphoid hyperplasia. Gastrointest. Endosc., 24:37, 1977.
24. Friedman, S. L., Wright, T. L., and Altman, D. F.: Gastrointestinal Kaposi's sarcoma in patients with acquired immunodeficiency syndrome. Gastroenterology, 89:102, 1985.
25. Gana, T. J., Soenen, G. M, and Koo, J.: A controlled study of human resting gastric mucosal blood flow by endoscopic laser-Doppler flowmetry. Gastrointest. Endosc., 36(3):264, 1990.
26. Gasparri, G., Caselegno, P. A., Camandona, M., Dei Poli, M., Salizzoni, M., Ferrarotti, G, and Bertero, D.: Endoscopic insertion of 248 prostheses in inoperable carcinoma of the esophagus and cardia: Short-term and Long-term results. Gastrointest. Endosc., 33:354, 1987.
27. Goldstein, D. P.: Acute and chronic pelvic pain. Adolesc. Gynecol., 36:573, 1989.
28. Graham, D. Y., Tabibian, N., Michaletz, P. A., Kinner, B. M., Schwartz, J. T., Heiser, M. C., Dixon, W. B., and Smith, J. L.: Endoscopic needle biopsy: A comparative study of forceps biopsy, two different types of needles, and salvage cytology in gastrointestinal cancer. Gastrointest. Endosc., 35(3):207, 1989.
29. Graham, D. Y., and Spjut, H. J.: Salvage cytology, A new alternative fiberoptic technique. Gastrointest. Endosc., 25:137, 1979.
30. Greenstein, A. J., Sachar, D. B., Smith, H., Janowicz, H. D., and Aufses, A. H., Jr.: A comparison of cancer risk in Crohn's disease and ulcerative colitis. Cancer, 48:2742, 1981.
31. Gueller, R., and Haddad, J. K.: Gastric carcinoids simulating benign polyps. Two cases diagnosed by endoscopic biopsy. Gastrointest. Endosc., 21:153, 1975.
32. Guillem, J. G., Forde, K. A., Treat, M. R., Neugut, A. I., and Bodian, C. A.: The impact of colonoscopy on the early detection of colonic neoplasms in patients with rectal bleeding. Ann. Surg., 206:606, 1987.
33. Hagenmueller, F., Sander, C., Sander, R., Ries, G., and Classen, M.: Laser and endoluminal 192-iridium radiation. Endoscopy, 19:16, 1987.
34. Hall, T. J., Donaldson, D. R., and Brennan, T. G.: The value of laparoscopy under local anesthesia in 250 medical and surgical patients. Br. J. Surg., 67:751, 1980.
35. Hall-Craggs, M. A., and Lees, W. R.: Fine needle biopsy: Cytology, Histology or both? Gut, 28:233, 1987.
36. Harashima, S., Hicata, M., and Masabuchi, K.: Cytology diagnosis of esophageal cancer by esophago-fiberscope. (Abstract) Proceedings of the Seventh International Congress of Cytology, Acta Cytol., 25:79, 1981.
37. Hardcastle, J. D., Winawer, S. J., Burt, R. W., Kronborg, O., and St. John, D. J. B.: Screening for colorectal neoplasia. Working Party Rep., Blackwell Scientific, Melbourne, 1990, pp. 27–35.
38. Hart, M. H., Vanderhoof, J. A., and Antonson, D. L.: Failure of blind small bowel biopsy in the diagnosis of intestinal lymphangiectasia. J. Pediatr. Gastroenterol. Nutr., 6:803, 1987.
39. Hennessy, T. P. J.: Choice of treatment in carcinoma of the esophagus. Br. J. Surg., 75:193, 1988.
40. Hirschowicz, B. I., Curtis, L. E., Peters, C. W., and Pollard, H. M.: Demonstration of a new gastroscope: the "fibrescope." Gastroenterology, 35:50, 1958.
41. Homes, G., Stokes, P., Sorahan, T., Prior, P., Waterhouse, J. A., and Cooke, W. T.: Coeliac disease, gluten-free diet, and malignancy. Gut, 17:612, 1978.
42. Hopkins, R., and Postelwait, R.: Caustic burns and carcinoma of the esophagus. Ann. Surg., 184:146, 1981.
43. Huibregtse, K.: Endoscopic biliary and pancreatic drainage. Georg Thieme Verlag, Stuttgart, 1988.
44. Hunt, R. H., Cotton, P. B., Crespi, M., Drago, J. R. Kawai, K., Lambert, R., Lightdale, C. J., Sanderson, D. R., and Stevenson, G. W.: Role of endoscopy in the diagnosis of cancer: a consensus statement prepared by a working parity of the International Union against cancer. Cancer Res., 49:6822, 1989.
45. Ichikawa, H.: Screening in Cancer. Genova, UICC, 1978.
46. Imaoka, W., Ida, K., and Katoh, T.: Is curative endoscopic treatment of early gastric cancer possible? Endoscopy, 19:1, 1986.
47. Johnson, M. G., and Jolly, P. C.: Analysis of a mass colorectal cancer screening program for cost-effectiveness. Am. J. Surg. 154:261, 1987.
48. Johnston, J. H., Fleisher, D., Petrini, J., and Nord, H. J.: Palliative bipolar electrocoagulation therapy of obstructing esophageal cancer. Gastrointest. Endosc., 33:349, 1987.
49. Kamiya, T., Morishita, T., Asa Kura, H., Miura, S., Munakata, Y., and Tsuchiya, M.: Long term followup study on gastric adenomas. Cancer, 50:2496, 1982.
50. Kayrim, K., Seidlitz, H. K., Hagenmüller, F., and Classen, M.: Videoendoscopes in comparison with fiberscopes: quantitative measurements of optical resolution. Endoscopy, 19:156, 1987.
51. Kiefhaber, P.: Indications for endoscopic neodymium—YAG laser treatment in the gastrointestinal tract. Twelve years experience. Scand. J. Gastroenterol., 2(Suppl. 139):53, 1987.
52. Kronborg, O., Hage, E., and Deichgraeber, E.: The clean colon: A prospective, partly randomized study of the effectiveness of repeated examinations of the colon after polypectomy and radical surgery for cancer. Scand. J. Gastroenterol., 16:879, 1981.
53. Kuyama, Y., Yamamoto, N., Takashimizu, Y., Tamura, Y., Sasabe, M., Kurosawa, H., Fujimoto, H., Nishiura, M., and Ohkusa, T.: Endoscopic microwave treatment. Gastrointest. Endosc., 33:229, 1987.
54. Lennard-Jones, J., Morson, B., Ritchie, J., Shove, D. C., and Williams, C. B.: Cancer in colitis: assessment of the individual risk by clinical and histological criteria. Gastroenterology, 73:1280, 1977.
55. Lewis, B. S., and Waye, J. D.: Total small bowel enteroscopy. Gastrointest. Endosc., 33:435, 1987.
56. Lightdale, C. J.: Clinical applications of laparoscopy in patients with malignant neoplasms. Gastrointest. Endosc., 28:99, 1982.
57. Lux, G., Wilson, D., Wilson, J., and Demling, L.: A cuffed tube for the treatment of oesophago-bronchial fistulae. Endoscopy, 19:28, 1987.
58. Maunoury, V., Brunetaud, J. M., Cochelard, D., Delette, O., Cortot, A., and Paris, J. C.: Palliative treatment of esophagogastric cancer by laser photoablation. Gastroenterol. Clin. Biol., 11:371, 1987.
59. McLean, G. K., and Burke, D. R.: Role of endoprosthesis in the management of malignant biliary obstruction. Radiology, 170:961, 1989.
60. Morson, B. C., Whiteway, J. E., Jones, E. A., Macrae, F. A., and Williams, C. B.: Histopathology and prognosis of colonrectal polyps treated by endoscopic polypectomy. Gut, 25(5):437, 1984.
61. Morson, B. C., and Dawson, I. P.: Non-epithelial tumours. In Gastrointestinal Pathology. Edited by B. C. Morson and I. P. Dawson. Oxford, Blackwell Scientific, pp. 187–199, 1979.
62. Nelson, R. S., and Lanza, F.: Malignant melanoma metastatic to the upper gastrointestinal tract. Gastrointest. Endosc., 24:156, 1978.

63. Northfield, T. C., Swain, C. P., Kirkham, J. S., Salmon, R. R., and Bown, S. G.: Controlled trial of Nd-YAG laser photocoagulation in bleeding peptic ulcers. Lancet, 1:1113, 1986.
64. Payne-James, J. J., Spiller, R. C., Misiewicz, J. J., and Silk, D. B. A.: Use of ethanol-induced tumor necrosis to palliate dysphagia in patients with esophagogastric cancer. Gastrointest. Endosc., 36:43, 1990.
65. Peetze, M. E., and Moseley, H. S.: Brunner's gland hyperplasia. Am. Surg., 55:474, 1989.
66. Pitt, H. A., Gomes, A. S., and Lois, J. F.: Does preoperative percutaneous biliary drainage reduce operative risk or increase hospital cost? Ann. Surg., 201:545, 1985.
67. Polydorou, A. A., Cairns, S. R., Dowset, J. F., Hatfield, A. R., Salmon, P. R., Cotton, P. B., and Russell, R. C.: Palliation of proximal malignant biliary obstruction by endoscopic endoprosthesis insertion. Gut, 32:685, 1991.
68. Qizibash, A., Castelli, M., Kowalsi, M., and Churly, A.: Endoscopic brush cytology and biopsy in the diagnosis of cancer of the upper gastrointestinal tract. Acta Cytol., 24:313, 1980.
69. Reddick, E. J., and Olsen, D. O.: Laparoscopic laser cholecystectomy. Surg. Endosc., 3:131, 1989.
70. Rey, J. F., Albuisson, M., Greff, M., Bidart, J. M., and Monget, J. M.: Electronic video endoscopy: Preliminary results of image modification. Endoscopy, 20:8, 1988.
71. Reynolds, J., Lukeman, J., and Fernandez, T.: Endoscopic cytology and biopsy diagnosis of esophageal carcinoma. South. Med. J., 75:1201, 1982.
72. Ritter, S., and Peterson, G.: Esophageal cancer hyperkeratosis, and oral leukoplakia: Occurrence in a 25-year-old woman. JAMA, 235:1723, 1978.
73. Ryan, M. E., Norfleet, R. G., Kirchner, J. P., Parent, K., Nunez, J. F., Rhodes, R., and Wyman, J.: The significance of diminutive colonic polyps found at flexible sigmoidoscopy. Gastrointest. Endosc., 35:85, 1989.
74. Sander, R., Poesl, H., Zuern, W., Spuhler, A. and Braida, M.: The water-jet guided Nd:YAG laser in the treatment of gastroduodenal ulcer with a visible vessel—a randomized controlled and prospective study. Endoscopy, 21:217, 1989.
75. Saw, E. C., Shields, S. J., Comer, T. P., and Huntington, R. W.: Granulomatous peritonitis due to coccidioides immitis. Arch. Surg., 108:369, 1974.
76. Schottenfeld, D., and Winawer, S.: Large intestine. In Cancer Epidemiology and Prevention. Edited by D. Schottenfeld and J. Fraumeni, Jr. Philadelphia, W. B. Saunders, 1982, pp. 703–727.
77. Schuman, B. M.: Diseases of the Duodenum. In Gastroenterologic Endoscopy. Edited by M. V. Sivak, Jr. Philadelphia, W. B. Saunders, 1987.
78. Shen, Q.: Diagnostic cytology and early detection. In Carcinoma of the Esophagus and Gastric Cardia. Edited by G. J. Huang and W. Y. Kai. Berlin, Springer Verlag, 1984, p. 156.
79. Shu, Y.-J.: Cytopathology of the esophagus. Acta Cytol., 27:7, 1983.
80. Silverstein, F. E., Martin, R. W., Kimmey, M. B., Jiranek, G. C., Franklin, D. W., and Proctor, A.: Experimental evaluation of an endoscopic ultrasound probe: In vitro and In vivo canine studies. Gastroenterology, 96:1058, 1989.
81. Sipponen, P., Kekki, M., Haapakoski, J., Ihamaki, T., and Siurala, M.: Gastric cancer risk in chronic atrophic gastritis: Statistical calculations of cross-sectional data. Int. J. Cancer, 35:173, 1985.
82. Sivak, M. V., Jr., and Jagelman, D. G.: Upper gastrointestinal endoscopy in polyposis syndromes: Familial Polyposis Coli and Gardner's syndrome. Gastrointest. Endosc., 30:102, 1984.
83. Sjogren, R., and Johnson, L.: Barrett's esophagus: A review. Am. J. Med., 74:313, 1983.
84. Spechler, S., Robbins, A., Bloomfield, R., Rubins, H. B., Vincent, M. E., Heeren, T., Doos, W. G., Colton, T., and Schimmel, E. M.: Adenocarcinoma and Barrett's esophagus: An overrated risk? Gastroenterology, 87:927, 1984.
85. Spechler, S.: Endoscopic surveillance for patients with Barrett's esophagus: Does the cancer risk justify the practice? Ann. Intern. Med., 106:902, 1987.
86. Stevenson, G.: Radiology in the detection of early gastric cancer. In Early Gastric Cancer. Edited by P. B. Cotton. Proceedings of the Second BSG SK&F International Workshop, 1981.
87. Suzuki, H., Miho, O., Watanabe, Y., Kohyama, M., and Nago, F.: Endoscopic laser therapy in the curative and palliative treatment of upper gastrointestinal cancer. World J., Surg., 13:158, 1989.
88. Tatsuta, M., Iishi, H., and Okuda, S.: Histological features and recurrence of completely and incompletely healed gastric ulcers classified by the methylene blue dye method. Endoscopy, 19:193, 1987.
89. Tepperman, B., and Fitzpatrick, P.: Second respiratory and upper digestive tract cancer after oral cancer. Lancet, 2:547, 1981.
90. Tio, T., Den Hartog Jager, F., and Tytgar, G.: Endoscopic ultrasonography of non-Hodgkin lymphoma of the stomach. Gastroenterology, 91:401, 1986.
91. Trier, J. S.: Complications of celiac sprue and potentially related diseases with similar intestinal histopathology. Gastroenterology, 75:314, 1978.
92. Tytgat, G.: Diagnosis and differential therapy of malignant esophageal stenosis. Internist, 23:251, 1982.
93. Tytgat, G. N. J.: Benign and malignant tumors of the esophagus. In Gastroenterologic Endoscopy. Edited by M. V. Sivak, Jr. Philadelphia, W. B. Saunders, 1987.
94. Wadas, D. D., Foutch, P. G., Manne, R. K., and Sanowski, R. A.: Endoscopic diagnosis of a duodenal gastrinoma. Gastrointest. Endosc., 34:430, 1988.
95. Watanabe, M., Takatori, Y., Ueki, K., Umekawa, Y., Yoshida, H., Kobatake, T., Hirakawa, H., Fukumoto, S., and Shimada, Y.: Pancreatic biopsy under visual control in conjunction with laparoscopy for diagnosis of pancreatic cancer. Endoscopy, 21:105, 1989.
96. Waye, J. D., and Braunfeld, S.: Surveillance intervals after colonoscopic polypectomy. Endoscopy, 14:79, 1982.
97. Weller, I. V. D.: AIDS and the gut. J. Gastroenterol., 81:619, 1986.
98. Williams, C. V., Macrae, F. A., and Bartram, C. I.: A prospective study of diagnostic methods in adenoma followup. Endoscopy, 14:74, 1982.
99. Wychulis, A., Woolam, G., and Anderson, H.: Achalasia and carcinoma of the esophagus. JAMA, 215:1638, 1971.

XI-2

Bronchoscopy

William J. Fulkerson, Jr.
Victor F. Tapson

Introduction

Bronchoscopy permits direct examination of the tracheobronchial tree and facilitates diagnosis and treatment of lung neoplasms and other pulmonary conditions that occur in patients with cancer or immune compromise.[1,2] The advent of flexible fiberoptics has greatly expanded the role and utility of bronchoscopy and allows outpatient procedures in many patients under topical anesthesia and minimal sedation. Indications for diagnostic and therapeutic bronchoscopy are listed in Table XI-2-1.

Tumors

Diagnostic flexible bronchoscopy is perhaps most valuable in evaluating patients with suspected lung cancer. Staging for resectability and tissue diagnosis are obtainable with one procedure. During bronchoscopy, the larynx and vocal cords are carefully examined, and suspicious lesions or vocal cord paralysis can be detected. Left vocal cord paralysis in patients with a left-sided lung mass is usually secondary to injury of the left recurrent laryngeal nerve by pathologic adenopathy in the mediastinum. This contraindicates surgical resection. Next, the proximal and distal trachea, and mainstem carina are examined. Involvement of these areas by endobronchial tumor or tumor in the mainstem bronchi within two centimeters of the mainstem carina also prohibit surgical resection. Edema, erythema, extrinsic compression, or splaying of the carina may also indicate submucosal tumor involvement and necessitate biopsy or needle aspiration.

The major mediastinal lymph node groups can be sampled transtracheally or transbronchially using a small biopsy needle attached to a flexible catheter.[23,25] The catheter can be passed through the channel of the bronchoscope, and the needle can penetrate the bronchial wall under direct vision to obtain cytologic samples of paratracheal or subcarinal lymph nodes (Figure XI-2-1). This yields accurate and defin-

Table XI-2-1.   Indications for Bronchoscopy

Diagnostic
    Persistent atelectasis
    Unresolved pneumonia
    Radiographic suspicion of neoplasia
    Persistent unexplained cough
    Hemoptysis
    Abnormal sputum cytology
    Diffuse lung disease
    Pulmonary infiltrate in immunocomprmised host

Therapeutic
    Foreign body aspiration
    Acute lobar collapse
    Potential laser therapy
    Endobronchial radiotherapy

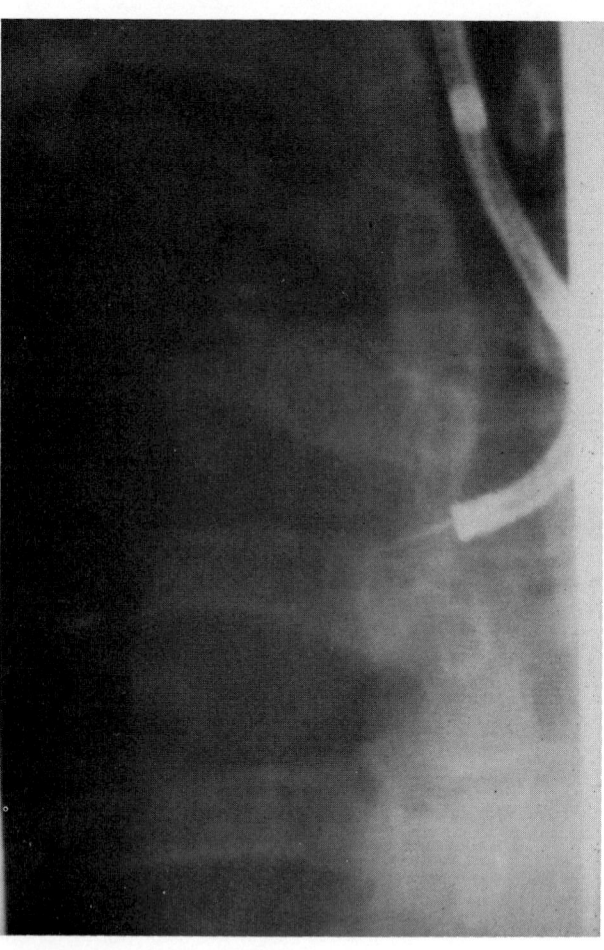

Figure XI-2-1. Transbronchial needle aspiration of a right paratracheal mass through the flexible bronchoscope.

itive information regarding staging of lung cancer. The sensitivity is comparable to CT scanning with superior specificity. Transbronchial needle aspiration (TBNA) of mediastinal nodes should be performed during diagnostic bronchoscopy for suspected malignancy whenever there is concern for nodal metastasis. Positive results make surgical staging procedures such as mediastinoscopy unnecessary, and thoracotomies for unresectable disease can be avoided.

Following examination of the main bronchi, a detailed inspection of all segmental and proximal subsegmental bronchi in each lung should be carried out. If endobronchial abnormalities are detected, the anatomic location and extent of a potential resection can be determined. Metachronous lung cancer may occur in as many as one percent to two percent of patients with bronchogenic carcinoma, and discovery of additional neoplasms almost always drastically changes patient management.[21]

The bronchoscopic yield for endobronchially visible carcinoma should exceed 90% (Figure XI-2-2).[8,19] More peripheral mass lesions may be approached by fluoroscopically directed transbronchial biopsy or needle aspiration, but the diagnostic success is less. Positive diagnoses of peripheral mass lesions in 60–70% of patients have been reported when combined transbronchial biopsy, cytologic brushings, and cytologic washings are reported.[6,19] Positive results are uncommon, however, for nodules less than 2 centimeters in diameter.

Transthoracic needle aspiration (TTNA) offers a higher yield than flexible bronchoscopy for diagnosing small peripheral mass lesions in the chest, but the pneumothorax complication rate is much higher. TTNA obviously supplies no information regarding endobronchial status, and aspiration of central or mediastinal masses is better performed transbronchially than transthoracically. Bronchoscopy is therefore the initial diagnostic procedure of choice for most patients with suspected lung cancer.

Pulmonary Infiltrates and Infections

Pulmonary infiltrates and pulmonary infections occur frequently in cancer patients who are immunocompromised secondary to chemotherapy-induced leukopenia, corticosteroids, or the primary disease process. Physicians must often decide between a course of empiric antibiotic therapy or an invasive diagnostic procedure. When the patient is ill and particularly when the infiltrates are diffuse and progressive, an invasive approach is often chosen. Bronchoscopy has been widely utilized in an attempt to bypass upper airway colonization and obtain diagnostic specimens in immunocompromised patients with pulmonary infiltrates. Several different techniques including the protected specimen brush (PSB), broncho-alveolar lavage (BAL), and transbronchial biopsy can be employed. The concept of the PSB is to avoid contamination during passage of the bronchoscope through the upper airway.[27] Using semi-quantitative cultures, results from the PSB have been accurate at diagnosing bacterial pneumonia in animal and clinical studies.[10,11,18,26]

BAL is a technique which, in conjunction with quantitative cultures of lavage fluid, has been utilized to distinguish pneumonia from bacterial colonization of the upper airways in intubated mechanically ventilated patients. The bronchoscope is wedged in a segment corresponding to the radiographic abnormality. In a patient with diffuse infiltrates, the right middle lobe, or lingula, is often used because of accessibility and because anatomic orientation favors recovery of fluid in the supine patient. Physiologic saline solution (100 ml–200 ml) is infused through the bronchoscope into the lung and subsequently suctioned out. Fever and increased

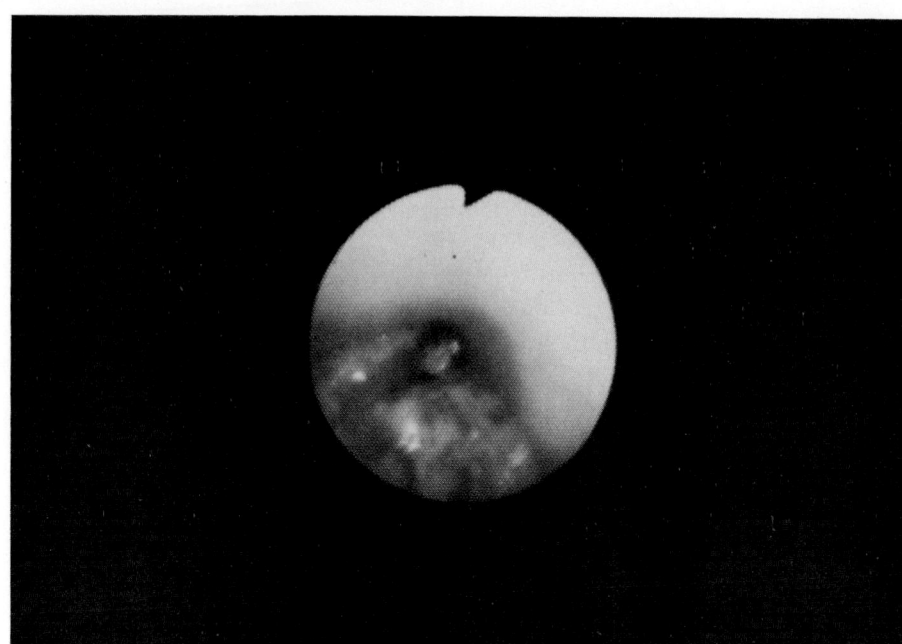

Figure XI-2-2. Endobronchial squamous cell carcinoma in the left upper lobe bronchus.

pulmonary infiltrates in the area of lavage have been reported, but blood cultures are usually negative. Hemorrhage is unusual and rarely significant. BAL has proven to be effective in diagnosing pneumonia due to *pneumocystis carinii* in patients with hematologic neoplasms and those with the acquired immunodeficiency syndrome with sensitivities ranging from 85–97%.[2,5,13] The culture of organisms such as *mycobacterium tuberculosis* and *legionella pneumophilia* is also diagnostic of infection, but quantitative cultures of BAL fluid are necessary to distinguish routine bacterial infections from colonization.[24] BAL may be useful for diagnosing fungal pneumonias in immunocompromised patients. Recovery of histoplasma organisms in BAL fluid is considered diagnostic of infection, but BAL may be less sensitive than transbronchial biopsy for diagnosing histoplasmosis. Candida species frequently colonize the respiratory tract of hospitalized patients, and positive cultures in BAL fluid for candida are not sufficiently diagnostic of true infection. Aspergillus species may also colonize the air passages of both normal and immunocompromised hosts without causing infection. Thus, a firm diagnosis of invasive aspergillus pneumonia requires demonstration of tissue invasion. Kahn and colleagues found that the presence of hyphae in BAL fluid in immunocompromised patients with new pulmonary infiltrates had a 53% sensitivity, a 97% specificity, and a 75% predictive value for invasive disease.[16] At the present time, a positive BAL smear from an immunocompromised host with prolonged neutropenia and focal infiltrate should warrant consideration of anti-fungal therapy. When possible, however, the patient should have direct biopsy evidence of tissue invasion.

The diagnosis of viral pneumonia may be difficult to make by BAL. Some clinicians accept the diagnosis if BAL fluid cultures reveal virus, but more conclusive information requires the addition of characteristic cytopathologic findings such as the intra-nuclear inclusions of cytomegalovirus infection. Crawford and co-workers found that viral cultures from rapid

centrifuges of BAL fluid from 33 bone marrow transplant recipients were positive in 96% of specimens.[7] Confirmatory lung tissue cultures were positive in all cases. The sensitivity of BAL fluid was thus 96%, and the specificity was 100%.

Transbronchial biopsy has been used to diagnose pulmonary infections. Critically ill patients may be more susceptible to bleeding, but the procedure can generally be safely performed if coagulation studies are normal and the platelet count is above 100,000/mm³. Mechanical ventilation may add a significant pneumothorax risk to the procedure. Hedemark and colleagues evaluated 39 renal allograft patients with fever and new pulmonary infiltrates using fiberoptic bronchoscopy.[15] Transbronchial biopsy was performed in 17 patients with specific diagnoses obtained in nine (53%). In three patients (18%) transbronchial biopsy was the only positive bronchoscopic specimen.

Diffuse or focal infiltrates in immunocompromised patients do not always represent infections. Pulmonary hemorrhage, pulmonary edema, lymphangitic carcinomatosis, radiation pneumonitis, and chemotherapy-induced lung disease may complicate the course and treatment of individual patients. Differentiation of these diagnoses from infection on the basis of clinical and radiographic findings is often impossible. Bronchoscopy and transbronchial biopsy will usually be diagnostic of lymphangitic carcinomatosis, but transbronchial biopsies will often only be suggestive or consistent with any of the alternative diagnoses. Open lung biopsy may be necessary when definitive information is necessary.

Therapeutic Bronchoscopy

The therapeutic role for flexible and rigid bronchoscopy is expanding. Aspirated foreign bodies in adults are often removable with flexible bronchoscopes using forceps to grasp objects or special basket attachments for retrieval. In small children and in some adults, rigid bronchoscopy is preferable. Lobar collapse in hospitalized patients due to retained mucus can often be resolved with bronchoscopic lavage and suctioning.

More appropriate to the cancer physician is the therapeutic role of bronchoscopy in managing endobronchial lesions. Successful treatment of airway obstruction due to benign and malignant lesions with a neodymium-YAG laser has been reported.[3,4] Airway caliber can be improved in 85–90% of patients with malignant airway obstruction. In addition to vaporizing airway lesions, hemostasis can be achieved in refractory bleeding lesions. The Nd-YAG laser can be used through a flexible bronchoscope. Most operators agree, however, that a rigid bronchoscope is safer and more effective for Nd-YAG laser therapy. Neodymium-YAG laser treatment of malignant airway lesions is effective but palliative treatment. Major complications include hemorrhage and broncho-pleural fistulae, but they are uncommon.

Successful phototherapy of unresectable endobronchial malignant neoplasms through the flexible bronchoscope with hematoporphyrin derivative (HpD) labelling and argon laser activation has been reported.[9,14] Occasional patients with small lesions, radiographically occult tumors, or carcinoma in situ have shown apparent cure through long term follow-up.[9] This methodology is currently being evaluated in multi-center trials and may be generally available soon.

Endobronchial irradiation brachytherapy with either implanted 198Au seeds or temporary indwelling catheters containing iridium 192 radioactive sources may also offer palliative relief of airway obstruction and control of tumor hemorrhage.[17,20] Objective evidence of airway improvement has been described in approximately 75% of patients. Radiation brachytherapy is easily performed through the flexible bronchoscope under minimal sedation. This treatment may be most appropriate for patients who have failed external beam therapy. Brachytherapy delivers an intensive short radiation dose to the surrounding area and minimizes potential radiation-induced damage to extra-pulmonary tissues. Combination of brachytherapy with Nd-YAG laser treatment may offer even greater palliation.[1,22]

Complications of Bronchoscopy

Complications from bronchoscopy are uncommon if patients are carefully selected and screened. Potential complications are listed in Table XI-2-2, and contraindications to the procedure are noted in Table XI-2-3. Problems related to medications are most often secondary to excessive dosage or underlying organ system dysfunction in the patient. Patients with significant respiratory or cardiac impairment pose an increased risk for subsequent complications, and the indi-

Table XI-2-2.   Complications of Bronchoscopy

Respiratory depression from over-medication
Laryngospasm
Bronchospasm
Hypoxemia
Cardiac arrhythmias
Fever
Pneumonia
Pneumothorax
Hemorrhage

Table XI-2-3.   Contraindications to Bronchoscopy

Routine
    Unstable asthma
    Severe hypoxemia
    Serious arrhythmia
    Unstable angina pectoris
    Poor cooperation

Biopsy Procedure
    Uncorrected bleeding diathesis
    Severe pulmonary hypertension
    Severe anemia

cations for procedures in these patients should be absolute and done under the most optimal conditions. In the average patient, the arterial partial pressure of oxygen will fall approximately 20 torr during flexible bronchoscopy. Fever occurs after bronchoscopy in 15–20% of patients, and radiographic and clinical evidence of pneumonia occurs in about 5%. Patients with near-obstructing endobronchial neoplasms are at increased risk for post-procedure pneumonia. Pneumothorax following transbronchial biopsy has been reported to occur in as many as 5% of patients, but our experience with routine use of fluoroscopic guidance reveals an incidence of less than 1%. Significant bleeding (greater than 50 ml) is uncommon after endobronchial or transbronchial biopsy in patients without evidence of an ongoing coagulopathy. Multiple antibiotics may qualitatively alter platelet function, and a pre-operative bleeding time is recommended in this patient population. All patients undergoing bronchoscopy should receive supplemental oxygen. Cardiac rhythm and arterial oxygen saturation should be continuously monitored throughout and immediately following the procedure.

References

1. Allen, M., Baldwin, J., Fish, V., Goffinet, D., Cannon, W., and Mark, J.: Combined laser therapy and endobronchial radiotherapy for unresectable lung carcinoma with bronchial obstruction. Am. J. Surg., 150:71, 1985.
2. Broaddus, C., Dake, M., Stulbarg, M., Blumfeld, W., Hadley, W., Golden, J., and Hopewell, P.: Bronchoalveolar lavage and transbronchial biopsy for the diagnosis of pulmonary infections in the acquired immunodeficiency syndrome. Ann. Intern. Med., 102:747, 1985.
3. Brutinel, W., Cortese, D., McDougall, J., Gillio, R., and Bergstral, H.: A two-year experience with the neodymium-YAG laser in endobronchial obstruction. Chest, 91:159, 1987.
4. Cavaliere, S., Foccoli, P., and Farina, P.: Nd:YAG laser bronchoscopy. A five year experience with 1,396 applications in 1,000 patients. Chest, 94:15, 1988.
5. Clement, M. J., Luce, J. M., and Hopewell, P. C.: Diagnosis of pulmonary disease. Clin. Chest Med., 9:497, 1988.
6. Cortese, D. A., and McDougall, J. C.: Biopsy and brushing of peripheral lung cancer with fluoroscopic guidance. Chest, 75:141, 1979.
7. Crawford, S., Bowden, R., Hackman, R., Gleaves, C., Meyers, J., and Clark, J.: Rapid detection of cytomegalovirus pulmonary infection by bronchoalveolar lavage and cyto-centrifugation culture. Ann. Intern. Med., 108:180, 1988.
8. Dreisin, R., Albert, R., Talley, P., Krygen, M., Scoggin, C., and Zwillich, C.: Flexible fiberoptic bronchoscopy in the teaching hospital: yield and complications. Chest, 74:144, 1978.
9. Edell, E., and Cortese, D.: Bronchoscopic phototherapy with hematoporphyrin derivative for treatment of localized bronchogenic carcinomas: a 5-year experience. Mayo. Clin. Proc., 62:8, 1987.
10. Fagon, J., Chastre, J., Domart, Y., Trouillet, J., Pierre, J., Darne, C., and Gibert, C.: Nosocomial pneumonia in patients receiving continuous mechanical ventilation. Am. Rev. Resp. Dis., 139:877, 1989.
11. Fagon, J. Y., Chastre, J., Hance, A., Guiget, M., Trouillet, J., Domart, Y., Pierre, J., and Gibert, C.: Detection of nosocomial lung infection in ventilated patients: use of a protected specimen brush and quantitative culture techniques in 147 patients. Am. Rev. Resp. Dis., 138:110, 1988.
12. Fulkerson, W. J.: Fiberoptic bronchoscopy. N. Eng. J. Med., 311:511, 1984.
13. Golden, J., Holander, H., Stulbarg, M., and Gamsu, G.: Bronchoalveolar lavage as the exclusive diagnostic modality for pneumocystis pneumonia: a prospective study among patients with acquired immunodeficiency syndrome. Chest, 90:18, 1986.
14. Hayata, Y., Kato, H., Konaka, C., Amemiya, R., Ono, J., Ogawa, I., Kinoshita, K., Sakai, H., and Takahashi, H.: Photoradiation therapy with hematoporphyrin derivative in early and stage 1 lung cancer. Chest, 86:169, 1984.
15. Hedemark, L., Kronenberg, R., Rasp, F., Simmons, R., and Peterson, P.: The value of

bronchoscopy in establishing the etiology of pneumonia in renal transplant recipients. Am. Rev. Resp. Dis., 126:981, 1982.

16. Kahn, F., Jones, J., and Englund, D.: The role of bronchoalveolar lavage in the diagnosis of invasive pulmonary aspergillosis. Am. J. Clin. Pathol., 86:518, 1986.

17. Mehta, M., Shahab, S., Jarjour, N., Steinmetz, M., and Kubsad, S.: Effect of endobronchial radiation therapy on malignant bronchial obstruction. Chest, 97:662, 1990.

18. Pollock, H. M., Hawkins, E. L., Bonner, J. R., Sparkman, T., and Bass, J. B.: Diagnosis of bacterial pulmonary infections with quantitative protective catheter cultures obtained during bronchoscopy. J. Clinic Microbiol., 17:255, 1983.

19. Popovich, J., Kvale, P., Eichenhorn, M., Radtke, J., Ohorodnik, J., and Fine, G.: Diagnostic accuracy of multiple biopsies from flexible fiberoptic bronchoscopy: a comparison of central vs peripheral carcinoma. Am. Rev. Resp. Dis., 125:521, 1982.

20. Rabie, T., Wilson, K., Easley, J., Teague, R., Bloom, K., Lawrence, C., and Ilaria, R.: Palliation of bronchogenic carcinoma with 198 Au implantation using the fiberoptic brochoscope. Chest, 90:641, 1986.

21. Rohmedder, J., and Weatherbee, L.: Multiple primary bronchogenic carcinoma with a review of the literature. Am. Rev. Resp. Dis., 109:435, 1974.

22. Schray, M., McDougall, J., Martinez, A., Cortese, D., and Brutinel, W.: Management of malignant airway compromise with laser and low dose rate brachytherapy. The Mayo Clinic experience. Chest, 93:264, 1988.

23. Shure, D., and Fedullo, P.: The role of transcarinal needle aspiration in the staging of bronchogenic carcinoma. Chest, 86:693, 1984.

24. Torres, A., Puig de la Bellacasa, J., Zaubet, A., Gonzalez, J., Rodriguez-Roisin, R., DeAnta, T., and Vidal, A.: Diagnostic value of quantitative cultures of bronchoalveolar lavage and telescoping plugged catheters in mechanically ventilated patients with bacterial pneumonia. Am. Rev. Resp. Dis., 140:306, 1989.

25. Wang, K., Brower, R., Haponik, E., and Siegelman, S.: Flexible transbronchial needle aspiration for staging bronchogenic carcinoma. Chest, 84:571, 1983.

26. Wimberly, N., Bass, J. B., Boyd, B. W., Kirkpatrick, M., Serio, R., and Pollock, H.: Use of a bronchoscopic protective catheter brush for the diagnosis of pulmonary infections. Chest, 81:556, 1982.

27. Wimberly, N., Faling, J. C., and Bartlett, J. G.: A fiberoptic bronchoscopy technique to obtain uncomplicated lower airway secretions for bacterial culture. Am. Rev. Resp. Dis., 199:337, 1979.

XI-3

Peritoneoscopy
Robert L. Fine

Introduction

Peritoneoscopy (laparoscopy) is an important tool in the diagnosis, planning and treatment of intra-abdominal cancer. Optical inspection of the abdominal cavity was initially reported by Ott in 1901 with a vaginal retractor and a head mirror for a light source.[66] In 1902, Kelling reported peritoneoscopic examinations using pneumoperitoneum induced by a needle and filtered air.[48] These early attempts were hampered by limited lens capabilities and insufficient light sources. In more modern times, technologic advances in fiber light transmission, wide angle lenses and less morbid peritoneal insufflation have made this procedure safe and relatively inexpensive. Though laparotomy offers wider diagnostic and therapeutic access than peritoneoscopy, peritoneoscopy is much less invasive and provides valuable information to the clinician that often can obviate the need for a laparotomy.

General Indications for Peritoneoscopy

Operability in Patients with Cancer

Peritoneoscopy yields important information to the clinician without making a large abdominal incision or exploratory laparotomy. Its major advantage in the work-up or staging of patients is to help decide which patients are inoperable, because of the presence of multiple liver metastases, peritoneal implants, malignant ascites or widespread carcinomatosis. Peritoneoscopy also defines which patients require laparotomy to further assess resectability including the subset that can undergo an attempt at curative surgery. Sugarbaker and Wilson have suggested that all patients who have advanced primary cancers, with statistically low cure rates, should undergo peritoneoscopy immediately preceding any surgery for curative intent.[90] They suggest that patients in this category might include those with pulmonary, esophageal, gastric, pancreatic, advanced endometrial, and rectal cancers. Patients with advanced colonic and gastric cancer may sometimes require surgical resection to circumvent obstruction and bleeding. Patients with primary colonic cancer do not benefit from preoperative peritoneoscopy since curative surgery is the intent, and resection will be performed in most cases. This is also true for primary ovarian cancer since debulking surgery together with chemotherapy has been shown to improve complete remission rates and survival.

Liver Metastases

The presence or absence of liver metastases significantly influences the course of patient management and therapy for a number of cancers. Non-invasive techniques such as ultrasound, computed tomography (CT) scan and magnetic resonance imaging (MRI) of the liver can detect lesions. Peritoneoscopy has the advantage of providing a diagnosis by biopsy and of detecting small metastatic sites on the liver surface and peritoneum not visualized by non-invasive techniques. The presence of small (<2 cm.) liver metastases in patients with lung cancer may be underestimated by CT scanning or ultrasound of the liver. In one series 11% of 140 patients who underwent curative resection for lung cancer had, at autopsy, within one month of surgery, metastatic disease in the liver not detected in the work-up.[59] In a series of 450 consecutive autopsies, Ozarda and Pickren found that in 89% of all cases with metastases to the liver at least one metastatic site was visible on the anterior surface of the liver.[67] Conversely, Hogg and Pack reported that if hepatic metastases were not found at laparotomy, then they were absent at autopsy in 95% of those patients.[41] Unfortunately, this type of study has not been reported for peritoneoscopy, but it is logical to assume that the greater the liver surface examined laparoscopically, the higher the likelihood of detecting hepatic metastases by peritoneoscopy.

Beside, blind percutaneous liver biopsy has been compared to peritoneoscopic guided liver biopsy for the detection of neoplastic lesions. The false negative rate for blind percutaneous liver biopsies for malignant lesions is high, sometimes approximating 50%.[60] Peritoneoscopically directed liver biopsies can double the detection rate of metastases compared to percutaneous liver biopsies in patients with Hodgkin's Disease,[3] hepatocellular carcinoma,[60] and various other cancers.[47] This is especially true if the lesions are small, single, or in the left lobe of the liver.

The diagnostic accuracy of peritoneoscopic liver biopsies in patients with cancers who have abnormal liver function tests and/or non-invasive test abnormalities approximates 90% in a number of series.[20,21,53] In patients with ascites from unknown origin peritoneoscopy diagnosed 80% of the cases.[84] Complication rates in this study were 4% or less and there was no mortality.

The relative diagnostic accuracy of peritoneoscopy compared to isotopic liver scans, ultrasound with fine needle biopsy, and CT scan has been addressed by a number of authors. In a study of 222 cases evaluated by liver (^{99}Tc-sulfur colloid) scanning and peritoneoscopy it was found that the liver scan had a true positive (sensitivity) rate of 79% with a false positive rate of 18%. Peritoneoscopy was virtually identical in the sensitivity rate but, as expected, had no false positives. These two techniques detected 123 cases of liver tumors (primary and metastatic), and 99 cases of benign conditions. All cases were confirmed by biopsy, laparotomy or autopsy.[81] Lightdale and colleagues reported similar results for liver scans in 100 consecutive patients with a clinical suspicion of liver neoplasia; they found an increased true positive rate for peritoneoscopy (92%) with no false positives.[54] Of the patients with a negative percutaneous blind liver biopsy, 38% were found to have neoplasm in the liver by peritoneoscopy. In the detection of liver neoplasms the liver scan is sensitive (80%), but specificity can vary significantly (50–82%);[92] while peritoneoscopy is sensitive (80–92%) with high specificity (100%). Based on these studies, liver scan should not be used alone for the proper work-up of neoplasms unless followed by peritoneoscopy.[12]

Peritoneoscopy vs. Sonography

A retrospective analysis of the merits of diagnosing hepatic neoplasms by ultrasound guided fine needle aspiration biopsy versus peritoneoscopy has shown equivalent sensitivity (75%) and overall accuracy (83%) for both procedures.[35] For small, deeply located and singular lesions ultrasound provided the most useful guide for biopsy while peritoneoscopy was superior for the diagnosis of cirrhosis and in lesions requiring more tissue for diagnosis or histologic architecture to differentiate subtypes of lymphoma. This is in agreement with a study by Prior and colleagues who demonstrated similar sensitivities in the procedures (approximately 85%).[74] However, a correct histologic diagnosis could only be made on 50% of the fine needle aspiration cytologies because of technical and methodologic difficulties. Obviously, the accuracy of cytology rests upon the experience of the cytopathologist, and the value of cytopathology is also dependent upon the type of tumor involved. Epithelial tumors can be accurately diagnosed on cytology, but this is not always true for lymphomas and sarcomas. Architecture is vital to the correct diagnosis of nodular and diffuse lymphomas and the cellular yield from aspirations of sarcomas may be poor.[17,22,34] Lymphoma classification can be made sometimes by cytology with immunocytochemical stains, but in general, the initial and, at times, relapse diagnosis (especially in low grade, nodular lymphomas) requires tissue that peritoneoscopy can offer. Suspected hepatocellular carcinoma is also best confirmed by tissue biopsy since regenerating hepatocytes in cirrhosis can mimic hepatoma cells.[82] Fine needle aspiration guided by ultrasound may not be the method of choice in patients for whom an exact histologic diagnosis is required as previously mentioned. However, for the staging and follow-up of known extrahepatic neoplasms, outside of lymphomas, sarcomas and, with some exceptions, hepatocellular carcinomas, fine needle aspiration guided by ultrasound is equivalent to peritoneoscopy.

Peritoneoscopy vs. CT Scans

Comparison studies between peritoneoscopy and CT scans for detection of hepatic neoplasms have been addressed in two studies, retrospectively, and each has shown distinct advantages for each procedure. The CT scan can display areas not routinely visualized by peritoneoscopy such as retroperitoneal structures, lymph nodes, skeletal structures, posterior and superior areas of the liver, kidneys and other viscera that may be inaccessible to the peritoneoscopist. Approximately 80% of the liver surface is visualized by peritoneoscopy, but deep seated lesions may be missed. In the study by Barth and colleagues, CT scan with guided thin needle biopsy and peritoneoscopy gave comparable results.[5] However, CT scans were superior for deep seated lesions and in patients with adhesions. A study involving 97 cases by Danielson and colleagues showed the sensitivity of CT scan and peritoneoscopy to be 89% and 62%, respectively; and their specificity 94% and 96%.[24] In 35% of biopsy-proven cases, the CT scan detected lesions not visible by peritoneoscopy and in 7% of the cases peritoneoscopy revealed lesions not seen on CT scan. The authors attributed the differences to the more frequent occurrence of lesions that were deep in the liver or obscured by adhesions. Of the lesions detected by peritoneoscopy and not CT scan, all were small surface or peritoneal implants too small for CT scan detection. In general, these studies suggest that CT scan analysis of the liver with a thin needle biopsy should be performed before peritoneoscopy, especially for deep seated lesions or in patients with lesions more accessible for CT scan detection. However, patients with negative CT scans or with positive CT scans but negative biopsies should undergo peritoneoscopy. Peritoneoscopy should be the first choice for biopsy if small peritoneal implants are suspected from the biology of the tumor.

In summary, radionuclide liver scan alone is not sufficient to diagnose hepatic neoplasms, either primary or metastatic, and should be followed by or replaced with a CT scan or peritoneoscopy. Ultrasound guided fine needle aspiration is equivalent to peritoneoscopy for sensitivity and accuracy but inferior in making a histologic diagnosis because of technical and cytological problems. Peritoneoscopy is preferred to ultrasound guided fine needle aspiration for tumors such as lymphomas requiring tissue rather than cytologic diagnosis.

The CT scan with biopsy should be performed initially in the work-up for hepatic lesions and should be followed by peritoneoscopy if the CT scan or biopsy is negative. Generally, the addition of peritoneoscopy to the staging work-up is mainly to negate the need for laparotomy by detecting small surface lesions on the liver, peritoneal implants, or malignant ascites. Peritoneoscopy allows for multiple biopsies of the liver. The usefulness of peritoneoscopy in specific cancers is discussed below.

Peritoneoscopy for Ovarian Cancer

The three major uses of peritoneoscopy in patients with ovarian cancer are: initial staging; surveillance to assess therapeutic response; and placement of a Tenckhoff catheter for intraperitoneal chemotherapy.

The indication for peritoneoscopy in the initial staging of ovarian cancer is limited to those patients who had an initial laparotomy but without a full assessment of the diaphragm. Bagley and colleagues performed peritoneoscopy on 14 patients that were referred to the National Cancer Institute (NCI) with ovarian carcinoma four weeks after diagnostic laparotomy.[4] They found that 11 of these patients had diaphragmatic metastases and none had any previous note of these sites from the referring physician. Diaphragmatic metastases were found in one patient who had apparently completely resected Stage IA disease and in 2 of 4 patients with Stage IIB disease, which upstaged them. In 7 of the 14 patients the diaphragm was the only site of cancer above the umbilicus. Also, small, superficial metastases on the liver serosa were found in 4 of the 10 patients whose livers were described as normal at initial laparotomy. Ozols and colleagues performed peritoneoscopy on 99 patients referred with ovarian cancer and found that 48% of these had new sites of disease undetected by conventional radiographic and isotopic procedures.[68] In 28% of patients referred with Stage I and II disease, upstaging occurred on the basis of diaphragmatic disease not described in the initial laparotomy but detected by peritoneoscopy. In addition, peritoneoscopy provided the only procedure to follow disease in 28% of the patients. Piver and colleagues have reported that 11% of Stage I and 23% of Stage II patients referred for presumed early stage disease had diaphragmatic metastases undetected at the initial laparotomy.[71] Most metastases in these patients were found on the right hemidiaphragm, and right and anterior abdominal walls. The lack of ascites does not exclude the presence of diaphragmatic metastases. The lymphatic drainage of the lower abdomen and pelvis is through diaphragmatic lymphatics and then up to retrosternal nodes.[4] Peritoneal washings and cytology are an additional means by which peritoneoscopy has upstaged patients who were thought to have early stage disease on their initial evaluation. Of the women with presumed Stage I and II disease, 32% and 12.5% respectively had malignant peritoneal washings found by peritoneoscopy.[71] In other studies, one-third to one-half of the positive peritoneoscopies were documented by cytologic washings only, since no disease could be visualized by peritoneoscopy or by laparotomy.[57,72] Other areas where sites of subclinical disease are underdiagnosed in early stage ovarian cancers are omen-

tum, aortic and pelvic lymph nodes. Peritoneoscopic biopsy or needle aspiration of an unruptured ovarian mass should not be done because malignant cells may spill into the peritoneum. Thus, peritoneoscopy and washings are important tools in the initial staging and work-up of patients with ovarian cancer if the diaphragm and peritoneal cytology have not been fully assessed at laparotomy.

The role of peritoneoscopy in the reevaluation of patients with ovarian cancer who have had initial chemotherapy with or without radiotherapy has been extensively researched. Early studies by many authors clearly demonstrated that second look peritoneoscopy can obviate the need for second look laparotomy in 30–50% of patients by finding residual disease, but that a negative peritoneoscopy is not sufficient to rule out persistent disease.[8,68,72,77] Ozols and colleagues found that 55% of patients with a negative second look peritoneoscopy nonetheless had residual cancer, found mainly in the pelvis and mesentery at laparotomy.[68] More recently, other studies utilizing peritoneoscopy with peritoneal washings have found similar results with respect to false negative second look peritoneoscopy.[51,75,79,100] The value of peritoneal cytology in patients with residual disease after therapy has recently come into question. Rubin and colleagues have found that approximately 70% of patients who have residual tumor found at second-look laparotomy had negative cytologies in their washings.[78]

Another test that may assist the clinician in the analysis of residual disease is the monoclonal antibody OC-125 (CA-125) described by Bast and colleagues.[6] Serum CA-125 levels less than 35 U/ml are predictive of a pathologic complete remission about 39–44% of the time. However, a value >35 has a positive predictive value of 96% for detecting cancer in the second-look operation.[7,50,65] An elevated CA-125 level may thus obviate the need for peritoneoscopy in this subset of patients. The usefulness of CA-125 in peritoneal fluid obtained during peritoneoscopic washings has been investigated by Allegra and colleagues.[1] All patients were pathologically staged with peritoneoscopy followed by laparotomy when the laparoscopy was negative. A peritoneal lavage (1,500 cc) was used to measure the CA-125 antigen. An antigen level higher than 33 U/ml accurately predicted the pathologic disease status 80% of the time. The predictive value of a positive test was 86% and for a negative test 72%. In 32 cases with concurrent serum and peritoneal CA-125 levels, the peritoneal antigen level was a more sensitive predictor of residual disease in six (19%). The peritoneal CA-125 level was elevated in 2 of 3 cases where peritoneoscopy was negative but laparotomy was positive. Based on this pilot study, the CA-125 level in peritoneal lavage fluid may help with greater precision to select patients who should go on to laparotomy after peritoneoscopy.

Peritoneoscopy can also be useful for the therapy of ovarian cancer by intraperitoneal (IP) chemotherapy. Peritoneoscopy is helpful in placing a Tenckhoff catheter or a subcutaneously implanted continuous infusion device into open areas of the peritoneum to ensure distribution of the antineoplastic agent. The topic of intraperitoneal chemotherapy is covered in Chapter XV-4. Some investigators have begun exploration of the potential of IP therapy via Tenckhoff catheter placed by peritoneoscopy as part of the primary induction therapy along with systemic therapy.

Peritoneoscopy for Lymphoma

Early studies by DeVita and colleagues in the staging of previously untreated patients with Hodgkin's disease demonstrated that peritoneoscopy may be an alternative to a staging laparotomy for evaluating the liver.[27] They found 16% of their patients to have positive liver biopsies (usually 6 biopsies performed), some of whom had had a previous negative percutaneous blind liver biopsy. Patients who had no intra-abdominal Hodgkin's disease by lymphangiogram or radiologic scans were extremely unlikely to have Hodgkin's in the liver. The authors stressed that a negative peritoneoscopy doesn't rule out disease in the spleen or lymph nodes (the spleen was visualized, but not biopsied) and it should be followed by a staging laparotomy if the lymphangiogram and abdominal CT scan were negative and regional therapy planned (see XXXVI-9). The yield of a positive liver biopsy in peritoneoscopy is significantly enhanced if CT scan and lymphangiogram suggest subdiaphragmatic disease. These initial recommendations for the role of peritoneoscopy were corroborated by other authors,[19,40] and now it is standard practice that if invasive subdiaphragmatic staging is to be undertaken, in the setting of a negative peritoneoscopy, lymphangiogram and CT scan, laparotomy should be performed for accurate staging in Hodgkin's disease. In a series by Veronesi and colleagues the sequential use of laparoscopy and laparotomy were studied in 102 patients with Hodgkin's and non-Hodgkin's lymphoma.[94] The percent positive for liver disease with Hodgkin's disease, either primary or relapsed, by peritoneoscopy and laparotomy were 1% and 7%, respectively. For splenic involvement it was 12% by peritoneoscopy and 42% by laparotomy. Thus, peritoneoscopy in Hodgkin's disease has a high false negative rate for the spleen. In patients with a negative lymphangiogram, CT scan, and peritoneoscopy, a laparotomy should be done to properly assess the spleen, liver, and lymph nodes. For non-Hodgkin's lymphoma the false negative rate is much lower.[94] The percent positive by peritoneoscopy and laparotomy for disease in the liver, both primary and relapsed, were 4% and 10%, respectively, while the percent found in the spleen by these two methods were 15% and 18%, respectively. These results have been substantiated by Chabner and colleagues[16] and others[63] who demonstrated that peritoneoscopy has a significant false negative rate for splenic Hodgkin's disease. However, concordance for the two procedures was found for non-Hodgkin's lymphoma, especially for splenic involvement (15% vs. 18%). Thus, current recommendations from these data suggest that if invasive staging is undertaken, peritoneoscopy can be used for both types of lymphoma with multiple liver biopsies and that laparotomy is reserved for patients with Hodgkin's disease who have a negative work-up including lymphangiogram, CT scan, and peritoneoscopy. For patients with non-Hodgkin's lymphoma, a peritoneoscopy without laparotomy is sufficient for staging.[16]

Peritoneoscopy for Gastrointestinal Tract Cancers

Hepatocellular Cancer

Hepatocellular cancer (HCC) is one of the most common cancers in the world, especially in the Orient and Africa. HCC is traditionally a highly fatal disease and because of this it is essential to delineate patients into those who can and cannot undergo curative resection.[55] HCC are generally hypervascular tumors that may be found in the presence of portal hypertension. Peritoneoscopy allows the operator the opportunity to biopsy less vascular regions of the tumor in an effort to decrease the risk of bleeding. In a series of 1,060 diagnostic peritoneoscopies reported by Jeffers and colleagues, 27 patients were identified with HCC.[46] All 27 had biopsies directly visualized and guided by peritoneoscopy. Cirrhosis was also found in 89% and malignant ascites was present in 78% of the patients. There were no significant complications to the procedure and all patients were deemed unresectable due to multiple lesions (78%), advanced cirrhosis (85%), and peritoneal metastases (7%). Peritoneoscopy was the procedure of choice for diagnosing HCC until recently, when ultrasound guided fine-needle biopsy was successful in obtaining diagnosis in about 90% of the cases. CT scan guided biopsy was approximately equal to ultrasound in diagnosing HCC. The remainder can be diagnosed by peritoneoscopy.[14,35,37] Ultrasonography can detect portal thrombosis, denoting advanced disease, while peritoneoscopy can detect peritoneal metastases and cirrhosis not visualized by ultrasonography. Ultrasonography, along with alpha-fetoprotein levels, are the initial exams of choice for screening high risk patients.[13] Peritoneoscopy should be performed if the ultrasound guided biopsy is negative, and if curative surgery is considered to rule out disseminated disease not detected by ultrasonography. Trials with magnetic resonance imaging have not yet been compared to ultrasonography or peritoneoscopy.

Gall Bladder Cancer

Carcinoma of the gall bladder is the most common cancer of the biliary tract. Resection is not possible in the majority of cases because of the silent progression to metastases. The majority of patients have metastatic tumor by the time ultrasound or CT scan can detect these tumors.[70,85] Bhargava and colleagues studied 23 patients with this disease by peritoneoscopy and all diagnoses were confirmed by either histology, cytology or laparotomy.[9] Cytology and/or biopsy from peritoneoscopy yielded a diagnosis in 86% of the patients. Peritoneoscopy avoided laparotomy in 39% of the patients by detecting multiple metastatic lesions over the liver serosa. Biopsies were taken from tumor nodules on the liver edge near the gall bladder or from a metastatic site. Cytologic brush samples were obtained from the gall bladder mass, but direct biopsy of the gall bladder was avoided so as to avoid spilling of bile or tumor cells into the peritoneum. In a study by Dagnani and colleagues, approximately 10% of the patients did not have signs of metastases by peritoneoscopy and subsequently underwent curative surgery by laparotomy.[23] Peritoneoscopy in this series allowed for the delineation of the few patients who could benefit from curative surgery, thereby circumventing unnecessary surgery for the other 90% of patients.

Esophageal and Gastric Cancer

Surgery for esophageal cancer has significant morbidity and mortality. In most series about 40% of lesions are resectable at presentation and only 15% of these patients become 5-year survivors.[33] Thus, it is important to differentiate resectable from non-resectable cancer with accuracy and safety. Carcinomas of the stomach are often different from esophageal carcinomas in that surgery is necessary in many cases of gastric carcinoma, even those that are widely metastatic, to provide palliation from gastric obstruction. The advent of percutaneous gastrointestinal feeding tubes can circumvent this problem in some patients. The major initial decision is whether or not patients with these tumors can undergo surgery with curative intent. Peritoneoscopy has been evaluated in Europe for this purpose; it has diagnosed 80–98% of unresectable cases correctly, obviating the need for laparotomy in patients with esophageal and gastric cancers.[83] Though some patients with gastric cancer required palliative surgery there were others whose problems of gastric obstruction was alleviated by percutaneous intestinal feeding tubes. The diagnosis of metastatic cancer by peritoneoscopy avoided surgery for 58% of patients. In another series, 360 patients with gastric carcinoma were evaluated for curability by liver scintigraphy, ultrasonography, serum alkaline phosphatase and peritoneoscopy. Peritoneoscopy was superior to the others for diagnosing metastases and liver involvement and had no morbidity or mortality. A negative peritoneoscopy led to a resection with curative intent in 64%.[73] In patients with widespread esophageal or gastric cancer, peritoneoscopic biopsy is diagnostic approximately 85% of the time. Common sites of metastasis are the liver, omentum and retroperitoneal nodes.[49] The diagnostic accuracy of peritoneoscopy, ultrasound and CT scan were compared in a recent study of 90 consecutive patients with esophageal and gastric cancer. Peritoneoscopy was significantly more sensitive and accurate (96%) than either ultrasound or CT scan with regard to hepatic status. Neither ultrasound nor CT scan detected peritoneal metastases, but peritoneoscopy discovered 98% of the cases.[98] Peritoneal carcinomatosis and resection site recurrence are the major causes for progression and relapse after surgery in patients with gastric cancer. Peritoneoscopy may assist in discovering these types of failure.

Pancreatic Cancer

At the time of diagnosis only 10–20% of cancers of the pancreatic head and even less for cancers of the body and tail can be cured by resection. Multiple staging procedures such as CT scanning, angiography, and ultrasound have approximately a 35% false negative rate when the patient undergoes laparotomy. The dismal surgical and chemotherapy cure rates have led investigators to use peritoneoscopy to identify resectable and non-resectable populations. Ishida and colleagues have developed a laparoscopic approach to the direct visualization and biopsy of the pancreas.[45] During peritoneoscopy, incision of the lesser omentum is made by forceps introduced through the scope, and

the scope is inserted into the lesser peritoneal sac (supragastric pancreascopy). The pancreas and surrounding lesions were biopsied with long Menghini needles 1.0 mm in diameter. This procedure led to a positive diagnosis of pancreatic cancer in five out of nine cases of carcinoma of the head and 13 out of 14 cases of carcinoma of the body and tail without complications. Subsequent studies after this initial report diagnosed 32% of carcinomas of the head and 85% of neoplasms of the body and tail of the pancreas, respectively, even in the presence of negative endoscopic retrograde cholangiopancreatography (ERCP) exams.[44] In another study peritoneoscopy was performed initially in 51 patients with pancreatic carcinoma who later underwent laparotomy. This study found that 42 patients were correctly judged to be inoperable by peritoneoscopy, but only four out of nine patients judged to be operable by peritoneoscopy were found to be operable at laparotomy.[97] Peritoneoscopy was extremely accurate in diagnosing peritoneal and omental metastases missed by hepatic radionuclide scan, ultrasound scanning of the pancreas and CT scan. In a prospective attempt to study the accuracy of preoperative staging techniques for assessing resectability of pancreatic and ampullary carcinoma, Warshaw and colleagues studied 88 patients with suspected pancreatic cancer, by contrast enhanced CT scan, MRI, angiography and peritoneoscopy.[96] CT scans were 92% accurate in predicting unresectability, but only 45% accurate in predicting resectability. MRI was similar to the CT scan and conferred no advantages for liver metastases or vascular encasement. Angiography was 95% accurate in predicting unresectability but only 54% in predicting resectability. Peritoneoscopy, used only for detecting hepatic and peritoneal metastases, discovered unresectability in 22 out of 23 cases (96%) and was 100% correct in showing no metastases in 24 localized cases. Overall, with all four procedures, 89% of unresectable cases were identified preoperatively with a 5% false resectable rate. Of the patients predicted to have resectable cancer (all tests negative), 78% of cancers of the head and 100% of ampullary cancers were resectable for cure. They concluded that the combined absence of any positive test results from these four exams is the prime index of resectability, and not the number of negative test results. Peritoneoscopy in this study was invaluable for detecting metastases commonly missed by CT scan, MRI, and angiography. The diagnosis, palliation and assessment of resectability in pancreatic cancer has changed from using laparotomy and palliative bypass of the biliary tree and/or duodenum to highly accurate tests and other safe procedures, such as stenting,[43,87] thereby obviating the morbidity and mortality of surgery. A tissue diagnosis can be made easily in most cases by percutaneous needle aspiration or biopsy.[28,86]

Peritoneoscopy for Other Cancers

Peritoneal Mesothelioma

Malignant peritoneal mesotheliomas form about 10% of all mesotheliomas. The diagnosis of this disease has usually been made by laparotomy because small (<2 cm) peritoneal implants may not be identified by CT scans. More recently, peritoneoscopy has been found to be a more sensitive diagnostic tool than any technique short of laparotomy.[61,91] The great majority of patients with peritoneal mesothelioma present with widespread, unresectable peritoneal tumor nodules with weight loss, abdominal pain and ascites. Cytology of the malignant ascites is often negative. Laparotomy for diagnosis should be avoided since the median survival is approximately 1 year.[101] Peritoneoscopy was studied as an alternative to laparotomy for diagnosis and found to be as sensitive as laparotomy for detecting mesothelioma.[69,91] Peritoneoscopy is now the procedure of choice in patients suspected to have malignant peritoneal mesothelioma. Intraperitoneal chemotherapy by Tenckhoff catheter placed during peritoneoscopy offers one therapeutic approach, especially in early stage patients.[2] Peritoneoscopy should be utilized in the diagnosis, possible placement of a Tenckhoff catheter for IP chemotherapy, and reassessment analysis of therapy in malignant peritoneal mesothelioma (see XXVIII-2).

Breast Cancer

Accurate staging of the patient with breast cancer is pivotal to the choice of a therapy plan that carries the highest likelihood of curing or palliating the patient. Metastatic breast cancer is a therapeutic challenge for the oncologist because of the incurability and relatively short median survival of patients at this stage. This is especially true when breast cancer is metastatic to the liver, which occurs in about 55–65% of patients.[80,95] Multimodality therapy to cure metastatic breast cancer to the liver is still under active investigation, but in general, this has not been achieved and, outside of the research setting, a palliative approach is warranted. The majority of metastatic lesions to the liver can be detected by a combination of liver function tests, ultrasound and contrast enhanced CT scanning. The small percentage of patients who are suspected of having hepatic metastases and an inconclusive work-up, or positive scans but negative biopsies (i.e., lesions <1 cm) can be accurately diagnosed with peritoneoscopy.[26,53,60,90] Peritoneoscopy has also been shown to provide an accurate assessment of tumor response to chemotherapy in patients with breast cancer metastatic within the peritoneal cavity.[10]

Lung Cancer

The lung cancers with a high proclivity for hepatic metastases are small cell, large cell and adenocarcinoma. Several diagnostic methods have been utilized to evaluate metastatic spread of lung cancer to the liver. Liver function tests (SGOT, LDH, and alkaline phosphatase) are highly predictive of the presence or absence of liver metastases only if *all* three tests are elevated or normal, respectively.[58] Non-invasive techniques such as liver scintigram and CT scan have been compared to peritoneoscopy for the evaluation of hepatic metastases in patients with small cell lung carcinoma.[64] Peritoneoscopy may be the most accurate method for diagnosing small cell lung cancer metastatic to the liver, when compared to CT scan or liver scintigraphy.[30,38,64] Ultrasonography with fine needle biopsy and peritoneoscopy were used concomitantly in 104 patients with small cell lung cancer to evaluate the liver. A total of 25% of the patients had hepatic involvement; peritoneoscopy confirmed 86% and ultrasound confirmed 79% of these cases. The difference

was not significant. The yield of positive biopsy by peritoneoscopy after a negative ultrasound was only 5%. It was recommended by these authors that ultrasonography with fine needle biopsy be used as the initial procedure in staging patients with small cell lung cancer and peritoneoscopy be reserved for those with positive ultrasounds but negative biopsies.[64] Thus, ultrasonography is a sensitive, highly accurate method to detect hepatic metastases from small cell lung cancer and should precede the use of peritoneoscopy.

Melanoma

Peritoneoscopy in patients with melanoma can detect hepatic metastases in 10% of patients thought not to have metastatic disease by the usual non-invasive tests.[15] Conversely, 10% of patients with positive liver scans or CT scans were found by peritoneoscopy to have benign hepatic lesions (i.e., cysts, and arteriovenous malformations).[15] The lesions detected by peritoneoscopy, but not by CT scan, ultrasound or liver scintigraphy, were usually less than 1 cm in diameter, or small peritoneal implants.[11,18,29,31] Ultrasound or CT scan guided biopsies in patients with melanoma should be the procedure of choice. Peritoneoscopy should be reserved for patients with negative biopsies of hepatic lesions and to document peritoneal disease histologically for a complete assessment of the patient.

Mycosis Fungoides

Though mycosis fungoides is a cutaneous T-cell lymphoma, it has become recognized as a clinicopathologic entity distinct from the classic lymphomas. Visceral involvement, lymphadenopathy and advanced skin disease are associated with shortened survival.[32,36] The liver is one of the most commonly involved organs in this disease and is positive in about 45% of patients.[52,56,76] In one series of patients who underwent staging laparotomy, 14% had hepatic metastases undetected by nonsurgical procedures.[93] Staging laparotomy is not necessary, however, to accurately stage patients with mycosis fungoides. In an autopsy series, hepatic and splenic involvement occurred with equal frequency.[93] In a peritoneoscopic study of this disease, all patients with splenic involvement had peripheral blood involvement and most had lymph node involvement.[42] Thus, laparotomy does not appear necessary to document extracutaneous disease if blood, nodes and liver are histologically examined. A study of hepatic involvement in 43 patients with mycosis fungoides was done by Huberman and colleagues which utilized liver function tests, liver scintigraphy, percutaneous liver biopsy and peritoneoscopy.[42] Multiple (six) liver biopsies by peritoneoscopy were positive in 7 of the 43 patients (16%) and percutaneous liver biopsy only detected three of these patients. The other exams were not helpful in predicting hepatic involvement, but all patients with hepatic disease also had leukocytosis, peripheral blood involvement, lymphadenopathy, and generalized erythroderma. The authors concluded that peritoneoscopy with multiple liver biopsies was the most effective and accurate assessment of liver involvement and could obviate the need for laparotomy, similar to the staging recommendations for non-Hodgkin's lymphoma.

Procedure

Peritoneoscopy

A standard, presurgical evaluation should be performed on all patients including chest roentgenogram, electrocardiogram, chemistries, complete urinalysis, blood count, prothrombin time and activated partial thrombin time. All patients should be independently evaluated by an anesthesiologist. If there are signs or symptoms of pulmonary compromise, a pulmonary function test should be performed, especially if the patient has recently undergone a lymphangiogram. If ascites is present, a paracentesis should be performed to minimize potential respiratory problems. In patients with significant mediastinal disease it is essential to rule out early superior vena cava syndrome by testing the ability to lie flat for one hour. Other contraindications to performing peritoneoscopy include: large abdominal masses, paralytic ileus, peritonitis, unstable angina, previous multiple abdominal operations and, of course, significant anemia, thrombocytopenia and clotting factor abnormalities. It is also imperative that preparations be made for emergency laparotomy prior to peritoneoscopy for the rare occurrence of uncontrolled bleeding after biopsy.

The patient is prepped in the standard fashion for abdominal surgery and sedated. A 2–4 cm incision is made through the skin at the lower edge of the umbilicus after local anesthesia in patients who have had no previous laparotomies. In patients with previous abdominal surgery, with possible adhesions around the entry site, an incision is made at the level of the umbilicus and immediately lateral to the right rectus muscle. The subcutaneous fat and fascia are dissected apart and the peritoneum is injected with local anesthesia. A spinal needle with a closed syringe is inserted carefully just into the peritoneum and aspirated to check for free air which, if present, can denote entry into a bowel loop that is tacked up to the anterior abdominal wall. If no air is present, then the peritoneum is punctured with a Verres needle when the patient extends his or her abdomen outward momentarily, and 2–4 liters of nitrous oxide are insufflated into the peritoneum under manometric control. The gas pressure is constantly monitored and should be below 15 cm of water with the patient relaxed. If the gas pressure gauge registers 20–30 cm of water, the needle could be within the space of Retzius in the subcutaneous tissue. If the gas pressure registers between 16 and 22 cm water, it is probably within the venules of the anterior abdominal wall.[89] After insufflation is completed, a spinal needle with a syringe half filled with sterile saline is introduced and aspirated downward and in all four quadrants to determine the largest air pocket space for entry of the trocar.

The trocar in the sleeve is introduced at a 45° angle to the abdominal wall and usually directed toward the pouch of Douglas. The trocar is removed and a rush of air should be heard before the peritoneoscope is advanced through the sleeve. If necessary, more nitrous oxide can be insufflated into the peritoneum through the scope to improve visualization. At this point, a second peritoneoscope can be inserted under direct visualization several inches below the xiphoid process, but away from the liver, which as an option, can improve the peritoneoscopic visualization of the inferior surface of the liver.[88] The second peritoneoscope is not necessary for the majority of patients when visualization from the first scope is adequate.

A complete visual exploration is attempted in all patients starting at the pelvis and proceeding in a clockwise fashion around the peritoneum (Figure XI-3-1). A Trendelenburg position is helpful for visualizing the pelvis and reverse Trendelenburg optimizes visualization of the upper abdomen. The operating table can be tilted to the left and right to help visualize the lateral aspect of the right lobe of the liver and spleen, respectively. Only small, thin adhesions not attached to bowel can be carefully dissected away by a pinch-biopsy forceps introduced into the scope. Percutaneous needle biopsies (i.e., Tru-Cut needle) of the liver can be directly visualized and guided by the scope to suspicious lesions (Figure XI-3-1). Bleeding from the liver biopsy sites should be monitored carefully until bleeding has ceased. It is not recommended to biopsy near the liver edge because the needle may traverse the liver and cause bleeding from the posterior aspect of the liver which is more difficult to monitor. Hepatic areas near the gall bladder and central veins should also be avoided. Biopsy of suspicious lesions on the diaphragm, hepatic serosa, visceral peritoneum lining the anterior or lateral abdominal wall, and omentum can be performed with a pinch biopsy forceps. In cases where peritoneal cytology is needed, 1,500 cc of pre-warmed dialysate (1.5% Impersol with 1,000 units of aqueous heparin per 2 liter bottle) or saline can be instilled at this time. The patient is tilted in all directions to maximize the cytologic yield and the fluid is aspirated with a cannula through the scope under direct visualization. At this point, a Tenckhoff silastic catheter with a dacron cuff can be placed safely under visualization for subsequent IP chemotherapy. Through a second trocar or stab incision the catheter is tunneled subcutaneously and it enters the peritoneum with the cuff extraperitoneal and subcutaneous, and the tip of catheter placed away from adhesions into the pelvic region by direct visualization (Figure XI-3-2).

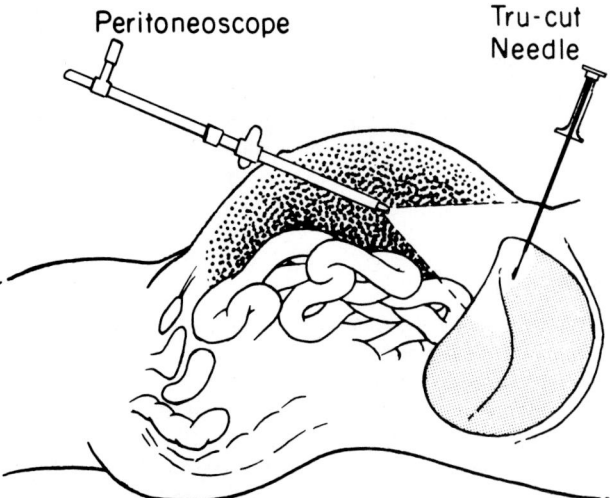

Peritoneoscope   **Tru-cut Needle**

Figure XI-3-1. Peritoneoscopy with an oblique view of the liver and percutaneous liver biopsy with a Tru-Cut needle under direct visualization.

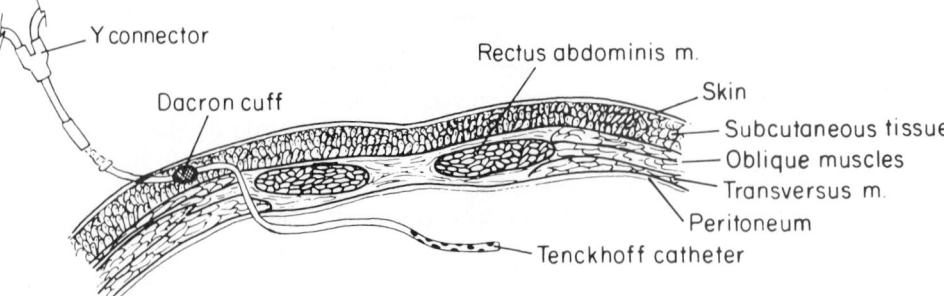

Figure XI-3-2. Tenckhoff catheter placement in the peritoneum with tunneling of the catheter and dacron cuff in the subcutaneous tissue.

After the procedure, gas and fluid are evacuated from the cavity and wound closure is obtained with subcuticular sutures. The patient's vital signs and hemoglobin are monitored and a chest x-ray is obtained. If the hemoglobin is stable, and there are no signs of pneumothorax or pneumomediastinum, the patient is discharged the next day.

Complications of Peritoneoscopy

In the series of ovarian cancer patients reported by Rosenoff and colleagues there was a 6% complication rate with no mortality.[77] The complications included: cellulitis,[1] pneumothorax,[1] and subcutaneous emphysema.[2] Ozols and colleagues reported similar findings in 99 patients with ovarian cancer.[68] Hypotension was the most common complication, but all patients recovered within 8 hours of the procedure and no long-term complications were observed. Hemorrhage from a liver biopsy site can be controlled in a number of ways without the need for surgical intervention. Direct, external tamponade of the thorax overlying the liver can sometimes stop bleeding and, if necessary, electrocoagulation through the peritoneoscope can stop superficial bleeding. For hemorrhage that is more deeply seated, hepatic angiography and clot embolization has been successful. Bleeding at the insertion site can be controlled by electrocoagulation or sutures.

A rare complication of peritoneoscopy is bowel perforation as the trocar is introduced into the abdominal cavity. This perforation usually occurs in the small intestine and is detected because of increasing subdiaphragmatic free air and signs of peritonitis. Immediate surgical intervention is always necessary.

Iatrogenic spread of tumor is a concern during any surgical procedure in a patient with cancer. Peritoneoscopy has been reported, in one case, to spread ovarian cancer at the puncture site, but otherwise this is an extremely rare event.[62]

Summary

Peritoneoscopy is an underutilized procedure that has many indications in the diagnosis and treatment of intra-abdominal cancers. Overall, it can delineate patients into resectable and non-resectable groups obviating the need for laparotomy. Peritoneoscopy has minimal morbidity and near zero mortality. In ovarian cancer, it is extremely helpful for patients who have an incomplete initial staging, for surveillance of therapy and for therapy of minimal, residual disease with intraperitoneal catheter chemotherapy. Peritoneoscopy can avoid laparotomy for patients with Hodgkin's disease and

provide information to complete the work-up of patients with non-Hodgkin's lymphoma and mycosis fungoides. It can complement the work-up of patients with hepatocellular, gastric, esophageal, pancreatic, breast, melanoma, and lung cancers, especially when an ultrasound or CT scan guided needle biopsy of a lesion is negative. Peritoneoscopy also obtains information not accessible from non-invasive techniques about peritoneal seeding and small hepatic lesions. Peritoneoscopy may be the procedure of choice for a suspected diagnosis and assessment of carcinoma of the gall bladder or malignant peritoneal mesothelioma. Peritoneoscopy will likely play a larger role in the diagnosis, staging for resectability and treatment of intra-abdominal cancers as more oncologists become familiar with its advantages.

References

1. Allegra, C. J., Fine, R. L., Behrens, B. C., Zweig, M. H., Ostchega, Y., Ozols, R. F., and Young, R. C.: CA-125 antigen levels in peritoneal lavage fluid: A useful staging tool in ovarian cancer. Proc. Amer. Soc. Clin. Oncol., 5:A118, 1986.
2. Antman, K. H., Osteen, R. T., Klegar, K. L., Pomfret, E. A., Amato, D. A., Larson, D. A., and Corson, J. M.: Early peritoneal mesothelioma: A treatable malignancy. Lancet, 2:977, 1985.
3. Bagley, C. M., Roth, J. A., and Thomas, L. B.: Liver biopsy in Hodgkin's disease; Clinicopathologic correlations in 127 patients. Ann. Int. Med., 76:219, 1972.
4. Bagley, C. M., Young, R. C., Schein, P. S., Chabner, B. A., and DeVita, V. T.: Ovarian carcinoma metastatic to the diaphragm: Frequently undiagnosed at laparotomy. Am. J. Obstet. Gynecol., 116:397, 1973.
5. Barth, R. A., Jeffrey, R. B., Moss, A. A., and Liberman, M. S.: A comparison study of computed tomography and laparoscopy in the staging of abdominal neoplasms. Dig. Dis. Sci., 26:253, 1981.
6. Bast, R. C., Klug, T. L., St. John, E., Jenison, E., Niloff, J. M., Lazarus, H., Berkowitz, R. S., Leavitt, T., Griffiths, C. T., Parker, L., Zurawski, V. R., and Knapp, R. C.: A radioimmunoassay using a monoclonal antibody to monitor the course of epithelial ovarian cancer. N. Engl. J. Med., 309:883, 1983.
7. Berek, J. S., Knapp, R. C., Malkasian, G. D., Lavin, P. T., Whitney, C., Niloff, J. M., and Bast, R. C.: CA-125 serum levels correlated with second look operations among ovarian cancer patients. Obstet. Gynecol., 67:685, 1986.
8. Berk, J. S., Griffiths, T., and Leventhal, J. M.: Laparoscopy for second look evaluation in ovarian cancer. Obstet. Gynecol., 58:192, 1981.
9. Bhargava, D. K., Sarin, S., Verma, K., and Kapur, B. M.: Laparoscopy in carcinoma of the gall bladder. Gastrointest. Endosc., 29:21, 1983.
10. Bleiberg, H., LaMeir, E., and Lejeune, F.: Laparoscopy in the diagnosis of liver metastases in 80 cases of malignant melanoma. Endoscopy, 12:215, 1980.
11. Bleiberg, H., Rozencweig, M., Gangji, D., and Heuson, J. C.: Peritoneoscopic evaluation of the effect of chemotherapeutic agents on liver metastases of breast cancer. Endoscopy, 8:217, 1976.
12. Boyd, W. P.: Relative diagnostic accuracy of laparoscopy and liver scanning techniques. Gastrointest. Endosc., 28:104, 1982.
13. Brady, P. G.: Laparoscopy and ultrasonography in the diagnosis of hepatocellular carcinoma. Gastrointest. Endosc., 35:577, 1989.
14. Buscarini, L., Sbolli, G., Cavanna, L., Civardi, G., Distasi, M., Buscarini, E., and Fornari, F.: Clinical and diagnostic features of 67 cases of hepatocellular carcinoma. Oncology, 44:93, 1987.
15. Caldironi, M. W., Nitti, D., Schiavon, M., Rossi, C. R., Aldinio, M. T., and Azzena, B.: Laparoscopy in the abdominal staging of melanoma. Eur. J. Cancer Clin. Oncol., 25:223, 1989.
16. Chabner, B. A., Johnson, R. E., Young, R. C., Canellos, G. P., Hubbard, S. P., Johnson, S. K., and DeVita, V. T.: Sequential nonsurgical and surgical staging of non-Hodgkin's lymphoma. Ann. Intern. Med., 85:149, 1976.
17. Christopherson, W. M.: Cytologic detection and diagnosis of cancer. Cancer, 51:1201, 1983.
18. Chuan Sheu, J., Low Sung, J., Sinn Chen, D., Jui-jun, Y., Hong-Wang, T., Tau-Su, C., and Ming-Tsang, Y.: Ultrasonography of small hepatic tumors using high resolution linear array real-time instruments. Radiology, 150:797, 1984.
19. Coleman, M., Lightdale, C. J., Vinciquerra, V. P., Degnan, T. J., Goldstein, M., Horwitz,

S. T., Winawer, S. J., and Silver, R. T.: Peritoneoscopy in Hodgkin's Disease. J.A.M.A., 236:2634, 1976.
20. Coupland, G., Townend, D. M., and Martin, C. J.: Peritoneoscopy-use in assessment of intra-abdominal malignancy. Surgery, 89:645, 1981.
21. Cuschieri, A.: Laparoscopy for pancreatic cancer: Does it benefit the patient? Europ. J. Surg. Oncol., 14:41, 1988.
22. Cusso, X., Marti-Vicente, A., Mones-Xiol, J., and Vilardell, F.: Laparoscopic cytology—an evaluation. Endoscopy, 20:102, 1988.
23. Dagnini, G., Marin, G., Patella, M., and Zotti, S.: Laparoscopy in the diagnosis of primary carcinoma of the gall bladder. Gastrointest. Endosc., 30:289, 1984.
24. Danielson, K. S., Sheedy, P. F., Stephens, D. H., Hattery, R. R., and La Russo, N. F.: Computed tomography and peritoneoscopy for detection of liver metastases: Review of Mayo Clinic experience. J. Comp. Assist. Tomog., 7:230, 1983.
25. deGraaf, P. W., Mellema, M. M., ten Bokkel Huinink, W. W., Aartsen, E. J., Dubbelman, R., Franklin, H. R., and Hart, A. A.: Complications of Tenckhoff catheter implantation in patients with multiple previous intraabdominal procedures for ovarian carcinoma. Gynecol. Oncol., 29:43, 1988.
26. DeSouza, L. J., and Shinde, S. R.: The value of laparoscopic liver examination in the management of breast cancer. J. Surg. Oncol., 14:97, 1980.
27. DeVita, V. T., Bagley, C. M., Goodell, B., O'Kieffe, D. A., and Trujillo, N.: Peritoneoscopy in the staging of Hodgkin's Disease. Cancer Res., 31:1746, 1971.
28. Dickey, J. E., Haaga, J. R., Stellato, T. A., Schultz, C. L., and Hainau, B. O.: Evaluation of computed tomography guided percutaneous biopsy of the pancreas. Surg. Gynecol. Obstet., 163:497, 1986.
29. Doiron, M., and Bernardino, M.: A comparison of non-invasive imaging modalities in melanoma patients. Cancer, 47:2581, 1981.
30. Dombernowsky, P., Hirsch, F., Hansen, H. H., and Hainau, B. O.: Peritoneoscopy in the staging of 190 patients with small cell anaplastic carcinoma of the lung with special reference to subtyping. Cancer, 41:2008, 1978.
31. Droese, M., Altmannsberger, M., Kehl, A., Lankisch, P. G., Weiss, R., Weber, K., and Osborn, M.: Ultrasound-guided percutaneous fine needle aspiration biopsy of abdominal and retroperitoneal masses. Acta Cytol., 28:368, 1984.
32. Epstein, E. H., Levin, D. L., Croft, J. D., and Lutzner, M. A.: Mycosis fungoides—survival prognostic features, response to therapy and autopsy findings. Medicine, 51:61, 1972.
33. Eurlam, R., and Cunha-Melo, J. R.: Oesphageal squamous cell carcinoma. I. A critical review of surgery. Brit. J. Surg., 67:381, 1980.
34. Ferruci, J. T., Wittenberg, J., Mueller, P. R., Simeone, J. F., Harbin, W. P., Kirkpatrick, R. H., and Taft, P. D.: Diagnoses of abdominal malignancy by radiologic fine needle aspiration biopsy. Am. J. Roentgenol., 134:322, 1980.
35. Fornari, F., Rapaccini, G. C., Cavanna, L., Civardi, G., Anti, M., Fedeli, G., and Buscarini, L.: Diagnosis of hepatic lesions: Ultrasonically guided fine needle biopsy or laparoscopy? Gastrointest. Endosc., 34:231, 1988.
36. Fuks, Z. Y., Bagshaw, M. A., and Farber, E. M.: Prognostic signs and the management of mycosis fungoides. Cancer, 32:1385, 1973.
37. Gandolfi, L., Muratori, R., Solmi, L., Rossi, A., and Leo, P.: Laparoscopy compared with ultrasonography in the diagnosis of hepatocellular carcinoma. Gastrointest. Endosc., 35:508, 1989.
38. Hansen, S. W., Jensen, F., Pederson, N. T., Pederson, A. G., and Hansen, H. H.: Detection of liver metastases in small cell lung cancer: A comparison of peritoneoscopy with liver biopsy and ultrasonography with fine needle aspiration. J. Clin. Oncol., 5:255, 1987.
39. Heintz, A. P., Van-Oosterom, A. T., Baptist, J., Baptist, J., Trimbos, J. B., Schaberg, A., Van der Velde, E., and Nooy, M.: The treatment of advanced ovarian carcinoma (II): Interval reassessment operations during chemotherapy. Gynecol. Oncol., 30:359, 1988.
40. Hoffman, K., and Schmidt, C. G.: Laparoscopy bei morbus Hodgkin. Deuts. Med. Wochenschr., 101:814, 1976.
41. Hogg, L., and Pack, G. T.: Diagnostic accuracy of hepatic metastases at laparotomy. Amer. Surg., 72:251, 1966.
42. Huberman, M. S., Bunn, P. A., Matthews, M. J., Ihde, D. C., Gazdar, A. F., Cohen, M. H., and Minna, J. D.: Hepatic involvement in cutaneous T-cell lymphomas: Results of percutaneous biopsy and peritoneoscopy. Cancer, 45:1683, 1980.
43. Huibregtse, K., Katon, R. M., Coene, P. P., and Tytgat, G. N.: Endoscopic palliative treatment in pancreatic cancer. Gastrointest. Endosc., 32:334, 1986.
44. Ishida, H.: Peritoneoscopy and pancreas biopsy in the diagnosis of pancreatic diseases. Gastrointest. Endosc., 29:211, 1983.
45. Ishida, H., Furukawa, Y., Kuroda, H., Kobayashi, M., and Tsuneoka, K.: Laparoscopic observation and biopsy of the pancreas. Endoscopy, 13:68, 1981.
46. Jeffers, L., Spieglman, G., Reddy, R., Dubow, R., Nadji, M., Ganjei, P., and Schiff, E. R.: Laparoscopically directed fine needle aspiration for diagnosis of hepatocelular carcinoma: A safe and accurate technique. Gastrointest. Endosc., 34:235, 1988.
47. Jori, G. P., and Peshle, C.: Combined peritoneoscopy and liver biopsy in the diagnosis of hepatic neoplasm. Gastroenterology, 63:1016, 1972.
48. Kelling, G.: Über Cesophagoskipie, Gastroskopie, Kollosiskopie. Muchen Med. Wenschr., 49:21, 1902.
49. Kriplani, A. K., and Sharma, L. K.: Peritoneoscopy in extrahepatic abdominal diseases. Arch. Surg., 121:818, 1986.
50. Lavin, P. T., Knapp, R. C., Malkalsean, G., Whitney, C. W., Berek, J. C., and Bast, R. C.: CA-125 for the monitoring of ovarian carcinoma during primary therapy. Obstet. Gynecol., 69:223, 1987.
51. Lele, S. B., and Piver, M. S.: Interval laparoscopy as predictor of response to chemotherapy in ovarian cancer. Obstet. Gynecol., 68:345, 1986.
52. Levi, J. A., and Wiernik, P. H.: Management of mycosis fungoides—current status and future prospects. Medicine, 54:73, 1975.
53. Lightdale, C. J.: Clinical applications of laparoscopy in patients with malignant neoplasms. Gastrointest. Endosc., 28:99, 1982.
54. Lightdale, C. J., Winawer, S. J., Kurtz, R. C., and Knapper, W. H.: Laparoscopic diagnosis of suspected liver neoplasms; value of prior liver scans. Dig. Dis. Sci., 24:588, 1979.
55. Lin, D. Y., Liaw, Y. F., Chu, C. M., Chevy-Chien, C. S., Wu, C. S., Chen, P. C., and Sheen, I. S.: Hepatocellular carcinoma in noncirrhotic patients—a laparoscopic study of 92 cases in Taiwan. Cancer, 54:1466, 1984.
56. Long, J. C., and Mihm, M.: Mycosis fungoides with extracutaneous dissemination: A distinct clincopathologic entity. Cancer, 34:1745, 1974.
57. Mangioni, C., Bolis, G., Molteni, P., and Belloni, C.: Indicating advantages and limitations of laparoscopy in ovarian cancer. Gynecol. Oncol., 7:47, 1979.
58. Margolis, R., Hansen, H. H., Muggia, F., and Kanhouwa, S.: Diagnosis of liver metastases in bronchogenic carcinoma. Cancer, 34:1825, 1974.
59. Matthews, M. J., Kanhouwa, S., Pickren, J., and Robinette, D.: Frequency of residual and metastatic tumor in patients undergoing curative surgical resection for lung cancer. Cancer Chemother. Rep., 4:63, 1973.
60. McCallum, R. W., and Berci, G.: Laparoscopy in hepatic disease. Gastrointest. Endosc., 23:20, 1976.
61. McCallum, R. W., Maceri, D. R., Jensen, D., and Berci, G.: Laparoscopic diagnosis of peritoneal mesothelioma. Dig. Dis. Sci., 24:170, 1979.
62. Miralles, R. M., Petit, J., Gine, L., and Balaguero, L.: Metastatic cancer spread at the laparoscopic puncture site. Report of a case in a patient with carcinoma of the ovary. Eur. J. Gynaec. Oncol., 10:442, 1989.
63. Miseria, S., Cetto, G., Cellerino, R., Martinelli, L., Tummarello, D., and Perona, G.: Assessment of liver and spleen involvement in Hodgkin's disease. Tumori, 70:147, 1984.
64. Mulshine, J. L., Makuch, R. W., Johnston-Early, A., Matthews, M. J., Carney, D. N., Ihde, D. C., Cohen, M. H., Bates, H. R., Dunnick, N. R., Minna, J. D., and Bunn, P. A.: Diagnosis and significance of liver metastases in small cell carcinoma of the lung. J. Clin. Oncol., 2:733, 1984.
65. Niloff, J. M., Bast, R. C., Schaetzl, E. M., and Knapp, R. C.: Predictive value of CA-125 antigen levels in second look procedures for ovarian cancer. Am. J. Obset. Gynecol., 151:981, 1985.
66. Ott, D.: Illumination of the abdomen (ventroscopy). Edited by J. Akush. Zhenak, Boleg, 15:1045, 1901.
67. Ozarda, A., and Pickren, J.: The topographic distribution of liver metastases—its relation to surgical and isotopic diagnosis. J. Nucl. Med., 3:149, 1962.
68. Ozols, R. F., Fisher, R. I., Anderson, T., Makuch, R., and Young, R. C.: Peritoneoscopy in the management of ovarian cancer. Am. J. Obstet. Gynecol., 140:611, 1981.
69. Piccigallo, E., Jeffers, L. J., Reddy, K. R., Caldironi, M. W., Parenti, A., and Schiff, E. R.: Malignant peritoneal mesothelioma: A clinical and laparoscopic study of 10 cases. Dig. Dis. Sci., 33:633, 1988.
70. Piehler, J. M., and Crichlow, R. W.: Primary carcinoma of the gall bladder. Surg. Gynecol. Obstet., 147:929, 1978.
71. Piver, M. S., Barlow, J. J., and Lele, S. B.: Incidence of subclinical metastases in Stage I and II ovarian carcinoma. Obstet. Gynecol., 52:100, 1978.
72. Piver, M. S., Lele, S. B., Barlow, J. J., and Gamarra, M.: Second look laparoscopy prior to proposed second look laparotomy. Obstet. Gynecol., 55:571, 1980.
73. Possik, R. A., Franco, E. L., Pires, D. R., Wohnrath, D. R., and Ferreira, E. B.: Sensitivity, specificity, and predictive value of laparoscopy for the staging of gastric cancer and for the detection of liver metastases. Cancer, 58:1, 1986.
74. Prior, C., Kathrein, H., Mikuz, G., and Judmaier, G.: Differential diagnosis of malignant intrahepatic tumors by ultrasonically guided fine needle aspiration biopsy and by laparoscopic/intraoperative biopsy: A comparative study. Acta Cytolog., 32:892, 1988.
75. Qu, J., Sun, A., and Lien, L.: Laparoscopy in the diagnosis and management of ovarian cancer. J. Reproduct. Med., 29:483, 1984.
76. Rappaport, H., and Thomas, L. B.: Mycosis fungoides: The pathology of extracutaneous involvement. Cancer, 34:1198, 1974.
77. Rosenoff, S. H., DeVita, V. T., Hubbard, S., and Young, R. C.: Peritoneoscopy in the staging and follow-up of ovarian cancer. Semin. Oncol., 2:223, 1975.
78. Rubin, S. C., Dulaney, E. D., Markman, M., Hoskins, W. J., Saigo, P. E., and Lewis, J. L.: Peritoneal cytology as an indicator of disease in patients with residual ovarian carcinoma. Obstet. Gynecol., 71:851, 1988.
79. Runowicz, C. D.: A critical assessment of the role of second-look surgery in ovarian carcinoma. Cancer Invest., 5:479, 1987.
80. Saphillo, O., and Parker, M. L.: Metastases of primary carcinoma of the breast with special reference to spleen, adrenal glands and ovaries. Arch. Surg., 42:1003, 1941.
81. Sauer, R., Fahrlauder, H., and Fridrich, R.: Comparison on the accuracy of liver scans and peritoneoscopy in benign and malignant primary and metastatic tumors of the liver. Scand. J. Gastroenterol., 8:387, 1973.
82. Schwerk, W. B., and Schmitz-Moorman, P.: Ultrasonically guided fine needle biopsies in neoplastic liver disease: Cytologic diagnoses and echo pattern lesions. Cancer, 48:1469, 1981.
83. Shandall, A., and Johnson, C.: Laparoscopy or scanning in oesophageal and gastric carcinoma? Brit. J. Surg., 72:449, 1985.
84. Sheth, S. S.: The place of laparoscopy in women with ascites. Brit. J. Obst. Gynec., 96:105, 1989.
85. Shieh, C. J., Dunn, E., and Standard, J. E.: Primary carcinoma of the gall bladder. Cancer, 47:966, 1981.
86. Silverstein, M. D., Richter, J. M., Podolsky, D. K., and Warshaw, A. L.: Suspected pancreatic cancer presenting as pain or weight loss: Analysis of diagnostic strategies. World J. Surg., 8:839, 1984.
87. Speer, A. G., Cotton, P. B., Russell, R. C., Mason, R. P., Hatfield, A. R., Leung, J. W., MacRae, K. D., Houghton, J., and Lennon, C. A.: Randomized trial of endoscopic versus percutaneous stent insertion in malignant obstructive jaundice. Lancet, 2:56, 1987.
88. Sugarbaker, P. H.: Optomizing peritoneoscopic visualization of the liver utilizing a double telescope technique. Surg. Gynecol. Obstet., 152:655, 1981.
89. Sugarbaker, P. H., and Roth, J. A.: Specialized Techniques of Cancer Management. *In* V. T. DeVita, S. Hellman, and S. A. Rosenberg. Cancer: Prnciples and Practice of Oncology, Third Edition. Philadelphia, J. B. Lippincott, 1989, pp. 423–440.
90. Sugarbaker, P. H., and Wilson, P. E.: Using celioscopy to determine stages of intra-abdominal malignant neoplasms. Arch. Surg., 111:41, 1976.
91. Van Gelder, T., Hoogsteden, H. C., Versnel, M. A., de Beer, P. H., Vanderbroucke, J. P., and Planteydt, H. T.: Malignant peritoneal mesothelioma: A series of 19 cases. Digestion, 43:222, 1989.
92. Van Waes, L., D'Haveloose, J., and Demeuhenaere, L.: Diagnostic accuracy of laparoscopy in the detection of liver metastases: A prospective study. Gastroenterology, 74:1107, 1978.
93. Variakojis, D., Rosas-Uribe, A., and Rappaport, H.: Mycosis fungoides: Pathologic findings in staging laparotomies. Cancer, 33:1589, 1974.

94. Veronesi, U., Spinelli, P., Bonnadonna, G., Gennari, L., Bajetta, E., Beretta, G., and Tancini, G.: Laparoscopy and laparotomy in staging Hodgkin's and non-Hodgkin's lymphoma. Am. J. Roentgenol., 127:501, 1976.

95. Warren, S., and Witman, E. M.: Studies on tumor metastases: The distribution of metastases in cancer of the breast. Surg. Gynecol. Obstet., 57:81, 1937.

96. Warshaw, A. L., Gu, Z. Y., Wittenberg, J., and Waltman, A. C.: Preoperative staging and assessment of resectability of pancreatic cancer. Arch. Surg., 125:230, 1990.

97. Watanabe, M., Takatori, Y., Ueki, K., Umekawa, Y., Yoshida, H., Kobatake, T., Hirakawa, H., Fukamoto, S., and Shimada, Y.: Pancreatic biopsy under visual control in conjunction with laparoscopy for diagnosis of pancreatic cancer. Endoscopy, 21:105, 1989.

98. Watt, I., Stewart, I., Anderson, D., Bell, G., and Anderson, J. R.: Laparoscopy, ultrasound and computed tomography in cancer of the oesophagus and gastric cardia: A prospective comparison for detecting intra-abdominal metastases. Brit. J. Surg., 76:1036, 1989.

99. Weiss, S. M., Skibber, J. M., Mohiuddin, M., and Rosato, F. E.: Rapid intra-abdominal spread of pancreatic cancer: Influence of multiple operative biopsy procedures. Arch. Surg., 120:415, 1985.

100. Xygakis, A. M., Politis, G. S., Michalas, S. P., and Kaskarelis, D. B.: Second look laparoscopy in ovarian cancer. J. Reproduct. Med., 29:583, 1984.

101. Young, J. R., and Reddy, E. R.: Peritoneal mesothelioma. Clin. Radiol., 31:243, 1980.

102. Zotti, S., Piccigallo, E., Rampinelli, L., Romagnoli, G., Tufano, A., and Dagnini, G.: Primary and metastatic tumors of the liver associated with cirrhosis. Gastrointest. Endosc., 32:91, 1986.

XII

Principles of Surgical Oncology

Donald L. Morton

Introduction

Surgery is the oldest and most frequently used modality in cancer therapy. More patients are cured of cancer by surgery alone than by any other single therapeutic modality. It is the treatment of choice for most localized, solid neoplasms, almost 90% of the 1,040,000 new cancer cases that presented during 1991 (ACS). The most common solid neoplasms arise in lung, colon, breast, and prostate. Although surgery is still preferred in a high percentage of cases, it is no longer considered the sole therapy for many neoplasms. Rather, surgery is increasingly combined with other treatment modalities. For this reason, it is essential that most patients with solid neoplasms have their treatment planned by an interdisciplinary team, which includes radiation and medical oncologists as well as surgical oncologists.

Over the years, the practices of the surgeon have come full circle. Originally, surgeons attempted to treat cancer conservatively by removing only the gross lesion. Unfortunately, this led to unacceptable rates of recurrence and patient mortality. In the late nineteenth century, surgeons first attempted complete en bloc resections and amputations of cancerous lesions. These techniques brought improved results, but the procedures were ablative and mutilating. Thus, it was with great trepidation that surgeons approached the management of the patient with neoplastic disease. The fear of postoperative death, coupled with the cosmetic mutilation necessary to rid the body of the lesion, often prejudiced the surgeon's judgment. Fortunately, during the past two decades, there have been major improvements in the surgical therapy of cancer, which have reduced the morbidity and mortality of surgical procedures and made surgery even more safe.

With the advent of other complementary treatment modalities—notably radiation therapy in the 1920s and chemotherapy in the 1940s—the attitude toward surgical resection is once again becoming conservative. Presently, the use of chemotherapy and radiation therapy in combination with surgery has considerably reduced the extent of surgery needed to manage many types of cancer. Improvements in conservative surgical therapy include breast salvage for carcinoma of the breast, limb salvage for the management of bone and soft tissue sarcomas, and preservation of sexual potency and urinary continence by improved operations for carcinoma of the prostate.

Although the most effective single treatment available, surgery has recognized limits in its applications to cancer treatment. At present, surgery is most efficacious in the treatment of local disease in the region of the primary tumor and in regional lymphatics. Radical resections and en bloc surgical procedures attempt to encompass gross and microscopic tumor in all adjacent, contiguous anatomic locations. Surgery is a local therapy, which primarily affects only the cells excised from the body. Surgery operates by zero order kinetics, meaning that 100% of cells excised are killed, whereas chemotherapy and radiation therapy operate by first order kinetics and are able to kill only a fraction of tumor cells with each treatment.

Adjuvant chemotherapy alone, or in combination with radiation therapy, has improved results in terms of disease-free survival and prolonged life for patients who have been rendered free of gross disease by surgery, but who have a high likelihood of recurrence due to subclinical, microscopic residual metastatic disease. Randomized clinical trials have demonstrated the benefit of adjuvant chemotherapy in a variety of tumors, including breast cancer, colon cancer, osteogenic sarcoma, testicular cancer, ovarian cancer, and certain types of lung cancer. Although in some cancers, such as colon cancers, the benefit of adjuvant therapy may be limited, in others, such as testicular and bone cancer, it has doubled or tripled survival rates.

Conventional logic would suggest that once a neoplasm has spread from the primary site to a distant organ, surgery should have little role in management of the disease. However, data from the management of a variety of tumors metastatic to the lung or liver have indicated that prolonged survival is possible following surgical resection of metastases. There are many examples of success for lung metastases of bone or soft tissue sarcomas, malignant melanoma, and other neoplasms (see XXVIII-5). Colon cancer with solitary metastasis in the liver has been found to be associated with a surprisingly high rate of five-year survival, up to 40% after surgical resection.

The above observations indicate the need to reassess the

traditional view of surgery as primarily a modality for localized cancer, which is therapeutic only when every last cancer cell is removed from the patient's body. To define the role of surgery in cancer therapy, thus, requires reevaluation of its mode of action.

The successful surgical oncologist must be able to coordinate and integrate the efforts of the entire oncologic team if he is to retain a primary role in the management of the cancer patient. The surgeon is no longer concerned solely with the mechanical aspects of surgery and treatment but must also understand and coordinate a specific multimodal approach, which includes the medical oncologist, the radiotherapist and the pathologist.

History of Surgical Oncology

Oncology (from the Greek words "onkos," meaning mass or tumor, and "logos," meaning study) is the study of neoplastic diseases. Cancer has plagued mankind, and indeed all multicellular organisms, since antiquity, although not always equally. Early authors suggested that certain families, races, and working classes were predisposed to neoplastic transformations. In 1862, Edwin Smith, an American Egyptologist, discovered the earliest writings on the surgical treatment of cancer.[3] Written in Egypt circa 1600 B.C., the treatise was based on teachings possibly dating back to 3000 B.C. The Egyptian author advised surgeons "to contend" with tumors that might be cured by surgery, but "not to treat" those lesions that might be fatal.

Hippocrates (460–375 B.C.) was the first to describe the clinical symptoms associated with cancer. He advised against treating terminal patients, who would enjoy a better quality of life without surgical intervention.[13] He also originated the terms carcinoma (crab legs tumor), and sarcoma (fleshy mass). In the second century A.D., Galen (129–199 A.D.) published his classification of tumors, describing cancer as a systemic disease caused by an excess of black bile.[11] Galen cautioned that as a systemic disease, cancer was not amenable to cure by surgical techniques and was, in fact, often followed by patient death. This strong admonition against surgery persisted for over 1,500 years until pathologists in the eighteenth century discovered that cancer often grew locally before spreading to other anatomic sites.

During the eighteenth and nineteenth centuries, advances in pathologic technique led to an increase in autopsies, which in turn resulted in a better understanding of human physiology. The early work of Morgagni, Le Dran and Da Salva indicated that there was an initial period of local tumor growth before dissemination. This led to the understanding that not all tumors are systemic and that certain lesions cause death solely by local invasive growth. Percival Pott (1714–1788) was the first to describe a specific etiological factor associated with cancer development. In 1775 he discovered a high incidence of cancer of the scrotum in chimney sweeps who had reached puberty and recommended a wide local resection to effect its cure. In 1829, Joseph Recamier (1774–1852), a French surgeon, was the first to describe the complicated process of tumor dissemination. The first recorded attempt at elective tumor surgery was performed in 1809 by Ephraim MacDowell, an American surgeon. He successfully removed a twenty-two pound ovarian tumor from a patient who subsequently survived 30 years. MacDowell's work, which included twelve more ovarian resections, encouraged greater interest in elective surgery for cancer patients.

Surgeons were originally hindered in their work by the extreme discomfort of patients during the surgical procedure and by the lack of agents that would reduce the incidence of infection. Dr. Crawford Long (1815–1878) was the first to use ether as a general anesthesia in 1842, but it was the reported work of Dr. John Collins Warren (1778–1856) and Dr. William T.G. Morton (1819–1868) that brought the potential of anesthesia to the public's attention. Dr. Joseph Lister (1827–1912) was the first to report the use of antisepsis during elective surgery. The work of these doctors opened new frontiers to surgical oncology in the late 1880s by freeing patients from pain and sepsis during and following their operations.

Even with the advent of antisepsis and general anesthesia, surgical oncology in the early twentieth century was still associated with a high incidence of patient mortality. Cancer was rarely diagnosed in the early stages, and thus few patients were considered candidates for curative surgery. Those surgeons who did attempt surgical excision of a cancerous lesion were hindered by poor anesthesia, which was associated with high patient mortality. Antibiotics were not yet available, and surgical instruments were crude. Also, the microscope was still rarely used to study frozen tissues or to evaluate the surgical margins, because surgeons had greater faith in their own assessment of the tumor. These conditions were not ideal and surgical oncology was associated with a high rate of patient mortality. A summary of major advances in surgical oncology is listed in Table XII-1-1.[11,13]

Surgical Therapy

Newer Concepts Regarding the Mechanism of Action

The current premise behind cancer surgery is that cancer begins as a local disease and then spreads in an orderly fashion from the primary site to adjacent tissues by direct extension, through the lymphatics to the regional lymph nodes, and via the vascular system to distant sites. The surgical procedure is designed to remove the primary neoplasm and the usual contiguous routes of spread; the aim is to ablate every cancer cell in the body. According to this view of surgical therapy, cure is achieved by the mechanical removal of every last cancer cell from the patient's body. However, compelling evidence suggests that this may be an incorrect assumption:

1) Cancer cells are frequently found in the washings of operative wounds or in postoperative wound drainage in patients undergoing definitive cancer surgery. The observation that many of these patients never develop recurrent cancer suggests the existence of host immune defenses, which destroy those tumor cells missed by the surgeon's knife.[22]

2) Apparently viable tumor cells frequently found in the blood or lymphatics of cancer patients seldom lead to meta-

Table XII-1-1.   Landmark Advances in Surgical Oncology

Year	Surgery/Discovery	Surgeon
1600 B.C	Edwin Smith Papyrus	Unknown
129 A.D.	Cancer as Systemic Disease	Galen of Pergamum
1543	De humani corporis fabrica	Andreas Vesalius
1775	Etiologic Cause of Cancer	Percival Pott
1809	Elective Oophorectomy	Ephraim McDowell
1829	Metastatic Process	Joseph Recamier
1846	Ether as Anesthesia	John Colins Warren
1867	Carbolic Acid as Antisepsis	Joseph Lister
1873	Laryngectomy	Albert Theodore Billroth
1878	Resection of Rectal Tumor	Richard von Volkman
1880	Esophagectomy	Albert Theodore Billroth
1881	Gastrectomy	Albert Theodore Billroth
1890	Radical Mastectomy	William Stewart Halsted
1904	Radical Prostatectomy	Hugh H. Young
1908	Abdominoperineal Resection	W. Ernest Miles
1910	Craniotomy	Harvey Cushing
1913	Thoracic Esophagectomy	Franz Torek
1927	Resection of Pulmonary Metastases	Georg Divis
1933	Pneumonectomy	Evarts Graham
1935	Pancreaticoduo-denectomy	Allen O. Whipple
1945	Adrenalectomy for Prostate Cancer	Charles B. Huggins

static lesions, and their presence cannot be correlated with prognosis. Since many of these patients never develop subsequent metastatic lesions, it is presumed that these tumor cells are destroyed by host defenses.[22]

3) Attempts to implant autologous tumor cells in man have been made by several investigators. Surprisingly, most attempts to implant human neoplasms from the primary site to intracutaneous or subcutaneous areas of the same patient fail to take. The incidence of successful tumor growth varies between 10% and 25%, even in patients with advanced malignant disease. Southam's studies suggest that this resistance is relative rather than absolute, since challenges of greater than 100 million tumor cells will often result in tumor growth.[25]

4) Ten to twenty years after successful treatment of the primary tumor, cancer sometimes recurs, with the development of rapidly progressive disease. During the long period of clinical remission, the tumor cells must have been inhibited in their growth by host defenses.

5) Many patients who have blood-borne metastases to distant organs, such as the lung or liver, can still be salvaged by resection of the metastases, even when they are multiple. If multiple metastatic lesions can be seen, there may be subclinical metastases at other sites and must have been other cells destroyed by host immune mechanisms.

6) Correlations between general immune competence of the patient and the results of cancer surgery:

Cell-mediated immune reactions of cancer patients have been measured by the ability of these patients to manifest delayed cutaneous hypersensitivity to a variety of common skin test antigens to which most normal persons are reactive by virtue of previous exposure, such as mumps, tuberculin, streptokinase, or streptodornase. In addition, the ability of these patients to manifest a primary immune response following initial exposure to a new antigen has been evaluated. An important method tests the ability of these patients to develop delayed cutaneous hypersensitivity to the contact sensitizer dinitrochlorobenzene (DNCB).

Studies have demonstrated a significant correlation between cell-mediated immunologic reactivity measured by the ability to manifest delayed cutaneous hypersensitivity following sensitization to DNCB, and the postoperative course of cancer patients.[15,19] It was found that more than 95% of normal control volunteers, patients with benign neoplasms and those free of disease for five years or more following cancer surgery, could be sensitized to this chemical. However, only 72% of all cancer patients who presented themselves as candidates for definitive cancer surgery were able to be sensitized to DNCB; the remaining 28% exhibited cutaneous anergy to this chemical. The anergic patients had a uniformly poor prognosis following surgical therapy. More than 95% of these patients either were found to have inoperable disease, because of local or metastatic spread, or had recurrent disease within 6 months after surgical resection.[8]

Most patients who were immunologically competent, as evidenced by their ability to be sensitized to DNCB, had a much improved prognosis. Eighty-four percent of these patients were found to have localized tumors that could be resected and were free of disease for at least six months following surgery. There appeared to be considerable differences, however, in the pattern of DNCB reactivity in patients with different histologic types of solid tumors. Patients with epidermoid carcinomas of either the cervix, mouth, pharynx, or larynx showed a very strong correlation between a positive DNCB response and a good prognosis following cancer surgery. Most patients with these neoplasms who could be sensitized to this chemical had operable disease and were free of disease for at least 6 months after surgery, whereas those who were anergic had a uniformly poor prognosis. In contrast, there appeared to be little correlation between positive DNCB tests and recurrence after surgery for skeletal and soft tissue sarcomas. Most sarcoma patients were immunologically competent regardless of whether they were free of disease at six months or had early recurrence.

Thus, it is evident that patients with severe impairment of the cell-mediated immune reaction, as exhibited by cutaneous anergy to 100 µg of DNCB, have a poor prognosis after surgical therapy, regardless of the histologic type of their neoplasm. However, the prognostic significance of an intact cellular immune response is very closely related to the histologic type of neoplasm being studied. The explanation for these differences in cutaneous reactivity with various tumor types is unknown, although it is possible that the patterns of cutaneous reactivity are indicative of some important differences in the effects of different types of neoplasms on the immune system.

Recent studies have done much to clarify the immunosuppression produced by malignant neoplastic disease.

Sequential evaluation of general immune competence in cancer patients revealed that variations in immune reactivity correlated with body burden of cancer. Patients who, on sequential testing with DNCB, converted from a reactive to an anergic status were usually found to have progressive cancer. Conversely, patients who converted from an anergic to a reactive status were observed to establish control of their tumor as frequently as those patients who were reactive initially and maintained their reactivity during the postsurgical observation period.[8] Thus, it was evident that the defect in systemic immunity was a result of the neoplastic process and that the immunosuppression could be reversed by successful therapy. Additional studies revealed that lymphocytes from cancer patients showed depressed functions when compared with those of normal individuals, and that the degree of depression correlated with the extent of the cancer.[10,14] Serum factors have also been found in cancer patients that inhibit the function of lymphocytes from normal individuals in culture. The factors undoubtedly contribute to the immunosuppression observed in cancer patients.[4,9] Thus, it appears that the immunosuppression caused by cancer is the result of a humoral factor released by the cancer cell itself, or a response by the body to the cancer cell, which is capable of depressing normal host cellular immunity, as measured by delayed cutaneous hypersensitivity and lymphocyte function.

Role of Surgery in Diagnosis and Staging

The histology of the primary lesion is of the utmost importance in accurately diagnosing and appropriately treating human neoplasms. Each specific human neoplasm has its own response to surgery, chemotherapy, and radiation therapy. Before planning the definitive treatment program, it is imperative to obtain a histologic diagnosis of the primary lesion.

Diagnosis of solid tumors depends upon locating and performing a biopsy of the lesion. This goal is most easily fulfilled when the tumor is near the body surface or involves one of the orifices of the body that can be examined with appropriate visual instruments, such as a bronchoscope, colonoscope, or cystoscope. Carcinomas of the breast, tongue, or rectum can be seen or palpated, and a portion can be excised for definitive diagnosis.

The most difficult cancers to diagnose, and unfortunately the most lethal ones, occur in the internal organs. Space-occupying lesions in the internal organs may grow quite large before causing symptoms. The newer techniques of ultrasonography and CT scans are the most useful techniques for localizing such lesions. They are important additions to older techniques such as barium sulfate opacification of the gastrointestinal tract, examination of the bronchial tree by iodinated oil bronchograms, selective arteriography of major vessels supplying internal organs, radioisotopes and radiopaque dyes that concentrate in various organs such as the liver, gallbladder, kidney, and lymph nodes. Although CT or sonographically directed needle biopsy may be useful in some patients, exploratory surgery is often required to obtain a biopsy and to confirm the exact histologic diagnosis.

Biopsy

It is imperative to obtain microscopic proof of malignant disease prior to institution of treatment, since significant morbidity and mortality may result from all forms of cancer therapy. The specific type of antitumor therapy depends on the histologic type of tumor, which must be established by biopsy. Significant errors have been made when biopsies have not been obtained; for example, radical mastectomies have been performed for fat necrosis. Even when biopsy reports from another hospital are available, the slides of the previous biopsy must be obtained and reviewed prior to the institution of therapy. This is essential, because not infrequently, and particularly in rare neoplasms, an erroneous interpretation may have been made. Definitive therapy cannot be planned rationally without knowing the nature of the neoplastic lesion.

Three methods for biopsy of suspicious tissue are commonly used. They are the needle, the incisional, and the excisional, or open, biopsy; each has its advantages and disadvantages. Regardless of the method used, the pathologic interpretation of the tumor mass can be valid only if a representative section of tumor is obtained. The oncologist must be aware that a sampling error can occur with needle and incisional biopsies when only a small portion of the total tumor mass is submitted for pathologic examination.

Needle Biopsy

This is the simplest method and may be used for the biopsy of subcutaneous masses, muscular masses, and some internal organs, such as liver, kidney and pancreas. Further, this method is inexpensive and causes minimal disturbance of the surrounding tissue. The danger of implanting tumor cells in a needle track during biopsy is extremely small and can be avoided if the location of the needle track is such that it can be excised easily at the time of the definitive surgical procedure. Needle biopsy may be disadvantageous when the specimen is small and not representative of the total tumor, or if the needle misses the space-occupying lesion. Hence, a needle biopsy requires experience to interpret. A negative report for malignant neoplastic disease is always viewed with skepticism and should be followed by incisional or excisional biopsy if there is any doubt. Stereotactic control of needle biopsies of the breast for mammographically demonstrable lesions should essentially eliminate geographic misses.

Needle biopsies can be of two types: fine needle aspiration biopsy or needle biopsy by a large bore needle such as the Vim Silverman or Tru Cut type. The latter actually obtains a small piece of tissue, which allows the pathologist to study the relationship between cancer cells and the surrounding tissue. The more frequent procedure is fine-needle aspiration cytology. In this procedure, a fine needle is inserted into the tumor, and strands of the single cells are obtained for cytologic diagnosis. This procedure is extremely useful for a number of tumors but requires considerable skill to interpret and should only be done by an experienced pathologist.

Incisional Biopsy

This involves the removal of only a portion of a tumor mass for pathologic examination. It is best performed under circumstances where, if tumor cells are spilled at the time of biopsy, the incisional wound can be encompassed and totally excised at the time of the definitive surgical procedure. Incisional biopsy includes the removal of portions of the tumor with forceps during endoscopic examination of the bronchus, esophagus, rectum and bladder, and by suction or curettage from the endometrium. Incisional biopsy is indicated for deeper subcutaneous or muscular tumor masses when needle biopsy fails to establish a diagnosis.

The incisional biopsy is also used when a tumor is so large that total local excision would expose wide tissue planes and prejudice any subsequent adequate wide, locally curative resection. If possible, such biopsy should take a deep section of tumor, as well as a margin of normal tissue. Incisional biopsies suffer from the same hazard as do needle biopsies: the removed portion may not be representative of all the involved tissue. Hence, a negative biopsy does not preclude the presence of cancer in the remaining mass. Another theoretical objection to the incisional method is the possibility that the surgeon may seed cancer cells into the operative wound or that transected lymphatics and blood vessels may transport the cells to distant sites. Despite these dangers, one must keep in mind that definitive surgical procedures cannot be planned rationally without knowing the nature of the neoplastic lesion.

Excisional Biopsy

This is the complete local removal of the tumor mass. It is used for small, discrete masses, 2–3 cm in diameter, when local removal will not interfere with the wider excision required for permanent local control. A major advantage of an excisional biopsy is that it allows the pathologist to examine the entire lesion. However, this method is contraindicated in large tumor masses because, again, the biopsy procedure often scatters tumor cells throughout a large incision that must be widely and totally encompassed by subsequent definitive surgical procedures. Therefore, excisional biopsy is usually contraindicated for skeletal and soft tissue sarcomas, although it is ideally suited for superficial squamous or basal cell carcinomas and malignant melanomas.

The excisional method is principally used for polypoid lesions of the colon, for thyroid and breast nodules, for small skin lesions, and when the pathologist cannot make a definitive diagnosis from tissue removed by incisional biopsy. An unbiopsied lump is surgically removed when the suspicious character of the lesion, the need for its removal (whatever the diagnosis), and the nonmutilating nature of the operation make such an approach reasonably definitive. Examples of such procedures include hemithyroidectomy for thyroid nodules and a right colectomy for a cecal mass that might be inflammatory or neoplastic. In the latter instance, colonoscopic biopsy is informative only if positive for neoplasm.

Surgeons should always mark the excisional biopsy margins with sutures so that if removal is incomplete and further excision is indicated, they will know where the tumor margin was positive. Biopsy incisions should be closed with meticulous hemostasis, since it may be possible for a collecting hematoma to extend tumor cell contamination by widespread infiltration of tissue planes. Contaminated instruments, gloves, gowns, and drapes should be discarded and replaced with noncontaminated substitutes when the definitive procedure is to follow immediately after the biopsy procedure.

Lymph nodes should be carefully selected for biopsy. Cervical lymph nodes should not be biopsied until a careful search for a primary tumor has been made. Nasopharyngoscopy, esophagoscopy, and bronchoscopy are all simple procedures with fiberoptic instruments. Thyroid scan may be required in the work-up. Enlargement of the upper cervical nodes by metastases is usually due to laryngeal, oropharyngeal, and nasopharyngeal primary neoplasms. Supraclavicular nodes are more frequently enlarged from metastases originating in the thoracic or abdominal cavity.

The specimen may be prepared for pathologic examination by either frozen or permanent sections. Frozen sections are made immediately, and pathologic diagnosis can be obtained within 10–20 minutes. Frozen sections are used when the diagnosis is required at the time of major surgery and when it is in the patient's best interests to have the definitive resectional surgery carried out at that time.

Occasionally, mediastinoscopy, laparoscopy (peritoneoscopy) exploratory thoracotomy or laparotomy is utilized and necessary to obtain adequate representative tissue samples for microscopic examination and confirmation of diagnosis. As a general rule, the neoplastic nature of the disease process must be confirmed by frozen section examination prior to closure of the wound, regardless of the suspected clinical picture. If the surgeon fails to obtain tissue for frozen section examination and proceeds immediately to major surgery, he risks mischaracterizing the neoplastic nature of the pathologic process, and the patient will experience the morbidity of operation without enjoying the benefits of an accurate diagnosis.

Staging of Tumors

Clinical evaluation of the extent of the patient's tumor at the time of initial presentation is called the clinical stage. In addition to making an exact histologic diagnosis of cancer, it is essential that the clinical stage of the disease be determined prior to making a decision regarding therapy. This is especially important when the patient initially presents for treatment, but it is also often desirable to repeat some of the diagnostic procedures periodically during the patient's course in order to assess his or her true status. The recognized importance of staging has led to a variety of international and national attempts to standardize the staging of the patient with cancer. To date, no single system has been universally accepted. The American Joint Committee on Cancer (AJCC) has recommended a staging system. Stage I usually indicates a neoplasm confined to its primary site of origin; Stage II indicates metastases to the regional lymph nodes; and Stage III often and Stage IV always indicate distant metastatic spread.

The Unio Internationale Contra Cancrum (UICC) has attempted to standardize one system for all nations. This has been called the TNM system because it relies on a statement of tumor extent in terms of the primary tumor (T), presence or absence of node metastases (N), and the presence or absence of distant metastases (M). The system was developed following careful analysis of the results of treatment in patients with various constellations of clinical findings. It was found that patients with larger tumors did less well than those with smaller tumors; hence, the separation of various stages on the basis of tumor size. Size criteria vary for different tumors, but in this system, decreasing prognosis is indicated by increasing numbers after the T, such as T_1, T_2, T_3, or T_4, for lesions of increasing size. The presence or absence of regional spread is usually indicated by variations in the secondary category, under N for nodes. The absence of nodal metastasis is designated as N_0; the presence of nodal metastasis is N_1; for more extensive nodal involvement, additional numbers may be used. Finally, distant metastases are indicated by adding a subscript 1 following M for metastases, or a subscript 0 for their absence. Thus, a small lesion that has neither spread to regional nodes nor metastasized would be designated as a T_1,N_0,M_0 lesion. A lesion that was larger and involved regional nodes but without distant metastases might be identified as a T_2,N_1,M_0 lesion. A larger neoplasm with both regional and distant metastases would be designated a T_3,N_1,M_1 lesion. For some tumor types, such as soft tissue sarcoma, a G for grade of malignancy is added. High-grade tumors are more anaplastic and tend to metastasize sooner.

The AJCC recognizes several types of cancer staging schemas (Table XII-1-2). The clinical-diagnostic staging (cTNM) represents the extent of the disease prior to first definitive treatment. Postsurgical resection-pathologic staging (pTNM) provides additional information after operation and is especially useful in planning adjuvant therapy for many types of tumors. Other staging types include surgical-evaluative staging (sTNM), usually after a disease-free interval, and autopsy staging (aTNM).

The importance of accurate staging when designating a therapeutic program for a patient with cancer cannot be overemphasized. It is an important consideration when comparing the results of therapy in different centers, and as therapeutic methods for cancer improve, it is only by comparison of neoplasms at equivalent stages that new forms of therapy can be appropriately evaluated.

Unfortunately, one of the great deficiencies of the present staging methods is their inability to indicate subclinical, microscopic metastatic lesions. Many patients who are treated for apparently localized cancers already have disseminated metastases. For example, about one-half of those patients who have cancer of the breast and who undergo mastectomy have subclinical distant metastasis at the time of the operation.

Selection of Appropriate Therapy: General Considerations

Today surgery and radiation represent the most successful means of treating cancer localized to the primary site and regional lymph nodes. Since these forms of therapy exert their effect locally, neither is usually considered curative once the disease has metastasized beyond the local region. Both methods are frequently useful as palliative treatments and occasional long-term survival follows surgical resection of metastases to single organs.

Unlike surgery and radiation therapy, chemotherapy and other forms of systemic therapy, including immunotherapy, hormonal therapy, and cytokines, represent systemic forms of treatment effective against tumor cells already metastatic to distant organ sites. These systemic therapeutic modalities have a greater chance of curing patients with a minimum number of tumor cells than those with clinically evident disease. Thus, though surgery and radiation therapy cannot be curative unless the tumor is confined locally or regionally, they can decrease the patient's tumor burden so that systemic therapy may become more effective. During the past several years, enough evidence has accumulated to suggest that treatments combining surgery, radiation therapy, and chemotherapy often significantly improve cure rates above those achievable with any single therapeutic modality.

Cancer treatment, therefore, should be approached in an interdisciplinary manner. Just as oncology should be approached as a unique field of study, so cancer should be regarded as a single but complex disease spectrum requiring a multidisciplinary approach. The practice of assigning certain types of neoplasms to surgery, radiation therapy, or medical oncology with a further division into various anatomically oriented specialties should be discontinued.

Goals of Therapy—Cure or Palliation?

Once the diagnosis of malignant neoplastic disease has been made and the extent of disease determined, a decision must be made about the specific therapy. Is the patient curable? This is the foremost question that must be answered before the physician recommends aggressive therapy with its attendant complications. The goals of therapy vary with the extent of the cancer. If the cancer is localized without evidence of spread, the goal is to eradicate the cancer and cure the patient. When the cancer is spread beyond local cure, the goal is to control the patient's symptoms and to

Table XII-1-2. Chronology and Types of Staging Recognized by the American Joint Committee on Cancer

Stage	Comment
cTNM	*Clinical-diagnostic staging:* The extent of disease using all information available prior to first definitive treatment, including pathologic confirmation of extent of disease by biopsy or invasive techniques
pTNM	*Postsurgical resection-pathologic staging:* The extent of disease using all data available at the time of surgery and on examination of a completely resected specimen
sTNM	*Surgical-evaluative staging:* The extent of disease using all clinical information available plus that obtained on surgical exploration: usually done for a few inaccessible tumors that are not amenable to definitive resection
rTNM	*Retreatment staging:* The classification when restaging is necessary for additional or secondary definitive treatment after a (disease-free) interval following first treatment
aTNM	*Autopsy staging:* Used only when the cancer is first diagnosed at autopsy

From Beahrs et al.[2] with permission

maintain maximum activity for the longest possible period of time. Palliation should be measured in terms of useful life. Diabetes is not cured, but the manifestations of the disease are controlled so that a patient has many years of active and useful life. Goals for the palliation of patients living with cancer are similar.

Patients are generally judged as incurable if they have distant metastases or evidence of extensive local infiltration of adjacent organs or structures. The most common criterion for incurability is distant metastases. However, some patients are potentially curable even if they have distant metastases. For example, patients with solitary pulmonary metastases may be curable by resection, and even those with widespread metastases who have choriocarcinoma may be curable with chemotherapy. Histologic proof of distant metastases should be obtained before the patient is assessed as incurable. Occasionally, an exploratory celiotomy or thoracotomy may be necessary to determine the nature of equivocal lesions in the lungs or liver. In rare situations, the clinical situation may point so overwhelmingly to distant metastases that the patient may safely be considered incurable without biopsy.

Local extension may be a criterion of incurability. For each anatomic site, there are certain local criteria that place the patient unequivocally in an incurable status, while others imply a poor prognosis but are not absolutely indicative of incurability. In equivocal situations after extensive studies have failed to demonstrate metastatic or incurable local extension, the patient deserves the benefit of doubt and should be treated for cure.

Choice of Therapy

Surgery, radiation therapy, and chemotherapy are the most frequently used therapeutic modalities in the fight against cancer. Each may play a role in both curative and palliative therapy. In choosing therapy, a variety of factors must be considered regardless of the disease, and the results obtained from each type of therapy must be known prior to choosing a modality or combination of modalities.

The patient's general condition and the presence of any coexisting disease must be considered in planning therapy. Surgery may be contraindicated in a patient who has recently experienced a myocardial infarction. A patient with preexisting diabetes will be much more susceptible to the toxic effects of hormonal therapy with corticosteroids. Renal disease may increase the toxicity of some of the chemotherapeutic drugs, such as methotrexate. In addition, evidence of infection or bleeding in a patient may make any form of cancer therapy dangerous, requiring vigorous treatment prior to the initiation of definitive therapy.

The psychological makeup of the patient and the patient's life situation must be considered. A patient who is unable to accept the realities of a given treatment should be offered an alternative approach when possible. Consultation with a psychiatrist experienced in cancer may be extremely helpful in helping patients deal with the reality. This is particularly true for surgical procedures that significantly alter the patient's appearance or that involve change of organ function requiring the patient's daily care, such as colostomy. Experimental

forms of therapy should also be avoided in some patients whose non-compliance might jeopardize themselves and the research. Obviously, a patient who is unwilling to tolerate the inconvenience of an intraarterial catheter and who thus might remove it without medical approval should not undergo such treatment.

Surgical Therapy: Introduction

Surgical treatment represents the most frequently used and the most successful single method of cancer therapy currently available. More patients are cured of cancer by surgery than by any other therapeutic modality. Only about one-third of cancer patients are cured by surgery alone, however; with a few notable exceptions, surgical therapy is curative only in those patients in whom the disease is localized to the primary site and regional nodes.

Advances in surgical techniques, anesthesia, and supportive care (blood transfusion, antibiotics, and fluid and electrolyte management) have permitted the development of more radical and extensive operative procedures. Ultraradical operations have been extended to their anatomic limits, permitting the surgical removal of nearly all organs. These advances have resulted in significant improvements in the cure rates for certain human neoplasms, such as the operation of pelvic exenteration for carcinoma of the cervix recurrent following radiation therapy. Unfortunately, for the most part, these more radical procedures have often failed significantly to increase cure rates for the common solid neoplasms.

Metastatic Routes of Spread of Primary Neoplasms

There are few subjects of greater importance to the surgical oncologist than the spread of cancer. Much is known about the routes of spread but little about the conditions that determine that spread. Some cancers are metastatic at the time of their clinical discovery, while others of the same type and in the same organ tissue may remain localized for years.

Metastases may entirely dominate the clinical picture, while the primary tumor remains latent and asymptomatic. Some patients present with metastatic cancer and no evidence of a primary site. For example, metastases to the brain secondary to silent cancers in the bronchus or the breast are often mistaken for primary brain tumors.

Knowledge of the particular manner in which different types of cancer spread is important in planning surgical therapy. In general, a malignant tumor may spread by four routes: directly by infiltrating surrounding tissue; via lymphatics; by vascular invasion; or by implantation in serous cavities (Figure XII-1-1). However, many cancers spread by more than one route, and an orderly course of metastases cannot be relied upon. For example, many patients with breast cancer, or melanoma, may manifest distant metastatic disease in the lungs, liver, or skeleton but never develop evidence of lymph node metastases. Metastatic patterns of various types of human tumors are summarized in Table XII-1-3.

Direct Extension. Cancer cells may spread by direct extension through tissue spaces. Some neoplasms, such as

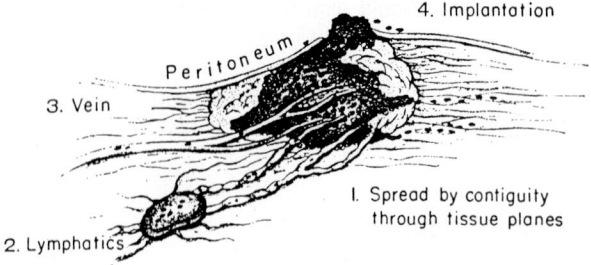

Figure XII-1-1. A diagrammatic illustration of the four mechanisms of the dissemination of cancer cells. The original tumor could be one of many organs with cells disseminating by the four mechanisms. (From Cole[6] with permission.)

Table XII-1-3. Estimated Frequency of Patterns of Neoplastic Spread for Some Common Human Cancers

Neoplasm	Hematogenous	Lymphatic	Local infiltration (expressed as local recurrence)
Adenocarcinoma			
Breast	4*	3	2
Endometrium	1	2	1
Ovary	2	3	4
Stomach	4	4	3
Pancreas	4	4	3
Colon	3	3	1
Kidney	2	2	2
Prostate	3	3	3
Liver	1	1	4
Epidermoid carcinoma			
Lung	4	3	2
Oropharynx	1	3	3
Larynx	1	3	2
Cervix	1	4	3
Transitional cell carcinoma			
Bladder	2	3	4
Cutaneous neoplasm			
Squamous cell carcinoma	1	2	1
Melanomas	3	3	2
Basal cell carcinomas	0	0	1
Sarcomas			
Bones	4	1	1
Soft tissue	4	1	3
Brain neoplasms	0	0	4

*0, Does not occur; 1, 1–15%; 2, 15–30%; 3, >30%; 4, >50%

soft tissue sarcomas and adenocarcinomas of the stomach or esophagus, may extend for considerable distances (10–15 cm) along tissue planes beyond the palpable tumor mass. Other neoplasms, such as a basal cell carcinoma of skin, rarely extend for more than a few millimeters beyond the visible margin. Even though some of the central nervous system tumors rarely metastasize, they may permeate nearby brain tissue, and their location can cause death by interfering with vital CNS functions.

Lymphatic Spread. Tumor cells can readily enter lymphatics and extend along these channels by permeation or embolism through the regional lymphatics to lymph nodes. Permeation is the growth of a colony of tumor cells along the course of the lymph vessel. This occurs commonly in the skin lymphatics in carcinoma of the breast and in the perineural lymphatics in carcinoma of the prostate.

Spread along the lymphatics by emoblism to the regional nodes or distant lymph nodes is of great importance. Lymph node metastases are first confined to the subcapsular space: at this stage the node is not enlarged and may appear normal to the naked eye. Gradually the tumor cells permeate the sinusoids and replace the parenchyma. There is little direct spread from node to node, because the capsule is not penetrated until a late stage. Tumor cells travel by anastomosing lymphatics, and spread generally occurs to other nodes proximally, sometimes skipping normal nodes, by way of collateral lymph channels. When a lymph node containing tumor is more than 3 cm in diameter, tumor has usually extended beyond the capsule into the perinodal fat, indicating an ominous prognosis.

The lymph from the abdominal organs and lower extremities drains into the cisterna chyli and then into the thoracic duct, which finally opens into the left jugular vein. Tumor cells probably pass freely from the lymph to the bloodstream. Originally, oncologists believed that solid neoplasms involved regional lymph nodes and then spread into the bloodstream by drainage through the lymphatics into the thoracic duct and to other parts of the body. An alternative explanation now favored by most oncologists assumes that the presence of cancer cells in regional lymph nodes indicates an unfavorable host-tumor relationship and the likelihood of distant metastases.

Lymphatic involvement is extremely common in epithelial neoplasms of all types, except basal cell carcinoma of the skin, which does not metastasize to regional lymphatics. Sarcomas metastasize to lymph nodes only 2–5% of the time.

Vascular Spread. Cancer cells may reach the bloodstream through the thoracic duct or by direct invasion of blood vessels. Capillaries are almost always invaded. Small veins are invaded frequently, the arteries rarely. The chief reason for the striking difference in characteristics of invasion between arteries and veins appears to be that veins form a plexus reaching to subendothelial regions, thus providing a portal of entry through the vein wall. When the vascular endothelium is destroyed, a thrombus forms that is quickly invaded by tumor. This combination of thrombus and tumor may detach to form large tumor emboli. Vascular invasion is commonly seen in both carcinomas and sarcomas and is associated with a poor prognosis. Some types of neoplasms have a remarkable tendency to grow as a solid column along the course of veins, for example, renal carcinomas and sarcomas. Renal carcinomas have been known to grow out of the renal vein into the inferior vena cava and up the inferior vena cava to the right atrium, where, amazingly, their removal may still result in long-term survival.

Spread Through Serous Cavities. Tumor cells occasionally gain entrance to serous cavities via direct growth of tumor through the wall of an organ. Many tumor cells are capable of growth in suspension without a supporting matrix and may grow and spread within the peritoneal cavity or attach to serous surfaces. In either case, it is common for tumor cells to spread widely when they encounter a space lined with a serous surface. Thus, widespread peritoneal seeding is commonly seen with gastrointestinal neoplasms and tumors of ovarian origin. A similar mechanism appears to operate in the case of malignant gliomas, which may spread widely within the central nervous system via cerebral spinal fluid.

Preoperative Preparation

Often, the patient's physical condition is relatively poor. Many malignant tumors appear to have a toxic effect on the host disproportionate to the size of the lesion. Patients may have a poor nutritional status because of interference with normal alimentary function, as is true with cancers of the mouth, pharynx, esophagus, intestinal tract and appended glandular organs. Pain may contribute to anorexia and severe electrolyte disorder. Anemia, vitamin deficiencies, and defects in the coagulation mechanisms must be corrected before an operation can be safely performed.

Every effort should be made to correct nutritional deficiencies, restore depleted blood volume, and correct hypoproteinemia prior to extensive surgical procedures. Total parenteral nutrition (TPN) can be used to prepare the malnourished patient for a major operation, although reconstitution is a slow process, and TPN may chiefly serve to interrupt further deterioration. Without correction of critical physiologic and biochemical deficiencies, the operative morbidity and mortality following extensive cancer operations will be excessive.

Cancer Surgery

Once the decision has been made to proceed with surgical therapy, the operative procedure should be planned carefully. It is essential to realize that the best, and often the only, opportunity for cure is at the time of the first operation. If the neoplasm is incompletely excised at that time, tissue planes, lymphatics, and blood vessels are violated and tumor cells are seeded throughout the wound. Any recurrence that follows may be difficult to separate from the inflammatory reaction and scarring that can distort tissue planes to a point where tumor margins are indistinct. Therefore, enucleation or incomplete excision of tumor masses is never indicated as a therapeutic measure.

Prevention of Tumor Cell Implantation During Surgery

Local recurrence of cancer following surgery may be due to incomplete removal or spillage of cancer cells into the operative area. The cancer surgeon must constantly be aware of the danger of possibly transferring cancer cells by inoculation into the surrounding tissues during the course of an operation. As soon as the incision is made, all edges of the wound should be protected with a plastic drape to prevent

tumor cell contamination (Figure XII-1-2). This precaution is exemplified best when laparotomy or thoracotomy is performed for malignant neoplastic disease within the abdomen or thorax.

Tumor cells may be inadvertently transplanted from the primary site to other sites during the surgical procedure. When preliminary biopsy has been done, the entire operative field should be reprepared after the biopsy incision is closed. The instruments and gloves used during the biopsy are not used again, because they may have been contaminated. Even the basin of saline solution in which the surgeon's gloved hand is dipped may be contaminated with cancer cells.

If the tumor is entered during an operative procedure with curative intent, the risk of implanting cancer cells into the wound is greatly increased. Should this happen, the operative field must be isolated; the cut surface of the tumor must be cauterized with the electrocautery and isolated from the remainder of the wound; and the contaminated knife, instruments, and gloves must be discarded. Then, and then only, can the operation continue through a new plane of dissection allowing a much wider margin around the tumor.

Many different cytotoxic solutions have been used to irrigate the wound following cancer surgery in an effort to sterilize the operative site. None has been effective in decreasing the local recurrence rate, with the exception of 0.5% formaldehyde used to prevent local recurrence from carcinoma of the cervix. Sodium hypochlorite solution, nitrogen mustard, and thiotepa have all been tried, with little success.

The rate of local recurrence in the suture line following resection for carcinoma of the colon is about 10%. There has been some success with various techniques to prevent this local recurrence. Ligation of the bowel with umbilical tape proximal and distal to the tumor, or irrigation of the cut ends of the colon with bichloride of mercury solution and then excision of the edge of each end of the bowel has been used and has decreased the recurrence rate to less than 2%. The use of closed anastomosis and iodized sutures has decreased the anastomotic recurrence rate in the laboratory.

Local recurrence can, however, occur despite every effort to isolate the tumor or avoid spilling cancer cells into the

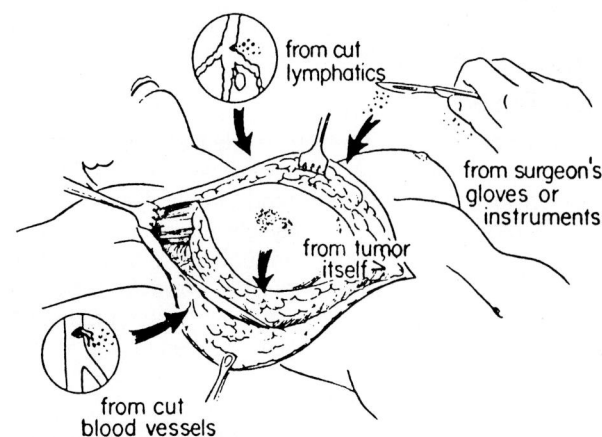

Figure XII-1-2. The seeding of cancer cells during the operative procedure. (From Cole[6] with permission.)

operative field. For example, tumor in local lymphatics may be unrecognized at the time of the initial operation, or blood-borne cells may implant the fresh wound. Usually a local recurrence is associated with systemic disease and is an unfavorable prognostic factor, but this is not always the case, because approximately 20% of the patients whose local recurrences are widely resected survive five years.

Prevention of Vascular Dissemination at Surgery

Blood-borne metastases are a major factor in the death of patients with most tumors. Although cancer cells have been identified in the blood of many cancer patients, only a small number of these circulating cancer cells survive because of host resistance and other factors. Thus, tumor embolism and metastases are not synonymous. In fact, there appears to be little difference in the prognosis of patients with or without tumor cells in their blood preoperatively. Furthermore, manipulation of the tumor at any time in the surgical procedure can greatly increase the number of cancer cells recovered from the blood. There have been reports of a correlation between prognosis and the presence of tumor cells in the blood during the operative procedure, which may be secondary to implantation and growth occurring as a result of the immunosuppression induced by the operation.

Definite measures should be taken to prevent the dissemination of tumor cells during the operation. These can include: avoiding manipulation of the tumor ("no-touch" technique), and early ligation of the vascular pedicle.

Since any manipulation of the tumor mass may result in exfoliation of tumor cells into the lymphatics and blood, such manipulation must be kept to a minimum prior to the operative procedure, during preparation of the skin with antiseptic agents, as well as during the operative procedure. Furthermore, it is imperative to use an incision of proper size to minimize unnecessary manipulation of the tumor. One that is too small will not permit the necessary wide excision without excessive handling. Turnbull has reported a significantly higher survival in left colon cancer using the no-touch technique, which combines minimal manipulation, early ligation of the vascular pedicle, and wide excision.[26] However, the importance of early ligation of the vascular pedicle has been questioned by other investigators, who reported similar results without the early ligation.

Types of Cancer Operations

Local Resection

Wide local resection in which an adequate margin of normal tissue is removed with the tumor mass may be adequate treatment for certain low-grade neoplasms that do not metastasize to regional nodes or widely infiltrate adjacent tissues. Basal cell carcinomas and the mixed tumors of the parotid gland are examples of such neoplasms. However, it is essential that at least some normal tissue surrounding the tumor is excised in order to prevent local recurrence.

Radical Local Resection

Some neoplasms may spread widely by infiltration into adjacent tissues. This is especially true for soft tissue sarcomas, and esophageal and gastric carcinomas. For this reason, it is necessary to remove a wide margin of normal tissue with the neoplasm in these cases. The wide normal-tissue margin between the line of excision and the tumor mass also acts as a protective barrier against tumor cell spill into the severed lymphatics and vessels. The greater the thickness of normal tissue between the plane of dissection and the tumor, the greater the likelihood of a complete local excision.

If the tumor was previously explored but not removed, or if an incisional biopsy was performed, there is a possibility that tumor cells may have been implanted in the incision at the time of this initial operation. It is therefore extremely important to remove a wide segment of skin and the underlying muscles, fat and fascia far beyond the limits of the original incision.

It must be constantly emphasized that malignant neoplasms are not well encapsulated. A pseudocapsule composed of a compression zone of neoplastic cells usually covers the tumor. This apparent encapsulation offers a great temptation for simple enucleation, because the tumor may be easily dislodged from its bed. This temptation must be resisted. The surgeon must cut through normal tissue at all times and should never encounter the neoplasm during its removal. Dissection should proceed with meticulous care to avoid tumor cell spill. Retraction always should be away from, rather than toward, the tumor. It is important for the surgeon to remember to make his incision as far as possible from the gross extent of the tumor on all sides, including the deep aspect. Skin, subcutaneous fat, and muscle usually can be sacrified with impunity and little functional loss. Involvement of major vessels, nerves, joints, or bones may require sacrifice of these structures and even amputation in order to obtain a curative result. When the only therapy is the surgical procedure, the extent of operation should be determined by the concern for adequate margins to achieve cure and not for planning of reconstruction and postoperative function. The problem of reconstruction should be approached as a separate specialized procedure, often requiring the assistance of plastic and reconstructive surgeons and perhaps other special surgical expertise.

The definition of adequate margins varies with the type of neoplasm; e.g., all deeply situated sarcomas lying between or within muscle groups require the removal of all muscle bundles from their origin to insertion within that particular fascial compartment; all surrounding or adjacent fascia, periosteum, vessels, nerves, and connective tissues; and all skin adjacent to the lesions. These procedures are imperative when surgery alone is used to treat sarcomas, because these lesions tend to infiltrate along fascial and muscle planes far beyond the palpable limits of the tumor. As surgeons proceed with the operation, they may be forced to alter their initial operative plan as they visualize the extent of tumor and as the pathology reports of frozen section examinations of surgical margins become available. Decisions regarding the extent of resection are difficult and require experienced judgment. In borderline situations, it is usually better to proceed with a potentially curative resection of the tumor mass unless there is histologic confirmation that the lesion has extended beyond the boundaries of possible surgical resection. Advances in the use of combined modality therapy for skeletal and soft tissue sarcomas have permitted the salvage rather than amputation of extremities for most patients.

Radical Resection with En Bloc Excision of Lymphatics

Since many neoplasms commonly metastasize by way of the lymphatics, operations have been designed to remove the primary neoplasm and the regional lymph nodes draining that area in continuity with all the intervening tissues. Conditions are best for this type of operation when the collecting nodes of the lymphatic channels draining the neoplasm lie adjacent to the primary site or when there is a single avenue of lymphatic drainage that can be removed without sacrificing vital structures. It is important to avoid cutting across involved lymphatic channels, because such action increases the possibility of local disease recurrence.

Individually Meyer and Halsted applied the principle of radical resection with en bloc excision of lymphatics to breast cancer at the turn of the century. This principle has formed the foundation of cancer surgery for many years. At the present time, it is generally agreed that en bloc regional lymph node dissections should be performed in patients having clinical involvement of nodes by metastatic tumor. In many cases, however, the tumor has already spread beyond the regional nodes. Although the cure rates following such procedures may be quite low (20–40%), undue pessimism should not prevent such patients from receiving surgical treatment. En bloc removal of the involved nodes offers the only chance for cure and provides significant palliation and local control. Therefore, the surgical oncologist should not view regional lymph node involvement as a contraindicator to surgery but as an indication for the use of additional systemic therapy such as chemotherapy.

Due to the high rate of local cancer recurrence following surgical resection when multiple lymph nodes are involved and the high error rate when palpation is used to assess the extent of the involvement, the routine dissection of regional nodes in close proximity to the primary tumor is recommended, even when they are not clinically involved. This procedure is supported by the microscopic evidence of tumor dissemination in 20–40% of carcinomas and melanomas. By resecting the subclinically involved lymph nodes before the disease has progressed to the palpably evident stage, some series suggest improved five-year survival rates.

This concept of elective, or prophylactic, lymph node dissection in cases where the regional nodes are not obviously involved has been challenged because it is not clear whether cure rates are improved if the nodes are removed before they are palpable. Controlled clinical trials directed toward this question in many types of neoplasms are currently underway. Regardless of direct therapeutic benefit, in many types of cancer foreknowledge of tumor in regional nodes does affect the staging of the patient, can alter the treatment, and can significantly influence prognosis. For example, patients with breast cancer who have metastases to regional nodes may benefit considerably from adjuvant chemotherapy or hormonal therapy. Also, some patients with deep melanomas may become candidates for investigational adjuvant trials only if lymph node metastases are present. Furthermore, a comparison of experimental results from one insti-

tution with those of another depends upon the accurate staging of each patient at the time of the initiation of therapy. For these reasons, the decision to recommend a prophylactic lymph node dissection must be based on the likelihood of benefit to the patient.

Extensive Surgical Procedures

Some slow growing primary tumors may reach enormous size and may locally infiltrate widely without developing distant metastases. Supraradical operative procedures can be undertaken for these extensive, nearly inoperable tumors, with cure of occasional patients. Although surgical care, anesthesia, blood replacement, and physiologic monitoring are much improved over the past, these operations should not be undertaken except by experienced surgeons who can select those patients most likely to benefit. Furthermore, these extensive surgical procedures sometimes offer a chance for a cure that is not possible by other means and are justified in selected situations when extensive work-up shows no evidence of distant metastases. However, the surgeon must be willing to accept the responsibility for the postoperative emotional rehabilitation of the patient before undertaking such extensive procedures as hemipelvectomy, forequarter amputation, mutilating operations for head and neck carcinomas, or pelvic exenteration.

For example, pelvic exenteration is a well-conceived operation capable of curing patients with radiation-treated recurrent cancer of the cervix and certain well-differentiated and locally extensive adenocarcinomas of the rectum. This operation removes the pelvic organs (bladder, uterus, and rectum) and all soft tissues within the pelvis. Bowel function is restored with colostomy. Urinary tract drainage is established by anastomosis of ureters into a segment of bowel (ileum or sigmoid colon). The five-year, relapse-free survival from pelvic exenteration is 25% in this situation.

Surgery of Recurrent Cancer

There is a definite role for surgical resection of localized recurrent neoplasms of low-grade malignancy and slow growth, when further resection may produce a long period of remission. Additional surgical procedures are frequently successful in controlling recurrent soft tissue sarcomas, anastomotic recurrences of colon cancer, certain basal and squamous carcinomas of skin, and breast cancer recurrent following lumpectomy.

Routine second-look operations to detect early recurrence of colon cancer were advocated by Gilbertsen and Wangensteen. The results of this second-look procedure have not been impressive and do not appear to justify its routine use. However, various tumor markers, such as CEA, have been extremely useful for selecting patients likely to benefit from reoperation. In general, a local recurrence can be treated surgically or with radiation. The surgeon must decide which form of treatment will achieve local control with the lowest morbidity.

Surgery for Metastatic Disease

Although logic would suggest that once a neoplasm has metastasized to a distant site it is no longer curable by sur-

Table XII-1-4. Neoadjuvant Chemotherapy and Radiation Therapy Trials for Extremity Soft Tissue Sarcoma at UCLA (1974–1987)*

Radiation Therapy	Year	No.	% Limb Salvage	% Local Recurrence	% Comp	% Path Necrosis
Control	1972–1976	63	40	24	20	—
3500 cGy	1974–1981	77	96	6	40	75
1750 cGy	1981–1984	137	95	15	20	50
2800 cGy	1984–1987	107	95	8	23	70

Control = no preoperative radiation therapy; 3500 cGy = Adriamycin + 350 cGy x-ray therapy × 10; Comp = complications requiring reoperation
*From Antman et al.[1] with permission

poor perfusion of chemotherapeutic agents and are frequently hypoxic and resistant to radiation therapy. Since surgery works by zero-order kinetics, it efficiently removes the residual cancer cells that are resistant to these other modalities in the local site. Another advantage of this altered sequence of therapy relates to the shrinkage of tumor mass that occurs with preoperative therapy due to the destruction of tumor cells sensitive to chemotherapy or radiation therapy. There have been promising results from preliminary trials using these concepts in bone and soft tissue sarcomas, locally advanced breast cancer, and other neoplasms. A major dividend is the frequent possibility of organ preservation because of a lesser need for radical surgery.

Surgery as Immunotherapy

Cancer surgery is perhaps the most frequently used form of immunotherapy. Present evidence suggests that the effectiveness of the host's immune defenses is limited because the growing neoplasm seems to be able to evade an immune attack by producing specific and nonspecific immunosuppression in the cancer patient to enhance its growth. The growing neoplasm constantly sheds soluble tumor-associated antigens into the blood, and these antigens circulate alone or as antigen-antibody complexes. These serum antigens can inhibit the lymphocyte-mediated destruction of tumor cells in vitro and may play a similar role in vivo.[12]

In addition to this tumor-antigen-specific blocking, a growing neoplasm often causes a nonspecific and generalized suppression of the cancer patient's immune competence. Humoral factors produced by, or in response to, the neoplasm can be found in the sera of cancer patients and are thought to be the cause of the general immune depression. The extent of the immunosuppression correlates with the stage of disease and level of tumor burden; it is reversible by removal of the growing neoplasm. Therefore, any therapeutic maneuver that lowers tumor burden may reverse both specific and nonspecific immunosuppression and alter the immune balance in favor of the patient. In this respect, cancer surgery is immunotherapy because it effectively removes the cancer cell mass that produces the immunodepression and allows the patient's immune responses to recover. The key to recovery of the balance in the host-tumor relationship depends on destruction or removal of the tumor cell "factory." These concepts are illustrated in Figure XII-1-5.

Once the tumor mass has been removed, the immune mechanisms may deal with the clinically silent micrometastases present in many patients with presumably localized solid tumors. These host defenses are quite capable of

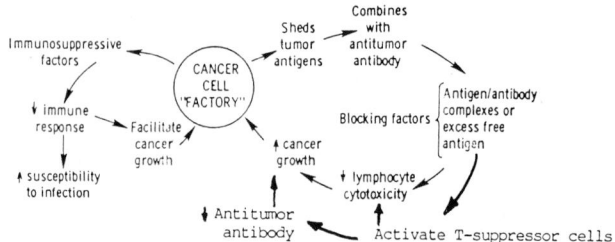

Figure XII-1-5. Cancer cell "factory" is depicted as a function of immunodepression in the host. Theoretically, cytoreductive cancer therapy interrupts this process, so that the host immune response returns to normal. (From Morton[19A] with permission.)

destroying small numbers of tumor cells on the order of 1–10 million, but not masses of 100 million or more. Unfortunately, the metastatic foci present in most patients are too great for the host's natural immune defenses and progressive growth will occur. Nonetheless, surgery for cancer becomes the first step in immunotherapy.

If this thesis is correct, it would follow that the approach to the surgical treatment for solid neoplasms must change dramatically. The future lies not in treating every patient with a solid neoplasm as one with localized disease, but in assuming that the local disease is merely a manifestation of a systemic illness, whether or not the patient has overt metastatic disease. Not until we accept surgery as merely one of the important modalities in the treatment of cancer, can we significantly improve our rates of cure. Therapeutic advances eventually must come from a multimethod combination of surgical therapy with radiotherapy, immunotherapy and/or chemotherapy. Unlike surgery and radiotherapy alone, which are both local treatments, the combinations represent a systemic treatment effective against tumor cells already metastatic to distant sites. However, at present, systemic therapeutic techniques have greater potential for curing those patients with a minimal number of tumor cells than those with clinically evident disease. Surgery for apparently localized tumors can favorably affect the host-tumor relationship and may even cure the patient with subclinical distant metastases. Debulking, or complete resection, of the recurrent neoplasm in the patient with metastatic disease is usually unsuccessful and rarely indicated, unless the entire tumor mass can be completely removed.

Surgical Techniques of the Future
Early Detection

One of the dilemmas facing the surgeon is the fact that approximately two-thirds of the growth of human neoplasms occurs before they are clinically detectable. Since cancer originates from a single cell, it takes approximately 30 exponential divisions to produce a 1 cm nodule. This represents about 1 billion neoplastic cells. After 40 exponential divisions, the patient is likely to be dead from the sheer bulk of the tumor mass. Based on growth dynamics, it is likely that most human cancers have been present in the body for at least one year and many for up to ten years prior to their clinical detection. There is ample evidence to suggest that 90% of solid neoplasms, whether they arise in the breast, colon, cervix, or other organs, are curable by surgical therapy at an early stage. Therefore, if tests can be perfected that detect the onset of neoplastic transformation, the surgeon and the oncologist would be better equipped to deal with human neoplasms. All therapeutic programs would benefit from battling a smaller colony of cancerous cells in a localized region.

Current methods for detecting such small neoplasms, however, are totally inadequate. With few outstanding exceptions such a mammography, it is impossible by current methodology to detect neoplasms smaller than 1 cm in size. A promising new technique that uses radioimaging techniques intraoperatively may be useful in this regard.

Radioimmunoguided Surgery Using Monoclonal Antibody

An exciting new surgical technique, radioimmunoguided surgery (RIGS), enables surgeons to localize and stage intra-abdominal disease during primary surgery. Basically, the surgeon guides a portable, hand-held gamma detection device that signals when it encounters radiolabelled monoclonal antibody conjugates that have bound to reactive antigen on the tumor cell surface. This allows the surgeon to seek out malignant lesions which might have escaped previous detection by CT scan or plain chest X-ray, and to examine more thoroughly those sites in which tumor cells may, or may not, be located. Although these techniques are in their infancy, they offer great promise for the future.

Technical Aspects of Radioimmunoguided Surgery. Murine monoclonal antibody B72.3 succeeds in identifying approximately 80% of gastrointestinal and ovarian tumors, as well as 80% of secondary colorectal carcinomas.[18] Basically, murine MAb B72.3 is an IgG which reacts with a 220–440 K glycoprotein complex.[5] B72.3 is then conjugated to ^{125}I, which has a half-life of about 60 days. The radiolabelled monoclonal antibody is administered to the patient intravenously anywhere from 5 to 42 days before surgery (average 15.5 days).[18] To avoid thyroid uptake of the free ^{125}I, patients are given a supersaturated solution of potassium iodide before they receive the B72.3 conjugate. During surgery, the surgeon manipulates the gamma-detecting device, consisting of a detection crystal, a preamplifier, and a signal processor with a digital readout. He responds to the audible and numerical displays, as the instrument encounters radiolabelled tumor cells. The device enables the surgeon to define tumor margins and identify subclinical disease intraoperatively, and the entire abdomen can be surveyed in less than five minutes.[21] Radioimmunoguided surgery is efficacious in localizing previously undetected malignant lesions and disseminated disease intraoperatively, and is especially effective in localizing primary and secondary colorectal, gastric and ovarian carcinomas.

Surgical Oncology as a Specialty

What is a surgical oncologist?[24] A surgical oncologist is a surgeon who devotes the majority of his time to the study and treatment of malignant neoplastic disease. He/she must possess the necessary knowledge, skills and clinical experience to perform the standard surgical procedures required by patients with cancer. The surgical oncologist must be able to diagnose all tumors accurately and to discern between aggressive neoplastic lesions and benign reactive processes. In addition, the surgical oncologist should have a firm understanding of radiation oncology, medical oncology, and hematology. He/she must also be capable of organizing interdisciplinary studies of cancer. The surgical oncologist should also be trained in pathology, since he/she will be called upon to decide surgical margins and to excise adequate tumor samples for the pathologist.

Unfortunately, the Accreditation Council for Graduate Medical Education has not yet granted subspecialty status to surgical oncology. This inaction has retarded growth in this field and, consequently, delayed progress in the treatment of solid neoplasms by surgical therapy. There is a great need for a larger number of trained surgical oncologists who will commit to comprehensive cancer research centers and will work together with other oncologists in multidisciplinary studies of combined modality treatment programs. In order to realize the full potential of surgery oncology, we need more trained surgical oncologists and the ACGME's recognition of its subspecialty status.

References

1. Antman, K. A., Eilber, F. R., and Shiu, M. H.: Soft tissue sarcomas: Current trends in diagnosis and management. Current Problems in Cancer, 13:339, 1989.
2. Beahrs, O. H., and Myers, M. H.: Manual for Staging of Cancer, 2nd Ed. Published for the American Joint Committee on Cancer. Philadelphia, Lippincott, 1983.
3. Breasted, J. H.: The Edwin Smith Surgical Papyrus. Chicago, University of Chicago Press, 1930.
4. Chretian, P. B., Catalona, W. G., Twomey, P. L., and Sample, W. F.: Correlation of immune reactivity and clinical status in cancer. Ann. Clin. Lab. Sci., 4:331, 1974.
5. Colchor, D., Zalutsky, M., Kaplan, W., Kufe, D., Austin, F., and Schlom, J.: Radiolocalization of human mammary tumors in athymic mice by a monoclonal antibody. Cancer Res., 43:736, 1983.
6. Cole, W. H., McDonald, G. O., Roberts, S. S., and Southwick, H. W.: Dissemination of Cancer. Prevention and Therapy. New York, Appleton-Century-Crofts, Inc., 1961.
7. Collins, V. P., Loeffler, R. K., and Tivey, H.: Observations on growth rates of human tumors. Amer. J. Roentgenol., 76:988, 1956.
8. Eilber, F. R., Nizze, A., and Morton, D. L.: Sequential evaluation of general immune competence in cancer patients: Correlation with clinical course. Cancer, 35:660, 1975.
9. Golub, S. H.: Host Immune Response to Human Tumor Antigens. New York, Plenum Press, 1976.
10. Gupta, R. K., and Morton, D. L.: Suggestive evidence for in vivo binding of specific antitumor antibodies of human melanomas. Cancer Res., 35:58, 1975.
11. Hayward, O. S.: The history of oncology. I. Early oncology and the literature of discovery. Surgery, 58:460, 1965.
12. Hellstrom, K. E., and Hellstrom, I.: Lymphocyte mediated cytotoxicity to tumor antigens. Adv. Immunol., 18:209, 1974.
13. Hill, G. J., 2nd: Historic milestones in cancer surgery. Sem. Oncol., 6:409, 1979.
14. Holmes, E. C., and Golub, S. H.: Immunologic defects in lung cancer patients. J. Thorac. Cardiovasc. Surg., 71:161, 1976.
15. Holmes, E. C., Roth, J. A., and Morton, D. L.: Delayed cutaneous hypersensitivity reactions to melanoma antigen. Surgery, 78:160, 1975.
16. Huth, J. F., Holmes, E. C., Vernon, S. E., Callery, C. D., Ramming, K. P., and Morton, D. L.: Pulmonary resection for metastatic sarcoma. Am. J. Surg., 140:90, 1980.
17. Joseph, W. J., Morton, D. L., and Adkins, P. C.: Prognostic significance of tumor doubling time in evaluating operability in pulmonary metastatic disease. J. Thorac. Cardiovasc. Surg., 61:23, 1971.
18. Martin, E. W., Jr., Mojzisik, C. M., Hinckle, G. H., Sampsel, J., Siddigi, M. A., Tuttle, S. E., Sidele-Santanello, B., Colchen, D., Thurston, M. O., Bell, J. G., Ferrara, W. B., and Schlom, J.: Radioimmunoguided surgery using monoclonal antibody. Am. J. Surg., 156:396, 1988.
19. Morton, D. L., Holmes, E. C., Eilber, F. R., and Wood, W. C.: Immunological aspects of neoplasia: A rational basis for immunotherapy. Ann. Intern. Med., 74:587, 1971.

19A.Morton, D. L., Holmes, E. C., Golub, S. H.: Immunologic aspects of lung cancer. Chest, 71:640, 1977.
20. Morton, D. L., Joseph, W. L., Ketcham, A. S., Geelhoed, G. W., and Adkins, P. C.: Surgical resection and adjunctive immmunotherapy for selected patients with multiple pulmonary metastases. Ann. Surg., 178:360, 1973.
21. Nieroda, C. A., Mojzsik, C., Sardi, A., Ferrara, P., Hinckle, G. R., Thurston, M. D., and Martin, E. W., Jr.: The impact of radioimmunoguided surgery (RIGS) on surgical decision making in colorectal cancer. Dis. Col. Rect., 32:927, 1989.
22. Roberts, S. S., Hengesh, J. W., McGrath, R. G., Valaitis, J., McGrew, E. A., and Cole, W. H.: Prognostic significance of cancer cells in circulating blood: A ten-year evaluation. Am. J. Surg., 113:757, 1967.
23. Schlom, J.: Radiolocalization of human mammary tumors in athymic mice by monoclonal antibody. Cancer Res., 43:736, 1983.
24. Schweitzer, R. J., Edwards, M. H., Lawrence, W., Jr., Mozden, P. J., Scanlon, E. F., and Leffal, L. D., Jr.: Training guidelines for surgical oncology. Cancer, 48:2336, 1981.
25. Southam, C. M., Brunschwig, W., Levin, A. G., and Dixon, Q. S.: The effect of leukocytes on transplantability of human cancer. Cancer, 19:1743, 1966.
26. Turnbull, R. B., Jr.: The no-touch isolation techniques of resection. JAMA, 231:1181, 1975.

Acknowledgments

I gratefully acknowledge the editorial assistance of Thomas Muzzonigro and Dr. Amy Walsh.

XIII

Principles of Radiation Oncology

XIII-1

Biological and Physical Basis to Radiation Oncology

Ralph R. Weichselbaum
Dennis E. Hallahan
George T.Y. Chen

Introduction

X-ray production by a cathode ray tube was first described in 1895 by Roentgen, and the production of gamma rays by radium was discovered in 1896 by the Curies. Curative radiotherapy for the treatment of cancer was first reported at the turn of the century. It was soon recognized that radiation not only led to tumor cures but also produced adverse effects on normal tissues. Radiobiology had its first clinical application in the 1920's when fractionation was first demonstrated in the successful treatment of laryngeal carcinoma. Supervoltage radiotherapy produced by Cobalt-60 sources and linear accelerators were introduced in the 1950's and increased the dose that could be delivered to deep tumors without excessive skin injury. Interstitial and intracavitary techniques of administering radiotherapy have been developed over the past 50 years and have resulted in the cure of tumors amenable to brachytherapy. Radiotherapy is likely to have a major impact on the future management of the systemic spread of cancer through treatment with radiolabeled monoclonal antibodies, and wide field radiotherapy and in combination with chemotherapy and biological response modifiers. In addition, technical improvements in radiotherapy will continue to provide for an increasing number of uncomplicated local cures.

Ionizing radiation produces its biological effects by imparting energy to body tissues. Radiations may be subdivided into indirectly and directly ionizing types. In either case, charged particles are ultimately set into motion through the interaction of radiation with matter, and result in the ionization and excitation of tissue atoms and molecules, causing biological damage.

Indirectly Ionizing Radiations

Photons

X-rays and gamma radiation are part of the electromagnetic spectrum which include radiowaves, infrared radiation, visible and ultraviolet light. Unlike these lower energy radiations, x- and gamma rays ionize the medium through which they travel. The distinction between x-rays and gamma radiation lies in their origin; gamma rays originate from excited or unstable nuclei while x-rays are produced by electron level transitions in an atom, or through high kinetic energy electrons which are rapidly decelerated. Photons have both wave and particle like properties. As such, x-rays are characterized with classical electromagnetic theory variables such as frequency and wavelength associated with the oscillating electric and magnetic vectors. In the quantum mechanical description, photons are considered to be packets of energy which are massless but have momentum. The energy of a photon is proportional to its frequency v:

$$E = hv$$

where h is Planck's constant. X-rays have frequencies of approximately 10^{20} cycles/sec. The energy of monochromatic photons are expressed in kiloelectron volts (keV) and million electron volts (MeV). Since therapeutic beams most commonly consist of a distribution or spectra of different energy photons, the highest energy photons are expressed in kVp (kilovolts peak) or MV (megavolts). In typical spectra, the average photon energy is approximately one third of the maximum. Radiations used in therapy span the energies from 50 kVp, (which penetrate superficially) to 25 MV or greater (for deep therapy). In this range, the relevant interactions of photons with matter[73,78] include the photoelectric effect, the Compton effect, and pair production. As a result of these interactions, electrons are set into motion, causing additional ionization and excitation of other atoms in the medium.

In the photoelectric effect, an incident photon is completely absorbed by an inner shell electron with the subsequent emission of a photoelectron. The kinetic energy of the ejected electron is equal to the incident photon energy less the electron binding energy. The probability of photoelectric interactions is proportional to Z^3/E^3, where Z is the atomic number of the material and E the photon energy. At low energies, differential absorption of radiation by high atomic number biological tissues such as bone, can be several times that of adjacent low Z soft tissues. At megavoltage energies, the probability of interaction through the photoelectric effect is small. A schematic representation of the photoelectric effect is shown in Figure XIII-1-1A.

The Compton effect is the dominant interaction in tissue for photons used in modern radiotherapy beams. In this interaction, the photon behaves like a particle, as it "collides" with an outer loosely bound orbital electron, scattering the incident photon and imparting kinetic energy to the electron. The angle of scatter and the energy of the scattered photon

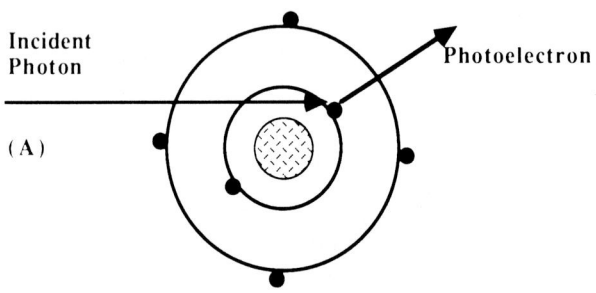

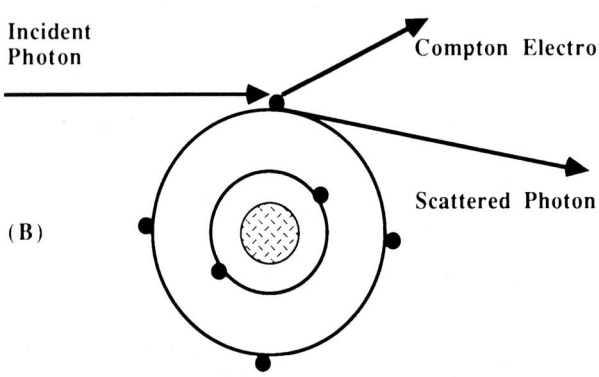

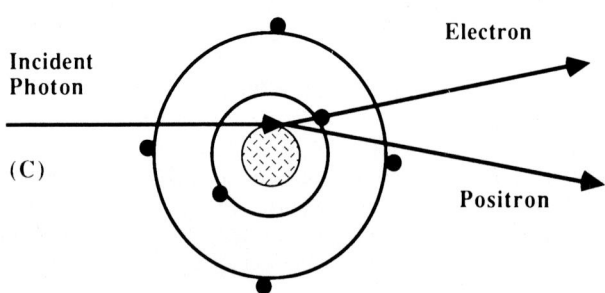

Figure XIII-1-1. Schematic representations of photon interactions with matter: A) photoelectric effect B) Compton effect and C) pair production.

are determined by the kinematics of an elastic collision, where both momentum and energy are conserved. Because the Compton electrons are energetic and are predominantly scattered in the forward direction, megavoltage photon beams exhibit skin sparing. In this effect, the first few millimeters of skin absorb less energy, thereby reducing skin erythema. The probability of interaction via the Compton process is independent of the atomic number of the material and decreases approximately as 1/E. The electron density (number of electrons/gm) is the dominant physical parameter in the attenuation of photons by the Compton effect. Since the Z/A (atomic number/atomic weight) ratio of soft tissue and bone are nearly the same, the energy imparted per gram to these tissues is nearly identical. A schematic representation of the Compton effect is shown in Figure XIII-1-1B.

At photon energies greater than 1.02 MeV, photons interacting near the strong electric field of the nucleus may lead to the creation of a positron electron pair, with the subsequent disappearance of the incident photon. This process is known as pair production, and increases with increasing energy and atomic number. Approximately 15% of the interactions of a 24 MV beam in water are due to pair production. In bone, this percentage rises to approximately 20%. A schematic representation of the pair production process is shown in Figure XIII-1-1C. After losing its kinetic energy, the positron is annihilated with an electron, producing two photons travelling in opposite directions.

As a photon beam passes through tissue, its intensity diminishes as a result of the interactions described above. A photon beam is attenuated according to an exponential attenuation law:

$$I(x) = I_oe^{-\mu x}$$

where I_o is the initial intensity of the photon beam, $I(x)$ the intensity after traversing a depth x, and μ is the linear attenuation coefficient. High energy beams are attenuated less than low energy beams, and thus are the choice for irradiation of deep seated tumors. The radiation intensity per unit area from a point source also diminishes as the inverse square of the distance from the source. This dependence is known as the inverse square law.

Free electrons formed by incident photons track through the cell nucleus producing clusters of ionizations by low energy secondary electrons. DNA damage is induced by ionizing radiation through direct and indirect interaction with these electrons. Direct damage occurs when the charged particle ionizes DNA without a free radical intermediate, whereas indirect damage occurs when water molecules are ionized, forming hydroxyl radicals which then ionize DNA. Ionization occurs primarily in cellular water which subsequently damages DNA.

Radiation Absorbed Dose

Approaches to the quantification of radiation for therapeutic purposes have evolved over time. Historically, in the early 20th century, units of skin erythema and the Roentgen, a measure of ionization produced in air, were used to quantify radiation. Today, the energy absorbed per unit mass, or dose, is used to relate a physically measurable quantity with biologic effect. In SI units, the unit of absorbed dose is the

Gray (Gy), which is defined as the absorption of 1 joule per kilogram. One gray is equivalent to 100 centigray (cGy) or 100 rads. Dose is plotted as a function of depth in water, and depth dose curves for different megavoltage energy beams are shown in Figure XIII-1-2.

Sources of Therapeutic Photon Beams

Therapeutic high energy photon beams (4 MV–25 MV) are produced by linear accelerators (Figure XIII-1-3). In these devices, electrons are accelerated to megavoltage energies by microwave power and the resulting electron beam is focused onto a high atomic number target, producing a forward peaked high energy photon beam. The photon beam is flattened to provide a large uniform radiation field (approximately 40 cm × 40 cm), which is then collimated by tungsten jaws to the desired rectangular field size. The gantry may be rotated about its axis to direct radiation to the target from the chosen angle. The patient is immobilized in a recumbent position, and is aligned to the radiation beam through optical positioning lasers. High dose rate beams are available, and typically, a treatment of 200 cGy is delivered to the tumor within a few minutes. Including setup and irradiation, a treatment session of average complexity requires approximately 20 minutes.

Cobalt-60 may also be used to provide megavoltage therapeutic beams (1.25 MeV). Cobalt-60 is artificially produced by irradiating cobalt-59 with neutrons from a nuclear reactor. The treatment head contains pellets of cobalt-60 packed in a stainless steel source housing. A shutter system controlled by a timer is used to determine radiation output. Cobalt units provide a dose rate of approximately 100 cGy/minute. Since the laws of radioactive decay govern the radiation output of a cobalt treatment unit, such units are considered more stable than complex linear accelerators. Because the source size is on the order of several cm in diameter, the beam scatter near the edge (penumbra) is large in comparison to the sharp penumbra of a linear accelerator beam. The pen-

etration of cobalt 60 beams is slightly less than that of a 4 MV linear accelerator beam.

Neutrons

A number of centers throughout the world are investigating the use of neutron beams for radiation therapy.[23] Therapeutic neutron beams are usually generated by bombarding a beryllium target with a cyclotron accelerated proton beam. Like photons, neutrons are indirectly ionizing radiation and are exponentially attenuated. Interactions of neutron beams with tissue include neutron proton collisions, and neutron–nuclei reactions, both of which set heavy charged particles in motion, as shown schematically in Figure XIII-1-4. The density of energy deposition along a charged particle track is quantified as its linear energy transfer or LET, and may be expressed in KeV/μ. In contrast to the electrons set into motion by photons, the heavy charged particles set into motion by neutrons ionize densely along their tracks, making neutrons a high LET radiation. High LET beams cause direct DNA damage, and exhibit a relative biological effectiveness (RBE) which is greater than that of low LET radiations such as photons or electrons.[61] The total dose for neutron beam therapy, therefore, is less than that required for x-irradiation for the same biological endpoint. Because neutrons interact primarily with hydrogen nuclei, resulting in proton ejection as opposed to electron ejection, a higher RBE is observed for tissues with a high hydrogen component such as the central nervous system and a lower RBE for tissues with few hydrogen nuclei such as bone. The concept of RBE is discussed more fully in the section on radiobiology.

Directly Ionizing Radiations

Charged particle beams, or charged particle radiations emitted from radioactive nuclei may be used for therapeutic applications. Unlike an exponentially attenuated photon beam, the depth of charged particle penetration can be controlled, and tissues beyond the chosen depth are not irradiated, thereby sparing distal normal tissues. The most common directly ionizing therapeutic beam is that of accelerated electrons and representative depth dose curves for electron beams are shown in Figure XIII-1-5. As shown after an initial buildup of dose, peaking at 3.0 cm depth, a 15 MeV electron beam dose falls to near zero after 6 cm (80% to 5% in 2 cm).

Proton and other heavy charged particle beams exhibit a Bragg peak, which is an increased dose near the end of particle range (Figure XIII-1-6). When a heavy charged particle Bragg peak is modified to encompass the tumor in depth, a high dose may be delivered to the target with reduced dose to the proximal tissues, and little dose to distal tissues. Charged particle beam penetration is much more sensitive to the presence of inhomogeneities (e.g., bone or air cavities) than photon beams, resulting in a technically more difficult treatment execution.[149] Energies of approximately 250 MeV are needed to generate proton beams of sufficient energy to reach deep tumors (25 cm range). Proton synchrotrons or cyclotrons are used to accelerate protons to these energy levels.[135] Currently, there are two proton therapy facilities in the United States, at the Harvard Cyclotron Laboratory (therapy in conjunction with the Department of Radiation Medi-

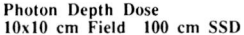

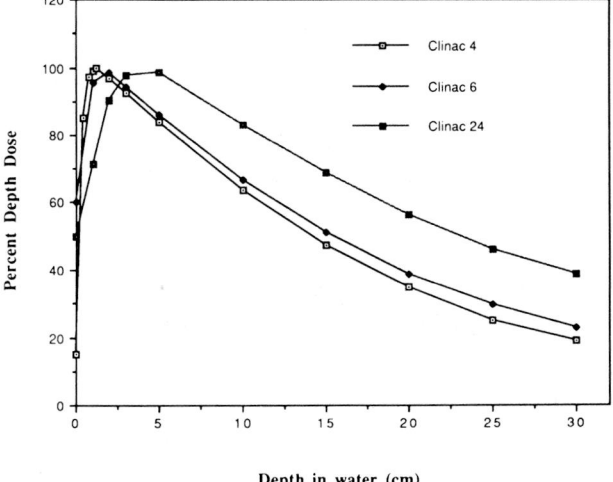

Figure XIII-1-2.   Percent depth dose curves for megavoltage photon radiation, including 4 MV, 6 MV and 24 MV beams.

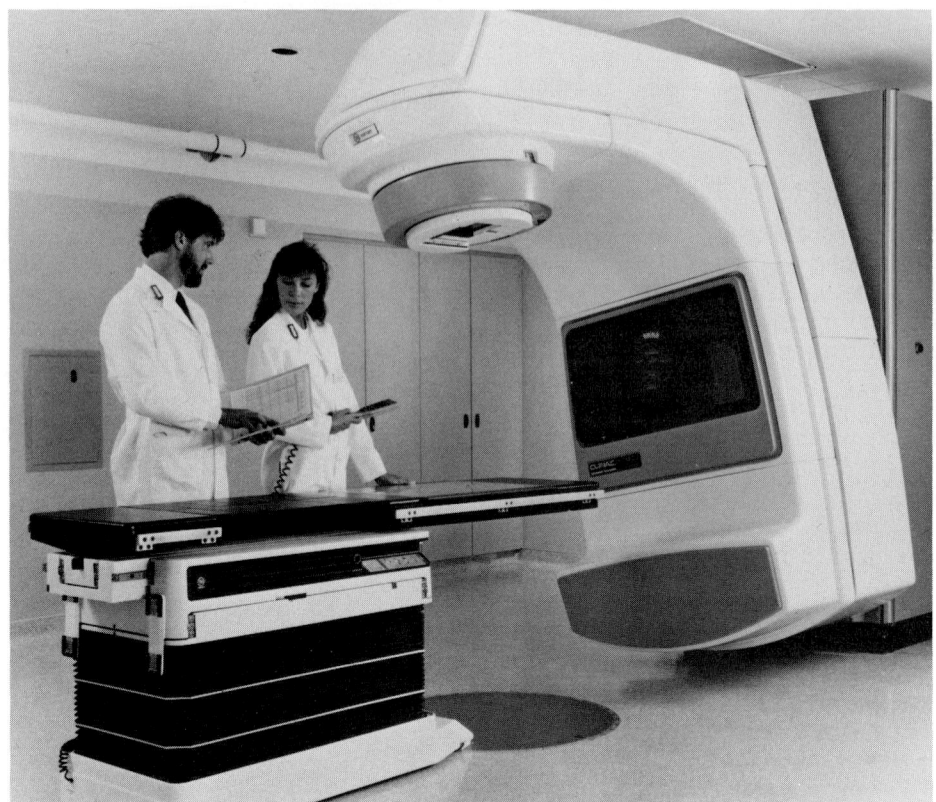

Figure XIII-1-3. A typical modern linear accelerator used in radiation therapy, which produces both photon and electron beams.

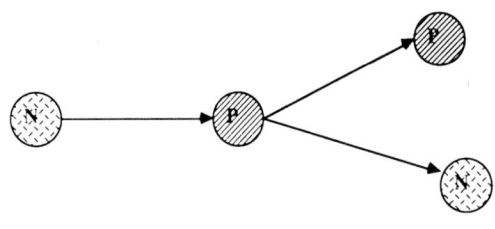

Elastic n,p scattering

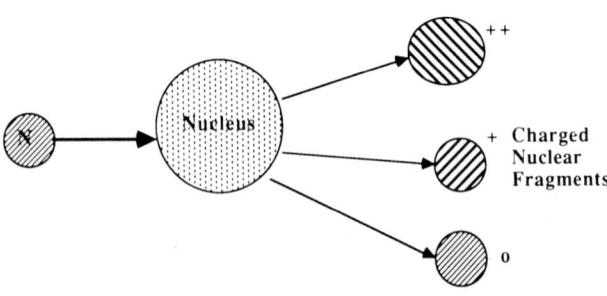

Nuclear Spallation

Figure XIII-1-4. Schematic representations of neutron interactions with matter. Heavy charged particles are set into motion, resulting in high LET energy deposition.

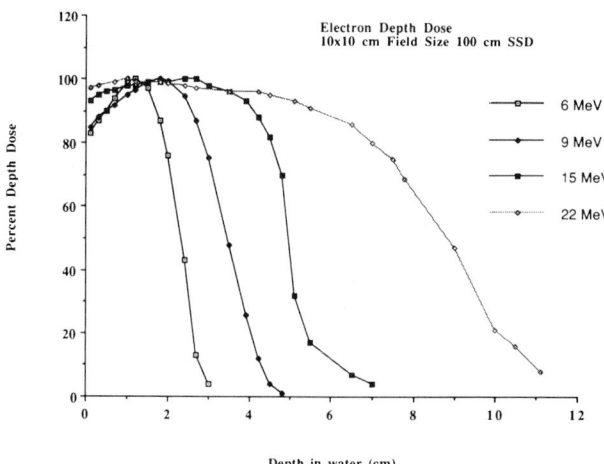

Figure XIII-1-5. Percent depth dose curves for megavoltage electron beams from a linear accelerator. Energies of electron beams range from 6 MeV to 22 MeV.

cine at Massachusetts General Hospital), and a new facility completing construction at Loma Linda Medical Center. In addition to the dose localization properties associated with the Bragg peak, beams of heavy ions (e.g., carbon or neon) also contain a high LET component. Heavy ion beams for radiation therapy clinical studies are available at the Lawrence Berkeley Laboratory, and a new accelerator for heavy ion radiotherapy is under construction at the National Institute of Radiological Sciences at Chiba, Japan.

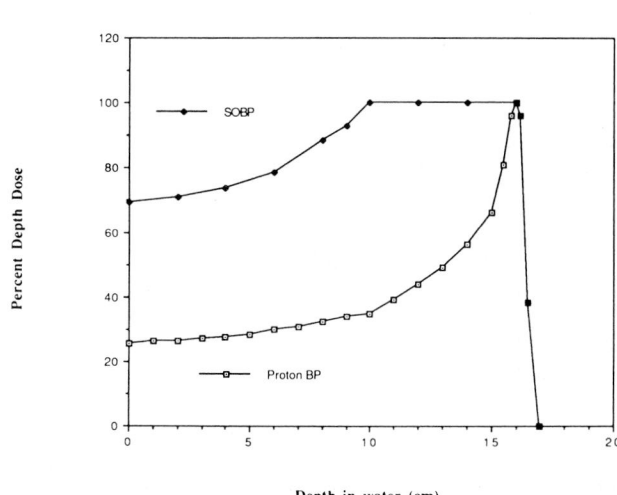

Proton Bragg Peaks

Figure XIII-1-6. Pristine proton Bragg peak (narrow peak) and a spread out Bragg peak beam (SOBP) used for radiation therapy. Maximum proton energy is 160 MeV. SOBP is generated by interposing variable absorber in the beam as a function of time.

Biological Basis of Radiotherapy

Radiation is randomly deposited within the cell, but the most critical target for cell killing is DNA. Radiation induced DNA damage includes single- or double-strand breaks in the sugar phosphate backbone of the DNA molecule and alterations or loss of nucleotide bases. Formation of cross links between DNA strands and chromosomal proteins also occur as a result of radiation exposure. Evidence implicating DNA as the principal target in radiation killing are:[61] 1) Cells are killed by radioactive tritiated thymidine incorporated into DNA. The range of the beta particles is very short and therefore localized in DNA; 2) Halogenated pyrimidines are selectively incorporated into DNA in place of thymine when substituted in cell culture medium; this incorporation greatly increases the radiosensitivity of cells.[79] Substituted deoxyuridines are not incorporated into DNA and do not affect radiosensitivity; and 3) There is a direct relationship between viral size and radiosensitivity which correlates with nucleic acid volume. The radiosensitivity of plants has been correlated with mean interphase volume which is defined as the ratio of nuclear volume to chromosome number.[61] The larger the mean chromosome number the greater the radiosensitivity. Taken together these data infer that DNA damage is the primary lethal event from radiotherapy.

The radiobiological definition of death is loss of reproductive integrity. Inhibition of the reproductive ability of cells is important to the cancer therapist because the aim of therapeutic radiation is sterilization of malignant tissue. Also, the major long-term effects of radiation on normal tissue result from killing of tissue stem cells and/or vascular endothelial cells. Most cell types do not show morphological evidence of radiation damage until they attempt to divide. Lethally irradiated cells may undergo several divisions before exhibiting metabolic death, and then disappearing from the population.[145] Exceptions are some populations of unstimulated lymphocytes and spermatogonia which undergo interphase

death at low doses. The concept that cell death may not be expressed for several cell divisions following radiation has clinical relevance in that very slowly proliferating tumors may persist for months and appear histologically viable. The histological appearance of malignancy may clear only after tumor cells have had an opportunity to divide. An example of a slowly proliferating tumor which may require up to 24 months after irradiation for accurate histological prediction of local control is prostate carcinoma.[30]

Radiation Survival Analysis

Puck and Marcus performed the first clonogenic in vitro radiation survival curves for HeLa cells in 1955.[115] Exponentially growing cells are irradiated, immediately trypsinized and a specific cell number is plated onto a dish. After 2–3 weeks, colonies are stained and those with greater than 50 cells are counted as representative of cells that are capable of infinite division (in the case of tumor cells). The surviving fraction is calculated by dividing the number of colonies by the plating efficiency of unirradiated cells. Radiation survival analysis is frequently represented by a graphic representation of the log of surviving fraction versus a linear plot of dose (Figure XIII-1-7). Resulting radiation survival curves are characterized by an initial shoulder followed by exponential killing at higher doses.

Radiation survival analysis can be studied both in vitro and in vivo. In vivo models examine both the inherent radiosensitivity of tumor cells and environmental influences such as hypoxia and host immunity. A commonly used model to

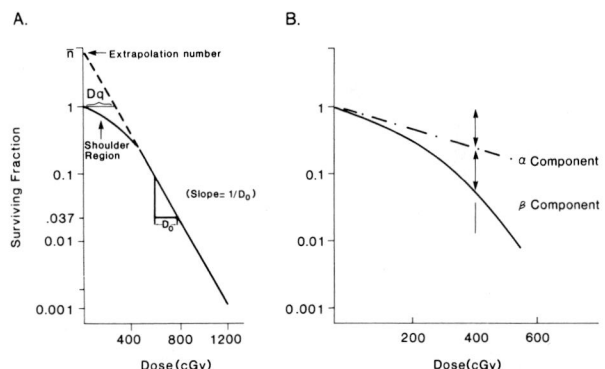

Figure XIII-1-7. Models for survival curve analysis. Experimental data are typically shown as the fraction of cells surviving a dose of radiation plotted on a logarithmic scale while the dosage of radiation is plotted on a linear scale. **A:** When using the multi-target model, the shoulder region is quantified by extrapolation of the exponential portion of the curve to the y-axis intercept. This point is referred to as n (extrapolation number) while a horizontal line drawn from 100% survival to the extrapolation line is referred to as D_q (or quasi-threshold dose). The slope of the terminal portion of the survival curve is quantified by the term, D_0, which is the inverse of the slope and designated as the radiosensitivity of the cells or tissue under study. **B:** When using the linear-quadratic models for survival analysis, there are two components for cell killing. The alpha component represents the initial slope while the beta component represents the terminal slope of the survival curve. The alpha component is proportional to the dose while the beta component is proportional to the square of the dose. The dose at which the alpha and beta components are equal is referred to as the alpha/beta ratio which, for example, is 400 cGy in **B**.

study radiation effects is the growth delay assay which measures the time interval required for a tumor exposed to radiation to regrow to a specified volume (Figure XIII-1-8).[6] An assay which analyzes the dose required to control 50% of tumors is the TCD 50 assay and has been widely employed to study tumors in a variety of experimental systems.[137] The radiobiological use of transplantable solid tumor systems in experimental animals is reviewed by Hall.[61] Radiation survival parameters can be assayed for normal tissues in vivo as well as for tumors. For acutely responding tissues, in vivo survival is measured by studying clones of normal tissues regrowing in situ (e.g., skin, or jejunal crypt cells) or cells transplanted to another site (bone marrow stem cells). To study radiation effects in late responding tissues, such as the nervous system, functional assays such as paralysis and death may be employed.

Models of Radiation Survival Curve Analysis

Radiation survival curves usually graph the dose of radiation on a linear scale and surviving fraction on a logarithmic scale as shown in Figure XIII-1-7. Two mathematical models are commonly employed to analyze radiation survival data. One analysis of radiation survival data is carried out by a two component or multitarget model. A two component survival curve derived from mammalian cells is characterized by an initial shoulder region followed by a terminal exponential region. The reciprocal of the slope is defined by a D_0 value (slope = $1/D_0$). The D_0 is referred to as the radiosensitivity of the cell population or tissue under investigation. The fraction of cells surviving the average of one lethal event per cell is defined by Poisson distribution to be $1/e$ or 37%. The D_0 is the dose required to reduce the surviving fraction to 37% in the exponential portion of the survival curve. The width of the shoulder region is represented by the quantity D_q. D_q is the quasi-threshold dose or the point at which killing becomes exponential. The term radiosensi-

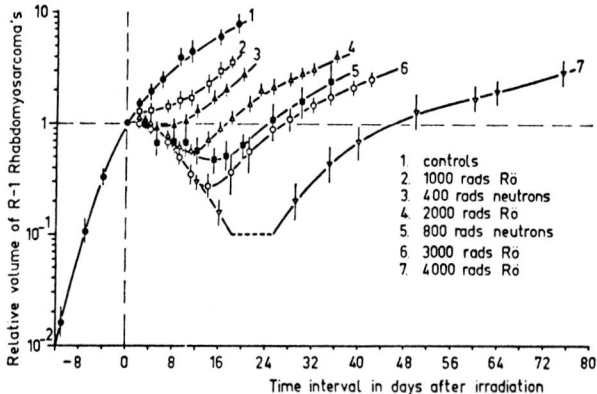

Figure XIII-1-8. The data points represent volume changes observed in tumors in animal models after irradiation. After an initial decrease in the volume size, tumors grow back to the original volume over a time interval referred to as the growth delay. Curve 1 is the growth of an unirradiated control tumor. Curves 2, 4, 6, and 7 represent the growth of tumors irradiated with 1,000, 2,000, 3,000, and 4,000 cGy of photons. Curves 3 and 5 represent the growth of tumors irradiated with 400 and 800 cGy of 15 MeV neutrons. Growth delay is prolonged with increasing dosage and more densely ionizing radiation such as neutrons. (From Barendsen et al.[6])

tive is frequently confused with radiocurability and radioresponsiveness. Radiocurability is defined as local control in a clinical (or laboratory) setting and implies that the therapeutic ratio is such that curative doses can be applied in a high percentage of cases. Radioresponsiveness refers to how rapidly a tumor disappears after initiation of radiotherapy and is a function of a variety of kinetic parameters such as the growth fraction as well as the radiobiological characteristics of the tumor cells. Small cell carcinoma of the lung is an example of a radioresponsive tumor that requires relatively high doses to be locally controlled. As mentioned previously, prostate carcinoma may regress slowly but is radiocurable in early stages. Therefore, radioresponsive tumors are not necessarily radiocurable and radiocurable tumors are not necessarily radioresponsive.[38,61,73]

The linear quadratic model (surviving fraction = $e^{\alpha D - \beta D^2}$) is used to fit radiation survival data to a continuously bending curve where D is dose and α/β are constants. The linear component, a measure of the initial slope, (termed alpha) represents single hit killing kinetics and dominates the radiation response at low doses. The quadratic component of cell killing (termed beta) represents multiple hit killing kinetics and causes the curve to bend at higher doses. The ratio alpha/beta is the dose at which the linear and quadratic components of cell killing are equal (Figure XIII-1-7). The more linear the response to killing of cells at low radiation dose the higher the value of alpha and the greater the radiosensitivity of cells (Figure XIII-1-7).[61,168] Neither the linear quadratic nor two component model has a firmly established biological basis. Therefore, they should be viewed only as convenient models for describing a survival curve mathematically. The concept of the mean inactivation dose (D) is an additional measure of intrinsic radiation sensitivity. The calculation of D involves a linear quadratic analysis of survival graphed on linear coordinates. The mean inactivation dose is equal to the area under the curve and is disproportionally influenced by surviving fractions obtained at 100–300 cGy.[38,43,146] Other authors suggest that the surviving fraction at 200 cGy is an important parameter when describing the radiobiological characteristics of human tumor cells because 200 cGy is a common daily dose used in radiotherapy.

The biological effectiveness of different types of radiation can be characterized by a parameter known as the relative biological effectiveness (RBE). RBE is defined as the ratio of a dose of a standard type of radiation to that of a test dose of a different type of radiation which gives the same biological effect (Figure XIII-1-9). High LET beams such as neutrons, cause direct DNA damage, and exhibit a relative biological effect (RBE) which is greater than that of low LET radiations such as photons or electrons. The total dose for neutrons to produce a biological effect, therefore, is less than that required for x-irradiation.[61,73]

Radiation Survival Parameters of Human Tumor Cells

A limitation of the study of in vitro radiobiological parameters of human tumor cells is that cells that grow in tissue culture might not be representative of the characteristics of clonogenic cells which comprise the host tumor. In addition, in vitro analysis may ignore physiological conditions within

Relative Biological Effect

Figure XIII-1-9. Survival curves from mammalian cells exposed to x-rays, neutrons, or alpha particles vary in the shoulder region and terminal slope. The relative biological effect (RBE) is a ratio of survival at a specific dose for different types of radiation.

the tumor such as hypoxia and cell cycle distribution. Nonetheless, the characterization of human tumor cells phenotypically resistant to chemotherapeutic agents in vitro has led to an increase in the understanding of the cellular and molecular biology of chemoresistance. Therefore, investigation of human tissue cell lines of differing radiosensitivity is useful to understand the basis of the cellular radiation response as one major determinant of clinical radiocurability.

Human tumor cell lines derived from various histologic tumor types have varying degrees of radiosensitivity.[50,77,100,155,157] Cellular radiosensitivity varies between and among tumor types. Most in vitro radiobiological data have been determined from cell lines passaged many times. To assess the in vitro radiobiological parameters of early passage human tumor cells derived from patients' tumors prior to radiotherapy, Weichselbaum and colleagues analyzed radiation survival data from 20 early passage epithelial tumor cell lines established from head and neck carcinoma patients and 13 early passage mesenchymal tumor lines established from patients with soft tissue sarcomas.[158,166] Both groups of patients were treated with curative intent radiotherapy and subsequently followed. Tumor cells cultured from head and neck cancer patients exhibited a relatively wide range of radiosensitivities with D_0's ranging from 100–330 cGy. Some patients whose tumors contained radioresistant tumor cells either had a rapid recurrence of their tumors and/or never had resolution of their disease with the exception of patients who underwent surgical resection of their tumors. Cell lines derived from patients with soft tissue sarcomas were more radiosensitive, and exhibited less heterogeneity of radiosensitivity than tumor cell lines derived from patients with head and neck carcinoma. This radiobiological characterization was true regardless of the method of radiobiological analysis. More infield recurrences occurred in head and neck cancer patients than in sarcoma patients. A larger number of patients with longer follow-up time is necessary to draw

conclusions about the predictive value of individual radiobiological parameters to local control following radiotherapy. However, the above data suggest that the inherent radiosensitivity/resistance of human tumor cells contributes to radiotherapy success or failure. This concept is supported by the fact that tumor cells cultured from patients' tumors who failed radiotherapy are more radioresistant as a group than normal fibroblasts (Figure XIII-1-10).[156,163,164] Thus, either radioresistant tumor cells are present at the beginning of therapy and radiosensitive cells are selected against during fractionated treatment, or genes are activated, amplified or mutated which render tumor cells radioresistant during fractionated treatment (Figure XIII-1-11).

Repair of Radiation Damage

Sublethal Damage Repair

When a population of cells is exposed to ionizing radiation, some cells may not receive damage in a site critical for cell division. Others may have accumulated enough damage in critical sites to be lethal and will die during subsequent mito-

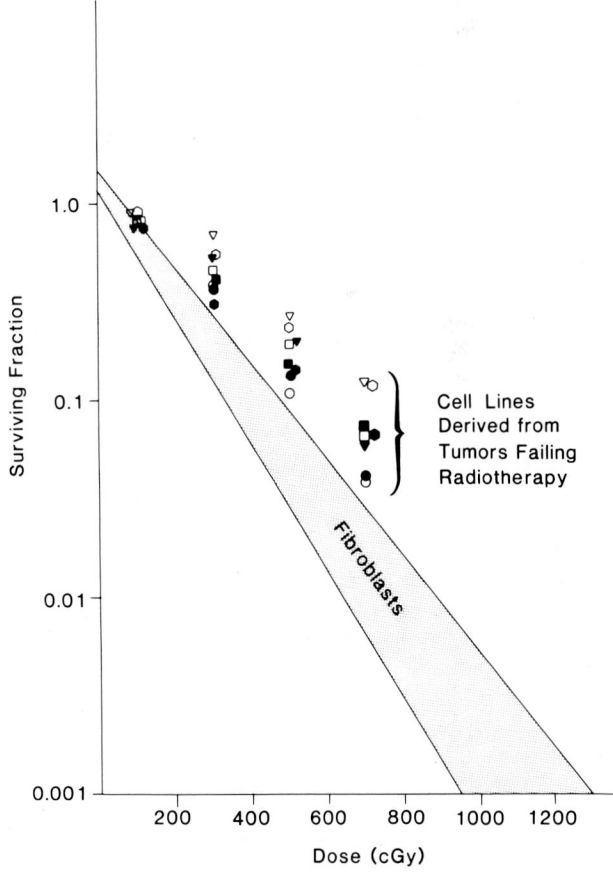

Figure XIII-1-10. The surviving fraction of cell lines derived from tumors that failed radiotherapy are plotted and compared to the range of survival for normal fibroblasts. Each symbol represents a different radioresistant cell line. The data indicate that cells derived from tumors following radiotherapy have survivals which are greater than that for normal fibroblasts. (Adapted from Weichselbaum et al.[163])

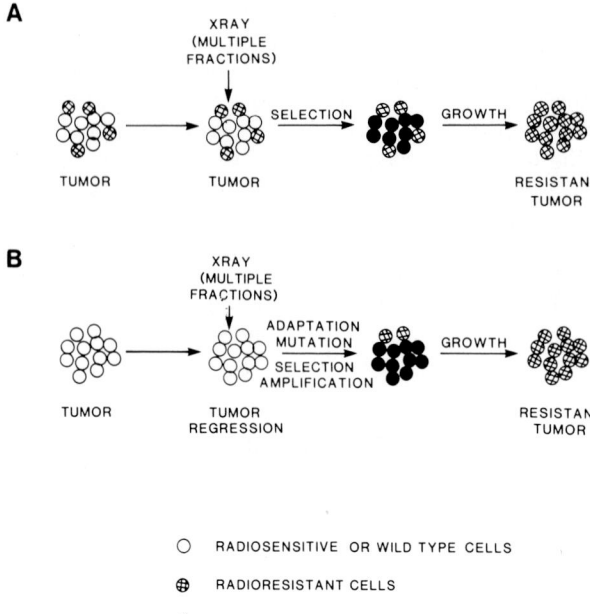

○   RADIOSENSITIVE OR WILD TYPE CELLS

⊕   RADIORESISTANT CELLS

●   KILLED CELLS

Figure XIII-1-11. Theoretical mechanisms of acquired radioresistance in tumors. In model A, radioresistant cells are present in a tumor cell population exposed to radiation. After multiple fractions of radiation, radioresistant cells are selected while sensitive cells are killed. After the radioresistant, clonogenic cells regrow, a resistant tumor population is present. In example B, radioresistant cells are not present prior to irradiation. Adaptation, mutation, and gene amplification may occur during multiple fractions of irradiation resulting in radioresistant cells. These cells regrow resulting in a resistant tumor population.

sis. An initial shoulder on a radiation survival curve suggests that sublethal damage must be accumulated prior to cell death. If additional radiation damage is accumulated before the first sublethal lesion is repaired, the two may interact resulting in cell death. Sublethal damage repair (SLDR) may be operationally defined as the enhancement in survival when a dose of radiation is separated over a period of time. SLDR may be represented by the extrapolation number (n) of the radiation survival curve when multitarget survival analysis is employed.[34,35,36,37,38]

Sublethal damage has been studied in vitro and in vivo. In general, SLDR experiments divide a single dose into two relatively equal doses spaced at variable time intervals. Elkind and colleagues investigated this phenomenon in great detail.[35–39] Figure XIII-1-12 shows the results representative of split dose experiments. An enhancement in survival following two doses separated in time is observed in exponentially growing Chinese hamster cells at 2 hours. This enhancement in survival is due to the rapid repair of SLD and is followed by a subsequent decline in survival at 5 hours and then another increase in survival at t = 8 hours. This variability in survival is due to synchronization of the exponentially growing cell populations by the first radiation dose and subsequent treatment with a second dose during the radioresistant S-phase (t = 2 hrs.) or radiosensitive G_2-M phase of the cell cycle (t = 6 hrs)[6,34,36,37,38] The concept of repair of SLD is important during a course of fractionated radiotherapy, because the shoulder region of the survival

curve is recapitulated due to SLDR (Figure XIII-1-12).[35] Fractionation magnifies the surviving fraction after each treatment to an exponent equal to the number of treatments (Table XIII-1-1). Therefore small differences in survival after each dose may have a great impact on treatment outcome. Most human tumor cell lines studied in vitro have relatively small shoulders (n = 1–3).[10,16,77,108,158,165] However, a large capacity for sublethal repair has been reported for some human tumor cell lines.[7,16]

The ability of tissues to repair sublethal damage has been demonstrated using a variety of normal tissue clonogenic or functional assays.[48,61,142] The capacity of different cell populations to repair SLD is reflected by the width of the shoulder (or initial slope) of their survival curve. An increase in the total dose required to give the same biological damage when a single dose (D_1) is split into two doses (total dose D_2) with a time interval between doses to obtain a single biological endpoint is the capacity of a normal tissue to repair SLD.

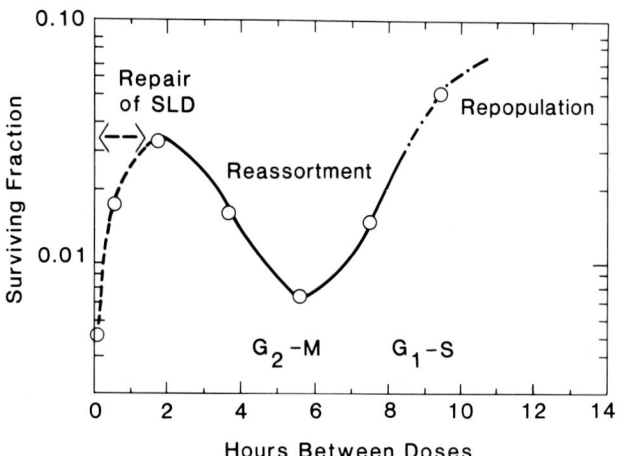

Figure XIII-1-12. The surviving fractions of Chinese hamster cells exposed to two doses of x-rays separated by various time intervals are shown. When the two doses are given together (time between doses = 0 hours), the surviving fraction is equal to that observed following the single larger dose of radiation. As the two doses are separated by time, an enhancement in survival occurs and is interpreted as the repair of sublethal damage (dashed line). Subsequent radiation doses result in a reduction in the surviving fraction. This reduction in survival occurs because of more sensitive phases of the cell cycle (G_2 and M). Later time points demonstrate increased surviving fractions due to radiation synchronization of cells and their entry into resistant phases of the cell cycle (G_1 and S). (Adapted from Elkind.[35,38])

Table XIII-1-1.   Calculated Cumulative Survival

Survival Fraction	X^{32*} X =	X^{20*} X =
10^{-11}	0.45	0.28
10^{-10}	0.49	0.32
10^{-9}	0.52	0.35
10^{-8}	0.56	0.40
10^{-7}	0.60	0.45
10^{-6}	0.65	0.50
10^{-5}	0.70	0.56

*Calculated cumulative survival fraction for either 32 or 20 equal fractions when the fractional survival is varied.
From Hellman[65A] with permission.

The difference in the two doses, $D_2 - D_1$, is a measure of SLDR by the tissue provided that the two doses are larger than those which generate the shoulder region of the survival curve[61,168,169] (see Figure XIII-1-13). $D_2 - D_1 = D_0$. If the D_0, is known then n can be calculated from the equation $\log_e n = D_q/D_0$.

A clinical example of exploiting the difference in the ability of various rapidly proliferating normal tissues to repair SLD is demonstrated by the application of fractionated TBI for bone marrow ablation delivered 2–3 times/day (separated by 4–6 hours, total dose 1,200–1,320 cGy) in preparation for bone marrow transplantation. The small bowel (n = 40) has a large shoulder compared to the bone marrow which has a small shoulder (n = 1).[48] Thus hematopoietic compartment is ablated while the gut is spared due to differences in the repair of SLD. Similar results are obtained at low dose rates.

Dose Rate Effect

Normal tissues tolerate relatively high doses of radiation (3,000–6,000 cGy) given over 2–7 days during brachytherapy with interstitial or intracavitary ^{137}Cs or ^{226}Ra. The dose rate is usually prescribed 40–50 cGy/hour at 0.5 cm from the sources. Conversely, ionizing radiation delivered at a higher dose rate (greater than 100 cGy/minute), as with external irradiation, must be fractionated over 5–7 weeks to be tolerated by normal tissues. Figure XIII-1-14 demonstrates that the D_0 is reduced by more than 2 and the shoul-

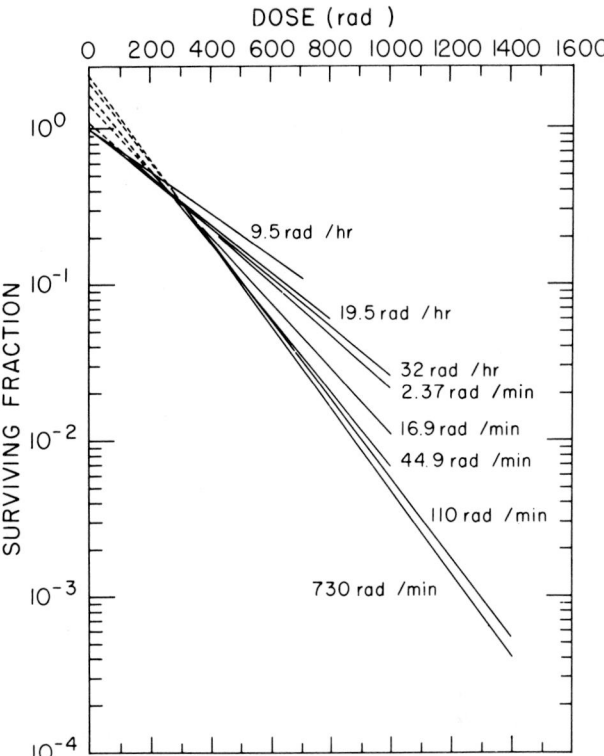

Figure XIII-1-14. The dose rate effect in HeLa cells. The slope of the survival curve steepens as the dose rate increases. The survival curves for HeLa cells exposed to x-rays given at various dose rates are shown. (From Hall.[60])

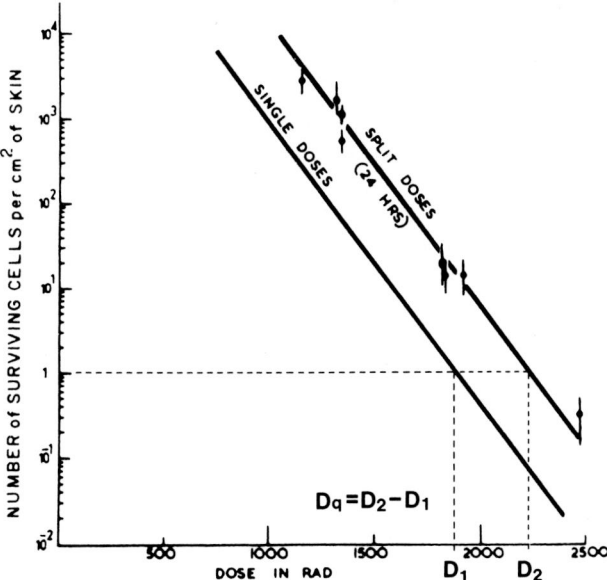

Figure XIII-1-13. Single-dose and two-doses survival curves, for epithelial cells. The D_0 is 135 Gy. The ordinate is not the surviving fraction, as in survival curves for cells cultured *in vitro*, but is the number of surviving cells per square centimeter of skin (the plating efficiency is obviously not known *in vivo*). In the two-dose survival curve the interval between dose fractions is 24 hours. Although the curves are parallel (similar D_0), their graphic horizontal separation is 350 cGy. This value corresponds to the D_q, the extrapolation number (n) may then be calculated from D_0 and D_q. (Adapted from Withers[168A] and Withers.[169A])

der on the survival curve is also decreased when dose rate is increased from 0.01 Gy to 1 Gy per minute in HeLa cells. This dose rate effect has also been demonstrated in normal tissue cell lines.[8,60]

Photon release from a radioisotope is a random event and is separated by random time intervals. Thus, reduced cell killing by low-dose-rate radiation represents sublethal damage repair and is analogous to irradiation with multiple small fractions. The shoulder region is recapitulated repeatedly with each dose delivered resulting in magnification of the shoulder region of the survival curve as demonstrated previously in Figure XIII-1-15. Constant, low dose rate radiation increases the therapeutic ratio during brachytherapy because tumor cells pass through relatively radiosensitive phases of the cell cycle. Also, surrounding tissues receive a lower dose rate than adjacent tumor cells because the dose rate falls off at a rate of the square of the distance from the isotope source. Whole-body, low dose rate radiation has been applied in bone marrow transplantation in a fashion similar to fractioned TBI to take advantage of the differentiated abilities of the gut and bone marrow to repair SLD.

Potentially Lethal Damage Repair

Varying environmental conditions can influence cell survival after a dose of x-rays. Thus, damage that is potentially lethal under a given set of conditions may not be lethal if post-irradiation conditions are altered.[111,162] The enhancement in survival seen following manipulation of post-irradi-

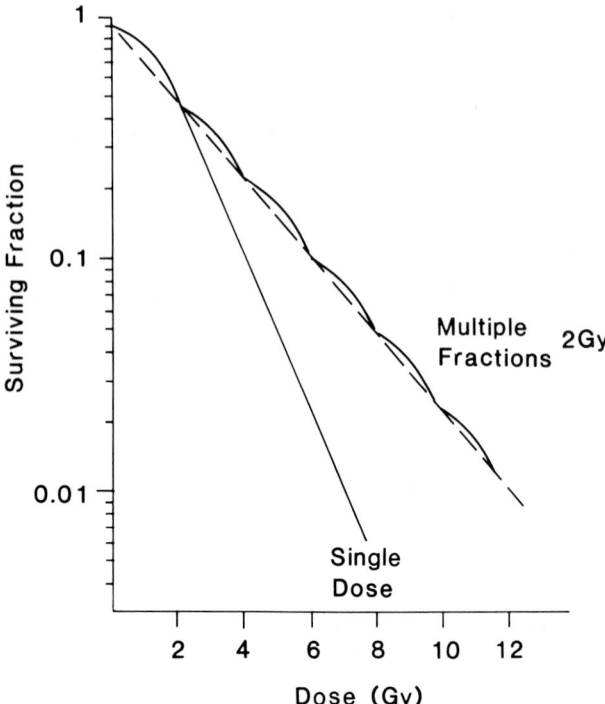

Figure XIII-1-15. Recapitulation of the shoulder on the survival curve during fractionation. When a single dose survival curve is performed, the terminal exponential region of the survival curve is reached. However, when multiple 2 Gy fractions are given, the shoulder region of the curve is reproduced following each dose due to the repair of sublethal damage. SLDR results in surviving fractions which are greater for a cumulative fractional dose compared to the same dose given in a single fraction.

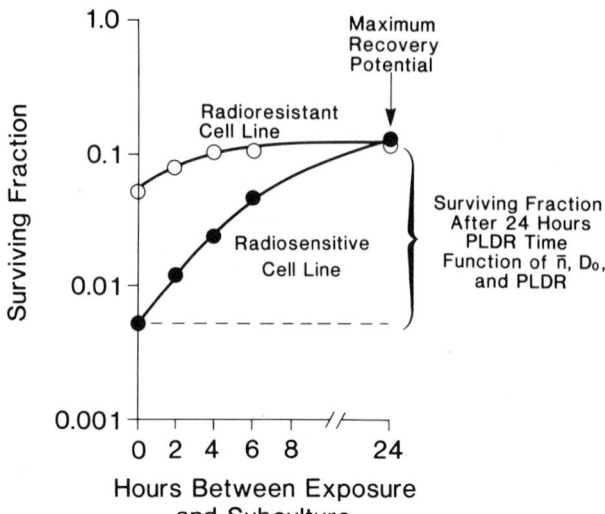

Figure XIII-1-16. The maximum recovery potential (MRP) for radioresistant and radiosensitive cells. Confluent cell lines (non-cycling) were irradiated and immediately subcultured which resulted in an initial surviving fraction (0 hr.) which is generally equal or slightly less than the surviving fraction of exponentially growing cells in tissue culture. However, when these irradiated confluent cells are not subcultured for the indicated time intervals, an enhancement in survival interpreted as STR repair of potentially lethal damage (PLDR) occurs. The surviving fraction of cells after a 24 hour delay in subculture (MRP) of confluent cells is dependent upon n, D_0, and PLDR. The initial surviving fraction of cells at 0 hr. is dependent upon n and D_0 but not PLDR.

ation conditions is referred to as the repair of potentially lethal damage (PLD). This phenomenon is analogous to liquid holding recovery observed in bacteria and yeast. Hahn and Little studied PLD repair in density-inhibited-stationary phase cultures which they considered more analogous to in vivo tumors than exponentially growing cells.[58,59] Quiescent cells were subcultured at varying time intervals after irradiation. Cells plated immediately after irradiation allow for no PLDR (Figure XIII-1-16). Delay in subculture allows quiescent cells to repair PLD resulting in a higher surviving fraction than immediate subculture. PLDR has also been shown to occur in vivo if the explant of an experimental animal tumor is delayed.[58,91,119] This effect is reported to be more pronounced in large tumors presumably because a large proportion of cells are in G_1 or G_0. PLDR has been described to occur principally in the G_1 phase of the cell cycle. Efficient PLDR occurs in a variety of human tumor cell lines in vitro.[80,115,159,164,166] Weichselbaum and colleagues,[159,160,164] and Guichard and colleagues[57] have suggested that PLDR contributes to radiotherapy failure under certain circumstances.

PLDR and/or SLDR may not be expressed under all conditions in vivo.[18] For example, cells must be genetically competent to repair these types of damages and the tumor environment may affect the proliferative status of tumor cells.[159,160,162] Also, radiation (or chemotherapy) may *induce* tumor proliferation which allows fixation of radiation damage

before PLDR or SLDR is complete.[159,162] Therefore, PLDR is likely to be most important in tumor cells of intermediate or high radiosensitivity when cells are quiescent between fractions. The 24 hr. PLDR surviving fraction following treatment of human tumor cells in plateau phase culture with a similar dose is referred to as the maximum recovery potential (MRP).[161] Figure XIII-1-16 shows that although two cell lines have different amounts of initial lethal damage induced by a constant radiation dose (a function of D_0 and n), the surviving fraction after a 24-hour delay in subculture (a function of n, D_0, and PLDR) may be similar.

The Cell Cycle and Radiation Killing

Radiation survival analysis of synchronously dividing cells demonstrated that cells irradiated during the G_2 and M phases of the cell cycle are more radiosensitive as compared to cells irradiated during G_1 and S (Figure XIII-1-17).[126] Thus, irradiation of an asynchronously dividing population of cells results in killing a greater proportion of cells in G_2 and M while surviving G_1 and S cells may progress into more sensitive phases. This phenomenon referred to as reassortment, results in increased cell killing when subsequent radiation doses are given during sensitive phases of the cell cycle as illustrated in Figure XIII-1-17.[126] Enhanced cell killing after synchronization and reassortment of irradiated tumor cells suggests a potential benefit from the fractionation of radiotherapy.

One consequence of x-ray exposure is the transient inhibition of cell cycle progression at the G_1/S and G_2/M interfaces of the cell cycle. Such delays likely represent active

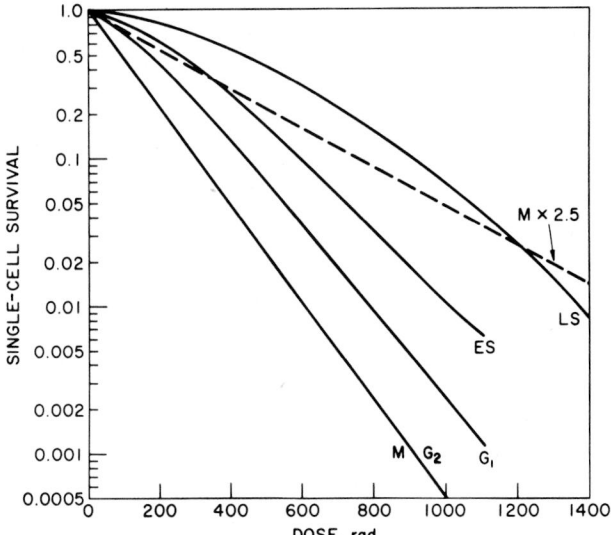

Figure XIII-1-17. Radiation survival curves for Chinese hamster cells irradiated at various stages of the cell cycle. Cells irradiated in G_2 and M are most radiation sensitive, followed by G_1, early S-phase (ES) and late S-phase (LS). The dashed line is the survival curve of mitotic cells under hypoxic conditions. (From Sinclair.[126])

processes and not simply the deleterious effects of DNA damage. For example, in the yeast Saccharomyces cerevisiae, the RAD-9 gene product is responsible for the arrest of cells in G_2 after radiation induced DNA damage.[167] It has been postulated that chromosomal reconstitution as well as fidelity of DNA replication requires the cell cycle arrest induced by the RAD-9 gene product. Yeasts which have the RAD-9 gene deleted do not undergo growth arrest and are more sensitive to the killing effect of x-rays than wild type yeast. This suggests that growth arrest is an important function during cellular repair of ionizing radiation damage. X-ray induced G_1/S cell cycle delays are also seen in mammalian cells, although specific genes associated with this phenotype have not been cloned. However, Fornance and colleagues have cloned several growth arrest DNA damage inducible genes, which are expressed following treatments with UV rays and alkylating agents in mammalian cells, some of which may be analogous in function to RAD-9 in yeast.[47] Potentially lethal damage repair discussed in the previous section may occur partially as a result of the effects of growth arrest genes. It is possible that combinations of growth arrest and repair gene products function to repair x-ray damage.

Molecular Aspects of Radioresistance

Common types of DNA damage induced by ionizing radiation include DNA base damage as well as DNA, single-strand and double-strand breaks. Unrepaired x-ray induced base damage is frequently mutagenic, whereas unrepaired x-ray induced DNA double-strand breaks are frequently lethal. Studies of x-ray sensitive rodent cell lines suggest that radiation killing is directly proportional to the rate of rejoining of DNA double-strand breaks.[72,133] Based on these data and data from lower organisms it is hypothesized that the initial number and/or the rate of rejoining (repair) of some classes

of DNA double-strand breaks may be important in cell survival following x-ray exposure. Schwartz and colleagues employed the DNA neutral filter elution assay to study repair of x-ray damage in human tumor cells and reported that radioresistant cell lines rejoined DNA double-strand breaks faster than more radiosensitive cell lines.[123] These data suggest that the neutral elution assay has promise as a rapid assay of human tumor radiosensitivity. Although this assay is relatively simple and rapid, it has been criticized because the doses of radiation employed are nonphysiological and it is difficult to distinguish various specific classes of DNA double strand-breaks. Only further investigation will clarify the use of neutral elution as a predictive assay of radiotherapy outcome.

Efforts to identify stress response genes have been successful for heat, alkylating agents and ultraviolet light in mammalian cells, whereas genes that repair gamma ray induced double-strand breaks or radiation base damage have not yet been successfully identified in higher eukaryotes. Well characterized genes that contribute to the repair of gamma induced radiation damage have been identified in bacteria, and lower eukaryotes.[9,24,153] For example, in E. coli various adverse stimuli can lead to the induction of stress related genes such as the ultraviolet and x-ray mediated sos-response.[153] In the sos-response, genes coding for DNA repair enzymes are coordinately induced after DNA damage. In this instance, DNA damage leads to activation of a specific proteinase function of the Rec-A protein that cleaves a repressor protein Lex-A. The Lex-A protein binds to the regulatory region of sos-genes and with its removal by activated Rec-A protein, transcription of these genes occurs. Many sos-genes encode for low abundance transcripts that are rapidly induced by 2- to 10-fold by activated Rec-A protein. The search for an sos-like response in mammalian cells has been limited since few DNA repair genes have been isolated. It is of interest that DNA damage inducible yeast genes RAD-6, -52, -54, play roles in x-ray damage repair, although RAD-52 is not x-ray inducible.[9,24] In mammalian cells, Herrlich and colleagues reported expression of damage inducible genes following UV-light exposure.[130] Induction of these genes is mediated by various transcription factors such as c-jun and NF-kB. Recently, Sherman and colleagues observed c-jun and c-fos to be transcriptionally induced by ionizing radiation in a human promyelocytic leukemia cell line.[125]

Molecular Radiation Oncology

The potential importance of identifying x-ray repair genes to radiotherapy is analogous to the importance of identifying genes that alter cell survival identification following exposure to chemotherapeutic agents.[19,91,124] Amplification of genes that repair DNA damage or induce growth arrest might be responsible for tumor radioresistance or indirectly influence tumor cell survival following radiation by altering cell cycle distribution. Manipulation of mammalian genes that repair different classes of x-ray induced DNA damage might increase the therapeutic ratio by increasing tumor cell kill as well as possibly decreasing normal tissue sequelae following radiotherapy. Identification of gamma DNA repair genes and the detection of amplification and/or overexpression of these genes may result in a rapid accurate prediction of clinical outcome in radiotherapy.

Oncogenes and the Cellular Response to Radiation

Fitzgerald and colleagues reported that leukemia cells transfected with the n-ras oncogene acquired radioresistance although the radioresistance was dose rate dependent.[45] Sklar reported that the intrinsic radiation resistance of NIH-3T3 cells was increased by transfection with ras-oncogenes activated by missense mutations.[127] Chang and colleagues transfected DNA from fibroblasts derived from members of a cancer prone family displaying the Li-Fraumeni syndrome into NIH 3T3 cells.[20] These transfections resulted in transformed colonies when compared to cells transfected with DNA from normal cells. This report was accompanied by the observation of Kasid and colleagues who reported that when DNA from a radioresistant human laryngeal carcinoma cell line was transfected into NIH 3T3 cells, a human c-raf transcript was identified in the subsequent transformants.[75] In the reports from Chang and colleagues and Kasid and colleagues, the human c-raf-1 oncogene appeared to be rearranged in transformed NIH-3T3 cells transfected with human DNA and retained the majority of a presumably unregulated kinase domain of the c-raf gene.[20,76] Kasid and colleagues followed this work by a report that anti-sense c-raf RNA partially reversed the radioresistant and tumorigenic phenotypes of raf-sense transfected human laryngeal carcinoma cells.[76] Pirollo and colleagues confirmed this observation and reported that activated c-raf-1 simultaneously conferred both the radioresistant and transformed phenotype on NIH 3T3 cells.[112] These investigators also observed that transfection with v-mos oncogene conferred radioresistance on 3T3 cells whereas transfection of cells with the v-fes and v-abl oncogenes did not. V-mos like c-raf is a serine threonine protein kinase, whereas v-fes and v-abl are tyrosine kinases. Pirollo and colleagues hypothesized that activated oncogenes whose protein products are related to serine and threonine phosphorylation effect radioresistance. They suggest that ras confers radioresistance because in addition to its role as a G-protein and affecting hydrolysis of phosphoinositides, ras transduces signals through a direct regulation of protein kinase-c, a serine threonine kinase.

Induction of Cytokines and the Radiation Response

Hallahan and colleagues proposed that a cytotoxic protein was induced by x-rays when media decanted following irradiation of tissue cultures of some human sarcoma cell lines was cytotoxic to these as well as other tumor cell lines.[63] ELISA analysis showed that the level of tumor necrosis factor alpha in the irradiated cultures was elevated over that of non-irradiated cells. This cytotoxicity was reversed by monoclonal antibodies to tumor necrosis factor alpha. Increased levels of TNF alpha mRNA were detected in TNF alpha producing cell lines. Nuclear run-on studies showed that radiation controlled TNF expression at the level of transcription. Because the media of irradiated cells was cytotoxic to other cell lines, a paracrine effect of TNF induction following x-rays was suggested. The authors proposed that intracellular

secretion of TNF following x-ray exposure may also produce autocrine effects on irradiated cells. TNF alpha is a polypeptide mediator of the cellular immune response with a wide range of activity. TNF has a direct effect on human cancer cell lines in vitro resulting in death and growth inhibition while in some normal cell lines growth stimulation is observed. The cytotoxic effect of TNF correlates with free radical formation, DNA fragmentation and microtubule destruction.[173,176] Radiation survival analyses conducted on cell lines which were TNF-producing as well as TNF-non-producing were carried out in the presence of varying concentrations of tumor necrosis factor.[63] In some cell lines, sublethal concentrations of TNF enhanced killing by radiation suggesting a radiosensitizing and synergistic effect between TNF and x-rays.[64] In other cell lines additive killing was observed. The interaction between TNF and ionizing radiation may be from saturation of radical scavenging systems within the cell. This fact is supported by reports that cell lines that are resistant to oxidative damage by TNF also have an elevated free radical buffering capacity. Thus cells that do not exhibit interactive killing between TNF and x-rays may be inherently more resistant to oxidative damage. Production of a cytokine (TNF-alpha in this instance) within irradiated cells may result in a greater biological effect after x-ray exposure than is observed from killing produced by the direct effects of ionizing radiation alone. It is also possible that if a cytokine is secreted into adjacent cells or the systemic circulation, its production may have paracrine and endocrine as well as autocrine effects. Further analysis will demonstrate whether TNF induction by x-rays is a common occurrence. However, TNF induction and secretion serves as a model for the general concept that radiation induced cytokines produce killing or protective effects in addition to effects predicted by direct effects of radiation on DNA.

The concept of release of growth factors from endothelial cells following irradiation was advanced by Witte and colleagues.[171] In their study, PDGF- and FGF-like growth factors were released following radiation treatment. These authors suggest that PDGF-like factors secreted from the intima of blood vessels may serve as paracrine factors for proliferation of smooth muscle cells observed in small arterioles after radiation in vivo. Similarly, FGF secreted after radiation may participate in abnormal proliferation of endothelial cells which obliterate the lumen of small caliber arterioles in various organs. Secretion of these growth factors may account for some of the long term effects of radiation secondary to small vessel obliteration. Woloschak and colleagues described transcriptional induction of IL-1 following x-ray exposure.[172] IL-1 is reported to be a radioprotector of hematopoietic cells in vivo.[99] The production of various growth factors and cytokines may explain some unusual effects of radiation such as the abscopal effect on hematopoietic cells or fatigue experienced by patients who undergo localized radiation therapy. Also, secretion of growth factors and cytokines may be an important step in radiation carcinogenesis in normal cells. Inhibition of molecular mediators of deleterious late radiation effects on the normal tissues may increase the therapeutic ratio and presents the possibility of genetic manipulation in clinical radiotherapy.

Cellular Radiation Response: Signal Transduction

Recent data suggest that radiation induction of the early response genes, c-jun, c-fos, and Egr-1 which act as transcription factors may initiate a cascade effect with pleiotropic cellular consequences.[65,125] At this time, the initiating events preceding early response gene induction are unknown although signaling in prokaryotes includes DNA strand breaks. Post translational modification of proteins which activate the early response genes are mediated in part through protein kinase-C.[65] Also, membrane changes induced by radiation may induce post-translational changes such as activation of tyrosine or serine/threonine protein kinases. Thus, biochemical changes within the cell may result in activation of protein kinase-C, the raf-1 protein or other related kinases which may activate early response genes and initiate DNA repair processes, cytokine production and cell cycle alteration. (Figure XIII-1-18). Several previously undescribed proteins induced by ionizing radiation have recently been described.[10] Also, activation of oncogenes by mutation or truncation (through deletion or inversion) may affect radioresistance especially throughout a fractionated course of radiotherapy. The investigation of the molecular aspects of radiobiology present exciting possibilities to enhance radiation therapy as a local and systemic modality.

PROPOSED RADIATION RESPONSE

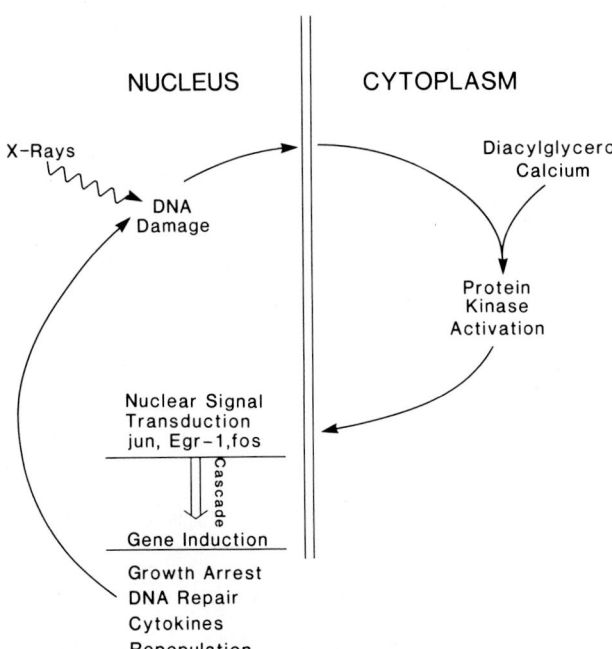

Figure XIII-1-18. The proposed radiation response cycle demonstrating nuclear and cytoplasmic components. Ionizing radiation damage of cellular components results in activation of kinases. Inhibition of these kinases results in attenuation of nuclear signal transduction. The transcription factor genes jun, Egr-1, and fos may be induced immediately after ionizing radiation damage. These transcription factors induce a cascade of molecular events leading to growth arrest, cytokine production and repopulation. Kinase activation may also lead to activation of DNA repair enzymes directly. The radiation response cycle is completed when repair enzymes repair DNA damage caused by ionizing radiation.

Growth and Regeneration Kinetics

The percentage of tumor cells detected to be in cycle is called the growth fraction. In human solid tumors, it is usually a small proportion of the total number of cells. If the growth fraction remains constant with time, the growth rate of the tumor is proportional to the growth fraction. If the growth fraction decreases with time, the rate of the tumor growth slows. Solid tumors usually grow at a slower rate as they enlarge and therefore growth is approximated by the Gompertzian equation.[70,168] In circumstances of equilibrium in normal tissues, each mitotic division results in the average of only one new cell. Usually, one daughter is lost by desquamation, apoptosis or metastasis. By definition, the cell loss factor in a steady state is one. Maximum growth occurs if the cell loss factor is reduced to zero. The only requirement for growth is a reduction from 1.0 in the cell loss factor, i.e., an average of less than 1 of 2 daughter cells of a division is lost. A cell loss factor of less than 1 is characteristic of both normal tissue regeneration and malignant growth. Tumor growth is usually characterized by cell loss factors that are closer to 1 than to 0.

An index for the potential regeneration of tumors and normal tissue populations is the proliferative activity of the cell population.[168] One common measurement of tumor growth is the potential doubling time and is defined as the time required to double the number of clonogenic cells if the cell loss factor decreased to 0. In this concept, the doubling time is equal to the cell cycle time. Tumors with a high rate of both cell production and loss have potential for early and rapid regeneration after irradiation or other cytotoxic treatment. Thus, even though a tumor may exhibit slow pretreatment growth, it may regenerate rapidly. Excessive protraction in the time of radiation fractionation or split course regimens may give inferior local control results if accelerated proliferation occurs during the time period when radiation is not given. Clonal proliferation during tumor regression after irradiation was demonstrated by Hermens and Barendsen who showed an exponential increase in clonogen number in a rat rhabdomyosarcoma during a time of tumor shrinkage (Figure XIII-1-19).[68] Thus clinical response may not be a good indication of the proliferative status of clonogenic tumor cells.

Tumor Hypoxia

As discussed earlier, ionizing radiation interacts with matter to produce short-lived free-radicals which results in oxidative damage to the cells. Anoxic cells require 2 to 3 times the radiation dose to produce the same amount of cell killing as well oxygenated cells.[143,144] As demonstrated in Figure XIII-1-20 the ratio of doses required to produce the same degree of cell killing in anoxic and oxygenated cells is referred to as the oxygen enhancement ratio (OER). The OER is 2.5–3 for x-rays but 1.6 for neutrons and 1.0 for alpha particles since these particulate forms of radiation directly damage DNA thus decreasing the need for oxygen fixation of DNA damage.

Thomlinson and Gray observed that tumors "outgrow" their vasculature resulting in necrotic areas (see I-11) and sug-

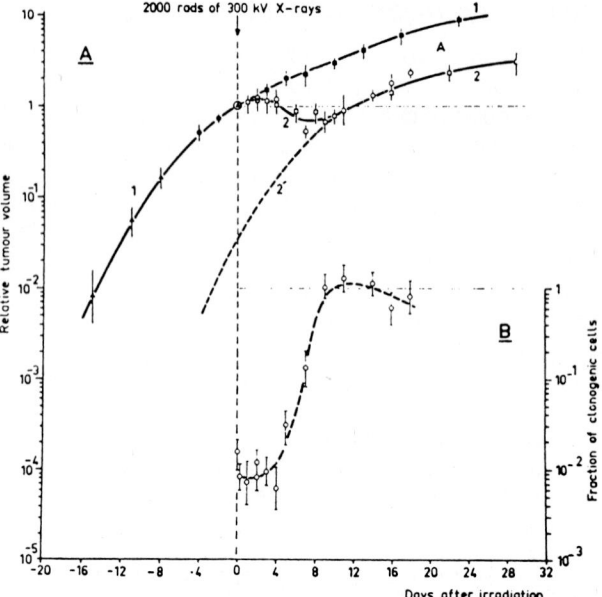

Figure XIII-1-19. Growth curves of rat rhabdomyosarcoma tumors irradiated in vivo demonstrating accelerated repopulation. Curve A shows the volume change in the tumor following a single dose of 2000 cGy. Curve 1 is the growth of an un-irradiated tumor. Curve 2 represents regression and regrowth of an irradiated tumor. Figure B shows the exponential increase in the fraction of clonogenic cells as a function of time after irradiation. Cells were obtained from the tumors irradiated in Figure A and the colony forming assay was used to determine clonogenic potential This figure demonstrates that there is an exponential increase in the number of clonogenic cells within 6 to 10 days after irradiating a tumor in vivo and that clonogens can repopulate during tumor regression. (From Hermens.[68])

gested that tumor cells adjacent to the anoxic region may be clonogenic but hypoxic.[143,144] As shown in Figure XIII-1-21 the oxygen tension within the tumor falls with the distance from the capillary producing a hypoxic region. In some experimental tumor systems, reoxygenation of hypoxic tumor cells occurs within 24 hours.[148] The physiological mechanism for reoxygenation may involve reduced oxygen utilization by radiation injured cells or the redistribution of blood flow within the tumor. The potential importance of reoxygenation during multifractionated radiotherapy is demonstrated when considering a theoretical tumor in which 90% of cells are well oxygenated and 10% are hypoxic. If reoxygenation did not occur, the percentage of hypoxic cells would eventually exceed that of aerated cells due to radioresistance of hypoxic cells. However, if reoxygenation occurs, the percentage of hypoxic cells remains constant (10%) and can eventually be eliminated.[74,148] Thus, reoxygenation provides an advantage to multifractionated radiotherapy by reducing the number of clonogenic hypoxic cells irradiated during each treatment. A theoretical model for tumor reoxygenation was proposed by Thomlinson (Figure XIII-1-22).[143,144] In this model small tumors have no hypoxic component (curve A) but the percent of hypoxic cells increases as the tumor grows (curve B). A steady state of hypoxia then develops (curve C). Immediately after irradiation, aerated cells are killed resulting in an increase in the percentage of hypoxic cells (curve D). Following a transient period of hypoxia (curve E), metabolism ceases and more oxygen is available to hypoxic cells (curve F). Tumor regrowth results in a return to the original percentage of hypoxic cells (curves G & I). Curve H represents the optimal time for the second radiation fraction (R_2).

A clinical observation which suggests that hypoxia participates in tumor radioresistance is that severe anemia is associated with worsened local control in a number of tumors. Several studies demonstrated improved survival in intermediate stage cervical carcinoma patients treated with radiotherapy when hemoglobin concentrations were above 11 grams as compared to patients with lower hemoglobin levels.[13,41,67] The reduction in survival associated with anemia during radiotherapy is also observed in other tumor types including endometrial, bladder and pharyngeal carcinomas.[103,117,121] Other clinical observations which suggest that

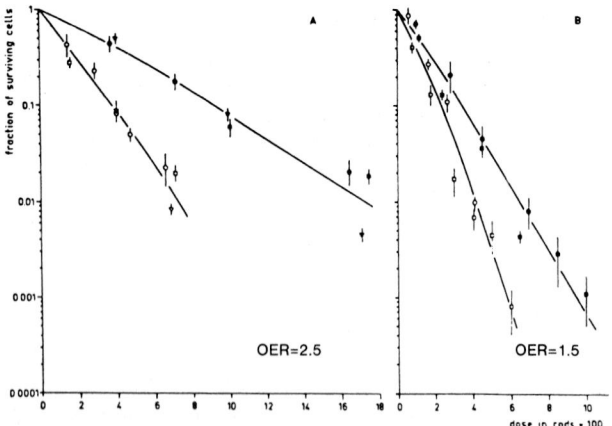

Figure XIII-1-20. Radiation survival curves for cells irradiated under hypoxic and aerated conditions demonstrating the oxygen enhancement ratio (OER). The OER is a ratio of the surviving fraction of cells following irradiation under hypoxic conditions. Figure A demonstrates the oxygen enhancement ratio for cells irradiated with x-rays. Curve B shows the oxygen enhancement ratio for cells irradiated with neutrons. (From Broerse et al.[11a])

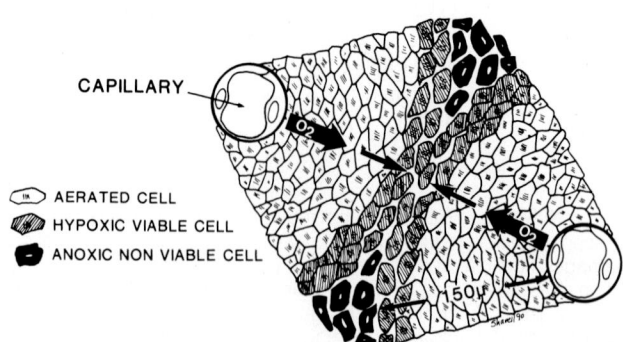

Figure XIII-1-21. Oxygen diffusion through tissue from a capillary resulting in hypoxic cells. Oxygen diffuses an average of 150 Ci from the capillary. Cells beyond this region are anoxic and nonviable. Cells at the periphery of this radius are hypoxic but viable.

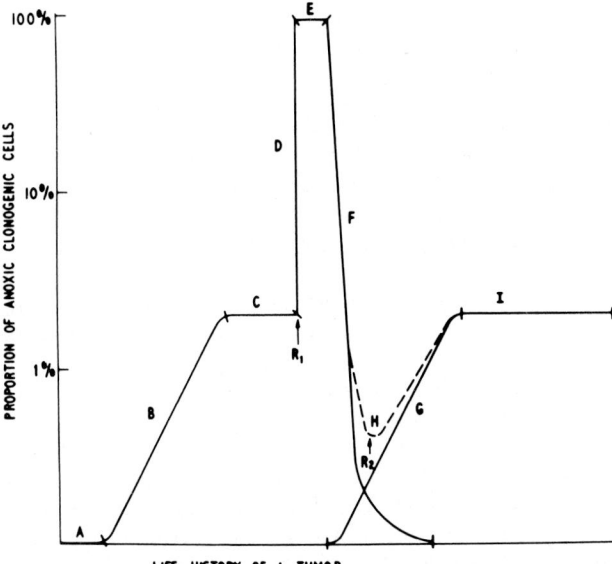

Figure XIII-1-22.   A theoretical model demonstrates that the percentage of viable hypoxic cells within a tumor varies as the tumor grows after irradiation. Curve A represents no hypoxic cells in a small tumor while Curve B shows the increase in hypoxic cells as the tumor "outgrows" its blood supply. This reaches a plateau region (Curve C) which frequently ranges from 10–20% in a tumor. R_1 represents the time at which this tumor is exposed to x-rays. This dosage of radiation kills most of the aerated cells while the hypoxic cells survive. Thus, Curve D represents the increase in the percentage of hypoxic cells which are clonogenic after irradiation. This increased percentage of hypoxic cells that persists for a short time period is represented by Curve E. Reoxygenation occurs and the proportion of hypoxic cells decreases (Curve F). Curve G represents regrowth of the tumor after irradiation and shows the increase in proportion of hypoxic cells in the growing tumor. Curve H is an extrapolation of the percentage of hypoxic cells due to reoxygenation and tumor regrowth. The plateau region is again obtained in Curve I. (From Thomlinson.[144])

hypoxia contributes to radioresistance include hyperbaric oxygen (HBO) which has been used to improve the therapeutic ratio during radiotherapy for hypoxic tumors. HBO was used during treatment of cervical carcinoma during a Medical Research Council (MRC) trial. The local control was improved by 25% (p = 0.0003) and survival improved by 12%.[32] The MRC trial of radiotherapy and HBO (O_2 at 3ATM) for head and neck cancer also demonstrated a significant improvement in local control and survival.[66] Despite the encouraging results, HBO is seldom used because of the technical difficulties associated with irradiating patients while they are in hyperbaric chambers. Also some hyperbaric oxygen trials have not shown an advantage to HBO compared to standard treatment.

Hypoxic Tumor Cell Radiosensitizers

Hypoxic tumor cell sensitizers are a class of electron affinic compounds which fix damage induced by ionizing radiation under hypoxic conditions thereby mimicking oxygen.[1] The prototypes of hypoxic cell sensitizers are the nitroimidazole compounds.[1,25-27] The nitroimidazole used in most clinical trials to date is misonidazole. Most studies have demon-

strated no benefit from misonidazole despite the fact it enhances cell killing under hypoxic conditions in vitro.[25–27] Possible reasons for the lack of efficacy are: neurotoxicity prevents obtaining adequate drug levels; misonidazole may not demonstrate adequate electron affinity; and hypoxia is not a cause of radioresistance in human tumors studied in sensitizer trials. Several recently developed nitroimidazole compounds may prove to have greater clinical efficacy because of less neurotoxicity. One such compound is SR-2508 (etanidazole) which can be given at five times greater dose than misonidazole; it has been used in Phase I and II trials.[25,26] Further clinical investigation with hypoxic cell sensitizers continues.

The importance of the role of hypoxic tumor cells in radiotherapy is a controversial subject because much of the clinical data comparing HBO and hypoxic cell sensitizers does not compare these modifiers to optimal fractionation schemes, or is negative. Theoretical calculations of potentially hypoxic tumor cells suggest that even a very small proportion of these cells would render most human tumors impossible to control with radiotherapy. It is likely, however, that tumor cell hypoxia plays a role in the failure of radiotherapy to sterilize some human tumors.

Radiation Protectors

A potential means of improving the therapeutic ratio is to develop drugs which protect normal tissues against ionizing radiation while not affecting tumor radiosensitivity.[174] One class of drugs under study are sulfhydryl containing compounds. A prototype compound is the sulfhydryl containing amino acid cysteine which demonstrates the property of being a free-radical scavenger. Cysteine experimentally protects mice from lethal doses of irradiation.[106,107] The proposed mechanisms by which sulfhydryls protect against radiation are at both the chemical level (free-radical scavenging, stabilization of chromatin, and hydrogen ion donation) and at the enzymatic level (enhanced DNA repair, and cell cycle delay).[53] Sulfhydryl compounds have been developed which are less toxic than cystine to humans. They include WR-2721 [S-2(3-aminopropylamino) ethylphosphoric acid] which reduces mucositis resulting from radiotherapy when applied topically.[83,175] Infusion of WR-2721 into rodents protected normal tissues while not affecting tumor control.[174] One clinical trial demonstrated protection of human bone marrow by WR-2721 in patients receiving hemibody irradiation.[28] The radioprotector WR-1065 has demonstrated protection against x-ray induced double-strand breaks, cytotoxicity and mutagenicity from Cisplatin.[98] Thus these protectors may be combined with radiotherapy or chemotherapy to reduce the risk of treatment related carcinogenesis.

Biological response modifiers which are demonstrated radioprotectors include Interleukin-1 (IL-1) and GM-CSF.[99,101] GM-CSF protects the bone marrow when added after irradiation, acting to enhance recovery of irradiated bone marrow. These agents are not classic radioprotectors since they do not directly scavenge free radicals but rather improve bone marrow tolerance, by expanding the hematopoietic compartment (IL-1 has been reported to induce free radical scavengers). IL-1 protects mice from lethal doses of radiation[101] and accelerates the recovery of CFU-E, GM-CFU, BFU-E, and CFU-Meg after irradiation. IL-1 also enhances the survival of lethally irradiated mice treated with allogenic bone marrow cells.[101]

Fractionation

Radiation therapy is usually delivered as a series of 180–300 cGy fractions in 5–6 days for 5–8 weeks. The use of fractionation arose from the empirical studies of European radiotherapists and radiobiologists in the early 20th century. Many modifications in fractionation have been attempted since these studies, but it is generally accepted that fractionation increases the therapeutic ratio.[48,137,142] The effects of fractionation on tumors and normal tissues depend upon the total dose, the fraction size (amount of radiation delivered per dose), the number of treatment sessions and the overall time of radiation delivery. Repair and regeneration (repopulation) discussed in the previous sections increase the total dose required to achieve a specific level of biological damage (referred to as an isoeffective dose) when radiation is fractionated.[137] Redistribution of cells to radiosensitive phases of the cell cycle, and reoxygenation of radioresistant hypoxic cells reduce the dose required for a specific level of biological damage. In general, the larger the fraction size, the more severe the late effects of radiotherapy on normal tissues. Acute reactions which are due to interruptions in relatively rapid cell renewal systems are not good indicators of late normal tissue effects and are usually not dose limiting in standard fraction schemes. Successful fractionation is a balance between delivery of a tumoricidal dose without causing acute reactions which are so severe that the duration of radiation therapy is excessively protracted or intolerable long term normal tissue damage occurs. Various mathematical models have been proposed to equate overall dose, time, fraction size and achieve an isoeffective dose. The clinical usefulness of these models is controversial.

Alterations in Fractionation

Historically, split course fractionated radiotherapy was one of the first alterations in fraction schedule attempted. A 2–3 week break was given in the middle of the treatment to allow tumor shrinkage and possible reoxygenation. However, clinical results obtained using split course radiotherapy are generally not superior to and in some instances worse than results obtained with continuous radiotherapy.[104] Accelerated fractionation decreases the overall treatment time to diminish clonogenic proliferation between doses. In accelerated fractionation schedules, treatment is given 2–4 times per day employing fractions of 150–200 cGy per treatment with 4–6 hours between fractions.[154,168] Thus, the daily dose is 300–600 cGy and the total dose is given in 3–4 weeks. Frequently, severe acute normal tissue reactions develop and a break in treatment is required.[110,168] Even when treatment interruption is necessary, the total treatment time is reduced from 6–8 weeks to 5–6 weeks. Tumors with a relatively short potential doubling time are the most suitable candidates for accelerated fractionation. Clinical gain from an accelerated fractionation schedule has been demonstrated in patients with Burkitt's lymphoma and promising results have been

obtained in patients with stages II and III head and neck cancer.[93,168]

Hyperfractionation employs relatively small doses per fraction usually 100–120 cGy administered 2–3 times per day.[93,168] This approach achieves a small decrease in the overall treatment time. Hyperfractionation delivers an increased number of treatments, 50–60 vs. 30–35. Thus relatively rapidly dividing cell populations may have a higher proportion of cells in the most sensitive phases of the cell cycle at each treatment. Cells in late responding normal tissues are slowly proliferating and therefore after a few fractions many surviving cells will be concentrated at the most resistant phases of the cell cycle. This concept provides a rationale for a potential differential response in normal tissue versus tumor in hyperfractionated regimens.

Vokes and colleagues and Taylor and colleagues have employed concomitant chemotherapy and radiotherapy on alternative weeks.[140,152] Preliminary data suggest that increased tumor cell kill achieved by concomitant radiotherapy and chemotherapy overcomes tumor cell proliferation between alternative week treatments. The goal of these trials will be to shorten the overall treatment time by manipulation of chemotherapy dose and radiotherapy fractionation. Hypofractionation or larger than standard fractions have been employed in melanoma, lung cancer and head and neck cancer.[164] Although tumor regressions are frequently more rapid with large fraction sizes, local control is not necessarily increased and in fact may be decreased under some circumstances. For example, Eichorn employed several fractionation schemes of 400–1,000 cGy in lung cancer compared to 200 cGy fraction sizes (but similar final doses) and found that an increased fraction size actually gave a decrease in tumor sterilization at the time surgery.[33] Byhard and Cox compared treatment five times per week to treatment three times per week with slightly larger fraction sizes and found decreased local control in the oral cavity and oropharynx with larger fraction sizes and a smaller number of fractions.[15] Increased PLDR at large fraction sizes is one reason suggested for the decrease in local control in these studies.[164]

Dose Response and the Therapeutic Ratio

Various levels of radiation yield different tumor control probabilities depending upon the size and anatomic extent of the lesion. The total number of surviving cells is proportional to the initial number and biological characteristics of clonogenic cells and the total cell kill achieved with a specified dose of radiation. Dose response relationships for local control of homogeneous tumor groups have been empirically determined. The higher the doses of radiation delivered the more likely tumor control (Table XIII-1-2).

The dose of radiation which can be delivered to a tumor is limited by the probability of serious normal tissue complications. Therefore choice of a tumor dose is based on the relative probability of tumor control and normal tissue complications. The potential therapeutic gain can be estimated for an average group of patients based on tumor size, histological type and the normal tissues which will be included in the treatment fields. Figure XIII-1-23 shows a theoretical dose response relationship for tumor control and normal tis-

Table XIII-1-2. Relationship of Tumor Diameter and Dose to Percent Local Control

Dose (5 × 200 cGy/wk)	% Control	
	Squamous Cell Carcinoma	Adenocarcinoma
5,000	>90% microfoci 50% 2–3 cm nodes	>90% subclinical
6,000	80–90% T$_1$ pharynx and larynx 50% T$_3$–T$_4$ tonsil	
7,000	90% 1–3 cm nodes 80% T$_3$–T$_4$ tonsil	90% axillary

Adapted from Fletcher[45a]

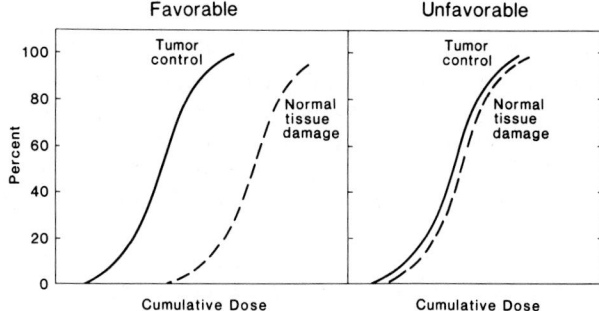

Figure XIII-1-23.   Dose control and complication curves in curable and noncurable tumors treated with radiotherapy. The percentage of tumor control and normal tissue damage are sigmoidal. In a radiocurable tumor, such as Hodgkin's disease, the dose required to control a tumor is less than the normal tissue tolerance. This results in a favorable therapeutic ratio. The dosage required to control an unfavorable tumor such as pancreatic carcinoma is approximately that of the normal tissue tolerance resulting in an unfavorable therapeutic ratio.

sue complications. The therapeutic ratio is defined as percentage of tumor cures which are obtained at a given level of toxicity for normal tissues. Tannock and Hill suggest that the therapeutic ratio is better defined in terms of a ratio of radiation doses required to produce a given percentage of tumor control and complications.[70] Figure XIII-1-23A depicts a favorable therapeutic ratio and Figure XIII-1-23B depicts an unfavorable therapeutic ratio. The greater the displacement between the two curves (in the favorable situation) the more radiocurable the tumor.

Chemotherapy X-Ray Interaction

The use of combined chemotherapy and radiation therapy aims to overcome lack of tumor radiocurability as a cause of local treatment failure and to eradicate distant micro- and/ or gross-metastases as a cause of systemic failure. Four theoretical types of interaction between radiation and chemotherapy can occur:[31,129,152] 1) "Spatial cooperation"; this term describes the independent activity of each treatment modality; for radiotherapy within the radiation treatment field against the primary site of disease, and for chemotherapy outside of the radiotherapy field against presumed metastatic disease. 2) "Toxicity independence"; in this concept, administration of each treatment modality at full or near full

dose without a significant increase in normal tissue damage might result in therapeutic enhancement. No interaction between the two therapy modalities is required and additive activity would be the expected clinical outcome. 3) The protection of normal tissues from radiation by a systemic agent might increase local control by allowing for the administration of higher doses of radiation. However, increased efficacy will result only if the tumor is exempted from the protective action of the drug. 4) Increased activity within the radiation field may result as a direct result of the interaction of chemotherapy with radiation. In this situation, the drug has been called a "sensitizer," "enhancer," or "potentiator" of radiation.[31,128,129,152]

Steel proposed terminology to characterize the type and extent of interaction between two agents in the laboratory.[128,129] These concepts are based on the availability of a dose-response curve for each of the single treatment modality agents and an isobologram analysis of their combined response. Where the drug is inactive by itself, a positive interaction with radiation is referred to as "sensitization" and a negative interaction as "protection." Where the drug has activity by itself and dose-response curves are available for both the drug and radiation, the interaction can be described as supra-additive (synergistic), additive, or subadditive.[31,129] One common definition of synergy is a reduction in the D$_0$ when the drug is added to radiation, while additivity is defined as a reduction in n with no change in D$_0$ when the drug is added.[31] Detailed dose response curves may be available for only one or none of the two agents. In these instances, a positive interaction is described as "enhancement" or "cooperation," and a negative interaction as "inhibition" or "antagonism," respectively. Vokes and Weichselbaum suggested the use of the term "enhancement" to describe an increase in the activity of radiation in the presence of chemotherapy, while not attempting to distinguish between additivity and synergy.[152]

Possible mechanisms of interaction between chemotherapeutic drugs and radiation have been previously reviewed in detail and include those listed in Table XIII-1-3.[152] These interactions may be based on differential activity of drug and

Table XIII-1-3. Interaction of Radiotherapy and Chemotherapy

Chemotherapy drug and radiation active against different tumor cell subpopulations based on hypoxia, cell cycle specificity, and pH

Decreased tumor cell repopulation following fractionated radiation due to effects of chemotherapy

Increased tumor cell recruitment from G$_0$ into a therapy-responsive cell cycle phase

Increased tumor cell oxygenation following radiation with improved drug or radiation activity

Improved drug delivery with shrinkage of tumor

Early eradication of tumor cells preventing emergence of drug and/ or radiation resistance

Eradication of cells resistant to one treatment modality by the other treatment

Cell cycle synchronization

Inhibition of repair of sublethal radiation damage or inhibition of recovery from potentially lethal radiation damage

Adapted from Vokes et al.[152]

radiation against specific tumor cell subpopulations, e.g., tumor cell hypoxia, and cell cycle phase sensitivity patterns, or on mechanical factors such as reduced tumor bulk leading to improved drug delivery to malignant cells. Other mechanisms require a direct interaction between drug and radiation and include inhibition of repair of radiation damage, cell cycle synchronization, or the elimination of inherently radioresistant cells. A major limitation to the effective combination of chemotherapy and radiotherapy is toxicity which limits potentially curative doses of either modality. A theoretical limitation to combined therapy is emergence of drug and/or x-ray resistant tumor cells which may occur as a result of gene alterations induced by drugs, x-rays or both. It has been suggested that chemotherapy administered concomitantly with radiotherapy may increase rather than decrease the incidence of distant metastases.[152]

The halogenated pyrimidines, iododeoxyuridine IUdR, and bromodeoxyuridine BUdR are analogs of thymidine which may be incorporated into DNA. The Vanderwaal forces surrounding the halogen approximate that of the methyl group of thymidine. DNA replaced with BUdR or IUdR are more susceptible to damage by ionizing radiation. Halogenated pyrimidines must be available to cells for several cell divisions prior to irradiation; radiosensitization increases as the percentage replacement of thymidine increases.[79,81] BUdR and IUdR demonstrate equal radiosensitization while BUdR produces more sensitization to fluorescent light and therefore, BUdR is used less frequently in clinical trials. Halogenated pyrimidines are under clinical investigation.

Basis for Combining Radiation and Surgery

Radical surgery frequently requires organ removal or amputation, while conservative surgery removes only clinically apparent tumor. Radiation therapy used in combination with conservative surgery eliminates residual microscopic tumor cell extension into normal tissues. The goal of conservative surgery combined with radiotherapy is to avoid the consequences of radical surgery and thus preserve organ function and cosmesis. These goals are achieved not only by reducing the extent of surgery but by reducing the radiation dose which would be required to control gross tumor. Examples of limited surgery and radiotherapy which have been shown to be effective in organ preservation and cosmesis are the treatment of localized limb sarcoma and breast cancer.[44,113]

Preoperative radiation therapy is given with the intention of reducing the quantity of viable tumor cells as well as the anatomic extent of tumor prior to surgery. Preoperative radiotherapy may diminish the risk of wound contamination by malignant cells and theoretically reduce the risk of metastases during tumor manipulation. Tumor regression subsequent to preoperative radiation therapy may increase the resectability of locally advanced disease. Limitations of preoperative irradiation are: 1) In general, higher radiation doses can be given postoperatively; 2) some patients within a disease category do not require radiotherapy but with current staging methods all patients treated would be (e.g., Duke's A, B$_1$, and D rectal cancer patients do not require radiotherapy but would likely be included in a preoperative radiotherapy protocol); and 3) examples of the use of preop-

erative radiation are the treatment of superior sulcus lung cancer, locally advanced rectal carcinoma and bladder carcinoma prior to cystectomy or interstitial implantation of radioactive sources.[11,69,147]

Indications for postoperative radiation therapy include known or suspected residual disease or anatomic sites with a high risk of local recurrence following surgery.[93,150] For example, anatomic sites within the upper aerodigestive tract with high incidence of local recurrence after resection are listed in Table XIII-1-4.[45,93] Table XIII-1-5 demonstrates the influence of surgical margins and postoperative radiotherapy on local recurrence.[93] Local recurrence increases significantly if the interval exceeds seven weeks.[93] Thus the interval should be as short as postoperative wound healing permits preferably within two weeks. The risk of poor wound healing increases with dose.[114,152]

Radiation Injury to Normal Tissue

The response of normal tissues to radiation may be categorized by the length of time after irradiation that damage is manifested. Acute radiation injury occurs hours to days after irradiation and is due to interruption of repopulation in rapidly proliferating tissues such as the oral mucosa or GI tract.[131] Subacute radiation injury occurs weeks to months after irradiation and is due to injury to cells such as the type II pneumocytes which manifest lethality or dysfunction during this time period.[29]

The pathogenesis of chronic radiation injury is multifactorial. 1) Microvascular destruction by radiation results in organ ischemia, fibrosis and necrosis; 2) stem cells required to replenish cell renewal systems can be sufficiently reduced in quantity to cause organ failure; and 3) the concept of the

Table XIII-1-4. Number of Patients with Negative Tumor Margins Who Develop Local Recurrences

Site	Total No.	No. Recurrences in Primary Site (%)
Tongue	510	166 (32.5)
Gingiva	134	42 (31.3)
Lip	81	7 (8.6)
Supraglottic larynx	167	42 (25.1)
Palate	137	57 (41.6)
Tonsil	147	61 (41.5)
Pharynx and pyriform sinus	183	68 (37.2)
Buccal mucosa	99	33 (33.3)
Floor of mouth	255	67 (26.3)

From Fletcher[45A]

Table XIII-1-5. Local Control is Dependent upon Status of Surgical Margins and Preoperative Radiotherapy

Status of Margin	Local Recurrence Without Radiotherapy (%)	Recurrence After Postoperative Radiotherapy (%)
No tumor	39*	2
In situ carcinoma	84.6	—
Close (within 5 mm)	73.7	—
Invasive cancer present	64–73	10.5

*See Table XIII-1-4 for recurrence rate for each site when margins are without tumor

Adapted from Looser[92] and Vikram[150]

functional unit theorizes that strategically placed cell death can result in dysfunction of the entire organ. Destruction of a functional unit produces significant morbidity for systems such as the spinal cord and the nephron. Injury to the renal tubule or glomerulus may cause dysfunction of the entire nephron. Myelopathy may result from injury to a microscopic cross section of the spinal cord and does not require injury to the entire organ. These processes act interdependently to cause the pathogenesis of chronic radiation injury. Thus, cell death can result in organ dysfunction if injuries are strategically placed.[110,168] Late tissue injury is usually the dose limiting event in radiotherapy, although acute and subacute reactions may be dose limiting under certain circumstances such as radiation pneumonitis, pericarditis, or severe mucositis.[29,131,132]

The shape of the radiation survival curve varies among normal tissues. The initial slopes and the terminal slopes are each different for early acute effects and late long term effects of responding tissues as illustrated in Figure XIII-1-24. For doses used during radiotherapy, the shape of the initial slope is extremely important. In general, early responding tissues have a steeper initial slope compared to late responding tissues. This results in a greater surviving fraction in late tissues as compared to early tissues.[168] During fractionation of radiotherapy these differences in surviving fractions are recapitulated daily, resulting in accentuation of the intial slope of the survival curve. Thus late responding tissues are spared by fractionation to a greater degree than early tissues.

The tumor curve dose versus normal tissue damage paradigm can be confusing. For example, to sterilize a gross tumor sufficient dose to kill 10^9 to 10^{11} cells must be delivered. A small volume of most normal tissue will tolerate such a dose depending upon the function of the organ. For example, the cervix tolerates much higher doses than the spinal cord because moderate fibrosis in the cervix usually does not result in severe functional consequences whereas a similar amount of damage in the spinal cord might be catastrophic. Also, fewer cells need to be killed to disrupt the functional unit of the spinal cord than to sterilize most tumors. Therefore, the volume of normal tissue exposed to radiation is critical and optimal treatment planning is necessary to maintain the most favorable therapeutic ratio possible in a specific clinical situation. The tolerance doses listed in Table XIII-1-6 are adapted and updated from Rubin.[119] The TD$_{5/5}$ is known from clinical studies in which 5% of patients develop the listed injury after the entire organ or a significant portion is irradiated using standard fractionation (200 cGy/day/5 days/week).

Clinical Treatment Planning

The goal in treatment planning is to uniformly irradiate the gross tumor volume and known or suspected routes of disease spread while sparing adjacent radiation sensitive tissues.[105] Treatment planning is the critical link between physics, biology, and clinical radiotherapy. The spatial distribution of radiation delivered is dependent upon the external patient contour, variations in tissue density which affect radiation transport, and the technical details of the planned irradiation, including beam energy and configuration of radiation portals. Because the gross tumor may be irregularly shaped, and a high dose margin around the tumor is needed to adequately treat microscopic disease and account for variations in daily patient setup, a three dimensional image-

Table XIII-1-6. Late Tissue Injury from Radiation

Organs	Injury	TD$_{5/5}$
Bone marrow (TBI)	Aplasia, pancytopenia	250
Liver	Acute and chronic	3000
Stomach	Perforation, ulcer,	4500
	hemorrhage	5000
Brain	Infarction, necrosis	6000
Spinal cord	Infarction, necrosis	4500
Heart	Pericarditis and	
	pancarditis	4500
Lung	Acute and chronic	
	pneumonitis	2000
Kidney	Acute and chronic	
	nephrosclerosis	2000
Esophagus	Ulceration	6000
Rectum	Ulcer, stricture	6000
Salivary glands	Xerostomia	5000
Bladder	Contracture	6000
Ureters	Stricture	7500
Testes	Sterilization	100
Ovary	Sterilization	200–300
Eye		
a) Retina	Blindness	5500
b) Cornea	Ulceration	5000
c) Lens	Cataract	500
Thyroid gland	Hypothyroidism	4500
Peripheral nerves	Neuropathy	6000

Normal tissue tolerance doses in cGy which produce injury in 5% (TD$_{5/5}$) within five years after irradiation. Modified from Rubin[119]

The Initial Slopes for Normal Tissues

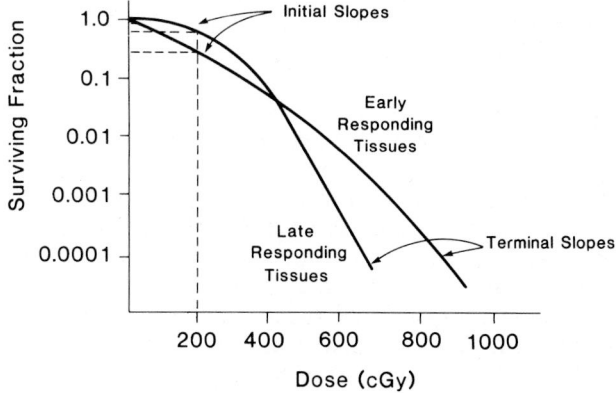

Figure XIII-1-24. The initial slopes and terminal slopes for early and late responding normal tissues. Late responding tissues have a small initial slope followed by a larger terminal slope of the survival curve. In contrast, early responding tissues have a larger initial slope and smaller terminal slope. Thus the surviving fraction of late responding tissues at 200 cGy is greater than that of early responding tissues. This difference in surviving fraction in the shoulder region of the survival curves of these two tissue types is recapitulated with each fraction of radiotherapy. This results in the risk of radiation injury to late responding tissues.

based approach is becoming increasingly important in radiation therapy planning.[51,52,90,95] As described in the previous section, limiting normal tissue volume irradiated is essential to decreasing complications. We describe both the basic concepts of treatment planning, and more advanced technical considerations in a three dimensional approach.

Imaging

Imaging plays a central role in radiotherapy, providing geometric information on external patient contour, tumor size, shape, and location relative to adjacent critical structures.[51] The process begins with the acquisition of a volumetric CT scan, where contiguous slices of transaxial image data are acquired with the patient in the treatment position. In a more conventional approach, information on tumor size, shape, and location are transferred from hardcopy films of the CT slices onto AP or lateral radiographs, using bony landmarks visualized on both CT and conventional radiographs. Mapping the target to oblique films is significantly more difficult to accomplish accurately.

To provide more flexible and precise treatment planning methods, image based treatment planning approaches which permit the graphic visualization of tumor and anatomy on computer workstations have been developed. Through interactive manipulations, these displays can provide insights into the optimal approaches for radiation portals. In a 3-D computerized planning approach, the image data set are read into the treatment planning computer, on which the radiation therapist identifies and outlines the target volume to be treated on each CT image. The external body outline and other critical structures are also defined. These contours are input into a Beam's Eye View (BEV) program, which permits display and inspection of the geometry from different viewpoints.

The radiotherapist views the target and adjacent critical structures and adjusts the viewpoint to identify beam orientations which fully irradiate the target volume but spare the most critical structure. Plate XIII-1-2 shows a tumor and adjacent normal anatomy from a superior anterior viewpoint. Viewing from obliques, the radiotherapist can find an angle which avoids irradiation of the spinal cord while adequately covering the target volume with the radiation portal. In addition to determining the optimal beam angle, BEV planning also permits the design of customized shielding blocks to spare uninvolved lung, heart, and cord. Alignment aids[52] may also be generated to assist in the accurate alignment of oblique fields at the time of treatment.

Multimodality Imaging

Although CT scanning is the primary imaging modality for radiation treatment planning, MRI provides important complementary information, especially for intracranial and head and neck tumors. Newer modalities such as PET or SPECT also provide complementary information.[2,87] Ideally, all imaging data can be cross correlated to transfer regions of interest from one study to another. For example, mapping the location of the tumor and critical organs from MRI studies to CT scans for treatment planning is desirable for accurate dose calculations and targetry. Other applications of image correlation in radiation oncology[21] include: the definition of

the pre-resection tumor volume and its transfer to post operative scans, in order to adequately treat the tumor bed; and the correlation of the three dimensional radiation dose distribution with post therapy imaging studies to evaluate the efficacy of therapy, tumor recurrence, or treatment related complication.

Image correlation methods for intracranial lesions have been developed by a number of investigators.[109,122] Approaches use either high precision localization masks, or depend on markers or surfaces (external or internal) to define the transformation. Plate XIII-1-1 shows the result of an image correlation technique used in radiation therapy planning, where the high intensity colored region indicating tumor and edema extracted from an MRI scan has been registered onto the corresponding CT image.

Interactive Treatment Planning

Once the tumor and normal anatomy have been defined, the planning process proceeds to choice of radiation type (photons, electrons, or both), radiation energy, and general arrangement of portals. This is performed interactively on a computer workstation. Variables in the development of a treatment plan include energy and modality of radiation beam, number of portals and their angulation, relative weights of radiation fields, and use of beam modifying devices (wedges, compensators). These parameters are adjusted interactively to generate an optimized isodose distribution. An optimized isodose distribution uniformly irradiates the target and minimizes dose to normal tissues.

The beam energy is chosen to match the scale of patient anatomy. High energy photon beams are appropriate for deep seated tumors in obese patients. Low megavoltage energy beams are appropriate for lesions of the head and neck. Superficial tumors may be treated with orthovoltage energy photon beams (100–250 kVp) or with electrons. The number of radiation fields to be used in a treatment plan is determined by physical considerations, such as the acceptability of the resulting dose distribution and radiobiological factors. Figure XIII-1-25 shows the irradiation of a pelvic tumor with one, two and four fields. In each plan, a dose of 100% is delivered to the tumor center. However, there is a significant dose non-uniformity within the target volume and regions of unacceptably high dose, as great as 130%, outside the target volume in the single field plan. The parallel opposed fields treatment plan irradiates the tumor uniformly, but irradiates tissues outside the target volume to an equally high dose. Finally, in the four field box plan, a greater volume of normal tissue is irradiated to a moderate dose level of 60% while the target is enclosed in a rectangular high dose region. In general, the greater number of radiation fields results in greater sparing of normal tissues from high doses if this field is treated every day. It was noted previously that an increase in the daily fraction size may dramatically increase tissue complications. In the case of the one field plan, normal tissues receive 30% more dose than that delivered to the target. Even if multiple fields are employed and only one field per day is treated (assuming the tumor receives 100% each day) the normal tissue will receive an unnecessarily large fraction size.

The radiation fields exiting from the linear accelerator are

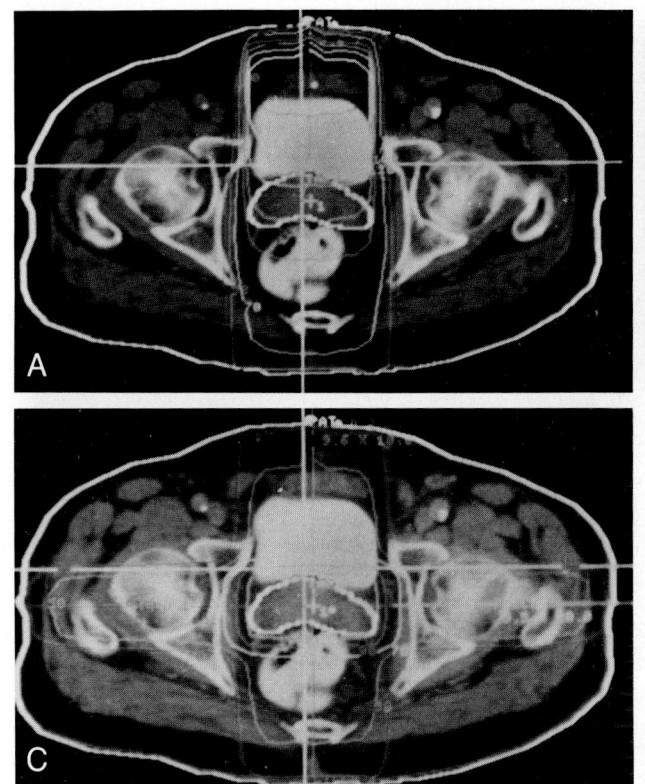

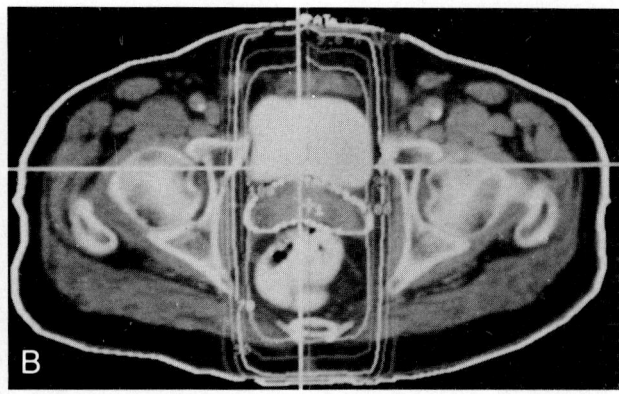

Figure XIII-1-25.   Isodose distributions as a function of number of radiation fields. A) Single field irradiation of the target volume (prostate) produces inhomogeneous distribution in the target and a high dose in normal tissues proximal to the target. For this reason, single fields are rarely used for more than very superficial targets. B) Two fields, parallel opposed, irradiate bladder and rectum to the same dose as the target. C) Four field irradiation of prostate results in high dose to target and spares normal tissues.

rectangular in shape and uniform across the field. The patient's external surface, tissue density differences, and shape and location of the target volume can be highly irregular in three dimensions. In order to achieve a uniform shaped high dose region confined to the target, the dose distribution is modified. In the plane perpendicular to the beam direction, high density low melting point blocks are individually shaped for each patient to include the target but exclude adjacent radiation sensitive tissues. Dose distribution in depth may be adjusted through the use of compensators which account for missing tissue, or through the use of wedges which vary the isodose shape.

Examples of Treatment Plans

Lung. Treatment of non-resectable lung tumors with radiation treatment is common. Figure XIII-1-26 shows a lung tumor (white outline) in the right lung, near the hilum. A treatment plan is designed to minimize dose to the spinal cord, normal lung, and heart within tolerable dose levels. Isodose lines indicate the relative dose distribution from a four field treatment plan. Both anterior/posterior opposed fields are used in addition to opposed oblique fields angled to avoid the spinal cord. Dose to the normal lung and spinal cord may be minimized by evaluating various radiation fields which irradiate normal tissues within the tolerance of the organs.

Head and Neck Tumors. Consider the nasopharyngeal carcinoma imaged by CT in Figure XIII-1-27. The gross mass is seen as an asymmetric fullness on the left side. Because of lymphatic drainage in this region, carcinoma of the nasopharynx metastasizes to regional cervical lymph nodes. The treatment volume therefore includes both the primary tumor

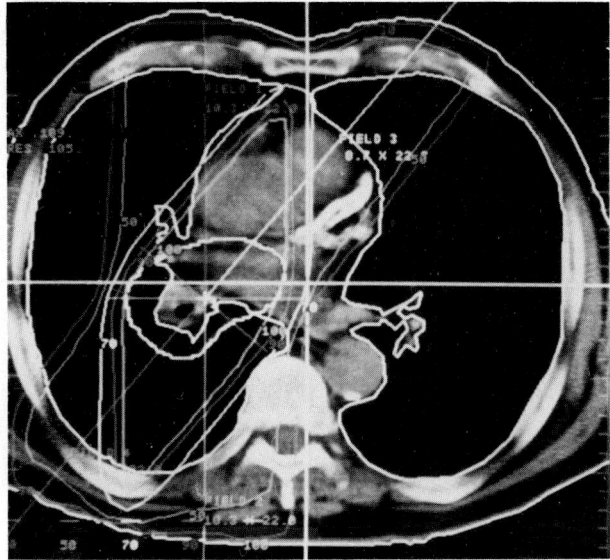

Figure XIII-1-26.   Representative lung treatment plan. Field configuration includes AP-PA and parallel opposed oblique portals.

and neck nodes. The initial target volume is treated with opposed lateral photon fields. Critical structures such as the eyes, portion of the tongue and brain are excluded from the port by shielding blocks. The initial dose distribution to the nasopharynx is shown in Figure XIII-1-27A. After an initial course of 45 Gy to control subclinical disease, the target is divided into a segment anterior to the cord and treated with opposed lateral photon beams for an additional 25 Gy (Fig-

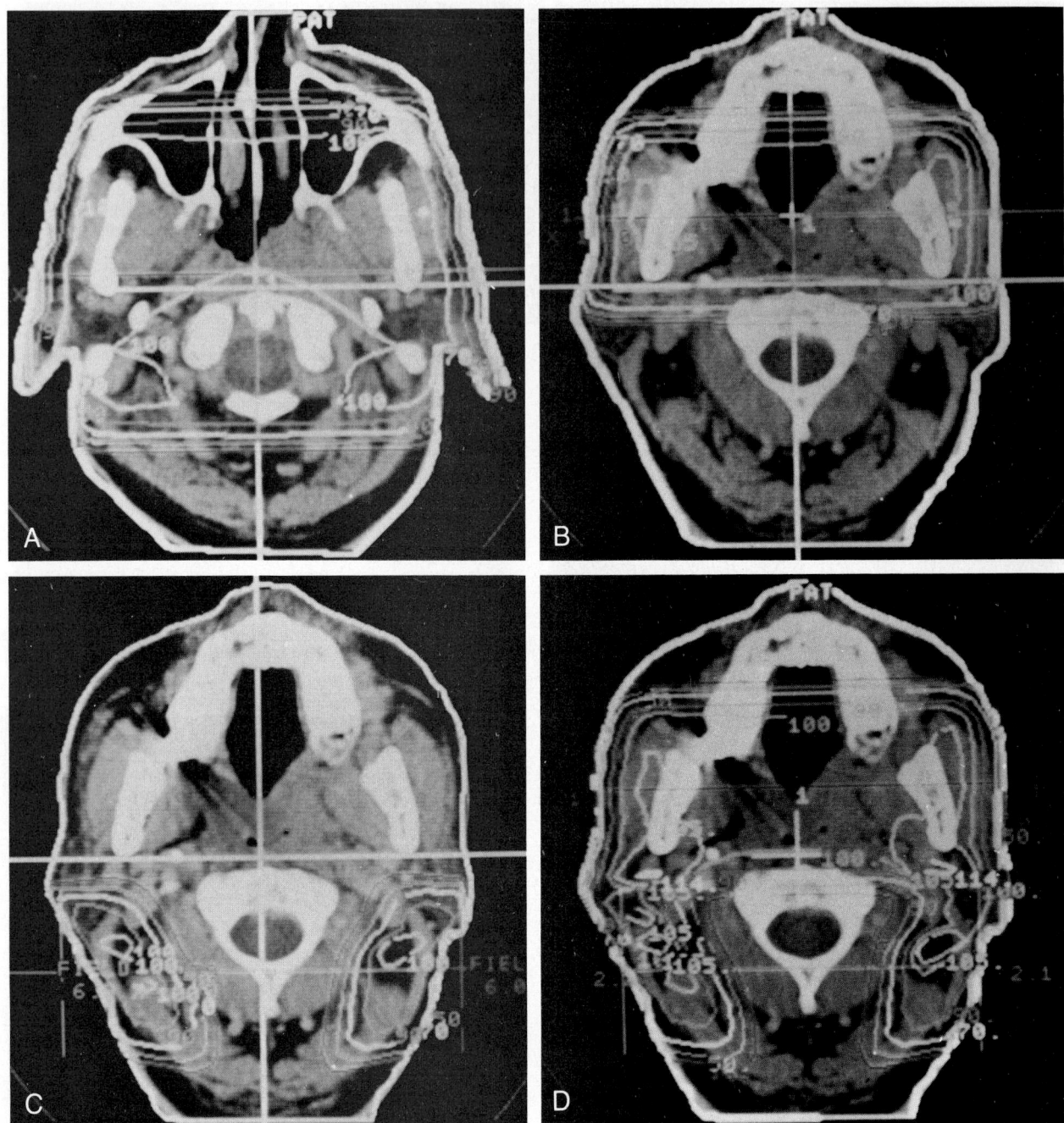

Figure XIII-1-27. Treatment plans for a head and neck case. The target area includes gross lesion and regional nodes, and is irradiated with opposed lateral photon fields to approximately 45 Gy (A). This is commonly followed by dividing the target volume into two regions, one anterior to the spinal canal, and the posterior neck nodes. The anterior target is irradiated with lateral opposed photon fields (B), and the neck nodes are irradiated with electron beams (C). A composite distribution is shown in (D).

ure XIII-1-27B). The posterior neck nodes are treated with electrons, matched to the photon fields, as shown in Figure XIII-1-27C. A composite dose distribution is shown in Figure XIII-1-27D.

Brachytherapy

Brachytherapy involves the use of sealed radioactive sources placed in proximity to the tumor (intracavitary technique) or within the tumor volume (interstitial treatment). In Greek, brachys means short, and brachytherapy implies a short distance between source and target.[71] Because the radioactive sources are placed in direct contact with the tumor, and the dose falls off as the square of the distance, the dose distribution is more localized than from external beam therapy. Brachytherapy has been used successfully in conjunction with external beam therapy in the curative treatment of tumors in a variety of primary sites, notably carcinoma of the cervix, bladder, breast, and head and neck cancers.

Brachytherapy was initially instituted with the use of naturally occurring isotopes such as radium or radon, but with the availability of artificially produced isotopes in the past few decades, has been practiced more frequently with cesium-137, iridium-198, and iodine-125. To illustrate one of the more common applications of brachytherapy, we describe the treatment technique of irradiation of carcinoma of the cervix with an intracavitary Fletcher-Suit applicator. Intracavitary insertion is the most commonly used brachytherapy technique, and can provide an excellent dose distribution for patients with early stage disease and normal anatomy.[49] The placement of this device is schematically shown in Figure XIII-1-28. The tubelike tandem is inserted into the uterus, and the colpostats are positioned against the lateral fornices. In general, the geometric distance of the isodose lines of radioactive material applied in this fashion is similar to the local spread of cervix cancer. The placement of the Fletcher Suit applicator is performed under anesthesia, with no sources loaded. After verification of proper placement, during which radiographs are taken with dummy sources, the radioactive sources are loaded into the applicator. This technique of

afterloading minimizes the radiation exposure to staff during the placement and positioning of the device. Representative dose distributions resulting from a standard loading of the applicator are shown in Figure XIII-1-29. A dose rate of approximately 40–50 cGy/hr at specified points is desirable. A boost dose of 25 Gy under this dose rate condition would require 50 hours of treatment, which is typical. Brachytherapy has also been used extensively in boosting the dose of tumors of the head and neck, breast, prostate, sarcomas, and recently the brain.[71] In these instances, plastic catheters are inserted into the target volume, guided by large gauge needles, followed by the placement of radioactive sources.

Newer Modalities for Radiation Therapy

While radiation therapy as sole treatment or in combination with chemotherapy and surgery is curative in a number of sites, a number of tumors are not well controlled. Investigational approaches to offer more effective radtiotherapy include techniques to increase the dose to tumor without increased morbidity through more effective dose localization, or through biologically more effective radiations such as high LET beams. These approaches will be discussed below.

Conformal Therapy

In the 1960's Takahashi proposed conformal therapy, a radiation therapy delivery technique, in which blocks, radiation field direction, and patient might be dynamically controlled during treatment in order to achieve a tightly con-

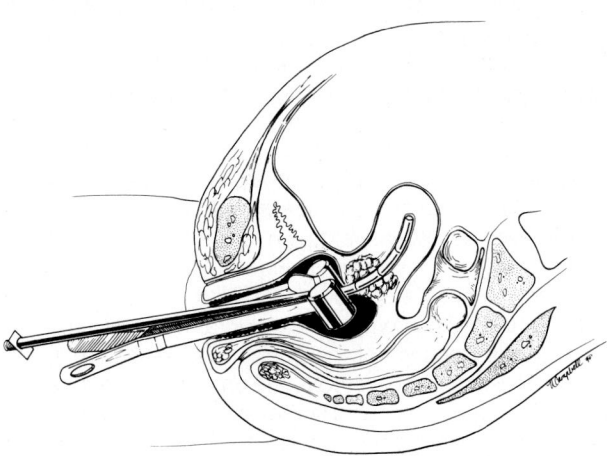

Figure XIII-1-28. Fletcher-Suit applicator. Typically, three sources are placed in the tandem (tube) and one source each into colpostats. (Photograph courtesy 3M Company.)

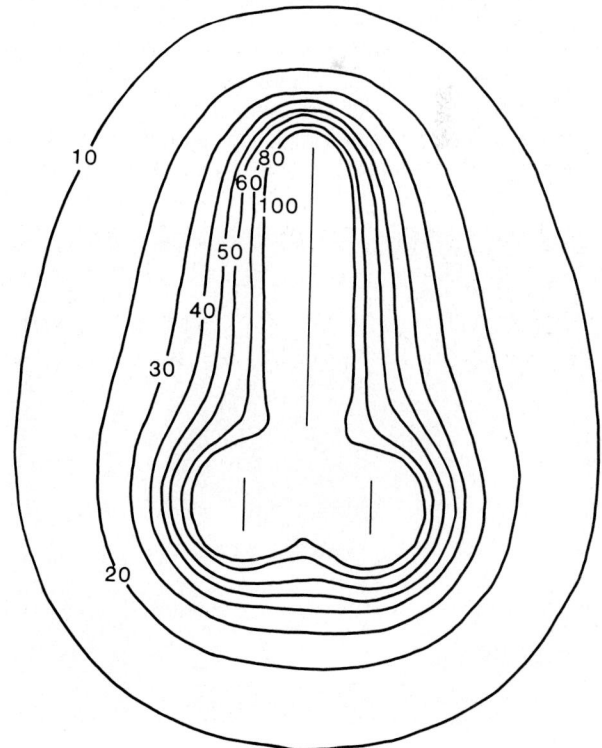

Figure XIII-1-29. Dose distribution from Fletcher Suit applicator, superimposed on anatomy, frontal view.

forming high dose region around the target volume.[138,139] More recently, three-dimensional computer simulations of conformal therapy[141] suggest that significant volumes of normal tissue can be spared. Conformal therapy is technically more feasible today with the wide availability of advanced imaging modalities and powerful minicomputers needed to calculate and control the complex movements of linear accelerator systems. Commercial availability of multivane collimators, which make feasible the numerous blocked fields needed to provide good dose localization (Figure XIII-1-30) and real time portal field imagers which verify the correct relationship between oblique non-coplanar radiation fields with computer calculations also make dynamic conformal therapy more feasible. Dynamic conformal radiation therapy is under study at a number of institutions, and is likely to be a technological focus for radiation therapy in the 1990's.

An example of the dose distributions achievable through computer controlled radiotherapy is shown in Figure XIII-1-31. In this example, the target is a sarcoma with a shell like volume in the left posterior retroperitoneal quadrant. The objective is to deliver a high dose to the target volume and to spare the bowel, spinal cord, and remaining kidney. In the implementation of this dynamic treatment plan, a collimator opening is modified at each gantry position.[22]

Charged Particle Therapy

If tumors are large, or are located near tissues damaged by relatively low doses of radiation, it becomes very difficult to deliver tumoricidal doses to the entire tumor volume without compromising the function of adjacent organs.[5,149] In some clinical situations, high energy proton beams are employed because of the ability to shape the high dose region in three dimensions.[4,149] Collimation of a proton beam in the plane perpendicular to the beam direction is achieved in the same manner as with photon beams; individually customized shielding blocks are used to shape the radiation portal. Treatment planning simulations suggest that greater doses may be delivered to a tumor with photon beams.[12]

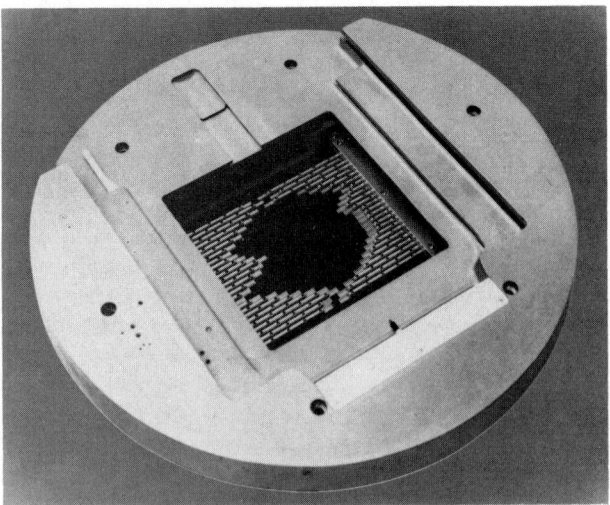

Figure XIII-1-30. Multivane (multileaf) collimator. Individual vanes are controlled by computer, and provide field shaping capabilities similar to blocks. (Photograph courtesy of Varian, Palo Alto, CA.)

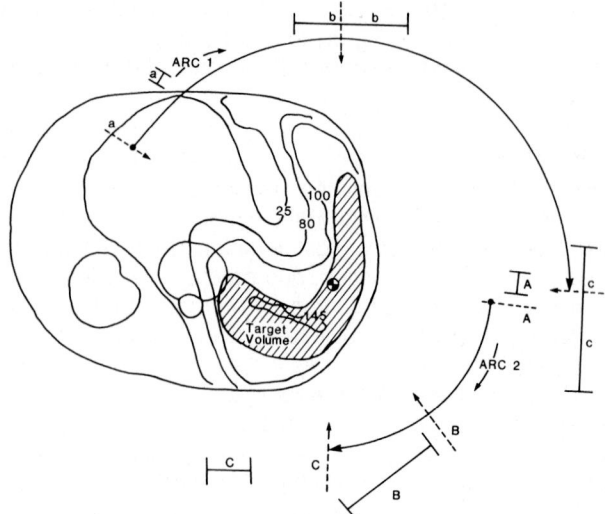

Figure XIII-1-31. Dose distribution from computer controlled radiotherapy. Two arcs are used to irradiate a sarcoma of the left posterior flank. Plan objective was to irradiate the target volume to a uniform dose and spare bowel, cord, and the remaining kidney.

However, because heavy charged particle beams have a well defined range in matter, a proton beam can also be shaped in depth, such that the Bragg peak region is stopped along the distal surface of a three dimensional target volume, with certain limitations imposed by different tissue densities.

Proton therapy has been shown to be successful in several clinical sites; examples are choroidal melanoma,[97] arteriovenous malformations (AVM's)[82] and juxtaspinal and base of skull tumors.[4,5] Over 1,300 patients have now been treated for choroidal melanomas at Harvard. In this technique, 70 Gy are delivered in five fractions. Munzenrider reported that the probability of retaining the eye after proton therapy is 89%, and that a large proportion of treated eyes retained useful vision.

Another site where success has been demonstrated for proton therapy has been in the treatment of chordomas and low grade chondrosarcomas of the base of the skull and cervical spine. Over 154 patients have been treated with proton therapy, with doses of approximately 69 Gy, a significantly higher dose than the usual 55 Gy delivered with photon beams. Local control rates were approximately 80% in comparison with 35% obtained with photon therapy. The higher dose delivered is a direct result of the depth dose properties of protons, which enable plans to be designed to treat the tumor and spare critical structures.

A representative treatment plan for proton irradiation of a juxtaspinal tumor[136] is shown in Figure XIII-1-32. The patient was found to have a chordoma causing a lytic destructive defect of C-2 with prominent extradural extension into the spinal canal. Because of the position of the lesion, a high dose is necessarily delivered to the anterior and right anterolateral region of the cord. The treatment plan included irradiation of the anterior portion of the tumor with lateral opposed proton fields, matched to a right posterior field to irradiate tumor excluded from the laterals. A total of 76 Gy equivalent was delivered to the tumor mass, with the mid-portion of the

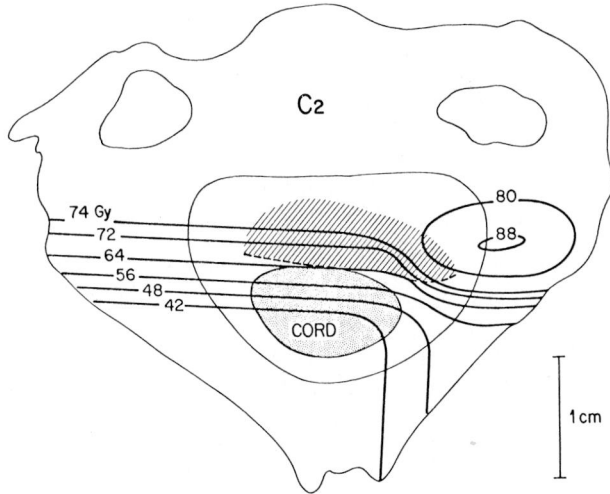

Figure XIII-1-32. Composite proton and photon beam dose distribution in the region of the cord. The darker area represents the tumor.

spinal cord receiving a dose less than 50 Gy. Setup verification films demonstrated a positional error of less than 1 mm.

Heavy charged particle radiotherapy with accelerated neon to argon ions has been under study for the past 15 years at the Lawrence Berkeley Laboratory.[18] Heavy charged particles not only have good Bragg peak dose localization properties, but also have high LET components in the beam, potentially important in radiotherapy. Light heavy ions such as helium have been used in the treatment of choroidal melanomas, juxtaspinal tumors and arteriovenous malformations.[17,18,42] Protocols are underway currently with heavier ions to study their efficacy in the treatment of advanced tumors of the lung and head and neck. Continued interest in particle therapy has resulted in a proposal for continued research into the 1990's.[135]

Neutron Therapy

In the past two decades, the NCI has supported the construction and development of isocentric neutron therapy centers. In the ensuing clinical trials, the biologic advantage of high LET radiations was assessed.[23,55,56] As described earlier, neutron beams are less dependent upon the presence of oxygen to effect cell kill. High LET particles induce irreparable and directly lethal changes in chromosome structure almost independent of cellular metabolism or biochemical state. For these reasons, tumors resistant to conventional radiotherapy are relatively more sensitive to high LET radiation. Neutron therapy is given as 2–3 fractions/week with fewer total fractions. Neutron irradiation may be beneficial for slowly proliferating tumors, hypoxic tumors and with inherently radioresistant tumors. Neutron irradiation has been shown to improve the local control and survival in patients with locally advanced prostate cancer[84,120] and unresectable salivary gland tumors.[54] Normal tissue tolerance to neutrons is dependent upon the RBE for that particular tissue and total dose delivered. In randomized clinical trials, irradiation of glioblastoma with neutron beams rather than photon beams

did not prolong survival. However, postmortem studies of the irradiated brain usually revealed widespread and often complete control of the tumor with an accompanying severe damage to normal brain. Dose searching with various mixtures of neutrons and photons failed to identify a therapeutic window in which normal tissue damage was acceptable.

Monoclonal Antibodies

Radioimmunotherapy utilizes antibodies with specificity against tumor associated antigens to carry radioactive nuclei to tumor. The concept was originally proposed in the late 1940's by Pressman, with renewed interest when Kohler and Millstein devised a technique to produce monoclonal antibodies in the quantities needed for therapy. A number of clinical trials using radiolabeled antibodies for both diagnosis and therapy have been conducted[40,46,85,86,88,102] and are reviewed in Section XVII-7.

Several aspects of radiolabeled monoclonal antibody therapy are appropriate to discuss within the context of radiation oncology. First, an understanding of the radiobiology of tumors and normal tissues is essential in the scientific study of this new modality. Traditionally, this scientific discipline has been an integral part of radiation oncology. Second, a detailed knowledge of the dosimetry of radiolabeled antibodies is essential in both the development and improvement of radioimmunotherapy. Radiation oncologists and therapy physicists have historically been involved with the development of dose calculations for therapeutic applications of radiation.

The dose to both tumor and normal tissues from radioimmunotherapy needs to be understood on a geometric scale ranging from tens of microns to centimeters. An example of this is the microdosimetry associated with alpha particle emitting radionuclides conjugated to antibodies. As the antibody/nuclide complex is distributed through the circulatory systems, it may preferentially accumulate in specific organs. Under these conditions, dose variations on the order of centimeters are important, and SPECT based treatment planning is needed. As the isotope distributes itself throughout the whole body, and irradiates radiation sensitive tissues such as bone marrow, whole body calculations become important. Within the next five years, techniques to calculate dose accurately for radioimmunotherapy appear to be within reach.

References

1. Adams, G. E.: Chemical Radiosensitization of Hypoxic Cells. Br. Med. Bull., 29:48, 1977.
2. Adler, L. P.: Consulting Reviewer, Oncology Overview, Selected Abstracts on *Newer Radionuclide Imaging Techniques in Oncology: PET and SPECT*, ICRBD, ICIC, US NCI Bethesda, MD.
3. Arundel, L. M., and Leith, J. T.: Effects on Nutritional State on Expression of Radiation Injury in Two Subpopulations Obtained from a Heterogeneous Colon Carcinoma. Int. J. Radiat. Oncol. Biol. Phys., 12:559, 1986.
4. Austin-Seymour, M., Munzenrider, J., Goitein, M., Verhey, L., Urie, M., Gentry, R., Birnbaum, S., Ruotolo, D., McManus, P., Skates, S., Ojemann, R. G., Rosenberg, A., Schiller, A., Koehler, A., and Suit, H. D.: Fractionated Proton Radiation Therapy of Chordoma and Low Grade Chondrosarcoma of the Base of Skull. J. Neurosurg., 70:13, 1989.
5. Austin-Seymour, M. M.: Particle Therapy, *In* Syllabus: Radiation Therapy in the 1990's. Rationale for the Emerging Modalities. Edited by E. J. Hall, and J. D. Cox. RSNA 1989 Categorical Course, pp. 35–38.
6. Barendsen, G. W., and Broerse, J. J.: Experimental Radiotherapy of a Rat Rhabdomyosarcoma with 15 MeV Neutrons and 300 kV X-rays. Europ. J. Cancer, 5:373, 1969.
7. Barranco, S. C., Romsdahl, N. M., and Humphrey, R. M.: The Radiation Response of Human Malignant Melanoma Cells Grown *In Vitro*. Cancer Res., 31:830, 1971.
8. Bedford, J. S., and Mitchell, J. B.: Dose Rate Effects in Synchronous Mammalian Cells in Culture. Radiat. Res., 54:316, 1973.

9. Bohr, V. A., Evans, M. K., and Fornace, A. J.: Biology of the DNA Repair and Its Pathogenetic Implications. Lab. Invest., 61:143, 1989.
10. Boothman, D. A., Bouvard, I., and Hughes, E. N.: Identification and Characterization of X-ray Induced Proteins in Human Cells. Cancer Res., 49:2871, 1989.
11. Boulis-Wassif, S., Langenhorst, B. L., and Hop, W. C. J.: The Contribution of Preoperative Radiotherapy in Borderline Operability Rectal Cancer. *In* Adjuvant Therapy Cancer. Edited by S. E. Jones, and S. E. Salmon. New York, Grune & Stratton, 1979, pp. 613-620.
11a. Broerse, J. J., Barendsen, G. W., and van Kersen, G. R.: Survival of Cultured Human Cells After Irradiation with Fast Neutrons of Different Energies in Hypoxic and Oxygenated Conditions. Int. J. Radiat. Biol. Relat. Stud. Phys. Chem. Med., 13:559, 1968.
12. Brown, A. P., Urie, M. M., Chisin, R., and Suit, H. D.: Proton Therapy for Carcinoma of the Nasopharynx: A Study in Comparative Treatment Planning. Int. J. Radiat. Oncol. Biol. Phys., 16:1607, 1989.
13. Bush, R. S., Jenkin, R. D. T., Allt, W. E. C., Beale, F. A., Beam, H., Dembo, A. J., and Pringle, J. F.: Definitive Evidence for Hypoxic Cells Influencing Cure in Cancer Therapy. Br. J. Cancer, 37(Suppl. III):302, 1978.
14. Byhardt, R. W., and Moss, W. T.: The Heart and Blood Vessels. *In* Radiation Oncology Rationale, Technique, Results. Edited by W. T. Moss, and J. D. Cox. St. Louis, Mosby, 1989, pp. 277–284.
15. Byhardt, R. W., Greenberg, M., and Cox, J. E.: Local Control of Squamous Carcinoma of the Oral Cavity and Oropharynx with 3 Versus 5 Treatment Fractions Per Week. Int. J. Radiat. Oncol. Biol. Phys., 2:415, 1977.
16. Carney, D. N., Mitchell, J. B., and Kinsella, T.: *In Vitro* Radiation and Chemotherapeutic Sensitivity of Established Cell Lines in Human Small Cell Lung Cancer and Large Cell Morphology Variants. Cancer Res., 43:2806, 1983.
17. Castro, J. R., Collier, J. M., Petti, P. L., Nowakowski, V., Chen, G. T., Lyman, J. T., Linstadt, D., Gauger, G., Gutin, P., Decker, M., Phillips, T. L., and Bakem, K.: Charged Particle Radiotherapy for Lesions Encircling the Brain Stem or Spinal Cord. Int. J. Radiat. Oncol. Biol. Phys., 17:477, 1989.
18. Castro, J. R., Chen, G. T. Y., and Blakely, E. A.: Current Considerations in Heavy Charged Particle Radiotherapy. Radiat. Res., 104:S263, 1985.
19. Chan, S. L. H., Thorner, P. S., Haddad, G., and Ling, V.: Immunohistochemical Detection of P-Glycoprotein: Prognostic Correlation in Soft Tissue Sarcoma of Childhood. J. Clin. Oncol., 8:689, 1990.
20. Chang, E. H., Pirollo, K. F., Zou, Z. Q., Cheung, H. Y., Lawler, E. L., Garner, R., White, E., Bernstein, W. B., Fraumeni, J. W., Jr., and Blattner, W. A.: Oncogenes in Radioresistant Non-Cancerous Skin Fibroblasts from a Cancer Prone Family. Science, 237:1036, 1987.
21. Chen, G. T. Y., Pelizzari, C. A., and Levin, D. N.: Image Correlation in Oncology. *In* Important Advances in Oncology, 1990, edited by V. T. DeVita, S. Hellman, and S. A. Rosenberg. Philadelphia, PA, J. B. Lippincott Co., 1990, pp. 131–141.
22. Chin, L. M., Kijewski, P. K., Svensson, G. K., and Bjarngard, B. E.: Dose Optimization with Computer-Controlled Gantry Rotation, Collimator Motion, and Dose-Rate Variation. Int. J. Radiat. Oncol. Biol. Phys., 9:723, 1983.
23. Cohen, L., and Awschalom, M.: Fast Neutron Radiation Therapy. Annl. Rev. Biophys. Bioeng., 11:359, 1982.
24. Cole, G., Schild, D., Lovett, S., and Mortimer, R. K.: Regulation of RAD-54 and RAD-52 Lac-Z Gene Fusions in Saccharomyes Cerevisiae in Response to DNA Damage. Mol. Cell. Biol., 7:1078, 1987.
25. Coleman, C. N., Bump, E. A., and Kramer, R. A.: Chemical Modifiers of Cancer Therapy. J. Clin. Oncol., 6:709, 1988.
26. Coleman, C. N., Wasserman, T. H., Urtasun, R. C., Halsey, J., Hirst, V. K., Hancock, S., and Phillips, T. L.: Phase I Trial of the Hypoxic Cells Radiosensitizer SR-2508: The Results of the Five to Six Week Drug Schedule. Int. J. Radiat. Oncol. Biol. Phys., 12:1105, 1986.
27. Coleman, C. N.: Modification of Radiotherapy by Radiosensitizers and Cancer Chemotherapy Agents. Semin. Oncol., 16:169, 1989.
28. Constine, L. S., Zagars, G., Rubin, P., and Kligerman, M. M.: Protection by WR-2721 of Human Bone Marrow Function Following Irradiation. Int. J. Radiat. Oncol. Biol. Phys., 12:1505, 1986.
29. Cox, J. D.: The Lung and Thymus. *In* Radiation Oncology, Rationale, Techniques, Results. Edited by W. T. Moss, and J. D. Cox. St. Louis, MO, C. V. Mosby, 1989, pp. 285–311.
30. Cox, J. D., and Kline, R. W.: Prostate Biopsies After Irradiation for Adenocarcinoma. Int. J. Radiat. Oncol. Biol. Phys., 9:229, 1983.
31. Dewey, W. C.: *In Vitro* Systems: Standardization of Endpoints. Int. J. Radiat. Oncol. Biol. Phys., 5:1165, 1979.
32. Dische, S., Anderson, P. J., Sealy, R., and Watson, E. R.: Carcinoma of the Cervix—Anaemia, Radiotherapy and Hyperbaric Oxygen. Br. J. Radiology, 56:251, 1983.
33. Eichorn, H. J.: Different Fractionation Schemes Tested by Histological Examination of Autopsy Specimens from Lung Cancer Patients. Br. J. Radiol., 54:132, 1981.
34. Elkind, M. M., and Sutton, H. G.: X-ray Damage and Recovery in Mammalian Cells in Culture. Nature, 184:1293, 1959.
35. Elkind, M. M.: Fractionated Dose Radiotherapy and Its Relationship to Survival Curve Shapes. Cancer Treat. Rev., 3:2, 1976.
36. Elkind, M. M., and Sutton, H.: Radiation Response of Mammalian Cells Grown in Culture I. Repair of X-ray Damage in Surviving Chinese Hamster Cells. Radiat. Res., 13:556, 1960.
37. Elkind, M. M., Sutton-Gilbert, H., Moses, W. B., Alescio, T., and Swan, R. B.: Radiation Response in Mammalian Cells in Culture V: Temperature Dependence of the Repair of X-ray Damage in Surviving Cells (Aerobic and Hypoxic). Radiat. Res., 25:359, 1965.
38. Elkind, M. M.: The Initial Part of the Survival Curve. Does It Predict Outcome of Fractionated Radiotherapy? Radiat. Res., 114:425, 1988.
39. Elkind, M. M., and Witmore, G. F.: Radiobiology of Cultured Mammalian Cells. New York, Gordon and Breach, 1967.
40. Epenetos, A. A., Britton, K. E., Mather, S., Shepherd, J., and Granowska, M.: Targeting of Iodine-123 Labeled Tumor-Associated Monoclonal Antibodies to Ovarian, Breast, and Gastrointestinal Tumors. Lancet, 2:999, 1982.
41. Evans, J. C., and Bergsio, P.: The Influence of Anemia on the Results of Radiotherapy in Carcinoma of the Cervix. Radiology, 84:709, 1965.
42. Fabrikant, J., Lyman, J. T., and Hosobuchi, Y.: Sterotactic Heavy Ion Bragg Peak Radiosurgery: Method for Treatment of Deep Arteriovenous Malformations. Br. J. Radiol., 57:479, 1984.
43. Fertil, B., and Malaise, E. P.: The Mean Activation Dose: Experimental versus Theoretical. Radiat. Res., 108:222, 1986.
44. Fischer, B., Bauer, M., Margolese, R., Poisson, R., Pilch, Y., Redmond, C., Fisher, E., Wolmark, N., Deutsch, M., Montague, E., Saffer, E., Wickerham, L., Lerner, H., Glass, A., Shibata, H., Deckers, P., Ketcham, A., Oishi, R., and Russell, I.: Five Year Results of Randomized Clinical Trial Comparing Total Mastectomy and Segmental Mastectomy with or without Radiation in the Treatment of Breast Cancer. N. Engl. J. Med., 312:665, 1985.
45. Fitzgerald, T. J., Daugherty, C., Kase, K., Rothstein, L. A., McKenna, M., and Greenberger, J. S.: Activated Human N-ras Oncogene Enhances X-irradiation Repair of Mammalian Cells *In Vitro* Less Effectively at Low Dose Rate. Implications for increased therapeutic ratio of low dose rate irradiation. Am. J. Clin. Oncol., 8:517, 1985.
45A. Fletcher, G. H.: Keynote Address: The Scientific Basis of the Present and Future Practice of Clinical Radiotherapy. Int. J. Radiat. Oncol. Biol. Phys., 9:1073, 1983.
46. Foon, K. A.: Monoclonal Antibodies in the Diagnosis and Treatment of Cancer. NeoRx Corp, Seattle, WA.
47. Fornace, A. J., Jr., Nebert, D. W., Hollander, M. C., Luethy, J. D., Papathanasiou M., Fargnoli, J., and Hollbrook, N. J.: Mammalian Genes Coordinately Regulated by Growth Arrest Signals and DNA Damaging Agents. Mol. Cell. Biol., 9:4196, 1989.
48. Fowler, J. F.: Review: Total Doses in Fractionated Radiotherapy. Int. J. Radiat. Biol., 2:103, 1984.
49. Fu, K. K., Sneed, P. K., Leibel, S. A., Nori, D., and Peschel, R. E.: Carcinoma of the Cervix in Interstitial Brachytherapy: Physical, Biological and Clinical Considerations, Interstitial Collaborative Working Group. Lowell L. Anderson, *et al.* Raven Press, 1990.
50. Gerwick, L. E., Kornblith, P., Burlett, P., Wang, J., and Seiger, S.: Radiation Sensitivity of Cultured Glioblastoma Cells. Radiol., 125:231, 1977.
51. Goitein, M., and Abrams, M.: Multidimensional Treatment Planning I: Delineation of Anatomy. Int. J. Radiat. Oncol. Biol. Phys., 9:777, 1983.
52. Goitein, M., Abrams, M., Rowell, D., Pollari, H., and Wiles, J.: Multidimensional Treatment Planning II: Beam's Eye View, Back Projection, and Projection Through CT Sections. Int. J. Radiat. Oncol. Biol. Phys., 9:789, 1983.
53. Grdina, D. J., and Sigdestad, C. P.: Radiation Protectors: The Unexpected Benefits. Drug Metabol. Rev., 20:13, 1989.
54. Griffin, T. W., Pajak, T. F., Laramiore, G. E., Duncan, W., Richter, M. P., Hendrickson, F. R., and Maor, M. H.: Neutron vs Photon Irradiation of Inoperable Salivary Gland Tumors: Results of an RTOG-MRC Cooperative Randomized Study. Int. J. Radiat. Oncol. Biol. Phys., 15:1085, 1988.
55. Griffin, T. W., Wambersie, A., Laramore, G., and Castro, J.: International Clinical Trials in Radiation Oncology. High LET: Heavy Particle Trials. Int. J. Radiat. Oncol. Biol. Phys., 14:S83, 1988.
56. Griffin, T. W.: Status of Clinical Trials with Neutron Irradiation. *In* Important Advances in Oncology, 1989. Edited by V. T. DeVita, S. Hellman, and S. A. Rosenberg. Philadelphia, J. B. Lippincott, 1989, pp. 221–234.
57. Guichard, M., Weichselbaum, R. R., Little, J. B., and Malaise, E. P.: Potential Lethal Damage as a Possible Determinant of Human Tumor Radiosensitivity. Radiother. Oncol., 1:263, 1984.
58. Hahn, G. M., Bagshaw, M. A., Evans, R. G., and Gordon, L. F.: Repair of Potentially Lethal Lesions in X-irradiated Density Inhibited Chinese Hamster Cells. Radiat. Res., 55:280, 1973.
59. Hahn, G. M., and Little, J. B.: Plateau Phase Cultures of Mammalian Cells: An *In Vitro* Model for Human Cancer. Curr. Top. Rad. Res., 8:39, 1972.
60. Hall, E. J.: Radiation Dose-rate: A Factor of Importance in Radiobiology and Radiotherapy. Br. J. Radiol., 45:81, 1972.
61. Hall, E. J.: Radiobiology for the Radiologist. Philadelphia, PA, J. B. Lippincott, 1988, pp. 17–160.
62. Hall, E. J., and Cox, J. D.: Syllabus. Radiation Therapy in the 1990's: Rationale for the Emerging Modalities. RSNA 1989 Categorical Course.
63. Hallahan, D. E., Spriggs, D. R., Beckett, M. A., Kufe, D. W., and Weichselbaum, R. R.: Increased Tumor Necrosis Factor Alpha mRNA After Cellular Exposure to Ionizing Radiation. Proc. Natl. Acad. Sci., 86:10104, 1989.
64. Hallahan, D. E., Beckett, M. A., Kufe, D., and Weichselbaum, R. R.: Interaction Between Recombinant Human Tumor Necrosis Factor and Radiation in 13 Human Tumor Cell Lines. Int. J. Radiat. Oncol. Biol. Phys., 19:69, 1990.
65. Hallahan, D. E., Sukhatme, V. P., Sherman, M. L., Virudachalam, S., Kufe, D. W., and Weichselbaum, R. R.: Protein Kinase C Mediates X-ray Inducibility of Nuclear Signal Transducers Egr-1 and c-jun. Proc. Natl. Acad. Sci. USA, 15:88, 1991.
65A. Hellman, S.: Cell Kinetics, Models and Cancer Treatment: Some Principles for the Radiation Oncologist. Radiology, 114:219, 1975.
66. Henk, J. M.: Does Hyperbaric Oxygen Have a Future in Radiation Therapy. Int. J. Radiat. Oncol. Biol. Phys., 7:1125, 1981.
67. Hierlihy, P., Jenkin, R. D. T., and Stryker, J. A.: Anemia as a Prognostic Factor in Cancer of the Cervix: A Preliminary Report. J. Cancer Med. Assoc., 100:1100, 1969.
68. Hermens, A. F., and Barendsen, G. W.: Changes of Cell Proliferation Characteristics Before and After X-irradiation. Europ. J. Cancer, 5:173, 1969.
69. Hilaris, B. S., and Martini, N.: Multimodality Therapy of Superior Sulcus Tumors. Adv. Pain. Res. Ther., 4:113, 1982.
70. Hill, R. P.: Experimental Radiotherapy. *In* The Basic Science of Oncology. Edited by I. F. Tannock, and R. P. Hill. Pergamon Press, Elmsford, NY, 1987.
71. Interstitial Brachytherapy: Physical, Biological and Clinical Considerations. Authored by the Interstitial Collaborative Working Group, Lowell L. Anderson, *et al.*, Raven Press, 1990.
72. Jeggo, P. A., and Kemp, L. M.: X-ray Sensitive Mutants of Chinese Hamster Ovary Cell Line. Isolation and Cross Sensitivity to Other DNA Damaging Agents. Mutat. Res., 112:313, 1983.
73. Johns, H. E., and Cunningham, J.: The Physics of Radiation Therapy. C. C Thomas Publishers, 1990.
74. Kallman, R. G.: Effects of Different Schedules of Dose Fractionation on the Oxygenation Status of a Transplantable Mouse Sarcoma. J. Natl. Cancer Inst., 44:369, 1970.
75. Kasid, U., Pfeifer, A., Brennan, T., Beckett, M., Weichselbaum, R. R., Dritschilo, A., and Mark, G. E.: Effect of Anti-sense c-raf-1 on Tumorigenecity and Radiation Sensitivity of a Human Squamous Cell Carcinoma. Science, 243:1354, 1989.
76. Kasid, U., Pfeifer, A., Weichselbaum, R. R., Dritschilo, A., and Mark, G. E.: The Raf-

Oncogene is Associated with a Radiation Resistant Human Laryngeal Cancer. Science, 237:1039, 1987.

77. Kelland, L. R., Bingle, L., Edwards, S., and Steele, G. G.: High Intrinsic Radiosensitivity of a Newly Established and Characterized Human Embryonal Rhabdomyosarcoma Cell Line. Br. J. Cancer, 59:160, 1989.

78. Khan, F. M.: The Physics of Radiation Therapy. Williams & Wilkins, 1984, Baltimore, MD.

79. Kinsella, T., Mitchell, J., Russo, A., Aiken, M., Morstyn, G., Hsu, S., Roland, J., and Gladstein, E.: Continuous Intravenous Infusions of Bromodeoxyuridine in a Clinical Radiosensitizer. J. Clin. Oncol., 2:1144, 1984.

80. Kinsella, T. J., Mitchell, J. B., McPherson, S., Miser, J., Triche, T., and Glatstein, E.: In Vitro Radiation Studies on Ewing Sarcoma Cell Lines and Human Bone Marrow: Application to the Clinical Use of Total Body Irradiation. Int. J. Radiat. Oncol. Biol. Phys., 10:10005, 1984.

81. Kinsella, T., Mitchell, J., Russo, A., Morstyn, G., and Gladstein, E.: The Use of Halogenated Thymine Analogs as Clinical Radiosensitizers. Rationale, Current Status in Future Prospects—Non-hypoxic Cell Sensitizers. Int. J. Radiat. Oncol. Biol. Phys., 10:1399, 1984.

82. Kjellberg, R. N., Hanamura, T., Davis, K. R., Lyons, S. L., and Adams, R. D.: Bragg Peak Proton Beam Therapy for Arteriovenous Malformations of the Brain. N. Engl. J. Med., 309:269, 1983.

83. Kligerman, M. M., Shaw, M. T., Slavik, M., and Yuhas, J. M.: Phase I Clinical Studies with WR-2721. Cancer Clin. Trials, 3:217, 1984.

84. Laramore, G. E., Griffin, T. W., and Maor, M. H.: Mixed Beam Radiation Therapy for Carcinoma of the Prostate: Results of a Randomized RTOG Study. Int. J. Radiat. Oncol. Biol. Phys., 11:1621, 1985.

85. Larson, S. M., Carrasquillo, J. A., Krohn, K. A., Brown, J. P., McGuffin, R. W., Ferens, J. M., Graham, M. M., Hill, L. D., Beaumier, P. L., Hellström, K. E., and Hellström, I.: Localization of 131-I Labeled p97-Specific Fab Fragments in Human Melanoma as a Basis for Radiotherapy. J. Clin. Invest., 72:2101, 1983.

86. Leibel, S. A., Klein, J. L., and Leichner, P. K.: Radioimmunotherapy: Current Results and Future Strategies. In Syllabus: Radiation Therapy in the 1990's: Rationale for the Emerging Modalities. Edited by E. J. Hall, and J. D. Cox. RSNA 1989 Categorical Course, pp. 39–44.

87. Levin, D. N., Hu, X., Tan, K., Galhotra, S., Pelizzari, C. A., Chen, G. T. Y., Beck, R. N., Chen, C. T., Cooper, M. D., Mullan, J. F., Hekmatpanah, J., and Spire, J. P.: The Brain: Integrated Three Dimensional Display of MRI and PET Images. Radiol., 172:783, 1989.

88. Leibel, S. A.: Targeted Radionuclides. In Innovations in Radiation Oncology. Edited by H. R. Withers, and L. J. Peters. Berlin/New York, Springer-Verlag, 1988, pp. 129–140.

89. Leith, G., Dexter, D. L., DeWyngaert, J., Zeman, E. M., Chu, M. Y., Calabresi, P., and Glicksman, A. S.: Differential Responses to X-irradiation of Subpopulations of Two Heterogeneous Human Carcinomas In Vitro. Cancer Res., 42:2556, 1982.

90. Lichter, A.: Clinical practice of modern radiation therapy treatment planning. In Syllabus: A Categorical Course in Radiation Therapy Treatment Planning. Edited by B. R. Paliway and M. L. Griem. RSNA, 1986.

91. Little, J. B., Hahn, G. M., Friendel, E., and Tubiana, M.: Repair of Potentially Lethal Radiation Damage In Vitro and In Vivo. Radiology, 106:689, 1973.

92. Looser, K. G., Shah, J. P., and Strong, E. W.: The Significance of Possible Margins in Surgically Resected Epidermoid Carcinoma. Head Neck Surg., 1:107, 1978.

93. Million, R. R., Cassissi, N. J., and Clark, J. R.: Cancer of the Head and Neck. In Cancer Principles and Practice of Oncology. Edited by V. T. DeVita, S. Hellman, and S. A. Rosenberg. Philadelphia, PA, J. B. Lippincott, 1989, pp. 488–580.

94. Mitchell, J. B., Morstyn, G., Russo, A., Kinsella, T. J., Fornance, A., McPherson, S., and Gladstein, E.: Changes of Cell Proliferation Characteristics Before and After X-irradiation. Int. J. Radiat. Oncol. Biol. Phys., 10:1447, 1983.

95. Mohan, R., Barest, G., Brewster, L. J., Chui, C. S., Kutcher, G. J., Laughlin, J. S., and Fuks, Z.: A Comprehensive Three Dimensional Radiation Treatment Planning System. Int. J. Radiat. Oncol. Biol. Phys., 15:481, 1988.

96. Moulder, J. E., and Rockwell, S.: Hypoxic Fractions of Solid Tumors: Experimental Techniques, Methods of Analysis, and a Survey of Existing Data. Int. J. Radiat. Oncol. Biol. Phys., 10:695, 1984.

97. Munzenrider, J. E., Gragoudas, E. S., McNulty, P., and Seddon, J. M.: Uveal Melanoma: Conservative Treatment with Radiation Therapy. In Innovations in Radiation Oncology. Edited by H. R. Withers, and L. J. Peters. Berlin/New York, Springer-Verlag, 1988, pp. 41–51.

98. Nagy, B., Dale, P. J., and Grdina, D. J.: Protection Against Cis-diamminedichloroplatinum Cytotoxicity and Mutagenicity in V79 Cells by 2[(aminopropyl)amino]ethanethiol. Cancer Res., 46:1132, 1986.

99. Neta, R., Oppenheim, J. J., and Douches, S. D.: Interdependence of the Radioprotective Effects of Human Recombinant Interleukin 1 Alpha Tumor Necrosis Factor Alpha, Granulocyte Colony Macrophage Colony Stimulating Factor. J. Immunol., 140:108, 1988.

100. Nilsson, S., Carlson, J., Larson, E., and Ponten, J.: Survival of Irradiated Giloma Cells Studied with a New Cloning Technique. Int. J. Radiat. Biol., 37:267, 1980.

101. Oppenheim, J. J., Neta, R., Tiberghien, P., Gress, R., Kenny, J. J., and Longo, D. L.: IL-1 Enhances Survival of Lethally Irradiated Mice Treated with Allogenic Bone Marrow Cells. Blood, 74:2257, 1989.

102. Order, S. E., Stillwagon, G. B., Klein, J. L., Leichner, P. K., Siegelman, S. S., Fishman, E. K., Ettinger, D. S., Haulk, T., Kopher, K., Finney, K., Surdyke, M., Self, S., and Leibel, S.: Iodine 131 Antiferritin, A New Treatment Modality in Hepatoma: A Radiation Therapy Oncology Group Study. J. Clin. Oncol., 3:1573, 1985.

103. Overgaard, J., SandHansen, H., Jorgensen, K., and Hjelm-Hansen, M.: Primary Radiotherapy of Larynx and Pharynx Carcinoma—An Analysis of Some Factors Influencing Local Control and Survival. Int. J. Radiat. Oncol. Biol. Phys., 12:515, 1986.

104. Overgaard, J., Hjelm-Hansen, M., Johansen, L. V., and Andersen, A. P.: Comparison of Conventional and Split-Course Radiotherapy as Primary Treatment in Carcinoma of the Larynx. Acta Oncol., 27:147, 1988.

105. Paliwal, B. R., and Griem, M. L.: Syllabus: A Categorical Course in Radiation Therapy Treatment Planning, RSNA, 1986.

106. Patt, H. M., Tyree, E. B., Straube, R. L., Smith, D. E., and Scystein, E.: Protection Against X-radiation. Science, 110:213, 1949.

107. Patt, H. M.: Protective Mechanisms in Ionizing Radiation Injury. Physiol. Rev., 33:35, 1953.

108. Peckham, M. J.: In The Biological Basis of Radiotherapy, Edited by G. G. Steele, and G. E. Adams, New York, Elsevier, 1983, pp. 1–15.

109. Pelizzari, C. A., Chen, G. T. Y., Spelbring, D., Weichselbaum, R. R., and Chen, C. T.: Three-dimensional Registration of CT, PET and or MRI Images of the Brain. J. Comp. Asst. Tomogr., 13:20, 1989.

110. Peters, L. J., Brock, W. A., and Travis, E. L.: Radiation Biology at Clinically Relevant Fractions, In Important Advances in Oncology. Philadelphia, PA, J. B. Lippincott, 1990, pp. 65–83.

111. Phillips, R. A., and Tolmach, L. J.: Repair of Potentially Lethal Damage in X-irradiated HeLa Cells. Radiat. Res., 29:413, 1966.

112. Pirollo, K. F., Garner, R., Yuan, Y. S., Blattner, W. A., and Chang, E. H.: Raf Involvement in the Simultaneous Genetic Transfer of the Radioresistant and Transforming Phenotypes. Int. J. Radiat. Biol., 55:783, 1989.

113. Potter, D. A., Glenn, J., Kinsella, T., Glatstein, E., Lack, E. E., Restrepo, C., White, D. E., Seipp, C. A., Wesley, R., and Rosenberg, S. A.: Patterns of Recurrence in Patients with High-Grade Soft-Tissue Sarcomas. J. Clin. Oncol., 3:353, 1985.

114. Powers, W. E., and Palmer, L. A.: Biological Basis of Preoperative Radiotherapy. Amer. J. Roentgenol., 102:176, 1968.

115. Puck, T. T., and Marcus, P. I.: Action of X-rays on Mammalian Cells. J. Exp. Med., 103:653, 1956.

116. Quillaret, P., Frelet, G., Nguyen, U. D., and Hofnung, M.: Detection of Ionizing Radiations with SOS Chemotest. Mutat. Res., 216:251, 1989.

117. Quilty, P. M., and Duncan, W.: The Influence of Hemoglobin Level on the Regression and Long Term Local Control of Transitional Cell Carcinoma of the Bladder Following Photon Irradiation. Int. J. Radiat. Oncol. Biol. Phys., 12:1735, 1986.

118. Rasey, J., and Nelson, N. J.: Discrepancies Between Patterns of Potentially Lethal Damage Repair in the RIF-1 Tumor System In Vitro and In Vivo. Radiat. Res., 93:157, 1986.

119. Rubin, P. J., Cooper, R., and Phillips, T. L.: Radiation Biology and Radiation Oncology Syllabus (Set RT 1: Radiation Oncology). Chicago, American College of Radiology, 1975.

120. Russell, K., Laramore, G. E., Krall, J. M., Thomas, F. J., Maor, M. H., Hendrickson, F. R., Krieger, J. N., and Griffin, T. W.: Eight Years Experience with Neutron Radiotherapy in the Treatment of Stages C and D Prostate Cancer: Updated Results of the RTOG 7704 Randomized Clinical Trial. Prostate, 11:183, 1987.

121. Rustowski, J., and Kupsc, W.: Factors Influencing the Results of Radiotherapy in Cases of Inoperable Endometrial Cancer. Gynecol. Oncol., 14:185, 1982.

122. Schad, L. R., Boesecke, R., Schlegel, W., Hartmann, G. H., Sturm, V., Strauss, L. G., and Lorenz, W. J.: Three-dimensional Image Correlation of CT, MR, and PET Studies in Radiotherapy Treatment Planning of Brain Tumors. J. Compt. Asst. Tomogr., 11:948, 1987.

123. Schwartz, J. L., Mustafi, R., Beckett, M. A., and Weichselbaum, R. R.: Prediction of Human Squamous Cell Carcinoma Line Radiosensitivity by DNA Filter Elution Measurements. Radiat. Res., 123:1, 1990.

124. Seeger, R. C., Brodeur, G. M., Sather, H., Dalton, A., Siegel, S. E., Wong, K. Y., and Hammond, D.: Association of Multiple Copies of the N-myc Oncogene with Rapid Progression of Neuroblastomas. N. Engl. J. Med., 313:1111, 1985.

125. Sherman, M. L., Datta, R., Hallahan, D. E., Weichselbaum, R. R., and Kufe, D. W.: Ionizing Radiation Regulates Expression of the c-jun Proto-oncogene. Proc. Natl. Acad. Sci., 87:5663, 1990, USA.

126. Sinclair, W. K.: Cyclic X-ray Responses in Mammalian Cells In Vitro. Radiat. Res., 33:620, 1968.

127. Sklar, M. D.: The Ras-Oncogenes Increase the Intrinsic Resistance of NIH-3T3 Cells to Ionizing Radiation. Science, 239:645, 1988.

128. Steele, G. G., and Peckham, M. J.: Exploitable Mechanisms and Combined Radiotherapy and Chemotherapy: The Concept of Additivity. Int. J. Radiat. Oncol. Biol. Phys., 5:85, 1979.

129. Steele, G. G.: Terminology in the Description of Drug Radiation Interactions. Int. J. Radiat. Oncol. Biol. Phys., 5:1145, 1979.

130. Stein, B., Rahmsdorf, F., Steffen, A., Litfin, M., and Herrlich, P.: UV-induced DNA Damage is an Intermediate Step in UV-induced Expression of Human Immunodeficiency Virus Type I, Collagenase, c-fos, and Mettalothionein. Mol. Cell. Biol., 9:5169, 1989.

131. Stevens, K. R.: The Stomach and Intestines. In Radiation Oncology, Rationale, Techniques. Edited by W. T. Moss, and J. D. Cox. St. Louis, C. V. Mosby, 1989, pp. 362–408.

132. Stewart, R., and Fajardo, L. F.: Dose Response in Human and Experimental Radiation-induced Heart Disease. Radiology, 99:403, 1971.

133. Stomato, T. D., Weinstein, R., Giaccia, A., and MacKinzie, L.: Isolation of Cell Cycle Dependent Gamma Ray Sensitive Chinese Hamster Ovary Cells. Somat. Cell Genet., 9:165, 1983.

134. Strandqvist, M.: Studien Uber Die Kumulative Wirkung Der Rontgenstrahlen Bei Fraktionierung. Acta Radiol., (Suppl) 55:1, 1944.

135. Suit, H. D., Griffin, T. W., Castro, J. R., and Verhey, L. J.: Particle Radiation Therapy Research Plan. Amer. J. Clin. Oncol., 11:330, 1988.

136. Suit, H. D., Goitein, M., Munzenrider, J., Verhey, L., Davis, K. R., Koehler, A., Linggood, R., and Ojemann, R. G.: Definitive Radiation Therapy for Chordoma and Chondrosarcoma of Base of Skull and Cervical Spine. J. Neurosurg., 56:377, 1982.

137. Suit, H., and Witte, R.: Radiation Dose Fractionation and Tumor Control Probability. Radiat. Res., 29:267, 1966.

138. Takahashi, S.: Conformation Radiotherapy. Rotation Techniques as Applied to Radiography and Radiotherapy of Cancer. Acta Radiol., 242:1, 1965.

139. Takahashi, S.: Conformation Radiotherapy. Acta Radiol. (Diag), S242, 1965.

140. Taylor, S. G., IV, Murthy, A. K., Showel, J. L., Caldarelli, D. D., Hutchinson, J. C., Jr., Holinger, L. D., Kramer, T., and Kiel, K.: Concomitant Therapy with Infusion at Cisplatin and 5-Fluorouracil Plus Radiation in Head and Neck Cancer. NCI Mono., 6:343, 1985.

141. Ten Haken, R. K., Perez-Tamayo, C., Tesser, R. J., McShan, D. L., Fraass, B. A., and Lichter, A. S.: Boost Treatment of the Prostate Using Shaped Fixed Fields. Int. J. Radiat. Oncol. Biol. Phys., 16:193, 1989.

142. Thames, H. D., and Henry, J. H.: Fractionation in Radiotherapy. London: Taylor & Francis, 1987.

143. Thomlinson, R. H., and Gray, L. H.: The Histological Structure of Some Human Lung Cancers and the Possible Implications for Radiotherapy. Br. J. Cancer, 9:539, 1955.

144. Thomlinson, R. H.: In Modern Trends in Radiotherapy, Vol. 1, Edited by T. J. Deelay, and C. A. P. Wood. London, Butterworths Scientific Publications, 1967, pp. 52–72.

145. Thompson, L. H., and Suit, H. D.: Proliferative Kinetics of X-irradiated Mouse L Cells Studies with Time Lapsed Photography. Int. J. Radiat. Biol., 13:391, 1967.

146. Tucker, S.: Is the Mean Inactivation Dose a Good Measure of Cell Radiosensitivity? Radiat. Res., 105:18, 1986.

147. vander Werf-Messing, B.: Carcinoma of the Urinary Bladder Treated by Preoperative Radiation. Int. J. Radiat. Oncol. Biol. Phys., 8:1849, 1982.

148. Van Putten, L. M.: Tumor Reoxygenation During Fractionated Radiotherapy. Europ. J. Cancer, 4:173, 1968.

149. Verhey, L., and Munzenrider, J. E.: Proton Beam Therapy. Annl. Rev. Biophys. Bioeng., 11:331, 1982.

150. Vikram, B., Strong, E. W., Shah, S. P., and Spiro, R.: Failure at the Primary Site Following Multimodality Treatment in Advanced Head and Neck Cancer. Head Neck Surg., 6:720, 1984.

151. Vokes, E. E., Panje, W. R., Weichselbaum, R. R., Schilsky, R. L., Moran, W. J., Awan, A. M., and Guarnieri, C. M.: Hydroxyurea, Fluorouracil, and Concomitant Radiotherapy and Poor Prognosis: Head and Neck Cancer. A Phase I, II, Study. J. Clin. Oncol., 7:761, 1989.

152. Vokes, E. E., and Weichselbaum, R. R.: Concomitant Chemo-radiotherapy: Rationale and Clinical Experience in Patients with Solid Tumors. J. Clin. Onc., 8:911 1990.

153. Walker, G. C.: Mutagenesis and Inducible Responses to Deoxyribonucleic Acid Damage in Escherichia Coli. Microbiol. Rev., 48:60, 1984.

154. Wang, C. C.: Cancer of the Head and Neck. In Clinical Radiation Oncology. Edited by C. C. Wang. PSG Publishing. Littleton MA, 1988, pp. 120–179.

155. Weichselbaum, R. R., Dahlberg, W., and Little, J. B.: Inherently Radioresistant Cells Exist in Some Human Tumors. Proc. Natl. Acad. Sci., USA, 82:4732, 1985.

156. Weichselbaum, R. R., Nove, J., and Little, J. B.: X-ray Sensitivity of 53 Human Diploid Fibroblast Cell Strains from Patients with Characterized Genetic Disorders. Cancer Res., 40:920, 1980.

157. Weichselbaum, R. R., Nove, J., and Little, J. B.: X-ray Sensitivity of Human Tumor Cells In Vitro. Int. J. Radiat. Oncol. Biol. Phys., 6:437, 1980.

158. Weichselbaum, R. R., Beckett, M. A., Vijayakumar, S., Simon, M. A., Awan, A. M., Nachman, J., Panje, W. R., Goldman, M. E., Tybor, A. G., Moran, W. J., Vokes, E. E., Ahmed-Swan, S., and Farhangi, E.: Radiobiological Characterization of Head and Neck and Sarcoma Cells Derived from Patients Prior to Radiotherapy. Int. J. Radiat. Oncol. Biol. Phys., 19:313, 1990.

159. Weichselbaum, R. R., Little, J. B., and Nove, J.: Response of Human Osteosarcoma In Vitro to Irradiation. Evidence for Unusual Cellular Repair Activity. Int. J. Radiat. Biol., 31:295, 1977.

160. Weichselbaum, R. R., Schmit, A., and Little, J. B.: Cellular Repair Factors Influencing Radiocurability of Human Malignant Tumors. Br. J. Cancer, 45:10, 1982.

161. Weichselbaum, R. R., and Beckett, M. A.: The Maximum Recovery Potential of Human Tumor Cells May Predict Clinical Outcome in Radiotherapy. Int. J. Radiat. Oncol. Biol. Phys., 13:709, 1987.

162. Weichselbaum, R. R., Nove, J., and Little, J. B.: Deficient Recovery from Potentially Lethal Radiation Damage in Ataxia Telangiectasia and Xeroderma Pigmentosum. Nature, 27:261, 1978.

163. Weichselbaum, R. R., Beckett, M. A., Schwartz, J. L., and Dritschilo, A.: Radioresistant Tumor Cells are Present in Head and Neck Carcinomas that Recur After Radiotherapy. Int. J. Radiat. Oncol. Biol. Phys., 15:575, 1988.

164. Weichselbaum, R. R.: The Role of DNA Repair Processes in the Response of Human Tumors to Fractionated Radiotherapy. Int. J. Radiat. Oncol. Biol. Phys., 10:1127, 1984.

165. Weichselbaum, R. R., Rotmensch, J., Ahmed-Swan, S., and Beckett, M. A.: Radiobiological Characterization of 53 Human Tumor Cell Lines. Int. J. Radiat. Biol., 56:553, 1989.

166. Weichselbaum, R. R., Dahlberg, W., Beckett, M. A., Karrison, T., Miller, D., Clark, J., and Ervin, T. J.: Radiation Resistant and Repair Proficient Human Tumor Cells May Be Associated with Radiotherapy Failure in Head and Neck Cancer Patients. Proc. Natl. Acad. Science, USA, 83:2683, 1986.

167. Weinert, T. A., and Hartwell, L. H.: The RAD-9 Gene Controls the Cell Cycle Response to DNA Damage in Saccharomyces Cervisiae. Science, 241:317, 1988.

168. Withers, H. R.: In Principles and Practice of Radiation Oncology. Edited by C. A. Perez, and L. W. Brady. J. B. Lippincott, Philadelphia, PA, 1987, pp. 67–98.

168A. Withers, H. R.: Recovery and Repopulation in vivo by Mouse Skin Epithelial Cells During Fractionated Irradiation. Radiat. Res., 32:227, 1967.

169. Withers, H. R.: Regeneration of Intestinal Mucosa After Irradiation. Cancer, 28:78, 1971.

169A. Withers, H. R.: The Dose-Survival Relationship for Irradiation of Epithelial Cells of Mouse Skin. Br. J. Radiol., 40:187, 1967.

170. Withers, H. R., Hunter, N., Barkley, H. T., and Reid, B. O.: Radiation Survival and Regeneration Characteristics of Spermatogenic Stem Cells of Mouse Testis. Radiat. Res., 57:88, 1974.

171. Witte, L., Fuks, Z., Haimovitz-Friedman, A., Vlodavsky, I., Goodman, D. S., and Eldor, A.: Effects of Radiation on the Release of Growth Factors from Cultured Bovine, Porcine, and Human Endothelial Cells. Cancer Res., 49:5066, 1989.

172. Woloschak, G. E., Liu, G. M. C., Jones, S., and Jones, C.: Modulation of Gene Expression in Syrian Hamster Embryo Cells Following Ionizing Radiation. Cancer Res., 50:339, 1990.

173. Yamauchi, N., Kuriyama, H., Wantanabe, N., Neda, H., Maeda, M., and Nittus, Y.: Intracellular Hydroxyl Radical Production Induced by Recombinant Human Tumor Necrosis Factor and Its Implication in the Killing of Tumor Cells In Vitro. Cancer Res., 49:1671, 1989.

174. Yuhas, J. M., and Storer, J. B.: Differential Chemoprotection of Normal and Malignant Tissues. J. Natl. Cancer Inst., 42:331, 1969.

175. Yuhas, J. M.: A More General Role for WR-2721 in Cancer Therapy. Br. J. Cancer, 41:832, 1980.

176. Zimmerman, R. J., Chan, A., and Leadon, S.: Oxidative Damage in Murine Tumor Cells Treated In Vitro by Recombinant Human Tumor Necrosis Factor. Cancer Res., 49:1644, 1989.

XIII-2

Principles of Hyperthermia

G. M. Hahn
D. S. Kapp
R. W. Carlson

Historical Perspective

Hyperthermia as a methodology to treat cancer has a long history. Many Greek and Roman physicians thought that if they could simply control body temperature, they could cure all diseases. Very likely this included cancer, because the pathology of tumor development had been described in the Greek literature. The modern use of this modality is based to a large extent on the well documented occurrences of spontaneous remissions in patients who had febrile episodes, and on extensive laboratory data obtained over the last few years. Initial attempts to take advantage of the anticancer activity of hyperthermia involved the use of pyrogens for the induction of high fevers in patients with cancer. Perhaps the best known of these studies were those of Coley in 1893,[8] who utilized bacterial toxins to raise the temperature in patients with osteosarcomas and soft tissue sarcomas. While he reported quite impressive results, it is not clear whether these involved primarily hyperthermia or, possibly, nonspecific host-immune responses. Perhaps more importantly, recent labortory studies have demonstrated that hyperthermia can inactivate cells, cause tumor regression, cause normal tissue damage, potentiate the effects of radiation therapy, and also enhance the action of many anticancer drugs.[12,15,31]

Biological Rationale

Heat Alone

The responses of tumors to hyperthermia involve both cellular and host-related factors. Experimentally it is frequently not easy to separate these. When cells are exposed to elevated temperatures, they are inactivated in a time- and temperature-dependent fashion. Inactivation starts at 40–41°C, at least for murine cells and tumors. At these low temperatures, cell inactivation continues for only a few hours. Beyond that time, the surviving cells appear resistant to prolonged exposure at these temperatures. Studies have shown that this is not a selection of heat-resistant subpopulations, but results from the induction of a temporary resistance to heat. This transient phenomenon is referred to as thermotolerance.

Above 43°C, for most rodent lines, inactivation is exponential with time, and thus resembles cell inactivation by ionizing radiations. Human cells tend to be more resistant, and this temperature threshold, in some human tumor cell lines, occurs at temperatures as high as 44.5°C. Hence, thermotolerance can develop during treatment of human lesions, since tumor temperatures only rarely exceed 44°C. At even higher temperatures, thermotolerance does not develop, but if the cells are returned to 37°C, within a few hours the surviving cells do become resistant.

The development of thermotolerance is accompanied by the preferential synthesis (or de novo synthesis) of a series of proteins referred to as heat shock proteins. These molecules are the subject of intense study, because of their importance in normal cell function and in various disease states.[30] In terms of survival, the effects of thermotolerance can be quite dramatic. For example, an exposure of 45 min to 45°C kills approximately 99.9% of Chinese hamster cells. If, however, such heating is preceded 4 h earlier by an exposure of 20 min at 45°C, then the 45 min 45°C treatment leaves about 50% of the cells as survivors. Clearly, thermotolerance must be taken into account when scheduling fractionated heat treatments of patients. Thermotolerance can also greatly modify the cells' response to some drugs, to heat and x-irradiation, but does not seem to have much effect on the cells' response to x-irradiation alone.

In addition to thermotolerance, there is also great variability in genetically determined heat-sensitivity of tumor cells. Heat-resistant variants of B16 melanoma cells and of a radiation-induced fibrosarcoma (RIF-1) have been isolated and characterized.[1,16] Very likely, many human neoplasms also contain subpopulations of resistant cells. The frequency of occurrence of such cells appears to be very low, however. There is no evidence of cross-resistance between heat-sensitivity and x-irradiation or most anticancer drugs. Hence, genetically heat-resistant cells may be of little importance during combination treatments with heat and radiation or chemotherapy.

Interestingly, when malignant cells and normal cells are tested under identical culture conditions, there is little or no difference in their response to heat. The old notion that cancer cells are necessarily more heat-sensitive than their normal counterparts does not appear to be correct.

The microenvironment of cells in solid tumors is particularly conducive to heat sensitivity, a finding that may be important in the treatment of such tumors. The combination of low pH, low oxygen tension, and lack of glucose and other nutrients tends to make cells extremely responsive to elevated temperatures.[15]

Heat and X-Irradiation

Heat enhances the cytotoxicity of X-rays, both in a super-additive and a complementary fashion. Superadditivity, that is, the increased cytotoxicity observed over that which would be expected on the basis of additivity of the two treatments, is maximum when these are given simultaneously. It decays with time when the treatments are separated more than one or two hours or, in some systems, even less. Complementarity results from the not unexpected findings that cells particularly resistant to radiation tend to be sensitive to heat. Lack of sufficient blood flow causes cells to become hypoxic, and hence, radiation resistant. This lack of blood flow also causes low pH and low nutrient availability, making the hypoxic cells highly susceptible to killing by hyperthermia. An additional feature of complementarity is related to the cells' age response. Cells in the late S-phase, i.e., cells that are in process of completing DNA replication, tend to be quite resistant to x-irradiation. These same cells, however, are particularly sensitive to heat. Overall, the results suggest strongly that tumors, providing they can be heated adequately, should be susceptible to the combination of x-irradiation and heat.[12,15,31]

Heat and Drugs

When cells are exposed to drugs at elevated temperatures, their response is frequently very different from that seen at 37°C. Drugs whose rate-limiting reaction is primarily chemical (i.e., not involving enzymes) would, on thermodynamic grounds, be expected to be more efficient at higher temperatures. The rates of alkylation of DNA, or of conversion of a nonreactive to a reactive species, can be expected to increase as the temperature increases. Tissue culture studies have shown this to be true for the nitrosoureas and cisplatin. For other drugs, there appears to be a threshold at or near 43°C. Below that temperature, drug activity is only mildly enhanced. At higher temperatures, however, cell killing proceeds at a greatly enhanced rate. Two such drugs are bleomycin and doxorubicin. For still other drugs, including most of the antimetabolites, cytotoxicity is not enhanced at elevated temperatures. Indeed, for the topoisomerase inhibitors, drug activity may be reduced at elevated temperatures. In addition, low pH can also enhance drug activity. The nitrosoureas and cisplatin are far more effective at low (~6.5) pH than they are at neutral pH. Tissue culture and animal studies indicate that heat and drug combinations should be quite effective against some tumors. The in vivo experiments show that effectiveness of such treatments can be further enhanced by blood flow manipulations to reduce pH.[18]

Physics and Physiology of Heating

Heating Methodologies

Whole Body Heating. Three major methods are now available to achieve reproducible, controlled whole body hyperthermia: thermal conduction (surface heating), extracorporeal induction, and radiant or electromagnetic induction.[28,37,47] The tolerance of liver and of brain limits the maximum temperature using whole body hyperthermia to 41.8–42.0°C, but this temperature may be maintained for several hours. All three methods of systemic hyperthermia require general anesthesia or sedation of the patient, careful monitoring for safety, and are all technically demanding.

Methods of whole body hyperthermia induction by direct thermal conduction have been developed using heated circulating water suits, heating blankets, or hot wax baths. Heating for 2–3.5 hours is required to achieve a core temperature of 41.8–42.0°C. Because the body surface is covered in this technique, access to temperature probes, EKG leads, and intravenous sites are limited. The use of extracorporeal induction requires both a high-flow arteriovenous shunt for vascular access and the availability of an extracorporeal heat exchanger. Extracorporeal heat exchangers, however, allow for the rapid induction of hyperthermia in only 30–60 minutes and for accurate temperature control. The patient is readily accessible for monitoring of vital signs and for initiation of supportive interventions.

Techniques are available using radiant heat, microwave radiation, infrared radiation or combinations of these to induce whole body hyperthermia with steady state temperatures of 41–42.0°C. While the power absorption patterns are nonuniform, redistribution of the thermal energy is rapid via the circulatory system.

The toxicities associated with whole body hyperthermia may be significant, and careful patient selection and supportive care are essential. Sedation or general anesthesia and continuous monitoring of vital signs, core body temperature, electrocardiogram, and urine output are necessary. Large fluid losses occur and require vigorous replacement. Electrolyte abnormalities, decreases in platelet count, and prolongation of coagulation are common; these changes may be more pronounced with the use of extracorporeal methods of hyperthermia induction. Elevation in liver function tests reflecting mild liver necrosis and increase in serum creatine phosphokinase reflecting skeletal muscle necrosis have also been observed. The physiologic response to hyperthermia includes an approximate doubling of cardiac output with an increase in pulse rate but little change in blood pressure. Cardiac arrhythmias, pulmonary edema, and seizures occur occasionally and may be life-threatening. Diarrhea, nausea and vomiting, post hyperthermia fever, and reactivation of herpes simplex infections are frequently observed.

Equipment Available for Localized (or Regional) Hyperthermia. While many heating modalities are discussed in the literature, almost all local heating is currently performed by microwave, radiofrequency or ultrasound equipment. Most microwave equipment works in the 100 MHz–3 GHz region (microwaves here is really a misnomer; strictly speaking, most of that range is termed ultra high frequency); radiofrequency systems work in the 500 kHz–15 MHz band, and ultrasound in the 300 kHz–2 MHz region. The relative merits of each of the techniques is presented in Table XIII-2-1. Other techniques (radiofrequency inductively coupled, ferromagnetic seeds, lasers) are either little used or in the developmental stage.[2,12,15,31]

Thermometry

Temperature measurements during heating are subject to two types of error. First, the measuring device may itself absorb energy, causing the temperature to rise in its immediate vicinity. The sensor may then record (correctly) the temperature but may overestimate tissue values. This problem can occur both with electromagnetic and ultrasound heating devices. In addition, electromagnetic energy may cause noise in the receiver, causing erroneous temperature readings. Optical temperature sensors can minimize or essentially eliminate this latter problem. Because temperature distributions in tumors and in normal tissue are usually anything but uniform, it is important to obtain many data points during treatment. One way of doing this is to implant one or more hollow catheters into the volume of tissue to be heated, and then pass a sensor through the catheter. Catheter material must be chosen carefully, particularly if ultrasound is used to heat the lesion. Automated samplers have been developed; these move the sensor at a predetermined rate so that measurement along a catheter can be made with essentially arbitrary frequency and spatial resolution.

Hyperthermic Dose

A serious problem in hyperthermia is the definition of "clinically meaningful dose." Deposition of energy, usually stated in terms of "specific absorption rate," while useful for quality control and intercomparison of equipment, is not necessarily related to tissue temperature and, therefore, not to cytotoxicity. The effect of nonuniform temperature distributions on cytotoxicity is amplified by the temperature threshold effect discussed earlier, which may vary from tumor to tumor and from normal tissue to tissue. Attempts to define a unifying biologically-based dose concept ("43°C equivalent minutes"),[40] have not been entirely satisfactory in part because of biological variations, and development of thermotolerance. Although cumbersome, it probably is best to describe treatments in terms of multiple local time-temperature profiles.

Clinical Experience

Heat Alone

Local-Regional Heating. In the 1970s, initial studies were undertaken utilizing hyperthermia alone primarily for the treatment of superficially-located, recurrent, or metastatic tumors. A detailed survey of these trials by Meyer revealed an overall complete response rate of 15%. The responses were typically of short duration.[27] Several studies (Table XIII-2-2) have suggested, however, that higher complete response rates and longer duration of response were associated with higher intratumoral temperatures. For example, Storm and colleagues reported tumor regressions in all of 12 patients in whom intratumoral temperatures of 46°C or greater were achieved.[46] A multi-institutional trial utilizing the annular phased array (BSD Medical Corporation, Salt Lake City, UT) reported only one complete and three partial responders among 47 patients treated with hyperthermia alone.[36]

Currently, local-regional hyperthermia is rarely employed as the sole treatment modality for advanced or recurrent cancer. One possible exception may be in the retreatment

Table XIII-2-1. Methods of Producing Local-Regional Hyperthermia

Heating Techniques	Advantages	Disadvantages	Applications (as described in the literature)	Commercial Availability
Microwaves	Technology very advanced. Heating of large volumes theoretically possible. Multiple applicators, coherent or incoherent, can be utilized. Specialized antennas for heating from body cavities have been developed. Skin cooling feasible. Interstitial use has been demonstrated.	Heating not localized at deph; limited penetration at high frequencies. Possible adverse effects on personnel. Shielding of treatment rooms required except at medically reserved frequencies (e.g., 915 MHz). Thermometry requires non-interacting probes. Temperature distributions subject to variations in localized blood flow. Commercial antennas available are of fixed length. Depth of tissue of implant alters specific absorption rate pattern.	Surface or near surface lesions. Lesions on breast, chest wall, extremities (external applicators). Bladder, prostate, esophagus; cervix, brain, head and neck with specialized or interstitial applicators.	USA—yes Japan—yes Europe—yes
Radiofrequency (direct current or capacitive coupling)	Equipment relatively simple. No specialized shielding required. Large volumes may be heated. Heating of deep-seated lesions sometimes possible. Interstitial use has been demonstrated. Electrodes not limited in size; insulation easily accomplished.	Fatty tissue may heat preferentially; current flow subject to local electrical tissue characteristics; temperature distribution additionally subject to blood flow variations. Heating regional with external applicators.	Large surface tumors; lesions in extremities, lung, pancreas, liver, bladder. Interstitial applications: chest wall, head and neck, prostate, uterine cervical cancer.	USA—no Japan—yes Europe—?
Ultrasound Single transducers	Readily focused in tissue. Heating possible to 5–10 cm depth with focused transducers. Dynamic systems have been demonstrated. Shielding not required, and no health hazards to personnel. Fat not treatment-limiting. In dynamic systems, effects of blood flow can be reduced by minimizing focal volume.	No penetration of tissue-air interfaces. "Shadowing" by bone. Bone tends to heat preferentially. Patients may experience pain during treatment.	Surface lesions; head and neck, and lesions in extremities.	USA—yes Japan—yes Europe—yes
Multiple transducers	Focusing and preferential heating to 20 cm depth has been demonstrated. Dynamic systems can heat larger volumes.	Same as above	Brain, prostate; head and neck.	USA—yes Japan—yes Europe—yes

of symptomatic recurrent chondrosarcomas. Delephin reported excellent tumor responses with decrease in tumor volumes noted, after six months, in four patients with pelvic chondrosarcoma treated with local-regional hyperthermia alone.[10] The relatively poor blood supply to tumor cells in chondrosarcomas may explain the response of such tumors to hyperthermia. Additional patient accrual and longer term follow-up will be needed before definitive conclusions can be reached concerning the role of hyperthermia alone in such selected tumors.

Whole Body Heating. Early attempts to induce systemic hyperthermia with pyrogens (e.g., Coley's toxin) resulted in occasional tumor responses, but the duration and height of temperature elevations were difficult to predict or control. Since the development of predictable, controlled whole body hyperthermia techniques, few studies using contemporary criteria of response have been reported. The available studies demonstrate no benefit of controlled whole body hyperthermia alone in the treatment of cancer.[4,6,44,51]

Hyperthermia as an Adjuvant

Radiation Therapy and Local Hyperthermia. The majority of clinical trials comparing hyperthermia as an adjunct to

Table XIII-2-4. Local Control Rates for Tumors Treated with Radiation Alone or in Combination with Hyperthermia

Author (Year)	Number of Fields	Time of Follow-up Months	Local Control (%)	
			Radiation Alone	Radiation plus Hyperthermia
A. Local-Regional Metastases from Breast Cancer				
LOW DOSE RADIATION				
Perez (1986)*	70	>6	31	61
Lindholm (1987)	34	12	30	53
		24	30	45
Gonzalez Gonzalez (1988)	18	>6	33†	78†
Kapp (1988)	85	24	N.P.	45
Dragovic (1989)	30	6–32	N.P.	43
Seegenschmiedt (1989)	95	≥6	N.P.	67
FULL DOSE RADIATION				
Scott (1984)	34	12	55	100
Perez (1986)**	95	>6	46	86
B. Advanced Neck Node Metastases from Head and Neck Cancers				
Scott (1984)	10	12	40	100
Arcangeli (1985)	81	24	14	58
Valdagni (1990)	36	36	23	83
			7‡	41‡
C. Superficially Located Metastases from Melanoma				
Gonzalez Gonzalez (1986)	24	≤36	17	83
Arcangeli (1987)	38	6–24	53	76
Overgaard (1987)	67	18	56	86
Emami (1988)	116	Not stated	21	57

*Dose <40 Gy; **Dose ≥40 Gy; †Maintained (CR plus PR); N.P. = not performed; ‡3-year survival rates

Table XIII-2-5. Survival or Local Control for Deep Seated Tumors Treated Either with Radiation Therapy or Combination Radiation Therapy and Hyperthermia

Author (Year)	Site and Number Patients (Fields or Lesions)	Type of Trial	Radiation Dose (Gy)	Follow-up Time (Years)	Survival Rate %		P-Value
					Radiation	Radiation plus Hyperthermia	
Sugimachi (1988)	Esophageal cancer: unresectable 31 (XRT plus bleomycin plus HT)	Historical controls 83 (XRT + bleomycin)	48	1 2	11 1	33 16	<0.05
	Esophageal cancer: preoperative 62 (XRT plus bleomycin plus HT)	Historical controls 121 (XRT + bleomycin)	30	1 3 5	45 20 15	66 43 43	<0.05
Sharma (1989)	Stage II and III SCC of uterine cervix 50	Prospectively randomized	70 or 45 plus 35 ICR	1.5	50*	70*	<0.05
Datta (1990)	Stage III and IV SCC of head and neck	Prospectively randomized	65	1.5	8	25	0.03

SCC, Squamous cell cancers; ICR, intracavitary radiation to point A; * Local tumor control colleagues demonstrated improved local tumor control in stage II and III squamous cell carcinomas of the uterine cervix with the addition of hyperthermia to standard radiation therapy treatment regimens.[41] Similarly, Datta and colleagues demonstrated improved survival at 18 months in stages III and IV squamous cell carcinoma of the head and neck with the addition of hyperthermia to external beam treatment (25%) compared with external beam treatment alone (8%).[9] In addition, a pilot study on the retreatment of locally recurrent prostatic cancer with external beam radiation therapy and hyperthermia has suggested that long term local control can be obtained.[20]

Multi-institutional studies have also suggested improved local control rates can be obtained when hyperthermia is utilized as an adjunct to radiation therapy for the treatment of deep-seated tumors. Petrovich and colleagues have reported the results of a 14-institutional trial conducted in the United States which employed the annular phased array system for regional hyperthermia production in 353 patients with advanced, recurrent, or persistent deep-seated tumors.[36] Hyperthermia was used in conjunction with radiation therapy, chemotherapy, chemotherapy and radiation therapy, or alone in 69%, 12%, 4%, and 13% of the patients respectively. Complete responses (10%) and partial responses (17%) were obtained, with the highest complete response rates noted in patients receiving radiation therapy in conjunction with their hyperthermia (12% vs. 2%; p = 0.003). There was a correlation between complete response rates and increasing radiation dose (p<0.001) but no correlation was noted between thermal dose and response. Of the 195 patients with pain present prior to treatment, 23% had complete pain resolution and 39% had partial pain relief. The treatment was, in general, well tolerated, but 35% of the patients had some pain during the treatment. Three percent of the patients had elevated heart rates, 2% had anxiety reactions, and 1% had claustrophobia noted during treatment. Only 1% of the patients developed infections in the sites of the catheters used for temperature monitoring, and 3% developed blisters within their hyperthermia treatment fields. A second generation phased array device (the Sigma-60, BSD-2000 system) has recently been developed (BSD Medical Corporation, Salt Lake City, UT) which should permit better power localization and possibly less patient discomfort. A multi-institutional Phase I/II trial is currently on-going in the United States employing this system while Phase III trials in patients with advanced bladder, rectal, and uterine cervical cancers are being conducted in Holland.

The preliminary results of a Japanese seven-institutional trial employing the Thermotron RF-8 capacitive heating device (Yamamoto Vinyter Co., Ltd., Osaka, Japan) are also noteworthy.[19] Treatment was given to 177 patients for deep-seated tumors utilizing hyperthermia in combination with radiation therapy (96 patients) or with chemotherapy (81 patients). Maximum intratumoral or intracavitary temperatures of greater than 42°C were obtained in 77% and 74% of the tumors, respectively. Response rates and symptomatic improvement were reported to be higher than expected for historical controls treated with radiation therapy or chemotherapy alone. No severe side effects were noted. Minor side effects were seen in 37 patients (21%) and consisted mainly of fatty indu-

ration, pain, and burns. Preliminary results of a prospectively randomized trial included in this report which compared preoperative radiation therapy (40 Gy) with or without hyperthermia in primary rectal cancers revealed statistically significant improved total response rates for patients with the addition of hyperthermia. Comparison of these results with historical controls treated with radiation (60 Gy) alone suggested a dose enhancement by hyperthermia of approximately 1.5 times. Further patient accrual and follow-up in this randomized study is awaited as is additional patient accrual utilizing this capacitive heating device in the treatment of other deeply situated tumors.

Interstitial Hyperthermia. Excellent results have been obtained utilizing interstitial hyperthermia techniques in conjunction with brachytherapy in the treatment of tumors at a variety of locations. Both radiofrequency local current field techniques and microwave antennas have been employed. Site-specific results of thermobrachytherapy for the more commonly treated sites (head and neck, pelvis, and breast and chest wall) are summarized in Table XIII-2-6. It should be borne in mind however, that high local control rates have also been reported utilizing brachytherapy without the addition of hyperthermia in similar tumors.[21] These results, therefore, await confirmation in randomized trials such as the study of patients randomized to brachytherapy with or without the addition of interstitial hyperthermia currently being performed by the Radiation Therapy Oncology Group (RTOG-84-19).

Chemotherapy. The compelling preclinical data that hyperthermia augments the antitumor activity of many chemotherapeutic agents has been tested in relatively few clinical trials. With rare exception the reported trials have not been disease specific, prospectively randomized clinical trials that compare chemotherapy alone versus chemotherapy plus hyperthermia. The inconvenience, required professional expertise, specialized equipment, expense, and potential toxicities require clear demonstration of benefit before hyperthermia should be adopted as a standard addition to chemotherapy.

At least four types of heat-drug interactions appear to occur in vitro (Table XIII-2-7).[15] The nature of the heat-drug interaction has important implications for the use of hyperthermia plus chemotherapy in the clinic. Hyperthermia, for instance, may not increase the cytotoxicity of some agents at temperatures that are tolerable using whole body hyperthermia. In addition, the heat-drug interaction may be influenced by blood flow, time to steady state temperature, tumor and normal tissue steady state temperatures, duration of heating, uniformity of heating, changes in drug pharmacokinetics, and the sequencing of the chemotherapy and hyperthermia.

Whole Body HT. The successful application of hyperthermia in the treatment of systemic neoplasms will require the application of whole body hyperthermia. Although a number of trials have tested the use of whole body hyperthermia plus chemotherapy, most trials are small and uncontrolled, include patients with multiple histologies, and utilize multiple different chemotherapy regimens.

The available studies document that combined whole body hyperthermia plus chemotherapy can be safely administered, although some drug toxicities do appear to be

Table XIII-2-6.   Interstitial Thermobrachytherapy: Site Specific Results

Author (Year)	HT System (Type; Frequency, MH$_z$)	Site Treated No. CR/Total No. Tumors (%)			
		Head & Neck	Pelvis	Breast & Chest Wall	Other
Surwit (1983)	RF, 0.5	—	7/21 (33)	—	—
Puthawala (1985)*	MW, 915	15/20 (75)	10/13 (77)	5/8 (63)	2/2 (100)
Vora (1988)	RF, 0.5	—	10/19 (53)	—	—
Gautherie (1989)	MW, 915	24/35 (69)	23/39 (59)	11/14 (79)	3/8 (39)
Rafla (1989)	MW, 915	8/15 (53)	8/14 (57)	3/6 (50)	—
Petrovich (1989)	MW, 915,630	16/23 (70)	3/4 (75)	7/9 (78)	2/8 (25)
Goffinet (1990)	RF, 0.5	5/5 (100)	3/5 (60)	—	—
Shimm (1990)	RF, 0.5	8/13 (61)	14/48 (29)	—	—
Phromratanapongse (1990)	MW, 915	22/30 (73)	7/11 (64)	0/2 (0)	2/2 (100)

*Local Control Rates; RF, Radiofrequency; MW, Microwaves; HT, Hyperthermia; CR, Complete response

Table XIII-2-7.   Types of Heat-Drug Interactions Observed In Vitro

Group		Examples
1	Linear increase in cytotoxicity	Thiotepa, cisplatin, mitomycin C, nitrosoureas
2	Threshold increase in cytotoxicity	Doxorubicin, bleomycin, actinomycin
3	Not cytotoxic at low temperature, becomes cytotoxic at high temperature	Lidocaine, amphotericin B
4	No effect on cytotoxicity	Methotrexate, 5-fluorouracil, vincristine

increased.[7,11,25,26,32,37] For instance, in a study of 11 patients with a variety of cancers treated with doxorubicin plus whole body hyperthermia, two partial responses were achieved, and there was a suggestion of enhanced anthracycline cardiac toxicity.[7] The same investigator has studied methyl-CCNU plus whole body hyperthermia in 12 patients with melanoma. Three partial responses were observed.

In a series of 132 patients with multiple tumor types treated with a variety of chemotherapeutic agents plus whole body hyperthermia, no relation between tumor histology or chemotherapeutic agent and response rates were observed.[26] The heterogeneous nature of the patient population and treatment, however, makes subset analysis difficult.

Preliminary results of a randomized study combining whole body hyperthermia plus doxorubicin, cyclophosphamide, and vincristine in the treatment of non-small cell lung cancer have been reported by Engelhardt.[11] Fifty-five patients were randomized and 44 patients were evaluable. The rates of response were 8/22 (36%) with chemotherapy alone and 15/22 (68%) with chemotherapy plus whole body hyperthermia. Mean duration of response was 105 days with chemotherapy alone and 130 days with the addition of hyperthermia.

Assessment of the impact of whole body hyperthermia added to chemotherapy in the treatment of cancer remains difficult because of the paucity of nonrandomized and randomized clinical trials. The use of whole body hyperthermia remains experimental until additional studies are performed.

Regional Perfusion Chemotherapy Plus Heat. Isolated hyperthermic perfusion chemotherapy has been utilized primarily in the treatment of malignant melanoma of the extremities.[14,24,39,42,43] Melphalan, cisplatin, nitrogen mustard, thiotepa, and actinomycin D have all been administered safely by hyperthermic isolated limb perfusion.[24] Most studies have utilized perfusion with melphalan, and all demonstrate benefit from the use of hyperthermic perfusion in association with surgical excision when compared with historical control groups. Limb perfusion requires isolation and cannulation of the arterial supply and venous drainage of the limb, the use of an extracorporeal blood oxygenator, and the use of a heating unit. The complication rates are low when the procedure is performed by an experienced team.[24]

With almost 6 years of follow-up, a randomized comparison of surgery with or without isolated hyperthermic limb perfusion of melphalan in patients with newly diagnosed intermediate and high risk malignant melanoma has documented the advantage of limb perfusion.[14] The use of hyperthermic limb perfusion decreased rates of recurrence (48% without perfusion, 11% with perfusion, p<0.001) and decreased the number of melanoma deaths (20% without perfusion, 6% with perfusion, p<0.01). The results of a second and larger, multi-institutional trial of the WHO, EORTC, and Melanoma Intergroup, testing the use of isolated, hyperthermic perfusion with melphalan is awaited with great interest.[49] If the second randomized trial also favors the use of perfusion, then an important role for perfusion chemotherapy will be clearly established in the treatment of intermediate risk melanoma of the extremity. The contribution of hyperthermia to these results needs to be explored.

Hyperthermic regional perfusion has also been utilized in the treatment of tumors of the liver, brain, breast and sarcomas of the extremity. The appropriate role of perfusion therapy in these sites and histologies, however, remains uncertain.

Regional Hyperthermia. The development of clinical systems capable of delivering controlled hyperthermia to local regions by ultrasound, microwaves, or radiofrequency energy has allowed the investigation of local-regional hyperthermia plus chemotherapy. A number of studies have been performed over the past decade. Unfortunately, none of the reported trials of combined chemotherapy plus local-regional hyperthermia are prospective, randomized trials.

Several series of patients with head and neck cancer treated with chemotherapy plus local hyperthermia have been reported. Fifteen patients with neck node metastasis were treated with either bleomycin or doxorubicin, with or without local hyperthermia.[3] All of the lymph node lesions treated with chemotherapy plus hyperthermia responded while only 25–50% of the lymph node lesions treated with doxorubicin or bleomycin alone responded. The rates of complete response also favored the use of hyperthermia. A series of 14 patients with recurrent head and neck cancers were treated with local hyperthermia plus a variety of chemotherapeutic agents.[29] Three of the patients experienced complete responses and one a partial response. In another series, 12 patients with pretreated, recurrent squamous cell cancer of the head and neck were treated with bleomycin, cisplatin, and 5-fluorouracil plus local hyperthermia simultaneous with the cisplatin.[44] A single patient achieved a complete response.

A series of 69 patients with primary or recurrent cancers of the vulva, vagina, uterine cervix, or ovary received chemotherapy with bleomycin or with peplomycin and mitomycin.[13] Forty-two of the patients received local hyperthermia concurrent with the chemotherapy. Most patients subsequently received additional surgery or radiation. Although the patients were not randomized to chemotherapy alone or to chemotherapy plus radiation, the rate of response was higher in those patients receiving hyperthermia (62% vs. 19%), as was survival.

Multiple similar series of patients treated with chemotherapy plus local-regional hyperthermia are available in the literature. The paucity of studies utilizing consistent chemotherapy in patients with tumors of the same histology and site prevent the formulation of even preliminary conclusions regarding the value of combination local-regional hyperthermia plus chemotherapy. Randomized clinical trials are clearly needed.

References

1. Anderson, R. L., Tao, T. W., Betten, D. A., and Hahn, G. M.: Heat shock protein levels are not elevated in heat-resistant B16 melanoma cells. Radiat. Res., 105:240, 1986.
2. Anderson, R. L., and Kapp, D. S.: Hyperthermia in cancer therapy: current status. Med. J. Aust., 152:310, 1990.
3. Arcangeli, G, Cividalli, A., Mauro, F, Nervi, C., and Pavin, G.: Enhanced effectiveness of Adriamycin and bleomycin combined with local hyperthermia in neck node metastases from head and neck cancers. Tumori, 65:481, 1979.
4. Barlogie, B., Corry, P. M., Yip, E., Lippman, L., Johnston, D. A., Khalil, K., Tenczynski, T. F., Reilly, E., Lawson, R., Dosik, G., Rigor, B., Han Kenson, R., and Freireich, E. J.: Total-body hyperthermia with and without chemotherapy for advanced human neoplasms. Cancer Res., 39:1481, 1979.
5. Barnett, T. A., Kapp, D. S., and Goffinet, D. R.: Adenoid cystic carcinoma of the salivary gland: management of recurrent, advanced, or persistent disease with hyperthermia and radiation therapy. Cancer, 65:2648, 1990.
6. Bull, J. M., Lees, D., Schuette, W., Whang-Peng, J., Smith, R., Bynum, G., Atkinson, E. R., Gottdiener, J. S., Gralnick, H. R., Shawker, T. H., and DeVita, V. T., Jr.: Whole body hyperthermia: A phase-I trial of a potential adjuvant to chemotherapy. Ann. Intern. Med., 90:317, 1979.
7. Bull, J. M. C.: A review of systemic hyperthermia. Front. Radiat. Ther. Oncol., 18:171, 1984.
8. Coley, W. B.: The treatment of malignant tumors by repeated inoculations of erysipelas, with a report of ten original cases. Am. J. Med. Sci., 105:488, 1893.
9. Datta, N. R., Bose, A. K., Kapoor, H. K., and Gupta, S.: Head and neck cancers: Results of thermoradiotherapy versus radiotherapy. Int. J. Hyperthermia, 6:479, 1990.
10. Delepine, N., Delepine, G., Desbois, J. C., Sidi, J., and Jasmin, C.: Treatment of pelvic chondrosarcoma by an external deep heating device in 12 cases. Abstracts of Papers for the 5th European BSD-Users Conference: Hyperthermia in Clinical Oncology. Rotterdam, The Netherlands, May 19, 1990.
11. Engelhardt, R.: Summary of recent clinical experience in whole-body hyperthermia combined with chemotherapy. Recent Results Cancer Res., 107:200, 1988.
12. Field, S. B., and Franconi, C.: Physics and Technology of Hyperthermia. Dordrecht, Boston, Lancaster, Martinus Nijhoff, 1987.
13. Fujiwara, K., Kohno, I., and Sekiba, K.: Therapeutic effect of hyperthermia combined with chemotherapy on vulvar and vaginal carcinoma. Acta Med. Okayama, 41:55, 1987.
14. Ghussen, F., Kruger, I., Smalley, R. V., and Groth, W.: Hyperthermic perfusion with chemotherapy for melanoma of the extremities. World J. Surg., 13:598, 1989.
15. Hahn, G. M.: Hyperthermia and Cancer. New York and London, Plenum Press, 1982.
16. Hahn, G. M., and van Kersen, I.: Isolation and initial characterization of thermoresistant RIF tumor cell strains. Cancer Res., 48:1803, 1988.
17. Hahn, G. M, Adwankar, M. K., Basrur, V. S., and Anderson, R. L.: Survival of cells exposed to anticancer drugs after stress. In Stress-Induced Proteins. UCLA Symposia on Molecular and Cellular Biology, Vol. 96. Edited by M. L. Pardue, J. R. Feramisco and S. Lindquist. New York, Alan R. Liss, Inc., 1989, p. 223.
18. Hiraoka, M., and Hahn, G. M.: Changes in pH and blood flow induced by glucose and their effects on hyperthermia with or without BCNU in RIF-1 tumours. Int. J. Hyperthermia, 6:97, 1990.
19. Kakehi, M., Ueda, K., Mukojima, T., Hiraoka, M., Seto, O., Akanuma, A., and Nakatsugawa, S.: Multi-institutional clinical studies on hyperthermia combined with radiotherapy or chemotherapy in advanced cancer of deep-seated organs. Int. J. Hyperthermia, 6:719, 1990.
20. Kaplan, I., Kapp, D. S., and Bagshaw, M. A.: Secondary external-beam radiotherapy and hyperthermia for local recurrence after 125-iodine implantation in adenocarcinoma of the prostate. Int. J. Radiat. Oncol. Biol. Phys., 20:551, 1991.
21. Kapp, D. S.: Site and disease selection for hyperthermia clinical trials. Int. J. Hyperthermia, 2:139, 1986.
22. Kapp, D. S., Cox, R. S., Fessenden, P., Meyer, J. L., Prionas, S. D., Lee, E. R., and Bagshaw, M. A.: Parameters predictive for complications of treatment with combined hyperthermia and radiation therapy. Int. J. Radiat. Oncol. Biol. Phys., In press, 1990.
23. Knox, S. J., and Kapp, D. S.: Hyperthermia and radiation therapy in the treatment of recurrent Merkel cell tumors. Cancer, 62:1479, 1988.
24. Krementz, E. T., Ryan, R. F., Carter, R. D. Sutherland, C. M., and Reed, R. J.: Hyperthermic regional perfusion for melanoma of the limbs. In Cutaneous Melanoma. Clinical Management and Treatment Results Worldwide. Edited by C. M. Balch, and G. W. Milton. Philadelphia, Lippincott Co., 1985, pp. 171.
25. Larkin, J. M.: A clinical investigation of total-body hyperthermia as cancer therapy. Cancer Res., 39:2252, 1979.
26. Maeta, M., Koga, S., Wada, J., Yokoyama, M., Kato, N., Kawahara, H., Sakai, T., Hino, M., Ono, T., and Yuasa, K.: Clinical evaluation of total-body hyperthermia combined with anticancer chemotherapy for far-advanced miscellaneous cancer in Japan. Cancer, 59:1101, 1987.
27. Meyer, J. L.: The clinical efficacy of localized hyperthermia. Cancer Res., 44(Suppl.):4745s, 1984.
28. Milligan, A. J.: Whole-body hyperthermia induction techniques. Cancer Res., 44(Suppl.):4869s, 1984.
29. Moffat, F. L., Rotstein, L. E., Calhoun, K., Langer, J. C., Makowka, L., Ambus, U., Palmer, J. A., Campbell, A., Howard, V., Mikkelsaar, R., Venturi, D., Laing, D., Falk, J. A., and Falk, R. E.: Palliation of advanced head and neck cancer with radiofrequency hyperthermia and cytotoxic chemotherapy. Can. J. Surg., 27:38, 1984.
30. Morimoto, R. I., Tissieres, A., and Georgopoulos, C.: Stress Proteins in Biology and Medicine. Cold Spring Harbor Press, 1990.
31. Paliwal, B. R., Hetzel, F. W., and Dewhirst, M. W.: Biological, Physical and Clinical Aspects of Hyperthermia. Am. Inst. Physics., 1988.
32. Parks, L. C., and Smith, G. V.: Systemic hyperthermia by extracorporeal induction. In Hyperthermia in Cancer Therapy. Edited by F. K. Strom. Boston, G. K. Hall, 1983.
33. Perez, C. A., Gillespie, B., Pajak, T., Hornback, N. B., Emami, B., and Rubin, P.: Quality assurance problems in clinical hyperthermia and impact on therapeutic outcome: A report by RTOG. Radiation Oncology Center Scientific Report, Mallinckrodt Institute of Radiology, 1987–1988, pp. 293.
34. Perez, C. A., Gillespie, B., Pajak, T., Hornback, N. B., Emami, B., and Rubin, P.: Quality assurance problems in clinical hyperthermia and impact on therapeutic outcome: a report by the Radiation Therapy Oncology Group. Int. J. Radiat. Oncol. Biol. Phys., 16:551, 1989.
35. Petersen, I. A., and Kapp, D. S.: Local hyperthermia and radiation therapy in the retreatment of superficially located recurrences in Hodgkin's disease. Int. J. Radiat. Oncol. Biol. Phys., 19:603, 1990.
36. Petrovich, Z., Langholz, B., Gibbs, F. A., Sapozink, M. D., Kapp, D. S., Stewart, R. J., Emami, B., Oleson, J., Senzer, N., Slater, J., and Astrahan, M.: Regional hyperthermia for advanced tumors: a clinical study of 353 patients. Int. J. Radiat. Oncol. Biol. Phys., 16:601, 1989.
37. Pettigrew, R. T.: Cancer therapy by whole body heating. In Proc. Int. Symp. on Cancer Therapy by Hyperthermia and Radiation. Edited by M. Wizenberg and S. F. Robinson. Baltimore, Amer. College Radiol. Press, 1975.
38. Robins, H. I., Hugander, A., and Cohen J. D.: Whole body hyperthermia in the treatment of neoplastic disease. Radiol. Clin. North Am., 27:603, 1989.
39. Rochlin, D. B., and Smart, C. R.: Treatment of malignant melanoma by regional perfusion. Cancer, 18:1544, 1965.
40. Sapareto, S. A., and Dewey, W. C.: Thermal dose determination in cancer therapy. Int. J. Radiat. Oncol. Biol. Phys., 10:787, 1984.
41. Sharma, S., Patel, F. D., Sandhu, A. P. S., Gupta, B. D., and Yadav, N. S.: A prospective randomized study of local hyperthermia as a supplement and radiosensitizer in the treatment of carcinoma of the cervix with radiotherapy. Endocuriether./Hyperther. Oncol., 5:151, 1989.
42. Shiu, M. H., Knapper, W. H., Fortner, J. G., Yeh, S., Horowitz, G., Schnog, J., Guerra, J., Gould-Rossbach, P., and Ray, C.: Regional isolated limb perfusion of melanoma intransit metastases using mechlorethamine (nitrogen mustard). J. Clin. Oncol., 4:1819, 1986.
43. Stehlin, J. S., Jr.: Hyperthermic perfusion for melanoma of the extremities: Experience with 165 patients, 1967 to 1979. Ann. NY Acad. Sci., 335:352, 1980.
44. Steindorfer, P., Jakse, R., Germann, R., Schneider, G., Berger, A., Mischinger, H. J., and Rehak P.: Hyperthermia as an adjuvant to radiation- and/or chemotherapy in far advanced recurrences of the head and neck region. Strahlentherapie und Onkologie, 163:449, 1987.

45. Stewart, J. R.: Past clinical studies and future directions. Cancer Res., 44(Suppl.):4902s, 1984.
46. Storm, F. K., Baker, H. W., Scanlon, E. F., Plenk, H. P., Meadows, P. M., Cohen, S. C., Olson, C. E., Thomson, J. W., Khandekar, J. D., Roe, D., Nizze, A., and Morton, D. L.: Magnetic-induction hyperthermia. Results of a 5-year multi-institutional national cooperative trial in advanced cancer patients. Cancer, 55:2677, 1985.
47. Storm, F. K.: Clinical hyperthermia and chemotherapy. Radiol. Clin. North Am., 27:621, 1989.
48. Sugimachi, K., Matsuda, H., Ohno, S., Fukuda, A., Matsuoka, H., Mori, M., and Kuwano, H.: Long term effects of hyperthermia combined with chemotherapy and irradiation

for the treatment of patients with carcinoma of the esophagus. Surg. Gynecol. Obstet., 167:319, 1988.
49. Sutherland, C. M., Krementz, E. T., Carter, R. D., and Muchmore, J. H.: Randomized trials of heated perfusion of extremity melanoma. Cancer Treat. Res., 43:173, 1988.
50. Valdagni, R., Amichetti, M., and Pani, G.: Radical radiation alone versus radical radiation plus microwave hyperthermia for N3 (TNM-UICC) neck nodes: a prospective randomized clinical trial. Int. J. Radiat. Oncol. Biol. Phys., 15:13, 1988.
51. van der Zee, J., van Rhoon, G. C., Wike-Hooley, J. L., Faithfull, N. S., and Reinhold, H. S.: Whole-body hyperthermia in cancer therapy: A report of a phase I-II study. Eur. J. Cancer Clin. Oncol., 19:1189, 1983.

XIII-3

Principles and Applications of Photodynamic Therapy

Thomas F. DeLaney
Eli Glatstein

Introduction

Optimal cancer treatment selectively destroys tumor without disrupting normal cell and tissue function. Recent laboratory and clinical work with light-activated photosensitizers demonstrates selective tumoricidal activity because of the preferential retention of the sensitizers in neoplastic tissue compared to certain normal tissues and the capability to selectively deliver light to tumors with lasers and optical fibers. This therapeutic strategy is generally referred to as photodynamic therapy (PDT), but has also been termed "photoradiation," "phototherapy," or "photochemotherapy."

Historical Observations

The earliest report on the action of light-activated chemicals in biologic systems was in 1900 by Raab who described the lethal effect of light on paramecium treated with an acridine dye.[16] Neither light nor dye alone had any apparent lethal effect on the cells but together were effectively cytotoxic with a dose dependent response demonstrable for each. Numerous other reports on sensitized photochemical processes in living systems have subsequently appeared but the majority of attention in the clinic to date has been focused on the porphyrins.[61] Policard reported reddish fluorescence in experimental rat sarcomas illuminated by a Wood's lamp, which he attributed to excitation of endogenous porphyrins accumulating at the tumor site.[53] Lipson and co-workers reported in 1961 on the use of hematoporphyrin derivative (HpD) for fluorescence detection of tumor tissue and subsequently on the treatment of a patient with recurrent breast cancer using HpD and localized exposure of the tumor to light.[40] Diamond and co-workers reported in 1972 on the destruction of glioma cells in tissue culture and subcutaneously transplanted gliomas in rats with hematoporphyrin and visible light.[15] Dougherty and co-workers at Roswell Park

reported in 1975 on the eradication of nearly 50% of subcutaneously transplanted tumors in mice and rats using intraperitoneally administered HpD and red light directed to the tumor. This was achieved without excessive damage to surrounding uninvolved skin in the light field.[16]

These encouraging early reports on the potential utility of HpD for tumor localization and treatment, as well as the recent development of appropriate high output laser and fiberoptic systems for light delivery, provided the impetus for the current interest in this field. Indeed, numerous clinical and experimental investigations with PDT have been pursued to examine efficacy in a variety of tumor sites. While the hematoporphyrins have been the principal photosensitizers evaluated to date in clinical trials, other promising agents have been studied in the laboratory. Before reviewing these studies, it would be helpful to examine the photochemistry and photobiology involved in photodynamic destruction of malignant tissue with this modality.

Photochemistry

PDT involves the interaction of photosensitizer, light, and oxygen. Sensitizer in a low energy (ground) state is initially excited by the absorption of light. In this energetic state, it can react directly through a free radical mechanism or indirectly via molecular oxygen which undergoes a spin-state transition to reactive singlet oxygen ($^1O_2$). Both pathways yield potentially cytotoxic compounds, although the singlet oxygen process is thought to predominate in PDT.[18] Oxygen has been shown to be critical for HpD photodynamic action in vitro,[15] consistent with the hypothesis that singlet oxygen is the mediator of photodynamic cytotoxicity.

De-excitation of activated sensitizer to ground state can also occur with either liberation of heat or emission of a photon. The latter process is termed fluorescence or phosphorescence, depending upon the spin state of the excited sensitizer. In the case of the HpD, fluorescence and phosphorescence yield light in the visible red range with a peak between 600 and 700 nm. Excitation with ultraviolet, blue, or green light produces pinkish-red fluorescence in tissue that has localized photosensitizer. This is the photochemical basis for the fluorescence detection of tumors. The first recent clinical use of HpD by Lipson and co-workers in 1961 was, in fact, for fluorescence detection of tumors via endoscopy in the trachea, esophagus, stomach and bronchial tree.[40] Fluorescence localization of transitional carcinoma and carcinoma in situ with subsequent histologic mapping of cystectomy specimens has been performed for lesions in the bladder.[7] Fluorescent areas were shown to represent either carcinoma or severe dysplasia in 15 patients studied after cystectomy, although faint fluorescence was occasionally seen in regenerative mucosa surrounding recent biopsy sites.

HpD is a complex mixture of porphyrins produced by the acetic acid-sulfuric acid treatment of hematoporphyrin, which in turn is manufactured commercially by the degradation of bovine hemoglobin. Lipson and co-workers demonstrated by using fluorescence detection that HpD localized better in malignant tissue than crude hematoporphyrin.[40] Consequently, the initial clinical work in PDT utilized HpD. Dougherty and co-workers later further purified from HpD a more active oligomeric porphyrin fraction with a high proportion of the active moiety, which has been proposed to be a dihematoporphyrin ether,[16] although an ester bond between the hematoporphyrin units has also been proposed.[38] This oligomeric porphyrin fraction, termed polyporphyrin or dihematoporphyrin ethers (DHE), provided a higher therapeutic ratio (tumor compared to skin response) in animal testing than the previously employed HpD. A preparation of dihematoporphyrin ethers is currently undergoing investigational clinical trials.

DHE has generally been administered by intravenous injection, followed 48–72 hours later by light delivery to the affected area. This schedule was developed empirically for the treatment of skin lesions, with the observation that tumor destruction relative to surrounding normal skin was greater when the time period between HpD injection and light delivery was increased from 24 to 72 hours. The optimal timing for light delivery to most anatomic sites in patients after drug injection remains uncertain. It is clear that in mice injected intraperitoneally (i.p.) with $[^{14}C]$HpD, there are high concentrations in the blood pool, tumors, and many normal tissues between 1 and 3 hours after injection.[20] In fact, there are up to 10-fold higher concentrations in liver and 4-fold higher in kidney and spleen than in tumors transplanted to the axillary regions of these mice during this time. The i.p. route of injection may enhance the relative hepatic, renal, and splenic drug levels. The relative concentration of drug in tumors compared to various normal tissues changes with time as the drug is cleared. The mechanism for selective retention in tumors compared to certain normal tissues is not known. In this mouse model, the maximum tumor to normal skin drug ratio of 2.5 occurs 24 hours after injection. Serum half-life of the HpD is 3 hours in mice and 25 hours in man. The whole body half-life of hematoporphyrin derivative has been measured at 396 hours.[9]

Because the HpD preparation currently in use is a complex mixture of porphyrin compounds, it has been difficult to study drug pharmacology and to assess photosensitizer levels in tumor and normal tissue in patients. Fluorescence assays have been examined but are complicated by autofluorescence of normal and tumor tissue. In addition, it is not clear whether the fluorescent moieties in HpD or DHE are those responsible for their photodynamic action. Thus, the schedules for light delivery after drug injection in patients remain empiric.

The ideal photosensitizer for clinical use would selectively localize in tumor, be nontoxic to normal tissue, be measurable in both normal tissue and tumor, and be photochemically active over a relatively narrow frequency range at a wavelength with appropriate tissue penetration. DHE fulfills some but not all of these criteria. It is photochemically activated to cause destruction of tumor, is preferentially retained by malignant compared to certain normal tissues (skin, brain, lung, muscle, colon) and has little serious systemic toxicity, although it induces cutaneous and ocular sensitivity to sunlight for four to six weeks after administration. Patients can avoid phototoxicity by shielding themselves appropriately from sunlight and can carry on normal daily activity under normal indoor lighting without risk. Since the liver is the primary metabolic and excretory organ for porphyrins (and the site of the highest accumulation of porphyrins after intraperitoneal HpD injection in mice), it has also been advised that the drug not be used in patients with compromised hepatic function.

HpD absorbs light most strongly in the ultraviolet/blue region around 400 nm, with other less prominent peaks seen at or near 514 nm (green), 540 nm, and 580 nm.[45] One of the least prominent of the excitation bands of the HpD is at 630 nm (red light) which, paradoxically, is most often utilized in the clinic. Red light is used because it has deeper tissue penetration than green or blue light. The absorption peaks in the blue-green range are not utilized for anti-tumor effect when red light is employed. Because HpD is retained in skin, however, this absorption in the blue-green range leaves the patient at increased risk for photosensitivity from sun exposure.

The penetration of red light in tissue is a complex phenomenon dependent upon many factors including tissue density, organ pigmentation, blood flow, surface geometry, and tissue interfaces. As a rough approximation, the optical power density falls off exponentially with the 1/e or 37% value occurring between 1 mm and 4 mm.[63] PDT with 630 nm light can produce tumor necrosis to a depth of 5–10 mm, depending on sensitizer concentration and light energy. Although certain carcinomas in situ, certain early stage invasive lesions, some dermal malignancies, and some intraperitoneal carcinomatoses may be confined to these dimensions, externally directed red light will not penetrate deeply enough to sterilize many tumors with a single treatment. Hence, effective use of hematoporphyrin PDT with red light in the clinic may require several external treatments, placement within the tumor of interstitial optical fibers, or combined modality therapy using surgery, radiotherapy, or chemotherapy to reduce the bulk of the tumor before using PDT to sterilize residual tumor.

Current research efforts include characterization of the active component(s) in HpD and attempted measurement of singlet oxygen levels to correlate drug and light dose with response. Singlet oxygen, the presumed final common mediator of photodynamic cytotoxicity, should reflect the combined effects of photosensitizer concentration and activity, light dose, and oxygen tension in tissue. Singlet oxygen fluoresces at 1,270 nm, which may permit detection in tissue but initial attempts at singlet oxygen level measurement have been hampered by a low signal to noise ratio.[49] Research directed at the development of new photosensitizers may yield clinically useful compounds which permit the use of longer wavelengths of light with deeper tissue penetration. Such compounds may be more amenable to pharmacokinetic studies and additionally may not be retained substantially in skin, thereby reducing the risk of systemic photosensitivity. Promising compounds include the phthalocyanines,[6] benzoporphyrins, chlorins, and metallopurpurin derivatives.

Light

PDT requires sufficient light to produce effective photosensitization. The energy and wavelength used are dictated by the photochemical properties of the photosensitizer, the biological and physical characteristics of the tumor and the mode of light delivery used. The amount of light energy delivered to a particular lesion is generally expressed in joules. It represents the product of light output or power in watts (joules/second) and the time of irradiation (in seconds). Light doses are also expressed as an energy density, such as joules/square centimeter (J/cm^2), or for interstitially placed fibers as the energy output per centimeter of light diffusing fiber (J/cm). Initial efforts with PDT used conventional wavelength-filtered lamps which, although generally inexpensive and reliable, were hampered by relatively low output and the inability to couple them to optical fibers, thereby making most deep lesions inaccessible. For treatment of most lesions, the lamp system required relatively long exposure times because of relatively low power outputs in the desired frequency range.

The combination of lasers and optical fibers has had a significant impact on the clinical development of PDT by permitting the effective delivery of light to deep-seated tumors using endoscopic, interstitial (placing optical fibers within the tumor), or intracavitary techniques. Significantly higher power densities can also be achieved. The use of the laser (light amplification by stimulated emission of radiation) for PDT differs somewhat from its use in other forms of medical therapy. The primary use of the laser in PDT is to provide high power densities of light at a desired wavelength in order to efficiently excite the photosensitizer present in tumor. Thermal effects, although potentially present in varying degrees depending on the technique of light delivery, are not necessary to effect treatment.

The laser systems for use in clinical PDT include the argon pumped dye laser and pulsed metal vapor lasers, which can yield 4–5 watts of usable light. A description of these systems is available in the literature.[71] More recently, solid state lasers have been developed which may offer greater reliability at lower cost than the currently employed systems.

Tissue Distribution of HpD

The mechanism of preferential localization of HpD in tumors is not understood. There is little doubt that differential fluorescence and cytotoxicity appears between tumor and certain normal tissues in vivo and in patients; this has been reported by many different independent investigators.[16,40] Attempts to study the phenomenon have been hindered by the fact that HpD represents a number of porphyrin compounds with differing photochemical and biologic activities. Gomer and co-workers examined the distribution of [^{3}H]- and [^{14}C]-labeled HpD in malignant and normal tissue in the mouse.[20] Interestingly, label counts were higher in tumor than in skin or muscle at all times sampled from 1–72 hours after injection. However, counts in liver, spleen, and kidney were consistently higher than those in the tumor.

Bugelski and co-workers examined the distribution of isotopically labeled HpD in murine normal and tumor tissue using autoradiography.[11] Tumor stroma contained more labelled HpD than did the tumor cells. They postulated that higher vascular permeability and inefficient lymphatic clearance seen in tumors might account for this distribution and the differential uptake between tumor and normal tissue.

Kessel and colleagues studied the localization of HpD in tumors and concluded that the most hydrophobic of the components in the preparation are involved in tumor localization.[37] Porphyrins bind to low density lipoproteins (LDL) in serum. Recently, it has been proposed that low density lipoprotein receptors may play a role in porphyrin localization in tumors.[5]

Photodynamic Effects on Cells In Vitro

The majority of work with in vitro cell lines indicates no clearly reproducible differences in the effects of photodynamic therapy on cell lines from tumors and normal tissue.[27] However, virus-induced tumorigenic thyroid cells are reported to be more sensitive to PDT than the normal parent line.[2] Bovine endothelial cells have been shown to be more sensitive than smooth muscle or fibroblast cells treated under identical conditions.[22] The association between the loss of cellular viability and inhibition of membrane transport as well as the localization of HpD fluorescence in a membrane fraction suggests that membrane targets are likely sites of cellular inactivation by the combination of HpD and light.[36] The actual target or site of inactivation, however, has not been identified. Many types of cellular injury have been reported,[47] but plasma membrane damage or mitochondrial injury[57] appear to be the most critical for cellular destruction. Studies by Gomer and co-workers of HpD photoradiation effects on Chinese hamster ovarian cells showed no mutagenic activity above background levels.[21] This suggests that DNA damage after HpD PDT might be relatively less pronounced than cytotoxic effects occurring elsewhere in the cell, although a recent report has described mutagenicity with DHE and red light in a mouse lymphoma cell line known to be deficient in repair of X-radiation-induced DNA double strand breaks.[55]

Photodynamic Effects on Tumors In Vivo

Differences in localization between tumors and normal tissue appear to occur at the tissue rather than the cellular level. Tumor destruction in vivo has been ascribed to both direct cytotoxicity on tumor cells as well as indirect cytotoxicity, possibly resulting from damage to vessels supplying the tumor. Tochner and co-workers sterilized an ascitic murine ovarian carcinoma implanted in the peritoneal cavity of mice using HpD and light introduced into the peritoneal cavity.[66] As the tumor cells in this model were essentially in a suspension of ascites fluid and not vascularized, the cytotoxic effects of photodynamic treatment appear to have been directly upon tumor cells.

Data from Henderson and co-workers from studies with murine tumors in vivo and in vitro suggested that mechanisms other than direct effects on tumor cells might also be responsible for the cytotoxicity seen with PDT.[28] When subcutaneous tumors were treated with PDT and then immediately explanted into tissue culture, tumor cell viability in a cell survival-clonogenicity assay was surprisingly found to be nearly the same as in untreated controls. If explantation and plating were delayed for varying lengths of time from 1–24 hours after light delivery to the subcutaneous tumors, tumor cell viability progressively fell with increasing exposure to the in situ environment after light treatment. This suggested that other host-related factors, such as photodynamic effects on vasculature, are involved in tumor cell death in vivo.

Work by Star and co-workers with tumors sandwiched in transparent observation chambers showed that blood vessels in the tumor began to empty with blanching of the tumor about 10–15 minutes after PDT.[62] Blood flow returned if the initial PDT were not too extensive; however, in cases where illumination was continued for long periods, circulation would slow, ultimately stop, and be followed by diffuse hemorrhage.

Currently, most investigators believe that photodynamic damage to tumor is a combination of direct anti-tumor cell effects and indirect effects produced by destruction of the vasculature.

Pre-clinical trials of PDT in animal models demonstrated efficacy in several anatomic sites including the urinary bladder, bronchus, eye, peritoneal cavity and central nervous system with destruction of tumor at doses of light that spared adjacent normal tissue, providing impetus for clinical trials in these sites.[16]

Clinical Experience with PDT

The clinical experience to date with PDT to date has been accumulated using either the HpD or the more active DHE. HpD is no longer commercially available in the United States while DHE is currently available only as an investigational drug. The first systematic use of PDT in the clinic was at Roswell Park beginning in 1976 by the group led by Dougherty.[16] Their initial efforts were with cutaneous and subcutaneous cancers. Since that time, several thousand patients have been treated worldwide for neoplasms involving various sites. For most patients, conventional treatment had failed or been refused. Few of the trials were controlled or randomized since investigators were still in the process of developing techniques to treat particular anatomic sites. As additional experience with this modality has been accumulated,

there has been increasing emphasis on the development of carefully controlled clinical studies to help define the role for the modality in the current management of patients with cancer.

Cutaneous and Subcutaneous Cancers

Malignant neoplasms involving the skin which have been treated with PDT include recurrent metastatic breast carcinoma, basal and squamous cell carcinomas, malignant melanomas, mycosis fungoides, and Kaposi's sarcomas (Table XIII-3-1).[4,16] Patients have generally received HpD by intravenous injection and have then been treated with red light, generally 72–96 hours after injection of HpD. Patients have been treated with external surface illumination, interstitial implantation for larger lesions, or some combination thereof. Most patients have had disease that had not been controlled by prior surgery, chemotherapy, and ionizing radiation. Although investigators have used different criteria to judge response, it is clear that responses have been obtained after extensive prior treatment. All reporting investigators have remarked upon the differential response seen between tumor and adjacent normal tissue within the light field. Treatment appears to be effective to a depth of 5–10 mm, depending on the drug and light dose delivered as well as the mode of light delivery. The recent discovery of photobleaching (photodestruction) of porphyrins during illumination has been an important development in the treatment of skin lesions.[42] By reducing the injected dose of photosensitizer, the drug concentration in the normal skin surrounding tumors may be low enough that any residual drug is photobleached and destroyed during light delivery. This permits large increases in light delivery to the tumors (which will still contain active photosensitizer) with much less risk of injury of normal skin.

For primary lesions involving skin, investigators report high complete response rates which are often durable.[16] Complete responses have been achieved lasting up to 4 years.[16] Bandieramonte and colleagues treated 43 basal cell carcinomas and 18 metastatic breast cancer lesions in 7 patients. A clinical complete response was seen in 26/61 while 16 had a partial response.[4] Waldow and colleagues reported treatment of 6 basal cell lesions and 3 Bowen's disease or squamous cell carcinomas.[68] All lesions had a clinical complete response with follow-up times of 8–24 months. Kennedy reported durable, complete responses of 38 primary basal cell carcinomas in 3 patients.[34] Pennington and colleagues, however, reported a less favorable experience in 53 primary basal cell or squamous cell skin tumors.[52] Using HpD 5 mg/kg and 30 J/cm^2, complete responses were achieved in 52% of the basal cell lesions and 81% of the squamous cell lesions. However, over one-half of the squamous lesions and most of the basal cell lesions recurred at the time of the six month follow-up visit. Recently the group at Roswell Park reported 133 complete and 18 partial responses in 151 basal cell lesions in 37 patients with acceptable normal tissue response and excellent cosme-

Table XIII-3-1.   The Results of Photodynamic Therapy for Cutaneous or Subcutaneous Tumors

Tumor Type	Pts./Sites	Light Dose J/cm²	Response Rate (%) CR	PR	NR	Comments	Ref.
Basal Cell	3/38	90	100			None recur at 35 m	34
Basal/SCCa	6/9	8–60	100			Follow-up 8–24 m	68
Basal/SCCa	6/53	30	68	NA	NA	Majority recur at 6 m	52
Basal/Breast	7/61	60–100	50	31	19	Follow-up 4–16 m	4
Basal/SCCa	37/151	52–216	88	12		61% PR retreated to CR	72
Breast	14/	26–288	15	69	15	Palliative, longest CR 6 m	35

Pts., patients; J, joules; CR, complete response, eradication of tumor; PR, partial response, greater than 50% reduction in tumor size; NR, no response; m, month(s); SCCa, squamous cell carcinoma; NA, not available.

sis.[72] Of particular interest, is the exciting finding by Kennedy that ALA (5-aminolevulinic acid), a precursor of protoporphyrin in the biosynthetic pathway for heme, can be applied topically to photosensitize skin tumors.[35] This permits photodynamic therapy to these lesions without causing systemic photosensitivity.

Dose seeking studies to determine the optimum treatment schedule for skin lesions are in progress. The best results for cutaneous and subcutaneous lesions will likely be seen in relatively thin (less than 5 mm), discrete lesions. For primary nonmelanotic skin cancers, it may prove to be curative in appropriately selected cases. Several investigators have noted excellent cosmetic results after the re-epithelialization of the treated lesions. Apart from cutaneous photosensitivity and some discomfort at the site of treatment, the therapy is well tolerated. The acceptability of PDT for skin lesions would be enhanced by the development of a topical formulation of the HpD, which is under investigation. Most lesions thicker than 1.0 cm will probably need several external treatments or treatment by interstitial technique unless photosensitizers with absorption at longer, more deeply penetrating wavelengths are employed.

Pigmented melanomas are almost completely unresponsive to PDT because of extremely efficient light absorption by melanin. Unpigmented lesions, however, can be effectively controlled by PDT. Control of Kaposi's sarcomas up to 3 cm in diameter has been reported.[16]

Schuh and colleagues reported treatment of 14 women with locally recurrent breast carcinoma on the chest wall which had not been controlled with radiation, chemotherapy, hormonal therapy, or additional surgery.[58] Thirty courses of treatment were given. Two treatments elicited complete clinical responses with resolution of all visible disease, although post-treatment biopsies were not performed. One of the two patients developed recurrent disease within four months, while the other patient remained disease-free at six months after treatment. Twenty-two treatments were felt to result in a partial response, considered to be a significant reduction of the amount of chest wall disease. The duration of response was most commonly 8–12 weeks but ranged from 8 weeks to 8 months. Thus, treatment of recurrent breast cancer on the chest wall with phototherapy appears to generally produce partial responses of short duration. The 5 mm light penetration is probably adequate for small nodules but will be insufficient to address the more commonly seen problem of diffuse skin and lymphatic involvement, which can permeate the entire thickness of a chest wall that is often 3–4

cm thick. Larger lesions will often be inadequately treated because of limited light penetration. Treated lesions often undergo necrosis after treatment and require dressings for several weeks until re-epithelialization occurs. Discomfort requiring oral narcotics is often seen after treatment of larger lesions. The literature suggests that patients who have received doxorubicin and prior irradiation to a given area may show increased normal tissue sensitivity to PDT.[16] Because of the limited light penetration, the role for photodynamic therapy for recurrent breast cancer on the chest wall will probably be limited to selected patients with focal areas of small nodular recurrences.

Head and Neck Tumors

Wile and co-workers reported on 21 patients with head and neck tumors recurrent in the primary site who were treated with HpD and red light (Table XIII-3-2).[70] The majority had squamous cell carcinomas refractory to conventional therapy. Complete responses were seen in 6 patients (29%) and partial responses were seen in 11 patients (52%). The complete responses were durable in 4 of the 6 cases at follow-up times from 8 to 18 months. These occurred in patients with tongue, soft palate, and nasopharyngeal lesions. In 10 patients with regional head and neck cancer recurrences in soft tissues, results were less favorable: two complete responses and three partial responses were seen. In these patients, however, tumor would often recur at the margins of the treated field; the overall disease process did not appear substantially altered by treatment.

Takata and Imakiire reported on six cases of squamous carcinomas involving larynx, oropharynx, or tongue treated with PDT.[64] They noted significant necrosis of tumor in each of the cases, but pathologic examination of biopsy and surgical specimens revealed nests of viable tumor below the mucosa, suggesting inadequate light delivery and dose inhomogeneity. They noted no deleterious effects on surrounding normal tissue, although localized edema was seen after the procedure, suggesting that tracheostomy for airway protection might be indicated in the case of laryngeal lesions.

Grossweiner and colleagues described 10 patients with either early stage squamous cell carcinoma of the head and neck region who had refused, or could not tolerate, conventional therapy, or with advanced or recurrent disease after conventional therapy who were treated with photodynamic therapy by superficial or interstitial illumination. With follow-up of 6–18 months, eight complete responses and

Table XIII-3-2. The Results of Photodynamic Therapy for Head and Neck Tumors

Tumor Type	Patients	Light Dose J/cm²	Response Rate (%)			Comments	Ref.
			CR	PR	NR		
Squamous	10	60–100	80	10	10	Early or advanced cancer	23
Squamous	17	NA	59	24	17	Early stage cancer	19
Squamous	21	17–91	29	52	19	Primary site	70
Squamous	10	17–91	20	30	50	Regional soft tissue	70
Squamous	6	34–390		100		Primary site	64

J, joules; CR, complete response, eradication of tumor; PR, partial response, greater than 50% reduction in tumor size; NR, no response; NA, not available.

one partial response were seen. One patient failed to respond to treatment.[23]

Recently, there have been several encouraging reports of the use of photodynamic therapy for early squamous carcinomas of the oropharynx and larynx, with control of tumor of up to two years. Gluckman and colleagues reported treatment of 17 patients with early lesions of the head and neck for whom conventional therapy was not possible. Ten complete and four partial responses were seen.[19] Photodynamic therapy should be a useful addition to head and neck oncology because of the accessibility of this area to endoscopy and laser light and because of the proclivity of these patients to develop multiple primary sites of cancer. Photodynamic therapy can be repeated when necessary and can be used in sites that have been previously irradiated. Another potential use for PDT in the head and neck is for detection and treatment of carcinoma in situ. In such a setting, one would be able to obtain optimal light distribution because of the minimal thickness of disease. One could hope to deliver effective local therapy with little risk of injury to normal tissue.

Photodynamic therapy has been shown to be effective in eradicating papillomas caused by papilloma virus in an animal model[60] and is thus being tested clinically for the eradication of laryngeal papillomatosis.

Central Nervous System Tumors

In view of the grim prognosis with high grade gliomas, there has been interest in PDT for these tumors (Table XIII-3-3). Diamond and co-workers reported the inactivation of glioma cells in tissue culture with hematoporphyrin and light, as well as significant destruction of gliomas transplanted subcutaneously in rats.[15] HpD, which is protein-bound in serum, does not appear to cross the normal blood-brain barrier in significant concentrations.[15] Indeed, a very favorable ratio of photosensitizer concentration in tumor compared to normal brain tissue of 20:1 has been reported in a brain tumor model in the rat.[41] However, some photosensi-

tization of normal mouse brain by HpD, has also been reported by Berenbaum, who attributed the phenomenon to localization of HpD in endothelial cells on the vascular side of the blood-brain barrier.[8]

Laws and co-workers from the Mayo Clinic, reported a Phase I feasibility study with PDT for the treatment of malignant brain tumors.[39] All patients were thought to be surgically incurable and had gross recurrent tumor after conventional therapy at the time of treatment. Five patients were studied, four of whom had primary brain tumors and one a metastatic lesion. After HpD administration, a single quartz fiber was stereotactically inserted into the tumor and 630 nm red light was delivered. The patients appeared to tolerate treatment well. Two of the patients showed a transient decrease in either the size of the mass or resultant mass effect on CT scans after the procedure. Needle aspiration specimens of tumor showed fluorescence under blue light; normal brain in the biopsy specimens did not fluoresce.

Two recent series have demonstrated that adjuvant photoradiation therapy can be delivered at the time of resection of cerebral gliomas with an acceptable level of risk, although increased intracranial pressure and cerebral edema may be seen in some patients.[31,46] Currently, investigators in this area are exploring the use of a light diffusing lipid solution, or a lipid filled balloon, to homogeneously illuminate the resection cavity to high dose.[60] However, the limited depth of photodynamic effects, ranging from 0.5–1.0 cm, which has been seen after illumination of the resection cavity, highlights the need for the development of photosensitizers and techniques to adequately treat deep-seated tumors and infiltrating glioma cells beyond the limits of grossly evident tumor. Multiple interstitial fibers are now being placed into the margins of the resection cavity in order to address this problem.[60] If these techniques can deliver adequate light doses to all areas of residual tumor, PDT may prove to be an effective adjuvant for the treatment of brain tumors. At this point, however, its efficacy remains to be determined.

Table XIII-3-3. The Results of Photodynamic Therapy for Brain Tumors

Tumor Type	Patients	Light Dose J/cm²	Response Rate (%)			Comments	Ref.
			CR	PR	NR		
Glioma/Met.	5	810 J	NA	NA	NA	No toxicity. Phase I	39
Glioma/Met.	23	70–230	NA	NA	NA	No toxicity. Phase I/II	31
Glioma	32	8–68	19	13	68	25% cerebral edema	46

J, joules; CR, complete response, eradication of tumor; PR, partial response, greater than 50% reduction in tumor size; NR, no response; Met., tumors metastatic to the brain.

Ocular Tumors

PDT has been attempted for control of choroidal malignant melanoma, a tumor managed traditionally by enucleation but increasingly treated in recent years by local radiation with scleral plaques or external particle beam irradiation in addition to laser photocoagulation or transscleral diathermy (Table XIII-3-4). Bruce reported treatment of 24 patients with red light 300–3,000 J/cm^2 delivered transcorneally, transsclerally, or via a combination of these approaches after intravenous administration of HpD. Post-treatment fluorescein angiograms showed dramatic reductions in the vascular supply to tumor. Tumor responses were scored according to tumor size: small ($\leq$ 500 mm^3), medium (500–1,000 mm^3), or large ($\geq$ 1,000 mm^3). Complete responses were seen in all of the patients with small or medium lesions, with the final appearance of the tumor that of a large chorioretinal scar. Tumor responses were incomplete in the large lesions even after re-treatment. With up to seven years of follow-up, ten patients required enucleation for recurrence of tumor and 3/24 died from metastatic melanoma.

Post-treatment complications included some degree of transient chemosis, iritis, and lid swelling in all patients, managed with cycloplegics and corticosteroid drops. Exudative retinal detachment worsened or developed in a majority of patients. Detachments were more extensive in patients with larger tumors. The detachments resolved within six weeks in approximately two-thirds of the cases. Other changes noted included choroidal detachment, cataract, vitreous hemorrhage, vitreous inflammatory reaction, and reduced visual acuity. The reduction in visual acuity occurred where tumor or retinal detachment involved the macula.

These investigators used high energy densities for treatment. There is no comment about the pigmentation in the lesions treated. Melanin is an efficient absorber of red light, so that high energy densities must be used if sufficient light is to reach the deepest portions of pigmented lesions. Thermal effects may have been present at the power densities (dose rates) employed. These doses of light may, however, increase the risk of damage to uninvolved normal tissue. Indeed, Murphree and Gomer treated seven patients with pigmented choroidal melanomas with PDT and achieved no complete responses. They suggested that pigmented melanomas of even modest height would not be adequately treated by conventional PDT alone and noted that the responses seen by other investigators may have resulted from the synergism of PDT with the secondary thermal effects seen at high power densities.[48] Nevertheless, there may be a role for PDT in the treatment of lesions $\leq$1,000 mm^3.

Photodynamic destruction of retinoblastoma cells in vitro has also been reported.[59] Moreover, eyes of athymic mice containing human retinoblastoma have been shown to retain higher concentrations of ^{3}H-HpD than control eyes. In vivo work has demonstrated regression of human retinoblastoma in the nude mouse after PDT. Murphree and Gomer noted initial complete responses to PDT in discrete retinoblastoma lesions in six patients but tumor regrowth occurred in every case within 3–4 months.[8] No responses were seen in lesions seeding the vitreous.

Cancers in the Thoracic Cavity

The earliest reported clinical use of HpD was for fluorescence detection of endobronchial tumor.[40] Several groups have more recently reported on the effective use of PDT for either palliative[3,50] or potentially curative[17,25] treatment of endobronchial tumors (Table XIII-3-5). Balchum reported on the palliative treatment with PDT of 35 patients with tumors of the tracheobronchial tree.[3] HpD was administered intravenously and then red light was delivered to the lesions using an optical fiber passed through the bronchoscope. Patients would undergo a second brochoscopy within two to three days of treatment in order to remove tumor debris. The majority of lesions treated were primary bronchogenic tumors, but several endobronchial metastases from other sites and one benign fibrous mass were also treated. Thirty-three of the 35 patients had tumors obstructing a bronchus. After one photodynamic treatment, the lumen reopened in 80% of cases in which tumor was confined to the bronchus. The remaining cases required two treatments to open the bronchus because of the extensive length involved or because multiple tumor sites were present. They were able to open the bronchus in all but one case. Bronchial inflammation after PDT was minimal and mucosal edema seldom occurred.

Complications included pneumothorax in two patients. Pulmonary hemorrhage led to death in 4 patients at 4–5 weeks after phototherapy. All had large necrotic tumors in the main stem bronchus. Autopsies were performed on two of these patients revealing necrosis of tumor in the medial aspect of the main stem bronchus and of tumor in the adjacent mediastinum. Because tumor necrosis was seen on bronchoscopy in these cases prior to PDT, it is not clear whether the treatment or the extent of tumor was responsible for the subsequent hemorrhage.

A randomized Phase III trial of PDT vs. Neodymium-YAG laser for relief of endobronchial obstruction in patients with recurrent, inoperable non-small cell lung cancer is currently in progress. In addition, a phase III randomized trial is comparing the effectiveness of radiation alone to radiation with PDT in patients undergoing radiation therapy for treatment of primary, non-small cell lung cancer.

The group at the Mayo Clinic reported on treatment results in 38 patients with 40 bronchogenic carcinomas involving

Table XIII-3-4.   The Results of Photodynamic Therapy for Ocular Tumors

Tumor Type	Pts./Eyes	Light Dose J/cm^2	Response Rate (%) CR	PR	NR	Comments	Ref.
Melanoma	24/24	300–3,000	41	6	53	CR's in small tumors	10
Melanoma	9/9	50–400	22	66	12	CR's non-pigmented	48
Retinoblast.	6/9	50–400	11	78	11	All later recurred	48

Pts., patients; J, joules; CR, complete response, eradication of tumor, PR, partial response, greater than 50% reduction in tumor size; NR, no response.

Table XIII-3-5.   The Results of Photodynamic Therapy for Lung and Bronchial Tumors

Tumor Type	Pts./Sites	Light Dose J/cm²	Response Rate (%) CR	PR	NR	Comments	Ref.
Lung	38/40	54–675	35	NA	NA	CR's in small lesions	17
Lung	8/8	120/240	75	25		Early stage lesions	25
Lung, Met.	10/13	250 J/cm	80% of bronchi re-opened after treatment				50
Lung, Met.	35/35	100 J/cm	If tumor endobronchial, 80% re-opened				3

Pts., patients; J, joules; CR, complete response, eradication of tumor; PR, partial response, greater than 50% reduction in tumor size; NR, no response; Met., metastatic lesion narrowing or obstructing the bronchus.

the tracheobronchial tree.[17] All patients had undergone previous pulmonary resection for another lung cancer or were considered inoperable for medical or technical reasons. In addition, these patients were ineligible for, or unresponsive to, conventional therapy with irradiation and chemotherapy. Patients were treated after HpD administration with 630 nm red light delivered via an optical fiber passed through the bronchoscope. A complete response to treatment was defined as the elimination of any evidence of tumor on chest roentgenogram, bronchoscopy, and bronchoscopic biopsies and washings. Complete responses were seen in 14 lesions in 13 patients, requiring one treatment in nine cases and two treatments in 5 cases. Eleven of the complete responses were maintained at follow-up periods ranging from 3–53 months, with a median of 29 months. Three of the lesions recurred at 9, 12, and 35 months. Of note, all of the tumors that showed a complete response were less than 2 cm² in surface area and radiographically occult, having been discovered on bronchoscopy. This indicates that use of this modality for curative treatment for lung lesions may be limited to carefully selected early cases.

The Mayo Clinic group also noted massive hemoptysis within weeks of PDT in 3 patients with large obstructing tumors. Pulmonary compromise was also seen in 2 patients with underlying pulmonary dysfunction; this was due to patient inability to clear necrotic debris after phototherapy. Bronchoscopy was required to ultimately do so. Cutaneous photosensitivity was seen in 3 patients early in their series, before patients were given explicit instructions to avoid sunlight exposure.

Hayata and co-workers reported on the treatment of 8 patients with early, centrally located squamous carcinomas of the lung with PDT.[25] These patients were all diagnosed by bronchoscopy. Five were treated with PDT alone, while the remaining three underwent surgical resection after phototherapy. A complete response endoscopically and histologically or cytologically was obtained in the five non-resected cases. These patients remained disease-free at 11–36 months after treatment. Of the three patients who underwent resection, one had a complete histologic response. The other two had no visible tumor at endoscopy prior to resection, but their resection specimens harbored microscopic residual tumor which was probably beyond the range of light penetration. One of these patients who had been treated for an early stage carcinoma of the lung with PDT because of poor pulmonary function was recently reported living beyond five years free of tumor.[30] These results again suggest that the PDT may be useful treatment for early or superficial lesions in the bronchus.

One area in which clinical investigation has recently begun is the use of PDT for diffuse malignant mesothelioma, a disease which is rarely treated effectively by conventional surgical, radiotherapeutic, or chemotherapeutic approaches.[51] Human malignant mesothelioma cells have been shown to be sensitive to PDT in vitro.[32] A phase I, light-dose escalation study of PDT delivered to the entire pleural surface intraoperatively following resection or debulking of tumor has been initiated by the Surgery and Radiation Oncology Branches of the National Cancer Institute.

Esophageal and Gastrointestinal Tract Cancers

PDT has been attempted for both cure and palliation of esophageal cancer (Table XIII-3-6). In the United States, where patients most often present with bulky tumor and adjacent nodal involvement indicative of advanced stage disease, investigators have reported palliation of esophageal obstruction using PDT. In Japan and China, where mass screening clinics have been able to detect early esophageal carcinomas, PDT has been attempted with curative intent.

McCaughan and co-workers reported on the treatment of 40 patients with esophageal tumors (19 adenocarcinomas, 19 squamous carcinomas, and 2 melanomas) in whom conventional treatments were unsuccessful.[43] Patients received HpD or DHE, followed by the delivery of red light via an optical fiber passed through a flexible endoscope. Four patients with stage I tumors had a complete response. One with squamous cancer subsequently died of recurrent disease at 18 months but two with adenocarcinoma were alive and free of disease at 11 and 23 months after treatment, while a third patient with melanoma died of another cancer 31 months after treatment. Of the 35 patients who could be evaluated one month after PDT, the average improvement in food intake was from a liquid to a soft diet. Of the 28 patients assessable one month after PDT, the average minimal esophageal diameter opening increased from 6 to 9 mm. Nine patients with complete obstruction were treated; of the seven survivors at one month, all were able to tolerate oral food. Side effects of treatment included six pleural effusions of which five resolved without treatment, six strictures requiring dilatation, three tracheo-esophageal fistulas (one in a patient with tracheal invasion and one in a patient who had had prior laryngeal surgery). Because of the advanced nature of most of their cases, overall survival was poor, averaging 7.7 months for patients with adenocarcinoma and 5.8 months for patients with squamous carcinomas.

Thomas and colleagues treated 14 patients with locally

Table XIII-3-6.   The Results of Photodynamic Therapy for Esophageal and Gastric Tumors

Tumor Type	Pts.	Light Dose J/cm^2	Response Rate (%) CR	PR	NR	Comments	Ref.
Esophagus	40	300–660 J/c	10	NA	NA	Majority improve swallowing	43
Esophagus	14	60–337	14	86		All improve swallowing	65
Esophagus	4	270–360	50	50		Early stage. CR's NED at 1,2 y	1
Esophagus	5	270–360		100		Advanced stage	1
Gastric	4	34–960	100			3/4 recur by 27 m	26
Gastric	12	34–960	Resected post PDT.			5/12 no tumor in specimen	26

Pts., patients; J, joules; J/c, joules/centimeter; CR, complete response, eradication of tumor; PR, partial response, greater than 50% reduction in tumor size; NR, no response; NED, no evidence of disease; y, years; m, months.

advanced esophageal cancer using high dose photodynamic therapy.[65] All patients achieved a measurable improvement in the severity of dysphagia persisting from 1–28 weeks. Two patients had a complete eradication of tumor proven by histologic examination of the subsequently resected esophagus. A complication rate of 16% was noted and included mediastinitis and broncho-esophageal fistula.

Aida and Hirashima treated four patients with superficial carcinomas of the esophagus.[1] Two had endoscopically complete responses and remained disease-free at one and two years after treatment. The other two patients went on to surgical resection and were found to have residual tumor cells in portions of the tumor thought to have been inadequately illuminated. Their advanced cases showed partial responses.

Hayata and co-workers in Japan have also treated 16 patients with early stage gastric carcinoma (Table XIII-3-6).[26] Four were treated by PDT alone because of medical inoperability or refusal of surgery, while the other 12 patients had resection after PDT. Complete disappearance by endoscopic visualization was obtained in all 4 patients treated with PDT alone. One patient remained disease-free at 30 months, one had a recurrence at 27 months and was retreated, and two patients died with recurrence of disease at 5 and 13 months. Of the 12 patients who had resection after PDT, there was no evidence of tumor in the operative specimen in five. Complications included epigastric pain and ulcer formation that were amenable to medical management.

PDT may thus have some applicability in early stage gastric cancer for patients who cannot undergo curative surgery. The shape of the stomach and deep rugae complicate the delivery of light. The technical aspects of light delivery must be addressed if adequate PDT is to be given. Because of the difficulty in diagnosing early stage cases and the propensity of gastric carcinomas to metastasize to adjacent lymph nodes, however, PDT for most gastric cancers in the United States will probably be limited to palliation of medically inoperable cases.

Genitourinary Cancer

The first reported use of PDT in a human was for a patient with transitional cell carcinoma of the bladder. Kelly and Snell observed destruction of tumor in the subsequent cystectomy specimen only in sites that had been illuminated.[33] This has been one of the most active areas of interest in PDT (Table XIII-3-7). Emphasis has been on treatment of superficial transitional cell cancers not involving the muscularis of the bladder (TIS, Ta, T1 tumors).

Benson and co-workers from the Mayo Clinic were able to demonstrate localization of HpD in transitional cell carcinoma in situ and severely dysplastic epithelium in the urinary bladder after intravenous administration and subsequent illumination of the bladder with violet light.[7] Their observations were confirmed at histologic examination of the bladders after cystectomy. Their only false-positive findings occurred where there was regenerative mucosal activity around healing biopsy sites.

The Mayo Clinic group initially reported biopsy-proven complete tumor responses in 4 patients with recurrent, previously treated transitional cell carcinomas of the bladder that were focally illuminated using optical fibers introduced through the cystoscope after intravenous HpD injection.[7] A collaborative group of American and Chinese urologists treated 50 papillary tumors and three areas of carcinoma in situ in 20 patients with focal PDT to the involved sites.[54] The carcinomas in situ were all eliminated and 74% of the papillary lesions had a complete response to treatment. The complete response rate was only 33% for lesions larger than 1.5 cm. Two groups from Japan reported that the highest complete remission rate was seen for lesions smaller than 1 cm.[29,67] Because of the tendency of tumors to later recur at other sites in the bladder that had not been illuminated, the Mayo Clinic group switched to using a modified optical fiber with a spherical diffusing bulb in order to illuminate the entire bladder.[7] They reported on treatment in this manner of 14 patients with diffuse resistant carcinoma in situ who had refused cystectomy. Initially using a dose of 50 J/cm^2 to the entire bladder for the first five patients, they noted severe bladder irritability. After scaling the dose back to 20 J/cm^2, treatment was better tolerated. In 10 patients with carcinoma in situ alone, biopsy and urinary cytology at follow-up examination three months after treatment showed complete disappearance of tumor. Two patients with both carcinoma in situ and papillary, noninvasive lesions were noted to have disappearance of the former but persistence of the latter. Of these 12 patients, three subsequently developed focal recurrent disease at 6 to 9 months after treatment. Two patients who had focal invasive carcinoma in addition to their in situ disease had persistent invasive disease after PDT, although their in situ disease was controlled. They subsequently underwent cystectomy.

Light dose and light delivery technique have been important in both tumor control and complication of treatment. High

Table XIII-3-7. The Results of Photodynamic Therapy for Urinary Bladder Tumors

Tumor Type	Pts./Sites	Light Dose J/cm²	Response Rate (%) CR	PR	NR	Comments	Ref.
TCCa	4/	F 150	100	—	—	CIS. Recur elsewhere in bladder	7
TCCa	8/	F 120–360	100	—	—	Ta-T2. Two recur at 6–18 m	67
TCCa	9/36	F 50–300	50	19	31	Ta, T1 tumors. All CR ≤ 2 cm	29
TCCa	19/50	F 100–200	24	50	26	Ta, T1, CIS tumors	54
TCCa	10/	WB 25–45	60	20	20	CIS or CIS and T2 tumors	7
TCCa	7/	WB 25 + F	78	—	22	4/7 develop contracted bladder	24

Pts., patients; J, joules; CR, complete response, eradication of tumor; PR, partial response, greater than 50% reduction in tumor size; NR, no response; TCCa, transitional cell carcinoma; m, month(s); F, focal; WB, whole bladder; CIS, carcinoma in situ; Ta, papillary tumor confined to mucosa; T1, tumor invading lamina propria; T2, tumor invading muscle superficially.

dose (100–200 J/cm²) focal light treatment delivered has been used to control papillary lesions. However, much lower doses (~20 J/cm²) have been used for the whole bladder treatment, which has been used to control either carcinoma in situ or microscopic disease after resection of papillary lesions. Of note, however, is the report from Harty and associates which describes the development of a contracted bladder with hydroureteronephrosis and vesicoureteral reflux in 4/7 patients treated with 25 J/cm² to the whole bladder, with or without additional focal treatment.[24] Deep bladder biopsies showed replacement of smooth muscle by fibrous tissue. Clearly, careful attention to light dose and treatment technique, as well as photosensitizer localization in tumor compared to normal bladder, will be important if this is to be a safe and effective treatment for superficial bladder cancer.

Ongoing clinical investigations in the U.S. and abroad for use of PDT in the bladder are currently focused on carcinoma in situ and multicentric, recurring papillary disease. In one trial patients with refractory or recurrent superficial transitional cell carcinoma in situ disease are being treated with PDT as an alternative to cystectomy. In a second trial, patients with high grade or recurrent, low grade papillary lesions are being randomized after complete transurethral resection to either observation or PDT in an attempt to assess its efficacy in preventing recurrences in this high risk population.

Gynecologic Cancer

The first report of the use of PDT for gynecologic cancers came from Australia in 1982, describing treatment of five patients with recurrent tumors involving the vaginal vault.[69] Two complete responses were seen, one in a patient with recurrent ovarian cancer and the other in a patient with melanoma. These were durable at 10 and 12 months. The only toxicity noted was cutaneous phototoxicity.

Multiple other reports have subsequently appeared, primarily in cases of gynecologic cancer recurring in the vagina or skin after conventional treatment (Table XIII-3-8).[44] Dahlman and associates reported the successful treatment of a patient with multiply recurrent carcinoma in situ of the vulva, whereas a second patient with cervical carcinoma recurrent in the vulva failed to respond.[13] Rettenmaier and co-workers reported treatment of 9 lesions in 6 patients with HpD and red light.[56] They obtained complete responses in 2 lesions

and partial responses in 4 others. The only toxicity noted was cutaneous phototoxicity.

Corti and co-workers treated 15 patients with vaginal recurrences of carcinoma of the cervix, endometrial carcinoma of the corpus uteri, and adenocarcinoma of the rectum.[12] Nine patients had superficial lesions that they treated with curative intent, while the other six had bulky lesions that were treated for palliation. They achieved eight complete responses, of which seven were in the patients with the superficial lesions. The duration of CR ranged from 2.5–25 months. They reported no treatment related morbidity.

PDT is also being investigated as an adjuvant therapy to be delivered to patients with ovarian cancer at the time of second look laparotomy. Tochner and co-workers were able to control an experimental murine ovarian ascites tumor in 17 of 20 animals using intraperitoneally administered HpD and four intraperitoneal light treatments.[66] On the basis of these experimental findings, a phase I study has been initiated in which PDT is administered to the peritoneal surface of patients with minimal thickness intraperitoneal tumor at the time of surgical resection. DeLaney and associates reported on treatment of three such patients with recurrent ovarian cancer in whom it was possible surgically to resect all gross disease at laparotomy and then deliver PDT to the entire peritoneal cavity.[14] In this Phase I light dose escalation study designed to determine feasibility and potential toxicity, such treatment was shown to be practical and tolerated at the initial light doses.

Summary

PDT represents another modality for the treatment of human cancer. Light activated photosensitizers have definite antitumor activity in both in vitro and in vivo experimental systems. Much of the early clinical work involved treatment of patients with advanced, recurrent disease who had not responded to conventional therapy. Because good responses with acceptable toxicity have been obtained in these patients, active investigation continues and is aimed at defining the most appropriate sites and applications for the technique. Because of the limited depth of light penetration in tissue, the most promising sites may be those where there is limited thickness of tumor, such as in superficial skin lesions or early stage carcinomas involving the aerodigestive tract, bronchial tree, or the genitourinary tract. Other potential uses include

Table XIII-3-8.   The Results of Photodynamic Therapy for Gynecologic Tumors

Tumor Type	Pts./Sites	Light Dose J/cm²	Response Rate (%) CR	PR	NR	Comments	Ref.
Vagina	5/5	NA	40	60	—	CR's durable at 10,12 m	69
Vulva	2/2	NA	50	—	50	CR in carcinoma in situ	13
Vagina/Per.	6/9	20–40	22	45	33	Treatment well tolerated	56
Vagina	15/15	60/240	53	40	7	Duration of CR 2.5–25 m	12
Vulva/Vagina	5/5	Variable	80	20	—	Follow-up 5–15 m	44

Pts., patients; J, joules; CR, complete response, eradication of tumor; PR, partial response, greater than 50% reduction in tumor size; NR, no response; Per., perineum; m, month(s); NA, not available.

those where PDT could be combined with surgical or chemotherapeutic debulking, such as pleural mesothelioma or advanced stage ovarian cancer. Whether PDT can be of benefit in surgical cases where the margins of resection are close is an interesting but speculative notion at the present time.

The hematoporphyrin derivative and the dihematoporphyrin ethers are currently only approved for use as investigational compounds in clinical studies. If ongoing trials of PDT in superficial bladder cancer, obstructing esophageal cancer, and non-small cell lung cancer show encouraging results, an application will be made to the Food and Drug Administration for approval of DHE as a photosensitizer for general clinical use for these indications. Laboratory work to better understand the mechanisms of action of HpD also continues, as well as investigations into alternative photosensitizers with improved tumor localization, less cutaneous photosensitivity, and absorption peaks at deeper penetrating wavelengths of light. Attempts at measurement of singlet oxygen, if successful, will permit the development of more meaningful dosimetry in order to correlate response with actual tissue levels of the purported cytotoxic agent. Hopefully, these and other developments in the field of PDT will improve the treatment for patients with cancer.

References

1. Aida, M., and Hirashima, T.: Cancer of the esophagus. In Lasers and Hematoporphyrin Derivative in Cancer. Edited by Y. Hayata and T. F. Dougherty. New York, Igaku-Shoin, 1983, p. 57.
2. Andreoni, A., Cubeddu, R., DeSilvestri, S., Laporta, P., Ambesi-Impiombato, F. S., Esposito, M., Mastrocinque, M., and Tramontano, D.: Effects of laser irradiation on hematoporphyrin-treated normal and transformed thyroid cells in culture. Cancer Res., 43:2076, 1983.
3. Balchum, O. J., and Doiron, D. R.: Photoradiation therapy of endobronchial lung cancer. Clin. Chest Med., 6:255, 1985.
4. Bandieramonte, C., Marchesini, R., Melloni, E., Andreoli, C., di Pietro, S., Spinelli, P., Fava, G., Zunino, Z., and Emanuelli, H.: Laser phototherapy following HpD administration in superficial neoplastic lesions. Tumori, 70:327, 1984.
5. Barel, A., Jori, G., Perin, A., Ramandini, P., Pagnan, A., and Biffanti, S.: Role of high, low and very low density lipoproteins in the transport and tumor delivery of hematoporphyrin in vivo. Cancer Lett., 32:145, 1986.
6. Ben-Hur, E., and Rosenthal, I.: The phthallocyanines: a new class of mammalian cell photosensitizers with a potential for cancer phototherapy. Int. J. Rad. Biol., 47:145, 1985.
7. Benson, R. C.: Laser photodynamic therapy for bladder cancer. Mayo. Clin. Proc., 61:859, 1986.
8. Berenbaum, M. C., Hall, G. W., and Hoyes, A. D.: Cerebral photosensitisation by hematoporphyrin derivative. Evidence for an endothelial site of action. Br. J. Cancer, 53:81, 1986.
9. Brown, S. B., Vernon, D. I., and Stribbling, S.: Fate of HPD after intravenous administration. Photochem. Photobiol., 51(supplement):97s, 1990 (abstract).
10. Bruce, R. A., Jr., and McCaughan, J. S.: Lasers in uveal melanoma. Ophthalm. Clin. of N. America, 2:597, 1989.
11. Bugelski, P. J., Porter, C. W., and Dougherty, T. J.: Autoradiographic distribution of HpD in normal and tumor tissue of the mouse. Cancer Res., 41:4606, 1981.
12. Corti, L., Tomio, L., Maluta, S., Stevanin, C., Iannone, T., and Calzavara, F.: Photodynamic therapy in gynecological cancer. Lasers Med. Sci., 4:155, 1989.
13. Dahlman, A., Wile, A. G., Burns, R. G., Mason, G. R., Johnson, F. M., and Berns, M. W.: Laser photoradiation therapy of cancer. Cancer Res., 43:430, 1983.
14. DeLaney, T. F., Sindelar, W., Smith, P., Friauf, W., Pass, H., Russo, A., Thomas, G.,
15. Dachowski, L., Cole, J., and Glatstein, E.: Initial Experience with Photodynamic Therapy for Intraperitoneal Carcinomatosis. In Ovarian Cancer: Biological and Therapeutic Challenges. Edited by F. Sharp, W. P. Mason, and R. E. Leake. London: Chapman and Hall Medical, 1990, p. 371.
15. Diamond, I., Granelli, S. G., McDonough, A. F., Nielsen, S., Wilson, C. B., and Jaenicke, R.: Photodynamic therapy of malignant tumours. Lancet, 2:1175, 1972.
16. Dougherty, T. J.: Photosensitization of malignant tumors. Sem. Surg. Oncol., 2:24, 1986.
17. Edell, E. S., and Cortese, D. A.: Bronchoscopic phototherapy with hematoporphyrin derivative for treatment of localized bronchogenic carcinoma: A 5-year experience. Mayo Clin. Proc., 62:8–14, 1987.
18. Foote, C. S.: Mechanisms of Photooxygenation. In Porphyrin Localization and Treatment of Tumors. Edited by D. R. Doiron, and C. J. Gomer. New York, Alan R. Liss, 1984, p. 3.
19. Gluckman, J. L., Waner, M., Shumrick, K., and Peerless, S.: Photodynamic therapy. A viable alternative to conventional therapy for early lesion of the upper aerodigestive tract. Arch. Otolaryngol. Head Neck Surg., 112:949, 1986.
20. Gomer, C. J., and Dougherty, T. J.: Determination of [³H] and [¹⁴C] hematoporphyrin derivative distribution in malignant and normal tissue. Cancer Res., 39:146, 1979.
21. Gomer, C. J., Rucker, N., Banerjee, A., and Benedict, W. F.: Comparison of mutagenicity and induction of sister chromatid exchange in chinese hamster cells exposed to hematoporphyrin derivative photoradiation, ionizing radiation, or ultraviolet radiation. Cancer Res., 43:2622, 1983.
22. Gomer, C. J., Rucker, N., and Murphree, A. L.: Differential cell photosensitivity following porphyrin photodynamic therapy. Cancer Res., 48:4539, 1988.
23. Grossweiner, L. I., Hill, J. H., and Lobraico, R. V.: Photodynamic therapy of head and neck squamous cell carcinoma: optical dosimetry and clinical trial. Photochem. Photobiol., 46:911, 1987.
24. Harty, J. I., Amin, M., Wieman, T. J., Tseng, M. T., Ackerman, D., and Broghamer, W.: Complications of whole bladder dihematoporphyrin ether photodynamic therapy. J. Urol., 141:1341, 1989.
25. Hayata, Y., Kato, H., Konaka, C., Amemiya, R., Ono, J., Ogawa, I., Kinoshita, K., Sakai, H., and Takahashi, H.: Photoradiation therapy with hematoporphyrin derivative in early and stage 1 lung cancer. Chest, 86:169, 1984.
26. Hayata, T., Kato, H., Okitsu, H., Kawaguchi, M., and Konaka, D.: Photodynamic therapy with hematoporphyrin derivative in cancer of the upper gastrointestinal tract. Sem. Surg. Oncol., 1:1, 1985.
27. Henderson, B. W., Bellinier, D. A., Ziring, B., and Dougherty, T. J.: Aspects of the cellular uptake and retention of hematoporphyrin derivative and their correlation with the biological response to PRT in vitro. In Porphyrin Photosensitization. Edited by D. Kessel and T. J. Dougherty. New York, Plenum Press, 1983, p. 129.
28. Henderson, B. W., Waldow, S. M., Mang, T. S., Potter, W. R., Malone, P. B., and Dougherty, T. J.: Tumor destruction and kinetics of tumor cell death in two experimental mouse tumors following photodynamic therapy. Cancer Res., 45:572, 1985.
29. Hisazumi, H., Misaki, T., and Miyoshi, N.: Photoradiation therapy of bladder tumors. J. Urol., 130:685, 1983.
30. Kato, H., Konaka, C., Kawate, N., Shinohara, H., Kinoshita, K., Noguchi, M., Ootome, S., and Hayata, Y.: Five-year disease-free survival of a lung cancer patient treated only by photodynamic therapy. Chest., 90:768, 1986.
31. Kaye, A. H., Morstyn, G., and Brownbill, D.: Adjuvant high-dose photoradiation therapy in the treatment of cerebral glioma: a Phase 1-2 study. J. Neurosurg., 67:500, 1987.
32. Keller, S. M., Taylor, D. D., and Weese, J. L.: In vitro killing of human malignant mesothelioma by photodynamic therapy. J. Surg. Res., 48:337, 1990.
33. Kelly, J. F., and Snell, M. E.: Hematoporphyrin derivative: A possible aid in the diagnosis and therapy of carcinoma of the bladder. J. Urol., 115:150, 1976.
34. Kennedy, J.: HPD Photoradiation Therapy for Cancer at Kingston and Hamilton. In Porphyrin Photosensitization. Edited by D. Kessel and T. J. Dougherty. New York, Plenum Press, 1983, p. 53.
35. Kennedy, J. C., Pross, D. C., and Pottier, R. H.: Topical application of 5-aminolevulinic acid selectively induces phototoxic concentrations of protoporphyrin IX in actinic keratoses, primary basal cell and squamous cell carcinomas, and transdermal secondaries of breast carcinoma. Presented at the International Photodynamic Association Meeting, Buffalo, New York, 1990.
36. Kessel, D.: Effects of photoactivated porphyrins at the cell surface of leukemia L-1210 cell. Biochemistry, 16:3443, 1977.
37. Kessel, D., and Chou, T.: Tumor-localizing components of the porphyrin preparation hematoporphyrin derivative. Cancer Res., 43:1994, 1983.
38. Kessel, D., Thompson, P., Musselman, B., and Chang, C. K.: Chemistry of hematoporphyrin-derived photosensitizers. Photochem. Photobiol., 46:563, 1987.
39. Laws, E. R., Jr., Cortese, D. A., Kinsey, J. H., Eagen, R. T., and Anderson, R. E.: Photoradiation therapy in the treatment of malignant brain tumors: A phase I (feasibility) study. Neurosurgery, 9:672, 1981.
40. Lipson, R. L., Baldes, E. J., and Olsen, E. M.: Hematoporphyrin derivative for detection and management of cancer. Proc IX Internat. Cancer Congr. 393, 1966.
41. Little, F. M., Gomer, C. J., Hyman, S., and Apuzzo, M. L. J.: Observations in studies

of quantitative kinetics of tritium labelled hematoporphyrin derivatives (HpD₁ and HpD₁₁) in the normal and neoplastic rat brain model. J. Neuro-Oncol., 2:361, 1984.

42. Mang, T. S., Dougherty, T. J., Potter, W. R., Boyle, D. G., Somer, S., and Moan, J.: Photobleaching of porphyrins used in photodynamic therapy and implications for therapy. Phototochem. Photobiol., 45:501, 1987.

43. McCaughan, J. S., Jr., Nims, T. A., Guy, J. T., Hicks, W. J., Williams, T. E., Jr., and Laufman, L. R.: Photodynamic therapy for esophageal tumors. Arch. Surg., 124:74, 1989.

44. McCaughan, J. S., Jr., Schellhas, H. F., Lomano, J., and Bethel, B. H.: Photodynamic therapy of gynecologic neoplasms after presentation with hematoporphyrin derivative. Lasers Surg. Med., 5:491, 1985.

45. Moan, J., and Sommer, S.: Action spectra for hematoporphyrin derivative and Photofrin II with respect to sensitization of human cells in vitro to photoinactivation. Photochem. Photobiol., 40:63, 1984.

46. Muller, P. J., and Wilson, B. C.: Photodynamic therapy of malignant primary brain tumors: Clinical effects, post-operative ICP, and light penetration of the brain. Photochem. Photobiol., 46:929, 1987.

47. Munson, B. R.: Photodynamic inactivation of mammalian DNA-dependent RNA polymerase by hematoporphyrin and visible light. Int. J. Biochem., 10:957, 1979.

48. Murphree, A. L., Cote, M., and Gomer, C. J.: The evolution of photodynamic therapy techniques in the treatment of intraocular tumors. Photochem. Photobiol., 46:919, 1987.

49. Parker, J. G.: Optical detection of singlet oxygen produced during the photodynamic treatment of subcutaneous murine tumors. Presented at Clayton Foundation Conference on Photodynamic Therapy, Los Angeles, CA, 1987.

50. Pass, H. I., DeLaney, T. F., Smith, P. D., Bonner, R., and Russo, A.: Bronchoscopic phototherapy at comparable dose rates: Early results. Ann. Thorac. Surg., 47:693, 1989.

51. Pass, H. I., Tochner, Z. A., DeLaney, T. F., Smith, P., Friauf, W., Glatstein, E., and Travis, W.: Intraoperative photodynamic therapy for malignant mesothelioma (letter). Ann. Thorac. Surg., 50:687, 1990.

52. Pennington, D. J., Waner, M., and Knox, A.: Photodynamic therapy for multiple skin cancers. Plastic and Reconst. Surg., 82:1067, 1987.

53. Policard, A.: Etude sur les aspects offerts part des tumeurs experimentales examinees a la lumiere de Wood. C. R. Soc. Biol., 91:1423, 1924.

54. Prout, G. R., Jr., Lin, C., Benson, R., Jr., Nseyo, U. O., Daly, J. J., Graffin, P. P, Kinsey, J., Tian, M., Lao, Y., Mian, Y., Chen, X., Ren, F., and Qiao, S.: Photodynamic therapy with hematoporphyrin derivative in the treatment of superficial transitional-cell carcinoma of the bladder. N. Engl. J. Med., 317:1251, 1987.

55. Rerko, R. M., Clay, M. E., Rodriquez-Antunez, A., Oleinick, N. L., and Evans, H. H.: Mutagenicity of Photofrin II in L5178Y mouse lymphoma cells. Photochem. Photobiol., 51(supplement):83s, 1990 (abstract).

56. Rettenmaier, M. A., Berman, M. L., Disaia, P. J., Burns, R. G., Weinstein, G. D., McCullough, J. L., and Berns, M. W.: Gynecologic Uses of Photoradiation Therapy. In Porphyrin Localization and Treatment of Tumors. Edited by D. R. Doiron, and C. J. Gomer. New York, Alan R. Liss, 1984, p. 767.

57. Sandberg, S., and Romsio, I.: Porphyrin-sensitized photodynamic damage of isolated rat liver mitochondria. Biochim. Biophys. Acta, 593:187, 1980.

58. Schuh, M., Nseyo, U. O., Potter, W. R., Dao, T. L., and Dougherty, T. J.: Photodynamic therapy for palliation of locally recurrent breast carcinoma. J. Clin. Onc., 5:1766, 1987.

59. Sery, T. W.: Photodynamic killing of retinoblastoma cells with hematoporphyrin and light. Cancer Res., 39:96, 1979.

60. Shikowitz, M. J., Steinberg, B. M., and Abramson, A. L.: Hematoporphyrin derivative therapy of papillomas: Experimental study. Arch. Otolaryngol. Head. Neck Surg., 112:42, 1986.

61. Spikes, J. D., and Straight, R.: Sensitized photochemical processes in biologic systems. Ann. Rev. Phys. Chem., 18:409, 1967.

62. Star, W. M., Marijinissen, J. P. A., van den Berg-Blok, A. E., Versteeg, J. A. C., Franken, K. A. P., and Reinhold, H. S.: Destruction of rat mammary tumor and normal tissue microcirculation by hematoporphyrin derivative photoradiation observed in vivo in sandwich observation chambers. Cancer Res., 46:2532, 1986.

63. Svaasand, L. O.: Optical dosimetry for direct and interstitial photoradiation therapy of malignant tumors. In Porphyrin Localization and Treatment of Tumors. Edited by D. R. Doiron, and C. J. Gomer. New York, Alan R. Liss, 1984, p. 91.

64. Takata, C., and Imakiire, M.: Cancer of the Ear, Nose, and Throat. In Lasers and Hematoporphyrin Derivative in Cancer. Edited by Y. Hayata and T. J. Dougherty. New York, Igaku-Shoin, 1983, 70.

65. Thomas, R. J., Abbott, M., Bhathal, P. S., St. John, D. J. B., and Morstyn, G.: High-dose photoradiation of esophageal cancer. Ann. Surgery, 206:193, 1987.

66. Tochner, Z., Mitchell, J. B., Smith, P., Harrington, F., Glatstein, E., Russo, D., and Russo, A.: Photodynamic therapy of ascites tumors within the peritoneal cavity. Br. J. Cancer, 53:733, 1986.

67. Tsuchiya, A, Obara, N., Miwa, M., Ohi, T., Kato, H., and Hayata, Y.: Hematoporphyrin derivative and laser photoradiation in the diagnosis and treatment of bladder cancer. J. Urol., 130:79, 1983.

68. Waldow, S. M, Lobraico, R. V., Kohler, I. K., Wallk, S., and Fritts, H. T.: Photodynamic therapy for treatment of malignant cutaneous lesions. Lasers Surg. Med., 7:451, 1987.

69. Ward, B. G., Forbes, I. J., Cowled, P. A., McEvoy, M. M., and Cox, L. W.: The treatment of vaginal recurrences of gynecologic malignancy with phototherapy following hematoporphyrin derivative in pretreatment. Am. J. Obstet. Gynecol., 142:356, 1982.

70. Wile, A. G., Novotny, J., Mason, G. R., Passy, V., and Berns, M. W.: Photoradiation Therapy of Head and Neck Cancer. In Porphyrin Localization and Treatment of Tumors. Edited by D. T. Doiron and C. J. Gomer. New York, Alan R. Liss, 1984, 681.

71. Wilson, B. C., and Patterson, M. S.: The physics of photodynamic therapy. Phys. Med. Biol., 31:327, 1986.

72. Wilson, B. D., Mang, T. S., Cooper, M., and Stoll, H.: A clinical evaluation of photodynamic therapy for the treatment of basal cell carcinoma. Presented at the International Photodynamic Association Meeting, Buffalo, New York, 1990.

XIV

Principles of Medical Oncology

James F. Holland
Emil Frei III
Robert C. Bast, Jr.
Donald W. Kufe

Introduction

A medical oncologist is an internist who has undergone additional specialized training. A good medical oncologist is one who applies the thoughtful approach to problem-solving learned as an internist to a body of knowledge that includes patients with cancer. Specific features about individual cancers and their treatments, and a reasonable familiarity with the origins, status and fruits of cancer research at clinical and preclinical levels are requisite.[12] More than in many specialties of internal medicine, a medical oncologist interacts with cognate brother and sister disciplines, particularly with surgical and radiation oncology, and pathology. The multiple other interfaces include diagnostic radiology, nursing oncology, pyscho-oncology, neuro-oncology, gynecologic oncology, rehabilitation medicine, and for young patients, pediatric oncology. Infectious diseases are common complications of cancers and their treatments, and the parallellism between use of antibiotics and chemotherapeutic agents forges a natural alliance with specialists in infectious disease.

The relationship of medical oncology to hematology is in a special category. Medical oncologists and hematologists both have legitimate interests in the neoplastic diseases of the hematopoietic tissues, one because of the commonality with other neoplasms, the other because of the organ system involved. There is a large segment of hematology which is not uniquely related to oncology, however, and the major segment of oncology is not in the province of hematology.

Medical oncology was established as a separate discipline by the American Board of Internal Medicine in 1971. More than 7,500 certified internists have been further certified in the subspecialty of medical oncology.[4] From time to time, since 1971, efforts have been made by others to re-amalgamate medical oncology and hematology. The content and orientation of the two subspecialties allow complementarity and coexistence, but the authors are disinclined to the sometime advocated homogenization. This reticence reflects the National Cancer Institute's separate identity from the National Heart, Lung and Blood Institute; the field of cancer research being far broader than just hematologic topics; and the patient mix in oncologic practice involving more than 80% of patients with diseases that arise from and affect other body systems. Although many topics and training programs elicit interests in common, the allocation of time to the two disciplines in those institutions that choose to maintain combined training programs should not obligatorily be equal. A separate hematology training track should be available to those whose interests do not focus on neoplasia; a separate medical oncology track should be available to those whose interests are primarily in cancer.[12]

The Medical Oncologist's Role

A medical oncologist must understand the pathophysiology of cancers of different sites. All cancers are not identical, and all patients who have cancer are not doomed. Indeed many patients live with cancer, and given the present state of our knowledge, many will have to do so until they die. Having cancer is not the same as having a cancer that will kill you, and not a few patients have a neoplastic disease which is relatively less important in their overall health than their cardiovascular disease or some other affliction. Faced with a diagnostic problem, oncologists must try to exclude cancer as the cause, recognizing that some other diseases can mimic cancer. In the endeavor to be certain not to miss the diagnosis of a nonmalignant disease, the medical oncologist must remember that cancer can "do anything." Cancer has replaced syphilis as the great imitator.[8] To ascribe a finding to cancer requires histologic proof on at least one occasion. For complex new syndromes appearing in a patient who once had cancer, or presenting de novo, such as pulmonary insufficiency, meningoencephalopathy, or inexplicable pain, it is prudent and usually indispensable to establish that cancer is the proximate cause.

Table XIV-1-1. Classification of Tumors By Chemotherapeutic Effects

	Curable	Subcurable	Precurable
Curability:	>50%	≤50%	Uncommon
Effects On:	Metastatic	Micrometastatic	Either
Susceptible Tumors:	Gigacytomas*	Megacytosis†	Neither
Regional Therapy:	Helpful	Essential	Insufficient
Drugs:	Single or combination	Combination	Mostly untried
Monitoring:	Biochemical, anatomic	Usually ineffective	Absent or ineffective

Tumors curable by chemotherapy are defined as >50% eradicable by drugs alone. Subcurability indicates the necessity for effective regional therapy in addition to chemotherapy to reach 50%, or in its absence, chemotherapeutic curability of less than 50%. Precurability defines the challenge that lies ahead. Most precurable tumors (except lung and metastatic breast cancer) have been poorly studied with respect to attempts to find more effective chemotherapeutic regimens. Most subcurable tumors, where population data of treated groups demonstrate convincing chemotherapeutic effect, are not susceptible to quantification or monitoring by chemical or present imaging methodology

*Tumor masses containing 10^9 cells (or more). Curability is much reduced when tumors reach 10^{12} cells

†Tumor masses $<10^9$, since clinically detectable metastastic tumors (usually 10^9 or 10^{10} cells) of these types of neoplasms preclude cure

For the patient in whom relatively asymptomatic findings lead to a diagnosis of cancer, it is useful to consider that the day before the discovery, the patient was also living with cancer. It is a source of some encouragement to patients to know that a diagnosis of cancer does not lead immediately nor inevitably to the end of life. The medical oncologist may be able to stress the long-term evolution of a cancer, the several stages which intervene between the carcinogenic stimulus, the mutation at a genetic level, the progressive selection of cells with a survival advantage, and the appearance of an autonomous neoplasm. Since this process usually takes years, and often decades, it is of use to place the neoplastic process in perspective.

The medical oncologist must distinguish between a neoplasm where a chance for cure exists with known information, where a chance for cure is possible in the context of current and ongoing research, or where our present ignorance precludes that likelihood. In this context, tumors can be classified therapeutically as curable and precurable (Table XIV-1-1).

There are probably few incurable tumors; the present state of our ignorance just obscures the proper approach to achieve cure.[10] It is an axiom that the day before the first metastatic choriocarcinoma was cured with high-dose methotrexate,[7,13] metastatic cancer in general was considered incurable by most observers. Similar circumstances apply to every neoplastic disease that is now curable (Table XIV-1-2). Other neoplasms are sub-curable by chemotherapy, insofar as the participation of surgery or radiotherapy is an intrinsic part of the therapeutic process (Table XIV-1-3).

The unexpected benefits of interferon therapy, and then of deoxycoformycin (pentostatin) and of chlorodeoxyadenosine in hairy-cell leukemia; the unique sensitivity of testicular

Table XIV-1-2. Chemotherapeutically Curable Cancers*

Choriocarcinoma
Acute lymphocytic leukemia of childhood
Burkitt's tumor
Hodgkin's disease
Acute promyelocytic leukemia
Large follicular center cell (diffuse histiocytic) lymphoma
Embryonal carcinoma of testis

*Defined as >50% curable by chemotherapy alone

Table XIV-1-3. Cancers Subcurable with Chemotherapy*

With Regional Therapy
  Wilms' Tumor
  Osteosarcoma
  Ewing's sarcoma
  Embryonal rhabdomyosarcoma
  Small cell carcinoma of lung
  Squamous cell carcinoma of upper aerodigestive tract
  Adenocarcinoma of ovary
  Adenocarcinoma of breast

Without Regional Therapy
  Acute lymphocytic leukemia of adulthood
  Acute myeloid leukemia
  Hairy cell leukemia (probable)

*Defined as ≤50% curable with chemotherapy alone; cure rates obtained with chemotherapy and regional therapy are significantly superior to those with regional therapy alone (i.e., chemotherapeutic cure of micrometastatic disease only)

tumors to cisplatin; the design of combination regimens which led to high cure rates in childhood cancers and in lymphomas; and the initial observations of some responses of renal cell carcinoma and malignant melanoma to interleukin 2 are examples of the unpredictability of the next place where dramatic change may become apparent. Old algorithms may fail, but new approaches and new drugs could provide dramatic opportunity for significant advance (Table XIV-1-4).

Clinical Responsibilities

The medical oncologist is often at the junction where final decisions concerning management are made, and the medical oncologist is frequently the final common pathway through which decisions are implemented. The timing of surgery and radiotherapy, the decisions whether to take curative or palliative approaches, and the decision that watchful waiting is the appropriate approach, or that vigorous action is necessary are often entrusted by the patient to the medical oncologist. He or she must have knowledge of the natural history of a disease so as to visualize the likely future, and its optimal organization for a specific patient. In addition to a personal library and selected reprints, a medical oncologist is well-advised to construct a database of patients seen. Not

Table XIV-1-4.   Discoveries That Could Lead To Major Advances In Cancer Therapy

1. Liposomes (to carry cytotoxic agents) that have selective affinity for tumor cells and not for organs that exhibit limiting toxicity
2. Monoclonal antibodies with exquisite specificity for tumor associated antigens, that are not absorbed non-specifically by other tissues, to carry toxins or radioisotopes, particularly those emitting alpha or beta particles
3. Drugs that suppress oncogene activity
    a. Gene repressors
    b. Antisense RNAs directed to oncogene messenger RNA
    c. Ribozymes that destroy mRNAs of oncogenes
    d. Monoclonal antibodies to gene products
4. Drugs that elicit tumor-suppressor gene activity
    a. Upregulators of suppressor gene function
    b. Polynucleotides that can imbue target cells with tumor supressor activity
    c. Polypeptide analogs of tumor suppressor gene products
5. Drugs that inhibit cellular repair mechanisms
    a. Inhibitors of specific and multidrug resistance genes, mRNAs, and derivative proteins
    b. Inhibitors of DNA polymerases, ligases and topoisomerases involved in DNA repair
    c. Drugs that deplete reductive detoxification processes in cancer cells
    d. Drugs that augment reductive detoxification processes in normal cells
6. Drugs that selectively induce programmed cell death (apoptosis) in tumor cells
7. Drugs that block autocrine, paracrine and endocrine stimulation
    a. Inhibitors of synthesis of, or inactivators of, secretory products that stimulate cancer cell growth
    b. Blockers of receptor sites for hormonal stimulation
    c. Blockers of receptor-stimulated phosphorylation cascades
8. Molecular alteration of cancer cells to initiate host immunologic response against them, and by simulating the untreated cancer cell membrane, also initiating lethal immunologic response against unaltered cancer cells not so altered
    a. By gene transfer into tumor cells
    b. By immunization with components of tumor-associated antigens
9. Use of cytokines in combination therapies
    a. Multiple cytokines
    b. Chemo-immunotherapy

a few of the editors now wish they could recount the details and locate the original charts on yesterday's remembered patients who are relevant to today's problem.

Patients are often influenced by their state of subjective well-being at the moment. It is the responsibility of an oncologist to recognize the often pernicious behavior of the neoplasm in its potential for recurrence and metastasis. In this context the medical oncologist must interact directly with the patient as well as with the chart, films, slides and other critical raw data. Only in such a fashion can advice be tendered with commitment, and with expectation that the patient can be guided to a proper choice. It is unrealistic to expect a patient with a neoplasm to make a choice (informed consent) that is cold and dispassionate, since the very fact of having cancer constitutes a serious emotional burden that may distort ordinary reason. By first hand intimacy with the diagnosis, the extent of the disease, and the patient's attitudes and infirmities, the medical oncologist can make rational plans and recommendations to the patient and to the other physicians involved.

Many of the other physicians involved with a particular patient may concentrate in fields other than surgical or radiation oncology. It is not uncommon, indeed it is often the case, that the patient has a primary family physician or internist who referred the patient to the medical oncologist. In some circumstances cardiologic, pulmonary disease or neurologic specialists may already have been involved with the patient prior to the recognition of a neoplastic disease. It is incumbent upon the medical oncologist to recognize their interests in, and their continuing role with respect to the management of patients with multi-system disease. An infectious disease specialist often becomes involved. In the absence of such consultants, however, the medical oncologist must also implement all aspects of internal medicine. Elsewhere this book contains descriptions in depth of various diseases, the therapies used in their treatment, the pharmacologic, immunologic, neurologic, psychologic, biochemical, epidemiologic and molecular-biologic aspects of cancers, and the complications that cancers cause. Oncologic emergencies, rehabilitation, and the oncologist's relationship to medical informatics, and to government are also presented. Familiarity with these topics constitutes a foundation for medical oncology from which the principles derive.

Cancer Prevention

Medical oncologists, because of their knowledge of neoplastic disease and because of their recognition of social, occupational, nutritional and sexual practices that contribute to neoplasia, have a special obligation among physicians to educate the general public, including other professionals with a lesser interest in cancer prevention. Smoking is the principal correctable cancer-inducing activity (see VI-1). Medical oncologists should not smoke. Medical oncologists should counsel patients and families about good nutrition (see VI-2 and VI-3) and healthy sexual practices (see XXXI-2 and XXXVII). Numerous publications that deal with cancer prevention are available for distribution to patients and families from the National Cancer Institute and the American Cancer Society. The Cancer Information Service (1-800-4-CANCER) will send available publications free of charge.

Familiarity with genetic predispositions to cancer is essential. Many family members immediately fear for their own safety when a relative is diagnosed with a neoplasm. This is entirely appropriate in those conditions known to predispose, but not for all types of cancer. It is usually the medical oncologist's responsibility to assess the risk for a particular disease, and to conduct the necessary surveillance. Cancer family syndromes and genetic predispositions are set forth in III-1.

Clinical Research

No cancer is so well-treated that an improvement in outcome or therapeutic approach cannot readily be imagined. Thus, research is imperative. Furthermore therapies that allow preservation of the involved organ are much to be desired, and investigations that have led in many patients to breast preservation, limb salvage, bladder conservation and avoidance of abdomino-perineal resection are major dividends in the treatment of cancers in these organs. Although in these instances it would appear self-evident, measuring the quality of life is now quantitatively valid, and has added major opportunity to reach value judgments (see XX).

Every established paradigm of medical oncologic management arose from some investigative effort. In many instances, these were one-armed studies that were so successful they became adopted. Examples are methotrexate for choriocarcinoma; vincristine and prednisone induction of acute lymphocytic leukemia; the MOPP regimen for Hodgkin's disease; araC and daunorubicin for acute myeloid leukemia; cisplatin, vinblastine and bleomycin for testicular cancer; leukovorin and fluorouracil for colon cancer; and many others. *After* the initial reports of activity, these regimens were often compared with standard programs and demonstrated not only to be highly active, but more active than the prevailing predecessor regimens. Thus there is a premium on good investigators conducting pioneering observational studies. This is not to say that chemotherapy in the hands of single institutions may not be different from that same regimen when applied by many cooperating physicians in a broad scale effort. Nonetheless, if a regimen is superior in the hands of many oncologists, it is likely that its utility and validity in the practice of medical oncology will be greater.

To ensure uniformity and reproducibility of procedures, research designs for studies of whatever size should be codified in a written protocol (see Table XIV-1-5). Long after a therapeutic program has been accepted into clinical practice the use of such protocols can be a great assistance in avoiding omissions, stipulating times for specific procedures, and ensuring that standard doses, thresholds and endpoints are used.

Every oncologist's office should be a research station. Every oncologist during his or her training was exposed to, and almost always was a participant in, clinical research. There is virtually no regimen or treatment for any tumor which is entirely satisfactory, and there is much reason to anticipate that progress would be more rapid if clinical research were accepted as an integral part of the practice of medical oncol-ogy with greater participation than is presently the case. The technology exists in medical informatics (see XLV) for community oncologists to ally themselves with their alma mater or other academic center to participate in diagnostic, preventive and therapeutic research trials using the convenience of the computer, the electronic mailbox, and facsimile transmission. Those oncologists who protest so serious a work overload that it prevents their devoting the necessary time to participate in clinical research need a partner, for they are depriving themselves, and perhaps their patients.

As a part of the commitment to medical oncology, a medical oncologist should reserve a certain number of hours per week for participation in clinical research. This has the virtue of maintaining greater currency with clinical investigation. Clinical investigation should serve as the bridge to fundamental science and the excitement in the new molecular biological understanding of the cancer cell. By such association, the medical oncologist in practice may also forestall the burn-out syndrome, which is discussed below.

It is not reasonable that an individual in practice devote the same time and energy to clinical research as one who serves on the faculty of a university, research institute, or hospital on a full-time basis. A set-aside for research, however, constitutes the same imperative commitment as a set-aside for education and updating. Initiation of one new patient on a protocol every other month should constitute a manageable burden of additional paperwork for a practicing oncologist, and using computer technology, even the paperwork can be diminished or eliminated. A patient every other month per medical oncologist would accelerate clinical cancer research by data acquisition on about 30,000 patients per year. Even a fraction of that newly generated information would seem like we'd hit the mother lode. Furthermore, participation in such a study would ordinarily guarantee the patient that he or she was getting a treatment equivalent to or already the best that is known. Patients with cancer are often apprehensive that they may not receive the best treatment. The medical oncologist can speak with greater authority when a deliberate comparison is being made, since the goal of such studies is toward improvement on the standard, not toward finding treatments that are equally good. Thus it is not onerous to offer the current best, or something possibly better.

Fundamental Science, Clinical Science and Medical Art

The medical oncologist serves as the principal interface between cancer research in the laboratory and cancer research implementation in the adult patient. Many early chapters in this treatise deal with the structure and aberrant function of the cancer cell, of the cancer process and of its dissection with molecular and chemical probes. Appreciation of this evolving understanding of science is incumbent on every medical oncologist. A patient with cancer should be viewed in the context of the etiology, pathogenesis, pathology and biochemistry of the particular neoplastic process. The effects of the tumor and its products on the structure and function of the patient's normal tissues, including the mind and emotions, define an understanding in depth of the

Table XIV-1-5. Topics To Be Covered in a Clinical Protocol

1. Cover sheet with names and emergency telephone numbers of responsible investigator(s)
2. Schema and synopsis
3. Objectives
4. Patient selection
5. Treatment plan, including changes in dose
6. Registration/randomization, stratification and data submission
7. Required data at entry, on study, and after
8. Expected toxicity and its treatment
9. Criteria for response, disease progression, and relapse
10. Removal of patients from protocol therapy
11. Drug formulation, availability, and preparation
12. Adverse drug reaction reporting
13. Ancillary therapy
14. Statistical considerations
15. References
16. Model consent form

disease process, and the patient in whom it takes place. It is not sufficient to order a therapy with the appropriate dose and schedule. A medical oncologist should understand the interaction, so far as is known, of the administered drug with target molecules, its metabolic pathways, and the chemical or immunological alteration that one seeks to make. Similarly, it is a given that there be a broad understanding of and attention to potential toxicities, which represent the drug effects on normal tissues. Therapies totally appropriate for someone whose disease might well be cured by judicious application of surgery, radiotherapy and/or chemotherapy would be unthinkable if applied to someone with widely metastatic disease for whom no known cure exists. Thus there is a time ordering of the sequence of therapeutic investigation. The intensity of therapy with curative intent, which may require a walk through the valley of the shadow of death, is ordinarily of short duration and high intensity. Conservatism means saving a life, not avoiding toxicity. Contrariwise, treatment for palliative purposes would not ordinarily condone similar risks and iatrogenic effects that diminished the quality of life, even temporarily.

Another world of scientific enterprise that materially affects the possibility for curative cancer therapy deals with host support. The availability of powerful antibiotics and the implementation of platelet transfusions were intrinsic to the early cures of the acute leukemias. The many new advances in colony stimulating factors (filgrastim, sargramostim) have already significantly altered the prospect of drug induced granulocytopenia (see XVIII-6). Continuing search for less cumbersome ways to deal with thrombocytopenia support the use of single donor pheresis. Evidence that interleukin 3 shortens drug-induced thrombocytopenia may have heuristic significance. The era of cytokines and their manipulation is just at its beginning; combinations have not been explored in depth (see XVIII-5). The impact of cytokines on circulating stem cells (CD34+) is major, making convenient the collection of such marrow repopulating precursors to allow autologous stem cell transfusions as a supplement to, or even as a substitute for autologous marrow transfusion (see XVIII-6 and XIX-1). New antibiotics make granulocytopenia less ominous, and studies of oral prophylaxis with antibiotics and antifungal agents appear to diminish hospital admissions (see XLI). All of these assets allow higher dose intensity chemotherapy, a characteristic of treatment with curative intent (see XV-3 and XV-1).

The availability of far better antiemetic control makes cancer chemotherapy less dreaded (see XL-3). The emergence of psycho-oncology as a widely recognized discipline has also made it possible for patients to strengthen their resolve to undertake approaches aimed at cure, or to accept the unlikelihood of curative therapy with greater serenity (see XX).

Chemotherapy Trials

A number of ethical issues are abrogated by the certainty that a specific patient is or is not potentially curable with the information presently known. For asymptomatic patients with indolent disease, knowledge of pre-curability eliminates the need to rush to treatment. Many problems are initially best approached by masterful observation, particularly where age, co-morbidity, and equanimity are present. Where rapid course, portending symptoms or inquietude prevail, however, therapy is indicated. In metastatic disease for which no cure is known, it is not only ethical but important that systematic designed investigation of new treatments be undertaken early in the course of the patient's disease to determine their activity before toxicities arise from conventional therapies that might limit dosing. Conventional therapies might also elicit resistance of one or another kind, or immunologic depression, which might foreclose the opportunity to recognize activity for the candidate compound. Compounds should likely not be investigated in man, however, before they have demonstrated in vitro activity against human cancer cells, and, ordinarily, activity in vivo against transplanted or spontaneous tumors. The predictive activity of human tumor xenografts in immunodeficient mice as contrasted to murine allografts, or autochthonous murine tumors has not been settled.[14]

By the same token, for diseases with especially unfavorable outlook and rare therapeutic success, delays before introducing candidate compounds to ensure that they have little or no risk of toxicity is an unwise investment of the public's wealth and time, let alone the patient's short-lived opportunity possibly to benefit. The outcome of unsuccessfully treated cancer is more ominous than the hazards of clinical investigation.

The design of chemotherapy trials is critical to the validity of the data produced. The essentials in the design of a protocol are provided in Table XIV-1-5. Statistical considerations in the design and interpretation of clinical research are detailed in the chapter on clinical trials (see V).

The conduct of clinical therapy using some locally toxic intravenous medications, and indeed the care of patients requiring much intravenous therapy commends the use of central venous access. Needle phobia is a perverse part of being under treatment, and it can largely be obviated by permanent venous access. Safe administration of the drugs and ready access to blood specimens are the rewards of the operative intervention that establishes central venous access, often with an implanted sub-cutaneous reservoir. This is particularly necessary when difficult venous access because of anatomy or obesity leads to major trauma and time loss in attempting peripheral venous access (see XXI).

Adjuvant and Neo-Adjuvant Chemotherapy

Most cancer chemotherapy is given to patients with clinically manifest cancer. In a few disease entities chemotherapy is curative. The advantage of treating patients with smaller body burdens of residual cancer has proved so persuasive that the profession and patients have accepted the technique of post-surgical chemotherapy, acknowledging that this entails the risk of treating some patients whose body burden is already zero. Thus adjuvant therapy after surgery has been demonstrated to be curative in several diseases where surgery alone has low cure rates and where chemotherapy alone can not cure in the manifest metastatic condition. Wilms' tumor and osteosarcoma are the prime examples. Although in many diseases there is evidence of prolonged disease-free survival and even of longer survival, it is still too recent in breast cancer and ovarian cancer to assert that greatly increased cure rates have been achieved, although this is likely. Since the adjuvant treatment is aimed at micrometastatic disease remote from the primary tumor, some exploration of applying chemotherapy before surgery has been undertaken in a few types of cancer. In addition to earlier application to the micrometastases, when they may be smaller, this neo-adjuvant, induction, or primary chemotherapeutic approach has two additional beneficial characteristics. First, regression of the primary lesion serves as a confirmatory bioassay that the micrometastases will also likely be sensitive.[15] Failure of the primary neoplasm to regress affords opportunity to shift chemotherapeutic treatment while there is still chance of affecting the micrometastases with a new regimen. Secondly, regression of the primary tumor may make primary surgery unnecessary, allowing curative radiotherapy, as in some head and neck cancers (see XXVII-1). In other instances, surgery may be technically easier, though not always less radical since there is no certainty that every cell has been eradicated at the original boundaries. Induction chemotherapy has allowed a major reduction in amputations, however, in favor of limb-sparing surgery (see XXV-1). Induction chemotherapy may also significantly augment the effectiveness of radiotherapy.

Surrogate Endpoints

The medical oncologist must be deeply interested in methods to measure disease progress that anticipate the appearance of symptoms. Recognizing that new therapies will always be forthcoming, it is prudent to anticipate methods to test them that do not depend on such primitive assays as bidimensional measurements of abdominal tumor masses, palpable nodes, and shadows on chest X-rays. These early methods have already been greatly improved by CT scanning, sonography, endoscopy and circulating tumor secretory products that represent marker molecules. Validation of each surrogate marker is desirable, but once established, as in hCG, α-fetoprotein, CEA, 5HIAA, calcitonin, PSA, and other similar compounds that correlate with specific tumor behaviors, the ability to monitor tumor activity is of major value. Recognizing disease progress by marker studies allows identification of inactive therapeutic regimens before clinical failure, and provides opportunity for alternative action before the patient has major additional tumor burden, and possibly before symptoms. Marker molecules are not infallible, however, and a tumor cell population may emerge in a cancer relapsing from prior therapy that fails to secrete the marker that had been monitored (see II).

Palliative therapy no longer requires the patient to have symptoms that require palliation. The more logical construction is to prevent symptoms from appearing, or reappearing, using more discriminant guideposts than palpable or painful tumor. In the future, after the initial treatment, we can confidently anticipate that cancer management will depend upon indirect measures of tumor activity. Thus major therapeutic efforts will be aimed at tumors when there are small body burdens and the medical oncologist will be assessing biochemical, molecular biological or immunologic surrogates for tumor presence. Some of the reasons for considering patients incurable are that therapeutic efforts have only been made when tumor body burdens exist that would prove too great for cure even for sensitive tumors. The demonstrated efficacy of adjuvant chemotherapy for breast cancer (see XXX-11) and of adjuvant chemoimmunotherapy for colon cancer (see XXIX-10) imply that small body burdens of these and other metastatic cancers detected only by markers, might be similarly sensitive even with today's therapies. A controlled clinical trial has been proposed in breast cancer manifested only by increased serum CA 15-3 levels.[6]

The Laws of Therapeutics

Certain principles govern the application of therapies no matter what the disease. These were enunciated more than half a century ago by the late Robert F. Loeb, Bard Professor of Medicine at Columbia University's College of Physicians and Surgeons (see Table XIV-1-6).

These simple rules have nearly universal applicability and profundity, and pertain to neoplastic diseases. They must be tempered, however, by an understanding of the neoplastic process. The first law is: *If what you're doing is doing good, keep doing it.* Vincristine and prednisone is an excellent induction treatment for acute lymphocytic leukemia of childhood. In 1968 the question was raised, why not keep administering this highly active induction regimen, rather than shifting to antimetabolite management? A cohort of children who were induced into remission by vincristine and prednisone were randomized to continue the induction treatment. They rapidly relapsed, whereas the favorable circumstances for antimetabolite treatment led some of the children randomized to these arms to long-term maintained remissions, and even cures.[2] Thus the first law of therapeutics does not always apply in the context of our knowledge, which is admittedly fragmentary, about the effect of successor treatment regimens in cancer. Much of curative oncology relates to the biology of the unseen tumor, for which current clinical status may be uninformative. The first law seems more applicable to clinically recognizable disease.

The second law of therapeutics does carry considerable universality, however: *If what you're doing is not doing good, stop doing it.* Most therapeutic regimens have little chance of success if the second monthly cycle of their application has failed to elicit therapeutic benefit. Indeed, most patients show incipient tumor regression after the first cycle, and apprehension rises if that is not so. It is nonetheless advantageous to undertake a second cycle in most instances since well documented early increase in tumor diameter on roentgenographic examinations or increased pain can indeed be followed by tumor regression. If, however, no therapeutic response attends this second cycle, which often represents a total observation-time of six weeks or longer, it is usually legitimate to infer that a third course will not likely be ben-

Table XIV-1-6. Loeb's Rules of Therapeutics

1. If what you are doing is doing good, keep doing it
2. If what you are doing is not doing good, stoping doing it
3. If you don't know what to do, do nothing
4. Never make the treatment worse than the disease

eficial. Before stopping treatment, however, corroborating information should be sought by direct measurements, by roentgenograms, or by biochemical markers. Increased bony uptake of radionuclides can be a sign of bone healing, even of a previously unsuspected lesion, and is not a suitable endpoint. The appearance of metastatic disease or its obviously increasing growth despite receiving chemotherapeutic treatment speaks against continuing a treatment, since at least one clone of metastatic cells is clinically resistant to it.

The second law of therapeutics does not extend to toxic effects, however, unless they are life-threatening or profoundly disabling. With the medications available today, complete avoidance of toxicity would doom many patients to death from their neoplasm who otherwise can sometimes obtain cure and oftentimes meaningful remission by accepting a transient effect of intensive therapy that kills tumor cells and normal cells alike. The patient almost always recovers, but the less resilient tumor may not. Hippocrates' admonition, *Primum non nocere* is also subject to reassessment in oncology.[10] To treat a population of patients at a dose that would avoid toxic harm (i.e., lethal jeopardy) to *any* patient would surely exact a higher price in depriving others of adequate dose to achieve maximum benefit. Curative cancer chemotherapy as we know it is always toxic, but rarely fatal. Attempts to abrogate toxicity by reducing the dose of an established regimen compromises the benefit for the majority.[5] Fortunately many other approaches to mitigating toxicity are now the substance of oncologic investigation (see XVIII-6).

The third law of therapeutics counsels against uninformed action: *If you don't know what to do, do nothing.* In many circumstances a rush to judgment, or worse, a rush to do something, anything, can be disastrous. Aside from oncologic emergencies (see XLII) there is rarely an occasion when observing the evolution of symptomatology and findings, or seeking consultation with another individual for a fresh viewpoint is contraindicated because of time loss. In the presence of pain, one should not delay pain relief, but other therapy may be delayed for the necessary *thinking* time. In the presence of a differential diagnosis which includes diseases other than cancer, particularly infections, one must be certain that delay does not risk mortality or morbidity from the other possible disorders. The time invested for observation and consultation should thus not be extravagant.

It is a rare exception, indeed, that a medical oncologist can countenance treatment without a histologic diagnosis. Cytologic diagnoses may provide sufficient information in the presence of unambiguous clinical syndromes, but cytology of the bronchus, stomach, cervix and body fluids has produced sufficient numbers of false positive identifications that corroborating clinical syndromes are essential. Still it is extremely useful to have histologic evidence whenever possible.

The fourth law of therapeutics: *Never make the treatment worse than the disease,* relates to total life equation and the price the oncologist knows the patient may be obliged to pay in side effects at present to attain real effects in the future. Often the patient's vision is foreshortened, since today's disease caused by drug toxicity can be more severe than the original symptomatology of the cancer, often excised,

for which the treatment is being given. The medical oncologist must ascertain the patient's concepts of the quality of life versus the duration of life. It is a medical oncologic responsibility to counsel the patient concerning this weighty topic. It is critical to distinguish therapy with curative intent from a palliative orientation. The proper equation is maximal life at maximal quality. It is a modification of the commentary that one should die young as late as possible. For some patients, the toxic effects of treatment outweigh the value of life. This is often directly related to age, and the treatments imperative for patients in their forties may be undesirable or even inappropriate for patients in their eighties. Pain and disability from the cancer temper the desirability of certain therapies which may not offer more than temporary partial relief.

It is inappropriate for the medical oncologist to substitute professional judgment for ardent patient wish, when the patient desires to terminate efforts, or when the patient passionately strives to accomplish something that is a reasonable therapeutic goal. The medical oncologist must serve as a bastion of reality, however, advising the patient of what is possible, and of what is likely. In the course of doing this, the laws of therapeutics and of humanity always include hope.

Truth Telling

Explanations of disease, of anticipated therapies, of protocols in which there is randomization, and of unknowns, must be tailored to the intellectual and emotional level of the particular patient. It is never permissible to lie, but it may be prudent not to deposit all the truth, let alone all at once, on a patient who cannot accept the full details and ramifications of diagnosis and management. "Your patient has no more right to all the truth you know than to all the medicine in your saddlebags" was a humane and ethical tenet when advanced by Oliver Wendell Holmes more than a century ago, and it does not seem to have changed.[11] It is dishonest to twist facts or to deny specific features such as the existence of metastases. By the same token it is wrong to deny a patient an opportunity to make final dispositions with respect to self, family, religion, the law, and business by falsely stating that a disease is benign or cured. Families who assert that the patient must not know because he or she could not stand it, are usually twice wrong: the patient often knows already, or may be more distraught by being excluded and not knowing; and the patient ordinarily incorporates the information into his or her life equation indistinguishably from other patients. A reading of Tolstoy's *The Death of Ivan Ilyich* should convince any doubting oncologist about the terror of uncertainty and the value of direct and honest yet humane interactions with the patient.

When a patient asks, "There is hope, isn't there?", the oncologist can always be enthusiastically positive. Hope is a uniquely human characteristic, which sustains the will to continue, and all oncologists and all patients do hope for a better outcome.

Resuscitation

Several states require 'Do not resuscitate' (DNR) orders be written on patient charts prior to death. In the absence of such orders, when a nurse finds a patient apparently dead she must by law initiate emergency calls for resuscitative efforts.

In circumstances where such laws exist, a medical oncologist should be meticulous in writing DNR orders, and in explaining them to the family. When death comes from cancer as the expected final event of a gradual deterioration of vital forces, resuscitative efforts do not succeed. If unable to keep someone alive, the likelihood of bring back meaningful life is infinitesimal. Resuscitative efforts should certainly be applied to patients with cancer who were not anticipated to die, since reversible phenomena such as pulmonary emboli, cardiac arrhythmias, aspiration and similar events can provoke unexpected death in a patient with a neoplasm just as in any other hospitalized or ambulatory patient. It is, however, in the circumstance of gradual decline and predictable disintegration of body functions that resuscitative efforts place great physical and emotional stress on nursing and ancillary personnel, house staff, the medical oncologist, and the distraught family. Many patients, particularly those apprised of the progress of their disease, and the elderly, can discuss the decision not to resuscitate with equanimity, and indeed with a certain personal satisfaction of avoiding the fruitless anguish that such a procedure entails for the surviving family. Many patients are eager to sign living wills or to appoint a health care proxy if these possibilities are presented to them.

Because of the medico-legal implications involved, where particular religious scruples obtain or where families have emotionally uncontrolled members who cannot accept the anticipated death of a loved one, the medical oncologist should spend considerable time in planning for the eventual death. Medical oncologists through their organizations should also invest effort to alter laws that place significant burdens on them and their colleagues and which infringe on the appropriate professional practice of medicine. DNR forms are a technique of documentation, and constitute a further evidence that society has moved medicine to a new plateau of accountability. The medical oncologist should, however, make known his or her intentions concerning the advisability of resuscitative efforts for each particular patient in advance, to forestall unnecessary trauma to patient, family and staff, to forestall litigation, and to settle in advance any serious disagreements with patient or family. An impasse might occasion a medical oncologist to find a suitable substitute physician if there is unresolvable conflict concerning the plans surrounding the anticipated death.

DNR orders do not imply that there be diminution of oncologic effort to control or palliate the disease before death. On the other hand, if good medicine indicates that continued efforts are fruitless, and only inflict suffering with no prospect of benefit, a discontinuation of active therapy should always be accompanied by DNR orders.

Burn-Out

A sense of frustration can affect any individual who encounters barriers to successful completion of an important task. This is particularly true of intellectual tasks and invisible barriers. When the barrier is a lethal disease about which the oncologist can do little that is effective, the frustration can be all-consuming. Oncologists who encounter several instances of recrudescent or refractory disease in a short time span (especially if punctuated by deaths of young or favorite patients uninterrupted by counterbalancing compensatory successes) may well experience frustration, a sense of inadequacy, and depression. Frequent repetition of this cyclic phenomenon not uncommonly leads to the syndrome of burn-out.

The medical oncologist knows that many of today's cancers are precurable. To the extent that he or she can be involved, actually and conceptually in the solution to that complex mystery, the frustration is lessened. Cancer research, whether at basic or clinical level, is held in high esteem by our fellow citizens. Group identity, being one of the team, helps to offset the self-deprecation when human tragedies mount despite one's best efforts. The camaraderie of other oncologists who battle the same enemy with the same primitive weapons helps. Another oncologist can understand the trauma and the distress; it is an encounter on familiar terrain.

The appreciation that the horizon is distant, and that oncologists are all working intently to proceed there, puts present frustration in a more appropriate perspective. Involvement in the systematized academic pursuit, whether in an academic setting, a medical school outreach, an oncologic society, or a local collaborative group, provides the security of collegial support, a buddy system, an anchor to windward.

A sound mind in a sound body implies rest, exercise, nutrition and enjoyment. To assure the last, the first three are prerequisites. Avocation and vacation are a portion of good mental health, included in the terms rest and exercise.

Donning the dress uniform of the grand enterprise against cancer, rather than the buckskin of the lone scout, can help imbue the oncologist with the identity and strength of the team. If these strategems do not assist the potentially burned out oncologist into a new orientation, and a more resilient response to the inevitable future traumas, he or she may well consider an alternative occupation. Many oncologists serve honorably in laboratory, administrative or pharmaceutical positions where they are insulated from the vagaries of patients' illnesses. it is better to have a happier oncologist aloof from patient contact than a depressed, and thus impaired, oncologist finally burnt out, still trying to perform at considerable personal discomfort and perhaps at some patient jeopardy.

Nomenclature: SI Units

A new system of quantitative nomenclature has recently come into use in the United States. Soon it will be impossible to read a medical journal without thorough familiarity with the SI (systeme internationale) units. They are presented in Table XIV-1-7 so that readers can have ready access to a source for translation from the old nomenclature which pervades this treatise.

Summary

The medical oncologist usually serves as the final common pathway for the application of cancer research to patients. A complex corpus of information is available, which expands

Table XIV-1-7. Representative SI (Systeme Internationale) Units for Laboratory Tests of Importance in Oncology

Component	Present reference interval	Present unit	SI conversion factor	SI reference intervals	Unit symbols
Albumin	4.0–6.0	g/dL	10.0	40–60	g/L
α-Fetoprotein, radioimmunoassay	0–20	ng/mL	1.00	0–20	μg/L
Bilirubin					
Total	0.1–1.0	mg/dL	17.10	2–18	μmol/L
Conjugated	0–0.2	mg/dL	17.10	0–4	μmol/L
Calcium	8.8–10.3	mg/dL	0.2495	2.20–2.58	mmol/L
Cholesterol	<200	mg/dL	0.02586	<5.20	mmol/L
Cortisol	4–19	μg/dL	27.59	110–520	nmol/L
Creatinine	0.6–1.2	mg/dL	88.40	50–110	μmol/L
Fibrinogen	200–400	mg/dL	0.01	2.0–4.0	g/L
Glucose	70–110	mg/dL	0.05551	3.9–6.1	mmol/L
Hemoglobin					
Male	14.0–18.0	g/dL	10.0	140–180	g/L
Female	11.5–15.5	g/dL	10.0	115–155	g/L
Immunoglobulins					
IgG	500–1200	mg/dL	0.01	5.00–12.00	g/L
IgA	50–350	mg/dL	0.01	0.50–3.50	g/L
IgM	30–230	mg/dL	0.01	0.30–2.30	g/L
IgD	<6	mg/dL	10	<60	mg/L
IgE	20–1000	ng/mL	1.00	20–1000	μg/L
Iron	80–180	μg/dL	0.1791	14–32	μmol/L
Iron-binding capacity	250–460	μg/dL	0.1791	45–82	μmol/L
Lipoproteins					
Low-density (LDL), as cholesterol	50–190	mg/dL	0.02586	1.30–4.90	mmol/L
High-density (HDL), as cholesterol	30–70	mg/dL	0.02586	0.80–1.80	mmol/L
Magnesium	1.8–3.0	mg/dL	0.4114	0.80–1.20	mmol/L
	1.6–2.4	mEq/L	0.500		
Metanephrines (as normetanephrine)	0–2.0	mg/24 hr	5.458	0–11.0	μmol/d
Osmolality	280–300	mOsm/kg	1.00	280–300	nmol/kg
Phosphate (as phosphorus, inorganic)	2.5–5.0	mg/dL	0.3229	0.80–1.60	mmol/L
Potassium	3.5–5.0	mEq/L	1.00	3.5–5.0	mmol/L
		mg/dL	0.2558		
Protein, total	6–8	g/dL	10.0	60–80	g/L
Serotonin (5-hydroxy-tryptamine)	8–21	μg/dL	0.05675	0.45–1.20	μmol/L
Thyroxine, free	0.8–2.8	ng/dL	12.87	10–36	pmol/L
Triiodothyronine (T$_3$)	75–220	ng/dL	0.01536	1.2–3.4	nmol/L
Urate (as uric acid)	2.0–6.0	mg/dL	59.48	120–360	μmol/L
Urea nitrogen	8–18	mg/dL	0.3570	3.0–6.5	mmol/L of urea
Vanillylmandelic acid (VMA)	<6.8	mg/24 hr.	5.046	<35	μmol/d

rapidly, both deeper into the nature of the cancer process, and higher into new approaches that provide demonstrated effectiveness in therapy, prevention or support.

The increasing appreciation that autocrine and paracrine secretions are seemingly ubiquitous, and influence the behavior of normal and neoplastic cells, provides a variety of new targets for therapy. Many products of oncogenes exert their activity through autocrine or paracrine effects. Tumor suppressor genes and their products offer exceptional promise of elucidating how cellular biochemistry is regulated, or is abnormally regulated in their absence, and thus may identify valuable targets for therapy. As a starter, the tumor suppressor gene products appear to be among nature's ways of controlling a cell from manifesting cancerous behavior. The tide of fundamental discoveries is already washing away many of the unknowns and the flyspeck observations. It is axiomatic that certain cancers can be cured today without knowing the intimate nature of neoplasia. How better the day, perhaps soon upon us, when we know what we are doing.

Clinical accomplishments have similarly been exceptionally productive in the 35 years since the first cancer was cured with drugs.[7,13] A large assortment of drugs has been provided. A wholly new array of genetically engineered drugs support host function, and others, that are cytokines with anti-cancer activity, are still early in their development. Imaging technologies have revolutionized the ability to detect, stage and monitor cancers. Biochemical markers of tumor behavior are a principal fruit of immunologic study, but immunotherapeutics also holds promise. The partition of the patient into a tumor bearing body that is exposed to highly intensive, even supralethal therapy, regaining viability through reassembly with unexposed marrow or peripheral stem cells extends even further the ability to deliver a potentially curative lethal injury to the tumor, and to salvage the host.

There is probably no cancer in which some progress in diagnosis or therapy has not been achieved in the last decade. Similar achievement has not attended our increased knowledge of cancer prevention. Oncologists must assume a greater responsibility for health preservation. Much could be accomplished by applying what is already known about diet, exercise, and lifestyle. Medical facts without political action have been slow to change the tax on health that tobacco levies.

The horizon has never been closer. Although still distant, there are enough promising paths to follow that one of them may prove considerably faster than even reasonable optimism would suppose. The information that serves as our foundation, its rate of accrual, its revelations, and the demonstrated success of translating science to clinical applications augur well for the future of medical oncology, and for the cancer patient.

References

1. Bhardwaj, S., Holland, J. F., and Norton, L.: An intensive sequence adjuvant chemotherapy regimen for breast cancer. Cancer Invest., 1993, In press.
2. Cancer and Leukemia Group B. Unpublished data.
3. Early Breast Cancer Trialists Collaborative Group: Systemic treatment of early breast cancer by hormonal, cytotoxic or immune therapy. Lancet, 339:1, 1992.
4. Frei, E., III: Combination cancer therapy: Presidential address. Cancer Res., 32:2593, 1972.
5. Frei, E., III, and Canellos, G. P.: Dose: A critical factor in cancer chemotherapy. Am. J. Med., 69:585, 1980.
6. Hayes, D.: Personal communication, 1992.
7. Holland, J. F: Methotrexate therapy of metastatic choriocarcinoma. Am. J. Obstet. Gynecol., 75:195, 1958.
8. Holland, J. F.: The diseases that cancer causes. J. Chron. Dis., 16:635, 1963.
9. Holland, J. F.: Ethics for a clinical investigator: Non primum non nocere. Am. J. Med., 66:554, 1979.
10. Holland, J. F.: Karnofsky Memorial Lecture. Breaking the cure barrier. J. Clin. Oncol., 1:75, 1983.
11. Holmes, O. W.: Medical Essays "The Young Practitioner."
12. Kennedy, B. J., Calabresi, P., Carbone, P. P., Frei, E., III, Holland, J. F., Owens, A. H., Jr. Sleisenger, M. H., and Beck, J. C.: Training Program in Medical Oncology. Ann. Int. Med., 78:127, 1973.
13. Li, M. C., Hertz, R., and Spencer, D. B.: Effect of methotrexate therapy upon choriocarcinoma and chorioadenoma. Proc. Soc. Exp. Biol. and Med., 93:361, 1956.
14. Martin, D. S., Balis, M. E., Fisher, B., Frei, E, Freireich, E. J., Heppner, G. H., Holland, J. F., Houghton, J. A., Houghton, P. J., Randall, K. J., Mittelman, A., Youcef, R., Sawyer, R. C., Schmid, F. A., Stolfi, R. L., and Young, C. W.: Role of murine tumor models in cancer treatment research. Cancer Res., 46:2189, 1986.
15. Rosen, G., Caparos, B, Huvos, A. G., Kosloff, C., Nirenberg, A., Cacavio, A., Marcove, R. C., Lane, J. M., Mehta, B., and Urba, C.: Preoperative chemotherapy for osteogenic sarcoma: Selection of post-operative adjuvant chemotherapy based upon the response of the primary tumor to pre-operative chemotherapy. Cancer, 49:1221, 1982.

XV

Principles of Chemotherapy

XV-1

Cytokinetics

Larry Norton
Antonella Surbone

Introduction: The Importance of Cytokinetics to the Oncologist

Growth is a fundamental attribute of life. As a medical discipline, oncology is distinguished by its primary concern not with organ dysfunction nor with foreign invasion but with the aberrant proliferation of the body's own cells. The study of the kinetics of growth, *cytokinetics,* is therefore central to clinical oncology. On the biological level, all of the cardinal features of a cancer—its proclivity to increase in size, to disseminate and to destroy the function of normal organs—are dependent on the reproduction of its cells. On the practical level, growth kinetic concepts pervade clinical thinking. Indeed, the everyday language of clinicians is replete with kinetic terms. Examples are: indolent growth, rapid growth, slow regression ("refractory to therapy"), and brisk regression ("responsive to therapy"). These terms, used as descriptions, have intuitive meanings, but an awareness of their biomathematic dimensions adds significantly to their value. This is especially so since there are now available practical methods for quantifying many of these terms in actual clinical practice. In addition to all of this, anticancer pharmacotherapy, because it is thought to work by disrupting mitosis, is productively viewed in the context of kinetic principles. This relates both to the impact of drugs on cancer cells and to their toxic effects on such rapidly proliferating host tissues as hematopoietic progenitors and gastrointestinal mucosa.

Recently, an exciting development has been the asking of kinetic questions in experimental treatment protocols. Can prognosis be predicted by pretreatment cytokinetic measurements? Does drug resistance emerge rapidly between diagnosis and the first opportunity to initiate chemotherapy? Is prognosis improved by shrinking a tumor mass as rapidly as possible, even before surgical removal? What is the optimal scheduling of non-cross resistant chemotherapies? What is the relationship between drug dose and the rate of tumor regression? These and many related issues are important to both the cytokineticist in the laboratory and the clinician at the bedside.

The field of cytokinetics is actually comprised of two related disciplines. The first is the study of cell proliferation, not in the biologic sense of examining how cells divide, but in the numeric sense of studying how fast they divide, how many are dividing and how biologic measurements—like DNA content per cell—relate to these kinetic processes. The second aspect of cytokinetics is growth curve analysis, the description of rates of change of cell number over time in both the unperturbed and perturbed (therapeutic) situation. The two disciplines are closely related in that the kinetics of cellular proliferation underlie the kinetics of tumor growth. In addition, both cellular proliferation and tumor growth are now thought to relate to many biological characteristics of a cancer, including its tendency to invade, to metastasize and to respond to drug therapy. Hence, this chapter will consider the two disciplines, their connections and their clinical implications.

Cell Proliferation

The Mitotic Cycle: PLM Curves

"Mitosis," or cell division, is the basic biological process that results in an increase in somatic cell numbers over time. The term "growth" applies to the increasing volume of a cellular population. This is largely the consequence of increasing numbers of cells, but also can be influenced by the increasing size of the individual cells as well as by such processes as edema, hemorrhage and infiltration by cells from another population. The term "proliferation" specifically applies to an increase in the number of cells. Cells divide by progressing through a sequence of steps that are collectively called the "mitotic cycle." Other names for mitotic cycle are "proliferative cycle" and "cell cycle." Classic autoradiographic techniques were first used to divide the cell cycle into four phases.[127,168] The terms for these phases, described below, are still used today, although the means of assessment is now often biochemical or biophysical, not biological as in the original usage.

The two key events in mitosis are the synthesis of DNA, which occurs mostly in the "S-phase" or *S* (for synthesis),

598

and the actual division of the parent cell into two daughters during "M-phase" or *M* (for mitosis). M-phase contains the metaphase plate which is visible microscopically. The time gap between cell division and DNA synthesis is "gap number one," or G_1. The time gap between DNA synthesis and cell division is "gap number two," or G_2. Although the term mitosis is often used to refer to M-phase, the adjective "mitotic" properly refers to all cells that are engaged in any portion of the whole process of self-replication. This whole process includes the submicroscopic events (G_1, S, G_2) that precede the M-phase, as well as the M-phase itself. This usage has the advantage of distinguishing cells that provide evidence of their intention to divide from those cells—G_0 cells—that do not express that intention.

Cell cycle phases are best understood in the context of their means of quantification. The venerable *mitotic index*, the counting of metaphase figures in histological slides, is of real value, but it is very labor-intensive, so it is now less popular than it should be.[11] An important variant of the mitotic index is the stathmokinetic technique, in which a mitotic poison is applied prior to counting.[86] Of all the older techniques, however, the most important by far is the thymidine labelling index.[286] In this method viable cells are exposed briefly in vitro to a radiolabelled precursor of DNA. The most common thymidine label is tritium (^{3}H), but carbon-14 has also been used. The percentage of tumor cells with autoradiographic grains over their nuclei estimates the fraction of cells that were in S-phase during the period of thymidine exposure. Newer variants use monoclonal antibodies directed against proteins expressed during growth (vide infra) to allow mitotic (i.e., cycling) cells to be identified visually.[4A,52,96] In all of the above techniques the microanatomy of the specimen is preserved so that the microscopist can actually know that the cell being counted is one of interest.

The highest refinement of the thymidine labelling index is the percentage of labeled mitoses (PLM) curve. This technique counts, as a function of time after exposure, the number of M-phases that contain radioactive label. This measures the cells presently in M-phase that had been in S-phase during the exposure to radioisotope. The PLM method had formerly been used to study human disease, but this application has been curtailed because it requires whole-body exposure to a long-lived radioisotope. In spite of its limitations the technique has been of fundamental importance in the field of cytokinetics because it directly estimates the durations of phases of the cell cycle. Its theory is illustrated schematically in Figure XV-1-1. In Figure XV-1-1A tritiated thymidine is administered as a pulse to label cells in S-phase. As time passes (Figure XV-1-1B) the labelled cells move beyond S and transverse G_2. At this moment no M-phase cells contain label, so the PLM is zero. Over the next short interval of time (Figure XV-1-1C) labelled cells enter M-phase. The PLM goes from zero to 100%, as shown in the graph at the bottom of Figure XV-1-1. The elapsed time from the pulse labelling to the achievement of 100% PLM is equivalent to the sum of the durations of G_2 and M. The time required for the PLM to drop down again to zero is the same as the time required for all of the cells labelled during S to pass through their M-phases: This is the same as the duration of S-phase (Figure XV-1-1D). If we follow the population

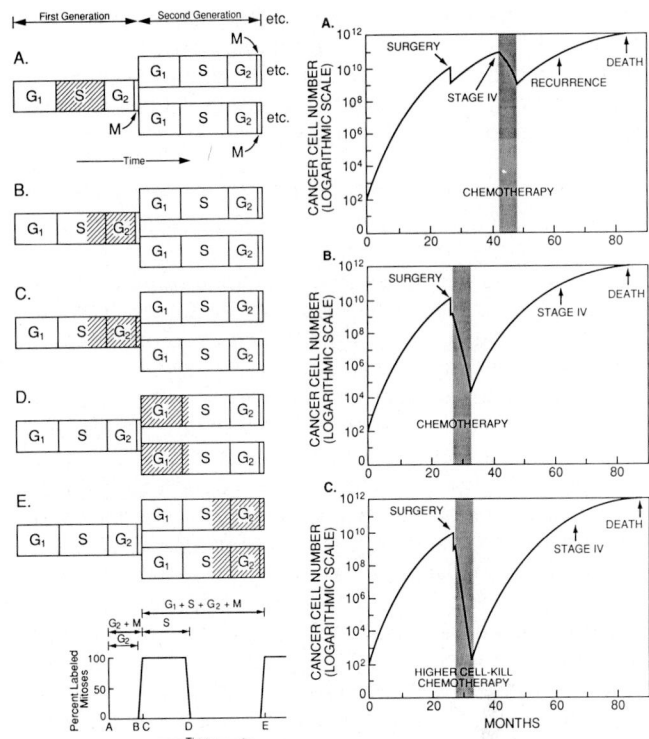

Figure XV-1-1. The mitotic cycle and percent labeled mitoses curve.

Figure XV-1-2. Gompertzian model of breast cancer growth.

through a second generation, the PLM will again rise from zero to 100% (Figure XV-1-1E). Figures XV-1-1C and XV-1-1E are the same except for a translocation in time which is equivalent to one full cell cycle.

Real PLM curves would be as sharp and as precise as is this hypothetical example were cycle lengths invariable, but, unfortunately, they are not. Another problem is that because of radiopharmacokinetic and other technical considerations, it is rare for label ever to be present in all M-phase cells. Hence, sophisticated mathematical methods must be used to estimate phase lengths by model-fitting.[273] Nevertheless, almost everything that we now know concerning cycle dynamics has been learned from the PLM method.

Cell Cycle Phases and DNA Content

At its birth a normal mammalian somatic cell contains a *diploid* number of chromosomes, and hence diploid (2N) DNA content. Following a successful cell division the new cell generally experiences a time gap before it begins to engage in measurable DNA synthesis. Some very primitive or embryonic cells enter DNA synthesis immediately, but these are exceptions to the usual pattern. We have termed this gap G_1, but a new cell is properly called G_1 only if it exhibits the biological intention of entering S-phase. Should the cell never actually progress to the point of starting DNA synthesis, it would have properly been classified as G_0. Since both G_0 and G_1 cells are diploid in DNA content, we avoid the presumption of prescience by considering the two phases together. In performing this grouping we recognize that the lengths of the G_0–G_1 phases are highly variable, fitting a lognormal probability distribution which is skewed markedly to the right. Since the cells on the far right end of the distribution will never divide within the lifespan of the host, they are the G_0 cells.

The distinction between G_0 and G_1 is biological as well as statistical. During G_0–G_1 cells prepare to enter S by progressing through defined stages which are dependent on protein synthesis.[230] These stages are regulated by kinases and other intracellular processes which are intrinsic but also sensitive to extracellular signals such as growth factors (platelet-derived, epidermal, insulin-like growth factors and insulin are some examples) and the supply of nutrients. Cancer cells may be less dependent on these external signals and conditions than normal cells, which may account for their ability to grow in suspension cultures without extracellular matrix. This ability may be related to the activity of oncogenes or to the deregulation of suppressor genes like p53 or the retinoblastoma gene. Cells in G_1 have already progressed beyond several preliminary steps to prepare for S-phase, whereas G_0 cells need further time to complete early synthetic events so that they can enter G_1. These differences can be exploited in the laboratory to discriminate G_0 from G_1 cells. G_0 cells tend to be smaller.[177] G_0 cells have lower RNA and protein contents than G_1 cells, as well as specific, characteristic mRNA's and proteins.[13,54] For example, the Ki67 antigen is present in all mitotic cells (G_1, S, G_2, M), but is not found in G_0 cells.[96] Also, G_0 cells do not metabolize the cationic dye rhodamide, which is thought, but not proven,[41] to reflect the cells' relatively low mitochondrial activity.[140] However G_0 cells, in spite of their distinctive biological characteristics, can be stimulated by external influences to proceed through the sequence of events that leads them into G_1 and eventually into S: This phenomenon is called "recruitment."

After M-phase, but before DNA synthesis begins in earnest, the cell either commits to proliferate by entering S-phase or stops dividing by differentiating into a nonmitotic cell. The ratio $G_1/(G_0 + G_1)$ at any one time defines the proportion of cells entering their next S-phase. A particular restriction point at the G_1–S interface, now called "Start," may be regulated by the p34^{cdc2} protein, which may couple with different cyclin proteins (whose levels vary within the cell cycle) to permit, alternatively, a cell's entry into S or its entry into M.[32] Normally, M-phase cannot take place unless S-phase is completed, and S-phase cannot take place unless M-phase is completed. Abnormalities in this system could result in an unblocking of the normal "block to re-replication" which prevents parts of the genome from being replicated more than once during a single S-phase.[207] Such abnormalities are one possible etiology for aberrant levels of DNA per neoplastic cell (vide infra). Once the cell enters S-phase its progression through the rest of the cycle is largely self-regulated.[117] This regulation involves direct controls, in which a step must be completed before the next step commences, as well as indirect feedback loops.[206]

The S-phase, lasting between 12 to 24 hours in mammalian cells, is generally much less variable than G_0–G_1. Specific regions of chromosomes replicate at specific times, clusters of replication units initiating synchronously, with the whole complex process transpiring in a highly orchestrated manner.[170] During S a cell's DNA contents should increase from 2N to 4N. A very small number of S_0 cells may actually stop synthesizing DNA before completing S.[55] Their ultimate fate is unclear, although it is likely that some can resume S, while others are prevented from proceeding by intrinsic blocks in their self-regulation. Cells completing S enter the second gap, marked by a dramatic diminution in the rate of DNA synthesis. G_2 usually lasts for about three hours in mammalian cells, ending when M-phase begins. Rarely, a cell can rest in G_2, and not proceed into actual cell division.[95] The initiation of M-phase may depend on the same molecular trigger as Start, but in a complex interplay with different cyclins and other factors that are actively under investigation.[225]

M-phase is composed of several parts. In *prophase* the cell assumes the shape of a sphere.[81] The microtubules and microfilaments of the cell's cytoskeleton rearrange, the Golgi apparatus disperses into small vesicles, protein synthesis drops, the dispersed chromosomes (duplicated during S-phase) cease metabolic activity and then condense into transportable units.[194] During *prometaphase* these units orient themselves linearly toward opposite ends of the cell and move to the midplane to form the *metaphase plate*. In *anaphase* spindle fibers attached to kinetochores on each chromosome guide them toward centrosomes in opposite ends of the cell. In *telophase* the nuclei reform, the chromosomes decondense and the cell normally divides into two approximately equal halves, one new nucleus per daughter cell. M is the phase that is least variable in length, lasting about one hour in most mammalian cells.

The total duration of the cell cycle, the "mitotic cycle time," also called the "generation time," varies considerably, but the average in human cancer is between 2 and 4 days. This is in marked contrast with the cell cycle in Drosophila, which may take minutes, or with that of mammalian embryos, which may take hours. Some normal cells, such as human neurons, may never divide at all. Cancer is not always a disease of rapid proliferation, but it is always one of persistent proliferation. If there are a large number of cancer cells dividing, even if they are dividing with deliberate speed, they will produce many offspring, which, by themselves dividing, will lead to an abnormal accumulation over time. For a given tissue, malignant or benign, the length of the cell cycle in vivo is fairly constant in spite of variations in the number of cycling cells in that population. However, subtle changes in cycle kinetics have been seen in cancers in laboratory animals that are allowed to grow large,[169,316] and phase lengths can shift significantly as cells are cultured in vitro.[14]

Flow Cytometry

The variation in cellular DNA content during the proliferative cycle can be exploited analytically by a collection of automated methods called "flow cytometry." Visual procedures, such as mitotic index, thymidine labelling index, and static Ki-67 staining, are slow, laborious and subjective. These negative features may change in the future with technological advances in assessing cellularity on slides and in the automated counting of visually distinctive cells.[145,263A] At present, however, flow methods are the most rapid and quantitative.[69] The major disadvantage of techniques like flow cytometry, in which the cells being analyzed are not visualized, is that normal stromal cells, normal blood cells, and tumor cells of various types and degrees of oxygenation are all counted together. Another disadvantage is that reliable flow cytometry requires meticulous technique and hence constant attention to quality control. Nevertheless, flow cytometry has become the most widely applied and hence the most productive method of cytokinetic assessment in the modern clinic.

In fluorescence-activated cell sorting a suspension of individual cells is automatically counted by being allocated into bins by DNA content, RNA content, cell size, antibody label or combination of such factors.[147,307] This can be performed on fresh tissue—leukemias, tumor cells in effusions or ascites, enzymatically dispersed solid tumors—or on cells recovered from paraffin-embedded specimens.[119] Enzymatic methods of dispersing fresh or fixed solid tumor specimens have been shown to produce high single-cell yields, representative of the tissue as a whole, with low degrees of contamination by cellular debris.[229]

Flow cytometry can be used to measure RNA per cell, which, as mentioned above, is helpful in distinguishing G_0 from G_1 cells. Various techniques of tagging cells for the purpose of sorting are being employed. For example, cells can be labelled by the Ki67 antibody (conjugated to a fluorescent dye).[96] Unfixed, viable cells can be exposed to bromodeoxyuridine, which is incorporated during S.[171] These cells will then react with an anti-bromodeoxyuridine antibody tagged with a fluorescent dye, a method that has proven reliable in the study of solid tumors.[201] Bromodeoxyuridine can also be administered intravenously to patients several hours prior to a biopsy. The tissue so recovered can then be examined for S-phase label, or can be exposed to tritiated thymidine to provide a double label, useful for examining phase durations, particularly in leukemia.[244]

The primary value of flow cytometry for cytokinetics is in its measurement of DNA content. DNA content is usually assessed by the use of intercalating or base-pair affinity dyes. The standard output of this technique is the DNA flow cytogram, also called a "DNA histogram." Standardization of the G_0–G_1 peak for DNA histograms uses diploid cells from the same species as the tissue being studied.[123] Human lymphocytes from normal donors are commonly used for many clinical applications. In the assessment of human breast cancer, lymphocytes are often obtained from normal lymph nodes removed at the time of primary surgery. The completed histogram graphs the relative proportions of cells with 2N DNA (i.e., diploid cells in G_0–G_1), 4N DNA (i.e., tetraploid cells in G_2–M) and DNA content between 2N and 4N, called the "S-Phase Fraction." Another cytometric term in common use is the "proliferative index," the fraction of cells that are in either S or G_2 or M.

By measuring DNA content per cell flow cytometry can also identify cells with abnormal amounts of DNA in the G_0–G_1 peak, termed *aneuploid*. Categories include near-diploid (2N ± 10%), hypodiploid (less than 2N), simple hyperdiploid (between 2N and 4N), tetraploid (4N), near-tetraploid (4N ± 10%), hypertetraploid (greater than 4N) or combinations,

called "multiploid." Each aneuploid G_0–G_1 peak is expected to have a corresponding G_2–M peak with twice as much DNA. The DNA Index is the ratio between the fluorescence channel of the malignant G_0–G_1 peak and the normal diploid G_0–G_1 peak: Less than 0.9 or greater than 1.1 is often considered abnormal. S-phase fraction may be impossible to measure in the presence of marked aneuploidy, especially if a diploid G_2–M peak overlaps with an aneuploid S. An overview of the literature suggests that ploidy can now be measured in more than 90% of solid tumors, and S-phase fraction in about 80% of specimens. However, the classification of DNA histograms is not well standardized at present, so interpretations are highly variable, especially when paraffin-embedded source material is used.[139]

Mitotic Compartments

When a cell divides the daughters must either remain in a mitotically quiescent state, or enter G_1, or die. There are no other possibilities. Entering G_1 means that the cell has positioned itself to divide again. Such a cell is thereby a member of the "proliferative fraction," also called the "growth fraction" or the "growth compartment."[197] The second possibility is that the cell enters a prolonged G_0 (or, rarely, S_0 or an arrested G_2), which means that the cell has joined the "nonproliferative" or "quiescent fraction." Classically, the growth fraction is measured by dividing the labelling index by the ratio of the durations of the S-phase and the total cycle time.[153]

The S-phase fraction as measured by flow cytometry includes S_0 cells in the quiescent fraction. For this and other technical reasons, the S-phase fraction is usually larger than the thymidine labelling index. S-phase fraction correlates with but is not equivalent to the growth fraction.[192] About 2–20% of cells in a typical cancer are in S at any point in time. Since S-phase occupies one-quarter to one-half of the cell cycle, the growth fraction is usually 4–80% with an average of less than 20%. Some normal tissues, such as bone marrow and alimentary mucosa, have larger growth fractions and shorter mitotic cycle times than many cancers, even cancers of those tissues.[125,240]

Nonproliferative cells fall into three types. Some highly differentiated cells, like neurons, are permanently nonproliferative but may survive as long as the life of the organism. In distinction, most terminally differentiated cells, like the polymorphonuclear leukocyte, have a finite life-span. The third type of nonproliferative cell is in an unstable G_0, which means that it may be recruited into G_1 on the proper extracellular signal. "Stem cells," like neurons, live as long as the organism, but, like unstable G_0 cells, they can periodically, or on demand, produce viable progeny.[34,295] The signal for stem cell recruitment is often from physiological changes in the environment, like cell death, cell injury, or extracellular influences like drugs or hormones. An operational definition of stem capacity is the ability to form colonies in soft agar.[113] Cell culture experiments have found that from 1% to less than 0.1% of the cells in many common tumors have this property, but this may be an underestimate, since in vitro conditions may be more austere than those occurring naturally in vivo. Yet, even though malignant stem cells are a minority population in a cancer, they are the prime target of anticancer therapy since they constantly replenish the whole population. If chemotherapy preferentially kills mitotic cells, termed the "mitotoxicity hypothesis," the ability of tumor stem cells to remain in G_0 for long periods may be one reason for therapeutic failure.[284]

The third possible fate for a cell is death. Cells lost from any phase of the cell cycle are collectively called the "cell loss fraction."[283] Cell loss is important because the growth rate is the difference between cell production and cell loss. Hence, a tumor with high cell loss may appear to be growing slowly, when in fact the rate of mitosis may be high. A well-known clinical example is basal cell epithelioma of the skin which grows slowly in spite of showing a large number of metaphase figures.

The significance of cell loss may be illustrated by a hypothetical numerical example. Let us imagine a tumor with a growth fraction of 100%, no cell loss and a mitotic cycle time of three days. This tumor will double in size each three days. In this case the generation time is equal to the doubling time, the time it takes the cell number to double in size. If, however, cells are lost from the tumor at one-half the rate of cell production, a cell loss fraction of 50%, the tumor will double in six rather than in three days. The importance of cell loss goes well beyond the determination of growth rate. Each mitotic cycle carries with it a finite probability of mutation.[223] It takes more mitotic cycles for the tumor with a cell loss of 50% to double in size than for the tumor with no cell loss. Hence the rate of cell loss relates directly to the rate of mutations toward biological properties of clinical importance.

Cytokinetics and Biological Diversity

Over the decade of the 1980's more than a thousand published studies have assayed the cytokinetics of clinical cancer. There have been major as well as minor applications. A relatively minor use has been in the screening of cytological specimens for malignant cells. This exercise exploits the observation that with few exceptions (noted below) normal cells are diploid while about 70% of clinical cancers are aneuploid. Screening, however, has been of secondary interest to the use of kinetic measurements for correlation with clinical course. S-phase fraction, thymidine labelling index and aneuploidy have all been evaluated as prognostic factors. Although S-phase fraction may be no higher in neoplastic than in some normal tissues, within a given histological type of cancer both high S-phase fraction and aneuploidy are frequently associated with growth that is relatively more rapid, malignant behavior that is relatively more aggressive and therapeutic response that is relatively poorer.

The reasons for the consistent association of aneuploidy with high S-phase fraction are conjectural. One possibility is that aneuploidy is caused by high S-phase activity because it is the consequence of errors in chromosomal construction. The reasoning in this regard is that a high S-phase fraction implies a large number of mitotic cycles per unit of time, which gives more opportunities for erroneous DNA replication. Against this argument is the observation that many normal tissues, such as bone marrow and epithelia, have high S-phase fractions but do not normally become aneuploid. This leaves another possibility, that high S-phase fraction is

not the cause of aneuploidy but rather the consequence of the chromosomal abnormalities reflected in the aneuploid state. Such abnormalities may be linked with oncogene activation or suppressor gene inactivation. Some clinically benign tumors are aneuploid, so chromosomal abnormalities do not always mean frank cancerous behavior. Yet aneuploidy is clearly a step in tumor progression: DNA errors lead to growth stimulation, high cell turnover results in more opportunities for error, errors produce increasing genetic aberrancy. The question of how fast mutations accumulate by this process is clinically relevant and will be discussed below in the context of growth curve models.

Regardless of the rate of mutations, however, the neoplastic process is so closely related to spontaneous genetic change that tumor progression toward increasing malignancy is regarded as an intrinsic property of cancer.[83,244] The clonal origin of tumors is well described.[129] It has been stated that over 80% of clinical cancers are monoclonal by glucose-6-phosphate dehydrogenase isotype or cytogenetics.[88] Yet clonal evoluation as the tumors evolve leads to heterogeneity in morphology, metastatic behavior, biochemistry, ploidy, immunogenicity, steroid and growth factor receptors, and drug sensitivity.[75] Metastases tend to grow faster than the primary tumors from which they arise.[40A,275] There is ample evidence that cytokinetics either underlies or is a direct covariate of tumor progression. That is, the mechanism relating aneuploidy with S-phase fraction also relates tumor progression to S-phase fraction. This will be illustrated below in the discussion of clinical correlates of cytokinetics and further below in the context of the doubling time and the Skipper-Schabel model.

As discussed theoretically above, the third determinant of growth rate, cell loss, is also relevant to the generation of genetic changes. High rates of cell turnover are implicated in carcinogenesis. Elevated levels of thyroid stimulating hormone predispose to thyroid cancer.[317] Chronic thermal injury with compensatory hyperplasia[211] and hyperplasia secondary to solar damage[110] lead to skin cancer. Hyperproliferation of the bone marrow in dysmyelopoiesis[107] and in chronic granulocytic leukemia[235] can result in acute leukemia. Hyperproliferation of the epithelium, as of the colon in inflammatory bowel disease and polyps,[231] and of the breast in murine models[59] and clinical specimens,[56,261] is also associated with neoplastic transformation. Indeed, chemical carcinogenesis requires a growth promoter.[258] It is possible that the hyperproliferation of cancer cells as a compensatory response to chronic antineoplastic drug treatment may predispose to the development of drug resistance in Hodgkin's lymphoma[100] and gastrointestinal cancer.[24]

All of the statistical associations between S-phase fraction, ploidy, cell loss fraction, and clinical behavior are of major scientific interest. It must be cautioned, however, that these associations are not always of practical importance, especially when kinetic parameters are highly correlated with more easily measured prognostic factors such as tumor size. As is seen with any weak prognostic factor, small studies are often falsely negative. Conversely, false-positive reports may arise via "data-driven subset analysis." For example, imagine that a population of patients is divisible into those with some arbitrary factor X and those without X, those with Y and those without Y, those with and without Z, and so on. A small study may show that aneuploidy means poor prognosis in patients with Y but good prognosis in patients without Y, whereas both X and Z seem unrelated to ploidy and prognosis. Here the subset allocation (by Y) is chosen because ploidy seems to be useful within the subset, not because there is a biological reason to suspect that ploidy and Y should be related. In fact, if ploidy carried no prognostic significance whatsoever, there is a real possibility that some other arbitrary division would distinguish the patients merely by chance. This other arbitrary division could be draped in the illusion of biologic tenability, but it would not prove reproducible in prospective confirmatory studies. Hence, purely statistical phenomena such as these should always be kept in mind when reading conflicting data concerning cytokinetics and clinical behavior.

Illustrative Clinical Correlates

Breast Cancer. Invasive adenocarcinomas (largely ductal) of the breast have received intensive cytokinetic scrutiny. Thymidine labelling indices of primary specimens have been shown to follow a log-normal probability distribution.[199] This means that while the majority of thymidine labelling indices are grouped about a median of 5–6%, some very large values are found in a few cases. Nuclear staining with the Ki-67 antigen correlates with thymidine labelling index.[146] Thymidine labelling indices from primary specimens correlate well with values determined from metastatic sites.[200] High thymidine labelling index predicts for the presence of necrosis in the tumor, low estrogen receptor content, anaplastic nuclear and histologic grade, and other predictors of poor clinical outcome. In locally advanced breast cancer high thymidine labelling index predicts high metastatic potential, short disease-free interval after intensive treatment and short survival.[271] The thymidine labelling index and S-phase fraction by flow cytometry show good correspondence.[193] As expected, therefore, high S-phase fraction in primary disease correlates with low estrogen and progesterone receptor content, high degree of nodal involvement, increasing nuclear anaplasia and aneuploidy.[70] In the subset of patients with estrogen receptor-negative stage II tumors, diploidy has been reported to be a positive prognostic factor.[165]

In node-negative breast cancer the presence of either high S-phase fraction or aneuploidy has been correlated with a higher probability of relapse.[44,198,270] However, this was only partially confirmed in a prospective series of node-negative breast cancer patients randomized to receive no postoperative adjuvant chemotherapy.[70] Ploidy (measured in 79% of cases) had no prognostic value. S-phase fraction (measured in 73% of patients) did, with low S-phase fraction predicting longer disease-free interval. However, low S-phase fraction correlated so well with small tumor size that its value as an independent predictor must be established by further study. It is also of interest to note that for the patients randomized to chemotherapy, treatment had a positive impact irrespective of the S-phase category.

Gastrointestinal Cancer. Aneuploidy is typical of premalignant colonic epithelial dysplasia in adenomas and inflammatory bowel disease. The majority of colorectal carcinomas are aneuploid, which correlates positively with high S-phase fraction and has been associated with poor prognosis, even within anatomical stages.[14A,298,319,323] However, as expected for a weak prognostic factor, the data are inconsistent. Cytometrics have been reported as very useful,[6,98,141,241,264A] slightly useful,[101] of secondary importance,[112] and of no value.[77,196] They may[9,138,157,265] or may not[23] relate to histopathology, and may[264] or may not[14A,156] have worth in advanced disease. In rectal carcinomas ploidy[142] and high S-phase fraction by Ki-67 immunohistology[269] may predict radiosensitivity. One-half of hepatocellular carcinomas have been reported as aneuploid, which seems to indicate worse prognosis.[93] The two-thirds of gastric cancers that are aneuploid fare worse than the diploid cases,[227,326,328] even in early disease.[288] The behavior of aneuploid gastric carcinomas may relate to their histology[158,159,212,327] and location. Most gastroesophageal-cardia lesions are aneuploid, compared with about half of lesions of the body-antrum, which have a better prognosis.[208] S-phase fraction via antibromodeoxyuridine correlates positively with degree of aneuploidy (the DNA index).[227A,325]

Genitourinary Cancer. In transitional cell carcinoma of the urinary bladder the presence of aneuploidy in voided cells has been used to screen for neoplasia, but this is of limited utility since only one third of cases are aneuploid.[111,188] When found, however, aneuploidy is a poor prognostic sign.[187,189,205] Tetraploidy may predict radiosensitivity.[136] In renal cell carcinoma aneuploidy is observed in two-thirds of cases.[53,243] Although ploidy may yield some prognostic information, nuclear grading appears to be of greater value.[4,155] In tumors of the renal pelvis, aneuploidy is related to histology, but may provide extra prognostic information in low-grade low-stage cases.[21] In prostate cancer one-quarter to one-half of cases are tetraploid, but other forms of aneuploidy are rare.[203,210,248] Results linking aneuploidy to prognosis are conflicting.[22,60,82,118]

Gynecological Cancer. About three-quarters of ovarian carcinomas are aneuploid.[91] This finding may[73] or may not[163] correlate positively with stage but the evidence suggests that it predicts shorter survival,[143] particularly in the presence of a high S-phase fraction.[154] In diploid tumors, a high S-phase fraction may be adverse.[144] In the presence of advanced disease the importance of ploidy wanes,[92] except, perhaps, in combination with morphologic characteristics (psammoma body content).[162] In endometrial carcinomas aneuploidy is observed in one-eighth of stage I cases.[31] Anaplasia may correlate with aneuploidy, high S-phase fraction and poor prognosis,[164,252] although this has not been found in all studies.[175] One-third to two-thirds of cervical carcinomas are aneuploid, which may[17,133–135,174,287] or may not[71] be prognostically inauspicious. Indeed, aneuploidy was a positive factor compared to diploidy and tetraploidy in one series.[256]

Pediatric Cancers. In neuroblastoma, in contrast to the general findings in other solid tumors, the discovery of aneuploidy seems to convey a positive prognostic influence.[228] Indeed, benign ganglioneuromas in children are frequently aneuploid.[293] This may be related to a positive association of N-myc amplification with near-diploidy and with an aggressive clinical course.[28,67] In children under one year of age, hyperdiploid tumors seem to respond to chemotherapy better than do diploid tumors.[182] Diploid medulloblastomas in children may have a greater tendency to metastasize than the half of tumors which are aneuploid.[324]

One-third of osteosarcomas are aneuploid.[15] Ploidy seems to be of prognostic value in young patients undergoing adjuvant chemotherapy for osteosarcoma of an extremity, with near-diploid status predicting for better outcome, even after adjustment for age.[184]

Miscellaneous Cancers. More than one-half of lung cancers (other than the small-cell variety) are aneuploid, which is related to poor outcome in all series[130,259,296,309–311,314] independent of stage[312] and age, sex, type of surgery, and site of involvement.[330] S-phase fraction also predicts for shorter survival.[313] Half of squamous cell carcinomas of the oral cavity are aneuploid, but the prognostic significance of this finding is equivocal.[302]

Up to one-half of thyroid malignancies are aneuploid, which, like high S-phase fraction, is a weak predictor of worse prognosis in papillary and follicular carcinomas.[300] The quarter of melanomas which are aneuploid may also experience a worse prognosis, even when stratified by the dominant factor of tumor thickness.[18,152] In high-grade soft tissue sarcomas ploidy may convey some prognostic information.[5] One-quarter of smooth muscle tumors of the stomach are aneuploid, but this does not distinguish benign from malignant cases.[299] However, aneuploid malignant leiomyosarcomas do fare worse. All oncocytic tumors of the salivary gland that have been studied have been diploid, but the one-quarter to one-half of oncocytic renal and thyroid cancers that are aneuploid seem to have a worse prognosis.[242] In glial brain tumors, flow-cytometry can be performed on stereotactic biopsies.[84] This is important because high Ki-67 staining, high bromodeoxyuridine labelling index, and aneuploidy all correlate with degree of histological malignancy and poor clinical outcome.[213] Ploidy was associated with degree of malignancy in a study of meningiomas.[279]

Hematological Neoplasms. In Hodgkin's disease, like neuroblastoma, aneuploidy, seen in 11% of cases, may predict for better survival.[204] Low S-phase fraction may also be favorable, but the effect of both ploidy and S-phase fraction are weak, and are confounded with routine histological classification. A quarter to a half of non-Hodgkin's lymphomas are aneuploid,[137] but this finding seems clinically insignificant compared to classic histopathology.[40,51] In contrast, S-phase fraction[42,176,329,247] and thymidine labelling index[166] correlate with anaplasia and aggressive natural history, and with poor response to therapy.[195,282] Cytokinetics may convey little additional information in subgroups already known to have unfavorable prognosis.[43,173]

The acute leukemias were one of the first diseases to be analyzed by autoradiographic techniques.[45] It was soon established that the thymidine labelling index of the malignant cells was higher in the marrow than in the peripheral blood, but lower than that of normal hematopoietic precursors.[191] A significant percentage of leukemic myeloblasts were found not be be cycling.[46] Leukemic lymphoblasts demonstrated a positive relationship between cell size and labelling,[149] which is now understood to reflect the volume diminution seen in early G_1 and G_0. Mitotic phase durations of chronic myelogenous leukemia cells are quite similar to those of normal marrow cells, with a smaller growth fraction than normal marrow, but a greatly expanded population size.[226,308]

DNA flow cytometry has been applied to human leukemia, but it has generally assumed a role secondary to immunophenotyping, gene rearrangement studies, and cytogenetic classification.[8] This may change as more interest develops in the relationship between oncogene expression and leukemia cell kinetics.[254] Oncogenes that code for membrane receptors and kinases, and those like c-myc that bind to the nucleus, seem to influence proliferation, and are expressed abnormally in hematopoietic cancer.[19]

S-phase fraction correlates positively with aneuploidy in acute lymphoblastic leukemia, but there is no firm evidence that pretreatment thymidine labelling index, S-phase fraction, or mitotic index have prognostic importance. In children with acute lymphoblastic leukemia, the presence of a single hyperdiploid population of blasts (DNA index >1.16, which correlates with a karyotype of >52 chromosomes) has been reported to predict for better response to chemotherapy, even after adjustment for other prognostic variables.[183] Late relapses are more common in patients whose leukemic blasts have lower DNA contents.[239]

In acute myeloid leukemia in adults, there is recent evidence that longer cell cycle time as determined by bromodeoxyuridine incorporation may correlate with longer complete remission duration.[201] Older studies had suggested that the labelling index of myeloid leukemia cells in the marrow correlated inversely with remission duration.[115] In all acute leukemias, high cellular RNA content (which measures the G_0–G_1 peak) predicts for high response rate but short response duration.[8]

Although the successful development of pioneering antileukemia chemotherapy programs was largely empirical, many of the fundamental principles of cell proliferation kinetics were originally formulated in an attempt to provide guidelines for improved treatment design.[10] The interactions of chemotherapy and cell proliferation have been reviewed.[290] High-dose cytosine arabinoside synchronizes myeloid leukemia cells in S-phase, doing so more predictably in children than in adults.[49] It is of interest that chemotherapy for acute myeloid leukemia decreases the S-phase fraction of residual bone marrow even when patients fail to attain complete remission.[7] A differentiating, antiproliferative action of chemotherapy beyond cell-kill has been observed.[253] The concept that chemotherapy may depress the cytokinetics of residual tumor cells may have therapeutic implications, which is discussed below in the context of the Norton-Simon model.

Growth Curve Analysis

The correlations between cytokinetics and clinical behavior support the concept that cell proliferation is intimately associated with the generation of tumor heterogeneity. Cell proliferation is, in addition, the primary mechanism for tumor growth. Anticancer therapy is, of course, intended to reverse growth by killing or removing cancer cells. Both upward and downward changes over time in the number of cells are described by a type of mathematic function called a "growth curve." These curves not only summarize clinical course but relate to the rate of emergence of mutations toward clinically-relevant cellular diversity. Through both of these attributes growth curves are proving useful in explaining human cancer and providing research directions toward improved cancer therapy.

The Skipper-Schabel-Wilcox Model

The Skipper-Schabel-Wilcox model or "log-kill model" was the original, and is still the preeminent, model of tumor growth and therapeutic regression.[276,277] It is based on the observation that leukemia L1210 in BDF$_1$ or DBA mice grows exponentially until it reaches a lethal tumor volume of 10^9 cells (one cubic centimeter).[274] Ninety percent of the leukemia cells divide every twelve to thirteen hours. This percentage is the same for a tiny tumor or a tumor close to the lethal volume. As a result the doubling time is always constant: If it takes 11 hours for 100 cells to grow into 200 cells, it will take 11 hours for 10^7 cells to grow into 2×10^7 cells. This pattern generalizes for any constant fractional increase: If it takes 40 hours for 10^3 cells to grow into 10^4 cells (an increase by a factor of ten), it will take 40 hours for 10^7 cells to grow into 10^8 cells.

Exponential growth and the concept of the doubling time have concrete clinical implications.[88] In the clinically observable range of tumor sizes there is great divergence between histologic types of cancer in their doubling times.[267] The most therapeutically-responsive human cancers, like testicular cancer and choriocarcinoma, tend to have doubling times which are less than one month long. Less responsive cancers like squamous cell cancer of the head and neck seem to double in about two months. The unresponsive cancers, like colon adenocarcinoma, tend to double each three months. Clearly, this clinical observation may relate to the relatively higher chemosensitivity of proliferating cells (vide infra). That is, if a tumor has a high fraction of dividing cells it will tend to grow faster and will also tend to be more responsive to drugs which kill dividing cells. Alternatively, tumors with a higher rate of cell loss will tend to have a relatively slower growth rate and also a higher rate of mutations toward drug-resistance. A combination of many such factors may be relevant. Regardless of the theoretical implications of the basic clinical observation, the unspoken assumption is that the fixed doubling time accurately summarizes the proliferative behavior of a given tumor. This assumption will be examined below.

Nevertheless, when a tumor that is growing exponentially and is homogeneous in drug sensitivity is treated with a specific chemotherapy regimen, the fraction of cells killed is always the same regardless of the initial size of the malignant population. If a given dose of a given drug reduces 10^6 cells to 10^5, the same therapy applied against 10^4 cells will result in 10^3 survivors. These two cytoreductions are both examples of "one-log" kill, which means a 90% decrease in cell number. It was shown quite early that for many drugs the log-kill increases with increasing dose.[105,250] Hence, it requires higher drug dosages to eradicate larger inoculum sizes of transplanted tumors. In addition, if two or more drugs are used, the log-kills are multiplicative: if a given dose of drug A kills 90% of the cells (a one-log kill) and a given dose of drug B kills 90%, drug A given with drug B should kill 90% of the 10% of cells left after B alone, resulting in a kill of 99%

of the cells (a two-log kill). As a numerical example, if treatment A given alone leaves 10^5 cells out of 10^6, and if treatment B given alone does the same, the combination A + B (at full doses of each) should be able to reduce 10^6 cells to 10^4. If treatment C is also a one-log kill therapy, A + B + C should leave only 10^3 cells. If A + B + C is used to treat 10^3 cells, only 10^0, or one, cell should remain! Hence, if enough drugs at adequate doses are applied against a tumor of sufficiently small size, the number of cells left after treatment should be smaller than one, which means that the tumor is cured. This concept was of major value in the design of early curative approaches to childhood leukemia.[126]

When the concept of fractional kill was applied to the postoperative adjuvant treatment of micrometastases, it engendered enormous optimism.[263,268] After all, micrometastases are very small collections of cancer cells. Indeed, very small solid tumors in the laboratory contain a higher percentage of actively dividing cells than their larger counterparts.[169,316] It is thought that most chemotherapeutic agents preferentially damage mitotic cells. Hence, the fraction of cells killed in a small tumor should actually be even greater than the fraction of cells killed in a histologically identical tumor of larger size. Therefore, according to the Skipper-Schabel-Wilcox model, if the log-kill estimate is wrong, the error should be in the direction of underestimating the impact of therapy against micrometastases. Small volume tumors should be even more promptly cured by aggressive combination chemotherapy than would be predicted by the model.

Clinical experience, unfortunately, has not entirely confirmed these optimistic predictions. An illustration is the postoperative adjuvant chemotherapy of early-stage breast cancer. Here drugs known to be active against advanced disease have a real impact, but a modest one.[72] Is this because the therapy is not being given for a long enough duration? Assume drug combination XYZ causes a one-log kill with each application. Six cycles of XYZ should cure tumors of fewer than 10^6 cells. For tumors of exactly 10^6 cells the six cycles will leave just one cell to regrow. If this were the case then merely extending the duration of treatment beyond six cycles should kill the remaining cell and thereby increase the cure rate. From a modelling perspective, this same argument generalizes for higher degrees of cell-kill and higher tumor cell burdens. Yet durations of exposure longer than 4–6 months do not improve results in adjuvant chemotherapy.[72] Hence, the prediction of the model does not match actual observations.

As a consequence, if we accept the basic tenets of the Skipper-Schabel-Wilcox model, the failure of adjuvant chemotherapy to cure all cases of early breast cancer compels consideration of another possibility for failure to cure. That other possibility is that some cells in the tumor are biochemically refractory to the applied dose-levels of the agents used. As we explore other models below we will see that it is not always necessary to hypothesize that absolutely refractory cells exist. Nevertheless, the inclusion of the concept of absolutely resistant cells in the Skipper-Schabel-Wilcox model can account for the phenomena. According to this reasoning, once all sensitive cells are eliminated by a certain duration X of treatment, continuing therapy for a longer duration will not give better results because all the cells left after X cannot be killed by the drugs. If we assume that such resistance is acquired during a cancer's growth history by tumor progression (vide infra), the only way to guarantee the absence of resistant cells is to initiate therapy at so small a tumor size that no recalcitrant mutants are as yet present. If this is true we need only answer two questions: When in the time-course of growth does resistance develop? Can tumors be diagnosed early enough to be able to start treatment when the tumor is still curable?[62]

The Delbruck-Luria Model

To answer these questions we must turn to quantitative models of the emergence of drug resistance. Drug resistance by myriad biochemical mechanisms was recognized quite early to be important in cancer therapeutics,[65] based originally on pioneering experiments in bacteriology. In 1943 Luria and Delbruck found that different bacterial cultures developed resistance to bacteriophage infection at random (and hence different) times in their growth histories, often long prior to exposure to the viruses.[186] They reasoned that those cultures that had experienced a mutation earlier in their histories had more time to develop a high percentage of resistant bacteria. If a bacterium mutates toward property X with probability x at each mitosis, the probability of the cell not developing property X in one mitosis is one minus x. In y mitoses, the probability of no mutations occurring is $(1-x)^y$. If each mitosis produces two viable cells (no cell loss), it takes $N-1$ mitoses (not $N-1$ generation times) for one cell to grow into N cells. That is, one mitosis produces two cells, each of these two cells undergoes mitosis (for a cumulative total of three mitoses) to produce four cells, each of these four divide (for a cumulative total of seven mitoses) to produce eight cells, and so on. Hence, the probability of not finding any bacteria with property X in N cells is

$$\exp[(N-1) * \ln(1-x)]$$

which is approximately $\exp[-x(N-1)]$ since x is small. A numerical example of the application of this formula is given below. Within a decade of the original observation in bacteria the same pattern was found to apply to the emergence of methotrexate resistance in L1210 cells.[172] Hence, antimetabolite resistance was reasoned to be a trait acquired spontaneously at random times in the pretreatment growth of this cancer.

The Goldie-Coldman Model

In a qualitative sense, these observations were highly influential in the genesis and development of the concept of combination chemotherapy.[36] If tumor cells could acquire resistance to a drug prior to exposure to that drug, then the therapist could be faced with a disease heterogeneous in drug sensitivity even at the time of first diagnosis. Only combinations of drugs could hope to eradicate all cells.[85] This concept formed the basis for the whole development of modern medical oncology. In a quantitative sense, the Delbruck-Luria model was applied again to human cancer in 1979 by Goldie and Coldman.[102,103] They later refined their original model to include multiple sublines with double or higher orders of drug resistance, and the presence of cell loss.[104]

Their analysis contended that there is a high probability that mutations arise over a two-log (100-fold) increase in tumor size. That is, using the expression $\exp[-x(N-1)]$ which was derived above, at a mutation rate x of 10^{-6} (which is tenable)[150] the probability of no mutants in 10^5 cells is $\exp[-10^{-6}(10^5-1)]$ which equals .905. Similarly, the probability of no mutants in 10^7 cells is .000045.

In this regard it should be noted that while Goldie and Coldman focused on the property of drug resistance, an even clearer illustration of their concept may perhaps be found in the acquisition of metastatic ability. The capacity to metastasize is now established to be a reflection of genetic lability.[237] The approximate volume of 10^7 packed cells is 0.01 cubic centimeters. If tumor cells are mixed with benign host tissue (including stromal cells, fibrosis, extracellular secretions, blood and lymphatic vessels, empty space, etc.) at a packing ratio of 1:10, 10^7 cancer cells would occupy a volume of 0.1 cubic centimeters. At a packing ratio of 1:100, which is more often realistic, 10^7 cancer cells would be found in a tumor volume of about 1.0 cubic centimeter. This example of scaling relates directly to clinical data. In primary breast cancer the best predictor of axillary metastases is tumor size. Only 17% of invasive ductal lesions under one centimeter in diameter are metastatic to the axilla, contrasted with 41% of lesions of two centimeters in diameter and 68% of tumors of five to ten centimeters.[209] For primary breast cancer that does not involve axillary lymph nodes, the probability of eventual metastatic spread increases sharply when the mass in the breast is greater than one centimeter in diameter.[251] Hence, metastatic ability is conspicuously more common in tumors larger than this critical size. A one centimeter spherical tumor contains a volume of slightly over 0.5 cubic centimeters, which is right in the middle of the range of 0.1 to 1.0 cubic centimeters described above. These calculations fit the model with reassuring precision, but they cannot be regarded as proof of the model, since other explanations are possible (see *Mitotoxicity Hypothesis* below).

Regarding drug sensitivity, the Goldie-Coldman model has generated specific, testable predictions. The model predicts that a cancer arising from a single, drug-sensitive malignant cell has a 90% chance of being curable at 10^5 cells. If it has a 90% chance of being curable at that size it will almost certainly become incurable by the time it grows to 10^7 cells. Hence, tumors larger than 0.1–1.0 cubic centimeters in size should always be incurable with any single agent. This leads to the conclusion that the best strategy is to treat as small a tumor size as possible as early as possible, i.e., perioperatively or even preoperatively. Once treatment is started, as many effective drugs as possible should be applied as soon as possible to prevent cells that are already resistant to one drug from mutating to resistance to others.

These recommendations are intuitive, conforming to established empiric principles of combination chemotherapy.[61] They differ from classic principles only in that they concentrate on the emergence of resistance during treatment, as contrasted with the likelihood that resistance is already present at the start of treatment. Most uniquely, they imply that if several drugs cannot be used simultaneously at good therapeutic levels (because of overlapping toxicity or competitive interference) they should be used in a strict alternating sequence. This recommendation is based on several assumptions: that cells sensitive to a given therapy A (and resistant to therapy B) are as sensitive to therapy A as cells sensitive to therapy B (but resistant to therapy A) are sensitive to therapy B; that the rate of mutation toward biochemical resistance is constant in both sublines (with cells sensitive to A mutating toward resistance to A, and cells sensitive to B mutating to resistance to B); and that the growth pattern and growth rates of the two sublines are equivalent.[47] These assumptions fit under the general mathematical term "symmetry." Critical appraisal of the various assumptions and conclusions of the Goldie-Coldman model have raised several interesting points. It would be informative to examine these in some detail to show the relevance of growth curve analysis to clinical problems.

The first assumption that we must question concerns the notion that all chemotherapeutic failure is rooted in absolute drug resistance. Contrary evidence is that lymphomas and leukemias frequently respond to the same chemotherapy when they relapse after the chemotherapeutic achievement of complete remission. Patients achieving complete remission from the combination chemotherapy of Hodgkin's disease who relapse 18 or more months later have an excellent chance of attaining complete remission again when the same chemotherapy is reapplied.[80] Similarly, breast adenocarcinomas frequently respond after they relapse from postoperative adjuvant chemotherapy. The Cancer and Leukemia Group B (CALGB) treated patients with advanced breast cancer with cyclophosphamide, adriamycin and 5-fluorouracil (CAF) with or without tamoxifen.[148] Although none of these patients had had prior chemotherapy for their advanced disease, some had had prior adjuvant chemotherapy. However, the response rate, response duration and overall survival were unaffected by a patient's past history of adjuvant chemotherapy. Similarly, patients on trials at the National Cancer Institute in Milan who progressed after adjuvant cyclophosphamide, methotrexate and 5-fluorouracil (CMF) responded as well to CMF for advanced disease as those who had been previously randomized to be treated with radical mastectomy alone.[303] Breast cancers that regrow after exposure to adjuvant CMF are not universally resistant to CMF.[304] Hence, all chemotherapeutic failure can not be due to permanent drug resistance. It is possible that some cancers escape cure because of a temporary absolute drug resistance that reverses over time. It is also possible, however, that cancers can escape cure even though some of their cells are not absolutely resistant. This theme will be developed further below as we consider other growth models.

Another prediction from the Goldie-Coldman model that is interesting to examine is that tumors larger than 1.0 cubic centimeter (10^7 cells at a packing ratio of 1:100) cannot be cured with single drugs. Two rapidly growing cancers, gestational choriocarcinoma and Burkitt's lymphoma, have been cured with single drugs[132] even when therapy is initiated at tumor sizes much larger than 1.0 cubic centimeter. Childhood acute lymphoblastic leukemias, other pediatric cancers, adult lymphomas and germ cell tumors of greater than 10^{10} cells are frequently cured with couplets and triplets of drugs. Hence, the size of 10^7 cells does not always mean incurability.

For the purposes of planning chemotherapy schedules the Goldie-Coldman model speculates that mutations develop rapidly during the treatable portion of a cancer's growth history. This may seem tenable since in our previous discussion of cell proliferation we have established that genetic lability is a key attribute of neoplasia. Yet, clinical observations hint at a deeper level of complexity. For example, let us examine metastatic ability as a measure of the rate of mutations. A primary breast cancer left untreated to grow in the breast, as was standard practice in the nineteenth century, always became metastatic.[20] Yet at thirty years of follow-up after radical mastectomy (with no adjuvant chemotherapy) more than 30% of patients are alive and free of disease.[2,74] The mortality rate drops gradually from about 10% per year in the first year to about 2% per year by year twenty-five,[114] but a plateau is reached after thirty years, with a rate of mortality indistinguishable from the general population.[30,257] This means that all breast cancers (as in the nineteenth century) have the potential for developing metastases, and many, but not all, have already done so by the time of initial presentation. Let us consider the case of a breast cancer that is diagnosed in the breast before it has developed metastatic ability. If the cancer cells in the breast are not completely removed or destroyed, will the residual cells mutate rapidly to produce metastatic clones? A protocol of the National Surgical Adjuvant Breast and Bowel Project (NSABP) asked this question.[78] Some patients with primary disease were treated by lumpectomy without radiotherapy. The local relapse rate was significant, indicating that residual tumor was left unchecked. Yet such patients did not have a higher metastatic rate (measured by the survival rate) than patients treated adequately de novo by lumpectomy plus immediate radiotherapy. Hence, this study indicates that tumor can remain in a breast, grow in the breast, and yet not develop cells with metastatic ability at a high rate. If metastases will ever develop, the odds are that they will have already done so before clinical presentation.

In a similar vein the Goldie-Coldman model concludes that chemotherapy must be started as soon as possible after diagnosis to be effective. There is, however, contradictory evidence. For example, in an early trial of the treatment of acute leukemia it was found that the response to an antimetabolite was the same if that drug was used first or sequentially after the use of a different antimetabolite.[85] In a randomized trial the International (Ludwig) Breast Cancer Study Group found that it was equally effective to give node-positive breast cancer patients either seven months of chemotherapy starting within 36 hours of surgery or six months of chemotherapy starting about four weeks later.[185] Another trial randomized patients with stage B nonseminomatous testicular cancer after retroperitoneal lymph node dissection to either two cycles of cisplatin combination chemotherapy or observation.[321] At a median follow-up of four years, 6% of patients randomized to adjuvant chemotherapy relapsed compared to 49% of patients randomized to observation. Yet because the response of relapsing cases to subsequent chemotherapy was excellent, there was no significant survival difference between the two approaches. Hence, most testicular carcinomas retained their chemosensitivity in spite of a prolonged period of unperturbed growth. We may conclude, therefore, that for both breast and testicular cancer, cells that are residual after surgery can grow unperturbed and yet not develop drug-resistant mutants at a fast rate.

If, as predicted by the Goldie-Coldman model, adjuvant treatment must be instituted as early as possible after surgery to be effective, all drugs in an adjuvant regimen must be introduced immediately to have a biological impact. This was questioned in a trial by the CALGB.[160,233] Node-positive patients with primary breast cancer were treated with eight months of an adjuvant CMF regimen (plus vincristine and prednisone) followed by either more CMFVP or six months of vinblastine, adriamycin, thiotepa and halotestin (VATH). Patients receiving the cross-over therapy had a significantly improved disease-free survival, especially those with four or more involved axillary nodes. Hence, dominant resistance to VATH did not develop rapidly in the cells left after treatment with CMFVP. It is of note that a trial in Milan found no advantage to adriamycin following CMF for patients with one to three involved nodes,[202] which corroborates the CALGB's finding of the relative inactivity of this approach for patients with low degrees of nodal involvement. The implications of the CALGB's results in patients with higher degrees of nodal involvement, including the issues of simultaneous vs. sequential therapies, dose-scheduling and optimal duration, are discussed in more detail below.

The assertion most singularly identified with the Goldie-Coldman model is the recommendation for alternating chemotherapy sequences. Has this strategy demonstrated unequivocal advantages? Numerous attempts at improving the prognosis of patients with small-cell lung cancer by using alternating chemotherapy sequences have resulted in no or little benefit.[315] In the treatment of diffuse aggressive non-Hodgkin's lymphoma the National Cancer Institute found no advantage to a ProMACE-MOPP hybrid, which delivered eight drugs during each monthly cycle, over a treatment plan delivering a full course of ProMACE (prednisone, methotrexate, adriamycin, cyclophosphamide, etoposide), which was then followed by MOPP.[180] For advanced Hodgkin's disease MOPP (mechlorethamine, vincristine, procarbazine, prednisone) has been compared with MOPP alternating with adriamycin, bleomycin, vinblastine and decarbazine (ABVD), an effective salvage regimen for patients refractory to MOPP.[26,262] Among chemotherapy-naive patients, MOPP-ABVD was found to be superior to MOPP in complete remission rate, freedom from progression and survival.[27A,305] However, the CALGB found that the complete remission rate and failure-free survival from MOPP-ABVD, although better than from MOPP alone, was not different from ABVD alone.[38] The superiority of MOPP-ABVD and ABVD over MOPP may have been due to differences in dose received, since only about 40% of MOPP patients received full doses of the cytotoxic agents by cycle three, whereas these percentages were greater than 70% on ABVD and on MOPP-ABVD. At comparable levels of received dose there were no clear advantages to the alternation of MOPP-ABVD over just ABVD alone. Similarly, the National Cancer Institute found no advantage to MOPP alternating with lomustine, adriamycin, bleomycin, and streptozocin over MOPP alone.[181] An American intergroup trial has found that a hybrid of MOPP-ABVD was superior in complete remission duration, failure-free survival and

overall survival to MOPP followed by ABVD.[99] As with MOPP-ABVD in the CALGB trial, it is possible that this result may be explained by the observation that patients treated with the hybrid regimen received higher doses because of the necessity to modify for toxicity the doses of MOPP in the regimen which delivered MOPP followed by ABVD. It is also possible that earlier introduction of adriamycin in the hybrid might have been advantageous because such an approach could diminish the adverse impact of the emergence of multidrug resistance. These points are discussed below in the context of the Norton-Simon model.

As with the lymphomas, in the treatment of breast cancer alternating cycles that have not resulted in a dosage difference have not proven advantageous. For example, the VATH regimen is active against tumors relapsing from or failing to respond to CMF, and thereby meets the noncross-resistance requirements of the Goldie-Coldman model.[116] In patients with advanced disease the CALGB found no advantage to CMFVP alternating with VATH over CAF or VATH alone.[3] A direct comparison of alternating vs. sequential chemotherapy in the adjuvant chemotherapy of breast cancer was conducted in Milan. This group had previously generated historically-controlled data which suggested a benefit from a sequential approach,[29] the rationale for which is discussed below.[216A] In the more recent study female patients with stage II breast cancer involving four or more axillary lymph nodes were randomized between two arms.[37] Arm I prescribed four three-week courses of adriamycin (A) followed by eight three-week courses of iv CMF (C), symbolized as AAAACCCCCCCC. Arm II stipulated the use of two courses of iv CMF alternated with one course of adriamycin four times for a total of twelve courses, symbolized as CCACCAC-CACCA. The total amount of adriamycin and CMF in both arms were equal, yet the patients who received arm I had a higher disease-free survival and a higher overall survival than those on arm II. With total dose controlled, alternating courses of chemotherapy were found to be inferior to a crossover therapy plan. This observation has major practical and theoretical implications.

The detailed examination of the Goldie-Coldman model which we have just completed illustrates the relevance of growth curve analysis to treatment design. The Goldie-Coldman model is mathematically sensible, and may well be applicable to some aspects of cancer biology. The model is also of major historical importance in that it has rekindled interest in the quantitative development of drug resistance. Several of its major predictions have not been sustained by clinical data, however. One common reason for a discrepancy between tenable theory and empirical results is the invalidity of underlying assumptions. An assumption of particular consequence concerns the concept of absolute drug resistance.

Implications of Relative Drug Resistance

It is now well established that much drug resistance is relative rather than absolute.[89] A cell that is absolutely resistant cannot be killed with any pharmacologic dose level of the agent. Relative drug resistance, on the other hand, depends upon the dose level employed. In terms of the Skipper-Schabel-Wilcox model one tumor may experience a log-kill of two (99% reduction in cell number) when it is exposed to a certain dose and duration of treatment. Another, more resistant, tumor may experience a log-kill of one (90% shrinkage) when it is treated with exactly the same therapy. However, if the dose-intensity of chemotherapy is increased against the relatively resistant tumor, the log-kill can increase as well.[33,109]

Clinically, even two-fold increases in dose level can have profound effects on the curative impact of chemotherapy,[87] although this is not always seen with all drugs in all diseases.[292] However, in retrospective analyses of the adjuvant chemotherapy of operable breast cancer[25,128] and the chemotherapy of advanced lymphoma[64] high dose seems to be a key beneficial variable. The validity of conclusions based on retrospective data has been questioned.[121,246] Hence, the results of ongoing prospective, randomized clinical studies are awaited anxiously.[35] Nevertheless, in randomized trials in childhood acute lymphoblastic leukemia,[236] adult germ cell tumors[260] and advanced breast cancer[291] the higher dose regimen has proven superior.

From a kinetic viewpoint the importance of dose is defensible. In many animal experiments the log-kill will be greater for the regimen with a higher dose-intensity.[33] The concept of dose intensity requires definition. It is not just the total amount of drug received, nor is it just the amount of drug received per unit of time, but rather a mathematical combination of both. If regimen I gives X amount of drug over Y days, and if regimen II gives 2X amount of drug over Y days, then regimen II is clearly more dose-intensive. Regimen III, giving X amount of drug over Y/2 days, is also more intensive than regimen I. Although the dose-rate of drug delivery of regimen III (2X/Y drug per day) is equivalent to regimen II, regimen II delivers more total drug and may thereby be superior to regimen III in clinical efficacy. Hence, dose-intensity alone may not account for clinical superiority. Yet sometimes, once a certain minimal total dose is achieved, further increases in total dose are unimportant. For example, a number of trials have shown that durations of adjuvant chemotherapy longer than four to six months do not improve clinical results in operable breast cancer.[27,120,249] Therefore, once the minimal total dose is determined empirically and adhered to, dose-intensity should be an important determinant of cell-kill.

A corollary of this argument is that clinical treatment failure may be the consequence of insufficient dose-intensity. A tumor may relapse because some of its cells, relatively but not absolutely insensitive to the agents applied, are not exposed to enough drug to be eradicated. This is analogous to a bacterial infection relapsing because an insufficient dose-intensity of an antibiotic is applied, even though the microorganisms are sensitive in vitro. In both infection and neoplasia, however, prolonged or repeated episodes of low-dose therapy can give rise to absolute resistance by the selection of biochemically resistant cells.

If insufficient dose-intensity is a major cause of failure to cure, then it is possible that increased dose-intensity itself can improve clinical results.[63,87] This statement is phrased as a possibility rather than a certainty because it is highly dependent on the shape ("steepness") of the dose-response curve for each agent for each disease. It is also dependent on the shape of the curve of tumor volume regression, which is considered in the next section.

The Gompertzian Model

The log-kill model was formulated from, and is expressed in terms of, exponential growth. Nodular pulmonary metastases and, much less commonly, measurable lesions in other sites do seem to follow exponential growth during periods of observation that are short in relationship to the total life histories of the tumors.[48,285,301] Doubling times, ranging from one week to one year, with a median of 1–3 months, correlate with histologic type, growth fraction and cell loss fraction. Yet many, if not all, human cancer do *not* grow exponentially with a constant doubling time.[58,281,289] A nonexponential growth pattern of major importance was first described by Gompertz in 1825.[167] In exponential growth the fixed doubling time means that the growth rate relative to tumor size always remains constant. In Gompertzian growth, however, the doubling time increases steadily as the tumor grows larger. Figure XV-1-2 illustrates a typical breast cancer (the specifics of this tumor's Gompertzian growth are detailed below). Between 10^2 cells and clinical appreciation at 10^{10} cells, the shape of the growth curve on the semilogarithmic plot deflects downward. An exponential curve would appear to follow a straight line. From the point of view of cell proliferation the progressive slowing of Gompertzian growth may be more the result of decreased cell production than increased cell loss in larger tumors.[169,316] A consequence is that if a Gompertzian tumor is erroneously assumed to be exponential, the doubling time during the preclinical phase of growth will be assumed to be too slow.[216] The assumption of exponentiality has led to some unrealistic estimates of the duration of time from carcinogenesis to the appearance of clinical disease.

Some of the important characteristics of Gompertzian growth will be illustrated below using a new model of human breast cancer.[218] In the nineteenth century breast cancer was often followed from diagnosis to death without surgery or any other effective treatment.[20] Speer, Retsky, and colleagues used survival histories for such patients, plus the growth histories of mammographic shadows[122] and also data for disease-free survival following mastectomy,[76] to fit a model in which tumors grow in randomly increasing steps of Gompertzian plateaus.[280] This work is interesting because it demonstrates that growth curves which deviate far from exponentiality can fit clinical data. However, the validity of the model has been challenged on several counts. Firstly, it is questionable if the temporary plateaus that are predicted by the model are ever actually observed.[219] Secondly, the Speer-Retsky model predicts that to maximize the efficacy of postsurgical adjuvant chemotherapy it should be applied intermittently over a prolonged duration so as to coincide with the presumed growth spurts. This approach, however, has proven ineffective in a clinical trial.[79] Thirdly, the same clinical data can be fit more parsimoniously, and with greater accuracy, by a family of simple Gompertzian curves.[218] A family of exponential curves could also be fit to these data, but the model that would result could not account for both disease-free survival and overall survival because the time from relapse to death would be too short. The curve used in Figure XV-1-2 is the median curve from the family of simple Gompertzian curves mentioned above.[218] Note that it takes just three and one-half months for the tumor to increase by two logs from 10^2 to 10^4. Yet it takes five and one-half months for 10^9 cells to grow just one log to 10^{10}. This is a relevant example of increasing doubling time with increasing tumor volume.

The Norton-Simon Model

The Skipper-Schabel-Wilcox model is so meaningful because it conceptualizes both tumor growth (exponential) and tumor regression (log-kill) in response to chemotherapy. We have already discussed the profound implications of the positive association between the rate of tumor regression and the dose-intensity of chemotherapy. Experimental and clinical data also indicate that the rate of tumor regression is positively related to the growth rate of the unperturbed tumor just prior to treatment.[214,215] This important observation is corroborated by data showing that the logarithm of the surviving fraction of an experimental neoplasm is negatively correlated with the logarithm of the tumor size at the time of treatment.[124]

This concept extends the Skipper-Schabel-Wilcox model. In exponential growth the growth rate is always *proportional* to tumor size. If a tumor at size X is growing at rate Y, the same tumor at size 2X would grow at rate 2Y. On a logarithmic scale these growth rates would appear to be the same since the rate of growth per tumor size (Y/X) is the same in both cases. A rate of regression proportional to growth rate is therefore also proportional to tumor size, which results in a constant proportional (or "log") kill. That is, if the tumor at size X shrinks at rate Z to achieve a size X/2 in one week (a change in size by the proportion of one-half), the tumor at size 2X treated with the same chemotherapy would shrink at rate 2Z to achieve size X in one week (also a change by the proportion of one-half). The absolute volume shrinkage would be X/2 in the first case and X in the second case, but the proportional change would be one-half in both cases (X to X/2; 2X to X). The distinction between the Skipper-Schabel-Wilcox model and the Norton-Simon model is that in Gompertzian growth, unlike exponential growth, the growth rate of the unperturbed tumor is always changing. That is, if tumor at size X grows at rate Y, the same tumor at size 2X would not grow at rate 2Y.

In Figure XV-1-2 a realistic numerical example illustrates the implications of Gompertzian regression. In Figure XV-1-2A the tumor is observed to grow to clinical diagnosis at 10^{10} cells (about 10 cc of packed tumor cells or about 100 cc at a packing ratio of 1:10). Let us assume for the purposes of this illustration that 90% of the tumor is in the breast and axillary lymph nodes, and about 10% of the cells are scattered in various micrometastatic sites. The mass in the breast itself would be about five centimeters in diameter. If this mass and the axillary contents are removed completely (or destroyed completely with radiotherapy) the total body's burden of tumor is reduced to the 10^9 metastatic cells. Since the 10^9 cancer cells are spread throughout the body, they are invisible to our diagnostic tests. No adjuvant therapy is given. The tumor grows for thirteen and a half months until it reaches about 10^{11} cells in total number, which is large enough for detection as metastases. At this time chemotherapy is employed,

reducing the total cell number to about 10^9 (a two-log kill). A period of remission is experienced but the tumor eventually relapses, leading to death at 10^{12} cells.

Figure XV-1-2B graphs the same tumor, but here the same chemotherapy is applied in the adjuvant setting at a total tumor size of 10^9 cells. The relative rate of growth (the slope of the curve on this semilogarithmic plot) is faster for the tumor at 10^9 cells than it would be for the same tumor at 10^{11} cells. This is clear by inspection of Figure XV-1-2A. According to the Norton-Simon model, the relative rate of regression of the 10^9-cell tumor will be faster as well even though the dose and schedule of chemotherapy are identical. Figure XV-1-2B shows that the chemotherapy which had caused a two-log kill of 10^{11} cells causes instead a five-log kill of 10^9 cells. The 10^4 cells which result regrow to relapse as stage IV disease at 10^{11} cells and to kill the patient at 10^{12} cells. Comparison of Figures XV-1-2A and XV-1-2B demonstrates a remarkable result. The time from surgery to stage IV is clearly longer when the adjuvant chemotherapy is applied. However, the time from surgery to death is identical! The greater fractional kill in the adjuvant setting is counterbalanced by a faster fractional regrowth. This may explain why the adjuvant chemotherapy of breast cancer has less impact on overall survival (a function of eventual tumor size) than on disease-free survival. It may also explain why the survival duration of patients with stage IV breast cancer has remained fairly stable in recent decades in spite of more aggressive approaches to management.[232,238,297]

What if another chemotherapy plan, more aggressive but still subcurative, is used in the adjuvant setting against the 10^9 cells? This is illustrated in Figure XV-1-2C. If 10^2 cells are left instead of 10^4 it will take only three and one-half months longer for the tumor to reach 10^{12}, since the growth from 10^2 cells to 10^4 cells is very rapid. Hence, adjuvant therapies can differ greatly in log-kill with only a slight impact on eventual clinical results measured years later. This slight impact could easily be lost in the "noise" caused by random fluctuations, especially in clinical data sets of small size. The pessimistic side of this observation is that more aggressive chemotherapy may produce little real clinical benefit. The optimistic side is that, if this model holds, current adjuvant chemotherapies for breast cancer are actually bringing us much closer to total cellular eradication than we might otherwise be led to suspect.

Survival can be improved to a significant degree only when tumor cell populations are actually eradicated or their regrowth is otherwise meaningfully impeded. In our previous discussion of cellular proliferation we concluded that heterogeneity in drug sensitivity is a characteristic of neoplasia. How can tumor cell eradication be accomplished in a heterogeneous cancer? Gompertzian regression means that slower growing collections of tumor cells will tend to regress more slowly in response to a given therapy than will the faster growing tumor cells treated at the same time.[217] In a heterogeneous cancer, therefore, the slower-growing clones are also the most kinetically resistant. These slower-growing cells should be in the minority by the time of diagnosis because they should by then have been overgrown by the faster-growing cells. The existance of a population of slow-growing cells may also be the consequence of the hypothetical ability of chemotherapy to differentiate cells that are not killed.[253] The best way to treat a heterogeneous population is to treat the dominant, faster-growing populations as efficiently as possible, and then to treat the numerically inferior, slower-growing populations as efficiently as possible.[216A] As in the Skipper-Schabel-Wilcox model, the most efficient therapy is the most dose-intense therapy, giving as much drug as possible over as short a period as possible. This is accomplished much better by crossover therapy than by strict alternation. For example, in the adjuvant breast cancer trial from Milan described above, the alternating plan, CCACCACCACCA, gave eight cycles of CMF over thirty weeks, and four cycles of adriamycin over thirty-three weeks. The crossover plan, AAAACCCCCCCC, gave eight cycles of CMF over thirty-three weeks, and four cycles of adriamycin over nine weeks. The dose-intensity of the CMF was almost the same, but for adriamycin it was significantly improved by the crossover. This by itself could account for the superiority of the crossover treatment. A similar result has been seen in the adjuvant chemotherapy of resected osteosarcoma: Adriamycin alone was superior to adriamycin alternating with high-dose methotrexate, presumably because the dose-intensity of the superior agent (adriamycin) was impaired by the alternation.[50]

In the breast cancer trial from Milan the use of adriamycin initially might have caused greater cell kill by avoiding the expression of the multidrug-resistance gene, which tends to progress over time, independent of treatment.[39,106] Conversely, the delayed use of adriamycin might have compromised the efficacy of two other regimens described previously: ABVD following prolonged MOPP for advanced Hodgkin's disease[99] and adriamycin following six months of CMF for primary breast cancer with low degrees of nodal involvement.[202] A pilot study in breast cancer used adriamycin following just 16 weeks of CMFVP in patients with node-positive primary disease.[16] The study has established the feasibility of this approach, but the determination of comparative efficacy awaits a randomized trial.

Although the invention and interpretation of clinical trials intended to test cytokinetic principles is fraught with subtleties and complexities, crossover therapy has been successful in the laboratory. The only way to cure 10^8 L1210 cells is by induction with cytosine arabinoside plus 6-thioguanine for two or three courses, followed by one course of high doses of cyclophosphamide and BCNU given simultaneously.[278] In the treatment of BDF$_1$ mice bearing the M5076 tumor the addition of one dose of L-phenylalanine mustard (L-PAM) (a drug which by itself is only weakly active) after four doses of methyl-CCNU doubles the complete remission rate and the median survival.[108] The presumed mechanism for this latter effect is that the few cells left after methyl-CCNU induction are L-PAM sensitive, whereas in the untreated situation most cells are methyl-CCNU sensitive, L-PAM resistant. In general, alkylating agents seem particularly helpful as the crossover therapy.

Goldie and Coldman's prediction of the superiority of alternating chemotherapy assumed stringent conditions of symmetrical tumor cell numbers, growth rates and mutation rates. Recently, Day performed computer simulations of mutation to drug resistance under asymmetrical conditions.[57] He came to a conclusion similar to the Norton-Simon model regarding

the expected superiority of a crossover plan.[222] By his "worst drug rule," in a coordinated two-regimen plan the therapy with a lower cell-kill per treatment (the worst drug) should be used either first or, if is used second, for a longer duration. However, the Norton-Simon model qualifies this to specify that the induction therapy must be sufficiently cytoreductive for the residual tumor cell burden to be low. This is another possible reason for the inferiority of ABVD following dose-reduced (and, hence, less cytotoxic) MOPP compared to a hybrid MOPP/ABV which could be delivered at fuller dosages.[99] The theoretical argument, therefore, would be in favor of an efficient induction followed by one or more aggressive chemotherapeutic crossovers. Indeed, in the treatment of acute lymphocytic leukemia in children, a classic trial demonstrated that induction by vincristine plus prednisone facilitates the anticancer activity of crossover methotrexate.[266] In the future, plans of this type could be facilitated by exploiting the ability of hematopoietic growth factors (like G-CSF and GM-CSF)[94] and other means of hematopoietic reconstitution[90,234] to permit dose intensification. For diffuse large cell lymphoma, induction adriamycin, vincristine, prednisone has been followed by sequential high-dose cyclophosphamide, then methotrexate (plus vincristine), then etoposide, then l-PAM (plus total body irradiation), all with GM-CSF support. In a randomized comparison against a standard aggressive combination the induction-intensification plan proved superior in complete remission rate, failure from relapse, failure from progression and event-free survival.[97] Such treatment plans merit scrutiny regarding both their practical utility and their theoretical implications.

The Mitotoxicity Hypothesis

Both the Skipper-Schabel-Wilcox and Norton-Simon models are based on the observation that the rate of tumor regression is positively related to the rate of unperturbed growth. The most obvious explanation for this observation is the mitotoxicity hypothesis: Tumors regress most rapidly when they are growing most rapidly because more of their cells are then synthesizing DNA and other macromolecules in preparation for mitosis; Such metabolically active cells are thereby at particular risk for cytotoxicity by drugs that interfere with such synthetic processes.[306] The intuitive notion is that poisoning S-phase renders cells incapable of progressing successfully through M-phase. This is a dominant idea in cytokinetic thinking, and it undoubtedly has considerable merit. Growth-stimulating substances (i.e., estradiol, epidermal growth factor) increase both cell proliferation and cell kill from adriamycin in MCF-7 cells in vitro.[128A] Pharmacologic concentrations of estradiol enhance the cytotoxicity of the chemotherapeutic agent melphalan in hormone-responsive cell lines.[228A] These observations have been applied clinically, and hormone recruitment schemes have indeed resulted in high local response rates in locally-advanced breast cancer.[49B,289A] However, such treatments have proven only slightly better or no better than chemotherapy alone in metastatic breast cancer, except in data-driven subsets.[49A,178A] Even when benefits have been seen, methodological issues have been raised regarding the analyzability of results.[177A]

We must be cautious, moreover, in interpreting laboratory

70. Dressler, L. G.: DNA flow cytometry measurements have significant prognostic impact in the node negative breast cancer patient: An intergroup study (INT 0076). Treatment of Early Stage Breast Cancer: Program and Abstracts. NIH Consensus Development Conference, National Cancer Institute and the Office of Medical Applications of Research of the National Institutes of Health, June 18–21, 1990, pp. 99–101.
71. Dyson, J. E., Joslin, C. A., Rothwell, R. I., Quirke, P., Khoury, G. G., and Bird, C. C.: Flow cytofluorometric evidence for the differential radioresponsiveness of aneuploid and diploid cervix tumours. Radiother. Oncol., 8:263, 1987.
72. Early Breast Cancer Trialists' Collaborative Group. Treatment of Early Breast Cancer: Worldwide Evidence in 1985–1990. A Systematic Overview of All Available Randomized Trials in Early Breast Cancer of Adjuvant Endocrine and Cytotoxic Therapy. Oxford University Press, New York, 1990.
73. Erba, E., Ubezio, P., Pepe, S., Vaghi, M., Marsoni, S., Torri, W., Mangioni, C., Landoni, F., and D'Incalci, M.: Flow cytometric analysis of DNA content in human ovarian cancers. Br. J. Cancer, 60:45, 1989.
74. Ferguson, D. J., Meier, P., Karrison, T., Dawson, P. J., Straus, F. H., and Lowenstein, F. E.: Staging of Breast Cancer and Survival Rates: An Assessment Based on 50 Years Experience with Radical Mastectomy. J. Am. Med. Assoc., 248:1337, 1982.
75. Fidler, I. J.: Tumor heterogeneity and the biology of cancer invasion and metastases. Cancer Res., 38:2651, 1978.
76. Fisher, B., Slack, N., Katrych, D., and Wolmark, N.: Ten-year follow-up results in patients with carcinoma of the breast in a cooperative clinical trial evaluating surgical adjuvant chemotherapy. Surg. Gynecol. Obstet., 140:528, 1975.
77. Fisher, E. R., Siderits, R. H., Sass, R., and Fisher, B.: Value of assessment of ploidy in rectal cancers. Arch. Pathol. Lab. Med., 113:525, 1989.
78. Fisher, B., Redmond, C., Poisson, R., Margolese, R., Wolmark, N., Wickerham, L., Fisher, E., Deutsch, M., Caplan, R., Pilch, Y.: Eight-year results of a randomized clinical trial comparing total mastectomy and lumpectomy with or without irradiation in the treatment of breast cancer. N. Engl. J. Med., 320:822, 1989.
79. Fisher, B., Brown, A. M., Dimitrov, N. V., Poisson, R., Redmond, C., Margolese, R. G., Bowman, D., Wolmark, N., Wickerham, D. L., Kardinal, G. C., Shibata, H., Paterson, A. H. G., Sutherland, C. M., Robert, N. J., Ager, P. J., Levy, L., Walter, J., Wozniak, T., Fisher, E. R., and Deutsch, M.: Two months of doxorubicin-cyclophosphamide with and without interval reinduction therapy compared with 6 months of cyclophosphamide, methotrexate, and fluorouracil in positive-node breast cancer patients with tamoxifen-nonresponsive tumors: Results from the National Surgical Adjuvant Breast and Bowel Project B-15. J. Clin. Oncol., 8:1483, 1990.
80. Fisher, R. I., DeVita, V. T., Hubbard, S. M., Simon, R., and Young, R. C.: Prolonged disease-free survival in Hodgkin's disease with MOPP reinduction after first relapse. Ann. Intern. Med., 90:761, 1979.
81. Folkman, J., and Moscona, A.: Role of cell shape in growth control. Nature, 273:345, 1978.
82. Fordham, M. V. P., Burdge, A. H., Matthews, J., Williams, G., and Cooke, T.: Prostatic carcinoma cell DNA content measured by flow cytometry and its relation to clinical outcome. Br. J. Surg., 73:400, 1986.
83. Foulds, L.: The histologic analysis of mammary tumors of mice. II. The histology of responsiveness and progression. The origins of tumors. J. Natl. Cancer Inst., 17:713, 1956.
84. Franzini, A., Broggi, G., Giorgi, C., Caiola, L., and Allegranza, A.: Predictive accuracy of cell kinetics data in glial tumors investigated by serial stereotactic biopsy. J. Neurosurg. Sci., 33:43, 1989.
85. Frei, E., III, Freireich, E. J., Gehan, E., Pinkel, D., Holland, J. F., Selawry, O., Haurani, F., Spurr, C. L., Hayes, D. M., James, G. W., Rothberg, H., Sodee, D. B., Rundles, R. W., Schroeder, L. R., Hoogstraten, B., Wolman, I. J., and Traggis, D. G.: Studies of sequential and combination antimetabolite therapy in acute leukemia: 6-mercaptopurine and methotrexate. Blood, 18:431, 1961.
86. Frie, E., III, Whang, J., Scoggins, R. B., van Scott, E. J., Rall, D. P., and Ben, M.: The stathmokinetic effect of vincristine. Cancer Res., 24:1918, 1964.
87. Frei, E., III, and Canellos, G. P.: Dose: A critical factor in cancer chemotherapy. Am. J. Med., 69:585, 1980.
88. Frei, E., III.: Models and the clinical dilemma. *In* Design of Models for Testing Therapeutic Agents. Edited by I. J. Fidler, and R. J. White. New York, Van Nostrand Reinhold, 1982, pp. 248–259.
89. Frei, E., Teicher, B. A., Holden, S. A., Cathcart, K. N., and Wang, Y. Y.: Preclinical studies and clinical correlation of the effect of alkylating dose. Cancer Res., 48:6417, 1988.
90. Frei, E., III, Antman, K., Teicher, B., Eder, P., and Schnipper, L.: Bone marrow autotransplantation for solid tumors—prospects. J. Clin. Oncol., 7:515, 1989.
91. Friedlander, M. L., Hedley, D. W., Taylor, I. W., Russell, P., Coates, A. S., and Tattersall, M. H. N.: Influence of cellular DNA content on survival in advanced ovarian cancer. Cancer Res., 44:397, 1984.
92. Friedlander, M. L., Hedley, D. W., Swanson, C., and Russell, P.: Prediction of long-term survival by flow cytometric analysis of cellular DNA content in patients with advanced ovarian cancer. J. Clin. Oncol., 6:282, 1988.
93. Fujimoto, J., Okamoto, E., Yamanaka, N., Fujiwara, S., Kato, T., Mitsunobu, M., and Toyosaka, A.: Nuclear DNA analysis of hepatocellular carcinoma. Journal of the Japanese Surgical Society, 90:1568, 1989.
94. Gabrilove, J. L.: Colony-stimulating factors: Clinical status. *In* Important Advances in Oncology 1991. Edited by V. T. DeVita, Jr., S. Hellman, and S. A. Rosenberg. Lippincott, New York, 1991, pp. 215–237.
95. Gelfant, S.: Cycling-noncycling cell transitions in tissue aging, immunological surveillance, transformation and tumor growth. Int. Rev. Cytol., 70:1, 1981.
96. Gerdes, J., Lemke, H., Brisch, H., Wacker, H. H., Schwab, U., and Stein, H.: Cell cycle analysis of a cell proliferation-associated human nuclear antigen defined by the monoclonal antibody Ki-67. J. Immunol., 133:1710, 1984.
97. Gianni, A. M., Bregni, M., Siena, S., Brambilla, C., Lombardi, F., Gandola, L., Tarella, C., Stern, A., Valagussa, P., and Bonadonna, G.: Prospective randomized comparison of MACOP-B vs. rhGM-CSF-supported high-dose sequential myeloablative chemoradiotherapy in diffuse large cell lymphoma. Proc. Am. Soc. Clin. Oncol., 10:951, 1991.
98. Givel, J. C., de Quay, N., Albe, X., and Vassilakos, P.: Prognostic value of DNA ploidy of colorectal tumor cells. Helvetica Chirurgica Acta, 55:679, 1989.
99. Glick, J., Tsiatis, A., Schilsky, R., Beck, T., Oken, M., Peterson, B., and Fisher, R.: A randomized phase III trial of MOPP/ABV hybrid vs. sequential MOPP-ABVD in advanced Hodgkin's disease: Preliminary results of the Intergroup Trial. Proc. Am. Soc. Clin. Oncol., 10:941, 1991.
100. Glicksman, A. S., Pajak, T. F., Gottlieb, A. J., Nissen, N., Stutzman, L., and Cooper, M. R.: Second malignant neoplasms in patients successfully treated for Hodgkin's disease: A Cancer and Leukemia Group B study. Cancer Treat. Rep., 66:1035, 1982.
101. Goh, H. S., Jass, J. R., Atkin, W. S., Cuzick, J., Northover, J. M.: Value of flow cytometric determination of ploidy as a guide to prognosis in operable rectal cancer: A multivariate analysis. Int. J. Color. Dis., 2:17, 1987.
102. Goldie, J. H., and Coldman, A. J.: A mathematic model for relating the drug sensitivity of tumors to their spontaneous mutation rate. Cancer Treat. Rep., 63:1727, 1979.
103. Goldie, J. H., and Coldman, A. J.: Application of theoretical models to chemotherapy protocol design. Cancer Treat. Rep., 70:127, 1986.
104. Goldie, J. H.: Scientific basis for adjuvant and primary (neoadjuvant) chemotherapy. Sem. Oncol., 14:1, 1987.
105. Goldin, A., Venditti, J. M., Humphreys, S. R., and Mantel, N.: Influence of the concentration of leukemic innoculum on the effectiveness of treatment. Science, 123:840, 1956.
106. Goldstein, L. J., Galski, H., Fojo, A., Willingham, M., Lai, S-L., Gazdar, A., Pirker, R., Green, A., Crist, W., Brodeur, G. M., Lieber, M., Cossman, J., Gottesman, M. M., and Pastan, I.: Expression of multidrug resistance gene in human tumors. J. Natl. Cancer Inst., 81:116, 1989.
107. Greenberg, P. L., and Mara, B.: The preleukemic syndrome: correlation of in vitro parameters of granulocytoloiesis with clinical features. Am. J. Med., 66:951, 1979.
108. Griswold, D. P., Schabel, F. M., Jr., Corbett, T. H., and Dykes, D. J.: Concepts for controlling drug-resistant tumor cells. *In* Design of Models for Testing Cancer Therapeutic Agents. Edited by I. J. Fidler, and R. J. White. New York, Van Nostrand Reinhold, 1982, pp. 215–224.
109. Griswold, D. P., Jr., Trader, M. W., Frei, E., III, Peters, W. P., Wolpert, M. K., and Laster, W. R., Jr.: Response of drug-sensitive and -resistant L1210 leukemias to high-dose chemotherapy. Cancer Res., 47:2323, 1987.
110. Groham, J. H., Helvig, E. B. *In* Dermal Pathology. Edited by J. H. Graham, W. C. Johnson, and E. B. Helvig. New York, Harper and Row, 1972, pp. 561–581.
111. Gustafson, H., Tribukait, B., and Esposti, P. L.: DNA profile and tumour progression in patients with superfical bladder tumours. Urol. Res., 10:13, 1982.
112. Halvorsen, T. B., and Johannesen, E.: DNA ploidy, tumour site, and prognosis in colorectal cancer. A flow cytometric study of paraffin-embedded tissue. Scand. J. Gastroenterol., 25:141, 1990.
113. Hamburger, A., and Salmon, S. E.: Primary bioassay of human myeloma stem cells. J. Clin. Invest., 60:846, 1977.
114. Harris, J. R., and Hellman, S.: Observations on survival curve analysis with particular reference to breast cancer. Cancer, 57:925, 1986.
115. Hart, J. S., George, S. L., Frei, E., III, Bodey, G. P., Nickerson, R. C., and Freireich, E. J.: Prognostic significance of pretreatment proliferative activity in adult acute leukemia. Cancer, 39:1603, 1977.
116. Hart, R., Perloff, M., and Holland, J.: One-day VATH (vinblastine, Adriamycin thiotepa, and halotestin) therapy for advanced breast cancer refractory to chemotherapy. Cancer, 48:1522, 1981.
117. Hartwell, L. H., and Weinert, T. A.: Checkpoints: Controls that ensure the order of cell cycle events. Science, 246:629, 1989.
118. Haugen, O. A., and Mjlnerd, O.: DNA-ploidy as prognostic factor in prostatic carcinoma. Int. J. Cancer, 45:224, 1990.
119. Hedley, D. W., Freidlander, M. L., Taylor, I. W., Rigg, C. A., and Musgrove, E. A.: Method for analysis of cellular DNA content of paraffin-embedded pathological material using flow cytometry. J. Histochem. Cytochem., 31:1333, 1983.
120. Henderson, I. C., Gelman, R. S., Harris, J. R., and Canellos, G. P.: Duration of therapy in adjuvant chemotherapy trials. Natl. Cancer Inst. Monograph, 1:95, 1986.
121. Henderson, I. C., Hayes, D. F., and Gelman, R.: Dose-response in the treatment of breast cancer: A critical review. J. Clin. Oncol., 6:1501, 1988.
122. Heuser, L., Spratt, J., and Polk, H.: Growth rates of primary breast cancer. Cancer, 43:1888, 1979.
123. Hiddeman, W. H., Schumann, J., Andreeff, M., Barlogie, B., Herman, C. J., Leif, R. C., Mayall, B. H., Murphy, R. F., and Sandberg, A. A.: Convention on nomenclature for DNA cytometry. Cytometry, 5:445, 1984.
124. Hill, R. P., and Stanley, J. A.: Pulmonary metastases of the Lewis lung tumor—cell kinetics and response to cyclophosphamide at different sizes. Cancer Treat. Rep., 61:29, 1977.
125. Hoffman, J., and Post, J.: *In vivo* studies of DNA synthesis in human normal and tumor cells. Cancer Res., 27:898, 1967.
126. Holland, J. F.: Clinical studies of unmaintained remissions in acute lymphocytic leukemia. *In* The Proliferation and Spread of Neoplastic Cells, Univ. of Texas M. D. Anderson Hospital and Tumor Institute at Houston, 21st Annual Symposium on Fundamental Cancer Research 1967. Baltimore, MD, Williams and Wilkins, 1968, pp. 453–462.
127. Howard, A., and Pelc, S. R.: Nuclear incorporation of ^{32}p as demonstrated by autoradiographs. Exp. Cell Res., 2:178, 1951.
128. Hryniuk, W. M.: The importance of dose intensity in the outcome of chemotherapy. *In* Important Advances in Oncology 1988. Edited by V. T. DeVita, Jr., S. Hellman, and S. A. Rosenberg. Philadelphia, J. B. Lippincott, 1988, pp. 121–141.
128A. Hug, V., Johnston, D., Finders, M., and Hortobagyi, G.: Use of growth-stimulating hormones to improve the *in vitro* therapeutic index of doxorubicin for human breast cancer. Cancer Res., 46:147, 1986.
129. Iannaccone, P. M., Weinberg, W. C., and Deamant, F. D.: On the clonal origin of tumors: A review of experimental models. Int. J. Cancer, 39:778, 1987.
130. Isobe, H., Miyamoto, H., Shimizu, T., Haneda, H., Hashimoto, M., Inoue, K., Mizuno, S., and Kwakami, Y.: Prognostic and therapeutic significance of the flow cytometric nuclear DNA content in non-small cell lung cancer. Cancer, 65:1391, 1990.
131. Isonishi, S., Andrews, P. A., and Howell, S. B.: Increased sensitivity to cis-diamminedichloroplatinum (II) in human ovarian carcinoma cells in response to treatment with 12-0-tetradecanoylphorbol-13-acetate. J. Biol. Chem., 265:3623, 1990.
132. Iversen, O. H., Iversen, U., Ziegler, J. L., and Bluming, A. Z.: Cell kinetics in Burkitt's lymphoma. Eur. J. Cancer, 10:155, 1974.
133. Jakobsen, A.: Ploidy level and short-time prognosis of early cervix cancer. Radiother. Oncol., 1:271, 1984.
134. Jakobsen, A.: Prognostic impact of ploidy level in carcinoma of the cervix. Am. J. Clin. Oncol., 7:475, 1984.
135. Jakobsen, A., Bichel, P., Kristensen, G. B., and Nyland, M.: Prognostic influence of ploidy level and histopathologic differentiation in cervical carcinoma stage Ib. Eur. J. Cancer Clin. Oncol., 24:969, 1988.
136. Jacobsen, A. B., Lunde, S., Ous, S., Melvik, J. E., Pettersen, E. O., Kaalhus, O., and Fossa, S. D.: T2/T3 bladder carcinomas treated with definitive radiotherapy with emphasis on flow cytometric DNA ploidy values. Int. J. Radiat. Oncol. Biol. Phys., 17:923, 1989.
137. Jalkanen, S., Joensuu, H., and Klemi, P.: Prognostic value of lymphocyte homing receptor and S phase fraction in non-Hodgkin's lymphoma. Blood, 75:1549, 1990.
138. Jass, J. R., Mukawa, K., Goh, H. S., Love, S. B., and Cepellaro, D.: Clinical importance of DNA content in rectal cancer measured by flow cytometry. J. Clin. Pathol., 42:254, 1989.

139. Joensuu, H., and Kallioniemi, O. P.: Different opinions on classification of DNA histograms produced from paraffin-embedded tissue. Cytometry, 10:711, 1989.
140. Johnson, L. V., Walsh, M. L., and Chen, L. B.: Localization of mitochondria in living cells with rhodamine 123. Proc. Natl. Acad. Sci. USA, 77:990, 1980.
141. Jones, D. J., Moore, M., and Schofield, P. F.: Refining the prognostic significance of DNA ploidy status in colorectal cancer: A prospective flow cytometric study. Int. J. Cancer, 41:206, 1988.
142. Jones, D. J., Zaloudik, J., James, R. D., Haboubi, N., Moore, M., and Schofield, P. F.: Predicting local recurrence of carcinoma of the rectum after preoperative radiotherapy and surgery. Br. J. Surg., 76:1172, 1989.
143. Kallioniemi, O. P., Punnonen, R., Mattila, J., Lehtinen, M., and Koivula, T.: Prognostic significance of DNA index, multiploidy, and S-phase fraction in ovarian cancer. Cancer, 61:334, 1988.
144. Kallioniemi, O. P., Punnonen, R., Mattila, J., Lehtinen, M., and Koivula, T.: Prognostic significance of DNA index, multiploidy, and S-phase fraction in ovarian cancer. Cancer, 61:334, 1988.
145. Kaman, E. J., Smeulders, A. W. N., Verbeek, P. W., Young, I. T., and Baak, J. P.: Image processing for mitoses in sections of breast cancer: A feasibility study. Cytometry, 5:244, 1984.
146. Kamel, O. W., Franklin, W. A., Ringus, J. C., and Meyer, J. S.: Thymidine labeling index and Ki-67 growth fraction in lesions of the breast. Am. J. Pathol., 134:107, 1989.
147. Kamensky, L. A., and Melamed, M. R.: Instrumentation for automated examination of cellular specimens. Proc. IEEE, 57:2007, 1969.
148. Kardinal, C. G., Perry, M. C., Korzun, A. H., Rice, M. A., Ginsberg, S., and Wood, W. C.: Responses to chemotherapy or chemohormonal therapy in advanced breast cancer patients treated previously with adjuvant chemotherapy: A subset analysis of CALGB study 8081. Cancer, 61:415, 1988.
149. Karle, H., Ernst, P., and Killman, S. A.: Changing cytokinetic patterns of human leukaemic lymphoblasts during the course of the disease, studied *in vivo*. Br. J. Haemat., 24:231, 1973.
150. Kendal, W. S., and Frost, P.: Metastatic potential and spontaneous mutation rates: Studies with two murine cell lines and their recently induced metastatic variants. Cancer Res., 46:6131, 1986.
151. Kennedy, S., Merino, M. J., Swain, S. M., and Lippman, M. E.: The effects of hormonal and chemotherapy on tumoral and nonneoplastic breast tissue. Hum. Pathol., 21:192, 1990.
152. Kheir, S. M., Bines, S. D., Vonroenn, J. H., Soong, S. J., Urist, M. M., and Coon, J. S.: Prognostic significance of DNA aneuploidy in stage I cutaneous melanoma. Ann. Surg., 207:455, 1988.
153. Killman, S. A.: Acute leukemia: The kinetics of leukemic blast cells in man. Series Hematologica, 1:38, 1968.
154. Klemi, P. J., Joensuu, H., Maenpaa, J., Kiiholma, P.: Influence of cellular DNA content on survival in ovarian carcinoma. Obstet. Gynecol., 74:200, 1989.
155. Kloppel, G., Klnofel, W. T., Baisch, H., and Otto, U.: Prognosis of renal cell carcinoma related to nuclear grade, DNA content and Robson stage. Eur. Urol., 12:426, 1986.
156. Kokal, W. A., Duda, R. B., Azumi, N., Sheibani, K., Kemeny, M. M., Terz, J. J., and Harada, J. R.: Tumor DNA content in primary and metastatic colorectal carcinoma. Arch. Surg., 121:1434, 1986.
157. Kokal, W. A., Gardine, R. L., Sheibani, K., Morris, P. L., Prager, E., Zak, I. W., and Terz, J. J.: Tumor DNA content in resectable, primary colorectal carcinoma. Ann. Surg., 209:188, 1989.
158. Korenaga, D., Okamura, T., Saito, A., Baba, H., and Sugimachi, K.: DNA ploidy is closely linked to tumor invasion, lymph node metastasis, and prognosis in clinical gastric cancer. Cancer, 62:309, 1988.
159. Korenaga, D., Haraguchi, M., Okamura, T., Baba, H., Saito, A., and Sugimachi, K.: DNA ploidy and tumor invasion in human gastric cancer. Histopathologic differentiation. Arch. Surg., 124:314, 1989.
160. Korzun, A., Norton, L., Perloff, M., Wood, W., Carey, R., Rice, M., Holland, J. F., Frei, E.: Clinical Equivalence Despite Dosage Differences of Two Schedules of Cyclophosphamide, Methotrexate, 5-Fluorouracil, Vincristine and Prednisone (CMFVP) For Adjuvant Therapy of Node-Positive Stage II Breast Cancer, Proc. Am. Soc. Clin. Oncol., 7:12, 1988.
161. Koury, M. J., and Bondurant, M. C.: Erythropoietin retards DNA breakdown and prevents programmed death in erythroid progenitor cells. Science, 248:378, 1990.
162. Kuhn, W., Kaufmann, M., Feichter, G. E., Schmid, H., Hanke, J., and Rummel, H. H.: Psammoma body content and DNA-flow cytometric results as prognostic factors in advanced ovarian carcinoma. Eur. J. Gynaecol. Oncol., 9:234, 1988.
163. Kuhn, W., Kaufmann, M., Feichter, G. E., Rummel, H. H., Schmid, H., and Heberling, D.: DNA flow cytometry, clinical and morphological parameters as prognostic factors for advanced malignant and borderline ovarian tumors. Gynecol. Oncol., 33:360, 1989.
164. Kuhn, W., Kaufmann, M., Feichter, G. E., Rummel, H. H., Abel, U., Heep, J., and von Minckwitz, G.: Prognostic significance of cell kinetic parameters of endometrial cancer. Geburtshilfe und Frauenheilkunde, 49:787, 1989.
165. Kute, T. E., Muss, H. B., Cooper, M. R., Case, L. D., Buss, D., Stanley, V., Gregory, B., Galleshaw, J., and Booher, K.: The use of flow cytometry for the prognosis of stage II adjuvantly treated breast cancer patients. Cancer, 66:1810, 1990.
166. Kvaly, S., Marton, P. F., Kaalhus, O., Hie, J., Foss-Abrahamsen, A., Godal, T.: 3H-thymidine uptake in B cell lymphomas—relationship to treatment response and survival. Scandinavian J. Haematology, 34:429, 1985.
167. Laird, A. K.: Dynamics of growth in tumors and normal organisms. Natl. Cancer Inst. Monogr., 30:15, 1969.
168. Lajtha, L. G., Oliver, R., and Ellis, F.: Incorporation of ^{32}p and adenine ^{14}C into DNA by human bone marrow cells *in vitro*. Br. J. Cancer, 8:367, 1954.
169. LaLa, P. K.: Age-specific changes in the proliferation of Ehrlich ascites tumor cells grown as solid tumors. Cancer Res., 32:628, 1972.
170. Laskey, R. A., Fairman, M. P., and Blow, J. J.: S phase of the cell cycle. Science, 246:609, 1989.
171. Latt, S. A.: Fluorometric detection of DNA synthesis; Possibilities for interfacing bromodeoxyuridine dye techniques with flow fluorometry. J. Histochem. Cytochem., 25:913, 1977.
172. Law, L. W.: Origin of resistance of leukaemic cells to folic acid antagonists. Nature, 169:628, 1952.
173. Lehtinen, T., Aine, R., Lehtinen, M., Kallioniemi, O., Leino, T., Hakala, T., Lienikki, P., and Alavaikko, M.: Flow cytometric DNA analysis of 199 histologically favourable or unfavourable non-Hodgkin lymphomas. J. Pathol., 157:27, 1989.
174. Leminen, A., Paavonen, J., Vesterinen, E., Forss, M., Wahlstrom, T., Kulomaa, P., and Lehtinen, M.: Deoxyribonucleic acid flow cytometric analysis of cervical adenocarcinoma: prognostic significance of deoxyribonucleic acid ploidy and S-phase fraction. Am. J. Obstet. Gynecol., 162:848, 1990.
175. Lindahl, B., Alm, P., Ferno, M., Killander, D., Langstrom, E., Norgren, A., and Trope, C.: Prognostic value of flow cytometrical DNA measurements in stage I–II endometrial carcinoma: correlations with steroid receptor concentration, tumor myometrial invasion, and degree of differentiation. Anticancer Res., 7:791, 1987.
176. Lindh, J., Jonsson, H., Lenner, P., and Roos, G.: Fraction of S-phase cells in blood mononuclear cells in non-Hodgkin's lymphomas—correlation with clinical features and prognosis. Eur. J. Hematol., 42:331, 1989.
177. Ling, M. R., and Kay, J. E.: Lymphocyte Stimulation. Elsevier, New York, 1965.
177A. Lippman, M. E., Cassidy, J., Wesley, M., and Young, R. C.: A randomized attempt to increase the efficacy of cytotoxic chemotherapy in metastatic breast cancer by hormonal synchronization. J. Clin. Oncol., 2:28, 1984.
178. Lippman, M. E., Dickson, R. B., Bates, S., Knabbe, C., Huff, K., Swain, S., McManaway, M., Bronzert, D., Kasid, A., and Gelmann, E. P.: Autocrine and paracrine growth regulation of human breast cancer. Breast Cancer Res. Treat., 7:59, 1986.
178A. Lippman, M. E.: Hormonal stimulation and chemotherapy for breast cancer (Editorial). J. Clin. Oncol., 5:331, 1987.
179. Lippman, M. E., and Dickson, R. B.: Growth control of normal and malignant breast epithelium. *In* Effects of Therapy on Biology and Kinetics of the Residual Tumor, Part A: Pre-Clinical Aspects. Edited by J. Ragaz, J. Simpson-Herren, M. E. Lippman, and B. Fisher. New York, Wiley-Liss, 1990, pp. 147–178.
180. Longo, D. L., DeVita, V. T., Jr., Duffey, P. L., Wesley, M. N., Ihde, D. C., Hubbard, S. M., Gilliom, M., Jaffe, E. S., Cossman, J., Fisher, R. I., and Young, R. C.: Superiority of ProMACE-CytaBOM over ProMACE-MOPP in the treatment of advanced diffuse aggressive lymphoma: Results of a prospective randomized trial. J. Clin. Oncol., 9:25, 1991.
181. Longo, D. L., Duffey, P. L., DeVita, V. T., Jr., Wiernik, P. H., Hubbard, S. M., Phares, J. C., Bastian, A. W., Jaffe, E. S., and Young, R. C.: Treatment of advanced-stage Hodgkin's disease: Alternating noncrossresistant MOPP/CABS is not superior to MOPP. J.Clin. Oncol., 9:1409, 1991.
182. Look, A. T., Hayes, F. A., Nitschke, R., McWilliams, N. B., and Green, A. A.: Cellular DNA content as a predictor of response to chemotherapy in infants with unresectable neuroblastoma. N. Engl. J. Med., 311:231, 1984.
183. Look, A. T., Robertson, P. K., Williams, D. L., Rivera, G., Bowman, W. P., Pui, C. H., Ochs, J., Abromowitch, M., Kalwinsky, D., Dahl, G. V., George, S., and Murphy, S. A.: Prognostic importance of blast cell DNA content in childhood acute lymphoblastic leukemia. Blood, 65:1079, 1985.
184. Look, A. T., Douglass, E. C., and Meyer, W. H.: Clinical importance of near-diploid tumor stem lines in patients with osteosarcoma of an extremity. N. Engl. J. Med., 318:1567, 1988.
185. Ludwig Breast Cancer Study Group. Combination adjuvant chemotherapy for node-positive breast cancer. N. Engl. J. Med., 319:677, 1988.
186. Luria, S. E., and Delbruck, M.: Mutations of bacteria from virus sensitivity to virus resistance. Genetics, 28:491, 1943.
187. Maier, G., Heissler, H. E., Blech, M., and Schroter, W.: DNA profile, recurrence rate and progression of superficial G2 cancer of the urinary bladder. Urologe-Ausgabe, 27:173, 1988.
188. Malmstrom, P. U.: Prognosis of transitional cell bladder carcinoma. With special reference to ABH blood group isoantigen expression and DNA analysis. Scand. J. Urol. Nephrol. Suppl., 112:1, 1988.
189. Malmstrom, P. U., Norlen, B. J., Andersson, B., and Busch, C.: Combination of blood group ABH antigen status and DNA ploidy as independent prognostic factor in transitional cell carcinoma of the urinary bladder. Br. J. Surg., 64:49, 1989.
190. Masui, H., Kawamoto, T., Sato, J. D., Wolf, B., Sato, G., and Mendelsohn, J.: Growth inhibition of human tumor cells in athymic mice by antiepidermal growth factor receptor monoclonal antibodies. Cancer Res., 44:1002, 1984.
191. Mauer, A. M., and Fisher, V.: Comparison of the proliferative capacity of leukemia cells in bone marrow and blood. Nature (Lond.), 193:1085, 1962.
192. McDivitt, R. W., Stone, K. R., and Meyer, J. S.: A method for dissociation of viable human breast cancer cells that produces flow cytometric kinetic information similar to that obtained by thymidine labeling. Cancer Res., 44:2628, 1984.
193. McDivitt, R. W., Stone, K. R., Craig, R. B., Palmer, J. O., Meyer, J. S., and Bauer, W. C.: A proposed classification of breast cancer based on kinetic information derived from a comparison of risk factors in 168 primary operable breast cancers. Cancer, 57:269, 1986.
194. McIntosh, J. R., and Koonce, M. P.: Mitosis. Science, 246:622, 1989.
195. McLaoughlin, P., Osborne, B. M., Johnston, D., Jennings, P., Butler, J. J., Cabanillas, F., and Barlogie, B.: Nucleic acid flow cytometry in large cell lymphoma. Cancer Res., 48:6614, 1988.
196. Melamed, M. R., Enker, W. E., Banner, P., Janov, A. J., Kessler, G., and Darzynkiewics, Z.: Flow cytometry of colorectal carcinoma with three years followup. Dis. Colon Rectum, 29:184, 1986.
197. Mendelsohn, M. L.: The growth fraction: A new concept applied to neoplasia. Science, 132:1496, 1960.
198. Meyer, J. S., Friedman, E., McCrate, M. M., and Bauer, W. C.: Prediction of early course of breast carcinoma by thymidine labeling. Cancer, 51:1879, 1983.
199. Meyer, J. S., Prey, M. U., Babcock, D. S., and McDivitt, R. W.: Breast carcinoma cell kinetics, morphology, stage, and host characteristics. A thymidine labeling study. Lab. Invest., 54:41, 1986.
200. Meyer, J. S., and McDivitt, R. W.: Reliability and stability of the thymidine labeling index of breast carcinoma. Lab. Invest., 54:160, 1986.
201. Meyer, J. S., Nauert, J., Koehm, S., and Hughes, J.: Cell kinetics of human tumors by in vitro bromodeoxyuridine labeling. J. Histochem. Cytochem., 37:1449, 1989.
202. Moliterni, A., Bonadonna, G., Valagussa, P., Ferrari, L., and Zambetti, M.: Cyclophosphamide, methotrexate, and fluorouracil with or without doxorubicin in the adjuvant treatment of resectable breast cancer with one to three positive axillary nodes. J. Clin. Oncol., 9:1124, 1991.
203. Montgomery, B. T., Nativ, O., Blute, M. L., Farrow, G. M., Myers, R. P., Zincke, H., Therneau, T. M., and Lieber, M. M.: Stage B prostate adenocarcinoma. Flow cytometric nuclear DNA ploidy analysis. Archives of Surgery, 125:327, 1990.
204. Morgan, K. G., Quirke, P., O'Brien, C. J., and Bird, C. C.: Hodgkin's disease: a flow cytometric study. J. Clin. Pathol., 41:365, 1988.
205. Murphy, W. M., Chandler, R. W., and Trafford, R. M.: Flow cytometry of deparaffinized nuclei compared to histological grading for the pathological evaluation of transitional cell carcinomas. J. Urol., 135:694, 1986.
206. Murray, A. W., and Kirschner, M. W.: Dominoes and clocks: The union of two views of the cell cycle. Science, 246:614, 1989.
207. Murray, A. W.: Remembrance of things past. Nature, 349:367, 1991.
208. Nanus, D. M., Kelsen, D. P., Niedzwiecki, D., Chapman, D., Brennan, M., Cheng, E., and Melamed, M.: Flow cytometry as a prognostic indicator in patients with operable gastric cancer. J. Clin. Oncol., 7:1105, 1989.

209. National Cancer Institute (USA): Surveillance, Epidemiology and End Results (SEER) Program, 1974–1987.
210. Nativ, O., Winkler, H. Z., Raz, Y., Therneau, T. M., Farrow, G. M., Myers, R. P., Zincke, H., and Lieber, M. M.: Stage C prostatic ademocarcinoma: flow cytometric nuclear DNA ploidy analysis. Mayo Clinic Proceedings, 64:911, 1989.
211. Neve, E. F.: Kangri-burn cancer. Br. Med. J., 2:1255, 1923.
212. Nishimura, M., Sowa, M., Chung, Y. S., Yoshino, H., Katoh, Y., Kubo, T., Maekawa, H., Umeyama, K.: An analysis of DNA histogram and the expression of carbohydrate antigens regarding the degree of malignancy in gastric cancer. Japanese Journal of Gastroenterology, 86:843, 1989.
213. Nishizaki, T., Orita, T., Furutani, Y., Ikeyama, Y., Aoki, H., and Sasaki, K.: Flow cytometric DNA analysis and immunohistochemical measurement of Ki-67 and BUdR labeling indices in human brain tumors. J. Neurosurg., 70:379, 1989.
214. Norton, L., and Simon, R.: Growth curve of an experimental solid tumor following radiotherapy. J. Natl. Cancer Inst., 58:1735, 1977.
215. Norton, L., and Simon, R.: Tumor size, sensitivity to therapy, and the design of treatment schedules. Cancer Treat. Rep., 61:1307, 1977.
216. Norton, L.: Mathematical interpretation of tumor growth kinetics. *In* Clinical Interpretation and Practice of Cancer Chemotherapy. Edited by E. M. Greenspan. New York, Raven, 1982. pp. 53–70.
216A. Norton, L.: Implications of kinetic heterogeneity in clinical oncology. Semin. Oncol., 12:231, 1985.
217. Norton, L., and Simon, R.: The Norton-Simon hypothesis revisited. Cancer Treat. Rep., 70:163, 1986.
218. Norton, L.: A Gompertzian model of human breast cancer growth. Cancer Res., 48:7067, 1988.
219. Norton, L.: (Reply to letter to the Editor.) Cancer Res., 49:6444, 1989.
220. Norton, L.: Biology of residual breast cancer after therapy: A kinetic interpretation. *In* Effects of Therapy on Biology and Kinetics of the Residual Tumor, Part A: Pre-Clinical Aspects. Edited by J. Ragaz, L. Simpson-Herren, M. E. Lippman, and B. Fisher. New York, Wiley-Liss, 1990, pp. 109–132.
221. Norton, L., Baselga, J., Masui, H., Hyman, J., Kumar, R., and Mendelsohn, J.: Growth factor perturbation: A therapeutically exploitable mechanism for chemotherapy action. Proc. Am. Soc. Clin. Oncol., 10:208, 1991.
222. Norton, L., and Day, R.: Potential innovations in scheduling in cancer chemotherapy. *In* Important Advances in Oncology 1991. Edited by V. T. DeVita, Jr., S. Hellman, and S. A. Rosenberg. New York, J. B. Lippincott, 1991, pp. 57–72.
223. Novick, A., and Szilard, L.: Experiments with the chemostat on spontaneous mutations of bacteria. Proc. Natl. Acad. Sci. USA, 36:708, 1950.
224. Nowell, P. C.: The clonal evolution of tumor cell populations. Science, 194:23, 1976.
225. O'Farrell, P. H., Edgar, B. A., Lakich, D., and Lehner, C. F.: Directing cell division during development. Science, 246:635, 1989.
226. Ogawa, M., Fried, J., Sakai, Y., Strife, A., and Clarkson, B. D.: Studies of cellular proliferation in human leukemia. VI. The proliferative activity, generation time, and emergence time of neutrophilic granulocytes in chronic granulocytic leukemia. Cancer, 25:1031, 1970.
227. Ohyama, S., Yonemura, Y., and Miyazaki, I.: Flow cytometric cell cycle analysis using a monoclonal antibody to bromodeoxyuridine on gastric cancers. Journal of the Japanese Surgical Society, 90:1848, 1989.
227A. Ohyama, S., Yonemura, Y., and Miyazaki, I.: Prognostic value of S-phase fraction and DNA ploidy studies with *in vivo* administration of bromodeoxyuridine in human gastric cancers. Cancer, 65:116, 1990.
228. Oppedal, B. R., Storm-Mathisen, I., Lie, S. O., and Brandtzaeg, P.: Prognostic factors in neuroblastoma: Clinical, histopathologic, and immunohistochemical features and DNA ploidy in relation to prognosis. Cancer, 62:772, 1988.
228A. Osborne, C. K., Kitten, L., and Arteaga, C. L.: Antagonism of chemotherapy-induced cytotoxicity for human breast cancer cells by antiestrogens. J. Clin. Oncol., 7:710, 1989.
229. Pallavicini, M. G.: Solid tissue dispersal for cytokinetic analyses. *In* Techniques for Analysis of Cellular Proliferation. Edited by J. W. Gray, and Z. Darzyniewicz. Clifton, NJ, Humana Press, 1986, pp. 139–162.
230. Pardee, A. B.: G_1 events and regulation of cell proliferation. Science, 246:603, 1989.
231. Parks, T. G., Bussey, H. J. R., and Lockhart-Mummery, H. E.: Familial polyposis coli associated with extracolonic abnormalities. Gut, 11:323, 1970.
232. Paterson, A. H. G., Lees, A. W., Hanson, J., Szafran, O., and Comish, F.: Impact of chemotherapy on survival in metastatic breast cancer. Lancet, 2:312, 1980.
233. Perloff, M., Norton, L., Korzun, A., Wood, W., Carey, R., Weinberg, V., and Holland, J. F.: Advantage of an adriamycin combination plus halotestin after initial CMFVP for adjuvant therapy of node-positive stage II breast cancer. Proc. Am. Soc. Clin. Oncol., 70:273, 1986.
234. Peters, W. P.: High dose chemotherapy and autologous bone marrow support for breast cancer. *In* Important Advances in Oncology 1991. Edited by V. T. DeVita, Jr., S. Hellman, and S. A. Rosenberg. New York, J. B. Lippincott, 1991, pp. 135–150.
235. Peterson, L. C., Bloomfield, C. D., and Brunning, R. D.: Blast crisis as an initial or terminal manifestation of chronic myeloid leukemia. Am. J. Med., 60:209, 1976.
236. Pinkel, D., Hernandez, K., Borella, L., Houlton, C., Aur, R., Samoy, G., and Pratt, C.: Drug dosage and remission duration in childhood lymphocytic leukemia. Cancer, 27:247, 1971.
237. Poste, G., and Fidler, I. J.: The pathogenesis of cancer metastases. Nature (London), 283:139, 1980.
238. Powles, T. J., Smith, I. E., Ford, H. T., Coombes, R. C., Jones, J. M., and Gazet, J. C.: Failure of chemotherapy to prolong survival in a group of patients with metastatic breast cancer. Lancet, 1:580, 1980.
239. Pui, C. H., Dodge, R. K., Look, A. T., George, S. L., Rivera, G. K., Abromowitch, M., Ochs, J., Evans, W. E., Crist, W. M., and Simone, J. V.: Risk of adverse events in children completing treatment for acute lymphoblastic leukemia: St. Jude tital therapy studies VIII, IX, and X. J. Clin. Oncol., 9:1341, 1991.
240. Quastler, H., and Sherman, F. G.: Cell population kinetics in the intestinal epithelium of the mouse. Exp. Cell Res., 17:420, 1959.
241. Quirke, P., Dixon, M. F., Clayden, A. D., Durdey, P., Dyson, J. E., Williams, N. S., and Bird, C. C.: Prognostic significance of DNA aneuploidy and cell proliferation in rectal adenocarcinomas. J. Pathol., 151:285, 1987.
242. Rainwater, L. M., Farrow, G. M., Hay, I. D., and Lieber, M. M.: Oncocytic tumours of the salivary gland, kidney, and thyroid: nuclear DNA patterns studied by flow cytometry. Br. J. Cancer, 53:799, 1986.
243. Rainwater, L. M., Hiosaka, Y., Farrow, G. M., and Lieber, M. M.: Well differentiated clear cell renal carcinoma: significance of nuclear deoxyribonucleic acid patterns studied by flow cytometry. J. Urol., 137:15, 1987.
244. Raza, A., Yasin, Z., and Grande, C.: A comparison of the rate of DNA synthesis in myeloblasts from peripheral blood and bone marrows in patients with acute nonlymphocytic leukemia. Exp. Cell Res., 176:13, 1988.
245. Raza, A., Preisler, H. D., Day, R., Yasin, Z., White, M., Lykins, J., Kukla, C., Barcos, M., Bennett, J., Browman, G., Goldberg, J., Grunwald, H., Larson, R., Vardiman, J., and Vogler, R.: Direct relationship between remission duration in acute myeloid leukemia and cell cycle kinetics: A Leukemia Intergroup study. Blood, 76:2191, 1990.
246. Redmond, C., Fisher, B., and Wieand, H. S.: The methodological dilemma in retrospectively correlating the amount of chemotherapy received in adjuvant therapy protocols with disease-free survival. Cancer Treat. Rep., 67:519, 1983.
247. Rehn, S., Glimelius, B., Strang, P., Sundstrom, C., and Tribukait, B.: Prognostic significance of flow cytometry studies in B-cell non-Hodgkin lymphoma. Hematol. Oncol., 8:1, 1990.
248. Ritchie, A. W., Dorey, F., Layfield, L. J., Hannah, J., Lovrekovich, H., and deKernion, J. B.: Relationship of DNA content to conventional prognostic factors in clinically localized carcinoma of the prostate. Br. J. Urol., 62:245, 1988.
249. Rivkin, S. E., Knight, W. A., McDivitt, R., Cruz, T., Foulkes, M., Osborne, C. K., Fabian, C. J., and Costanzi, J. J.: Adjuvant therapy for breast cancer with positive axillary nodes designed according to estrogen receptor status. World J. Surg., 9:723, 1985.
250. Roosa, R., Weaver, C. F., and DeLamater, E. D.: Importance of transplant size in chemotherapeutic assay with the use of the Gardner lymphosarcoma. Proc. Am. Assoc. Cancer Res., 2:243, 1957.
251. Rosen, P. P., and Groshen, S.: Factors influencing survival and prognosis in early breast carcinoma (T1N0M0-T1N1M0): Assessment of 644 patients with median follow-up of 18 years. Surg. Clin. North Am., 70:937, 1990.
252. Rosenberg, P., Wingren, S., Simonsen, E., St'al, O., Risberg, B., and Nordenskjold, B.: Flow cytometric measurements of DNA index and S-phase on paraffin-embedded early stage endometrial cancer: an important prognostic indicator. Gynecol. Oncol., 35:50, 1989.
253. Ross, D. W., and Capizzi, R. L.: Differentiation vs. cytoreduction during remission induction in acute nonlymphoblastic leukemia treated with sequential high-dose ara-c and asparaginase. Cancer, 53:1651, 1984.
254. Ross, D. W.: Luekemia, oncogenes and cell cycle kinetics (editorial). Nouv. Rev. Fr. Hematol., 30:135, 1988.
255. Rowley, J. D., Golomb, A. M., and Vardiman, J. W.: Nonrandom chromosomal abnormalities in acute leukemia and dysmyelopoietic syndromes in patients with previously treated malignant disease. Blood, 58:759, 1981.
256. Rutgers, D. H., van der Linden, P. M., and van Peperzeel, H. A.: DNA-flow cytometry of squamous cell carcinomas from the human uterine cervix: the identification of prognostically different subgroups. Radiother. Oncol., 7:249, 1986.
257. Rutqvist, L. E., Wallgren, A., and Nilsson, B.: Is breast cancer a curable disease? A study of 14,731 women with breast cancer from the Cancer Registry of Norway. Cancer, 53:1793, 1984.
258. Ryser, H. J. P.: Chemical carcinogenesis. N. Engl. J. Med., 285:721, 1971.
259. Sahin, A. A., Ro, J. Y., el-Naggar, A. K., Lee, J. S., Ayala, A. G., Teague, K., and Hong, W. K.: Flow cytometric analysis of the DNA content of non-small cell lung cancer. Ploidy as a significant prognostic indicator in squamous cell carcinoma of the lung. Cancer, 65:530, 1990.
260. Samson, M. K., Rivlin, S. E., Jones, S. E., Constanzi, J. J., LoBuglio, A. F., Stephens, R. L., Gehan, E. A., and Cummings, G. D.: Dose-response and dose-survival advantage for high- vs. low-dose Cisplatin combined with vinblastine and bleomycin in disseminated testicular cancer. Cancer, 53:1029, 1984.
261. Sandison, A. T.: An autopsy study of the adult human breast: with special reference to the proliferative epithelial changes of importance in the pathology of the breast. Natl. Cancer Inst. Monograph., 8:1, 1962.
262. Santoro, A., Bonfante, V., Viviani, S., Valagussa, P., and Bonadonna, G.: Salvage chemotherapy in relapsing Hodgkin's disease. Proc. Am. Soc. Clin. Oncol., 3:254, 1984.
263. Schabel, F. M.: Concepts for the systemic treatment of micrometastases. Cancer, 35:15, 1975.
263A. Schipper, N. W., Smeulders, A. W., and Baak, J. P.: Automated estimation of epithelial volume in breast cancer sections. A comparison with the image processing steps applied to gynecological tumors. Pathol. Res. Pract., 186:737, 1990.
264. Schutte, B., Reynders, M. M., Wiggers, T., Arends, J. W., Volovics, L., Bosman, F. T., and Blijham, G. H.: Retrospective anlaysis of the prognostic significance of DNA content and proliferative activity in large bowel carcinoma. Cancer Res., 47:5494, 1987.
264A. Scott, N. A., Wiand, H. S., Moertel, C. G., Cha, S. S., Beart, R. W., and Lieber, M. M.: Colorectal cancer. Dukes' stage, tumor site, preoperative plasma CEA level, and patient prognosis related to tumor DNA ploidy pattern. Arch. Surg., 122:1375, 1987.
265. Scott, N. A., Rainwater, L. M., Wiand, H. S., Weiland, L. H., Pemberton, J. H., Beart, R. W., Jr., and Lieber, M. M.: The relative prognostic value of flow cytometric DNA analysis and conventional clinicopathologic criteria in patients with operable rectal carcinoma. Dis. Colon Rectum, 30:513, 1987.
266. Selawry, O. S., Hananian, J., Wolman, I. J., Abir, E., Chevalier, L., Gourdeam, R., Denton, R., Gussoff, B. D., Levy, R., Burgert, O., Jr., Mills, S. D., Blom, J., Jones, B., Patterson, R. B., McIntyre, O. R., Haurnai, F. I., Moon, J. H., Hoogstraten, B., Kung, F. H., Sheehe, P. R., Frie, E., III, and Holland, J. F.: New treatment schedule with improved survival in childhood leukemia. J. Am. Med. Assoc., 194:187, 1965.
267. Shackney, S. E., McCormack, G. W., and Cuchural, G. J., Jr.: Growth rate patterns of solid tumors and their relation to responsiveness to therapy: An analytical review. Ann. Int. Med., 89:107, 1978.
268. Shapiro, D. M., and Fugmann, R. A.: A role for chemotherapy as an adjunct to surgery. Cancer Res., 17:1098, 1957.
269. Shepherd, N. A., Richman, P. I., and England, J.: Ki-67 derived proliferative activity in colorectal adenocarcinoma with prognostic correlations. J. Pathol., 155:213, 1988.
270. Silvestrini, R., Daidone, M. G., and Gasparini, G.: Cell kinetics as a prognostic marker in node-negative breast cancer. Cancer, 56:78, 1985.
271. Silvestrini, R., Daidone, M. G., Valagussa, P., Salvadori, B., Rovini, D., and Bonadonna, G.: Cell kinetics as a prognostic marker in locally advanced breast cancer. Cancer Treat. Rep., 71:375, 1987.
272. Silvestrini, R., Daidone, M. G., Valagussa, P., Di Fronzo, G., Mezzanotte, G., Mariani, L., and Bonadonna, G.: 3H-thymidine labeling index as a prognostic indicator in node-positive breast cancer. J. Clin. Oncol., 8:1321, 1990.
273. Simon, R. M., Stroot, M. T., and Weiss, G. H.: Numerical inversion of Laplace transforms with application to percent labelled mitoses experiments. Comput. Biomed. Res., 5:596, 1972.
274. Simpson-Herren, L., and Lloyd, H. H.: Kinetic parameters and growth curves for experimental tumor systems. Cancer Chemother. Rep., 54:143, 1970.
275. Simpson-Herren, L., Sanford, A. H., and Holmquist, J. P.: Cell population kinetics of transplanted and metastatic Lewis lung carcinoma. Cell Tissue Kinet., 7:349, 1974.
276. Skipper, H. E., Schabel, F. M., Jr., and Wilcox, W. S.: Experimental evaluation of potential anticancer agents XIII: On the criteria and kinetics associated with "curability" of experimental leukemia. Cancer Chemother. Rep., 35:1, 1964.

277. Skipper, H. E.: Laboratory models: The historical perspective. Cancer Treat. Rep., 70:3, 1986.
278. Skipper, H. E.: Analyses of multiarmed trials in which animals bearing different burdens of L1210 leukemia cells were treated with two, three, and four drug combinations delivered in different ways with varying dose intensities of each drug and varying average dose intensities. Southern Research Institute Booklet 7, 42:87, 1986.
279. Spaar, F. W., Ahyai, A., and Blech, M.: DNA-fluorescence-cytometry and prognosis (grading) of meningiomas—a study of 104 surgically removed tumors. Neurosurg. Rev., 10:35, 1987.
280. Speer, J. F., Petrovsky, V. E., Retsky, M. W., and Wardwell, R. H.: A stochastic numerical model of breast cancer that simulates clinical data. Cancer Res., 44:4124, 1984.
281. Spratt, J. S., Greenberg, R. A., and Heuser, L. S.: Geometry, growth rates and duration of cancer and carcinoma in situ of the breast before detection by screening. Cancer Res., 46:970, 1986.
282. Srigley, J., Barlogie, B., Butler, J. J., Osborne, B., Blick, M., Johnston, D., Kantarjian, H., Reuben, J., Batsakis, J., and Freireich, E. J.: Heterogeneity of non-Hodgkin's lymphoma probed by nucleic acid cytometry. Blood, 65:1090, 1985.
283. Steel, G. G.: Cell loss as a factor in the growth rate of human tumors. Eur. J. Cancer, 3:381, 1967.
284. Steel, G. G., and Lamerton, L. F.: Cell population kinetics and chemotherapy. In Human Tumor Cell Kinetics. Edited by S. Perry. Natl. Cancer Inst. Monograph, 30:29, 1968.
285. Steel, G. G.: Growth Kinetics of Tumours—Cell Population Kinetics in Relation to the Growth and Treatment of Cancer. Oxford, Clarendon Press, 1977, pp. 46–52.
286. Steel, G. G.: Autoradiographic analysis of the cell cycle: Howard and Pelc to the present day. Int. J. Radiat. Biol., 49:227, 1986.
287. Strang, P., Eklund, G., Stendahl, U., and Frankendal, B.: S-phase rate as a predictor of early recurrences in carcinoma of the uterine cervix. Anticancer Res., 7:807, 1987.
288. Sugiyama, K., Yonemura, Y., Nishimura, K., Hashimoto, T., Hijimura, T., Miwa, K., and Miyazaki, I.: Malignancy of gastric cancer according to DNA ploidy pattern and tumor markers. Journal of the Japanese Surgical Society, 88:1430, 1987.
289. Sullivan, P. W., and Salmon, S. E.: Kinetics of tumor growth and regression in IgG multiple myeloma. J. Clin. Invest., 51:1697, 1972.
289A. Swain, S. M., Sorace, R. A., Bagley, C. S., Danforth, D. N., Jr., Bader, J., Wesley, M. N., Steinberg, S. M., and Lippman, M.E.: Neoadjuvant chemotherapy in the combined modality approach of locally advanced nonmetastatic breast cancer. Cancer Res., 47:3889, 1987.
290. Tannock, I. F.: Experimental chemotherapy and concepts related to the cell cycle. Int. J. Radiat. Biol. Relat. Stud. Phy. Chem. Med., 49:335, 1986.
291. Tannock, I. F., Boyd, N. F., DeBoer, G., Erlichman, C., Fine, S., Larocque, G., Mayers, C., Perrault, D., and Sutherland, H.: A randomized trial of two dose levels of cyclophosphamide, methotrexate, and fluorouracil chemotherapy for patients with metastatic breast cancer. J. Clin. Oncol., 6:1377, 1988.
292. Tattersall, M. H. N., Parker, L. M., Pitman, S. W., and Frei, E., III.: Clinical pharmacology of high-dose methotrexate. Cancer Chemother. Rep., Part 3, 6:25, 1975.
293. Taylor, S. R., Blatt, J., Constantino, J. P., Roederer, M., and Murphy, R. F.: Flow cytometric DNA analysis of neuroblastoma and ganglioneuroma: A 10-year retrospective study. Cancer, 62:749, 1988.
294. Teicher, B. A., Herman, T. S., Holden, S. A., Wang, Y., Pfeffer, M. R., Crawford, J. W., and Frei, E., III: Tumor resistance to alkylating agents conferred by mechanisms operative only in vivo. Science, 247:1457, 1990.
295. Till, J. E., McCulloch, G. A., Phillips, R. A., and Siminovitch, L.: Aspects of the regulation of stem cell function. In The Proliferation and Spread of Neoplastic Cells, Univ. of Texas M. D. Anderson Hospital and Tumor Institute at Houston, 21st Annual Symposium on Fundamental Cancer Research 1967. Baltimore, MD, Williams and Wilkins, 1968, pp. 235–244.
296. Tirindelli-Danesi, D., Teodori, L., Mauro, F., Modini, C., Botti, C., Cicconetti, F., and Stipa, S.: Prognostic significance of flow cytometry in lung cancer. A 5-year study. Cancer, 60:844, 1987.
297. Tormey, D., Carbone, P., and Band, P.: Breast cancer survival in single and combination chemotherapy trials since 1968. Proc. Am. Assoc. Cancer Res., 18:64, 1977.
298. Tsushima, K., Nagorney, D. M., Rainwater, L. M., Adson, M. A., Faroow, G. M., Ilstrup, D. M., and Lieber, M. M.: Prognostic significance of nuclear deoxyribonucleic acid ploidy patterns in resected hepatic metastases from colorectal carcinoma. Surgery, 102:635, 1987.
299. Tsushima, K., Rainwater, L. M., Goellner, J. R., van Heerden, J. A., and Lieber, M. M.: Leiomyosarcomas and benign smooth muscle tumors of the stomach: nuclear DNA patterns studied by flow cytometry. Mayo Clinic Proceedings, 62:275, 1987.
300. Tsuchiya, A., Sekikawa, K., Kimijima, I., Suzuki, S., Nihei, M., Rokkaku, Y., and Abe, R.: Flow cytometric DNA measurements of thyroid carcinomas. Japanese Journal of Cancer Clinics, 35:886, 1989.
301. Tubiana, M.: Tumor cell proliferation kinetics and tumor growth rate. Acta Oncol., 28:113, 1989.
302. Tytor, M., Franzen, G., and Olofsson, J.: DNA ploidy in oral cavity carcinomas, with special reference to prognosis. Head & Neck, 11:257, 1989.
303. Valagussa, P., Tancini, G., and Bonadonna, G.: Salvage treatment of patients suffering relapse after adjuvant CMF chemotherapy. Cancer, 58:1411, 1986.
304. Valagussa, P., Brambilla, C., Zambetti, M., and Bonadonna, G.: Salvage treatment after first relapse of breast cancer: A review. Third International Conference on Adjuvant Therapy of Primary Breast Cancer, St. Gallen, Switzerland, 1988, p. 9.
305. Valagussa, P., Santoro, A., Boracchi, P., Viviani, S., and Bonadonna, G.: 9-year results of two randomized studies with MOPP and ABVD in Hodgkin's disease: Multiple regression analysis. Proc. Am. Soc. Clin. Oncol., 8:976, 1989.
306. Valeriote, F., and van Putten, L.: Proliferation-dependent cytotoxicity of anticancer agents: A review. Cancer Res., 35:2619, 1975.
307. VanDilla, M. A., Trujillo, T. T., Mullaney, P. F., and Coulter, J. R.: Cell microfluorometry: A method for rapid fluorescence measurement. Science, 169:1213, 1969.
308. Vincent, P.C., Cronkite, E. P., Greenberg, M. L., Kirsten, C., Schiffer, L. M., and Stryckmans, P. A.: Leukocyte kinetics in chronic myeloid leukemia. I. DNA synthesis time in blood and marrow myelocytes. Blood, 33:843, 1969.
309. Volm, M., Drings, P., Mattern, J., Sonka, J., Vogt-Moykopf, I., and Wayss, K.: Prognostic significance of DNA patterns and resistance-predictive tests in non-small cell lung carcinoma. Cancer, 56:1396, 1985.
310. Volm, M., Drings, P., Kleine, W., and Maltern, J.: Flow cytometry as a tool for the prognostic assessment of patients with lung and ovarian carcinomas. Strahlentherapie und Onkologie, 163:791, 1987.
311. Volm, M., Mattern, J., Muller, T., and Drings, P.: Flow cytometry of epidermoid lung carcinomas: relationship of ploidy and cell cycle phases to survival. A five-year follow up study. Anticancer Res., 8:105, 1988.
312. Volm, M., Hahn, E. W., Mattern, J., Muller, T., Vogt-Moykopf, I., and Weber, E.: Five-year follow-up study of independent clinical and flow cytometric prognostic factors for the survival of patients with non-small cell lung carcinoma. Cancer Res., 48:2923, 1988.
313. Volm, M.: Prognostic significance of DNA ploidy and distribution of cell cycle phases in non-small cell bronchial cancer. A 5-year survival study. Versicherungsmedizin, 41:2, 1989.
314. Volm, M., Kayser, K., and Mattern, J.: Demonstration of independent cellular prognostic factors in squamous cell carcinoma of the lung. Strahlentherapie und Onkologie, 165:587, 1989.
315. Wampler, G. L., Heim, W. J., Ellison, N. A., Ahlgren, J. D., and Fryer, J. G. for the Mid-Atlantic Oncology Program: Comparison of cyclophosphamide, doxorubicin, and vincristine with an alternating regimen of methotrexate, etoposide, and cisplatin/cyclophosphamide, doxorubicin, and vincristine in the treatment of extensive-disease small-cell lung cancer. J. Clin. Oncol., 9:1438, 1991.
316. Watson, J. V.: The cell proliferation kinetics of the EMT6/M/AC mouse tumor at four volumes during unperturbed growth in vivo. Cell Tissue Kinet., 9:147, 1976.
317. Wegelin, C.: Malignant disease of the thyroid gland and its relations to goitre in man and animals. Cancer Rev., 3:297, 1928.
318. Weinberg, R. A., Bishop, J. M., Minna, J. D., and Sharp, P. A.: Gene regulation and oncogenes: AACR special conference in cancer research. Cancer Res., 49:2188, 1989.
319. Wiggers, T., Arends, J. W., Schutte, B., Volovics, L., and Bosman, F. T.: A multivariate analysis of pathologic prognostic indicators in large bowel cancer. Cancer, 61:386, 1988.
320. Williams, G. T., Smith, C. A., Spooncer, E., Dexter, T. M., and Taylor, D. R.: Haemopoietic colony stimulating factors promote cell survival by suppressing apoptosis. Nature, 343:76, 1990.
321. Williams, S., Stablein, D., Einhorn, L., Muggia, F., Weiss, R., Donohue, J., Paulson, D., Brunner, K., Jacobs, E., Spaulding, J., DeWys, W., and Crawford, E.: Immediate adjuvant chemotherapy versus observation with treatment at relapse in pathological stage II testicular cancer. N. Engl. J. Med., 317:1433, 1987.
322. Wilson, A. J., Baum, M., Brinkley, D. M., Dossett, J. A., McPherson, K., Patterson, J. S., Rubens, R. D., Smiddy, F. G., Stoll, B. A., Richards, D., and Ellis, S. H.: Six-year result of a controlled trial of tamoxifen as single adjuvant agent in management of early breast cancer. World J. Surg., 9:756, 1985.
323. Wolley, R. C., Schreiber, K., Koss, L. G., Karas, M., and Sherman, A.: DNA distribution in human colon carcinomas and its relationship to clinical behavior. J. Natl. Cancer Inst., 69:15, 1982.
324. Yasue, M., Tomita, T., Engelhard, H., Gonzalez-Crussi, F., McLone, D. G., and Bauer, K. D.: Prognostic importance of DNA ploidy in medulloblastoma of childhood. J. Neurosurg., 70:385, 1989.
324A. Yee, D., Rosen, N., Favoni, R. E., and Cullen, K. J.: The insulin-like growth factors, their receptors, and their binding proteins in human breast cancer. Cancer Treat. Res., 53:93, 1991.
325. Yonemura, Y., Sugiyama, K., Makata, T., Fijimura, T., Yamaguchi, A., Miwa, K., and Miyazaki, I.: Malignancy in gastric carcinoma, with special reference to the DNA ploidy and proliferative activity. Journal of the Japanese Surgical Society, 89:1175, 1988.
326. Yonemura, Y., Ooyama, S., Sugiyama, K., Kamata, T., De Aretxabala, X., Kimura, H., Kosaka, T., Yamaguchi, A., Miwa, K., and Miyazaki, I.: Retrospective analysis of the prognostic significance of DNA ploidy patterns and S-phase fraction in gastric carcinoma. Cancer Res., 50:509, 1990.
327. Yonemura, Y., Sugiyama, K., Kamata, T., Kosaka, T., Yamaguchi, A., Miwa, K., De Aretxeblala, X., and Miyazaki, I.: Correlation of DNA ploidy and clinical outcome in early gastric carcinoma. Oncology, 47:49, 1990.
328. Yoshino, H.: A study of DNA ploidy patterns of gastric cancers. Journal of the Japanese Surgical Society, 89:522, 1988.
329. Young, G. A., Hedley, D. W., Rugg, C. A., Iland, H. J.: The prognostic significance of proliferative activity in poor histology non-Hodgkin's lymphoma: A flow cytometry study using archival material. Eur. J. Cancer Clin. Oncol., 23:1497, 1987.
330. Zimmerman, P. V., Hawson, G. A., Bint, M. H., and Parsons, P. G.: Ploidy as a prognostic determinant in surgically treated lung cancer. Lancet, 2:530, 1987.
331. Zuckiet, G., and Tritton, T. R.: Adriamycin causes up-regulation of epidermal growth factor receptors in actively growing cells. Exp. Cell Res., 148:155, 1983.

XV-2

Drug Resistance and Its Clinical Circumvention

Charles S. Morrow
Kenneth H. Cowan

Introduction

Systemic therapy with cytotoxic drugs is the basis for the most effective treatment of disseminated cancers. Additionally, adjuvant chemotherapy can offer a significant survival advantage to selected patients following the treatment of localized disease with surgery or radiotherapy, presumably by eliminating undetected minimal or microscopic residual tumor. However, the responses of tumors to chemotherapeutic regimens vary and failures are frequent owing to the emergence of drug resistance. Patterns of treatment response and tumor sensitivity are conveniently divided into three groups. First, with modern treatments, prompt cytoreduction and cures are common for some intrinsically drug-sensitive tumors such as childhood acute lymphoblastic leukemia (ALL), Hodgkin's disease, some non-Hodgkin's lymphomas, and testicular cancer. A second group, including tumors such as breast carcinomas, small cell lung cancers, and ovarian carcinomas, is also usually highly responsive to initial treatments but more often becomes refractory to further therapy. Relapses in either group of tumors, particularly during or shortly after the completion of therapy, generally herald the emergence of tumor cells that are resistant to the antineoplastic agents used initially and often to drugs to which the patient was never exposed. Therefore, success with conventional salvage chemotherapies has been limited. Finally, a third common pattern of drug sensitivity is found in tumors that are intrinsically resistant to most chemotherapeutic agents. This group is represented by malignancies such as non-small cell lung cancers, malignant melanoma, and colon cancer. For these tumors, the number of active antineoplastic agents is few and significant chemotherapeutic responses are effected in a minority of cases.

The phenomenon of clinical drug resistance has prompted studies to clarify mechanisms of drug action and identify mechanisms of antineoplastic resistance. It is expected that through such information drug resistance may be circumvented by rational design of new non-cross-resistant agents, by novel delivery or combinations of known drugs, and by the development of other treatments that may augment the activity of or reverse resistance to known antineoplastics. Multiple mechanisms of antineoplastic failure have been identified using in vitro (tissue culture) and in vivo (animal and xenograft) models of antineoplastic failure. A list of these general mechanisms of drug resistance are categorized in Table XV-2-1. Considered are mechanisms involving anatomic, pharmacologic, and host-drug-tumor interactions that are uniquely pertinent to patients and to in vivo models of drug resistance as well as cellular mechanisms that can be

Table XV-2-1. General Mechanism of Drug Resistance

Cellular and Biochemical Mechanisms
  Decreased drug accumulation
    Decreased drug influx
    Increased drug efflux
    Altered intracellular trafficking of drug
  Decreased drug activation
  Increased inactivation of drug or toxic intermediate
  Increased repair of drug-induced damage to:
    DNA
    Protein
    Membranes
  Drug targets altered (quantitatively or qualitatively)
  Altered cofactor or metabolite levels
  Altered gene expression
    DNA mutation, amplification, or deletion
    Altered transcription, post-transcription processing or translation
    Altered stability of macromolecules
Mechanisms Relevant In Vivo
  Pharmacologic and anatomic drug barriers (tumor sanctuaries)
  Host–drug interactions
    Increased drug inactivation by normal tissues
    Decreased drug activation by normal tissues
    Relative increase in normal tissue drug sensitivity (toxicity)
  Host–tumor interactions

described at the molecular level. These mechanisms are frequently interrelated as, for example, altered gene expression must ultimately underlie most of the cellular and biochemical mechanisms listed in Table XV-2-1. Furthermore, multiple independent mechanisms of antineoplastic resistance may coexist in a population of tumor cells.

While mechanisms of drug resistance have been largely determined in experimental systems, many have been implicated in at least some examples of clinical chemotherapeutic failure. Evidence that bears upon these mechanisms of resistance and strategies to circumvent them are discussed below. First, we discuss the general mechanisms of cellular drug resistance and then some specific examples in the sections that follow. Additionally, the important concept of resistance to multiple antineoplastic agents, resistance to specific classes of drugs, and resistance mechanisms unique to in vivo situations are discussed.

General Mechanisms of Drug Resistance

Experimental selection of drug resistance by repeated exposure to single antineoplastic agents will generally result in cross-resistance to some related agents of the same drug class. This phenomenon is explained on the basis of shared drug transport carriers, drug-metabolizing pathways, and intracellular cytotoxic targets of these structurally and biochemically similar compounds. Generally, the resistant cells retain sensitivity to drugs of different classes with alternative mechanisms of cytotoxic action.[77,137] Thus cells selected for resistance to alkylating agents or antifolates will usually remain sensitive to unrelated drugs such as anthracyclines. Exceptions include emergence of cross-resistance to multiple, structurally and functionally unrelated drugs to which the patient or cancer cells were never exposed during the initial drug treatment. Despite apparent differences in the families of drugs associated with multiple drug resistance phenotypes, when the mechanisms underlying these phenotypes are identified, we frequently discover that the involved antineoplastic agents share common metabolic pathways, efflux transport systems, or sites of cytotoxic action. Conceptually then, the targets of multiple drug resistance mechanisms are similar to the targets of single-agent resistance mechanisms.

In this section we describe broadly defined processes related to drug resistance and a few specific examples. A more comprehensive discussion follows in the sections on resistance to specific classes of drugs.

Decreased Drug Accumulation

Decreased intracellular levels of cytotoxic agents is one of the most common mechanisms of drug resistance. This may result from decreased drug influx due to a defective carrier-mediated transport system. Decreased influx via a high-affinity folate-transport system is a well-described cause of methotrexate resistance.[8,75,130] A deficient membrane transport system has similarly been identified in cells resistant to nitrogen mustard.[62] Enhanced drug efflux may also lower intracellular steady-state levels of drugs. Cells that are multiply resistant to antineoplastic drugs due to overexpression of the P-glycoprotein drug efflux pump, classical multidrug resistance (MDR), represent the most important example of this mechanism of resistance.[50]

Altered Drug Metabolism

Modified drug activation, drug inactivation, or cofactors can confer resistance to selected antineoplastic agents. For example, many antimetabolites and some alkylating agents (e.g., cyclophosphamide) are administered as prodrugs, which must be activated to their cytotoxic forms by the targeted tumor or by other tissues. Resistance to some nucleobase drugs has been associated with decreased conversion of these analogs to their cytotoxic nucleoside and nucleotide derivatives by kinases and phosphoribosyl transferase salvage enzymes.[20,45] Furthermore, enhanced inactivation of pyrimidine and purine analogs by elevated deaminases has been linked to resistance toward these agents.[81,133] Finally, cofactor levels may modify drug toxicity. For example, optimal formation of inhibitory complexes between 5-fluorodeoxyuridine monophosphate (FdUMP) and its target enzyme, thymidylate synthase, requires the cofactor 5,10-methylene tetrahydrofolate.[80]

Increased Repair

Cells contain multiple complex systems involved in the repair of membrane and DNA damage. Because such damage may occur as a direct or secondary consequence of cytotoxic drug action, altered intrinsic repair mechanisms can influence drug sensitivity. For example, resistance to cisplatin, a drug whose cytotoxic action is thought to involve intrastrand DNA cross-linkages (see below), has been associated with altered activities presumed to reflect increased DNA repair.

Altered Drug Targets

The mechanisms of cell kill of several antineoplastic drugs involve interactions between the drug and an essential intracellular enzyme. These interactions result in alteration or inhibition of normal functions. Quantitative or qualitative changes in these enzyme targets of antineoplastic drugs can compromise drug efficacy. These changes have been demonstrated in several enzymes associated with drug resistance cells including dihydrofolate reductase, thymidylate synthetase, and topoisomerase II.[10,72,115]

Altered Gene Expression

The cellular mechanisms of drug resistance outlined above depend upon altered levels or function of key gene products. These alterations may result from changes that occur at any point along the transduction pathway of genetic information. Indeed, multiple molecular processes have been shown to be involved in examples of drug resistance, including: DNA mutation, deletion, or amplification; altered transcriptional or posttranscriptional control of RNA levels; and altered posttranslational modifications of proteins. The prevalence of these changes reflects the phenotypic and genetic instability of cancer cells under the selective, and perhaps mutagenic, pressures of xenobiotic toxin and drug exposure.

Resistance to Multiple Drugs

De novo and acquired cross-resistance to multiple antineoplastic agents can result from several alternative factors and processes. Accordingly, we have grouped the major patterns of cross-resistance into three categories based upon their presumed underlying mechanisms: classical or P-glycoprotein-dependent MDR, MDR confined to drugs that are topoisomerase II poisons, and MDR in which the pattern of cross-resistance to particular agents may resemble the other two groups but apparently occurs independently of P-glycoprotein or topoisomerase II functions. Additionally, more speculative mechanisms of multidrug resistance mediated by nonspecific xenobiotic metabolizing enzymes and cell-to-cell transfer of genetic information are discussed separately.

Classical (P-Glycoprotein-Dependent) MDR

An in vitro model of MDR was described by Biedler and coworkers over two decades ago.[19] In these studies cultured cells selected for resistance by exposure to actinomycin D developed cross-resistance to a surprising array of structurally diverse compounds including Vinca alkaloids, puromycin, daunomycin, and mitomycin C. Subsequently, induction of this pattern of cross-resistance has been observed by numerous investigators who have selected cells in the presence of the same and other drugs. Generally, exposure of cells to any of the drugs (many of which are listed in Table XV-2-2) related to this MDR phenotype can result in cross-resistance to all other members of the phenotype.[50] Drug transport studies using parental and MDR cells have demonstrated that the reduced cytotoxicity of these drugs is the result of decreased drug accumulation secondary to enhanced drug efflux.[85,120] Furthermore, the emergence of MDR has been associated with increased levels of a membrane-bound glycoprotein, P-glycoprotein (P-170 or MDR-associated protein).

The consensus view that P-glycoprotein is the energy-dependent drug efflux pump responsible for MDR is supported by pharmacologic, genetic, and biochemical data. First, the expression of P-glycoprotein is associated with concomitant increases in drug efflux and resistance that are sensitive to metabolic poisons. Furthermore, gene transfer experiments have shown that the expression of P-glycoprotein genes is sufficient to confer drug resistance.[69,145] P-glycoproteins are encoded by members of a multigene family. Analyses of these *mdr* genes have revealed a striking sequence homology between P-glycoproteins and several bacterial transport proteins.[31,70] The deduced amino acid sequences of P-glycoproteins predict the presence of two pairs of six transmembrane domains and two adenosine triphosphate (ATP) binding sites (Figure XV-2-1). Photoaffinity labeling experiments have demonstrated direct binding of drugs to P-glycoprotein.[123] The existence of multiple drug binding sites likely contributes to the capacity of P-glycoprotein to process the structurally diverse drugs associated with MDR. Finally, the distribution of P-glycoprotein on the luminal surfaces of normal tissues including renal tubules, colon, small intestine, and bile canaliculi is consistent with its proposed role in excretory transport.[66] Thus, P-glycoprotein appears to fulfill the requirements predicted of a membrane-bound energy-dependent drug carrier.

P-glycoprotein-associated MDR is subject to significant phenotypic heterogeneity. The relative degree of cross-resistance to the drugs listed in Table XV-2-2 will vary depending upon the cell line and the selecting drug. While the level of drug resistance is roughly correlated with the level of P-glycoprotein expression, protein and RNA levels may be disproportionately higher or lower than expected for the level of resistance observed. Similarly, the magnitude of the drug accumulation defect may appear insufficient to account for the degree of resistance. The phenotypic variability may result from the expression of alternative *mdr* alleles or by differential expression of the different members of the *mdr* gene family. Indeed, the human genome contains two closely related *mdr* genes. However, only one of these genes, *mdr-1*, has been shown to confer drug resistance in humans.[50] Mutations in the coding region of the *mdr-1* gene have been reported to alter the relative resistance patterns of cells.[35] Posttranslational modifications of P-glycoprotein may also alter pump function. For example, P-glycoprotein can be phosphorylated by protein kinase C and by a novel membrane-associated protein kinase.[29,132] Activation of protein kinase C by a phorbol ester was associated with altered ^{3}H-vinblastine accumulation when cells were incubated in the presence of the MDR reversing agent verapamil.[29] While the function of P-glycoprotein phosphorylation is poorly understood, these results suggest that altered kinase activities may influence drug resistance and MDR phenotypic diversity. Other cofactors involved in augmentation of P-glycoprotein function have been proposed but not yet identified.[54] Lastly, other mechanisms of drug resistance may coexist with classical MDR.

A thorough understanding of the regulation of P-glycoprotein production and the means to suppress its expression might significantly influence future cancer treatment strategies. Studies addressing this issue have shown that high levels of P-glycoprotein expression in vitro are often associated with *mdr* gene amplification and transcriptional activation.[50] Increased expression of P-glycoprotein can also be stimulated by heat shock, heavy metals, cytotoxic drugs, toxic and ablative liver insults, differentiating agents, and by repeated exposure to ionizing radiation.[14,33,34,53,76,103,140] However, the responses to these treatments appear to vary between species and are cell line specific. Thus, predictable modulation of *mdr* gene expression is not yet possible.

A considerable literature has accumulated that concerns the importance of P-glycoprotein in human cancer. P-glycoprotein RNA or protein has been detected in tumor specimens derived from patients with acute and chronic leukemias,[95,122,124] ovarian cancer,[16] multiple myeloma,[42] breast cancer,[87,125] neuroblastoma,[64] soft tissue sarcomas,[30] renal cell carcinoma,[102] and others.[65] Although the numbers of patients with particular tumors in these studies were small, the results have tended to link P-glycoprotein expression with a history of prior therapy (usually with MDR-associated drugs) or toxin exposure, emergence of intrinsic or acquired drug resistance, and treatment outcome. Ma and colleagues reported that in two patients with acute nonlymphoblastic leukemia (ANLL), disease progression with treatment (including an anthracycline), was associated with increasing P-glycoprotein levels in leukemic blasts.[95] In a study of 15 additional patients with ANLL, Sato and colleagues found

Table XV-2-2.   Cross-resistance Pattern of Classical MDR

Class	Drug
Anthracyclines	Doxorubicin
	Daunorubicin
	Mitoxantrone
Antibiotics	Actinomycin D
	Plicamycin
Antimicrotubule drugs	Vincristine
	Vinblastine
	Colchicine
Epipodophyllotoxins	Etoposide
	Teniposide

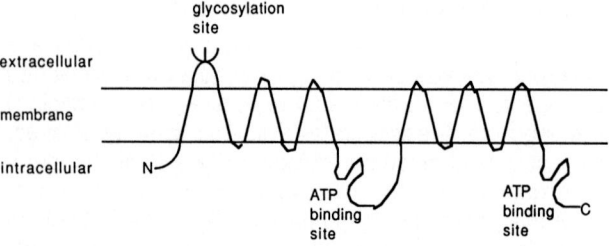

Figure XV-2-1.   Model of P-glycoprotein.

that P-glycoprotein was commonly present in leukemic blasts but more prevalent in blasts derived from patients of poor prognostic groups including those with a history of prior toxin exposure.[124] Although P-glycoprotein was frequently present in tumor specimens from both treated and untreated patients with neuroblastoma, P-glycoprotein RNA tended to be higher in patients treated with regimens including doxorubicin than in untreated patients.[64] In tumor specimens obtained from patients with childhood ALL and soft tissue sarcomas, the presence of P-glycoprotein was associated with anthracycline pre-treatment, increased rate of remission induction failure, and increased frequency of relapse.[30,122] Over 400 tumor specimens were tested for P-glycoprotein RNA levels in a recent large study.[65] Increased levels of P-glycoprotein RNA were more prevalent in tumors that tend to be intrinsically resistant to therapy (colon, renal, adrenal, hepatic, and pancreatic cancers) compared with intrinsically sensitive tumors. Furthermore, P-glycoprotein RNA was often increased in tumors at relapse (acute leukemias, breast cancer, neuroblastoma, pheochromocytoma, and nodular poorly differentiated lymphoma). Additional and prospective studies will be required to confirm the clinical significance of P-glycoprotein in human cancer. However, these preliminary results indicate that P-glycoprotein overexpression is associated with clinical evidence of drug resistance and treatment failure in a significant number of patients. Determinations of P-glycoprotein levels in patients at diagnosis or relapse may have a major role in the design of future treatment protocols.

Similar phenotypes of multiple resistance to antineoplastic agents have been described that are associated with the expression of other membrane proteins. In many of these examples resistance occurs independently of P-glycoprotein expression.[32,97,98,100,112] The mechanisms of multidrug resistance in these cell lines and whether these membrane proteins are directly involved in drug sensitivity or are merely markers of the resistant phenotype are subjects of current investigations.

Multidrug Resistance Associated With Topoisomerase Poisons

Topoisomerases are nuclear enzymes that catalyze the formation of transient single- or double-stranded DNA breaks, facilitate the passage of DNA strands through these breaks, and promote rejoining of the DNA stands.[94,148] As a consequence of these activities, topoisomerases are thought to be critical for DNA replication, transcription, and recombination. The cytotoxicity of drugs that target topoisomerases (topoisomerase poisons) is thought to depend upon the DNA cleavage activities of topoisomerases. There are two classes of mammalian enzymes, topoisomerases I and II. Topoisomerase I catalyzes the formation of single-stranded DNA breaks while topoisomerases II catalyze both single- and double-stranded breaks. During the cleavage reactions reversible DNA-topoisomerase complexes (cleavable complexes) can be stabilized by interactions with topoisomerase poisons. The formation of these stabilized DNA-topoisomerase-drug complexes is thought to initiate the production of lethal DNA strand breaks. Of the chemotherapeutic drugs that affect topoisomerase activities, the topoisomerase II poi-

sons have been the most important clinically. A partial list of these agents, which include DNA intercalating and nonintercalating drugs appears in Table XV-2-3.

Several laboratories have described an MDR pattern characterized by resistance of cells to several or all of the drugs listed in Table XV-2-3.[61,71] It is readily apparent that many of these topoisomerase II-targeting drugs are also members of the classical MDR phenotype (Table XV-2-2). However, the pattern of the topoisomerase II-related multidrug resistance differs from the pattern of P-glycoprotein-associated MDR in several important ways. First, resistance to these drugs is not usually associated with a drug transport defect or P-glycoprotein expression. Exceptions to this rule have been described and probably reflect the presence of multiple simultaneous mechanisms of resistance. Additionally, cells that display this topoisomerase II-related resistance phenotype are usually sensitive to antimicrotubule drugs associated with classical MDR including Vinca alkaloids and colchicine unless a concomitant drug transport or microtubule alteration exists. The mechanism of resistance to topoisomerase II poisons is thought to involve altered topoisomerase II activity. Both qualitative and quantitative changes in enzyme activity have been demonstrated in resistant cell lines. Reduced levels of topoisomerase activity have been associated with decreased drug-induced DNA strand breaks as well as reduced drug cytotoxicity[44,114] Other studies have implicated intrinsic changes in drug-induced catalytic properties or associated cofactors as the basis of drug resistance in some cells.[43,60,115,149] The nature of the topoisomerase II alterations may influence the cross-resistance patterns observed. For example, cells that develop alterations in topoisomerase II following exposure to m-AMSA (amsacrine) may show cross-resistance to other intercalating topoisomerase II poisons but not to epipodophyllotoxins.[149] Collectively, these data indicate that reduced topoisomerase protein levels or selectively altered enzyme activities influencing drug-enzyme interactions may render cells relatively more resistant to drugs by interfering with the formation of stable cleavable complexes and hence cytotoxic DNA strand breaks. Indeed, the normal down regulation of topoisomerase II in nondividing cells may explain the relative insensitivity to topoisomerase II-poisons of some solid tumors containing a large proportion of quiescent cells.[94]

The cytotoxic agent camptothecin has been shown to enhance topoisomerase I-mediated strand breaks. Until recently host toxicity has prohibited the clinical use of such topoisomerase I poisons. However, the prospect of less toxic analogs of this drug that maintain a high level of activity

Table XV-2-3. Topoisomerase II Poisons

	Class	Drugs
Nonintercalators	Epipodophyllotoxins	Etoposide
		Teniposide
Intercalators	Anthracyclines	Doxorubicin
		Daunorubicin
	Acridine	m-AMSA (amsacrine)
	Anthracenedione	Mitoxantrone
	Antibiotic	Actinomycin D
	Ellipticine	9-Hydroxyellipticine

against topoisomerase I-rich human cancer cells has renewed interest in the clinical application of this class of compounds.[59] Consequently, the emergence of resistance to these agents may become an increasingly important consideration. This problem is illustrated in a report by Andoh and colleagues, who have characterized a resistant leukemia cell line expressing defective topoisomerase I activity that mediates reduced camptothecin-induced DNA strand breaks.[7]

Multidrug Resistance Associated With Altered Expression of Drug-Metabolizing Enzymes

The emergence of acquired drug resistance may be viewed as an acute or chronic adaptive response of tumor cells to environmental stress, primarily in the form of drug challenge. As discussed above, rapid transient induction of P-glycoprotein may sometimes be mediated by an acute insult such as cytotoxic drug exposure, heavy metal exposure, or heat shock. Alternatively, chronic or repeated exposure to drugs may enhance P-glycoprotein levels by complex, stable genetic changes. In other models and tumor cells, challenges with cytotoxic agents result in alterations in the expression of several genes including those involved in drug metabolism. In the Solt-Farber model of chemical carcinogenesis, treatment of rats with various cytotoxins followed by partial hepatectomy results in the appearance of multiple preneoplastic nodules.[55] A number of biochemical changes occur in these nodules including the overexpression of P-glycoprotein, the induction of several phase II drug-metabolizing (drug-conjugating) enzymes, and the down-regulation of some phase I drug-metabolizing (cytochrome P450-dependent mixed function oxidases) enzymes.[53,140] These drug-metabolizing enzymes are generally considered to be involved in the sequential oxidation of xenobiotics to more electrophilic, reactive intermediates followed by the formation of less toxic conjugated compounds, which may be further metabolized or excreted (Figure XV-2-2). A similar pattern of P-glycoprotein expression, phase I enzyme suppression, and phase II enzyme induction has been shown in a human breast cancer cell line made multidrug resistant by chronic doxorubicin exposure.[37,52] The emergence of this phenotype appears to represent a programmed cellular stress response that might offer generalized protection from a variety of exogenous toxins via increased drug efflux secondary to P-glycoprotein expression, decreased drug activation due to reduced phase I enzymes, and increased drug inactivation by phase II enzymes. Of the phase II enzymes, the glutathione S-transferases (GSTs) have been the most extensively studied.

GSTs are comprised of multiple soluble and membrane-associated isozymes which catalyze the conjugation of elec-

trophilic, hydrophobic compounds (R-X) with the thiol, glutathione (GSH):[96,107,142]

$$R\text{-}X + GSH \xrightarrow{GST} R\text{-}SG + HX$$

Circumstantial evidence has linked the increase in specific GST isozymes or bulk GST activity in cells with resistance to alkylating agents, doxorubicin, and other drugs.[107,142] However, direct evidence that GSTs are responsible for altering drug sensitivities is limited. Another catalytic activity, selenium-independent glutathione peroxidase activity, has been attributed to some isozymes of GST:

$$R\text{-}O\text{-}OH + 2GSH \xrightarrow{GST} R\text{-}OH + GSSG + H_2O$$

This and other GST-mediated reactions are of interest because of their potential to detoxify oxidative damage to membranes and DNA.

Studies using cell-free preparations of GSTs have identified a limited number of antineoplastic drug substrates of these enzymes. These drugs and other substrates possibly associated with drug-mediated oxidative damage are listed in Table XV-2-4. Whether GST levels in tumor cells are sufficient to detoxify antineoplastic drugs to a clinically significant extent is a matter of considerable debate. Gene transfer experiments using recombinant GST genes and tissue culture cells have suggested that some GST isozymes may confer a very modest level of resistance to melphalan, chlorambucil, cisplatin, and doxorubicin.[110,119] Other experiments have failed to confirm any consistent resistance to doxorubicin, cisplatin, or melphalan in breast cancer cells transfected with the pi class isozyme of GST.[108] Clearly, additional studies are necessary to clarify the role of GSTs in drug resistance.

Emergence of Refractory Tumors Associated With Multiple Resistance Mechanisms

The backbone of many treatment protocols designed to circumvent the proliferation of resistant tumor cells is the administration of multiple drugs with different structural properties and mechanisms of action. The approach supposes that if enough carefully selected drugs are delivered at optimal doses and intervals, individual clones of cells resistant to one class of drug will be effectively killed by another drug in the regimen. The rapid appearance of refractory tumors despite an initially favorable cytoreductive response suggests that the emergence of multiply resistant tumor cell clones is a common clinical occurrence. We have seen how a single genetic change such as increased P-glycoprotein or altered topoisomerase II can mediate cross-resistance to

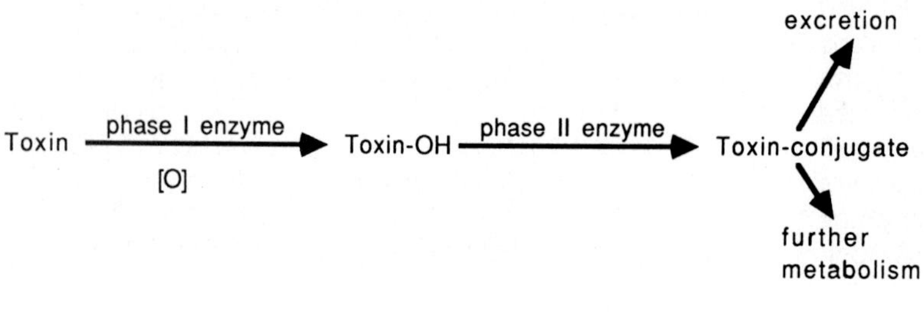

Figure XV-2-2. Phases I and II drug-metabolizing enzymes.

Toxin $\xrightarrow[\text{[O]}]{\text{phase I enzyme}}$ Toxin-OH $\xrightarrow{\text{phase II enzyme}}$ Toxin-conjugate

excretion

further metabolism

Table XV-2-4.   Some Important Substrates of GSTs Related to Drug Detoxification and Repair of Drug-Mediated Damage

Antineoplastic drugs	Products of membrane and DNA
Nitrogen mustards	oxidation
Chlorambucil	Fatty acid hydroperoxides
Melphalan	4-Hydroxy alkenals
Cyclophosphamide	?DNA hydroperoxides
Nitrosoureas	
1,3-bis(2-chloroethyl)-1-	
nitroso urea (BCNU)	
Anthracenedione	
Mitoxantrone	

Table XV-2-5.   Approaches to Overcome or Circumvent Drug Resistance

Prevention
  Aggressive multiple agent therapy
  Appreciation of factors that induce resistance mechanisms
Circumvention
  Drug-screening programs and rational drug design
  Circumvention of drug uptake defects
    Dose escalation
    Drugs that use alternative transport mechanisms
  Agents that reverse increased efflux
  Cofactors that augment drug activation or efficacy
  Inhibition of drug inactivation
  Novel treatment modalities
    Immunotherapy

several, but not all useful antineoplastic drugs. Although these mechanisms provide a molecular explanation for broad-spectrum resistance, it is clear that many refractory tumor clones must simultaneously develop multiple resistance mechanisms. These mechanisms may arise from multiple independent genetic changes in single cell clones or, as suggested by Cadman, from cell-to-cell transfer of genetic information.[24]

Resistance Factors Unique to Tumor Cells In Vivo: Host-Tumor-Drug Interactions

The failure of chemotherapy to eradicate a tumor in vivo despite exquisite sensitivity to drug in vitro may be due to anatomic or pharmacologic sanctuaries. For example, the failure to deliver adequate amounts of many drugs across blood-brain and -testicular barriers probably accounts for the relatively high frequency of ALL relapse at these sites.[116] In large solid tumors, chemotherapeutic failures are frequently attributed to decreased drug delivery to a tumor that has overgrown its vascular supply. Additionally, development of acidosis and hypoxia in poorly perfused areas of large tumors may interfere with the cytotoxicity of some drugs. Altered prodrug activation by liver or other normal tissues may profoundly influence the efficacy of drugs such as cyclophosphamide.

A recent report by Teicher and colleagues suggests that tumor-host interactions may influence drug pharmacokinetics and tumor resistance in unexpected ways.[138] In this study, tumor cells selected for cyclophosphamide and cisplatin resistance in vivo were normally sensitive to drugs in vitro. When the tumor cells were reimplanted into nude mice in vivo drug resistance was restored. These results suggest that resistant tumors may harbor cellular resistance factors that are operative only in conjunction with host factors and therefore mediate resistance by altered drug pharmacokinetics in vivo only. If this novel host-dependent mechanism of tumor resistance proves common, these results would provide one explanation for the failure of conventional in vitro testing to predict clinical responsiveness in all cases.

Approaches to Overcoming Resistance to Specific Groups of Drugs

Approaches to overcoming chemotherapeutic failures include efforts to prevent the emergence of drug resistance (Table XV-2-5). An appreciation of factors which induce resistance mechanisms may lead to the choice of more efficacious treatment regimens. For example, drugs that may have only sporadic activity against a specific tumor yet are likely to select for cross-resistance to more active agents would be avoided. It is hoped that aggressive combination chemotherapy with non-cross-reacting drugs will eliminate tumor rapidly enough to prevent the selection of multiply resistant tumor cell clones. Failures of the preventative approach require the incorporation of specific measures aimed at reversing or circumventing drug resistance.

Drugs Associated With P-Glycoprotein-Mediated Resistance

Prior to the original descriptions of P-glycoprotein, Tsuruo and coworkers noted that treatment with verapamil of leukemia cells made drug resistant by selection in vincristine or doxorubicin could partially restore antineoplastic drug sensitivity.[144] Furthermore, this verapamil-enhanced antineoplastic cytotoxicity, which was specific for drug-resistant but not sensitive parental cells, was associated with increased accumulation of vincristine and doxorubicin. These results suggested that in the drug-resistant cells vincristine and doxorubicin share a common transport system that is sensitive to modulation by verapamil. This transport system has now been identified as the P-glycoprotein drug efflux pump. Subsequently, numerous agents have been studied that can partially reverse the drug accumulation defects in classically multidrug-resistant cells including several calcium channel blockers, calmodulin inhibitors such as phenothiazines, and other drugs.[2,134] Although the mechanism(s) by which these agents reverse MDR is incompletely understood, it is believed that a direct interaction between these agents and P-glycoprotein interferes with antineoplastic drug efflux activity. Since a considerable clinical experience in the use of MDR reversing agents has existed for the treatment of other disorders, these agents have been included in several clinical trials designed to enhance the antitumor activity of conventional cancer drugs in refractory human neoplasms.

An early clinical trial examined the effect of diltiazem on vincristine cytotoxicity in patients with refractory childhood ALL.[18] A significant cytolytic response was seen in four of five patients who received the drugs on schedule. Although no complete responses were seen, these results indicated that further studies using this approach to the reversal of clinical drug resistance were warranted. Presant and colleagues evaluated the utility of verapamil in the treatment of patients with a variety of advanced malignancies.[117] Four of the patients had been pretreated with and found refractory to doxorubicin. Of these, one patient achieved a transient partial response and two patients transient minimal responses. A second study using verapamil in combination with vincristine and etoposide showed that 8 of 11 pediatric patients with leukemia refractory to MDR-associated drugs achieved partial responses.[25] While the responses were measured as decreased peripheral blast counts in most patients, one patient with acute myeloblastic leukemia (AML) demonstrated significant objective improvement by bone marrow analysis. In contrast, Ozols and co-workers failed to demonstrate antitumor responses in eight patients with refractory ovarian carcinoma treated with verapamil and doxorubicin.[113] Furthermore, unacceptable cardiotoxicity was reported, indicating the need for better tolerated reversing agents in future clinical trials. The influence of the phenothiazine, trifluoperazine on doxorubicin efficacy was studied in 36 patients whose tumors displayed acquired (previously responsive but later refractory) or intrinsic (not previously responsive) resistance to doxorubicin.[104] Sedation and extrapyramidal effects were the dose limiting toxicities. While no benefit of treatment was seen for any of the patients with intrinsically resistant tumors, favorable responses, including one complete response, were seen in 7 of 21 patients whose tumors displayed acquired resistance. In the studies described above, P-glycoprotein levels in tumors were not measured. Thus, the relationship between *mdr* gene expression and efficacy of reversing agents could not be assessed. To address this issue, Dalton and colleagues examined eight patients with myelomas and lymphomas refractory to regimens containing vincristine and doxorubicin.[41] Patient tumors were analyzed for the presence of P-glycoprotein RNA and protein as well as for their responses to treatment regimens consisting of verapamil administered with vincristine, doxorubicin, and dexamethasome. Three patient tumors responded to the verapamil-containing regimens (two transient PRs and one transient CR) and all of these responding tumors were P-glycoprotein-positive. Collectively, these trials suggest that the use of MDR-reversing agents may be of some benefit to selected patients with P-glycoprotein positive refractory tumors. Needed before such reversing drugs can be recommended are additional clinical trials that correlate antitumor response with the presence of P-glycoprotein, identification of reversing agents with less toxicity, and determinations of optimal dosages and schedules. Additionally, preclinical studies indicate that anti-P-glycoprotein antibodies, either covalently linked to cellular toxins or used in conjunction with complement, can specifically reduce the burden of P-glycoprotein-positive tumor cells.[57,141] The clinical utility of these immunologic reagents is a matter for future investigation.

Topoisomerase II Poisons

As discussed above, resistance to topoisomerase II poisons may occur as a consequence of P-glycoprotein overexpression or altered topoisomerase II activities. However, neither of these mechanisms will necessarily result in cross-resistance to all of the topoisomerase II-directed drugs listed in Table XV-2-3. For example, resistance to epipodophyllotoxins and anthracyclines on the basis of increased P-glycoprotein is not usually associated with resistance to the acridine derivative amsacrine. Conversely, resistance to amsacrine and other intercalating drugs due to alterations in topoisomerase II protein is not always associated with resistance to the nonintercalating, epipodophyllotoxin class of topoisomerase II poisons.[149] Therefore, these data derived from in vitro studies suggest a rationale for administering an alternative class of topoisomerase II poison in selected cases of clinical resistance to another class of topoisomerase II-directed drug.

Recently, the cross resistance patterns of several multidrug resistant human leukemia cell lines to a series of amsacrine analogs has been reported.[12,56] In these studies resistant cells were selected in the presence of amsacrine or doxorubicin. When compared with their parental cell lines, the resistant cells displayed multiple patterns of cross-resistance to the panel of drugs tested. Most significantly, for some cell lines resistant or cross-resistant to amsacrine, analogs of amsacrine were identified to which resistant cells showed increased sensitivity that approached the level of parental cell sensitivity. Although the precise changes in the resistant cells were not determined, the authors suggested that an altered topoisomerase II with reduced capacity to form stable ternary complexes with drugs and DNA might underlie one resistance pattern. Furthermore, some specific modifications in the putative drug-binding portion of the amsacrine analogs were associated with increased toxicity of the drugs toward amsacrine-resistant cells displaying this pattern. It was suggested that rational design of such analogs might enhance drug interaction with the altered topoisomerase II and thereby augment the clinical efficacy of these drugs in some resistant tumor cells.

Resistance to Free Radical-Mediated Drug Cytotoxicity

Several antineoplastic agents form free radical intermediates that are thought to contribute to drug cytotoxicity. Anthracyclines, such as doxorubicin, are among the most important members of this class of compound. While DNA-intercalating anthracyclines can damage cells by multiple mechanisms including inhibition of nucleic acid synthesis, induction of topoisomerase II-mediated DNA strand breaks, and perturbation of cell membranes; these quinone-hydroquinone compounds can also generate toxic free radical species that may cause cell death. As represented in Figure XV-2-3, doxorubicin and related drugs can undergo one-electron reductions in reactions catalyzed by a variety of enzymes.[109,128] The semiquinone radical so generated may either form a covalently binding free radical derivative, or in the presence of oxygen may be reoxidized to the quinone species in a reaction producing superoxide anion. Decomposition of hydrogen peroxide formed by dismutation of superoxide anion produces the highly reactive hydroxyl radical, which may directly damage DNA, lipid, and protein. Thus cellular factors that limit hydrogen peroxide production or repair peroxidative damage to macromolecules could theoretically confer some resistance to anthracyclines.

The pathways depicted in Figure XV-2-3 suggest several

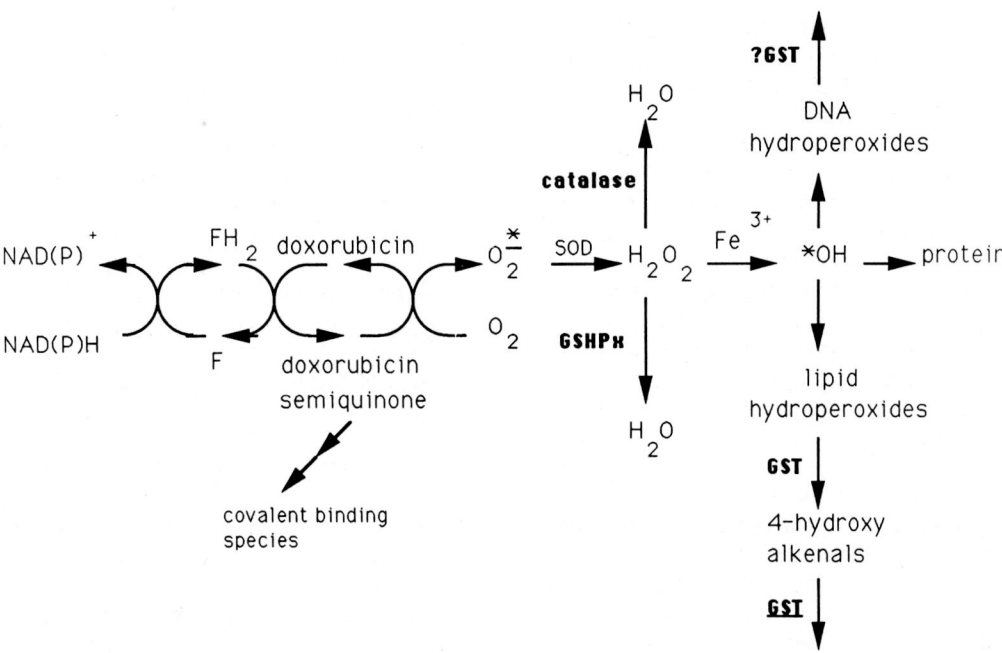

Figure XV-2-3. Mechanisms of free-radical-dependent doxorubicin toxicity and its reversal. GST, glutathione S-transferase; GSHPx, glutathione peroxidase, SOD, superoxide dismutase.

mechanisms by which tumor cells may become resistant to anthracycline-mediated free radical damage. First, superoxide anion formation is limited in poorly vascularized, relatively hypoxemic tissues such as may exist in the centers of large solid tumors. Second, increased intracellular levels of catalase and glutathione peroxidase (GSHPx) can deplete hydrogen peroxide, thus reducing the formation of toxic hydroxyl radicals. Indeed, in comparing parental and MDR MCF-7 cells, Sinha and coworkers have reported an association between increased GSHPx activity and reduced doxorubicin-stimulated hydroxyl radical formation.[129] Furthermore, lowering GSHPx activity by depleting the enzyme's cosubstrate, GSH resulted in enhanced doxorubicin-dependent free radical formation and cytotoxicity.[47] Additionally, Kramer and colleagues found that GSH depletion with buthionine sulfoximine (BSO) could partially restore the doxorubicin sensitivity of MDR MCF-7 cells, presumably by interfering with GSH-dependent reactions including those catalyzed by GSHPx.[90] While these results are consistent with the importance of hydrogen peroxide and hydroxyl radical formation in anthracycline cytotoxicity in MCF-7 cells, other investigators have noted that increased catalase, GSH, and GSHPx levels are not always protective of some cells from doxorubicin-mediated damage.[88] Finally, increased repair of peroxidative damage to DNA and unsaturated lipids represents another potentially protective mechanism against doxorubicin-dependent hydroxyl radical toxicity. For example, some isozymes of GST exhibit significant lipid hydroperoxidase activity and may also contain limited DNA hydroperoxidase activity.[89] Additionally, the highly toxic 4-hydroxy alkenals formed from the decomposition of lipid hydroperoxides are relatively good substrates for some GSTs.[3] Thus overexpression of particular GST isozymes could conceivably contribute to doxorubicin resistance.

The relative importance of free radical generation in tumor cell kill is unknown and the protective mechanisms outlined above are speculative. Nevertheless, the GSH-dependent detoxification pathways are of particular interest as they are subject to pharmacologic manipulation. GSHPx and GST activities can be secondarily reduced by depleting tissue GSH with BSO treatment. Furthermore, the activity of GSTs can be inhibited by the administration of competitive substrates such as ethracrynic acid.[139] Such clinical manipulations may enhance tumorcidal activity of doxorubicin but must be viewed cautiously as they may also potentiate drug toxicity towards normal tissues.

Alkylating Agents and Platinum Compounds

Resistance to alkylating agents and platinum compounds can be described by at least three broad mechanistic categories including decreased drug accumulation, increased drug inactivation, and enhanced repair of DNA damage. Preclinical studies have indicated that the latter two mechanisms may be circumvented by pharmacologic manipulations. Reactions of electrophilic alkylating agents with thiol-containing compounds represent a relatively general mechanism of antineoplastic inactivation or detoxification. For example, GSH forms conjugates with a variety of alkylating agents in both non-enzymatic and in GST-dependent reactions. Table XV-2-4 lists some of the compounds whose conjugation with GSH is catalyzed by GSTs in vitro.[107] Several laboratories have demonstrated an association between increased bulk GST levels or specific GST isozymes with resistance to drugs such as nitrosoureas, chlorambucil and other nitrogen mustards.[21,51,91,119,121,147] Additionally, increased GSH levels have been correlated with resistance to alkylating agents and cisplatin.[73,131] While the electrophilic cisplatin compound can react directly with GSH, it is unknown whether

GSTs can catalyze this reaction. This issue is unresolved by conflicting results, which show a correlation between elevated expression of the pi isozyme of GST and resistance to cisplatin in some cells but not others.[105,108,111]

The correlations between GSH or GST levels and drug resistance are variable. Indeed, some investigators have been unable to demonstrate a relationship between the overexpression of multiple isozymes of GST and antineoplastic resistance.[54,92,108] In other studies that have compared paired parental and resistant cell lines, the magnitude of alkylating agent resistance associated with increased GST activity is often modest. While the clinical importance of GST and GSH in alkylating resistance is accordingly debated, existing preclinical data have prompted phase I trials using GST inhibitors or the GSH synthesis inhibitor BSO in conjunction with alkylating agents.

Aldehyde dehydrogenase is another drug-metabolizing enzyme that has been linked to cyclophosphamide resistance in a murine leukemia model.[36,78] This enzyme converts a metabolite of cyclophosphamide, aldophosphamide to the inactive compound carboxyphosphamide, thereby preventing the decomposition of aldophosphamide to its cytotoxic derivative, phosphoramide mustard. Increased expression of aldehyde dehydrogenase has been associated with resistance to cyclophosphamide in vitro. Whether inhibitors of aldehyde dehydrogenase such as disulfiram and diethylaminobenzaldehyde can be used therapeutically to enhance the antitumor effect of cyclophosphamide without undue host toxicity remains to be explored.

Cisplatin toxicity is thought to be mediated primarily by the formation of lethal intrastrand DNA cross links. Recently, several reports have suggested that increased DNA repair is associated with resistance to this compound. For example, unscheduled DNA synthesis, which is thought to be indicative of DNA repair, is relatively increased in response to cisplatin treatment in cisplatin-resistant ovarian cancer cells when compared with drug-sensitive parental cells.[99] In a murine leukemia model, cells selected for cisplatin resistance showed enhanced ability to repair cisplatin-induced intrastrand DNA cross links.[48,127] Aphidicolin can inhibit an enzyme implicated in DNA repair, DNA polymerase alpha. Treatment of ovarian carcinoma cells with aphidicolin potentiated the toxicity of cisplatin in resistant but not sensitive cells.[99] These results suggest that the coadministration of DNA polymerase alpha inhibitors with cisplatin may be useful in overcoming cisplatin resistance. The results of ongoing phase I trials using the analog aphidicolin glycinate should help clarify the feasibility of this approach.

Antimetabolites

The antimetabolites are a clinically important group of cancer drugs used in the treatment of a variety of solid tumors and hematologic malignancies. The cytotoxicities of the antimetabolites stem from their abilities to interfere with key enzymatic steps in nucleic acid metabolism. The discussion that follows concerns three particularly well-studied compounds, the antifolate methotrexate (MTX) and the pyrimidine analogs 5-fluorouracil (5-FU) and cytosine arabinoside (ara-C, 1-β-D-arabinofuranosylcytosine, cytarabine). Strategies designed to overcome the multiple described mechanisms of cellular

resistance to these compounds include dose escalation, pharmacologic manipulation of drug metabolism, and rational design of new antimetabolites.

The clinically important antifolate MTX displays significant tumoricidal activity against a variety of human neoplasms such as acute leukemia, osteogenic sarcoma, choriocarcinoma, breast cancer, head and neck cancers, and others.[39] Consideration of MTX metabolism and sites of action (Figure XV-2-4) serves as the basis for understanding mechanisms of methotrexate resistance. Following uptake by the folate transport system, MTX can bind avidly to and inhibit its primary enzyme target, dihydrofolate reductase (DHFR). In the presence of adequate thymidylate synthase activity, inhibition of DHFR results in depletion of the reduced folate pools essential for thymidylate and de novo purine synthesis. The cytotoxicity of MTX is significantly influenced by intracellular polyglutamation. MTX polyglutamates are retained preferentially by cells and bind more effectively to DHFR. Additionally, these polyglutamyl derivatives can inhibit other folate-dependent enzymes including thymidylate synthase and 5-aminoimidazole carboxamide ribotide (AICAR) transformylase, enzymes involved in thymidylate and de novo purine synthesis, respectively.[4,5] Therefore, resistance to MTX can result from a number of alternative mechanisms including reduced MTX uptake via a defective folate transport system,[130] reduced polyglutamation leading to decreased drug retention as well as reduced inhibition of thymidylate synthase and AICAR transformylase,[38] and either elevated levels of DHFR or reduced affinity of DHFR for MTX.[6,58,63,101] While all of these mechanisms have been described in examples of experimental resistance of cultured cells to MTX, increased DHFR levels secondary to gene amplification is the only mechanism identified to date that has been associated with clinical MTX resistance.[28,40,143]

The use of high-dose MTX (HDMTX) with subsequent rescue of normal tissues by administration of the reduced folate, leucovorin (N^5-formyl tetrahydrofolate) has been advocated as an approach that could theoretically circumvent most mechanisms of MTX resistance. At high systemic drug concentrations, cytocidal levels can be achieved by passive diffusion of drug into transport-defective resistant cells. Furthermore, prolonged exposure of cells to high extracellular concentrations of drug can maintain cytotoxic intracellular drug levels in the face of a drug retention defect secondary to decreased polyglutamation. Finally, increased intracellular MTX delivered by HDMTX therapy can saturate DHFR in cells whose resistance is due to amplification of the DHFR gene or due to lowered affinity of DHFR for MTX. Although HDMTX is of proven value in the treatment of ALL and perhaps osteogenic sarcoma, the rationale for the use of this modality in the treatment of other cancers has been recently questioned.[1,86] Indeed, some tumors, as well as normal tissues, are rescued from HDMTX toxicity by leucovorin. In these and other cases, the use of HDMTX with leucovorin rescue offers no therapeutic advantage over regimens that use conventional MTX doses. While early studies suggested that HDMTX improved response rates to chemotherapy of osteogenic sarcoma, the contribution of HDMTX therapy to the success of recent multiagent adjuvant protols is unclear.[83] In contrast, HDMTX is indisputably efficacious in the treat-

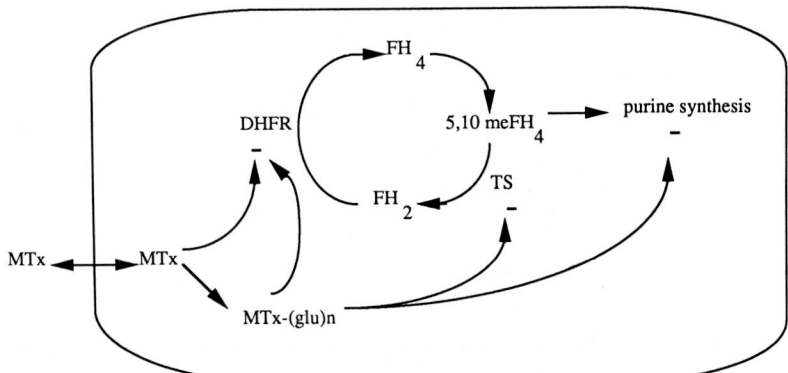

Figure XV-2-4. Methotrexate metabolism and toxicity. MTx, methotrexate; MTx-(glu)n, polyglutamated methotrexate; DHFR, dihydrofolate reductase; TS, thymidylate synthase; FH_2, dihydrofolate; FH_4, tetrahydrofolate; 5,10 meFH_4, 5,10-methylene tetrahydrofolate.

ment of ALL. The success of HDMTX in this setting is probably due to the penetration of drug across anatomic and pharmacologic barriers into tumor sanctuaries such as testes and, at very high MTX doses, the central nervous system.[116]

In an effort to improve drug efficacy, other inhibitors of DHFR such as trimetrexate and piritrexim have been developed.[17,46,93] These lipid-soluble drugs are taken up by cells independently of the folate-carrier system; consequently their use might obviate transport-mediated antifolate resistance. However, cells that are resistant to MTX on the basis of amplified DHFR will be cross-resistant to trimetrexate. The utility of trimetrexate is further limited by the association of classical MDR with cross-resistance to trimetrexate.[11] These results suggest that trimetrexate and drugs of the MDR phenotype share the same P-glycoprotein efflux pump.

Other antifolate compounds capable of inhibiting folate-dependent enzymes besides DHFR have been investigated. One drug, 10-propargyl-5,8-dideazafolate, has shown promise as a thymidylate sythase inhibitor.[82] Another drug with potential clinical utility, 5,10-dideazatetrahydrofolate, is an effective inhibitor of glycinamide ribonucleoside transformylase, the first folate-dependent enzyme in de novo purine synthesis.[15] As these and related antifolates pass through preclinical and clinical testing, they may assume important roles as cytotoxic agents for the treatment of tumors refractory to the conventional antifolate MTX. Cells resistant to MTX by virtue of increased DHFR expression would be expected to remain sensitive to these novel antifolates.

The pyrimidine base 5-FU and its deoxynucleoside metabolite 5-fluoro-2'-deoxyuridine (FdUrd) have been used in the treatment of gastrointestinal tumors, breast cancer, and some other malignacies. The metabolism of 5-FU is complex and

is partially shown in Figure XV-2-5.[10] The best characterized mechanism of fluoropyrimidine cytotoxicity involves the inhibition of thymidylate synthase by 5-fluoro-2'-deoxyuridine monophosphate (FdUMP). Additionally, the incorporation of the metabolite, 5-fluorouridine triphosphate (FUTP), into RNA has been correlated with cytotoxicity in some systems. While 5-fluoro-2'-deoxyuridine triphosphate (FdUTP) can be incorporated into DNA, the relationship between this process and the cytocidal activity of fluoropyrimidines remains undetermined. Resistance to 5-FU may be conferred by alterations in enzymes involved in fluoropyrimidine metabolism, particularly those reactions associated with the conversion of 5-FU to the thymidylate synthase inhibitor FdUMP.[10] Furthermore, changes in thymidylate synthase level or its affinity for FdUMP have been associated with 5-FU resistance.[13,84,118]

Several strategies to improve fluoropyrimidine efficacy and overcome resistance have been advanced. It has been suggested that tumor cell killing may be improved by prolonged or continuous exposure to drug.[26,126] Other studies have advocated the coadministration with 5-FU of the reduced folate leucovorin. The efficacy of this combination stems from leucovorin-dependent increases in intracellular 5,10-methylene tetrahydrofolate (5,10-meTHF), a cofactor that stabilizes the FdUMP-thymidylate synthase inhibitor complex.[9,67] Synergy between 5-FU and other agents that might be exploited clinically has also been studied. For example, pretreatment of cells with methotrexate enhances the toxicity of 5-FU subsequently administered. Such pretreatment with methotrexate, an inhibitor of de novo purine synthesis (see above) has been shown to increase the level of phosphoribosyl pyrophosphate (PRPP). Thus, the expanded pool of PRPP is available for conversion of 5-FU to FUMP and FUTP (Figure XV-2-5). It has been suggested that the increased

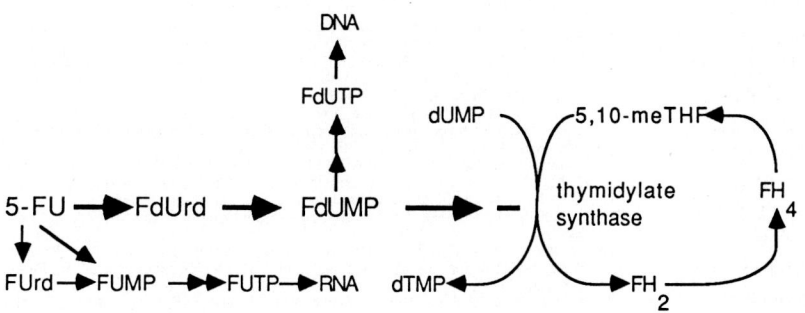

Figure XV-2-5. 5-Fluorouracil metabolism and toxicity. 5-FU, 5-fluorouracil; FdUrd, 5-fluoro-2'-deoxyuridine; FdUMP and FdUTP, 5-fluoro-2'-deoxyuridine mono- and triphosphate; FUrd, 5-fluorouridine; FUMP and FUTP, 5-fluorouridine mono- and triphosphate.

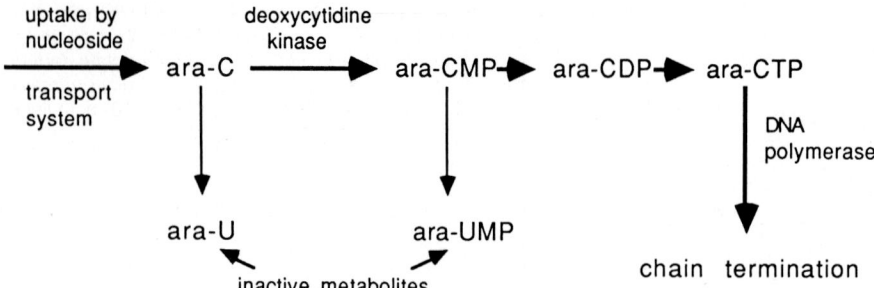

Figure XV-2-6. Cytosine arabinoside (ara-c) metabolism and toxicity.

incorporation of FUTP into RNA that results is responsible for the improved cytotoxicity.[22,23] The inhibitor of de novo pyrimidine synthesis, phosphonacetyl-L-aspartate (PALA), has been used with 5-FU in an effort to reduce pyrimidine metabolites that compete for the targets of fluoropyrimidine toxicity.[68] Finally, the synergistic interaction between interferon and halogenated pyrimidines has been recently investigated.[49]

Ara-C is an important nucleoside antineoplastic agent effective in the treatment of acute leukemias. The metabolism and mechanism of cytotoxicity of ara-C are represented in Figure XV-2-6.[106] Following its uptake by the nucleoside transport system, ara-C is activated by a series of kinases to ara-CTP, a substrate of DNA polymerase that is incorporated into nascent DNA causing premature chain termination and ultimately cell death. The rate-limiting step in ara-C activation is the S-phase specific reaction catalyzed by deoxycytidine kinase. The cytotoxic compound ara-CTP or its precursors (ara-CMP and ara-CDP) can be catabolized by phosphatases or they (ara-C and ara-CMP) can be inactivated by deaminases. Several mechanisms of cancer cell resistance to ara-C have been demonstrated including, but not confined to the following. Because ara-C activation is cell-cycle-dependent, quiescent cells or cells that fail to enter S-phase during the interval of treatment escape the cytotoxicity of ara-C. At suboptimal doses otherwise drug-sensitive tumor cells located in pharmacologic or anatomic sanctuaries may survive ara-C treatment[27] Decreased nucleoside transport has also been implicated in ara-C resistance.[146] Additionally, resistance may be conferred by altered drug metabolism such as decreased activation by deoxycytidine kinase,[106] increased inactivation by cytidine deaminase,[133] or altered DNA polymerase affinity for ara-C.[136]

Administration of high-dose ara-C represents one approach to overcoming resistance to the drug and has been clinically useful in the treatment of some leukemias refractory to conventional doses of ara-C. Resistance based upon diminished nucleoside transport and pharmacologic/anatomic sanctuaries can be circumvented with high-dose drug treatment.[27] In resistance secondary to increased drug inactivation by cytidine deaminase, coadministration with ara-C of a cytidine deaminase inhibitor such as tetrahydrouridine may reverse this mode of drug resistance.[79] The alternative pyrimidine analog, ara-AC (arabinofuranosyl-5-azacytosine, fazarabine), has shown activity against a broad range of tumor cells in preclinical testing and has been the subject of two recently completed phase I clinical trials.[74,135] This compound contains a triazine ring that is resistant to deamination and therefore, should theoretically be effective against tumors

that are resistant to ara-C due to increased cytidine deaminase activity.

Conclusions and Future Directions

Through the kinds of studies done largely in vitro described in this chapter, many of the mechanisms of antineoplastic drug resistance have been identified. While several of these processes operate in vivo, their relative clinical importance must be better clarified in controlled, prospective examinations of patient tumor specimens and correlations with therapeutic responses to chemotherapy. Nevertheless, these mechanisms have suggested potentially useful approaches to overcoming clinical drug resistance. These approaches include the rational choice of conventional agents or design of novel drugs that are less likely to share resistance mechanisms. Additionally, many of the pathways of antineoplastic drug inactivation or transport are targets for pharmacologic manipulations that may reverse or circumvent the resistance of tumors to some drugs. Despite these efforts, many tumors will remain refractory to conventional chemotherapeutic drugs. Their successful treatment may require novel modalities such as biologic response modifiers. For example, the use of cytokines alone or in combination with adoptive immunotherapy, differentiating agents like retinoic acid, and pharmacologic agents capable of altering the responses of tumors to exogenous and autocrine growth factors may hold promise for the treatment of some cancers. Finally, dose escalation of conventional agents followed by hematologic rescue with cytokines or bone marrow transplantation is assuming a greater role in protocols designed to treat a variety of cancers.

References

1. Ackland, S. P., and Schilsky, R. L.: High-dose methotrexate: A critical reappraisal. J. Clin. Oncol., 5:2017, 1987.
2. Akiyama, S., Shiraishi, N., Kuratomi, Y., Nakagawa, M., and Kuwano, M.: Circumvention of multidrug resistance in P388 murine leukemia and its circumvention by calcium antagonists. Cancer Res., 45:1687, 1985.
3. Alin, P., Danielson, U. H., and Mannervick, B.: 4-Hydroxyalk-2-enals are substrates for glutathione transferases. FEBS Lett., 179:267, 1985.
4. Allegra, C. J., Chabner, B. A., and Drake, J. C.: Enhanced inhibition of thymidylate synthase by methotrexate polyglutamates. J. Biol. Chem., 260:9720, 1985.
5. Allegra, C. J., Drake, J. C., Jolivet, J., and Chabner, B. A.: Inhibition of phosphoribosyl aminoimidazole carboxamide transformylase by methotrexate and dihydrofolic acid polyglutamates. Proc. Natl. Acad. Sci. USA, 82:4881, 1985.
6. Alt, F. W., Kellems, R. E., Bertino, J. R., and Schimke, R. T.: Selective multiplication of dihydrofolate reductase genes in methotrexate resistant variants of cultured murine cells. J. Biol. Chem., 253:1357, 1978.
7. Andoh, T., Ishii, K., Suzuki, Y., Ikegami, Y., Kusunoki, Y., and Okada, K.: Characterization of a mammalian mutant with a camptothecin-resistant DNA topoisomerase I. Proc. Natl. Acad. Sci. USA, 84:5565, 1987.
8. Anthony, A. C., Kane, M. A., Portillo, R. M., Elwood, P. C., and Kolhouse, J. F.: Studies of the role of a particulate folate-binding protein in the uptake of 5-methyltetrahydrofolate by cultured human KB cells. J. Biol. Chem., 260:14911, 1985.
9. Arbuck, S. G.: 5-FU/leucovorin: Biochemical modulation that works. Oncology, 1:61, 1987.
10. Armstrong, R. A.: Fluoropyrimidine activity and resistance at the cellular level. In Resistance to Antineoplastic Drugs. Edited by D. Kessel. Boca Raton, FL, CRC Press, 1989, p. 317.
11. Assaraf, Y. G., Molina, A., and Schimke, R. T.: Cross-resistance to the lipid soluble

antifolate trimetrexate in human carcinoma cells with the multidrug-resistant phenotype. J. Natl. Cancer Inst., 81:290, 1989.
12. Baguley, B. C., Holdaway, K. M., and Fray, L. M.: Design of DNA intercalators to overcome topoisomerase II-mediated multidrug resistance. J. Natl. Cancer Inst., 82:398, 1990.
13. Bapat, A. R., Zarow, C., and Danenberg, P. V.: Human leukemic cells resistant to FdUrd contain a thymidylate synthase with lower affinity for nucleotides. J. Biol. Chem., 258:4130, 1983.
14. Bates, S. E., Mickley, L. A., Chen, Y.-N., Richert, N., Rudick, J., Biedler, J. L., and Fojo, A. T.: Expression of a drug resistant gene in human neuroblastoma cell lines: Modulation by retinoic acid-induced differentiation. Mol. Cell. Biol., 9:4337, 1989.
15. Beardsley, G. P., Moroson, B. A., Taylor, E. C., and Moran, R. G.: A new folate antimetabolite, 5,10-dideaza-5,6,7,8-tetrahydrofolate is a potent inhibitor of de novo purine synthesis. J. Biol. Chem., 264:328, 1989.
16. Bell, D. R., Gerlach, J. H., Kartner, N., Buick, R. N., and Ling, V.: Detection of P-glycoprotein in ovarian cancer: A molecular marker associated with multidrug resistance. J. Clin. Oncol., 3:311, 1985.
17. Bertino, J. R.: Folate antagonists: Toward improving the therapeutic index and development of new analogs. J. Clin. Pharmacol., 30:291, 1990.
18. Bessho, F., Kinumaki, H., Kobayashi, M., Habu, H., Nakamura, K., Yokota, S., Tsuruo, T., and Kobayashi, N.: Treatment of children with refractory acute lymphocytic leukemia with vincristine and diltiazem. Med. Pediatr. Oncol., 13:199, 1985.
19. Biedler, J. L., and Riehm, H.: Cellular resistance to actinomycin D in Chinese hamster ovary cells in vitro: Cross resistance, radioautographic, and cytogenetic studies. Cancer Res., 30:1174, 1970.
20. Brockmann, R. W.: Mechanisms of resistance to the anticancer agents. Adv. Cancer Res., 7:129, 1963.
21. Buller, A. L., Clapper, M. L., and Tew, K. D.: Glutathione S-transferases in nitrogen mustard-resistant and -sensitive cell lines. Mol. Pharmacol., 31:1987.
22. Cadman, E., Heimer, R., and Davis, L.: The influence of methotrexate pretreatment on 5-fluoroucil metabolism in L1210 cells. J. Biol. Chem., 256:1695, 1981.
23. Cadman, E., Heimer, R., and Davis. L.: Enhanced 5-fluorouracil nucleotide formation after methotrexate: Explanation for drug synergism. Science, 205:1135, 1979.
24. Cadman, E. C.: The selective transfer of drug-resistant genes in malignant cells. *In* Resistance to Antineoplastic Drugs. Edited by D. Kessel. Boca Raton, FL, CRC Press, 1989, p. 167.
25. Cairo, M. S., Siegel, S., Arias, N., and Sender, L.: Clinical trial of continuous infusion verapamil, bolus vinblastine and continuous infusion VP-16 in drug-resistant pediatric tumors. Cancer Res., 49:1063, 1989.
26. Calabro-Jones, P. M., Byfield, J. E., Ward, J. F., and Sharp, T. R.: Time-dose relationship for 5-fluorouracil toxicity against human epithelial cancer cells in vivo. Cancer Res., 42:4413, 1982.
27. Capizzi, R. L., Yang, J. I., Rathmell, J. P., White, J. C., Cheng, E., Cheng, Y. C., and Kute, T.: Dose-related pharmacologic effects of high-dose ARA-C and its self potentiation. Semin. Oncol., 12 (Suppl. 3):65, 1985.
28. Carman, M. D., Schornagel, J. H., Rivest, R. S., Srimatkandada, S., Portlock, C. S., Duffy, T., and Bertino, J. R.: Resistance to methotrexate due to gene amplification in a patient with acute leukemia. J. Clin. Oncol., 2:16, 1984.
29. Chambers, T. C., McAvoy, E. M., Jacobs, J. W., and Eilon, G.: Protein kinase C phosphylates P-glycoprotein in multidrug resistant human KB carcinoma cells. J. Biol. Chem., 265:7679, 1990.
30. Chan, H. S., Thorner, P. S., Haddad, G., and Ling, V.: Immunohistochemical detection of P-glycoprotein: Prognostic correlation in soft tissue sarcoma of childhood. J. Clin. Oncol., 8:689, 1990.
31. Chen, C., Chin, J. E., Ueda, K., Clark, D. P., Pastan, I., Gottesman, M. M., and Roninson, I. B.: Internal depletion and homology with bacterial transport proteins in the mdr 1 gene for multidrug-resistant human cells. Cell, 47:381, 1986.
32. Chen, Y.-N., Mickley, L. A., Schwartz, A. M., Acton, E. M., Hwang, J., and Fojo, A. T.: Characterization of Adriamycin resistant human breast cancer cells which display overexpression of a novel resistance-related membrane protein. J. Biol. Chem., 265:10073, 1990.
33. Chin, K., Tanaka, S., Darlington, G., Pastan, I., and Gottesman, M. M.: Heat shock and arsenate increase expression of multidrug resistance (MDR 1) gene in human renal carcinoma cells. J. Biol. Chem., 265:221, 1990.
34. Chin, K.-V., Chauhan, S. S., Pastan, I., and Gottesman, M. M.: Regulation of mdr RNA levels in response to cytotoxic drugs in rodent cells. Cell Growth Differ., 1:361, 1990.
35. Choi, K. H., Chen, C. J., Kriegler, M., and Roninson, I. B.: An altered pattern of cross-resistance in multidrug-resistant human cells results from spontaneous mutations in the mdr1 (P-glycoprotein) gene. Cell, 53:519, 1988.
36. Colvin, M., Russo, J. E., Hilton, J., Dulik, D. M., and Fenselau, C.: Enzymatic mechanisms of resistance to alkylating agents in tumor cells and normal tissues. Adv. Enz. Regul., 27:211, 1988.
37. Cowan, K. H., Batist, G., Tulpule, A., Sinha, B. K., and Myers, C. E.: Similar biochemical changes associated with multidrug resistance in human breast cancer cells and carcinogen-induced resistance to xenobiotics in rats. Proc. Natl. Acad. Sci. USA, 83:9328, 1986.
38. Cowan, K. H., and Jolivet, J.: A methotrexate resistant human breast cancer cell line with multiple defects including diminished formation of methotrexate polyglutamates. J. Biol. Chem., 259:10793, 1984.
39. Curt, G. A., and Allegra, C. J.: Methotrexate resistance: Mechanisms and implications. *In* Resistance to Antineoplastic Drugs. Edited by D. Kessel. Boca Raton, FL, CRC Press, 1989, p. 369.
40. Curt, G. A., Carney, D. N., Cowan, K. H., Jolivet, J., Bailey, B. D., Drake, J. C., Kao-Shan, C. S., Minna, J., and Chabner, B. A.: Unstable methotrexate resistance in human small cell carcinoma associated with double minute chromosomes. N. Engl. J. Med., 308:199, 1983.
41. Dalton, W. S., Grogan, T. M., Meltzer, P. S., Scheper, R. J., Durie, B. G., Taylor, C. W., Miller, T. P., and Salmon, S. E.: Drug resistance in multiple myloma and non-Hodgkin's lymphoma: Detection of P-glycoprotein and potential circumvention by addition of verapamil to chemotherapy. J. Clin. Oncol., 7:415, 1989.
42. Dalton, W. S., Grogan, T. M., Rybski, J. A., Scheper, R. J., Richter, L., Kailey, J., Broxterman, H. J., Pinedo, H. M., and Salmon, S. E.: Immunohistochemical detection and quantitation of P-glycoprotein in multiple drug-resistant human myeloma cells: association with level of drug resistance and drug accumulation. Blood, 73:747, 1989.
43. Danks, M. K., Schmidt, C. A., Cirtain, M. C., Suttle, D. P., and Beck, W. T.: Altered catalytic activity of and DNA cleavage by DNA topoisomerase II from human leukemia cells selected for resistance to VM-26. Biochemistry, 27:8861, 1988.
44. Deffie, A. M., Batra, J. K., and Goldenberg, G. J.: Direct correlation between DNA topoisomerase II activity and cytotoxicity in Adriamycin-sensitive and resistant P388 leukemia cell lines. Cancer Res., 49:58, 1989.
45. Drahovsky, D., and Kreis, W.: Studies on drug resistance. II. Kinase Patterns in P815 neoplasms sensitive and resistant to 1-β-D-arabinofuranosyl cytosine. Biochem. Pharmacol, 19:940, 1970.
46. Duch, D. S., Edelstein, M. P., Bowers, S. W., and Nichol, C. A.: Biochemical and chemotherapeutic studies on 2,4-diamino-6-(2,5-dimethoxybenzyl)-5-methylpyrido-[2,3-d] pyrimidine (BW 301U), a novel lipid-soluble inhibitor of dihydrofolate reductase. Cancer Res., 42:3987, 1982.
47. Dusre, L., Mimnaugh, E. G., Myers, C. E., and Sinha, B. K.: Potentiation of doxorubicin cytoxicity by butathionine sulfoximine in multidrug-resistant human breast cancer cells. Cancer Res., 49:511, 1989.
48. Eastman, A., and Schulte, N.: Enhanced DNA repair as a mechanism of resistance to cis-diammine dichloroplatinum (II). Biochemistry, 27:4730, 1988.
49. Elias, L., and Crissman, H. A.: Interferon effects upon the adenocarcinoma MCA 38 and HL-60 cell lines. Antiproliferative responses and synergistic interactions with halogenated pyrimidine antimetabolites. Cancer Res., 48:4868, 1988.
50. Endicott, J. A., and Ling, V.: The biochemistry of P-glycoprotein-mediated multidrug resistance. Annu. Rev. Biochem, 58:137, 1989.
51. Evans, C. G., Bodell, W. J., Tokuda, K., Doane-Setzer, P., and Smith, M. T.: Glutathione and related enzymes in rat brain tumor cell resistance to 1,3-bis(2-chloroethyl)-1-nitrosourea and nitrogen mustard. Cancer Res., 47:2525, 1987.
52. Fairchild, C. R., Ivy, S. P., Kao-Shaw, C.-S., Whang-Peng, J., Rosen, N., Israel, M. A., Melera, P. W., Cowan, K. H., and Goldsmith, M. E.: Isolation of amplified and overexpressed DNA sequences from adriamycin-resistant human breast cancer cells. Cancer Res., 47:5141, 1987.
53. Fairchild, C. R., Ivy, S. P., Rushmore, T., Lee, G., Koo, P., Goldsmith, M. E., Myers, C. E., Farber, E., and Cowan, K. H.: Carcinogen-induced mdr overexpression is associated with xenobiotic resistance in rat preneoplastic liver nodules and hepatocellular carcinomas. Proc. Natl. Acad. Sci. USA, 84:7701, 1987.
54. Fairchild, C. R., Moscow, J. A., O'Brien, E. E., and Cowan, K. H.: Multidrug resistance in cells transfected with human genes encoding a variant P-glycoprotein and glutathione S-transferase-pi. Mol. Pharmacol., 37:801, 1990.
55. Farber, E.: Cellular biochemistry of the stepwise development of cancer with chemicals. Cancer Res., 44:5463, 1984.
56. Finlay, G. J., Baguley, B. C., Snow, K., and Judd, W.: Multiple patterns of resistance of human leukemia cell sublines to amsacrine analogues. J. Natl. Cancer Inst., 82:662, 1990.
57. Fitzgerald, D. J., Willingham, M. C., Cardarelli, C. O., Hamada, H., Tsuruo, T., Gottesman, M. M., and Pastan, I.: Monoclonal antibody–Pseudomonas toxin conjugate that specifically kills multidrug-resistant cells. Proc. Natl. Acad. Sci. USA, 84:4288, 1987.
58. Flintoff, W. F., and Essani, K.: Methotrexate-resistant Chinese hamster ovary cells contain a dihydrofolate reductase with an altered affinity for methotrexate. Biochemistry, 19:4321, 1980.
59. Giovanella, B. C., Stehlin, J. S., Wall, M. E., Wani, M. C., Nicholas, A. W., Liu, L. F., Silber, R., and Potmesil, M.: DNA topoisomerase I-targeted chemotherapy of human colon cancer in xenografts. Science, 246:1046, 1989.
60. Glisson, B., Gupta, R., Smallwood-Kentro, S., and Ross, W.: Characterization of acquired epipodophyllotoxin resistance in a Chinese hamster ovary cell line: Loss of drug-stimulated DNA cleavage activity. Cancer Res., 46:1934, 1986.
61. Glisson, B. S.: Multidrug resistance mediated through alterations in topoisomerase II. Cancer Bull., 41:37, 1989.
62. Goldenberg, G. J., Vanstone, C. L., Isreals, L. G., Isle, D., and Bihler, D.: Evidence for a transport carrier of nitrogen mustard in nitrogen mustard-sensitive and -resistant L5178Y lymphoblasts. Cancer Res., 30:2285, 1970.
63. Goldie, J. H., Krystal, G., Hartley, D., Gudauskas, G., and Dedhar, S.: A methotrexate insensitive variant of folate reductase present in two lines of methotrexate resistant L5178Y cells. Eur. J. Cancer, 16:1539, 1980.
64. Goldstein, L. J., Fojo, A. T., Ueda, K., Crist, W., Green, A., Brodeur, G., Pastan, I., and Gottesman, M. M.: Expression of the multidrug resistant, MDR1, gene in neuroblastoma. J. Clin. Oncol., 8:128, 1990.
65. Goldstein, L. J., Galski, H., Fojo, A., Willingham, M., Lai, S.-L., Gazdar, A., Pirker, R., Green, A., Crist, W., Brodeur, G. M., Lieber, M., Cossman, J., Gottesman, M. M., and Pastan, I.: Expression of a multidrug resistance gene in human cancers. J. Natl. Cancer Inst., 81:116, 1989.
66. Gottesman, M. M., and Pastan, I.: Resistance to multiple chemotherapeutic agents in human cancer cells. Trends Pharmacol. Sci., 9:54, 1988.
67. Grem, J. L., Hoth, O. F., Hamilton, J. M., King, S. A., and Leyland-Jones, B.: Overview of current status and future direction of clinical trials with 5-fluorouracil in combination with folinic acid. Cancer Treat. Rep., 71:1249, 1987.
68. Grem, J. L., King S.A., O'Dwyer, P. J., and Leyland-Jones, B.: Biochemistry and clinical activity of N-(phosphonacetyl)-L-aspartate: A review. Cancer Res., 48:4441, 1988.
69. Gros, P., Ben Neriah, Y., Croop, J. M., and Houseman, D. E.: Isolation and expression of a complementary DNA that confers multidrug resistance. Nature, 323:728, 1986.
70. Gros, P., Croop, J., and Houseman, D.: Mammalian multidrug resistant gene: Complete cDNA sequence indicates strong homology to bacterial transport proteins. Cell, 47:371, 1986.
71. Gupta, R. S.: Genetic, biochemical, and cross-resistance studies with mutants of Chinese hamster ovary cells resistant to anticancer drugs, VM-26 and VP-16-213. Cancer Res., 43:1568, 1983.
72. Haber, D. A., Beverly, S. M., Kiely, M. L., and Schimke, R. T.: Properties of altered dehydrofolate reductase encoded by amplified genes in cultured mouse fibroblasts. J. Biol. Chem., 256:9501, 1981.
73. Hamilton, T. C., Ozols, R. F., and Dabrow, M. B.: Multidrug resistance to alkylating agents and platinum compounds: State of our knowledge. Oncology, 4:101, 1990.
74. Heideman, R. L., Gillespie, A., Ford, H., Reaman, G. H., Balis, F. M., Tan, C., Sato, J., Ettinger, L. W., Packer, R. J., and Poplack, D. G.: Phase I trial and pharmacokinetic evaluation of fazarabine in children. Cancer Res., 49:5213, 1989.
75. Hill, B. T., Bailey, B. D., White, J. C., and Goldman, I. D.: Characteristics of transport of 4-amino antifolates and folate compounds by two cell lines of LY5178Y lymphoblasts, one with impaired transport of methotraxate. Cancer Res., 39:2440, 1979.
76. Hill, B. T., Deuchars, K., Hosking, L. K., Ling, V., and Whelan, R. D.: Overexpression of P-glycoprotein in mammalian tumor cell lines after fractionated X irradiation in vitro. J. Natl. Cancer Inst., 82:607, 1990.
77. Hill, B. T., Price, L. A., and Goldie, J. H.: The value of adriamycin in overcoming resistance to methotrexate in cell culture. Eur. J. Cancer, 12:541, 1976.
78. Hilton, J.: Role of aldehyde dehydrogenase in cyclophosphamide-resistant L1210 leukemia. Cancer Res., 44:5156, 1984.
79. Ho, D. H., Carter, C. J., Brown, N. S., Hester, J., McCredie, K., Benjamin, R. S., Freireich, E. J., and Bodey, G. P.: Effects of tetrahydrouridine on the uptake and

metabolism of 1-β-D-arabinofuranosylcytosine in human normal and leukemic cells. Cancer Res., 40:2441, 1980.
80. Houghton, J. A., Maroda, S. J., Phillips, J. O., and Houghton, P. J.: Biochemical determents of responsiveness to 5-fluorouracil and its derivatives in xenografts of human colorectal adenocarcinomas in mice. Cancer Res., 41:144, 1981.
81. Hunt, S. W., and Hoffee, P. A.: Amplification of adenosine deaminase gene sequence in deoxycoformycin-resistant rat hepatoma cells. J. Biol. Chem., 258:13185, 1983.
82. Jackson, R. C., Jackman, A. L., and Calvert, A. H.: Biochemical effects of a quinazoline inhibitor of thymidylate synthase, CB3717, on human lymphoblastoid cells. Biochem. Pharmacol., 32:3783, 1983.
83. Jaffe, N., Link, M. P., Cohen, D., Traggis, D., Frei, E., Watts, H., Beardsley, G. P., and Abelson, H. T.: High dose methotrexate in osteogenic sarcoma. NCI Monogr., 56:201, 1981.
84. Jenh, C. H., Geyer, P. K., Baskin, F., and Johnson, L. F.: Thymidylate synthase gene amplification in fluorodeoxyuridine resistant mouse cell lines. Mol. Pharmacol., 28:80, 1985.
85. Juliano, R. L., and Ling, V.: A surface glycoprotein modulating drug permeability in Chinese hamster ovary cell mutants. Biochem. Biophys. Acta, 455:1252, 1976.
86. Kamen, B. A., and Winick, N. J.: High dose methotrexate therapy: Insecure rationale? Biochem. Pharmacol., 37:2713, 1988.
87. Keith, W. N., Stallard, S., and Brown, R.: Expression of mdr1 and GST π in human breast tumors: Comparison to in vitro sensitivity. Br. J. Cancer, 61:712, 1990.
88. Keizer, H. G., Rijn, J., Pinedo, H. M., and Joenje, H.: Effect of endogenous glutathione, superoxide dismutase, catalase, and glutathione peroxidase on Adriamycin tolerance of Chinese hamster ovary cells. Cancer Res., 48:4493, 1988.
89. Ketterer, B., Tan, K. H., Meyers, D. J., and Coles, B.: Glutathione transferases: A possible role in the detoxification of DNA and lipid hydroperoxides. *In* Glutathione S-transferases and Carcinogenesis. Edited by T. J. Mantle, C. Pickett, and J. D. Hayes. London, Taylor and Francis, 1987, p. 149.
90. Kramer, R. A., Zakher, J., and Kim, G.: Role of glutathione redox cycle in acquired and de novo multidrug resistance. Science, 241:694, 1988.
91. Lewis, A. D., Hickson, I. D., Robson, C. N., Harris, A. L., Hayes, J. D., Griffiths, S. A., Manson, M. M., Hall, A. E., Morris, J. E., and Wolf, C. R.: Amplication and increased expression of alpha class glutathione S-transferase-encoding genes associated with resistance to nitrogen mustards. Proc. Natl. Acad. Sci. USA, 85:8511, 1988.
92. Leyland-Jones, B. R., Townsend, A. J., Tu, C.D., Cowan, K. H., and Goldsmith, M. E.: Antineoplastic drug sensitivity of human MCF-7 breast cancer cells stably transfected with a human alpha class glutathione S-transferase gene. Cancer Res., 51:587, 1991.
93. Lin, J. T., and Bertino, J. R.: Trimetrexate: a second generation folate antagonist in clinical trial. J. Clin. Oncol., 5:2032, 1987.
94. Liu, L.: DNA topoisomerase poisons as antitumor drugs. Annu. Rev. Biochem., 58:351, 1989.
95. Ma, D. D., Scurr, R. D., Davey , R. A., Mackertich, S. M., Dowden, G., and Bell, D. R.: Detection of a multidrug resistant phenotype in acute non-lymphoblastic leukaemia. Lancet, 1:135, 1987.
96. Mannervik, B., and Danielson, U. H.: Glutathione transferases-structure and catalytic activity. Crit. Rev. Biochem., 23:283, 1988.
97. Marquardt, D., McCrone, S., and Center, M. S.: Mechanisms of multidrug resistance in HL60 cells: Detection of resistance-associated proteins with antibodies against synthetic peptides that correspond to the deduced sequences of P-glycoprotein. Cancer Res., 50:1426, 1990.
98. Marsh, W., and Center, M.: Adriamycin resistance in HL60 cells and accompanying modification of a surface membrane protein contained in drug-sensitive cells. Cancer Res., 47:5080, 1987.
99. Masuda, H., Ozols, R. F., Gi-Ming, L., Fojo, A., Rothenberg, M., and Hamilton, T. C.: Increased DNA repair as a mechanism of acquired resistance to cis-diamminedichloroplatinum (II) in human ovarian cancer cell lines. Cancer Res., 48:1988.
100. McGrath, T., Latoud, C., Arnold, S. T., Safa, A. R., Felsted, R. L., and Center, M. S.: Mechanisms of multidrug resistance in HL60 cells. Analysis of resistance associated membrane proteins and levels of mdr gene expression. Biochem. Pharmacol., 38:3611, 1989.
101. Melera, P. W., Lewis, J. A., Biedler, J. L., and Hession, C.: Antifolate resistant Chinese hamster cells. J. Biol. Chem., 255:7024, 1980.
102. Mickisch, G., Bier, H., Bergler, W., Bak, M., Tschada, R., and Alken, P.: P-170 glycoprotein, glutathione and associated enzymes in relation to chemoresistance of primary human renal cell carcinomas. Urol. Int., 45:170, 1990.
103. Mickley, L. A., Bates, S. E., Richert, N. D., Currier, S., Tanaka, S., Foss, F., Rosen, N., and Fojo, A. T.: Modulation of the expression of a multidrug resistance gene (mdr1/P-glycoprotein) by differentiating agents. J. Biol. Chem., 264:18031, 1989.
104. Miller, R. L., Bukowski, R. M., Budd, G. T., Purvis, J., Weick, J. K., Shepard, K., Midha, K. K., and Ganapathi, R.: Clinical modulation of deoxorubicine resistance by the calmodulin-inhibitor trifluoperazine: A phase I/II trial. J. Clin. Oncol., 6:880, 1988.
105. Miyazaki, M., Kohno, K., Saburi, Y., Matsuo, K., Ono, M., Kuwano, M., Tsuchida, S., Sato, K., Sakai, M., and Muramatsu, M.: Drug resistance to cis-diammine dichloroplatinum (II) in Chinese hamster ovary cell lines transfected with glutathione S-transferase pi gene. Biochem. Biophys. Res. Commun., 166:1358, 1990.
106. Momparle, R. L., and Oretto-Pothier, N.: Drug Resistance to Cytosine Arabinoside. *In* Resistance to Antineoplastic Drugs. Edited by D. Kessel. Boca Raton, FL, CRC Press, 1989, p. 353.
107. Morrow, C. S. and Cowan, K. H.: Glutathione S-transferases and drug resistance. Cancer Cells, 2:15, 1990.
108. Moscow, J. A., Townsend, A. J., and Cowan, K.H.: Elevation of the π class glutathione S-transferase activity in human breast cancer cells by transfection of the GSTπ gene and its effect on sensitivity to toxins. Mol. Pharmacol., 36:22, 1989.
109. Myers, C. E., Mimnaugh, E., Yeh, G., and Sinha, B. K.: Biochemical mechanisms of tumor cell kill by the anthracyclines. *In* Anthracyclines and Anthracenedione-Based Anticancer Agents. Edited by J. W. Lown. Amsterdam, Elsevier, 1988.
110. Nakagawa, K., Saijo, N., Tsuchida, S., Sakai, M., Tsunokawa, Y., Yokota, J., Muramatsu, M., Sato, K., Tekada, M., and Tew, K. D.: Glutathione S-transferase π as a determinant of drug resistance in transfectant cell lines. J. Biol. Chem., 265:4296, 1990.
111. Nakagawa, K., Yokota, J., Wada, M., Sasaki, Y., Fujiwara, Y., Saki, M., Muramatsu, M., Terasaki, T., Tsunokawa, Y., Terada, M., and Saijo, N.: Levels of glutathione S-transferase pi mRNA in human lung cancer cell lines correlate with the resistance to cisplatin and carboplatin. Jpn. J. Cancer Res., 79:301, 1988.
112. Ohtsu, T., Ishida, Y., Tobinai, K., Minato, K., Hamada, H., Ohkodu, E., Tsuruo, T., and Shimoyama, M.: A novel multidrug resistance in cultured leukemia and lymphoma cells detected by a monoclonal antibody to 85kDa protein, MRK20. Jpn. J. Cancer Res., 80:1133, 1989.
113. Ozols, R. F., Cunnion, R. E., Klecker, R. W., Hamilton, T. C., Ostchega, Y., Parrillo, J. E., and Yang, R. C.: Verapamil and Adriamycin in the treatment of drug-resistant ovarian cancer patients. J. Clin. Oncol., 5:641, 1987.
114. Per, S.-R., Mattern, M. R., Mirabelli, C. K., Drake, F. H., Johnson, R. K., and Crooke, S. T.: Characterization of a subline of P388 leukemia resistant to amsacrine: Evidence of altered topoisomerase II function. Mol. Pharmacol., 32:17, 1987.
115. Pommier, Y., Kerrigan, D., Schwartz, R. E., Swack, J. A., and A., M.: Altered DNA topoisomerase II activity in Chinese hamster cells resistant to topoisomerase II inhibitors. Cancer Res., 46:3075, 1986.
116. Poplack, D. G., and Reaman, G.: Acute lymphoblastic leukemia in childhood. Pediatr. Clin. North Am., 35:903, 1988.
117. Presant, C. A., Kennedy, P. S., Wiseman, C., Gala, K., Bouzaglon, A., Wyres, M., and Naessig, V.: Verapamil reversal of clinical doxorubicin resistance in human cancer. A Wilshire Oncology Medical Group pilot phase I-II study. Am. J. Clin. Oncol., 9:355, 1986.
118. Priest, D. G., Ledford, B. E., and Day, M. T.: Increased thymidylate synthase in FdUrd resistant cultured hepatoma cells. Biochem. Pharmacol., 29:1549, 1980.
119. Puchalski, R. B., and Fahl, W. E.: Expression of recombinant glutathione S-transferase π, Ya or Yb1 confers resistance to alkylating agents. Proc. Natl. Acad. Sci. USA, 87:2443, 1990.
120. Riordan, J. R., and Ling, V.: Genetic and biochemical characterization of multidrug resistance. Pharmacol. Ther., 28:51, 1985.
121. Robson, C. N., Lewis, A. D., Wolf, C. R., Hayes, J. D., Hall, A., Proctor, S. J., and Harris, A. L. Hickson, I. D.: Reduced levels of drug-induced DNA cross-linking in nitrogen mustard-resistant Chinese ovary cells expressing elevated glutathione S-transferase activity. Cancer Res., 47:6022, 1987.
122. Rothenberg, M. L., Mickley, L. A., Cole, D. E., Balis, F. M., Tsuruo, T., Poplack, D., and Fojo, A. T.: Expression of the mdr1 gene/P-170 gene in patients with acute lymphoblastic leukemia. Blood, 74:1388, 1989.
123. Safa, A. R., Glover, C. J., Meyers, M. B., Biedler, J. L., and Felsted, R. L.: Vinblastine photoaffinity labeling of a high molecular weight surface membrane glycoprotein specific for multidrug-resistant cells. J. Biol. Chem., 261:6137, 1986.
124. Sato, H., Gottesman, M. M., Goldstein, L. J., Pastan, I., Block, A., Sandberg, A. A., and Preisler, H. D.: Expression of the multidrug reistance gene in myeloid leukemias. Leuk. Res., 14:11, 1990.
125. Schneider, J., Bak, M., Efferth, T. H., Kaufmann, M., Mattren, J., and Volm, M.: P-glycoprotein expression in treated and untreated breast cancer. Br. J. Cancer, 60:815, 1989.
126. Seifert, P., Baker, L. H., Reed, M. L., and Vaitkevicious, V. K.: Comparison of continuously infused FUra with bolus injection in treatment of patients with colorectal carcinoma. Cancer, 36:123, 1975.
127. Sheibani, N., Jennerwein, M. M., and Eastman, A.: DNA repair in cells sensitive and resistant to cis-diamine dichloroplatinum (II): host cell reactivation of damaged plasmid DNA. Biochemistry, 28:3120, 1989.
128. Sinha, B. K.: Free radicals in anticancer drug pharmacology. Chem. Biol. Interact., 69:293, 1989.
129. Sinha, B. K., Katki, A. G., Batist, G., Cowan, K. H., and Myers, C. E.: Differential formation of hydroxy radicals by Adriamycin in sensitive and resistant MCF-7 human breast cancer tumor cells: Implications for the mechanism of action. Biochemistry, 26:3776, 1987.
130. Sirotnak, F. M., Moccio, D. M., Kelleher, L. E., and Goutsas, L. J.: Relative frequency and kinetic properties of transport defective phenotypes among methotrexate-resistant L1210 clonal cell lines derived in vivo. Cancer Res., 41:4447, 1981.
131. Somfai-Relle, S., Suzukake, K., Vistica, B. P., and Vistica, D. T.: Reduction in cellular glutathione by buthionine sulfoximine and sensitization of murine tumor cells to L-phenylalamine mustard. Biochem. Pharmacol., 33:485, 1984.
132. Staats, J., Marquardt, D., and Center, M. S.: Characteristics of a membrane-associated protein kinase of multidrug-resistant HL60 cells which phosphorylates P-glycoprotein. J. Biol. Chem., 265:4084, 1990.
133. Steuart, C. D., and Burke, P. J.: Cytidine deaminase and the development of resistance to cytosine arabinoside. Nature New Biol., 233:109, 1971.
134. Stewart, D. J., and Evans, W. K.: Non-chemotherapeutic agents that potentiate chemotherapy efficacy. Cancer Treat. Rev., 16:1, 1989.
135. Surbone, A., Ford, H., Jr., Kelley, J. A., Ben-Baruch, N., Thorn, R. V., Fine, R., and Cowan, K. H.: Phase I and pharmacokinetic study of arabinofuranosyl-5-azacytosine (fazarabine, NSC 281272). Cancer Res., 50:1220, 1990.
136. Tanaka, M., and Yoshida, S.: Altered sensitivity to 1-β-D-arabinofuranosylcytosine 5′-triphosphate of DNA polymerase from leukemia blasts of acute lymphoblastic leukemia. Cancer Res., 42:649, 1982.
137. Teicher, B. A., Cucchi, C. A., Lee, J. B., Flatow, J. L., Rosowsky, A., and Frei, E., III: Alkylating agents : In vitro studies of cross-resistance patterns in human cell lines. Cancer Res., 46:4379, 1986.
138. Teicher, B. A., Herman, T. S., Holden, S. A., Wang, Y., Pfeffer, M. R., Crawford, J. W., and Frei, E., III: Tumor resistance to alkylating agents conferred by mechanisms operative only in vivo. Science, 247:1457, 1990.
139. Tew, K. D., Bomber, A. W., and Hoffman, S. J.: Ethracrynic acid and piriprost as enhancers of cytotoxicity in drug resistant cell lines. Cancer Res., 48:3622, 1988.
140. Thorgeirsson, S. S., Huber, B. E., Sorrel, S., Fojo, A., Pastan, I., and Gottesman, M. M.: Expression of the multidrug-resistant gene in hepatocarcinogenesis and regenerating liver. Science, 236:1120, 1987.
141. Tong, A. W., Lee, J., Wang, R-M., Dalton, W. S., Tsuruo, T., Fay, J.W., and Stone, M. J.: Elimination of chemoresistant multiple myeloma clonogenic colony forming cells by combined treatment with a plasma cell-reactive monoclonal antibody and a P-glycoprotein-reactive monoclonal antibody. Cancer Res., 49:4829, 1989.
142. Townsend, A. J., and Cowan, K. H.: Glutathione S-transferases and antineoplastic drug resistance. Cancer Bull., 41:31, 1989.
143. Trent, J. M., Buick, R. N., Olson, S., Horns, R. C., and Schimke, R. T.: Cytologic evidence for gene amplification in methotrexate resistant cells obtained from a patient with ovarian adenocarcinoma. J. Clin. Oncol., 2:8, 1984.
144. Tsuruo, T., Iida, H., Yamashiro, M., Tsukagoshi, S., and Sakurai, Y.: Enhancement of vincristine- and adriamycin-induced cytoxicity by verapamil in P388 leukemia and its sublines resistant to vincristine and adriamycin. Biochem. Pharmacol., 31:3138, 1982.
145. Ueda, K., Cardarelli, C., Gottesman, M. M., and Pastan, I.: Expression of a full-length cDNA from the human mdr 1 gene confers resistance to colchicine, doxorubicin, and vinblastine. Proc. Natl. Acad. Sci. USA, 84:3004, 1987.

146. Wiley, J. S., Jones, S. P., Sawyer, W. H., and Paterson, A. R.: Cytosine arabinoside influx and nucleoside transport sites in acute leukemia. J. Clin. Invest., 69:479, 1982.
147. Wolf, C. R., Hayward, I. P., Lawrie, S. S., Buckton, K., McIntyre, M. A., Adams, D. J., Lewis, A. D., Scott, A.R., and Smyth, J.F.: Cellular heterogeneity and drug resistance in two ovarian adenocarcinoma cell lines derived from a single patient. Int. J. Cancer, 39:695, 1987.
148. Zhang, H., D'Arpa, P., and Liu, L. F.: A model for tumor cell killing by topoisomerase poisons. Cancer Cells, 2:23, 1990.
149. Zwelling, L. A., Hinds, M., Chan, D., Mayes, J., Sie, K. L., Parker, E., Silberman, L., Radcliffe, A., Beran, M., and Blick, M.: Characterization of an amsacrine-resistant line of human leukemia cells. Evidence for a drug-resistant form of topoisomerase II. J. Biol. Chem., 264:16411, 1989.

XV-3

Combination Chemotherapy, Dose, and Schedule

Emil Frei III
Karen H. Antman

Introduction

The identification of novel, clinically active agents has been central to progress in cancer chemotherapy. The optimal use of such agents, of which some forty have been identified over the past thirty years, has been crucial.

Dose can be a critical determinant of the antitumor activity and toxicology for most chemotherapeutic agents.[26] This is not true for the majority of hormonal agents; the situation with biotherapeutics is complex (see below).

The schedule of drug administration may be important to the therapeutic index, independent of dose. For example, cytokinetic studies of experimental and clinical leukemia have led to the improved use of agents such as arabinosyl-cytosine.[60,61]

Finally, combination chemotherapy has been critical to the development of curative regimens for the hematologic malignancies, for pediatric solid tumors, for testis cancer, and for many adjuvant and neoadjuvant regimens.[21] Combination chemotherapy trials have derived from studies of the development of drug resistance.[36] Thus, clinical trials conducted in the 1950s of combination antimicrobial therapy for tuberculosis,[48] and an emerging understanding of tumor cell heterogeneity particularly with respect to drug resistance,[56] have influenced cancer therapeutic strategy, particularly including combination chemotherapy.

Dose

Dose must be expressed per unit time—that is, dose intensity or dose rate.[35] Dose intensity is a deceptively simple concept. There are numerous factors which influence the dose effect. The major ones are illustrated in Figure XV-3-1, A through J and are considered below.

Cytokinetics of the Bone Marrow. Because of its cytokinetic activity, bone marrow toxicity is dose limiting for many cancer chemotherapeutic agents. The effect of a cell cycle specific agent (CSA) such as ara-C, given for 24 hours to mice, produces in the spleen colony assay the curves presented in Figure XV-3-1A.[8] With increasing doses, the ara-C effect plateaus at approximately 10% because that proportion of bone marrow stem cells is out of mitotic cycle during any given 24 hour period in the mouse. This applies not only to ara-C but to other cell cycle specific agents as well. On the other hand, agents which are non-cycle dependent such as the alkylating agents and many of the antitumor antibiotics produce a steep dose response curve that is maintained through multiple logs of normal bone marrow stem cell kill (Figure XV-3-1A).[8]

Dose Schedule. The effect of the schedule of ara-C is presented in Figure XV-3-1B. The top curve is a repeat of the top curve in Figure XV-3-1A. If ara-C, on the other hand, is continued for three days, a greater bone marrow stem cell kill occurs, presumably as a result of a greater flux of cells into mitotic cycle during the longer exposure. This is true as well for the other cell cycle specific agents.

Tumor Cell vs. Normal Stem Cell. In Figure XV-3-1C, non cell cycle specific agents, and perhaps cell cycle specific agents administered over a matter of days, may produce a linear dose response curve with a greater effect on tumor stem cells as compared to bone marrow stem cells. This presumably reflects intrinsically greater sensitivity on the part of tumor cells—therefore a better therapeutic index. On the other hand, when the bone marrow stem cells and the tumor stem cells are equally sensitive (Figure XV-3-1D), the situation is less favorable.[8]

Intrinsic Tumor Cell Sensitivity. The effect of agents on an insensitive tumor are compared to those on a sensitive tumor in Figure XV-3-1E.[23,26] If unit dose produces a 0.5 log kill, then a doubling of that dose may produce a 1.0 log kill—a limited achievement at best. Clinically, it would represent a partial remission. A doubling of the dose could markedly increase toxicity. On the other hand, in a sensitive tumor wherein unit dose produces a 2 log kill, a doubling of the dose may produce a 3–4 log kill.[60] This is a major achievement in terms of a complete response and duration of complete response and, most importantly, is on the way to cytoeradication—that is, cure. These data may explain why clinical studies generally demonstrate a major dose effect for sensitive hematologic and embryonal neoplasms as compared to the less sensitive common epithelial tumors where the dose effect is less evident.

Drug Resistance. Drug resistance may have a profound

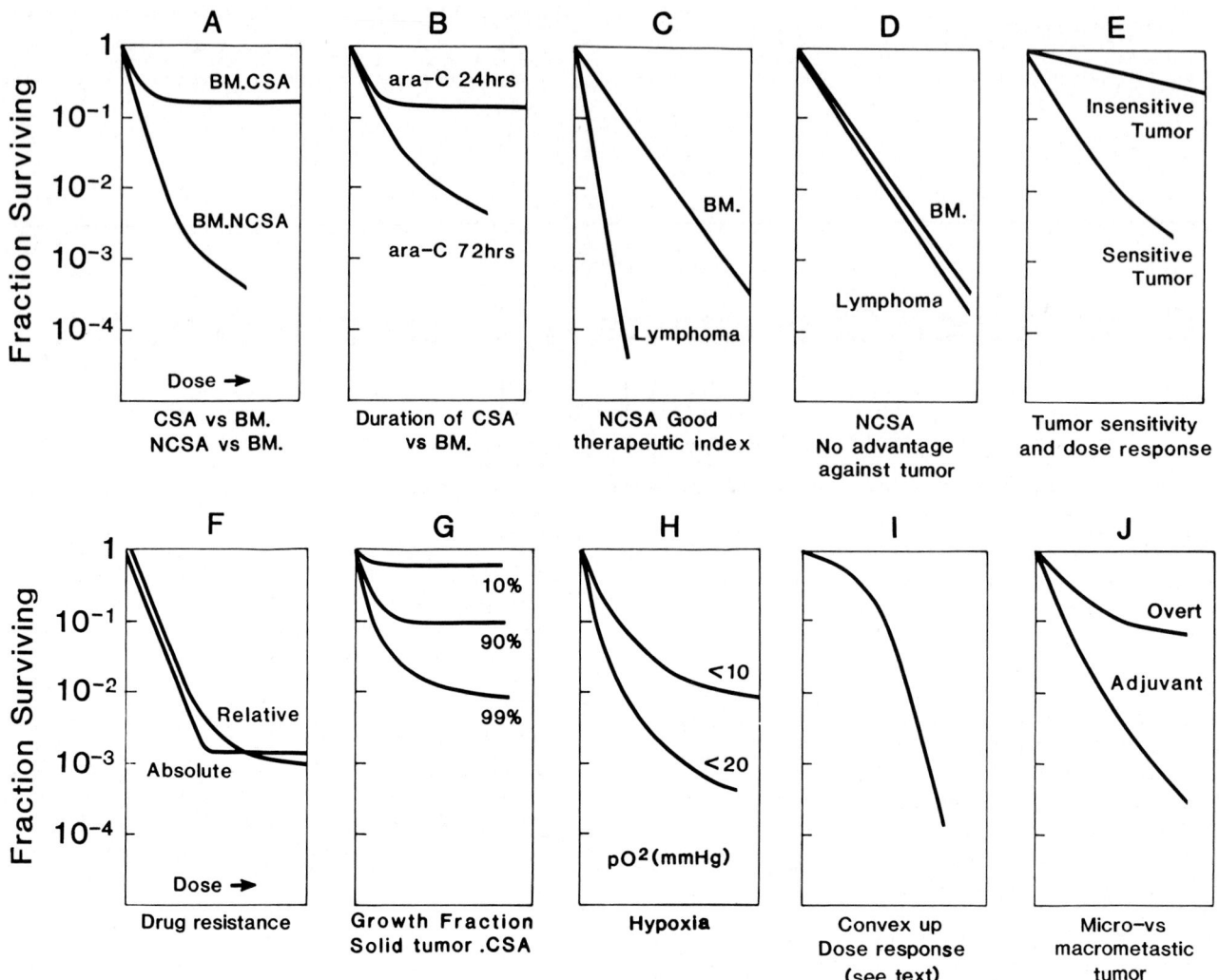

Figure XV-3-1. Some of the variables that influence the dose effect. The ordinate represents the fraction of tumor cells or bone marrow stem cells surviving. The abscissa is labelled and generally represents linear increase in dose. For some of the boxes, the data are direct, such as boxes A, B, and C which are taken from Bruce;[6] the fractional surviving stem cells represent spleen colonies. For the other boxes, the data are representative of a composite of studies. See text for details. CSA = cell cycle specific agent, e.g., ara-C Mtx, hydroxyurea; NCSA = noncycle specific agent, e.g., alkylating agents; BM = bone marrow.

Drug Resistance. Drug resistance may have a profound influence on the dose effect (Figure XV-3-1F). Theoretical calculations of the impact of drug resistance on the dose effect often assume that resistance is total, irreversible, and occurs as a result of selection. These considerations for a situation where one cell in 1000 (10^{-3}) were resistant would lead to the absolute resistance curve (Figure XV-3-1F). Resistance is almost always dose related. Indeed, in vivo and in patients, the two- or three-fold increase in resistance may render the tumor refractory. Given the fact that tumor cell resistance is variable with respect to dose and quite certainly variable with respect to reversibility, the more damped curve (relative resistance) in Figure XV-3-1F is more appropriate.[27]

Growth Fraction. The effect of growth fraction on dose curves is presented in Figure XV-3-1G. Tritiated thymidine autoradiographic studies of experimental tumors found that the volume doubling time was in excess of the generation time of cycling cells.[42] This led to the observation that many

cells within tumors are "non-cycling," that is, in G1 or G0 or commonly, particularly after injury, in G2. This was referred to as "low" growth fraction.[41] Such cells would be markedly less sensitive to cell cycle specific agents and variably less sensitive to other cancer chemotherapeutic agents. In Figure XV-3-1G, for a solid tumor with a growth fraction of, for example, 10%, cell cycle specific agents would be minimally effective, killing approximately 10% of the cells. Alkylating agents on the other hand might produce a somewhat greater log kill but still with an attenuated curvilinear killing rate. High growth fractions (90%, 99%) are associated with greater log kill with cell cycle specific chemotherapy. The growth fraction may be improved experimentally by reducing tumor size with, for example, alkylating agents. The resultant smaller tumors have a disproportionately better blood supply. As result, the growth fraction increases, and the tumor becomes more sensitive to chemotherapy.[41]

Hypoxia. As solid tumors increase in size, there is a relative decrease in blood supply.[22] This will result in a slower growth curve) due presumably to a limitation in oxygen and metabolite supply. This is the major reason for the low growth fraction. Correction of hypoxia increases sensitivity to radiotherapy some three- to five-fold. More recently, this has been found to be true for a number of chemotherapeutic agents. In Figure XV-3-1H, the control curve and the curve after correction of hypoxia experimentally with perfluorocarbon oxygen breathing is presented.[65,66]

Convex-Up Curves. A convex upward curve, representing an increasing fractional tumor cell kill with increasing dose, is presented in Figure XV-3-1I. Such curves have rarely been observed experimentally and rarely occur clinically though they probably would be missed in vivo. Such curves might result from pharmacokinetic factors. For example, if a drug inactivation process becomes saturated, the area under the plasma curve (AUC) of the active agent would increase disproportionately with dose, and the curve as seen in Figure XV-3-1I could occur. Such pharmacology has been observed with fluorouracil.[12,53]

Clinically, for slow-growing tumors, reduction in tumor size as a function of treatment may be delayed and have the appearance of the curve in Figure XV-3-1I. On the other hand, where tumor stem cell assays have been employed, the curve is log linear with dose.[62] This presumably results in the delay and clearing of dead tumor and related stromal tissues. It is also true that for many agents, tumor cells can be rendered clonogenically dead and may undergo several cycles of replication before delayed death and resorption occurs.

Thirdly, the curve in Figure XV-3-1I resembles x-ray survival curves, somewhat, wherein the shoulder is a function of DNA repair. Potential lethal damage repair has been described for a variety of preclinical models and could explain a curve such as that in Figure XV-3-1I.[68]

Finally, there could be a microenvironmental effect. If treatment reduces tumor size only slightly with resultant improvement in growth fraction and oxygen saturation, increasing sensitivity could be observed. This would probably be seen with successive cycles of chemotherapy, however, and not within one cycle.

Adjuvant Chemotherapy

It is almost axiomatic for neoplasia that the greater the tumor burden, the worse the prognosis. This is because macroscopic tumor burdens are, as a function of increasing size, increasingly adversely affected by essentially all factors including tumor cell number, growth fraction, hypoxia, diminished blood supply, heterogeneity, and drug resistance. In the adjuvant situation where chemotherapy addresses micrometastatic disease, however, these factors are eliminated or very much reduced (Figure XV-3-1J). Accordingly, much more effective killing curves can be achieved in experimental in vivo studies and may be inferred from clinical studies.[23]

Hryniuk has conducted a number of sophisticated retrospective studies of dose intensity for a variety of tumors. He has found steep dose response curves in essentially all situations including sensitive hematologic neoplasms but also in the relatively less sensitive tumors such as breast cancer. These results await confirmatory prospective studies.[34,35]

There have been relatively few clinical studies wherein dose intensity was an independent randomized variable. The first such study was performed in patients with Hodgkin's disease and non-Hodgkin's lymphoma wherein patients were randomized to full dose or to half dose of an alkylating agent. It was found that full dose was significantly superior, producing a 60% objective response rate as compared to 10% for half dose. Toxicity was also increased.[7] A similar study with similar results was conducted in patients with lymphoma using folic acid antagonists.[28] In acute lymphocytic leukemia, it was found that the dose rate of maintenance chemotherapy had a major impact on the duration of response.[47] Similarly, in studies of combination chemotherapy of small-cell lung cancer, the dose effect was major.[11] On the other hand, the dose effect is more difficult to achieve in patients with chemotherapy-resistant epithelial solid tumors for reasons presented in Figure XV-3-1E. A recent comparative study in patients with metastatic breast cancer provided evidence for improved response and quality of life in patients randomized to the higher dose.[64] Two randomized comparative studies of dose in the breast cancer adjuvant situation are ongoing.[9,44]

Autologous Bone Marrow Transplantation

Perhaps the most compelling evidence with respect to dose response relates to bone marrow transplantation (Table XV-3-1).[24,67] The alkylating agents and total body radiotherapy are most commonly employed in this situation since dose limiting toxicity is myelosuppressive. Thus, a major (5–20-fold) increase in dose intensity can be delivered before non-myelosuppressive toxicity becomes dose limiting (Table XV-3-1). In this setting, 40–60% of patients with metastatic melanoma and colorectal cancer respond to alkylating agents as compared to standard response rates of 10–20%.[15] In the transplant situation, total body radiotherapy plus cyclophosphamide produces a 50% cure rate in selected patients in first complete remission with acute myelogenous leukemia as do intensification programs involving, for example, busulphan plus cyclophosphamide.[51] Allogeneic (see XIX-2) or autologous bone marrow transplantation (See XIX-1) produces significant disease-free survival plateaus (cures) in patients with previously treated Hodgkin's disease (see XIX-9), non-Hodgkin's lymphoma (See XIX-10), and acute lymphocytic leukemia (See XIX-5). This approach is currently being employed in patients with metastatic breast cancer, high risk primary breast cancer, testis cancer, ovarian cancer, and small-cell lung cancer. It may be concluded from these latter studies in solid tumor patients that high response rates, including complete response rates, can be achieved. Improved survival has not yet been demonstrated however. Toxicity can be major, and this approach should be limited to specialized centers.[3,4,24,32,45]

From the practical point of view, the clinical take-home message is that dose deserves major emphasis in diseases wherein curative intent treatment is possible. Thus for the leukemias, the lymphomas, testis cancer, childhood solid tumors, and the adjuvant treatment of, for example, breast cancer, every effort should be made not to compromise dose

Table XV-3-1. Dose: Standard and Intensive with Marrow Transplantation

| Agent | Dose (MG/M²) | | | Disease | Response (CR + PR) | | |
	Standard	Transplant	Ratio		Standard Dose %	Transplant Dose %	(CR)
BCNU	150	600–900	5	Melanoma	17	40–70	(10%)
PAM	35	180–240	6	Melanoma	12	40–60	(15%)
PAM	35	180–240	6	Colorectal	<10	40–50	(5%)
CPA	600	5,000–7,000	10	—	—	—	—
TSPA	50	900–1,150	20	Melanoma	10	50	(11%)
TBI & CPA	—	—	>5	AML	0	50	CURE
CPA & Busulfan	—	—	>5	AML	0	50	CURE

From Dicke,[15] Frei,[24] Santos,[51] and Thomas[67]

even at the risk of significant toxicity. On the other hand, with the more resistant tumors where palliative intent chemotherapy is underway, dose should be adjusted primarily on the basis of side effects (toxicity). With the major dose increases made possible by bone marrow transplantation, significant cure rates can be achieved in some patients who have relapsed after standard therapy.

Schedule of Drug Administration

Prior to 25 years ago, it was generally thought that chemotherapy should be delivered at maximum safe doses—that is, to definite (albeit limited) toxicity, and that the schedule of administration made little difference. Experimentalists had long known that the therapeutic index of chemotherapeutic agents could be affected by the schedule of drug administration.[29]

Cytarabine. Skipper and Schabel performed elegant, quantitative studies in L1210 mouse leukemia of the prototype cell cycle phase specific agent arabinosyl-cytosine (ara-C).[60,61] They observed that the generation time of the L1210 cells was 12 hours; that the growth fraction approached 100%; and thus, that treatment over a 24 hour period would allow for essentially all of the leukemia cells to enter S—that is, the ara-C sensitive phase of the cycle. They and others observed that ara-C given over a 24 hour period resulted in a plateau of the dose toxicity curve (Figure XV-3-1B), presumably because of resting cells in the bone marrow, and that by 3–4 days the marrow completely recovered. Twenty-four hour continuous exposure to ara-C at 4-day intervals did not produce cumulative toxicity.[60] This schedule, presumably for these cytokinetic reasons, produced a far greater therapeutic index for ara-C in mouse in vivo L1210 leukemia than, for example, longer durations of treatment or other schedules such as daily administration. Clarkson observed that 5–7 days of continuous infusion of tritiated thymidine to patients with AML resulted in the labelling of well over 90% of leukemic cells, indicating that this fraction had entered DNA synthesis some time over the 5–7 day period.[10] Thus for AML continuous infusion for 5–7 day courses, with a 2–3 week interrupt, was extrapolated from the aforementioned preclinical and cytokinetic studies. This treatment produced a 30–40% complete remission rate, as compared to 10% for other schedules such as daily intravenous administration.[5,19]

Methotrexate. Five day courses of intensive methotrexate were developed by Li for gestational choriocarcinoma and proved curative.[38] Goldin demonstrated in L1210 mouse leukemia that intermittent methotrexate was superior to continuous (daily) methotrexate.[29] In a randomized comparative study of patients with acute lymphocytic leukemia (ALL) in complete remission, intermittent methotrexate proved to be significantly superior to daily therapy.[58] This observation, empirical at the time, is consistent with recent findings by Schimke indicating that for methotrexate, continuous exposure is the most effective way of producing drug resistance as compared to intermittent methotrexate. Moreover, with continuous infusion, the resistance relates to gene amplification as compared to a transport defect following intermittent methotrexate.[50,54]

Fluoropyrimidines. In clinical studies, fluorouracil (FU) has classically been administered by daily pulse doses for five days. When treatment is given by continuous infusion over five days, twice the dose can be delivered, and mucositis and diarrhea become dose limiting as compared to bone marrow suppression.[57] Fluorodeoxyuridine (FUDR) delivered by continuous infusion is much more toxic. For example, doses in the range of 30–50 mg/M² per day produce toxicity. The biochemical basis for these schedule differences is speculative. There is some evidence that FUDR, given by continuous infusion, has a greater effect on DNA synthesis, whereas the other schedules have a relatively greater effect on host tissue RNA and RNA synthesis.[31] There are, however, relatively few data to the effect that these differences in schedule make a difference with respect to therapeutic index. (For modulation with leucovorin, see below.) Longer durations of systemic administration are under study.[40]

Anthracyclines. Cardiotoxicity is an important form of delayed toxicity for the anthracyclines. There is experimental evidence to the effect that peak concentrations are more likely to produce cardiotoxicity than lower concentrations given on a more continuous basis. The first clinical trial suggesting a dose schedule effect was the observation by Weiss that weekly administration of adriamycin produced less cardiotoxicity per given total dose than the standard tri-weekly regimens.[69] Benjamin has demonstrated that the continuous administration of adriamycin for 2–4 day courses every three weeks is less cardiotoxic.[37] These approaches allow for a 30–50% increase in total dose. There is experimental evidence that liposomal adriamycin is less cardiotoxic.

Alkylating Agents. Most of the data with respect to the

alkylating agents suggests that they are schedule independent—that is, the antitumor and host effects are dose related, independent of schedule.

Nausea and Vomiting. There is evidence that the emetogenic effect of some agents relates to peak concentration. This is particularly true for azacytidine which, at 150 mg/M²/day × 5d, produces major nausea and vomiting. The same dose rate given as a continuous infusion for 120 hours is well tolerated and produces the same antileukemic effect. There is evidence that continuous infusion cisplatin may be less emetogenic than the same total dose given by bolus injection.[30]

Intermittent Intensive Treatment

In experimental systems and in man there is evidence that, for most chemotherapeutic agents used alone or in combination, intermittent courses of treatment are superior to continuous, i.e., daily treatment. Though definitive studies have not been performed in most instances, data supporting this position exist with respect to cyclophosphamide and methotrexate in Burkitt's lymphoma,[21] methotrexate and actinomycin D in choriocarcinoma,[21] melphalan in myeloma, ara-C in acute myelocytic leukemia, and methotrexate in remission maintenance in acute lymphocytic leukemia.[47] It is also true for most combination regimens, such as MOPP treatment for Hodgkin's disease,[14] combination chemotherapy for acute myelocytic leukemia,[5] and the combination chemotherapy (usually including cyclophosphamide, actinomycin D, and vincristine) for childhood solid tumors (see XXXV-1, XXXIX-1A, and XXXIX-8).

Experimental and clinical studies indicate superiority of intermittent intensive treatment for the rapidly proliferating tumors. There is evidence that continuous treatment may be superior for the more slow-growing, low-growth fraction tumors, but more definitive studies are needed.[40]

In addition to the foregoing cytokinetic and pharmacologic rationale, there is evidence that immunologic factors may, in part, explain the superior effect of intermittent treatment. The various facets of immune response, as affected by five-day courses of intensive single-agent or combination chemotherapy given every three to four weeks, have been studied.[6,33] Although the various parameters of immune response were reported to be greatly suppressed by five-day courses of intensive treatment, immunologic recovery was brisk and usually complete by the tenth day following treatment. For continuous daily treatment with cancer chemotherapeutic agents, immunosuppression initially is less intense, but tends to be sustained and progressive.[33] Consistent with these reports is the evidence that intermittent treatment results in fewer infections with organisms of low pathogenicity.

Combination Chemotherapy

Rationale

The most compelling pragmatic rationale for combination chemotherapy has been its success. Essentially all curative regimens for clinically overt neoplasia involve combinations.[21] This is true for the acute leukemias, Hodgkin's and non-Hodgkin's lymphoma, testis cancer, and the childhood

solid tumors. In addition, in the adjuvant situation, combination chemotherapy would appear to be superior to single agents for breast cancer and definitely for osteogenic sarcoma.[21]

Criteria for the definition of combination chemotherapy and for its effectiveness are important. In the clinic, combinations often include agents whose toxicity is qualitatively different and therefore not additive, whereas the therapeutic effect is additive. For example, prednisone and 6-mercaptopurine (6-MP) can be delivered at full doses in combination to children with acute lymphocytic leukemia. The complete response rate for 6-MP is 35%, for prednisone, 50%, and for the combination, 83%. Thus the therapeutic effect is additive, the toxicity is non-additive, and the end result has been called either synergistic or additive.[20] It is important that the therapeutic effect be expressed for equal cost in toxicity. There are some circumstances where combinations have produced a greater therapeutic effect than a single component of the combination, but the cost in toxicity for the combination was greater. Under those circumstances, both the therapeutic effect and the toxicity may be additive, but the overall therapeutic effect inferior.

In experimental systems, elaborate and mathematical approaches to defining additive effects, synergy, antagonism, and other results have been developed. The isobologram is an in vitro approach to the evaluation of two agents employed in combination (Figure XV-3-2). Equi-cytotoxic effect doses (ED) of drugs 1 and 2 are expressed on the coordinates. A straight line between the extremes, wherein ED_{50} of drug 1 + ED_{50} of drug 2 is always the total of ED_{50} of

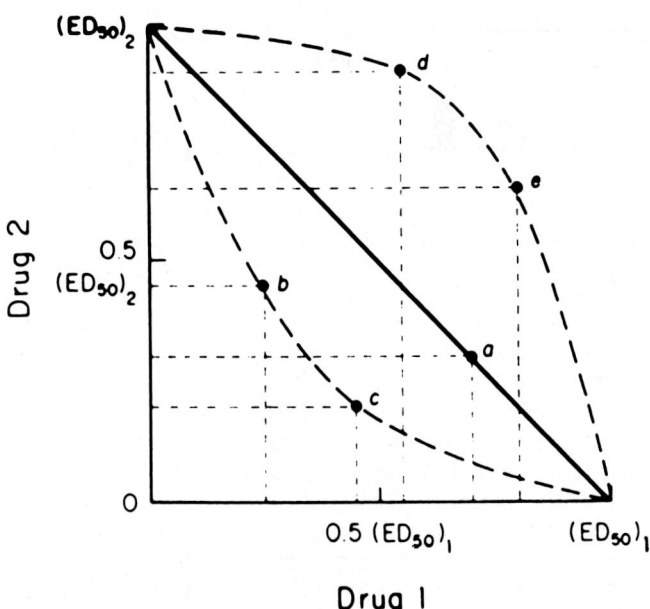

Figure XV-3-2. The classical ED_{50}-isobologram depicting the additive, synergistic, and antagonistic effects of two drugs. When an experimental combination data point falls on the hypotenuse, e.g., point *a*, the effects of two drugs are additive. If experimental combination data points fall in the lower left, e.g., *b* and *c*, then the effects of the two drugs are synergistic. If the data points fall in the upper right, e.g., *d* and *e*, the effects of the two drugs are antagonistic.

either drug 1 or 2, is additive. A concave curve is synergistic and a convex, antagonistic. This technique allows for looking at different ratios of combinations (Figure XV-3-2). The isobologram has been modified in a number of ways, particularly in the direction of simplicity for the evaluation of in vivo studies. This literature has been superbly reviewed recently by Rideout and Chou.[49]

Additional Rationale

There are several other compelling components of the rationale for combination chemotherapy:

Biochemistry. Metabolic pathways to essential cellular constituents such as nucleic acids can be blocked at sequential points or at concurrent points in two biochemical pathways. Complementary blockade is defined as inhibition of the metabolic pathway, as well as damage to the final product by a second agent. Such considerations provide a major conceptual framework for combination chemotherapy. Unfortunately, with relatively few exceptions, this approach has not provided greater selectively, i.e., a greater toxic effect to tumor as compared to host.[52] For other biochemical approaches, see Modulation below.

Tumor Cell Heterogeneity and Drug Resistance. The most compelling basic rationale for combination chemotherapy (or any form of systemic therapy, e.g., endocrine, biotherapy) is tumor cell heterogeneity. While tumors are clonal in origin, the increasing DNA instability that accompanies the onset of neoplasia, leads to increased variation of daughter cells with selection of tumor cells with greater survival capacity, such as greater metastatic or invasive potential, and of tumor cells with a higher proliferative thrust. Heterogeneity among tumor cells with respect to a target site for chemotherapy (for example, dihydrofolate reductase) will lead to the selection of resistant clones. Such heterogeneity has also been demonstrated for hormone receptors and for surface antigens. Thus the selection of resistant cell lines by systemic hormonal manipulation and by biotherapeutics including monoclonal antibody therapy is likely. It used to be thought that monodrug resistance occurred, that is, resistance obtained only for the selecting agent. The recognition of multidrug resistance requires a re-examination of the approach to combination chemotherapy.[39] Thus P-glycoprotein multidrug resistance relates almost exclusively to natural products, but there is increasing evidence that glutathione transferase and topoisomerase II alterations may also be associated with multidrug resistance. It still remains to be determined whether such multidrug resistance is operational at the low levels of resistance (2- to 4-fold) necessary for clinical relevance. (See XV-2).[56]

In support of the combination chemotherapy approach, clinical trials indicate that combinations of agents are essential to prevent the development of resistance in tuberculosis and to provide a markedly improved therapeutic effect.[48] The same is true in a number of other infectious disease situations.

Assume that drug A results in the selection of one resistant tumor cell out of a total of 10^4 cells (10^{-4}). A second drug B produces a similar effect. The same with drug C. Then theoretically, drug A plus B plus C at full doses (and assuming no cross resistance) would produce a $(10^{-4})^3$, i.e., a 10^{-12}

effect. If, on the other hand, drugs A and B and C are totally cross resistant, then A plus B plus C would still select 10^{-4} resistant tumor cells, and the maximal tumor cell reduction would be 10^{-4}. In experimental systems, data suggest that the truth is in between, in part because of partial, perhaps multidrug, cross resistance.[39,55] Clearly, experimental studies concerning mechanisms of sensitivity and resistance, and particularly cross resistant patterns, will increasingly influence the construct of combination chemotherapy, including modulation (see below).

Dose Preservation. Dose is a critical factor in the therapeutic effect. If, on the other hand, one has to modify dose substantially for agents used in combination, the potential advantage gained by the combination may be lost because of suboptimal dose. Accordingly, drugs with non-overlapping dose-limiting toxicity, wherein dose can be maintained in the combination, may be required for full realization of potential of the combination.[26] This was first appreciated in acute lymphocytic leukemia where the combination of methotrexate and 6-mercaptopurine produced a slight increase in complete response rate but required a 50% dose reduction for each agent because of overlapping myelosuppression. On the other hand, vincristine and prednisone, and 6-mercaptopurine and prednisone, could be combined at full dose resulting in a 90% complete response rate—a synergistic effect.[21] The MOPP program in Hodgkin's disease, the PEB (cisplatin, etoposide, bleomycin) program for testis cancer, and the programs employed for non-Hodgkin's lymphoma commonly use agents which can be employed at full or nearly full doses because of non-additivity of toxicity.[21]

These two factors, dose preservation and tumor cell heterogeneity, provide the most important basis for the success of combination chemotherapy.

Cytokinetics. The appreciation that solid tumors contained a large number of potentially clonogenic cells that were in G1 or G0, provided a basis for combination chemotherapy.[63] (See tumor hypoxia and growth fraction above.) Thus cell cycle specific agents were employed for cytotoxicity to mitotically active cells, and agents that were not cell cycle specific such as BCNU were added to damage the non-cycling portion of the growth fraction.

Recruitment. Experimentally in vivo, one can "recruit" tumor cells into cycle by reducing tumor size with non-cell-cycle specific chemotherapy. This probably results from a relative improvement in blood supply and therefore an increased growth fraction. This increases susceptibility to cell cycle specific agents. While this approach has been widely employed, it is not proven that such sequential scheduling does in fact provide an improvement in the therapeutic index.

Synchronization. It is possible with inhibitors of DNA synthesis, or with drugs that arrest cells in mitosis, to synchronize cells in vitro and experimentally in vivo, and to exploit this synchronization with a cell cycle phase specific agent. Unfortunately, such approaches may synchronize host target cells such as the bone marrow as well, thus providing no improvement in the therapeutic index.

A rationale for recruitment and perhaps synchronization is provided by hormone dependent tumors. Thus Allegra has conducted several studies in patients with metastatic breast cancer where the cells were arrested cytokinetically with tamoxifen, then pulse-stimulated into cycle with an estrogen. There is experimental and limited clinical evidence that some degree of synchrony of tumor cells follows this hormonal manipulation. Chemotherapy is ideally delivered at the time of maximum synchronization into mitosis. However, the heterogeneity of human tumors with respect to the time course of synchronization and recruitment has been a major problem and this approach remains experimental.[2]

Pharmacologic Rationale for Combination Chemotherapy. Perhaps the first important clinical example here was the use of leucovorin to supply the product of the enzyme dihydrofolate reductase when inhibited by methotrexate. There is no question that this approach does in fact rescue the host and allows for the delivery of gram quantities of methotrexate safely, provided that the patient is carefully monitored and that rescue with leucovorin is applied appropriately. More commonly, intermediate doses (in the range of 200–400 mg/M^2) are employed. There is only one disease, osteogenic sarcoma, wherein methotrexate with leucovorin rescue is clearly superior to standard methotrexate. High-dose methotrexate with rescue is not only highly effective against the primary tumor and against metastatic disease, but it also provides a core component of the highly successful adjuvant approach.[1,25] (See XXXV-1.)

Non-Hodgkin's lymphoma provides a setting for understanding the methotrexate rescue approach. Skarin demonstrated in patients with advanced refractory non-Hodgkin's lymphoma that high-dose methotrexate with rescue produced a 50–60% response rate and a low complete response rate.[59] This was comparable in terms of response rate to older studies using methotrexate only. However, if properly monitored pharmacologically and toxicologically, the high-dose methotrexate leucovorin rescue can be delivered without toxicity and particularly without important myelosuppression. This was the basis for combining it with other combination chemotherapy regimens (M-BACOP, m-BACOP). While the response rate for single institution studies of this program was superior to BACOP or CHOP, this difference has not been confirmed by comparative studies though the latter are difficult to interpret because of several variables. In diseases such as breast cancer or head and neck cancer, high or intermediate dose methotrexate with rescue is effective and when integrated with combination chemotherapy, might be more effective. However, such has not been conclusively demonstrated. Indeed, studies in patients with head and neck cancer comparing high-dose methotrexate with intermediate or even low-dose methotrexate have not shown an advantage for the former (see XXVII-1).

Leucovorin rescue after methotrexate, properly applied, precludes toxicity. This is true if rescue is delivered by 24 hours. At 36 or 42 hours, such rescue is often incomplete and toxicity can be major. The biochemical and biological rationale for high-dose methotrexate with rescue has been the subject of several studies and much discussion, but remains uncertain.[1]

Sanctuary Sites. Sanctuary sites such as the central nervous system may be a basis for combination chemotherapy. Thus, intrathecal methotrexate and whole brain irradiation has been effective in markedly reducing the incidence of meningeal leukemia.[46] This can also be accomplished, perhaps not quite as well, with high-dose methotrexate and LCV rescue which provides cytotoxic concentrations in the cerebrospinal fluid. It can also be accomplished with combination intrathecal therapy.[46]

Modulation. Of ascending importance has been the modulation approach. A modulator ideally is an agent which of itself is non-toxic, but which, based generally on a biochemical rationale, may improve the therapeutic index of a given chemotherapeutic agent.

A clinically successful example is fluorouracil modulated by leucovorin. The biochemical rationale is that the product of FU, FdUMP, binds to the substrate site of thymidylate synthase, thus inhibiting DNA synthesis and therefore cellular replication. The stability and duration of this inhibition is directly related to a third agent, 5–10 methylene-tetrahydrofolate, a metabolic product of leucovorin, which also binds to thymidylate synthase producing the so-called ternary complex (FdUMP-TS-5-10 methylene-tetrahydrofolate). In preclinical systems in vitro and in vivo, leucovorin can favorably modulate the therapeutic index of fluorouracil. In clinical trials, four studies comparing FU to FU + leucovorin indicate an advantage for the latter in patients with metastatic colorectal cancer. In this setting, FU produces a 5–15% response rate and FU + leucovorin a 30–50% response rate; two studies indicate improved survival.[16] There is now uncontrolled evidence in patients with head and neck cancer and with metastatic breast cancer that FU modulated with leucovorin is superior to FU alone.[17] Leucovorin moderately increases the host effect in the form of mucositis and diarrhea. This promising approach is now being applied to other tumors. Why there should be an increase in therapeutic effect as compared to toxicity is not known.

Another interesting approach to modulation involves multidrug resistance. Verapamil and a number of other lipid soluble heterocycle drugs can inhibit p-glycoprotein and thus decrease efflux of a number of natural antitumor products (doxorubicin, vincristine, and others) from the cell, thereby increasing the cytotoxicity. An increase in p-glycoprotein has been demonstrated in patients with B cell tumors, acute myeloid leukemia, and sarcoma. A clinical study in myeloma wherein patients refractory to vincristine and adriamycin with increased p-glycoprotein were treated with the same combination plus verapamil will be watched with considerable interest.[13]

The modulation of alkylating agents and cisplatin is under study. Glutathione may combine chemically with alkylating agents, thus diminishing their activity. Glutathione production can be decreased by the inhibitor buthionine sulfoximine—an approach which preclinically improves the therapeutic index of a number of alkylating agents.[43] Similarly, glutathione transferase, which mediates the aforementioned conjugation, can be inhibited by several agents. Hypoxia in solid tumors can be modulated experimentally by perfluorocarbon-oxygen breathing and by oxygen mimics such as the nitroimidazoles (see XIII). Finally, inhibitors of DNA repair will increase the effectiveness of alkylating agents experimentally.[18]

Biotherapeutics and Endocrine Therapy

The effect of dose schedule and combination therapy for biotherapeutics is under study and will be represented elsewhere and discussed briefly here (see XVIII). The mechanisms of antitumor action of biological agents such as tumor necrosis factor, the interferons, and IL-2, are complex. The effects on immune and inflammatory response may be responsible for their antitumor effects. In addition, the interferons and TNF are directly cytotoxic to tumor cells in culture, and thus, in addition to immune and inflammatory modulation, these agents have a direct cancer cell antiproliferative effect. While it was hoped that these agents might be employed with limited or no toxicity in the clinic, such has not proven to be the case. Indeed for most of these agents (IL2, interferons, and TNF) there is a positive correlation between dose and toxicity and, where antitumor effect has been observed, a dose effect can be demonstrated. It has been demonstrated that for the interferons, randomization to two dose levels produces significantly greater toxicity at the higher dose, but also a significantly greater antitumor effect for Kaposi's sarcoma in HIV infected patients (see XXXVII) and for patients with hairy cell leukemia (see XXXVI-8). The absence of clinical antitumor activity for TNF precludes evidence for a dose effect. Clinical toxicity is clearly dose related. In experimental tumors, there is a steep dose tumor response curve for TNF (see XVIII-4).

There are a number of experimental circumstances where cytokines employed in combination or in combination with chemotherapeutic agents have proven synergistic. These studies are in process of being extrapolated to the clinic (see XVIII).

Endocrine Therapy

The dose response curves for hormonal agents are not as steep as for most chemotherapeutic agents, and may be complex. For example, low doses of estrogens may stimulate estrogen receptor positive breast cancer, whereas higher doses may cause tumor regression. This subject is covered elsewhere (see XVII).

References

1. Ackland, S. P., and Schilsky, R. L.: High dose methotrexate: A critical reappraisal. J. Clin. Oncol., 5:2017, 1987.
2. Allegra, C. J.: Antifolates. In Cancer Chemotherapy: Principles and Practice. Edited by B. A. Chabner and J. M. Collins. Philadelphia, J. B. Lippincott Company, 1990, p. 110.
3. Antman, K., Ayash, L., Elias, A., Wheeler, C., Hunt, M., Eder, J. P., Teicher, B. A., Critchlow, J., Bibbo, J., Schnipper, L. E., and Frei, E., III: A phase II study of high dose cyclophosphamide, thiotepa, and carboplatin with autologous marrow support in women with measurable advanced breast cancer responding to standard dose therapy. J. Clin. Oncol., (In Press.)
4. Antman, K., Eder, J. P., and Frei, E., III: High-dose chemotherapy with bone marrow support for solid tumors. In Important Advances in Oncology. Edited by V. T. DeVita, Jr., S. Hellman, and S. A. Rosenberg. Philadelphia, J. B. Lippincott, 1987, p. 221.
5. Bodey, G. P., and Coltman, C. A.: Arabinosyl cytosine (ara-C) vs. combination chemotherapy (COAP) for adult acute leukemia. Proc. Amer. Assoc. Res., 13:107, 1972.
6. Bodey, G. P., and Hersh, E. M.: The problem of infection in patients with malignant disease. In Neoplasia in Childhood. Chicago, Year Book Publishers, 1969, p. 135.
7. Brindley, C. A., Salvin, L. G., Lipowska, B., Shnider, B. I., Regelson, W., and Colsky, J.: Further comparative trial of thiophosphoro-amide and mechlorethamine in patients with melanoma and Hodgkin's disease. J. Chronic Dis., 17:19, 1964.
8. Bruce, W. R., Meeker, R. E., and Valeriote, F. A.: Comparison of the sensitivity of normal hematopoietic and transplanted lymphoma colony-forming cells to chemotherapeutic agents administered in vivo. J. Natl. Cancer Inst., 37:233, 1966.
9. Budman, D., Wood, W., and Henderson, I. C.: Dose study in the adjuvant chemotherapy of breast cancer. CALGB ongoing study, 1991.
10. Clarkson, B. D., Sakai, Y., Kimura, T., Ohkita, T., and Fried, J.: Studies of cellular proliferation in human leukemia II. Variability in rates of growth and cellular differentiation in acute myelomonoblastic leukemia and effects of treatment. In The Proliferation and Spread of Neoplastic Cells. Baltimore, Williams & Wilkins Co., 1968, p. 295.
11. Cohen, M. H., Creaven, P. J., Fossieck, E. B., Jr., Broder, L. E., Selawry, O. S., Johnston, A. V., Williams, C. L., and Minna, J. D.: Intensive chemotherapy of small cell bronchogenic carcinoma. Cancer Treat. Rep., 61:349, 1977.
12. Collins, J. M., Dedrick, R., King, F., Speyer, J., and Myers, C.: Nonlinear pharmacokinetic models for 5-fluorouracil in man; Intravenous and intraperitoneal routes. Clin. Pharmacol. Ther., 28:235, 1980.
13. Dalton, W. S., Grogan, T. M., Meltzer, P. S., Scheper, R. J., Durie, B. G. M., Taylor, C. W., Miller, T. P., and Salmon, S. E.: Drug resistance and multiple myeloma in non-Hodgkin's lymphoma: Detection of p-glycoprotein and potential circumvention by the addition of verapamil to chemotherapy. J. Clin. Oncol., 7:415, 1989.
14. DeVita, V. T., Jr., Serpick, A. A., and Carbone, P. P.: Combination chemotherapy in the treatment of advanced Hodgkin's disease. Ann. Intern. Med., 73:881, 1970.
15. Dicke, K. A., Spitzer, D., and Zander, A. R.: Autologous Bone Marrow Transplantation. Proceedings of the First International Symposium. Houston, The University of Texas M. D. Anderson Hospital and Tumor Institute at Houston, 1985.
16. Doroshow, J. H., Multhauf, P., Leong, L., Margolin, K., Litchfield, T., Akman, S., Carr, B., Bertrand, M., Goldberg, D., Blayney, D., Odujinrin, O., DeLap, R., Shuster, J., and Newman, E.: Prospective randomized comparison of fluorouracil versus fluorouracil and high-dose continuous infusion leucovorin calcium for the treatment of advanced measurable colorectal cancer in patients previously unexposed to chemotherapy. J. Clin. Oncol., 8:491, 1990.
17. Dreyfuss, A. I., Clark, J. R., Wright, J. E., Norris, C. M., Jr., Busse, P. M., Lucarini, J. W., Fallon, B. G., Casey, D., Andersen, J. W., Klein, R., Rosowsky, A., Miller, D., and Frei, E., III: Continuous infusion high-dose leucovorin with 5-fluorouracil and cisplatin for untreated stage IV carcinoma of the head and neck. Ann. Intern. Med., 112:167, 1990.
18. Eder, J. P., Teicher, B. A., Holden, S. A., Cathcart, K. N., Schnipper, L. E., and Frei, E., III: Effect of novobiocin on the antitumor activity and tumor cell and bone marrow survivals of three alkylating agents. Cancer Res., 49:595, 1989.
19. Ellison, R. R., Holland, J. F., Weil, M., Jacquillat, C., Boiron, M., Bernard, J., Sawitsky, A., Rosner, F., Gussoff, B., Silver, R. T., Karanas, A., Cuttner, J., Spurr, C. L., Hayes, D. M., Blom, J., Leone, L. A., Haurani, F., Kyle, R., Hutchison, J. L., Forcier, J., and Moon, J. H.: Arabinosyl cytosine: A useful agent in the treatment of acute leukemia in adults. Blood, 32:507, 1968.
20. Frei, E., III: Combination cancer therapy: Presidential address. Cancer Res., 32:2593, 1972.
21. Frei, E., III: Curative cancer chemotherapy. Cancer Res., 45:6523, 1985.
22. Frei, E., III: Pathobiology of cancer. In Scientific American Medicine, 1988, 12:III, p. 1.
23. Frei, E., III, Antman, K., and Teicher, B.: Dose in the adjuvant setting: Experimental and clinical considerations. In Adjuvant Chemotherapy of Cancer VI. Edited by S. E. Salmon. Philadelphia, W. B. Saunders Company, 1990, p. 39.
24. Frei, E., III, Antman, K., Teicher, B., Eder, P., and Schnipper, L.: Bone marrow autotransplantation for solid tumors—prospects. J. Clin. Oncol., 7:515, 1989.
25. Frei, E., III, Blum, R. H., Pitman, S. W., Kirkwood, J. M., Henderson, I. C., Skarin, A. T., Mayer, R. J., Bast, R. C., Garnick, M. B., Parker, L. M., and Canellos, G. P.: High dose methotrexate with leucovorin rescue. Rationale and spectrum of antitumor activity. Am. J. Med., 68:370, 1980.
26. Frei, E., III, and Canellos, G. P.: Dose: a critical factor in cancer chemotherapy. Am. J. Med., 69:585, 1980.
27. Frei, E., III, Cucchi, C. A., Rosowsky, A., Tantravahi, R., Bernal, S., Ervin, T. J., Ruprecht, R. M., and Haseltine, W. A.: Alkylating agent resistance: In vitro studies with human cell lines. Proc. Natl. Acad. Sci. USA, 82:2158, 1985.
28. Frei, E., III, Spurr, C. L., Brindley, C. O., Selawry, O., Holland, J. F., Rall, D. P., Wasserman, L. R., Hoogstraten, B., Shnider, B. I., McIntyre, O. R., Matthews, L. B., Jr., and Miller, S. P.: Clinical studies of dichloromethotrexate (NSC 29630). Clin. Pharm. Ther., 6:160, 1965.
29. Goldin, A., Vendetti, J. M., Humphreys, S. B., and Mantel, N.: Modification of treatment schedules in the management of advanced mouse leukemia with amethopterin. J. Natl. Cancer Inst., 17:203, 1956.
30. Gralla, R. J.: Nausea and Vomiting. In Cancer, Principles and Practice of Oncology. Edited by V. T. DeVita, Jr., S. Hellman and S. A., Rosenberg. J. B. Lippincott Co., 1989, p. 2137.
31. Grem, J. L.: Fluorinated pyrimidines. In Cancer Chemotherapy: Principles and Practice. Edited by B. A. Chabner and J. M. Collins. Philadelphia, J. B. Lippincott Co., 1990, p. 180.
32. Henderson, I. C., Hayes, D. F., and Gelman, R.: Dose-response in the treatment of breast cancer: A critical review. J. Clin. Onc., 6:1501, 1988.
33. Hersh, E. M., Whitecar, J. P., McCredie, K. B., Bodey, G. P., and Freireich, E. J.: Chemotherapy, immunocompetence, immunosuppression and prognosis in acute leukemia. N. Engl. J. Med., 285:1211, 1971.
34. Hryniuk, W. M.: The importance of dose intensity in the outcome of chemotherapy. In Important Advances in Oncology 1988. Edited by V. T. DeVita, Jr., S. Hellman, and S. A. Rosenberg. Philadelphia, J. B. Lippincott Co., 1988, p. 121.
35. Hryniuk, W., and Bush, H.: The importance of dose intensity in chemotherapy of metastatic breast cancer. J. Clin. Oncol., 2:1281, 1984.
36. Law, L. W.: Origin of the resistance of leukemic cells to folic acid antagonists. Nature (Lond), 169:268, 1956.
37. Legha, S. S., Benjamin, R. S., Mackay, B., Ewer, M., Wallace, S., Valdivieso, M., Rasmussen, S. L., Blumenschein, G. R., and Freireich, E. J.: Reduction doxorubicin and cardiotoxicity by prolonged continuous intravenous infusion. Ann. Intern. Med., 96:133, 1982.
38. Li, M. C., Hertz, R., and Spencer, D. V.: Effect of Methotrexate Upon Choriocarcinoma and Chorioadenoma. Proc. Soc. Exp. Biol. Med., 93:361, 1956.
39. Ling, V., Kartner, N., Sudo, T., Siminovitch, L., and Riordan, J. R.: Multidrug resistance phenotype in Chinese hamster ovary cells. Cancer Treat. Rep., 67:869, 1983.
40. Lokich, J. J.: In Cancer Chemotherapy by Infusion. Edited by J. J. Lokich. Chicago, Precept Press, Inc., 1987, p. 1.
41. Mendelsohn, M. L.: The growth fraction: A new concept applied to tumors. Science, 132:1496, 1960.
42. Mendelsohn, M. L.: Autoradiographic analysis of cell proliferation in spontaneous

breast cancer of C3H mouse. III. The growth fraction. J. Natl. Cancer Inst., 28:1015, 1962.

43. Ozols, R. F., Hamilton, T. C., Masuda, H., and Young, R. C.: Manipulation of cellular thiols to influence drug resistance. *In* Mechanisms of Drugs Resistance in Neoplastic Cells. Bristol-Myers Cancer Symposia, Vol 9. Edited by P. V. Woolley, III and K. D. Tew. San Diego, Academic Press, Inc., 1988, p. 289.

44. Peters, W. P.: Personal communication, 1991.

45. Peters, W. P., Eder, J. P., Henner, W. D., Schryber, S., Wilmore, D., Finberg, R., Schoenfeld, D., Bast, R., Gargone, B., Antman, K., Anderson, J., Anderson, K., Kruskall, M. S., Schnipper, L., and Frei, E., III: High-dose combination alkylating agents with autologous bone marrow support: A phase I trial. J. Clin. Oncol., 4:646, 1986.

46. Pinkel, D.: The ninth annual David Karnofsky Lecture: Treatment of acute lymphocytic leukemia. Cancer, 48:1128, 1979.

47. Pinkel, D., Hernandez, K., Borella, L., Holton, C., Aur, R., Samoy, G., and Pratt, C.: Drug dosage and remission duration in childhood lymphocytic leukemia. Cancer, 27:247, 1971.

48. Report to the British Medical Research Council by their Tuberculosis Chemotherapy Trials Committee: Various combinations of isoniazid with streptomycin or with PAS in the treatment of pulmonary tuberculosis. Brit. Med. J., 435:4911, 1955.

49. Rideout, D. C., and Chou, T. C.: Synergism, potentiation, and antagonism in chemotherapy: An overview. *In* Synergism and Antagonism in Chemotherapy. Edited by T. C. Chou, and D. C. Rideout. Academic Press, Inc., 1991, p. 3.

50. Rath, H., Tlsty, T., and Schimke, R. T.: Rapid emergence of methotrexate resistance in cultured mouse cells. Cancer Res., 44:3303, 1984.

51. Santos, G. W., Tutschka, P. J., Brookmeyer, R., Saral, R., Beschorner, W. E., Bias, W. B., Braine, H. G., Burns, W. H., Elfenbein, G. J., Kaizer, H., Mellits, D., Sensenbrenner, L. L., Stuart, R. K., and Yeager, A. M.: Marrow transplantation for acute nonlymphocytic leukemia after treatment with busulfan and cyclophosphomide. N. Engl. J. Med., 309:1347, 1983.

52. Sartorelli, A. C., and Caresy, W. A.: Combination chemotherapy. *In* Cancer Medicine, 2nd Edition. Edited by J. F. Holland, and E. Frei, III. Philadelphia, Lea & Febiger, 1982, p. 720.

53. Schaaf, L. J., Dobbs, B. R., Edwards, T. R., and Perrier, D. G.: Nonlinear pharmacokinetic characteristics of 5-fluorouracil in colorectal cancer patients. Eur. J. Clin. Pharmacol., 32:411, 1987.

54. Schimke, R. T., Roos, D. S., and Brown, P. C.: Amplification of genes in somatic mammalian cells. Methods in Enzymology, 151:85, 1987.

55. Schimke, T. T., Sherweed, S., Johnston, R., Hill, A., Rice, G., Hoy, C., Feder, J., and Farnham, P.: On the mechanism of induced gene amplification in mammalian cells.

In Mechanisms of Drug Resistance in Neoplastic Cells. Edited by P. V. Woolley, III, and K. D. Tew. San Diego, Academic Press, Inc., 1988, p. 29.

56. Schnipper, L. E.: Clinical implications of tumor-cell heterogeneity. N. Engl. J. Med., 314:1423, 1986.

57. Seifert, P., Baker, L., Reed, M. L., and Vaitkevicius, V. K.: Comparison of continuously infused 5-fluorouracil with bolus injection in treatment of patients with colorectal adenocarcinoma. Cancer, 36:123, 1975.

58. Selawry, O. S., Hananian, J., Wolman, I. J., Abir, E., Chavalier, L., Gourdeau, R., Denton, R., Gussoff, B. D., Levy, R., Burgert, O., Jr., Mills, S. D., Blom, J., Jones, B., Patterson, R. B., McIntyre, O. R., Haurani, F. I., Moon, J. H., Hoogstraten, B., Kung, F. H., Sheehe, P. R., Frei, E., III, and Holland, J. F. (Acute Leukemia Group B): New treatment schedule with improved survival in childhood leukemia. J.A.M.A., 194:715, 1965.

59. Skarin, A. T., Zuckerman, K. S., Pitman, S. W., Rosenthal, D. S., Moloney, W., Frei, E., III, and Canellos, G. P.: High-dose methotrexate with folinic acid in the treatment of advanced non-Hodgkin lymphoma including CNS involvement. Blood, 50:1039, 1977.

60. Skipper, H. E., Schabel, F. M., Jr., and Wilcox, W. S.: Experimental evaluation of potential anticancer agents. XIII. On the criteria and kinetics associated with "curability" of experimental leukemia. Cancer Chemother. Rep., 35:1, 1964.

61. Skipper, H. E., Schabel, F. M., Jr., and Wilcox, W. S.: Experimental evaluation of potential anticancer agents. XXI. Scheduling of arabinosyl cytosine to take advantage of its S-phase specificity against leukemia cells. Cancer Chemother. Rep., 51:125, 1967.

62. Steel, G. G.: Growth Kinetics of Tumors; Cell Population Kinetics in Relation to the Growth in Premedic Cancer. Oxford, Clarendon Press, 1977.

63. Tannock, I.: Cell kinetics in chemotherapy: A critical review. Cancer Treat. Rep., 62:1117, 1978.

64. Tannock, I. F., Boyd, N. F., DeBoer, G., Erlichman, C., Fine, S., Larocque, G., Mayers, C., Perrault, D., and Sutherland, H.: A randomized trial of two dose levels of CMF chemotherapy for patients with metastatic breast cancer. J. Clin. Oncol., 6:1377, 1988.

65. Teicher, B. A., and Holden, S. A.: A Survey of the effect of adding fluosol-DA 20%/O2 to treatment with various chemotherapeutic agents. Cancer Treat. Rep., 71:173, 1987.

66. Teicher, B. A., and Rose, C. M.: Perfluorochemical emulsions can increase tumor radiosensitivity. Science, 223:934, 1984.

67. Thomas, E. D.: Current status of bone marrow transplantation. Transplantation Proceedings, 17:428, 1985.

68. Weichselbaum, R. R., Schmit, A., and Little, J. B.: Cellular repair factors influencing radiocurability of human malignant tumours. Brit. J. Cancer, 44:10, 1982.

69. Weiss, A. J., and Manthel, R. W.: Experience with the use of adriamycin in combination with other anticancer agents using a weekly schedule, with particular reference to lack of cardiac toxicity. Cancer, 40:2046, 1977.

Regional Chemotherapy

Stephen B. Howell

Introduction

Regional chemotherapy refers to the local instillation of drug into a tumor-containing region of the body to increase the ratio of drug exposure for the tumor relative to that for other parts of the body. The amount of tumor cell kill achieved with a dose of drug is a function of how much drug actually reaches critical targets in the tumor cell, and how long cytotoxic concentrations of the drug remain in the environment of the cell. As for cell lines and xenografts, virtually all tumors show increasing cell kill with dose; for most human tumors the problem is that, in the clinical setting, the doses required to produce enough cell kill to be scored as a useful response are often well above what is tolerated by marrow, gut, and other drug-sensitive normal tissues. The rationale for the use of regional chemotherapy is its potential for increasing the ratio of drug exposure for the tumor relative to that for dose-limiting normal tissues of the body. The clinically useful forms of regional chemotherapy rely either on specific anatomic compartments or localized intra-arterial administration to create a differential drug exposure for tumor and normal tissues.

Pharmacologic Principles of Regional Chemotherapy

Pharmacologic Principles of Intracavitary Therapy

The behavior of a drug administered into an extravascular cavity is conveniently described by a two-compartment model (Figure XV-4-1).[16] The first compartment represents the tumor-containing cavity, and the second the vascular volume and all the other tissues of the body that are in direct contact with the bloodstream. Total drug exposure is defined as the integral of the area under the concentration times time curve, and is abbreviated AUC. The relative advantage of administering a drug by the intracavitary route is determined by the cavity/plasma AUC ratio following intracavitary versus intravenous injection, assuming that drug in cavity fluid and plasma have equal access to the target tumor cell.

Relative Clearances and First Pass Metabolism. Following rapid intracavitary instillation, the concentration of a drug falls as drug leaks or is pumped into the plasma, or as it is metabolized in the cavity. Most chemotherapeutic agents undergo little metabolism in the cavity, and for such agents the rate at which concentration decreases is a function of the volume of the fluid in the cavity, the surface area through which the drug diffuses out of the cavity, the permeability of this surface, and the difference in free drug concentration between the cavity and the plasma. Under steady-state con-

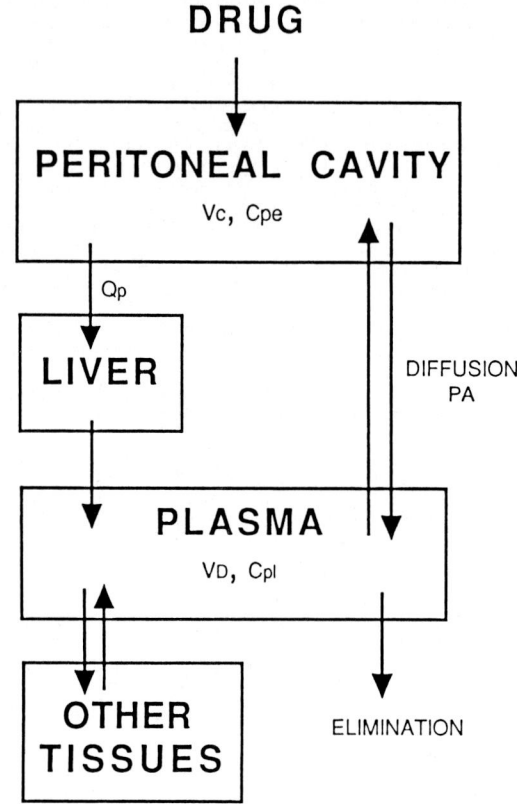

DRUG

PERITONEAL CAVITY
V_c, C_{pe}

Q_p

LIVER

PLASMA
V_D, C_{pl}

DIFFUSION
PA

OTHER TISSUES

ELIMINATION

Figure XV-4-1. Compartmental model of intraperitoneal chemotherapy. V_c, volume of the cavity; C_{pe}, concentration in the peritoneal cavity; Q_p, portal blood flow; PA, permeability area product; V_D, apparent plasma volume of distribution; C_{pl}, concentration in the plasma.

ditions the cavity-to-plasma concentration ratio is given by Equation 1.

$$\frac{C_c}{C_p} = \frac{\text{Plasma clearance} + (\text{Cavity clearance})}{(\text{Cavity clearance})} \qquad \text{Eq. 1}$$

Since AUC is a function of the product of concentration and time, the clearances also determine the AUC ratio, and anything that either reduces the cavity clearance or increases the plasma clearance will increase the pharmacologic advantage of intracavitary instillation. Thus, the smaller the clearance from the cavity and the greater the clearance from the plasma the higher the AUC ratio. An optimal drug would be one that leaves the cavity very slowly but that is promptly removed from the plasma once it reaches the systemic circulation so that it has little time to circulate to the bone marrow and gut, the two most commonly dose-limiting normal tissues. As a general rule, drugs that have a hard time getting across lipid membranes because they are large, highly ionized, or not very lipid soluble will have low cavity clearances. However, the advantage of intracavitary administration cannot be predicted by these characteristics alone because they also affect plasma clearance, and it is the cavity clearance relative to plasma clearance that determines the pharmacokinetic advantage. Equation 1 permits reasonably accurate predictions of the relative advantage of intracavitary instillation.

The AUC ratio is also influenced by the anatomic route of drug absorption from the cavity because this can influence the extent to which the drug is metabolized to an inactive form during transit between the cavity and the systemic compartment. Inactivation of a drug after it has left the tumor-containing cavity but before it reaches the systemic compartment has the same effect on the AUC ratio as increasing the plasma clearance. The route of absorption is different for each of the major cavities for which regional chemotherapy is used. In the case of the pleural and pericardial cavities, drug is absorbed directly into the systemic circulation. In the case of the peritoneal cavity, however, most drugs in the molecular weight range of the commonly used antitumor drugs are absorbed primarily via the portal circulation. The majority of peritoneal perfusion comes from the splanchnic circulation, and the structures that account for most of the surface area of the peritoneum, including the visceral peritoneum, the omentum, and the mesentery, drain into the portal circulation. Only the parietal peritoneum drains directly into the systemic circulation, and although a rich network of diaphragmatic lymphatics drains the peritoneal cavity, for drugs with molecular weights less than 1,000 Daltons the flow in the lymphatic channels is so much less than portal flow that quantitatively this probably does not constitute an important route of drug absorption. Drugs that have extensive first-pass metabolism in the liver, such as cytarabine, 5-fluorouracil, 6-thioguanine, and floxuridine have very much higher AUC ratios following intraperitoneal instillation than drugs with little hepatic metabolism such as cisplatin (Table XV-4-1).

Tumor Penetration. A chemotherapeutic agent administered by the intracavitary route may have direct access to single cells free in the cavity, but therapeutic efficacy requires that it enter the tumor mass. Figure XV-4-2 shows a schematic drawing of a tumor nodule growing on a serosal surface. As the drug begins to penetrate from the free surface it is at risk for being removed or inactivated by: 1) metabolism in the extracellular fluid; 2) uptake and metabolism in cells; and 3) diffusion into capillaries that enter the nodule from the systemic circulation. Each of these acts as a "sink" reducing the amount of drug available to penetrate deeper into the interstitium. Pharmacokinetic modelling suggests that the capillary area and permeability, blood flow, and the diffusion coefficient of the drug in the tumor are particularly important variables. Tumor capillaries are abnormal and have higher permeability than capillaries in normal tissues resulting in increased interstitial fluid formation and pressure.[37]

Table XV-4-1.   Ratio of Peritoneal to Plasma Area Under the Curve of Concentration Times Time (AUC)

Drug	Mean AUC Ratio	Major Toxicities
Bleomycin	4	Peritonitis, fever
Carboplatin	6–10	Myelosuppression
Cisplatin	12	Nephrotoxicity
Cytarabine	300–1000	Myelosuppression
Doxorubicin	400	Peritonitis
Etoposide	65	Myelosuppression
Fluorodeoxyuridine	440–1300	Myelosuppression
Fluorouracil	400–2500	Peritonitis and myelosuppression
r-IFN alpha 2	Unknown	Flu-like syndrome
IFN beta	Unknown	Flu-like syndrome
r-IFNgamma	Unknown	Flu-like syndrome
IL2	200–1000	Peritoneal sclerosis
Melphalan	65	Myelosuppression
Methotrexate	92	Myelosuppression
Mitomycin	32	Myelosuppression and peritonitis
Mitoxantrone	1400	Myelosuppression and peritonitis
Teniposide	9.6	Myelosuppression
6-Thioguanine	1800	Myelosuppression capillary leak syndrome
ThioTEPA	4.3	Myelosuppression

Since tumor nodules generally have poorly formed or non-functional lymphatics, interstitial fluid moves in a radial direction toward the edge of the nodule. Thus, to enter a tumor nodule from the periphery, a drug must move upstream against this convective flow. Since diffusion coefficients for the available chemotherapeutic drugs are low, these considerations lead to the prediction that tumor volume will have a major influence on the success of intracavitary chemotherapy. One can also predict that the profile of drug concentration as a function of distance into the tumor nodule will be more favorable for non-metabolized drugs entering poorly vascularized nodules, and that the cavity to plasma AUC ratio will exceed the tumor to plasma AUC ratio.

Clinical experience confirms that tumor volume is a very important determinant of the efficacy of intracavitary chemotherapy. In the case of ovarian carcinoma, intraperitoneal chemotherapy can produce significant increases in survival for patients whose largest tumor nodule is less than 2 cm, but not in patients with larger volume disease.[33] Direct measurement of cisplatin penetration into millimeter sized murine colon carcinoma nodules indicates that the advantage of an intraperitoneal over an intravenous injection is limited to approximately the first 1.5 mm depth into the tumor from the surface, that a peritoneal to plasma AUC ratio of 12–15 is associated with a 1.7-fold increase in drug delivery to such nodules, and that even in nodules of a few millimeters there is marked heterogeneity of actual drug delivery.[42]

The significance of the drug "sink" produced by capillary blood flow is given credence by the clinical observation that intraperitoneal chemotherapy produces very little damage

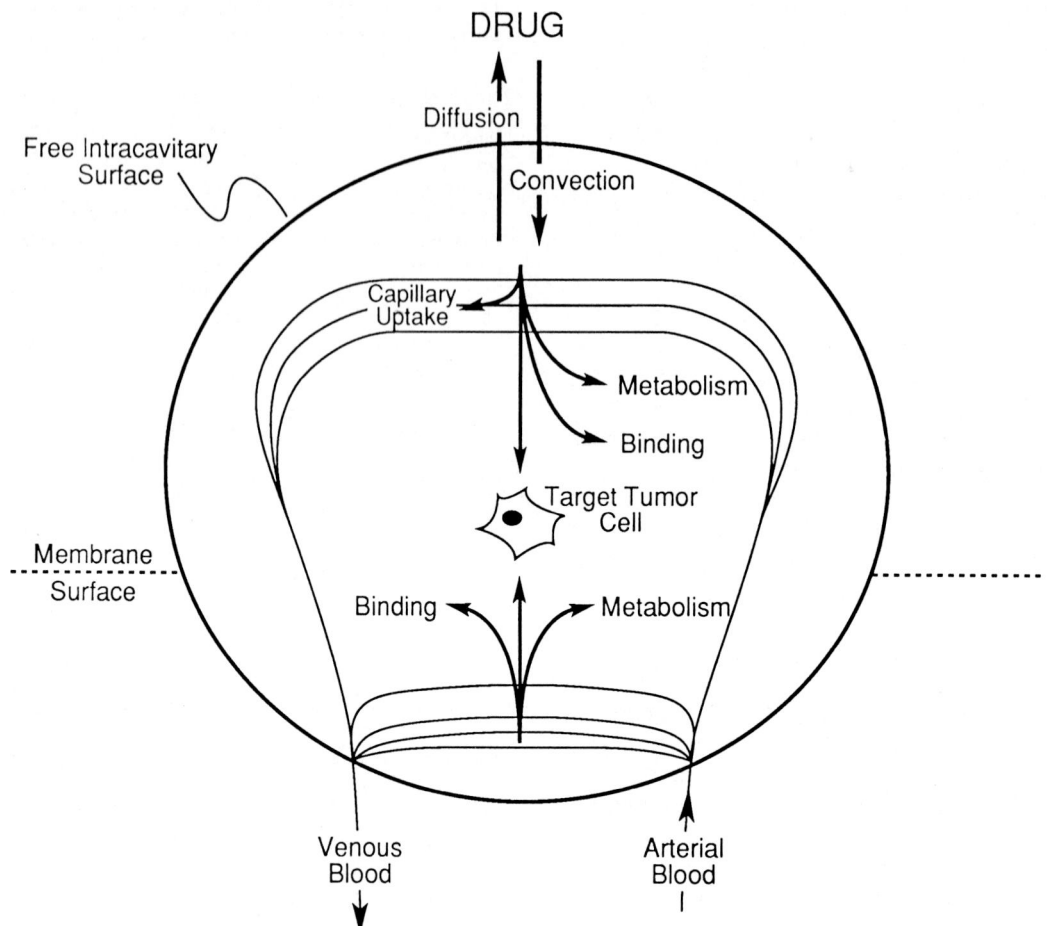

Figure XV-4-2. Schematic diagram of a tumor nodule growing on a serosal surface, and the processes that control delivery of drug to the target tumor cell by free surface diffusion or systemic capillary blood flow.

to gut even when drug doses are high enough to cause serious bone marrow and other systemic toxicity. Since the crypt cells of the intestinal epithelium are rarely more than 1 mm from the visceral peritoneum, one might expect very high concentrations of drug in the peritoneal cavity to kill these critical stem cells. It is probably the presence of a rich capillary network with relatively high flow rates that protects the gut by siphoning off drug before it can reach the crypt cells.

Intracavitary Drug Distribution. If drugs administered via the intracavitary route are to be effective they must reach the surface of the tumor. This is often a problem, particularly for intraperitoneal and intrapleural therapy, since tumors in these cavities frequently produce compartmentalizing adhesions. In the peritoneal cavity, adequate drug distribution to even accessible surfaces requires the instillation of large volumes (e.g., 1.4 L/m^2) of drug-containing fluid. The poor results obtained with early attempts at intraperitoneal therapy can be accounted for in part by the use of small volumes of injection. It is currently unclear how best to obtain good drug distribution in the pleural cavity where instillation of large volumes can result in collapse of the lung. Poor distribution probably contributes to the relative lack of success with intrapleural relative to intraperitoneal chemotherapy.

Principles for the Selection of Drugs for Intracavitary Administration. It is unlikely that a single intracavitary instillation of any drug will be curative; the successful clinical programs depend on being able to instill drugs repeatedly. In this regard it is a basic pharmacologic principle of intracavitary therapy that one should use drugs or doses that do not cause extensive chemical injury to the surfaces of the cavity. Such injury is usually associated with fibrosis and adhesion formation which limits drug access on subsequent administrations.

It is also a basic pharmacologic principle of intracavitary chemotherapy that one should use drugs that have as high a cavity to plasma AUC ratio as possible, but whose intracavitary dose is limited by a toxicity that results from drug entering the systemic circulation rather than by local compartmental toxicity. This strategy has important advantages. It permits intracavitary dose escalation to the point where the amount of drug leaking into the systemic circulation is equivalent to the systemic AUC that could be produced by an intravenous injection. Thus there is no compromise of drug delivery to those parts of the tumor nodule distant from a free surface, while those portions near the surface receive drug by both capillary flow and free surface diffusion. One would expect this to result in greater total drug delivery, and better distribution throughout the nodule. Stated another way, if a drug has a high AUC ratio, for a given amount of systemic toxicity, one can obtain a substantially greater AUC for the surface of the tumor without reducing capillary drug delivery by using an intracavitary rather than an intravenous injection.

Neutralizing Agents. One tactic that can further increase the therapeutic index of intracavitary therapy is to inject a second drug into the systemic compartment that can either neutralize the chemotherapeutic agent before it damages normal cells, or rescue such cells even after the target molecules in the cell have been affected. However, since the neutralizing or rescue agent has the potential of entering the cavity from the systemic compartment, and entering the tumor via capillary flow, the success of this approach depends critically on the concentration of the chemotherapeutic and protective agents actually attained in the tumor, and on the protective agent being a competitive rather than non-competitive antagonist. This approach is facilitated by using an antagonist whose ability to interfere with the cytotoxicity of the agonist is overcome by relatively small increases in the concentration of the agonist. The methotrexate/leucovorin pair is one that is often used.[30] Studies with human bone marrow indicated that a concentration of leucovorin that prevents the toxicity of 1 μM methotrexate will not protect against 10 μM methotrexate. Thus, even if the leucovorin equilibrates into the cavity, as long as the intracavitary concentration of methotrexate can be maintained at a level 10-fold higher than that in plasma, the leucovorin should not interfere with the antitumor activity of methotrexate in the cavity.

When sufficient leucovorin is introduced into the systemic circulation to antagonize the effect of methotrexate on bone marrow, it may also be sufficient to antagonize the effect of methotrexate delivered to the tumor nodule by capillary flow. Another tactic is to use a neutralizing agent that is relatively specific for the most sensitive organ in the body. This principle is exemplified by the use of intravenous thiosulfate in combination with intraperitoneal cisplatin. Thiosulfate is a competitive antagonist that reacts with cisplatin to form a covalently linked product that is neither nephrotoxic nor cytotoxic to the tumor. At the concentrations of both agents usually attained in the plasma, the rate of reaction is much slower than the rate of clearance of free cisplatin through reaction with plasma proteins. In contrast, thiosulfate is extensively concentrated in the kidneys. The result is that when cisplatin is administered in large doses intraperitoneally and thiosulfate intravenously, there is little neutralization of the cisplatin in the plasma, but excellent protection of the kidneys.[32] This tactic reduces the concern that delivery of the neutralizing agent to the tumor by capillary flow may interfere with the effectiveness of the chemotherapeutic agent.

Pharmacologic Principles of Intrathecal Chemotherapy

Figure XV-4-3 shows a compartmental model of drug transport between the CNS and other parts of the body. Since both the volume of the CNS and clearance of drug from the

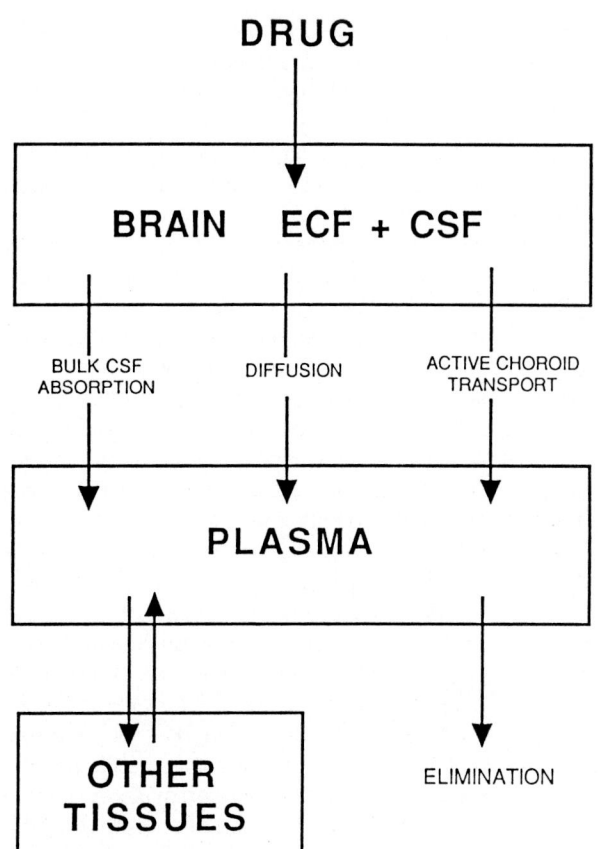

Figure XV-4-3. Compartmental model of intrathecal chemotherapy and routes by which drug leaves the CSF.

CNS are relatively small, extraordinarily high CSF/plasma AUC ratios can be attained by IT drug administration. Unlike the situation in other cavities, where relatively homogeneous drug distribution is attained by flooding the compartment with drug-containing fluid, drugs can only be administered into the CSF in small volumes (5–18 ml). Drug injected via an Ommaya reservoir into a lateral ventricle must be distributed to the rest of the CSF by bulk flow, and thence by diffusion into the extracellular spaces of the brain. Bulk flow carries drug from the ventricle to the cisterna magnum and then up over the cerebrum to the arachnoid granulations where the CSF is reabsorbed into the venous system. Drug is also circulated down over the spinal cord to the lumbar sac. Drug introduced into the lumbar sac is carried by bulk flow to the cisterna magnum; it eventually reaches the ventricles where, in the case of methotrexate, it peaks at 4–8 hours. Abnormalities of CSF flow have been reported in 70% of patients with meningeal neoplasia, and may impair drug distribution.[27] Drug can leave the CSF/brain ECF compartment by: 1) bulk flow transport along with CSF into the plasma at the arachnoid granulations; 2) diffusion into brain and choroid plexus capillaries; or 3) metabolism within the CSF/brain compartment. In the case of methotrexate and cytarabine, which are the two agents most commonly used by the intrathecal route, bulk flow accounts for the majority of the clearance. Neither drug is significantly metabolized in the CSF compartment. The CSF has a volume of approximately 140 ml in subjects more than 3 years old, and the bulk flow absorption of CSF has been reported to be 31.2 ml/hr.[8] Data from preclinical studies in monkeys indicates that bulk flow dominates the clearance of other water soluble chemotherapeutic agents, resulting in similar CSF half-lives for many of these drugs.[12]

The extent to which anticancer agents in the CSF penetrate into the brain and spinal cord is unknown. Early studies suggested that penetration is limited to a few millimeters.[5,6,22,50] More recent studies based on quantitative autoradiography in rabbits have shown deeper penetration,[11] but whether cytotoxic concentrations are attained more than a few millimeters from the surface has not been established. It is clear that penetration is not homogeneous; gray matter regions of both the brain and spinal cord contained higher concentrations than white matter tracks.

The administration of very high doses of drug by the IV route provides a strategy for increasing drug penetration into the CSF to therapeutically effective levels. Although this approach voids the differential drug exposure attainable with IT injection, the presence of meningeal disease often signals the need for systemic therapy as well. This strategy permits more uniform distribution of drug throughout the neuraxis, and, since continuous IV infusion is more readily accomplished than frequent IT dosing, longer duration of drug exposure. This approach can be used effectively with both methotrexate and cytarabine.

Pharmacologic Principles of Intra-Arterial Chemotherapy

There is a voluminous literature on IA therapy. Some aspects of the pharmacokinetic principles underlying IA infusion are counter-intuitive, however, accounting in part for the confusion that is prevalent in this field. Many claims for efficacy of IA therapy are not substantiated by adequate pharmacologic data. The overall relative advantage of an IA compared to an IV injection of the same drug (R_d) is a composite of the advantage from the point of view of the tumor (R_t) and from the point of view of the systemic circulation (R_s).[17] The reason for considering R_t and R_s separately is that they are controlled by entirely different factors.

Figure XV-4-4 presents a flow diagram that illustrates the factors that determine the pharmacokinetic advantage of an IA infusion.[15] When drug is infused at a constant rate until steady-state is reached, then the relative advantage of an IA infusion from the point of view of the tumor located in the infused volume is given by Equation 2.

$$R_t = 1 + \frac{CL_{tb}}{Q} \qquad \text{Eq. 2}$$

where CL_{tb} is the total body clearance during an intravenous infusion, and Q is the blood flow to the region. Under the same conditions, the relative advantage from the point of view of the systemic circulation, R_s, is given by Equation 3.

$$R_s = 1 - E \qquad \text{Eq. 3}$$

where E is the extraction ratio, or the fraction of drug entering the perfused organ that is permanently inactivated, bound, or excreted and thus fails to enter the systemic circulation. Equations 2 and 3 can be combined to yield an expression for the overall relative advantage of an IA infusion (Equation 4).

$$R_d = 1 + \frac{CL_{tb}}{Q(1 - E)} \qquad \text{Eq. 4}$$

Equation 4 provides a remarkably simple and powerful tool that allows reasonably accurate prediction of pharmacologic advantage if CL_{tb}, Q, and E are known or can be measured.[13] Equation 4 is derived from considerations of the mass of drug moving into and out of the perfused region under steady-state conditions, but is equally valid for predicting the advantage of an IA infusion on the basis of total drug exposure (area under the curve of concentration times time) when clearances are independent of concentration (i.e., when the pharmacokinetics are linear). Table XV-4-2 lists R_d as a function of flow rate (Q) for some commonly used chemotherapeutic agents.

All of the pharmacokinetic advantage of an IA injection devolves from exposure that occurs during the first pass of the drug through the tumor. Once the drug reaches the venous circulation, then subsequent exposure for the tumor is the same irrespective of whether the drug was injected IA or IV. Equation 2 indicates that the relative advantage from the point of view of the tumor is controlled solely by total body clearance and the blood flow to the region perfused. This means that R_t values substantially greater than 1 will be obtained only for drugs with relatively high CL_{tb}, and for tumors in regions receiving relatively low blood flow. This relationship is illustrated in Figure XV-4-5. The lower the blood flow and the larger the total body clearance, the greater the advantage; the relationship is hyperbolic so that while a decrement in blood flow to a well perfused organ will have little effect on R_t, the same absolute decrement in flow to a poorly perfused organ can strikingly increase R_t. Organ blood flows range from 100–1,500 ml/min in man, leading to the predication that one must select drugs with relatively high total body clearance before R_t can be expected to be very significant.

In contrast to R_t, Equation 3 indicates that the only factor influencing the relative advantage from the point of view of the systemic circulation is the extraction ratio. The smaller the fraction of drug injected by the IA route that reaches the venous circulation, the greater the advantage. Overall, predicated R_d values are greatest for the IA treatment of tumors in organs with very low blood flows using drugs with high total body clearances and extraction ratios.

Equation 4 results in a number of counter-intuitive predictions. First, if the extraction ratio is low, as it is for most anticancer drugs injected into organs other than the liver or kidney, then the use of the IA route is of no advantage at all from the point of view of decreasing toxicity to tissues in contact with the systemic circulation. On the other hand, if the target tissue is the only organ that clears the drug from

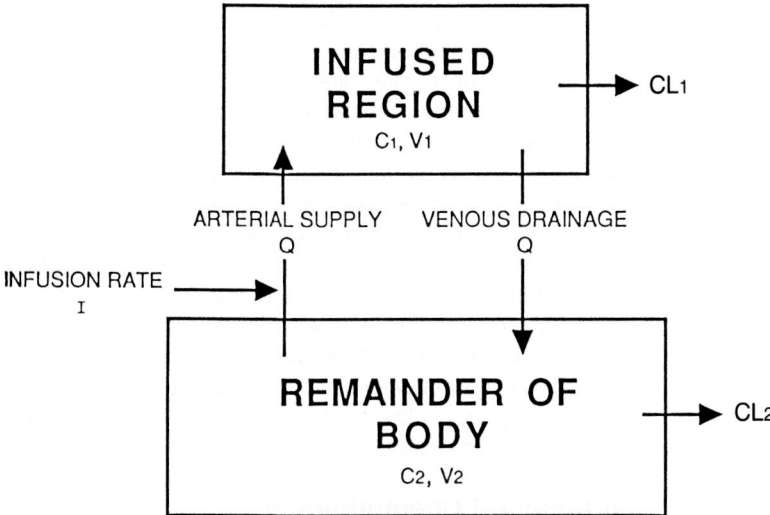

Figure XV-4-4. Flow diagram illustrating the pharmacokinetics of intra-arterial drug administration. C is the drug concentration in the blood; V is the volume of distribution; CL is the clearance; Q is the blood flow rate; and I is the infusion rate of the drug. Subscripts 1 and 2 refer to the infused region and the remainder of the body respectively. Redrawn from Dedrick.[15]

Table XV-4-2. R_d **as a Function of Flow Rate for Some Commonly Used Chemotherapeutic Agents**

Drug	CL_{tb} ml/min	R_d			
		Q = 1	Q = 10	Q = 100	Q = 1000
Carmustine	1,000	1,001	101	11	2
Cisplatin	400	401	41	5	1.4
Cytarabine	3,000	3,001	301	31	4
Doxorubicin	900	901	91	10	1.9
Floxuridine	25,000	25,001	2,501	251	26
5-fluorouracil	4,000	4,001	401	41	5
Methotrexate	200	201	21	3	1.2

CL_{tb} = total body clearance of drug
R_d = relative advantage compared to intravenous administration of same drug
Q = blood flow in ml/min. for tumor bed under consideration
From Eckman[15]

the body, then clearance from the rest of the body is zero and R_d is equal to 1. Under this circumstance one can anticipate reduced systemic toxicity but no increase in therapeutic response. This has particular relevance for the use of drugs such as floxuridine by hepatic arterial infusion. Another surprising prediction is that R_d is independent of infusion rate and of infusion duration. Although both of these will alter peak regional and plasma drug concentration, R_d varies with regional concentration only to the extent that regional concentration alters the extraction ratio. Thus, the ratio of peak regional to peak plasma concentrations is not an appropriate descriptor of relative advantage.

In using Equation 4 to predict the relative advantage of an IA infusion it is important to recognize that the derivation of the equation is based on the total rate of delivery of biologically active drug to the perfused region. If biologically active drug is carried only in the plasma phase, then it is the plasma flow and clearance that are the relative parameters; if active drug is partitioned between plasma and blood cells, then total blood flow and blood clearance must be used for prediction. Equation 4 is also based on the assumption that the drug is well mixed in the artery at the site of infusion. Recent studies indicate that streaming of drug is common, that it is critically dependent on catheter position, and can

result in marked inhomogeneity of tumor exposure following IA injection.[15] Finally, the rate at which concentration changes is a function of the volume of the region and flow rate. Since the volumes of perfused organs are much less than total body volume, concentrations in the perfused organ tend to change more rapidly than plasma concentration.

In addition to permitting predications about the relative advantage of an IA infusion, Equation 4 also points to a number of strategies that can be used to increase R_d. Blood flow to an organ can potentially be decreased through the use of balloon catheters or IA injected particles. Total body clearance can be increased through the use of concurrently administered neutralizing agents or devices that remove drug from the systemic circulation. Finally, isolation of the perfused organ from the systemic circulation has the effect of increasing tumor exposure relative to systemic exposure.

Intraperitoneal Chemotherapy

Chemotherapeutic agents can be instilled IP via a catheter placed through the skin into the cavity, but it is more common to place a catheter surgically leading from the cavity up through the fascial planes, and then to a port located in a subcutaneous pocket over the lower anterior rib cage. This type of totally implanted access device permits drug instil-

Table XV-4-3. Recommended Intrathecal Methotrexate Dose as a Function of Age

Patient age (years)	Dose (mg)
<1	6
1	8
2	10
≥3	12

From Bleyer[7]

vomiting, and CSF pleocytosis within a matter of hours to several days after drug injection. In some cases this may be due to changes in CSF flow dynamics induced by the presence of neoplastic meningitis. Methotrexate can also cause subacute deficits consisting of paresis and paraplegia, cranial nerve palsies, ataxia, visual impairment, altered mentation, and convulsions that evolve over a few days to a week after starting therapy. Necrotizing leukoencephalopathy can develop as a late complication and may vary in severity from mild changes in cognitive functions to dysarthria, dysphagia, spasticity, ataxia, dementia, and coma. Concurrent cranial radiation in children appears to enhance the neurotoxicity of intrathecal methotrexate.

Cytarabine

Although pharmacokinetic principles indicate that cytarabine dose, like that for methotrexate, should be based on CNS volume according to age rather than body surface area, the relative lack of cytarabine toxicity permits more latitude. In practice IT cytarabine is administered in doses of 30–100 mg/m[2], generally once or twice weekly. Although pharmacokinetically and cytokinetically sound, multiple dose or continuous delivery schedules have not been extensively explored.

When given by injection into a lateral ventricle in a dose of 30 mg the peak ventricular CSF concentration was in excess of 2 mM, and the terminal half-life was 3.4 hours.[66] A cytarabine concentration cytotoxic for murine lymphoblasts (0.4 μM) was found to be present in the CSF for more than 24 hours, and no drug was detected in the plasma. Clearance of cytarabine from the CSF is almost entirely by bulk flow; in contrast to plasma, there is very little conversion of cytarabine to uracil arabinoside in the CSF. Following iV injection, cytarabine enters the CSF more readily than methotrexate, and because of the difference in cytidine deaminase activity, the half-life of cytarabine in the CSF is substantially longer than its half-life in plasma. The CSF cytarabine concentration increases linearly with IV dose. When cytarabine was given at a dose of 3 g/m[2] over 3 hours, the mean lumbar CSF concentration of 4.4 μM was 12% of simultaneous plasma concentration;[52] when given at the same dose over 1 hour the mean ventricular level was 2.1 μg/ml or 7% of the plasma concentration.[41] In the latter case the CSF half-life was 140 ± 45 minutes as compared to a plasma half-life of 17 ± 2 minutes, suggesting that a therapeutic concentration of cytarabine would be present in the CSF continuously when high dose IV cytarabine was given every 12 hours. Figure XV-4-7 shows that, as a result of extensive deamination of cytarabine in the liver, both plasma and CSF

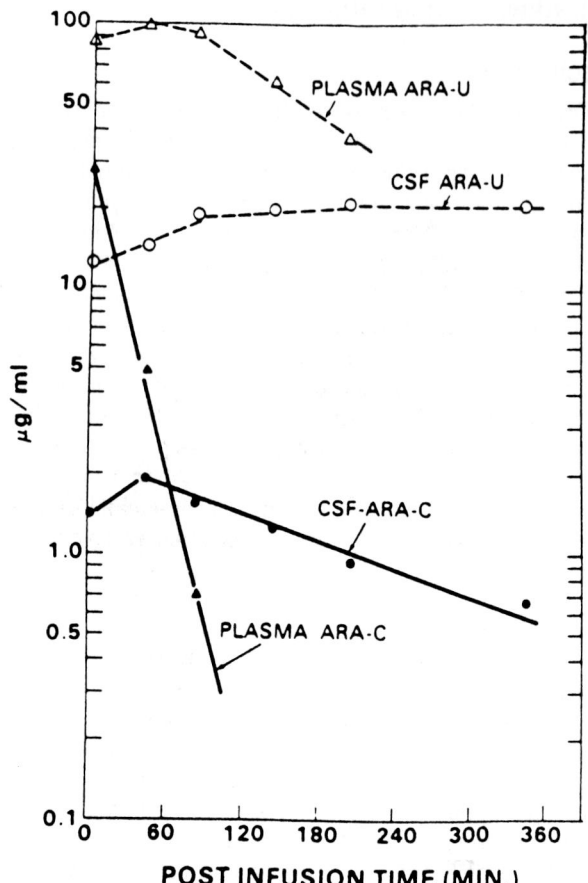

Figure XV-4-7. Plasma and CSF cytosine arabinoside (ara-C) and uracil arabinoside (ara-U) concentration in plasma and CSF following IV administration of cytosine arabinoside 3 g/m[2] over 1 hour. (From Lopez.[41])

levels of the nearly inactive deamination product uracil arabinoside are even higher than the cytarabine concentration.

In general the toxicity of IT cytarabine is less than that of methotrexate. The common toxicities of IT cytarabine include nausea and vomiting, headache, and fever; paraparesis, paraplegia, and seizures have been reported in patients receiving very high dose rates.

Other Drugs

Hydrocortisone has been added to regimens containing methotrexate and cytarabine in an attempt to reduce the incidence of arachnoiditis. No pharmacokinetic studies of IT administration have been reported, and no information is available on its activity against meningeal neoplasia.

Although thioTEPA has activity when given IT, recent pharmacokinetic studies have called into question the rationale for the use of this route.[57] ThioTEPA is quite lipid soluble, and when injected IV both the native drug and its active metabolite, TEPA, enter the CNS well. TEPA has a substantially longer plasma half-life than thioTEPA and thus accounts for a significant fraction of the total CNS drug exposure following IV dosing. Monkey studies indicate equivalent AUC in the plasma and both lumbar and ventricular CSF.[57] Although ventricular injection of 10 mg of thioTEPA in a patient with meningeal leukemia produced a ventricular exposure that was 273 times higher than plasma exposure, monkey studies suggest that distribution of drug from the ventricles to the lumbar CSF is poor, probably related to the fact that the transcapillary clearance of the drug is greater than CSF bulk flow. In addition, thioTEPA is not converted to TEPA in the CSF, limiting total CNS exposure to active forms of the drug. When thioTEPA is injected IT its major toxicity is myelo-suppression; it can produce mild lower extremity paras-thesias shortly following lumbar instillation.

Therapeutic Results

Intrathecal therapy with methotrexate is highly effective in the treatment of leukemic meningitis in children with acute lymphoblastic leukemia, or in the prophylaxis against its development, either when used alone or in combination with cranial radiation.[1,7] In combination with either radiation or other drugs it can induce remissions in patients with menin-geal lymphoma, and provide prophylaxis against the devel-opment of this complication.[51] Cytarabine is also active against meningeal leukemia when administered IT, even in patients failing IT methotrexate.[60] Current regimens usually combine methotrexate with hydrocortisone and cytarabine.[10] Recent randomized trials have suggested that the use of triple IT chemotherapy is able to obviate the need for cranial radiation in children with acute lymphoblastic leukemia and improve overall survival.[59] Several reports have documented the activity of high dose IV methotrexate or cytarabine against menin-geal leukemia and lymphoma.[1,24,45]

Intrathecal treatment of meningeal carcinomatosis has been much less successful. Response is often difficult to evaluate in these patients since, even with substantial tumor cell kill, fixed neurologic deficits may not improve. In most centers meningeal carcinomatosis is treated with a combination of intrathecal drugs and cranial radiation. Response rates range from 40–65%, but relapse is common and median survival is only in the range of 1–5 months.[29,61,65] A single randomized study with a relatively small number of patients indicated that cytarabine did not improve the response rate in patients with meningeal carcinomatosis when added to IT methotrexate.[29] Intrathecal thioTEPA has produced responses in patients with meningeal neoplasia, but the small numbers of patients studied precludes any useful assessment of its activity rel-ative to that of methotrexate or cytarabine. Assessment of response in patients with meningeal neoplasia is difficult in many studies because concurrent IV therapy was used to treat systemic disease. There is little information from ran-domized trials on the relative efficacy of single agents or of single agents versus combinations.

Intrapericardial Chemotherapy

Malignant pericardial effusions are commonly treated with one of five modalities of therapy: pericardiocentesis, peri-cardial sclerosis, systemic chemotherapy, radiation therapy, or surgical creation of a pericardial window. Malignant per-icardial effusion often occurs in the setting of widespread carcinomatosis, and one or more of these modalities is usu-ally effective in controlling the effusion for the short subse-quent lifespan. Regional chemotherapy has not been exten-sively utilized, although intrapericardial administration of cisplatin, methotrexate, 5-fluorouracil, bleomycin, or thio-TEPA appears to be safe and effective in at least some cases. Pharmacologic information is available only for meth-otrexate where pericardial to plasma AUC ratios were found to average 434.[30]

Intra-Arterial Chemotherapy

The most extensive use of IA therapy has been for the treatment of primary and metastatic disease in the liver. Since the liver is the primary site of metabolism of 5-fluorouracil and floxuridine, intra-hepatic infusion of these agents rep-resents a special circumstance where there is no increased advantage from the point of view of the tumor, but where extensive first pass metabolism limits the amount of drug reaching the systemic circulation. This permits very long duration perfusions, which, in principle, should improve the therapeutic effectiveness of these cell cycle phase specific drugs. The subject of intra-hepatic arterial infusion is dealt with in XXIX-4 elsewhere in this book. IA therapy has also been used in the treatment of limb sarcomas, carcinomas of the head and neck, and carcinomas of the lung.

Intra-Arterial Chemotherapy for Soft Tissue Sarcoma and Osteosarcoma of the Extremities

Pre-operative IA therapy with doxorubicin (30 mg/day for 3 days by continuous infusion) followed by radiation and surgery for the treatment of limb soft tissue sarcomas has been studied in a series of randomized trials from a single institution over the past 15 years. This strategy has resulted in a local recurrence rate of only 2.7%, but has not changed the rate of failure due to pulmonary metastases when com-pared to historical controls.[19,21] However, doxorubicin must be infused into large arteries in order to avoid vasculitis, and since doxorubicin has little tissue extraction and a relatively long plasma half-life, the rationale for the IA use of this drug is questionable. Preliminary results of a trial randomizing patients to IA or IV doxorubicin followed by radiation and surgery indicate no superiority for the IA route of adminis-tration.[20] The value of the use of systemic doxorubicin in combination with radiation and surgery has also not been established. There is little experience with IA infusion of any other agents for the treatment of soft tissue sarcomas, but a number of studies have been done using isolation/perfu-sion (vide infra).

There is a current surge of interest in the use of IA cisplatin for the pre-operative treatment of osteogenic sarcoma. Using catheters positioned in the brachial or femoral arteries, it was found that cisplatin doses of 150 mg/m^2 could be delivered in 3% saline over two hours on an every other week schedule when very large volume forced diuresis was employed to protect the kidneys.[34] This represents an extraordinary high dose rate for cisplatin, and this program proved more effective than high dose methotrexate for induction of initial response.[36] The extent of tumor response is greater in patients receiving more than four cycles of treatment, pulmonary metastases have responded in some patients, and the rate of limb salvage in treated patients is high.[35] The predicted advantage for an IA infusion of cisplatin into a high flow vessel is not very great, however, and it is unclear whether the IA route is a crucial component of the program. Pharmacokinetic data from an ongoing randomized trial comparing IA versus IV cisplatin as pre-operative treatment for osteogenic sarcoma demonstrated no difference in plasma AUC, renal platinum excretion, or tumor platinum content.[4]

Intra-Arterial Chemotherapy for Carcinomas of the Head and Neck

Intra-arterial chemotherapy for head and neck carcinomas is attractive because this tumor is often localized, and obtains most of its blood supply from the external carotid artery.[64] There is a long history of attempts at IA therapy, but widespread acceptance has been hampered by a high catheter complication rate, progression of tumor outside the infused volume, and the lack of cogent pharmacokinetic data and randomized trials. Comparison of patients receiving cisplatin 50 mg/m² as a 1 or 6 hour infusion IA or IV showed no difference in plasma AUC or tumor platinum content as a function of route of administration.[26] Local toxicity rates have also been high. For cisplatin these include hemi-alopecia, cranial nerve palsies, visual disturbances and seizures. Several recent studies have identified tactics for decreasing the rate of catheter complications, and have established that the dose intensity of IA cisplatin can be increased to 100 mg/m² IA every 7–14 days for three doses.[46] This offers the possibility of completing a course of pre-operative chemotherapy in a period of less than one month compared with the three months required with standard IV administration of cisplatin and 5-fluorouracil. It has also been possible to combine IA cisplatin with 14-day infusions of floxuridine, an agent for which the predicted advantage of regional delivery is very high.[23] There have been no randomized studies comparing IA and IV therapy for head and neck carcinoma.

Intra-Arterial Chemotherapy for Lung Cancer

Blood flow in the bronchial arteries constitutes only a small fraction of cardiac output, predicting a relatively large pharmacokinetic advantage for IA infusion via these arteries for the treatment of small cell and non-small cell lung cancer. However, the pharmacology is complicated by an unknown but presumably variable effect of pulmonary arterial blood flow, and the risk of damage to normal lung tissue; no pharmacokinetic data have been published. There is a modest but poorly documented clinical experience with bronchial artery infusions, particularly with doxorubicin, mitomycin, and cisplatin.[62] This approach is capable of producing responses, particularly in squamous cell carcinomas, but the existing published information does not permit an assessment of whether such responses increase resectability or alter survival.

Intra-Arterial Therapy for Primary Central Nervous System Tumors

The treatment of brain tumors poses a special challenge for IA therapy related to the fact that a variable portion of the tumor is protected from even high capillary drug concentrations by the blood-brain barrier, and to the marked regional and clonal heterogeneity of drug sensitivity found in glioblastoma multiforme.[54] Injection of drug in the carotid artery limits the pharmacologic advantage because of high blood flow; in principle the use of highly selective supra-ophthalmic injections can improve the pharmacologic advantage somewhat. A number of phase I and II trials using BCNU or cisplatin alone or in combination have been reported, and it is clear that IA administration results in novel ipsilateral brain and eye toxicities including hemiparesis, aphasias, seizures, leukoencephalopathy, brain necrosis, blurring of vision and blindness.[2] Ocular toxicity may be decreased by administration of the IA injection above the ophthalmic artery.[14] Although the occurrence of such regional toxicities strongly suggests increased drug delivery, the actual pharmacologic advantage or survival benefit attained for either of these drugs has not been well documented.[53]

The extent to which the blood-brain barrier is disrupted in brain tumors appears to be quite variable, but drug delivery to most tumors is probably at least partially impeded by tight endothelial junctions that limit drug diffusion. The blood-brain barrier can be transiently opened by the use of hyperosmolar agents such as mannitol,[47] or by the chemotherapeutic agent etoposide.[56] In experimental systems, opening the barrier just prior to chemotherapeutic drug administration can increase drug delivery to the brain, but has the potential of increasing delivery to both normal and malignant brain tissue, a situation which yields no increase in selectivity.[54] A 30 minute IA infusion of mannitol serves to open the blood-brain barrier as documented by the entry of ⁹⁹Tc, and this strategy has been used in combination with BCNU and cisplatin in phase II trials.[48] However, this approach is associated with significant morbidity due to local toxicity, and convincing evidence for net therapeutic benefit is still lacking.

Isolation-Perfusion Chemotherapy for Melanoma and Soft Tissue Sarcoma

This strategy for differentially increasing total drug exposure involves cannulating the major artery and vein for all or a portion of a limb, and connecting a pump oxygenator to create a closed circuit into which drug is introduced. Leakage from this closed circuit into the systemic circulation is limited by the application of a constricting bandage at the base of the limb. Although a large number of variations have been employed, by far the greatest experience is with the use of hyperthermic isolation/perfusion with melphalan for the prevention of recurrence of limb melanomas following wide local excision with or without lymph node dissection. A commonly used program involves heating of the blood in the extracorporeal circuit to 39–42° C with careful thermistor monitoring of limb temperature. Melphalan is introduced into the circuit as the temperature rises, and perfusion is continued for 1 hour. The extracorporeal circuit is then rinsed with new blood or dextran solution to remove the melphalan, and the vessels are repaired.

Early studies used melphalan dosing regimens that were based on body weight or surface area; a dose of 1–1.5 mg/kg was commonly employed. However, neither body weight nor surface area are good predictors of the blood volume of a limb, and selection of dose based on direct measurement of limb volume,[63] or indirect estimation of limb blood volume results in smaller patient to patient variance.[39] Melphalan has a terminal half-life of 53 minutes in the extracorporeal circuit, and total drug exposure for the circuit ranges from 1,000 to nearly 4,000 ug·min/ml.[3] For comparison, IV injection of a maximum tolerated dose of melphalan produces an AUC in the range of 55 ug·min/ml. Although generally 5–12% of the volume of the albumin in the extracorporal circuit leaks into the systemic circulation during a 1 hour perfusion,[25,40] systemic melphalan exposure is insufficient to cause myelosupression in more than a small fraction of the patients treated.

Although melphalan hyperthermic isolation/perfusion has established activity against advanced limb melanomas and soft tissue sarcomas, its major use has been as an adjuvant to wide local resection of early stage disease. Despite more than 30 years of experience, only one prospective randomized trial has been completed.[25] This study showed a significant decrease in relapse rate (11% vs. 48%) and increase in both disease free and total survival for patients with operable limb melanomas undergoing melphalan hyperthermic isolation/perfusion. A number of retrospective analyses have shown minimal or no benefit, however, and this form of treatment remains controversial.[18,40] Acute complications of isolation/perfusion include edema, nerve palsy, and skin toxicity, but significant long-term sequelae other than limitation of motion at distal joints is unusual. While a number of other drugs besides melphalan have been administered by limb isolation/perfusion, including imidazole, carboxamide, doxorubicin, cisplatin, etoposide, mechlorethamine, and actinomycin D, pharmacokinetic information is lacking and no comparative studies of efficacy have been conducted.

Overview

Regional therapy is currently part of standard treatment only for the prophylaxis or management of meningeal metastases; the extent to which other forms of regional therapy should be part of standard treatment has not yet been clearly defined. One criticism of regional therapy is that it usually cannot deal with all of the disease in the body. However, tumor burden is an important determinant of treatment outcome for many types of cancer, and under circumstances where regional therapy actually increases drug delivery to the tumor, there is a high probability that the regional approach will improve the chances that concurrent or subsequent systemic therapy will cure the disease. The pharmacologic advantage of regional therapy can be enhanced by a variety of currently available tactics, such as the use of systemic neutralizing agents and modulation of tumor blood flow and regional clearances. Newly evolving technologies for creating slow-release forms of drug promise additional improvements in the efficacy of regional therapy in the future.

References

1. Abromowitch, M., Ochs, J., Pui, C., Kalwinsky, D., Rivera, G. K, Fairclough, D., Look, A. T., Hustu, H. O., Murphy, S. B., Evans, W. E., Dahl, G. V., and Bowman, W. P.: High-dose methotrexate improves clinical outcome in children with acute lymphoblastic leukemia: St. Jude total therapy study X. Med. Ped. Oncol., 16:297, 1988.
2. Bashir, R., Hochberg, F. H., Linggood, R. M., and Hottleman, K.: Pre-irradiation internal cartoid artery BCNU in treatment of glioblastoma multiforme. J. Neurosurg., 68:917, 1988.
3. Benckhuijsen, C., Varossieau, F. J., Hart, A. A. M., Weiberdink, J., and Noordhoek, J.: Pharmacokinetics of melphalan in Isolated perfusion of the limbs. J. Pharm. Exp. Therap., 237:583, 1986.
4. Bielack, S. S., Erttmann, R., Looft, G., Purfurst, C., Delling, G., Winkler, K., and Landbeck, G.: Platinum disposition after intraarterial and intravenous infusion of cisplatin for osteosarcoma. Cancer Chemother. Pharmacol., 24:376, 1989.
5. Blasberg, R., Patlak, C. S., and Fenstermacher, J. D.: Intrathecal chemotherapy: Brain tissue profiles after ventriculocisternal perfusion. J. Pharmacol. Exp. Ther., 195:73, 1975.
6. Blasberg, R., Patlak, C. S., and Shapiro, W. R.: Distribution of methotrexate in the cerebrospinal fluid and brain after intraventricular administration. Cancer Treat. Rep., 61:633, 1977.
7. Bleyer, W. A., Coccia, P. F., Sather, H. N., Level, C., Lukens, J., Neibrugge, D. J., Siegel, St., Littman, P. S., Leikin, S. L., Miller, D. R., Chard, R. L., Hammond, G. D., and the Childrens Cancer Study Group: Reduction in central nervous system leukemia with a pharmacokinetically derived intrathecal methotrexate dosage regimen. J. Clin. Oncol., 1:317, 1983.
8. Bleyer, W. A., and Dedrick, R. L.: Clinical pharmacology of intrathecal methotrexate. I. Pharmacokinetics in nontoxic patients after lumbar injection. Cancer Treat. Rep., 614:703, 1977.
9. Bleyer, W. A., Poplack, D. G., and Simon, R. M.: "Concentration × Time" methotrexate via a subcutaneous reservoir: A less toxic regimen for intraventricular chemotherapy of central nervous system neoplasms. Blood, 51:835, 1978.
10. Buchanan, G. R., Rivera, G. K., Boyett, J. M., Chauvenent, A. R., Crist, W. M., and Vietti, T. J.: Reinduction therapy in 297 children with acute lymphoblastic leukemia in first bone marrow relapse: A pediatric oncology group study. Blood, 72:1286, 1988.
11. Burch, P. A., Grossman, S. A., and Reinhard, C. S.: Spinal cord penetration of intrathecally administered cytarabine and methotrexate: A quantitative autoradiographic study. J. Natl. Cancer Inst., 80:1211, 1988.
12. Collins, J. M.: Pharmacokinetics of intra-ventricular administration. J. Neuro-Oncol., 1:283, 1983.
13. Collins, J. M.: Pharmacologic rationale for regional drug delivery. J. Clin. Oncol., 2:498, 1984.
14. Clayman, D. A., Wolpert, S. M., and Heros, D. O.: Superselective arterial BCNU infusion in the treatment of patients with malignant gliomas. A.J.N.R., 10:767, 1989.
15. Dedrick, R. L.: Review: Arterial drug infusion: Pharmacokinetic problems and pitfalls. J. Natl. Cancer Inst., 802:84, 1988.
16. Dedrick, R. L., Myers, C. E., Bungay, P. M., and DeVita, V. T.: Pharmacokinetic rationale for peritoneal drug administration in the treatment of ovarian cancer. Cancer Treat. Rep., 62:1, 1978.
17. Eckman, W. W., Patlak, C. S., and Fenstermacher, J. D.: A critical evaluation of the principles governing the advantages of intra-arterial infusions. J. Pharmacokinet. Biopharm., 2:257, 1974.
18. Edwards, M. J., Soong, S., Boddie, A. W., Balch, C. M., and McBride, C. M.: Isolated limb perfusion for localized melanoma of the extremity. Arch. Surg., 125:317, 1990.
19. Eilber, F. R., Guiliano, A. E., Huth, A., Mirra, J., and Morton, D. L.: Limb salvage for high-grade soft tissue sarcomas of the extremity: Experience at the University of California. Cancer Treat. Symp., 3:49, 1985.
20. Eilber, F. R., Giuliano, A. E., Huth, J. F., Weisenburger, T., and Eckardt, J.: Intravenous IV vs. intra-arterial IA adriamycin, 2800r radiation and surgical excision for extremity soft tissue sarcomas: A randomized prospective trial. Proc. Am. Soc. Clin. Oncol., 9:309, 1990.
21. Eilber, F. R., Morton, D. L., Eckardt, J., Grant, T., and Weisenburger, T.: Limb salvage for skeletal and soft tissue sarcomas. Cancer 53:2579, 1984.
22. Fenstermacher, J. D., Blasberg, R. G., and Patlak, C. S.: Methods for quantifying the transport of drugs across brain barrier systems. Pharmacol. Ther., 14:217, 1981.
23. Forastiere, A. A., Baker, S. R., Wheeler, R., and Medvec, B. R.: Intra-arterial cisplatin and FUDR in advanced malignancies confined to the head and neck. J. Clin. Oncol., 5:1601, 1987.
24. Freeman, A. I., Weinberg, V., Brecher, M. L., Jones, B., Glicksman, A. S., Sinks, L. F., Weil, M., Pleuss, H., Hananian, J., Burgert, E. O., Gilchrist, G. S., Necheles, T., Harris, M., Kung, F., Patterson, R. B., Maurer, H., Leventhal, B., Chevalier, L., Forman, E., and Holland, J. F.: Comparison of intermediate-dose methotrexate with cranial irradiation for the post-induction treatment of acute lymphocytic leukemia in children. N. Eng. J. Med., 308:477, 1983.
25. Ghussen, F., Kruger, I., Smalley, R. V., and Groth W.: Hyperthermic perfusion with chemotherapy for melanoma of the extremities. World J. Surg., 13:598, 1989.
26. Gouyette, A., Apchin, A., Foka, M., and Richards, J.: Pharmacokinetics of intra-arterial and intravenous cisplatin in head and neck cancer patients. Eur. J. Cancer Clin. Oncol., 22:257, 1986.

27. Grossman, S. A., Trump, D. L., Chen, D. C. P., Thompson, G., and Camargo, E. E.: Cerebrospinal fluid flow abnormalities in patients with neoplastic meningitis. Amer. J. Med., 73:641, 1982.

28. Hausheer, F. H., and Yarbro, J. W.: Diagnosis and treatment of malignant pleural effusions. Semin. Oncol., 12:54, 1985.

29. Hitchins, R. N., Bell, D. R., Woods, R. L., and Levi, J. A.: A prospective randomized trial of single-agent versus combination chemotherapy in meningeal carcinomatosis. J. Clin. Oncol., 5:1655, 1987.

30. Howell, S. B., Chus, B. C. F., Wung, W., Metha, B., and Mendolsohn, J.: Long duration intracavitary infusion of methotrexate with systemic leucovorin protection in patients with malignant effusions. J. Clin. Invest., 67:1167, 1981.

31. Howell, S. B., Kirmani, S., Lucas, W. E., Zimm, S., Goel, R., Kim, S., Horton, C., McVey, L., Morris, J., and Weiss, R. J.: A phase II trial of intraperitoneal cisplatin and etoposide for primary treatment of ovarian epithelial cancer. J. Clin. Oncol., 8:137, 1990.

32. Howell, S. B., Pfeifle, C. E., Wung, W. E., Olshen, R. A., Lucas, W. E., Yong, J. L., and Green, M.: Intraperitoneal cisplatin with systemic thiosulfate protection. Ann. Int. Med., 97:845, 1982.

33. Howell, S. B., Zimm, S., Markman, M., Abramson, I. S., Cleary, S., Lucas, W. E., and Weiss, R. J.: Long term survival of advanced refractory ovarian carcinoma patients with small volume disease treated with intraperitoneal chemotherapy. J. Clin. Oncol., 5:1607, 1987.

34. Jaffe, N., Knapp, J., Chuang, V. P., Wallace, S., Ayala, A., Murray, J., Cangir, A., Wang, A., and Benjamin, R. S.: Osteosarcoma: intra-arterial treatment of the primary tumor with cis-diammine-dichloroplatinum II (CDP). Cancer 51:402, 1983.

35. Jaffe, N., Raymond, A. K., Ayala, A., Carasco, C. H., Wallace, S., Robertson, R., Griffiths, M., and Wang, Y.: Effect of cumulative courses of intraarterial cis-diammi-nedichloroplatin-II on the primary tumor in osteosarcoma. Cancer, 63:63, 1989.

36. Jaffe, N., Robertson, R., Ayala, A., Wallace, S., Chuang, V., Anzai, T., Cangir, A., Wang, Y., and Chen, T.: Comparison of intra-arterial cis-diamminedichloroplatinum II with high-dose methotrexate and citrovorum factor rescue in the treatment of primary osteosarcoma. J. Clin. Oncol., 3:1101, l985.

37. Jain, R. K.: Transport of molecules across tumor vasculature. Cancer Metastasis Reviews, 6:559, 1987.

38. Kieffer, S. A., Wolff, J. M., Prentice, W. B., and Loken, M. K.: Scinticisternography in individuals without known neurological disease. Amer. J. Roentgen., 112:225, 1971.

39. Lejeune, F. J., and Ghanem, G. E.: A simple and accurate new method for cytostatics dosimetry in isolation perfusion of the limbs based on exchangeable blood volume determination. Cancer Res., 47:639, 1987.

40. Lejeune, F. J., Lienard, D., El Douaihy, M., Seyedi, J., and Ewalenko, P.: Results of 206 isolated limb perfusions for malignant melanoma. Eur. J. Surg. Oncol., 15:510, 1989.

41. Lopez, J. A., Nassif, E., Vannicola, P., Krikorian, J. G. and Agarwal, R. P.: Central nervous system pharmacokinetics of high-dose cytosine arabinoside. J. Neuro-Oncol. 3:119, 1985.

42. Los, G., Mutsaers, P. H., van der Vijgh, W. J., Baldew, G. S., de Graaf, P. W., and McVie, J. G.: Direct diffusion of cis-diamminedichloroplatinum(II) in intraperitoneal rat tumors after intraperitoneal chemotherapy: a comparison with systemic chemotherapy. Cancer Res., 49:3380, 1989.

43. Markman, M., Cleary, S., Pfeifle, C., and Howell, S. B.: Cisplatin administered by the intracavitary route as treatment for malignant mesothelioma. Cancer, 58:18, 1986.

44. Montaldo, P. G., Figoli, F., Zanette, M. L., Sorio, R., Zucchetti, M., Tirelli, U., and D'Incalci, M.: Pharmacokinetic of intrapleural versus intravenous etoposide (VP16) and teniposide (VM26) in patients with malignant pleural effusion. Oncol., 47:55, 1990.

45. Morra, E., Lazzarino, M., Inverardi, D., Brusamolino, E., Orlandi, E., Canevari, A., Pagnucco, G., and Bernasconi, C.: Systemic high-dose ara-C for the treatment of meningeal leukemia in adult acute lymphoblastic leukemia and non-Hodgkin's lymphoma. J. Clin. Oncol., 4:1207, 1986.

46. Mortimer, J. E., Taylor, M. E., Schulman, S., Cummings, C., Weymuller, E., and Laramore, G.: Feasibility and efficacy of weekly intraarterial cisplatin in locally advanced (stage III and IV) head and neck cancers. J. Clin. Oncol., 6:969, 1988.

47. Neuwelt, E. A., Barnett, P. A., Bigner, D. D., and Frenkel, E.P.: The effects of osmotic modification of the blood brain barrier and adrenal steroid administration on methotrexate delivery of gliomas in rats: the blood brain barrier is a factor. Proc. Natl. Acad. Sci., 79:4420, 1982.

48. Neuwelt, E. A., Howieson, J., Frenkel, E. P., Specht, H. D., Weigel, R., Buchan, C. G., and Hill, S. A.: Therapeutic efficacy of multiagent chemotherapy with drug delivery enhancement by blood-brain barrier modification in glioblastoma. Neurosurg., 19:573, 1986.

49. Ostrowski, M. J.: Intracavitary therapy with bleomycin for the treatment of malignant pleural effusions. J. Surg. Oncol., 1(Suppl.):7, 1989.

50. Patlak, C. S., and Fenstermacher, J. D.: Measurements of dog blood-brain transfer constants by ventriculocisternal perfusion. Am. J. Physio., 229:877, 1975.

51. Recht, L., Straus, D. J., Cirrincione, C., Thaler, H., and Posner, J. B.: Central nervous system metastases from non-Hodgkin's lymphoma: treatment and prophylaxis. Am. J. Med., 84:425, 1988.

52. Selvin, M. L., Piall, E. M., Aherne, G. W., Harvey, V. J., Johnston, A., and Lister, T. A.: Effect of dose and schedule on pharmacokinetics of high-dose cytosine arabinoside in plasma and cerebrospinal fluid. J. Clin. Oncol. 1:546, 1983.

53. Shani, J., Bertram, J., Russell, C., Dahalan, R., Chen, D. C. P., Parti, R., Ahmadi, J., Kempf, R. A., Kawada, T. K., Muggia, F. M., and Wolf, W.: Noninvasive monitoring of drug biodistribution and metabolism: studies with intraarterial Pt-195m-cisplatin in humans. Cancer Res., 49:1877, 1989.

54. Shapiro, W. R., and Shapiro, J. R.: Principles of brain tumor chemotherapy. Semin. Oncol., 13:56, 1986.

55. Shapiro, W. R., Young, D. F., and Mehta, B. M.: Methotrexate: Distribution in cerebrospinal fluid after intravenous, ventricular and lumbar injections. N. Engl. J. Med., 293:161, 1975.

56. Spigelman, M. K., Zappulla, R. A., Strauchen, J. A., Feuer, E. J., Johnson, J., Goldsmith, S. J., Malis, L. I., and Holland, J. F.: Etoposide induced blood-brain barrier disruption in rats: Duration of opening and histological sequelae. Cancer Res., 46:1453, 1986.

57. Strong, J. M., Collins, J. M., Lester, C., and Poplack, D. G.: Pharmacokinetics of intraventricular and intravenous N,N′,N″-triethylenethiophosphoramide (thiotepa) in rhesus monkeys and humans. Cancer Res., 46:6101, 1986.

58. Strother, D. R., Glynn-Barnhart, A., Kovnar, E., Gregory, R. E., and Murphy, S. B.: Variability in the disposition of intraventricular methotrexate: a proposal for rational dosing. J. Clin. Oncol., 7:1741, 1989.

59. van Eys, J., Berry, D., Crist, W., Doering E., Fernbach, D., Pullen, J., Shuster, J., and Wharam, M.: A comparison of two regimens for high-risk acute lymphocytic leukemia in childhood. A Pediatric Oncology Group Study. Cancer, 63:23, 1989.

60. Wang, J. J., and Pratt, C. B.: Intrathecal arabinosyl cytosine in meningeal leukemia. Cancer, 25:531, 1970.

61. Wasserstrom, W. R., Glass, J. P., and Posner, J. B.: Diagnosis and treatment of leptomeningeal metastases from solid tumors: experience with 90 patients. Cancer, 49:759, 1982.

62. Watanabe, Y., Shimizu, J., Murakami, S., Yoshida, M., Tsubota, M., Iwa, T., Kitagawa, M., Mizukami, Y., Nonomura, A., and Matsubara, F.: Reappraisal of bronchial arterial infusion therapy for advanced lung cancer. Jap. J. Surg., 20:27, 1990.

63. Wieberdink, J., Benckhuysen, C., Braat, R. P., Van Slooten, E. A., and Olthuis, G. A. A.: Dosimetry in isolation perfusion of the limbs by assessment of perfused tissue volume and grading of toxic tissue reactions. Eur. J. Cancer Clin. Oncol., 18:905, 1982.

64. Wheeler, R. H., Ziessman, H. A., Medvec, B. R., Juni, J. E., Thrall, J. H., Keyes, J. W., Pitt, S. R., and Baker, S. R.: Tumor blood flow and systemic shunting in patients receiving intraarterial chemotherapy for head and neck cancer. Cancer Res., 46:4200, 1986.

65. Yap, H. Y., Rasmussen, S., Levens, M. E., Hortobagyi, G. N., Bulmenschein, G. R., and Yap, B. S.: The treatment for meningeal carcinotosis in breast cancer. Cancer, 50:219, 1982.

66. Zimm, S., Collins, J. M., Miser, J., Chatterji, D., and Poplack, D. G.: Cytosine arabinoside cerebrospinal fluid kinetics. Clin. Pharmacol. Ther., 35:826, 1984.

Animal Models in Drug Development

Samir N. Khleif
Gregory A. Curt

Introduction

The process of cancer drug discovery may begin with either empiric screening or rational drug design. In either case, the necessary steps in drug development which follow the identification of an interesting lead require appropriate animal model systems. Just as screening systems and rational drug design have benefited from recent advances in cell culture technique and molecular biology, so too has the role of animal model systems in drug development. Beyond simply predicting dose-limiting toxicity, drug metabolism or tissue and compartment distribution, animal models are increasingly being used to guide dose escalation in Phase I trials and provide tumor microenvironments which mimic the clinical situation. The processes of cancer drug discovery and drug development have evolved, and will continue to change, since the first successful use of drugs to treat systemic cancer more than 50 years ago. This chapter will discuss the history and future of cancer drug discovery and drug development with special emphasis on the role of animal models in the process.

The Role of Animal Models in Drug Discovery

Drug Screening

The idea that systemic drugs could treat, and possibly cure, systemic cancer is relatively new in medicine. In the mid 1940's, Gilman's treatment of lymphomas with alkylating agents at Yale, and Farber's induction of short remissions in leukemia with antifolates at Harvard led the National Cancer Institute (NCI) to begin a major effort in cancer drug discovery and development. Stated in its simplest terms, the purpose of the initial NCI screen was to select and prioritize drugs for clinical trial.[4–6,17–23,33,38,78,113,168,169]

In 1955, murine leukemia models, P388 and L1210 were selected as the initial system in which potential agents would need to demonstrate activity before further development. The reason for this selection was simple. Murine leukemia and lymphoma models were relatively inexpensive and allowed for a relatively high throughput of compounds. Indeed, from the inception of the mouse screen until its first modifications in the mid 1970's, more than 400,000 compounds passed through this screen.

At first, this mouse screening system was empiric. Over time, however, this empiricism became more enlightened with the development of the NCI Drug Information System. This computer-based inventory maintains the structure of each compound screened and its activity in murine model systems. This system has been used to limit the screening of analogs while turning greater attention to novel structures. Importantly, the Drug Information System also maintains discrete databases on compounds provided to NCI on a proprietary basis by pharmaceutical companies, allowing open access of the screen to industry.

From the beginning, however, it was obvious that this system had serious limitations. While most of the active drugs currently used in the treatment of leukemia and lymphoma were initially screened in the L1210 system, screening against rapidly growing leukemic cells could bias selection toward compounds that are preferentially active against rapidly growing tumors with essentially a 100% growth fraction. In fact, it was found that plateau phase cultures were less sensitive to cycle specific agents than log phase culture, while some classes of clinically useful drugs, such as the alkylators, were active in plateau phase cell lines. The development of drugs active against the solid tumors of adulthood would presumably require a different approach.

The availability of new rodent models enabled the NCI to take further steps toward rational drug screening in 1975.[63] Instead of a single hurdle of activity in murine leukemia, compounds active in this system were subsequently tested against a panel that included transplantable murine tumor models designed to resemble common human solid tumors (including melanoma and lung, colon and breast cancer) both in histology and cell kinetics. In a step which would presage later changes in the NCI screen, the availability of athymic (nude) mice also allowed the screening of drugs against transplantable human tumors as well.[138,162] Initially, these human tumor xenografts included lung, colon and breast cancer.[52,97,121]

Overall, these changes took the NCI screen from a compound-oriented toward a more tumor-specific approach. However, the high cost of the transplantable mouse and human xenograft systems (approximately $5,000 per compound) was unsuitable for high capacity screening. Instead, the NCI designed a two stage system in which the murine leukemia model was maintained as a Stage I "prescreen." Compounds entering the system were first tested against

spontaneous or artificially transplanted systems. Solid tumors are usually transplanted by the inoculation of cell suspensions either by the subcutaneous (SC), intradermal (ID), intramuscular (IM), intraperitoneal (IP) or intravenous (IV) routes. Leukemia models are transplanted only by the SC, IV or IP routes.

The spontaneous tumor models which are either idiopathic or arise following carcinogenic,[28,29] or viral exposure mimic the clinical situation most closely. Spontaneous tumors are usually measurable only late in their course. Their metastatic pattern is not uniform and their response to therapy is generally poor. They also resemble human cancers in kinetics and antigenicity.

However, there are significant obstacles to the use of such model systems. For example, a relatively small percentage of animals may develop disease following exposure to carcinogen or virus and the tumors may have a variable natural course. In addition, the inability to establish accurate staging makes these models quantitatively unsuitable for assessing therapeutic response to an agent given in a uniform fashion. Generally speaking, spontaneous tumor models have their greatest role in studying the biology of carcinogenesis. In the future, they may also be important in the development of chemopreventive or chemosuppressive drugs.

The models with the widest use in experimental therapeutics are the transplanted animal tumor models and the human tumor xenografts. These will be discussed in some detail below.

Transplantable Animal Tumor Models

Early passages of transplanted tumors resemble spontaneous cancer most closely. These early passages show significant heterogeneity in cell kinetics and histology.[101,151] Despite these limitations, such models have been used in drug screening. Because established transplantable tumor models are well characterized and reproducible, they have traditionally been the foundation of cancer drug development.[108,131,132,144] How good are they in predicting clinical activity?

Multiple studies have been undertaken to assess the ability of preclinical animal activity to predict antitumor response in man.[11,14,89] Marsoni and co-workers evaluated the activity of all cytotoxic drugs introduced into Phase II clinical trial by the NCI between 1970–1985.[99] Of the 75 drugs entered into clinical trial during this period, 24 showed some evidence for clinical activity. One interpretation of these data is that the screen is highly predictive for clinical activity. Approximately 30% of drugs taken to clinical trial showed some evidence of activity. However, 74% of the drugs were active against lymphoma and 35% were active against leukemia. Only minimal activity was observed against solid tumors including those represented in the Phase II portion of the screen. Indeed, analysis showed a poor correlation between preclinical in vivo and clinical activity in the same tumors. One must conclude that either animal model systems using transplantable tumors do not predict for clinical activity or that the P388 prescreen effectively selected against compounds specifically active in human solid tumors. The new in vitro human cell line screen will be important in answering these questions, since the initial identification of activity is in a human solid tumor rather than a murine leukemia-lymphoma model system.

Tumor Response Evaluation in Animal Models

A range of methods can be used to evaluate drug effect on tumors in animal models. Tumor size and tumor weight or volume changes are simple and easily reproducible parameters. Morphologic changes and alterations in tumor immunogenicity or invasiveness are other markers of response.[62]

In addition, many specific assays have been developed for the measurement of treatment effects on tumors. This section will discuss some assays that can be used to judge tumor response.

Excision Clonogenic Assay

This assay has been used widely as a method to assess what fraction of cells in a tumor population retain proliferative capability after being exposed to a chemotherapeutic agent. This assay is based on the assumption that the proliferative or clonogenic potential of tumor cells reflects the in vivo tumorigenicity of the tumor stem cell.[149,152] Thus, colony number is assumed to be proportionate to the number of viable cells.

The assay itself is straightforward. Tumor-bearing animals are tested with the drug under evaluation. At 24 hours, the tumors are excised from treated and untreated animals. A cell suspension is prepared from every tumor. The proliferative capacity of the cells in each suspension is evaluated by either in vivo inoculation intravenously into test animals of a selected cell suspension dilution,[76,153] or by plating the cells in liquid or agar medium.[26,75,133] If an animal model is used, colony count is then performed in specific tissues at necroscopy. The lung, liver and spleen are commonly used for this purpose. If the cells were plated in agar, a colony count is performed in the dish. Colony-forming efficiency (CE) of the inoculated cells is calculated to assess the efficacy of treatment in terms of cell survival.

$$CE = \frac{\text{Number of tumor colonies counted}}{\text{Number of tumor cells plated}}$$

The ratio of the CE treated to the CE control is called surviving fraction (SF).

$$SF = \frac{CE \text{ treated}}{CE \text{ control}}$$

SF is the best parameter for expressing cell survival results from the excisional biopsy.[92,154]

This assay has the advantage of placing the treated and untreated tumors in identical environments. It is also able to select a resistant population of cells within the tumor at a low drug dose. In addition, excising the tumor 24 hours after exposing the animal to the cytotoxic agent allows giving doses up to the transplant range, which has important implications for the selection of agents for bone marrow transplantation.

TD$_{50}$ (Endpoint Dilution Assay)

TD$_{50}$[74,77,93] is the tumor cell inoculum that produces tumor growth in 50% of inoculated animals or sites. It is a measurement of the number of cells required to produce tumors from inocula in vivo. The assay is based on the same principles as that of colony formation. A cell suspension is prepared from both treated and untreated animals, with ranges of dilutions for each tumor depending on the expected value of TD$_{50}$. The suspension is inoculated into groups of test animals subcutaneously, intramuscularly or intradermally for solid tumors and intraperitoneally or intravenously for leukemias. The percentage of tumor take versus cell number inoculated for each treatment is determined and compared to control animals to determine TD$_{50}$.[49]

Tumor Growth Delay Assay

Cytotoxic treatment can slow tumor growth and delay disease progression. These effects are measured by the tumor growth delay assay.[9,10,157] Tumor delay by definition is the time required for the treated tumor to reach a specific size minus the time for the untreated tumor to reach that certain size. This assay involves a very simple technique, little equipment, and can be completed for many types of tumors before animals are lost to metastasis or disease progression. Unlike the survival time assay discussed later, this evaluation does not require death as an endpoint.

The correlation between the growth delay and the amount of cell kill varies with the growth rate of the tumor.[10] Thus, when a treatment effect on tumors with different growth rates is assessed, a comparison of absolute growth delay between tumor models is misleading. Therefore, a specific growth delay (growth delay/doubling time of the tumor) reflects more accurately the differences in cell kill. Figure XV-5-3 illustrates the concept of specific growth delay.

The Survival Time Assay

Another parameter that can be used to assess the effect of a drug on tumor in the animal model is the survival time. Survival time is an obvious endpoint, since it combines the sum total of interactions between tumor, drug and host. Since drug toxicity and tumor growth both have independent effects on survival, a judgment can be made about therapeutic index. However, this approach cannot directly assess cell kill or time-dependent cytotoxicity.

The therapeutic efficacy can be assessed by determining the increase in survival as an effect of the escalating dose of the studied drug. As the dose of an active drug increases, the survival time increases because of increasing logarithmic tumor cell kill. Survival time reaches a maximum point as the toxic effect of the drug outweighs the therapeutic effect and survival times diminish.[145] The maximum point of survival is called the optimal point (OP) or the maximum increase in life span (IL). The higher the OP the better the given intervention's therapeutic efficacy. This model also helps in assessing the safety of certain drugs by measuring the therapeutic ratio (TR), that is, the ratio between the optimal dose and that dose which leads to a specific increase in survival time (e.g., IL 20, IL 40, etc.). Therefore, in comparing drugs with the same maximum survival (optimal point), the higher the therapeutic ratio, the safer the drug.[145]

A common use of survival to assess drug efficacy or increase in life span is the T/C percent ratio. This is defined as the ratio of the survival time of treated animals to the survival time of control, expressed as a percentage. This parameter has been used by the NCI for decision-making, setting specific criteria of activity before further development is undertaken. A T/C of >120 in the solid tumor panel has been used as the benchmark for clinical development (Figure XV-5-1).[15,16,100,122]

Animal Tumor Xenografts

Prior to the availability of athymic or nude mice, human tumors were xenografted in mice immunocompromised by irradiation, thymectomy, or steroids.[32,158,159] The first nude mice arose spontaneously in a closed, but not inbred colony of albino mice in a virus laboratory in Ruchill Hospital, Glasgow, Scotland,[134] and were described by Isaacson and Cattancer as lacking fur.[84] The first xenograft in nude mice was performed by Rygaard and Povlsen in 1969 using a human colon adenocarcinoma.[136]

Flanagan initially described the genetic component of immunodeficiency in this important model. He found that the mutant gene (nu: for nude) is present on chromosome 11, as an autosomal recessive gene.[50] It is responsible for the absence of hair in addition to other abnormalities including retarded growth, low fertility, and short life span (100% mortality within 25 weeks of birth and 45% mortality within 2 weeks of birth).[134] It was not until 1968 that Panetlouris noted that some of the nude mice lacked a thymus gland. These mice were found to have a homozygous mutation nu/nu, while both the phenotypically normal +/+, and the heterozygous nu/+ had a thymus.[124] Immunologically, the nu/nu athymic mice have a small number of T cells that are residual after transplacental passage from heterozygous mothers. However, these T cells do not affect the rejection of tissue transplants (or other markers of T cell function).[129] These animals preserve B cell function[147] and exhibit a higher activity of natural killer cells.[73,80] These characteristics led to widespread use of nude mice in tissue transplantation and other areas of biomedical research,[50,53,82,118,135,137] including their use in human tumor transplantation.

The success of human tumor xenografting into the nude mice, and the ability to maintain the histologic and biologic identity of tumors through successive passages in vivo revolutionized many aspects of cancer research, including drug development.[83,114,128,140] Transplantation of tumor cell lines into nude mice can be accomplished via multiple routes: subcutaneous, intraperitoneal,[59] intravenous, intracranial,[58] intrasplenic, renal subcapsular, or through a new orthotopic model by site-specific organ inoculation. Each site has specific advantages and limitations.

Subcutaneous implantation is the predominant site for transplantation of human tumor into the nude mouse because of its simplicity and easy access to tumor. Indeed, it provides the mainstay for in vivo testing of the drug discovery and screening program of the NCI.[120]

A tumor cell suspension is usually injected into the flank of the animal. Depending on the clonogenic potential of the tumor, between 10^6–10^7 cells are required for successful

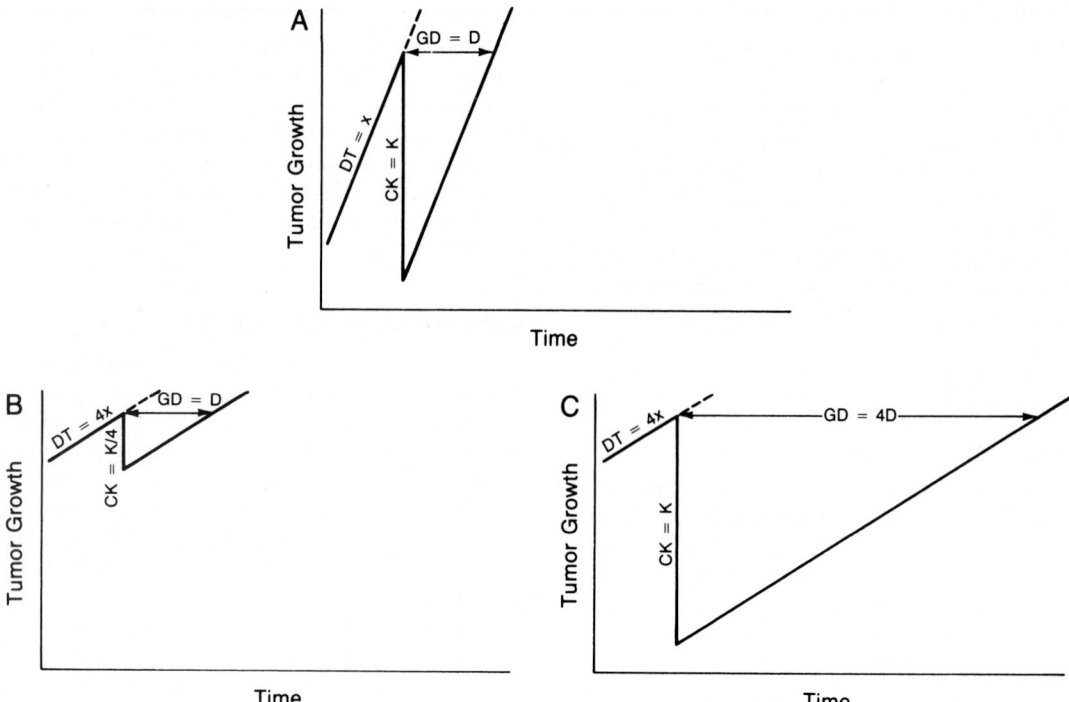

Figure XV-5-3. Tumor growth in relation to time before and after treatment (A). A 4-fold doubling time requires 1/4 of cell kill for the same growth delay (B). The same amount of cell kill results in 4-fold increase in growth delay (C). DT = Doubling time, CK = Cell kill, GD = Growth delay, K = Relative cell kill, D = Relative growth delay over time.

engraftment. Tumors usually require between a few days to a few months to grow depending on the growth rate of the cell line used. Many human tumor xenografts have been established to date including those from most of the solid tumors affecting adults. Human colon cancer and melanoma have been passaged for the longest time in vivo. Brain tumors have proven the most difficult to maintain.[40,47] Approximately one-half of the brain tumor cell lines have been successfully xenografted into athymic mice.[40]

Of interest, subcutaneous xenografts metastasize infrequently and seldom invade adjacent tissues. This may be because of the retention of some host defenses, especially natural killer cell activity.[73,80] Thus, animal survival is not a feasible endpoint for assessing drug efficacy in nude mice, since large tumor burdens prior to death may be associated with discomfort. Instead, the growth delay or the clonogenic assay would be more appropriate in this model. However, it is possible to select primary tumors or perturb the host defense mechanisms to develop models which are locally invasive or metastatic. Metastasis can be enhanced with the depletion of NK cells by pretreating the mice with cyclophosphamide, beta estradiol, or other agents.[44,48,94]

Human tumor cells undergo kinetic changes after transplantation and passage in the nude mice. Most frequently, the transplanted tumor adapted to growth in animals has a shorter doubling time than the original tumor isolated from a patient.[149] Growth rates increase further during subsequent passages.[35,150] The vascularity of the primary and transplanted tumor also differ with transplanted tumors showing better blood supply and less necrosis. This difference could be due to selection of the most rapidly growing cells from a

heterogeneous primary animal, secretion of paracrine growth factors which induce neovascularization, or simply tumor size.

Despite these changes in kinetic of invasive potential, the majority of the xenografted human tumors maintain the morphologic and biochemical characteristics of their original tumors. Therefore, it is expected that chemosensitivity would be similar in both the original and the xenografted human tumor, and that this correlation would predict for both active single agents and active drug combinations. In fact, excellent correlations can be made between average growth delay for human tumors in nude mice treated with the best available drug combinations and complete clinical response rates.[46,61] In increasing order of responsiveness, these correlations have been shown for human xenografts of non-small cell lung cancer,[114,142] colon cancer,[119] breast cancer,[60] small cell lung cancer,[30] and malignant melanoma.[51]

Renal Subcapsular Assay (RSC)

Unlike the subcutaneous xenograft assay, the renal subcapsular assay has a relatively short and constant period between tumor inoculation and the appearance of a grossly palpable mass. Tumors can usually be assessed in a period of six days.[3] Therefore, this model is particularly appropriate when a short term in vivo assay is required. Cells are inoculated as a tumor fragment, usually 1 mm in size, under the kidney capsule of the nude mouse, as first described by Bodgen and colleagues in 1978.[15] These tumors maintain true morphologic, functional and growth characteristics of the original tumor from which they were derived.[2] For example, they preserve cell-cell contact, maintain the spatial relationship of the tumor, and form a more representative model of human metastasis than the subcutaneous xenograft. Therefore, tumor response can be subsequently assessed by measuring tumor size (growth assay), colony formation by surviving cells (the clonogenic assay), or simply animal survival.[1,14,39,42,156]

While appealing in many ways, the renal subcapsular assay has limitations. The subcapsular area of the kidney is not a totally immunoprivileged site. When sectioned and examined microscopically, variable amounts of tumor mass represent invading lymphocytes.[49,98,160] Thus, the immunogenicity of a given tumor in a given animal model is an important variable to control and considerable controversy surrounds the use of this assay.[1] However, as will be discussed later, it might be an ideal orthotopic model for renal cell carcinoma (see below).[111]

Intraperitoneal, Microencapsulated Tumor Assay

Because of the limitations of the renal subcapsular assay, and its specific poor adaptability to slow-growing tumors,[2,12,43] alternative short-term in vivo assays have been developed. One of the more interesting is the microencapsulated tumor assay which depends on microencapsulation technology. Tumor cells are encapsulated in semipermeable gels that can be formed into microcapsules of (0.05–1 mm).[90] These microcapsules can be inoculated into the peritoneal space of experimental animals. Under typical assay conditions using mice, approximately 600 microcapsules are injected into the peritoneum. The semi-permeability of the capsule protects the tumor cells from host cell-mediated immune cytotoxicity, so that athymic (nude) mice need not be used. At the same time, it allows nutrients and systemic cytotoxic agents to diffuse and reach the tumor cells. Anticancer effect is assessed by recovering microcapsules and counting viable tumor cells in treated vs. control animals (Figure XV-5-4).[67,68]

The microencapsulation assay is simple, rapid and relatively inexpensive. For a given analysis, it requires fewer mice when compared to the subcutaneous transplanted tumor assay.[68] By definition, tumor cells are evaluated after exposure to drug concentrations which are obtainable in vivo. In addition, the system is adaptable to most solid tumors and, unlike the subcutaneous transplanted tumor assay, uses immunocompetent mice. For these reasons, the microencapsulated tumor assay is being evaluated by the NCI screening program as an in vivo second line screen to follow initial drug leads that pass the in vitro screening system previously described.[20]

Orthotopic Xenograft Model

In 1889, after analyzing autopsies from patients with metastatic breast cancer, Paget concluded that metastasis is not a random phenomenon. Rather, he concluded the malignant cells have special affinity for growth in the environment of certain organs, the familiar seed and soil hypothesis.[123] Certainly, there exist organ site specific interactions which are essential for optimal growth and progression of cancer in vivo.[77,106,117,126,127] The orthotopic xenograft model is a system in which tumor cells are implanted at the site of the organ of origin. This organ-specific site presumably provides the tumor cells with an optimal environment for growth and progression. Because of its relevant expense and novelty, this model has as yet not been used widely by the NCI drug screening program. However, it is being used extensively to explore its role as an in vivo evaluation model for cytotoxic agents specific for organ sites such as lung cancer.

Multiple tumor xenografts have already been developed using nude mice, including renal cell carcinoma,[44,45,112] pancreatic carcinoma,[136] certain brain tumors,[139] prostate, colon, and to a larger extent lung cancer (Table XV-5-2).[102] All of these models are potentially amenable to orthotopic development.

The lung tumor model is the predominant orthotopic model that has been explored by the NCI[102,105] and application of other models is currently underway. In the case of lung can-

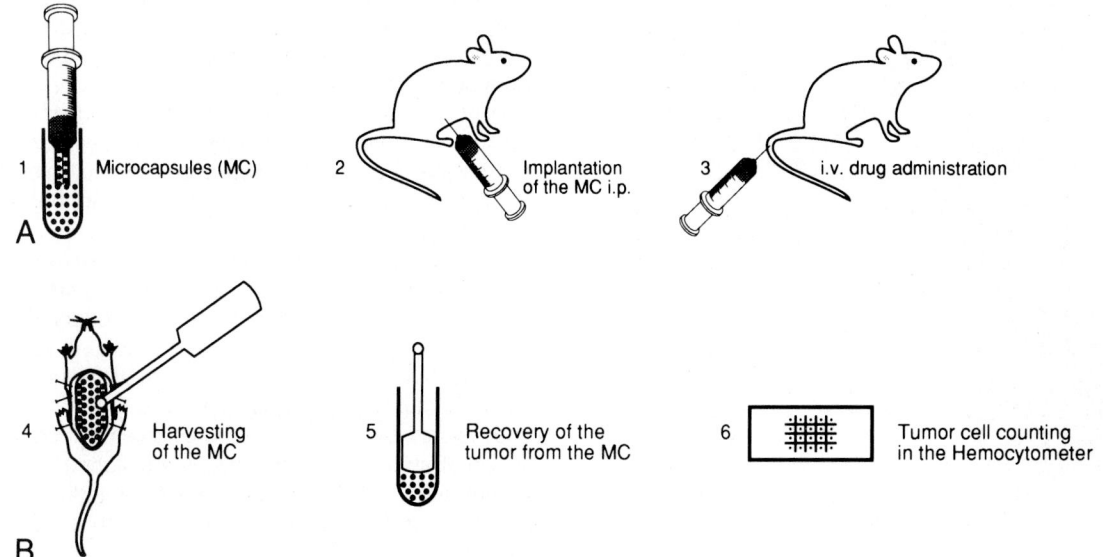

Figure XV-5-4. Intraperitoneal microencapsulated tumor assay.

Table XV-5-2.   Orthotopic Models for Study of Human Cancers Grown in Athymic Nude Mice

Human cancer organ site of origin	Implantation site in nude mice	Nomenclature
Central nervous system	Percutaneous intracranial implantation into cerebral cortex	Intracranial model
Colon	Wall of cecum	Intracolonic model
Lung	(a) Intrabronchially into right mainstem bronchus	Intrapulmonary model
	(b) Percutaneously into right pleural space	Percutaneous intrathoracic model
Pancreas	Pancreas parenchyma	Intrapancreatic model
Renal	(a) Subrenal capsule	Subrenal capsule model
	(b) Kidney parenchyma	Intrarenal model

cer, tumor cells in suspension are inoculated through the right main stem bronchus into the right lung in a lightly anesthetized animal (Figure XV-5-5). Tumor response can be evaluated by sacrificing the animal and histologically quantifying tumor growth, or as shown in Figure XV-5-6, noninvasive chest x-ray may be sufficient to provide interim evaluation of tumor response.[104]

Another approach towards establishing a lung tumor orthotopic model is through percutaneous intrathoracic implantation (Figure XV-5-7).[102] A disadvantage to this model is the finding that as many as 30% of the inoculated tumor grows outside the lung parenchyma, either in the pleural space or the chest wall. Tumor related mortality from the intrabronchial model is higher than that of intrathoracic implantation. Both orthotopic approaches have a much higher

Lung carcinoma cell suspension

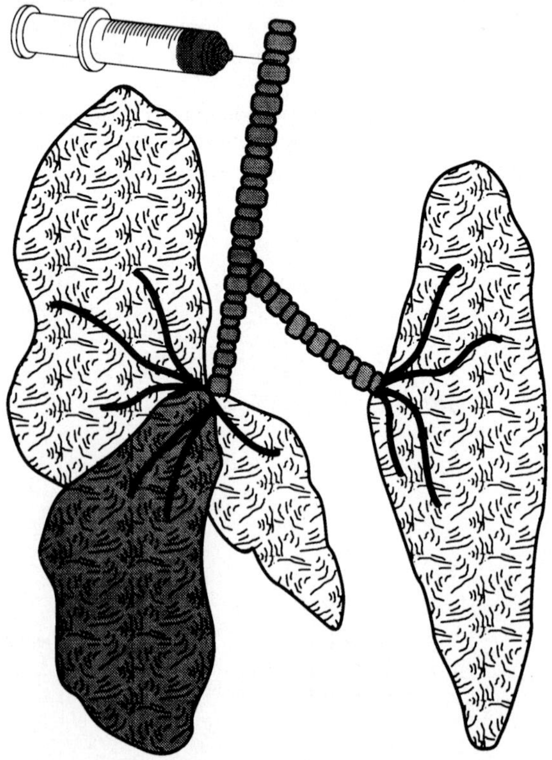

Figure XV-5-5. Orthotopic in vivo human lung cancer model in athymic nude mice. Intrabronchial tumor cell inoculations. Tumor shown as shaded area.

tumor mortality than the subcutaneous model of the same tumor cell line.[102] The far greater aggressiveness of identical inoculates of lung cancer injected into the bronchus compared with subcutaneous injection is a reflection of Paget's early observation on tumor cell tissue tropism and suggests that orthotopic models may reflect the clinical situation most closely.[69,95,110,116]

Limitations of Animal Models

Immunogenicity

The development of immunogenicity to a transplantable tumor model can complicate interpretation of treatment results. The cell kill and animal survival can become exaggerated as a result of this potential for genetic drift over time. Therefore, periodic monitoring is important to quality assurance in maintaining a stable animal model with consistent predictability.

Infection

Several viral infections are difficult to control in laboratory animals and require constant vigilance. These infections not only cause a decrease in the reproductive capacity but also can limit the tolerance of the animal to both tumor inoculation and therapeutic interventions. Many of the effects of viral infection: wasting, cachexia, or growth retardation can mimic the dose-limiting toxicities of anticancer drugs. The most common viruses that affect laboratory mice are the mouse hepatitis virus (MHV), the Sendai virus, and the pneumonia virus of the mouse (PVM).

MHV is a major cause of death among nude mice.[41] Infection can be fatal and usually[55,56] produces cachexia and necrotizing hepatitis. Infected mice may not tolerate drugs which require hepatic clearance or which are hepatotoxic in themselves.

The Sendai virus is a common murine respiratory virus. It causes a wasting syndrome and death in immunocompromised mice.[13,41,166] It also causes pulmonary vein thrombosis, suppurative rhinitis and otitis media. In addition, this virus can lead to squamous metaplasia of the lung that might cause confusion in assessing tumors in these animals.[130] Subclinical infection of breeding colonies can occur with no apparent symptoms,[56] continuous monitoring of animals is essential. Like the Sendai virus, PVM can induce squamous cell changes in the bronchus similar to squamous cell cancer.[115]

Another virus that can affect athymic mice is the mouse leukemia virus that can cause erythroleukemia. Reovirus,

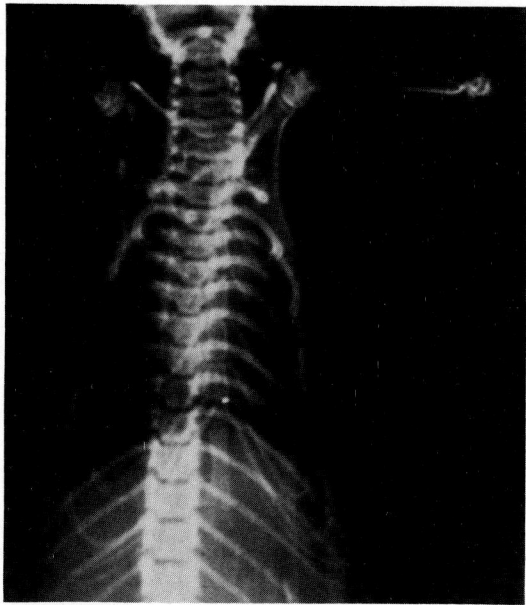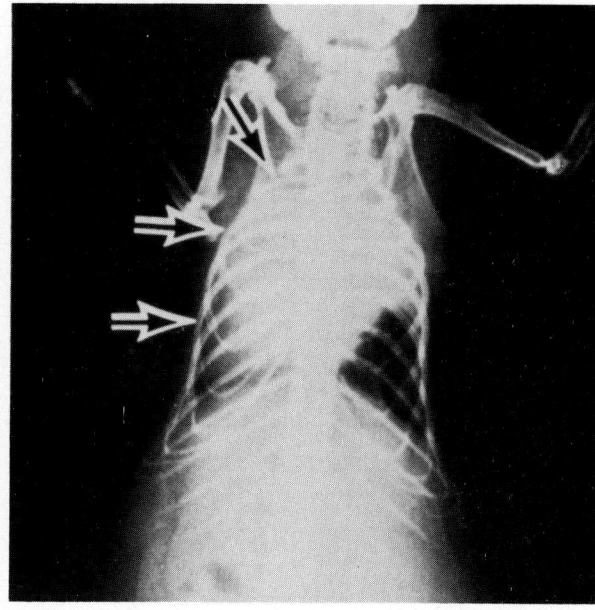

Figure XV-5-6.   X-ray of a lung field of a normal athymic mouse (left) and an x-ray showing a right lung carcinoma resulted from intrabronchial inoculation of human lung cancer cell line (right). Arrows indicate tumor site.

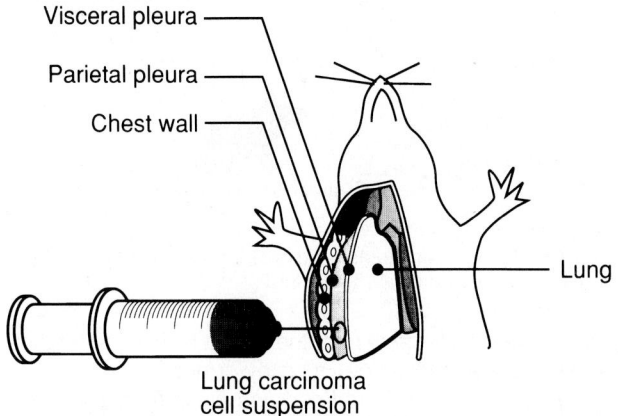

Figure XV-5-7.   Orthotopic in vivo human lung cancer model in athymic nude mice. Percutaneous tumor cell inoculation.

polyomavirus and ectomelia are other pathogens that can affect lab animals.

Because of the high susceptibility of the nude mice for infection, strict isolation and exclusion of infected animals from experiments is essential. In addition, microbiological monitoring is important to maintain any reproducible experimental animal model system. Microbiological monitoring includes routine viral isolation and serological studies on the breeding colonies.

Other Animal Models

Transgenic and Chimeric Mice

The transgenic mouse is the resultant progeny of the pronucleus of a fertilized egg that is injected with a foreign gene. This progeny then carries and expresses this exogenous gene and passes it on in a Mendelian fashion to its descen-

dants.[25] Genes can be transferred to the pronucleus by microinjection,[24,66,79,85] retroviral infection,[86–89,146] or embryonal stem cell (ESC) transfer (Figure XV-5-8).[36,81,96] By far, the most efficient of these three strategies is microinjection. ESC provides a means to manipulate and select cells containing the transferred gene in culture prior to insertion into animals. This is accomplished by transferring the gene into ES cells, which are then transplanted into the blastocyst to create a chimeric mouse. If reproductive tissues derived from the embryonal stem cell contribute to the germ line, a transgenic mouse is established from the progeny of the chimeric animals (Figure XV-5-9).[65]

The ability to integrate a gene of interest into the genome of an animal which then expresses it provides a novel approach for cancer investigation. Tumorigenesis can be studied through a better understanding of interactions between regulation of expressed cellular and viral oncogenes.[21] Transgenic mice are excellent models for studying the consequences of oncogene expression in animals, the effect of oncogenes on growth and differentiation, and their potential for cellular transformation. These mice also provide an in vivo preclinical model for gene therapy and gene transfer.

An example of how this technique can be applied to drug development is the recent introduction of drug resistance genes into transgenic animals. These genes include the multiple drug resistance (or mdr gene) which confirms resistance to a variety of important drugs of the natural product class including VP-16, adriamycin, and the vinca alkaloids.[20]

Because normal cells from transgenic mice transected with the mdr gene express the same surface glycoprotein which confers drug resistance to tumor cells, they are able to tolerate normally lethal doses of anticancer drugs of the natural product class with toxicity. Such animal models may have unique roles in cancer drug development.[57,109] For example, they could be used, in an in vivo system, to screen

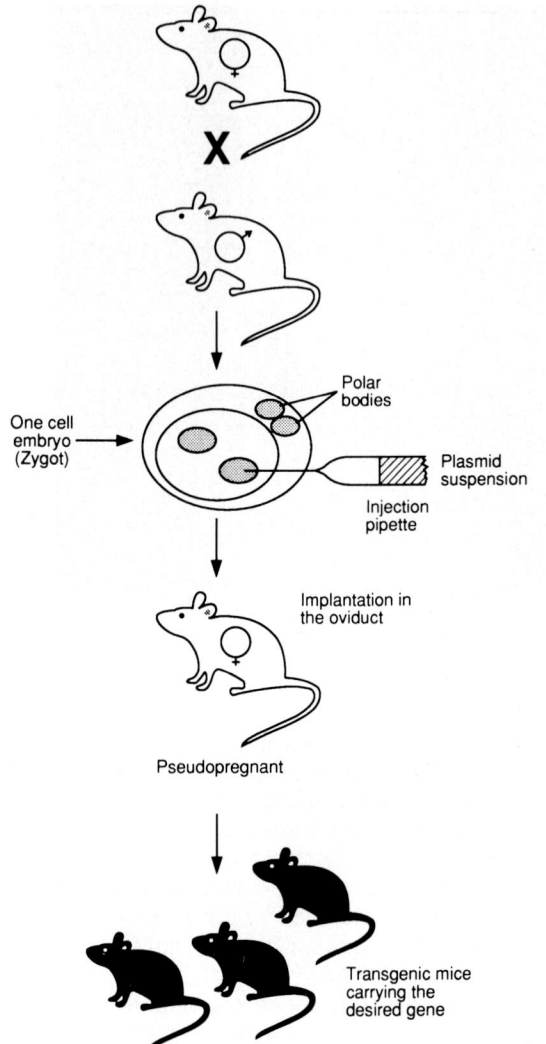

Figure XV-5-8.   Transgenic mice production by pronuclear microinjection.

or further evaluate drugs capable of reversing the resistance phenotype.

Animal Models in Cancer Drug Development

The previous section of this chapter has reviewed the role of animal models in cancer drug discovery. Following identification of a compound of interest, animal models continue to be important to the process of cancer drug development, specifically in the area of preclinical toxicology. These studies are done with a two-fold purpose: 1) to estimate a safe starting dose for Phase I clinical trials in man, and 2) to predict acute and chronic toxicities in a relevant preclinical animal model. The role of the animal model has evolved in this area as well.

In the 1970's, the NCI used only dogs and monkeys in its preclinical toxicology protocols. Lethal and non-lethal doses were established in both models and chronic toxicity studies undertaken only in dogs. Starting doses for patient studies

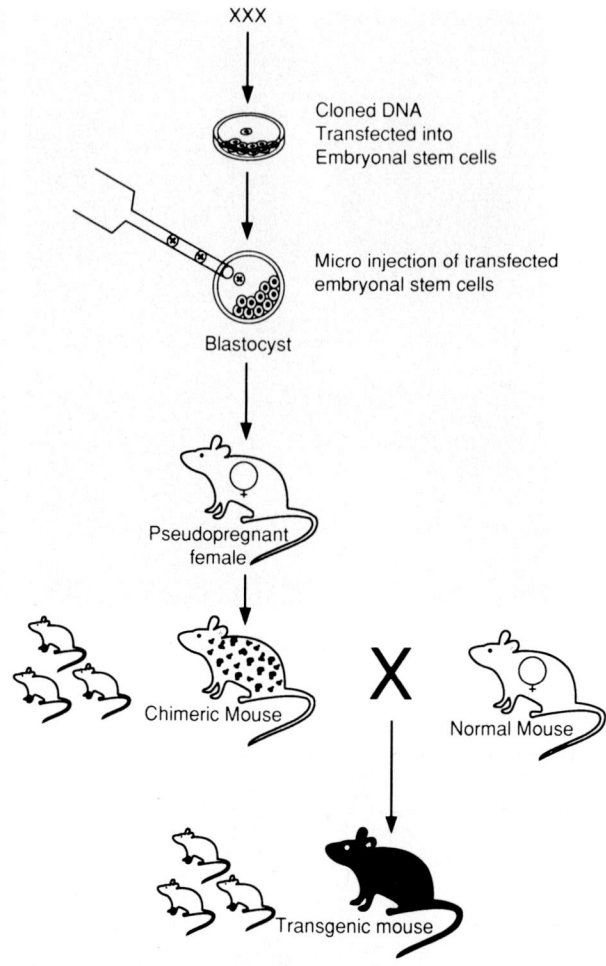

Figure XV-5-9.   Chimeric transgenic mice derived from transfected embryonal stem cell mediated transfer.

were calculated as one-third of the lowest toxic dose for the most sensitive animal model, monkey or dog.[70]

In 1979, the NCI and the Food and Drug Administration reviewed existing data and agreed that toxicity studies performed largely in mice could safely replace the more costly and time-consuming large animal studies in dog and monkey models.

Currently, the LD_{10} (the dose of drug lethal to 10% of animals) in mice is tested in a dog model using an $MELD_{10}$ or mouse equivalent LD_{10}. This dose can be estimated from a conversion equation:

Dose in mg/m² in dogs

$$= \frac{Km \ dog}{Km \ mouse} \times Dose \ in \ mg/m^2 \ in \ mouse$$

where Km is the surface area to weight ratio in each species.[54] This is an important equation for dose conversion between species for cancer drug development (Table XV-5-3). In the absence of severe toxicity in dogs, Phase I trials in humans may begin at one-tenth the LD_{10} in mice. Of course, if severe toxicity is observed in dogs at the mouse LD_{10}, doses are de-escalated to determine the minimally toxic dose

Table XV-5-3. Surface Area to Weight Ratios (Km) of Various Species

Species	Body Weight (kg)	Surface Area	Surface Area to Weight Ratio (Km)
Mouse	0.02	0.0066	3.0
Rat	0.15	0.025	5.9
Monkey	3	0.24	12
Dog	8	0.40	20
Human			
Child	20	0.80	25
Adult	60	1.6	37

in dogs. Clinical studies may then begin at one-third of this dose derived in dogs. Overall, the new NCI toxicology protocol has performed well in predicting safe initial doses for clinical trials, while reducing the reliance on and cost of preclinical large animal toxicology.

A new use of animals in preclinical drug development beyond simple prediction of toxicity has recently gained momentum. This is the use of preclinical pharmacology to guide dose escalation during the conduct of Phase I clinical trials. As Collins and co-workers note in a recent excellent review of this concept,[27] the rationale for pharmacologically guided dose escalation derives from the simple assumption that similar toxicities will occur at similar drug levels in mice and man. Since both toxicity and efficacy of anticancer drugs is related to total drug exposure, the area under the pharmacokinetic curve (AUC) has been proposed for this purpose.

In essence, the AUC is measured in mice following treatment with a given drug at the LD_{10} dose. This is compared to the AUC in patients entering the first dose of the Phase I study, which, as previously discussed, is usually one-tenth the mouse LD_{10}. If the AUC in man is significantly lower than that observed at the LD_{10} in mice, dose escalation can be accelerated beyond the standard Fibonacci schema. The speed with which dose can be escalated depends upon the therapeutic index of a given agent, but two escalation schemas have been proposed. The first, a geometric mean approach, uses a dose escalation factor equal to the square root of the ratio of the AUC at the mouse LD_{10} to the AUC in man at the entry dose level. The second schema continues to double doses at each escalation until the AUC in man approaches that seen in the mouse at the LD_{10}. Drug levels would continue to be monitored in all patients on study to be certain that non-linear kinetics would not cause unexpected toxicities.

This hypothesis, of course, assumes that drug metabolism and end organ sensitivity to both parent drug and metabolites are similar in mouse and man. As Collins and others have convincingly demonstrated, these assumptions generally are true so that this approach could potentially save significant time in clinical drug development. In fact, pharmacologically directed dose escalation has been successfully used to accelerate dose escalation in a number of anticancer drugs in Phase I clinical trials, including HMBA, merbarone, piraxantrone and lodoxorubicin.

Conclusions

The use of animals in cancer drug discovery and development has evolved to become both more sophisticated and efficient over the past four decades. Despite contemporary interests and pressure to decrease animal use in research, it is likely that animal models will play an increasingly important role in both cancer drug discovery and development.

To be sure, it is likely that the broad-based in vivo mouse screen using sensitive murine tumor cell lines, and which required several million mice during each year of operation, has been supplanted by more targeted screening systems which no longer require an in vivo model. The current NCI human tumor cell line screen has the theoretic advantage of being able to identify compounds specifically active in a given tumor type (e.g., breast, colon, lung) or histology (e.g., adenocarcinoma or squamous cell cancer). In addition, the assay conditions of the screen will hopefully allow the identification and characterization of new natural products from novel sources.

There are other screening models which require neither animals nor living cells. These screens select biochemical targets which can be purified and then inhibited as part of a screen. Examples include the P170 glycoprotein (screening for compounds which displace active drugs from the binding site, and which could reverse the multiple drug resistance phenotype), inhibitors of DNA topoisomerases or drugs which bind to specific growth factor receptors.

While these new screening systems are now possible because of a better understanding of the biology and growth requirements of cancer cells, they do not supplant animals entirely. Once a screen of any kind has identified an interesting lead, intermediate steps requiring animals will still be required prior to clinical trials in man.

These studies at a minimum include confirming activity against a given tumor in a relevant animal model: growth delay or improved survival in nude mice, inhibition of orthotopic tumor growth, or significant cell kill in the microencapsulation model. The animal model is critical in taking the screen one step closer to the clinic. It confirms that the drug and/or its metabolites reach their target and demonstrate a positive and reproducible therapeutic effect.

While this chapter has focused on cancer drug discovery and development, animal models have a special role in the development of biological agents. Here the relevant biologic endpoints may not cross species. For example, G-CSF does not affect bone marrow function in mice, while GM-CSF treatment induces a profound leucocytosis in mice. These agents may require animal models closer to man (non-human primates) or other systems, such as the SCID (severe combined immunodeficiency) mouse model, in which the human immune system can be selectively introduced and the effects of biological agents monitored in a controlled, yet essentially human, milieu.

Just as the role of animals in cancer drug discovery has become more refined over time, so too has their role in drug development. The general convertability of doses between species has decreased the need for larger animals (non-human primates and dogs) during preclinical toxicology. The incorporation of pharmacokinetics into preclinical toxicology has become routine and is appealing for a number of reasons. Such studies provide insights into drug metabolism as it relates to end organ toxicity and can determine whether saturable (non-linear) kinetics contribute to the therapeutic index. Perhaps most interesting is the recent successful application of pharmacologically directed dose escalation to Phase I studies in man and the refinement that this approach will give to what has been a largely empiric area of clinical research.

Appropriate use of animal models is essential to the successful, efficient and safe discovery and development of new treatments for patients with cancer. The lessons learned will hopefully have a positive influence on the development of new therapies for other diseases as well.

References

1. Aamdal, S., Fostad, O., Kaalhus, O., and Phil, A.: Chemosensitivity profiles of human cancers assessed by the 6-day SRC assay on serially xenografted tumors. Int. J. Cancer, 37:579, 1986.
2. Aamdal, S., Fodstad, O., and Phil, A.: Human tumor xenografts transplanted under the renal capsule of conventional mice. Growth rates and host immune response. Int. J. Cancer, 34:725, 1984.
3. Aamdal, S., Fodstad, O., and Phil, A.: Methodological aspects of the 6-day subrenal capsule assay for measuring response of human tumors to anticancer agents. Anticancer Res., 5:329, 1985.
4. Ad Hoc review committee proceedings for National Cancer Institute. In Vitro/In Vivo Disease-oriented Screening Project. NIH, Bethesda, MD, September 23–24, 1985. Sponsored by Developmental Therapeutics Program, Division of Cancer Treatment, National Cancer Institute.
5. Ad Hoc review committee proceedings for National Cancer Institute. In Vitro/In Vivo Disease-oriented Screening Project. NIH, Bethesda, MD, December 8–9, 1986. Sponsored by Developmental Therapeutics Program, Division of Cancer Treatment, National Cancer Institute.
6. Ad Hoc review committee proceedings for National Cancer Institute. In Vitro/In Vivo Disease-oriented Screening Project. NIH, Bethesda, MD, December 8–9, 1989. Sponsored by Developmental Therapeutics Program, Division of Cancer Treatment, National Cancer Institute.
7. Alley, M. C., Hursey, M. L., Pacula-Cox, C. M., Stinson, S. F., McLemore, T. L., and Boyd, M. R.: Suitability of multicellular growth units in soft agar culture for experimental drug evaluations and morphologic examinations. Proc. Am. Assoc. Cancer Res., 30:529, 1989.
8. Alley, M. C., Scudiero, D. A., Monks, A., Hursey, M. L., Czerwinski, M. J., Fine, D. L., Abbott, B. J., Mayo, J. G., Shoemaker, R. H., and Boyd, M. R.: Feasibility of drug screening with panels of human tumor cell lines using a microculture tetrazolium assay. Cancer Res., 48:589, 1988.
9. Begg, A. C.: Analysis of growth delay data. Potential pitfalls. Brit. J. Cancer, 41 (Suppl. IV):93, 1980.
10. Begg, A. C.: Principles and Practices of the Tumor Growth Delay Assay. *In* Rodent Tumor Models in Experimental Cancer Therapy. Edited by R. F. Kallman. New York, Pergamon Press, 1987, p. 114.
11. Bellet, R. E., Danna, V., Mastrangelo, M. J., and Berd, D.: Evaluation of a nude mouse-human tumor panel as a predictive secondary screen for cancer chemotherapeutic agents. J. Natl. Cancer Inst., 63:1185, 1979.
12. Bennett, J. A., Pilon, V. A., and MacDowell, R. T.: Evaluation of growth and histology of human tumor xenografts implanted under the renal capsule of immunocompetent and immunodeficient mice. Cancer Res., 45:4963, 1985.
13. Blandford, G., Cureton, R. J., and Heath, R. B.: Studies of the immune response in Sendai virus infection of mice. J. Med. Microbiol., 4:351, 1971.
14. Bogden, A. E., Griffin, W., Reich, S. D., Constanza, M. E., and Cobb, W. R.: Predictive testing with the subrenal capsule assay. Cancer Treat. Rev., 11:113, 1984.
15. Bogden, A. E., Haskell, P. M., LePage, D. J., Kelton, D., Cobb, W. R., and Esber, H. J.: Growth of human tumor xenografts implanted under the renal capsule of normal immunocompetent mice. Exp. Cell Biol., 47:218, 1979.
16. Bogden, A. E., Kelton, D. E., Cobb, W. R., and Esber, H. J.: *In* Proceedings of the Symposium on the Use of Athymic (Nude) Mice in Cancer Research. Edited by D. P. Houchens, and A. A. Ovejera. New York, Gustav Fisher, 1978, p. 231.
17. Boyd, M. R.: National Cancer Institute drug discovery and development. *In* Accomplishments in Oncology Vol. 1, No. 1, Cancer Therapy: Where Do We Go From Here? Edited by E. Frei and E. J. Freireich. Philadelphia, J. B. Lippincott, Co., 1986.
18. Boyd, M. R.: NIH new drug program. Proceedings of the IV World Conference on Lung Cancer, Toronto, Canada, August 25–30, 1985, Chest, 89:355S, 1986.
19. Boyd, M. R.: Status of implementation of the NCI human tumor cell line in vitro primary drug screen. Proc. Am. Assoc. Cancer Res., 30:652, 1989.
20. Boyd, M. R.: Status of the NCI preclinical antitumor drug discovery screen. *In* Principles and Practice of Oncology Updates. Edited by V. T. DeVita, S. Hellman, and S. A. Rosenberg. Philadelphia, J. B. Lippincott, 1981.
21. Boyd, M. R., Shoemaker, R., Alley, M., et al.: New NCI disease-oriented drug screening program. *In* Proceedings of the 5th NCI-EORTC Symposium on New Drugs Cancer Therapy. Amsterdam, 1986.
22. Boyd, M. R., Shoemaker, R. H., Cragg, G. M., and Suffness, M.: New avenues of investigation of marine biologicals in the anticancer drug discovery program of the National Cancer Institute. *In* Pharmaceuticals and the Sea. Edited by C. W. Rinehart, K. L. Rinehart, and L. S. Shields. Lancaster, Technomic Publishing AG, 1988.
23. Boyd, M. R., Shoemaker, R. H., McLemore, T. L., et al.: New drug development. *In* Thoracic Oncology. Edited by J. Roth, J. C. Ruckdescel, and T. H. E. Weisenburger. Philadelphia, W. B. Saunders, 1989.
24. Brinster, R. L., Chen, H. Y., Trumbauer, M. E., Yagle, M. K., and Palmiter, R. D.: Factors affecting the efficiency of introducing foreign DNA into mice by microinjecting eggs. Proc. Natl. Acad. Sci., USA, 82:4438, 1985.
25. Brinster, R. L., and Palmiter, R. D.: Introduction of genes into germ line of animals. The Harvey Lectures, 80:1, 1985.
26. Bruce, W. R., Meeker, B. E., and Valeriote, F. A.: Comparison of the sensitivity of normal hematopoietic and transplanted lymphoma colony-forming cells to chemotherapeutic agents administered in vivo. J. Natl. Cancer Inst., 37:233, 1966.
27. Collins, J. M., Grieshaber, C. K., and Chabner, B. A.: Pharmacologically guided Phase I clinical trials based on preclinical drug development. J. Natl. Cancer Inst., 82:1321, 1990.
28. Corbett, T. H., Griswold, D. P., Jr., Roberts, B. J., Peckham, J. C., and Schabel, F. M., Jr.: Tumor induction relationships in development of transplantable cancers of the colon in mice for chemotherapy assays, with a note on carcinogen structure. Cancer Res., 35:2434, 1975.
29. Corbett, T. H., Roberts, B. J., Leopold, W. R., Peckham, J. C., Wilhoff, L. J., Griswold, D. P., Jr., and Schabel, F. M., Jr.: Induction and chemotherapeutic response of two transplantable ductal adenocarcinomas of the pancreas in C57B2/6 mice. Cancer Res., 44:717, 1984.
30. Corbett, T. H., Valeriote, F. A., and Baker, L. H.: Is the P388 murine tumor no longer adequate as a drug discovery model? Investigational New Drugs, 5:3, 1987.
31. Danks, M. K., Yalowich, J. C., and Bech, W. T.: Atypical multiple drug resistance in a human leukemic cell line selected for resistance to teniposide (VM-26). Cancer Res., 47:1297, 1987.
32. Davis, A. J. S., Leuchars, E., Wallis, V., and Koler, P. C.: The mitotic response of thymus-derived cells to antigenic stimulus. Transplantation, 4:4348, 1966.
33. DeVita, V. T., Oliverio, V. T., Muggia, F. M., et al.: The drug development and clinical trials programs of the Division of Cancer Treatment. National Cancer Institute, Cancer Clin. Trials, 2:195, 1979.
34. DeVita, V. T., and Schein, P. S.: The use of drugs in combination for the therapy of cancer. N. Engl. J. Med., 288:998, 1973.
35. Division of Cancer Treatment Board approves new screening program, natural products concepts. Cancer Lett., 11:4, 1985.
36. Doetschman, T. C., Eistetter, H., Katz, M., Schmidt, W., and Kemler, R.: The in vitro development of blastocyst-derived embryonic stem cell lines: Formation of visceral yolk sac, blood islands and myocardium. J. Embryol. Exp. Morphol., 87:27, 1985.
37. Donovick, R., Alley, A. M., Stinson, S., McLemore, T., Mayo, J., Shoemaker, R., Fiebig, H., and Boyd, M.: Current status and future development of "disease-oriented" panels of human tumor cell lines for use in the NCI anticancer drug screen. Proc. Am. Assoc. Cancer Res., 30:611, 1989.
38. Driscoll, J. S.: The preclinical new drug research program of the National Cancer Institute. Cancer Treat. Rep., 68:63, 1984.
39. Dumont, P., VanderEsch, E. P., Jabri, M., Lejeune, F., and Atassi, G.: Chemosensitivity of human melanoma xenografts in immunocompetent mice and its histological evaluation. Int. J. Cancer, 33:447, 1984.
40. Dykes, D. J., Mayo, J. G., Abbott, B. J., Harrison, S. D., Jr., Laster, W. R., Jr., Simpson-Herren, L., Griswold, D. P., Jr., and Boyd, M. R.: In vivo growth characteristics of human tumor xenografts from the NCI in vitro "disease-oriented" drug discovery program. Proc. Am. Assoc. Cancer Res., 30:614, 1989.
41. Eaton, G. J., Outzen, H. C., Custer, R. P., and Johnson, F. N.: Husbandry of the "nude" mouse in conventional and germ-free environments. Lab. Anim. Sci., 25:309, 1975.
42. Edelstein, M. B., Smink, T., Ruiter, D. J., Visser, W., and Van Putten, L. M.: Improvements and limitations of the subrenal capsule assay for determining tumour sensitivity to cytostatic drugs. Europ. J. Cancer Clin. Oncol., 20:1549, 1984.
43. Edelstein, M. D., Fiebig, H. H., Smink, T., Van Putten, L. M., and Schuchhardt, C.: Comparison between macroscopic and microscopic evaluation of tumor responsiveness using the subrenal capsule assay. Europ. J. Cancer Clin. Oncol., 19:995, 1983.
44. Fidler, I. J.: Rationale and methods for the use of nude mice to study the biology and therapy of human cancer metastasis. Cancer Metastasis Rev., 5:29, 1986.
45. Fiebig, H. H., Weigeldt, H., Schuchhardt, C., Zeschnigk, C., and Lohr, G. W.: Transplantation of human tumors under the renal capsule of nude, immunocompetent and preirradiated normal mice. *In* Advances in the Chemotherapy of Gastrointestinal Cancer. Edited by H. D. Klein and H. Kohn. Erlanden: perimed Fachbuch-Verlagsgesellschaft, 1984, p. 27.
46. Fiebig, H. H., Schuchhardt, C., Henss, H., Fiedler, L., and Lohr, G. S.: Comparison of tumor response in nude mice and in the patients. Behring Inst. Mitt., 74:343, 1984.
47. Fiebig, H. H., Winterhalter, B., Berger, D., Wittekind, C., Bender, K., Selby, M., Bittner, C., Alley, M., and Boyd, M.: Properties of 6 human tumor xenografts in vivo from which cell lines were developed. Proc. Am. Assoc. Cancer Res., 30:612, 1989.
48. Fine, D. L., Shoemaker, R., Gazdar, A., Mayo, J. G., Fodstad, O., Boyd, M. R., Abbott, B. J., and Donovan, P. A.: Metastatic models of human tumors in athymic mice: useful models for drug development. Cancer Detect. Prev. Suppl., 1:291, 1987.
49. Finney, D. J.: Statistical Method in Biological Assay, 2nd ed. Charles Griffin and Co., London, 524, 1964.
50. Flanagan, S. P.: Nude, a new hairless gene with pleiotropic effects in the mouse. Genet. Res., 8:295, 1966.
51. Fodstad, O., Aas, N., and Phil, A.: Response to chemotherapy of human, malignant melanoma xenografts in athymic, nude mice. Int. J. Cancer, 25:453, 1980.
52. Fogh, J., and Trempe, G.: *In* Human Cells in Vitro New Human Tumor Cell Line. Edited by J. Fogh. New York, Plenum, 1975, p. 115.
53. Fogh, J., and Giovanella, B. C. (eds.): The Nude Mouse in Experimental and Clinical Research. New York, Academic Press, 1978.
54. Freireich, E. J., Gehan, E. A., Rall, D. P., Schmidt, L. H., and Skipper, H. E.: Quantitative comparison of toxicity of anticancer agents in mouse, rat, hamster, dog, monkey and man. Cancer Chemother. Rep., 50:219, 1966.
55. Fujiwara, K.: Spontaneous virus infections of nude mice. *In* The Nude Mouse in Experimental and Clinical Research. Edited by J. Fogh and B. C. Giovalla. 2:1, 1982.
56. Fujiwara, K., Takenaka, S., and Shumiya, S.: Carrier state of antibody and viruses in a mouse breeding colony persistently infected with Sendai and mouse hepatitis viruses. Lab. Anim. Sci., 26(2 Pt.1):153, 1976.

57. Galski, H., Sullivan, M., Willingham, M. C., Chin, K.-V., Gottesman, M. M., Pastan, I., and Merlino, G. T.: Expression of a human multidrug resistance cDNA (MDR1) in the bone marrow of transgenic mice: Resistance to daunomycin-induced leukopenia. Mol. Cell. Biol., 9:4357, 1989.
58. Gazdar, A. F. Carney, D. N., Sims, H. L., and Simmons, A.: Heterotransplantation of small cell carcinoma of the lung into nude mice: Comparison of intracranial and subcutaneous route. Int. J. Cancer, 28:777, 1981.
59. Gazdar, A. F., Shoemaker, R., Mayo, J., Oie, H. K., Donovan, P., and Fine, D.: Human lung cancer xenografts and metastases in athymic (nude) mice. *In* Immune-deficient animals in biomedical research, 5th International Workshop. Edited by N. Rygaard, N. Brunner, N. Graem, and M. Spang-Thornsen. Basel: Karger Publications, 1987, p. 277.
60. Giovanella, B. C., Stehlin, J. S., and Shepard, R. C.: Experimental chemotherapy of human breast carcinomas heterotransplanted in nude mice. *In* Proc. Second Internat. Workshop on Nude Mice. University of Tokyo Press, Tokyo, 1977, p. 475.
61. Giovanella, B. C., Stehlin, J. S., Shepard, R. C., and Williams, L. J.: Correlation between response to chemotherapy of human tumors in patients and in nude mice. Cancer, 52:1146, 1983.
62. Goldin, A., and Carter, S. K.: Screening and Evaluation of Antitumor Agents. *In* Cancer Medicine. Edited by J. F. Holland and E. Frei III. Philadelphia, Lea & Febiger, 1982, p. 633.
63. Goldin, A., Schepartz, S. A., Venditti, J. M., et al.: Historical development and current strategy of the National Cancer Institute Drug Development Program. *In* Methods of Cancer Research vol XVI, Cancer Drug Development. Edited by V. T. DeVita, and H. Busch. New York, Academic Press, 1979, p. 165.
64. Goldin, A., Venditti, J. M., Macdonald, J. S., Muggia, F. M., Henney, J. E., and DeVita, V. T., Jr.: Current results of the screening program at the Division of Cancer Treatment, National Cancer Institute. Europ. J. Cancer, 17:129, 1981.
65. Gordon, J. W.: Transgenic Animals. Int. Rev. Cytol., 115:171, 1989.
66. Gordon, J. W., and Ruddle, F. H.: Gene transfer into mouse embryos: production of transgenic mice by pronuclear injection. Methods Enzymol., 101:411, 1983.
67. Gorelik, E., Alley, M., and Shoemaker, R.: A new in vivo short-term assay for evaluation of antitumor chemotherapeutic drugs. Proc. Am. Assoc. Cancer Res., 27:389, 1986.
68. Gorelik, E., Ovejera, A., Shoemaker, R., Jarvis, A., Alley, M., Doff, R., Mayo, J., Herberman, R., and Boyd, M.: Microencapsulated tumor assay: New short-term assay for in vivo evaluation of the effects of anticancer drugs on human tumor cell lines. Cancer Res., 47:5739, 1987.
69. Goustin, A. S., Leof, E. B., Shipley, G. D., and Moses, H. L.: Growth factors and cancer. Cancer Res., 46:1015, 1986.
70. Grieshaber, C. K., and Marsoni, S.: Relation of preclinical toxicology to findings in early clinical trials. Cancer Treatment Reports, 70:65, 1986.
71. Gupta, R. S.: Genetic, biochemical and cross-resistance studies with mutants of Chinese hamster ovary cells resistant to the anticancer drugs, VM-26 and VP16-213. Cancer Res., 43:1568, 1983.
72. Hart, I. R.: 'Seed and soil' revisited: Mechanisms of site-specific metastasis. Cancer Met. Rev., 1:5, 1982.
73. Herberman, R. B.: Natural cell-mediated cytotoxicity in nude mice. *In* The Nude Mouse in Experimental and Clinical Research. Edited by J. Fogh and B. C. Herbeman. New York, Academic Press, 1978, p. 135.
74. Hill, R. P.: An appraisal in vivo assays of excised tumours. Brit. J. Cancer, 41(Suppl. IV):230, 1980.
75. Hill, R. P.: Excision Assay. *In* Rodent Tumor Models in Experimental Cancer Therapy. Edited by R. F. Kallman. New York, Pergamon Press, 1987, p. 67.
76. Hill, R. P.: The assay of tumour colonies in the lung. *In* Cell Clones: A Manual of Mammalian Cell Techniques. Edited by C. Potten, and J. H. Hendry. Churchill-Livingstone, London, Edinburgh, 1985, p. 208.
77. Hill, R. P.: The TD_{50} assay for tumour cells. *In* Cell Clones: A Manual of Mammalian Cell Techniques. Edited by C. Potten, and J. H. Hendry. Churchill-Livingstone, London, Edinburgh, 1985, p. 223.
78. Hirschberg, E.: Patterns of response of animal tumors to anticancer agents. Cancer Res., 23:(Suppl. 5, Part 2):521, 1963.
79. Hogan, B., Constantini, F., and Lacy, E.: Manipulating the mouse embryo: a laboratory manual. Cold Spring Harbor Laboratory Manual. New York, Cold Spring Harbor. D. Hanahan, (ed.), 1986.
80. Holden, H. T., Herberman, R. B., Santoni, A., et al.: Natural cell-mediated cytotoxicity in nude mice. *In* Proceedings of the Symposium on the Use of Athymic Nude Mice in Cancer Research. Edited by D. P. Houchens and A. A. Ovejera. New York, Gustav Fischer, 1978, p. 81.
81. Hooper, M., Hardy, K., Handyside, A., Hunter, S., and Monk, M.: HPRT-deficient (Lesch-Nyhan) mouse embryos derived from germline colonization by cultured cells. Nature, 326:292, 1987.
82. Houchens, D. P., and Ovejera, A. A. (eds.).: Proceedings of the Symposium on the Use of Athymic Nude Mice in Cancer Research. New York, Gustav Fischer, 1978.
83. Houghton, J. A., and Taylor, D. M.: Growth characteristics of human colorectal tumours during serial passage in immune-deprived mice. Brit. J. Cancer, 37:213, 1978.
84. Isaacson, J. H., and Cottanach, B. M.: Report. Mouse Newsletter, 27:31, 1962.
85. Jaenisch, R.: Infection of mouse blastocysts with SV40 DNA: normal development of the infected embryos and persistence of SV40-specific DNA sequences in the adult animals. Cold Spring Harb. Symp Quant. Biol., 39:375, 1975.
86. Jaenisch, R.: Retroviruses and embryogenesis: Microinjection of Moloney leukemia virus into midgestation mouse embryos. Cell, 19:181, 1980.
87. Jaenisch, R., Kahner, D., Nobis, P., Simon, I., Lohler, J., Harbers, K., and Grotkopp, D.: Chromosomal position and activation of retroviral genomes inserted into the germ line of mice. Cell, 24:519, 1981.
88. Jaenisch, R., and Mintz, B.: Simian virus 40 DNA sequences in DNA of healthy adult mice derived from preimplantation blastocysts infected with viral DNA. Proc. Nat. Acad. Sci., USA, 71:1250, 1974.
89. Jahner, D., and Jaenisch, R.: Integration of Moloney leukaemia virus into the germ line of mice: Correlation between site of integration and virus activation. Nature, 287:456, 1980.
90. Jarvis, A. P., and Grdina, T. A.: Production of biologicals from microencapsulated living cells. Biotechniques, 1:22, 1983.
91. Johnson, R. D., and Goldin, A.: The clinical impact of screening and other experimental tumor studies. Cancer Treat. Rev., 2:1, 1975.
92. Jung, H., Beck, H. P., Brammer, I., and Zywietz, F.: Depopulation and repopulation of R1H rhabdomyosarcoma of the rat after X-irradiation. Europ. J. Cancer, 17:375, 1981.
93. Kallman, R. F., Silini, G., and Van Putten, L. M.: Factors influencing the quantitative estimation of the in vivo survival of cells from solid tumors. J. Natl. Cancer Inst., 39:539, 1967.
94. Kerbel, R. S., Frost, P., Liteplo, R., Carlow, D. A., and Elliot, B. E.: Possible epigenetic mechanism of tumor progression: Induction of high-frequency heritable but phenotypically unstable changes in the tumorigenic and metastatic properties of tumor cell populations by 5-azacytidine treatment. J. Cell Physiol. Suppl., 3:87, 1984.
95. Korman, L. Y., Carney, D. N., Citron, M. L., and Moody, T. W.: Secretin/vasoactive intestinal peptide-stimulated secretion of bombesin/gastrin releasing peptide from human small cell carcinoma of the lung. Cancer Res., 46:1214, 1986.
96. Kuehn, M. R., Bradley, A., Robertson, E. J., and Evans, M. J.: A potential animal model for Lesch-Nyhan syndrome through introduction of HPRT mutations into mice. Nature, 326:295, 1987.
97. Lee, S. S., Giovanella, B. C., Stehlin, J. S., Jr., and Brunn, J. C.: Progression of human tumors established in nude mice after continuous infusion of thymidine. Cancer Res., 39:2928, 1979.
98. Levi, F. A., Blum, J. P., Lemaigre, G., Bourut, C., Reinberg, A., and Mathe, G.: A four-day subrenal capsule assay for testing the effectiveness of anticancer drugs against human tumors. Cancer Res., 44:2660, 1984.
99. Marsoni, S., Hoth, D., Simon, R., Leyland-Jones, B., De Rosa, M., and Wittes, R. E.: Clinical Drug Development: An Analysis of Phase II Trials, 1970–1985. Cancer Treat. Rep., 71:71, 1987.
100. Martin, D. S., Fugmann, R. A., Stolfi, R. L., and Hayworth, P. E.: Solid tumor animal model therapeutically predictive for human breast cancer. Cancer Chemother. Rep., Part 2, 5:89, 1975.
101. McCredie, J. A., Inch, W. R., and Sutherland, R. M.: Differences in growth and morphology between the spontaneous C3H mammary carcinoma in the mouse and its syngeneic transplants. Cancer, 27:635, 1971.
102. McLemore, T. L., Abbott, B. J., Mayo, J. G., and Boyd, M. R.: Development and application of new orthotopic in vivo models for use in the U.S. National Cancer Institute's drug screening program. *In* 6th International Workshop on Immunodeficient Animals in Biomedical Research. Edited by B. Wu and J. S. Zheng. Basel: S. Karger, A. G., 1988.
103. McLemore, T., Alley, M., Liu, M., Hubbard, W., Adelberg, S., Czerwinski, M., Yu, S., Stinson, S., Storeng, R., Eggleston, J., and Boyd, M.: Histopathologic, biochemical and molecular genetic characterization of four newly established human pulmonary carcinoma cell lines. Proc. Am. Assoc. Cancer Res., 30:225, 1989.
104. McLemore, T. L., Eggleston, J. C., Shoemaker, R. H., Abbott, B. J., Bohlman, M. E., Liu, M. C., Fine, D. L., Mayo, J. G., and Boyd, M. R.: Comparison of intrapulmonary, percutaneous intrathoracic and subcutaneous models for the propagation of human pulmonary and nonpulmonary cancer cell lines in athymic nude mice. Cancer Res., 48:2880, 1988.
105. McLemore, T. L., Liu, M. C., Blacker, P. C., Gregg, M., Alley, M. C., Abbott, B. J., Shoemaker, R. H., Bohlman, M. E., Litterst, C. C., and Hubbard, W. C.: Novel intrapulmonary model for orthotopic propagation of human lung cancers in athymic nude mice. Cancer Res., 47:5132, 1987.
106. McLemore, T. L., Liu, M. C., Blacker, P. C.: Comparison of intrapulmonary, percutaneous intrathoracic and subcutaneous models for the propagation of human pulmonary and non-pulmonary cancer cell lines in athymic nude mice. Cancer Res., 48:2880, 1988.
107. McLemore, T., Storeng, R., Adelberg, S., Czerwinski, M., Yu, S., Nhamburo, P., Gonzalez, F., Hines, R., and Boyd, M.: Expression of different cytochrome P450 genes in human lung cancer cell lines. Proc. Am. Assoc. Cancer Res., 30:11, 1989.
108. McNally, N. J., and DeRonde, J.: Radiobiological studies of tumours in situ compared with cell survival. Brit. J. Cancer, 41 (Suppl. IV):259, 1980.
109. Mickisch, G. H., Merlino, G. T., Galski, H., Gottesman, M. M., and Pastan, I.: Transgenic mice that express the human multidrug-resistance gene in bone marrow enable a rapid identification of agents that reverse drug resistance. Proc. Natl. Acad. Sci., 88:547, 1991.
110. Moody, T. W., Pert, C. B., Gazdar, A. F., Carnay, D. N., and Minna, J. D.: High levels of intracellular bombesin characterize human small cell lung carrcinoma. Science, 214:1246, 1986.
111. Naito, S., von Eschenhach, A. C., and Fidler, I. J.: Different growth patterns and biologic behavior of human renal cell carcinoma implanted into different organs of nude mice. J. Natl. Cancer Inst., 78:377, 1987.
112. Naito, S., von Eschenbach, A. C., Giavazzi, R., and Fidler, I. J.: Growth and metastasis of tumor cells isolated from a human renal cell carcinoma implanted into different organs of nude mice. Cancer Res., 46:4109, 1986.
113. National Cancer Institute planning to switch drug development emphasis from compound to human cancer-oriented strategy. Cancer Lett., 10:1, 1984.
114. Neeley, J. E., Ballard, E. T., Britt, A. L., and Workman, L.: Characteristics of 85 pediatric tumors heterografted into nude mice. Exp. Cell Biol., 51:217, 1983.
115. Nettesheim, P., Schreiber, H., Creasia, D. A., and Richter, C. B.: Respiratory infections and the pathogenesis of lung cancer. Recent Results Cancer Research, 44:138, 1974.
116. Nicolson, G.: Tumor cell instability, diversification, and progression to metastatic phenotype: from oncogene to oncofetal expression. Cancer Res., 47:1473, 1987.
117. Nicolson, G. L.: Organ colonization and the cell surface properties of malignant cells. Biochem. Biophys. Acta, 695:113, 1982.
118. Nomura, T., Oshawa, N., Tamaoki, N., et al.: Proceedings of the Second International Workshop on Nude Mice. Tokyo, Univ. of Tokyo Press, 1977.
119. Nowak, K., Peckham, M. J., and Steel, G. G.: Variation in response of xenografts of colorectal carcinoma to chemotherapy. Brit. J. Cancer, 37:576, 1978.
120. Ovejera, A. A.: The Use of Human Tumor Xenografts in Large-Scale Drug Screening. *In* Rodent Tumor Models in Experimental Cancer Therapy. Edited by R. F. Kallman. 1987, p. 218.
121. Ovejera, A. A., and Houchens, D. P.: Human tumor xenografts in athymic nude mice as a preclinical screen for anticancer agents. Semin. Oncol., 8:386, 1981.
122. Ovejera, A. A., Johnson, R. K., and Goldin, A.: Growth characteristics and chemotherapeutic response of intravenously implanted Lewis lung carcinoma. Cancer Chemother. Rep., Part 2, 5:111, 1975.

123. Paget, S.: The distribution of secondary growths in cancer of the breast. Lancet, 1:571, 1889.
124. Pantelouris, E. M.: Absence of a thymus in a mouse mutant. Nature, 217:370, 1968.
125. Pattengale, P. K., Stewart, T. A., Leder, A., Sinn, E., Muller, W., Tepler, I., Schmidt, E., and Leder, P.: Animal models of human disease. Pathology and molecular biology of spontaneous neoplasms occurring in transgenic mice carrying and expressing activated cellular oncogenes. American Journal of Pathology, 135:39, 1989.
126. Poste, G.: Experimental systems for analysis of the malignant phenotype. Cancer Met. Rev., 1:141, 1982.
127. Poste, G., and Fidler, I. J.: The pathogenesis of cancer metastasis. Nature, 283:139, 1980.
128. Povlsen, C. O., and Rygaard, J.: Heterotransplantation of human adenocarcinoma of the colon and rectum to the nude mouse. A study of nine consecutive transplantations. Acta Pathol. Microbiol. Scand., 79:159, 1971.
129. Raff, M. C., and Wortis, H. H.: Thymus dependence of Theta-bearing cells in the peripheral lymphoid tissue of mice. Immunology, 18:1931, 1970.
130. Richter, C. B.: In "Morphology of Experimental Respiratory Carcinogenesis." AEC Symposium Series, 21:365, 1971.
131. Rockwell, S.: In vivo-in vitro models for studying the response of tumors to therapy. Lab. Anim. Sci., 27:831, 1977.
132. Rockwell, S.: In vivo-in vitro tumour cell lines: Characteristics and limitations as models for human cancer. Brit. J. Cancer, 41(Suppl. IV):118, 1980.
133. Rockwell, S. C., Kallman, R. F., and Fajardo, L. F.: Characteristics of a serially transplanted mouse mammary tumor and its tissue-culture adapted derivative. J. Natl. Cancer Inst., 49:735, 1972.
134. Rygaard, J., and Povlsen, C. O.: Athymic (nude) mice. In The Mouse in Biochemical Research, Vol. VI. Edited by H. L. Foster, J. D. Small, and J. G. Fox. New York, Academic Press, 1982, p. 51.
135. Rygaard, J., and Povlsen, C. O. (Eds.): Bibliography of the Nude Mouse, Stuttgart/New York, Gustav Fischer Verlag, 1977.
136. Rygaard, J., and Povlsen, C. O.: Heterotransplantation of a human malignant tumor in nude mice. Acta Pathol. Microbiol. Scand., 77:758, 1969.
137. Rygaard, J., and Povlsen, C. O. (Eds.): Proceedings of the First International Workshop on Nude Mice, Stuttgart, Gustav Fischer Verlag, 1974.
138. Schepartz, S. A.: Memorandum to suppliers of compounds. In Methods of Development of New Anticancer Drugs, National Cancer Institute Monograph 45, DHEW Publication No. (NIH), 76-1037, 155, 1977.
139. Shapiro, W. R., Basler, G. A., Chernick, N. L., and Posner, J. B.: Human brain tumor transplantation into nude mice. J. Natl. Cancer Inst., 62:447, 1979.
140. Sharkey, F. E., Fogh, J., Hajdu, S., Fitzgerald, P., and Fogh, J.: Experience in surgical pathology with human tumor growth in the nude mouse. In The Nude Mouse in Experimental and Clinical Research. Edited by J. Fogh and B. Giovanella. New York, Academic Press, 1978, 188.
141. Shoemaker, R. H., Monks, A., Alley, M. C., et al.: Development of human tumor cell line panels for use in disease-oriented drug screening. In Prediction of Response to Cancer Chemotherapy. Edited by T. Hall. New York, Alan Liss, 1988.
142. Shorthouse, A. J., Peckham, M. J., Smyth, J. F., and Steel, G. G.: The therapeutic response of bronchial carcinoma xenografts: A direct patient-xenograft comparison. Brit. J. Cancer, 41(Suppl. IV):142, 1980.
143. Shorthouse, A. J., Smyth, J. F., Steel, G. G., Ellison, M., Mills, J., and Peckham, M. J.: The human tumour xenograft—a valid model in experimental chemotherapy? Br. J. Surg., 67:715, 1980.
144. Siemann, D. W.: Satisfactory and unsatisfactory tumor models: Factors influencing the selection of a tumor model for experimental evaluation. In Rodent Tumor Models in Experimental Cancer Therapy. R. F. Kallman, (ed.) 12, 1987.
145. Skipper, H. E., and Schmidt, L. H.: Background: description of criteria, and presentation of quantitative therapeutic data on various classes of drugs obtained in diverse experimental tumor systems. Cancer Chemother. Rep., 17:1, 1962.
146. Soriano, P., and Jaenisch, R.: Retroviruses as probes for mammalian developments: Allocation of cells to the somatic and germ cell lineages. Cell, 46:19, 1986.
147. Sprent, J., and Miller, J.: Thoracic duct lymphocytes from nude mice: Migratory properties and life span. Eur. J. Immunol., 2:384, 1972.
148. Staquet, M. J., Byar, D. P., Green, S. B., and Rozencweig, M.: Clinical predictivity of transplantable tumor systems in the selection of new drugs for solid tumors: Rationale for a three-stage strategy. Cancer Treat. Rep., 67:753, 1983.
149. Steel, G. G.: Growth Kinetics of Tumours. Oxford University Press, Oxford, 1977.
150. Steel, G. G., Courtenay, V. D., and Peckham, M. J.: The response to chemotherapy of a variety of human tumour xenografts. Brit. J. Cancer, 47:1, 1983.
151. Steel, G. G., Adams, K., Hodgett, J., and Janik, P.: Cell population kinetics of a spontaneous rat tumor during serial transplantation. Brit. J. Cancer, 25:802, 1971.
152. Steel, G. G., and Stephens, T. C.: Stem cells in tumours. In Stem Cells: Their Identification and Characterization. Edited by C. S. Pottern. Churchill-Livingstone, London, 1983, p. 271.
153. Stephens, T. C.: Measurement of tumor cell surviving faction and absolute numbers of clonogens per tumor in excision assays. In Rodent Tumor Models in Experimental Cancer Therapy. Edited by R. F. Kallman. 1987, p. 90.
154. Stephens, T. C., Currie, G. A., and Peacock, J. H.: Repopulation of irradiated Lewis lung carcinoma by malignant cells and host macrophage progenitors. Brit. J. Cancer, 38:573, 1978.
155. Stinson, S. F., Alley, M. C., Kenney, S., Fiebig, S., and Boyd, M. R.: Morphologic characterization of human carcinoma cell lines. Proc. Am. Assoc. Cancer Res., 30:613, 1989.
156. Stratton, J. A., Kucera, P. R., Micha, J. P., Rettenmaier, M. A., Braly, P. S., Berman, M. L., and Di Saia, P. J.: The subrenal capsule tumor implant assay as predictor of clinical response to chemotherapy: 3 years of experience. Gynecol. Oncol., 19:336, 1984.
157. Thomlinson, R. H.: An experimental method for comparing treatments of intact malignant tumours in animals and its application to the use of oxygen in radiotherapy. Brit. J. Cancer, 14:555, 1980.
158. Toolan, H. W.: Successful subcutaneous growth and transplantation for human tumors in X-irradiated laboratory animals. Proc. Soc. Exp. Biolg. Med., 77:572, 1951.
159. Toolan, H. W.: Transplantable human neoplasms maintained in cortisone-treated laboratory animals: HS #1, HEP #1, HEP #2, HEP #3, and HENBRH #1. Cancer Res., 14:660, 1954.
160. Tueni, E. A., Dumont, P., Jacobovitz, D., Massi, G., Rocmans, P., Lejeune, F., de Franquer, P., Semal, P., and Klastersky, J.: Subrenal capsule assay for fresh human tumors in immunocompetent mice; an inappropriate technique for non-small cell lung cancer. Europ. J. Cancer Clin. Oncol., 23:1163, 1987.
161. Uvarov, O.: Research with animals: Requirements, responsibilities, welfare. Lab. Animal, 19:51, 1985.
162. Venditti, J. M.: Foreword. In Proceedings of the Symposium on the Use of Athymic Nude Mice in Cancer Research. Edited by D. P. Houchens, and A. A. Ovejera. New York, Gustav Fischer, 1978, p. ix.
163. Venditti, J. M.: Preclinical drug development: Rationale and methods. Semin. Oncol., 8:349, 1981.
164. Venditti, J. M.: The model's dilemma. In Design of Models for Testing Cancer Chemotherapeutic Agents. Edited by I. J. Fidler, and R. J. White. New York, Van Nostrand Reinhold, 1981, p. 80.
165. Venditti, J. M.: The National Cancer Institute Drug Discovery Program current and future perspectives. A commentary. Cancer Treat. Rep., 67:767, 1983.
166. Ward, J. M., Houchens, D. P., Collins, M. J., Young, D. M., and Reagan, R. L.: Naturally-occurring Sendai virus infection of athymic nude mice. Vet. Pathol., 13:36, 1976.
167. Workshop on "Disease-oriented Antitumor Drug Discovery and Development," NIH, Bethesda, MD, January 9–10, 1985. Sponsored by Developmental Therapeutics Program, Division of Cancer Treatment, National Cancer Institute.
168. Zubrod, C. G.: Chemical control of cancer. Proc. Natl. Acad. Sci., 69:1042, 1972.
169. Zubrod, C. G., Schepartz, S., Leiter, J., et al.: The Chemotherapy Program of the National Cancer Institute: History, analysis and plans. Cancer Chemother. Rep., 50:349, 1966.

XV-6

In Vitro and In Vivo Predictive Tests

A.-R. Hanauske
D. D. Von Hoff

Introduction

The majority of patients with cancer will require treatment with chemotherapeutic agents at some point in the course of their disease. Current treatment recommendations rest on carefully designed clinical studies in large patient populations and provide an individual patient with a probability for reponse based on clinically observed response rates. This approach has led to major progress in clinical oncology and has helped to identify curative therapeutic regimens for testicular cancer, some leukemias, some malignant lymphomas, and childhood tumors. Successful regimens are now also available for the adjuvant treatment of breast cancer, osteogenic sarcoma, and colorectal cancer. However, there are still a large number of cancers for which there is only marginal treatment. For this reason, numerous attempts have been made to develop in vitro or in vivo assays that might predict individual response or resistance.[22a,25,39,47]

Conceptually, there are a number of problems with predictive assays which are independent of the type of experimental system used. These include: the choice of drug concentrations relevant for the clinical situation; intratumor and intertumor heterogeneity in the tumor specimen: interference of experimental conditions with the usual physiological microenvironment of tumor cells as they existed in the patient; and selection pressure on tumor cells by the experimental system used. The relationship between inhibition of tumor growth in vitro and a patient's response to chemotherapy (and survival) is obviously quite complex.

Chemosensitivity assays only would be helpful in patients with curable diseases receiving known effective first-line chemotherapy if they had an excellent predictivity allowing for identification of the rare patient with primary resistant disease. There is no convincing evidence that any chemosensitivity assay has such a predictive power. However, in the clinical setting of patients with refractory disease where palliation is the goal they certainly might help avoid toxic side effects of agents which are unlikely to be clinically effective. At present, there is no convincing evidence that such assay-guided chemotherapy is superior to a treatment recommendation by an experienced oncologist with regard to patient survival. There is, however, recent evidence that clinical response rates may be superior for in vitro assays-directed chemotherapy versus chemotherapy selected by a clinician.[48]

Table XV-6-1 lists the various in vitro and in vivo tests which have been used to predict patient response or lack of response. Details on these assays are provided below.

In Vitro Techniques

Early attempts to establish predictive tests were dependent on the availability of cell culture techniques in the 1950's. The procedures used included evaluation of cell morphology, exclusion of vital dyes, activity of various enzymes, and incorporation of radioactive precursor molecules after incubation of tumor cells with anticancer agents.[5,17,52] However, subsequent correlative studies showed that only a minority of tests were of predictive value.[39,53] Potential problems which

Table XV-6-1.   Different Techniques Utilized for Predictive Tests

I. In Vitro Systems
A. Dye exclusion
B. Explant (organoid) cultures
C. Precursor incorporation
D. Fluorescence
E. Cellular adhesive matrix
F. Human tumor cloning assay
G. Intracellular drug concentrations
II. In Vivo Systems
A. Subrenal capsule
B. Nude mouse xenograft

may have confounded the predictive value included a lack of standardization, and an inability to accurately distinguish growth of malignant and non-malignant cells in explant cultures from primary tumors. In addition, some assays (e.g., tests for oxygen consumption by tumor cells) proved to be too complicated for routine use.[33]

Some techniques continue to be of interest for the prediction of clinical response (see Table XV-6-1).

Dye Techniques

Early attempts to use exclusion of vital dyes like trypan blue, eosin, or nigrosin to predict chemosensitivity were unsuccessful. More recently, Weisenthal and colleagues, and others have used a combination of fast green dye and eosin-hematoxylin with more promising results particularly in patients with hematologic malignancies such as CLL.[31,45,50,51] No prospective trial of the Weisenthal assay has yet been performed, however, to demonstrate its ability to predict for response or lack of response.

Another assay currently used at the National Cancer Institute to screen for anticancer activity of new chemicals may have some predictive value in hematologic neoplasms.[30] It is based on the ability of vital cells to reduce a tetrazolium compound to a blue formazan product which can be measured by photometry in a semiautomated fashion. This assay is relatively simple and rapid and may be used conveniently in screening cell lines in the setting of drug development. However, at the present time there are not sufficient data from primary tumor specimens available to reach a final conclusion with regard to its predictive value.

Explant (Organoid) Cultures

During the early years of development of chemosensitivity, short term organ cultures and explant cultures were used to assess anticancer effects of clinically used drugs.[2,54] Despite some reports on positive clinical correlations, most investigators have subsequently abandoned these techniques because of technical problems and lack of standardization. More recently, staining of tumor cell clusters with fluorescein diacetate has been reported to be predictive for clinical response in a series of 50 patients with a specificity of 84% and a sensitivity of 100%.[41] However, again, those results need to be confirmed in larger prospective studies.

Precursor Incorporation

Incorporation of radiolabeled precursor molecules into cellular macromolecules has long been used to measure cell proliferation and cell death. Specifically, [^{3}H]thymidine incorporation has been used to determine directly the extent of DNA replication. This can be either done autoradiographically or by liquid scintillation counting. Autoradiographic determination of the thymidine labeling index is more specific for malignant cells but too time consuming for general use. However, it will provide information on tumor growth kinetics. DNA histograms might also be used and have the advantage of providing information on the ploidy status. The value of overall determination of [^{3}H]precursor incorporation by liquid scintillation spectrometry after short term incubation has been heavily debated.[15,35,39,43] Encouraging clinical correlations in retrospective clinical trials still need to be confirmed by prospective, randomized correlative studies. Precursor incorporation assays are rapid, relatively inexpensive, and are feasible in the majority of tumor types. However, they will not differentiate between malignant and non-malignant cells and might lead to false negative predictions if lethally damaged cells undergo a final division.

Fluorescence

As stated above, fluorescent dyes may be used in conjunction with microscopic evaluation methods as an in vitro chemosensitivity assay.[41] For this assay, tumor biopsies are not completely disintegrated into single cells. In order to allow for cell-cell interactions to continue, clusters of tumor tissues—termed 'micro-organs'—are prepared using mild mechanical or enzymatic techniques. This method has not had a prospective clinical trial yet.

In another approach, cells from primary tumors may be exposed to propidium iodide after drug exposure and the resulting fluorescence determined by flow cytometry.[22] This also allows for the determination of cell kinetic parameters of individual tumor specimens. Because of technical difficulties in applying flow cytometry to primary tumor specimens, however, data on the predictive value for clinical response are too scarce to permit definitive conclusions.

Cellular Adhesive Matrix

The adhesive tumor cell culture system represents a variation of chemosensitivity testing in monolayer cell cultures. Single cells are prepared from biopsies or effusions and seeded with medium in multiwell dishes. Adherent cells are exposed to antineoplastic agents for several days. Selectivity for malignant cells is achieved by preparation of the underlying plastic surface with a solution containing fibronectin and fibrinopeptides.[3] At the end of the culture period, cells are fixed and stained. The total number of cells is determined and expressed relative to control dishes. In one retrospective series good clinical correlations were obtained with the assay.[1] Three-dimensional matrices have also been used to culture tumor cells for drug testing but no definitive clinical trial has been published on their predictive value.

Intracellular Drug Concentrations

Only limited information is available on using intracellular drug concentrations to predict patient response. Determination of intracellular drug concentration requires sophisticated methods specific for each compound under investigation. In previously untreated acute non-lymphocytic leukemia, cellular retention of arabinosyl cytidine triphosphate (Ara-CTP) has been reported to correlate with longer remission duration in vivo.[38] Retention by leukemic cells of less than 20% of ara-CTP four hours after removal of arabinosyl cytosine from the medium was correlated with a median clinical remission duration of three months. For retention of more than 20% of ara-CTP by leukemic blasts, median remission duration was 45 months. Other investigators have not been able to find any correlation between clinical response or remission duration and formation of ara-CTP.[37,40,42]

There is no definitive evidence for the predictive value of intracellular concentrations of other antineoplastic agents. Determining the predictive value of intracellular drug con-

centrations is difficult if the compound is clinically used as part of a combination regimen. Effects on tumor response and patient survival might be caused by other components of the combination and does not provide stringent evidence for sensitivity to the drug under investigation.

Specific Molecular Markers for Resistance

While no molecular markers to predict sensitivity to a specific drug have been identified, great progress has been made to elucidate the molecular mechanisms underlying inherent or acquired resistance to chemotherapeutic agents. Interference with these mechanisms is of potential clinical value since it may offer a specific approach to predict and possibly overcome resistance and may obviate the need for cell culture techniques. Still, this approach would not tell the clinician to which agents a patient's tumor is sensitive and could only be used to exclude drugs from any planned regimen. Table XV-6-2 summarizes important molecular mechanisms of drug resistance. At present, there are no definitive clinical trials available describing how accurately these mechanisms reflect clinical resistance.

Human Tumor Cloning Assay

Clonogenic assays are used to determine the effect of anticancer agents on actively growing tumor cells.[28] Contrary to most other assays, inhibition of cellular proliferation is directly used as the experimental endpoint.[12,26] Single cell suspensions are prepared from tumor biopsies and exposed to anticancer agents. After the cells are washed, they are seeded in a semisolid medium (agar or methylcellulose) to prevent proliferation of non-malignant cells in the specimen. After 14–28 days, some cells will have undergone several divisions and have formed tumor colonies which can be quantified in a visual or semiautomated fashion.

No other in vitro test system has been investigated as thoroughly as have clonogenic assays. As a result, the potentials and limitations are best known for these types of assays. Retrospective and prospective clinical correlative trials have been performed in more than 2,000 patients. Table XV-6-3 summarizes the cumulative results of 2,300 correlations.[47] From these data, there is a 69% probability for a patient to have at least a partial response if the tumor specimen is sensitive to the drug in vitro. On the other hand, if a tumor is resistant in vitro, there will be a 91% chance for clinical resistance. These results are comparable to other clinically accepted laboratory tests, e.g., determination of estrogen or progesterone receptor status in breast cancer patients to predict response to endocrine therapy. Of course, the accuracy of the prediction of clinical resistance depends on the actual response rates in vivo.[46] Recently, a prospective, randomized trial of assay-guided chemotherapy versus a clinician's choice of drugs in patients with a variety of cancers has shown higher response rates when test results were used in patient management.[48] Patients with disseminated malignancies were stratified for performance status, tumor type, and prior chemotherapy. They were then randomized to single agent chemotherapy which was either recommended by a physician or determined by the cloning assay. If progression occurred, patients were crossed over to the other treatment option. A total of 65 patients were

Table XV-6-2. Molecular Mechanisms of Drug Resistance Which Might Be Helpful for the Prediction of Clinical Response

Molecular Alteration	Mechanism	Drug Affected	Reference
1. Alteration of drug transport			
1.1. Expression of P-170 glycoprotein	Increased drug efflux	Miscellaneous	23
	("pleiotropic drug resistance")		
2. Increased enzyme activity			
2.1. Glutathione-S-transferase	Drug inactivation	Alkylating agents	27
2.2. Aldehyde dehydrogenase	Drug inactivation	Cyclophosphamide	29
2.3. Guanine-O^6-alkyl transferase	DNA repair	Nitrosoureas	20
2.4. Ribonucleotide reductase	Increase of binding sites	Hydroxyurea	10
3. Decreased enzyme activity			
3.1. Deoxycytidine kinase	Drug activation	AraC	18
3.2. Pyrimidine salvage pathways	Drug activation	5-Fluorouracil	36
3.3. Topoisomerase II	Decrease of binding sites	Anthracyclines	16
		Epipodophyllotoxins	24
4. Gene amplification			
4.1. Dihydrofolate reductase	Increase of binding sites	Methotrexate	13
4.2. Ribonucleotide reductase	Increase of binding sites	Hydroxyurea	11

Table XV-6-3. Cumulative Results from 2,300 Clinical Correlations Using Clonogenic Assays to Predict Clinical Treatment Outcome[47]

		N	%
True Positive	:	512	69
True Negative	:	1427	91
False Positive	:	226	31
False Negative	:	135	9
TOTAL	:	2300	
Sensitivity[a]	:		79
Specificity[b]	:		86
Positive Predictive Value[c]	:		69
Negative Predictive Value[d]	:		91

$$^a Sensitivity = \frac{True\ Positives}{True\ Positives + False\ Negatives}$$

$$^b Specificity = \frac{True\ Negatives}{True\ Negatives + False\ Positives}$$

$$^c Positive\ Predictive\ Value = \frac{True\ Positives}{True\ Positives + False\ Positives}$$

$$^d Negative\ Predictive\ Value = \frac{True\ Negatives}{True\ Negatives + False\ Negatives}$$

randomized to the clinician's choice while 68 patients were randomized to the assay's choice. However, due to a variety of reasons only 36 and 19 patients, respectively, actually received the treatment they were assigned to and were evaluable for response. In the assay-guided arm the largest group of patients inevaluable for response were those with inevaluable in vitro growth. For evaluable patients, one partial response (3%) was noted in the clinician's choice and four in the assay's choice (21%). The difference was statistically significant at 0.04. Twenty-six percent of the patients in the assay's choice arm had stable disease as compared to 8% in the clinician's choice arm. There was no difference in the survival curves either for the whole group of randomized patients or for the group of actually treated patients who were therefore evaluable for response. This study does provide an encouraging lead for future clinical trials. It pinpoints the need for further improvements in the methodology of cloning assays. Also, it may be of interest to determine the value of assay-guided chemotherapy in less refractory tumors.

Traditional clonogenic systems suffer from a number of significant technical problems including lack of growth in 40–60% of all specimens and a long incubation time (at least 14 days) before results can be made available to the clinician. Furthermore, insufficient data are available on the effect of assay-guided chemotherapy on patient survival. Since most clinically observed responses are partial responses, a significant increase in overall survival is not to be expected.

A combination of [^{3}H]thymidine incorporation and cloning techniques has shown promise by increasing the number of evaluable specimens (80–90% of patient specimens are evaluable) and decreasing the incubation time.[44] With this variation of tumor cloning techniques, the experimental endpoint no longer is direct visualization of clonal proliferation. Instead, the amount of trichloroacetic acid precipitable radioactivity is determined and taken as representative for cell growth. The relationship between colony counts and tritiated thymidine incorporation is non-linear and an algorithm has been developed for conversion.[32] However, no prospective clinical trials of that improved system to predict patients' response or lack of response has been performed.

In Vivo Techniques

The two most commonly used in vivo systems to predict clinical drug activity are the subrenal capsule assay and transplantation of tumor cells into nude mice. Advantages of in vivo techniques include: feasibility of testing agents that require metabolic activation and the preservation of three-dimensional tumor structure with cell-cell-interactions. Also, drug effects on cell growth can be determined over several cell cycles and the effects of drug combinations may be studied. Significant disadvantages include the necessity of an animal facility as well as high costs. Extrapolation of assay results to the clinical setting may be hampered by the fact that treatment in animals is usually started at a low tumor burden while patients usually are treated in an advanced stage when the tumor burden is rather high.

Subrenal Capsule Assay

The subrenal capsule assay was developed by Bogden and coworkers for drug testing.[7,8] In principle, small pieces of tumors are implanted under the renal capsule of athymic or of immunocompetent mice. The animals are then treated with chemotherapy and after four to eleven days size determinations of tumor transplants are performed. Active anticancer agents lead to a decrease in size of tumor transplant relative to untreated controls. Evaluability rates range from 60–80% which is somewhat better than evaluability rates in conventional clonogenic assays.[6] However, evaluability depends on the tumor type tested. Some tumors will not grow in this system.[14,19] Retrospective and prospective correlating trials have reported true positives for the assay in the 60–83% range and true negatives in the 66–95% range.[34] In one study, Favre and coworkers compared retrospective and prospective clinical correlations.[21] In the retrospective analysis, true correlation with clinical sensitivity was observed in 8/11 (72%) and true correlation with clinical resistance in 45/45 (100%) assays. In the prospective series, true prediction for clinical resistance was observed in 26/27 (96%) assays and true prediction for clinical sensitivity was found in 19/23 (82%) tests. The cumulative analysis gave 98% true resistant correlations and 82% true sensitive correlations.

Nude Mouse Xenografts

Heterotransplantation of human tumors into athymic nude mice has been extensively used in cancer research. Experimental endpoints are a decrease in size of tumor nodules and the prolongation of survival. These endpoints may not correlate with each other. Except for work with cell lines, this assay is too laborious and expensive for routine predictive drug testing. The yield of growing tumors is quite low (15–40%) when primary cells are used.[4,9,35] In contrast to the subrenal capsule assay, tumors implanted in nude mice may require two to three months to be evaluable for drug testing, a lag time usually not acceptable in the clinical setting. Because of these difficulties there have only been a handful of attempted clinical correlations with the nude mouse xenograft system. None of the studies has been definitive.

Summary

In summary, an ideal predictive chemosensitivity assay should be simple, rapid, reproducible, applicable to all tumor types, and inexpensive. At present, no such system is available. Even the most extensively studied assays will more often identify agents which will NOT work in an individual patient than agents that will. Clearly, the lack of active agents in cancer chemotherapy is an important factor in this context pointing at the dire need to identify new and more active agents. The most important contribution of chemosensitivity assays still lies in the area of research and not in routine clinical use.

References

1. Ajani, J. A., Baker, F. L., Spitzer, G., Kelly, A., Brock, W., Tomasovic, B., Singletary, S. E., McMurtrey, M., and Plager, C.: Comparison between clinical response and in vitro drug sensitivity of primary human tumors in the Adhesive Tumor Cell Culture System. J. Clin. Oncol., 5:1912, 1987.
2. Ambrose, E. J., Andrews, R. D., Easty, D. M., Field, E. O., and Wylie, J. A.: Drug assays on cultures of human tumour biopsies. Lancet, 1:24, 1962.
3. Baker, F. L., Spitzer, G., Ajani, J. A., Brock, W. A., Lukeman, J., Pathak, N., Tomasovic, B., Thieldvoldt, D., Williams, M., Vines, C., and Tofilon, P.: Drug and radiation sensitivity measurements of successful primary monolayer culturing of human tumor cells using cell-adhesive matrix and supplemented medium. Cancer Res., 46:1263, 1986.
4. Bellet, R. E., Danna, V., Mastrangelo, M. J., and Berd, D.: Evaluation of a "nude" mouse-human tumor panel as a predictive secondary screen for cancer chemotherapeutic agents. J. Natl. Cancer Inst., 63:1185, 1979.
5. Black, M. M., and Speer, F. D.: Further observations on the effects of cancer chemotherapeutic agents on the in vitro dehydrogenase activity of cancer tissue. J. Natl. Cancer Inst., 14:1147, 1954.
6. Bogden, A. E.: The subrenal capsule assay (SRCA) and its predictive value in oncology. Ann. Chir. Gynaecol., 74(Suppl. 199):12, 1985.
7. Bogden, A. E., Haskell, P. M., LePage, D. J, Kelton, D. E., Cobb, W. R., and Esber, H. J.: Growth of human tumor xenografts implanted under the renal capsule of normal immunocompetent mice. Exp. Cell Biol., 47:281, 1979.
8. Bogden, A. E., Kelton, D. E., Cobb, W. R., and Esber, H. J.: A rapid screening method for testing chemotherapeutic agents against human tumor xenografts. In Proceedings of the symposium on the use of athymic (nude) mice in cancer research. Edited by D. P. Houchens, and A. A. Ovejera. New York, G. Fischer, 1978, pp. 231–250.
9. Braakhuis, B. B., and Snow, G. B.: Nude Mice Model as a Predictive Assay in Head and Neck Cancer. In Head and Neck Cancer, Vol. 1. Edited by P. B. Chretien, M. E. Johns, D. E. Shedd, F. W. Strong, and P. H. Ward. Philadelphia, B. C. Decker, Inc., 1985, pp. 421–424.
10. Choy, B. K., Mc Clarty, G. A., Chan, A. K., Thelander, L., and Wright, J. A.: Molecular mechanisms of drug resistance involving ribonucleotide reductase: hydroxyurea resistance in a series of clonally related mouse cell lines selected in the presence of increasing drug concentrations. Cancer Res., 48:2029, 1988.
11. Cocking, J. M., Tonin, P. N., Stokoe, N. M., Wensing, E. J., Lewis, W. H., and Srinivasan, P. R.: Gene for M1 subunit of ribonucleotide reductase is amplified in hydroxyurea-resistant hamster cells. Somatic Cell Mol. Genet., 13:221, 1987.
12. Courtenay, V. D., and Mills, J.: An in vitro colony assay for human tumours grown in immune-suppressed mice and treated in vivo with cytotoxic agents. Brit. J. Cancer, 37:261, 1978.
13. Cowan, K. H., Goldsmith, M. E., Levine, R. M., Aitken, S. T., Douglass, E., Clendeninn, N., Nienhuis, A. W., and Lippman, M. E.: Dihydrofolate reductase gene amplification and possible rearrangement in estrogen-responsive methotrexate-resistant human breast cancer cells. J. Biol. Chem., 257:15079, 1982.
14. Cunningham, D., Jack, A., McMurdo, D. F., Soukop, H., McArdle, C. S., Carter, D. C., and Kaye, S. B.: The 6-day subrenal capsule assay is of no value with primary surgical explants from gastric cancer. Br. J. Cancer, 54:519, 1986.
15. Daidone, M. G., Silvestrini, R., Sanfilippo, O., Zaffaroni, N., Varini, M., and De Lena, M.: Reliability of an in vitro short-term assay to predict the drug sensitivity of human breast cancer. Cancer, 56:450, 1985.
16. Deffie, A. M., Batra, J. K., and Goldenberg, G. G.: Direct correlation between DNA topoisomerase II activity and cytotoxicity in adriamycin-sensitive and -resistant P388 leukemia cell lines. Cancer Res., 49:58, 1989.
17. Dendy, P. P.: Human Tumors in Short-Term Culture. New York, Academic Press, 1976.
18. Drahovsky, D., and Kreis, W.: Studies on drug resistance: II. Kinase patterns in P815 neoplasms sensitive and resistant to 1-beta-D-arabinofuranosylcytosine. Biochem. Pharmacol., 19:940, 1970.
19. Edelstein, M. B.: The subrenal capsule assay: a critical commentary. Eur. J. Cancer Clin. Oncol., 22:757, 1986.
20. Ewig, R. A. G., and Kohn, K. W.: DNA damage and repair in mouse leukemia L 1210 cells treated with nitrogen mustard, 1,3-bis(2-chloroethyl)-1-nitrosourea, and other nitrosoureas. Cancer Res., 37:2114, 1977.
21. Favre, R., Mariota, L., Drancourt, M., Jaquemier, J., Delpero, J. R., Guerinel, G., and Carcassonne, Y.: 6-day subrenal capsule assay (SRCA) as a predictor of the response of advanced cancers to chemotherapy. Eur. J. Cancer, 22:1171, 1986.
22. Funa, K., Dawson, N., Jewett, P. B., Agren, H., Ruckdeschel, J. C., Bunn, P. A., Jr., and Gazdar, A. F.: Automated fluorescent analysis for drug-induced cytotoxicity assays. Cancer Treat. Rep., 70:1147, 1986.
22a. Gellhorn, A., and Hirschberg, E. (Eds.): Investigation of diverse systems for cancer chemotherapy screening. Cancer Res., 3(Suppl.):1, 1955.
23. Gerlach, J. H., Kartner, N., Bell, D. R., and Ling, V.: Multidrug resistance. Cancer Surveys, 5:25, 1986.
24. Glisson, B., Gupta, R., Hodges, P., and Ross, W.: Cross-resistance to intercalating agents in an epipodophyllotoxin-resistant Chinese hamster ovary cell line: evidence for a common intracellular target. Cancer Res., 46:1939, 1986.
25. Hamburger, A. W.: Use of in vitro tests in predictive cancer chemotherapy. J. Natl. Cancer Inst., 66:981, 1981.
26. Hamburger, A. W., and Salmon, S. E.: Primary bioassay of human tumor stem cells. Science, 197:461, 1977.
27. Hamilton, T. C., Winker, M. A., Louie, K. G., Batist, G., Behrens, B. G., Tsuruo, T., Grotzinger, K. R., McKoy, W. M., Young, R. C., and Ozols, R. F.: Augmentation of adriamycin, melphalan, and cisplatin toxicity in drug resistant and -sensitive human ovarian cancer cell lines by buthionine sulfoximine mediated glutathione depletion. Biochem. Pharmacol., 34:2583, 1985.
28. Hanauske, A.-R., Hanauske, U., and Von Hoff, D. D.: The human tumor cloning assay in cancer research and therapy. Curr. Probl. Cancer, 9:1, 1985.
29. Hilton, J.: Role of aldehyde dehydrogenase in cyclophosphamide-resistant L1210 leukemia. Cancer Res., 44:5156, 1984.
30. Hongo, T., Fujii, Y., and Igarashi, Y.: An in vitro chemosensitivity test for the screening of anti-cancer drugs in childhood leukemia. Cancer, 65:1263, 1990.
31. Ihde, D., Russell, E., Oic, H. K., et al.: Prospective clinical trial of individualized chemotherapy based on in vitro drug sensitivity testing in extensive stage small cell lung cancer. In Adjuvant Therapy of Cancer V. Edited by S. E. Salmon. Orlando, Fla., Grune & Stratton, 1987, pp. 201–207.
32. Kern, D. H., and Weisenthal, L. M.: Highly specific prediction of antineoplastic drug resistance with an in vitro assay using suprapharmacologic drug exposures. J. Natl. Cancer Inst., 7:582, 1990.
33. Laszlo, J., Stengle, J., Wight, K., and Burk, D.: Effects of chemotherapeutic agents on metabolism of human acute leukemia cells in vitro. Proc. Soc. Exp. Biol. Med., 97:127, 1958.

34. Maeenpaeae, J., Kangas, L., and Groenroos, M.: The subrenal capsule assay for chemosensitivity testing of tumors. A review. Zentralbl. Gynaecol., 110:989, 1988.

35. Mattern, J., and Volm, M.: Clinical relevance of predictive tests for cancer chemotherapy. Cancer Treat. Rev., 9:267, 1982.

36. Mulkins, M. A., and Heidelberger, C.: Isolation of fluoropyrimidine-resistant murine leukemic cell lines by one-step mutation and selection. Cancer Res., 42:956, 1982.

37. Plunkett, W., Iacobini, S., and Keating, M. J.: Cellular pharmacology and optimal therapeutic concentrations of 1-beta-D-arabinofuranosylcytosine 5'-triphosphate in leukemic blasts during treatment of refractory leukemia with high-dose 1-beta-D-arabinofuranosylcytosine. Scand. J. Haematol., 34:51, 1986.

38. Preisler, H. D., Rustum, Y., and Priore, R. L.: Relationship between leukemic cell retention of cytosine arabinoside triphosphate and the duration of remission in patients with acute non-lymphocytic leukemia. Eur. J. Cancer Clin. Oncol., 21:23, 1985.

39. Roper, P. R., and Drewincko, B.: Comparison of in vitro methods to determine drug-induced cell lethality. Cancer Res., 36:2182, 1976.

40. Ross, D. D., Thompson, B. W., Joneckis, C. C., Akman, S. A., and Schiffer, C. A: Metabolism of ara-C by blast cells from patients with ANLL. Blood, 68:76, 1986.

41. Rotman, B.: Fluorescent cytoprinting: A simple nondestructive process for assessing chemosensitivity in micro-organcultures. Proc. Amer. Assoc. Cancer Res., 30:654, 1989.

42. Rustum, Y. M., Riva, C., and Preisler, H. D.: Pharmacokinetic parameters of 1-beta-D-arabinofuranosylcytosine and their relationship to intracellular metabolism of ara-C, toxicity, and response of patients with acute non-lymphocytic leukemia treated with conventional and high dose ara-C. Semin. Oncol., 14:141, 1987.

43. Sanfilippo, O., Silvestrini, R., Zaffaroni, N., Piva, L., and Pizzocaro, G.: Application of an in vitro antimetabolic assay to human germ cell testicular tumors for the preclinical evaluation of drug sensitivity. Cancer, 58:1441, 1986.

44. Tanigawa, N., Kern, D. H., Hikasa, Y., and Morton, D. L.: Rapid assay for evaluating the chemosensitivity of human tumors in soft agar culture. Cancer Res., 42:2159, 1982.

45. Tidefelt, U., Sundman-Engberg, B., Rhedin, A.-S., and Paul, C.: In vitro drug testing in patients with acute leukemia with incubations mimicking in vivo intracellular drug concentrations. Eur. J. Haematol., 43:374, 1989.

46. Twentyman, P. R.: Predictive chemosensitivity testing. Br. J. Cancer, 51:295, 1985.

47. Von Hoff, D. D.: He's not going to talk about in vitro predictive assays again, is he? J. Natl. Cancer Inst., 1990.

48. Von Hoff, D. D., Sandbach, J. F., Clark, G. M., Turner, J. N., Forseth, B. F., Piccart, M. J., Colombo, N., and Muggia, F. M.: Selection of cancer chemotherapy for a patient by an in vitro assay versus a clinician. J. Natl. Cancer Inst., 82:110, 1990.

49. Von Hoff, D. D., and Weisenthal, L.: In vitro methods to predict for patient response to chemotherapy. Adv. Pharmacol. Chemother., 17:133, 1980.

50. Weisenthal, L. M., Dill, P. L., and Lippman, M. E.: Comparison of dye exclusion assays with a clonogenic assay in the determination of drug-induced cytotoxicity. Cancer Res., 43:258, 1983.

51. Weisenthal, L. M., Marsden, J. A., Dill, P. L., and Macaluso, C. K.: A novel dye exclusion method for testing in vitro chemosensitivity of human tumors. Cancer Res., 43:749, 1983.

52. Wright, J. C., Plummer-Cobb, J., Gumport, S., Golomb, F. M., and Safadi, D.: Investigation of the relation between clinical and tissue culture response to chemotherapeutic agents on human cancer. N. Engl. J. Med., 257:1207, 1957.

53. Wright, J. C., Plummer-Cobb, J., Gumport, S. L., Safadi, D., Walker, D. G., and Golomb, F. M.: Further investigation of the relation between the clinical and tissue culture response to chemotherapeutic agents on human cancer. Cancer, 15:284, 1962.

54. Yarnell, M., Ambrose, E. J., Shepley, K., and Tchao, R.: Drug assays on organ culture of biopsies from human tumours. Br. Med. J., 2:490, 1964.

XV-7

Pharmacology

Mark J. Ratain
Richard L. Schilsky

For many years the clinical pharmacology of anti-cancer drugs was poorly understood due primarily to the lack of sensitive and specific assays for measuring the concentration of these compounds in biological fluids. The recent development and widespread application of high performance liquid chromatography and other sophisticated analytical tools now allows plasma drug level monitoring to be performed with a high degree of precision and efficiency. Clinical pharmacokinetic studies of anticancer drugs, particularly new agents, are now performed routinely. Although the pharmacokinetic characteristics of many drugs have been well-defined, the application of this information to the clinical care of individual patients still lags far behind other areas in medicine. Plasma concentrations of digoxin, theophylline, aminoglycosides, phenytoin and many other drugs are monitored routinely to optimize efficacy and reduce toxicity, yet the measurement of doxorubicin or 5-fluorouracil (5-FU) concentrations in plasma is virtually meaningless since there are no established relationships between pharmacokinetics and clinical effects for these or most other commonly used anti-cancer drugs. A notable exception is methotrexate where delayed clearance has clearly been related to an increased risk of severe toxicity.

Pharmacokinetic-pharmacodynamic relationships are difficult to develop for many reasons. For most antineoplastic agents there is a delay of days to weeks between measurement of drug concentrations and clinical effect. It is therefore necessary to observe patients frequently following chemotherapy administration to accurately assess the drug effect. The maximum observed effect may be significantly less than the true maximum effect unless patients are seen daily. Although the desired effect of cancer chemotherapy is a reduction in tumor volume, usually optimized by maximizing the dose, the narrow therapeutic index of antineoplastic drugs requires that most dosing strategies focus on minimizing toxicity rather than on optimizing efficacy. Despite these difficulties, significant progress has recently been made in understanding the clinical pharmacodynamics of anti-cancer drugs and further studies in this area will no doubt lead to more rational administration of cancer chemotherapy.

This chapter will focus on the principles of clinical pharmacology as they apply to cancer chemotherapy and will attempt to illustrate how an understanding of clinical pharmacokinetics and pharmacodynamics can optimize the therapeutic index of cancer chemotherapy.

General Mechanisms of Drug Action

The initial requirement for drug action is adequate drug delivery to the target site. This depends largely on blood flow in the tumor bed and the diffusion characteristics of the drug in tissue. However, delivery may also be influenced by the extent of plasma protein binding and, for orally administered drugs, by absorption and first pass metabolism in the liver (Figure XV-7-1). Blood flow across a capillary bed is directly proportional to the arteriovenous pressure difference and inversely proportional to the geometric and viscous resistances. The geometric resistance to blood flow increases with increasing tumor size, a factor that may limit drug and oxygen delivery to large tumors and thereby diminish the effectiveness of treatment with chemotherapy or radiation.[125]

Membrane Transport

In order to produce cytotoxicity, most anticancer drugs require uptake into the cell. A number of mechanisms exist for the passage of drugs across the plasma membrane including passive diffusion, facilitated diffusion and active transport systems (Figure XV-7-2).[50] Passive diffusion of drugs through the lipid bilayer structure of the plasma membrane is a function of the size, lipid solubility and charge of the drug molecule. If the extracellular drug concentration is constant, then drug accumulation by the cell will continue until the rate of drug uptake from the extracellular space is equal to the rate of drug efflux from the cell. At this point, a dynamic equilibrium is reached and intracellular and extracellular drug concentrations are equal. As drug is cleared from the extracellular space, intracellular drug levels will decline if the drug is not bound or metabolized intracellularly. An important feature of the passive diffusion process is that it does not saturate. That is, as the extracellular drug concentration increases, influx into the cell increases proportionally and high intracellular drug levels can be achieved. Passive diffusion, how-

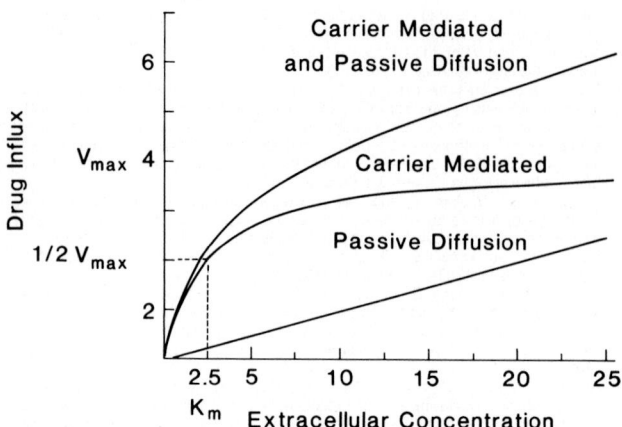

Figure XV-7-2. Relationship between drug influx rate and extracellular concentration. The lower line illustrates the linear relationship for a passive diffusion process that does not saturate. For carrier-mediated processes, initial influx is rapid; K_m is equal to the extracellular concentration at which the influx rate is ½ maximal. Saturation occurs at high extracellular concentrations. For transport processes with a component of carrier-mediated influx and passive diffusion, the diffusion process dominates once saturation of the carrier occurs.

ever, is a highly inefficient and non-specific process that may be a particularly important mechanism of drug uptake when carrier-mediated processes are nonfunctional, such as occurs in some cases of methotrexate resistance.

The passage of physiologically important hydrophilic compounds across the plasma membrane is usually mediated by a specific receptor, or carrier, in the plasma membrane that facilitates the translocation of the substance into or out of the cell. Carrier-mediated transport systems are distinguished from passive diffusion by having a high degree of specificity and by being saturable at high extracellular drug concentrations due to the presence of a finite number of receptor molecules within the membrane. Once all carrier sites become occupied, further increases in extracellular drug concentration will not produce further increments in drug influx unless a component of passive diffusion comes into play. The affinity of the carrier for the substrate can be estimated from the Km, the drug concentration at which the influx rate is one-half maximal; the lower the Km, the higher the carrier affinity.

While all carrier-mediated systems enhance the rate of influx into the cell, not all carriers are able to translocate compounds against electrochemical forces and ultimately develop gradients such that the intracellular concentration exceeds the extracellular drug level. To do so requires the expenditure of energy and the coupling of carrier-mediated transport to an energy-requiring reaction, usually hydrolysis of adenosine triphosphate (ATP).

Many antineoplastic drugs, particularly those that are structural analogs of natural compounds, gain entry into the cell by carrier-mediated mechanisms. Naturally occuring nucleosides are transported by facilitated diffusion along both Na+-dependent and Na+-independent pathways while nucleoside analogs such as cytosine arabinoside (ara-C) appear to utilize primarily Na+-independent pathways.[23,63,64,149] Transport of reduced folates and methotrex-

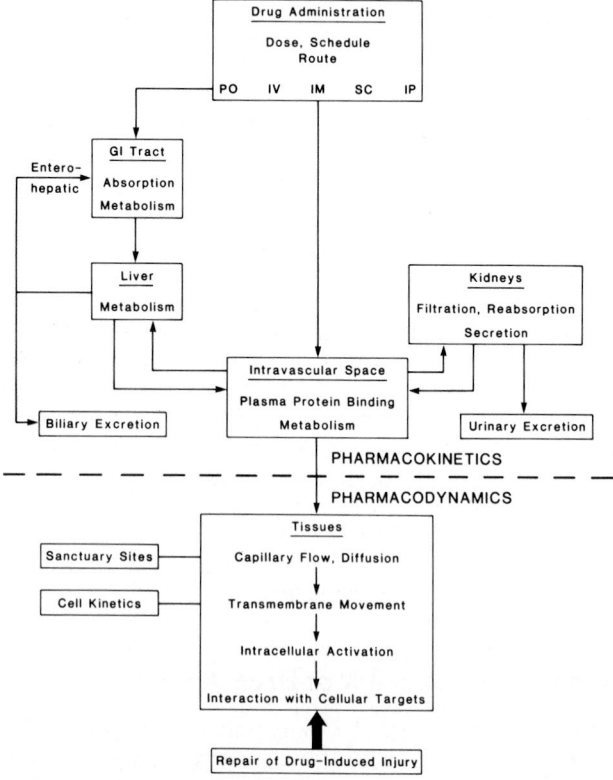

Figure XV-7-1. Schematic representation of pharmacokinetics and pharmacodynamics. Pharmacokinetics represents the distribution, metabolism and elimination of drugs from the body. Pharmacodynamics describes the interaction of drugs with target tissues.

ate is an active energy-dependent process mediated by specific folate binding proteins in the plasma membrane.[39,79,126] L-phenylalanine mustard utilizes at least two amino acid transport systems and its influx can be inhibited by the amino acid substrates specific for these transport carriers.[48]

The importance of transmembrane movement of a drug to its pharmacologic effect depends on several factors including the rate of drug delivery to the tissue, the affinity of the transport process, and the nature of the intracellular biochemical events required for drug action. Though membrane transport can be the rate-limiting step in drug action if it limits the rate at which the drug reaches intracellular targets, this is not always the case. If drug delivery to a cell is slow relative to the influx rate then the drug effect will be limited primarily by extracellular concentration, i.e., blood flow and diffusion of the drug. Similarly, if a drug requires intracellular activation, such as phosphorylation, before it can exert a cytotoxic effect, then the rate limiting step in drug action could be activation rather than transport if the rate of activation is slow relative to the rate of influx into the cell.

Finally, it is important to recognize that membrane transport is frequently bidirectional with the final drug concentration in the cell representing the balance between drug influx and drug efflux. These processes may utilize different carrier systems and operate at different rates. One efflux system that appears to have great importance in cancer chemotherapy is the P-glycoprotein system that mediates a form of multi-drug resistance.[8] (See XV-2.)

Intracellular Activation

Many anticancer drugs require activation before they are able to exert a cytotoxic effect. The activation process may involve chemical or enzymatic reactions in either normal or tumor tissues (Table XV-7-1). Cisplatin, for example, undergoes a chemical reaction with water molecules intracellularly resulting in the generation of a positively charged aquated species that attacks nucleophilic sites on DNA.[78] In contrast, the activation of cyclophosphamide is mediated by hepatic

XV-7-1. Activation of Anticancer Drugs

Activation Reaction*	Drug
Polyglutamylation	Methotrexate
Phosphorylation	Cytosine arabinoside, 5-fluorouracil, 6-mercaptopurine, 6-thioguanine, fludarabine
Microsomal oxidation	Cyclophosphamide, ifosfamide, procarbazine
Microsomal reduction	Bleomycin
Demethylation	Dacarbazine, hexamethylmelamine
Acetylation	Amonafide
Aquation	Cisplatin

*Reaction necessary for formation of active cytotoxic drug metabolite or for production of a more potent metabolite

microsomal mixed function oxidases resulting in the release of active alkylating species into the systemic circulation.[21]

Intracellular activation by tumor cells is a critical determinant of effect for virtually all antimetabolites. Ara-C, 5-FU and the purine antimetabolites (6-mercaptopurine and 6-thioguanine) all require phosphorylation to active nucleotide forms before they are able to exert a cytotoxic effect. While methotrexate (MTX) is an effective enzyme inhibitor in its native form, intracellular conversion of the drug to polyglutamate metabolites significantly increases its potency and facilitates its binding to a number of enzymatic sites.[5,66]

The rate of formation of the activated drug species in the cell depends on a number of variables: The rate of transmembrane influx of the drug, the amount and affinity of the activating enzyme(s) in the cell, the extent of competition by the naturally occurring substrates of the activating enzymes, and the rate of degradation of the activated drug by catabolic enzymes. For most antimetabolites, membrane transport is rapid relative to enzymatic activation and is therefore not rate limiting. Once inside the cell, antimetabolites must compete with the natural enzyme substrates for binding and activation. Finally, the activated drug then becomes a substrate for catabolic enzymes in the cell that tend to degrade it to the parent compound or to an inactive metabolite. The concentration of active cytotoxic drug in the cell is the result of all these processes. An excellent example of this is the pyrimidine nucleoside analog, ara-C. After gaining entry to the cell, ara-C is metabolized in three successive phosphorylation reactions to the active triphosphate derivative, ara-CTP. The first activating enzyme, deoxycytidine kinase, is found in lowest concentration in cells and is believed to be the rate limiting step in drug activation. At each phosphorylation step, ara-C competes with endogenous substrates for enzyme binding. In the case of deoxycytidine kinase, the affinity of the enzyme for ara-C ($Km = 20$ μM) is lower than for the natural substrate, deoxycytidine ($Km = 7.8$ μM).[19] However, the enzyme is strongly inhibited by dCTP but weakly inhibited by ara-CTP, allowing accumulation of ara-CTP to higher concentrations.[95] Opposing the activation of ara-C are two deaminases, cytidine deaminase and dCMP deaminase that convert ara-C and ara-CMP, respectively, to inactive uracil derivatives. The balance of these processes is crucial in determining the cytotoxicity of ara-C. In human leukemic blasts, the persistence of ara-CTP concentrations of at least 75 μM correlates strongly with the probability of achieving a complete remission.[96] Loss or diminished affinity of an activating enzyme or enhanced activity of a catabolic enzyme may be responsible for drug resistance. In the case of ara-C, cells selected in vitro for drug resistance have demonstrated both loss of deoxycytidine kinase activity and increased deaminase activity as potential causes of drug resistance.[11,84] Recent studies of acute lymphoblastic leukemia cell lines derived from patients clinically resistant to ara-C therapy suggest that decreased or absent deoxycytidine kinase activity may be a major mechanism of clinical resistance.[69]

Drug Targets

While anticancer drugs have traditionally been classified based on their mechanism of action or their origins, they can also be grouped based upon the target of drug action. There are essentially five potential targets of drug action: Nucleic acids, enzymes, membranes, microtubules, and hormone/growth factor receptors. When nucleic acids are the target, it is generally DNA rather than RNA binding that is presumed to cause cell death. There are several mechanisms by which drugs can bind DNA, the most well understood being alkylation of nucleophilic sites within the double helix. Most alkylating agents have two moieties capable of developing a charged carbon that binds covalently to negatively charged sites on DNA such as the O6 or N7 positions of guanine. The crosslinking of the two strands of DNA produced by the bifunctional alkylating agents prevents the use of that DNA as a template for further DNA synthesis leading to inhibition of cell replication and death.[13,71] Although alkylating agents are among the most widely used drugs in clinical oncology, the relationship of pharmacologic parameters to clinical effects has not been well-defined for these agents. In part, this has been due to the lack of sensitive and specific techniques to detect drug-DNA binding in clinical specimens. Recent studies of chlorambucil-DNA binding in the tumor cells of patients with chronic lymphocytic leukemia have demonstrated considerable heterogeneity in drug-DNA binding among patient samples, but no clear correlations between amount of drug bound and disease stage or sensitivity to treatment have been shown.[7] By contrast, cisplatin binding to DNA has been shown to correlate with cell kill in mammalian tumor cell lines.[139] Reed and colleagues have recently utilized an ELISA assay based on a polyclonal anti-cisplatin-DNA antiserum to quantitate platinum-DNA adduct formation in peripheral white blood cells of patients receiving cisplatin chemotherapy.[110] Adduct formation appears to correlate with the cumulative cisplatin dose received by the patient and, perhaps, with the response of the tumor to chemotherapy but not with the extent of leukopenia observed. Platinum-DNA adduct levels greater than 160 amol/mcg DNA (1 attomol = 10^{-18} mol) seem be associated with the greatest probability of tumor regression.[109] As new analytical methods become available, further studies will be necessary to confirm and expand on these initial observations.

A second mechanism of drug binding to nucleic acids is intercalation, the insertion of a planar ring structure between two adjacent nucleotide bases of DNA. This mechanism is characteristic of many antitumor antibiotics. The antibiotic molecule is non-covalently, although firmly, bound to DNA and distorts the shape of the double helix resulting in inhibition of RNA or DNA synthesis.[94,150] Recent data suggest that many classical intercalating agents such as doxorubicin may in fact be inhibitors of the enzyme topoisomerase II, and may produce DNA strand breaks by inhibition of the reannealing function of this enzyme.[114,140] Indeed, a direct correlation has been noted between DNA topoisomerase II activity and cytotoxicity in doxorubicin-sensitive and resistant P388 leukemia cells.[25]

A third mechanism of nucleic acid damage is illustrated by the anticancer drug bleomycin. The amino terminal tripeptide of the bleomycin molecule appears to intercalate between guanine-cytosine base pairs of DNA. The opposite end of the bleomycin peptide binds Fe (II) and serves as a ferrous oxidase, able to catalyze the reduction of molecular oxygen to superoxide or hydroxyl radicals that produce DNA strand scission.[47,138]

Enzymes represent the second general category of targets for chemotherapeutic agents. Antimetabolites function as inhibitors of key enzymes in the purine or pyrimidine biosynthetic pathways or as inhibitors of DNA polymerase. Since most of these enzymes are highly active during DNA synthesis, antimetabolites tend to be cytotoxic only when present in sufficient concentration during the vulnerable S phase of the cell cycle. These drugs are thus frequently referred to as S phase-specific. The effectiveness of enzyme inhibitors also depends on the amount and affinity of the target enzyme and on the extent of competition by natural substrates for enzyme binding. In the case of MTX, for example, complete saturation of all dihydrofolate reductase binding sites is required before the enzyme is effectively inhibited. As MTX inhibits enzymatic activity, dihydrofolate, the natural substrate, accumulates behind the metabolic block and is able to effectively compete with MTX for further enzyme binding.[148] Thus, large amounts of MTX, well in excess of the enzyme binding capacity, are required to effectively inhibit dihydrofolate reductase activity. Similarly, in the case of 5-FU, the dUMP/FdUMP ratio may be an important determinant of optimal inhibition of thymidylate synthase and high ratios have been associated with lack of tumor response.[131–133]

In addition to the enzymes required for purine and pyrimidine biosynthesis, the topoisomerases have recently been identified as important targets of several antineoplastic agents. Both topoisomerase I and II catalyze the passage of DNA strands through single or double-strand breaks in the DNA molecule by nicking then reannealing the DNA strands. Topoisomerase inhibitors bind to the enzyme and stabilize the enzyme-DNA cleavable complex resulting in DNA strand breaks that are lethal to the cell. The epipodophyllotoxins, etoposide and teniposide, are potent inhibitors of topoisomerase II as are a number of DNA intercalating agents including doxorubicin, actinomycin D and amsacrine.[113,114,140] Recently, camptothecin, a natural product derived from the Asian tree, *Camptotheca acuminata,* has been shown to be a potent inhibitor of topoisomerase I and one of its derivatives, hycamptamine, is now undergoing clinical trial (see XVI-5, 6, 7, 8).[65]

The microtubule spindle structure provides a third target for chemotherapeutic agents, classically the vinca alkaloids, VCR and VLB. The vinca alkaloids exert their cytotoxic effects by binding to specific sites on tubulin causing inhibition of assembly of tubulin into microtubules and ultimately leading to dissolution of the mitotic spindle structure.[90] The microtubule system in cells performs a variety of other important functions including transport of solutes, cell movement and provides structural integrity, any one of which could potentially be disrupted by tubulin binding agents.[14] Taxol, a novel plant alkaloid, inhibits cell division by enhancing the formation and stability of microtubules and stimulating tubulin synthesis.[116] Taxol-treated cells contain large numbers of microtubules, free and in bundles, that result in disruption of microtubule function and, ultimately, cell death.[80,122] Initial clinical trials in patients with refractory acute leukemia have demonstrated a clear relationship between susceptibility to bundle formation in leukemic blasts and anti-tumor effect.[115]

The drug has also shown promise in the treatment of advanced ovarian cancer.[81]

The search for specific inhibitors of hormone and growth factor receptors has been ongoing since the demonstration that antiestrogens can be effective treatment for breast cancers that contain the estrogen receptor. Recent studies have also demonstrated an important role for the antiandrogen flutamide in the treatment of prostate cancer.[24] As more information becomes available concerning the growth regulatory properties of peptide oncogene products and their cellular receptors, these molecules are likely to become increasingly important targets of novel chemotherapeutic agents.[49] One such drug appears to be the polysulfonated naphthylurea, suramin, which has been shown to block the binding of a range of tumor growth factors including platelet-derived growth factor (PDGF), transforming growth factor-beta (TGF-β) and epidermal growth factor (EGF) to their cellular receptors.[134] Recent clinical trials have demonstrated that treatment with suramin can induce anti-tumor effects in patients with adrenocortical carcinoma, renal cell carcinoma and prostate cancer.

Repair of Drug-Induced Injury

Cells that have been damaged by cytotoxic drugs exhibit a variety of repair mechanisms. Indeed the cytotoxic effects of a drug often represent the balance between injury and repair, and amplified repair mechanisms may account for cellular resistance to certain drugs. The cytotoxicity of alkylating agents reflects the balance between DNA crosslink formation and removal by cellular repair processes. Many cells contain specific enzymes able to remove alkyl moieties from DNA thereby repairing drug damage. A specific example is the protein O^6-alkyl-guanine transferase (AGT) that repairs DNA injury produced by chloroethyl-nitrosoureas. Cells containing large amounts of this protein tend to be relatively resistant to these chemotherapeutic agents. Depletion of AGT activity by exposure of cells to modified purine bases such as O^6-methylguanine may be effective in circumventing this mechanism of resistance.[26,28]

Cells also contain a variety of free radical scavenging systems that protect them from the effects of ionizing radiation and drugs that generate oxygen free radicals intracellularly. Catalase, superoxide dismutase and glutathione peroxidase, key enzymes in the detoxification of reactive oxygen species, may be deficient in some tissues, like cardiac muscle, leading to excessive drug toxicity or increased in others leading to relative drug resistance.[31] Some doxorubicin-resistant cells have been shown to have increased activity of superoxide dismutase and sodium dependent glutathione peroxidase and diminished susceptibility to oxygen radical injury.[86] Other recent studies suggest that expansion of intracellular reduced glutathione pools or increased expression of glutathione transferase may be important mechanisms of alkylating agent resistance in animal and human tumors.[3,52,87]

Finally, cells may be able to circumvent drug-induced injury by increased production of target enzymes. In experimental models, exposure of cells to MTX or 5-FU can be shown to stimulate production of dihydrofolate reductase or thymidylate synthase respectively.[29,137] New enzyme production occurs within minutes to hours of drug exposure and is presumed to represent enhanced translation of existing mRNA rather than transcription of additional message. Overexpression of DNA also occurs, however, and may be a fundamental mechanism of cellular resistance to antimetabolites and natural products due to increased constitutive production of target enzymes or P-glycoprotein.[124]

As mentioned earlier, a prerequisite to drug effect at the target tissue is adequate drug delivery. Pharmacokinetics describes the concentration-time history of a drug in the body and can be used to answer fundamental questions concerning the optimal route and schedule of drug administration. The remainder of this chapter will present the principles of pharmacokinetics and pharmacodynamics and illustrate their importance in cancer chemotherapy.

Principles of Pharmacokinetics

Definitions

Pharmacokinetics is the study of drug absorption, distribution, metabolism and excretion. A fundamental concept in pharmacokinetics is drug clearance, i.e., elimination of drugs from the body, analogous to the concept of creatinine clearance. In clinical practice, clearance of a drug is rarely measured directly but is calculated as either

$$\text{Clearance} = \text{Dose/AUC} \qquad \text{(eq. 1)}$$

or

$$\text{Clearance} = \text{Infusion rate}/C_{ss} \qquad \text{(eq. 2)}$$

The area under the concentration-time curve (AUC) represents the total drug exposure integrated over time and is an important parameter for both pharmacokinetic and pharmacodynamic analyses. As indicated in equation 1, the clearance is simply the ratio of the dose to the AUC, so that the higher the AUC for a given dose, the lower the clearance. If a drug is administered by continuous infusion *and* steady-state is achieved, the clearance can be estimated from a single measurement of the plasma drug concentration (C_{ss}) as per equation 2.

Clearance can conceptually be considered to be a function of both distribution and elimination. In the simplest pharmacokinetic model,

$$\text{Clearance} = \text{V K} \qquad \text{(eq. 3)}$$

V is the volume of distribution and K is the elimination constant. V is the volume of fluid in which the dose is initially diluted, and thus the higher the V, the lower the initial concentration. K is the elimination constant, which is inversely proportional to the half-life, the period of time that must elapse to reach a 50% decrease in plasma concentration. When the half-life is short, K is high and plasma concentrations decline rapidly. Thus both a high V and a high K result in relatively low plasma concentrations and a high clearance.

Linear Pharmacokinetic Models

Although pharmacokinetic analysis can be conducted without specifying any mathematical models (noncompartmental methods), it is helpful to use such models as guides in therapeutic decision making. There are several important properties of drugs that have linear pharmacokinetics (Table XV-7-2). The key feature of a linear pharmacokinetic model is that

$$\frac{dC}{dt} = -KC \qquad \text{(eq. 4)}$$

This indicates that the instantaneous rate of change in drug concentration depends only on the current concentration. The half-life will remain constant, no matter how high the concentration.

One implication of this principle is that the drug exposure (AUC) is not affected by changes in drug schedule. For example, the AUC after a 60 mg/m² bolus dose of doxorubicin equals the total AUC for 3 daily (or weekly) bolus doses of 20 mg/m², which equals the AUC for the same dose administered as a 96 hour infusion. A second implication is that the AUC is proportional to the dose. Thus, if one measures the AUC for a 60 mg/m² dose, one can estimate the AUC for a 90 mg/m² dose in the same patient as being 50% higher.

The simplest linear pharmacokinetic model is

$$C(t) = \frac{Dose}{V} e^{-kt} \qquad \text{(eq. 5)}$$

shown graphically in Figure XV-7-3. This model assumes that the drug is administered as an instantaneous bolus, and that complete distribution of the drug is also instantaneous.

These assumptions are often not valid. If the drug is administered as a slow bolus or infusion, the model must be cor-

Table XV-7-2. Characteristics of Drugs with Linear Pharmacokinetics

Half-life is independent of concentration
Clearance is independent of dose
Clearance is independent of schedule

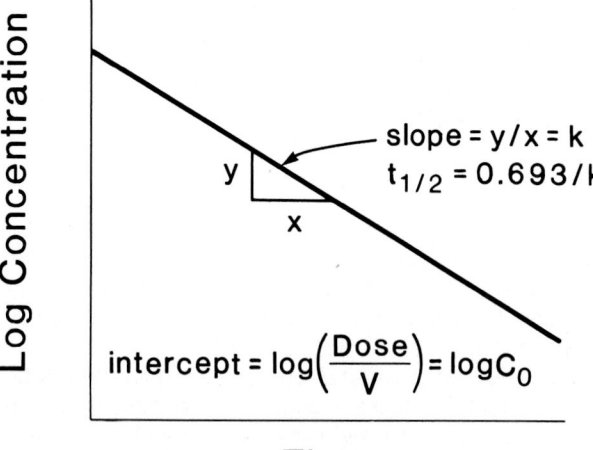

Time

Figure XV-7-3. Concentration-time plot for 1-compartment linear pharmacokinetic mode. C_0 represents the initial concentration, assuming instantaneous administration and distribution. The half-life is $\log_e(2)/k$.

rected for the infusion duration. During the administration of the drug the concentration is increasing:

$$C(t) = \frac{Dose}{VKT} (1 - e^{-kt}) \qquad \text{(eq. 6)}$$

After the infusion is terminated, the drug concentration decays at the same rate as if it had been administered as an instantaneous bolus. Thus, if T represents the infusion time, then the post-infusion drug concentrations can be represented as

$$C'(t) = C(T)e^{-k(t-T)} \qquad \text{(eq. 7)}$$

Often, the pharmacokinetic data are more complex than those shown in Figure XV-7-3, and may be optimally fitted to a multi-compartment model, usually two or three compartments (Figure XV-7-4). It must be emphasized that the compartments are theoretical, and do not necessarily correlate with any anatomic space or physiologic process.

With the widespread availability of nonlinear regression programs, it has become relatively easy to analyze pharmacokinetic data.[45] Standard pharmacokinetic modeling programs are also available.[83] The details of pharmacokinetic modeling are outside the scope of this chapter, although there are several caveats that should be emphasized.[82] The validity of pharmacokinetic modeling depends to a large extent on the quality of the data entered into the model. Thus, drug infusions must be precisely timed, plasma samples must be obtained on schedule, and analytical methods must be sensitive and specific. The data must be properly weighted to avoid bias due to the increased probability of analytical errors at drug concentrations near the detection limit of the assay. Results obtained using a specific model should be compared to those using noncompartmental methods. Extrapolation of models outside the known time points must be done with great caution.

Nonlinear Pharmacokinetic Models

Nonlinear pharmacokinetic models imply that some aspect of the pharmacokinetic behavior of the drug is saturable. The mathematics of nonlinear models are beyond the scope of this chapter, but the principles are very relevant to several anticancer agents.[46,147] In contrast to drugs with linear pharmacokinetics, alteration of the schedule of administration of drugs that display nonlinear kinetics may markedly affect the AUC and potentially alter clinical effects.

Nonlinear pharmacokinetic behavior commonly occurs when there is saturation of a major metabolic pathway. This results in decreased clearance at higher doses, with a greater than proportional increase in the AUC. The AUC will also increase if the infusion duration is shortened, due to slower clearance at the higher peak plasma concentrations. This is clearly the case for 5-FU, probably due to saturation of its conversion to dihydrofluorouracil by the enzyme dihydrouracil dehydrogenase.[20,88,121,146] Schaaf and colleagues demonstrated that doubling of the 5-FU dose from approximately 7.5 mg/kg to 15 mg/kg (by i.v. bolus) resulted in a 135% increase in the mean AUC.[121] Since 5-FU is used on a variety of schedules, its nonlinear pharmacokinetic behavior may be one factor in its highly schedule-dependent effects.

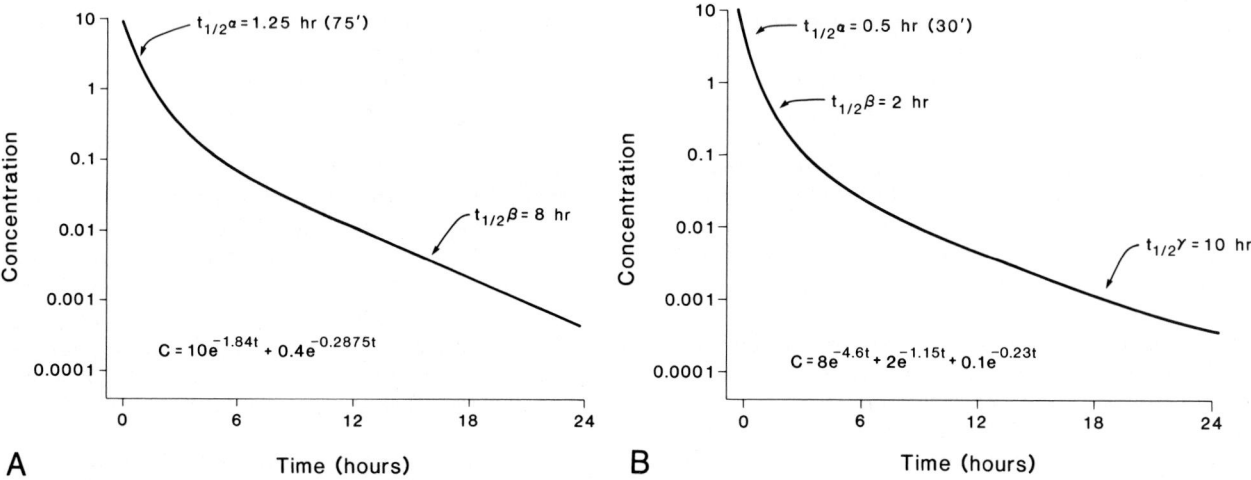

Figure XV-7-4. Concentration-time plots for representative 2-compartment (A) and 3-compartment (B) linear pharmacokinetic models. The two curves are very similar, with C_0 ~10 for both models. Note that for each "compartment" there is one term, and the corresponding half-life equals $\log_e(2)/k^n$, where k^n is the nth term.

The opposite situation arises when a drug's absorption from the gastrointestinal tract (or renal tubular reabsorption) is saturable. In this case, an increase in dose results in a less than proportional increase in the AUC. Gastrointestinal absorption of drugs that resemble natural compounds is frequently mediated by active transport processes in the gastrointestinal tract that display saturable kinetics. Folate analogues such as MTX or leucovorin and amino acid analogues such as melphalan are examples of drugs with saturable absorption.[4,17,136] Cisplatin appears to have nonlinear pharmacokinetics due to saturation of its renal tubular reabsorption.[44,107] Forastiere and colleagues demonstrated that free plasma platinum is increased by 42% when the drug is given as a 24 hr continuous infusion, rather than as a 20 min infusion.[44] Prolonged infusion was also associated with a greater than 3-fold increase in the free platinum half-life.

Interpatient Pharmacokinetic Variability

In describing a drug's pharmacokinetics, it is important to consider the extent of interpatient variability, often represented as the coefficient of variation (ratio of standard deviation to mean). Interpatient pharmacokinetic variability may be due to genetic differences in drug metabolism, or may result from acquired abnormalities.[142,144] Cancer patients may have significant hepatic or renal dysfunction, as well as other abnormalities that lead to alterations in pharmacokinetic parameters (Table XV-7-3). Genetic differences in drug metabolism may be particularly relevant to clinical trials of amonafide, a new intercalating agent that is metabolized by N-acetylation.[43,53] Acetylation phenotype is genetically determined and recent data suggest that rapid acetylators of amonafide are at greatest risk for bone marrow toxicity from this agent.[98]

An understanding of interpatient pharmacokinetic variability is potentially of great importance for optimizing antineoplastic therapy. Variability in gastrointestinal absorption is generally not considered in the use of orally administered antineoplastic agents even though drugs such as chlorambucil and melphalan are commonly administered orally

Table XV-7-3. Potential Sources of Interpatient Pharmacokinetic Variability in Cancer Patients

Abnormalities of Absorption
 Nausea/vomiting
 Prior surgery, radiotherapy, or chemotherapy
 Concurrent antiemetics affecting gut motility
 Patient compliance

Abnormalities of Distribution
 Weight loss
 Obesity
 Decreased body fat (lipophilic drugs)
 Pleural effusions or ascites (methotrexate)

Abnormalities of Elimination
 Hepatic dysfunction due to tumor replacement or prior
  (or concurrent) therapy
 Renal dysfunction due to malignant involvement or prior
  (or concurrent) therapy

Abnormalities in Protein-binding
 Hypoalbuminemia
 Concomitant medications

for treatment of chronic lymphocytic leukemia or multiple myeloma. The percentage of a drug absorbed is referred to as its bioavailability, i.e., the ratio of the plasma AUC after oral administration to the plasma AUC after intravenous administration of the same dose. Bioavailability may be influenced by drug metabolism in the gastrointestinal tract or liver as well as by absorption. The (6S) isomer of leucovorin, for example, has limited bioavailability due primarily to its rapid conversion to 5-methyl tetrahydrofolate prior to reaching the systemic circulation.[123] By contrast, the bioavailability of (6R) leucovorin is limited due primarily to poor absorption. The bioavailability of some agents, such as melphalan, etoposide, and 6-mercaptopurine is highly variable and unpredictable, and may be accentuated by concomitant administration of other chemotherapeutic agents, particularly those that produce toxicity to the gastrointestinal mucosa.[17,151]

Variability in drug distribution may be attributed to changes in body size or to the ratio of fat to total mass.[16] In the latter case, there may be altered distribution of lipophilic drugs—which includes most of the natural product anticancer drugs and their analogs. The most well-described example of abnormal drug distribution is delayed clearance of methotrexate due to accumulation and slow release of the drug from ascites or pleural effusions.[15] The terminal elimination half-life of doxorubicin, cyclophosphamide and ifosfamide is prolonged in obese patients.[77,112] In the case of doxorubicin and cyclophosphamide this appears to be due to a reduction in clearance whereas in the case of ifosfamide, it is related to an increased volume of distribution of the drug.[77]

Many patients with advanced cancer have abnormalities of liver function tests or known mass lesions within the liver, often in association with significant malnutrition. Given that many antineoplastic agents are metabolized or excreted by the liver, recognizing altered elimination by the liver becomes important in the optimization of chemotherapy dosing. Unfortunately, altered hepatic elimination or metabolism of drugs is not easily predictable. Clearly, patients with severe hyperbilirubinemia due to parenchymal replacement or obstruction are likely to have altered elimination. However, it is not often recognized that many patients with normal serum bilirubin levels may have a low drug clearance resulting in a high AUC and corresponding toxicity. A decrease in serum albumin (in patients with normal serum bilirubin concentrations) has been associated with a decrease in the hepatic elimination of antipyrine—a commonly used marker drug—and of VLB and trimetrexate.[12,42,105,130] Thus, patients with a serum albumin less than 2.5 g/dl may be at increased risk of toxicity, and are potentially candidates for dose reduction of agents requiring hepatic metabolism or excretion. At present, there are few firm guidelines useful for accurate dosing of antineoplastics in the setting of obvious hepatic disease.

In contrast, alterations in renal function generally correlate with renal clearance of drugs, since renal drug clearance tends to correlate with creatinine clearance. This has been well established for carboplatin, where a firm relationship exists between renal function and carboplatin clearance that can be used prospectively to modify the carboplatin dose and avoid excessive toxicity.[35,59]

Abnormalities of protein binding are common, but rarely impact upon clinical outcome. Many anticancer drugs, such as the vinca alkaloids and etoposide, are highly protein-bound.[30,135] Changes in protein binding may affect drug clearance.[128] Most importantly, abnormal protein binding must be considered in the interpretation of measured total plasma drug concentrations, since a decrease in protein binding will result in a relative increase in the pharmacologically active free drug.[99]

Intrapatient Pharmacokinetic Variability

Although it is well established that interpatient pharmacokinetic variability may be significant, the importance of intrapatient variability (within a single patient) is less clear. Oncologists are commonly faced with the clinical situation of increasing myelosuppression after repetitive dosing. This is generally assumed to be due to the cumulative effects of chemotherapy, making the patient more sensitive to subsequent doses. However, it is also possible that the patient's

clearance of the drug(s) may have decreased, resulting in increased drug exposure.

Such a situation may arise when either hepatic or renal function changes. Renal function may change due to progressive disease (ureteral obstruction), complications of therapy (volume depletion), or as a direct toxic effect of therapy (cisplatin). Similarly, renal function may improve over time, reducing the actual drug exposure. Hepatic function may also change, producing changes in drug clearance which may result in the appearance of increased toxicity over time, as is the case for VLB administered by prolonged continuous infusion.[105] Thus, clinicians should carefully review the outcome of prior doses to minimize the risk of an undesirable outcome due to intrapatient pharmacokinetic variability.

Another potential source of intrapatient pharmacokinetic variability is an individual's circadian rhythm. The best-studied drugs in this regard are 5-FU and 5-fluorodeoxyuridine.[62] Petit and colleagues evaluated circadian variability of 5-FU plasma concentrations during a five-day infusion at a constant dose and demonstrated greater than a 2-fold difference between maximum and minimum values.[93] Similar results were obtained by Harris and colleagues who demonstrated an inverse correlation between plasma 5-FU concentration and the activity of dihydropyrimidine dehydrogenase, a major catabolic enzyme for 5-FU.[60]

Principles of Pharmacodynamics

Definitions

In a general sense, pharmacodynamics is the study of dose-response relationships. Thus, any laboratory or clinical study employing different doses of an agent is addressing a pharmacodynamic question. Examples include the exposure of tumor cells in vitro to varying doses of a new agent to evaluate its dose-response relationship, or a phase I clinical trial to define the maximally tolerated dose and dose-limiting toxicities in patients.

In the clinical setting, the results of treatment depend on both pharmacokinetics and pharmacodynamics (Figure XV-7-1). A patient may have excessive toxicity at the usual dose for one of two reasons. If the patient's pharmacokinetics are different from those of the usual patient (e.g., decreased renal clearance of carboplatin), there may be decreased total body clearance resulting in a higher than expected drug exposure. The second possibility is that the patient might simply be more sensitive to an average drug exposure—due to prior therapy, poor nutrition or other less well-defined reasons. It is important to distinguish between these two possibilities. In the first case, lowering the dose will result in an "average" drug exposure, whereas in the second case lowering the dose will result in a lower than average drug exposure. Therefore, in the setting of dose reduction, there is a greater possibility of a response in the patient with abnormal pharmacokinetics than in the "sensitive" patient with abnormal pharmacodynamics.

General Pharmacodynamic Principles

In the most general sense, any drug may be considered to have a maximal effect and a median dose, i.e., that required for 50% of the maximal effect. Wagner proposed a generalized sigmoidal model of drug effect (Figure XV-7-5), derived from the hypothesis that all drug effects require an initial interaction with a receptor.[145]

Most studies addressing pharmacodynamic modeling of anticancer agents have addressed phase–specific agents separately.[67,91] It may be adequate to use a simple log-linear model for non-phase-specific agents:[68,127]

Survival fraction (SF)

$$= \frac{\text{No. of treated cells}}{\text{No. of control cells}} = e^{-KC} \quad \text{(eq. 8)}$$

This may be referred to as a steep dose-response curve, since the effect continues to increase proportionally as the concentration (C) increases. For any K (in equation 8), an increase in C by 2.3/K will result in a 1-log increase in antitumor effect (Figure XV-7-6A).

The dose-response relationships for phase-specific agents, such as the antimetabolites, are much more complicated. By definition, some cells are out of "phase" and therefore not sensitive (or relatively insensitive) to the effects of the drug during the period of drug exposure. This is not nec-

essarily overcome by increasing the dose, but could be overcome by increasing the duration of drug exposure. The result is the appearance of a plateau in the dose-response curve (Figure XV-7-6B).

The effects of some antineoplastic agents depend on both the drug concentration and the duration of exposure to that concentration. For some agents, the effect is a function of the product of the concentration and exposure time, analogous to the AUC.[38] However, for antimetabolites and other phase-specific agents, the mathematical relationships are much more complex.[37,67,91] Drug effect tends to be related to duration of exposure above a threshold concentration.

Plasma concentrations may be an inadequate predictor of clinical effect for those agents that undergo intracellular anabolism to active metabolites such as the case for ara-C.[76] Plasma ara-C concentrations do not appear to correlate with the rate of cellular ara-CTP accumulation or peak ara-CTP concentration in leukemic cells, although the intracellular concentration of ara-CTP is an important determinant of treatment outcome. Thus, knowledge of the plasma pharmacokinetics of ara-C is not likely to be a useful predictor of treatment outcome for individual patients. Pharmacogenetic evaluation may be potentially useful for modeling relationships between 6-mercaptopurine pharmacokinetics and clinical effects, as this drug's conversion to active intracellular 6-thioguanine metabolites by thiopurine methyltransferase is genetically determined.[75] Recent studies in children with acute lymphoblastic leukemia suggest that intracellular levels of 6-thioguanine nucleotides may be an independent predictor of remission duration.[74]

Pharmacodynamic Modeling of Cancer Chemotherapy

The introduction of pharmacodynamic modeling into clinical oncology has been a slow process. The relationship between toxicity subsequent to high-dose MTX and delayed MTX clearance has led to the routine use of therapeutic drug monitoring of plasma MTX concentrations to guide leucovorin dosing.[2] However, studies of other drugs have not clearly resulted in a change in clinical practice, although there has been a recent increase in clinical research in this area.[100]

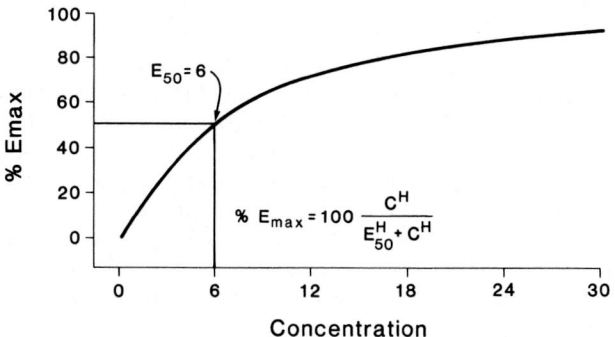

Figure XV-7-5. Example of E_{max} model as proposed by Wagner.[145] The maximum effect is 100%, and a concentration of 6 results in 50% effect. The exponent H, also known as the Hill constant, determines the shape of the curve and is usually between 1 and 2.

$$\% \, E_{max} = 100 \, \frac{C^H}{E_{50}^H + C^H}$$

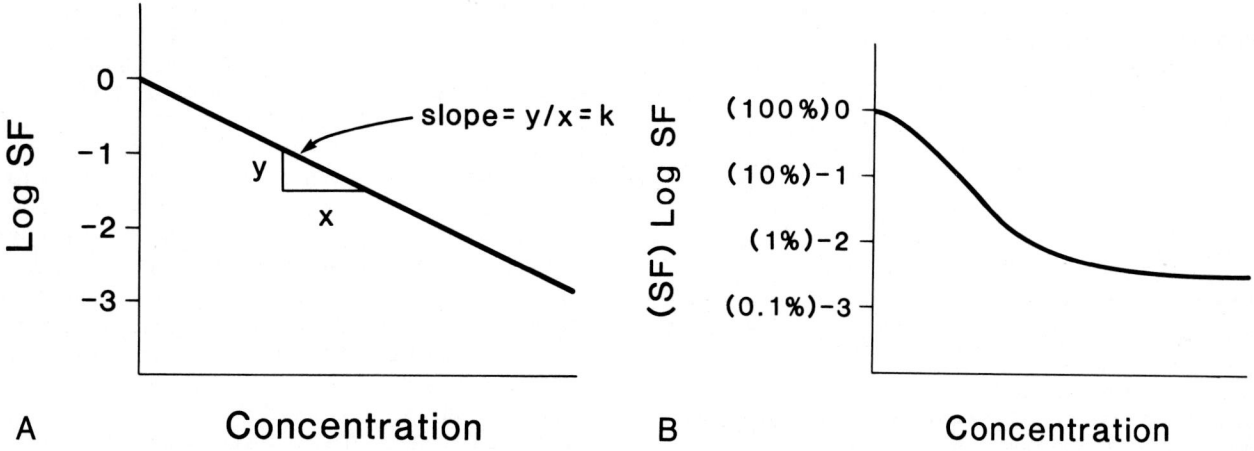

Figure XV-7-6. Pharmacodynamic plots for drugs with non-saturable (A) and saturable (B) effects. In the simplest pharmacodynamic model (A), there is a linear relationship between dose and log kill. In B, there is a maximal effect, resulting in a plateau in the dose-response curve.

Most pharmacodynamic studies to date have addressed relationships between measurements of drug exposure (AUC, C_{ss}) and toxicity. Hematologic toxicity (Table XV-7-4) has been easier to model than non-hematologic toxicity (Table XV-7-5).

The best characterized drug is carboplatin, an analog of cisplatin. Unlike cisplatin, the dose-limiting toxicity of carboplatin is thrombocytopenia, which is a function of drug dose, renal function, pre-treatment platelet count, and prior therapy.[35] The platelet nadir produced by a dose of carboplatin is related to the carboplatin clearance which is directly proportional to creatinine clearance. Thus, patients at high risk of severe thrombocytopenia following carboplatin therapy can be identified prospectively and the drug doses can be modified by monitoring creatinine clearance.

Etoposide has also been the subject of extensive evalu-

Table XV-7-4. Pharmacodynamic Studies of Hematologic Toxicity[a]

Drug	Reference	Pharmacokinetic Parameter[c]	Toxicity[d]
Carboplatin	Egorin[35]	AUC	P
	Newell[89]	AUC	W
DADAG[b]	Kerpel-Fronius[70]	AUC	P
Doxorubicin	Ackland[1]	C_{ss}	W
Etoposide	Bennett[10]	C_{ss}	W
	Ratain[99]	C_{ss}	W
5-Fluorouracil	Au[6]	C_{ss}	W
HMBA[b]	Egorin[34]	AUC	P
	Rowinsky[117,118]	C_{ss}, AUC	P
Iproplatin	Pendyala[92]	AUC	P
Menogaril	Egorin[32,36]	AUC	W, N
	Dodion[27]	AUC, SP	W, N
Trimetrexate	Fanucchi[42]	AUC	P
	Reece[106]	AUC, C_{ss}	P
	Grochow[56,57]	AUC, SP	P, W
Vinblastine	Ratain[103]	C_{ss}	W

[a]Adapted from Ratain[100]

[b]DADAG, diacetyldianhydrogalactitol; HMBA, hexamethylene bisacetamide

[c]AUC, area under the curve; C_{ss}, "steady-state" concentration during continuous infusion; SP, single point

[d]P, thrombocytopenia; W, leukopenia; N, neutropenia

Table XV-7-5. Pharmacodynamic Studies of Non-hematologic Toxicity[a]

Drug	Reference	Pharmacokinetic Parameter[c]	Toxicity[d]
Busulfan	Grochow[55]	AUC	H
Cisplatin	Reece[108]	SP, AUC	R
DCMTX[b]	Hantel[58]	AUC	H
5-Fluorouracil	Thyss[141]	AUC	NS
	van Groeningen[143]	AUC	NS
NMF[b]	Rowinsky[119]	AUC	H, NVM
SR2508	Coleman[18]	AUC	PN

[a]Adapted from Ratain[100]

[b]DCMTX, dichloromethotrexate; NMF, N-methylformamide

[c]AUC, area under the curve; C_{ss}, "steady-state" concentration during continuous infusion; SP, single point

[d]R, nephrotoxicity; NS, not specified; H, hepatotoxicity; NVM, nausea-vomiting-malaise symptom complex; PN, peripheral neuropathy

ation. Pharmacodynamic modeling of etoposide is complicated by the need to either measure free etoposide directly, or to estimate the free etoposide concentration on the basis of measured total plasma etoposide concentration, albumin, and/or bilirubin.[99,135] Several studies have now demonstrated that the extent of leukopenia/neutropenia is correlated with etoposide exposure.[10,85,99] Furthermore, interpatient pharmacodynamic variability may be significant and needs to be considered in future modeling of etoposide and potentially in other drugs.[99]

There is an expanding interest in trying to optimize cancer chemotherapy by individualizing dosing on the basis of measurements of plasma or tissue drug concentrations. One recent example is the titration of carboplatin dosing discussed above. Other investigators have attempted to optimize the dosing of etoposide, hexamethylene bisacetamide, and 5-FU, by measuring plasma drug concentrations during continuous infusion, then using the information obtained to modify the total dose of chemotherapy administered in an attempt to avoid severe toxicity.[22,99,120] Although it has not yet been established in a prospective randomized study that this approach will improve the therapeutic index, the studies to date have been very encouraging. Santini and colleagues have demonstrated that therapeutic monitoring of 5-FU reduces toxicity and increases response rate to cisplatin/5-FU in head and neck cancer compared to historical controls.[120] Ratain and colleagues have conducted two prospective randomized studies of the role of therapeutic monitoring of etoposide.[99] In the first study, these investigators were unable to show an advantage for this approach compared to standard dosing due to extensive unexpected interpatient pharmacodynamic variability. This variability was taken into account in a revised model that was applied in a second study.[101] A preliminary report of that study suggests that the use of the refined model allows the mean delivered dose to be increased significantly, without a significant increase in severe toxicity.

The Future Role of Anticancer Pharmacodynamics

Should the clinical oncologist care about pharmacodynamics? Will therapeutic drug monitoring of antineoplastics be as useful as monitoring of theophylline or aminoglycoside dosing? How will these studies improve the therapeutic index? These are important issues that are currently being addressed.

Our true understanding of dosing of most antineoplastic drugs is primitive. Body surface area is generally the only value used to determine initial dosing, and even this has recently been questioned.[54] Prior toxicity may be used to adjust dosing for subsequent cycles, although doses are more often reduced than escalated and the magnitude of dose changes is determined empirically and often arbitrarily.

For drugs with a relatively broad therapeutic index and/or minimal interpatient pharmacokinetic or pharmacodynamic variability, these strategies may not be necessary. As an example, therapeutic drug monitoring of interferon alfa in hairy cell leukemia is unlikely to be useful.[51] In contrast, therapeutic drug monitoring of doxorubicin in the adjuvant treatment of breast cancer may potentially help to ensure adequate drug exposure and minimize the risk of life-threatening toxicity.

Most of the pharmacodynamic studies to date have focused on toxicity as an endpoint, primarily due to the patient populations studied; i.e., patients with refractory tumors enrolled in Phase I clinical trials. The potential usefulness of this area is underscored by several studies correlating the clearance of MTX, teniposide, and 6-mercaptopurine with response or survival in acute lymphocytic leukemia.[40,61,72,111] Prospective evaluation of plasma concentrations in conjunction with Phase II clinical trials may improve our understanding of the relationship between clinical pharmacology and drug efficacy for other tumors as well.[98] Although most studies to date have utilized continuous infusion chemotherapy, recent strategies have been developed with the aim of optimizing dosing after conventional bolus administration.[33,73,102,104] It may eventually become possible to dose routinely towards a target AUC or C_{ss}, using principles of therapeutic drug monitoring to guide dosing.

The next challenge will be optimizing the use of combination chemotherapy. A prospective randomized study is in progress at St. Jude Children's Research Hospital which is designed to show that individualized dosing of ara-C, teniposide, and high-dose MTX is superior to conventional dosing for treatment of childhood acute leukemia.[41] As studies of the pharmacodynamics of single agents are completed it will become possible to evaluate the pharmacodynamics of drug combinations. As an example, Belani and colleagues recently demonstrated that etoposide does not significantly affect the pharmacodynamics of carboplatin-induced thrombocytopenia.[9]

In conclusion, it is hoped that a better understanding of the clinical pharmacology of antineoplastics will improve the care of patients with cancer. At a minimum, clinicians should understand the basic principles, realizing the limitations of our current approaches.

References

1. Ackland, S. P., Ratain, M. J., Vogelzang, N. J., Choi, K. E., Ruane, M., and Sinkule, J. A.: Pharmacokinetics and pharmacodynamics of long-term continuous-infusion doxorubicin. Clin. Pharmacol. Ther., 45:340, 1989.
2. Ackland, S. P., and Schilsky, R. L.: High-dose methotrexate: A critical reappraisal. J. Clin. Oncol., 5:2017, 1987.
3. Ahmad, S., Okine, L., Le, B., Najarian, P., and Vistica, D. T.: Elevation of glutathione in phenylalanine mustard-resistant murine L1210 leukemia cells. J. Biol. Chem., 262:15048, 1987.
4. Alberts, D. S., Chang, S. Y., Chen, H.-S. G., Evans, T. L., and Moon, T. E.: Oral melphalan kinetics. Clin. Pharmacol. Ther., 26:737, 1979.
5. Allegra, J. C., Chabner, B. A., Drake, J. C., Lutz, R., Rodbard, D., and Jolivet, J.: Enhanced inhibition of thymidylate synthase by methotrexate polyglutamates. J. Biol. Chem., 260:9720, 1985.
6. Au, J. L.-S., Rustum, Y. M., Ledesma, E. J., Mittelman, A., and Creaven, P. J.: Clinical pharmacological studies of concurrent infusion of 5-fluorouracil and thymidine in the treatment of colorectal carcinoma. Cancer Res., 42:2930, 1982.
7. Bank, B. B., Kanganis, D., Liebes, L. F., and Silber, R.: Chlorambucil pharmacokinetics and DNA binding in chronic lymphocytic leukemia lymphocytes. Cancer Res., 49:554, 1989.
8. Beck, W. T.: The cell biology of multiple drug resistance. Biochem. Pharmacol., 36:2879, 1987.
9. Belani, C. P., Egorin, M. J., Abrams, J., Hiponia, D., Eisenberger, M., Aisner, J., and Van Echo, D. A.: A novel pharmacodynamic approach to dose optimization of carboplatin when used in combination with etoposide. J. Clin. Oncol., 7:1896, 1989.
10. Bennett, C. L., Sinkule, J. A., Schilsky, R. L., Senekjian, E., and Choi, K. E.: Phase I clinical and pharmacological study of 72-hour continuous infusion of etoposide in patients with advanced cancer. Cancer Res., 47:1952, 1987.
11. Bhalla, K., Nayak, R., and Grant, S.: Isolation and characterization of a deoxycytidine kinase-deficient human promyelocytic leukemic cell line highly resistant to 1-β-D-arabinofuranosylcytosine. Cancer Res., 44:5029, 1984.
12. Branch, R. A., Herbert, C. M., and Read, A. E.: Determinants of serum antipyrine half-lives in patients with liver disease. Gut, 14:569, 1973.
13. Brookes P., and Lawley, P. D.: The reaction of mono- and bifunctional alkylating agents with nucleic acids. Biochem. J., 80:496, 1961.
14. Cass, C. E., and Beck, W. T.: Vinca Alkaloid Pharmacology and Resistance. In Resistance to Antineoplastic Drugs. Edited by D. Kessel. Boca Raton, CRC Press, Inc., 1989, p. 141.
15. Chabner, B. A., Stoller, R. G., Hande, K., Jacobs, S., and Young, R. C.: Methotrexate disposition in humans: Case studies in ovarian cancer and following high-dose infusion. Drug Metab. Rev., 8:107, 1978.
16. Cheymol, G.: Drug pharmacokinetics in the obese. Fundam. Clin. Pharmacol., 2:239, 1988.
17. Choi, K. E., Ratain, M. J., Williams, S. F., Golick, J. A., Beschorner, J. C., Fullem, L. J., and Bitran, J. D.: Plasma pharmacokinetics of high-dose oral melphalan in patients treated with trialkylator chemotherapy and autologous bone marrow reinfusion. Cancer Res., 49:1318, 1989.
18. Coleman, C. N., Halsey, J., Cox, R. S., Hirst, V. K., Blaschke, T., Howes, A. E., Wasserman, T. H., Urtasun, R. C., Pajak, T., Hancock, S., Phillips, T. L., and Noll, L.: Relationship between the neurotoxicity of the hypoxic cell radiosensitizer SR 2508 and the pharmacokinetic profile. Cancer Res., 47:319, 1987.
19. Coleman, C. N., Stoller, R. G., Drake, J. C., and Chabner, B. A.: Deoxycytidine kinase: Properties of the enzyme from human leukemic granulocytes. Blood, 46:791, 1975.
20. Collins, J., Dedrick, R., King, F., Speyer, J., and Myers, C.: Nonlinear pharmacokinetic models for 5-fluorouracil in man: Intravenous and intraperitoneal routes. Clin. Pharmacol. Ther., 28:235, 1980.
21. Colvin, M., Padgett, C. A., and Fenselau, C.: A biologically active metabolite of cyclophosphamide. Cancer Res., 33:915, 1973.
22. Conley, B. A., Forrest, A., Egorin, M. J., Zuhowski, E. G., Sinibaldi, V., and Van Echo, D. A.: Phase I trial using adaptive control dosing of hexamethylene bisacetamide (NSC 95580). Cancer Res., 49:3436, 1989.
23. Crawford, C. R., Ng, C. Y. C., Noel, L. D., and Belt, J. A.: Nucleoside transport in L1210 murine leukemia cells. J. Biol. Chem., 265:9732, 1990.
24. Crawford, E. D., Eisenberger, M. A., McLeod, D.G., Spaulding, J. T., Benson, R., Dorr, F. A., Blumenstein, B. A., Davis, M. A., and Goodman, P. J.: A controlled trial of leuprolide with and without flutamide in prostate carcinoma. N. Engl. J. Med., 321:419, 1989.
25. Deffie, A. M., Batra, J. K., and Goldenberg, G. J.: Direct correlation between DNA topoisomerase II activity and cytotoxicity in Adriamycin-sensitive and resistant P388 leukemia cell lines. Cancer Res., 49:58, 1989.
26. Dexter, E. U., Yamashita, T. S., Donovan, C., and Gerson, S. L.: Modulation of O^6-alkylguanine-DNA alkyltransferase in rats following intravenous administration of O^6 methylguanine. Cancer Res., 49:3520, 1989.
27. Dodion, P., de Valeriola, D., Crespeigne, N., Peeters, B., Wery F., Van Berchem, C., Piccart, M., Tueni, E., Joggi, J., and Kenis, Y.: Phase I clinical and pharmacokinetic trial of oral menogaril administered on three consecutive days. Eur. J. Cancer Clin. Oncol., 24:1019, 1988.
28. Dolan, M. E., Young, G. S., and Pegg, A. E.: Effect of O^6-alkylguanine pretreatment on the sensitivity of human colon tumor cells to the cytotoxic effects of chloroethylating agents. Cancer Res., 46:4500, 1986.
29. Domin, B. A., Grill, S. P., Bastow, K. F., and Cheng, Y. C.: Effect of methotrexate on dihydrofolate reductase activity in methotrexate resistant human KB cells. Mol. Pharmacol., 21:478, 1982.
30. Donigian, D. W., and Owellen, R. T.: Interaction of vinblastine, vincristine and colchicine with serum proteins. Biochem. Pharmacol., 22:2113, 1973.
31. Doroshow, J. H., Locker, G. Y., and Myers, C. E.: Enzymatic defenses of the mouse heart against reactive oxygen: Alterations produced by doxorubicin. J. Clin. Invest. 65:128, 1980.
32. Egorin, M. J., Conley B. A., Forrest, A., Zuhowski, E. G., Sinibaldi, V., and Van Echo, D. A.: Phase I study and pharmacokinetics of menogaril (NSC 269148) in patients with hepatic dysfunction. Cancer Res., 47:6104, 1987.
33. Egorin, M. J., Forrest, A., Belani, C. P., Ratain, M. J., Abrams, J. S., and Van Echo, D. A.: A limited sampling strategy for cyclophosphamide pharmacokinetics. Cancer Res., 49:3129, 1989.
34. Egorin, M. J., Sigman, L. M., Van Echo, D. A., Forrest, A., Whitacre, M. Y., and Aisner, J.: Phase I clinical and pharmacokinetic study of hexamethylene bisacetamide (NSC 95580) administered as a five-day continuous infusion. Cancer Res., 47:617, 1987.
35. Egorin, M. J., Van Echo, D. A., Tipping, S. J., Olman, E. A., Whitacre, M. Y., Thompson, B. W., and Aisner, J.: Pharmacokinetics and dosage reduction of cis-diammine (1,1-cyclobutanedicarboxylato)-platinum in patients with impaired renal function. Cancer Res., 44:5432, 1984.
36. Egorin, M. J., Van Echo, D. A., Whitacre, M. Y., Forrest, A., Sigman, L. M., Engisch, K. L., and Aisner, J.: Human pharmacokinetics, excretion, and metabolism of the anthracycline menogaril (7-OMEN, NSC 269148) and their correlation with clinical toxicities. Cancer Res., 46:1513, 1986.
37. Eichholtz, H., and Trott, K. R.: Effect of methotrexate concentration and exposure time on mammalian cell survival in vitro. Br. J. Cancer, 41:277, 1980.
38. Eichholtz-Wirth, H.: Dependence of the cytostatic effect of adriamycin on drug concentration and exposure time in vitro. Br. J. Cancer, 41:886, 1980.
39. Elwood, P. C., Kane, M. A., Portillo, R. M., and Kolhouse, J. F.: The isolation, characterization, and comparison of the membrane-associated and soluble folate-binding proteins from human KB cells. J. Biol. Chem., 261:15416, 1986.
40. Evans, W. E., Crom, W. R., Abromowitch, M., Dodge, R., Look, A. T., Bowman, W. P., George, S. L., and Pui, C.-H.: Clinical pharmacodynamics of high-dose methotrexate in acute lymphocytic leukemia. N. Engl. J. Med., 314:471, 1986.
41. Evans, W. E., Rodman, J. H., Petros, W. P., Madden, T., Crom, C. R., Relling, M. V., Rivera, G. K., Kalwinsky, D. K., and Crist, W. M.: Individualized doses of chemotherapy for children with acute lymphocytic leukemia. Proceedings of the American Society of Clinical Oncology, 9:69, 1990.
42. Fanucchi, M. P., Walsh, T. D., Fleisher, M., Lokos, G., Williams, L., Cassidy, C., Vidal, P., Chou, T.-C., Niedzwiecki, O., and Young, C. W.: Phase I and clinical pharmacology study of trimetrexate administered weekly for three weeks. Cancer Res., 47:3303, 1987.
43. Felder, T. B., McLean, M. A., Vestal, M. L., Lu, K., Farquhar, D., Legha, S. S., Shah, R., and Newman, R. A.: Pharmacokinetics and metabolism of the anticancer drug amonafide (NSC-308847) in humans. Drug Metab. Dispos., 15:773, 1987.
44. Forastiere, A. A., Belliveau, J. F., Goren, M. P., Vogel, W. C., Posner, M. R., and O'Leary, G. P., Jr.: Pharmacokinetics and toxicity evaluation of five-day continuous

infusion versus intermittent bolus cis-diamminedichloroplatinum (II) in head and neck cancer patients. Cancer Res., 48:3869, 1988.
45. Garcia-Pena, J., and Azen, S. P.: A user's experience with a standard non-linear regression program (BMDP 3R). Comput. Programs Biomed., 10:185, 1979.
46. Gibaldi, M., and Perrier, D.: Pharmacokinetics, 2nd Edition. New York, Marcel Dekker, 1982.
47. Giloni, L., Takeshita, M., Johnson, F., Iden, C., and Grollman, A. P.: Bleomycin induced strand scission of DNA: mechanism of deoxyribose cleavage. J. Biol. Chem., 256:8608, 1981.
48. Goldenberg, A., Masui, H., Divgi, C., Kamrath, H., Pentlow, K., and Mendelsohn, J.: Imaging of human tumor xenografts with an indium-111-labeled anti-epidermal growth factor receptor monoclonal antibody. J. Natl. Cancer Inst., 81:1616, 1989.
49. Goldenberg, G. J., and Begleiter, A.: Membrane transport of alkylating agents. Pharmacol. Ther., 8:237, 1980.
50. Goldman, I. D.: Pharmacokinetics of Antineoplastic Agents at the Cellular Level. In Pharmacologic Principles of Cancer Treatment. Edited by B. A. Chabner. Philadelphia, W. B. Saunders, 1982, p. 15.
51. Golomb, H. M., Jacobs, A., Fefer, A., Ozer, H., Thompson, J., Portlock, C., Ratain, M., Golde, D., Vardiman, J., Burke, J. S., Brady, J., Bonnem, E., and Spiegel, R.: Alpha-2 interferon therapy of hairy cell leukemia: A multicenter study of 64 patients. J. Clin. Oncol., 4:900, 1986.
52. Green, J. A., Vistica, D. T., Young, R. L., Hamilton, T. C., Rogan, A. M., and Ozols, R. F.: Potentiation of melphalan cytotoxicity in human ovarian cancer cell lines by glutathione depletion. Cancer Res., 44:5427, 1984.
53. Grever, M. R., Staubus, A. E., and Malspeis, L.: Correlation of N-acetylation phenotype with plasma levels of the N-acetyl metabolite of amonafide (NSC 308847). Proceedings of the American Association for Cancer Research, 31:178, 1990.
54. Grochow, L. B., Baraldi, C., and Noe, D.: Is dose normalization to weight or body surface area useful in adults? J. Natl. Cancer. Inst., 82:323, 1990.
55. Grochow, L. B., Jones, R. J., Brundrett, R. B., Braine, H. G., Chen, T.-L., Saral, R., Santos, G. W., and Colvin, M. O.: Pharmacokinetics of busulfan: Correlation with veno-occlusive disease in patients undergoing bone marrow transplantation. Cancer Chemother. Pharmacol., 25:55, 1990.
56. Grochow, L. B., Noe, D. A., Dole, G. B., Rowinsky, E. K., Ettinger, D. S., Graham, M. L., McGuire, W. P., and Donehower, R. C.: Phase I trial of trimetrexate glucuronate on a five-day bolus schedule: Clinical pharmacology and pharmacodynamics. J. Natl. Cancer Inst., 81:124, 1989.
57. Grochow, L. B., Noe, D. A., Ettinger, D. S., and Doehower, R. C.: A phase I trial of trimetrexate glucuronate (NSC 352122) given every 3 weeks: Clinical pharmacology and pharmacodynamics. Cancer Chemother. Pharmacol., 24:314, 1989.
58. Hantel, A., Rowinsky, E. K., Noe, D. A., McGuire, W. P., Grochow, L. B., Vito, B. L., Ettinger, D. S., and Donehower, R. C.: Clinical and pharmacologic reappraisal of dichloromethotrexate. J. Natl. Cancer Inst., 80:1547, 1988.
59. Harland, S. J., Newell, D. R., Siddik, Z. H., Chadwick, R., Calvert, A. H., and Harrap, K. R.: Pharmacokinetics of cis-diammine-1,1-cyclobutane dicarboxylate platinum (II) in patients with normal and impaired renal function. Cancer Res., 44:1693, 1984.
60. Harris, B. E., Song, R., Soong, S. J., and Diasio, R. B.: Relationship between dihydropyrimidine dehydrogenase activity and plasma 5-fluorouracil levels with evidence for circadian variation of enzyme activity and plasma drug levels in cancer patients receiving 5-fluorouracil by protracted continuous infusion. Cancer Res., 50:197, 1990.
61. Hayder, S., Lafolie, P., Bjork, O., and Peterson, C.: 6-mercaptopurine plasma levels in children with acute lymphoblastic leukemia: Relation to relapse risk and myelotoxicity. Ther. Drug Monit., 11:617, 1989.
62. Hrushesky, W. J. M., von Roemeling, R., Lanning, R. M., and Rabatin, J. T.: Circadium-shaped infusions of floxuridine for progressive metastatic renal cell carcinoma. J. Clin. Oncol., 8:1504, 1990.
63. Jamieson, G. P., Snook, M. B., Bradley, T. R., Bertoncello, I., and Wiley, J. S.: Transport and metabolism of 1-β-D-arabinofuranosylcytosine in human ovarian adenocarcinoma cells. Cancer Res., 49:309, 1989.
64. Jarvis, S. M., and Young, J. D.: Nucleoside transport in rat erythrocytes: Two components with differences in sensitivity to inhibition by nitrobenzylthioinosine and p-chloro-mercuriphenyl sulfonate. J. Membr. Biol., 93:1, 1986.
65. Jaxel, C., Kohn, K. W., Wani, M. C., Wall, M. E., and Pommier, Y.: Structure-activity study of the actions of camptothecin derivatives on mammalian topoisomerase I: Evidence for a specific receptor site and relation to antitumor activity. Cancer Res., 49:1465, 1989.
66. Jolivet, J., Schilsky, R. L., Bailey, B. D., Drake, S. C., and Chabner, B. A.: Synthesis, retention and biological activity of methotrexate polyglutamates in cultured human breast cancer cells. J. Clin. Invest., 70:351, 1982.
67. Jusko, W. J.: A pharmacodynamic model for cell-cycle-specific chemotherapeutic agents. J. Pharmacokinet. Biopharm., 1:175, 1973.
68. Jusko, W. J.: Pharmacodynamics of chemotherapeutic effect: Dose-time-response relationships for phase-nonspecific agents. J. Pharm. Sci., 60:892, 1987.
69. Kees, U. R., Ford, J., Dawson, V. M., Piall, E., and Ahern, G. W.: Development of resistance to 1-β-D-arabinofuranosylcytosine after high dose treatment in childhood lymphoblastic leukemia: analysis of resistance mechanisms in established cell lines. Cancer Res., 49:3015, 1989.
70. Kerpel-Fronius, S., Erdelyi-Toth, V., Gyergyay, F., Hindy, I., Mechl, Z., Nekulova, M., Somfai-Relle, S., Kovacs, P., Ujj, G., Kanyer, B., and Eckhardt, S.: Relation between dose, plasma concentration and toxicity in a phase I trial using high dose intermittent administration of an alkylating agent, diacetyldianhydrogalactitol (DADAG). Cancer Chemother. Pharmacol., 16:264, 1986.
71. Kohn, K. W., Spears, C. L., and Doty, P.: Inter-strand crosslinking of DNA by nitrogen mustard. J. Mol. Biol., 19:266, 1966.
72. Koren, G., Ferrazini, G., Sulh, H., Langevin, A. M., Kapelushnik, J., Klein, J., Giesbrecht, E., Soldin, S., and Greenberg, M.: Systemic exposure to mercaptopurine as a prognostic factor in acute lymphocytic leukemia in children. N. Engl. J. Med., 323:17, 1990.
73. Launay, M. C., Milano, G., Iliadis, A., Frenay, M., and Namer, N.: A limited sampling procedure for estimating adriamycin pharmacokinetics in cancer patients. Br. J. Cancer, 60:89, 1989.
74. Lennard, L., and Lilleyman, J. S.: Variable mercaptopurine metabolism and treatment outcome in childhood lymphoblastic leukemia. J. Clin. Oncol., 7:1816, 1989.
75. Lennard, L., Lilleyman, J. S., Van Loon, J., and Weinshilboum, R. M.: Genetic variation in response to 6-mercaptopurine for childhood acute lymphoblastic leukaemia. Lancet, 336:225, 1990.
76. Liliemark, J. O., Plunkett, W., and Dixon, D. O.: Relationship of 1-β-D-arabinofuranosylcytosine in plasma to 1-β-D-arabinofuranosylcytosine-5'-triphosphate levels in leukemic cells during treatment with high dose 1-β-D-arabinofuranosylcytosine. Cancer Res., 45:5952, 1985.
77. Lind, M. J., Margison, J. M., Cerny, T., Thatcher, N., and Wilkinson, P. M.: Prolongation of ifosfamide elimination half-life in obese patients due to altered drug distribution. Cancer Chemother. Pharmacol., 25:139, 1989.
78. Lippard, S. J.: New chemistry of an old molecule: Cis (Pt $(NH_3)_2$ Cl_2). Science, 218:1075, 1982.
79. Luhrs, C. A., Pitiranggon, P., DaCosta, M., Rothenberg, S. P., Slomiany, B. L., Brink, L., Tous, G. I., and Stein, S.: Purified membrane and soluble folate-binding proteins from cultured KB cells have similar amino acid compositions and molecular weights but differ in fatty acid acylation. Proc. Natl. Acad. Sci. U. S. A., 84:6546, 1987.
80. Manfredi, J. J., and Horwitz, S. B.: Taxol: An antimitotic agent with a new mechanism of action. Pharmacol. Ther., 25:83, 1984.
81. McGuire, W. P., Rowinsky, E. P., Rosenshein, N. B., Grumbine, F. C., Ettinger, D. S., Armstrong, D. K., and Donehower, R. C.: Taxol: A unique antineoplastic with significant activity in advanced ovarian epithelial neoplasms. Ann. Intern. Med., 111:273, 1989.
82. Metzler, C. M.: Estimation of pharmacokinetic parameters: Statistical Considerations. Pharmacol. Ther., 13:543, 1981.
83. Metzler, C. M., Elfring, G. L., and McEwen, A. J.: A User's Manual for NONLIN and Associated Programs. Michigan, The Upjohn Co., 1974.
84. Meyers, R., Malathi, V. G., Cox, R. P., and Silber R.: Studies on nucleoside deaminase. Increase in activity in Hela cell cultures caused by cytosine arabinoside. J. Biol. Chem., 248:5909, 1973.
85. Miller, A. A., Stewart, C. F., and Tolley, E. A.: Clinical pharmacodynamics of continuous-infusion etoposide. Cancer Chemother. Pharmacol., 25:361, 1990.
86. Mimnaugh, E. G., Dusre, L., Atwell, J., and Myers, C. E.: Differential oxygen radical susceptibility of Adriamycin-sensitive and resistant MCF-7 human breast tumor cells. Cancer Res., 49:8, 1989.
87. Moscow, J. A., Fairchild, C. R., Madden, M. J., Ransom, D. T., Wieand, H. S., O'Brien, E. E., Poplack, D. G., Cossman, J., Myers, C. E., and Cowan, K. A.: Expression of anionic glutathione-S-transferase and P-glycoprotein genes in human tissues and tumors. Cancer Res., 49:1422, 1989.
88. Mukherjee, K., and Heidelberger, C.: Studies on fluorinated pyrimidines, IX. The degradation of 5-fluorouracil-6-C^{14}. J. Biol. Chem., 235:433, 1960.
89. Newell, D. R., Siddik, Z. H., Gumbrell, L. A., Boxall, F. E., Gore, M. E., Smith, I. E., and Calvert, A. H.: Plasma free platinum pharmacokinetics in patients treated with high dose carboplatin. Eur. J. Cancer Clin. Oncol., 23:1399, 1987.
90. Owellen, R. J., Hartke, C. A., Dickerson, R. M., and Hains, F. O.: Inhibition of tubulin-microtubule polymerization by drugs of the Vinca alkaloid class. Cancer Res., 36:1499, 1976.
91. Ozawa, S., Sugiyama, Y., Mitsuhashi, J., and Inaba, M.: Kinetic analysis of cell killing effect induced by cytosine arabinoside and cisplatin in relation to cell cycle phase specificity in human colon cancer and Chinese hamster cells. Cancer Res., 49:3823, 1989.
92. Pendyala, L., Madajewicz, S., and Creaven, P. J.: Effect of renal function on impairment of iproplatin pharmacokinetics and relation to toxicity. Cancer Res., 45:5936, 1985.
93. Petit, E., Milano, G., Levi, F., Thyss, A., Bailleul, F., and Schneider, M.: Circadian rhythm-varying plasma concentration of 5-fluorouracil during a five-day continuous venous infusion at a constant rate in cancer patients. Cancer Res., 48:1676, 1988.
94. Pigram, W. J., Fuller, W., and Hamilton, L. D.: Stereochemistry of intercalation: interaction of daunomycin with DNA. Nature New Biol., 235:17, 1972.
95. Plagemann, P. G. W., Marz, R., and Wohlhueter, R. M.: Transport and metabolism of deoxycytidine and 1-β-D-arabinofuranosylcytosine into cultured Novikoff rat hepatoma cells, relationship to phosphorylation, and regulation of triphosphate synthesis. Cancer Res., 38:978, 1978.
96. Plunkett, W., Iacoboni, S., Estey, E., Danhauser, L., Liliemark, J. O., and Keating, M. J.: Pharmacologically-directed ara-C therapy for refractory leukemia. Semin. Oncol., 12(Suppl 3):20, 1985.
97. Powis, G., Reece, P., Ahmann, D. L., and Ingle, J. N.: Effect of body weight on the pharmacokinetics of cyclophosphamide in breast cancer patients. Cancer Chemother. Pharmacol., 20:219, 1987.
98. Ratain, M. J., Propert, K., Costanza, M., Allen, S., Berezin, F., Schilsky, R. L., and Van Echo, D. A.: Population pharmacodynamic study of amonafide: CALGB 8862. Proceedings of the American Association for Cancer Research, 31:181, 1990.
99. Ratain, M. J., Schilsky, R. L., Choi, K. E., Guarnieri, C., Grimmer, D., Vogelzang, N. J., Senekjian, E., and Liebner, M. A.: Adaptive control of etoposide administration: Impact of interpatient pharmacodynamic variability. Clin. Pharmacol. Ther., 45:226, 1989.
100. Ratain, M. J., Schilsky, R. L., Conley, B. A., and Egorin, M. J.: Pharmacodynamics in cancer therapy. J. Clin. Oncol., 8:1739, 1990.
101. Ratain, M. J., Schilsky, R. L., Vogelzang, N. J., Berezin, F. S., and Mick, R.: Adaptive control dosing of etoposide: A means of safely increasing dose-intensity. Clin. Pharmacol. Ther., 47:206, 1990.
102. Ratain, M. J., Staubus, A. E., Schilsky, R. L., and Malspeis, L.: Limited sampling models for amonafide (NSC 308847) pharmacokinetics. Cancer Res., 48:4127, 1988.
103. Ratain, M. J., and Vogelzang, N. J.: Phase I and pharmacological study of vinblastine by prolonged continuous infusion. Cancer Res., 46:4827, 1986.
104. Ratain, M. J., and Vogelzang, N. J.: A limited sampling model for vinblastine pharmacokinetics. Cancer Treat. Rep., 71:935, 1987.
105. Ratain, M. J., Vogelzang, N. J., and Sinkule, J. A.: Interpatient and intrapatient variability in vinblastine pharmacokinetics. Clin. Pharmacol. Ther., 41:61, 1987.
106. Reece, P. A., Morris, R. G., and Bishop, J. F.: Pharmacokinetics of trimetrexate administered by five-day continuous infusion to patients with advanced cancers. Cancer Res., 47:2996, 1987.
107. Reece, P. A., Stafford, I., Russell, J., and Gill, P. G.: Nonlinear renal clearance of ultrafilterable platinum in patients treated with cis-dichloradiammine platinum (II). Cancer Chemother. Pharmacol., 15:295, 1985.
108. Reece, P. A., Stafford, I., Russell, J., Khan, M., and Gill, P. G.: Creatinine clearance

as a predictor of ultrafilterable platinum disposition in cancer patients treated with cisplatin: Relationship between peak ultrafilterable platinum plasma levels and nephrotoxicity. J. Clin. Oncol., 5:304, 1987.

109. Reed, E., Ozols, R. F., Tarone, R., Yuspa, S. H., and Poirier, M. C.: Platinum-DNA adducts in leukocyte DNA correlate with disease response in ovarian cancer patients receiving platinum-based chemotherapy. Proc. Natl. Acad. Sci. U. S. A., 84:5024, 1987.

110. Reed, E., Yuspa, S. H., Zwelling, L. A., Ozols, R. F., and Poirier, M. C.: Quantitation of cis-diamminedichloroplatinum II-DNA-intrastrand adducts in testicular and ovarian cancer patients receiving cisplatin chemotherapy. J. Clin. Invest., 77:545, 1986.

111. Rodman, J. H., Abromowitch, M., Sinkule, J. A., Rivera, G. K., and Evans, W. E.: Clinical pharmacodynamics of continuous infusion teniposide: Systemic exposure as a determinant of response in a Phase I trial. J. Clin. Oncol., 5:1007, 1987.

112. Rodvold, K. A., Rushing, D. A., and Tewksbury, D. A.: Doxorubicin clearance in the obese. J. Clin. Oncol., 6:1321, 1988.

113. Ross, W., Rowe, T., Glisson, B., Yalowich, J., and Liu, L.: Role of topoisomerase II in mediating epipodophyllotoxin-induced DNA cleavage. Cancer Res., 44:5857, 1984.

114. Ross, W. E., and Bradley, M. O.: DNA double-stranded breaks in mammalian cells after exposure to intercalating agents. Biochim. Biophys. Acta, 654:129, 1981.

115. Rowinsky, E. K., Burke, P. J., Karp, J. E., Tucker, R. W., Ettinger, D. S., and Donehower, R. C.: Phase I and pharmacodynamic study of taxol in refractory acute leukemias. Cancer Res., 49:4640, 1989.

116. Rowinsky, E. K., Cazenave, L. A., and Donehower, R. C.: Taxol: A novel investigational antimicrotubule agent. J. Natl. Cancer Inst., 82:1247, 1990.

117. Rowinsky, E. K., Ettinger, D. S., Grochow, L. B., Brundrett, R. B., Cates, A. E., and Donehower, R. C.: Phase I and pharmacologic study of hexamethylene bisacetamide in patients with advanced cancer. J. Clin. Oncol., 4:1835, 1986.

118. Rowinsky, E. K., Ettinger, D. S., McGuire, W. P., Noe, D. A., Grochow, L. B., and Donehower, R. C.: Prolonged infusion of hexamethylene bisacetamide: A phase I and pharmacological study. Cancer Res., 47:5788, 1987.

119. Rowinsky, E. K., Noe, D. A., Orr, D. W., Grochow, L. B., Ettinger, D. S., and Donehower, R. C.: Clinical pharmacology of oral and i.v. N-methylformamide: A pharmacologic basis for lack of clinical antineoplastic activity. J. Natl. Cancer Inst., 80:671, 1988.

120. Santini, J., Milano, G., Thyss, A., Renee, N., Ayela, P., Schneider, M., and Demard, F.: 5-FU therapeutic monitoring with dose adjustment leads to improved therapeutic index in head and neck cancer. Br. J. Cancer, 59:287, 1989.

121. Schaaf, L. J., Dobbs, B. R., Edwards, I. R., and Perrier, D. G.: Nonlinear pharmacokinetic characteristics of 5-fluorouracil (5-FU) in colorectal cancer patients. Eur. J. Clin. Pharmacol., 32:411, 1987.

122. Schiff, P. B., and Horwitz, S. B.: Taxol stabilizes microtubules in mouse fibroblast cells. Proc. Natl. Acad. Sci. U. S. A., 77:1561, 1980.

123. Schilsky, R. L., and Ratain, M. J.: Clinical pharmacokinetics of high dose leucovorin calcium after intravenous and oral administration. J. Natl. Cancer Inst., 82:1411, 1990.

124. Schimke, R. T.: Gene amplification, drug resistance and cancer. Cancer Res., 44:1735, 1984.

125. Sevick, E. M., and Jain, R. K.: Geometric resistance to blood flow in solid tumors perfused ex vivo: Effects of tumor size and perfusion pressure. Cancer Res., 49:3506, 1989.

126. Sirotnak, F. M.: Correlates of folate analog transport, pharmacokinetics and selective antitumor action. Pharmacol. Ther., 8:71, 1980.

127. Skipper, H. E., Schabel, F. M., Mellett, L. B., Montgomery, J. A., Wilkoff, L. J., Lloyd, H. H., and Brockman, R. W.: Implications of biochemical, cytokinetic, pharmacologic, and toxicologic relationships in the design of optimal therapeutic schedules. Cancer Chemother. Rep., 54:431, 1970.

128. Smallwood, R. H., Mihaly, G. W., Smallwood, R. A., and Morgan, D. J.: Effect of a protein binding change on unbound and total plasma concentrations for drugs of intermediate hepatic extraction. J. Pharmacokinet. Biopharm., 16:529, 1988.

129. Smyth, R. D., Pfeffer, M., Scalzo, A., and Comis, R. L.: Bioavailability and pharmacokinetics of etoposide (VP-16). Semin. Oncol., 12:48(suppl 2):51, 1985

130. Sotaniemi, E. A., Pelkonen, R. O., Mokka, R. E., Huttunen, R., and Viljakainen, E.: Impairment of drug metabolism in patients with liver cancer. Eur. J. Clin. Invest., 7:269, 1977.

131. Spears, C. P., Gustavsson, B. G., Berne, M., Frosing, R., Bernstein, L., and Hayes, A. A.: Mechanisms of innate resistance to thymidylate synthase inhibition after 5-fluorouracil. Cancer Res., 49:5894, 1988.

132. Spears, C. P., Hayes, A. A., Shahinian, A. H., and Danenberg, P. V.: Deoxyuridylate effects on thymidylate synthase-5-fluoro-deoxyuridylate-folate ternary complex formation. Biochem. Pharmacol., 38:2985, 1989.

133. Spears, C. P., Waugh, W., Leichman, L., Leichman, C. G., Jeffers, S., Gustavsson, B. G., and Muggia, F. M.: Salvage therapy of breast cancer with fluorouracil and high dose leucovorin: Response correlations with tumor pharmacodynamics. Proceedings of the American Society of Clinical Oncology, 9:73, 1990.

134. Stein, C. A., LaRocca, R. V., Thomas, R., McAtee, N., and Myers, C. E.: Suramin: An anticancer drug with a unique mechanism of action. J. Clin. Oncol., 7:499, 1989.

135. Stewart, C. F., Pieper, J. A., Arbuck, S. G., and Evans, W. E.: Altered protein binding of etoposide in patients with cancer. Clin. Pharmacol. Ther., 45:49, 1989.

136. Straw, J. A., Szapary, D., and Wynn, W. T.: Pharmacokinetics of the diastereoisomers of leucovorin after intravenous and oral administration to normal subjects. Cancer Res., 44:3114, 1984.

137. Swain, S. M., Lippman, M. E., Egan, E. F., Drake, J. C., Steinberg, S. M., and Allegra, C. J.: Fluorouracil and high dose leucovorin in previously treated patients with metastatic breast cancer. J. Clin. Oncol., 7:890, 1989.

138. Takeshita, M., Grollman, A. P., Ohtsubo, E., and Ohtsubo, H.: Interaction of bleomycin with DNA. Proc. Natl. Acad. Sci. U. S. A., 75:5983, 1978.

139. Terheggen, P. M. A. B., Emondt, J. Y., Floot, B. G. J., Dijkman, R., Schrier, P. I., and den Engelse, L.: Correlation between cell killing by cis-diamminedichloroplatinum (II) in six mammalian cell lines and binding of a cis-diamminedichloroplatinum (II) DNA antiserum. Cancer Res., 50:3556, 1990.

140. Tewey, K. M., Rowe, T. C., Yang, L., Halligan, B. D., and Liu, L. F.: Adriamycin-induced DNA damage mediated by mammalian DNA topoisomerase II. Science, 226:466, 1984.

141. Thyss, A., Milano, G., Renee, N., Vallicioni, J., Schneider, M., and Demard, F.: Clinical pharmacokinetic study of 5-FU in continuous 5-day infusions for head and neck cancer. Cancer Chemother. Pharmacol., 16:64, 1986.

142. Urber, W. W., and Hein, D. W.: N-acetyltation pharmacogenetics. Pharmacol. Rev., 37:25, 1985.

143. van Groeningen, C. J., Pinedo, H. M., Heddes, J., Kok, R. M., de Jong, A. P. J. M., Wattel, E., Peters, G. J., and Lankelma, J.: Pharmacokinetics of 5-fluorouracil assessed with a sensitive mass spectrometric method in patients on a dose escalation schedule. Cancer Res., 48:6956, 1988.

144. Vesell, E. S.: Pharmacogenetic perspectives gained from twin and family studies. Pharmacol. Ther., 41:535, 1989.

145. Wagner, J. G: Kinetics of pharmacologic response: I. Proposed relationships between response and drug concentration in the intact animal and man. J. The. Biol., 20:173, 1968.

146. Wagner, J. G., Gyves, J. W., Stetson, P. L., Walker-Andrews, S. C., Wollner, I. S., Cochran, M. K., and Ensminger, W. D.: Steady-state nonlinear pharmacokinetics of 5-fluorouracil during hepatic arterial and intravenous infusions in cancer patients. Cancer Res., 46:1499, 1986.

147. Wagner, J. G., Szpunar, G. J., and Ferry, J. J.: A nonlinear physiologic pharmacokinetics model: I. Steady-state. J. Pharmacokinet. Biopharm., 13:73, 1985.

148. White, J. C., and Goldman, I. D.: Mechanism of action of methotrexate. IV. Free intracellular methotrexate required to suppress dihydrofolate reduction to tetrahydrofolate by Ehrlich ascites tumor cells in vitro. Mol. Pharmacol., 12:711, 1976.

149. Wiley, J. S., Jones, S. P., Sawyer, W. D., and Paterson, A. R. P.: Cytosine arabinoside influx and nucleoside transport sites in acute leukemia. J. Clin. Invest., 69:479,1982.

150. Young, R. C., Ozols, R. F., and Myers, C. E.: The anthracycline antineoplastic drugs. N. Engl. J. Med., 305:139, 1981.

151. Zimm, S., Collins, J. M., Riccardi, E., O'Neill, D., Narang, P. K., Chabner, B., and Poplack, D. G.: Variable bioavailability of oral mercaptopurine: Is maintenance chemotherapy in acute lymphoblastic leukemia being optimally delivered? N. Engl. J. Med., 308:1005, 1983.

XV-8

Toxicology by Organ System

Michael R. Grever
Charles K. Grieshaber

Introduction

The treatment of cancer may involve the use of various modalities including surgery, radiation, and chemotherapy. Each form of therapeutic intervention has the potential for producing adverse effects on normal host tissues, and some of these toxicities may be accentuated in the face of combined modality therapy. While other chapters have been devoted to specific classes of agents utilized in the treatment of cancer, the purpose of this contribution is to discuss the generalizations regarding evaluation of toxicity and the organ specificity of the adverse effects of cancer treatment.

The antineoplastic chemotherapeutic drugs are of widely diverse chemical structures capable of inducing varying degrees of cell destruction by distinct mechanisms of action. They are divided into arbitrary classes based on a combination of their mechanisms of cytotoxicity, chemical structure, and source. The effective clinical use of these antineoplastic agents requires an understanding of toxicology in order to maximize the adverse effects against the tumor cells and minimize the damage to the normal host tissue. For example, antimetabolites and other direct cytotoxic agents, which interfere with cell division, have the greatest effect on rapidly dividing cells. Thus, cytotoxic effects will be observed on both the tumor cells and those normal host cells with rapid cell cycle kinetics. The blood forming hematopoietic cells and gastrointestinal mucosal cells that have rapid doubling times are the targets of cytotoxic chemotherapy. These antineoplastic agents, therefore, frequently produce leukopenia, anemia, thrombocytopenia, and mucosal ulceration.

The objective of this chapter is to discuss the basic principles of antineoplastic drug toxicology learned in the rapidly growing fields of experimental oncology and drug development. As such, the purpose is not to solely catalog the myriad of toxic effects associated with the use of the commonly employed anticancer chemotherapeutic agents but to describe the principles and the procedures through which toxic responses can be anticipated, understood, and possibly surmounted. While the number and the types of agents under development change rapidly and constantly, the basic principles involved in toxicology evolve and change more slowly. Therefore, a clear understanding of the latter enables one to maintain pace with the former.

Basic Principles of Preclinical Toxicology

Chemotherapeutic Agents

Following the demonstration of encouraging preclinical antitumor activity involving either in vitro or in vivo tumor models, pharmacologic and toxicologic investigations are targeted to optimize the proposed clinical trials in man. The goals of the preclinical toxicology studies are to establish the safety of new agents in experimental animals and to predict primary toxicities as doses are escalated.

Preclinical toxicology testing is the final step in the progression of a chemotherapeutic drug from discovery to initial human studies. While the major goals of preclinical studies are to define a safe starting dose and to predict the qualitative toxicities that may be encountered with subsequent dose escalation in patients, the toxicologic findings may also result in a decision to forego further investigation of a new anticancer agent. In general, toxicities are expected to occur with the administration of effective agents, however, the definition of the therapeutic to toxic ratio has a major impact on the final decision to pursue new agents into clinical trials.

Approximately 16 chemotherapeutic agents have been dropped from further evaluation because of the results of the preclinical toxicologic studies. There were a variety of reasons for the decisions to discontinue investigation of those anticancer agents. The reasons reflected irreversible or serious degrees of toxicity in a dose range that was dangerously close to the targeted therapeutic levels. Furthermore, the

appearance of an unacceptable systemic complication (e.g., disseminated intravascular coagulation) has also resulted in discontinuation of evaluation for several agents. The appearance of a significant toxic effect in the preclinical setting (e.g., hepatotoxicity or a seizure) does not necessarily preclude entering clinical trial, but should result in vigorous efforts to further investigate both the cause and the potential for circumventing the toxicity (e.g., dose adjustment or schedule variation).

The observation that prolonged phase I clinical studies was in large part attributable to the empiric dose escalation procedures compounded by safe but ineffective starting doses prompted reassessment of the preclinical pharmacologic and toxicologic protocols.[23] A commitment was made to expedite the process of preclinical toxicologic assessment with a focus on determining the toxicities likely to be encountered at the proposed clinical doses with less attention on defining the highly lethal doses. Therefore, the current protocols determine the maximum tolerable doses and the dose-limiting toxicities in rodents and a second species on the schedule that is planned to enter the clinical studies. In addition, the pharmacologic parameters (e.g., area under the plasma concentration-time curve) are correlated with the toxicologic data to provide the basis for subsequent pharmacologically-guided dose escalation in patients during the phase I trial.[23,24]

The actual protocols for performing preclinical toxicology have changed significantly over the past two decades.[51,81] Numerous schedules of drug administration were examined in a variety of species in the 1972–1980 era. The emphasis from 1980, however, focused on initial mouse lethality studies to define the general toxic dose ranges followed by further studies in rats and dogs on relatively fixed schedules to refine the various dose levels associated with lethal and nonlethal toxicities. The revised protocols did expedite the preclinical evaluation, and in general (with the exception of fludarabine phosphate), were successful in providing safe starting doses for phase I studies.[51] The predicted acute organ toxicities demonstrated a reasonable correlation between the preclinical and clinical data.[23,39,51,80,81,111,115]

Retrospective analyses of preclinical and clinical correlations have confirmed that expressing the dose of a chemotherapeutic agent in mass units per body surface area (e.g., mg/m^2) improves the predictive relationship between dose and toxicity across species.[39] The quantitative assessment of toxicity with respect to dose of drug administered is accurately determined using small animal models.[39,115] Furthermore, the use of small animals may make a significant contribution to providing an early assessment of the therapeutic to toxic ratio because the xenograft models for antitumor activity have been primarily established in the murine species.[115] The subsequent investigation of qualitative toxicity is better defined by using larger animals that can be carefully assessed for specific organ toxicities by serial blood tests and tissue examinations.[80,111]

While further information is occasionally acquired by completing additional large animal studies (e.g., monkeys), the majority of agents are adequately characterized with a single large animal model. In general, dogs provide better organ specific toxicity information for predicting human toxicity than mice.[51,80] Myelosuppression and gastrointestinal toxicity are most often identified as correlating well between dog and human toxicity profiles. Hepatotoxicity and nephrotoxicity are predicted less well by the dogs. Pancreatic, cardiac, and pulmonary toxicities are potentially demonstrable, but have been underpredicted in the acute toxicity studies. The identification of neurologic and cutaneous toxicities are probably the least well-predicted from the preclinical models. This reflects the obvious difficulties in assessing the cognitive functions of an animal in contrast to man. The sole evidence of neurologic toxicity may be manifest at relatively high doses in the animals associated with gross neurologic dysfunctions (e.g., seizures or hind-limb paralysis). Finally, agents that produce local discomfort or skin irritation may be extremely difficult to evaluate in an animal model.

The preclinical identification of either cardiac or pulmonary toxicity has been attempted by using specific animal models, but these usually require specialized maneuvers (e.g., determining the specific weight of an organ; utilizing physiologic monitoring with blood pressure, pulse, and electrocardiogram; or measuring a biochemical parameter associated with toxic injury, for example, hydroxyproline in the lungs following bleomycin).[115] Therefore, the use of specialized manipulations or determinations add significantly to the time and cost involved in completing the routine toxicologic studies, and may be better utilized in comparing various analogs within a chemical class to identify the agent likely to produce the minimum of toxicity in a specific target organ.

There has been a substantial interest in the development of in vitro test systems that would predict organ specific toxicities. The in vitro evaluation of murine and human colony forming assays is being attempted to assess the relative myelotoxicity of various experimental agents.[33,34,50] This type of analysis might have predicted the unanticipated, severe myelosuppression associated with fludarabine monophosphate administration in the early phase I clinical trials. In addition, efforts are underway using either single cell suspensions (e.g., cardiac cells) or organ slices (e.g., liver) to develop models for either toxicity or metabolic studies relative to new agents.[37,74] The use of these innovative approaches will hopefully enhance the ability to derive additional predictive information regarding qualitative toxicities (e.g., mechanism of toxicity), but will not likely replace the need for continued use of the whole animal in preclinical toxicologic studies.

Biologic Agents

This diverse category of antineoplastic agents includes: monoclonal antibodies both labeled and unlabeled with radioactive nuclides, and conjugated and unconjugated to toxin molecules; cytokines including the numerous interleukins, interferons, tumor necrosis factor (TNF), the myriad of growth factors both unconjugated and conjugated to toxin molecules; cytokines in combination with target immunocompetent effector cells (e.g., LAK and TIL cells); and the numerous potential combinations of these biologic products either with each other or in combination with cytotoxic chemotherapy or hormonal therapy. The advent of biologic therapy originally had promised to usher in relatively well-tolerated and novel modalities for treating malignancy. In fact, the observations

of significant toxicities in clinical trials are not now surprising and in many cases are still being defined.

The development of recommendations for conducting preclinical toxicologic evaluations for this group of novel therapeutic products is quite challenging.[44,120,127] These products may be highly specific in their targeted interaction, and thus, can make the choice of an appropriate preclinical animal model difficult. For example, a monoclonal antibody directed against a specific antigen found exclusively in primates could make testing in small animals unproductive. Assessment of the effects of a growth factor in a species unlikely to have responsive tissue with the appropriate receptor represents an analogous dilemma.

The observation that the optimal immunomodulatory dose of a biologic product is not likely to be identical to the maximal tolerated dose adds substantial complexity to the development of an optimal toxicologic protocol.[127] Furthermore, the development of the optimal therapeutic protocol requires both definition of these important parameters and confirmation that the desired biologic effect has indeed been produced. Adding to the complexity of defining the optimal dose, schedule, and route of administration, the proper sequence of administration of the biologic product(s) must be determined.[44]

Despite the inherent complexity of determining the preclinical toxicologic and pharmacologic data relevant to these biologic products, the acquisition of this information should enhance the likelihood that the subsequent therapeutic trial will be successful.[120] In particular, the preclinical demonstration of enhanced antitumor activity with combination therapies suggests that an attempted evaluation of enhanced toxicity is also warranted. For example, the in vitro combination of TNF and gamma interferon produced enhanced tumor cell cytotoxicity with human colon and pancreatic carcinoma cell lines.[110,113,114] Since the initial phase I clinical evaluations of each agent administered individually demonstrated tolerable side effects, the two agents were combined in a clinical protocol that had to be discontinued quite early because of unacceptable toxicity of the combination.[1] The doses of each agent in the combination were empirically modified to avoid excessive toxicity but the toxic effects were still observed. Optimal doses and schedules of agents in novel combinations might be determined by utilizing a preclinical in vivo model. While substantial research is needed in this area, the basic approach should include provision for preclinical toxicologic testing in appropriate animal models whenever feasible.[120]

Hormonal Agents

The number of effective hormonal agents introduced for the treatment of cancer has been somewhat limited. In general, the administration of the currently effective hormonal agents involve long-term exposure to the drugs. The use of estrogen-blocking agents in the treatment of breast cancer has been extended to involve years of therapy.[16] Furthermore, the treatment of prostatic carcinoma with either estrogenic agents or androgenic blocking agents also involves prolonged drug administration. Consequently, the type of toxicologic evaluation that must be considered in dealing with hormonal agents would involve an assessment of both the acute and chronic toxicities that may be attributable to these products. One report suggested a possible increase in endometrial cancer in patients receiving tamoxifen, but the role of this agent in the development of this outcome was not clear.[66]

The preclinical toxicologic evaluation of a hormonal agent, which is likely to be administered for a protracted period, includes both the short and long-term administration of the drug to a group of animals. There has been a tendency to administer high doses of these agents in this setting to maximize the likelihood of identifying various toxic events. However, this approach carries a risk that the exaggerated doses may unmask toxicities that are unlikely to occur at the intended therapeutic doses, and will miss subtle toxicities resulting from low dose prolonged drug exposure.

The type of toxic event that results from the long-term exposure to a hormonal agent may not be evident for an extended period of time (e.g., the development of gynecologic malignancies in the offspring of women treated with stilbesterol appeared decades after exposure in utero).[56] The cardiovascular effects and the enhancement of a risk for thromboembolic events subsequent to estrogenic agents would have been very difficult to assess in a preclinical model.[8,14] Likewise, the effects of endocrine blockade in producing premature menopausal symptoms or decrease in libido would not be readily assessed in a preclinical model. Therefore, the assessment of the acute and chronic toxic events subsequent to the administration of hormonal agents (e.g., in particular on suspected targeted tissues or the liver) presents a challenge in animal toxicologic protocol design, and yet the full toxicity profile ultimately involves completion of the evaluation in a careful long-term study in man.

Toxicology: The Bridge Between Preclinical and Clinical Oncology

The clinical relevance of a toxicologic evaluation rests equally with qualitative and quantitative findings. The qualitative findings describe the adverse effects of a drug on the organ systems of the host species, whereas the quantitative data focus on the determination of doses which produce a specific adverse effect. For example, the dose which produces lethality in 10% of the test animals is identified as the LD10. In addition, the highest dose which is non-toxic is also quite important. Whereas in the past, substantial efforts were directed at determining the doses of the drug which produced lethality in specific fractions of the test animals (i.e., LD10, LD50, and LD90), the current emphasis is concentrated on defining the maximum tolerable dose, thereby estimating the LD10. In contrast, the highly lethal doses (i.e., LD50 and LD90) provide little useful information for further human investigation. More attention is now given to carefully assessing the qualitative toxicities that are likely to be observed at doses slightly higher than the highest non-toxic dose.

A critical element, which is essential for both safety and efficacy, is the selection of the initial human starting dose. The usual determinant of the clinical starting dose is based upon the LD10 determined from the murine acute toxicity studies.[23,39,111] The LD10 dose is then converted on the basis of of body surface area for interspecies equivalency and termed the MELD10 dose (i.e., the murine equivalent LD10 dose). In fact, it has been postulated that the MELD10 dose in mice and the maximum tolerable dose (MTD) in humans are equitoxic endpoints.[23] In retrospective analyses of data at the National Cancer Institute, the risk of exceeding the human maximum tolerable dose in phase I clinical trials is approximately 1% if the initial starting dose is based on the MELD10 data.[111]

Since there may be substantial variation between species for tolerance of specific anticancer drugs, a safety factor is used to empirically reduce the probability that the starting dose will be unsafe. The selected starting dose in humans is frequently 10% of the MELD10. Prior to administering the drug to humans, however, the safety of the projected starting dose is confirmed in a second species, notably beagle dogs. If there are no unacceptable toxicities, human trials are scheduled to begin using this dose. On the other hand, if the 0.1MELD10 dose is toxic in dogs, the entry dose in human trials is lowered to a confirmed non-toxic dose, usually by an additional factor of three (i.e., 1/30 MELD10).

In recent years, the approach to dose escalation in human phase I clinical trials has been based on pharmacologic data derived during the preclinical study combined with the data from the initial patient pharmacokinetic profile obtained in early phase I trial.[23,24] Therefore, the toxicologic studies performed in preparation for human investigation will be complemented by studies designed to provide the area under the plasma-concentration time curve at the MELD10 in mice. These data will provide a target for dose escalation maneuvers in patients being treated on the phase I clinical trials.

The majority of the new chemotherapeutic agents have been customarily tested clinically on two relatively fixed schedules: single bolus intravenous dosing once every 3–4 weeks and five consecutive days of treatment repeated at 3–4 week intervals. Thus, the established, traditional protocols for preclinical toxicology reflect each of these schedules. New, more unique schedules of drug administration are coming into fashion in clinical practice (e.g., continuous intravenous infusion for several hours or days or prolonged oral administration). There are neither official nor traditional requirements for preclinical toxicity testing using unique administration schedules to possibly uncover unanticipated human toxicities. Good preclinical practice, however, encompasses the testing of drugs for toxic effects on the planned schedules for clinical administration. Thus, close collaboration between the preclinical toxicologist and the clinical investigator is essential.

Evaluation of Toxicity in Man

Generalizations Regarding the Toxicologic Information Derived from Organized Clinical Trials

Adverse effects emanating from the administration of a therapeutic agent may be either acutely observed or delayed in onset. A correlation may exist between the dose of the drug and the toxic effects. Furthermore, the adverse effects may be related to various factors: the peak plasma concentration, rate of drug delivery, cumulative dose, schedule, or route of drug delivery. Therefore, a complete definition of the toxicity profile of an antineoplastic agent involves observation for both acute and chronic toxicities, and a correlation of the toxicologic and pharmacologic data.

Various well-defined phases of clinical investigation have been established to provide an organized approach to the drug evaluation process. At each step in the developmental process the toxicity profile is more accurately defined. In the phase I clinical trial, the ultimate goal is to define the toxicity and the pharmacology of a new agent. The dose-limiting toxicity(ies) (DLT) and the maximum tolerable dose (MTD) on a particular schedule are established. The dose-limiting toxicity is that adverse effect which limits the further escalation of the dose. The maximum tolerable dose has been defined differently in various phase I trials, but in general, is the dose that results in either serious (i.e., life-threatening) or irreversible toxicity in a predetermined percentage of patients.

The phase II clinical investigation is designed primarily to assess the potential for the new agent to produce a response in a specific type of cancer. There is a strict requirement for evaluable and measurable disease. In general, the patients have good performance status and may have had minimal previous treatment for their cancer. These patients are more frequently treated with multiple courses of the new agent at therapeutic levels based on the information derived from the phase I trial. Thus, the potential exists for recognizing additional toxicities associated with prolonged drug administration (i.e., cumulative toxicity) during this phase of clinical evaluation.

In a phase III clinical investigation, the major objective is a comparison of both the efficacy and the toxicity of a new therapy with standard treatment. In this phase of investigation, the new agent may be either tested alone or in a combination with other chemotherapeutic agents. The enrollment in phase III trials is much larger than the other phases of clinical investigation, and thus, permits a more accurate assessment of the frequency and characterization of treatment-induced toxicities. Furthermore, this large accrual permits recognition of the rare toxic events (e.g., idiosyncratic-type drug-related toxicities or hypersensitivity reactions). Therefore, a relatively complete toxicity profile of a new agent may be constructed following completion of these organized phases of clinical investigation.

Actual Conduct of the Phase I Trial in Man

During the phase I investigation, the acute toxicities are identified. The potential duration and reversibility of the toxicities are defined. While patients with malignancy that have limited therapeutic options may be offered an opportunity to participate in these trials, the selection of appropriate patients to accurately evaluate toxicity in a phase I clinical investigation is extremely important. In general, patients should have reasonably good performance status and basically normal organ function. Since the major objective of this phase of clinical investigation is to define the organ toxicity, patients with significant pre-treatment organ dysfunction will be unevaluable for assessing toxic events. In addition, abnormal organ function may increase the risk of participation in this early phase of investigation. After the pharmacologic and toxicologic profiles of a new agent have been characterized,

patients with impaired organ function can be entered with appropriate modification of the dose and schedule to further elucidate the appropriate use of the agent under these altered circumstances.

As previously stated, the selection of a starting dose in human trials is based on consideration of several preclinical animal models. Every effort is made to select a safe starting dose, but this conservative approach usually results in an initial dose which is sub-therapeutic. Since patients entering onto these trials are confronted with lethal diseases, it is imperative that every effort be made to arrive as quickly as possible at doses which approximate a biologically effective dose. The procedure for dose escalation of new anticancer agents in the past was simply based on predetermined fixed increments without a biological or pharmacologic basis. The current effort stresses the use of pharmacologically-guided dose escalation to expedite arrival at an effective, yet safe, anticancer dose.

Extensive efforts are made to document and characterize the toxicity observed at each dose level. Cohorts of three to six patients are entered at each dose level on a specific schedule of drug administration. In addition to defining the clinical toxicity, the majority of these patients are concurrently participating in detailed pharmacologic studies. The pharmacokinetic parameters and metabolites of the new agent are identified. Important correlations are made between the toxicologic and pharmacologic data.

The procedure for demonstrating the MTD involves the careful escalation of doses from an initial starting dose until dose-limiting toxicity is achieved. The phase I investigation is considered to be successfully completed when both the DLT and the MTD on a specific schedule have been identified. The recommendation of a dose and schedule for further phase II testing should result from the data derived from the phase I trial.

Assessment of Delayed Toxicity

The potential for delayed-onset toxicity must always be appreciated. For example, in a recent phase I trial of a promising new agent, fludarabine monophosphate, the acute dose-limiting toxicity in patients with solid tumors was reversible myelosuppression.[48,59] The doses were subsequently escalated in patients with refractory forms of leukemia, and a delayed-onset of serious neurologic toxicity was observed.[21,48,138] Approximately 4–6 weeks after administration of high doses of this agent, cortical blindness and coma developed in the patients. Therefore, myelosuppression was the dose-limiting toxicity in the low-dose range, and delayed neurologic toxicity was dose-limiting at the high-dose range.

Delayed-onset toxicity is not always recognized easily during the phase I clinical investigation. The characteristics of this patient population frequently result in relatively few courses of drug actually being administered. Many of these patients have advanced or refractory disease that is unresponsive to chemotherapy. In the interest of safety, there is also a definite potential for sub-therapeutic doses to be delivered during the early portions of the trial. Therefore, many patients who are registered on the phase I clinical investigation receive only one or two courses of the new agent, and consequently

Table XV-8-1.   Cardiotoxicity

Drug	Toxic Dose[a,b] Range	Comment
Doxorubicin	> 550 mg/m^2 (Total dose)	Congestive heart failure (cumulative toxic effect)
		Arrhythmias
	< 550 mg/m^2 (Total dose)	Cardiac toxicity/with additional risk factors
Daunorubicin	> 550 mg/m^2 (Total dose)	Same toxicity as doxorubicin
Mitoxantrone	> 100–140 mg/m^2 (Total dose)	Congestive heart failure
		Decrease in LVEF
Cyclophosphamide	> 100–120 mg/kg over 2 days	Congestive heart failure
		Hemorrhagic myocarditis/pericarditis/necrosis
5-Fluorouracil	Conventional Dose	Angina/myocardial infarction
Vincristine	Conventional Dose	Myocardial infarction
Vinblastine	Conventional Dose	Myocardial infarction
Busulfan	Conventional Oral Daily Dose	Endocardial fibrosis
Mitomycin C	Conventional Dose	Myocardial damage/like radiation-induced injury
Cisplatin	Conventional Dose	Acute myocardial ischemia
Amsacrine	Conventional Dose	Ventricular arrhythmias
Taxol	Conventional Dose	Bradycardia
Interferons	Conventional Dose	Exacerbates underlying cardiac disease
Interleukin-2	Conventional Dose	Acute myocardial injury
		Ventricular arrhythmias
		Hypotension

[a]Route of administration is IV unless otherwise indicated
[b]Conventional dose is commonly accepted therapeutic range

phamide in bone marrow transplant dose regimens) and chronically with the administration of the anthracyclines.[10,90] Significant information exists regarding the mechanism and clinical characteristics of myocardial injury following the use of doxorubicin. In general, the incidence of congestive heart failure increases significantly when the total dose of doxorubicin exceeds 550 mg/m^2. Other factors that also increase the risk include a past history of cardiac disease, and prior exposure to either chemotherapy or radiation therapy to the mediastinal region.[17,90] In patients with additional risk factors, the total cumulative dose of doxorubicin that can be considered safe is less than 500 mg/m^2. The decision to utilize an anthracycline in an individual patient involves a comprehensive assessment of the relative importance of the drug in the cancer treatment regimen and the degree of cardiac impairment.

The actual mechanism of cardiotoxicity has been felt to result from the generation of reactive oxygen radicals within the cardiac tissue.[90] Studies have demonstrated that either ICRF-187 administration or a change in the schedule of drug delivery may reduce the potential for cardiotoxicity associated with anthracycline administration.[117,123,129] Furthermore, evidence exists that modification of the chemical structure of the anthracycline may reduce the propensity for producing cardiac toxicity. The clinical investigation of agents (e.g., epirubicin or 4'-deoxy-doxorubicin) have demonstrated some potential for a reduction in drug-induced cardiotoxicity.[93,130,134,135] These agents were not, however, completely devoid of cardiotoxic effects. The true advantage of these agents over doxorubicin will require further assessment in phase II and III comparative trials.

The contribution of radiation to enhancing the potential for cardiac toxicity may involve several different mechanisms of tissue injury. The combination of thoracic radiation and chemotherapy has been felt to increase the risk of coronary artery disease. Pericardial injury may also be observed in patients with a previous exposure to combined modality therapy. Therefore, a careful balance of patients with similar cardiac risk factors must be achieved to eliminate these variables in any comparative assessment of drug-induced cardiotoxicity.

Monitoring the dose of an anthracycline to avoid cardiac toxicity can best be accomplished by considering the individual patient risk factor(s). The serial performance of radionuclide angiocardiography and more invasive cardiac monitoring (e.g., endomyocardial biopsy) may enable the clinician to administer the maximum dose for the individual patient. While no monitoring system can guarantee perfect predictability for the development of cardiotoxicity, the aggressive use of these devices may enable additional anthracycline to be administered to those patients who are continuing to derive additional antitumor effect from the antineoplastic drug.[13,133,142]

The major objective in developing mechanisms to reduce the cardiotoxic potential of antineoplastic therapy will be to enable dose-escalation for those agents demonstrating a significant dose-response relationship. Preclinical predictive animal models do exist for evaluating cardiotoxicity, and should be utilized to evaluate the effectiveness of new approaches.[60]

Nephrotoxicity Associated With Chemotherapy

In general, renal damage secondary to chemotherapeutic agents is predominantly a result of injury to the renal tubules. (Table XV-8-2) Substantial information has been developed to explain the pathophysiology of the renal injury resulting from chemotherapeutic agents, and clinical approaches have been discovered which may lessen the damage.[28]

Cisplatin, an important chemotherapeutic agent in the treatment of ovarian cancer, lung cancer, head and neck, and bladder cancer has been demonstrated to produce nephrotoxicity which is dose-related.[28] This drug-induced

Table XV-8-2.   Renal Toxicity

Drug	Toxic Dose[a,b] Range	Comment
Cisplatin	50–200 mg/m²	Nephrotoxicity dose limiting
		Dose-related/cumulative effects on renal tubules
		Hypomagnesemia/Hypocalcemia
Carboplatin	Conventional Dose	Renal dysfunction less common than with cisplatin
Carmustine (BCNU)	> 1,200 mg/m² (Total dose)	Renal dysfunction/cumulative dose effect
		Glomerular sclerosis/tubular atrophy
		Interstitial fibrosis
Streptozotocin	Conventional Dose	Dose-related/cumulative nephrotoxicity
		Proteinuria early sign nephropathy
		Interstitial nephritis
		Tubular atrophy
Cyclophosphamide	> 50 mg/kg	Hemorrhagic cystitis (may occur with low dose daily administration)
		Tubular injury/water retention
Ifosfamide	1.2 gm/m²/day × 5 days	See cyclophosphamide
Methotrexate	Variable	Related to drug and metabolite precipitation
		Excretion, renal route
Mitomycin C	> 30 mg/m² (total dose)	Renal insufficiency/hemolytic uremic syndrome
Interferons	Conventional Dose	Renal tubular injury

[a]Route of administration is IV unless otherwise indicated
[b]Conventional dose is commonly accepted therapeutic range

nephrotoxicity is due to a direct injury involving both the proximal and distal tubules. In addition, there may be an element of vasoconstriction superimposed on the tubular injury. The exact cellular target for the toxicity has not been identified. There is evidence that cellular proteins excreted in the urine of patients experiencing tubular injury include beta-2-microglobulin, alanine aminopeptidase, and leucine aminopeptidase, which are enzymes specifically located in the proximal tubular cells. Detection of increased excretion of these proteins has been utilized as a marker of subclinical renal damage related to the drug.

Certain parameters correlated with the degree of nephrotoxicity include: drug dose, state of hydration, and concomitant administration of additional nephrotoxic agents (e.g., aminoglycosides). Empirically defined measures for reducing the toxicity of the cisplatin include the administration of mannitol, adequate hydration, and utilization of hypertonic saline. Experimental evidence has demonstrated that the administration of thiols and thio-ethers may reduce the nephrotoxicity without impairing the antitumor response in animal models.[68]

Carboplatin, a structural analogue of cisplatin, has been associated with less nephrotoxicity than the parent compound.[137] However, it has been demonstrated that carboplatin may produce renal damage in patients with underlying damage secondary to previous cisplatin.[105] Therefore, caution should be exercised in particular when large doses of carboplatin are administered.

While heavy metal compounds have been associated with renal tubular damage, other agents are also capable of producing intrinsic renal injury (e.g., nitrosoureas, biologic agents including interferons alpha and gamma, and IL-2).[6,7,69,116,141]

The use of either cisplatin or mitomycin alone or in combination with other agents has been associated with an infrequent type of renal injury characterized as a microangiopathic-hemolytic process.[61,82] Recognition of this complication

is important because it may be reversible with discontinuation of the responsible agent, and possibly additional benefit is obtainable if the patient is subjected to plasmapheresis. In general, this type of nephrotoxicity is associated with additional evidence of a hemolytic anemia characterized by mechanical red cell fragmentation.

The use of high-dose cytotoxic agents such as ifosfamide has also been associated with toxicity to both the kidney and bladder.[5] The discovery of mesna has remarkably reduced the genitourinary toxicity associated with the administration of alkylating agents, but predictably has unmasked additional dose-limiting toxicity of these agents by permitting larger doses of alkylators to be administered.

Hepatic Toxicity Associated With Chemotherapy

Despite the predominant role that the liver plays in drug detoxification, the organ is frequently the site of drug-induced toxicity (Table XV-8-3). Hepatotoxicity, however, is frequently reversible with discontinuation of the responsible agent. A myriad of chemotherapeutic agents are capable of producing acute and reversible drug-induced hepatic cell toxicity.[125] The histologic pattern of hepatic cell injury associated with most chemotherapeutic agents is more often found in the centrilobular location, and the clinical manifestation of the injury is an elevation of hepatic enzymes. Several agents have the potential for producing a specific cholestatic pattern of injury (e.g., anabolic steroids and mercaptopurine), and will have an expected increase in alkaline phosphatase and bilirubin.

In addition, a rare but serious hypersensitivity-type hepatocellular injury has been described with dacarbazine which has characteristic histologic features including eosinophilic infiltration of the hepatic vessels with centrilobular necrosis. The clinical picture is associated with acute onset of upper abdominal pain, ascites, jaundice, and elevation of aminotransferases.[125] Early recognition and intervention with cor-

Table XV-8-3. Hepatic Toxicity

Drug	Toxic Dose[a,b] Range	Comment
L-Asparaginase	Conventional dose	Elevation of transaminases/alkaline phosphatase
		Diffuse fatty metamorphosis
		Decreased clotting factors (II, V, VII, IX, X)
Nitrosoureas	Conventional dose	Elevation of transaminases/alkaline phosphatase
6-Mercaptopurine	Conventional dose	Elevation of transaminases/alkaline phosphatase
		Hepatocellular disease
Methotrexate	Conventional dose	Elevation of transaminases
		Portal fibrosis/cirrhosis after total dose > 1.5 gm
Cytosine Arabinoside	Conventional dose	Elevation of transaminases
Hydroxyurea	Conventional dose	Elevation of transaminases/alkaline phosphatase
Mithramycin (Plicamycin)	> 30 μg/kg/day or > 10 doses	Elevation of transaminases/alkaline phosphatases
		Hemorrhagic diathesis/dose-related decrease in clotting factors (II, V, VII, X)
Dacarbazine	Conventional dose	Elevation of transaminases
		Hepatocellular necrosis
		Hepatic vein thrombosis

[a]Route of administration is I.V. unless otherwise indicated
[b]Conventional dose is commonly accepted therapeutic range

ticosteroids and discontinuation of the dacarbazine are necessary to avoid fatal complications.

Both acute and chronic hepatotoxicity have been clearly documented with methotrexate, and the chronic toxicity appears to be related to the duration of exposure and to the total cumulative dose administered.[64,128] The histologic feature frequently observed with the chronic hepatotoxicity is periportal fibrosis leading to cirrhosis.[96] Many other agents are capable of producing dose-related acute hepatotoxicity, and the potential for inducing chronic toxicity is probably underappreciated since many of the cancer patients do not receive chronic drug administration. In contrast, patients with inflammatory joint and skin diseases who receive methotrexate for prolonged periods develop hepatotoxicity.[19,121,132]

An important clinicopathologic entity called veno-occlusive disease (VOD) of the liver has been associated with the administration of high-doses of chemotherapy alone and in association with radiation to the liver.[107,125] The occurrence of VOD has been described in association with bone marrow transplantation, and is felt to result from the high-doses utilized for the preparative regimen.[84,85] The temporally-related onset of VOD is observed within the first three to five weeks after the preparative regimen. The clinical features of this complication include acute onset of pain in the upper abdomen, ascites, weight gain, and jaundice. The pathologic features may be difficult to demonstrate during the acute setting because of the associated thrombocytopenia and coagulation defects. However, in those patients who die during the first week of the illness, the liver demonstrates marked centrilobular necrosis. Furthermore, in those patients who either survive or die later, the characteristic histopathologic lesion is obliteration of the vascular lumen of the central venules.

The frequency of VOD in conjunction with bone marrow transplantation is 20% with death from complications of this entity occurring in approximately 7–50%.[107] Pre-existing liver disease with abnormalities of liver enzymes result in a 3.4 fold increase in the risk of developing VOD.[84] The advent of the use of autologous bone marrow transplantation and hematopoietic growth factors to enhance the intensity of che-

motherapy and combined modality therapy administration warrant observation for an increase in the frequency of this complication.

Neurotoxicity Associated With Chemotherapy

In general, antineoplastic agents have produced either peripheral (sensory and/or motor) or central neuropathic findings (Table XV-8-4) The tubulin binding agents have been known to produce peripheral neuropathy, and taxol, the newest active agent from this class is no exception.[108] The tubulin binding agents demonstrate a dose-dependent relationship to this toxicity, and usually result in reversible injury if the drug is discontinued.

Heavy metal intoxication has been associated with peripheral neuropathy.[92] Cisplatin was the first heavy metal compound demonstrating substantial anticancer activity, and its potential for producing neurotoxicity was initially described in 1978.[63] Neurologic toxicity is actually the dose-limiting toxicity associated with cisplatin in the treatment of some cancers.[43,54,87] The patterns of neurotoxicity are both peripheral and central in distribution with patients developing paresthesias, loss of proprioception or vibration sensation, retrobulbar neuritis, seizures, and ototoxicity. Over the past 10 years little progress was made in ameliorating the neurologic toxicity associated with the administration of this agent. A recent discovery has demonstrated that a peptide may actually prevent or attenuate the neurotoxicity without adversely affecting the cytotoxic effect of the drug.[43]

Central nervous system toxicity associated with chemotherapeutic agents may be transient or devastating in nature. The observation that high-dose cytosine arabinoside produces remarkable results in refractory forms of aggressive leukemia resulted in the widespread application of the high-dose regimens. The cerebellar and cerebral toxic events of repeated doses greater than 2–3 gram/m² have been clearly identified as being dose-related.[35,58,76,91,109] Recently, the association of age and renal function on the incidence of the serious degrees of cytosine arabinoside-induced neurologic toxicity have been better defined.[27] Consequently,

Table XV-8-4. Neurotoxicity

Drug	Toxic Dose[a,b] Range	Comment
Methotrexate	> 12 mg/m² I.T.	Acute meningeal irritation Arachnoiditis/paraplegia Necrotizing leukoencephalopathy
Cytosine Arabinoside	> 100 mg/m² I.T. > 3 gm/m² I.V.	Necrotizing leukoencephalopathy Cerebral/cerebellar dysfunction
5-Fluorouracil	Conventional dose	Acute cerebellar syndrome
Vincristine	Conventional dose	Symmetric sensory/motor peripheral neuropathy Cranial nerve motor neuropathy
Cisplatin	Conventional dose	Peripheral neuropathy Ototoxicity
Deoxycoformycin (Pentostatin)	High dose therapy	Central nervous system toxicity (seizure/coma)
Ifosfamide	High dose therapy	Central nervous system toxicity (somnolence/confusion/ coma)
Fludarabine	Low dose	Peripheral neuropathy/possible central nervous system toxicity
	High dose	Delayed-onset central nervous system toxicity (cortical blindness/coma)
Taxol	Conventional dose	Peripheral neuropathy
Interferons	Conventional dose	Decreased mental status/dizziness and paresthesias
Interleukin-2	Conventional dose	Altered mental status/somnolence

[a]Route of administration is I.V. unless otherwise indicated
[b]Conventional dose is commonly accepted therapeutic range

appropriate dose reductions can be employed for those patients with renal dysfunction or advanced age.

Another promising antimetabolite, fludarabine monophosphate, was demonstrated to have dose-dependent neurotoxic potential. The serious central nervous system toxicity appeared to be associated with a demyelinating process that was clinically delayed in onset.[138] The observation of cortical blindness, coma, and death associated with the high-dose administration of this agent almost precluded completion of an assessment of the drug's clinical utility. The demonstration of antitumor activity at lower doses fortunately saved this drug from abandonment. The potential for low-doses of this agent to produce neurologic toxicity has not yet been totally assessed.[48,86] Therefore, caution will need to be exercised with this agent until the total experience with it broadens.

Other Toxicities Associated With Chemotherapy

The chemotherapeutic agents associated with pulmonary toxicity have, in general, resulted in the production of interstitial lung injury (Table XV-8-5).[25] These toxic effects frequently are dose-related, but may be enhanced by prior radiation therapy to the thorax. While idiosyncratic or hypersensitivity reactions may be the cause of pulmonary toxicity in any given patient, it is necessary to review all the medications being administered to the patient as several agents can contribute to the overall toxicity.

The earliest clinical manifestations of pulmonary toxicity may be subtle (e.g., nonspecific cough), and early recognition may prevent the irreversible consequences of continued drug administration. Careful monitoring of patients receiving agents known to produce pulmonary toxicity is also warranted.

Table XV-8-5. Pulmonary Toxicity

Drug	Toxic Dose[a,b] Range	Comment
Bleomycin	> 400 Units (total dose)	Interstitial pneumonitis/fibrosis Dyspnea/cough early symptoms Fine rales early sign/decreased lung volume and vital capacity Toxicity dose and age-related
Mitomycin C	Conventional dose	Interstitial pneumonitis
Carmustine (BCNU)	> 1 gm/m² (total dose)	Interstitial pneumonitis Delayed pulmonary fibrosis
Busulfan	Conventional dose	Bronchopulmonary dysplasia/fibrosis onset delayed months to years
Cyclophosphamide	High dose therapy	Interstitial pneumonitis/fibrosis
Chlorambucil	Conventional dose	Interstitial pneumonitis/fibrosis
Melphalan	High dose therapy	Interstitial pneumonitis
Cytosine Arabinoside	Conventional dose	Pulmonary edema
Methotrexate	Conventional dose	Interstitial pneumonitis

[a]Route of administration is I.V. unless otherwise indicated
[b]Conventional dose is commonly accepted therapeutic range

Table XV-8-6.   Gastrointestinal Toxicity

Drug	Toxic Dose[a,b] Range	Comment
Methotrexate	Variable	Nausea and vomiting Mucositis and ulceration
5-Fluorouracil	Conventional dose	Nausea and vomiting Mucositis and bloody diarrhea
Cisplatin	Conventional dose	Severe nausea and vomiting
Cyclophosphamide	Conventional dose	Nausea and vomiting Diarrhea
Vincristine	Conventional dose	Dose-related constipation/abdominal cramps/ adynamic ileus
Doxorubicin	Conventional dose	Nausea and vomiting Mucositis
Hydroxyurea	Conventional dose	Nausea and vomiting Mucositis
Dacarbazine	Conventional dose	Nausea and vomiting
Nitrosoureas	Conventional dose	Nausea and vomiting
Cytosine Arabinoside	Conventional dose	Nausea and vomiting Diarrhea and mucositis

[a]Route of administration is I.V. unless otherwise indicated
[b]Conventional dose is commonly accepted therapeutic range

Table XV-8-7.   Hematologic Toxicity

Drug	Level of WBC Suppression	Maximum Suppression (Days)	Time to Recovery (Days)
Busulfan	Severe	11–30	30–60
Carmustine (BCNU)	Severe	28–42	35–90
Lomustine (CCNU)	Severe	28–42	35–90
Semustine (Methyl-CCNU)	Severe	28–42	35–90
Chlorambucil	Severe	7–14	14–28
Cyclophosphamide	Severe	7–14	21–28
Dacarbazine (DTIC)	Severe	16–25	25–35
Ifosfamide	Severe	10–20	21–35
Mechlorethamine (HN2)	Severe	7–14	14–28
Melphalan (l-PAM)	Severe	7–14	14–28
Carboplatin	Severe	21	28
Cytosine Arabinoside	Severe	12–24	21–30
5-Fluorouracil	Severe	9–14	21–30
Fludarabine	Severe	7–14	14–21
Methotrexate	Severe	7–14	14–21
Daunorubicin	Severe	10–14	21–28
Doxorubicin	Severe	10–14	21–28
Taxol	Severe	8–11	15–21
Hydroxyurea	Moderate	7–10	14–21
Vinblastine	Moderate	5–10	10–21
Mitoxantrone	Moderate	7–14	14–28
Mitomycin C	Moderate	21–42	35–70
Cisplatin	Mild	18–23	21–40

The most frequent toxicities encountered with standard chemotherapeutic agents include the gastrointestinal and hematologic toxicities outlined in Tables XV-8-6 and XV-8-7. The recent application of intensive principles of antiemetic therapy and the utilization of colony stimulating factors may permit significant dose intensification of these agents.[29,52,57,89,119] Perhaps, the positive contribution of these improved supportive care measures to lessen the toxicity and permit dosing on time will be as important as the actual dose increment achieved.

The toxicologic effects of chemotherapeutic agents on gonadal tissue is critically important to those patients in the child-bearing years. The cumulative effect of specific agents on testicular function indicate that certain combination regimens may be more detrimental than others. The teratogenic effects of chemotherapy have been recognized, but the long-term followup in the children of cancer patients subsequent to the administration of chemotherapy remains largely unknown. In fact, the long-term consequences of chemotherapy administration to cancer patients with respect to the development of secondary neoplasms is an area requiring intensive study. The problem of defining the long-term toxic

Table XV-8-8.   Guide To The Design of Preclinical Toxicology Studies in Support of Early Clinical Investigations on New Anticancer Agents

	Stage 1	Stage 2
Species	Mice	Mice and appropriate second species
Purpose	To establish potential clinical entry dose	To determine the safety of the clinical entry dose
	To determine plasma elimination kinetics and concentration dependency of agent	To forecast the potential toxicities likely to be encountered
		To establish presence of dose dependent toxicity
		To relate plasma pharmacokinetics to predictable biological effects
Design	Determine MTD (LD10) following bolus dosing and potential clinical schedule	Determine toxicity at MTD and 0.1 MTD on bolus administration and repeated dose scheduling
	Determine plasma elimination kinetics following bolus dosing and continuous administration	Establish relationship between pharmacokinetics and toxicity observed

effects of chemotherapy should be recognized as a product of success deserving careful scrutiny to avoid unnecessary, additional risks without compromising therapeutic intent.

Conclusion

This chapter has presented an overview of the basic principles of toxicologic investigation of antineoplastic agents. The appropriate utilization of animal models will permit reasonable quantitative and qualitative predictions of the toxicities that may be anticipated in humans. In Table XV-8-8, the basic approach to initiating the necessary preclinical studies for subsequent trials in humans is summarized. The process of defining the comprehensive toxicity profile of a new agent will encompass both extensive preclinical and clinical investigations as previously described in detail.

The study of human toxicology has contributed significantly to the current therapeutic approach to the management of cancer patients. The discovery and development of novel therapeutic agents, the combination of biologic products with cytotoxic agents, and the utilization of differentiating agents open new areas for toxicologic investigation. The correlation of pharmacologic data with toxicity and efficacy, and the willingness to implement newer approaches to predicting human toxicity should enhance the contributions yet to be made by this discipline.

References

1. Abbruzzese, J. L., Levin, B., Ajani, J. A., Faintrich, J. S., Pazdur, R., Saks, S., Edwards, C., and Gutterman, J. U.: A Phase II trial of recombinant human interferon-gamma and recombinant tumor necrosis factor in patients with advanced gastrointestinal malignancies: results of a trial terminated by excessive toxicity. J. Biol. Resp. Modifiers, 9:522, 1990.
2. Akoun, G. M., and White, J. P.: Treatment-Induced Respiratory Disorders. Edited by M. N. G. Dukes. New York, Elsevier, 1989, p. 60.
3. Andreeff, M., and Welte, K.: Hematopoietic colony-stimulating factors. Semin. Oncol., 16:211, 1989.
4. Andrieu, J.-M., Ifrah, N., Payen, C., Fermanian, J., Coscas, Y., and Flandrin, G.: Increased risk of secondary acute nonlymphocytic leukemia after extended-field radiation therapy combined with MOPP chemotherapy for Hodgkin's disease. J. Clin. Oncol., 8:1148, 1990.
5. Antman, K. H., Elias, A., and Ryan, L.: Ifosfamide and mesna: response and toxicity at standard and high-dose schedule. Semin. Oncol., 17 (Suppl. 4):68, 1990.
6. Ault, B. H., Stapleton, F. B., Gaber, L., Martin. A., Roy, S., and Murphy, S. B.: Acute renal failure during therapy with recombinant human gamma interferon. N. Engl. J. Med., 319:1397, 1988.
7. Averbuch, S. D., Austin, H. A., Sherwin, S. A., Antonovych, T., Bunn, P. A., and Longo, D. L.: Acute interstitial nephritis with the nephrotic syndrome following recombinant leukocyte A interferon for mycosis fungoides. N. Engl. J. Med., 310:32, 1984.
8. Bailar, J. C., III, and Byar, D. P.: Estrogen treatment for cancer of prostate: early results with three doses of diethylstilbesterol and placebo. Cancer, 26:257, 1970.
9. Balis, F. M., and Poplack, D. G.: Central nervous system pharmacology of antileukemia drugs. Am. J. Pediatr. Hematol. Oncol., 11:74, 1989.
10. Baverman, A. C., Antin, J. H., Plappert, M. T., Cook, E. F., and Lee, R. T.: Cyclophosphamide cardiotoxicity in bone marrow transplantation. J. Clin. Oncol., 9:1215, 1991.
11. Bender, K. S., Shematek, J. P., Leventhal, B. G., and Kan, J. S.: QT interval prolongation associated with anthracycline cardiotoxicity. J. Pediatr., 105:442, 1984.
12. Berry, J., Jacobs, C., Sikic, B., Halsey, J., and Borch, R. F.: Modification of cisplatinum toxicity with diethyldithiocarbamate. J. Clin. Oncol., 8:1585, 1990.
13. Billingham, M. E., and Bristow, M. R.: Evaluation of anthracycline cardiotoxicity: predictive ability and functional correlation of endomyocardial biopsy. Cancer Treat. Symp. 3:71, 1984.
14. Blackard, C. E., Byar, D. P., and Jordan, W. P.: Orchiectomy for advanced prostate carcinoma: a re-evaluation. Urology, 1:553, 1973.
15. Bookman, M. A., Longo, D. L., and Young, R. C.: Late complications of curative treatment in Hodgkin's disease. J.A.M.A., 260:680, 1988.
16. Breast Cancer Trials Committee, Scottish Cancer Trials Office (MRC): Adjuvant tamoxifen in the management of operable breast cancer in the Scottish trial. Lancet, 2:171, 1987.
17. Bristow, M. R.: Toxic cardiomyopathy due to doxorubicin. Hosp. Pract., 17:12, 1982.
18. Brock, N., Pohl, J., and Stekar, J.: Detoxification of urotoxic oxazaphosphorines by sulfhydryl compounds. J. Cancer Res. Clin. Oncol., 100:311, 1981.
19. Chassagne, P., Levesque, H., and Moore, N.: Methotrexate. Pharmacology applied to the treatment of rheumatoid arthritis. Therapie, 45:499, 1990.
20. Chaudary, S., Song, S. Y. T., and Jaski, B. E.: Profound, yet reversible, heart failure secondary to 5-fluorouracil. Am. J. Med., 85:454, 1988.
21. Chun, H. G., Leyland-Jones, B. R., Caryk, S. M., and Hoth, D. F.: Central nervous system toxicity of fludarabine phosphate. Cancer Treat. Rep., 70:1225, 1986.
22. Cimino, G., Papa, G., Tura, S., Mazza, P., Rossi Ferrini, P. L., Bosi, A., Amadori, S., Lo Coco, F., D'Arcangelo, E., Giannarelli, D., and Mandelli, F.: Second primary cancer following Hodgkin's disease: updated results of an Italian multicentric study. J. Clin. Oncol., 9:432, 1991.
23. Collins, J. M., Zaharko, D. S., Dedrick, R. L., and Chabner, B. A.: Potential roles for preclinical pharmacology in Phase I clinical trials. Cancer Treat. Rep., 70:73, 1986.
24. Collins, J. M., Grieshaber, C. K., and Chabner, B. A.: Pharmacologically guided Phase I clinical trials based upon preclinical drug development. J. Natl. Cancer Inst., 82:1321, 1990.
25. Cooper, J. A. D., Jr., and Matthay, R. A.: Pneumonitis induced by cytotoxic drugs. In Treatment-Induced Respiratory Disorders, Vol. 3. Edited by G. M. Akoun, J. P. White. New York, Elsevier, 1989, p. 51.
26. Dameshek, W., and Gunz, F.: Leukemia, 2nd Edition. New York, Grune & Stratton, 1964.
27. Damon, L. E., Mass, R., and Linher, C. A.: The association between high-dose cytarabine neurotoxicity and renal insufficiency. J. Clin. Oncol., 7:1563, 1989.
28. Daugaard, G.: Cisplatin nephrotoxicity: experimental and clinical studies. Dan. Med. Bull., 37:1, 1990.
29. Demetri, G. D., and Griffin, J. D.: Hematopoietic growth factors and high-dose chemotherapy: will grams succeed where milligrams fail? J. Clin. Oncol., 8:761, 1990.
30. DeSouza, J. J. V., Grever, M. R., Neidhart, J. A., Staubus, A. E., and Malspeis, L.: Comparative pharmacokinetics and metabolism of fludarabine phosphate (NSC 312887) in man and dog. Proc. Am. Assoc. Cancer Res., 25:361, 1984.
31. Dixon, A. C., Nakamura, J. M., Oishi, N., Wachi, D. H., and Fukuyama, O.: Angina pectoris and therapy with cisplatin, vincristine, and bleomycin. Ann. Intern. Med., 111:342, 1989.
32. Doll, D. C., List, A. F., Greco, F. A., Hainsworth, J. D., Hande, K. R., and Johnson, D. A.: Acute vascular ischemic events after cisplatinum-based combination chemotherapy for germ-cell tumors of the testes. Ann. Intern. Med., 105:48, 1986.
33. Du, D.-L, Volpe, D. A., Grieshaber, C. K., and Murphy, M. J., Jr.: Comparative toxicity of fostriecin, hepsulfam, and pyrazine diazohydroxide to human and murine hematopoietic progenitor cells in vitro. Invest. New Drugs, 9:149, 1991.
34. Du, D.-L, Volpe, D. A., Grieshaber, C. K., and Murphy, M. J., Jr.: Effects of L-phenylalanine mustard and L-buthionine sulfoximine on murine and human hematopoietic progenitor cells in vitro. Cancer Res., 50:4038, 1990.
35. Early, A. P., Preisler, H. D., Slocum, H., and Rustum, Y. M: A pilot study of high-dose a-β-D-arabinofuranosylcytosine for acute leukemia and refractory lymphoma: clinical response and pharmacology. Cancer Res., 42:1587, 1982.
36. El Dareer, S. M., Struck, R. F., Tillery, K. F., Rose, L. M., Brockman, R. W., Montgomery, J. A., and Hill, D. L.: Disposition of 9-β-D-arabinofuranosyl-2-fluoroadenine in mice, dogs, and monkeys. Drug Metab. Dispos., 8:60, 1980.
37. Frazier, J. M., Tyson, C. A., McCarthy, C., McCormack, J. J., Meyer, D., Powis, G., and Ducat, L.: Contemporary issues in toxicology: Potential use of human tissues for toxicity research and testing. Toxicol. Appl. Pharmacol., 97:387, 1989.
38. Freeman, N., and Costanza, M.: 5-Fluorouracil associated cardiotoxicity. Cancer, 61:36, 1988.

39. Freireich, E. J., Gehan, E. A., Rall, D. P., Schmidt, L. H., and Skipper, H. E.: Quantitative comparison of toxicity of anticancer agents in mouse, rat, hamster, dog, monkey, and man. Cancer Chemother. Rep., 50:219, 1966.
40. Gandara, D. R., Perez, E. A., Wiebe, U., and DeGregorio, M. W.: Cisplatin chemoprotection and rescue: pharmacologic modulation of toxicity. Semin. Oncol., 18(Suppl. 3):49, 1991.
41. Gaynor, E. R., Vitek, L., Sticklin, L., Creekmore, S. P., Ferraro, M. E., Thomas, J. X., Jr., Fisher, S. G., and Fisher, R. I.: The hemodynamic effects of treatment with interleukin-2 and lymphokine-activated killer cells. Ann. Intern. Med., 109:953, 1988.
42. Kragel, A. H., Travis, W. D., Feinberg, L., Pittaluga, S., Striker, L. M., Roberts, W. C., Lotze, M. T., Yang, J. J., and Rosenberg, S. A.: Pathologic findings associated with interleukin-2-based immunotherapy for cancer: a postmortem study of 19 patients. Hum. Pathol., 21:493, 1990.
43. Gerritsen van der Hoop, R., Vecht, C. J., van der Burg, M. E. L., Elderson, A., Boogerd, W., Heimans, J. J., Vries, E. P., van Houwelingen, J. C., Jennekens, F. G. I., Gispen, W. H., and Neijt, J. P.: Prevention of cisplatin neurotoxicity with an ACTH(4-9) analogue in patients with ovarian cancer. N. Eng. J. Med., 322:89, 1990.
44. Gilewski, T., and Golomb, H. M.: Design of combination biotherapy studies: future goals and challenges. Semin. Oncol., 17(Suppl. 1):3, 1990.
45. Ginsberg, S. J., and Comis, R. L.: The pulmonary toxicity of antineoplastic agents. Semin. Oncol., 9:34, 1982.
46. Grever, M. R., Siaw, M. F. E., Jacob, W. F., Neidhart, J. A., Miser, J. S., Coleman, M. S., Hutton, J. J., and Balcerzak, S. P.: The biochemical and clinical consequences of 2′-deoxycoformycin in refractory lymphoproliferative malignancy. Blood, 57:406, 1981.
47. Grever, M. R., Staubus, A. E., and Malspeis, L.: Correlation of N-acetylation phenotype with plasma levels of the N-acetylmetabolite of amonafide (NSC 308847). Proc. Am. Assoc. Cancer Res., 31:178, 1990.
48. Grever, M., Leiby, J., Kraut, E., Metz, E., Neidhart, J., Balcerzak, S., and Malspeis, L.: A comprehensive Phase I and II clinical investigation of fludarabine phosphate. Semin. Oncol., 17(Suppl. 8):39, 1990.
49. Grever, M. R., Leiby, J. M., Kraut, E. A., Wilson, H. E., Neidhart, J. A., Wall, R. L., and Balcerzak, S. P.: Low-dose deoxycoformycin in lymphoid malignancy. J. Clin. Oncol., 3:1196, 1985.
50. Grieshaber, C. K.: Predictions of human toxicity from animal studies. *In* Mechanisms of Toxicity of Anticancer Drugs: A Study in Human Toxicity. Edited by G. Powis, M. Hacket. New York, Pergamon Press, 1991, p. 10.
51. Grieshaber, C. K., and Marsoni, S.: Relation of preclinical toxicology to findings in early clinical trials. Cancer Treat. Rep., 70:65, 1986.
52. Griffin, J. D.: Hemopoietins in oncology: factoring out myelosuppression. J. Clin. Oncol., 7:151, 1989.
53. Gutierrez, M. L., and Crooke, S. T.: Mitotane (o,p-DDD). Cancer Treat. Rev., 7:49, 1980.
54. Hansen, S. W., Helweg-Larsen, S., and Trojaborg, W.: Long-term neurotoxicity in patients treated with cisplatin, vinblastine, and bleomycin for metastatic germ cell cancer. J. Clin. Oncol., 7:1457, 1989.
55. Hawkins, M. M.: Second primary tumors following radiotherapy for childhood cancer. Int. J. Radiat. Oncol. Biol. Phys., 19:1297, 1990.
56. Herbst, A. L., Ulfelder, H., and Poskunzes, D. C.: Adenocarcinoma of the vagina: association of maternal stilbestrol therapy with tumor appearance in young women. N. Engl. J. Med., 11:284, 1971.
57. Herrimann, F., Schulz, G., Wieser, M., Kolbe, K., Nicolay, U., Noack, M., Lindemann, A., and Mertelsmann, R.: Effect of granulocyte-macrophage colony-stimulating factor on neutropenia and related morbidity induced by myelotoxic chemotherapy. Am. J. Med., 88:619, 1990.
58. Herzig, R. H., Hines, J. D., Herzig, G. P., Wolff, S. N., Cassileth, P. A., Lazarus, H. M., Adelstein, D. J., Brown, R. A., Coccia, P. F., Strandjord, S., Massa, J. J., Fay, J., and Phillips, G. L.: Cerebellar toxicity with high-dose cytosine arabinoside. J. Clin. Oncol., 5:927, 1987.
59. Hutton, J. J., Von Hoff, D. D., Kuhn, J., Phillips, J., Hersh, M., and Clark, G.: Phase I clinical investigation of 9-β-D-arabinofuranosyl-2-fluoroadenine 5′-monophosphate (NSC 312887), a new purine antimetabolite. Cancer Res., 44:4183, 1984.
60. Iatropoulos, M. J.: Anthracycline cardiomyopathy: predictive value of animal models. Cancer Treat. Symp. 3:3, 1984.
61. Jackson, A. M., Rose, B. D., Graff, L. G., Jacobs, J. B., Schwartz, J. H., Strauss, G. M., Yang, J. P. S., Rudnick, M. R., Elfenbein, I. B., and Narins, R. G.: Thrombotic microangiopathy and renal failure associated with antineoplastic chemotherapy. Ann. Intern. Med., 101:41, 1984.
62. Jordan, V. C., Fritz, N. F., and Tormey, D. C.: Endocrine effects of adjuvant chemotherapy and long-term tamoxifen administration on node-positive patients with breast cancer. Cancer Res., 47:624, 1987.
63. Kedar, A., Cohen, M. E., and Freeman, A. I.: Peripheral neuropathy as a complication of cis-dichlorodiamine platinum (II) treatment: a case report. Cancer Treat. Rep., 62:819, 1978.
64. Keim, D., Ragsdale, C., Heidelberger, K., and Sullivan, D.: Hepatic fibrosis with the use of methotrexate for juvenile rheumatoid arthritis. J. Rheumatol., 17:846, 1990.
65. Kellie, S. J., and Kingston, J. E.: Letter to the Editor: Ovarian failure after high-dose melphalan in adolescents. Lancet, 1:1425, 1987.
66. Killackey, M. A., Hakes, T. B., and Pierce, V.: Endometrial adenocarcinoma in breast cancer patients receiving antiestrogens. Cancer Treat. Rep., 69:237, 1985.
67. Kirk, J. A., Raghupathy, P., Stevens, M. M., Cowell, C. T., Menser, M. A., Bergin, M., Tink, A., Vines, R. H., and Silink, M.: Growth failure and growth-hormone deficiency after treatment for acute lymphoblastic leukemia. Lancet, 1:190, 1987.
68. Kobayashi, H., Hasuda, K., Aoki, K., Taniguchi, S., and Baba, T.: Systemic chemotherapy in tumor-bearing rats using high-dose cis-diamminedichloroplatinum(II) with low nephrotoxicity in combination with angiotensin II and sodium thiosulfate. Int. J. Cancer, 45:940, 1990.
69. Kramer, R., and Boyd, M. R.: Nephrotoxicity of 1-(2-chloroethyl)-3-(trans-4-methylcyclohexyl)-1-nitrosourea (MeCCNU) in the fischer 344 rat. J. Pharmacol Exp. Ther., 227:409, 1983.
70. Kraut, E. H., Bouroncle, B. A., and Grever, M. R.: Low-dose deoxycoformycin in the treatment of hairy cell leukemia. Blood, 68:1119, 1986.
71. Kraut, E. H., Fleming, T., Segal, M., and Neidhart, J. A.: Phase II study of pibenzimol in pancreatic carcinoma. A Southwest Oncology Group study. Invest. New Drugs, 9:95, 1991.
72. Krischer, J., Land, V. J., Civin, C. I., Ragub, A. H., Mahoney, D. M., and Frankel, L. S.: Evaluation of AMSA in children with acute leukemia. Cancer, 54:207, 1984.
73. Laghi Pasini, F., Perri, T. D. I., van der Plas, K., Palmer, P., and Franks, C. R.: Myocardial injury after interleukin-2 therapy. Lancet, 1:674, 1989.
74. Lampidis, T. L., Henderson, I. C., Israel, M., and Canellos, G. P.: Structural and functional effects of adriamycin on cardiac cells *in vitro*. Cancer Res., 40:3901, 1980.
75. LaRocca, R. V., Stein, C. A., Danesi, R., and Jamis-Dow, C. A.: Suramin in adrenal cancer: modulation of steroid hormone production, cytotoxicity *in vitro*, and clinical antitumor effect. J. Clin. Endocrinol. Metab., 71:497, 1990.
76. Lazarus, H. M., Herzig, R. H., Herzig, G. P., Phillips, G. L., Roessmann, U., and Fishman, D. J.: Central nervous system toxicity of high-dose systemic cytosine arabinoside. Cancer, 48:2577, 1981.
77. Legha, S. S., Benjamin, R. S., Mackay, B., Ewer, M., Wallace, S., Valdivieso, M., Rasmussen, S. L., Blumenschein, G. R., and Freireich, E. J.: Reduction of doxorubicin cardiotoxicity by prolonged continuous intravenous infusion. Ann. Intern. Med., 96:133, 1982.
78. Legha, S. S., Ring, S., Raber, M., Felder, T. B., Newman, A., and Krakoff, I. H.: Phase I clinical investigations of benzisoquinolinedione. Cancer Treat. Rep., 71:1165, 1987.
79. Leiby, J. M., Malspeis, L., Staubus, A. E., Kraut, E. H., and Grever, M. R.: Amonafide (NSC 308847): a clinical Phase I study of two schedules of administration. Proc. Am. Assoc. Cancer Res., 29:278, 1990.
80. Lowe, M. C.: Large animal toxicological studies of anticancer drugs. *In* Fundamentals of Cancer Chemotherapy. Edited by K. Hellman, and S. Carter. New York, McGraw Hill, 1987, p. 236.
81. Lowe, M. C., and Davis, R. D.: The current toxicology protocol of the National Cancer institute. *In* Fundamentals of Cancer Chemotherapy. Edited by K. Hellman, S. Carter. New York, McGraw Hill, 1987, p. 228.
82. Lyman, N. W., Michaelson, R., Viscuso, R. L., Winn, R., Mulgaonkar,S., and Jacobs, M. G.: Mitomycin-induced hemolytic-uremic syndrome. Arch. Intern. Med., 143:1617, 1983.
83. Malspeis, L., Grever, M. R., Staubus, A. E., and Young, D.: Pharmacokinetics of 2-F-ara-A (9-β-D-arabinofuranosyl-2-fluoroadenine) in cancer patients during the Phase I clinical investigation of fludarabine phosphate. Semin. Oncol., 17(Suppl. 8):18, 1990.
84. McDonald, G. B., Sharma, P., Matthews, D. E., Shulman, H. M., and Thomas, E. D.: Venocclusive disease of the liver after bone marrow transplantation: diagnosis, incidence, and predisposing factors. Hepatology, 4:116, 1984.
85. McDonald, G. B., Shulman, H. M., Wolford, J. L., and Spencer, G. D.: Liver disease after human marrow transplantation. Semin. Liver Dis., 7:210, 1987.
86. Merkel, D. E., Griffin, N. L., Kagan-Hallet, K., and Von Hoff, D. D.: Central nervous system toxicity with fludarabine. Cancer Treat. Rep., 70:1449, 1986.
87. Mollman, J. E.: Cisplatin neurotoxicity. N. Engl. J. Med., 322:126, 1990.
88. Monk, M. R., Sanchez, J. D., Phelps, C. D., and Miller, D. M.: Myocardial ischemia with fluorouracil and floxuridine therapy. Clin. Pharmacy, 6:659, 1987.
89. Morstyn, G., Campbell, L., Lieschke, G., Layton, J. E., Maher, D., O'Connor, M., Green, M., Therdan, W., Vincent, M., Alton, K., Souza, L., McGrath, K., and Fox, R. M.: Treatment of chemotherapy-induced neutropenia by subcutaneously administered granulocyte colony-stimulating factor with optimization of dose and duration of therapy. J. Clin. Oncol., 7:1554, 1989.
90. Myers, C. E., McGuire, W. P., Liss, R. H., Ifrim, I., Grotzinger, K., and Young, R. C.: Adriamycin: the role of lipid peroxidation in cardiac toxicity and tumor response. Science, 197:165, 1977.
91. Nand, S., Messmore, H. L., Jr., Patel, R., Fisher, S. G., and Fisher, R. I.: Neurotoxicity associated with systemic high-dose cytosine arabinoside. J. Clin. Oncol., 4:571, 1986.
92. Needleman, H. L., Schell, A., Bellinger, D., Leviton, A., and Allred, E. N.: The long-term effects of exposure to low doses of lead in childhood: an 11-year follow-up report. N. Engl. J. Med., 322:83, 1990.
93. Nielssen, D., Jensen, J. B., Dombernowsky, P., Munck, O., Fogh, J., Brynjolf, I., Havsteen, H., and Hansen, M.: Epirubicin cardiotoxicity: a study of 135 patients with advanced breast cancer. J. Clin. Oncol., 8:1806, 1990.
94. Noker, P. E., Duncan, G. F., El Dareer, S. M., and Hill, D. L.: Disposition of 9-β-D-arabinofuranosyl-2-fluoroadenine 5′-monophosphate in mice and dogs. Cancer Treat. Rep., 67:445, 1983.
95. Nora, R., Abrams, J. S., Tait, N. S., Hiponia, D. J., and Silverman, H. J.: Myocardial toxic effects during recombinant interleukin-2 therapy. J. Natl. Cancer Inst., 81:59, 1989.
96. O'Connor, G. T., Olmstead, E. M., Zug, K., Baughman, R. D., Beck, J. R., Dunn, J. L., Seal, P., and Lewandowski, J. F.: Detection of hepatotoxicity associated with methotrexate therapy for psoriasis. Arch. Dermatol., 125:1209, 1989.
97. Osanto, S., Cluitmans, F. H. M., Franks, C. R., Bosker, H. A., and Cleton, F. J.: Myocardial injury after interleukin-2 therapy. Lancet, 2:48, 1988.
98. Patel, S. R., Kvols, L. K., Rubin, J., O'Connell, M. J., Edmonson, J. H., Ames, M. M., and Kovach, J. S.: Phase I-II study of pibenzimol hydrochloride (NSC 322921) in advanced pancreatic carcinoma. Invest. New Drugs, 9:53, 1991
99. Pedersen-Bjergaard, J., Specht, L., Larsen, S. O., Ersboll, J., Struck, J., Hansen, M. M., Hansen, H. H., and Nissen, N. I.: Risk of therapy-related leukemia and preleukaemia after Hodgkin's disease. Lancet, 2:83, 1987.
100. Poplack, D. G., Sallan, S. E., Rivera, G., Holcenberg, J., Murphy, S. B., Blatt, J., Lipton, J. M., Venner, P., Glaubiger, D. L., Ungerleider, R., and Johns, D.: Phase I study of 2′-deoxycoformycin in acute lymphoblastic leukemia. Cancer Res., 41:3343, 1981.
101. Ratain, M. J., Mick, R., Berezin, F., Janisch, L., Shilsky, R. L., Williams, S. F., and Smiddy, J.: Prospective correlation of acetylation phenotype with amonafide toxicity. Proc. Am. Soc. Clin. Oncol., 10:101, 1991.
102. Ratain, M. J., Propert, K., Costanza, M., Allen, S., Berezin, F., Shilsky, R. L., and Van Echo, D. A.: CALGB-population pharmacodynamic study of amonafide CALGB 8862. Proc. Am. Assoc. Cancer Res., 31:181, 1990.
103. Ratain, M. J., Staubus, A. E., Shilsky, R. L., and Malspeis, L.: Limited sampling models for amonafide (NSC 308847) pharmacokinetics. Cancer Res., 48:4127, 1988.
104. Ravdin, P. M., Fritz, N. F., Tormey, D. C., and Jordan, V. C.: Endocrine status of premenopausal node-positive breast cancer patients following adjuvant chemotherapy and long-term tamoxifen. Cancer Res., 48:1026, 1988.

105. Reed, E., and Jacob, J.: Carboplatin and renal dysfunction. Ann. Int. Med., 110:409, 1989.

106. Rivkees, S. A., and Crawford, J. D.: The relationship of gonadal activity and chemotherapy-induced gonadal damage. JAMA, 259:2123, 1988.

107. Rollins, R. J.: Hepatic veno-occlusive disease. Am. J. Med., 81:297, 1986.

108. Rowinsky, E. K., Cazenave, L. A., and Donehower, R. C.: Taxol: a novel investigational antimicrotubule agent. J. Natl. Cancer Inst., 82:1247, 1990.

109. Rudnick, S. A., Cadman, E. C., Capizzi, R. L., Skeel, R. T., Bertino, J. R., and McIntosh, S.: High dose cytosine arabinoside (HDARAC) in refractory acute leukemia. Cancer, 44:1189, 1979.

110. Salmon, S. E., Young, L., Scuderi, P., and Clark, B.: Antineoplastic effects of tumor necrosis factor alone and in combination with gamma interferon on tumor biopsies in clonogenic assay. J. Clin. Oncol., 5:1816, 1987.

111. Schein, P., and Anderson, T.: The efficacy of animal studies on predicting clinical toxicity of cancer chemotherapeutic drugs. Int. J. Clin. Pharmacol., 8:228, 1973.

112. Schein, P. S., Winokur, S., MacDonald, J. S., and Woolley, P. V.: Long-term complications of cytotoxic and immunosuppressive chemotherapy. In Cancer Medicine, 2nd Edition. Edited by J. F. Holland, and E. Frei, III. Philadelphia, Lea & Febiger, 1982, p. 759-774.

113. Schiller, J. H., Bittner, G., Storer, B., and Willson, J. K. V.: Synergistic antitumor effects of tumor necrosis factor and γ interferon on human colon carcinoma cell lines. Cancer Res., 47:2809, 1987.

114. Schmiegel, W. H., Caesar, J., Kalthoff, H., Greten, H., Schreiber, H. W., and Thiele, H. G.: Antiproliferative effects exerted by recombinant human tumor necrosis factor α (TNFα) and interferon-γ (IFN-γ) on human pancreatic tumor cell lines. Pancreas, 3:180, 1988.

115. Schurig, J. E., and Bradner, W. T.: Small animal toxicology of cancer drugs. In Fundamentals of Cancer Chemotherapy. Edited by K. Hellman, and S. Carter. New York, McGraw Hill, 1987, p. 248.

116. Shalmi, C. L., Dutcher, J. P., Feinfeld, D. A., Chun, K. J., Saleemi, K. R., Freeman, L. M., Lynn, R. I., and Wiernik, P. H.: Acute renal dysfunction during interleukin-2 treatment: suggestion of an intrinsic renal lesion. J. Clin. Oncol., 8:1839, 1990.

117. Shapira, J., Gottfried, M., Lishner, M., and Ravid, M.: Reduced cardiotoxicity of doxorubicin by a 6-hour infusion regimen. Cancer, 65:870, 1990.

118. Shapiro, S., and Mealey, J., Jr.: Late anaplastic gliomas in children previously treated for acute lymphoblastic leukemia. Pediatr. Neurosci., 15:176, 1989.

119. Sheridan, W. P., Wolf, M., Lusk, J., Layton, J. E., Souza, L., Morstyn, G., Dodds, A., Maher, D., Green, M. D., and Fox, R. M.: Granulocyte colony-stimulating factor and neutrophil recovery after high-dose chemotherapy and autologous bone marrow transplantation. Lancet, 2:891, 1989.

120. Sherwin, S. A., Foon, K. A., and Oldham, R. K.: Animal tumor models for biological response modifier therapy: an approach to the development of monoclonal antibody therapy in humans. In Fundamentals of Cancer Chemotherapy. Edited by K. Hellman, and S. Carter. New York, McGraw Hill, 1987, p. 202.

121. Singh, G., Fries, J. F., Williams, C. A., Zatarain, E., Spitz, P., and Bloch, D. A.: Toxicity profiles of disease modifying antirheumatic drugs in rheumatoid arthritis. J. Rheumatol., 18:188, 1991.

122. Smyth, J. F., Paine, R. M., Jackman, A., Harrap, K. R., Chassin, M. M., Adamson, R. H., and Johns, D. G.: The clinical pharmacology of the adenosine deaminase inhibitor 2'-deoxycoformycin. Cancer Chemother. Pharmacol., 5:93, 1980.

123. Speyer, J. L., Green, M. D., Kramer, E., Rey, M., Sanger, J., Ward, C., Dubin, N., Ferrans, V., Stecy, P., Zeleniuch-Jacquotte, A., Wernz, J., Feit, F., Slater, W., Blum, R., and Muggia, F.: Protective effect of the bispiperazinedione ICRF-187 against

124. Steuber, C. P., Holbrook, T., Cumitta, B., Land, V. J., Sexauer, C., and Krischer, J.: Toxicity trials of amsacrine (AMSA) and etoposide +/- azacitidine (AZ) in childhood acute non-lymphocytic leukemia (ANLL): a pilot study. Invest. New Drugs, 9:181, 1991.

125. Sznol, M., Ohnuma, T., and Holland, J. F.: Hepatic toxicity of drugs used for hematologic neoplasia. Semin. Liver Dis., 7:237, 1987.

126. Talcott, J., and Herman, T. S.: Acute ischemic vascular events and cisplatin. Ann. Intern. Med., 107:122, 1987.

127. Talmadge, J. E.: Therapeutic potential of cytokines: a comparison of preclinical and clinical studies. Prog. Exp. Tumor Res., 32:154, 1988.

128. Tolman, K. G.: Hepatotoxicity of antirheumatic drugs. J. Rheumatol. Suppl., 22:6, 1990.

129. Torti, F. M., Bristow, M. R., Howes, A. E., Aston, D., Stockdale, F. E., Carter, S. K., Kohler, M., Brown, B. W., and Billingham, M. E.: Reduced cardiotoxicity of doxorubicin delivered on a weekly schedule. Ann. Intern. Med., 99:745, 1983.

130. Torti, F. M., Bristow, M. M., Lum, B. L., Carter, S. K., Howes, A. E., Aston, D. A., Brown, B. W., Hannigan, J. F., Meyers, F. J., Mitchell, E. P., and Billingham, M. E.: Cardiotoxicity of epirubicin and doxorubicin: assessment by endomyocardial biopsy. Cancer Res., 46:3722, 1986.

131. Trump, D. L., Tutsch, K. D., Willson, J. K. V., Remick, S., Simon, K., Alberti, D., Grem, J., Loeller, J., and Tormey, D. C.: Phase I clinical trial and pharmacokinetic evaluation of acodazole (NSC 305884), an imidazoquinoline derivative with electrophysiological effects on the heart. Cancer Res., 47:3895, 1987.

132. Tung, J. P., and Maibach, H. I.: The practical use of methotrexate in psoriasis. Drugs, 40:697, 1990.

133. Unverferth, D. V.: Evaluation of anthracycline-induced cardiotoxicity. Cancer Treat. Symp., 3:67, 1984.

134. Villani, F., Comazzi, R., Genitoni, V., Lacaita, G., Guindani, A., Crippa, F., Monti, E., Piccinini, F., Rozza, A., Lanza, E., and Favalli, L.: Preliminary evaluation of myocardial toxicity of 4'-deoxydoxorubicin: experimental and clinical results. Drugs Exptl. Clin. Res., 11:223, 1985.

135. Villani, F., Galimberi, M., Comazzi, R., Crippa, F., Bonfante, V., Ferrari, L., and Pacciarini, M. A.: Clinical evaluation of the cardiac toxicity of 4'-deoxy-doxorubicin. Int. J. Clin. Pharmacol. Ther. Toxicol., 26:185, 1988.

136. Von Hoff, D. D., Layard, M. W., Basa, P., Davis, H. L., Jr., Von Hoff, A. L., Rozencweig, M., and Muggia, F. M.: Risk factors for doxorubicin-induced congestive heart failure. Ann. Intern. Med., 91:710, 1979.

137. Wagstaff, A. J., Ward, A., Benfield, P., and Heel, R. C.: Carboplatin: a preliminary review of its pharmacodynamic and pharmacokinetic properties and therapeutic efficacy in the treatment of cancer. Drugs, 37:162, 1989.

138. Warrell, R. P. Jr., and Berman, E.: Phase I and II study of fludarabine phosphate in leukemia: therapeutic efficacy with delayed central nervous system toxicity. J. Clin. Oncol., 4:74, 1986.

139. Watson, A. R., Rance, C. P., and Bain, J.: Long term effects of cyclophosphamide on testicular function. Br. Med. J., 29:1457, 1985.

140. Waxman, J., Terry, Y., Rees, L. H., and Lister, T. A.: Gonadal function in men treated for acute leukaemia. Br. Med. J., 287:1093, 1983.

141. Weiss, R. B., Posada, J. G., Kramer, R. A., and Boyd, M. R.: Nephrotoxicity of semustine. Cancer Treat. Rep., 67:1105, 1983.

142. Zaret, B. L., Schwartz, P. E., Berger, H. J., and Schwartz, R. G.: Evaluation of doxorubicin cardiotoxicity with radionuclide angiocardiography at rest. Cancer Treat. Symp., 3:61, 1984.

doxorubicin-induced cardiac toxicity in women with advanced breast cancer. N. Engl. J. Med., 319:745, 1988.

XVI

Chemotherapeutic Agents

XVI-1

Folate Antagonists

Joseph R. Bertino
Antonella Romanini

Introduction

Folate antagonists act as antineoplastic agents by interfering with one or more biosynthetic steps involving folate coenzymes of the tumor cell. Theoretically, a folate antagonist might act in one of several ways, e.g., competition with folates for uptake into cells, inhibition of the formation of folate coenzymes, or inhibition of one or more reactions that are folate coenzyme-mediated. Thus far, however, all the clinically important folate antagonists that have been developed appear to act primarily by inhibiting the enzyme dihydrofolate reductase (DHFR) of the neoplastic cell, thereby inhibiting the formation of the coenzyme tetrahydrofolate. During recent years several folate antagonists that target different folate requiring enzymes have been developed and are now in clinical trial (vide infra).

The availability of crystalline pteroylglutamic acid (PGA, folic acid), resulting from a series of research efforts involving several research groups, prompted investigators to test this compound as well as its diglutamate and triglutamate form for possible antineoplastic activity. It was soon recognized that administration of these substances was not only ineffective, but possibly even accelerated the course of the disease of patients with chronic myelocytic leukemia and acute leukemia.[74,96] Efforts to treat these leukemias thus turned to creating folate deficiency, and some encouraging results were obtained through use of folate-deficient diets, either alone or in combination with a weak folate antagonist, "x-methyl" folic acid (probably 7-methyl PGA). Soon after, aminopterin (4-amino-4-deoxy PGA) was synthesized and found by Farber and his co-investigators to be effective in producing remissions in acute leukemia.[74] This demonstration was a landmark in cancer chemotherapy: it provided the first demonstration that an antimetabolite could be an effective antineoplastic agent, and provided the stimulus for the development of other antimetabolites as possible antitumor agents.

Since the initial study demonstrating the usefulness of aminopterin in the treatment of acute leukemia of childhood, there has been a sustained interest in, and a continued re-evaluation of this and other folate antagonists. In studies with mice bearing the L1210 leukemia, methotrexate (4-amino-4-deoxy-10-methyl PGA; amethopterin) (MTX) was found to have a more favorable therapeutic index than aminopterin, and during the past decade, MTX has largely supplanted aminopterin in the clinic. In recent years an ever broadening use for MTX has evolved: This drug has been used not only for the treatment of neoplastic diseases, but also for the treatment of certain non-neoplastic conditions, e.g., rheumatoid arthritis, generalized psoriasis and as an immuno-suppressive agent.[5,215,246,267] Although details of therapeutic use are given elsewhere in this text, the broad spectrum of use of this drug deserves emphasis. MTX is the drug of choice in the treatment of choriocarcinoma, where its use provided the first demonstration of drug cure of cancer, and approximately 50% of these patients appear to be cured with the use of MTX alone. MTX is used in curative combination regimens to treat patients with acute lymphocytic leukemia (ALL) and lymphoma, and in combination regimens to treat advanced breast cancer, bladder cancer and cancer of the head and neck. The drug is also used in high dose with leucovorin (LV) rescue as a component of adjuvant therapies for breast cancer and osteosarcoma. In addition to the clinical usefulness of MTX and other folate antagonists, knowledge of the mechanism of action and the pharmacology of these agents has yielded important additional dividends in terms of information on important principles of cancer chemotherapy and mechanism of drug resistance of general applicability to all types of antineoplastic agents. MTX, the prototype folate antagonist, has probably been studied as intensively as any drug employed in present-day clinical medicine.

Chemistry

The two clinically studied 4-aminofolate antagonists, MTX and aminopterin (Figure XVI-1-1), resemble pteroylgluta-

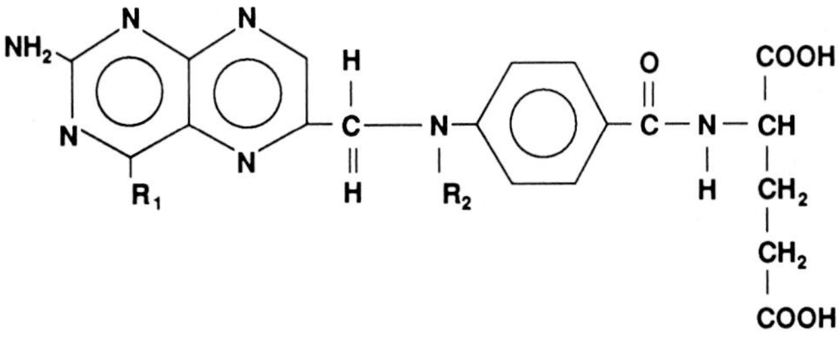

	R_1	R_2
Folic Acid	OH	H
Aminopterin	NH_2	H
MTX	NH_2	CH_3

Figure XVI-1-1. Structure of folic acid (PGA), aminopterin, and MTX.

Table XVI-1-1. Absorption Maxima (nm) and Molar Extinction Coefficients (ϵ) of Aminopterin and Methotrexate in 0.1 N Sodium Hydroxide Solution

Aminopterin		MTX	
λ_{max}	$\epsilon \times 10^{-3}$	λ_{max}	$\epsilon \times 10^{-3}$
(nm)		(nm)	
260	28.5	257	23.0
284	26.2	302	22.4
370	8.5	370	7.0

mate in many of their physical and chemical properties.[217,218] The free acids form yellow or yellowish-orange microcrystals, and are practically insoluble in most organic solvents and sparingly soluble in water. The disodium salts are extremely water-soluble, however, and are the most convenient form for parenteral administration. Like pteroylglutamic acid, the folic acid antagonists decompose without melting at about 200°C. Both antagonists have characteristic absorption spectra in ultraviolet and visible region, convenient for identification and for quantitation. The absorption maxima for aminopterin and MTX in dilute alkaline solution (0.1 N sodium hydroxide) are listed in Table XVI-1-1. Aminopterin, like folic acid, gives a positive Bratton-Marshall reaction after reductive cleavage at the C^9-N^{10} bond; MTX however, having a methyl substituent on the N^{10}-nitrogen, does not yield a primary aromatic amine on cleavage, and thus does not give this color reaction. Alkaline hydrolysis of aminopterin in the absence of oxygen results in deamination at the 4-position, yielding folic acid. Like the parent compound, pteroylglutamate, both compounds are subject to reduction of the pyrazine ring to the dihydro and tetrahydro stage by the use of reducing agents such as sodium hydrosulfite and sodium borohydride; unlike pteroylglutamate, however, they do not appear to undergo such reduction in vivo. If protected from light both compounds are stable for several days in aqueous solution as the sodium salts; however, on prolonged storage in solution, they undergo both cleavage and condensation reactions. For most purposes, the purity of commercial preparations is adequate if solutions are freshly prepared. For studies in which a high degree of purity is required, purification treatment by high performance liquid chromatography or other means is advisable.[189,210,255]

Mechanism of Action

MTX powerfully inhibits a key enzyme in the thymidylate cycle, dihydrofolate reductase (DHFR (Figure XVI-1-2)).[181,190] The formation of thymidylate is a key step in the synthesis of DNA, and is the only folate coenzyme-mediated one carbon transfer reaction in which dihydrofolate, rather than tetrahydrofolate, is the product. Regeneration of tetrahydrofolate is accomplished by DHFR, thus allowing thymidylate and purine biosynthesis to continue. In rapidly dividing cells, inhibition of thymidylate biosynthesis leads to a decrease in thymidine triphosphate pools, a decrease in DNA synthesis, and eventually cell death.[32,86,252] Inhibition of tetrahydrofolate formation leading to inhibition of purine synthesis and rapid cell death has been described to occur in lymphoblasts treated with high doses of MTX.[5,107]

Important to the present understanding of MTX action is the concept that MTX in molar excess to the target enzyme, DHFR, is required to shut off tetrahydrofolate synthesis.[228,265] Although the binding of MTX is essentially stoichiometric under ideal conditions (i.e., pH 6.0 and low levels of substrate), in the intact cell, the pH is higher, and blockade of the enzyme results in elevated levels of dihydrofolate and its polyglutamates, thus decreasing the binding of inhibitor to the enzyme.[17,177,264] Inasmuch as DHFR is in excess in most cells, only a small fraction of the total enzyme need remain catalytically functional to maintain the intracellular reduced folate pool.[5,16]

In recent years, the important role of polyglutamylation as a determinant in MTX sensitivity has been elucidated (Figure XVI-1-3).[88,90,119,129,139,140,151,157,211,215,266] A single enzyme, folylpolyglutamate synthetase, appears to be responsible for adding glutamates in gamma-carboxyl linkage to both folate coenzyme and methotrexate and other analogs with a glutamate moiety.[36-38,41,165,175,176] This enzyme process by which up to 7 or 8 additional glutamate molecules are added to folate coenzymes or MTX, serves to add additional negative charges to these molecules, and thus efflux is markedly reduced.[9] In addition, MTX polyglutamates bind as tightly to DHFR as MTX, and may dissociate less rapidly than MTX.[40,127,145] Certain human cancer cell lines naturally resistant to MTX, especially to short term exposures, have been found to have a low capacity to form long chain MTX polyglutamates.[48,49] In addition, fresh human tumor cells from patients with acute myelocytic leukemia and soft tissue sarcoma, tumors usually refractory to MTX therapy, are unable to form long chain MTX polyglutamates.[149] MTX polyglutamates are also potent inhibitors of other folate requiring enzymes including glycinamide ribonucleotide (GAR) and aminoimidazole carboximide ribonucleotide (AICAR) transformylases and thymidylate synthase.[5] Dihydrofolate polyglutamates, and the formylated form of this coenzyme (10-formyl dihydrofolate), which increase after MTX blockage of DHFR, are also potent inhibitors of thymidylate synthase and GAR transformylase.[5,11]

Biologic Activity

Inhibition of DNA synthesis by MTX and its polyglutamate forms results in "megaloblast" or giant cell formation, followed by cell death with continued inhibition. Mammalian cells require reduced folate coenzymes for replication, and it is perhaps not surprising that MTX is capable of preventing DNA synthesis in both normal and neoplastic cells.

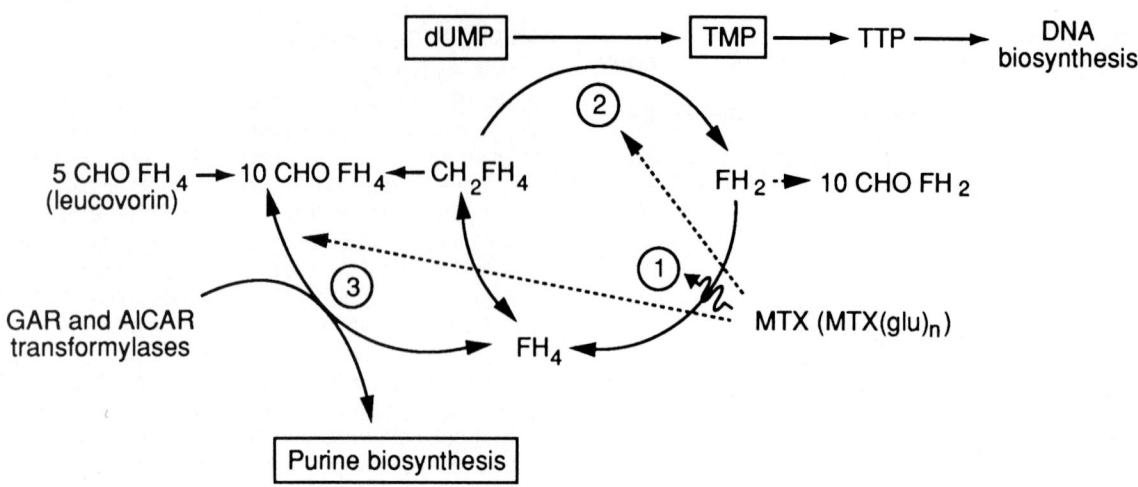

Figure XVI-1-2. Sites of action of MTX and MTX polyglutamates (MTX(glu)$_N$). MTX and its polyglutamates are potent inhibitors of DHFR (1); in addition MTX polyglutamates and dihydrofolate polyglutamates (FH$_2$(glu)$_N$) are also inhibitors of thymidylate synthase (2) and GAR and AICAR transformylase (3). Abbreviations used are FH$_2$, dihydrofolate; FH$_4$, tetrahydrofolate; CH$_2$FH$_4$, N^5, N^{10}-methylene tetrahydrofolate; 10 CHOFH$_4$, 10-formyl tetrahydrofolate; 5CHO-FH$_4$, 5 formyl tetrahydrofolate (leucovorin, folinic acid); dUMP, deoxyuridylate; TMP, thymidine-monophosphate; TTP, thymidine triphosphate.

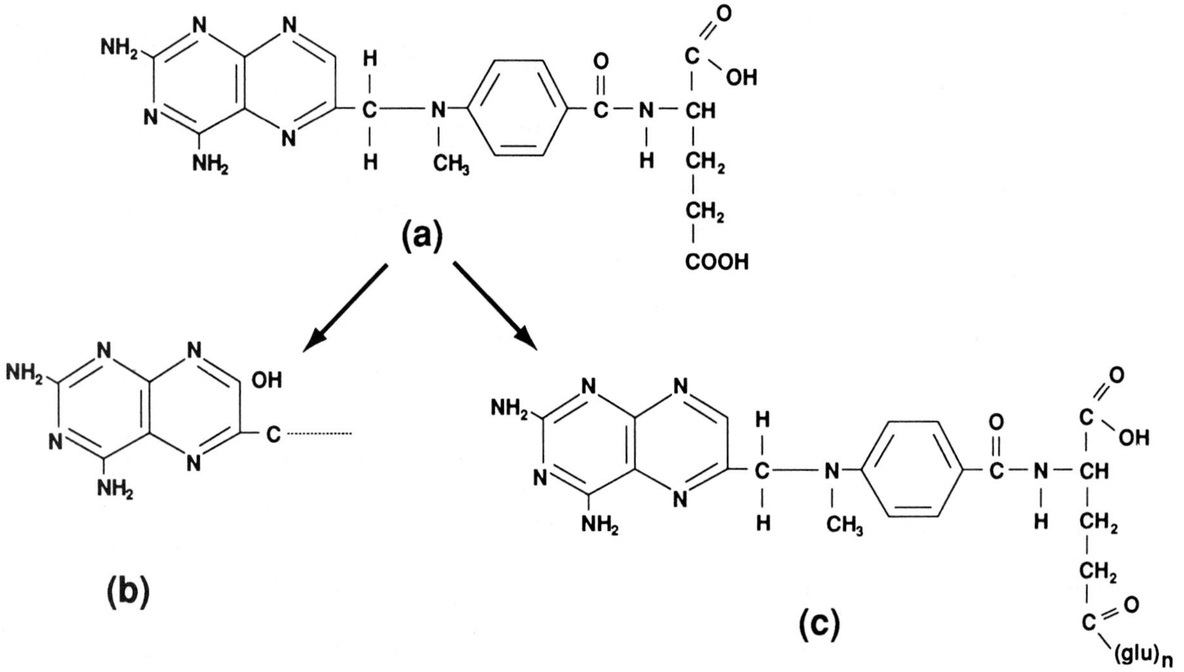

(a)

(b)

(c)

Figure XVI-1-3. Catabolism of MTX. (a) Methotrexate; (b) Liver converts MTX to 7-OH MTX; (c) Bowel bacteria convert MTX to DAMPA (see text).

As a result of the inhibition of DNA synthesis, cell populations are reduced by MTX in proportion to the dose of drug administered and to the duration of exposure to the drug in relation to the growth kinetics of the cell.[193] A cell population that has relatively few "resting" or G$_0$ cells and that accumulates MTX readily as a consequence of polyglutamylation, will be severely affected by a dose of MTX delivered over a period exceeding the generation time of the cell population, assuming the drug gets to the target site in sufficient concentration to inactivate the enzyme.[78,109] A cell population with a large number of G$_0$ cells would be less affected by

the same concentration and time of exposure to MTX, if this G$_0$ fraction is able to enter the proliferating pool when the drug is removed. Thus MTX, like other inhibitors of DNA synthesis, is most effective when it is employed in the treatment of neoplastic disease characterized by rapidly growing populations with a small percentage of cells in the resting or G$_0$ phase. Some selectivity, and thus successful use of this drug in certain cancers, has attended the use of high intermittent pulses of the drug, which has little effect on bone marrow and the gastrointestinal tract, organs which, if normal, are characterized by having a substantial number of stem cells "out of cycle" or in the so-called G_0 state. This relative kinetic selectivity may be lost when either the bone marrow or gastrointestinal mucosa is compromised by previous X-ray or drug therapy, or infiltration with tumor cells or infection.

The effectiveness of MTX against certain tumors (e.g., carcinoma of breast, osteogenic sarcoma) is difficult to explain on the basis of a rapid growth rate. In the latter condition, high dose therapy appears to be necessary, with LV (folinic acid, citrovorum) rescue. High plasma levels of MTX may lead, by passive diffusion, to a greater intracellular concentration of the drug, resulting in polyglutamate formation. The process results in retention of a high concentration of MTX polyglutamates, thus leading to prolonged inhibition of DHFR. In contrast, normal gut and marrow progenitor cells appear to have limited capacity to polyglutamate and thus retain MTX.[71,143]

Other factors that may modify the activity of MTX, in addition to the growth rate of the tumor and retention via polyglutamylation, are the transport characteristics of MTX into cells, its interaction with DHFR, and the rate of turnover of this enzyme.[142,215,227,228] In cells with a rapid turnover of enzyme and limited ability to form MTX polyglutamates, e.g., acute granulocytic leukemia blasts, an increase in DHFR may occur, presumably due to decreased degradation of this protein because MTX and MTX polyglutamates are bound to it.[18] These cells may be able to withstand exposure to MTX because this increase in inhibitor bound DHFR leads to generation of free enzyme as MTX (Glu_2 or less) rapidly effluxes from cells as the plasma concentration decreases.

Structure-Activity Relationships

The relationships between structure of folate antagonists and their antitumor activity have been ably summarized, and the relationship between structure and tightness of binding to the DHFR has also been comprehensively reviewed and discussed.[166-168,180,269] Differences between DHFR from mammalian and non-mammalian species, including differing susceptibility to enzyme inhibitors, have been extensively studied, and have led to development of effective antibacterial and antiprotozoal agents.[104,215,245]

A great many inhibitors of DHFR have been described which, unlike aminopterin and MTX, show little or no resemblance to the classic 4-amino-4-deoxypteroylglutamate structure. These include the lipid-soluble antimalarial pyrimethamine (Daraprim), 2,4-diamino-5-(3',4'-dichlorophenyl)-6-methyl-pyrimidine (DDMP), "Baker's antifol" (triazinate), and two compounds now in phase II clinical trials, trimetrexate and piritrexim (Figure XVI-1-4). These "nonclassical" inhibitors bind tightly to this enzyme via hydrophobic interaction as well as via the 2,4-diaminopyrimidine motif.[215]

Resistance To Antifolates

Although the development of effective chemotherapeutic regimens including MTX has significantly improved the therapy of a variety of malignancies (Table XVI-1-2), achieving actual cures is still difficult even in chemotherapy-sensitive diseases. The two problems that represent the major obstacles to the effective treatment of neoplastic disease with MTX as well as with most other antineoplastic agents are toxicity and resistance. Resistance to MTX can be either natural or

Table XVI-1-2. Sensitivity of Neoplastic Diseases to MTX

Sensitive[a]	Moderately Sensitive[b]	Not Sensitive
Acute lymphocytic leukemia	Head and neck cancer	Acute myelocytic leukemia
Burkitt's lymphoma	Breast cancer	Colon cancer
Choriocarcinoma	Bladder cancer	Renal cell cancer
Diffuse large cell lymphoma		

[a]Cures disease or is part of curative regimen.
[b]Greater than 15% response.

may be acquired after initial response to the drug.[149,234] Resistance to antifolates is also observed in bacteria and protozoa and often limits the usefulness of these drugs as anti-infectives.[215]

Acquired Resistance To MTX

Along with natural resistance, acquired drug resistance remains a major obstacle to effective chemotherapy. For example, 90% of patients with ALL achieve a complete remission with drug combinations that include MTX. However, 5-year disease-free survival rates are only 50–60%. Retreatment of these patients with the same agents is less effective because of the development of drug resistance.

Four major mechanisms of resistance to MTX have been described in experimental tumors: An increase in DHFR activity due to amplification of this gene, a decrease in uptake of MTX either due to a decreased influx or a decrease of long chain polyglutamate formation, or a mutation that results in an altered DHFR with decreased binding to DHFR.[5,16] Other mechanisms for MTX resistance are also possible, however.[133]

Amplification of the DHFR gene resulting in increased levels of the enzyme has been identified as a common mechanism of acquired MTX resistance. Since the original description of DHFR gene amplification in MTX-resistant mouse tumor cells,[7] a number of mouse, hamster, and human MTX-resistant cell lines have been described with increased DHFR and amplification of the DHFR gene as a mechanism of MTX resistance.[43,79,200,239] Unstable or reversible resistance due to gene amplification has usually been associated with the presence of "double minute" or centromereless chromosomes containing the DHFR amplicon, while high level stable resistance has been associated with an abnormal banding region, often referred to as a homogenous staining region (HSR).[13,135-137] It has also been demonstrated that gene amplification occurs in some patients treated with MTX, although the relative frequency of this event in patients whose tumors are resistant to MTX is not known.[29,47,105,257]

Transport resistance as well as gene amplification is often found as the mechanism of acquired resistance in experimental systems.[80,206,214] MTX utilizes the reduced folate carrier system for influx, and uptake is a function of both influx and efflux, as well as polyglutamylation, that leads to retention.[34,55,88,99-101,183,184] The relationship between the reduced folate carrier system and a folate binding protein present in some epithelial cells is not clear.[131]

Although defects in polyglutamylation have been described in several MTX-resistant cell lines, the resistance of these cells has usually been found to be due to a combination of mechanisms.[44,207] Recently, cell lines have been described that are resistant to MTX solely due to impaired polyglutamylation.[196] These cells were obtained by a more clinically relevant selection schedule consisting of short-term, high

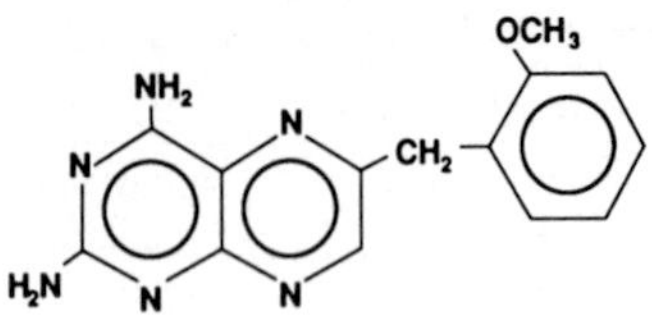

Pyritrexim

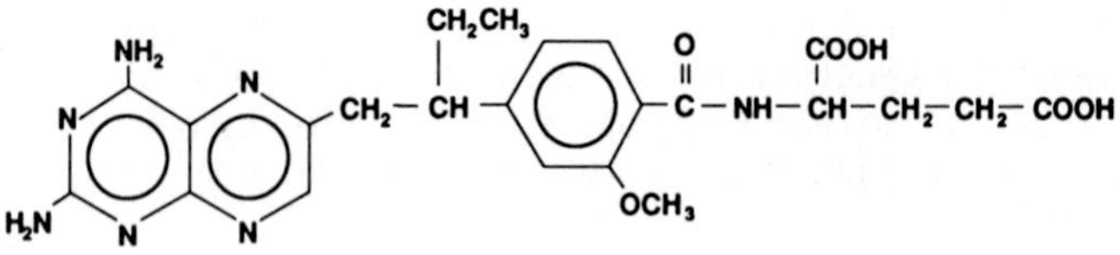

10-Ethyl, 10-Deaza-aminopterin

(10-EDAM)

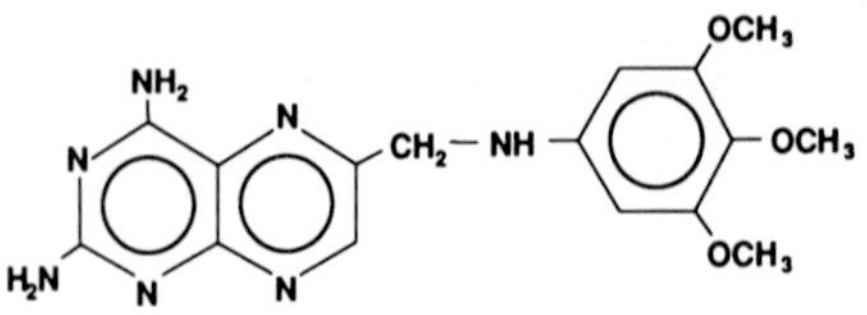

Trimetrexate

Inhibitors of Dihydrofolate Reductase

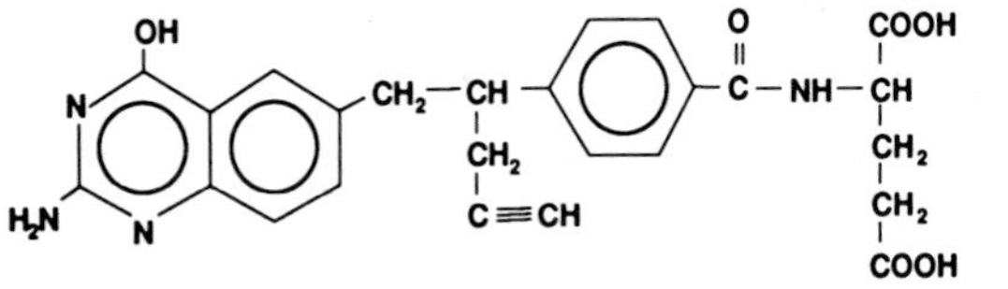

5, 10, Deaza, 10-Propargylfolic acid

(CB3717)

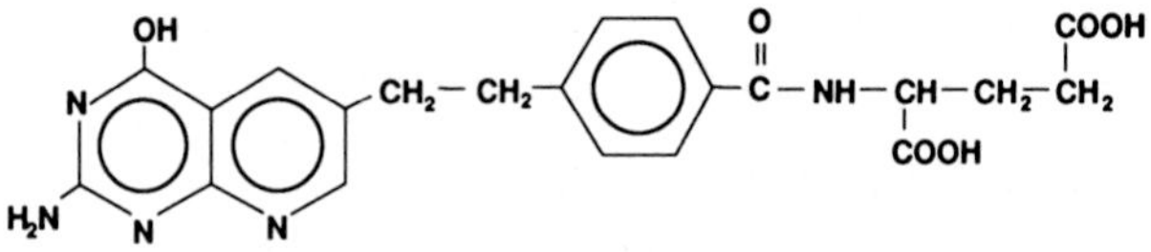

5, 10-Dideazatetrahydrofolate

(DDTHF)

Inhibitors of other Folate Enzymes

Figure XVI-1-4.   New folate antagonists of current interest.

dose treatments with MTX rather than to continuous exposure to this drug. Recent studies have indicated that the basis of the defect in these cells is an alteration in the enzyme folyl-polyglutamate synthetase.[162]

Although several MTX-resistant cell lines have been found to possess an altered DHFR that has a decreased affinity for MTX, only few altered human DHFRs have been characterized in any detail.[53,54,58,82,93,94,118,170,171,239] Point mutations in several cell lines, including human cells, have been detected that cause a change in the binding of MTX to the enzyme, and have usually involved amino acids that bind to the inhibitor by hydrophobic interaction.[215] Evidence for mutations in the gene for DHFR as a mechanism for resistance in blast cells from patients has not yet been documented, but sensitive methodology (polymerase chain reaction, amplification of DHFR cDNA) to allow sequencing and detection of possible mutations has only been recently avail-

able.[56,215] It may be possible to develop antifolates with specificity for altered DHFR enzymes.[52,188,215] These efforts will be guided by a detailed knowledge of the structure of this enzyme, and its interaction with substrates and inhibitors.[158-160,197,215,257] It may be also possible to convert normal marrow to a state of resistance to MTX by transfection with an altered DHFR in a viral vector.[114,268]

Pharmacokinetics of MTX

Absorption. In contrast to older studies that demonstrated good absorption at low doses of MTX , recent studies have emphasized the relatively poor and unpredictable nature of absorption of this drug after oral administration.[10,35,98,133,237] The extent of absorption may be <50%, even at low doses ($\leq$15mg/m^2). Absorption decreases with increasing oral doses. Following oral administration, peak plasma concentrations may occur 1–5 hours after a dose (15–30 mg/m^2). Food, non-absorbable antibiotics, bile salts and a shortened intestine transit time may decrease the rate and extent of MTX absorption.[209,241] The marked intra- and interpatient variability of MTX absorption may explain the wide variation in oral doses of MTX observed in leukemia patients in remission required to maintain the WBC between 2,000 and 4,000 µL. Therefore, while oral use of MTX is convenient, IM or SC administration may be preferable since absorption from these routes is complete.

Distribution. After IV administration, MTX distributes within an initial volume approximately of 18% (0.18 L/kg of body weight), with a variable steady state volume of 40–80% of body weight.[112,222] The distribution phase (α) t1/2 is 30–45 min, the renal clearance phase (β) t1/2 is 3–4 hrs, and the t1/2 of the third phase, representing reabsorption from the gut and excretion, is 6–20 hrs.[222,241] MTX binding to plasma proteins, especially to albumin, is approximately 50%.[240] The 7-hydroxymetabolite of MTX is 90% bound to plasma proteins, but apparently does not interfere with MTX binding to plasma proteins at concentrations found in patients. The highest tissue to plasma concentrations found in man are in liver and kidney, followed by the gastrointestinal tract. Higher plasma levels in man, as compared to the mouse, are attributed to less rapid excretion in the bile and by the kidney, and a longer residue time in the small intestine.[32,144,248,249] Prolonged plasma levels after high dose MTX infusions in man have been attributed to decreased transit rate secondary to gastrointestinal obstruction.

Patients with pleural or peritoneal effusions may be at increased risk for developing toxicity to high dose MTX as a result of "third spacing", or MTX trapping in the infusion, and slow release leading to sustained MTX concentrations in serum.[261] This phenomenon is more of a problem when high doses of the drug are administered. In these circumstances higher doses and prolonged rescue with leucovorin may be necessary, until the serum level of MTX decreases to $<5 \times 10^{-8}$ M.

After high doses of MTX (>6 gm/m^2), serum concentrations in the range of 10^{-3} to 10^{-4} M are achieved.[1,5,15,25,70,75,141] At these concentrations, the active transport of this drug is saturated, limiting further influx of drug to passive diffusion. These high extracellular MTX concentrations inhibit the uptake of reduced folates, including exogenous administered LV, explaining the need for larger doses of LV to reverse MTX action, because of the competitive nature of this interaction at the transport level. Selectivity to high dose MTX regimens likely depends on the intracellular concentration of MTX achieved in the tumor, and subsequent polyglutamylation and retention. Bone marrow and intestinal mucosa have a limited capacity to retain MTX, explaining in part the selectivity of this drug for certain tumors. Even with intravenous administration, there is a wide range in the area under the plasma curve (AUC) produced by a given dose in patients.[24,68,70,141]

The passage of MTX from plasma to cerebrospinal fluid (CSF) is poor, and MTX does not achieve cytocidal concentrations in the CSF ($\geq 5 \times 10^{-8}$ M) after conventional doses (15–30 mg/m^2).[67,69,221] CSF concentrations after MTX administration are dose related, and cytocidal levels are obtained with doses of 500 mg/m^2 and higher. After high dose systemic MTX administration, lumbar CSF and ventricular CSF concentrations were similar. When MTX is given by the lumbar route into the CSF, it distributes unreliably into the ventricles while MTX given by a indwelling ventricular shunt provides reproducible therapeutic drug concentrations ($>10^{-6}$ M) for at least 48 hrs.[169] An improved dose schedule utilizing administration of multiple small doses of MTX has been suggested.[20] Following intrathecal administration, MTX slowly exits into the systemic circulation with a t1/2 of 8–10 hrs.[23] The pharmacology of intrathecal methotrexate may be altered by overt meningeal leukemia, and efflux may be impaired.

Among experimental agents, DDMP is highly lipid soluble and crosses the blood-brain barrier readily giving high CNS levels.[103] Other antifolates including trimetrexate and piritrexim are only poorly transported into the CNS.[115]

The clinical observation that irradiation followed by MTX treatment may predispose patients to neurotoxicity (*vide infra*) may be a consequence of the effect of radiation therapy on the blood brain barrier.[247]

Metabolism. The major metabolite of MTX is 7-hydroxy MTX (Figure XVI-1-3).[65,147,235,243] This hydroxylation process is due to hepatic aldehyde oxidase, and results in a much less active form of MTX, as it is only one percent as potent an inhibitor of DHFR as is MTX.[73,125,126,198] The 7-hydroxymetabolite is less water soluble than MTX, and may contribute to the renal toxicity frequently seen after high doses of the antifolate.[120]

A second less important pathway of metabolism of MTX occurs in the intestine, and the drug is hydrolysed by bacteria to the pteroate (4-amino-4-deoxy-N^{10}-methyl pteroic acid, DAMPA) and glutamic acid (Figure XVI-1-3).[60,258] DAMPA, like 7-OH MTX, is also a relatively inactive metabolite with approximately 1/200th the affinity of MTX for DHFR. DAMPA excretion in the urine accounts for only a small percentage of the dose administered ($<5\%$).

As mentioned, the third metabolic product of MTX that occurs via intracellular conversion is polyglutamylation. MTX polyglutamates are at least as potent inhibitors of DHFR as MTX, and have a slower rate of disassociation from DHFR than does MTX.[127] MTX polyglutamates are not found in plasma or urine because of the activity of hydrolase(s) (conjugase) in plasma that convert folyl and MTX polyglutamates to monoglutamates. Like MTX, 7-OH MTX is also polyglutamylated intracellularly, and retention of these polyglutamate forms could contribute to MTX cytotoxicity.[72,164,199]

Biliary Excretion. Following IV administration of doses of 30 to 80 mg/m^2, 0.4–20% of the administered dose can be recovered in bile and less than 10% of MTX is recovered in the feces collected over 24 hrs.[45,186,247] The enterohepatic recycling of MTX has been estimated using the D-isomer as a reference marker for non-absorbable drug.[97]

Inadvertent Drug Interactions

Several drugs used in cancer patients, including antibiotics, may increase toxicity when used with MTX, and should be avoided if possible.[115,116] Obviously, drugs that increase the possibility of bleeding in patients who are at risk of thrombocytopenia should be avoided, e.g., aspirin. During recent years deleterious and even fatal reactions have been reported between MTX and non-steroidal anti-inflammatory drugs, in particular with Naproxen and Ketoprofen.[8,51,226,254] This increased toxicity may be due to decreased renal elimination, possibly due to competition for renal secretion.[110] Other commonly used organic drugs may also potentiate MTX toxicity, such as phenylbutazone, salicylate and probenecid.[3,150] Probenecid increased the efficacy of MTX in tumor bearing mice, but it has not been used clinically with this goal in mind.[230,231]

Increased toxicity has also been reported when trimethoprim, the antibacterial agent, has been used together with MTX; presumably this antifolate, with only weak binding affinity to mammalian DHFR, lowers folate stores, especially in patients with subclinical folate deficiency, making marrow cells more susceptible to MTX-induced toxicity.[155,256] Alcohol should also be avoided in patients receiving MTX because of the risk of hepatic fibrosis and cirrhosis.

Clinical Application

Clinical Dosage Schedules

MTX has been administered in a variety of dosage schedules, since its introduction into the clinic over 30 years ago (Table XVI-1-3). Remarkably, there are few carefully controlled studies comparing different dose regimens. The importance of dose scheduling has been recently emphasized by an experimental study showing that resistance to high dose pulse MTX may not extend to continuous low dose exposure.[196] Tumor cells capable of long chain MTX polyglutamate formation may be more selectively treated with high dose pulse MTX; examples are ALL, and possibly some osteosarcomas and head and neck cancers.[255] The marked sensitivity of choriocarcinoma to MTX has also been attributed to the ability of this tumor to form and retain long chain MTX polyglutamates.[5] The relative lack of toxicity of normal renewal tissues to high dose MTX regimens with LV rescue may reflect the inability of progenitor cells from these tissues to form long chain polyglutamates of MTX.[71,143]

Optimum dose scheduling of MTX is complicated by the use of this drug in combination, thus making generalizations as to what dose schedule is best, difficult. Sequencing appears to be important when MTX is used with 5-fluorouracil (5-FU) (24 hr pretreatment with MTX appears to be best), with l-asparaginase (again 24 hr pretreatment is best), and probably with cytosine arabinoside (concurrent treatment may be optimal) and 6-mecaptopurine (pretreatment with MTX may be optimal). Table XVI-1-4 summarizes the use of drug combinations that include MTX.

Current Uses for MTX in the Treatment of Neoplastic Disease

Acute Leukemia. Although aminopterin was initially used as a single agent to induce remissions in children with acute leukemia, MTX is now used as part of combination regimens to treat this disease, especially as treatment during remission, and as intrathecal administration for prophylaxis of, as well for treatment of meningeal leukemia. Early studies by the Acute Leukemia B Group showed that twice weekly therapy (20 mg/m²) was superior to continuous daily oral administration for treatment during remission.[2] Other dose schedules appear to be even more beneficial, including 5 day courses administered every 3–4 weeks, or high dose regimens with LV rescue.[75,83,85] Methotrexate and L-asparaginase and MTX/6-mercaptopurine combinations are now commonly employed as part of the treatment of ALL.[111,153,271] Optimum use of these two combinations requires adequate dosing and correct sequencing.[28,147]

MTX has limited value in the treatment of acute non-lymphocytic leukemia. High dose regimens with LV rescue have a transient but rapid effect on the peripheral blood count without producing marrow remissions in the large majority of these patients.[15,108] The lack of efficacy of this drug in this disease has been attributed to poor retention of the drug due to lack of polyglutamylation, and an increase of the target enzyme DHFR following treatment with this drug.[18,149]

Lymphoma. Based on phase II studies that indicated that high doses of MTX with LV rescue could produce transient regressions in patients with large cell lymphoma, MTX in high doses (200 mg/m²–3 gm/m²) with LV rescue have been added to combination regimens for intermediate grade and high grade lymphomas.[201] In certain of these regimens (M-BACOD), MTX is used with LV during the leukopenic phase of drug treatment, since the MTX/LV combination has little marrow toxicity.[223] Based on experimental studies showing that MTX and cytosine arabinoside produce additive and possibly synergistic effects, this combination has also been utilized in regimens to treat this disease (e.g., COMLA; cyclophosphamide, vincristine, methotrexate, cytosine arabinoside and LV).[14,62]

Choriocarcinoma. This neoplasm is unique in that single drug treatment with either MTX or actinomycin D produces a substantial number of cures.[102] The basis for the unusual sensitivity of this tumor to MTX is not entirely clear, but choriocarcinoma cells may accumulate and retain this drug effectively by synthesizing long chain polyglutamates.[5] Single agent curative treatment with intensive 5 day courses of MTX has not resulted in secondary neoplasias in long term survivors.[208] Thus MTX is not considered to be carcinogenic. Current programs for the treatment of this malignancy utilize

Table XVI-1-3.   Dosage Schedules Used for MTX

	Comment
I. Oral Use	*Comment*
a. Daily continuous (5–10 mg/day)	Not used anymore
b. Weekly, biweekly (15–25 mg in single or divided doses)	Used mainly to treat psoriasis or rheumatoid arthritis
c. Twice weekly (20–30 mg/m²)	Used in maintainance treatment of ALL
II. Parenteral Use	*Comment*
a. Pulse weekly (IV) 30–60 mg/m²	"Conventional dose" MTX
Daily × 5 days 10–20 mg/m²	Used to treat choriocarcinoma, maintainance in ALL
b. Weekly intermediate dose MTX (120–500 mg/m²), or as part of *m* BACOD given between cycles (200 mg/m²), or as a modulating agent (24 h before 5FU, 240 mg/m²). In FAMTX combination, MTX (1000 mg/m²) is used as modulating agent, followed in one hour by 5FU (1500 mg/m²)	Requires leucovorin "rescue," 10–15 mg/m² q 6h for 6-8 doses beginning 24–42 h after MTX
c. High dose MTX (greater than 500 mg/m²)	Used in treatment of osteosarcoma (adjuvant) and in ALL. (See Table XVI-1-5)

Table XVI-1-4. Combination Chemotherapy with Methotrexate

Used With	Result
5-Fluorouracil	Synergistic if MTX precedes 5-fluorouracil by 24 h[19,59,76,80,156,185,270]
L-Asparaginase	Synergistic if MTX precedes L-asparaginase by 24 h (null and T cell leukemia); antagonizes MTX action if used together[28,111,128,153,271]
Cytosine arabinoside	Additive or synergistic if used together[14,62]
6-Mercaptopurine	Sequencing may be important (MTX increases 6MP nucleotide levels)[22]
Cyclophosphamide	Additive cytotoxicity if used together[212]
Cisplatin	MTX should precede cisplatin because of renal toxicity of cisplatin
Corticosteroids	Synergistic when used together in treatment of ALL
Vinca alkaloids	Additive effects when used together[33,89,91,146,262]
Bleomycin	Additive effects when used together; mucosal cell toxicity increased[233]
Anthracyclines	Additive effects when used together

MTX in combination with other drugs, especially for "poor risk" patients.[179]

Breast Cancer. MTX as a single agent causes regressions of this tumor in approximately 30% of patients. No single dose schedule has emerged as the optimum treatment when the drug is used as a single agent, including high dose treatment with LV rescue. When used with fluorouracil, sequential use of this combination has improved response rates to 50%, and this sequential combination has improved disease free survival when used as adjuvant therapy (see also XXXII).[81] The most frequently used combination regimen to treat advanced breast cancer, and as adjuvant therapy, is cyclophosphamide, MTX and 5-FU (CMF).

Gastrointestinal Cancer. MTX as a single agent has limited effectiveness in the treatment of GI malignancies. Its role in the treatment of these diseases is mainly to modulate and possibly improve the effectiveness of 5-FU. In the treatment of gastric cancer, an alternating regimen of doxorubicin with high dose MTX followed by high dose 5-FU and LV rescue has resulted in a 35% response rate with 10% long time survivors. Data from recent trials using this sequence in colon cancer emphasizes the need for a 7–24 hr interval between MTX and 5-FU administration, presumably to optimize increases in phospho-ribosyl-pyrophosphate (PRPP) that occur as a consequence of MTX inhibition of purine biosynthesis, to increase FU nucleotide formation (*vide supra*).[27,156,185,270] The sequential use of MTX followed by 5-FU 24 hours later has increased the response rate over that of 5-FU alone, with results comparable to other regimens that "modulate" 5-FU activity with less or comparable toxicity.[156]

Genitourinary Cancer. MTX (100 mg/m^2) without or with high doses (>0.5 gm/m^2) with LV rescue is clearly active in the treatment of advanced bladder cancer. The response rate reported (*ca* 30%) is similar to the response rate of the other most active single drug, cisplatin. Combinations of drugs including MTX with cisplatin, vinblastine and doxorubicin (M-VAC) has resulted in a substantial number of long term clinical remissions.[242] This combination is now being further modified and tested as predefinitive (neoadjuvant) treatment in an attempt to improve cure rates of patients with bladder cancer, and possibly to avoid cystectomy.

Head and Neck Cancer. MTX and cisplatin are the two most active single agents for the treatment of patients with advanced carcinoma of the head and neck region. High dose MTX regimens with LV rescue appear to improve response rates from 30 to 50%, but remission duration and survival are not improved.[26] MTX has also been used with 5-FU in this disease, and response rates of 50–60% have been reported, but the sequence and timing of drug administration has not been shown to affect the response rate, although different patterns of toxicity were observed.[26]

Lung Cancer. MTX as a single agent in conventional doses, or in high doses with LV rescue, has only marginal activity in non-small cell lung cancer.[236] This drug does have activity in small cell lung cancer, and has been used in combination regimens to treat this disease (see XXVIII-2).

Osteogenic Sarcoma. After studies were reported indicating that high dose MTX with LV rescue could cause regressions in patients with advanced osteogenic sarcoma, the drug was tested as adjuvant therapy in patients with disease following resection of the tumor with encouraging results.[121,122] Recent randomized trials of pre- and post-definitive treatment have demonstrated the beneficial effect of chemotherapy that includes high dose MTX with LV rescue.[63,152]

Adverse Effects

Hematologic Toxicity. Tissues that are self renewing, i.e., the bone marrow and epithelial cells, are at highest risk for damage by the folate antagonists. Bone marrow progenitor cells of all lineage are affected by MTX, but neutropenia usually predominates. Recovery after a single dose is usually rapid, occuring 14–21 days following a nadir that occurs 10 days after drug administration. The effects on marrow are dose related, but there is considerable variability encountered between patients. Subclinical folate deficiency usually due to poor nutrition, impaired renal function (pre-treatment with cisplatin is a risk factor); and a stressed marrow due to previous x-ray treatment, chemotherapy or infection may predispose patients to hematologic (and gastrointestinal) toxicity to this drug. Young patients usually tolerate this drug better than older individuals, presumably related to clearance of the drug by the kidneys. The administration of LV, before 42 hours have elapsed, if given in appropriate dose, may prevent or lessen MTX toxicity, and allow larger doses of the antifolate to be administered.[15,146]

Gastrointestinal Toxicity. Mucositis is a common side effect of MTX treatment, and usually is manifest 3–5 days following a dose or course of the drug. This is an early sign of MTX toxicity, and the drug should be discontinued when it occurs. Subsequent doses should not be increased unless the mucositis is grade 1 or less. More severe gastrointestinal toxicity is manifest by diarrhea, which may progress to severe bloody diarrhea. When this occurs in association with neutropenia, these patients are at high risk of sepsis and death. These patients should be hospitalized and managed vigorously with fluids and antibiotics. These severe side effects usually occur in a setting of renal damage, usually a consequence of high doses of MTX, but may also occur in patients treated with conventional doses. MTX blood levels and serum creatinine levels should be followed, and appropriate doses of LV administered, along with the supportive measures instituted (*vide infra*). Nausea and vomiting, even with high doses of MTX is usually mild to moderate, and most patients will not require antinausea medication.

Renal Toxicity. Conventional dose MTX regimens, not requiring LV, were occasionally reported to cause renal toxicity, presumably as a direct effect of MTX on renal tubular epithelium.[42] With the introduction of high dose regimens requiring LV rescue, renal toxicity leading to delayed MTX clearance and severe marrow and gastrointestinal toxicity and fatalities became a problem especially in adults. This toxicity is believed to be due to precipitation of MTX and its less soluble metabolite, 7-OH MTX, in the tubules, as well as a possible direct effect of this drug on the renal tubule.[120] The use of vigorous hydration and alkalinization of urine to increase solubility of MTX and 7-OH MTX has markedly ameliorated this problem. Occasional patients, even with this regimen (Table XVI-1-5), manifest renal impairment. Through careful monitoring of MTX and creatinine serum levels, these patients may be identified and larger doses and prolonged duration of LV employed to prevent toxicity.

Extremely high levels of MTX ($>1 \times 10^{-5}$ M) are difficult to rescue even with high doses of leucovorin.[1,5,192] Hemodialysis and peritoneal dialysis have proved ineffective in substantially lowering MTX plasma levels.[95] Charcoal hemoperfusion columns have been used successfully in a small number of patients.[57] Oral charcoal and cholestyramine have also been used to bind MTX in the gut, and limit enterohepatic recirculation and toxicity.[62,161] Thymidine ($1–3$ mg/m^2/day) is also capable of rescuing patients from MTX toxicity, but this metabolite is not generally available.[64,106,251] Car-

---

Table XVI-1-5. Regimen for High Dose MTX Treatment (>0.5 gm/m^2).[a] Prehydration and Alkalinization of Urine[b]

8-12 h before treatment, patients should receive 1.5 L/m^2 of saline or 5% glucose with 100 mEq HCO$_3^-$ and 20 mEq KCl/L. Continue until pH of urine is 7.0 or greater at time of MTX administration.

MTX Administration

(1) 0.5 gm to 3.0 gm/m^2 as 20–30 minute bolus. At 24 h begin leucovorin 15 mg/m^2 q 6 h × 6 doses.

(2) Jaffe regimen: 1.2–6 gm/m^2 over 6 h IV, with continued IV hydration for an additional 18 h. Begin leucovorin 2 h after end of MTX infusion, 15 mg/m^2 q 6 h × 7 doses.

(3) 36 hour infusion: MTX, 50 mg/m^2, is given as bolus, followed by infusion of MTX over 36 h at dose of 1.5 gm/m^2. Leucovorin rescue is started at end of infusion: 200 mg/m^2 over 12 h as infusion, then 25 mg/m^2 IM q 6 h × 6.

Drug Monitoring

MTX levels should be monitored at 24 hrs for regimen 1, or 48 h for regimens 2 and 3. Serum creatinine levels pretreatment and at 24 and 48 h should also be performed.

For regimen 1, 24 h levels of MTX of greater than 1×10^{-6}M require additional leucovorin rescue; for regimens 2 and 3, 48 h blood levels above 5×10^{-7}M should receive additional leucovorin rescue. The dose of leucovorin should be increased to 100 mg/m^2 q 6 h for blood levels of 1×10^{-6}M to 5×10^{-6}M; blood levels above 5×10^{-6}M should receive doses of 200 mg/m^2 or higher. Drug levels should be monitored daily, and leucovorin continued (in decreasing doses as the MTX blood levels fall), until the plasma concentration of MTX is below 1×10^{-8}M.

[a]See references 70,75,168,176,182,194,195,244.
[b]See references 1,5,9.

---

boxypeptidase G$_1$, an enzyme capable of cleaving the peptide bond in MTX resulting in glutamate and DAMPA (Figure XVI-1-3), has also been used to lower MTX levels, but DAMPA is even less soluble than MTX.[163] This enzyme has also been proposed for use as a "rescue" agent, based upon studies in experimental tumors.[31]

Hepatotoxicity. Chronic low dose continuous treatment with MTX has been associated with portal fibrosis and in some patients frank cirrhosis.[272] The basis for this liver damage is not known, but may be due to interference with choline synthesis; acute MTX hepatotoxicity in rats is reversed by choline administration.[84] Cirrhosis has been reported in patients with psoriasis, rheumatoid arthritis and ALL treated with long term continuous oral MTX.[154] Alcohol and other hepatotoxic drugs should be avoided in this patient population. Intermittent schedules with pulse therapy appear to decrease the incidence of fibrosis and cirrhosis.[50]

Acute elevations of liver enzymes (SGOT) commonly occur several days after treatment with high dose MTX, but rapidly return to normal, and do not appear to predict for chronic liver toxicity.[263]

Central Nervous System Toxicity. Although intrathecal MTX has been used extensively to treat patients with meningeal leukemia, its use has been associated with neurotoxicity, ranging from mild to severe. In cases of inadvertent overdosing (>100 mg), fatalities have been reported.

The most common side effect of intrathecal MTX administration, manifest by severe headache, fever, meningismus, vomiting and CSF pleocytosis, is thought to be due to a chemical arachnoiditis. Dosage adjustment or switching to cytosine arabinoside may be required if these symptoms persist.

More serious neurotoxicity has been observed in 5–10% of patients receiving 12–15 mg/m^2 of MTX intrathecally, consisting of motor paralysis of the extremities, cranial nerve palsies, seizures and even coma. Inasmuch as these signs occur mainly in adult patients with active meningeal disease, it is often difficult to distinguish these side effects from meningeal leukemia. This subacute toxicity usually occurs during the second or third week of intrathecal treatment, and has been attributed to slow CSF clearance of MTX.[20]

A severe chronic demyelinating encephalopathy has also been observed in children treated prophylactically with intrathecal MTX, and who have also received prophylactic cranial irradiation ($>2,000$ rads).[220] These patients develop dementia and limb spasticity, and even coma months or years after intrathecal MTX treatment. CT scans show cortical thinning, ventricular enlargement, and diffuse intracerebral calcifications.[191] Rarely, encephalopathy has been reported in patients treated only with high dose intravenous MTX. Acute transient cerebral dysfunction occurring several days after high dose systemic MTX treatment has also been reported; in these patients signs (paresis, aphasia, seizures) usually resolve within 2–3 days.[87,123]

In patients who receive a MTX overdose intrathecally (>100 mg), immediate CSF removal with ventriculumbar perfusion is indicated.[238] Recently, intrathecal use of carboxypeptidase G$_2$ has been shown to markedly decrease mortality in animals given a lethal dose of MTX intrathecally and may be the preferred treatment for this complication when available.[2a] Intrathecal or systemic LV is not indicated in these cases, since it is unlikely that this toxicity is due to inhibition of DHFR.

Pulmonary Toxicity. Although uncommon, pulmonary toxicity due to MTX has been described and has been noted even in patients receiving low-dose oral MTX for RA.[30,39,216,237] The clinical picture usually consists of cough, dyspnea, fever and hypoxemia. Chest x-ray films are nonspecific but show patchy interstitial infiltrates. Pneumocystis carinii must be ruled out, especially in patients also receiving steroids. Histologic examinations show diffuse interstitial lymphocytic infiltrates, giant cells, and noncaseating granulomas. In some patients a peripheral eosinophilia is observed, raising the possibility that this is an allergic pneumonitis. The process may progress to fibrosis, and it is important to discontinue the drug when pulmonary toxicity is reversible. Some patients have been retreated without recurrence of the problem.

Skin Toxicity. Skin toxicity to MTX occurs in 5–10% of patients, consisting of an erythematous rash, characteristically noted on the neck and upper trunk. The rash may be pruritic and relatively insignificant, and usually lasts for several days. In other instances, especially when related to other signs of severe MTX toxicity, it may progress to severe bullous formation and desquamation.[61]

Teratogenic and Mutagenic Effects. MTX is known to be a potent abortifacient, especially if administered during the first trimester of pregnancy. However, there is no indication of a higher than normal incidence of fetal abnormalities in women who have been successfully treated with MTX for choriocarcinoma. These women also have not had a higher than normal incidence of secondary malignancies. Thus far, there is no evidence that MTX has any mutagenic or carcinogenic effects.[219]

Miscellaneous Toxicity. Osteoporosis has been reported with chronic low-dose MTX administration.[178] Fever, seizures, recall of radiation toxicity or phototoxicity, and anaphylactoid reactions have been reported with high-dose administration.[92] Pleuritic and left upper quadrant pain, presumably due to splenic capsule inflammation, has been reported with a moderately high-dose regimen.

New Folate Antagonists Now in Clinical Trial

Inhibitors of DHFR. MTX is an extremely potent inhibitor of DHFR, and while it may be possible to develop inhibitors that are more tightly bound or may irreversibly inactivate this enzyme, unless these compounds possess other advantages, i.e., more avid uptake and/or more efficient retention by malignant cells vs. normal cells, selectivity may not improve. Two types of second generation folate antagonists are now in clinical trial, "classic" antagonists, i.e., whose structure resembles the metabolite folic acid, and "non-classic" agents, whose structure is markedly different than the substrate.

10-Ethyldeazaaminopterin (10-EDAM, Figure XVI-1-4), developed by Sirotnak and associates, was chosen for clinical trial after detailed structure activity studies demonstrated that hydrophobic substitutions at the N-10 position of aminopterin resulted in improved uptake and retention (polyglutamylation) by tumor cells as compared to normal cells.[212,232] The drug is now under active clinical investigation, and encouraging response rates have been noted in patients with non-small cell lung cancer, head and neck cancer, and breast cancer.[31,213,224] One limitation to its use may be that it may be relatively ineffective against MTX-resistant cells, since it utilizes the same carrier mechanism for transport, and is polyglutamylated by the same enzyme as is MTX.

In contrast, the non-classical antifolates, trimetrexate and piritrexim (Figure XVI-1-4), currently in phase II trials, are also potent inhibitors of DHFR, but enter cells by passive or facilitative diffusion rather than by the reduced folate transport carrier.[115,132,187,225] Consequently, these antifolates are still effective cytotoxic agents against MTX resistant cells if the mechanism of resistance is impaired transport, decreased polyglutamylation, or even low level amplification of DHFR.[134,172,202,203,253] Cells resistant to MTX due to a mutation in the enzyme leading to decreased binding of the inhibitor may or may not be cross-resistant to trimetrexate, depending on the nature of the mutation.[215] These drugs also differ from MTX in that they are not substrates for polyglutamate synthetase; therefore retention depends on other factors. Certain sensitive tumor cells appear to retain trimetrexate in concentrations that are in excess of that required to completely inhibit DHFR, after efflux in drug free medium. The mechanism of this retention has not been determined. Another intriguing possibility currently under investigation is that some human tumors may resemble the Pneumocystis organism in that they are unable to transport reduced folates and MTX well.[4] Similar to the approach currently being taken to treat Pneumocystis infections, co-administration of trimetrexate and LV would be non-toxic to the host, but could be cytotoxic to such tumors.[6,149,151]

Inhibitors of Other Folate Enzymes. During recent years, other targets for development of folate antagonists have been identified, including thymidylate synthase, GAR and AICAR transformylase, and methionine synthetase.[5] Potent inhibitors of thymidylate synthase and GAR transformylase have been synthesized, and are now under active investigation (Figure XVI-1-4). The quinazoline inhibitors, IAHQ and CB3717, both showed antitumor activity in experimental systems, and CB3717 also demonstrated activity in phase II clinical trials in breast and ovarian cancer, but renal and hepatic toxicity precluded further testing.[77,117,130]

Based on a series of structure-activity studies, and toxicity studies in animals, another analog (N-(5-[N-(3,4-dihydro-2-methyl-4-oxoquinolin-6-ylmethyl)-N-methylamino]-2-thenoyl)-L-glutamic acid (D1694) has been chosen for further clinical trials.[124] Of interest is that these drugs, even more so than MTX, are "pro-drugs," in that polyglutamylation increases cytotoxicity. The potential advantages of folate inhibitors of thymidylate synthase over 5-FU are that these agents are not incorporated into RNA, and that the increase in dUMP levels that may result as a consequence of inhibition of this enzyme might increase, rather than decrease, the inhibition of thymidylate synthase produced.[77]

5-10 Dideazatetrahydrofolate (DDTHF) is also undergoing clinical trials (Figure XVI-1-4). This drug is also a prodrug, and the addition of glutamates to the molecule markedly increases the inhibition of GAR transformylase.[12] DDTHF is extremely potent, and low doses of this agent have produced delayed and prolonged marrow suppression in early clinical trials, not predicted by rodent toxicity data.[46]

The identification of these and other folate mediated enzymes as targets for new folate inhibitors, and the demonstration of the antitumor properties of the compounds mentioned, have provided a new impetus for drug development in this field. This work undoubtedly will be guided by computer graphics using crystallographic data on these target enzymes.[215]

References

1. Ackland, S. P., and Schilsky, R. L.: High dose methotrexate: A critical reappraisal. J. Clin. Oncol., 5:2017, 1987.
2. Acute Leukemia Group B: New treatment schedule with improved survival in childhood leukemia. Intermittent parenteral versus daily oral administration of methotrexate for maintenance of induced remission. J.A.M.A., 194:75, 1965.

2a. Adamson, P. C., Balis, F. M., McCully, C. L., et al.: Rescue of experimental intrathecal methotrexate with carboxypeptidase G_2. J. Clin. Oncol., 9:670–674, 1991.

3. Aherne, G. N., Prall, E., Marks, V., Mould, G., and White, W. F.: Prolongation and enhancement of serum methotrexate concentrations by probenicid. B.M.J., 1:1097, 1978.
4. Alberto, P., Peytremann, R., Modenica, R., and Beretta-Piccoli, M.: Initial clinical experience with a simultaneous combination of 2-4-diamino 5 (3′,4′-dichlorophenyl)6-methyl pyrimidine (DDMP) with folinic acid. Cancer Chemother. Pharmacol., 1:101, 1978.
5. Allegra, C. J.: Antifolates. *In* Cancer Chemotherapy: Principles and Practice. Edited by B.A. Chabner and J.M. Collins. Philadelphia, J.B. Lippincott, 1990, p. 110.
6. Allegra, C. J., Chabner, B. A., Tuazon, C. U. Ogata-Araki, D., Baird, B., Drake, J. C., Simmons, J. T., Lack, E. E., Shelhamer, J. H., and Balis, F.: Trimetrexate, a novel and effective agent for the treatment of pneumocystis carinii pneumonia in patients with acquired immunodeficiency syndrome. N. Engl. J. Med., 317:978, 1987.
7. Alt, F. W., Kellems, R. E., Bertino, J. R., and Schimke, R. T.: Selective multiplication of dihydrofolate reductase genes in methotrexate-resistant variants of cultured murine cells. J. Biol. Chem., 253:1357, 1978.
8. Badr, M.Z., and Theresa, S.C.: Potentiation of methotrexate induced gastrointestinal toxicity by non-steroidal anti-inflammatory drugs (NSAIDs) and vincristine. Toxicology, 29:333, 1985.
9. Balinska, M., Galivan, J., and Coward, J. K.: Efflux of methotrexate and its polyglutamate derivatives from hepatic cells in vitro. Cancer Res., 41:2751, 1981.
10. Balis, F. M., Savitch, J. L., and Bleyer, W. A.: Pharmacokinetics of oral methotrexate in children. Cancer Res., 43:2342, 1983.
11. Baram, J., Chabner, B. A., Drake, J. C., Fitzhugh, A. L., Sholar, P. W., and Allegra, C. J.: Identification and biochemical properties of 10-formyl dihydrofolate, a novel folate found in methotrexate-treated cells. J. Biol. Chem., 263:7105, 1988.
12. Beardsley, G. P., Moroson, B., Taylor, E. C., and Moran, R. G.: Deaza derivatives of tetrahydrofolic acid: A new class of folate antimetabolite. J. Biol. Chem., 264:328, 1989.
13. Beidler, J. L., and Spengler, B. A.: Metaphase chromosome anomaly: Association with drug resistance and cell-specific products. Science, 191:185, 1976.
14. Berd, D., Cornog, J., DeConti, R. C., Levitt, M., and Bertino, J. R.: Long term remission in diffuse histiocytic lymphoma treated with combination sequential chemotherapy. Cancer, 35:1050, 1975.
15. Bertino, J. R.: "Rescue" techniques in cancer chemotherapy: Use of leucovorin and other rescue agents after methotrexate treatment. Semin. Oncol., 2:203, 1977.
16. Bertino, J. R.: The General Pharmacology of Methotrexate. *In* Methotrexate Therapy in Rheumatic Diseases. Edited by W. S. Wilke. New York, Marcel Dekker, Inc., 1989, p. 11.
17. Bertino, J. R., Boothe, B. A., Cashmore, A., Bieber, A. L., and Sartorelli, A. C.: Studies of the inhibition of dihydrofolate reductase by the folate antagonists. J. Biol. Chem., 239:479, 1964.
18. Bertino, J. R., Sawicki, W. L., Cashmore, A. R., Cadman, E. C., and Skeel, R. T.: Natural resistance to methotrexate in human acute non-lymphocytic leukemia. Cancer Treat. Rep., 61:667, 1977.
19. Bertino, J. R., Sawicki, W. L., Lindquist, C. A., and Gupta, V. S.: Schedule dependent antitumor effects of methotrexate and 5-fluorouracil. Cancer Res., 37:327, 1977.
20. Bleyer, W. A., Drake, J. C., and Chabner, B. A.: Neurotoxicity and elevated cerebrospinal fluid methotrexate concentration in meningeal leukemia. N. Engl. J. Med., 289:770, 1973.
21. Bleyer, W. A., Poplack, D. G., and Simon, R. M.: "Concentration × time" methotrexate via a subcutaneous reservoir: A less toxic regimen for intraventricular chemotherapy of central nervous system neoplasms. Blood, 51:835, 1978.
22. Bokkerink, J. P. M., Bakker, M. A. H., Hulscher, T. W., and De Abreu, R. A.: Purine de novo synthesis as the basis of synergism of methotrexate and 6-mercaptopurine in human malignant lymphoblasts of different lineages. Biochem. Pharmacol., 37:2321, 1988.
23. Bode, U., Magrath, I. T., Bleyer, U. A., Poplack, D. G., and Glaubiger, D. L.: Active transport of methotrexate from cerebrospinal fluid in humans. Cancer Res., 40:2184, 1980.
24. Borsi, J. D., and Moe, P. J.: Systemic clearance of methotrexate in the prognosis of acute lymphoblastic leukemia in children. Cancer, 60:3020, 1987.
25. Borsi, J. D., Sager, E., Romelo, I., and Moe, P. J.: Rescue after intermediate and high-dose methotrexate. Pediatric Hematology and Oncology, 7:347, 1990.
26. Browman, G. P., Levine, M. N., Goodyear, M. D., Russell, R., Archibald, S. D., Jackson, B. S., Young, J. E. M., Basrur, V., and Johanson, C.: Methotrexate-fluorouracil scheduling influences normal tissue toxicity but not antitumor effects in patients with squamous cell head and neck cancer: Results from randomized trial. J. Clin. Oncol., 6:963, 1988.
27. Cadman, E., Heimer, R. and Davis, L.: Enhanced 5-fluorouracil nucleotide formation after methotrexate administration. Explanation for drug synergism. Science, 205:1135, 1979.
28. Capizzi, R. L.: Schedule-dependent synergism and antagonism between methotrexate and L-asparaginase. Biochem. Pharmacol., 23: 151, 1974.
29. Carman, M. D., Schornagel, J. H., Rivest, R. S., Srimatkandata, S., Portlock, C. S., Duffy, T., and Bertino, J. R.: Resistance to methotrexate due to gene amplification in a patient with acute leukemia. J. Clin. Oncol., 2:16, 1984.
30. Carson, C. W., Cannon, G. W., Egger, J. M., Ward, J. R., and Clegg, D. O.: Pulmonary disease during the treament of rheumatoid arthritis with low-dose pulse methotrexate. Semin. Arthritis Rheum., 16:186, 1987.
31. Chabner, B. A., Johns, D. G., and Bertino, J. R.: Enzymatic cleavage of methotrexate provides a method for prevention of drug toxicity. Nature, 239:395, 1972.
32. Chabner, B. A., and Young, R. C.: Threshold methotrexate concentration for in vivo inhibition of DNA synthesis in normal and tumorous target issues. J. Clin. Invest., 52:1804, 1973.
33. Chello, P. L., and Sirotnak, F. M.: Increased schedule dependent synergism of vindisine versus vincristine in combination with methotrexate against L1210 leukemia. Cancer Treat. Rep., 65:1049, 1981.
34. Chello, P. L., Sirotnak, F. M., and Dorick, D. M.: Alterations in the kinetics of methotrexate transport during growth of L1210 murine leukemia cells in culture. Mol. Pharmacol., 18:274, 1980.
35. Chungi, V. S., Bourne, D. W. A., and Dittert, L. W.: Drug absorption: Kinetics of GI absorption of methotrexate. J. Pharm. Sci., 67:560, 1978.
36. Cichowicz, D. J. and Shane, B.: Mammalian folylpoly-γ-glutamate synthetase: 1. Purification and general properties of the hog liver enzyme. Biochemistry, 26:504, 1987.
37. Cichowicz, D. J. and Shane, B.: Mammalian folyl-γ-glutamate synthetase: 2. Substrate specificity and kinetic properties of the hog liver enzyme. Biochemistry, 26:513, 1987.
38. Clarke, L., and Waxman, D. J.: Human liver folylpolyglutamate synthetase: Biochemical characterization and interactions with folates and folate antagonists. Arch. Biochem. Biophys., 256:585, 1987.
39. Clarysse, A. M., Catney, W. J., Cartwright, G. E., and Wintrobe, M. M.: Pulmonary disease complicating intermittent therapy with methotrexate. J.A.M.A., 209:1861, 1969.
40. Clendeninn, N. J., Drake, J. C., Allegra, C. J., Welch, A. D., and Chabner, B. A.: Methotrexate (MTX) polyglutamates have a greater affinity and more rapid on-rate for purified human dihydrofolate reductase (DHFR) than MTX. Proceedings of the American Association for Cancer Research, 26:232, 1985.
41. Cook, J. D., Cichowicz, D. J., George, S., Lawler, A., and Shane, B: Mammalian folylpoly-γ-glutamate synthetase: 4. In vitro and in vivo metabolism of folates and analogues and regulation of folate homeostasis. Biochemistry, 26:530, 1987.
42. Condit, P. T., Chanes, R. E., and Joel, W.: The renal toxicity of methotrexate. Cancer, 23:126, 1969.
43. Cowan, K. H., Goldsmith, M. E., Levine, R. M., Aitken, S. C., Douglass, E., Clendenin, N., Neinhuis, A. W., and Lippman, M. E.: Dihydrofolate reductase gene amplification and possible rearrangement in estrogen-responsive methotrexate-resistant human breast cancer cells. J. Biol. Chem., 257:15079, 1982.
44. Cowan, K. H., and Jolivet, J.: A methotrexate-resistant human breast cancer cell line with multiple defects, including diminished formation of methotrexate polyglutamates. J. Biol. Chem., 259:10793, 1984.
45. Creaven, P. J., Hansen, H. H., Alfred, D. A., and Allen, L. M.: Methotrexate in liver and bile after intravenous dosage in man. Br. J. Cancer, 28:589, 1973.
46. Currie, V. E., Warrell, R. P., Arlin, Z., Tan, C., Sirotnak, F. M., Greene, G., and Young, C. W.: Phase I trial of 10-deaza-aminopterin in patients with advanced cancer. Cancer Treat. Rep., 67:149, 1983.
47. Curt, G. A., Carney, D. N., Cowan, K. H., Jolivet, J., Bailey, B. D., Drake, J. C., Chiensong, R. S., Minna, J. D., and Chabner, B. A.: Unstable methotrexate resistance in human small cell cancer associated with double minute chromosomes. N. Engl. J. Med., 308:199, 1983.
48. Curt, G. A., Jolivet, J., Bailey, B. D., Carney, D. N., and Chabner, B. A.: Synthesis and retention of methotrexate polyglutamates by human small cell lung cancer. Biochem. Pharmacol., 33:1682, 1984.
49. Curt, G. A., Jolivet, J., Carney, D. N., Bailey, B. D., Drake, J. C., Clendenin, N. J., and Chabner, B. A.: Determinants of the sensitivity of human small-cell lung cancer cell lines to methotrexate. J. Clin. Invest. 76:1323, 1985.
50. Dahl, M. G. C., Gregory, M. M., and Scheuer, P. J.: Methotrexate hepatotoxicity in psoriasis—comparison of different dose regimens. B.M.J., 1:654, 1972.
51. Daly, H., Boyle, J., Roberts, C., and Scott, G.: Interaction between methotrexate and non-steroidal antiinflammatory drugs. Lancet, 1:8480, 1986.
52. Dedhar, S., Freisheim, J. H., Hynes, J. B., and Goldie, J. H.: Further studies on substituted quinazolines and triazines as inhibitors of a methotrexate-insensitive murine dihydrofolate reductase. Biochem. Pharmacol., 35:1143, 1986.
53. Dedhar, S., and Goldie, J. H.: Overproduction of two antigenically distinct forms of dihydrofolate reductase in a highly methotrexate-resistant mouse leukemia cell line. Cancer Res., 43:4863, 1983.
54. Dedhar, S., Hartley, D., Fitz-Gibbons, D., Phillips, G., and Goldie, J. H.: Heterogeneity in the specific activity and methotrexate sensitivity of dihydrofolate reductase from blast cells of acute myelogenous leukemia patients. J. Clin. Oncol., 3:1545, 1985.
55. Dembo, M., Sirotnak, F. M., and Moccio, D. M.: Effects of metabolic deprivation on methotrexate transport in L1210 cells: Further evidence for separate influx and efflux systems with different energetic requirements. J. Membr. Biol., 78:9, 1984.
56. Dicker, A., Volkenandt, M., Adamo, A., Barreda, C., and Bertino, J. R.: Sequence analysis of a human gene responsible for drug resistance: A rapid method for manual and automated direct sequencing of products generated by the polymerase chain reaction. Biotechniques, 7:830, 1989.
57. Djerassi, I.: Removal of methotrexate by filtration absorption using charcoal filters or by hemodialysis. Cancer Treat. Rep., 61:751, 1977.
58. Domin, B. A., Cheng, Y., and Hakala, M. T.: Properties of dihydrofolate reductase from a methotrexate-resistant subline of human KB cells and comparison with enzyme from KB parent cells and mouse S180 AT/3000 cells. Mol. Pharmacol., 21:231, 1982.
59. Donehower, R. C., Allegra, J. C., Lippman, M. E., and Chabner, B. A.: Combined effects of methotrexate and 5-fluoropyrimidine on human breast cancer cells in serum-free cultures. Eur. J. Cancer, 16:655, 1980.
60. Donehower, R. C., Hande, K. R., Drake, J. C., and Chabner, B. A.: Presence of 2,4-diamino-N^{10}-methyl pteroic acid after high-dose methotrexate. Clin. Pharmacol. Ther., 26:63, 1979.
61. Doyle, L. A., Berg, C., Bottino, G., and Chabner, B. A.: Erythema and desquamation after high-dose methotrexate. Ann. Intern. Med., 98:611, 1983.
62. Edelstein, M., Vietti, T., and Valeriote, F.: The enhanced cytotoxicity of 1 β-D-arabinosylcytosine and methotrexate. Cancer Res., 35:1555, 1975.
63. Eilber, F., Guliano, A., Eckart, J., Patterson, K., Mosely, S., and Goodnight, J.: Adjuvant chemotherapy for osteosarcoma: A randomized prospective trial. J. Clin. Oncol., 5:21, 1987.
64. Ensminger, W. D., and Frei, E., III: The prevention of methotrexate toxicity by thymidine infusions in humans. Cancer Res., 37:1857, 1977.
65. Erttman, R., Bielack, S., and Landbeck, G.: Kinetics of 7-hydroxy-methotrexate after high-dose methotrexate therapy. Cancer Chemother. Pharmacol., 15:101, 1985.
66. Erttman, R., and Landbeck, G.: Effect of oral cholestyramine on the elimination of high-dose methotrexate. J. Cancer Res. Clin. Oncol., 110:48, 1985.
67. Ettinger, L. J., Chervinsky, D. S., Freeman, A., and Creaven, P. J.: Pharmacokinetics of methotrexate following intravenous and intraventricular administration in acute lymphocytic leukemia and non-Hodgkin's lymphoma. Cancer, 50:1676, 1982.
68. Evans, W. E., Crom, W. R., Abromowitch, M., Dodge, R., Look, A. T., Bowman, W. P., George, S. L., and Pui, C. H.: Clinical pharmacodynamics of high-dose methotrexate in acute lymphocytic leukemia: Identification of a relation between concentration and effect. N. Engl. J. Med., 314:471, 1986.
69. Evans, W. E., Hutson, P. R., Stewart, C. F., Cairnes, D. A., Bowman, W. P., Rivera, G., and Crom, W. R.: Methotrexate cerebrospinal fluid and serum concentrations after intermediate dose methotrexate infusion. Clin. Pharmacol. Ther., 33:301, 1983.

70. Evans, W. E., Pratt, C. B., Taylor, H., Barker, L. F., and Crom, W. R.: Pharmacokinetic monitoring of high-dose methotrexate. Cancer Chemother. Pharmacol., 3:161, 1979.
71. Fabre, I., Fabre, G., and Goldman, I. D.: Polyglutamylation, an important element in methotrexate cytotoxicity and selectivity in tumor versus murine granulocytic progenitor cells in vitro. Cancer Res., 44:3190, 1984.
72. Fabre, G., Fabre, I., Matherly, L. H., Cano, J. P., and Goldman, I. D.: Synthesis and properties of 7-hydroxymethotrexate polyglutamyl derivatives in Ehrlich ascites tumor cells in vitro. J. Biol. Chem., 259:5066, 1984.
73. Fabre, G., Seither, R., and Goldman, I. D.: Hydroxylation of 4-amino-antifolates by partially purified aldehyde oxidase from rabbit liver. Biochem. Pharmacol., 35:1325, 1986.
74. Farber, S., Diamond, L. K., Mercer, R. D., Sylvester, R. F., Jr., and Wolff, J. A.: Temporary remissions in acute leukemia in children produced by folic acid antagonist, 4-aminopteroyl-glutamic acid (aminopterin). N. Engl. J. Med., 238:787, 1948.
75. Favre, R., Monjanel, S., Alfonsi, M., Pradora, J. P., Bagarry-Liegey, D., Clement, S., Imbert, A. M., Lena, N., Colonida d'Istria, J., Cano, J. P., and Carcassonne, Y: High-dose methotrexate: A clinical and pharmacokinetic evaluation. Chemother. Pharmacol., 9:156, 1982.
76. Fernandes, D. J., Bertino, J. R., and Hynes, J. B.: Biochemical and antitumor effects of 5,8-dideazaisopteroylglutamate, a unique quinazoline inhibitor of thymidylate synthetase. Cancer Res., 43:1117, 1983.
77. Fernandes, D. J., Sur, P., Kute, T. E., and Capizzi, R. L.: Proliferation-dependent cytotoxicity of methotrexate in murine L5178Y leukemia. Cancer Res., 48:5638, 1988.
78. Fernandez, D. J., and Bertino, J. R.: 5-fluorouracil-methotrexate synergy. Enhancement of 5-fluorodeoxyuridylate binding to thymidylate synthase by dihydropteroylpolyglutamates. Proc. Natl. Acad. Sci, USA, 77:5663, 1980.
79. Fischer, G. A.: Increased levels of folic acid reductase as a mechanism of resistance to amethopterin in leukemic cells. Biochem Pharmacol., 7:75, 1961.
80. Fischer, G. A.: Defective transport of amethopterin (methotrexate) as a mechanism of resistance to the antimetabolite in L5178Y leukemic cells. Biochem. Pharmacol., 11:1233, 1962.
81. Fisher, B., Redmond, C., Dimitrov, N. U., Bowman, D., Legault-Poisson, S., Wickerham, D. L., Wolmack, N., Fisher, E. R., Margolese, R., Sutherland, C., Glass, A., Foster, R., and Caplan, R.: A randomized clinical trial evaluating sequential methotrexate and fluorouracil in the treatment of patients with node negative breast cancer who have estrogen receptor tumors. N. Engl. J. Med., 320:473, 1969.
82. Flintoff, W. F., and Essani, K.: Methotrexate-resistant Chinese hamster ovary cells contain a dihydrofolate reductase with an altered affinity for methotrexate. Biochemistry, 19:4321, 1980.
83. Frankel, L. S., Wang, Y. M., Shuster, J., Nitschke, R., Doering, E. J., and Pullen, J..: High dose methotrexate as part of remission maintenance therapy for childhood acute lymphocytic leukemia: A pediatric oncology group pilot study. J. Clin. Oncol., 1:804, 1983.
84. Freeman-Narrod, M., Narrod, S. A., and Custer, R. P.: Chronic toxicity of methotrexate in rats: Partial to complete protection of the liver by choline: Brief communication. J. Natl. Cancer Inst., 59:1013, 1977.
85. Frei, E., III, Blum, R. H., Pitman, S. W., Kirkwood, J. M., Henderson, I. C., Skarin, A. T., Mayer, R. J., Bast, R. C., Garnick, M. B., Parker, L. M., and Canellos, G. P.: High dose methotrexate with leucovorin rescue. Rationale and spectrum of antitumor activity. Am. J. Med., 68:370, 1980.
86. Fridland, A.: Effect of methotrexate on deoxynucleotide pools and DNA synthesis in human lymphocyte cells. Cancer Res., 34:1883, 1974.
87. Fritsch, G., and Urban, C.: Transient encephalopathy during the late course of treatment with high-dose methotrexate. Cancer, 53:1849, 1984.
88. Fry, D. W., Anderson, L. A., Borst, M., and Goldman, I. D.: Analysis of the role of membrane transport and polyglutamation of methotrexate in gut and Ehrlich tumor in vivo as factors in drug sensitivity and selectivity. Cancer Res., 43:1087, 1983.
89. Fry, D. W., Yalowich, J. C., and Goldman, I. D.: Augmentation of the intracellular levels of polyglutamyl derivatives of methotrexate by vincristine and probenecid in Ehrlich ascites tumor cells. Cancer Res., 42:25323, 1982.
90. Fry, D. W., Yalowich, J. C., and Goldman, I. D.: Rapid formation of poly-γ-glutamyl derivatives of methotrexate and their association with dihydrofolate reductase as assessed by high-pressure liquid chromatography in Ehrlich ascites tumor cell in vitro. J. Biol. Chem., 259:257, 1982.
91. Fyfe, M. J., and Goldman, I. D.: Characteristics of the vincristine-induced augmentation of methotrexate uptake in Ehrlich ascites tumor cells. J. Biol. Chem., 248:5067, 1973.
92. Goldberg, N. H., Romolo, J. L., Austin, E. H., Drake, J., and Rosenberg, S. A.: Anaphylactoid type reactions in two patients receiving high-dose intravenous methotrexate. Cancer, 41:52, 1978.
93. Goldie, J. H., Dedhar, S., and Krystal, G.: Properties of a methotrexate-insensitive variant of dihydrofolate reductase from methotrexate-resistant L5178Y cells. J. Biol. Chem. 256:11629, 1981.
94. Goldie, J. H., Krystal, G., Hartley, D. Gudauskas, G., and Dedhar, S.: A methotrexate-insensitive variant of folate reductase present in two lines of methotrexate-resistant L5178Y cells. Eur. J. Cancer, 16:1539, 1980.
95. Hande, K. R., Balow, D. E., Drake, J. C., Rosenberg, S. A., and Chabner, B. A.: Methotrexate and hemodialysis. Ann. Intern. Med., 87:495, 1977.
96. Heinle, R. W., and Welch, A. D.: Experiments with pteroylglutamic acid and pteroylglutamic acid deficiency in human leukemia. J. Clin. Invest., 27:539, 1948.
97. Hendel, J., and Brodthagen, H.: Entero-hepatic cycling of methotrexate estimated by use of the D-isomer as a reference marker. Eur. J. Clin. Pharmacol., 26:103, 1984.
98. Henderson, E. S., Adamson, R. H., and Oliverio, V. T.: The metabolic fate of tritiated methotrexate: 2. Absorption and excretion in man. Cancer Res., 25:1018, 1965.
99. Henderson, G. B., and Tsuji, J. M.: Methotrexate efflux in L1210 cells: kinetic and specificity properties of the efflux system sensitive to bromosulfophtalein and its possible identity with a system which mediates the efflux of 3′,5′-cyclic AMP. J. Biol. Chem., 262:13571, 1987.
100. Henderson, G. B., Tsuji, J. M., and Kumar, H. P.: Characterization of the individual transport routes that mediate the influx and efflux of methotrexate in CCRF-CEM human lymphoblastic cells. Cancer Res., 46:1633, 1986.
101. Henderson, G. B., Tsuji, J. M., and Kumar, H. P.: Transport of folate compounds by leukemic cells: evidence for a single influx carrier for methotrexate, 5-methyltetrahydrofolate, and folate in CCRF-CEM human lymphoblasts. Biochem. Pharmacol., 36:3007, 1987.
102. Hertz, R., Lewis, J. Jr., and Lipsett, M. B.: Five years experience with the chemotherapy of metastatic choriocarcinoma and related trophoblastic tumors in women. Am. J. Obstet. Gynecol., 82:631, 1961.
103. Hill, B. T., and Price, L. A.: DDMP (2,4-diamino-5-(3′,4′- dichlorophenyl)-methylpyrimidine. Cancer Treat. Rev., 7:95, 1980.
104. Hitchings, G. H., Burchall, J. J., and Ferone, R.: The comparative enzymology of dihydrofolate reductase and the design of chemotherapeutic agents. Symposium of the Society of General Microbiology, XVI:294, 1966.
105. Horns, R. C., Jr., Dower, W. J., and Schimke, R. T.: Gene amplification in a leukemic patient treated with methotrexate. J. Clin. Oncol., 2:2, 1984.
106. Howell, S. B., Ensminger, W. D., Krishan, A., and Frei, E., III: Thymidine rescue of high-dose methotrexate in humans. Cancer Res., 38:325, 1978.
107. Hryniuk, W. M.: Purineless death as a link between growth rate and cytotoxicity of methotrexate. Cancer Res., 32:1506, 1972.
108. Hryniuk, W. M., and Bertino, J. R.: Treatment of leukemia with large doses of methotrexate and folinic acid: Clinical-biochemical correlates. J. Clin. Invest., 48:2140, 1969.
109. Hryniuk, W. M., Fischer, G. A., and Bertino, J. R.: S-phase cells of rapidly growing and resting populations. Differences in response to methotrexate. Mol. Pharmacol., 5:557, 1969.
110. Huang, K. C., Wenczak, B. A., and Liu, Y. K.: Renal tubular transport of methotrexate in the rhesus monkey and dog. Cancer Res., 39:4843, 1979.
111. Hudson, M. M., Dahl, G. U., Kalminsky, D. K., and Pui, C. H.: Methotrexate plus asparaginase. An active combination for children with acute non-lymphocytic leukemia. Cancer, 65:2615, 1990.
112. Huffman, D. H., Wan, S. H., Azaranoff, D. L., and Hogstraten, B.: Pharmacokinetics of methotrexate. Clin. Pharmacol. Ther., 14:572, 1973.
113. Isacoff, W. H., Morrison, P. F., Aroessty, J., Willis, K. L., Block, J. B., and Lincoln, T. L.: Pharmacokinetics of high-dose methotrexate with citrovorum factor rescue. Cancer Treat. Rep., 61:1665, 1977.
114. Isola, L. M., and Gordon, J. W.: Systemic resistance to methotrexate in transgenic mice carrying a mutant dihydrofolate reductase gene. Proc. Natl. Acad. Sci. USA, 83:9621, 1986.
115. Iven, H., and Brasch, H.: Influence of the antibiotics piperacillin deoxycycline and tobramycin on the pharmacokinetics of methotrexate in rabbits. Cancer Chemother. Pharmacol., 17:218, 1986.
116. Iven, H., and Brasch, H.: The effects of antibiotics and uricosuric drugs on the renal elimination of methotrexate and 7-hydroxymethotrexate in rabbits. Cancer Chemother. Pharmacol., 21: 337, 1988.
117. Jackman, A. L., Jones, T. R., and Calvert, A. H.: Thymidylate Synthetase Inhibitors: Experimental and Clinical Aspects. *In* Experimental and Clinical Progress in Cancer Chemotherapy. Edited by F. Mussia. Boston, Martinus Nijhoff, 1985, p. 155.
118. Jackson, R. C., Hart, L. I., and Harrap, K. R.: Intrinsic resistance to methotrexate of cultured mammalian cells in relation to the inhibition kinetics of their dihydrofolate reductase. Cancer Res., 36:1991, 1980.
119. Jacobs, S. A., Derr, C. J., and Johns, D. G.: Accumulation of methotrexate diglutamate in human liver during methotrexate therapy. Biochem. Pharmacol. 26:2310, 1977.
120. Jacobs, S. A., Stoller, R. G., Chabner, B. A., and Johns, D. G.: 7-hydroxymethotrexate as a urinary metabolite in human subjects and rhesus monkeys receiving high dose methotrexate. J. Clin. Invest., 57:534, 1976.
121. Jaffe, N., Frei, E., III, Traggis, D., and Bishop, Y.: Adjuvant methotrexate and citrovorum-factor treatment of osteogenic sarcoma. N. Engl. J. Med., 291:994, 1974.
122. Jaffe, N., and Paed, D.: Recent advances in the chemotherapy of metastatic osteogenic sarcoma. Cancer, 30:1627, 1972.
123. Jaffe, N., Takaue, Y., and Anzai, T.: Transient neurologic disturbances induced by high-dose methotrexate treatment. Cancer, 56:1356, 1985.
124. Jodrell, D. I., Newell, D. R., Calvete, J. A., Stephens, T. C., and Calvert, A. H.: Pharmacokinetic and toxicity studies with the novel quinazoline inhibitor, D 1694. Proceedings of the American Association for Cancer Research, 31:341, 1990.
125. Johns, D. G., Iannotti, A. T., Sartorelli, A. C., Booth, B. A., and Bertino, J. R.: The identity of rabbit-liver methotrexate oxidase. Biochim. Biophys. Acta, 105:380, 1965.
126. Johns, D. G., and Loo, T. L.: The metabolite of 4-amino-4-deoxy- N^{10}-methylpteroylglutamic acid (methotrexate). J. Pharm. Sci. 56:356, 1967.
127. Jolivet, J., and Chabner, B. A.: Intracellular pharmacokinetics of methotrexate polyglutamates in human breast cancer cells: Selective retention and less dissociable binding of 4-NH_2-10-CH_3-pteroylglutamate$_4$ and 4-NH_2-10-CH_3-pteroylglutamate$_5$ to dihydrofolate reductase. J. Clin. Invest., 72:773, 1983.
128. Jolivet, J., Cole, D. E., Holcenberg, J. S., and Poplack, D. G.: Prevention of methotrexate cytotoxicity by asparaginase inhibition of methotrexate polyglutamate formation. Cancer Res., 45:217, 1985.
129. Jolivet, J., Schilsky, R. L., Bailey, B. D., Drake, J. C., and Chabner, B. A.: Synthesis, retention, and biological activity of methotrexate polyglutamates in cultured human breast cancer cells. J. Clin. Invest., 70:351, 1982.
130. Jones, T. R., Calvert, A. H., Jackman, A. L., Brown, S. J., Jones, M., and Harrap, K. R.: A potent antitumor quinazoline inhibitor of thymidylate synthetase: synthesis, biological properties and therapeutic results in mice. Eur. J. Cancer, 17:11, 1981.
131. Kamen, B. A., and Capdevila, A.: Receptor-mediated folate accumulation regulated by the cellular folate content. Proc. Natl. Acad. Sci. USA, 83:5983, 1986.
132. Kamen, B. A., Eibl, B., Cashmore, A., and Bertino, J. R.: Uptake and efficacy of trimetrexate (TMQ, 2,4-diamino-5-methyl-6-[3,4,5- trimethoxy-anilino)-methyl] quinazoline), a non-classical antifolate in methotrexate-resistant leukemia cells in vitro. Biochem. Pharmacol., 33:1697, 1984.
133. Kamen, B. A., Whyte-Bauer, W., and Bertino, J. R.: A mechanism of resistance to methotrexate: NADPH but not NADH stimulation of methotrexate binding to dihydrofolate reductase. Biochem. Pharmacol., 32:1837, 1983.
134. Kano, Y., Ohnuma, T., and Holland, J. F.: Folate requirements of methotrexate-resistant human acute lymphoblastic leukemia cell lines. Blood, 68:586, 1986.
135. Kaufman, R. J., Bertino, J. R., and Schimke, R. T.: Quantitation of dihydrofolate reductase in individual parental and methotrexate-resistant murine cells: Use of a fluorescence activated cell sorter. J. Biol. Chem., 253:5852, 1978.
136. Kaufman, R. J., Brown, P. C., and Schimke, R. T.: Loss and stabilization of amplified dihydrofolate reductase genes in mouse sarcoma S-180 cell lines. Mol. Cell. Biol., 1:1084, 1981.
137. Kaufman, R. J., and Schimke, R. T.: Amplification and loss of dihydrofolate reductase genes in a Chinese hamster ovary cell line. Mol. Cell. Biol., 1:1069, 1981.
138. Kearney, P. J., Light, P. A., Preece, A., and Mott, M. G.: Unpredictable serum levels after oral methotrexate in children with acute lymphoblastic leukemia. Cancer Chemother. Pharmacol., 3:117, 1979.
139. Kennedy, D. G., Van den Berg, H. W., Clark, R., and Murphy, R. F.: The effect of the rate of cell proliferation on the synthesis of methotrexate poly-gamma-glutamates in two human breast cancer cell lines. Biochem. Pharmacol., 34:3087, 1985.
140. Kennedy, D. G., van den Berg, H. W., Clarke, R., and Murphy, R. F.: The effect of leucovorin on the synthesis of methotrexate poly-gamma-glutamates in the MCF-7 human breast cancer cell line. Biochem. Pharmacol., 34:2897, 1985.
141. Kerr, I. G., Jolivet, J., Collins, J. M., Drake, J. C., and Chabner, B. A.: Test dose for predicting high-dose methotrexate infusions. Clin. Pharmacol. Ther., 33: 44, 1983.

Purine and Pyrimidine Antimetabolites

Robert E. Handschumacher
Yung Chi Cheng

Introduction

Development of purine and pyrimidine analogs as potential antineoplastic agents evolved from an early presumption that nucleic acids are involved in growth control. Among the first analogs produced and tested for biological activity were the 5-halogenated pyrimidines, 5-chloro, 5-bromo-, and 5-iodouracil. Although in original concept these agents were targeted toward the malarial parasite, G. H. Hitchings and his colleague G. B. Elion recognized that these compounds might be of value in the treatment of cancer, a disease then correctly perceived as a disease of inappropriate growth.[59,134] These early studies were primarily focused on the incorporation of analog nucleic acid bases into RNA or DNA of bacterial species.[89] Concurrent studies on the metabolic activation of these heterocycle analogs, as well as their biochemical targets for growth inhibition, and the study of resistance to them afforded many new insights into the intermediary metabolism responsible for the synthesis of DNA and RNA precursors. Subsequently it was recognized that control of these biosynthetic pathways afforded additional targets for therapeutic intervention.

Further development of these analogs was stimulated by the demonstration of quantitative, but not qualitative, differences in the activity of these pathways in normal versus neoplastic tissue. It was also realized that rapid catabolism of these agents to inactive compounds could severely limit anabolic conversion to fraudulent nucleotides. This in itself affords targets for modulation of cytotoxic activity on a tissue-specific basis.

A virtually complete understanding of the enzymes involved in the biosynthesis of purine and pyrimidine nucleotide precursors of RNA and DNA is now at hand.[107,155] This intricate matrix of metabolic reactions is under a complex web of positive and negative feedback controls. Since most purine or pyrimidine analogs are active only after metabolic activation to the nucleotide form, these fraudulent nucleotides may not only be incorporated but also can mimic the natural effector compounds in regulatory pathways. Alternatively, they may deplete critical intermediates, thereby generating enlarged pools of the natural precursors behind a metabolic block, effects that can cause a distortion of the balance of ribo- and deoxyribonucleoside triphosphates. A target of even greater complexity is the polymerization of triphosphates into DNA or RNA and subsequent modification of these macromolecules. It is the existence of subtle differences in the specificity and function of the polymerases that generates the selectivity of certain purine and pyrimidine nucleotides as anticancer and, more importantly, as antiviral agents.

It must be recognized that the demonstration of inhibition of specific enzyme reactions by analog pyrimidine or purine nucleotides does not assure that these reactions are rate limiting for tumor growth or are responsible for cytotoxicity to either normal or neoplastic tissues. Even though several inhibitory sites have been identified, some with greater apparent sensitivity than others, attribution of an effect to inhibition of a specific reaction in general is difficult. Similarly, analogs may be incorporated into nucleic acids and either inhibit subsequent replication cycles or result in miscoding, but these mechanisms must be balanced against activity of the DNA editing and repair reactions that can minimize the effects of incorporation.

In addition to purine and pyrimidine analogs, other agents have been developed that inhibit biosynthetic reactions that lead to the ultimate nucleic acid precursors. These include PALA, brequinar, acivicin, and hydroxyurea.

Another factor that may affect the action of nucleoside analogs is the rate and nature of transport systems for both normal and analog nucleosides in and out of host versus neoplastic tissues. A wide range of neoplastic cell lines have been shown to have a saturable system responsible for the facilitated diffusion of ribo- and deoxyribonucleosides.[223] This system essentially equilibrates the cytoplasm with the extracellular milieu. More recently, Na^+-dependent active transport systems for purine and pyrimidine nucleosides have been found in a variety of normal tissues.[68,173,253] In neoplastic cell lines and some tumors, the Na^+-dependent concentrative mechanisms, if they exist, are nullified by the facilitated diffusion mechanism. These effects are particularly evident with uridine which is 3–10-fold concentrated in normal tissues and may be responsible for the selectivity of some antimetabolites.

Pyrimidine Analogs

Fluorouracil

Background and Properties. A major motivation for the development of pyrimidine analogs of uracil was the early observation that preneoplastic rat liver and hepatomas more actively incorporated uracil than normal liver.[246] Although this may also reflect a difference in the relative degradative capacity of these different tissues for uracil, it provided a focus for the synthetic efforts of Dushinsky and Heidelberger that led to 5-fluorouracil (5-FU) (Figure XVI-2-1), and a family of related fluorinated pyrimidines.[81] This specific site of substitution on the pyrimidine ring was selected because it might inhibit the subsequent conversion of a uracil nucleotide to thymine nucleotides. Since insertion of the methyl group occurs on the 5-position, halogen replacement of hydrogen in that position was felt to have a greater chance of inhibiting DNA synthesis and thus growth. The selection of fluorine to replace the hydrogen in uracil was based on the similar Van der

Waals radii (F = 1.35 Å and H = 1.20 Å). Unlike earlier syntheses of halogenated pyrimidines that involved simple displacement of the hydrogen with the other halogens, chlorine, bromine or iodine, 5-FU was originally synthesized from an acyclic precursor. This synthesis permitted the formation of the corresponding 5-fluoroorotic acid; subsequently the ribosides and deoxyribosides of FU were prepared. More recently a direct means of fluorinating FU has been developed that permits positron emission tomography (PET) studies with 18F-FU (Figure XVI-2-1).[288]

As anticipated, the pKa of FU (8.1) is more acidic than is that of uracil (9.6); thus under physiological conditions, FU exists partially as an anionic species. This is undoubtedly important to the metabolic activation to the nucleotide form via the orotidylate pyrophosphorylase reaction. This uridylate analog, 5-fluorouridylic acid (FUMP), can then substitute for UMP in a wide spectrum of intermediary reactions. The product of one of these, fluorodeoxyuridylate (FdUMP) plays a major role by inhibiting displacement of hydrogen from the 5-position of deoxyuridylate and its replacement with a methyl group via a tetrahydrofolate catalyzed reaction.[247] Many of the properties predicted for FU were seen in early studies of bacterial and model tumor systems. A remarkably rapid progression to a clinical trial occurred within two years of its synthesis.[128] These early clinical studies showed enough promise in colon cancer and other solid tumors to sustain 35 subsequent years of further development. A primary focus of this research has been to reduce its very real toxicity for a variety of normal tissues while retaining antitumor activity. FU remains today an important component of the therapy of selected solid tumors, not only as a single agent but also in combination with agents that modulate directly or indirectly the metabolism of pyrimidine nucleotides.

Cellular Entry and Efflux Mechanisms. Limited evidence suggests that FU enters cells by a carrier-mediated transport mechanism. Early reports suggested that a specific mechanism for the transport of uracil existed in the intestine. These studies, however, used methods that made it difficult to distinguish between transport and metabolism. In the Novikoff hepatoma, evidence has been presented for a nonconcentrative transporter that exhibits competitive kinetics between uracil and FU.[291] Under conditions in which the FU ring is minimally ionized, enhanced entry of FU occurs if cells were preloaded with uracil, a result consistent with a counter transport mechanism. To date no evidence suggests that an alteration of FU entry into cells is responsible for natural or acquired resistance.

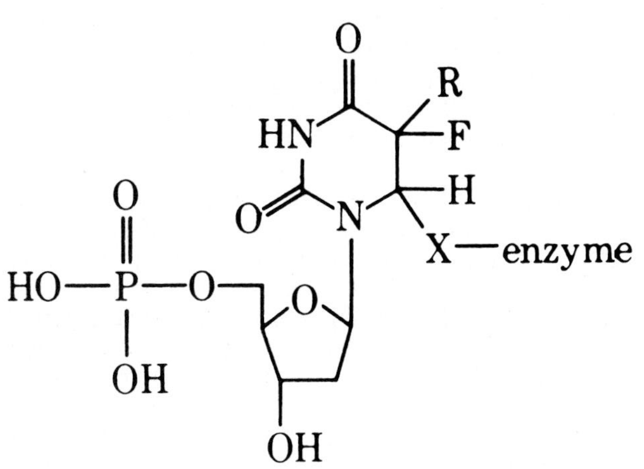

In contrast to FU, the entry of fluorodeoxyuridine (FdUrd) (Figure XVI-2-1) into most neoplastic cells involves the saturable but non-concentrative mechanism responsible for the facilitated diffusion of a wide spectrum of nucleosides.[27] This transporter has been quantified in several cell lines by titration with p-nitrobenzylthioinosine (NBMPR). The deletion of this transport mechanism is the basis for resistance to FdUrd[264] or to purine nucleoside analogs[43] in at least two cell lines. Such a deletion makes the cells collaterally sensitive to methotrexate and other inhibitors of thymidylate synthase since they are unable, or limited in their ability, to salvage thymidine, whether naturally available or administered.[265] Fluorouridine and FdUrd released from 5-fluorouridylic and 5-fluorodeoxyuridylic by phosphatase action exit the cell via this same facilitated diffusion transporter. Thus, agents that affect this transporter may selectively affect FU cytotoxicity by a differential effect on specific normal or neoplastic cell types. The facilitated diffusion mechanism may play a secondary role in the modulation of FU action in vivo by uridine since this normal nucleoside but not fluorouridine or fluorodeoxyuridine is actively concentrated by a Na+-dependent system.[70] Neoplastic cells appear to be less capable of this transport and are not protected.

Anabolism. Once inside the cell there are several possibilities for the activation of FU to nucleotide form. In normal tissues the predominant mechanism appears to be competition with orotate for the condensation with pyrophosphorylribose-5-PO4 (PRPP) via orotidylate pyrophosphorylase to form 5-fluorouridylate.[242] In mammalian cells, this protein is a bifunctional enzyme that also catalyzes the decarboxylation of orotidylate to 5'-uridylic acid.[242] FU can successfully compete with the very low concentrations of orotate in this reaction because of its acidic pKa = (8.1) which generates a significant amount of anionic species.

Alternative routes of activation of FU follow the salvage pathways for uracil and thymine but are presumed to be less important in most tissues.[65,140,231] The first enzyme, uridine phosphorylase, condenses ribose-1-P with uracil or FU in a reaction that energetically favors synthesis but normally is probably catabolic in the cell because of further reactions such as PRPP synthesis and phosphatases that reduce the concentration of ribose-1-P. The corresponding reaction for thymine utilizes deoxyribose-1-P, but it is not considered a significant contribution to FU activation in current therapeutic regimens. After formation of the nucleoside, phosphorylation by uridine kinase and ATP forms 5-fluorouridine-5-P (FUMP) (Figure XVI-2-2). Further phosphorylation of FUMP to FUDP by nucleotide kinase provides a branch point in FU anabolism.[127] Additional phosphorylation of a major portion of FUDP to FUTP provides the substrate for RNA polymerases with consequent incorporation into several forms of RNA.[114] Alternatively FUDP can be reduced to FdUDP which is hydrolyzed to FdUMP, the covalent inhibitor of thymidylate synthase.[247] Some FdUDP is phosphorylated to FdUTP which is an alternate substrate for dTTP in DNA polymerase reactions; however, the presence of high dUTP pyrophosphatase activity converts most of the FdUTP to FdUMP.[149] When FU is incorporated into DNA, uracil N-glycosylase removes it

Figure XVI-2-1. Covalent thymidylate synthase-FdUMP complex; R = H or CH2FH4 = Methylene tetrahydrofolate. From Santi.[247]

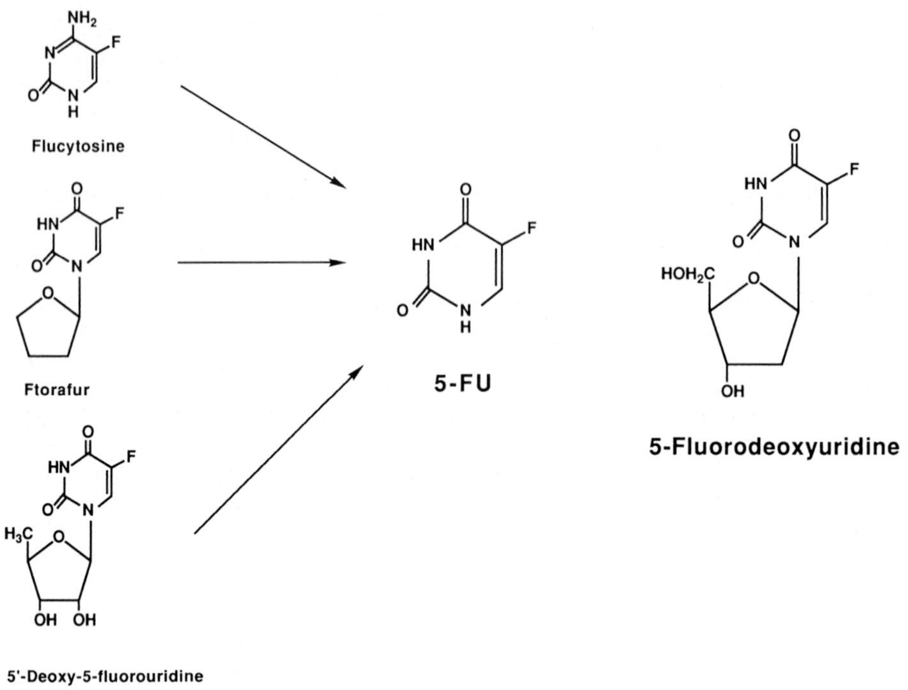

Figure XVI-2-2. 5-Fluorouracil and analog structures.

leaving an apyrimidinic sugar for the process of DNA repair, an additional basis for cytotoxicity.[149]

Minor amounts of FUDP sugar derivatives have been detected as anabolic products but their inhibitory potential for cell growth or toxicity has not been documented.[228,229] In some of the above reactions, the analog FU nucleotides are better substrates than the corresponding uracil derivatives.

Pharmacokinetics. Consideration of the pharmacokinetics of FU must focus primarily on the balance between anabolism and catabolism. The conversion to nucleotide derivatives is responsible for most, if not all, of its antineoplastic activity even though it accounts for a very minor portion of the administered drug. Catabolism via the normal degradation pathway for uracil is the immediate fate of more than 80% of an administered dose of FU.[77] Slight alterations in this pathway can, therefore, greatly affect the very limited amount that is available for conversion to nucleotide form.

Because of great variability and limited bioavailability via the oral route (10–25%),[57] FU is generally administered intravenously. Dosage is dependent upon the schedule of administration.[9] The most common dosage schedules are a monthly course of five daily doses given as an IV bolus of 400–600 mg/m[2], or the same dosage given as a single bolus on a weekly basis.[98] The limiting toxicity of these regimens is generally myelosuppression or mucositis. When continuous intravenous infusion is employed, higher doses are required (1,000–2,000 mg/m[2]/day) to sustain steady state concentrations of FU in plasma (1–5 uM) adequate to achieve therapeutic effects.[254] With this route, toxicity is most frequently mucositis with minimal myelosuppression. It was found that during continuous IV infusions plasma concentrations of FU varied by as much as 10-fold, and subsequent studies have demonstrated that variations in dihydropyrimidine dehydrogenase may be responsible for this effect.[124] Since in current practice FU is most often used in combination with other agents such as leukovorin and methotrexate, it is important in each case to modify dosage to limit, but not eliminate,

host toxicity. It is generally felt that therapeutic benefit requires a dosage intensity that causes significant host toxicity, a result documented by studies with colorectal cancer.[144]

Administered FU has a volume of distribution (Vd) of 0.20–0.25 l/kg which suggests distribution into the extracellular space.[105,179] Good penetration into cerebrospinal fluid, lymph and neoplastic effusions has been documented.[60] As noted above, there is no apparent selective concentration of free drug in any cell type, nor active secretion into bile or urine. Since the drug apparently freely permeates cells in culture, it is not clear why the volume of distribution approximates the extracellular space.

The rate of plasma clearance is generally first order with a t½ of 10–20 minutes and ranges between 500 and 1,500 ml/min.[77] Above a dosage of 800 mg/m[2] clearance may decrease rapidly. In a recent study, using the much more sensitive GC-MS method, an additional elimination phase in humans has been detected with t½ of several hours.[284] This may reflect the release of FU from nucleotide forms in tissues. Since the primary fate of the drug is catabolism, the decreased clearance undoubtedly reflects saturation of these reactions.[190] The circulating concentrations of the initial metabolite, dihydro-5-FU, can be much greater than that of FU and the fate of this metabolite may affect pharmacokinetics and response to FU.

Intra-arterial infusion of FU has been used with some success in patients with isolated hepatic metastases. As with systemic therapy, extensive single pass clearance is achieved (19–51%), but saturation of catabolism is seen when doses are elevated.[96] Nevertheless, hepatic concentrations of FU considerably in excess of that tolerated systemically can be achieved. The limiting factor in high dose regimens is cholestatic jaundice and evidence of chemical hepatitis.

FdUrd, the 2′-deoxyriboside of FU, is a very much more potent inhibitor of cell growth in culture than FU in cell culture.[281] This presumably reflects the ease with which this compound can be activated by thymidine kinase in a single step to FdUMP, the titrating inhibitor of thymidylate synthase, which after further phosphorylation can also be incorporated into DNA. In man or animals, intravenous bolus injection of FdUrd gives a dose-response that is essentially that of FU, because it is rapidly cleaved to an equivalent amount of FU which subsequently experiences the same metabolic fate as directly injected FU. If, however, FdUrd is given by a 14-day continuous infusion the maximum tolerated dose is approximately 100-fold less;[270] however, its therapeutic index is not significantly better than FU alone. It can be used, however, for isolated hepatic metastases of colon cancer by hepatic artery infusion since approximately 90% of the drug is cleared in a single pass by the liver, thus reducing systemic effects.[96] By this route, major increases in the hepatic concentrations of intact drug are achieved relative to systemic targets of toxicity.

The only other approved preparation of FU is in a 2% or 5% formulation in ethylene glycol or a water-based cream, for topical application to treat epithelial dysplasias, particularly actinic keratoses and early basal cell carcinomas.[84] Vulvar and vaginal epithelial neoplasms and genital condylomas are also responsive to this treatment.[167,259] Insufficient drug is absorbed from these preparations to cause systemic effects, and reports of local drug kinetics are limited. It is not clear which, if any, of the biochemical mechanisms detailed above are responsible for this therapeutic effect nor has the reason for the rather selective action on lesions been established except for their presumed more rapid cell kinetics.

Although not of direct use in the treatment of cancer, the 4-amino derivative of FU, 5-fluorocytosine (flucytosine; Figure XVI-2-2), is a valuable antifungal agent for systemic infections that are a common complication of antineoplastic therapy.[250] 5-Fluorocytosine is relatively non-toxic in mammalian systems because it cannot be activated by direct condensation with pyrophosphoryl ribose 5-phosphate (PRPP) and, like uracil, it is poorly anabolized by uridine-cytidine phosphorylase. However, pathogenic fungi, including Candida and Cryptococcal species, deaminate 5-fluorocytosine to FU which is lethal to the organisms by the same mechanisms as in mammalian cells.[136] Although resistant strains emerge rapidly, combination therapy with amphotericin B is valuable in systemic fungal infections caused by the above organisms. Unfortunately, some 5-fluorocytosine appears to be converted to FU in the host, presumably by intestinal organisms, and causes bone marrow depression (leukopenias and thrombocytopenia).[76] Evidence for its relative stability in humans, however, is the observation that about 80% of an oral dose is excreted in the urine unchanged compared to about 5% of a comparable dose of FU.

Several other compounds that serve as prodrugs of FU have been developed. These include ftorafur, a 1-(2-tetrahydrofuranyl) derivative of FU that is metabolized to free FU in liver by both P450 and cytoplasmic activation.[13] This agent (Figure XVI-2-1) appears to have less myelosuppression but mucositis and CNS toxicity are dose limiting.[8] In controlled clinical trials, this agent appears to be equal to or somewhat less effective than FU at a comparable dose.[238] However, the favorable bioavailability of the oral formulation has sustained interest in this compound.

Another FU derivative, 5′-deoxy-5-fluorouridine (Figure XVI-2-2), is cleaved by uridine phosphorylase to liberate FU.

Since some studies suggest higher levels of phosphorylase are present in neoplastic tissues than their normal counterpart, selectivity might be expected.[11] Clinical trials revealed activity in breast and colorectal neoplasms but neuro- and cardiotoxicity have limited further studies.[7,129]

Catabolic Reactions. The primary mode of clearance of FU is via catabolism along the degradative pathway for uracil.[77] Since the products of this pathway are not U.V. absorbing, GC-MS, or radioisotopic methods must be employed. The initial reaction is reduction by dihydrouracil dehydrogenase. The liver is a major site of FU metabolism. This is particularly true when it is given orally, intraperitoneally or by intrahepatic artery infusion. It is now recognized, however, that metabolism in the lung and kidneys may be of equal or even greater importance after IV administration.[179] These findings have therapeutic relevance since it was previously felt that hepatic metastases might compromise FU clearance and limit dosage.

In recent years, marked circadian variations in the metabolism of FU have been detected and related to 24-hour cyclic variations in dihydrouracil dehydrogenase activity.[87,124] These changes are reflected in the inverse variations in plasma concentrations of FU during intravenous infusions in humans.[124,248] Means to employ these differences in the design of clinical protocols have been outlined.[143] In a related finding, familial deficiency of dihydropyrimidine dehydrogenase activity causes severe FU toxicity in patients with this genetic defect.[75]

The subsequent metabolic step catalyzed by dihydropyrimidinase yields β-fluoroureidopropionic acid. In contrast to the dehydrogenase, this enzyme may be rate-limiting in most normal tissues for the degradation of uracil (and presumably FU).[206] A wide variety of tumors apparently express high levels of this activity since they accumulate the subsequent degradation products β-ureidopropionic acid and β-alanine.

α-Fluoro-β-alanine, the counterpart to the final product of uracil catabolism, β-alanine, is the major urinary excretion product of FU.[126] In cancer patients, this has been shown to be conjugated with bile acids and constitutes the primary biliary secretion product of FU.[271] It has been suggested that the chenodeoxycholate conjugate may be responsible for the biliary toxicity seen after intrahepatic infusion of large doses of FU, and cholestasis associated with this conjugate has been demonstrated in isolated perfused rat livers. A summary of FU metabolism is shown in Figure XVI-2-3.

Mechanisms of Action

Experimental evidence has suggested numerous sites for the biological action of FU (Figure XVI-2-2). The relative importance of each of these vary widely among different normal tissues and neoplasms. Commonly, the effects are divided into DNA or RNA "directed" toxicity.

RNA. FUTP, the predominant phosphorylated nucleoside of FU, is as good a substrate for several RNA polymerase reactions as is UTP. The degree of FUTP incorporation into RNA bears a direct relationship to its concentration relative to the concentration of the normal substrate, UTP. In cell lines greater incorporation is associated with reduced clonogenic survival.[114,168] Very substantial amounts of FU replacement of uracil have been reported in each of the RNA species. The highest degree of incorporation is generally seen in the 4S-RNA.[114] There is some evidence to suggest that with a given cell type the proportion of RNA incorporation

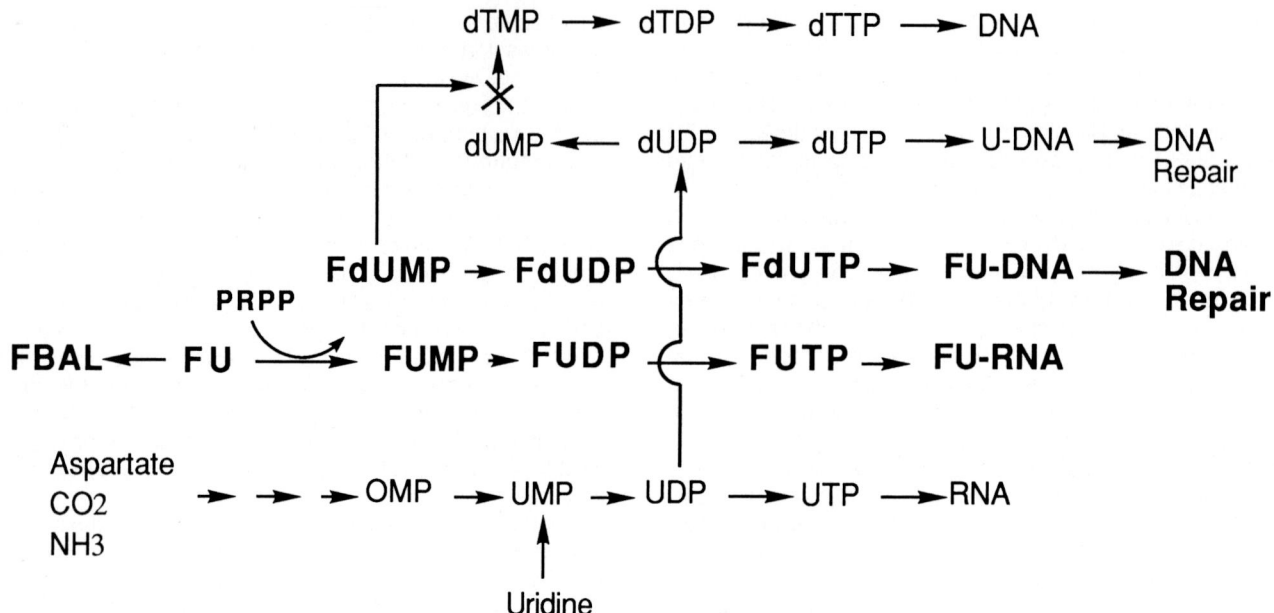

Figure XVI-2-3.   Metabolic activation and targets of fluorinated pyrimidines. dT = thymidine (thymine deoxyriboside); MP, DP, TP = mono-, di-, and triphosphate; dTMP also called thymidylate; dU = deoxyuridine; FdU = fluorodeoxyuridine; dUMP and FdUMP also called deoxyuridylate and fluorodeoxyuridylate; FBAL = fluoro-β-alanine; FU = fluorouracil; FUMP also called fluorouridylate; O = orotidine; U = uridine (uracil riboside); OMP also called orotidylate; UMP also called uridylate.

in different species depends on the available form of the analog (FU vs. FUrd), a result that suggests compartmentalization or channeling of the analog en route to incorporation.[257]

What is less clear is the relative contribution to cytotoxicity of incorporation into RNA. Earlier studies indicated effects on t-RNA acceptor activity, miscoding of protein synthesis and inhibition of the maturation or processing of ribosomal RNA.[183] More recently attention has focused on inhibition of the processing of nuclear RNA to smaller molecular weight species.[218] Other post-transcriptional effects of FU include inhibition of polyadenylation of mRNA and effects on DNA primase. In some model tumors and tumor lines, there is persuasive evidence that these RNA-directed events can be associated with cytotoxicity, particularly when effects of extended exposure are monitored.[102,187]

Thymidylate Synthase. The target site that can be defined most clearly is the covalent inactivation of thymidylate synthase by 5-FdUMP. This fluorinated deoxyuridylate analog is formed via reduction of FUDP by ribonucleotide reductase and dephosphorylation.[160] Alternatively, it can be directly formed from 5-FdUrd by thymidine kinase[123] when this FU deoxynucleoside is regionally infused. The earliest studies by Heidelberger indicated that in selected cell lines growth inhibition could be prevented by thymidine but not by uridine.[281] Direct inhibition of the enzyme responsible for the 1-carbon transfer confirmed this site of action.[63,125] Subsequent research identified specific steps in the reaction in which a methylene group from 5-10-methylene-tetrahydrofolate is transferred to the 5-position of 2'-deoxyuridylate.[247] These studies elegantly established the formation of a stable ternary covalent complex between the 5'-fluoro-analog of deoxyuridylate, the reduced folate derivative and the enzyme, thymidylate synthase. The obvious consequence of this inhibition is an induced enzyme deficiency, depletion of dTTP

and the accumulation of dUMP behind the blockade.[22,204] More recently it has been realized that in some but not all tumors or normal tissues the rate limiting factor in the formation of the abortive ternary complex with FdUMP is the availability of the reduced folate derivative.[101,141] When this cofactor is limiting it is possible to enhance inhibition by administration of leucovorin.[191] The consequence of dTTP depletion is generally considered to be unbalanced growth consequent to reduced DNA synthesis. As might be anticipated, this mode of inhibition would be nullified if thymidine were supplied since after phosphorylation by thymidine kinase it would circumvent the site of inhibition. However, thymidine administration in vivo can actually increase the cytotoxic effects of FU in vivo by inhibiting FU catabolism.[14]

DNA. Initially, the incorporation of FU into DNA was not detected and was assumed to be prevented by the active dUTP phosphatases that also dephosphorylate FdUTP as it is formed.[149] Subsequently, small quantities of FU could be detected in internucleotide linkage in DNA.[169,275] Although FdUTP like dUTP, when it is available, is fully active as a substrate for the several DNA polymerases, a very active glycosylase is present in most cells that excises any FU or uracil that is incorporated in the place of thymine.[140,149] Mutants have been found that are relatively deficient in this editing function. It may be that incorporation per se is not the cytotoxic event but that the excision and repair that involves a pyrimidine endonuclease generates opportunities for error-prone repair that might again re-incorporate FU or uracil instead of thymine nucleotides.[39,82,150] Since considerable accumulation of dUMP occurs behind the blockade of thymidylate synthase, higher concentrations of dUTP are generated which, along with any FdUTP, increase the need for the editing function to remove incorporated uracil. Examination of the kinetics of the excision reaction indicates that uracil is removed as much as 30 times more rapidly than FU.

Similar elevation of dUTP concentrations can be achieved by methotrexate therapy via secondary inhibition of thymidylate synthase.[115] Under these conditions as well, uracil incorporation into DNA is increased and the potential for error-prone repair is enhanced.

It is not possible to rank the importance of these different potential mechanisms of cytotoxicity (RNA incorporation, dTTP depletion by thymidylate synthase inhibition, DNA incorporation, or damage to DNA consequent to excision of uracil or FU). In fact, in different cell types the relative importance of each of these sites may vary. Evidence for high sensitivity to RNA-directed effects is seen in some tumor lines by the inability of thymidine to overcome growth inhibition despite the presence of an active thymidine kinase.[180,281] In these same lines, uridine rescue is more successful than in other lines where thymidine effectively prevents cytotoxicity presumably by repleting dTTP.

Resistance

As with most drugs, partial or complete responses of human cancer to FU generally are followed by the eventual regrowth of tumor despite sustained or even increased dosages. Understanding some of the factors that contribute to natural or acquired resistance has stimulated some of the approaches to modulation of FU therapy. The most prominent mechanism seen in experimental tumors is reduced anabolism of the analog to nucleotide form.[202,203] This may reflect altered condensation with PRPP or activation via the two-stage salvage pathway involving ribose 1-phosphate or deoxyribose 1-phosphate and the appropriate nucleoside phosphorylase with subsequent phosphorylation of the resultant nucleoside by the uridine or thymidine kinase. Alternatively, lack of sensitivity has been correlated with an increased rate of disappearance of FU nucleotides, documented in one case to reflect enhanced nucleotide phosphatase activity.[103] Other well-documented mechanisms of resistance reflect changes in the thymidylate synthase, with reduced affinity for FdUMP,[17] or increases in the rate of synthesis and activity of the enzyme, possibly associated with gene amplification or altered enzyme turnover rates.[23] Finally, effective deletion of the facilitated diffusion transport of FdUrd has been shown to confer resistance to this FU derivative but not to FU in a human colon cancer cell line.[264]

Modulation of FU Therapy

In an effort to improve the limited response rate to therapy with FU (10–25% in most cancers), various biochemical strategies have been investigated.

The degree of activation of FU by orotidylate pyrophosphorylase is affected by the available concentrations of PRPP. Since alterations of traffic along both the purine and pyrimidine nucleotide biosynthetic pathway affect the available concentrations of PRPP, several drug or metabolite combinations have been shown to modify the activation of FU presumably by altering the concentration of this ribose-5'-phosphate donor.[35,252,290]

Others have explored depletion of pyrimidine nucleotides by inhibitors of the de novo synthesis of pyrimidines.[216] A major focus has been placed on enhancing the efficiency with which the covalent complex of FdUMP with the folate cofactor and thymidylate synthase is formed by supplementation with the reduced folate cofactor.[280]

Several current efforts seek to alter the amount of uridine available to normal tissues that are the target of FU toxicity, either by administration of large doses of uridine or by inhibiting its degradation by uridine phosphorylase.[71,164] These efforts were stimulated by the improved therapeutic index of FU when plasma concentrations of uridine were elevated.[185] Some selectivity is achieved presumably because of the ability of uridine to affect selectively the anabolism of FU nucleotides and thus its cytotoxic activity, as well as the existence in most normal tissues of a Na^+-dependent concentrative mechanism for uridine that is either minimal or absent in neoplastic cell lines, and perhaps in malignant tumors.

PALA. Modulation of the action of FU might be expected if the concentration of normal uracil nucleotides with which it competes in tumors was reduced. Phosphonacetyl-L-aspartic acid (PALA) (Figure XVI-2-4), has been documented to deplete pyrimidine nucleotide pools of most cell types and was a logical candidate to enhance the cytostatic action of FU.

This agent was designed as a transition state analog of the intermediate in the condensation of carbamylphosphate with L-aspartic acid.[64] Early studies demonstrated its effective depletion of cellular pools of pyrimidine nucleotides and as a cytostatic agent for cells in culture.[272] Effective reversal of the biochemical and cytotoxic effects could be achieved by supplying uridine to replete pyrimidine nucleotide pools via the salvage pathway.[152] The sensitivity to growth inhibition was inversely related to the aspartate transcarbamylase activity of the cell line in question.[151,153] Conversely, cell lines selected for resistance often displayed gene amplified enhancement of enzyme activity.[159] In naturally occurring solid tumors, however, such a correlation was not observed.[151] The most consistent correlation appeared to be the capacity of the tumor tissue to salvage preformed pyrimidines.

Despite the extreme sensitivity of the target enzyme to PALA, relatively large doses of this agent were required in animals and in clinical trials to reach dose limiting toxicity, 1.2–6 g/m^2.[4] This undoubtedly reflects poor penetration of this highly charged molecule into cells. It may also reflect the degree of inhibition required to make this the rate limiting reaction in the de novo pathway. Nevertheless, marked reductions of pyrimidine nucleotides were seen in some biopsy specimens of tumors.[4] Strong inhibition of the target enzyme was also observed. The drug accumulates in bone but does not cause myelosuppression. This persistence in bone and the lack of perceptible metabolism in animals or man achieves

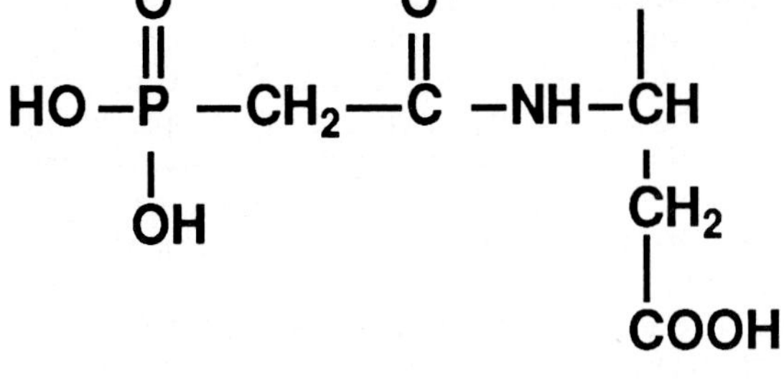

Figure XVI-2-4. PALA [N-(phosphonacetyl)-L-aspartic acid].

a prolonged biochemical effect on pyrimidine metabolism. The primary limiting toxicity is associated with epithelial tissues (skin rash, diarrhea, and mucositis) but neurotoxicity has also been noted. Despite its potency in animal tumor models, PALA, as a single agent, was found to have minimal antitumor effects on human disease.[4]

It was appreciated, however, that this agent, with its profound effect on pyrimidine synthesis de novo, could modulate the action of other agents. Combination therapy with FU was tested as a means to reduce the pools of pyrimidine nucleotides with which FU nucleotides would compete. Early studies employed high doses of PALA and though biochemically successful[42] encountered serious toxicity and limited therapeutic effects.[99] More recent trials have achieved significant increases in the number of responses in colorectal cancer with much lower doses of PALA (400 mg/m^2, 10–20% of the MTD) given daily in 5-day courses,[10,216] Under these conditions, FU is reduced to 150–350 mg/m^2/d given in the same 5-day course. As discussed in XXIX-10, this combination has approximately doubled the response rate in colorectal cancer without serious increase in toxicity.

Brequinar. A similar approach to modulation employs brequinar (DUP-785) an inhibitor of dihydroorotate dehydrogenase. This quinolone carboxylic acid derivative is unique in that it inhibits the only enzyme in the de novo pyrimidine pathway found in the mitochondria, and does it in a noncompetitive manner.[48,225] Good activity against a variety of solid tumors in mice was observed,[225] and inhibition could be completely overcome by supplementation with uridine as anticipated by its site of inhibition. Though minimal clinical activity has been demonstrated when used as a single agent,[62,198] the compound can depress pools of pyrimidine nucleotides in tumors for longer periods than in normal tissues. This had led to treatment with brequinar prior to FU.[234] In low-dose experimental regimens, this strategy improves the tumor suppression seen in multicourse FU therapy of experimental colon neoplasms. Clinical trials of this combination are in progress.

Pyrazofurin and Azauridine. Other inhibitors of de novo pyrimidine synthesis have been examined as single agents, and to a limited degree in combination with the major antimetabolites FU and Ara C. Pyrazofurin[34] and 6-azauridine,[263] after conversion to their respective monophosphates are potent inhibitors of the final reaction in the de novo pathway, orotidylate decarboxylase. This enzyme is a dual function protein which also catalyzes the preceding step in the pathway, condensation of orotate with phosphoribosyl pyrophosphate (PRPP).

Inhibition by either of these agents results in accumulation of orotic acid and orotidine, the dephosphorylation product of orotidylate, in blood and urine.[34] The degree of this accumulation caused by pyrazofurin has been used to quantify effects of agents that may inhibit earlier steps in the pathway.[201,225] As single agents, both azauridine, administered orally as the triacetyl derivative to facilitate rapid absorption, and pyrazofurin showed limited activity. With both agents, epithelial and erythropoietic toxicity limited their clinical usefulness. The potential use of these compounds in combination with FdUDR might be considered since thymidine kinase or transport deficient cells that are resistant to FdUrd would show enhanced sensitivity to inhibitors of de novo synthesis.

Allopurinol. Modulation has also been achieved by co-administration of allopurinol and FU. Allopurinol, after oxidation and conversion to oxypurinol ribonucleotide effectively inhibits orotidylate decarboxylase,[19,112] with accumulation of PRPP and orotate behind the target enzyme, a result manifest as orotinuria in patients.[19] This accumulation is apparently somewhat tissue-specific and may selectively enhance the toxicity of FU to neoplastic tissues.[251] Initial clinical trials indicated increased clearance of FU without loss of the antitumor activity,[108,142] but further studies have not been as encouraging.[295]

Acivicin. Another approach to modulation of pyrimidine nucleotide biosynthesis would be to inhibit the generation of carbamyl phosphate, a substrate in the first reaction of the de novo pathway. Acivicin, a glutamine antagonist that blocks the carbamylation of phosphate by covalent alkylation of the enzyme to achieve this goal, and elevates PRPP pools that would favor FU activation. Acivicin also inhibits conversion of UTP to CTP and several amide transfer steps in purine biosynthesis because it is a general glutamine analog.[4] No clinical benefits were observed as a single agent, but combination studies with FU or other pyrimidine analogs have been limited thus far.

Methotrexate. Modulation of FU therapy with methotrexate has been widely documented to increase the cytotoxicity of FU in cell culture and the inhibition of tumor growth in animal models. Optimal effects have been observed when FU follows the administration of methotrexate (MTX) by one to three hours, an interval that appears to be longer in human colorectal cancer (greater than six hours to achieve up to 48% complete and partial responses).[25]

The biochemical basis for this enhanced response is commonly attributed to the expansion of pools of PRPP generated by inhibition of purine synthesis in cells pre-exposed to MTX.[35] This favors greater activation of FU to nucleotide form and subsequent conversion to FdUMP. An augmenting effect is the depletion of thymidylate nucleotides achieved by MTX via depletion of tetrahydrofolate derivatives. Reversing the sequence, FU before MTX, decreases cytotoxicity in tumor cell lines and is less effective in model tumor systems, presumably because the consumption of tetrahydrofolates for thymidylate synthesis is blocked by the FU effect on the synthase.[24] Consequently, more reduced folate is available for other reactions. Results from large scale clinical trials now in progress with MTX followed by FU will determine the ultimate value of this combination and may motivate future efforts to define with greater certainty the responsible biochemical mechanisms.

Folinic Acid. Formation of the ternary complex of FdUMP, thymidylate synthase and folate coenzymes may be limited by the availability of reduced folates in some cell lines and tumors.[67,139] To optimize formation of the covalent complex, administration of large doses of leucovorin (D,L N5-formyl tetrahydrofolate) has been employed to saturate target enzymes with L-5-10-methylene-tetrahydrofolate via conversion of the L-isomer of leucovorin to 5-methyl-tetrahydrofolate.[162]

Sound experimental evidence supports the logic of this approach to modulation. Early studies demonstrated that optimal FU cytotoxicity in cell lines was achieved only when cells were supplemented with folates to concentrations that were much greater than required for optimal growth.[102,280]

These effects were directly related to the quantity of the ternary complex formed within the cells. The importance of sustaining the folate levels to stabilize the ternary complex could be seen in xenografts of human tumors in which only transient inhibition of thymidylate synthase with FU would be expected unless supplemental reduced folates were present.[138,280] The importance of polyglutamylation to enhance binding to thymidylate synthase in retaining folates within cells has been documented using cells that are defective in polyglutamate synthase.[244]

If modulation by leucovorin in human disease is to be successful, it is important that enhancement of ternary complex formation be selective for tumor tissue. In a murine tumor model, leucovorin could be shown to expand reduced folate pools in the tumor but not in bone marrow.[296] This result was consistent with the antitumor effect seen without increased host toxicity. In other model systems; however, a consistent improvement in therapeutic index is not seen. Because of the enhanced inhibition of thymidylate synthase when prior supplementation with leucovorin is employed, doses of FU must be reduced about 20%.[98] Under these conditions, diarrhea and mucositis remain the limiting toxicity.

A wide range of clinical studies have, in general, confirmed the increased response rate to FU therapy in colorectal cancer when supplemented by leucovorin.[191,212] Evidence for increased survival in these trials is limited, however.[98] In breast and stomach cancer, the response rate in patients not previously treated with FU appears to be increased by addition of leucovorin. Data for other diseases are insufficient to draw conclusions. The generally favorable results obtained in these studies have led to a rather universal addition of leucovorin to FU trials in combination with other drugs. Particularly promising are three studies of combinations of 5-FU-leucovorin with cisplatin in head and neck cancer.[191] Despite these positive results, carefully controlled studies are needed to assure the validity of this mode of modulation, particularly as other new drugs are combined with FU-leucovorin regimens.

Thymidine and Uridine. One of the earliest attempts to modulate FU toxicity employed thymidine.[215] It might be expected that this nucleoside, after conversion to the nucleotide form by thymidine kinase, would be able to rescue tissues from inhibition of thymidylate synthase. Such a circumvention of the blockade was documented in some but not all cell lines.[281] The in vivo extension of these cell culture studies suffered from two limitations. First, thymidine phosphorylase activity in many normal tissues is high. Consequently, the plasma half life is short at doses below 45 g/m²/day,[215] and large quantities were needed to sustain plasma concentrations used in the cell culture experiments. A far more serious limitation in the use of thymidine was the competition for catabolism between FU and the large amounts of thymine generated by phosphorolysis.[14] The net effect of thymidine given in large doses was not rescue but rather prolongation of the pharmacokinetics of FU without an improved therapeutic effect in most circumstances. It is of interest that myelosuppression replaced mucositis as the dose-limiting toxicity.[294]

Modulation of FU therapy with uridine has shown more promise in model systems but the clinical value of this combination has not been fully tested. In a limited number of cell lines, uridine can prevent the toxicity of FU.[227] In vivo studies

of uridine modulation established not only the value of uridine rescue but the importance of a delay in uridine administration for up to 24 hours after FU.[185] When given simultaneously in experimental animals, uridine can actually increase the toxicity of FU, presumably because it inhibits FU catabolism. Other studies with animal tumor models confirmed that delayed uridine could reduce toxicity without impairing antitumor activity.[165,226] Large doses of uridine were required because of the very short half life (t½ = 3–10 minutes). Several mechanisms have been postulated for these effects based on changes in uridine nucleotide pools. Thus, one might invoke competition of the enhanced UTP pools with FU nucleotides that had been formed in the period before uridine administration. Tumor tissues that were less able to augment their uridine nucleotide pool would remain susceptible. In support of this observation is the documentation of a Na⁺-dependent concentrative transport system for uridine in a variety of normal tissues.[265] Concentrations of uridine that range from 5–10-fold greater than in plasma are present in liver, spleen, kidney and, to a lesser degree, the intestine. Of potential therapeutic importance is the lack of such elevated uridine pools in neoplastic cell lines examined. Preliminary studies indicate experimental rodent and human tumors in general do not have elevated uridine pools. These observations may, to some degree, contribute to the tumor specificity of FU. Fluorouridine and FdUrd are very poor substrates for this transport system[70] in normal cells.

Clinical trials with very large doses of uridine administered 3–24 hours after FU by intermittent intravenous infusion achieved millimolar concentrations of uridine. The leukopenia but not the thrombocytopenia associated with weekly bolus doses of FU was prevented.[283] However, these patients require hospitalization and experience fever and phlebitis. Oral uridine (8–12 g/m²) achieves much lower plasma concentrations (50–80 μM), but the dose-limiting toxicity was diarrhea not fever.[285] Further clinical evaluation of uridine rescue after FU is in progress.

The practical difficulties posed by administering extremely large doses of uridine suggested the value of inhibiting its phosphorolysis. Benzylacyclouridine (BAU), originally synthesized as a potential antiviral agent was found to be a potent inhibitor of uridine phosphorylase.[210] Administration of BAU to experimental animals greatly expanded the pool of free uridine in normal tissues but had a minimal effect on pools in murine colon tumor 38.[69] This alteration of uridine homeostasis after FU therapy achieved a better therapeutic effect in this tumor model than the same dose of FU alone, and actually reduced host toxicity. Clinical trials are planned for this combination, possibly in conjunction with reduced doses of uridine, a combination that has been shown to improve therapy with FU in a murine breast tumor model.[186]

Other Modulators. Modulation of nucleoside transport has been considered as another approach to improve FU therapy. The facilitated diffusion mechanism for many natural nucleosides as well as analog derivatives has been shown to be the primary mode of entry and exit of uridine in most neoplastic cell lines.[223] Very effective inhibition of this process in vitro by nitrobenzylthioinosine (nitrobenzyl mercaptopurine riboside, NBMPR) has been extended to in vivo studies by use of the corresponding 5'-phosphate derivative that improves solubility and is hydrolyzed to NBMPR. The vasodilatory drug, dipyridamole, also inhibits this transporter and has been used in combination with FU.[116] The rationale is that access of circulating uridine to the neoplastic cell would be limited and that loss of any fluorouridine formed by phosphatase action on FU nucleotides from the target cell would be restricted. Considerable potentiation of FU action by dipyridamole was seen in culture.[117] Limited clinical studies indicate this agent can also affect FU clearance but it is not established whether an improvement in the therapeutic index of FU can be achieved.[116,239]

Two agents that can modulate host defense mechanisms, levamisole and interferon, have been documented to enhance clinical responses to FU. It is not clear, however, that the effectiveness of these combinations can be attributed to their activity as immunomodulators.

Levamisole, originally employed as an anthelminic agent, was an attractive candidate to augment antineoplastic therapy because of its ability to increase the number of functional T cells and to activate macrophages in model systems.[241] It should be recognized, however, that levamisole has a wide spectrum of activity on the autonomic and central nervous systems. Although it has limited activity as a single drug, when combined with FU there is convincing evidence from two randomized studies that the rate of postsurgical recurrence of disease in patients with stage C colorectal cancer is reduced and survival increased.[170,193] In general the toxicity of the combination reflects that of FU with mucositis and moderate myelosuppression. There is an increase in nausea and diarrhea and mild CNS disturbances, but the combination was, in general, well tolerated. At the present time no clear mechanistic explanation of the basis of the therapeutic effects can be given. Evaluation of this combination in other tumors in which FU has marginal activity is certainly warranted.

The interferons have been evaluated as a means to recruit host defense mechanisms during FU therapy. Synergistic effects of interferon combined with FU have been observed with human tumor cell cultures[208] and xenografts in nude mice.[200] The enhancement generated by α-interferon has been attributed to the activation of macrophages in a species specific manner (mouse α-interferon in mice). α-Interferon has also engendered interest since it appears to enhance accumulation of FdUMP in HL 60 cells.[88] Limited clinical studies have been reported with α-interferon in combination with FU. Although initial response rates of 76% were reported in colorectal cancer,[289] major increases in both mucositis and granulocytopenia required dose reductions of FU and interferon. Subsequent confirmatory studies yield only 26–35% response rates.[224]

Cytosine Arabinoside

Background. Cytosine arabinoside (Cytarabin, araC, Cytosar[R]), is a nucleoside analog of deoxycytidine first synthesized in 1950 and introduced into clinical medicine in 1963.[274] It is one of the most important drugs in the treatment of acute myeloid leukemia. It is also active against acute lymphocytic leukemia and, to a lesser extent, is useful in chronic myelocytic leukemia and non-Hodgkin's lymphoma.[46] It has not proven to be particularly useful in the treatment of nonhematological neoplasms. Myelosuppression and gastrointestinal epithelial injury are the primary toxic effects of araC. Using high-dose araC regimens, additional toxic effects such as intrahepatic cholestasis and central nervous system toxicity are frequently observed.[36]

Metabolism. AraC is rapidly deaminated by cytidine deaminase systemically to a much less active compound, arabinosyluracil (araU).[45,50,55] AraC enters cells through a carrier mediated process or simple diffusion.[161,222] At low concentrations of araC (<2 μM), the carrier mediated process predominates. The efficiency of this transport process depends on the binding affinity of araC for the carrier, the number of molecules of the carrier in the membrane and the presence of competing nucleosides sharing the same system. Once it enters the cells, it is metabolized primarily by the enzymes which normally metabolize deoxycytidine or, in some instances, cytidine (Figure XVI-2-5).

The enzyme responsible for AraCMP synthesis is cytoplasmic deoxycytidine kinase. Mitochondrial deoxypyrimidine nucleoside kinase, which can phosphorylate deoxycytidine and thymidine, does not efficiently phosphorylate araC.[51] The activity of the cytoplasmic deoxycytidine kinase is higher in the S phase of the cell cycle. The amount of araCMP formed depends on the relative activity of cytoplasmic deoxycytidine kinase and cytidine deaminase. Tetrahydrouridine (THU) is a potent inhibitor of cytidine deaminase with a KI value of 10-8M.[45,292] Potentiation of the cytotoxic effect of low concentration of AraC by THU underscores the role of cytidine deaminase in araC metabolism. The enzyme responsible for conversion of araCMP to araCDP is CMP-UMP-dCMP kinase. There are two forms of this enzyme and both are capable of phosphorylating araCMP. It has been suggested that araCMP could be deaminated to araUMP by dCMP deaminase.[182] Whether this pathway is functional in cells is questionable since araCMP is a very poor substrate for dCMP deaminase in comparison to dCMP. Several mammalian cell lines are partially resistant to araC due to decreased activity of dCMP deaminase.[73,74] The enzymes responsible for the phosphorylation of araCDP to araCTP are nucleoside diphosphate kinases (NDP kinases). There are multiple species of NDP kinase activities in human cells.[52] Whether there is a preference of one isozyme over another for the phosphorylation of araCDP is unclear. The formation of araCDP choline in human cells incubated with araC has been reported.[38,171] The enzyme which catalyzes this reversible

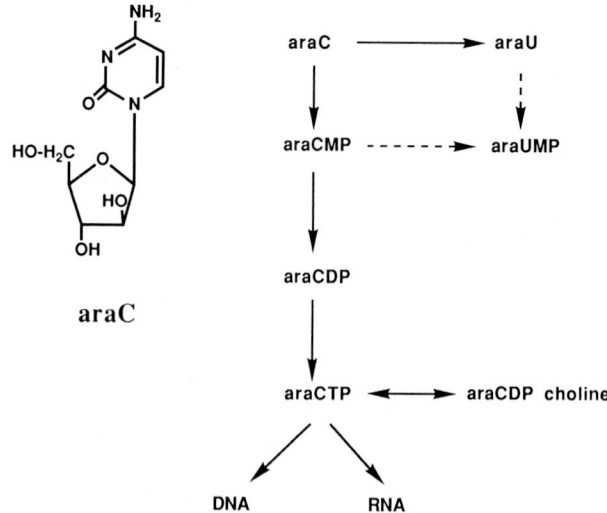

Figure XVI-2-5. Structure and metabolism of Ara C (arabinosyl cytosine).

process is phosphorylcholine cytidyltransferase. Both CDP choline and dCDP choline serve as donors of the phosphorylcholine moiety in phosphatidylcholine synthesis. Whether araCDP choline participates in or interferes with this reaction is not clear.

Major attention has been focused on the incorporation of AraCTP into DNA in competition with dCTP.[111,194,282] Elongation of DNA by polymerase α is retarded considerably by incorporation of araCMP whereas no significant impact on elongation by DNA polymerase β could be seen after incorporation of a single araC nucleoside residue. However, neither polymerase alone could appreciably elongate the DNA if two consecutive araCMP residues were incorporated. Thus the behavior of araCTP on DNA polymerase is not only polymerase dependent but also sequence dependent.[217,278]

Mechanism of Action. The primary action of araC is inhibition of nuclear DNA synthesis.[15,195] Mitochondrial DNA synthesis is not affected by araC even at concentrations 10 times greater than that required to inhibit cell growth by 50%.[49] Three mechanisms have been suggested to account for the inhibition of nuclear DNA synthesis by araC. The relative importance of each mechanism could be dependent on the intracellular concentration of araCTP. The first mechanism is inhibition of the initiation of new replication units in chromosomes[109] consequent to the incorporation of araC into the replicon initiation primer. The second mechanism is the retardation of DNA chain elongation as the result of the incorporation of araC into DNA.[111,194] This effect is DNA polymerase and sequence dependent as discussed above. Reactions catalyzed by DNA polymerase α and perhaps DNA polymerase δ are more susceptible than other DNA polymerase activities. The third mechanism, which may become important only when a high dosage araC protocol is used, is the inhibition of DNA primase.[219] AraCTP can inhibit the formation of the RNA oligomer required for the initiation of DNA synthesis with KI values of 25–125 μM depending on the template used. Although there is no evidence that araCMP could be incorporated into an RNA oligomer in vitro, it was found that some of the araC associated with DNA was alkaline labile.[181] This indicates the possibility that araC is incorporated into the RNA primer of DNA and requires further investigation. In general, inhibition of cell growth correlates well with the degree of incorporation of araC into cellular DNA. The majority of the incorporated araCMP is in internucleotide linkage in DNA. The relative ratio of araC in internucleotide compared to chain terminal positions is dependent on the concentration of araC. The higher the concentration of araC to which cells are exposed, the lower the relative amount of internucleotide araC residues. This could be the result of the higher probability of consecutive araCMP's being incorporated into DNA which stops further DNA chain elongation catalyzed by DNA polymerase α as well as by DNA polymerase β. The amount of araCMP incorporated into DNA is also dependent on the relative ratio of araCTP to dCTP. Decreases in the pool of dCTP intracellularly can increase the amount of araCMP incorporated.

Among other potential targets, araCTP is not a potent inhibitor of ribonucleotide reductase, a key enzyme early in the course of dCTP formation.[47] AraCTP can act in lieu of dCTP to activate dCMP deaminase for the deamination of dCMP to dUMP, the substrate for dTMP synthesis. Since araCMP is a poor substrate for dCMP deaminase, the accumulation of araCTP enhances the deamination of dCMP and subsequently decreases the intracellular dCTP pool.[182] This could "self-potentiate" the incorporation of araCTP into DNA. This hypothesis is based on enzyme studies in vitro, but is substantiated by the observation that cells become resistant to araC as the result of decreased dCMP deaminase activity.[74]

The mechanism of action of araC may be dosage dependent. At noncytotoxic concentration, araC can cause human promyeloblast HL-60 cell lines to differentiate. It has been suggested that the success of low dosage araC therapy of patients with myelodysplastic syndrome may be consequent to the differentiation effects of araC.[15] High doses of araC given to leukemic patients cause rapid tumor cell lysis.[38] Whether additional mechanisms of araC start to play an important role in this protocol is also unclear. In patients treated with high dose araC, the concentration of araU, the deamination product of araC, can exceed 100 μM in plasma of patients receiving high dosage araC treatment.[37] The high concentrations of araU may act in concert with araC and may also affect cell growth by mechanisms that have not yet been established.[298]

Mechanism of Resistance. Cells could become resistant to araC due to the decrease of carrier for araC transport, the decreased level of cytoplasmic deoxycytidine kinase, the increased activity of the catabolism of araC through the action of cytidine deaminase, the increase of the formation of dCTP through the action of ribonucleotide reductase and nucleoside diphosphate kinase, or the decreased activity of dCMP deaminase which could lead to the increase of dCTP in competition with araCTP for incorporation into DNA. An increased activity of 3' to 5' exonuclease which could remove the araCMP from the DNA chain terminus has also been suggested.[172]

5-Azacytidine

Background. 5-Azacytidine (5-AC) was first synthesized in 1963 and later isolated as a natural product from fungal cultures.[122,266] The clinical utility of this cytidine analog is primarily in the treatment of acute myelocytic leukemia and myelodysplastic syndrome. Occasionally, clinical response has been observed in patients with solid tumors. This compound can promote the expression of genes which are suppressed due to hypermethylation of specific genes.[1,154] This activity suggested use in some genetic diseases such as sickle cell anemia and thalassemia, but its usefulness in the treatment of these diseases is limited by its bone marrow toxicity and concerns about its carcinogenic potential. The major toxicity of 5-AC is leukopenia and, to a lesser degree, thrombocytopenia. Hepatotoxicity has also been reported, particularly in patients with preexisting hepatic dysfunction.[46]

Metabolism. The replacement of carbon in position 5 of the heterocyclic ring of cytidine by nitrogen results in a marked chemical instability. The product of the ring opening, N-formylamidinoribofuranosylguanylurea, may recycle to form the parent compound but it is also susceptible to further decomposition. This tendency to decompose not only may play a role in its mechanism of action but also is troublesome in its clinical use.[20] Although 5-AC can be deaminated by cytidine deaminase to 5-AU, a less toxic compound, the efficiency of this deamination by cytidine deaminase is less than for cytidine. Nevertheless, inhibition of the deamination by tetrahydrouridine can enhance 5-AC toxicity. 5-AC enters mammalian cells by a facilitated nucleoside transport mechanism shared with other nucleosides.[235] The initial step in its activation is the conversion to 5-ACMP by uridine-cytidine kinase.[79] 5-ACMP is further phosphorylated to 5-AC di- and triphosphate by CMP-UMP-dCMP kinases and nucleoside diphosphate kinases respectively. 5-AC triphosphate, the predominant form of the metabolites in cells treated with 5-AC for a few hours, can be incorporated into RNA, but its pathway for incorporation into DNA is not well defined. It is likely that 5-ACDP is reduced by ribonucleotide reductase to the corresponding deoxynucleotide diphosphate which is phosphorylated to 5-AdCTP by nucleoside diphosphate kinases. 5-AdCTP can be incorporated into DNA efficiently by DNA polymerase α and β. The incorporated 5-AdCMP at the 3' terminus of DNA has less effect on subsequent DNA chain elongation than the incorporated araCMP at the 3' terminus of DNA. It was observed that 5-AdC was stabilized against hydrolytic degradation by incorporation into DNA. This could be due in part to hydrophobic shielding of the triazine ring from water and other polar nucleophiles within the DNA double helix.[277,278]

A summary of 5-AC metabolism is shown in Figure XVI-2-6. 5-AC is most cytotoxic to cells in the DNA synthetic phase of the cell cycle, but the exact mechanism of its cytotoxic action has not been well established. It could inhibit both DNA and RNA synthesis. The incorporation into RNA can lead to the inhibition of the process of ribosomal RNA synthesis from higher molecular weight species, disassembly of polyribosomes and marked inhibition of protein synthesis. Its incorporation into DNA could also inhibit DNA synthesis.[58,176,177,287] An important, well-documented effect is the inhibition of DNA methylation as a result of stoichiometric binding with DNA-methyltransferase after its incorporation. The methylation of cytosine residues in DNA is responsible for inactivation of specific genes. Thus, treatment of cells with 5-AC leads to a reduction in cytosine methylation and enhanced expression of selected genes that are normally suppressed. 5-AC, at minimally cytotoxic concentration, stimulates differentiation of some tumor cell lines in culture and has been suggested for the treatment of genetic diseases associated with hypermethylation (see XXXVI-1).[1,154]

Mechanism of Resistance. Cells become resistant to 5-AC by reduction or elimination of uridine-cytidine kinase. Decreased nucleoside transport by the facilitated diffusion

mechanism can also decrease sensitivity to 5-AC. Cytosine deaminase may also play an important role in cell sensitivity to 5-AC. It has been observed that tumor cells resistant to araC because of deletion of cytoplasmic deoxycytidine kinase activity, a frequent mechanism of cellular resistance to araC, are more susceptible to 5-AC than the parent tumor line in animal models. Sequential treatment with araC and then 5-AC bears further study, particularly in patients who become refractory to araC.

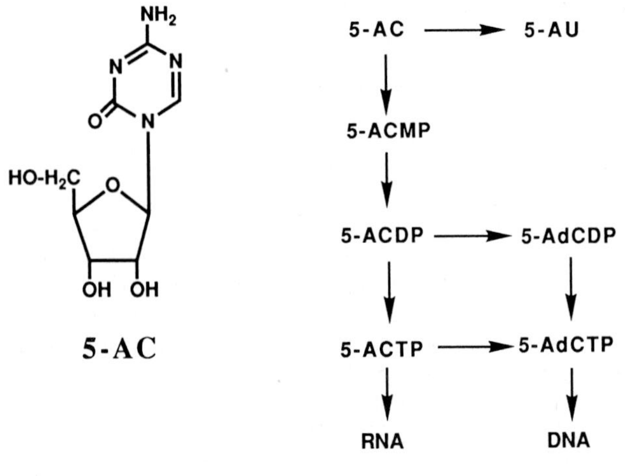

Purine Analogs

Introduction

The original syntheses of purine antimetabolites focused on isosteric replacement of O, C, or N in the purine ring and were predicted on the same logic as that used for pyrimidines.[134] C-N or O-N substitutions gave 8-azaguanine and 2-6-diaminopurine. The first clinically useful agent was 6-mercaptopurine (6-MP),[33] in which the 6-OH of hypoxanthine was replaced with a thiol group (Figure XVI-2-7). Subsequently, the equivalent analog of guanine, 6-thioguanine, was prepared.[90] Two glutamine analogs, 6-diazo-5-oxo-L-norleucine (DON) and azaserine, also made major contributions to our understanding of the purine biosynthetic pathways during that period but were not found to be clinically useful.[4] Studies of these initial analogs established many of the relevant issues addressed in the subsequent development of purine and pyrimidine analogs.[221]

Early studies with 6-MP in model systems quickly established the dependence of inhibitory activity on metabolic conversion to the corresponding analog nucleotides by identification of metabolites and characterization of resistance mechanisms.[92] Of equal importance to the activity of many purine analogs has been an understanding of catabolic reactions that limit their availability. Xanthine oxidase which inactivates 6-mercaptopurine and thioguanine,[221] and adenosine deaminase,[2] which is the target for deoxycoformycin and limits the action of arabinosyl adenosine are of particular relevance.

Two more recently developed purine analogs, acyclovir and ganciclovir, are acyclic nucleoside derivatives and valuable antiviral agents. These agents, along with arabinosyl adenine, are activated by kinase reactions but exert their effects on the same spectrum of biochemical reactions exerted by purine base analogs. Their role in cancer therapy remains to be established.

6-Mercaptopurine

6-Mercaptopurine was among the first purine analogs that demonstrated antineoplastic activity; it remains a useful agent in the treatment of acute leukemia.[276] This derivative of hypoxanthine is a relatively insoluble amphoteric compound that is stable except in alkaline solutions. Metabolic activation occurs primarily by reaction with 1-pyrophosphoryl-ribose-5-phosphate (PRPP) via hypoxanthine-guanine pyrophosphorylase (HGPRT) to form 6-mercaptopurine riboside 5'-phosphate, more properly called thioinosine monophosphate (TIMP).[91]

TIMP is believed to exert its major effect on purine nucleotide metabolism by inhibition of the first step in purine biosynthesis, the formation of 1-NH$_2$-ribose-5-PO$_4$, via a pseudo-feedback inhibition in which TIMP mimics the regulatory action of adenine or guanine nucleoside monophosphates.[104,132,262]

Figure XVI-2-6. Structure and metabolism of 5-AC (5-azacytidine).

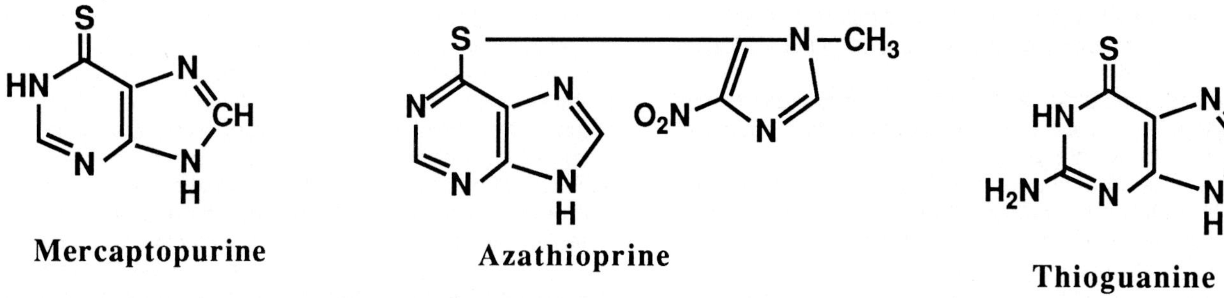

Mercaptopurine   **Azathioprine**   **Thioguanine**

Figure XVI-2-7.   Purine antimetabolites.

An early precursor of purine biosynthesis, 5 amino imidazol-4-carboxamide, which can be converted to the corresponding ribonucleotide, protects cells in culture against growth inhibition by 6-MP. This finding is consistent with the view that the primary site of action is limitation of an early step in de novo synthesis. TIMP also blocks the subsequent metabolism of inosinic acid, the initial purine nucleotide, to adenylic acid by inhibiting adenosylsuccinate synthase.[91] Similarly, synthesis of guanine nucleotides is reduced by inhibition of the oxidation of inosinic acid to xanthylic acid. Although TIMP is not incorporated into nucleic acids as such, minor amounts are converted to thioguanylic acid which is incorporated into RNA and DNA. It is not established that this incorporation is of significance to the toxic or antineoplastic actions of 6-MP. A summary of 6-MP metabolism is presented in Figure XVI-2-8.

6-MP is generally administered orally (90 mg/m²) for sev-

eral weeks. Absorption is variable and incomplete and associated with a t½ of 20–45 minutes in the plasma where it is minimally bound to serum proteins.[302] The rapid turnover is largely the result of oxidation by xanthine oxidase which converts it to inactive thiouric acid, the primary urinary excretion product.[94] In patients receiving allopurinol to control uricemia, the dosage of 6-MP must be reduced by about 75% since drug catabolism is sharply reduced with the attendant risks of toxicity.[12] No selective advantage in tumor therapy is achieved by this combination. Another metabolite, the S-methyl derivative of 6-mercaptopurine, is found in cells as methyl mercaptopurine ribonucleotide where it is inhibitory of purine metabolism; it is excreted in urine.[24]

The dose-limiting toxicity of 6-MP is myelosuppression which is slow in onset (2–4 weeks) and is rapidly reversed after dosage is reduced or discontinued.[100,230] All formed elements, thrombocytes, granulocytes, and erythrocytes, can be affected. Although gastrointestinal mucositis or stomatitis

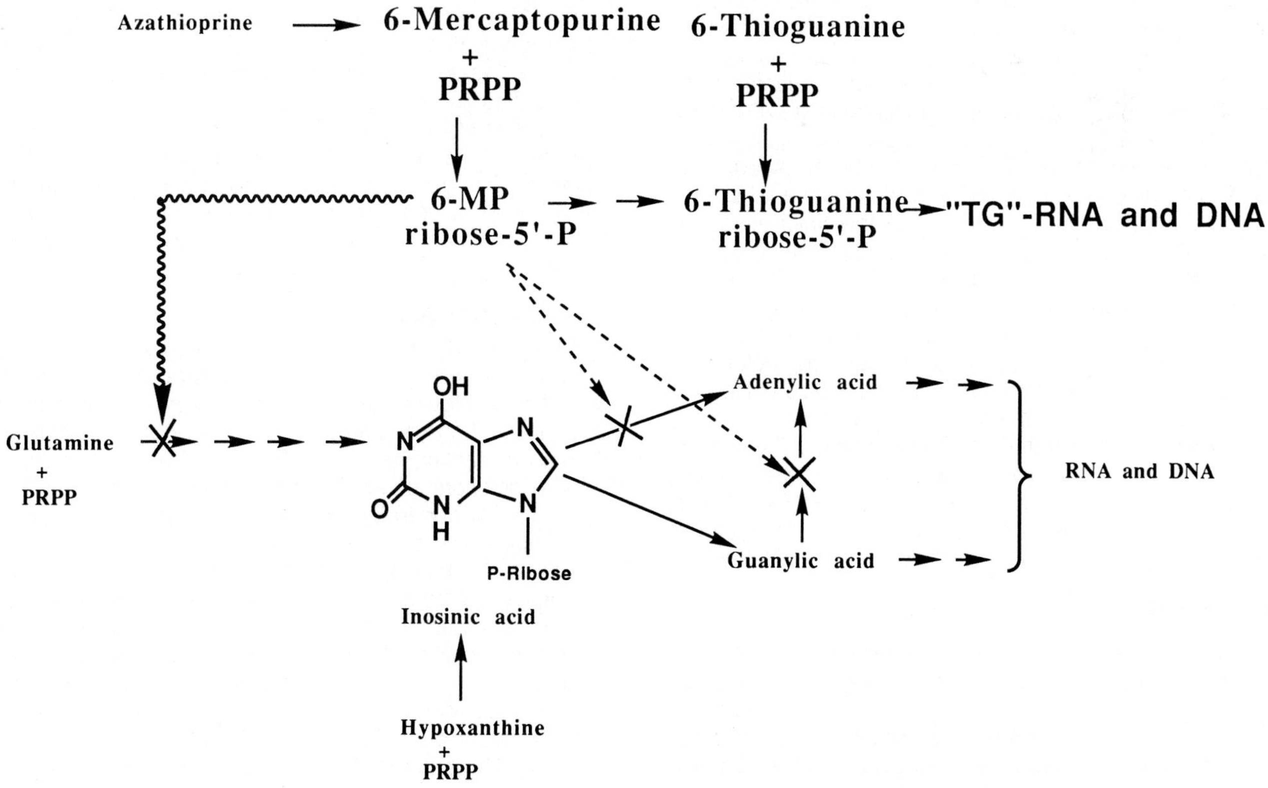

Figure XVI-2-8.   Metabolic activation and targets of thiopurines.

is minimal, about one-quarter of treated patients experience nausea, vomiting and anorexia, and a small number display hepatotoxicity.[86]

The therapeutic action is dependent upon formation of the nucleotide, 6-mercaptopurine ribonucleoside monophosphate. In experimental tumor systems, resistance is commonly associated with a decreased rate of activation to the nucleotide form consequent to deletion or modification of HGPRT activity. Limited studies in humans, however, suggest that resistance is caused by increased activity of a 5'-phosphatase that limits the concentration and duration of intracellular 6-mercaptopurine ribonucleotide.[249]

6-Mercaptopurine was found to be effective in combination with prednisone in the induction of remission in acute lymphoblastic leukemia of children. Currently it is a regular component of consolidation and maintenance therapy for this disease (see XXXIX-3). It is also of some value in adult acute lymphocytic leukemias (see XXXVI-5). It is no longer commonly used in myeloid leukemias of adults, although it has modest activity in combination therapy (see XXXVI-2).

Although a large number of 6-mercaptopurine derivatives have been synthesized and evaluated in model systems, only one, azathioprine (Imuran[R]), is available at this time. This methyl-nitro-imadazole derivative of the thiol group on 6-mercaptopurine is cleaved in vivo, presumably by thiols, to liberate 6-mercaptopurine. It is generally not used in cancer therapy but remains an important element of immunosuppressant therapy for allograft transplantation and selected autoimmune states.[133]

Thioguanine

Thioguanine (Figure XVI-2-8) is the 6-thiol derivative of guanine corresponding to 6-MP and also depends upon activation via HGPRT.[276] Unlike 6-MP, however, di- and triphosphates of thioguanine ribonucleotide are formed and incorporated into RNA. After conversion to thioguanine deoxynucleotide triphosphate it can substitute for dGTP in DNA polymerase reactions.[174] This incorporation is thought to be the primary mechanism of cytotoxicity.[209] Even though thioguanylate monophosphate is the predominant acid-soluble nucleotide, it does not appear to exert the major effects on de novo purine synthesis observed with 6-MP nor to deplete pools of normal purine nucleotides.

Like 6-MP, thioguanine, after deamination to thioxanthine by guanase, is readily catabolized to thiouric acid by xanthine oxidase. S-methylation is also observed, yielding S-methyl-thioguanine and thioxanthine. Dethiolation also contributes to metabolism as evidenced by urinary excretion of ^{35}S-SO_4 after administration of ^{35}S-thioguanine. The primary use of thioguanine is in acute myeloid leukemia where it may be combined with arabinosyl cytosine; however, recent studies question its value in this disease.[83,188] A summary of thioguanine metabolism is presented in Figure XVI-2-8.

Allopurinol

Allopurinol (4-hydroxypyrazalo-3,4-d-pyrimidine) is an important adjuvant to antineoplastic therapy (Figure XVI-2-9). This agent as well as its primary metabolite, oxipurinol are potent inhibitors of xanthine oxidase.[93,267] As such they limit the formation of uric acid from the degradation of purine nucleotides and nucleic acids. It is of interest that oxipurinol is formed by the target enzyme xanthine oxidase and is a potent inhibitor of this enzyme. In addition to this mechanism, allopurinol has been shown to inhibit purine nucleotide biosynthesis by feedback inhibition of the first reaction in the pathway and to deplete pyrophosphoryl ribose-5-PO4, presumably by formation of the corresponding allopurinol and oxypurinol ribonucleotides.[85] These nucleotides also are inhibitors of orotidylate decarboxylation and result in excretion of urinary orotate and orotidine.[158] These actions may relate to the ability of allopurinol to selectively reduce the toxicity of FU to some normal tissues as previously described.

Although originally synthesized as an antineoplastic agent, allopurinol is widely used in the treatment of hyperuricemia associated with gout and other metabolic disorders.[243] Certain neoplastic states, particularly lympho- and myeloproliferative diseases, also generate hyperuricemia and allopurinol is an effective means to avoid the associated episodes of gout or uric acid nephropathy.[121] This is of particular importance in leukemias, lymphomas and in other patients with bulky disease when chemotherapy produces rapid tumor lysis with attendant release of purine bases from the nucleic acids.

Oral doses of 300–800 mg daily have been recommended and are generally well tolerated. Skin rashes and gastrointestinal disturbances are common and of increased frequency and severity when the allopurinol is given together with ampicillin but rarely limit therapy.[26] Severe drug induced fever, vasculitis and blood dyscrasias of a hypersensitivity nature have occurred infrequently.[260] Since allopurinol also reduces the rate of metabolic inactivation of oral 6-mercaptopurine and azathioprine, doses of these purine antimetabolites must be reduced by 50–75% to avoid excessive toxicity.[302] Although oxidation by xanthine oxidase is the primary route of allopurinol metabolism and the relevant site of its action, allopurinol can also inhibit metabolism of drugs such as cyclophosphamide by the mixed function oxidases.[286]

The elevation of hypoxanthine and xanthine concentrations in plasma by inhibition of xanthine oxidase is less dangerous than elevated uric acid since these purines are more soluble and less likely to form stones or cause gout. Nevertheless, it is generally recommended that patients treated with allopurinol for hyperuricemia also be hydrated and alkalinized when uric acid concentrations are significantly elevated.

Deoxycoformycin

Background. Deoxycoformycin (pentostatin) is a natural product isolated in 1974 from the culture of *streptomyces antibioticus* (Figure XVI-2-9).[256] Its structure mimics the transitional state form of adenosine in an adenosine deaminase catalyzed reaction, and it was found to be one of the most potent inhibitors of adenosine deaminase known (KI = 10^{-10}–10^{-12}M depending on the source of the enzyme).[293] Since adenosine deaminase is not essential for cell growth in culture, this compound did not show antitumor activity in the preclinical screens. The initial clinical development of deoxycoformycin centered on its activity as an adenosine deaminase inhibitor for the potentiation of adenosine arabinoside which was also deaminated to yield less toxic compounds by adenosine deaminase. In early phase I studies of deoxycoformycin, the profound lymphotoxic effect of the compound was noted. Others had described a congenital syndrome of severe combined immunodeficiency associated with low or undetectable levels of adenosine deaminase

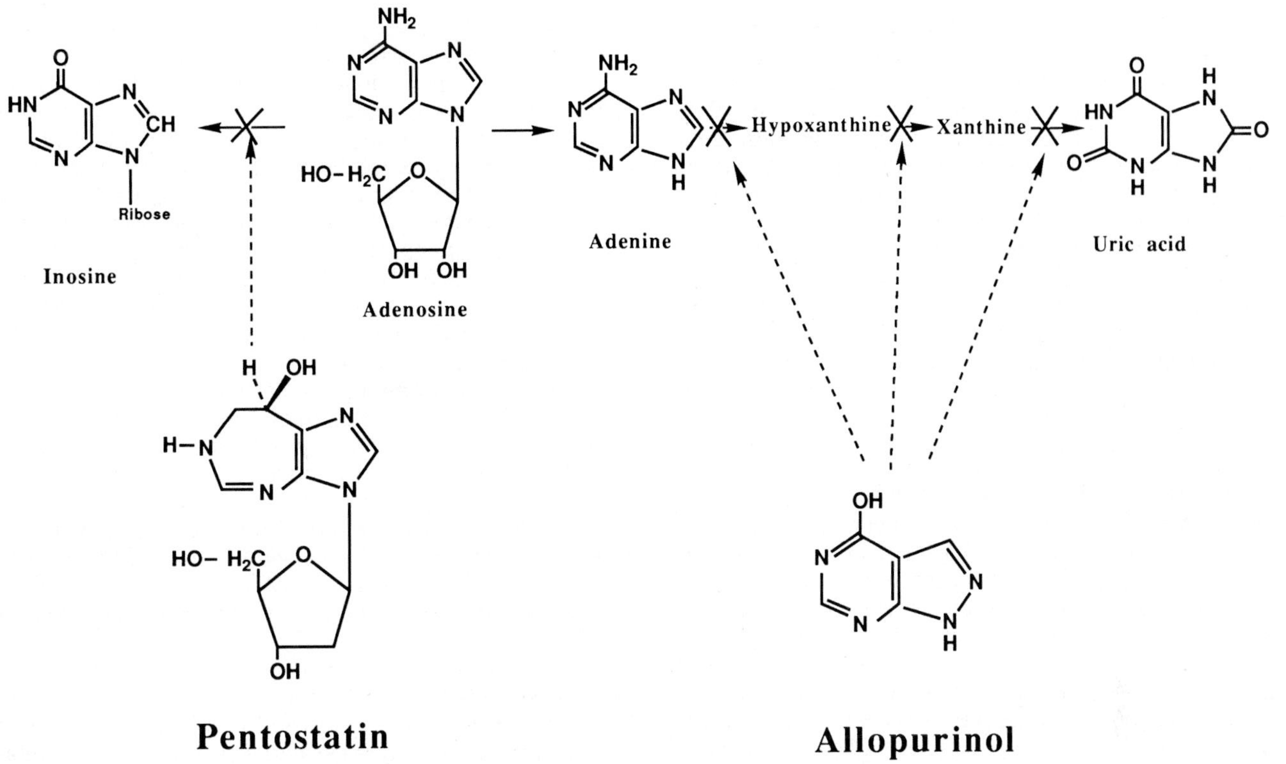

Figure XVI-2-9. Inhibitors of purine nucleoside catabolism.

in lymphocytes.[110] These results suggested the importance of adenosine deaminase in lymphocyte function and led to intensive development of deoxycoformycin as a single agent for the treatment of lymphoproliferative diseases. The most responsive tumor identified is hairy cell leukemia, in which durable remissions are achieved in more than 90% of patients with a relatively brief course of treatment (see XXXVI-8).[166,268] Other responsive lymphoid diseases include chronic lymphocytic leukemia (see XXXVI-7), prolymphocytic leukemia (see XXXVI-7), mycosis fungoides (see XXXVI-11), and acute T-cell leukemia/lymphoma (see XXXVI-6).[72,118] Considerable variability has been seen in the susceptibility of patients to deoxycoformycin toxicity. This includes immunosuppression,[213,214] central nervous system disturbances, impaired renal function, conjunctivitis, and muscle and joint pain. Impaired renal function and poor performance status place patients at high risk for toxicity even at low dosage of the drug.

Metabolism. Deoxycoformycin enters the cell through the facilitated diffusion nucleoside carrier. It can be phosphorylated to mono-, di- and triphosphate nucleotides. Significant incorporation of deoxycoformycin into DNA but not RNA has been observed.[166] Adenosine kinase and deoxycytidine kinase[258] do not appear to be responsible for the initial phosphorylation but reversal of the 5'-nucleotidase reaction is a potential basis for nucleotide formation. Definitive statements cannot be made about the enzymology of deoxycoformycin metabolism at this time.

Mechanism of Action and Resistance. The primary site of action of deoxycoformycin is the inhibition of adenosine deaminase. As the result of the inhibition of adenosine deaminase in vivo, deoxyadenosine and adenosine cannot be

catabolized efficiently. Consequently, deoxyadenosine phosphorylated metabolites accumulate in many cell types.[192] This imbalance in adenosine derivatives is known to be toxic to cells and the antitumor activity of deoxycoformycin may result from the combination of direct effects of deoxycoformycin and its metabolites as well as the expanded pools of deoxyadenosine. The failure of deoxyadenosine to accumulate in cultures treated with deoxycoformycin is the reason deoxycoformycin was not identified to be a potential antitumor compound in cell culture systems. The degree of dATP accumulation correlated well with cell death caused by deoxycoformycin. Thus, dATP, known to be an allosteric inhibitor of ribonucleotide reductase, could result in growth inhibition by generation of an imbalance of pools of deoxynucleotide triphosphates. However, additional sites of action of deoxycoformycin and deoxyadenosine are suggested by the observation that deoxycoformycin and deoxyadenosine are cytotoxic to nondividing cells which do not require the function of ribonucleotide reductase. One potential site is the depletion of nicotinamide adenine dinucleotide (NAD) in deoxycoformycin and deoxyadenosine treated cells. NAD is required for the formation of poly-ADP ribosylation essential for maintenance of the integrity of DNA and its repair process. Depletion of NAD could reduce the capacity for DNA repair, a constant process in cells, and cause DNA breaks as well as cell death.[255,301] The second suggested site is inhibition of S-adenosyl homocysteine hydrolase by deoxyadenosine.[131] Inhibition of this enzyme decreases the capacity of cells to perform transmethylation, a reaction critical for certain macromolecular functions. This mechanism does not require deoxyadenosine to be phosphorylated and may play an important role in the toxicity of deoxycoformycin in non-proliferating tissues such as liver and central nervous system. Deoxycoformycin and deoxyadenosine have also been demonstrated to decrease ATP levels in some cell systems. In mice, hemolysis after treatment with deoxycoformycin is related to ATP depletion. Deoxycoformycin has also been shown to form phosphorylated metabolites that can be incorporated into DNA. Whether these metabolites contribute to deoxycoformycin action is not clear.[214]

The mechanism of resistance to deoxycoformycin has not been defined. This is due to the fact that deoxycoformycin is not cytotoxic in cell culture. Since the action of deoxycoformycin in vivo is due to the combined action of deoxycoformycin and deoxyadenosine, the mechanism of the cellular resistance to deoxyadenosine should be applicable. This could include deficiency in adenosine kinase or alteration of ribonucleotide reductase in quality or quantity.

2-Fluoroadenosine-5′-Phosphate

Background. In the search for compounds more effective than adenine arabinoside (araA, vidarabine), which had limited clinical usefulness because of its rapid deamination by adenosine deaminase, 2-fluoroadenosine arabinoside (fludarabine) (9-β-D-arabinofuranosyl-2-fluoradenine) was synthesized and found to be relatively resistant to adenosine deaminase. This compound was shown to have impressive antitumor activities in vivo as well as in cell culture. However, its limited solubility and consequent difficulties in formulation, led to the synthesis of the prodrug, the 5′-monophosphate of 2-F-araA (Fludara I.V.). Fludara I.V. entered clinical trials in 1982. It is one of the most active agents in the treatment of chronic lymphocytic leukemia (CLL).[119,157] A high level of activity was also observed in a variety of indolent lymphoproliferative neoplasms including low-grade non-Hodgkin's lymphoma (NHL), cutaneous T-cell lymphoma, macroglobinemia and hairy cell leukemia.[54,135,156] The dose-limiting toxicity in phase I trials is myelosuppression and leukopenia. Delayed onset of severe neurotoxicity was noted with doses ≥ 96 mg/m²/d for 5–7 days. Other toxicities noted in phase 1 trials included somnolence, mild to moderate nausea and vomiting, and rare but reversible interstitial pneumonitis. Fludara I.V. is converted to 2-F-araA within several minutes of injection by the action of phosphatases; it is not further catabolized in plasma. The majority of 2-F araA in plasma remains as F-araA.

Metabolism. Transport of F-araA into mouse L1210 cells was shown to be mediated by nonconcentrative high affinity and low affinity systems.[261] In contrast to these leukemia cells, epithelial crypt cells from mouse intestine possess only a low affinity system.[18] This difference in transport could be partly responsible for the favorable therapeutic index of F–araA against sensitive tumor cells in mice. In future human studies, the potential role of transport systems in determining the sensitivity to 2-F-araA should be considered. Once 2-F araA is taken up by cells, it is phosphorylated to 2-F araAMP, not like araA as a substrate of adenosine kinase, but by cytoplasmic deoxycytidine kinase.[30] Tumor cells lacking cytoplasmic deoxycytidine kinase are resistant to F-araA. Intracellular F-araAMP can be further phosphorylated to F-araADP, but it is not clear which enzyme is responsible for this reaction. It is likely that AMP kinases may be responsible for the further phosphorylation of F-araADP to F-araATP. Nucleoside diphosphate kinases may be the predominant enzyme species responsible for this conversion. F-araATP can be incor-

porated into DNA in competition with dATP by DNA polymerases. Although DNA polymerase α, β, γ, and δ are all capable of utilizing F-araATP as a substrate, DNA polymerase α has a greater affinity for F-araATP than other DNA polymerases.[236,279] Once F-araAMP is incorporated into the terminus of the growing chain of DNA, the next step of DNA chain elongation is retarded, regardless which DNA polymerase is employed.[148,279] F-araA has also been shown to be incorporated into RNA;[147,269] which RNA polymerase is responsible has not been established. The incorporation of F-araA into poly(A+) RNA was 12 fold greater than that into poly (A−) RNA. A summary of metabolism of 2F-araA is shown in Figure XVI-2-10.

Mechanism of Action. The major site of growth inhibition by F-araA is inhibition of DNA synthesis. Treatment of cells with F-araA is associated with the accumulation of cells at the G1/S phase boundary and in S phase; thus, it is a cell cycle S phase-specific drug. Incorporation of the active metabolite, F-araATP, retards DNA chain elongation. The degree of incorporation of the analog nucleotide is dependent not only on the type of DNA polymerase but also the amount of intracellular dATP that competes with F-araATp for incorporation.

Among DNA polymerases in human cells, DNA polymerase α, which is the critical enzyme in nuclear DNA synthesis, is more susceptible to incorporation of F-araATP. A consequence of this analog nucleotide incorporation is the retardation of DNA chain elongation.

F-araATP is also a potent inhibitor of ribonucleotide reductase, the key enzyme responsible for the formation of dATP. This causes a decrease of deoxynucleotides in 2F-araA treated cells which enhances the incorporation of F-araATP into DNA. This may be considered "self potentiation" of the inhibition

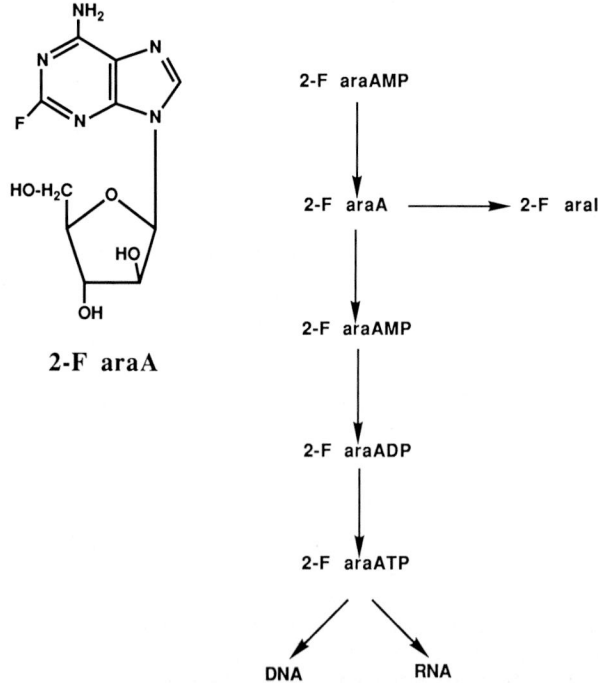

Figure XVI-2-10. Structure and metabolism of 2-F-Ara A (2-fluoro-arabinosyladenine). 2-F araI represents the dominated inosine derivative.

of DNA synthesis by F-araATP. In addition, F-araATP was found to be an inhibitor of DNA primase which is responsible for Okazaki fragment synthesis,[219] an important step for DNA synthesis. The inhibition of RNA primer formation for DNA synthesis by F-araATP was also recently demonstrated.[44] The inhibition of Okazaki fragment formation by F-araATP could conceivably play a role in the inhibition of DNA synthesis by F-araA. F-araA can also inhibit mitochondrial DNA synthesis at concentrations similiar to those that cause cytotoxicity; however, inhibition of mitochondrial DNA synthesis does not affect cell growth for several cell generations.[44] Thus, cytotoxicity of F-araA, which is usually estimated by continuous exposure of cells to drugs for three to four generations, is not likely due to the inhibition of mitochondrial DNA. It has also been reported that the incubation of normal lymphocytes for 24 hours with 10 μM F-araA but not 1 μM F-araA, caused a decrease in both cytoplasmic NAD and ATP concentrations, that could be correlated with a decrease in cellular viability.[28] The mechanism of the depletion of NAD and ATP by F-araA is not clear. Whether inhibition of mitochondrial DNA synthesis by F-araA or the depletion of NAD and ATP is responsible for the delayed onset of toxicity of F-araA observed clinically has not been established.

Resistance to F-araA may occur as the result of decrease uptake, the lack of deoxycytidine kinase, an increase in the intracellular concentration of dATP, a decrease of the susceptibility of activity of ribonucleotide reductase, decrease of the affinity of DNA polymerase for F-araATP, or increase of efficient removal of F-araATP from the 3' terminus where incorporated into DNA. The potential role of the 3'–5' exonuclease activity of DNA polymerase δ and other 3'–5' exonuclease activities in removal of the incorporated F-araAMP remains to be defined as a possible mechanism of resistance.

2-Chlorodeoxyadenosine

Background. 2-chlorodeoxyadenosine (Cl-dAdo) was synthesized and found to be resistant to adenosine deaminase.[1,154] This compound was shown to be highly cytotoxic to a variety of cell lines in culture, and demonstrated to have potent antileukemic activity in mice.[40,145] Recently, this compound was also shown to have potent and lasting effects in the treatment of low grade B-cell neoplasms such as chronic lymphocytic leukemia, non-Hodgkins' lymphoma, and hairy-cell leukemia.[41,232,233] The spectrum of clinical activity is similar to that of Fludara I.V. The major toxicity encountered is bone marrow suppression. The degree of suppression was related to the rate of administration, cumulative dosage and tumor burden at the start of therapy.[41]

Metabolism. The mechanism responsible for transport of 2-Cl-dAdo into a variety of human hematopoietic cell lines was explored using nucleoside transport inhibitors such as dipyridamole and NBTI. It can be concluded that the transport mechanism of 2-Cl-dAdo appears to be different in different cell lines based on their differential response to nucleoside transport inhibitors.[16] Both NBTI sensitive and insensitive nucleoside transporters are involved. Once it enters cells, it can be phosphorylated by dCyd kinase to 2-Cl-dAMP.[120] Subsequently, 2-Cl-dAMP is phosphorylated to 2-Cl-dADP and then to 2-Cl-dATP. The enzymes involved are not clear. As 2-Cl-dATP, it can be incorporated into DNA through the action of DNA polymerases by competing with dATP.[120,121]

The structure and metabolism of 2-Cl dAdo are shown in Figure XVI-2-11.

Mechanism of Action and Resistance. 2-Cl-dAdo can inhibit DNA synthesis in growing cells as well as DNA repair in resting cells.[146] When growing cells were treated with 2-Cl-dAdo, accumulation of cells in S-phase was observed, suggesting that inhibition of DNA synthesis could be responsible for the cell killing effect of the drug. The active metabolite of the compound is 2-Cl-dATP which can compete with dATP to be incorporated into the 3' end of the growing DNA chain. Elongation beyond the incorporated analog was significantly retarded. This could contribute partly to its inhibitory activity against DNA synthesis. Furthermore, 2-Cl-dATP is a potent inhibitor of ribonucleotide reductase.[220] Intracellular deoxynucleoside triphosphates were found to decrease in cells after exposure to 2-Cl-dAdo.[120] This could also contribute to its antitumor activity.

The mechanism of resistance is not clear and could be similar to that of 2-F araA. It should be pointed out that although 2-F araA and 2-Cl-dAdo share many similar features, there are also differences in their metabolism and mechanism of action.

Hydroxyurea

Background. Although it was first synthesized in 1869,[80] the biological activity of hydroxyurea was not recognized until 60 years later when it was found that hydroxyurea could produce leukopenia, anemia, and megaloblastic changes in the bone marrow of rabbit.[245] This simple molecule (Figure XVI-2-12) has been evaluated in a number of types of cancer, but its principal uses are in myeloproliferative diseases. Currently it is an initial therapy of choice for chronic myelogenous leukemia (CML); it is also used as a therapy for polycythemia vera and hypereosinophilic syndrome. Activity against solid tumors has been demonstrated, but it is generally used in combination with other anticancer agents or with radiation for the treatment of carcinomas.[78]

Hydroxyurea can be taken orally and the half-life in plasma is about four hours.[21] It readily crosses the blood-brain barrier. It is excreted predominantly in urine; the interpatient variability is significant. The full extent and significance of hydroxyurea metabolism in humans has not been well established. It can be degraded by intestinal bacterial urease to form hydroxylamine (NH_2OH) which can interact with acteyl-coenzyme A to form acetohydroxamic acid. This metabolite is found in the plasma of patients receiving hydroxyurea therapy.[106]

The dose limiting toxicity of hydroxyurea is myelosuppression. This is due to inhibition of DNA synthesis in bone marrow. This toxicity begins within two to five days and its duration is short once the drug is discontinued. Gastrointestinal side effects are frequently seen but rarely require discontinuation of therapy at the doses commonly used. Some dermatologic changes such as hyperpigmentation can also occur in patients after extended therapy.[78]

Mechanism of Action and Resistance. Hydroxyurea is considered to enter cells by passive diffusion.[273] It inhibits cellular DNA synthesis through inhibition of ribonucleotide reductase, the key enzyme responsible for the synthesis of deoxynucleotides; the building blocks of DNA. The substrates for this reaction are the four ribonucleoside diphosphates; other substrates of the reaction are 5-FUDP, 5-azaCDP and 6-ThioGDP. The activity of ribonucleotide reductase is

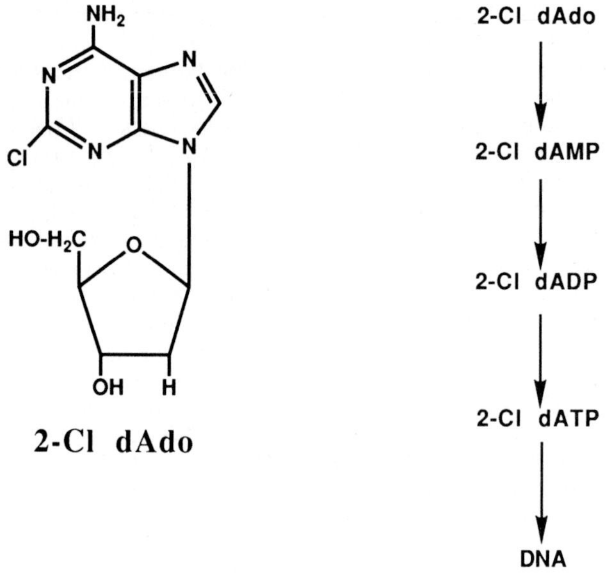

Figure XVI-2-11. Structure and metabolism of 2-Cl-dAdo (2-chlorodeoxyadenosine).

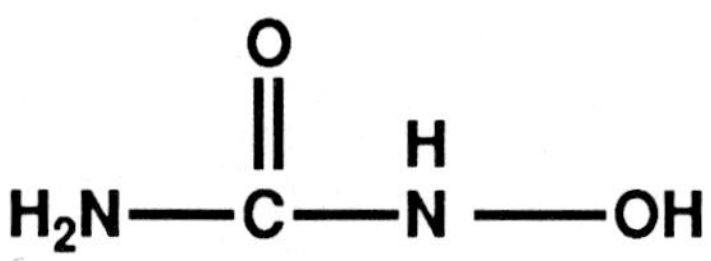

Figure XVI-2-12. Hydroxyurea.

highly regulated by the intracellular concentration of ribonucleoside and deoxyribonucleoside triphosphates. Two models, sequential and intercalating, are proposed for the interplay of ribonucleotide reductase and deoxynucleoside triphosphates.[211] The metabolites of deoxynucleoside analogs, such as 2F-araATP and araATP are also potent inhibitors of this enzyme. The activity of this enzyme plays a key role in controlling the intracellular concentrations of deoxynucleotide triphosphates, and, thus, can influence the activation or incorporation of deoxynucleoside antimetabolites such as araC, FUdR, and 2F-araA into DNA. Inhibition of ribonucleotide reductase by hydroxyurea would not affect the incorporation of these antimetabolites and, thus, could potentiate their action. Ribonucleotide reductase is composed of two types of protein subunits, M1 and M2. These two proteins are coded by two different chromosomes. M1 protein, which is coded by chromosome 11 and has a molecular weight of 170KD, does not vary with cell cycle and is responsible for the interaction with nucleotides.[29,184] M2 protein, which is coded by a gene on chromosome 2 in close proximity to the ornithine decarboxylase gene, has a molecular weight of 88KD, and fluctuates throughout the cell cycle with peak activity in S phase. The alteration of ribonucleotide reductase activity through the cell cycle is primarily controlled by the amount of M2 protein which binds a stoichiometric amount of iron and a stable organic free radical localized to a tyrosine residue.[95,97,300] Hydroxyurea inhibits ribonucleotide reductase through inactivation of the tyrosyl free radical on the M2 subunit. This inactivation can be partially prevented by ferrous iron.[5] The concentration of hydroxyurea required to inhibit human ribonucleotide reductase by 50% is about 0.5 μM.

As the result of the inhibition of ribonucleotide reductase by hydroxyurea, pools of deoxynucleotide triphosphates decrease, with concomitant inhibition of DNA synthesis. The cytotoxicity of hydroxyurea is dosage and time dependent. Most cells are accumulated in S phase and the G1-S boundary under the influence of hydroxyurea.[163,199]

Cells can become resistant to hydroxyurea as the result of increased ribonucleotide reductase activity primarily consequent to an increase in the M2 protein. M1 protein increases only when high levels of resistance to hydroxyurea are generated. The increase of M1 or M2 proteins is generally due to the overexpression of the proteins as the result of gene amplification.[56,61,175,189,297] Since ribonucleotide reductase is also responsible for the antitumor activity of some antimetabolites, such as thioguanine, the increment of ribonucleotide reductase in hydroxyurea resistant cells could render these cells more sensitive to those antimetabolites.[53] Alternating usage of hydroxyurea with those antimetabolites warrants further exploration for cancer treatment.[53]

References

1. Adams, R. L., and Burdon, R. H.: DNA methylation in eukaryotes. CRC Crit. Rev. Biochem., 13:349, 1982.
2. Agarwal, R. P., Spector, T., and Parks, R. E., Jr.: Tight-binding inhibitors: IV. Inhibition of adenosine deaminase by various inhibitors. Biochem. Pharmacol., 26:359, 1977.
3. Agarwal, R. P., Spector, T., and Parks, R. E., Jr.: Tight-binding inhibitors: IV. Inhibition of adenosine deaminase by various inhibitors. Biochem. Pharmacol., 26:359, 1977.
4. Ahluwalia, G. S., Grem, J. L., Hao, Z., and Cooney, D.: Metabolism and action of amino acid analog anti-cancer agents. Pharmac. Ther., 46:243, 1990.
5. Akerblom, L., Ehrenberg, A., Graslsund, A., Lankinen, H., Reichard, P., and Thelander, L.: Overproduction of the free radical of ribonucleotide reductase in hydroxyurea-resistant mouse fibroblast 3T6 cells. Proc. Natl. Acad. Sci., U.S.A., 78:2159, 1981.
6. Albert, A., and Brown, D. J.: Purine studies. Part I. Stability to acid and alkali. Solubility. Ionization. Comparison with pteridines. J. Chem. Soc., Part II:2060, 1954.
7. Alberto, P., Mermillod, B., Wever, W., Joss, R., and Cavalli, F.: A randomized comparison of doxifluridine and fluorouracil in advanced colorectal cancer. Proc. Am. Soc. Clin. Oncol., 5:94, 1986.
8. Ansfield, F. J., Kallas, G. J., and Singson, J. P.: Phase I-II studies or oral tegafur (ftorafur). J. Clin. Oncol., 1:107, 1983.
9. Ansfield, R., Klotz, J., Nealon, T., Ramirez, G., Minton, J., Hill, G., Wilson, W., Davis, H., Jr., and Cornell, G.: A Phase III study comparing the clinical utility of four regimens of 5-fluorouracil. Cancer, 39:34, 1977.
10. Ardalan, D., Singh, G., and Silberman, H.: A randomized Phase I and II study of Short-Term infusion of high-dose fluorouracil with or without N- (phosphonacetyl)-L-Aspartic acid in patients with advanced pancreatic colorectal cancers. J. Clin. Oncol., 6:1053, 1988.

11. Armstrong, R. D., and Diasio, R. B.: Metabolism and biological activity of 5′-deoxy-5-fluorouridine, a novel fluoropyrimidine. Cancer Res., 40:3333, 1980.
12. Ascione, F. J.: Allopurinol with mercaptopurine. Drug Ther., 7:69, 1977.
13. Au, J. L., Wu, A. T., Friedman, M. A., and Sadée, W.: Pharmacokinetics and metabolism of ftorafur in man. Cancer Treat. Rep., 63:343, 1979.
14. Au, J. L., Rustum, Y. M., Ledesma, E. J., Mittelman, A., and Greaven, P. J.: Clinical pharmacological studies of concurrent infusion of 5-fluorouracil and thymidine in treatment of colorectal carcinoma. Cancer Res., 42:2930, 1982.
15. Aul, C., and Schnider, W.: The role of low-dosage cytosine arabinoside and aggressive chemotherapy in advanced myelodysplastic syndomes. Cancer, 64:1812, 1989.
16. Avery, T. L., Rehg, J. E., Lumm, W. C., Harwood, F. C., Santana, V. M., and Blakly, R. L.: Biochemical pharmacology of 2-chlorodeoxyadenosine in malignant human hematopoietic cell lines and therapeutic effects of 2-bromodeoxyadenosine in drug combinations in mice. Cancer Res., 49:4972, 1989.
17. Bapat, A. R., Zarow, C., and Danenberg, P. V.: Human leukemic cells resistant to 5-fluoro-2′-deocyuridine contain a thymidylate synthase with a lower affinity for nucleotides. J. Biol. Chem., 258:4130, 1983.
18. Barrueco, J. R., Jacobsen, D. M., Chang, C. H., Brockman, R. W., and Sirotnak, F. M.: Proposed mechanism of therapeutic selectivity of 9-β-D-arabinofuranosyl-2-fluoradenine against murine leukemia based upon lower capacities for transport and phosphorylation in proliferative intestinal epithelium compared to tumor cells. Cancer Res., 47:700, 1987.
19. Beardmore, T. D., and Kelley, W. N.: Effects of Allopurinol and Oxipurinol on Pyrimidine Biosynthesis in Man. *In* Purine Metabolism in Man. Edited by O. Sperling, S. DeVries, and J. B. Wyngaarden. New York, Plenum Publishing Corp., 1974, p. 609.
20. Beisler, J.: Isolation, characterization, and properties of labile hydrolysis product of the antitumor nucleoside, 5-azacytidine. J. Med. Chem., 21:204, 1978.
21. Belt, R. J., Haas, C. D., Kennedy, J., and Taylor, S.: Studies of hydroxyurea administered by continuous infusion: Toxicity, pharmacokinetics, and cell synchronization. Cancer, 46:455, 1980.
22. Berger, S. H., and Hakala, M. T.: Relationship of dUMP and free FdUMP pools to inhibition to thymidylate synthase by 5-fluorouracil. Mol. Pharmacol., 25:303, 1984.
23. Berger, S. H., Jenh, C.-H., Johnson, L. F., and Berger, F. G.: Thymidylate synthase overproduction and gene amplification in fluorodeoxyuridine-resistant human cells. Mol. Pharmacol., 28:461, 1985.
24. Bertino, J. R., Mini, E., and Fernandes, D. J.: Sequential methotrexate and 5-fluorouracil: Mechanisms of synergy. Semin. Oncol., 10:2, 1983.
25. Bertino, J. R., and Mini, E.: Does Modulation of 5-Fluorouracil by Metabolites or Antimetabolites Work in the Clinic? *In* New Avenues in Developmental Cancer Chemotherapy. Edited by D. S. Martin. New York, Academic Press, 1987.
26. Boston Collaborative Drug Surveillance Program: Excess of ampicillin rash associated with allopurinol or hyperuricemia. N. Engl. J. Med., 286:505, 1972.
27. Bowen, D., Diasio, R. B., and Goldman, I. D.: Distinguishing between membrane transport and intracellular metabolism of fluorodeoxyuridine in Ehrlich ascites tumor cells by application of kinetic and high-performance liquid chromatographic techniques. J. Biol. Chem., 254:5333, 1979.
28. Brager, P. M., Grever, M. R.: 9-β-D-arabinofuranosyl-2-fluoradenine reduces NAD in normal lymphocytes and neoplastic cells in CLL. Proc. Am. Assoc. Cancer Res., 27:21, 1986.
29. Brissenden, J. R., Caras, I., Thelander, L., and Francke, U.: The structural gene for the M1 subunit of ribonucleotide reductase maps to chromosome II, band 15 in human and to chromosome 7 in mouse. Exp. Cell Res., 174:302, 1988.
30. Brockman, R. W., Cheng, Y. C., Schabel, F. M., Jr., and Montgomery, J. A.: Metabolism and chemotherapeutic activity of 9-β-D-arabinofuranosyl-2-fluoradenine against murine leukemia L1210 and evidence for its phosphorylation by deoxycytidine kinase. Cancer Res., 40:3610, 1980.
31. Brockman, R. W.: Mechanism of resistance to anticancer agents. Adv. Cancer Res., 7:129, 1963.
32. Brockman, R. W., Schabel, F. M., Jr., and Montgomery, J. A.: Biologic activity of 9-β-D-arabinofuranosyl-2-fluoradenine, a metabolically stable analog of 9-β-D-arabinofuranosyl-adenine. Biochem. Pharmacol., 26:2193, 1977.
33. Burchenal, J. H., Murphy, M. L., Ellison, R. R., Sykes, M. P., Tan, T. C., Leone, L. A., Darnofsky, D. A., Craver, L. F., Dargeon, H. W., and Rhoads, C. P.: Clinical evaluation of a new antimetabolite, 6-mercaptopurine, in the treatment of leukemia and allied diseases. Blood, 8:965, 1953.
34. Cadman, E. C., Dix, D. E., and Handschumacher, R. E.: Clinical, biological and biochemical effects of pyrazofurin. Cancer Res., 38:682, 1978.
35. Cadman, E., Davis, L., and Heimer, R.: Enhanced 5-fluorouracil nucleotide formation following methotrexate: biochemical explanation for drug synergism. Science, 205:1135, 1979.
36. Calabresi, P., and Chabner, B. A.: Antineoplastic Agents. *In* The Pharmacological Basis of Therapeutics, Eighth Edition. Edited by A. G. Gilman, T. W. Rall, A. S. Nies, and P. Taylor. New York, Pergamon Press, 1990, pp. 1231-1232.
37. Capizzi, R. L., Yang, J.-L., Cheng, E., and Bjornsson, T., Sahasrabudhe, D., Tan, R. -S., and Cheng, Y. C.: Alteration of the Pharmacokinetics of High-Dose Ara-C by Its Metabolite, High Ara-U in Patients with Acute Leukemia. J. Clin. Oncol., 1:763, 1983.
38. Capizzi, R. L., and Cheng, Y. C.: Sequential high-dose cytosine arabinoside and asparaginase in refractory actue leukemia. Medical and Pediatric Oncology, 10(S1):221, 1982.
39. Caradonna, S. J., and Cheng, Y.-C.: The role of deoxyuridine triphosphate nucleotidohydrolase, uracil-DNA glycosylase, and DNA polymerase in the metabolism of FUdR in human tumor cells. Mol. Pharmacol., 18:513, 1980.
40. Carson, D. A., Wasson, D. B., Kaye, J., Ullman, B., Martin, D. W., Jr., Robins, R. K., and Montgomery, J. A.: Deoxyadenosine kinase-mediated toxicity of deoxyadenosine analogs toward malignant human lymphoblasts in vitro and toward murine L1210 leukemia in vivo. Proc. Natl. Acad. Sci., U.S.A., 77:6865, 1980.
41. Carson, D. A., Wasson, D. B., and Beutler, E.: Antileukemic and immunosuppressive activity of 2-chloro-2′ deoxyadenosine. Proc. Natl. Acad. Sci., U.S.A., 81:2232, 1984.
42. Casper, E. S., Vale, K., Williams, L. J., Martin, D. S., and Young, C. W.: Phase I and clinical pharmacological evaluation of biochemical modulation of 5-fluorouracil with N-(phosphonacetyl)-L-aspartic acid. Cancer Res., 43:2324, 1983.
43. Cass, C. E., Kolassa, N., Uehara, Y., Dahlig-Harley, E., Harley, E., and Paterson, A. R. P.: Absence of binding sites for the transport inhibitor nitrobenzylthioinosine on nucleoside transport-deficient mouse lymphoma cells. Biochim. Biophys. Acta, 649:769, 1981.
44. Catapano, C. V., Chandler, K. B., Fernandes, D. J.: Effects of anticancer agents on primer RNA formation in human leukemia cells. Proc. Am. Assoc. Cancer Res., 31:420, 1990.
45. Chabner, B. A., Johns, D. G., Coleman, N., Drake, J. C., and Evans, W. G.: Purification and properties of cytidine deaminase from normal and leukemic granulocytes. J. Clin. Invest., 53:922, 1974.
46. Chabner, B. A.: Cytidine Analogues. *In* Cancer Chemotherapy: Principles and Practice. Edited by B. A. Chabner and J. M. Collins. Philadelphia, J. B. Lippincott Co., 1990, pp. 154–179.
47. Chang, C.-H., and Cheng, Y.-C.: Effects of Nucleoside Triphosphates on Human Ribonucleotide Reductase from Molt-4F Cells. Cancer Res., 39:5087, 1979.
48. Chen, S.-F., Ruben, R. L., and Dexter, D. L.: Mechanism of action of the novel anticancer agent 6-fluoro-2-(2′-fluoro-1,1′-biphenyl-4-yl)-3-methyl-4-quinolinecarboxylic acid sodium salt (NSC-368390): Inhibition of de novo pyrimidine nucleotide biosynthesis. Cancer Res., 46:5014, 1986.
49. Chen, C.-H., Vazquez-Padua, M., and Cheng, Y.-C.: The effect of anti-HIV nucleoside analogs on mitochondrial DNA and its implication on delayed toxicity. Molec. Pharmacol., 39:27, 1991.
50. Cheng, Y.-C., Tan, R.-S., Ruth, J. L., and Dutschman, G. E.: Cytotoxicity of 2′-fluoro-5-iodo-1-β-D-arabinofuranosylcytosine and its relationship to deoxycytidine deaminase. Biochem. Pharmacol., 32:726, 1983.
51. Cheng, Y. C., Domin, B., and Lee, L.-S.: Human deoxycytidine kinase. Purification and characterization of the cytoplasmic and mitochondrial isozymes derived from blast cells of acute myelocytic leukemia patients. Biochem. Biophys. Acta., 481:481, 1977.
52. Cheng, Y. C., Agarwal, P., and Parks, R. E.: Erythrocytic nucleoside diphosphokinase IV. Evidence for electrophoretic heterogeneity. Biochemistry, 10:2139, 1971.
53. Cheng, Y. C., and Brockman, R. W.: Mechanisms of Drug resistance and collateral sensitivity: Bases for development of chemotherapeutic agents. *In* Development of Target Oriented Anticancer Drugs. Edited by Y. C. Cheng, B. Goz, and M. Minkoff. New York, Raven Press, 1983, pp. 107–117.
54. Cheson, B. D.: Issues for the Future Development of Fludarabine Phosphate. *In* Seminars in Oncology, Vol. 17, No. 5. Edited by J. W. Yarbro, R. Bornstein, M. J. Mastrangelo. Philadelphia, PA, W. B. Saunders Company, 1990.
55. Chou, T. C., Arlin, Z., Clarkson, B. D., and Phillips, F. S.: Metabolism of 1-β-D-arabinofuranosylcytosine in human leukemic cells. Cancer Res., 37:3561, 1977.
56. Choy, B. K., McClarty, G. A., Chan, A. K., Thelander, L., and Wright, J. A.: Molecular mechanisms of drug resistance involving ribonucleotide reductase: Hydroxyurea resistance in a series of clonally related mouse cell lines selected in the presence of increasing drug concentrations. Cancer Res., 48:2029, 1988.
57. Christophidis, N., Vajda, F. J. E., Lucas, I., Drummer, O., Moon, W. J., and Louis, W. J.: Fluorouracil therapy in patients with carcinoma of the large bowel: a pharmacokinetic comparison of various rates and routes of administration. Clinical Pharmacokinetics, 3:330, 1978.
58. Cihak, A., and Vesely, J.: Prolongation of the lag period preceding the enhancement of thymidine and thymidylate kinase activity in regenerating rat liver by 5-azacytidine. Biochem. Pharmacol., 21:3257, 1972.
59. Clarke, D. A., Elion, G. B., Hitchings, G. H., and Stock, C. C.: Structure-activity relationships among purines related to 6-mercaptopurine. Cancer Res., 18:445, 1958.
60. Clarkson, B., O'Connor, A., Winston, L., and Hutchinson, D.: The physiologic disposition of 5-fluorouracil and 5-fluoro-2′-deoxyuridine in man. Clin. Pharmacol. Ther., 5:581, 1964.
61. Cocking, J. M., Tonin, P. N., Stokoe, N. M., Wensing, E. J., Lewis, W. H., and Srinivasan, P. R.: Gene for M1 subunit of ribonucleotide reductase is amplified in hydroxyurea-resistant hamster cells. Somat. Cell Mol. Genet., 13:221, 1987.
62. Cody, R., Stewart, D., deForni, M., Moore, M., Neidhart, J., Maurer, H., Dallaire, B., and Grillo-Lopez, A.: A phase II study of brequinar sodium (DuP 785, NSC 368390) in breast cancer. Proc. Am. Assoc. Cancer Oncol., 10:61, 1991.
63. Cohen, S. S., Flaks, J. G., Barner, H. D., Loeb, M. R., and Lichtenstein, J.: The mode of action of 5-fluorouracil and its derivatives. Proc. Nat. Acad. Sci. (Wash.), 44:1004, 1958.
64. Collins, K. D., and Stark, G. R.: Aspartate transcarbamylase interaction with the transition state analog N-(phosphonacetyl)-L-aspartate. J. Biol. Chem., 246:6599, 1971.
65. Cory, J., Breland, J. B., and Carter, G. L.: Effect of 5-fluorouracil on RNA metabolism in Novikoff hepatoma cells. Cancer Res., 39:4905, 1979.
66. Cory, J. G.: Role of ribonucleotide reductase in cell division. *In* Inhibitors of Ribonucleoside Diphosphate Reductase Activity. Edited by J. G. Cory and A. H. Cory. New York, Pergamon Press, 1989, pp. 1–16.
67. Danenberg, P. V., and Danenberg, K. D.: Effect of 5,10-methylenetetrahydrofolate and the dissociation of 5-fluorodeoxyuridylate binding of human thymidylate synthetase: Evidence for an ordered mechanism. Biochemistry, 17:4018, 1978.
68. Darnowski, J. W., and Handschumacher, R. E.: Tissue uridine pools. Evidence in vivo of a concentrative mechanism for uridine uptake. Cancer Res., 46:3490, 1986.
69. Darnowski, J. W., and Handschumacher, R. E.: Tissue-specific enhancement of uridine utilization of 5-fluorouracil therapy in mice by benzylacyclouridine. Cancer Res., 45:5364, 1985.
70. Darnowski, J. W., Holdridge, C., and Handschumacher, R. E.: Concentrative uridine transport by murine splenocytes: kinetics, substrate specificity, and sodium dependency. Cancer Res., 47:2614, 1987.
71. Darnowski, J. W., and Handschumacher, R. E.: Enhancement of fluorouracil therapy by the manipulation of tissue uridine pools. Pharmac. Ther., 41:381, 1989.
72. Dearden, C. E., Hoffbrand, A. V., Ganeshaguru, K., Brozovic, M., Williams, H. J., Traub, N., Mills, M., Linch, D. C., and Catovsky, D.: Membrane phenotype and response to deoxycoformycin in mature T-cell malignancies. Br. Med. J., 295:873, 1987.
73. De Saint Vincent, B. R., Dechamps, M., and Butlin, G.: The modulation of the thymidine triphosphate pool of chinese hamster cells by dCMP deaminase and UDP reductase. J. Biol. Chem., 255:162, 1980.
74. De Saint Vincent, B. R., and Buttin, G.: Studies on 1-β-D-Arabinofuranosyl-cytosine resistant mutants of Chinese Fibroblasts. III. Joint Resistance to Arabino-furanosylcytosine and to Excess Thymidine—A Semidominant Manifestation of Deoxyctidine Triphosphate Pool Expansion. Somat. Cell Genet., 5:67, 1979.
75. Diasio, R. B., Beavers, T. I., and Carpenter, J. T.: Familial deficiency of dihydropyrimidine dehydrogenase. Biochemical basis for familial pyrimidemia and severe 5-fluorouracil-induced toxicity. J. Clin. Invest., 81:447, 1988.
76. Diasio, R. B., Lakings, D. E., and Bennett, J. E.: Evidence for conversion of 5-fluorocytosine to 5-fluorouracil in humans: possible factor in 5- fluorocytosine clinical toxicity. Antimicrob. Agents Chemother., 14:903, 1978.
77. Diasio, R. B., and Harris, B. E.: Clinical pharmacology of 5-fluorouracil. Clinical Pharmacokinetics, 16:215, 1989.
78. Donehower, R. C.: Hydroxyurea. *In* Cancer Chemotherapy: Principles and Practice. Edited by B. A. Chabner, and J. M. Collins. J. B. Lippincott Co., Philadelphia, 1990, pp. 154-179.
79. Drake, J. C., Stoller, R. G., and Chabner, B. A.: Characteristics of the enzyme uridine-cytidine kinase isolated from a cultured human cell line. Biochem. Pharmacol., 26:64, 1977.

80. Dresler, W. F. C., and Stein, R.: Über den Hydroxylharnstoff. Justus Leibigs Ann. Chem., 150:242, 1869.
81. Duschinsky, R., Pleven, E., and Heidelberger, C.: The synthesis of 5-fluoropyrimidines. J. Amer. Chem. Soc., 79:4559, 1957.
82. Dusenbury, C. E., Davis, M. A., Lawrence, T. S., and Maybaum, J.: Induction of megabase DNA fragments by 5-fluorodeoxyuridine in human colorectal tumor (HT29) cells. Molecular Pharmacology, 39:285, 1990.
83. Dutcher, J. P., Wiernik, P. H., Markus, S., Weinberg, V., Schiffer, C. A., and Harwood, K. V.: Intensive maintenance therapy improves survival in adult acute nonlymphocytic leukemia: An eight-year follow up. Leukemia, 2:413, 1988.
84. DuVivier, A.: Topical cytostatic drugs in the treatment of skin cancer. Clin. Exp. Dermatol., 7:89, 1982.
85. Edwards, N. L., Recker, D., Airozo, D., and Fox, I. H.: Enhanced purine salvage during allopurinol therapy: An important pharmacologic property in humans. J. Lab. Clin. Med., 98:673, 1981.
86. Einhorn, M., and Davidsohn, I.: Hepatotoxicity of 6-mercaptopurine. JAMA, 188:802, 1964.
87. el Kouni, M. H., Naguib, F. N. M., and Cha, S.: Circadian rhythm of dihydrouracil dehydrogenase (DHUDase), uridine phosphorylase (UrdPase), and thymidine phosphorylase (dThdPase) in mouse liver. FASEB J., 3:A397, 1989.
88. Elias, L., and Sandoval, J. M.: Interferon effects upon fluorouracil metabolism by HL-60 cells. Biochem. Biophys. Res. Commun., 163:867, 1989.
89. Elion, G. B., Hitchings, G. H., and Vander-Werff, H.: Antagonists of nucleic acid derivatives. VI. Purines. J. Biol. Chem., 192:505, 1951.
90. Elion, G. B., and Hitchings, G. H.: The synthesis of 6-thioguanine. J. Am. Chem. Soc., 77:1676, 1955.
91. Elion, G. B.: Biochemistry and pharmacology of purine analogs. Fed. Proc., 26:898, 1967.
92. Elion, G. B., and Hitchings, G. H.: Azathioprine, *In* Handbook of Experimental Pharmacology. Edited by A. C. Sartorelli and D. G. Johns. Berlin, Springer-Verlag, 1975, p. 404.
93. Elion, G. B.: Enzymatic and metabolic studies with allopurinol. Ann. Rheum. Dis., 25:608, 1966.
94. Elion, G. B., Callahan, S., Rundles, R. W., and Hitchings, G. H.: Relationship between metabolic fates and antitumor activities of thiopurines. Cancer Res., 23:1207, 1963.
95. Engstrom, Y., Eriksson, S., Jildevik, I., Skog, S., Thelander, L., and Tribukait, B.: Cell cycle-dependent expression of mammalian ribonucleotide reductase. Differential regulation of the two subunits. J. Biol. Chem., 260:9114, 1985.
96. Ensminger, W. D., Rosowsky, A., Raso, V., Levin, D. C., Glode, M., Come, S., Steel, G., and Frei, E., 3rd: A clinical pharmacological evaluation of hepatic arterial infusion of 5-fluoro-2′-deoxyuridine and 5-fluorouracil. Cancer Res., 38:3784, 1978.
97. Eriksson, S., Graslund, A., Skog, S., Thelander, A., and Tribukait, B.: Cell cycle dependent regulation of mammalian ribonucleotide reductase. J. Biol. Chem., 259:11695, 1984.
98. Erlichman, C., Fine, S., and Wong, A.: A randomized trial of fluorouracil and folinic acid in patients with metastatic colorectal carcinoma. J. Clin. Oncol., 6:469, 1988.
99. Erlichman, C., Donehower, R. C., Speyer, J. L., Klecker, R., and Chabner, B. A.: Phase I-Phase II trial of N-phosphonacetyl-L-aspartic acid given by intravenous infusion and 5-fluorouracil given by bolus injection. J. Natn. Cancer Inst., 68:227, 1982.
100. Esterhay, R. J., Jr., Aisner, J., Levi, J. A., and Wiernik, P. H.: High-dose 6-mercaptopurine in advanced refractory cancer. Cancer Treat. Rep., 62:1229, 1978.
101. Evans, R. M., Laskin, J. D., and Hakala, M. T.: Assessment of growth-limiting events caused by 5-fluorouracil in mouse cells and in human cells. Cancer Res., 40:4113, 1980.
102. Evans, R. M., Laskin, J. D., and Hakala, M. T.: Effect of excess folates and deoxyinosine on the activity and site of action of 5-fluorouracil. Cancer Res., 41:3288, 1981.
103. Fernandes, D. J., and Carroll, C. C.: Multiple modes of resistance of human CCRF-CEM leukemic cells to 5-fluoro-2′-deoxyuridine. Cancer Res., 24:283, 1983.
104. Fernandes, J. F., LePage, G. A., and Lindner, A.: The influence of azaserine and 6-mercaptopurine on the in vivo metabolism of ascites tumor cells. Cancer Res., 16:154, 1956.
105. Finch, R. E., Bending, M. R., and Lant, A. F.: Plasma levels of 5-fluorouracil after oral and intravenous administration in cancer patients. Br. J. Clin. Pharmacol., 7:613, 1979.
106. Fishbein, W. N., and Carbone, P. P.: Hydroxyurea: mechanisms of action. Science, 142:1069, 1963.
107. Fox, I. H.: Metabolic basis for disorders of purine nucleotide degradation. Metabolism, 30:616, 1981.
108. Fox, R. M., Woods, R. L., Tattersall, M. H. N., Piper, A. A., and Sampson, D.: Allopurinol modulation of fluorouracil toxicity. Cancer Chemother. Pharmacol., 5:151, 1981.
109. Fridland, A.: Effect of cytosine arabinoside on replicon initiation in human lymphoblasts. Biochem. Biophys. Res. Commun., 74:72, 1977.
110. Fritsch, G. L.: Adenosine deaminase in disorders of purine metabolism and immune deficiency. Ann. NY Acad. Sci., 451:1, 1985.
111. Furth, J. T., and Cohen, S. S.: Inhibition of mammalian DNA polymerase by 1-β-D-arabinofuranosylcytosine and the 5′-triphosphate of 9-β-D-arabinofuranosyladenine. Cancer Res., 28:2061, 1968.
112. Fyfe, J. A., Miller, R. L., and Krenitsky, T. A.: Kinetic properties and inhibition of orotidine 5′-phosphate decarboxylase. J. Biol. Chem., 248:3801, 1973.
113. Gandhi, V., and Plunkett, W.: Modulation of arabinosylnucleoside metabolism by arabinosylnucleotides in human leukemia cells. Cancer Res., 48:329, 1988.
114. Glazer, R. I., and Lloyd, L. S.: Association of cell lethality with incorporation of 5-fluorouracil and 5-fluorouridine into nuclear RNA in human colon carcinoma cells in culture. Mol. Pharmacol., 21:468, 1982.
115. Goulian, M., Bleile, B., and Tseng, B. Y.: Methotrexate-induced misincorporation of uracil into DNA. Biochemistry, 77:1956, 1980.
116. Grem, J. L., and Fischer, P. H.: Enhancement of 5-Fluorouracil's anticancer activity by dipyridamole. Pharmac. Ther., 40:349, 1989.
117. Grem, J. L., and Fischer, P. H.: Augmentation of 5-fluorouracil cytotoxity in human colon cancer cells by dipyridamole. Cancer Res., 45:2967, 1985.
118. Grever, M. R., Chapman, R. A., Ratanatharathorn, V., and Slease, R. B.: An investigation of deoxycoformycin in advanced cutaneous T-cell lymphoma. Blood, 66(suppl 1):215a, 1986.
119. Grever, M. R., Kopecky, K. J., Coltman, C. A., Files, J. C., Greenberg, B. R., Hutton, J. J., Talley, R., Von Hoff, D. D., and Balcerzak, S. P.: Fludarabine monophosphate: A Potentially Useful Agent in Chronic Lymphocytic Leukemia. Nouv. Rev. Fr. Hematol., 30:457, 1988.
120. Griffig, J., Koob, R., and Blakley, R. L.: Mechanism of inhibition of DNA synthesis by 2-chlorodeoxyadenosine in human lymphoblastic cells. Cancer Res., 49:6923, 1989.
121. Hande, K., Hixon, C., and Chabner, B.: Postchemotherapy purine excretion in lymphoma patients receiving allopurinol. Cancer Res., 41:2273, 1981.
122. Hanka, L. J., Evans, J. S., Mason, D. J., and Dietz, A.: Microbiological production of 5-azacytidine: I. Production and biological activity. Antimicrob. Agents Chemother., 6:619, 1966.
123. Harbers, E., Chaudhuri, N. K., and Heidelberger, C.: Studies on fluorinated pyrimidines. VIII. Further biochemical and metabolic investigations. J. Biol. Chem., 234:1255, 1959.
124. Harris, B. E., Ruiling, S., Soong, S., and Diasio, R. B.: Relationship between dihydropyrimidine dehydrogenase activity and plasma 5-fluorouracil levels with evidence for circadian variation of enzyme activity and plasma drug levels in cancer patients receiving 5-fluorouracil by protracted continuous infusion. Cancer Res., 50:197, 1990.
125. Hartmann, K. U., and Heidelberger, C.: Studies on fluorinated pyrimidines. VIII. Inhibition of thymidylate synthetase. J. Biol. Chem., 236:3006, 1961.
126. Heggie, G. D., Sommadossi, J.-P., Cross, D. S., Huster, W. J., and Diasio, R. B.: Clinical pharmacokinetics of 5-fluorouracil and its metabolites in plasma, urine, and bile. Cancer Res., 47:2203, 1987.
127. Heidelberger, C., Danenberg, P. V., and Moran, R. G.: Fluorinated pyrimidines and their nucleosides. Adv. Enzymol. 54:57, 1983.
128. Heidelberger, C., Chaudhuri, N. K., Danneberg, P., Mooreh, D., Griesbach, L., Duschinsky, R., Schnitzer, R. J., and Pleven, E.: Fluorinated pyrimidines, a new class of tumor-inhibitory compounds. Nature, 179:663, 1957.
129. Heier, M. S., and Fossa, S. D.: Wernicke-Korsakoff-like syndrome in patients with colorectal carcinoma treated with high-dose doxifluridine. Acta Neurol. Scand., 73:449, 1986.
130. Helland, S., and Ueland, P. M.: Effect of 2′-deoxycoformycin infusion on S-adenosylhomocysteine hydrolase and the amount of S-adenosylhomocysteine and related compounds in tissues of mice. Cancer Res., 43:4142, 1983.
131. Hershfeld, M. S.: Apparent suicide inactivation of human lymphoblast S-adenosylhomocysteine hydrolase by 2′-deoxyadenosine and adenine arabinoside: a basis for direct toxic effects of analogs of adenosine. J. Biol. Chem., 254:22, 1979.
132. Hill, D. L., and Bennett, L. L., Jr.: Purification and properties of 5-phosphoribosyl pyrophosphate amidotransferase from adenocarcinoma 758 cells. Biochemistry, 8:122, 1969.
133. Hillman, R. S.: Hematopoietic agents: Growth factors, minerals and vitamins. Goodman & Gilman Ch. 54, p. 1277.
134. Hitchings, G. H., and Elion, G. B.: The chemistry and biochemistry of purine analogs. Ann. N. Y. Acad. Sci., 60:195, 1954.
135. Hochster, H., and Cassileth, P.: Fludarabine Phosphate Therapy of Non-Hodgkin's Lymphoma. *In* Seminars in Oncology. Edited by J. W. Yarbro, R. Bornstein, M. J., Mastrangelo. W. B. Saunders Company, Philadelphia, PA, 1990, Vol. 17, No. 5.
136. Holt, R. J., and Newman, R. L.: The antimycotic activity of 5-fluorocytosine. J. Clin. Pathol., 26:167, 1973.
137. Houghton, J. A., Weiss, K. D., Williams, L. G., Torrance, P. M., and Houghton, P. J.: Relationship between 5-fluoro-2′-deoxyuridylate, 2′-deoxyuridylate, and thymidylate synthase activity subsequent to 5-fluorouracil administration in xenografts of human colon adenocarcinomas. Biochem. Pharmacol., 35:1351, 1986.
138. Houghton, J. A., Williams, L. G., Radparvar, A., and Houghton, P. J.: Characterization of the pools of 5,10-methylenetetrahydrofolates and tetrahydrofolates in xenografts of human colon adenocarcinoma. Cancer Res., 48:3062, 1988.
139. Houghton, J. A., Torrance, P. M., Radparvar, S., Williams, L. G., and Houghton, P. J.: Binding of 5-fluorodeoxyuridylate to thymidylate synthetase in human colon adenocarcinoma xenografts. Eur. J. Cancer Clin. Oncol., 22:505, 1986.
140. Houghton, J. A., and Houghton, P. J.: Elucidation of pathways of 5-fluorouracil metabolism in xenografts of human colorectal adenocarcinoma. Eur. J. Clin. Oncol., 19:807, 1983.
141. Houghton, J. A., Maroda, S. J., Jr., Phillips, J. O., and Houghton, P. J.: Biochemical determinants of responsiveness to 5-fluorouracil and its derivatives in xenografts of human colorectal adenocarcinomas in mice. Cancer Res., 41:144, 1981.
142. Howell, S. B., Wung, W. E., Taetle, R., Hussain, F., and Romine, J. S.: Modulation of 5-fluorouracil toxicity by allopurinol in man. Cancer, 48:1281, 1981.
143. Hrushesky, W.: Circadian timing of cancer chemotherapy. Science, 228:73, 1985.
144. Hryniuk, W. M.: The importance of dose intensity in the outcome of chemotherapy. Important Adv. Oncol., p. 121, 1988.
145. Huang, M.-C., Avery, T. L., Blakley, R. L., Secrist, J. A., III, and Montgomery, J. A.: Improved synthesis and antitumor activity of 2-bromo-2′-deoxyadenosine. J. Med. Chem., 27:800, 1984.
146. Huang, M.-C., Ashmun, R. A., Avery, T. L., Kuehl, M., and Blakley, R. L.: Effects of cytotoxicity of 2-chloro-2′-deoxyadenosine and 2-bromo-2′-deoxyadenosine on cell growth, clonogenicity, DNA synthesis, and cell kinetics. Cancer Res., 46:2362, 1986.
147. Huang, P., and Plunkett, W.: Preferential incorporation of arabinofuranosyl-2-fluoradenine into poly (A+) RNA and its inhibitory effects on transcription and translation. Proc. Am. Assoc. Cancer Res., 27:21, 1986.
148. Huang, P., Chubb, S., and Plunkett, W.: Incorporation of 9-β-D-arabinofuranosyl-2-fluoradenine into DNA and its chain termination effect on DNA synthesis. J. Biol. Chem., 265:16617, 1990.
149. Ingraham, H. A., Tseng, B. Y., and Goulian, M.: Mechanism for exclusion of 5-fluorouracil from DNA. Cancer Res., 40:998, 1980.
150. Ingraham, H. A., Tseng, B. Y., and Goulian, M.: Nucleotide levels and incorporation of 5-fluorouracil and uracil into DNA of cells treated with 5-fluorodeoxyuridine. Mol. Pharmacol., 21:211, 1981.
151. Jayaram, H. N., Cooney, D. A., Vistica, D. T., Kariya, S., and Johnson, R. K.: Mechanisms of sensitivity of resistance of murine tumors to N- (phosphonacetyl)-L-aspartate (PALA). Cancer Treat. Rep., 63:1291, 1979.
152. Johnson, R. K., Swyryd, E. A., and Stark, G. R.: Reversal of toxicity and antitumor activity of N-(phosphonacetyl)-L-aspartate by uridine or carbamyl-DL-aspartate in vivo. Biochem. Pharmac., 26:81, 1977.
153. Johnson, R. K., Swyryd, E. A., and Stark, G. R.: Effects of N-(phosphonacetyl)-L-aspartate on murine tumors and normal tissues in vivo and in vitro and the relationship of sensitivity to rate of proliferation and levels of aspartate transcarbamylase. Cancer Res., 38:371, 1978.
154. Jones, P. A., Taylor, S. M., and Wilson, V.: DNA modification, differentiation, and transformation. J. Exp. Zool., 228:287, 1983.
155. Jones, M. E.: Pyrimidine nucleotide biosynthesis in animals: genes, enzymes, and regulation of UMP biosynthesis. Ann. Rev. Biochem., 49:253, 1980.
156. Kantarjian, H. M., Redman, J. R., and Keating, M. J.: Fludarabine Phosphate Therapy in Other Lymphoid Malignanices. *In* Seminars in Oncology. Edited by J. W. Yarbro, R. Bornstein, M. J. Mastrangelo. W. B. Saunders Company, Philadelphia, PA, 1990, Vol. 17, No. 5.
157. Keating, M.: Fludarabine Phosphate in the treatment of chronic lymphocytic leukemia. *In* Seminars in Oncology. Edited by J. W. Yarbro, R. Bornstein, M. J. Mastrangelo. W. B. Saunders Company, Philadelphia, PA, 1990, Vol. 17, No. 5. pp. 49-62.

158. Kelley, W., and Beardmore, T.: Allopurinol: alteration in pyrimidine metabolism in man. Science, 169:388, 1970.
159. Kempe, T. D., Swyryd, E. A., Bruist, M., and Stark, G. R.: Stable mutant mammalian cells that overproduce the first three enzymes of pyrimidine nucleotide biosynthesis. Cell, 9:541, 1976.
160. Kent, R. J., and Heidellberger, C.: Fluorinated pyrimidines, ribonucleotide reductase. Molec. Pharmacol., 8:465, 1972.
161. Kessel, D., Hall, T. C., and Wodinsky, I.: Transport and phosphorylation as factors in the antitumor action of cytosine arabinoside. Science, 156:1240, 1967.
162. Keyomarsi, K., and Moran, R.: Folinic acid augmentation of the effects of fluoropyrimidines on murine and human leukemic cells. Cancer Res., 46:5229, 1986.
163. Kim, J. H., Gelbard, A. S., and Perez, A. G.: Action of hydroxyurea on the nucleic acid metabolism and viability of HeLa cells. Cancer Res., 27:1301, 1967.
164. Klubes, P., and Leyland-Jones, B.: Enhancement of the antitumor activity of 5-fluorouracil by uridine rescue. Pharmac. Ther., 41:289, 1989.
165. Klubes, P. K., and Cerna, I.: Use of uridine rescue to enhance the antitumor selectivity of 5-fluorouracil. Cancer Res., 43:3182, 1983.
166. Kraut, E. H., Bouroncle, B. A., and Grever, M. R.: Low-dose deoxycoformycin in the treatment of hairy cell leukemia. Blood, 68:1119, 1986.
167. Krebs, H. B.: The use of topical 5-fluorouracil in the treatment of genital condylomas. Obstet. Gynecol. Clin. North Am., 14:559, 1987.
168. Kufe, D. W., and Major, P. P.: 5-Fluorouracil incorporation into human breast carcinoma RNA correlates with cytotoxicity. J. Biol. Chem., 256:9802, 1981.
169. Kufe, D. W., Major, P. P., Egan, E. M., and Loh, E.: 5-Fluoro-2′-deoxyuridine incorporation in L1210 DNA. J. Biol. Chem., 256:8885, 1981.
170. Laurie, J. A., Moertel, C. G., Fleming, T. R., Wieand, H. S., Leigh, J. E., Rubin, J., McCormack, G. W., Gerstner, J. B., Krook, J. E., Malliard, J., Twito, D. I., Morton, R. F., Tschetter, L. K., and Barlow, J. F.: Surgical adjuvant therapy of large-bowel carcinoma: an evaluation of levamisole and the combination of levamisole and fluorouracil. J. Clin. Oncol., 7:1447, 1989.
171. Lauzon, G. J., Paran, J. H., and Paterson, A. R. P.: Formation of l-β-D-arabinofuranosylcytosine diphosphate choline in cultured human leukemic RPMI6410 cells. Cancer Res., 38:1723, 1978.
172. Leclerc, J. M., and Cheng, Y.-C.: Demonstration of activities in leukemic cells capable of removing 1′-β-D-arabinofuranosyl cytosine (araC) from araC incorporated DNA. Proc. Amer. Assoc. Cancer Res., 25:19, 1984.
173. Lee, C. W., Cheeseman, C. I., and Jarvis, S. M.: Na+ – and K+ – dependent uridine transport in rat renal brush-border membrane vesicles. Biochim. Biophys. Acta, 942:139, 1988.
174. LePage, G. A.: Basic biochemical effects and mechanism of action of 6-thioguanine. Cancer Res., 23:1202, 1963.
175. Lewis, W. H., and Wright, J. A.: Altered ribonucleotide reductase activity in mammalian tissue culture cells resistant to hydroxyurea. Biochem. Biophys. Res. Commun., 60:926, 1974.
176. Li, L. H., Olin, E. J., Fraser, T. J., and Bhuyan, B. K.: Phase specificity of 5-azacytidine against mammalian cells in tissue culture. Cancer Res., 30:2770, 1970.
177. Li, L. H., Olin, E. J., Buskirk, H. H., and Reineke, L. M.: Cytotoxicity and node of action of 5-azacytidine on L1210 leukemia. Cancer Res., 30:2760, 1970.
178. Liliemark, J., and Juliusson, G.: On the Pharmacokinetics of 2-chloro-2′-deoxyadenosine in Humans. Cancer Res., 51:5570, 1991.
179. MacMillan, W. E., Wolberg, W. H., and Welling, P. G.: Pharmacokinetics of fluorouracil in humans. Cancer Res., 38:3479, 1978.
180. Madoc-Jones, H., and Bruce, W. R.: On the mechanism of the lethal action of 5-fluorouracil on mouse L cells. Cancer Res., 28:1976, 1968.
181. Major, P. P., Egan, E. M., Beardsley, G. P., Minden, M. D., and Kufe, D. W.: Lethality of human myeloblasts correlates with the incorporation of arabinofuranosylcytosine into DNA. J. Biol. Chem., 78:3235, 1981.
182. Mancini, W. R., and Cheng, Y.-C.: Human Deoxycytidylate Deaminase. Substrate and Regulator Specificities and Their Chemotherapeutic Implications. Molec. Pharmacol., 23:159, 1983.
183. Mandel, H. G.: The incorporation of 5-fluorouracil into RNA and its molecular consequences. Prog. Mol. Subcell. Biol., 1:82, 1969.
184. Mann, G. J., Musgrove, E. A., Fox, R. M., and Thelander, L.: Ribonucleotide reductase M1 subunit in cellular proliferation, quiescence, and differentiation. Cancer Res., 48:5151, 1988.
185. Martin, D. S., Stolfi, R. L., Sawyer, R. C., Spiegelman, S., and Young, C. W.: High-dose 5-fluorouracil with delayed uridine 'rescue' in mice. Cancer Res., 42:3964, 1982.
186. Martin, D. S., Stolfi, R. L., and Sawyer, R. C.: Utility of oral uridine as a substitute for parenteral uridine rescue of 5-fluorouracil therapy, with and without the uridine phosphorylase inhibitor 5-benzylacyclouridine. Cancer Chemother. Pharmacol. 24:9, 1989.
187. Maybaum, J., Ullman, B., Mandel, H. G., Day, J. L., and Sadee, W.: Regulation of RNA- and DNA-directed actions of 5-fluoropyrimidines in mouse T-lymphoma (S-49) cells. Cancer Res., 40:4209, 1980.
188. Mayer, R. J.: Current chemotherapeutic treatment approaches to the management of previously untreated adults with de novo acute myelogenous leukemia. Seminars in Oncology, 14:384-396, 1987.
189. McClarty, G. A., Chan, A. K., Engstrom, Y., Wright, J. A., and Thelander, L.: Elevated expression of M1 and M2 components and drug-induced posttranscriptional modulation of ribonucleotide reductase in a hydroxyurea-resistant mouse cell line. Biochemistry, 26:8004, 1987.
190. McDermott, B. J., van der Berg, H. W., and Murphy, R. F.: Nonlinear pharmacokinetics for the elimination of 5-fluorouracil after intravenous administration in cancer patients. Pharmacology, 9:173, 1982.
191. Mini, E., Trave, F., Rustum, Y. M., and Bertino, J. R.: Enhancement of the antitumor effects of 5-fluorouracil by folinic acid. Pharmac. Ther., 47:1, 1990.
192. Mitchell, B. S., Edwards, N. L., and Koller, C. A.: Deoxyribonucleoside triphosphate accumulation by leukemic cells. Blood, 62:419, 1983.
193. Moertel, C. G., Fleming, T. R., MacDonald, J. S., Haller, D. G., Laurie, J. A., Goodman, P. J., Ungerleider, J. S., Emerson, W. A., Tormey, D. C., Glick, J. H., Veeder, M. H., and Mailliard, J. A.: Levamisole and fluorouracil for adjuvant therapy of resected colon carcinoma. N. Engl. J. Med., 322:352, 1990.
194. Momparler, R. L.: Kinetic and template studies with 1-β-D-arabinofuranosylcytosine 5′-triphosphate and mammalian deoxyribonucleic acid polymerase. Mol. Pharmacology, 8:362, 1972.
195. Momparler, R. L.: Effect of cytosine arabinoside 5′-triphosphate on mammalian DNA polymerase. Biochem. Biophys. Res. Commun., 34:465, 1969.
196. Montgomery, J. A.: The chemistry and biology of purines and ring analogues. *In* Nucleosides, Nucleotides, and their Biological Applications. Edited by J. Ridout, D. W. Henry, and L. M. Beacher, III. New York, Academic Press, Inc., 1984, pp. 19-46.
197. Moore, E. C., Friedman, J., Valdivieso, M., Plunkett, W., Marti, J. R., Russ, J., and Loo, T. L.: Aspartate carbamoyltransferase activity, drug concentrations, and pyrimidine nucleotides in tissue from patients treated with N-(phosphonacetyl)-L-aspartate. Biochem. Pharmac., 31:3317, 1982.
198. Moore, R., Robert, F., Cripps, M., Ruckdeschel, J., Neidhart, J., Natale, R., Dallaire, D., and Gyves, J.: A phase II study of brequinar solium (DuP 785, NSC 368390) in gastrointestinal (GI) cancers. Proc. ASCO, 10:152, 1991.
199. Moran, R. E., and Straus, M. J.: Cytokinetic analysis of L1210 leukemia after continuous infusion of hydroxyurea in vivo. Cancer Res., 39:1616, 1979.
200. Morikawa, K., Fan, D., Denkins, Y. M., Levin, B., Gutterman, J. U., Walker, S. M., and Fidler, I. J.: Mechanisms of combined effects of τ-interferon and 5-fluorouracil on human colon cancer implanted into nude mice. Cancer Res., 49:799, 1989.
201. Moyer, J. D., and Handschumacher, R. E.: Selective inhibition of pyrimidine synthesis and depletion of nucleotide pools by N-(phosphonacetyl)-L-aspartate. Cancer Res., 39:3089, 1979.
202. Mulkins, M. A., and Heidelberger, C.: Isolation of fluoropyrimidine-resistant murine leukemic cell lines by one-step mutation and selection. Cancer Res., 40:1431, 1982.
203. Mulkins, M. A., and Heidelberger, C.: Biochemical characterization of fluoropyrimidine-resistant murine leukemic cell lines. Cancer Res., 42:965, 1982.
204. Myers, C. E., Young, R. C., Johns, D. G., and Chabner, B. A.: Assay of 5-fluorodeoxyuridine 5′-monophosphate and deoxyuridine 5′-monophosphate pools following 5-fluorouracil. Cancer Res., 34:2682, 1974.
205. Myers, C. E., Young, R. C., and Chabner, B. A.: Biochemical determinants of 5-fluorouracil response in vivo: the role of deoxyuridylate pool expansion. J. Clin. Invest., 56:1231, 1975.
206. Naguib, F. N. M., el Kouni, M. H., and Cha, S.: Enzymes of uracil catabolism in normal and neoplastic human tissues. Cancer Res., 45:5405, 1985.
207. Nakajima, T., Takahashi, T., Takagi, K., Kuno, K., and Kajitani, T.: Comparison of 5-fluorouracil with ftorafur in adjuvant chemotherapies with combined inductive and maintenance therapies for gastric cancer. J. Clin. Oncol., 2:1366, 1984.
208. Namba, M., Miyoshu, T., Kanamori, T., Nobuhara, M., Kimoto, T., and Ogawa, S.: Combined effects of 5-fluorouracil and interferon on proliferation of human neoplastic cells in culture. Gann, 73:819, 1982.
209. Nelson, J. A., Carpenter, J. W., Rose, L. M., and Adamson, D. J.: Mechanisms of action of 6-thioguanine, 6 mercaptopurine and 8-azaguanine. Cancer Res., 35:2782, 1975.
210. Niedzwicki, J. G., Chu, S. H., el Kouni, M. H., Rowe, E. C., and Cha, S.: 5-Benzylacyclouridine and 5-benzyloxybenzylacyclouridine, potent inhibitors of uridine phosphorylase. Biochem. Pharmac., 31:1857, 1982.
211. Nutter, L. M., and Cheng, Y. C.: Nature and properties of mammalian ribonucleoside diphosphate reductase. *In* Inhibitors of Ribonucleoside diphosphate reductase activity. Edited by J. G. Cory, A. H. Cory. Pergamon Press, New York, 1989, pp. 37-54.
212. O'Connell, M. J.: A phase III trial of 5-fluorouracil and leucovorin in the treatment of advanced colorectal cancer. Cancer, 63:1026, 1989.
213. O'Dwyer, P. J., and Marsoni, S.: Conference on deoxycoformycin: Current status and future directions. Cancer Treatment Symposium, 2:1, 1984.
214. O'Dwyer, P. J., Wagner, B., Leyland-Jones, B., Wittes, R. E., Cheson, B. D., and Hoth, D. F.: 2′Deoxycoformycin (Pentostatin) for lymphoid malignancies. Ann. Intern. Med., 108:733, 1988.
215. O'Dwyer, P. J., King, S. A., Hoth, D. F., and Leyland-Jones, B.: Role of thymidine in biochemical modulation: A review. Cancer Res., 47:3911, 1987.
216. O'Dwyer, P. J., Paul, A. R., Walczak, J., Weiner, L. M., Litwin, S., and Comic, R. L.: Phase II study of biochemical modulation of fluorouracil by low dose PALA in patients with colorectal cancer. J. Clin. Oncol., 8:1497, 1990.
217. Ohno, Y., Spriggs, D., Matsukage, A., and Kufe, D.: Effects of 1-β-D-Arabinofuranosylcytosine Incorporation on elongation of specific DNA sequences by DNA polymerase β. Cancer Res., 48:1494, 1988.
218. Parker, W. B., and Cheng, Y. C.: Metabolism and mechanism of action of 5-fluorouracil. Pharmac. Ther., 48:381, 1990.
219. Parker, W. B., and Cheng, Y. C.: Inhibition of DNA primase by nucleoside triphosphates and their arabinofuranosyl analogs. Mol. Pharmacol., 31:146, 1987.
220. Parker, W. B., Bapat, A. R., Shen, J. X., Townsend, A. J., and Cheng, Y. C.: Interaction of 2-halogenated dATP analogs (F, Cl and Br) with human DNA polymerases, DNA primase, and ribonucleotide reductase. Mol. Pharmacol., 34:485, 1988.
221. Paterson, A. R. P., and Tidd, D. M.: 6-Thiopurines. *In* Handbook of Experimental Pharmacology. Edited by A. D. Sartorelli and D. G. Johns. Berlin, Springer-Verlag, 1975, 384.
222. Paterson, A. R. P., and Oliver, U. M.: Nucleoside transport. II. Inhibition by p-Nitrobenzylthioguanosine and related compounds. Can. J. Biochem., 49:271, 1971.
223. Paterson, A. R. P., Kolassa, N., and Cass, C. E.: Transport of nucleoside drugs in animal cells. Pharmacol. & Ther., 12:515, 1981.
224. Pazdur, R., Ajani, J. A., Patt, Y. Z., Winn, R., Jackson, D., Shepard, B., DuBrow, R., Campos, L., Quaraishi, M., Faintuch, J., Abbruzzese, J. L., Gutterman, J., and Levin, B.: Phase II study of fluorouracil and recombinant interferon α-2a in previously untreated advanced colorectal carcinoma. J. Clin. Oncol., 8:2027, 1990.
225. Peters, G. J., Sharma, S. L., Laurensse, E., and Pinedo, H. M.: Inhibition of pyrimidine de novo synthesis by DUP-785 (NSC 368390). Invest. New Drugs, 5:235, 1987.
226. Peters, G. J., van Dijk, J., van Groeningen, C. J., Laurensse, E. J., Leyva, A., Lankelma, J., and Pinedo, H. M.: Toxicity and antitumor effect of 5-fluorouracil and its rescue by uridine. Adv. Exp. Med. Biol., 195B:121, 1986.
227. Peters, G. J., van Dijk, J., Laurensse, E., van Groeningen, C. J., Lankelma, J., Leyva, A., Nadal, J. C., and Pinedo, H. M.: In vitro biochemical and in vivo biological studies of the uridine 'rescue' of 5-fluorouracil. Br. J. Cancer, 57:259, 1988.
228. Peters, G. J., Laurensse, E., Lankelma, J., Leyva, A., and Pinedo, H. M.: Separation of several 5-fluorouracil metabolites in various melanoma cell lines: evidence for the synthesis of 5-fluorouracil-nucleotide sugars. Eur. J. Cancer Clin. Oncol., 20:1425, 1984.
229. Peterson, M. S., Ingraham, H. A., and Goulian, M.: 2′-Deoxyribosyl analogues of UDP-N-acetylglucosamine in cells treated with methotrexate or 5-fluorodeoxyridine. J. Biol. Chem., 258:10831, 1983.
230. Philips, F. S., Sternberg, S. S., Hamilton, L., and Clarke, D. A.: The toxic effects of 6-mercaptopurine and related compounds. Ann. N. Y. Acad. Sci., 60:283, 1954.
231. Piper, A. A., and Fox, R. M.: Biochemical basis for the differential sensitivity of human T- and B-lymphocyte lines to 5-fluorouracil. Cancer Res., 42:3753, 1982.
232. Piro, L. D., Carrera, C. J., Carson, D. A., and Beutler, E.: Lasting remissions in hairy-cell leukemia induced by a single infusion of 2-chlorodeoxyadenosine. N. Engl. J. Med., 322:1117, 1990.
233. Piro, L. D., Carrera, C. J., Beutler, E., and Carson, D. A.: 2-Chloro-deoxyadenosine: an effective new agent for the treatment of chronic lymphocytic leukemia. Blood, 72:1069, 1988.
234. Pizzorno, G., Wiegand, R. A., Lentz, S. K., and Handschumacher, R. E.: Brequinar potentiates 5-fluorouracil antitumor activity in a murine model colon 38 tumor by

tissue specific modulation of uridine nucleotide pools. Cancer Res.,:(in press) 2, 1992.
235. Plagemann, P. G. W., Behrens, M., and Abraham, D.: Metabolism and cytotoxicity of 5-azacytidine in cultured Novikoff rat hepatoma and P388 mouse leukemia cells and their enhancement by preincubation with pyrazofurin. Cancer Res., 38:2458, 1978.
236. Plunkett, W., Huang, P., and Gandhi, V.: Metabolism and action of fludarabine phosphate. Semin. Oncol., 17(Suppl. 8):3, 1990.
237. Plunkett, W., and Saunders, P. P.: Metabolism and action of purine nucleoside analogs. Pharmac. Ther., 49:239-268, (1991).
238. Queisser, W., Schnitzler, G., Schaefer, J., Arnold, H., Drings, P., Fritze, D., Geldmacher, J., Hartwich, G., Herrmann, R., Kempf, P., Konig, H., Meiser, R. J., Nedden, R., von Oldershausen, H. F., Pappas, A., Sievers, H., Wahrendorf, J., Westerhausen, M., and Witte, S.: Comparison of ftorafur with 5-fluorouracil in combination chemotherapy of advanced gastrointestinal carcinoma. Recent Results Cancer Res., 79:82, 1981.
239. Remick, S. C., Grem, J. L., Fischer, P. H., Tutsch, K. D., Alberti, D. B., Nieting, L. M., Tombes, M. D., Bruggink, J., Willson, J. K. V., and Trump, D. L.: Phase I trial of 5-fluorouracil and dipyridamole administered by seventy-two-hour concurrent continuous infusion. Cancer Res., 50:2667, 1990.
240. Remy, C. N.: Metabolism of thiopyrimidines and thiopurines: S-methylation with S-adenosylmethionine transmethylase and catabolism in mammalian tissues. J. Biol. Chem., 238:1078, 1963.
241. Renoux, G.: The general immunopharmacology of levamisole. Drugs, 19:89, 1980.
242. Reyes, P., and Guganig, M. E.: Studies on a pyrimidine phosphoribosyltransferase from murine leukemia P1534J. J. Biol. Chem., 250:5097, 1975.
243. Rodnan, G. P., Robin, J. A., Tolchin, S. F., and Elion, G. B.: Allopurinol and gouty hyperuricemia. JAMA, 231:1143, 1975.
244. Romanini, A., Lin, J. T., Niedzwiecki, D., Bunni, M., Priest, D. G., and Bertino, J. R.: Role of folypolyglutamates in biochemical modulation of fluoropyrimidines by leucovorin. Cancer Res., 51:789, 1991.
245. Rosenthal, F., Wislicki, L., and Koller, L.: Über die Beziehungen von schwertsen Blutgiften zu Abbauprodukten des Einweisses: ein Beitrag zum Enstehungmechanismus der pernizosen Anemie. Klin. Wochenschr., 7:972, 1928.
246. Rutman, R. J., Cantarow, A., and Paschkis, K.: Studies in 2-acetylaminofluorene carcinogenesis. III. The utilization of uracil-2-C14 by preneoplastic rat liver and rat hepatoma. Cancer Res., 14:119, 1954.
247. Santi, D. V., McHenry, C. S., and Sommer, H.: Mechanism of interaction of thymidylate synthetase with 5-fluorodeoxyuridylate. Biochemistry, 13:471, 1974.
248. Schneider, M.: Circadian rhythm-varying plasma concentration of 5-fluorouracil during a five-day continuous venous infusion at a constant rate in cancer patients. Cancer Res., 48:1676, 1988.
249. Scholar, E. M., and Calabresi, P.: Increased activity of alkaline phosphates in leukemic cells from patients resistant to thiopurines. Biochem. Pharmacol., 28:445, 1979.
250. Scholer, J. J.: Flucytosine. *In* Antifungal Chemotherapy. Edited by D. C. E. Speller. New York, Wiley, 1980, p. 35.
251. Schwartz, P. M., Dunigan, J. M., Marsh, J. C., and Handschumacher, R. E.: Allopurinol modification of the toxicity and antitumor activity of 5-fluorouracil. Cancer Res., 40:1885, 1980.
252. Schwartz, P. M., Dunigan, J. M., Marsh, J. C., and Handschumacher, R. E.: Allopurinol modification of the toxicity and antitumor activity of 5-fluorouracil. Cancer Res., 40:1885, 1980.
253. Schwenk, M., Hegazy, E., and Lopez Del Pino, V.: Uridine uptake by isolated intestinal epithelial cells of guinea pig. Biochim. Biophys. Acta, 805:370, 1984.
254. Seifert, P., Baker, L., Reed, M. L., and Vaitkevicius, V. K.: Comparison of continuously infused 5-fluorouracil with bolus injection in treatment of patients with colorectal adenocarcinoma. Cancer, 36:123, 1975.
255. Seto, S., Carrera, C. J., Kubota, M., Wasson, D. B., and Carson, D. A.: Mechanism of deoxyadenosine and 2-chlorodeoxyadenosine toxicity to non-dividing human lymphocytes. J. Clin. Invest., 75:377, 1985.
256. Seto, S., Carrera, C. J., Wasson, D. B., and Carson, D. A.: Inhibition of DNA repair by deoxyadenosine in resting human lymphocytes. J. Immunol., 136:2839, 1986.
257. Shani, J., and Danenberg, P. V.: Evidence that intracellular synthesis of 5-fluorouridine-5′-phosphate from 5-fluorouracil and 5-fluorouridine is compartmentalized. Biochem. Biophys. Res. Commun., 122:439, 1984.
258. Siaw, M. F., and Coleman, M. S.: In vitro metabolism of deoxycoformycin in human T lymphoblastoid cells. Phosphorylation of deoxycoformycin and incorporation into cellular DNA. J. Bio. Chem., 259:9426, 1984.
259. Sillman, F. H., Sedlis, A., and Boyce, J. G.: A review of lower genital intraepithelial neoplasia and the use of topical 5-fluorouracil. Obstet. Gynecol. Surv., 40:190, 1985.
260. Singer, J., and Wallace, S. L.: The allopurinol hypersensitivity syndrome: unnecessary morbidity and mortality. Arthritis Rheum., 29:82, 1986.
261. Sirotnak, F. M., Chello, P. L., Dorick, D. M., and Montgomery, J. A.: Specificity of systems mediating transport of adenosine, 9-β-D-arabinofuranosyl-2-fluoradenine, and other purine nucleoside analogues in L1210 cells. Cancer Res., 43:104, 1983.
262. Skipper, H. E.: On the mechanism of action of 6-mercaptopurine. Ann. N. Y. Acad. Sci., 60:315, 1954.
263. Skoda, J.: Azapyrimidine nucleosides. *In* Antineoplastic and Immunosuppressive Agents. Edited by A. C. Sartorelli, and D. G. Johns. Berlin, Springer-Verlag, 1975, p. 348.
264. Sobrero, A. F., Moir, R. D., Bertino, J. R., and Handschumacher, R. E.: Defective facilitated diffusion of nucleosides, a primary mechanism of resistance to 5-fluoro-2′-deoxyuridine in the HCT-8 human carcinoma line. Cancer Res., 45:3155, 1985.
265. Sobrero, A. F., Handschumacher, R. E., and Bertino, J. R.: Highly selective drug combinations for human colon cancer cells resistant in vitro to 5-fluoro-2′-deoxyuridine. Cancer Res., 45:3161, 1985.
266. Sorm, F., Piskala, A., Cihak, A., and Vesely, J.: 5-Azacytidine, a new highly effective cancerostatic. Experientia, 20:202, 1964.
267. Spector, T., and Johns, D. G.: Stoichiometric inhibition of reduced xanthine oxidase by hydroxypyrazolo (3,4-d) pyrimidines. J. Biol. Chem., 239:2570, 1964.
268. Spiers, A. S., Moore, D., Cassileth, P. A., Harrington, D. P., Cummings, F. J., Neiman, R. S., Bennett, J. M., and O'Connell, M. J.: Remissions in hairy-cell leukemia with pentostatin (2′-deoxycoformycin). N. Engl. J. Med., 316:825, 1987.
269. Spriggs, D., Robbins, G., Mitchell, T., and Kufe, D.: Incorporation of 9-β-D-arabinofuranosyl-2-fluoradenine into HL-60 cellular RNA and DNA. Biochem. Pharmacol., 35:247, 1986.
270. Sugarbaker, P. H., Klecker, R. W., Gianola, F. J., and Speyer, J. C.: Prolonged treatment schedules with intraperitoneal 5-fluorouracil diminish the local-regional nature of drug distribution. Am. J. Clin. Oncol., 9:1, 1986.
271. Sweeny, D. J., Barnes, S., Heggie, G. D., and Diasio, R. B.: Metabolism fluorouracil N-choly-2-fluoro-a-alanine conjugate: previously unrecognized role for bile acids in drug conjugation. Proc. Natl. Acad. Sci. USA, 84:5439, 1987.
272. Swyryd, E. A., Seaver, S. S., and Stark, G. R.: N-(Phosphonacetyl)-L-aspartate, a potent transition state analog inhibitor as aspartate transcarbamylase, blocks proliferation of mammalian cells in culture. J. Biol. Chem., 249:6945, 1974.
273. Tagger, A. V., Boux, J., and Wright, J. A.: Hydroxy [^{14}C] urea uptake by normal and transformed human cells: evidence for a mechanism of passive diffusion. Biochem. Cell Biol., 65:925, 1987.
274. Talley, R. W., and Vaitkevicius, V. K.: Megaloblastosis produced by a cytosine antagonist, 1-β-D-arabinofuranosylcytosine. Blood, 21:252, 1963.
275. Tanaka, M., Kimura, K., and Yoshida, S.: Increased incorporation of 5-fluorodeoxyuridine into DNA of human T-lymphoblastic cell lines. Gann, 75:986, 1984.
276. Tidd, D. M.: Antipurines. *In* Handbook of Experimental Pharmacology. Edited by B. W. Fox, and M. Fox. Springer-Verlag, Berlin, 1984, p. 445.
277. Townsend, A., Leclerc, J.-M., Dutschman, G., Cooney, D., and Cheng, Y.-C.: Metabolism of 1-β-D-Arabinofuranosyl-5-Azacytosine and Incorporation into DNA of Human T-Lymphoblastic Cells (Molt-4). Cancer Res., 45:3522, 1985.
278. Townsend, A. J., and Cheng, Y.-C.: Sequence-specific Effects of ara-5-aza-CTP and ara-CTP on DNA Synthesis by Purified Human DNA Polymerases in vitro: Visualization of Chain Elongation on a Defined Template. Mol. Pharmacol., 32:330, 1987.
279. Tseng, W. C., Derse, D., Cheng, Y. C., Brockman, R. W., and Bennett, L. L., Jr.: In vitro activity of 9-β-D-arabinofuranosyl-2-fluoradenine and the biochemical actions of its triphosphate on DNA polymerases and ribonucleotide reductase from HeLa cells. Mol. Pharmacol., 21:474, 1982.
280. Ullman, B., Lee, M., Martin, D. W., Jr., and Santi, D. V.: Cytotoxicity of 5-fluoro-2′-deoxyuridine: requirement for reduced folate cofactors and antagonism by methotrexate. Proc. Natl. Acad. Sci., USA, 75:980, 1978.
281. Umeda, M., and Heidelberger, C.: Comparative studies of fluorinated pyrimidines with various cell lines. Cancer Res., 28:2529, 1968.
282. Valeriote, F.: Cellular aspects of the action of cytosine arabinoside. Medical and Pediatric Oncology, 10(S1):221, 1982.
283. van Groeningen, C. J., Peters, G. J., Leyva, A., Laurensse, E., and Pinedo, H. M.: Reversal of 5-fluorouracil-induced myelosuppression by prolonged administration of high-dose uridine. J. Natl. Cancer Inst., 81:157, 1989.
284. van Groeningen, C. J., Pinedo, H. M., Heddes, J., Kok, R. M., de Jong, A. P. J. M., Wattel, E., Peters, G. J., and Lankelma, J.: Pharmacokinetics of 5-fluorouracil assessed with a sensitive mass spectrometric method in patients on a dose escalation schedule. Cancer Res., 48:6956, 1988.
285. van Groeningen, C. J., Peters, G. J., Nadal, J. C., Laurensse, E., and Pinedo, H. M.: Clinical and pharmacologic study of orally administered uridine. J. Natl. Cancer Inst., 83:437, 1991.
286. Vesell, E. S., Passananti, G. T., and Greene, F.: Impairment of drug metabolism in man by allopurinol and nortriptyline. N. Eng. J. Med., 283:1484, 1970.
287. Vesely, J., and Cihak, A.: 5-Azacytidine: Mechanism of action and biological effects in mammalian cells. Pharmacol. Ther., 2:813, 1978.
288. Vine, E. N., Young, D., Vine, W. H., and Wolf, W.: An improved synthesis of ^{18}F-5-fluorouracil. International Journal of Applied Radiation and Isotopes, 30:401, 1979.
289. Wadler, S., Schwartz, E. L., Goldman, M., Lyver, A., Rader, M., Zimmerman, M., Itri, L., Weinberg, V., and Wiernik, P. H.: Fluorouracil and recombinant α-2a-interferon: An active regimen against advanced colorectal carcinoma. J. Clin. Oncol., 7:1769, 1989.
290. Washtien, W. L.: Comparison of 5-fluorouracil metabolism in two human gastrointestinal tumor cell lines. Cancer Res., 44:909, 1984.
291. Wohlhueter, R. M., McIvor, R. S., and Plagemann, P. G. W.: Facilitated transport of uracil and 5-fluorouracil, and permeation of orotic acid into cultured mammalian cells. J. Cell. Physiol., 104:309, 1980.
292. Wolfenden, R., and Wentworth, D. F.: On the interaction of 3, 4, 5, 6-tetrahydrouridine with human liver cytidine deaminase. Biochemistry, 14:5099, 1975.
293. Woo, P. W., Dion, H. W., Lange, S. M., Dahl, L. F., and Durham, L. J.: A Novel adenosine and araA inhibitor, (R)-3-(2-deoxy-βD-erythropento-furanosyl)-3, 6, 7, 8-tetrahydroimidazo (4, 5-d) (1, 3) diazepin-8-o1. J. Heterocyclic Chen., 11:64, 1974.
294. Woodcock, T. M., Martin, D. S., Damin, L. A. M., Kemeny, N. E., and Young, C. W.: Combination clinical trials with thymidine and fluorouracil: a Phase I and clinical pharmacologic evaluation. Cancer, 45:1135, 1980.
295. Woolley, P. V., Ayoob, M. J., Smith, F. P., Lakey, J. L., DeGreen, P., Marantz, A., and Schein, P. S.: A controlled trial of the effect of 4-hydroxypyrazolopyrimidine (allopurinol) on the toxicity of a single bolus dose of 5-fluorouracil. J. Clin. Oncol., 3:103, 1985.
296. Wright, J. E., Dreyfuss, A., El-Magharbel, I., Trites, D., Jones, S. M., Holden, S. A., Rosowsky, A., and Frei, E., III.: Selective expansion of 5, 10-methylenetetrahydrofolate polls and modulation of 5-fluorouracil antitumor activity by leucovorin in vivo. Cancer Res., 49:2592, 1989.
297. Wright, J. A., Alam, T. G., McClarty, G. A., Tagger, A. Y., and Thelander, L.: Altered expression of M1 and M2 gene amplification in hydroxy-urea resistant hamster, mouse, rat, and human cell line. Somat. Cell Mol. Genet., 13:155, 1987.
298. Yang, J. L., Chang, E. H., and Capizzi, R. L.: Effect of uracil arabinoside on metabolism and cytotoxicity of cytosine arabinoside in 25178Y murine leukemia. J. Clin. Invest., 75:141, 1985.
299. Yang, S.-W., Huang, P., Plunkett, W., Becker, F. F., and Chan, J. Y. H.: Dual Mode of Inhibition of Purified DNA Ligase I from Human Cells by 9-β-D-arabinofuranosyl-2-Fluoroadenosine Triphosphate. JBC, In Press.
300. Yang-Feng, T. L., Barton, D. E., Thelander, L., Lewis, W. H., Srinivasan, P. R., and Francke, U.: Ribonucleotide reductase M2 subunit sequences mapped to four different chromosomal sites in humans and mice: functional locus identified by its amplification in hydroxyurea-resistant cell lines. Genomics, 1:77, 1987.
301. Yu, J., Matsumoto, S. S., and Yu, A. L.: Inhibition of transcription as a mechanism of lymphocytotoxicity induced by deoxyadenosine and 2′-deoxycoformycin. Cancer Treat. Symp., 2:75, 1984.
302. Zimm, S., Collins, J. M., Riccardi, R., O'Neill, D., Narang, P. K., Chabner, B., and Poplack, D. G.: Variable bioavailability of oral mercaptopurine. Is maintenance chemotherapy in acute lymphoblastic leukemia being optimally delivered? N. Engl. J. Med., 308:1005, 1983.
303. Zimm, S., Collins, J., O'Neill, D., Chabner, B. A., and Poplack, D. G.: Inhibition of first-pass metabolism in cancer chemotherapy: interaction of 6-mercaptopurine and allopurinol. Clin. Pharmacol. Ther., 34:810, 1983.

Alkylating Agents and Platinum Antitumor Compounds

Michael Colvin

Introduction

The alkylating agents and the platinum antitumor compounds form strong chemical bonds with electron rich atoms (nucleophiles), such as sulfur in proteins and nitrogen in DNA. While these compounds react with many biological molecules, the primary cytotoxic actions of both classes of agents appear to be the inhibition of DNA replication and cell division produced by their reactions with DNA. However, the chemical differences between these two classes of agents produce significant differences in their antitumor and toxic effects.

The Alkylating Agents

The alkylating agents were the first nonhormonal drugs to be used effectively in the treatment of cancer, and the story behind the recognition of the antitumor effects of these compounds is a remarkable one. During World War I toxic gases were used as military weapons. The most devastating of these gases was sulfur mustard (Figure XVI-3-1). The compound was used as a weapon because of its vesicant effects, which produce skin irritation, blindness, and pulmonary damage. However, it was observed that troops and civilians who were exposed to sulfur mustard also developed bone marrow suppression and lymphoid aplasia. Because of these findings, sulfur mustard was evaluated as an antitumor agent.[3] The closely related, but less toxic, nitrogen mustards were selected for further study. Trials in patients with lymphoma demonstrated regression of tumors, with relief of symptoms in some patients.[174,232,380] These results encouraged the search for nitrogen mustards which were more effective and less toxic, and stimulated efforts to find other chemicals with antitumor activity.

Chemistry of the Alkylating Agents

The alkylating agents are compounds which react with electron rich atoms in biological molecules to form covalent bonds. Traditionally, these agents have been divided into two types, those which react directly with biological molecules, and those which form a reactive intermediate which then reacts with the biological molecules. These types are termed S_N1 and S_N2, respectively, and are illustrated in Figure XVI-3-2. The terms refer to the kinetics of the reactions; the rate of reaction of an S_N1 agent is dependent only on

$$RX \longrightarrow R^+ + X^- \xrightarrow{Y^-} RY + X^-$$

$$S_N1 \text{ Reaction}$$

$$RX + Y^- \longrightarrow [Y \cdots \overset{\delta^-}{R} \cdots \overset{\delta^-}{X}] \longrightarrow RY + X^-$$

$$S_N2 \text{ Reaction}$$

Figure XVI-3-2. S_N1 and S_N2 reactions of alkylating agents.

the concentration of the reactive intermediate, while the rate of reaction of an S_N2 agent is dependent on the concentration of the alkylating agent and of the molecule with which it is reacting. This distinction has important implications in understanding the cellular and molecular pharmacology of specific alkylating agents. The nitrogen mustards and nitrosoureas are examples of S_N1 agents, while busulfan is an S_N2 agent.

A large number of chemical compounds are alkylating agents under physiological conditions, and a variety of such compounds have been found to have antitumor activity. While it is not possible to describe all of the compounds which have been used clinically, those compounds which are currently used extensively, look promising in clinical trials, or represent a type of alkylating agent will be discussed.

Types of Alkylating Agents

Nitrogen Mustards. The most widely used alkylating agents are the nitrogen mustards. While thousands of nitrogen mustards have been synthesized and tested, only five are commonly used in cancer therapy today. These are mechlorethamine (the original "nitrogen mustard"), cyclophosphamide, ifosfamide, melphalan and chlorambucil, and are illustrated in Figure XVI-3-3. The characteristic chemical constituent of the nitrogen mustards is the bischloroethyl group and all of the nitrogen mustards react through an aziridinium intermediate as shown in Figure XVI-3-4. The remainder of the molecule is important in determining the physical properties of the molecule and affects the transport, distribution, and reactivity of the specific agents. The importance of the total molecule is demonstrated by cyclophosphamide.

Cyclophosphamide is not a reactive compound, but undergoes activation in the body. The complex activation scheme[90] is shown in Figure XVI-3-5. The initial activation reaction is carried out by microsomal oxidation in the liver to produce 4-hydroxycyclophosphamide, which is in spontaneous equilibrium with the tautomer, aldophosphamide. At physiological pH, this equilibrium is predominantly in the

$$ClCH_2CH_2-S-CH_2CH_2Cl$$

Figure XVI-3-1. Structure of sulfur mustard (bischloroethylsulfide).

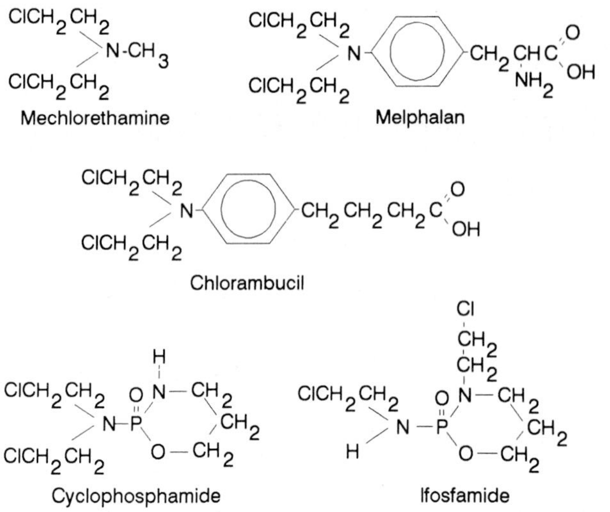

Figure XVI-3-3. Structures of nitrogen mustards currently used in therapy.

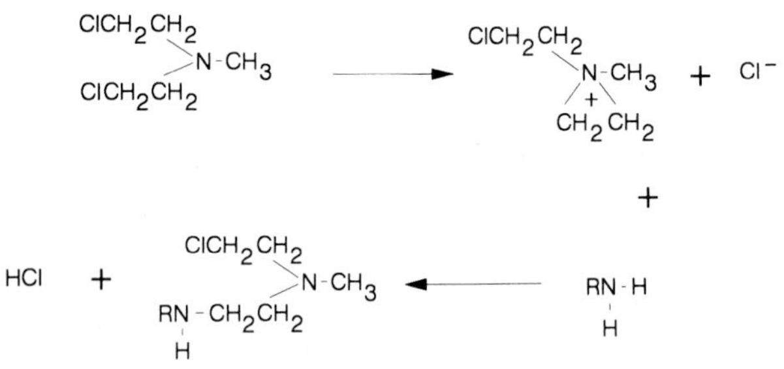

Figure XVI-3-4. Alkylation mechanism of nitrogen mustards.

form of 4-hydroxycyclophosphamide.[484] This equilibrium mixture diffuses from the hepatocyte into the plasma and is distributed throughout the body. Since 4-hydroxycyclophosphamide is relatively nonpolar, it enters target cells readily by diffusion. Aldophosphamide spontaneously decomposes to produce phosphoramide mustard, which is the first reactive alkylating agent produced in the metabolism of cyclophosphamide. While phosphoramide mustard is also produced extracellularly, this compound is very polar, enters cells poorly, and appears to play relatively little role in the therapeutic and toxic effects of cyclophosphamide. Thus, 4-hydroxycyclophosphamide/aldophosphamide serves as an efficient mechanism to deliver the alkylating phosphoramide mustard into cells. The major reason that cyclophosphamide is the most widely used alkylating agent is that it produces less gastrointestinal and hematopoietic toxicity than other alkylating agents. The basis for this decreased toxicity is the enzyme aldehyde dehydrogenase. This enzyme oxidizes aldophosphamide to carboxyphosphamide, an inactive product, which is excreted in the urine and accounts for about 80% of an administered dose of cyclophosphamide in any species. This enzyme is found in high concentration in the hepatic cytosol, in primitive hematopoietic cells, and in the stem cells and mucosal absorptive cells in the intestine.[396] Administration of an inhibitor of this enzyme to an animal markedly increases the hematopoietic and gastrointestinal toxicity of cyclophosphamide.[396]

Ifosfamide is a structural isomer of cyclophosphamide which is being used increasingly in the treatment of testicular tumors and sarcomas.[19,284,364] This compound undergoes the same metabolic reactions as cyclophosphamide, but the location of the chloroethyl group on the ring nitrogen produces quantitative changes in the metabolism of the drug[88] and subtle changes in the chemical properties of the reactive metabolite, ifosfamide mustard, so that it is less reactive than phosphoramide mustard.[51] The primary metabolite, aldoifosfamide, is a substrate for aldehyde dehydrogenase, so that the bone marrow and gastrointestinal tract sparing properties are similar to those of cyclophosphamide. The oxidation of the chloroethyl side chains to produce choroacetaldehyde is a minor metabolic pathway for cyclophosphamide (~10% of dose), but is increased to as much as 50% for ifosfamide. The increased production of chloracetaldehyde has been implicated in the neurotoxicity of ifosfamide,[175] and may also contribute to the greater renal and bladder toxicity of ifosfamide. The greater side chain oxidation of ifosfamide and the lesser reactivity of the ifosfamide mustard are consistent with the fact that higher doses of ifosfamide than cyclophosphamide are used clinically.

Melphalan is an alkylating agent which has been used extensively in the treatment of multiple myeloma,[30,94] ovarian cancer,[153,462,480] and breast cancer.[144,382] Melphalan is an amino acid analog which has been shown to enter cells and cross the blood-brain barrier through active transport systems. The natural substrates for these systems are amino acids,[37,170,464] and the entry of melphalan into cells[465] and the central nervous system[182] can be modulated by the presence of certain amino acids in the extracellular fluid.

Chlorambucil has been used extensively for the treatment of chronic lymphocytic leukemia,[152,194,395] ovarian carcinoma,[197,476] and lymphoma,[172,363] but has been used less often in high dose combination therapies than the other nitrogen mustards which are described here. This agent is well tolerated by most patients, and can be used in patients who have severe nausea and vomiting with cyclophosphamide or melphalan.

Aziridines and Epoxides. Closely related to the nitrogen mustards are the aziridines, which are represented in current therapy by thiotepa, mitomycin C, and AZQ, illustrated in Figure XVI-3-6. These agents presumably alkylate by the same mechanism as the aziridinium intermediates produced by the nitrogen mustards, but the aziridine rings in these compounds are uncharged and not very reactive in vitro.

Thiotepa (triethylene thiophosphoramide) has been used particularly in the treatment of carcinomas of the breast and ovary and for the intrathecal therapy of meningeal carcinomatosis. Thiotepa is oxidatively desulfurated by hepatic microsomes to produce TEPA.[322A] While TEPA is cytotoxic, it is less so than Thiotepa.[307A,437A] After the clinical administration of thiotepa, both thiotepa and TEPA are found in the blood,[191B,205A] and the concentration and AUC exposure to TEPA may exceed those of thiotepa.[191B] The AUC exposure to thiotepa has been shown to correlate with the degree of myelosuppression in patients, while the AUC exposure to TEPA did not.[191A] Some studies have suggested that a metabolite is produced which is more reactive than the parent compound.[126,439] However, such a metabolite has not been characterized, and the activity of thiotepa may be enhanced by low pH within tumor cells. At the lower pH, the aziridine ring will be protonated and more reactive.

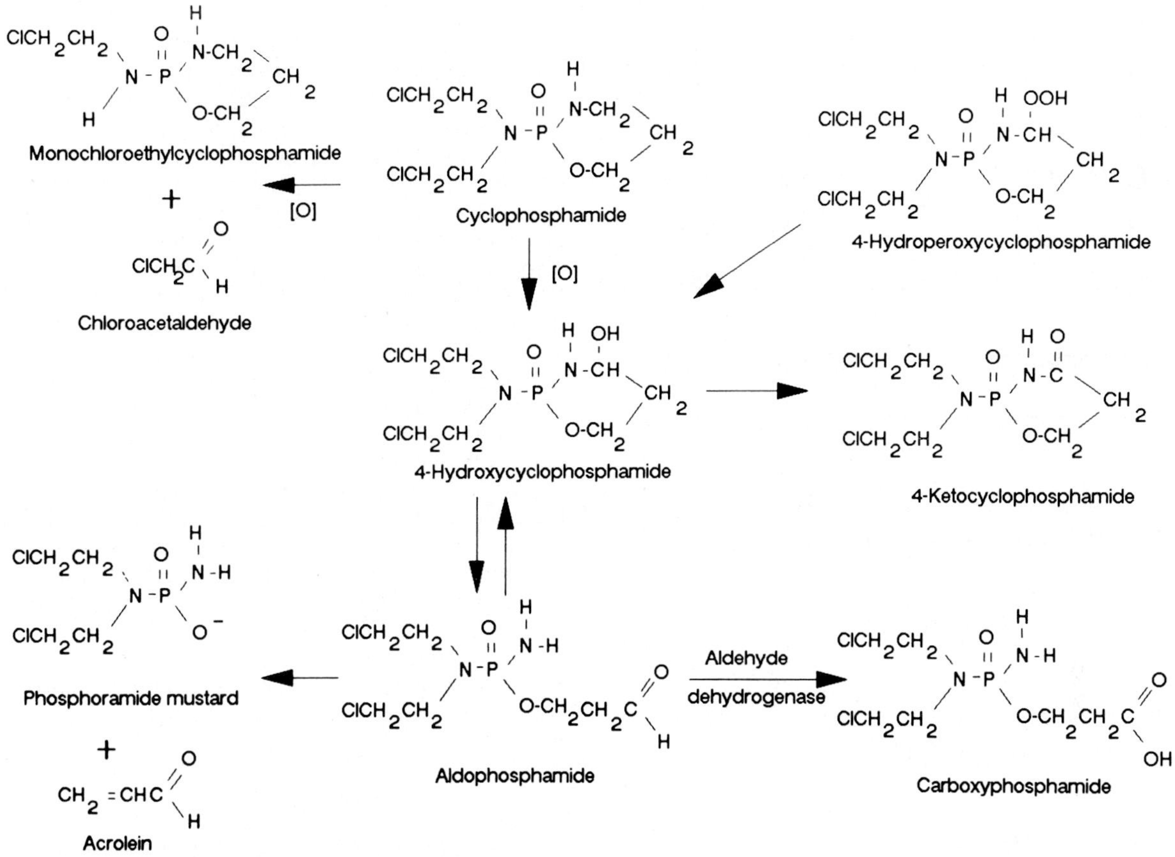

Figure XVI-3-5.   Metabolism of cyclophosphamide.

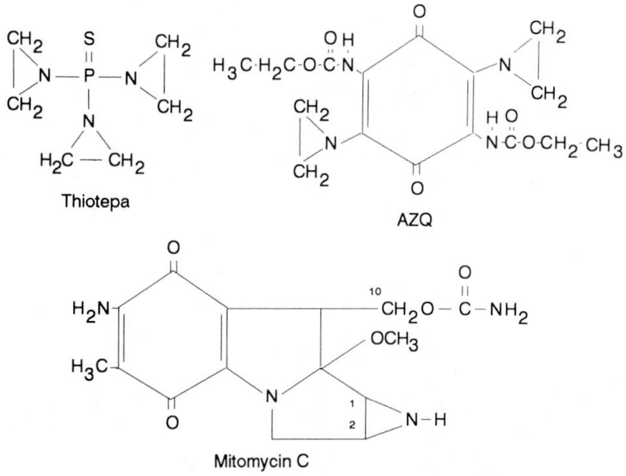

Figure XVI-3-6.   Structures of aziridine alkylating agents.

Mitomycin C is a natural product which has been used in the treatment of breast cancer and cancers of the gastro-intestinal tract.[21,287,305,475] This compound contains an aziridine ring, and appears to exert its cytotoxic effect through the crosslinking of DNA.[112,117,250] Mitomycin C undergoes reduction in the cell, with enhancement of the affinity of the carbon 1 atom of the aziridine ring for nucleophiles, such as the extracyclic nitrogen atom on guanylic acid in DNA. Fol-

lowing this alkylation, there is displacement of the activated carbamate group on the 10 carbon atom of mitomycin C by an extracyclic amino nitrogen of a guanylic acid molecule on the complementary DNA strand to produce an interstrand DNA crosslink.[59,60,229]

AZQ (diazoquone) was designed to be sufficiently lipophilic to readily cross the blood-brain-barrier for the treatment of central nervous system tumors.[251] It has demonstrated clinical activity against brain tumors,[98,482] other solid tumors, and leukemia.[137] AZQ has been shown to undergo reduction of the quinone ring in cells. This reduction results in protonation of the aziridine rings and enhancement of reactivity of the compound.[187,392]

The epoxides, such as *dianhydrogalactitol*[78,189] (Figure XVI-3-7), are chemically related to the aziridines and alkylate through a similar mechanism of attack of a nucleophile, such as an amino nitrogen, on a carbon of a strained three member ring. *Dibromodulcitol*[444] is hydrolysed to dianhydrogalactitol and thus is a prodrug to an epoxide.[408]

Alkyl Sulfonates. The alkyl alkane sulfonate, *busulfan* (Figure XVI-3-8), was one of the earliest alkylating agents.[190] This compound is one of the few currently used agents which clearly alkylates through an S_N2 reaction, as shown in Figure XVI-3-9. Hepsulfam, an alkyl sulfamate analog of busulfan with a wider range of antitumor activity in preclinical studies,[338] is currently in clinical trials. Busulfan has a most interesting, but poorly understood, selective toxicity for early myeloid precursors.[131,154] This selective effect is probably

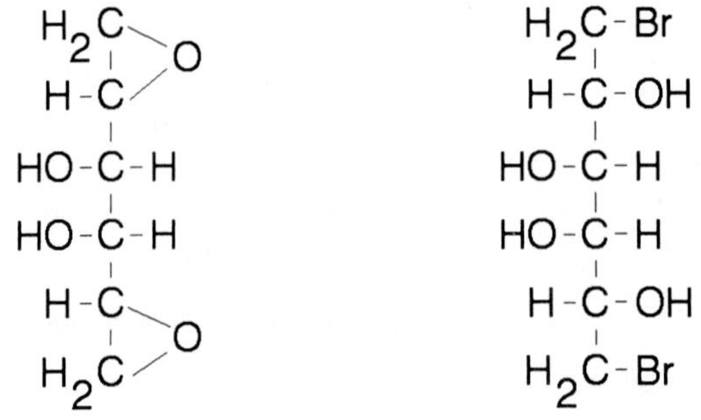

Dianhydrogalactitol   Dibromodulcitol

Figure XVI-3-7. Structures of an epoxide alkylating agent (dianhydrogalactitol) and an epoxide prodrug (dibromodulcitol).

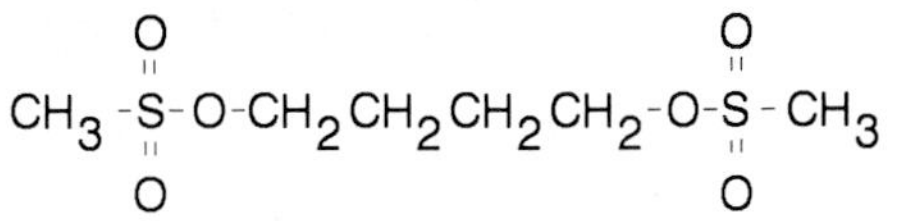

Busulfan

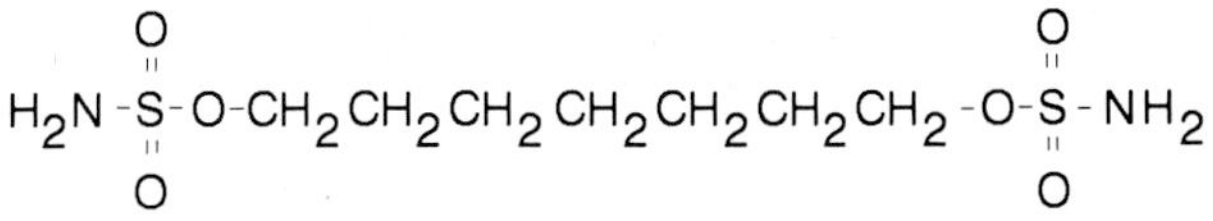

Hepsulfam

Figure XVI-3-8. Structure of alkyl sulfonate (busulfan) and alkyl sulfamate (hepsulfam) agents.

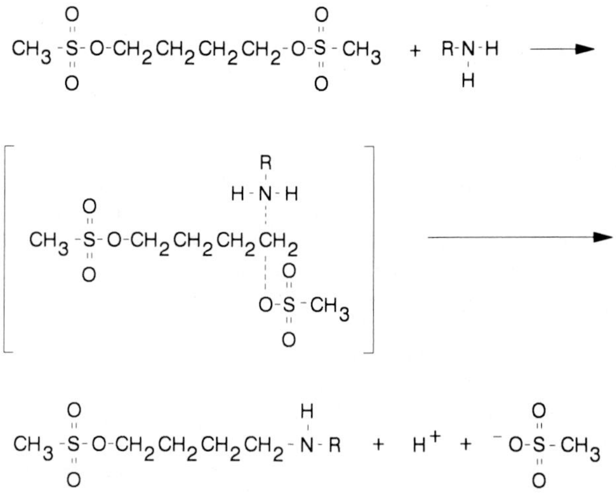

Figure XVI-3-9. Mechanism of alkylation by busulfan.

responsible for its activity against chronic myelocytic leukemia[158] and its successful use as a component of bone marrow ablative regimens for bone marrow transplantation of acute myeloid leukemia.[399]

Nitrosoureas. The nitrosoureas are a class of alkylating agents which have received considerable attention during the past three decades.[106,227,402] Several nitrosoureas currently in clinical use or clinical trials are shown in Figure XVI-

3-10. These compounds decompose to produce alkylating compounds under physiological conditions. While there are several mechanisms by which this may occur, the predominant mechanism is probably that shown in Figure XVI-3-11, a base catalyzed decomposition to a chloroethyl diazonium moiety,[89] which has been shown to react with DNA,[257,286] as discussed below. *BCNU* (carmustine) was the first agent to demonstrate significant activity against a preclinical model of intracerebral tumor[402] and is currently used for the treatment of primary brain tumors[84,471] and in the treatment of multiple myeloma.[116,458] *CCNU* (lomustine) and *methyl CCNU* (semustine) demonstrated greater activity against solid tumors in preclinical studies.[401] CCNU is used in the treatment of CNS tumors[265,272] and lymphomas,[230,274] and methyl CCNU has been used particularly in the treatment of gastrointestinal tumors.[2,83,162,457] *ACNU*, which is more water soluble than most of the nitrosoureas, has been employed for the intraarterial and intrathecal treatment of CNS tumors[22,276,385] and for solid tumors.[237] The clinical use of the nitrosoureas has been limited by marked and prolonged hematopoietic toxicity and by renal toxicity. The development of nitrosoureas with a higher therapeutic index remains a very active area of endeavor.[201,233,243,359,434,474]

Other nitrogen containing compounds spontaneously decompose or can be metabolized to produce alkyl diazo-

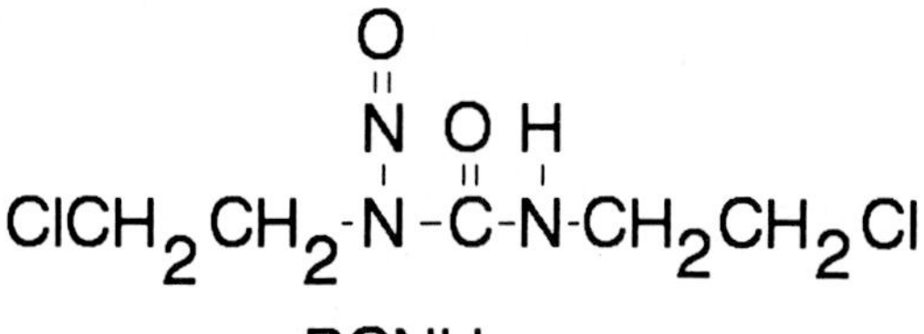

BCNU

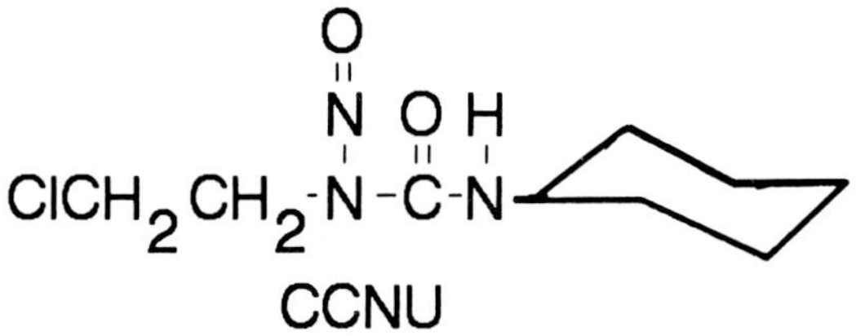

CCNU

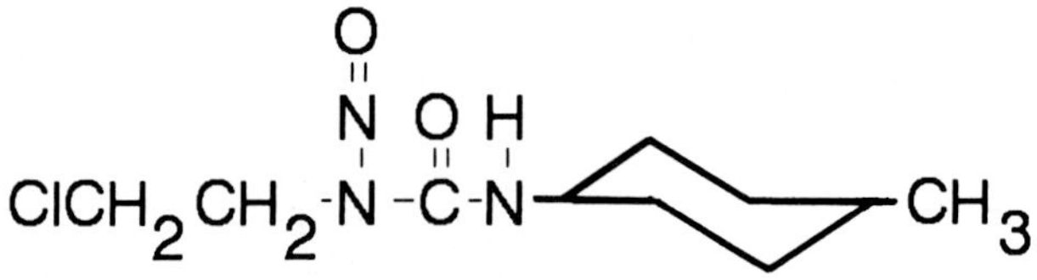

4-Methyl CCNU

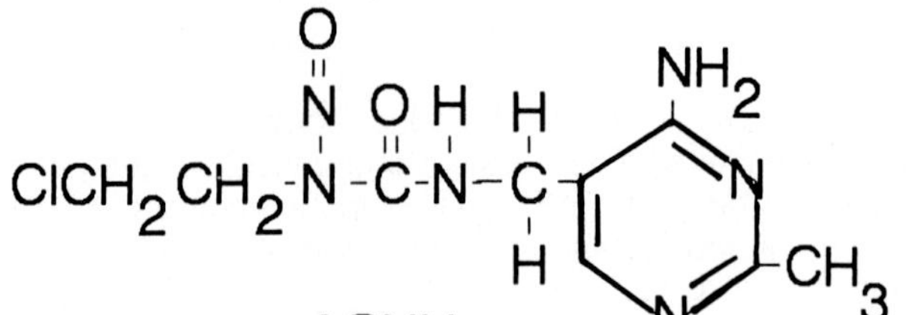

ACNU

Figure XVI-3-10. Structures of nitrosoureas.

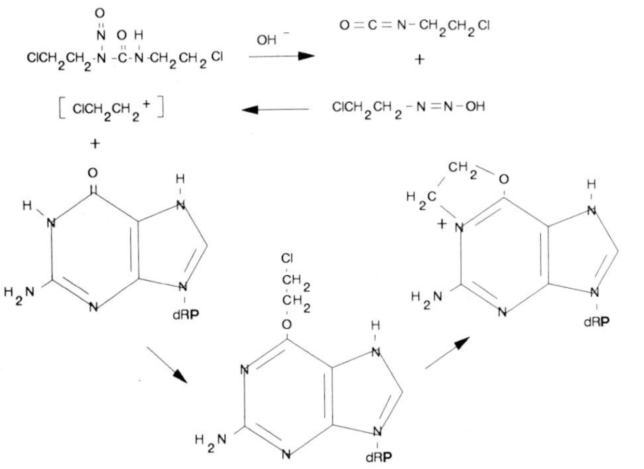

Figure XVI-3-11. Mechanism of nitrosourea activation and alkylation of deoxyguanylic acid.

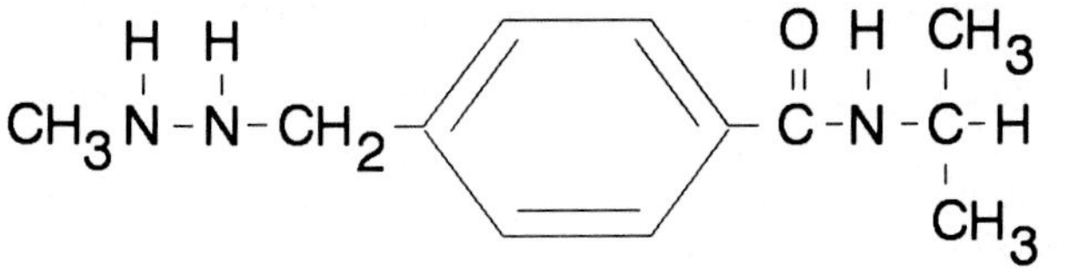

Procarbazine

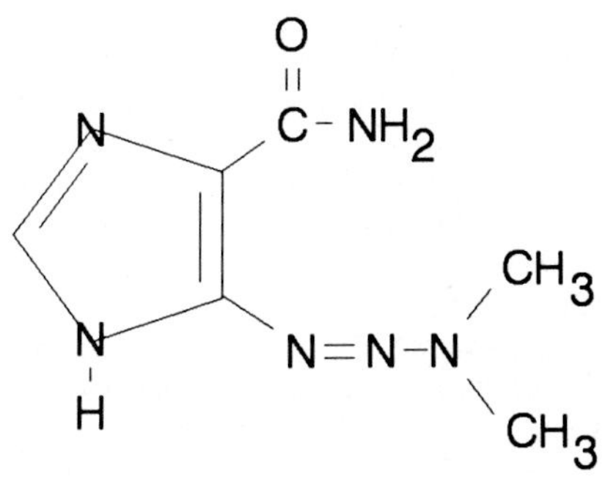

Dacarbazine

Figure XVI-3-12. Structures of monofunctional alkylating agents.

nium intermediates which alkylate biological molecules. *Procarbazine* and *dacarbazine* which are illustrated in Figure XVI-3-12, are metabolized to reactive intermediates which decompose to produce methyl diazonium, which methylates DNA.[25] Both procarbazine and dacarbazine are used in the treatment of Hodgkin's Disease,[57,107] procarbazine is a component of combination regimens used for the treatment of primary brain tumors,[278] and dacarbazine has a role in the treatment of melanoma (see XVI-4).[146,253] Procarbazine was originally developed as a monomine oxidase inhibitor, and can produce central nervous system depression and acute hypertensive reactions after the ingestion of tyramine rich foods.[25]

Decomposition and Metabolism

The alkylating agents react with water, and are inactivated by this hydrolysis. The alkylating agents also are inactivated by reaction with thiols, such as glutathione. The reaction of alkylating agents with glutathione can be increased by the enzyme glutathione S-transferase, as will be discussed below in mechanisms of cellular resistance. The alkylating agents also undergo microsomal and other types of xenobiotic metabolism. Such metabolism may activate agents, as described above, inactivate them, or change their physical properties without inactivating them. Nitrosoureas are denitrosated and inactivated by microsomal metabolism.[213,279] Chlorambucil is metabolized to bischoroethylphenylacetic acid, which is an active alkylating agent, and probably contributes to the therapeutic and toxic effects of chlorambucil.[6,135,304]

Mechanism of Cytoxicity

While the alkylating agents react with a number of biological molecules, including amino acids, thiols, RNA, and DNA, a number of lines of evidence have led to the generally accepted conclusion that the cytotoxic effects of the agents are due to reactions with DNA. Bifunctional agents are much more effective antitumor agents than monofunctional agents, but addition of more than two alkylating groups does not further increase the cytotoxic activity. These observations,[285] and the early studies of Brookes and Lawley[65,66] led to the suggestion that interstrand cross-linking of DNA was responsible for the cytotoxic activity of the bifunctional alkylating agents. A good correlation has been shown between cytotoxicity and the formation of interstrand crosslinks by bifunctional alkylating agents. The alkaline elution technique developed by Kohn[136] has been especially important in these studies. More recently, nitrogen mustard interstrand crosslinks in oligonucleotides have been chemically characterized.[307,330]

While the alkylating agents can react with virtually all the nitrogens in the DNA bases, there is selectivity, based on the electron density of the nitrogens and the local structure of the DNA. The nitrogen mustards react most readily with the N-7 position of guanylic acid.[368] This nitrogen atom has a high electron density, which appears to be enhanced by base stacking in the DNA helical structure.[65] Brookes and Lawley suggested that the nitrogen mustard crosslink in DNA was between the N-7 guanine atoms in base paired G-C sequences in DNA.[65] However, two recent studies which examined the crosslinking of oligonucleotides have found the interstrand crosslink of mechlorethamine to occur between the N-7 atoms of guanylic acids in a G-X-C sequence, as illustrated in Figure XVI-3-13.[307,330] The crosslinking of mitomycin C between two extracyclic guanylic acid amino groups is described above.[59] This site of crosslinking may be determined by the orientation of mitomycin C in the minor groove of DNA.[60] The reactive species of the nitrosoureas is more reactive than the aziridiniums of the nitrogen mustards, and appears to initially alkylate the 0-6 position of guanylic acid.[133,341] According to a mechanism proposed by Ludlum, after a series of rearrangements involving a reactive cyclic 5 membered intermediate of the N-1, C-6, and O-6 atoms of guanylic acid and two carbons from the chloroethyl group of the nitrosourea (see Figure XVI-3-11), a crosslink is formed between N-1 of guanylic acid and N-3 of a cytidylic acid on the complementary DNA strand.[53,288]

Some alkylating agents, such as procarbazine and dacarbazine, are not bifunctional, but are cytotoxic. The cytotoxic effects of these agents are probably produced by the alkyl-

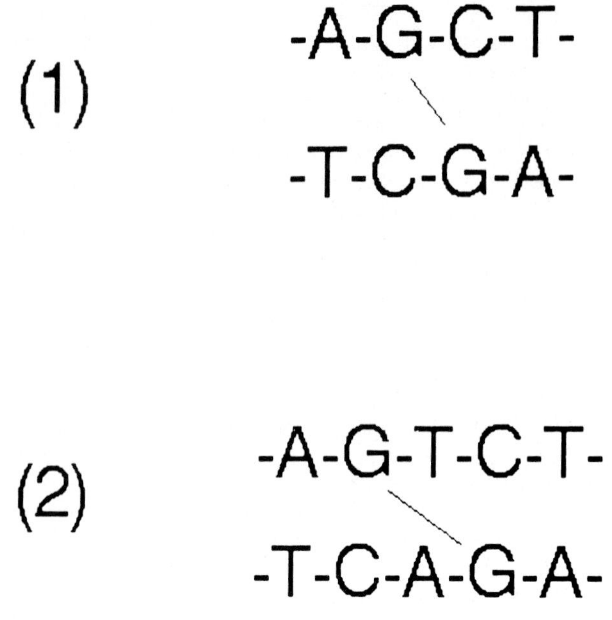

(1)

-A-G-C-T-

-T-C-G-A-

(2)

-A-G-T-C-T-

-T-C-A-G-A-

Figure XVI-3-13.   Interstrand crosslinking of DNA by nitrogen mustards. (1) Site of crosslinking proposed by Brookes.[65] (2) Site of crosslinking found by Loechler[330] and Hopkins.[307]

ation of guanylic acid with the subsequent depurination and production of single strand DNA breaks.[459,460] Bifunctional agents also produce monofunctional alkylations, depurination, and single strand breaks, but these compounds are cytotoxic at concentrations below those necessary to produce the degree of single strand breaks associated with cytotoxic levels of monofunctional agents.

Cellular Resistance to Alkylating Agents

Cellular resistance to antitumor agents is a critical determinant of the effectiveness of therapy. Resistance mechanisms in normal tissues provide selectivity and an improved therapeutic index. Resistance of tumor cells allows these cells to escape the effects of therapy. Consideration of the pharmacology and chemistry of the alkylating agents predicts three general types of cellular resistance to alkylating agents (Figure XVI-3-14). These are: 1) decreased uptake of agents into or increased export out of the cell; 2) increased inactivation of agents in the cell; and 3) enhanced repair of the DNA damage produced by the alkylating agents. All three of these mechanisms have now been shown to occur. Resistance of tumor cells to mechlorethamine can occur on the basis of decreased transport into the cell[171,477] and it has also been demonstrated that certain cells resistant to melphalan have decreased active transport of the agent and of amino acids.[99,371] Most alkylating agents enter cells by diffusion, however, and the alkylating agents, with the exception of mitomycin C, are not substrates for the multiple drug resistance (mdr) export system. It seems unlikely therefore, that decreased cellular uptake or increased export of alkylating agents will prove to be major mechanisms of resistance to most of the alkylating agents.

The second mechanism of cellular resistance to alkylating agents is intracellular inactivation of the agent. As discussed above, the enzyme aldehyde dehydrogenase detoxifies the primary metabolites of cyclophosphamide and ifosfamide,

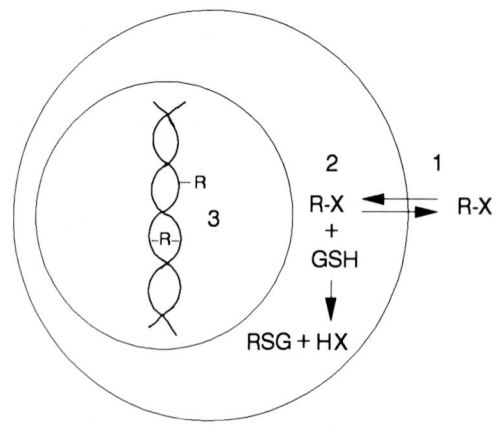

1. Decreased entry into or increased exit of agent from cell

2. Inactivation of agent in cell

3. Enhanced repair of DNA lesions produced by alkylation

Figure XVI-3-14.   Mechanisms of resistance to alkylating agents.

and the presence of this enzyme in the bone marrow and gastrointestinal system protects these organs from toxicity of the agents. Aldehyde dehydrogenase has also been demonstrated to be a mechanism of cyclophosphamide resistance of murine,[214] rat,[256] and human leukemia cells,[91] and human ovarian cancer cells.[342] An association between cellular resistance to alkylating agents and increased cellular levels of glutathione,[72,430] and the enzyme glutathione transferase has been described by a number of investigators.[70,318,369,384] Glutathione is a thiol containing tripeptide which is present at millimolar concentrations in many cells, reacts with electrophilic (electron deficient) molecules, and protects cells from such electrophiles. While most electrophiles of biologic significance react spontaneously with glutathione, glutathione S-transferase catalyzes the reaction between glutathione and electrophiles. The glutathione conjugates of several alkylating agents have been characterized[114,115,481] and their formation shown to be enhanced by glutathione S-transferase.

There are a number of isozymes of glutathione S-transferase, and recent studies indicate that different isozymes may catalyse the conjugation of different alkylating agents.[56,82,417] At this time it seems evident that glutathione alone or glutathione plus an appropriate glutathione S-transferase can render cells resistant to alkylating agents, and that this mechanism is probably an important mechanism of resistance to electrophilic antitumor drugs, such as the alkylating agents. The quantitative aspects of this type of resistance, and the characterization of the isozymes of glutathione S-transferase associated with resistance to specific agents are currently areas of intense investigation.

Several investigators have demonstrated that buthionine sulfoxime (BSO), an inhibitor of glutathione synthesis, can reduce cellular glutathione levels and sensitize tumors to alkylating agents in vitro and in vivo.[156,263,336] However, normal cells can also be sensitized by BSO administration[155,228,416] to produce significant toxicity. BSO in combination with alkylating agents is now undergoing clinical trials. Inhibitors of glutathione S-transferase have been shown to enhance the cytotoxicity of melphalan on cells resistant to alkylating agents[440] and such inhibitors are being examined in clinical trials.

Since the cytotoxicity of the alkylating agents appears to be mediated through the alkylation of DNA, the repair of alkylation lesions is an obvious mechanism of resistance to these agents, and has been the subject of intense investigation. The best defined DNA repair resistance to alkylating agents is resistance to the nitrosoureas and other compounds which alkylate the O6 position of guanylic acid in DNA. The protein O-6-alkylguanine-alkyltransferase has been shown to remove alkyl groups from the O6 position of guanine, and thus prevent the formation of the interstrand crosslink.[53,133,345] The alkyl group is covalently and irreversibly bound to the alkyltransferase, so that the protein can catalyse the removal of only one alkyl molecule. A strong association has now been shown between the presence of high levels of this protein in certain normal and tumor cells and the resistance of these cells to nitrosoureas. In particular, it seems clear that elevated O-6-alkylguanine-DNA-alkyltransferase is a mechanism of resistance to nitrosoureas in human glioma[9,53,405] and rhabdomyosarcoma.[63] As described above, the less reactive alkylating agents do not produce DNA crosslinks through the O-6 position of guanylic acid, and elevated alkyltransferase does not confer resistance to these agents.

Removal of interstrand crosslinks from DNA in cells can be shown to occur, in studies using alkaline elution and other techniques.[96,258,394] However, a mammalian tumor cell which is resistant to alkylating agents on the basis of enhanced crosslink repair has not been definitively described. There is increasing evidence that cells which remain in a quiescent phase following alkylating agent damage are able to repair lesions and are more resistant than cells which enter into a proliferative stage following such damage. This phenomenon probably provides a degree of tumor specificity to the alkylating agents. Inhibitors of DNA repair have been shown to enhance the cytoxicity of alkylating agents[100,124,454] and some of these inhibitors are being examined in clinical trials. It seems likely that increased understanding of the DNA repair process will allow more effective utilization of alkylating agents.

In Vivo Resistance. Several investigators have reported tumors which are resistant in vivo, but are found to be sensitive in vitro.[437] Definitive reasons for this phenomenon have not been established. There may be changes in known cellular resistance factors in the in vivo condition, as opposed to the in vitro situation. Changes in the cell membrane, poor perfusion of the tumor, and changes in cellular pH[235] are other possible explanations. Another possibility is that the capillary endothelial cells, which proliferate under drug exposure along with the tumor cells, may be selected for mechanisms of inactivation or decreased transport of the antitumor agents.

Clinical Pharmacology

Accurate data on the clinical pharmacology of the alkylating agents has become available only in recent years, and still remains limited. This is because the newer accurate and definitive methods, such as gas chromatography-mass spectrometry and high performance liquid chromatography, are necessary for many of these measurements.

Cyclophosphamide. After the administration of a systemic dose of 50 mg/kg, plasma levels of the parent compound of up to 400 micromolar may be achieved and decay with a half-life of 3–10 hours.[125,238,241,427] The rate of metabolism of the parent compound varies considerably between individuals, and can be modulated by the administration of compounds which affect the rate of microsomal metabolism, such as phenobarbital[236] or a previous dose of cyclophosphamide.[110,134] However, the clearance rate of the parent compound does not appear to significantly affect the toxicity or therapeutic effect of the agent.[413] This independence of effect from the rate of metabolism is probably because the parent compound is not rapidly excreted and continues to be activated, so that the area under the curve (AUC) for systemic exposure to the active metabolites is similar after a given dose. Plasma concentrations of 4-hydroxycyclophosphamide/aldophosphamide, the metabolite which appears to be responsible for the principal therapeutic effects, reach maximum levels of 1-20 micromolar, and this compound has a plasma half-life of 1–6 hours.[140,414,427,469] After doses of 20 mg/kg of cyclophosphamide, Wagner and colleagues found an AUC of concentration times time of 16.7 micromolar hours for 4-hydroxycyclophosphamide.[468] Sladek and colleagues studied patients who were receiving 50 mg/kg of cyclophosphamide and found a mean AUC for 4-hydroxycyclophosphamide of 80 micromolar hours.[414] Struck and coworkers, using a different analytic technique, measured an AUC of 2 micromolar hours after doses of 30 mg/kg.[427] The majority of a dose of cyclophosphamide (~70%) is excreted in the urine as the inactive metabolite, carboxyphosphamide.[29,238,428] Renal function does not significantly affect the toxicity of cyclophosphamide,[225] most likely because spontaneous decomposition, and not renal excretion, determines the clearance of the principal active metabolites. The clinical pharmacology of ifosfamide is similar to that of cyclophosphamide, except that microsomal activation is somewhat slower, and chloroethyl side chain oxidation plays a greater role in its metabolism.[61,320,327,468] Thus, for a dose of ifosfamide, lower systemic concentrations of the 4-hydroxy metabolite are achieved than for the same dose of cyclophosphamide.[468] Both cyclophosphamide and ifosfamide are well absorbed after oral administration.[240,427]

Melphalan. Alberts and colleagues found that peak plasma levels of 4–13 micromolar were present after intravenous administration of a 0.6 mg/kg dose of melphalan, and the half-life (t½β) was 1.8 hours.[7] At this dose, the mean AUC for melphalan was 8 micromolar hours. After conventional oral doses of 0.25 mg/kg, peak plasma levels of up to 0.625 micromolar were found.[339] There is variable systemic availability after oral dosing,[5,79,435] and it has been shown that oral administration of L-leucine or food with melphalan will inhibit absorption of the agent.[373,375] It has been reported that myelosuppression from melphalan is increased in patients with decreased renal function.[93] The half-life of melphalan is prolonged in anephric dogs,[8] and significant renal clearance of the parent compound in patients has been shown by Reece and colleagues.[374]

Chlorambucil. After the oral administration of 0.6 mg/kg of chlorambucil, peak levels of 2–6 micromolar parent compound were found at 1 hour by Alberts and colleagues.[5,6] Peak plasma levels of phenylacetic acid mustard of 2–4 micromolar occurred at 2–4 hours after chlorambucil administration. The plasma half-life (t½β) of chlorambucil was 92 minutes, and that of phenylacetic acid mustard 145 minutes. At a dose of 0.6 mg/kg of chlorambucil, the plasma AUC of

in serum osmolality and sodium concentration. Pericardial and pleural effusions may be seen, and seizures due to hyponatremia have occurred in children after cyclophosphamide therapy,[198] especially if low sodium replacement fluids have been administered. This antidiuretic syndrome appears to be due to an effect of cyclophosphamide metabolites on the distal renal tubule, and is self-limited, with the excess fluid excreted over a period of about 12 hours. Administration of furosemide will promote free water clearance and ameliorate the syndrome.[179]

Renal Toxicity. Renal toxicity has proven to be a serious toxicity of the nitrosoureas.[199,403] This effect is dose-related and may produce severe renal failure and death after administration of more than 1,200 mg of BCNU. Elevation of serum creatinine and other clinical evidence of renal toxicity may not be seen until after the completion of therapy. The histology of the kidneys in patients with renal nitrosourea damage is similar to that in radiation nephritis. A case of acute renal failure after melphalan therapy has been reported,[246] and increase in creatinine has been described when melphalan was added to high doses of alkylating agents.[18]

Alopecia. While the association between an alkylating agent and alopecia was first described with busulfan therapy,[46] this toxicity has been predominantly associated with cyclophosphamide and ifosfamide therapy. The alopecia produced by these agents may be quite severe, especially if the agent is given in combination with vincristine or doxorubicin. Regrowth of the hair occurs after cessation of therapy, and may be associated with a change in the texture and color of the hair.[160] The structure-function studies of Feil and Lamoureaux suggest that this toxicity is due to the entry of lipophilic metabolites into the hair follicles.[139] This suggestion is consistent with the fact that busulfan, vincristine, and adriamycin are all lipophilic molecules.

Allergic and Hypersensitivity Reactions. Since the alkylating agents react with many biological molecules, it is not surprising that they would serve as haptenes and produce allergic reactions.[92,268,393] The most frequent reactions which have been reported have been cutaneous hypersensitivity. Anaphylactic reactions are rare, but have occurred.[244] Patterns of cross-reactivity have not been carefully defined, but cross-reactivity between agents of similar structure, such as the nitrogen mustards, have been described.[252,393]

Cardiotoxicity. The dose limiting toxicity of cyclophosphamide is cardiac toxicity.[68,415,423] The fulminant syndrome has been seen most frequently in patients receiving a total dose of cyclophosphamide greater than 200 mg/kg, preparatory to bone marrow transplantation. The clinical course of the syndrome consists of the rapid onset of severe heart failure, which is fatal within 10–14 days. The hearts of such patients are dilated, with patchy transmural hemorrhage and pericardial effusion. The microscopic findings consist of interstitial hemorrhage and edema, myocardial necrosis and vacuolar changes, and specific changes in the intramural small coronary vessels.[415] Decreased electrocardiographic voltage and a transient increase in heart size is seen in high dose cyclophosphamide patients without clinical symptoms, and the characteristic pathological findings are present in such patients who die of other causes. Cardiotoxicity and cardiomegaly have been seen in patients receiving lower doses of cyclophosphamide in combination with other alkylating agents.[18,20] Age greater than 50 and previous adriamycin exposure appears to increase the risk of cyclophosphamide cardiotoxicity.[423]

Neurotoxicity. In preclinical studies of alkylating agents, convulsions have often been seen.[422] At the usual clinical doses of these agents, frank neurotoxicity is not usually seen but drowsiness and alterations of consciousness can be seen.[44] With the increasing use of higher doses of alkylating agents and combinations of alkylating agents, more clinical neurotoxicity is being seen.[123] At BCNU doses of 1,200 mg/m^2 severe central nervous system toxicity has been seen[431] and the intracarotid administration of BCNU has produced severe eye pain and blindness.[479] High dose busulfan therapy produces seizures and anticonvulsants are often used prophylactically in these patients.[455]

Teratogenecity. Studies carried out in vivo and in embryo cultures have demonstrated that virtually all of the alkylating agents are teratogenic.[54,316] The teratogenic effect is probably due to cytotoxic effects on the embryo by the same mechanisms by which the compounds are toxic to tumor cells.[167,192,283,310] The available clinical information indicates that there is a definite risk of a malformed infant if the mother is treated with an alkylating agent during the first trimester of pregnancy.[161,421,443] In a review of the literature, Nicholson found that, of 25 women who had received alkylating agents during the first trimester of pregnancy, there were four fetal malformations.[324] However, the administration of alkylation agents during the second and third trimesters is not associated with an increased risk of fetal malformation.[275,324,332]

Carcinogenesis. Since the initial reports of acute leukemia occurring in patients treated with alkylating agents,[217,266,389,390] it has become increasingly obvious that this type of oncogenesis is a significant complication of alkylating agent therapy (see XL-17). Several studies have indicated that rate of acute leukemia after alkylating agent therapy may be 10% or higher in certain groups of patients.[127,377,447] Procarbazine and other methylating agents appear to be the most potent oncogens,[111] and melphalan appears to produce a higher rate of acute leukemia than cyclophosphamide.[180] The lesser leukemogenic potential of cyclophosphamide may well be related to the hematopoietic stem cell sparing effect of this agent.[396] An increased rate of solid tumors is also seen in patients treated with alkylating agents.[128,348,447] Although sufficient data are not yet available to be certain, it appears that high dose alkylating agent therapy administered in intermittent pulses over a relatively short period of time is less oncogenic than prolonged alkylating agent therapy.

Immunosuppression. The immunosuppressive effect of alkylating agents was first described by Hektoen and Corper for sulfur mustard.[207] Cyclophosphamide is particularly immunosuppressive[291] and is used for the treatment of autoimmune diseases.[31,270,445] Cyclophosphamide is also used in preparative regimens for allogeneic transplantation, because of its immunoablative activity.[398] Low doses of cyclophosphamide and melphalan can enhance the immune response by selectively inhibiting the immune suppressor cells.[42,113,334] Because of this effect moderate doses of cyclophosphamide have been used in conjunction with immunotherapy and biological response modifiers, such as interleukin-2.[41,311]

The clinical significance of the immunosuppression produced by alkylating agents in their role as antitumor agents is not certain. The two major concerns are susceptibility to infection in the immunosuppressed host and the potential interference with a host immune response to the tumor. The available evidence indicates that most intermittent antitumor regimens do not produce a profound or prolonged immunosuppression.[314]

The Platinum Antitumor Compounds

The platinum antitumor agents are complexes of platinum with ligands which can be displaced by nucleophilic (electron rich) atoms to form strong bonds with covalent characteristics. Thus, like the alkylating agents, the platinum agents form strong chemical bonds with thiol sulfurs and amino nitrogens in proteins and nucleic acids.

The first platinum antitumor compound was discovered by Rosenberg and colleagues while studying the effects of electric current on bacterial growth.[387] The growth inhibition observed was found to be caused by a platinum complex of ammonia and chloride, which was produced in the medium from the platinum electrode. These investigators found several such compounds to have antitumor activity against murine tumors in vivo.[388] The most active of these compounds was the one now known as cisplatin (Figure XVI-3-17).

Cisplatin went into clinical trials in the early 1970's,[210,211,260,281,432] and was found to have significant antitumor activity against testicular cancer, lymphoma, squamous cell carcinoma of the head and neck, ovarian cancer, and bladder cancer. Because of its significant therapeutic effect in these tumors, and activity against a number of other solid tumors, it has subsequently become the most frequently used antitumor agent.

Chemistry

The platinum compounds which are active antitumor agents can have either four or six ligands (Figure XVI-3-17), with a square planar or hexahedral configuration, respectively. Those with four ligands have an oxidation state of $+2$, and those with six ligands an oxidation state of $+4$. The chloride ligands of cisplatin and the other complexes with the $+2$ oxidation state can be exchanged for nucleophilic atoms in the biological milieu, including the nitrogens of the DNA bases. The chloride ligands of the $+4$ compounds are much less reactive than those of the $+2$ compounds,[200] and it is likely that the $+4$ compounds are reduced in vivo to produce the reac-

tive $+2$ complexes.[49,346,347] The ligand substitution reactions of the square planar complexes occur with retention of the configuration of the platinum complex.[200] Since the trans-platinum compounds are essentially inactive as antitumor compounds, the ability of the cis compounds to form certain stereospecific cross-links probably accounts for their antitumor activity.

In some cis-platinum compounds in clinical use the Cl leaving ligands are replaced with carboxyl ester groups, as in carboplatin (Figure XVI-3-17). These ligands are less readily displaced, and thus these compounds require higher concentrations for cytotoxicity. The decreased renal and neurologic toxicity of these compounds is also probably due to the fact that they are less chemically reactive than cisplatin.

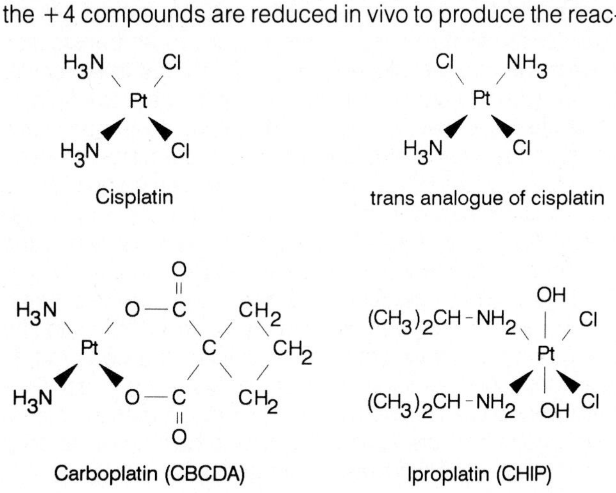

Cellular and Molecular Pharmacology

While the Cl and carboxyester ligands can probably be directly displaced by biological atoms, it is likely that, in the biological milieu, the chloride or carboxy ligands are displaced by water molecules to form the aquo ligand, which is a better leaving group than the chloride or carboxy groups.[297] The high chloride content of the extracellular fluid maintains the platinum compounds in the chloride and less reactive form. However, in the lower chloride content of the cell the more reactive aquo species is formed. The loss of a proton produces the hydroxy ligand, which is unreactive.[297] The proposed aquation pathway for cisplatin is shown in Figure XVI-3-18. The platinum compounds react with many biological molecules, but there is considerable evidence that these compounds, like the bifunctional alkylating agents, exert their cytotoxic effect by reacting with DNA and interfering with DNA replication and cell division. Roberts and Pera and colleagues demonstrated that the amount of platinum bound to DNA was directly related to the degree of toxicity of platinum compounds.[383] Zwelling and coworkers demonstrated that the degree of DNA interstrand cross-linking in vitro and in vivo was directly related to the degree of cytoxicity in rodent tumor cells.[485]

The cis-platinum compounds, like the alkylating agents,[119,120,142] react with nitrogen atoms of DNA and preferentially react with the N7 atom of deoxyguanylic acid. Specific adducts of Pt compounds with DNA have now been characterized and studied. The consensus of the studies is

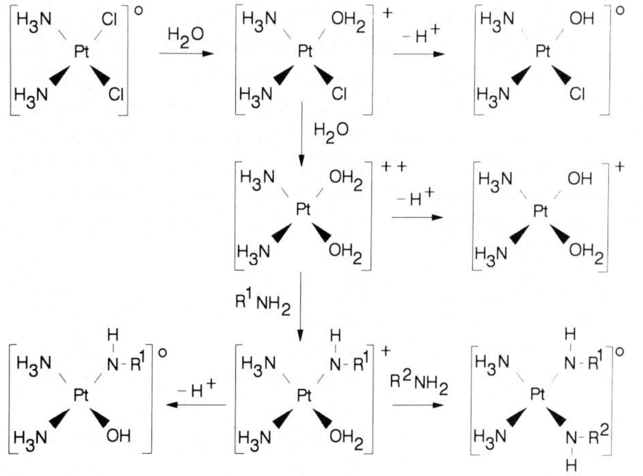

Figure XVI-3-17. Structures of platinum antitumor agents.

Figure XVI-3-18. Aquation of platinum compounds and reaction with nucleophiles.

that the most frequent adducts are dGpdG and dApdG (Figure XVI-3-19), which result from the cis-platinum complex binding to adjacent deoxyguanylates or an adjacent deoxyadenylate and deoxyguanylate in a strand of DNA, to produce an intrastrand crosslink in both situations. A less common, but perhaps more critical, lesion is the one which results from binding of the platinum atom to the N7 of a deoxyguanylate in one strand of DNA and to the N7 atom of a deoxyguanylate in the complementary strand of DNA, thereby producing an interstrand crosslink (Figure XVI-3-19). Repair of these lesions does occur, and the cytotoxicity to the cell is probably determined by the resultant of the formation and repair of the lesions. As mentioned above, a close correlation between interstrand DNA cross-linking has been demonstrated, but equally precise methods for quantifying intrastrand cross-links in whole cells after drug exposure are not available. Thus, intrastrand DNA cross-links might correlate equally well or better with cytotoxicity. The DNA adducts formed by Pt compounds other than cisplatin have been less well studied, but appear to be the same as those formed by cisplatin.[255,358,429]

While there is considerable evidence that the formation of DNA adducts is responsible for the cytotoxicity of the platinum antitumor agents, the mechanism through which the cytotoxic effects are mediated is not established. Evidence has been presented that the platinum adducts inhibit replication.[356,463] In a recent paper, Lippard and colleagues have demonstrated that as few as two platinum adducts per genome were sufficient for inhibition of DNA replication by cisplatin.[206] Sorenson and Eastman found that cytoxicity with cisplatin was correlated with the duration of arrest in the G_2 phase of the cell cycle and postulated that the G_2 arrest was due to the inability of the cells to transcribe the Pt damaged DNA and produce the mRNA essential for mitosis.[418]

Mechanisms of Cellular Resistance to Platinum Agents

A number of mechanism of cellular resistance to platinum compounds have been described. These mechanisms include decreased uptake of the platinum compound into resistant cells, inactivation of the drug by cellular thiol compounds, and enhanced repair of the platinum related DNA damage.

Decreased cellular uptake of cisplatin by cells resistant to the compound has been described by several investigators.[15,224,306,438,473] The uptake of cisplatin into cells is linear for over an hour and does not appear to be an active transport process, although it is partially inhibited by metabolic inhibitors.[15] No increase in the efflux of cisplatin has been seen thus far in resistant cells. Howell and colleagues could not demonstrate changes in the physical properties of the cell membrane of the resistant cells.[293] Thus, while decreased cellular accumulation of the platinum compounds appears

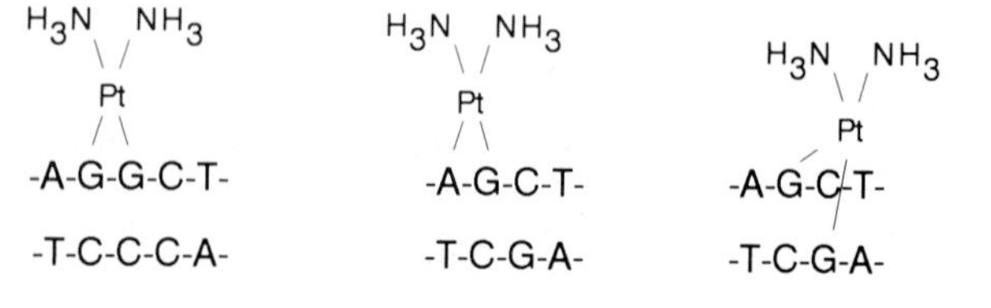

to be one type of cellular resistance, the mechanism of this type of resistance remains undefined, and may be related to altered binding of the agents to cellular proteins, rather than alteration of passage through the cell membrane.[409]

A number of investigators have demonstrated that both rodent and human tumor cells which are selected in vitro or in vivo by exposure to the platinum antitumor compounds frequently demonstrate elevated glutathione levels in association with resistance to these drugs.[13,32,35,36,38,150,220,221,223,337,407] Tumor cell lines derived from patients resistant to therapy with cisplatin have also been found to have elevated glutathione levels.[45,108] In one report the resistant cell line was also found to have elevated activity of gamma-glutamyl transpeptidase, an enzyme in glutathione synthesis.[45]

Further evidence that glutathione is involved in resistance to platinum compounds can be inferred from the fact that several investigators have shown that tumor cells can be sensitized to the platinum agents by depletion of cellular glutathione by treatment with buthionine sulfoximine, an inhibitor of glutathione synthesis.[11,14,193,223]

The mechanism(s) through which glutathione associated resistance is mediated have not been definitively elucidated. Andrews and colleagues demonstrated that cisplatin binds to glutathione,[11] and Borch and coworkers have studied the reaction rates of cisplatin with various thiols, including glutathione, and characterized a reaction product in which two glutathiones appeared to be found to each platinum through the cysteine residues of the glutathiones.[102] The thiol platinum ligand is very stable and thus will not react further. Eastman has presented evidence that glutathione may react with monofunctional adducts on DNA to quench the second reactive ligand and prevent cross-link formation.[121] Resistance to cisplatin has also been associated with elevation of glutathione transferase enzyme activity, increased levels of the pi (acidic) isozyme of the protein, and increased levels of the mRNA for the pi isozyme.[36,319,397,472] However, the catalysis of the conjugation of glutathione with platinum agents by this enzyme has not been characterized.

Cellular resistance to platinum agents has also been associated with another sulfhydryl containing protein, metallothionein. Several investigators have found that tumor cells exposed to heavy metals, such as cadmium, develop resistance to cisplatin which is associated with increased cellular levels of metallothionein.[12,132,249] In one report, transfection of cells with the metallothionein gene resulted in increased metallothionein levels and resistance of the cells to cisplatin, melphalan, and chlorambucil.[249] Imura and colleagues have reported that administration of bismuth subnitrate to mice produced increased levels of metallothionein in the kidneys and resulted in protection of the mice from the renal and gastrointestinal toxicity of cisplatin, but did not affect the response of transplanted tumors to cisplatin in the mice.[317] Cisplatin binds to metallothionein in Ehrlich ascites tumor cells[261] and in the liver and kidney of rats,[409,483] and the systemic administration of cisplatin or its hydrolysed product can induce metallothionein in liver and kidney.[138] These findings indicate that metallothionein can protect both tumor and normal cells from cisplatin, although the binding of the drug to this protein has not been characterized.

As with the alkylating agents, there is extensive evidence that enhanced DNA repair can be responsible for resistance

Figure XVI-3-19. Platinum-DNA adducts.

to the platinum compounds, and recent work has begun to define specific enzymes involved in this type of resistance. Roberts and colleagues first reported that caffeine, a known inhibitor of DNA repair, potentiated cytotoxicity and chromosomal damage in mammalian cells,[449] and shortly thereafter demonstrated that excision repair of cisplatin-damaged DNA does occur in treated cells.[151] Many subsequent studies have demonstrated that cells deficient in DNA repair, such as those from patients with xeroderma pigmentosum or Fanconi's anemia, are very sensitive to cisplatin.[80,109,196,299,360,361]

Agents which are known to inhibit the activity of enzymes involved in the repair of DNA, such as aphidocolin and novobiocin, have been shown to sensitize cells to cisplatin and to reverse the resistance of repair resistant cell lines.[75,124,248,298] The antitumor agents hydroxyurea and cytosine arabinoside, which inhibit DNA repair synthesis, both produce a synergistic cytotoxic effect with cisplatin.[145,446]

Studies in E. coli have shown that the uvrABC excinuclease is involved in the removal of cisplatin adducts from plasmids which have been treated with the agent and transfected into E. coli with known repair enzyme deficits.[33,226] In one study,[33] it was demonstrated that the repair nuclease complex cut the DNA at the eighth phosphodiester bond 5′ to a GG pair crosslinked by Pt and at the fourth phosphodiester bond 3′ to the Pt lesion, and excised this fragment.

Subsequent studies have demonstrated that very sensitive tumor cells may have a decreased ability to remove DNA interstrand cross-links[34] and that tumor cells resistant to cisplatin may have increased DNA repair capacity.[38,298,410] Other reports have found increased activity of repair enzymes, such as DNA polymerase beta, in cisplatin resistant cells.[262] Recently, factors in resistant cells which will recognize and bind to Pt damaged DNA have been described.[81] Reed and colleagues have found that transfection into tumor cells of the human DNA repair gene ERCC-1, which appears to be a homolog of the uvrA gene in E. coli, confers resistance to cisplatin and enhances the ability of the cells to remove cisplatin from DNA.[376] A very interesting report by Scanlon and colleagues has described increased levels of dehydrofolate reductase, thymidine synthetase, thymidine kinase, and the DNA polymerases alpha and beta in human colon tumor cells, as well as the oncogenes c-fos and c-H-ras.[400] This combination of increased enzymes could account for the observations that certain cell lines resistant to platinum compounds were cross-resistant to methotrexate, and had alteration of folate disposition.[322,391] One of the cell lines was also resistant to 5-fluorouracil.[322]

While it is clear that each of these mechanisms can be associated with the resistance of tumor and normal cells to the platinum agents, the relative roles of these mechanisms in the resistance of tumors to treatment in patients have not been established. Such studies, and attempts to overcome resistance with BSO and inhibitors of DNA repair are currently in progress.

Clinical Pharmacology

Analogs in Clinical Use. Cisplatin continues to be the most frequently used platinum antitumor agent. While a number of analogs are currently being investigated, the two compounds which have received the most clinical evaluation are carboplatin and iproplatin (CHIP).[149A,442] Both of these compounds have shown activity similar to that of cisplatin in

clinical trials and both have predominantly hematopoietic toxicity, with much less renal, auditory, neurologic, and gastrointestinal toxicity than cisplatin.[4,10,24,77,97,149,292,302,340,452] In preclinical studies there have been indications that there might not be complete cross-resistance between the various platinum analogs,[406] but such lack of cross-resistance has not been seen in clinical trials. Carboplatin has now been licensed in the United States and is being used increasingly. In particular, it is currently being used in situations where non-hematopoietic toxicity should be avoided, such as with bone marrow support,[17,448] or with hematopoietic stimulatory factors. If carboplatin proves to be as effective in various tumors as cisplatin, but with marked reduction in the toxicities other than hematopoietic, it seems likely that its use, and that of other second and third generation platinum complexes, will surpass that of cisplatin.

Pharmacokinetics. Platinum antitumor compounds have been measured in human plasma and other human tissues as total platinum, as ultrafilterable platinum, and as the specific parent compounds. Total platinum can be measured by using compounds containing the radioactive 193Pt or 195Pt isotopes,[105,269] by trapping the platinum with an ultraviolet absorbing ligand, such as diethyldithiocarbamate, or by flameless atomic absorption spectroscopy.[101,168] Ultrafiltration of plasma and other biologic fluids separates the free platinum compounds from those bound to protein. The protein-bound species are biologically inactive, and essentially irreversibly bound to the protein.[378] Both cisplatin and carboplatin have been measured specifically by separation from other species on HPLC columns and detection by electrochemical detection or by collecting fractions and quantifying the total platinum in each fraction.[344,372] The cisplatinum concentration has been found to be consistently between 60–80% of the ultrafilterable platinum, and to follow the same kinetics as the ultrafilterable platinum (Figure XVI-3-20).[215,344] Carboplatinum represents a higher percentage of the ultrafilterable platinum and follows kinetics similar to the ultrafilterable platinum. Because of the sensitivity, accuracy, and convenience of the method, flameless atomic absorption spectroscopy is the most common technique used to measure the platinum agents. Furthermore, since measuring filterable species appears to measure the reactive com-

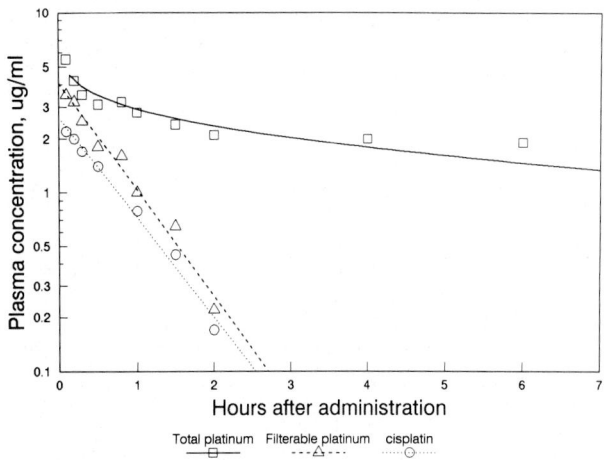

Figure XVI-3-20.   Clinical pharmacokinetics of cisplatin after single injection of 100 mg/m². (Adapted from Patton et al.[344])

pounds, and to approximate closely the measurement of the parent compounds, measurement of ultrafilterable platinum is most commonly used in pharmacokinetic studies.

In pharmacokinetic studies after cisplatin administration, total platinum in the plasma follows a triphasic pattern, with the first phase t½ about 30 minutes, the second phase t½ about 60 minutes, and the third phase phase t½ greater than 24 hours.[39,101,215] Measurements of the ultrafilterable platinum indicate that the initial, more rapid clearance phases are due to the renal clearance of filterable platinum, the majority of which is the parent compound.[344] Carboplatin exhibits similar pharmacokinetics, except that the initial half lives are somewhat longer, less of the total platinum is protein bound, and a greater percentage of the agent is excreted by the kidneys.[328,372] The pharmacokinetics of total and filterable platinum after iproplatin administration appears to be similar to those of carboplatin.[97] Decreased creatinine clearance results in higher plasma levels of both cisplatin and carboplatin and potentially greater toxicity.[126A]

After bolus administration of 100 mg/m^2 of cisplatin, initial peak plasma concentrations of 3–5 µg/ml are achieved,[344] with this value decreasing to less than 0.2 microgram/ml at two hours (Figure XVI-3-20). After the usual clinical dose of about 300 mg/m^2 of carboplatin, peak plasma levels of about 30 µg/ml are reached, declining to about 5 µg/ml at 2 hours.[328,372]

In typical clinical use, usually in combination with other agents, the platinum antitumor agents are given intravenously, either as a single dose or daily for several days, with repeat courses at three to four weeks. The agents are given as an infusion over several hours rather than as a bolus dose, and, especially with very high doses, may be given as 24 hour or longer infusions.

Cisplatin and carboplatin have also been administered regionally. There has been considerable experience with the intraperitoneal route, particularly in the treatment of ovarian cancer.[303,351,354,419] Very high intraperitoneal concentrations can be obtained, and systemic toxicities can be reduced by the concomitant systemic administration of thiosulfate.[222,295] Cisplatin has also been administered intra-arterially for the treatment of tumors in the extremities,[26,71,234,245] brain tumors,[147,273,424] carcinoma of the head and neck,[28,313] carcinoma of the liver,[247] and carcinoma of the bladder.[118,231] Intra-vesicular instillation of cisplatin has been used for the treatment of superficial cancers of the bladder.[50,219,280] Cisplatin has also been instilled into the pericardial sac for the treatment of malignant pericardial effusions.[143,296]

Toxicities

Renal. The most serious, and usually dose limiting, toxicity of cisplatin is renal.[176,355] This toxicity is manifested clinically by elevated BUN and creatinine, is cumulative with continued cisplatin exposure, and is potentiated by other nephrotoxins.[104] Decreases in serum electrolytes have been associated with platinum renal toxicity, including symptomatic hypomagnesemia.[404] While the toxicity may remain subclinical, or the renal function return to normal, significant pathological damage appears to persist.[173] The pathology of the renal damage is characterized by focal acute tubular necrosis, dilatation of convoluted tubules, thickened tubular basement membranes, formation of casts, and epithelial atypia of the collecting ducts.[173,289] High fluid intake with forced diuresis[76,205] can reduce the incidence and severity of the

renal toxicity. Systemic administration of thiols can reduce renal toxicity of cisplatin in animal models, and in a clinical trial systemic diethyldithiodicarbamate appeared to reduce nephrotoxicity without affecting ototoxicity or myelosuppression.[43] The nephrotoxicity of the second generation platinum complexes, such as carboplatin and iproplatin, is markedly less than that of cisplatin.

Ototoxicity. Ototoxicity has been a significant problem with cisplatin. This toxicity is characterized by tinnitus and hearing loss.[210,211,281,412] The hearing loss is usually in the high frequency range, 4,000–8,000 Hz, but may occur in the lower ranges, which include the speech frequencies.[264,412] Since the higher frequencies are usually involved, the hearing loss may not be symptomatic. Vestibular toxicity does not usually occur, but can be seen.[47,478] The ototoxicity of cisplatin is dose related, and is usually cumulative with subsequent courses of the agent.[191,461] Radiation prior to or simultaneous with the cisplatin administration enhances the toxicity,[178,470] but this additive effect may be less if the cisplatin precedes the radiation.[264]

The pathological findings associated with ototoxicity, in both experimental animals and patients, are selective damage to the outer hair cells of the cochlea, and lesions in the organ of Corti, the spiral ganglion and cochlear nerve, and the stria vascularis.[55,259,312,425] In studies of organ cultures of the cochlear structures the hair cells are very sensitive to very low concentrations of cisplatin.[16] Vestibular toxicity is associated with degeneration of the maculae and cristae.[478]

Neurotoxicity. The neurotoxicity seen with the administration of cisplatin consists principally of peripheral neuropathy involving both the upper and lower extremities, with paresthesias, weakness, tremors, and loss of taste.[466] Seizures and leucoencephalopathy have also been described.[157,362] The neurotoxicity may be persistent[195] and may progress after cessation of cisplatin therapy.[186] The quantitative determination of vibratory perception threshold has been reported to correlate with cisplatin neurotoxicity.[130]

Particularly severe neurotoxicity has been reported after intraarterial infusions of cisplatin, with cranial nerve paralysis occurring after intraarterial infusions for head and neck cancer[157,362] and severe peripheral neuropathy after lower limb perfusion.[69] In experimental animals, severe CNS toxicity was seen when compounds which open the blood brain barrier were administered prior to systemic cisplatin treatment, and intracarotid cisplatin produced damage to the blood brain barrier and severe neurotoxicity.[321] However, severe neurotoxicity was not seen in patients treated with intracarotid cisplatin for primary brain tumors.[290] The neurotoxicity of ifosfamide has been reported to be enhanced by prior treatment with cisplatin.[365]

Since various pharmacologic maneuvers have been able to control or reduce the nephrotoxicity and severe nausea and vomiting produced by cisplatin, neurotoxicity has become the dose limiting toxicity of cisplatin.[335] An interesting observation is that treatment of animals with an ACTH analog will prevent neurotoxicity from cisplatin, and will facilitate the recovery of established neurotoxicity,[450A] but does not interfere with the antitumor effect of the agent. In a randomized, placebo controlled clinical trial, this compound appeared to prevent or ameliorate the neurotoxicity of cisplatin.[450a] Neither carboplatin or iproplatin appear to produce significant neurotoxicity, even with high doses used with autologous bone marrow transfusion.[4,77,323,340,442,453]

Gastrointestinal Toxicity. Severe nausea and vomiting have been a significant problem with cisplatin, occurring in almost all patients receiving the drug.[260,367] The cause of this toxicity is not firmly established. Work in animal models indicate that abdominal visceral innervation and 5-hydroxytryptamine receptors on visceral afferent nerves play a role in mediating this toxicity,[204] but there is also evidence that the chemoreceptor trigger zone in the medulla plays a role.[212,300] The use of a dopamine antagonist, metoclopramide, prior to and during cisplatin administration has been effective in controlling this toxicity,[177,242] and the steroids dexamethasone or methylprednisolone alone or in combination with metoclopramide have also been useful.[1,40,164] More recently antiserotonin analogs such as ondansetron and granisetron have proven highly effective in controlling nausea and vomiting (see XL-3). The gastrointestinal toxicities of carboplatin and iproplatin are much less than those of cisplatin.[23,129,169]

Immune Effects. In contrast to the alkylating agents, many of which are significantly immunosuppressive, cisplatin appears to have no immunosuppressive effect at the usual clinical doses, and may even augment immune function at these doses.[376] Monocyte-mediated cytotoxicity was found to be increased in ovarian cancer patients after cisplatin treatment,[254] and OKT8+ cytotoxic cells were increased in patients after cisplatin therapy.[331]

References

1. Aapro, M. S., Plezia, P. M., Alberts, D. S., Graham, V., Jones, S. E., Surwit, E. A., and Moon, T. E.: Double-blind crossover study of the antiemetic efficacy of high-dose dexamethasone versus high-dose metoclopramide. J. Clin. Oncol., 2:466, 1984.
2. Abdi, E. A., Hanson, J., Harbora, D. E., Young, D. G., and McPherson, T. A.: Adjuvant chemoimmuno- and immunotherapy in Dukes' stage B2 and C colorectal carcinoma: A 7-year follow-up analysis. J. Surg. Oncol., 40:205, 1989.
3. Adair, C. P. J., and Bogg, H. J.: Experimental and clinical studies on the treatment of cancer by dichloroethylsulfide (mustard gas). Ann. Surg., 93:190, 1931.
4. Adams, M., Kerby, I. J., Rocker, I., Evans, A., Johansen, K., and Franks, C. R.: A comparison of the toxicity and efficacy of cisplatin and carboplatin in advanced ovarian cancer. Acta Oncol., 28:57, 1989.
5. Alberts, D. S., Chang, S. Y., Chen, H.-S. G., Larcom, B. J., and Evans, T. L.: Comparative pharmacokinetics of chlorambucil and melphalan in man. Recent Results Cancer Res., 74:124, 1980.
6. Alberts, D. S., Chang, S. Y., Chen, H.-S. G., Larcom, B. J., and Jones, S. E.: Pharmacokinetics and metabolism of chlorambucil in man: A preliminary report. Cancer Treat. Rev., 6(Suppl.):9, 1979.
7. Alberts, D. S., Chang, S. Y., Chen, H.-S. G., Moon, T. E., Evans, T. L., Furner, R. L., Himmelstein, K., and Gross, J. F.: Kinetics of intravenous melphalan. Clin. Pharmacol. Ther., 26:73, 1979.
8. Alberts, D. S., Chen, H.-S. G., Benz, D., and Mason, N. L.: Effect of renal dysfunction in dogs on the disposition and marrow toxicity of melphalan. Br. J. Cancer, 43:330, 1981.
9. Ali-Osman, F., Srivenugopal, K., Berger, M. S., and Stein, D. E.: DNA interstrand crosslinking and strand break repair in human glioma cell lines of varying {1,3-bis(2-chlorethyl)-1-nitrosourea} resistance. Anticancer Res., 10:677, 1990.
10. Anderson, H., Wagstaff, J., Crowther, D., Swindell, R., Lind, M. J., McGregor, J., Timms, M. S., Brown, D., and Palmer, P.: Comparative toxicity of cisplatin, carboplatin (CBDCA) and iproplatin (CHIP) in combination with cyclophosphamide in patients with advanced epithelial ovarian cancer. Eur. J. Cancer Clin. Oncol., 24:1471, 1988.
11. Andrews, P. A., Murphy, M. P., and Howell, S. B.: Differential sensitization of human ovarian carcinoma and mouse L1210 cells to cisplatin and melphalan by glutathione depletion. Mol. Pharmacol., 30:643, 1986.
12. Andrews, P. A., Murphy, M. P., and Howell, S. B.: Metallothionein mediated cisplatin resistance in human ovarian carcinoma cells. Cancer Chemother. Pharmacol., 19:149, 1987.
13. Andrews, P. A., Murphy, M. P., and Howell, S. B.: Characterization of cisplatin-resistance COLO 316 human ovarian carcinoma cells. Eur. J. Cancer Clin. Oncol., 25:619, 1989.
14. Andrews, P. A., Schiefer, M. A., Murphy, M. P., and Howell, S. B.: Enhanced potentiation of cisplatin cytotoxicity in human ovarian carcinoma cells by prolonged glutathione depletion. Chem. Biol. Interact., 65:51, 1988.
15. Andrews, P. A., Velury, S., Mann, S. C., and Howell, S. B.: cis-Diamminendichloroplatinum (II) accumulation in sensitive and resistant human ovarian carcinoma cells. Cancer Res., 48:68, 1988.
16. Anniko, M., and Sobin, A.: Cisplatin: evaluation of its ototoxic potential. Am. J. Otolaryngol., 7:276, 1986.
17. Antman, K., Eder, J. P., Elias, A., Ayash, L., Shea, T. C., Weissman, L., Critchlow, J., Schryber, S. M., Begg, C., Teicher, B. A., Schnipper, L. E., and Frei, E., III: High-dose thiotepa alone and in combination regimens with bone marrow support. Semin. Oncol., 17(Suppl. 3):33, 1990.
18. Antman, K., Eder, J. P., Elias, A., Shea, T., Peters, W. P., Andersen, J., Schryber, S., Henner, W. D., Finberg, R., and Wilmore, D.: High-dose combination alkylating agent preparative regimen with autologous bone marrow support: The Dana-Farber Cancer Institute/Beth Israel Hospital Experience. Cancer Treat. Rep., 71:119, 1987.
19. Antman, K. H., Elias, A., and Ryan, L.: Ifosfamide and mesna: Response and toxicity at standard- and high-dose schedules. Semin. Oncol., 17:68, 1990.
20. Appelbaum, F., Strauchen, J. A., Graw, R. G., Jr., Savage, D. D., Kent, K. M., Ferrans, V. J., and Herzig, G. P.: Acute lethal carditis caused by high-dose combination chemotherapy: A unique clinical and pathological entity. Lancet, 1:58, 1976.
21. Arbuck, S. G., Silk, Y., Douglass, H. O., Jr., Nava, H., Rustum, Y. M., and Milliron, S.: A phase II trial of 5-fluorouracil, doxorubicin, mitomycin C, and leucovorin in advanced gastric carcinoma. Cancer, 65:2442, 1990.
22. Arita, N., Ushio, Y., Hayakawa, T., Nagatant, M., Huang, T. Y., Izumoto, S., and Mogami, H.: Intrathecal ACNU—a new therapeutic approach against malignant leptomingeal tumors. J. Neurooncol., 6:221, 1988.
23. Arseneau, J., Blessing, J. A., Stehman, F. B., and McGehee, R.: A phase II study of carboplatin in advanced squamous cell carcinoma of the cervix (a Gynecologic Oncology Group Study). Invest. New Drugs, 4:187, 1986.
24. Ashbury, R. F., Kramer, A., Green, M., Qazi, R., Skeel, R. T., and Haller, D. G.: A phase II study of carboplatin and CHIP in patients with metastatic colon carcinoma. Am. J. Clin. Oncol., 12:416, 1989.
25. Auerbuch, S. D.: Nonclassic alkylating agents. *In* Cancer Chemotherapy: Principles and Practice. Edited by B. A. Chabner, and J. M. Collins. J. B. Lippincott, Philadelphia, 1990, pp. 314-328.
26. Bacci, G., Picci, P., Ruggieri, P., Mercuri, M., Avella, M., Capanna, R., Brach-Del-Prever, A., Mancini, A., Gherlinzoni, F., Padovani, G., Leonossa, C., Biagini, R., Ferraro, A., Ferruzi, A., Cazzola, A., Manfrini, M., and Campanacci, I.: Primary chemotherapy and delayed surgery (neoadjuvant chemotherapy) for osteosarcoma of the extremities. The Instituto Rissoli Experience in 127 patients treated preoperatively with Intravenous methotrexate (high versus moderate doses) and intraarterial cisplatin. Cancer, 65:2539, 1990.
27. Bailey, C. C., Marsden, H. B., and Jones, P. H.: Fatal pulmonary fibrosis following 1,3-bis(2-chloroethyl)-1-nitrosourea (BCNU) therapy. Cancer, 42:74, 1978.
28. Baker, S. R., and Wheeler, R.: Intraarterial chemotherapy for head and neck cancer, Part 2: Clinical experience. Head-Neck Surg., 6:751, 1984.
29. Bakke, J. E., Feil, V. J., Fjelstul, C. E., and Thacker, E. J.: Metabolism of cyclophosphamide by sheep. J. Agric. Food Chem., 20:384, 1972.
30. Barlogie, B., Jagannath, S., Dixon, D. O., Cheson, B., Smallwood, L., Hendrickson, A., Purvis, J. D., Bonnem, E., and Alexanian, R.: High-dose melphalan and granulocyte-macrophage colony-stimulating factor for refractory multiple myeloma. Blood, 76:677, 1990.
31. Barratt, T. M., and Soothill, J. F.: Controlled trial of cyclophosphamide in steroid-sensitive relapsing nephrotic syndrome of childhood. Lancet, 2:279, 1970.
32. Batist, G., Behrens, B. C., Makuch, R., Hamilton, T. C., Katki, A. G., Louie, K. G., Meyers, C. E., and Ozols, R. F.: Serial determinations of glutathione levels and glutathione-related enzyme activities in human tumor cells in vitro. Biochem. Pharmacol., 35:2257, 1986.
33. Beck, D. J., Popoff, S., Sancar, A., and Rupp, W. D.: Reactions of the UVRABC excision nuclease with DNA damaged by diamminedichloroplatinum (II). Nucleic Acids Res., 13:7395, 1985.
34. Bedford, P., Fichtinger-Schepman, A. M., Shellard, A. A., Walker, M. C., Masters, J. R., and Hill, B. T.: Differential repair of platinum-DNA adducts in human bladder and testicular tumor continuous cell lines. Cancer Res., 48:3019, 1988.
35. Bedford, P., Shellard, S. A., Walker, M. C., Whelan, R. D., Masters, J. R., and Hill, B. T.: Differential expression of collateral sensitivity or resistance to cisplatin in human bladder carcinoma cell lines pre-exposed in vitro to either x-irradiation or cisplatin. Int. J. Cancer, 40:681, 1987.
36. Bedford, P., Walker, M. C., Sharma, H. L., Perera, A., McAuliffe, C. A., Masters, J. R., and Hill, B. T.: Factors influencing the sensitivity of two human bladder carcinoma cell lines to cis-diamminedichloroplatinum (II). Chem. Biol. Interact., 61:1, 1987.
37. Begleiter, A., Lam, H.-Y. P., Grover, J., Froese, E., and Goldenberg, G. J.: Evidence for active transport of melphalan by two amino acid carriers in L5178Y lymphoblasts *in vitro*. Cancer Res., 39:353, 1979.
38. Behrens, B. C., Hamilton, T. C., Masuda, H., Grotzinger, K. R., Whang-Peng, J., Louie, K. G., Knutsen, T., McKoy, W. M., and Young, R. C.: Characterization of a cis-diamminedichloroplatinum (II)-resistant human ovarian cancer cell line and its use in evaluation of platinum analogues. Cancer Res., 47:414, 1987.
39. Belt, R. J., Himmelstein, K. J., Patton, T. F., Bannister, S. J., Sternson, L.A., and Repta, A. J.: Pharmacokinetics of non-protein-bound platinum species following administration of cis-dichlorodiammineplatinum (II). Cancer Treat. Rep., 63:1515, 1979.
40. Benrubi, G. I., Norvell, M., Nuss, R. C., and Robinson, H.: The use of methylprednisolone and metoclopramide in control of emesis in patients receiving cis-platinum. Gynecol. Oncol., 21:306, 1985.
41. Berd, D., and Mastrangelo, M. J.: Active immunotherapy of human melanoma exploiting the immunopotentiating effects of cyclophosphamide. Cancer Invest., 6:337, 1988.
42. Berd, D., and Mastrangelo, M. J.: Effect of low dose cyclophosphamide on the immune system of cancer patients: depletion of CD4+, 2H4+ suppressor-inducer T-cells. Cancer Res., 48:1671, 1988.
43. Berry, J. M., Jacobs, C., Sikic, B., Halsey, J., and Borch, R. F.: Modification of cisplatin toxicity with diethyldithiocarbamate. J. Clin. Oncol., 8:1585, 1990.
44. Bethlenfalvay, N. C., and Bergin, J. J.: Severe cerebral toxicity after intravenous nitrogen mustard therapy. Cancer, 29:366, 1972.
45. Bier, H., Bergler, W., Mende, S., and Ganzer, U.: Glutathione content and gamma-glutamyltranspeptidase activity in squamous cell head and neck cancer xenografts. Arch. Otorhinolaryngol., 245:166, 1988.
46. Bierman, H. R., Kelly, K. H., Knudson, A. G., Jr., Maekawa, T., and Timmis, G. M.: The influence of 1,4-dimethylsulfonoxy-1,4-dimethylbutane (CB 2348, di-methyl Myleran) in neoplastic disease. Ann. N. Y. Acad. Sci., 68:1211, 1958.
47. Black, F. O., Myers, E. N., Schramm, V. L., Johnson, J., Sigler, B., Thearle, P. B., and Burns, D. S.: Cisplatin vestibular ototoxicity: Preliminary report. Laryngoscope, 92:1363, 1982.
48. Blake, D. B., Heller, R. H., Hsu, S. H., and Schacter, B. Z.: Return of fertility in a

patient with cyclophosphamide-induced azoospermia. Johns Hopkins Med. J., 139:20, 1976.

49. Blatter, E. E., Vollano, J. E., Krishnan, B. S., and Dabrowiak, J. C.: Interaction of the Antitumor Agents cis,cis,trans-Pt(NH3)C12(OH)2 and cis,cis,trans-Pt IV{(CH3)2CHNH2}2C12(OH)2 and their reduction products with PM2 DNA. D1. Biochemistry, 23:4817, 1984.
50. Blumenreich, M. S., Needles, B., Yagoda, A., Sogani, P., Grabstald, H., and Whitmore, W. F., Jr.: Intravesical cisplatin for superficial bladder tumors. Cancer, 50:863, 1982.
51. Boal, J. H., Williamson, M., Boyd, V. L., Ludeman, S. M., and Egan, W.: PNMR studies of the kinetics of bisalkylation by isophosphoramide mustard: Comparisons with phosphoramide mustard. J. Med. Chem., 32:1768, 1989.
52. Bode, U., Seif, S. M., and Levine, A. A.: Studies on the antidiuretic effect of cyclophosphamide: Vasopressin release and sodium excretion. Med. Pediatr. Oncol., 8:295, 1980.
53. Bodell, W. J., Tokuda, K., and Ludlum, D. B.: Differences in DNA alkylation products formed in sensitive and resistant human glioma cells treated with N-(2-chloroethyl)-N-nitrosurea. Cancer Res., 48:4489, 1988.
54. Bodenstein, D., and Goldin, A.: A comparison of the effects of various nitrogen mustard compounds on embryonic cells. J. Exp. Zool., 108:75, 1948.
55. Boheim, K., and Bichler, E.: Cisplatin-induced ototoxicity: audiometric findings and experimental cochlear pathology. Arch. Otorhinolaryngol., 242:1, 1985.
56. Bolton, M. G., Colvin, O. M., and Hilton, J.: Specificity of isozymes of murine hepatic glutathione S-transferase for the conjugation of glutathione with melphalan. Cancer Res., 51:2410, 1991.
57. Bonadonna, G., Valgussa, P., Santoro, A., Viviani, S., Bonfante, V., and Banfi, A.: Hodgkin's disease: The Milan Cancer Institute experience with MOPP and ABVD. Recent Results Cancer Res., 117:169, 1989.
58. Borison, H. L., Brand, E. D., and Orland, R. K.: Emetic action of nitrogen mustard (Mechlorethamine hydrochloride) in dogs and cats. Am. J. Physiol., 192:410, 1968.
59. Borowy-Borowski, H., Lipman, R., Chowdary, D., and Tomasz, M.: Duplex oligodeoxyribonucleotides cross-linked by mitomycin C at a single site: Synthesis, properties, and cross-link reversibility. Biochemistry, 29:2992, 1990.
60. Borowy-Borowski, H., Lipman, R., and Tomasz, M.: Recognition between mitomycin C and specific DNA sequences for cross-link formation. Biochemistry, 29:2999, 1990.
61. Brade, W. P., Herdrich, K., and Varini, M.: Ifosfamide—pharmacology, safety and therapeutic potential. Cancer Treat. Rev., 12:1, 1985.
62. Brandt, S. J., Peters, W. P., Atwater, S. K., Kurtzberg, J., Borowitz, M. J., Jones, R. B., Shpall, E. J., Bast, R. C., Jr., Gilbert, C. J., and Oette, D. H.: Effect of recombinant human granulocyte-macrophage colony-stimulating factor on hemotopoietic reconstitution after high-dose chemotherapy and autologous bone marrow transplantation. N. Engl. J. Med., 31:869, 1988.
63. Brent, T. P., Houghton, P. J., and Houghton, J. A.: 06-Alkylguanine-DNA alkyltransferase activity correlates with the therapeutic response of human rhabdomyosarcoma xenografts to 1-(2-chlorethyl)-3-(trans-4-methylcyclohexyl)-1-nitrosourea. Proc. Natl. Acad. Sci. U. S. A., 82:2985, 1985.
64. Brock, N.: The development of mesna for the inhibition of urotoxic side effects of cyclophosphamide, ifosfamide, and other oxazaphosphorine cytostatics. Recent Results Cancer Res., 74:270, 1980.
65. Brookes, P., and Lawley, P. D.: The reaction of mono- and difunctional alkylating agents with nucleic acids. Biochem. J., 80:486, 1961.
66. Brookes, P., and Lawley, P. D.: The action of alkylating agents on deoxyribonucleic acid in relation to biological effects of the alkylating agents. Exp. Cell Res., 9(Suppl.):512, 1963.
67. Bruck, W., Heise, E., and Friede, R. L.: Leukoencephalopathy after cisplatin therapy. Clin. Neuropathol., 8:263, 1989.
68. Buckner, C. D., Rudolph, R. H., Fefer, A., Clift, R. A., Epstein, R. B., Funk, D. D., Neiman, P. E., Slichter, S. J., Storb, R., and Thomas, E. D.: High dose cyclophosphamide therapy for malignant disease. Cancer, 29:357, 1972.
69. Busse, O., Aigner, K., and Wilimzig, H.: Peripheral nerve damage following isolated extremity perfusion with cis-platinum. Recent Results Cancer Res., 86:264, 1983.
70. Butler, A. L., Clapper, M. L., and Tew, K. D.: Glutathione S-transferase in nitrogen mustard-resistant and -sensitive cell lines. Mol. Pharmacol., 31:575, 1987.
71. Calabro, A., Singletary, S. E., Carrasco, C. H., and Legha, S. S.: Intraarterial infusion chemotherapy in regionally advanced malignant melanoma. J. Surg. Oncol., 43:239, 1990.
72. Calcutt, G., and Conners, T. A.: Tumor sulfhydryl levels and sensitivity to the nitrogen mustard merophan. Biochem. Pharmacol., 12:839, 1963.
73. Carden, P. A., Mitchell, S. L., Waters, K. D., Tiedemann, K., and Ekert, H.: Prevention of cyclophosphamide/cytarabine-induced emisis with ondansetron in children with leukemia. J. Clin. Oncol., 8:1531, 1990.
74. Cattaneo, M. T., Filipazzi, V., Piazza, E., Damiani, E., and Mancarella, G.: Transient blindness and seizure associated with cisplatin therapy. J. Cancer Res. Clin. Oncol., 114:528, 1988.
75. Chao, C. C., Lee, Y. L., and Lin-Chao, S.: Phenotypic reversion of cisplatin resistance in human cells accompanies reduced host cell reactivation of damaged plasmid. Biochem. Biophys. Res. Commun., 170:851, 1990.
76. Chary, K. K., Higby, D. J., Henderson, E. S., and Swinerton, K. D.: Phase I study of high-dose cis-dichlorodiammineplatinum (II) with forced diuresis. Cancer Treat. Rep., 61:367, 1977.
77. Chawla, S. P., Yap, B. S., Tenney, D. M., Bodey, G. P., and Benjamin, R. S.: Phase I study of weekly-administered iproplatin (cis-dichloro-trans-dithydroxy-bis-isopropylamine platin {chip, JM9}). Invest. New Drugs, 6:311, 1988.
78. Chiuten, D. F., Roseneweig, M., Von Hoff, D. D., and Muggia, F. M.: Clinical trials with hexitol derivatives in the U.S. Cancer, 47:442, 1981.
79. Choi, K. E., Ratain, M. J., Williams, S. F., Golick, J. A., Beschorner, J. C., Fullem, L. J., and Bitran, J. D.: Plasma pharmacokinetic of high-dose oral melphalan in patients treated with trialkylator chemotherapy and autologous bone marrow. Cancer Res., 49:1318, 1989.
80. Chu, G., and Berg, P.: DNA cross-linked by cisplatin: a new probe for the DNA repair defect in xeroderma pigmentosum. Mol. Biol. Med., 4:277, 1987.
81. Chu, G., and Chang, E.: Cisplatin-resistant cells express increased levels of a factor that recognizes damaged DNA. Proc. Natl. Acad. Sci. USA, 87:3324, 1990.
82. Ciaccio, P. J., Tew, K. D., and Lacreta, F. P.: The spontaneous and glutathione S-transferase mediated reaction of chlorambucil with glutathione. Cancer Commun., 2:279, 1990.
83. Clark, J. L., Barcewicz, P., Nava, H. R., Goodwin, P. S., and Douglass, H. O., Jr.: Adjuvant 5-FU and MeCCNU improves survival following curative gastrectomy for adenocarcinoma. Am. Surg., 56:423, 1990.
84. Clayman, D. A., Wolpert, S. M., and Heros, D. O.: Superselective arterial BCNU infusion in the treatment of patients with malignant giomas. AJNR, 10:767, 1989.
85. Codling, B. W., and Chakera, T. M.: Pulmonary fibrosis following therapy with melphalan for multiple myeloma. J. Clin. Pathol., 25:668, 1972.
86. Cohen, B. E., Egorin, M. J., Kohlhepp, E. A., Aisner, J., and Gutierrez, P. L.: Human plasma pharmacokinetics and urinary excretion of thiotepa and its metabolites. Cancer Treat. Rep., 70:859, 1986.
87. Cole, R. C., Myers, T. J., and Klatsky, A. U.: Pulmonary disease with chlorambucil therapy. Cancer, 41:455, 1978.
88. Colvin, M.: The comparative pharmacology of cyclophosphamide and ifosfamide. Semin. Oncol., 9:2, 1982.
89. Colvin, M., Brundrett, R. B., Cowens, W., Jardine, E., and Ludlum, D. B.: A chemical basis for the antitumor activity of chloroethylnitrosoureas. Biochem. Pharmacol., 25:695, 1976.
90. Colvin, M., and Chabner, B. A.: Alkylating agents. *In* Cancer Chemotherapy: Principles and Practice. Edited by B. A. Chabner, and J. M. Collins. J. B. Lippincott, Philadelphia, 1990, pp. 276-313.
91. Colvin, M., Russo, J. E., Hilton, J., Dulik, D. M., and Fenselau, C.: Enzymatic mechanisms of resistance to alkylating agents in tumor cells and normal tissues. *In* Advances in Enzyme Regulation, Vol. 27, 1988, pp. 211-221.
92. Cornwell, G. G., III, Pajak, T. F., and McIntyre, O. R.: Hypersensitivity reactions to i.v. melphalan during treatment of multiple myeloma: Cancer and Leukemia Group B experience. Cancer Treat. Rep., 63:399, 1979.
93. Cornwell, G. C., III, Pajak, T. F., McIntyre. O. R., Kochna, S., and Dosik, H.: Influence of renal failure on myelosuppressive effects of melphalan: Cancer and leukemia group B experience. Cancer Treat. Rep., 66:475, 1982.
94. Costa, G., Engle, R. L., Jr., Schilling, A., Carbone, P., Kochna, S., Nachman, R. L., and Glidewell, O.: Melphalan and prednisone: An effective combination for the treatment of multiple myeloma. Am. J. Med., 54:589, 1973.
95. Cox, P. J.: Cyclophosphamide cystitis—identification of acrolein as the causative agent. Biochem. Pharmacol., 28:2045, 1979.
96. Crathorne, A. R., and Roberts, J. J.: Mechanism of the cytotoxic action of alkylating agents in mammalian cells and evidence for the removal of alkylated groups from deoxynucleic acid. Nature, 211:150, 1966.
97. Creaven, P. J., Pendyala, L., and Madajewicz, S.: Clinical development of iproplatin (CHIP). Drugs Exp. Clin. Res., 12:287, 1986.
98. Curt, G. A., Kelley, J. A., Kufta, C. V., Smith, B. H., Kornblith, P. L., Young, R. C., and Collins, J. M.: Phase II and pharmacokinetic study of aziridinylbenzoquinone {2,5-diazirindinyl-3,6-bis(carboethoxyamino)-1,4-benzoquinone, diaziquone, NSC 182986} in high-grade gliomas. Cancer Res., 43:6102, 1983.
99. Dantzig, A. H., Fairgrieve, M., Slayman, C. W., and Adelberg, E. A.: Isolation and characterization of a CHO amino acid transport mutant resistant to melphalan (L-phenylalanine mustard). Somat. Cell Mol. Genet., 10:113, 1984.
100. Das, S. K., Lau, C. C., and Pardee, A. B.: Comparative analysis of caffeine and 3-aminobenzamide as DNA repair inhibitors in Syrian baby hamster kidney cells. Mutat. Res., 131:71, 1984.
101. DeConti, R. C., Toftness, B. A. U., Lange, R. C., and Creasey, W. A.: Clinical and pharmacological studies with cis-diamminedichloroplatinum (II). Cancer Res., 33:1310, 1973.
102. Dedon, P. C., and Borch, R. F.: Characterization of the reactions of platinum antitumor agents with biologic and nonbiologic sulfur-containing nucleophiles. Biochem. Pharmacol., 36:1955, 1987.
103. DeFronzo, R. A., Braine, H. G., Colvin, M., and Davis, P. J.: Water intoxication in man after cyclophosphamide therapy. Ann. Intern. Med., 78:861, 1973.
104. Dentino, M., Luft, F. C., Yum, M. N., Williams, S. D., and Einhorn, L. H.: Long term effect of cis-diamminedichloride platinum (CDDP) on renal function and structure in man. Cancer, 41:1274, 1978.
105. DeSimone, P. A., Yancey, R. S., Coupal, J. J., Butts, J. D., and Hoeschel, J. D.: Effect of a forced diuresis on the distribution and excretion (via urine and bile) of 195m platinum when given as 195m platinum cis-dichlorodiammineplatinum (II). Cancer Treat. Rep., 63:951, 1979.
106. DeVita, V. T., Carbone, P. P., Owens, A. H., Jr., Gold, G. L., Krant, M. J., and Edmonson, J.: Clinical trials with 1,3-bis(2-chloroethyl)-1-nitrosourea, NSC-409962. Cancer Res., 25:1876, 1965.
107. DeVita, V. T., Serpick, A. A., and Carbone, P. P.: Combination chemotherapy in the treatment of advanced Hodgkin's disease. Ann. Intern. Med., 73:881, 1970.
108. de Vries, E. G., Jeijer, C., Timmer-Bosscha, H., Berendsen, H. H., de Leij, L., Scheper, R. J., and Mulder, N. H.: Resistance mechanisms in three human small cell lung cancer cell lines established from one patient during clinical follow up. Cancer Res., 49:4175, 1989.
109. Dijt, F. J., Fichtinger-Schepman, A. M., Berends, F., and Reedijk, J.: Formation and repair of cisplatin-induced adducts to DNA in cultured normal and repair-deficient human fibroblasts. Cancer Res., 48:6058, 1988.
110. D'Incalci, M., Bolis, G., Facchinetti, T., Mangioni, C., Morasca, L., Morazzoni, P., and Salmona, M.: Decreased half-life of cyclophosphamide in patients under continual treatment. Eur. J. Cancer, 19:7, 1979.
111. Dorr, F. A., and Coltman, C. A., Jr.: Second cancers following antineoplastic therapy. Curr. Probl. Cancer, 9:1, 1985.
112. Dorr, R. T., Bowden, G. T., Alberts, D. S., and Liddil, J. D.: Interactions of mitomycin C with mammalian DNA detected by alkaline elution. Cancer Res., 45:3510, 1985.
113. Dray, S., and Mokyr, M. B.: Cyclophosphamide and melphalan as immunopotentiating agents in cancer therapy. Med. Oncol. Tumor Pharmacother., 6:77, 1989.
114. Dulik, D. M., Colvin, O. M., and Fenselau, C.: Characterization of glutathione conjugates of chlorambucil by fast atom bombardment and thermospray liquid chromatography/mass spectrometry. Biomed. Environ. Mass. Spectrom., 19:248, 1990.
115. Dulik, D. M., Fenselau, C., and Hilton, J.: Characterization of melphalan-glutathione adducts whose formation is catalysed by glutathione S-transferase. Biochem. Pharmacol., 35:3405, 1986.
116. Durie, B. G., Dixon, D. O., Carter, S., Stephens, R., Rivkin, S., Bonnet, J., Salmon,

S. E., Dabich, L., Files, J. C., and Costanzi, J. J.: Unimproved survival duration with combination chemotherapy induction for multiple myeloma: A Southwest Oncology Group Study. J. Clin. Oncol., 4:1227, 1986.

117. Dusre, L., Covey, J. M., Collins, C., and Sinha, B. K.: DNA damage, cytotoxicity and free radical formation by mitomycin in human cells. Chem. Biol. Interact., 71:63, 1989.

118. Eapen, L., Stewart, D., Danjoux, C., Genest, P., Futter, N., Moors, D., Irvine, A., Crook, J., Aitken, S., Gerig, L., Peterson, R., and Rasuli, P.: Intraarterial cisplatin and concurrent radiation for locally advanced bladder cancer. J. Clin. Oncol., 7:230, 1989.

119. Eastman, A.: Characterization of the adducts produced in DNA by cis-Diamminedichloroplatinum (II) and cis-Dichloro (ethylenediamine) platinum (II). Biochemistry, 22:3927, 1983.

120. Eastman, A.: Re-evaluation of interaction of cis-dichloro(ethylenediamine)platinum (II) with DNA. Biochemistry, 25:3912, 1986.

121. Eastman, A.: Cross-linking of glutathione to DNA by cancer chemotherapeutic platinum coordination complexes. Chem. Biol. Interact., 61:241, 1987.

122. Eder, J. P., Antman, K., Peters, W., Henner, W. D., Elias, A., Shea, T., Schryber, S., Anderson, J., Come, S., Schnipper, L., Frei, E., III, and Antman, K.: High-dose combination alkylating agent chemotherapy with autologous bone marrow support for metastatic breast cancer. J. Clin. Oncol., 4:1592, 1986.

123. Eder, J. P., Elias, A., Shea, T. C., Schryber, S. M., Teicher, B. A., Hunt, M., Burke, J., Siegel, R., Schnipper, L. E., Frei, E., III, and Antman, K.: A phase I-II study of cyclophosphamide, thiotepa, and carboplatin with autologous bone marrow transplantation in solid tumor patients. J. Clin. Oncol., 8:1239, 1990.

124. Eder, J. P., Teicher, B. A., Holden, S. A., Cathcart, K. N., and Schnipper, L. E.: Novobiocin enhances alkylating agent cytotoxicity and DNA interstrand crosslinks in a murine model. J. Clin. Invest., 79:11524, 1987.

125. Egorin, M. J., Forrest, A., Belani, C. P., Ratain, M. J., Abrams, J. S., and Van Echo, D. A.: A limited sampling strategy for cyclophosphamide pharmacokinetics. Cancer Res., 49:3129, 1989.

126. Egorin, M. J., and Snyder, S. W.: Characterization of nonexchangeable radioactivity in L1210 cells incubated with (14C) thiotepa: Labeling of phosphatidylethanolamine. Cancer Res., 50:4044, 1990.

126A. Egorin, M. J., Van Echo, D. A., Olman, E. A., Whitacre, M. Y., Forrest, A., and Aisner, J.: Prospective validation of a pharmacologically based dosing scheme for the cis-diamminedichloroplatinum (II) analogue. Cancer Res., 45:6502, 1985.

127. Einhorn, N.: Acute leukemia after chemotherapy (melphalan). Cancer, 41:444, 1978.

128. Einhorn, N., Eklund, G., and Lambert, B.: Solid tumours and chromosome aberrations as late side effects of melphalan therapy in ovarian carcinoma. Acta Oncol., 27:215, 1988.

129. Eisenberger, M., Hornedo, J., Silva, H., Donehower, R., Spaulding, M., and Van Echo, D.: Carboplatin (NSC-241-240): an active platinum analog for the treatment of squamous-cell carcinoma of the head and neck. J. Clin. Oncol., 4:1506, 1986.

130. Elderson, A., Gerritsen van der Hoop, R., Haanstra, W., Neijt, J. P., Gispen, W. H., and Jennekens, F. G.: Vibration perception and thermoperception as quantitative measurements in the monitoring of cisplatin induced neurotoxicity. J. Neurol. Sci., 93:167, 1989.

131. Elson, L. A.: Hematological effects of the alkylating agents. Ann. N. Y. Acad. Sci., 68:826, 1958.

132. Endresen, L., Schjerven, L., and Rugstad, H. E.: Tumours from a cell strain with a high content of metallothionein show enhanced resistance against cis-dichlorodiammineplatinum. Acta Pharmacol. Toxicol. (Copenh.), 55:183, 1984.

133. Erickson, L. C., Laurent, G., Sharkey, N. A., and Kohn, K. W.: DNA cross-linking and monoadduct repair in nitrosourea-treated human tumour cells. Nature, 288:727, 1980.

134. Erlichman, C., Soldins, S. J., Hardy, R. W., Thiessen, J. J., Sturgeon, J. F., Fine, S., and Baskerville, T.: Disposition of cyclophosphamide on two consecutive cycles of treatment in patients with ovarian carcinoma. Arzneim. -Forsch./Drug Res., 38:839, 1988.

135. Everett, J. C., Roberts, J. J., and Ross, W. C. J.: Aryl-2-halogenoalkylamines: Part XII. Some carboxylic derivatives of N,N-di-2-chloroethylaniline. J. Chem. Soc., 3:2386, 1953.

136. Ewig, R. A. G., and Kohn, K. W.: DNA damage and repair in mouse leukemia L1210 cells treated with nitrogen mustard. 1,3-bis(2-chloroethyl)-1-nitrosourea, and other nitrosoureas. Cancer Res., 37:2114, 1977.

137. Falletta, J. M., Cushing, B., Lauer, S., Bell, B., Mahoney, D. H., Castleberry, R., and Krance, R. A.: Phase I evaluation of diaziquone in childhood cancer. A Pediatric Oncology Group study. Invest. New Drugs, 8:167, 1990.

138. Farnworth, P. G., Hillcoat, B. L., and Roos, I. A.: Metallothionenin induction in mouse tissues by cis-dichlorodiammineplatinum (II) and its hydrolysis products. Chem. Biol. Interact., 69:319, 1989.

139. Feil, V. S., and Lamoureaux, C. J. H.: Alopecia activity of cyclophosphamide metabolites and related compounds in sheep. Cancer Res., 34:2596, 1974.

140. Fenselau, C., Kan, M. N., Rao, S. S., Myles, A., Friedman, O. M., and Colvin, M.: Identification of aldophosphamide as a metabolite of cyclophosphamide *in vitro* and *in vivo* in humans. Cancer Res., 37:2538, 1977.

141. Fetting, J. H., McCarthy, L. E., Borison, H. L., and Colvin, M.: Vomiting induced by cyclophosphamide and phosphoramide mustard in cats. Cancer Treat. Rep., 66:1625, 1982.

142. Fichtinger-Schepman, A. M. J., van der Veer, J. L., den Hartog, J. H. J., Lohman, P. H. M., and Reedijk, J.: Adducts of the antitumor drug cis-diamminedichloroplatinum (II) with DNA: Formation, identification, and quantitation. Biochemistry, 24:707, 1985.

143. Fiorentino, M. V., Daniele, O., Morandi, P., Aversa, S. M., Ghiotto, C., Paccagnella, A., and Fornasiero, A.: Intrapericardial instillation of platin in malignant pericardial effusion. Cancer, 62:1904, 1988.

144. Fisher, B., Sherman, B., Rockette, H., Redmond, C., Margolese, R., and Fisher, E. R.: L-phenylalanine mustard (L-PAM) in the management of premenopausal patients with primary breast cancer. Cancer, 44:847, 1979.

145. Fisher, R. I., and Erickson, L. C.: 1-beta-D-arabinofuranosylcytosine and hydroxyurea production of cytotoxic synergy with cis-diamminedichloroplatinum (II) and modification of platinum-induced DNA interstrand cross-linking. Cancer Res., 49:1383, 1989.

146. Flaherty, L. E., Redman, B. G., Chabot, G. G., Martino, S., Gualdoni, S. M., Heilbrun, L. K., Valdivieso, M., and Bradley, E. C.: A phase I-II study of dacarbazine in combination with outpatient interleukin-2 in metastatic malignant melanoma. Cancer, 65:2471, 1990.

147. Follezou, J. Y., Fauchon, F., and Chiras, J.: Intraarterial infusion of carboplatin in the treatment of malignant gliomas: A phase II study. Neoplasma, 36:349, 1989.

148. Forni, A. M., Koss, L. G., and Geller, W.: Cytological study of the effect of cyclophosphamide on the epithelium of the urinary bladder in man. Cancer, 17:1348, 1964.

149. Foster, B. J., Clagett-Carr, K., Leyland-Jones, B., and Hoth, C.: Results of NCI-sponsored phase I trials with carboplatin. Cancer Treat. Rev., Suppl. A-43, 1985.

149A. Foster, B. J., Harding, B. J., Wolpert-DeFilippes, M. K., Rubinstein, L. Y., Clagett-Carr, K., and Leyland-Jones, B.: A strategy for the development of two clinically active cisplatin analogs: CBDCA and CHIP. Cancer Chemother. Pharmacol., 25:395, 1990.

150. Fram, R. J., Woda, B. A., Wilson, J. M., and Robichaud, N.: Characterization of acquired resistance to cis-diamminedichloroplatinum (II) in BE human colon carcinoma cells. Cancer Res., 50:72, 1990.

151. Fravel, H. N., and Roberts, J. J.: Excision repair of cis-diamminedichloroplatinum (II)-induced damage to DNA of Chinese hamster cells. Cancer Res., 39:1793, 1979.

152. The French Cooperative Group on Chronic Lymphocytic Leukemia: A randomized clinical trial or chlorambucil versus COP in stage chronic lymphocytic leukemia. Blood, 75:1422, 1990.

153. Frick, J. C., Tretter, P., Tretter, W., and Hyman, G. A.: Disseminated carcinoma of the ovary treated by L-phenylalanine mustard. Cancer, 21:508, 1968.

154. Fried, W., Kede, A., and Barone, J.: Effects of cyclophosphamide and busulfan on spleen-colony-forming units and on hematopoietic stroma. Cancer Res., 37:1205, 1977.

155. Friedman, H. S., Colvin, O. M., Aisaka, K., Popp, J., Bossen, E. H., Reimer, K. A., Powell, J. B., Hilton, J., Gross, S. S., Levi, R., Bigner, D. D., and Griffith, O. W.: Glutathione protects cardiac and skeletal muscle from cyclophosphamide-induced toxicity. Cancer Res., 50:2455, 1990.

156. Friedman, H. S., Colvin, O. M., Griffith, O. W., Lippitz, B., Elion, G. B., Schold, S. C., Jr., Hilton, J., and Bigner, D. D.: Increased melphalan activity in intracranial human medulloblastoma and glioma xenografts following buthionine sulfoximine-mediated glutathione depletion. J. Natl. Cancer Inst., 81:524, 1989.

157. Frustaci, S., Barzan, L., Comoretto, R., Tumolo, S., LoRe, G., and Monfardini, S.: Local neurotoxicity after intra-arterial cisplatin in head and neck cancer. Cancer Treat. Rep., 71:257, 1987.

158. Galton, D.: Myleran in chronic myeloid leukaemia. Lancet, 1:208, 1953.

159. Galton, D. A. G., Till, M., and Wiltshaw, E.: Busulfan (1,4-dimethyl-sulfonoxy-butane, Myleran): Summary of clinical results. Ann. N. Y. Acad. Sci., 68:967, 1958.

160. Ganci, L., and Serrou, B.: Changes in hair pigmentation associated with cancer chemotherapy. Cancer Treat. Rep., 64:193, 1980.

161. Garrett, M. J.: Teratogenic effects of combination chemotherapy. Ann. Intern. Med., 80:667, 1974.

162. Gerard, A., Metzger, U., and Buyse, M.: Adjuvant therapy in colorectal cancer. Anticancer Res., 9:1033, 1989.

163. Not used.

164. Gez, E., Ben Yosef, R., Catane, R., Brufman, G., and Biran, S.: Chlorpromazine and dexamethasone versus high-dose metoclopramide and dexamethasone in patients receiving cancer chemotherapy, particularly cis-platinum: A prospective randomized crossover study. Oncology, 46:150, 1989.

165. Gez, E., Sulkes, A., Ochayon, L., Gera, C., Nathan, S., Cass, Y., Rubello, E., and Biran, S.: Methylprednisolone versus metochlopramide as antiemetic treatment in patients receiving adjuvant cyclophosphamide, methotrexate, 5-fluorouracil (CMF) chemotherapy: A randomized crossover blind study. J. Chemother., 1:365, 1989.

166. Gianni, A. M., Bregni, M., Siena, S., Orazi, A., Stern, A. C., Gandola, L., and Bonadonna, G.: Recombinant human granulocyte-macrophage colony-stimulating factor reduces hematologic toxicity and widens clinical applicability of high-dose cyclophosphamide treatment in breast cancer and non-Hodgkin's lymphoma. J. Clin. Oncol., 8:768, 1990.

167. Gibson, J. E., and Becker, B. A.: Teratogenicity of structural truncates of cyclophosphamide in mice. Teratology, 4:141, 1971.

168. Goel, R., Andrews, P. A., Pfeifle, C. E., Abramson, I. S., Kirmani, S., and Howell, S. B.: Comparison of the pharmacokinetics of ultrafilterable cisplatin species detectable by derivatization with diethyldithiocarbamate or atomic absorption spectroscopy. Eur. J. Cancer, 26:21, 1990.

169. Goldenberg, A. S., Kelsen, D., Dougherty, J., and Magill, G.: Phase II study of CHIP chemotherapy in advanced adenocarcinomas of the upper gastrointestinal tract. Invest. New Drugs, 8:71, 1990.

170. Goldenberg, G. J., Lee, M., Lam, H.-Y. P., and Begleiter, A.: Evidence for carrier-mediated transport of melphalan by L5178Y lymphoblasts *in vitro*. Cancer Res., 37:755, 1977.

171. Goldenberg, G. J., Vanstone, C. L., Israels, L. G., Iise, D., and Bihler, I.: Evidence for a transport carrier of nitrogen mustard in nitrogen mustard-sensitive and -resistant L51784 lymphoblasts. Cancer Res., 30:2285, 1970.

172. Galton, D. A. G., Israels, L. S., Nabarro, J. D. N., and Till, M.: Clinical trials of p-(di-2-chlorethylamino)-phenylbutyric acid (CB 1348) in malignant lymphoma. Br. Med. J., 2:172, 1955.

173. Gonzales-Vitale, J. C., Hayes, D. M., Cvitkovic, E., and Sternberg, S. S.: The renal pathology in clinical trials of cis-platinum (II) diamminedichloride. Cancer, 39:1362, 1977.

174. Goodman, L. S., Wintrobe, M. M., Dameshek, W., Goodman, J. J., Gilman, A., and McLennan, M. T.: Use of methyl-bis(beta-chlorethyl)amine hydrochloride for Hodgkin's disease, lymphosarcoma, leukemia. J.A.M.A., 132:263, 1946.

175. Goren, M. P., Wright, R. K., Pratt, C. B., and Pell, F. E.: Dechlorethylation of ifosfamide and neurotoxicity. Lancet, 2:1219, 1986.

176. Gottlieb, J. A., and Drewinko, B.: Review of the current clinical status of platinum coordination complexes in cancer chemotherapy. Cancer Chemother. Rep., 59:621, 1975.

177. Gralla, R. J., Itri, L. M., Pisko, S. E., Squillante, A. E., Kelsen, D. P., Braun, D. W., Jr., Bordin, L. A., Braun, T. J., and Young, C. W.: Antiemetic efficacy of high-dose metoclopramide: Randomized trials with placebo and prochlorperazine in patients with chemotherapy-induced nausea and vomiting. N. Engl. J. Med., 305:905, 1981.

178. Granowetter, L., Rosenstock, J. G., and Packer, R. J.: Enhanced cis-platinum neurotoxicity in pediatric patients with brain tumors. J. Neurooncol., 1:293, 1983.

179. Green, T. P., and Mirkin, B. L.: Prevention of cyclophosphamide-induced antidiuresis by furosemide infusion. Clin. Pharmacol. Ther., 29:634, 1981.
180. Green, M. H., Harris, E. L., Gershenson, D. M., Malkasian, G. D. Jr., Melton, L. J., III, Dembo, A. J., Bennett, J. M., Moloney, W. C., and Boice, J. D., Jr.: Melphalan may be a more potent leukemogen than cyclophosphamide. Ann. Intern. Med., 105:360, 1986.
181. Greenspan, E. M.: Thio-TEPA and methotrexate chemotherapy of advanced ovarian carcinoma. J. Mount Sinai Hosp. N. Y., 35:52, 1968.
182. Greig, N. H., Momma, S., Sweeney, D. J., Smith, Q. R., and Rapoport, S. I.: Facilitated transport of melphalan at the rat blood-brain barrier by the large neutral amino acid carrier system. Cancer Res., 47:1571, 1987.
183. Grochow, L. B., Jones, R. J., Brundrett, B. R., Braine, H. G., Chen, T. L., Saral, R., Santos, G. W., and Colvin, O. M.: Pharmacokinetics of busulfan: correlation with veno-occulusive disease in patients undergoing bone marrow transplantation. Cancer Chemother. Pharmacol., 25:55, 1989.
184. Grochow, L. B., Krivit, W., Whitley, C. B., and Blazar, B.: Busulfan disposition in children. Blood, 75:1723, 1990.
185. Grunberg, S. M.: Advances in the management of nausea and vomiting induced by non-cisplatin containing chemotherapeutic regimens. Blood Rev., 3:216, 1989.
186. Grunberg, S. M., Sonka, S., Stevenson, L. L., and Muggia, F. M.: Progressive paresthesias after cessation of therapy with very high-dose cisplatin. Cancer Chemother. Pharmacol., 25:62, 1989.
187. Gutierrez, P. L.: Mechanism(s) of bioreductive activation. The example of diaziquone (AZQ) Free Radic. Biol. Med., 6:405, 1989.
188. Gutin, P. H., Levi, J. A., Wiernik, P. H., and Walker, M. D.: Treatment of malignant meningeal disease with intrathecal thioTEPA: A phase II study. Cancer Treat. Rep., 61:885, 1977.
189. Haas, C. D., Stephens, R. C., Hollister, M., and Hoogstraten, B.: Phase I evaluation of dianhydrogalactitol (NSC-132313). Cancer Treat. Rep., 60:611, 1976.
190. Haddow, A., and Timmis, G. M.: Myeleran in chronic myeloid leukemia—chemical constitution and biological action. Lancet, 1:207, 1953.
191. Hadjilaskari, P., Fengler, R., Hartmann, R., and Henze, G.: Ototoxicity of cisplatin in children with malignant diseases. Klin. Padiatr., 201:316, 1989.
191A. Hagen, B.: Pharmacokinetics of thio-TEPA and TEPA in the conventional dose-range and its correlation to myelosuppressive effects. Cancer Chemother. Pharmacol., 27:373, 1991.
191B. Hagen, B., Neverdal, G., Walstad, R. A., and Nilsen, O. G.: Long-term pharmacokinetics of thio-TEPA, TEPA and total alkylating activity following i. v. bolus administration of thio-TEPA in ovarian cancer patients. Cancer Chemother. Pharmacol., 25:257, 1990.
192. Hales, B. F.: Effects of phosphoramide mustard and acrotein, cytotoxic metabolites of cyclophosphamide, on mouse limb development *in vitro*. Teratology, 40:11, 1989.
193. Hamilton, T. C., Winker, M. A., Louie, K. G., Batist, G., Behrens, B. C., Tsuruo, T., Grotzinger, K. R., McKoy, W. M., Young, R. C., and Ozols, R. F.: Augmentation of adriamycin, melphalan, and cisplatin cytotoxicity in drug-resistant and sensitive human ovarian carcinoma cell lines by buthionine sulfoximine mediated glutathione depletion. Biochem. Pharmacol., 34:2583, 1985.
194. Han, T., and Rai, K. R.: Management of chronic lymphocytic leukemia. Hematol. Oncol. Clin. North Am., 4:431, 1990.
195. Hansen, S. W., Helweg-Larsen, S., and Trojaborg, W.: Long-term neurotoxicity in patients treated with cisplatin, vinblastine, and bleomycin for metastatic germ cell cancer. J. Clin. Oncol., 7:1457, 1989.
196. Hansson, J., and Wood, R. D.: Repair synthesis by human cell extracts in DNA damaged by cis- and trans-diamminedichloroplatinum (II). Nucleic Acids Res., 117:8073, 1989.
197. Harding, M., Kennedy, R., Mill, L., MacLean, A., Duncan, I., Kennedy, J., Soukop, M., and Kaye, S. B.: A pilot study of carboplatin (JM8, CBDCA) and chlorambucil in combination for advanced ovarian cancer. Br. J. Cancer, 58:640, 1988.
198. Harlow, P. J., DeClerck, Y. A., Shore, N. A., Ortega, J. A., Carraza, A., and Heuser, E.: A fatal case of inappropriate ADH secretion induced by cyclophosphamide therapy. Cancer, 44:896, 1979.
199. Harmon, W. E., Cohen, H. J., Schneeberger, E. E., and Grupe, W. E.: Chronic renal failure in children treated with methyl CCNU. N. Engl. J. Med., 300:1200, 1979.
200. Hartley, F. R.: The Chemistry of Platinum and Palladium, Chapter 11. New York, Wiley Press, 1973.
201. Hartley-Asp, B., Christensson, P. I., Gunnarsson, K., Gunnarsson, P. O., Jensen, G., Polacek, J., and Stamvik, A.: Anti-tumour, toxicological and pharmacokinetic properties of a novel taurine-based nitrosourea (TCNU). Invest. New Drugs, 6:19, 1988.
202. Hartvig, P., Simonsson, B., Oberg, G., Wallin, I., and Ehrsson, H.: Inter- and intraindividual differences in oral chlorambucil pharmacokinetics. Eur. J. Clin. Pharmacol., 35:551, 1988.
203. Hassan, M., Oberg, G., Ehrsson, H., Ehrnebo, M., Wallin, I., Smedmyr, B., Toherman, T., Eksborg, S., and Simonsson, B.: Pharmacokinetic and metabolic studies of high-dose busulfan in adults. Eur. J. Clin. Pharmacol., 36:525, 1989.
204. Hawthorn, J., Ostler, K. J., and Andrews, P. L.: The role of the abdominal visceral innervation and 5-hydroxytryptamine M-receptors in vomiting induced by the cytotoxic drugs cyclophosphamide and cis-platin in the ferret. Q. J. Exp. Physiol., 73:7, 1988.
205. Hayes, D. M., Cvitkovic, E., Golbey, R. B., Scheiner, E., Helson, L., and Krakoff, I. H.: High-dose cis-platinum diammine dichloride: amelioration of renal toxicity by mannitol diuresis. Cancer, 39:1372, 1977.
205A. Heideman, R. L., Cole, D. E., Balis, F., Sato, J., Reaman, G. H., Packer, R. J., Singher, L. J., Ettinger, L. J., Gillespie, A., Sam, J., and Poplack, D. G.: Phase I and pharmacokinetic evaluation of thiotepa in the cerebrospinal fluid and plasma of pediatric patients: evidence for dose-dependent plasma clearance of thiotepa. Cancer Res., 49:736, 1989.
206. Heiger-Bernays, W. J., Essigmann, J. M., and Lippard, S. J.: Effect of the antitumor drug cis-diamminedichloroplatinum (II) and related platinum complexes on eukaryotic DNA replication. Biochemistry, 29:8461, 1990.
207. Hektoen, L., and Corper, H. J.: The effect of mustard gas (dichloroethyl-sulphide) on antibody formation. J. Infect. Dis., 28:279, 1921.
208. Henner, W. D., Peters, W. P., Eder, J. P., Antman, K., Snipper, L., and Frei, E., III: Pharmacokinetics and immediate effects of high-dose carmustine in man. Cancer Treat. Rep., 70:877, 1986.
209. Henner, W. D., Shea, T. C., Furlong, E. A., Flaherty, M. D., Eder, J. P., Elias, A., Begg, C., and Antman, K.: Pharmacokinetics of continuous-infusion high-dose thiotepa. Cancer Treat. Rep., 71:1043, 1987.
210. Higby, D. J., Wallace, H. J., Jr., Albert, D. J., and Holland, J. F.: Diaminodichloroplatinum: A phase I study showing responses in testicular and other tumors. Cancer, 33:1219, 1974.
211. Higby, D. J., Wallace, H. J., Jr., and Holland, J. F.: Cis-diamminedichloroplatinum (NSC-119875): A phase I study. Cancer Chemother. Rep., 57:459, 1973.
212. Higgins, G. A., Kilpatrick, G. J., Bunce, K. T., Jones, B. J., and Tyers, M. B.: 5-HT3 receptor antagonists injected into the area postrema inhibit cisplatin-induced emesis in the ferret. Br. J. Pharmacol., 97:247, 1989.
213. Hill, D. L., Kirk, M. C., and Struck, R. F.: Microsomal metabolism of nitrosoureas. Cancer Res., 35:296, 1975.
214. Hilton, J.: Role of aldehyde dehydrogenase in cyclophosphamide-resistant L1210 leukemia. Cancer Res., 44:5156, 1984.
215. Himmelstein, K. J., Patton, T. F., Belt, R. J., Taylor, S., Repta, A. J., and Sternson, L. A.: Clinical kinetics on intact cisplatin and some related species. Clin. Pharmacol. Ther., 29:658, 1981.
216. Hinkes, E., and Plotkin, D.: Reversible drug-induced sterility in a patient with acute leukemia. J.A.M.A., 223:1490, 1973.
217. Hochberg, M. C., and Shulman, L. E.: Acute leukemia following cyclophosphamide therapy for Sjogren's syndrome. Johns Hopkins Med. J., 142:211, 1978.
218. Holoye, P. Y., Jenkins, D. E., and Greenberg, S. D.: Pulmonary toxicity in long-term administration of BCNU. Cancer Treat. Rep., 60:1691, 1976.
219. Horn, Y., Eidelman, A., Walach, N., Waron, M., and Barak, F.: Intravesical chemotherapy of superficial bladder tumors in a controlled trial with cis-platinum versus cis-platinum versus cis-platinum plus hyaluronidase. J. Surg. Oncol., 28:304, 1985.
220. Hospers, G. A., Meijer, C., de Leij, L., Uges, D. R., Mulder, N. H., and de Vries, E. G.: A study of human small-cell lung carcinoma (hSCLC) cell lines with different sensitivities to detect relevant mechanisms of cisplatin (CDDP) resistance. Int. J. Cancer, 46:138, 1990.
221. Hospers, G. A., Mulder, N. H., de Jong, B., de Ley, L., Uges, D. R., Fichtinger-Schepman, A. M., Scheper, R. J., and De Vries, E. G.: Characterization of a human small cell lung carcinoma cell line with acquired resistance to cis-diamminedichloroplatinum (II) *in vitro*. Cancer Res., 48:6803, 1988.
222. Howell, S. B.: Intraperitoneal chemotherapy: The use of concurrent systemic neutralizing agents. Semin. Oncol., 12:17, 1985.
223. Hromas, R. A., Andrews, P. A., Murphy, M. P., and Burns, C. P.: Glutathione depletion reverses cisplatin resistance in murine L1210 leukemia cells. Cancer Lett., 34:9, 1987.
224. Hromas, R. A., North, J. A., and Burns, C. P.: Decreased cisplatin uptake by resistant L1210 leukemia cells. Cancer Lett., 36:197, 1987.
225. Humphrey, R. L., and Kvols, L. K.: The influence of renal insufficiency on cyclophosphamide-induced hematopoietic depression and recovery. Proc. Am. Assoc. Cancer Res., 15:84, 1974.
226. Husain, I., Chaney, S. G., and Sancar, A.: Repair of cis-platinum-DNA adducts by ABC excinuclease *in vivo* and *in vitro*. J. Bacteriol., 163:817, 1985.
227. Hyde, K. A., Acton, E., Skinner, W. A., Goodman, L., Greenberg, J., and Baker, B. R.: Potential anticancer agents-LX11. The relationship of chemical structure to antileukemia activity with analogues of 1-methyl-3-nitro-1-nitrosoguanidine (NSC-9369). II. J. Med. Pharmaceutical. Chem., 5:1, 1962.
228. Ishikawa, M., Sasaki, K., and Takayanagi, Y.: Injurious effect of buthionine sulfoximine, an inhibitor of glutathione biosynthesis, on the lethality and urotoxicity of cyclophosphamide in mice. Jpn. J. Pharmacol., 51:146, 1989.
229. Iyer, V. N., and Szybalski, W.: Mitomycin and porfiromycin: Chemical mechanisms of activation and cross-linking of DNA. Science, 145:551, 1964.
230. Jackson, D. V., Jr., Craig, J. B., Spurr, C. L., White, D. R., Muss, H. B., Cruz, J. M., Richards, F., and Powell, B. L.: Vincristine infusion with CHOP-CCNU in diffuse large-cell lymphoma. Cancer Invest., 8:7, 1990.
231. Jacobs, S. C., and Menashe, D. S.: Intraarterial chemotherapy for bladder cancer. Prog. Clin. Biol. Res., 350:101, 1990.
232. Jacobson, L. P., Spurr, C. L., Barron, E. S. G., Smith, T., Lushbaugh, C., and Dick, G. F.: Studies on the effect of methyl-bis(beta-chloroethyl)amine hydrochloride on neoplastic diseases and allied disorders of the hemapoietic system. J.A.M.A., 132:263, 1946.
233. Jacquillat, C., Khayat, D., Banzet, P., Weil, M., Avril, M. F., Fumoleau, P., Namer, M., Bonneterre, J., Kerbrat, P., Bonerandi, J. J., Bugat, R., Monteuquet, P., Audhuy, B., Cupissol, D., Lauvin, R., Grosshans, E., Vilmer, C., Prache, C., and Bizzari, J. P.: Chemotherapy by fotemustine in cerebral metastases of disseminated malignant melanoma. Cancer Chemother. Pharmacol., 25:263, 1990.
234. Jaffe, N., Raymond, A. K., Ayala, A., Carrasco, C. H., Wallace, S., Robertson, R., Giffiths, M., and Wang, Y. M.: Effect of cumulative courses of intraarterial cis-diamminedichloroplatin-II on the primary tumor in osteosarcoma. Cancer, 63:63, 1989.
235. Jahde, E., Glusenkamp, K. H., and Rajewsky, M. F.: Protection of cultured malignant cells from mitoxantrone cytotoxicity by low extracellular pH: A possible mechanism for chemoresistance *in vivo*. Eur. J. Cancer, 26:101, 1990.
236. Jao, J. Y., Jusko, W. J., and Cohen, J. L.: Phenobarbital effects on cyclophosphamide pharmacokinetics in man. Cancer Res., 32:2761, 1972.
237. Japan Radiation—ACNU Study Group: A randomized prospective study of radiation versus radiation versus plus ACNU Study Group. Cancer, 63:249, 1989.
238. Jardine, I., Fenselau, C., Appler, M., Kan, M.-N., Brundrett, R. B., and Colvin, M.: Quantitation by gas chromatography-chemical ionization mass spectrometry of cyclophosphamide, phosphamide mustard, and nornitrogen mustard in the plasma and urine of patients receiving cyclophosphamide therapy. Cancer Res., 38:408, 1978.
239. Jones, R. J., Lee, K. S., Beschorner, W. E., Vogel, V. G., Grochow, L. B., Braine, H. G., Vogelsang, G. B., Sensenbrenner, L. L., Santos, G. W., and Saral, R.: Venoocclusive disease of the liver following bone marrow transplantation. Transplantation, 44:778, 1987.
240. Juma, F. D., Rogers, H. J., and Trounce, J. R.: Pharmacokinetics of cyclophosphamide and alkylating activity in man after intravenous and oral administration. Br. J. Clin. Pharmacol., 8:209, 1979.
241. Juma, F. D., Rogers, H. J., and Trounce, J. R.: The pharmacokinetics of cyclophosphamide, phosphoramide mustard and nor-nitrogen mustard studied by gas chro-

matography in patients receiving cyclophosphamide therapy. Br. J. Clin. Pharmacol., 10:327, 1980.

242. Kahn, T., Elias, E. G., and Mason, G. R.: A single dose of metoclopramide in the control of vomiting from cis-dichlorodiammineplatinum (II) in man. Cancer Treat. Rep., 62:1106, 1978.
243. Kaleagasioglu, F., Berger, M. R., Schmahl, D., and Elsenbrand, G.: In vitro evaluation of 1-(2-chloroethyl)-1-nitroso-3-(2-hydroxyethyl) urea linked to 4-acetoxy-bisdes-methyltamoxifen, estradiol and dihydrotestosterone. Arzneimitteiforschung, 40:603, 1990.
244. Karchmer, R. K., and Hansen, B. L.: Possible anaphylactic reaction to intravenous cyclophosphamide. J.A.M.A., 237:475, 1977.
245. Kashdan, B. J., Sullivan, K. L., Lackman, R. D., Shapiro, M. J., Bonn, J., Weiss, A. J., and Gardiner, G. A., Jr.: Extremity osteosarcomas: intraarterial chemotherapy and limb-sparing resection with 2-year follow up. Radiology, 177:95, 1990.
246. Kashimura, M., Kondo, M., Abe, T., Shinohara, M., and Baba, S.: A case report of acute renal failure induced by melphalan in a patient with ovarian cancer. Gan. No. Rinsho., 34:2015, 1986.
247. Kasugai, H., Kojima, J., Tatsuta, M., Okuda, S., Sasaki, Y., Imaoka, S., Fujita, M., and Ishiguro, S.: Treatment of hepatocellular carcinoma by transcatheter arterial cisplatin and ethiodized oil. Gastroenterology, 97:965, 1989.
248. Katz, E. J., Andrews, P. A., and Howell, S. B.: The effect of DNA polymerase inhibitors on the cytoxicity of cisplatin in human ovarian carcinoma cells. Cancer Commun., 2:159, 1990.
249. Kelley, S. L., Basu, A., Teicher, B. A., Hacker, M. P., Hamer, D. H., and Lazo, J. S.: Overexpression of metallothionein confers resistance to anticancer drugs. Science, 241:1813, 1988.
250. Kennedy, K. A., McGuirl, J. D., Leondaridis, L., and Alabaster, O.: pH dependence of mitomycin C-induced cross-linking activity in tumor cells. Cancer Res., 45:3541, 1985.
251. Khan, A. S., and Driscoll, J. S.: Potential central nervous system antitumor agents. J. Med. Chem., 19:313, 1976.
252. Kim, H. C., Kesarwala, H. H., Colvin, M., and Saidi, P.: Hypersensitivity reaction to a metabolite of cyclophosphamide. J. Allergy Clin. Immunol., 76:591, 1985.
253. Kirkwood, J. M., Ernstoff, M. S., Giuliano, A., Gams, R., Robinson, W. A., Costanzi, J., Pouillart, P., Speyer, J., Grimm, M., and Spiegel, R.: Interferon alpha-2a and dacarbazine in melanoma. J. Natl. Cancer Inst., 82:1062, 1990.
254. Kleinerman, E. S., and Zwelling, L. A.: The effect of cis-diamminedichloroplatinum (II) on immune function in vitro and in vivo. Cancer Res., 40:3099, 1980.
255. Knox, R. J., Friedlos, F., Lydall, D. A., and Roberts, J. J.: Mechanism of cytotoxicity of anticancer platinum drugs: Evidence that cis-diamminedichloroplatinum (II) and cis-diammine-(1,1-cyclobutanedicarboxylato) platinum (II) differ only in the kinetics of their interaction with DNA. Cancer Res., 46:1972, 1986.
256. Koelling, T. M., Yeager, A. M., Hilton, J., Haynie, D. T., and Wiley, J. M.: Development and characterization of a cyclophosphamide-resistant subline of acute myeloid leukemia in the Lewis and Brown Norway hybrid rat. Blood, 76:1209, 1990.
257. Kohn, K. W.: Interstrand cross-linking of DNA by 1,3-bis(2-chloroethyl)-1-nitrosourea and other 1-(2-chloroethyl)-1-nitrosourea and other 1-(2-haloethyl)-1-nitrosoureas. Cancer Res., 37:1450, 1977.
258. Kohn, K. W., Steigbigel, N. H., and Spears, C. L.: Cross-linking and repair of DNA in sensitive and resistant strains of E. coli treated with nitrogen mustard. Proc. Natl. Acad. Sci., U. S. A., 53:1154, 1965.
259. Kohn, S., Fradis, M., Pratt, H., Zidan, J., Podoshin, L., Robinson, E., and Nir, I.: Cisplatin ototoxicity in guinea pigs with special reference to toxic effects in the stria vascularis. Larynogoscope, 98:665, 1988.
260. Kovach, J. S., Moertel, C. G., Schutt, A. J., Reitemeier, R. G., and Hahn, R. G.: Phase II study of cis-diamminedichloroplatinum (NSC-119875) in advanced carcinoma of the large bowel. Cancer Chemother. Rep., 57:357, 1973.
261. Kraker, A., Schmidt, J., Krezoski, S., and Petering, D. H.: Binding of cis-dichloro-diammine platinum (II) to metallothionein in Ehrlich cells. Biochem. Biophys. Res. Commun., 130:786, 1985.
262. Kraker, A. J., and Moore, C. W.: Elevated DNA polymerase beta activity in a cis-diamminedichloroplatinum (II) resistant P388 murine leukemia cell line. Cancer Lett., 38:307, 1988.
263. Kramer, R. A., Greene, K., Ahmad, S., and Vistica, D. T.: Chemosensitization of L-phenylalaline mustard by the thiol-modulating agent buthionine sulfoximine. Cancer Res., 47:1593, 1987.
264. Kretschmar, C. S., Warren, M. P., Lavally, B. L., Dyer, S., and Tarbell N. J.: Ototoxicity of preradiation cisplatin for children with central nervous system tumors. J. Clin. Oncol., 8:1191, 1990.
265. Krouwer, D., McDermott, M., and Prados, M.: Postoperative radiotherapy and radiotherapy combined with CCNU chemotherapy for treatment of brain gliomas. J. Neurooncol., 8:189, 1990.
266. Kyle, R. A., Pierce, R. V., and Bayrd, E. D.: Multiple myeloma and acute myelomonocytic leukemia. N. Engl. J. Med., 283:1121, 1970.
267. Kyoma, H., Wada, T., Nishizawa, T., Iwanaga, T., and Aoki, Y.: Cyclophosphamide induced ovarian failure and its therapeutic significance in patients with breast cancer. Cancer, 39:1403, 1977.
268. Lakin, J. D., and Cahill, R. A.: Generalized urticaria to cyclophosphamide: Type I hypersensitivity to an immunosuppressive agent. J. Allergy Clin. Immunol., 58:160, 1976.
269. Lange, R. C., Spencer, R. P., and Harder, H. C.: The antitumor agent cis-P + $(NH_3)_2Cl_2$ distribution studies and dose calculations for 193m Pt. J. Nucl. Med., 14:191, 1973.
270. Laros, R. K., Jr., and Penner, J. A.: "Refractory" thrombocytopenic purpura treated successfully with cyclophosphamide. J.A.M.A., 215:445, 1971.
271. Lee, F. Y., Workman, P., Roberts J. T., and Bleehen, N. M.: Clinical pharmacokinetics of oral CCNU (lomustine). Cancer Chemother. Pharmacol., 14:125, 1985.
272. Lefkowitz, I. B., Packer, R. J., Sielgel, K. R., Sutton, L. N., Schut, L., and Evans, A. E.: Results of treatment of children with recurrent medulloblastoma/primitive neuroectodermal tumors with lomustine, cisplatin, and vincristine. Cancer, 65:412, 1990.
273. Lehane, D. E., Bryan, R. N., Horowitz, B., DeSantos, L., Ehni, G., Zubler, M. A., Moiel, R., Rudolph, L., Aldama-Leubbert, A., Mahoney, D., and Harper, R.: Intraarterial cisplatinum chemotherapy for patients with primary and metastatic brain tumors. Cancer Drug Deliv., 1:69, 1983.
274. Lennard, A. L., Carey, P. J., Jackson, G. H., and Proctor, S. J.: An effective oral combination in advanced relapsed Hodgkin's disease prednisolone, etoposide, chlorambucil and CCNU. Cancer Chemother. Pharmacol., 26:301, 1990.
275. Lergier, J. E., Jiminez, E., Maldonado, N., and Veray, F.: Normal pregnancy in multiple myeloma treated with cyclophosphamide. Cancer, 34:1018, 1974.
276. Levin, V. A., Chamberlain, M., Silver, P., Rodriguez, L., and Prados, M.: Phase I/II study of intraventricular and intrathecal ACNU for leptomeningeal neoplasia. Cancer Chemother. Pharmacol., 23:301, 1989.
277. Levin, V. A., Hoffman, W., and Weinkam, R. J.: Pharmacokinetics of BCNU in man: A preliminary study of 20 patients. Cancer Treat. Rep., 62:1305, 1978.
278. Levin, V. A., Silver, P., Hannigan, J., Wara, W. M., Gutin, P. H., David, R. L., and Wilson, C. B.: Superiority of post-radiotherapy adjuvant chemotherapy with CCNU, procarbazine, and vincristine (PCV) over BCNU for anaplastic gliomas. Int. J. Radiat. Oncol. Biol. Phys., 18:321, 1990.
279. Levin, V. A., Stearns, J., Byrd, A., Finn, A., and Weinkam, R. J.: The effect of phenobarbital on the antitumor activity of 1,3-bis(2-chlorethyl)-1-nitrosourea (BCNU), 1-(2-chlorethyl)-3-cyclohexyl-1-nitrosourea (CCNU) and 1-(2-chlorethyl)-3-(2,6-dioxo)-3-piperidyl-1-nitrosourea (PCNU), and on the plasma pharmacokinetics and biotransformation of BCNU. J. Pharmacol. Exp. Ther., 208:1, 1979.
280. Liopis, B., Gallego, J., Mompo, J. A., Boronat, F., and Jimenez, J. F.: Thiotepa versus adriamycin versus cis-platinum in the intravesical prophylaxis of superficial bladder tumors. Eur. Urol., 11:73, 1985.
281. Lippman, A. J., Helson, C., Helson, L., and Krakoff, I. H.: Clinical trials of cis-diamminedichloroplatinum (NSC-119875). Cancer Chemother. Rep., 57:191, 1973.
282. Litam, J. P., Dail, D. H., Spitzer, G., Vellekoop, L., Verma, D. S., Zander, A. R., and Dicke, K. A.: Early pulmonary toxicity after administration of high-dose BCNU. Cancer Treat. Rep., 65:39, 1981.
283. Little, S. A., and Mirkes, P. E.: DNA cross-linking and single-strand breaks induced by teratogenic concentrations of 4-hydroperoxycyclophosphamide and phosphoramide mustard in postimplantation rat embryos. Cancer Res., 47:5421, 1987.
284. Loehrer, P. J., Sr., Lauer, R., Roth, B. J., Williams, S. D., Kalasinski, L. A., and Einhorn, L. H.: Salvage therapy in recurrent germ cell cancer: Ifosfamide and cisplatin plus either vinblastine or etoposide. Ann. Intern. Med., 109:540, 1988.
285. Loveless, A., and Ross, W. C. J.: Chromosome alteration and tumour inhibition by nitrogen mustards: The hypothesis of cross-linking alkyation. Nature, 155:111, 1950.
286. Ludlum, D. B., Kramer, B. S., Wang, J., and Fenselau, C.: Reaction of 1,3-bis(2-chloroethyl)-1 nitrosourea with synthetic polynucleotides. Biochemistry, 14:5480, 1975.
287. Lyss, A. P., Luedke, S. L., Einhorn, L., Luedke, D. W., and Raney, M.: Vindesine and mitomycin C in metastatic breast cancer. A Southeastern Cancer Study Group Trial. Oncology, 46:357, 1989.
288. MacFarland, J. G., Kirk, M. C., and Ludlum, D. B.: Mechanism of action of the nitrosoureas—IV. Synthesis of the 2-haloethylnitrosourea-induced DNA cross-link 1-(3-cytosinyl),2-(1-guanyl)ethane. Biochem. Pharmacol., 39:33, 1990.
289. Madias, N. E., and Harrington, J. T.: Platinum nephrotoxicity. Am. J. Med., 65:307, 1978.
290. Mahaley, M. S., Jr., Hipp, S. W., Dropcho, E. J., Bertsch, L., Cush, S., Tirey, T., and Gillespie, G. Y.: Intracarotid cisplatin chemotherapy for recurrent gliomas. J. Neurosurg., 70:371 1989.
291. Makinodan, T., Snatos, G. W., and Quinn, R. P.: Immunosuppressive drugs. Pharmacol. Rev., 22:189, 1970.
292. Mangioni, C., Bolis, G., Pecorelli, S., Bragman, K., Epis, A., Favalli, G., Gambino, A., Landoni, F., Presti, M., Torri, W., Vassena, L., Zanaboni, F., and Marsoni, S.: Randomized trial in advanced ovarian cancer comparing cisplatin and carboplatin. J. Natl. Cancer Inst., 81:1464, 1989.
293. Mann, S. C., Andrews, P. A., and Howell, S. B.: Comparison of lipid content, surface membrane fluidity, and temperature dependence of cis-diamminedichloroplatinum (II) accumulation in sensitive and resistant human ovarian carcinoma cells. Anticancer Res., 8:1211, 1988.
294. Mark, G. J., Lehimgar-Zadeh, A., and Ragsdale, B. D.: Cyclophosphamide pneumonitis. Thorax, 33:89, 1978.
295. Markman, M., Cleary, S., and Howell, S. B.: Nephrotoxicity of high-dose intracavitary cisplatin with intravenous thiosulfate protection. Eur. J. Cancer Clin. Oncol., 21:1015, 1985.
296. Markman, M., and Howell, S. B.: Intrapericardial instillation of cisplatin in a patient with a large malignant effusion. Cancer Drug Deliv., 2:49, 1985.
297. Martin, R. B.: Hydrolytic equilibria and N7 versus N1 binding in Purine Nucleosides of cis-Diamminedichloroplatinum (II). *In* Platinum, Gold, and Other Metal Chemotherapeutic Agents. Edited by the American Chemical Society, Washington, D. C., 1983, p. 231.
298. Masuda, H., Ozols, R. F., Lai, G. M., Fojo, A., Rothenberg, M., and Hamilton, T. C.: Increased DNA repair as a mechanism of acquired resistance to cis-diamminedichloroplatinum (II) in human ovarian cancer cell lines. Cancer Res., 48:5713, 1988.
299. Maynard, K. R., Hosking, L. K., and Hill, B. T.: Use of host cell reactivation of cisplatin-treated adenovirus 5 in human cell lines to detect repair of drug-treated DNA. Chem. Biol. Interact., 71:353, 1989.
300. McCarthy, L. E., and Borison, H. L.: Cisplatin-induced vomiting eliminated by ablation of the area postrema in cats. Cancer Treat. Rep., 68:401, 1984.
301. McElwain, T. J., Hedley, D. W., Gordon, M. Y., Jarman, M., Millar, J. L., and Pritchard, J.: High dose melphalan and non-cryopreserved autologous bone marrow treatment of malignant melanoma and neuroblastoma. Exp. Hematol., 7(Suppl. 5):360, 1979.
302. McGuire, W. P., 3rd, Arseneau, J., Blessing, J. A., Disaia, P. J., Hatch, K. D., Given, F. T., Jr., Teng, N. N., and Creasman, W. T.: A randomized comparative trial of carboplatin and iproplatin in advanced squamous carcinoma of the utrine cervix: A Gynecologic Oncology Group Study. J. Clin. Oncol., 7:1462, 1989.
303. McLay, E. F., and Howell, S. B.: A review: Intraperitoneal cisplatin in the management of patients with ovarian cancer. Gynecol. Oncol., 36:1, 1990.
304. McLean, A., Woods, R. C., Catovsky, D., and Farmer, P.: Pharmacokinetics and metabolism of chlorambucil in patients with malignant disease. Cancer Treat. Rev., 6(Suppl.):33, 1979.
305. Menichetti, E. T., Silva, R. R., Tummarello, D., Miseria, S., Torresi, U., and Cellerino, R.: Etoposide and mitomycin-C in pretreated metastatic breast cancer. Tumori, 75:473, 1989.
306. Metcalfe, S. A., Cain, K., and Hill, B. T.: Possible mechanism for diferences in sensitivity to cis-platinum in human prostate tumor cell lines. Cancer Lett., 31:163, 1986.
307. Millard, J. T., Raucher, S., and Hopkins, P. B.: Mechlorethamine cross links deoxy-

guanosine residues of 5' GNC sequences in duplex DNA fragments. J. Am. Chem. Soc., 112:2459, 1990.
307A. Miller, B., Teneholz, T., Egorin, M. J., Sosnovsky, G., Rao, N. U., and Gutierrez, P. L.: Cellular pharmacology of N,N', N''-triethylene thiophosphoramide. Cancer Lett., 41:157, 1988.
308. Miller, D. G.: Alkylating agents and human spermatogenesis. J.A.M.A., 217:1662, 1971.
309. Miller, J. J., Williams, G. F., and Leissring, J. C.: Multiple late complications of therapy with cyclophosphamide, including ovarian destruction. Am. J. Med., 50:530, 1971.
310. Mirkes, P. E.: Cyclophosphamide teratogenesis: A review. Teratogenesis Carcinog. Mutagen., 5:75, 1985.
311. Mitchell, M. S., Kempf, R. A., Harel, W., Shau, H., Bosell, W. D., Lind, S., and Bradley, E. C.: Effectiveness and tolerability of low-dose cyclophosphamide and low-dose intravenous interleukin-2 in disseminated melanoma. J. Clin. Oncol., 6:409, 1988.
312. Moroso, M. J., and Blair, R. L.: A review of cis-platinum ototoxicity. J. Otolaryngol., 12:365, 1983.
313. Mortimer, J. E., Taylor, M. E., Schulman, S., Cummings, C., Weymuller, E., Jr., and Laramore, G.: Feasibility and efficacy of weekly intraarterial cisplatin in locally advanced (stage III and IV) head and neck cancers. J. Clin. Oncol., 6:969, 1988.
314. Mullins, G. M., Anderson, P. N., and Santos, G. W.: High dose cyclophosphamide therapy in solid tumors. Cancer, 36:1950, 1975.
315. Mullins, G. M., and Colvin, M.: Intensive cyclophosphamide therapy in solid tumors. Cancer Chemother. Rep., 59:411, 1975.
316. Murphy, M. L., Del Moro, A., and Lacon, C.: The comparative effects of five polyfunctional alkylating agents on the rat fetus, with additional notes. Ann. N. Y. Acad. Sci., 68:762, 1958.
317. Naganuma, A., Satoh, M., and Imura, N.: Prevention of lethal and renal toxicity of cis-diamminedichloroplatinum (II) by induction of metallothione in synthesis without compromising its antitumor activity in mice. Cancer Res., 47:983, 1987.
318. Nakagawa, K., Saijo, N., Tsuchida, S., Sakal, M., Tsunokawa, Y., Yokota, J., Muramatsu, M., Sato, K., Terada, M., and Tew, K. D.: Glutathione-S-transferase pi as a determinant of drug resistance to transfectant cell lines. J. Biol. Chem., 265:4296, 1990.
319. Nakagawa, K., Yokota, J., Wada, M., Sasaki, Y., Fujiwara, Y., Sakai, M., Muramatsu, M., Terasaki, T., Tsunokawa, Y., Terada, M., and Saijo, N.: Levels of glutathione S-transferase pi mRNA in human lung cancer cell lines correlate with the resistance to cisplatin and carboplatin. Jpn. J. Cancer Res., 79:301, 1988.
320. Nelson, R. L., Allen, L. M., and Creaven, P. J.: Pharmacokinetics of divided-dose ifosfamide. Clin. Pharmacol. Ther., 19:365, 1976.
321. Neuwet, E. A., Glasberg, M., Frenkel, E., and Barnett, P.: Neurotoxicity of chemotherapeutic agents after blood-brain barrier modification: Neurophathological studies. Ann. Neurol., 14:316, 1983.
322. Newman, E. M., Lu, Y., Kashani-Sabet, M., Kesavan, V., and Scanlon, K. J.: Mechanisms of cross-resistance to methotrexate and 5-fluorouracil in an A2780 human ovarian carcinoma cell subline resistant to cisplatin. Biochem. Pharmacol., 37:443, 1988.
322A. Ng, S. F., and Waxman, D. J.: N,N'N''-triethylenethiophosphoramide (thio-TEPA) oxygenation by constitutive hepatic P450 enzymes and modulation of drug metabolism and clearance in vivo by P450-inducing agents. Cancer Res., 51:2340, 1991.
323. Nichols, C. R., Tricot, G., Williams, S. D., van Besien, K., Loehrer, P. J., Roth, B. J., Akard, L., Hoffman, R., Goulet, R., Wolff, S. N., Giannone, L., Greer, J., Einhorn, L. H., and Jansen, J.: Dose-intensive chemotherapy in refractory germ cell cancer—a phase I/II trial of high-dose carboplatin and etoposide with autologous bone marrow transplantation. J. Clin. Oncol., 7:932, 1989.
324. Nicholson, H. O.: Cytotoxic drugs in pregnancy. J. Obstet. Gynaecol. Br. Commonw., 75:307, 1968.
325. Nimer, S. D., Milewicz, A. L., Champlin, R. E., and Busittil, R. W.: Successful treatment of hepatic venoocclusive disease in a bone marrow transplant patient with orthotopic liver transplantation. Transplantation, 49:819, 1990.
326. Nissen-Meyer, R., and Host, H.: A comparison between the hematological side effects of cyclophosphamide and nitrogen mustard. Cancer Chemother., 9:51, 1960.
327. Norpoth, K.: Studies on the metabolism of isophosphamide (NSC-109724) in man. Cancer Treat. Rep., 60:437, 1976.
328. Oguri, S., Sakakibara, T., Mase, H., Shimizu, T., Ishikawa, K., Kimura, K., and Smyth, R. D.: Clinical pharmacokinetics of carboplatin. J. Clin. Pharmacol., 28:208, 1988.
329. Oliner, H., Schwartz, R., Rubio, F., Jr., and Dameshek, W.: Interstitial pulmonary fibrosis following busulfan therapy. Am. J. Med., 31:134, 1961.
330. Ojwang, J. D., Grueneberg, D. A., and Loechler, E. L.: Synthesis of a duplex oligonucleotide containing a nitrogen mustard interstrand DNA-DND cross-link. Cancer Res., 49:6529, 1989.
331. Onsrud, M., Bosnes, V., and Graham, I.: cis-Platinum as adjunctive to surgery in early stage ovarian carcinoma: Effects on lymphoid cell subpopulations. Gynecol. Oncol., 23:323, 1986.
332. Ortega, J.: Multiple agent chemotherapy including bleomycin of non-Hodgkin's lymphoma during pregnancy. Cancer, 40:2829, 1977.
333. Orwoll, E. S., Kiessling, P. J., and Patterson, J. R.: Interstitial pneumonia from mitomycin. Ann. Intern. Med., 89:352, 1978.
334. Ozer, H., Cowens, J. W., Colvin, M., Nussbaum-Blumenson, A., and Sheedy, D.: In vitro effects of 4-hydroperoxycyclophosphamide on human immunoregulatory T subset function. 1. Selective effects of lymphocyte function in T-B cell collaboration. J. Exp. Med., 155:276, 1982.
335. Ozols, R. F.: Cisplatin dose intensity. Semin. Oncol., 16:22, 1989.
336. Ozols, R. F., Louie, K. G., Plowman, J., Behrens, B. C., Fine, R. L., Dykes, D., and Hamilton, T. C.: Enchanced melphalan cytotoxicity in human ovarian cancer in vitro and in tumor-bearing nude mice by buthionine sulfoximine depletion of glutathione. Biochem. Pharmacol., 36:147, 1987.
337. Ozols, R. F., Masuda, H., and Hamilton, T. C.: Mechanisms of cross-resistance between radiation and antineoplastic drugs. NCI Monogr., 6:159, 1988.
338. Pacheco, D. Y., Stratton, N. K., and Gibson, N. W.: Comparison of the mechanism of action of busulfan with hepsulfam, a new antileukemic agent, in the L1210 cell line. Cancer Res., 49:5108, 1989.
339. Pallante, S. L., Fenselau, C., Mennel, R. G., Brundrett, R. B., Appler, M., Rosenshein, N. B., and Colvin, M.: Quantitation by gas chromatography-chemical ionization-mass spectrometry of phenylalanine mustard in plasma of patients. Cancer Res., 40:2268, 1980.
340. Paolozzi, F. P., Gaver, R., Poiesz, B. J., Louie, A., Difino, S., Comis, R. L., Newman, N., and Ginsberg, S.: Phase I—preliminary phase II trial of iproplatin, a cisplatin analogue. Invest. New Drugs, 6:199, 1988.
341. Parker, S., Kirk, M. C., and Ludlum, D. B.: Synthesis and characterization of 06-(2-chloroethyl)guanine: A putative intermediate in the cytotoxic reaction of chloroethylnitrosoureas with DNA. Biochem. Biophys. Res. Commun., 148:1124, 1987.
342. Parsons, P. G., Lean, J., Kable, E. P. W., Favier, D., Khoo, S. K., Hurst, T., Holmes, R. S., and Bellet, A. J. D.: Relationship between resistance to cross-linking agents and glutathione metabolism, aldehyde dehydrogenase isozymes and adenovirus replication in human tumor all lines. Biochem. Pharmacol., 40:2641, 1990.
343. Patel, A. R., Shah, P. C., Rhee, H. L., Sassoon, H., and Rao, K. P.: Cyclophosphamide therapy and interstitial pulmonary fibrosis. Cancer, 38:1542, 1976.
344. Patton, T. F., Repta, A. J., and Sternson, L. A.: Clinical pharmacology of cisplatin. *In* Pharmacokinetics of Anticancer Agents in Humans. Edited by M. M. Ames, G. Powis, and J. S. Kovach. New York, Elsevier, 1983.
345. Pegg, A. E.: Mammalian 06—alkylguanine-DNA alkyltransferase: Regulation and importance in response to alkylating carcinogenic and therapeutic agents. Cancer Res., 50:6119, 1990.
346. Pendyala, L., Cowens, J. W., Chheda, G. B., Dutta, S. P., and Creaven, P. J.: Identification of cis-dichloro-bis-isopropylamine platinum (II) as a major metabolite of iproplatin in humans. Cancer Res., 48:3533, 1988.
347. Pendyala, L., Walshm, J. R., Huq, M. M., Arakali, A. V., Cowens, J. W., and Creaven, P. J.: Uptake and metabolism of iproplatin in murine L1210 cells. Cancer Chemother. Pharmacol., 25:15, 1989.
348. Penn, I.: Second malignant neoplasma associated with immunosuppressive medications. Cancer, 37:1024, 1976.
349. Perloff, M., Hart, R. D., and Holland, J. F.: Vinblastine, adrimycin, thio-TEPA, and Holotestin (VATH). Cancer, 42:2534, 1978.
350. Peters, W. P., Eder, J. P., Henner, W. D., Schryber, S., Wilmore, D., Finberg, R., Schoenfeld, D., Bast, R., Gargone, B., Antman, K., Anderson, J., Anderson, K., Kruskall, M. S., Schnipper, L., and Frei, E., III: High-dose combination alkylating agents with autologous bone marrow support. A Phase I trial. J. Clin. Oncol., 4:646, 1986.
351. Pfeiffer, P., Bennedbaek, O., and Bertelsen, K.: Intraperitoneal carboplatin in the treatment of minimal residual ovarian cancer. Gynecol. Oncol., 36:306, 1990.
352. Philips, F. S., Sternberg, S. S., Cronin, A. P., and Vidal, P. M.: Cyclophosphamide and urinary bladder toxicity. Cancer Res., 21:1577, 1961.
353. Phillips, G. L., Fay, J. W., Herzig, G. P., Herzig, R. H., Weiner, R. S., Wolff, S. N., Lazarus, H. M., Karanes, C., Ross, W. E., and Kramer, B. S.: Intensive 1,3-bis(2-chloroethyl)-1-nitrosourea (BCNU), NSC #4366650 and cryopreserved autologous marrow transplantation for refractory cancer. A Phase I-II study. Cancer, 51:1792, 1983.
354. Piccart, M. J., Abrams, J., Dodion, P. F., Crespeigne, N., and Schulier, J. P.: Intraperitoneal chemotherapy with cisplatin and melphalan. J. Natl. Cancer Inst., 80:1118, 1988.
355. Piel, I. J., and Perlia, C. P.: Phase II study of cis-dichlorodiammineplatinum (II) (NSC-119875) in combination with cyclophosphamide (NSC-26271) in the treatment of human malignancies. Cancer Chemother. Rep., 59:995, 1975.
356. Pinto, A. L., and Lippard, S. J.: Sequence-dependent termination of *in vitro* DNA synthesis by cis- and trans-diamminedichloroplatinum (II). Proc. Natl. Acad. Sci., U. S. A., 82:4616, 1985.
357. Plooy, A. C., van Dijk, M., Berends, F., and Lohman, P. H.: Formation and repair of DNA interstrand cross-links in relation to cytotoxicity and unscheduled DNA synthesis induced in control and mutant human cells treated with cis-diamminedichloroplatinum (II). Cancer Res., 45:4178, 1985.
358. Poirier, M. C., Egorin, M. J., Fichtinger-Schepman, A. M., Yushpa, S. H., and Reed, E.: DNA adducts of cisplatin and carboplatin in tissues of cancer patients. *In* Damaging Agents in Humans: Applications in Cancer Epidemiology and Prevention (IARC Scientific Publication No. 89). Edited by H. Bartsch, K. Hemminke, and I. K. O'Neill. 1988, p. 313.
359. Poisson, M., Chiras, J., Fauchon, F., Debussche, C., and Delattre, J. Y.: Treatment of malignant recurrent glioma by intra-arterial infraophthalmic infusion of HECNU 1-(2-chloroethyl)-1-nitroso-3-(2-hydroxyethyl) urea. A phase II study. J. Neurooncol., 8:255, 1990.
360. Poll, E. H., Abrahams, P. J., Arwert, F., and Eriksson, A. W.: Host-cell reactivation of cis-diamminedichloroplatinum (II)-treated SV40 DNA in normal human, Fanconi anaemia and xeroderma pigmentosum fibroblasts. Mutat. Res., 132:181, 1984.
361. Poll, E. H., Arwert, F., Joenje, H., and Eriksson, A. W.: Cytogenetic toxicity of antitumor platinum compounds in Fanconi's anemia. Hum. Genet., 61:228, 1982.
362. Pomes, A., Frustaci, S., Cattaino, G., DeGrandis, D., Bongiovanni, L. G., Tumolo, S., and Quadu, G.: Local neurotoxicity of cisplatin after intra-arterial chemotherapy. Acta Neurol. Scand., 73:302, 1986.
363. Portlock, C. S., Fischer, D. S., Cadman, E., Lundberg, W. B., Levy, A., Bobrow, S., Bertino, J. R., and Farber, L.: High-dose pulse chlorambucil in advanced, low-grade non-Hodgkin's lymphoma. Cancer Treat. Rep., 71:1029, 1987.
364. Pratt, C. B., Douglass, E. C., Etcubanas, E., Goren, M. P., Green, A. A., Hayes, F. A., Horowitz, M. E., Meyer, W. H., Thompson, E. L., and Wilimas, J. A.: Clinical studies of ifosfamide/mesna at St. Jude Children's Research Hospital, 1983-1988. Semin. Oncol., 16:51, 1989.
365. Pratt, C. B., Goren, M. P., Meyer, W. H., Singh, B., and Dodge, R. K.: Ifosfamide neurotoxicity is related to previous cisplatin treatment for pediatric solid tumors. J. Clin. Oncol., 8:1399, 1990.
366. Pratt, C. B., Horowitz, M. E., Meyer, W. H., Etcubanas, E., Thompson, E. L., Douglass, E. C., Wilimas, J. A., Hayes, F. A., and Green, A. A.: Phase II trial of ifosfamide in children with malignant solid tumors. Cancer Treat. Rep., 71:131, 1987.
367. Prestayko, A. W.: Cisplatin and analogues: A new class of anticancer drugs. *In* Cancer and Chemotherapy, Vol. III, Antineoplastic Agents. Edited by S. T. Crooke, and A. W. Prestayko. Academic Press, New York, 1981, p. 133.
368. Price, C. C., Gaucher, G. M., Koneru, P., Shibakawa, R., Sowa, J. R., and Yamaguchi, M.: Relative reactivities for monofunctional nitrogen mustard alkylation of nucleic acid components. Biochim. Biophys. Acta, 166:327, 1968.
369. Puchalski, R. B., and Fahl, W. E.: Expression of recombinant glutathione-S-transferase

pi, Ya and Yb1 confers resistance to alkylating agents. Proc. Natl. Acad. Sci. U. S. A., 87:2443, 1990.
370. Radin, A. E., Haggard, M. E., and Travis, L. B.: Lung changes and chemotherapeutic agents in childhood. Am. J. Dis. Child., 120:337, 1970.
371. Redwood, W. R., and Colvin, M.: Transport of melphalan by sensitive and resistant L1210 cells. Cancer Res., 40:1144, 1980.
372. Reece, P. A., Bishop, J. F., Olver, I. N., Stafford, I., Hillcoat, B. L., and Morstyn, G.: Pharmacokinetics of unchanged carboplatin (CBDCA) in patients with small cell lung carcinoma. Cancer Chemother. Pharmacol., 19:326, 1987.
373. Reece, P. A., Dale, B. M., Morris, R. G., Kotasek, G., Gee, D., Rogerson, S., and Sage, R. E.: Effect of L-leucine on oral melphalan kinetics in patients. Cancer Chemother. Pharmacol., 20:256, 1987.
374. Reece, P. A., Hill, H. S., Green, R. M., Morris, R. G., Dale, B. M., and Kotasek, D.: Renal clearance and protein binding of melphalan in patients with cancer. Cancer Chemother. Pharmacol., 22:348, 1988.
375. Reece, P. A., Kotasek, D., Morris, R. G., Dale, B. M., and Sage, R. E.: The effect of food on oral melphalan absorption. Cancer Chemother. Pharmacol., 16:194, 1986.
376. Reed, E., and Kohn, K. W.: Platinum Analogues in Chabner, B. A., and Collins, J. M.: *In* Cancer Chemotherapy: Principles and Practice. J. B. Lippincott, Philadelphia, 1990, p. 475.
377. Reimer, R. R., Hoover, R., Fraumeni, J. F., Jr., and Young, R. C.: Acute leukemia after alkylating-agent therapy of ovarian cancer. N. Engl. J. Med., 297:177, 1977.
378. Repta, A. J., and Long, D. F.: Cisplatin: Current Status and New Developments. Edited by A. W. Prestayko, S. T. Crooke, and S. K. Carter. New York, Academic Press, 1980, p. 285.
379. Reyes, E. S., Talley, R. W., O'Bryan, R. M., and Gastesi, R. A.: Clinical evaluation of 1,3-bis-(2-chloroethyl)-1-nitrosourea (BCNU; NSC-409962) with fluoxymesterone (NSC-12165) in the treatment of solid tumors. Cancer Chemother. Rep., 57:225, 1973.
380. Rhoads, C. P.: Nitrogen mustards in treatment of neoplastic disease. J.A.M.A., 131:656, 1946.
381. Rhodes, D. F., Lee, W. M., Wingard, J. R., Pavy, M. D., Santos, G. W., Shaw, B. W., Wood, R. P., Sorrell, M. F., and Markin, R. S.: Orthotopic liver transplantation for graft-versus-host disease following bone marrow transplantation. Gastroenterology, 99:536, 1990.
382. Rivkin, S. E., Green, S., Metch, B., Glucksberg, H., Gad-el-Mawla, N., Constanzi, J. J., Hoogstraten, B., Athens, J., Maloney, T., Osborne, C. K., and Vaughn, C. B.: Adjuvant CMFVP versus melphalan for operable breast cancer with positive axillary nodes: 10-year results of a Southwest Oncology Group Study. J. Clin. Oncol., 7:1229, 1989.
383. Roberts, J. J., and Pera, M. F.: DNA as a target for anticancer coordination compounds. *In* Platinum, Gold, and the Metal Chemotherapeutic Agents. Edited by J. J. Lippard. American Chemical Society, Washington, D. C., 1983, p. 3.
384. Robson, C. N., Lewis, A. D., Wolf, C. R., Hayes, J. D., Hall, A., Proctor, S. J., Harris, A. L., and Hickson, I. D.: Reduced levels of drug-induced DNA cross-linking in nitrogen mustard-resistant Chinese hamster ovary cells expressing elevated glutathione S-transferase activity. Cancer Res., 47:6022, 1967.
385. Roosen, N., Kiwit, J. C., Lins, E., Schirmer, M., and Bock, W. J.: Adjuvant intraarterial chemotherapy with nimustine in the management of World Health Organization Grade IV gliomas of the brain. Cancer, 64:1984, 1989.
386. Rose, D. P., and Davis, T. E.: Ovarian function in patients receiving adjuvant chemotherapy for breast cancer. Lancet, 1:1174, 1977.
387. Rosenberg, B., Van Camp, L., and Krigas, T.: Inhibition of Cell Division in *Escherichia coli* by Electrolysis Products from a Platinum Electrode. Nature, 205:698, 1965.
388. Rosenberg, B., Van Camp, L., Trosko, J. E., and Mansour, V. H.: Platinum Compounds: a new class of potent antitumour agents. Nature, 222:385, 1969.
389. Rosner, F., and Grunwald, H.: Multiple myeloma terminating in acute leukemia. Am. J. Med., 57:927, 1974.
390. Rosner, F., and Grunwald, H.: Hodgkin's disease and acute leukemia. Am. J. Med., 58:339, 1975.
391. Rosowsky, A., Wright, J. E., Cucchi, C. A., Flatow, J. L., Trites, D. H., Teicher, B. A., and Frei, E., 3rd: Collateral methotrexate resistance in cultured human head and neck carcinoma cells selected for resistance to cis-diamminedichloroplatinum (II). Cancer Res., 47:5913, 1987.
392. Ross, D., Siegel, D., Gibson, N. W., Pacheco, D., Thomas, D. J., Reasor, M., and Wierda, D.: Activation and deactivation of quinones catalyzed by DT-diaphorase. Evidence for bioreductive activation of diaziquone (AZQ) in human tumor cells and detoxification of benzene metabolites in bone marrow stroma. Free Radic. Res. Commun., 6:373, 1990.
393. Ross, W. E., and Chabner, B. A.: Allergic reaction to cyclophosphamide in a mechlorethamine-sensitive patient. Cancer Treat. Rep., 61:495, 1977.
394. Ross, W. E., Ewig, R. A., and Kohn, K. W.: Differences between melphalan and nitrogen mustard in the formation and removal of DNA cross-links. Cancer Res., 38:1502, 1978.
395. Rundles, R. W., Striggle, J., Bell, W., Corley, C. C., Frommeyer, W. B., Jr., Greenberg, B. G., Huguley, C. M., Jr., James, G. W., Jones, R., Jr., Larsen, W. E., Loe, B. V., Leone, L. A., Palmer, J. G., Riser, W. E., Jr., and Wilson, S. J.: Comparison of chlorambucil and Myleran in chronic lymphocytic and granulocytic leukemia. Am. J. Med., 27:424, 1959.
396. Russo, J. E., Hilton, J., and Colvin, O. M.: The role of aldehyde dehydrogenase isoenzymes in cellular resistance to the alkylating agent cyclophosphamide. *In* Enzymology and Molecular Biology of Carbonyl Metabolism, Vol. 2. Alan R. Liss, New York. 1989, p. 65.
397. Saburi, Y., Nakagawa, M., Ono, M., Sakai, M., Muramatsu, M., Kohno, K., and Kuwano, M.: Increased expression of glutathione S-transferase gene in cis-diamminedichloroplatinum (II)-resistant variants of a Chinese hamster ovary cell line. Cancer Res., 49:7020, 1989.
398. Santos, G. W., Sensenbrenner, L. L., Anderson, P. N., Burke, P. J., Kelin, D. L., Slavin, R. E., Schacter, B., and Borgaonkar, D. S.: HLA-identical marrow transplants in aplastic anemia, acute leukemia, and lymphosarcoma employing cyclophosphamide. Transplant. Proc., 8:607, 1976.
399. Santos, G. W., Tutschka, P. J., Brookmeyer, R., Saral, R., Beschorner, W. E., Bias, W. B., Braine, H. G., Burns, W. H., Elfenbein, G. J., Kaizer, H., Mellits, D., Sensenbrenner, L. L., Stuart, R. K., and Yeager, A. M.: Marrow transplantation for acute nonlymphocytic leukemia after treatment with busulfan and cyclophosphamide. N. Engl. J. Med., 309:1347, 1983.
400. Scanlon, K. J., Kashani-Sabet, M., and Sowers, L. C.: Overexpression of DNA replication and repair enzymes in cisplatin-resistant human colon carcinoma HCT8 cells and circumvention by azidothymidine. Cancer Commun., 1:269, 1989.
401. Schabel, F. M., Jr.: Nitrosoureas: A review of experimental anti-tumor activity. Cancer Treat. Rep., 60:665, 1976.
402. Schable, F. M., Jr., Johnston, T. P., McCaleb, G. S., Montgomery, J. A., Laster, W. R., and Skipper, H. E.: Experimental evaluation of potential anticancer agents: VIII. Effects of certain nitrosoureas on cerebral L1210 leukemia. Cancer Res., 23:725, 1963.
403. Schacht, R. G., and Baldwin, D. S.: Chronic interstitial nephritis and renal failure due to nitrosourea (NU) therapy. Kidney Inst., 14:661, 1978.
404. Schilsky, R. L., and Anderson, T.: Hypomagnesemia and renal magnesium wasting in patients receiving cisplatin. Ann. Intern. Med., 90:929, 1979.
405. Schold, S. C., Jr., Brent, T. P., von Hofe, E., Friedman, H. S., Mitra, S., Bigner, D. D., Swenberg, J. A., and Kleihues, P.: 06-alkylguanine-DNA-alkyltransferase and sensitivity to procarbazine in human brain-tumor xenografts. J. Neurosurg., 70:573, 1989.
406. Schroyens, W., Dodion, P., and Rozencweig, M.: Comparative effect of cisplatin, spiroplatin, carboplatin and iproplatin in a human tumor clonogenic assay. J. Cancer Res. Clin. Oncol., 116:392, 1990.
407. Sekiya, S., Oosaki, T., Andoh, S., Susuki, N., Akaboshi, M., and Takamizawa, H.: Mechanisms of resistance to cis-diamminedichloroplatinum (II) in vitro. Cancer Res., 48:6803, 1988.
408. Sellei, C., Ecklardt, I. P., Horvath, I. P., Kralovanszky, J., and Institoris, L.: Clinical and pharmacologic experience with dibromodulcitol (NSC-104800), a new antitumor agent. Cancer Chemother. Rep., 53:377, 1969.
409. Sharma, R. P., and Edwards, I. R.: cis-Platinum: Subcellular distribution and binding to cytosolic proteins. Biochem. Pharmacol., 32:2665, 1983.
410. Sheibani, N., Jennerwin, M. M., and Eastman, A.: DNA repair in cells sensitive and resistant to cis-diamminedichloroplatinum (II): host cell reactivation of damaged plasmid DNA. Biochem., 28:3120, 1989.
411. Sherins, R. J., and DeVita, V. T.: Effect of drug treatment for lymphoma on male reproductive capacity. Ann. Intern. Med., 79:216, 1973.
412. Skinner, R., Pearson, A. D., Amineddine, H. A., Mathias, D. B., and Craft, A. W.: Ototoxicity of cisplatinum in children and adolescents. Br. J. Cancer, 61:927, 1990.
413. Sladek, N.: Therapeutic efficacy of cyclophosphamide as a function of its metabolism. Cancer Res., 32:535, 1972.
414. Sladek, N. E., Doeden, D., Powers, J. F., and Krivit, W.: Plasma concentrations of 4-hydroxyclophosphamide and phosphoramide mustard in patients repeatedly given high doses of cyclophosphamide in preparation for bone marrow transplantation. Cancer Treat. Rep., 68:1247, 1984.
415. Slavin, R. E., Millan, J. C., and Mullins, G. M.: Pathology of high dose intermittent cyclophosphamide therapy. Hum. Pathol., 6:693, 1975.
416. Smith, A. C., Liao, J. T., Page, J. G., Wientjes, M. G., and Grieshaber, C. K.: Pharmacokinetics of buthionine sulfoximine (NSC 326231) and its effect on melphalan-induced toxicity in mice. Cancer Res., 49:5385, 1989.
417. Smith, M. T., Evans, C. G., Doane-Setzer, P., Castro, V. M., Tahir, M. K., and Mannervik, B.: Denitrosation of 1,3-bis(2-chlorethyl)-1-nitrosourea by class mu glutathione transferases and its role in cellular resistance in rat brain tumor cells. Cancer Res., 49:2621, 1989.
418. Sorenson, C. M., and Eastman, A.: Influence of cis-diamminedichloroplatinum (II) on DNA synthesis and cell cycle progression in excision repair proficient and deficient Chinese hamster ovary cells. Cancer Res., 48:6703, 1988.
419. Speyer, J. L., Beller, U., Colombo, N., Sorich, J., Wernz, J. C., Hochster, H., Green, M., Porges, R., Muggia, F. M., Canetta, R., and Beckman, E. M.: Intraperitoneal carboplatin: favorable results in women with minimal residual ovarian cancer after cisplatin therapy. J. Clin. Oncol., 8:1335, 1990.
420. Spitz, S.: The histological effects of nitrogen mustards on human tumors and tissues. Cancer, 1:383, 1948.
421. Steege, J. F., and Caldwell, D. S.: Renal agenesis after first trimester exposure to chlorambucil. South. Med. J., 73:1414, 1980.
422. Steinberg, S. S., Philips, F. S., and Scholler, J.: Pharmacological and pathological effects of alkylating agents. Ann. N. Y. Acad. Sci., 68:811, 1958.
423. Steinherz, L. J., and Steinherz, P. G.: Cyclophosphamide cardiotoxicity. Cancer Bull., 37:231, 1985.
424. Stewart, D. J., Grahovac, Z., Hugenholtz, H., Russell, N., Richard, M., and Benoit, B.: Combined intraarterial and systemic chemotherapy for intracerebral tumors. Neurosurgery, 21:207, 1987.
425. Strauss, M., Towfighi, J., Lord, S., Lipton, A., Harvey, H. A., and Brown, B: Cis-platinum ototoxicity: Clinical experience and temporal bone histopathology. Laryngoscope, 93:1554, 1983.
426. Strong, J. M., Collins, J. M., Lester, C., and Poplack, D. G.: Pharmacokinetics of intraventricular and intravenous N, N′, N″-triethylenethiophosphoramide (thiotepa) in rhesus monkeys and humans. Cancer Res., 46:6101, 1986.
427. Struck, R. F., Alberts, D. S., Horne, K., Phillips, J. G., Peng, Y. M., and Roe, D. J.: Plasma pharmacokinetics of cyclophosphamide and its cytotoxic metabolites after intravenous versus oral administration in a randomized, crossover trial. Cancer Res., 47:2723, 1987.
428. Struck, R. F., Kirk, M. C., Mellett, L. B., et-Dareer, S., and Hill, D. L.: Urinary metabolites of the antitumor agent cyclophosphamide. Mol. Pharmacol., 7:519, 1971.
429. Sundquist, W. I., Lippard, S. J., and Stollar, B. D.: Monoclonal antibodies to DNA modified with cis- or trans-diamminedichloroplatinum (II). Proc. Natl. Acad. Sci., U. S. A., 84:8225, 1987.
430. Suzukaka, D., Petro, B. J., and Vistica, D. T.: Reduction in glutathione content of L-PAM resistant L1210 cell confers drug sensitivity. Biochem. Pharmacol., 31:121, 1982.
431. Takvorian, T., Parker, L. M., Hochberg, F. H., Zervas, N. P., Frei, E., III, and Canellos, G. P.: Single high dose of BCNU with autologous bone marrow (ABM). Proc. A. A. C. R. and Am. Soc. Clin. Oncol., 21:341, 1980.
432. Talley, R. W., O'Bryan, R. M., Gutterman, J. U., Brownlee, R. W., and McCredie, K. B.: Clinical evaluation of toxic effects of cis-diamminedichloroplatinum (NSC-119875)—phase I clinical study. Cancer Chemother. Rep., 57:465, 1973.
433. Talmadge, J. E., Tribble, H., Pennington, R., Bowersox, O., Schneider, M. A., Castelli,

P., Black, P. L., and Abe, F.: Protective, restorative and therapeutic properties of recombinant colony-stimulating factors. Blood, 73:2093, 1989.
434. Tapiero, H., Yin, M. B., Catalin, J., Paraire, M., Deloffre, P., Rustum, Y., Bizzari, J. P., and Tew, K. D.: Cytotoxicity and DNA damaging effects of a new nitrosourea, fotemustine, diethyl-1-(3-{2-chloroethyl}-3-nitrosoureido) ethylphosphonate-S10036. Anticancer Res., 9:1617, 1989.
435. Tattersall, M. H. N., and Weinberg, A.: Pharmacokinetics of melphalan following oral or intravenous administration in patients with malignant disease. Eur. J. Cancer, 14:507, 1978.
436. Taylor, K. M., Jagannath, S., Spitzer, G., Spinolo, J. A., Tucker, S. L., Fogel, B., Cabanillas, F. F., Hagemeister, F. B., and Souza, L. M.: Recombinant human granulocyte colony-stimulating factor hastens granulocyte recovery after high-dose chemotherapy and autologous bone marrow transplantation in Hodgkin's disease. J. Clin. Oncol., 7:1791, 1989.
437. Teicher, B. A., Herman, T. S., Holden, S. A., Wang, Y. Y., Pfeffer, M. R., Crawford, J. W., and Frei, E., III: Tumor resistance to alkylating agents conferred by mechanisms operative only in vivo. Science, 24:1457, 1990.
437A. Teicher, B. A., Holden, S. A., Eder, J. P., Herman, T. S., Antman, K. H., and Frei, E.: Preclinical Studies Relating to the Use of Thiotepa in the High-Dose Setting Alone and in Combination. Semin. Oncol., 1(Suppl. 3):18, 1990.
438. Teicher, B. A., Holden, S. A., Kelley, M. J., Shea, T. C., Cucchi, C. A., Rosowsky, A., Henner, W. D., and Frei, E., 3rd: Characterization of a human squamous carcinoma cell line resistant to cis-diamminedichloroplatinum (II). Cancer Res., 47:388, 1987.
439. Teicher, B. A., Waxman, D. J., Holden, S. A., Wang, Y. Y., Clarke, L., Alvarez-Sotomayor, E., Jones, S. M., and Frei, E. 3rd: Evidence for enzymatic activation and oxygen involvement in cytotoxicity and antitumor activity of N,N,N triethylenethiophosphoramide. Cancer Res., 49:4996, 1989.
440. Tew, K. D., Bomber, A. M., and Hoffman, S. J.: Ethacrynic acid and piriprost as enhancers of cytotoxicity in drug resistant and sensitive cell lines. Cancer Res., 48:3622, 1988.
441. Thatcher, D., Lind, M., Morgenstern, G., Carr, T., Chadwick, G., Jones, R., and Craig, P.: High-dose, double alkylating agent chemotherapy with DTIC, melphalan, or ifosfamide and marrow rescue for metastatic malignant melanoma. Cancer, 63:1296, 1989.
442. Thatcher, N., and Lind, M.: Carboplatin in small cell lung cancer. Semin. Oncol., 17:40, 1990.
443. Toledo, T. M., Harper, R. C., and Moser, R. H.: Fetal effects during cyclophosphamide and irradiation therapy. Ann. Intern. Med., 74:87, 1971.
444. Tormey, D. C., Falkson, G., and Simon, R. M.: A randomized comparison of two sequentially administered regimens to a single regimen in metastatic breast cancer. Cancer Clin. Trials, 2:247, 1979.
445. Townes, A. S., Sowa, J. M., and Schuman, L. E.: Controlled trial of cyclophosphamide in rheumatoid arthritis (RA): An 11-month double-blind crossover study. Arthritis Rheum., 15:129, 1972.
446. Trujillo, J. M., and Yang, L. Y.: Synergism of 1-beta-D-arabinofuranosylcytosine and cis-diamminedichloroplatinum in their lethal efficacies against seven established cancer cell lines of gastrointestinal origin. Anticancer Res., 9:197, 1989.
447. Tucker, M. A., Coleman, C. N., Cox, R. S., Varghese, A., and Rosenberg, S. A.: Risk of second cancers after treatment for Hodgkin's disease. N. Engl. J. Med., 318:76, 1988.
448. van Besien, K., Nichols, C. R., Tricot, G., Langefeld, C., Miller, M. E., Akard, L., English, D. K., Graves, V. L., Cheerva, A., McCarthy, L. J., et al.: Characteristics of engraftment after repeated autologous bone marrow transplantation. Exp. Hematol., 18:785, 1990.
449. Van Den Berg, H. W., and Roberts, J. J.: Post-replication repair of DNA in Chinese hamster cells treated with cis platinum (II) diamine dichloride. Enhancement of toxicity and chromosome damage by caffeine. Mutat. Res., 33:279, 1975.
450. van der Hoop, R., deKoning, P., Boven, E., Neijt, J. P., Jennekens, F. G., and Gispen, W. H.: Efficacy of the neuropeptide ORG 2766 in the prevention and treatment of cisplatin-induced neurotoxicity in rats. Eur. J. Cancer Clin. Oncol., 24:637, 1988.
450A. van der Hoop, R. G., Vecht, C. J., van der Burg, M. E., Elderson, A., Boogerd, W., Heimans, J. J., Vries, E. P., and van Houwelingen, J. C.: Prevention of cisplatin neurotoxicity with an ACTH(4-9) analogue in patients with ovarian cancer. N. Engl. J. Med., 322:89, 1990.
451. Van Dyk, J. J., Falkson, H. C., Van der Merwe, A. M., and Falkson, G.: Unexpected toxicity in patients treated with iphosphamide. Cancer Res., 32:921, 1972.
452. van Glabbeke, M., Renard, J., Pinedo, H. M., Cavalli, F., Vermorken, J., Sessa, C., Abele, R., Clavel, M., and Monfardini, S.: Iproplatin and carboplatin induced toxicities: Overview of phase II clinical trial conducted by the EORTC Early Clinical Trials Cooperative Group (ECTG). Eur. J. Cancer Clin. Oncol., 24:255, 1988.
453. van Zandwijk, N., ten Bokkel Huinink, W. W., Wanders, J., Simonetti, G., Dubbelman, R., Franklin, H., van Tinteren, H., and McVie, J. G.: Dose-finding studies with carboplatin, ifosfamide, etoposide, and mesna in non-small cell lung cancer. Semin. Oncol., 17:16, 1990.
454. van Zeeland, A. A., Bussmann, C. J., Degrassi, F., Filon, A. R., van Kasteren-van Leeuwen, A. C., Palitti, F., and Natarajan, A. T.: Effects of aphidicolin on repair replication and induced chromosomal aberrations in mammalian cells. Mutat. Res., 92:379, 1982.
455. Vassal, G., Deroussent, A., Hartmann, O., Challine, D., Benhamou, E., Valiteau-Couanet, D., Brugleres, L., Kalifa, C., Gouyette, A., and Lemerle, J.: Dose-dependent neurotoxicity of high-dose-busulfan in children: a clinical and pharmacological study. Cancer Res., 50:6203, 1990.
456. Vassal, G., Gouyette, A., Hartmann, O., Pico, J. L., and Lemerle, J.: Pharmacokinetics of high-dose busulfan in children. Cancer Chemother. Pharmacol., 24:386, 1989.
457. Vaughan, C., Chapman, J., Chinn, B., Ward, D., Groshko, G., Maniscalco, B., Reznik, S., and Piper, D.: Activity of 5-fluorouracil, mitomycin C, and methyl CCNU in inoperable adenocarcinoma of pancreas. Am. J. Clin. Oncol., 12:49, 1989.
458. Ventura, G. J., Barlogie, B., Hester, J. P., Yau, J. C., LeMaistre, C. F., Wallerstein, R. O., Spinolo, J. A., Dicke, K. A., Horwitz, L. H., and Alexantan, R.: High dose cyclophosphamide, BCNU and VP-16 with autologous blood stem cell support for refractory multiple myeloma. Bone Marrow Transplant., 5:265, 1990.
459. Verly, W. G.: Monofunctional alkylating agents and apurinic sites in DNA. Biochem. Pharmacol., 23:3, 1974.
460. Verly, W. G., and Paquette, Y.: An endonuclease for depurinated DNA in Escherichia coli B. Can. J. Biochem., 50:217-224, 1972.
461. Vermorken, J. B., Kapteijn, T. S., Hart, A. A., and Pinedo, H. M.: Ototoxicity of cis-diamminedichloroplatinum (II): influence of dose, schedule and mode of administration. Eur. J. Cancer Clin. Oncol., 19:53, 1983.
462. Viens, P., Maraninchi, D., Legros, M., Oberling, F., Philips, T., Herve, P., Plagne, R., Dufour, P., Bergerat, J. P., Guastalla, J. P., Rozenbaum, A., and Carcassonne, Y.: High dose melphalan and autologous marrow rescue in advanced epithelial ovarian carcinomas: a retrospective analysis of 35 patients treated in France. Bone Marrow Transplant. 5:227, 1990.
463. Villani, G., Hubscer, U., and Butour, J. L.: Sites of termination of in vitro DNA synthesis on cis-diamminedichloroplatinum treated single stranded DNA: a comparison between E. coli DNA polymerase I and eucaryotic DNA polymerases alpha. Nucleic Acids Res., 16:4407, 1988.
464. Vistica, D. T., Rabon, A., and Rabinowitz, M.: Effects of L-alpha-amino-gamma-guanidinobutyric acid on melphalan therapy of the L1210 murine leukemia. Cancer Lett., 6:345, 1979.
465. Vistica, D. T., Toal, J. N., and Rabinowitz, M.: Amino acide conferred protection against melphalan: Characterization of melphalan transport and correlation of uptake with cytotoxicity in cultured L1210 murine leukemia cells. Biochem. Pharmacol., 27:2865, 1978.
466. Von Hoff, D. D., Schilsky, R., Reichert, C. M., Reddick, R. L., Rozencweig, M., Young, R. C., and Muggia, F. M.: Toxic effects of cis-diamminedichloroplatinum (II) in man. Cancer Treat. Rep., 63:1527, 1979.
467. Wadler, S., Egorin, M. J., Zuhowski, E. G., Tororello, L., Salva, K., Runowicz, C. D., and Wiernik, P. H.: Phase I clinical and pharmacokinetic study of thiotepa administered intraperitoneally in patients with advanced malignancies. J. Clin. Oncol., 7:132, 1989.
468. Wadler, T., Heydrich, D., Jork, T., Voelker, G., and Hohorst, H. J.: Comparative study of human pharmacokinetics of activated ifosfamide and cyclophosphamide by a modified fluorometric test. Cancer Res. Clin. Oncol., 100:95, 1981.
469. Wagner, T., Heydrich, D., Voelcker, G., and Hohorst, H. J.: Characterization and quantitative estimation of activated cyclophosphamide in blood and urine. Cancer Res. Clin. Oncol., 96:79, 1980.
470. Walker, D. A., Pillow, J., Waters, K. D., and Keir, E.: Enhanced cis-platinum ototoxicity in children with brain tumours who have received simultaneous or prior cranial irradiation. Med. Pediatr. Oncol., 17:48, 1989.
471. Walker, M. D., Alexander, E., Jr., Hunt, W. E., MacCarty, C. S., Mahaley, M. S., Jr., Mealey, J., Jr., and Norrell, H. A., Owens, G., Ransohoff, J., Wilson, C. B., Gehan, E. A., and Strike, T. A.: Evaluation of BCNU and/or radiotherapy in the treatment of anaplastic gliomas. A cooperative clinical trial. J. Neurosurg., 49:333, 1978.
472. Wang, Y. Y., Teicher, B. A., Shea, T. C., Holden, S. A., Rosbe, K. W., al-Achi, A., and Henner, W. D.: Cross-resistance and glutathione-S-transferase-pi levels among four human melonoma cell lines selected for alkylating agent resistance. Cancer Res., 49:6185, 1989.
473. Waud, W. R.: Differential uptake of cis-diamminedichloroplatinum (II) by sensitive and resistant murine L1210 leukemia cells. Cancer Res., 47:6549, 1987.
474. Whittle, I. R., MacPherson, J. S., Miller, J. D., and Smyth, J. F.: The disposition of TCNU (tauromustine) in human malignant glioma. J. Neurosurg., 72:721, 1990.
475. Wils, J., and Bleiberg, H.: Current status of chemotherapy for gastric cancer. Eur. J. Cancer Clin. Oncol., 25:3, 1989.
476. Wiltshaw, E.: Chlorambucil in the treatment of primary adenocarcinoma of the ovary. J. Obstet. Gynecol. Br. Commonw., 72:586, 1964.
477. Wolpert, M. K., and Ruddon, R. W.: A study on the mechanisms of resistance to nitrogen mustard (HN2) in Ehrlich ascites tumor cells: Comparison of uptake of HN2-^{14}C. Cancer Res., 29:873, 1969.
478. Wright, C. G., and Schaefer, S. D.: Inner ear histopathology in patients treated with cis-platinum. Laryngoscope, 92:1408, 1982.
479. Yamada, K., Bremer, A. M., West, C. R., Ghoorah, J., Park, H. C., and Takita, H.: Intra-arterial BCNU therapy in the treatment of metastatic brain tumor from lung carcinoma. Cancer, 44:2000, 1979.
480. Young, R. C., Walton, L. A., Ellenberg, S. S., Homesley, H. D., Wilbanks, G. D., Decker, D. G., Miller, A., Park, R., and Major, F., Jr.: Adjuvant therapy in stage I and stage II epithelial ovarian cancer. N. Engl. J. Med., 322:1021, 1990.
481. Yuan, Z. M., Fenselau, C., Dulik, D. M., Martin, W., Emary, W. B., Brundrett, R. B., Colvin, O. M., and Cotter, R. J.: Laser desorption electron impact: application to a study of the mechanism of conjugation of glutathione and cyclophosphamide. Anal. Chem., 62:868, 1990.
482. Yung, W. K., Harris, M. I., Bruner, J. M., and Feun, L. G.: Intravenous BCNU and AZQ in patients with recurrent malignant gliomas. N. Neurooncol., 7:237, 1989.
483. Zelazowski, A. J., Garvey, J. S., and Hoeschele, J. D.: In vivo and in vitro binding of platinum to metallothionein. Arch. Biochem. Biophys., 229:246, 1984.
484. Zon, G., Ludeman, S. M., Brandt, J. A., Boyd, V. L., Ozkan, G., Egan, W., and Shao, K. L.: NMR spectroscopic studies of intermediary metabolites of cyclophosphamide. A comprehensive kinetic analysis of the interconversion of cis- and trans-4-hydroxycyclophosphamide with aldophosphamide and the concomitant partitioning of aldophosphamide between irreversible fragmentation and reversible conjugation pathways. J. Med. Chem., 27:466, 1984.
485. Zwelling, L. A., Anderson, T., and Kohn, K. W.: DNA-protein and DNA interstrand cross-linking by cis- and trans-platinum (II) diamminedichloride in L1210 mouse leukemia cells and relation to cytotoxicity. Cancer Res., 39:365, 1979.

Dacarbazine, Procarbazine, Hexamethylmelamine

Steven D. Averbuch

Introduction

The classical alkylating agents discussed in Chapter XVI-3 are commonly used drugs that usually contain two chloroethyl groups and their biological activity is a result of bifunctional alkylation of DNA. In contrast, there is a distinct group of less commonly used but clinically important compounds that have monofunctional covalent binding capacity. These compounds include dacarbazine, procarbazine, and hexamethylmelamine. They are often referred to as "non-classical alkylating agents." Although they are structurally dissimilar, they share a common structural feature in a N-methyl group which is important for activity.[143]

Historically, each of these agents arose from chemical synthetic programs based on rationales that were somewhat different from the end result. Dacarbazine was synthesized in the late 1950s as an analogue of 5-amino-imidazole-4-carboxamide (AIC), an intermediate in purine ring synthesis, as an attempt to develop agents capable of interfering with endogenous synthesis of purines.[139] Procarbazine was synthesized as part of an effort to develop new monoamine oxidase inhibitors and was found to have antitumor activity in preclinical testing.[15,16,210] Hexamethylmelamine, a structural analogue of the alkylating agent, triethylenemelamine, was synthesized in the early 1950's and it was initially shown to have activity against experimental rodent sarcomas.[31,109]

Dacarbazine (5-(3,3-Dimethyl-1-triazeno)-imidazole-4-carboxamide, DTIC, DIC, NSC-45388)

Chemistry and Structure Activity Relationships

The 5-diazoimidazole derivative of the purine precursor 5-amino-imidazole-4-carboxamide (AIC) has antitumor activity. The addition of a dimethyl substituted third nitrogen group to form the triazene analogue, dacarbazine, results in a stable, but light sensitive derivative that has clinical activity (Figure XVI-4-1).[177] N-substitution of the triazeno group results in analogues which are active in preclinical testing; however, increasing the alkyl side-chain length beyond pentyl weakened the antitumor activity against Ehrlich carcinoma.[177,205] Lipophilic and steric properties caused by triazene structural alterations also may determine its oxidative metabolism and antitumor activity.[155,190,206] At the present time, dacarbazine remains the only dimethyl-triazene available for clinical use.

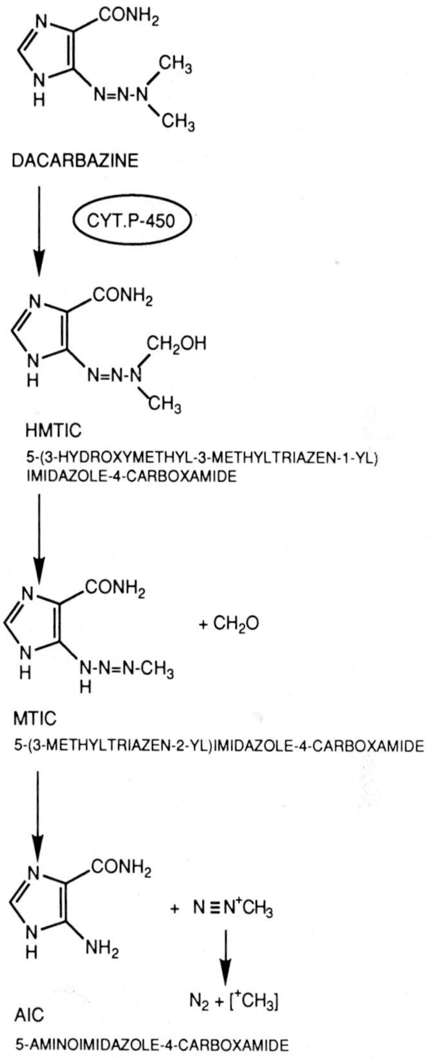

Cellular Pharmacology

Mechanisms of Action. Most studies in tissue culture show that the parent dacarbazine compound has little activity; and it is fairly well established that host metabolic activation to a methylating species is necessary for antitumor activity.[9,43,67,135,166,168,172,183] Alkylation of nucleic acids and the production of alkali-labile DNA lesions have been dem-

Figure XVI-4-1. Pathway for metabolic activation of dacarbazine. Brackets indicate postulated but unidentified reactive intermediate.

onstrated in vitro, and ^{14}C labeled 7-methylguanine has been recovered from urine in humans following ^{14}C labeled dacarbazine administration.[124,141,166,183]

Early studies showing direct cytotoxicity with dacarbazine were most likely the result of light activation of the parent compound to toxic species in vitro.[9,135,166,167] However, dacarbazine may have direct DNA damaging effects in the presence of functioning DNA polymerase α.[123] The mechanism for cellular uptake of dacarbazine or its activated metabolic intermediates has not been studied. Dacarbazine appears to be active in all phases of the cell cycle and it may cause progression delay through G2.[167,207]

In addition to its cytotoxic activity, dacarbazine can inhibit metastatic spread of experimental tumors and increase survival time in vivo.[169] These effects may be related to a multiplicity of immunogenic properties ascribed to the triazenes.[19,71,85,130,169]

Mechanisms of Resistance. Knowledge regarding the mechanisms of cellular resistance to dacarbazine is incomplete. Tumor cell resistance to triazenes in vitro has been associated with an increase in calmodulin mediated DNA excision-repair enzymes or a decrease in DNA polymerase α.[100,167] As for procarbazine (*vide infra*), several recent studies suggest that increased levels of the DNA repair enzyme O^6-alkylguanine-DNA alkyltransferase may be a determinant of tumor cell resistance to dacarbazine.[74,128,133]

Metabolism and Clinical Pharmacology

The metabolic pathway for dacarbazine is shown in Figure XVI-4-1. Dacarbazine activation requires an initial oxidation of a N-methyl group by microsomal NADPH cytochrome P-450 mixed-function oxidase to form the hydroxymethyl metabolite HMTIC.[190,197] Loss of formaldehyde results in the formation of the monomethyl metabolite MTIC, which then spontaneously tautomerizes to AIC and the methyldiazonium ion, $CH_3N^+{\equiv}N$, which is the active methylating agent.[43,67,135,168,183] The question has been raised as to whether nucleophilic alkylation by MTIC directly may explain the antitumor specificity of dacarbazine.[67,102]

The major metabolite of dacarbazine found in plasma and urine is AIC (Figure XVI-4-1), with cumulative excretion in the urine accounting for 9–20% of parent compound in several patients that were studied.[22,105,183,184] AIC is also formed from dacarbazine in the presence of liver microsomes and by some tumor cells in vitro.[124] A small fraction of radiolabeled dacarbazine recovered as expired radiolabeled CO_2 is presumably derived from formaldehyde produced in the course of dacarbazine catabolism.[105,185]

Dacarbazine pharmacokinetics and metabolism have been studied utilizing radiochemical, colorimetric, HPLC, and mass spectroscopic methods producing variable results.[12,22,67,70,105,183-186] After oral administration, the drug is absorbed slowly and variably; therefore, intravenous administration is the preferred route.[125,186] Following intravenous administration of dacarbazine, Breithaupt and coworkers found a biphasic plasma disappearance of the parent drug with a distribution half-life of 3 min. and an elimination half-life of 41 min.[22] Approximately 20% of dacarbazine is loosely bound to plasma protein.[125] The mean volume of distribution for dacarbazine was 0.6 liter per kg, a volume exceeding total body water, and the total body clearance was 15.4 ml per kg × min.[22] Approximately 50% of an intravenous dose of dacarbazine was recovered in the urine and the renal clearance was calculated to be between 5 and 10 ml per kg × min, consistent with earlier reports that tubular secretion may be involved in the renal excretion of dacarbazine.[22,125,186] Altered schedules of intravenous drug administration did not change the area under the curve (concentration × time), confirming a lack of schedule dependence for dacarbazine pharmacokinetics.[22]

Hepatobiliary excretion of dacarbazine is probably of some importance, but this has not been adequately studied. A patient with hepatic and renal dysfunction was reported to have an increased dacarbazine plasma half-life.[124] In several species, dacarbazine shows poor penetration into the cerebrospinal fluid with a ratio between plasma and spinal fluid of 1:7.[125] This finding is surprising considering that dacarbazine has activity against some CNS tumors in mice and that the drug may have activity against primary and metastatic brain tumors in humans.[42,63,66,169,198]

Toxicity and Drug Interactions

The most frequent toxicity of dacarbazine treatment is moderately severe nausea and vomiting, which occurs in 90% of patients.[126,140] These symptoms appear soon after infusion and they may persist for up to 12 hours. The severity of gastrointestinal toxicity may decrease with successive doses when the drug is given on a five-day schedule.[140] Following rapid infusion of a high dose of dacarbazine (>1,380 mg/M^2), hypotension may occur.[32]

Myelosuppression is a common, dose-related toxicity of dacarbazine when given above 1000 mg/M^2. The degree of leukopenia and thrombocytopenia is variably mild to moderate with sufficient recovery so that dacarbazine may be administered every 21–28 days. Occasionally, marrow recovery may take up to six weeks.[126] Less frequent toxicities include a flu-like syndrome of fever up to 39°C, myalgias, and malaise lasting several days after dacarbazine treatment. Headache, facial flushing, facial paresthesias, pain along the injection vein, alopecia, and abnormal hepatic and renal function tests rarely occur.

Photosensitivity to dacarbazine has been reported in several patients, especially after high dose therapy.[32,176] This toxicity was reproduced in an animal model and it is probably due to the fact that dacarbazine is photodecomposed to toxic intermediates.[57] Therefore, patients should be advised to avoid sunlight exposure for several days after dacarbazine therapy. Recently, cases of hepatic vascular toxicity associated with fever, eosinophilia, hepatic necrosis and death, have been attributed to dacarbazine as a distinct clinical pathological syndrome.[90,131,134]

Dacarbazine has mutagenic, carcinogenic, and teratogenic properties in experimental systems.[10,172,194] It is not known whether dacarbazine is carcinogenic for humans. In a retrospective analysis of patients receiving dacarbazine-containing chemotherapy for Hodgkin's disease, Valagussa and colleagues reported no treatment associated secondary cancers.[196] Isolated cases of acute leukemia occurring after dacarbazine therapy have been reported but a causal association with dacarbazine was not established.[28,33] Teratogenic effects were observed following dacarbazine administration to pregnant rats and rabbits, however, the implications of these observations for human teratogenicity is unknown.[195]

In regard to drug interactions, patients receiving Corynebacterium parvum adjuvant immunotherapy did have a prolongation of dacarbazine serum half-life consistent with C. parvum's ability to depress hepatic microsomal N-demethylation of a variety of drugs.[12,121] The interaction of phenobarbital or other commonly used cytochrome P-450 inducing agents with dacarbazine has not been reported.

Dacarbazine activity against L1210 murine leukemia was potentiated by melphalan and by doxorubicin.[139] Activity was also enhanced when dacarbazine was combined with the nitrosoureas, BCNU or CCNU. The mechanism(s) for the potentiation observed using these combinations has not been studied, yet it is of interest that these combinations have clinical activity against Hodgkin's disease, sarcoma, and melanoma. Preliminary results suggest that the combination of dacarbazine with biological agents such as recombinant alpha interferon or interleukin-2 may have enhanced activity against metastatic melanoma.[72,200]

Clinical Use

Dacarbazine is supplied in sterile vials containing 100 mg or 200 mg of dacarbazine for intravenous administration. After reconstitution the drug should be protected from light. It is most frequently used at a dose of 250 mg/M² daily for five days every three to four weeks.[32,126,149] The latter schedule was developed in an attempt to minimize the gastrointestinal toxicity. However, most studies fail to show any significant schedule dependency with respect to antitumor efficacy or toxicity.[149] There are no specific guidelines for dacarbazine dosing in hepatic or renal dysfunction. However, dose modifications may be necessary in some patients with moderately severe liver and/or renal abnormalities.

Dacarbazine is an active single agent in the treatment of metastatic malignant melanoma, producing remissions in the range of 16–31% of patients with this disease.[42] It is also active as a single agent in pretreated patients with Hodgkin's disease.[78] Thus, in the United States, dacarbazine is approved for use in these two diseases. It is frequently used alone or in combination with a variety of agents, such as, nitrosoureas, bleomycin, and vinca alkaloids in the treatment of melanoma, and it is commonly used as part of the ABVD regimen for Hodgkin's disease.[17,18,34,63,119,149] Dacarbazine has demonstrated activity in the treatment of sarcomas, childhood neuroblastoma, primary brain tumors, and it may be the most active agent alone or in combination for the treatment of malignant APUD and other neuroendocrine tumors.[6,7,66,69,88,95,111,126] Dacarbazine has also been used by intra-arterial infusion for the regional treatment of malignant melanoma with high response rates in uncontrolled series.[1,64] These results are difficult to interpret since dacarbazine requires metabolic activation in the liver for its antitumor activity.

Procarbazine: (N-isopropyl-alpha-(2-methylhydrazine)-p-toluamide, Ibenzmethyzin, Natulan, Matulane, NSC-77213)

Chemistry and Structure Activity Relationships

Procarbazine is a structural modification of 1-methyl-2-benzyl hydrazine, a monoamine oxidase inhibitor found to have potent antitumor activity.[16] It exists as the hydrochloride salt which is unstable in aqueous solutions. In the presence of light specific breakdown products appear.[89,145,150,201] The route of chemical decompostion is not important for the biological activity of procarbazine which must undergo cytochrome P-450 mediated metabolism to cytotoxic species in vivo (Figure XVI-4-2).[61,94,115,137,150,151,201] The N-methyl structure is a prerequisite for activity and among hydrazine analogs with this structure, the presence of a benzyl ring appears to confer the highest antitumor properties.[210]

Cellular Pharmacology

Mechanisms of Action. Most of the studies on procarbazine mechanism of action have focused on intermediates produced by hepatic or erythrocyte microsomal metabolism.

Some of these metabolites have been proposed as the active species capable of covalently binding cellular macromolecules, although It is not clear which of the many identified metabolic products are responsible for this cytotoxic activity.[46,143,150,179]

The production of alkylating intermediates appears to be necessary for procarbazine's anticancer activity. These alkylating species have not been clearly identified, although a methyl carbonium and/or a benzaldehyde derivative have been proposed.[138,150] The methylation of nucleic acid bases occurs through direct transfer of the N-methyl group and may also occur through folate incorporation during de novo purine synthesis.[113] A methyl radical or a carbon-centered free radical may also be involved in mediating procarbazine's anticancer activity.[138,182]

Several additional cellular effects of procarbazine and its metabolites have been demonstrated, although it is unclear whether these contribute directly to cytotoxicity. Procarbazine and its metabolites are capable of causing chromatid and single strand DNA breaks in murine tumor cells in vitro.[65,150] Procarbazine can also inhibit DNA, RNA, and protein synthesis in vitro and in vivo.[94,165] Procarbazine appears to inhibit normal tRNA methylation and the resulting altered tRNA synthesis and function may well account for some of the effects on nucleic acid and protein synthesis.[113]

The parent drug procarbazine is taken up into cells by passive diffusion.[117] Since procarbazine activation occurs following hepatic metabolism its cellular uptake is probably not important, except for the observation that human leukemia cells are capable of metabolizing procarbazine to cytotoxic species.[192]

Mechanisms of Resistance. Resistance develops rapidly in tumor cells following exposure to procarbazine and one study suggested a direct correlation between the rate of DNA synthesis and the rapidity of resistance development.[15,94] As for dacarbazine (vide supra), cellular levels of O⁶-alkylguanine-DNA alkyltransferase, an enzyme involved in DNA repair, may be a determinant in tumor sensitivity to procarbazine.[173] Procarbazine is not cross-resistant to alkylating agents or other major classes of anticancer agents.[187]

Metabolism and Clinical Pharmacology

The metabolism and pharmacokinetics of procarbazine have been studied mostly in laboratory animals and, to a lesser extent in humans, by high pressure liquid chromatography (HPLC) and mass spectroscopy.[8,46,58,61,89,115,145,151,154,174,179,201]

The complex pharmacokinetic and excretion characteristics of procarbazine reflect the rapid and extensive enzymatic metabolism of this compound which is necessary for antitumor activity and presumably for host organ toxicities. The oxidation of procarbazine to azoprocarbazine occurs by microsomal cytochrome P-450 oxidoreductase or by mitochondrial monoamine oxidase enzymatic conversion (Figure XVI-4-2).[8,44,61,152] Several lines of evidence have confirmed that the liver is the predominant site of the initial metabolism of procarbazine.[61,65,115,137,150,151] Subsequent N-oxidation results in the formation of methylazoxy and benzylazoxy isomers (Figure XVI-4-2).[46,61,153] It has been proposed that carbon hydroxylation of either azoxyisomer results in unstable compounds that react to produce a reactive alkylating alkyldiazonium ion. It now appears that the methylazoxy isomer is probably the metabolite which accounts for procarbazine's

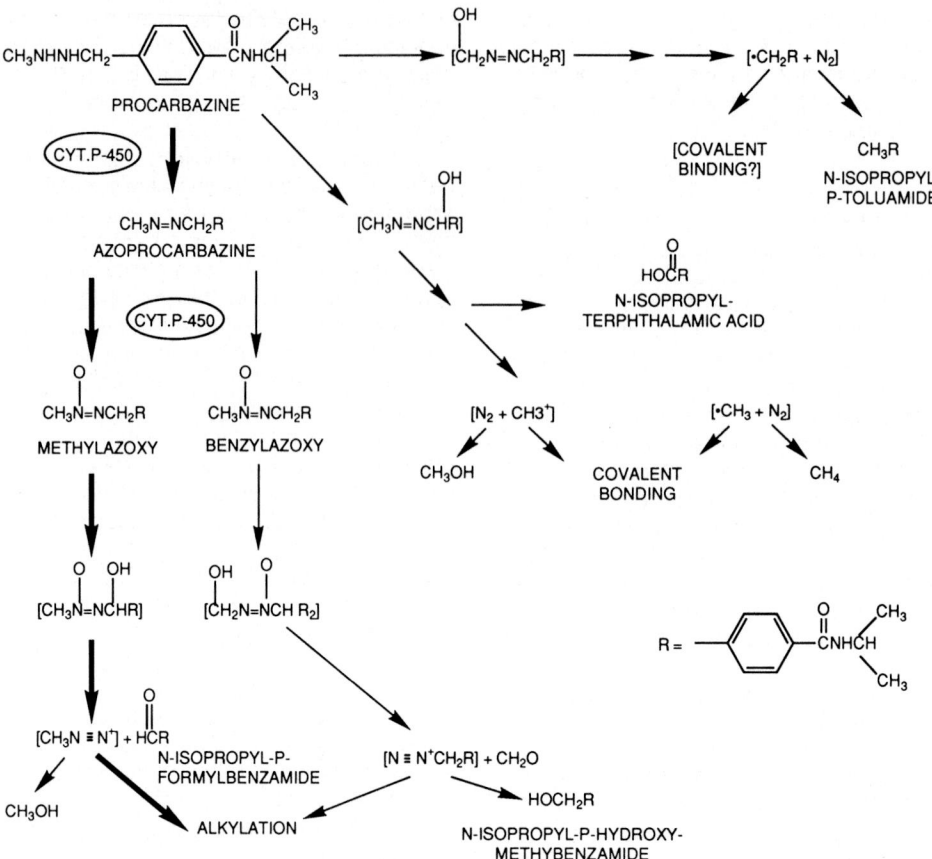

Figure XVI-4-2. Possible pathways for metabolic activation of procarbazine. The pathway indicated by bold arrows is the one most likely responsible for the alkylating activity of procarbazine. Brackets indicate postulated but unidentified reactive intermediates.

cytotoxicity.[65,193] Further microsomal metabolism of the azoxy compounds results in formation of N-isopropyl-p-formylbenzamide or N-isopropyl-p-hydroxymethylbenzamide and these compounds are then oxidized to the major urinary metabolite, N-isopropyl-terephthalamic acid.[46,150,154,179] Alternative pathways involving oxidation of the benzyl carbon atom or the methyl carbon adjacent to the azo function have also been proposed for metabolic activation of procarbazine (Figure XVI-4-2).[8,58,83,138,150,174,201]

Following oral administration, the drug is rapidly and completely absorbed from the gastrointestinal tract. The biodistribution of procarbazine is not well studied. There is rapid equilibration between plasma and cerebrospinal fluid in dogs and humans.[145] Following the intravenous administration of 150 mg ^{14}C-procarbazine, the plasma half-life of parent drug was approximately 7 minutes in humans.[154] Since single bolus intravenous doses of procarbazine produce a spectrum of toxicity, primarily neurotoxicity, distinct from the myelosuppression seen after oral administration, it is likely that a "first pass" effect of the drug through the portal circulation significantly influences drug metabolism and pharmacokinetics.[37] Preliminary data in humans show that the methylazoxy isomer is the major plasma metabolite following a single 250 mg/kg oral dose of procarbazine. This compound peaks at approximately 90 minutes and appears to have an initial plasma half-life of approximately 60 minutes. Azoprocarbazine and the benzylazoxy isomer are present in relatively equal but lesser concentrations compared to the meth-

ylazoxy isomer. Procarbazine treatment may alter its own metabolism which is reflected by increased azoprocarbazine plasma concentrations following repeated dosing.[179,180]

The major urinary metabolite of procarbazine is the biologically inactive N-isopropyl-terephthalamic acid (Figure XVI-4-2).[8,145,154,174] Approximately 70% of adminstered procarbazine is recovered, primarily as the acid, in the urine during the first 24 hours. There is minimal fecal excretion (4–12% over 96 hours) and approximately 30% of radioactivity labeled in the N-methyl group appears as respiratory CO_2.[82,174]

Toxicity and Drug Interactions

Following intravenous administration, procarbazine causes neurotoxicity which is dose-limiting.[36,37] Since this route does not offer any benefit over oral administration, procarbazine is not used intravenously. Following oral administration, procarbazine causes anorexia, mild nausea and vomiting, probably of central origin, which often abates with continued use.[48] In some patients it is often helpful to escalate the dose in a stepwise fashion over the first several days of drug administration in order to minimize these gastrointestinal side effects. Mild to moderate myelosuppression in the form of reversible leukopenia and thrombocytopenia is the most common dose limiting toxicity of procarbazine given orally. Depression of peripheral leukocyte and platelet counts become apparent after one week of therapy and may persist for two weeks or longer after discontinuation of the drug.[103]

Procarbazine may also cause hemolysis in individuals with glucose-6-phosphate dehydrogenase deficiency.[189]

Patients receiving procarbazine orally may occassionally experience neurotoxicity manifest by drowsiness, depression, agitation, paresthesias of the extremities and reversible orthostatic hypotension.[164,203] These effects are likely a result of central monoamine oxidase inhibition and may be related to drug-induced depletion of pyridoxal phosphate.[36,38,49] The peripheral neuropathy caused by procarbazine may be prevented by administration of pyridoxine. Procarbazine may also cause hypersensitivity reactions including maculopapular skin rash, hypereosinophilia, pulmonary infiltrates, or, rarely, transient hepatic dysfunction.[24,27,132,203] The skin rash usually responds to concomitant glucocorticosteroid treatment and the procarbazine may be continued. In contrast, procarbazine-induced interstitial pneumonitis usually requires discontinuation of the drug.

Procarbazine has potent immunosuppressive properties which may contribute to the infectious complications that patients experience as a result of myelosuppressive antineoplastic chemotherapy.[122] Although these immunosuppressive properties were useful in the past for the treatment of lupus erythematosus and in the suppression of graft versus host disease following bone marrow transplantation, procarbazine should not be used for non-neoplastic diseases since superior alternatives for immunosuppressive therapy are available.[191]

Chronic and late toxicities of procarbazine result from its profound azospermic, teratogenic, mutagenic and carcinogenic properties.[40,41,81,110,148,181] Over 90% of men receiving procarbazine in combination with classical alkylating agents, such as in MOPP combination chemotherapy for Hodgkin's disease, have prolonged or irreversible azoospermia while approximately 50% of women have permanent drug-induced ovarian failure.[39,104,170,171] Since procarbazine causes congenital skeletal and central nervous system abnormalities in pregnant animals, women of child-bearing capacity should be advised against pregnancy while receiving procarbazine.[40,108]

Mutagenesis and carcinogenesis resulting from procarbazine have been demonstrated experimentally.[81,110] The increased incidence of secondary leukemias and other cancers in patients following treatment with MOPP combination chemotherapy has accordingly implicated procarbazine as the responsible oncogen.[86,101] Since this regimen also contains an alkylating agent with oncogenic properties it is difficult to assign a direct causal effect to procarbazine alone.[87,101]

Other drugs inactivated by microsomal metabolism may be inhibited in the presence of procarbazine; therefore, patients taking barbiturates, phenothiazines, narcotics and other hypnotics or sedatives may experience potentiated effects of these agents.[118,145,156] Conversely, drugs which affect hepatic metabolism, may increase or decrease procarbazine metabolism and thereby alter procarbazine activity and toxicity.[98,175] For example, phenobarbital or phenytoin pretreatment increased the survival of tumor-bearing mice treated with procarbazine, presumably due to microsomal enzyme induction resulting in increased production of active procarbazine metabolites.[180] It is not known whether this biochemical modulation of procarbazine activity would offer similar therapeutic advantage in humans.

The CNS depression caused by procarbazine-induced monoamine oxidase inhibition and pyridoxal phosphate depletion may also potentiate the sedative effects of other CNS depressants.[38,49] The inhibition of monoamine oxidase also predisposes patients to acute hypertensive reactions following concomitant therapy with tricyclic antidepressants and sympathomimetic drugs as well as following ingestion of tyramine-rich containing foods, such as, red wine, bananas, ripe cheese, and yogurt. A disulfiram-like reaction, manifest by sweating, facial flushing, and headache may occur in patients who ingest alcohol while taking procarbazine.

Clinical Use

Procarbazine hydrochloride is supplied in capsules containing the equivalent of 50 mg. of the base for oral administration. As a single agent, the usual dose is 100–200 mg/M^2 of body surface area given daily until myelosuppression occurs. As part of the MOPP combination regimen for Hodgkin's disease, the daily dose of procarbazine is 100 mg/M^2 of body surface area daily for 14 days.[50]

Early clinical trials demonstrated significant efficacy for procarbazine in the treatment of Hodgkin's Disease and lymphomas with little activity shown against most carcinomas.[27,132,164,188] It is still widely used in combination with other agents in the treatment of Hodgkin's and non-Hodgkin's lymphomas, and it is used to a lesser extent in brain tumors, small cell lung carcinoma, and melanoma.[35,47,50,51,82,127]

Hexamethylmelamine: (HMM, NSC-13875)

Chemistry and Structure Activity Relationships

Hexamethylmelamine (HMM) is a dimethylamino substituted s-triazine analogue (Figure XVI-4-3). The urinary metabolite, pentamethylmelamine (PMM) has a therapeutic index equal to HMM in rodents but it causes significant toxicity in humans.[75] For these compounds the in vivo antitumor activity declines as a function of the number of methyl groups.[45,116] Thus, tetramethylmelamine retained some activity, but trimethylmelamine was inactive, and substitution of the methyl group with ethyl or other constituents also rendered the compound inactive.[161] A symmetrical trimethyl trihydroxymethyl analogue that does not require metabolic activation, has been synthesized and has been shown to possess equivalent or superior activity to HMM in preclinical studies.[21,45,162]

Cellular Pharmacology

Mechanisms of Action. Since N-methyl substitution is a requirement for activity, it was originally thought that the HMM methyl groups were the source of reactive alkylating species. However, neither HMM nor its metabolites showed reactivity with 4-(p-nitrobenzyl)pyridine, an acceptor for alkylating species, in a chemical assay.[208] HMM undergoes extensive demethylation with the formation of formaldehyde in vivo (Figure XVI-4-3).[160,161,162,208,209] It is unlikely that the formaldehyde formed from HMM metabolism is responsible for cytotoxicity.[158,159,162] Alternatively, the N-hydroxy metabolite, N-hydroxymethyl-pentamethyl-melamine (HMPMM) has been suggested as an active intermediate that has cytotoxic activity in vitro and antitumor activity in vivo.[52,136,158,161] HMPMM has been identified as a metabolite of HMM both in vitro and in vivo.[59,84] HMM and HMPMM have also been shown to inhibit DNA and RNA synthesis.[159]

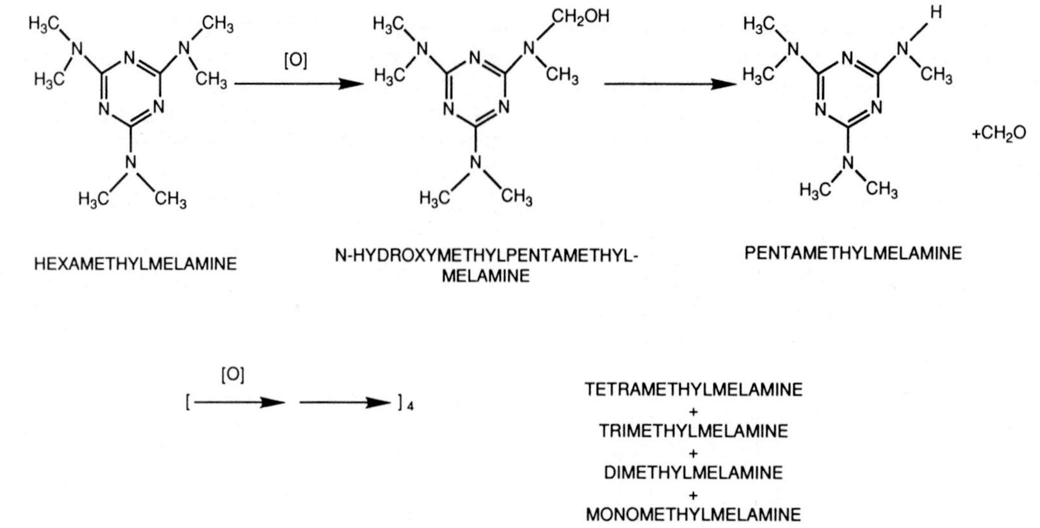

Figure XVI-4-3.   Metabolic pathway for hexamethylmelamine resulting in demethylated metabolites.

HMM appears to enter cells by simple diffusion and some tumor cells have been shown to metabolize HMM and PMM in vitro, while others do not seem to have this property.[11,52,136,160]

Mechanisms of Resistance. Very little is known about cellular mechanisms of HMM resistance except for the fact that, clinically, many alkylator resistant tumors do not exhibit cross resistance to HMM, and that Chinese Hamster Ovary cells with a multidrug resistant phenotype do not exhibit cross-resistance to HMM.[93,106,146,199]

Metabolism and Clinical Pharmacology

Studies in multiple species have demonstrated rapid and extensive metabolism of HMM.[2,11,20,23,59,84,99,112,136,147,158,161,162,208,209] The metabolic route based on these studies is summarized in Figure XVI-4-3. Sequential microsomal N-demethylation takes place following hydroxylation of the methyl group. The latter reaction is catalyzed by inducible, NADPH-dependent cytochrome P-450 which appears to be regulated by cellular glutathione.[20,23] Mitochrondial metabolism of HMM has also been demonstrated in hepatic and intestinal preparations. In contrast to 5-azacytidine, the s-triazine ring of HMM is not metabolically cleaved.[209]

The metabolism and pharmacokinetics of HMM have been studied extensively in experimental animals and in humans using several analytical techniques.[3,20,30,59] Following oral administration, HMM was shown to have an extremely variable bioavailability with a 100-fold variation in peak blood levels.[53] This variable bioavailability is probably due to extensive first-pass hepatic metabolism or intestinal wall metabolism, rather than poor absorption.[2,112] In patients, the peak plasma levels were achieved 0.5–3 hours after the oral dose with concentrations ranging between 0.2– 20.8 μg/ml The initial half-life of parent drug plasma disappearance in one study was 0.5 hours and in several studies, the terminal half-life varied between 4.7–13 hours.[53,54,76,244] Approximately 94% of HMM is highly bound to serum protein.[23] Benvenuto and coworkers have shown considerable variation in the pharmacokinetic behavior of each demethylated HMM metabolite.[13]

Following an oral dose in a small series of patients, the highest concentration of HMM was found in tissues containing significant fat content while lower concentrations (equal to plasma) were found in primary tumor.[55] Small metastatic deposits contained signficantly higher HMM concentrations compared to larger metastases or primary tumor. In one patient, HMM measured in cerebrospinal fluid was found to be 6% of the plasma concentration while the less methylated melamine metabolites were found in the CSF in higher concentrations with CSF/plasma ratios approaching 1.[56]

The major elimination route for HMM is hepatic metabolism, with less than 1% of parent compound found in the urine.[2,4,208,209] The majority (approximately 70–90%) of administered drug was ultimately accounted for in the urine when radiolabel recovery of total drug and metabolites were measured.[2] Up to 30% of the administered dose was recovered as respiratory $^{14}CO_2$ only if the N-methyl group contained the radiolabel rather than the triazene ring.[208] There is minimal fecal elimination of HMM.

Toxicity and Drug Interactions

The major toxicity of HMM is dose-limiting gastrointestinal toxicity consisting of nausea and vomiting, anorexia, and diarrhea, which may worsen with cumulative dosing.[75,76,106,204] The mechanism for this toxicity is most likely due to CNS effects. Another consequence of high CNS drug and metabolite concentrations is a 25% or greater incidence of neurotoxicity (consisting of mood changes, such as lethargy, depression, agitation, hallucinations, and peripheral neuropathy).[75,76,204]

Prolonged administration of HMM also results in myelosuppression with leukopenia observed more frequently than thrombocytopenia.[204] This is rarely a dose-limiting toxicity and it may be avoided with shorter courses of treatment. Cutaneous hypersensitivity is rarely observed after HMM. The immunologic, mutagenic, and carcinogenic activities of HMM have not been well studied and its association with secondary cancers is not established.[5,91,107]

In rodents, pretreatment with phenobarbital enhances HMM microsomal metabolism and antagonizes HMM antitumor activity.[147] Whether similar effects occur in humans is not known. Hande and coworkers recently showed that cimetidine, through inibition of microsomal metabolism, causes a dose-dependent prolongation of HMM half-life which was associated with increased toxicity.[99] HMM pharmacokinetics are not altered by concomitant doxorubicin or cyclophosphamide administration.[54]

Clinical Use

Because of its poor aqueous solubility, HMM is supplied in capsules of 50 mg and 100 mg for oral administration. To overcome the highly variable bioavailability of oral HMM, a parenteral formulation has been developed and is currently undergoing clinical evaluation.[4] Usual doses are 4–12 mg per kg daily for 14–21 days each month, although longer periods of continuous administration have been used.[76,106] In December 1990, HMM was approved by the FDA for use in the United States. As a single agent, HMM has activity against advanced ovarian cancer with an overall objective response rate of 21%.[14,76] In selected, previously untreated patients, the response rate exceeds 30%, with some patients observed to have pathologically proven complete remissions of modest duration.[204] The precise role for HMM in combination chemotherapy regimens for advanced ovarian cancer remains controversial, although these regimens clearly have high activity.[25,26,62,76,77,96,97,142] As second line therapy in ovarian carcinoma, HMM has demonstrated activity in patients previously treated with alkylating agents or cisplatin.[106,129,146,157,199] HMM may have activity against non small cell and small cell lung carcinoma, breast cancer, endometrial cancer, refractory lymphomas, bilharzial bladder carcinoma, and, when combined with prednisone, possibly against multiple myeloma.[76,79,144]

References

1. Aigner, K., Hild, P., Henneking, K., Paul, E., and Hundeiker, M.: Regional perfusion with cisplatinum and dacarbazine. Recent Results. Cancer Res., 86:239, 1983.
2. Ames, M. M., Powis, G., Kovach, J. S., and Eagan, R. T.: Disposition and metabolism of pentamethylmelamine and hexamethylmelamine in rabbits and humans. Cancer Res., 39:5016, 1979.
3. Ames, M. M., and Powis, G.: Determination of pentamethylmelamine and hexamethylmelamine in plasma and urine by nitrogen-phosphorous gas-liquid chromatography. J. Chromatog., 174:245, 1979.
4. Ames, M. M., Richardson, R. L., Kovach, J. S., Moertel, C. G., and O'Connell, M. J.: Phase I and clinical pharmacological evaluation of a parenteral hexamethylmelamine formulation. Cancer Res., 50:206, 1990.
5. Ashby, J., Callander, R. D., and Rose, F. L.: Weak mutagenicity to salmonella of the formaldehyde-releasing anti-tumor agent hexamethylmelamine. Mutat. Res., 142:121, 1985.
6. Averbuch, S. D., Steakley, C. S., Young, R. C., Gelmann, E. P., Goldstein, D. S., Stull, R.S., and Keiser, H. R.: Malignant pheochromocytoma: Effective treatment with a combination of cyclophosphamide,vincristine, and dacarbazine. Ann. Int. Med., 109:267, 1988.
7. Averbuch, S., Wu, L., Pertsemlidis, D., and Drakes, T.: Cyclophosphamide (C), Vincristine (V), and Dacarbazine (D) for advanced neuroendocrine carcinomas. Proc. Am. Soc. Clin. Oncol., 9:A382, 1990.
8. Baggliolini, M., Bickel, H. M., and Messiha, F. S.: Demethylation in vivo of Natulan, a tumor-inhibiting methylhydrazine derivative. Experientia, 21:334, 1965.
9. Beal, D. D., Skibba, J. L., Whitnable, K. K., and Bryan, G. T.: Effects of 5-(3,3-dimethyl-1-triazeno)-imidazole-4-carboxamide and its metabolites on Novikoff hepatoma cells. Cancer Res., 36:2827, 1976.
10. Beal, D.D., Skibba, J. L., Croft, W. A., Cohen, S. M., and Bryan, G. T.: Carcinogenicity of the antineoplastic agent, 5-(3,3-dimethyl-1-triazeno)-imidazole-4-carboxamide, and its metabolites in rats. J. Natl. Cancer Inst., 54:951, 1975.
11. Begleiter, A., Grover, J., and Goldenberg, G. J.: Uptake and metabolism of hexamethylmelamine and pentamethylmelamine L5178Y lymphoblasts in vitro. Cancer Res., 40:4489, 1980.
12. Benvenuto, J. A., Hall, S. W., Farquhar, D., Lu, K., and Loo, T. L.: High-pressure liquid chromatography in pharmacological studies of anticancer drugs. Chromatogr. Sci., 10:377, 1979.
13. Benvenuto, J. A., Stewart, D. J., Benjamin, R. S., and Loo, T. L.: Pharmacology of pentamethylmelamine in humans. Cancer Res., 41:566, 1981.
14. Blum, R. H., Livingston, R. B., and Carter, S. K.: Hexamethylmelamine–a new drug with activity in solid tumors. Eur. J. Cancer, 9:195, 1973.
15. Bollag, W., and Grunberg, E.: Tumour inhibitory effects of a new class of cytotoxic agents: methylhydrazine derivatives. Experientia (Basel), 19:130, 1963.
16. Bollag, W.: The tumor-inhibitory effects of the methylhydrazine derivative Ro 4-6467/1 (NSC-77213). Cancer Chemother. Rep., 33:1, 1963.
17. Bonadonna, G., Zucali, R., Monfardini, S., De Lena, M., and Uslenghi, C.: Combination chemotherapy of Hodgkin's disease with adriamycin, bleomycin, vinblastive and imidazole carboxamide versus MOPP. Cancer, 36:252, 1975.
18. Bonadonna, G., Valagussa, P., and Santoro, A.: Alternating non-cross-resistant com-
19. bination chemotherapy or MOPP in stage IV Hodgkin's disease: A report of 8-year results. Ann. Intern. Med., 104:739, 1986.
19. Bonmassar, E., Bonmassar, A., Vadlamudi, S., and Goldin, A.: Immunological alteration of leukemic cells in vitro after treatment with an antitumor drug. Proc. Natl. Acad. Sci. U.S.A., 66:1089, 1970.
20. Borm, P. J. A., Mingels, M. J. J., Frankhuijzen-Sierevogel, A. C., van Graft, M., Hulshoff, A., and Noordhoek, J.: Cellular and subcellular studies of the biotransformation of hexamethylmelamine in rat and isloated hepatocytes and intestinal epithelial cells. Cancer Res., 44:2820, 1984.
21. Boven, E., Nauta, M. M., Schluper, H. M. M., Erkelens, C. A. M., and Pinedo, H. M.: Superior efficacy of trimelamol to hexamethylmelamine in human ovarian cancer xenografts. Cancer Chemother. Pharmacol., 18:124, 1986.
22. Breithaupt, H., Dammann, A., and Aigner, K.: Pharmacokinetics of dacarbazine (DTIC) and its metabolite 5-aminoimidazole-4-carboxamide (AIC) following different dose schedules. Cancer Chemother. Pharmacol., 9:103, 1982.
23. Broggini, M., Colombo, T., D'Incalci, M., Donellis, M. G., Gescher, A., and Garattini, S.: Pharmacokinetics of hexamethylmelamine and pentamethylmelamine in mice. Cancer Treat. Rep., 65:669, 1981.
24. Brooks Jr., B. J., Hendler, N. B., Alvarez, S., Anealmo, N., and Grinton, S. F.: Delayed life-threatening pneumonitis secondary to procarbazine. Am. J. Clin. Oncol., 13:244, 1990..
25. Bruckner, H. W.: Role of hexamethylmelamine in the treatment of ovarian cancer: Where is the needle in the haystack? Cancer Treat. Rep., 71:666, 1987.
26. Bruckner, H. W., Cohen, C. J., Feuer, E., and Holland, J. F.: Modulation and intensification of a cyclophosphamide, hexamethylmelamine, doxorubicin, and cisplatin ovarian cancer regimen. Obstet. Gynecol., 73:349, 1989.
27. Brunner, K. W., and Young, C. W.: A methylhydrazine derivative in Hodgkin's disease and other malignant neoplasms: Therapeutic and toxic effects studies in 51 patients. Ann. Int. Med., 63:69, 1965.
28. Brusamolino, E., Papa, G., Valagussa, P., Mandelli, F., Bernasconi, C., Marmont, A., Bonadonna, G., Tura, S., Bosi, A., Mango, G., Mazza, P., Rossi,. E, Leoni, F., D'Onofrio, G., and D'Arcangelo, S.: Treatment-related leukemia in Hodgkin's disease: A multi-institution study on 75 cases. Hematol. Oncol., 5:83, 1987.
29. Bryan, G. T., Worzalla, J. F., Gorske, A. L., and Ramirez, G.: Plasma levels and urinary excretion of hexamethylmelamine following oral administration to human subjects with cancer. Clin. Pharmacol. Ther., 9:777, 1968.
30. Bryan, G. T., and Gorske, A. L.: Use of ion-exchange chromatography in the spectrophotometric assay for the antineoplastic agent, hexamethylmelamine, in biological fluids. J. Chromatog., 34:67, 1968.
31. Buckley, S. M., Srock, C. C., Crossley, M. L., and Rhoads, C. P.: Inhibition of the Crocker mouse sarcoma 180 by certain ethylenimine derivatives and related compounds. Cancer, 5:144, 1952.
32. Buesa, J. M., Gracia, M., Valle, M., Estrada, E., Hidalgo, O. F., and Lacave, A. J.: Phase I trial of intermittent high-dose dacarbazine. Cancer Treat. Rep., 68:499, 1984.
33. Carey, R. W., and Kunz, V. S.: Acute nonlymphocytic leukemia (ANLL) following treatment with dacarbazine for malignant melanoma. Amer. J. Hematol., 25:119, 1987.
34. Carey, R. W., Anderson, J. R., Green, M., Ellison, R. R., Nathanson, L., and Kennedy, B. J.: Treatment of metastatic malignant melanoma with vinblastine, dacarbazine, and cisplatin: A report from the cancer and leukemia group B. Cancer Treat. Rep., 70:329, 1986.
35. Carmo-Pereira, J., Costa, F. O., and Henriques, E.: Combination cytotoxic chemotherapy with procarbazine, vincristine, and lomustine in disseminated malignant melanoma: 8 years follow-up. Cancer Treat. Rep., 68:1211, 1984.
36. Casimir, A., Kavanagh, J., Liu, F., Hester, J., Bodey, G., and Valdivieso, M.: Phase I trial of intravenous procarbazine administered as a 5 day continuous infusion. Correlation with plasma levels of pyridoxal phosphate. Proc. Amer. Assoc. Cancer Res., 24:144, 1983.
37. Chabner, B. A., Sponzo, R., Hubbard, S., Canellos, G. P., Young, R. C., Schein, P. S., and DeVita, V. T.: High dose intermittent intravenous infusion of procarbazine (NSC-77213). Cancer Chemother. Rep., 57:361, 1973.
38. Chabner, B. A., DeVita, V. T., Considine, N., and Oliverio, V. T.: Plasma pyridoxal phosphate depletion by the carcinostatic procarbazine. Proc. Soc. Exp. Biol. Med., 132:1119, 1969.
39. Chapman, R. M.: Effect of cytotoxic therapy on sexuality and gonadal function. Sem. Oncol., 9:84, 1982.
40. Chaube, S., and Murphy, M.: Fetal malformations produced in rats by procarbazine. Teratology, 2:23, 1969.
41. Chryssanthou, C. P., Wallach, R. C. and Atchison, M.: Meiotic chromosomal changes and sterility produced by nitrogen mustard and procarbazine in mice. Fertil. Steril., 39:97, 1983.
42. Comis, R. L.: DTIC (NSC 45388) in malignant melanoma: A perspective. Cancer Treat. Rep., 60:165, 1976.
43. Connors, T. A., Goddard, P. M., Merai, K., Ross, W. C. J. and Wilman, D. E. V.: Tumour inhibitory triazenes: Structural requirements for an active metabolite. Biochem. Pharmacol., 25:241, 1976.
44. Coomes, M. W., and Prough, R. A.: The mitochondrial metabolism of 1,2-disubstituted hydrazines, procarbazine and 1,2-dimethylhydrazine. Drug Metab. Dispos., 11:550, 1983.
45. Cumber, A. J., and Ross, W. C. J: Analogues of hexamethylmelamine. The antineoplastic activity of derivatives with enhanced water solubility. Chem. Biol. Interact., 17:349, 1977.
46. Cummings, S. W., Guengerich, F. P., and Prough, R. A.: The characterisation of N-isopropyl-p-hydroxymethylbenzamide formed during the oxidative metabolism of azoprocarbazine. Drug Metab. Dispos., 10:459, 1982.
47. Daniels, J. R., Chak, L. Y., Sikic, B. I., Lockbaum, P., Kohler, M., Carter, S. K., Reynolds, R., Bohnen, R., Gandara, D., and Yu, J.: Chemotherapy of small cell carcinoma of lung. A randomized comparison of alternating and sequential combination chemotherapy programs. J. Clin. Oncol., 2:1192, 1984.
48. DeVita, V., Serpick, and Carbone, P.: Preliminary clinical studies with ibenzmethyzin. Clin. Pharmacol. Ther., 7:542, 1966.
49. DeVita, V., Hahn, M., and Oliverio, V.: Monoamine oxidase inhibition by a new carcinostatic agent, procarbazine. Proc. Soc. Exp. Biol. Med., 120:561, 1965.
50. DeVita, V. T., Serpick, A. A., and Carbone, P. P.: Combination chemotherapy in the treatment of advanced Hodgkin's disease. Ann. Int. Med., 73:881, 1970.
51. DeVita, V. T., Hubbard, S. M., and Longo, D. L.: The chemotherapy of lymphomas: Looking back, moving forward–The Richard and Hinda Rosenthal Foundation award lecture. Cancer Res., 47:5810, 1987.
52. D'Incalci, M., Erba, E., Balconi, G., Morasca, L., and Garattini, S.: Time dependence of the in vitro cytotoxicity of hexamethylmelamine and its metabolites. Br. J. Cancer, 41:630, 1980.

53. D'Incalci, M., Bolis, G., Mangioni, C., Morasca, L., and Garattini, S.: Variable oral absorption of hexamethylmelamine in man. Cancer Treat. Rep., 62:2117, 1978.
54. D'Incalci, M., Beggiolin, G., Sessa, C., and Mangioni, C.: Influence of ascites on the pharmacokinetics of hexamethylmelamine and N-demethylated metabolites in ovarian cancer patients. Eur. J. Clin. Oncol., 17:1331, 1981.
55. D'Incalci, M., Farina, P., Sessa, C., Mangioni, C., and Garattini, S.: Hexamethylmelamine distribution in patients with ovarian and other pelvic cancers. Cancer Treat. Rep., 66:231, 1982.
56. D'Incalci, M., Sessa, C., Begglilin, G., and Mangioni, C.: Cerebrospinal fluid levels of hexamethylmelamine and N-demethylated metabolites. Cancer Treat. Rep., 65:350, 1981.
57. Dorr, R. T., Soble, M., Alberts, D. S., Einspahr, J., Mason, N. L., and Liddil, J. D.: Experimental dacarbazine (DTIC) antitiumor activity and skin toxicity in relation to light exposure and pharmacologic antidotes. Cancer Treat. Rep., 71:267, 1987.
58. Dost, F. N., and Reed, D. J.: Methane formation in vivo from N-isopropyl-alpha-(2-methylhydrazino)-p-toluamide hydrochloride, a tumor-inhibiting methylhydrazine derivative. Biochem. Pharmacol., 16:1741, 1967.
59. Dubois J, Atassi G, Hanocq M and Abikhalil F: Pharmacokinetics and metabolism of hexamethylmelamine in mice bearing renal cell tumors. Cancer Chemother. Pharmacol., 22:282, 1988.
60. Dunagin, W.G.: Clinical toxicity of chemotherapeutic agents: Dermatologic toxicity.Sem Oncol 9:14, 1982.
61. Dunn, D. L., Lubet, R. A., and Prough, R. A.: Oxidative metabolism of N-isopropyl-alpha-(2-methyl-hydrazino)-p-toluamide hydrochloride (procarbazine) by rat liver microsomes. Cancer Res., 39:4555, 1979.
62. Edmonson, J. H., Wieand, H. S., and McCormack, G. W.: Role of hexamethylmelamine in the treatment of ovarian cancer: Where is the needle in the haystack? J. Natl. Cancer Inst., 80:1172, 1988.
63. Einhorn, L. H., and Furnas, B.: Combination chemotherapy for disseminated melanoma with DTIC, vincristine, and methyl-CCNU. Cancer Treat. Rep., 61:881, 1977.
64. Einhorn, L. H., McBride, C. M., Luke, J. K., Caoili, E., and Gottlieb, J. A.: Intra-arterial infusion therapy with 5-(3,3-dimethyl-1-triazeno)imidazole-4-carboxamide (NSC-45388) for malingnant melanoma. Cancer, 32:749, 1973.
65. Erikson, J. M., Tweedie, D. J., Ducore, J. M., and Prough, R. A.: Cytotoxicity and DNA damage caused by the azoxy metabolites of procarbazine in L1210 tumor cells. Cancer Res., 49:127, 1989.
66. Eyre, H. J., Eltringham, J. R., Gehan, E. A., Vogel, F. S., Al-Sarraf, M., Talley, R. W., Costanzi, J. J., Athens, J. W., Oishi, N., and Fletcher, W. S.: Randomized comparisons of radiotherapy and carmustine versus procarbazine versus dacarbazine for the treatment of malignant gliomas following surgery: A Southwest Oncology Group Study. Cancer Treat. Rep., 70:1085, 1986.
67. Farina, P., Benfenati, B. R., Torti, L., D'Incalci, M., Threadgill, M. D., and Gescher, A.: Metabolism of the anticancer agent 1-(4-acetylphenyl)-3,3-dimethyltriazene. Biomed. Mass Spectrom., 10:485, 1983.
68. Farina, P., Gescher, A., Hickman, J. A., Horton, J. K., D'Incalci, M., Ross, D., Stevens, M. F. G., and Torti, L.: Studies of the mode of action of the antitumour triazenes and triazines-IV. The metabolism of 1-(4-acetylphenyl)-3,3-dimethyltriazene. Biochem. Pharmacol., 31:1887, 1982.
69. Finklestein, J. Z., Klemperer, M. R., Evans, A., Bernstein, I., Leikin, S., McCreadie J., Grosfeld, J., Hittle, R., Weiner, J., Sather, H., and Hammond, D.: Multiagent chemotherapy for children with metastatic neuroblastoma: A report from Childrens Cancer Study Group. Med. Pediatr. Oncol., 6:179, 1979.
70. Fiore, D., Jackson, A. J., Didolkar, M. S., and Dandu, V. R.: Simultaneous determination of dacarbazine, its photolytic degradation product, 2-azahypoxanthine, and the metabolite 5-aminoimidazole-4-carboxamide in plasma and urine by high-pressure liquid chromatography. Antimicrob. Agents Chemother., 27:977, 1985.
71. Fioretti, M. C., Nardelli, B., Bianchi, R., Nisi, C., and Sava, G.: Antigenic changes of a murine lymphoma by in vivo treatment with triazene derivatives. Cancer Immunol. Immunother., 11:283, 1981.
72. Flaherty, L., Redman, B., Chabot, G., Martino, S., Valdivieso, M., and Bradley, E.: Combination of dacarbazine (DTIC) and interleukin-2 (IL-2) in metastatic malignant melanoma (MMM). Proc. Amer. Soc. Clin. Oncol., 7:254, 1988.
73. Fosch, P. J., Cazarnetzki, B. M., Macher, E., Grundmann, E., and Gottshalk, I.: Hepatic failure in a patient treated with DTIC for malignant melanoma. J. Cancer Res. Clin. Oncol., 95:281, 1979.
74. Foster, B. J., Newell, D. R., Lunn, J. M., Jones, M., and Calvert, A. H.: Correlation of dacarbazine and CB10-277 activity against human melanoma xenografts with O_6 alkyltransferase. Proc. Amer. Assoc. Cancer Res., 31:401, 1990.
75. Foster, B. J., Clagett-Carr, K., Hoth, D., and Leyland-Jones, B.: Pentamethylmelamine: review of an aqueous analog of hexamethylmelamine. Cancer Treat Rep 70:383, 1986.
76. Foster, B. J., Harding, B. J., Leyland-Jones, B., and Hoth, D.: Hexamethylmelamine: A critical review of an active drug. Cancer Treat. Rev., 13:197, 1986.
77. Foster, B. J., Clagett-Carr, K., Marsoni, S., Simon, R., and Leyland-Jones, B.: Role of hexamethylmelamine in the treatment of ovarian cancer: Where is the needle in the haystack? Cancer Treat. Rep., 70:1003, 1986.
78. Frei E., Luce J. K., Talley R. W., Vaitkevicius V. K., and Wilson H. E.: 5-(3,3-Dimethyl-1-triazeno)imi-dazole-4-carboxamide (NSC 45388) in the treatment of lymphoma. Cancer Chemother. Rep., 56:667, 1972.
79. ad-el-Mawla, N., Ziegler, J. L., Hamza, R., Elserafi, M., and Khaled, H.: Randomized phase II trial of hexamethylmelamine versus pentamethylmelamine in carcinoma of the Bilharzial bladder. Cancer Treat. Rep., 68:793, 1984.
80. Gale, G. R., Simpson, J. G., and Smith, A. B.: Studies of the mode of action of N-isopropyl-alpha-(2-methylhydrazino)-p-toluamide. Cancer Res., 27:1186, 1967.
81. Gatehouse, D. G., and Paes, D. J.: A demonstration of the in vitro bacterial mutagenicity of procarbazine, using the microtitre fluctuation test and large concentrations of S9 fraction. Carcinogenesis, 4:347, 1983.
82. Gersel Pedersen, A., Sorenson, S., Aabo, K., Dombernowsky, P., and Hansen, H. H.: Phase II study of procarbazine in small cell carcinoma of the lung. Cancer Treat. Rep., 66:273, 1982.
83. Gescher, A., and Raymont, C.: Studies of the metabolism of N-methyl containing antitumor agents. $^{14}CO_2$ breath analysis after administration of ^{14}C-labelled N-methyl drugs, formaldehyde and formate in mice. Biochem. Pharmacol., 30:1245, 1981.
84. Gescher, A., D'Incalci, M., Fanelli, R., and Farina, P.: N-hydroxymethylpenta-methylmelamine, a major in vitro metabolite of hexamethylmelamine. Life Sciences, 26:147, 1979.
85. Giraldi, T., Sava, G., Persissin, L., and Zorzet, S.: Role of host responses in the drug treatment of metastasis. Adv. Exp. Med. Biol., 233:351, 1988
86. Glicksman, A. S., Pajak, T. F., Gottlieb, A., Nissen, N., Stutzman, L., and Cooper, M. R.: Second malignant neoplasms in patients successfully treated for Hodgkin's disease: A Cancer and Leukemia Group B study. Cancer Treat. Rep., 66:1035, 1982.
87. Goldstein, L. S.: Dominant lethal mutations induced in mouse spermatogonia by mechlorethamine, procarbazine, and vincristine administered in 2-drug and 3-drug combinations. Mutat. Res., 191:171, 1987.
88. Gottlieb, J. A., Benjamin, R. S., Baker, L. H., O'Bryan, R. M., Sinkovics, J. G., Hoogstraten, B., Quagliana, J. M., Rivkin, S. E., Bodey, G. P., Rodriguez, V., Blumenschein, G. R., Saiki, J. H., Coltman Jr., C., Burgess, M. A., Sullivan, P., Thigpen, T., Bottomley, R., Balcerzak, S., and Moon, T. E.: Role of DTIC (NSC-45388) in the chemotherapy of sarcoma. Cancer Treat. Rep., 60:199, 1976.
89. Gorsen, R. M., Weiss, A. J., and Manthei, R. W.: Analysis of procarbazine and metabolites by gas chromatography-mass spectrometry. J. Chromatog., 221:309, 1980.
90. Greenstone, M. A., Dowd, P. M., Mikhailidis, D. P., and Scheuer, P. J.: Hepatic vascular lesions associated with dacarbazine treatment. Brit. Med. J., 282:1744, 1981.
91. Grubb, B. P., and Thant, M.: Case report: Acute myelocytic leukemia in a patient treated with hexamethylmelamine. Am. J. Med. Sci., 292:393, 1986.
92. Grunwald, H. W., and Rosner, F.: Acute myeloid leukemia following treatment of Hodgkin's disease. Cancer, 50:676, 1982.
93. Gupta, R. S.: Genetic, biochemical, and cross-resistance studies with mutants of chinese hamster ovary cells resistant to the anticancer drugs VM-26 and VP16-213. Cancer Res., 43:1568, 1983.
94. Gutterman, J., Huang, A. T., and Hochstein, P.: Studies on the mode of action of N-isopropyl-alpha-(2-methylhydrazine)-p-toluamide. Proc. Soc. Exp. Biol. Med., 130:797, 1969.
95. Hahn, R. G., Cnaan, A., Kessinger, A., Foley J. F., Doyal, Y., Petrelli, N.,Tormey, D., and Smith, T.: A phase II study of DTIC in the treatment of non-resectable islet cell carcinoma: An ECOG treatment protocol. Proc. Am. Soc. Clin. Oncol., 9:A417, 1990.
96. Hainsworth, J. D., Grosh, W. W., Burnett, L. S., Jones, H. W. III, Wolf, S. N., and Greco, F. A.: Advanced ovarian cancer: long-term results of treatment with intensive cisplatin-based chemotherapy of brief duration. Ann. Intern. Med., 108:165, 1988.
97. Hainsworth, J. D., Johnson, D. H., and Greco, F. A.: A retrospective comparison of hexamethylmelamine, cyclophosphamide, doxorubicin, and cisplatin (H-CAP) versus cyclophosphamide, doxorubicin, and cisplatin (CAP) in advanced ovarian cancer. Proc. Amer. Soc. Clin. Oncol., 9:161, 1990.
98. Hande, K. R., and Noone, R. M.: Cimetidine prolongs the half-life of procarbazine and hexamethylmelamine. Proc. Amer. Assoc. Cancer Res., 24:287, 1983.
99. Hande, K., Combs, G., Swingle, R., Combs, G. L., and Anthony, L.: Effect of cimetidine and ranitidine on the metabolism and toxicity of hexamethylmelamine. Cancer Treat. Rep., 70:1443, 1986.
100. Hayward, I. P., and Parson, P. G.: Epigenetic effects of the methylating agent 5-(3-methyl-1-triazeno)-imidazole carboxamide in human melanoma cells. Austr. J. Exp. Biol. Med. Sci., 62:597, 1984.
101. Henry-Amar, M.: Quantitative risk of second cancer in patients in first complete remission from early stages of Hodgkin's disease. N. C. I. Monogr., 6:65, 1988.
102. Hickman, J. A.: Investigation of the mechanism of action of antitumour dimethyltriazenes. Biochimie, 60:997, 1978.
103. Hoagland, H. C.: Hematologic complications of cancer chemotherapy. Sem. Oncol., 9:95,1982.
104. Horning, S. J., Hoppe, R. T., Kaplan, H. S., and Rosenberg, S. A.: Female reproductive potential after treatment for Hodgkin's disease. N. Engl. J. Med., 304:1377, 1981.
105. Householder, G. E., and Loo, T. L.: Disposition of 5-(3,3-dimethyl-1-triazeno)imidazole-4-carboxamide, a new antitumor agent. J. Pharmacol. Exp. Ther., 179:386, 1971.
106. Johnson, B. L., Fisher, R. I., Bender, R. A., DeVita, V. T., Chabner, B. A., and Young, R. C.: Hexamethylmelamine in alkylating agent-resistant ovarian carcinoma. Cancer, 42:2157, 1978.
107. Johnson, D. H., Porter, L. L., List, A. F., Hande, K. R., Hainsworth, J. D., and Greco, F. A.: Acute nonlymphocytic leukemia after treatment of small cell lung cancer. Am. J. Med., 81:962, 1986.
108. Johnson, J. M., Thompson, D. J., Haggerty, G. C., Dyke, I. L., and Lower, C. E.: The effect of prenatal procarbazine treatment on brain development in the rat. Teratology, 32:203, 1985.
109. Kaiser, D. W., Thurston, J. T., Dudley, J. R., Schaefer, F. C., Heckenbleikner, I., and Holm-Harsen, D.: Cyanuric chloride derivatives: II, Substituted melamines. J. Amer. Chem. Soc., 73:2984,1951.
110. Kelly, M. G., O'Gara, R. W., Yancey, S. T., Gadekar, K., Botkin, C., and Oliverio, V. T.: Comparative carcinogenicity of N-isopropyl-alpha-(2-methylhydrazino)-p-toluamide HCl (procarbazine hydrochloride), its degradation products, other hydrazines, and isonicotinic acid hydrazide. J. N. C. I., 42:337, 1969.
111. Kessinger, A., Foley, J. F., and Lemon, H. M.: Therapy of malignant APUD cell tumors. Effectiveness of DTIC. Cancer, 51:790, 1983.
112. Klippert, P. J., Hulshoff, A., Mingels, M. J. J., Hofman, G., and Noordhoek, J.: Low oral bioavailability of hexamethylmelamine in the rat due to simultaneous hepatic and intestinal metabolism. Cancer Res., 43:3160, 1983.
113. Kreis, W.: Metabolism of an antineoplastic methylhydrazine derivative in a P815 mouse neoplasm. Cancer Res., 30:82, 1970.
114. Kumar, A. R., Renaudin, J., Wilson, C. B., Boldrey, E. B,, Enot, K. J., and Levin, V. A.: Procarbazine hydrochloride in the treatment of brain tumors. J. Neurosurg., 40:365, 1974.
115. Kuttab, S. H., Tanglerpaibul, S., and Vouros, P.: Studies on the metabolism of procarbazine by mass spectroscopy. Biomed. Mass. Spectrom., 9:78, 1982.
116. Lake, L. M., Grunden, E. E., and Johnson, B. M.: Toxicity and antitumor activity of hexamethylmelamine and its N-demethylated metabolites in mice with transplantable tumor. Cancer Res., 35:2858, 1975.
117. Lam, H., Begleiter, A., Stein, W., Lam, H. Y. P., Begleiter, A., Stein, W., and Goldenberg, G. J.: On the mechanism of uptake of procarbazine by L5178Y lymphoblasts in vivo. Biochem. Pharmacol., 27:1883, 1978.
118. Lee, I. P., and Lucier, G. W.: The potentiation of barbiturate-induced narcosis by procarbazine. J. Pharmacol. Exp. Ther., 196:586, 1976.
119. Legha, S. S., Ring, S., Papadopoulos, N., Plager, C., Chawla, S., and Benjamin, R.: A prospective evaluation of a triple-drug regimen containing cisplatin, vinblastine, and dacarbazine (CVD) for metastatic melanoma. Cancer, 64:2024, 1989.
120. Levin, V. A., Rodriguez, L. A., Edwards, M. S. B., Wara, W., Liu, H., Fulton, D., Davis, R. L., Wilson, C. B., and Silver, P.: Treatment of medulloblastoma with procarbazine, hydroxyurea, and reduced radiation dose to whole brain and spine. J. Neurosurg., 68:383, 1988.
121. Lipton, A., Hepner, G. W., White, D. S., and Harvey, H. A.: Decreased hepatic drug demethylation in patients receiving chemo-immunotherapy. Cancer, 41:1680, 1978.
122. Liske, R.: A comparative study of the action of cyclophosphamide and procarbazine on the antibody production in mice. Clin. Exp. Immunol., 15:271, 1973.
123. Lonn, U., and Lonn, S.: Prevention of dacarbazine damage of human neoplastic cell DNA by aphidicolin. Cancer Res., 47:26, 1987.

124. Loo, T. L., Householder, G. E., Gerulath, A. H., Saunders, P. H., and Farguhar, D.: Mechanism of action and pharmacology studies with DTIC (NSC-45388). Cancer Treat. Rep., 60:149, 1976.
125. Loo, T. L., Luce, J. K., Jardine, H., and Frei, E.: Pharmacologic studies of the antitumor agent 5-(dimethyl-triazeno)imidazole-4-carboxamide. Cancer Res., 28:2448, 1968.
126. Luce, J. K., Thurman, W. G., Isaacs, B. L., and Talley, R. W.: Clinical trials with the antitumor agent 5-(3,3-dimethyl-1-triazeno)imidazole-4-carboxamide (NSC-45388). Cancer Chemother. Rep., 54:119, 1970.
127. Luce, J. K.: Chemotherapy of malignant melanoma. Cancer, 30:1604, 1972.
128. Lunn, J. M., and Harris, A. L.: Cytotoxicity of 5-(3-methyl-1-triazeno)imidazole-4-carboxamide (MTIC) on Mer $^+$, Mer$^+$Rem$^-$ and Mer$^-$ cell lines: Differential potentiation by 3-acetamidobenzamide. Brit. J. Cancer, 57:54, 1988.
129. Manetta, A., MacNeill, C., Lyter, J. A., Scheffler, B., Podczaski, E. S., Larson, J. E., and Schein, P.: Hexamethylmelamine as a single second-line agent in ovarian cancer. Gynecol. Oncol., 36:93, 1990.
130. Marelli, O., Canti, G., Franco, P., Prandoni, N., Ricci, L., and Nicolin, A.: L1210/DTIC antigenic subline: Studies at the clone level. Eur. J. Cancer Clin. Oncol., 22:1401, 1986.
131. Marsh, J. C.: Hepatic vascular toxicity of dacarbazine (DTIC): Not a rare complication. Hepatol., 9:790, 1989.
132. Martz, G., D'Allessandri, A., Keel, H. J., and Bollag, W.: Preliminary clinical results with a new anti-tumor agent Ro4-6467 (NSC-77213). Cancer Chemother. Rep., 33:5, 1963.
133. Maynard, K., Parsons, P. G., Cerny, T., and Margison, G. P.: Relationships among cell survival O^6–alkytransferase activity, and reaction of methylated adenovirus 5 and Herpes Simplex virus type 1 in human melanoma cell lines. Cancer Res., 49:4813, 1989.
134. McClay,. E, Lusch, C. J., and Mastrangelo, M. J.: Allergy-induced hepatic toxicity associated with dacarbazine. Cancer Treat. Rep., 71:219, 1987.
135. Metelmann, H. R., and Von Hoff, D. D.: Application of a microsomal drug activation system in a human tumor cloning assay. Invest. New Drugs, 1:27, 1983.
136. Miller, K. J., McGovern, R. M., and Ames, M. M.: Effect of a hepatic activiation system on the antiproliferative activity of hexamethylmelamine against human tumor cell lines. Cancer Chemother. Pharmacol., 15:49, 1985.
137. Molony. S. J., and Prough, R. A.: Studies on the pathway of methane formation from procarbazine, a 2-methylbenzyl hydrazine derivative, by rat liver microsomes. Arch. Biochem. Biophys., 221:577, 1983.
138. Moloney, S. J., Wiebkin, P., Cummings, S. W., and Prough, R. A.: Metabolic activation of the terminal N-methyl group of N-isopropyl-alpha-(2-methylhydrazino)-p-toluamide hydrochloride (procarbazine). Carcinogenesis, 6:397, 1985.
139. Montgomery, J. A.: Experimental studies at Southern Research Institute with DTIC (NSC-45388). Cancer Treat. Rep., 60:125, 1976.
140. Moore, G. E., and Meiselbaugh, D.: DTIC (NSC 45388) toxicity. Cancer Treat. Rep., 60:219, 1976.
141. Nagasawa, H. T., Shirota, F. N., and Mizuno, N. S.: The mechanism of alkylation of DNA by 5-(3-methyl-1-triazeno)imidazole-4-carboxamide (MIC), a metabolite of DIC (NSC-45388). Chem. Biol. Interact., 8:403, 1974.
142. Neijt, J. P., ten Bokkel Huinink, W. W., van der Burg, M. E. L., van Oosterom, A. T., Willemse, P. H. B., Heintz, A. P. M., van Lent, M., Trimbos, J. B., Vermorken, J. B., and van Houwelingen, J. C.: Randomized trial comparing two combination chemotherapy regimens (CHAP-5 v CP) in advanced ovarian carcinoma. J. Clin. Oncol., 5:1157, 1987.
143. Newell, D., Gescher, A., Harland, S., Ross, D., and Rutty, C.: N-Methyl antitumor agents. A distinct class of anticancer drugs? Cancer Chemother. Pharmacol., 19:91, 1987.
144. Oken, M. M., Lenhard, R. E., Tsiatsis, A. A., Glick, J. H., and Silverstein, M. N.: Contribution of prednisone to the effectiveness of hexamethylmelamine in multiple myeloma. Cancer Treat. Rep., 71:807, 1987.
145. Oliverio, V. T., Denham, C., Devita, V. T., and Kelly, M. G.: Some pharmacologic properties of a new antitumor agent, N-isopropyl-alpha-(2-methylhydrazino)-p-toluamide hydrochloride (NSC-77213). Cancer Chemother. Rep., 42:1, 1964.
146. Omura, G. A., Greco, F. A., and Birch, R.: Hexamethylmelamine in mustard-resistant ovarian adenocarcinoma. Cancer Treat. Rep., 64:530, 1980.
147. Paoline, A., D'Incalci, M.: Effect of phenobarbital pretreatment on the metabolism and antitumor activity of hexamethylmelamine. Cancer Treat. Rep., 70:513, 1986.
148. Parvinen, L.: Early effects of procarbazine (N-isopropyl-L-(2methylhydrazino)-p-toluamidehydrochloride) on rat spermatogenesis. Exp. Mol. Pathol., 30:1, 1979.
149. Pritchard, K. I., Quirt, I. C., Cowan, D. H., Osoba, D., and Kutas, G. J.: DTIC therapy in metastatic melanoma: A simplified dose schedule. Cancer Treat. Rep., 64:1123, 1980.
150. Prough, R. A., and Tweedie, D. J.: Procarbazine. *In* Metabolism and action of anticancer drugs. Edited by G. Powis and R. A. Prough. London, Taylor & Francis, 1987, p. 29.
151. Prough, R. A., Wittkop, J. A., and Reed, D. J.: Evidence for the hepatic metabolism of some mono-alkylhydrazines. Arch. Biochem. Biophys., 131:369, 1969.
152. Prough, R. A., Coomes, M. L., and Dunn, D. L.: The microsomal metabolism of carcinogenic and/or therapeutic hydrazines. *In* Microsomes and Drug Oxidations. Edited by V. Ullrich, I. Roots, A. Hildebrandt, R. Estabrook, A. H. Conney. Oxford, Pergamon Press, 1977, p. 500.
153. Prough, R. A., Brown, M. I., Dannan, G. A., and Guengerich, F. P.: Major isozymes of rat liver microsomal cytochrome P-450 involved in the N-oxidation of N-isopropyl-alpha-(2 methyl-azo)-p-toluamide, the azo derivative of procarbazine. Cancer Res. 44:543, 1984.
154. Raaflaub, J., and Schwartz, D. E.: Uber den Metabolismus eines cytostatisch wirksamen methylhydrazin-derivates (Natulan). Experientia, 21:44, 1965.
155. Ray, S., Basak, S., Raychaudhury, C., Roy, A. B., and Ghosh, J. J.: The utility of information content, hydrophobicity, and van der Waals volume in the design of barbiturates and tumor inhibitory triazenes: A comparative study. Arzheim Forsch, 33:352, 1983.
156. Reed, D. J.: Effects in vivo of lymphoma ascites tumors and procarbazine, alone and in combination, upon hepatic drug-metabolizing enzymes of mice. Biochem. Pharmacol., 25:153, 1976.
157. Rosen, G. F., Lurain, J. R., and Newton, M.: Hexamethylmelamine in ovarian cancer after failure of cisplatin-based multiple-agent chemotherapy. Gynecol. Oncol., 27:173, 1987.
158. Ross, D., Langdon, S. P., Gescher, A., and Stevens, M. F. G.: Studies of the mode of action of antitumor triazenes and triazines–V. The correlation of the in vitro cytotoxicity and in vivo antitumor activity of hexamethylmelamine analogues with their metabolism. Biochem. Pharmacol., 33:1131, 1984.
159. Ross, W. E., McMillan, D. R., and Ross, C. F.: Comparison of DNA damage by methylmelamines and formaldehyde. J. N. C. I., 67:217, 1981.
160. Rutty, C. J., and Connors, T. A.: In vitro studies with hexamethylmelamine. Biochem. Pharmacol., 26:2385, 1977.
161. Rutty, C. J., Abel, G., and Harrap, K. R.: In vitro cytotoxicity of hexamethylmelamine and its analogues. Br. J. Cancer, 40:317, 1979.
162. Rutty, C. J., Connors, T. A., Hoang-Nam, N., Cao-Thang, D., and Hoellinger, H.: In vivo studies with hexamethylmelamine. Eur. J. Cancer, 14:713, 1978.
163. Rutty, C. J., Judson, I. R., Abel, G., Goddard, P. M., Newell, D. R., and Harrap, K. R.: Preclinical toxicology, pharmacokinetics and formulation of N_2, N_4, N_6-trihydroxymethyl-N_2, N_4, N_6-trimethylamine (Trimelamol), a water-soluble cytotoxic s-triazine which does not require metabolic activiation. Cancer Chemother. Pharmacol., 17:251, 1986.
164. Samuels, M. L., Leary, W. V., Alexanian, R., Howe, C. D., and Frei, E.: Clinical trials with N-isopropyl-(2-methylhydrazino)-p-toluamide hydrochloride in malignant lymphoma and other disseminated neoplasia. Cancer, 20:1187, 1967.
165. Sartorelli, A. C., and Tsunamura, S.: Studies on the biochemical mode of action of a cytotoxic methylhydrazine derivative, N-isopropyl-alpha-(2-methylhydrazino)-p-toluamide. Mol. Pharmacol., 2:275, 1966.
166. Saunders, P. P., and Chao, L. Y.: Fate of the ring moiety of 5-(3,3-dimethyl-1-triazeno)-imidazole-4-carboxamide in mammalian cells. Cancer Res., 34:2464, 1974.
167. Saunders, P. P., DeChang, W., and Chao, L. Y.: Mechanisms of 5-(3,3-dimethyl-1-triazeno)imidazole-4-carboxamide (dacarbazine) cytotoxicity toward Chinese hamster ovary cells in vitro are dictated by incubation conditions. Chem. Biol. Interactions, 58:319, 1986.
168. Sava, G., Giraldi, T., Lassiani, L., Nisi, C., and Farmer, P. B.: Mechanism of the antileukemic effects of 1-p-carboxamidophenyl-3,3-dimethyltriazene and its in vitro metabolites. Biochem. Pharmacol., 31:3629, 1982.
169. Sava, G., Giraldi, T. Perissin, L., Zorzet, S,, Mallardi, F., and Grill, V.: Infiltration of liver and brain by tumor cells in leukemic mice: Prevention by dimethyltriazenes and cyclophosphamide. Tumori, 70:477, 1984.
170. Schilsky, R. L., Lewis, B. J., Sherins, R. J., and Young, R. C.: Gonadal dysfunction in patients receiving chemotherapy for cancer. Ann. Intern. Med., 93:109, 1980.
171. Schilsky, R. L., Sherins, R. J., Hubbard, S. M., Wesley, M. N., Young, R. C., and DeVita, V. T.: Long-term follow up of ovarian function in women treated with MOPP chemotherapy for Hodgkin's disease. Am. J. Med., 71:552, 1981.
172. Schmid, F. A., and Hutchison, D. J.: Chemotherapeutic, carcinogenic, and cell-regulatory effects of triazenes. Cancer Res., 34:1671, 1974.
173. Schold, Jr., S. C., Brent, T. P., von Hofe, E., Friedman, H. S., Mitra, S., Bigner, D. D., Swenberg, J. A., and Kleihues, P.: O^6-Alkylguanine-DNA alkyltransferase and sensitivity to procarbazine in human brain-tumor xenografts. J. Neurosurg., 70:573, 1989.
174. Schwartz, D. E., Bollag, W., and Obrecht, P.: Distribution and excretion studies of procarbazine in animals and man. Arzneimittel-Forsch, 17:1389, 1967.
175. Schwartz, D. E.: Comparative metabolic studies with natulan, methylhydrazine, and methylamine in rats. Experientia (Basel), 22:212, 1966.
176. Serrano, G., Aliaga, A., Febrer, I., Pujol, C., Camps C., and Godes, M.: Dacarbazine-induced photosensitivity. Photodermatol., 6:140, 1989.
177. Shealy, Y. F., Montgomery, J. A., and Laster, W. R., Jr.: Antitumor activity of triazenoimidazoles. Biochem. Pharmacol., 11:674,1962.
178. Shealy, Y. F.: Synthesis and biological activity of 5-amino imidazoles and 5-triazenoimidazoles. J. Pharm. Sci., 59:1533, 1970.
179. Shiba, D. A., and Weinkam, R. J.: Quantitative analysis of procarbazine, procarbazine metabolites and chemical degradation products with application to pharmacokinetic studies. J. Chromatogr., 229:397, 1982.
180. Shiba, D. A., and Weinkam, R. J.: The in vivo cytotoxic activity of procarbazine and procarbazine metabolites against L1210 ascites leukemia cells in CDF1 mice and the effects of pretreatment with procarbazine, phenobarbital, diphenylhydantoin, and methylprednisolone upon in vivo procarbazine activity. Cancer Chemother. Pharmacol., 11:124, 1983.
181. Sieber, S. M., Correa, P., Dalgard, D. W., and Adamson, R.H.: Carcinogenic and other adverse effects of procarbazine in nonhuman primates. Cancer Res., 38:2125, 1978.
182. Sinha, B. K.: Metabolic activation of procarbazine. Evidence for carbon-centered free radical intermediates. Biochem. Pharmacol., 33:2777, 1984.
183. Skibba, J. L., Beal, D. D., Ramirez, G., and Bryan, T.: N-Demethylation of the antineoplastic agent 4(5)-(3,3-dimethyl-1-triazeno)imidazole-5(4)-carboxamide by rats and man. Cancer Res., 30:147, 1970.
184. Skibba, J. L., and Bryan, G. T.: Methylation of nucleic acids and urinary excretion of ^{14}C-labelled-7-methylguanine by rats and man after administration of 4(5)-(3,3-dimethyl-1-triazeno)imidazole-5(4)-carboxamide. Toxicol. Appl. Pharmacol., 18:707, 1971.
185. Skibba, J. L., Ramirez, G., Beal, D. D., and Bryan, G. T.: Metabolism of 4(5)-(3,3-dimethyl-1-triazeno)-imidazole-5(4)-carboxamide to 4(5)amino-imidazole-5(4)-carboxamide in man. Biochem. Pharmacol., 19:2043, 1970.
186. Skibba, J. L., Ramirez, G., Beal, D. D., and Bryan, G. T.: Preliminary clinical trial and the physiologic disposition of 4(5)-(3,3-dimethyl-1-triazeno)imidazole-5(4)-carboxamide in man. Cancer Res., 29:1944,1969.
187. Skipper, H. E., Hutchison, D. J., Schabel, F. M., Jr., Schmidt, L. H., Goldin, A., Brockman, R. W., Venditti, J. M., and Wodinsky, I.: A quick reference chart on cross resistance between anticancer agents. Cancer Chemother. Rep., 56:493, 1972.
188. Spivack, S. D.: Procarbazine. Ann. Int. Med., 81:795, 1974.
189. Sponzo, R. W., Arseneau, J., and Canellos, G. P.: Procarbazine-induced oxidative haemolysis: Relationship to in vivo red cell survival. Brit. J. Haematol., 27:587, 1974.
190. Stevens, M. F. G.: DTIC: A springboard to new antitumour agents. *In* Structure Activity Relationships of Antitumour Agents. Edited by D. W .Reinhoudt, T. A. Connors, H. M. Pinedo, K. W. van de Poll. The Hague, Martinus Nijhoff, 1983, p. 183.
191. Sullivan, K. M., Shulman, H. M., Storb, R., Weiden, P. L., Witherspoon, R. P., McDonald, G. B., Schubert , M. M., Atkinson, K., and Thomas, E. D.: Chronic graft-versus-host disease in 52 patients: Adverse natural course and successful treatment with combination immunosuppression. Blood, 57:267, 1981.
192. Swaffar, D. S., Harker, W. G., Pomerantz, S., Nelson, C., and Yost, G. S.: In vitro bioactivation of procarbazine to cytotoxic species in human leukemia cells. Proc. Amer. Assoc. Cancer Res., 31:384, 1990.
193. Swaffar, D. S., Horstman, M. G., Jaw, J. Y., Thrall, B. D., Meadows, G. G., Harker, W. G., and Yost, G. S.: Methazoxyprocarbazine, the active metabolite responsible for the anticancer activity of procarbazine against L1210 leukemia. Cancer Res., 49:2442, 1989.
194. Tamaro, M., Dolzani, L., Monti-Bragadin, C., and Sava, G.: Mutagenic activity of the dacarbazine analog p-(3,3-dimethyl-1-triazeno)benzoic acid potassium salt in bacterial cells. Pharmacol. Res. Comm., 18:491, 1986.
195. Thompson, D. J., Molello, J. A., Sterbing, R. J., and Dyke, I. L.: Reproduction and teratology studies with oncolytic agents in the rat and rabbits. II. 5-(3,3-dimethyl-1-triazeno)-imidazole-4-carboxamide (DTIC). Toxicol. Appl. Pharmacol., 33:281, 1975.
196. Valagussa, P., Santoro, A., Fossati-Bellani, F., Franchi, F., Banfi, A., and Bonadonna,

    G.: Absence of treatment-induced second neoplasms after ABVD in Hodgkin's disease. Blood, 59:488,1982.
197. Vaughan, K., Tang, Y., Llanos, G., Horton, J. K., Simmonds, R. J., Hickman, J. A., and Stevens, M. F. G.: Studies of the mode of action of antitumor triazenes and triazines. 6. 1-Aryl-3-(hydroxymethyl-3-methyltriazenes: synthesis, chemistry and antitumor properties. J. Med. Chem., 27:357, 1984.
198. Venditti, J. M.: Antitumor activity of DTIC (NSC 45388) in animals. Cancer Treat. Rep., 60:135, 1976.
199. Vogl, S. E., Pagano, M., Davis, T. E., Einhorn, N., Tunca, J. C., Kaplan, B. H., and Arseneau, J. C.: Hexamethylmelamine and cisplatin in advanced ovarian cancer after failure of alkylating-agent therapy. Cancer Treat. Rep., 66:1285, 1982.
200. Vorobiof, D. A., Falkson, G., and Voges, C. W.: DTIC versus DTIC and recombinant interferon alfa 2b in the treatment of patients with advanced malignant melanoma. Proc. A. S. C. O., 8:284, 1989.
201. Weinkam, R. J., and Shiba, D. A.: Metabolic activation of procarbazine. Life Sci., 22:937, 1978.
202. Weiss, R. B., and Baker, J. R.: Hypersensitivity reactions from antineoplastic agents. Cancer Metastasis Rev., 6:413, 1987.
203. Weiss, H. D., Walker, M. D., and Wiernik, P. H.: Neurotoxicity of commonly used antineoplastic agents. N. Engl. J. Med., 291:127, 1974.

204. Wharton, J.., Rutledge, F., Smith, J.., Herson, J., and Hodge, M.,P.: Hexa-methyl-melamine: an evaluation of its role in the treatment of ovarian cancer. Am. J. Obstet. Gynecol., 133:833, 1979.
205. Wilman, D. E. V., and Goddard, P. M.: Tumor inhibitory triazenes. 2. Variation of antitumor activity within an homologous series. J. Med. Chem., 23:1052, 1980.
206. Wilman, D. E. V., Cox, P. J., Goddard, P. M., Hart, L. I., Merai, K., and Newell, D. R.: Tumor inhibitory triazenes. 3. Dealkylation within an homologous series and its relation to antitumor activity. J. Med. Chem., 27:870, 1984.
207. Wodinsky, I., Swiniarski, J., and Kensler, C. J.: Spleen colony studies of leukemia L1210. IV. Sensitivities of L1210 and L1210/6-MP to triazenoimidazole carboxamides–a preliminary report. Cancer Chemother. Rep., 52:393, 1968.
208. Worzalla, J. F., Johnson, B. M., Ramirez, G., and Bryan, G. T.: N-demethylation of the antineoplastic agent hexamethylmelamine by rats and man. Cancer Res., 33:2810, 1973.
209. Worzalla, J., Kaiman, B. D., Johnson, B. M., Ramirez, G., and Bryan, G. T.: Metabolism of hexamethylmelamine-ring-C^{14} in rats and man. Cancer Res., 34:2669, 1974.
210. Zeller, P., Gutmann, H., Hegedus, B., Kaiser, A., Langemann, A., and Muller, M.: Methylhydrazine derivatives, a new class of cytotoxic agents. Experientia (Basel), 19:129, 1963.

XVI-5

Anthracyclines and DNA Intercalators

Charles Myers

Historical Background

DNA intercalators represent one of the most important classes of anticancer drugs, second only to the alkylating agents in their overall utility in clinical oncology (Table XVI-5-1). The term, DNA intercalation, is used to describe the process by which drugs with a planar aromatic ring structure insert themselves in the space between the successive DNA base pairs. This binding is reversible and is stabilized by the hydrophobic interaction between the opposed aromatic rings of the drug and those of the adjacent DNA bases. In addition, the binding may be enhanced by ionic binding between the drug and charge centers on the DNA double helix. The first intercalator to reach wide usage in oncology was actinomycin D, followed by daunorubicin.[5,32] However, interest in this drug class really may be dated from the discovery of doxorubicin. While actinomycin D and daunorubicin were each antitumor agents with utility in a narrow spectrum of tumors, doxorubicin soon proved its value in a wide range of cancers including such common neoplasms as carcinoma of the breast, ovary, and lung, as well as both lymphomas and sarcomas. This discovery was followed by much theoretical work on structural requirements for DNA intercalation and the development of ground rules for the rational synthesis of DNA intercalating agents.[5,32] It is ironic that while this rational approach has led to the development of agents such as amsacrine and mitoxantrone, none of these agents has matched the broad antitumor spectrum of doxorubicin.[5,32]

Mechanism of Action

Efforts to understand the basis for the antitumor activity of the anthracyclines naturally included a focus on the impact of drug intercalation upon DNA double helix structure (Table XVI-5-2). Normally, the spacing between base pair planes in the DNA double helix is approximately 2.5 Å. The planar aromatic chromophore of doxorubicin is itself approximately 2.5 Å in thickness. Thus, intercalation of doxorubicin between base pair planes results in at least a doubling of the usual spacing between them. As a direct consequence of this spreading of base pair planes, the DNA helix undergoes unwinding. If the DNA exists in a supercoiled state, the supercoiling will also undergo a degree of unwinding. Thus, one invariant consequence of intercalation is an alteration of DNA topology. DNA intercalators may be characterized by a range of physical properties including unwinding angle, binding affinity, kinetics of DNA association and dissociation. Within a family of drugs, such as the anthracyclines, loss of

Table XVI-5-1.   DNA Intercalators in Clinical Use

1. Daunorubicin
2. Doxorubicin
3. Epirubicin
4. Idarubicin
5. Dactinomycin
6. Mitoxantrone
7. Amsacrine

Table XVI-5-2.   Characteristics Shared by Most Clinically Used DNA Intercalators

1. Possess at least 3 planar aromatic rings
2. Trigger topoisomerase II-associated DNA breaks
3. Exhibit redox metabolism
4. Cross resistance based on *mdr* gene expression or altered topoisomerase II
5. High tissue-to-plasma ratios
6. Most intracellular drug is nuclear in location
7. Terminal half-life of 25–50 hours
8. Radiation sensitization

activity may be observed when the ability to intercalate is lost. However, in general, the correlation between any of these physical constants and clinical utility of intercalators has been disappointing. Thus, DNA intercalators have been synthesized with much greater affinity for DNA than the intercalators in current clinical use, but these high affinity binders almost always have been potent cytotoxins without a useful therapeutic index. For example, cyanomorpholino-doxorubicin binds covalently to the minor groove of DNA and this results in a marked increase in cytotoxicity to tumor cells in tissue culture compared with doxorubicin, but the overall efficacy is not improved because toxicity also increases.[26,99]

For the above reasons, much of the work in intercalator development has focused on the impact of intercalators on DNA function rather than its structure.[32] These drugs were quickly shown to alter the function of DNA and RNA polymerases in a range of experimental models. The drug concentrations required to elicit these effects, however, were uniformly outside the clinically useful range. The only exception to this appears to be actinomycin D, where inhibition of RNA synthesis and, secondarily, protein synthesis appears to be the major mechanism of tumor cell kill, although this drug does trigger topoisomerase II-associated DNA breaks. There followed a series of studies which documented effects of these drugs on nucleolar structure and in chromosomal organization. Again, however, a convincing relationship was never established between these effects and clinical utility of a given intercalator.

The degree of DNA supercoiling has been shown to play an important role in chromosomal structure and gene activity. As might be expected, the degree of DNA supercoiling is therefore under the control of enzymes. Because one major effect of all intercalators is to alter DNA supercoiling, it should not be surprising that this effect should trigger activity of the enzymes responsible for regulating DNA topology. One enzyme so affected is topoisomerase II (Figure XVI-5-1). This enzyme helps control the topology of DNA by allowing one strand to pass through the other.[5,101] This strand passing is also important in the decatenation of chromosomes after DNA replication but prior to mitosis. The steps in this process include first the establishment of a protein-DNA covalent bond between a tyrosine in the enzyme and phosphates in the backbone of the DNA helix (Figure XVI-5-1). This is followed by a double stranded cut with the cut strands held together by the protein-DNA covalent bond until strand passing has completed. This is followed by rejoining of the cut DNA strands and dissociation of the enzyme. In mammalian cells, one major function of topoisomerase II is the decatenation of daughter strands after DNA replication in preparation for mitosis. Amsacrine, the anthracyclines and other intercalators have been shown to arrest this process after formation of the protein associated double strand cut.[5,101] The net effect is the formation of stable protein associated double stranded cuts. In addition to these intercalators, nonintercalating drugs such as etoposide and teniposide also cause similar topoisomerase II associated double strand breaks (see XVI-7). There is now strong evidence that topoisomerase-mediated DNA damage is one of the major mechanisms by which DNA intercalators kill cells. First, topoisomerase-mediated DNA damage is triggered by drug concentrations that are clinically relevant. Second, there is a good correlation between cytotoxicity and DNA damage. Third, cell lines that have altered topoisomerase II activity are resistant to a wide range of intercalating agents.

Most of the clinically useful intercalators also possess the capacity to undergo metabolism which leads to the generation of free radicals; one of the most difficult issues in this field has been to determine the relative contribution of drug-induced free radical formation and DNA intercalation to both antitumor activity and host toxicity (Table XVI-5-1).[32] There are several reasons for the free radical generating properties of these agents.[71] Some, such as the anthracyclines, are quinones, which in general are easily reduced to the corresponding semiquinone free radicals. This chemistry has been best worked out for anthracyclines, where it leads to a rich range of products including potential DNA alkylating structures and a range of reactive oxygen products including superoxide, hydrogen peroxide and the hydroxyl radical (Figure XVI-5-2). These compounds are able to cause severe cell injury by damaging membranes. Oxygen radical damage to membranes can occur in at least two sites. First, oxygen radicals attack and destroy the double bonds in unsaturated fatty acids. Within the phospholipids of the cell membrane, the fatty acids at the 2 position are predominantly unsaturated and are the major site of free radical attack. This process is called lipid peroxidation in that one of the intermediate products is a lipid peroxide. There is a wide range of proteins which are critical to membrane structure. Some of these contain thiol groups very sensitive to oxidation and these have been shown to also be destroyed by free radical attack. In addition, some of these agents form complexes with transition metal ions such as iron and copper, and the resulting metal complexes can act as redox catalysts. This has been demonstrated for the anthracyclines (Figure XVI-5-3). Finally, aromatic hydrocarbons are frequently disposed of by the microsomal mixed function oxidases.[71] This process can result in the formation of quinones, diols and epoxides all of which can be chemically quite reactive with DNA and other cellular constituents and which thus can cause cell kill or sublethal injury leading to carcinogenesis. The latter has been demonstrated for 9-methoxyellipticine, one of the early intercalators introduced into clinical trial. There is general agreement that free radical formation forms the basis for anthracycline cardiac toxicity. This is reviewed in more detail below. For doxorubicin, there is strong evidence that free radical formation is involved in the ability of the drug to kill breast cancer cell lines in vitro.[85] Two of the clinically useful DNA intercalators, amsacrine[75,80] and mitoxantrone,[60,61,74] are much less active in redox reactions and this has been proposed as one of the reasons for the lower frequency of cardiomyopathy in patients treated with these agents.

Cross resistance between intercalators is a common event. Resistance to anthracyclines, mitoxantrone, amsacrine, and actinomycin D has been associated with expression of the *mdr* gene product.[9,57,58] This membrane protein mediates drug efflux and is a common basis for cross resistance (see XV-2). As might be expected from the importance of topoisomerase II in tumor cell kill, altered topoisomerase II has also been reported to be the basis for broad resistance to agents including intercalators.[9]

Anthracyclines

The anthracyclines are second only to the alkylating agents in the breadth of their antitumor spectrum. Their discovery

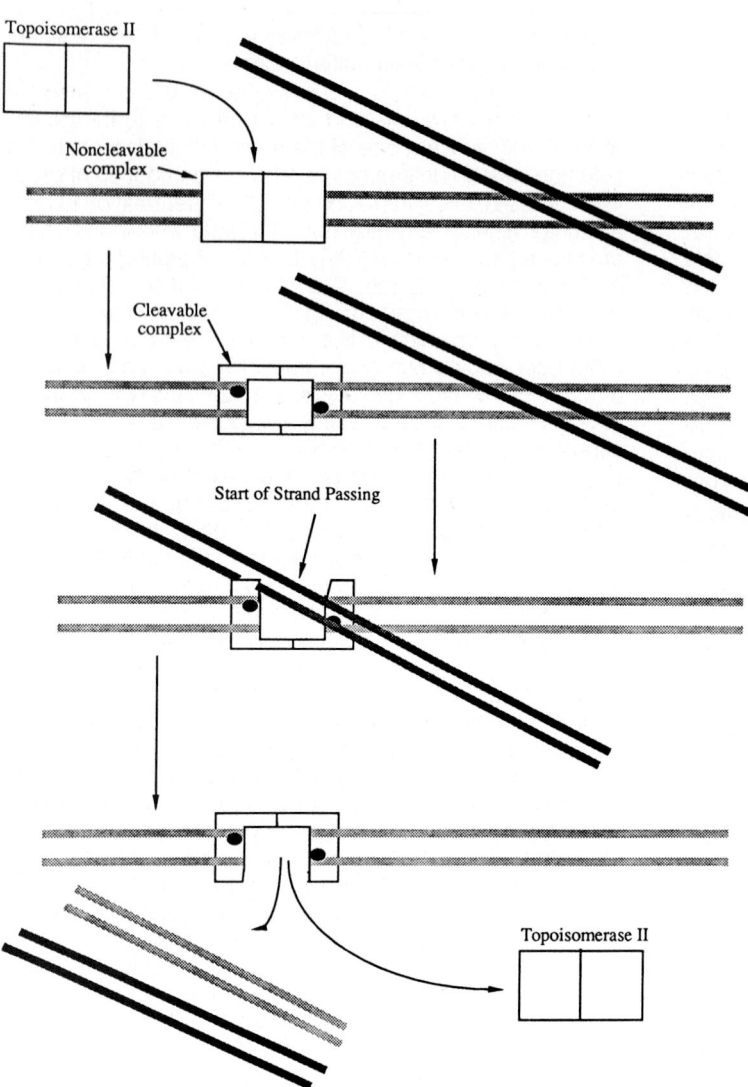

Topoisomerase II

Noncleavable complex

Cleavable complex

Start of Strand Passing

Topoisomerase II

Figure XVI-5-1. Action of topoisomerase II. The enzyme forms a covalent bond with DNA, creating first a noncleavable, then a cleavable, complex. DNA intercalators arrest the enzyme at this stage creating protein-associated DNA breaks. Under normal conditions, topoisomerase II will then allow one strand to pass through the other and then reseal the break. (See XVI-6-1.)

and the initial description of their biology was made by Di Marco and Arcamore.[1,33] The initial clinical investigations were conducted by Bonadonna.[15a] Both are antibiotics produced by Streptomyces species. Daunorubicin was named for the Daunos tribe, native to the region where the original soil sample was obtained. The commercial name for doxorubicin, Adriamycin, derives from the soil sample which came from the Adriatic shore. The structures of the clinically used anthracyclines are shown in Figure XVI-5-4. These drugs are composed of a four ring chromophore attached to the amino sugar, daunosamine. The chromophore is composed of three planar rings which are responsible for the ability of the drug to intercalate. In addition, the chromophore contains an hydroxyquinone functionality on the middle two rings. It is this hydroxyquinone functionality which is responsible for the intense color of these compounds, their intense fluorescence, their free radical properties and their ability to chelate transition metal ions (Figure XVI-5-3).[48]

Routes of Administration, Schedule, and Pharmacokinetics

The clinically used anthracyclines have poor or erratic oral bioavailability and thus are traditionally given parenterally.

The only exception to this is idarubicin which appears to have good bioavailability and to be well tolerated orally.[42,89] When extravasated, the anthracyclines cause extensive local injury, which renders them appropriate only for intravenous use. Within three hours of administration, tissue levels exceed that of plasma reaching tissue-to-plasma ratios as high as 100.[39,87,95] Within cells, greater than 80% of the drug is found within the nucleus.[22] The anthracyclines are highly fluorescent and cells exposed to anthracyclines typically show an intense nuclear fluorescence.

Thus, within a short time of administration, a bulk of the administered dose of drug in the body is bound to DNA from which it is only slowly released. All anthracyclines undergo, to a variable degree, reduction of the side chain to the corresponding alcohol, daunorubicinol or doxorubicinol, within the liver.[47,98] In the case of daunorubicinol, the formation of this metabolite is rapid enough that daunorubicinol concentrations usually exceed those of the parent daunorubicin. These events dominate the plasma pharmacokinetics of the anthracyclines. The plasma disappearance curve for the anthracyclines is typically sharply biphasic with a rapid early distributive phase. This is followed by a terminal phase with

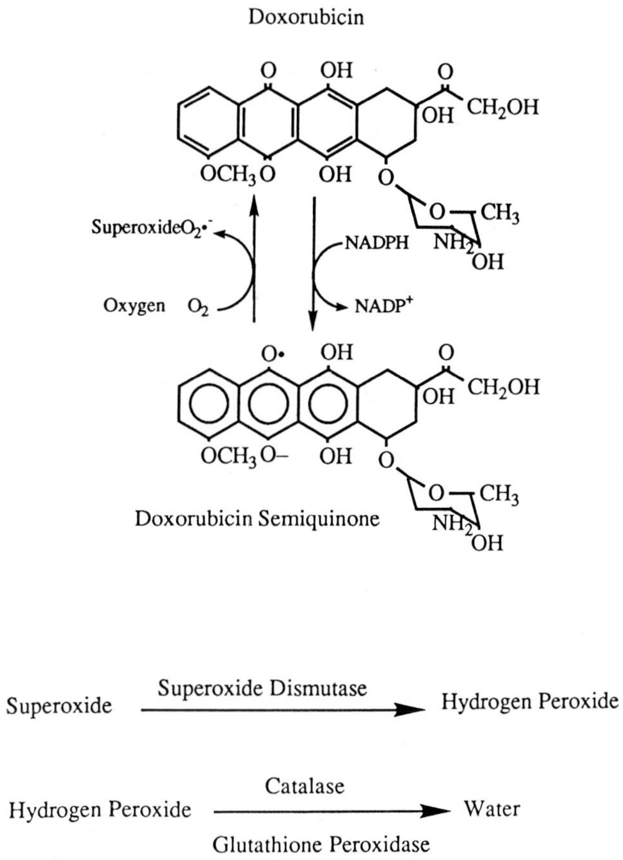

Doxorubicin

Doxorubicin Semiquinone

Superoxide $\xrightarrow{\text{Superoxide Dismutase}}$ Hydrogen Peroxide

Hydrogen Peroxide $\xrightarrow[\text{Glutathione Peroxidase}]{\text{Catalase}}$ Water

Figure XVI-5-2. Doxorubicin redox cycle and detoxification pathway. The upper portion of the figure shows the one electron reduction of doxorubincin to its corresponding semiquinone. This drug-free radical then donates this extra electron to molecular oxygen generating superoxide. The lower portion of the figure shows the enzymatic pathways for detoxification of superoxide and hydrogen peroxide to water.

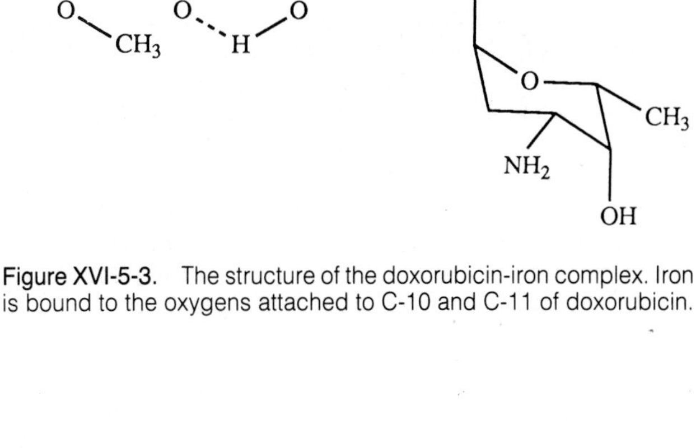

Figure XVI-5-3. The structure of the doxorubicin-iron complex. Iron is bound to the oxygens attached to C-10 and C-11 of doxorubicin.

half-lives on the order of 24–48 hours that is dominated by the slow release of drug bound to DNA.[17,19] During this time period, plasma levels are usually much lower than simultaneously measured tissue levels.[87,95] Renal elimination is not quantitatively significant for the anthracyclines. The liver is known to be a major site of metabolism, with the major metabolites being the reduction of the side chain ketone to an alcohol. For epirubicin, hepatic glucuronidation also appears to be important.[79] Despite the major role played by the liver in drug clearance, it is not clear that drug dosages need to be reduced in the face of abnormal liver functions.

Anthracyclines have been given by a range of schedules including bolus administration every 28 days, once a week, daily for 3–4 days and by continuous infusion for various times.[55,90] The drug dose tolerated appears to be relatively independent of schedule. For example, 60 mg/M² of doxorubicin results in similar overall toxicity whether given by bolus or by 96-hour infusion.[55] The specific dose limiting toxicity does shift, however. With bolus administration of doxorubicin, dose limiting toxicity is generally myelosuppression, while with a 96-hour infusion, mucositis becomes more of a problem. There is clinical trial evidence to suggest that prolonged infusions may be less cardiotoxic than large monthly bolus dose administration.[55,90,95] The effect of schedule on antitumor activity is less clear. Available evidence does not suggest a difference in response rate in breast cancer if the drug is given by either monthly or weekly bolus or 96-hour infusion.

While dose-intensification has been extensively applied to the use of alkylating agents, anthracyclines have been subjected to only limited study.[56A] One recent trial has suggested that with coadministration of G-CSF, it may be possible to administer much larger doses of doxorubicin: patients with breast cancer tolerated as much as 180 mg/M² of doxorubicin every 2 weeks as a single agent with a response rate of 80%.[18,19]

Patterns of Toxicity

The major toxicities of the anthracyclines include myelosuppression, mucositis, hair loss, cardiac toxicity and severe local injury upon extravasation.

Cardiac Toxicity. Of the possible toxicities, cardiac toxicity has been the most studied and, as a result, the mechanism of this side effect is known and means are available for its prevention.

The cardiac toxicity of the anthracyclines can manifest in two distinct clinical syndromes. The drugs can precipitate an acute myocarditis-pericarditis syndrome in which the patient develops rapidly progressive heart failure and arrhythmias that can be associated with fever and pericarditis. This syndrome can appear after only 1–3 doses of doxorubin and can result in sudden death within 7–14 days after a dose of an anthracycline. The second manifestation of cardiac toxicity is a gradual loss of myocardial function with cumulative dosage of anthracycline. Endocardial biopsies performed after various total dosages of doxorubicin suggest a linear relationship between total dose administered and the amount of cardiac tissue lost.[14] However, the incidence of clinically evident congestive heart failure increases exponentially with total dose of anthracycline administered.[96,97] This may result from the fact that the heart has physiologic reserves that must be exceeded before clinically evident congestive heart failure is manifest. Each anthracycline appears to have its

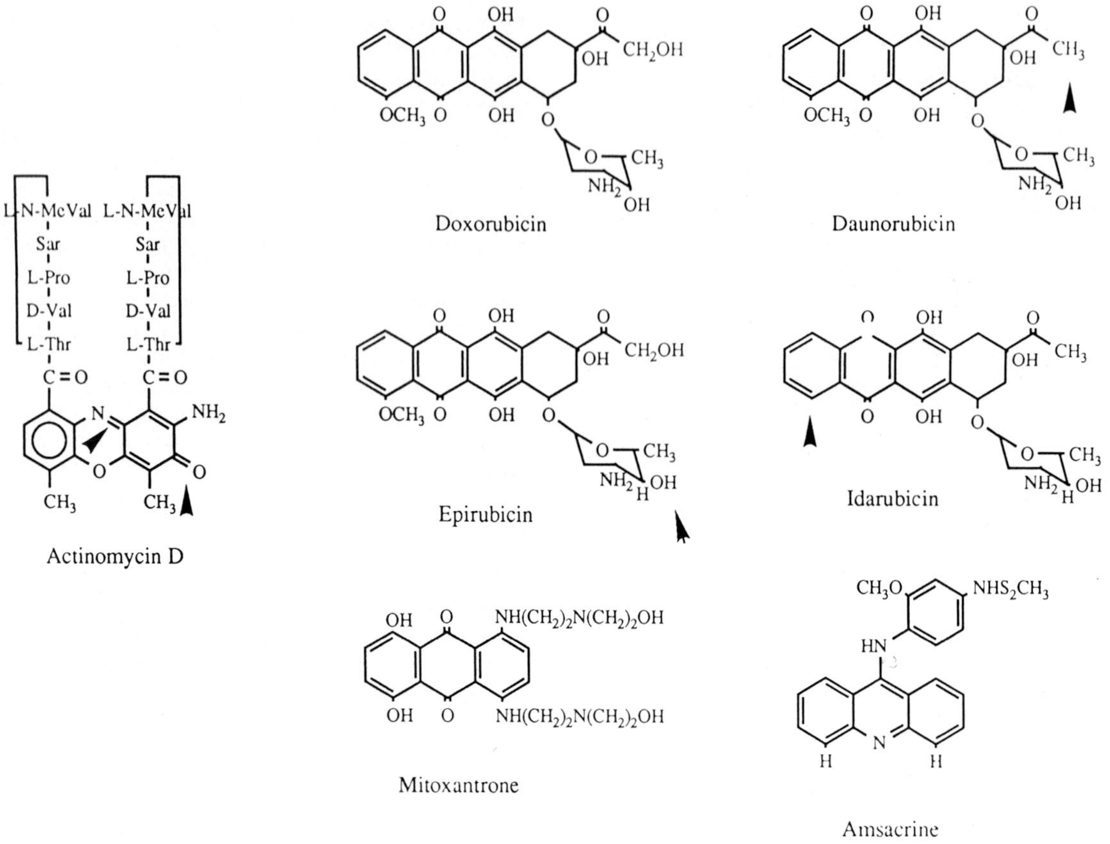

Figure XVI-5-4. DNA intercalators in clinical use. The arrows on actinomycin D show sites of potential redox cycling. The arrows on the anthracyclines show step by step the changes in structure compared to doxorubicin.

own unique quantitative relationship between total dose and degree of myocardial damage so that 550 mg/M² of doxorubicin is equivalent to 900 mg/M² of daunorubicin, both giving an approximate risk of congestive heart failure of 5%.[96,97] Each of the anthracyclines also differ in their potency as anticancer agents and when this is taken into consideration, the clinically used anthracyclines appear to be equally cardiotoxic when given at doses of equivalent therapeutic effectiveness.

In the face of the above information, it has been the custom to limit the total dose of anthracycline administered. These limits have been usually set at a risk of 5% or the equivalent of 550 mg/M² of doxorubicin. This practice has been useful in limiting the risk of cardiac toxicity. However, there is considerable individual variation in susceptibility to anthracycline cardiac toxicity with some individuals developing cardiac toxicity at total doxorubicin doses below 300 mg/M² while others are without symptoms at doxorubicin doses above 800 mg/M².[14,88] It is clear that optimum practice requires monitoring each patient for cardiac toxicity and individualizing the use of the drug. Two techniques have been accepted for this purpose. Endocardial biopsies may be made and used to quantify the degree of cardiac damage pathologically. A useful alternate to this is to measure the ejection fraction with an ECG-gaited blood pool scan.[14,88]

The role of this redox chemistry in anthracycline cardiac toxicity is well worked out and illustrative of how drug-induced free radical damage can occur. The flavin-centered reduc-

tases are the enzyme family most commonly associated with the reduction of the anthracyclines to their corresponding semiquinone free radicals.[4] These enzymes include cytochrome P450 reductase, xanthine oxidase, and mitochondrial NADH oxidase. Cardiac tissue is a rich source of these enzymes with doxorubicin free radical formation being demonstrated in both cardiac cytosol and mitochondrial fractions.[34-36] However, these enzymes are so widely distributed in normal tissue that presence or absence of these enzymes is not sufficient to explain the unusual sensitivity of cardiac tissue. Superoxide and hydrogen peroxide are generated at many points in normal intermediary aerobic metabolism. As a result, all aerobic organisms possess enzymatic machinery to detoxify these reactive oxygen species. The detoxification pathway involves the sequential conversion of each of these reactive species to water (Figure XVI-5-2). The first step in this process is the conversion of superoxide to hydrogen peroxide by the enzyme superoxide dismutase. The second step is the conversion of hydrogen peroxide to water. This step can be accomplished by either catalase or the enzyme, glutathione peroxidase. The latter uses the thiol-containing tripeptide, glutathione, to reduce hydrogen peroxide to water. Cardiac tissue is relatively unusual in that it contains very little catalase and seems to be solely dependent upon glutathione peroxidase for the reduction of hydrogen peroxide to water.[37] However, following the administration of doxorubicin, there is a rapid reduction in glutathione peroxidase activity.[37] Thus, at the same time that doxorubicin initiates the formation of both superoxide and hydrogen peroxide, it abrogates the major means available for cardiac tissue to dispose of these reactive oxygen species.

The first indication that the above picture was not the complete explanation for anthracycline cardiac toxicity came from the observation that agents which are active free radical scavengers, such as N-acetyl cysteine, were not able to block chronic cardiac toxicity in humans.[70] The missing factor proved to be the interaction of doxorubicin and other anthracyclines with iron.[70] These drugs are powerful chelators of iron, with measured affinity constants of 10^{33}. In addition, the resulting iron complexes are able to bind to cell membranes and DNA and cause extensive local free radical damage through hydroxyl radical formation.[43,49–51,68,69,72,73] Because hydroxyl radical formation occurs in the immediate vicinity of the biologic target, general free radical scavengers such as N-acetyl-cysteine and vitamin E are destined to be inefficient. Instead, the only successful approach appears to make the iron unavailable to the anthracycline.[28–31,50,94] ICRF-187, ADR 529 or dexrazoxane, as it is now known, is an EDTA derivative in which the metal chelating structures of EDTA have been fused into amide rings creating a nonchelating nonpolar drug which readily diffuses throughout the body (Figure XVI-5-5). In the presence of the doxorubicin-iron complex, ADR 529 undergoes prompt hydrolysis to the corresponding carboxylamine which accepts the iron from the anthracycline-iron complex with the regeneration of

free doxorubicin.[52,53] As a result, ADR 529 is effective in preventing iron-mediated free radical damage initiated by doxorubicin.[88]

The pathology and physiology of anthracycline cardiac toxicity is distinctive. In the normal cardiac contractile cycle, the wave of electrical depolarization passes down the sarcoplasmic reticulum. This results in release of the calcium bound to the sarcoplasmic reticulum that then diffuses to the contractile elements and triggers mechanical contraction by activating a calcium-dependent ATPase. The subsequent relaxation involves rebinding of the calcium by the sarcoplasmic reticulum. The sarcoplasmic reticulum has been shown to be a site of avid anthracycline free radical formation.[34–36] This free radical formation results in oxidative damage to the sarcoplasmic reticulum membrane and thus defective calcium binding.[84] The result is defective relaxation following contraction and an elevated level of free calcium.[84] As with skeletal muscles, heart muscle contains proteases activated by elevated calcium. This sequence of events results in the loss of muscle fibers and consequently myocardial contractility seen following anthracycline administration. In addition, it explains the pathologic hallmarks of this toxicity which includes dilation of the sarcoplasmic reticulum and fragmentation and loss of myofibrils.[14]

At present, there are two approaches which appear to successfully limit the severity of anthracycline cardiac toxicity. First, the cardiac toxicity of these drugs appears to be

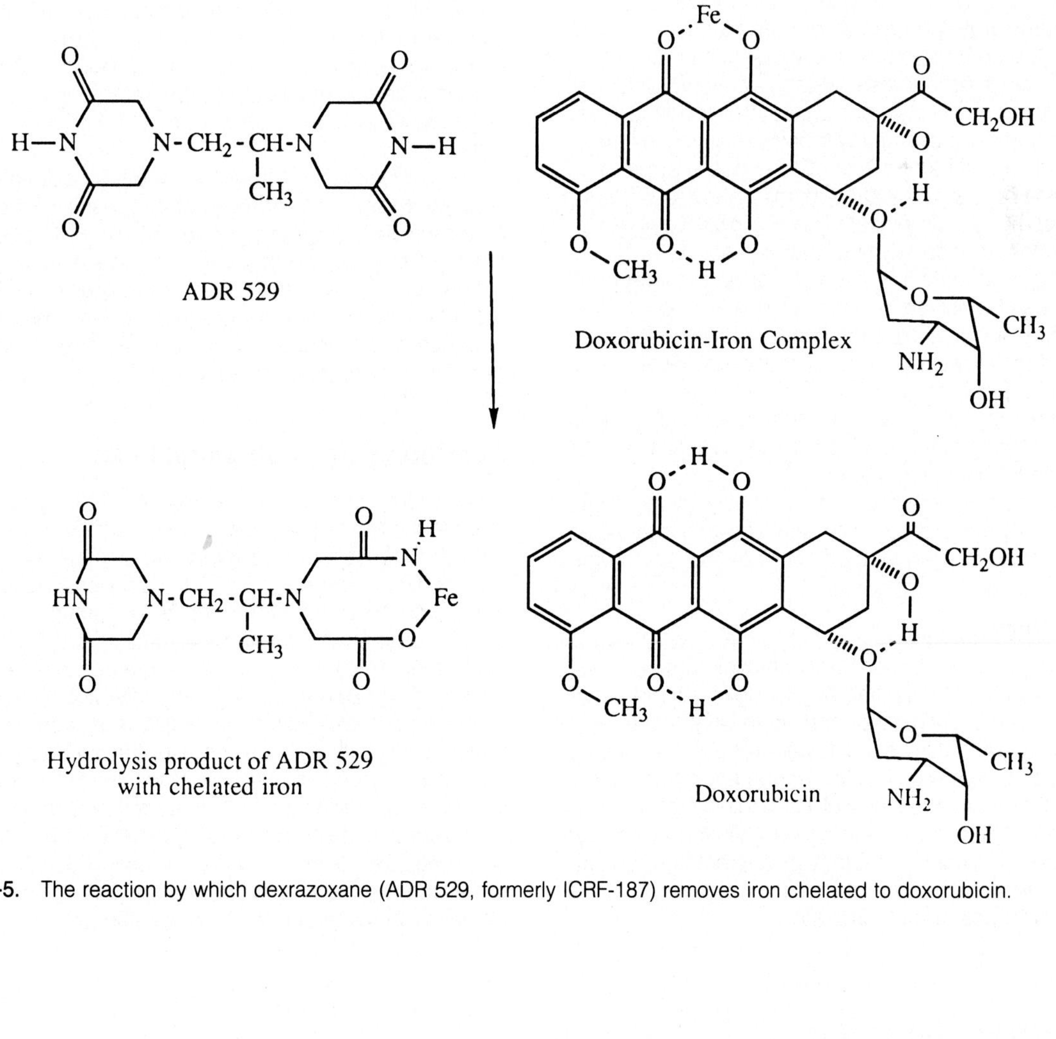

Figure XVI-5-5. The reaction by which dexrazoxane (ADR 529, formerly ICRF-187) removes iron chelated to doxorubicin.

related to peak drug level; thus bolus administration every four weeks results in a greater risk of cardiac toxicity than weekly bolus administration or 96-hour infusions.[55,90] The second approach is dependent upon coadministration of the drug ADR 529, formerly ICRF 187. This agent is an analog of EDTA and is an effective chelator of transition metal ions such as iron and copper. Since these transition metal ions are critical catalysts of oxygen free radical reactions, it has been proposed that ADR 529 lessens the cardiac toxicity of the anthracyclines by limiting free radical damage to the heart. At present, it is not clear which of these two approaches is more effective.

Myelosuppression. In clinical practice, the most common dose-limiting toxicity of the anthracyclines is granulocytopenia. Although lymphopenia, thrombocytopenia and anemia also occur, they are less severe and rarely dose-limiting. While the precise mechanism of this hematopoietic toxicity has not been determined, ADR 529 did not alter the lymphocytopenia and granulocytopenia and thus has been assumed not to be due to free radical formation by the drug, but rather as a consequence of DNA intercalation.[88] One clinical trial has suggested that G-CSF may be highly effective in treating granulocytopenia, thereby allowing a doubling in the maximum tolerated dose intensity of doxorubicin, but not the total dose, which is determined by cardiotoxicity.[18,19]

Mucositis. Drugs of this family can cause inflammation and ulceration of oropharynx, esophagitis, colitis and, occasionally, vulvitis. When doxorubicin is given by 96-hour infusion rather than bolus administration, mucositis rather than hematopoietic toxicity may become dose limiting.[55,90]

Extravasation Injury. Leakage of currently used anthracyclines into the subcutaneous tissues results in the development of local tissue necrosis which heals only with difficulty (Plate XVI-5-1).[39] In severe cases, the resulting ulcer can continue to extend over many months resulting in severe disability, and even loss of a limb. This process appears to depend on the fact that the drug binds tightly to the subcutaneous tissues causing local injury. Following cell death, the drug is released and binds to the next tissue layer and the process thus repeats itself. A wide range of therapeutic approaches have been advocated ranging from cold compresses to wide surgical excision of involved tissue followed by skin grafting. However, none of these proposals have been subjected to rigorous clinical trial. The best approach appears to be prevention by making sure that the drug is administered through a freely flowing intravenous line or indwelling central venous catheter.

Hair Loss. The mechanism by which anthracyclines cause hair loss, a nearly universal toxicity, is unknown. Local scalp hypothermia has been advocated, but has not seen wide use.

Antitumor Spectrum

The most important activities for Adriamycin are in breast cancer, sarcoma, Hodgkin's and non-Hodgkin's lymphoma, pediatric solid tumors, myeloma, and acute lymphocytic and myeloid leukemias. It has definite, albeit, less compelling activity in stomach, small cell, ovary, endometrial, transitional cell and thyroid carcinomas, as well as carcinoid, and malignant thymoma. Doxorubicin is uncommonly used alone, but is a component of many combination chemotherapy regimens, particularly with cyclophosphamide, cisplatin, the vinca alkaloids, fluorouracil or methotrexate.

Daunorubicin is currently used in combination with cytosine arabinoside in the treatment of acute myeloid leukemia, and with vicristine and prednisone in acute lymphocytic leukemia.

Idarubicin has recently been approved for the same indications as daunorubicin because of a series of randomized clinical trials indicating superior results with idarubicin compared with daunorubicin in the treatment of leukemia.[3,11,12,23,24] In addition, it has shown activity in non-Hodgkin's lymphomas. Orally administered idarubicin has proven active in breast cancer.[7,8,42] Its value for this indication as compared to epirubicin or doxorubicin is not clear, except for the availability of an oral route of administration. Activity has also been seen in non-small cell carcinoma of the lung.[1]

Epirubicin has antitumor activity similar to doxorubicin in breast cancer.[77] Its activity against other tumors is less clearly defined, but responses have been seen in acute leukemias, sarcomas and carcinomas of the lung and ovary.[6,15,25,66,67] It has been claimed to possess reduced cardiac toxicity compared with doxorubicin and this assertion has been contested.[66,67] Until this issue is settled, epirubicin seems to offer no significant advantage over doxorubicin.

Interactions

Anthracyclines can sensitize normal tissues to radiation damage.[32] This effect appears to be fairly general, but is a particular problem in certain treatment situations. First, doxorubicin has been shown to increase the severity of radiation pneumonitis. Second, exposure of the heart to greater than 2,000 cGy effectively doubles the cardiac toxicity of a given cumulative dose of doxorubicin.[13] Third, doxorubicin has been shown to worsen the severity of radiation damage to oral and esophageal mucosa. Fourth, anthracyclines can trigger radiation recall in the skin with resultant erythema and folliculitis.

The anthracyclines may be readily coadministered with most other anticancer drugs without significant problem—a factor which has played a role in their wide use in combination chemotherapy. In experimental animals and in tissue culture, exposure to doxorubicin and drugs, such as BCNU or acetaminophen, that deplete tissue thiols, has been reported to cause acute death of liver cells. To date, this interaction has not been noted clinically.

Dactinomycin (Actinomycin D)

Dactinomycin consists of two symmetric polypeptide chains attached to a phenoxazone, a planar three ring system (Figure XVI-5-4). As might be expected, it is the planar aromatic phenoxazone ring system which is responsible for the ability of this compound to intercalate DNA. Dactinomycin exhibits considerable DNA sequence specificity, with the most stable DNA complexes forming with the sequence dATGCAT.[21,64,81,91] This binding appears to be highly effective at blocking RNA synthesis with elongation of RNA strands more affected than chain initiation or release. As with the anthracyclines, dactinomycin also exhibits redox chemistry.[46,81,82] In this case, the drug possesses a quinone-imine functionality which can be reduced to the corresponding semiquinone. Little is known about the consequences of this reduction, but antitumor activity in a series of dactinomycin analogs correlated with redox potential rather than DNA binding affinity.

Routes of Administration, Schedule, and Pharmacokinetics

Dactinomycin may only be administered intravenously. The drug crosses cell membranes by free diffusion, although in the presence of the *mdr* gene product the drug is susceptible to active efflux.[16] Within cells, most of the drug is tightly bound to DNA. As with the anthracyclines, DNA binding dominates the pharmacokinetics of actinomycin D. The initial phase of actinomycin D plasma clearance involves rapid distribution of the drug to tissues.[10,93] The second phase has a half-life of 36 hours and is determined by the slow dissociation of the DNA bound drug. While no metabolites have been detected, urinary and biliary clearance of parent drug accounts for less than half the administered dose. From this it is clear that our knowledge of the pharmacokinetics of actinomycin D is far from complete. The usual clinical dose is 10–15 μg/kg/day for 5 days.

Patterns of Toxicity

Dactinomycin causes nausea, vomiting, diarrhea, mucositis, and alopecia. The most common dose limiting toxicity is granulocytopenia and thrombocytopenia with a nadir 10–14 days following drug administration. As with the anthracyclines, extravasation of actinomycin D is associated with severe local injury.

Antitumor Spectrum

At present, the use of actinomycin D is limited to pediatric cancers. Useful activity is seen in Wilms' tumor, rhabdomyosarcoma, Ewing's sarcoma and neuroblastoma, and has been described in gestational choriocarcinoma, and embryonal carcinoma.[44,63,92,100]

Interactions

Dactinomycin causes radiation sensitization.[27,64] In addition, it can trigger a recall phenomenon at sites of previous radiation therapy. This can result in severe skin reactions or compromise of organ function. Corticosteroids have been used to treat these complications.

Mitoxantrone

Mitoxantrone (Figure XVI-5-4) is a member of the anthracenedione family of DNA intercalators. This drug class is completely synthetic in origin and was developed as part of the search for analogs of anthracyclines. As with the anthracyclines, mitoxantrone has a chromophore composed of three planar aromatic rings. Also, as with the anthracyclines, the chromophore is an hydroxyquinone. In place of the daunosamine sugar characteristic of the anthracyclines, mitoxantrone has two identical aminoalkyl side chains. As a result, mitoxantrone possesses the ability to intercalate into DNA and to trigger topoisomerase II dependent DNA cleavage, and this is probably the mechanism of tumor cell kill.[41] While it can undergo reduction to the corresponding semiquinone, the redox potential for this reaction is such that it is not favored.[60,61,74] In addition, while mitoxantrone is able to bind copper and iron as can the anthracyclines, the resultant complexes appear unable to catalyze free radical damage to cell membranes. As a result, mitoxantrone does not cause lipid peroxidation in cardiac tissue and is less cardiotoxic than doxorubicin.[54]

Routes of Administration, Schedule, and Pharmacokinetics

Mitoxantrone appears to enter cells by free diffusion. Inside cells, most of the drug exists bound to DNA. As with the anthracyclines, DNA binding dominates the pharmacokinetics of mitoxantrone. The initial distribution of the drug occurs with a half-life of 1–2 hours followed by a terminal half-life of 23–42 hours limited by the slow dissociation of the drug from DNA40. Parent drug eliminated in urine and stool accounts for less than 30% of the drug administered. While the metabolism of this drug is incompletely described, side chain oxidation to inactive mono and dicarboxylic acid metabolites has been described. Common schedules of administration appear to be patterned after those used for the anthracyclines. For acute nonlymphocytic leukemia, a dose of 12 mg/M^2/day for three days has been used in combination with cytosine arabinoside. For carcinoma of the breast, the typical schedule is 12–14 mg/M^2 once every 3 weeks. In lymphocytic neoplasms, 10–15 mg/M^2/day for three days in association with vincristine and prednisone have been used.

Patterns of Toxicity

Dose-limiting toxicity is granulocytopenia with recovery typically complete by day 14 after usual doses. The drug also can cause thrombocytopenia, nausea and vomiting. Because of its intense blue color, the drug can cause bluish discoloration of the sclera, fingernails and urine. In contrast to the anthracyclines, extravasation injury is uncommon. While cardiac toxicity has been seen in patients receiving mitoxantrone, this has been most common in patients previously treated with doxorubicin or daunorubicin.[54] Previous chest wall irradiation and underlying cardiac disease are other risk factors associated with cardiac toxicity of mitoxantrone. Liver injury can also occur and this has been associated with lipid peroxidation and other in vitro evidence of free radical injury.[40,65] The enzymatic basis for such free radical formation is not clear. Mucositis is similar to the anthracyclines, but alopecia, nausea and vomiting are less.

Antitumor Spectrum

Antitumor activity of mitoxantrone appears to be limited to breast cancer, leukemias and lymphomas.

Interactions

Synergy between cytosine arabinoside and mitoxantrone has been reported in acute nonlymphocytic leukemia.

Amsacrine

Amsacrine (m-AMSA) is a derivative of acridine and thus, as with mitoxantrone, a totally synthetic drug. Again, as with the other drugs in this family, the ability of this drug to intercalate into DNA depends upon the presence of a three ring planar aromatic chromophore (Figure XVI-5-4). This drug is effective at triggering topoisomerase II-dependent protein-associated DNA breaks; available evidence strongly suggests that this is the mechanism of tumor cell kill.[59] While this drug can cause cardiac toxicity, it is likely that this side effect is not the result of drug-induced free radical production, since amsacrine is a poor substrate for one electron reduction.[2,45,83] Hypokalemia potentiates the cardiac arrhythmias. There is evidence that drug metabolism may play a part in maximizing DNA breakage, but the nature of such a metabolite has yet to be identified.[102]

Routes of Administration, Schedule, and Pharmacokinetics

As with the other DNA intercalators, m-AMSA rapidly enters cells where the bulk of the drug may be found bound to DNA. As a result, tissue concentrations are typically 3–10 times higher than those of plasma. The pharmacokinetics of m-AMSA are very different from the other drugs in this class.[20,56,75,76] The terminal half life is on the order of 4–8 hours rather than the 25–50 hour half lives found for the anthracyclines, dactinomycin and mitoxantrone. In addition, there is strong evidence that glutathione conjugation by glutathione transferase plays an important role in drug inactivation.[75,80] First, drugs which inhibit the steps in glutathione conjugation significantly alter drug clearance. Second, in rodents 70–80% of the administered dose appears in the bile and 70–80% of the drug in the bile appears as a glutathione conjugate. In addition, drug administration results in sufficient glutathione consumption to cause depletion of hepatic glutathione. Finally, an m-AMSA resistant breast cancer cell line exhibited a nearly 10-fold increase in the expression of glutathione transferase π in the absence of expression of the *mdr* gene product. Because of the importance of hepatic metabolism, dose of this drug should be adjusted in the presence of liver function abnormalities.[75,80] This usual dose is 120 mg/M² iv daily for five days. In addition, 75–150 mg/M² has been administered as a continuous infusion over 72 hours without any significant alteration in the pattern of toxicity or loss in antitumor efficacy.

Patterns of Toxicity

The most common dose limiting toxicities of m-AMSA are mucositis and myelosupression with relative platelet sparing. Alopecia, and mild to moderate nausea and vomiting are also common. Hepatic toxicity has been noted, but usually is limited to asymptomatic transaminitis. This may be the consequence of the extensive hepatic metabolism of m-AMSA.[75,80] Amsacrine also can cause cardiac toxicity.[2,45,78,83] This can manifest as two distinct syndromes. First, patients who have had previous exposure to anthracyclines can have a cardiomyopathy precipitated by m-AMSA administration. Second, the drug can result in a wide range of arrhythmias. The risk of the latter appears to be markedly diminished if normal serum potassium levels are maintained.

Antitumor Spectrum

This drug has its major use in the treatment of the acute myeloid leukemias. Activity has also been noted in a range of lymphomas, but it has not seen wide use in their treatment.

Interactions

The drug–drug interactions have not been clearly defined in man. However, in view of the clear documentation of the role of hepatic metabolism in drug clearance, caution should be excised with coadministration of this drug with certain other agents. In animal models, cimetidine and phenobarbital, two drugs which alter microsomal mixed function oxidases, clearly alter m-AMSA clearance[75,80] Buthionine sulfoximine, an agent which blocks glutathione synthesis, also alters m-AMSA clearance. Coadministration of m-AMSA with drugs which alter hepatic glutathione should be approached with caution. The nitrosoureas block glutathione reduction and thus are potentially a problem. In addition, acetaminophen is well known to deplete hepatic glutathione and should be used with caution.

Bibliography

1. Arcamone, F., Cassinelli, G., Fantini, G., Grein, A., Orezzi, P., Pol, C., and Spalla, C.: Adriamycin, 14-hydroxy daunomycin, a new antitumor antibiotic from S. peucetius var. Caesius. Biotechnol. Bioeng., 11:1101, 1969.
1A. Ardizzoni, A., Pennucci, C., Fusco, V., Gulisano, M., Bonavia, M., Pronzato, P., De Palma, M., Serrano, J., and Rosso, R.: Oral chemotherapy for poor risk small-cell lung cancer patients with combined idarubicin and etoposide. Anticancer Res., 9:937, 1989.
2. Arlin, Z., Mehta, R., Feldman, E., Sullivan, P., and Pucillo, A.: Amsacrine treatment of patients with supraventricular arrhythmias and acute leukemia. Cancer Chemother. Pharmacol., 19:163, 1987.
3. Arlin, Z. A.: Idarubicin in acute leukemia: An effective new therapy for the future. Semin. Oncol., 16:35, 1989.
4. Bachur, N. R., Gordon, S. L., and Gee, M. V.: Anthracycline antibiotic augmentation of microsomal electron transport and free radical formation. Mol. Pharmacol., 13:901, 1977.
5. Baguley, B. C.: DNA intercalating anti-tumour agents. Anticancer Drug Des., 6:1, 1991.
6. Banham, S. W., Henderson, A. F., Bicknell, S., Hughes, J., Milroy, R., and Monie, R. D.: High dose epirubicin chemotherapy in untreated poorer prognosis small cell lung cancer. Respir. Med., 84:241, 1990.
7. Bastholt, L., Dalmark, M., Jakobsen, A., Gadeberg, C. C., Sandberg, E., and Mouridsen, H. T.: Oral idarubicin in the treatment of advanced breast cancer. Acta Oncol., 28:893, 1989.
8. Bastholt, L., Dalmark, M., Jakobsen, A., Gadeberg, C. C., Sandberg, E., and Mouridsen, H. T.: Weekly oral idarubicin in postmenopausal women with advanced breast cancer. A phase II study. Acta Oncol., 29:143, 1990.
9. Beck, W. T.: Mechanisms of multidrug resistance in human tumor cells. The role of P-glycoprotein, DNA topoisomerase II, and other factors. Cancer Treat. Rev., 17 (Suppl. A):11, 1990.
10. Benjamin R. S., H. S., and Burgass, M. A.: A pharmacokinetically based phase 1-2 study of single dose actinomycin D (NSC-3053). Cancer Treat. Rep., 60:289, 1976.
11. Berman, E., Heller, G., Santorsa, J., McKenzie, S., Gee, T., Kempin, S., Gulati, S., Andreeff, M., Kolitz, J., Gabrilove, J., et al.: Results of a randomized trial comparing idarubicin and cytosine arabinoside with daunorubicin and cytosine arabinoside in adult patients with newly diagnosed acute myelogenous leukemia. Blood, 77:1666, 1991.
12. Berman, E., Raymond, V., Daghestani, A., Arlin, Z. A., Gee, T. S., Kempin, S., Hancock, C., Williams, L., Stevens, Y. W., Clarkson, B. D., and Young, C.: 4-demethoxydaunorubicin (idarubicin) in combination with 1-beta-D-arabinofuranosylcytosine in the treatment of relapsed or refractory acute leukemia. Cancer Res., 49:477, 1989.
13. Billingham, M. E., Bristow, M. R., Glatstein, E., Mason, J. W., Masek, M. A., and Daniels, J. R.: Adriamycin cardiotoxicity: endomyocardial biopsy evidence of enhancement by irradiation. Am. J. Surg. Pathol., 1:17, 1977.
14. Billingham, M. E., Mason, J. W., Bristow, M. R., and Daniels, J. R.: Anthracycline cardiomyopathy monitored by morphologic changes. Cancer Treat. Rep., 62:865, 1978.
15. Blackstein, M., Eisenhaver, E. A., Wierzbick, R., and Yoshida, S.: Epirubicin in extensive small-cell lung cancer: a phase II study in previously untreated patients: a National Cancer Institute of Canada Clinical Trials Group Study (see comments). J. Clin. Oncol., 8:385, 1990.
15A. Bonadonna, G., Monfardini, S., De Lena, M., and Fossati-Bellani, F.: Clinical evaluation of adriamycin, a new antitumor antibiotic. Br. Med. J., 3:503, 1969.
16. Bowen, D., and Goldman, I. D.: The relationship among transport, intracellular binding, and inhibition of RNA synthesis by actinomycin D in Ehrlich ascites tumor cells in vitro. Cancer Res., 35:3054, 1975.
17. Brenner, D. E., Wiernik, P. H., Wesley, M., and Bachur, N. R.: Acute doxorubicin toxicity. Relationship to pretreatment liver function, response, and pharmacokinetics in patients with acute nonlymphocytic leukemia. Cancer, 53:1042, 1984.
18. Bronchud, M. H., Howell, A., Crowther, D., Hopwood, P., Souzal, L., and Dexter, T. M.: The use of granulocyte colony-stimulating factor to increase the intensity of treatment with doxorubicin in patients with advanced breast and ovarian cancer. Br. J. Cancer, 60:121, 1989.
19. Bronchud, M. H., Margison, J. M., Howell, A., Lind, M., Lucas, S. D., and Wilkinson, P. M.: Comparative pharmacokinetics of escalating doses of doxorubicin in patients with metastatic breast cancer. Cancer Chemother. Pharmacol., 25:435, 1990.
20. Brons, P. P., Wessels, J. M., Linssen, P. C., Haanen, C., and Speth, P. A.: Determination of amsacrine in human nucleated hematopoietic cells. J. Chromatogr., 422:175, 1987.
21. Brown, S., Mullis, K., Levenson, C., and Shafer, R. H.: Aqueous solution structure of an intercalated actinomycin D-dATGCAT complex by two dimensional and one dimensional proton NMR. Biochemistry, 23:403, 1984.
22. Calendi, E., DiMarco, A., Reggiani, M., Scarpinato, B., and Valentini, L.: On physicochemical interactions between daunomycin and nucleic acids. Biochim. Biophys. Acta, 103:25, 1965.
23. Carella, A. M., Berman, E., Maraone, M. P., and Ganzina, F.: Idarubicin in the treatment of acute leukemias. An overview of preclinical and clinical studies. Haematologica, 75:159, 1990.
24. Carella, A. M., Pungolino, E., Piatti, G., Gaozza, E., Nati, S., Spriano, M., Giordano, D., D'Amico, T., and Damasio, E.: Idarubicin in combination with intermediate-dose cytarabine in the treatment of refractory or relapsed acute leukemias. Eur. J. Haematol., 43:309, 1989.
25. Casadio, M., Lelli, G., Giordani, S., Beltri, B., Blotta, A., Busutti, L., Ramini, R., Falcone, F., and Pannuti, F.: Small cell bronchogenic carcinoma: a cyclical alternating combination of epirubicin plus cisplatin and cyclophosphamide plus etoposide. J. Chemother., 2:199, 1990.
26. Cramer, S. C., Rhodes, R. H., Acton, E. M., and Tokes, Z. A.: Neurotoxicity and dermatotoxicity of cyanomorpholinyl adriamycin. Cancer Chemother. Pharmacol., 23:71, 1989.
27. D'Angio, G. J., Farber, S., and Maddock, C. L.: Potentiation of x-ray effects by actinomycin D. Radiology, 73:175, 1959.
28. Demant, E. J. F.: Binding of adriamycin-FE³⁺ complex to membrane phospholipids. Eur. J. Biochem., 142:571, 1984.
29. Demant, E. J. F.: Mobilization of ferritin-iron by adriamycin. FEBS Lett., 176:97, 1984.
30. Demant, E. J. F.: Transfer of ferritin-bound iron to adriamycin. FEBS Lett., 176:97, 1984.

31. Demant, E. J. F., and Nørskov-Lauritsen, N.: Binding of transferrin-iron by adriamycin at acidic pH. FEBS Lett., 196:321, 1986.
32. Denny, W. A.: DNA-intercalating ligands as anti-cancer drugs: prospects for future design. Anticancer Drug Des., 4:241, 1989.
33. DiMarco, A., Gaetani, M., Orezzi, P., Scarpinato, B., Silvestrini, R., Soldati, M., Dasdia, T., and Valentini, L.: Daunomycin, a new antibiotic of the rhodomycin group. Nature, 201:706, 1964.
34. Doroshow, J. H.: Anthracycline antibiotic-stimulated superoxide, hydrogen peroxide, and hydroxyl radical production by NADH dehydrogenase. Cancer Res., 43:4543, 1983.
35. Doroshow, J. H.: Effect of anthracycline antibiotics on oxygen radical formation in rat heart. Cancer Res., 43:460, 1983.
36. Doroshow, J. H., and Davies, K. J.: Comparative cardiac oxygen radical metabolism by anthracycline antibiotics, mitoxantrone, bisantrene, 4′-(9-acridinylamino)-methanesulfon-m-anisidide, and neocarzinostatin. Biochem. Pharmacol., 32:2935, 1983.
37. Doroshow, J. H., Locker, G. Y., and Myers, C. E.: The enzymatic defenses of the mouse heart against reactive metabolites. J. Clin. Invest., 65:128, 1980.
38. Dorr, R. T.: Antidotes to vesicant endomyocardial extravasations. Blood Rev., 4:41, 1990.
39. Dorr, R. T., Dordal, M. S., Koenig, L. M., Taylor, C. W., and McCloskey, T. M.: High levels of doxorubicin in the tissues of a patient experiencing extravasation during a 4-day infusion. Cancer, 64:2462, 1989.
40. Duthie, S. J., and Grant, M. H.: The toxicity of menadione and mitoxantrone in human liver-derived Hep G2 hepatoma cells. Biochem. Pharmacol., 38:1247, 1989.
41. Ehninger, G., Schuler, U., Proksch, B., Zeller, K. P., and Blanz, J.: Pharmacokinetics and metabolism of mitoxantrone. A review. Clin. Pharmacokinet., 18:365, 1990.
42. Elbaek, K., Ebbehoj, E., Jakobsen, A., Juul, P., Rasmussen, S. N., Bastholt, L., Dalmark, M., and Steiness, E.: Pharmacokinetics of oral idarubicin in breast cancer patients with reference to antitumor activity and side effects. Clin. Pharmacol. Ther., 45:627, 1989.
43. Eliot, H., Gianni, L., and Myers, C.: Oxidative destruction of DNA by adriamycin-iron complex. Biochemistry, 23:928, 1984.
44. Farber, S.: Chemotherapy in the treatment of leukemia and Wilm's tumor. JAMA, 198:826, 1966.
45. Feldman, E. J., Arlin, Z. A., Sullivan, P., and Engelking, C.: Preventing amsacrine-induced cardiac arrhythmias. (Letter) J. Clin. Oncol., 5:2041, 1987.
46. Flitter, W. D., and Mason, R. P.: The enzymatic reduction of actinomycin D to a free radical species. Arch. Biochem. Biophys., 267:632, 1988.
47. Forrest, G. L., Akman, S., Krutzik, S., Paxton, R. J., Sparkes, R. S., Doroshow, J., Felsted, R. L., Glover, C. J., Mohandas, T., and Bachur, N. R.: Induction of a human carbonyl reductase gene located on chromosome 21. Biochim. Biophys. Acta, 1048:149, 1990.
48. Gianni, L., et al.: The biochemical basis of anthracycline toxicity and antitumor activity. *In* Reviews in Biochemical Toxicology. Edited by E. Hodgson, J. R. Bend, and R. M. Philport. Elsevier, Amsterdam, 1983, p. 1.
49. Gianni, L., Vigano, L., Lanzi, C., Niggeler, M., and Malatesta, V.: Role of daunosamine and hydroacetyl side chain in reaction with iron and lipid peroxidation by anthracyclines. J. Natl. Cancer Inst., 80:1104, 1988.
50. Gianni, L., Vigano, L., Niggeler, M., Levi, S., and Arosio, P.: Human ferritin (HLF) as iron source for lipid peroxidation by adriamycin(Adr). San Francisco, Proc. A.A.C.R., 1988.
51. Gianni, L., Zweier, J. L., Levy, A., and Myers, C. E.: Characterization of iron-mediated electron transfer from adriamycin to molecular oxygen. Biol. Chem., 260:6820, 1985.
52. Hasinoff, B. B.: The interaction of the cardioprotective agent ICRF-187 ((+)-1,2-bis(3,5,-dioxopiperazinyl-1-yL)propane); its hydrolysis product (ICRF-198); and other chelating agents with the Fe(III) and Cu(II) complexes of adriamycin. Agents Actions, 26:378, 1989.
53. Hasinoff, B. B., and Davey, J. P.: The iron(III)-adriamycin complex inhibits cytochrome c oxidase before its inactivation. Biochem. J., 250:827, 1988.
54. Henderson, I. C., Allegra, J. C., Woodcock, T., Wolff, S., Bryan, S., Cartwright, K., Dukart, G., and Henry, D.: Randomized clinical trial comparing mitoxantrone with doxorubicin in previously treated patients with metastatic breast cancer. J. Clin. Oncol., 7:560, 1989.
55. Hortobagyi, G. N., Frye, D., Buzdar, A. V., Ewer, M. S., Fraschini, G., Hug, V., Ames, F., Montague, E., Carrasco, C. H., MacKay, B., and Benjamin, R. S.: Decreased cardiac toxicity of doxorubicin administered by continuous intravenous infusion in combination chemotherapy for metastatic breast carcinoma. Cancer, 63:37, 1989.
56. Jehn, U., and Heinemann, V.: Intermediate-dose Ara-C/m-AMSA for remission induction and high-dose Ara-C/m-AMSA for intensive consolidation in relapsed and refractory adult acute myelogeneous leukemia. Hamatol. Bluttransfus., 33:333, 1990.
56A. Jones, R. B., Holland, J. F., Bhordwaj, S., Norton, L., Wilfinger, C., and Strashun, A.: A phase I-II study of intensive-dose adriamycin for advanced breast cancer. J. Clin. Oncol., 5:172, 1987.
57. Juranka, P. F., Zastawny, R. L., and Ling, V.: P-glycoprotein: multidrug-resistance and a superfamily of membrane-associated transport proteins. Faseb J., 3:2583, 1989.
58. Kane, S. E., Pastan, I., and Gottesman, M. M.: Genetic basis of multidrug resistance of tumor cells. J. Bioenerg. Biomembr., 22:593, 1990.
59. Kawamata, J., and Imanishi, M.: Interaction of actinomycin with DNA. Nature, 187:1112, 1960.
60. Kharasch, E. D., and Novak, R. F.: Bis(alkylamino)anthracenedione antineoplastic agent metabolic activation by NADPH-cytochrome P-450 reductase and NADH dehydrogenase: Diminished activity relative to anthracyclines. Arch. Biochem. Biophys., 224:682, 1983.
61. Kharasch, E. D., and Novak, R. F.: Mitoxantrone and ametantrone inhibit hydroperoxide-dependent initiation and propagation reactions in fatty acid peroxidation. J. Biol. Chem., 260:10645, 1985.
62. Lefevre, D., Riou, J. F., Ahomadegbe, J. C., Zhou, D. Y., Bernard, J., and Riou, G.: Study of molecular markers of resistance to m-AMSA in a human breast cancer cell line. Decrease of topoisomerase II and increase of both topoisomerase I and acidic glutathione S transferase. Biochem. Pharmacol., 41:1967, 1991.
63. Lewis, J.: Chemotherapy of gestational choriocarcinoma. Cancer, 30:1517, 1972.
64. Littman, P., Rosenstock, J. G., and Bailey, C.: Radiation myelitis following craniospinal irradiation with concurrent actinomycin D therapy. Oncol., 5:145, 1978.
65. Llesuy, S. F., and Arnaiz, S. L.: Hepatotoxicity of mitoxantrone and doxorubicin. Toxicology, 63:187, 1990.
66. Macchiarini, P., Chella, A., Riva, A., Mengozzi, G., Silvano, G., Solfanelli, S., and Angeletti, C. A.: Phase II feasibility study of high dose epirubicin-based regimens for untreated patients with small-cell lung cancer. Am J. Clin. Oncol., 13:495, 1990.
67. Macchiarini, P., Danesi, R., Mariotti, R., Marchetti, A., Fazzi, P., Bevilacqua, G., Mariani, M., Giuntini, C., Del Tacca, M., and Angeletti, C. A.: Phase II study of high-dose epirubicin in untreated patients with small-cell lung cancer. Am. J. Clin. Oncol., 13:302, 1990.
68. Muindi, J., Sinha, B. K., Gianni, L., and Myers, C.: Thiol dependent DNA damage produced by anthracycline-iron complexes: The structure activity relationships and molecular mechanisms. Mol. Pharm., 27:356, 1985.
69. Muindi, J. R. F., Sinha, B. K., Gianni, L., and Myers, C. E.: Hydroxyl radical production and DNA damage induced by anthracycline iron complex. FEBS Lett., 172:226, 1984.
70. Myers, C. E., Borow, R., Palmeri, S., Jenkins, J., Gorden, B., Locker, G., Doroshow, J., and Epstein, S.: A randomized controlled trial assessing the prevention of doxorubicin cardiomyopathy by N-acetylcysteine. Semin. Oncol., 10:53, 1983.
71. Myers, C. E., Cowan, K., Sinha, B., and Chabner, B.: The Phenomenon of Pleiotropic Drug Resistance. *In* Important Advances in Oncology. Edited by V. T. DeVita, S. Rosenberg, and S. Hellman. Philadelphia, J. B. Lippincott Co., 1987, p. 27.
72. Myers, C. E., Gianni, L., Simone, C. B., Klecker, R., and Greene, R.: Oxidative destruction of erythrocyte ghost membranes catalyzed by the doxorubicin-iron complex. Biochemistry, 21:1707, 1982.
73. Myers, C. E., Gianni, L., Zweier, J., Muindi, J., Sinha, B. K., and Eliot, H., The role of iron in adriamycin biochemistry. Fed. Proc., 45:2792, 1986.
74. Novak, R. F., and Kharasch, E. D.: Mitoxantrone: Propensity for free radical formation and lipid peroxidation—implications for cardiotoxicity. Invest. New Drugs, 3:95, 1985.
75. Paxton, J. W., Evans, P. C., and Hardy, J. R.: The effect of cimetidine, phenobarbitone and buthionine sulphoximine on the disposition of N-5-dimethyl-9-[(2-methoxy-4-methylsulphonylamino)phenylamino]-4-acridinecarboxamide (CI-921) in the rabbit. Cancer Chemother. Pharmacol., 23:291, 1989.
76. Petros, W. P., Rodman, J. H., Mirro, J., Jr., and Evans, W. E.: Pharmacokinetics of continuous-infusion amsacrine and teniposide for the treatment of relapsed childhood acute nonlymphocytic leukemia. Cancer Chemother. Pharmacol., 27:397, 1991.
77. Porzsolt, F., Kreuser, E. D., Meuret, G., Mende, S., Buchelt, L., Redenbacher, M., Heissmeyer, H. H., Strigl, P., Hiemeyer, V., Krause, H. H., Fleischer, K., Saumweber, G., Leichtle, R., Matischok, B., Gaus, W., and Heimpel, H.: High-intensity therapy versus low-intensity therapy in advanced breast cancer patients. Cancer Treat. Rev., 17:287, 1990.
78. Puccio, C. A.: Amsacrine is safe in patients with ventricular ectopy. Am. J. Hematol., 28:197, 1988.
79. Robert, J., David, M., and Granger, C.: Metabolism of epirubicin to glucuronides: Relationship to the pharmacodynamics of the drug. Cancer Chemother. Pharmacol., 27:147, 1990.
80. Robertson, I. G., Kestell, P., Dormer, R. A., and Paxton, J. W.: Involvement of glutathione in the metabolism of the anilinoacridine antitumour agents CI-921 and amsacrine. Drug Metabol. Drug Interact., 6:371, 1988.
81. Sehgal, R. K., Sengupta, S. K., Waxman, D. J., and Tauber, A. I.: Enzymic and chemical reduction of 2-deaminoactinomycins to free radicals. Anticancer Drug Des., 1:13, 1985.
82. Sengupta, S. K., Kelly, C., and Sehgal, R. K.: Reverse: and symmetrical: analogues of actinomycin D: metabolic activation and in vitro and in vivo tumor growth inhibitory activities. J. Med. Chem., 28:620, 1985.
83. Shinar, E., and Hasin, Y.: Acute electrocardiographic changes induced by amsacrine. Cancer Treat. Rep., 68:1169, 1984.
84. Singal, P. K., and Pierce, G. N.: Adriamycin stimulates low affinity CA^{2+} binding and lipid peroxidation but depresses myocardial function. Am. J. Physiol., 250:H419, 1986.
85. Sinha, B. K., Katki, A. G., Batist, G., Cowan, K. H., and Myers, C. E.: Adriamycin-simulated hydroxyl radical formation in human breast tumor cells. Biochem. Pharm., 36:793, 1987.
86. Sobell, H. M., and Jain, S. C.: Stereochemistry of actinomycin D binding to DNA: II. Detailed molecular model of actinomycin-DNA complex and its implications. J. Mol. Biol., 68:21, 1972.
87. Speth, P., Linssen, P. C. M., Holdrinet, R. S. G., and Haanen, C.: Plasma and cellular adriamycin concentrations in patients with myeloma treated with 96 hour continuous infusion. Clin. Pharmacol. Ther., 41:661, 1987.
88. Speyer, J. L., Green, M. D., Kramer, E., Rey, M., Sanger, J., Ward, C., Dubin, N., Ferrans, V., Stecy, P., Zeleniuch-Jacquotte, A., Wernz, J., Feit, F., Slater, W., Blum, R., and Muggia, F.: Protective effect of the bispiperazinedione, ICRF-187, against doxorubicin-induced cardiac toxicity in women with advanced breast cancer. N. Engl. J. Med., 319:745, 1988.
89. Stewart, D. J., Grewaal, D., Green, R. M., Verma, S., Maroun, J. A., Redmond, D., Robillard, L., and Gupta, S.: Bioavailability and pharmacology of oral idarubicin. Cancer Chemother. Pharmacol., 27:308, 1991.
90. Sweatman, T. W., Lokich, J. J., and Israel, M.: Clinical pharmacology of continuous infusion doxorubicin. Ther. Drug Monit., 11:3, 1989.
91. Takusagawa, F., Goldstein, B. M., Youngster, S., Jones, R. A., and Berman, H. M.: Crystallization and preliminary x-ray study of a complex between dATGCAT and actinomycin D. J. Biol. Chem., 259:4714, 1984.
92. Tan, C. T., Dargen, H. W., and Burchenal, J. H.: The effect of actinomycin D on cancer in childhood. Pediatrics, 24:544, 1959.
93. Tattersall, M. H., Sodergren, J. E., Sengupta, S. K., Trites, D. H., Modest, E. J., and Frei, E., III: Pharmacokinetics of actinomycin D in patients with malignant melanoma. Clin. Pharmacol. Ther., 17:701, 1975.
94. Thomas, C. E., and Aust, S. D.: Release of iron from ferritin by cardiotoxic anthracycline antibiotics. Arch. Biochem. Biophys., 248:684, 1986.
95. Timour, Q., et al.: Doxorubicin concentrations in plasma and myocardium and their respective roles in cardiotoxicity. Cardiovasc. Drugs Ther., 1:559, 1988.
96. Von Hoff, D. D., Layard, M. W., Basa, P., Davis, H. L., Jr., Von Hoff, A. L., Rozencweig, M., and Muggia, F. M.: Risk Factors for doxorubicin-induced congestive heart failure. Ann. Intern. Med., 91:710, 1979.
97. Von Hoff, D. D., Rozencweig, M., Layard, M., Slavik, M., and Muggia, F. M.: Daunomycin-induced cardiotoxicity in children and adults. Am. J. Med., 62:200, 1977.
98. Wermuth, B.: Aldo-keto reductases. Prog. Clin. Biol. Res., 174:209, 1985.
99. Westendorf, J., Aydin, M., Groth, G., Weller, O., and Marquardt, H.: Mechanistic aspects of DNA damage by morpholinyl and cyanomorpholinyl anthracyclines. Cancer Res., 49:5262, 1989.
100. Wolf, J. A., D'Angio, G., Hartman, J., Krivit, W., and Newton, W. A., Jr.: Long-term evaluation of single vs multiple courses of actinomycin D therapy of Wilms' tumor. N. Engl. J. Med., 290:84, 1974.
101. Zhang, H., D'Arpa, P., and Lui, L. F.: A Model for Tumor Cell Killing by Topoisomerase Poisons. Cancer Cells, 2:23, 1990.
102. Zwelling, L. A., Slovak, M. L., Doroshow, J. H., Hinds, M., Chan, D., Parker, E., Mayes, J., Sic, K. L., Meltzer, P. S., and Trent, J. M.: HT1080/DR4: A P-glycoprotein-negative human fibrosarcoma cell line exhibiting resistance to topoisomerase II-reactive drugs despite the presence of a drug-sensitive topoisomerase II. J. Natl. Cancer Inst., 82:1553, 1990.

Epipodophyllotoxins

Antoinette Wozniak
Warren E. Ross

Introduction

The epipodophyllotoxins etoposide (VP-16) and tenipo-side (VM-26) are semisynthetic derivatives of podophyllo-toxin. Both of these compounds exhibit a wide spectrum of antitumor activity and the former, in particular, is now widely used in the treatment of both hematological and solid neo-plasms. In the past decade a great deal has been learned of the mechanism of action, disposition, and clinical role of the epipodophyllotoxins. This chapter will focus mainly on etoposide since that has been the compound commercially available in the U.S. and the one which has received the most extensive clinical testing.

History of Development

The history of the discovery of the epipodophyllotoxins is of considerable interest and has been recently reviewed.[36] The parent compound, podophyllotoxin, is derived from the American mandrake *Podophyllum peltatum*. Extracts from the root of this plant were used in Europe and the U.S. in the early 19th century and were valued for their activity as cathartics and anthelminthics. The principal active species of these extracts, podophyllotoxin, was structurally charac-terized in 1951. By this time its medicinal use was limited to the treatment of condylomata acuminata. Chemists at San-doz Laboratory hypothesized that glucoside derivatives of podophyllotoxin might be less toxic and more active than the parent compound and in 1954 succeeded in identifying such glucosides in the podophyllum plants. Some of these glucosides fulfilled the expectations regarding activity and toxicity and further synthetic efforts led to the compound demethylepipodophyllotoxin-benzylidene-glucoside (DETBG). This compound was significant for not only having excellent activity against leukemia animal models, but also for the fact that its mechanism of action differed from that of podo-phyllotoxin. As early as 1946, the action of podophyllum, the extract containing podophyllotoxin, was identified as the arrest of cells in metaphase of mitosis. This results from the binding of podophyllotoxin to tubulin, causing the inhibition of micro-tubule assembly. In contrast, DETBG and the epipodophyl-lotoxins which followed, inhibit the entry of cells into mitosis. Further synthetic efforts by the Sandoz group led to the syn-thesis of teniposide in 1955 and two years later, etoposide. Although the former was marketed in Europe in the mid-1970's, its place in antitumor therapy has been eclipsed by that of etoposide whose development was facilitated by San-doz licensing the compound to Bristol Myers in 1978. It was not until 1983, however, sixteen years after its synthesis, that etoposide was approved by the FDA for treatment of testic-ular cancer.

Mechanism of Action

The mechanism of the epipodophyllotoxin's antineoplastic effect is based principally on a unique interaction with the nuclear enzyme DNA topoisomerase II which leads to DNA damage.[30,31] This enzyme catalyzes the double stranded breaking and resealing of DNA, thereby allowing the pas-sage of one double helical segment of DNA through another (Figure XI-6-1). The enzyme's actions are adenosine tri-phosphate (ATP) dependent and result in changes in DNA topology, such as unknotting, relaxation, and decatenation. The principal cellular function of this enzyme is to catalyze the separation of daughter DNA strands just prior to mitosis. Like the DNA intercalating agents, the epipodophyllotoxins interact with DNA topoisomerase II and/or DNA in such a way as to prevent the DNA resealing action, thereby creating a DNA-protein crosslink for as long as drug is present. This crosslink has been designated a "cleavable complex" because when exposed to denaturing agents, a frank DNA double stranded break is revealed (Figure XVI-6-2). The pre-cise mechanism by which the epipodophyllotoxins inhibit the resealing action is unknown.

As a drug target, DNA topoisomerase II occupies a unique niche in antineoplastic therapy. Cytotoxicity results not from inhibition of enzyme activity, but rather from the creation of a form of DNA damage by virtue of the drug's perturbation of enzyme function. One consequence of this, addressed below, is that drug potency increases in parallel with intra-cellular enzyme content.

The cellular consequences of cleavable complex forma-tion include chromosomal aberrations, arrest of cell cycle progression in G2 phase, and finally cell death. Maximal cytotoxicity is observed when cells are treated in S phase.[12] Quiescent cells are usually less sensitive than proliferating ones owing principally to reduction in intracellular topoiso-merase II content accompanying quiescence.[38]

Structure activity relationships of the epipodophyllotoxins are of particular interest when compared to the parent podo-phyllotoxin since they have quite different mechanisms of action (Figure XVI-6-3). The three structural differences between podophyllotoxin and its semisynthetic derivatives which are responsible for the change in drug target from tubulin to DNA topoisomerase II include; demethylation at position 4′, epimerization in position C-4, and the presence of a glucopyranose at C-4. It is of note that these two mech-anisms of action form the poles of a continuum and a number of structural congeners share both mechanisms. Neither eto-poside nor teniposide exhibit significant tubulin binding. Computer assisted comparisons of the structures of the epi-podophyllotoxins to intercalating agents suggest consider-able similarity and that the relationship of the glucopyranose

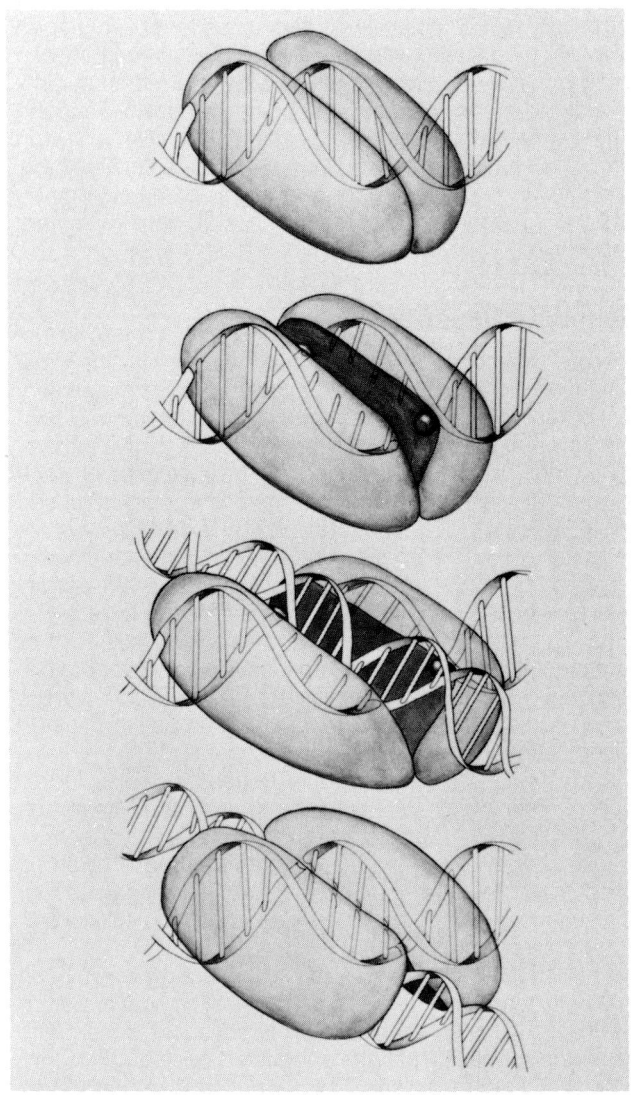

Figure XVI-6-1. A schematic representation of steps leading to DNA strand passage by topoisomerase II. (Only the presumed catalytic area of the enzyme is shown for simplicity.) Following noncovalent attachment, the enzyme cleaves the sugar phosphate backbone and becomes covalently attached at the 5′ termini of the break site. The dimeric structure of the enzyme appears well-suited for allowing passage of a second DNA duplex through the break site. (See XVI-5-1.)

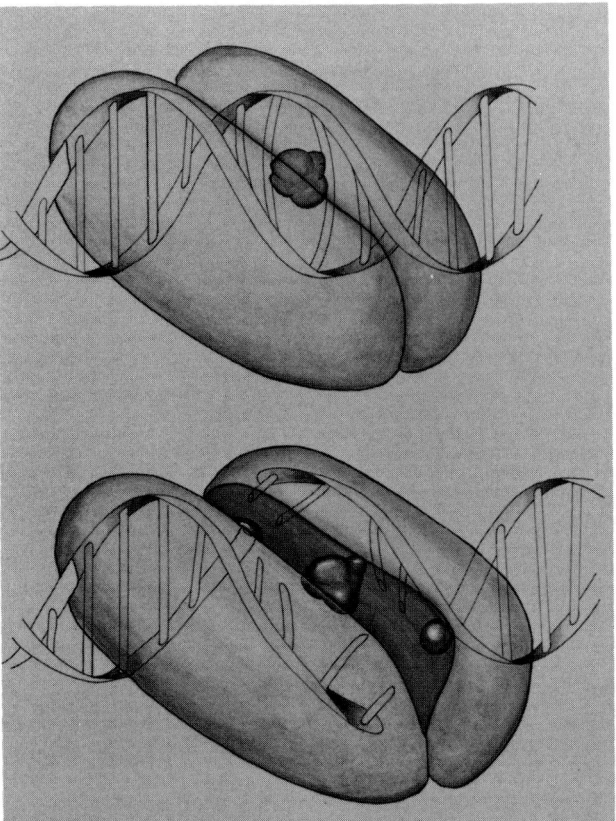

Figure XVI-6-2. A proposed model of how the presence of drug may independently affect topoisomerase II-mediated DNA cleavage and strand passage. Drug binding to DNA is presumed. Cleavable complex formation could result from an altered relationship between the cleaved DNA strands and the catalytic center for the enzyme.

ring and the pendant E-ring to the polycyclic array represented by rings A–D are of importance in the interaction of drug with topoisomerase II and DNA.[23]

Cellular resistance to epipodophyllotoxins can occur for a variety of reasons. The drugs are one of the known substrates for the *mdr* protein which actively pumps drugs out of cells. This phenomenon, described elsewhere in this book, can occur as a result of cellular exposure to epipodophyllotoxins or a variety of other known substrates for the transport protein. Resistance can also result from a decrease in intracellular topoisomerase II content, either as a natural consequence of cellular quiescence, or from loss of one of the two alleles encoding the enzyme. Alterations in the topoisomerase molecule conferring drug resistance, presumably resulting from genetic mutation, can also give rise to cellular

resistance.[37] Each of the above mechanisms have been studied in experimental cell culture systems. Studies of human tumor cells of hematopoetic origin indicate that intracellular topoisomerase II content is highly variable and that this heterogeneity could account in part for differences in tumor response.[4,28]

Pharmacokinetics

The majority of pharmacokinetic studies done with etoposide show a biexponential decay following bolus intravenous (IV) administration.[11] The terminal elimination half-life is 4–8 hours and is independent of the dose. The volume of distribution of etoposide is 7–17 L/m² in adults.[9] Inter- and intra-patient variability exists with regard to these pharmacokinetic parameters. Both the area under the concentration versus time curve (AUC) and the peak plasma concentration of etoposide are dose dependent. There is no drug accumulation with consecutive daily dosing of the drug. Whether the drug is given in bolus or by continuous infusion, there is essentially no change in the pharmacokinetics.

Etoposide is also available in oral form. There have been different formulations including a drink ampule, a lipophilic capsule, and a hydrophilic soft gelatin capsule. The time to peak drug concentration occurs at approximately one hour after administration. The bioavailability of the drug is about

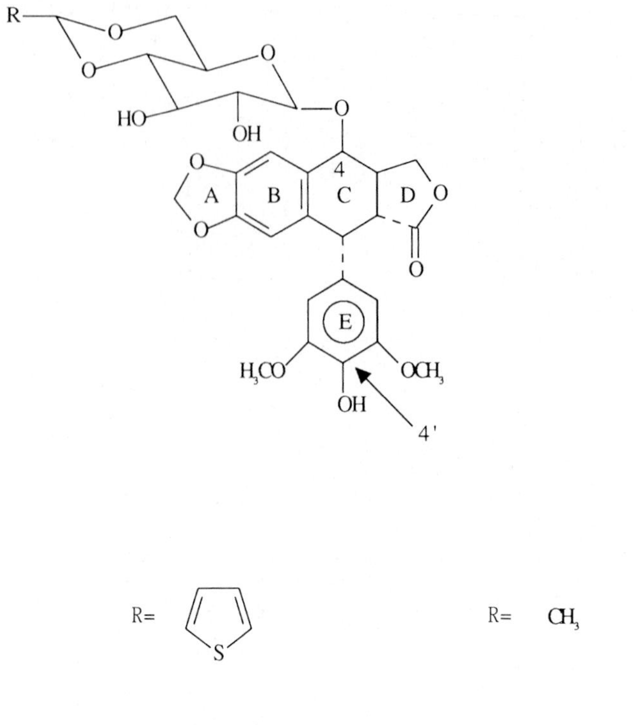

$R=$ (thiophene structure) S $R=$ CH_3

Teniposide   Etoposide

Figure XVI-6-3.   Chemical structure of podophyllotoxin derivatives.

50%. There are no statistically significant differences in any pharmacokinetic parameters when the IV and oral routes of administration are compared.[35] It is suggested that when doses of etoposide above 200 mg are administered orally, they should be divided to allow for maximum absorption.[20] Food does not interfere with etoposide absorption.[19]

Approximately 30–50% of etoposide is recovered in the urine as unchanged drug. Fecal elimination may account for 16% of the administered dose but biliary excretion is minimal.[11] Etoposide is highly protein bound and is metabolized by the liver. A number of metabolites, none of therapeutic importance, have been discovered including the hydroxy-acid derivatives, cis(picro)-lactone, and the glucuronide and sulfate conjugates of the parent compound.[9] One cannot account for the majority of the etoposide dose. Etoposide has very poor penetration into the cerebrospinal fluid.

There are no specific dose reductions that are recommended for etoposide in patients with hepatic dysfunction. There is a suggestion that the clearance of the drug is reduced in patients with renal insufficiency.[3] Although there are no specific guidelines for dose reduction, it is recommended that patients with renal insufficiency be closely monitored for excessive toxicity.

Teniposide is available only in the intravenous form. Depending on the study, teniposide was found to follow either a two or three compartment model. The elimination half-life varies according to the compartment model (6–10 hours versus 20–48+ hours).[9] The volume of distribution of teniposide is 8–30 L/m^2. The drug is highly protein bound. Both the plasma clearance and the renal clearance are greater for etoposide than for teniposide. The majority of the initial dose of etoposide (30–70%) is accounted for by excretion

but only 5–20% of teniposide is accounted for as unchanged drug. Biliary excretion is minimal. The differences between the two drugs has been explained by the reduced renal clearance of teniposide as compared to etoposide, and the higher protein binding of teniposide.[2] Very little is known about the metabolism of the drug. Various metabolites have been described including the hydroxy acid, the cis-isomer, and the aglycone glucuronide. Teniposide penetrates very poorly into the cerebrospinal fluid.

Schedule Dependence

There have been several studies dealing with the dose scheduling of etoposide. Table XVI-6-1 contains a summary of the Phase I etoposide studies. Based on these and subsequent studies, it appears more efficacious to give the etoposide daily for 3–5 days rather than giving it once or twice a week. In the Cavalli study the response rate increased (20–65%) when the etoposide was given for 3 days as opposed to a single weekly dose.[7] Slewin conducted a randomized trial to evaluate the effect of schedule on the activity of etoposide in small cell lung cancer.[33] Patients received either etoposide 500 mg/m^2 as a continuous infusion over 24 hours or 100 mg/m^2 as a 2 hour infusion daily for 5 days. There was a marked difference in response rate, 10% versus 89%. The pharmacokinetics were similar in both arms indicating the superiority of the 5 day schedule.

Interest in etoposide schedule dependence has led to trials of chronic daily oral administration. The maximally tolerated dose is 50 mg/m^2 daily for 21 days.[17] The spectrum of toxicity is similar to that seen when the drug is given by other schedules and routes. Early evidence suggests that this schedule may evoke responses in patients failing etoposide given by traditional dosing schemes.

The scheduling of teniposide in humans has not been studied extensively. There is some suggestion in animal studies that the dosing of teniposide is schedule dependent. Based on a Phase I trial the suggested dose is 67 mg/m^2 intravenously once a week. Teniposide has also been given on a daily schedule and by continuous infusion.

Toxicities

The primary dose limiting toxicity of etoposide is hematologic. Neutropenia occurs in 7 to 10 days with complete recovery usually by day 20. Thrombocytopenia also occurs but is less frequent. There is no cumulative bone marrow toxicity.

Table XVI-6-1.   Summary of Phase 1 Studies with Etoposide

Schedule	Reference
290 mg/m^2 IV weekly	Creaven[11]
200–250 mg/m^2 IV weekly	Cavalli[7]
69–86 mg/m^2 IV twice weekly for 3 weeks	Nissen[25]
125–140 mg/m^2 IV QOD for 3 days	Eagan[13]
45 mg/m^2 IV daily for 7 days	Nissen[25]
60 mg/m^2 IV daily for 5 days	Tucker[39]
125 mg/m^2 daily as continuous infusion for 5 days	Aisner[1]
300–400 mg/m^2 PO (capsule) over 5 days	Falkson[15]
120 mg/m^2 PO (drinking ampule) daily for 5 days	Nissen[24]
100–130 mg/m^2 PO (capsule) daily for 5 days	Lau[22]

Gastrointestinal toxicities occur in about 20% of the patients and can include nausea, vomiting, diarrhea, and anorexia. The nausea and vomiting is usually mild and can be controlled with antiemetics. There is more gastrointestinal toxicity associated with the oral formulation of the drug. Mucositis is unusual at conventional doses; however, when etoposide is used in high doses (greater than one gram/m^2), oropharyngeal mucositis is the dose limiting toxicity.[27] Transient elevation in bilirubin, alkaline phosphatase, and aminotransferase levels can occur with the administration of etoposide in high doses.

Alopecia is frequent and reversible. Occasionally acute side effects including fever, chills, hypotension, bronchospasm, anaphylaxis and vasomotor response have been attributed to etoposide. The hypotension can be associated with the rate of administration of the drug.

Peripheral neuropathy is uncommon but may increase in frequency when etoposide is administered with a vinca alkaloid. There have been case reports of phlebitis, acute dystonia, and radiation recall.[16]

Cardiac toxicity has been reported; however, the patients involved had previous histories of cardiac disease and mediastinal radiation so that the importance of etoposide-induced cardiac toxicity is unknown.[1,32]

The major toxicities of teniposide parallel those of etoposide and include leukopenia, thrombocytopenia, alopecia, gastrointestinal and neurotoxicities, and acute hypersensitivity reactions. There has been a report of hyaline membrane disease.[10]

Clinical Spectrum of Activity

Etoposide has a wide range of activity. Composite single agent response rates of greater than 20% for etoposide have been reported in small cell lung cancer, testicular cancer, gestational choriocarcinoma, Hodgkin's and non-Hodgkin's lymphomas, acute myelogenous leukemia, acute myelomonocytic leukemia, Kaposi's sarcoma, neuroblastoma, Ewing's sarcoma, Wilms' tumor, and rhabdomyosarcoma.[21] In combination with other agents, etoposide is used first line in the treatment of a number of malignancies.

Small Cell Lung Cancer. Etoposide is the single most active agent in the treatment of small cell lung cancer and is generally utilized in combination with other drugs. Some of the more common treatment regimens are listed in Table XVI-6-2. The combination of etoposide and cisplatin yields responses that are equivalent or better than non-etoposide containing regimens. This drug combination has also produced encouraging responses in previously treated patients.[14] Oral etoposide has been used in the treatment of small cell lung cancer in elderly patients with good response rates and acceptable toxicity.[34]

Testicular Cancer. Etoposide has proven to be a very useful agent in the treatment of testicular cancer. Interest in using it as a first line agent grew when it was reported to produce responses in tumors that were resistant to standard PVB (cisplatin, vinblastine, bleomycin) chemotherapy. Etoposide containing regimens have been proven to produce better response rates and improved survival particularly among patients with advanced disease.[40] The two-drug combination of etoposide and cisplatin is being evaluated as first-line therapy for patients with low volume metastatic disease. VIP

Table XVI-6-2. Common Etoposide-Containing Regimens for Small Cell Lung Cancer

CAE	
Cyclophosphamide	1,000 mg/m^2 IV day 1
Doxorubicin (Adriamycin)	45 mg/m^2 IV day 1
Etoposide (VP-16)	50 mg/m^2 IV days 1–5
Repeat cycle every 3 weeks	
CEV	
Cyclophosphamide	1,000 mg/m^2 IV day 1
Etoposide	50 mg/m^2 IV day 1; 100 mg/m^2 PO days 2–5
Vincristine	1.4 mg/m^2 IV day 1
Repeat cycle every 3 weeks	
VAM	
Etoposide	200 mg/m^2 IV day 1
Doxorubicin	50 mg/m^2 IV day 1
Methotrexate	30 mg/m^2 IV day 1
Repeat cycle every 3 weeks	
CAVE	
Cyclophosphamide	1,000 mg/m^2 IV day 1
Doxorubicin	50 mg/m^2 IV day 1
Vincristine	1.5 mg/m^2 IV day 1
Etoposide	60 mg/m^2 IV days 1–5
Repeat cycle every 3 weeks	
EP	
Etoposide	100 mg/m^2 IV days 1–3 or 50–100 mg/m^2 IV days 1–5
Cisplatin	25 mg/m^2 IV days 1–3 or 20 mg/m^2 IV days 1–5 or 75–100 mg/m^2 day 1
Repeat cycle every 3 weeks	
CAV/EP	
Cycle of CAV (Cyclophosphamide, Doxorubicin, Vincristine) alternating every 3 weeks with a cycle of EP	

(VP-16, ifosfamide, cisplatin) is an important salvage regimen in the treatment of refractory testicular cancer.

Hematologic Malignancies. Etoposide has been used in combination with other drugs to treat acute non-lymphocytic leukemia (ANLL) in children and adults. It may prove to be useful in treating refractory AML because of its lack of cross resistance with the anthracycline and cytarabine. Many of the multidrug regimens that are being used to treat non-Hodgkin's lymphoma also contain etoposide. Etoposide is clearly active, but exactly what it adds to the treatment of this disease remains to be resolved.

Other Malignancies. There is high single agent activity for etoposide in epidemic Kaposi's sarcoma. The drug is being evaluated in the treatment of breast cancer, hepatocellular carcinoma, head and neck cancer, gliomas, gestational choriocarcinoma, ovarian cancer, and histiocytosis X.

Bone Marrow Transplantation. Etoposide is an ideal candidate for use in bone marrow transplantation because its only major life threatening toxicity is bone marrow and it has activity in a number of hematologic malignancies. In a Phase I study of autologous bone marrow transplantation (ABMT) in advanced refractory neoplasms 2,400 mg/m^2 was the maximally tolerated dose and recovery from myelosuppression occurred within 16 days of bone marrow infusion.[41] High dose etoposide with ABMT has been most successfully utilized in the treatment of Hodgkin's disease. Etoposide (60 mg/kg) and total body irradiation have been used with good preliminary results in allogeneic bone marrow transplantation of patients with hematologic malignancies.[5] There were no unusual acute or long term toxicities. Additional studies need to be done comparing the use of etoposide with cyclophosphamide with regard to disease relapse, toxicity, and immunosuppressive potency of the two drugs. Etoposide has also been used as an in vitro purging agent for the treatment of acute leukemia with ABMT.[8]

Teniposide

Teniposide is an investigational drug that has been used primarily in the pediatric population probably as a result of its course of development rather than its activity as an antineoplastic agent. Teniposide has received its most extensive evaluation in childhood leukemia, particularly acute lymphocytic leukemia (ALL). It has very modest activity as a single agent. Teniposide has primarily been used in combination with cytosine arabinoside because some preclinical data suggests there is synergistic activity when the two drugs are administered together.[29] There have clearly been responses in patients with ALL who have failed previous therapy. Teniposide is being utilized in many multi-drug protocols for the treatment of both childhood and adult leukemia. The drug's impact on this disease, however, is still to be determined.[18] Teniposide has also been incorporated in ablation regimens prior to bone marrow transplantation. It is an active agent in other hematologic malignancies such as Hodgkin's and non-Hodgkin's lymphoma.

Teniposide has been shown to be very active in small cell lung cancer when used in untreated patients.[6] It is unclear as to whether it offers any advantage over other drugs in the treatment of this disease.

Although teniposide penetrates poorly into the cerebrospinal fluid it can accumulate in brain tumor tissue and responses have been observed in brain tumors. It has been used in combination with cisplatin in the treatment of neuroblastoma.[26] Teniposide is currently being evaluated in Phase II trials to determine its activity in other malignancies.

The Future of Epipodophyllotoxins

There is good reason to believe that the clinical role of epipodophyllotoxins will expand considerably in the next few years. The recent availability of an oral preparation, concomitant with a better appreciation of the drug's schedule dependency, could increase the drug's spectrum of activity as suggested by the early data with chronic oral administration. Further understanding of its mechanism of cytotoxicity may also yield methods of modulating activity to advantage. Finally, it is worth noting that the structure-activity relationships of epipodophyllotoxin congeners, especially with respect to topoisomerase inhibition, are only beginning to be explored. Similarities in structure with intercalating agents, a class of drugs sharing the epipodophyllotoxin's mechanism of action, hint at potentially useful synthetic pathways. Undoubtedly other opportunities will be apparent as more effort is invested.

References

1. Aisner, J., Van Echo, D. A., Whitacre, M., and Wiernik, P. H.: A phase I trial of continuous infusion VP16-213 (etoposide). Cancer Chemother. Pharmacol., 7:157, 1982.
2. Allen, L. M., and Creaven, P. J.: Comparison of the human pharmacokinetics of VM-26 and VP-16, two antineoplastic epipodophyllotoxin glucopyranoside derivatives. Eur. J. Cancer, 11:697, 1975.
3. Arbuck, S. G., Douglass, H. O., Crom, W. R., Goodwin, P., Silk, Y., Cooper, C., and Evans, W. E.: Etoposide pharmacokinetics in patients with normal and abnormal organ function. J. Clin. Oncol., 4:1690, 1986.
4. Bakic, M., Beran, M., Andersson, B. S., Silberman, L., Estey, E., and Zwelling, L. A.: The production of topoisomerase II-mediated DNA cleavage in human leukemia cells predicts their susceptibility to 4'-(9-acridinylamino)methanesulfon-m-anisidide (m-AMSA). Biochem. Biophys. Res. Commun., 134:638, 1986.
5. Blume, K. G., Forman, S. J., O'Donnell, M. R., Doroshow, J. H., Krance, R. A., Nademanee, A. P., Snyder, D. S., Schmidt, G. M., Fahey, J. L., Metter, G. E., Hill, L. R., Findley, D. O., and Sniecinski, I. J.: Total body irradiation and high-dose etoposide: A new preparatory regimen for bone marrow transplantation in patients with advanced hematologic malignancies. Blood, 69:1015, 1987.
6. Bork, E., Hansen, M., Dombernowsky, P., Hansen, S. W., Pedersen, A. G., and Hansen, H. H.: Teniposide (VM26) an overlooked highly active agent in small-cell lung cancer. Results of a phase II trial in untreated patients. J. Clin. Oncol., 4:524, 1986.
7. Cavalli, F., Sonntag, R. W., Jungi, F., Senn, H. J., and Brunner, K. W.: VP-16-213 monotherapy for remission induction of small cell lung cancer: A randomized trial using three dosage schedules. Cancer Treat. Rep., 62:473, 1978.
8. Ciobanu, N., Paietta E., Andreef, M., Papenhausen, P., and Wiernik, P. H.: Etoposide as an in vitro purging agent for the treatment of acute leukemias and lymphomas in conjunction with autologous bone marrow transplantation. Exp. Hematol., 14:626, 1986.
9. Clark, P. I., and Slevin, M. L.: The clinical pharmacology of etoposide and teniposide. Clin. Pharmacokinet., 12:223, 1987.
10. Commers, J. R., and Foley, J. F.: Pulmonary hyaline membrane disease occuring in the course of VM-26 therapy. Cancer Treat. Rep., 63:2093, 1979.
11. Creavan, P. J., and Allen, L. M.: EPEG: A new antineoplastic epipodophyllotoxin. Clin. Pharmacol. Ther., 18:221, 1975.
12. Drewinko, B., and Barlogie, B.: Survival and cycle-progression delay of human lymphoma cells in vitro exposed to VP-16-213. Cancer Treat. Rep., 60:1295, 1976.
13. Eagan, R. T., Ahmann, D. L., Hahn, R. G., and O'Connell, M. J.: Pilot study to determine an intermittent dose schedule for VP-16-213. Proceedings of AACR, 16:55, 1985.
14. Evans, W. K., Osoba, D., Feld, R., and Shepard, F. A., Bazos, M. J., and Deboer, G.: Etoposide (VP-16) and cisplatin: An effective treatment for relapse of small cell lung cancer. J. Clin. Oncol., 3:65, 1985.
15. Falkson, G., Van Dyk, J. J., Van Eden, E. B., Van Der Merwe, A. M., Van Den Bergh, J. A., and Falkson, H. C.: A clinical trial of the oral form of 4'-demethylepipodophyllotoxin-B-D-ethydine glucoside (NSC 141540) V.P.16-213. Cancer, 35:1141, 1975.
16. Fleming, R. A., Miller, A. A., and Stewart, C. F.: Etoposide: An update. Clin. Pharm., 8:274, 1989.
17. Greco, F. A., Johnson, D. H., and Hainsworth, J. D.: Chronic daily administration of oral etoposide. Semin. Oncol., 17(Suppl. 2):71, 1990.
18. Grem, J. L., Hoth, D. F., Leyland-Jones, B., King, S. A., Ungerleider, R. S., and Wittes, R. E.: Teniposide in the treatment of leukemia: A case study of conflicting priorities in the development of drugs for fatal diseases. J. Clin. Oncol., 6:351, 1988.
19. Harvey, V. J., Slevin, M. L., Joel, S. P., Johnston, A., and Wrigley, P. F. M.: The effect of food and concurrent chemotherapy on the bioavailability of oral etoposide. Br. J. Cancer, 52:363, 1985.
20. Harvey, V. J., Slevin, M. L., Joel, S. P., Johnston, A., and Wrigley, P. F. M.: The effect of dose on the bioavailability of oral etoposide. Cancer Chemother. Pharmacol., 16:178, 1986.
21. Issell, B. F., Rudolph, A. R., and Louie, A. C.: An Overview. In Etoposide (VP-16) Current Status and New Developments, Issell ed. London, Academic Press, Inc., 1984.
22. Lau, M. E., Hansen, H. H., Nissen, N. I., and Pederson, H.: Phase I trial of a new form of an oral administration of VP 16-213. Cancer Treat. Rep., 63:485, 1979.
23. Macdonald, T. L., Lehnert, E. K., Loper, J. T., Chow, K.-C., and Ross, W. E.: On the Mechanism of Interaction of DNA Topoisomerase II with Chemotherapeutic Agents. In DNA Topoisomerases in Cancer Chemotherapy, Potmesil ed. London, Oxford Press, 1989.
24. Nissen, N. I., Dombernowsky, P., Hansen, H. H., and Larsen, V.: Phase I clinical trial of an oral solution of V.P.16-213. Cancer Treat. Rep., 60:943, 1976.
25. Nissen, N. I., Larsen, V., Pedersen, H., and Thomsen, K.: Phase I clinical trial of a new antitumor agent, 4'-demethylepipodophyllotoxin 9-(4,6-0-ethylidene-B-D-glucopyranoside) (NSC 141540; VP-16-213). Cancer Chemother. Rep., 56:769, 1972.
26. O'Dwyer, P. J., Alonso, M. T., Leyland-Jones, B., and Marsoni, S.: Teniposide: A review of 12 years experience. Cancer Treat. Rep., 68:1455, 1984.
27. Postmus, P. E., Mulder, N. H., Sleijfer, D. T., Meinesz, A. F., Vriesendorp, R., and de Vries, E. G.: High-dose etoposide for refractory malignancies: A phase I study. Cancer Treat. Rep., 68:1471, 1984.
28. Potmesil, M., Hsiang, Y. H., Liu, L. F., Bank, B., Grossberg, H., Kirschenbaum, S., Forlenza, T. J., Penziner, A., Kanganis, D., and Knowles, D., Traganos, F., and Silber, R.: Resistance of human leukemic and normal lymphocytes to drug-induced DNA cleavage and low levels of DNA topoisomerase II. Cancer Res., 48:3537, 1988. Erratum in Cancer Res., 48:4716, 1988.
29. Rivera, G., Avery, T., and Roberts, D.: Response of L1210 to combinations of cytosine arabinoside and VM-26 or VP-16-213. Eur. J. Cancer, 11:639, 1975.
30. Ross, W. E., Rowe, T., Yalowich, J., Glisson, B., and Liu, L.: Role of topoisomerase II in mediating epipodophyllotoxin-induced DNA cleavage. Cancer Res., 44:5857, 1984.
31. Ross, W. E., Sullivan, D. M., and Chow, K.-C.: Altered Function of DNA Topoisomerases as a Basis for Antineoplastic Drug Action. In Important Advances in Oncology. Edited by V. DeVita. Phildadelphia, J.B. Lippincott Company, 1988.
32. Schechter, J. P., Jones, S. E., and Jackson, R. A.: Myocardial infarction in a 27-year old woman: Possible complication of treatment with VP-16-213 (NSC-141540), mediastinal irradiation or both. Cancer Chemother. Rep., 59:887, 1975.
33. Slevin, M. L., Clark, P. I., Joel, S. P., Malik, S., Osborne, R. J., Gregory, W. M., Lowe, D. G., Reznek, R. H., and Wrigley, P. F.: A randomized trial to evaluate the effect of schedule on the activity of etoposide in small-cell lung cancer. J. Clin. Oncol., 7:1333, 1989.
34. Smit, E. F., Carney, D. N., Harford, P., Sleijfer, D. T., and Postmus, P. E.: A phase II study of oral etoposide in elderly patients with small cell lung cancer. Thorax, 44:631, 1989.
35. Smyth, R. D., Pfeffer, M., Scalzo, A., and Comis, R. L.: Bioavailability and pharmacokinetics of etoposide (VP-16). Semin. Oncol., 12(Suppl. 2):48, 1985.
36. Stahelin, H., and von Wartburg, A.: From podophyllotoxin glucoside to etoposide. Prog. Drug Res., 33:169, 1989.
37. Sullivan, D. M., Latham, M. D., and Ross, W. E.: Proliferation dependent topoisomerase II content as a determinant of anti-neoplastic drug action. Cancer Res., 47:3973, 1987.

38. Sullivan, D. M., Latham, M. D., Rowe, T. C., and Ross, W. E.: Purification and characterization of an altered topoisomerase II from a drug resistant Chinese hamster ovary cell line. Biochem., 28:5680, 1989.
39. Tucker, R. D., Ferguson, A., Van Wyk, C., Sealy, R., Hewitson, R., and Levin, W.: Chemotherapy of small cell carcinoma of the lung with V.P.-16-213. Cancer, 41:1710, 1978.
40. Williams, S. D., Birch, R., Einhorn, L. H., Irwin, L., Greco, F. A., and Loehrer, P. J.: Treatment of disseminated germ-cell tumors with cisplatin, bleomycin and either vinblastine or etoposide. N. Engl. J. Med., 316:1435, 1987.
41. Wolff, S. N., Mckay, C. M., Fer, M. F., Hande, K. R., Hainsworth, J. D., and Greco, F. A.: High dose VP-16-213 and autologous bone marrow transplantation for refractory malignancies: A phase I study. J. Clin. Oncol., 1:701, 1983.

XVI-7

DNA Topoisomerase I Inhibitors

Robert Silber
Milan Potmesil

Introduction

DNA topoisomerases are enzymes that change the topology of DNA in the course of replication and transcription, by two different mechanisms: topoisomerase I introduces breaks in one strand of DNA, whereas topoisomerase II cleaves both strands of the helix. In either case, the breaks are transient.[35] Although this catalytic activity is important for various cellular functions, topoisomerase inhibitors exert their therapeutic action through a more complex process.

Topoisomerase inhibitors block the rejoining of broken DNA and reversibly trap a covalent enzyme–DNA complex. Studies of mammalian cells have suggested that the collision between the trapped complex and DNA replication forks is responsible for the S- and G_2-phase arrest of cells treated with these drugs. This, and additional not fully understood events, result in cell death.[19] While several inhibitors of topoisomerase II are used in clinical medicine (see XVI-5), camptothecin, a plant alkaloid, and its semisynthetic or totally synthetic analogs are the only well-characterized inhibitors of topoisomerase I. The enzyme is a 100-kd monomeric protein encoded by a single gene located on human chromosome 20q12-13.2.[18,19]

In the late 1950s during screening of plant products, extracts from the stemwood of an oriental tree (Camptotheca acuminata) were noted for their antitumor activity. The active agent, camptothecin, was isolated and its structure defined in 1965.[34] It was soon recognized that the compound inhibits both DNA and RNA synthesis and causes reversible fragmentation of DNA in cultured mammalian cells.[11] The impressive activity against mouse L1210 leukemia, rat Walker carcinosarcoma, and other experimental tumors, led to brief clinical trials, which were conducted in the early 1970s in several medical centers in the United States.[1,30]

Early Clinical Studies

A water-soluble sodium salt of camptothecin was used in three phase-I and phase-II clinical trials.[9,20,22] The first phase-I study included 18 patients with advanced tumors. Since the primary purpose of any phase-I trial is to determine drug toxicity, therapeutic responses could be evaluated only in some patients. A partial remission, defined as >50% tumor shrinkage, was noted in 5 patients on the weekly treatment schedule, with evidence of a lesser objective response in an additional six. The brief improvement of a median duration of 2 months occurred mainly in patients with advanced gastrointestinal carcinoma refractory to other treatments.[9]

Another study compared weekly and daily treatments in 15 cancer patients. In 2 of 10 patients whose response could be evaluated, objective improvement followed weekly courses of treatment.[22] In a phase-II study, only 2 of 32 patients with advanced gastrointestinal cancer responded to the weekly schedule by >50% reduction in tumor size.[20]

Dose- and schedule-related hematologic toxicity consisted of neutropenia and mild thrombocytopenia. Neutropenia was more severe following daily as compared to weekly treatments. With higher daily doses, the pattern of hematologic toxicity became unpredictable. Alopecia, mild gastrointestinal toxicity, and severe hemorrhagic cystitis were also noted among patients with either schedule of treatment.[9,22] Hemorrhagic cystitis continued to be a problem particularly in patients with insufficient hydration. This unexpected complication may have discouraged further clinical studies.

Recent Preclinical and Clinical Studies

Many chemical and preclinical investigations of camptothecin and its analogs have been conducted over the last decade. The research is now being extended to the clinical level. A better understanding of camptothecin cytotoxicity and the structural requirements for the synthesis of active analogs has resulted from this effort. Topoisomerase I is the sole known target for the cytotoxic action of camptothecin.[12,13] The drug exists in the active lactone form or as the less active hydrolyzed and water-soluble sodium salt (Figure XVI-7-1). There is a pH-dependent hydrolysis of the lactone (E) ring, which results in an equilibrium of biologically active drug molecules with the closed and inactive forms with the open E ring.[10] Among the two optical isomers, 20(S) and 20(R), only the former is biologically active.

Since the isolation of camptothecin, numerous analogs have been developed. Biologically active compounds require

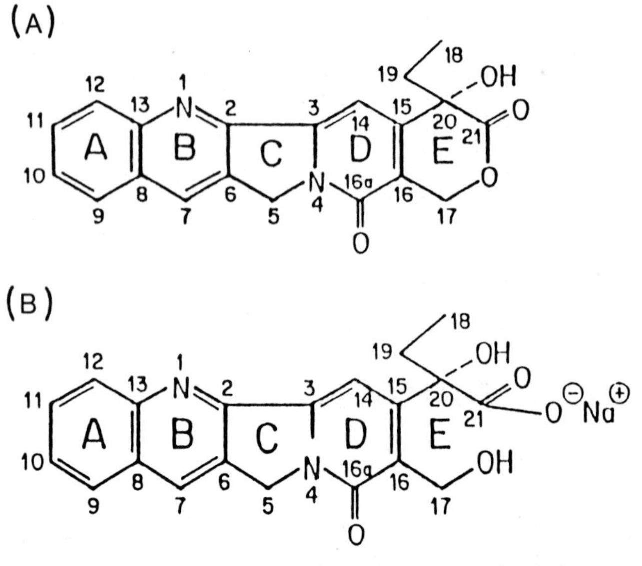

(A)

(B)

Figure XVI-7-1. Structural formulas of the camptothecin lactone form (A) and a camptothecin sodium salt (B).

the presence of the carbonyl oxygen, the 20-OH group, and the lactone-ring oxygen.[33,36–38] Substitution at the C-9, C-10, and/or C-11 positions of the A ring substantially improves drug effectiveness.[14,15] Part of the synthetic effort was directed toward water-soluble derivatives. Two of those, hycamptamine (SK&F 104864), a product of the Smith Kline Beecham Corporation, and CPT-11 (7-ethyl-10-[4-(1-piperidino)-1-piperidino]carbonyloxycamptothecin), a product of Yakult Honsha Company, Japan, are being tested in phase-I or phase-II clinical trials. Hycamptamine was given as a single iv dose repeated every 3 weeks,[31] or as an infusion over a span of several days.[29] Among 12 patients with refractory solid tumors treated with 19 courses of an iv bolus, a minor response was seen in a patient with squamous lung carcinoma. Hematologic toxicities occurred at each dose level, but were limited only to pretreated patients. Non-hematologic toxicities were sporadic and did not include hemorrhagic cystitis.[31] Pharmacokinetic studies showed that the biologically active lactone form was predominant during injection.[17] However, lactone hydrolysis was rapid, and 50% of the drug was converted into the inactive carboxylate form within 15 minutes.

Another water-soluble analog of camptothecin, CPT-11, was tested in Japan in phase-II studies of patients with non-small-cell lung cancer.[3] The drug was given by a weekly 90 minute iv infusion, and responses to treatment were assessed after four cycles. Nine of 22 patients achieved a partial remission, which lasted on average 9 weeks. Among the responders, there were patients with squamous cell and large cell carcinoma and adenocarcinoma. Side effects included leukopenia, alopecia and gastrointestinal toxicity. CPT-11 is a prodrug that is hydrolyzed in the liver—at least in the mouse—to its biologically active metabolite SN-38.[16] While the clinical study of hycamptamine is still at an early stage, the effects of CPT-11 against non-small cell lung cancer are probably better than most single or combination treatments tested in this type of cancer.

A rationale for the testing of two lipophilic camptothecin analogs against human colon cancer xenografts in immu-

nodeficient mice was based on the finding of significantly increased concentrations of topoisomerase I in tumors obtained from patients with advanced stages of colon adenocarcinoma as well as in human colon cancer xenografts. On average, the enzyme was increased 14–16-fold in cancerous tissue of patients with lymph node involvement and/or distant metastases over the levels detected in normal colonic mucosa.[8,23,25] When compared to normal human lymphocytes, elevated topoisomerase I levels were also detected in several types of non-Hodgkin's lymphoma and B-CLL lymphocytes.[24] Synthetic analogs of camptothecin were then tested with purified topoisomerase I and tissue culture screens. The two most effective drugs, 9-amino-20 (RS) and 10,11-methylenedioxy-20 (RS) camptothecins, are lipophilic. Their overall in vivo efficacy surpasses that of their water-soluble congeners.[14] A suitable formulation form was found, which allowed the use of either iv, sc or im routes of drug application.[5]

To test the hypothesis that elevated topoisomerase I levels in human cancers could provide a therapeutic advantage, three subcutaneous xenograft lines of human colon cancer (HT-29, CASE, and SW-48) were carried in immunodeficient mice.[8,23] Representative results of treatment are shown in Figure XVI-7-2. Among ten commonly used anticancer agents, only marginal growth-retardation of tumor implants was noticed in some cases (Figures XVI-7-2A and B). This part of the experiment confirmed earlier results showing the ineffectiveness of tested drugs against 14 human colorectal xenograft lines.[6] In contrast, one or two courses of treatment of CASE (Figure XI-7-2B and C) or SW-48 tumors (Figure XVI-7-2D) with 9-amino-20 (RS) camptothecin resulted in tumor regression in all mice treated.

Advanced SW-48 tumors were also selected for treatment with 9-amino-20 (RS) camptothecin. The disparity of tumor sizes between the control and treated groups is intentional (Figure XVI-7-2D); the largest tumors available were selected for treatment with six doses of the 9-amino-20 (RS) analog. There was a notable 91% reduction in the volume of the tumors in treated mice. Drug toxicity, evaluated in all experiments, was minimal and gastrointestinal toxicity or hemorrhagic cystitis absent.

Long term survival was observed in mice implanted with SW-48 or CASE tumor lines and treated with 9-amino-20 (RS) camptothecin (Figures XVI-7-2C and D). At present, mice included in this experiment are approaching their natural life expectancy.[23] Their overall performance status is unimpaired and there are no apparent signs of delayed or chronic toxicities.

Since metastatic spread to liver is commonly seen in patients with advanced colon cancer, drug treatments of established metastases were also studied. A cell suspension of a human colon cancer xenograft line McCN was injected into the spleen, forcing the inoculum retrograde through the vessels of the splenic pedicle. The resulting liver metastases were treated with 10,11-methylenedioxy-20 (RS) camptothecin starting on day 7 following tumor cell injection. The treatment continued for several days. Control and drug-treated mice were inspected on day 28. While massive tumor infiltration of the liver was seen in the controls, the tumor involvement was substantially reduced in drug-treated animals. The treatment doubled the survival time of experimental animals compared to treatment with 5-fluorouracil (5-FU) which was ineffective.[7,23]

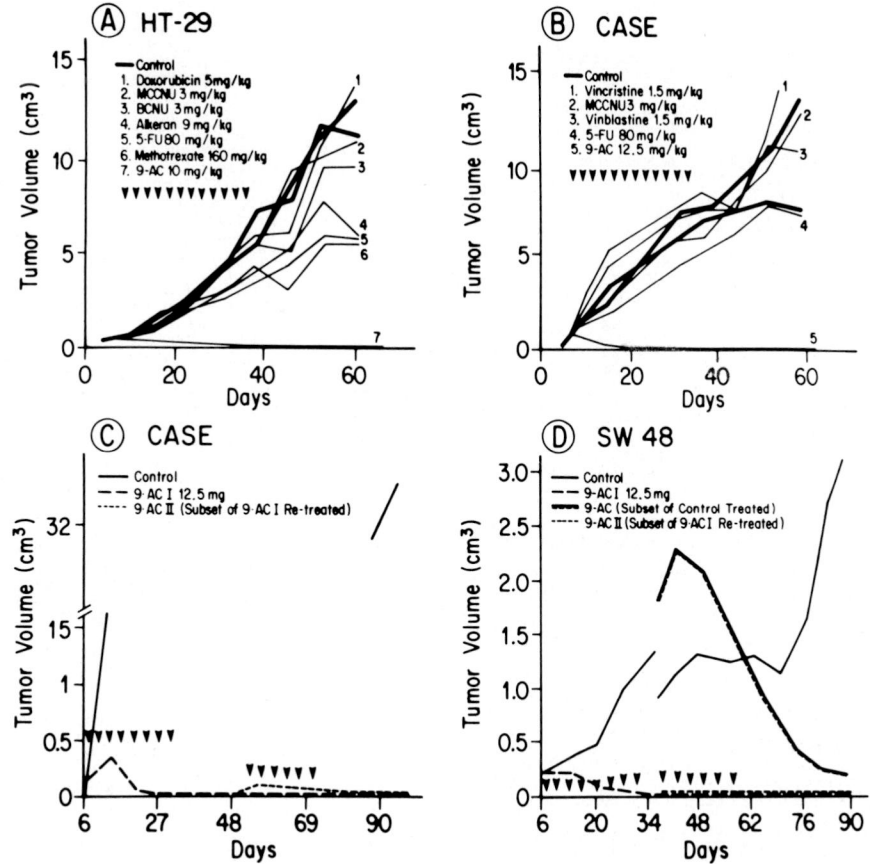

Figure XVI-7-2. Treatment of human colon cancer xenografts HT-29, CASE and SW-48 carried by immunodeficent NIH-1 mice. Each control (A,B) or drug treated (C, D) group included six males; tumor fragments were implanted on day 0. For an implant, 50 mg wet weight of finely minced tumor tissue was injected under the skin over the right dorsal chest region. The treatments started on day 7 and continued twice a week for 3 to 6 weeks. The drugs were formulated in Tween 80:0.15 M NaCl and injected subcutaneously, except for doxorubicin, which was injected intravenously. Controls were treated with the solvent only. The tumors were measured in three dimensions with a caliper, and the tumor volumes were calculated. Means of tumor volumes in centimeters cubed were plotted against time; SD of the means were less than 15% of the value. The arrowheads indicate the time of injections. All mice were treated at the same time; two control groups are shown in (A) and (B) to indicate variability. Variation between the two groups was statistically insignificant (P>0.1, t test) at any point of the measurements. All indicated drug doses represent each single treatment. Abbreviations: 9-AC, 9-amino-20(RS)-camptothecin; BCNU, 1, 3-bis(2-chlorethyl-1-nitrosurea); 5-FU, 5-fluorouracil; MCCNU, methyl-1(2-chlorethyl)-3-cyclo-hexyl-1-nitrosourea.

To determine whether the "classic" multidrug resistance (mdr) phenotype can be bypassed by camptothecin or its analogs, a "wild" KB-3-1 ovarian cancer cell line and a mutant line (KB-V1) expressing the mdr gene, resistant to colchicine, doxorubicin, or vinblastine, were compared.[2,21,27] The finding of high resistance against colchicine, doxorubicin, and vinblastine with no resistance to camptothecin and its 9-amino-20 (RS) analog demonstrates that the two drugs overcome mdr 1-related cell resistance.[23,26]

Camptothecin was cytotoxic to phytohemagglutinin (PHA)-stimulated normal human lymphocytes.[17] In a recent study, 10,11-methylenedioxy-20 (RS)-camptothecin was significantly more active against interleukin-2-stimulated B-CLL lymphocytes than its parent drug.[28] This finding raises the possibility that this analog–unlike camptothecin–is also active against G_0/G_1 cells.

Further studies of 9-amino-20 (RS)-camptothecin and 10,11-methylenedioxy-20 (RS)-Camptothecin are necessary to evaluate their clinical usefulness. Recent improvements in the total synthesis procedure now permit the 20 (RS) analogs

to be prepared in the pure and more effective 20(S) form.[32] 9-Amino-20 (RS) camptothecin was recently selected by the Decision Network of the National Cancer Institute, Division of Cancer Treatment, for clinical trials.

Present Status and Perspectives

There has been a resurgence of interest in a new class of anticancer drugs, analogs of camptothecin, which interact with DNA topoisomerase I. Studies of their mechanism of cytotoxicity have provided valuable information on structure–function relationships. Two of the semisynthetic analogs are in phase-I or phase-2 clinical studies and their therapeutic potential remains to be assessed. Several totally synthetic analogs were evaluated in nude mice. They showed unprecedented efficacy against human colon cancer xenografts. Their overall low toxicity and effectiveness against experimental liver metastases and cancer cells with the multidrug resistance phenotype may indicate a potential usefulness in the clinic.

References

1. DeWys, W. D., Humphreys, S. R., and Goldin, A.: Studies on therapeutic effectiveness of drugs with tumor weight and survival time indices of Walker 256 carcinosarcoma. Cancer Chemother. Rep., 52:229, 1968.
2. Fline, R. L.: Multidrug Resistance. In Cancer Chemotherapy and Biological Response Modifiers, Annual 10. Edited by H. M. Pinedo, D. L. Longo, and B. A. Chabner. New York, Elsevier Amsterdam, 1988, p. 73.
3. Fukuoka, M., Negoro, S., Niitani, H., and Taguchi, T.: A phase II study of a new camptothecin derivative, CPT-11 in previously untreated non-small cell lung cancer. Proc. Am. Assoc. Canc. Res., Abstract #873, 9:226, 1990.
4. Gallo, R. C., Whang-Peng, J., and Adamson, R. H.: Studies on the antitumor activity, mechanism of action, and cell cycle effects of camptothecin. J. Natl. Cancer Inst., 46:789, 1971.
5. Giovanella, B. C.: Unpublished data, 1990.
6. Giovanella, B. C., Stehlin, J. S., Jr., Shepard, R. C., and Williams, L. J., Jr.: Correlation between response to chemotherapy of human tumors in patients and in nude mice. Cancer, 52:1146, 1983.
7. Giovanella, B. C., Stehlin, J. S., Vardeman, D., Wall, M. E., Wani, M. C., Silber, R., and Potmesil, M.: DNA topoisomerase-I targeted chemotherapy of human colon cancer metastases in xenografts. Proc. Am. Assoc. Canc. Res., Abstract #2661, 31:448, 1990.
8. Giovanella, B. C., Wall, M. E., Wani, M. C., Nicholas, A. W., Liu, L. F., Silber, R., and Potmesil, M.: Highly effective topoisomerase-I targeted chemotherapy of human colon cancer in xenografts. Science, 246:1046, 1989.
9. Gottlieb, J. A., Guarino, A. M., Call, J. B., Olivierio, V. T., and Block, J. B.: Preliminary pharmacological and clinical evaluation of camptothecin sodium (NSC-100880). Cancer Chemoth. Rep., 54:461, 1970.
10. Hertzberg, R. P., Caranfa, M. J., Holden, K. G., Jakas, D. R., Gallagher, G., Mattern, M. R., Mong, S.-M., Bartus, J. O., Johnson, R. K., and Kingsbury, W. D.: Modification of the hydroxy lactone ring of camptothecin: Inhibition of mammalian topoisomerase I and biological activity. J. Med. Chem., 32:715, 1989.
11. Horwitz, S. B.: Camptothecin. In Antibiotics: Mechanism of Action of Antimicrobial and Antitumor Agents, Volume 3. Edited by J. W. Corcoran, and F. E. Hahn. New York, Springer-Verlag, 1975, p. 48.
12. Hsiang, Y.-H., Hertzberg, R., Hecht, S., and Liu, L. F.: Camptothecin induced protein-linked DNA breaks via mammalian DNA topoisomerase I. J. Biol. Chem., 260:14873, 1985.
13. Hsiang, Y.-H., and Liu, L. F.: Identification of mammalian topoisomerase I as an intracellular target of the anticancer drug camptothecin. Cancer Res., 48:1722, 1988.
14. Hsiang, Y.-H., Liu, L. F., Wall, M. E., Wani, M. C., Kirschenbaum, S., Silber, R., and Potmesil, M.: DNA topoisomerase I-mediated DNA cleavage and cytotoxicity of camptothecin analogs. Cancer Res., 49:4385, 1989.
15. Jaxel, C., Kohn, K. W., Wani, M. C., Wall, M. E., and Pommier, Y.: Structure-activity study of the actions of camptothecin derivatives on mammalian topoisomerase I. Evidence for a specific receptor site and for a relation to antitumor activity. Cancer Res., 49:1465, 1989.
16. Kaneda, N., Nagata, H., Furuta, T., and Yokokura, T.: Metabolism and pharmacokinetics of the camptothecin analogue CPT-11 in the mouse. Cancer Res., 50:1715, 1990.
17. Kuhn, J., Burris, S., Wall, J., Brown, T., Cagnola, J., Havlin, K., Weiss, G., Koeller, J., Rodriguez, G., Smith, B., Johnson, R., and Von Hoff, D.: Pharmacokinetics of the topoisomerase I inhibitor, SK&F 104864. Proc. Am. Assoc. Canc. Res., Abstract #269, 9:70, 1990.
18. Liu, L. F.: DNA poisons as antitumor drugs. Annu. Rev. Biochem., 58:351, 1989.

19. Liu, L. F.: Anticancer Drugs That Convert DNA Topoisomerases into DNA Damaging Agents. In DNA Topology and Its Biological Effects. Edited by N. R. Cozzarelli, and J. C. Wang. Cold Spring Harbor, NY, Cold Spring Harbor Press, 1990, p. 371.
20. Moertel, C. G., Schutt, A. J., Reitemeier, R. J., et al.: A phase II study of camptothecin (NSC-100880) in gastrointestinal cancer. Cancer Chemother. Rep., 56:95, 1972.
21. Moscow, J. A., and Cowan, K. H.: Multidrug Resistance. J. Natl. Cancer Inst., 80:14, 1988.
22. Muggia, F. M., Creaven, P. J., Hansen, H. H., Cohen, M. N., and Selawry, O. S.: Phase I clinical trials of weekly and daily treatment with camptothecin (NSC-100880): Correlation with clinical studies. Cancer Chemoth. Rep., 56:515, 1972.
23. Potmesil, M., Giovanella, B. C., Liu, L. F., Wall, M. E., Silber, R., Stehlin, J. S., Hsiang, Y.-H., and Wani, M. C.: Preclinical Studies of DNA Topoisomerase I-Targeted 9-Amino and 10,11-Methylenedioxy Camptothecins. In DNA Topoisomerases in Cancer. Edited by M. Potmesil, K. W. Kohn, L. F. Liu, W. Ross, R. Silber, and F. Muggia. New York, Oxford University Press, 1990. In press.
24. Potmesil, M., Hsiang, Y.-H., Liu, L. F., Bank, B., Grossberg, H., Kirschenbaum, S., Penzinger, A., Kanganis, D., Knowles, D., Traganos, F., and Silber, R.: Resistance of human leukemic and normal lymphocytes to drug-induced DNA cleavage and low levels of DNA topoisomerase II. Cancer Res., 48:3537, 1988.
25. Potmesil, M., and Silber, R.: DNA Topoisomerases in Clinical Oncology. In DNA Topology and Its Biological Effects. Edited by N. R. Cozzarelli, and J. C. Wang. Cold Spring Harbor, NY, Cold Spring Harbor Press, 1990, p. 391.
26. Potmesil, M., Wall, M. E., Wani, M. C., Silber, R., Cordon-Cardo, C., Stehlin, J. S., Kozielski, A., and Giovanella, B. C.: DNA topoisomerase-I targeted chemotherapy of human colon cancer xenografts with mdr phenotype. Proc. Am. Assoc. Canc. Res., Abstract #2602, 31:438, 1990.
27. Shen, D.-W., Fojo, A., Chin, J. E., Roninson, I. B., Richert, N., Pastan, I., and Gottesman, M. M.: Human multidrug-resistant cell lines: Increased mdr1 expression can precede gene amplification. Science, 232:643, 1986.
28. Silber, R., Shen, T., Wall, M. E., Wani, M. C., Hawkins, I., Canellikis, Z. N., and Potmesil, M.: 20(RS)-9-amino (9-AC) and 20(RS)-10,11-methylenedioxy (10,11-MDC) camptothecins are cytotoxic to chronic lymphocytic leukemia (CLL) lymphocytes. Proc. Am. Assoc. Canc. Res., Abstract #2601, 31:438, 1990.
29. ten Bokkel Huinink, W. W.: Unpublished data, 1990.
30. Venditti, J. M., and Abbott, B. J.: Studies on oncolytic agents from natural sources. Correlations of activity against animal tumors and clinical effectiveness. Lloydia, 30:332, 1967.
31. Wall, J., Havlin, K., Burris, H., Weiss, G., Brown, T., Brown, J., Kuhn, J., Johnson, R., Mann, W., Webb, D., and Von Hoff, D.: Phase I study of SK&F 104864, a novel topoisomerase I inhibitor. Proc. Am. Assoc. Canc. Res., Abstract #336, 9:86, 1990.
32. Wall, M. E.: Unpublished data, 1990.
33. Wall, M. E., Wani, M. C., Natschke, S. M., and Nicholas, A. V.: Plant antitumor agents. 22. Isolation of 11-hydroxycamptothecin from Camptotheca acuminata Decne: Total synthesis and biological activity. J. Med. Chem., 29:1553, 1986.
34. Wall, M. E., Wani, M. C., Cooke, C. E., Palmer, K. H., McPhail, A. T., and Slim, G. A.: Plant antitumor agents. I. The isolation and structure of camptothecin, a novel alkaloidal and antitumor inhibitor from Camptotheca acuminate. J. Am. Chem. Soc., 88:3888, 1966.
35. Wang, J. C.: DNA topoisomerases. Annu. Rev. Biochem., 54:665, 1985.
36. Wani, M. C., Nicholas, A. W., and Wall, M. E.: Total synthesis and antitumor activity of 20(S) and 20(R) camptothecins. J. Med. Chem., 30:2317, 1987.
37. Wani, M. C., Ronman, P. E., Lindley, J. T., and Wall, M. E.: Plant antitumor agents. 18. Synthesis and biological activity of camptothecin analogues. J. Med. Chem., 23:554, 1980.
38. Wani, M. C., and Wall, M. E.: The structure of two new alkaloids from Camptotheca acuminate. J. Org. Chem., 34:1364, 1969.

XVI-8

Anticancer Drugs From Plants: *Vinca* Alkaloids and Taxol

William T. Beck
Carol E. Cass
Peter J. Houghton

Introduction

The treatments of many diseases owe much to the important medicines that have been derived from plants, and the therapy of cancer is no exception. Unique classes of natural product anticancer drugs have been derived from plants. As distinct from those agents derived from bacterial and fungal sources, the plant products, represented by the *Vinca* and *Colchicum* alkaloids, as well as other plant-derived products such as taxol and podophyllotoxin, do not target DNA. Rather, they either interact with intact microtubules, integral components of the cytoskeleton of the cell, or with their subunit molecules, the tubulins. In this chapter, we will focus attention on the clinically useful plant products: The *Vinca* alkaloids, primarily vinblastine (VLB) and vincristine (VCR), as well as taxol, which is presently undergoing clinical trial. It is usual in chapters on plant alkaloids to include the epipodophyllotoxins, teniposide (VM-26) and etoposide (VP-

16-213), as they are semisynthetic derivatives of podophyllotoxin. However, while podophyllotoxin has essentially the same mechanism of action as colchicine, it is not an alkaloid (it has no nitrogen). Further, the antitumor mechanism of the epipodophyllotoxins is distinct from that of the parent compound: while podophyllotoxin inhibits microtubule polymerization, its glucoside derivatives, teniposide and etoposide, target DNA, and in fact inhibit the essential nuclear enzyme, DNA topoisomerase II.[142,265] Because of these facts and because of their clinical importance, the epipodophyllotoxins are considered elsewhere. (See XVI-6.)

The major areas of *Vinca* alkaloid pharmacology that require updating from the previous edition of this volume are those concerning the mechanisms by which tumor cells express resistance to these agents, their clinical pharmacology and usage. Clinical studies with newer *Vinca* alkaloids will also be discussed, and we will identify the important place of the *Vinca* alkaloids in clinical oncology. We will also provide an overview of the current knowledge of the pharmacology, pharmacokinetics, toxicity and usefulness of taxol and discuss the interest it has generated in recent clinical trials.

Vinca Alkaloids

History and Chemistry

By now the history of the *Vinca* alkaloids and the story of their discovery is well-known.[118,119] Because of a folklore that had developed about the oral hypoglycemic properties of extracts of the periwinkle plant, they were studied independently by two different laboratories. The plants had no antidiabetic actions, but were shown to cause granulocytopenia, bone marrow depression in rats, and were subsequently found to prolong the life of mice bearing a transplantable lymphocytic leukemia. The investigators quickly saw the possibilities and began vigorous development of these agents, and in a relatively short time VCR and VLB were isolated and put in clinical trials.

The chemistry of the *Vinca* alkaloids has been reviewed extensively.[51,154,189] Suffice to say here that they are derived from the periwinkle plant *Catharanthus roseus* G. Don (frequently known as *Vinca rosea* Linn). They are considered to be dimeric compounds in which indole and dihydroindole nuclei are joined together with other complex ring systems. Modifications have been made on both the velbanamine (catharanthine) and vindoline moieties.[189] The basic structures of the major (in terms of clinical utility) *Vinca* alkaloids, VCR, VLB, and semisynthetic derivatives, vindesine (VDS), vinzolidine, and vinorelbine, are shown in Figure XV1-8-1. Note that VCR and VLB differ only in the presence of a formyl or methyl group, respectively, in the vindoline moiety. As will be seen later, this apparently modest difference in structure, which does not alter in any fundamental way the mechanism of action of and binding to tubulin, has considerable significance with regard to the clinical spectrum of antitumor efficacy and clinical toxicity of these drugs.

Mechanism of Action

Among the many biochemical effects seen after exposure of cells and tissues to the *Vinca* alkaloids are: disruption of microtubules, inhibition of synthesis of proteins and nucleic acids; elevation of oxidized glutathione; alteration of lipid metabolism and the lipid content of membranes; elevation of cAMP; and inhibition of calcium-calmodulin regulated cAMP

phosphodiesterase.[6,45,54,55,125,126,150,157,190,204,213, 222,256,261,262] The *Vinca* alkaloids are relatively hydrophobic molecules that partition into lipid bilayers in the uncharged state, altering the structure and function of membranes.[129,180,239,240] Of these diverse effects, their only well-documented direct action is disruption of microtubules resulting from their reversible binding to tubulin, the subunit protein of microtubules. At pharmacologically active concentrations, most of the biochemical effects associated with exposure to the *Vinca* alkaloids are probably secondary to disruption of microtubules, although it is possible that drug-induced changes in lipid bilayers may alter some membrane-dependent processes. At high intracellular concentrations, these compounds induce formation of large crystalline aggregates that are composed of tubulin and drug.[20,21,31] Despite their many biochemical actions, the antineoplastic activity of the *Vinca* alkaloids is usually attributed to their ability to disrupt microtubules, causing dissolution of mitotic spindles and metaphase arrest in dividing cells.[30,83,110,131,139, 150,186,248] However, disruption of microtubules also leads to toxicity in non-mitotic neoplastic cells and while the *Vinca* alkaloids are classified as "mitotic inhibitors," their antineoplastic activity in clinical treatment of cancer probably arises from perturbation of a variety of microtubule-dependent processes.[132,148,149,220,221]

Microtubules are involved in many cellular processes besides mitosis, and exposure to *Vinca* alkaloids gives rise to diverse biological effects, many of which could impair essential functions, both in dividing and non-dividing cells.[67] Morphological changes and cell death after treatment with VCR or VLB have been seen in non-dividing normal and leukemic lymphocytes, in cultured leukemic cells during interphase, and in G1- and S-phase cells.[132,148,149,220,221] Chemotaxis in human monocytes and directional migration of cultured tumor cells are inhibited by *Vinca* alkaloids.[155,270] Microtubules are required for the transport of various metabolites and the movement of organelles, including mitochondria and secretory granules, along neuronal processes.[210] Exposure of nervous tissue to *Vinca* alkaloids inhibits axonal transport, causing neurotoxicity.[42,92] The *Vinca* alkaloids also inhibit secretory processes, apparently as a result of perturbations in membrane trafficking with disruption of the cytoskeleton.[232] Platelets, which depend on integrity of the peripheral ring of microtubules for their discoidal shape, become spherical after treatment with *Vinca* alkaloids.[16,259] These few examples illustrate that the *Vinca* alkaloids exert a variety of potentially cytotoxic effects that are unrelated to mitotic inhibition.

While the effects of the *Vinca* alkaloids on organization and function of microtubules have been characterized extensively, establishing the nature and number of *Vinca* alkaloid binding sites on tubulin has been difficult because of methodological problems.[67,261,262] However, it appears that each heterodimer of α-β tubulin possesses a single "Vinca-specific" site of high intrinsic affinity and an unknown number of non-specific sites of low affinity.[171,228] Attempts to compare the tubulin-binding capabilities of different *Vinca* alkaloids are also complicated by differences in assay conditions and methods of analysis of ligand-binding data.[96,171,172,228] Nevertheless, some generalizations can be made. For example, the relative strength of drug binding to *Vinca*-specific sites on the α-β heterodimers of tubulins is VCR > vindesine > VLB.[136,180,183] Also, VCR and VLB are more potent inhibitors

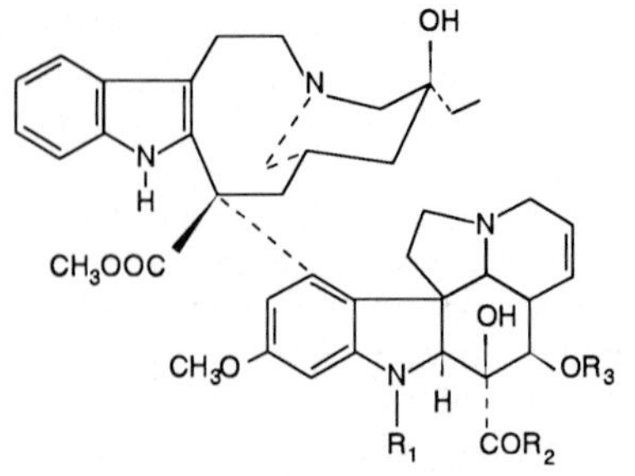

	R₁	R₂	R₃
Vinblastine	-CH₃	-OCH₃	-COCH₃
Vincristine	-CHO	-OCH₃	-COCH₃
Vindesine	-CH₃	-NH₂	-H

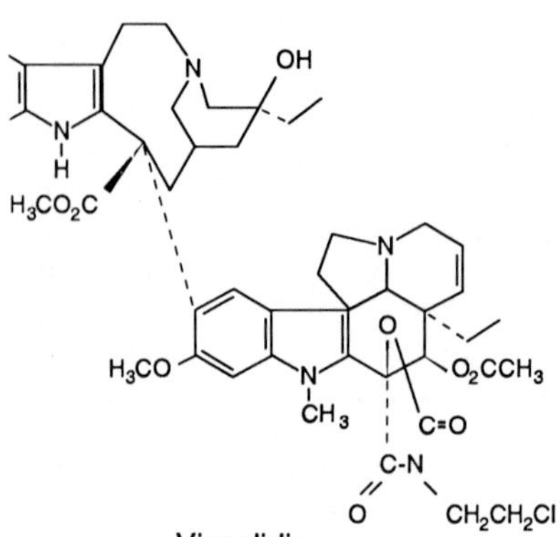

Figure XVI-8-1. Chemical structures of *Vinca* alkaloids.

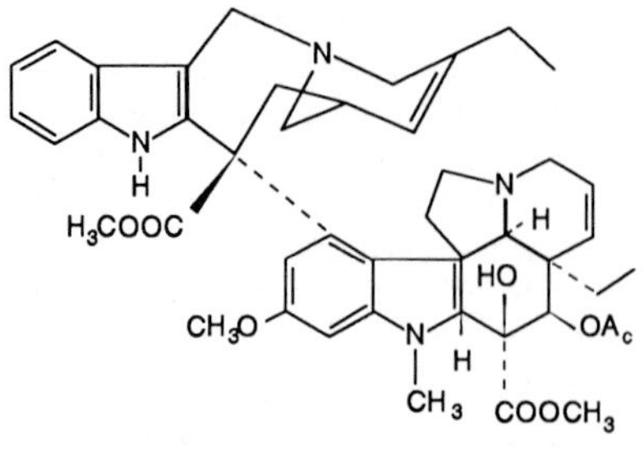

of in vitro assembly than vinrelbine.[72] It should also be noted that both the velbanamine and vindoline moieties are required for site-specific binding of the *Vinca* alkaloids to tubulin.[180]

From the several effects of VLB on assembly of microtubules in vitro, it is generally assumed that the *Vinca* alkaloids disrupt microtubules by more than one mechanism.[121,263] At low concentrations, VLB inhibits microtubule formation in a "substoichiometric" fashion in that assembly is blocked by binding of only a few molecules to high-affinity sites on tubulin heterodimers located at the ends of microtubules.[263] It has been estimated that binding of *Vinca* alkaloids by this mechanism to only 1–2% of total tubulin could reduce microtubules by 50%.[261] At higher concentrations, disassembly results from binding of VLB to tubulin heterodimers located along the microtubule surface, through stoichiometric interaction with *Vinca*-specific sites of reduced affinity and/or nonspecific ionic interaction.[229,263] According to current theories of microtubule assembly, microtubules are dynamic, inherently polar structures that rapidly assemble and disassemble, depending on conditions at the ends.[101,163–165] In cells, one end is usually anchored to an organizing center and the other end may be either slowly growing by addition of tubulin heterodimers, or rapidly shrinking.[209] Conversion between the two states, which is thought to be controlled by specialized proteins, occurs infrequently. At any given time, cells contain mixed populations of microtubules of different stability, and in at least one experimental system, there are differences among these populations in intrinsic sensitivity to *Vinca* alkaloids.[24,162,223]

While there is no question that the *Vinca* alkaloids disrupt microtubules, the biological mechanisms underlying the antineoplastic activity of these drugs are less certain. In actively proliferating cells, the mechanism of cytotoxicity of the *Vinca* alkaloids is usually considered to be disruption of the mitotic spindle, resulting in metaphase arrest and, ultimately, cell death.[30,83,131,150,186] In support of this mechanism, correlations have been shown in studies with cultured cells between dissolution of mitotic spindles and cytotoxicity, and between the accumulation of mitotic figures and the concentration and duration of drug exposure.[30,110,139,248] Among anticancer drugs, the *Vinca* alkaloids are classified as "mitotic inhibitors", with their primary site of action being M phase of the cell cycle, although it is by no means certain that mitotic inhibition is the predominant cytotoxic mechanism in vivo.

The many biological actions of the clinically active *Vinca* alkaloids are seen over a wide range of drug concentrations, and there are selective effects in various normal and neoplastic tissues. Since VCR, vindesine and VLB exhibit similar potencies against preparations of tubulin isolated from the same tissue, in vivo differences in biological activity must be due either to heterogeneity of expression of various tubulin isoforms in different tissues and/or to differences in processes that influence interaction with tubulin, by affecting drug binding (e.g., microtubule-associated proteins, cytoplasmic cofactors) or by limiting the availability of drug (e.g., permeation).[28,66,73,100,105,120,181] A key determinant of the pharmacological activity of the *Vinca* alkaloids in different tissue types appears to be cellular retention of drug. For example, greater retention of VCR through stronger binding to tubulin of neoplastic tissues, relative to normal tissues, is responsible for the selective action of VCR against xenografts of human rhabdomyosarcoma.[106–108] The greater potency of VCR, relative to VLB, can be explained by differences in cellular retention of the two drugs, particularly during drug exposures of limited duration.[73,74,91,138] VCR and VLB are equitoxic against cultured leukemic cells during continuous exposures, whereas VCR is more potent during exposures of short duration, because cellular retention of VCR is greater than that of VLB.[73,90]

Vinca Alkaloid Resistance

Resistance of tumor cells to the cytotoxic actions of the *Vinca* alkaloids has been well-described experimentally, and appears to have clinical correlates.[7–9,38,58,87] In nearly all instances, *Vinca* alkaloid resistance derived in cells in culture is associated with cross resistance to a variety of natural product antitumor drugs of different structure and mechanisms of action. For example, as seen in Table XVI-8-1, human leukemic lymphoblasts selected for resistance to VLB are cross-resistant to other *Vinca* alkaloids and colchicine, but not to another tubulin-binding drug, podophyllotoxin. Of

Table XVI-8-1. Cross-resistance of CEM/VLB$_{100}$ Human Leukemic Lymphoblasts Selected for Resistance to Vinblastine

Drug	Degree of Resistance*
Vinblastine	186
Vincristine	2023
Vindesine	1186
Colchicine	20
Podophyllotoxin	0.8
Etoposide	44
Teniposide	32
Doxorubicin	152
Daunorubicin	44
Mitoxantrone	21
Dactinomycin	49
Bleomycin	3.2
*Bis*chloroethylnitrosourea	0.5
Methotrexate	2.1
6-Mercaptopurine	1.0

*Drug-sensitive CEM and MDR CEM/VLB$_{100}$ cells were tested for their sensitivity to the drugs shown in a 48-hr growth-inhibition assay, and the 50% inhibitory concentrations (IC$_{50}$) were determined. The degree of resistance is the ratio of the IC$_{50}$ for the resistant cells over that of the sensitive cells.

Data compiled from Danks[59] and Beck[15] with permission.

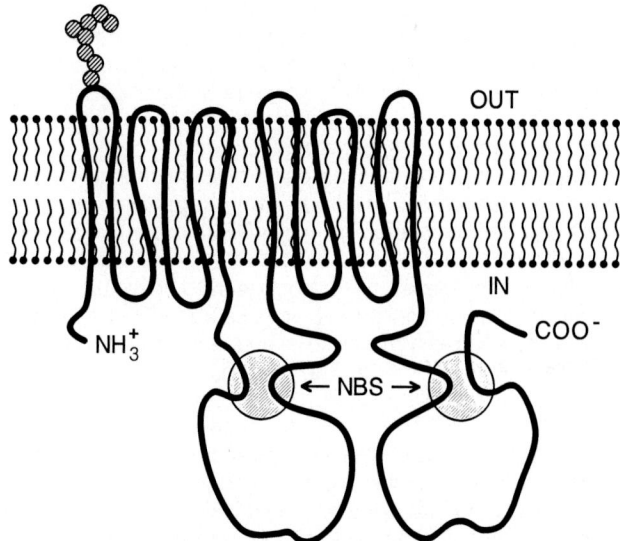

Figure XVI-8-2. Proposed model of P-glycoprotein in the cell membrane. The protein spans the membrane 12 times, has a major glycosylation site near the amino-terminus, and has two potential ATP (nucleotide) binding sites. NBS, nucleotide binding site. Adapted from Chen[43] and Gros.[93]

interest, however, is the fact that the cells are cross-resistant to the podophyllotoxin derivatives, teniposide and etoposide. They are also cross-resistant to the DNA intercalators, doxorubicin, daunorubicin, dactinomycin and mitoxantrone, but no cross resistance is seen to other agents that damage DNA either directly (BCNU, bleomycin) or indirectly (methotrexate, 6-mercaptopurine). This profile of cross-resistance properties typifies the "classic" multidrug resistance (MDR) phenotype.[14,59] MDR associated with overexpression of P-glycoprotein (Pgp-MDR) is the subject of several recent reviews.[69,167,251]

Although the *Vinca* alkaloids bind to tubulin and disrupt microtubules, most tumor cells express resistance to these agents through a mechanism that does not appear to involve alterations in tubulin binding. In all instances where it has been studied in tumor cells in vitro, resistance to the *Vinca* alkaloids appears to be due to their decreased accumulation and retention.[8] The altered cellular pharmacology is mediated by the action of a protein, termed P-glycoprotein (Pgp or P170), that is expressed in the plasma membranes of the drug-resistant tumor cells.[7,9,38] This protein (Figure XVI-8-2), encoded by the *mdr1* gene, spans the membrane 12 times and most likely forms a pore or channel in the membrane through which drugs are transported.[43,76,85,93] P-glycoprotein appears to bind the *Vinca* alkaloids and extrudes them from the tumor cell through a process that requires energy.[8,13,48,49,206,230] This is the most likely mechanism behind the cross-resistance to the other natural product drugs listed in Table XVI-8-1, although alternative mechanisms have been proposed.[9] It is now known that many of the drugs that can circumvent *Vinca* alkaloid resistance or MDR (see below) also bind to P-glycoprotein and compete with the anticancer drug for binding to this protein.[191,192,205,269] The putative binding sites on P-glycoprotein for *Vinca* alkaloids, other anticancer drugs, and modulators of MDR are not known, but it is clear that the process of drug export from the P-glyco-

protein-expressing tumor cell requires energy derived from ATP, which also binds to this protein.[8,50,60,104] Hydrolysis of ATP or phosphorylation of P-glycoprotein may cause a conformational change in the protein which, in turn, could affect drug binding or even provide energy to actively extrude the *Vinca* alkaloid from the cell.

As will be discussed below, MDR due to overexpression of the *mdr1* gene may have clinical correlates, as P-glycoprotein is expressed in many different tumors.[87] Also, certain classes of clinically available membrane-active drugs have been shown to be able to "reverse" or overcome this form of drug resistance in vitro, and efforts are underway to determine whether such reversal can be achieved clinically.[10,11]

Of considerable interest, and in marked contrast to *Vinca* alkaloid resistant murine tumors developed experimentally, a human rhabdomyosarcoma xenograft selected for VCR resistance in vivo did not express P-glycoprotein.[104] Rather, this tumor was shown to express an altered β-tubulin, which most likely accounted for the decreased VCR binding.[104] An alteration in tubulin isoforms has only been shown in vitro in rodent cells selected for resistance to taxol and colchicine and griseofulvin, but no evidence was presented that those cells expressed P-glycoprotein.[33,34,124] As will be detailed in the section on taxol, the mechanism behind selection of one form of resistance versus another is not immediately apparent.

Modulation of *Vinca* Alkaloid Resistance

This subject has been reviewed in substantial detail recently, and will only be summarized here.[10–12,79] One of the first compounds shown to reverse what we now know to be Pgp-MDR was a detergent, Tween 80.[189] However, interest in modulation of MDR grew after the important observation by Tsuruo and colleagues that verapamil, a membrane-active drug used in cardiology, could sensitize VCR-resistant cells to the cytotoxic actions of VCR and VLB, both in vitro and in mice bearing VCR-resistant Ehrlich ascites tumors.[247]

Because verapamil blocks the voltage-gated Ca^{2+} current (the slow calcium channels) in excitable tissues, other "calcium channel blockers" and calmodulin antagonists were quickly studied for their ability to circumvent Pgp-MDR. Many, if not most, of these agents were found to have varying degrees of activity in experimental systems.

Drugs belonging to the classes of "calcium channel blockers" and "calmodulin inhibitors" do not appear to reverse *Vinca* alkaloid resistance or Pgp-MDR through direct inhibition of either voltage-gated calcium channels or calmodulin activity.[137,173,264] Where it has been examined, these and other classes of compounds shown to reverse Pgp-MDR all appear to work by competing with the anticancer drug for binding to P-glycoprotein.[10,12,48] Indeed, verapamil and progesterone, another modulator of Pgp-MDR, both bind directly to P-glycoprotein.[112,191,192,205,269] As a consequence of this competition, the efflux of the anticancer drug, e.g., VCR, from the resistant tumor cell is blocked, and its levels in the cell rise to levels that are apparently cytotoxic.[15,247]

There are many clinically available compounds that modulate or circumvent experimental Pgp-MDR, and therefore *Vinca* alkaloid resistance, and they reflect a variety of chemical structures and different drug classes that include: detergents, progestational and antiestrogenic agents, antibiotics, antihypertensives, antimalarials, and immunosuppressives. The specific compounds are discussed in recent reviews and will not be detailed here.[10–12] Suffice to say that at this writing several clinical trials of modulators of MDR are ongoing. While this is an important and active field of research, there are some serious concerns that may limit its full development.[11] P-glycoprotein, which is central to *Vinca* alkaloid resistance and MDR, is also expressed in such normal tissues as liver, kidney, small intestine, and colon.[47,241] Drugs that bind to and inhibit tumor cell P-glycoprotein will also do the same to the P-glycoprotein of these normal tissues, consequently increasing their levels of the anticancer drug and causing unacceptable tissue toxicities. Indeed, using VCR-treated mice bearing human tumor xenografts, Horton and colleagues showed that administration of verapamil at levels necessary to reverse MDR in vitro caused substantial increases in VCR levels in kidney, small intestine, and liver, and increased the overall toxicity of VCR to the mice.[102] This important observation draws attention to the potential problems associated with circumvention of *Vinca* alkaloid resistance, and provides a challenge not only to design creative therapeutic protocols to obtund the potential toxicities associated with the use of modulators, but also to devise new strategies to circumvent Pgp-MDR.[11]

Pharmacology/Pharmacodynamics

The pharmacokinetics of the *Vinca* alkaloids in humans have been determined by detection in body fluids of ³H-labeled drugs and their derivatives, and by immunoassay using antiserum raised against *Vinca* alkaloids.[18,26,29, 113,128,145,174,176,182,218,225,226] These approaches differ in their resolution and reliability. Interpretation of results obtained with ³H-labeled *Vinca* alkaloids is compromised by their chemical instability. For example, both VLB and VCR undergo spontaneous degradation under relatively mild conditions, forming a variety of structurally related products that can be separated using high performance liquid chromatography.[227,243] The extent to which formation of degradation products, some of which have biological activity (e.g., 4-deace-tylvinblastine), occurs in vivo is unknown. Detection of *Vinca* alkaloids by radioimmunoassay, which has been used most frequently in pharmacokinetic studies, has the advantage of greater sensitivity, allowing detection of material in body fluids at nanomolar concentrations.[177,179,193,224] However, because the polyclonal antisera raised against the *Vinca* alkaloids, usually VLB, cannot distinguish between parent drug and its structurally related derivatives, the various radioimmunoassays currently in use for pharmacokinetic studies cannot provide information on formation of degradative products and/or metabolites.

When administered by intravenous bolus injection, the normal route of administration, the *Vinca* alkaloids exhibit triphasic serum decay patterns in humans.[26,174–176] The pharmacokinetic parameters for the various *Vinca* alkaloids are summarized in Table XVI-8-2. In adult cancer patients, the mean half-lives of the first two phases are about the same for VCR, VLB, vindesine and vinorelbine (1–5 min and 1–2 hr), whereas that of the terminal phase differs by ≈4-fold for VCR (≈85 hr), vinorelbine (≈40 hr), VLB (≈25 hr) and vindesine (≈24 hr). The initial rapid clearance of the *Vinca* alkaloids from plasma is due to uptake of drug by various tissues, particularly blood elements such as platelets.[18,26,182] The terminal phase of clearance from plasma represents the slow release of drug from various tissues, where it has been sequestered, presumably through binding to tubulin. The range of values obtained for the terminal clearance phase, particularly with VCR, is large.[174,176] The greater potency of VCR has been attributed to prolonged exposures of sensitive tissues resulting from its slow clearance, relative to that of the other *Vinca* alkaloids.[29,174,176] At the doses currently used in therapy of adults, the plasma peak concentrations, which persist for only a few minutes, are between 100 and 500 nM, and the steady state concentrations are 1–2 nM.[26,174] The values found for the volumes of the central compartment differ significantly: Vindesine is equivalent to the plasma volume (5.4% of body weight), whereas VCR and VLB greatly exceed the plasma volume (32.8 and 70% of body weight, respectively).[174,176]

Excretion of the *Vinca* alkaloids is primarily by the hepatobiliary route.[113,130,184] Cancer patients with impaired liver function exhibit reduced clearance of VCR, resulting in higher steady state concentrations of drug and prolongation of the terminal elimination phase.[63,250] In such patients, reduction in drug dosage is recommended to reduce VCR-related neurotoxicity.[63]

The *Vinca* alkaloids are sometimes given by continuous intravenous infusion in an effort to achieve longer periods during which pharmacologically effective drug levels are maintained in serum. Although a variety of different sched-

Table XVI-8-2.   Pharmacokinetic Values for Parenteral Administration of *Vinca* Alkaloids in Humans

Parameter	VCR	VLB	VDS	VRB	VZL
$T_{1/2}$ α (min)	2–6	2–6	1–3	1–3	0.39
$T_{1/2}$ β (hr)	2.27	1.64	0.91	1.9	1.8
$T_{1/2}$ γ (hr)	85	24.8	24.2	40	159
V_{ss} (1/kg)	8.42	27.3	8.84	27	11.4
Clearance (1/kg/hr)	0.106	0.252	0.74	0.8	0.06
Urinary elimination (%)	10–20	<10	<10	<8	13.6

Data from Armand,[2] Kreis,[127] and Nelson.[176]

ules have been used, the administration of VCR, VLB or vindesine by infusion generally results in steady-state concentrations of drug that are higher than those achieved after intravenous bolus injection.[115,116,145,177,195,268]

The pharmacokinetics of vinzolidine have been studied after either oral administration or intravenous bolus injection of tritium-labeled drug.[128,218] After oral administration, vinzolidine is rapidly absorbed with an absorption half-life of 1 hr and a peak at 4 hr. The serum decay curve is biphasic, with half-lives of 10.5 and 172 hr. After intravenous administration, the pharmacokinetics of vinzolidine resemble those of VLB, except that volume of distribution is much larger (about 15–20 times the blood volume). The terminal half-life for elimination of vinzolidine from plasma is about 23 hr.

Toxicities and Doses

The toxicities of the *Vinca* alkaloids in humans are well documented and are related to the drug, route of administration, and dose.[29,52,53,123,158] The toxicities of the *Vinca* alkaloids differ significantly, despite similarities in biochemical activities. The dose-limiting toxicity of VCR is neurologic, with extensive peripheral neuropathy occuring at higher doses.[199,211] Similar neurotoxicity is also seen with VLB, but, at the dosages used clinically, to a much lesser extent since its dose-limiting toxicity is myelosuppression. Early symptoms of neurotoxicity are numbness and painful paresthesias in the fingers and toes and depression of the Achilles tendon reflex, followed, if treatment continues, with severe muscle weakness and uncoordinated movements. The dose-limiting toxicity of VLB is myelosuppression, with the nadir of leukopenia 5–9 days after administration and recovery within 14–21 days. Myelosuppression is rare with VCR, probably because dosages are limited by neurotoxicity. Vindesine is both myelosuppressive and neurotoxic, and the neurotoxicity is less severe than that seen with VCR.[29,39] Vinorelbine is myelosuppressive with mild, reversible neurotoxicity.[23] Nausea and vomiting are frequently seen in patients receiving VLB or vindesine, and constipation, resulting from neurotoxicity, can occur in patients receiving VCR. In elderly patients, particularly those with a tendency toward constipation, prophylactic cathartics are indicated. Alopecia and irritation at sites of intravenous administration are also common. For all of the *Vinca* alkaloids, dose reduction should be considered in patients with impaired liver function since the primary excretory route is hepatobiliary.[113,130,184] Toxicities, particularly neurotoxicity and myelosuppresion, are increased when the *Vinca* alkaloids are administered by continuous intravenous infusion. Severe neurologic and hematologic toxicity is seen with infusion of high doses of VCR, although lower doses are reasonably well tolerated.[114,116,255] Neurotoxicity is seen during infusion of VLB and vindesine, and the major toxicity during infusion of VLB is myelosuppression.[177,195,268] It is now appropriate to discuss specific toxicities in relation to drug and dose.

VCR and VLB are most frequently administered by direct intravenous injection or through tubing of a running intravenous infusion. Administration is complete within one minute. Extravasation may cause irritation, and the local application of hyaluronidase and moderate heat to the area of leakage helps dispersion of drug and may minimize discomfort and the possibility of cellulitis. Both agents are given at intervals of seven days until moderate or limiting toxicity occurs. In preclinical models the scheduling of VCR has

been shown to affect antitumor activity markedly.[105] The usual dose of VCR in adults is 1.4 mg/M^2 and 2 mg/M^2 in children (>10 kg). For smaller children a dose of 0.05 mg/kg every seven days is used. The dose of VCR is reduced by 50% for patients having direct serum albumin values above 3 mg/100 mL.[64] For VLB usual doses are 4–5 mg/M^2 every week, although because of variable leukopenia an escalating schedule has been suggested. Alternative routes of administration of both VLB and VCR have been reported. Oral administration of VLB was unpredictable, not very effective and potentially severely toxic.[70] VLB, 1.4–2.0 mg/M^2/day administered as a 5-day continuous intravenous infusion resulted in unacceptable myelosuppression at dose rates above 1.8 mg/M^2/day in patients with refractory breast cancer.[268] A similar study in testicular cancer patients (3 mg/M^2/day) resulted in frequent non-hematologic toxicity including inappropriate ADH secretion, paralytic ileus, mucositis, neuropathy and Raynaud's syndrome.[44] Nonhematologic toxicity was correlated directly with steady state plasma levels. Toxicity was greater in patients with plasma levels of 8.5 ng/mL compared to a group where the mean steady-state level was 5.8 ng/mL. VCR given as continuous infusion for up to 5 days has caused primarily neuropathy, hyponatremia and leukopenia, with dose-limiting toxicity occurring at 0.5 mg/M^2/day.[117] Although responses have been reported in a number of hematologic and solid tumors, the value of prolonged infusion of VLB and VCR relative to bolus administration remains to be demonstrated conclusively at both the preclinical and clinical levels.

Most studies with vindesine have used this agent at weekly intervals at a dose level between 2 and 5 mg/M^2. Exceptions have been in acute lymphoblastic leukemia (ALL) where in one study 2 mg/M^2 was administered daily for 5 days, and in another 0.5 mg/M^2 was given every 12 hours for 5 days.[151,236] There is some suggestion that continuous infusion vindesine may be superior to bolus administration in terms of therapeutic efficacy. Five day continuous infusion of vindesine (1.0–1.4 mg/M^2/day) gave an objective response rate of 25% in refractory breast cancer, whereas bolus administration (3–4 mg/M^2) yielded a 7% response rate. Further, 4 of 11 patients who progressed on bolus vindesine, achieved partial remission when treated with continuous infusion.[266] A similar observation has been made in patients with ALL.[160]

Phase II studies of intravenous vinorelbine were initiated at 30 mg/M^2 weekly until either disease progression or severe toxicity occurred. Leukopenia and neutropenia have been the most significant side effects, the latter being observed in 42% of cycles. However, the neutropenia was not cumulative and was of short duration.[156] Preclinical studies indicated that vinorelbine retained both toxicity and antitumor activity when given orally. The maximum tolerated dose of oral vinorelbine in Phase I trial was determined to be approximately 80 to 100 mg/M^2.[71,249] Again noncumulative leukopenia was limiting, with no unpredictable toxicities. Nausea, vomiting, and neurotoxicity were mild and did not alter drug administration or absorption.[2]

Pharmacokinetics of parenterally administered *Vinca* alkaloids has been determined either using a sensitive radioimmunoassay or radiolabeled material. Bolus administration is characterized by a rapid initial elimination from serum, tight tissue binding, and a relatively long terminal half-life.

Pharmacokinetic parameters are summarized in Table XVI-8-2.[127,156,176]

Clinical Uses: VCR, VLB and Newer *Vinca* Alkaloids

Vinca alkaloids have been incorporated into combination chemotherapy protocols, based not only on their lack of cross resistance with drugs that alkylate DNA, but also because of their different mechanism of action. VCR has the added advantage that its limiting toxicity is peripheral neuropathy, whereas VLB may cause additive myelosuppression with other myelosuppressive agents. The use of VCR and VLB in combination therapy extends beyond the spectrum of cancers for which definitive activity has been demonstrated. VCR is approved as a component of combination therapy for use in Hodgkin's lymphoma, non-Hodgkin's lymphomas (including lymphocytic, mixed cell, histiocytic, undifferentiated, nodular and diffuse), rhabdomyosarcoma of childhood, neuroblastoma and Wilms' tumor (nephroblastoma).[3,65,144,146,233,253,233A] VLB has a similar spectrum of activity for Hodgkin's and non-Hodgkin's lymphomas, and has been used in advanced mycosis fungoides, advanced carcinoma of testis, Kaposi's sarcoma and histiocytosis X.[36,37,169,254]

Four new *Vinca* alkaloids, vindesine, vinzolidine, vinepedine and vinorelbine have been introduced into clinical treatment of cancer. Vindesine (4-desacetylvinblastine carboxy amide; Figure XV-8-1), the most extensively studied of these analogs, was selected for clinical evaluation based upon its VCR-like spectrum of activity against murine tumors, and its greater activity against the murine B16 melanoma.[86] Preclinical data also suggested that cross-resistance between VCR and vindesine was not absolute. It has been shown clinically that vindesine has activity against hematologic malignancies, causing responses in VCR-resistant disease. Mathé and colleagues initially reported six complete responses in fifteen patients with VCR-resistant acute lymphocytic leukemia.[160] Of interest was that two complete responses were obtained by administration of vindesine as a 48 hour infusion in patients not responsive to bolus administration of this agent. Several other studies have confirmed the lack of complete cross-resistance with VCR in hematologic malignancies, although this is less apparent in therapy of solid tumors.[133,151,231,252] Vindesine has also shown activity against resistant hematologic malignancies, breast carcinoma, malignant melanoma and adenocarcinoma of the lung.[75,81,109,133,151,178,196,231,252]

Vinzolidine (3'(2-chloroethyl)-3-de(methoxycarbonyl)-3-deoxy-2', 4'-dioxospiro[oxazoladine-5'', 3-vincaleukoblastine]) was developed for clinical trial because it had greater therapeutic activity in murine tumors than either VCR or VLB. In rhesus monkeys, bioavailability was 2.5-fold that of VLB after oral administration.[32] Vinzolidine has a substituted oxazolidine dione ring at the 4' position of the vindoline moiety. The β-chloroethyl side chain is non-functional with respect to alkylation, but increases the lipophilicity of the molecule. In vitro studies of vinzolidine activity suggested a lack of cross resistance with VLB, and potential activity in gastrointestinal, breast and lung carcinoma and in melanoma.[135,235] Phase I studies have revealed primarily hematologic, gastrointestinal and neurologic toxicities.[32,204] Hematologic toxicities have been dose-limiting and marked variation in tolerance between patients was observed. Unpredictable and severe toxicity of oral dosing schedules has led to early closure of several studies. Variable toxicity appears to relate to marked differences either in the terminal half life of vinzolidine in patients (35–100 hours), or in erratic absorption. Early trials using oral administration demonstrated some activity in both Hodgkin's and non-Hodgkin's lymphoma, Kaposi's sarcoma, adenocarcinoma of pancreas, breast, and both squamous cell- and adeno-carcinoma of lung.[32,204,212] Parenteral trials have shown more predictable toxicity, which has been predominantly hematologic, with responses reported in melanoma, renal and breast carcinoma.[237]

Vinca alkaloids with modifications of the velbanamine (catharanthine) moiety have generally been associated with reduced potency. For example, the natural alkaloids, 4'-deoxyvinblastine and 4'-deoxyleurosidine were less active mitotic inhibitors in vitro, and were less potent against rodent tumors in vivo. Leurosidine (epimeric at C-4') was also less potent than VLB against P-1534 leukemia in mice. However, leurosidine and 4'-deoxyleurosidine demonstrated high therapeutic index against P-1534 leukemia and B16 melanoma, with activity equal or superior to that of VLB.[119] Vinepidine, 4'deoxyepivincristine, epimeric at C-4', differs from deoxyleurosidine in substitution of a formyl group at the N-atom of the vindoline moiety. These modifications to the velbanamine moiety imparted some new activities for a *Vinca* alkaloid. In mice, vinepidine was more potent than VCR, and in vitro vinepidine demonstrated 50- to 100-fold less potency in the rat mid-brain cell culture assay, which has an excellent correlation with *Vinca* alkaloid induced neuropathy in man.[25,244] Vinepidine was therefore selected for clinical evaluation based upon a VCR-like preclinical spectrum of activity in vivo, and lack of potential neurotoxicity determined using an in vitro assay. However, in clinical studies using a weekly administration schedule, neurotoxicity was observed and this drug was not evaluated further.[170] Whether neurotoxicity was due to cumulative effects caused by slower elimination or metabolism using this schedule is not known. Preclinical data indicated that drug was accumulated in tumor tissue even at very low plasma concentrations, raising the possibility that continuous infusion may achieve adequate levels in tumor, but reduce the incidence of toxicity to the host.[170]

Vinorelbine (Navelbine; 3',4'-didehydro-4-deoxy-C'-nor-vincaleucoblastine; 5'-nor-anhydrovinblastine) demonstrated a profile of activity against murine tumors similar to that of other *Vinca* alkaloids, and also showed activity against five human tumor xenografts in nude mice. Further, no neurotoxicity, demyelination or muscle degeneration was observed in monkeys.[156] In Phase I evaluation, dose limiting toxicity was leucopenia, and two of 16 patients with refractory lymphomas experienced partial responses.[159] Vinorelbine has shown considerable activity in non small cell lung cancer when administered weekly at 30 mg/M². The overall objective response rate was 33%.[62] Significant activity of intravenous vinorelbine was demonstrated against predominantly untreated advanced breast carcinoma (52% objective responses) with 4/24 patients having a complete response.[35] The response rate in heavily pretreated patients was 38%.[157] The response rate of advanced (Stage III, IV) previously untreated Hodgkin's lymphoma was 90%, and 5/25 evaluable patients with previously treated ovarian cancer had objective responses.[82,156] Preclinical and clinical studies have shown that vinorelbine is absorbed well following oral dosing, and has not been associated with erratic or unpredictable toxicities, as was found with vinzolidine.[71]

Clinical Resistance

In cell culture systems, cross-resistance between *Vinca* alkaloids is common, although not absolute; the degree of resistance may depend on the specific agent. In patients, drug effectiveness may also be a function of dose, route of administration, and pharmacokinetic factors, all of which compound the difficulties in interpreting whether cross-resistance between *Vinca* alkaloids occurs in clinical cancer. VCR-resistant acute lymphoblastic leukemia was shown to be responsive to vindesine, and several other studies support this.[160] Vindesine infusion was also active in some patients who did not respond to bolus administration, and similar observations have been made with VCR and VLB. This suggests that, as in vitro, the degree of resistance between *Vinca* alkaloids may differ, and that dose and intensity of therapy may determine the response rate in *Vinca*-resistant disease.

Several mechanisms of resistance to *Vinca* alkaloids have been discussed above. The best characterized is that mediated by P-glycoprotein, thought to act as an energy dependent drug efflux pump. There are now many reports documenting the presence of P-glycoprotein in patients' tumors by analysis of RNA transcripts or using immunologic methods.[4,17,27,40,41,58,77,78,84,87,88,122,147,168,208,219] The presence of P-glycoprotein has been correlated with poor outcome in childhood rhabdomyosarcoma and neuroblastoma, but definitive relationships have not been established for other tumor types.[40,41] The incidence of P-glycoprotein-positive human cancers is summarized in Table XVI-8-3. The apparent differences in detection of Ppg may reflect the sensitivity of RNA analysis compared to immunological techniques. At this time there is limited information regarding the significance of these data. However, several clinical trials have been initiated using agents that have reversed P-glycoprotein-mediated multidrug resistance in cultured cells, as recently summarized by Beck.[12] Initial studies with verapamil showed that concentrations of modulator required in vitro (5–10 uM) could not be sustained in patients.[22,185] The use of this slow calcium channel blocker was limited by its intrinsic pharmacological activity, causing heart block. Transient responses were observed in pediatric patients treated with 6-day continuous infusion of verapamil (0.005 mg/kg/min) with bolus VLB (2 mg/M^2) and 5-day continuous infusion of VP-16 (200 mg/M^2/day). However, the study design prevented conclusions regarding the role of verapamil. In P-glycoprotein-positive, drug-resistant myeloma, there is some indication that simultaneous infusion of verapamil with VCR and doxorubicin may elicit transient responses in some patients.[57] Other modulators of P-glycoprotein-mediated multidrug resistance currently in clinical trial include Bepridil, R-verapamil, trifluoperazine, cyclosporine A, acrivastine and amiodarone. Clearly, this concept of modulation should be thoroughly evaluated in controlled, randomized trials. However, there are few preclinical data to support therapeutic selectivity, and P-glycoprotein may play an important role in protecting certain normal tissues in man and rodents.[56,89,102]

Taxol

History and Chemistry

Taxol was isolated in 1971 from the Western Yew, *Taxus brevifolia* Nut (Taxaceae) and was found to have antitumor and antileukemic activity.[103] It has subsequently been found in the roots, leaves and stems of this tree and related members of the yew family.[103] As seen in Figure XVI-8-3, taxol is a complex ester with an unusual structure, consisting of a an oxetan ring attached to a derivative of taxane. Because of its unusual mechanism of action, it has become an important tool to investigate mictotubule function. Importantly, its unique action and spectrum of antitumor activity have earned it a place in experimental therapeutics and it is presently undergoing clinical trials. The major barrier to taxol's clinical development is its low abundance in the yew trees, since chemical synthesis has not been possible. Thus, there simply has not been enough taxol to do the appropriate trials. Fortunately, however, this situation is changing, as considerable effort is now being expended to make analogs and derivatives of this agent.

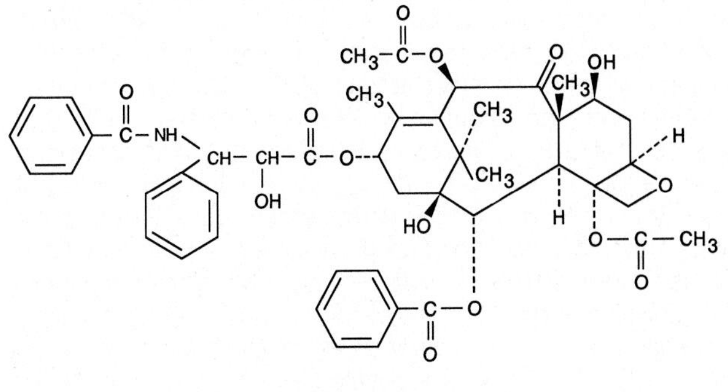

Table XVI-8-3. Incidence of Detection of Biochemical Markers of P-glycoprotein Mediated Multidrug Resistance in Human Cancer

| Tumor | Treatment Status (positive/total) | | | Method |
	Untreated	Treated	Not Defined	
Breast CA	2/12	8/11	5/16	I
	9/57	2/2	0/5	R
Colon CA			6/54	I/W
	35/41		10/20	R
Ovarian CA		2/5	6/66	I/W
	0/56	3/10	0/16	R
Renal Cell CA	0/4		3/13	I
	72/88		7/8	R
Lung CA	0/19			R
(NSCLC)	7/19			R
Neuroblastoma	35/78	32/52		R
Myeloma	4/7	7/13		I
Sarcoma	0/11	4/4		R
			9/30	I
Pheochromocytoma	25/34			R

I: Detection by immunocytochemistry; W: Western blot; R: RNA slot blot.
Data compiled from refs. 4, 17, 40, 58, 77, 78, 84, 87, 88, 122, 147, 168, 208, 219

Taxol

Figure XVI-8-3. The chemical structure of taxol.

Mechanism of Action

Among antineoplastic drugs that interfere with microtubules, taxol exhibits a unique mechanism of action and, for this reason, has been studied extensively.[19,103,152,200] Taxol promotes assembly of microtubules by shifting the equilibrium between soluble tubulin and microtubules toward assembly, reducing the critical concentration of tubulin required for assembly.[215,216] The result is stabilization of microtubules, even in the presence of conditions (e.g., low temperature, high calcium) that normally promote disassembly of microtubules.[134,207,215,216,245] The remarkable stability of microtubules induced by taxol is damaging to cells because of the perturbation in the dynamics of various microtubule-dependent cytoplasmic structures that are required for such functions as mitosis, maintenance of cellular morphology, shape changes, neurite formation, locomotion, and secretion.[5,61,80,99,111,124,140,141,158,166,194,198,201,203,216,246] Microtubules are the only known biochemical targets of taxol, and the many biological effects observed in taxol-treated cells are thought to arise from perturbations of microtubule dynamics.

Interaction of taxol with microtubules occurs by reversible, high-affinity binding of the drug to polymerized microtubules.[46,134,153,187,188] The stoichiometry of binding is approximately 1 mole of taxol per mole of polymerized tubulin, and the binding site for taxol is distinct from the binding sites for the *Vinca* alkaloids, colchicine or podophyllotoxin.[134,188,217] Cells treated with pharmacological levels of taxol (0.1–10 μM) are arrested in the G2 + M phases of the cell cycle and contain disorganized arrays of microtubules, often aligned in parallel bundles.[80,98,99,201,216] Treatment of mitotic cells with taxol results in the formation of abnormal spindle asters.[61,166,201] Studies of the effects of low concentrations (0.25 μM) of taxol on cultured cells, under conditions of minimal inhibition of DNA, RNA and protein synthesis, demonstrated that taxol specifically blocks progression of cells through the cell cycle at M-phase, indicating that mitosis exhibits high sensitivity to taxol.[215] Higher concentrations of taxol result in damage to interphase cells, with formation of microtubule bundles and loss of a variety of cell functions known to be dependent on microtubules.

Resistance to Taxol

Taxol resistance has been described in cells in culture, and it appears to take two forms. In one, resistance is associated with alterations or mutations in α and β tubulins, whereas in another, taxol resistance is associated with overexpression of P-glycoprotein and the MDR phenotype.[33,94,95,202,218] Whether these distinct lesions co-exist in the same cell is not known; the cross-resistance properties of the tubulin mutants were not examined, and in the P-glycoprotein mutants, tubulins were not examined. The taxol-resistant cells that express altered tubulins were selected after mutagenesis of the cells by ultraviolet irradiation, whereas the taxol resistant cells that overproduced P-glycoprotein were selected for resistance by long-term growth in sublethal concentrations of the drug.[33,94,95,202,218] However, it is unlikely that the selection conditions played a major role in the type of resistance obtained, since other cell lines that expressed a "classic" Pgp-MDR phenotype were selected for resistance after mutagenesis by exposure to ethylmethanesulfonate.[1] It should be noted, however, that those cells were not examined for tubulin isoforms or P-glycoprotein expression.

Dose and Pharmacokinetics

Taxol is formulated in dehydrated alcohol, cremophor EL (1:1), at a concentration of 6 mg/mL. The drug is diluted to a final concentration of 0.03–0.6 mg/mL in 0.9% sodium chloride or 5% dextrose solution. In the concentration range 0.3–1.2 mg/mL taxol is stable for at least 12 hours. The frequency of hypersensitivity reactions appeared to relate to the rate of admininistration during infusion. Schedules, recommended doses and limiting toxicities of taxol derived from Phase I studies, are given in Table XVI-8-4. Based upon this information, the National Cancer Institute recommended that Phase II trials utilize 24 hour infusion, with prophylactic premedication with dexamethasone (20 mg) given 14 and 7 hours prior to taxol, diphenhydramine (50 mg i.v) and cimetidine or ranitidine (300 or 50 mg i.v) given 30 minutes before taxol. For treatment of renal cell carcinoma the dose was 250 mg/M² every 3 weeks.[242] In patients with refractory ovarian carcinoma, whose hematopoietic tolerance is reduced, dose escalation has started at 110 mg/M². Of significance is that responses have occurred at this relatively low dose, whereas dose levels of 200–250 mg/M² appear to be safe in previously untreated patients.

Pharmacokinetic parameters for taxol have been obtained in several clinical trials, and are summarized in Table XVI-8-5. Taxol is extensively bound to plasma proteins (95–98%), but is readily eliminated from plasma in a biphasic manner, with a $t\frac{1}{2}\alpha$ of 0.29 hours and $t\frac{1}{2}\beta \approx 5$ hours. Renal elimination of taxol in urine appears to be low (1.4–6.6%) and contributes minimally to systemic clearance. Detailed clinical pharmacology of taxol is ongoing, but high taxol concentrations and an unidentified metabolite have been detected in bile of two patients with a biliary catheter.[200]

Clinical Toxicity of Taxol

Dose limiting and other toxicities of taxol are listed in Table XVI-8-4. The onset of neutropenia, which is not schedule-dependent, usually begins by day 8; the nadir of neutrophil counts is seen around days 8–11, with rapid recovery by day 21. The incidence of fever and sepsis has been infrequent. Although neutropenia does not appear to be cumulative, severe neutropenia has been reported consistently in heavily pretreated ovarian cancer patients.[161] Significant anemia and thrombocytopenia appear to occur infrequently. Type I hypersensitivity reactions occurred in early phase I trials, the predominant manifestations being hypotension, dyspnea with bronchospasm, and urticaria. Other adverse effects included abdominal and extremity pain, angioedema, diaphoresis, generalized erythema and pruritus. It is possible that the hypersensitivity reactions are caused by formulation of taxol with cremophor, as other agents with similar formulation (teniposide, cyclosporine) have also been associated with reactions attributed to the release of histamine.[143]

Clinical Use and Clinical Resistance

Taxol entered clinical Phase I trials in 1983. A high incidence of acute hypersensitivity reactions necessitated discontinuation of many trials. However, concomitant administration of steroids, histamine H$_1$- and H$_2$-antagonists, and prolonged infusion (6–24 hrs), have been used successfully. In early phase I trials, significant activity has been demonstrated in refractory ovarian carcinoma, breast carcinoma, melanoma, non-small cell lung carcinoma, and adenocar-

Table XVI-8-4. Phase I Studies of Taxol

Schedule	Maximum Tolerated Dose (mg/m^2)	Recommended Phase II Dose (mg/m^2)	Dose-limiting Toxic Effect	Other Principal Effects
1- to 6-hr infusion every 21 days	265	210	Neutropenia	Neuropathy, mucositis, arthralgias/ myalgias, hypersensitivity reactions
1- to 6-hr infusion every 21 days	275	250	Neutropenia Neuropathy	Hypersensitivity reactions, alopecia, mucositis
24-hr infusion every 21 days	275	250	Neutropenia Neuropathy	Hypersensitivity reactions
3-hr infusion every 21 days	190		Hypersensitivity reactions	Leukopenia, nausea, alopecia
6-hr infusion every 21 days	275	225	Neutropenia	Arthralgias/myalgias, mucositis, alopecia, neuropathy, hypersensitivity reactions
24-hr infusion every 21 days	200		Neutropenia	Alopecia, nausea, vomiting
1-hr infusion × 5 days every 21 days	40	20	Neutropenia	Alopecia, diarrhea
1- to 6-hr infusion × 5 days every 21 days	40	30	Neutropenia	Hypersensitivity reactions, nausea, vomiting, alopecia, mucositis, thrombocytopenia
24-hr infusion every 14–21 days	390	310	Mucositis	Neutropenia, hypersensitivity reactions, neuropathy
24 hr infusion plus cisplatin every 21 days	135–170 +75 (cisplatin)	135–170 +75 (cisplatin)	Neutropenia	Arthralgias/myalgias, alopecia, cardiac, hypersensitivity reactions, neuropathy

From Rowinsky.[200]

Table XVI-8-5. Taxol Pharmacokinetic Parameters

Schedule	Model	T$_{1/2}\alpha$ (hr)	T$_{1/2}\beta$ (hr)	Cl (mL/min/m^2)	C$_p$ μmol/L	C$_p$ Dose (mg/m^2)	VD$_{ss}$ (L/m^2)	MRT (hr)	Urine (% dose)
6-hr infusion	Biphasic	0.32	8.6	100	3.2–8.1	175–275	55	8.6	5.2
24-hr infusion	Biphasic	0.27	3.9	993	0.6–0.94	200–275	182	19.9	1.4
1- to 6-hr infusion × 5 days	Biphasic	—	1.3	833	0.06–0.37	15–40	81	—	6.6
1- to 6-hr infusion	Biphasic	0.27	6.4	253	1.3–13.0	60–265	67	5.6	5.9
24-hr infusion	—	—	—	—	1.6–3.5	250–390	—	—	—
6-hr infusion	Biphasic	—	4.8	300	2.3–4.6	175–275	167	11.8	—
Mean	—	0.29	5.0	496	—	—	110	11.5	4.8
SD		0.03	2.7	392			59	6.2	2.3

CL, systemic clearance; C$_p$, peak plasma concentration; VD$_{ss}$, volume of distribution of steady state; MRT, mean resonance time.
From Rowinsky.[200]

cinoma of unknown origin. Minor responses were observed in gastric, colon, and head and neck carcinomas as well as lymphoblastic and myeloblastic leukemias as reviewed by Rowinsky and colleagues.[200] Phase II trials are ongoing in refractory ovarian carcinoma, where an objective response rate of 30% has been reported.[161] Confirmatory studies have reported a 37% response rate, and 33% of patients with documented platinum resistance have responded. Taxol has limited value in renal cell carcinoma, where no responses were observed in 18 patients receiving high doses of this drug.[68]

Relatively little information is available currently to determine cross-resistance patterns to taxol in human tumors.

However, as preclinical studies have demonstrated that taxol resistance is associated with the multidrug resistance phenotype, one would anticipate cross-resistance with *Vinca* alkaloids, and possibly epipodophyllotoxins and certain other natural products.[94,95,202] A relatively high response rate in ovarian carcinoma refractory to cisplatin, suggests little or no cross resistance between this agent and taxol.

Summary

It is clear that the *Vinca* alkaloids are important oncolytic agents that have an important place in the chemotherapy of many neoplastic diseases. In this chapter we have updated current knowledge about *Vinca* alkaloid action and reviewed the current status of clinical trials with newer *Vinca* alkaloids. Using VCR and VLB as a paradigm, it is evident that small modifications of the chemical structure of these agents have substantial effects on their clinical efficacy and toxicity without altering in any fundamental way their mechanism of action, binding to tubulin and causing mictotubule depolymerization. Toxicity of the *Vinca* alkaloids is also related to dose and route of administration. Since the last edition of this volume, much has been learned about the mechanisms of resistance to these agents. It is abundantly clear that resistance to *Vinca* alkaloids in vitro is due to overexpression of the *mdr1* gene and its product, P-glycoprotein. *Vinca* alkaloid resistance is associated with a broad cross-resistance to many natural product compounds, and this is called multidrug resistance. Expression of P-glycoprotein is seen in a number of different types of tumors from patients, and it is frequently seen to increase after therapy that can include *Vinca* alkaloids. Efforts over the next few years will focus not only on the development of newer, non-cross-resistant *Vinca* alkaloids, but also on the development of agents that may be effective in circumventing clinical multidrug resistance. We have also included in this chapter a section on taxol, another plant product with a unique mechanism of action, stabilization of microtubules. This agent has shown activity against a number of tumors, and clinical trials are ongoing. Unfortunately, taxol's low yield from natural sources and its difficult chemical synthesis currently restrict its full development.

References

1. Akiyama, S. I., Fojo, A., Hanover, J. A., Pastan, I., and Gottesman, M. M.: Isolation and genetic characterization of human KB cell lines resistant to multiple drugs. Somatic Cell. Genet., 11:117, 1985.
2. Armand, J. P., and Marty, M.: Navelbine: A new step in cancer chemotherapy? Semin. Oncol., 2:41, 1989.
3. Bagley, C. M., Jr., DeVita, V. T., Jr., Berard, C. W., and Canellos, G. P.: Advanced lymphosarcoma: Intensive cyclical chemotherapy with cyclophosphamide, vincristine, and prednisone. Ann. Intern. Med., 76:227, 1972.
4. Baker, R. M., Fredericks, W. J., Chen, Y., Murawski, M. J., Meegan, R. L., Rustum, Y. M., Karakousis, C., and Piver, M. S.: Detection of P-glycoprotein in human tumors by immunoblot analysis. *In* Drug resistance mechanisms and reversal. Edited by E. Mihich. John Libbey, 1990, p. 167.
5. Baum, S. G., Wittner, M., Nadler, J. P., Horwitz, S. B., Dennis, J. E., Schiff, P. B., and Tanowitz, H. B.: Taxol, a microtubule stabilizing agent, blocks the replication of Trypanosoma cruzi. Proc. Natl. Acad. Sci. USA, 78:4571, 1981.
6. Beck, W. T.: Increase by vinblastine of oxidized glutathione in cultured mammalian cells. Biochem. Pharmacol., 29:2333, 1980.
7. Beck, W. T.: Vinca alkaloid-resistant phenotype in cultured human leukemic lymphoblasts. Cancer Treat. Rep., 67:875, 1983.
8. Beck, W. T.: Cellular pharmacology of Vinca alkaloid resistance and its circumvention. Adv. Enzyme Regul., 22:207, 1984.
9. Beck, W. T.: The cell biology of multiple drug resistance. Biochem. Pharmacol., 36:2879, 1987.
10. Beck, W. T.: Multidrug resistance and its circumvention. Eur. J. Cancer, 26:513, 1990.
11. Beck, W. T.: Strategies to circumvent multidrug resistance due to P-glycoprotein or to altered DNA topoisomerase II. Bull. Cancer, 77:1131, 1990.
12. Beck, W. T.: Modulators of P-glycoprotein-associated multidrug resistance. *In* Molecular and Clinical Advances in Anticancer Drug Resistance. Edited by R. F. Ozols. Norwell, MA, Kluwer Academic Publishers, 1991, p. 151.
13. Beck, W. T., Cirtain, M. C., and Lefko, J. L.: Energy-dependent reduced drug binding as a mechanism of Vinca alkaloid resistance in human leukemic lymphoblasts. Mol. Pharmacol., 24:485, 1983.
14. Beck, W. T., Cirtain, M. C., Danks, M. K., Felsted, R. L., Safa, A. R., Wolverton, J. S., Suttle, D. P., and Trent, J. M.: Pharmacological, molecular, and cytogenetic analysis of "atypical" multidrug-resistant human leukemic cells. Cancer Res., 47:5455, 1987.
15. Beck, W. T., Cirtain, M. C., Look, A. T., and Ashmun, R. A.: Reversal of Vinca alkaloid resistance but not multiple drug resistance in human leukemic cells by verapamil. Cancer Res., 46:778, 1986.
16. Behnke, O.: An electron microscope study of the rat megacaryocyte. II. Some aspects of platelet release and microtubules. J. Ultrastruct. Res., 26:111, 1969.
17. Bell, D. R., Gerlach, J. H., Kartner, N., Buick, R. N., and Ling, V.: Detection of P-glycoprotein in ovarian cancer: a molecular marker associated with multidrug resistance. J. Clin. Oncol., 3:311, 1985.
18. Bender, R. A., Castle, M. C., Margileth, D. A., and Oliverio, V. T.: The pharmacokinetics of [^{3}H]-vincristine in man. Clin. Pharmacol. Therap., 22:430, 1977.
19. Bender, R. A., Hamel, E., and Hande, K. R.: Plant alkaloids. *In* Cancer Chemotherapy. Principals and Practice. Edited by B. A. Chabner and J. M. Collins. Philadelphia, J.B. Lippincott, 1990, p. 253.
20. Bensch, K. G., and Malawista, S. E.: Microtubule crystals: A new biophysical phenomenon induced by Vinca alkaloids. Nature, 218:1176, 1968.
21. Bensch, K. G., and Malawista, S. E.: Microtubular crystals in mammalian cells. J. Cell Biol., 40:95, 1969.
22. Benson, A. B., Trump, D. L., Koeller, J. M., Egorin, M. I., Olman, E. A., Witte, R. S., Davis, T. E., and Tormey, D. C.: Phase I study of vinblastine and verapamil given by concurrent i.v infusion. Cancer Treat. Rep., 69:795, 1985.
23. Besenval, M., Delgado, M., Demarez, J. P., and Krikorian, A.: Safety and tolerance of navelbine in Phase I-II clinical studies. Semin. Oncol., 16:37, 1989.
24. Binet, S., Fellous, A., Lataste, H., Krikorian, A., Couzinier, J. P., and Meininger, V.: In situ analysis of the action of navelbine on various types of microtubules using immunofluorescence. Semin. Oncol., 16:5, 1989.
25. Boder, G. B., Bromer, W. W., Poore, G. A., Thompson, G. L., and Williams, D. C.: Comparative cellular responses to semisynthetic and natural vinca alkaloids. Proc. Am. Assoc. Cancer Res., 23:201, 1982.
26. Bore, P., Rahmani, R., van Cantfort, J., Focan, C., and Cano, J. P.: Pharmacokinetics of a new anticancer drug, navelbine, in patients. Cancer Chemother. Pharmacol., 23:247, 1989.
27. Bouris, J., Benard, J., Hartman,O., Boccon-Gibod, L., Lemerle, J., and Riou, G.: Correlation of MDR1 gene expression with chemotherapy in neuroblastoma. J. Natl. Cancer Inst., 81:1401, 1989.
28. Bowman, L. C., Houghton, J. A., and Houghton, P. J.: GTP influences the binding of vincristine in human tumor cytosols. Biochem. Biophys. Res. Commun., 135:695, 1986.
29. Brade, W.: Critical review of pharmacology, toxicology, pharmacokinetics of vincristine, vindesine, vinblastine. *In* Proceedings of the International Vinca Alkaloid Symposium–Vindesine. Edited by W. Brade, G. A. Nagel, and S. Seeber. Basel, S. Karger, 1980, p. 95.
30. Bruchovsky, N., Owen, A. A., Becker, A. J., and Till, J. E.: Effects of vinblastine on the proliferative capacity of L cells and their progress through the division cycle. Cancer Res., 25:1232, 1965.
31. Bryan, J.: Vinblastine and microtubules. II. Characterization of two protein subunits from the isolated crystals. J. Mol. Biol., 66:157, 1972.
32. Budman, D. R., Schulman, P., Marks, M., Vinciguerra, V., Weiselberg, L., Kreis, W., and Degnan, T. J.: Phase I trial of vinzolidine. Cancer Treat. Rep., 68:979, 1984.
33. Cabral, F., Abraham, I., and Gottesman, M. M.: Isolation of a taxol-resistant Chinese hamster ovary cell mutant that has an alteration in α-tubulin. Proc. Natl. Acad. Sci. USA, 78:4388, 1981.
34. Cabral, F., Sobel, M. E., and Gottesman, M. M.: CHO mutants resistant to colchicine, colcemid or griseofulvin have an altered α-tubulin. Cell, 20:29, 1980.
35. Cannobio, L., Pastorino, G., Gasparini, G., Brema, F., Fosser, V., and Boccardo, F.: Phase II study of navelbine in advanced breast cancer patients. Second International Congress of Neo-Adjuvant Chemotherapy (Paris), 1988, p. 15.
36. Carbone, P. P., Kaplan, H. S., Musshoff, K., Smither, D. W., and Tubiana, M.: Report of the committee on Hodgkin's disease staging classification. Cancer Res., 31:1860, 1971.
37. Carter, S. K. and Livingston, R. B.: Single-agent therapy for Hodgkin's disease. Arch. Intern. Med., 131:377, 1973.
38. Cass, C. E. and Beck, W. T.: Vinca alkaloid pharmacology and resistance. *In* Resistance to Antineoplastic Drugs. Edited by D. Kessel. CRC Press, Boca Raton, 1989, p. 141.
39. Cersosimo, R. J., Bromer, R., Licciardello, J. T. W., and Hong, W. K.: Pharmacology, clinical efficacy and adverse effects of vindesine sulfate, a new Vinca alkaloid. Pharmacotherapy, 3:259, 1983.
40. Chan, H. S. L., Thorner, P. S., Haddad, G., DeBoer, G., Lin, S., Yeger, H., Ondrusek, N., and Ling, V.: Increased P-glycoprotein expression in advanced neuroblastoma correlates with adverse outcome of therapy. Proc. Am. Assoc. Cancer Res., 31:372, 1990.
41. Chan, H. S. L., Thorner, P. S., Haddad, G., and Ling, V.: Immunohistochemical detection of P-glycoprotein: prognostic correlation in soft tissue sarcoma of childhood. J. Clin. Oncol., 8:689, 1990.
42. Chan, S. Y., Worth, R., and Ochs, S.: Block of axoplasmic transport in vitro by Vinca alkaloids. J. Neurobiol., 11:251, 1980.
43. Chen, C-J., Chin, J. E., Ueda, K., Clark, D. P., Pastan, I., Gottesman, M. M., and Roninson, I. B.: Internal duplication and homology with bacterial transport proteins in the mdr1 (P-glycoprotein) gene from multidrug-resistant human cells. Cell, 47:381, 1986.
44. Chong, D. C. K., Logothetis, C. J., Savaraj, N., Fritsche, H. A., Gietner, A. M., and Samuels, M. L.: The correlation of vinblastine pharmacokinetics to toxicity in testicular cancer patients. J. Clin. Pharmacol., 28:714, 1988.
45. Cline, M. J.: Effect of vincristine on synthesis of ribonucleic acid and protein in leukaemic leucocytes. Br. J. Haematol., 14:21, 1968.
46. Collins, C. A., and Vallee, R. B.: Temperature-dependent reversible assembly of taxol-treated microtubules. J. Cell Biol., 105:2847, 1987.
47. Cordon-Cardo, C., O'Brien, J. P., Casals, D., Rittman-Grauer, L., Biedler, J. L., Melamed, M. R., and Bertino, J. R.: Multidrug resistance gene (P-glycoprotein) is expressed by endothelial cells at blood-brain barrier sites. Proc. Natl. Acad. Sci. USA, 86:695, 1989.
48. Cornwell, M. M., Pastan, I., and Gottesman, M. M.: Certain calcium channel blockers bind specifically to multidrug-resistant human KB carcinoma membrane vesicles and inhibit drug binding to P-glycoprotein. J. Biol. Chem., 262:2166, 1987.
49. Cornwell, M. M., Safa, A. R., Felsted, R. L., Gottesman, M. M., and Pastan, I.: Membrane vesicles from multidrug-resistant human cancer cells contain a specific 150- to 170-kDa protein detected by photoaffinity labeling. Proc. Natl. Acad. Sci. USA, 83:3847, 1986.
50. Cornwell, M. M., Tsuruo, T., Gottesman, M. M., and Pastan, I.: ATP-binding properties of P-glycoprotein from multidrug-resistant KB cells. FASEB J., 1:51, 1987.
51. Creasey, W. A.: Vinca alkaloids and colchicine. *In* Antineoplastic and Immunosuppressive Agents. II. Edited by A. C. Sartorelli, and D. G. Johns. Berlin, Springer-Verlag, New York, 1975, p. 670.
52. Creasey, W. A.: The Vinca alkaloids. *In* Antibiotics, V-2. Edited by F. E. Hahn. Berlin, Springer-Verlag, 1979, p. 414.
53. Creasey, W. A.: The Vinca alkaloids and similar compounds. *In* Cancer and Chemotherapy 3. Edited by S. T. Crooke, and A. W. Prestayko. New York, Academic Press, 1981, p. 79.
54. Creasey, W. A., and Markiw, M. E.: Biochemical effects of the Vinca alkaloids. II. A comparison of the effects of colchicine, vinblastine and vincristine on the synthesis of ribonucleic acids in Ehrlich ascites carcinoma cells. Biochem. Biophys. Acta, 87:601, 1964.
55. Creasey, W. A., and Markiw, M. E.: Biochemical effects of the Vinca alkaloids-III. The synthesis of ribonucleic acid and the incorporation of amino acids in Ehrlich ascites cells in vitro. Biochem. Biophys. Acta, 103:635, 1965.
56. Croop, J. M., Raymond, M., Haber, D., DeVault, A., Arceci, R. J., Gros, P., and

Housman, D. E.: The three mouse multidrug resistance (mdr) genes are expressed in a tissue-specific manner in mouse normal tissues. Mol. Cell. Biol., 9:1346, 1989.
57. Dalton, W. S., Grogan, T. M., Meltzer, P. S., Scheper, R. J., and Salmon, S. E.: Drug-resistance in multiple myeloma and non-Hodgkin's lymphoma: detection of P-glycoprotein and potential circumvention by addition of verapamil to chemotherapy. J. Clin. Oncol., 7:415, 1989.
58. Dalton, W. S., Grogan, T. M., Rybski, J. A., Scheper, J., Richter, L., Kailey, J., Broxterman, H. J., Pinedo, H. M., and Salmon, S. E.: Immunohistochemical detection and quantitation of P-glycoprotein in multiple drug-resistant human myeloma cells: association with level of drug resistance and drug accumulation. Blood, 73:747, 1989.
59. Danks, M. K., Yalowich, J. C., and Beck, W. T.: Atypical multiple drug resistance in a human leukemic cell line selected for resistance to teniposide (VM-26). Cancer Res., 47:1297, 1987.
60. Danø, K.: Active outward transport of daunomycin in resistant Ehrlich ascites tumor cells. Biochim. Biophys. Acta, 323:466, 1973.
61. De Brabander, M., Geuens, G., Nuydens, R., Willebrords, R., and De Mey, J.: Taxol induces the assembly of free microtubules in living cells and blocks the organizing capacity of the centrosomes and kinetochore. Proc. Natl. Acad. Sci. USA, 78:5608, 1981.
62. Depierre, A., Lemarie, E., Dabouis, G., Samak, R., Krikorian, A., and Besenval, M.: Phase II study of navelbine (NVB) in non small cell lung cancer (NSCLC). Proc. Am. Soc. Clin. Oncol., 7:201, 1988.
63. Desai, Z. R., Van den Berg, H. W., Bridges, J. M., and Shanks, R. G.: Can severe vincristine neurotoxicity be prevented? Cancer Chemother. Pharmacol., 8:211, 1981.
64. DeVita, V. T., Jr., Hellman, S., and Rosenberg, S. A.: Cancer, Principles and Practice of Oncology, 2nd edition. Philadelphia, J. B. Lippincott, 1985.
65. DeVita, V. T., Jr., Serpick, A. A., and Carbone, P. P.: Combination chemotherapy in the treatment of advanced Hodgkin's disease. Ann. Intern. Med., 73:881, 1970.
66. Donoso, J. A., Haskins, K. M., and Himes, R. H.: Effect of microtubule-associated proteins on the interaction of vincristine with microtubules and tubulin. Cancer Res., 39:1604, 1979.
67. Dustin, P.: Microtubules, Second Edition. Berlin, Springer-Verlag, 1984.
68. Einzig, A. I., Gorowski, E., Sasloff, J., and Wiernik, P. H.: Phase II trial of taxol in patients with renal carcinoma. Proc. Am. Assoc. Cancer Res., 29:884,1988.
69. Endicott, J. A., and Ling, V.: The biochemistry of P-glycoprotein-mediated multidrug resistance. Ann. Rev. Biochem., 58:137, 1989.
70. Falkson, G., Van Dyk, J. J., and Falkson, F. C.: Oral vinblastine sulfate (NSC49842) in malignant disease. S. Afr. Cancer Bull., 12:78, 1968.
71. Favre, R., Delgado, M., Besenval, M., Saraga, J., Danet, S., and Krikorian, A.: Phase I trial of escalating doses of orally administered navelbine (NVB): Part II–clinical results. Proc. Am. Soc. Clin. Oncol., 8:A246, 1989.
72. Fellous, A., Ohayon, R., Vacassin, T., Lataste, H., Krikorian, H., Couzinier, J. P., and Meininger, V.: Biochemical effects of navelbine on tubulin and associated proteins. Semin. Oncol. 2(Suppl. 4):9, 1989.
73. Ferguson, P. J., and Cass, C. E.: Differential cellular retention of vincristine and vinblastine by cultured human promyelocytic leukemia HL-60/C1 cells: The basis of differential toxicity. Cancer Res., 45:5480, 1985.
74. Ferguson, P. J., Phillips, J. R., Selner, M., and Cass, C. E.: Differential activity of vincristine and vinblastine against cultured cells. Cancer Res., 44:3307, 1984.
75. Ferrazzi, E., Zagonel, V., Vinante, O., Galligioni, E., Pappagallo, G. L., and Cartei, G.: Vindesine in the treatment of squamous cell carcinoma (WHO I), adenocarcinoma (WHO III), and large cell carcinoma (WHO IV) of the lung. Tumori, 68:531, 1982.
76. Ferro-Luzzi Ames, G.: The basis of multidrug resistance in mammalian cells: Homology with bacterial transport. Cell, 47:323, 1986.
77. Fojo, A. T., Shen, D-W., Mickley, L. A., Pastan, I., and Gottesman, M. M.: Intrinsic drug resistance in human kidney cancer is associated with expression of a human multidrug-resistance gene. J. Clin Oncol., 5:1922, 1987.
78. Fojo, A. T., Ueda, K., Slamon, D. J., Poplack, D. G., Gottesman, M. M., and Pastan, I.: Expression of a multidrug-resistance gene in human tumors. Proc. Natl. Acad. Sci., 84:265, 1987.
79. Friche, E., Skovsgaard, T., and Dano, K.: Multidrug resistance: Drug extrusion and its counteraction by chemosensitizers. Eur. J. Haematol., 42:59, 1989.
80. Fuchs, D. A., and Johnson, R. K.: Cytologic evidence that taxol, an antineoplastic agent from Taxus brevifolia, acts as a mitotic spindle poison. Cancer Treat. Rep., 62:1219, 1978.
81. Garewal, H. S., Brooks, R. J., Jones, S. E., and Miller, T. P.: Treatment of advanced breast cancer with mitomycin C combined with vinblastine or vindesine. J. Clin. Oncol., 1:772, 1983.
82. George, M., Heron, J. F., Kerbrat, P., Chauvergne, J., Lebrun, D., and Guastalla, J. P.: Phase II study of navelbine (NVB) in advanced ovarian cancer (ADOVA). Proc. Am. Soc. Clin. Oncol., 7:A553, 1988.
83. George, P., Journey, L. J., and Goldstein, M. N.: Effect of vincristine on the fine structure of HeLa cells during mitosis. J. Nat. Cancer Inst., 35:355, 1965.
84. Gerlach J. H., Bell, D. R., Karakousis, C., Slocum, H. K., Kartner, N., Rustum, Y. M., Ling, V., and Baker, R. M.: P-glycoprotein in human sarcoma: Evidence for multidrug resistance. J. Clin. Oncol., 5:1452, 1987.
85. Gerlach, J. H., Endicott, J. A., Juranka, P. F., Henderson, G., Sarangi, F., Deuchars, K. L., and Ling, V.: Homology between P-glycoprotein and a bacterial haemolysin transport protein suggests a model for multidrug resistance. Nature, 324:485, 1986.
86. Gerzon, K.: *In* Anticancer agents based on natural products. Edited by J. M. Cassidy, and J. D. Douros. Academic Press, 1980, p. 271.
87. Goldstein, L. J., Fojo, A. T., Ueda, K., Crist, W., Green, A., Brodeur, G., Pastan, I., and Gottesman, M. M.: Expression of the multidrug resistance, MDR1, gene in neuroblastomas. J. Clin. Oncol., 8:128, 1990.
88. Goldstein, L. J., Galski, H., Fojo, A., Willingham, M., Lai, S-L., Gazdar, A., Pirker, R., Green, A., Crist, W., Brodeur, G. M., Lieber, M., Cossman, J., Gottesman, M. M., and Pastan, I.: Expression of a multidrug resistance gene in human cancers. J. Natl. Cancer Inst., 81:116, 1989.
89. Gottesman, M. M. and Pastan, I.: The multidrug transporter, a double-edged sword. J. Biol. Chem., 263:12163, 1988.
90. Gout, P. W., Noble, R. L., Bruchovsky, N., and Beer, C. T.: Vinblastine and vincristine-growth-inhibitory effects correlate with their retention by cultured Nb2 node lymphoma cells. Int. J. Cancer, 34:245, 1984.
91. Gout, P. W., Wijcik, L. L., and Beer, C. T.: Differences between vinblastine and vincristine in distribution in the blood of rats and binding by platelets and malignant cells. Eur. J. Cancer, 14:1167, 1978.
92. Green, L. S., Donoso, J. A., Heller-Bettinger, I. E. and Samson, F. E.: Axonal transport disturbances in vincristine-induced peripheral neuropathy. Ann. Neurol., 1:255, 1977.
93. Gros, P., Croop, J., and Housman, D.: Mammalian multidrug resistance gene: Complete cDNA sequence indicates strong homology to bacterial transport proteins. Cell, 47:371, 1986.
94. Gupta, R. S.: Taxol resistant mutants of Chinese hamster ovary cells: Genetic biochemical, and cross-resistance studies. J. Cell. Physiol., 114:137, 1983.
95. Gupta, R. S.: Cross-resistance of vinblastine- and taxol resistant mutants of Chinese hamster ovary cells to other anticancer drugs. Cancer Treat. Rep., 69:515, 1985.
96. Hains, F. O., Dickerson, R. M., Wilson, L., and Owellen, R. J.: Differences in the binding properties of Vinca alkaloids and colchicine to tubulin by varying protein sources and methodology. Biochem. Pharmacol., 27:71, 1978.
97. Hande, K., Gay, J., Gober, J., and Greco, F. A.: Toxicity and pharmacology of bolus vindesine injection and prolonged vindesine infusion. Cancer Treat. Rev., 7:25, 1980.
98. Hausmann, K., Linnenbach, M., and Patterson, D. J.: The effects of taxol on microtubular arrays: In vivo effects on heliozoan axonemes. J. Ultrastruc. Res., 82:212, 1983.
99. Herman, B., Langevin, M. A., and Albertini, D. F.: The effects of taxol on the organization of the cytoskeleton in cultured ovarian granulosa cells. Eur. J. Cell Biol., 31:34, 1983.
100. Himes, R. H., Kersey, R. N., Heller-Bettinger, I., and Samson F. E.: Action of the Vinca alkaloids vincristine, vinblastine, and desacetyl vinblastine amide on microtubules in vitro. Cancer Res., 36:3798, 1976.
101. Horio, T. and Hotani, H.: Visualization of the dynamic instability of individual microtubules by dark-field microscopy. Nature, 321:605, 1986.
102. Horton, J. K., Thimmaiah, K. N., Houghton, J. A., Horowitz, M. E., and Houghton, P. J.: Modulation by verapamil of vincristine pharmacokinetics and toxicity in mice bearing human tumor xenografts. Biochem. Pharmacol., 38:1727, 1989.
103. Horwitz, S. B., Liao, L.-L., Greenberger, L., and Lothstein, L.: Mode of action of taxol and characterization of a multidrug-resistant cell line selected with taxol. *In* Resistance to Antineoplastic Drugs. Edited by D. Kessel. CRC Press, Boca Raton, 1989, p. 109.
104. Houghton, J. A., Houghton, P. J., Hazelton, B. J., and Douglass, E. C.: In situ selection of a human rhabdomyosarcoma resistant to vincristine with altered α-tubulins. Cancer Res., 45:2706, 1985.
105. Houghton, J. A., Meyer, W. H., and Houghton, P. J.: Scheduling of vincristine: Drug accumulation and response of xenografts of childhood rhabdomyosarcoma determined by frequency of administration. Cancer Treat. Rep., 71:717, 1987.
106. Houghton, J. A., Williams, L. G., Dodge, R. K., George, S. L., Hazelton, B. J., and Houghton, P. J.: Relationship between binding affinity, retention and sensitivity of human rhabdomyosarcoma xenografts to Vinca alkaloids. Biochem. Pharmacol., 36:81, 1987.
107. Houghton, J. A., Williams, L. G., and Houghton, P. J.: Stability of vincristine complexes in cytosols derived from xenografts of human rhabdomyosarcoma and normal tissues of the mouse. Cancer Res., 45:3761, 1985.
108. Houghton, J. A., Williams, L. G., Torrance, P. M., and Houghton, P. J.: Determinants of intrinsic sensitivity to Vinca alkaloids in xenografts of pediatric rhabdomyosarcomas. Cancer Res., 44:582, 1984.
109. Houwen, B., Ockhuizen, Th., Marrink, J., and Nieweg, H. O.: Vindesine therapy in melphalan-resistant multiple myeloma. Eur. J. Cancer Clin. Oncol., 17:227, 1981.
110. Howard, S. M. H., Theologides, A., and Sheppard, J. R.: Comparative effects of vindesine, vinblastine, and vincristine on mitotic arrest and hormonal response of L1210 leukemia cells. Cancer Res., 40:2695, 1980.
111. Howell, S. L., Hii, C. S., Shaikh, S., and Tyhurst, M.: Effects of taxol and nocodazole on insulin secretion from isolated rat islets of Langerhans. Biosci. Rep., 2:795, 1982.
112. Huang Yang, C-P., DePinho, S. G., Greenberger, L. M., Arceci, R. J., and Horwitz, S. B.: Progesterone interacts with P-glycoprotein in multidrug-resistant cells and in the endometrium of gravid uterus. J. Biol. Chem., 264:782, 1989.
113. Jackson, D. V., Jr., Castle, M. C., and Bender, R. A.: Biliary excretion of vincristine. Clin. Pharmacol. Ther., 24:101, 1978.
114. Jackson, D. V., Jr., Chauvenet, A. R., Callahan, R. D., Atkins, J. N., Trahey, T. F., and Spurr, C. L.: Phase II trial of vincristine infusion in acute leukemia. Cancer Chemother. Pharmacol., 14:26, 1985.
115. Jackson, D. V., Jr., Sethi, V. S., Long, T. R., Muss, H. B., and Spurr, C. L.: Pharmacokinetics of vindesine bolus and infusion. Cancer Chemother. Pharmacol., 13:114, 1984.
116. Jackson, D. V., Jr., Sethi, V. S., Spurr, C. L., White, D. R., Richards, F., 2nd, Stuart, J. J., Muss, H. B., Cooper, M. R., and Castle, M. C.: Pharmacokinetics of vincristine infusion. Cancer Treat. Rep., 65:1043, 1981.
117. Jackson, D. V., Jr., Sethi, V. S., Spurr, C. L., Willard, V., White, D. R., Richards, F. 2nd, Stuart, J. J., Muss, H. B., Cooper, M. R., Homesley, H. D., Jobson, V. W., and Castle, M. C.: Intravenous vincristine infusion: Phase I trial. Cancer, 48:2559, 1981.
118. Johnson, I. S.: Historical background of Vinca alkaloid research and areas of future interest. Cancer Chemother. Rep., 52:455, 1968.
119. Johnson, I. S., Armstrong, J. G., Gorman, M., and Burnett, J. P., Jr.: The Vinca alkaloids: A new class of oncolytic agents. Cancer Res., 23:1390, 1963.
120. Jordan, M. A., Himes, R. H., and Wilson, L.: Comparison of the effects of vinblastine, vincristine, vindesine, and vinepidine on microtubule dynamics and cell proliferation in vitro. Cancer Res., 45:2741, 1985.
121. Jordon, M. A., Margolis, R. L., Himes, R. H. and Wilson, L.: Identification of a distinct class of vinblastine binding sites. Cancer Chemother. Pharmacol., 8:215, 1982.
122. Kanamaru, H., Kalehi, Y., Yoshida, O., Nakanishi, S., Pastan, I., and Gottesman, M. M.: MDR1 RNA levels in human renal cell carcinomas: Correlation with grade and prediction of reversal of doxorubicin resistance by quinidine in tumor explants. J. Natl. Cancer Inst., 81:844, 1989.
123. Kaplan, R. S., and Wiernik, P. H.: Neurotoxicity of antineoplastic drugs. Semin. Oncol., 9:103, 1982.
124. Keller, H. U., and Zimmermann, A.: Shape changes and chemokinesis of Walker 256 carcinosarcoma cells in response to colchicine, vinblastine, nocodazole and taxol. Invasion Metastasis, 6:33, 1986.
125. Kennedy, M. S., and Insel, P. A.: Inhibitors of microtubule assembly enhance beta-adrenergic and prostaglandin E1-stimulated cyclic AMP accumulation in S49 lymphoma cells. Mol. Pharmacol., 16:215, 1979.
126. Kotani, M., Koizumi, Y., Yamada, T., Kawasaki, A., and Akabane, T.: Increase of cyclic adenosine 3′:5′-monophosphate concentration in transplantable lymphoma cells by Vinca alkaloids. Cancer Res., 38:3094, 1978.
127. Kreis, W., Budman, D. R., Freeman, J., Milazzo, J., Bergstrom, R. F., and Nelson, R.: Clinical pharmacology studies with i. v. administered 3H-vinzolidine. Proc. Am. Assoc. Cancer Res., 29:216, 1988.
128. Kreis, W., Budman, D. R., Schulman, P., Freeman, J., Greist, A., Nelson, R. L., Marks, M., and Kevill, L.: Clinical pharmacology of vinzolidine. Cancer Chemother. Pharmacol., 16:70, 1986.
129. Kremmer, T., and Holczinger, L.: Investigation of Vinca alkaloid-plasma membrane interactions by detergent gel chromatography. J. Chromatogr., 191:287, 1980.
130. Krikorian, A., Rahmani, R., Bromet, M., Bore, P., and Cano, J. P.: Pharmacokinetics and metabolism of navelbine. Semin. Oncol., 16:21, 1989.

131. Krishan, A.: Time-lapse and ultrastructure studies on the reversal of mitotic arrest induced by vinblastine sulfate in Earle's L-cells. J. Natl. Cancer Inst., 41:581, 1968.

132. Krishan, A., and Frei, E., III: Morphological basis for the cytolytic effect of vinblastine and vincristine on cultured human leukemic lymphoblasts. Cancer Res., 35:497, 1975.

133. Krivit, W., Chilcote, R., Pyesmany, A., Anderson, J., and Hammond, D.: An initial report of a phase III trial comparing vindesine and vincristine for acute lymphocytic leukemia of childhood. Cancer Chemother. Pharmacol., 2:267, 1979.

134. Kumar, N.: Taxol-induced polymerization of purified tubulin. J. Biol. Chem., 256:10435, 1981.

135. Lathan, B., Von Hoff, D. D., Melink, T. J., and Kisner, D. L.: Screening phase I drugs in the human tumor cloning system (HTCS) to pinpoint areas of emphasis in phase II studies. In Human Tumor Cloning. Edited by S. E. Salmon, and J. M. Trent, Grune and Stratton, 1984, p. 669.

136. Lee, J. C., Harrison, D., and Timasheff, S. N.: Interaction of vinblastine with calf brain microtubule protein. J. Biol. Chem., 250:9276, 1975.

137. Lee, S. C., Deutsch, C., and Beck, W. T.: Comparison of ion channels in multidrug-resistant and -sensitive human leukemic cells. Proc. Natl. Acad. Sci. USA, 85:2019, 1988.

138. Lengsfeld, A. M., Dietrich, J., and Schultze-Maurer, B.: Accumulation and release of vinblastine and vincristine by HeLa cells: Light microscopic, cinematographic, and biochemical study. Cancer Res., 42:3798, 1982.

139. Lengsfeld, A. M., Schultze, B., and Maurer, W.: Time-lapse studies on the effect of vincristine on HeLa cells. Eur. J. Cancer, 17:307, 1980.

140. Letourneau, P. C., and Ressler, A. H.: Inhibition of neurite initiation and growth by taxol. J. Cell Biol., 98:1355, 1984.

141. Letourneau, P. C., Shattuck, T. A., and Ressler, A. H.: Branching of sensory and sympathetic neurites in vitro is inhibited by treatment with taxol. J. Neurosci., 7:1912, 1986.

142. Loike, J. D., and Horwitz, S. B.: Effects of VP-16-213 on the intracellular degradation of DNA in HeLa cells. Biochemistry, 15:5443, 1976.

143. Lorenz, W., Reiman, H. J., Schmal, A., Dormann, P., Neugebauer, E., and Doenicke, A.: Histamine release in dogs by cremophor EL and its derivatives: Oxyethylated oleic acid is the most effective constituent. Agents Actions, 7:63,1977.

144. Lowenbraun, S., DeVita, V. T., Jr., and Serpick, A. A.: Combination chemotherapy with nitrogen mustard, vincristine,procarbazine, and prednisone in lymphosarcoma, and reticulum cell sarcoma. Cancer, 25:1018, 1970.

145. Lu, K., Yap, H.-Y., and Loo, T. L.: Clinical pharmacokinetics of vinblastine by continuous intravenous infusion. Cancer Res., 43:1405, 1983.

146. Luce, J. K., Gamble, J. F., Wilson, H. E., Monto, R. W., Isaacs, B. L., Palmer, R. L., Cottman, C. A., Jr., Hewlett, J. S., Gehan, E. A., and Frei, E., III: Combined cyclophosphamide, vincristine and prednisone therapy of malignant lymphoma. Cancer, 28:306, 1971.

147. Ma, D. D., Davey, R. A., Harman, D. H., Isbister, J. P., Scurr, R. D., Mackertich, S. M., Dowden, G., and Bell, D. R.: Detection of a multidrug resistant phenotype in acute non-lymphoblastic leukaemia. Lancet, 1:135, 1987.

148. Madoc-Jones, H., and Mauro, F.: Interphase action of vinblastine and vincristine: Differences in their lethal action through the mitotic cycle of cultured mammalian cells. J. Cell. Physiol., 72:185, 1968.

149. Madoc-Jones, H., and Mauro, F.: Site of action of cytotoxic agents in the cell life cycle. In Antineoplastic and Immunosuppressive Agents, Part 1, Handbook of Experimental Pharmacology XXXVIII/1. Edited by A. C. Sartorelli, and D. G. Johns. Berlin, Springer-Verlag, 1974, p. 205.

150. Malawista, S. E., Bensch, K. G., and Sato, H.: Vinblastine and griseofulvin reversibly disrupt the living mitotic spindle. Science, 160:770, 1968.

151. Mandelli, F., Amadori, S., Giona, F., Antonietta, M., Spiriti, A., Pastore, S., Meloni, G., and Paolucci, G.: Vindesine in the treatment of refractory hematologic malignancies: a phase II study. Leuk. Res., 6:649, 1982.

152. Manfredi, J. J., and Horwitz, S.B.: Taxol: An antimitotic agent with a new mechanism of action. Pharmacol. Ther., 25:83, 1984.

153. Manfredi, J.J., Parness, J., and Horwitz, S. B.: Taxol binds to cellular microtubules. J. Cell Biol., 94:688, 1982.

154. Marantz, R., Ventilla, M., and Shelanski, M.: Vinblastine-induced precipitation of microtubule protein. Science, 165:498, 1969.

155. Mareel, M. M., Storme, G. A., De Bruyne, G. K., and Van Cauwenberge, R. M.: Vinblastine, vincristine and vindesine: Anti-invasive effect on MO4 mouse fibrosarcoma cells in vitro. Eur. J. Cancer Clin. Oncol., 18:199, 1982.

156. Marty, M., Extra, J. M., Leandri, S., Besenval, M., and Krikorian, A.: Advances in vinca-alkaloids: Navelbine. Nouv. Rev. Fr. Hematol., 31:77, 1989.

157. Marty, M., Leandri, S., Extra, J. M., Espie, M., and Besenval, M.: A phase II study of vinorelbine (NVB) in patients (PTS) with advanced breast cancer (BC). Proc. Am. Assoc. Cancer Res., 30:256, 1989.

158. Masurovsky, E. B., Peterson, E. R., Crain, S. M., and Horwitz, S. B.: Morphological alterations in dorsal root ganglion neurons and supporting cells of organotypic mouse spinal cord-ganglion cultures exposed to taxol. Neuroscience, 10:491, 1983.

159. Mathe, G., Delgado, M., Ribaud, P., and Gouveia, J.: Discovery of a new vinca alkaloid: Navelbine (NVB). J. Chemother. Infect. Dis. Malignancies, 1:A478, 1989.

160. Mathe, G., Misset, J. L., De Vassal, F., Gouveia, J., Hayat, M., Machover, D., Belpomme, D., Pico, J. L., Schwarzenberg, L., Ribaud, P., Musset, M., Jasmin, C., and De Luca, L.: Phase II clinical trial with vindesine for remission induction in acute leukemia, blastic crisis of chronic myeloid leukemia, lymphosarcoma, and Hodgkin's disease: Absence of cross resistance with vincristine. Cancer Treat. Rep., 62:805, 1978.

161. McGuire, W. P., Rowinsky, E. K., Rosenshein, N. B., Grundine, F. C., Ettinger, D. S., Armstrong, D. K., and Donehower, R. C.: Taxol: A unique antineoplastic agent with significant activity in advanced ovarian epithelial neoplasms. Ann. Intern. Med., 111:273,1989.

162. Meininger, V., Binet, S., Chaineau, E., and Fellous, A.: In situ response to vinca alkaloids by microtubules in cultured post-implanted mouse embryos. Biol. Cell, 68:21, 1990.

163. Mitchison, T., and Kirschner, M.: Dynamic instability of microtubule growth. Nature, 312:237, 1984.

164. Mitchison, T., and Kirschner, M.: Microtubule assembly nucleated by isolated centrosomes. Nature, 312:232, 1984.

165. Mitchison, T. J.: Microtubule dynamics and kinetochore function in mitosis. Ann. Rev. Cell Biol., 4:527, 1988.

166. Mole-Bajer, J., and Bajer, A. S.: Action of taxol on mitosis: Modification of microtubule arrangements and function of the mitotic spindle in Haemanthus endosperm. J. Cell Biol., 96:527, 1983.

167. Moscow, J. A., and Cowan, K. H.: Multidrug resistance. J. Natl. Cancer Inst., 80:14, 1988.

168. Moscow, J. A., Fairchild, C. R., Madden, M. J., Ransom, D. T., Wieand, H. S., O'Brien, E. E., Poplack, D. G., Cossman, J., Myers, C. E., and Cowan, K. H.: Expression of anionic glutathione-S-transferase and P-glycoprotein genes in human tissues and tumors. Cancer Res., 49:1422, 1989.

169. Muggia, F. M.: New drugs in the treatment of testicular cancer. In Therapeutic progress in ovarian cancer, testicular cancer and the sarcomas. Edited by A. T. Van Oosterom, and F. M. Muggia. Martinus Nijhoff, 16:507, 1979.

170. Mullin, K., Houghton, P. J., Houghton, J. A., and Horowitz, M. E.: Studies with 4'-deoxyepivincristine (vinepidine) a semi synthetic vinca alkaloid. Biochem. Pharmacol., 34:1975, 1985.

171. Na, G. C., and Timasheff, S. N.: Interaction of vinblastine with calf brain tubulin: Multiple equilibria. Biochemistry, 25:6214, 1986.

172. Na, G. C., and Timasheff, S. N.: Interaction of vinblastine with calf brain tubulin: Effects of magnesium ions. Biochemistry, 25:6222, 1986.

173. Nair, S., Samy, T. S., and Krishan, A.: Calcium, calmodulin, and protein content of adriamycin-resistant and -sensitive murine leukemic cells. Cancer Res., 46:229, 1986.

174. Nelson, R. L.: The comparative clinical pharmacology and pharmacokinetics of vindesine, vincristine, and vinblastine in human patients with cancer. Med. Pediatr. Oncol., 10:115, 1982.

175. Nelson, R. L., Dyke, R. W., and Root, M. A.: Clinical pharmacokinetics of vindesine, Cancer Chemother. Pharmacol., 2:243, 1979.

176. Nelson, R. L., Dyke, R. W., and Root, M. A.: Comparative pharmacokinetics of vindesine, vincristine and vinblastine in patients with cancer. Cancer Treat. Rev., 7:17, 1980.

177. Ohnuma, T., Norton, L., Andrejczuk, A., and Holland, J. F.: Pharmacokinetics of vindesine given as an intravenous bolus and 24-hour infusion in humans. Cancer Res., 45:464, 1985.

178. Osterlind, K., Horbov, S., Dombernowsky, P., Rorth, M., and Hansen, H. H.: Vindesine in the treatment of squamous cell carcinoma, adenocarcinoma, and large cell carcinoma of the lung. Cancer Treat. Rep., 66:305, 1982.

179. Owellen, R. J., Blair, M., Van Tosh, A., and Hains, F. C.: Determination of tissue concentrations of Vinca alkaloids by radioimmunoassay. Cancer Treat. Rep., 65:469, 1981.

180. Owellen, R. J., Donigian, D. W., Hartke, C. A., and Hains, F. O.: Correlation of biologic data with physico-chemical properties among the Vinca alkloids and their congeners. Biochem. Pharmacol., 26:1213, 1977.

181. Owellen, R. J., Hartke, C. A., Dickerson, R. M., and Hains, F. O.: Inhibition of tubulin-microtubule polymerization by drugs of the Vinca alkaloid class. Cancer Res., 36:1499, 1976.

182. Owellen, R. J., Hartke, C. A., and Hains, F. O.: Pharmacokinetics and metabolism of vinblastine in humans. Cancer Res., 37:2597, 1977.

183. Owellen, R. J., Owens, A. H., Jr., and Donigian, D. W.: The binding of vincristine, vinblastine and colchicine to tubulin. Biochem. Biophys. Commun., 47:685, 1972.

184. Owellen, R. J., Root, M. A., and Hains, R. O.: Pharmacokinetics of vindesine and vincristine in humans. Cancer Res., 37:2603, 1977.

185. Ozols, R. F., Cunnion, R. E., Klecker, R. W., Jr, Hamilton, T. C., Ostchega, Y., Parillo, J. E., and Young, R. C.: Verapamil and adriamycin in the treatment of drug-resistant ovarian cancer patients. J. Clin. Oncol., 5:641, 1987.

186. Palmer, C. G., Livengood, D., Warren, A. K., Simpson, P. J., and Johnson, I. S.: The action of vincaleukoblastine on mitosis in vitro. Exp. Cell Res., 20:198, 1960.

187. Parness, J., Asnes, C. F., and Horwitz, S. B.: Taxol binds differentially to flagellar outer doublets and their reassembled microtubules. Cell Motility, 3:123, 1983.

188. Parness, J., and Horwitz, S. B.: Taxol binds to polymerized tubulin in vitro. J. Cell Biol., 91:479, 1981.

189. Pearce, H. L.: Medicinal chemistry of bisindole alkaloids from Catharanthus. In The Alkaloids, Vol. 37. Edited by A. Brossi. Orlando, Academic Press, Inc., 1990, p. 145.

190. Pike, M. C., Kredich, N. M., and Snyderman, R.: Influence of cytoskeletal assembly on phosphatidylcholine synthesis in intact phagocytic cells. Cell, 20:373, 1980.

191. Qian, X.-D., and Beck, W. T.: Binding of an optically pure photoaffinity analogue of verapamil, LU-49888, to P-glycoprotein from multidrug-resistant human leukemic cell lines. Cancer Res., 50:1132, 1990.

192. Qian, X.-D., and Beck, W. T.: Progesterone photoaffinity labels P-glycoprotein in multidrug resistant human leukemic lymphoblasts. J. Biol. Chem., 265:18753, 1990.

193. Rahmani, R., Martin, M., Barket, J., and Cano, J. P.: Radioimmunoassay and preliminary pharmacokinetic studies in rats of 5'-noranhydrovinblastine (navelbine). Cancer Res., 44:5609, 1984.

194. Rainey, W. E., Kramer, R. E., Jason, J. I., and Shay, J. W.: The effects of taxol, a microtubule-stabilizing drug, on steroidogenic cells. J. Cell. Physiol., 123:17, 1985.

195. Ratain, M. J. and Vogelzang, N. J.: Phase I and pharmacological study of vinblastine by prolonged continuous infusion. Cancer Res., 46:4827, 1986.

196. Retsas, S., Newton, K. A., and Westbury, G.: Vindesine as a single agent in the treatment of advanced malignant melanoma. Cancer Chemother. Pharmacol., 2:257, 1979.

197. Riehm, H., and Biedler, J. L.: Potentiation of drug effect by Tween 80 in Chinese hamster cells resistant to actinomycin D and daunomycin. Cancer Res., 32:1195, 1972.

198. Roberts, R. L., Nath, J., Friedman, M. M., and Gallin, J. I.: Effects of taxol on human neutrophils. J. Immunol., 129:2134, 1982.

199. Rosenthal, S., and Kaufman, S.: Vincristine neurotoxicity. Ann. Int. Med., 80:733, 1974.

200. Rowinsky, E. K., Cazenave, L. A., and Donehower, R. C.: Taxol: a novel investigational antimicrotubule agent. J. Natl. Cancer Inst., 82:1247, 1990.

201. Rowinsky, E. K., Donehower, R. C., Jones, R. J., and Tucker, R. W.: Microtubule changes and cytotoxicity in leukemic cell lines treated with taxol. Cancer Res., 48:4093, 1988.

202. Roy, S. N., and Horwitz, S. B.: A phosphoglycoprotein associated with taxol resistance in J774.2 cells. Cancer Res., 45:3856, 1985.

203. Roytta, M., Laine, K.-M., and Harkonen, P.: Morphological studies on the effect of taxol on cultured human prostatic cancer cells. The Prostate, 11:95, 1987.

204. Rudolph, S., Greengard, P., and Malawista, S. E.: Effect of colchicine on cyclic AMP levels in human leukocytes. Proc. Nat. Acad. Sci. USA, 74:3404, 1977.

205. Safa, A. R.: Photoaffinity labeling of the multidrug-resistance-related P-glycoprotein with photoactive analogs of verapamil. Proc. Natl. Acad. Sci. USA, 85:7178, 1988.

206. Safa, A. R., Glover, C. J., Meyers, M. B., Biedler, J. L., and Felsted, R. L.: Vinblastine photoaffinity labeling of a high molecular weight surface membrane glycoprotein specific for multidrug-resistant cells. J. Biol. Chem., 261:6137, 1986.

207. Salmon, E. D. and Wolniak, S. M.: Taxol stabilization of mitotic spindle microtubules: analysis using calcium-induced depolymerization. Cell Motility, 4:155, 1984.

208. Salmon, S. E., Grogan, T. M., Miller, T., Scheper, R., and Dalton, W. S.: Prediction of doxorubicin resistance in vitro in myeloma, lymphoma, and breast cancer by P-glycoprotein staining. J. Natl. Cancer Inst., 81:696, 1989.

209. Sammak, P. J., and Borisy, G. G.: Direct observation of microtubule dynamics in living cells. Nature, 332:724, 1988.
210. Samson, F. E., Jr.: Mechanism of axoplasmic transport. J. Neurobiol., 2:347, 1971.
211. Sandler, S. G., Tobin, W., and Henderson, E. S.: Vincristine-induced neuropathy. A clinical study of fifty leukemic patients. Neurology, 19:367, 1969.
212. Sarna, G., Mitsuyasu, R., Figlin, R., Ambersely, J., and Groopman, J.: Oral vinzolidine as therapy for Kaposi's sarcoma and carcinomas of lung, breast, and colon/rectum. Cancer Chemother. Pharmacol., 14:12, 1985.
213. Schellenberg, R. R., and Gillespie, E.: Effects of colchicine, vinblastine, griseofulvin and deuterium oxide upon phospholipid metabolism in concanavalin A-stimulated lymphocytes. Biochim. Biophys. Acta, 619:522, 1980.
214. Schibler, M. J., and Cabral, F.: Taxol-dependent mutants of Chinese hamster ovary cells with alterations in α- and β-tubulin. J. Cell Biol., 102:1522, 1986.
215. Schiff, P. B., Fant, J., and Horwitz, S. B.: Promotion of microtubule assembly in vitro by taxol. Nature, 277:665, 1979.
216. Schiff, P. B., and Horwitz, S. B.: Taxol stabilizes microtubules in mouse fibroblast cells. Proc. Natl. Acad. Sci. USA, 77:1561, 1980.
217. Schiff, P. B., and Horwitz, S. B.: Taxol assembles tubulin in the absence of exogenous guanosine 5'-triphosphate or microtubule-associated proteins. Biochemistry, 10:3247, 1981.
218. Schilber, M. J., and Cabral, F.: Taxol-dependent mutants of Chinese hamster ovary cells with alterations in α- and β-tubulin. J. Cell Biol., 102:1522, 1986.
219. Schneider, J., Bak, M., Efferth, Th., Kaufmann, M., Mattern, J., and Volm, M.: P-glycoprotein expression in treated and untreated human breast cancer. Br. J. Cancer, 60:815, 1989.
220. Schrek, R.: Cytotoxicity of vincristine to normal and leukemic cells. Am. J. Clin. Pathol., 62:1, 1974.
221. Schrek, R., and Stefani, S. S.: Toxicity of microtubular drugs to leukemic lymphocytes. Exp. Mol. Pathol., 34:369, 1981.
222. Schroeder, F., Fontaine, R. N., Feller, D. J., and Weston, K. G.: Drug-induced surface membrane phospholipid composition in murine fibroblasts. Biochim. Biophys. Acta, 643:76, 1981.
223. Schulze, E., and Kirschner, M.: New features of microtubule behaviour observed in vivo. Nature, 324:356, 1988.
224. Sethi, V. S., Burton, S. S., and Jackson, D. V.: A sensitive radioimmunoassay for vincristine and vinblastine. Cancer Chemother. Pharmacol., 4:183, 1980.
225. Sethi, V. S., Jackson, D. V., Jr., White, D. R., Richards, F., II, Stuart, J. J., Muss, H. B., Cooper, M. R., and Spurr, C. L.: Pharmacokinetics of vincristine sulfate in adult cancer patients. Cancer Res., 41:3551, 1981.
226. Sethi, V. S., and Kimball, J. C.: Pharmacokinetics of vincristine sulfate in children. Cancer Chemother. Pharmacol., 6:111, 1981.
227. Sethi, V. S., and Thimmaiah, K. N.: Structural studies on the degradation products of vincristine dihydrogen sulfate. Cancer Res., 45:5386, 1985.
228. Singer, W. D., Hersh, R. T., and Himes, R. H.: Effect of solution variables on the binding of vinblastine to tubulin. Biochem. Pharmacol., 37:2691, 1988.
229. Singer, W. D., Jordan, M. A., Wilson, L. A., and Himes, R. H.: Binding of vinblastine to stabilized microtubules. Mol. Pharmacol., 36:366, 1989.
230. Skovsgaard, T.: Mechanism of cross-resistance between vincristine and daunorubicin in Ehrlich ascites tumor cells. Cancer Res., 38:4722, 1978.
231. Smith, I. E., Hedley, D. W., Powles, T. J., and McElwain, T. J.: Vindesine: A phase II study in breast carcinoma, malignant melanoma, and other tumors. Cancer Treat. Rep., 62:1427, 1978.
232. Sterle, M., and Pipan, N.: Influence of antimicrotubular drugs on the Golgi apparatus of stomach secretory mucoid cells and small intestine absorptive cells. Virchows Archiv. B. Cell. Pathol., 58:317, 1990.
233. Sullivan, M. P., Nora, A. H., Kulapongs, P., Lane, D. M., Windmiller, J., and Thurman, W. G.: Evaluation of vincristine sulfate and cyclophosphamide chemotherapy for metastatic neuroblastoma. Pediatrics, 44:685, 1969.
233A. Sutow, W. W., and Sullivan, M. P.: Successful chemotherapy for childhood rhabdomyosarcoma. Tex. Med., 66:78, 1970.
234. Takasugi, B. J., Jones, S. E., and Robertone, A. B.: Phase II trial of vinzolidine, an oral vinca alkaloid, in Hodgkin's disease and non-Hodgkin's lymphoma. Cancer Treat. Rep., 68:1399, 1984.
235. Takasugi, B. J., Salmon, S. E., Nelson, R. L., Young, L., and Liu, R. M.: Antitumor activity of vinzolidine in the human tumor clonogenic assay and comparison with vinblastine. Invest. New Drugs, 2:49, 1984.
236. Tan, C.: Clinical and pharmacokinetic studies of vindesine in 50 children with malignant disease. In Current Chemotherapy (Proceedings of the 10th Int. Congress of Chemotherapy). Edited by W. Siegenthaler, and R. Luthy. Washington, DC, American Society of Microbiology. Volume 2, p. 1326.
237. Taylor, C. W., Salmon, S. E., Satterlee, W. G., Alberts, D. S., Robertone, A. B., and Peng, Y. M.: Intravenous vinzolidine (IV VZL): A phase I and pharmacokinetic study. Proc. Am. Assoc. Cancer Res., 29: 325, 1988.
238. Taylor, C. W., Salmon, S. E., Satterlee, W. G., Robertone, A. B., McCloskey, T. M., Holdsworth, M. T., Plezia, P. M., and Alberts, D. S.: A phase I and pharmacokinetic study of intravenous vinzolidine. Invest. New Drugs, 8:S51, 1990.
239. Ter-Minassian-Saraga, L., and Madelmont, G.: Enhanced hydration of dipalmitoyl-phosphatidylcholine multibilayer by vinblastine sulphate. Biochim. Biophys. Acta, 728:394, 1983.
240. Ter-Minassian-Saraga, L., Madelmont, G., Hort-Legrand, C., and Metral, S.: Vinblas-

tine and vincristine action on gel-fluid transition of hydrated DPPC. Biochem. Pharmacol., 30:411, 1981.
241. Thiebaut, F., Tsuruo, T., Hamada, H., Gottesman, M. M., Pastan, I., and Willingham, M. C.: Immunohistochemical localization in normal tissues of different epitopes in the multidrug transport protein P170: Evidence for localization in brain capillaries and cross reactivity of one antibody with a muscle protein. J. Histochem. Cytochem., 37:159, 1989.
242. Thigpen, T., Blessing, J., Ball, H., Hummel, S., and Barret, R.: Phase II trial of taxol as second-line therapy for ovarian carcinoma: A gynecologic oncology group study. Proc. Am. Soc. Clin. Oncol., 9:604, 1990.
243. Thimmaiah, K. N., and Sethi, V. S.: Chemical characterization of the degradation products of vinblastine dihydrogen sulfate. Cancer Res., 45:5382, 1985.
244. Thompson, G. L., Boder, G. B., Bromer, W. W., Grindey, G. B., and Poore, G. A.: A novel potent vinca analog with unique biological properties. Proc. Am. Assoc. Cancer Res., 23:201, 1982.
245. Thompson, W. C., Wilson, L., and Purich, D. L.: Taxol induces microtubule assembly at low temperature. Cell Motility, 1:445, 1981.
246. Thuret-Carnahan, J., Bossu, J.-L., Feltz, A., Langley, K., and Aunis, D.: Effect of taxol on secretory cells: functional, morphological, and electrophysiological correlates. J. Cell Biol., 100:1863, 1985.
247. Tsuruo, T., Iida, H., Tsukagoshi, S., and Sakurai, Y.: Overcoming of vincristine resistance in P388 leukemia in vivo and in vitro through enhanced cytotoxicity of vincristine and vinblastine by verapamil. Cancer Res., 41:1967, 1981.
248. Tucker, R. W., Owellen, R. J., and Harris, S. B.: Correlation of cytotoxicity and mitotic spindle dissolution by vinblastine in mammalian cells. Cancer Res., 37:4346, 1977.
249. Tueni, E., Dodion, P., Piccart, M., Wery, F., Kerger, J., and Delgado, M.: A new oral phase I trial with navelbine (NVB) administered on a weekly schedule. Proc. Am. Assoc. Cancer Res., 31:207, 1990.
250. Van den Berg, H. W., Desai, Z. R., Wilson, R., Kennedy, G., Bridges, J. M., and Shanks, R. G.: The pharmacokinetics of vincristine in man: Reduced drug clearance associated with raised serum alkaline phosphatase and dose-limited elimination. Cancer Chemother. Pharmacol., 8:215, 1982.
251. van der Bliek, A. M., and Borst, P.: Multidrug resistance. Adv. Cancer Res., 52:165, 1989.
252. Vats, T. S., Mehta, P., Trueworthy, R. C., Smith, S. D., and Klopovich, P.: Vindesine and prednisone for remission induction in children with acute lymphocytic leukemia. Cancer, 47:2789, 1981.
253. Vietti, T. J., Sullivan, M. P., Haggard, M. E., Holcomb, T. M., and Berry, D. H.: Vincristine sulfate and radiation therapy in metastatic Wilm's tumor. Cancer, 25:12, 1970.
254. Volberding, P. A., Abrams, D., Conant, M., Kaslow, K., Vranizan, K., and Ziegler, J.: Vinblastine therapy for Kaposi's sarcoma in the acquired immunodeficiency syndrome. Ann. Intern. Med., 103:335, 1985.
255. Watanabe, K., and West, W. L.: Calmodulin, activated cyclic nucleotidephosphodiesterase, microtubules, and Vinca alkaloids. Fed. Proc., 41:2292, 1982.
256. Watanabe, K., Williams, E. F., Law, J. S., and West, W. L.: Effects of Vinca alkaloids on calcium-calmodulin regulated cyclic adenosine 3',5'-monophosphate phosphodiesterase activity from brain. Biochem. Pharmacol., 30:335, 1981.
257. Weber, W., Nagel, G. A., Nagel-Studer, E., and Albrecht, R.: Vincristine infusion: a phase I study. Cancer Chemother. Pharmacol., 3:49, 1979.
258. Weiss, H. D., Walker, M. D., and Wiernik, P. H.: Neurotoxicity of commonly used antineoplastic agents. N. Engl. J. Med., 291:127, 1974.
259. White, J. G.: Effects of colchicine and Vinca alkaloids on human platelets. I. Influence on platelet microtubules and contractile function. Am. J. Pathol., 53:281, 1968.
260. Wilbur, J. R., Sutow, W. W., Sullivan, M. P.: Successful treatment of rhabdomyosarcoma with combination chemotherapy and radiotherapy. Proc. Am. Soc. Clin. Oncol., 1971.
261. Wilson, L.: Microtubules as drug receptors: pharmacological properties of microtubule protein. Ann. N. Y. Acad. Sci., 253:213, 1975.
262. Wilson, L., Bamburg, J. R., Mizel, S. B., Grisham, L. M., and Creswell, K. M.: Interaction of drugs with microtubule proteins. Fed. Proc., 33:158, 1974.
263. Wilson, L., Jordan, M. A., Morse, A., and Margolis, R. L.: Interaction of vinblastine with steady-state microtubules in vitro. J. Mol. Biol., 159:125, 1982.
264. Yamashita, N., Hamada, H., Tsuruo, T., and Ogata, E.: Enhancement of voltage-gated Na+ channel current associated with multidrug resistance in human leukemia cells. Cancer Res., 47:3736, 1987.
265. Yang, L., Rowe, T. C., and Liu, L. F.: Identification of DNA topoisomerase II as an intracellular target of antitumor epipodophyllotoxins in Simian virus 40-infected monkey cells. Cancer Res., 45:5872, 1985.
266. Yap, H. Y., Blumenschein, G. R., Bodey, G. P., Hortobagyi, G. N., Buzdar, A. U., and DiStefano, A.: Vindesine in the treatment of refractory breast cancer: improvement in therapeutic index with continuous 5-day infusion. Cancer Treat. Rep., 65:775, 1981.
267. Yap, H. Y., Blumenschein, G. R., Keating, M. J., Hortobagyi, G. N., Tashima, C. K., and Loo, T. L.: Vinblastine given as a continuous 5-day infusion. Cancer Treat. Rep., 64:279, 1980.
268. Young, J. A., Howell, S. B., and Green, M. R.: Pharmacokinetics and toxicity of 5-day continuous infusion of vinblastine. Cancer Chemother. Pharmacol., 12:43, 1984.
269. Yusa, K., and Tsuruo, T.: Reversal mechanism of multidrug resistance by verapamil: Direct binding of verapamil to P-glycoprotein on specific sites and transport of verapamil outward across the plasma membrane of K562/ADM cells. Cancer Res., 49:5002, 1989.
270. Zakhireh, B., and Malech, H. L.: The effect of colchicine and vinblastine on the chemotactic response of human monocytes. J. Immunol., 125:2143, 1980.

Asparaginase

Robert L. Capizzi
John Stanley Holcenberg

Introduction and History

"Enzymes far exceed man-made catalysts in their reaction specificity, their catalytic efficiency, and their capacity to operate under mild conditions of temperature and hydrogen-ion concentration."[81] As drugs, enzymes also have unique disadvantages. They must be extensively purified to eliminate contaminating toxic materials such as endotoxins; they are often rapidly degraded in the body; they have limited distribution because of their size; and they are often antigenic. Despite these problems E. coli and Erwinia asparaginase have become major components in the treatment of acute lymphoblastic leukemia.

Asparaginase enzymes catalyze the conversion of the amino acid L-asparagine to aspartic acid and ammonia. Although L-asparagine is commonly a non-essential amino acid, some types of leukemia and cancer lack this synthetic capacity and are thus dependent on extracellular sources of asparagine for protein synthesis. While the enzyme does not enter the cell, asparaginase degrades all the circulating asparagine to aspartic acid which, in turn, cannot be converted to asparagine by these cancers. In contrast, most normal cells can synthesize asparagine from aspartic acid. Thus, asparaginase exploits a metabolic difference between normal and cancer cells and provides a relative degree of pharmacologic selectivity. However, as will be noted in the toxicity profile for the drug, this metabolic difference between normal and neoplastic cells is not absolute.

The potential for asparaginase treatment stemmed from the observation of Kidd in that certain mouse and rat lymphomas were destroyed by guinea pig serum, a property that was not shared by rabbit or horse serum. In these experiments, the guinea pig serum was used as a source of complement to enhance the antigen-antibody reaction between tumor cells and rabbit antilymphoma antiserum.[73] Other unrelated developments during this period provided further intriguing information. Certain experimental neoplasms, the Walker carcinosarcoma 256 and the L5178Y leukemia, were found to require asparagine, an amino acid previously considered non-essential, to support growth in tissue culture.[20,34] When Broome proved that asparaginase was the active antitumor component of the guinea serum,[11] many investigators screened microorganisms for a more practical source of this enzyme. The next major advance came in 1964 when asparaginase from E. coli was shown to be as effective as guinea pig serum in treating these tumors.[89] This finding allowed the production of large quantities of pure enzyme for preclinical and clinical trials.[15,60,119,142] Preparations were sought with the following properties: high activity and stability in blood; low Km for asparagine since circulating levels of this amino acid are only about 40 μM; selective hydrolysis of asparagine; no inhibition or reversibility by the high concentrations of products of the enzyme reaction that build up in the circulation; slow clearance from the circulation; easy purification and elimination of endotoxin; and no or low antigenicity. While very effective drugs have been discovered, not all of these properties have been universally achieved.

Asparaginase was found to have antitumor activity against more than 50 mouse neoplasms, rat Murphy-Sturm and canine lymphosarcomas, rat fibrosarcoma, Walker carcinosarcoma 256, and Jensen sarcoma.[20,22,146,147] The initial clinical trials in acute lymphocytic leukemia using partially purified guinea pig serum and E. coli asparaginase were very promising.[40,57,98] Although occasional patients with acute myelogenous leukemia, non-Hodgkin's lymphoma, and chronic leukemias responsed, most solid tumors are not affected by asparaginase treatment.[32,37,88,90] Laboratory observations of the marked sensitivity of T-cell-derived tumor cells relative to the less sensitive B-cell neoplasms[75,100] have not been explored in clinical trial. Extensive monographs detailing the early development of asparaginase are available.[20,34]

Sources and Chemistry

Although asparaginase enzymes have been isolated and characterized from many gram-negative bacteria, mycobacteria, yeasts, molds, plants and vertebrates,[146,147,149] not all asparaginases were found to have oncolytic activity. Only the asparaginase derived from the serum of the guinea pig and other members of the superfamily Cavioidea and bacterial asparaginase from E. coli, Erwinia chrysanthemi (formerly called Erwinia carotovora), Vibrio succinogenes, and Serratia marcescens had activity against lymphomas.[39,139] At present, only the enzymes from E. coli and Erwinia chrysanthemi are used clinically. The properties of these enzymes are shown in Table XVI-9-1.

These asparaginases are composed of four identical subunits with one active site per subunit. The asparaginases from two Erwinia chrysanthemi strains and E. coli and Acinetobacter glutaminase-asparaginase have been sequenced and the crystallographic structure is being determined.[87,93,134] The deduced sequence from Erwinia asparaginase indicates that they have a leader peptide that signals export from the bacteria to the periplasmic space. There is considerable homology between these sequences. The threonine that covalently binds the glutamine analogue DON (6-diazo-5-oxo-L-norleucine) to two glutaminase-asparaginase enzymes lies within an N-terminal 8-amino acid segment of 5 different asparaginase and glutaminases.[63,134] A threonine at residue 118 of E. coli asparaginase that is part of the binding site of the asparagine analogue DONV (5-diazo-4-

Table XVI-9-1.   Properties of Therapeutic Asparaginases

	Activity,* (I.U./mg protein)	Km (μM)		Ratio Maximal Activity L-Gln/L-Asn	Molecular Weight	pI	Half-life, (hrs.)
		L-Asn	L-Gln				
E. coli	280–400	12	3,000	0.03	141,000	5.0	8–44
Erwinia	650–700	15	1,400	0.10	138,000	8.7	7–13

L-Asn, L-Gln and pI refer to L-asparagine, L-glutamine and isoelectric point, respectively.
*One IU hydrolyzes one micromole of asparagine per minute.

oxo-L-norvaline) is conserved in the three enzymes that have been sequenced through this region.[107]

E. coli and Erwinia asparaginase differ greatly in isoelectric point. Chemical modifications of Erwinia asparaginase that decrease the isoelectric point prolong its half-life in animals.[121] The substrate specificity of both enzymes is restricted to four- and five-carbon L- or D-amino acids. Enzyme activity does not appear to be affected by high levels of the products of asparagine hydrolysis, aspartic acid and NH_3.[124] The purification[147] and properties of these enzymes have been extensively reviewed.[20,22,34,142,147] These enzymes have most of the ideal properties that were sought. They have high activity and stability, they have a low Km for asparagine, they are not inhibited by aspartic acid or ammonia[124] and they are readily purified and freed from endotoxin. These enzymes are similar in size to gamma globulins. Both enzymes hydrolyze L-glutamine as well as L-asparagine. Although the maximal rate of hydrolysis of L-glutamine is only 3–9% of the activity for L-asparagine and the Km is 100 times greater or more, high doses of these enzymes will deplete circulating glutamine in animals and patients.[92]

Therapeutic trials of amidohydrolases with high glutaminase and asparaginase activities have shown a wider spectrum of antitumor activity. Acinetobacter glutaminase-asparaginase was chemically modified with succinic anhydride to prolong its half-life in the circulation. This enzyme causes more neurotoxicity and inhibition of protein synthesis than the asparaginase enzymes with low glutaminase activity.[62,127,140] Thus, some of the toxicity of these asparaginase enzymes may be caused by glutamine depletion. Furthermore, L-glutamine is a competitive substrate for these asparaginases. Since the plasma levels of L-glutamine are 10 times higher than L-asparagine, the relative effect on plasma asparagine is greater for those enzymes that hydrolyze both substrates. Thus, an enzyme with no glutaminase activity may have more selectivity and less toxicity. Guinea pig asparaginase has no glutaminase activity but insufficient quantities are available for clinical trials. Vibrio succinogenes asparaginase was originally reported to have very low glutaminase activity but further studies showed that this activity was similar to the E. coli enzyme.

Biochemical Pharmacology and Resistance

The antitumor activity of asparaginase enzymes is mediated by the depletion of asparagine from the plasma, which in turn, deprives auxotrophic cells and tissues from their only source of the amino acid. The most prompt biochemical effect of asparaginase is the hydrolysis of plasma asparagine to aspartic acid and ammonia. Plasma asparagine is essentially undetectable throughout the entire period in which asparaginase is present. The plasma level of asparagine is normally tightly controlled by the liver,[144,145] and there appears to be a rigorous homeostatic control of the plasma concentration of the amino acid in a variety of disease states by endogenous asparaginase activity in the liver and kidneys. Many normal and neoplastic cells concentrate asparagine by an active transport process to levels 2–10 times that in the plasma. Most normal human cells have the ability to synthesize asparagine by induction of the enzyme asparagine synthetase.[55,111] Tumors sensitive to asparaginase lack this enzyme activity and are dependent on exogenous sources of L-asparagine. Most tissues have low or undetectable asparagine synthetase activity. This is caused by a feedback control of its synthesis by the high asparagine concentrations in the circulation and in cells. As the circulating levels of asparagine fall following asparaginase treatment, asparagine synthetase activity is induced in normal tissues. Asparagine synthetase activity in asparaginase-resistant tumors may be present before treatment or be induced by treatment. Thus, measurement of asparagine synthetase prior to treatment with asparaginase is usually not predictive of response. Mammalian asparagine synthetase has been cloned and sequenced.[3,49] This gene has been identified as one of the causes of temperature-sensitive growth arrest and appears to be regulated in the cell cycle. Methylation of cytosine residues in DNA appears to be related to the degree of expression of this enzyme. For example, cells with high asparagine synthetase activity have the 5′ region of the gene less methylated than those with low activity. 5-azacytidine, which decreases methylation of cytosine residues in genes, can reactivate asparagine synthetase activity in cells. Nyce[97] and Avramis and coworkers[35] have recently shown that cytosine arabinoside and other antitumor drugs can increase the methylation of cytosines in DNA. These drugs may be able to lower the activity of asparagine synthetase and thus enhance sensitivity to asparaginase treatment. This effect may relate the observed pre-clinical[125] and clinical[23] synergy noted between high dose ara-C and asparaginase.

Broome showed that at 1 and 3 hours after treatment, the free asparagine concentration in both asparaginase-sensitive and -resistant murine lymphomas fell to about one-sixth of the normal level.[12] Protein synthesis rapidly decreased followed by a fall in DNA and RNA synthesis. While these parameters remained suppressed in the asparaginase-sensitive tumors, in asparaginase-resistant tumor cells, asparagine concentration increased within 1–2 days and the rate of protein synthesis recovered. This change corresponds to the time course of induction of asparagine synthetase activity.[144] Similar effects on macromolecular synthesis occurred in normal tissues; protein synthesis recovered as asparagine synthetic activity increased.

Half-maximal growth of an asparaginase-sensitive lymphoma occurred at extracellular asparagine concentrations of about 1μM. This is 3% of normal circulating levels and the lower level of detection by most methods of amino acid analysis.[136] It is not known how much lower asparagine levels must be for optimal kill of circulating cells. The concentration of asparagine in intercellular spaces may be of even greater importance. Since asparaginase is largely confined to the vascular space, asparagine is primarily depleted in interstitial spaces by diffusion of the amino acid into the circulation. Because of the intrinsic glutaminase activity of asparaginase, plasma levels of glutamine are temporarily depressed or eliminated and the levels of glutamic acid and ammonia are correspondingly elevated.[34]

Clinical Pharmacology

In man, asparaginase enzymes from E. coli and Erwinia chrysanthemi have a wide range of circulating half-lives (7–44 hours). The current commercial E. coli preparation (#Elspar, Merck®) has a longer half-life (mean = 23 hours) than earlier E. coli preparations from Bayer (mean = 11 hours) or the Erwinia chrysanthemi enzyme (mean = 10 hours).[21,22,52–54,60,101,124] The half-life is independent of the dose administered, age, sex, disease status, hepatic or renal function.[124,146] Various chemical modifications have been employed in order to alter the half-life in the circulation and mask the antigenic determinants. The most extensively studied altered enzyme is PEG-asparaginase. This is formed by covalent attachment through succinate linkages of monomethoxypolyethylene glycol (PEG) to E. coli asparaginase. PEG-asparaginase has similar kinetic properties as the native E. coli enzyme but has decreased immunogenicity and a prolonged serum half-life.[1,58,138] Initial clinical trials show that it is safe and effective even in patients with prior allergy to the native enzyme.[71,78] The prolonged half-life of PEG-asparaginase allows lower doses and less frequent administration.

Eighteen to 24 hours after intravenous injection of 10, 200, 1,000, and 5,000 IU/kg of the E. coli enzyme, plasma levels of 0.1–0.4, 2–6, 14–27, and 57–70 IU/ml are achieved, respectively.[21,124] Daily administration of the same dose achieves a sustained or slightly cumulative plasma level, and after cessation of therapy measurable plasma levels may persist for 10 or more days. If administered intramuscularly, the peak plasma level is about one-half that of intravenously administered asparaginase.[22] The volume of distribution is slightly greater than the plasma volume. The enzyme activity in lymphatic fluid is 5–20% that of plasma. Interstitial fluid is about 10% and cerebrospinal fluid less than 0.5% of plasma.[59,117]

Simultaneous measurement of enzyme activity and asparagine concentrations in plasma during asparaginase treatment of mice and humans showed that asparagine concentration is not detectable (greater than 1μM) when the asparaginase activity was greater than 0.02 IU/ml.[61] Since 1 μM is less than 10% of the Km for asparagine, the actual enzyme activity is only 0.002 μmoles/min/ml at this concentration. A mathematical model was developed to predict optimal dose and dosing interval to keep the asparagine concentration below 1 μM.[61,64] The model utilizes the kinetic properties of the enzyme, an exponential equation for its disappearance from the plasma and an input function for the entrance of asparagine into the circulation. The maximal input rate of asparagine should be equal to the asparaginase

activity that maintains an undetectable asparagine concentration, i.e., 0.002 μmoles/min/ml. The change in asparagine concentration with time is equal to the sum of the input of asparagine and the enzyme activity. The disappearance of the enzyme from the plasma is much slower than its catalytic rate or the rate of input. Thus, the equation can be simplified to:

$$\frac{(Asn) \cdot Vmax}{Km + (Asn)} \cdot e^{-0.693 \ T/t1/2} = Imax$$

where (Asn) is the concentration of asparagine in plasma, Km and Vmax are kinetic constants for asparaginase, t½ is the half-life of the enzyme in circulation and Imax is the maximal rate of input of asparagine from the tissues. T is the duration of depletion of asparagine.

This model was confirmed in a recent clinical trial (Enzon ASP-301) by Dr. S. Sallan, Dana Farber Cancer Institute, comparing Erwinia (Erwinase®), native E. coli (Elspar®) and PEG-asparaginase. The half-lives of the three enzymes were 0.6, 1.2, and 5.8 days, respectively. Following injection of each enzyme, the plasma concentration of asparagine remained undetectable as long as the asparaginase activity was greater than 0.03 IU/ml. At levels of asparaginase less than 0.02 IU/ml, asparagine reappeared in the plasma. The asparaginase activity reached 0.03 IU/ml after 6, 14, and >28 days with Erwinia, E. coli and PEG-asparaginase. These data suggest that the three enzymes have similar distribution in the body. The area under the plasma concentration curve (AUC) was similar with 25,000 IU/m² of native E. coli and 2,500 IU/m² of the PEG-asparaginase. The AUC for 25,000 IU/m² of Erwinia asparaginase was less than one-half the value of the other two products. Since the AUC should be proportional to effect, this indicates that much lower doses of the PEG-asparaginase can be given.

The model predicts that with standard doses that produce peak plasma activity of 2 IU/ml, native E. coli asparaginase would deplete plasma asparagine for about six days while the PEG-asparaginase would deplete it for about a month. Similar calculations indicate that cerebrospinal fluid asparagine is depleted as long as the asparaginase activity in blood is greater than 0.1 IU/ml. The model would predict that E. coli asparaginase would deplete cerebrospinal fluid asparagine for four days while PEG-asparaginase would deplete it for over two weeks.[61] Because of these considerations, three injections per week of native E. coli asparaginase are needed to maintain high enough enzyme activity to deplete asparagine in the circulation, interstitial fluids and in cerebrospinal fluid. Doses of PEG-asparaginase could be given every two weeks. Asselin and coworkers have recently suggested that in vitro sensitivity to asparaginase of lymphoblasts from patients correlates with their clinical response.[4] This test is complicated by the greater glutamine depletion that occurs in tissue culture than in the patient with any dose of asparaginase.

Antineoplastic Activity

The first demonstration of the clinical utility of asparaginase occurred in 1966 when an 8 year old boy with acute lymphoblastic leukemia (ALL) achieved a clinical response with partially purified guinea pig asparaginase.[40] Further clinical trials with the enzyme from E. coli documented clinical responses primarily in patients with acute lymphoblastic leukemia.[57] There have been isolated reports of responses in patients with acute myeloblastic leukemia, non-Hodgkin's lymphoma, chronic lymphocytic leukemia, and chronic myelogenous leukemia. The enzyme has not been extensively studied in adults with solid tumors.

Response rates from asparaginase treatment of ALL as a single agent have ranged from 25% to over 60% in patients who had relapsed after conventional therapy.[21,32,37,54,67,98,103,130,133,143] Higher response rates were seen in children with ALL than in adults. In responders, there was a rapid decrease in lymphoblast count and organomegaly and lymphadenopathy.[5,21,32] The addition of asparaginase to the combination of vincristine and prednisone improved the re-induction rate for relapsed patients to approximately 75%.[30,77,131,132] A four drug regimen of asparaginase, vincristine, prednisone, and daunomycin induces complete second remission in up to 90% of these children.[13,116] Asparaginase is an ideal drug for induction therapy since it is highly active and causes very little myelosuppression. There is no reported cross-resistance with other effective antileukemia agents.

Approximately 90–95% of newly diagnosed children with ALL achieve a complete remission when asparaginase is used in combination with vincristine and prednisone for induction therapy.[110] The most effective induction regimens currently in use for childhood ALL add an anthracycline to this combination.[118,128] An early study suggested that the delayed administration of asparaginase after three weeks of corticosteroid and vincristine improved remission duration compared to pre-treatment or concurrent treatment with corticosteroid and vincristine;[70] however, this interesting study requires confirmation.

Asparaginase also has value during consolidation and maintenance therapy of ALL. An early study from the Children's Cancer Study Group indicated that patients who received asparaginase as a maintenance agent had a median duration of remission one-third longer than patients without such therapy. These data suggested that asparaginase remained effective during prolonged use.[94] A more recent study showed that the administration of 25,000 IU asparaginase/m^2/week after remission induction for a median of 20 doses per patient significantly improved the event-free survival of children with acute lymphoblastic leukemia.[33,38] These interesting results await confirmation in a randomized trial. Unfortunately, the poorer tolerance of adults to protracted asparaginase therapy prohibits the testing of this procedure in older patients with ALL. Other studies have used pulses of vincristine, prednisone and asparaginase during maintenance therapy.[110,118]

Asparaginase also has been shown to be effective against meningeal leukemia.[21,56] The enzyme can be given intrathecally but this is usually not needed since asparagine is depleted from the cerebrospinal fluid by diffusion into the circulation as a result of the concentration gradient between the plasma and CSF.[117] Doses of asparaginase have ranged from 200 IU/kg (approximately 6,000 IU/m^2) to approximately 425,000 IU/m^2.[22,95,110,112] Most studies have administered asparaginase for periods of at least three weeks. A dose of 6,000 IU/m^2 given intramuscularly three times a week for a total of nine doses has become one of the most common

schedules during induction therapy of ALL. Intravenous administration is associated with a higher incidence of hypersensitivity reactions. Because of its longer half-life, PEG-asparaginase has been administered IM every two weeks.[78]

Both the E. coli and Erwinia-derived enzymes have comparable enzymatic, therapeutic, and toxicologic properties; however, their antigenic determinants are sufficiently different so that they generally do not cross react immunologically. Thus, patients allergic to the E. coli enzyme may be successfully treated with the Erwinia enzyme without the immediate appearance of an anaphylactic or other allergic reaction.[20,72,102] However, with continued use, the Erwinia enzyme is just as allergenic as the E. coli variant (see below).

Inhibition of protein synthesis secondary to the deletion of an essential amino acid[27] or the administration of a protein synthesis inhibitor attenuates the cytotoxic effects of a variety of cancer therapeutic agents including radiation therapy.[18,82] These laboratory experiments have implications for clinical combination chemotherapy. The inclusion of asparaginase in multidrug programs for the treatment of ALL fulfills many of the standard criteria for combination chemotherapy (see XV-3), however, the schedule-dependent drug-drug interactions noted in the laboratory should be considered in this process. A series of laboratory and clinical investigations with asparaginase in combination with methotrexate (MTX) or cytosine arabinoside (ara-C) illustrate these interactions. Inhibition of protein synthesis due to the deletion of asparagine from culture medium or treatment with asparaginase attenuates the cytotoxic effect of MTX or ara-C both in vitro[27,125] as well as in vivo.[17,125] Conversely, the delayed administration of asparaginase following the administration of either of these antimetabolites resulted in pharmacologic synergy.[17,125] In leukemic mice, the delayed administration of asparaginase after MTX permitted tolerance of larger doses of MTX by attenuating the toxic effects of MTX on the gastrointestinal tract & bone marrow.[18,19] These schedule and time-dependent effects between a preceding dose of asparaginase and a subsequent dose of MTX appear to be related to asparaginase effect on MTX polyglutamylation,[47,69,129] a biochemical effect linked to the cellular retention of MTX and its ultimate cytotoxic effect.[6,47,48,91]

By monitoring asparaginase effect on the ability of MTX to inhibit the incorporation of deoxyuridine into DNA, the optimal time interval between asparaginase and a subsequent dose of MTX was found to be 9–10 days.[17] Figure XVI-9-1 illustrates this effect. Inhibition of deoxyuridine [^{3}H]dUrd incorporation into DNA reflects the inhibitory effect of MTX on dihydrofolate reductase, an effect which impacts on the synthesis of thymidylate and ultimately DNA synthesis. As noted in Figure XVI-9-1, the inhibitory effect of MTX on [^{3}H]dUrd incorporation into the DNA of bone marrow leukemic cells was assayed before and at various times after the administration of a single i.v. dose of asparaginase. As previously noted in murine leukemia, the inhibitory effect of MTX was decreased after asparaginase treatment; however, seven days after asparaginase treatment, MTX effect was the same as that before asparaginase, and on the ninth day the cells were even more sensitive to MTX inhibition. Consequently, on the 10th day a single i.v. dose of 80 mg/m^2 of MTX was given, followed by a single dose of 500 IU asparaginase/kg 24 hours later. The 10-day cycle was repeated and with each subsequent course the patient received an increasingly larger dose of MTX. After a second dose of 800

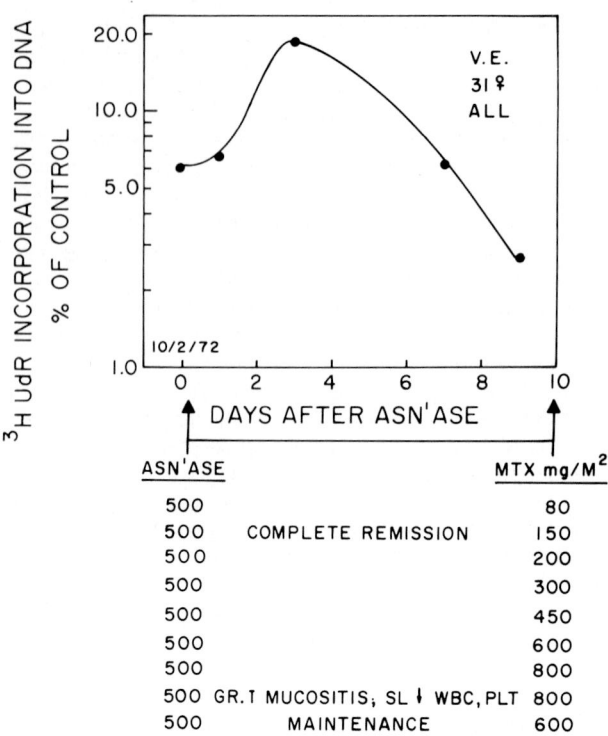

ASN'ASE		MTX mg/M^2
500		80
500	COMPLETE REMISSION	150
500		200
500		300
500		450
500		600
500		800
500	GR.1 MUCOSITIS; SL ↓ WBC, PLT	800
500	MAINTENANCE	600

Figure XVI-9-1.   Asparaginase pretreatment of a patient with acute lymphoblastic leukemia (ALL): Inhibitory effect of MTX on DNA synthesis in vitro, and the patient's subsequent tolerance to MTX in vivo. Biochemical studies were performed after the first dose of asparaginase (IU/kg). The first dose of MTX was administered 10 days later, and asparaginase was repeated 24 hr after MTX. Thereafter, the interval between asparaginase and each succeeding dose of MTX was 10 days. The asparaginase of a new cycle was administered 24 hr after each dose of MTX. (From Capizzi, R.L.: Schedule-dependent synergism and antagonism between methotrexate and asparaginase. Biochem. Pharmacol., (Suppl. 2)23:151, 1974.)

mg/m^2, or 1.2 g for this patient, slight erythema of the oral mucosa was noted along with a 50% decrease in peripheral white count and platelet count. Subsequently, the patient received a maintenance dose of MTX at 600 mg/m^2 (900 mg total), approximately five times larger than that which was previously tolerated. The patient was treated continuously with the combination at 10-day intervals. She died approximately two years later of cerebral gliosis and at autopsy there was no evidence of recurrent leukemia.

Similar effects of MTX on [^{3}H]dUrd incorporation into DNA have been noted in other patients with refractory ALL with a relatively consistent temporal relationship of 9–10 days between the antecedent dose of asparaginase and subsequent dose of MTX. These data would suggest, then, that weekly courses of MTX and asparaginase might be less effective than an every 9- or 10-day schedule. Thus, the protocol outlined in Table XVI-9-2 was developed.[19] This remission induction and maintenance protocol is reasonably well tolerated, such that in most instances it can readily be administered on an outpatient basis.

A summary of five clinical trials, in which this combination has been used for the treatment of children and adults with refractory ALL, is shown in Table XVI-9-3. Almost one-half of the 36 adults had been previously treated with MTX; none had prior exposure to asparaginase. Twenty-three of the 36

Table XVI-9-2.   Sequential MTX→Asparaginase Protocol: Acute Lymphocytic Leukemia (ALL)*

Initial Phase		
Day 0	Asparaginase	6,000 IU/m^2 i.m.
Continuation		
Day 10	MTX	60 mg/m^2 i.v.
Day 11	Asparaginase	6,000 IU/m^2 i.m.

Repeat MTX-asparaginase every 9-10 days: Monday–Tuesday alternating with Thursday–Friday

MTX Dose Escalation
    Increase dose of MTX by 25–50% with each course to point of minimal toxicity, then maintain with a 25% reduction

*Adapted from Capizzi[19]

adult patients (64%) responded with a complete remission.[24,148] Of the 10 adults initially reported,[24] nine had relapsed on MTX-containing combinations. Of 39 children who had extensive prior exposure to both MTX and asparaginase, approximately 50% have entered complete remission.[2,51,85] In several of these reports, a 7-day interval between courses was used, in contrast to the 9- or 10-day interval that was suggested by the biochemical studies. The shorter treatment interval may have several disadvantages: the MTX may be given at a time when the previous dose of asparaginase may block MTX effect on the tumor cell; and host toxicity may actually be enhanced by the shorter interval, since recovery of normal organs from asparaginase effect may be at its peak at this time. This might explain the lower maximally tolerated dose of MTX reported for those patients treated with the 7-day interval compared to the 10- to 14-day interval between courses. This lower dose of MTX may, in turn, affect remission duration if tumor cell kill follows a dose-response relationship.

The addition of vincristine, or prednisone and vincristine to sequential MTX/asparaginase has resulted in similarly good induction rates[43] and remission duration in ALL.[8,43] As noted above, asparaginase affects MTX polyglutamylation of MTX, an effect that is more prominent in gastrointestinal mucosa than in leukemia cells.[128] This biochemical effect appears to have impact on the therapeutic index of MTX.[18,19] In view of the steep dose-response relationship for MTX, it is highly probable that the larger doses of MTX made possible by asparaginase-protection of normal organs[18] accounts, at least in part, for the improved therapeutic responses associated with this combination.

Schedule-dependent pharmacologic synergy associated with the sequential administration of high dose ara-C (HiDAC) and asparaginase[125] has also been noted clinically in adult[23,25,26] and pediatric AML.[141] A comparative trial of HiDAC alone vs sequential HiDAC/asparaginase showed superior results from the combination in adult patients with refractory AML with equivalent toxicity to normal organs in both arms (Table XVI-9-4).[23] These data suggest the capacity for asparaginase to improve the therapeutic index for HiDAC in this group of patients.

Toxicity

The toxic effects of asparaginase are related to immunologic reactions to this foreign protein and/or the effects of asparagine depletion with its consequent inhibition of protein synthesis. Table XVI-9-5 presents the combined data on the

Table XVI-9-3.   MTX-Asparaginase Treatment of Refractory ALL

	No. of Patients	Complete Response	Previous Therapy MTX	Asparaginase	Maximum Tolerated Dose of MTX (mg/m²)	Series Reference
Adults						
Capizzi	10	8	96	0	350	24
Yap	26	15	7	0	200	148
Children						
Lobel	12	4	11	8	361	85
	40	Maint.**	37	5	—	
Amadori*	17	10	17	17	Not stated	2
Harris	10	6	10	9	230	51
	4	Maint.**	4	4	—	

*Median age for group, 11 year (range 4–31)
**MTX-asparaginase used to maintain complete remission induced by other agents

Table XVI-9-4.   Phase III Trial: HiDAC→Asparaginase v HiDAC Complete Remission Rates According to Prior Response and Age in 195 Adults with AML

	Refractory		Relapsed	
Age (yr)	HiDAC/ASNase	HiDAC	HiDAC/ASNase	HiDAC
<60	54%	18%	37%	33%
≥60	31%	0%	43%	21%

HiDAC = high dose ara-C; ASNase = asparaginase
From Capizzi[23]

Table XVI-9-5.   Toxicity From E. coli and Erwinia Asparaginase

	E. Coli		Erwinia	
	Number[1]	%	Number[1]	%
Allergic Reactions	103/971	11	10/547	1.9
Hyperglycemia (requiring insulin)	30/682	4.4	1/483	0.2
Pancreatitis	21/971	2.2	0/483	0
Hypofibrinogenemia (grade 4)	6/275	2.2	2/483	0.4
Coagulopathy (grade 4)	22/861	2.6	16/483	3.3
Neurologic Dysfunction	23/861	3.4	10/483	2.1

[1]Number reactions/number of patients observed for this toxicity

major grade 3 and 4 toxicities of asparaginase in three large clinical trials in ALL with asparaginase used alone and in combination therapy of ALL.[33,42,79] Unlike most antineoplastic-drugs, asparaginase has a minimal effect on the bone marrow and is not cytotoxic to oral and intestinal mucosa or hair follicles.

Both E. coli and Erwinia asparaginase enzymes can induce immune responses; the antibodies to either species are usually not cross-reactive.[21,102] Reported hypersensitivity reactions vary from localized erythema and rash at the site of injection to generalized urticaria, bronchospasm, laryngeal edema and full blown anaphylaxis.[21,44,54,74,120,130,133] These allergic reactions are unpredictable and for that reason a physician should always be in attendance when the drug is administered and appropriate supportive care measures must

be available. In most instances, the reaction is effectively aborted with an intravenous injection of 0.2–0.4 ml of a 1:1000 dilution of aqueous epinephrine. However, an occasional death due to anaphylaxis has been reported. A recent review of ALL treatment protocols of the Pediatric Oncology Group (POG) and Childrens Cancer Study Group (CCSG) showed an incidence of hypersenstivity reactions to E. coli asparaginase ranging from 3–73%. The highest incidence occurred in children receiving asparaginase during maintenance therapy or for re-induction following a relapse. The incidence of severe allergic reaction to Erwinia asparaginase was only 10/547 (1.9%) in children during induction treatment (Table XVI-9-5).[41] In contrast, it increased to 9/54 (17%) and 16/90 (18%) in children with prior allergy to E. coli asparaginase.[33,84]

The majority of reactions consist of local reactions and/or urticaria; life threatening anaplylaxis was less frequent. The incidence of hypersensitivity reactions is known to be lower in patients receiving combination chemotherapy than in those receiving the drug as a single agent. This is a presumed consequence of the immunosuppressive effects of the accompanying chemotherapy.[44,94,99] Asparaginase-specific IgG antibodies appear to correlate better with clinical reactions than IgE antibodies and clinical hypersensitivity reactions appear to be mediated by the complement pathway.[45] Neither skin test nor measurement of antibody levels are sufficiently reliable to predict allergic reactions.[21,31]

The incidence of reactions appears to be greater in protocols using higher doses of the drug (greater than 6,000 IU/m² per dose), in those using intravenous rather than intramuscular administration and with repeated courses of treatment.[66,94,99,135] In a CCSG investigation, there was a significantly lower incidence of anaphylaxis in patients treated with IM compared to IV enzyme; the overall incidence of other toxic manifestations was the same with IM and IV doses.[42,94] Consequently, the most common form of administration of asparaginase on current ALL treatment protocols is the intramuscular (IM) route. With IM administration, the incidence of severe hypersensitivity reactions is substantially less frequent than that associated with intravenous administration.[94] However, localized reactions of swelling, redness and pain are problematic and frequently require either discontinuation of the drug or more commonly switching a patient from E. coli asparaginase to Erwinia asparaginase. Although there is lack of immunologic cross-reactivity between the two available enzyme preparations, hypersensitivity reactions frequently develop to the alternate source of the enzyme.[41,106]

The absence of acute allergic reactions following IV or IM administration of asparaginase does not mean that an immune response has not occurred. Early clinical studies noted that some patients without acute allergic reactions developed anti-asparaginase antibodies that were associated with the rapid clearance of the enzyme from the circulation (Figure XVI-9-2).[21,101] Rapid immune clearance of the enzyme may be a cause of drug resistance. Undoubtedly, "silent" immune response still occurs and may account for apparent acquired drug resistance. With IM injections, the antibodies may delay or prevent absorption of the asparaginase. Thus, an unknown number of patients who receive asparaginase may not benefit from it because of rapid clearance or poor bioavailability. The only way to discern this is to monitor the plasma levels of the enzyme.

PEG-asparaginase is less immunogenic than the native enzyme and can be given safely to children with prior acute

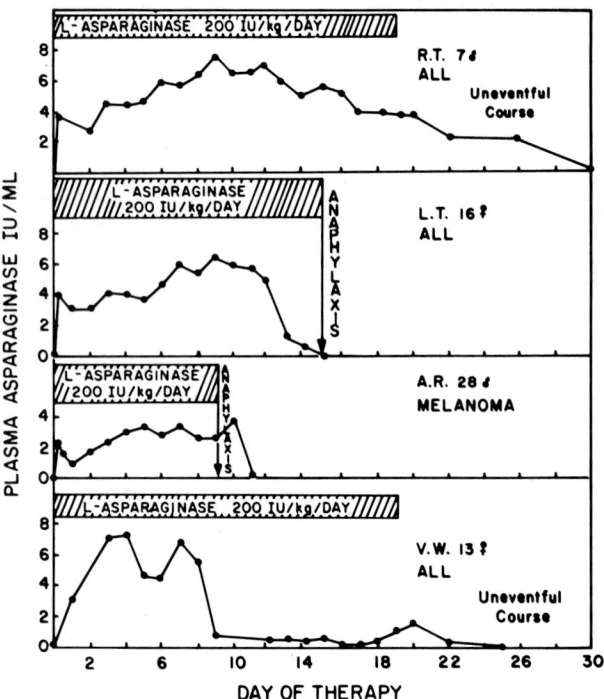

Figure XVI-9-2. Patients received a daily intravenous injection of asparaginase 200 IU/kg/day. Plasma asparaginase levels were measured on a daily basis. Patient RT had sustained plasma concentrations of asparaginase throughout the 21 day uneventful course. Patient LT had the rapid clearance of plasma asparaginase which coincided with the appearance of passive hemagglutinating antibodies to asparaginase. This rapid clearance preceded the development of anaphylaxis by several days. Patient AR had an anaphylactic reaction in association with the rapid clearance of enzyme from the plasma and increasing passive hemagglutinating antibodies titers. Patient VW had a "silent" immunological reaction wherein the L-asparaginase was rapidly cleared from the plasma despite the daily administration of drug. This patient completed a 21-day course without any evidence of allergy. However, plasma asparaginase was undetectable from day 9 on through the remaining 12 days of therapy. This "silent" immune reaction could be a means for drug resistance. (From Capizzi, R.L., et al.: L-asparaginase: Clinical biochemical, pharmacological and immunological studies. Ann. Intern. Med., 74:893, 1971.)

allergic reactions to E. coli and Erwinia asparaginase.[78] Studies of IgG titers and enzyme activity in these patients with prior allergic reactions indicate that about one-half the patients analyzed had persistent asparaginase activity throughout the 14 day dosing interval. The other patients had an increase in antibody titer and accelerated clearance of asparaginase activity starting 3–5 days after administration of this enzyme preparation. Thus, PEG-asparaginase appears to prevent this "silent allergy" in about 50% of hypersensitive patients. These observations indicate that asparaginase activity should ideally be monitored during prolonged or repeated asparaginase treatment to be sure that the enzyme has not been cleared from the blood or poorly absorbed from IM sites. Unfortunately, convenient assay methods are not available for routine use.

The other major group of side effects associated with asparaginase is related to the drug's inhibitory effects on protein synthesis. While inhibition of protein synthesis in normal organs is usually a transient phenomenon, it may be sufficiently severe to warrant discontinuation of the drug. These effects are especially evident on the liver, pancreas, and protein factors involved in blood coagulation. On rare occasions, the toxicity may be severe and totally unexpected suggesting that a genetic difference may indeed exist in the ability of that individual to respond to asparagine depletion. For that individual, asparagine may truly be an essential amino acid. Decreased serum concentrations of insulin, albumin, and lipoproteins are commonly observed.[86,99,143] In a rare patient, the level of serum insulin may drop precipitously and has resulted in severe complications from nonketotic, hyperosmolar hyperglycemia which if unrecognized can be fatal. Prior to therapy, patient and parents should be altered to the early signs and symptoms of hyperglycemia. Hyperglycemia appears to be more severe and prolonged in regimens that combine asparaginase with high doses of a glucocorticoid.[104,131] Hyperglycemia can be controlled with small doses of insulin. Close monitoring of blood sugar is essential in order to avoid hypoglycemia secondary to recovery of the synthesis of endogenous insulin.[10] Bleeding and/or peripheral or cerebral thrombosis may occur from deficiencies and imbalances in coagulation factors (fibrinogen, factors II, VI, VII, VIII, X, antithrombin III, and protein-C).[7,28,29,46,65,76,80,83,105,108,113–115,123,126,137] Many patients show laboratory evidence of coagulopathy or abnormal platelet aggregation without symptomatology. Furthermore, the changes are usually reversible within a few weeks even if the asparaginase is continued.[21] This recovery is probably due to induction of asparagine synthetase in normal tissues. Only a minority of patients (1–2%) develop severe complications like hemorrhagic infarction in the central nervous system and thromboses in the extremities.[114,126]

Acute pancreatitis occurs in approximately 1–2%.[50,122] Symptoms range from mild nausea and anorexia to vomiting, abdominal pain and full blown hemorrhagic pancreatitis with shock hypocalcemia, hyperamylasemia, lipemia and pseudocyst formation.[9,16,36,96] Hepatic dysfunction characterized by elevation in the AST, ALT, alkaline phosphatase, and bilirubin is believed to result both from a decrease in protein synthesis and from fatty metamorphosis and infiltration within the liver. Severe or fatal hepatic dysfunction is extremely unusual.[68] The blood ammonia level may be as high as

700–900 ug/dl but of itself it appears to have no relationship to cerebral function. Most patients have a slight rise in the blood urea nitrogen. This is usually of pre-renal origin.

Somnolence, lethargy or confusion have been observed in up to 25% of patients.[109] These effects appear to be worse in older patients. Personality changes, seizures and coma are rare. Other than small intracranial hemorrhages,[14] biochemical mechanisms for the neurologic dysfunction are not well elucidated but may be related to combined alterations in asparagine, aspartate, glutamate, glutamine or ammonia metabolism in the brain.

The rapid lysis of lymphoblasts (tumor lysis syndrome) in regimens containing asparaginase can lead to severe renal and metabolic abnormalities caused by the large load of potassium, phosphorus, and nucleic acids released from these cells. Rarely, renal failure can occur from urate and xanthine nephropathy (when taking allopurinol). The differential diagnosis is often difficult in patients with leukemic infiltrates of the kidneys. These problems can be lessened by hydration, allopurinol and careful monitoring of serum potassium levels and fluid balance.

Nausea, vomiting, malaise and lassitude may relate to the multiplicity of events noted above. In general, these effects are more marked in adult patients, especially the elderly, compared to children with ALL.

The dose, route of administration and type of asparaginase administered appear to affect the incidence of these toxicities. There is both preclinical and clinical evidence that the type of asparaginase preparation also influences the incidence of observed toxicity. Studies by the British Medical Research Council suggest that the Erwinia preparations have a lower incidence of toxicities than E. coli preparations (Table XVI-9-5). The results of this study, however, have not been prospectively tested in a randomized trial.

In summary, asparaginase plays a pivotal role in the induction therapy of patients with ALL. Its lack of overlapping toxicity with other drugs allows administration of full doses. However, schedule-dependent interactions between asparaginase and antimetabolites should be kept in mind during combination chemotherapy. Continued administration during remission may prolong remission duration, but this remains to be proven in a randomized trial. Also, its potential benefit must be weighed against unusual toxicities related to chronic inhibition of protein synthesis. The usage of asparaginase for the treatment of solid tumors, especially those that afflict adults, has not been thoroughly explored to date. Preliminary studies suggest potential utility in collagen vascular diseases.

References

1. Abuchowski, A., Kazo, G. M., Verhoest, C. J., Jr., Vanes, T., Kafkewitz, D., Nucci, M. L., Viau, A. T., and Davis, F. F.: Cancer therapy with chemical modified enzymes. I. antitumor properties of polyethylene glycol-asparaginase conjugates. (Abstract) Cancer Biochem. Biophys., 7:175, 1984.
2. Amadori, S., Tribalto, M., Pacilli, L., DeLaurentis, C., Papa, G., and Mandelli, F.: Sequential combination of methotrexate and asparaginase in the treatment of refractory acute leukemia. Cancer Treat. Rep., 64:939, 1980.
3. Andrulis, I. L., and Barrett, M. T.: DNA methylation patterns associated with asparagine synthetase expression in asparagine-overproducing and -auxotrophic cells. Mol. Cell Biol., 9:2922, 1989.
4. Asselin, B. L., Ryan, D., Frantz, C. N., Bernal, S. D., Leavitt, P., Sallan, S. E., and Cohen, H. J.: In vitro and in vivo killing of acute lymphoblastic leukemia cells by L-asparaginase. Cancer Res., 49:4363, 1989.
5. Aur, R. J. A., Simone, J. V., and Pratt, C. B.: Successful remission induction in children with acute lymphocytic leukemia at high risk for treatment failure. Cancer, 27:1332, 1971.
6. Balinska, M., Galivan, J., and Coward, J. K.: Efflux of methotrexate and its polyglutamate derivatives from hepatic cells in vitro. Cancer Res., 41:2751, 1981.
7. Babrui, T., Finazzi, G., Vigano, S., and Mannucci, P. M.: L-Asparaginase lowers protein C antigen. Thromb. Haemostas., 52:216, 1984.
8. Baum, E., Nachman, J., Ramsay, N., Weetman, B., Neerhout, R., Littman, P., Griffin, T., Norris, D., and Sather, H.: Prolonged second remissions in childhood acute lymphocytic leukemia: A report from the Childrens Cancer Study Group. Med. Pediat. Oncol., 11:1, 1983.
9. Bertolone, S. J., Fuenfer, M. M., Groff, D. B., and Patel, C. C.: Delayed pancreatic pseudocyst formation. Cancer, 50:2964, 1982.
10. Boston, B., Rosen, M., and Capizzi, R. L.: Autoregulation of L-asparaginase-induced diabetes mellitus. Cancer Treat. Rep., 61:1607, 1977.
11. Broome, J. D.: Evidence that the L-asparaginase of guinea pig serum is responsible for its antilymphoma effects. J. Exp. Med., 118:99, 1963.
12. Broome, J. D.: Studies on the mechanism of tumor inhibition by L-asparaginase. J. Exp. Med., 127:1055, 1968.
13. Buchanan, G. R., Boyett, J. M., and Rivera, G. K.: Reinduction therapy in 273 children with acute lymphoblastic leukemia (ALL) in first bone marrow (BM) relapse: A Pediatric Oncology Group Study. (Abstract) Proc. Am. Soc. Clin. Oncol., 6:146, 1987.
14. Cairo, M. S., Lazarus, K., Gilmore, R. L., and Baehner, R. L.: Intracranial hemorrhage and focal seizures secondary to use of L-asparaginase during induction therapy of acute lymphocytic leukemia. J. Pediatr., 97:829, 1980.
15. Campbell, H. A., Mashburn, L. T., Boyse, E. A., and Old, L. J.: Two L-asparaginase from E. coli B., their separation, purification and antitumor activity. Biochem. Genet., 6:721, 1967.
16. Caniano, D. A., Browne, A. F., and Bole, E. T., Jr.: Pancreatic pseudocyst complicating treatment of acute lymphoblastic leukemia. J. Pediatr. Surg., 20:452, 1985.
17. Capizzi, R. L.: Schedule-dependent synergism and antagonism between methotrexate and asparaginase. Biochem. Pharmacol., 23(Suppl. 2):151, 1974.
18. Capizzi, R. L.: Improvement in the therapeutic index of methotrexate (NSC-740) by L-asparaginase (NSC-109229). Cancer Chemother. Rep., 6:37, 1975.
19. Capizzi, R. L.: Asparaginase-methotrexate in combination chemotherapy: schedule-dependent differential effects on normal versus neoplastic cells. Cancer Treat. Rep., 65(Suppl. 4):115, 1981.
20. Capizzi, R. L., Bertino, J. R., and Handschumacher, R. E.: L-asparaginase. Ann. Rev. Med., 21:433, 1970.
21. Capizzi, R. L., Bertino, J. R., Skeel, R. T., Creasey, W. A., Zanes, R., Olayon, C., Peterson, R. G., and Handschumacher, R. E.: L-asparaginase: Clinical, biochemical, pharmacological and immunological studies. Ann. Intern. Med., 74:893, 1971.
22. Capizzi, R. L., and Cheng, Y.-C.: Therapy of neoplasia with asparaginase. In Enzymes as Drugs. Edited by J. S. Holcenberg and J. Roberts. New York, J. Wiley & Sons, 1981, p. 1.
23. Capizzi, R. L., Davis, R., Powell, B., Cuttner, J., Ellison, R. R., Cooper, M. R., Dillman, R., Major, W. B., Dupre, E., and McIntyre, O. R.: Synergy between high-dose cytarabine and asparaginase in the treatment of adults with refractory and relapsed acute myelogenous leukemia—a Cancer and Leukemia Group B Study. J. Clin. Oncol., 6:499, 1988.
24. Capizzi, R. L., Keiser, L. W., and Sartorelli, A. C.: Combination chemotherapy—Theory and practice. Semin. Oncol., 4:227, 1977.
25. Capizzi, R. L., Poole, M., Cooper, M. R., Richards, F., 2d., Stuart, J. J., Jackson, D. V., Jr., White, D. R., Spurr, C. L., Hopkins, J. O., Muss, H. B., Rudnick, S. A., Wells, R., Gabriel, D., and Ross, D.: Treatment of poor risk acute leukemia with sequential high dose ara-C and asparaginase. Blood, 63:694, 1984.
26. Capizzi, R. L., and Powell, B. L.: Sequential high dose ara-C and asparaginase versus high dose ara-C alone in the treatment of patients with relapsed and refractory acute leukemias. Semin. Oncol., 14(Suppl. 1):40, 1987.
27. Capizzi, R. L., Summers, W. P., and Bertino, J. R.: L-asparaginase-induced alteration of amethopterin (methotrexate) activity in mouse leukemia L5178Y. Ann. N. Y. Acad. Sci., 186:302, 1971.
28. Cappellato, M. G., Rosolen, A., Zanesco, L., and Girolami, A.: Clotting complications of L-asparaginase therapy in children with ALL. Blut, 80:377, 1986.
29. Casonato, A., Lazzaro, A. R., Rosolen, A., and Girolami, A.: Factor VIII/von Willebrand factor abnormalities during L-asparaginase treatment in patients with acute lymphoblastic leukemia. Acta Haematol., 80:190, 1988.
30. Chessells, J. M., and Cornbleet, M.: Combination chemotherapy for bone marrow relapse in childhood lymphoblastic leukemia. Med. Pediat. Oncol., 6:359, 1979.
31. Cheung, N. K. V., Chau, I. Y., and Coccia, P. F.: Antibody response to Escherichia coli L-asparaginase: Prognostic significance and clinical utility of antibody measurement. Am. J. Pediatr. Hematol., 8:99, 1986.
32. Clarkson, B., Krakoff, I., Burchenal, J., Karnofsky, D., Golbey, R., Dowling, M., Oettgen, H., and Lipton, A.: Clinical results of treatment with E. coli L-asparaginase in adults with leukemia, lymphoma, and solid tumors. Cancer, 25:279, 1970.
33. Clavell, L. A., Gelber, R. D., Cohen, H. J., Hitchcock-Bryan, S., Cassady, J. R., Tarbell, N. J., Blattner, S. R., Tantravahi, R., Leavitt, P., and Sallan, S. E.: Four-agent induction and intensive asparaginase therapy for treatment of childhood acute lymphoblastic leukemia. N. Engl. J. Med., 315:657, 1986.
34. Cooney, D. A., and Handschumacher, R. E.: L-asparaginase and L-asparagine metabolism. Ann. Rev. Pharmacol., 10:421, 1970.
35. Crane, L. R., Jackson, R., and Avramis, V. I.: DNA hypermethylation studies in CEM/O cells after treatment with therapeutic and sub-therapeutic concentrations of cytosine arabinoside (ara-C). (Abstract) Proc. Am. Assoc. Cancer Res., 30:496, 1989.
36. Cremer, P., Lakomek, M., Beck, W., and Prindull, G.: The effect of L-asparaginase on lipid metabolism during induction chemotherapy of childhood lymphoblastic leukaemia. Eur. J. Pediatr., 147:64, 1988.
37. Crowther, D.: L-asparaginase and human malignant disease. Nature, 229:168, 1971.
38. Desai, S. J., Barr, R. D., Andrew, M., De Veber, L. L., and Pai, M. K. R.: Management of Ontario children with acute lymphoblastic leukemia by the Dana-Farber Cancer Institute protocols. Canad. Med. Assoc. J., 141:693, 1989.
39. Distasio, J. A., Niederman, R. A., Kafkewitz, D., and Goodman, D.: Purification and characterization of L-asparaginase with anti-lymphoma activity from Vibrio succinogenes. J. Biol. Chem., 251:6929, 1976.
40. Dolowy, W. C., Hensen, D. V. M., Cornet, J., and Sellin, H.: Toxic and antineoplastic effects of L-asparaginase. Cancer, 19:1813, 1966.
41. Eden, O. B., Shaw, M. P., Lilleyman, J., and Richards, J.: L-asparaginase: decreased toxicity with Erwinia Asparaginase used in MRC UKALL VIII. Proc. SIOP, Trondheim, 1988.

Antitumor Activity of Polyanions

Charles Myers
Michael Cooper
Malcolm Ranson
Oliver Sartor
Edward Sausville

Introduction

Interest in polyanions as possible antineoplastic agents has recently been stimulated by studies which indicate that suramin has antitumor activity both in vitro and in vivo. These are not new drugs, however, and their history is tied to the development of modern pharmacology and modern concepts of drug development. In the first decade of this century, Paul Ehrlich conducted a series of investigations which led to the idea that a drug's specificity is the result of a match between its three dimensional structure and that of its cellular receptor.[20] During that same time period, he also played a major role in the development of the concepts of drug screening and preclinical drug development. These twin developments paved the way for the modern concept of drug efficacy which involves minimizing toxicity while maximizing therapeutic efficacy. When Ehrlich initiated his program to test dyes for therapeutic activity, one of the targets he selected was trypanosomiasis. By 1904, he had identified the sulfonated cotton dye, trypan red, as an agent with considerable activity. The major disadvantage of trypan red was that it stained the mice an intense red. This observation triggered an extensive search for a better compound and by 1908, trypan blue had emerged as a second agent with worthwhile activity. However, this agent stained mice blue. The focus then shifted to finding related structures which were colorless, but that preserved the antitrypanosomal activity of these two dyes. Bayer & Co. screened in excess of 1,000 structures for antitrypanosomal activity before coming upon suramin in 1917, some two years after Dr. Ehrlich's death.[19] The sequence of structures leading to the synthesis of suramin are shown in Figure XVI-10-1. Since that time, it has been estimated that more than 2,500 additional structural variations have been synthesized without the emergence of an analog superior to suramin in the treatment of trypanosomiasis.

The activity of suramin in trypanosomiasis immediately triggered a wide range of interest in other potential therapeutic uses of sulfonated dyes and other polyanions that has been ably reviewed by Regelson.[77,78] Between 1908 and 1924, both sulfonated dyes and naturally occurring polysulfated polymers such as the glycosaminoglycan, chondroitin sulfate, were tested for antitumor activity. Unfortunately, the results were inconsistent and there followed a waning of interest in the antitumor activity of these compounds. However, there continued to be scattered observations of antitumor potential of polyanionic compounds, such

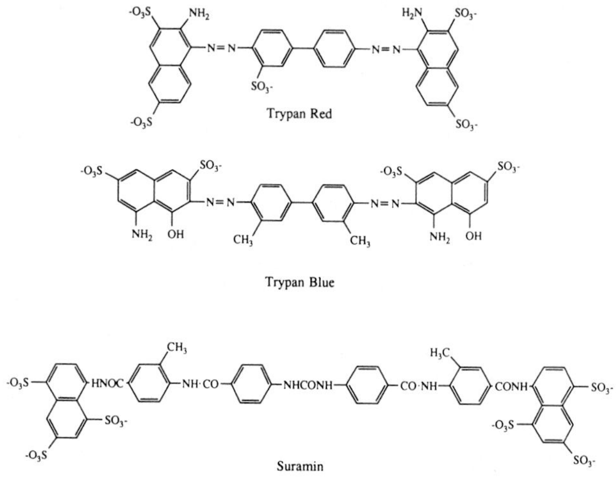

Figure XVI-10-1. The development of suramin. Trypan red was the first in a series of dyes active against trypanosomiasis. This was followed by the development of trypan blue and, finally, suramin. A major theme common to all three compounds is the presence of sulfonic acid groups.

as the demonstration in 1937 by Peters that suramin had activity in murine lymphosarcoma.[77,78]

In the late 1960's, interest in polyanions was renewed and advances in animal tumor models allowed for more comprehensive preclinical evaluation.[77,78] Several compounds elicited interest including dextran sulfate, heparinoids of various types and pyran copolymer among others. While none of these survived to become clinically useful anticancer drugs, perhaps some reevaluation of their activity may be in order given the advances in supportive care and clinical pharmacology which have made suramin administration possible.

Mechanism of Action

Naturally Occurring Polyanions Regulating Cell Growth and Differentiation

The antitumor activity of suramin and other polyanion drugs are best understood by considering first the naturally occurring polyanions which control cell growth and differentiation. The most prominent of these are the heparan sulfate proteoglycans, a diverse family of anionic macromolecules involved in the regulation of cell growth and differentiation.[15,32,47,52,56,57,80,91,92]

Proteoglycans consist of a core protein to which glycosaminoglycan chains are covalently linked. In broad terms, the core proteins have importance for intracellular trafficking and the localization of the mature proteoglycan, while the glycosaminoglycan chains, being anionic and hydrophilic, are frequently involved in interactions with a variety of proteins including enzymes, growth factors and components of the extracellular matrix.

The sulfated polysaccharide chains of heparan sulfate consist almost entirely of alternating N-acetylglucosamine and uronic acid moieties (glucuronic and iduronic acid). During biosynthesis a number of chemical and configurational modifications are imposed upon these units leading to a wide range of potential structures. Importantly, rather than being modified at random, the mature glycosaminoglycan chains have been shown to exist as ordered polymeric structures with regions of high and low sulfation along the chain. A schematic representation of the formation of these domains is shown in Figure XVI-10-2.

The regions of most extensive modification have been identified as being involved in many of the biological activities of heparan sulfates. It is clear that remarkable specificity in structure-activity relationships can occur. An example of such specificity may be seen by comparing a pentasaccharide sequence which has little anticoagulant action but which exhibits antiangiogenic activity, to a similar pentasaccharide sequence which has anticoagulant activity by its

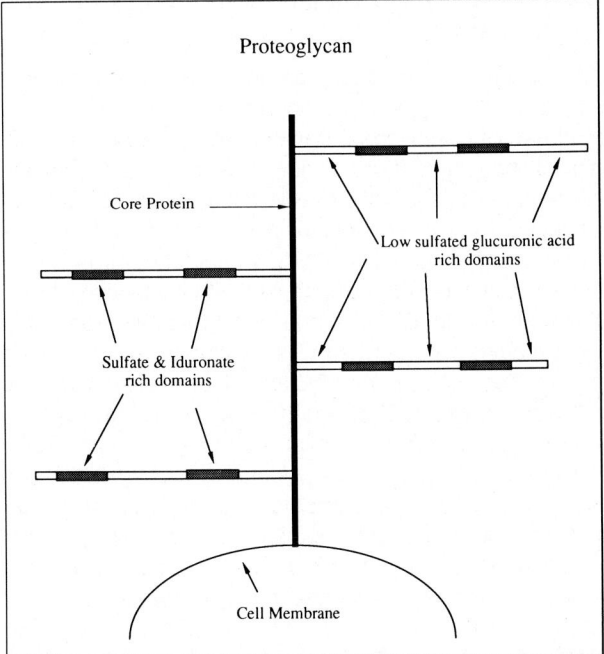

Figure XVI-10-2. Structure of heparan sulfate-containing proteoglycans. The core protein is anchored to the cell membrane. The heparan sulfate chains are attached to the core protein at various points along the protein chain. Within the heparan sulfate chains, there are regions rich in both sulfate and iduronate separated by regions low in sulfate and rich in glucuronic acid. Most of the biologic activity of the heparan sulfates appear to arise from the highly sulfated regions.

ANTIANGIOGENIC PENTASACCHARIDE

ANTITHROMBIN III BINDING PENTASACCHARIDE

Figure XVI-10-3. Heparan sulfate structure determines biologic activity. The pentasaccharide sequence shown at the top has been reported to inhibit angiogenesis, but does not alter coagulation. The lower pentasaccharide shows high affinity for antithrombin III. The arrows show the only site where these two pentasaccharides differ.

Table XVI-10-1. Biologic Actions of Heparan Sulfate

1. Extracellular matrix organization
2. Basement membrane organization and regulation of permeability
3. Cell attachment, spreading, and migration
4. Growth and differentiation
5. Membrane localization of enzymes (e.g., acetylcholine esterase, lipoprotein lipase)
6. Localization of cytokines in pericellular domain (IL-3, GM-CSF, bFGF, TGF-β)
7. Anticoagulation
8. Modulation of angiogenesis

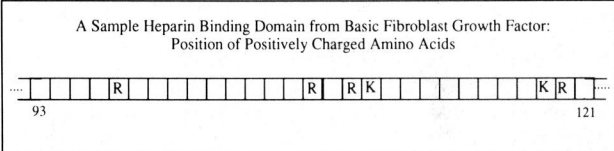

A Sample Heparin Binding Domain from Basic Fibroblast Growth Factor: Position of Positively Charged Amino Acids

Figure XVI-10-4. Heparan sulfate binding region of basic fibroblast growth factor. The postively charged amino acids are arginine[(R)] and lysine[(K)]. Since heparan sulfate binding to a protein is likely to involve interactions between the negatively charged sulfates in heparan and positively charged amino acids, we have shown the positions of lysine and arginine; it is likely that one or more of these positively charged amino acids are also involved in the binding to suramin through the drug's sulfonic acid groups.

ability to interact with antithrombin III (Figure XVI-10-3).[3,4,11,12,26,34,67,72,73,82,99]

Heparan sulfate and heparin contain the same disaccharide repeat structure of N-acetylglucosamine and uronic acid, but differ in the extent of N-sulfation with heparan sulfates typically exhibiting 45–55% N-sulfation compared to >80% for heparin. Both polymers may contain similar functional domains such as are illustrated in Figure XVI-10-3 and have similar biological effects (Table XVI-10-1). For example, the antithrombin III-binding sequence shown in Figure XVI-10-3 represents approximately 10% of heparin, but can also be found in many heparan sulfate preparations. Thus, while the two families of polymers may be distinguished based upon degree of sulfation, they can have similar effects when added to biological systems and are often used interchangeably.

The binding of anionic polysaccharide chains to proteins typically involves the interaction between negatively charged groups on the carbohydrate and positively charged amino acids in the protein ligand. Sequences of amino acids that have affinity for heterogeneous populations of heparan sulfate or heparin have been identified for a number of proteins. Figure XVI-10-4 shows one such amino acid sequence identified in basic fibroblast growth factor, an important mitogen for endothelial cells.[5,25] However, the structural features of the binding of glycosaminoglycan oligosaccharides have yet to be characterized in many instances because of the lack of any simple, widely available means for the sequence determination of sulfated oligosaccharides.

A detailed consideration of the biology of heparan sulfates (Table XVI-10-1) is beyond the scope of this chapter and the reader is referred to several recent comprehensive reviews on the subject.[15,32,47,52,56,57,80,91,92] We confine ourselves here to some of the growth regulatory effects of these molecules which have particular bearing on the observed antiproliferative activity of suramin in cancer patients.

Direct nuclear actions of heparan sulfates have been proposed in hepatocytes, where an accumulation of oligosaccharides enriched in an unusual glucuronic acid 2-sulfate residue were preferentially translocated to the nucleus following endocytosis of the proteoglycan.[23,24,42,81] Increased levels of this nuclear-targeted heparan sulfate was accompanied by an arrest in cell cycle at the G1 to S transition.

An extensive and growing list of growth factors have been found to display an affinity for either heparan sulfate or heparin (Table XVI-10-2). In some instances, the interaction between cytokine and polysaccharide has functional impor-

tance. For example, bone marrow stromal heparan sulfate is capable of binding and presenting the growth factors IL-3 and GM-CSF in active form to hemopoietic progenitor cells.[79] It has been proposed that heparan sulfates in the bone marrow act to localize and present these cytokines in a paracrine fashion.

The sequestration and localization of basic fibroblast growth factor, an important mitogen for endothelial cells, in basement membranes and extracellular matrix has also been documented and this interaction restricts the bioavailability of the cytokine while simultaneously protecting it from enzymatic degradation.[5,25,47,91,92] Recently, it has been shown that both the interaction of basic fibroblast growth factor with its high affinity receptor and its mitogenic activity in vitro requires the association of the cytokine with a heparin-like molecule.[100]

A further novel mechanism for modulation of growth factor activity by heparan sulfate has been suggested by studies involving transforming growth factor-β (TGF-β).[61] A variable proportion of serum TGF-β is bound in an inert complex with alpha-s-macroglobulin. Heparinoids lead to the dissociation of active TGF-β from the complex making the cytokine available for interaction with cell surface receptors.

As these examples serve to illustrate, heparan sulfates are important constituents of the cell membrane and the pericellular matrix. They are thus ideally placed to regulate the availability of a range of polypeptides to cell surface receptors.

Autocrine Growth Stimulation and Malignant Transformation

One of the most important advances in cancer research over the past 15 years has been the identification of the genetic basis of malignant transformation, i.e., the identification of oncogenes. This has been followed by a description of some of the mechanisms by which the oncogenes accomplish malignant transformation. An important step in this process was the proposal in 1980 of autocrine growth as a mechanism of malignant transformation.[86] In autocrine growth, a cell normally dependent upon growth signals from other cells becomes independent of such control by producing the cytokines needed to stimulate its own growth (Figure XVI-10-5). An example of this mechanism is the transformation of fibroblasts by the simian sarcoma virus. Fibroblasts have receptors for platelet-derived growth factor (PDGF) and this cytokine will stimulate fibroblast growth. The simian sarcoma virus possesses the *sis* oncogene and expression of this oncogene results in the production of the *sis* gene product, a protein similar in structure to the β chain of PDGF.[33,97] This protein then binds to the PDGF receptor and stimulates growth and transformation, both of which are reversed by addition of anti-PDGF antibody. Of the cytokines listed in Table XVI-10-2, several fibroblast growth factor family members, epidermal growth factor family, IL-3, GM-CSF and insulin-like growth factor 2 as well as PDGF have been shown to mediate transformation by autocrine mechanisms. A significant majority of those cytokines documented to be involved in autocrine growth are heparin-binding growth factors.

Table XVI-10-2.   Cytokines Which Bind to Heparan Sulfate

Growth Factor	Reference
Fibroblast growth factor (FGF) family	
Acidic FGF	46
Basic FGF	5
Int-2	9
Hst/K-FGF	18
FGF-5	103
FGF-6	60
KGF	28
Epidermal Growth Factor (EGF) Family	
Amphiregulin	83
Heparin binding EGF-like GF	38
Platelet Derived Growth Factor (PDGF)	59
Macrophage Inflammatory Peptide-2 family	98
Neuronal Growth Factors	
Schwann cell mitogen	74
Glial maturation factor-β	55
Hemopoietic Growth Factors	
Interleukin-3	79
GM-CSF	79
Leukemia-Derived Transforming GF	102
Insulin-like Growth Factor 2	65
Hepatocyte Growth Factor	35
Midkine Factor Family	
Heparin binding growth-associated molecule	62
Pleiotropin	53
Heparin-binding neurotropic factor	49
OSF-1	88
Retinoic acid induced heparin-binding protein	90
Heparin-binding growth factor-8	64

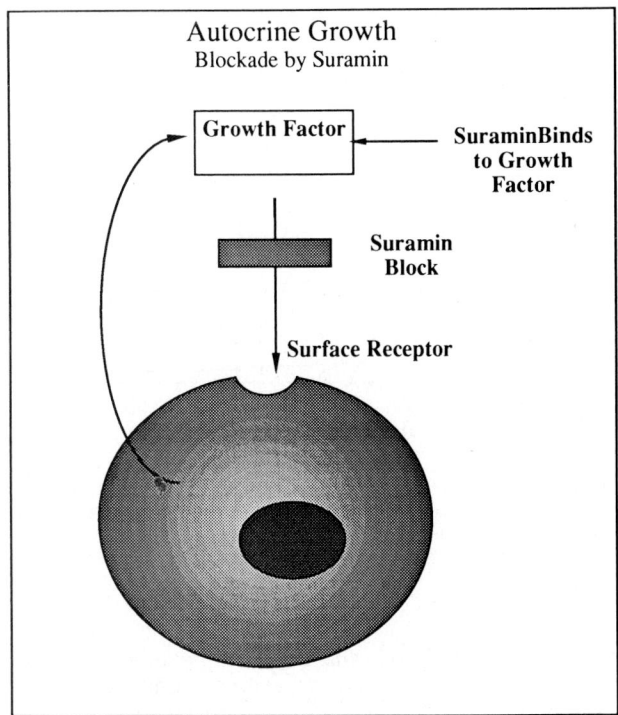

Figure XVI-10-5. The mechanism by which autocrine growth occurs. The cell in question elaborates and secretes into the surrounding medium a peptide growth factor for which it possesses a functional receptor. The consequence is self-stimulation of cellular proliferation. For a majority of the peptide growth factors where such a process has been invoked, suramin binds to the growth factor in question and prevents its association with its cell surface receptor.

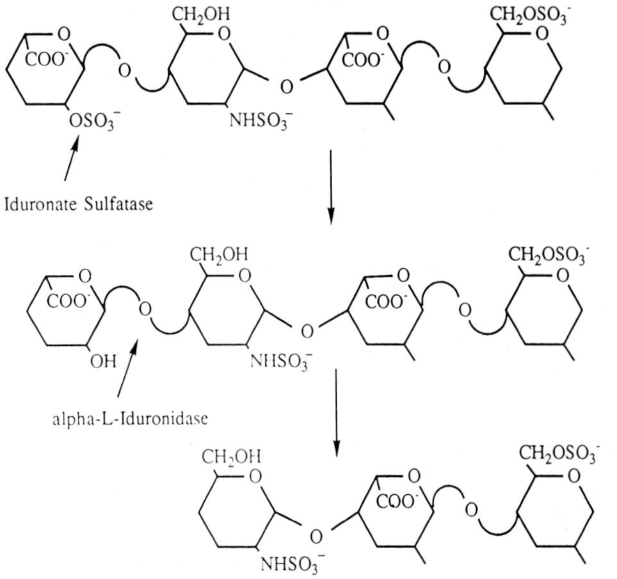

Figure XVI-10-6. Inhibition of heparan sulfate and dermatan sulfate degradation by suramin. The first step in the degradation of the iduronate containing regions is an O-desulfation reaction involving the enzyme iduronate sulfatase. The next step involves cleavage of the carbohydrate chain by alpha-L-iduronidase. Suramin arrests this process by inhibiting iduronate sulfatase. The result is a relative sparing of the highly sulfated regions. Hunter's syndrome is an inborn error in glycosaminoglycan degradation characterized by a lack of this same enzyme. Both Hunter's syndrome and suramin administration result in accumulation of the two glycosaminoglycans possessing sulfated iduronic acid residues, heparan sulfate and dermatan sulfate.

Relationship of Heparan Sulfate Biology to Suramin Action

The ability of the *sis* oncogene to transform fibroblasts by an autocrine mechanism was first reported in 1984. Within that same year, it was shown that suramin was able to promptly reverse the transformation of fibroblasts by this oncogene. Suramin has been shown to bind to PDGF and to the *sis* oncogene and thus to prevent these peptides from binding to the cell surface receptor.[7,29,33,41,44,45,96,97] Suramin has subsequently been shown to reverse malignant transformation by hst/K-fgf as well as the *v-sis* gene product.[66] This observation has led to the suggestion that suramin acts as an analog of heparan sulfate. Indeed, a comparison of the known effects of suramin suggest that it acts as an agonist or antagonist of heparan sulfate for most of the functions listed in Table XVI-10-1. In this hypothesis, the sulfonic acid groups of suramin must substitute for the sulfate groups on heparan sulfate.

The ability of suramin to bind to heparin-binding sites within proteins may account for suramin's ability to inhibit a number of glycosaminoglycan degradative enzymes. An important step in the degradation of functionally important iduronate and sulfate-rich regions of heparan sulfate is desulfation by iduronate sulfatase. This is then followed by enzymatic cleavage of the carbohydrate chain (Figure XVI-10-6). In vitro, suramin has been shown to be a powerful inhibitor of iduronate sulfatase. A genetic defect in this enzyme results in Hunter's syndrome, a mucopolysaccharidosis that is asso-

ciated with the accumulation of heparan and dermatan sulfate. This has enabled Brady and coworkers to create an animal model for mucopolysaccharidosis by administering suramin to rats.[16,75,76] We have noted that suramin administration to patients also results in elevated heparan and dermatan sulfate levels in blood and urine.[40] Under certain conditions, this can become severe enough to result in anticoagulation, although in most cases the anticoagulation seen with suramin is due to a direct action of the drug. Also, since iduronate sulfatase is a lysosomal enzyme and heparan degradation normally occurs within the lysosome, suramin administration results in accumulation of both heparan and dermatan sulfate within the lysosomes throughout the body.[39,40,75,76]

Since heparan sulfate may either inhibit or stimulate cell growth, the accumulation of heparan sulfate seen in patients receiving suramin might either enhance or antagonize the antitumor activity of suramin. For this reason, we have isolated heparan sulfate from patients undergoing treatment with suramin. This material has considerable activity against a range of human tumor cells in vitro.

In Vitro Antitumor Activity of Suramin

The antitumor activity of suramin has been reported in a wide range of tumor types in vitro, with most impressive activity being reported in carcinomas of the prostate, stomach, endometrium, ovary and lung (nonsmall cell), glioma, melanoma, rhabdomyosarcoma, osteogenic sarcoma and nonHodgkin's lymphomas.[2,13,17,22,30,48,51,68-70,85,93,95,101] In cell cultures, one striking property is that maximal antitumor activity requires prolonged contact. For prostate cancer, which we have recently studied in some depth, drug effects are reversible after three days exposure. After six days, however, cells proceed to die even days after drug removal.

In general, caution must be applied when considering the relevance of in vitro antitumor activity to clinical cancer treatment. This is especially so for suramin. The activity of this drug may be due to its action on cytokines and little is known about how well the cytokine levels in vitro match those in patients. It is particularly likely that tissue culture media are lacking growth factors present in patients that might plausibly alter the effectiveness of suramin. The only solution presently available is to perform phase 2 trials in each of the tumors listed above.

Routes of Administration, Distribution, Pharmacokinetics and Implications for Scheduling

This drug is not absorbed after oral administration and so must be given parenterally. Suramin is chemically stable in all commonly used intravenous infusion media.[6] In all current trials of suramin as an anticancer agent, therapy has been administered intravenously. The administered drug binds tightly to plasma proteins and is greater than 99.7% protein bound at blood levels below 200 μg/ml.[8] As blood levels increase above 200 μg/ml, free drug levels increase rapidly as does toxicity of the drug. In addition to extensive binding to plasma proteins, animal studies of suramin administration have shown that the drug accumulates in tissues, particularly the kidney and adrenal gland. The levels of suramin in most other tissues reflect circulating plasma levels.

The plasma pharmacokinetics of suramin may be accounted for by a three compartment model. In 71 patients studied at NCI, total body clearance was 0.331 ± 0.138 ml/hr/Kg with a volume of distribution at steady state of 32.2 ± 11.8 L. The alpha, beta and gamma half lives were 2.2 ± 0.48 hours, 1.3 ± 0.47 days and 42 ± 23 days. For each of these values, there is significant variation and this leads to considerable patient to patient variability in blood levels attained following any given drug dose. As a result, current treatment protocols require drug level monitoring in order to ensure safe drug administration. Figure XVI-10-7 illustrates how suramin levels typically decline after a bolus dose, with a rapid early decline reflecting the two early compartments followed by a very gradual decline which can be followed for months. It is conventional wisdom that with a drug with a terminal half life of this length, it should be relatively easy to maintain consistent blood levels with an intermitent bolus schedule. Figure XVI-10-7 illustrates nicely how the rapid early decline in blood levels due to the three compartment behavior makes this more complicated than the long terminal half life might indicate. At present, there is no known drug metabolism and renal elimination of the parent drug is the only documented pathway of drug clearance.

In early trials with suramin, the drug was administered as a weekly bolus at a fixed dose rate. These trials revealed an unacceptable frequency of neurotoxicity associated with blood levels above 350 μg/ml. After the patient-to-patient variability in drug disposition became apparent, it became customary to measure blood levels after initial drug administration and adjust subsequent dosing to keep blood levels below 300

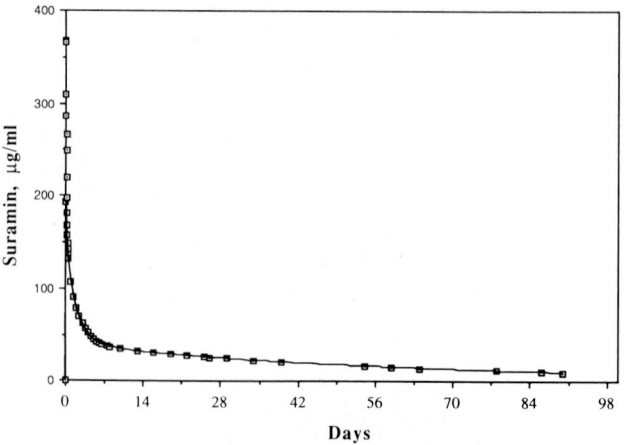

Figure XVI-10-7.   An example of the three compartment behavior of suramin. This a computer simulation of the blood levels to be expected after a single bolus dose of 1500 mg of suramin to a patient who weighs 70 kg and who has pharmacokinetic parameters of the average patient.

μg/ml. Initially, drug dose was adjusted, based upon a simple nomogram constructed from a one compartment model. The pharmacokinetic data arising from these early trials allowed documentation of three compartment behavior of suramin's pharmacokinetics and a determination of the variability of each pharmacokinetic parameter.[14,87] This information has allowed a more sophisticated approach to dose adjustment. Currently, best control of suramin blood levels has been obtained by two groups using Bayesian techniques.[43,54] A full discussion of the Bayesian approach is beyond the scope of this chapter and the reader is referred to several recent reviews.[71] This is an approach to estimation of individual pharmacokinetic behavior wherein the patient is assumed to behave like the average patient until sufficient information is accumulated to prove otherwise. The result is that an extreme response to possibly erroneous early drug measurements is effectively prevented. A recently developed computer program which operates on desk top computers makes Bayesian control of drug administration practical for most cancer centers.

The clinical protocols yielding the highest response rate appear to be those which give prolonged exposure to drug levels in excess of 100 μg/ml. This has been accomplished by either bolus or continuous infusion protocols in which the drug is administered for as long as eight weeks.

Patterns of Toxicity

Most anticancer agents are limited by toxicity that is evident in a few organs which are consistently involved when full doses of the drug is administered. In contrast, suramin can cause a wide range of toxicities, but it is uncommon for a patient to manifest all or even most of the possible side effects. In addition, the toxicity of the drug appears to be dependent upon blood drug level and to escalate rapidly at blood levels in excess of 200–225 μg/ml. In an elderly male population with prostate cancer, drug levels below 200 μg/ml are associated with a frequency of serious or life-threatening side effects of less than 20%, while at blood levels between 275–300 μg/ml the frequency may reach as high as 70–80%.

Adrenal Cortical Failure

Suramin can cause destruction of the normal adrenal cortex in both man and in a wide range of experimental animals.[27] Adrenal medullary function is preserved. Suramin accumulates within the adrenal gland and this probably plays some role in the development of this toxicity. The natural history of this toxicity has not been documented, but individual patients have had recovery of apparently normal adrenal function six or more months after suramin administration was discontinued.

Neurotoxicity

This drug causes three distinct patterns of neurotoxicity. The first to be noted was an acute demyelinating peripheral neuropathy resembling acute Guillain-Barré syndrome seen only in patients with prolonged blood levels in excess of 350 μg/ml.[87] Blood levels between 200–300 μg/ml are associated with stocking-glove paresthesias very similar to those caused by the vinca alkaloids. Regardless of severity, this neuropathic syndrome improves, usually dramatically, over 6–12 months following discontinuation of suramin.

A third neuropathic syndrome has been seen only in protocols where drug administration has continued beyond one month. This syndrome presents as proximal muscle weakness suggestive of a myopathy, but markers of muscle injury are absent and nerve conduction changes are observed. This neuropathic syndrome typically continues to progress after drug administration has been discontinued, sometimes for more than a month. Recovery is very gradual over 4–9 months.

Renal Injury

Suramin causes a 25–50% decline in creatinine clearance in most patients. There is usually complete or nearly complete recovery in patients who have normal renal function to start with. More severe renal functional abnormalities have been noted in patients who become septic during suramin administration. However, in such cases the patients have usually been hypotensive and have received aminoglycoside antibiotics. From such cases, it is difficult to determine the relative contribution of suramin.

In addition, suramin may cause proteinuria. This rarely exceeds 1 gm per 24 hours and does not result in a nephrotic syndrome.

As mentioned above, suramin accumulates in the kidneys to a considerable degree. While the mechanism of this accumulation is not known, it undoubtedly plays a role in the nephrotoxicity observed. The drug has been shown to accumulate within the renal tubular lysosomes and this is followed by the degeneration of the renal tubular cells.

Anticoagulation

Suramin inhibits factors V, VIII, IX, X, XI and XII, while thrombin, prothrombin and factor VII are unaffected. The inhibition of factor V is irreversible, while the effect of suramin on the other coagulation factors is readily reversible upon dilution.

As a result of these changes, patients with suramin often experience prolongation of prothrombin time, activated partial thromboplastin time, and thrombin clotting times. An unusual aspect is that the thrombin clotting time abnormalities caused by suramin do not correct with toluidine blue, while those caused by heparin do.

In practice, we have found that the risk of hemorrage is markedly reduced if administration of suramin is discontinued when the prothrombin time exceeds 17 seconds. Tumor-induced diffuse intravascular coagulation can be a problem with prostate carcinoma. At present, guidelines have not been developed for safe use of suramin in this situation.

Bacterial Infections

While suramin may induce neutropenia, it is uncommon for the absolute neutrophile count to drop below 1,000 cells/ml. Nevertheless, it is apparent that prolonged exposure to suramin levels of 270–300 μg/ml is associated with an increased risk of bacterial infections. In our prostate cancer population, these have typically arisen from either the urinary tract or the catheter used for intravenous drug administration. Catheter-related infections appear to be less frequent when suramin is given by intermittent IV bolus administration compared to continuous intravenous infusion.

Suramin has been demonstrated to impair both the rate of phagocytosis and killing of bacteria by neutrophils, and this may be the mechanism underlying the increase in bacterial infections.[36,37,84,89,94]

Lymphocytopenia

Lymphocytopenia occurs in up to 80% of the patients exposed to blood levels of 275–300 μg/ml and seems to be selective for T cells. Nevertheless, opportunistic infections have been relatively uncommon in patients treated with suramin. Suramin binds IL-2 and prevents its association with the T cell receptor. Since T cells undergo programmed cell death in vitro when IL-2 is removed, this provides a possible explanation and a mechanism for blocking the toxicity of suramin for T cells. In fact, addition of excess IL-2 does dramatically lessen the toxicity of suramin for T cells.[63]

Thrombocytopenia

Suramin may induce thrombocytopenia; platelet counts below 50,000 are relatively uncommon, however. In addition, thrombocytopenia is usually self-limiting and resolves despite persistent blood levels of suramin. Bone marrow biopsies in patients with suramin-induced thrombocytopenia reveal normal megakaryocytes with normal budding, suggesting that the thrombocytopenia results from an accelerated peripheral clearance of platelets. Suramin-induced thrombocytopenia is usually a dose limiting toxicity only in patients with pre-existing thrombocytopenia due to marrow replacement, previous radiation or chemotherapy or tumor-induced diffuse intravascular coagulation.

Vortex Keratopathy

Suramin-induced lysosomal accumulation of heparan and dermatan sulfate occurs in the corneal epithelium.[39] As a result, every patient receiving suramin has a vortex keratopathy which can be detected by slit lamp examination. In most cases, the only symptom associated with this is the appearance of a ring around bright lights. In an occasional patient, pitting of the corneal epithelium occurs resulting in a gritty sensation, photophobia and excess tearing. This complication has resolved completely in every case without residual eye damage. Until the corneal epithelium has healed, symptomatic relief may be given with dark glasses, methyl cellulose eye drops and soft contact lenses.

Skin Rash

Suramin induces a skin rash in a majority of the patients who receive the drug. This rash is a mildly pruritic, erythematous, macular eruption which typically starts on the chest and back and can spread to involve the extremities. The rash usually presents during the first two weeks following initiation of suramin treatment. This toxicity is nearly always self-limiting and resolves in the face of continued suramin administration. In the occasional severe case, the rash can be severe enough to lead to desquamation. In such severe cases, the rash is associated with fever and thrombocytopenia.

Edema

Ankle edema has developed in individual patients with intact lymphatic and venous drainage to the lower extremities and with a serum albumin within the normal range. Edema can become a significant problem if the patient also has any of these other problems. The physiologic basis for this complication is unknown.

Liver Injury

Suramin may cause mild elevation of the hepatic enzymes and bilirubin, but rarely causes severe injury in the absence of other sources of liver injury. Patients with ongoing liver injury from other causes can exhibit a marked decline in liver function with suramin administration, however.

Antitumor Spectrum

The efficacy of suramin in prostate cancer has received the greatest attention. In patients with measurable soft tissue disease, the combined PR and CR rate has ranged between ~15% to greater than 50%. However, soft tissue involvement is seen in only 15% of patients with prostate cancer. In the more common presentation of bone involvement alone, the major evidence of suramin's antitumor activity has been the decline seen in prostate specific antigen (PSA). In the initial trial of suramin in prostate cancer at the NCI, approximately one third of the patients experienced a decline of their pretreatment PSA of 75% or greater by 8 weeks after therapy was initiated. Declines of PSA of this magnitude were associated with a dramatic shift in survival, with greater than 80% of the patients alive at one year and greater than 60% alive at two years for the responders compared to a median survival of less than 40 weeks for nonresponders. In this trial, the drug was infused over a two week period. Subsequent trials have reported response rates between 40–60%.[1,21] These phase 2 results are sufficiently promising that suramin should receive additional evaluation in the treatment of metastatic prostate carcinoma.

Since suramin induces depletion of splenic lymphocytes and thymic atrophy in mice, it is perhaps not surprising that suramin has shown clear activity against a range of lymphomas. The first response was noted in the trial of suramin as an agent to treat AIDS.[10] In that trial, a patient with non-Hodgkin's lymphoma went into complete response which has continued for more than four years. We have treated 10 patients with nodular lymphomas who had been heavily pretreated and have seen five partial responses. In addition, we have treated two patients with thymoma who had failed radiation therapy and conventional chemotherapy programs, both of whom experienced PRs on suramin. Finally, one out of five patients with HTLV-1 associated T cell leukemia experienced a PR from suramin as a single agent which lasted nearly five months.[50]

Early in our work with suramin, we evaluated suramin in adrenal carcinoma and observed a response rate below 20%. It is now possible to administer suramin in a much more dose-intense fashion, however, and its activity in this disease should probably be reevaluated.

Suramin has not been subjected to phase 2 trial in most of the tumor types against which it exhibits activity in vitro.

Interactions

Suramin has been shown to interact synergistically with alkylating agents with regard to antitumor activity murine models, without evidence of additive toxicity.[70] There is more extensive information about the interaction of suramin with doxorubicin.[22,31,70] Here again, there does not appear to be additive toxicity, but antitumor activity of the two compounds range from additive to synergistic over a range of tumor types including human breast cancer and prostate cancer cell lines. Synergy has also been seen with tumor necrosis factor, but not with gamma-interferon.[31,58]

Summary

A nearly infinite number of anionic polyelectrolytes can be synthesized. The understanding of suramin's mechanism of action by electrostatic association with highly charged basic proteins offers the possibility that designer molecules could be synthesized (or may already exist in nature or in polymer inventories) with more selective anti-neoplastic action.

References

1. Ahmann, F. R., Schwartz, J., Dorr, R., and Salmon, S.: Suramin in Hormone Resistant Metastatic Prostate Cancer: Significant Anticancer Activity but Unanticipated toxicity. (Abstract). Proc. Am. Soc. Clin. Oncol., 10:574, 1991.
2. Alberts, D., Miranda, E., Dorr, R., Nichols, N., Ketcham, M., MacNeal, W., Hatch, K., Surwit, E., Childers, J., Taylor, C., Ahmann, R., and Salmon, S.: Phase II, pharmacokinetic and human tumor cloning assay study of suramin in advanced ovarian cancer. (Abstract). Proc. Am. Soc. Clin. Oncol., 10:609, 1991.
3. Barzu, T., Lormeau, J. C., Petitou, M., Michelson, S., and Choay, J.: Heparin-derived oligosaccharides: Affinity for acidic fibroblast growth factor and effect on its growth-promoting activity for human endothelial cells. J. Cell Physiol., 140:538, 1989.
4. Beguin, S., Choay, J., and Hemker, H. C.: The action of a synthetic pentasaccharide on thrombin generation in whole plasma. Thromb. Haemost., 61:397, 1989.
5. Baird, A., Schubert, D., Ling, N., and Guillemin, R.: Receptor- and heparin-binding domains of basic fibroblast growth factor. Proc. Natl. Acad. Sci. USA, 85:2324, 1988.
6. Beijnen, J. H., van Gijn, R., Horenblas, S., and Underberg, W. J.: Chemical stability of suramin in commonly used infusion fluids. DICP, 24:1056, 1990.
7. Betsholtz, C., Johnsson, A., Heldin, C. H., and Westermark, B.: Efficient reversion of simian sarcoma virus-transformation and inhibition of growth factor-induced mitogenesis by suramin. Proc. Natl. Acad. Sci. USA, 83:6440, 1986.
8. Bos, O. J., Vansterkenburg, E. L., Boon, J. P., Fischer, M. J., Wilting, J., and Janssen, L. H.: Location and characterization of the suramin binding sites of human serum albumin. Biochem. Pharmacol., 40:1595, 1990.
9. Burgess, W. H., and Maciag, T.: The heparin binding (fibroblast) growth factor family of proteins. Annu. Rev. Biochem., 58:575, 1989.
10. Cheson, B. D., Levine, A. M., Mildvan, D., Kaplan, L. D., et al.: Suramin therapy in AIDS and related disorders. Report of the US Suramin Working Group. Jama, 258:1347, 1987.
11. Choay, J.: Chemically synthesized heparin-derived oligosaccharides. Ann. N. Y. Acad. Sci., 556:61, 1989.
12. Choay, J.: Structure and activity of heparin and its fragments: An overview. Semin. Thromb. Hemost., 15:359, 1989.
13. Coffey, R. J., Goustin, A. S., Soderquist, A. M., Shipley, G. D., et al: Transforming growth factor alpha and beta expression in human colon cancer lines: Implications for an autocrine model. Cancer Res., 47:4590, 1987.
14. Collins, J. M., Klecker, R. J., Yarchoan, R., Lane, H. C., et al.: Clinical pharmacokinetics of suramin in patients with HTLV-III/LAV infection. J. Clin. Pharmacol., 26:22, 1986.

15. Conrad, H. E.: Structure of heparan sulfate and dermatan sulfate. Ann. N. Y. Acad. Sci., 556:18, 1989.
16. Constantopoulos, G., Rees, S., Cragg, B. G., Barranger, J. A., et al.: Suramin-induced storage disease. Mucopolysaccharidosis. Am. J. Pathol., 113:266, 1983.
17. Culouscou, J. M., Garrouste, F., Remacle-Bonnet, M., Bettetini, D., Marvaldi, J., and Pommier, G.: Autocrine secretion of a colorectum-derived growth factor by HT-29 human colon carcinoma cell line. Int. J. Cancer, 42:895, 1988.
18. Delli-Bovi, P., Basilico, C.: Isolation of a rearranged human transforming gene following transfection of Kaposi sarcoma DNA. Proc. Natl. Acad. Sci. USA, 84:5660, 1987.
19. Dressel, J., Oesper, R. E.: The Discovery of Germanin by Oskar Dressel and Richard Kothe. J. Chem. Educ., 38:620, 1961.
20. Reference not used.
21. Eisenberger, M., Jodrell, D., Sinibaldi, V., Zuhowski, E., Jacobs, S., Egorin, M., and Van Echo, D. A.: Preliminary Evidence of Antitumor Activity Against Prostate Cancer Observed in a Phase 1 Trial with Suramin. (Abstract) Proc. Am. Soc. Clin. Oncol., 10:537, 1991.
22. Favoni, R. E., Russo, R., Pirani, P., Repetto, L., Nicolin, A., Miglietta, L.: Synergistic activity of suramin and doxorubicin on human breast cancer cell lines. Proc. Am. Ass. Cancer Res., 32:2282, 1991.
23. Fedarko, N. S., and Conrad, H. E.: A unique heparan sulfate in the nuclei of hepatocytes: structural changes with the growth state of the cells. J. Cell Biol., 102:587, 1986.
24. Fedarko, N. S., Ishihara, M., and Conrad, H. E.: Control of cell division in hepatoma cells by exogenous heparan sulfate proteoglycan. J. Cell Physiol., 139:287, 1989.
25. Feige, J. J., Bradley, J. D., Fryburg, K., Farris, J., Cousens, L. C., Barr, P. J., and Baird, A.: Differential effects of heparin, fibronectin, and laminin on the phosphorylation of basic fibroblast growth factor by protein kinase C and the catalytic subunit of protein kinase A. J. Cell Biol., 109:3105, 1989.
26. Ferro, D. R., Provasoli, A., Ragazzi, M., Casu, B., Torri, G., Bossennec, V., Perly, B., Sinay, P., Petitou, M., and Choay, J.: Conformer populations of L-iduronic acid residues in glycosaminoglycan sequences. Carbohydr. Res., 195:157, 1990.
27. Feuillan, P., Raffeld, M., Stein, C. A., Lipford, N., et al.: Effects of suramin on the function and structure of the adrenal cortex in the cynomolgus monkey. J. Clin. Endocrinol. Metab., 65:153, 1987.
28. Finch, P., Rubin, J., Miki, T.: Human KGF in FGF-related with properities of a paracrine effector of epithelial cell growth. Science, 245:752, 1988.
29. Fleming, T. P., Matsui, T., Molloy, C. J., Robbins, K. C., and Aaronson, S. A.: Autocrine mechanism for v-sis transformation requires cell surface localization of internally activated growth factor receptors. Proc. Natl. Acad. Sci. USA, 86:8063, 1989.
30. Forgue-Lafitte, M. E., Coudray, A. M., Breant, B., and Mester, J.: Proliferation of the human colon carcinoma cell line HT29: Autocrine growth and deregulated expression of the c-myc oncogene. Cancer Res., 49:6566, 1989.
31. Fruehauf, J. P., Myers, C. E., and Sinha, B. K.: Synergistic activity of suramin with tumor necrosis factor alpha and doxorubicin on human prostate cancer cell lines. J. Natl. Cancer Inst., 82:1206, 1990.
32. Gallagher, J. T., Turnbull, J. E., and Lyon, M.: Heparan sulphate proteoglycans. Biochem. Soc. Trans., 18:207, 1990.
33. Garrett, J. S., Coughlin, S. R., Niman, H. L., Tremble, P. M., et al.: Blockade of autocrine stimulation in simian sarcoma virus-transformed cells reverses down-regulation of platelet-derived growth factor receptors. Proc. Natl. Acad. Sci. USA, 81:7466, 1984.
34. Gettins, P., and Choay, J.: Examination, by 1H-n.m.r. spectroscopy, of the binding of a synthetic, high-affinity heparin pentasaccharide to human antithrombin III. Carbohydr. Res., 185:69, 1989.
35. Gohda, E., Tsubouchi, H., Nakayama, H. et al.: Purification and partial characterization of hepatocyte growth factor from plasma of a patient with fulminant hepatic failure. J. Clin. Invest., 81:414, 1988.
36. Hart, P. D., Young, M. R., Jordan, M. M., Perkins, W. J., et al.: Chemical inhibitors of phagosome-lysosome fusion in cultured macrophages also inhibit saltatory lysosomal movements. A combined microscopic and computer study. J. Exp. Med., 158:477, 1983.
37. Heyneman, R. A.: Inhibition by suramin of the NADPH oxidase from horse polymorphonuclear leukocytes. Vet. Res. Commun., 11:149, 1987.
38. Higashiyama, S., Abraham, J. A., Miller, J., Fiddes, J. C., and Klagsbrun, M.: A heparin binding growth factor secreted by macrophage cells that is related to EGF. Science, 251:936, 1991.
39. Holland, E. J., Stein, C. A., Palestine, A. G., LaRocca, R., Chan, C. C., Kuwabara, T., Myers, C. E., Thomas, R., McAtee, N., and Nussenblatt, R. N.: Suramin keratopathy. Am. J. Ophthalmol., 106:216, 1988.
40. Horne, M. K., 3rd, Stein, C. A., LaRocca, R. V., and Myers, C. E.: Circulating glycosaminoglycan anticoagulants associated with suramin treatment. Blood, 72:273, 1988.
41. Huang, S. S., and Huang, J. S.: Rapid turnover of the platelet-derived growth factor receptor in sis-transformed cells and reversal by suramin. Implications for the mechanism of autocrine transformation. J. Biol. Chem., 263:12608, 1988.
42. Ishihara, M., Fedarko, N. S., and Conrad, H. E.: Transport of heparan sulfate into the nuclei of hepatocytes. J. Biol. Chem., 261:13575, 1986.
43. Jodrell, D., Zuhowski, E., Egorin, M., Sinibaldi, V., Forrest, A., and Eisenberger, M.: Intermitent bolus dosing with suramin: The use of adaptive control with Feedback. (Abstract) Proc. Am. Soc. Clin. Oncol., 10:237, 1991.
44. Johnsson, A., Betsholtz, C., Heldin, C. H., and Westermark, B.: The phenotypic characteristics of simian sarcoma virus-transformed human fibroblasts suggest that the v-sis gene product acts solely as a PDGF receptor agonist in cell transformation. Embo. J., 5:1535, 1986.
45. Keating, M. T., Escobedo, J. A., Fantl, W. J., and Williams, L. T.: Ligand activation causes a phosphorylation-dependent change in platelet-derived growth factor receptor conformation. Trans. Assoc. Am. Physicians, 101:24, 1988.
46. Klagsbrun, M., and Shing, Y.: Heparin affinity of anionic and cationic capillary endothelial cell growth factors: analysis of hypothalamus-derived growth factors and fibroblast growth factors. Proc. Natl. Acad. Sci. USA, 82:805, 1985.
47. Klagsbrun, M.: The affinity of fibroblast growth factors (FGFs) for heparin; FGF-heparan sulfate interactions in cells and extracellular matrix. Curr. Opin. Cell Biol., 2:857, 1990.
48. Kopp, R., and Pfeiffer, A.: Suramin alters phosphoinositide synthesis and inhibits growth factor receptor binding in HT-29 cells. Cancer Res., 50:6490, 1990.
49. Kovesdi, I., Fairhurst, J. L., Kretschmer, P. J., and Bohlem, P.: Heparin-binding neurotrophic factor and MK. Members of a new family of homologous, developmentally regulated proteins. Biochem. Biophys. Res. Commun., 172:850, 1990.
50. LaRocca, R. V., Myers, C. E., Stein, C. A., Cooper, M. R., and Uhrich, M.: Effect of Suramin in Patients with Refractory Nodular Lymphomas Requiring Systemic Therapy. (Abstract) Proc. Am. Soc. Clin. Oncol., 9:1041, 1990.
51. LaRocca, R. V., Cooper, M. R., Uhrich, M., Danesi, R., et al.: Use of suramin in treatment of prostatic carcinoma refractory to conventional hormonal manipulation. Urol. Clin. North. Am., 8:123, 1991.
52. Leblond, C. P., and Inoue, S.: Structure, composition, and assembly of basement membrane. Am. J. Anat., 185:367, 1989.
53. Li, Y. S., Milner, P. G., Chauhan, A. K., Watson, M. A., Hoffman, R. M., Kodner, C. M., Milbrandt, J., and Deuel, T. F.: Cloning and expression of a developmentally regulated protein that induces mitogenic and neurite outgrowth activity. Science, 250:1690, 1990.
54. Lieberman, R., Katzper, M., Cooper, M.: Nonmem Population Pharmacokinetic Analysis and Bayesian Forecasting During Suramin Therapy in Prostate Cancer: One-versus two compartment PK models. Proc. Ass. Clin. Oncol., 9:262, 1990.
55. Lim, R., Miller, J. F., and Zaheer, A.: Purification and characterization of glia maturation factor beta: A growth regulator for neurons and glia. Proc. Natl. Acad. Sci., 86:3901, 1989.
56. Lindahl, U.: Approaches to the synthesis of heparin. Haemostasis, 1:146, 1990.
57. Lindahl, U., Kusche, M., Lidholt, K., and Oscarsson, L G.: Biosynthesis of heparin and heparan sulfate. Ann. N. Y. Acad. Sci., 556:36, 1989.
58. Liu, S., Ewing, M. W., Anglard, P., Trahan, E., LaRocca, R. V., Myers, C. E., and Linehan, W. M.: The effect of suramin, tumor necrosis factor and interferon gamma on human prostate carcinoma. J. Urol., 145:389, 1991.
59. Marez, A., N'Guyen, T., Chevallier, B., et al.: Platelet derived growth factor is present in human placenta: purification from an industrially processed fraction. Biochemie, 69:125, 1987.
60. Marics, I., Adelaide, J., Raybaud, F., Mattei, M. G., Coulier, F., Planche, J., de Lapeyriere, O., and Birnbaum, D.: Characterization of the HST-related FGF-6 gene, a member of the fibroblast growth factor family. Oncogene, 4:335, 1989.
61. McCaffrey, T. A., Falcone, D. J., Brayton, C. F., Agarwal, L. A., Welt, F., and Weksler, B. B.: TGF-β activity is potentiated by heparin via dissociation of TGF-β-alpha 2 macroglobulin inactive complex. J. Cell Biol., 109:441, 1988.
62. Merenmies, J., and Rauvala, H.: Molecular cloning of the 18 kDa growth associated protein of developing brain. J. Biol. Chem., 265:16721, 1990.
63. Mills, G. B., Zhang, N., May, C., Hill, M., and Chung, A.: Suramin prevents binding of interleukin 2 to its cell surface receptor: A possible mechanism for immunosuppression. Cancer Res., 50:3036, 1990.
64. Milner, P. G., Li, Y. S., Hoffman, R. M., Kodner, C. M., Siegel, N. R., and Deuel, T. F.: A novel 17 kD heparin-binding growth factor (HBGF-8) in bovine uterus: Purification and N-terminal amino acid sequence. Biochem. Biophys. Res. Commun., 165:1096, 1989.
65. Mohan, S., Jennings, J. C., Linkhart, T. A., and Baylink, D. J.: Primary structure of human skeletal growth factor: Homology with IGF-II. Biochim. Biophys. Acta, 966:44, 1988.
66. Moscatelli, D., and Quarto, N.: Transformation of NIH 3T3 cells with basic fibroblast growth factor of the hst/K-fgf oncogene causes down regulation of the fibroblast growth factor receptor: reversal of morphological changes and restoration of receptor number by suramin. J. Cell Biol., 109:2519, 1989.
67. Mourey, L., Samama, J. P., Delarue, M., Choay, J., Lormeau, J. C., Petitou, M., and Moras, D.: Antithrombin III: Structural and functional aspects. Biochimie, 72:599, 1990.
68. Nakajima, M., DeChavigny, A., Johnson, C. E., Hamada, J., Stein, C. A., and Nicolson, G. L.: Suramin. A potent inhibitor of melanoma heparanase and invasion. J. Biol. Chem., 266:9661, 1991.
69. Olivier, S., Formento, P., Fischel, J. L., Etienne, M. C., and Milano, G.: Epidermal growth factor receptor expression and suramin cytotoxicity in vitro. Eur. J. Cancer, 26:867, 1990.
70. Osswald, H., and Youssef, M.: Suramin enhancement of the chemotherapeutic actions of cyclophosphamide or adriamycin of intramuscularly-implanted Ehrlich carcinoma. Cancer Lett., 6:337, 1979.
71. Peck, C. C., and Rodman, J. H.: Analysis of Pharmacokinetic Data for Individualizing Patient Dosage Regimens. *In* Applied Pharmacokinetics: The Principles of Therapeutic Drug Monitoring. Edited by W. E. Evans, J. J. Schentag, and W. J. Jusko. Vancouver, WA, Applied Therapeutics, 1986, p. 55.
72. Petitou, M., Lormeau, J. C., and Choay, J.: Chemical synthesis of glycosaminoglycans: New approaches to antithrombotic drugs. Nature, 350:30, 1991.
73. Ragazzi, M., Ferro, D. R., Perly, B., Sinay, P., Petitou, M., and Choay, J.: Conformation of the pentasaccharide corresponding to the binding site of heparin for antithrombin III. Carbohydr. Res., 195:169, 1990.
74. Ratner, N., Hong, D. M., Lieberman, M. A., Bunge, R. P., and Glaser, L.: The neuronal cell-surface molecule mitogenic for Schwann cells is a heparin-binding protein. Proc. Natl. Acad. Sci, USA, 895:6992, 1988.
75. Rees, S., Constantopoulos, G., and Brady, R.: The suramin-treated rat as a model of mucopolysaccharidosis: reversibility of biochemical and morphological changes in the liver. Virchows Arch. [b], 51:235, 1986.
76. Rees, S., Constantopoulos, G., and Brady, R. O.: The suramin-treated rat as a model of mucopolysaccharidosis. Variation in the reversibility of biochemical and morphological changes among different organs. Virchows Arch [b], 52:259, 1986.
77. Regeleson, W.: The Biologic Activity of Polyanions: Past History and New Prospectives. J. Polymer Sci, 1979:483, 1979.
78. Regelson, W.: The Antimitotic Activity of Polyanions. Adv. In Chemother, 3:303, 1968.
79. Roberts, R., Gallagher, J., Spooncer, E., Allen, T. D., Bloomfield, F., and Dexter, T. M.: Heparan sulfate bound growth factors: A mechanism for stromal cell mediated hematopoiesis. Nature, 332:376, 1988.
80. Rosenberg, R. D.: Biochemistry of heparin antithrombin interactions, and the physiologic role of this natural anticoagulant mechanism. Am. J. Med., 87:25, 1989.
81. Shaklee, P. N., Glaser, J. H., and Conrad, H. E.: A sulfatase specific for glucuronic acid 2-sulfate residues in glycosaminoglycans. J. Biol. Chem., 260:9146, 1985.

82. Shore, J. D., Olson, S. T., Craig, P. A., Choay, J., and Bjork, I.: Kinetics of heparin action. Ann. N. Y. Acad. Sci., 556:75, 1989.

83. Shoyab, M., Plowman, G. D., McDonald, V. L., Bradley, J. G., and Todaro, G. J.: Structure and function of human amphiregulin. A member of the EGF family. Science, 243:1074, 1989.

84. Sipka, S., Danko, K., Nagy, P., Taskov, V., Denes, L., Czirjak, L., and Szegedi, G.: Effects of suramin on phagocytes in vitro. Ann. Hematol., 63:45, 1991.

85. Spigelman, Z., Dowers, A., Kennedy, S., DiSorbo, D., et al.: Antiproliferative effects of suramin on lymphoid cells. Cancer Res., 47:4694, 1987.

86. Sporn, M. B., and Todaro, G. J.: Autocrine secretion and malignant transformation of cells. N. Engl. J. Med., 303:878, 1980.

87. Stein, C. A., LaRocca, R. V., Thomas, R., McAtee, N., and Myers, C. E.: Suramin: An anticancer drug with a unique mechanism of action. J. Clin. Oncol., 7:499, 1989.

88. Tezuka, K., Takeshita, S., Hakeda, Y., Kumegawa, M., Kikuno, R., and Hashimoto-Gotoh, T.: Isolation of mouse and human cDNA clones encoding a protein expressed specifcally in osteoblasts and brain tissue. Biochem. Biophys. Res. Commun., 173:246, 1990.

89. Toshkov, A., Neychev, H., and Dimov, V.: Suramin increases the nonspecific anti-bacterial resistance through macrophage activation. Acta. Microbiol. Bulg., 19:13, 1986.

90. Tsutsui, J., Uehara, K., Kadomatsu, K.: A new family of heparin-binding factors: strong conservation of midkine (MK) sequences between the human and the mouse. Biochem. Biophys. Res. Commun., 176:792, 1990.

91. Vlodavsky, I., Fuks, Z., Ishai-Michaeli, R., Bashkin, P., Levi, E., Korner, G., Bar-Shavit, R., and Klagsbrun, M.: Extracellular matrix-resident basic fibroblast growth factor: Implication for the control of angiogenesis. J. Cell Biochem., 45:167, 1991.

92. Vlodavsky, I., Korner, G., Ishai, M. R., Bashkin, P.: Extracellular matrix-resident growth factors and enzymes: Possible involvement in tumor metastasis and angiogenesis. Cancer Metastasis Rev., 9:203, 1990.

93. Walz, T. M., Abdiu, A., Wingren, S., Smeds, S., Larsson, S. E., and Wasteson, A.: Suramin inhibits growth of human osteosarcoma xenografts in nude mice. Cancer Res., 51:3585, 1991.

94. Warr, G. A., and Jakab, G. J.: Lung macrophage defense responses during suramin-induced lysosomal dysfunction. Exp. Mol. Pathol., 38:193, 1983.

95. Wellstein, A., Zugmaier, G., Califano, J. A., 3rd., Kern, F., Paik, S., and Lippman, M. E.: Tumor growth dependent on Kaposi's sarcoma-derived fibroblast growth factor inhibited by pentosan polysulfate. J. Natl. Cancer Inst., 83:716, 1991.

96. Westermark, B., and Heldin, C. H.: Platelet-derived growth factor as a mediator of normal and neoplastic cell proliferation. Med. Oncol. Tumor Pharmacother., 3:177, 1986.

97. Williams, L. T., Tremble, P. M., Lavin, M. F., and Sunday, M. E.: Platelet-derived growth factor receptors from a high affinity state in membrane preparations. Kinetics and affinity cross-linking studies. J. Biol. Chem., 259:5287, 1984.

98. Wolpe, S. D., and Cerami, A.: Macrophage inflammatory proteins 1 and 2: Members of a novel superfamily of cytokines. FASEB J., 3:2565, 1989.

99. Wright, T. C., Jr., Castellot, J. J., Jr., Petitou, M., Lormeau, J. C., and Karnovsky, M. J.: Structural determinants of heparin's growth inhibitory activity. Interdependence of oligosaccharide size and charge. J. Biol. Chem., 264:1534, 1989.

100. Yayon, A., Klagsbrun, M., Esco, J. D., Leder, P., and Ornitz, D. M.: Cell surface heparin-like molecules are required for binding of basic fibroblast growth factor to its high affinity receptor. Cell, 64:841, 1991.

101. Zabrenetzky, V. S., Kohn, E. C., and Roberts, D. D.: Suramin inhibits laminin- and thrombospondin-mediated melanoma cell adhesion and migration and binding of these adhesive proteins to sulfatide. Cancer Res., 50:5937, 1990.

102. Zack, J., Smith, R. G., Ozanne, B.: Characterization of a leukemia-derived transforming growth factor. 1:737, 1987.

103. Zhan, X., Bates, B., Hu, X. G., and Goldfarb, M.: The human FGF-5 oncogene encodes a novel protein related to fibroblast growth factor. Mol. Cell. Biol., 88:3487, 1988.

XVII

Principles of Endocrine Therapy

XVII-1

Steroid Hormone Binding and Hormone Receptors

Elwood V. Jensen
Eugene R. DeSombre

Introduction

It has long been recognized that some human cancers are "hormone-dependent" in that their growth is influenced by variations in levels of steroid sex hormones, and they undergo regression after removal of glands producing these supporting agents. In the case of breast cancer, as early as 1836 Cooper observed a correlation between tumor growth and the menstrual cycle,[20] and in 1896 Beatson reported the regression of metastatic lesions after oophorectomy in some premenopausal patients.[8] For postmenopausal women, where breast cancer occurs most frequently, Huggins and Bergenstal demonstrated in 1952 that excision of the adrenal glands can provide significant remission of metastatic disease;[48] shortly thereafter Luft and Olivecrona obtained similar regression after hypophysectomy.[72] For prostatic cancer, Huggins and Hodges reported in 1941 that most patients with advanced disease show striking remissions after orchiectomy or administration of estrogenic hormones.[49]

Hormone deprivation, by the surgical ablation of steroidogenic glands, or alteration of the endocrine milieu, by administration of hormones, hormone antagonists or inhibitors of hormone biosynthesis, provides effective palliative treatment for patients whose metastatic tumors are of the hormone-dependent type. In contrast to prostatic cancer, in which the majority of tumors respond to endocrine therapy, less than one-third of the patients with advanced breast cancer show objective remission to hormonal manipulation. Thus, there has been need for some means to predict which breast tumors are hormone-dependent, so that endocrine therapy can be restricted to those persons it can help, and patients with non-dependent tumors can be placed directly on other treatments.

Recognition that steroid sex hormones exert their actions in so-called target tissues in combination with intracellular receptor proteins, and that non-target tissues generally contain only small amounts of such receptors, offered an approach to predicting hormone dependency in breast cancers.[50] In the early 1970s, it was reported that determination of the estrogen receptor content of an excised specimen of a primary or metastatic tumor predicts the likelihood of response to endocrine therapy for the majority of breast cancer patients.[29,51,68,73] Tumors with estrogen receptors were then shown to have a better chance of response if they also contain progestin receptors.[46] It was also found that the receptor content of a primary breast cancer is a valuable indicator of the risk of cancer recurrence in mastectomy patients with no evident metastases.[63,109] Thus, determination of estrogen and progestin receptors in primary and metastatic breast cancers, as a guide to prognosis and therapy selection, has become standard medical practice.[25] There is also a relation between the presence of estrogen receptors in the primary tumor and the site where the first metastases are likely to appear.[102]

Receptor Proteins in Steroid Hormone Action

During the three decades since the discovery of steroid hormone receptors, much progress has been made toward an understanding of the nature of receptor proteins and of their role in the action of these hormones in target cells.[7,12,94,112] Receptor proteins were first discovered for the estrogens by the ability of target tissues, especially the rodent uterus, to take up and bind labeled estradiol without chemical alteration of the steroid itself.[52] Similar binding studies, both in vivo and in vitro, soon established the presence of specific receptors in target tissues for all classes of steroid hormones.[36,69] Unlike receptors for peptide hormones, which are located in the cell membrane and require a second messenger to transmit the regulatory signal to the eventual site of action, receptors for steroid hormones reside within the target cell. Here they are loosely held until association with the hormone converts them to a form that can bind tightly in the genome to stimulate RNA synthesis.

During recent years, techniques of molecular biology and immunology have provided detailed knowledge about receptor structure and function.[31,53,66] Cloning of the cDNAs for various steroid hormone receptors has led to elucidation of their primary structures. With the aid of deletion mutants, individual domains in the molecule have been identified and correlated with different aspects of receptor function. Steroid receptors belong to a general family of intracellular proteins

815

that mediate the actions of many important cell regulators, including the gonadal and adrenal hormones (Figure XVII-1-1), vitamin D, ecdysone, thyroid hormone, and retinoic acid.[86] Although these receptor proteins vary in size from 427 amino acids for vitamin D to 984 for mineralocorticoid, corresponding to molecular weights of 47.5–107 KDa, they are composed of comparable units. Each contains a DNA-binding domain of 66–68 amino acids (C), showing a high degree of homology throughout the family, a ligand-binding domain (E) with some homology, a small hinge region (D) joining these two domains, and variable regions (A/B, F) showing little homology. Avian and human progestin receptors are unique in that they come in two sizes; the B form consists of the A protein plus an additional unit at the N-terminus. Through a pair of zinc fingers in the C-region, the steroid-receptor complex, in dimeric form, binds to a hormone response element (HRE), located upstream from the transcription site, to enhance RNA synthesis in target genes.

The hormone-induced conversion of the native receptor protein to a functional transcription factor has been the subject of much investigation,[40] for this concept of receptor transformation[54] identified, for the first time, a biochemical role for the steroid. It is now established that transformation involves the removal of a dimeric heat shock protein that obscures the DNA-binding region in the native receptor, as well as of other macromolecular and micromolecular factors that participate in this association.[40,53,92] Just how the interaction with steroid hormone effects this disaggregation within the cell is not clear, nor is the precise mechanism by which transformed receptor enhances transcription in target genes at a site distant from the hormone response element.

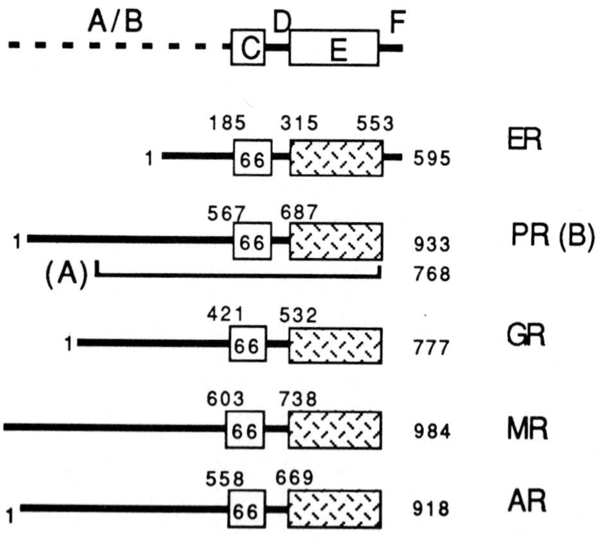

Figure XVII-1-1. Structures of human receptor proteins for gonadal and adrenal hormones. The top diagram shows the six functional domains: A/B, F, modulating regions; C, DNA-binding region; D, "hinge" region; E, hormone-binding region. Boxes indicate highly conserved domains; thin black lines are regions of low homology. The position of each domain boundary is given as the number of amino acids from the amino terminus (left). For these receptors the C-domain contains 66 amino acids. Receptors are: ER, estrogen; PR, progestin (A and B forms); GR, glucocorticoid; MR, mineralocorticoid; AR, androgen.

Measurement of Estrogen and Progestin Receptors

Steroid Binding Methods

The first correlations of receptors with breast cancer response to endocrine therapy involved the uptake of radioactive hormone by tumor tissue after administration of tritiated hexestrol to patients,[34] or on incubation of excised tumor slices with tritiated estradiol at 37°C, in the presence and absence of either excess unlabeled hormone or an antiestrogen, to distinguish between specific and nonspecific binding.[51,58] When it was found that, before exposure to hormone, the receptor in target cells is not tightly held and appears in the high speed supernatant (cytosol) fraction of tissue homogenates, this protein could be measured conveniently by adding excess tritiated estradiol to tumor cytosol and counting the radioactivity bound to the receptor.

Several procedures have been developed for distinguishing between receptor-bound steroid and the excess unbound hormone. These include the identification of the steroid-receptor complex by ultracentrifugation (sedimentation) in sucrose gradients,[51,55] or by electrophoresis[107] or isoelectric focusing[111] on gels; the precipitation of the complex with protamine sulfate[14] or adsorption on hydroxylapatite;[35,45] and the removal of unbound hormone by adsorption on Dextran-coated charcoal (DCC)[65] or immobilized antibody to the steroid.[13,33] Each of these techniques has advantages and drawbacks.

Many of the earlier measurements of receptors in breast cancers were done with the sedimentation technique. This procedure, while informative, is too costly and time consuming to be employed for routine assays. Moreover, the values as originally obtained, though self-consistent, did not indicate directly the total binding capacity of the cytosol, although they can be readily corrected to provide this value.[55] As receptor assays were undertaken on a larger scale, most laboratories adopted the Dextran-coated charcoal (DCC) method to remove unbound hormone. Because DCC causes some dissociation of steroid from the receptor, the preferred technique involves incubating cytosol aliquots with several hormone concentrations, in each case plotting the ratio of bound to free steroid against the amount bound, according to the method of Scatchard (Figure XVII-1-2).[99] The intercept of the straight line plot with the abscissa gives the total binding capacity, and the reciprocal of the slope indicates the dissociation constant of the complex, thus distinguishing high affinity binding to receptor from any weaker, nonspecific binding. Scatchard plots are also used in the hydroxylapatite assay. A disadvantage of these titration procedures is that they often require a larger tumor specimen than is available, especially with metastatic cancers. For such cases, a single high concentration of hormone can be employed, although such saturation assays are less accurate or informative than are multipoint determinations.

In general, the foregoing assay procedures were developed for estrogen receptors, but many of them have been extended to the measurement of progestin receptors as well. For the most part, progestin receptors have been determined by the DCC technique, and to a lesser extent by sedimentation in sucrose gradients where the progesterone-receptor complex is somewhat less stable than that of the estrogen receptor.

All steroid-binding procedures suffer from two inherent

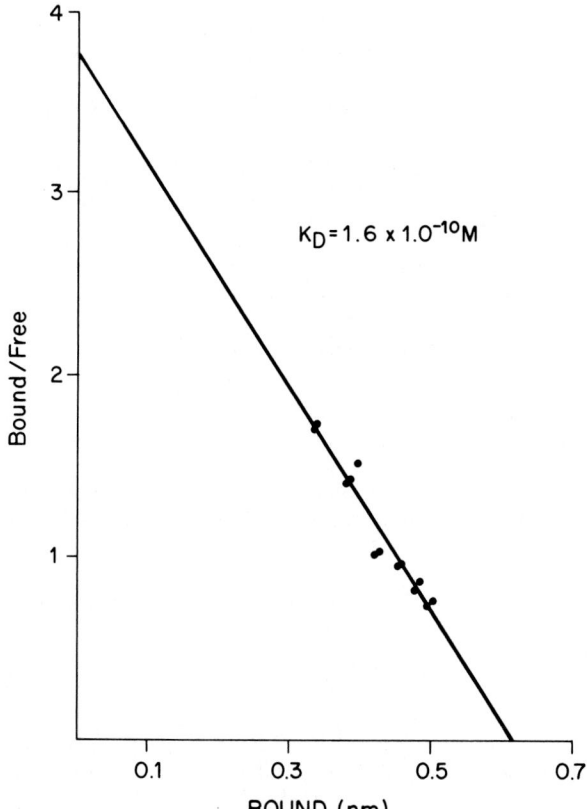

$$K_D = 1.6 \times 1.0^{-10} M$$

Figure XVII-1-2. Scatchard plot of the binding of tritiated estradiol to receptors in cytosol of hormone-dependent rat mammary tumor. Aliquots of cytosol were incubated for 16 hours at 2°C with various concentrations of tritiated estradiol (0.2 to 1.0 nM). After treatment with Dextran-coated charcoal and centrifugation at 2°C to remove unbound (free) steroid, the macromolecularly bound estradiol remaining in each supernatant was determined by scintillation counting. The amount of free estradiol is the difference between the total and the bound steroid in each mixture. The receptor capacity is 0.62 nmoles.

disadvantages; 1) steroid hormone receptors are labile proteins that easily lose binding capacity during storage and processing of the tumor specimen, and 2) unless some kind of ligand-exchange procedure is included, they do not detect receptor that is already occupied by endogenous hormone or by endocrine agents used in therapy. Binding loss can be minimized by rapidly cooling the specimen after excision, storage at −80°C or below, pulverization of the specimen in liquid nitrogen, and homogenizing briefly in a Polytron apparatus, with efficient cooling, in medium containing traces of sulfhydryl compounds to protect against heavy metals. Although techniques for exchanging endogenous ligand have been developed, these can lead to some loss of binding capacity, and they introduce an additional step in the assay procedure.

Immunochemical Methods

With the availability of monoclonal antibodies to human estrogen[37] and progestin[30,38] receptors, it became possible to utilize the techniques of immunochemistry and immunocytochemistry for measuring these proteins in breast cancers. Because these antibodies recognize occupied as well as unoccupied receptor, and, in some instances, receptor

that has lost ability to bind steroid, immunochemical methods overcome many of the difficulties inherent in binding techniques, and they eliminate the use of radioactivity. Two types of immunochemical analyses have been developed: a sandwich-type enzyme immunoassay (EIA),[56,84] for measuring receptor in tumor cytosols, and an immunocytochemical assay (ICA),[56,61] that detects receptor in individual cells of a tumor section or fine needle aspirate. Kits for both types of analyses are now available from Abbott Laboratories and are widely used throughout the world. Early experience with the use of these immunoassays for estrogen receptor is summarized in a supplemental issue of Cancer Research,[93] whereas immunocytochemical assay for estrogen and progestin receptors is discussed in detail in a recent monograph.[88]

In the enzyme immunoassay for estrogen and progestin receptors in tumor cytosol, one monoclonal antibody,* bound to a polystyrene bead, adsorbs the receptor from the diluted cytosol (Figure XVII-1-3). The immobilized receptor is then treated with a second monoclonal antibody, which binds to a different region of the receptor molecule and is linked to an enzyme (horseradish peroxidase) that gives rise to a yellow color when exposed to substrate (hydrogen peroxide plus o-phenylenediamine). The color intensity is read in a colorimeter, and the receptor content of the cytosol calculated from a standard curve obtained with lyophylized cytosol from MCF-7 breast tumor cells for estrogen receptor and from T47D cells for progestin receptor. The steroid-binding capacity of each reference standard is originally determined by DCC assay. Because the cytosol can be diluted extensively, analyses can be carried out with very small tumor samples, even with fine needle aspiration biopsies.[75] Immunoassay can be carried out on specimens from patients receiving tamoxifen therapy, where steroid-binding techniques usually fail to detect receptor.[75]

The immunocytochemical assays employ the peroxidase-

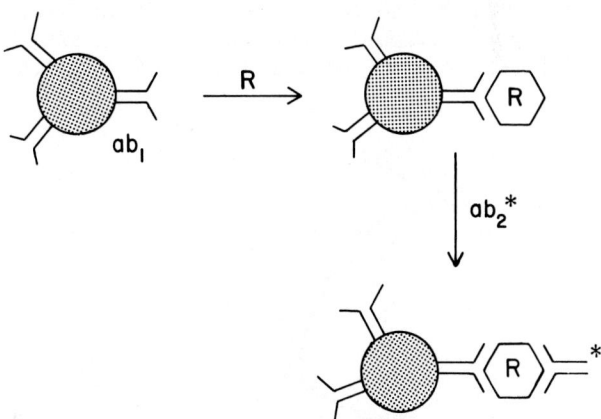

Figure XVII-1-3. System for the immunochemical determination of receptors. A polystyrene bead, coated with one monoclonal antibody preparation, adsorbs the receptor (R, occupied or unoccupied) from the diluted cytosol. The receptor thus bound adsorbs a second monoclonal antibody that has been labeled with an enzyme(*) that serves as the basis for a colorimetric assay. From Greene et al.[39]

*In the original Abbott EIA for estrogen receptor,[84] antibody D547[37] was used to adsorb the receptor, and D75 served as the enzyme-labeled reagent; more recently, D75 has been replaced by H222[39,56] as the labeled antibody. In the EIA for progestin receptor, antibodies KD68 and JZB39[38] are used as the anchor and label, respectively.

antiperoxidase method of Sternberger, in which frozen tumor sections, after gentle fixation, are treated, first with an anti-receptor antibody, then with a bridging antibody (goat anti-rat immunoglobulin), and finally with peroxidase-antiperoxidase (PAP) reagent.[104] Subsequent treatment with hydrogen peroxide and p-diaminobenzidine produces a brown stain in the nuclei of cells where the receptor has retained the antibody and, thereby, the PAP reagent (Figure XVII-1-4). Abbott immunocytochemical assays for estrogen (ERICA) and progestin (PRICA) receptors use antibodies H222 and KD68, respectively. Counterstaining is with hematoxylin to delineate cell nuclei (XVII-1-Plates 1 and 2).

Because immunocytochemical procedures detect receptors in individual cells, they can be used with very small tumor sections or fine needle aspiration biopsies of either tumor[11,41,77,110] or bone marrow.[9] For estrogen receptor, the ICA technique is most dependable and sensitive with frozen sections of tumors, although it has been used successfully with paraffin-embedded specimens if the tissue is fixed in a special way with cold buffered formalin[100] or Bouin's solution.[24,91] Specimens fixed in formalin in the usual way often yield erratic results, so that negative staining patterns are of questionable significance. However, subjecting the section to enzymatic digestion with trypsin,[4,44] pronase,[16] or DNase[101] permits the use of conventionally fixed tissues and thus the assay of archival samples of breast cancers. In contrast, ICA analysis of progestin receptor is reported to work well with embedded specimens without the need for special fixation procedures.[83] With embedded specimens, monoclonal antibody D75 appears to be especially favorable with estrogen receptor and KD68 with progestin receptor.

In attempts to quantify the results of immunocytochemistry, staining descriptions have been proposed that consider both the proportion of receptor-containing cells and the degree of staining. These include the H-Score[76] and the staining intensity index (SII),[78] in which individual cells are assigned to different staining categories and the percentage of cells in each group, multiplied by an intensity factor, is totaled. Such characterization of tumors has proved quite successful

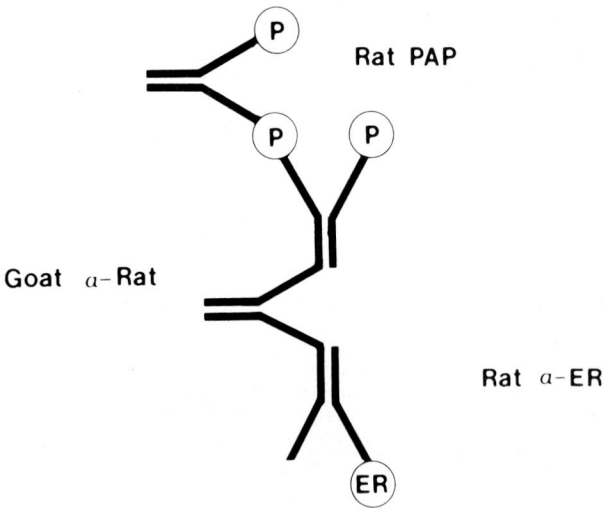

Figure XVII-1-4. Schematic representation of the immunocytochemical assay for estrogen receptor (ERICA), using goat anti-rat immunoglobulin as a bridge between the monoclonal antibody to ER and the rat peroxidase/antiperoxidase reagent (P).

in predicting prognosis for recurrence and response to therapy. More recent developments, involving use of automated optical instrumentation, are the SAMBA computerized image analysis[15,19] and the receptogram,[88,103] each of which yields characteristic patterns derived from a combination of receptor concentration (measured optical density, MOD) and receptor content (integrated optical density, IOD) of individual tumor cells.

Receptors and Response to Endocrine Therapy

Estrogen Receptors (ER)

The rationale of estrogen receptor determination to identify hormone-dependent breast cancers originated in the observations of uptake and binding of tritiated estrogens by female reproductive tissues of experimental animals, and the subsequent realization that steroid hormones require receptor proteins to exert their biological actions. Early studies demonstrated that, when injected with tritiated hexestrol, patients who then responded favorably to adrenalectomy incorporated more radioactivity into their tumors than those who did not respond.[34] With the advent of techniques for determining estrogen binding by tissues in vitro, and then by receptor in the cytosol fraction of tissue homogenates, it became possible to examine excised specimens of breast cancers for the correlation of receptor levels with clinical response. Four early reports established that patients whose tumors lack detectable ER rarely respond either to endocrine ablation or to hormone administration (3/71 = 4%), whereas most patients with ER-containing cancers (42/49 = 86%) benefit from such treatment.[29,51,68,73] In 1974, investigators from 14 groups in various countries reported similar findings at a workshop sponsored by the Breast Cancer Task Force of the U.S. National Cancer Institute.[79] Despite the variety of procedures used for determining estrogen binding, the conclusions were in substantial agreement: about 60% of patients with ER-positive cancers showed objective remission to some type of endocrine therapy, as compared to fewer than 10% of those with ER-negative tumors.

As methods for the measurement of receptor proteins became more sensitive, it was evident that most breast cancers contain small amounts of estrogen receptor. However the tumors with lower receptor content rarely respond to endocrine therapy, so that quantitative ER levels are important.[26,55,57,67,85,87] For example, of 160 treated patients studied from 1966–1976 at the University of Chicago,[27] very few objective remissions (4%) were observed in those whose tumors contained less than a certain amount of receptor (Figure XVII-1-5). This critical level appears to be lower in premenopausal patients, either because some of the receptor is occupied by endogenous hormone and is not detected by binding assay or because the actual production of receptor may be reduced in the presence of higher serum levels of hormone.[42] Because tumors with lower receptor content rarely respond to endocrine manipulation, it is advantageous to classify patients as "receptor-rich" or "receptor-poor," rather than positive or negative. If the low receptor cancers are transferred from the positive category to the ER-poor group, the remaining ER-rich cancers show a response rate to endocrine ablation of 71% as compared with 3% in the ER-poor group.[27]

When determination of estrogen receptors in breast can-

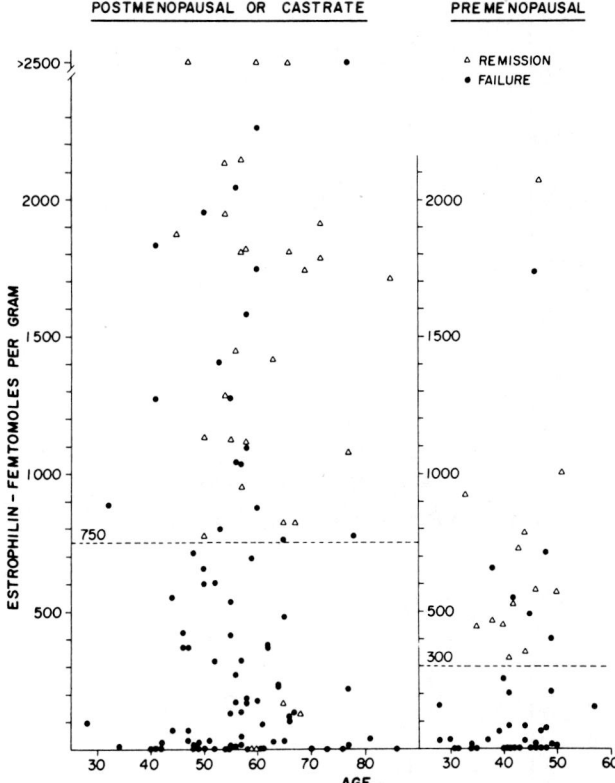

POSTMENOPAUSAL OR CASTRATE   PREMENOPAUSAL

△ REMISSION
● FAILURE

Figure XVII-1-5. Correlation of cytosol ER content with objective remissions to endocrine therapy for 160 patients with metastatic breast cancer. Assays were carried out by sucrose gradient ultracentrifugation using non-saturating concentrations of tritiated estradiol. When receptor values are corrected to saturation,[55] the division between receptor-rich and receptor-poor tumors occurs at about 2.5 pmoles per gram tumor for postmenopausal patients and 1.0 pmole/g for premenopausal. Considering the amounts of protein usually found in breast tumor cytosols, these results suggest that for postmenopausal patients the optimal dividing level is at least 50 fmole ER per mg cytosol protein. From DeSombre et al.[27]

cers became a routine clinical procedure, the correlations with patient response generally were not as favorable as those just described or those in the original reports. A somewhat higher proportion of patients with ER-negative tumors were found to respond to endocrine therapy, probably because assays carried out in central laboratories on specimens sent in from different sources provide more chance for the labile receptor protein to lose its binding capacity during tissue collection, storage and processing. The lower response rate among the so-called positive tumors (often quoted as 50% or less) is due at least in part to the way positivity has been defined. For reasons more of convenience than of scientific merit, receptor content is expressed in relation to total cytosol protein, a parameter that varies with the serum content of the tumor. Despite evidence that breast cancers with low receptor levels rarely respond to endocrine therapy, tumors originally were considered to be ER-positive if they contain at least 3 fmole of receptor per milligram of cytosol protein, about the level of detectability. With this definition, many investigators found that 70–80% of breast cancers were called ER-positive, not a very useful criterion in attempting to predict which patients will respond

to a treatment known to benefit fewer than 35% of the total. Accordingly some groups readjusted the dividing value, first to 10 fmole/mg cytosol protein and later to 20 and even 30 fmole. This is an improvement, although the data in Figure XVII-1-5 suggest that a more appropriate value would be even higher, at least in postmenopausal patients. Of more than 1,300 breast cancers analyzed at the University of Chicago, about two-thirds had detectable estrogen receptor, but only 35% contained sufficient amounts to be classified as ER-rich.

No matter what the optimal cut-off level should be, it is apparent that some cancers with high receptor content still do not respond to hormonal manipulation.[74] Explanations include the possibility that the receptor protein in these tumors binds hormone but is otherwise non-functional, that tumor cells may escape from hormone dependency without shutting down receptor synthesis (this appears to be the case in some autonomous rat mammary tumors[6]), or that the cancer is a mixture of hormone-dependent and autonomous cells, with the former responsible for a positive receptor assay but the latter precluding a significant response to endocrine therapy. Both by multiple sampling[22,106] and by immunocytochemistry[56,61] (XVII-1-Plates 1 and 2) it has been found that many, if not most, breast cancers are heterogeneous, showing both ER-containing and non-containing cells. A good response may be observed only with tumors in which the proportion of ER-containing cells is so great that their regression following endocrine treatment results in a significant remission of the overall cancer.

The immunocytochemical procedure for determining steroid receptors in tumor specimens not only has the advantage of being applicable to small tissue samples, but, by identifying receptor in individual cells, it gives a valuable indication of the relative proportion of ER-positive and ER-negative cells in the tumor. The presence of a high proportion of negative cells is associated with poor prognosis.[108] When semi-quantitative criteria for distinguishing between positive and negative tumors are employed, ICA appears to be somewhat superior to biochemical methods,[78,89] giving response rates 72 or 80% in the ER-positive group as compared to 4 or 8%, respectively, in those with low staining indices. In 336 patients studied in nine different laboratories, the overall response rate in the ER-positive group was 74% by ERICA, as compared to 65% by DCC assay.[3] Included in this summary are results obtained with fine needle aspiration biopsy.[9,11]

Because many patients with advanced breast cancer do not have readily accessible metastatic lesions for analysis, it was of interest to determine whether ER determination on the primary tumor at the time of mastectomy could predict response to endocrine therapy if the cancer recurs in disseminated form. Early studies indicated that metastases generally resemble the primary cancer in their receptor content, and that the mastectomy specimen can be used for prediction of response to therapy at a later time.[10,26,85] These conclusions have been confirmed by many investigators, and analysis of primary tumors at the time of mastectomy is done routinely.

Early studies on patients being treated with cytotoxic chemotherapy suggested that those with ER-negative breast cancers may respond more favorably to chemotherapy than do those with ER-positive cancers.[70,71] Although some laboratories reported similar findings, which are consistent with the impression that ER-negative tumors are more aggressive, less differentiated, and more rapidly growing, most workers could not confirm these observations. Not only did several investigators find no correlation of receptor status with response to chemotherapy,[43,59,95,96] but others actually observed a higher response rate among the ER-positive group.[21,60,98] The significance of some of these studies is limited by their use of either 3 or 5 fmoles/mg protein as the definition of an ER-positive tumor, but others employed more reasonable criteria, so one must conclude that an inverse relation between ER positivity and response to cytotoxic chemotherapy has not been established.

Progestin Receptors (PR)

Since the failure of some ER-containing breast cancers to respond to endocrine treatment might result from the receptor being non-functional, it was proposed that progestin receptor, known to be produced by estrogen action in many female reproductive tissues, might serve as a measure of functional estrogen receptor.[46] It was found that breast cancers containing both estrogen and progestin receptors show a higher response rate (81%) than those having ER alone (41%).[80] Similar findings have been reported from many laboratories.[80,81,85] In most of these studies, the ER-positive category has included receptor-poor cancers, which do not respond, so part of the effect may result from the fact that PR-positive tumors in general are those which also have a higher ER content. Nonetheless, the determination of PR in addition to ER appears to be of value, and analysis of both receptors is generally recommended.[25]

Receptors and Prognosis for Cancer Recurrence

The observation that mastectomy patients with ER-positive primary tumors show a lower incidence of recurrence of advanced disease, and a longer disease-free interval if they do recur, opened a new dimension in the application of hormone receptor analyses to the clinical management of breast cancer (Figure XVII-1-6).[63,109] This prognostic criterion appears to be independent of tumor size or nodal status and permits the classification of patients into four groups as to the risk of recurrence: low (ER-positive, node-negative), intermediate (ER-negative, node-negative; ER-positive, node-positive), and high (ER-negative, node-positive).[17,28] This information is of value in the choice of adjuvant or prophylactic therapy after mastectomy. Patients in the high-risk group can justifiably be treated aggressively with cytotoxic chemotherapy, while those in the low-risk group can be spared this discomfort and receive either no treatment or a nontraumatic endocrine therapy, such as tamoxifen. The presence of progesterone receptors was also found to predict disease-free survival and may be superior to estrogen receptor,[90] especially with stage II primary cancers.[18,81]

Although a relation between the presence of ER and/or PR and the duration of the disease-free interval has been observed in many laboratories,[17,18] other investigators failed to confirm these findings,[2,23,32,47,97] while others concluded that only ER and not PR is of prognostic value.[105] It has also been observed that differences in disease-free survival, observed during the first few years after mastectomy, disappear after a longer time.[1] Thus, there has been some

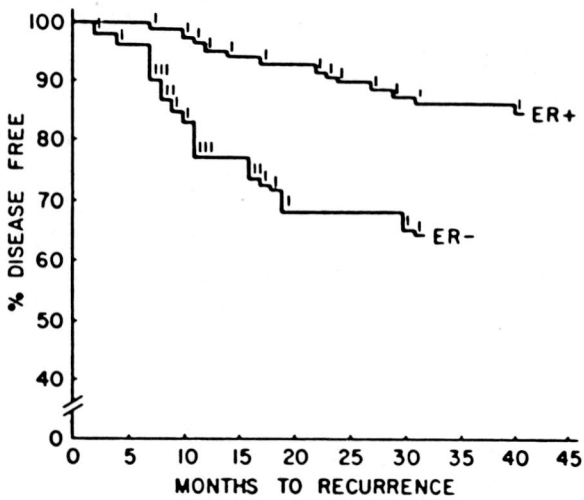

Chart 1. ER and recurrence in all patients.

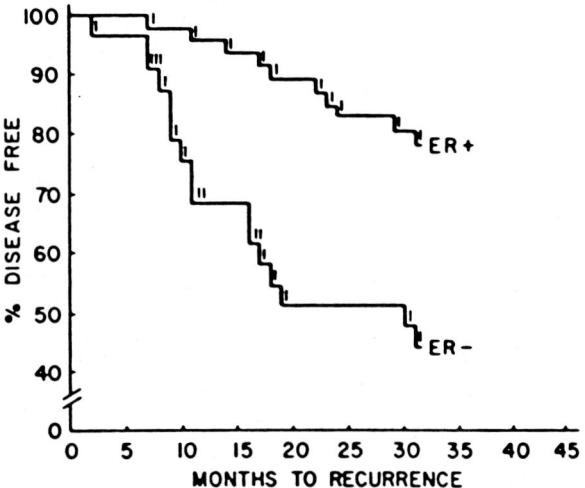

Chart 2. ER and recurrence in axillary node-positive patients.

Figure XVII-1-6. Relation of ER status of the primary tumor to the time of appearance of first metastases after mastectomy. Chart 1: 145 patients irrespective of nodal involvement. Chart 2: 74 patients with one or more positive axillary nodes. ER negative = <10 fmole/mg cytosol protein by DCC assay. From Knight et al.[63]

controversy over the value of receptor assays in the prognostication for cancer recurrence. It has been suggested that, for the best prediction now available, one should consider a combination of receptor content with other parameters, such as nuclear grade, tumor size, and ploidy.[82]

As in the case of response to therapy, the usefulness of biochemical receptor assays for prognostic information has been hampered by arbitrary definitions of positive and negative tumors and by the fact that most cancers are mixtures of receptor-containing and non-containing cells. With immunocytochemical procedures, which consider both the staining intensity and the number of cells stained, the prognostic value of receptor determinations appears to be greatly enhanced. The ERICA procedure was found to be equivalent,[5,28] or superior,[3,62] to biochemical ER determination, and after a five-year observation period, the ICA, but not the DCC

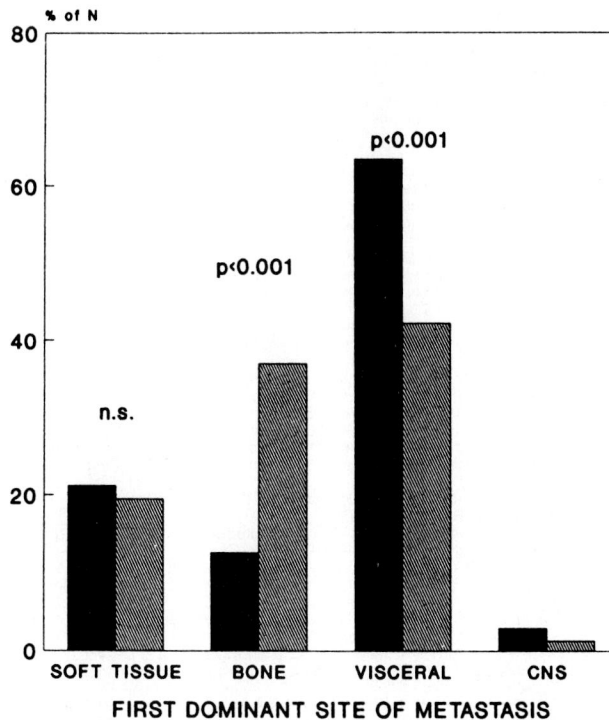

% of N

p<0.001

p<0.001

n.s.

FIRST DOMINANT SITE OF METASTASIS

SOFT TISSUE   BONE   VISCERAL   CNS

■ ER-NEGATIVE n=104   ▨ ER-POSITIVE n=154

Figure XVII-1-7. The location of first metastases in relation to the estrogen receptor status of the primary breast cancer. ER negative = <10 fmole/mg cytosol protein by DCC assay. From Koenders et al.[64]

assay, was still able to distinguish between higher and lower risk groups.[62] In these studies, ER rather than PR had the highest prognostic significance.

Receptors and Site of First Metastases

Not only do estrogen and progestin receptor assays on primary breast cancers furnish useful information about the prognosis for recurrence and the response of metastases to endocrine therapy, but they also provide a clue as to the most probable location where the first metastases will appear. The early observation that ER-positive primary tumors show a greater tendency to spread to bone, and ER-negative cancers to lung and liver,[102,109] has been widely confirmed,[64] with only a few dissenting reports. Although both estrogen and progestin receptors show similar patterns, ER appears to be the only independent prognostic factor for this phenomenon (Figure XVII-1-7).

Summary

Determination of estrogen and progestin receptors in excised breast cancer tissue provides information concerning the response of the patient to endocrine therapy, the risk of recurrence of advanced disease, and the probable site of first metastases. Such assays have been of considerable value, but their usefulness has been limited by the lability of the steroid-binding capacity of the receptor, the heterogeneity of many tumor specimens, and the use of less than

optimal definition of receptor positivity. Recent development of immunochemical receptor assays, and especially of immunocytochemical techniques that identify receptor with individual cancer cells, promises to overcome many of these deficiencies and to enhance the utility of receptor measurements in the clinical management of breast cancer patients.

References

1. Aamdal, S., Børmer, O., Jørgensen, O., Høst, H., Eliassen, G., Kaalhus, O., and Pihl, A.: Estrogen receptors and long-term prognosis in breast cancer. Cancer, 53:2525, 1984.
2. Alanko, A., Heinonen, E., Scheinin, T., Tolppanen, E.-M., and Vihko, R.: Significance of estrogen and progesterone receptors, disease-free interval, and site of first metastasis on survival of breast cancer patients. Cancer, 56:1696, 1985.
3. Allred, D. C., Bustamante, M. A., Daniel, C. O., Gaskill, H. V., and Cruz, A. B., Jr.: Immunocytochemical analysis of estrogen receptors in human breast carcinomas. Arch. Surg., 125:107, 1990.
4. Andersen, J., Ørntoft, T. F., and Poulsen, H. S.: Immnohistochemical demonstration of estrogen receptors (ER) in formalin-fixed, paraffin-embedded human breast cancer tissue by use of a monoclonal antibody to ER. J. Histochem. Cytochem., 36:1553, 1988.
5. Andersen, J., Thorpe, S. M., King, W. J., Rose, C., Christensen, I., Rasmussen, B. B., and Poulsen, H. S.: The prognostic value of immunohistochemical estrogen receptor analysis in paraffin-embedded and frozen sections versus that of steroid-binding assays. Eur. J. Cancer, 26:442, 1990.
6. Arbogast, L. Y., and DeSombre, E. R.: Estrogen-dependent in vitro stimulation of RNA synthesis in hormone-dependent mammary tumors of the rat. J. Nat. Cancer Inst., 54:483, 1975.
7. Beato, M.: Gene regulation by steroid hormones. Cell, 56:335, 1989.
8. Beatson, G. T.: On the treatment of inoperable cases of carcinoma of the mamma: suggestions for a new method of treatment with illustrative cases. Lancet, 2:104, 1896.
9. Berger, U., Mansi, J. L., Wilson, P., and Coombes, R. C.: Detection of estrogen receptor in bone marrow from patients with metastatic breast cancer. J. Clin. Oncol., 5:1779, 1987.
10. Block, G. E., Ellis, R. S., DeSombre, E., and Jensen, E.: Correlation of estrophilin content of primary mammary cancer to eventual endocrine treatment. Ann. Surg., 188:372, 1978.
11. Burton, G. V., Flowers, J. L., Cox, E. B., Leight, G. S., Dent, G. A., Geisinger, K. R., McCarty, K. S., and McCarty, K. S., Jr.: Estrogen receptor determination by monoclonal antibody in fine needle aspiration breast cancer cytologies: a marker of hormone response. Breast Cancer Res. Treat., 10:287, 1987.
12. Carson-Jurica, M. A., Schrader, W. T., and O'Malley, B. W.: Steroid-receptor family: structure and functions. Endocrine Rev., 11:201, 1990.
13. Casteñeda, E., and Liao, S.: The use of antisteroid antibodies in the characterization of steroid receptors. J. Biol. Chem., 250:883, 1975.
14. Chamness, G. C., Huff, K., and McGuire, W. L.: Protamine-precipitated estrogen receptor: a solid-phase ligand exchange assay. Steroids, 25:627, 1975.
15. Charpin, C., Martin, P.-M., Jacquemier, J., Lavaut, M. N., Pourreau-Schneider, N., and Toga, M.: Estrogen receptor immunocytochemical assay (ER-ICA): Computerized image analysis system, immunoelectron microscopy, and comparisons with estradiol binding assays in 115 breast carcinomas. Cancer Res., 46:4271s, 1986.
16. Cheng, L., Binder, S. W., Fu, Y. S., and Lewin, K. J.: Demonstration of estrogen receptors by monoclonal antibody in formalin-fixed breast tumors. Lab. Invest., 58:346, 1988.
17. Clark, G. M., and McGuire, W. L.: Steroid receptors and other prognostic factors in the treatment of breast cancer. Semin. Oncol., 15:20, 1988.
18. Clark, G. M., McGuire, W. L., Hubay, C. A., Pearson, O. H., and Marshall, J. S.: Progesterone receptors as a prognostic factor in stage II breast cancer. N. Engl. J. Med., 309:1343, 1983.
19. Cohen, O., Brugal, G., Seigneurin, D., and Demongeot, J.: Image cytometry of estrogen receptors in breast carcinomas. Cytometry, 9:579, 1988.
20. Cooper, A. P.: The Principles and Practice of Surgery. London, E. Cox, 1836, pp. 333–335.
21. Corle, D. K., Sears, M. E., and Olson, K. B.: Relationship of quantitative estrogen-receptor level and clinical response to cytotoxic chemotherapy in advanced breast cancer. Cancer, 54:1554, 1984.
22. Davis, B. W., Zava, D. I., Locher, G. W., Goldhirsch, A., and Hartmann, W. H.: Receptor heterogeneity of human breast cancer as measured by multiple intratumoral assays of estrogen and progesterone receptor. Eur. J. Cancer Clin. Oncol., 20:375, 1984.
23. Daxenbichler, G., Forsthuber, E.-P., Marth, C., Kemmler, G., Wiegele, J., Margreiter, R., Müller, L., Hausmaninger, H., Manfreda, D., and Dapunt, O.: Steroid hormone receptors and prognosis in breast cancer. Breast Cancer Res. Treat., 12:267, 1988.
24. De Rosa, C. M., Ozzello, L., Greene, G. L., and Habif, D. V.: Immunostaining of estrogen receptor in paraffin sections of breast carcinomas using monoclonal antibody D75P3Y: Effects of fixation. Am. J. Surg. Pathol., 11:943, 1987.
25. DeSombre, E. R., Carbone, P. P., Jensen, E. V., McGuire, W. L., Wells, S. A., Jr., Wittliff, J. L., and Lipsett, M. B.: Steroid receptors in breast cancer. N. Engl. J. Med., 301:1011, 1979.
26. DeSombre, E. R., and Jensen, E. V.: Estrophilin assays in breast cancer: Quantitative features and applications to the mastectomy specimen. Cancer, 46:2783, 1980.
27. DeSombre, E. R., Greene, G. L., and Jensen, E. V.: Estrophilin and endocrine responsiveness of breast cancer. In Progress in Cancer Research and Therapy. Vol. 10: Hormones, Receptors and Breast Cancer. Edited by W. L. McGuire. New York, Raven Press, 1978, pp. 1–14.
28. DeSombre, E. R., Thorpe, S. M., Rose, C., Blough, R. R., Andersen, K. W., Rasmussen, B. B., and King, W. J.: Prognostic usefulness of estrogen receptor immunocytochemical assays for human breast cancer. Cancer Res., 46:4256s, 1986.
29. Englesman, E., Persijn, J. P., Korsten, C. B., and Cleton, F. J.: Oestrogen receptors in human breast cancer tissue and response to endocrine therapy. Brit. Med. J., 2:750, 1973.
30. Estes, P. A., Suba, E. J., Lawler-Heavner, J., Elashry-Stowers, D., Wei, L. L., Toft, D. O., Sullivan, W. P., Horwitz, K. B., and Edwards, D. P.: Immunologic analysis of human breast cancer progesterone receptors. 1. Immunoaffinity purification of transformed receptors and production of monoclonal antibodies. Biochemistry, 26:6250, 1987.
31. Evans, R. M.: The steroid and thyroid hormone receptor superfamily. Science, 240:889, 1988.

32. Fisher, B., Redmond, C., Fisher, E. R., and Caplan, R.: Relative worth of estrogen or progesterone receptor and pathologic characteristics of differentiation as indicators of prognosis in node negative breast cancer patients: Findings from National Surgical Adjuvant Breast and Bowel Project protocol B-06. J. Clin. Oncol., 6:1076, 1988.
33. Fishman, J., Fishman, J. H., Nisselbaum, J. S., Menendez-Botet, C., Schwartz, M. K., Martucci, C., and Hellman, L.: Measurement of the estradiol receptor in human breast tissue by the immobilized antibody method. J. Clin. Endocrinol. Metab., 40:724, 1975.
34. Folca, P. J., Glascock, R. F., and Irvine, W. T.: Studies with tritium-labelled hexoestrol in advanced breast cancer. Comparison of tissue accumulation of hexoestrol with response to bilateral adrenalectomy and oophorectomy. Lancet, 2:796, 1961.
35. Garola, R. E., and McGuire, W. L.: A hydroxylapatite micromethod for measuring estrogen receptor in human breast cancer. Cancer Res., 38:2216, 1978.
36. Gorski, J., and Gannon, F.: Current models of steroid hormone action: A critique. Annu. Rev. Physiol., 38:425, 1976.
37. Greene, G. L., Nolan, C., Engler, J. P., and Jensen, E. V.: Monoclonal antibodies to human estrogen receptor. Proc. Natl. Acad. Sci. U. S. A., 77:5115, 1980.
38. Greene, G. L., Harris, K., Bova, R., Kinders, R., Moore, B., and Nolan, C.: Purification of T47D human progesterone receptor and immunochemical characterization with monoclonal antibodies. Mol. Endocrinol., 2:714, 1988.
39. Greene G. L., Sobel, N. B., King, W. J., and Jensen, E. V.: Immunochemical studies of estrogen receptors. J. Steroid Biochem., 20:51, 1984.
40. Grody, W. W., Schrader, W. T., and O'Malley, B. W.: Activation, transformation, and subunit structure of steroid hormone receptors. Endocrine Rev., 3:141, 1982.
41. Hawkins, R. A., Sangster, K., Tesdale, A., Levack, P. A., Anderson, E. D. C., Chetty, U., and Forrest, A. P. M.: The cytochemical detection of oestrogen receptors in fine needle aspirates of breast cancer; correlation with biochemical assay and prediction of response to endocrine therapy. Br. J. Cancer, 58:77, 1988.
42. Helin, H. J., Isola, J. J., Helle, M. J., and Adlercreutz, H.: Influence of endocrine status on biochemical and immunocytochemical estrogen and progesterone receptor assays in breast cancer patients. Breast Cancer Res. Treat., 12:67, 1988.
43. Hilf, R., Feldstein, M. L., Savlov, E. D., Gibson, S. L., and Seneca, B.: The lack of relationship between estrogen receptor status and response to chemotherapy. Cancer, 46:2797, 1980.
44. Hiort, O., Kwan, P. W. L., and DeLellis, R. A.: Immunohistochemistry of estrogen receptor protein in paraffin sections. Am. J. Clin. Pathol., 90:559, 1988.
45. Hoffman, P. G., Jones, L. A., Kuhn, R. W., and Siiteri, P. K.: Progesterone receptors: Saturation analysis by a solid phase hydroxylapatite adsorption technique. Cancer, 46:2801, 1980.
46. Horwitz, K. B., McGuire, W. L., Pearson, O. H., and Segaloff, A.: Predicting response to endocrine therapy in human breast cancer: a hypothesis. Science, 189:726, 1975.
47. Howat, J. M. T., Harris, M., Swindell, R., and Barnes, D. M.: The effect of oestrogen and progesterone receptors on recurrence and survival in patients with carcinoma of the breast. Br. J. Cancer, 51:263, 1985.
48. Huggins, C., and Bergenstal, D. M.: Inhibition of human mammary and prostatic cancer by adrenalectomy. Cancer Res., 12:134, 1952.
49. Huggins, C., and Hodges, C. V.: Studies on prostatic cancer. 1. The effect of castration, of estrogen and of androgen injection on serum phosphatases in metastatic carcinoma of the prostate. Cancer Res., 1:293, 1941.
50. Jensen, E. V., DeSombre, E. R., and Jungblut, P.W.: Estrogen receptors in hormone-responsive tissues and tumors. *In* Endogenous Factors Influencing Host Tumor Balance. Edited by R. W. Wissler, T. L. Dao, and S. Wood, Jr. Chicago, University of Chicago Press, 1967, pp. 15–30, 68.
51. Jensen, E. V., Block, G. E., Smith, S., Kyser, K., and DeSombre, E. R.: Estrogen receptors and breast cancer response to adrenalectomy. Natl. Cancer Inst. Monograph, 34:55, 1971.
52. Jensen, E. V., and Jacobson, H. I.: Basic guides to the mechanism of estrogen action. Recent Prog. Hormone Res., 18:387, 1962.
53. Jensen, E. V.: Steroid hormone receptors. Current Topics Pathol., 83:365, 1991.
54. Jensen, E. V., and DeSombre, E. R.: Estrogen-receptor interaction. Science, 182:126, 1973.
55. Jensen, E.V., Smith, S., and DeSombre, E. R.: Hormone dependency in breast cancer. J. Steroid Biochem., 7:911, 1976.
56. Jensen, E. V., Greene, G. L., and DeSombre, E. R.: The estrogen-receptor immunoassay in the prognosis and treatment of breast cancer. Lab. Management, 24:25, 1986.
57. Jensen, E. V., Polley, T. Z., Smith, S., Block, G. E., Ferguson, D. J., and DeSombre, E. R.: Prediction of hormone dependency in human breast cancer. *In* Estrogen Receptors in Human Breast Cancer. Edited by W. L. McGuire, P. P. Carbone, and E. P. Vollmer, New York, Raven Press, 1975, pp. 37–56.
58. Johansson, H., Terenius, L., and Thorén, L.: The binding of estradiol-17β to human breast cancers and other tissues *in vitro*. Cancer Res., 30:692, 1970.
59. Jonat, W., Maass, H., Stolzenbach, G., and Trams, G.: Estrogen receptor status and response to polychemotherapy in advanced breast cancer. Cancer, 46:2809, 1980.
60. Kiang, D. T., Frenning, D. H., Goldman, A. I., Ascensao, V. F., and Kennedy, B.J.: Estrogen receptors and responses to chemotherapy and hormonal therapy in advanced breast cancer. N. Engl. J. Med., 299:1330, 1978.
61. King, W. J., DeSombre, E. R., Jensen, E. V., and Greene, G. L.: Comparison of immunocytochemical and steroid-binding assays for estrogen receptor in human breast tumors. Cancer Res., 45:293, 1985.
62. Kinsel, L. B., Szabo, E., Greene, G. L., Konrath, J., Leight, G. S., and McCarty, K. S., Jr.: Immunocytochemical analysis of estrogen receptors as a predictor of prognosis in breast cancer patients: comparison with quantitative biochemical methods. Cancer Res., 49:1052, 1989.
63. Knight, W. A., III, Livingston, R. B., Gregory, E. J., and McGuire, W. L.: Estrogen receptor as an independent prognostic factor for early recurrence in breast cancer. Cancer Res., 37:4669, 1977.
64. Koenders, P. G., Beex, L. V. A. M., Langens, R., Kloppenborg, P. W. C., Smals, A. G. H., and Benraad, Th. J.: Steroid hormone receptor activity of primary human breast cancer and pattern of the first metastasis. Breast Cancer Res. Treat., 18:27, 1991.
65. Korenman, S. G., and Dukes, B. A.: Specific estrogen binding by the cytoplasm of human breast carcinoma. J. Clin. Endocrinol. Metab., 30:639, 1970.
66. Kumar, V., Green, S., Stack, G., Berry, M., Jin, J.-R., and Chambon, P.: Functional domains of the human estrogen receptor. Cell, 51:941, 1987.
67. Leclercq, G., Heuson, J. C., Deboel, M. C., and Mattheiem, W. H.: Oestrogen receptors in breast cancer: a changing concept. Brit. Med. J., 1:185, 1975.
68. Leung, B. S., Fletcher, W. S., Lindell, T. D., Wood, D. C., and Krippaehne, W. W.: Predictability of response to endocrine ablation in advanced breast carcinoma. Arch. Surg., 106:515, 1973.
69. Liao, S.: Cellular receptors and mechanisms of action of steroid hormones. Internat. Rev. Cytol., 41:87, 1975.
70. Lippman, M. E., Allegra, J. C., Thompson, E. B., Simon, R., Barlock, A., Green, L., Huff, K. K., Do, H. M. T., Aitkin, S. C., and Warren, R.: The relation between estrogen receptors and response rate to cytotoxic chemotherapy in metastatic breast cancer. N. Engl. J. Med., 298:1223, 1978.
71. Lippman, M. E., and Allegra, J. C.: Quantitative estrogen receptor analyses: The response to endocrine and cytotoxic chemotherapy in human breast cancer and the disease-free interval. Cancer, 46:2829, 1980.
72. Luft, R., and Olivecrona, H.: Experiences with hypophysectomy in man. J. Neurosurg., 10:301, 1953.
73. Maass, H., Engel, B., Hohmeister, L., Lehmann, F., and Trams, G.: Estrogen receptors in human breast cancer tissue. Am. J. Obstet. Gynecol., 113:377, 1972.
74. Maass, H., Jonat, W., Stolzenbach, G., and Trams, G.: The problem of nonresponding estrogen receptor-positive patients with advanced breast cancer. Cancer, 46:2835, 1980.
75. Magdelenat, H., Merle, S., and Zajdela, A.: Enzyme immunoassay of estrogen receptors in fine needle aspirates of breast tumors. Cancer Res., 46:4265s, 1986.
76. McCarty, K. S., Jr., Szabo, E., Flowers, J. L., Cox, E. B., Leight, G. S., Miller, L., Konrath, J., Soper, J. T., Budwit, D. A., Creasman, W. T., Seigler, H. F., and McCarty, K. S., Sr.: Use of a monoclonal anti-estrogen receptor antibody in the immunohistochemical evaluation of human tumors. Cancer Res., 46:4244s, 1986.
77. McClelland, R. A., Berger, U., Wilson, P., Powles, T. J., Trott, P. A., Easton, D., Gazet, J.-C., and Coombes, R. C.: Presurgical determination of estrogen receptor status using immunocytochemically stained fine needle aspirate smears in patients with breast cancer. Cancer Res., 47:6118, 1987.
78. McClelland, R. A., Berger, U., Miller, L. S., Powles, T. J., and Coombes, R. C.: Immunocytochemical assay for estrogen receptor in patients with breast cancer: relationship to a biochemical assay and to outcome of therapy. J. Clin. Oncol., 4:1171, 1986.
79. McGuire, W. L., Carbone, P. P., and Vollmer, E. P.: Estrogen Receptors in Breast Cancer. New York, Raven Press, 1975.
80. McGuire, W. L.: Hormone receptors: Their role in predicting prognosis and response to endocrine therapy. Semin. Oncol., 5:428, 1978.
81. McGuire, W. L., Clark, G. M., Dressler, L. G., and Owens, M. A.: Role of steroid hormone receptors as prognostic factors in primary breast cancer. NCI Monogr., 1:19, 1986.
82. McGuire, W. L., and Clark, G. M.: Prognostic factors for recurrence and survival in axillary node-negative breast cancer. J. Steroid Biochem., 34:145, 1989.
83. Müller-Holzner, E., Zeimet, A., Müller, L. C., Daxenbichler, G., and Dapunt, O.: Monoclonal technique to aid decision on endocrine therapy in breast cancer. Lancet, 1:1147, 1989.
84. Nolan, C., Przywara, L. W., Miller, L. S., Suduikis, V., and Tomita, J. T.: A sensitive solid-phase enzyme immunoassay for human estrogen receptor. *In* Current Controversies in Breast Cancer. Edited by F. C. Ames, G. R. Blumenschein, and E. D. Montague. Austin, University of Texas Press, 1984, pp. 433–441.
85. Osborne, C. K., Yochmowitz, M. G., Knight, W. A., III and McGuire, W. L.: The value of estrogen and progesterone receptors in the treatment of breast cancer. Cancer, 46:2884, 1980.
86. Parker, M.: Nuclear Hormone Receptors. London, Academic Press, 1991.
87. Paridaens, R., Sylvester, R. J., Ferrazzi, E., Legros, N., Leclercq, G., and Heuson, J. C.: Clinical significance of the quantitative assessment of estrogen receptors in advanced breast cancer. Cancer, 46:2889, 1980.
88. Pertschuk, L. P.: Immunocytochemistry tor Steroid Receptors. Boca Raton, CRC Press, 1990.
89. Pertschuk, L. P., Eisenberg, K. B., Carter, A. C., and Feldman, J. G.: Immunohistologic localization of estrogen receptors in breast cancer with monoclonal antibodies. Correlation with biochemistry and clinical endocrine response. Cancer, 55:1513, 1985.
90. Pichon, M.-F., Pallud, C., Brunet, M., and Milgrom, E.: Relationship of presence of progesterone receptors to prognosis in early breast cancer. Cancer Res., 40:3357, 1980.
91. Poulsen, H. S., Ozzello, L., King, W. J., and Greene, G. L.: The use of monoclonal antibodies to estrogen receptors (ER) for immunoperoxidase detection of ER in paraffin sections of human breast cancer tissue. J. Histochem. Cytochem., 33:87, 1985.
92. Pratt, W. B., Sanchez, E. R., Bresnick, E. H., Meshinchi, S., Scherrer, L. C., Dalman, F. C., and Welsh, M. J.: Interaction of the glucocorticoid receptor with the M_r90000 heat shock protein: an evolving model of ligand-mediated receptor transformation and translocation. Cancer Res., 49:2222s, 1989.
93. Pusztay, H. M., and McDonald, E. M., editors: Symposium on estrogen receptor determination with monoclonal antibodies. Cancer Res., 46:4231s, 1986.
94. Ringold, G. M.: Steroid hormone regulation of gene expression. Annu. Rev. Pharmacol. Toxicol., 25:529, 1985.
95. Rosenbaum, C., Marsland, T. A., Stolbach, L. L., Raam, S., and Cohen, J. L.: Estrogen receptor status and response to chemotherapy in advanced breast cancer. Cancer, 46:2919, 1980.
96. Rubens, R. D., and Hayward, J. L.: Estrogen receptors and response to endocrine therapy and cytotoxic chemotherapy in advanced breast cancer. Cancer, 46:2922, 1980.
97. Rydén, S., Fernö, M., Borg, Å., Hafström, L., Möller, T., and Norgren, A.: Prognostic significance of estrogen and progesterone receptors in stage II breast cancer. J. Surg. Oncol., 37:221, 1988.
98. Samal, B. A., Brooks, S. C., Cummings, G., Franco, L., Hire, E. A., Martino, S., Singhakowinta, A., and Vaitkevicius, V. K.: Estrogen receptors and responsiveness of advanced breast cancer to chemotherapy, Cancer, 46:2925, 1980.
99. Scatchard, G.: The attraction of proteins for small molecules and ions. Ann. N. Y. Acad. Sci., 51:660, 1949.
100. Shimada, A., Kimura, S., Abe, K., Nagasaki, K., Adachi, I., Yamaguchi, K., Suzuki, M., Nakajima, T., and Miller, L. S.: Immunocytochemical staining of estrogen receptor in paraffin sections of human breast cancer by use of monoclonal antibody: comparison with that in frozen sections. Proc. Natl. Acad. Sci. U.S.A., 82:4803, 1985.
101. Shintaku, I. P., and Said, J. W.: Detection of estrogen receptors with monoclonal antibodies in routinely processed formalin-fixed paraffin sections of breast carcinoma. Am. J. Clin. Pathol., 87:161, 1987.
102. Singhakowinta, A., Potter, H. G., Buroker, T. R., Samal, B., Brooks, S. C., and Vaitkevicius, V. K.: Estrogen receptor and natural course of breast cancer. Ann. Surg., 183:84, 1976.
103. Sklarew, R. J., Bodmer, S. C., and Pertschuk, L. P.: Quantitative imagining of immunocytochemical (PAP) estrogen receptor staining patterns in breast cancer sections. Cytometry, 11:359, 1990.
104. Sternberger, L. A.: Immunocytochemistry. New York, Prentice-Hall, 1974.
105. Sutton, R., Campbell, M., Cooke, T., Nicholson, R., Griffiths, K., and Taylor, I.: Predictive power of progesterone receptor status in early breast carcinoma. Br. J. Surg., 74:223, 1987.

106. van Netten, J. P., Algard, F. T., Coy, P., Carlyle, S. J., Brigden, M. L., Thornton, K. R., Peter, S., Fraser, T., and To, M. P.: Heterogeneous receptor levels detected via multiple microsamples from individual breast cancers. Cancer, 56:2019, 1985.
107. Wagner, R. K.: Characterization and assay of steroid hormone receptors and steroid-binding serum proteins by agargel electrophoresis at low temperature. Hoppe-Seyler's Z. Physiol. Chem., 353:1235, 1972.
108. Walker, K. J., Bouzubar, N., Robertson, J., Ellis, I. O., Elston, C. W., Blamey, R. W., Wilson, D. W., Griffiths, K., and Nicholson, R. I.: immunocytochemical localization of estrogen receptor in human breast tissue. Cancer Res., 48:6517, 1988.
109. Walt, A. J., Singhakowinta, A., Brooks, S. C., and Cortez, A.: The surgical implications of estrophile protein estimations in carcinoma of the breast. Surgery, 80:506, 1976.
110. Weintraub, J., Weintraub, D., Redard, M., and Vassilakos, P.: Evaluation of estrogen receptors by immunocytochemistry on fine-needle aspiration biopsy specimens from breast tumors. Cancer, 60:1163, 1987.
111. Wrange, Ö, Nordenskjöld, B., and Gustafsson, J.-Å.: Cytosol estradiol receptor in human mammary carcinoma: An assay based on isoelectric focusing in polyacrylamide gel. Analyt. Biochem., 85:461, 1978.
112. Yamamoto, K. R.: Steroid receptor regulated transcription of specific genes and gene networks. Annu. Rev. Genet., 19:209, 1985.

Acknowledgment

Preparation of this chapter was supported by a grant (RDP-53B) from the American Cancer Society.

XVII-2

Hormone Physiology and Endocrine Ablation

B. J. Kennedy

Introduction

The removal of endogenous hormones can significantly alter the course of cancer. The ablation of an endocrine gland may result in the decrease or disappearance of one or more hormonal factors essential in the continuing growth of the neoplasm. Because of the biologic differences of tumors within a specific type, not all patients respond favorably to hormonal manipulation. Therefore, it is desirable that a careful recording of the patient's previous cancer history be made, noting the response to other hormonal therapies, so that judicious selection of the patient can be made for the approporiate ablative procedure.

Female Breast Cancer

The estrogenic hormone is a major factor in the stimulation and growth of some breast cancers. When estrogens are first employed in the treatment of menopausal symptoms, careful examination of the breasts during the first few months is recommended, since an existing small cancer could be stimulated by such hormonal therapy. The administration of androgens can also stimulate the growth of breast cancer, since the hormone is converted to small amounts of estrogen. This accounts for the induction of hypercalcemia in the initial treatment of patients with advanced osseous metastases.

Administration of small physiologic doses of estrogenic hormone in premenopausal women may also stimulate breast cancer growth as with the use of contraceptive estrogens. The administration of massive doses of estrogen may cause tumor regression in all ages, but in the postmenopausal patient estrogenic hormone in a large dose (e.g., greater than 3 mg daily of diethylstilbesterol) is a major therapy for advanced disease. Although androgenic hormones and progestogens also produce suppression of tumor growth, the estrogenic hormone is more effective. The estrogen antagonists (e.g., tamoxifen) also play a major role in breast cancer management. The utilization of administered hormones and antagonists is an essential part of the selective sequential use of hormonal therapies.

Since the biologic behavior of carcinoma of the breast in some females is dependent on hormonal factors, their alteration can stimulate or inhibit growth of the cancer. By measuring estrogen receptors of primary breast cancer and its metastases, the response to hormone manipulation can be predicted with reasonable accuracy. Those with positive receptors are candidates for hormonal therapies. Tumors that lack receptors or have low receptor levels have a less than 3% chance of responding to ablative therapy.[6]

The removal of hormonal factors involved in the stimulation or maintenance of tumor growth may result in tumor regression. This can be accomplished by ablating hormone production directly or indirectly. Three ablative procedures are available.

Ovariectomy

In approximately one-third of premenopausal women with breast cancer, the estrogenic hormones in physiologic amounts produced by the patient are a significant factor in the maintenance of tumor growth. Removal of these hormones by bilateral ovariectomy may produce objective improvement in breast cancer.

Castration was employed first in 1896, but only recently has the role of this procedure been clarified in the sequential selection of therapies for breast cancer. That castration should be carried out at the time of recurrence of breast cancer (therapeutic castration) rather than at the time of the initial mastectomy ("prophylactic" or adjuvant castration) has been established.[4] A comparison of patients undergoing castration at the time of mastectomy to those undergoing therapeutic castration when the disease was recurrent demonstrated that survival from mastectomy to death was not different between the two groups. Although castration at the time of mastectomy did delay the onset of metastases, it did not prevent the recurrence of the cancer. In this sense it was a form of adjuvant therapy. Furthermore, when the disease recurred in these patients, the interval from recurrence to death was much shorter than that of patients having a therapeutic castration. Hence, castration at the time of mastectomy has not increased the curability of breast cancer by conventional surgical methods. Castration is of benefit, however, in that the survival period of castrated patients has been greater than that of noncastrated patients.

When "prophylactic" castration is carried out and the cancer later recurs, there is no information available regarding the hormonal characteristics of the tumor. This index of the biologic nature of the cancer is lost. Without this information of the hormonal characteristics of the tumor, an appropriate selection of future therapies was formerly impossible. With the knowledge of the estrogen receptor content of the tumor and with the response to castration, a high response rate to hypophysectomy, adrenalectomy, or antiestrogen therapy is assured. A new biopsy for estrogen and progesterone receptor data at the time of relapse is advantageous, since a tumor that lacked receptors would have a low rate of response to ablative procedures. To carry out a castration at the time of mastectomy is therefore disadvantageous for the patient.

Castration is primarily of value in premenopausal women with advanced primary, recurrent, or distant metastatic cancer of the breast. The nature of the tumor response to therapeutic castration consists of a decrease in size of skin, liver, or lung metastases, recalcification of osseous lesions, and decrease in size of a primary tumor. Central nervous system metastases are less likely to respond. The reported rates of regression in premenopausal women vary from 24.5–50%. The culling of results of twelve different studies revealed an average regression rate of 40%. By limiting ovariectomy to those patients whose cancers expressed high levels of estrogen receptor (ER), the objective response rate can be almost doubled to approximately 64%. The median duration of such improvement is nine months, with ranges from four months to six years. Patients who respond to therapeutic castration live longer than do nonresponders. Although some investigators have reported regression of tumor following castration in postmenopausal women, in most of these patients it is less than two years since the last menstrual period. Castration is of no value in truly postmenopausal women.

The presence of estrogen receptor and the type of tumor response to therapeutic castration are significant indices of the nature of the breast cancer and provide a guide to the selection of other hormonal therapies. In non-responders to castration, the formidable methods of secondary hormonal ablative therapy may be avoided. Patients who do not respond to therapeutic castration become candidates for chemotherapy and other supportive measures. Patients who demonstrate an unequivocally objective response following a therapeutic castration are, upon reactivation of the disease, candidates for hypophysectomy, bilateral adrenalectomy, aminoglutethimide, adrenal cortical hormone administration, or estrogen antagonists.

The procedure of bilateral ovariectomy is relatively simple. A hysterectomy need not be performed concomitantly. Although castration can be performed by radiotherapy, surgical ovariectomy is complete and removes any doubt that the ovaries might have a residual function. Furthermore, for complications such as hypercalcemia or severe bone pain, which require an immediate antitumor effect, surgical castration is preferable. A rapid response will occur in contrast to radiotherapeutic castration wherein a response could be delayed several weeks.

Castration in premenopausal women induces an artificial menopause. This is frequently more intense than the spontaneous menopause, but of shorter duration. In those patients responding to castration, no replacement therapy with estrogenic or androgenic hormones should be undertaken. Even women who had ER-negative tumors and were castrated should not be given estrogenic hormones.

In a patient who undergoes ovariectomy, but whose cancer fails to improve, it could be implied that the estrogenic hormone plays no role in the growth pattern of that disease. Once this has been established, replacement therapy with estrogenic hormone might seem appropriate to relieve the patient of severe menopausal symptoms. However, such therapy could be detrimental to the course of the patient's disease.

Most breast cancers are a mixture of ER-positive and ER-negative cells. This has been clearly demonstrated with the monoclonal assay method for measuring estrogen receptors immunocytochemically. Hence, the administration of estrogens for the menopausal symptoms could result in stimulating those few receptor-positive cells that exist in an apparently ER negative tumor. If the menopausal symptoms are sufficiently severe to require hormonal therapy, the use of a progestogen may be effective.

The role of Tamoxifen in lieu of oophorectomy has been considered in receptor positive patients. Oophorectomy would be preferable, especially in younger women, whereas Tamoxifen can still be employed for later relapses.

Adrenalectomy

Bilateral adrenalectomy has been performed for the management of advanced breast cancer in the female. Removal of estrogenic hormone produced by the adrenals can result in a further antitumor effect, especially in patients previously demonstrating a response to castration, as premenopausal women, or to hormone administration in postmenopausal patients.

Bilateral adrenalectomy was first introduced in 1951, and hypophysectomy as an alternative to adrenalectomy was introduced in 1954. Both procedures have been employed in similar circumstances. The degree of morbidity, the mortality, and the regression rates have been factors in determining which of these ablative procedures is preferred. Whether adrenalectomy or hypophysectomy should be selected for a given patient depends in part on the availability of the proper surgeon. The tumor site may also be a factor in selecting one of these procedures. For example, a patient with extensive skull metastases is a better candidate for adrenalectomy. A patient with abdominal metastases would probably withstand hypophysectomy more easily. In this era of medical science, the mortality rate for both procedures is low.

The results of adrenalectomy for female breast cancer reported by several investigators have been comparable. A collaborative study comparing bilateral adrenalectomy and hypophysectomy revealed a regression rate of 28.4% and 32.6% respectively.[8] The difference was not significant. Fracchia had a regression rate of 32.4% following adrenalectomy.[2] These figures reflect the overall regression rate in breast cancer without specific selection of the patient as a candidate for the procedure on the basis of prior response to other hormone therapy.

Currently, with knowledge of estrogen receptor contents of the tumors plus the observations of the response to endocrine therapies, it can be predicted what type of patient will benefit from adrenalectomy. By discreet selection of patients, a higher rate of improvement can be expected than by random use of the procedure. The premenopausal patient with a long cancer-free interval following mastectomy, who has mainly osseous or soft tissue disease and who has responded favorably to therapeutic castration is most likely to benefit from adrenalectomy. The postmenopausal women who developed primary breast cancer before the menopause and women responding to hormone therapy also have a high rate of regression following adrenalectomy. Utilization of adrenalectomy in advanced cancer was recommended primarily for those female patients whose disease had reactivated following objective improvement as the result of castration or estrogen therapy and in whom the estrogen receptor was positive. In view of the low response rate (16% or less) in patients failing to respond to castration and the lack of the response in ER-negative tumors, the employment of this formidable procedure in this type of patient for such a low improvement rate hardly seemed of value to the patients.

Aminoglutethimide inhibits the biosynthesis of adrenocortical steroids. It also appears to block the peripheral conversion of androstendione to estrone. This "medical adrenalectomy" has been employed in lieu of the surgical procedure, making adrenalectomy a procedure of the past.[10]

Hypophysectomy

Hypophysectomy had a specific role in the management of advanced female breast cancer.[5] The utilization of hypophysectomy is dependent on the selection of patients in an attempt to avoid employing the procedure needlessly in patients who would not respond because of the known characteristics of their disease. Only patients with ER-positive tumors should be considered for this procedure. In female breast cancer, hypophysectomy was carried out at the time of reactivation of the disease in premenopausal women who had responded favorably to surgical castration or postmenopausal patients who had responded to estrogen therapy. The presence of ER-positive metastases plus a response to prior endocrine therapy almost assures a response to hypophysectomy.

Hypophysectomy removes adrenocorticotropic and gonadotropic hormones and secondarily eliminates adrenal functions. Therefore, the expected antitumor results of hypophysectomy and adrenalectomy have been similar. Approximately 20% of patients who had undergone oophorectomy followed by adrenalectomy had a subsequent remission after hypophysectomy, suggesting that prolactin may be a factor in tumor growth. However, the employment of these two major procedures seems excessive medical therapy and is not indicated.

The conventional transfrontal craniotomy is formidable. Transsphenoidal cryophypophysectomy or similar techniques afford a simplified procedure and shorter hospitalization.[1] These newer techniques resulted in decreasing utilization of the direct craniotomy or adrenalectomy procedures. The results of the various techniques for pituitary destruction appear to give comparable clinical alterations in the course of breast cancer.

The previous response to hormone therapy is a factor in the subsequent response to hypophysectomy. More than 55% of patients responding to therapeutic castration can be expected to improve after hypophysectomy.[5] In postmenopausal women who experienced a response to estrogenic or androgenic therapy, more than 70% can be expected to improve. With more specific selection of patients by the added information of estrogen receptor content of the tumor, these figures can be even greater.

Patients who have had clinical responses to hormonal therapies, and in whom prior determinations of estrogen receptors were positive, have an exceedingly high chance of having an objective regression after hypophysectomy. This emphasizes the great importance of establishing the estrogen receptor values in patients with breast cancer at all stages of the disease, primary and recurrent.

As with adrenalectomy, the use of aminoglutethimide and hydrocortisone has replaced the use of hypophysectomy. The use of these two major ablative procedures represent a historical era in the evolution of hormonal therapies in breast cancer. The sequential use of endocrine therapies plays a significant role in the overall management of breast cancer.[9]

Male Breast Cancer

Carcinoma of the male breast is effectively controlled by hormonal measures. The low incidence of this disease does not allow accurate data for incidence of regression. Since growth of male breast cancer is in part dependent on androgenic hormones, the antitumor measures of advanced disease are directed toward removal of androgenic hormones.

Orchiectomy is reserved for recurrent or advanced cancer in men of any age. With removal of the androgenic hormones, primary tumor masses, node and skin metastases, and lung lesions decrease in size or disappear. Osseous lesions recalcify. Central nervous system lesions are less apt to respond. The response to castration in male breast cancer with a regression rate of 68% is almost twice that in females.[11]

Adrenalectomy and hypophysectomy offer a further method of control of male breast cancer. Although the results of these ablative procedures have been derived from a small number of patients, the data seem to indicate that hypophysectomy or adrenalectomy may offer a greater response rate in males (50% and 53% respectively) than in females.[7] Remissions following adrenalectomy or hypophysectomy have been observed in patients who did not respond to orchiectomy.

A sequential pattern for the management of advanced male breast cancer was developed. Orchiectomy should be the first approach. When the cancer relapses after orchiectomy, hypophysectomy, adrenalectomy, or aminoglutethimide could be considered. The use of aminoglutethimide has largely replaced the use of these ablative procedures. In patients at high risk for operative mortality or in whom urgent need for improvement is required, massive doses of corticosteroids may be employed. Subsequently, aminoglutethimide could be added. Furthermore, response to antiestrogens or LHRH agents and flutamide, may also occur.

In males with carcinoma of the breast, androgenic hormones are never employed in treatment of this disease, since stimulation of the cancer may occur.

Cancer of the Prostate

The growth of carcinoma of the prostate is dependent on androgenic hormones. The removal of androgens results in tumor regression; administration of androgens stimulates the growth of the cancer. Hence, hormonal therapy is essential in the management of this tumor.

synthesis, furnished the evidence for the theory of neuro-humoral control of the pituitary gland put forward by Harris and others.[41,103] Hypothalamic hormones are known to influence growth, reproduction, lactation, metabolism, gastrointestinal function and the response to stress. Basal release of some hypothalamic hormones, including luteinizing hormone-releasing hormone (LH-RH), into hypophysial portal blood is pulsatile, but surges occur before events like ovulation.[56] LH-RH pulses are activated at the time of puberty. Some hypothalamic peptide hormones are also produced in the extra-hypothalamic brain areas (where they may serve as neurotransmitters) and in endocrine-like cells of non-neural tissues. Thus, somatostatin is present in discrete cells of the pancreas, gastric mucosa, duodenum and other tissues, and may, through paracrine control, play an important role in the regulation of the endocrine pancreas and gastrointestinal tract. The understanding of neurohumoral functions combined with the ready availability of synthetic hypothalamic hormones and their analogs should enable the clinician to diagnose and treat a variety of diseases much more successfully than in the past.

Agonists of Luteinizing Hormone-Releasing Hormone (LH-RH)

Early Studies and the Basis of Oncological Applications. Nineteen years have passed since the laboratory of one of us(AVS) accomplished the isolation, determination of structure and synthesis of the hypothalamic hormone controlling the secretion of both LH and FSH from the anterior pituitary gland.[108] The discovery of LH-RH also called gonadotropin-releasing hormone (Gn-RH) has led to many practical clinical uses.[106,108] Since 1972, systematic work has been proceeding to synthesize agonistic and antagonistic analogs of LH-RH. A strong interest in medical applications of LH-RH derivatives stimulated this undertaking. However, at that time we could not imagine the impact and the variety of applications, including major uses in oncology that LH-RH analogs would eventually have. It was not until the late 1970's, after more than two decades of involvement in the work on hypothalamic hormones, that one of us (AVS), influenced profoundly by the high activity of some peptide analogs, decided to investigate their possible effects on various cancers. In the past 18 years, more than 3,000 analogs of LH-RH have been synthesized.[106] Many agonistic analogs more potent than the parent hormone have been made.[106]

A number of LH-RH analogs substituted in positions 6, 10 or both are much more active than LH-RH.[106] Among the agonists being used clinically are: [D-Trp[6]]LH-RH (Decapeptyl, Triptorelin), [D-Leu[6], Pro[9]-NHEt]LH-RH (Leuprolide, Lupron), [D-Ser(Bu[t])[6], Pro[9]-NHEt]-LH-RH (Buserelin), [D-Ser(Bu[t])[6], Aza-Gly[10]]LH-RH (Goserelin, Zoladex, I.C.I. 118630), and [D-Nal(2)[6]]LH-RH (Nafarelin) (Table XVII-3-1), These agonists are 50 to 100 times more potent than LH-RH and also possess prolonged activity.[106]

Although an acute injection of superactive agonists of LH-RH induces a marked and sustained release of LH and FSH, chronic administration produces inhibitory effects through a process of "down regulation" of pituitary receptors for LH-RH, desensitization of the pituitary gonadotrophs, and reduction in gonadal receptors for LH and FSH.[100,106,115] Continuous administration of high doses of LH-RH agonists causes a suppression of circulating levels of LH (bioactive but not always radioimmunoactive and of sex steroid levels.[72]

The inhibition of pituitary and gonadal function that occurs after chronic administration of agonists of LH-RH with the creation of a state of sex steroid deprivation and elimination of stimulatory effects of estrogen or testosterone is the basis for oncological application of LH-RH analogs.[106,107,110]

Development of Sustained Delivery Systems. Initially, superagonists of LH-RH were given daily by the subcutaneous or intranasal route.[72,106] However, intranasal absorption is only about 2% and daily injections are inconvenient. Subsequently, long-acting delivery systems for [D-Trp[6]]LH-RH and other agonists in microcapsules of poly (DL-lactide-co-glycolide) (PLG) or different polymers designed to release a controlled dose of the peptide over a 30-day period were developed.[69,81,94] These microcapsules contain 2–6% analog and 94–98% of biodegradable, biocompatible polymer (DL-lactide-co-glycolide).Spherical microcapsules are prepared by a phase separation process.

Another form of sustained delivery system consists of microparticles (microgranules) containing the peptide analogs. The microparticles were obtained by cryogenic grinding of extruded polymer containing the homogeneously dispersed peptide, grinding, and sieving of the particles. This process results in particles of amorphous shape in a large variety of sizes, but it does not involve the use of solvents like freon which may be banned in the future on environmental grounds. For administration, the microcapsules or microgranules are suspended in an injection vehicle containing 2% carboxymethylcellulose and 1% Tween 20 or 80 in water and injected once-a-month intramuscularly through an 18 gauge needle. Depot preparations consisting of cylindrical rods of the polymer PLG with 3.6 mg Zoladex (Goserelin) injectable through a 14 or 16 gauge needle, and polyhydroxybutyrate tablets containing 5 mg Buserelin which are implantable s.c. are also available.

The mechanism of peptide release from sustained delivery systems (microcapsules and microgranules) after intramuscular injection, was studied by histological and immunohistochemical approaches.[22] It was determined that the diffusion of the peptides from the aqueous channels in PLG was negligible and that the peptide release from the PLG microcapsules and microparticles was controlled mostly by the speed of the biodegradation of the polymer matrix.[22] Sustained delivery formulations are capable of maintaining therapeutic levels of peptides for 4 weeks. Delayed delivery systems (microcapsules, microparticles or implants) developed for monthly administration are efficacious, reliable, convenient, and also increase the patient's compliance.

Current Uses of LH-RH Agonists. Chronic administration of LH-RH agonists is being utilized to induce the regression of endocrine-dependent malignant neoplasms, especially prostate and breast cancer and more recently, ovarian carcinoma.[106] LH-RH agonists are under study for the treatment of exocrine pancreatic cancer and endometrial cancer.[38] Reduction of sex steroid levels by LH-RH agonists can be also used for treatment of idiopathic precocious puberty. The inhibition of LH and ovarian steroidogenesis provides the basis for the therapeutic use of LH-RH agonists in diseases and conditions which result from inappropriate hormone levels or which can be treated by suppression of estrogens. These applications include endometriosis, uterine fibroids (leiomyomas), polycystic ovarian disease (PCOD), dysfunctional uterine bleeding, and hirsutism. LH-RH agonists are

Table XVII-3-1. LH-RH Agonists in Clinical Use

LH-RH	Structure									
	1	2	3	4	5	6	7	8	9	10
	pyro-Glu	His	Trp	Ser	Tyr	Gly	Leu	Arg	Pro	Gly-NH$_2$
Buserelin (Hoechst)	|------					---- D-Ser(Bu^t) -----				------Ethylamide
Nafarelin (Syntex)	|------					---- D-(2-Nal) ----				------|
Leuprolide (Abbott-Takeda)	|------					--- D-Leu ---				------Ethylamide
Zoladex; Goserelin (ICI)	|------					--- D-Ser(Bu^t) ---				-- Az-Gly-NH$_2$
Decapeptyl Tryptorelin; (Debiopharm; Ferring; Ache; Ipsen-Beaufour)	|------					--- D-Trp---				------|

The abbreviations of the amino acids are in accord with the recommendations of the IUPAC-IUB JCBN. In addition: LH-RH, luteinizing hormone-releasing hormone; Az-Gly = AZA-Glycine; Nal(2) = 3-(2-naphthyl)alanine; Bu^t = o-tert butyl; Ethylamide, -NH-CH$_2$-CH$_3$; (NHEt in text).

also used for in vitro fertilization, and embryo transfer (IVF-ET), gamete intrafallopian transfer (GIFT), and the development of new contraceptive methods.[106]

Pharmacokinetics and Metabolism. LH-RH agonists are degraded and eliminated from plasma several times more slowly than natural LH-RH.[8,106] The binding affinity of some LH-RH agonists to LH-RH receptors is about 10 times higher than that of LH-RH.[49,104,106] In normal volunteers, plasma half-life of D-Trp-6-LH-RH was 19 min for the fast and 50 min for the slower component.[8] The plasma clearance of D-Trp-6-LH-RH was reported to be 161–508 ml/min.[8] A single i.m. injection of the 3.75 mg of depot preparation of microcapsules of D-Trp-6-LH-RH liberating 100 µg/day results, after an initial peak, in D-Trp-6-LH-RH concentrations of 200–500 pg/ml lasting for about 4–5 weeks.[37] Labelled LH-RH analogs accumulate primarily in the liver and kidneys (the main degrading organs) and the pituitary, the biological target.[106]

Side Effects and Toxicology. The main side effects caused by chronic administration of LH-RH agonists are those that can be attributed to sex-hormone deficiency.[104,106] These consist of impotence and loss of libido in men and "hot flashes", climacteric-like vasomotor phenomena in both sexes. Episodes of temporary "flare-up" in disease manifested by an increase in bone pain during the first week of administration have been reported in 2–20% of patients with prostate cancer. None of the patients with prostate cancer develop gynecomastia or thromboembolic episodes in contrast to treatment with diethylstilbestrol. The acute toxicity of LH-RH agonists is extremely low.

LH-RH Antagonists

Theoretical Considerations and Early Studies. LH-RH antagonists represent another class of peptide analogs that may be useful for treatment of hormone-dependent cancers.[106] These antagonists act on the same receptor sites as LH-RH and cause an immediate inhibition of the release of gonadotropins and sex steroids.[106] While repeated administration of LH-RH agonists is necessary for inhibition of LH and sex steroids, this effect can be induced with a single injection of a potent LH-RH antagonist.[104,106] During agonist

administration, a transient LH and sex steroid release which precedes the secretion blockade may result in a flare-up of disease, whereas the antagonists induce an immediate suppression. The use of antagonists should prevent flare-up phenomena, which can occur in some cancer patients.[104,106] Antagonistic analogs of LH-RH were developed for contraception.[49,104,106] Modern antagonists possess modifications in positions 1, 2, 3, 6, 10 and others. Since 1972, hundreds of LH-RH antagonists have been synthesized and assayed in animals. Some of the more potent early antagonists were also tested in human beings.[104,106] [D-Phe^2, D-Trp^3, D-Phe^6]-LH-RH was the first inhibitory analog found to be active in human beings.[104,106] Insertion of D-arginine, in position 6 of LH-RH antagonists increases the inhibitory activity. [Ac-D-(4Cl)-Phe^{1,2}, D-Trp^3, D-Arg^6, D-Ala^{10}]LH-RH exhibited antiovulatory activity at a dose of 1–3 mg in rats.[49,104,106] However, antagonists with D-Arg or related basic residues in position 6 induce histamine liberation resulting in transient edema and other anaphylactoid reactions. In preliminary human tolerance studies in Europe, erythema at the site of subcutaneous injection was observed in some women after administration of antagonists. These side effects delayed clinical use of earlier LH-RH antagonists in humans.

Modern LH-RH Antagonists. In order to eliminate the undesirable edematogenic effect of the LH-RH antagonists containing basic D-amino acids at position 6, new analogs with D-ureidoalkyl amino acids such as D-Cit, D-Hci, (Table XVII-3-2) at position 6 were synthesized in our laboratory and tested in several in vitro and in vivo systems.[3,6] These antagonists included [Ac-D-Nal(2)^1, D-Phe(4Cl)^2, D-Trp^3, D-Hci^6, D-Ala^{10}]-LH-RH (SB-29); [Ac-D-Nal(2)^1, D-Phe(4Cl)^2, D-Trp^3, D-Cit^6, D-Ala^{10}]-LH-RH (SB-30); [Ac-D-Nal(2)^1, D-Phe(4Cl)^2, D-Pal(3)^3, D-Cit^6, D-Ala^{10}]-LH-RH (SB-75); [Ac-D-Nal(2)^1, D-Phe(4Cl)^2, D-Pal(3)^3, D-Hci^6, D-Ala^{10}]-LH-RH (SB-88) (Table XVII-3-2). In vivo, the most active antagonists SB-29, SB-30, SB-75, and SB-88 caused complete inhibition of ovulation in cycling rats in doses of 1.5–3 mg and suppressed the LH level in castrated rats for 24–48 hours when administered at levels of 5–25 mg. These peptides did not exert any ede-

Table XVII-3-2. Modern LH-RH Antagonists

Trivial Name	
SB-29	[Ac-D-Nal(2)^1, D-Phe(4Cl)^2, D-Trp^3, D-Hci^6, D-Ala^{10}]LH-RH
SB-30	[Ac-D-Nal(2)^1, D-Phe(4Cl)^2, D-Trp^3, D-Cit^6, D-Ala^{10}]-LH-RH
SB-75	[Ac-D-Nal(2)^1, D-Phe(4Cl)^2, D-Pal(3)^3, D-Cit^6, D-Ala^{10}]LH-RH
SB-88	[Ac-D-Nal(2)^1, D-Phe(4Cl)^2, D-Pal(3)^3, D-Hci^6, D-Ala^{10}]LH-RH
Antide	[N-Ac-D-Nal(2)^1, D-Phe(4Cl)^2, D-Pal(3)^3, Lys(Nic)^5, D-Lys(Nic)^6, Lys(iPr)^8, D-Ala^{10}]LH-RH
Nal-Glu Antagonist	[Ac-D-Nal(2)^1, D-Phe(4Cl)^2, D-Pal(3)^3, Arg^5, D-Glu^6(AA), D-Ala^{10}]LH-RN

Abbreviations: The abbreviations of the amino acids are in accord with the recommendations of the IUPAC-IUB JCBN. In addition: LH-RH, luteinizing hormone-releasing hormone; D-Glu^6(AA), 4-(p-methoxy-benzoyl)-D-2-aminobutyric acid; Cit, citrulline (2-amino-5-ureidopentanoic acid); Hci, homocitrulline (2-amino-6-ureidohexanoic acid); Nal(2), 3-(2-naphyl)alanine; Pal(3), 3-(3-pyridyl)alanine; Phe(4Cl), 4-chlorophen-ylalanine; Ac, acetyl; Lys(Nic), N$^\epsilon$-nicotinoyllysine; Lys-(iPr), N$^\epsilon$-isopropyllysine.

For comparison with the amino acids sequence of LH-RH, see Table XVII-3-1.

matogenic effects even at a dose of 1.5 mg/kg.[3,6] These properties of the D-Cit/D-Hci^6 antagonists may make them useful clinically.

Other groups have also reported different structural modifications which diminish anaphylactoid toxicity, in particular the histamine releasing activity of the D-Arg^6 antagonists.[64,97] Analogs like antide [N-Ac-D-Nal(2)^1, D-Phe(4Cl)^2, D-Pal(3)^3, Lys (Nic)^5, D-Lys (Nic)^6, Lys (iPr)^8, D-Ala^{10}]-LH-RH) and Nal-Glu antagonist ([Ac-D-Nal(2)^1, D-Phe (4Cl)^2, D-Pal(3)^3, Arg^5, D-Glu^6(AA), D-Ala^{10}]LH-RH (Table XVII-3-2) are highly potent and relatively free of side-effects in animal studies.[97]

Current Status of LH-RH Antagonists. Ongoing phase I clinical studies indicate that new antagonists like SB-75 inhibit LH and FSH release in hypergonadotropic women for more than 20 hours when given in doses of 300–600 mg, and cause no edematogenic side effects on acute or chronic administration.[39] Normal men showed an 80% fall in total and free serum testosterone levels 12 hours after s.c. administration of 300 mg SB-75.[39] Preliminary results in patients with advanced prostate carcinoma (D$_2$) treated with 300–500 mg SB-75 b.i.d. indicate persistent inhibition of serum LH and FSH levels and a fall in serum testosterone levels.[39] Several prototypes of sustained delivery systems (microcapsules and microgranules) of antagonist SB-75 have already been produced.

Antagonist SB-75 in microcapsules inhibited the growth of carcinogen-induced pancreatic cancers in hamsters, transplanted mammary cancers in mice, and Dunning R3327 rat prostate cancers.[111] Some of the antitumor effects of SB-75 could be direct since the growth of estrogen-independent MDA-MB-231 mammary cancer cell line in vitro can be suppressed by SB-75.[111]

Antagonists like Nal-Glu LH-RH were also shown to suppress pituitary and gonadal function in normal men.[85] However the efficacy of modern LH-RH antagonists like SB-75 in patients with sex-hormone dependent tumors still remains to be demonstrated and is the subject of intensive current investigations. The LH-RH antagonists could be particularly useful for patients with metastases in brain, liver, bone marrow and other sites in whom the agonists cannot be used, or who are presently excluded from clinical protocols for the use of LH-RH agonists, because of the possibility of flare-up.

LH-RH Analogs Carrying Cytotoxic Radicals

Additional new classes of antitumor drugs are being developed based on LH-RH analogs bearing various cyto-

toxic radicals such as melphalan (Mel), metal complexes related to cisplatin, and other chemotherapeutic agents. LH-RH agonists and antagonists carrying various cytotoxic radicals are designed as targeted chemotherapeutic agents intended for treatment of cancers that contain receptors for LH-RH. Early compounds of this class were already reported by us.[4,5] Such analogs exert the effect of LH-RH agonists or antagonists and, at the same time, might act as chemotherapeutic agents targeted to the tumor cells by their peptide portions for which binding sites are present on the tumor cell membranes. It is assumed that a peptide containing a nitrogen mustard compound such as Mel or another radical can be bound to the membrane receptors and internalized. After endocytosis, such a compound could interfere with intracellular events in cancer cells. The damage inflicted by cytotoxic analogs to pituitary LH- and FSH-secreting cells would not be deleterious to the cancer patient, since hypophysectomy has been used for treatment of some cancers. A possible damage to other cells, e.g., corticotrophs, thyrotrophs could be alleviated by replacement therapy. The agonistic and antagonistic analogs containing cytotoxic radicals show high biological activity in vitro and in vivo. Some agonists and antagonists containing cytotoxic radicals were found to bind with high affinity to the LH-RH receptors in human breast cancers and prostate cancers. In cytotoxicity tests in cultures of human breast cancer and prostate cancer cell lines, some analogs containing cytotoxic groups powerfully inhibited the ^{3}H-thymidine incorporation into DNA. Some of these compounds are being tested in vivo. Because the antitumor action may be exerted to a greater degree locally or at least at more selective sites that have the cell membrane receptors, the peripheral toxicity would be reduced. In addition to prostate and breast cancers such compounds could be tried for treatment of ovarian, endometrial and pancreatic cancer. The availability of cytotoxic compounds linked to hormonal peptides like LH-RH, that can be targeted to certain cancers possessing receptors for those peptides, and therefore more selective for killing cancer cells, could be of significant practical therapeutic importance. This approach might extend the utility of hormonal analogs of LH-RH from the current palliation toward an eventual cure.

Mode of Action of LH-RH Analogs

Pituitary-Gonadal Axis. LH-RH analogs are widely used in oncology, but their mode of action is not completely understood. However, many of the effects of these analogs are the result of a chemical gonadectomy. We will discuss the mode of action from the standpoint of gonadal suppression and then point to some inconsistencies with that concept which if resolved might extend therapy beyond the effects of castration.

When various LH-RH agonist analogs became available, the hope that these drugs would be useful in increasing fertility in both sexes required reevaluation.[100,104,106,115] Chronic administration diminished fertility in both sexes.

In the female rat, administration of LH-RH agonists gave results dependent on the dose schedule. Acute administration of agonist analogs paralleled the LH release effect of the native LH-RH. In contrast, continued high dose administration of agonist decreased the mass of estrogen target organs, the concentration of plasma estradiol, prolactin, and progesterone, and reduced the growth of DMBA-induced estradiol-receptor positive mammary tumors.[18,78] The effects of chronic administration of agonist analogs were identical to those of ovariectomy and suggested a non-surgical type of endocrine treatment for breast cancer.

Administration of LH-RH agonists to male rats also resulted in the expected acute response followed by decreased plasma gonadotropin and androgen as well as atrophy of gonadal tissue.[2] Atrophy of prostatic tissue suggested that chronic administration of agonist analogs of LH-RH might mimic the effects of orchidectomy in prostatic cancer.

Chronic administration of LH-RH agonist analogs to pre-menopausal women results in a predictable endocrine response. At the start of treatment, gonadotropin plasma levels are increased with concomitant but small increases in estradiol and progesterone. However, after 3–4 weeks of administration, sex steroid levels are in the postmenopausal range.[78] The fall in estradiol and progesterone is not as rapid as occurs after ovariectomy where postmenopausal levels are achieved in a week.[130] It is of interest that plasma estrone, androstenedione, and testosterone while decreased are somewhat above the levels in ovariectomized or postmenopausal women.[45,77] The main effects of LH-RH analogs are similar in Decapeptyl, Zoladex, Buserelin, and Leuprolide, although chronic administration of Zoladex is said to reduce plasma prolactin, an effect not noted in Buserelin or Lupron.[78] The response to analogs will vary as a function of potency, binding to specific receptors, and to pharmacokinetic factors. The use of timed release preparations can be expected to have large effects on biological response.[94,99]

Chronic administration of agonist analogs to the human male results in the expected early rise of FSH, LH, and testosterone which occasionally results in increased symptoms or "flare." After 4–6 weeks of treatment, plasma testosterone levels are at the castrate level.[2] The exact mechanism of the down-regulation is not clear. Pituitary desensitization accounts for the chemical castration but immunoassayable LH does not decrease sufficiently to account for the lowering of testosterone.[11] The disparity is partly explained by LH-RH treatment causing secretion of an LH with decreased biological potency; bioassay of serum LH gives concentrations which parallel the fall in testosterone.[11] The chemical changes in LH producing a disparity between RIA and bioassay also occur in women but have been studied in males in more detail.

Currently, the mode of action of LH-RH agonists is explained in terms of down-regulation of the pituitary LH-RH receptors and subsequent decrease in gonadotropin secretion result-ing in chemical castration. The mechanism of pituitary LH release is not completely understood, but involves the interplay of calcium, calmodulin, phosphoinositides, and protein kinase C.[16] The possibility of direct effects of LH-RH agents on tumor cells is considered below.

The mode of action of LH-RH antagonists may differ in some respects from that of the agonists; down-regulation of receptors was reported not to occur with antagonists.[16] Therefore it was surmised that the agent must be present at all times to compete with the native hormone. However, recent evidence indicates that prolonged treatment with relatively high doses of the LH-RH antagonist SB-75 released from microcapsules down-regulates pituitary LH-RH receptors in rats.[116] The antagonists reduce plasma gonadotropin and gonadal steroid concentration within hours of administration. They cause more rapid gonadal atrophy than agonists and are free of the risks of tumor flare which may occur in the early gonadotropin release phase of agonist action. They are considered elsewhere.

Direct Effects. Clinical evidence in both sexes suggests that chemical castration in both sexes by LH-RH analogs must account for most of the benefit derived from the chronic administration of these analogs to patients with advanced breast or prostate cancer. Elsewhere we compare the results of therapy for these diseases with the results of gonadectomy; there is no striking difference in response rate or time to failure with current agents and protocols. However, there are compelling reasons to believe that direct effects of LH-RH agents on tumor cells exist and that exploiting these effects may improve the results of therapy. All present LH-RH analog treatments mimic the effects of gonadectomy. If direct effects exist this limitation would be surpassed. To assess the possibility of such effects, we must examine inconsistencies between clinical results and those of gonadectomy.

Chemical castration should not benefit postmenopausal women. However, Harris and colleagues reported that 7 of 28 postmenopausal women with advanced breast cancer had either PR or stabilization of disease with Zoladex treatment.[43] Schwartz and colleagues, and Plowman and colleagues also report such effects.[88,112] Harvey and colleagues obtained 16% benefit in postmenopausal women treated with Leuprolide.[47] Anecdotal reports of benefits from LH-RH analog treatment in orchiectomy relapse prompted Ostenson to demonstrate inhibition of growth of human prostatic cancer cell lines in castrated nude mice by Leuprolide.[80] This interesting result is reminiscent of the work of Sundaram and colleagues who demonstrated inhibition of steroid-induced growth of accessory sex glands by an LH-RH analog in hypophysectomized, gonadectomized rats.[120]

Chemical castration should not benefit patients with receptor negative tumors. However, Zoladex therapy of 118 premenopausal women with advanced breast cancer showed response in 49.3% ER-positive, 45.3% PR-positive, 33% ER-negative, and 48% PR-negative tumors.[50] Manni and colleagues also noted benefits in receptor-negative premenopausal patients treated with Leuprolide.[68]

Receptors for LH-RH in Various Tumors. Direct effects of LH-RH analogs could be mediated by receptors found on tumor cells. Specific membrane receptors for LH-RH have been found in various animal and human cancers. Both Dunning rat prostate cancers and specimens of human prostate cancers exhibited two types of receptors for D-Trp-6-LH-RH, one with high affinity and low capacity and one with low affinity and high capacity.[27]

Miller and colleagues, Eidne and colleagues, and Butzow and colleagues found LH-RH receptors in human mammary carcinoma cell lines.[13,25,74] In 260 of 500 samples of human breast cancer (52%), two classes of D-Trp-6-LH-RH membrane receptor sites were also detected, one class showing high affinity and low capacity, and the other class showing low affinity and high capacity.[28] MXT rat mammary cancers also show low affinity and high capacity receptors for D-Trp-6-LH-RH.[121] Low affinity binding sites for [125I]-[D-Ala6-des-Gly10]LH-RH ethylamide were reported in human ovarian epithelial cancers.[26] However, using D-Trp-6-LH-RH as a ligand, we have recently found both high affinity and low affinity LH-RH receptors in human ovarian cancers.[118] In human endometrial carcinomas, the presence of a single, class of high affinity membrane receptors for D-Trp-6-LH-RH was established.[119] LH-RH receptors were also demonstrated in BOP-induced pancreatic cancers in hamsters and in specimens of human pancreatic cancers.[29] These findings provide a rationale for the use of therapeutic approaches based on LH-RH analogs in malignancies in which specific receptors for LH-RH are found.

Effects on Cell Lines. Very compelling, are observations on growth inhibition of cultured tumor cells. The literature is controversial but on balance, significant inhibition of human breast and prostatic cells is well documented.[12,31,34,44,54,73,80,102,114] All of these results suggest a significant, regulatory role of LH-RH-like substances in growth control. Since hypothalamic hormones are not present in the general circulation in significant concentrations, investigators have sought some local form of these substances. Butzow has found immunoreactive LH-RH-like substances and chorionic gonadotropin on cultured breast cancer cells.[13] If such substances have regulatory functions, exploiting them may lead to improved therapy. The presence of LH-RH immunoreactivity and mRNA in human mammary cancer cells suggests that LH-RH may play a role in the growth of mammary tumors.[44]

Somatostatin Analogs

Tetradecapeptide somatostatin (Figure XVII-3-1) has many biological actions, inhibits a large variety of cells and appears to be an endogenous antiproliferative agent.[105] The clinical potential of somatostatin has been appreciated for more than 15 years. Various studies demonstrated inhibitory effects of somatostatin in patients with acromegaly, endocrine pancreatic tumors such as insulinomas and glucagonomas, ectopic tumors like gastrinomas and vasoactive intestinal peptide (VIP) producing tumors.[105] However, the half-life of somatostatin is very short, so that its therapeutic use is impractical.[105]

Several groups designed and synthesized somatostatin analogs with more selective and prolonged activities.[9,14,128] Veber et al., carried out conformational analysis, and designed several analogs by replacing 9 of the 14 amino acids of somatostatin with a single proline residue (Figure XVII-3-1).[128] Some of the resulting hexapeptide analogs, including cyclo (-Pro-Phe-D-Trp-Lys-Thr-Phe), and subsequently cyclo (N-Me-Ala-Tyr-D-Trp-Lys-Val-Phe) were much more potent than somatostatin in inhibiting GH, insulin and glucagon release.[105,128] However, some of these analogs did not reveal

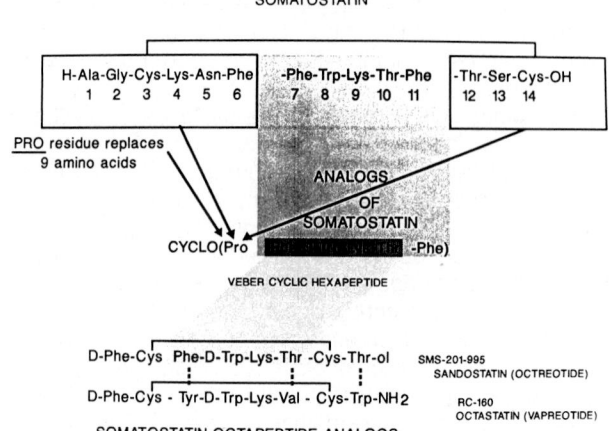

Figure XVII-3-1. Somatostatin and its analogs.

antitumor activities in various tumor models.[105] Bauer and colleagues synthesized another series of highly potent octapeptide analogs of somatostatin.[9] They incorporated the sequence 7–10 of somatostatin, Phe-D-Trp-Lys-Thr, proposed as essential by Veber and colleagues into a series of cystine-bridged analogs of which D-Phe-Cys-Phe-D-Trp-Lys-Thr-Cys-Thr-OL, containing a C-terminal amino alcohol was the most active (Figure XVII-3-1).[9,128] This analog, designated SMS-201-995 (Sandostatin) was 45–70 times more potent than somatostatin in tests on inhibition of GH secretion, and more selective.

Our analogs were designed specifically for antitumor activity. Nearly 300 analogs of somatostatin were synthesized by us by solid-phase methods.[14,105] The activity of some somatostatin analogs was enhanced by incorporation of Tyr and Val in positions corresponding to residue 7 and 10 respectively, of Somatostatin-14. Thus the analogs, D-Phe-Cys-Tyr-D-Trp-Lys-Val-Cys-Thr-NH2 (RC-121) and D-Phe-Cys-Tyr-D-Trp-Lys-Val-Cys-Trp-NH2 (RC-160) (Figure XVII-3-1) were about 100 times more potent than SS-14 in tests for inhibition of growth hormone release in vivo in rats and possessed a prolonged duration of action. We have demonstrated that our somatostatin analog RC-160, alone or in combination with LH-RH agonist D-Trp-6-LH-RH can inhibit the growth of N-Nitrosobis(2-oxopropyl)amine (BOP)-induced ductal pancreatic cancers in hamsters, Dunning prostate tumors in rats and MXT mammary tumors in mice.[109,121,124]

Analog SMS-201-995 (Sandostatin) and other somatostatin analogs have been used for the treatment of acromegaly, endocrine tumors of the gastroenteropancreatic system including carcinoid tumors, insulinomas, glucagonomas, gastrinomas and VIPomas.[59,105] Attempts are being made to use modern somatostatin analogs for the therapy of human breast cancer, prostate cancer and carcinoma of exocrine pancreas.[105]

Mechanisms of Antitumoral Action of Somatostatin Analogs. It is likely that somatostatin analogs, by virtue of having a wide spectrum of activities, which include the suppression of the secretions of the pituitary, pancreas, stomach, and gut, interference with growth factors, and possible direct antiproliferative effects on some tissues, inhibit various tumors through multiple mechanisms.[105] The fall in GH levels induced by somatostatin analogs could, through mechanisms involving endogenous growth factors, especially insulin-like growth factor (IGF-I), be of major importance for the inhibition of growth of various tumors. IGF-I and II and other growth factors including epidermal growth factor (EGF), and transforming growth factor (TGF-α) appear to be involved in the proliferation of both normal and neoplastic cells.[40,105]

In the Mia PaCa-2 human pancreatic cancer cell line, somatostatin reverses the stimulatory effect of EGF on the phosphorylation of the tyrosine kinase portion of the EGF receptor and on cell growth.[63] Superactive octapeptide analogs RC-160 and RC-121 but not SMS-201-995 exhibit high activity on dephosphorylation of EGF receptor and inhibit the EGF-induced growth of cultured MIA PaCa-2 cells more powerfully than somatostatin.[63] These observations indicate that some somatostatin analogs act as growth inhibitors in cancer cells through the activation of tyrosine phosphatase.[63,105] Somatostatin analogs appear to inhibit the action of other endogenous growth factors by mechanisms involving interference with transmission of intracellular signals that regulate cell growth.[63,105] Another possible mechanism by which somatostatin analogs might inhibit tumor growth is the interference with the synthesis of autocrine growth factors by tumor cells. Thus, the action of somatostatin analogs could involve the inhibition of not only endocrine, but also paracrine and autocrine-mediated effects of growth factors. Somatostatin analogs might also inhibit oncogene products, several of which are similar to growth factors or their receptors.[63,105] The product of viral oncogene erbB is a truncated receptor for EGF.[23] The sequence encoded in erbB corresponds to the transmembrane and cytoplasmic portions of the EGF receptors.[23] Therefore, oncological applications of somatostatin analogs are based on multiple effects, and several mechanisms of action are possible.

Receptors for Somatostatin. Direct antiproliferative actions of somatostatin analogs could be also mediated by specific receptors located on tumor cells.[111,117] High or low affinity SS-14 receptors were identified in various normal human tissues, human brain tumors including meningiomas, pituitary tumors, hormone producing gastrointestinal tumors, human breast cancers, small cell lung carcinoma cell lines, human pancreatic cancer specimens, human prostate cancers and in human ovarian cancers.[111,117] Radioiodinated analogs of somatostatin can be used for localization of endocrine-related tumors containing receptors for somatostatin.[57] The binding affinities of various analogs are different for diverse tumors.[117] The analog SMS 201-995 binds well to some normal tissues where it is a good anti-secretory agent, but poorly to most tumors.[117] It is possible that some octapeptide analogs of somatostatin, selected in part on the basis of binding studies, could be potentially useful for the treatment of various neoplasms.

Side effects of somatostatin analogs consist mainly of steatorrhea, which can be controlled, and malabsorption.[105] Consequently, somatostatin analogs should be less toxic than adjuvant chemotherapy.

Antagonists of Bombesin and Gastrin Releasing Peptide (GRP). Antagonists of other peptide growth factors such as amphibian tetradecapeptide bombesin and its 27-amino acid mammalian counterpart gastrin releasing peptide (GRP) (Table XVII-3-3), may have antitumor activity in small cell lung carcinoma (SCLC), which accounts for 20–25% of all cases of lung cancer.[75] GRP has a carboxy-terminal decapeptide fragment which is identical to the carboxy-terminus of bombesin except for Gln/His interchange at positions 7 and 20 in bombesin and GRP, respectively and which has all the biological and immunological activity. Recent evidence indicates that SCLC may be hormone-dependent.[75,76] SCLC produces bombesin or GRP which act as autocrine growth factors. SCLC cell lines also have receptors for bombesin/GRP, and their clonal growth is stimulated by bombesin.[75,76] Consequently, the development of hormonal therapy for SCLC based on bombesin antagonists is being tried by several groups. The first competitive and specific receptor antagonist of bombesin/GRP was pseudo tetradecapeptide [Leu13, ψCH2NHLeu14]bombesin.[19] Subsequently, short-chain bombesin (6–14) nonapeptide analogs with a reduced peptide bond (CH2-NH) and higher potency were reported.[20] Our group synthesized more than 40 pseudo [ψ] 13–14 bombesin (6–14) analogs with different modifications at positions 6, 7 and 14. These antagonists inhibit the binding of 125I-GRP (14-27) in a receptor binding assay on intact Swiss 3T3 cells.[111] Some of these GRP antagonists inhibited the response to GRP (14–27) measured as incorporation of 3H-Thymidine in 3T3 fibroblasts and in SCLC H-345 cells. Certain GRP/bombesin antagonists are active in vivo. Future studies will determine the possible application of bombesin/GRP antagonists in the treatment of SCLC.

The Treatment of Various Tumors with Peptide Analogs

The Treatment of Advanced Prostatic Cancer with LH-RH Analogs

Eligibility for Hormone Treatment. At this writing, radical prostatectomy or radical prostatic irradiation are the only treatments for prostatic cancer offering a reasonable probability for cure. Before recommending palliative treatment, one must ensure that the tumor is correctly staged C or D and that therefore surgery or curative intensive irradiation is contraindicated. In addition to histological proof of prostatic cancer by needle biopsy, an ultrasound study with a rectal probe, a chest film, and bone scan should be done. The ultrasound study will often reveal extension not appreciated by digital examination which will alter the staging, and therefore indicate hormonal treatment. The role of radiation in the treatment of stages A, B and C disease is discussed elsewhere.

Choice of Hormone Treatment. A major goal of research on the endocrinology of prostatic cancer is the conversion of present useful palliation to cure. There are many unanswered questions; patients should be encouraged to enroll in randomized studies which will lead to improved therapy. Clearly, patients with symptoms require and will accept palliation. We do not know the optimal time to begin treatment in asymptomatic patients; the question is decided on an individual basis or by enrollment in ongoing randomized studies.

With the exception of some symptomatic stage B or C disease which may be helped by radiation, palliative treatment involves androgen deprivation therapy. It is frustrating to realize that orchiectomy, estrogens, anti-androgens, and LH-RH analogs with or without additional agents all give a 60–70% remission rate lasting only 1–3 years. Aside from the vascular complications of estrogen therapy there are few adverse effects of any of the treatments; all with the possible exception of flutamide impair sexual potency. The patient

Table XVII-3-3. Bombesin and Gastrin Releasing Peptide

Bombesin

pGlu	-	Gln	-	Arg	-	Leu	-	Gly	-	Asn	-	Gln	-	Trp	-	Ala	-	Val	-	Gly	-	His	-	Leu	-	Met	-	NH$_2$
1		2		3		4		5		6		7		8		9		10		11		12		13		14		

Gastrin releasing peptide (Human)

Val - Pro - Leu - Pro - Ala - Gly - Gly - Gly - Thr - Val - Leu - Thr - Lys -

Met	-	Tyr	-	Pro	-	Arg	-	Gly	-	Asn	-	His	-	Trp	-	Ala	-	Val	-	Gly	-	His	-	Leu	-	Met	-	NH$_2$
14		15		16		17		18		19		20		21		22		23		24		25		26		27		

In analogs ψ (psi) indicates a reduced (pseudo) peptide bond (-CH$_2$-NH-).

should be given the choice of treatments which do not differ in efficacy but which do differ with respect to the impact on his life style. We now discuss the practical use of LH-RH analogs in therapy.

LH-RH Agonistic Analogs in Prostatic Cancer. Based on the finding of Redding and Schally in 1981 that D-Trp-6-LH-RH inhibited the growth of transplantable rat prostatic cancer, the first demonstration of successful palliation in humans by LH-RH analogs was done in a collaborative trial at the Royal Victoria Hospital in Montreal by Tolis and collaborators.[92,125] This demonstration that LH-RH analogs were safe and effective alternatives to orchiectomy was followed by many confirmations which have been reviewed.[115] The peptides could be administered intranasally but were more effective by subcutaneous injection.[110] However, early daily injections are inconvenient and may produce compliance problems. The development of long-acting biodegradable sustained release formulations permitted excellent results with injections on a monthly basis.[1,37,48,69,81,94,98,104,106,110,113] We will review large collaborative studies which will demonstrate that LH-RH agonist analog treatment gives the same benefit as orchiectomy or estrogen with minimal adverse effects.

A collaborative study involving daily subcutaneous injections of 1 mg/day leuprolide compared with 3 mg/day of diethylstilbestrol orally enrolled 199 patients with carcinoma of the prostate and bone metastases, lymph node metastases above the aortic bifurcation, or metastases to other soft tissues (Stage D2); and two measurable or evaluable manifestations.[62] The subjects had no previous systemic or radiation treatment except for local radiotherapy to non-indicator regions. Plasma testosterone was decreased by both treatments so that in 4 weeks both groups were at the castrate level (>1 ng/ml). There was, however, a significant delay of about 1 week for the steroid level in the leuprolide group to fall. The testosterone level actually rises during the early stage of LH-RH treatment. This rise in testosterone may increase pain in bony metastases or injure adjacent nervous tissue. Such a "flare" can be prevented in several ways to be discussed later. Response was evaluated by the National Prostatic Cancer Project (NPCP) criteria. Suppression of testosterone, dihydrotestosterone, and of the elevated acid phosphatase were equivalent in the two groups. The leuprolide group had an overall 86% response rate (complete 1%, partial 37%, stable disease 48%) compared with an 85% response rate in the DES group (complete 2%, partial 44%, stable 39%). Survival rates at one year were 87% for leuprolide and 78% for DES (p=0.17). The leuprolide group had hot flashes, and loss of libido and potency. Patients receiving DES had more gynecomastia and thromboem-

bolism as well as loss of potency.[62] This study showed leuprolide to be a safe, effective alternate to DES treatment when administered as a daily subcutaneous injection.

In another study, Leuprolide was administered in the form of microcapsules of a biodegradable copolymer of lactic and glycolic acids.[113] A single injection of 7.5 mg leuprolide in depot formulation every 4 weeks produced a chemical castration. Median time to lower testosterone to castration level with the depot preparation was 21 days. Mean testosterone levels increased during the first week, peaking at day 4, and then fell to the castration level which was steadily maintained. The response rate was 81% in 53 evaluable patients. The response and adverse effect rates were similar to those in the group on daily leuprolide.[113]

A Phase III study of depot goserelin (Zoladex) was done in the U.K. comparing a 3.6 mg implant of goserelin every 28 days with 3 mg DES daily and with orchiectomy.[86] No significant differences were found in response rate, time to treatment failure, or survival. The LH-RH agonist was considered superior to DES because 15% of patients in the DES group stopped treatment due to side effects; no patient dropped out of the goserelin group.[86]

One may conclude that potent LH-RH agonists in a depot formulation can be easily administered in dosages which match the endocrine and clinical results of orchiectomy. Aside from the expected loss of libido and potency, the only serious adverse effect is the flare in symptoms observed in the early phase of treatment. During the first few weeks, plasma testosterone rises because of increased LH release from the pituitary in response to the releasing hormone. In general, increased symptoms are not seen but since expanding tumor may cause spinal cord or cauda equina damage with irreversible neurological loss, the flare should be prevented. Administration of DES 1 mg/day for 7 days before and during the first 14 days of LH-RH therapy will prevent flare.[66] Administration of flutamide 250 mg every 8 hours starting 7 days before LH-RH treatment and continuing for 2 weeks after starting LH-RH will also prevent flare.[60] The antiandrogen nilutamide can similarly prevent flare.[58]

Monitoring the Effects of Treatment. The response to LH-RH treatment in terms of decreased plasma testosterone and gonadotropins is so universal that these parameters are not usually monitored except in investigative work. In patients who fail to respond to treatment, one should ensure that plasma testosterone is at the castration level, however.

During treatment, the tumor response can be followed by appropriate clinical measurement and imaging. Two markers are commonly used to detect response and treatment failure. Prostatic acid phosphatase is elevated in 7% of normal males and is a more specific marker when measured by RIA rather than by enzymatic activity. It may be useful to detect impending relapse.[17] Prostatic specific antigen is elevated in benign prostatic hyperplasia as well as in cancer and it is very useful in following the response to therapy.[52]

Combination of LH-RH Agonists with Other Agents. We have mentioned addition of the pure antiandrogen flutamide with LH-RH agonists to prevent flare. There is a controversial literature advocating continuing flutamide treatment indefinitely along with LH-RH agonists. The basic concept is that adrenal androgen may initiate growth of residual tumor in a subset of patients. Presumably this subset is small or else adrenalectomy would be a better treatment for orchiectomy relapse. Recently, in a double blind study, 603 men with D2 prostatic cancer were randomized between leuprolide and leuprolide plus flutamide. There was a small but significant increase in progression-free survival and median length of survival.[21] It is quite possible that a subset of patients would show a very significant difference due to total blockade.

Combinations of LH-RH agonists with a somatostatin analog RC-160 produced encouraging results in a rat prostatic cancer model.[109,110,111] However, this combination has not been tested clinically.

Relapse from Androgen Control. In general, after relapse from any androgen control treatment, the next treatment is far less likely to be of benefit. Iverson and colleagues treated 56 previously untreated patients with advanced prostatic cancer with monthly depot Zoladex.[48] Of 53 evaluable patients, 27 achieved partial remissions, and seven were stable. Only one of 32 patients who underwent bilateral orchiectomy following treatment failure with Zoladex achieved a second partial remission.[48] Many studies of patients in relapse give rise to controversial reports of second remissions by additional androgen control with agents like aminoglutethimide, ketoconazole, and anti-androgens. Drago and colleagues treated 43 previously castrated patients in relapse with aminoglutethimide and cortisol.[24] There were six partial responses, one complete long-term response, and 10 patients who showed stable disease.[24] There is no agreement on this or on other treatment attempts after relapse, however. The controversial results may suggest that we are dealing with many subsets of disease and identification of these may lead to the far more frequent second remissions seen in advanced breast cancer.

The hypothesis that somatostatin analogs may delay or prevent the relapse still remains to be tested clinically.[110]

Possibilities for Improvement of LH-RH Analogs. Progress has been made in developing analogs which safely produce chemical castration. If this is the only mechanism by which these substances work, making more LH-RH agonists will clearly not be productive. In the section on mode of action of LH-RH analogs, we discuss the possibility of direct effects on prostatic cancer, and if these exist one would expect that differences among agonists would be found beyond those involving dose or affinity for the receptor. LH-RH antagonists are already developed and may offer advantages in therapy beyond speed of action or avoidance of flare.[3,6,39,64,85,97,111] Further studies should reveal effective combinations of peptides which will enhance tumoricidal effects. Our lack of progress in developing a specific, effective chemotherapeutic agent has been a real deterrent. Newer methods to use LH-RH analogs as carriers for alkylating agents, or platinum derivatives or other cytotoxic radicals

may open up a new area of research and bring nearer the possibility for eventual cure.[4,5,111]

Breast Cancer

Approximately 30% of breast cancers in women are estrogen-dependent. The antiestrogen, tamoxifen, provides effective therapy in premenopausal women with advanced breast cancer, but does not completely antagonize the effects of estrogen.[101] Various experimental studies in rat and mouse models of mammary tumors suggest that analogs of LH-RH, by creating a state of sex-steroid deficiency, might be useful for treatment of estrogen-dependent breast cancer.[77,78,107] Clinical trials conducted since 1982 with Decapeptyl, Buserelin, Zoladex or Leuprolide in premenopausal and postmenopausal women with metastatic breast cancer are encouraging.[46,47,53,68,71,88,89,131,133,134] Responses to LH-RH analogs in a small percentage of postmenopausal women were incompletely understood but tentatively explained by a hypothesis of direct effects of LH-RH agonists on tumors.[46,133] Subsequently, LH-RH agonists have been shown to have direct inhibitory effects on human breast cancer cell lines in vitro and receptors for LH-RH have been demonstrated in cell lines and in primary breast tumors.[12,13,25,28,31,54,73,74,102] Consequently, various LH-RH agonists are being evaluated in postmenopausal women with breast cancer, on the assumption of direct antitumor effects.[88,133] However, LH-RH agonists are mainly targeted at premenopausal women with breast cancer, in whom a clear suppression of ovarian estrogen can be obtained.[78] Mathé and colleagues treated 23 patients with advanced breast cancer, 35–85 years of age, with the sustained release formulation of D-Trp-6-LH-RH designed to release 100 mg/day.[71] The patients were first treated with daily subcutaneous injections of 500 mg D-Trp-6-LH-RH for 7 days, followed by treatment with microcapsules every 28 days. Eight patients were premenopausal and fifteen postmenopausal. Five of eight premenopausal patients were estrogen receptor (ER)-positive, three of these responded (2 CR, 1 PR).[71] Three of fifteen postmenopausal patients also responded; two of these were ER-positive; there was one CR and one PR. These results indicate that the treatment with D-Trp-6-LH-RH is more efficacious in ER-positive patients. The findings recorded in postmenopausal patients imply that D-Trp-6-LH-RH may have a direct antitumoral action. However, recently Harris and colleagues reported that in postmenopausal women with breast cancer, responders and nonresponders showed similar reduction in estradiol.[43] This suggests that LH-RH analogs act indirectly via changes in peripheral hormones, rather than directly on LH-RH receptors on the tumors.[43]

Williams and colleagues observed tumor remissions after Zoladex therapy in 31% of patients.[134] Regressions occurred primarily in women with well-differentiated, slow-growing and ER-positive disease (53%). A large recent trial by Kaufmann and colleagues in premenopausal women with breast cancer, utilizing depot implants of Zoladex, demonstrated 53% objective tumor responses.[51] Santen and colleagues summarized these various studies and calculated a 41% objective response rate in unselected premenopausal patients and 51% in women with ER-positive tumors.[101] Overall results suggest that "medical oophorectomy" with LH-RH analogs is effective in women with estrogen-dependent breast cancers.

There was a remarkable lack of significant clinical toxicity with LH-RH agonists. The phenomenon of tumor flare has not been clearly documented in women with breast cancer during therapy with LH-RH agonists.[101]

Combination Therapy and LH-RH Antagonists. The combination of LH-RH analog with an antiestrogen in the treatment of breast cancer might provide complete "estrogen blockade." Klijn et al. and Walker et al. have reported that combination of Buserelin or Zoladex, in long acting depot preparations, and tamoxifen can be safely used in premenopausal women with breast cancer.[55,132] Significantly greater lowering of serum estradiol and FSH was obtained with the combination.[132]

In addition to growth factors like epidermal growth factor (EGF) and insulin-like growth factor (IGF-I), both growth hormone (GH) and prolactin (PRL) may be involved in breast cancer growth.[40,105,107,117,121] Manni and colleagues evaluated the effects of combined somatostatin analog SMS 201-995 and bromocriptine therapy in postmenopausal women with advanced breast cancer to suppress both GH and PRL secretion.[67] They concluded that combined SMS 210-995 and bromocriptine therapy can suppress GH, IGF-I and PRL secretion in most patients.[67] Since only one patient experienced disease stabilization, its efficacy in the treatment of metastatic breast cancer should be tested in patients with less advanced disease. Vennin and colleagues treated sixteen postmenopausal advanced breast cancer patients with somatostatin analog, SMS 201-995 (Sandostatin).[129] They noted tumor stabilization in three patients after a 90 day treatment period, and some decrease in plasma IGF-I. Side effects were very mild.[129]

Recently it was reported that the presence of receptors for somatostatin (SS-R) in human breast cancer is associated with a good prognosis.[32,96] The relapse-free survival for the 15% of patients with tumors containing SS-R was significantly longer than for patients with SS-R-negative tumors; after 5 years 82% versus 46% were disease free.[32] Estrogen deprivation, interference with growth factors and inhibition of GH and PRL could be produced by treatment with D-Trp-6-LH-RH in combination with somatostatin analog RC-160.[105] This treatment causes reduction of tumor weight and volume in animal models of breast cancer.[121] These results suggest therapeutic trials with a combination of LH-RH agonists and somatostatin analogs in patients.

New antagonistic analogs of LH-RH cause an immediate inhibition of the pituitary-gonadal axis and avoid the initial stimulatory effects on tumor growth.[3,6,39,64,97,111] In addition, in vitro studies on breast cancer cell lines suggest that LH-RH antagonists may directly inhibit cell proliferation.[111,114] The LH-RH antagonist SB-75, free of edematogenic effects, administered to mice bearing transplanted hormone-sensitive MXT mammary tumors caused 84% inhibition of tumor weight.[122] LH-RH antagonist SB-75 proved to be superior to the agonist D-Trp-6-LH-RH, to tamoxifen, and even surgical ovariectomy.[122] Thus, the antagonist SB-75 could be of potential clinical value in the treatment of breast cancer.

Uterine Fibroids (Leiomyoma)

Uterine leiomyoma is the most common solid tumor of the female genital tract and is often associated with pelvic pain, abnormal uterine bleeding, infertility, and spontaneous abortion.[30,35,65,87,126] Surgical myomectomy is not always feasible and therefore, medical management may be needed. Fibroids contain high-affinity estrogen receptors and depend on estrogen for their growth.[135] The estrogen dependence of fibroids is also indicated by their degeneration and atrophy after the menopause.[135] The induction of a hypoestrogenic state by chronic administration of LH-RH agonists in patients with uterine fibroids can lead to shrinkage of the tumors.[104,106] Various investigators have reported beneficial effects of [D-Trp6]-LH-RH (Decapeptyl) and other LH-RH agonists in the treatment of patients with leiomyomas.[30,35,65,87,126] Overall results suggest that LH-RH agonist-induced hypoestrogenism may be a useful method for management of uterine myomas, as a primary therapy or as an adjunct to surgical leiomyomectomy. This new approach could be particularly valuable in those cases where hysterectomy is not desirable, for instance in young women who have not yet completed their families and in patients with symptomatic myomas approaching the menopause.

Epithelial Ovarian Cancer

Gonadotropins have been implicated in ovarian carcinogenesis.[104,106,107,111] Experimental and clinical findings indicate that suppression of the secretion of gonadotropins produced by LH-RH agonists may inhibit the growth of ovarian epithelial cancers.[82–84,104,106,107,111]

Parmar and colleagues were the first to report that chronic treatment with D-Trp-6-LH-RH microcapsules induced the regression of an inoperable, bilateral, serous cystadenocarcinoma of the ovary in a 78-year-old woman.[82] Recently, these findings were confirmed and extended in 40 unselected patients 42–49 years old with advanced epithelial ovarian cancer (FIGO Stage III or IV).[83,84] There was a marked suppression of LH and FSH in response to D-Trp-6-LH-RH and about 30% of patients showed partial remission or stabilization of disease.[83,84] Benefit of therapy with microcapsules of D-Trp-6-LH-RH in ovarian carcinoma is encouraging. This treatment offers a non-toxic alternative in patients who do not tolerate chemotherapy or who have progressive disease following chemotherapy.[82,83,84] Some of the inhibitory effects of LH-RH agonists could be direct since human ovarian epithelial cancers have LH-RH binding sites.[26,118] Membrane receptors for somatostatin and EGF have also been found in human ovarian cancers.[111,117] Combination of somatostatin analogs such as RC-160 with LH-RH agonists might improve the clinical response.[111] LH-RH antagonists also await clinical trial.

Endometrial Carcinoma

The involvement of estrogens in the pathogenesis of endometrial adenocarcinoma is well recognized.[104,107,111,119] About 80% of human endometrial carcinomas of different histological types show specific high affinity membrane receptors for LH-RH and EGF.[119] The functional role of the receptors for D-Trp-6-LH-RH in human endometrial carcinoma is not clear, but this finding provides an additional rationale for the use of therapeutic approaches based on LH-RH analogs in this cancer.[104,119] The principal mechanism by which LH-RH analogs could influence endometrial cancer may be estrogen deprivation, although the incidence of this neoplasm is much higher in postmenopausal women. Direct effect of LH-RH analogs on tumors must be also considered.[119] At this writing only a few cases of successful use of the LH-RH agonists in the treatment of endometrial carcinoma have been reported.[104,109] LH-RH agonists and antagonists could be also tried for the therapy of carcinoma of the uterine cervix. Human papillomavirus (HPV) has been implicated in the pathogenesis of human cervical squamous carcinoma. Mathé and colleagues showed that treatment with Decapeptyl produced a reduction in lesions in condylomas related to papillomaviruses.[70]

Exocrine Pancreatic Cancer

Carcinoma of the pancreas has a very poor prognosis and the 5-year survival rate is about 2%.[15,105,106,107] Only 15–20% of tumors are resectable and radiation and chemotherapy are of limited effectiveness.[15,105,106,107] All potential avenues of treatment must be explored in order to devise a more effective therapy. Exocrine pancreatic cancer has not been considered as a classical hormone-dependent neoplasm, but recent experimental and clinical findings indicate that it may be sensitive to sex steroids, gastrointestinal hormones, and growth factors. These studies have been reviewed extensively.[15,91,105,106,107,111] Various experimental results also indicate that the growth of pancreatic tumors can be inhibited by hormonal manipulations.[15,63,105,124] Inhibition of growth of pancreatic acinar and ductal carcinomas in animal models by analogs of LH-RH and somatostatin was first reported by Redding and Schally in 1984.[93] A variety of experimental and clinical studies performed since then, support the view that it might be possible to develop a hormonal therapy for exocrine cancer of the pancreas based on new somatostatin analogs in combination with LH-RH agonists or antagonists.[63,105,106,107,111,123,124] Somatostatin analogs suppress the secretion and/or action of gastrointestinal hormones (gastrin, secretin, and cholecystokinin), which might influence the growth of the malignant cells of the pancreas.[105] In addition, Somatostatin analogs inhibit the action or secretion of growth factors such as EGF, TGF-α and IGF-I, which appear to be involved in neoplastic processes.[63,105,106] Sex steroids may also play a role in the growth of the cancerous pancreas.[42] The therapeutic effect of LH-RH-agonists could be explained in part by the creation of a state of sex steroid deprivation.[106] A direct effect of LH-RH analogs on the tumor cells is also possible since D-Trp-6-LH-RH receptors are present in pancreatic cancers.[29] Direct antiproliferative actions of somatostatin analogs are similarly mediated by specific high affinity receptors located on pancreatic tumor cells.[63,117] A marked inhibition of tumor growth occurs in hamsters with BOP-induced pancreatic cancer after treatment with microcapsules of somatostatin analog RC-160 or D-Trp⁶-LH-RH.[105,124] The combination of both peptides produced the best results in terms of prolongation of survival, elimination of ascites and histological regression signs.[105,124] The increase of the dosage of RC-160 from 25 to 48 mg/day led to greater regression of tumors and in combination with D-Trp-6-LH-RH produced an 85% reduction in tumor weight. The tumors of hamsters treated with analogs showed striking histological regressive changes characteristic of apoptosis.[124] Chronic treatment with LH-RH antagonist SB-75 also causes a powerful inhibition of pancreatic tumor growth.[123]

On the basis of experimental observations that administration of D-Trp-6-LH-RH inhibits the growth of pancreatic cancers, this analog was tried clinically in five patients with inoperable stage III and IV pancreatic cancer.[38] Therapy with D-Trp-6-LH-RH was started at a daily dose of 1 mg subcutaneously for the first seven days, after which it was reduced to 100 μg daily. All five patients showed clinical improvement,

and a reduction in tumor mass in one.[38] During the 16 months of treatment with D-Trp-6-LH-RH, this patient continued to show clinical improvement. In a more recent study involving 16 patients with advanced pancreatic cancer (stage IV disease), a subjective improvement (decreased pain) and increased appetite as well as a reduction in bilirubin and increase in hemoglobin values were observed in 12 patients after three weeks of D-Trp-6-LH-RH administration.[36] This improvement in the quality of life persisted until the clinical relapse occurred about two weeks before death. The median survival time after treatment with D-Trp-6-LH-RH was 7.2 months.[36] The median survival time of the 12 patients who responded was 9.3 months vs. 2.1 months for the nonresponders ($p > 0.05$).

In cooperative trials, RC-160 is being tried clinically in England and France as a single drug in patients with advanced inoperable pancreatic cancer. Preliminary results based on a dose of 500 mg RC-160 t.i.d. indicate clinical improvement, dramatic decrease in doses of analgesics, and occasional reduction in tumor mass in some patients.[90] Side effects including cramps and diarrhea were minimal. Seven of 14 patients showed improved Karnofsky scores and a tendency toward an increased survival rate was observed.[90] The combination of somatostatin analogs and D-Trp-6-LH-RH might be even more efficacious in treating patients with cancer of the pancreas than single peptides and such trials are planned, but the clinical efficacy of the combined treatment still remains to be assessed.

Colorectal Cancer

Colorectal cancer is the second most common malignant tumor in the United States.[10] Sex steroids, G.I. hormones, especially gastrin and growth factors such as EGF, IGF-I and TGF-α, may be involved in tumorigenesis of the colon.[105] The incidence of colon cancer is increased in acromegalics, suggesting that excessive secretion of GH or IGF-I may be a factor.[105] IGF-I receptors were found in human colon carcinomas.[105] Consequently, an approach similar to that on pancreatic cancer and based on hormonal manipulations such as the use of analogs of somatostatin and LH-RH agonists or antagonists and aimed at inhibiting sex steroids, G.I. hormones and growth factors could also be tested in colorectal cancer. Bombesin antagonists could be also tried since they might interfere with gastrin secretion.[111] However, additional experimental studies are needed to substantiate (validate) these approaches. Although clinical trials have been started or planned, no data are at present available.

Brain Tumors

Therapeutic modalities for primary brain tumors such as malignant astrocytomas (glioblastomas) or even benign tumors like meningiomas need to be improved. That meningiomas and other brain tumors are hormone-sensitive, is supported by epidemiologic, clinical, and laboratory evidence.[79] The presence of estrogen-binding and progesterone-binding proteins in meningiomas has been documented.[79] The presence of receptors for EGF and IGF-I and II in human brain tumors was also established.[105] Thus, sex-steroids and growth factors may be involved in the proliferation of brain tumors. Various brain tumors including astrocytomas and meningiomas, have been found to contain significant levels of high affinity receptors for somatostatin.[61,95,117] These findings suggest the merit of investigations to determine whether somatostatin analogs could inhibit the growth of brain tumors.[105] We have recently established that somatostatin octapeptide analogs such as RC-160 penetrate the blood brain barrier.[7] Radioiodinated somatostatin analogs can label somatostatin receptors in various tumors including meningiomas and astrocytomas in vivo and can therefore be used for tumor localization.[57] Somatostatin analogs could be considered for the development of new approaches to the treatment of some brain tumors. There are also anecdotic reports of symptomatic relief of meningioma by therapy with buserelin.[127] All these results support the need of further studies of hormonal manipulation as another mode of treatment for brain tumors.

Small Cell-Lung Carcinomas

Lung cancer is the leading cause of cancer-related deaths in the USA and in the western world. Small-cell lung carcinoma (SCLC) accounts for 20–25% of all cases of lung cancer.[75] Most cases of SCLC are already metastatic at the time of diagnosis and although chemotherapy can be used, long-term survival is infrequent and new therapeutic modalities are needed.[75]

The development of hormonal therapy could be considered for SCLC, since bombesin/GRP-like peptides function like autocrine growth factors which are secreted by the tumors and which stimulate their own growth.[75,76,111] One of the hormonal approaches is based on bombesin/GRP antagonists.[19,20,111] These peptide analogs should have markedly reduced side effects as compared to combination chemotherapeutic agents. Potent bombesin/GRP analogs active in vitro and in vivo have been synthesized.[19,20,111] Future studies will determine their possible application in the treatment of SCLC.

In addition, somatostatin analogs should also be investigated as possible inhibitors of SCLC since they reduce the secretion of bombesin and GRP and might also inhibit tumor growth by interfering with the synthesis of autocrine growth factors by tumor cells.[105] Somatostatin analogs could be also tried in squamous and other non-small cell lung carcinomas because of high EGF receptor expression in these tumors.

References

1. Ahmann, F. R., Citrin, D. L., deHaan, H. A., Guinan, P., Jordan, V. C., Kreis, W., Scott, M., and Trump, D. L.: Zoladex: A sustained-release, monthly luteinizing hormone-releasing hormone analogue for the treatment of advanced prostate cancer. J. Clin. Oncol., 5:912, 1987.
2. Auclair C., Kelly P. A., Coy D. H., Schally A. V., Labrie F.: Potent inhibitory activity of (D-Leu-6-Des-Gly-NH_2) LHRH ethylamide on LH/hCG and PRL testicular receptor levels in the rat. Endocrinology, 101:1890, 1977.
3. Bajusz, S., Csernus, V. J., Janaky, T., Bokser, L., Fekete, M., and Schally, A. V.: New antagonists of LHRH: II. Inhibition and potentiation of LHRH by closely related analogues. Int. J. Peptide Prot. Res., 32:425, 1988.
4. Bajusz, S., Janaky, T., Csernus, V. J., Bokser, L., Fekete, M., Srkalovic, G., Redding, T. W., and Schally, A. V.: Highly potent analogues of luteinizing hormone-releasing hormone containing D-phenylalanine nitrogen mustard in position 6. Proc. Natl. Acad. Sci. U.S.A., 86:6318, 1989.
5. Bajusz, S., Janaky, T., Csernus, V. J., Bokser, L., Fekete, M., Srkalovic, G., Redding, T. W., and Schally, A. V.: Highly potent metallopeptide analogues of luteinizing hormone-releasing hormone. Proc. Natl. Acad. Sci. U.S.A., 86:6313, 1989.
6. Bajusz, S., Kovacs, M., Gazdag, M., Bokser, L., Karashima, T., Csernus, V. J., Janaky, T., Guoth, J., and Schally, A. V.: Highly potent antagonists of luteinizing hormone-releasing hormone free of edematogenic effects. Proc. Natl. Acad. Sci. U.S.A., 85:1637, 1988.
7. Banks, W. A., Schally, A. V., Barrera, C. M., Fasold, M. B., Durham, D. A., Csernus, V. J., Groot, K., and Kastin, A. V.: Permeability of the murine blood-brain barrier to some octapeptide analogs of somatostatin. Proc. Natl. Acad. Sci. U.S.A., 87:6762,1990.
8. Barron, J. L., Millar, R. P., and Searle, D. I.: Metabolic clearance and plasma half-disappearance time of D-Trp^6 and exogenous luteinizing hormone-releasing hormone. J. Clin. Endocr. Metab., 54:1169, 1982.
9. Bauer, W., Briner, U., Doepfner, W., Haller, R., Huguenin, R., Marbach, P., Petcher, T. J., and Pless, J.: SMS-201-995: A very potent and selective octapeptide analogue of somatostatin with prolonged action. Life Sci., 31:1133, 1982.
10. Beart, Jr., R. W.: Colon, rectum, and anus. Cancer, 33:684, 1990.
11. Bhasin S. and Swerdloff R. S.: Mechanisms of gonadotropin-releasing hormone agonist action in the human male. Endocrine Reviews, 7:106, 1986.
12. Blankenstein, M. A., Hankelman, M. S., and Klijn, J. G.: Direct inhibitory effect of a luteinizing hormone-releasing hormone agonist on MCF-7 human breast cancer cells. Eur. J. Cancer Clin. Oncol., 21:1493, 1985.
13. Butzow R., Huktaniemi I., Clayton R., Wahlstrom T., Andersson L. C., and Seppala M.: Cultured mammary carcinoma cells contain gonadotropin-releasing hormone-like immunoreactivity, GNRH binding sites and chorionic gondadotropin. Intl. J. Cancer, 39:498, 1987.
14. Cai, R. Z., Szoke, B., Lu, R., Fu, D., Redding, T. W., and Schally, A. V.: Synthesis and biological activity of highly potent octapeptide analogs of somatostatin. Proc. Natl. Acad. Sci. U.S.A., 83:1896, 1986.
15. Comaru-Schally, A. M., and Schally, A. V.: LH-RH agonists as adjuncts to somatostatin analogs in the treatment of pancreatic cancer. *In* Gn-RH analogues in cancer and human reproduction, Volume III. Benign and Malignant tumors. Edited by B. Lunenfeld and V. Vickery. Dordrecht/Boston, Kluwer Academic Publishers, p. 203, 1990
16. Conn P. M.: The molecular basis of gonadotropin-releasing hormone action. Endocrine Reviews, 7:3, 1986.
17. Cooper, J. F.: Current experience with radioimmunoassay techniques for prostatic acid phosphatase. Urol. Clin. North Amer., 7:653, 1980.
18. Corbin A., Beattie C. W., Tracy J., Jones R., Foell T. J., Yardley J., and Rees R. W. A.: The anti-reproductive pharmacology of LHRH and antagonistic analogs. Intl. J. Fert., 23:81, 1978.
19. Coy, D. H., Heinz-Erian, P., Jiang, J., Sasaki, Y., Taylor, J., Moreau, J. P., Wolfrey, W. T., Gardner, J. D., and Jensen, R. T.: Probing peptide backbone function in bombesin. A reduced peptide bond analogue with potent and specific receptor antagonist activity. J. Biol. Chem., 263:5056, 1988.
20. Coy, D. H., Taylor, J. E., Jiang, N.-Y, Kim, S. H., Wang, L.-H, Huang, S., Moreau, J. P., Gardner, J. D., and Jensen, R. T.: Short-chain pseudopeptide bombesin receptor antagonists with enhanced binding affinities for pancreatic acinar and Swiss 3T3 cells display strong antimitotic activity. J. Biol. Chem., 264:14691, 1989.
21. Crawford, E. D., Eisenberger, M. A., McLeod, D. G., Spaulding, J. T., Benson, R., Dorr, F. A., Blumenstein, B. A., Davis, M. A., and Goodman, P. J.: A controlled trial of leuprolide with and without flutamide in prostatic carcinoma. N.Engl. J. Med., 321:419, 1989.
22. Csernus, V. J., Szende, B., and Schally, A. V.: Release of peptides from sustained delivery systems (microcapsules and microparticles) in vivo: A histological and immunohistological study. Int. J. Peptide Prot. Res., 35:557, 1990.
23. Downward, J., Yarden, Y., Mayes, E., Scrace, G., Totty, N., Stockwell, P., Ulrich, A., Schlessinger, J., and Waterfield, M. D.: Close similarity of epidermal growth factor receptor and v-erb-B oncogene protein sequences. Nature (London), 307:521, 1984.
24. Drago, J. R., Santen, R. J., Lipton, A., Worgul, T. J., Harvey, H. A., Boucher, A., Manni, A., and Rohner, T.: Clinical effect of aminoglutethimide, medical adrenalectomy, in treatment of 43 patients with advanced prostatic carcinoma. Cancer, 53: 1447, 1984.
25. Eidne K. A., Flanagan C. A., Harris N. S., and Millar R. P.: Gonadotropin-releasing hormone (GnRH)-binding sites in human breast cancer cell lines and inhibitory effects of GnRH antagonists. J. Clin. Endocrin. Metab., 64:425, 1987.
26. Emons G., Pahwa G. S., Brack C., Sturm R., Oberheuser F., and Knuppen R.: Gonadotropin releasing hormone binding sites in human epithelial ovarian carcinomata. Eur. J. Cancer Clin. Oncol., 25:215, 1989.
27. Fekete M., Redding T. W., Comaru-Schally A. M., Pontes A. E., Connelly R. W., Srkalovic G., and Schally A. V.: Receptors for luteinizing hormone-releasing hormone, somatostatin, prolactin and epidermal growth factor in rat and human prostate cancers and in benign prostatic hyperplasic. Prostate, 14:191, 1989.
28. Fekete M., Wittliff J. L., and Schally A. V.: Characteristics and distribution of receptors for [D-Trp^6]-luteinizing hormone-releasing hormone, somatostatin, epidermal growth factor, and sex steroids in 500 biopsy samples of human breast cancer. J. Clin. Lab. Anal., 3:137, 1989.
29. Fekete M., Zalatnai A., Comaru-Schally A. M., and Schally A. V.: Membrane receptors for peptides in experimental and human pancreatic cancers. Pancreas, 4:521, 1989.
30. Filicori, M., Hall, D. A., Loughlin, J. S., Rivier, J., Vale, W., and Crowley, W. F.: A conservative approach to the managmement of uterine leiomyomas: Pituitary desensitization by a luteinizing hormone-releasing hormone analogue. Am. J. Obstet. Gynecol., 147:726, 1983.
31. Foekens, J. A., Henkelman, M. S., Bolt-de-Vries, J., Portengen, H., Fukkink, J. F., Blankenstein, M. A., vanSteengrugge, G. J., Mulder E., and Klijn, J. G. M.: Direct effects of LHRH analogs on breast and prostate tumor cells. *In* Proceedings of the International Symposium on Hormonal manipulations of cancer: peptides, growth factors and new (anti)steroidal agents Edited by J. G. M. Klijn, R. Paridaens, J. A. Foekens. EORTC Monograph Series. New York, Raven Press, vol. 18, pp. 369, 1987.
32. Foekens, J. A., Portengen, H., van Putten, W. L. J., Trapman, A. M. A. C., Reubi, J. C., Alexieva-Figusch, J., and Klijn, J. G. M.: Prognostic value of receptors insulin-like growth factor 1, Somatostatin, and epidermal growth factor in human breast cancer. Cancer Res., 49:7002, 1989.
33. Gammeltoft, A., Ballotti, R., Kowalski, A., Westermark, B, and van Obberghen, E.: Expression of two types of receptors for insulin-like growth factors in human malignant glioma. Cancer Res., 48:1233, 1988.
34. Gattani A., Brower S., Platica M., Schally A. V., and Hollander V.: The inhibition of thymidine incorporation by LHRH and Somatostatin analogs on prostatic cancer line LNCaP in culture (meeting abstract). Proceedings of Annual Meeting of American Association of Cancer Research, 1299:219, 1990.
35. George, M., Lhomme, C., Lefort, J., Gras, C., Comaru-Schally, A. M., and Schally, A. V.: Long term use of an LHRH agonist in the management of uterine leiomyomas: A study of 17 cases. Int. J. Fertil., 34:19, 1989.
36. Gonzalez-Barcena, D., Ibarra-Olmos, M. A., Garcia-Carrasco, F., Gutierrez-Samperio, C., Comaru-Schally, A. M., and Schally, A. V.: Influence of D-Trp-6-LH-RH on the survival time in patients with advanced pancreatic cancer. Biomed. & Pharmacother., 43:313, 1989.
37. Gonzalez-Barcena, D., Perez-Sanchez, P. L., Graef, A., Gomez, A. M., Berea, H., Comaru-Schally, A. M., and Schally A. V.: Inhibition of the pituitary-gonadal axis by a single intramuscular administration of D-Trp-6-LH-RH (Decapeptyl) in a sustained-release formulation in patients with prostatic carcinoma. Prostate, 14:291, 1989.
38. Gonzalez-Barcena, D., Rangel-Garcia, N. E., Nerez-Sanchez, P. L., Gutierrez-Damperio, C., Garcia-Carrasco, F., Comaru-Schally, A. M., and Schally, A. V.: Response to D-Trp-6-LH-RH in advanced adenocarcinoma of pancreas. Lancet, 2:154, 1986.
39. Gonzalez-Barcena, D., Vadillo-Buenfil, M., Guerra-Arguero, L., Carreno, J., Comaru-Schally, A. M., and Schally, A. V.: Potent antagonistic analog of LH-RH (SB-75) inhibits LH, FSH, and testosterone levels in human beings. Program, 72nd Annual Meeting, Endocrine Society, Atlanta, Ga., Abstr. No. 1318, p. 354, June 20-23, 1990.
40. Goustin, A. S., Loef, E. B., Shipley, G. S., and Moses, H. L.: Growth factors and cancer. Cancer Res., 46:1015, 1986.

41. Green, J. D., Harris, G. W.: The neurovascular link between the neurohypophysis and adenohypophysis. J. Endocrinol., 5:136, 1947
42. Greenway, B. A.: Carcinoma of the exocrine pancreas: a sex hormone responsive tumor? Br. J. Surg., 74:441, 1987.
43. Harris, A. L., Carmichael, J., Cantwell, B. M. J., and Dowsett, M.: Zoladex: Endocrine and therapeutic effects in post-menopausal breast cancer. Br. J. Cancer, 59:97, 1989.
44. Harris, N. S., Wilcox, J. N., Dutlow, C. M., Flanagan, C.A., Prescott, R.A., Roberts, J.L., Eidne, K.A., and Millar, R.P.: A putative autocrine role for GnRH in mammary carcinoma cell lines. In Progress in Cancer Research and Therapy, Volume 35: Hormones and Cancer 3. Edited by F. Bresciani, R.J.B. King, M.E. Lippman, and J.P. Raynaud. New York, Raven Press, Ltd., 1988, p. 174.
45. Harvey H. A.: Luteinizing hormone-releasing hormone agonist in the therapy of breast cancer. In Endocrine Therapies in Breast and Prostate Cancer. Edited by C.K. Osborne. Boston, Kluwer Academic Publishers, 1988, p. 39.
46. Harvey, H. A., Lipton, A., and Max, D.: LH-RH analogs for human mammary carcinoma. In LH-RH and its analogs- contraceptive and therapeutics applications. Edited by B. H. Vickery, J. J. Nestor, Jr., E. S. E. Hafez. Boston/Lancaster, MTP Press, 1984, p. 329.
47. Harvey H. A., Lipton A., Santen R. J., Escher G. C., Hardy M. N., Glode I. M., Segaloff A., Landau R. Z., Schneir H., and Max D. T.: Phase I study of a gonadotropin-releasing hormone analogue (Leuprolide) in postmenopausal advanced breast cancer patients. Proceedings of American Association of Cancer Research, Abstract, 22:44, 1981.
48. Iversen, P., Rose, C., Stage, J. G., Iversen, H. G., Hansen, R. I., Hvidt, V., Mogensen, P., Pedersen, T., and Hansen, J. B.: LHRH analogue as a depot preparation (Zoladex) in the treatment of advanced carcinoma of the prostate followed by orchiectomy as a second line therapy – a Phase II study. Scand. J. Urol. Nephrol., 23:177, 1989.
49. Karten, M. J., and Rivier, J. E.: Gonadotropin-releasing hormone analog design. Structure-function studies toward the development of agonists and antagonists: Rationale and perspective. Endocr. Rev., 7:44, 1986.
50. Kaufmann M.: GNRH-agonists (Zoladex) therapy in premenopausal women with metastasizing breast carcinoma.: Hormone Res, 32 (suppl. I):202, 1989.
51. Kaufmann, M., Jonat, W., Kleeburg, U., Eirmann, W., Janicke, F., Hilfrich, J., Kreienberg, R., Albrecht, M., Weitzel, H. K., Schmid, H., Strunz, P., Schachner-Wunschmann, E., Bastert, G., Maass, H.: The German zoladex trial group: Goserelin, a depot gonadotropin releasing hormone agonist in the treatment of premenopausal patients with metastatic breast cancer. J. Clin. Oncol., 7:1113, 1989.
52. Killian C. S., Yang M. C., Emrich, L. J., Vargas, F. P., Manabu K., Wang M. C., Slack N. H., Papsidero L. D., Murphy G. P., Chu T. M., and the Investigators of The National Prostatic Cancer Project.: Prognostic importance of prostate specific antigen for monitoring patients with stages B_2 to D_1 prostate cancer. Cancer Res, 45:886, 1985.
53. Klijn, J. G. M., and de Jong, F. H.: Treatment with a luteinizing hormone-releasing hormone analogue (Buserelin) in premenopausal patients with metastatic breast cancer. Lancet, 1:1213, 1982.
54. Klijn J. G. M., de Jong F. H., Lamberts F. W., and Blankenstein M. A.: LHRH agonist treatment in clinical and experimental human breast cancer. J. Ster. Biochem., 23:867, 1985.
55. Klijn, J.G.M., van Geel, A.N., Sandow, J., and deJong, F.H.: Treatment with high dose LH-RH-agonist (Buserelin) plus tamoxifen and with buserelin implants in premenopausal patients: an endocrine and pharmacokinetic study. In: Progress in Cancer Research and Therapy, Volume 35, Hormones and Cancer 3. Edited by F. Bresciani, R.J.B. King, M.E. Lippman, and J.P. Raynaud. New York, Raven Press, Ltd., 1988, p. 365.
56. Knobil, E.: The neuroendocrine control of the menstrual cycle. Recent Prog. Horm. Rec. 36:53, 1980.
57. Krenning, E.P., Breeman, W.A.P., Kooij, P.P.M., Lameris, J.S., Bakker, W.H., Koper, J.W., Ausema, L., Reubi, J.C., and Lamberts, S.W.J.: Localisation of endocrine-related tumors with radioiodinated analogue of somatostatin. The Lancet, 1:242, 1989.
58. Kuhn, J. M., Billebaud, T., Navratil, H., Moulonguet, A., Fiet, J., Grise, P., Louis, J. F., Costa, P., Husson, J. M., Dahan, R., Bertagna, C., and Edelstein, R.: Prevention of the transient adverse effects of a gonadotropin-releasing hormone analogue (buserelin) in metastatic prostatic carcinoma by administration of an antiandrogen (nilutamide). N. Engl. J. Med., 321:413, 1984.
59. Kvols, L.D., Moertel, C.G., O'Connell, M.J., Schutt, A.J., Rudin, J., Hahn, R.G.: Treatment of the malignant carcinoid syndrome. N Engl J Med, 315:663, 1986.
60. Labrie, F., Dupont, A., Belanger, A., and Lachance, R.: Flutamide eliminates the risk of disease flare in prostatic cancer patients treated with a luteinizing hormone-releasing hormone agonist. J. Urol., 138:804, 1987.
61. Lambert, S. W. J., Koper, J. W., and Reubi, J. C.: Potential role of somatostatin analogues in the treatment of cancer. Eur. J. Clin. Invest., 17:281, 1987.
62. The Leuprolide Study Group: Leuprolide versus diethylstilbestrol for metastatic prostate cancer. N. Engl. J. Med., 311:1281, 1984.
63. Liebow, C., Reilly, C., Serrano, M., and Schally, A. V.: Somatostatin analogues inhibit growth of pancreatic cancer by stimulating tyrosine phosphatase. Proc. Natl. Acad. Sci. U.S.A., 86:2003, 1989.
64. Ljungqvist, A., Feng, D. M., Hook, W., Shen, Z. X., Bowers, C., and Folkers, K.: Antide and related antagonists of luteinizing hormone release with long action and oral activity. Proc. Natl. Acad. Sci. U.S.A., 85:8236, 1988.
65. Maheux, R., Guilloteau, C., Lemay, A., Bastide, A., and Fazekas, A. T. A.: Luteinizing hormone-releasing hormone agonist and uterine leiomyoma: A pilot study. Am. J. Obstet. Gynecol., 152:1034, 1985.
66. Mahler, C., and Denis, L.: Simultaneous administration of a luteinizing hormone releasing hormone agonist and diethylstilbestrol in the initial treatment of prostatic cancer. Am. J. Clin. Oncol., 11 Suppl 2:127, 1988.
67. Manni, A., Boucher, A. E., Demers, L. M., Harvey, H. A., Lipton, A., Simmonds, M. A., and Bartholomew, M.: Endocrine effects of combined somatostatin analog and bromocriptine therapy in women with advanced breast cancer. Breast Cancer Res. Treat., 14:289, 1989.
68. Manni A., Santen R., Harvey H., Lipton A., and Max D.: Treatment of breast cancer with gonadotropin-releasing hormone. Endocrine Rev., 7:89, 1986.
69. Mason-Garcia, M., Vigh, S., Comaru-Schally, A. M., Redding, T. W., Somogyvari-Vigh, A., Horvath, J., and Schally, A. V.: Radioimmunoassay for D-Trp^6 analog of luteinizing hormone-releasing hormone: measurement of serum levels after administration of long-acting microcapsules formulation. Proc. Natl. Acad. Sci. U.S.A., 82:1547, 1985.
70. Mathé, G., Busuttil, M., Reynes, M., Hagipantelli, R., Mauvernay, Y., and Schally, A. V.: Triptorelin in treatment of cervical and vaginal dysplasia related to papillomavirus. Lancet, 1:819, 1988.
71. Mathé, G., Keiling, R., Prevot, G., Vo Van, M. L., Gastiaburu, J., Vannetzel, J. M., Despax, R., Jasmin, C., Levi, F., Musset, M., Machover, D., Ribaud, R., Misset, J. L.: LH-RH agonist: Breast and prostate cancer. *In* Hormonal manipulation of cancer: Peptides, growth factors, and new (anti) steroidal agents. Edited by J. G. M. Klijn, R. Paridaens, J. A. Foekens. New York, Raven Press, 1987, p. 315.
72. Meldrum, D. R., Tasao, Z., Monroe, S. E., Braustein, G. D., Sladek, J., Lu, J. K. H., Vale, W., Rivier, J., Judd, H. L., and Chang, R. J.: Stimulation of LH fragments with reduced bioactivity following GnRH agonist administration in women. J. Clin. Endocrinol. Metab., 58:755, 1984.
73. Miller, E. R., Scott, W. N., Fraser, H. M., and Sharpe, R. M.: Direct inhibition of human breast cancer cell growth by an LHRH agonist. Monograph Series European Organ Research for Treatment of Cancer, 18:357, 1987.
74. Miller, E. R., Scott W. N., Morris R., Fraser, H. M., and Sharpe R. M.: Growth of human breast cancer cells inhibited by a luteinizing hormone-releasing hormone agonist. Nature, 313:231, 1985.
75. Minna, J. D.: Neoplasms of the lung. *In* Harrison's Principles of Internal Medicine, 11th Edition. Edited by E. Braunwald, K.J. Isselbacher, R. G. Petersdorf, J. D. Wilson, J. B. Martin, and A. S. Fauci. New York, McGraw Hill, 1987, p. 1115.
76. Moody, T. W., Carney, D. N., Cuttitta, F., Quattrocchi, K., and Minna, J. D.: High affinity receptors for bombesin/GRP-like peptides on human small cell lung cancer. Life Sci., 37:105, 1985.
77. Nicholson R. I., Walker K. J., Turkes A., Turkes, A. O., Dyas, J., Blamey, R. W., Campbell, F. C., Robinson, M. R. C., and Griffiths, K.: Therapeutic significance and mechanism of action of the LHRH agonist ICI 118630 in breast and prostate cancer. J. Ster. Biochem., 20:129, 1984.
78. Nicholson R. I., Walker K. J., Walker R. F., Read G. F., Turkes A., Robertson J. F. R., and Blamey R. W.: Review of the endocrine actions of LHRH analogs in premenopausal women in breast cancer. Hor. Res., 32:198, 1989.
79. Olson, J. J., Beck, D. W., MacIndoe, J. W., and Min-Loh, P.: Androgen receptors in meningiomas. Cancer, 61:952, 1988.
80. Ostenson R., and Loop S.: Direct in vitro and in vivo inhibition of human prostate carcinoma cell lines by the luteinizing hormone-releasing hormone (LHRH) agonist Leu-6-LH-RH. Proceedings of Annual Meeting of American Society of Clinical Oncology, Abstract, 6:A60, 1987.
81. Parmar, H., Lightman, S. L., Allen, L., Phillips, R. H., Edwards, L., and Schally, A. V.: Randomised controlled study of orchidectomy vs, long-acting D-Trp-6-LH-RH microcapsules in advanced prostatic carcinoma. Lancet, 2:1202, 1985.
82. Parmar, H., Nicoll, J., Stockdale, A., Cassoni, A., Phillips, R. H., Lightman, S. L., and Schally A. V.: Advanced ovarian carcinoma: response to the agonist [D-Trp^6]LHRH. Cancer Treat. Rep., 69:1341, 1985.
83. Parmar, H., Phillips, R. H., Rustin, G., Hanham, I. W., Schally, A. V., and Lightman, S. L.: Response to [D-Trp^6]LHRH (Decapeptyl) microcapsules in advanced ovarian cancer. Br. Med. J., 296:1229, 1988.
84. Parmar, H., Phillips, R. H., Rustin, G., Lightman, S. L., and Schally, A. V.: Therapy of advanced ovarian cancer with D-Trp^6-LH-RH (decapeptyl) microcapsules. Biomed. & Pharmacotherapy, 42:531, 1988.
85. Pavlou, S. N., Wakefield, G., Schlechter, N. L., Lindner, J., Souza, K. H., Kamilaris, T. C., Konidaris, S., Rivier, J. E., Vale, W. W., and Toglia, M.: Mode of suppression of pituitary and gonadal function after acute or prolonged administration of a luteinizing hormone-releasing hormone antagonist in normal men. J. Clin. Edocr. Metab., 68:446, 1989.
86. Peeling, W. B.: Phase III studies to compare goserelin (Zoladex) with orchiectomy and with diethylstilbestrol in treatment of prostatic carcinoma. Urology, 33:45, 1989.
87. Perl, V., Marquez, J., Schally, A. V., Comaru-Schally, A. M., Leal, G., Zacharias, S., Gomez-Lira, C.: Treatment of leiomyomata uteri with D-Tpr-6-LH-RH. Fertil. Steril., 48:383, 1987.
88. Plowman P. N., Nicholson R. I., and Walker K. J.: Responses in post-menopausal breast cancer with an LH-RH analog (ICI 118,630). Eur. J. Cancer and Clin. Oncol., 22:746, 1986.
89. Plowman, P. N., Nicholson, R. I., and Walker, K. J.: Remission of postmenopausal breast cancer during treatment with the luteinizing hormone releasing hormone agonist ICI 118630. Brit. J. Cancer, 54:903, 1986.
90. Poston, G. J., Davies, N., Schally, A. V., Schally, A. M., Gastiaburu, J., and Guillou, P. J.: Phase one B study of somatostatin analogue RC-160 in the treatment of patients with advanced exocrine pancreatic cancer. Abstract, European Pancreatic Club, Basel, Switzerland. October 15-17, 1990. Digestion, 46:170, 1990.
91. Poston, G. J., Gillespie, J., and Guillou, P. J.: The biology of pancreatic cancer. Gut, 32:800, 1991.
92. Redding, T. W., and Schally, A. V.: Inhibition of prostate tumor growth in two rat models by chronic administration of D-Trp-6-LH-RH. Proc. Natl. Acad. Sci. U.S.A., 78:6509, 1981.
93. Redding, T. W., and Schally, A. V.: Inhibition of growth of pancreatic carcinomas in animal models by analogs of hypothalamic hormones. Proc. Natl. Acad. Sci. U.S.A., 81:248, 1984.
94. Redding, T. W., Schally, A. V., Tice, T. R., and Meyers, W. E.: Long-acting delivery systems for peptides: Inhibition of rat prostate tumors by controlled release of (D-Trp-6-) luteinizing hormone-releasing hormone from injectable microcapsules. Proc. Natl. Acad. Sci. U.S.A., 81:5845, 1984.
95. Reubi, J. C., Maurer, R., Klijn, J. G. M., Stefanko, S. Z., Foekens, J. A., Blaauw, G., Blankenstein, M. S., and Lamberts, S. W. J.: High incidence of somatostatin receptors in human meningiomas: biochemical characterization. J. Clin. Endocrinol. Metab., 63:433, 1986.
96. Reubi, J. C., and Torhorst, J.: The relationship between somatostatin, epidermal growth factor, and steroid hormone receptors in breast cancer. Cancer, 64:1254, 1989.
97. Rivier, J. E., Porter, J., Rivier, C. L., Perrin, M., Corrigan, A., Hook, W. A., Siraganian, R. P., and Vale, W. W.: New effective gonadotropin releasing hormone antagonists with minimal potency for histamine release in vitro. J. Med. Chem., 29:1846, 1986.
98. Roger, M., Duchier, J., Lahlou, N., and Schally, A. V.: Treatment of prostatic cancers by periodic administration of a delayed-release preparation of D-Trp(6)-LHRH. Ann. Urology (Paris), 20:109, 1986.
99. Sandow J., Seidel H. R., Krauss B., and Jerabek-Sandow G.: Pharmacokinetics of LHRH agonists in different delivery systems and the relation to endocrine function. *In* Hormonal manipulation of cancer: peptides, growth factors, and new steroidal agents. Edited by J. G. M. Klijn, R. Paridaens, J. A. Foekens. New York, Raven Press, 1987, p. 203.
100. Sandow, J., von Rechenberg, W., Jerzabek, G., Stoll, W.: Pituitary gonadotropins inhibition by a highly active analog of luteinizing hormone-releasing hormone. Fertil. Steril., 30:205, 1978.
101. Santen, R. J., Manni, A., Harvey, H., and Redmond, C.: Endocrine treatment of breast cancer in women. Endoc. Rev., 11:221, 1990.
102. Scambia G., Panici P. B., Baiocchi G., Perrone L., Gaggini C., Jacobelli S., Mancuso S.: Growth inhibitory effect of LHRH analogs on human breast cancer cells. Anticancer Research, 8:187-190, 1988.

103. Schally, A. V.: Aspects of hypothalamic regulation of the pituitary gland. Science, 202:18-28, 1978.

104. Schally, A. V.: The use of LH-RH analogs in Gynecology and Tumor Therapy. In Advances in Gynecology and Obstetrics, Volume 6, General Gynecology. Edited by P. Belfort, J. A. Pinotti. Carnforth, England, Parthenon Publishing, 1989, p.3.

105. Schally, A. V.: Oncological application of somatostatin analogues. Cancer Res., 48:6977, 1988.

106. Schally, A. V., Bajusz, S., Redding, T. W., Zalatnai, A., Comaru-Schally, A. M.: Analogs of LHRH: The present and the future. In GnRH analogues in cancer and in human reproduction, Basic Aspects. Edited by B. H. Vickery and V. Lunenfeld. Dordrecht/Boston/London, Kluwer Academic Publishers, Vol. I, p. 5, 1989.

107. Schally, A. V., Comaru-Schally, A. M., and Redding, T.: Antitumor effects of analogs of hypothalamic hormones in endocrine-dependent cancers. Proc. Soc. Exp. Biol. Med., 175:259, 1984.

108. Schally, A. V., Kastin, A. J., Arimura, A.: Hypothalamic FSH and LH-regulating hormone: Structure, physiology and clinical studies. Fertil. Steril., 22:703, 1971.

109. Schally, A. V., and Redding, T. W.: Somatostatin analogs as adjuncts to agonists of luteinizing hormone-releasing hormone in the treatment of experimental prostate cancer. Proc. Natl. Acad. Sci. U.S.A., 84:7275, 1987.

110. Schally, A. V., Redding, T. W., Paz-Bouza, J. I., Comaru-Schally, A. M., and Mathe, G.: Current concept for improving treatment of prostate cancer based on combination of LHRH agonists with other agents. In Prostate Cancer Part A: Research, Endocrine Treatment and Histopathology. Edited by G. P. Murphy, S. Khoury, R. Kuss, C. Chatelain, L. Denis. New York, Alan R. Liss, Inc., 1987, p. 173.

111. Schally, A. V., Srkalovic, G., Szende, B., Redding, T. W., Janaky, T., Juhasz, T., Korkut, E., Cai, R. Z., Szepeshazi, K., Radulovic, S., Bokser, L., Groot, K., Serfozo, P., and Comaru-Schally, A. M.: Antitumor effects of analogs of LH-RH and Somatostatin: Experimental and clinical studies. Int. J. Steroid Biochem., 37:1061, 1990.

112. Schwartz, L., Guiochet, N., Keiling, R: Two partial remissions induced by LHRH analog in two postmenopausal women with metastatic breast cancer. Cancer, 62: 2498, 1988.

113. Sharifi, R., Soloway, M., Leuprolide Study Group: Clinical study of leuprolide depot formulation in the treatment of advanced prostate cancer. J. Urology, 143:68, 1990.

114. Sharoni Y., Bosin E., Miinster A., Levy J., and Schally A. V.: Inhibition of growth of human mammary tumor cells by potent antagonists of luteinizing hormone-releasing hormone. Proceedings of the National Academy Science (U.S.A.), 86:1648, 1989.

115. Sogani, P. C., Fair, W. R.: Treatment of Advanced Prostatic Cancer. Urol. Clin. North Am., 14:253-271, 1987.

116. Srkalovic G., Bokser L., Radulovic S., Korkut E., and Schally A. V.: Receptors for luteinizing hormone-releasing hormone (LH-RH) in Dunning R3327 prostate cancers and rat anterior pituitaries after treatment with a sustained delivery system of LH-RH antagonist SB-75. Endocrinology, 127:3052, 1990.

117. Srkalovic, G., Cai, R. Z., and Schally, A. V.: Evaluation of receptors for somatostatin in various tumors using different analogs. J. Clin. Endocrin. Metab., 70:661, 1990.

118. Srkalovic G., Schally A. V., Wittliff, J., Day, T. G., Jenison, E. L.: Presence and characteristics of receptors for [D-Trp⁶]-luteinizing hormone releasing hormone and epidermal growth factor in human ovarian carcinoma. Cancer Res. (In Press).

119. Srkalovic G., Wittliff J. L., and Schally A. V.: Detection and partial characterization of receptors for [D-Trp-⁶]-luteinizing hormone-releasing hormone and epidermal growth factor in human endometrial carcinoma. Cancer Res., 50:1841, 1990.

120. Sundaram K., Cao Y. Q., Wang N. G., Bardin C. W., Rivier J., and Vale W.: Inhibition of the action of sex steroids by gonadotropin-releasing hormone (GnRH agonists: A new biological effect. Life Science, 28:83, 1981.

121. Szende, B., Lapis, K., Redding, T. W., Srkalovic, G., and Schally, A. V.: Growth inhibition of MXT mammary carcinoma by enhancing programmed cell death (apoptosis) with analogs of LH-RH and somatostatin. Breast Canc. Res. Treat., 14:307, 1989.

122. Szende, B., Srkalovic, G., Groot, K., Lapis, K., and Schally, A. V.: Growth inhibition of mouse MXT mammary tumor by the luteinizing hormone-releasing hormone antagonist SB-75. J. Natl. Cancer Inst., 82:513, 1990.

123. Szende, B., Srkalovic, G., Groot, K., Lapis, K., and Schally, A. V.: Regression of nitrosamine-induced pancreatic cancers in hamsters treated with LH-RH antagonists or agonists. Cancer Res., 50:3716, 1990.

124. Szende, B., Srkalovic, G., Schally, A. V., Lapis, K., and Groot, K.: Inhibitory effects of analogs of luteinizing hormone-releasing hormone (LH-RH) and somatostatin on pancreatic cancers in hamsters: Events which accompany tumor regression.Cancer, 65:2279, 1990.

125. Tolis, G., Ackman, D., Stellos, A., Mehta, A., Labrie, F., Fazekas, A., Comaru-Schally, A. M., and Schally, A. V.: Tumor growth inhibition in patients with prostatic carcinoma treated with luteinizing hormone-releasing agonists. Proc. Natl. Acad. Sci. U.S.A., 79:1658, 1982.

126. Van Leusden, H. A. I. M.: Rapid reduction of uterine myomas after short-term treatment with microencapsulated D-Trp-6-LH-RH. Lancet, 2:1213, 1986.

127. van Seters, A. P., van Dulken, H., deKeizer, R. J. W., and Vielvoye, G. J.: Symptomatic relief of meningioma by buserelin maintenance therapy. Lancet, i:564, 1989.

128. Veber, D. F., Freidinger, R. M., Schwenk-Perlow, D., Paleveda, W. J., Jr., Holly, R. W., Strachan, R. G., Nutt, R. F., Arison, B. H., Homnick, C., Randall, W. C., Glitzer, M. S., Saperstein, R., and Hirschmann, R.: A potent cyclic hexapeptide analogue of somatostatin. Nature (London), 292:55, 1981.

129. Vennin, P. H., Peyrat, J. P., Bonneterre, J., Louchez, M. M., Harris, A. G., and Demaille, A.: Effect of the long-acting somatostatin analogue SMS 201-995 (Sandostatin) in advanced breast cancer. Anticancer Res., 9:153, 1989.

130. Vermeulen, A.: The hormonal activity of the postmenopausal ovary. J. Clin. Endocrinol. Metab., 42:247, 1976.

131. Walker, K. J., Turkes, A., Williams, M. R., Blamey, R. W., and Nicholson, R. I.: Preliminary endocrinological evaluation of a sustained-release formulation of the LH-Releasing hormone agonist D-Ser(Buᵗ)⁶Azgly¹⁰LH-RH in premenopausal women with advanced breast cancer. J. Endocr., 111:349, 1986.

132. Walker, K. J., Walker, R. F., Turkes, A., Robertson, J. R F., Blamey, R. W., Griffiths, K., and Nicholson, R. I.: Endocrine effects of combination antioestrogen and LH-RH agonist therapy in premenopausal patients with advanced breast cancer. Eur. J. Cancer Clin. Oncol., 25:651, 1989.

133. Waxman, J. H., Harland, S. J., Coombes, R. C., Wrigley, P. F. M., Malpas, J. S., Powles, T., Lister, T. A.: The treatment of postmenopausal women with advanced breast cancer with buserelin. Cancer Chemother. Pharmacol., 15:171, 1985.

134. Williams, M. R., Walker, K. J., Turkes, A., Blamey, R. W., and Nicholson, R. I.: The use of an LH-RH agonist (ICI 118630, Zoladex) in advanced premenopausal breast cancer. Brit. J. Cancer, 53:629, 1986.

135. Wilson, E. A., Yang, F., Rees, E. D.: Estradiol and progesterone binding in uterine leiomyomata and in normal uterinetissues. Obstet. Gynecol., 55:20, 1980.

XVII-4

Medical Management of Thyroid Nodules

Enrico Macchia
Leslie J. DeGroot

Introduction

Thyroid nodules are a common finding in endocrine pathology. Up to 4 percent of the population living in iodine sufficient areas have clinically detectable thyroid nodules and the prevalence of nodular thyroids is higher in iodine deficient areas. Of these nodular thyroids, one half are considered uninodular and one half multinodular.[13,14] The frequency increases with age and the female/male ratio is considered to be 5:1.[3] A much higher prevalence of thyroid nodules is obtained in studies of consecutive autopsy series. In one series reported in 1955, half of the thyroids were found to harbor nodules and 12 of 100 contained a solitary nodule.[9] Ultrasonography studies revealed nodules in 13–40% of patients evaluated for non-thyroid problems.[2,7] Thus, the true prevalence of thyroid nodules is clearly higher than that rec-ognized by physical examination. More than 95% of thyroid nodules are benign.[6] The incidence of clinically evident thyroid cancer in the general population is considered to be 0.004%.[3,12] The availability of new preoperative techniques able to distinguish between benign and malignant lesions has produced a seven-fold increase in the surgical incidence of thyroid cancer. In fact, at present 10–30% of solitary thyroid nodules submitted for surgical resection are malignant neoplasms.[8,10,11] Moreover, a high incidence of thyroid cancer is found in autopsy series. Despite this relatively high incidence of thyroid cancer, only an estimated 1,000 deaths are due to thyroid carcinoma each year in the United States.

In view of their large number, the physician might choose to take a conservative approach in the management of thyroid nodules. The following are the main reasons in favor of this strategy: very few thyroid nodules are malignant; malignant nodules are rarely lethal; the highly lethal anaplastic carcinomas are surgically incurable; the growth of differentiated thyroid cancer can be blocked by suppressive L-T4 therapy; and surgical complications have to be considered, and surgical treatment has to be integrated with medical therapy.

On the other hand, there are several reasons to favor surgery in those nodules which seem more likely to be cancerous:

1) the clinical behavior of differentiated thyroid carcinoma is relatively aggressive in 10–20% of patients; thus differentiated cancer may not be lethal but can cause highly invasive lesions.
2) thyroidectomy in differentiated thyroid carcinoma, followed by other appropriate therapeutic measures, often cures the illness.

The above considerations lead one to conclude that the correct management of thyroid nodules is to select carefully the higher risk thyroid nodules for surgery on the basis of an appropriate and precise diagnostic protocol, leaving the other nodules for periodic medical observation.

Classification of Thyroid Nodules

Human thyroid neoplasms of follicular cell origin are divided into adenomas, differentiated carcinomas and undifferentiated carcinomas (Table XVII-4-1). About 60% of malignant lesions of the thyroid are papillary carcinomas, about 30% are follicular and 5% are medullary carcinomas.

Thyroid nodules are the clinical manifestation of different pathological processes. A solitary nodule may be found in a gland of normal morphology or in a diffuse goiter. Frequently, especially in iodine deficient areas, the thyroid is enlarged and contains multiple nodules. One of them, however, may become clinically dominant. One classification of thyroid nodules, based on pathological and clinical criteria, divides all nodules into non-neoplastic nodules, benign neo-

plasms, malignant neoplasms, and non-thyroidal lesions. Table XVII-4-2 lists the thyroid abnormalities that may appear as a nodule.

Non-Neoplastic Nodules

Some nodules consist of areas of glandular hyperplasia as a result of a process of unknown origin or as a compensatory phenomenon after partial thyroidectomy. Degenerative nodules normally develop in old goiters, are rarely solitary, and represent the evolution of colloid goiter in areas of hemorrhage, infarction, fibrosis and calcification. Nodules associated with Hashimoto's thyroiditis are areas of lymphocytic infiltration, scattered through the damaged follicles. In subacute thyroiditis the structure of the gland is disrupted and typical granulomata are present.

Benign Neoplasms

Benign neoplasms are classically divided into non-functioning nodules and autonomously functioning nodules. Nonfunctioning nodules appear "cold" on the scintiscan and may be solid, cystic or partially cystic (mixed). Autonomously functioning nodules appear "hot" on the scintiscan: they may be typical adenomas (surrounded by a capsule and derived from a single cell, i.e., monoclonal) or areas of polyclonal thyroid tissue functioning independent of pituitary control mechanisms.

Malignant Neoplasms

The majority of malignant thyroid neoplasms are well differentiated carcinomas and are further divided into papillary

Table XVII-4-1. Pathological Classification of Thyroid Neoplasms

Benign	Malignant
Adenoma	Carcinoma
Follicular	Follicular carcinoma
colloid (macrofollicular)	pure follicular adenocarcinoma
embryonal (trabecular)	
fetal (microfollicular)	clear cell carcinoma
Hurthle cell	Hurthle (oxyphil) cell carcinoma
Papillary (?)	Papillary adenocarcinoma
Atypical	pure papillary adenocarcinoma
Teratoma	mixed papillary and follicular carcinoma
	Medullary carcinoma
	Undifferentiated carcinoma
	Epidermoid carcinoma
	Other malignant tumors
	Lymphoma
	Sarcoma
	Metastatic tumor
	Fibrosarcoma

Table XVII-4-2. Lesions that May Appear as a Thyroid Nodule

Non-neoplastic nodules
  Nodular goiter
  Thyroid hemiagenesis
  Effect of prior operation or ^{131}I therapy
  Hashimoto's thyroiditis
  Subacute thyroiditis
  Infections
  Granulomatous diseases

Benign neoplasms
  Cyst
  Adenoma (non-functioning or functioning)
  Parathyroid cyst or adenoma
  Thyroglossal cyst

Malignant neoplasms
  Thyroid carcinoma
  Metastatic cancer

Nonthyroidal lesions
  Inflammatory or neoplastic nodes
  Cystic hygroma
  Aneurysm
  Bronchocele
  Laryngocele
  Thyroglossal duct cyst

and follicular carcinomas. As with the other tumors, the etiology is largely unknown. At least two factors contribute to the development of these neoplasms: radiation and chronic stimulation of the thyroid by TSH. Medullary carcinoma derives from parafollicular cells, represents 4–8% of thyroid cancer and is familial in 20% of cases. Undifferentiated anaplastic carcinoma of the thyroid is extremely malignant, occurs more commonly in elderly females, grows rapidly and usually leads to the death of the patient within a few months as a consequence of massive hemorrhage or suffocation.

Diagnostic Protocol

The main aim of the diagnostic studies is to differentiate between malignant and benign nodules. At the same time, diagnostic studies must be able to reveal obstructive symptoms, which are an indication for surgical therapy, regardless of the nature of the thyroid nodules.

History

When there is a history of external irradiation to the neck and head during childhood or infancy, an aggressive approach to the thyroid nodule must be taken. Several studies demonstrated a linear relationship between radiation dose to the neck and the incidence of malignant thyroid nodules, which are commonly multifocal. The earlier the age at exposure to radiation the higher the risk of thyroid neoplasia.[4] Sex and age are also important elements to be considered in the evaluation. In children the presence of a thyroid nodule is highly suspicious, regardless of sex. A single thyroid nodule in an adult man is rare and must always be considered suspicious. Benign nodules are much more frequent in women and in elderly people, but undifferentiated thyroid carcinoma is normally found in patients over 60 years of age. Other important elements in the history of a thyroid nodule are the pattern of growth, the duration of the lesion and the presence of local symptoms. The family history may reveal a case of familial medullary carcinoma; 20% of medullary carcinomas are familial. Some of these patients have multifocal medullary carcinomas as part of familial multiple endocrine tumor syndromes. Symptoms of thyrotoxicosis can direct the diagnosis toward a toxic adenoma of the thyroid.

Physical Examination

A single nodule in an otherwise normal gland is more suspicious than one which is part of a goiter, especially if multinodular. The size of the nodule is not a criterion for malignancy. However, larger nodules, if malignant, are more likely to lead to local or distant invasion. Tenderness or pain of the nodule has to be taken into consideration, because rapidly growing cancers can be painful, even if most malignancies are painless. Hardness, irregularity and fixation to surrounding structures are highly indicative of malignancy. Cord paralysis on the side of the nodule often indicates a malignant nodule. Locally enlarged lymph nodes suggest thyroid malignancy with regional metastases. Firm, smooth, resilient nodules are often cystic.

Laboratory Tests

Tests of thyroid function are of little help in the differential diagnosis of thyroid nodules. However elevated values of serum thyroid hormones may confirm the diagnosis of toxic adenoma, whereas reduced values of these hormones may suggest the presence of a nodular Hashimoto's thyroiditis. The finding of circulating anti-thyroid antibodies indicates the presence of an autoimmune thyroid disease, but a malignancy cannot be excluded on the basis of positive evidence for thyroiditis. The assay of thyroglobulin is a very useful marker in the follow up of differentiated thyroid cancer treated with total thyroidectomy. This assay is, however, not useful in the differential diagnosis between benign and malignant thyroid nodules. Elevation of serum calcitonin in the presence of a thyroid nodule is specific for the diagnosis of medullary carcinoma of the thyroid. Thus the assay of calcitonin is an obligatory step in the diagnostic protocol of thyroid nodules if this cancer is suggested by history.

Diagnostic Studies In Vivo

Thyroid scintiscan provides some help in differential diagnosis. Nodules that are hyperfunctional and produce hyperthyroidism ("hot" nodules) are rarely malignant. They represent less than 10% of the adenomas and typically have grown to more than 3 cm in diameter. The nodules that accumulate iodine in concentrations equal to the surrounding tissue are usually benign. Most thyroid cancers appear as inactive areas on the scan ("cold" nodules), but the great majority of cold nodules are benign.

Imaging using ultrasound can differentiate solid from cystic nodules or mixed cystic and solid structures, which are usually, but not always, associated with a benign process. Ultrasonography may be used to detect multinodularity, detect small thyroid nodules in the presence of metastatic cervical lymphadenopathy, to monitor the size of a nodule, and to guide needle biopsy.

Fine needle aspiration biopsy (FNA) with cytology has been used with a high degree of accuracy during the last decade on a large number of patients with thyroid nodules. The diagnostic accuracy of FNA depends on the experience of the physician performing the biopsy and of the pathologist examining the specimen. The cytologic examination of the specimen may provide a diagnosis ranging from "inadequate for diagnosis," "benign," "suspicious for malignancy," to "malignant." Patients with lesions diagnosed as malignant or suspicious, or those with hypercellular follicular cytological patterns are sent to surgery. If all "suspicious" nodules are taken to surgery, the sensitivity of FNA is more than 90%, with a specificity of about 70%.[4,15] Lesions with benign cytology at the first biopsy occasionally may give a malignant pattern at a subsequent aspiration. It is therefore advisable to repeat the FNA at some point in the follow up of thyroid nodules. In particular, "mixed" nodules require careful follow up. Difficulties in interpreting biopsy specimens involve the differentiation of: 1) follicular adenomas from carcinomas, 2) Hurthle cell tumors from other histotypes; and 3) Hashimoto's disease from lymphoma. Solid nodules which are more than 4 cm or less than 1 cm in diameter are associated with an increased error in collecting a reliable sample. In expert hands, however, few false positive diagnoses are made and false negative diagnoses are very uncommon. Thus, at present the needle biopsy with cytologic examination plays a central role in the differential diagnosis of thyroid nodules and must always be performed in the presence of thyroid nodules. A chest and neck radiograph is useful because it can demonstrate: 1) metastatic pulmonary disease; 2) tracheal displacement or compression; 3) fine speckled deposits of calcium within a thyroid nodule, suggesting papillary cancer; 4) and eggshell-like calcifications, indicative of a benign nodule. Computerized tomography (CT) is recommended in patients with substernal extension of nodules or metastases.

Differential Diagnosis

The differential diagnosis to be considered when examining a patient with a thyroid nodule includes thyroid carcinoma, adenoma, nodular goiter, cyst, thyroiditis, irregular regrowth of tissue after previous surgery, thyroid hemiagenesis and other problems noted in Table XVII-4-2. The protocol described above permits effective diagnosis of a thyroid nodule in the majority of cases. The distinction between follicular adenomas and well-differentiated follicular carcinomas is a challenge and a precise differential diagnosis can be achieved only after a careful histological examination of a surgical specimen documenting the presence of vascular or capsular invasion by the tumor. Another controversial topic is the malignant potential of histologically benign Hurthle cell adenomas. Among the factors to be considered in the management of thyroid nodules is the age and sex of the patient. A solitary nodule in patients under 25 and older than 60 is highly suspect of being malignant and nodules in men carry a far greater risk of malignancy than do nodules in women. Other factors include the family history of the patient, a history of exposure to radiation, growth and duration of the lesion, local symptoms, physical characteristics of the gland, signs of abnormal thyroid status, laboratory studies and fine needle biopsy. Table XVII-4-3 summarizes the major factors to be considered in distinguishing benign from malignant nodules. Obviously, enlarged regional lymph nodes suggest malignant disease.

Therapeutic Approaches

The therapeutic approach to a thyroid nodule must be preceded by a complete diagnostic evaluation. History, physical examination, laboratory evaluation, scintiscan, ultrasound and fine needle biopsy will orient the therapeutic strategy to simple follow up, medical treatment or surgery.

The primary strategy is to select nodules for surgery which are probably malignant. Table XVII-4-4 synthesizes this management strategy. The patient is referred for operation if the thyroid nodule is malignant or suspicious or if it compresses neck organs. In the case of toxic adenoma two therapeutic alternatives are available: radioiodine or surgery. Table XVII-4-5 indicates the advantages, disadvantages and indications of these two forms of therapy. If the final decision is not to pursue surgical exploration and the nodule is not autonomously functioning, two possible strategies may be followed: simple observation or thyroid hormone administration. The aim of the medical therapy is to suppress the pituitary secretion of thyroid stimulating hormone (TSH). The rational basis of this treatment derives from experiments in rats fed iodine-deficient diets. Lack of iodine causes a functional failure of the thyroid gland, which in turn stimulates TSH secretion. The excess of TSH produces thyroid hyperplasia and the formation of nodules. The administration of thyroid hormone (levo-thyroxine) at suppressive doses can occasionally produce their complete regression. If the nodules have been established for some time, the suppressive therapy may determine a partial regression or at least block further growth and avoid the appearance of other nodules.

Medical Therapy of Solid, "Cold," Cytologically Benign Thyroid Nodules

If an adequate specimen is obtained for cytology and the patient is euthyroid, conservative medical treatment is indicated. Levo-thyroxine is administered at a dose able to suppress TSH secretion from the pituitary. Table XVII-4-6 summarizes the aims, the plan of treatment and the contraindications. The treatment is recommended on a long-term basis, but is contraindicated in the elderly. The patient must be re-examined at annual intervals and a new biopsy must be performed periodically. We usually perform a re-biopsy during the second to third and fifth to sixth years of follow up. The risk of false negative needle biopsy diagnosis is always present. Therefore, when the behavior of the nodule or the new cytology make it evident that a malignancy may have been overlooked, the patient should undergo surgery.

Therapy of an Autonomously Functioning Thyroid Nodule

The incidence of cancer in functioning nodules is so rare that the therapeutic approach depends on the metabolic

Table XVII-4-3. Risk Factors Useful in Distinguishing Benign from Malignant Thyroid Nodules

	More Likely Benign	More Likely Malignant
History	Family history of benign goiter Residence in endemic goiter area	Family history of medullary cancer of thyroid Previous irradiation of head and neck Recent growth of nodule Hoarseness, dysphagia, dysphonia
Physical characteristics	Older women Soft nodule Multinodular goiter	Child, young adult, male Solitary, firm nodule Vocal cord paralysis, firm lymph nodes
Laboratory findings	Presence of thyroid autoantibodies	Elevated serum calcitonin
Scintiscan	"Hot nodule"	"Cold nodule"
Echo scan	Pure cyst	Solid or semicystic
Biopsy (FNA)	Benign appearance	Suggestion of malignancy

Table XVII-4-4.   Management of Thyroid Nodules

Toxic hot nodule	$\longrightarrow$	Surgery or ^{131}I
Cystic nodule	$\longrightarrow$	Aspiration for diagnosis and therapy; reaspirate as needed; surgery if multiple recurrences
Other nodules →	Fine needle aspiration cytology	a. Probable cancer → Surgery
		b. Suspicious → Reaspiration or surgery
		c. Inadequate spec → Reaspiration
		d. Benign → Follow on T_4 therapy

Table XVII-4-5.   Therapeutic Alternatives of Toxic Adenoma

Radioiodine	Surgery
ADVANTAGES	
Low cost	Normal thyroid tissue present after treatment
Safety in patients with heart disease	
DISADVANTAGES	
Persistence of nodule	High cost
Age limits	Surgical complications
	Not feasible in patients with contraindications
INDICATIONS	
Adult or old age	Young age
Patients with cardiac or vascular disease or contraindications to surgery	Presence of obstructive symptoms
	Large adenomas

Table XVII-4-6.   Medical Therapy of Solid, "Cold," Cytologically Benign Thyroid Nodule

Theoretical aims
   Obtain reduction of size
   Block further growth
   Avoid the appearance of other nodules

Plan of treatment
   Levothyroxine at a dose able to suppress pituitary TSH secretion to 0.3-0.5 μU/ml
   The dose must be adjusted after 4-6 months by assay of basal TSH level

Contraindications
   Autonomous function of the thyroid (TSH pre-therapy)
   Cardiac and vascular diseases

status of the patient. Eighty percent of autonomously functioning thyroid nodules are associated with euthyroidism. Generally their size is less than 3 cm. The therapeutic approach is conservative: no treatment, but periodic observation. If the "hot" nodule causes hyperthyroidism, two therapeutic options are available: surgery or radioiodine. See Table XVII-4-5 for further details.

Therapy of the Thyroid Cyst

Simple thyroid cysts are often successfully cured by aspiration of the fluid, but not infrequently they recur after several aspirations. The character of the fluid may allow the distinction between thyroid and parathyroid cysts. In the latter, the fluid is crystal clear. The evaluation of parathormone levels in the cyst fluid is decisive for the diagnosis. Cysts more than 4 cm in diameter that recur after two or more aspirations are usually sent to surgery, especially if the fluid is hemorrhagic or some residual tissue is still present in the nodule after drainage.

Management of Inflammatory Nodules of Hashimoto's Thyroiditis and Subacute Thyroiditis

If a certain diagnosis of Hashimoto's thyroiditis or subacute thyroiditis has been made, the nodules most probably have an inflammatory origin. A biopsy is, however, necessary, taking into account the infrequent, but still possible, presence of a thyroid cancer or lymphoma in a lymphocytic thyroiditis. If the cytology confirms the diagnosis of thyroiditis, the therapy will be that specific for each form of thyroiditis.

Management of Nodules for Which FNA Can Neither Exclude Nor Establish a Diagnosis of Malignancy

In the case of microfollicular or trabecular adenoma (with or without Hurthle cells) biopsy findings are often unable to exclude a malignancy. Thus a surgical approach is suggested: lobectomy and contralateral sub-total thyroidectomy with careful examination of the surgical specimen. If the nodule is malignant, operation should be followed by ^{131}I thyroid ablation. On FNA these lesions are found to have a highly cellular pattern, but not to be diagnostic of malignancy.

Management of Nodules for Which an Adequate Biopsy Specimen is Not Obtained

The specimen for cytological examination may be unsatisfactory for several reasons. The nodule may contain only degenerative material without cells. Alternatively, the physician performing the biopsy and/or the pathologist may not have sufficient experience. In any case, FNA must be repeated. If unsatisfactory specimens continue to be obtained, the diagnosis and the management have to be based on clinical and laboratory criteria. If the nodule is not suspicious for malignancy, suppressive therapy with levo-thyroxine is started, but usually surgical resection is favored.

Therapy of Malignant Thyroid Nodules

All malignant nodules require surgical treatment. In the case of papillary or follicular carcinomas, the procedure of choice is near-total thyroidectomy, followed by ^{131}I thyroid ablation and systemic ^{131}I therapy if needed. A cytology positive for medullary carcinoma requires pre-operative screening for pheochromocytoma and parathyroid adenoma. If a diagnosis of undifferentiated carcinoma or lymphoma is made the patient is referred to an oncologist for the appropriate treatment. Surgical treatment is limited to debulking procedures in order to prevent airway obstruction.

Final Considerations on the Response of Thyroid Nodules to Suppressive Therapy with L-T$_4$

Because the growth of some thyroid nodules is thought to be dependent on TSH stimulation, thyroid nodules which are not selected for surgery or radioiodine treatment and are not autonomously functioning are usually treated medically with doses of L-T$_4$ capable of suppressing the secretion of TSH. The dose of thyroid hormone is adjusted to keep serum TSH at 0.3-0.5 μU/ml, a level below the normal range but not equivalent to that observed in thyrotoxosis. It must, however, be emphasized that a lack of growth or even a partial reduction of a nodule under L-T$_4$ at suppressive doses is no guarantee that the nodule is benign (15). The effectiveness of long-term suppressive therapy with L-T$_4$ is debated. Often the results obtained are the blocking of further growth of the nodule or the prevention of the formation of new nodules. A clear decrease in size of a nodule is infrequent. Conversely, enlargement of a nodule in spite of treatment with L-T$_4$ does not always indicate malignancy. Other causes may be responsible for the enlargement including an autonomously functioning thyroid nodule, hemorrhage or inflammation. In any case a new needle biopsy should be performed. If no specific and clear explanation is found, it may be prudent to remove the nodule.

References

1. Ahmann, A. J., and Wartofsky, L.: The Thyroid Nodule. In Principles and Practice of Endocrinology and Metabolism, Part III. Edited by K. L. Becker. Philadelphia, J.B. Lippincott Company, 1990, p. 312.
2. Carrol, B. A.: Asymptomatic thyroid nodules: incidental sonographic detection. A.J.R., 133:499, 1982.
3. Clark, O. H.: Thyroid nodules and thyroid cancer. In Endocrine Surgery of the Thyroid and Parathyroid Glands. Edited by O. H. Clark. St. Louis, The C.V. Mosby Company, 1985, p. 56.
4. DeGroot, L. J., Reilly, M., Pinnameneni, K., and Refetoff, S.: Retrospective and prospective study of radiation-induced thyroid disease. Am. J. Med., 74:852, 1983.
5. Goellner, J. R., Gharib, H., Grant, C. S., and Johnson, D. A.: Fine needle aspiration cytology of the thyroid, 1980 to 1986. Acta Cytologica, 31:587, 1987.
6. Hamburger, J. I.: The discrete or dominant thyroid nodule. In Management of Thyroid Patients, Vol. 1. Edited by J. L. Hamburger. Southfield, MI., J. I. Hamburger, 1985, p. 132.
7. Horlocker, T. T., Haye, J. E., James, E. M., et al.: Prevalence of incidental nodular thyroid disease detected during high-resolution parathyroid ultrasonography. In Frontiers in Thyroidology, Vol 1. Edited by G. Medeiros-Neto, and E. Gaitan, New York, Plenum Press, 1986, p. 1309.
8. Liechty, R. D., Stoffel, P. T., Zimmermann, D. E., and Silverberg, S. G.: Solitary thyroid nodules. Arch. Surg., 112:59, 1977.
9. Mortensen, J. D., Woolner, L. B., and Bennett, W. A.: Gross and microscopic findings in clinically normal thyroid glands. J. Clin. Endocrin. Metab., 15:1270, 1955.
10. Psarras, A., Papadopulos, S. H., Livadas, D., Pharmakiotis, A. D., and Koutras, D. A.: The single thyroid nodule. Br. J. Surg., 59:545, 1972.
11. Robinson, E., Horn, Y., and Hochmann, A.: Incidence of cancer in thyroid nodules. Surg. Gynecol. Obstet., 123:1024, 1966.
12. Thompson, N. W.: The thyroid nodule—surgical management. In Endocrine Surgery. Edited by I. D. A. Johnston, and N. W. Thompson. London, Butterworths, 1983, p. 14.
13. Vander, J. B., Gaston, E. A., and Dawber, T. R.: Significance of solitary nontoxic thyroid nodules. N. Engl. J. Med., 251:970, 1954.
14. Vander, J. B., Gaston, E. A., and Dawber, T. R.: The significance of nontoxic thyroid nodules: Final report of a 15-year study of the incidence of thyroid malignancy. Ann. Intern. Med., 69:537, 1968.
15. VanHerle, A. J., Rich, P., Ljung, B. E., et al.: The thyroid nodule. Ann. Intern. Med., 96:221, 1982.

Acknowledgments

From the Institute of Endocrinology at the University of Pisa and the Thyroid Study Unit, Department of Medicine, The University of Chicago

Supported by United States Public Health Service Grants DK13377 and DK27384, The March of Dimes Birth Defects Foundation Grant No. 1-1166, The Boots Pharmaceutical Company, and the David Wiener Research Fund.

XVII-5

Corticosteroids

John A. Cidlowski
Robert A. Schwartzman

Hormones of the Adrenal Cortex

For over 30 years cortisol and its synthetic analogs have been in widespread clinical use. A great deal of knowledge has been gained on the physiology, biochemistry, and pharmacology of steroids over this period and numerous publications discuss the therapeutic uses and toxicological hazards of corticosteroids. This chapter will review the physiological and pharmacological actions of corticosteroids and then discuss the use of these agents in the treatment of various neoplasms. Finally, the mechanism of action of these hormones will be considered in the context of their therapeutic efficacy.

The necessity of functional adrenal glands for survival was discovered in the 1850s based on observations by Addison of patients with destructive diseases of the adrenal gland and experiments done by Brown-Sequard on adrenalectomized animals.[2,18] By the 1930s it was noted that the effects of adrenal insufficiency could be divided into two categories: those due to electrolyte imbalances and those resulting from altered carbohydrate metabolism.[16,72] In 1932 Cushing described the syndrome of hypercorticism.[35] In the 1940s and 1950s the discovery of adrenocorticotropic hormone (ACTH) in the adrenal pituitary and its role in the stimulation of the adrenal cortex was made.[9,94] The regulation of ACTH release was found to depend on a precise balance between the negative feedback of adrenal corticosteroids and positive stimulation from the nervous system, both effects being mediated at the level of the hypothalamus.[82] During these same years several bioactive steroids were isolated from the adrenal cortex and their structures elucidated, including the principle active corticosteroids in humans, cortisol and aldosterone.[117,134]

In 1949, Hench announced the dramatic effects of cortisol and ACTH in the treatment of rheumatoid arthritis.[76] This observation evoked wide interest and therapeutic applications of these hormones were subsequently extended to a wide variety of diseases. This surge in clinical investigation prompted an equally large amount of study on the basic sciences of these compounds. During the 1950s most of the biochemistry involved in the synthesis and metabolism of adrenocortical steroids was elucidated and most of the synthetic analogs available today were developed. Along with these advances, practical methods for plasma cortisol determinations were developed allowing rapid advances in the field of corticosteroid therapy.

Synthetic analogs of the adrenocortical steroids were eventually developed that separated the anti-inflammatory potency of these compounds from their effects on electrolyte metabolism. However, chemists have not been able to separate desirable clinical effectiveness from toxicity. Consequently, these drugs are very powerful but have slow cumulative toxic side effects on many tissues, which may not be apparent until made manifest in a catastrophic manner.

Adrenal Anatomy. The adrenal cortex is composed of three zones, whose divisions are not clear-cut in humans. The outer zone is the zona glomerulosa which is responsible for aldosterone synthesis and which is controlled both morphologically and biochemically by sodium, potassium, and angiotensin levels. Cortisol is produced in the inner zones, the zona fasciculata and the zona reticularis, which, along with the zona glomerulosa to a lesser extent, are regulated primarily by ACTH from the pituitary.

Secreted Steroids. All five classes of steroid hormones are produced in the adrenal cortex in varying amounts: the glucocorticoids, mineralocorticoids, and progestins, which contain 21 carbons; the androgens, which contain 19 carbons; and the estrogens, which contain 18 carbons. The amounts of progestins, androgens, and estrogens produced in the adrenal cortex represent only a minor percentage of the total amount of each steroid synthesized in the body; thus they will not be discussed further in this chapter. The glucocorticoids and the mineralocorticoids are made almost exclusively in the adrenal cortex and therefore represent its major biological product. The physiological role of glucocorticoids includes the control of glucose metabolism, gluconeogenesis and modulation of the immune system. The major human form is cortisol and to a lesser extent corticosterone. The mineralocorticoids are crucial in mineral and water metabolism and the major bioactive forms in humans are aldosterone and deoxycorticosterone.

Biosynthetic Pathways. The steps in the biosynthesis of corticosteroids have been elucidated and are presented in simplified form in Figure XVII-5-1. The synthesis of all steroids begins with cholesterol,[26] which is converted to various steroid molecules in a series of reactions that are mediated by several cytochrome P-450 enzymes.[89] The adrenal cortex can synthesize cholesterol to some extent; however 60–80% of the cholesterol used in steroid synthesis originates from sources outside the adrenal.[67] This cholesterol is derived primarily from the cholesterol that is circulating in plasma bound to low density lipoproteins, for which the adrenal cortex has a large number of receptors. Once synthesized, the corticosteroids are not stored within the adrenal cortex but are rapidly secreted. The adrenal contains only enough steroid to maintain normal serum corticosteroid levels for a few minutes once synthesis is halted. Therefore, the rate of corticosteroid synthesis is essentially equal to the rate of secretion from the adrenal gland.

Control of Corticosteroid Secretion

Glucocorticoids. The rate of synthesis of corticosteroids is controlled by the peptide hormone ACTH.[88] This hormone, synthesized and secreted from the corticotrophs (basophilic cells) of the anterior pituitary, affects all three zones of the adrenal cortex. High levels of ACTH can lead to hyperplasia and hypertrophy of the adrenal cortex and a continuous high output of cortisol and corticosterone. A lack of ACTH results in atrophy of the cortex and decreased secretion of both cortisol and corticosterone. In contrast, aldosterone levels are not significantly affected by changes in ACTH because the zona glomerulosa is least affected by ACTH. ACTH acts through the classical mechanism of action of peptide hormones; i.e., ACTH binds to specific receptors that are located in the adrenal cell membrane and subsequently exerts its effects through an increase in intracellular cyclic adenosine monophosphate (cAMP) and other second messengers.[73] ACTH acts on the adrenal cortex to increase steroid synthesis and secretion, at least in part by increasing the number of LDL receptors.[17] The principal site of action of ACTH is on the side chain cleavage reaction that converts cholesterol to pregnenolone. ACTH stimulates the rate of this reaction by increasing the availability of cholesterol as a substrate for this enzymatic reaction as well as by increasing the synthesis of the cytochrome P-450 side chain cleavage enzyme.[68,133]

ACTH secretion from the anterior pituitary is positively regulated by corticotropin releasing factor (CRF) which is secreted from the median eminence of the hypothalamus.[66] Neural signals converge on the hypothalamus to cause the release of CRF, which travels via a vascular connection to the pituitary where it stimulates the synthesis and release of the polyprotein precursor to ACTH, pro-opiomelanocortin (POMC). The POMC protein is cleaved into several bioactive peptides that are secreted from the corticotrophs along with ACTH, including β-lipotropin and β-endorphin. Negative feedback control is exerted on ACTH levels by glucocorticoids, which act at the level of both the pituitary and the hypothalamus.[58] Glucocorticoids suppress POMC synthesis and decrease ACTH stores in secretory granules. High levels of glucocorticoids cause corticotropic cell degeneration. Following adrenalectomy or in patients with Addison's disease, when glucocorticoid levels are low, the concentration of ACTH in the plasma remains high. ACTH levels can, however, still be stimulated by CRF, indicating that ACTH remains under nervous control in the absence of negative feedback.

Frequent measurement of plasma cortisol levels has revealed that the level of this steroid fluctuates irregularly.[152] These spontaneous changes are the result of rapid increases in the cortisol secretion rate that occur 7–13 times a day. These increases, although irregular, occur in a reproducible pattern for any given person. The slope of the rise in secretion rate is constant for any individual and averages around 50 µg/min. The decline of these peaks of cortisol levels occurs in a semilog fashion indicating that this spontaneous secretion occurs in an "on/off" manner. Thus, the total amount of cortisol secreted throughout the day reflects the number of episodes of high secretion that occur rather than changes in the secretion rate. This spontaneous rhythm of cortisol secretion results in minimal plasma cortisol levels 1–2 hours after the onset of sleep, with a rise occurring during sleep to maximum levels at the time of awakening and a fall in

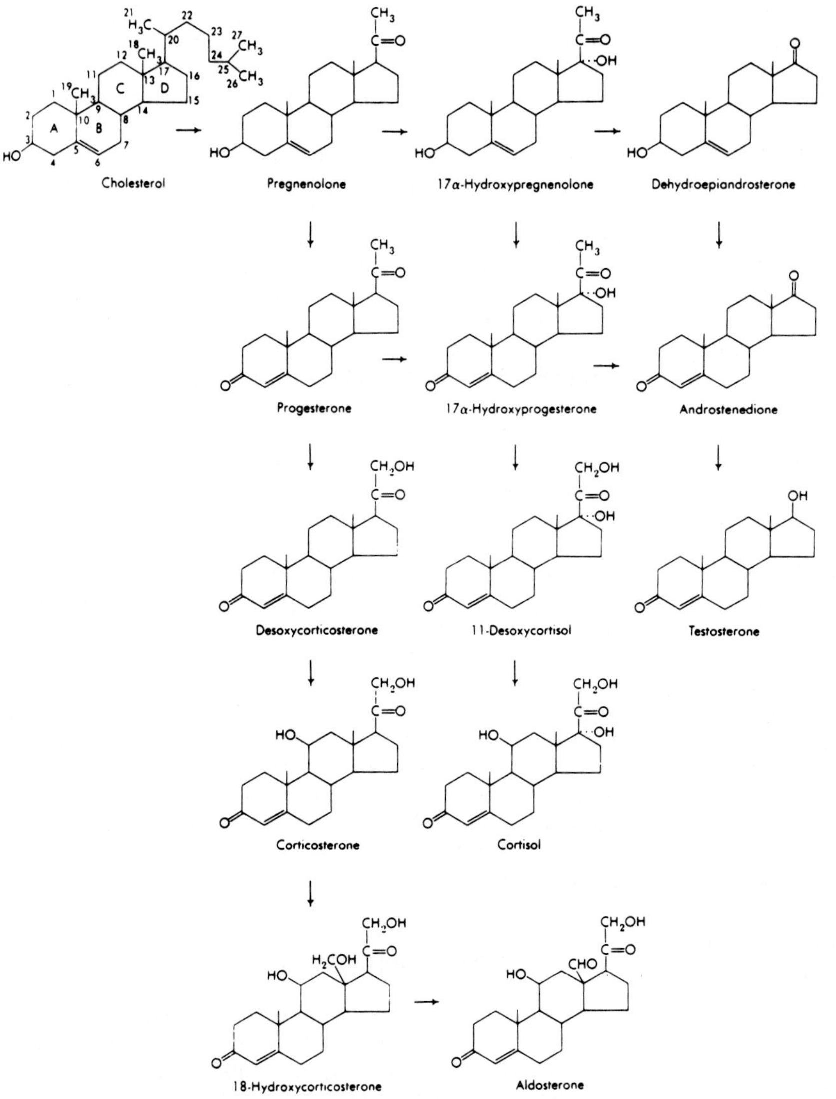

Figure XVII-5-1. Principal pathways for biosynthesis of adrenocorticosteroids. From Haynes and Murad.[74]

plasma levels during the day. This secretion pattern is due to an intrinsic function of the hypothalamus and is not subject to glucocorticoid induced negative feedback. Although the specific mechanism responsible for this intrinsic rhythm is unknown, the major factors that affect the pattern appear to be timing of sleep, feeding, and exposure to light.

Stress also causes a stimulation of ACTH production and subsequent adrenal steroid secretion.[36] These stimuli can be psychological (e.g., anticipation, fear, depression) or physical (e.g., exercise, hypoglycemia, surgery, burns, cold, hypotension). If the sensory connections that mediate these stimuli are blocked, no adrenal stimulation occurs.[60] There is a quantitative relationship between the intensity of the stressful stimulus and the adrenal response;[144] however, pretreatment with glucocorticoid can inhibit this effect through negative feedback mechanisms.[33]

Mineralocorticoids. The major physiological regulator of aldosterone levels is the renin-angiotensin system.[38] Renin, a protein made in the kidney, converts angiotensinogen to angiotensin I, a tetradecapeptide that is subsequently converted by other factors to the active peptides angiotensin II and angiotensin III. Angiotensin II and III stimulate aldos-

terone biosynthesis through interaction with cell surface receptors in the zona glomerulosa. This effect is mediated by changes in intracellular calcium but not by changes in cAMP levels.[44] Another effect of angiotensin is to increase peripheral arterial resistance, which in turn increases blood pressure.[11] Changes in blood pressure then feed back on renin secretion, whose control mechanism has not been established but which appears to involve kidney baroreceptors as well as sympathetic innervation and serum sodium and potassium levels.

A second control of mineralocorticoid synthesis is serum sodium and potassium levels. Increases in serum potassium increase aldosterone secretion. Potassium acts directly on the adrenal gland to stimulate some of the early steps in steroid biosynthesis and may also affect renin release.[22] Low serum sodium also increases aldosterone secretion but its action does not appear to be a major regulator of mineralocorticoid secretion since serum sodium concentration changes little with changes in total volume.

Pharmacokinetics of Corticosteroids

Rate of Secretion. Cortisol, the major glucocorticoid in humans, is secreted at a rate of 15–20 mg/day in men and

fore, glucose and triglyceride accumulation would occur in response to the rise in insulin levels. In contrast, fat cells containing higher levels of receptor (perhaps in the periphery) would respond to the high glucocorticoid level by decreasing glucose uptake and would not accumulate triglycerides. Alternatively, cells in the extremities may be less sensitive to insulin.[47] The mobilization of fat from peripheral depots by epinephrine and other lipolytics is severely blunted in the absence of glucocorticoids.[129] Cortisol facilitates the response of adipocytes to the rise in cAMP induced by these agents rather than creating a larger increase in the amount of cAMP.

Electrolyte and Water Balance. The major effect of mineralocorticoids is the regulation of electrolyte excretion in the kidney.[110] Aldosterone treatment results in increased sodium reabsorption from tubular fluid and an increase in excretion of potassium and hydrogen. Similar effects on cation transport in most other tissues account for all the systemic activity of mineralocorticoids. The primary features of excess mineralocorticoids are positive sodium balance, increase in extracellular fluid volume, normal or slightly high plasma sodium, hypokalemia, and alkalosis. Under conditions of hypocorticism there is renal loss of sodium, hyponatremia, hyperkalemia, a decrease in extracellular fluid volume and cellular hydration. The 1% decrease in sodium reabsorption that occurs in hypocorticism is enough to cause profound cardiovascular changes, resulting in circulatory collapse, renal failure, and ultimately in death. Aldosterone modulates sodium levels by acting through mineralocorticoid receptors, located in the distal tubules of the kidney, to increase the permeability of the apical membrane of the cells lining the cortical collecting tube. Aldosterone also increases activity of the sodium/potassium-ATPase in the serosal membrane.[103] These changes allow more sodium to be reabsorbed and generates a higher negative potential in the lumen, which is the driving force for increased potassium and hydrogen excretion. Mineralocorticoids also increase calcium and magnesium excretion, probably due to volume expansion. Prolonged aldosterone treatment results in sodium "escaping," a cessation of sodium changes while potassium and hydrogen loss continues to occur. The mechanism for this effect is unknown, but may involve mineralocorticoid receptor downregulation and subsequent cessation of hormonal responsiveness.

Glucocorticoids have effects on the kidney that differ from the effects of mineralocorticoids. Glucocorticoids increase water diuresis, glomerular filtration rate, and renal plasma flow. Although increases in sodium retention and potassium excretion occur with cortisol there seems to be no increase in hydrogen excretion. The major renal complications of glucocorticoid therapy are nephrocalcinosis, nephrolithiasis, and increased stone formation from the increase in urinary concentrations of calcium and uric acid.[90]

Electrolyte changes also occur in tissues other than the kidney in response to mineralocorticoid treatment. These affected tissues include: gastrointestinal mucosa,[49] salivary and sweat glands,[12] and exocrine pancreas. In these tissues a longer onset period is required to detect significant responses to aldosterone and no sodium "escape" occurs after prolonged hormone administration. Aldosterone apparently does not cause changes in intestinal electrolyte absorption,[28] but glucocorticoids increase sodium and water absorption and potassium secretion. Both glucocorticoid and mineralocorticoid receptors are present in the mucosa but dexamethasone can bind to both receptor types while aldosterone can only bind to its own receptor. Cortisol also increases gastric acid secretion and blood flow to the gastric mucosa while decreasing the rate of gastric cell proliferation. High doses of glucocorticoids may cause peptic ulceration or aggravate pre-existing ulcers.

Endocrine System. In addition to the effects on ACTH secretion previously described, corticosteroids influence the action of several other hormones. Cortisol increases growth hormone secretion in patients with acromegaly.[15] In contrast, the spontaneous secretion of growth hormone is inhibited in hypercorticism.[139] Growth failure is observed with prolonged glucocorticoid treatment in children. This response is apparently due to decreased maturation of the epiphyseal plates and a decrease in long bone growth.[98] Corticosteroids depress the secretion of thyroid-stimulating hormone in patients with myxedema,[153] and reduce the physiological effectiveness of thyroxine.[21] High doses of steroid decrease leutinizing hormone release in response to leutinizing hormone-releasing hormone.[126] Corticosteroids also have been shown to potentiate the β-adrenergic effects of catecholamines and stimulate the synthesis of epinephrine from norepinephrine.[45] Other systemic effects of high doses of glucocorticoids include adrenocortical insufficiency upon glucocorticoid removal,[32] steroid-induced diabetes,[3] hyperlipidemia,[114] high glucagon levels,[107] and hypocalcemia.[42]

Cardiovascular System. The major effects of corticosteroids on the cardiovascular system are due to their influence on plasma volume, electrolyte retention, epinephrine synthesis, and angiotensin levels, which together result in the maintenance of normal blood pressure and cardiac output. However, the hypotension that occurs from corticosteroid deficiency cannot be totally explained by these factors. Corticosteroids have effects on myocardial responsiveness, arteriolar tone, and capillary permeability. Hypocorticism leads to increased capillary permeability, inadequate vasomotor response, and decrease in cardiac output and cardiac size. Hypercorticism leads to chronic arterial hypertension.[92] The mechanism responsible for this effect is unclear but it is specific for mineralocorticoid activity and may be due to prolonged, excessive sodium retention. Hypertension can also be induced by glucocorticoids. The mechanism for this response is also unknown but glucocorticoids influence many factors, including increased filtration fraction and glomerular hypertension, increased angiotensinogen synthesis, decreased prostaglandin synthesis that leads to decreased vasodilation, increased responsiveness to vasopressors and increased synthesis of atrial natriuretic peptide. There is a fair amount of evidence that glucocorticoids potentiate atherosclerosis and thromboembolic complications.[37,86]

Musculoskeletal System. Normal corticosteroid levels are required for muscle maintenance; however, either excess glucocorticoid or mineralocorticoid can lead to muscle abnormalities.[4,101] High aldosterone levels cause muscle weakness due to hypokalemia. High glucocorticoid levels cause muscle wasting due to catabolic effects on protein metabolism as described previously. Corticosteroid insufficiency results in decreased work capacity of striated muscle, weakness, and fatigue. This response reflects an inadequacy of the circulatory system rather than electrolyte and carbohydrate imbalances. The most debilitating effect of glucocorticoids on bone is induction of osteoporosis.[120] This response results from a decrease in osteoblast activity as well as from a decrease in gastrointestinal absorption of calcium. The decrease in serum calcium causes increased secretion of parathyroid hormone, which in turn stimulates osteoclast activity. Therefore, glucocorticoids act to decrease bone formation as well as to increase bone resorption. Other effects of high doses of glucocorticoids on the musculoskeletal system include aseptic necrosis and spontaneous tendon rupture,[37,118] presumably through an effect on collagen metabolism.

Central Nervous System. Corticosteroids affect the nervous system indirectly in a number of ways by maintaining normal plasma glucose levels, adequate circulation, and normal electrolyte levels. Direct effects of corticosteroids on the central nervous system are not well defined; however changes in corticosteroid levels do influence mood, behavior, electroencephalograph patterns, and brain excitability. Chronic glucocorticoid treatment has been shown to cause cell death in hippocampal neurons in rats, but it is unknown if such a response occurs in humans.[104] Addison's patients are subject to apathy, depression, irritability, and psychosis.[24] These symptoms are alleviated by glucocorticoid treatment but not by mineralocorticoids. Individuals with Cushing's disease are known to develop neuroses and psychoses that are reversible with removal of excess hormone.[69] Increases in brain excitability in hypercorticism and following mineralocorticoid treatment are due to electrolyte imbalances. However, the increase in brain excitability induced by cortisol is not due to changes in sodium concentration. Chronic glucocorticoid treatment can also result in pseudotumor cerebri, primarily in children.[150]

Hematologic Effects. Corticosteroids increase hemoglobin and red cell content of blood as demonstrated by the occurrence of polycythemia in Cushing's disease and mild normochromatic anemia in Addison's disease. These steroids may retard erythrophagocytosis. Corticosteroids also affect circulating white cells.[34] Glucocorticoid treatment results in increased polymorphonuclear leukocytes in blood as a result of increased rate of entrance from marrow and a decreased rate of removal from the vascular compartment. In contrast, the lymphocytes, eosinophils, monocytes, and basophils decrease in number after administration of glucocorticoids. A single dose of cortisol results in a 70% decrease in lymphocytes and a 90% decrease in monocytes, which occurs 4–6 hours after treatment and persists for about 24 hours. The decrease in lymphocytes, monocytes, and eosinophils is thought to be due to redistribution of these cells rather than to their destruction, although recent data suggest that certain lymphocyte subpopulations are lysed in response to glucocorticoids.[54,56] The T-lymphocytes are more sensitive to glucocorticoids than B-lymphocytes and certain T-cell subpopulations are more sensitive to glucocorticoids than others. The decrease in basophils occurs by an unknown mechanism.

Anti-Inflammatory Effects. Glucocorticoids prevent or suppress the full inflammatory reaction to infectious, physical, or immunological agents. The local heat, redness, swelling, and tenderness typically associated with an inflammatory response do not develop. The glucocorticoids inhibit the early events in the process, including edema, cellular exudation, fibrin deposition, capillary dilatation, migration of leukocytes into the area and phagocytic activity. Later events are also inhibited, including capillary and fibroblast proliferation, deposition of collagen and cicatrization. The mechanism is not clearly understood but it is of great therapeutic relevance.

A major effect of glucocorticoids on the inflammatory process is inhibition of recruitment of neutrophils and monocytes.[113] The tendency of neutrophils to adhere to capillary endothelial cells, which is mediated by prostaglandins, is also decreased. Glucocorticoids decrease the synthesis and release of prostaglandins by inducing a protein (lipocortin) that inhibits phospholipase A_2, which is an enzyme involved in the synthesis of prostaglandins. Glucocorticoids also inhibit synthesis of plasminogen activator and migration inhibitory factor,[6,63] stabilize lysosomes, thereby decreasing the release of irritating hydrolytic enzymes and histamine,[124,136] and also decrease binding of chemotactic peptides that attract white blood cells.[135] Glucocorticoids slow wound healing by blocking the normal inflammatory reaction of breaking down and disorganizing collagen.

Immune System. It has been known for a long time that hypocorticism results in hypertrophy of lymphoid tissue (i.e., thymus, spleen, lymph nodes) and that hypercorticism leads to decreases or total loss of these tissues.[48] Glucocorticoids induce rapid lysis of lymphatic tissue in rats and mice but these effects occur only at suprapharmacological doses in man. The effects that are seen in humans, therefore, may be due to changes in the rate of formation or destruction of lymphoid cells which only become manifest over a longer period of time. More acute effects of glucocorticoid on lymphoid cells in man are probably due to sequestration of the cells rather than to cell lysis, although recent reports suggest that certain types of activated T-lymphocytes are susceptible to glucocorticoid-induced lysis.[54] In contrast to normal human lymphocytes, acute lymphocytic leukemias and other malignancies respond to glucocorticoid treatment with lymphocytolysis as is seen in rodents. Glucocorticoids decrease the secretion of interleukin-1 and other mediators of immune response and inhibit lymphocyte participation in delayed hypersensitivity reactions and interfere with the rejection of immunologically incompatible graft tissue.[62] This is probably due to decreases in leukocyte recruitment. High doses of glucocorticoids inhibit immunoglobulin synthesis, kill B-cells,[65] and decrease production of certain components of the complement system.[23]

Other Effects. Other effects of prolonged glucocorticoid therapy include ophthalmologic problems (posterior subcapsular cataracts,[97] increased intraocular pressure[61]) and dermatologic problems (redistribution of subcutaneous fat, hirsutism, alopecia, impaired wound healing, purpura, purple striae, and acneiform eruptions).[143]

Corticosteroids in the Treatment of Neoplasms

Once corticosteroids became available, many experiments were done to test the effect of these compounds on experimental neoplasms. It was first discovered that cortisone caused tumor regression in a transplantable mouse lymphosarcoma,[75] and this finding was soon extended to a wide variety of mouse lymphatic tumors. The effects of corticosteroids were also evaluated on many nonendocrine and nonlymphoid transplantable rodent tumors. Pharmacological doses of steroid inhibited growth of various tumor systems.[146] Tissue culture studies subsequently confirmed that lymphoid cells were the most sensitive to glucocorticoids and responded to treatment with decreases in DNA, RNA, and protein synthesis.[7] Studies of proliferating human leukemic lymphoblasts supported the hypothesis that glucocorticoids have preferential lymphocytolytic effects.[46] The mechanism of action was initially thought to be due to a decrease in glucose transport and/or phosphorylation, which would lead to decreased energy utilization from the lack of glucose.[123] However, it has recently been discovered that glucocorticoids induce a specific form of death called apoptosis, or programmed cell death, in certain lymphoid cell populations.[30] Despite a lack of understanding of the mechanism of action of glucocorticoids, it is clear that these steroids have great clinical value in the treatment of neoplasms of lymphoid origin and, to a much lesser extent, other endocrine-responsive cancers. Glucocorticoids also serve a function in the treatment of several frequently occurring side effects of malignancies as well as for general palliative therapy.

Neoplasms Treated With Corticosteroids

Acute Lymphoblastic Leukemia. Early studies of acute lymphocytic leukemia treated with prednisone alone showed that 50% of the affected children responded with prompt clinical improvement and remission.[145] However, the duration of remission was short (<1 year) and relapse was inevitable, often coinciding with the appearance of steroid resistance. For these reasons multiple drug therapy was initiated which involves combining prednisone with other cytotoxic agents. Today more than 90% of children and 60–80% of adults achieve remission with regimens that contain vincristine and prednisone or prednisolone.[27] The inclusion of other agents, such as anthracyclines, L-asparaginase, and cyclophosphamide, may or may not increase this rate of remission but does appear to prolong remission.

Once remission is achieved, a 2–3 year program of maintenance therapy follows which involves regular intensive chemotherapy sessions that include glucocorticoids.[125] With this approach more than 50% of children appear to be cured (no relapse within 5 years). The success rate is considerably lower in adults; only 15–30% of adults appear to be cured.

Acute Myeloid Leukemia. Glucocorticoids appear to have little if any value in the treatment of acute myeloid leukemia. Use of glucocorticoids as a single agent results in <10% complete remission.[96] Although glucocorticoids are sometimes included in combination chemotherapies, their value in such treatments is questionable given the current data.

Chronic Lymphocytic Leukemia. Typical B-cell chronic lymphocytic leukemia in the early stage of progression responds well to combination chemotherapy including an alkylating agent (usually chlorambucil) plus prednisolone.[50] Advanced stages of the disease usually require the addition of an anthracycline and a vinca alkaloid for successful therapy. Corticosteroids are particularly useful if the neoplasm is associated with autoimmune hemolytic anemia, neutropenia, and thrombocytopenia with hemorrhagic complications.[83] Glucocorticoids alleviate the lymphadenopathy and hepatosplenomegaly that are often associated with this condition. The more rare forms of chronic lymphocytic leukemia are more difficult to treat effectively. Both B-cell prolympho-

cytic leukemia and lymphosarcoma cell leukemia show poor response to chemotherapy.[57] In contrast, hairy-cell leukemia has a better prognosis. Combined chemotherapy with chlorambucil and prednisolone can work successfully although recent studies suggest even more encouraging results with interferon and deoxycoformycin.[137,140] T-cell chronic lymphocytic leukemias may respond to the same treatment as B-cell chronic lymphocytic leukemia but they are normally more difficult to treat.

Chronic Myeloid Leukemia. Chronic myeloid leukemia progresses in three phases. In the chronic phase, which generally lasts 3–4 years, symptoms are controlled easily with cytotoxic therapy. The next stage, blast transformation, is characterized by increased splenomegaly, bone pain, and deposits of leukemia outside the lymphohematopoietic system. Approximately 20–30% of cases show blast cells that resemble those of acute lymphoblastic leukemia. The remainder of cases are myeloblastic although a proportion have phenotypic features of both types.

Transformed lymphoblastic cells generally respond to the same treatments that are employed in acute lymphoblastic leukemia. Some patients enter complete remission but most return to the chronic phase. This chronic phase is brief; blastic transformation reappears and becomes increasingly difficult to treat, perhaps due to the development of resistant cell types.

Hodgkin's Lymphoma. Hodgkin's lymphoma is a solid tumor early found to be curable by chemotherapy. Corticosteroids alone were found to achieve worthwhile objective results in 66% of Hodgkin's lymphoma patients resistant to alkylating agents.[70] Combination chemotherapy, with MOPP (mustine, vincristine, procarbazine, prednisone), was the first treatment to effectively cause complete remission, and probably cures, in a majority of patients.[39] Since then other regimens have been found to be equally effective as MOPP.[81] One of these, ABVD (doxorubicin, bleomycin, vinblastine, dacarbazine), which is at least as effective as MOPP and has a lower incidence of certain side effects, contains no glucocorticoid component.[13]

Non-Hodgkin's Lymphoma. Corticosteroids used as single agent therapy produce temporary responses in patients with non-Hodgkin's lymphoma and they are therefore included in virtually every complex regimen used for the treatment of non-Hodgkin's lymphoma.[95] These regimens differ according to lymphoma histologic subtypes (see XXXVI-10). Complete response rates are in the range of 60–80%. Patients treated with recent generations of drug combinations have 3–4 year survival rates of 60–70%.[84,100] If the tumor is located within the central nervous system dexamethasone is preferred instead of prednisone to decrease tumor swelling.[95]

Multiple Myeloma. The standard therapy for multiple myeloma is melphalan and prednisone, which results in a 75% response rate.[130] However, a complete cure is rare and less than 10% of patients show a 99% tumor cell kill. Very high doses of glucocorticoids alone are indicated in cases of progressive or resistant disease, or if bone marrow reserve is limited. These doses can be as high as 1 g/m²/day for prednisone and 40 mg/m²/day for dexamethasone.

Breast Cancer. Glucocorticoids are never used as the sole treatment for breast cancer because of the low response rate (<25%) and the deleterious side effects that result from the high doses needed.[101] Nevertheless, glucocorticoids are included in various regimens of combination chemotherapy. The CMF (cyclophosphamide, methotrexate, 5-fluorouracil) type regimens, with and without other drugs such as prednisone, result in tumor regression in 50–80% of patients and complete response in 15–20%.[77] Although palliation of symptoms occurs in a majority of patients only a small percentage benefit by prolonged survival. The impact on median survival is no more than 2–3 months.

The role of prednisone in the effectiveness of the CMFP regimen is unclear. Some trials comparing CMF and CMFP found that the response to CMFP in premenopausal, node-positive women was not different from the response to CMF.[99,41] Another comparison trial of CMF versus CMFP found that the inclusion of prednisone resulted in a longer time to treatment failure and longer survival time.[40] However, this may be due to the higher average dose of CMF in the CMFP patients. A trial of radiation treatment plus or minus prednisone found that radiation and prednisone together had a significant increase over radiation alone in disease-free and overall survival in premenopausal women over 45.[106] A trial of high dose chemotherapy involving an 11 drug combination including prednisone resulted in a very high response rate (overall response, 92%; complete response, 73%) but median survival time was not markedly increased from other studies.[141] The efficacy of the glucocorticoids may be due, at least in part, to the improved tolerance of cytotoxic drugs.

Other Uses. Hydrocortisone replacement (approximately 40 mg/day) is indicated after either surgical adrenalectomy or medical adrenalectomy via steroid synthesis inhibitors is performed to eliminate circulating steroids in cases of breast cancer, prostate cancer, and ectopic ACTH excess.[64,102,109] Thymomas are sometimes treated with glucocorticoids if the tumor is unresectable or is unresponsive to radiation treatment.[112]

Symptomatic Uses of Corticosteroids

Palliative Care. Glucocorticoid treatment produces rapid symptomatic improvements in critically ill patients, including temporary relief of fever, sweats, lethargy, weakness, and other non-specific effects of cancer. Glucocorticoids also cause mild euphoria, a general feeling of well being, and a stimulation of appetite. These effects are transient and only short term treatment is possible due to side effects of the high doses. Also when glucocorticoids are withdrawn adrenocortical insufficiency and patient discomfort can occur. For these reasons corticosteroid treatment is normally reserved for patients whose life expectancy is brief (a few weeks or less). Doses of 25 mg/day prednisolone are used initially with a decrease to 7.5–15 mg/day for maintenance of effects.

Hypercalcemia. Hypercalcemia is a common complication of many malignancies.[5] It is caused in many cases by increased bone resorption and renal calcium reabsorption and is thought to be due to many factors which may be secreted by various tumors (see XVII-10 and XL-6), especially those of lymphoid origin. Although glucocorticoids do not lower normal calcium levels, glucocorticoids in large doses have been used for treatment of hypercalcemia (100 mg/day prednisolone, 400 mg/day hydrocortisone). The mechanisms by which glucocorticoids reduce serum calcium are thought to be the cytolytic action on lymphoid cells, the decrease in lymphokine secretion, and the inhibition of vitamin D action on calcium metabolism. Glucocorticoids are most effective on hypercalcemia that is secondary to high

vitamin D levels. They are less effective in patients with solid tumors. The results in treatment of patients with multiple myeloma have been inconsistent. Glucocorticoids are therefore a poor choice except in cases of vitamin D-mediated hypercalcemia.

Central Nervous System Tumors. Neurological symptoms from primary and metastatic brain and spinal cord tumors are partially due to peritumoral edema.[43] Glucocorticoids can ameliorate these symptoms in about 70% of cases after several days of treatment.[151] There is evidence that glucocorticoids cause both a decrease in edema production and an increase in edema reabsorption. Dexamethasone is the recommended steroid for this treatment because it contains no mineralocorticoid activity and is highly potent. A dose of 16 mg/day is used with an increase to 100 mg/day if no response occurs. This dose is continued until the maximum response is obtained. Doses are then decreased gradually and are maintained at the smallest effective dose. Glucocorticoid effects on the brain and spinal cord are short lived and only increase survival time slightly unless other measures, such as radiotherapy and surgery, are taken. Glucocorticoids are often administered during these therapies to alleviate the edema that is normally induced by these treatments. Some preliminary evidence suggests that glucocorticoids might decrease the amount of cytotoxic drug that gets to the tumor by decreasing capillary permeability. Because of the extensive use of glucocorticoids in treating central nervous system tumors this issue must be studied further.

Antiemetic Action. Glucocorticoids have been shown to decrease the severity of chemotherapy-induced emesis.[1] Both dexamethasone (8–20 mg) and methylprednisolone (125–250 mg) have been used successfully, with vomiting episodes reduced by as much as 74%. Glucocorticoids are most effective when used at low doses to enhance the antiemetic efficacy of other drugs. The mechanism by which antiemesis occurs is unknown but it may be associated with decreases in prostaglandin synthesis. Alternatively, glucocorticoids may act directly on the chemoreceptor trigger zone by modifying capillary permeability or stabilizing lysosomal membranes.

Dyspnea Due To Lymphangitic Carcinomatosis. The dyspnea due to lymphangitic carcinomatosis may be a result of tumor edema and is effectively relieved in most cases by glucocorticoid treatment.[59] If the primary tumor is chemosensitive, then cytotoxic agents are also given. Prednisone is initially given at a dose of 60–100 mg/day and is then reduced rapidly to the minimum level that maintains the response. The benefits of this treatment may be short lived and high doses may be indicated with the attendant danger of long term complications.

Mechanism of Glucocorticoid Action

The biological effects of all of the steroid hormones are mediated by intracellular receptor proteins that are specific for each steroid.[25] The glucocorticoid receptor, a cytoplasmic protein of approximately 98 kD is present in all tissues that are targets of glucocorticoid action.[19] The concentration of glucocorticoid receptors in a given cell depends on many factors, including cell type, state of differentiation, phase of the cell cycle, endocrine status, and age. Glucocorticoid receptors are required for glucocorticoid-induced changes to occur but hormonal sensitivity is not guaranteed by the presence of receptors. There is, in general, a good correlation between the concentration of glucocorticoid receptors in a cell and the cellular sensitivity to glucocorticoids. However, other factors may modulate glucocorticoid sensitivity, including the presence of nonfunctional or modified receptors and other cellular factors that modify receptor function.

The current model for glucocorticoid action (Figure XVII-5-2) starts with the passive diffusion of glucocorticoids into the cell. The steroid then binds noncovalently and with high affinity to the glucocorticoid receptor in the cytoplasm. Ligand binding causes the receptor to undergo a process called activation or transformation in which a conformational change in the receptor is thought to occur (see XVII-1). The receptor dissociates from the nonsteroid-binding subunits with which it is normally associated, unmasking the DNA binding domain of the receptor protein. The steroid-receptor complex then translocates to the nucleus where it binds to specific DNA sequences called glucocorticoid-regulatory elements (GREs). After binding to a GRE, the steroid-receptor complex alters the transcription rate of specific genes near or in which the GRE is located. A typical glucocorticoid-responsive gene is shown in Figure XVII-5-3. The GRE, shown with the consensus DNA sequence, is located in the 5' regulatory region of the gene where a glucocorticoid receptor bound to the GRE can interact with transcription factors that bind to other regulatory elements, such as the TATA and CAAT boxes, which are also present in this region. In this fashion glucocorticoids increase or decrease the amount of messenger RNA and ultimately the level of protein that is synthesized from these genes, and thus alter cellular functions. It should be noted that glucocorticoids do not cause genes to turn on and off but rather they modulate the expression of genes that are already expressed at a certain level.

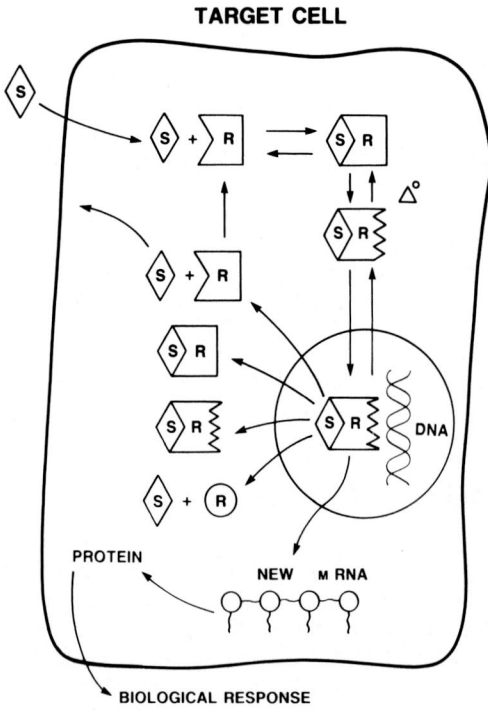

TARGET CELL

Figure XVII-5-2. Mechanism of action of steroid hormones. S, steroid; R, receptor.

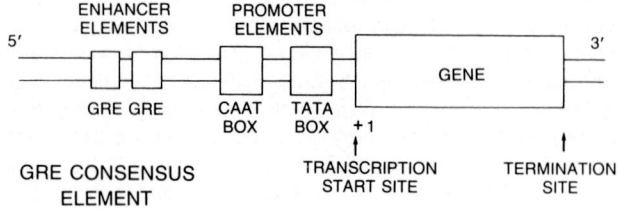

TYPICAL GLUCOCORTICOID RESPONSIVE GENE

GGTACANNNTGTTCT

Figure XVII-5-3. Structural requirements for glucocorticoid regulation of gene transcription.

One important aspect of receptor regulation that is especially relevant to glucocorticoid therapy is glucocorticoid-induced down regulation (tachyphylaxis) of the glucocorticoid receptor. The ability of glucocorticoid to down regulate its own receptor is mediated by the receptor itself.[20] The maximum effect is a 50–75% decrease in receptor protein, which is reflected by a decrease in receptor messenger RNA that occurs within 24 hours of treatment. Long-term administration of glucocorticoids is not only associated with down regulation of the glucocorticoid receptor but also with decreased function of other genes that are glucocorticoid sensitive.[10] This phenomenon implies that continuous glucocorticoid treatment can have widespread deleterious effects on cell function and may explain why alternate day glucocorticoid therapy is associated with a lesser risk of unwanted side effects.[149] These results indicate that it may be important, in terms of efficacy and safety, to administer therapeutic doses of glucocorticoids in a manner that simulates the natural diurnal rhythm of glucocorticoid secretion.

Anticorticosteroids

Steroid receptor antagonists have been synthesized that inhibit the action of receptor ligands. Most of these antagonists are modified steroids that are competitive inhibitors of the receptor. The antagonist forms a complex with the receptor and then interferes with one or more of the normal functions of a ligand-bound receptor by not translocating to the nucleus, not binding to the appropriate DNA sequences with high affinity, or not affecting transcription rates. The best characterized antiglucocorticoids are the steroid metabolite cortexolone (11-deoxycortisol) and the antiprogestin RU-486.[51] The antiprogestin effects of RU-486 are used clinically for the induction of abortions. Perhaps the antiglucocorticoid effects of this drug will also be applied in the treatment of hypercorticism.[53] Spironolactone is a commonly used antimineralocorticoid. Recent reports suggest that antimineralocorticoids may be useful in the treatment of diseases involving blood pressure and body fluid regulation.[147]

Corticosteroid Resistance

Since it was discovered that glucocorticoids have a specific cytolytic effect on human leukemic and lymphomatous tissue, the medical significance of glucocorticoid receptors in these tissues has been studied. The fact that not all leukemia patients respond to glucocorticoid treatment combined with the observation that some patients cease to respond during therapy has prompted investigators to try to identify a relationship between glucocorticoid receptor concentration and clinical responsiveness.[105,115] Various human and mouse lymphoid cell lines, including CEM-C7,[71] P1798,[138] and S49.1,[131] have been extensively studied to determine how these cells become resistant to glucocorticoids. In almost every single case of resistance in mouse cells, the cause is a defective glucocorticoid receptor or a large decrease in receptor number.[132] However, resistant human leukemia cells have not been found to contain major receptor defects such as those described in mouse lymphoma cell lines.[80] No consistent relationship has been found between glucocorticoid receptor number and sensitivity to lymphocytolysis.[85] The correlation is strongest for acute lymphocytic leukemia and non-Hodgkin's lymphoma.[116] Other diseases, notably acute myeloid leukemia,[91] have no correlation at all. For chronic lymphocytic leukemia the results are inconsistent.[79] The lack of a consistent relationship between receptor number and sensitivity to glucocorticoid therapy suggests that some factor(s) other than the presence of glucocorticoid receptors may mediate the susceptibility of lymphoid cells to glucocorticoid-induced lymphocytolysis.

Glucocorticoid-Induced Lymphocytolysis

For many years it has been known that glucocorticoids induce massive lymphocytolysis in rats and mice, resulting in significant reductions in the size of lymphoid tissues, including thymus, spleen, and lymph nodes. This phenomenon has been widely studied, especially in rodent thymus, where immature thymocytes are available in high number and die rapidly after glucocorticoid treatment. This form of cell death has been found to be identical both morphologically and biochemically with a specific form of cell death known as apoptosis, or programmed cell death.[52] Apoptosis is associated with many physiological processes, including embryogenesis, morphogenesis, normal tissue turnover and cell-mediated immunity, and is induced by many different signals in these various systems.[148] Morphological characteristics of apoptosis include cellular condensation and internucleosomal chromatin degradation followed by fragmentation into apoptotic bodies that are phagocytosed by neighboring cells or circulating macrophages.

Recent studies have shown that glucocorticoid-induced apoptosis occurs only in lymphocytes and is mediated by the glucocorticoid receptor.[31,127] Not all lymphocytes are sensitive, however. Immature T-cells, and some B-cells, are very sensitive to apoptosis while mature T-cells are not. Those cells that are responsive start to die within 8 hours of glucocorticoid treatment in vivo. Nearly all immature thymocytes are dead within 48 hours of treatment.

In contrast, the sensitivity of human lymphocytes to glucocorticoid-induced apoptosis appears to be quite different. Although these cells do respond to glucocorticoids they do not lyse rapidly or do not die at all after glucocorticoid treatment. The marked lymphocytopenia observed after glucocorticoid treatment is mostly due to redistribution of lymphocytes into other tissues and is returned to normal within 24 hours. This difference in species sensitivity to lymphocytolysis may reflect differences in the predominant glucocorticoid in each species, the major circulating glucocorticoid in man is cortisol while in rats and mice it is corticosterone.

Although human lymphocytes are generally resistant to lymphocytolysis, certain subpopulations do lyse in response to glucocorticoids. These include lymphocytes in nonperipheral blood compartments and certain activated lympho-cytes.[54,55] More importantly, several malignant lymphoid cells are sensitive to glucocorticoid-induced apoptosis. Several investigators have demonstrated that some human leukemic cells, notably acute and chronic lymphocytic leukemia and acute myeloid leukemia, show morphological and biochemical signs of apoptosis upon death.[8,55] The difference between normal and malignant human lymphocytes that causes the increased susceptibility of malignant cells to apoptosis is unknown but may eventually be exploited in the treatment of lymphoid neoplasms.

References

1. Aapro, M. S.: Corticosteroids as antiemetics. Recent Results Cancer Res., 108:102, 1988.
2. Addison, T.: On the constitutional and local effects of disease of the suprarenal capsules. Samual Highly, London, 1855.
3. Alavi, I. A., Sharma, B. K., and Pillay, V. K. G.: Steroid-induced diabetic ketoacidosis. Am. J. Med. Sci., 262:15, 1971.
4. Askari, A., Vignos, P. J., and Moskowitz, R. W.: Steroid myopathy in connective tissue disease. Am. J. Med., 61:485, 1976.
5. Attie, M. F.: Treatment of hypercalcemia. Endocrinol. Metab. Clin. North Am., 18:807, 1987.
6. Balow, J. E., and Rosenthal, A. S.: Glucocorticoid suppression of macrophage migration inhibitory factor. J. Exp. Med., 137:1031, 1973.
7. Baxter, G. D., Collins, R. J., Harmon, B. V., Kumar, S., Prentice, R. L., Smith, P. J., and Lavin, M. F.: Cell death by apoptosis in acute leukemia. J. Pathol., 158:123, 1989.
8. Baxter, J. D., Harris, A. W., Tomkins, G. M., and Cohn, M.: Glucocorticoid receptors in lymphoma cells in culture: relationship to glucocorticoid killing activity. Science, 171:189, 1971.
9. Bell, P. H., Howard, K. S., Shepherd, R. G., Finn, B. M., and Misenhelder, J. H.: Studies with corticotropin. II. Pepsin degradation of β-corticotropin. J. Am. Chem. Soc., 78:5059, 1956.
10. Berkovitz, G. D., Carter, K. M., Migeon, C. J., and Brown, T. R.: Down-regulation of the glucocorticoid receptor in cultured human skin fibroblasts: implications for the regulation of aromatase activity. J. Clin. Endocrinol. Metab., 66:1029, 1988.
11. Blair-West, J. R., Coghlan, J. P., Denton, D. A., Fei, D. T. W., Hardy, K. J., Scoggins, B. A., and Wright, R. D.: A dose-response comparison of the actions of angiotensin II and angiotensin III in sheep. J. Endocrinol., 87:409, 1980.
12. Blair-West, J. R., Coghlan, J. P., Denton, D. A., Goding, J. R., and Wright, R. D.: The effect of adrenal corticoid steroids on parotid salivary secretion. In Salivary Glands and Their Secretions. Proceedings of International Conference, Washington, D.C., Aug., 1962. New York, Pergamon Press, 1964, p. 253.
13. Bonadonna, G., Santoro, A., Bonfante, V., and Valagussa, P.: Cyclic delivery of MOPP and ABVD in stage IV Hodgkin's disese: Rationale, background studies, and recent results. Cancer Treat. Rep., 66:881, 1982.
14. Bondy, P. K.: The Adrenal Cortex. In Metabolic Control and Disease, 8th Ed. Edited by P. K. Bondy, and L. E. Rosenberg. Philadelphia, W. B. Saunders, 1980, p. 1427.
15. Bridson, W. E., and Kohler, P. O.: Cortisol stimulation of growth hormone production by human pituitary tissue in culture. J. Clin. Endocrinol. Metab., 30:538, 1970.
16. Britton, S. W., and Silvette, H.: Some effects of corticoadrenal extract and other substances on adrenalectomized animals. Am. J. Physiol., 99:15, 1931.
17. Brown, M. S., Kovanen, P. T., and Goldstein, J. L.: Receptor-mediated uptake of lipoprotein-cholesterol and its utilization for steroid synthesis in the adrenal cortex. Recent Prog. Horm. Res., 35:215, 1979.
18. Brown-Sequard, C. E.: Recherches experimentales sur la physiologie et la pathologie des capsules surrénales. C. R. Acad. Sci. [D] (Paris), 43:422, 1856.
19. Burnstein, K. L., and Cidlowski, J. A.: Regulation of gene expression by glucocorticoids. Annu. Rev. Physiol., 51:683, 1989.
20. Burnstein, K. L., Jewell, C. M., and Cidlowski, J. A.: Human glucocorticoid receptor cDNA contains sequences sufficient for receptor down-regulation. J. Biol. Chem., 265:7284, 1990.
21. Burr, W. A., Ramsden, D. B., Griffiths, R. S., Black, E. G., Hoffenberg, R., Meinhold, H., and Wenzel, K. W.: Effect of a single dose of dexamethasone on serum concentrations of thyroid hormones. Lancet, 2:58, 1976.
22. Cannon, P. J., Ames, R. P., and Laragh, J. H.: Relation between potassium balance and aldosterone secretion in normal subjects and in patients with hypertensive or renal tubular disease. J. Clin. Invest., 45:865, 1966.
23. Caren, L. D., and Rosenberg, L. T.: Steroids and serum complement in mice: influence of hydrocortisone, diethylstilbestrol, and testosterone. Science, 152:782, 1966.
24. Carpenter, W. T., and Gruen, P. H.: Cortisol's influence on human mental functioning. J. Clin. Psychopharmacol., 2:91, 1982.
25. Carson-Jurica, M. A., Schrader, W. T., and O'Malley, B. W.: Steroid receptor family: structure and functions. Endocr. Rev., 11:201, 1990.
26. Caspi, E., Dorfman, R. I., Khan, B. T., Rosenfeld, G., and Schmid, W.: Degradation of corticosteroids. VI. Origin of the carbon atoms of steroid hormones biosynthesized in vitro in the bovine adrenal from acetate-1-C14. J. Biol. Chem., 237:2085, 1962.
27. Champlin, R., and Gale, R. P.: Acute lymphoblastic leukemia: recent advances in biology and therapy. Blood, 73:2051, 1989.
28. Charney, A. N., Kinsey, M. D., Myers, L., Giannella, R. A., and Gots, R. E.: Na+-K+-activated adenosine triphosphatase and intestinal electrolyte transport. J. Clin. Invest., 56:653, 1975.
29. Cheng, S. C., Harding, B. W., and Carballeira, A.: Effects of metyrapone on pregnenolone biosynthesis and on cholesterol-cytochrome P-450 interaction in the adrenal. Endocrinology, 94:1451, 1974.
30. Cohen, J. J.: Lymphocyte Death Induced by Glucocorticoids. In Anti-inflammatory Steroid Action Basic and Clinical Aspects. Edited by R. P. Schleimer, H. N. Claman, and A. L. Oronsky. San Diego, Academic Press, 1989, p. 110.
31. Compton, M. M., and Cidlowski, J. A.: Rapid in vivo effects of glucocorticoids on the integrity of rat lymphocyte genomic deoxyribonucleic acid. Endocrinology, 118:38, 1986.
32. Cope, C. L.: The adrenal cortex in internal medicine. Br. Med. J., 2:847, 1966.
33. Copinschi, G., L'Hermite, M., LeClerq, R., Golstein, J., Vanhaelst, L., Virasoro, E.,

and Robyn, C.: Effects of glucocorticoids on pituitary hormone responses to hypoglycemia. Inhibition of prolactin release. J. Clin. Endocrinol. Metab., 40:442, 1975.
34. Cupps, T. R., and Fauci, A. S.: Corticosteroid-mediated immunoregulation in man. Immunol. Rev., 65:1133, 1982.
35. Cushing, H.: The basophil adenomas of the pituitary body and their clinical manifestations. Bull. Johns Hopkins Hosp., 50:137, 1932.
36. Czeisler, C. A., Ede, M. C. M., Regenstein, Q. R., Kisch, E. S., Fang, V. S., and Ehrlich, E. N.: Episodic 24-hour cortisol secretory patterns in patients awaiting elective cardiac surgery. J. Clin. Endocrinol. Metab., 42:273, 1976.
37. David, D. S., Grieco, M. H., and Cushman, P. Jr.: Adrenal glucocorticoids after twenty years—a review of their clinically relevant consequences. J. Chron. Dis., 22:637, 1970.
38. Davis, J. D.: Regulation of Aldosterone Secretion. *In* The Adrenal Cortex. Edited by A. B. Eisenstein. Little, Brown, and Co., Boston, 1967, p. 203.
39. DeVita, V. T., Serpick, A. A., and Carbone, P. P.: Combination chemotherapy in the treatment of advanced Hodgkin's disease. Ann. Intern. Med., 73:881, 1970.
40. Eastern Cooperative Oncology Group: Adjuvant Systemic Therapy in Premenopausal (CMF, CMFP, CMFPT) and Postmenopausal (Observation, CMFP and CMFPT) Women with Node Positive Breast Cancer. *In* Adjuvant Therapy of Cancer, IV. Edited by S. E. Jones, and S. E. Salmon. Orlando, Grune & Stratton, 1984, p. 359.
41. Eastern Cooperative Oncology Group: Comparison of induction chemotherapies for metastatic breast cancer. Cancer, 50:1235, 1982.
42. Eberlein, W. R., Bongiovannia, A. M., and Rodriguez, C. S.: The complications of steroid treatment. Pediatrics, 40:279, 1967.
43. Edwards, M. S. B., and Prados, M.: Current management of brain stem gliomas. Pediatr. Neurosci., 13:309, 1987.
44. Elliot, M. E., Alexander, R. C., and Goodfriend, T. L.: Aspects on angiotensin action in the adrenal. Key roles for calcium and phosphatidylinositol. Hypertension, 4:52, 1982.
45. Ellul-Micallef, R., and Fenech, F. F.: Effect of intravenous prednisolone in asthmatics with diminished adrenergic responsiveness. Lancet, 2:1269, 1975.
46. Ernst, P., and Killman, S.: Perturbation of generation of human leukemic blast cells by cytostatic therapy in vivo: effect of corticosteroids. Blood, 36:689, 1970.
47. Fain, J. N., and Czech, M. P.: Glucocorticoid Effects on Lipid Mobilization and Adipose Tissue Metabolism. *In* Adrenal Gland, Vol. 6, Sect. 7, Endocrinology. Handbook of Physiology. Edited by H. Blashko. American Physiology Society, Washington, D.C., 1975, p. 169.
48. Fauci, A. S., Dale, D. C., and Balow, J. E.: Glucocorticosteroid therapy: mechanisms of action and clinical considerations. Ann. Int. Med., 84:304, 1976.
49. Foster, E. S., Zimmerman, T. W., Hayslett, J. P., and Binder, H. J.: Corticosteroid alteration of active electrolyte transport in rat distal colon. Am. J. Physiol., 245:6668, 1983.
50. French Cooperative Group on Chronic Lymphocytic Leukemia: Therapy of chronic lymphocytic leukemia patients. Results from the French cooperative trials. Nouv. Rev. Fr. Hematol., 30:443, 1988.
51. Gagne, D., Pons, M., and Philbert, D.: RU 38486: A potent antiglucocorticoid *in vitro* and *in vivo*. J. Steroid Biochem., 23:247, 1985.
52. Gaido, M. L., Schwartzman, R. A., Caron, L. M., and Cidlowski, J. A.: Glucocorticoids and Cell Death: Biochemical Mechanisms. *In* Molecular Biology of Aging. Edited by C. E. Finch, and T. E. Johnson. New York, Wiley-Liss, 1990, p. 299.
53. Gaillard, K., Poffet, D., Riondel, A., and Saurat, J.-H.: RU486 inhibits peripheral effects of glucocorticoids in humans. J. Clin. Endocrinol. Metab., 61:1009, 1985.
54. Galili, N., Galili, U., Klein, F., Rosenthal, I., and Nordenskjold, B.: Human T lymphocytes become glucocorticoid sensitive upon immune activation. Cell. Immunol., 50:440, 1980.
55. Galili, U., Leizerowitz, R., Moreb, J., Gamliel, H., Gurfel, D., and Polliack, A.: Metabolic and ultrastructural aspects of the *in vitro* lysis of chronic lymphocytic leukemia cells by glucocorticoids. Cancer Res., 42:1433, 1982.
56. Galili, U.: Glucocorticoid induced cytolysis of human normal and malignant lymphocytes. J. Steroid Biochem., 19:483, 1983.
57. Galton, D. A., Goldman, J. M., Wiltshaw, E., Catovsky, D., Henry, K., and Goldenberg, G. J.: Prolymphocytic leukemia. Br. J. Haematol., 27:7, 1974.
58. Gann, D. S., Dallman, M. F., and Engleland, W. C.: Reflex control and modulation of ACTH and corticosteroids. Int. Rev. Physiol., 24:157, 1981.
59. Geimer, N. F., and Donegan, W. L.: Role and mechanism of corticosteroid therapy in breast cancer. Rev. Endocrine-Related Cancer, 6:5, 1980.
60. George, J. M., Reier, C. E., Lanese, R. R., and Rower, J. M.: Morphine anesthesia blocks cortisol and growth hormone response to surgical stress in humans. J. Clin. Endocrinol. Metab., 38:736, 1974.
61. Giles, C. L.: The ocular complications of steroid therapy. Mich. Med., 66:298, 1967.
62. Gillis, S., Crabtree, G. R., and Smith, K. A.: Glucocorticoid-induced inhibition of T cell growth factor. J. Immunol., 123:1632, 1979.
63. Granelli-Piperno, A., Vassali, J. D., and Reich, E.: Secretion of plasminogen activator by human polymorphonuclear leukocytes. Modulation by glucocorticoids and other effectors. J. Exp. Med., 146:1693, 1977.
64. Grayhack, J. T., Keeler, T. C., and Kozlowski, J. M.: Carcinoma of the prostate: Hormonal therapy. Cancer, 60:589, 1987.
65. Grayson, J., Dooley, N. J., Koski, I. P., and Blaese, R. M.: Immunoglobulin production induced in vitro by glucocorticoid hormones. T cell-dependent stimulation of immunoglobulin production without B cell proliferation in cultures of human peripheral lymphocytes. J. Clin. Invest., 68:1539, 1981.
66. Grossman, A., Perry, L., Schally, A. V., Rees, L. H., Nieuwenhuyzen Krusemann, A. C., Tomlin, S., Coy, D. H., Comaru-Schally, A. M., and Besser, G. M.: New hypothalamic hormone, corticotropin-releasing factor, specifically stimulates the release of adrenocorticotropic hormone and cortisol in man. Lancet., 1:921, 1982.
67. Gwynne, J. T., and Strauss, J. F. III: The role of lipoprotein in steroidogenesis and cholesterol metabolism in steroidogenic glands. Endocr. Rev., 3:299, 1982.
68. Gwynne, J. T., Mahaffee, D., Brewer, H. B., and Ney, R. L.: Adrenal cholesterol uptake from plasma lipoproteins; regulation by corticotropin. Proc. Natl. Acad. Sci. U.S.A., 73:4329, 1976.
69. Hall, R. C. W., Popkin, M. K., Stickney, S. K., and Gardner, E. R.: Presentation of the steroid psychoses. J Nerv. Ment. Dis., 167:229, 1979.
70. Hall, T. C., Choi, O. S., Abadi, A., and Krant, M. J.: High-dose corticoid therapy in Hodgkin's disease and other lymphomas. Ann. Inter. Med., 66:1144, 1967.
71. Harmon, J. M., Thompson, E. B., and Baione, U. A.: Analysis of glucocorticoid-resistant human leukemic cells by somatic cell hybridization. Cancer Res., 45:1587, 1955.
72. Harrop, G. A., Soffer, L. J., Ellsworth, R., and Ney, R. L.: Studies on the suprarenal cortex. III. Plasma electrolytes and electrolyte excretion during suprarenal insufficiency in the dog. J. Exp. Med., 58:17, 1933.
73. Haynes, R. C. Jr.: The activation of adrenal phosphorylase by the adrenocorticotropic hormone. J. Biol. Chem., 233:1220, 1958.
74. Haynes, R. C. Jr., and Murad, F.: Adrenocorticotropic Hormone; Adrenocortical Steroids and their Synthetic Analogs; Inhibitors of Adrenocortical Steroid Biosynthesis. *In* Goodman and Gilman's The Pharmacological Basis of Therapeutics, 7th Edition. Edited by A. G. Gilman, L. S. Goodman, T. W. Rall, and F. Murad. New York, Macmillan, 1985, p. 1459.
75. Heilman, F. R., and Kendall, E. C.: The influence of 11-dehydro-17-hydroxycorticosterone (compound E) on the growth of malignant tumor in the mouse. Endocrinology, 34:416, 1944.
76. Hench, P. S., Kendall, E. C., Slocumb, C. H., and Polley, H. F.: The effect of a hormone of the adrenal cortex (17-hydroxy-11-dehydrocorticosterone; compound E) and of pituitary adrenocorticotropic hormone on rheumatoid arthritis. Proc. Staff Meet. Mayo Clin., 24:181, 1949.
77. Henderson, I. C., Hayes, D. F., Come, S., Harris, J. R., and Canellos, G.: New agents and medical treatments for advanced breast cancer. Semin. Oncol., 14:34, 1987.
78. Hogan, T. F., Citrin, D. L., Johnson, B. M., Nakamura, S., Davis, T. E., and Borden, E. C.: o,p'-DDD (mitotane) therapy of adrenal corticol carcinoma. Cancer, 42:2177, 1978.
79. Homo, F., Durant, S., Duval, D., Marie, J. P., Zittoun, R., and Harrouseau, J. L.: Glucocorticoid receptors and hormonal responsiveness of human blood and bone-marrow cells in non-lymphocytic leukemia. J. Steroid Biochem., 15:479, 1981.
80. Homo-Delarche, F.: Glucocorticoid receptors and steroid sensitivity in normal and neoplastic human lymphoid tissues: a review. Cancer Res., 44:431, 1984.
81. Hoppe, R. T.: The contemporary management of Hodgkin disease. Radiology, 169:297, 1988.
82. Ingle, D. J., Higgins, G. M., and Kendall, E. C.: Atrophy of the adrenal cortex in the rat produced by administration of large amounts of cortin. Anat. Rec., 71:363, 1938.
83. Johnson, L. E.: Chronic lymphocytic leukemia. Am. Fam. Physician, 38:167, 1988.
84. Juliusson, G., Abrahamsen, A. F., Cavallin-Stahl, E., Goldstone, A. H., Lister, T. A., Nissen, N., Robert, K.-H., Singer, C. R. J., Somers, R., Ost, A., and Gahrton, G.: Management of non-Hodgkin lymphoma in adults in Scandinavia, United Kingdom, and the Netherlands. Acta Oncol., 28:135, 1989.
85. Junker, K.: Glucocorticoid receptors on lymphoid cells. Cell biological and clinical aspects. Dan. Med. Bull., 1:12, 1986.
86. Kalbak, K.: Incidence of arteriosclerosis in patients with rheumatoid arthritis receiving long-term corticosteroid therapy. Ann. Rheum. Dis., 31:196, 1972.
87. Kaplan, S. A., and Nagareda Shimizu, C. S.: Effects of cortisol on amino acids in skeletal muscle and plasma. Endocrinology, 72:267, 1963.
88. Kimura, T.: ACTH stimulation of cholesterol side chain cleavage activity of adrenocortical mitochondria. Mol. Cell. Biochem., 36:105, 1981.
89. Kimura, T., and Suzuki, K.: Components of the electron transport system in adrenal steroid-hydroxylase. J. Biol. Chem., 242:485, 1967.
90. Kobayashi, O., Wada, H., and Utsumi, J.: Urinary lithiasis in children treated with adrenocorticosteroid hormone. Acta Med. Biol., 15:91, 1967.
91. Koeffler, H. P., Golde, D. W., and Lippman, M. E.: Glucocorticoid sensitivity and receptors in cells of human myelogenous leukemia lines. Cancer Res., 40:563, 1980.
92. Krakoff, L. R.: Glucocorticoid excess syndromes causing hypertension. Cardiol. Clin., 6:537, 1988.
93. Lecocq, F. R., Mebane, D., and Madison, L. L.: The acute effect of hydrocortisone on hepatic glucose output and peripheral glucose utilization. J. Clin. Invest., 43:237, 1964.
94. Li, C. H., Evans, H. M., and Simpson, M. E.: Adrenocorticotropic hormone. J. Biol. Chem., 149:413, 1943.
95. Longo, D. L., and Hathorn, J.: Current therapy for diffuse large-cell lymphoma. Prog. Hematol., 15:115, 1987.
96. Lowenthal, R. M., and Jestrimski, K. W.: Corticosteroid drugs: Their role in oncological practice. Med. J. Austr., 144:81, 1986.
97. Lubkin, V. L.: Steroid cataract—a review and a conclusion. J. Asthma Res., 14:55, 1977.
98. Lucky, A. W.: Principles of the use of glucocorticoids in the growing child. Pediatr. Dermatol., 1:226, 1984.
99. Ludwig Breast Cancer Study Group: A randomized trial of adjuvant combination chemotherapy with or without prednisone in premenopausal breast cancer patients with metastases in one to three axillary lymph nodes. Cancer Res., 45:4454, 1985.
100. Lymphoma Study Group: Chemotherapeutic results and prognostic factors of patients with advanced non-Hodgkin's lymphoma treated with VEPA or VEPA-M. J. Clin. Oncol., 6:128, 1988.
101. Mandel, S.: Steroid myopathy. Postgrad. Med., 72:207, 1982.
102. Manni, A.: Endocrine therapy of breast and prostate cancer. Endocrinol. Metab. Clin. North Am., 18:569, 1989.
103. Marver, D.: Aldosterone action in target epithelia. Vitam. Horm., 38:57, 1980.
104. Masters, J. N., Finch, C. E., and Sapolsky, R. M.: Glucocorticoid endangerment of hippocampal neurons does not involve deoxyribonucleic acid cleavage. Endocrinology, 124:3083, 1989.
105. McCaffrey, R., Lillquist, A., and Bell, R.: Abnormal glucocorticoid receptors in acute leukemia cells. Blood, 59:393, 1982.
106. Meakin, J. W., Allt, W. E. C., and Beale, F. A.: Ovarian irradiation and prednisone following surgery and radiotherapy for carcinoma of the breast. Breast Cancer Res. Treat., 3(Suppl.):45, 1983.
107. Melby, J. C.: Clinical pharmacology of systemic corticosteroids. Annu. Rev. Pharmacol. Toxicol., 17:511, 1977.
108. Miller, L. K., Kral, J. G., Strain, G. W., and Zumoff, B.: Differential binding of dexamethasone to ammonium sulfate precipitates of human adipose tissue cytosols. Steroids, 49:507, 1987.
109. Misbin, R. I., Canary, J., and Williard, D.: Aminoglutethimide in the treatment of Cushing's syndrome. J. Clin. Pharmacol., 16:645, 1976.
110. Mulrow, P. J., and Forman, B. H.: The tissue effects of mineralocorticoids. Am. J. Med., 53:561, 1972.
111. New, M. I., Seaman, M. P., and Peterson, R. E.: A method for the simultaneous determination of the secretion rates of cortisol, 11-desoxycortisol, corticosterone, 11-desoxycorticosterone and aldosterone. J. Clin. Endocrinol. Metab., 29:514, 1969.
112. Papatestas, A. E., Pozner, J., Genkins, G., Kornfeld, P., and Matta, R. J.: Prognosis in occult thymomas in myasthenia gravis following transcervical thymectomy. Arch. Surg., 122:1352, 1987.
113. Parrillo, J. E., and Fauci, A. S.: Mechanisms of glucocorticoid action on immune processes. Annu. Rev. Pharmacol. Toxicol., 19:179, 1979.
114. Pennisi, A. J., Fiedler, J., Lipsey, A., Mickey, R., Melekzadeh, M. H., and Fine, R. N.: Hyperlipidemia in pediatric renal allograft patients. J. Pediatr., 87:249, 1975.
115. Pui, C. H., Dahl, G. V., Rivera, G., Murphy, S.-B., and Costlow, M. E.: The relationship

of blast cell glucocorticoid receptor levels to response to single-agent steroid trial and remission response in children with ALL. Leuk. Res., 8:579, 1984.

116. Quddus, F. F., Levanthal, B. G., Boyet, J. M., Pullen, D. J., Crist, N. M., and Borowitz, M. J.: Glucocorticoid receptors in immunological subtypes of childhood acute lymphocytic leukemia cells: a pediatric oncology group study. Cancer Res., 45:482, 1985.

117. Reichstein, T., and Shoppee, C. W.: The hormones of the adrenal cortex. Vitam. Horm., 1:346, 1943.

118. Richards, J. M., Santiago, S. M., and Klanstermeyer, W. B.: Aseptic necrosis of the femoral head in corticosteroid-treated pulmonary disease. Arch. Intern. Med., 140:1473, 1980.

119. Rimsza, M. E.: Complications of corticosteroid therapy. Am. J. Dis. Child., 132:806, 1978.

120. Ringe, J. D.: Glucocorticoid-induced osteoporosis. Clin. Rheumatol., 2(Suppl. 8):109, 1989.

121. Rizza, R. A., Mandarino, L. J., and Gerich, J. E.: Cortisol-induced insulin resistance in man: impaired suppression of glucose production and stimulation of glucose utilization due to a post receptor defect of insulin action. J. Clin. Endocrinol. Metab., 54:132, 1982.

122. Rose, L. I., and Saccar, C.: Choosing corticosteroid preparations. Am. Fam. Physician, 17:198, 1978.

123. Rosen, J. M., Fina, J. J., Millholland, R. J., and Rosen, F.: Inhibition of glucose uptake in lymphosarcoma 1798 by cortisol and its relationship to the biosynthesis of deoxyribonucleic acid. J. Biol. Chem., 245:2074, 1970.

124. Saavedra-Delgado, A. M., Mathews, K. P., Pan, P. M., Kay, D. R., and Muilenberg, M. L.: Dose-response studies of the suppression of whole blood histamine and basophil counts by prednisone. J. Allergy Clin. Immunol., 66:464, 1980.

125. Sabbath, K. D., Weitberg, A. B., and Calabresi, P.: Potentially curable neoplasms. Dis. Mon., 32:593, 1986.

126. Sakakura, M., Takebe, K., and Nakagawa, S.: Inhibition of leutinizing hormone secretion by synthetic LHRH by long-term treatment with glucocorticoids in human subjects. J. Clin. Endocrinol. Metab., 40:774, 1975.

127. Schwartzman, R. A., and Cidlowski, J. A.: Internucleosomal DNA cleavage activity in apoptotic thymocytes: detection and endocrine regulation. Endocrinology, 128:1190, 1991.

128. Scurry, M. T., and Sheart, L.: Stop-flow analysis of the reabsorption of cortisol. Endocrinology, 84:681, 1969.

129. Shafrir, E., and Steinberg, D.: The essential role of the adrenal cortex in the response of plasma free fatty acids, cholesterol and phospholipids to epinephrine injection. J. Clin. Invest., 39:310, 1960.

130. Shopper, L. P.: Immunoproliferative disorders: detection, prevention and therapeutics. Amer. Pharm., NS29:31, 35, 1989.

131. Sibley, C. H., and Tomkins, G. M.: Mechanisms of steroid resistance. Cell, 2:221, 1974.

132. Sibley, C. H., and Yamamoto, K. R.: Mouse Lymphoma Cells: Mechanism of Resistance to Glucocorticoids. In Glucocorticoid Hormone Action. Edited by J. D. Baxter, and G. G. Rousseau, Heidelberg, Springer-Verlag, 1979, p. 357.

133. Simpson, E. R., Mason, J. I., John, M. E., Zuber, M. X., Rodgers, R. J., and Waterman, M. R.: Regulation of the biosynthesis of steroidogenic enzymes. J. Steroid Biochem., 27:801, 1987.

134. Simpson, S. A., Tait, J. F., Wettsteon, A., Neher, R., Euw, J. V., Schindler, O., and

Reichstein, T.: Konstitution de aldosterons des neuen mineralocorticoids. Experientia, 10:132, 1954.

135. Skubitz, K. M., Craddock, P. R., Hammerschmidt, D. E., and August, J. T.: Corticosteroids block binding of chemotactic peptide to its receptor on granulocytes and cause disaggregation of granulocyte aggregates in vitro. J. Clin. Invest., 68:13, 1981.

136. Spath, J. A., and Lefer, A. M.: Effects of dexamethasone on myocardial cells in the early phase of acute myocardial infarction. Am. Heart J., 90:50, 1975.

137. Spiers, A. S. D., Moore, D., Cassileth, P. A., Harrington, D. P., Cummings, F. J., Neiman, R. S., Bennett, J. M., and O'Connell, M. J.: Remissions in hairy-cell leukemia with pentostatin (2'-deoxycoformycin). N. Eng. J. Med., 316:825, 1987.

138. Stevens, J., Stevens, Y.-N., and Haabenstock, H.: Molecular Basis of Glucocorticoid Resistance in Experimental and Human Leukemia. In Biochemical Actions of Hormones. Edited by G. Litwack. New York, Academic Press, 1983, 10:383.

139. Stiel, J. N., Island, D. P., and Liddle, G. W.: Effect of glucocorticoids on plasma growth hormone in man. Metabolism, 19:158, 1970.

140. Talpaz, M., Kantarjian, H. M., McCredie, K., Trujillo, J. M., Keating, M. J., and Gutterman, J. U.: Hematologic remission and cytogenetic improvement induced by recombinant human interferon alpha in chronic myelogenous leukemia. N. Engl. J. Med., 314:1065, 1986.

141. Tormey, D. C., Kline, J. C., and Palta, M.: Short term high density systemic therapy for metastatic breast cancer. Breast Cancer Res. Treat., 5:177, 1985.

142. Touitou, Y., Bogdan, A., Legrand, J. C., and Desgrez, P.: Aminoglutethimide and glutethimide's effects on 18-hydroxycorticosterone biosynthesis by human and sheep adrenals in vitro. Acta Endocrinol., 80:517, 1975.

143. Truhan, A. P., and Ahmed, A. R.: Corticosteroids: a review with emphasis on complications of prolonged systemic therapy. Ann. Allergy, 62:375, 1989.

144. Vaugan, G. M., Becker, R. A., Allen, J. P., Goodwin, C. W. Jr., Pruitt, B. A. Jr., ad Mason, A. D. Jr.: Cortisol and corticotrophin in burned patients. J. Trauma, 22:263, 1982.

145. Vietti, T. J., Sullivan, M. P., Berry, D. H., Haddy, T. B., Haggard, M. E., and Blattner, R. J.: The response of acute childhood leukemia to an initial and a second course of prednisone. J. Pediatr., 66:18, 1965.

146. Vollmer, E. P.: A viewpoint on animal tumors as test systems for steroids. In Hormonal Steroids, Biochemistry, Pharmacology, and Therapeutics. Proc. First Int. Cong. on Horm. Steroids, 2:351, 1965.

147. Waeber, B., Nussberger, J., and Brunner, H. R.: Clinical applications of antimineralocorticoids. J. Steroid Biochem., 31:739, 1988.

148. Walker, N. I., Harmon, B. V., Gobe, G. C., and Kerr, J. F. R.: Patterns of cell death. Methods Achiev. Exp. Pathol., 13:18, 1988.

149. Walton, J., Watson, B. S., and Ney, R. L.: Alternate-day versus shorter-interval steroid administration. Arch. Intern. Med., 126:601, 1970.

150. Weisberg, L. A., and Chatorian, A. M.: Pseudotumor cerebri of childhood. Am. J. Dis. Child., 131:1243, 1977.

151. Weissman, D. E.: Glucocorticoid treatment for brain metasteses and epidural spinal cord compression: a review. J. Clin. Oncol., 6:543, 1988.

152. Weitzman, E. D., Fukushima, D., Nogeire, C., Roffwarg, H., Gallagher, T. F., and Hellman, L.: Twenty-four hour pattern of the episodic secretion of cortisol in normal subjects. J. Clin. Endocrinol. Metab., 33:14, 1971.

153. Wilber, J. F., and Utiger, R. D.: The effect of glucocorticoids on thyrotropin secretion. J. Clin. Invest., 48:2096, 1969.

Acknowledgments

The authors thank Lu-Ann Caron-Leslie, Deborah Bellingham, and Dr. Kerry Burnstein for editorial assistance, and Tobi Schwartzman for manuscript preparation.

XVII-6

Estrogens and Antiestrogens

V. Craig Jordan

Introduction

It has been known since the turn of the century[9] that approximately one third of premenopausal women with advanced breast cancer will respond to oophorectomy. Advances in the understanding of reproductive endocrinology, and steroid biochemistry, during the early decades of the twentieth century permitted the development of specific strategies to restrict the availability of estrogen, the hormone widely believed[40] to be responsible for the development of breast carcinoma. Breast cancer in postmenopausal women will respond to hypophysectomy[85] and adrenalectomy[43] but paradoxically high dose therapy with synthetic estrogens like diethylstilbestrol (DES)[21] and trianisylchorethylene (TACE)[103] cause breast tumor regression[38,111] (Figure XVII-6-1). However it was unclear which patient would respond until the discovery of the estrogen receptor (ER)[47,105] and the development of models[35,48] to describe the subcellular actions of estrogen in its target tissues, i.e., uterus, vagina, pituitary gland and some breast cancers.[78]

The studies of the structure activity relationships of estrogens have provided the medical community with cheap simple molecules that have proved to have powerful biological effects in a woman's target tissues. The wide application of estrogens in the gynecological community has resulted in the realization that estrogens might cause a number of cancers in target tissues.[40]

As early as 1936, Lacassagne predicted that a therapeutic agent might be found that could block the stimulatory effects of estrogen in breast tissue.[63] The nonsteroidal antiestrogen MER25 (Figure XVII-6-2) was first described by Lerner and coworkers in 1958.[66] This discovery provoked clinical testing

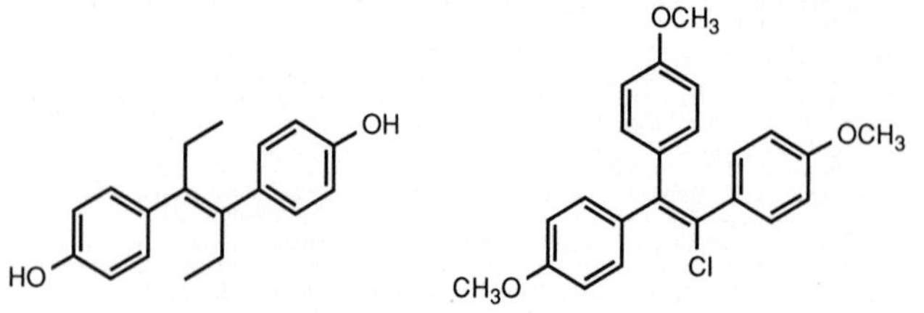

Diethylstilbestrol (DES)   TACE

Figure XVII-6-1. The structure of synthetic estrogens.

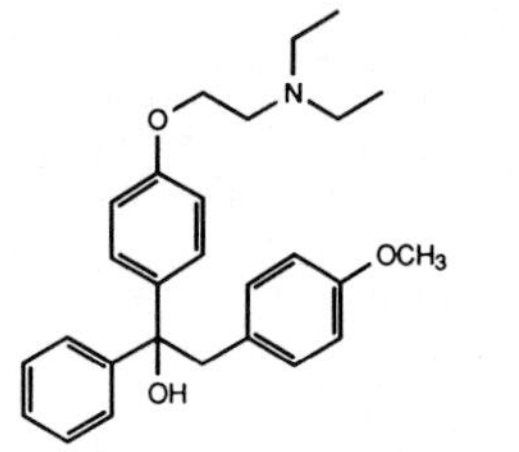

Ethamoxytriphetol (MER 25)

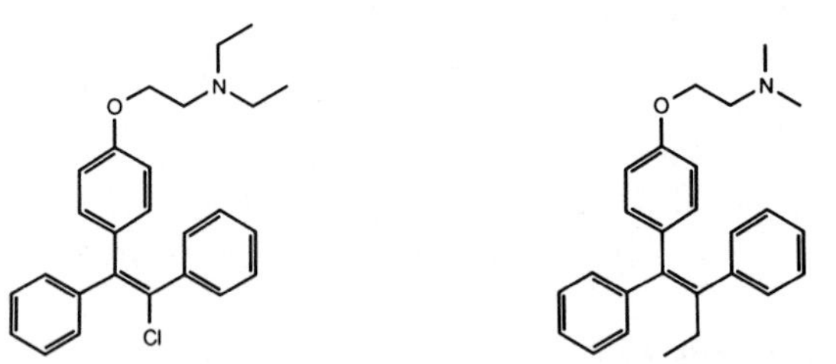

Clomiphene (cis and trans isomers)   Tamoxifen (trans isomer)

Figure XVII-6-2. The structure of non-steroidal antiestrogens.

for a variety of applications but trials were stopped because of toxic side effects.[65] Nevertheless, and in response to the encouraging clinical findings, the pharmaceutical industry synthesized a wide range of compounds in the 1960s but regrettably there were few clinical successes. One notable exception was Clomid®, (Figure XVII-6-2) a mixture of *cis* and *trans* geometric isomers of a substituted triphenyl-ethylene (note the similarity to the structure of TACE). Although clomiphene is an antifertility agent in rodents[42] the compound was shown to induce ovulation in women.[37] Clomid is used routinely as a profertility agent in subfertile women with a functioning hypothalamo-pituitary-ovarian axis.[44]

For obvious reasons several antiestrogens[64] were tested as therapeutic agents to control the growth of advanced breast cancer in postmenopausal women but only tamoxifen (ICI46,474)[14,112] was developed further because of demonstrated efficacy and a low incidence of side effects.

Tamoxifen: General Pharmacology in the Laboratory

Tamoxifen is the *trans* geometric isomer of a substituted triphenylethylene with well characterized antifertility[39] and antitumor[55] activity in the rat. As a group, the triphenylethylene-type antiestrogens have an extremely interesting species specific pharmacology.[34] In short term tests in the mouse, tamoxifen can cause increases in uterine wet weight and

vaginal cornification. In contrast tamoxifen is classified as a pure antiestrogen in the chick. Tamoxifen exhibits the properties of a partial estrogen agonist/antagonist in rats and women. It is this balance of biological properties that is key to the current strategies for the use of tamoxifen.

Mode of Action in Breast Cancer

Tamoxifen is a competitive inhibitor of estradiol binding to the ER.[52] Estradiol causes the proliferation of ER positive breast cancer cells in culture and tamoxifen can reversibly prevent estrogen-stimulated growth.[70] Similarly, tamoxifen will prevent estrogen-stimulated growth of ER positive breast cancer cells transplanted into immune deficient (athymic) mice.[83]

Estrogens are believed to modulate cell growth by causing an increase in stimulatory growth factors (e.g., transforming growth factor α) and a decrease in inhibitory growth factors (e.g., the family of transforming growth factor β's).[20] These growth factors are thought to initiate, or prevent, progress through the cell cycle by interaction with their respective membrane receptors. The regulatory mechanism functions as an autocrine loop. There are also paracrine (cell to cell) influences of growth factors (e.g., insulin-like growth factor 1) that can play a role in modulating the replication of epithelial cells.

Antiestrogens negate the stimulatory effects of estrogen by blocking the ER causing the cell to be held at the G1 phase of the replicative cycle (Figure XVII-6-3).[82] Tamoxifen also causes a decrease in the circulating levels of insulin-like growth factor 1.[15]

A variety of alternate, non-ER mediated biochemical interactions have been described for antiestrogens that might also contribute to the antitumor activity of tamoxifen. This topic has recently been reviewed.[56]

Clinical Pharmacology

Tamoxifen (Nolvadex®) is available in 10 mg tablets as the citrate salt. Treatment schedules vary depending upon the country and their initial clinical trials to evaluate the drug. Schedules of 10 mg b.i.d. are recommended in the United States although 10 mg t.i.d. and 20 mg b.i.d. are routinely used in other countries. Doses over 100 mg b.i.d. have been used to treat breast cancer, but retinal degeneration has been reported.[60] In general the high therapeutic index has permitted such wide variations in dosage. There is a low incidence of side effects, the most frequent of which is hot flashes.[34]

Tamoxifen is rapidly absorbed and attains steady state serum levels within 4–6 weeks.[50] The drug is extensively metabolized (Figure XVII-6-4) to N-desmethyltamoxifen (major metabolite) and 4-hydroxy-tamoxifen (minor metabolite). Both metabolites have the potential[92] to be converted to 4-hydroxy-N-desmethyltamoxifen which is also a minor metabolite.[68,69] Nevertheless 4-hydroxylated triphenylethylenes have high affinity for the ER[54] and may play a significant role in the antitumor actions of tamoxifen.[25]

Tamoxifen has a long serum half-life (7 days) and N-desmethyltamoxifen has a serum half-life of 14 days.[84] This long serum half-life is probably why a clinical response has not been routinely documented when tamoxifen therapy is discontinued.

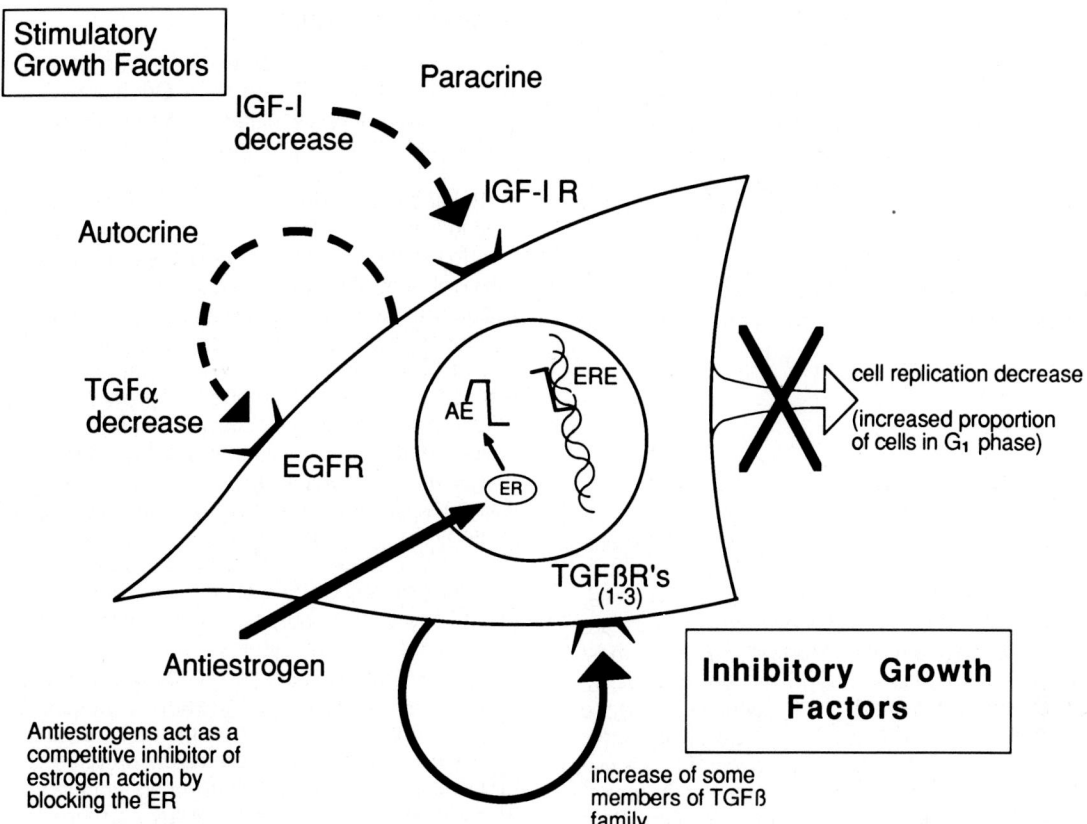

Figure XVII-6-3. The mode of action of antiestrogens to inhibit replication in a breast cancer cell. Antiestrogens (AE) can bind to the estrogen receptor (ER). This produces an incomplete change in the tertiary structure of the ER[52] so that there is an altered interaction with the estrogen response elements (ERE) on the DNA. As a response to the binding in AE to ER there is a decrease in the production of transforming growth factor α (TGF α) but there is an increase in the production of some members of the transforming growth factor β (TGF β) family. Antiestrogens also cause a decrease in insulin-like growth factor-1 (IGF-1)[15] that may stimulate cell replication from adjacent cells (paracrine) or organs (endocrine). Cell culture studies have demonstrated that antiestrogens cause an arrest in the G_1 phase of the cell cycle.[82]

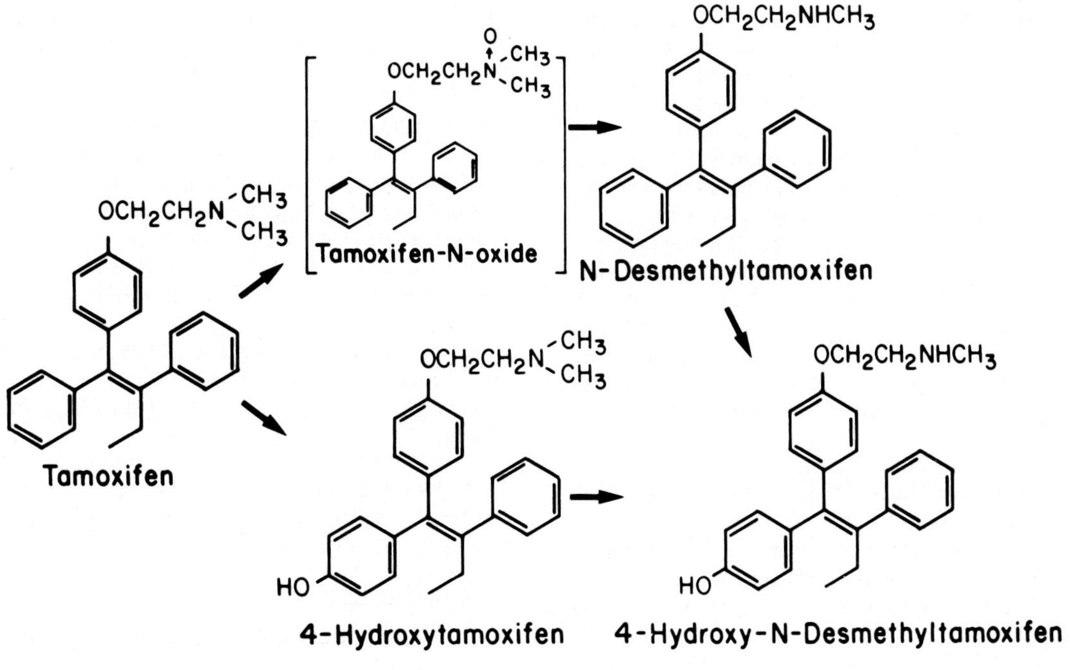

Figure XVII-6-4. The metabolites of tamoxifen.

Tamoxifen exhibits weak estrogen-like properties in post-menopausal women.[34,56] There is a partial decrease in LH and FSH, increases in sex hormone binding globulin, decreases in antithrombin III, some changes in vaginal cytology and hyperplasia of the endometrium (although this is not consistently reported). Tamoxifen causes ovarian stimulation in premenopausal women with ovulatory cycles and increases in steroidogenesis.[77,88,98,99] Women are at risk for pregnancy during tamoxifen therapy. Tamoxifen is not recommended if a woman is pregnant and patients should be counseled about the requirement for barrier contraception. Clinical cases of teratogenesis have not been reported with tamoxifen.

Advanced Breast Cancer

Tamoxifen is the endocrine treatment of choice for metastatic disease in postmenopausal patients.[34] Approximately one third of patients respond and the response rate is similar to that seen with DES therapy.[45] However side effects are reported to be lower with tamoxifen than with DES. The most prevalent side effects noted with DES are nausea (51%), edema (53%), vaginal bleeding (15%), and incontinence (10%). In contrast, hot flashes (29%) is the side effect most reported during tamoxifen therapy. Patients with ER positive disease are more likely to benefit from tamoxifen therapy.[34] Correlation of clinical response and ER status indicates that 48% (159/333) of patients with ER positive disease have partial or complete responses whereas only 13% (17/129) of ER negative patients have responses. A variety of combinations of other hormonal agents and combination chemotherapy have been examined[34] but tamoxifen is usually administered as a monotherapy. Prospective randomized clinical trials of tamoxifen vs either megestrol acetate[79] (40 mg 4 x daily) or medroxyprogesterone acetate[109] (300 mg 3 x daily) indicate similar response rates but the authors recommend tamoxifen as first-line endocrine therapy based upon side effects and time to progression. Amino-glutethimide[2] (+ hydrocortisone) produces response rates similar to tamoxifen and a combination is not superior to either agent alone. However, toxicity is significantly greater in patients taking aminoglutethimide. Aminoglutethimide can be an effective second-line agent following tamoxifen.[101]

Tamoxifen is effective in the treatment of advanced disease in premenopausal women.[77,98] Small randomized trials have demonstrated that tamoxifen produces a response rate and overall survival similar to oophorectomy.[12,46] Regrettably, the patient population is too small to demonstrate whether any benefit would preferentially accrue from one treatment approach over the other. However tamoxifen does cause increases in circulating estradiol levels[77,88,98,99] that could potentially reduce the efficacy of the antiestrogen. Recent studies in the laboratory[53] have, however, demonstrated that much higher levels of estradiol than are noted clinically are required to reverse the actions of tamoxifen. Nevertheless, combinations of tamoxifen and LHRH agonists (to reduce ovarian steroidogenesis by preventing LH release from the pituitary gland) are being evaluated.[91] Tamoxifen is currently available in the United States to treat ER+ disease in premenopausal women.

Adjuvant Therapy

The low incidence of side effects was an important factor when the Eastern Cooperative Oncology Group (ECOG) established their adjuvant trial[17] of tamoxifen in elderly patients who would be unable to cope with the rigors of chemotherapy. Similar adjuvant trials with tamoxifen were conducted in the United Kingdom,[1,4,5,6,89,90] Canada[87] and some countries in Europe.[76,94,96]

In the main, a conservative course of one or two years of adjuvant tamoxifen was selected. However, this decision was based upon a number of reasonable concerns. Patients with advanced disease usually respond to tamoxifen for perhaps one or two years so that it was expected that ER negative disease would be encouraged to grow prematurely during adjuvant therapy. If this occurred, then the physician would have already used a valuable palliative drug and only have combination chemotherapy to slow the relentless growth of recurrent disease. A related argument involved the changing strategy for the application of combination chemotherapy. Recurrent treatment cycles (2 years) were found to be of no long-term benefit for the patient. The strategy was formulated that an aggressive course of short term treatment (6 months), with the most active cytotoxic drugs, could have the best chance to kill tumor cells before the premature development of drug resistance. Using the same argument there was an intuitive reluctance to use long-term tamoxifen therapy because this would lead to premature drug resistance. Longer might not be better. Finally there was a sincere concern about the side effects of adjuvant therapy and the ethical issue of treating patients who "might" not recur. Although this argument primarily focused on chemotherapy and node negative patients, it is fair to say that very few patients in the mid 1970s had received extended therapy with tamoxifen so that long term side effects were in the main unknown. The majority of tamoxifen-treated patients, up to that point, had only received about two years of treatment for advanced disease before drug resistance occurred. Potential side effects of thrombosis, osteoporosis, etc. were only of secondary importance. The use of tamoxifen in the disease free patient would change that perspective.

The overall success of one or two years of adjuvant tamoxifen therapy has recently been evaluated in the overview analysis of randomized clinical trials.[22] Two conclusions can be drawn. Tamoxifen confers a survival advantage to postmenopausal women whereas combination chemotherapy confers a survival advantage to premenopausal women. Unfortunately, it is not possible to draw a definite conclusion about whether 1 year or 2 years of tamoxifen therapy is of value.

Based upon laboratory studies[51] that demonstrate the value of long-term or indefinite tamoxifen therapy clinical trials organizations are in the process of evaluating this treatment strategy.

Clinical experience with long-term tamoxifen therapy has been garnered from nation-wide clinical trials with and without chemotherapy in pre- and postmenopausal patients with node positive and negative disease.

Chemotherapy Plus Tamoxifen

The ECOG has evaluated the duration of tamoxifen therapy in postmenopausal patients all of whom received combination chemotherapy (CMF). An early analysis[26] has demonstrated an increase in disease free survival with 5 years vs 1 year of tamoxifen. The 5 year arm has now gone through a second randomization to evaluate the value of indefinite tamoxifen therapy.

The National Surgical Adjuvant Breast and Bowel Project (NSABP) clinical trials organization has conducted a registration study of two years of combination chemotherapy (L-PAM, 5-FU) and tamoxifen plus an additional year of tamoxifen alone[31] to build on the successes of their earlier trials that demonstrated the efficacy of tamoxifen in receptor positive postmenopausal patients. Overall these investigators conclude that 3 years of tamoxifen confers a significant advantage over two years of tamoxifen.

A recent report[8] from Italy has demonstrated that the addition of combination chemotherapy (CMF 6 cycles followed by 4 courses of epirubicin) to long-term tamoxifen (5 years) for the treatment of ER and node-positive disease does not seem to improve significantly the clear cut effectiveness of tamoxifen alone to prevent recurrence.

Tamoxifen Alone

Although the 2 year adjuvant tamoxifen study conducted by the NATO demonstrates[5,6] a survival advantage for women, current clinical trials are evaluating a longer duration of tamoxifen therapy. A small randomized[19] clinical trial comparing 3 years of tamoxifen to no treatment has demonstrated a survival advantage for ER positive patients receiving tamoxifen. Similarly the Scottish trial,[10] that has compared 5 years of tamoxifen to no treatment, has demonstrated a survival advantage for patients taking tamoxifen. The Scottish trial is particularly interesting because it addresses the question of whether to administer tamoxifen early or save the drug until recurrence. Most patients in the control arm received tamoxifen at recurrence. Since an overall survival advantage is observed for the patients receiving adjuvant tamoxifen this demonstrates that early resistance to tamoxifen does not occur. The Scottish study included a mixture of node positive and node negative patients, but the greatest effect was observed in the node positive cohort. The problem with being able to demonstrate a significant advantage for the node negative group is the statistical power necessary to show an effect based upon the low incidence of recurrence.

The NSABP has focused attention upon the use of adjuvant tamoxifen to delay the recurrence of ER positive node negative disease.[30] Tamoxifen increases the disease free survival and, perhaps most importantly, the antiestrogen is active in premenopausal women. The NSABP protocol B_{14} used an initial treatment period of 5 years of tamoxifen but the patients will now continue tamoxifen for another 5 years. At present no overall survival advantage has been noted, but the preliminary analysis at 4 years is probably premature.

In summary, multiple clinical trials have demonstrated the effectiveness and safety of long-term tamoxifen therapy for treating breast cancer. The trials that are currently underway will provide additional reassurance to both patients and physicians about the safety of tamoxifen in node negative disease where only a minority of patients will have a recurrence.[53]

Toxicological Considerations in Postmenopausal Women

Several concerns have been expressed about the biological consequences of long-term tamoxifen treatment for women with breast cancer. In the main, these concerns (Table XVII-6-1) are minor compared with the ability of tamoxifen to control the recurrence of a fatal disease.

Ophthalmic

Triphenylethylenes are known to cause cataracts in rats during long-term therapy. Clomiphene is particularly active and ocular effects have been noted with tamoxifen.[34]

A recent evaluation[72] of patients receiving 10 mg tamoxifen for up to two years has noted no ocular changes. Nevertheless high-dose tamoxifen therapy has been associated with retinal changes[60] (keratopathy and multiple paramacular refractile lesions in the nerve fiber and inner plexiform layers) and it may be possible that accumulated toxicity will occur with decades of tamoxifen therapy. At present there appears to be little evidence that severe ocular changes occur. Regular eye examinations are not recommended although patients should be questioned about changes in visual acuity.

Antiestrogenic Effects

Osteoporosis. Estrogen is important to maintain bone in premenopausal women. After menopause, hormone replacement therapy (HRT) is often recommended to prevent the development of osteoporosis. Clearly the long-term administration of an antiestrogen has the potential to precipitate premature osteoporosis.

Some but not all animal studies show that tamoxifen creates estrogenic effects on bone.[27,59,107] Preliminary clinical evaluations have confirmed that tamoxifen does not cause osteoporosis. Clinical studies show that 2 years of adjuvant tamoxifen does not decrease bone density[28,74,86,106] and there is anecdotal evidence to suggest that tamoxifen is beneficial and may replace bone.

Fornander and colleagues[33] have evaluated the impact of either two or five years of adjuvant tamoxifen therapy on bone mineral density at two levels of the distal forearm representing cortical and trabecular bone. The results did not indicate an accelerated bone loss.

Atherosclerosis. Estrogen lowers low density lipoprotein (LDL) cholesterol and raises high density lipoprotein (HDL) cholesterol. It is possible that this change in blood lipids is responsible for the decrease in myocardial infarction observed in premenopausal women when compared to men. Following menopause, women develop the same risk for coronary heart disease as men. It can be argued that the long-term administration of an antiestrogen could produce a population at

Table XVII-6-1. Potential Concerns About the Use of Long-term Tamoxifen Therapy in Postmenopausal Patients.

Ophthalmic
Antiestrogenic effects
a) Osteoporosis
b) Atherosclerosis
Estrogenic effects
a) Thromboembolic disorders
b) Uterine stimulation
c) Liver carcinogenesis

risk for premature coronary heart disease. However the estrogen-like effects of tamoxifen[34] lower the circulating levels of cholesterol in female patients.[3,7,11,13,75,95] Unfortunately HDL cholesterol does not consistently increase during tamoxifen therapy[75] and this may be significant for the overall beneficial effect of long-term adjuvant therapy.

Estrogenic Effects

Clearly the fact that tamoxifen has an appropriate level of estrogenic activity may become a two edged sword. The administration of estrogen to women is known to cause an increased risk for thrombosis and endometrial carcinoma. Clearly, information is required to evaluate the safety of long-term tamoxifen therapy.

Thromboembolic Disorders. There are several anecdotal reports associating the administration of tamoxifen for advanced breast cancer with subsequent thromboembolic episodes.[41,71,80] Similarly an association between adjuvant tamoxifen therapy, given with chemotherapy, and thrombosis has been reported.[26] However there are really no reports of a serious increase in thromboembolic disorders during long-term tamoxifen monotherapy. Nevertheless decreases in antithrombin III have been noted in postmenopausal patients treated with tamoxifen for advanced[23] or node positive breast cancer[57] although the majority of patients have values well within the normal range. Decreases in antithrombin III are rarely below the level of clinical concern (>30% decrease). However, patients who have a known history of thromboembolic disorders should be carefully evaluated before a decision is made to use long-term tamoxifen therapy.

Uterine Stimulation. Tamoxifen is known to produce some estrogen-like effects in postmenopausal women[34] but very little is known about the long-term stimulatory effects of tamoxifen on the human uterus.[16,81]

One particular focus of current research is the effect of tamoxifen on endometrial carcinoma. Tamoxifen does have some efficacy in the treatment of endometrial carcinoma.[102] Nevertheless the findings that ER and PgR positive human endometrial carcinoma can have enhanced growth in athymic mice with tamoxifen[97] and other antiestrogens has raised justifiable concerns about the safety of long-term tamoxifen therapy. Indeed animals bitransplanted with an MCF-7 breast tumor and endometrial carcinoma EnCa101 demonstrate target site specific effects with tamoxifen. Estradiol stimulated growth of the breast tumor is controlled by tamoxifen whereas the endometrial tumor grows more rapidly.[36]

The clinical situation is more complex. Only about one-third of endometrial tumors are hormone responsive although it is widely believed[40] that estrogen stimulation is responsible for the promotion of all early disease. Endometrial carcinoma has been reported to occur in patients who are receiving adjuvant tamoxifen therapy[62] but this is unremarkable as breast and endometrial carcinoma are known to be associated. Nevertheless, one randomized adjuvant clinical trial result reported by Fornander and colleagues[32] in Sweden has demonstrated a significant increase in endometrial carcinoma in those patients receiving tamoxifen for between 2 and 5 years. There were 13 endometrial tumors identified in patients (N=931) taking tamoxifen and 2 in the control arm (N=915). Interestingly enough there was a significant decrease in second primary breast tumors (tamoxifen arm 18, control arm 32). The dose of tamoxifen used, 20 mg b.i.d., is larger than the dose, 10 mg b.i.d, used in other major clinical studies in Europe and the United States. In this regard an increase in endometrial carcinoma has not been reported from either the Scottish trial[10] (5 years tamoxifen) or the NSABP trial B_{14}[30] (5–10 years tamoxifen). Nevertheless physicians should remain vigilant to the possibility of endometrial stimulation by tamoxifen that might encourage the growth of occult endometrial carcinomas. All cases of persistent vaginal bleeding should be followed up with a gynecological examination and an endometrial biopsy. It is clear though that patients should not be denied the advantages of tamoxifen to control the recurrence of breast cancer because of the potential complications of endometrial carcinoma which has a good prognosis.

Liver Carcinogenesis. Estrogens are known to act as promoters of rat liver carcinogenesis. Similarly tamoxifen will produce liver tumors in rats if large dose or extended administration schedules are used (ICI Pharmaceutical unpublished toxicology data). To date there have been no reports of a significant increase in liver tumor incidence in tamoxifen-treated patients. A recent clinical study to evaluate the use of tamoxifen in the treatment of hepatocellular carcinoma demonstrated that this therapeutic approach was not beneficial.[24] Conversely the authors did not comment that tamoxifen exacerbated the course of the disease as four patients continued to have long term survival. Clearly this area of concern needs to be monitored carefully by the clinical community.

Prevention of Breast Cancer

Tamoxifen will prevent carcinogenesis in rodent models of mammary cancer.[49,58,113] These laboratory data, the efficacy of tamoxifen to produce a significant survival advantage in postmenopausal women[22] and to prevent[10,30,32] the appearance of second primary breast cancers (Table XVII-6-2) has increased enthusiasm to use tamoxifen as a chemosuppressive agent (i.e., to prevent the appearance of occult disease) in postmenopausal women at risk for breast cancer.[18,29,73] The carcinogenic insult that initiates breast cancer probably occurs during the reproductive years. Tamoxifen could not be used as a true preventive because the timing of the event is unknown and the unrestricted use of tamoxifen in young women of reproductive age (20–40 years) would be unwise. Women would be at risk for pregnancy and tamoxifen should not be administered during pregnancy. Postmenopausal women who are at increased risk to develop breast cancer would be a suitable population to conduct a clinical evaluation of the concept of chemosuppression that was developed in the laboratory.[51,58,59]

Table XVII-6-2. The Numbers of Second Primary Breast Cancers in Patients Treated With and Without Adjuvant Tamoxifen Therapy.

Trial (number of patients)	Treatment Schedule	New Breast Tumors			
		Tamoxifen	Control	P	Ref.
Stockholm Trial (1,846)	40 mg qd x 2–5 years	18	32	0.05	32
NSABP B_{14} (2,644)	20 mg qd x 5 years	13	29	0.009	30
Scottish Trial (1,312)	20 mg qd x 5 years	7	7	NS	10

A preliminary pilot study in healthy women has proved successful,[86] although compliance is seen to be the major obstacle to conducting a successful nationwide clinical trial in tens of thousands of women.

New Agents

The success of tamoxifen in the treatment of all stages of breast cancer has focused attention on the possibility of developing additional drugs with different pharmacological properties. Several novel compounds are being evaluated in the laboratory and the clinic,[56] but only two compounds, toremifene and ICI 164,384 (Figure XVII-6-5) merit comment at present.

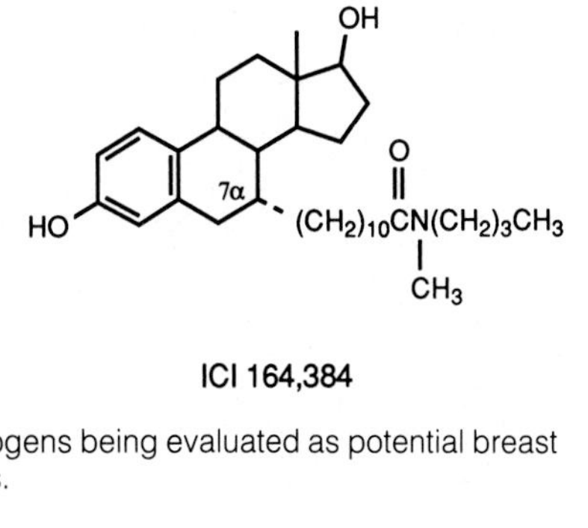

Toremifene

Toremifene is a structural derivative of tamoxifen with similar antiestrogenic and estrogenic properties in laboratory animals. The drug is active against carcinogen-induced rat mammary tumors and exhibits the properties of a tumoristatic agent.[61,93] Interestingly toremifene has been reported to have activity against a hormone-independent mouse uterine sarcoma. However, no antitumor action can be demonstrated in hormone independent breast tumors.

The metabolism of toremifene has been described in both animals and patients. In general toremifene is highly protein bound which can explain the long serum half-life. The principal metabolite of toremifene is N-desmethyltoremifene. 4-Hydroxytoremifene is a minor metabolite but has a high affinity for the ER.[100] Toremifene is less potent than tamoxifen and consequently clinical studies are using a higher dose than during tamoxifen therapy. Phase II studies indicate that 60 mg of toremifene as single daily dose is effective for the treatment of ER positive advanced breast cancer.[108] Currently clinical trials are evaluating high dose (100–240 mg/day) toremifene therapy. Interestingly enough no liver toxicity has been described during laboratory tests. This property may ultimately make toremifene the agent of choice should the studies to prevent (chemosuppress) breast cancer with tamoxifen prove to be successful but are terminated if an unacceptably high incidence of hepatocellular carcinoma (or some other side effect) is detected.

Pure Antiestrogens

ICI 164,384, the 7α-alkylamine derivative of 17β estradiol is a steroidal antiestrogen[110] specifically designed to eliminate partial agonist activity to reduce the risks of toxicity associated with the estrogenic action of tamoxifen.[34] This compound binds to the ER with high affinity and has all the characteristics of a pure antiestrogen. It completely inhibits estrogen or tamoxifen-induced uterine growth in immature rats and mice and produces a reduction in mature uterine weight, almost equivalent to the effect with ovariectomy. By itself, the drug does not stimulate progesterone receptor synthesis. Studies in vitro demonstrate that ICI 164,384 is more effective than tamoxifen in inhibiting breast cancer cell proliferation and invasion.[104]

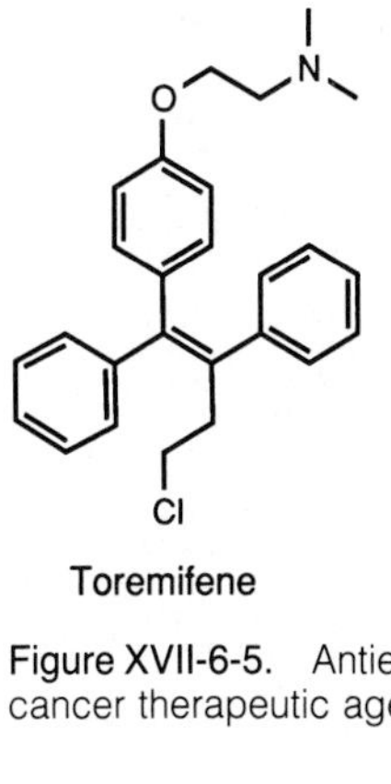

The pure antiestrogens may offer clinical advantages over tamoxifen by decreasing tumor cell invasion, tumor flare (that is especially problematic in patients with bone metastases) and the stimulation of occult endometrial carcinoma. Overall this class of drugs could have a role as a second line therapy in patients who eventually fail primary tamoxifen treatment. Long-term application as an adjuvant in node negative disease appears unlikely because of the high probability of developing early atherosclerosis and osteoporosis.

Conclusion

The past twenty years have seen the development of antiestrogens as an important new class of drugs.[67] Tamoxifen has found ubiquitous applications as the front line endocrine therapy in the treatment of all stages of breast cancer. Current clinical and laboratory research is focused on the evaluation of long term adjuvant therapy. It is possible that a clinical trials organization will conduct an evaluation of tamoxifen to prevent the development of breast cancer in postmenopausal women. Several novel antiestrogens with different pharmacological properties will become available for clinical evaluating during the next five years.

Figure XVII-6-5.   Antiestrogens being evaluated as potential breast cancer therapeutic agents.

References

1. Abram, W. P., Baum, M., Berstock, D. A., and members of the CRC Adjuvant Trial Working Party: Cyclophosphamide and tamoxifen as adjuvant therapies in the management of breast cancer. Br. J. Cancer, 57:604, 1988.
2. Alonso-Munoz, M. C., Ojeda-Gonzalez, M. B., Beltron-Fabregat, M., Dorca-Ribugent, J., López-Lopez, L., Borras-Balada, J., Cardenal-Alemany, F., Gomez-Batiste, X., Fabregat-Mayol, J., and Viladiu-Quemada, M.: Randomized trial of tamoxifen versus aminoglutethimide and versus combined tamoxifen and aminoglutethimide in advanced postmenopausal breast cancer. Oncology, 45:350, 1988.
3. Bagdade, J. D., Wolter, J., Subbaiah, P. V., and Ryan, W.: Effect of tamoxifen treatment on plasma lipids and lipoproteins lipid composition. J. Clin. Endocrinol. Metab., 70:1132, 1990.
4. Baum, M. and other members of the Nolvadex Adjuvant Trial Organization: Controlled trial of tamoxifen as single adjuvant agent in management of early breast cancer. Lancet, 1:257, 1983.
5. Baum, M. and other members of the Nolvadex Adjuvant Trial Organization: Controlled trial of tamoxifen as single adjuvant agent in management of early breast cancer. Lancet, 1:836, 1985.
6. Baum, M. and other members of the Nolvadex Adjuvant Trial Organization: Controlled trial of tamoxifen as a single adjuvant agent in management of early breast cancer. Br. J. Cancer, 57:608, 1988.
7. Bertelli, G., Pronzato, P., Amoroso, D., Cusimano, M. P., Conte, P. F., Montagma, G., Bertolini, S., and Rosso, R.: Adjuvant tamoxifen in primary breast cancer: influence on plasma lipids and antithrombin III levels. Breast Cancer Res. Treat., 12:307, 1988.
8. Boccardo, F., Rubagotti, A., Bruzzi, P., Cappellini, M., Isola, G., Nenci, I., Piffanelli, A., and other members of the Breast Cancer Adjuvant Chemo-Hormone Therapy Cooperative Group: Chemotherapy versus tamoxifen versus chemotherapy plus tamoxifen in node-positive, estrogen receptor-positive breast cancer patients: results of a multicentric Italian Study. J. Clin. Oncol., 8:1310, 1990.
9. Boyd, S.: On oophorectomy in cancer of the breast. Br. Med. J., ii:1161, 1900.
10. Breast Cancer Trials Committee, Scottish Cancer Trials Office (MRC): Adjuvant tamoxifen in the management of operable breast cancer: the Scottish Trial. Lancet, 2:171, 1987.
11. Bruning, P. F., Banfrer, J. M. G., Hart, A. A. M., de Jorg-Bakker, M., Linders, D., Van Loor, J., and Nooyen, W.J.: Tamoxifen, serum lipoproteins and cardiovascular risk. Br. J. Cancer, 58:497, 1988.
12. Buchanan, R. B., Blamey, R. W., Durrent, K. R., Howell, A., Paterson, A. G., Preece, P. E., Smith, D. C., Williams, C. J. and Wilson, R. G.: A randomized comparison of tamoxifen with surgical oophorectomy in premenopausal patients with advanced breast cancer. J. Clin. Oncol., 4:1326, 1986.
13. Caleffi, M., Fentiman, I. S., Clark, G. M., Wang, D. Y., Needham, J., Clark, K., LaVille, A., and Lewis, B.: Effect of tamoxifen on estrogen binding, lipid and lipoprotein concentrations and blood clotting parameters in premenopausal women with breast pain. J. Endocrinol., 119:335, 1988.
14. Cole, M. P., Jones, C. T. A., and Todd, I. D. H.: A new antioestrogenic agent in late breast cancer. An early clinical appraisal of ICI46,474. Br. J. Cancer, 25:270, 1971.
15. Colletti, R. B., Roberts, J. D., Devlin, J. T., and Copeland, K. C.: Effect of tamoxifen

on insulin-like growth factor 1 in patients with breast cancer. Cancer Res., 49:1882, 1989.
16. Cross, S. S., and Ismail, S. M.: Endometrial hyperplasia in an oophorectomized woman receiving tamoxifen therapy. Case report. Br. J. Obst. Gynaecol., 97:190, 1990.
17. Cummings, F. J., Gray, R., Davis, T. E., Tormey, D. C., Harris, J. E., Falkson, G., and Arsenau, R.: Adjuvant tamoxifen treatment of elderly women with stage II breast cancer. Ann. Int. Med., 103:324, 1985.
18. Cuzick, J., Wang, D. Y., and Bulbrook, R. D.: The prevention of breast cancer. Lancet, 1:83, 1986.
19. Delozier, T., Julien, J. P., Juret, P., Veyret, C., Covette, J. E., Grai, Y., Olliver, J. M., and deRanieri, E.: Adjuvant tamoxifen in postmenopausal breast cancer: preliminary results of a randomized trial. Breast Cancer Res. Treat., 7:105, 1986.
20. Dickson, R. B., and Lippman, M. E.: Estrogenic regulation of growth and polypeptide growth factor secretion in human breast carcinoma. Endo. Rev., 8:29, 1987.
21. Dodds, E. C., Lawson, W., and Noble, R. L.: Biological effects of the synthetic oestrogenic substance 4:4′-dihydroxy-α:β diethylstilbene. Lancet, 1:1389, 1938.
22. Early Breast Cancer Trialists' Collaborative Group: Effect of adjuvant tamoxifen and of cytotoxic therapy on mortality in early breast cancer. N. Engl. J. Med., 319:1681, 1988.
23. Enck, R. E., and Rios, C. N.: Tamoxifen treatment of metastatic breast cancer and antithrombin III levels. Cancer, 53:2607, 1984.
24. Engstrom, P. F., Levin, B., Moertel, C. G., and Schutt, A.: A phase II trial of tamoxifen in hepatocellular carcinoma. Cancer, 65:2641, 1990.
25. Etienne, M. C., Milano, G., Fischel, J. L., Frenay, M., François, E., Formento, J. L., Gioanni, J., and Namer, M.: Tamoxifen metabolism: pharmacokinetics and *in vitro* study. Br. J. Cancer, 60:30, 1989.
26. Falkson, H. C., Gray, R., Wolberg, W. H., Gilchrist, K. W., Harris, J. E., Tormey, D. C., and Falkson, G.: Adjuvant trial of 12 cycles of CMFPT followed by observation or continuous tamoxifen versus four cycles of CMFPT in postmenopausal women with breast cancer: an ECOG Phase III study. J. Clin. Oncol., 8:599, 1990.
27. Feldman, S., Minne, H. W., Parvizi, S., Pfeifer, M., Lempert, U. G., Bauss, F., and Ziegler, R.: Antiestrogen and antiandrogen administration reduce bone mass in the rat. Bone and Mineral, 7:245, 1989.
28. Fentiman, I. S., Caleffi, M., and Rodin, A.: Bone mineral content of women receiving tamoxifen for mastalgia. Br. J. Cancer, 60:262, 1989.
29. Fentiman, I. S., and Powles, T. J.: Tamoxifen and benign breast problems. Lancet, 2:1070, 1987.
30. Fisher, B., Costantino, J., Redmond, C., and other members of the NSABP.: A randomized clinical trial evaluating tamoxifen in the treatment of patients with node-negative breast cancer who have estrogen receptor positive tumors. N. Engl. J. Med., 32:479, 1989.
31. Fisher, B., and other NSABP Investigators: Prolonging tamoxifen for primary breast cancer. Findings from the National Surgical Adjuvant Breast and Bowel Project Clinical Trial. Ann. Int. Med., 106:649, 1987.
32. Fornander, T., Rutqvist, L. E., Cedermark, B. V., Glas, U., Mattson, A., Silversward, J. D., Skoog, L., Somell, A., Theve, T., Wilking, N., Askergren, J., and Hjolmar, M. L.: Adjuvant tamoxifen in early breast cancer: occurrence of new primary cancers. Lancet, 1:117, 1989.
33. Fornander, T., Rutqvist, L. E., Sjöberg, H. E., Blomqvist, L., Mattsson, A., and Glas, U.: Long-term adjuvant tamoxifen in early breast cancer: effect on bone mineral density in postmenopausal women. J. Clin. Oncol., 8:1019, 1990.
34. Furr, B. J. A., and Jordan, V. C.: The pharmacology and clinical uses of tamoxifen. Pharmacol. Ther., 25:127, 1984.
35. Gorski, J., Welshons, W., and Sakai, D.: Remodeling the estrogen receptor model. Mol. Cell. Endocr., 36:11, 1984.
36. Gottardis, M. M., Robinson, S. P., Satyaswaroop, P. G., and Jordan, V. C.: Contrasting actions of tamoxifen on endometrial and breast tumor growth in the athymic mouse. Cancer Res., 48:812, 1988.
37. Greenblatt, R. B., Barfield, W. E., Jungck, E. C., and Ray, A. W.: Induction of ovulation with MRL-41. Preliminary report. JAMA, 178:101, 1961.
38. Haddow, A., Watkinson, J. M., and Paterson, E.: Influence of synthetic oestrogens upon advanced malignant disease. Br. Med. J., ii:393, 1944.
39. Harper, M. J. K., and Walpole, A. L.: A new derivative of triphenylethylene: effect on implantation and mode of action in rats. J. Reprod. Fertil., 13:101, 1967.
40. Henderson, B. E., Ross, R., and Bernstein, L.: Estrogens as a cause of human cancer: The Richard and Hilda Rosenthal Foundation Award Lecture. Cancer Res., 48:246, 1988.
41. Hendrick, A., and Subraminian, V.: Tamoxifen and thromboembolism. JAMA, 243:514, 1980.
42. Holtkamp, D. E., Greslin, J. G., Root, C. A., and Lerner, L. J.: Gonadotrophin inhibiting and antifecundity effects of chloramiphene. Proc. Soc. Exp. Biol. Med., 105:197, 1960.
43. Huggins, C., and Bergenstad, D. M.: Inhibition of human mammary and prostatic cancers by adrenalectomy. Cancer Res., 12:134, 1952.
44. Huppert, L. C.: Induction of ovulation with clomiphene citrate. Fertil. Steril., 31:1, 1979.
45. Ingle, J. N., Ahmann, D. L., Green, S. J., Edmonson, J. H., Bisel, H. F., Kvols, L. K., Nichols, W. C., Creagon, E. T., Hahn, R. G., Rubin, J., and Frytack, S.: Randomized clinical trial of diethylstilbestrol versus tamoxifen in postmenopausal women with advanced breast cancer. N. Engl. J. Med., 304:16, 1981.
46. Ingle, J. N., Krook, J. E., Green, S. J., Kukista, T. P., Everson, L. K., Ahman, D. L., Chang, M. N., Bisel, H. F., Windschitl, H. E., Twito, D. I., and Pfeiffe, M. M.: Randomized trial of bilateral oophorectomy versus tamoxifen in premenopausal women with metastatic breast cancer. J. Clin. Oncol., 4:4178, 1986.
47. Jensen, E. V., and Jacobson, H. I.: Basic guides to the mechanism of estrogen action. Recent Prog. Horm. Res., 18:387, 1962.
48. Jensen, E. V., Suzuki, T., Kawashima, T., Stumpf, W. E., Jungblut, P. W., and DeSombre, E. R.: A two step mechanism for the interaction of estradiol with rat uterus. Proc. Natl. Acad. Sci. USA, 59:632, 1968.
49. Jordan, V. C.: Effect of tamoxifen (ICI 46,474) on initiation and growth of DMBA-induced rat mammary carcinomata. Eur. J. Cancer, 12:419, 1976.
50. Jordan, V. C.: Metabolites of tamoxifen in animals and man: identification, pharmacology and significance. Breast Cancer Res. Treat., 2:123, 1982.
51. Jordan, V. C.: Laboratory studies to develop general principles for the adjuvant treatment of breast cancer with antiestrogens: problems and potential for future clinical applications. Breast Cancer Res. Treat., 3(Suppl. 1):73, 1983.
52. Jordan, V. C.: Biochemical pharmacology of antiestrogen action. Pharm. Rev., 36:245, 1984.
53. Jordan, V. C.: Long-term adjuvant tamoxifen therapy for breast cancer. Breast Cancer Res. Treat., 15:125, 1990.
54. Jordan, V. C., Collins, M. M., Rowsby, L., and Prestwich, G.: A monohydroxylated metabolite of tamoxifen with potent antioestrogenic activity. J. Endocrinol., 75:305, 1977.
55. Jordan, V. C., and Dowse, L. J.: Tamoxifen as an antitumour agent: effect on oestrogen binding. J. Endocrinol., 68:297, 1976.
56. Jordan, V. C., and Murphy, C. S.: Endocrine pharmacology of antiestrogens as antitumor agents. Endocr. Rev. 11:578, 1990.
57. Jordan, V. C., Fritz, N. F., and Tormey, D. C.: Long-term adjuvant therapy with tamoxifen: Effects on sex hormone binding globulin and antithrombin III. Cancer Res., 47:4517, 1987.
58. Jordan, V. C., Lababidi, M. K., and Mirecki, D. M.: The antiestrogenic and antitumor properties of prolonged tamoxifen therapy in C3H/OUJ mice. Eur. J. Cancer, 26:718, 1990.
59. Jordan, V. C., Phelps, E., and Lingren, J. U.: Effect of antiestrogens on bone in castrated and intact female rats. Breast Cancer Res. Treat., 10:31, 1987.
60. Kaiser-Kupfer, M. L., and Lippman, M. E.: Tamoxifen retinopathy. Cancer Treat. Rep., 62:315, 1978.
61. Kangas, L., Nieminen, A. L., Blaco, G., Grontroos, M., Kallico, S., Karjalianen, M., Perila, M., Sondervall, M., and Toivola, T.: A new triphenylethylene compound Fc-1157a II. Antitumor effects. Cancer Chemother. Pharmacol., 17:109, 1986.
62. Killackey, M. A., Hakes, T. B., and Pierce, V. K.: Endometrial adenocarcinoma in breast cancer patients receiving tamoxifen. Cancer Treat. Rep., 69:237, 1985.
63. Lacassagne, A.: Hormonal pathogenesis of adenocarcinoma of the breast. Am. J. Cancer, 27:217, 1936.
64. Legha, S. S., and Carter, S. K.: Antiestrogens in the treatment of breast cancer. Cancer Treat. Rev., 3:205, 1976.
65. Lerner, L. J.: The First Non-Steroidal Antioestrogen-MER-25. *In:* Non-Steroidal Antioestrogens: Molecular Pharmacology and Antitumour Activity. Edited by R. L. Sutherland, and V. C. Jordan. Sydney, Australia, Academic Press, 1981, p.1.
66. Lerner, L. J., Holthaus, F. J., Jr., and Thompson, C. R.: A non-steroidal estrogen antagonist 1-(p-2-diethylaminoethoxyphenyl)-1-phenyl-2-p-methoxyphenylethanol. Endocrinology, 63:295, 1958.
67. Lerner, L. J., and Jordan, V. C.: Development of antiestrogens and their use in breast cancer: Eighth Cain Memorial Award Lecture. Cancer Res., 50:4177, 1990.
68. Lien, E. A., Solheim, E., Kvinnsland, S., and Veland, P. M.: Identification of 4-hydroxy N-desmethyltamoxifen as a metabolite in human bile. Cancer Res., 48:2304, 1988.
69. Lien, E. A., Solheim, E., Lea, O. A., Lundgren, S., Kvinnsland, S., and Ueland, P. M.: Distribution of 4-hydroxy-N-desmethyl tamoxifen and other tamoxifen metabolites in human biological fluids during tamoxifen treatment. Cancer Res., 49:2175, 1989.
70. Lippman, M. E., and Bolan, G.: Oestrogen-responsive human breast cancer in long term tissue culture. Nature, 256:592, 1975.
71. Lipton, A., Harvey, H. A., and Hamilton, R. W.: Venous thrombosis as a side effect of tamoxifen treatment. Cancer Treat. Rep., 68:887, 1984.
72. Longstaff, S., Sigurdson, H., O'Keefe, M., Ogston, S., and Preece, P.: A controlled study of the ocular effects of tamoxifen in conventional dosage in the treatment of breast carcinoma. Eur. J. Cancer Clin. Oncol., 25:1805, 1989.
73. Love, R. R.: Prospect for antiestrogen chemoprevention of breast cancer. J.N.C.I., 90:18, 1990.
74. Love, R. R., Mazess, R. B., Tormey, D. C., Barden, H. S., Newcomb, P. A., and Jordan, V. C.: Bone mineral density in women with breast cancer treated for at least two years with tamoxifen. Breast Cancer Res. Treat., 12:297, 1988.
75. Love, R. R., Newcomb, P. A., Wiebe, D. A., Surawicz, T. S., Jordan, V. C., Carbone, P. P., and DeMets, D. L.: Lipid and lipoprotein effects of tamoxifen therapy in postmenopausal patients with node negative breast cancer. J.N.C.I., 82:1327, 1990.
76. Ludwig Breast Cancer Group: Randomized trial of chemoendocrine therapy, endocrine therapy and mastectomy alone in postmenopausal patients with operable breast cancer and axillary node metastases. Lancet, 1:1256, 1984.
77. Manni, A., and Pearson, O. H.: Antiestrogen-induced remission in premenopausal women with stage IV breast cancer: effects on ovarian function. Cancer Treat. Rep., 64:779, 1980.
78. McGuire, W. L., Carbone, P. P., and Vollmer, E. P.: Estrogen Receptors in Human Breast Cancer. New York, Raven Press, 1975.
79. Muss, H. B., Wells, H. B., Paschold, E. H., Black, W. R., Cooper, M. R., Capizzi, R. L., Christian, R., Cruz, J. M., Jackson, D. V., Powell, B. L., Richards, R., White, D. R., Zekan, P. J., Spurr, C. L., Pope, E., Case, D., and Morgan, T. M.: Megestrol acetate versus tamoxifen in advanced breast cancer 5-year analysis—a phase III trial of the Piedmont Oncology Association. J. Clin. Oncol., 6:1098, 1988.
80. Nevasaari, K., Heikkimein, M., and Taskinen, P.: Tamoxifen and thrombosis. Lancet, 2:946, 1978.
81. Neven, P., DeMuylder, X., Von Belle, Y., Vanderick, G., and De Muylder, E.: Hysteroscopic follow-up during tamoxifen treatment. Eur. J. Obstet. Gynecol. Reprod. Biol., 35:235, 1990.
82. Osborne, C. K., Boldt, D. H., Clark, G. M., and Trent, J. M.: Effects of tamoxifen on human breast cancer cell kinetics: Accumulation of cells in early G_1 phase. Cancer Res., 43:3583, 1983.
83. Osborne, C. K., Hobbs, K., and Clark, G. M.: Effect of estrogens and antiestrogens on growth of human breast cancer cells in athymic mice. Cancer Res., 45:584, 1985.
84. Patterson, J. S., Settatree, R. S., Adam, A. K., and Kemp, J. V.: Serum concentrations of tamoxifen and major metabolites during long-term Nolvadex therapy, correlated with clinical response. *In:* Breast Cancer—Experimental and Clinical Aspects. Edited by H. T. Mouridsen, and T. Palshoff. Oxford, Pergamon Press, 1980, p. 89.
85. Pearson, O. H., Ray, B. S., and Harold, C. C.: Hypophysectomy in the treatment of advanced cancer. JAMA, 161:17, 1956.
86. Powles, T. J., Hardy, J. R., Ashley, S. E., Farrington, G. M., Cosgrove, D., Davey, J. B., Dowsett, M., McKinna, J. A., Nash, A. G., Sinnett, H. D., Tillyer, C. R., and Treleven, J. G.: A pilot trial to evaluate the acute toxicity and feasibility of tamoxifen for prevention of breast cancer. Br. J. Cancer, 60:126, 1989.
87. Pritchard, K. I., Meakin, J. W., Boyd, N. F., Ambus, K., DeBoer, G., Dembo, A. J., Paterson, A. H. G, Sutherland, D. J. A, Wilkinson, R. H., Bassett, A. A., Evans, W. K., Beale, F.A., Clark, R. M., and Keane, T. J.: A randomized trial of adjuvant tamoxifen in postmenopausal women with axillary node positive breast cancer. *In:* Adjuvant Therapy of Breast Cancer IV. Edited by S. E. Jones, and S. E. Salmon. New York, Grune & Stratton, 1984, p. 339.
88. Ravdin, P. M., Fritz, N. F., Tormey, D. C., and Jordan, V. C.: Endocrine status of premenopausal node positive breast cancer patients following adjuvant chemotherapy and long-term tamoxifen. Cancer Res., 48:1026, 1988.
89. Ribeiro, G., and Palmer, M. K.: Adjuvant tamoxifen for operable carcinoma of the breast: Report of a clinical trial by the Christie Hospital and Holt Radium Institute. Br. Med. J., 286:827, 1983.
90. Ribeiro, G., and Swindell, R.: The Christie Hospital tamoxifen (Nolvadex) adjuvant

trial for operable breast carcinoma—seven year results. Eur. J. Cancer Clin. Oncol., 21:897, 1985.

91. Robertson, J. F. R., Walker, K. J., Nicholson, R. I., and Blamey, R. W.: Combined endocrine effects of LH-RH agonist (Zoladex®) and tamoxifen (Nolvadex®) therapy in premenopausal women with breast cancer. Br. J. Surg., 76:1262, 1989.

92. Robinson, S. P., Langan-Fahey, S. M., and Jordan, V. C.: Implications of tamoxifen metabolism in the athymic mouse for the study of antitumor effects upon human breast cancer xenografts. Eur. J. Cancer Clin. Oncol., 25:1769, 1989.

93. Robinson, S. P., Mauel, D. A., and Jordan, V. C.: Antitumor actions of toremifene in the 7,12 dimethylbenzanthracene (DMBA)-induced rat mammary tumor model. Eur. J. Cancer Clin. Oncol., 24:1817, 1988.

94. Rose, C., Thorpe, S. M., Andersen, K. W., Pederson, B. V., Mouridsen, H. T., Blicher-Toft, M., and Rasmussen, B. B.: Beneficial effect of adjuvant tamoxifen therapy in primary breast cancer patients with high oestrogen receptor values. Lancet, 1:16, 1985.

95. Rossner, S., and Wallgren, A.: Serum lipoproteins after breast cancer surgery and effects of tamoxifen. Atherosclerosis, 53:339, 1984.

96. Rutqvist, L. E., Cedermark, B., Glas, U., Johansson, H., Nordenskjold, B., Skoog, L., Sommell, A., Theve, T., Friberg, S., and Askergren, J.: The Stockholm trial on adjuvant tamoxifen in early breast cancer. Breast Cancer Res. Treat., 10:255, 1987.

97. Satyaswaroop, P. G., Zaino, R. J., and Mortel, R.: Estrogen-like effects of tamoxifen on human endometrial carcinoma transplanted into nude mice. Cancer Res., 44:4006, 1984.

98. Sawka, C. A., Pritchard, K. I., Paterson, D. J. A., Thomsen, D. B., Shelley, W. E., Myers, R. E., Mobbs, B. G., Malkin, A., and Meakin, J. W.: Role and mechanism of action of tamoxifen in premenopausal women with metastatic breast cancer. Cancer Res., 46:3152, 1986.

99. Sherman, B. M., Chapler, F. K., Crickard, K., and Wycoff, D.: Endocrine consequences of continuous antiestrogen therapy with tamoxifen in premenopausal women. J. Clin. Invest., 64:398, 1979.

100. Sipila, H., Kangas, L., Vuorilehto, L., Kalapudas, A., Eloranta, M., Sondervall, M., Toivola, R., and Antila, M.: Metabolism of toremifene in the rat. J. Steroid. Biochem., 36:211, 1990.

101. Smith, I. E., Harris, A. L., Morgan, M., Ford, H. T., Gazet, J.-C., Harmer, C. L., White, H., Parsons, C. A., Villardo, A., Walsh, G., and McKinna, J. A.: Tamoxifen versus aminoglutethimide in advanced breast carcinoma: a randomized crossover trial. Br. Med. J., 283:1432, 1981.

102. Swenerton, K. D.: Treatment of advanced endometrial adenocarcinoma with tamoxifen. Cancer Treat. Rep., 64:805, 1980.

103. Thompson, C. R., and Werner, H. W.: Studies of estrogen tri-p-anisylchlorethylene. Proc. Soc. Exp. Biol. Med., 77:494, 1951.

104. Thompson, E. W., Katz, D., Shima, T. B., Wakeling, A. E., Lippman, M. E., and Dickson, R. B.: ICI164,384 a pure antagonist of estrogen-stimulated MCF-7 cell proliferation and invasion. Cancer Res., 49:6929, 1989.

105. Toft, D., and Gorski, J.: A receptor molecule for estrogens: isolation from the rat uterus and preliminary characterization. Proc. Natl. Acad. Sc. USA, 55:1574, 1966.

106. Turken, S., Siris, E., Seldin, E., Seldin, D., Flaster, E., Hyman, G., and Lindsay, R.: Effects of tamoxifen on spinal bone density in women with breast cancer. J. Natl. Cancer Inst., 81:1086, 1989.

107. Turner, R. T., Wakley, G. K., Hannon, K. S. and Bell, N. A.: Tamoxifen prevents the skeletal effects of ovarian hormone deficiency in rats. J. Bone Min. Res., 2:449, 1987.

108. Valavaara, R., Pyrhonen, S., Heikkinen, M., Rissanen, P., Blanco, G., Tholix, E., Nordman, E., Taskinen, P., Holsi, L., and Hajba, A.: Toremifene a new antiestrogenic compound for the treatment of advanced breast cancer. Phase II Study. Eur. J. Cancer Clin. Oncol., 24:785, 1988.

109. VanVeelen, H., Willemse, P. H. B., Tjabbes, T., Sweitzer, M. J. H., and Sleijfer, D. T.: Oral high-dose medroxyprogesterone acetate versus tamoxifen. Cancer, 58:7, 1986.

110. Wakeling, A. E., and Bowler, J.: Biology and mode of action of pure antiestrogens. J. Steroid Biochem., 30:141, 1988.

111. Walpole, A. L. and Paterson, E.: Synthetic oestrogens in mammary cancer. Lancet, 2:783, 1949.

112. Ward, H. W. C.: Antioestrogen therapy for breast cancer: a trial of tamoxifen at two dose levels. Br. Med. J., i:13, 1973.

113. Welsch C. W., Goodrich-Smith, M., Brown, C. K., Miglorie, N., and Clifton, K. H.: Effect of an estrogen antagonist (tamoxifen) on the initiation and progression of γ irradiated induced mammary tumors in female Sprague Dawley rats. Eur. J. Cancer, 17:1255, 1981.

XVII-7

Clinical Use of Aromatase Inhibitors in Breast Carcinoma

Richard J. Santen

Introduction

Physiology of Aromatase Enzyme

The rate-limiting step in estrogen biosynthesis, the conversion of androstenedione to estrone, is catalyzed by the enzyme aromatase. This enzyme consists of a complex containing a cytochrome P_{450} protein as well as the flavoprotein, NADPH cytochrome P_{450} reductase.[73] The gene coding for the cytochrome P_{450} (P_{450} AROM) has been cloned and codes for a protein of 503 amino acids. The structure of the aromatase protein, which is deduced from its gene, has sequence homology in certain regions with a variety of cytochrome P_{450}-mediated steroid hydroxylating enzymes. The greatest homology with other P_{450} enzymes is in the region of heme binding. However, P_{450} AROM overall exhibits 31% or less homology with other cytochrome P_{450} species. On this basis, P_{450} AROM has been designated as the first member of a new gene family within the overall superfamily of genes known collectively as cytochrome P_{450}, namely gene family CYP-19 or P_{450} XIX.[73]

Aromatase catalyzes three separate steroid hydroxylations involved in the conversion of androstenedione to estrone. Each utilizes NADPH as cofactor and the aromatase-specific P_{450} to insert molecular oxygen into the steroid structure. Two of these hydroxylations take place at the C_{19} carbon position. The site of the last step is controversial and not fully established. After the three hydroxylations are completed, a non-enzymatic condensation takes place which releases formic acid and results in the formation of estrone.[16,29] The enzyme, 17β-hydroxysteroid dehydrogenase, then converts estrone to estradiol. Aromatase also catalyzes the conversion of testosterone to estradiol but the enzyme has higher affinity for androstenedione. Under most circumstances, higher amounts of androstenedione are present as substrate than testosterone. For these reasons, the preferred pathway for estradiol synthesis is via androstenedione to estrone to estradiol.

The aromatase enzyme is present in many organs, including ovary, placenta, hypothalamus, liver, muscle, fat tissue and hair follicles.[73] In the ovary, the amount of enzyme present is stimulated by FSH. Regulation of extragonadal aromatase is less clear. In vitro, glucocorticoids, cyclic AMP analogs, and growth factors can enhance enzymatic activity.

Sites of Estrogen Biosynthesis

Ovary. During the mid- and late follicular and luteal phases of the menstrual cycle in premenopausal patients, estradiol is synthesized predominantly in the ovary (Figure XVII-7-1A). This endocrine gland can be considered as having two separate compartments.[23] In one, the interstitial compartment, LH controls the production of androstenedione by stromal cells. In the other, the granulosa cell compartment, FSH pos-

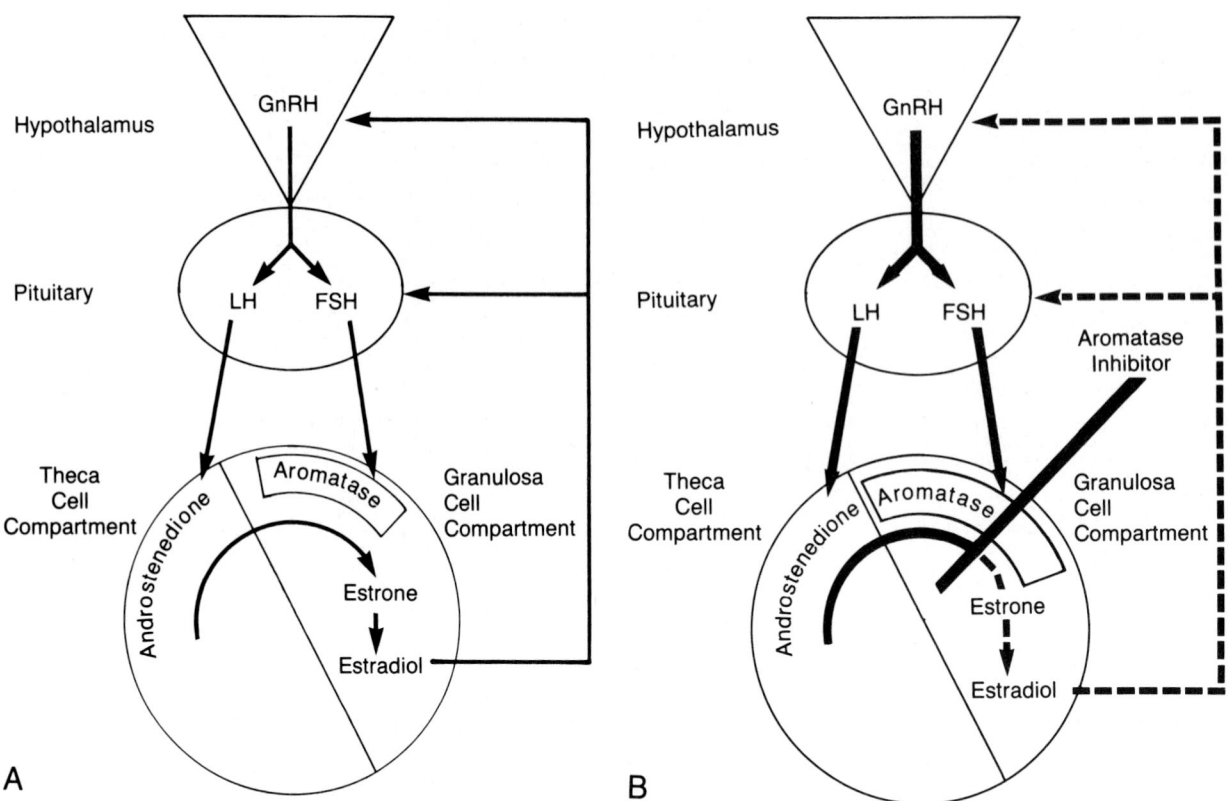

Figure XVII-7-1. A. Diagrammatic representation of the hypothalamic-pituitary-ovarian axis. The triangle represents the hypothalamus; the ovoid, the pituitary; and the circle, the ovary. GnRH, gonadotropin releasing hormone; LH, luteinizing hormone; FSH, follicle stimulating hormone. As indicated, the ovary is divided into the theca cell compartment where androstenedione is synthesized and the granulosa cell compartment which contains the majority of the aromatase enzyme. B. Blockade of aromatase interrupts the negative feedback inhibition of GnRH, LH and FSH by estradiol. Consequently, LH increases and stimulates greater production of androstenedione. FSH stimulates increased production of the aromatase enzyme. These two actions are generally sufficient to overcome the inhibitory effects of most aromatase inhibitors.

itively regulates the amount of aromatase enzyme present. Acting in concert, LH stimulates the substrate for aromatase and FSH increases the amount of the enzyme aromatase so that estradiol production can increase by 8–10-fold at the time of ovulation.

Because of the complexity of regulation in the ovary, pharmacologic blockade of ovarian aromatase has been difficult in patients. Interruption of estrogen biosynthesis reduces the tonic inhibitory action of estradiol on LH and FSH secretion. The reflex rise in FSH stimulates production of new aromatase enzyme. The LH increment results in enhanced ovarian steroidogenesis in the thecal compartment, and specifically in higher amounts of the aromatase substrate, androstenedione. These two effects tend to counteract the inhibitory actions of nonsteroidal aromatase blocking drugs on the ovary (Figure XVII-7-1B).[65]

Extraglandular Aromatase. In postmenopausal women, the granulosa cell compartment of the ovary is lost and aromatase activity there is markedly reduced. Estrogen synthesis takes place nearly exclusively in extraglandular tissues in such individuals (Figure XVII-7-2).[72] During menses and in the early follicular phase of the menstrual cycle in premenopausal women, extraglandular aromatase also is predominant. Under these circumstances, the adrenal directly secretes androstenedione (A) which enters tissue for aromatization to estrone (E_1). The enzyme, 17β-hydroxysteroid dehydrogenase, then converts estrone to estradiol (E_2). It

should be noted that a small fraction of androstenedione is secreted by the ovaries as well.[41] For that reason, precise measurement of estrogens reveals slightly lower values in surgically oophorectomized than in spontaneously menopausal woman.[56] Through the androstenedione to estrone pathway, postmenopausal women produce approximately 100 μg of estrone/day and more, if obese.[42] A substantial fraction of estrone is converted to estradiol to produce circulating concentrations of 10–20 pg/ml.

Local Estrogen Synthesis in Breast Tumors. The levels of estradiol in human breast tumor tissues are an order of magnitude higher than in plasma.[27,28] The mechanisms responsible for maintenance of high tissue estradiol concentrations are not clearly defined at present but could potentially involve local production of estradiol via either aromatase or sulfatase[57] in the tumor or in tissue surrounding the tumor (Figure XVII-7-3). Our studies suggest that conversion of estrone sulfate (E_1S) to estrone via sulfatase may be the most important pathway for local estrogen synthesis in human tumors. Several investigative groups including our own have also identified aromatase activity in human breast tumors.[1,45,53] Compared to human placenta, absolute levels of activity are relatively low, ranging from 5–80 pmol/g protein/hour. Bradlow regarded this degree of activity to be too low for a meaningful level of estradiol to be synthesized locally.[8] Aromatase, however, could be localized to specific cell types such as adipose cells, stroma or certain epithelial

Sources of Estrogen in Postmenopausal Women

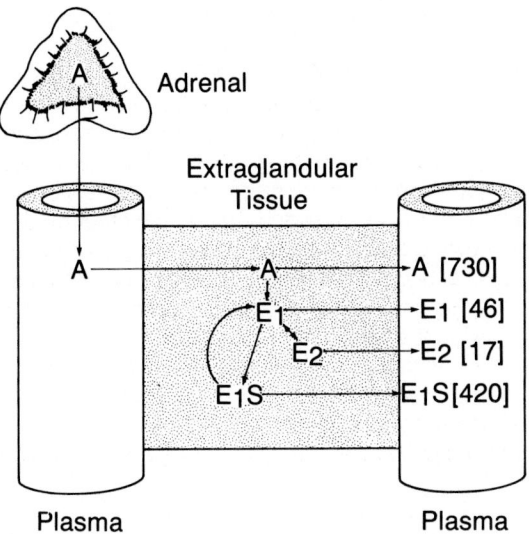

Figure XVII-7-2. Diagrammatic representation of the source of estrogen in postmenopausal women. The adrenal secretes androstenedione (A) which enters plasma and then tissue. The extraglandular tissues contain the enzymes necessary to convert A to estrone (E_1) and to estradiol (E_2) or to estrone sulfate (E_1S). These steroids then reenter plasma to circulate at levels indicated within the brackets and expressed as pg/ml.

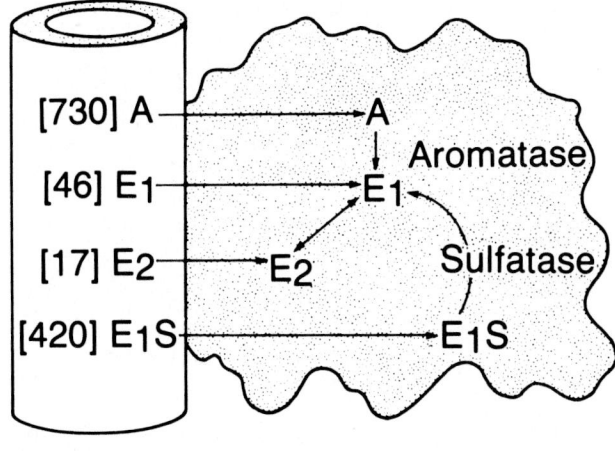

Figure XVII-7-3. Diagrammatic representation of the biosynthetic pathways for estrogen production locally in breast tumors. The shaded area indicates breast tumor tissue. Symbols are the same as in Figure XVII-7-2.

tumor cells.[53] If correct, biochemical measurement of total aromatase activity would underestimate the levels of enzyme activity present, for example, in isolated epithelial tumor cells. Miller and O'Neill measured aromatase activity in fat tissue contiguous to and in the quadrants opposite from human breast carcinomas.[49] The finding of higher aromatase in regions contiguous to the tumor supported the possibility that fat tissue might synthesize estradiol which would then act in a paracrine fashion to stimulate nearby breast tumor cells. Provided that this hypothesis is correct, the aromatase

enzyme could play an important role in local estrogen synthesis in human breast tumors.

The biologic importance of *tumor* aromatase rests in the concept that aromatase inhibitors could block estradiol synthesis directly at the site of the tumor. Indirect support for this hypothesis comes from preliminary studies correlating tumor aromatase activity with clinical responses to aromatase inhibition.[6,49] Prospective trials of responses to aromatase inhibition in aromatase-rich and aromatase-poor tumors are now required to critically examine this issue. The author of this review favors the argument of Bradlow that tumor aromatase activity is too low for biologic significance.[8] Local estrogen production is more likely to result from conversion of estrone sulfate to estrone via the enzyme, sulfatase.[57] Nonetheless, production of estrone sulfate in *peripheral tissues* still requires aromatase as the rate-limiting enzymatic step.

Development of the First-Generation Aromatase Inhibitor—Aminoglutethimide

Background

Inhibition of Aromatase. Aminoglutethimide was initially used as an anticonvulsant, and later recognized to be an inhibitor of cytochrome P_{450}-mediated steroid hydroxylations, particularly those involving the cholesterol side-chain cleavage enzyme.[15] The first clinical use of aminoglutethimide for breast cancer attempted to produce a "medical adrenalectomy" by blocking cholesterol side-chain cleavage.[31,58] Replacement glucocorticoid was added to compensate for the inhibition of cortisol biosynthesis. After initial clinical reports, Siiteri and colleagues and Chakraborty and colleagues directed attention to the aromatase inhibitory properties of aminoglutethimide and confirmed its potency in vitro.[18,79] Direct isotopic kinetic studies in patients then confirmed the inhibitory activity of aminoglutethimide as an aromatase inhibitor in vivo.[59] A dose of 1,000 mg of aminoglutethimide daily produced 95–98% inhibition of aromatase in postmenopausal women with breast cancer.

The regimen of aminoglutethimide plus hydrocortisone inhibited plasma and urinary estradiol to levels comparable to those observed following surgical adrenalectomy[60] or hypophysectomy in patients with breast cancer.[35] The primary effect of this drug in lowering estrogen production was shown to be inhibition of the aromatase enzyme (Figure XVII-7-4—*step 6*). This conclusion was inferred from the observation that androstenedione levels were unchanged (or even increased), whereas estrogen levels fell profoundly during administration of aminoglutethimide and hydrocortisone.[61] The lack of a decrease in androstenedione was initially unexpected since blockade of cholesterol side-chain cleavage activity should lower androstenedione levels (Figure XVII-7-4—*step 1*). However, this preservation of androgen secretion, which included testosterone and dihydrotestosterone as well as androstenedione, was later explained by the blocking effect of aminoglutethimide on another cytochrome P_{450}-mediated step, the 11β-hydroxylase enzyme (Figure XVII-7-4—*step 4*).[82] Enhanced conversion of delta-5 to delta-4 steroids was also reported to occur (Figure XVII-7-4—*step 7*).[4]

Other Endocrine Effects. Comprehensive studies of the endocrine effects of aminoglutethimide plus hydrocortisone identified several additional actions (Table XVII-7-1, Figure

XVII-7-4). These included blockade of aldosterone and thyroxine synthesis as well as enhancement of estrone sulfate metabolic clearance rate.[47] The latter effect has been proposed as an additional mechanism for lowering of plasma estrogen levels. Estrone sulfate can be converted to estrone through the enzyme, sulfatase. Lowering of estrone sulfate levels through enhancement of clearance should result in a reduction in the amount of substrate available for sulfatase, and thus the amount of estrone produced through this mechanism.

Clinical Efficacy

An overall compilation of clinical responses to aminoglutethimide plus glucocorticoid in women with breast cancer reveals results similar to those expected with other forms of endocrine therapy (Figure XVII-7-5). Approximately one-third of women experience either complete or partial tumor regression whereas 54% with estrogen receptor positive tumors respond with objective regressions.[54] Responses persist for

a mean of 13 months and patients survive for an average of 20 months. By site of disease, soft tissues respond most frequently followed by lymph nodes, bone, lung/pleura, viscera, and liver.

Randomized comparative trials of aminoglutethimide/hydrocortisone vs. other endocrine therapies provide a more precise assessment of efficacy. When compared to surgical adrenalectomy[60] or tamoxifen (Table XVII-7-2) in controlled trials, aminoglutethimide/hydrocortisone produces responses as frequently, and for a similar duration, as the other modalities. A trend toward greater healing of osteolytic lesions was observed with aminoglutethimide/hydrocortisone than with tamoxifen but this finding has not reached statistical significance in individual small trials.

Although the efficacy of aminoglutethimide/hydrocortisone is similar to that of other agents, cross-resistance between aminoglutethimide/hydrocortisone and tamoxifen or progesterone therapy is not complete. Overall, 31% of patients treated

Table XVII-7-1.   Endocrine and Metabolic Effects of Aminoglutethimide

Metabolic Step	Action	Measurable Results	Clinical Import	Clinical Implications	Ref
Aromatase enzyme	Inhibition	Reduction estrogen synthesis	Major	Mechanism of action -breast tumor regression	79, 59
Estrone sulfate metabolic clearance	Acceleration	Reduction plasma estrone levels	Uncertain	Additional mechanism -breast tumor regression	47
CSCC	Inhibition	Reduction of cortisol biosynthesis	Major	Requirement for GC replacement although effect usually overcome by reflex ↑ in ACTH (with AG, 1000 mg alone)	40
11-OHase	Inhibition	↑ 17α-OH-prog, Δ_4-A, T, DHT in absence of exogenous GC administration	Virilization can occur when AG given without exogenous GC	Explains lack of Δ_4-A suppression with combination AG + GC	82
C-21-OHase	Inhibition	↑ 17α-OH prog levels	Minor	None	40, 31
C-18-OHase	Inhibition	Partial reduction in aldosterone levels	Major	One-third of patients require mineralocorticoid replacement	80
3βol dehydrogenase $\Delta_5 \rightarrow \Delta_4$ isomerase	Enhanced $\Delta_5 \rightarrow \Delta_4$ conversion	↑ ratios Δ_4/Δ_5 steroidal pairs	Minor	None	4
Hepatic 6β-hydroxylase	Enhanced 6β hydroxylation synthetic glucocorticoids	Accelerated metabolic clearance rate-dexamethasone	Enhanced requirement for synthetic GC	3 mg dexamethasone needed as GC replacement in patients receiving AG	70
Thyroxine biosynthesis	Inhibition	Lowered thyroxine, ↑ TSH levels	5% of pts develop hypothyroidism	Must monitor thyroid function in patients on AG	62
Coumadin metabolism	Acceleration	Prothrombin time lowered in pts receiving coumarin	Drug-drug interaction	Coumadin dose adjustment to compensate	48
Prostaglandin biosynthesis	Inhibition	In vitro only	Uncertain	May partially explain relief of bone pain in patients with breast cancer metastases	33
2-hydroxylase	Inhibition	In vitro only	Uncertain	Uncertain	83
AG metabolism	Accelerated	Reduces AG blood levels	Major	Gradual dose escalation advised	50

CSCC, cholesterol side-chain cleavage; 11-OHase, 11-hydroxylase; C_{21}-OHase, 21-hydroxylase; C_{18}-OHase, 18-hydroxylase; 17OH-prog, 17-hydroxyprogesterone; GC, glucocorticoids; Δ_4-A, androstenedione; T, testosterone; DHT, dihydrotestosterone; AG, aminoglutethimide.

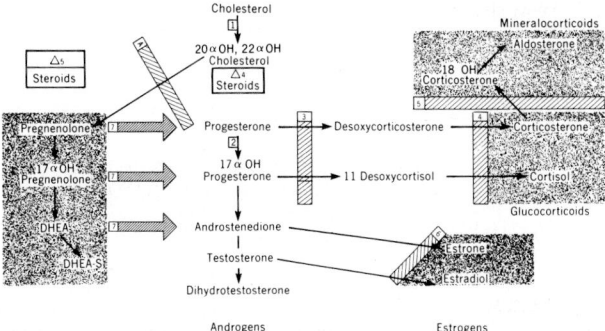

Figure XVII-7-4. Effects of aminoglutethimide on various steroidogenic steps. The numbers in boxes identify several enzymes: 1) 20- and 22-hydroxylase; 2) 17α-hydroxylase; 3) 21-hydroxylase; 4) 11-hydroxylase; 5) 18-hydroxylase; 6) aromatase; 7) 3β-ol-dehydrogenase/delta-4,delta-5-isomerase. Aminoglutethimide blocks several of these steps which can lower the levels of the steroids shown in the shaded boxes. The primary effect of aminoglutethimide is to block step 6—the aromatase enzyme, which converts androgens to estrogens.

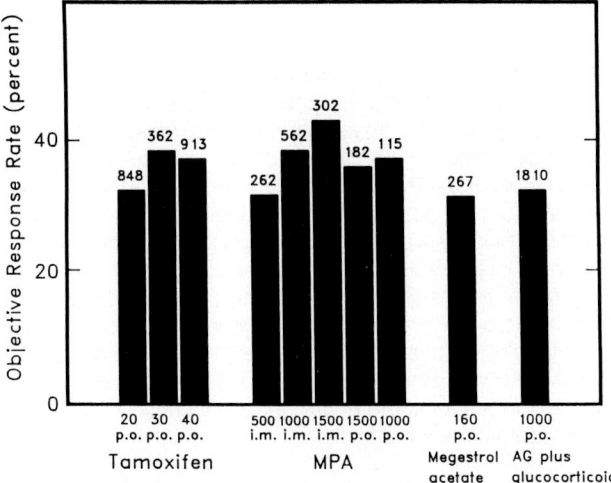

Figure XVII-7-5. Comparative rates of objective responses (i.e., complete and partial objective regression) to various endocrine therapies. Data are from non-randomized trials and represent patients receiving first-line or subsequent endocrine therapy. The numbers above the bars represent the number of patients in each category. Adapted from Petru and colleagues.[54]

initially with tamoxifen later responded objectively to aminoglutethimide/hydrocortisone. Patients can be subdivided into those initially responding to tamoxifen with later relapse, and those with initial progression. Fifty percent of patients initially responding objectively to tamoxifen and then relapsing later experience an objective response to aminoglutethimide/hydrocortisone (Figure XVII-7-6). On the other hand, only 25% of tamoxifen non-responders were objectively benefited by aminoglutethimide/hydrocortisone. Although somewhat controversial, responders to progestin therapy also may benefit from aminoglutethimide/hydrocortisone upon relapse.

Side Effects

Patients receiving standard dose aminoglutethimide experience a wide range of side effects during the induction of therapy (Figure XVII-7-7). The major problems encountered include drug rash, fever, and lethargy. These precluded continuing treatment in 8–15% of patients and particularly in elderly women. Many of these symptoms resolve completely or diminish in severity with treatment for longer than six weeks (Figure XVII-7-7). One possible basis for the reduction in side effects over time is the fact that aminoglutethimide accelerates its own metabolism from 12 hours to approximately 7 hours, presumably through hepatic enzyme induction.[50]

Skin rash is a particularly important side effect but resolution occurs spontaneously in the majority of patients without discontinuation of therapy. Approximately one-third of women require mineralocorticoid replacement with 9α-fluoro-hydrocortisone (Florinef®) because of the inhibition of aldosterone production.[60] Another 5% of patients require thyroxine supplementation because of the effects of aminoglutethimide to inhibit thyroid hormone synthesis.[62] In the remainder, TSH levels increase sufficiently to completely overcome the blockade of thyroxine biosynthesis. The frequency and severity of side effects, particularly when compared to tamoxifen administration, has led to attempts to reduce aminoglutethimide dosage and to develop second and third generation aromatase inhibitors.

Selection of Patients for Aromatase Inhibition Therapy

Postmenopausal Women. Endocrine therapy is often chosen for patients with recurrent disease who have estrogen receptor and/or progesterone receptor positive tumors or whose tumor receptor content is unknown. Clinical features suggesting a favorable response in addition to receptors include a long disease-free interval after initial surgery or the presence of soft tissue, bone and lung but not CNS metastases. The decision to choose one endocrine therapy over another depends upon considerations of efficacy, ease of administration, side effects, cost and menopausal status of the patient.[63] Data on the comparative efficacy of various forms of endocrine therapy in postmenopausal women are available from a compilation of results of uncontrolled studies over the past four decades (Figure XVII-7-5). Information obtained from these studies suggest that each therapy, with the possible exception of androgens and glucocorticoids, is equally efficacious.

More critical data are available from numerous randomized controlled trials. On practical grounds, no one study can compare all forms of endocrine therapy in similar groups of patients. Nonetheless, individual comparisons of each of the therapies with one another allow the reasonably firm conclusion that most endocrine therapies are equally efficacious.[63] Choice of therapy is then predicated upon considerations of ease of administration, side effects and cost rather than efficacy. Of all the endocrine therapies, tamoxifen is associated with the fewest side effects. This aspect favors tamoxifen as the endocrine therapy of first choice. Aromatase inhibitors are then considered either as second or third line endocrine approaches. At the present time, randomized trials are ongoing to compare various agents as second line therapy. The major choices at present are between megestrol acetate or medroxyprogesterone acetate and aromatase inhibitor therapy with aminoglutethimide. Because of the associated lethargy and skin rash attributable to aminoglutethimide, most clinicians would choose progestin therapy as second line and aminoglutethimide/hydrocortisone as third

Table XVII-7-2.   Randomized Trials Comparing Aromatase Inhibition With Tamoxifen

Reference	Treatments	Patients n	Complete and partial responses n (%)	Remarks
Tamoxifen vs. Aromatase Inhibition				
Lipton et al.[46]	Tamoxifen (20 mg BID)	39	15 (38)	Bone responses greater with AG (33%) than with tamoxifen (15%).
	vs.			
	AG (250 QID) plus HC (20 mg BID)	36	13 (36)	
Smith et al.[74]	Tamoxifen (10 mg BID)	60	18 (30)	AG regimen more toxic; bone responses greater with AG (35%) than with tamoxifen (17%)
	vs.			
	AG (250 QID) plus HC (20 mg BID)	57	17 (30)	
Alonso-Munoz et al.[2]	Tamoxifen (20 mg BID)	34	18 (53)	AG regimen more toxic
	vs.			
	AG (250 mg QID) plus HC (20 mg BID)	31	15 (48)	

AG, Aminoglutethimide; HC, hydrocortisone

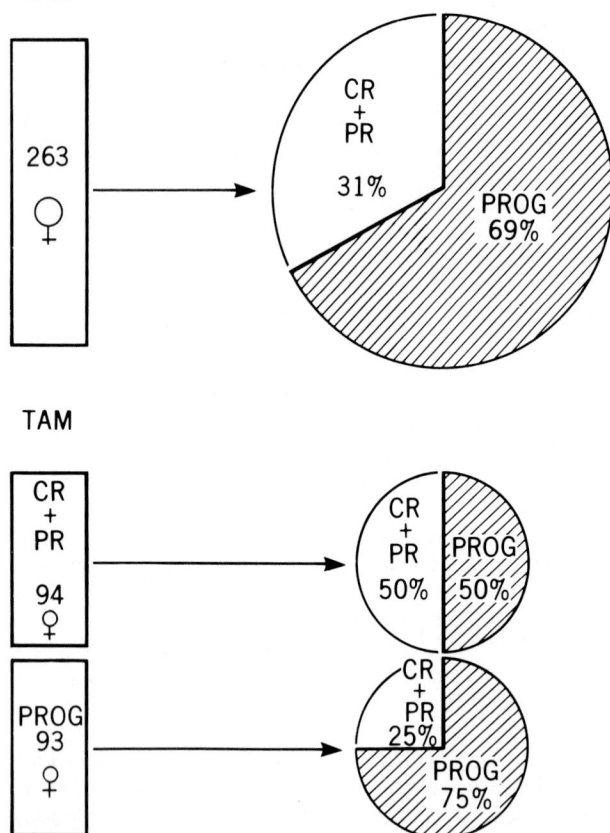

Figure XVII-7-6.   The rectangles represent patients with metastatic breast cancer initially treated with TAM (tamoxifen) and the circles, patients then crossed over to aminoglutethimide/hydrocortisone. CR, complete objective tumor regression; PR; partial objective tumor regression; PROG, progression. Data represent a compilation of several non-randomized studies.[3]

line treatment. An exception to this might be individuals with severe bone pain and lytic metastases in whom aminoglutethimide/hydrocortisone may be more efficacious in relieving pain. This clinical observation has not been established unambiguously.

Premenopausal Patients. Considerations of efficacy, cost, toxicity and ease of administration also dictate the choice of endocrine therapy in premenopausal patients. On these bases, first line therapy would include either tamoxifen or oophorectomy. Aromatase inhibitors can only be used after surgical oophorectomy in premenopausal patients because of the resistance of the ovary to aromatase inhibition as discussed above.[65] As with postmenopausal patients, oral progestins such as megestrol acetate, are generally chosen prior to the use of aromatase inhibitors.

Low Dose Aminoglutethimide with Hydrocortisone

The limitations of aromatase inhibitor therapy at the present time are the side effects and lack of specificity of ami-

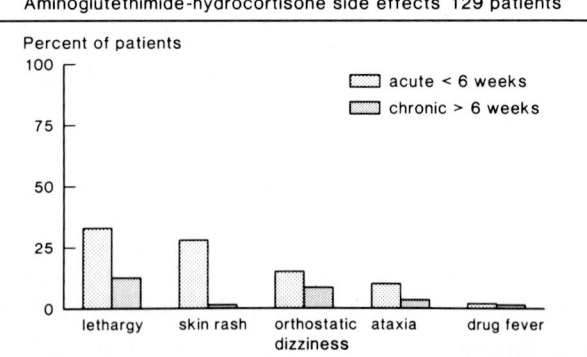

Figure XVII-7-7.   Side effects observed in patients receiving 1,000 mg of aminoglutethimide and 40 mg of hydrocortisone daily. Signs or symptoms scored in patients receiving the drug for <6 weeks and >6 weeks. (Reproduced with permission from Santen et al.[61]).

noglutethimide. Two approaches have been taken to improve the utility of such agents. One is to systematically evaluate lower doses of aminoglutethimide; the second is to develop more specific and less toxic aromatase inhibitors.

In seeking lower doses of aminoglutethimide to reduce side effects, several investigators conducted dose-response studies using complete aromatase inhibition as the endpoint to judge sufficiency of dosage.[24,63,77,78] With this criterion, 125 mg of aminoglutethimide daily blocked aromatase significantly and 250–500 mg daily produced maximum inhibition. Studies which were predominantly non-randomized then compared 250, 500, and 1,000 mg of aminoglutethimide daily in combination with hydrocortisone (Table XVII-7-3). No major differences were observed among the various doses. The idiosyncratic reactions such as skin rash occurred as commonly with low as with high dose therapy (Table XVII-7-4). Side effects such as lethargy, fatigue, and drowsiness, which could be attributed to the CNS sedative properties were still reported but somewhat less frequently with lower

doses (Table XVII-7-4). No cases of agranulocytosis were observed in patients receiving 250 mg of aminoglutethimide daily[14,32,51] whereas 1–2% of patients receiving 1,000 mg of aminoglutethimide daily experienced this toxicity.[88] Clinical responses to low dose aminoglutethimide plus hydrocortisone appeared equal to those observed with higher doses of aminoglutethimide (Table XVII-7-3).

Low Dose Aminoglutethimide without Hydrocortisone

Reduction of aminoglutethimide dosage sufficiently should abrogate inhibitory effects on cholesterol side-chain cleavage and other enzymes involved in cortisol biosynthesis and eliminate need for replacement glucocorticoid. This strategy would provide pure aromatase inhibition and eliminate need for exogenous hydrocortisone. Two studies (Table XVII-7-3) utilized this strategy and employed 125 mg twice daily of aminoglutethimide without glucocorticoid.[14,51] Plasma estro-

Table XVII-7-3.   Studies of Varying Doses of Aminoglutethimide with and without Glucocorticoid

Regimen	Number of Patients	Overall Objective Responses (%)	Mean Duration Responses (mo)	Mean Duration Survival (mo)	Ref	Comments
Study Design—Nonrandomized: Aminoglutethimide without Glucocorticoid						
AG, 250 mg	25	16	—	—	14	(*18% with objective response to dose escalation to 1000 AG, 40 mg HC)
AG, 250 mg	57	19	8+	—	51	(23% with objective response to dose escalation to 750 AG, 37.5 mg cortisol acetate)
AG, 250 mg	57	19	—	—	51	
AG, 375 mg	19	26	—	—	14	
AG, 500 mg	27	33	—	—	14	
AG, 1,000 mg	38	13	13	—	39	Extensively pretreated patients
Aminoglutethimide with Glucocorticoid						
AG, 250 mg HC, 40 mg	101	25	12 (median)	18 (median)	32	73% with prior endocrine therapy; 56% response rate in patients with no prior endocrine therapy
AG, 500 mg HC, 40 mg	76	33	—	—	52	
AG, 500 mg HC, 40 mg	73	19	—	—	7	Similar response as in patients randomized to 1000 mg AG, 40 mg HC (i.e., 24%)
AG, 1,000 mg Glucocorticoid, 20–50 mg	1,810	33	13	20	54	Compilation of data from multiple studies
Study Design— Randomized Aminoglutethimide with and without Glucocorticoid						
AG, 500 mg vs.	73	41	11	26	17	Randomized trial First-line therapy
AG, 500 mg HC, 40 mg	75	45	13	27		

Table XVII-7-4.　Dose-Related Side Effects and Toxicity of Aminoglutethimide

	Aminoglutethimide without Hydrocortisone				Aminoglutethimide with Hydrocortisone				
	250 mg		500 mg	1,000 mg	250 mg	500 mg		1,000 mg	
Signs/Symptoms (%)									
Rash	15	16	12	23	22	4	6	23	11
Drowsiness, fatigue, lethargy	31	0	40	62	9	9	23	33	17
Nausea	12	4	4	26	9	4	3	15	8
Ataxia	0	0	0	32	4	3	0	4	6
Drugs Discontinued (%)	8	1	0	9	1	5	0	5	7
Number of Patients	65	57	28	47	101	78	29	213	83
Study Reference	77	51	17	39	32	7	17	34	7

gens fell to the same extent as had been demonstrated in prior studies with high doses of aminoglutethimide plus hydrocortisone. However, objective tumor regressions occurred in only 16–19% of patients and response rates appeared somewhat lower than expected. In addition, dose escalation either to 750 or 1,000 mg of aminoglutethimide with addition of glucocorticoid produced additional responses in 18–23% of patients.[14,51] Further data were provided by Dowsett and colleagues, who suggested that addition of hydrocortisone to 250 mg of aminoglutethimide daily produced greater suppression of estrogens than did aminoglutethimide alone.[25] They attributed this reduction of estrogens to an effect of hydrocortisone to lower the levels of androstenedione as substrate in a setting of incomplete aromatase inhibitory doses of aminoglutethimide (i.e., 250 mg). However, other studies demonstrated equal estrogen suppression with and without hydrocortisone supplementation and this issue remains controversial.

A recent study compared the use of aminoglutethimide with and without hydrocortisone in a randomized, controlled trial.[17] Five hundred mg of aminoglutethimide alone was compared with 500 mg of aminoglutethimide plus 40 mg of hydrocortisone as first-line therapy in estrogen receptor positive or unknown patients. Estrogen levels fell similarly with either regimen. Complete and partial objective regression did not differ (i.e., 45% AG + HC; 41% AG alone) nor did duration of remission and survival. These data suggest that addition of hydrocortisone adds little to the therapeutic efficacy of the aromatase inhibitor given alone provided that the dosage of aromatase inhibitor is sufficient.

In summary, the optimal aminoglutethimide regimen is not yet clearly established. The author favors starting with 125 mg of aminoglutethimide twice daily in combination with 20 mg of hydrocortisone twice daily with escalation of the aminoglutethimide dosage to 250 mg twice daily after two weeks. Glucocorticoid is used since anecdotal reports suggested that adrenal insufficiency can occur in patients receiving low-dose aminoglutethimide alone.[51] This phenomenon might be attributed to retarded aminoglutethimide metabolism and higher drug blood levels in some patients. This approach also takes into account the fact that aminoglutethimide accelerates its own metabolism and that patients better tolerate escalating doses of aminoglutethimide. Generally, the aminoglutethimide can be continued in patients who develop drug rash as this side effect will resolve spontaneously. Measurements of plasma estrogens are not necessary since suppression is generally uniform at this dosage.

Development of Improved Aromatase Inhibitors

Background

The successful use of aminoglutethimide provided an impetus to investigate further the concept of inhibiting estrogen biosynthesis as a means of treating breast cancer. The problems with the multiple actions of aminoglutethimide and its associated side effects spurred interest in the aromatase inhibitors. Originally studied by Brodie and colleagues, compounds such as 4-hydroxyandrostenedione were designed as selective inhibitors of aromatase with greater potency than aminoglutethimide.[9] A wide variety of compounds including 4-hydroxyandrostenedione are now under study (Table XVII-7-5).[5] A convenient classification divides inhibitors into the mechanism based or "suicide inhibitors" and those of the competitive type. Suicide inhibitors initially complete with the natural substrate (i.e., androstenedione and testosterone) for binding to the active site of the enzyme. The enzyme, then, specifically acts upon the inhibitor to yield reactive alkylating species which can form covalent bonds at or near the active site of the enzyme. Through this mechanism, the enzyme is irreversibly inactivated. Competitive inhibitors, on the other hand, bind reversibly to the active site of the enzyme and prevent product formation only as long as the inhibitor occupies the catalytic site. Whereas mechanism-based inhibitors are exclusively steroidal in type, competitive inhibitors consist both of steroidal and nonsteroidal compounds.

Mechanism-based or suicide inhibitors should be preferable to competitive inhibitors because of their irreversible nature. Theoretically, their duration of action in vivo should be prolonged and related primarily to the rate at which new enzyme can be synthesized. These concepts require experimental verification.[43]

Specificity of inhibition as well as intrinsic biologic activity are important considerations regarding aromatase inhibitors.[5] In general, nonsteroidal inhibitors are more likely than are steroidal compounds to lack specificity since they have a potential for blocking several cytochrome P_{450}-mediated steroid hydroxylations. On the other hand, steroidal inhibitors or their metabolites have greater potential for producing estrogen, androgen, glucocorticoid or progestin agonist or antagonistic effects through the inherent properties of their structures. The aromatase inhibitors presently in clinical trials are indicated in Table XVII-7-6.

4-Hydroxyandrostenedione

This compound competitively inhibits aromatase in vitro and exhibits mechanism-based inactivation with a K inact of

Table XVII-7-5.   Partial List of Aromatase Inhibitors

Type of Inhibition	Type of Compound	Name of Compound	Ki[a]	K inact[c]	Ref
Mechanism Based	Steroid	1,4,6-androsta-triene-3,17-dione		$1.1 \times 10^{-3}S^{-1}$	5
	Steroid	4-OH-androstene-dione		$4.5 \times 10^{-3}S^{-1}$	10
	Steroid	4-androstene-3,6,17-trione		$4.03 \times 10^{-3}S^{-1}$	13
	Steroid	testolactone		$5.5 \times 10^{-4}S^{-1}$	5, 13
	Steroid	10β-propargylestr-4-ene-3,17-dione		$1.11 \times 10^{-3}S^{-1}$	5
	Steroid	7α(4'-amino)phenyl-thio,1,4-androsta-diene-3,17-dione		$8.4 \times 10^{-3}S^{-1}$	5, 75
	Steroid	1-methyl-androsta-1,4-diene,3,17-dione		$1.8 \times 10^{-4}S^{-1}$	37
Competitive	Steroid	6α-bromo-androstene-dione	3.4 nM		5
	Steroid	7α(4'-amino)phenyl thio-4-androstene-3,17-dione	18 nM		5
	Non-steroid	aminoglutethimide	540 nM		66
	Non-steroid	pyridoglutethimide	1100 nM		5
	Imidazole	CGS 16949A	0.19 nM		66
	Imidazole	R-76713	0.70 nM		86
	Imidazole	CGS 20267	—		81
	Imidazole	econazole	0.06 μM[b]		5

[a]Ki—inhibitory constant
[b]IC50
[c]K inact—rate constant for inactivation of the enzyme
S, seconds

$4.1 \times 10^{-3}S^{-1}$. 4-Hydroxyandrostenedione effectively blocks estradiol production in vivo. Extensive studies revealed no estrogenic, antiestrogenic, or antiandrogenic properties.[5,10,11,84] However, transformation to 4-hydroxytestosterone occurs and androgenic effects can be demonstrated under certain circumstances.[12] This action is biologically important under circumstances where LH and FSH feedback loops are intact. As an example, 4-hydroxyandrostenedione markedly lowers ovarian estradiol production during the estrous cycle in rats but does not result in reflex increments in LH and FSH as would be expected. Wing and colleagues provided evidence that an androgenic effect of 4 hydroxyandrostenedione was responsible for the inhibitory effect on gonadotropin secretion.[84]

This agent has been studied extensively in postmenopausal women with breast cancer. In the initial endocrine study, postmenopausal women received 500–1,000 mg of 4-hydroxyandrostenedione by weekly intramuscular injection.[19,20] Although the drug has a short plasma half-life, concentrations of drug during chronic therapy and one week after the last injection, ranged from 0.7–23.2 (mean = 7.8 ± 1.1) ng/ml. During therapy, plasma estradiol levels fell from 7.2 ± 0.8 (SEM) pg/ml to 2.6–2.8 pg/ml from 1 to >4+ months after initiating treatment.

Preliminary clinical data with 4-hydroxyandrostenedione (Table XVII-7-7) demonstrated a 33% objective regression rate of breast cancer in postmenopausal patients previously treated with multiple endocrine therapies. An insufficient number of patients were evaluable to determine the predictive nature of estrogen receptor status or the sites more favorable to response to 4-hydroxyandrostenedione. Toxicity included six patients with sterile abscesses due to intramuscular injections, two of sufficient severity to warrant discontinuation of therapy. No androgenic effects were observed

and particularly, no regression of LH or FSH over basal postmenopausal values.

4-Hydroxyandrostenedione has also been given orally.[26] Even though there is a marked first-pass effect with conversion in the liver to a glucuronidated derivative, oral doses of 250 mg reduce plasma estradiol by 53%[26] and doses up to 1,000 mg produce no further suppression. The response rate after three months of therapy was 33% when this agent was administered via the oral route. The only serious side effect from the oral dosage was leukopenia in a single patient.[21]

Hoffken and colleagues recently conducted a large trial of 4-hydroxyandrostenedione administration in postmenopausal women.[38] Patients initially received 500 mg intramuscularly every two weeks for six weeks and then 250 mg every two weeks thereafter. Plasma estradiol levels fell from baseline values of 10–11 pg/ml to levels of approximately 4 pg/ml for up to seven months of therapy. The drug appeared specific since no reduction of cortisol or symptoms of cortisol deficiency were observed. Of 86 evaluable patients, there were two complete and 19 partial remissions (21/86 = 24%) and 26 with disease stabilization (30%). Side effects included minor systemic symptoms in 11%, hot flashes, constipation, alopecia and pruritus in two patients each, and local symptoms in 8% (three pruritus, one local pain, and one erythema). These resulted in discontinuation of therapy in only 2% of patients. Phase III trials are now ongoing to compare this inhibitor with standard endocrine therapies.

1-Methyl-1,4-androstadiene-3,17-dione is also a mechanism-based inhibitor and has been studied in patients. Single dose administration reveals a major reduction of plasma estrogens with this compound.[37]

Competitive Inhibitors

A variety of steroidal inhibitors of aromatase are currently under investigation (Tables XVII-7-5 and XVII-7-6). Pyrido-

Table XVII-7-6. New Aromatase Inhibitors Reaching Clinical Trial

Name of Compound	Type of Inhibitor	Potency for Aromatase		Inhibition of Other Enzymes				
		Ki[a]	K inact[c]	CSCC	C17–20 lyase	C-11 hydrox-ylase	C-21 hydroxylase	Aldosterone inhibition
1-methyl-1,4-androstadiene-3,17-dione	Mechanism-based		$1.8 \times 10^{-4} S^{-1}$	—	—	—	—	—
4-OH-androstene-dione	Mechanism-based		$4.1 \times 10^{-3} S^{-1}$	—	—	—	—	—
10β-propargyl-estr-4-ene-3,17-dione	Mechanism-based		$1.11 \times 10^{-3} S^{-1}$	—	—	—	—	—
Pyridoglutethimide	Competitive	1100 nM	—	—	?	?	?	?
CGS-16949A	Competitive	0.19 nM	—	—	—	+	?	+
CGS-20267	Competitive	—	—	—	—	—	—	—
R-76713	Competitive	0.70 nM	—	—	±	±	—	—

a = See Table XVII-7-5 for definition
b = androgenic
c = See Table XVII-7-5 for definition
Reprinted with the permission from Santen et al.[63]

glutethimide is a non-steroidal compound resulting from modifications of the structure of aminoglutethimide to enhance specificity and to reduce side effects.[5,20] This agent has a Ki for aromatase (1,100 nM), somewhat higher than does aminoglutethimide (600 nM), but does not inhibit cholesterol side-chain cleavage at concentrations of up to 50 μg/ml. Tests of CNS activity in animals suggest that sedative properties, so prominent with aminoglutethimide, are lacking. This agent reduces the growth of NMU-induced mammary tumors in rats. Further studies with this compound are ongoing and new, more potent, congeners are being developed.

The imidazole compounds have potent effects on a number of cytochrome P_{450}-mediated steroid hydroxylation steps. Ketoconazole, for example, blocks C_{17-20} lyase at low concentrations and aromatase at high concentrations.[85] This observation suggests that compounds can be found which exert relatively specific effects on certain P_{450}-mediated steroid hydroxylations with little activity on others. This appears to be the case since CGS 16949A and R76713 are both potent competitive inhibitors of aromatase but lack significant cholesterol side-chain cleavage activity.[71,76,86] Specificity is not absolute since high concentrations of drug may block other P_{450}-mediated steps as well. Development of CGS 16949A has progressed furthest as this agent is now in Phase III testing.

CGS 16949A 4-(5,6,7,8-tetrahydroimidazo[1,5a]-pyridin-5yl)benzonitrile monohydro-chloride, is a highly potent inhibitor of aromatase with a Ki of 0.19 nM (vs. 600 nM for aminoglutethimide).[76,66] Cholesterol side-chain cleavage activity is minimal but C_{11}-hydroxylase inhibitory effects are observed in vitro at high drug concentrations (i.e., 10^{-6} M). Negligible toxicity was observed in animal studies.[71]

Initial dose seeking studies were conducted in patients which suggested effective aromatase inhibition at doses of 1.8–4.0 mg daily.[22,67] A phase II study then compared doses of 0.6 mg three times daily, 1 mg twice daily, and 2 mg twice daily.[68] Maximal suppression of plasma and urinary estrogens occurred at a dosage of 1.0 mg twice daily and minimal effects on cortisol secretion were observed. Basal cortisol

and ACTH levels were unaffected and cortisol levels increased to >20 μg/dl after exogenous synthetic c_{1-24} ACTH (Cortrosyn®) administration in all patients. Basal levels of aldosterone also remained stable upon administration of all three drug dosages. No change in urinary or plasma sodium or potassium were observed, nor changes in standing blood pressure to suggest a clinical state of aldosterone deficiency. However, cortrosyn-stimulated aldosterone levels were significantly blunted at all three doses.[69]

The antitumor activity of CGS 16949A in patients is not as yet precisely defined since available clinical data are limited. In the 54 patients treated in a phase II trial, objective regressions were recorded in 11 of 54 (20%).[36] Twenty-eight percent of 18 patients treated by Possinger and colleagues experienced objective tumor regression as well.[55] All of the patients entered had been pretreated with at least one, and as many as 4 endocrine treatments. The potency of the compound, its relatively specific effects on aromatase and its lack of toxicity suggest that it may represent a major improvement over aminoglutethimide for treatment of patients with breast cancer.

R76713 represents another highly potent and specific aromatase inhibitor with little toxicity in animal studies.[86] The Ki for placental aromatase is 0.8 nM and this agent is approximately 500-fold more potent than aminoglutethimide. From animal data, R76713 appears to be highly specific for aromatase without major effects on other cytochrome P_{450}-mediated steroid hydroxylations. Phase I clinical studies revealed an acute reduction of plasma estradiol to undetectable levels in normal men receiving one 10-mg dose and a 64% reduction in premenopausal women.[87] Clinical trials in patients with breast cancer have not, as yet, been reported.

CGS 20267 is another imidazole aromatase inhibitor effective in suppressing estrogens in male volunteers at doses as little as 20 μg.[81] Maximal suppression of estrogens is achieved with doses of 250 μg. The agent appears to be specific for aromatase since their were no changes in aldosterone or cortisol at any of the time points studied. This

Table XVII-7-6.   New Aromatase Inhibitors Reaching Clinical Trial (continued)

Steroid Agonist or Antagonist Properties	Phase I Trials	Phase II Trials	Phase III Trials	Major Sides Effects	Comments
Unknown	+	—	—	—	Lowers estrogen levels in male volunteers
A[b]	+	+	—	—	Active in producing tumor regression (see Table XV)
—	+	—	—	—	Human data unpublished
—	+	—	—	—	Clinical data preliminary
—	+	+	+	—	Active in producing tumor regression
—	+	—	—	—	Active in men in microgram doses
—	+	—	—	—	Studies in monkeys demonstrate blockade of aromatase with isotopic methods

Table XVII-7-7.   Non-Randomized Studies of 4-Hydroxyandrostenedione in Postmenopausal Women with Breast Carcinoma

Dose	Number of Patients	Overall Objective Responses	Median Duration Response	Mean Duration Survival	Comments	Ref
250 mg I.M. every other week	55	33%	12 mo	—		20
500 mg I.M. weekly	52	33%	10 mo	—	Dose escalated to 1000 mg weekly in 11 non-responders; sterile abscesses in 6 patients	20
500 mg I.M. every other week	86	24%	13+	—	Dose reduced to 250 I.M. every other week after 6 weeks. No significant toxicity and side effects minimal	38
500 mg p.o. daily	24	33%	—	—		20

agent is highly promising as a potent, selective, long-acting and very well tolerated aromatase inhibitor.

Perspectives

Availability of newer aromatase inhibitors with high potency and specificity and lack of side effects should allow wider use of these agents for patients with breast cancer. Application in women with benign disorders such as dysfunctional uterine bleeding and leiomyomata uteri requires blockade of ovarian as well as extraglandular aromatase. The challenge will be to develop sufficiently potent inhibitors to block ovarian estrogen biosynthesis even in the face of reflex gonadotropin increments. A wide range of estrogen-dependent disorders might then be amenable to treatment with aromatase inhibitors.

Aromatase inhibitors and agents designed to block androgen biosynthesis more specifically for men with prostate cancer are being evaluated at the present time. While beyond the scope of this chapter, a recent review details these approaches in-depth.[89]

References

1. Abul-Hajj, Y. J., Iverson, R., and Kiang, D. T.: Aromatization of androgens by human breast cancer. Steroids, 33:205, 1979.
2. Alonso-Munoz, M. C., Ojeda-Gonzalez, M. B., Beltran-Fabregat, M., Dorca-Ribugent, J., Lopez-Lopez, L., Borras-Balada, J., Cardenal-Alemany, F., Gomez-Batiste, X., Fabregat-Mayol, J., and Viladiu-Quemada, P.: Randomized trial of tamoxifen versus aminoglutethimide and versus combined tamoxifen and aminoglutethimide in advanced postmenopausal breast cancer. Oncology, 45:350, 1988.
3. Aromatase: New Perspective for Breast Cancer meeting. Key Biscayne, FL, December 6–9, 1981.
4. Badder, E. M., Lerman, S., and Santen, R. J.: Aminoglutethimide stimulates extra adrenal delta-4 androstenedione production. J. Surg. Res., 34:380, 1983.
5. Banting, L., Nicholls, P. J., Shaw, M. A., and Smith, H. J.: Recent developments in aromatase inhibition as a potential treatment for oestrogen-dependent breast cancer. Prog. Med. Chem., 26:253, 1989.
6. Bezwoda, W. R., Mansoor, N., and Dansey, R.: Correlation of breast tumour aromatase activity and response to aromatase inhibition with aminoglutethimide. Oncology, 44:345, 1987.
7. Bonneterre, J., Coppens, H., Mauriac, L., Metz, M., Roesse, J., Armand, J. P., Fargeot, P., Mothieu, M., Tubiana, M., and Cappelaere, P.: AG in advanced breast cancer: Clinical results of a French multicentre randomized trial comparing 500 mg and 1g/day. Eur. J. Cancer Clin. Oncol., 21:1153, 1985.
8. Bradlow, H. L.: A reassessment of the role of breast tumor aromatization. Cancer Res., 42:3382S, 1982.
9. Brodie, A. M. H., and Santen, R. J.: Aromatase in breast cancer and the role of aminoglutethimide and other aromatase inhibitors. Crit. Rev. Oncol./Hematol., 5:361, 1986.
10. Brodie, A. M. H., Schwarzel, W. C., Shaikh, A. A., and Brodie, H. J.: The effect of an aromatase inhibitor 4-hydroxy-4-androstene-3,17-dione, on estrogen-dependent processes in reproduction and breast cancer. Endocrinology, 100:1684, 1977.
11. Brodie, A. M. H., and Longcope, C.: Inhibition of peripheral aromatization by aromatase inhibitors, 4-hydroxy- and 4-acetoxy-androstene-3,17-dione. Endocrinology, 106:19, 1980.
12. Brodie, A. M. H., Romanoff, L. D., and Williams, K. I. H.: Metabolism of the aromatase inhibitor 4-hydroxy-4-androstene-3,17-dione by male rhesus monkeys. J. Steroid Biochem., 14:693, 1981.
13. Brodie, A. M. H.: personal communication.
14. Bruning, P. F., Bonfrer, J. M. G., Hart, A. A. M., Van Der Linden, E., De Jong-Bakker, M., Moolenaar, A. J., and Nooijen, W. J.: Low dose aminoglutethimide without hydrocortisone for the treatment of advanced postmenopausal breast cancer. Eur. J. Cancer Clin. Oncol., 25:369, 1989.
15. Cash, R., Brough, A. J., Cohen, M. N. P., and Satoh, P. S.: Aminoglutethimide (Elipten-CIBA) as an inhibitor of adrenal steroidogenesis. Mechanism of action and therapeutic trial. J. Clin. Endocrinol. Metab., 27:1239, 1967.

16. Caspi, E., and Njar, V. C. O.: Concerning the pathway from 19-oxoandrost-4-ene-3,17-dione to estrone. Steroids, 50:347, 1987.
17. Ceci, G., Cocconi, G., Bisagni, G., Franciosi, V., Bartolucci, R., Bacchi, M., Boni, C., Carpi, A., Gori, S., Indelli, M., Padalino, D., and Passalacqua, R.: Aminogluethimide with and without hydrocortisone as a first-line endocrine therapy in metastatic breast carcinoma. A prospective randomized trial. Presented at the Third IST International Symposium on Biology and Therapy of Breast Cancer, Genoa, Italy. Abstr 26/36, 1989. Data from Table XII obtained from copies of posters, courtesy of Dr. Cocconi.
18. Chakraborty, J., Hopkins, R., and Parke, D.: Inhibition studies on the aromatization of androst-4-ene-3,17-dione by human placental microsomes. Biochem. J., 130:19, 1972.
19. Coombes, R. C., Goss, P. E., Dowsett, M., Gazet, J.-C., and Brodie, A. M. H.: 4-Hydroxy-androstenedione in treatment of postmenopausal patients with advanced breast cancer. Lancet, 2:1237, 1984.
20. Coombes, R. C., and Stein, R. C.: Aromatase inhibitors in human breast cancer. Proc. Royal Soc. Edinburgh, 95B:283, 1989.
21. Coombes, R. C., Powles, T. J., Goss, P. E., Cunningham, D., Hutchison, G., Dowsett, M., and Brodie, A. M. H.: Clinical studies with 4-hydroxyandrostenedione in breast cancer patients. *In* Hormonal Manipulation of Cancer, Peptides, Growth Factors, and New (Anti)Steroidal Agents, EROTC Monograph Series, Vol 18. Edited by J. G. M. Klijn, R. Paridaens, and J. A. Foekens. New York, Raven Press, 1987, p. 81.
22. Demers, L. M., Melby, J. C., Wilson, T. E., Lipton, A., Harvey, H. A., and Santen, R. J.: The effects of CGS 16949A, an aromatase inhibitor on adrenal mineralocorticoid biosynthesis. J. Clin. Endocrinol. Metab., 70:1162, 1990.
23. Dorrington, J. H., and Armstrong, D. T.: Effects of FSH on gonadal functions. Rec. Progr. Horm. Res., 35:301, 1979.
24. Dowsett, M., Santner S. J., Santen, R. J., Jeffcoate, S. L., and Smith, I. E.: Effective inhibition by low dose aminoglutethimide of peripheral aromatization in postmenopausal breast cancer patients. Br. J. Cancer, 52:31 1985.
25. Dowsett, M., Harris, A. L., Stuart-Harris, R., Hill, M., Cantwell, B. M. J., Smith, I. E., and Jeffcoate, S. L.: A comparison of the endocrine effects of low dose aminoglutethimide with and without hydrocortisone in postmenopausal breast cancer patients. Br. J. Cancer, 52:525, 1985.
26. Dowsett, M., Cunningham, D. C., Stein, R. C., Evans, S., Dehennin, L., Hedley, A., and Coombes, R. C.: Dose-related endocrine effects and pharmacokinetics of oral and intramuscular 4-hydroxyandrostenedione in postmenopausal breast cancer patients. Cancer Res., 49:1306, 1989.
27. Edery, M., Goussard, J., Dehennin, L., Scholler, R., Reiffsteck, J., and Drosdowsky, M. A.: Endogenous oestradiol 17β concentration in breast tumours determined by mass fragmentography and radioimmunoassay: Relationship to receptor content. Eur. J. Cancer, 17:115, 1981.
28. Fishman, J., Nisselbaum, J. S., Menendez-Botet, C. J., and Schwartz, M. K.: Estrone and estradiol content in human breast tumors: Relationship to estradiol receptors. J. Steroid. Biochem., 8:893, 1977.
29. Fishman, J., and Hahn, E. F.: The nature of the final oxidative step in the aromatization sequence. Steroids, 50:339, 1987.
30. Gower, D. B.: Modifiers of steroid-hormone metabolism: A review of their chemistry, biochemistry and clinical applications, J. Steroid Biochem., 5:501, 1974.
31. Griffiths, C. T., Hall, T. C., Saba, Z., Barlow, J. J., and Nevinny, H. B.: Preliminary trial of aminoglutethimide in breast cancer. Cancer, 32:31, 1973.
32. Harris, A. L., Cantwell, B. M. J., Carmichael, J., Dawes, P., Robinson, A., Farndon, J., and Wilson, R.: Phase II study of low dose aminoglutethimide 250 mg/day plus hydrocortisone in advanced postmenopausal breast cancer. Eur. J. Cancer. Clin. Oncol., 25:1105, 1989.
33. Harris, A. L., Mitchell, M. D., Smith, I. E., and Powles, T. J.: Suppression of plasma G-keto-prostaglandin F_{1a} and 13,14-dihydro-15-keto-prostaglandin F_{2a} by aminoglutethi-mide in advanced breast cancer. Br. J. Cancer, 48:595, 1983.
34. Harris, A. L., Powles, T. J., Smith, I. E., Coombes, R. C., Ford, H. T., Gazet, J. C., Harmer, C. L., Morgan, M., White, H., Parsons, C. A., and McKinna, J. A.: AG for the treatment of advanced postmenopausal breast cancer. Eur. J. Cancer Clin. Oncol., 19:11, 1983.
35. Harvey, H. A., Santen, R. J., Osterman, J., Samojlik, E., White, D., and Lipton, A.: A comparative trial of transsphenoidal hypophysectomy and estrogen suppression with aminoglutethimide in advanced breast cancer. Cancer, 43:2207, 1979.
36. Harvey, H. A., Lipton, A., Santen, R. J., Demers, L., Henderson, I. C., Miller, A. A., Navari, R., Mulagha, M. T., and Hanagan, J.: Clinical trials with the aromatase inhibitor CGS 16949A in advanced breast cancer: The U.S. experience. Program of a Symposium, Aromatase Inhibition: Past, Present and Future, Hamburg, Germany, 1990, Abstr.
37. Henderson, D., Norbisrath, G., and Kreb, U.: 1-Methyl-1,4,-androstadiene-3,17-dione (SH 489): Characterization of an irreversible inhibitor of estrogen biosynthesis. J. Steroid Biochem., 24:303, 1986.
38. Hoffken, K., Jonat, W., Possinger, K., Kolbel, M., Kunz, T. H., Wagner, H., Becher, R., Callies, R., Friederich, P., Willmanns, W., Maass, H., and Schmidt, C. G.: Aromatase inhibition with 4-hyroxyandrostenedione in the treatment of postmenopausal patients with advanced breast cancer: A phase II study. J. Clin. Oncol., 8:875, 1990.
39. Hoffken, K., Kempf, H., Miller, A. A., Miller, B., Schmidt, C. G., Faber, P., and Kley, H. K.: Aminoglutethimide without hydrocortisone in the treatment of postmenopausal patients with advanced breast cancer. Cancer Treat. Rep., 70:1153, 1986.
40. Hughes, S. W. M., and Burley, D. M.: Aminoglutethimide: a "side-effect" turned to therapeutic advantage. Postgrad. Med. J., 46:409, 1970.
41. Judd H. L., Judd, G. E., Lucas, W. E., and Yen, S. S. C.: Endocrine function of the postmenopausal ovary: Concentration of androgens and estrogens in ovarian and peripheral vein blood. J. Clin. Endocrinol. Metab., 39:1020, 1974.
42. Kirschner, M. A., Schneider, G., Ertel, N. H., and Worton, E.: Obesity, androgens, estrogens, and cancer risk. Cancer. Res., 42(Suppl):3281s, 1982.
43. Klein, H., Bartsch, W., Niemand, A., Sturenburg, H. J., and Voigt, K. D.: Inhibition of human placental aromatase in a perfusion model. Comparison with kinetic cell-free experiments. J. Steroid Biochem., 29:161, 1988.
44. Krekels, M. D., Wouters, W., and De Coster, R.: Aromatase inhibition by R76713: A kinetic analysis in rat ovarian homogenates. Steroids, 52:69, 1990.
45. Lipton, A., Santner, S. J., Santen, R. J., Harvey, H. A., Feil, P. D., White-Hershey, D., Bartholomew, M. J., and Antle, C. E.: Aromatase activity in primary and metastatic human breast cancer. Cancer, 59:779, 1987.
46. Lipton, A., Harvey, H. A., Santen, R. J., Boucher, A., White, D., Bernath, A., Dixon, R., Richards, G., and Shafik, A.: Randomized trial of aminoglutethimide versus tamoxifen in metastatic breast cancer. Cancer Res., 42(Suppl):3434s, 1982.
47. Lonning, P. E., Dowsett, M., and Powles, T. J.: Treatment of breast cancer with aromatase inhibitors—Current status and future prospects. Brit. J. Cancer, 60:5, 1989.
48. Lonning, P. E., Ueland, P. M., and Kvinnsland, S.: The influence of a graded dose schedule of aminoglutethimide on the disposition of the optical enantiomers of warfarin in patients with breast cancer. Cancer Chemother. Pharmacol., 17:177, 1986.
49. Miller, W. R., and O'Neill, J.: The importance of local synthesis of estrogen within the breast. Steroids, 50:537, 1987.
50. Murray, F. T., Santner, S., Samojlik, E., and Santen, R. J.: Serum aminoglutethimide levels: Studies of serum half-life, clearance and patient compliance. J. Clin. Pharmacol., 19:704, 1979.
51. Murray, R., and Pitt P.: Low-dose aminoglutethimide without steroid replacement in the treatment of postmenopausal women with advanced breast cancer. Eur. J. Cancer Clin. Oncol., 21:19, 1985.
52. Nemoto, T., Rosner, D., Patel, J. K., and Dao, T. L.: Aminoglutethimide in patients with metastatic breast cancer. Cancer, 63:1673, 1989.
53. O'Neill, J. S., and Miller, W. R.: Aromatase activity in breast adipose tissue from women with benign and malignant breast diseases. Br. J. Cancer, 56:601, 1987.
54. Petru, E., and Schmahl, D.: On the role of additive hormone monotherapy with tamoxifen, medroxyprogesterone acetate and aminoglutethimide, in advanced breast cancer. Klin. Wochenshr., 65:959, 1987.
55. Possinger, K.: The role of aromatase inhibitors in the treatment of breast cancer. (Abstract) Program of a Symposium, Aromatase Inhibition: Past, Present and Future, Hamburg, Germany.
56. Samojlik, E., Veldhuis, J. D., Wells, S. A., and Santen, R. J.: Preservation of androgen secretion during estrogen suppression with aminoglutethimide in the treatment of metastatic breast carcinoma. J. Clin. Invest., 65:602, 1980.
57. Santen, R. J., Leszczynski, D., Tilson-Mallet, N., Feil, P. D., Wright, C., Manni, A., and Santner, S. J.: Enzymatic control of estrogen production in human breast cancer: Relative significance of aromatase vs. sulfatase pathways. *In* Endocrinology of the Breast: Basic and Clinical Aspects, Vol. 464. Edited by A. Angeli, H. L. Bradlow, and L. Dogliotti. New York, Acad. Sci., 1986, p. 126.
58. Santen, R. J., Lipton, A., and Kendall, J.: Successful medical adrenalectomy with aminoglutethimide: Role of altered drug metabolism. JAMA, 230:1661, 1974.
59. Santen, R. J., Santner, S. J., Davis, B., Veldhuis, J., Samojlik, E., and Ruby, E.: Aminoglutethimide inhibits extraglandular estrogen production in postmenopausal women with breast carcinoma. J. Clin. Endocrinol. Metab., 47:1257, 1978.
60. Santen, R. J., Worgul, T. J., Samojlik, E., Interrante, A., Boucher, A. E., Lipton, A., Harvey, H. A., White, D. S., Smart, E., Cox, C., and Wells, S. A.: A randomized trial comparing surgical adrenalectomy with aminoglutethimide plus hydrocortisone in women with advanced breast cancer. N. Engl. J. Med., 305:545, 1981.
61. Santen, R. J., Worgul, T. J., Lipton, A., Harvey, H. A., Boucher, A., Samojlik, E., and Wells, S. A.: Aminoglutethimide as treatment of postmenopausal women with advanced breast carcinoma: Correlation of clinical and hormonal responses. Ann. Intern. Med., 96:94, 1982.
62. Santen, R. J., Wells, S. A., Cohn, N., Demers, L. M., Misbin, R., and Foltz, E. L.: Compensatory increase in TSH secretion without effect on prolactin secretion in patients treated with aminoglutethimide. J. Clin. Endocrinol. Metab., 45:739, 1977.
63. Santen, R. J., Manni, A., Harvey, H., and Redmond, C.: Endocrine treatment of breast cancer in women. Endocr. Rev., 11:221, 1990.
64. Santen, R. J., Boucher, A. E., Santner, S. J., Henderson, I. C., Harvey, H., and Lipton, A.: Inhibition of aromatase as treatment of breast carcinoma in postmenopausal women. J. Lab. Clin. Med., 109:278, 1987.
65. Santen, R. J., Samojlik, E., and Wells, S. A.: Resistance of the ovary to blockade of aromatization with aminoglutethimide. J. Clin. Endocrinol. Metab., 51:473, 1980.
66. Santen, R. J., Langecker, P., Santner, S., Sikka, S., Rajfer, J., and Swerdloff, R.: Potency and specificity of CGS-16949A as an aromatase inhibitor. Endocr. Res., 16:77, 1990.
67. Santen, R. J., Demers, L. M., Adlercreutz, H., Harvey, H. A., Santner, S., Sanders, S., and Lipton, A.: Inhibition of aromatase with CGS-16949A in postmenopausal women. J. Clin. Endocrinol. Metab., 68:99, 1989.
68. Santen, R. J., Demers, L., Lipton, A., Harvey, H. A., Hanagan, J., Mulagha, M., Navari, R. M., Henderson, I. C., Garber, J. E., and Miller, A. A.: Phase II study of the potency and specificity of a new aromatase inhibitor—CGS 16949A. Clin. Res., 37:535A, 1989.
69. Santen, R. J., Demers, L. M., Lynch, J., Harvey, H., Lipton, A., Mulagha, M., Hanagan, J., Garber, J. E., Henderson, I. C., Navari, R. M., and Miller, A.: Specificity of low dose fedrozole hydrochloride (CGS 16949A) as an aromatase inhibitor. J. Clin. Endocrinol. Metab., 73:99–106, 1991.
70. Santen, R. J., and Misbin, R. I.: Aminoglutethimide: Review of pharmacology and clinical use. Pharmacotherapy, 1:95, 1981.
71. Schieweck, K., Bhatnagar, A. S., and Matter, A.: CGS 16949A, a new nonsteroidal aromatase inhibitor: effects on hormone-dependent and -independent tumors in vivo. Cancer Res., 48:834, 1988.
72. Siiteri, P. K., and MacDonald, P. C.: Role of extraglandular estrogen in human endocrinology. *In* Handbook of Physiology, vol. II, part 1. Edited by S. R. Geiger, E. B. Astwood, and R. O. Greep. Baltimore, American Physiological Society, 1973, p. 615.
73. Simpson, E. R., Merrill, J. C., Hollub, A. J., Graham-Lorence, S., and Mendelson, C. R.: Regulation of estrogen biosynthesis by human adipose cells. Endocr. Rev., 10:136, 1989.
74. Smith, I. E., Harris, A. L., Morgan, M., Ford, H. T., Gazet, J. C., Harmer, C. L., White, H., Parsons, C. A., Villardo, A., Walsh, G., and McKinna, J. A.: Tamoxifen versus aminoglutethimide in advanced breast carcinoma: A randomized cross-over trial. Brit. Med. J., 283:1432, 1981.
75. Snider, C. E., and Brueggemeier, R. W.: Potent enzyme-activated inhibition of aromatase by a 7α-substituted C_{19} steroid. J. Biol. Chem., 262:8685, 1987.
76. Steele, R. E., Mellor, L. B., Sawyer, W. K., Wasvary, J. M., and Browne, L. J.: In vitro and in vivo studies demonstrating potent and selective estrogen inhibition with the nonsteroidal aromatase inhibitor CGS 16949A. Steroids, 50:147, 1987.
77. Stuart-Harris, R., Dowsett, M., Bozek, T., McKinna, J. A., Gazet, J. C., Jeffcoate, S. L., Kurkure, A., Carr, L., and Smith, I. E.: Low-dose aminoglutethimide in treatment of advanced breast cancer. Lancet, 2:604, 1984.
78. Stuart-Harris, R., Dowsett, M., D'Souza, A., Donaldson, A., Harris, A. L., Jeffcoate, S. L., and Smith, I. E.: Endocrine effects of low dose aminoglutethimide as an aromatase inhibitor in the treatment of breast cancer. Clin. Endocrinol., 22:219, 1985.
79. Thompson, E. A., and Siiteri, P. K.: The involvement of human placental microsomal cytochrome P-450 in aromatization. J. Biol. Chem., 249:5373, 1974.
80. Touitou, Y., Bogdan, A., Legrand, J. C., and Desgrez, P.: Aminoglutethimide and

Glutethimide: Effects on 18-hydroxycorticosterone biosynthesis by human and sheep adrenals in vitro. Acta Endocrinol., 80:517, 1975.

81. Trunet, P., Muller, P., Bhatnagar, A., Chaudri, H., Beh, I., and Monnet, G.: Phase I study in healthy male volunteers with the non-steroidal aromatase inhibitor, CGS 20267. Proceedings of the Second International Symposium on "Hormonal Manipulation of Cancer: Peptides, Growth Factors and New (Anti)Steroidal Agents," April 9–11, 1990. Rotterdam, The Netherlands, Astr. 109, p. 50.

82. Vermeulen, A., Paridaens, R., and Heuson, J. C.: Effects of aminoglutethimide on adrenal steroid secretion. Clin. Endocrinol., 19:673, 1983.

83. Weisz, J., et al., personal communication.

84. Wing, L. Y. C., Hammond, J. O., and Brodie, A. M. H.: Differential responses of sex steroid target tissues of rats treated with 4-hydroxyandrostenedione. Endocrinology, 122:2418, 1988.

85. Wouters, W., De Coster, R., Goeminne, N., Beerens, D., and Van Dun, J.: Aromatase inhibition by the antifungal ketoconazole. J. Steroid Biochem., 30:387, 1988.

86. Wouters, W., De Coster, R., Krekels, M., Van Dun, J., Beerens, D., Haelterman, C., Raeymaekers, A., Freyne, E., Van Gelder, J., Venet, M., and Janssen, P. A. J.: R 76713, A new specific non-steroidal aromatase inhibitor. J. Steroid Biochem., 32:781, 1989.

87. Wouters, W., De Coster, R., Tuman, R. W., Bowden, C. R., Bruynseels, J., Vanderpas, H., Van Rooy, P., Amery, W. K., and Janssen, P. A. J.: Aromatase inhibition by R76713: Experimental and clinical pharmacology. J. Steroid Biochem., 34:427, 1989.

88. Young, J. A., Newcomer, L. N., and Keller, A. M.: Aminoglutethimide-induced bone marrow injury. Cancer, 54:1731, 1984.

89. Santen, R. J.: Endocrine aspects of prostate cancer. In Principles and Practice of Endocrinology and Metabolism. Edited by K. L. Becker. Philadelphia, J. B. Lippincott Co., 1990, p. 1656.

XVII-8

Progestins

Kenneth S. McCarty, Jr.
Kenneth S. McCarty, Sr.

Introduction

The naturally occurring progestin is progesterone. In non-gravid women it is principally derived from the corpus luteum of the ovary. This changes dramatically during pregnancy where the major source of progesterone becomes the placenta. The corpus luteum is the source of progesterone in the first eight weeks of pregnancy. At this time progesterone is required for the development of a secretory endometrium in which the blastocyst can implant. The trophoblast becomes dominant in progesterone production after the eighth week of gestation. Progesterone is also synthesized by the adrenal through conversion of pregnenolone. In the luteal phase of the menstrual cycle progesterone levels of 25 ng/ml are usual, while levels to 150 ng/ml are typical of pregnancy at term. Such high levels of progesterone as are seen in term pregnancy are associated with a number of effects with implications for other conditions. Among these are progesterone associated inhibition of T-lymphocyte cell-mediated immune response, inhibition of prostaglandin formation, and inhibition of smooth muscle contractility through binding to receptors in the uterine smooth muscle.

Progestins are widely utilized in contraceptive preparations. They have emerged as anti-neoplastic agents in uterine and breast cancer, have been tested with promising results in meningiomas and pulmonary lymphangiomyomatosis and have been studied for anti-neoplastic potential against other neoplasms.

The use of progestins or anti-progestins in contraceptive preparations is the area in which the greatest effort has been applied to understanding the pharmacology and mechanism of action of progesterone and the various synthetic progestins and anti-progestins. Recommendations for progestin replacement therapy in the climacteric places new emphasis on understanding the mechanism of progesterone action in settings other than contraception, particularly in populations with a significant incidence of endometrial cancer, breast cancer, and other neoplasms.

Target cells must not only distinguish progesterone in the presence of other steroids present in small amounts, but also distinguish progesterone from other hydrophobic molecules that are frequently found in 10^6 to 10^9 fold excess. This high degree of discrimination is limited to differentiated cells that possess progesterone receptor proteins (PR) and progesterone responsive elements (PRE) in their genome.[90]

The regulation of the target gene mRNA level is primarily dependent on progesterone activation of PR that results in a complex series of events.[50] The biochemical mechanism of this cellular response to progesterone is prototypical as PR is a member of a superfamily of transcriptional regulatory proteins.[18] As with other members of this superfamily, activated PR acquires the capacity to modulate the activity of specific target genes. Some target genes under the regulation of both PR and glucocorticoid receptor (GR) include: estrogen receptor,[79] human metallothionein IIA,[77] uteroglobin,[19] vitellogenin,[86] and human pregnancy specific beta glycoprotein.[75] The molecular mechanism to provide discrimination is dependent on a highly specific protein-DNA interaction that involves specific amino acid residues of the PR and nucleotide residues of the target genes. The amino acid residues of the PR are defined as the "DNA binding domain" (DBD), and the DNA elements of these target genes as "progesterone responsive elements" (PRE). In fact, the PRE sequences of a whole network of target genes are recognized by the trans-activated PR.[3] These PRE gene sequences are further characterized as "enhancer-like" in that neither their precise orientation nor position appear to be critical.[84] The PREs that are recognized by the DBD are confined, however, to the 5' upstream end of the genes, near the promoter regions of all progesterone responsive target genes examined to date.[23,47] The critical role of both the hormone and its receptor in this function makes it a worthy candidate for careful review.

The precise protein-DNA interaction of the trans-activated PR with specific target genes is the critical feature that determines its specificity. This mechanism of hormone induction is common to the whole superfamily of steroid receptors.[32,90]

The progesterone PR-complex[93] activates the positively charged cysteine-rich amino acid residues of the DBD,[32] which in turn function to increase its binding affinity for specific PRE residues of target genes.[16,70] This activation is often referred to as "trans-activation" denoting that its function spans many amino acid residues.[29] The precise molecular mechanism is dependent on: hormone recognition, activation of the DBD, and interaction of the DBD with chromosomal DNA target gene PRE sequences.[3,9,15,46]

DNA sequence analysis also demonstrates that most progesterone responsive target genes not only have multiple PRE copies, but also have other hormone responsive elements (HRE), including in particular, glucocorticoid responsive elements (GRE). Many of these HREs have the capacity to modify the function of the PR. This observation of the existence of multiple PRE and HRE elements in combination provides for the first time a plausible mechanism to account for a long standing clinical observation that both the dose and prior hormone history have a profound effect on the clinical response of patients to hormone therapy of cancer. Thus it is frequently observed that the administration of different levels of progesterone enhances the cooperative binding to HREs and also that a number of hormone combinations both down- and up-regulate the progesterone responsive gene.[21,23]

In addition, the role played by the chromosomal DNA target gene configuration is a critical factor in gene response that includes many proteins (RNA polymerase II enzyme complexes, and specific proteins essential for RNA polymerase function).[8,73,80,82] Thus any inappropriate DNA hypermethylation and/or heterochromatin configuration is likely to exert a profound effect on the PR response and may in some tumors account for clinical failures. This failure to respond must also be passed to the metastatic tumor by maintenance methylase.[80]

For those who wish to have more details with regard to the structure and function that contribute to receptor-ligand interactions at the molecular level, might consider a number of reviews.[18,36,38,59,61,64,82,90]

The first part of this discussion considers some aspects of the pharmacology of progestogens. This is followed by a discussion of some of the functions of progesterone receptors in terms of genetic structure, differentiation, synthesis, post-synthetic modification, and intracellular location. The third part will consider some aspects of the clinical response to progestins of specific neoplasms. Excluded from consideration will be progesterone induction of proto-oncogenes and modulation of cell cycle activity,[11,27,31] as these are considered elsewhere in this volume.

Pharmacology of Progestogens

Progestogens are properly classified as natural or synthetic. Progesterone is the only natural progestogen of clinical importance. Progesterone occupies a position early in the scheme of the synthetic pathway involving the conversion of precursor cholesterol to the production of adrenal cortical derived hormones including androgens and estrogens. After menopause and in the absence of hormone replacement, the adrenal is the critical source of these sex steroids.

Progesterone is poorly absorbed orally, and when injected must be used with an oil carrier. In contrast, a number of synthetic progestogens are available which are well absorbed orally. Synthetic progestogens are derivatives of the steroid structure of either progesterone or testosterone. Knowledge of this derivative relationship provides the basis for the classification of the synthetic progestogens. The synthetic progestogen steroids which are most often encountered include 17 hydroxyprogesterone, medroxyprogesterone (Provera), medroxyprogesterone acetate, megestrol acetate (Megace), norethindrone, norethindrone enanthate, norethindrone acetate, norethynodrel, norgestrol, desogestrel, and gestodene. In view of their importance in contraception as well as their therapeutic use in the climacteric and neoplastic disease, new synthetic progestational compounds are under continued development and evaluation.

Progesterone may be administered either intramuscularly or may be taken orally. Oral progesterone, however, as noted above is associated with relatively poor bio-availability when compared to intramuscular administration of progesterone. The issue of bio-availability with oral agents has been overcome with some of the synthetic progestogens, but at a cost of adverse effects on plasma lipid levels.[66] Medroxyprogesterone (Provera) given as a single intramuscular injection of 25–50 mg shows an effect on estrogen stimulated endometrium for just over two weeks, although increases in basal body temperature from such treatment may last six or more weeks. Depo-provera has a period of action which is considerably longer. Oral medroxyprogesterone (Provera) and oral megestrol acetate (Megace) are well absorbed. Medroxyprogesterone produces a luteal effect in anovulatory patients with an oral dose of 5 mg daily for five days. A dose of 5–10 mg/day for five days is typically recommended in anovulatory patients and in programs of cyclic estrogen/progesterone therapy for the climacteric.

The 19-norsteroid, RU 486 is among the first available true anti-progesterones. This agent opens a new vista for therapeutic intervention in progesterone response. This compound is effectively absorbed orally and appears to bind to the progesterone receptor with high affinity.[7] RU 486 also has significant anti-glucocorticoid activity as well as weak anti-androgen activity.[7]

PR concentration is increased in target cells by the preovulatory surge of estrogen. Target cells are thus primed to respond to progesterone subsequent to ovulation, when progesterone is secreted by the corpus luteum. Loss of the function of the corpus luteum (luteolysis) is associated with a rapid decrease of progesterone and estradiol. Following this, there is a disintegration of the endometrium. Since progesterone activity is dependent on intact functional progesterone receptor, one molecular mechanism proposed for RU 486 action is a modulation of PR function. This mechanism suggests that RU 486 facilitates the binding of a heat shock protein (Hsp-90) to the PR as a post-synthetic modification.[6] The Hsp-90 when bound to the PR keeps it in an inactive configuration preventing its interaction with the target genes. Some aspects of the Hsp-90 proteins with hormone receptors will be discussed below under post-synthetic modifications. It is becoming increasingly evident that heat shock proteins are likely to represent an important component of the normal function of PR and will be significant in future studies.

In developing treatment strategies using progestogens, effects on bone metabolism, water retention, lipid metabolism and the central nervous system must all be considered, although the impact on growth, differentiation and neoplastic transformation of specific target tissues is the central theme of the present discussion.

Function of Progesterone Receptors

Progesterone response is totally dependent on the presence of functionally intact PR. This activity is only initiated when the steroid is bound to the carboxyl terminal or progesterone binding domain PBD[83] to induce trans-activation at the DBD.[79] An absence of hormone response usually results from either the absence of the PR or its failure to bind the steroid binding domain SBD.[94] Many tumors lack PR, but there is also evidence of point mutations or total deletions in the SBD of the PR from some neoplasms.

If one considers the complexity of the multilevel controls to include defects at the level of: recognition of the PRE in the selective transcription of the target gene heterogeneous nuclear RNA (hnRNA);[50] processing of this messenger RNA (mRNA);[94] transport from the nucleus to the cytoplasm of this mRNA;[1] and/or modulation of the mRNA half-life,[4] there is the potential for multiple defects to account for clinical resistance to progestins.

Differentiation and Receptor Synthesis

Presence of Two Progesterone Receptors. In the human, PR is unique among steroid receptors in that it is composed of two hormone binding proteins A and B. PR-B is slightly larger than PR-A.[22] Both are synthesized from a single mRNA, where the PR-A corresponds to the smaller N-terminally truncated form of the PR-B that is cleaved at an internal methionine residue. The amino terminal of PR specifies target gene activity. There appears to be a functional difference between PR-A and PR-B in the transcriptional activation of target genes. If the function of the PR-A does indeed differ from that of the PR-B, the potential is at hand to explain a number of clinical observations.

Progesterone Receptor Synthesis. In the breast, differentiation is dependent on the synthesis and activation of both PR and estrogen receptor (ER). The synthesis of either PR or ER requires both a specific signal response and a "permissive chromosomal configuration" in the region of the steroid receptor gene within the nucleus. To attain this permissive state requires a number of nuclear events including: the synthesis of trans-activating nuclear proteins; demethylation of the DNA; estrogen modulation of PR and post-synthetic modification a number of specific nuclear proteins.[81] PR and ER activation then is not only dependent on receptor synthesis and ligand binding affinity, but equally dependent on associations with at least five additional proteins including a 45Kd and a 35Kd protein and two classes of heat shock proteins.

Modulation of Receptor Activity. The progesterone response mediated by trans-activated PR represents critical interactions with chromatin and its complement of associated proteins. Most abundant among these are the histones,[40,49,85] and the HMG1 and HMG2 chromosomal proteins,[14] which have been shown to interact directly with steroid receptors. These proteins are post-synthetically modified by both histone kinases and acetylases. A mechanism for the modulation of specific gene activity has been proposed.[60]

PR not only functions in its binding to cis-activating PRE elements at the 5′ upstream DNA sequences of a number of progesterone responsive genes, it also has the capacity to function as a down-regulator of the synthesis of other HRs (e.g., ER).[62,73] PR should be considered a target gene for estrogen response in that a functional ER is required to up-regulate the synthesis of PR.[33] This mechanism may also account for the modulation of PR synthesis in response to glucocorticoid,[61,65,88] modulating the binding affinity of PREs on PR target genes.

Post-synthetic modifications involve very subtle alterations in the PR structure, as well as cis- and trans-acting factors. Modifications include: 1) phosphorylation and acetylation of chromosomal proteins such as histones HMG1 and HMG2, 2) post-synthetic modification of the binding of heat-shock proteins to PR; and 3) the phosphorylation of both of these proteins. In addition to the multiple cis-activating components described for HRE, trans-acting elements are also required for RNA transcription that is critical for the hormone response.[21]

Structure, Sequence of Hormone and DNA-Binding Residues

Progesterone Receptor as a Superfamily Member. The superfamily of receptor proteins that interact with many lipophilic ligands have a number of features in common with PR.[36] Examples are the ligand and DNA binding that were delineated in early studies using proteolytic digestion of progesterone receptor proteins.[25,39] These early studies demonstrated a loss of DNA binding in spite of a retention of the specific ligand binding.[25] These proteolytic receptor digests were referred to as "mero" receptor fragments.[39]

Cloning of receptor proteins has permitted a rapid advance in understanding the structure of receptors for estrogen,[51,55,87] progesterone,[21,26] and glucocorticoid.[78,88] There is a striking homology of PR with other hydrophobic signal proteins including thyroid receptor, three forms of retinoic acid receptors, and vitamin D3 receptor.[90] A number of highly conserved regions for these genes are observed.[21,30,44,89]

Structure of the DNA Binding Domain. The DNA binding domain of all of the receptors that are known to respond to lipophilic signals are defined as a highly conserved sequence. The consensus sequence cores involved in DNA binding are composed of approximately 70 amino acids that include 9 perfectly conserved cysteines. There are two "zinc fingers" in which each finger has 1 zinc coordinated with 4 cysteines. As described for GR, one of these fingers appears to be involved in dimer formation and the other is needed for recognition of PREs of the DNA of progesterone responsive genes in a complex series of reactions.[9,24,28,30,37,59,68,69] Transactivation appears to be a positive modification that "unmasks" the DNA binding domain.[42] Steroid receptors function as dimers, with one of the fingers interacting in the wide DNA groove while the other maintains the dimer configuration.

Target Genes and Progesterone Responsive Elements. The DNA binding mechanism of the PR resembles that of other steroid receptors. Thus, the ability to discriminate between different hormone responsive elements must depend on a limited number of subtle modifications such as post-synthetic modification of the protein or the presence of trans-acting elements.[9]

Perturbation of the amino acid sequence, post-synthetic modification of the amino acid sequence, interaction with other proteins, deletion or mutations in the PRE, changes in the open configuration of the chromatin, or ligand competition will alter the delicate balance required that determines the affinity or specificity of DNA binding. Target genes can have at least two HREs with competitive binding for more than one type of activated receptor.[30] Examples of this type of competitive binding include ER and GR. The PREs of hormone responsive genes must be maintained in an open chromatin configuration. These PRE sequences are located 5′ to the DNA promoter region of the progesterone responsive genes.

Receptor Protein Target Gene Interactions. Experiments that most clearly define the precise mechanism of HR enhancer element interaction are based on observations using solution nuclear magnetic resonance spectroscopy (NMR) and distance geometry.[42] These experiments utilized a purified DNA binding fragment (residues 440–510) obtained from a rat glucocorticoid receptor (GR) expressed in *E. coli*.[42] Convincing evidence was obtained the GR-protein binds as a dimer to the DNA glucocorticoid responsive elements (GREs). This model is consistent with previous results that define the importance of specific amino acid residues in interaction of protein with DNA GRE elements and in dimer formation. (See Figure XVII-8-1.) Protein-protein contacts appear to be essential for dimer formation and are very likely to involve a segment of the receptor that is important for its cooperativity. This provides a plausible mechanism as to how a limited, subtle conformational distortion of amino acid residues at one end of the receptor in the ligand binding region, could exert such a profound effect on the DNA binding domain. Since PR is also a member of the HR superfamily, the mechanism of dimer formation is likely to resemble that of GR. The critical role of one of the zinc fingers in dimer formation, and the other zinc finger in specificity of gene recognition and activation is apparent.[42] (See Figure XVII-8-1.)

Intracellular Localization and Post-Synthetic Modifications. As a hydrophobic signal, progesterone is unrestricted by plasma or nuclear membranes and is free to diffuse through membranes to interact with specific proteins which are confined to the nucleus. Whereas it is clear that the specificity attained by hydrophilic signals is dependent on its interaction with cell surface receptors, the precise intracellular localization of all hydrophobic steroid molecules is unresolved. The use of anti-receptor antibodies to PR and estrogen receptor (ER) demonstrates these proteins in the nucleus, whereas immunoreactive glucocorticoid receptors (GR) in the absence of ligand are found in the cytoplasm. All steroid receptors after complexing with their specific ligands are only detected in the nucleus. The presence of the specific ligand is a primary signal for nuclear translocation.

Prior to hormone activation, when receptors are isolated under low ionic conditions, steroids form large oligomeric complexes (~9S). As a large complex, these receptors lack the capacity to bind DNA. Oligomers appear to be complexed with a specific protein detected immunologically as a 90kD heat shock protein (Hsp90). When the Hsp90 is complexed to the PR, DNA binding is prevented. Hsp90 binds as a dimer at the carboxyl terminal of a single PR molecule. The Hsp dimer PR complex may maintain an inactive configuration in the absence of progesterone. Such post-synthetic modifications function to modify both the initial activation of PR, the hormone receptor, and secondary hormone

receptor-HRE interactions. Many of the enzymes involved in these post-synthetic modifications are also under hormone control. These include, for example, heat shock proteins,[5,10,17,34,67,71,72,89] kinases,[92] and RNA transcription factors.[8]

Clinical Observations on Progestin Receptor and Target Tissue Response to Progestins

Progesterone is associated with a number of biologic activities which include: a critical role in the support of the products of conception; the differentiation of the endometrium and the promotion of the secretory phase of the endometrium following the estrogen-induced proliferative phase; maturation and cornification of the vaginal mucosal epithelium; suppression of ovulation; inhibition of gonadotropin release; proliferation of breast epithelium; secretory activity in breast epithelium; and a naturietic effect on the kidney. A number of these biologic effects of progesterone are seen only in concert with priming of the target tissues with estrogen, whereas other effects appear to be interrelated with the actions of other steroid hormones, peptide hormones and/or growth factors. Both progesterone and estrogen influence the response when super-pharmacologic doses are used. Possible interactions between progesterone, estrogen, and growth factors must be taken into account when constructing treatment strategies.

Uterus

Normal Uterus. The cyclic response of the uterus to estrogen and progesterone is among the best studied examples of hormonal modulation of tissue response. There is clear evidence for cyclic regulation of estrogen and progesterone receptor proteins in the endometrial epithelium, the myometrium and the endometrial stroma. The induction of progesterone receptor by estrogen has been shown both in vitro and in vivo. An increase in progesterone receptor at the end of the proliferative phase of the menstrual cycle occurs in the stromal/myometrial tissue 24–48 hrs before the observed peak of progesterone receptor levels in endometrial epithelial tissue.[52] This cyclic change can be aborted by the administration of 10 mg of provera for 5–10 days, associated with regression of the epithelium. Epithelial hyperplasia of the uterus exposed to progestins first shows acanthomatous changes (a change wherein the cells resemble squamous cells) followed by secretory differentiation and finally regression of the hyperplastic change with eventual atrophy after 10–14 days.

Uterine Carcinoma. Uterine carcinoma is observed as a localized disease in the majority of cases. In clinical practice there is an increased incidence of adenocarcinoma of the uterus when a woman is given unopposed estrogen in physiologic doses and this increased frequency is significantly reduced if progestins are also given. Progestins can be given for the last 10 days of the estrogen replacement cycle or at a lower dose throughout the cycle.

When diagnosed, adenocarcinoma of the uterus is cured by local therapy in 80% of cases. In the event of recurrence, exogenous progestin is an effective treatment in a significant fraction of cases with more than 30% of patients with recurrent disease demonstrating objective response to exogenous progestins. ER and PR can be measured in these tumors and the presence of these receptors correlates with differ-

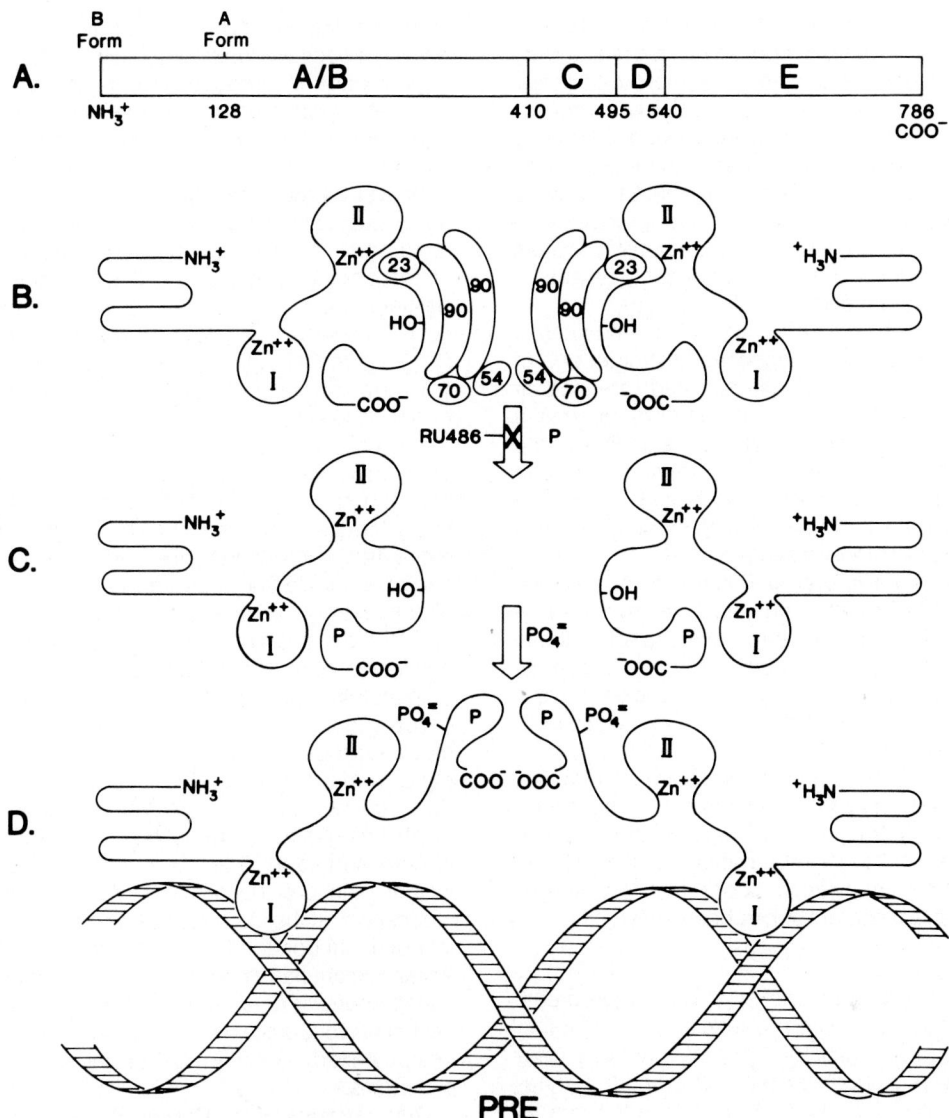

Figure XVII-8-1A. Schematic representation of the linear amino acid sequence of the progesterone receptor illustrating the relation of the functional domains. Progesterone receptor-B (PR-B) is composed of a total of 786 amino acids. Progesterone receptor-A (PR-A) consists of 658 amino acids representing a truncated form of the progesterone receptor lacking 128 amino acids of the amino terminal of PR-B. Both PR-B and its truncated form PR-A are synthesized from same mRNA as described in the text.

The A/B domain extends from the amino terminal end to amino acid residue 410 and functions in tissue-cell specificity. The C domain (residues 410–495) function as the DNA binding domain (DBD) required for recognition of the target gene Progesterone responsive elements (PREs). The D domain (residues 495–540) is often referred to as the "hinge" region to designate its functional interaction with heat shock protein (Hsp 90) and other proteins 23, 70, and 54. The function of the E domain or Steroid binding domain (SBD) (residues 540–786) is to bind PR and trans-activate the DBD.

B–D. This is a diagram outlining PR interaction with the target gene PRE and DNA elements. The inactive form of the PR sediments as an inactive 8S complex, composed of Hsp 90 dimer, Hsp 70 and at least two other proteins, 23kD and 70kD. The present concept suggests that in the absence of progesterone (P), the Hsp 90 dimer is associated with the D domain or hinge region. The function of this complex is to maintain the PR in its inactive configuration. The binding of P in the hinge or E domain induces the release of the Hsp 90 dimer (and possibly the 23, 70, and 54) as the first step in the trans-activation of the C region or DBD domain, Figure 1B. When progesterone anagonist as RU486 binds to the SBD the heat shock protein 90 dimer fails to be released from the hinge region D and the inactive 8S PR complex fails to become trans-activated to the 4S PR configuration **C** and **D.**

Recent evidence also implicates phosphorylation as an essential final step of trans-activation of the DBD. As diagramed in **D,** the progesterone bound trans-activated PR requires phosphorylation in order to assume its function as a Protein-DNA-PRE complex. In its active configuration, the PR is maintained as a dimer, with the zinc finger region I interacting through a charge interaction with the DNA of the PRE in the major groove. The second zinc finger II appears to function to stabilize the PR dimer configuration as described in the text.

entiation of the tumor, prognosis for the patient and response to progestins. The duration of response is not predicted by the presence of receptor and varies from months to years. Tumors that lack ER and PR respond objectively to progestins in less than 10% of cases. Tumors that have been treated with radiotherapy have a greater tendency to be progesterone receptor negative than tumors that have not been treated with radiation. Because of the low toxicity of progestins, a trial of progestin therapy is often warranted, even if receptors have not been measured in the tumor or appear to be absent in recurrent or inoperable endometrial carcinoma.

The effective use of progestins in treating endometrial hyperplasia associated with "unopposed" estrogen and in patients with receptor rich well-differentiated adenocarcinomas further supports the role of progestins in suppressing proliferation of the endometrium. While a reduction in the incidence of endometrial carcinoma is associated with including progestins in estrogen replacement regimes, it remains to be determined whether adding cyclic progestins is helpful or harmful in breast disease.

Other Neoplasms of the Uterus. Pharmacologic progestin has a clearly beneficial effect on uterine leiomyomas and significant levels of PR have been demonstrated in these proliferations of mesenchymal origin.[54] Uterine sarcomas, including stromal sarcomas and leiomyosarcomas, have a variable response to progesterone.[48] PR is not consistently observed in these tumors.

PR has been reported in some studies of squamous carcinoma of the uterine cervix (41% of tumors).[45] Cervical epithelial maturation was correlated with progesterone secretion (ovulation). PR was not found in the majority of tumors in other studies and no firm evidence for clinical or histologic correlation of the presence of PR has been shown.[20]

Breast

Normal Breast. Progestin response in the human breast is complex and influences both proliferation and differentiated function. The luteal phase of the menstrual cycle (progesterone dominant) is characterized both by active secretion and by the peak of proliferative activity in the normal breast.[56] Epidemiologic data appear to implicate progestins in proliferative disorders and cancers of the breast in a more direct fashion than had been previously thought.[56] It has been recognized from the earliest studies of ER and PR in breast epithelial systems that progesterone action, mediated through PR, resulted in the down regulation of the estrogen receptor in breast epithelium. This observation suggested that the influence of estrogen would be to stimulate proliferation of the breast epithelium and that the effect of progesterone might be to inhibit proliferation similar to the effect seen in the uterus. While the effect on regulation of ER appears to be similar, the effect of progestins and specifically progesterone in physiologic amounts is not similar. The assumption that progestins will act to reduce "estrogen associated" proliferative change does not appear to be valid. This must be considered in recommending sex steroid replacement therapy in the climacteric. Thought should be given to the fact that adding progestogen to estrogen replacement therapy does not reduce the risk of breast cancer and may actually increase it.[56] Three factors support this consideration: 1) ovarian hormones are critical to breast cancer risk; 2) inclusion of progestin in combination oral contraceptive pills does not effectively oppose the risk of cancer; and 3)

in individuals who have had surgical oophorectomy, even daily unopposed conjugated estrogens at a dose of 1.25 mg/day does not produce risk comparable to that associated with prolonged years of "normal" menstrual cycles or with replacement therapy with estrogen and progestin in the climacteric.

Breast Cancer. Progesterone receptors have been extensively studied in human breast cancer. Patients whose tumors are progesterone receptor positive have a higher probability of responding to endocrine therapy (not necessarily progestins), and in most series show a somewhat better prognosis both with respect to survival and disease free interval.[11] Progesterone receptor, in contrast to estrogen receptor, does not show increasing levels with increasing age of the population studied.[57]

Progestin therapy in metastatic breast cancer has been principally used as a second-line therapy following Tamoxifen. The principal progestin used has been megestrol acetate (Megace). The response of metastatic breast cancer to megestrol is predicted by the presence of estrogen receptor and/or progesterone receptor, but is best predicted by the observation of objective response to prior hormonal therapy.[74] One of the more interesting aspects of progestin therapy for metastatic breast cancer is the observation of a dose response increase in efficacy. Patients who have relapsed or progressed on conventional therapeutic doses of medroxyprogesterone (100–200 mg/day) or megestrol (160 mg/day) may show additional response with increased dose (to 2,000 mg/day for medroxyprogesterone or to 1,600 mg/day for megestrol). A beneficial side-effect of the progestin is increased appetite and weight gain, although some of the weight gain can be associated with fluid retention.[2] The mechanism of the increased appetite and actual weight gain is poorly understood although this property of appetite enhancement has been used clinically to treat cancer-associated anorexia and cachexia. There are a number of other central nervous system effects of progestins which have been characterized including beneficial effects on climacteric symptoms.[53]

Other Tumors of the Breast. Progesterone receptors have been reported in fibroadenomas, cystosarcoma phylloides and breast sarcomas. There is no convincing evidence for a biologic response of either cystosarcoma phylloides or stromal sarcoma of the breast to progestin manipulation.

Ovary

Epidemiologic data have shown a decrease in the incidence of ovarian epithelial carcinoma in patients who have used estrogen/progesterone preparations to inhibit ovulation. This reduction in tumor incidence does not appear to be a direct effect of the sex steroids on the ovarian epithelium but rather is mediated through FSH/LH or other factors associated with ovulation. Progesterone receptor is observed in 30–40% of ovarian carcinomas. While some studies have observed a trend toward better survival in patients with progesterone receptor positive carcinomas,[38] no data to indicate objective response to progestin therapy have been reported.

Other Tissues

Progesterone receptor and response to progestins has been reported in meningiomas, pulmonary lymphangioleiomyomatosis, renal cell carcinomas, and squamous cell carcinoma of the head and neck. The presence of progestin receptors in meningiomas is consistently observed and in some trials a response to progestin has been suggested,[41] although insufficient data exist to indicate what proportion of "receptor positive" meningiomas respond objectively to progestin therapy. In squamous cell carcinoma of the head and neck the presence of progestin receptors has been detected but in these tumors, as in renal cell carcinoma, objective response to progestin treatment has not been observed.[12] In contrast, progestin therapy has become a mainstay in the treatment of pulmonary lymphangioleiomyatosis which was a uniformly fatal condition before progestin/hormonal therapy was shown to be effective.[13] In patients with pulmonary lymphangiomyomatosis treated early in the course of the disease, before extensive chylous effusion is present, objective response to continued progesterone therapy is noted in the majority of patients. This response continues only so long as the progestin is continued. Responses of greater than 5 years have been observed, although in some patients the disease progresses after a period of remission despite continued progesterone.

Conclusion

Progesterone and the various synthetic progestins have a role in the treatment of a number of neoplasms, in particular tumors of the endometrium and breast. Study of the biochemistry of the progesterone receptor and the cellular mechanisms of progesterone action are prototypes for the study of the sex steroid hormone receptors. Further such studies are prerequisite to understanding the relationship of these hormones to development, differentiation and neoplasia in their target tissues.

References

1. Agutter, P. S.: Nucleo-cytoplasmic transport of mRNA: Its relationship to RNA metabolism, subcellular structures and other nucleocytoplasmic exchanges. *In* Progress in Molecular and Subcellular Biology. Edited by P. Jeanteur, Y. Kuchino, W. E. G. Muller, and P. L. Paine. New York, Springer-Verlag, 1988, pp. 15–96.
2. Aisner, J., Simon, T., Moody, M., and Tait, N.: High-dose megestrol acetate for the treatment of advanced breast cancer: dose and toxicities. Seminars in Hematology, 24:48, 1987.
3. Bagchi, M. K., Elliston, J. F., Tsai, S. Y., Edwards, D. P., Tsai, M. J., and O'Malley, B. W.: Steroid hormone-dependent interaction of human progesterone receptor with its target enhancer element. Mol. Endocrinol., 2:1221, 1988.
4. Bagchi, M. K., Tsai, S. Y., Weigel, N. L., Tsai, M. J., and O'Malley, B. W.: Regulation of in vitro transcription by progesterone receptor characterization and kinetic studies. J. Biol. Chem., 265:5129, 1990.
5. Baulieu, E. E.: RU486 (an anti-steroid hormone) receptor structure and heat shock protein mol. wt 90,000 (hsp 90). Hum. Reprod., 3:541, 1988.
6. Baulieu, E. E.: A novel approach to human fertility control: contragestion by the antiprogesterone RU 486. Eur. J. Obstet. Gynecol. Reprod. Biol., 28:125, 1988.
7. Baulieu, E. E.: Contragestion and other clinical applications of RU 486, an antiprogesterone at the receptor. Science, 245:1351, 1989.
8. Bautz, K. F., and Petersen, G.: Eukaryotic RNA polymerases. *In* Molecular Biology of Chromosome Function. Edited by K. W. Adolph. New York, Springer-Verlag, 1989, pp. 157–206.
9. Beato, M.: Gene regulation by steroid hormones.Cell, 56:335, 1989.
10. Ben-Ze'ev, A., and Amsterdam, A.: Regulation of heat shock protein synthesis by gonadotropins in cultured granulosa cells. Endocrinology, 124:2584, 1989.
11. Benner, S. E., Clark, G. M., and McGuire, W. L.: Steroid receptors, cellular kinetics, and lymph node status as prognostic factors in breast cancer. Am. J. Med. Sci., 296:59, 1988.
12. Berg, N. J., Colvard, D. S., Neel, H. B., III, Weiland, L. H., and Spelsberg, T. C.: Progesterone receptors in carcinomas of the upper aerodigestive tract. Laryngol. Head Neck Surgery, 101: 527,1989.
13. Berger, U., Khaghani, A., Pomerance, A., Yacoub, M. H., and Coombes, R. C.: Pulmonary lymphangioleiomyomatosis and steroid RE receptors. An immunocytochemical study. Am. J. Clin. Pathol., 93:609, 1990.
14. Bernues, J., and Querol, E.: Non-random reconstitution of HMG1 and HMG2 in chromatin. Determination of the histone contacts. Biochimica et Biophysica Acta, 1008:52, 1989.
15. Bocquel, M. T., Kumar, V., Stricker, C., Chambon, P., and Gronemeyer, H.: The contribution of the N- and C-terminal regions of steroid receptors to activation of transcription is both receptor and cell-specific. Nucleic Acids Res., 17:2581, 1989.
16. Bradshaw, M. S., Tsai, M. J., and O'Malley, B. W.: A steroid response element can function in the absence of a distal promoter TX 77030. Mol. Endocrinol., 2:1286, 1988.
17. Carson-Jurica, M. A., Lee, A. T., Dobson, A. W., Conneely, O. M., Schrader, W. T.,

and O'Malley, B. W.: Interaction of the chicken progesterone receptor with heat shock protein (HSP) 90. J. Steroid. Biochem., 34:1, 1989.
18. Carson-Jurica, M. A., Schrader, W. T., and O'Malley, B. W.: Steroid receptor family: Structure and functions. Endocr. Rev., 11:201, 1990.
19. Chilton, B. S., Mani, S. K., Bullock, D. W.: Servomechanism of prolactin and progesterone in regulating uterine gene expression. Mol. Endocrin., 2:1169, 1988.
20. Ciocca, D. R., Puy, L. A., and Fasoli, L. C.: Study of estrogen receptor, progesterone receptor, and the estrogen-regulated mr 24,000 protein in patients with carcinomas of the endometrium and cervix. Cancer Res., 49:4298, 1989.
21. Conneely, O. M., Dobson, A. D., Carson, M. A., Maxwell, B. L., Tsai, M. J., Schrader, W. T., and O'Malley, B. W.: Structure-function relationships of the chicken progesterone receptor. Biochem. Soc. Trans., 16:683, 1988.
22. Conneely, O. M., Kettelberger, D. M., Tsai, M. J., Schrader, W. T., and O'Malley, B. W.: The chicken progesterone receptor A and B isoforms are products of an alternate translation initiation event. J. Biol. Chem., 264:14062, 1989.
23. Dean, D. C., Knoll, B. J., Riser, M. E., and O'Malley, B. W.: A 5'-flanking sequence essential for progesterone regulation of an ovalbumin fusion gene. Nature, 305:551, 1983.
24. Dobson, A. D., Conneely, O. M., Beattie, W., Maxwell, B. L., Mak, P., Tsai, M. J., Schrader, W. T., and O'Malley, B. W.: Mutational analysis of the chicken progesterone receptor. J. Biol. Chem., 264:4207, 1989.
25. Duffy, M. J.: Biochemical markers as prognostic indices in breast cancer. Clin. Chem., 36:188, 1990.
26. Dufrene, L., Pageaux, J. F., Fanidi, A., Renoir, J. M., Laugier, C., and Baulieu, E. E.: Biochemical characterization and subunit structure of quail oviduct progesterone receptor. J. Steroid. Biochem., 32:703, 1989.
27. Eilers, M., Picard, D., Yamamoto, K. R., and Bishop, J. M.: Chimaeras of myc oncoprotein and steroid receptors cause hormone-dependent transformation of cells foundation. Nature, 340:66, 1989.
28. Eul, J., Meyer, M. E., Tora, L., Bocquel, M. T., Quirin-Stricker, C., Chambon, P., and Gronemeyer, H.: Expression of active hormone and DNA-binding domains of the chicken progesterone receptor in E. coli. EMBO J., 8:83, 1989.
29. Evans, R. M., and Hollenberg, S. M.: Cooperative and positional independent transactivation domains of the human glucocorticoid receptor. Cold Spring Harbor Symp. Quant. Biol., 53:813, 1988.
30. Evans, R. M., and Hollenberg, S. M.: Zinc fingers: gilt by association. Cell, 52:1, 1988.
31. Fink, K. L., Wieben, E. D., Woloschak, G. E., and Spelsberg, T. C.: Rapid regulation of c-myc protooncogene expression by progesterone in the avian oviduct. Proc. Natl. Acad. Sci. U.S.A., 85:1796, 1988.
32. Freedman, L. P., Yoshinaga, S. K., Vanderbilt, J. N., and Yamamoto, K. R.: In vitro transcription enhancement by purified derivatives of the glucocorticoid receptor. Science, 245:298, 1989.
33. Gasc, J. M., and Baulieu, E. E.: Regulation by estradiol of the progesterone receptor in the hypothalamus and pituitary: an immunohistochemical study in the chicken. Endocrinology, 122:1357, 1988.
34. Gasc, J. M., Renoir, J. M., Faber, L. E., Delahaye, F., and Baulieu, E. E.: Nuclear localization of two steroid receptor-associated proteins, hsp90 and p59. Exp. Cell Res., 186:362, 1990.
35. Gompel, A., Malet, C., Spritzer, P., Lalardrie, J. P., Kuttenn, F., and Mauvais-Jarvis, P.: Progestin effect on cell proliferation and 17 beta-hydroxysteroid dehydrogenase activity in normal human breast cells in culture. J. Clin. Endocrin. Metab., 63:1174, 1986.
36. Green, S., and Chambon, P.: A superfamily of potentially oncogenic hormone receptors. Nature, 324:615, 1986.
37. Green, S., and Chambon, P.: Oestradiol induction of a glucocorticoid-responsive gene by a chimaeric receptor. Nature, 325:75, 1987.
38. Green, S., and Chambon, P.: Nuclear receptors enhance our understanding of transcription regulation. TIG, 4:309, 1988.
39. Gronemeyer, H.: The Chicken Progesterone Receptor. *In* Affinity Labelling and Cloning of Steroid and Thyroid Hormone Receptors. Edited by H. Gronemeyer, USA and Canada, Ellis Horwood, 1988, pp. 55-67.
40. Grunstein, M., Han, M., Kim, U., Schuster, T., and Kayne, P.: Histone and Nucleosome Function in Yeast. *In* Molecular Biology of Chromosome Function. Edited by K. W. Adolph. New York, Springer-Verlag, 1989, pp. 347–365.
41. Halper, J., Colvard, D. S., Scheithauer, B. W., Jiang, N-S., Press, M. F., Graham, M. L., Riehl, E., Laws, E. R., and Spelsberg, T. C.: Estrogen and progesterone receptors in meningiomas: comparison of nuclear binding, dextran-coated charcoal and immunoperoxidase staining assays. Neurosurgery, 25:546, 1989.
42. Hard, T., Kellenbach, E., Boelens, R., Maler, B. A., Dahlman, K., Freedman, L., Carlstedt-Duke, J., Yamamoto, K. R., Gustafsson, J., and Kaptein, R.: Solution structure of the glucocorticord receptor DNA-binding domain. Science, 249:157, 1990.
43. Harding, M., Cowan, S., Hole, D., Cassidy, L., Kitchener, H., Davis, J., and Leake, R.: Estrogen and progesterone receptors in ovarian cancer. Cancer, 65:486, 1990.
44. Horwitz, K. B., and Francis, M. D. Photoaffinity Labeling of the Human Progesterone Receptor. *In* Affinity Labelling and Cloning of Steroid and Thyroid Receptors. Edited by H. Gronemeyer. USA and Canada, Ellis Horwood, 1988, pp. 186–198.
45. Hunter, R. E., Longcope, C., and Keough, P.: Steroid hormone receptors in carcinoma of the cervix. Cancer; 60:392, 1987.
46. Isola, J. J.: Distribution of estrogen and progesterone receptors and steroid-regulated gene products in the chick oviduct. Mol. Cell. Endocrinol., 69:235, 1990.
47. Kastner, P., Krust, A., Turcotte, B., Stropp, U., Tora, L., Gronemeyer, H., and Chambon, P.: Two distinct estrogen-regulated promoters generate transcripts encoding the two functionally different human progesterone receptor forms A and B. EMBO J., 9:1603, 1990.
48. Keen, C. E., and Philip, G.: Progestogen-induced regression in low-grade endometrial stromal sarcoma. Case report and literature review. Br. J. Obstet. Gynaecol., 96:1435, 1989.
49. Kelner, D. N., and McCarty, K. S., Sr.: Porcine liver nuclear histone acetyltransferase: partial purification and basic properties. J. Biol. Chem., 259:3413, 1984.
50. Klein-Hitpass, L., Tsai, S. Y., Weigel, N. L., Allan, G. F., Riley, D., Rodriguez, R., Schrader, W. T., Tsai, M. J., and O'Malley, B. W.: The progesterone receptor stimulates cell-free transcription by enhancing the formation of a stable preinitiation complex. Cell, 60:247, 1990.
51. Kumar, V., Green, S., Stack, G., Berry, M., Jin, J. R., and Chambon, P.: Functional domains of the human estrogen receptor. Cell, 51:941, 1987.
52. Lessey, B. A., Metzger, D. A., Haney, A. F., and McCarty, K. S., Jr.: Immunohistochemical analysis of estrogen and progesterone receptor in endometriosis: Comparison with normal endometrium during the menstrual cycle and the effect of medical therapy. Fertil. Steril., 51:409, 1989.
53. Lobo, R. A., and Gibbons, W. E.: The role of progestin therapy in breast disease and central nervous system function. J. Reprod. Med., 27:515, 1982.

54. Maheux, R.: Treatment of uterine leiomyomata: past, present and future. Horm. Res., 32:125, 1989.
55. Maxwell, B. L., McDonnell, D. P., Conneely, O. M., Schulz, T. Z., Greene, G. L., and O'Malley, B. W.: Structural organization and regulation of the chicken estrogen receptor. Mol. Endocrinol., 1:25, 1987.
56. McCarty, K. S., Jr.: Proliferative stimuli in the normal breast: Estrogens or progestins. Hum. Pathol., 20:1137, 1989.
57. McCarty, K. S., Jr., Silva, J. S., Cox, E. B., Leight, G. S., Jr., Wells, S. A., and McCarty, K. S., Sr.: Relationship of age and menopausal status to estrogen receptor content in primary carcinoma of the breast. Ann. Surg., 197:123, 1983.
58. Meyer, M. E., Gronemeyer, H., Turcotte, B., Bocquel, M. T., Tasset, D., and Chambon, P.: Steroid hormone receptors compete for factors that mediate their enhancer function. Cell, 57:433, 1989.
59. Miesfeld, R. L.: The structure and function of steroid receptor proteins. Crit. Rev. Biochem. Mol. Biol., 24:101, 1989.
60. Mold, D. E., and McCarty, K. S., Sr.: A chinese hamster ovary cell histone deacetylase that is associated with a unique class of mononucleosomes. Biochemistry, 26:8257, 1987.
61. Moore, D. D.: Promiscuous behaviour in the steroid hormone receptor superfamily. Trends Neurosci., 12:165, 1989.
62. Nardulli, A. M., Greene, G. L., O'Malley, B. W., and Katzenellenbogen, B. S.: Regulation of progesterone receptor messenger ribonucleic acid and protein levels in mcf-7 cells by estradiol: analysis of estrogen's effect on progesterone receptor synthesis and degradation. Endocrinology, 122:935, 1988.
63. Nickerson, J. A., Krochmalnic, G., Wan, K. M., and Penman, S.: Chromatin architecture and nuclear RNA. Proc. Natl. Acad. Sci. U.S.A., 86:177, 1989.
64. O'Malley, B. W.: The steroid receptor superfamily: more excitement predicted for the future. Mol. Endocrinol., 4:353, 1990.
65. Oro, A. E., Hollenberg, S. M., and Evans, R. M.: Transcriptional inhibition by a glucocorticoid receptor-beta-galactosidase fusion protein studies. Cell, 55:1109, 1988.
66. Ottosson, U. B., Johansson, B. G., and Shultz, B.: Subfraction of high density lipoprotein cholesterol during estrogen replacement therapy: a comparison between progestogen and natural progesterone. Am. J. Obstet. Gynecol., 6:746, 1985.
67. Picard, D., Salser, S. J., and Yamamoto, K. R.: A movable and regulable inactivation function within the steroid binding domain of the glucocorticoid receptor. Cell, 54:1073, 1988.
68. Pinney, K. G., Carlson, K. E., and Katzenellenbogen, J. A.: A high affinity ligand and novel photoaffinity labeling reagent for the progesterone receptor. J. Steroid Biochem., 35:179, 1990.
69. Power, R. F., Conneely, O. M., McDonnell, D. P., Clark, J. H., Butt, T. R., Schrader, W. T., and O'Malley, B. W.: High level expression of a truncated chicken progesterone receptor in Escherichia coli. J. Biol. Chem., 265:1419, 1990.
70. Pratt, W. B., Jolly, D. J., Pratt, D. V., Hollenberg, S. M., Giguere, V., Cadepond, F. M., Schweizer-Groyer, G., Catelli, M. G., Evans, R. M., and Baulieu, E. E.: A region in the steroid binding domain determines formation of the non-DNA-binding, 9 S glucocorticoid receptor complex. J. Biol. Chem., 263:267, 1988.
71. Pratt, W. B., Redmond, T., Sanchez, E. R., Bresnick, E. H., Meshinchi, S., and Welsh, M. J.: Speculations on the Role of the 90 kDa Heat Shock Protein in Glucocorticoid Receptor Transport and Function. In The Steroid/Thyroid Hormone Receptor Family and Gene Regulation. Edited by J. Carlstedt-Duke, H. Eriksson, and J. A. Gustafsson. Basel: Birkhauser Verlag, 1989, pp. 109–126.
72. Radanyi, C., Renoir, J. M., Sabbah, M., and Baulieu, E. E.: Chick heat-shock protein of Mr = 90,000, free or released from progesterone receptor, is in a dimeric form. J. Biol. Chem., 264:2568, 1989.
73. Ree, A. H., Landmark, B. F., Eskild, W., Levy, F. O., Lahooti, H., Jahnsen, T., Aakvaag, A., and Hansson, V.: Autologous down-regulation of messenger ribonucleic acid protein levels for estrogen receptors in MCF-7 cells: An inverse correlation to progesterone receptor levels. Endocrinology, 124:2577, 1989.
74. Robertson, J. F. R., Williams, M. R., Todd, J., Nicholson, R. I., Morgan, D. A. I., and Blamey, R. W.: Factors predicting the response of patients with advanced breast cancer to endocrine (megace) therapy. Eur. J. Clin. Oncol., 25:469, 1989.
75. Rye, P. D., and Walker, R. A.: Analysis of glycoproteins released from benign and malignant human breast: changes in size and fucosylation with malignancy. Eur. J. Cancer Clin. Oncol., 25:65, 1989.
76. Sasano, H., Comerford, J., Wilkinson, D. S., Schwartz, A., and Garrett, C. T.: Serous papillary adenocarcinoma of the endometrium: Analysis of proto-oncogene amplification, flow cytometry, estrogen and progesterone receptors, and immunohistochemistry. Cancer, 65:1545, 1990.
77. Slater, E. P., Cato, A. C., Karin, M., Baxter, J. D., and Beato, M.: Progesterone induction of metallothionein-IIA gene expression. Mol. Endocrin., 2:485, 1988.
78. Schena, M., Freedman, L. P., and Yamamoto, K. R.: Mutations in the glucocorticoid receptor zinc finger region that distinguish interdigitated DNA binding and transcriptional enhancement activities. Genes Dev., 3:1590, 1989.
79. Smanik, E. J., Calderon, J. J., Muldoon, T. G., and Mahesh, V. B.: Effect of progesterone on the activity of occupied nuclear estrogen receptor in vitro. Mol. Biol., 64:111, 1989.
80. Spelsberg, T. C., Graham, M. L., Berg, N. J., Umehara, T., Riehl, E., Coulam, C. B., and Ingle, J. N.: A nuclear binding assay to assess the biological activity of steroid receptors in isolated animal and human tissues. Endocrinology, 121:631, 1987.
81. Spelsberg, T. C., Rories, C., Rejman, J. J., Goldberger, A., Fink, K., Lau, C. K., Colvard, D. S., and Wiseman, G.: Steroid action on gene expression: possible roles of regulatory genes and nuclear acceptor sites. Biol. Reprod., 40:54, 1989.
82. Spelsberg, T. C., Ruh, T., Ruh, M., Goldberger, A., Horton, M., Hora, J., and Singh, R.: Nuclear acceptor sites for steroid hormone receptors: comparisons of steroids and antisteroids. J. Steroid. Biochem., 31:579, 1988.
83. Tora, L., Gronemeyer, H., Turcotte, B., Gaub, M. P., and Chambon, P.: The N-terminal region of the chicken progesterone receptor specifies target gene activation. Nature, 333:185, 1988.
84. Tsai, S. Y., Tsai, M. J., and O'Malley, B. W.: Cooperative binding of steroid hormone receptors contributes to transcriptional synergism at target enhancer elements. Cell, 57:443, 1989.
85. Ueda, K., Isohashi, F., Okamoto, K., Yoshikawa, K., and Sakamoto, Y.: Interaction of rat liver glucocorticoid receptor with histones. Endocrinology, 124:1042, 1989.
86. Wahli, W.: Evolution and expression of vitellogenin genes. Trends Genet., 4:227, 1988.
87. Walter, P., Green, S., Greene, G. L., Krust, A., Bornert, J., Jeltsch, J., Staub, A., Jensen, E., Scrace, G., Waterfield, M., and Chambon, P.: Cloning of the human estrogen receptor cDNA. Proc. Natl. Acad. Sci. U.S.A., 82:7889, 1985.
88. Webster, N. J. G., Green, S., Jin, J. R., and Chambon, P.: The hormone-binding domains of the estrogen and glucocorticoid receptors contain an inducible transcription activation function. Cell, 54:199, 1988.
89. Weigel, N. L., Schrader, W. T., and O'Malley, B. W.: Antibodies to chicken progesterone receptor peptide 523-536 recognize a site exposed in receptor-deoxyribonucleic acid complexes but not in receptor-heat shock protein-90 complexes. Endocrinology, 125:2494, 1989.
90. Weinberger, C., and Bradley, D. J.: Gene regulation by receptors binding lipid-soluble substances. Ann. Rev. Physiol., 52:823, 1990.
91. Weissbach, A., Ward, C., and Bolden, A.: Eukaryotic DNA methylation and gene expression. Curr. Top. Cell Regul., 30:1, 1989.
92. Williams, J. A., Schlichter, D., and Wicks, W. D.: Progesterone decreases DNA binding factor activity and the expression in xenopus oocytes of a cAMP responsive gene from rat liver. Second Messengers and Phosphoproteins, 12:261, 1989.
93. Yamamoto, K. R., Godowski, P. J., and Picard, D.: Ligand-regulated nonspecific inactivation of receptor function: a versatile mechanism for signal transduction. Cold Spring Harbor Symp. Quant. Biol., 53:803, 1988.
94. Zeitlin, S., Parent, A., Silverstein, S., and Efstratiadis, A.: Pre-mRNA splicing and the nuclear matrix. Mol. Cell. Biol., 7:111, 1987.

XVII-9

Androgens and Antiandrogens

Nicholas Bruchovsky

Introduction

The collective title for compounds which resemble testosterone in biological action is the term androgen, derived from the Greek andros, genitive of aner (man) and gennan (to produce). The actual isolation and characterization of naturally occurring androgens in the 1930's was the crowning point of a process of observation and discovery which started at an early time in history, when primitive man first became aware of the more obvious effects of removing the testes from animals not excluding members of his own species. Castration is found in mythology, was a feature of certain religions, used as an instrument of punishment and revenge in many societies, and served to guarantee the supply of eunuchs for guard duty in harems, and of male sopranos for the embellishment of devout and secular music to the end of the 19th century.[22,30,93] Aristotle was the first to make castration the subject of enquiry describing its effect in considerable detail and recognizing that the testes were essential for the virility and fertility of an animal.[93] The first experimental demonstration that the testes contributed an endocrine factor to the bloodstream was made by John Hunter in 1794 when he showed that the spur of a hen would undergo masculine development if transplanted into the leg of a cock.[22] In 1849, Berthold reported that the secondary sexual characteristics of capons could be restored on transplantation of the testes from cocks.[7] In 1889, at the age of 72 years, Brown-Sequard gave himself subcutaneous injections of extracts from the testes of dogs and guinea pigs and reported an increased bodily and mental vigor which he correctly hesitated to ascribe to his preparation.[22] The first objective evidence of a hormonal rejuvenating factor was provided by Pezard in 1911 who showed that simple extracts of porcine testes contained active material.[22,30] Two decades later the first androgen, androsterone, was purified from human urine by Butenandt.[22,30] In 1935 David and colleagues isolated an androgenic compound from fresh testicular tissue more potent than androsterone which they named testosterone.[22] Shortly thereafter, the synthesis of testosterone from cholesterol by Ruzicka and Wettstein and Butenandt and Hanisch paved the way for the preparation of artificial androgens.[22] These achievements were succeeded by a long period of vigorous investigation of many aspects of the production, excretion, relative biological activity and clinical usefulness of androgenic compounds, including applications to the treatment of breast cancer.[92]

Opportunities for studying the molecular action of androgens emerged in the 1960's when radioactive compounds suitable for experimentation were initially introduced. In 1968, Bruchovsky and Wilson,[12] and Anderson and Liao[2] reported that dihydrotestosterone is the active intracellular form of testosterone, and receptors for dihydrotestosterone were demonstrated for the first time.[13] Subsequent attempts to purify the androgen receptor were met with little or no success; however in 1988, Trapman and colleagues,[102] Chang and colleagues,[24] and Lubahn and colleagues[59] cloned the androgen receptor complementary DNA and deduced the amino acid sequence of the receptor protein. Not only did these results confirm that the androgen receptor belongs to a superfamily of regulatory thyroid and steroid binding proteins, but also they provided exciting new clues to the relationship between primary structural changes in the androgen receptor and disorders of male sexual differentiation.

With the development of bioassays to measure androgenic activity, a large number of compounds with inhibitory action were found. In 1962 Dorfman suggested that substances with antiandrogenic activity might be useful in the treatment of hirsutism and androgen-dependent prostatic tumors.[31] Two years later, Lerner formalized the concept of hormone inhibition specifying that "an antagonist is a compound that inhibits the activity of a hormone at one or more sites without regard to the route of administration or the dose employed" and noted that antiandrogenic substances might be employed clinically to alleviate a number of pathological conditions.[57] In the next decade, the prototype antiandrogens cyproterone acetate[67] and flutamide[65] were synthesized and, as predicted, have been successfully applied to the treatment of a variety of androgen-dependent conditions.

Androgens

Mechanism of Action

The basic steps of androgen action on a target cell are outlined in Figure XVII-9-1. In the blood, testosterone, the principal male sex hormone secreted by the testes, circulates in association with two major plasma proteins, sex-hormone binding globulin (SHBG) and albumin.[33] Under equilibrium conditions, only 2% of the testosterone is unbound and available for diffusion into the target cell where it is immediately converted to dihydrotestosterone by the enzyme 5α-reductase.[12] Dihydrotestosterone binds with high affinity and specificity to a receptor protein in the cytoplasm to form an androgen-receptor complex which is then translocated into the target cell nucleus.

The androgen receptor itself is a transcription enhancer factor characterized by three major functional domains: a carboxyl (C)-terminal steroid binding domain, an N-terminal region involved in the activation of transcription, and an intermediate DNA-binding domain. The latter contains nine molecules of the amino acid cysteine, eight of which contribute to the formation of two finger-like projections each containing one molecule of zinc. The zinc finger couplet is thought to specify the particular hormone response element located in genomic DNA adjacent to target genes to which the androgen receptor binds. This binding reaction triggers a cascade of transcriptional events underlying a given biological response.

Under physiological conditions, not only is most of the dihydrotestosterone in the cell concentrated in the nucleus,[17] but also, in the presence of dihydrotestosterone, most of the androgen receptor in the cell is nuclear bound. Entry of dihydrotestosterone into the nucleus appears to depend largely on a non-receptor mediated transport process since the accumulation of dihydrotestosterone is 10- to 30-fold greater than that of receptor.[17,18]

Following orchiectomy or equivalent androgen withdrawal therapy the intranuclear concentration of dihydrotestosterone drops by about 90%, and most of the androgen receptor appears to leave the nucleus.[85] Formerly it was believed that all of the receptor is discharged into the cytoplasm, but a more up-to-date view is that at least some of it is retained in the nucleus in an inactive modified state which precludes the binding of either radioactive ligand or specific antibody and makes detection impossible.

Although the native androgen receptor possesses a molecular weight of 117,000 (4–5 S), the principal form recovered from the nucleus is a proteolytic fragment with a molecular weight of about 33,000 (3–4 S) which lacks the N-terminus but retains the steroid-binding properties of the native receptor.[20] As yet no functional role has been assigned to this fragment.

Biological Effects

The androgenic regulation of a target tissue is characterized by three broadly defined responses as shown in Figure XVII-9-2 for prostate.[16] In the presence of androgen, undifferentiated or involuted cells initiate new rounds of DNA synthesis and cell proliferation; the DNA initiation response (i.e., androgen sensitivity) is an example of positive gene regulation by androgens.[4] When the tissue becomes normal in size, a negative-feedback mechanism comes into play and shuts down DNA synthesis and cell proliferation. This distinctive "wearing-off" effect is a consequence of negative-gene regulation by androgens, i.e., transcription is inhibited in the presence of a rising concentration of hormone.[4] Withdrawal of androgen brings on autophagic lysis (apoptosis), which actively reduces the size of the prostate to a basal level. This manifestation of programmed cell death (i.e., androgen dependence) involves a number of androgen-repressed genes[63,84] which become active when androgens are withdrawn. A functional androgen-receptor mechanism is clearly essential for each type of response, but the manner

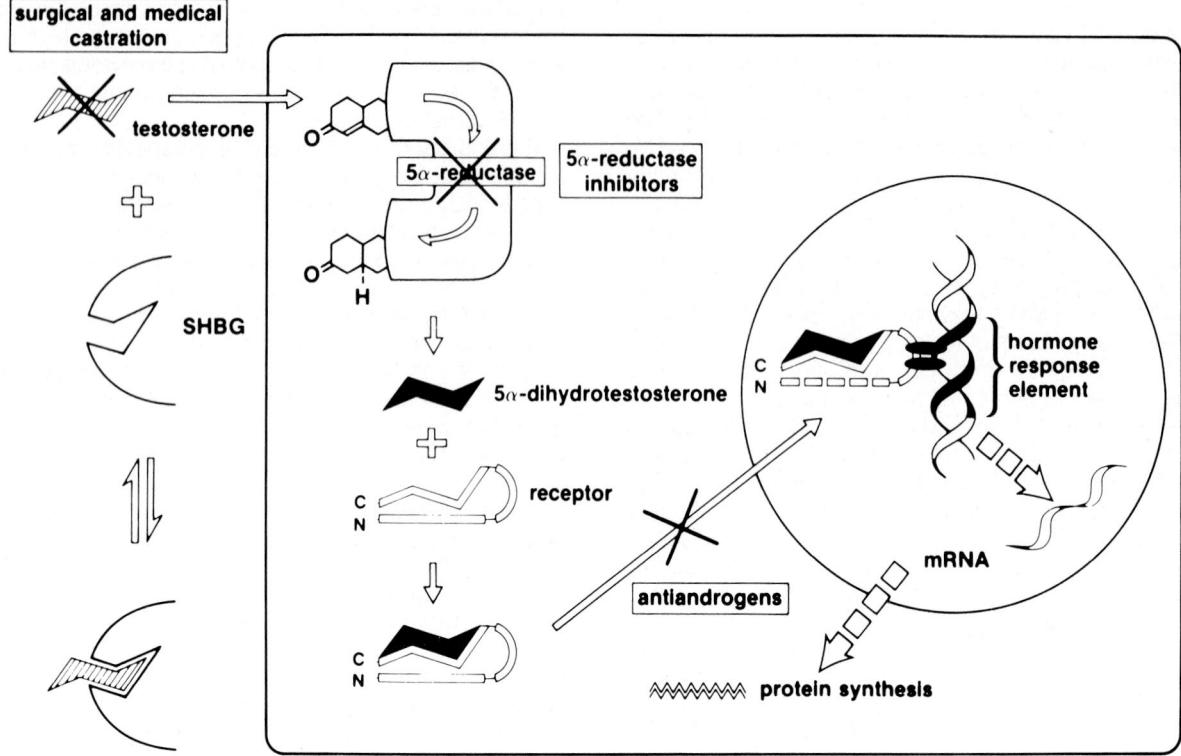

Figure XVII-9-1. The mechanism of action of androgens and types of androgen withdrawal therapy.

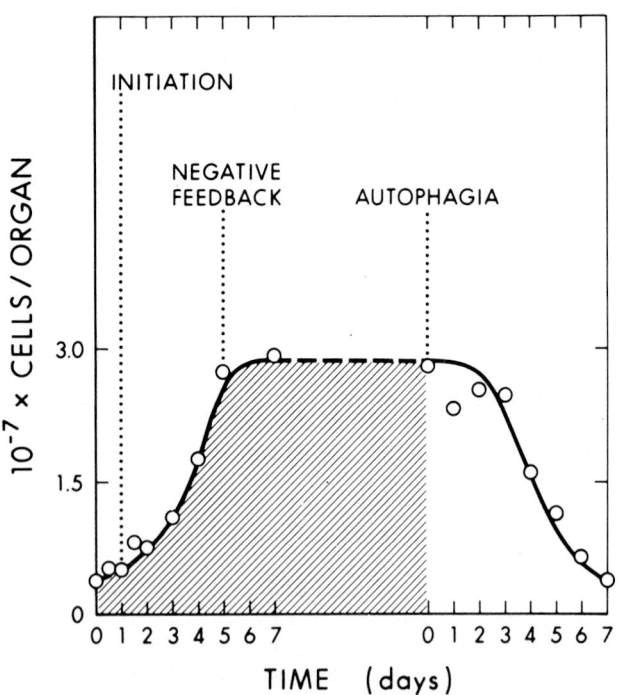

Figure XVII-9-2. Androgenic regulation of the prostate: 1) initiation of DNA synthesis and cell proliferation by androgens; 2) negative feedback; 3) autophagic lysis (apoptosis).[16]

in which the three levels of gene regulation is achieved by the androgen receptor acting as a single transcription regulatory factor has yet to be worked out.

Malignant transformation of a target cell is associated with progressive stepwise loss of hormonal regulation.[14] Deletion of the negative type of gene regulation (i.e., control over negative feedback) results in an androgen-sensitive, androgen-dependent tumor. Deletion of both the negative and androgen-repressed types of gene regulation (i.e., control over negative feedback and autophagic lysis) produces an androgen-sensitive, androgen-independent tumor. With further progression, positive-gene regulation (i.e., control over DNA initiation) disappears as well and the tumor, now androgen-insensitive and androgen-independent, is characterized by completely autonomous growth. Since all androgen-dependent and some androgen-independent tumors retain androgen-sensitivity, any treatment which elevates the concentration of plasma testosterone carries the risk of accelerated tumor growth and clinical manifestations of a flare reaction. Optimum therapeutic results will be observed when androgen withdrawal therapy has the double effect of arresting the initiation of DNA synthesis and inducing autophagic cell death. Withdrawal-induced killing of cells follows zero-order kinetics;[11] the one-time total cell kill is probably related but not proportional to the decrease in intranuclear concentration of dihydrotestosterone.

The system of androgen regulation described above for prostate is also observed in male breast cancer which responds to both orchiectomy and antiandrogens,[35,58] and is duplicated in the androgen-dependent Shionogi mouse mammary carcinoma.[19] In contrast, since female breast cancer is brought into remission by the administration of androgens, it is highly unlikely that the same regulatory mechanisms apply. In fact, androgen-induced responses appear to be mediated by the estrogen receptor, and the need for prior aromatization to estrogen has not been ruled out. Other less direct effects on growth factors, growth inhibitors and differentiation of malignant stem cells are also possible.

Description of Agents

A large number of androgens are available in potent forms for oral or parenteral administration; generally speaking, lower doses are anabolic, higher doses both anabolic and androgenic.[39] In recent years, such agents have gained notoriety owing to sensational revelations of improper usage in competitive sports where it is often taken for granted, rightly or wrongly, that an athlete's level of performance is improved by androgenic steroids, sometimes taken in massive doses.[109]

Ironically, as androgen misuse has become more prevalent, clinical interest in such compounds has waned. Once somewhat popular for the treatment of breast cancer, only a small number of androgens remain in use for this purpose. The most commonly used oral compounds are fluoxymesterone (10–20 mg/day) and methyltestosterone (50–100 mg/day); for intramuscular administration, nandrolone phenpropionate (25–50 mg/week) is sometimes tried. Agents are better tolerated if started at a lower dose and gradually increased until a clinical response is evident.

Clinical Applications

Breast Cancer. In previous detailed studies on the therapeutic effects of androgenic compounds in breast cancer, an objective response was observed in about 20% of women irrespective of menopausal status, and patients with objective remissions survived significantly longer than patients who did not respond.[1,92] From the outset, however, the use of androgens for treating breast cancer was not strongly endorsed owing to distressing physiological changes caused by therapy, i.e., deepening of the voice, hirsutism, acne, and seborrhea, increased libido, clitoral hypertrophy, alopecia and increased muscle mass.[1] In addition, treatment was sometimes complicated by hypercalcemia and symptomatic flare-up of disease.[103] Increasing use of tamoxifen, megestrol acetate, aminoglutethimide and cytotoxic drugs further reduced the need for androgens, now considered suitable only for third or fourth line therapy.[78]

Notwithstanding the disadvantages of androgens when administered at therapeutic doses, a more conservative regimen sometimes will produce minor but beneficial results; these include reduction of bone pain, augmented energy, improved appetite, and increased hemoglobin. Occasionally there is evidence of healing of bone metastases but in this respect androgens are probably no better than standard therapy.[1,97] Treatment can be started with a small amount of androgen (fluoxymesterone 5 mg/day) and gradually increased to a dose which restores the patient's sense of well-being but avoids virilization.

When fluoxymesterone (20 mg/day) and tamoxifen are given together, the objective response rate and time to progression are increased relative to results obtained with tamoxifen alone.[101] However, no significant differences between the two treatments with regard to duration of response or survival have been observed,[48] and in one study, monotherapy with tamoxifen was superior.[107] Owing to the lack of demonstrable effect on survival and the increased incidence of side effects, the combination of tamoxifen plus fluoxymesterone (20 mg/day) is not recommended for routine use in the treatment of breast cancer.[48] However, in certain situations the combination of low-dose fluoxymesterone (5–10 mg/day) with tamoxifen or megestrol acetate can be rationalized by the clinical value of the minor benefits related to the androgenic component of the treatment.

Androgenic agents, especially fluoxymesterone, continue to be included in multiple-drug chemotherapy regimens for advanced breast cancer. In studies by Tormey and colleagues, the addition of androgen was associated with maintenance of higher blood counts, better tolerance of chemotherapy and a longer time to treatment failure.[100] Thus, it may be possible to bring about a greater degree of cell kill if the bone marrow is supported by androgens. The dose of fluoxymesterone used in such protocols is usually 20 mg/day but lower doses might be tried to keep side-effects to a minimum.

Prostate Cancer. In the past, testosterone was given occasionally as initial hormonal therapy of prostate cancer,[10,37,79] and also as a form of "shock" therapy to re-establish the estrogen-responsiveness of a tumor.[74] More recently, it has been used as a priming agent to increase the rate of proliferation of advanced (androgen-sensitive, androgen-independent) prostate cancer. In theory, since the uptake of lethal radioactive isotopes and cytotoxic drugs is greater in rapidly dividing cells than in slowly growing or resting cells, there should be a proportional increase in cell kill. Unfortunately, the high incidence of bone pain, urinary obstruction, spinal cord compression and other adverse responses has discouraged acceptance of this approach.[36,62,98]

It has been pointed out that androgen priming might be more beneficial if instituted 2–3 months after orchiectomy when tumor burden has reached a nadir.[62] Not only would there be less chance of major side-effects, but, in theory, chemotherapy should be more effective in the presence of minimal disease.[11] An attractive alternative to priming with exogenous androgen is self-priming,[40] a stratagem which relies on the gradual recovery of testicular function after the interruption of certain types of androgen withdrawal therapy (Table XVII-9-1) where the suppressive effects are completely reversible. It should be emphasized that the potential of such applications remains to be fully explored, and, as yet, there are no clear indications for the use of androgens in prostate cancer treatment.

Antiandrogens

Description of Agents

According to Dorfman, "antiandrogens are substances which prevent androgens from expressing their activity at target sites."[32] He suggested that the inhibitory effect of these substances should be differentiated from compounds which decrease the secretion of hypothalamic releasing factors and anterior pituitary hormones, particularly luteinizing hormone. He also excluded materials which act directly on the gonads to inhibit synthesis and secretion of androgens. From a practical point of view, it is difficult to adhere to this definition. On the one hand, antiandrogens with a progestin-like

Table XVII-9-1. Androgen Withdrawal Therapies

Type	Supplied	Administration	Dose
Standard			
Orchiectomy[47]			
Diethylstilbestrol (DES)[99]	Tablet	p.o.	1 mg t.i.d.
Steroidal antiandrogens			
Cyproterone acetate (Androcur)[72]	Tablet	p.o.	100 mg b.i.d.
Megestrol acetate (Megace)[38]	Tablet	p.o.	160 mg q.d.
Nonsteroidal antiandrogens			
Flutamide (Eulevin)[80]	Tablet	p.o.	250 mg t.i.d.
Nilutamide (Anandron)[6]	Tablet	p.o.	100 mg t.i.d.
ICI 176,334 (Casodex)[61]	Tablet	p.o.	50 mg q.d.
LHRH agonists			
Leuprolide (Lupron)[99]	Aqueous solution	s.c.	1.0 mg q.d.
	Suspension of microcapsules	i.m.	7.5 mg q.4 w.
Goserelin (Zoladex)[28]	Cylindrical implant	s.c.	3.6 mg q.4 w.
Buserelin (Suprefact)[55]	Aqueous solution	s.c.	200 μg q.d.
		i.n.	400 μg t.i.d.
Nafarelin (Synarel)[76]	Aqueous solution	i.n.	200 μg b.i.d.
Tryptorelin (Decapeptyl)[42]	Suspension of microcapsules	i.m.	2.8 mg q.4 w.
5α-reductase inhibitors			
Finasteride (Proscar)[106]		p.o.	5 mg q.d.
Adrenalectomy			
Medical (aminoglutethimide)[46]			
Surgical[43]			
Steroidogenesis inhibitors			
Aminoglutethimide (Cytadren)[46]	Tablet	p.o.	250 mg b.i.d.
Ketoconazole (Nizoral)[104]	Tablet	p.o.	400 mg t.i.d.

Combinations
A. *Concurrent*
      Orchiectomy + cyproterone acetate (p.o. 50 mg b.i.d.)[90]
      Orchiectomy + nilutamide (p.o. 50 mg t.i.d.)[6]
      Cyproterone acetate (p.o. 100 mg b.i.d.) + low-dose DES (p.o. 0.1 mg q.d.)[41]
      Megestrol acetate (p.o. 120 mg q.d.) + low-dose DES (p.o. 0.1 mg q.d.)[105]
      Leuprolide (s.c. 1.0 mg q.d.) + flutamide (p.o. 250 mg t.i.d.)[26]
      Goserelin (s.c. 3.6 mg q.4w.) + flutamide (p.o. 250 mg t.i.d.)[50]
      Buserelin (s.c. 500 μg q.d.) + nilutamide (p.o. 100 mg q.d.)[56]
      Buserelin (s.c. 1.5 mg q.d.) + cyproterone acetate (50 mg t.i.d.)[87]

B. *Sequential* (to eliminate flare reaction)
      DES (p.o. 1 mg t.i.d.) + leuprolide (s.c. 1 mg q.d.)[96]
      Cyproterone acetate (p.o. 100 mg t.i.d.) + buserelin (s.c. 1.5 mg q.d.)[8]
      Cyproterone acetate (p.o. 50 mg b.i.d.) + low-dose DES (p.o. 0.1 mg q.d.) + goserelin (s.c. 3.6 mg q.4w)[15]

ring structure are both antigonadotropic and antiandrogenic and would not meet Dorfman's criteria. On the other hand, a 5α-reductase inhibitor might qualify under a liberal interpretation of the criteria, but in the mechanistic sense is not an antiandrogen. Since antiandrogens are frequently combined with LHRH agonists and other agents, their individual effects may be of little relevance in therapeutic situations.

Until recently, androgen withdrawal therapy was restricted to a choice between bilateral orchiectomy or estrogens usually in the form of diethylstilbestrol. When these measures failed, adrenalectomy was occasionally tried, seldom yielding an objective response.[43,64] The advent of antiandrogens and luteinizing-hormone releasing-hormone (LHRH) agonists has greatly increased the number of options which are now available for suppressing the influence of androgens on the growth of prostate cancer (Table XVII-9-1).

Mechanism of Action

The effectiveness of an antiandrogen either alone or in combination with other agents is related to its ability to reduce the amount of functionally active androgen receptor in the nucleus of the target cell (Figure XVII-9-1).[85] This is accomplished therapeutically to varying degrees by medical or surgical castration, the inhibition of 5α-reductase activity, and the blockade of receptor translocation into the nucleus by steroidal and nonsteroidal antiandrogens. The nuclear depletion of androgen receptor is thought to be more complete with those types of androgen-withdrawal therapy that combine medical or surgical castration with a steroidal or nonsteroidal antiandrogen; however, there is no direct experimental evidence showing that this assumption is correct.[89] Each particular type of treatment has both advantages and disadvantages which are related to effects on both the target cell and the hypothalamic-pituitary-gonadal axis of the endocrine system. Some of the main changes for several representative treatments are described below.

Normal Regulation

The normal pathways of the neuroendocrine control of gonadal function are summarized in Figure XVII-9-3A. Testicular synthesis of testosterone accounts for 90% or more of the dihydrotestosterone formed in the prostate,[85] the remainder being derived from the weak adrenal androgens androstenedione and dehydroepiandrosterone,[21] and dietary sources. Testosterone provides a negative-feedback signal to the hypothalamus regulating the secretion of LHRH and thereby of luteinizing hormone (LH). Negative feedback regulation of the hypothalamus by testosterone also involves the release of endogenous opioid peptides which act as inhibitory factors to suppress the intrahypothalamic release of catecholamines (norepinephrine and dopamine); the amount of LHRH secreted is directly proportional to the concentration of catecholamines in the hypothalamus.[81]

Orchiectomy

The principal result of bilateral orchiectomy, as shown in Figure XVII-9-3B, is the elimination of the testicular source of testosterone. Not only does this result in lowering of the concentration of dihydrotestosterone in the prostate but it also eliminates the negative-feedback regulation of the hypothalamus. Resultant increases in the circulating levels of LHRH and LH are probably without significance except for their indirect association with vasomotor symptoms. Since the concentration of testosterone-dependent opioid peptide decreases, catecholamine levels in the hypothalamus increase with consequent stimulation of the thermal regulatory centre.[81]

Radio-orchiectomy for the treatment of metastatic prostatic carcinoma was first described by Keyes and Ferguson in 1936,[94] and surgical orchiectomy by Huggins and Hodges in 1941;[47] the latter procedure has withstood the test of time and remains the standard therapy for advanced prostate cancer. All patients are rendered impotent and hot flashes are experienced by many.

Estrogens

As depicted in Figure XVII-9-3C, estrogenic compounds such as diethylstilbestrol substitute for testosterone in the negative-feedback inhibition of the hypothalamus. The resultant suppression of both LHRH and LH is accompanied by marked lowering of the concentration of plasma testosterone (radioimmunoassay measures total of bound and free) into the castrate range. Estrogens were used for the treatment of prostate cancer as early as 1935[94] and diethylstilbestrol continues to be employed as a cost-effective drug for this condition. Loss of libido and potency, gynecomastia, breast tenderness, cardiovascular complications, edema, deep vein thrombosis and pulmonary embolus are the chief side-effects.[23,99]

Cyproterone Acetate

Cyproterone acetate, derived from 17α-hydroxyprogesterone, is characterized by progestin-like activity in addition to being a potent antiandrogen; the resultant dual mode of action[66,67,72] is illustrated in Figure XVII-9-3D. Owing to its progestational properties, cyproterone acetate simulates the negative feedback inhibition of the hypothalamus by testosterone; in addition to lowering the concentration of testosterone in the blood, it is active at the peripheral level where it inhibits the translocation of androgen receptor from cytoplasm to nucleus in the prostate and other target tissues.[85] Hot flashes are rarely experienced since the antigonadotropic negative-feedback of testosterone is replaced by that of cyproterone acetate. The most frequently recorded adverse effects of treatment are those related to hormone deprivation, namely loss of libido, impotence, reduced energy and weakness. Drug related effects include nipple tenderness, breast swelling, shortness of breath and thrombosis, but the complication rate is low relative to that observed with diethylstilbestrol.[27,41] Megestrol acetate,[38] another member of the large steroidal antiandrogen group of compounds,[82] is similar in action to cyproterone acetate.

Flutamide

The action of nonsteroidal antiandrogens of the flutamide type[65,88] is illustrated in Figure XVII-9-3E. Flutamide inhibits the translocation of androgen receptor from cytoplasm to nucleus in target tissues including both the prostate and the hypothalamus. Negative-feedback signals provided by testosterone are no longer registered in the hypothalamus with resultant increases in the secretion of LHRH and LH. The testis is stimulated to increase its production of testosterone resulting in an elevation of plasma testosterone.[53,60,73] The mean concentration increases slowly to a peak 50% above the mean normal value after 6 months of treatment; a gradual decline follows such that after 12 months a normal baseline value is again observed.[60] Corresponding fluctuations are likely to take place in the concentration of dihydrotestosterone in tissue[85] and there is some doubt whether the rising titers of testosterone and dihydrotestosterone are wholly offset by the peripheral antiandrogenic action of the drug.[88] Indeed, the observation that the plasma testosterone level declines after 6 months implies that the negative-feedback effect of testosterone on the hypothalamus is re-established at this time owing to diminished effectiveness of the flutamide-dependent receptor blockade. Persistence of normal or elevated levels of plasma testosterone probably account for the low incidence of hot flashes and the preservation of potency in 70–80% of men receiving the agent.[73,80,95] About one-half of all patients are already impotent at the time when they first require systemic therapy for metastatic prostate cancer; thus the benefit of flutamide in maintaining potency is limited to the other one-half, or about 40% of the total number.

Another consequence of the excessive production of testosterone is a higher level of estrogen in the bloodstream[53] with the attendant side effect of gynecomastia in 60–70% of patients.[73,80,95] Occasionally severe and painful, the gynecomastia can be averted by prior irradiation of breast tissue. Other side effects in order of importance include diarrhea, nausea, vomiting and reversible abnormalities of liver enzymes. The related agent, nilutamide, in addition causes visual disturbances and alcohol intolerance both of which to some extent limit its usefulness.[6]

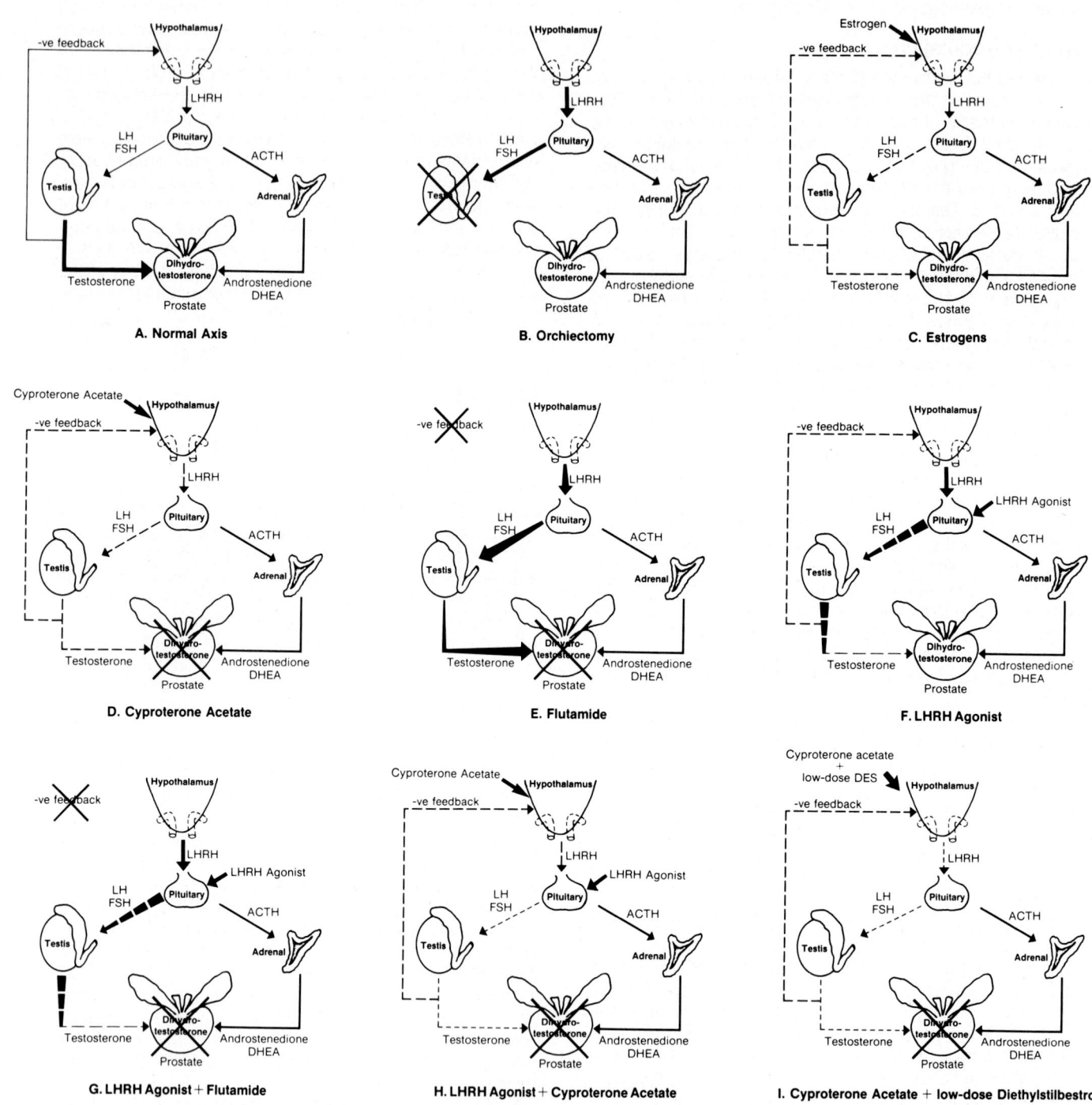

Figure XVII-9-3. Effects of antiandrogens on the hypothalamic-pituitary-gonadal axis of the endocrine system.

LHRH Agonists

The inhibitory action of an LHRH agonist is characterized by many changes in the hypothalamic-pituitary-gonadal axis as shown in Figure XVII-9-3F. The pituitary is normally stimulated by the pulsatile release of LHRH from the hypothalamus; when this periodicity is effaced by the continuous infusion of an exogenous LHRH agonist the pituitary becomes refractory to hypothalamic regulation. Gonadotropin secretion initially rises and then tapers off as does the secretion of testosterone by the testis. Associated with the initial transient surge in plasma testosterone is an acute exacerbation of clinical symptoms and signs (flare reaction) in 5–10% of patients.[103] In addition transient prostatic enlargement may occur in 30–50% of men [54,76] and presumably tumor growth is temporarily stimulated with similar frequency. Thus, until it is definitely known whether or not an LHRH agonist causes early flare-related progression of disease, the assumption that LHRH agonist monotherapy is equivalent to conventional treatment of prostate cancer should be accepted with caution.[29] LHRH agonists generally do not produce any side effects except for hot flashes in 60–70% of patients and loss of libido and potency in all patients.

LHRH Agonist and Flutamide. In attempts to cancel out the adverse features of nonsteroidal antiandrogens and LHRH agonists, the agents have been combined to achieve a better balance of control of testicular function as shown in Figure XVII-9-3G.[26] On the one hand, the LHRH agonist prevents the rise in the titer of plasma testosterone caused by flutamide or similar antiandrogen (i.e., nilutamide). On the other hand, flutamide reduces the risk of a flare reaction that may occur during the surge in the concentration of plasma testosterone caused by the LHRH agonist.

Since adrenal androgens have yet to be implicated in the recurrent growth of prostate cancer,[68,89,90] the strongest justification for combining an antiandrogen with an LHRH agonist is to avert symptoms, signs and other untoward side-effects of a flare reaction. Moreover, once the concentration of plasma testosterone is in the castrate range and the danger of a flare reaction has passed, it is probably unnecessary to continue the antiandrogenic component of therapy. This conclusion is supported by the failure of combined therapy with an LHRH agonist and flutamide (i.e., complete androgen blockade) to improve survival over that observed with standard therapy of orchiectomy alone.[50,86] Side effects associated with treatment are loss of libido and potency in all patients, and hot flashes in 60–70%.

LHRH Agonist and Cyproterone Acetate. As shown in Figure XVII-9-3H the combination of an LHRH agonist and cyproterone acetate preserves the negative-feedback mechanism in the hypothalamus owing to the progestational action of cyproterone acetate.[87] Furthermore, if cyproterone acetate is administered for several days prior to the first administration of LHRH agonist, the plasma concentrations of LH and testosterone will be suppressed, eliminating the risk of a biochemical or clinical flare reaction.[8] Longer term administration of cyproterone acetate (100 mg/day) reduces the incidence of hot flashes.[81] All patients are rendered impotent by therapy.

Cyproterone Acetate and Low-Dose Diethylstilbestrol

One of the shortcomings of androgen withdrawal therapy with either cyproterone acetate or megestrol acetate is that the suppression of hypothalamic function is incomplete and the testis thus continues to synthesize a small amount of testosterone. In therapeutic situations, this may not be important in view of the peripheral antiandrogenic action of these agents; nonetheless, in order to reinforce the central inhibitory action of the antiandrogens on the hypothalamus (Figure XVII-9-3I), they may be combined with a very small amount of an estrogen such as diethylstilbestrol (0.1 mg/day) if plasma testosterone is to be maintained in the castrate range.[38,41,105] The cyproterone acetate (100–200 mg/day) and low-dose diethylstilbestrol (0.1 mg/day) combination has been shown to have a rapid onset of action significantly lowering the concentration of plasma testosterone within 1 day, and down to the castrate range within 1 week.[41] Side effects are similar to those reported for cyproterone acetate alone.

Other Actions

In experimental situations, both steroidal and nonsteroidal antiandrogens sometimes demonstrate anomalous activity and appear to behave as weak androgens.[3,108] Cyproterone acetate is known to have virilizing effects during fetal development of some animal species, and at very high doses will delay the involution of the prostate in castrated rats.[34] Since glucocorticoids in high doses will also retard the involution of prostatic tissue,[83] the slowing action of cyproterone acetate is probably an indication of slight glucocorticoid activity related to its structural similarity to progesterone. Detailed information on such effects is available, and there are no findings indicative of a potential hazard or limitation with respect to the clinical use of steroidal antiandrogens such as cyproterone acetate in prostate cancer.[45]

Both steroidal and nonsteroidal antiandrogens have also been found to stimulate the growth of prostatic cells in tissue culture.[69,108] The mechanism of this effect has not been explained but may be related to a direct or indirect effect on negative-gene regulation (Fig. 2) rather than a direct effect on cell proliferation. While such paradoxical effects in experimental systems will undoubtedly provide more insight into the mechanisms which regulate the growth and maintenance of prostate, in the more physiological setting of normal or abnormal prostate function, the possibility of any clinical significance is remote.

Clinical Applications

Breast Cancer. Experience with antiandrogens in the treatment of breast cancer in women is limited but promising results have been obtained in male breast cancer. Responses were observed in 7 of 11 male patients with breast cancer who were treated with cyproterone acetate at a dose of 200 mg/day.[58] In a study of 33 women with breast cancer, flutamide at a dose of 750 mg/day yielded only 1 brief partial response.[75] Further studies are needed to determine if antiandrogens are as effective as antiestrogens in the treatment of the condition when it occurs in males. Until this point is clarified, sequential therapy with tamoxifen[71] followed by cyproterone acetate might be tried before proceeding to orchiectomy.[5]

Prostate Cancer. There are several options for first-line therapy of stage D2 prostate cancer: orchiectomy, diethylstilbestrol, cyproterone acetate, cyproterone acetate and low-dose diethylstilbestrol, megestrol acetate and low-dose diethylstilbesterol, and LHRH agonist and flutamide (or another antiandrogen). The choice of a procedure or an agent for first-line therapy will rest on a number of factors including acceptance by the patient, preference of attending physician, availability, expense, and other concurrent health problems. Treatment is clinically indicated when evidence is found of (symptomatic or life-threatening) metastases to lymph nodes and/or bone in addition to local disease. With all first-line therapies the response rate is between 60–90%. Treatments which combine different modalities such as orchiectomy and antiandrogen, LHRH agonist and antiandrogen or cyproterone acetate and low-dose diethylstilbestrol, tend to yield a response rate at the high end of the range and a slight increase in time to progression. On the other hand, the rate of survival is approximately the same with all treatments, i.e., 80%, 60%, 40% and 20% after 1, 2, 3 and 5 years respectively.[6,23,40,50,72,90] A complete response is more likely to be observed when the initial tumor burden is relatively small and limited to prostate and lymph nodes, and is a favorable prognostic sign. In contrast, extensive skeletal metastases are indicative of a poor prognosis.[41]

The majority of men, especially elderly patients, will likely accept bilateral orchiectomy as initial therapy. Although the use of diethylstilbestrol at a conventional dose of 3 mg/day is associated with a high incidence of gynecomastia and an increased risk of cardiovascular complications, it is inexpensive, effective and well-tolerated by some men.

Cyproterone acetate has been shown to be equally as effective as standard therapy and is associated with a lower incidence of side effects compared to diethylstilbestrol. Owing to the uncertain effects of an elevated plasma testosterone on the growth of prostate cancer, nonsteroidal antiandrogens such as flutamide should be used with caution especially in situations where the agent will be used over an extended period of time. If maintenance of libido and potency are a major consideration, the use of flutamide may have some appeal.

Monotherapy with an LHRH agonist carries the risk of a flare reaction and on rare occasions will precipitate acute urinary retention, hydronephrosis and spinal cord compression in patients with a large tumor burden. In addition, there is circumstantial evidence suggesting that earlier progression of disease may occur owing to the initial LHRH agonist-induced increase in plasma testosterone concentration. By combining an LHRH agonist with an antiandrogen (e.g., leuprolide and flutamide), the risk of a flare reaction is reduced or eliminated. Few if any cardiovascular side-effects are observed and hence this option is indicated for patients with cardiovascular or peripheral vascular disease who are not candidates for surgical orchiectomy and in whom diethylstilbestrol is contraindicated. There has been considerable interest in the possibility that the "complete androgen blockade" achieved by the combination of LHRH agonist and antiandrogen might prove superior to conventional androgen withdrawal therapy which ignores the potential effect of adrenal androgens on growth of prostate cancer. However, a number of clinical trials testing this hypothesis have failed to produce any conclusive evidence for the involvement of adrenal androgens in prostate cancer.[86] The only supportive results at the present time, provided by the U.S.A. National Cancer Institute Intergroup Study INT 0036 of leuprolide versus leuprolide and flutamide, are consistent with the conclusion that treatment with leuprolide and flutamide is supe-

rior to treatment with leuprolide alone when the end points of median progression-free survival and median overall survival are compared.[26] However, no concurrent study was done to prove that leuprolide monotherapy was equivalent to standard therapy thus leaving the question open whether combination treatment is indeed superior to surgical orchiectomy or estrogen therapy.[29] In fact, no significant differences in time to progression and survival have been found in the equivalent European trials of goserelin and flutamide versus orchiectomy.[50,86]

The progestational antiandrogen, cyproterone acetate, produces a therapeutic effect similar to that of the combination of an LHRH agonist and a nonsteroidal antiandrogen. When it is combined with low-dose diethylstilbestrol (0.1 mg/day), castrate levels of plasma testosterone are uniformly achieved and the long term maintenance of plasma testosterone within the castrate range is more reliable. Owing to the synergistic action of low-dose diethylstilbestrol, cyproterone acetate can be used at a reduced dose of 100 mg/day, and the comparable agent megestrol acetate, at a dose of 120 mg/day, making these antiandrogens the most cost-effective after diethylstilbestrol.

Some of the androgen withdrawal therapies listed in Table XVII-9-1 are not ideally suited for first-line therapy. The combination of orchiectomy and antiandrogen (flutamide, nilutamide or cyproterone acetate) has not proven to be superior to orchiectomy alone and thus need not be considered as an option. At the present time, it is not known whether the 5α-reductase inhibitor, finasteride,[106] is effective against prostate cancer but in view of its mechanism of action, it could be a promising agent for this purpose. In the absence of a scientifically validated rationale for an adrenal contribution to the growth of prostate cancer, neither surgical,[64] nor medical adrenalectomy procedures should be considered for first-line therapy.[46] The steroidogenesis inhibitor, ketoconazole,[104] characterized by gastrointestinal side effects, skin reactions, gynecomastia and severe asthenia, should only be considered for use in emergency situations requiring an acute reduction in the concentration of plasma testosterone.

Prevention of Flare Reaction. A flare reaction usually begins with symptoms of localized or low back pain which starts 1–3 days after the administration of an LHRH agonist and resolves after another 1–4 days. Biochemical manifestations include temporary increases in the plasma levels of LH, testosterone, prostatic acid phosphatase and prostate specific antigen (PSA) lasting 7–14 days. Transient stimulation of tumor growth may also take place leading to urinary and neurological complications. The flare phenomenon has been implicated in the early progression of disease by the results of the Leuprolide Study Group Trial comparing leuprolide versus diethylstilbestrol,[99] and those of the N.C.I. INT 0036 study comparing leuprolide with, and without, flutamide.[26] In the former clinical trial, treatment was considered to have failed at the 3 month time-point in 10 patients receiving leuprolide as compared with 2 receiving diethylstilbestrol because of early progression of disease. In the latter trial, a 2.6 month gain in median time-to-progression was observed in the group receiving leuprolide and flutamide. This advantage was already evident at the 3 month time-point implying that there was earlier progression of disease in the leuprolide monotherapy group.

The flare reaction can be avoided with any one of several methods. Cyproterone acetate (preferably in combination with low-dose diethylstilbestrol) given as "lead-in" therapy for 3–4 weeks prior to the first dose of LHRH agonist will presuppress the pituitary and completely eliminate any possiblity of a flare reaction.[15] Alternatively, flutamide, nilutamide,[56] or cyproterone acetate[87] given concurrently with the first administration of LHRH agonist will safely blunt the reaction. Prior administration of diethylstilbestrol at doses of 1 mg or 3 mg daily for 1 week has proven to be less effective.[96] Since the danger of a flare reaction abates in the second week following LHRH agonist administration, there is no strong reason for continuing antiandrogens much beyond this time, and such antiflare treatment can safely be stopped after 1 month provided that the plasma testosterone is in the castrate range.

Second-Line Therapy. In patients relapsing after a response to first-line therapy, the probability of an objective response to a second androgen-withdrawal procedure is less than 10%.[120] Before steps are taken to introduce second-line therapy, it is necessary to measure the plasma testosterone level to determine whether there has been an escape from primary therapy. The choice of a second-line option will be determined to some extent by the original treatment as shown in Table XVII-9-2.

Following orchiectomy, it is unlikely that the plasma testosterone concentration will be elevated but nevertheless a trial of cyproterone acetate or flutamide for a period of 3 months is reasonable; the PSA level in the blood should be followed for any indication of a response. A common mistake is to administer LHRH agonist monotherapy after failure of orchiectomy; such treatment is totally ineffective in the absence of the testes.

An elevated plasma testosterone is more likely to be seen with diethylstilbestrol owing to incomplete absorption of tablet preparations or non-compliance. In this case the second-line treatment should be effective in lowering plasma testosterone and cyproterone acetate, LHRH agonist or orchiectomy will suffice for this purpose.

Plasma testosterone may be incompletely suppressed if cyproterone acetate is used as monotherapy and thus the addition of low-dose diethylstilbestrol (0.1 mg/day) should be tried first, with the other options being an LHRH agonist or orchiectomy. A patient who progresses while taking flutamide will invariably be found to have a normal or elevated level of plasma testosterone. The option selected for second-line therapy in this situation should result in a lowering of plasma testosterone to castrate levels; this can be achieved with cyproterone acetate, an LHRH agonist or orchiectomy.

If LHRH agonist monotherapy has been used as first-line therapy, antiandrogen should be tried for a short period of time followed by orchiectomy if no effect is observed.

In the event that a patient progresses while receiving the combination of LHRH agonist and antiandrogen as first-line therapy, a switch to an alternative antiandrogen will occasionally result in lowering of the PSA tumor marker. Otherwise, the orchiectomy option is indicated.

There is no evidence that second-line therapy increases the 6–12 month median survival time between progression and death.[25,51]

Management of Hormone Resistant Disease. Advanced prostate cancer which has become refractory to primary androgen-withdrawal therapy has a poor prognosis and the question arises whether the patient would benefit from continuation of such treatment. Owing to the retained androgen-sensitivity of androgen-independent malignancy (Figure XVII-9-2), there is a strong possibility that termination of medical castration therapy will result in an acceleration of tumor growth. This is particularly the situation where flutamide has been used as monotherapy, since the acceleration of growth may start very shortly after the drug has been discontinued. Two factors contribute to this acute complication: first, the half-life of flutamide in plasma is 5–6 hours and quite short; second, with clearance of flutamide, the normal or elevated level of plasma testosterone is no longer countered by antiandrogen. Thus in the face of progressive disease in patients who have not been surgically castrated, therapy with LHRH agonists and/or antiandrogens should probably be continued.

Intermittent Therapy. The reversibility of new types of androgen withdrawal therapy based on the use of antiandrogens and LHRH agonists makes it possible to alternate a patient between periods of treatment and no treatment. Potential advantages of this approach include recovery of sexual function, prolongation of the androgen-dependent condition of a tumor and sensitization of a tumor to chemotherapy during periods of hormonal rebound and self-priming. Clinical results based on the use of diethylstilbestrol suggest that satisfactory palliation of disease is achieved in selected patients with intermittent therapy.[52] Currently available forms of androgen withdrawal therapy (Table XVII-9-1) are better suited to a cyclic regimen owing to more reliable suppression of plasma testosterone and fewer side effects as compared with diethylstilbestrol. Moreover, careful sequential monitoring of plasma testosterone and PSA makes it possible to track successive periods of response and progression with considerable precision. Each cycle can be started with any treatment that reduces plasma testosterone into the castrate range and should be interrupted only after the PSA level has been normal for at least 4 months. Treatment is restarted when the PSA concentration reaches the lesser of the pre-treatment value or a value of 10–20 µg/L. This regimen has been used in preliminary studies in which the on- and off-treatment periods lasted about 6 months each; complete cycles were repeated up to 4 times with no loss of androgen dependency of PSA.[40]

Table XVII-9-2. Options for Second-line Therapy of Prostate Cancer

First-line Option	Second-line Options
Orchiectomy	Cyproterone acetate, flutamide
Diethylstilbestrol	Cyproterone acetate, LHRH agonist, orchiectomy
Cyproterone acetate	Cyproterone acetate + low-dose diethylstilbestrol, LHRH agonist, orchiectomy
Flutamide	Cyproterone acetate, LHRH agonist, orchiectomy
LHRH agonist	Cyproterone acetate, flutamide, orchiectomy
LHRH agonist + flutamide	LHRH agonist + cyproterone acetate, orchiectomy
LHRH agonist + cyproterone acetate	LHRH agonist + flutamide, orchiectomy

Neoadjuvant Therapy. A better understanding of the biology of prostate cancer has highlighted the fact that the risk of systemic spread is already appreciable at the time of initial diagnosis. Under such conditions, the results of radical prostatectomy will be less than optimal although it may still be indicated for control of local-regional disease. Preoperative treatment for 3–4 months with a reversible androgen withdrawal agent affords the possibility of downstaging the primary tumor,[91] reducing the incidence of positive margins, and eradicating micrometastases. Theoretically, this approach should result in improved survival and is a subject of several preliminary trials. The same principle has been used in the cytoreduction of prostate cancer prior to external beam irradiation.[44,77]

Adjuvant Treatment. It is intuitively evident, but not proven that adjuvant therapy in conjunction with radical prostatectomy should be beneficial when there is evidence of positive margins of resection, histological evidence of lymph node involvement or a failure of the PSA to fall to zero.[9] Experimental data from studies on animal models of prostate cancer indicate that androgen withdrawal therapy is more effective when started early in the treatment history of a tumor.[49] Although the clinical applications of adjuvant hormonal therapy are subject to controversy,[9] men with pathological stage C disease appear to have a lower local recurrence rate with the combination of radical prostatectomy and simultaneous androgen-withdrawal therapy.[110] Furthermore, men with diploid prostate cancer (pathological stage D1) who receive early androgen withdrawal therapy following radical prostatectomy, survive longer than men with non-diploid or aneuploid cancer who receive no early endocrine therapy.[111] Such results suggest that both DNA ploidy pattern and response to androgen-withdrawal therapy are major prognostic factors for patients with operable disease.

The optimum duration of adjuvant hormonal therapy has not been established. In advanced disease, regression of soft tissue tumor and normalization of PSA are usually observed within 3–6 months of starting therapy suggesting that 6–12 months of adjuvant treatment may be sufficient; this period is consistent with the observed rate of regression of prostate cancer after orchiectomy.[54]

The reversibility of some types of androgen withdrawal therapy (Table XVII-9-1) adds to the appeal of adjuvant hormonal therapy, since even if there is a recurrence of malignancy after therapy has been interrupted, the tumor is likely to be androgen-dependent and respond again to the first-line agent.

Treatment of Emergency Conditions. Urinary retention is a common presenting sign in patients with prostate cancer and is rapidly relieved by catheterization and subsequent transurethral resection. Androgen withdrawal therapy which results in a rapid decline of plasma testosterone may also be used to bring about regression of the obstructing lesion, especially in a high risk surgical patient or the individual with extensive local disease. If orchiectomy is not indicated, agents such as cyproterone acetate (200 mg/day), preferably with diethylstilbestrol (0.1 mg/day) or ketoconazole (1,200 mg/day) may be used as alternatives. In situations where there are signs of impending or early spinal cord compression, it is reasonable to add to conventional management with the administration of a steroidal or nonsteroidal antiandrogen. The use of an LHRH agonist is not advised since any acute elevation of plasma testosterone may stimulate tumor growth and exacerbate the condition.

Treatment of Hot Flashes. Hot flashes can be blocked by the administration of central antiadrenergic medication (clonidine)[70] or steroids with central inhibitory action which reduce the concentration of catecholamines in the hypothalamus. Cyproterone acetate owing to its partial progestational action has been successful in significantly suppressing hot flashes with minimum side effects at a dose of 100 mg/day.[81] Nonsteroidal antiandrogens which lack a central antigonadotropic effect cannot be used for this purpose.

Summary

The history of androgens is old and prodigious, yet the hormonal nature of androgens was not discovered until the earlier part of this century. Clinical testing of testosterone and other androgenic compounds began soon after their isolation and synthesis. Although breast cancer proved responsive to such therapy, the virilization induced by androgens and the introduction of antiestrogens caused a marked decline in the use of androgens for this purpose. Additive therapy with androgens is not indicated in the treatment of prostate cancer. This is in contrast to various types of androgen withdrawal therapies including orchiectomy, steroidal and nonsteroidal antiandrogens, LHRH agonists and others, which have become increasingly accepted as conventional treatment for prostate cancer. Reversible androgen withdrawal therapies based on the use of antiandrogens and LHRH agonists have found a number of applications in the treatment of prostate cancer at different stages offering flexibility and many new potential approaches. Of considerable interest is the application of reversible androgen withdrawal therapy to conventional treatment-regimens which might be enhanced by neoadjuvant or adjuvant endocrine therapy. Intermittent therapy with reversible modalities based on antiandrogens and LHRH agonists offer potential for long-term control of prostate cancer while minimizing side effects, especially suppression of libido and potency, in the younger male patient. In the near future, it is likely that the indications for the use of antiandrogens will expand and that the number of antiandrogenic agents available for treating prostate cancer will increase.

References

1. American Medical Association Council on Drugs.: Androgens and estrogens in the treatment of disseminated mammary carcinoma. JAMA, 172:1271, 1960.
2. Anderson, K. M., and Liao, S.: Selective retention of dihydrotestosterone by prostatic nuclei. Nature, 219:277, 1968.
3. Bardin, C. W., Brown, T., Isomaa, V. V., and Janne, O. A.: Progestins can mimic, inhibit and potentiate the actions of androgens. Pharmacol. Therap., 23:443, 1984.
4. Beato, M., Chalepakis, G., Schauer, M., and Slater E. P.: DNA regulatory elements for steroid hormones. J. Steroid Biochem., 32:737, 1989.
5. Becher, R., Hoeffken, K., Pape, H., and Schmidt, C.-G.: Tamoxifen treatment before orchiectomy in advanced breast cancer in men. N. Engl. J. Med., 305:169, 1981.
6. Beland, G., Elhilali, M., Fradet, Y., Laroche, B., Ramsey, E. W., Trachtenberg, J., Venner, P. M., and Tewari, H. D.: A controlled trial of castration with and without nilutamide in metastatic prostatic carcinoma. Cancer, 66(suppl.):1074, 1990.
7. Berthold, A. A.: Uber Die Transplantation Der Hoden. *In* Male Reproduction. Edited by B. P. Setchell. New York, Van Nostrand Reinhold Company Inc., 1984, p. 225.
8. Boccon-Gibod, L., Laudat, M. H., Dugue, M. A., and Steg, A.: Cyproterone acetate lead-in prevents initial rise of serum testosterone induced by luteinizing hormone-releasing hormone analogs in the treatment of metastatic carcinoma of the prostate. Eur. Urol., 12:400, 1986.
9. Bosch, R., and Schroeder, F. H.: Radical Prostatectomy and Adjuvant Endocrine Treatment: A Review. *In* EORTC Genitourinary Group Monograph 8: Treatment of Prostatic Cancer—Facts and Controversies. Edited by F. H. Schroeder. New York, Wiley-Liss, Inc., 1990, p. 239.
10. Brendler, H., Chase, W. E., and Scott, W. W.: Prostatic cancer, further investigation of hormonal relationships. Arch. Surg., 61:433, 1950.
11. Bruchovsky, N., and Goldie, J. H.: Basis for the Use of Drug and Hormone Combinations in the Treatment of Endocrine-Related Cancer. *In* Drug and Hormone Resistance in Neoplasia, Volume II, Clinical Concepts. Edited by N. Bruchovsky and J. H. Goldie. Boca Raton, CRC Press, 1983, p. 129.

12. Bruchovsky, N., and Wilson, J. D.: The conversion of testosterone to 5α-androstan-17β-ol-3-one by rat prostate in vivo and in vitro. J. Biol. Chem., 243:2012, 1968.

13. Bruchovsky, N., and Wilson, J. D.: The intranuclear binding of testosterone and 5α-androstan-17β-ol-3-one by rat prostate. J. Biol. Chem., 243:5953, 1968.

14. Bruchovsky, N., Brown, E. M., Coppin, C. M., Goldenberg, S. L., Le Riche, J. C., Murray, N. C., and Rennie, P. S.: The Endocrinology and Treatment of Prostate Tumor Progression. In Current Concepts and Approaches to the Study of Prostate Cancer. Edited by D. S. Coffey, N. Bruchovsky, W. A. Gardner, Jr., M. I. Resnick, and J. P. Karr. New York, Alan R. Liss, Inc., 1987, p. 347.

15. Bruchovsky, N., Goldenberg, S. L., Rennie, P. S., and Coppin, C. M.: Pre-suppression of the pituitary: An adjunct to LHRH agonist therapy of prostatic cancer. Clin. Invest. Med., 12:R-478, 1989.

16. Bruchovsky, N., Lesser, B., Van Doorn, E., and Craven, S.: Hormonal effects on cell proliferation in rat prostate. Vitam. Horm., 33:61, 1975.

17. Bruchovsky, N., Rennie, P. S., and Vanson, A.: Studies on the regulation of the concentration of androgens and androgen receptors in nuclei of prostatic cells. Biochim. Biophys. Acta, 394:248, 1975.

18. Bruchovsky, N., Rennie, P. S., and Wilkin, R. P.: New Aspects of Androgen Action in Prostatic Cells: Stromal Localization of 5α-Reductase, Nuclear Abundance of Androstanolone and Binding of Receptor to Linker Deoxyribonucleic Acid. In Steroid Receptors, Metabolism and Prostatic Cancer. Edited by F. H. Schroeder, and H. J. de Voogt. Amsterdam, Excerpta Medica, 1980, p. 57.

19. Bruchovsky, N., Rennie, P. S., Coldman, A. J., Goldenberg, S. L., To, M., and Lawson, D.: Effects of androgen withdrawal on the stem cell composition of the Shionogi carcinoma. Cancer Res., 50:2275, 1990.

20. Bruchovsky, N., Rennie, P. S., To, M. P., Snoek, R., Lefebvre, Y. A., and Golsteyn, E. J.: Chemical demonstration of nuclear androgen receptor following affinity chromatography with immobilized ligands. The Prostate, 10:207, 1987.

21. Bruchovsky, N.: Comparison of the metabolites formed in rat prostate following the in vivo administration of seven natural androgens. Endocrinology, 89:1212, 1971.

22. Burrows, H.: Biological Actions of Sex Hormones. Cambridge, University Press, 1949, p. 176.

23. Byar, D. P., and Corle, D. K.: Hormone therapy for prostate cancer: results of the Veterans Administration cooperative urological research group studies. N.C.I. Monogr., 7:165, 1988.

24. Chang, C., Kokontis, J., and Liao, S.: Molecular cloning of human and rat complementary DNA encoding androgen receptors. Science, 240:324, 1988.

25. Collste, L. G.: Second Line Treatment of Hormone Refractory Prostatic Cancer Patients. In EORTC Genitourinary Group Monograph 7: Prostatic Cancer and Testicular Cancer. Edited by D. W. W. Newling and W. G. Jones. New York, Wiley-Liss, Inc., 1990, p. 29.

26. Crawford, E. D., Eisenberger, M. A., McLeod, D. G., Spaulding, J. T., Benson, R., Dorr, A., Blumenstein, B. A., Davis, M. A., and Goodman P. J.: A controlled trial of leuprolide with and without flutamide in prostatic carcinoma. N. Engl. J. Med., 321:419, 1989.

27. De Voogt, H. J., Smith, P. H., Pavone-Macaluso, M., De Pauw, M., Suciu, S., and Members of the European Organization for Research on Treatment of Cancer Urological Group: Cardiovascular side effects of diethylstilbestrol, cyproterone acetate, medroxyprogesterone acetate and estramustine phosphate used for the treatment of advanced prostatic cancer: results from European Organization for Research on Treatment of Cancer trials 30761 and 30762. J. Urol., 135:303, 1986.

28. Debruyne, F. M. J., Denis, L., Lunglmayer, G., Mahler, C., Newling, D. W. W., Richards, B., Robinson, M. R. G., Smith, P. H., Weil, E. H. J., and Whelan, P.: Long-term therapy with a depot luteinizing hormone-releasing hormone analogue (Zoladex) in patients with advanced prostatic carcinoma. J. Urol., 140:775, 1988.

29. Denis, L.: Conclusions of the American Cancer Society Workshop on Combined Castration and Androgen Blockade Therapy in Prostate Cancer. Cancer, 66(Suppl.):1086, 1990.

30. Dorfman, R. I., and Shipley, R. A.: Androgens, Biochemistry, Physiology, and Clinical Significance. New York, John Wiley & Sons, Inc., 1956, p. 5.

31. Dorfman, R. I.: Anti-Androgenic Substances. In Methods in Hormone Research, Volume II. Edited by R. I. Dorfman. New York, Academic Press, 1962, p. 315.

32. Dorfman, R. I.: Biological activity of antiandrogens. Brit. J. Derm., 82:supplement 6, 3, 1970.

33. Dunn, J. F., Nisula, B. C., and Rodbard, D.: Transport of steroid hormones: binding of 21 endogenous steroids to both testosterone-binding globulin and corticosteroid-binding globulin in human plasma. J. Clin. Endocrinol. Metab., 53:58, 1981.

34. El Etreby, M. F., Habenicht, U.-F., Louton, T., Nishino, Y., and Schroeder, H. G.: Effect of cyproterone acetate in comparison to flutamide and megestrol acetate on the ventral prostate, seminal vesicle, and adrenal glands of adult male rats. The Prostate, 11:361, 1987.

35. Everson, R. B., and Lippman, M. E.: Male Breast Cancer. In Breast Cancer 3, Advances in Research and Treatment. Edited by W. L. McGuire. New York, Plenum Medical Book Company, 1979, p. 239.

36. Fowler, J. E., Jr., and Whitmore, W. F., Jr.: Considerations for the use of testosterone with systemic chemotherapy in prostatic cancer. Cancer, 49:1373, 1982.

37. Fowler, J. E., Jr., and Whitmore, W. F., Jr.: The response of metastatic adenocarcinoma of the prostate to exogenous testosterone. J. Urol., 126:372, 1981.

38. Geller, J., Albert, J., and Yen, S. S. C.: Treatment of advanced cancer of prostate with megestrol acetate. Urology, 12:537, 1978.

39. Goldenberg, I. S., and Segaloff, A.: Androgens. In Cancer Medicine, 2nd Edition. Edited by J. F. Holland, and E. Frei, III. Philadelphia, Lea & Febiger, 1982, p. 990.

40. Goldenberg, S. L., and Bruchovsky, N.: The use of cyproterone acetate in prostate cancer. Urologic Clinics of North America, 18:111, 1991.

41. Goldenberg, S. L., Bruchovsky, N., Rennie, P. S., and Coppin, C. M.: The combination of cyproterone acetate and low dose diethylstilbestrol in the treatment of advanced prostatic carcinoma. J. Urol., 140:1460, 1988.

42. Gonzalez-Barcena, D., Perez-Sanchez, P. L., Graef, A., Gomez, A. M., Berea, H., Comaru-Schally, A. M., and Schally, A. V.: Inhibition of the pituitary-gonadal axis by a single intramuscular administration of D-trp-6-LH-RH (Decapeptyl) in a sustained-release formulation in patients with prostatic carcinoma. The Prostate, 14:291, 1989.

43. Grayhack, J. T.: Adrenalectomy and hypophysectomy for carcinoma of the prostate. JAMA, 210:1075, 1969.

44. Green, N., Bodner, H., Broth, E., Chiang, C., Garrett, J., Goldstein, A., Goldberg, H., Gualtieri, V., Gray, R., Jaffe, J., Kaplan, R., Polse, S., Ross, S., Skaist, L., Treible, D., Vatz, A., and Wallack, H.: Improved control of bulky prostate carcinoma with sequential estrogen and radiation therapy. Radiat. Oncol. Biol. Phys., 10:971, 1984.

45. Habenicht, U.-F., Schroeder, F. H., El Etreby, M. F., and Neumann, F.: Advantages and Disadvantages of Pure Antiandrogens and of Antiandrogens of the Cyproterone Acetate—Type in the Treatment of Prostatic Cancer. In Management of Advanced Cancer of Prostate and Bladder. Edited by P. H. Smith, and M. Pavone-Macaluso. New York, Alan R. Liss, Inc., 1988, p. 63.

46. Havlin, K. A., and Trump, D. L.: Aminoglutethimide: Theoretical Considerations and Clinical Results in Advanced Prostate Cancer. In Endocrine Therapies in Breast and Prostate Cancer. Edited by C. Kent Osborne. Boston, Kluwer Academic Publishers, 1988, p. 83.

47. Huggins, C., and Hodges, C. V.: Studies on prostate cancer: I. Effect of castration, estrogen, and androgen injection on serum phosphatases in metastatic carcinoma of the prostate. Cancer Res., 1:293, 1941.

48. Ingle, J. N., Twito, D. I., Schaid, D. J., Cullinan, S. A., Krook, J. E., Mailliard, J. A., Marschke, R. F., Long, H. J., Gerstner, J. G., Windschitl, H. E., Everson, L. K., and Pfeifle, D.M.: Randomized clinical trial of tamoxifen alone or combined with fluoxymesterone in postmenopausal women with metastatic breast cancer. J. Clin. Oncol., 6:825, 1988.

49. Isaacs, J. T.: The timing of androgen ablation therapy and/or chemotherapy in the treatment of prostatic cancer. The Prostate, 5:1, 1984.

50. Iversen, P., Suciu, S., Sylvester, R., Christensen, I., and Denis, L.: Zoladex and flutamide versus orchiectomy in the treatment of advanced prostatic cancer. A combined analysis of two European studies, EORTC 30853 and DAPROCA86. Cancer, 66(Suppl.):1067, 1990.

51. Jacobi, G. H.: Second-Line Endocrine Treatment. In The Medical Management of Prostate Cancer. Edited by L. Denis. Berlin, Springer-Verlag, 1988, p. 73.

52. Klotz, L. H., Herr, H. W., Morse, M. J., and Whitmore, W. F., Jr.: Intermittent endocrine therapy for advanced prostate cancer. Cancer, 58:2546, 1986.

53. Knuth, U. A., Hano, R., and Nieschlag, E.: Effect of flutamide or cyproterone acetate on pituitary and testicular hormones in normal men. J. Clin. Endocrinol. Metab., 59:963, 1984.

54. Kojima, M., Watanabe, H., Ohe, H., Miyashita, H., and Inaba, T.: Kinetic evaluation of the effect of LHRH analog on prostatic cancer using transrectal ultrasonotomography. The Prostate, 10:11, 1987.

55. Koutsilieris, M., Faure, N., Tolis, G., Laroche, B., Robert, G., and Ackman, C. F. D.: Objective response and disease outcome in 59 patients with Stage D2 prostatic cancer treated with either buserelin or orchiectomy. Urology, 27:221, 1986.

56. Kuhn, J.-M., Billebaud, T., Navratil, H., Moulonguet, A., Fiet, J., Grise, P., Louis, J.-F., Costa, P., Husson, J.-M., Dahan, R., Bertagna, C., and Edelstein, R.: Prevention of the transient adverse effects of a gonadotropin-releasing hormone analogue (Buserelin) in metastatic prostatic carcinoma by administration of an antiandrogen (Nilutamide). N. Engl. J. Med., 321:413, 1989.

57. Lerner, L. J.: Hormone antagonists: Inhibitors of specific activities of estrogen and androgen. Rec. Prog. Horm. Res., 20:435, 1964.

58. Lopez, M., Di Lauro, L., Lazzaro, B., and Papaldo, P.: Hormonal treatment of disseminated male breast cancer. Oncology, 42:345, 1985.

59. Lubahn, D. B., Joseph, D. R., Sullivan, P. M., Willard, H. F., French, F. S., and Wilson, E. M.: Cloning of human androgen receptor complementary DNA and localization to the X chromosome. Science, 240:327, 1988.

60. Lund, F., and Rasmussen, F.: Flutamide versus stilboestrol in the management of advanced prostatic cancer, a controlled prospective study. Brit. J. Urol., 61:140, 1988.

61. Lungmayr, G.: Casodex (ICI 176,334), A new, non-steroidal anti-androgen. Early clinical results. Horm. Res., 32(Suppl. 1):77, 1989.

62. Manni, A., Santen, R. J., Boucher, A. E., Lipton, A., Harvey, H., Simmonds, M., White-Hershey, D., Gordon, R. A., Rohner, T. J., Drago, J., Wettlaufer, J., and Glode, L. M.: Androgen priming and response to chemotherapy in advanced prostatic cancer. J. Urol., 136:1242, 1986.

63. Montpetit, M. L., Lawless, K. R., and Tenniswood, M.: Androgen-repressed messages in the rat ventral prostate. The Prostate, 8:25, 1986.

64. Morales, P. A., Brendler, H., and Hotchkiss, R. S.: The role of the adrenal cortex in prostatic cancer. J. Urol., 73:399, 1955.

65. Neri, R., Florance, K., Koziol, P., and Van Cleave, S.: A biological profile of a non-steroidal antiandrogen, SCH 13521 (4'-nitro-3'-trifluoromethylisobutyranilide). Endocrinology, 91:427, 1972.

66. Neumann, F., Humpel, M., Senge, T., Schenck, B., and Tunn, U.: Cyproterone Acetate—Biochemical and Biological Basis for Treatment of Prostatic Cancer. In Prostate Cancer. Edited by G. H. Jacobi, and R. Hohenfellner. Baltimore, MD, Williams & Wilkins, 1982, p. 269.

67. Neumann, F., von Berswordt-Wallrabe, R., Elger, W., Steinbeck, H., Hahn, J. D., and Kramer, M.: Aspects of androgen-dependent events as studied by antiandrogens. Rec. Prog. Horm. Res., 26:337, 1970.

68. Oesterling, J. E., Epstein, J. I., and Walsh, P. C.: The inability of adrenal androgens to stimulate the adult human prostate: an autopsy evaluation of men with hypogonadotropic hypogonadism and panhypopituitarism. J. Urol., 136:1030, 1986.

69. Olea, N., Sakabe, K., Soto, A. M., and Sonnenschein, C.: The proliferative effect of "anti-androgens" on the androgen-sensitive human prostate tumor cell line LNCaP. Endocrinology, 126:1457, 1990.

70. Parra, R. O., and Gregory, J. G.: Treatment of post-orchiectomy hot flashes with transdermal administration of clonidine. J. Urol., 143:753, 1990.

71. Patterson, J. S., Battersby, L. A., and Bach, B. K.: Use of tamoxifen in advanced male breast cancer. Cancer Treat. Rep., 64:801, 1980.

72. Pavone-Macaluso, M., De Voogt, H. J., Viggiano, G., Barasolo, E., Lardennois, B., De Pauw, M., and Sylvester, R.: Comparison of diethylstilbestrol, cyproterone acetate and medroxyprogesterone acetate in the treatment of advanced prostatic cancer: final analysis of a randomized phase III trial of the European Organization for Research on Treatment of Cancer Urological Group. J. Urol., 136:624, 1986.

73. Pavone-Macaluso, M., Pavone, C., Serretta, V., and Daricello, G.: Antiandrogens alone or in combination for treatment of prostate cancer: the European experience. Urology, 34(Suppl.):27, 1989.

74. Pedrotti, R., and Frizzi, V.: Treatment of prostatic carcinoma by hormonal shock as suggested by Mayor. Cancer Chemotherap. Abst., 7:100, 1966.

75. Perrault, D. J., Logan, D. M., Stewart, D. J., Bramwell, V. H. C., Paterson, A. H. G., and Eisenhauer, E. A.: Phase II study of flutamide in patients with metastatic breast cancer. A National Cancer Institute of Canada Clinical Trials Group study. Invest. New Drugs, 6:207, 1988.

76. Peters, C. A., and Walsh, P. C.: The effect of nafarelin acetate, a luteinizing-hormone-releasing hormone agonist, on benign prostatic hyperplasia. N. Engl. J. Med., 317:599, 1987.

77. Porter, A. T., and Venner, P. M.: The Role of Cytoreduction Prior to Definitive Radiotherapy in Locally Advanced Prostate Cancer—The Canadian Perspective. In EORTC Genitourinary Group Monograph 8: Treatment of Prostatic Cancer—Facts and Controversies. Edited by F. H. Schroeder. New York, Wiley-Liss, Inc., 1990, p. 231.

78. Pritchard, K. I., and Sutherland, D. J.: The use of endocrine therapy. Hematology/Oncology Clinics of North America, 3:765, 1989.

79. Prout, G. R., Jr., and Brewer, W. R.: Response of men with advanced prostatic carcinoma to exogenous administration of testosterone. Cancer, 20:1871, 1967.
80. Prout, G. R., Jr., Keating, M. A., Griffin, P. P., and Schiff, S. F.: Long-term experience with flutamide in patients with prostatic carcinoma. Urology, 34(Suppl.):37, 1989.
81. Radlmaier, A., Bormacher, K., and Neumann, F.: Hot Flushes: Mechanism and Prevention. In EORTC Genitourinary Group Monograph 8: Treatment of Prostatic Cancer—Facts and Controversies. Edited by F. H. Schroeder. New York, Wiley-Liss, Inc., 1990, p. 131.
82. Raynaud, J.-P., and Ojasoo, T.: The design and use of sex-steroid antagonists. J. Steroid Biochem., 25:811,1986.
83. Rennie, P. S., Bowden, J.-F., Freeman, S. N., Bruchovsky, N., Cheng, H., Lubahn, D. B., Wilson, E. M., French, F. S., and Main, L.: Cortisol alters gene expression during involution of the rat ventral prostate. Mol. Endocrinol., 3:703, 1989.
84. Rennie, P. S., Bruchovsky, N., Buttyan, R., Benson, M., and Cheng, H.: Gene expression during the early phases of regression of the androgen-dependent Shionogi mouse mammary carcinoma. Cancer Res., 48:6309, 1988.
85. Rennie, P. S., Bruchovsky, N., Goldenberg, S. L., Lawson, D., Fletcher, T., and Foekens, J. A.: Relative effectiveness of alternative androgen withdrawal therapies in initiating regression of rat prostate. J. Urol., 139:1337, 1988.
86. Robinson, M. R. G.: Reasons Against Total Androgen Suppression. In EORTC Genitourinary Group Monograph 8: Treatment of Prostatic Cancer—Facts and Controversies. Edited by F. H. Schroeder. New York, Wiley-Liss, Inc., 1990, p. 117.
87. Schroeder, F. H., Lock, T. M. T. W., Chadha, D. R., Debruyne, F. M. J., Karthaus, H. F. M., de Jong, F. H., Klijn, J. G. M., Matroos, A. W., and de Voogt, H. J.: Metastatic cancer of the prostate managed with buserelin versus buserelin plus cyproterone acetate. J. Urol., 137:912, 1987.
88. Schroeder, F. H.: Pure antiandrogens as monotherapy in prospective studies of prostatic carcinoma. In EORTC Genitourinary Group Monograph 8: Treatment of Prostatic Cancer—Facts and Controversies, New York, Wiley-Liss, Inc., 1990, p. 93.
89. Schulze, H., Oesterling, J. E., Isaacs, J. T., and Coffey, D. S.: Hormonal Therapy of Prostate Cancer: Limitations in the Total Androgen Ablation Concept. In A Multidisciplinary Analysis of Controversies in the Management of Prostate Cancer. Edited by D. S. Coffey, M. I. Resnick, F. A. Dorr, and J. P. Karr. New York, Plenum Press, 1986, p. 215.
90. Schulze, H., Isaacs, J., and Senge, T.: Inability of complete androgen blockade to increase survival of patients with advanced prostatic cancer as compared to standard hormonal therapy. J. Urol., 137:909, 1987.
91. Scott, W. W., and Boyd, H. L.: Combined hormone control therapy and radical prostatectomy in the treatment of selected cases of advanced carcinoma of the prostate: a retrospective study based upon 25 years of experience. J. Urol., 101:86, 1969.
92. Segaloff, A.: Results of studies of the cooperative breast cancer group—1961–63. Cancer Chemotherap. Rep., 41:1, 1964.
93. Setchell, B. P.: Introduction. In Male Reproduction. Edited by B. P. Setchell. New York, Van Nostrand Reinhold Company Inc., 1984, p.1.
94. Sharifi, R., and Kiefer, J.: History of endocrine manipulation in the treatment of carcinoma of the prostate—who was first? J. Endocrinol. Invest., 10(Suppl. 2):91, 1987.
95. Sogani, P. C., Vagaiwala, M. R., and Whitmore, W. F. Jr.: Experience with flutamide in patients with advanced prostatic cancer without prior endocrine therapy. Cancer, 54:744, 1984.
96. Stein, B. S., and Smith, J. A.: DES lead-in to use of luteinizing hormone releasing hormone analogs in treatment of metastatic carcinoma of prostate. Urology, 25:350, 1985.
97. Stoll, B. A.: Hormonal Therapy—Pain Relief and Recalcification. In Bone Metastasis, Monitoring and Treatment. Edited by B. A. Stoll and S. Parbhoo. New York, Raven Press, 1983, p. 321.
98. Suarez, A. J., Lamm, D. L., Radwin, H. M., Sarosdy, M., Clark, G., and Osborne, C. K.: Androgen priming and cytotoxic chemotherapy in advanced prostatic cancer. Cancer Chemotherap. Pharmacol, 8:261, 1982.
99. The Leuprolide Study Group: Leuprolide versus diethylstilbestrol for metastatic prostate cancer. N. Engl. J. Med., 311:1281, 1984.
100. Tormey, D. C., Gelman, P. R., Band, P. R., Sears, M., Bauer, M., Arseneau, J. C., and Falkson, G.: A prospective evaluation of chemohormonal therapy remission maintenance in advanced breast cancer. Breast Cancer Res. Treat., 1:111, 1981.
101. Tormey, D. C., Lippman, M. E., Edwards, B. K., and Cassidy, J. G.: Evaluation of tamoxifen doses with and without fluoxymesterone in advanced breast cancer. Ann. Int. Med., 98:139, 1983.
102. Trapman, J., Klaassen, P., Kuiper, G. G. J. M., van der Korput, J. A. G. M., Faber, P. W., van Rooij, H. C. J., van Kessel, A. G., Voorhorst, M. M., Mulder, E., and Brinkmann, A. O.: Cloning, structure and expression of a cDNA encoding the human androgen receptor. Biochem. Biophys. Res. Commun., 153:241, 1988.
103. Vallis, K., and Waxman, J.: Tumour Flare in Hormonal Therapy. In Endocrine Management of Cancer 2, Contemporary Therapy. Edited by B. A. Stoll. Basel, S. Karger AG, 1988, p. 144.
104. Vanuytsel, L., Ang, K. K., Vantongelen, K., Drochmans, A., Baert, L., and Van Der Schueren, E.: Ketoconazole therapy for advanced prostatic cancer: feasibility and treatment results. J. Urol., 137:905, 1987.
105. Venner, P. M., Klotz, P. G., Klotz, L. H., Stewart, D. J., Davis, I. R., Orovan, W. L., and Ramsey, E. W.: Megestrol acetate plus minidose diethylstilbestrol in the treatment of carcinoma of the prostate. Sem. Oncol., 15(Suppl. 1):62, 1988.
106. Vermeulen, A., Giagulli, V. A., De Schepper, P., Buntinx, A., and Stoner, E.: Hormonal effects of an orally active 4-azasteroid inhibitor of 5α-reductase in humans. The Prostate, 14:45, 1989.
107. Westerberg, H.: Tamoxifen and fluoxymesterone in advanced breast cancer: A controlled clinical trial. Cancer Treat. Rep., 64:117, 1980.
108. Wilding, G., Chen, M., and Gelmann, E. P.: Aberrant reponse in vitro of hormone-responsive prostate cancer cells to antiandrogens. The Prostate, 14:103, 1989.
109. Wilson, J. D.: Androgen abuse by athletes. Endocrine Rev., 9:181, 1988.
110. Zincke, H.: Bilateral pelvic lymphadenectomy and radical prostatectomy for stage C or D1 adenocarcinoma of the prostate: possible beneficial effect of adjuvant treatment. N.C.I. Monogr., 7:109, 1988.
111. Zincke, H.: Extended experience with surgical treatment of stage D1 adenocarcinoma of prostate: significant influences of immediate adjuvant hormonal treatment (orchiectomy) on outcome. Urology, 33(Suppl.):27, 1989.

XVII-10

Ectopic Hormones and Humoral Syndromes of Cancer

William D. Odell

Introduction

In addition to producing symptoms by direct invasion or tumor mass, cancers also produce symptoms distant from the tumor site by production of humoral substances that circulate in blood. Although humoral syndromes of cancer were considered rare in past years, as better understanding of the pathophysiology has been gained, it is now realized that such manifestations of cancer are common and may, in fact, be associated with all cancers.[75] The mechanisms by which cancers produce their distant symptoms are, with rare exception, caused by tumor production of one or more proteins. For the endocrine syndromes (often called ectopic hormone syndromes), studies from our laboratory and from several others, have shown that many of the hormones and hormone precursors produced by cancers are also produced in small amounts by virtually all normal non-endocrine tissues. Thus the cancers produce the same substances in larger quantities or convert biologically weak or inactive precursors to biologically active substances. It is in this context that we believe ectopic hormone production is not ectopic.[73,75] The neurological syndromes associated with cancer are, for the most part, produced by tumor antigen stimulation of antibody production. The antibody in turn reacts with a normal tissue such as the cerebellum or retina. Table XVII-10-1 lists the humoral syndromes of cancer.

Cancer Hormone Production and Hormone-Like Syndromes

The number of protein hormones or protein-hormone precursors produced by cancers is large. Table XVII-10-2 lists these hormones. Table XVII-10-2 also includes the steroids estrone and estradiol. With the exception of neoplasms originating in steroid secreting tissues (e.g., adrenal, ovary, tes-

Table XVII-10-1. Spectrum of Humoral Syndromes of Cancer

Humoral substances
   Protein hormones and hormone precursors
   Metabolism of steroids
Paraneoplastic syndromes of the nervous system
   Cerebellar syndromes
      Cerebellar cortical degeneration
      Myoclonic encephalopathy
   Subacute sensory neuropathy
   Visual paraneoplastic syndrome
   Limbic and bulbar encephalitis
   Multifocal leukoencephalopathy
Skeletal muscle syndromes
   Polymyositis-dermatomyositis
   Carcinomatous neuromyopathy
   Myasthenic syndromes (e.g., Eaton-Lambert syndrome)
Miscellaneous syndromes
   Anorexia
   Fever
   Glomerular kidney disease
   Enzyme production (e.g., alkaline phosphatase, thymidine kinase)
   Fetal protein production (α-fetoprotein, carcinoembryonic antigen)
   Digital clubbing—pulmonary osteoarthropathy
   Hematologic syndromes (e.g., ITP)

Modified from Odell[71A]

Table XVII-10-2. Hormones and Hormone Precursors Reported to be Produced by Neoplasms

1. Pro-opiomelanocortin and related peptides
2. Corticotropin-releasing hormone
3. Chorionic gonadotropin and its subunits (α and β)
4. Vasopressin
5. Growth factors (e.g., TGF-β, EGF, IGF-II)
6. Parathyroid hormone-like protein
7. Erythropoietin
8. Eosinophilopoietin
9. Growth hormone
10. Growth hormone-releasing hormone
11. Prolactin
12. Gastrin
13. Gastrin-releasing peptide (and bombesin)
14. Secretin
15. Glucagon
16. Calcitonin
17. Renin
18. Vasoactive intestinal peptide
19. Somatostatin
20. Hypophosphatemia-producing factor
21. Estrone and estradiol

Modified from Odell and Appleton[72]

tes), cancers do not synthesize and secrete steroids de novo. Rarely, however, a cancer may convert a steroid precursor to a biologically active steroid. For example, Kew and colleagues demonstrated that an hepatic cancer converted dehydroepiandyosteyone to estrone and estradiol to produce feminization.[52]

In this section on protein hormone production by cancers, we discuss three common syndromes in adequate detail to develop the hypothesis that cancers produce protein hormones or hormone-like proteins that are normally produced in small quantities by normal cells. Thus the term ectopic production is not a correct one. The three examples are: 1) ACTH and related peptides; 2) chorionic gonadotropin; and 3) hypercalcemia and cancers. Some other protein hormone syndromes of cancer will be very briefly summarized, because adequate space to discuss them in detail is not available.

Cancer Production of ACTH and Related Peptides

Cushing's syndrome associated with cancer was first described in 1928, and was the second (after hypercalcemia) hormonal syndrome of cancer to be described. In the 1960's, Liddle and colleagues[6] published their studies of 88 patients with cancer and Cushing's syndrome which demonstrated that the primary cancer and its metastases contained large amounts of biologically active ACTH. Several hundred patients with this syndrome have now been reported. The types of neoplasms which produce biologically active ACTH are listed in Table XVII-10-3. The production of Cushing's syndrome by a cancer can generally be distinguished from a pituitary ACTH-producing adenoma or pituitary dependent Cushing's disease by several findings: 1) hypokalemia is common in the cancer-induced Cushing's syndrome, and unusual in Cushing's disease; 2) serum and urine cortisol concentrations are usually markedly elevated in cancer-induced Cushing's syndrome, but high-normal without diurnal variation, or modestly above normal in Cushing's disease; 3) plasma ACTH is usually very highly elevated in cancer-induced Cushing's syndrome, but is normal or slightly elevated in Cushing's disease; 4) suppression of ACTH and cortisol by large doses of dexamethasone (e.g., 2 mg Q.6H) is unusual in cancer-induced Cushing's syndrome, but is expected in Cushing's disease.[70] An increase in plasma ACTH/cortisol in response to corticotropin-releasing hormone (CRH) stimulation is present in Cushing's disease, but is usually not seen in cancer-induced Cushing's syndrome. Occasionally, however, the cancer-ACTH syndrome is subtle and the tumor is small. In such patients diagnosis must be made by metabolic criteria, followed by a careful search for the primary tumor. CT scan of chest and abdomen, as well as venous catheterization (at times including the petrosal veins), may be required to identify the tumor.

Table XVII-10-3. Types of Neoplasms that Produce Biologically Active ACTH

Type of Neoplasm	Approximate Percentage of Cases
Carcinoma of the lung (predominantly small or oat cell)	50
Carcinoma of the thymus	10
Carcinoma of the pancreas (including carcinoid and islet cell)	10
Pheochromocytoma, neuroblastoma, ganglioma and paraganglioma	5
Medullary carcinoma of the thyroid	5
Bronchial adenoma and carcinoid	2
Miscellaneous carcinomas* or hematologic malignancies	18

*e.g., carcinoma of the ovary, prostate, breast, thyroid, kidney, salivary glands, testes, stomach, colon, gall bladder, esophagus, appendix, acute myeloblastic leukemia.
Modified from Odell and Appleton[72]

Table XVII-10-4. Types of Neoplasms Associated with Hypercalcemia

Type of Neoplasm	Approximate Percentage of Cases
Carcinomas	
Carcinoma of the lung	35
Carcinoma of the kidney	24
Carcinoma of the ovary	8
Miscellaneous carcinomas*	<2 each
Hematologic malignant neoplasms	
Multiple myeloma	7
T-cell lymphoma	2
Other	1
Tumors with bony metastases	
Breast carcinoma	Not included in
Others	frequency estimates

*This includes almost every type of carcinoma (e.g., pancreas, urinary bladder, colon, prostate, penis, esophagus, parotid glands, testes, liver, stomach).
Modified from Odell[71A]

Patients with bronchial carcinoid or carcinoma of the thymus (see Table XVII-10-3) causing Cushing's syndrome are particularly difficult to distinguish from those with Cushing's disease. Suppression of ACTH/cortisol with high dose dexamethasone is seen in 40–50% of the carcinoid produced Cushing's syndrome and is expected in Cushing's disease.[48,61,72] Response to corticotropin-releasing hormone (CRH) is brisk in Cushing's disease, and is usually absent in Cushing's syndrome caused by bronchial carcinoid, although some patients with bronchial carcinoid do show CRH stimulation.[48,61,76]

The precursor molecule of ACTH is a glycoprotein proopiomelanocortin (POMC). POMC contains the amino acid sequences of lipotropin, melanocyte stimulating hormone (MSH), the endorphins and enkephalins and of ACTH itself.[69] In 1977[75] and 1979,[74,110] Odell and colleagues reported that *extracts* of all carcinomas of several histological types, from patients without signs of Cushing's syndrome (i.e, cancers not producing biologically active ACTH), contained large amounts of both ACTH and lipotropin as measured by immunoassay. Furthermore, in prospective clinical studies it was shown that an immunoactive ACTH-like material was present *in plasma* in amounts greater than found in patients without cancer.[74,110] This ACTH-like material showed no biological activity as assessed by in vitro radioreceptor assay and had a larger size than the 4,500 daltons of biologically active ACTH. Subsequently, Odell and colleagues showed that nonendocrine tissues from humans without cancer, as well as normal tissues from rats, all contained a 26,000 Da glycoprotein which possessed both ACTH and lipotropin immunoactivities.[73,83] This molecule contained no biological ACTH activity as assessed by in vitro dispersed adrenal cell assays. However, a biologically active 4,500 d ACTH was produced by treatment of the glycoprotein with trypsin in vitro. This precursor ACTH molecule resembled POMC. Odell and colleagues hypothesized that the same molecule was synthesized in greatly increased quantities by all carcinomas, and that a subset of carcinomas metabolized this ACTH precursor to biologically active ACTH to produce the so-called ectopic ACTH syndrome.[72,73,75]

Chorionic Gonadotropin (CG) Production by Cancers

Human CG is a glycoprotein composed of single alpha and beta chains linked by charge-charge interaction. The alpha chain of CG is identical in amino acid sequence to the alpha of three other human glycoprotein hormones, thyrotropin (TSH), luteinizing hormone (LH) and follicle stimulating hormone (FSH).[77] In the 1960's, it was generally believed that CG was produced solely by the trophoblast cell during normal pregnancy, by gestational trophoblastic neoplasms derived from these cells, or rarely by teratomas containing trophoblast cells. Between 1949 and 1972, some 8 patients were reported who had non-trophoblastic carcinomas (malignant melanoma, adrenocortical carcinoma, renal carcinoma, breast carcinoma, carcinoma of the lung), which appeared to produce a CG-like hormone.[72] In 1972, Vaitukaitis and colleagues reported the development of the beta CG assay, an assay with increased ability to distinguish CG from its very close biochemical relative LH.[105] Using this assay, Braunstein and colleagues studied serum samples from a large number of patients with a wide variety of carcinomas, including carcinoma of the lung, stomach, colon and pancreas.[15] They found 6–13% of their patients had increased blood CG concentrations.

In 1977 and 1979, Odell and colleagues and Yoshimoto et al.[113] reported that when extracts of carcinomas were studied, all contained a CG-like material as assessed by both the beta CG immunoassay and by CG radioreceptor assays.[75] In addition, these workers showed (similar to the story for ACTH) that a CG-like material was also extractable from normal human tissues.[75,111,112] Furthermore, this CG-like material bound to testicular LH/CG receptors; judged by binding to concanavalin-A (CON-A), a plant lectin which binds glycoproteins containing mannose and glycopyranose sugars, the CG-like material was shown to have carbohydrate structure strikingly different from placental CG. The normal tissue CG-like material showed little or no binding to CON-A, while placental CG was 95–100% bound to CON-A. Furthermore, the molecular weight of the normal tissue CG-like material was less than that of placental CG and was similar to carbohydrate-free placental CG.[73] The CG-like material in blood of patients with carcinomas and in extracts of carcinomas had variable CON-A binding, ranging from 4–5% (similar to normal tissue CG) to 85% (similar to placental CG).

Alteration or removal of carbohydrate from placental CG alters biological activity by changing the metabolic degradation rate. For example, desialated CG has a half time of degradation (t½) in humans of 3.6 minutes, whereas carbohydrate-rich CG has a t½ of approximately nine hours.[80] In essence, the degradation of carbohydrate-poor CG is so rapid, it is unlikely the blood concentrations would be increased to detectable levels.

Odell and colleagues hypothesized that all carcinomas and normal human tissues produce CG.[73,75,112] Those carcinomas associated with increased blood concentrations of CG either produced very large quantities of this normal tissue CG and/or glycosylated the CG, transforming it into a hormone with longer half-life and increased biological activity in vivo.

Hypercalcemia and Cancer

Hypercalcemia is a relatively common manifestation of cancer. For example, hypercalcemia occurs in 20–40% of patients with multiple myeloma,[67] in over 50% of patients with type C virus-induced T-cell lymphoma,[20] and in 12.5% of patients with bronchogenic carcinoma.[10] Among patients with bronchogenic carcinoma, the frequency of hypercalcemia varies with histological type: 23% with epidermoid carcinoma, 13% with large cell anaplastic carcinoma, and 2% with adenocarcinoma.[10] The mechanisms producing hypercalcemia are several and can be divided into three major categories. Table XVII-10-4 lists these categories along with the approximate percentage that each represents as percent of total patients reported in the literature. Hypercalcemia is associated with poor life expectancy in cancer patients. Ralston and colleagues reviewed their experience with 126 patients treated for hypercalcemia caused by cancer.[79] Irrespective of the response of serum calcium, the median survival was 30 days. The pathophysiology of hypercalcemia will be described first for solid tumors and then for the hematologic neoplasms (see Table XVII-10-4).

Solid tumors without evidence of bony metastases, or with minimal metastatic disease, appear to synthesize and secrete a protein which binds to the parathormone receptor.[22,63,66,96,98] The syndrome of hypercalcemia associated with solid tumors was the earliest of the hormonal syndromes of cancer to be reported, by Zondek in 1924.[114] Albright discussed such a patient in a 1941 clinical conference and first postulated that these tumors produced a parathormone-like substance.[4] The patient Albright discussed had hypercalcemia and hypophosphatemia with normal parathyroid glands at autopsy. Several publications employing early generation parathormone radioimmunoassays reported increased parathormone in blood of such patients.[13,18,89,99] As assay methods improved, however, it became clear that parathormone per se was rarely produced by such tumors. Federman reported a patient in 1971, also at a clinical pathological conference, who had squamous cell carcinoma, hypercalcemia and hypophosphatemia, but no detectable plasma parathormone.[30] In 1973, Powell and colleagues studied 11 patients with cancer and no bony metastases, who had hypercalcemia and hypophosphatemia.[78] Treatment of the tumor restored calcium to normal in nine of the patients. Using several parathormone immunoassays designed to react with parathormone fragments, as well as intact parathormone, no parathormone was detectable in either tumor extracts or blood. In extracts of all 11 tumors, however, a substance was detected that caused resorption of calcium from mouse calvaria incubated in vitro. In 1983, Simpson and colleagues studied five human and three animal cancers producing hypercalcemia using a sensitive and specific hybridization assay with parathormone messenger RNA.[91] No parathormone message was detected in these eight tumors. These studies suggested that a substance with parathormone-like biological properties was produced, but that this substance was not structurally identical to parathormone.

Subsequently, a number of investigators purified the proteins responsible for tumor hypercalcemia, sequenced the proteins, and identified the responsible gene.[62,101,103] The results show that a single gene appears to be expressed as three different proteins by alternative splicing.[101,103] The most abundant protein contains 139 amino acids of which the amino terminal portion shows 70% homology with parathormone.[101] It is this amino acid sequence, however, which is required for binding to the parathormone receptor. The 139 amino acid protein has been shown to have biological properties very similar to parathormone, but the potency relative to parathormone varies with different tissues or assays employed.[103] The gene for this protein, which has been called Parathyroid Hormone-Related Protein (PTHRP), is expressed in normal lactating mammary tissue[100] and possibly in normal keratinocytes.[65] Thus the ectopic hormone syndrome of hypercalcemia in carcinomas is another example of cancers expressing in greater amounts, a function of normal tissues. Recently, three groups of investigators[19,21,47] have developed standard immunoassays as well as immunoradiometric assays for PTHRP and have shown that PTHRP concentrations are increased in most patients with solid tumors and hypercalcemia. Increased PTHRP concentrations correlate with increased urinary cyclic AMP excretion. Plasma from normal subjects contains low or undetectable PTHRP. Since the normal lactating breast produces large amounts of PTHRP, the mechanism of hypercalcemia in patients with breast cancer has been reevaluated. Henderson and colleagues[47] have shown that 39% of 31 patients with breast cancer had elevated blood PTHRP.

The hematologic malignancies produce hypercalcemia by different mechanisms. In 1974 Mundy and colleagues reported that a bone resorbing substance produced by myeloma cells was similar to osteoclast-activating factor (OAF), a substance also produced by normal leukocytes activated in vitro.[68] Subsequently, it has appeared likely that OAF is not a single substance, but a group of substances which include lymphotoxin (produced by normal lymphocytes) and tumor necrosis factor ((also called cachectin) (produced by normal monocytes)).[2] Both substances are potent stimulators of bone resorption in vitro. Garret and colleagues reported that cultured myeloma cells secrete lymphotoxin and that this production is related to the hypercalcemia caused by myeloma.[35]

The hypercalcemia caused by type C virus-induced T-cell lymphoma, and occasionally by other neoplasms, is caused by still another mechanism. Breslau and colleagues[16] and Rosenthal and colleagues[81] demonstrated that these patients have increased quantities of 1,25 dihydroxy-vitamin D (1,25-D) in their blood. Helikson and colleagues described a patient with a large plasma cell myeloma and hypercalcemia who had increased blood 1,25-D.[46] Following tumor resection, 1,25-D concentrations returned to normal. The resected tumor was shown to convert 25 hydroxy vitamin D to 1,25-D. Hypercalcemia with increased 1,25-D in blood has also been reported in a patient with leiomyoblastoma and one with Hodgkin's disease. The patients with the carcinomas with hypercalcemia previously discussed do not have elevated blood 1,25-D.

Vasopressin (Antidiuretic Hormone) Production by Cancers

In 1957, Schwartz and colleagues first described the syndrome of hyponatremia, renal sodium loss, hypervolemia, and inappropriately high urine osmolality in association with cancer.[85] They attributed this syndrome to vasopressin (antidiuretic hormone, ADH) production by the cancer. Subsequently, several investigators verified that ADH could be

most part, these are less well understood than the hormone syndromes discussed in the first section. Anorexia is a common symptom in patients with cancer, especially in subjects with lung carcinoma, hypernephroma and carcinoma of the pancreas. This has been attributed to tumor production of the protein tumor necrosis factor (TNF), also called cachectin. This protein has a MW of 17,000,[14,24,88] and it has been speculated that the tumor induces TNF production by host cells. In 1985, Aderka and colleagues reported TNF was produced by peripheral blood mononuclear cells in patients with cancer.[1] Balkwill and colleagues reported in 1987 that 114 of 226 (50%) freshly obtained sera from patients with cancer had detectable TNF.[6] In contrast, only one of 32 samples from normal controls and only seven of 39 samples (18%) from asymptomatic cancer patients had detectable TNF. In contrast to these suggestive findings of Balkwill, four groups,[86,87,92,108] have reported that TNF is not detectable in sera of patients with cancer and cachexia. The explanation for the differences in these findings is uncertain. Balkwill and colleagues emphasized the importance of using freshly obtained serum samples,[6] but Selby and colleagues did use fresh samples and still did not detect TNF.[87]

While it is attractive to postulate that TNF/cachectin produced in response to a cancer is the cause of cancer-associated anorexia and weight loss, the data do not support such a view.

Fever and Cancer

Fever may be seen in patients with cancer in the absence of evidence of infection. It is estimated, for example, that 18% of patients with renal adenocarcinoma have fever.[59] Hodgkin's disease can also be associated with fever in the absence of an infection. Fever could be produced by either tumor induction of pyrogen formation by host white cells or by direct tumor production of a pyrogen. Pyrogen production by human tumor cell lines grown in vitro has been reported.[11]

Hematologic Syndromes

Idiopathic thrombocytopenic purpura (ITP), pure red cell aplasia, and aplastic anemia have all been reported to be associated with a variety of carcinomas and with lymphatic neoplasms. Kim and Boggs reviewed 10 patients with this syndrome.[53] Four of the 10 had lymphoid neoplasms. In 7 patients ITP occurred at the same time the cancer was diagnosed or following its recognition. Subsequently, 3 patients (2 with multiple myeloma and 1 with endometrial carcinoma) were reported to have ITP and circulating anti-platelet antibodies.[34,106] It was not possible to prove the tumor induced these antibodies. In 1987, however, Aghai and colleagues reported a patient with ITP and hepatic lymphoma.[3] Removal of the hepatic lymphoma was the only effective way of treating the ITP, and this was associated with return of platelet count to normal.

References

1. Aderka, D., Fisher, S., Levo, Y., Holtmann, H., Hahn, T., and Wallach, D: Cachectin/tumour-necrosis-factor production by cancer patients. Lancet, 2:1190, 1985.
2. Aggarwal, B. B., Henzel, W. J., Moffat, B., Kohr, W. J., and Hawkins, R. N.: Primary structure of human lymphotoxin derived from 1788 lymphoblastoid cell line. J. Biol. Chem., 260:2334, 1985.
3. Aghai, E., Quitt, M., Lurie, M., Antal, S., Cohen, L., Bitterman, H., and Froom, P.: Primary hepatic lymphoma presenting as symptomatic immune thrombocytopenic purpura. Cancer, 60:2308, 1987.
4. Albright, F.: Case records of the Massachusetts General Hospital case 27461. N. Engl. J. Med., 225:789, 1941.
5. Anderson, N. E., Rosenblum, M. K., Graus, F., Wiley, R. G., and Posner, J. B.:
Autoantibodies in paraneoplastic syndromes associated with small-cell lung cancer. Neurology, 38:1391, 1988.
6. Balkwill, F., Osborne, R., Burke, F., Naylor, S., Talbot, D., Durbin, H., Tavernier, J., and Fiers, W.: Evidence for tumour necrosis factor/cachectin production in cancer. Lancet, 2:1229, 1987.
7. Barkan, A. L., Shenker, Y., Grekin, R. J., Vale, W. W., Lloyd, R. B., and Beals, T. F.: Acromegaly due to ectopic growth hormone (GH)-releasing hormone (GHRH) production: dynamic studies of GH and ectopic GHRH secretion. J. Clin. Endocrinol. Metab., 63:1057, 1986.
8. Barnes, B. E., and Mawr, B.: Dermatomyositis and malignancy. A review of the literature. Ann. Intern. Med., 84:68, 1976.
9. Beck, C., and Burger, H. G.: Evidence for the presence of immunoreactive growth hormone in cancers of the lung and stomach. Cancer, 30:75, 1972.
10. Bender, R. A., and Hansen, H.: Hypercalcemia in bronchogenic carcinoma. Ann. Int. Med., 80:205, 1974.
11. Bernheim, H. A., Block, L. H., and Atkins, E.: Fever: pathogenesis, pathophysiology, and purpose. Ann. Int. Med., 91:261, 1979.
12. Berson, E. L., and Lessell, S.: Paraneoplastic night blindness with malignant melanoma. Am. J. Ophthalmol., 106:307, 1988.
13. Berson, S. A., and Yalow, R. S.: Parathyroid hormone in plasma in adenomatous hyperparathyroidism, uremia, and bronchogenic carcinoma. Science, 154:907, 1966.
14. Beutler, B., and Cerami, A.: Cachectin: more than a tumor necrosis factor. N. Engl. J. Med., 316:379, 1987.
15. Braunstein, G. D., Vaitukaitis, J. L., Carbore, P. D., and Ross, G. T.: Ectopic production of human chorionic gonadotropin by neoplasms. Ann. Int. Med., 78:39, 1973.
16. Breslau, N. A., McGuire, J. L., Zerwekh, J. E., Frenkel, E. P., and Pak, C. Y.: Hypercalcemia associated with increased serum calcitriol levels in three patients with lymphoma. Ann. Intern. Med., 100:1, 1984.
17. Buchanan, T. A., Gardiner, T. A., and Archer, D. B.: An ultra-structural study of retinal photoreceptor degeneration associated with bronchial carcinoma. Am. J. Ophthalmol., 97:277, 1984.
18. Buckle, R. M., McMillan, M., and Mallinson, C.: Ectopic secretion of parathyroid hormone by a renal adenocarcinoma in a patient with hypercalcemia. Br. Med. J., 4:724, 1970.
19. Budayr, A. A., Nissenson, R. A., Klein, R. F., Pun, K. K., Clark, O. H., Diep, D., Arnaud, C. D., and Strewler, G. J.: Increased serum levels of a parathyroid hormone-like protein in malignancy-associated hypercalcemia. Ann. Intern. Med., 111:807, 1989.
20. Bunn, P. A., Jr., Schechter, G. P., Jaffe, E., Blayney, D., Young, R. C., Matthews, M. J., Blattner, W., Broder, S., Robert-Guroff, M., and Gallo, R. C.: Clinical course of retrovirus-associated adult t-cell lymphoma in the United States. N. Engl. J. Med., 309:257, 1983.
21. Burtis, W. J., Brady, T. G., Orloff, J. J., Ersbak, J. B., Warrell, R. P., Jr., Olson, B. R., Wu, T. L., Mitnick, M. E., Broadus, A. E., and Stewart, A. F.: Immunochemical characterization of circulating parathyroid hormone-related protein in patients with humoral hypercalcemia of cancer. N. Eng. J. Med., 322:1106, 1990.
22. Burtis, W. J., Wu, T., Buch, C., Wysolmerski, J. J., Ingogna, K. L., Weir, E. C., Broadus, A. E., and Stewart, A. F.: Identification of a novel 17,000-dalton parathyroid hormone-like adenylate cyclase-stimulating protein from a tumor associated with humoral hypercalcemia of malignancy. J. Biol. Chem., 262:7151, 1987.
23. Cameron, D. P., Burger, H. G., DeKretzer, D. M., Catt, K. J., and Best, J. B.: On the presence of immunoreactive growth hormone in a bronchogenic carcinoma. Aust. Ann. Med., 18:143, 1969.
24. Cerami, A., Tracey, K. J., Lowry, S. F., and Beutler, B.: Cachectin: a pluripotent hormone released during the host response to invasion. Rec. Prog. Horm. Res., 43:99, 1987.
25. Crofts, J. W., Bachynski, B. N., and Odel, J. G.: Visual paraneoplastic syndrome associated with undifferentiated endometrial carcinoma. Can. J. Ophthalmol., 23:128, 1988.
26. Dabek, J. T.: Bronchial carcinoid tumour with acromegaly in two patients. J. Clin. Endocrinol. Metab., 38:329, 1974.
27. Daughaday, W. H., Emanuele, M. A., Brooks, M. H., Barbato, A. L., Kapadia, M., and Rotwein, P.: Synthesis and secretion of insulin-like growth factor II by a leiomyosarcoma with associated hypoglycemia. N. Eng. J. Med., 319:1434, 1988.
28. Dropcho, E. J., Chen, Y. T., Posner, J. B., and Old, L. J.: Cloning of a brain protein identified by autoantibodies from a patient with paraneoplastic cerebellar degeneration. Proc. Natl. Acad. Sci. USA, 84:4552, 1987.
29. Dropcho, E. J., Stanton, C., and Oh, S. J.: Neuronal antinuclear antibodies in a patient with Lambert-Eaton myasthenic syndrome and small-cell lung carcinoma. Neurology, 39:249, 1989.
30. Federman, D. D.: Case records of the Massachusetts General Hospital Case 15-1971. N. Engl. J. Med., 284:839, 1971.
31. Field, J. B., Keen, H., Johnson, P., et al.: Insulin-like activity of non-pancreatic tumors associated with hypoglycemia. J. Clin. Endocrinol. Metab., 23:1229, 1963.
32. Froesch, E. R., Zapf, J., and Widmer, U.: Hypoglycemia associated with non-islet-cell tumor and insulin-like growth factors. N. Eng. J. Med., 306:1178, 1982.
33. Frohman, L. A., Szabo, M., Berelowitz, M., and Stachura, M. E.: Partial purification and characterization of a peptide with growth hormone-releasing activity from extrapituitary tumors in patients with acromegaly. J. Clin. Invest., 65:43, 1980.
34. Furie, B.: Case records of the Massachusetts General Hospital. Case 8-1988. N. Engl. J. Med., 318:500, 1988.
35. Garrett, I. R., Durie, B. G. M., Nedwin, G. E., Gillespie, A., Bringman, A. T., Sabatini, M., Bertolini, D. R., and Mundy, G. R.: Production of lymphotoxin, a bone-resorbing cytokine, by cultured human myeloma cells. N. Engl. J. Med., 317:526, 1987.
36. George, J. M., Capen, C. C., and Phillips, A. S.: Biosynthesis of vasopressin in vitro and ultrastructure of a bronchogenic carcinoma. Patient with the syndrome of inappropriate secretion of antidiuretic hormone. J. Clin. Invest., 51:141, 1972.
37. Gilby, E. D., Rees, L. H., and Bondy, P. K.: Advances in Tumour Prevention, Detection and Characterization. Edited by W. Davis, and C. Maltoni. In Proceedings of the 6th International Symposium on Biology and characterization of human tumours, Copenhagen, 1975. Vol. 3. New York, American Elsevier, 1976, p. 132.
38. Gorden, P., Hendricks, C. M., Kahn, C. R., Megyesi, K., and Roth, J.: Hypoglycemia associated with non-islet-cell tumor and insulin-like growth factors. A study of the tumor types. N. Engl. J. Med., 305:1452, 1981.

39. Graus, F., Cordon-Cardo, C., and Posner, J. B.: Neuronal anti-nuclear antibody in sensory neuronopathy from lung cancer. Neurology, 35:538, 1985.
40. Graus, F., Elkon, K. B., Cordon-Cardo, C., and Posner, J. B.: Sensory neuronopathy and small cell lung cancer. Antineuronal antibody that also reacts with the tumor. Amer. J. Med., 80:45, 1986.
41. Graus, F., Elkon, K. B., Lloberes, P., Ribalta, T., Torres, A., Ussetti, P., Valls, J., Obach, J., and Agusti-Vidal, A.: Neuronal anti-nuclear antibody (anti-Hu) in paraneoplastic encephalomyelitis simulating acute polyneuritis. Acta Neurol. Scand., 75:249, 1987.
42. Greenlee, J. E., and Brashear, H. R.: Antibodies to cerebellar Purkinje cells in patients with paraneoplastic cerebellar degeneration and ovarian carcinoma. Ann. Neurol., 14:609, 1983.
43. Greenlee, J. E., and Sun, M.: Immunofluorescent labeling of non-human cerebellar tissue with sera from patients with systemic cancer and paraneoplastic cerebellar degeneration. Acta Neuropathol., 67:226, 1985.
44. Grunwald, G. B., Klein, R., Simmonds, M. A., and Kornguth, S. E.: Autoimmune basis for visual paraneoplastic syndrome in patients with small-cell lung carcinoma. Lancet, 1:658, 1985.
45. Hamilton, B. P. M., Upton, G. V., and Amatrude, T. T., Jr.: Evidence for the presence of neurophysin in tumors producing the syndrome of inappropriate antidiuresis. J. Clin. Endocrinol. Metab., 35:764, 1972.
46. Helikson, M. A., Havey, A. D., Zerwekh, J. E., Breslau, N. A., and Gardner, D. W.: Plasma-cell granuloma producing calcitriol and hypercalcemia. Ann. Intern. Med., 105:379, 1986.
47. Henderson, J. E., Shustik, C., Kremer, R., Rabbani, S. A., Hendy, G. N., and Goltzman, D.: Circulating concentrations of parathyroid hormone-like peptide in malignancy and in hyperparathyroidism. J. Bone Miner. Res., 5:105, 1990.
48. Howlett, T. A., Drury, P. L., Perry, L., Donlach, I., Rees, L. H., and Besser, G. M.: Diagnosis and management of ACTH-dependent Cushing's syndrome: Comparison on the features in ectopic and pituitary ACTH production. Clin. Endocrinology, 24:699, 1986.
49. Kaganowicz, A., Farkouh, H., Frantz, A. G., and Blaustein, A. U.: Ectopic human growth hormone in ovaries and breast cancer. J. Clin. Endocrinol. Metab., 48:5, 1978.
50. Kearsley, J. H., Johnson, P., and Halmagyi, G. M.: Paraneoplastic cerebellar disease. Remission with excision of the primary tumor. Arch. Neurol., 42:1208, 1985.
51. Keltner, J. L., Roth, A. M., and Chang, R. S.: Photoreceptor degeneration. Possible autoimmune disorder. Arch. Ophthalmol., 101:564, 1983.
52. Kew, M. C., Kirschner, M. A., Abrahams, G. E., and Katz, M.: Mechanisms of feminization in primary liver cancer. N. Engl. J. Med., 296:1084, 1977.
53. Kim, H. D., and Boggs, D. R.: A syndrome resembling idiopathic thrombocytopenic purpura in 10 patients with diverse forms of cancer. Am. J. Med., 67:371, 1979.
54. Klingele, T. G., Burde, R. M., Rappazzo, J. A., Isserman, M. J., Burgess, D., and Kantor, O.: Paraneoplastic retinopathy. J. Clin. Neuro. Ophthalmol., 101:239, 1984.
55. Kornguth, S. E., Kalinke, T., Grunwald, G. B., Schutta, H., and Dahl, D.: Anti-neurofilament antibodies in the sera of patients with small cell carcinoma of the lung and with visual paraneoplastic syndrome. Cancer Res., 46:2588, 1986.
56. Kornguth, S. E., Klein, R., Appen, R., and Choate, J.: Occurrence of anti-retinal ganglion cell antibodies in patients with small cell carcinoma of the lung. Cancer, 50:1289, 1982.
57. Kyle, C. V., Evans, M. C., and Odell, W. D.: Growth hormone-like material in normal human tissues. J. Clin. Endocrinol. Metab., 53:1138, 1981.
58. Lakhanpal, S., Bunch, T. W., Ilstrup, D. M., and Melton, L. J., III: Polymyositis-dermatomyositis and malignant lesions: Does an association exist? Mayo Clin. Proc., 61:645, 1986.
59. Laski, M. E., and Vugrin, D.: Paraneoplastic syndromes in hypernephroma. Semin. Nephrol., 7:123, 1987.
60. Liddle, G. W., Nicholson, W. E., Island, D. P., Orth, D. N., Abe, K., and Lowder, S. C.: Clinical laboratory studies of "ectopic" hormonal syndromes. Rec. Prog. Horm. Res., 25:283, 1969.
61. Malchoff, C. D., Orth, D. N., Abhoud, C., Carney, J. A., Pairolcro, P. C., and Corey, R. M.: Ectopic ACTH syndrome caused by a bronchial carcinoid tumor responsive to dexamethasone, metyrapone and corticotropin-releasing factor. Am. J. Med., 84:760, 1988.
62. Mangin, M., Ikeda, K., Dreyer, B. E., and Broadus, A. E.: Two distinct tumor-derived, parathyroid hormone-like peptides result from alternative RNA processing. Program of the 70th Annual Meeting of the Endocrine Society, 1988, p. 26, Abstract 21.
63. Mangin, M., Sebb, A. C., Dreyer, B. E., et al.: Identification of a cDNA encoding a parathyroid hormone-like peptide from a human tumor associated with humoral hypercalcemia of malignancy. Proc. Natl. Acad. Sci. U.S.A., 85:597, 1988.
64. Melmed, S., Ezrin, C., Kovacs, K., Goodman, R. S., and Frohman, L. A.: Acromegaly due to secretion of growth hormone by an ectopic pancreatic islet-cell tumor. N. Engl. J. Med., 312:9, 1985.
65. Merendino, J. J., Jr., Insogna, K. L., Miltone, L. M., Broadus, A. E., and Stewart, A. F.: A parathyroid hormone-like protein from cultured human keratinocytes. Science, 231:388, 1986.
66. Moseley, J. M., Kubota, M., Diefenbach-Jagger, H., Wettenhall, R. E., Kemp, B. E., Suva, L. J., Rodda, C. P., Ebeling, P. R., Hudson, P. J., Zajac, J. D., et al.: Parathyroid hormone-related protein purified from a human lung cancer cell line. Proc. Natl. Acad. Sci. U.S.A., 84:5048, 1987.
67. Mundy, G. R.: Pathogenesis of hypercalcemia of malignancy. Clin. Endocrinol., 23:705, 1985.
68. Mundy, G. R., Raisz, L. G., Cooper, R. A., Schechter, G. P., and Salmon, S. E.: Evidence for the secretion of an osteoclast stimulating factor in myeloma. N. Engl. J. Med., 291:1041, 1974.
69. Nakanishi, S., Inove, A., Kita, T., Nakamura, M., Chang, A. C., Cohen, S. N., and Numa, S.: Nucleotide sequence of a cloned cDNA for bovine corticotropin-β-lipotropin precursor. Nature, 278:423, 1979.
70. Nieman, L. K., Chrousos, G. P., Oldfield, E. H., Augerinos, P. C., Cutler, G. B., and Loriaux, D. C.: The ovine corticotropin-releasing hormone stimulation test and the dexamethasone suppression test on the differential diagnosis of Cushing's syndrome. Ann. Int. Med., 105:862, 1986.
71. North, W. G., LaRochelle, F. T., Jr., Melton, J., et al.: Human neurophysins (HNPs) as potential tumor markers for small-cell carcinoma (SCC). Clin. Res., 26:536A, 1978.
71A. Odell, W. D.: Paraendocrine syndromes of cancer. *In* Advances in Internal Medicine, Vol. 34. Edited by G. H. Stollerman, W. J. Harrington, J. T. LaMont, et al. Chicago, Year Book Medical Publishers, 1989, p. 325.
72. Odell, W. D., and Appleton, W. S.: Hormonal manifestations of cancer. *In* Williams Textbook of Endocrinology, 8th Edition. Edited by J. D. Wilson, and D. W. Foiter. Philadelphia, W. B. Saunders Co., In press, 1990.
73. Odell, W. D., and Saito, E.: Protein hormone-like materials from normal and cancer cells—"Ectopic" hormone production. *In* 13th International Cancer Congress, Part E, Cancer Management. Edited by E. A. Mirand, W. B. Hutchinson, and E. Mihich. New York, Alan R. Liss, Inc., 1983, pp. 247–248.
74. Odell, W. D., Wolfsen, A. R., Bachelot, I., and Hirose, F. M.: Ectopic production of lipotropin by cancer. Am. J. Med., 66:631, 1979.
75. Odell, W. D., Wolfsen, A., Yoshimoto, Y., Weitzman, R., Fisher, D., and Hirose, F.: Ectopic peptide synthesis. A universal concomitant of neoplasia. Trans. Assoc. Am. Phys., 90:204, 1977.
76. Pass, H. I., Doppmon, J. L., Nieman, L., Stouroff, M., Vetto, J., Norton, J. A., Travis, W., Chrousos, G. P., Oldfield, E. H., and Cutler, G. B., Jr.: Management of the ectopic ACTH syndrome due to thoracic carcinoids: The NIH experience and review of the world literature annals of thoracic surgery. Ann. Thoracic Surg., 50:52, 1990.
77. Pierce, J. G., and Parsons, T. F.: Glycoprotein hormones: Structure and function. Ann. Rev. Biochem., 50:465, 1981.
78. Powell, D., Singer, F. R., Murray, T. M., Minkin, C., and Potts, J. T., Jr.: Nonparathyroid humoral hypercalcemia in patients with neoplastic diseases. N. Engl. J. Med., 289:176, 1973.
79. Ralston, S. H., Gallacher, S. J., Patel, U., Campbell, J., and Boyle, I. T.: Cancer-associated hypercalcemia: Morbidity and mortality. Clinical experience in 126 treated patients. Ann. Int. Med., 112:499, 1990.
80. Rosa, C., Amr, S., Birken, S., Wehmann, R., and Nisula, B.: Effect of desialylation of human chorionic gonadotropin on its metabolic clearance rate in humans. J. Clin. Endocrinol. Metab., 59:1215, 1984.
81. Rosenthal, N., Insogna, K. L., Godsall, J. W., Smaldone, L., Waldron, J. A., and Stewart, A. F.: Elevations in circulating 1,25-dihydroxyvitamin D in three patients with lymphoma-associated hypercalcemia. J. Clin. Endocrinol. Metab., 60:29, 1985.
82. Saeed uz Zafar, M., Mellinger, R. C., Fine, G., Szabo, M., and Frohman, L. A.: Acromegaly associated with a bronchial carcinoid tumor: evidence for ectopic production of growth hormone-releasing activity. J. Clin. Endocrinol. Metab., 48:66, 1979.
83. Saito, E., and Odell, W. D.: Corticotropin/lipotropin common precursor-like material in normal rat extrapituitary tissues. Proc. Natl. Acad. Sci. U.S.A., 80:3792, 1983.
84. Sawyer, R. A., Selhorst, J. B., Zimmerman, L. E., and Hoyt, W. F.: Blindness caused by photoreceptor degeneration as a remote effect of cancer. Am. J. Ophthalmol., 81:606, 1976.
85. Schwartz, W. B., Bennett, W., Curelop, S., et al.: A syndrome of renal sodium loss and hyponatremia probably resulting from inappropriate secretion of antidiuretic hormone. Am. J. Med., 23:529, 1957.
86. Scuderi, P., Sterling, K. E., Lam, K. S., Finley, P. R., Ryan, K. J., Ray, C. G., Petersen, E., Slymen, D. J., and Salmon, S. E.: Raised serum levels of tumour necrosis factor in parasitic infections. Lancet, 2:1364, 1986.
87. Selby, P., Hobbs, S., Viner, C., Jackson, E., Jones, A., Newell, D., Calvert, A. H., McElwain, T., Fearon, K., Humphreys, J., et al.: Tumour necrosis factor in man: clinical and biological observations. Br. J. Cancer, 56:803, 1987.
88. Shear, M. J., Turner, F. C., Perrault, A., et al.: Chemical treatment of tumors. V. Isolation of the hemorrhage-producing fraction from serratia marcescens (bacillus prodigiosus) culture filtrate. HNCI, 4:81, 1943.
89. Sherwood, L. J., O'Riordan, J. L. H., Aurbach, G. D., and Potts, J. T.: Production of parathyroid hormone by nonparathyroid tumors. J. Clin. Endocrinol. Metab., 27:140, 1967.
90. Shirabe, T., Hirokawa, M., Yasuda, T., et al.: An autopsy case of carcinoma of the lung associated with subacute cerebellar degeneration and Eaton-Lambert syndrome. Kawasaki Med. J., 7:177, 1981.
91. Simpson, E. L., Mundy, G. R., D'Souza, S. M., Ibbotson, K. J., Bockman, R., and Jacobs, J. W.: Absence of parathyroid hormone messenger RNA in non-parathyroid tumor associated with hypercalcemia. N. Engl. J. Med., 309:325, 1983.
92. Socher, S. H., Martinez, D., Craig, J. B., Kuhn, J. G., and Oliff, A.: Tumor necrosis factor not detectable in patients with clinical cancer cachexia. JNCI, 80:595, 1988.
93. Stefansson, K., Marton, L. S., Dieperink, M. E., Molnar, G. K., Schlaepfer, W. W., and Helgason, C. M.: Circulating autoantibodies to the 200,000-dalton protein of neurofilaments in the serum of healthy individuals. Science, 228:1117, 1985.
94. Steiner, H., Dahlback, O., and Waldenstrom, J.: Ectopic growth-hormone production and osteoarthropathy in carcinoma of the bronchus. Lancet, 1:783, 1968.
95. Steven, M. M., Mackay, I. R., Carnegie, P. R., Bhathal, P. S., and Anderson, R. M.: Cerebellar cortical degeneration with ovarian carcinoma. Postgrad. Med. J., 58:47, 1982.
96. Strewler, G. J., Stern, P. H., Jacobs, J. W., Eveloff, J., Klein, R. F., Leung, S. C., Rosenblatt, M., and Nissenson, R. A.: Parathyroid hormone-like protein from human renal carcinoma cells. Structural and functional homology with parathyroid hormone. J. Clin. Invest., 80:1803, 1987.
97. Sparagana, M., Phillips, G., Hoffman, C., and Kucera, L.: Ectopic growth hormone syndrome associated with lung cancer. Metabolism, 20:730, 1971.
98. Suva, L. J., Winslow, G. A., Wettenhall, R. E., Hammonds, R. G., Moseley, J. M., Diefenbach-Jagger, H., et al.: A parathyroid hormone-related protein implicated in malignant hypercalcemia: cloning and expression. Science, 237:893, 1987.
99. Tashjian, A. H., Jr., Levine, L., and Munson, P. L.: Immunochemical identification of parathyroid hormone in non-parathyroid neoplasms associated with hypercalcemia. J. Exp. Med., 119:467, 1964.
100. Thiede, M. A., and Rodan, G. A.: Expression of a calcium-mobilizing parathyroid hormone-like peptide in lactating mammary tissue. Science, 242:278, 1988.
101. Thiede, M. A., Strewler, G. J., Nissenson, R. A., Rosenblatt, M., and Rodan, G. A.: Human renal carcinoma expresses two messages encoding a parathyroid hormone-like peptide: Evidence for the alternative splicing of a single-copy gene. Proc. Natl. Acad. Sci. U.S.A., 85:4605, 1988.
102. Thirkill, C. E., Roth, A. M., and Keltner, J. L.: Cancer-associated retinopathy. Arch. Ophthalmol., 105:372, 1987.
103. Thorikay, M., Kramer, S., Reynolds, F. H., et al.: Synthesis of a gene encoding parathyroid hormone-like protein-(1-141): Purification and biological characterization of the expressed protein. Endocrinology, 124:111, 1989.

104. Trotter, J. L., Hendin, B. A., and Osterland, C. K.: Cerebellar degeneration with Hodgkin's disease. An immunological study. Arch. Neurol., 33:660, 1976.

105. Vaitukaitis, J. V., Braunstein, G. D., and Ross, G. T.: A radioimmunoassay which specifically measures human chorionic gonadotropin in the presence of human luteinizing hormone. Am. J. Obstet. Gynecol., 113:751, 1972.

106. Verdirame, J. D., Feagler, J. R., and Commers. J. R: Multiple myeloma associated with immune thrombocytopenic purpura. Cancer, 56:1199, 1985.

107. Vorherr, H., Massry, S. G., Utiger, R. D., and Kleeman, C. R.: Antidiuretic principle in malignant tumor extracts from patients with inappropriate ADH syndrome. J. Clin. Endocrinol. Metab., 28:162, 1968.

108. Waage, A., Espevik, T., and Lamvik, J.: Detection of tumour necrosis factor-like cytotoxicity in serum from patients with septicaemia but not from untreated cancer patients. Scand. J. Immunol., 24:739, 1986.

109. Widmer, U., Zapf, J., and Froesch, E. R.: Is extrapancreatic tumor hypoglycemia associated with elevated levels of insulin-like growth factor II? J. Clin. Endocrinol. Metab., 55:833, 1982.

110. Wolfsen, A. R., and Odell, W. D.: ProACTH: Use for early detection of lung cancer. Am. J. Med., 66:765, 1979.

111. Yoshimoto, Y., Wolfsen, A., Hirose, F., and Odell, W. D.: Human chorionic gonadotropin-like material: Presence in normal human tissue. Am. J. Obstet. Gynecol., 134:729, 1979.

112. Yoshimoto, Y., Wolfsen, A. R., and Odell, W. D.: Human chorionic gonadotropin-like substance in non-endocrine tissues of normal subjects. Science, 197:575, 1977.

113. Yoshimoto, Y., Wolfsen, A. R., and Odell, W. D.: Glycosylation, a variable in the production of hCG by cancers. Am. J. Med., 67:414, 1979.

114. Zondek, H., Petow, H., and Siebert, W: Die bedeutungder calcium best immung in blute fur dic diagnose der niereninsuffizieuz. Ztshr f. klin med Berl, 99:129, 1924.

XVIII

Principles of Biotherapeutics

XVIII-1

Immunostimulants

Robert C. Bast, Jr.
Donald L. Morton

Introduction

Bacteria and their products have been used to treat cancer patients for more than a hundred years. During the last two decades of the 19th century, physicians and surgeons in Europe and in the United States had observed tumor regression associated with successful resolution of erysipelas.[125] Based upon these observations, William B. Coley had utilized culture supernatants from *Micrococcus pyogenes* and *Serratia marcescens* to treat cancer patients with impressive, albeit anecdotal responses.[24] Coley's mixed bacterial vaccine (MBV) was given to several hundred patients and activity was observed against a variety of human cancers.[120] A formal clinical trial of MBV was undertaken more recently in patients with nodular non-Hodgkin's lymphoma to compare chemotherapy with and without the addition of the bacterial immunostimulants. In an early analysis, MBV appeared to enhance the results of conventional chemotherapy,[73] but improvement was not maintained during subsequent followup.[74] A carefully controlled trial in hepatocellular carcinoma has also been reported where MBV appeared to improve the survival of patients who received cisplatin chemotherapy, but the differences between the immuno-chemotherapy and chemotherapy groups did not achieve statistical significance.[176]

Many different immunostimulants and immunomodulators have been evaluated in preclinical studies and in clinical trials. Contact allergens, Bacillus Calmette Guérin, muramyl dipeptide, *Corynebacterium parvum* and levamisole have received particular attention. In addition, certain cancer chemotherapeutic agents thought to act by direct cytotoxicity have been shown to modulate the immune response.[32] Notable among these are 6-mercaptopurine,[156] doxorubicin,[31] cisplatin,[97] and cyclophosphamide.[59,131] When given in high doses, cyclophosphamide can inhibit both T-cell and B-cell mediated reactions, but in low doses this agent can eliminate suppressor cells and act as an immunostimulant in a fraction of trials.[59,131] This chapter will focus upon those immunostimulants for which reproducible antitumor activity has been

documented against human cancer, although a number of other immunopotentiators have been evaluated.[38,123,148,162]

Contact Allergens

The intense delayed hypersensitivity evoked by contact allergens has been used to treat cutaneous neoplasms.[79,80] Primary squamous and basal cell carcinomas have regressed following application of contact allergens such as dinitrochlorobenzene (DNCB) or triethylene-iminobenzoquinone. Patients with multiple basal and squamous cell carcinomas have been sensitized to contact allergens. Dilutions of the contact allergens have then been found that would not produce reactivity on normal skin. When these were applied to tumor bearing areas, both neoplastic and pre-neoplastic lesions developed marked erythema and regressed. Complete control of tumor growth has been obtained in some patients for more than four years. In dermatologic practice, topical application of efudex (5-fluorouracil; 5-FU) has proven as effective. Here, direct cytotoxic activity as well as contact allergy are probably important.

Contact allergens have also been used to treat gynecologic neoplasms. Topical application of DNCB or 5-FU has been evaluated in patients with vulvar, vaginal and cervical carcinomas.[46,47,62,87,106,140,141] DNCB induced regression of vulvar carcinoma in situ in as many as 60% of patients in early studies, although lower response rates have been observed in more recent series. Topical DNCB achieved long term control of disease in 26% of 180 patients with positive cervical cytologies in the absence of demonstrably invasive cancer.[47] Use of DNCB has, however, been associated with marked vulvar discomfort and 5-FU may be somewhat better tolerated.[62] In small series, topical 5-FU has eradicated vaginal carcinoma in situ or cervical intraepithelial neoplasia in a majority of cases.[140,141] Given the efficacy of alternative methods for managing these lesions, contact allergens are still not sufficiently reliable to provide the treatment of choice for many patients. Studies with contact allergens in dermatologic and gynecologic practice have, however, provided excellent examples of the antitumor activity of delayed cutaneous reactivity when it can be focused on tumor tissue.

Bacillus Calmette Guérin (BCG)

BCG is an attenuated strain of *Mycobacterium bovis* that has been widely used as a tuberculosis vaccine.[45,104] Vaccination with BCG induces intense and prolonged reactivity to PPD, precluding use of tuberculin skin tests to document exposure to virulent mycobacteria. With the development of effective anti-tuberculous chemotherapy, BCG has been used less frequently for the prevention of tuberculosis in the United States.

In animals, BCG can delay or prevent the development of cancers induced with chemical carcinogens, oncogenic viruses or radiation.[5] Treatment with BCG can also delay the onset of leukemias[93] and mammary cancers[194] in animals genetically predisposed to the development of these neoplasms.

The incidence of acute leukemia appeared to be decreased in children who had had BCG vaccination.[27,145] Prospective confirmatory trials were discouraged by other retrospective trials that suggested BCG vaccination in Puerto Rico was associated with a slight excess of lymphomas.[26,163]

In tumor transplant models, pretreatment with BCG has inhibited or suppressed progressive tumor growth when tumor cells were subsequently injected.[129] Growth of established tumor transplants could also be inhibited. Systemic treatment with BCG has been most effective when treatment with the immunostimulant has been combined with more conventional modalities such as surgical excision, cytotoxic chemotherapy, hormonal manipulation or radiotherapy.[5] In animal models and in the clinic, the most dramatic effects have been obtained with direct intralesional injection of BCG.[119,208] The efficacy of intralesional therapy has related to contact between tumor cells and micro-organisms, the size of the tumor, the dose of BCG, the immunocompetence of the host and, possibly, to the immunogenicity of the tumor cells.[5] intralesional injection of BCG has eliminated regional lymph node metastases of a poorly immunogenic guinea pig hepatoma and has established systemic immunity.[208]

Several mechanisms have been proposed for the activity of BCG in animal models. Tumor cells can be eliminated by the development of a specific T-cell mediated response to tumor associated antigens (see XVIII-2) or can be killed as "bystanders" at the site of an intense host response to the mycobacteria. Chronic macrophage mediated cytotoxicity may be particularly important for bystander killing. Activated histiocytes have been found in close association with degenerating tumor cells.[50] Antigenic mycobacterial products such as PPD can specifically stimulate T-lymphocytes that can attract, arrest and activate macrophages through the release of different cytokines including interferon-gamma. Once activated, macrophages can control the growth of phagocytized micro-organisms and can kill adjacent tumor cells.[112] Tumor necrosis factor, reactive oxygen species and reactive nitrogen species may all be important mediators of macrophage cytotoxicity in different systems. NK cells,[105] lymphotoxin,[135] antibodies[119] and microvascular damage[5] may also contribute to the antitumor activity of BCG. Production of cytokines

such as IL-2 that augment inducer function is likely to facilitate the development of T-cell mediated immunity against tumor associated antigens. Suppressor cells can, however, also be induced by treatment with BCG.

Cutaneous metastases from malignant melanoma have regressed following intralesional injection of BCG.[119] In patients who are immunocompetent, more than 90% of cutaneous melanoma metastases have regressed after direct intralesional injection. Overall, more than 60% of cutaneous lesions have responded.[5] In addition, 15% of noninjected lesions have also regressed, consistent with a systemic antitumor effect.[5,119] Cutaneous lesions have responded most frequently, regional node metastases have been controlled less often and visceral metastases have regressed only on rare occasions.

A large number of studies have been undertaken to demonstrate the systemic impact of cutaneous administration of BCG on a variety of human cancers. Despite promising early reports using BCG with or without tumor cells as a vaccine,[48,108] most carefully controlled studies have failed to document a therapeutic effect following the systemic administration of BCG.[5,56,125,178] Possible exceptions include intravenous administration of BCG to patients with acute myeloid leukemia[196] and the intralesional administration of BCG to patients with primary melanoma.[144] In the latter study, intratumoral injection of BCG was associated with a significant fraction of long term survivors. An initial observation that intrapleural administration of BCG prolonged survival of patients with resectable lung cancer[109,110] was not confirmed in a larger subsequent trial.[103]

Local complications of BCG administration have included erythema, induration, pruritus, and ulceration at injection sites, associated with regional lymphadenopathy.[5] Systemic reactions have been observed more frequently after intralesional injection than following intradermal administration of the vaccine. Chills, fever and malaise have been observed after repeated injections.[168] Rarely, erythema nodosum, granulomatous hepatitis, anaphylaxis, and shock associated with DIC have been observed. Progressive BCG infection has occurred in a small number of profoundly immunosuppressed patients. When recognized, BCG infection has responded to treatment with multiple anti-tuberculous drugs. In a comparison of intralesional treatment of melanoma metastases with BCG and DNCB, the two agents were similarly effective in controlling injected lesions, but the contact allergen was significantly less toxic.[23]

The major clinical application of BCG has been in the treatment of bladder cancer by intravesical administration of the agent.[88,118,139] Regional administration of BCG permits direct contact between the micro-organisms and superficial lesions on the bladder mucosa. BCG may bind selectively to fibronectin exposed on disrupted urothelial surfaces.[61] In collected series, BCG administered therapeutically has produced complete regression of Ta, T1 or Tis lesions in 71% of cases.[52] Moreover, intravesical BCG administered prophylactically has significantly delayed disease progression, prolonged the period of bladder preservation and increased overall survival in a randomized concurrently controlled study.[53] In direct comparisons and in meta-analysis of intravesical therapy, BCG has proven superior to cytotoxic drugs including thiotepa, doxorubicin and mitomycin C.[52,90] In addition BCG has produced a complete response in up to 50% of patients who have failed intravesical thiotepa or mitomycin C.[164]

The intense inflammation evoked by the intravesical administration of BCG can produce dysuria, frequency, urgency and hematuria, but severe cystitis has occurred in less than 10% of patients in large series.[52,132] Systemic reactions have generally been mild with fever >103°F in <4% of patients. Less than 1% of those treated with intravesical BCG have experienced pneumonitis, hepatitis, arthralgia, arthritis, skin rash, ureteral obstruction, epididymo-orchitis or bladder contracture.[89] Monthly maintenance therapy has not improved the results obtained with six weekly treatments, but did increase local toxicity including dysuria, frequency and urgency.[3]

Following intravesical administration of BCG, several cytokines including IL-1, IL-2, and TNF can be detected in the urine.[11] Urinary levels of IL-2 and of an IL-2 inhibitor have both correlated with a favorable response to BCG.[35] As the inhibitor can neutralize IL-2 activity, correlation of both markers with prognosis calls into question the importance of urinary IL-2 in controlling tumor growth. Both markers might, however, reflect the intensity of local inflammation.

Chemically Defined Components of Mycobacterial Immunostimulants

Much of the local antitumor and systemic adjuvant activity of BCG is maintained in the mycobacterial cell walls when they are presented to the host on the surface of oil droplets. Intralesional injection of such preparations can produce local regression of guinea pig hepatoma transplants or primary autochthonous tumors of the lid and conjunctiva in cattle.[42,81] Muramyl dipeptide (MDP) and trehalose dimycolate (TDM) are components of mycobacteria that have been analyzed in greatest depth.[92] MDP is the smallest compound identified to date that retains the adjuvant properties of whole mycobacteria in Freund's complete adjuvant. MDP can activate macrophages, stimulate NK cells and modify T- and B-cell reactivity to unrelated antigens. MDP has stimulated the expression of IL-6,[154] membrane associated IL-1,[4,152] and paf-Acether[152] by macrophages. Oral administration of MDP has primed mice for the release of tumor necrosis factor.[122] MDP has augmented the effect of interferon-gamma on macrophages,[165,188] as well as the effects of IL-2 and IL-4 on B-cells.[166] TDM is closely related to the "cord factor" of virulent mycobacteria that prevents fusion of lysosomes with endosomal vacuoles.[167] A combination of MDP and TDM is required to produce regression of guinea pig hepatoma transplants after intralesional injection.[111,207]

Following parenteral administration, MDP is cleared from the circulation within 60 minutes, an interval that does not permit systemic activation of macrophages.[36,134] When contained in negatively charged liposomes, MDP is preferentially localized in macrophages and released slowly.[133] MDP in liposomes can produce regression of pulmonary metastases in several murine models.

Greater antitumor activity has been obtained with muramyl tripeptide phosphatidylethanolamine (MTP-PE), a lipophilic derivative of water-soluble MDP, that can associate more effectively with liposomes. MTP-PE in liposomes has activated macrophages in T-cell deficient hosts.[75] Additional macrophage activation has been achieved when MTP-PE and interferon-γ have been combined within liposomes. The combination of MTP-PE and interferon-gamma has proven particularly effective for eradicating pulmonary metastases in a murine melanoma model.[133] In a concurrently controlled trial of liposome encapsulated MTP-PE following resection of primary autochthonous canine osteosarcomas, MTP-PE prolonged median survival from 77 to 222 days and produced disease free survivors at one year.[133] Phase I trials in cancer patients have demonstrated the ability of MTP-PE to modify human macrophage function, but have not yet detected anti-tumor activity.[82,187] Of importance for future trials, the optimal dose of MTP-PE for stimulating macrophage function was several fold lower than the maximally tolerated dose,[82] a property that is shared with several other biological response modifiers.

Corynebacterium parvum (Propionobacterium acnes)

C. parvum is an anaerobic gram positive bacillus that can modulate a number of host immune functions. Non-viable C. parvum can exert antitumor activity, avoiding the possibility of progressive growth of the bacteria in immunocompromised patients. Both local and systemic effects have been observed in experimental systems. Systemic administration of the agent has produced regression of established murine tumor transplants.[49,113,198] Intraperitoneal treatment with C. parvum has cured mice bearing >10^5 syngeneic ovarian carcinoma cells.[7,83] Intralesional injection has been particularly effective in producing regression of well established tumor transplants and inducing systemic anti-tumor immunity.[86,99,100,157]

C. parvum can affect T-cell, B-cell, NK cell, macrophage and granulocyte function.[6,72,95,98,124] T-cell mediated reactions can be stimulated or suppressed. Incubation of C. parvum with human peripheral blood mononuclear cells can induce interferon-γ,[55,58] and tumor necrosis factor-α.[147] As in the case of BCG, C. parvum is thought to kill tumor cells as bystanders at sites of intense local inflammation and also to induce specific T-cell mediated immunity that can be expressed systemically. Macrophages, granulocytes and NK cells may be most important as effectors of local bystander killing by C. parvum. In contrast to BCG, the antitumor activity of C. parvum is only partially reduced in T-cell deficient hosts.[157,199] C. parvum can induce tumoricidal activity in different macrophage populations by T-cell dependent[21] or independent[72] mechanisms. Contact between C. parvum and tumor cells can also induce specific immunity toward tumor associated antigens mediated by T-cells.[182,183] Potentiation of B-cell activity has also been observed.[124] Treatment with C. parvum restored the impaired accessory cell function of adherent splenocytes from mice bearing transplants of EL4 lymphoma and partially restored the ability of tumor bearing mice to produce antibodies against exogenous antigens.[128]

In the clinic, the systemic administration of C. parvum has failed to affect tumor growth reproducibly in advanced disease or in adjuvant trials.[30,34,57,125,137,191,200] One possible exception to this generalization has been raised by the long term analysis of two concurrently controlled, randomized trials that had compared subcutaneous injection of *C. parvum* and intradermal injection of BCG as adjuvant immunotherapy for stage II melanoma.[101] If data from the two trials were pooled, patients treated with *C. parvum* enjoyed significantly greater disease-free survival and overall survival than did those treated with BCG. Subcutaneous injection of *C. parvum* has produced local inflammation, swelling, low grade fever, and chills. Intravenous administration has been associated with more severe side effects including high fever, rigors, headache, cyanosis, blanching, mild hypertension, more severe hypotension, nausea, and vomiting.[17,33,39,40]

The most convincing clinical activity of *C. parvum* has been observed after regional administration of the agent into the pleura or peritoneum to control malignant effusions.[15,107,114,146,193] In one study of lung and breast cancer patients, three weekly intrapleural injections of *C. parvum* produced total resolution in 50 of 53 malignant pleural effusions.[15] Toxicity was limited to fever, pleuritic pain, and cough judged less intense than that produced by other agents.[15] Sequential studies of pleural fluid have been performed in a limited number of patients.[15,146] At 6–72 hours after treatment granulocytes, lymphocytes and macrophages appeared in increased numbers associated with tumor necrosis.[15] By one week, decreased fluid accumulation was associated with a decrease in the concentration of leukocytes in the pleural fluid.[146] On a percentage basis, granulocytes were persistently elevated, whereas lymphocytes and macrophages had decreased. At this late interval, NK activity and interferon levels did not differ from baseline.

Consistent with earlier studies in a murine model,[7,83] intraperitoneal injection of *C. parvum* produced regression of small tumor nodules (<1 cm) in 30% of ovarian cancer patients.[8,9] Intraperitoneal injection of the agent attracted and activated macrophages and NK cells capable of more effective tumor cell killing in the absence or presence of antibodies against tumor associated antigens.[8,9,96] Intense inflammation and formation of adhesions has, however, limited the use of *C. parvum* for the treatment of ovarian cancer. More recent phase I studies of intraperitoneal immunotherapy have tested purified cytokines including the interferons[10] and IL-2.[170,186] Intraperitoneal injection of interferon-α has, in general, been well tolerated and has been substantially more effective than systemic injection of the same agent in controlling ovarian tumor growth.[12] Use of IL-2 in this setting may be limited by the same regional toxicity observed with *C. parvum*.

Other Bacterial Vaccines

Systemic administration of *Nocardia rubra* cell wall skeletons (N-CWS) has suppressed the growth of murine leukemia transplants.[68] Intralesional injection of N-CWS produced regression of autochthonous bovine lymphosarcomas.[130] Administration of N-CWS induced tumoricidal macrophages[63,65] and augmented the production of several cytokines by peritoneal cells including IL-1,[64] TNF[67] and interferons-α, β and γ.[66] N-CWS has also induced the local accumulation of NK cells[150] as well as precursors for lymphokine activated killer (LAK) cells which may contribute to synergistic interactions with IL-2.[116] Intratumor injection of murine and rat fibrosarcomas has augmented specific concomitant immunity that is apparently mediated through T-cells[71] or macrophages.[126]

In clinical studies, N-CWS has augmented human NK activity,[202] ADCC effector function,[202] interferon production,[202] and granulocyte cytostatic activity.[158] N-CWS has also activated human pleural macrophages to inhibit lung cancer cells[151] and potentiated the production of human LAK cells in the presence of suboptimal concentrations of IL-2.[160] During a concurrently controlled adjuvant trial in patients with operable lung cancer, intrapleural injection of N-CWS prolonged remission, decreased the incidence of systemic or local recurrence and prolonged survival in a subset of patients.[204] In lung cancer patients with malignant pleural effusions, regional administration of N-CWS and doxorubicin produced better local control than did doxorubicin alone.[127] A concurrently controlled clinical trial has also been conducted in 213 patients with gastric cancer treated with gastrectomy to compare immuno-chemotherapy with N-CWS and tegafur to chemotherapy alone.[84] Survival was significantly prolonged by immunochemotherapy. Administration of N-CWS has been well tolerated, with fever most frequently observed after intratumoral and intrapleural injection.[203] Erythema, induration and sterile abscesses have occurred at intradermal injection sites.[203]

OK-432 (picibanil) has been prepared from a strain of group A *Streptococcus pyogenes* by treatment with heat and penicillin. The preparation has activated NK effectors and high density T-cells that kill both autologous tumor cells[25,184,185,189] and drug resistant allogeneic tumor cells.[1] OK-432 has also activated macrophages[20,206] and potentiated the effect of IL-2 for generating LAK cells from human peritoneal precursors.[14] Treatment of lymphoid populations with OK-432 has induced the production of interferon-α, interferon-γ and IL-2.[22] The latter cytokines may be particularly important for the activation of NK cells by OK-432.[205]

OK-432 has inhibited the growth of several murine tumors.[20] Intralesional injection of human hepatomas with OK-432 increased the levels of peripheral blood LAK cells in 7 of 12 patients. Among the seven patients with enhanced LAK activity, three partial responses and one complete response were observed.[159] Intralesional injection of OK-432 into bladder cancers has increased the number of NK and T-cells infiltrating tumor nodules.[181] In a concurrently controlled trial with 382 cervical cancer patients, the repeated intradermal injection of OK-432 significantly prolonged recurrence free interval in stage II disease, but not in Stage III. In those stage II patients who had undergone radical hysterectomy and pelvic lymphadenectomy in addition to radiotherapy, treatment with OK-432 significantly prolonged survival.[121]

Lentinan is a beta (1–3) glucan with beta (1–6) branches. Both T-cell and macrophage function have been stimulated by lentinan, as was the production of several cytokines such as IL-1, IL-3, and interferon-γ.[18,37,115] In murine systems, endogenous production of LAK cells by IL-2 was potentiated by treatment with lentinan in vivo, but not in vitro.[174] Lentinan can prime macrophages for more effective ADCC mediated by monoclonal antibodies.[51] Growth of syngeneic tumor transplants has been suppressed in mice[173] and rats[70] by the administration of lentinan. A randomized clinical trial in patients with advanced or recurrent gastric cancer has compared chemo-immunotherapy with lentinan and tegafur to chemotherapy with tegafur alone.[175] Significant prolongation of survival was observed in the chemo-immunotherapy group. Similarly, the addition of lentinan to 5-FU and mitomycin C significantly prolonged the survival of patients with advanced gastric and colorectal cancer.[192] Each of these trials awaits further confirmation.

Levamisole

Levamisole is a low molecular weight anti-helminthic agent with immunomodulatory activity.[19,69] Levamisole has affected T-cell, macrophage, and granulocyte function in some reports.[172,190] Suboptimal immune function has been restored more often than normal function has been stimulated. Many studies were performed more than decade ago, antedating our current understanding of lymphocyte phenotype, immunoregulation, cytokine production, and intra-cellular signalling. A more recent attempt failed to demonstrate the immunostimulatory or immunorestorative activity of levamisole in vitro over a broad range of concentrations using a comprehensive battery of phenotypic and functional studies.[155] Animal models have detected limited activity against tumor transplants. In some models, antitumor activity has been critically dependent upon dosage.[153] The most effective approaches have combined levamisole with chemotherapy or radiotherapy.

In cancer patients, levamisole has augmented or restored delayed cutaneous hypersensitivity.[94,180] The maximally tolerated dose of levamisole (150 mg daily) has produced blood levels of 1 μg/ml or less.[190] When observed, the optimal modulation of immune function has been achieved in vitro with levels of 20–400 μg/ml. Several potential explanations have been suggested for this discrepancy including induction of an endogenous immunostimulant, transformation to a more potent metabolite, inhibition of an endogenous immunosuppressant or modulation of cholinergic receptors.[190]

In clinical trials, conflicting results have been obtained when levamisole has been added to other modalities for the treatment of melanoma,[41,69,102,142,169] breast cancer,[60,76,77,78,143,171,179] lung cancer,[2,16,28,54,136,138,195,201] and colon cancer.[13,29,44] Among these studies, the most reproducible activity appears to have been obtained in Duke's C colon cancer,[44] where three randomized clinical trials have demonstrated that adjuvant treatment with 5-FU (450 mg/m² qd × 5 once followed by weekly 5-FU starting on day 28) and levamisole (150 mg p.o. 3 days a week every other week) for 1 year significantly prolonged survival.[91,117,197] In one of the three trials, subgroup analysis was required to demonstrate an effect.[91,161] In previous adjuvant trials, 5-FU alone has generally failed to affect survival of patients with resected colorectal cancer. Whether the more intensive 5-FU regimens used in combination with levamisole would have impacted on survival cannot be determined. Although 5-FU is an immunosuppressive agent, it is not certain that immunomodulation is responsible for the antitumor activity observed. Direct toxic

effects of levamisole on colon cancer cell lines have, however, been found only with supra-pharmacologic concentrations of the drug.[43]

Levamisole has been well tolerated with gastrointestinal distress and fatigue reported most frequently. The most significant toxicity associated with levamisole has been granulocytopenia in 2–13% of patients which has usually resolved when the drug was discontinued.[149] IgM antibodies against human granulocytes have been detected in sera from patients who developed granulocytopenia after treatment with levamisole.[177]

Conclusion

Immunostimulants and immunorestorative agents have demonstrated significant antitumor activity when used locally and regionally. Application to clinical practice has, however, generally been limited to the treatment of cutaneous neoplasms, superficial bladder cancers and malignant effusions. Local or regional control of cancer can usually be achieved with more conventional agents, but elimination of systemic metastases remains the major barrier to the cure of many epithelial neoplasms. Recent results with levamisole and 5-FU could contribute to the control of visceral metastases from a frequently occurring human cancer.

Given the complex interactions of cells and factors that regulate the immune response to specific tumor associated antigens, "stimulating" immunity nonspecifically might amplify inappropriate signals that suppress a response to tumor associated antigens. On the other hand, intralesional injection of BCG, mycobacterial products or C. parvum has stimulated systemic tumor specific immunity in a number of animal models. Regression of non-injected lesions has been observed in patients treated with BCG for metastatic melanoma, consistent with the stimulation of specific immunity to tumor associated antigens. In the past, a major obstacle to more specific active immunotherapy has been the difficulty in identification and isolation of relevant antigens. Using techniques of molecular biology it has now been possible to characterize and clone several tumor associated antigens. Having identified these molecular targets, vaccines can now be prepared. Appropriate regulation of the immune response to these vaccines must still be achieved and immunostimulants may well have a role as adjuvants in this setting.

References

1. Allavena, P., Peccatori, F., Maggioni, D., Pirovano, P., and Mantovani, A.: Killing of tumor cells with pleiotropic drug resistance by OK432-activated effector cells. Immunopharmacol. Immunotoxicol., 11:257, 1989.
2. Amery, W. K.: Final results of a multicenter placebo-controlled levamisole study of resectable lung cancer. Cancer Treat. Rep., 62:1677, 1978.
3. Badalament, R. A., Herr, H. W., Wong, G. Y., Gnecco, C., Pinsky, C. M., Whitmore, W. F., Jr., Fair, W. R., and Oettgen, H. F.: A prospective randomized trial of maintenance versus nonmaintenance intravesical Bacillus Calmette-Guérin therapy of superficial bladder cancer. J. Clin. Oncol., 5:441, 1987.
4. Bahr, G. M., Chedid, L. A., and Behbehani, K.: Induction, in vivo and in vitro, of macrophage membrane interleukin-1 by adjuvant-active synthetic muramyl peptides. Cell. Immunol., 107:443, 1987.
5. Bast, R. C., Jr., Zbar, B., Borsos, T., and Rapp, H. J.: BCG and cancer. N. Engl. J. Med., 290:1413, 1974.
6. Bast, R. C., Jr., and Bast, B. S.: Critical review of previous reported animal studies of tumor immunotherapy with nonspecific immunostimulants. Ann. New York Acad. Sci., 227:60, 1976.
7. Bast, R. C., Jr., Knapp, R. C., Mitchell, A. K., Thurston, J. G., Tucker, R. W., and Schlossman, S. F.: Immunotherapy of a murine ovarian carcinoma with Corynebacterium parvum and specific heteroantiserum. I. Activation of peritoneal cells to mediate antibody-dependent cytotoxicity. J. Immunol., 123:1945, 1979.
8. Bast, R. C., Jr., Berek, J. S., Obrist, R., Griffiths, C. T., Berkowitz, R. S., Hacker, N.

F, Parker, L., Lagasse, L. D., and Knapp, R. C: Intraperitoneal immunotherapy of human ovarian carcinoma with *Corynebacterium parvum.* Cancer Res., 43:1395, 1983.

9. Berek, J. S., Knapp, R. C., Hacker, N. F., Lichtenstein, A., Jung, T, Spina, C., Obrist, R., Griffiths, C. T., Berkowitz, R. S., Parker, L., Zighelboim, J., and Bast, R. C., Jr.: Intraperitoneal immunotherapy of epithelial ovarian carcinoma with *Corynebacterium parvum.* Am. J. Obstet. Gynecol., 152:1003, 1985.
10. Berek, J. S., Hacker, N. F., Lichtenstein, A., Jung, T., Spina, C., Knox, R. M., Brady, J., Greene, T., Ettinger, L. M., Logasse, L. D., Bonnem, E. M., Spiegel, R. J., and Zighelboim, J.: Intraperitoneal recombinant alfa-interferon for "salvage" immunotherapy in stage III epithelial ovarian cancer: A Gynecologic Oncology Group study. Cancer Res., 45:4447, 1985.
11. Böhle, A., Nowc, C., Ulmer, A. J., Musehold, J., Gerdes, J., Hofstetter, A. G., and Flad, H. D.: Detection of urinary TNF, IL 1, and IL 2 after local BCG immunotherapy for bladder carcinoma. Cytokine, 2:175, 1990.
12. Bookman, M. A., and Bast, R. C., Jr.: The immunobiology and immunotherapy of ovarian cancer. Semin. Oncol., 18:270, 1991.
13. Borden, E. C., Davis, T. E., Crowley, J. J., Wolberg, W. H., McKnight, B., and Chirigos, M. A.: Interim analysis of a trial of levamisole and 5-fluorouracil in metastatic colorectal carcinoma. *In* Immunotherapy of Human Cancer. Edited by W. D. Terry, and S. A. Rosenburg. New York, Excerpta Medica, 1982, p. 231.
14. Boyer, P. J., Berek, J. S., and Zighelboim, J.: Lymphocyte activation by recombinant interleukin-2 in ovarian cancer patients. Obstet. Gynecol., 73:793, 1989.
15. Casali, A., Gionfra, T., Rinaldi, M., Tonachella, R., Tropea, F., Venturo, I., De Martino, C., and Curcio, C. G.: Treatment of malignant pleural effusions with intracavitary Corynebacterium parvum. Cancer, 62:806, 1988.
16. Chahinian, A. P., Goldberg, J., Holland, J. F., Reisman, A., Jaffrey, I. S., and Mandel, E. M.: Chemotherapy versus chemoimmunotherapy with levamisole or Corynebacterium parvum in advanced lung cancer. Cancer Treat. Rep., 66:1291, 1982.
17. Cheng, V. S. T., Suit, H. D., Wang, C. C., and Cummings, C.: Nonspecific immunotherapy by Corynebacterium parvum. Phase I toxicity study in 12 patients with advanced cancer. Cancer, 37:1687, 1976.
18. Chihara, G., Hamuro, J., Maeda, Y., Shiio, T., Suga, T., Takasuka, N., and Sasaki, T.: Antitumor and metastasis-inhibitory activities of lentinan as an immunomodulator: An overview. Cancer Detect. Prev. Suppl., 1:423, 1987.
19. Chirigos, M. A., and Mastrangelo, M. J.: Immunorestoration by chemicals. *In* Immunological Approaches to Cancer Therapeutics. Edited by E. Mihich. New York, John Wiley & Sons, 1982, p. 191.
20. Chirigos, M. A., Saito, T., Talmadge, J. E., Budzynski, W., and Gruys, E.: Cell regulatory and immunorestorative activity of picibanil (OK432). Cancer Detect. Prev., 1(Suppl.):317, 1987.
21. Christie, G. H., and Bomford, R.: Mechanisms of macrophage activation by Corynebacterium parvum. I. In vitro experiments. Cell. Immunol., 17:141, 1975.
22. Christmas, S. E., Meager, A., and Moore, M.: Studies of the enhancement of natural cytotoxicity by the streptococcal immunopotentiator OK432. Int. J. Immunopharmacol., 8:83, 1986.
23. Cohen, M. H., Jessup, J. M., Felix, E. L., Weese, J. L., and Herberman, R. B.: Intralesional treatment of recurrent metastatic cutaneous malignant melanoma: a randomized prospective study of intralesional Bacillus Calmette-Guérin versus intralesional dinitrochlorobenzene. Cancer, 41:2456, 1978.
24. Coley, W. B.: Treatment of inoperable malignant tumors with the toxins of erysipelas and the bacillus prodigiosus. Trans. Am. Surg. Assoc., 12:183, 1894.
25. Colotta, F., Rambaldi, A., Colombo, N., Tabacchi, L., Introna, M., and Mantovani, A.: Effect of a streptococcal preparation (OK432) on natural killer activity of tumour-associated lymphoid cells in human ovarian carcinoma and on lysis of fresh ovarian tumour cells. Br. J. Cancer, 48:515, 1983.
26. Comstock, G. W., Martinez, I., and Livesay, V. T.: Efficacy of BCG vaccination in prevention of cancer. J. Natl. Cancer Inst., 54:835, 1975.
27. Davignon, L., Robillard, P., Lemonde, P., and Frappier, A.: BCG vaccination and leukemia mortality. Lancet, 2:638, 1970.
28. Davis, S., Mietlowski, W., Rohwedder, J. J., Griffin, J. P., and Neshat, A. A.: Levamisole as an adjuvant to chemotherapy in extensive bronchogenic carcinoma: A Veterans Administration Lung Cancer Group Study. Cancer, 50:646, 1982.
29. Davis, T. E., Borden, E. C., Wolberg, W. H., and Crowley, J. J.: Levamisole and 5-fluorouracil in metastatic colorectal carcinoma. Proc. Am. Soc. Clin. Oncol., 1:102, 1982.
30. DiSaia, P. J., Bundy, B. N., Curry, S. L., Schlaerth, J., and Thigpen, J. T.: Phase III study on the treatment of women with cervical cancer, Stage IIB, IIIB, and IVA (confined to the pelvis and/or periaortic nodes), with radiotherapy alone versus radiotherapy plus immunotherapy with intravenous Corynebacterium parvum: A Gynecologic Oncology Group Study. Gynecol. Oncol., 26:386, 1987.
31. Ehrke, M. J., Tomazic, V., Ryoyama, K., Cohen, S. A., and Mihich, E.: Adriamycin induced immunomodulation: Dependence upon time of administration. Int. J. Immunopharmacol., 5:43, 1983.
32. Ehrke, M. J., and Mihich, E.: Immunoregulation by cancer chemotherapeutic agents. *In* The Reticuloendothelial System: A Comprehensive Treatise. Volume 8, Pharmacology. Edited by J. W. Hadden, and A. Szentivanyi. New York, Plenum Press, 1985, p. 309.
33. Fisher, B., Rubin, H., Sartiano, G., Ennis, L., and Wolmark, N.: Observations following Corynebacterium parvum administration to patients with advanced malignancy. A phase I study. Cancer, 38:119, 1976.
34. Fisher, B., Brown, A., Wolmark, N., Fisher, E. R., Redmond, C., Wickerham, L., Margolese, R., Dimitrov, N., Pilch, Y., Glass, A., Sutherland, C., and Foster, R.: Evaluation of the worth of Corynebacterium parvum in conjunction with chemotherapy as adjuvant treatment for primary breast cancer. Cancer, 66:220, 1990.
35. Fleischmann, J. D., Toossi, Z., Ellner, J. J., Wentworth, D. B., Ratliff, T. L., and Imbembo, A. L.: Urinary interleukins in patients receiving intravesical Bacillus Calmette-Guérin therapy for superficial bladder cancer. Cancer, 64:1447, 1989.
36. Fogler, W. E., Wade, R., Brundish, D. E., Fidler, I. J: Distribution and fate of free and liposome-encapsulated [^{3}H]nor-muramyl dipeptide and [^{3}H] muramyl tripeptide phosphatidylethanolamine in mice. J. Immunol., 135:1372, 1985.
37. Fruehauf, J. P., Bonnard, G. D., and Herberman, R. B.: The effect of lentinan on production of interleukin-1 by human monocytes. Immunopharmacology, 5:65, 1982.
38. Fudenberg, H. H., and Whitten, H. D.: Immunostimulation: Synthetic and biological modulators of immunity. Ann. Rev. Pharmacol. Toxicol., 24:147, 1984.
39. Gall, S. A., DiSaia, P. J., Schmidt, H., Mittelstaedt, L., Newman, P., and Creasman, W.: Toxicity manifestations following intravenous Corynebacterium parvum administration to patients with ovarian and cervical carcinoma. Am. J. Obstet. Gynecol., 132:555, 1978.
40. Gill, P. G., Morris, P. J., and Kettlewell, M.: The complications of intravenous Corynebacterium parvum infusion. Clin. Exp. Immunol., 30:229, 1977.
41. Gonzalez, R. L., Spitler, L. E., and Sagebiel, R. W.: Effect of levamisole as a surgical adjuvant therapy for malignant melanoma. Cancer Treat. Rep., 62:1703, 1978.
42. Gray, G. R., Ribi, E., Granger, D., Parker, R., Azuma, I., and Yamamoto, K.: Immunotherapy of cancer: Tumor suppression and regression by cell walls of Mycobacterium phlei attached to oil droplets. J. Natl. Cancer Inst., 55:727, 1975.
43. Grem, J. L., and Allegra, C. J.: Toxicity of levamisole and 5-fluorouracil in human colon carcinoma cells. J. Natl. Cancer Inst., 81:1413, 1989.
44. Grem, J. L.: Levamisole as a therapeutic agent for colorectal carcinoma. Cancer Cells, 2:131, 1990.
45. Guérin, C.: The history of BCG. *In* BCG Vaccination Against Tuberculosis. Edited by S. R. Rosenthal. Boston, Little, Brown and Company, 1957, p. 48.
46. Guthrie, D., and Way, S.: Immunotherapy of non-clinical vaginal cancer. Lancet, 2:1242, 1975.
47. Guthrie, D., and Way, S.: Failure of topical DNCB immunotherapy in most patients with non-clinical carcinoma of the cervix. Br. J. Cancer, 39:445, 1979.
48. Gutterman, J. U., Mavligit, G., McBride, C., Frei, E., III, Freireich, E. J., and Hersh, E. M.: Active immunotherapy with BCG for recurrent malignant melanoma. Lancet, 1:1208, 1973.
49. Halpern, B. N., Biozzi, G., Stiffel, C., and Mouton, D.: Inhibition of tumour growth by administration of killed Corynebacterium parvum. Nature, 212:853, 1966.
50. Hanna, M. G., Jr., Zbar, B., and Rapp, H. J.: Histopathology of tumor regression after intralesional injection of Mycobacterium bovis. I. Tumor growth and metastasis. J. Natl. Cancer Inst., 48:1441, 1972.
51. Herlyn, D., Kaneko, Y., Powe, J., Aoki, T., and Koprowski, H.: Monoclonal antibody-dependent murine macrophage-mediated cytotoxicity against human tumors is stimulated by lentinan. Jpn. J. Cancer Res., 76:37, 1985.
52. Herr, H. W., and Laudone, V. P.: Intravesical therapy for superficial bladder cancer. *In* Cancer: Principles & Practice of Oncology: Updates 2. Edited by V. T. DeVita, Jr., S. Hellman, and S. A. Rosenberg. New York, J. B. Lippincott, 1988a, p. 1.
53. Herr, H. W., Laudone, V. P., Badalament, R. A., Oettgen, H. F, Sogani, P. C., Freedman, B. D., Melamed, M. R., and Whitmore, W. F., Jr.: Bacillus Calmette-Guérin therapy alters the progression of superficial bladder cancer. J. Clin. Oncol., 6:1450, 1988b.
54. Herskovic, A., Bauer, M., Seydel, H. G., Yesner, R., Doggett, R. L. S., Perez, C. A., Durbin, L. M., and Zinninger, M.: Post-operative thoracic irradiation with or without levamisole in non-small cell lung cancer: Results of a radiation therapy oncology group study. Int. J. Radiat. Oncol. Biol. Phys., 14:37, 1988.
55. Hertzog, P. J., Cheetham, B. F., Sexton, J. L, Linnane, A. W.: Characterization of interferons produced by peripheral blood mononuclear cells from healthy subjects in response to *Corynebacterium parvum* or poly I: poly C. Biochem. Int., 19:1427, 1989.
56. Heyn, R., Borges, W., Joo, P., Karon, M., Nesbit, M., Shore, N., Breslow, N., and Hammond, D.: BCG in the treatment of acute lymphocytic leukemia (ALL). Proc. Am. Assoc. Cancer Res., 14:45, 1973.
57. Hilal, E. Y., Pinsky, C. M., Hirshaut, Y., Wanebo, H. J., Hansen, J. A., Braun, D. W., Jr., Fortner, J. G., and Oettgen, H. F.: Surgical adjuvant therapy of malignant melanoma with Corynebacterium parvum. Cancer, 48:245, 1981.
58. Hirt, H. M., Schwenteck, M., Becker, H., and Kirchner, H.: Interferon production and lymphocyte stimulation in human leucocyte cultures stimulated by Corynebacterium parvum. Clin. Exp. Immunol., 32:471, 1978.
59. Hoon, D. S., Foshag, L. J., Nizze, A. S., Bohman, R., and Morton, D. L.: Suppressor cell activity in a randomized trial of patients receiving active specific immunotherapy with melanoma cell vaccine and low dosages of cyclophosphamide. Cancer Res., 50:5358, 1990.
60. Hortobagyi, G. N., Gutterman, J. U., Blumenschein, G. R., Tashima, C. K., Buzdar, A. U., and Hersch, E. M.: Levamisole in the treatment of breast cancer. Prog. Cancer Res. Ther., 7:131, 1978.
61. Hudson, M. L. A., Brown, E. J., Ritchey, J. K., and Ratliff, T. L.: Modulation of fibronectin-mediated Bacillus Calmette-Guérin attachment to murine bladder mucosa by drugs influencing the coagulation pathways. Cancer Res., 51:3726, 1991.
62. Hull, M. G., Bowen-Simpkins, P., and Paintin, D. B.: 5-Fluorouracil versus immunotherapy for non-clinical vaginal cancer. Lancet, 1:588, 1976.
63. Inamura, N., Fujitsu, T., Nakahara, K., Abiko, M., Horii, Y., Hashimoto, S., and Aoki, H.: Potentiation of tumoricidal properties of murine macrophages by Nocardia rubra cell wall skeleton (N-CWS). J. Antibiot., 37:244, 1984.
64. Inamura, N., Nakahara, K., Kuroda, Y., Yamaguchi, I., Aoki, H., and Kohsaka, M.: Effect of Nocardia rubra cell wall skeleton on interleukin-1 production from mouse peritoneal macrophages. Int. J. Immunopharmacol., 10:547, 1988.
65. Ito, M., Iizuka, H., Masuno, T., Yasunami, R., Ogura, T., Yamamura, Y., and Azuma, I.: Killing of tumor cells in vitro by macrophages from mice given injections of squalene-treated cell wall skeleton of Nocardia rubra. Cancer Res., 41:2925, 1981.
66. Izumi, S., Ueda, H., Okuhara, M., Aoki, H., and Yamamura, Y.: Effect of Nocardia rubra cell wall skeleton on murine interferon production in vitro. Cancer Res., 46:1960, 1986.
67. Izumi, S., Hirai, O., Hayashi, K., Konishi, Y., Okuhara, M., Kohsaka, M., Aoki, H., and Yamamura, Y.: Induction of a tumor necrosis factor-like activity by Nocardia rubra cell wall skeleton. Cancer Res., 47:1785, 1987.
68. Izumi, S., Ogawa, T., Miyauchi, M., Fujie, K., Okuhara, M., and Kohsaka, M.: Antitumor effect of Nocardia rubra cell wall skeleton on syngeneically transplanted P388 tumors. Cancer Res., 51:4038, 1991.
69. Janssen, P. A. J.: Levamisole as an adjuvant in cancer treatment. J. Clin. Pharmacol. 31:396, 1991.
70. Jeannin, J. F., Lagadec, P., Pelletier, H., Reisser, D., Olsson, N. O., Chihara, G., and Martin, F.: Regression induced by lentinan of peritoneal carcinomatoses in a model of colon cancer in rat. Int. J. Immunopharmacol., 10:855, 1988.
71. Kawase, I., Uemiya, M., Yoshimoto, T., Ogura, T., Hirao, F., and Yamamura, Y.: Effect

of Nocardia rubra cell wall skeleton on T-cell-mediated cytotoxicity in mice bearing syngeneic sarcoma. Cancer Res., 41:660, 1981.
72. Keller, R., Keist, R., Van der Meide, P. H., Groscurth, P., Aguet, M., and Leist, T. P.: Induction, maintenance, and reinduction of tumoricidal activity in bone marrow-derived mononuclear phagocytes by Corynebacterium parvum. Evidence for the involvement of a T cell- and Interferon-γ-independent pathway of macrophage activation. J. Immunol., 138:2366, 1987.
73. Kempin, S., Cirrincione, C., Straus, D. S., Gee, T. S., Arlin, Z., Koziner, B., Pinsky, C., Nisce, L., Myers, J., Lee, B. J., III, Clarkson, B. D., Old, L. J., and Oettgen, H. F.: Improved remission rate and duration in nodular non-Hodgkin lymphoma (NNHL) with the use of mixed bacterial vaccine (MBV). Proc. Am. Soc. Clin. Oncol., 22:514, 1981.
74. Kempin, S., Cirrincione, C., Myers, J., Lee, B., III, Straus, D., Koziner, B., Arlin, Z., Gee, T., Mertelsmann, R., Pinsky, C., Comacho, E., Nisce, L., Old, L., Clarkson, B., and Oettgen, H.: Combined modality therapy of advanced nodular lymphomas (NL): The role of nonspecific immunotherapy (MBV) as an important determinant of response and survival. Proc. Am. Soc. Clin. Oncol., 24:56, 1983.
75. Key, M. E., Talmadge, J. E., Fogler, W. E., Bucana, C., and Fidler, I. J.: Isolation of tumoricidal macrophages from lung melanoma metastases of mice treated systemically with liposomes containing a lipophilic derivative of muramyl depeptide. J. Natl. Cancer Inst., 69:1189, 1982.
76. Klefström, P.: Combination of levamisole immunotherapy and polychemotherapy in advanced breast cancer. Cancer Treat. Rep., 64:65, 1980.
77. Klefström, P., Gröhn, P., Heinonen, E., Holsti, L., and Holsti, P.: Adjuvant postoperative radiotherapy, chemotherapy, and immunotherapy in stage III breast cancer. II. 5-Year results and influence of levamisole. Cancer, 60:936, 1987.
78. Klefström, P., and Nuortio, L.: Levamisole in the treatment of advanced breast cancer. A Ten-Year follow-up of a randomized study. Acta Oncol., 30:347, 1991.
79. Klein, E.: Hypersensitivity reactions at tumor sites. Cancer Res., 29:2351, 1969.
80. Klein, E.: Introduction: Immunotherapy of cancer in man, a reality. Natl. Cancer Inst. Monogr., 39:139, 1973.
81. Klein, W. R., Ruitenberg, E. J., Steerenberg, P. A., De Jong, W. H., Kruizinga, W., Misdorp, W., Bier, J., Tiesjema, R. H., Kreeftenberg, J. G., Teppema, J. S., and Rapp, H. J.: Immunotherapy by intralesional injection of BCG cell walls or live BCG in bovine ocular squamous cell carcinoma: A preliminary report. J. Natl. Cancer Inst., 69:1095, 1982.
82. Kleinerman, E. S., Murray, J. L., Snyder, J. S., Cunningham, J. E., and Fidler, I. J.: Activation of tumoricidal properties in monocytes from cancer patients following intravenous administration of liposomes containing muramyl tripeptide phosphatidylethanolamine. Cancer Res., 49:4665, 1989.
83. Knapp, R. C., and Berkowitz, R. S.: Corynebacterium parvum as an immunotherapeutic agent in an ovarian cancer model. Am. J. Obstet. Gynecol., 128:782, 1977.
84. Koyama, S., Ozaki, A., Iwasaki, Y., Sakita, T., Osuga, T., Watanabe, A., Suzuki, M., Kawasaki, T., Soma, T., Tabuchi, T., Nakayama, M., Koizumi, S., Yokoyama, K., Uchida, T., Orii, K., and Tanaka, T.: Randomized controlled study of postoperative adjuvant immunotherapy with Nocardia rubra cell wall skeleton (N-CWS) and Tegafur for gastric carcinoma. Cancer Immunol. Immunother., 22:148, 1986.
85. Krauss, S., Comas, F., Perez, C., Gordon, D., Philpott, G., Broun, G., Mill, W., Robbins, R., Smalley, R., Mendiondo, O., DeSimone, P., McLaren, J., Keller, J., Durant, J., Birch, R., and Buchanan, R.: Treatment of inoperable non-small cell carcinoma of the lung with radiation therapy, with or without levamisole. A randomized trial of the Southeastern Cancer Study Group. Am. J. Clin. Oncol., 7:405, 1984.
86. Kreider, J. W., Bartlett, G. L., Purnell, D. M., and Webb, S.: Immunotherapy of an established rat mammary adenocarcinma (13762A) with intratumor injection of Corynebacterium parvum. Cancer Res., 38:689, 1978.
87. Krupp, P. J., and Bohm, J. W.: 5-Fluorouracil topical treatment of in situ vulvar cancer. A preliminary report. Obstet. Gynecol., 51:702, 1978.
88. Lamm, D. L., Thor, D. E., Harris, S. C., et al.: Intravesical and percutaneous BCG immunotherapy of recurrent superficial bladder cancer. *In* Immunotherapy of Human Cancer. Edited by W. D. Terry, and S. A. Rosenberg. New York, Elsevier, North Holland, 1982, p. 315.
89. Lamm, D. L., Thor, D. E., Winters, W. D., Stogdill, V. D., and Radwin, H. M.: BCG immunotherapy of bladder cancer: Inhibition of tumor recurrence and associated immune responses. Cancer, 48:82, 1985.
90. Lamm, D. L., Crossman, J., Blumenstein, B., Crawford, E. D., Montie, J., Scardino, P., Grossman, H. B., Stanisic, T., Smith, J., Sullivan, J., and Sarosdy, M.: Adriamycin versus BCG in superficial bladder cancer: A Southwest Oncology Group study. Prog. Clin. Biol. Res., 310:263, 1989.
91. Laurie, J. A., Moertel, C. G., Fleming, T. R., Wieand, H. S., Leigh, J. E., Rubin, J., McCormack, G. W., Gerstner, J. B., Krook, J. E., Malliard, J., Twito, D. I., Morton, R. F., Tschetter, L. K., and Barlow, J. F.: Surgical adjuvant therapy of large-bowel carcinoma: An evaluation of levamisole and the combination of levamisole and fluorouracil. J. Clin. Oncol., 7:1447, 1989.
92. Lederer, E., and Chedid, L.: Immunomodulation by synthetic muramyl peptides and trehalose diesters. *In* Immunological Approaches to Cancer Therapeutics. Edited by E. Mihich. New York, John Wiley & Sons. 1982, p. 107.
92. Lemonde, P., Dubreuil, R., Guindon, A., and Lussier, G.: Stimulating influence of Bacillus Calmette-Guérin on immunity to polyoma tumors and spontaneous leukemia. J. Natl. Cancer Inst., 47:1013, 1971.
94. Lewinski, U. H., Mavligit, G. M., and Hersh, E. M.: Cellular immune modulation after a single high dose of levamisole in patients with carcinoma. Cancer, 46:2185, 1980.
95. Lichtenstein, A., Bick, A., Cantrell, J., and Zighelboim, J.: Augmentation of NK activity by Corynebacterium parvum fractions in vivo and in vitro. Int. J. Immunopharmacol., 5:137, 1983.
96. Lichtenstein, A., Berek, J., Bast, R., Spina, C., Hacker, N., Knapp, R. C., and Zighelboim, J.: Activation of peritoneal lymphocyte cytotoxicity in patients with ovarian cancer by intraperitoneal treatment with *Corynebacterium parvum*. J. Biol. Response Mod., 3:371, 1984.
97. Lichtenstein, A. K, and Pende, D.: Enhancement of natural killer cytotoxicity by cis-diamminedichloroplatinum (II) in vivo and in vitro. Cancer Res., 46:639, 1986.
98. Lichtenstein, A., Seelig, M., Berek, J., and Zighelboim, J.: Human neutrophil-mediated lysis of ovarian cancer cells. Blood, 74:805, 1989.
99. Likhite, V. V.: Rejection of tumors and metastases in Fischer 344 rats following intratumor administration of killed Corynebacterium parvum. Int. J. Cancer, 14:684, 1974a.
100. Likhite, V. V., and Halpern, B. N.: Lasting rejection of mammary adenocarcinoma cell tumors in DBA-2 mice with intratumor injection of killed Corynebacterium parvum. Cancer Res., 34:341, 1974b.
101. Lipton, A., Harvey, H. A., Balch, C. M., Antle, C. E., Heckard, R., and Bartolucci, A. A.: Corynebacterium parvum versus Bacille Calmette-Guérin adjuvant immunotherapy of Stage II malignant melanoma. J. Clin. Oncol., 9:1151, 1991.
102. Loutfi, A., Shakr, A., Jerry, M., Hanley, J., and Shibata, H. R.: Double blind randomized prospective trial of levamisole/placebo in stage I cutaneous malignant melanoma. Clin. Invest. Med., 10:325, 1987.
103. Ludwig Lung Cancer Study Group (LLCSG): Immunostimulation with intrapleural BCG as adjuvant therapy in resected non-small cell lung cancer. Cancer, 58:2411, 1986.
104. Mande, R.: BCG Vaccination. London, Dowsons of Pall Mall. 1968.
105. Mandeville, R., Sombo, F.-M., and Rocheleau, N.: Natural cell-mediated cytotoxicity in normal human peripheral blood lymphocytes and its in vitro boosting with BCG. Cancer Immunol. Immunother., 15:17, 1983.
106. Mansell, P. W., Litwin, M. S., Ichinose, H., and Krementz, E. T.: Delayed hypersensitivity to 5-fluorouracil following topical chemotherapy of cutaneous cancers. Cancer Res., 35:1288, 1975.
107. Mantovani, A., Sessa, C., Peri, G., Allavena, P., Introna, M., Polentarutti, N., and Mangioni, C.: Intraperitoneal administration of Corynebacterium parvum in patients with ascitic ovarian tumors resistant to chemotherapy: Effects on cytotoxicity of tumor-associated macrophages and NK cells. Int. J. Cancer, 27:437, 1981.
108. Mathé, G., Amiel, J. L., Schwarzenberg, L., Schneider, M., Cattan, A., Schlumberger, J. R., Hayat, M., and De Vassal, F.: Active immunotherapy for acute lymphoblastic leukaemia. Lancet, 1:697, 1969.
109. McKneally, M. F., Maver, C., and Kausel, H. W.: Regional immunotherapy of lung cancer with intrapelural BCG. Lancet, 1:377, 1976.
110. McKneally, M. F., Maver, C., Lininger, L., Kausel, H. W., McIlduff, J. B., Older, T. M., Foster, E. D., and Alley, R. D.: Four-year follow-up of the Albany experience with intrapleural BCG in lung cancer. J. Thorac. Cardiovasc. Surg., 81:485, 1981.
111. McLaughlin, C. A., Schwartzman, S. M., Horner, B. L., Jones, G. H., Moffatt, J. G., Nestor, J. J., Jr., and Tegg, D.: Regression of tumors in guinea pigs after treatment with synthetic muramyl dipeptides and trehalose dimycolate. Science, 208:415, 1980.
112. Meltzer, M. S., and Nacy, C. A.: Delayed-type hypersensitivity and the induction of activated, cytotoxic macrophages. *In* Fundamental Immunology. Second Edition. Edited by W. E. Paul. New York, Raven Press, 1989, p. 765.
113. Milas, L., Hunter, N., Basic, I., and Withers, H. R.: Complete regression of an established murine fibrosarcoma induced by systemic application of Corynebacterium granulosum. Cancer Res., 34:2470, 1974.
114. Millar, J. W., Hunter, A. M., and Horne, N. W.: Intrapleural immunotherapy with Corynebacterium parvum in recurrent malignant pleural effusions. Thorax, 35:856, 1980.
115. Miyakoshi, H., and Aoki, T.: Acting mechanisms of lentinan in human-II. Enhancement of non-specific cell-mediated cytotoxicity as an interferon inducer. Int. J. Immunopharmacol., 6:373, 1984.
116. Miyazaki, K., Yasumoto, K., Yano, T., Matsuzaki, G., Sugimachi, K., and Nomoto, K.: Synergistic effect of Nocardia rubra cell wall skeleton and recombinant interleukin 2 for in vivo induction of lymphokine-activated killer cells. Cancer Res., 51:5261, 1991.
117. Moertel, C. G., Fleming, T. R., MacDonald, J. S., Haller, D. G., Laurie, J. A., Goodman, P. J., Ungerleider, J. S., Emerson, W. A., Tormey, D. C., Glick, J. H., Veeder, M. H., and Mailliard, J. A: Levamisole and Fluorouracil for adjuvant therapy of resected colon carcinoma. N. Engl. J. Med., 322:352, 1990.
118. Morales, A., Eidenger, D., and Bruce, A. W.: Intracavitary Bacillus Calmette-Guérin in the treatment of superficial bladder tumors. J. Urol., 116:180, 1976.
119. Morton, D. L., Eilber, F. R., Malmgren, R. A., and Wood, W. C.: Immunological factors which influence response to immunotherapy in malignant melanoma. Surgery, 68:158, 1970.
120. Nauts, H. C.: The beneficial effects of bacterial infections of host resistance to cancer. End results in 449 cases. New York, Cancer Research Institute, Monograph No. 8, 1980.
121. Noda, K., Teshima, K., Tekeuti, K., Hasegawa, K., Inoue, K.-Y., Yamashita, K., Sawaragi, I., Nakajima, T., Takashima, E., Ikeuchi, M., Sekiba, K., Okuda, H., Ichijo, J., Saito, T., Ozawa, M., Tamura, H., Chihara, T., Kuzuya, K., Ozaki, M., Inagaki, M., and Tominaga, S.: Immunotherapy using the streptococcal preparation OK-432 for the treatment of uterine cervical cancer. Gynecol. Oncol., 35:367, 1989.
122. Noso, Y., Parant, M., Parant, F., and Chedid, L.: Production of tumor necrosis factor in nude mice by muramyl peptides associated with bacterial vaccines. Cancer Res., 48:5766, 1988.
123. Oates, K. K., Sztein, M. B., and Goldstein, A. L.: Mechanism of action of the thymosins: Modulation of lymphokines, receptors, and T-cell differentiation antigens. *In* Cell Surface Antigen Thy-1: Immunology, Neurology, and Therapeutic Applications. Edited by A. E. Reif, and M. Schlesinger. New York, Marcel Dekker, Inc., 1989, p. 273.
124. Oettgen, H. F., Pinsky, C. M., and Delmonte, L.: Treatment of cancer with immunomodulators. Corynebacterium parvum and levamisole. Med. Clin. North Am., 60:511, 1976.
125. Oettgen, H. F., and Old, L. J.: The history of cancer immunotherapy. *In* Biologic Therapy of Cancer. Edited by V. T. DeVita, Jr., S. Hellman, and S. A. Rosenberg. Philadelphia, J. B. Lippincott Co., 1991, p. 87.
126. Ogura, T., Hara, H., Yokota, S., Hosoe, S., Kawase, I., Kishimoto, S., and Yamamura, Y.: Effector mechanism in concomitant immunity potentiated by intratumoral injection of Nocardia rubra cell wall skeleton. Cancer Res., 45:6371, 1985.
127. Ogura, T., and Sakatani, M.: Randomized controlled study on adjuvant immunotherapy for unresectable lung cancer with Nocardia rubra cell wall skeleton. Nippon Kyobu Shikkan Gakkai Zasshi, 23:62, 1985.
128. Okuda, S., Taniguchi, K., Kubo, C., and Nomoto, K.: Accessory cell function in tumor-bearing mice and effects of Corynebacterium parvum. J. Natl. Cancer Inst., 69:1293, 1982.
129. Old, L. J., Benacerraf, B., Clarke, D. A., Carswell, E. A., and Stockert, E.: The role of the reticuloendothelial system in the host reaction to neoplasia. Cancer Res., 21:1281, 1961.
130. Onuma, M., Yamamoto, M., Yasutomi, Y., Takahashi, K., Kawakami, Y., and Azuma, I.: Regression of bovine lymphosarcoma by treatment with cell-wall skeleton of Nocardia rubra. Vaccine, 7:121, 1989.
131. Oratz, R., Dugan, M., Roses, D. F., Harris, M. N., Speyer, J. L., Hochster, H., Weiss-

man, J., Henn, M., and Bystryn, J. C.: Lack of effect of cyclophosphamide on the immunogenicity of a melanoma antigen vaccine. Cancer Res., 51:3643, 1991.
132. Orihuela, E., Herr, N. W., Pinsky, C. M., and Whitmore, W. F., Jr.: Toxicity of intravesical BCG and its management in patients with superficial bladder tumors. Cancer, 60:326, 1987.
133. Pak, C. C., and Fidler, I. J.: Liposomal delivery of biological response modifiers to macrophages. Biotherapy, 3:55, 1991.
134. Parant, M., Parant, F., Chedid, L., Yapo, A., Petit, J. F., and Lederer, E.: Fate of the synthetic immunoadjuvant, muramyl dipeptide (^{14}C-labeled) in the mouse. Int. J. Immunopharmacol., 1:35, 1979.
135. Parr, I. B., Jackson, L. E., and Alexander, P.: Role of "lymphotoxin" in the local antitumor action associated with inflammation caused by delayed hypersensitivity responses or intralesional BCG. I. Variations in response of different synegeneic mouse tumours. Br. J. Cancer, 48:385, 1983.
136. Perez, C. A., Bauer, M., Emami, B. N., Byhardt, R., Brady, L. W., Doggett, R. L. S., Gardner, P., and Zinninger, M.: Thoracic irradiation with or without levamisole (NSC #177023) in unresectable non-small cell carcinoma of the lung: A phase III randomized trial of the RTOG. Int. J. Radiat. Oncol. Biol. Phys., 15:1337, 1988.
137. Petersen, E., Hokland, P., and Ellegaard, J.: Adjuvant immune stimulation with Corynebacterium parvum during maintenance chemotherapy of acute myeloid leukemia. A prospective randomized study. Cancer Immunol. Immunother., 16:88, 1983.
138. Pines, A.: BCG plus levamisole following irradiation of advanced squamous bronchial carcinoma. Int. J. Radiat. Oncol. Biol. Phys., 6:1041, 1980.
139. Pinsky, C. M., Camacho, F. J., Kerr, D., Braun, D. W., Jr., Whitmore, W. F., Jr., and Oettgen, H. F.: Treatment of superficial bladder cancer with intravesical BCG. *In* Immunotherapy of Human Cancer. Edited by W. D. Terry, and S. A. Rosenberg. New York, Elsevier North Holland, Inc. Exerpta Medica, 1982, p. 309.
140. Piver, M. S., Barlow, J. J., Tsukada, Y., Gamarra, M., and Sandecki, A.: Postirradiation squamous cell carcinoma in situ of the vagina: Treatment by topical 20 percent 5-fluorouracil cream. Am. J. Obstet. Gynecol., 135:377, 1979.
141. Pride, G. L., and Chuprevich, T. W.: Topical 5-fluorouracil treatment of transformation zone intraepithelial neoplasia of cervix and vagina. Obstet. Gynecol., 60:467, 1982.
142. Quirt, I. C., Shelley, W. E., Pater, J. L., Bodurtha, A. J., McCulloch, P. B., McPherson, T. A., Paterson, A. H. G., Prentice, R., Silver, H. K. B., Willan, A. R., Wilson, K., and Zee, B.: Improved survival in patients with poor-prognosis malignant melanoma treated with adjuvant levamisole: A phase III study by the National Cancer Institute of Canada Clinical Trials Group. J. Clin. Oncol., 9:729, 1991.
143. Rojas, A. F., Feierstein, J. N., Glait, H. M., and Olivari, A. J.: Levamisole action in breast cancer stage III. *In* Immunotherapy of Cancer: Present Status of Trials in Man. Edited by: W. D. Terry, and D. Windhorst. New York, Raven Press, Progress in Cancer Research and Therapy, 1978, p. 696.
144. Rosenberg, S. A., Rapp, H., Terry, W., Zbar, B., Costa, J., Seipp, C., and Simon, R.: Intralesional BCG therapy of patients with primary stage I melanoma. *In* Immunotherapy of Human Cancer. Edited by W. D. Terry, and S. A. Rosenberg. New York, Excerpta Medica, 1982, p. 239.
145. Rosenthal, S. R., Crispen, R. G., Thorne, M. G., Piekarski, N., Raisys, N., and Rettig, P. G.: BCG vaccination and leukemia mortality. J.A.M.A., 222:1543, 1972.
146. Rossi, G. A., Felletti, R., Balbi, B., Sacco, O., Cosulich, E., Risso, A., Melioli, G., and Ravazzoni, C.: Symptomatic treatment of recurrent malignant pleural effusions with intrapleurally administered Corynebacterium parvum. Clinical response is not associated with evidence of enhancement of local cellular-mediated immunity. Am. Rev. Respir. Dis., 135:885, 1987.
147. Rossol, S., Voth, R., Brunner, S., Müller, W. E. G., Büttner, M., Gallati, H., Meyer zum Büschenfelde, K.-H., and Hess, G.: Corynebacterium parvum (Propionibacterium acnes): An inducer of tumor necrosis factor-α in human peripheral blood mononuclear cells and monocytes in vitro. Eur. J. Immunol., 20:1761, 1990.
148. Ruszala-Mallon, V., Linn, Y.-I. Durr, F. E., and Wang, B. S.: Low molecular weight immunopotentiators. Int. J. Immunopharmacol., 10:497, 1988.
149. Ruuskanen, O., Remes, M., Makela, A. L., Isomaki, H., and Toivanen, A.: Levamisole and agranulocytosis. Lancet, 2:958, 1976.
150. Saijo, N., Ozaki, A., Beppu, Y., Irimajiri, N., Shibuya, M., Shimizu, E., Takizawa, T., Taniguchi, T., and Hoshi, A.: In vivo and in vitro effects of Nocardia rubra cell wall skeleton on natural killer activity in mice. Gann, 74:137, 1983.
151. Sakatani, M., Ogura, T., Masuno, T., Kishimoto, S., and Yamamura, Y.: Effect of Nocardia rubra cell wall skeleton on augmentation of cytotoxicity function in human pleural macrophages. Cancer Immunol. Immunother., 25:119, 1987.
152. Salem, P., Deryckx, S., Dulioust, A., Vivier, E., Denizot, Y., Damais, C., Dinarello, C. A., and Thomas, Y.: Immunoregulatory functions of paf-Acether. IV. Enhancement of IL-1 production of muramyl dipeptide-stimulated monocytes. J. Immunol., 144:1338, 1990.
153. Sampson, D., Peters, T. G., Lewis, J. D., Metzig, J., and Kurtz, B. E.: Dose dependence of immunopotentiation and tumor regression induced by levamisole. Cancer Res., 37:3526, 1977.
154. Sancéau, J., Falcoff, R., Beranger, F., Carter, D. B., and Wietzerbin, J.: Secretion of interleukin-6 (IL-6) by human monocytes stimulated by muramyl dipeptide and tumour necrosis factor alpha. Immunology, 69:52, 1990.
155. Schiller, J. H., Lindstrom, M., Witt, P. L., Hank, J. A., Mahvi, D., Wagner, R. J., Sondel, P., and Borden, E. C.: Immunological effects of levamisole in vitro. J. Immunother., 10:297, 1991.
156. Schwartz, R. S.: Immunosuppressive drugs. Prog. Allergy, 9:246, 1965.
157. Scott, M. T.: Corynebacterium parvum as a therapeutic antitumor agent in mice. II. Local injection. J. Natl. Cancer Inst., 53:861, 1975.
158. Shimizu, E., Saijo, N., Shibuya, M., Takizawa, T., and Hoshi, A.: The analysis of cytostatic activity of human peripheral blood granulocytes and its augmentation with Nocardia rubra cell wall skeleton (N-CWS). J. Cancer Res. Clin. Oncol., 106:130, 1983.
159. Shirai, M., Watanabe, S., and Nishioka, M.: Intratumoral injection of OK432 and lymphokine-activated killer activity in peripheral blood of patients with hepatocellular carcinoma. Eur. J. Cancer, 26:965, 1990.
160. Shirasaka, T., Kawase, I., Okada, M., Kitahara, M., Ikeda, T., Komuta, K., Hosoe, S., Yokota, S., Masuno, T., and Kishimoto, S.: Augmentative effect of Nocardia rubra cell-wall skeleton on the induction of human lymphokine-activated killer (LAK) cells by the production of LAK cell helper factor(s). Cancer Immunol. Immunother., 30:195, 1989.
161. Skillings, J. R., Levine, M., Rayner, H. L., Eisenhauer, E., Erlichman, C., Germond, C., Kerr, I., Lofters, W., Maroun, J., and Yoshida, S.: Levamisole and 5-fluorouracil therapy for resected colon cancer: A new indication. Can. Med. Assoc. J., 144:297, 1991.
162. Smalley, R. V., and Oldham, R. K.: Chemical inducers of lymphokines. *In* Principles of Cancer Biotherapy. Edited by R. K. Oldham. New York, Raven Press, Ltd., 1987, p. 223.
163. Snider, D. E., Comstock, G. W., Martinez, I., and Caras, G. J.: Efficacy of BCG vaccination in prevention of cancer: An update. J. Natl. Cancer Inst., 60:785, 1978.
164. Soloway, M. S., and Perry, A.: Bacillus Calmette-Guérin for treatment of superficial transitional cell carcinoma of the bladder in patients who have failed thiotepa and/or mitomycin C. J. Urol., 137:871, 1987.
165. Sone, S., Lopez-Berestein, G., and Fidler, I. J.: Potentiation of direct antitumor cytotoxicity and production of tumor cytolytic factors in human blood monocytes by human recombinant interferon-gamma and muramyl depeptide derivatives. Cancer Immunol. Immunother., 21:93, 1986.
166. Souvannavong, V., Brown, S., and Adam, A.: Muramyl dipeptide (MDP) synergizes with Interleukin 2 and Interleukin 4 to stimulate, respectively, the differentiation and proliferation of B cells. Cell. Immunol., 126:106, 1990.
167. Spargo, B. J., Crowe, L. M., Ioneda, T., Beaman, B. L., and Crowe, J. H.: Cord factor (α, α-trehalose 6,6′-dimycolate) inhibits fusion between phospholipid vesicles. Proc. Natl. Acad. Sci. USA, 88:737, 1991.
168. Sparks, F. C., Silverstein, M. J., Hunt, J. S., Haskell, C. M., Pilch, Y. H., and Morton, D. L.: Complications of BCG immunotherapy in patients with cancer. N. Eng. J. Med., 289:827, 1973.
169. Spitler, L. E.: A randomized trial of levamisole versus placebo as adjuvant therapy in malignant melanoma. J. Clin. Oncol., 9:736, 1991.
170. Steis, R. G., Urba, W. J., VanderMolen, L. A., Bookman, M. A., Smith, J. W., Clark, J. W., Miller, R. L., Crum, E. D., Beckner, S. K., McKnight, J. E., Ozols, R. F., Stevenson, H. C., Young, R. C., and Longo, D. L.: Intraperitoneal lymphokine-activated killer-cell and Interleukin-2 therapy for malignancies limited to the peritoneal cavity. J. Clin. Oncol., 8:1618, 1990.
171. Stephens, E. J. W., Wood, H. F., and Mason, B.: The influence of levamisole on the survival of patients with disseminated mammary carcinoma treated with chemotherapy. *In* Immunotherapy of Human Cancer. Edited by W. D. Terry, and S. A. Rosenberg. New York, Elsevier, North Holland, Inc., Excerpta Medica, 1982, p. 199.
172. Stevenson, H. C., Green, I., Hamilton, J. M., Calabro, B. A., Parkinson, D. R.: Levamisole: Known effects on the immune system, clinical results and future applications to the treatment of cancer. J. Clin. Oncol., 9:2052, 1991.
173. Suga, T., Shiio, T., Maeda, Y. Y., and Chihara, G.: Antitumor activity of lentinan in murine syngeneic and autochthonous hosts and its suppressive effect on 3-methylcholanthrene-induced carcinogenesis. Cancer Res., 44:5132, 1984.
174. Suzuki, M., Higuchi, S., Taki, Y., Taki, S., Miwa, K., and Hamuro, J.: Induction of endogenous lymphokine-activated killer activity by combined administration of lentinan and interleukin 2. Int. J. Immunopharmacol., 12:613, 1990.
175. Taguchi, T.: Clinical efficacy of lentinan on patients with stomach cancer: End point results of a four-year follow-up survey. Cancer Detect. Prev., 1(Suppl.):333, 1987.
176. Tang, Z. Y., Zhou, H. Y., Zhao, G., Chai, L. M., Zhou, M., Lu, J. Z., Liu, K. D., Havas, H. F., Nauts, H. C.: Preliminary results of mixed bacterial vaccine as adjuvant treatment of hepatocellular carcinoma. Med. Oncol. Tumor Pharmacother., 8:23, 1991.
177. Thompson, J. S., Herbick, J. M., Klassen, L. W., Severson, C. D., Overlin, V. L., Blaschke, J. W., Silverman, M. A., and Vogel, C. L.: Studies on levamisole-induced agranulocytosis. Blood, 56:388, 1980.
178. Treatment of acute lymphoblastic leukaemia: Comparison of immunotherapy (BCG), intermittent methotrexate, and no therapy after a five-month intensive cytotoxic regimen (Concord trial): Preliminary report to the Medical Research Council by the Leukaemia Committee and the Working Party on Leukaemia in Childhood. Br. Med. J., 4:189, 1971.
179. Treurniet-Donker, A. D., Meischke-De Jongh, M. L., van Putten, W. L. J.: Levamisole as adjuvant immunotherapy in breast cancer. Cancer, 59:1590, 1987.
180. Tripodi, D., Parks, L. C., and Brugmans, J.: Drug-induced restoration of cutaneous delayed hypersensitivity in anergic patients with cancer. N. Engl. J. Med., 289:354, 1973.
181. Tsujihashi, H., Matsuda, H., Uejima, S., Akiyama, T., and Kurita, T.: Immunocompetence of tissue infiltrating lymphocytes in bladder tumors. J. Urol., 140:890, 1988.
182. Tuttle, R. L., and North, R. J.: Mechanisms of antitumor action of Corynebacterium parvum: The generation of cell-mediated tumor specific immunity. J. Reticuloendothelial Soc., 20:197, 1976.
183. Tuttle, R. L., and North, R. J.: Mechanisms of antitumor action of Corynebacterium parvum: Replicating short-lived T cells as the mediators of potentiated tumor-specific immunity. J. Reticuloendothelial Soc., 20:209, 1976.
184. Uchida, A., Micksche, M., and Hoshino, T.: Intrapleural administration of OK432 in cancer patients: Augmentation of autologous tumor killing activity of tumor-associated large granular lymphocytes. Cancer Immunol. Immunother., 18:5, 1984.
185. Uchida, A.: Augmentation of autologous tumor killing activity of tumor-associated large granular lymphocytes by the streptococcal preparation OK432. Methods Find. Exp. Clin. Pharmacol., 8:81, 1986.
186. Urba, W. J., Clark, J. W., Steis, R. G., Bookman, M. A., Smith, J. W., II, Beckner, S., Maluish, A. E., Rossio, J. L., Rager, H., Ortaldo, J. R., Longo, D. L.: Intraperitoneal lymphokine-activated killer cell-interleukin-2 therapy in patients with intra-abdominal cancer: Immunologic considerations. J. Natl. Cancer Inst., 81:602, 1989.
187. Urba, W. J., Hartmann, L. C., Longo, D. L., Steis, R. G., Smith, J. W., II, Kedar, I., Creekmore, S., Sznol, M., Conlon, K., Kopp, W. C., Huber, C., Herold, M., Alvord, W. G., Snow, S., and Clark, J. W.: Phase I and immunomodulatory study of a muramyl peptide, muramyl tripeptide phosphatidylethanolamine. Cancer Res., 50:2979, 1990.
188. Utsugi, T., and Sone, S.: Comparative analysis of the priming effect of human interferon-γ, α, and β on synergism with muramyl dipeptide analog for anti-tumor expression of human blood monocytes. J. Immunol., 136:1117, 1986.
189. Vanky, F., Uchida, A., Klein, E., and Willems, J.: Lysis of autologous tumor cells by high-density lymphocytes is potentiated by the streptococcal preparation OK432 (Picibanil). Int. J. Cancer, 37:531, 1986.
190. Van Wauwe, J., Janssen, P. A. J.: Review article on the biochemical mode of action of levamisole: An update. Int. J. Immunopharmacol., 13:3, 1991.
191. Vogl, S. E., Schoenfeld, D. A., Kaplan, B. H., Lerner, H. J., Horton, J., Creech, R. H.,

Barnes, L. E.: Methotrexate alone or with regional subcutaneous Corynebacterium parvum in the treatment of recurrent and metastatic squamous cancer of the head and neck. Cancer, 50:2295, 1982.

192. Wakui, A., Kasai, M., Konno, K., Abe, R., Kanamura, R., Takahashi, K., Nakai, Y., Yoshida, Y., Koie, H., and Masuda, H.: Randomized study of lentinan on patients with advanced gastric and colorectal cancer. Gan To Kagaku Ryoho, 13:1050, 1986.

193. Webb, H. E., Oaten, S. W., Pike, C. P.: Treatment of malignant ascitic and pleural effusion with Corynebacterium parvum. Br. Med. J., 1:338, 1978.

194. Weiss, D. W., Lavrin, D. H., Dezfulian, M., Vaage, J., Blair, P. B.: Studies on the immunology of spontaneous mammary carcinomas of mice: In Viruses Inducing Cancer. Edited by W. J. Burdette, Salt Lake City, University of Utah Press, 1966, p. 138.

195. White, J. E., Chen, T., Reed, R., Mira, J., Stuckey, W. J., Weatherall, T., O'Bryan, R., Samson, M. K., and Seydel, H. G.: Limited squamous cell carcinoma of the lung: A Southwest Oncology Group randomized study of radiation with or without doxorubicin chemotherapy and with or without levamisole immunotherapy. Cancer Treat. Rep., 66:1113, 1982.

196. Whittaker, J. A., Bailey-Wood, R., and Hutchins, S.: Active Immunotherapy for the treatment of acute myelogenous leukemia: The use of intravenous BCG and a comparison between BCG and irradiated leukemic blast cells. In Immunotherapy of Human Cancer. Edited by W. D. Terry, and S. A. Rosenberg. New York, Experta Medica, 1982, p. 23.

197. Windle, R., Bell, P. R. F., and Shaw, D.: Five year results of a randomized trial of adjuvant 5-fluorouracil and levamisole in colorectal cancer. Br. J. Surg., 74:569, 1987.

198. Woodruff, M. F. A., and Boak, J. L.: Inhibitory effect of injection of Corynebacterium parvum on the growth of tumour transplants in isogenic hosts. Br. J. Cancer, 20:345, 1966.

199. Woodruff, M., Dunbar, N., and Ghaffar, A.: The growth of tumours in T-cell deprived mice and their response to treatment with Corynebacterium parvum. Proc. R. Soc. Lond. B., 184:97, 1973.

200. Woodruff, M., and Walbaum, P.: A phase-II trial of Corynebacterium parvum as adjuvant to surgery in the treatment of operable lung cancer. Cancer Immunol. Immunother., 16:114, 1983.

201. Wright, P. W., Hill, L. D., Peterson, A. V., Jr., Pinkham, R., Johnson, L., Ivey, T., Bernstein, I., Bagley, C., and Anderson, R.: Preliminary results of combined surgery and adjuvant Bacillus Calmette-Guérin plus levamisole treatment of resectable lung cancer. Cancer Treat. Rep., 62:1671, 1978.

202. Yamakido, M., Ishioka, S., Onari, K., Matsuzaka, S., Yanagida, J., and Nishimoto, Y.: Changes in natural killer cell, antibody-dependent cell-mediated cytotoxicity and interferon activities with administration of Nocardia rubra cell wall skeleton to subjects with high risk of lung cancer. Gann, 74:896, 1983.

203. Yamamura, Y., Ogura, T., Hirao, F., Yasumoto, K., Sawamura, K., Hattori, S., Hayata, Y., Kishimoto, S., Yamada, K., Niitani, H., and Masaoka, T.: Phase I study with cell wall skeleton of Nocardia rubra. Cancer Treat. Rep., 65:707, 1981.

204. Yamamura, Y., Ogura, T., Sakatani, M., Hirao, F., Kishimoto, S., Fukuoka, M., Takada, M., Kawahara, M., Furuse, K., Kuwahara, O., Ikegama, H., and Ogawa, N.: Randomized controlled study of adjuvant immunotherapy with Nocardia rubra cell wall skeleton for inoperable lung cancer. Cancer Res., 43:5575, 1983.

205. Yamaue, H., Tanimura, H., Iwahashi, M., Tani, M., Tsunoda, T., Tabuse, K., Kuribayashi, K., and Saito, K.: Role of interleukin-2 and interferon-gamma in induction of activated natural killer cells from mice primed in vivo and subsequently challenged in vitro with the streptococcal preparation OK432. Cancer Immunol. Immunother., 29:79, 1989.

206. Yanagawa, E., Uchida, A, Moore, M., and Micksche, M.: Autologous tumor killing and natural cytotoxic activity of tumor-associated macrophages in cancer patients. Cancer Immunol. Immunother., 19:163, 1985.

207. Yarkoni, E., Lederer, E., and Rapp, H. J.: Immunotherapy of experimental cancer with a mixture of synthetic muramyl dipeptide and trehalose dimycolate. Infect. Immun., 32:273, 1981.

208. Zbar, B., Bernstein, I. D., Bartlett, G. L., Hanna, M. G., Jr., and Rapp, H. J.: Immunotherapy of cancer: Regression of intradermal tumors and prevention of growth of lymph node metastases after intralesional injection of living Mycobacterium bovis. J. Natl. Cancer Inst., 49:119, 1972.

XVIII-2

Active Specific Immunotherapy with Vaccines

Donald L. Morton
Mepur H. Ravindranath

Introduction

The clinical use of vaccines to treat cancer was initiated at the turn of the century. Success of vaccines in inducing prophylactic immunity against infectious diseases prompted clinical trials with cancer vaccines. In contrast to vaccines against infectious agents, cancer vaccines were generally administered *after* the advent of disease, rather than *before* the disease developed. Both types of vaccines utilized killed whole cells, cell walls, specific antigens, or nonpathogenic strains of living organisms to stimulate the patient's own immune system to fight the disease.[70] The specific goals of active immunotherapy with cancer vaccines have been: 1) to overcome the immunosuppression produced by tumor-derived factors; 2) to stimulate specific immunity that will destroy tumor cells; and 3) to enhance the immunogenicity of tumor associated antigens.

Several observations support the potential value of active specific immunotherapy for the treatment of cancer including 1) vaccine-induced immunity against cancer in animal models, 2) the regression and eradication of tumors injected directly with immunostimulants,[19,167,223,224,254] 3) occasional regression of noninjected tumors after the intralesional injection of bacillus Calmette-Guérin (BCG),[150,151,161,163,168,173,203] and 4) the development of anti-tumor antibodies. This chapter will discuss theoretical requirements for tumor vaccines and review the outcome of vaccine trials.

Tumor/Host Interactions

TAAs as Targets for Immunotherapy. Tumor cells express potentially immunogenic molecules that are commonly referred to as tumor associated antigens (TAAs). TAAs can be grouped into three categories. The first includes *neoantigens*[202] that are not expressed by the normal cells from which the cancer cells are derived, but that can be found in other normal tissues. For example, the human melanoma associated ganglioside GD_2, which is expressed on the surface of human melanomas[24,196] but not on normal melanocytes,[24] is a ganglioside found in human brain and spinal cord. A second group of TAAs include *oncofetal antigens* that are not expressed by any normal tissues but that may be expressed on fetal tissues. Finally, a small group of antigens appear to be *tumor specific antigens* in that they are not found in normal adult or fetal tissues. Examples include O-acetylated GD_3 on the surface of melanoma cells[194,196] and gangliosides containing N-glycolylneuraminic acid in human gastric, liver, and colon cancers as well as lymphoma.[110] Under appropriate conditions, antigens of all three groups can serve as targets for active immunotherapy with cancer vaccines.

If TAAs are found in normal cells, why doesn't the host

recognize these antigens immunologically?[102] The TAA may be cryptic on the normal cell due to: 1) the orientation or physical conformation of the antigen on the cell surface, 2) a physical separation by cell membranes, or 3) to masking by other normal cell surface components. The density of the antigen on a normal cell may be lower than a threshold level required for recognition by the immune system.[246] The pattern of surface distribution of the antigen may differ between normal and tumor cells.[28,29] Immunorecognition of tumor specific antigens (such as O-AcGD$_3$ or N-glycolylneuraminic acid-containing gangliosides) may also involve secondary recognition of neoantigens. Thus, antibodies produced against O-AcGD$_3$ in melanoma patients after active specific immunotherapy also selectively cross-react with the progenitor of the antigen, namely GD$_3$.[195]

Host Immunosuppression by Shed TAAs. One common explanation for a failure of the host to reject tumors is that the TAAs may be continuously shed from the tumor cell surface[22,39,88,89,119,120,158,188,192] and bind to reticuloendothelial cells and antibodies causing immunosuppression.[14,39,94,119,187] Thus repeated washing of the peripheral blood lymphocytes from cancer patients restored and enhanced the ability of the lymphocytes to kill tumor cells.[39]

In contrast to peripheral blood lymphocytes, tumor infiltrating lymphocytes proliferate less readily in response to IL-2 or mitogens.[248] Similarly, peripheral blood lymphocytes exposed to tumor cells or to their shed products show significantly reduced proliferation.[150] A gradient of suppression in the lymph node lymphocytes of melanoma patients correlates inversely with distance from the tumor mass.[32] Although further characterization of the immunosuppressive substances produced by tumors is needed, there is impressive evidence that shed tumor associated gangliosides are involved in blocking the functions of lymphocytes.[14,94,187]

The degree to which immune recognition is suppressed correlates with the stage of disease and overall tumor burden.[50,78,250] The presence of circulating TAA-antibody complexes in cancer patients who have not received immunotherapy suggests that an antibody response against some TAAs is initiated early during tumor growth.[43,81] Such antitumor antibodies may be masked by shed antigens during tumor progression.[126] Such suppression may be reversed by removing the growing neoplasm.[159] When serum samples were analyzed for antitumor antibodies before and after surgery for primary sarcoma,[50] successful resection of tumor was associated with a four-fold rise in antitumor antibody titer. In contrast, most patients who had no antitumor antibodies before or after surgery developed recurrences within six months. Patients who had developed pulmonary metastasis postoperatively showed a progressive decline in their antitumor antibody titers. Studies of complement fixing antibody titers in patients with sarcomas[50] and melanomas[78,236,250] have shown that complement fixing antibodies are masked by the shed TAAs neutralizing antitumor activity.

Antigenic Alteration and Immunological Heterogeneity. Although a malignant neoplasm usually evolves from a single transformed cell, most cancers are composed of genetically unstable populations of proliferating cells that become heterogeneous over time.[86,176] Heterogeneity enables subsets of the tumor cell population to evade the host's immune response as well as to resist chemical, physical and biological therapies.[151,176] Tumors recurring at the resection site of a primary neoplasm can differ antigenically from the primary tumor.[182] This is consistent with the possibility that antigenic variants have been selected for their ability to escape from immune surveillance. The biochemical profile of gangliosides in human melanoma provides a classic example of heterogeneity in antigen expression.[196] GM$_3$ constitutes >95% of the gangliosides on melanocytes, the progenitors of human melanoma.[24] During the early, radial phase of migration, neoplastically transformed melanocytes express more GD$_3$, a derivative of GM$_3$, than do normal progenitors.[89,194] After the appearance of GD$_3$, the tumor cells begin to migrate vertically. Subsequently, levels of GD$_3$ continue to increase[89,194] and other derivatives of GD$_3$, namely GD$_2$ and O-AcGD$_3$, begin to appear.[195–197] These alterations in gangliosides correlate with and may facilitate invasion and metastasis. Similar alterations are observed during melanoma progression in MHC antigens (HLA-DR), cell adhesion molecules (ICAM-I) and mucins (MUC18).[220]

Cell surface sialic acid can mask TAAs.[128,130,132,207] Sialylated TAAs are only weakly immunogenic. Removal of sialic acid with neuraminidase can enhance immune recognition and tumor cell destruction.[7,92,227] *Vibrio cholera* neuraminidase (VCN) has been used to remove cell surface sialic acids from autologous and allogenic tumor cells before immunization.[58,92,215,229]

Heterogeneity in the expression of TAAs within a given tumor poses a significant obstacle to vaccine therapy. Elimination of cells that bear a single major antigen can still permit the survival of a subpopulation that expresses a minor antigenic variant.[67] Antigenic heterogeneity may reflect the selective elimination of immunogenic cells leading to the outgrowth of less immunogenic subpopulations. To compensate for heterogeneity in antigen expression, several antigenically distinct tumor cell lines can be combined within a single tumor cell vaccine (TCV) or combinations of purified antigens can be used, so that the vaccine collectively expresses all the TAAs contained within a given neoplasm.[158]

Strategies for Increasing the Immunogenicity of Vaccines. The goals of active immunotherapy are: 1) to combat the decreasing immunocompetence that results from an interaction of tumor-related products with components of the immune system during tumor progression, and 2) to eliminate the diverse clones within a tumor cell population by the augmentation of cellular and/or humoral immunity. A tumor vaccine should have the ability: 1) to stimulate the clearance of immunosuppressive TAAs from the circulation;[14,94,187,188] 2) to minimize the immunosuppressive activity of suppressor T-cells and suppressor inducer cells;[8–10,12,155,164,167] 3) to activate the antigen presenting function of macrophages, monocytes, histiocytes and dendritic cells;[1,82–84] 4) to elicit an antibody response against TAAs on the tumor cell surface,[164,167] not only to clear the shed TAAs but also to kill tumor cells; 5) to stimulate the generation of newly activated T cells capable of killing tumor cells;[37] and 6) to direct the migration of these lymphocytes into metastatic tumors[10,179] that rarely contain lymphocytes.[10,17]

Optimal vaccines have contained whole autologous or allogeneic tumor cells mixed with appropriate adjuvants such as virus,[4] whole bacteria (BCG, *C. parvum, Salmonella minnesota),* or bacterial components including cell wall skeleton, trehalose dimycotate, and monophosphoryl lipid A. Bacterial adjuvants have evoked tumor specific cellular[44,45,55,68,69,239,240] and humoral [78,195,250] immune responses. Several strategies have been utilized to augment tumor cell immunogenicity.

Modify the Composition of Allogeneic Tumor Cell Vaccines. By exposing the patient's immune system to diverse TAAs from different tumor cell lines, Morton and colleagues[164,167,170] nearly doubled the fraction of patients who developed a humoral response to tumor cell vaccines.

Diminish Generation of Suppressor T Cells. Suppressor T cells interfere with B cell production of antibodies and with other immunoregulatory functions. Cyclophosphamide has been shown to reduce suppressor cell functions and to enhance the antibody response leading to immunity to TAAs.[8-13,20,21,155,164,167]

Combine Adjuvants with Tumor Cell Vaccines. (Table XVII-2-1). Repeated efforts have been made to increase the immunogenicity of tumor vaccines by adding an adjuvant. Adjuvants used in clinical trials have included live vaccinia virus, *Salmonella* extracts, viable BCG and BCG derivatives[156,239,240] such as cell wall skeleton, trehalose dimycolate, muramyl dipeptide and glycolipids. Table XVII-2-1 lists the tumor vaccines and immunopotentiators used to date in clinical trials for the treatment of different cancers. Data obtained in clinical trials and in animal models underline the importance of the ratio of tumor cells to adjuvant as well as the sequence and site of administration of the tumor cell preparation and the adjuvant.

Protein Adjuvants. Addition of a highly antigenic carrier protein to an otherwise nonantigenic substance can often evoke an immune response. The antibodies formed against this complex are specifically directed against the previously nonantigenic substance, as well as against the foreign protein in the complex. Early reports[36,42] using rabbit gamma globulin attached to proteins of autologous tumor cells reported some therapeutic benefit, but the efficacy of this type of treatment has not been confirmed.

Viral Adjuvants. There is convincing evidence in animal models that infection of tumor cells by certain viruses augments the immunogenicity of tumor antigens.[91,115] Based on animal models, randomized clinical trials have been undertaken with allogeneic or autologous tumor cells infected with Newcastle disease virus,[25,26] vesicular stomatitis virus,[129] and vaccinia virus[91,209,241-244] in patients with melanoma and osteosarcoma.[76]

Bacterial Adjuvants. Immunologic adjuvants, such as BCG, *Salmonella minnesota, C. parvum,* MER (methanol extractable residue of tubercle bacillus), and Freund's adjuvant (Table XVII-2-1), are potent immunostimulants in animal systems, capable of enhancing the humoral and cellular immune response to a variety of antigens.

Chemical Adjuvants. TAAs in human tumor cells can also be modified in a variety of ways by chemicals such as iodoacetate and cholesteryl hemisuccinate,[208,209,213,214] which increase the immunogenicity of tumor cells. Certain enzymes, such as neuraminidase, enhance the immunoresponse to neoplasms by chemically altering the surface glyco-conjugates.[7,58,215,227,229] Repeated intradermal immunization with neuraminidase-treated allogeneic acute myeloid leukemic cells prolonged disease-free survival in patients treated with chemotherapy.[92]

Whole Cell Tumor Vaccines

Many vaccines have been prepared from whole tumor cells. In animal models, injection of living autologous tumor cells in numbers too small to cause progressive tumor growth has generally provided the most effective immunogen.[77A] For the treatment of certain tumors that share common TAAs, such as melanomas, one patient could be immunized with an allogeneic vaccine of living tumor cells from another patient.[133,156A,165] An immune response should develop against the foreign major histocompatibility complex antigens on the transplanted tumor cells causing their rejection. In addition, the immune response to the foreign MHC antigens may provide help, inducing a strong immune response against the common cross-reacting TAA.

The possibility that viable autologous tumor cells could result in tumor growth at the inoculation site has precluded the use of such vaccines in man. For this reason, vaccines composed of tumor cells inactivated by a variety of different methods, including irradiation, mitomycin C, freezing and thawing or heat treatment have been used. Such treatments

Table XVIII-2-1.   Different Kinds of Tumor Specific Vaccine Used in Clinical Trials to Promote Immunogenicity of Tumor-Associated-Antigens

Kinds of Vaccine
1. Autologous tumor cells
i) Whole cells alone[238]
ii) Whole cells + BCG[11,95,122,123,134]
iii) Whole cells + *Cornyebacterium parvum*[118,148,206]
iv) Whole cells + PPD + *Candida albicans*[191,228,233]
v) Whole cells-cholesteryl hemisuccinate (CHS)[213,214]
vi) Whole cells-Muramyl dipeptide and TDM[46]
vii) Whole cells-neuraminidase treated + Freund's (C)[227]
viii) Cell Extract + PPD[228,237]
ix) Oncolysate-VSV[129]
2. Allogeneic tumor cells
i) Whole cells alone[30,80,157]
ii) Whole cells + BCG[133,162,198,199,249]
iii) Whole cells + *Cornyebacterium parvum*[64,131,152]
iv) Whole cells + BCG-CWS[251]
v) Whole cells + Cholesterol hemisuccinate[208,209]
vi) Whole cells + Muramyl dipeptide and TDM[46]
vii) Whole cells-neuraminidase treated + BCG[7,58,215,229]
viii) Cell Extract[201]
ix) Cell Extract + Freund's adjuvant[93,222,227]
x) Cell Extract + BCG-CWS + TDM-MPL[155]
xi) Oncolysate-NDV[25,26]
xii) Oncolysate-Vaccinia[91,209,241-244]
3. Purified tumor associated antigens
i) Gangliosides-*Salmonella minnesota* R595[128]
ii) Gangliosides-BCG[129,130]
ii) Gangliosides-MPL[130]

BCG, *Bacillus Calmette-Guérin*; FC, Freund's complete adjuvant; PPD, purified protein derivative (tuberculin) from *Mycobacterium tuberculosis*; CWS, Mycobacterial cell wall skeleton; TDM, Trehalose dimycocholate; MPL, Monophosphoryl lipid A extracted from a gram negative Bacteria *Salmonella minnesota* R595; VSV, Vesicular stomatitis virus; NDV, Newcastle disease virus; VV, vaccinia virus may, however, chemically alter tumor antigens and diminish the effectiveness of the vaccine.

Advantages of Autologous and Allogeneic Vaccines

Numerous trials have utilized autologous tumor cells alone, without the addition of adjuvants. Since autologous tumor cells express the same blood group and histocompatibility antigens as the host, they are considered ideal for tumor cell vaccines. The restricted availability of autologous tumor tissues limits, however, the amount of vaccine, and thus, the number of immunizations possible. Moreover, antigen expression may vary from site to site and a vaccine prepared from autologous cells isolated from any particular nodules may not have the same TAA profile as tumor at another metastatic site.

Allogeneic tumor grown in cell culture can provide sufficient vaccine for multiple injections. Mixtures of cells from different tumors can provide a spectrum of TAAs. On the other hand, passage of tumor cells in culture may introduce contaminants and favor the growth of subpopulations that diverge from the antigenic phenotype of the original cancer. Fetal bovine serum (FBS), for example, is widely used in culture media. Often the proteins and glycolipids in FBS are incorporated into tumor cells and function as xenogeneic antigens.[63] Patients who receive tumor cells grown in FBS develop an antibody response against FBS components.[21,137,138] Serum-free media or media that contain human serum are considered ideal for the preparation of tumor cell vaccines. Tumor cells grown in culture may also undergo antigenic alterations similar to those documented for ganglioside profiles of human melanoma[194,232] and glioma.[61] In some cases, these alterations have been used to advantage by mixing different cell lines with increased TAA expression to prepare allogeneic tumor cell vaccines.[164,167]

Clinical Trials of Tumor Vaccines

The history of vaccine therapy can be divided into two phases that reflect different levels of understanding of the immune response.[37]

Early Vaccine Trials

Therapy with tumor cell vaccines was first described in 1902 by von Leyden and Blumenthal,[238] followed shortly thereafter by other reports.[31,237] Coca and colleagues attributed several instances of tumor regression (5/48) to the repeated administration of viable autologous and allogeneic tumor cells in large numbers at 14-day intervals.[30,31] Risley immunized tumor-bearing patients with large volumes of autologous or allogeneic tumor cell extract every 14 days without apparent benefit.[201] Vaughan administered tumor extracts intraperitoneally and recognized that "the best results were obtained in cases in which the amount of tumor tissue present was small, and in which the differential leucocyte count of the patient show[ed] a decided reaction following administration of the cancer protein."[235] Kellock and co-workers irradiated the site of live-tumor-cell immunization in an attempt to reduce the risk of tumor growth at the implantation site.[111] Later, irradiated tumor cells were used in patients

with malignant melanoma.[73] Graham and Graham reported that the administration of a tumor cell vaccine to patients from whom tumor had been removed "appeared to radio-sensitize the residual disease."[73]

Later Vaccine Trials

Since 1960, greater emphasis has been given to tumor cell antigens in various forms and to the use of different adjuvants mixed with tumor cell vaccine. Finney, Byers and Wilson[57] administered a tumor cell homogenate admixed with complete Freund's adjuvant (containing components of *Mycobacterium bovis*) intramuscularly to patients with a variety of malignant tumors and found that all treated patients developed antibodies against tumor cells. Injecting these antibodies, after purification, into subcutaneous nodules produced dramatic, albeit temporary, regression of tumor.

Czajkowski and colleagues chemically coupled rabbit gamma globulin to human tumor cells and found that it enhanced the immunogenicity of the tumor cell vaccine.[42] Cunningham and co-workers treated 42 cancer patients with autologous TCV-rabbit gamma globulin vaccine.[36] In another study, responders showed DTH responses to the TCV-adjuvant complex, suggesting that the vaccine had evoked cell-mediated immunity.[99]

There have been conflicting reports regarding the value of vaccine therapy (Table XVIII-2-5). Frequent immunization with allogeneic tumor cells did prolong the period of remission and the survival times of patients with acute lymphoblastic leukemia.[144] Autoimmunization was also found to augment both circulating antibodies, and specifically, cytotoxic lymphocytes.[40,100] The first report[163] on the regression of cutaneous metastases of melanoma following intralesional injection of live BCG not only redirected the course of immunotherapy trials (Table XVIII-2-2) but also rekindled interest in combining tumor cell vaccines with extrinsic adjuvants such as BCG for active specific therapy.

Goodnight and Morton have addressed this area in detail and identified several factors that limit interpretation of trials with tumor vaccines.[70,71] These include: 1) The variability of human cancer and thus the need for precise definitions of the population of patients chosen to enter a clinical trial; and 2) The need for appropriate randomly selected controls. The problems of experimental design and performance of clinical trials for immunotherapy are not fundamentally different from those encountered more generally in cancer clinical trials. The principles and approaches to designing clinical trials are presented in V.

Current Status of Vaccine Therapy for Different Human Cancers

The current status of active immunotherapy can be understood best from the results of past clinical trials conducted in different forms of cancer.[160] Table XVIII-2-5 represents the condensed results of the trials classified according to Goodnight and Morton.[70,71] Among patients with different forms of cancer, those with malignant melanoma seem to have accrued the most benefit from active immunotherapy, as shown by tumor regression and increased disease-free survival. Some of the results obtained in other forms of cancer are also encouraging. The success of the therapy in the hands of

Table XVIII-2-2. Response to Intralesional Administration of BCG in Melanoma Patients

Strain of BCG	Patients (n)	Responders Complete + Partial	Regression at Non-Injected Sites	References
Glaxo	8	5	2/5	156A
	1	0	0	125
	22	11	0/11	208
	8	3	0/3	109
Tice	9	2 + 5	2/7	173
	19	5	na	16
	7	3	1/3	216
	2	1	0/1	5
	36	6 + 9	6/25	161
	22 (intratumor)	3 + 7	3/10	174
	22 (intraderm)	0 + 2	0/2	174
	25	6 + 15	0/21	33
	15	2 + 3	na	141
Tice/Glaxo	29	2 + 13	2/15	184
	6	3 + 1	2/4	127
Connaught	3	2	1/2	112
Pasteur	11	7	0/7	104
Not specified	4	1	1/4	116
	8	2	0/8	154
	50	19	2/19	59
	19	4 + 14	na	218
	13	3 + 4	na	200
Methanol extract	18	8 + 4	na	117
	101	61	na	210
	6	2 + 2	na	135
	19	14 + 1	5/15	185

some and failure in the hands of others, however, requires that positive results be viewed with caution. Several factors may have influenced the outcome of different trials including the source of vaccine, method of preparation, and schedule of administration as well as the patients' tumor burdens prior to therapy. There is no doubt that reduction of the tumor burden would enhance the success rate of immunotherapy. Appropriate use of adjuvants also seems to be important. Treatment with an immunopotentiator like BCG or *C. parvum* may result in significantly increased response rates or survival in some trials and failure in others (Table XVIII-2-5). The quality and quantity of the immunopotentiator, route of administration, disease status, duration of treatment, effects of other therapies, and degree of immunological impairment influence the outcome of trials.

Malignant Melanoma. Morton and co-investigators were the first to demonstrate complete regression of metastatic tumor nodules after intralesional injection of living BCG; 90% of 184 melanoma metastases in 8 patients regressed.[163] Many clinical trials have subsequently confirmed this observation (Table XVIII-2-2). Contact between tumor cells and BCG appears to have produced systemic immunity evidenced by: 1) regression of noninjected nodules at sites distant from intralesional injections (Table XVIII-2-2); 2) the relationship between the clinical course of disease and the in vitro cytotoxicity of the patient's lymphocytes in the presence of the patient's serum;[16] and 3) the regression of a pulmonary metastasis in a patient treated for multiple intradermal metastasis.[141] The interaction of BCG with tumor cells may facilitate the infiltration into tumor nodules of antigen-presenting cells and lymphocytes. Antibodies may be directed against some common antigenic determinants shared by BCG and tumor cells,[153,163] or the administration of BCG may enable the patient's immune system to recognize the TAAs on tumor cells more effectively.

In animal models, Hanna and co-workers observed that histiocytes infiltrated lesions in response to BCG infection.[82–84] Barlett and Zbar tested this possibility by mixing irradiated tumor cells with BCG before administration and confirmed that the mixture evoked a better anti-tumor response than did either component.[6] Similarly, Morton and colleagues admixed TCV with BCG and administered it intradermally to melanoma patients (Tables XVIII-2-3 and XVIII-2-4). They noted an increase in the number of disease-free survivors and a lengthening of disease free intervals, but found no striking difference from BCG alone.[161,165,170] Recent observations of Ratliff and coworkers have shown that tumor cells which are able to fuse with BCG in the presence of fibronectin[98] elicit better immune responses than did tumor cells which were not capable of fusing with BCG.[193] After Zbar and co-workers administered irradiated tumor cells admixed with BCG intradermally to animals and showed antigen specificity of the therapeutic effect of tumor cell-BCG vaccine, a number of investigators (Table XVIII-2-4) have undertaken clinical trials with tumor cell vaccines.[6,252-254] These have included both autologous and allogeneic tumor cells with or without different immunomodulators.

Leukemia. Promising results were obtained by Mathe and

Table XVIII-2-3.   Disease-Free Survival of Melanoma Patients after Administration of BCG

	No. of Patients			Disease-Free Survivors			
Route	Control	BCG	BCG + TCV	Control	BCG	BCG + TCV	References
Intralesional	13	13	na	3	8	na	204
Intradermal	46	45	49	19	19	26	165

na: not applicable; TCV: tumor cell vaccine

Table XVIII-2-4.   A Survey of Clinical Trials Involving Active Specific Immunotherapy of Metastatic Melanoma with Vaccines

Stage	Nature of Vaccine	Adjuvant	Route	Patients (n)	Response (%)	Survival % (yrs)	References
II	Allo/whole	BCG	i.d.	28		60 (1)	80
	Asialo-allo/whole*	BCG	i.d.	166		45 (3)	58
	Asialo-allo/whole*	BCG	s.c.	846		(Contrl) 33 (3)	215
						(1 node) 53 (5)	
						(<4 node) 43 (5)	
						(>4 node) 25 (5)	
	Allo/whole (Cy)		i.d.	68		52 (<2)	161
	Allo/extract	FC	i.d.	16	69		93
	Allo/lysate	NDV	s.c.	32		88 (3)	25
	Allo/lysate	NDV	s.c.	21		71 (<3)	26
	Allo/lysate	VV	i.d.	38		55 (1)	244
				39		(hist. Cntl) 25 (1)	
	Allo/lysate	VV	i.d.	90		75 (2)	91
				56		(Contrl) 47 (2)	
	Allo/extract (Cy)	CWS/TDM/MPL	i.d.	5			155
	Allo/subcell (Cy)	alum	i.d.	36			21
	Allo/subcell (Cy)	alum	i.d.	63		(23 DTH+)52 (5)	21
						(40 DTH−)26 (5)	
	Auto/extract/Chem	PPD	s.c.	5			228
III	Auto/whole	BCG	i.d.	18	22		122
	Auto/whole	BCG	i.d.	5			123
	Auto/whole	BCG	i.d.	13	0		134
	Auto/whole (Cy)	BCG	i.d.	33	12		12
	Allo/whole	BCG	i.d.	22	0		133
	Allo/whole		i.l.	34	26		245
	Allo/whole	BCG	i.d.	139		(Contrl) 41 (5)	170
						(BCG) 53 (5)	
						(BCG-TCV)52 (5)	
	Allo/extract	FC	i.d.	23	35		93
	Auto/lysate	VSV	s.c.	11	0		129
	Allo/lysate	VSV	s.c.	13	0		
	Allo/extract (Cy)	CWS/TDM/MPL	i.d.	17	29		155

*Vibrio cholerae neuraminidase treated tumor cells; BCG, *Bacillus Calmette-Guérin*; FC, Freund's complete adjuvant; PPD, purified protein derivative (tuberculin) from *Mycobacterium tuberculosis*; CWS, mycobacterial cell wall skeleton; TDM, Trehalose dimycolate, diglucose containing glycolipid extracted from CWS; MPL, Monophosphoryl lipid A extracted from *Salmonella minnesota* R595; TCV, Tumor cell vaccine; VSV, Vesicular stomatitis virus; NDV, New Castle disease virus; VV, Vaccinia virus; i.d., intradermal; i.l., intralymphatic; s.c., Subcutaneous; DTH, Delayed type of hypersensitivity response; Contrl, Control; Hist Contl, Historical control; Response refers to clinical response. Cy, Cyclophosphamide

co-workers when they administered both BCG and allogeneic leukemic cells to patients with acute lymphoblastic leukemia of childhood.[144] The long-term clinical follow-up of the 20 original patients treated with immunotherapy found that eight were alive in remission, with seven in their first complete remission.[145] Mathe and colleagues reported the overall five year survival for a larger group of 100 patients treated with BCG plus allogeneic leukemic cells was approximately 50%.[146] Unfortunately, several similar clinical trials could not confirm the findings of Mathe and co-workers, possibly related to differences in immunotherapy protocols.[172] Immunotherapy involving BCG and allogeneic leukemic cells has also been used for the maintenance of patients with acute myeloid leukemia (AML).[35] No difference was noted in the duration of remission between the two groups of patients, although the patients who received BCG plus irradiated tumor cells had longer remissions than did those maintained on either BCG or tumor cells alone. Powles and colleagues reported that the 45 of 107 leukemic patients who received BCG-TCV achieved complete remission with a median duration of 70 weeks.[190] A long-term follow-up of the trial, which closed in 1973,[189] reported that the actual median remission for patients receiving maintenance chemotherapy was 191 days versus 305 days for those receiving chemoimmunotherapy (not statistically significant). The median survival was, however, significantly improved by active specific immunotherapy (270 versus 510 days [P = 0.03]).[62] In a similar study involving irradiated allogeneic AML blast cells and BCG (Glaxo), therapy was most successful when administered to patients with low tumor burdens (Table XVIII-2-5).[62]

In another study, 191 adults with AML were first treated with combination chemotherapy consisting of daunorubicin and cytosine arabinoside.[85] Sixty-three patients achieved remission and were admitted to one of the three arms of active immunotherapy: immunotherapy alone, immunotherapy (following the protocol of Freeman and colleagues[62]) with maintenance chemotherapy, or no treatment. By contrast to immunotherapy plus chemotherapy, immunotherapy alone was associated with easy and repeated reinduction of remission and marked prolongation of survival after first relapse. Whittaker and coworkers compared the therapeutic effects of BCG alone and BCG plus allogeneic blast cells in a large patient population (n = 182) and found that BCG alone was as effective as BCG plus tumor cells.[249] Reizenstein and colleagues reported that 57% of 195 patients with acute non-lymphocytic leukemia entered complete remission after treatment with chemotherapy and BCG plus tumor cells.[199] After remission, the patients were randomized to maintenance with chemotherapy alone or chemotherapy in combination with active specific immunotherapy, involving weekly administration of frozen, non-irradiated allogeneic blast cells with BCG. The median survival in the chemoimmunotherapy group (n = 40) was 690 days vs. 408 days in the group with chemotherapy alone (n = 36). The survival difference was significant (P<0.01) according to the log rank test. Immunotherapy of AML using allogeneic cells with *C. parvum* showed no detectable impact on either remission rate or duration of survival.[64] Table XVIII-2-5 surveys various other clinical trials conducted on patients with AML and ALL.

The treatment of tumor cells with neuraminidase to remove sialic acids has yielded cells with increased immunogenicity.[7,92] A randomized clinical trial was initiated to compare chemotherapy alone, neuraminidase treated-allogeneic myeloblasts and neuraminidase treated myeloblasts plus methanol extract of BCG (MER).[92] Patients received 10^{10} asialo-myeloblasts injected at 50 sites draining into node-bearing regions at one session. A total dose of 1 mg MER was distributed in five equal injections. All immunotherapy was given at the midpoint between courses of chemotherapy. The median duration of remission for each immunotherapy arm was >78 weeks compared to 20 weeks for the group treated with chemotherapy alone. The survival for those who received immunotherapy and for those with chemotherapy alone was quite different: 27 of 32 patients treated with immunotherapy were alive compared with only 4 of 21 controls.[92] In other trials of active specific immunotherapy, BCG and cultured cell lines were administered intradermally to 15 patients with uncomplicated Philadelphia chromosome positive chronic myeloid leukemia (CML).[217] The CML patients who received immunotherapy survived twice as long as historical controls treated in the same institution.

Lung Cancer. More than 35% of lung cancer patients undergoing pulmonary resection harbor residual tumor cells within the thorax or at distant sites. Most lung cancer patients experience immunosuppression accompanying tumor growth and surgical intervention. In the postoperative interval Stewart and colleagues injected intracutaneously a vaccine composed of purified antigenic extracts from autochthonous lung cancer cells in combination with complete Freund's adjuvant.[222] Survival in Stage I patients treated with immunotherapy was superior to that in nonrandomized controls. The studies showed increases in cell-mediated immunity to antigenic tumor preparations when tested by DTH responses in the skin. Takita and coworkers treated 15 stage III lung cancer patients with complete Freund's adjuvant in combination with antigens extracted from autochthonous tumor.[227] The survival rate for this group increased to 63% at 2 years (Table XVIII-2-5). Reid and colleagues randomized 45 Stage I and 6 Stage II patients with operable non-small cell lung cancer to receive a) no further therapy after resection, b) BCG alone or c) BCG plus allogeneic tumor cells administered intradermally twice monthly for 2 years.[198] They found that BCG or BCG-TCV is of marginal benefit in patients with resected lung cancer. Another study investigated the effects of a) methotrexate alone (n = 8), b) immunotherapy with a homogenate of soluble tumor cell vaccine admixed with Freund's complete adjuvant (n = 15), and c) a combination of chemoimmunotherapy (n = 13). Survival in immunized patients was significantly prolonged (P<0.01; Wilcoxon). Takita and colleagues randomized patients after resection into three different groups:[226] group 1 received no treatment; group 2 received tumor antigens admixed with Freund's adjuvant intradermally 3 times; and group 3 received only Freund's adjuvant. Actuarial analysis yielded estimates of three-year survival of 34% for group 1, 84% for group 2, and 89% for group 3. The difference in survival rates between the control arm and each of the immunotherapy arms is statistically significant (P<0.05). These studies, together with those reviewed in Table XVIII-2-5, suggest that immunonpotentiation of patients with adjuvant alone or adjuvant with tumor cells may be beneficial.

Sarcoma. Evidence of immunogenic TAAs in human and animal sarcomas prompted the initiation of trials with tumor vaccines. Morton and colleagues administered an admixture of BCG and 5 to 75 × 10^6 irradiated autologous tumor cells to 15 patients with various histological types of sarcomas.[157] Vaccine recipients had an increase in complement fixing and cytotoxic antibodies concomitant with a slowing of the progression of tumor. A year later, Morton and colleagues,[169] reported encouraging results combining immunotherapy with surgical resection of pulmonary nodules. The eight vaccine recipients had a modest prolongation of survival compared to the nine nonrandomized patients who received surgery alone. Most patients with slowly growing tumors (doubling time over 40 days) did well after surgery, with no apparent benefit from immunotherapy.

Currie described the recovery of immunological competence in a patient treated monthly with BCG plus irradiated autologous cells.[38] Similarly, Green and coworkers observed higher titers of antitumor cytotoxic antibodies and improved in vitro cellular immunity to tumor in patients with osteosarcoma administered with irradiated autologous or allogenic cells infected with influenza virus.[76] No clinical benefit was derived from the irradiated whole cell vaccine or cell lys-

Table XVIII-2-5.   Results of Some of the Clinical Trials Using Immunotherapy as a Modality of Cancer Treatment (Melanoma Excluded)

Kinds of Tumor	Type of Vaccine	Route	Outcome	References
Brain	TCV			72
	TCV			56
	TCV (autologous)	i.d.	nil	15
	TCV			137
	TCV (mitomycin + auto + allo + MDP + TDM)	s.c.	+ cell respns.	46
Colo-rectal	TCV (auto) + BCG	i.d.	DTH + (16/24)	95, 96
Gynecologic	TCV (allo)	i.d.	no respns.	73
	TCV (allo) + BCG	i.d.	+ respns.	101
	TC antigen + BCG + Chemotherapy	i.d.	no respns.	181
	TCV + BCG + Chem.	i.d.	+ respns.	97
Genitourinary	TCV (auto)	i.d.	+ respns.	191
	TCV (auto) + *C. parvum*	i.d.	25% respns.	147, 148
	TCV (auto) + *C. parvum*	i.d.	+ respns.	206
	TCV (auto/allo) + *C. parvum*	i.d.	24% respns.	118
	TCV (auto/all) + PPD + *Candida albicans*	i.d.	+ respns.	227
	TCV (auto) + PPD + *C. albicans*	i.d.	+ respns.	228
	TCV + PPD + PHA	i.d.	+ respns.	175
Leukemia (ALL)	TCV (allo) + BCG	i.d.	+ survival	144–146
	TCV (allo) + BCG-MeOH extrct.	i.d.	no respns.	124
	TCV (allo) + BCG + Chemo.	i.d.	no respns.	186
	TCV (allo) + BCG	i.d.	− respns.	180
(AML)	TCV (allo) + BCG + Chemo.	i.d.	Signf. surv.	189
	TCV (allo) + BCG	i.d.	Signf. surv.	190
	TCV (allo) + BCG	i.d.	+ respns.	62
	TCV (allo) + BCG + Chemo.	i.d.	Signf. surv.	247
	TCV (asialo-allo) + BCG	i.d.	Signf. respns.	92
	TCV (allo) + BCG	i.d.	Signf. respns.	85
	TCV (allo) + BCG	i.d.	Signf. surv.	249
	TCV (allo) + BCG	i.d.	Signf. surv.	199
	TCV (allo) + *C. parvum*	i.d.	no respns.	64
Lung	TC antigen + Chem.	i.d.	+ surv.	22
	TCV (asialo-allo)	i.d.	+ surv.	226–227
	TCV extrct.	i.d.	no respns.	2
	TCV + BCG	i.d.	no respns.	198
Sarcoma (osteo)	TCV (allo-extrct)	i.d.	+ respns.	140
	TCV (allo) + BCG	i.d.	no respns.	51
	TCV (allo) + BCG	i.d.	+ surv.	157
	TCV (allo) + BCG	i.d.	+ respns.	217
	TCV (allo) + BCG	i.d.	+ respns.	231
	TCV (allo) + BCG + vironcolysate + Chemo.	i.d.	+ respns.	212
	Viral oncolysate	i.d.	no respns.	76

TCV, tumor cell vaccine; TCV-asialo, Neuraminidase treated TCV free of sialic acids; MDP, muramyl dipeptide; TDM, Trehalose mycolate; BCG-MetOH ext, Methanol extract of BCG; Chemo, chemotherapy; i.d., intradermal; s.c., subcutaneous; i.les, intralesional; nil, no effect; + cell respns., positive cellular response; respns, response; surv, survival; PHA, phytohemagglutinin. (For further details see Refs. 70 and 71) ates.[139] Sokal and Aungst treated patients who had undergone resection of primary osteosarcoma with vaccines that contained autologous or allogeneic tumor cells and BCG, two were free of disease at 13 and 18 months and a third developed pulmonary metastases shortly after initiation of therapy.[217] Townsend and colleagues reported clinical benefit for sarcoma patients of active specific immunotherapy consisting of tine-administered Tice BCG, initially given at multiple sites weekly, then every two weeks.[231] Cultured allogeneic sarcoma cells were given concurrently by intradermal injection at five separate sites. The control group consisted of nine patients who refused therapy. Eight of the nine patients (89%) relapsed with no evidence of clinical benefit. With follow-up of up to 3.5 years, 11 of 18 patients (61%) who received treatment remained disease-free, but only 5 of the 15 (33%) treated by surgery alone escaped recurrence.

Breast Cancer. Intralesional injection of BCG has produced regression of skin metastases from breast carcinoma. Complete regression was observed in 7 of 8 patients in one study,[216] and in 7 of 14 patients in another.[113] Failure to respond is not uncommon.[65] The administration of irradiated autologous tumor vaccine after radical mastectomy for breast carcinoma showed no therapeutic benefit.[3] Several clinical trials have attempted combination immunotherapy and chemotherapy.[103,183]

Genitourinary Cancer. Active immunotherapy of renal cell carcinoma has been thoroughly reviewed.[47,74,225,234] Tumor cell vaccines with or without adjuvants have been administered in renal cell carcinoma.[108,148,233] McCune and colleagues administered weekly intracutaneous injections of autologous irradiated tumor cells admixed with *C. parvum* in five patients with residual renal carcinoma.[148] In another study, autologous tumor cell vaccine with *C. parvum* was administered to 14 patients with metastatic renal carcinoma; 4 of the 14 patients had objective responses and a fifth had prolonged stabilization. Responding patients generally had an excellent performance status and received greater than 2×10^8 cells.

In a concurrently controlled study, Tykka demonstrated a significant increase in survival for Stage IV renal cell carcinoma patients treated with a vaccine that contained autologous tumor polymerized with ethylchlorformate and PPD or *Candida albicans*.[233] Among 71 patients with advanced renal adenocarcinoma treated by Tallberg and colleagues with polymerized autologous tumor cell vaccine, 13 remained alive with at least three years follow-up, compared to only three survivors among 56 patients treated by the best conventional measures.[228] Similarly, Prager and colleagues observed a significant increase in survival among recipients of autologous tumor cell vaccines compared to that of controls who had not received vaccine.[191] Neidhart reported two complete responses and two partial responses among 30 patients treated with autologous tumor using tuberculin or phytohemagglutinin as an adjuvant.[175]

In an attempt to increase immunogenicity by abrogating the T suppressor cell activity, Sahasrabudhe and coworkers administered cyclophosphamide before vaccination using tumor cells admixed with *C. parvum*.[206] Of the 20 patients thus treated, five had responses, of which one was complete and four were partial. Four of the 15 patients developed DTH

responses to autologous renal carcinoma cells. Of these four, three had clinical responses. Of the eleven patients who failed to develop DTH, only one had a clinical response. The results of this study are consistent with the possibility that inhibiting suppressor function during active specific immunotherapy can enhance T-helper function, induce a DTH response to autologous tumor cells, and induce objective regression of metastases. More recently, Kurth and colleagues reported 33 patients with metastatic renal cell carcinoma who were treated monthly after palliative nephrectomy or excision of metastases using an intradermal injection of an autologous or allogeneic irradiated tumor cell preparation mixed with *C. parvum*.[118] Antitumor activity was evident in 8 TCV-recipients (one complete, four partial and three minor responses) for a 24% response rate. The median survival for responding patients was 32 months, whereas it was 17 months for all patients. Considering the median survival of non-responders, this difference was not significant statistically. In summary, most trials of active specific immunotherapy for renal cancer have demonstrated low toxicity, reasonable responses, and lengthened survival times.

Autopheresis involves the pheresis of lymphocytes from a patient, incubation of the cells with autologous or heterologous tumor antigens, and reinfusion of the cells. In theory, the incubated cells will be specifically activated by TAA and will be further stimulated by endogenous lymphokines to destroy antigenic tumor cells in vivo. Treatment can be performed in outpatient facilities and toxicity is minimal. Carpinito and colleagues used autopheresis combined with cimetidine to abrogate suppressor cell activity in 16 patients.[23] The objective response rate was 19% (3/16). In a later series of patients with renal cell carcinoma, the survival rate was 25% at 24 months, compared with historical survival of 5% to 10% at 24 months.[74]

Perhaps the most dramatic and consistent benefits of BCG have been reported in its use in carcinoma in *situ* of the bladder.[18,90,121] (See XVIII-1 and XXX-3.)

Gynecological Cancers. A preliminary report indicated that administration of tumor cell vaccine admixed with BCG, but not with tumor cells alone,[73] may have benefited patients with ovarian carcinoma.[101] Hudson and coworkers found that patients with advanced ovarian carcinoma who received a combination of BCG, tumor cell vaccine and chemotherapy lived longer than patients who received chemotherapy alone.[97]

Colorectal Cancer. One of the most interesting and well designed clinical studies of active, specific immunotherapy is that of Hoover and colleagues in colorectal cancer.[96] Following standard surgical resection, patients who were at high risk for recurrence were randomized to receive postoperative follow-up or active specific immunotherapy using 10^7 irradiated, autologous tumor cells mixed with 10^7 BCG organisms at weekly intervals for three weeks. DTH to the autologous tumor cells developed in 67% of patients following immunization but in none of the controls.[95] After follow-up of 2–3 years, patients who received active specific immunotherapy had fewer recurrences and deaths than patients who were not immunized.[96] By contrast, the oral administration of BCG has been reported to have produced no significant results.[71]

Glioblastoma. There has recently been increased interest in the evaluation of immunotherapy for glioma and glioblastomas. In a phase I pilot study, selected patients (n = 19) with anaplastic gliomas were immunized with allogeneic human glioma cell lines.[137,138] One patient showed antibody against glioma antigen after absorption with FBS, human platelets and other allogenic glioma cell lines.[137,138] In another study, Eggers and co-workers were able to immunize a patient with glioblastoma in vivo with a mixture of autologous and allogeneic cells inactivated with mitomycin and coupled to muramyl dipeptide and trehalose dimycolate (TDM).[46] Immune activity of peripheral blood lymphocytes was measured in a short-term chromium release assay against autologous tumor target cells. The patient developed cell-mediated cytotoxicity against TAAs, which appeared to be T cell mediated.

Future Directions

Problems Associated with Vaccine Therapy

Both obstacles and opportunities are associated with vaccine therapy. A large tumor burden significantly compromises immunotherapy. Reduction of the tumor burden should precede immunotherapy. An inverse relationship between the tumor burden and therapeutic outcome is indicated in animal models. A tolerable tumor burden in a mouse generally does not exceed a million cells. If results in murine models can be extrapolated to humans,[142] a tolerable tumor burden for a 70 kg man would be 3.5×10^9 tumor cells with a spherical tumor volume of about 2.5 cm^3 and a diameter of about 1.5 cm. The human immune response should then be capable of rejecting a small, but clinically evident, tumor.

Spontaneous regression of large visceral metastases of malignant melanoma and of accidentally transplanted allogeneic tumors suggests that the human immune response may sometimes be capable of eliminating larger tumor nodules. Mastrangelo and colleagues argue that, given the proper circumstances, such as depletion of suppressor T-cells, tumor specific immunity can cope with much larger tumor burdens than is generally appreciated.[142] The combination of vaccines with more conventional modes of therapy could enable tumor specific immunity to cope with greater numbers of tumor cells. Immunotherapy in combination with chemotherapy has shown promise for the treatment of leukemia, lung cancer and melanoma.[229]

Another problem encountered in previous studies is the application of the same immunomodulator for all kinds of cancers. For example, BCG is useful in melanoma and bladder cancer but does not provide much benefit to other forms of cancer. BCG is known to activate histiocytes, macrophages with little phagocytic activity. It is not clear whether BCG, or its low molecular weight derivatives, can efficiently activate macrophages in every organ. The mechanism of antigen presentation by the different macrophages could vary from tissue to tissue. Antigen presentation is known to vary with different kinds of TAAs. Consequently, different immunopotentiators might prove optimal for different cancers that arise or metastasize to different sites.

New Approaches

Future directions in the active specific immunotherapy of cancer depend on understanding the *modus operandi* of

adjuvants administered with tumor cell vaccines. While BCG has proven to be an excellent non-specific immunopotentiator, immunoregulation and trafficking of cells within the immune system are not well understood. The role of various components of BCG and other mycobacteria, such as BCG cell walls, trehalose dimycolate, muramyl dipeptide, and nontoxic derivatives from lipopolysaccharides of gram-negative bacteria in augmenting immunogenicity of tumor-cell vaccines requires further study.

Melanoma patients can be classified into different groups based on the distribution of four biosynthetically related tumor associated glycolipids.[197] Vaccine treatment can be adjusted depending upon antigenic profile of biopsied tumor cells. Different combinations of tumor cell vaccines may prove optimal for different groups of patients. A similar strategy has been utilized to choose appropriate monoclonal antibodies for serotherapy in melanoma.[10] In the future, the ultimate success of immunotherapy depends on a better understanding of the heterogeneity of TAAs for the preparation of tumor cell vaccines, as well as the role of immunopotentiators in rectifying the immunodeficiency encountered in patients with different kinds of cancer.

Infiltration with T cells may be required for immunologically mediated regression of human cancer. Factors favoring T-cell infiltration must be identified. The absence of infiltrating T cells in metastatic tumors excised from cancer patients[171] and their presence in metastatic tumors after immunotherapy[10,179] suggest that vaccines may have a role in potentiating the appropriate migration of cytotoxic effectors.

Modification of response to genetically altered tumor vaccines is under study. Interleukin-4 participates in the regulation, growth and differentiation of B cells and T cells and in the generation of cytotoxic lymphocytes. A renal cell carcinoma has been transfected with the IL-4 gene permitting the tumor cells to secrete large amounts of the cytokine. IL-4 transfected tumor cells are rejected by the host associated with the development of tumor-specific immunity mediated primarily by CD8-positive T cells. Furthermore, tumor cells that lacked IL-4 expression could then be rejected.[69A] Consequently, transfection of genes encoding different cytokines into autologous or allogeneic tumor cells should provide a novel approach to immunopotentiation within vaccines. Fearon and colleagues have transfected the IL-2 gene to tumor cells, thereby significantly enhancing cytolytic T cell recruitment to the tumor, leading to cell killing.[55A] Related approaches involving the genetic engineering of tumor infiltrating lymphocytes with cytokine-producing genes such as TNF are subjects of current and future studies.[204A,B]

References

1. Alexander, P.: Activated macrophages and the antitumor action of BCG. Natl. Cancer Inst. Monogr., 39:127, 1973.
2. Alth, G., Denck, H., Fischer, M., Karrer, K., Kokron, O., Korizek, E., Micksche, M., Ogris, E., Reider, C., Titscher, R., and Wrba, H.: Aspects of the immunologic treatment of lung cancer. Cancer Chemother. Rep., 4:271, 1973.
3. Anderson, J. M., Kelly, F., Wood, S. E., and Holnan, K. E.: Stimulatory immunotherapy in mammary cancer. Br. J. Surg., 61:778, 1974.
4. Austin, F. C., and Boone, C. W.: Virus augmentation of the antigenicity of tumor cell extracts. Adv. Cancer Res., 30:301, 1979.
5. Baker, M. A., and Taub, R. N.: BCG in malignant melanoma. Lancet, 1:1117, 1973.
6. Bartlett, G. L., and Zbar, B.: Tumor-specific vaccine containing Mycobacterium bovis and tumor cells; safety and efficacy. J. Natl. Cancer Inst., 46:1709, 1972.
7. Bekesi, J. G., St. Arneault, G., Walter, L., Holland, J. F.: Immunogenicity of leukemia L1210 cells after neuraminidase treatment. J. Natl. Cancer Inst., 49:107, 1972.
8. Berd, D., Herlyn , M., Koprowski, H., Mastrangelo, M. J.: Flow cytometric determi-

nation of the frequency and heterogeneity of expression of human melanoma-associated-antigens. Cancer Res., 49:6840, 1989.
9. Berd, D., Maguire, H. C., Jr., and Mastrangelo, M. J.: Induction of cell-mediated immunity to autologous melanoma cells and regression of metastases after treatment with a melanoma cell vaccine preceded by cyclophosphamide. Cancer Res., 46:2572, 1986.
10. Berd, D., Maguire, H. C., Jr., McCue, P., and Mastrangelo, M. J.: Treatment of metastatic melanoma with an autologous tumor-cell vaccine: Clinical and immunological results in 64 patients. J. Clin. Oncol., 8:1858, 1990.
11. Berd, D., and Mastrangelo, M. J.: Effect of low dose cyclophosphamide on the immune system of cancer patients: Reduction of T suppressor function without depletion of the CD8+ subset. Cancer Res., 47:3317, 1987.
12. Berd, D., and Mastrangelo, M. J.: Active immunotherapy of human melanoma exploiting the immuno-potentiating effects of cyclophosphamide. Cancer Invest., 6:335, 1988.
13. Berd, D., and Mastrangelo, M. J.: Effect of low dose cyclophosphamide on the immune system of cancer patients: Depletion of CD4+2H4+ suppressor-inducer T-cells. Cancer Res., 48:1671, 1988.
14. Bergelson, L. D., and Dyatlovitzkaya,, E V.: Gangliosides and antitumor immunity. J. Cancer Res. Clin. Oncol., 116 (Suppl.):1159,1990.
15. Bloom, W. H., Peckham, M. J., Richardson, A. E., Alexander, P. A., and Payne, P. M.: Glioblastoma multiforme: A controlled trial to assess the value of specific active immunotherapy in patients treated by radical surgery and radiotherapy. Br. J. Cancer, 27:253, 1973.
16. Bornstein, R. S., Mastrangelo, M. J., and Sulit, H.: Immunotherapy of melanoma with intralesional BCG. Cancer Inst. Monogr., 39:213, 1973.
17. Brocker, E. B., Zwaldo, G., Holzmann, B., Macher, E., and Sorg, C.: Inflammatory cell infiltration in human melanoma at different stages of tumor progression. Int. J. Cancer, 41:562, 1989.
18. Brosman, S. A.: BCG in the management of superficial bladder cancer. Urology, 23 (4 Suppl.):82, 1984.
19. Burdick, J. F., Wells, S. A., and Herberman, R. B.: Immunologic evaluation of patients with cancer by delayed hypersensitivity reaction. Collective review. Surg. Gynecol. Obstet., 141:779, 1975.
20. Bystryn, J-C., Jacobsen, S., Harris, M., Roses, D., Speyer, J., and Levin, M.: Preparation and characterization of a polyvalent human melanoma antigen vaccine. J. Biol. Res. Mod., 5:211, 1986.
21. Bystryn, J-C., Oratz, R., Harris, M. N., Roses, D. F., Golomb, F. M., and Speyer, J. C.: Immunogenicity of a polyvalent melanoma antigen vaccine in humans. Cancer, 61:1065, 1988.
22. Bystryn, J-C., Tedholm, C. A., and Heaney-Kieras, J.: Release of surface macromolecules by human melanoma and normal cells. Cancer Res., 41:91, 1981.
23. Carpinto, G. A., Levine, S., Hamilton, H., Krane, R. J., and Osband, M. E.: Successful adoptive immunotherapy of cancer using in vitro immunized autologous lymphocytes and cimetidine. Surg. Forum., 37:418, 1986.
24. Carubia, J. M., Yu, R. K., Macala, L. J., Kirkwood, J. M., and Varga, J. M.: Gangliosides of normal and neoplastic human melanocytes. Biochem. Biophys. Res. Commun., 120:500, 1984.
25. Cassel, W. A., Murray, D. R., and Phillips, H. S.: A phase II study on the postsurgical management of stage II malignant melanoma with a Newcastle disease virus oncolysate. Cancer, 52:856, 1983.
26. Cassel, W. A., Weidenheim, K. M., Campbell, W. G., and Murray, D. R.: Malignant melanoma: inflammatory mononuclear cell infiltrates in cerebral metastases during concurrent therapy with viral oncolysate. Cancer, 57:1302, 1986.
27. Chassot, P. G., Guttmann, R. D., Beaudoin, J. G., Morehouse, D. D., Gonda, A., and MacLean, L. D.: Cancer in renal allograft recipients. Prog. Exp. Tumor. Res., 19:91, 1974.
28. Cheung, N. K., Lazarus, H., Miraldi, F. D., Abramowsky, C. R., Kallick, S., Saarinen, U. M., Spitzer, T., Strandojord, S. E., Coccia, P. F., and Berger, N. A.: Ganglioside GD2 specific monoclonal antibody 3F8: A phase I study in patients with neuroblastoma and malignant melanoma. J. Clin. Oncol., 5:1430, 1987.
29. Cheung, N. K., and Miraldi, F. D.: Iodine 132 labelled GD2 monoclonal antibody in the diagnosis and therapy of human neuroblastoma. Prog. Clin. Biol. Res., 27:595, 1988.
30. Coca, A. F., Dorrance, G. M., and Lebredo, M. G.: Vaccination in cancer: A report of the results of vaccination therapy as applied to seventy-nine cases of human cancer. Z. immun. exp. Ther., 13:543, 1912.
31. Coca, A. F., and Gilman, G.: The specific treatment of carcinoma. Phil. J. Sci. Med., 4:381, 1909.
32. Cochran, A. J., Pihl, E., Wen, D-R., Hoon, D. B. S., Korn, L.: Zoned immune suppression of lymph nodes draining malignant melanoma. Histologic and immunohistologic studies. J. Natl. Cancer Inst., 78:399, 1987.
33. Cohen, M. H., Jessup, J. M., Felix, E. L., Wesse, J. L., and Herberman, R. B.: Intralesional treatment of recurrent metastatic cutaneous malignant melanoma: A randomized prospective study of intralesional bacillus Calmette-Guérin versus intralesional dinitrochlorobenzene. Cancer, 41:2456, 1978.
34. Cole, W. H.: Spontaneous regression of cancer: The metabolic triumph of the host. Ann. N. Y. Acad. Sci., 230:111, 1974.
35. Crowther, D., Powles, R. L., Bateman, C. J. J., Beard, M. E. J., Gauci, C. L., Wrigley, P. F. M., Malpas, J. S., Fairley, G. H., and Scott, R. B.: Management of adult acute myelogenous leukemia. Br. Med. J., 1:131, 1973.
36. Cunningham, T. J., Olson, K. B., Laffin, R., Horton, J., and Sullivan, J.: Treatment of advanced cancer with active immunization. Cancer, 24:932, 1969.
37. Currie, G. A.: Eighty years of immunotherapy: A review of immunological methods used for the treatment of human cancer. Br. J. Cancer, 26:141, 1972.
38. Currie, G. A.: Effect of active immunization with irradiated tumor cells on specific serum inhibition of cell-mediated immunity in patients with disseminated cancer. Br. J. Cancer, 28:25, 1973.
39. Currie, G. A., and Basham, S.: Serum mediated inhibition of the immunological reactions of the patient to his own tumor. A possible role of circulating antigen. Br. J. Cancer, 26:427, 1972.
40. Currie, G. A., Lejeune, F., and Fairley, G. H.: Immunization with irradiated tumor cells and specific lymphocyte cytotoxicity in malignant melanoma. Br. Med. J., 2:305, 1971.
41. Cuttner, J., Glidewell, O., and Holland, J. F.: A controlled trial of chemoimmunotherapy of acute myelogenous leukemia with the methanol extraction residue of tubercle Bacilli (MER) *In* Immunotherapy of Human Cancer. Edited by W. D. Terry and S. A. Rosenberg, New York, Excerpta Medica, 1982, p. 33.
42. Czajkowski, N. P., Rosenblatt, M., Wolf, P. L., and Vasquez, J.: A new method of active immunization to autologous human tumour tissue. Lancet, 2:905, 1967.
43. de Kernion, J. B., Ramming, K. P., and Gupta, R. K.: The detection and clinical significance of antibodies to tumor associated antigens in patients with renal cell carcinoma. J. Urol., 111:330, 1974.
44. Dufour, F. D., and Morton, D. L.: Induction of melanoma specific monocyte cytotoxicity in patients receiving BCG immunotherapy. Surg. Forum., 28:165, 1977.
45. Edwards, F. R., and Whitwell, F.: Use of BCG as an immunostimulant in the surgical treatment of carcinoma of the lung.Thorax, 29:654, 1974.
46. Eggers, A. E., Tarmin, L., and Gamboa, E. T.: In vivo immunization against autologous glioblastoma-associated antigens. Cancer Immunol. Immunother., 19:43, 1985.
47. Eidinger, D.: Genitourinary cancer. *In* Clinical Immunotherapy. Edited by A. F. Lobuglio. New York, Marcel Dekker, 1980, p. 243.
48. Eilber, F. R., Holmes, E. C., and Morton, D. L.: Immunotherapy experiments with a methylcholanthrene-induced guinea pig liposarcoma. J. Natl. Cancer Inst., 46:803, 1971.
49. Eilber, F. R., and Morton, D. L.: Impaired immunologic reactivity and recurrence following cancer surgery. Cancer, 25:362, 1970.
50. Eilber, F. R., Nizze, A., and Morton, D. L.: Sequential evaluation of general immune competence in cancer patients: Correlation with clinical course. Cancer, 35:660, 1975.
51. Eilber, F. R., Townsend, C. M., Jr., and Morton, D. L.: Osteosarcoma: Results of treatment employing adjuvant immunotherapy. Clin. Orthop. Relat. Res., 111:94, 1975.
52. Ekert, H., and Jose, D. G.: Chemotherapy and BCG in acute lymphocytic leukemia. Lancet, 2:713, 1975.
53. Everson, T. C., and Cole, W. H.: Spontaneous regression of cancer. Philadelphia, W. B. Saunders Co., 1966, p. 11.
54 .Fairlamb, D. J.: Spontaneous regression of metastases of renal cancer: A report of two cases including the first recorded regression following irradiation of a dominant metastasis and review of the world literature. Cancer, 47:2102, 1981.
55. Falk, R. E., MacGregor, A. B., Landi, S., Ambus, U., and Langer, B.: Immunostimulation with intraperitoneally administered bacillus Calmette-Guérin for advanced malignant tumors of the gastrointestinal tract. Surg. Gynecol. Obstet., 142:363, 1976.
55A.Fearon, E. R., Pardoll, D. M., Itaya,T., Golumbek, P., Levitsky, H. I., Simons, J. W., Karasuyama, H., Vogelstein, B., and Frost, P.: Interleukin-2 production by tumor cells bypasses T helper function in the generation of an antitumor response. Cell, 60:397, 1990.
56. Febvre, H., Maunoury, R., Constans, J. P., and Trouillas, P.: Réactions d'hypersensibilité retardée avec des lignées de cellules tumorales humaines cultivées in vitro chez des malades porteurs de tumeurs cerebrales malignes. Int. J. Cancer, 10:221, 1972.
57. Finney, J. W., Byers, E. H., and Wilson, R. H.: Studies in tumour auto-immunity. Cancer Res., 20:351, 1960.
58. Fisher, R. I., Terry, W. D., Nodes, R. J., Rosenberg, S. A., Makuch, R., Gordon, H. G., and Fisher, S. G.: Adjuvant immunotherapy or chemotherapy for malignant melanoma. Surg. Clin. N. Am., 61:1267, 1981.
59. Fortner, J. G., Booker, R. J., and Pack, G. T.: Results of groin dissection for malignant melanoma in 200 patients. Surgery, 55:485, 1964.
60. Fortner, J. G., and Shiu, M. H.: Organ transplantation and cancer. Surg. Clin. North Am., 54:871, 1974.
61. Fredman, P., von Holst, H., Collins, V. P., Ammar, A., Delheden, B., Wahren, B., Granholm, L., and Svennerholm, L.: Potential ganglioside antigens associated with human gliomas. Neurol. Res., 8:123, 1986.
62. Freeman, C. B., Harris, R. G., Colin, G., Leyland, M. J., MaCiver, J. E., and Delamore, I. W.: Active immunotherapy used alone for the maintenance of patients with acute myeloid leukaemia. Br. Med. J., 4:571, 1973.
63. Furukawa, K., Yamaguchi, H., Oettgen, H. F., Old, L. J., and Lloyd, K. O.: Analysis of the expression of N-glycolylneuraminic acid-containing gangliosides in cells and tissues using two human monoclonal antibodies. J. Biol. Chem., 236:18507, 1988.
64. Gale, R. P., Foon, K. A., Yale, C., and Zighelboim, J.: Immunotherapy of acute myelogenous leukemia using Corynebacterium parvum and allogeneic cells. *In* Immunotherapy of Human Cancer. Edited by W. D. Terry and S. A. Rosenberg. New York, Excerpta Medica, 1982, p. 40.
65. Garas, J., Besbeas, S., Papmatheakis, J., Gropas, G., Maragoudakis, S., Katsenis, A., Kiparissiadis, P., Konstadakos, P., and Georgaka, A.: Attempt with immunotherapy to control metastatic skin nodules from breast cancer by BCG. Panminerva Med., 17:193, 1975.
66. Gatti, R. A., and Good, R. A.: Occurrence of malignancy in immunodeficiency diseases. A literature review. Cancer, 28:89, 1971.
67. Ghosh, S., White, L. M., Ghosh, R., and Bankert, R. B.: Vaccination with membrane associated idiotype provides greater and more prolonged protection of animals from tumor challenge than the soluble form of idiotype. J. Immunol., 145:365, 1990.
68. Golub, S. H., Forsythe, A. B., and Morton, D. L.: Sequential examination of lymphocyte proliferative capacity in patients with malignant melanoma receiving BCG immunotherapy. Int. J. Cancer, 19:18, 1977.
69. Golub, S. H., Roth, J. A., Forsythe, A., and Morton, D. L.: In vitro monitoring of cellular function during BCG immunotherapy. Bibl. Hematol., 43:270, 1976.
69A.Golumbek, P. T., Lazenby, A. J., Levitsky, H. I., Jaffee, L. M., Karasuyama, H., Baker, M., and Pardoll, D. M.: Treatment of established renal cancer by tumor cells engineered to secrete interleukin-4. Science, 254:713, 1991.
70. Goodnight, J. E., and Morton, D. L.: Immunotherapy for malignant disease. Ann. Rev. Med., 29:231, 1978.
71. Goodnight, J. E., and Morton, D. L.: Immunotherapy of cancer: Current status. Prog. Exp. Tumor Res., 25:61, 1980.
72. Grace, J. T., Jr., Perese, D. M., Metzgar, R. S., Sasabe, T., and Holdridge, B.: Tumor autograft responses in patients with glioblastoma multiforme. J. Neurosurg., 18:159, 1961.
73. Graham, J. B., and Graham, R. M.: Autologous vaccine in cancer patients. Surg. Gynec. Obstet., 109:121, 1962.
74. Graham, S. D., Jr.: Immunotherapy of renal cell carcinoma. Sem. Urol., 7:215, 1989.

75. Grant, R. M., Mackie, R., Cochran, A. J., Murray, E. L., Hoyle, D., and Ross, C.: Results of administering BCG to patients with melanoma. Lancet, 2:1096, 1974.
76. Green, A. A., Pratt, C., Webster, R. G., and Smith, K.: Immunotherapy of osteosarcoma patients with virus-modified tumor cells. Ann. N. Y. Acad. Sci., 277:396, 1976.
77. Greene, M. H., Young, T. I., and Clark, W. H., Jr.: Malignant melanoma in renal transplant recipients. Lancet, 1:1196, 1981.
77A. Gross, L.: Intradermal immunization of C3H mice against a sarcoma that originated in an animal of the same line. Cancer Res., 3:326, 1943.
78. Gupta, R. K., Golub, S. H., and Morton, D. L.: Correlation between tumor burden and anticomplementary activity in sera from patients. Cancer Immunol. Immunother., 6:63, 1979.
79. Gutterman, J. U., Mavligit, T. J., Burgess, M. A., Cardenas, J. O., Blumenschein, G. R., Gottlieb, J. A., McBride, C. M., McCredie, K. B., Bodey, G. P., Rodriquez, V., Freireich, E. J., and Hersh, E. M.: Immunotherapy of breast cancer, malignant melanoma, and acute leukemia with BCG: Prolongation of disease-free interval and survival. Cancer Immunol. Immunother., 1:99, 1976.
80. Hadley, D. W., McElwain, T. J., Currie, G. A.: Specific active immunotherapy does not prolong survival in surgically treated patients with stage IIB malignant melanoma and may promote early recurrence. Br. J. Cancer, 37:491, 1978.
81. Hakansson, L., Fredman, P., and Svennerholm, L.: Gangliosides in serum immune complexes from tumor-bearing patients. J. Biochem., 98:843, 1985.
82. Hanna, M. G., Jr., Snodgrass, M. J., Zbar, B., and Rapp, H.: Histopathology of tumor regression after intralesional injection of mycobacterium bovis. IV. Development of immunity to tumor cells and BCG. J. Natl. Cancer Inst., 51:1897, 1973.
83. Hanna, M. G., Jr., Zbar, B., and Rapp, H. J.: Histopathology of tumor regression and intralesional injection of Mycobacterium bovis. I. Tumor growth and metastasis. J. Natl. Cancer Inst., 48:1441, 1972.
84. Hanna, M. G., Jr., Zbar, B., and Rapp, H. J.: Histopathology of tumor regression after intralesional injection of mycobacterium bovis. II. Comparative effects of vaccinia virus, oxazolone, and turpentine. J. Natl. Cancer Inst., 48:1697, 1972.
85. Harris, R., Zuhrie, S. Z., Freeman, C. B., Read, A. P., Maclver, J. E., Geary, C. G., Delamore, I. W., and Tooth, J. A.: A successful randomized trail of immunotherapy alone versus no maintenance treatment in Acute myelogenous leukemia. *In* Immunotherapy of Human Cancer. Edited by W. D. Terry and S. A. Rosenberg. New York, Excerpta Medica, 1982, p. 11.
86. Heppner, G. H.: Tumor heterogeneity. Cancer Res., 44:2259, 1984.
87. Herlyn, M., Guerry, D., and Koprowski, H.: Recombinant gamma-interferon induces changes in expression and shedding of antigens associated with normal human melanocytes, nevus cells and primary and metastatic melanoma. J. Immunol., 134:4226, 1985.
88. Herlyn, M., Rodeck, U., and Koprowski, H.: Shedding off human tumor associated antigens in vitro and in vivo. Adv. Cancer Res., 49:189, 1987.
89. Herlyn, M., Thurin, J., Balaban, G., Bennicelli, J. L., Herlyn, D., Elder, D. E., Bondi, E., Guerry, D., Nowell, P., Clark, W. H.; and Koprowski, H.: Characteristics of cultured human melanocytes isolated from different stages of tumor progression. Cancer Res., 45:5670, 1985.
90. Herr, H. W., Pinsky, C. M., Whitmore, W. F., Jr., Sogani, P. C., Oettgen, H. F., and Melamed, M. R.: Long-term effect of intravesical bacillus Calmette-Guérin on flat carcinoma in situ of the bladder. J. Urol., 135:265, 1986.
91. Hersey, P., Edwards, A., Coates, A., Shaw, H., McCarthy, W. H., and Milton, G. W.: Evidence that treatment with vaccinia melanoma cell lysates (VMCL) may improve survival of patients with stage II melanoma. Cancer Immunol. Immunother., 25:257, 1987.
92. Holland, J. F., Bekesi, J. G., and Cuttner, J.: Chemoimmunotherapy for acute myelocytic leukemia. *In* Immunotherapy of Human Cancer. New York, Raven Press, 1978, p. 237.
93. Hollinshead, A., Arlen, M., Yonemoto, R., Cohen, M., Janner, K., Kundin, W. D., and Scherrer, J.: Pilot studies using melanoma tumor-associated antigens (TAA) in specific active immunochemotherapy of malignant melanoma. Cancer, 49:1387, 1982.
94. Hoon, D. S. B., Irie, R. F., and Cochran, A. J.: Gangliosides from melanoma immunomodulate response of T-cells to interleukin-2. Cell Immunol., 111:1, 1988.
95. Hoover, H. C., Jr., Surdyke, M., Dangel, R. B., Peter, L. C., and Hanna, M. G., Jr.: Delayed cutaneous hypersensitivity to autologous tumor cells in colorectal cancer patients immunized with an autologous tumor cell: Bacillus Calmette-Guérin vaccine. Cancer Res., 44:1671, 1984.
96. Hoover, H. C., Jr., Surdyke, M. G., Dangel, R. B., Peters, L. C., and Hanna, M. G., Jr.: Prospectively randomized trial of adjuvant active-specific immunotherapy for human colorectal cancer. Cancer, 55(6):1236, 1985.
97. Hudson, C. N., McHardy, J. E., Curling, O. M., English, P. E., Levin, L., Poulton, T. A., Crowther, M., and Leighton, M.: Active specific immunotherapy for ovarian cancer. Lancet, 2:877, 1976.
98. Hudson, M. A., Richey, J. K., Catalona, W. J., Brown, E. J., and Ratliff, T. L.: Comparison of the fibronectin-binding ability and antitumor efficacy of various mycobacteria. Cancer Res., 50:3843, 1990.
99. Hughes, L. F., Kearney, R., and Tully, M.: A study in clinical cancer immunotherapy. Cancer, 26:269, 1970.
100. Ikonopisov, R. L., Lewis, M. G., Hunter-Craig, I. D., Bodenham, D. C., Phillips, T. M., Cooling, C. I., Proctor, J., Hamilton-Fairley, G., and Alexander, P.: Autoimmunization with irradiated tumor cells in human malignant melanoma. Br. Med. J., 2:752, 1970.
101. Imperato, S., Rossi, R., Ermiglia, G., De Marini, M., and Cassolino, A.: Active specific immunotherapy with immunological monitoring in late stage ovarian cancers. Acta Eur. Fertil., 5:25, 1974.
102. Irie, R. F., and Ravindranath, M. H.: Gangliosides as targets for monoclonal antibody therapy of cancer. *In* Therapeutic monoclonal antibodies. Edited by C. A. K. Borrebaeck and J. W. Larrick. New York, Stockton Press, 1990, p. 75.
103. Israel, L.: Report on 414 cases of human tumors treated with Corynebacteria. *In* Corynebacterium Parvum: Applications in Experimental and Clinical Oncology. Edited by B. Halpern. New York, Plenum Press, 1975, p. 389.
104. Israel, L., de Pierre, A., and Edelstein, R.: Effect of intranodal BCG in 22 melanoma patients. Proc. IVth Int. Symp. Locoregional Treatment of Tumors.Turin, Italy, IUCC, 1973.
105. Israel, L., Edelstein, R., de Pierre, A., and Dimitrov, N.: Daily infusions of Corynbacterium parvum in twenty patients with disseminated cancer: A preliminary report of clinical and biological findings. J. Natl. Cancer Inst., 55:29, 1975.
106. Janik, P.: Cell proliferation during the course of immunological rejection of Ehrlich ascites tumor cells. Cell Tissue Kinet., 4:69, 1971.
107. Janik, P., and Steel, G. G.: Cell proliferation during immunological perturbation in three transplanted tumours. Br. J. Cancer, 26:108, 1972.
108. Juillard, G. J. K., Boyer, P. J. J., and Yamashiro, C. H.: A phase I study of active specific intralymphatic immunotherapy (ASILI). Cancer, 41:2215, 1978.
109. Karakousis, C. P., Douglass, H. O., Yeracaris, P. M., and Holyoke, E. D.: BCG immunotherapy in patients with malignant melanoma. Arch. Surg., 111:716, 1976.
110. Kawai, T., Kato, A., Higashi, H., Kato, S., and Naiki, M.: Quantitative determination of N-glycolylneuraminic acid expression in human cancerous tissues and avian lymphoma cell lines as a tumor associated sialic acid by gas chromatography-mass spectrometry. Cancer Res., 51:1242, 1991.
111. Kellock, T. H., Chambers, H., and Russ, S.: An attempt to procure immunity to malignant disease in man. Lancet, 1:217, 1922.
112. Klein, E., and Holterman, O. A.: Immunotherapeutic approaches to the management of neoplasms. Natl. Cancer Inst. Monogr., 35:379, 1972.
113. Klein, E., Holterman, O., Milgrom, H., Case, R. W., Klein, D., Rosner, D., and Djerassi, I.: Immunotherapy for accessible tumors utilizing delayed hypersensitivity reactions and separated components of the immune system. Med. Clin. North Am., 60:389, 1976.
114. Kleinschuster, S. J., Rapp, H. J., and Lueker, D. C., et al.: Regression of bovine ocular carcinoma by treatment with mycobacterial vaccine. J. Natl. Cancer Inst., 58:1805, 1977.
115. Kobayashi, H.: Immunological xenogeneration of tumor cells. Tokyo, Japan Scientific Societies, 1979.
116. Krementz, E. T., Samuels, M. S., Wallace, J. H., and Benes, E. N.: Clinical experiences in immunotherapy of cancer. Surg. Gynecol. Obstet., 133:209, 1971.
117. Krown, S. E., Hilal, E. Y., Pinsky, C. M., Hirshaut, Y., Wanebo, H. J., Hansen, J. A., Huvos, A. G., and Oettgen, H. F.: Intralesional injection of the methanol extraction residue of bacillus Calmette-Guérin (MER) into cutaneous metastases of malignant melanoma. Cancer, 42:2648, 1978.
118. Kurth, K. H., Marquet, R., Zwartendijk, J., and Warnar, S. O.: Autologous anticancer antigen preparation for specific immunotherapy in advanced renal cell carcinoma. Eur. Urol., 13:103, 1987.
119. Ladisch, S.: Tumor gangliosides: Shedding, structural characterization and immunosuppressive activity. *In* Gangliosides and Cancer. Edited by H. F. Oettgen. New York, VCH Publishers, N.Y., 1989, p. 219.
120. Ladisch, S., Wu, Z. L., Feig, S., Ulsh, L., Schwartz, E., Floutsis, G., Wiley, F., Lenarsky, C., and Seeger, R.: Shedding of GD2 gangliosides by human neuroblastoma. Int. J. Cancer, 39:73, 1987.
121. Lamm, D. L., Blumenstein, B., Crawford, E. D., Montie, J. E., Scardino, P., Stanisic, T. H., and Grossman, H. B.: South-west Oncology Group comparison of bacillus Calmette-Guérin and doxorubicin in the treatment and prophylaxis of superfical bladder cancer. J. Urol., 137:178A, 1987.
122. Laucius, J. F., Bodurtha, A. J., Mastrangelo, M. J., and Bellet, R. E.: A phase II study of autologous irradiated tumor cells plus BCG in patients with metastatic malignant melanoma. Cancer, 40:2091, 1977.
123. Leong, S. P. L.: Detection of human malignant melanoma antigens by immunofluorescence and autologous postimmune antimelanoma sera. Ann. N. Y. Acad. Sci., 420:237, 1983.
124. Leventhal, B. G., LePourheit, A., Halterman, R. H., Henderson, E. S., and Herberman, R. B.: Immunotherapy in previously treated acute lymphatic leukemia. Natl. Cancer Inst. Monogr., 39:177, 1973.
125. Levy, N. L., Mahaley, M. S., Jr., and Day, E. D.: Serum-mediated blocking of cell-mediated anti-tumor immunity in a melanoma patient: Association with BCG immunotherapy and clinical deterioration. Int. J. Cancer, 10:244, 1972.
126. Lewis, M. G., Phillips, T. M., Cook, K. B., and Blake, J.: Possible explanation for loss of detectable antibody in patients with disseminated malignant melanoma. Nature (Lond.), 232:52, 1971.
127. Lieberman, R., Wybran, J., and Epstein, W.: The immunologic and histopathologic changes of BCG-mediated tumor regression in patients with malignant melanoma. Cancer, 35:756, 1975.
128. Livingston, P. O.: The basis for ganglioside vaccines in melanoma. *In* Human Tumor Antigens and Specific Tumor Therapy (UCLA Symposia on Molecular and Cellular Biology; new ser. vol. 99). Edited by R. S. Metzgar and M. S. Mitchell. New York, Alan Liss, 1989, p. 287.
129. Livingston, P. O., Albino, A. P., Chung, T. J. C., Real, F. X., Houghton, A. N., Oettgen, H. F., and Old, L. J.: Serological response of melanoma patients to vaccines prepared from VSV lysates of autologous and allogeneic cultured melanoma cells. Cancer, 55:713, 1985.
130. Livingston, P. O., Calves, M. J., and Natoli, E. J.: Approaches to augmenting the immunogenicity of the ganglioside GM2 in mice: Purified GM2 is superior to whole cells. J. Immunol., 138:1524, 1987.
131. Livingston, P. O., Kaelin, K., Pinsky, C. M., Oettgen, H. R., and Old, L. J.: The serological response of patients with stage II melanoma to allogeneic melanoma cell vaccines. Cancer, 56:2194, 1985.
132. Livingston, P. O., Natoli, E. J., Calves, M. J., Stockert, E., Oettgen, H. F., and Old, L. J.: Vaccines containing purified GM2 ganglioside elicit GM2 antibodies in melanoma patients. Proc. Natl. Acad. Sci. USA, 84:2911, 1987.
133. Livingston, P. O., Takeyama, H., Pollack, M. S., Houghton, A., Albino, A., Oettgen, H. F., and Old, L. J.: Serological responses of melanoma patients to vaccines derived from allogeneic cultured melanoma cells. Int. J. Cancer, 31:567, 1983.
134. Livingston, P. O., Watanabe, T., Shiku, H., Houghton, A. N., Albino, A.,Takahashi, T., Resnick, L. A., Pinsky, C. M., Oettgen, H. F., and Old, L. J.: Serological response of melanoma patients receiving melanoma cell vaccines. 1. Autologous cultured melanoma cells. Int. J. Cancer, 30:413, 1982.
135. Lokich, J. J., Garnick, M. B., and Legg, M.: Intralesional immune therapy: Methanol extraction residue of BCG or purified protein derivative. Oncology, 36:236, 1979.
136. Ludwig, G., Jentzsch, R., and Nuri, M.: Spontanregression von Lungenmetastasen beim Hypernephroma. Med. Klin., 21:173, 1978.
137. Mahaley, M. S., Jr., Bigner, D. D., Dudka, L. F., Wilds, P. R., Williams, D. H., Bouldin, T. W., Whitaker, J. N., and Bynum, J. M.: Immunobiology of primary intracranial tumors. Part 7: Active immunization of patients with anaplastic human glioma cells: a pilot study. J. Neurosurg., 59:201, 1983.
138. Mahaley, M. S., Jr., Gillespie, G. Y., Gillespie, R. P., Watkins, P. J., Bigner, D. D., Wikstrand, C. J., MacQueen, J. M., and Sanfilippo, F.: Immunobiology of primary

intracranial tumors. Part 8: Serological responses to active immunization of patients with anaplastic gliomas. J. Neurosurg., 59:208, 1983.

139. Marcove, R. C.: A clinical trial of autogenous vaccines in the treatment of osteogenic sarcoma. In Investigation and Stimulation of Immunity in Cancer Patients. Edited by G. Mathe and R. Weiner. New York, Springer-Verlag, 1974, p. 488.

140. Marcove, R. C., Southam, C. M., Levin, A., Mike, V., and Huvos, A.: A clinical trial of autogenous vaccine in osteogenic sarcoma in patients under the age of twenty-five. Surg. Forum, 22:434, 1971.

141. Mastrangelo, M. J., Bellet, R. E., Berkelhammer, J., and Clark, W. H., Jr.: Regression of pulmonary metastatic disease associated with intra-lesional BCG therapy of intra-cutaneous melanoma metastases. Cancer, 36:1305, 1975.

142. Mastrangelo, M. J., Berd, D., and Maguire, H. C.: Current condition and prognosis of tumor immunotherapy: A second opinion. Cancer Treat. Rep., 68:207, 1984.

143. Mastrangelo, M. J., Sulit, H. L., Prehn, L. M., Bornstein, R. S., Yarbo, J. W., and Prehn, R. T.: Intralesional BCG in the treatment of metastatic malignant melanoma. Cancer, 37:684, 1976.

144. Mathe, G., Amiel, J. L., and Schwarzenberg, L.: Active immunotherapy for acute lymphoblastic leukaemia. Lancet, 1:697, 1969.

145. Mathe, G., Pouillart, P., Schwarzenberg, L., Amiel, J. L., Schneider, M., Hayat, M., De Vassal, F., Jasmin, C., Rosenfeld, C., Weiner, R., and Rappaport, H.: Attempts at immunotherapy of 100 patients with acute lymphoid leukemia: Some factors influencing results. Natl. Cancer Inst. Monogr., 35:361, 1972.

146. Mathe, G., Schwarzenberg, L., de Vassal, F., Delgado, M., Pena-Angulo, J., Belpomme, D., Pouillart, P., Machover, D., Misset, J. L., Pico, J. L., Jasmin, C., Hayat, M., Schneider, M., Cattan, A., Amiel, J. L., Musset, M., and Rosenfeld, C.: Chemotherapy followed by active immunotherapy (A.I.) in the treatment of acute lymphoid leukemias (A.L.L.) for patients of all ages. In Immunotherapy of Cancer: Present Status of Trials in Man. Edited by W. D. Terry and E. Windhorst. New York, Raven, 1978, p. 451.

147. McCune, C. S., and Marquis, D. M.: Interleukin I as an adjuvant for active specific immunotherapy in a murine tumor model. Cancer Res., 50:1212, 1990.

148. McCune, C. S., Patterson, W. B., and Henshaw, E. C.: Active specific immunotherapy with tumor cells and Corynebacterium parvum. A phase I study. Cancer, 43:1619, 1979.

149. McCune, C. S., Schapira, D. V., and Henshaw, E. C.: Specific immunotherapy of advanced renal carcinoma: Evidence for polyclonality of metastases. Cancer, 47:1984, 1981.

150. Miescher, S., Whiteside, T. L., Carrel, S., and von Fliedner, V.: Functional properties of tumor-infiltrating and blood lymphocytes in patients with solid tumors: Effect of tumor cells and their supernatants on proliferative responses of lymphocytes. J. Immunol., 136(5):1899, 1986.

151. Miller, B. E., Miller, F. R., Leith, J., and Heppner, G. H.: Growth interaction in vivo between tumor subpopulations derived from a single mouse mammary tumor. Cancer Res., 40:3977, 1980.

152. Miller, G. A., Pontes, J. E., Huber, R. P., and Goldrosen, M. H.: Humoral immune response of patients receiving specific active immunotherapy for renal cell carcinoma. Cancer Res., 45:4478, 1985.

153. Minden, P.: Shared antigens between animal and human tumors and microorganisms. In BCG in Cancer Immunotherapy. Edited by G. Lamoureux, R. Turcotte and V. Portelance. New York, Grune & Stratton, 1976, p. 73.

154. Minten, J. P.: Mumps virus and BCG vaccine in metastatic melanoma. Arch. Surg., 106:503, 1973.

155. Mitchell, M. S., Kan-Mitchell, J., Kempf, R. A., Harel, W., Shau, H., and Lind, S.: Active specific immunotherapy for melanoma: Phase I trial of allogeneic lysates and a novel adjuvant. Cancer Res., 48:5883, 1988.

156. Moertel, C. G., Ritts, R. E., Jr., Schutt, A. J., and Hahn, R. G.: Clinical studies of methanol extraction residue fraction of bacillus Calmette-Guérin as an immunostimulant in patients with advanced cancer. Cancer Res., 35:3075, 1975.

156A. Moore, G. E., and Germen, R. E.: Cancer immunity—hypothesis and clinical trial of lymphocytotherapy for malignant diseases. Ann. Surg., 172:733, 1970.

156B. Morton, D. L., Eilber, F. R., Malmgren, R. A., Wood, W. C.: Immunological factors which influence response to immunotherapy in malignant melanoma. Surgery, 68:158,1970.

157. Morton, D. L.: Immunotherapy of human melanomas and sarcomas. J. Natl. Cancer Inst., 35:375, 1972.

158. Morton, D. L.: Cancer immunotherapy: An overview. Sem. Oncol., 1:297, 1974.

159. Morton, D. L.: Changing concepts of cancer surgery: Surgery as immunotherapy. Am. J. Surg., 135:367, 1978.

160. Morton, D. L.: Active immunotherapy against cancer: Present status. Sem. Oncol., 13(2):180, 1986.

161. Morton, D. L., Eilber, F. R., Holmes, E. C., Hunt, J. S., Ketcham, A. S., Silverstein, M. J., and Sparks, F. C.: BCG immunotherapy of malignant melanoma: Summary of a seven year experience. Ann. Surg., 180:635, 1974.

162. Morton, D. L., Eilber, F. R., Holmes, E. C., Sparks, F. C., and Ramming, K. P.: Present status of BCG immunotherapy of malignant melanoma. Cancer Immunol. Immunother., 1:93, 1976.

163. Morton, D. L., Eilber, F. R., Malmgren, R. A., and Wood, W. C.: Immunological factors which influence response to immunotherapy in malignant melanoma. Surgery, 68:158,1970.

164. Morton, D. L., Foshag, L. J., Nizze, J. A., Gupta, R. K., Famatiga, E., Hoon, D. S. B., and Irie, R. F.: Active specific immunotherapy in Malignant melanoma. Sem. Surg. Oncol., 5:420, 1989.

165. Morton, D. L., Holmes, E. C., Eilber, F. R., and Ramming, K. P.: Adjuvant immunotherapy of malignant melanoma: Results of a randomized trial in patients with lymph node metastases. In Immunotherapy of Human Cancer. Edited by W. D. Terry and S. A. Rosenberg. New York, Excerpta Medica, 1982, p. 245.

166. Morton, D. L., Holmes, E. C., Eilber, F. R., and Wood, W. C.: Immunological aspects of neoplasia: A rational basis for immunotherapy. Ann. Intern. Med., 74:587, 1971.

167. Morton, D. L., Hoon, D. S. B., Gupta, R. G., Nizze, A. J., Famatiga, E., Foshag, L. J., Furutani, S., and Irie, R. F.: Treatment of malignant melanoma by active specific immunotherapy in combination with biological response modifiers. In New Horizons of Tumor Immunotherapy. Edited by M. Torisu and T. Yoshida. Amsterdam and New York, Elsevier Science Publishers, B. V., 1989, p. 665.

168. Morton, D. L., Hunt, K. K., Bauer, R. L., and Lee, J. D.: Immunotherapy by active

immunization of the host using mono-specific agents. In Biologic Therapy of Cancer. Edited by V. T. DeVita, Jr., S. Hellman, and S. A. Rosenberg. Philadelphia, J. B. Lippincott, 1991, p. 627.

169. Morton, D. L., Joseph, W. L., Ketcham, A. S., Geedhold, G. W., and Adkins, P. C.: Surgical resection and adjunctive immunotherapy for selected patients with pulmonary metastasis. Ann. Surg., 178:1118, 1973.

170. Morton, D. L., Nizze, J. A., Gupta, R. K., Famatiga, E., Hoon, D. S. B., and Irie, R. F.: Active specific immunotherapy of malignant melanoma. In Current Status of Cancer Control and Immunobiology. Edited by J. P. Kim, B. S. Kim, and J. G. Park. Seoul, 1987, p. 152.

171. Morton, D. L., and Wells, S. A., Jr.: Immunobiology of neoplastic disease. In Christopher's Text Book of Surgery. Edited by D. C. Sabiston. Philadelphia, Saunders, 1972, p. 542.

172. Murphy, S., and Hersh, E.: Human Leukemia. In Clinical Immunotherapy. Edited by A. F. LuBuglio. New York, Marcel Dekker, 1980, p.73.

173. Nathanson, L.: Regression of intradermal malignant melanoma after intralesional injection of Mycobacterium bovis strain BCG. Cancer Chemother. Rep., 56:659, 1972.

174. Nathanson, L., Schoenfeld, D., Regelson, W., Colsky, J., and Mittelman, A.: Prospective comparison of intralesional and multipuncture BCG in recurrent intradermal melanoma. Cancer, 46:1640, 1979.

175. Neidhart, J. A., Murphy, S. G., Hennick, L. A., and Wise, H. A.: Active specific immunotherapy of stage IV renal carcinoma with aggregated tumor antigen adjuvant. Cancer, 46:1126, 1980.

176. Nowell, P. C.: Mechanisms of tumor progression. Cancer Res., 46:2203, 1986.

177. Oettgen, H. F.: Immunotherapy of cancer. N. Engl. J. Med., 297:484, 1977.

178. Oldham, R. K.: Biologicals and biological response modifiers: Fourth modality of cancer treatment. Cancer Treat. Rep., 68:221, 1984.

179. Oratz, R., Cockrell, C., Speyer, J. L., Harris, M., Roses, D., and Bystryn, J.-C.: Induction of tumor-infiltrating lympho-cytes in human malignant melanoma metastases by immunization to melanoma antigen vaccine. J. Biol. Res. Mod., 8:355, 1989.

180. Otten, J.: Immunotherapy of Cancer: Present Status of Trials in Man. Edited by W. D. Terry and D. Windhorst. New York, Raven Press, 1977.

181. Patillo, R. A.: Immunotherapy and chemotherapy of gynecologic cancers. Am. J. Obstet. Gynecol., 124:808, 1976.

182. Pimm, M. V., and Baldwin, R. W.: Antigenic differences between primary methylcholanthrene-induced rat sarcoma and post-surgical recurrences. Int. J. Cancer, 20:37, 1977.

183. Pinsky, C. M., DeJager, R. L., Whittes, R. E., Wong, P. P., Kaufman, R. J., Mike, V., Hansen, J. A., Oettgen, H. F., and Krakoff, I. H.: Corynebacterium parvum as adjuvant to combination chemotherapy in patients with advanced breast cancer: Preliminary results of a prospective randomized trial. In Immunotherapy of Cancer: Present Status of Trials in Man. Edited by W. D. Terry and D. Windhorst. New York, Raven Press, 1978, p. 647.

184. Pinsky, C. M., Hirshaut, Y., and Oettgen, H. F.: Treatment of malignant melanoma by intratumoral injection of BCG. Natl.Cancer Inst. Monogr., 39:225, 1973.

185. Plesnicar, S., and Rudolf, Z.: Combined BCG and irradiation treatment of skin metastases originating from malignant melanoma. Cancer, 50:1100, 1982.

186. Poplack, D. G., Graw, R. G., Pomeroy, T. C., Henderson, E. S., and Leventhal, B. G.: Chemotherapy (CT) vs. chemotherapy and immunotherapy (CT + IMT) in childhood acute lymphatic leukemia (ALL). Proc. Am. Soc. Clin. Oncol., 16:230, 1975.

187. Portoukalian, J.: Immunoregulatory activity of gangliosides shed by melanoma tumors. In Gangliosides and Cancer. Edited by H. F. Oettgen. New York, VCH Publishers, 1989, p. 209.

188. Portoukalian, J., Zwinglestein, G., Abdul-Malek, N., and Dore, J. F.: Alteration of gangliosides in plasma and red cells of human bearing melanoma tumors. Biochem. Biophys. Res. Commun., 85:916, 1978.

189. Powles, R. L.: Immunologic maneuvers in the management of acute leukemia. Med. Clin. N. Am., 60:463, 1976.

190. Powles, R. L., Crowther, D., Bateman, C. J. T., Beard, M. E. J., McElwain, T. J., Russel, J., Lister, T. A., Whitehouse, J. M. A., Wrigley, P. F. M., Pike, M., Alexander, P., and Hamilton-Fairley, G.: Immunotherapy for acute myelogenous leukaemia. Br. J. Cancer, 28:365, 1973.

191. Prager, M. D., Baechtel, F. S., Peters, P. C., Brown, G. L., and Greene, C. L.: Specific immunotherapy of human metastatic renal cell carcinoma. Proc. Am. Assoc. Cancer Res., 22:163, 1981.

192. Rahman, A. F. R., Liao, S. K., and Dent, P.: Characterization of human malignant melanoma cell lines. VII Glycoprotein synthesis and shedding as revealed by (3H) glucosamine labelling. In Vitro, 13:580, 1977.

193. Ratliff, T. L., Kavoussi, L. R., and Catalona, W. J.: Role of fibronectin in intravesical BCG therapy for superficial bladder cancer. J. Urol., 139:410, 1988.

194. Ravindranath, M. H., and Irie, R. F.: Gangliosides as antigens of human melanoma. In Malignant Melanoma: Biology, Diagnosis and Therapy. Edited by L. Nathanson. Boston, Kluwer Academic Publishers, 1988, p. 14.

195. Ravindranath, M. H., Morton, D. L., and Irie, R. F.: An epitope common to gangliosides O-AcGD3 and GD3 recognized by antibodies in melanoma patients after active specific immunotherapy. Cancer Res., 49:3891, 1989.

196. Ravindranath, M. H., Paulson, J. C., and Irie, R. F.: Human melanoma associated antigen O-acetylganglioside GD3 is recognized by cancer antennarius lectin. J. Biol. Chem., 260:8838, 1985.

197. Ravindranath, M. H., Tsuchida, T., Morton, D. L., and Irie, R. F.: Gangliosides GM3:GD3 ratio as an index for management of melanoma. Cancer, 67:1, 1991.

198. Reid, J. W., Perlin, E., Oldham, R. K., Weese, J. L., Heim, W., Mills, M., Miller, C., Blom, J., Green, D., Ballinger, S., Cannon, G. B., Law, I., Connor, R., and Herberman, R. B.: Immunotherapy of carcinoma of the lung with intradermal BCG and allogeneic tumor cells. In Immunotherapy of Human Cancer. Edited by W. D. Terry and S. A. Rosenberg. New York, Excerpta Medica, 1982, p. 147.

199. Reizenstein, P., Anderssorn, B., Bjorkholm, M., Brenning, G., Engstedt, L., Gahrton, G., Hat, R., Holm, G., Hornsten, P., Killander, A., Lantz, B., Lindemalm, Ch., Lockner, D., Lonnqvist, B., Mellstedt, H., Palmblad, J., Paul, C., Simonsson, B., Sjogren, A.-M., Stalfelt, A.-M., Uden, A.-M., Wadman, B., Oberg, G., and Osby, E.: BCG plus leukemic cell therapy in patients with acute nonlymphoblastic leukemia: Effect in groups with high and low remission rates. In Immunotherapy of Human Cancer. Edited by W. D. Terry and S. A. Rosenberg. New York, Excerpta Medica, 1982, p. 17.

200. Richman, S. P., Gutterman, J. U., Hersh, E. M., and Ribi, E. E.: Phase I-II study of

intratumor immunotherapy with BCG cell wall skeleton plus P3. Cancer Immunol. Immunother., 5:41, 1978.

201. Risley, E. H.: The Gilman-Coca vaccine emulsion treatment of cancer. Boston Med. Surg. J., 165:784, 1911.

202. Roitt, I., Brostoff, J., and Male, D.: Immunology. St. Louis, MO., C. V. Mosby, 1985.

203. Rosenberg, S. A., and Rapp, H. J.: Intralesional immunotherapy of melanoma with BCG. Med. Clin. N. Am., 60:419, 1976.

204. Rosenberg, S. A., Rapp, H., Terry, W. D., Zbar, B., Costa, J., Seipp, C., and Simon, R.: Intralesional BCG therapy of patients with primary stage I melanoma. In Immunotherapy of Human Cancer. Edited by W. D. Terry and S. A. Rosenberg. New York, Excerpta Medica, 1982, p. 239.

204A. Rosenberg, S. A.: Adoptive Immunotherapy for cancer using lymphokine activated killer cells and IL2. In Important Advances in Oncology. Edited by H. DeVita and S. A. Rosenberg. Lippincott, 1986, p. 55.

204B. Rosenberg, S. A., Spiess, P., and Lutuvenieve, R. A.: A new approach to the adoptive immunotherapy of cancer with tumor infiltrating lymphocytes. Science, 233:1318, 1986.

205. Rudowski, W.: Two cases of spontaneous neoplasm regression extending over many years. Nowotwory, 28:173, 1978.

206. Sahasrabudhi, D. M., de Kernion, J. B., Pontes, J. E., Ryan, D. M., O'Donnell, R. W., Marquis, D. M., Mudholkar, G. S., and McCune, C. S.: Specific immunotherapy with suppressor function inhibition for metastatic renal cell carcinoma. J. Biol. Res. Mod., 5:581, 1986.

207. Schauer, R.: Sialic acids. Adv. Carbohydr. Chem. Biochem., 40:131, 1982.

208. Seigler, H. F., Buckley, C. E., Sheppard, L. D., Horne, B. J., and Shingleton, W. W.: Adoptive transfer and specific active immunization of patients with malignant melanoma. Ann. N. Y. Acad. Sci., 277:522, 1976.

209. Seigler, H. F., Shingleton, W. W., Metzgar, R. S., Buckley, C. E., Bergoc, P. M., Miller, D. S., Fetter, B. G., and Phaup, M. D.: Nonspecific and specific immunotherapy in patients with melanoma. Surg., 72:162, 1972.

210. Seigler, H. F., Shingleton, W. W., and Pickrell, K. I.: Intralesional BCG, intravenous immune lymphocytes and immunization with neuraminidase-treated tumor cells to manage melanoma: A clinical assessment. Plast. Reconstr. Surg., 55:294, 1975.

211. Simmons, R. L., Rios, A., and Ray, P. R., et al.: Effect of neuraminidase on growth of a 3-methylcholanthrene-induced fibrosarcoma in normal and immunosuppressed syngeneic mice. J. Natl. Cancer Inst., 47:1087, 1971.

212. Sinkovics, J. G.: Immunotherapy with viral oncolysates for sarcoma. J.A.M.A., 237:869, 1977.

213. Skornick, Y., Danciger, E., Rozin, R. R., and Shinitzky, M.: Postitive skin tests with autologous tumor cells of increased membrane viscosity. First report. Cancer Immunol. Immunother., 11:93, 1981.

214. Skornick, Y. G., Rong, G. H., Sindelar, W. F., Richert, L., Klausner, J. M., Rozin, R. R., and Shinitzky, M.: Active immunotherapy of human solid tumor with autologous cells treated with cholesteryl hemisuccinate. A phase I study. Cancer, 58:650, 1986.

215. Slingluff, C. L., Vollmer, R., and Seigler, H. F.: Stage II malignant melanoma: Presentation of a prognostic model and assessment of specific active immunotherapy in 1,273 patients. J. Surg. Oncol., 39:139, 1988.

216. Smith, G. V., Morse, P. A., Deraps, G. D., Raju, S., and Hardy, J. D.: Immunotherapy of patients with cancer. Surgery, 74:59, 1973.

217. Sokal, J. E., and Aungst, C. W.: Immunization with cultured cell-BCG mixtures. In Investigation of Immunity of Cancer Patients. Edited by G. Mathe and R. Weiner. New York, Springer-Verlag, 1974, p. 488.

218. Sopkova, B., and Kolar, V.: Intralesional BCG application in malignant melanoma. Neoplasma, 23:421, 1976.

219. Sorg, C., Bruggen, J., Seibert, E., and Macher, E.: Membrane-associated antigens of human malignant melanoma VI: Changes in expression of antigens on cultured melanoma cells. Cancer Immunol. Immunother., 3:259, 1978.

220. Stade, B. G., Lehmann, J., Riethmoller, G., and Johnson, J. P.: Markers for melanoma progression. J. Cancer Res. Clin. Oncol., 166(Suppl.):784, 1990.

221. Steel, G. G.: Cell loss from experimental tumours. Cell Tissue Kinet., 1:193, 1968.

222. Stewart, T. H. M., Hollinshead, A. C., Harris, J. E., and Raman, S.: Specific active immunotherapy of Stage II lung cancer patients. In Immunotherapy of Cancer. Edited by W. D. Terry and S. A. Rosenberg. New York, Excerpta Medica, 1982, p. 153.

223. Steward, T. H. M., and Orizaga, M.: The presence of delayed hypersensitivity reactions in patients toward cellular extracts of their malignant tissues. 3. The frequency, duration and cross reactivity of this phenomenon in patients with breast cancer, and its correlation with survival. Cancer, 28:1472, 1971.

224. Stjernsward, J., and Levin, A.: Delayed hypersensitivity-induced regression of human neoplasms. Cancer, 28:628, 1971.

225. Swanson, D. A.: Systemic treatment for renal cell carcinoma: An overview. In Urooncology: Current Status and Future Trends. New York, Wiley-Liss, 1990, p. 201.

226. Takita, H., Hollinshead, A. C., Bhayana, J. N., Edgerton, F., Conway, D., Moskowitz, R. M., Adler, R. H., Ramundo, M., Han, T., Rao, U., Vincent, R. G., Federico, A., Takita, L., and Smith, R.: Specific active immunotherapy of squamous cell lung carcinoma. In Immunotherapy of Human Cancer. Edited by W. D. Terry and S. A. Rosenberg. New York, Excerpta Medica, 1982, p. 159.

227. Takita, H., Takada, M., Minowada, J., Han, T., and Edgerton, F.: Adjuvant immunotherapy of stage III lung carcinoma. In Immunotherapy of Cancer: Present Status of Trials in Man. Edited by W. D. Terry and D. Windhorst. New York, Raven Press, N. Y. 1978, p. 217.

228. Tallberg, T., Kalimo, T., Halttunen, P., Tykka, H., Mahlberg, K., Matous, B., and Sundell, B.: Postoperative active specific immunotherapy with supportive measures in patients suffering from recurrent metastasized melanoma: Case reports of six patients. J. Surg. Oncol., 33:115, 1986.

229. Terry, W. D., Hodes, R. J., Rosenberg, S. A., Fisher, R. I., Makuch, R., Gordon, H. G., and Fisher, S. G.: Treatment of stage I and II malignant melanoma with adjuvant immunotherapy or chemotherapy: Preliminary analysis of a prospective randomized trial. In Immunotherapy of Human Cancer. Edited by W. D. Terry and S. A. Rosenberg. New York, Excerpta Medica, 1982, p. 251.

230. Terry, W. D., and Rosenberg, S. A.: Immunotherapy of Human Cancer. New York, Excerpta Medica, 1982.

231. Townsend, C. M., Eilber, F. R., and Morton, D. L.: Skeletal and soft tissue sarcomas. J. A. M. A., 236:2187, 1976.

232. Tsuchida, T., Ravindranath, M. H., Saxton, R. E., and Irie, R. F.: Gangliosides of human melanoma: Altered expression in vivo and in vitro. Cancer Res., 47:1278, 1987.

233. Tykka, H.: Active specific immunotherapy with supportive measures in the treatment of advanced palliatively nephrectomized renal adenocarcinoma. A controlled clinical study. Scand. J. Urol. Nephrol., 63:1, 1981.

234. van der Meijden, A. P. M., Debruyne, F. M. J., Steerenberg, P. A., and de Jong, W. H.: Aspects of non-specific immunotherapy with BCG in superficial bladder cancer: An overview. In EORTC Genitourinary Group Monograph 6: BCG in Superficial Bladder Cancer. New York, Alan Liss, 1989, p. 11.

235. Vaughan, J. W.: Cancer vaccine and anti-cancer globulin as an aid in the surgical treatment of malignancy. J. A. M. A., 63:1258, 1914.

236. Vlock, D. R., and Kirkwood, J. M.: Serial studies of autologous antibody reactivity to melanoma. Relationship to clinical course and circulating immune complexes. J. Clin. Invest., 76:849, 1985.

237. von Dungren, E.: Über Immunität gegen Geschwulst. Munch. Med. Wschr., 56:1099, 1909.

238. von Leyden, V. E., and Blumenthal, F.: Vorlautige Mitteilungen übber einige Ergebnisse der Krebsforschung auf den 1. medizinischen Klinik. Dt. Med. Wschr., 28:637, 1902.

239. Vosika, G. J.: Clinical immunotherapy trials of bacterial components derived from mycobacteria and Nocardia. J. Biol. Res. Mod., 2:321, 1983.

240. Vosika, G. J., Schmidtke, J. R., Goldman, A., Parker, R., and Gray, G.R.: Intralesional immunotherapy of malignant melanoma with Mycobacterium smegmatis cell wall skeleton combined with trehalose dimycotate (P3). Cancer, 44:495, 1979.

241. Wallack, M. K.: Specific immunotherapy with vaccinia oncolysates. Cancer Immunol. Immunother., 12:1, 1981.

242. Wallack, M. K., Bash, J., Leftheriotis, E., Seigler, H., Bland, K., Wanebo, H., Balch, C., and Bartolucci, A. A.: Positive relationship of clinical and serologic responses to vaccinia melanoma oncolysate. Arch. Surg., 122:1460, 1987.

243. Wallack, M. K., McNally, K., Leftheriotis, E., Seigler, H., Balch, C., Wanebo, H., Bartolucci, A. A., and Bash, J. A.: A Southeastern Cancer Study Group phase I/II trial with vaccinia melanoma oncolysates. Cancer, 57:649, 1986.

244. Wallack, M. K., Meyer, M., Bourgoin, A., Dore, J.-F., Leftheriotis, E., Carcagne, J., and Koprowski, H.: A preliminary trial of vaccinia oncolysates in the treatment of recurrent melanoma with serologic responses to the treatment. J. Biol. Res. Mod., 2:586, 1983.

245. Weisenburger, T. H., Jones, P. C., Ahn, S. C., Irie, R. F., and Juillard, G. J. F.: Active specific intralymphatic immunotherapy in metastatic malignant melanoma: Evidence of clinical response. J. Biol. Response Modif., 1:57, 1982.

246. Welt, S., Carswell, E. A., Vogel, C. W., Oettgen, H. F., and Old, L. J.: Immune and nonimmune effector functions of IgG3 mouse monoclonal antibody R24 detecting the disialoganglioside GD3 on the surface of melanoma cells. Clin. Immunol. Immunopathol., 45:214, 1987.

247. Whiteside, M. G., Cauchi, M. N., Paton, C., and Stone, J.: Chemoimmunotherapy for maintenance in acute myeloblastic leukemia. Cancer, 38:1581, 1976.

248. Whiteside, T. L., Miescher, S., Hurlimann, J., Moretta, L., and von Fliedner, V.: Separation, phenotyping and limiting dilution analysis of lymphocytes infiltrating human solid tumors. Int. J. Cancer, 37:803, 1986.

249. Whittaker, J. A., Bailey-Wood, R., and Hutchins, S.: Active immunotherapy for the treatment of acute myelogenous leukemia: The use of intravenous BCG and a comparison between BCG and irradiated leukemic blast cells. In Immunotherapy of Human Cancer. Edited by W. D. Terry and S. A. Rosenberg. New York, Excerpta Medica, 1982, p. 23.

250. Wile, A. G., Sparks, F. C., and Morton, D. L.: Monitoring immunotherapy with bacillus Calmette-Guérin by antibody titer. Cancer Res., 37:2251, 1977.

251. Yamamura, Y., Yoshizaki, K., Azuma, I., Yagura, T., and Watanabe, T.: Immunotherapy of human malignant melanoma with oil-attached BCG cell-wall skeleton. Gann, 66:355, 1975.

252. Zbar, B.: Tumor regression mediated by mycobacterium bovis (strain BCG). Natl. Cancer Inst. Monogr., 35:341, 1972.

253. Zbar, B., Bernstein, I. D., Bartlett, G. L., Hanna, M. G., Jr., and Rapp, H. J.: Immunotherapy of cancer: Regression of intradermal tumors and prevention of growth of lymph node metastases after intralesional injection of living mycobacterium bovis. J. Natl. Cancer Inst., 49:119, 1972.

254. Zbar, B., Ribi, E., and Rapp, H. J.: An experimental model for immunotherapy for cancer. Natl. Cancer Inst. Monogr., 39:3, 1973.

255. Zbar, B., and Tanaka, T.: Immunotherapy of cancer: Regression of tumors after intralesional injection of living mycobacterium bovis. Science, 172:271, 1971.

Acknowledgements

We thank Judith Ann Nizze and Dr. Amy Walsh for critically reviewing the manuscript and for editorial assistance.

Interferons

Ernest C. Borden

Introduction

Interferons (IFNs) are now licensed in more than forty countries for antiviral and antitumor use. IFNs have been a prototype for dissecting biological and clinical effects of cytokines. Like other cytokines, IFNs are a family of molecules which includes more than twenty different proteins coded on human chromosome 9 (except IFN-γ on chromosome 12). Cellular action follows binding to a relatively small (<2000/cell) number of high-affinity receptors. Although signal transduction pathways for IFN cellular response remain poorly defined, positive and negative nuclear regulatory proteins which modulate gene expression, resulting in production of induced proteins, have been identified. Cellular proteins induced by IFNs underlie the pleiotropic biological effects which include virus inhibition, immunomodulation, slowing of cell proliferation, oncogene suppression, and alterations in differentiation. However, which cellular proteins result in the various biological and therapeutic effects remain undefined as do cellular mechanisms of antitumor action.

In more than a dozen cancers, IFNs result in regression or control of disease process (Table XVIII-3-1). The spectrum of single-agent activity of IFNs compares favorably with other systemic antitumor modalities. Like many other drugs, IFNs are more active against hematologic malignancies than solid tumors. Greater therapeutic benefit will undoubtedly come by combining IFNs with other cancer-treatment modalities. Antitumor effects of IFNs can be enhanced in experimental tumor models when given with cytotoxic compounds, radiation and other biologicals. Emerging clinical results suggest that IFNs, when used in combination, will have substantially broader clinical impact in the future.

Molecules: Their Induction and Receptors

IFNs are a family of proteins, each residing at a specific genetic locus which has been retained through evolution. Three major classes of IFNs (α, β, γ) were initially defined on the basis of chemical, antigenic, and biologic differences. These have now been confirmed to result from significant differences in primary amino-acid sequence. With the advances in molecular biology and sequencing technology, complete nucleotide sequences for more than 15 human

IFNs have been defined.[100,114,150] Human IFNs α and β are structurally similar and located on chromosome 9. Both IFN α and IFN β are 166 amino acids in length with an additional 20 amino-acid secretory peptide present on the amino-terminal end. Comparison of the sequences of IFN α and IFN β has defined approximately 45% homology of nucleotides and 29% homology of amino acids. Each of the nonallelic human IFN α genes differ by approximately 10% in nucleotide sequence and 15% to 25% in amino-acid sequence (Table XVIII-3-2). IFN γ, 143 amino acids in length, is located on chromosome 12 and also contains a 20 amino acid secretory peptide.[54,124] IFN γ has only minimal sequence homology with IFN α or IFN β (Table XVIII-3-2). A fourth IFN class, ω, has recently been defined.[1,28] Although IFN β and IFN γ, produced by eukaryotic cells, are glycosylated, biological differences from the unglycosylated proteins produced in *E. coli* have not yet been identified. All IFNs retain the fundamental biological property of induction of cellular resistance to replication of both RNA and DNA viruses.

It is important to conceptually distinguish IFN production and action (Figure XVIII-3-1). IFNs were initially identified in vitro after exposure of cells to virus. Viruses remain the prototypic producer of IFN α and IFN β. Although not exhaustively studied, all body cells probably have the capacity to produce IFN α and IFN β. IFN γ was identified after exposure of lymphocytes to mitogens or sensitized lymphocytes to specific antigens. IL-2 and TNF are also potent inducers of IFN γ, under some circumstances resulting in substantial IFN titers.[70,86,173] Production of IFNs are part of host defense mechanisms for response to pathogens and neoplasia. Experimental suppression of IFN production in mice results in increased lethality from both tumors and viruses.[57,59]

Molecular mechanisms underlying cellular production of IFNs have been partially dissected by use of a series of promoter sequence mutations. Positive and negative nuclear

Table XVIII-3-1. Interferons: Current Status

High quality products from recombinant DNA technology
Biological response modulatory effects defined in man
Phase II antitumor activity confirmed in more than twelve human cancers
Effectiveness of other treatment approaches enhanced

Table XVIII-3-2. The Family of Interferon Molecules

Family	Chr (Hu)	Types (n)	Amino Acids N	Homology* %
Alpha**	9	>14	166	75–85
Beta	9	1	166	30
Gamma	12	1	143	1
Omega	9	>1	173	50

*Compared to IFN α

**The IFN, licensed for clinical use and produced by recombinant DNA technology, is IFN α2. IFN α2a (Hoffmann LaRoche) differs from IFN α2b (Schering-Plough) by a single amino acid at amino acid 23 (lysine in IFN α2a; arginine in IFN α2b). IFN α2 is 165 amino acids, with a deletion at amino acid 44 of an aspartate residue

therapy by utilizing monoclonal antibodies as a carrier for radionuclides or cytotoxic agents.

The enzymes 2',5' oligoadenylate synthetase (2–5A synthetase), a protein kinase, and indoleamine 2,3 dioxygenase (IDO) are induced by IFNs (Table XVIII-3-3).[115,130] 2–5A synthetase has been shown to transfer a nucleoside 5' monophosphate to the 2' position of an accepting chain. 2–5A synthetase is a relatively specific marker of IFN system activation. A latent ribonuclease is activated by 2–5A; the result of induction of these enzymes is in part inhibition of DNA and protein synthesis. The degradation of tryptophan to kynurenine by IDO has been implicated in protein synthesis inhibition and antiproliferative effects as a result of depletion of tryptophan.[27,111,152,172] Low tryptophan levels and increased kynurenine excretion have occurred in patients treated with IFNs. Depletion of this essential amino acid may be related to both IFN action and side effects of treatment. Production of neopterin, a metabolite of GTP, is increased in serum following IFNs and is catalyzed by an induced enzyme GTP cyclohydrolase I.[67,80]

Induced proteins and their products can be identified on cells and in serum of treated patients (Table XVIII-3-4). Their measurement or the quantitation of immune effector cell function can be used to define biologically active molecules, doses, schedules and routes of administration. Most biological response modulatory effects peak at 24–48 hours which contrast with maximal serum levels in pharmacokinetic studies.[51,95] After intravenous bolus administration, the $t\frac{1}{2}$ of IFN $\alpha 2$ is short (<60 minutes); mean terminal half-life is 4–5 hours with no serum levels measurable at 12 hours. After intramuscular or subcutaneous administration, peak levels are 6–10 hours.[61,171] The pharmacologic hallmark of IBN β is virtual absence of serum levels with subcutaneous or intramuscular administration; yet biological response modulatory and therapeutic effects occur.[51,63] These findings suggest traditional measurements of serum levels may not be the best guide for clinical trial design with IFNs.

Antiproliferative and Differentiative Effects

In addition to immune effector cells, IFNs regulate function and proliferation of somatic cells (Table XVIII-3-3). IFNs retard growth and proliferation of tumor cells and normal cells by prolonging the cell cycle. Diploid cells are somewhat less sensitive to the antiproliferative effects of IFNs than are aneuploid cells. Substantial differences exist among normal as well as tumor cells in their sensitivity to direct antiproliferative actions, with some being extremely sensitive and others completely resistant.[140,143,162] For example, the human lymphoblastoid β-cell lines transformed by Epstein-Barr virus (EBV) are extraordinarily sensitive to the antiproliferative action of IFN α and IFN β but not IFN γ. Another EBV-transformed lymphoblastoid cell line (Namalwa), a vigorous producer of IFN α subtypes, is essentially resistant to the action of IFNs. IFN-resistant mutant cells can be isolated from IFN-sensitive cell lines. Since the resistant mutants can sometimes retain their antiviral sensitivity,[84] the resistance is not necessarily due to the reduced number or absence of IFN receptors but points to some other mechanism of resistance.

IFNs α and β can affect all phases of the cell cycle, M, G_1, and G_2. When fibroblasts are stimulated to grow by serum, epidermal growth factor, insulin or vasopressin, IFNs cause a prolongation of the G_1 phase, a reduced rate of entry into the S phase and a lengthening of the S and the G_2 phases.[8,144,145] The cumulative effects of prolongation of the cell cycle of both normal and tumor cells by IFNs results in cytostasis, increase in cell size, and occasionally cell death.[49,116]

IFNs alter differentiation of many cell types. IFN α, IFN β, and IFN γ induced B-cell blast transformation as well as plasmacytoid differentiation in chronic lymphocytic leukemic cells.[38,110] IFNs α and β induce differentiation of multilineage colony-forming cells in hairy-cell leukemia[96] and IFN γ induces differentiation of monocytes.[138] Treatment of HL-60 promyelocytic leukemia cells with IFN α alone or in combination with retinoic acid resulted in enhancement of differentiation.[83] Melanoma cells were differentiated by IFN β, an effect which did not correlate directly with an antiproliferative effect.[44] Human IFN α, given to nude mice bearing xenografts of human osteosarcoma, inhibited tumor growth. In some cases, the sarcoma was replaced by normal bone and marrow, an effect possibly explained by tumor differentiation.[22]

Several other observations have raised the possibility that IFNs may progressively cause reversion of the transformed phenotype. When radiation-transformed mouse fibroblasts were cultivated and passaged in the continuous presence of mouse IFN α/β: the cells no longer produced tumors in nude mice and their morphology changed from fibroblastic to epithelioid. When IFN treatment ceased, cells reverted to the transformed phenotype and became tumorigenic.[24] Mouse 3T3 cells transformed with the human HA-ras-1 gene and cultured continuously in the presence of murine IFN α/β produced revertant colonies in which transcription of the ras gene was inhibited. Most cells retained the revertant phenotype during many cell generations despite renewed high levels of transcription of the ras gene and of p21 ras protein.[137] However, one line of bladder tumor cells seemed to become more tumorigenic in nude mice than cells not treated with IFN.[23] Thus, it has not yet been possible to predict what change in phenotype may occur by long-term in vitro exposure to interferon.

Antitumor Activity in Humans

IFNs as single agents are active in inducing regressions in more than a dozen different malignancies (Table XVIII-3-5). IFN $\alpha 2$ was the first previously unlicensed therapeutic, produced by recombinant DNA technology, to be approved for marketing by the U.S. Food and Drug Administration.[16,50,75] Large-scale trials of IFNs as treatment for malignancies began in 1979 with the American Cancer Society program. The IFN α used in that program, produced from buffy coat leukocytes by the pioneering program of Cantell of the Finnish State Serum Institute and National Red Cross, was only a partially purified preparation which by today's standards was quite crude. The American Cancer Society program did, however, confirm the activity of this IFN α preparation in inducing disease regression in multi-institutional studies. With this evidence in hand, the infant biotechnology industry was willing to make the commitment to cloning and large-scale production of recombinant IFNs.

Table XVIII-3-5.   Antitumor Effectiveness of Interferon Alpha in Phase II Trials*

Chronic leukemias
  Myeloid*
  Hairy cell*
  Lymphocytic
Lymphomas
  Nodular*
  T-cell*
Multiple myeloma
Renal carcinoma
Malignant melanoma
Mid-gut carcinoids
Gliomas
Kaposi's sarcoma
Ovarian carcinomas
Basal cell carcinomas**
Bladder carcinomas**

*Response rates >40%
**Intralesional or regional administration

Hematologic Malignancies

The degree of activity and improvement in quality of life of patients with hairy cell leukemia resulted in the first licensed approval for an IFN in the United States. More than 85% of patients have objective evidence of partial or complete hematologic response to IFN α2.[45,118] Following IFNs, there is a gradual decrease in bone-marrow infiltration with malignant cells as well as a normalization of peripheral hematologic parameters. This has resulted in reduced morbidity from the disease process: a reduction in red cell and platelet transfusion requirements and a decreased frequency of infection.[52] Reduction of hairy cells in peripheral blood may occur in <1 month but improvement in peripheral cytopenias may take much longer—from 2 to 8 months in marrow and peripheral blood. Responses may occur at doses as low as 0.2×10^6 units/M^2 but more slowly than at the more conventional dose of 2×10^6 units/M^2. Although duration of optimal treatment remains uncertain, the time required to induce objective response and persistence of hairy cells in the bone marrow even after 6 months suggests a need for relatively continuous treatment.[125] Some evidence suggests that with the exquisite sensitivity of hairy cell leukemia to IFNs, maintenance treatment can be given as infrequently as one or two times per week. IFN β and IFN γ are both also active in the disease but their roles remain under investigation.

In chronic myelogenous leukemia, IFN α results in therapeutic response in a majority (>75%) of patients.[3,112,154] Untreated patients or patients with disease of less than one-year duration are more likely to respond.[153] A higher dose ($\geq 5 \times 10^6$ units/M^2) than required for hairy cell leukemia is needed to achieve the best therapeutic control. Frequency of administration for optimal clinical effect has not been critically examined but higher response rates have been reported with daily rather than 3 × week, subcutaneous administration. In addition to reduction in leukemic cell mass, a gradual reduction has occurred in frequency of cells bearing the underlying 9–22 chromosomal translocations. A complete cytogenetic response can occur in >50% of patients who clinically respond; suppression of these clones of cells sug-

gests a profound change in the neoplastic process. To sustain hematologic and cytogenetic response in myeloproliferative disorders, continued treatment seems to be required. IFN γ can also result in complete and partial responses in CML.[78] Thrombocytosis associated with myeloproliferative disorders, whether Philadelphia chromosome positive or negative, can be effectively controlled by IFN α2.[87,155]

Response rates of 10%–20% occur in patients with advanced multiple myeloma treated with various schedules.[29,117,168] When patients who received 12×10^6 units/M^2 of IFN α2a intramuscularly daily were analyzed according to prior therapy, 50% of previously untreated patients had responded.[117] Similarly, patients who had received only phenylalanine mustard and prednisone had a 40% response rate.[29] In patients who had a tumor response, levels of serum immunoglobulins were restored, an effect infrequently seen with chemotherapy.[117] Complete responses can be sustained for more than two years, an unusual event in myeloma. Thus, IFNs will probably eventually become part of the treatment of various stages of multiple myeloma.

In chronic lymphocytic leukemia, previously treated patients received either 50×10^6 units/M^2 or 5×10^6 units/M^2 of IFN α2a, a dose based upon pretreatment platelet count.[46] Of patients at the higher dose, 2 of 12 responded vs 0 of 6 at the lower dose. However, in other trials, 30–35% of patients receiving 2–5×10^6 units/M^2, 3 × week or daily responded.[156,168] Of possible importance is schedule; response in 2 patients could not be sustained on a weekly schedule.[108] Intensive treatment with IFNs in chronic lymphocytic leukemia merits further evaluation.

In lymphomas of various histologies and of both B- and T-cell phenotypes, IFN α may have a therapeutic role. IFN α2a, 50×10^6 units 3 × week, was effective in 45% of patients with advanced cutaneous T-cell lymphoma;[25] responses lasted from 3 months to >25 months (median, 5 months). Partial response to IFN β occurs in T-cell leukemias.[157] IFNs may prove to be more effective for cutaneous T-cell lymphomas and leukemias than any other reported agent. In nodular, poorly differentiated B-cell lymphomas, a greater than 45% response frequency has occurred with IFN α2.[47,108,168] Many responding patients have been pretreated with combination chemotherapy. Responses can persist for >6 months after cessation of therapy. Patients who have relapsed after IFN was discontinued, have subsequently responded to second courses. Doses of 50×10^6 units/M^2 intramuscularly 3 × weekly, a dose which required at least 50% reduction within 4 weeks in all patients, and a much lower dose, 2×10^6 units/ M^2 3 × weekly, have been effective. Thus, as in hairy cell leukemia, objective response can be achieved at lower doses.

Solid Tumors

For some solid tumors, IFN α has resulted in response rates equivalent to the best chemotherapeutic approaches. Response rates of metastatic melanoma to IFN α have ranged from 2–29%; the cumulative response totaled from 3 recent series of 124 patients involving patients utilizing recombinant IFN α2 was 15% (10% partial and 5% complete), a level comparable to results with cytotoxic agents.[30,32,134] Response has been correlated with better performance status, no prior chemotherapy and low volume of visceral disease. Response has not yet been clearly correlated with dose. For example, IFN α2a at 50 x 10⁶ units/M² intramuscularly 3 × week resulted in partial or complete responses in 7 of 31 (23%) patients. This dose resulted in >80% of patients developing deterioration in performance status. A lower dose (12 x 10⁶ units/ M² given 3 × week) was used in a subsequent trial. Although fewer complete responses occurred, results were statistically indistinguishable (6 of 30 responses) from the prior trial.[30,32] Response rates to IFN γ have been reported between 6 and 11%.[31,41]

Metastatic renal cell carcinoma has a response rate to cytotoxic agents of less than 10%. Response rates from 4–26% have been reported in trials of recombinant IFN α2 in this disease, with a mean response of 15% in cumulative summary of several trials.[103] In one of the initial trials, either 2 or 20 x 10⁶ units/M² was administered daily.[120] No objective responses occurred at the lower dose, but at the high dose, 4 of 15 patients responded. Subsequently, 26 additional patients were treated at 20 x 10⁶ units/M² with 8 of 26 responses; median duration of response was 3 months and dose reduction was required in more than half the patients.[121] To ameliorate toxicity, IFN α2 was evaluated in a schedule of gradual dose escalation from 3 to 36 x 10⁶ units intramuscularly over a 10-day period.[74] Patients were maintained at 36 x 10⁶ units daily for 9 weeks after which responding and stable patients continued on a thrice-weekly schedule. In 62 evaluable patients, 7 partial responses were observed. By gradually increasing the dose, the acute toxicity of fever and chills was lessened, with <10% of patients developing fever greater than 38.5°C. However, dose reduction for granulocytopenia, fatigue, and anorexia to 18 x 10⁶ units was required in many patients. A more favorable response has been observed in patients who have had resection of bulky primary disease; lung metastases appear to respond better than disease at other sites. Two studies of IFN γ or combinations of IFN α and γ have had response rates of 9–30% (CR plus PR) in renal cell carcinoma.[6,119,127] The response rate of 30% occurred in patients receiving IFN γ at a biologically effective but low dose (1 x 10⁶ units weekly).[6]

Response rates for recombinant IFN α2 in Kaposi's sarcoma have had a mean of 33%.[34,60,77,81,126,131,165] A dose-response effect has been identified and responses have been seen in patients with visceral and nodal disease. Responses occur in the skin, nodes and gastrointestinal tract with a mean duration of 13 months. The rate of opportunistic infection has been less after IFN α administration to responding patients, but no overall decrease in infection frequency has been identified.[60,77]

Clinical trials of IFN α in endocrine pancreatic tumors have reported a high objective rate (>75%) of response (decrease in tumor-produced peptides).[40,105] In addition, a partial response has occurred in approximately one-third of patients. IFN α has also been useful in decreasing the severe diarrhea common in pancreatic endocrine tumors. Midgut carcinoid tumors, although often behaving in an indolent fashion, produce symptoms such as flushing and diarrhea which may interfere with daily activities. In trials of recombinant IFN α, a mean response rate [improvement in symptoms or decrease in 5 hydroxyindoleacetic acid (5HIAA)] of approximately 50% has been reported.[98,106,107] The decrease in 5HIAA has been

correlated with lessened symptoms; rebound of 5HIAA levels frequently occurred when IFN was discontinued or with development of antibodies to the administered IFN α2.[106] Objective tumor regression occurs less frequently being observed in approximately 20% of patients, but can include both primary tumors and hepatic metastases.

Other solid tumors, such as gliomas, ovarian, bladder and basal cell carcinomas, have responded to IFN α administered regionally. Trials have defined an objective response rate of up to 40% for IFN β given by combined intratumor and/or systemic administration.[99,174] Systemic injection of IFN α has also resulted in partial responses in patients with malignant gliomas.[88] Recurrent and persistent ovarian carcinoma presents an opportunity for local therapy because of its predilection for intra-abdominal serosal surfaces. To reach IFN levels which are inhibitory for ovarian carcinoma cell proliferation in vitro, trials with all three IFN types have been conducted with intraperitoneal (i.p.) administration.[169] In 14 patients with persistent disease at second-look laparotomy, who received weekly i.p. IFN α2 postoperatively, 4 complete and 1 partial response were documented in the 11 patients who underwent laparotomy following IFN treatment.[12] An additional patient was considered a complete responder on the basis of physical examination alone. In 8 patients receiving intraperitoneal IFN β, 4 experienced resolution of ascites.[123] IFN γ was administered intraperitoneally to 27 patients with residual carcinoma following combination chemotherapy; no responses occurred.[33] In superficial bladder carcinoma (carcinoma in situ or noninvasive, low-grade transitional cell carcinoma), IFN α2 gave a greater than 40% objective response and was effective in patients with large disease volumes. A dose-response correlation and higher response rates with intraepithelial neoplasia than with frank bladder carcinoma were identified.[161,170] Intralesional treatment for another intraepithelial neoplasm, basal cell carcinoma, has also been effective in yielding a high (>75% CR) objective response frequency.[55]

Combinations

Greater effectiveness of IFNs with tumor cell burden first reduced by surgery or chemotherapy has been demonstrated for established murine tumors.[58] Immunomodulatory effects may be greater when tumor cell mass is reduced.[69] The pioneering studies of IFNs in osteosarcoma involved this clinical setting.[149] Randomized trials are currently underway in the U.S. with IFNs α being used as adjuncts to surgery in melanoma and renal carcinoma. The melanoma trials all prospectively randomize the high-risk individual with melanoma after surgery to standard treatment (regular medical evaluation) or to IFNs. Together with a similar ongoing study in renal carcinoma, these trials should begin to establish whether IFN α is effective in the minimal tumor burden setting.

Trials in myeloma are prototypes for the approaches being used for combination of IFNs with chemotherapy. In Phase II trials of the Eastern Cooperative Oncology Group (ECOG), both complete response and 2-year survival with the IFN α2a and chemotherapy are better than historical controls.[109] This IFN combination, which involves alternate cycles of IFN α2 and chemotherapy, is currently being compared in prospectively randomized trials to chemotherapy alone by ECOG.

A similar alternating therapy program in hairy cell leukemia shows promise of resulting in sustained responses.[93] An Italian multi-institutional study has identified prolonged survival when 3×10^6 units/M^2, $3 \times$ weekly of IFN α2b was used as maintenance therapy for patients stable or responding to 1 year of induction chemotherapy. Median duration of response for the IFN-α2b-treated patients was 26 months (compared to 14 months for the untreated patients, p = 0.0002) and median survival was 52 months for treated patients and 39 months for controls (p = 0.05).[91]

IFNs α and β have potentiated 5-fluorouracil (5FU) in preclinical, antiproliferative and antitumor experimental models.[39,147,148] Combining 5FU with IFN α or IFN β may lead to potentiated clinical results. This combination has been used at maximal doses of both 5FU and IFN α2a and has resulted in an 80% objective response rate.[167] Some responses have been sustained for more than a year. Interestingly, IFNs used in mice not only increased therapeutic effectiveness, but also protected from lethal toxicities of 5FU.[148]

For rational pharmacology, complementary mechanisms can be used to develop effective combination therapies.[14,17] Because of their pleiotropic regulatory effects on cell function, IFN combinations may have potent inhibitory effects in both viral and neoplastic diseases. For example, the differing mechanisms of inhibition of HIV replication may result in greater therapeutic effectiveness when combined with zidovudine for AIDS.[73,76] Not only do IFNs potentiate cytotoxic drugs, but also radiation and the effects of other cytokines.[53,139] To dissect logical strategies for biochemical or cellular inhibition with other molecules, expanded preclinical research will be required. Dose, route and schedule will become increasingly important considerations.

Side Effects

Like other potent physiologic products such as glucocorticoids, IFNs have toxicities when administered with pharmacologic intent (Table XVIII-3-6). Side effects with the initial dose are predominantly constitutional. These are dominated by malaise, fever, and chills which begin a few hours after the commonly used subcutaneous route and last for 2–8 hours. These influenza-like symptoms occur uniformly following the initial injection with subsequent development of tachyphylaxis with subsequent daily injections. The rapidity of tachyphylaxis is dependent upon type of IFN, dose, route, and schedule. Flu-like symptoms which occur despite increases in endogenous glucocorticoids[104,141] can be par-

tially controlled with aspirin or acetaminophen. The chronic fatigue may necessitate dose reduction; tolerance can be improved with lower doses and intermittent scheduling. Fatigue and anorexia are the dose-limiting toxicities with chronic administration; weight loss occurs and may be significant (>10%). Any nausea and vomiting have usually been mild and of short duration. The most frequent neurologic side effect (other than the possible relationship of the fatigue) is somnolence and confusion which may result from a diffuse slowing seen on EEG. In general, older patients tolerate these side effects less well than younger patients.

Hematologic effects include mild granulocytopenia with a reduction in counts by 40–60% followed by rapid rebound to normal after discontinuation of therapy. No increase in infectious sequelae has occurred during IFN-induced leukopenia, and granulocytopenia is rarely dose-limiting. Anemia occurs with chronic therapy but is rarely severe. This may reflect an influence on the erythropoiesis because recovery of normal hematocrit has often required weeks or months. Mild thrombocytopenia has been reported in 5–50% of patients and is influenced by marrow infiltration with tumor.

Elevation of transaminases, usually mild, has occurred more commonly in the presence of pretreatment hepatic abnormalities and is dose-related. Cholesterol levels decrease, often accompanied by a rise in triglycerides. LDL commonly declines and HDL both increases and decreases, depending on dose and type of IFN.[94,135] A statistically significant, though rarely clinically important, hypocalcemic effect occurs. The decrease in calcium is out of proportion to mild declines in albumin. Creatinine does not change. The most common renal toxicity described has been mild proteinuria, but nephrotic syndrome and acute renal insufficiency have been rarely reported.[7,142] Although little or no IFN can be identified in urine, nephrectomy in the rat reduces but does not eliminate clearance, suggesting catabolism by renal tubular cells is one degradative pathway.[151,160] Although occasional patients may develop alterations in thyroid function,[26] in general, no residual toxicities in parenchymal organ function have been identified.[122] With improved understanding of mechanism of action and clinical introduction of other members of the IFN α family,[62,66] it can be anticipated that the therapeutic index of IFNs will improve.

With chronic administration, a minority of patients develop neutralizing antibody to the administered IFN.[68,82,166] Antibody development is a function of dose, schedule, route and possibly underlying disease. Antibodies have rarely been identified with <4 months of IFN administration and are not

Table XVIII-3-6. Clinical Side Effects of Interferon*

Acute	Chronic
Fever	Fatigue
Chills	Anorexia
Malaise	Weight loss
Myalgias	Mild neutropenia
Headache	Transaminase elevations
Nausea	Diarrhea
	Depression
	Less common: mental slowing, confusion, hair shedding, thrombocytopenia, diarrhea, nausea and vomiting

*See Quesada, et al.[122]

Table XVIII-3-7. Studies Resulting in More Effective Use of Interferons in Cancer

Molecules	Mechanism of action
Inducers	Protein modulation
Structure-function relationships	Immunomodulatory effects
	Antiproliferative/differentiation
Effects of new types	Angiogenesis inhibition
Cellular activation mechanisms	Clinical strategies
Receptors	Dose/schedule optimization
Signal transduction	Combination therapies
Function-induced proteins	New disease targets

clearly related to IFN type or preparation. Particularly when present in high titer, they may be correlated with disease progression.[48,166]

Perspective

IFNs have improved therapeutic approaches for viral diseases and malignancies. They are the first human proteins to be effective as a cancer-treatment modality. The full spectrum of actions and interactions, mechanism of antitumor effects, and optimal dose, schedule and type of IFN for specific clinical indications has not yet been fully delineated (Table XVIII-3-7). IFNs, both themselves and as a prototype for other biological response modifiers, have opened a new era in oncologic treatment. The groundwork has been laid for the use of IFNs to modulate specific gene regulation, oncogene expression, cell proliferation and differentiation, and immunological function. This must be complemented by studies dissecting other aspects of IFNs' cellular and clinical actions (Table XVIII-3-7). In combination with other lymphokines, monoclonal antibodies, and cytoreductive approaches, IFNs should continue to reduce morbidity from cancer.

References

1. Adolf, G. R.: Antigenic structure of human interferon omega$_1$ (interferon alpha II$_1$): Comparison with other human interferons. J. Gen. Virol., 68:1669, 1987.
2. Aguet, M., Dembic, Z., and Merlin, G.: Molecular cloning and expression of the human interferon-γ receptor. Cell, 55:273, 1988.
3. Alimena, G., Morra, E., Lazzarino, M., Liberati, A. M., Montefusco, E., Inverardi, D., Bernasconi, P., Mancini, M., Donti, E., Grignani, F., Bernasconi, C., Dianzani, F., and Mandelli, F.: Interferon alpha-2b as therapy for Ph-positive chronic myelogenous leukemia: a study of 82 patients treated with intermittent or daily administration. Blood, 72:642, 1988.
4. Anderson, P., Yip, Y. K., and Vilcek, J.: Specific binding of ^{125}I-human interferon-gamma to high affinity receptors on human fibroblasts. J. Biol. Chem., 257:11301, 1982.
5. Arenzana-Seisdedos, F., Virelizier, J. L., and Fiers, W.: Interferons as macrophage-activating factors III. Preferential effects of interferon-gamma on the interleukin 1 secretory potential of fresh or aged human monocytes. J. Immunol., 134:2444, 1985.
6. Aulitzky, W., Gastl, G., Aulitzky, W. E., Herold, M., Kemmler, J., Mull, B., Frick, J., and Huber, C.: Successful treatment of metastatic renal cell carcinoma with a biologically active dose of recombinant interferon-gamma. J. Clin. Oncol., 7:1875, 1989.
7. Averbach, S. D., Austin, H. A., III, Sherwin, S. A., Antonovych, T., Bunn, P. A., Jr., and Longo, D.L.: Acute interstitial nephritis with nephrotic syndrome following recombinant leukocyte A IFN therapy for mycosis fungoides. N. Engl. J. Med., 310:32, 1984.
8. Balkwill, F., and Taylor-Papadimitriou, J.: Interferon affects both G$_1$ and S + G$_2$ in cells stimulated from quiescence to growth. Nature, 274:798, 1978.
9. Balkwill, F. R., Moodie, E. M., Freedman, V., and Fantes, K. H.: Human interferon inhibits the growth of established human breast tumors in the nude mouse. Int. J. Cancer, 30:231, 1982.
10. Basham, T. Y., Bourgeade, M. F., Creasey, A. A., and Merigan, I.: Interferon increases HLA synthesis in melanoma cells: interferon-resistant and sensitive cell lines. Proc. Natl. Acad. Sci. (U.S.A.), 79:3625, 1982.
11. Belardelli, F., Gresser, I., Maury, C., and Maunoury, M. T.: Antitumor effects of interferon in mice injected with interferon-sensitive and interferon-resistant Friend leukemia cells. II. Role of host mechanisms. Int. J. Cancer, 30:821, 1982.
12. Berek, J. S., Hacker, N. F., Lichtenstein, A., Jung, T., Spina, C., Knox, R. M., Brady, J., Greene, T., Ettinger, L. M., Lagasse, L. D., Bonnem, E. M., Spiegel, R. J., and Zighelboim, J.: Intraperitoneal recombinant alpha-interferon for "salvage" immunotherapy in stage III epithelial ovarian cancer: A Gynecologic Oncology Group study. Cancer Res., 45:4447, 1985.
13. Billard, C., Sigaux, F., Castaigne, S., Valensi, F., Flandrin, G., Degos, L., Falcoff, E., and Aguet, M.: Treatment of hairy cell leukemia with recombinant alpha IFN: II. In vivo down-regulation of alpha IFN receptors on tumor cells. Blood, 67:821, 1986.
14. Borden, E. C.: Interferons and cancer: How the Promise is Being Kept. In Interferons, Vol. 5. Edited by I. Gresser. London, Academic Press, 1984, p. 43.
15. Borden, E. C.: Augmented tumor-associated antigen expression by interferons. J. Natl. Cancer Inst., 80:148, 1988.
16. Borden, E. C.: Effects of interferons in neoplastic diseases of man. Pharmacol. Therap., 37:213, 1988.
17. Borden, E. C., and Hawkins, M. J.: Biologic response modifiers as adjuncts to other therapeutic modalities. Semin. Oncol., 13:144, 1986.
18. Borden, E. C., Hawkins, M. J., Sielaff, K. M., Storer, B. M., Schiesel, J. D., and Smalley, R. V.: Clinical and biological effects of recombinant interferon-beta administered intravenously daily in Phase I trial. J. Interferon Res., 8:357, 1988.
19. Borden, E. C., Sidky, Y., Erturk, E., Wierenga, W., and Bryan, G. T.: Protection from carcinogen-induced murine bladder carcinoma by interferons and an oral interferon-inducing pyrimidinone, bropirimine. Cancer Res., 50:1071, 1990.
20. Borden, E. C., Verma, A. J., and Wolberg, W. H.: Potential role of polyribonucleotides in human neoplastic diseases. J. Biol. Response Mod., 4:676, 1985.
21. Branca, A. A., and Baglioni, C.: Evidence that types I and II interferons have different receptors. Nature, 294:768, 1981.
22. Brosjö, O., Bauer, H. C. F., Broström, L. A., Nilsson, O. S., Reinholt, F. P., and Tribukait, B.: Growth inhibition of human osteosarcomas in nude mice by human interferon-α: Significance of dose and tumor differentiation. Cancer Res., 47:258, 1987.
23. Brouty-Boye, D.: Interferon and the tumour cell phenotype. In Interferon, Vol. 7. Edited by I. Gresser. London, Academic Press, 1986, p. 145.
24. Brouty-Boye, D., and Gresser, I.: Reversibility of the transformed and neoplastic phenotype. I. Progressive reversion of the phenotype x-ray-transformed C3H/10T½ cells under prolonged treatment with interferon. Int. J. Cancer, 28:165, 1981.
25. Bunn, P. A., Foon, K. A., Ihde, D. C., Longo, D. L., Zeffren, J., Sherwin, S. A., and Oldham, R. K.: Recombinant leukocyte A interferon: an active agent in advanced cutaneous T-cell lymphomas. Ann. Intern. Med., 101:484, 1984.
26. Burman, P., Totterman, T. H., Oberg, K., and Karlsson, K. A.: Thyroid autoimmunity in patients on long-term therapy with leukocyte-derived interferon. J. Clin. Endocrinol. Metab., 63:1086, 1986.
27. Byrne, G. I., Lehmann, L. K., Kirschbaum, J. G., Borden, E. C., Lee, C. M., and Brown, R. R.: Induction of tryptophan degradation in vitro and in vivo: a gamma-interferon-stimulated activity. J. Interferon Res., 6:389, 1986.
28. Capon, D. J., Shepard, H. M., and Goeddel, D. V.: Two distinct families of human and bovine interferon-alpha genes are coordinately expressed and encode functional polypeptides. Mol. Cell. Biol., 5:768, 1985.
29. Costanzi, J. J., Cooper, M. R., Scarffe, J. H., Ozer, H., Grubbs, S. S., Ferraresi, R. W., Pollard, R. B., and Spiegel, R. J.: Phase II study of recombinant alpha-2 interferon in resistant multiple myeloma. J. Clin. Oncol., 3:654, 1985.
30. Creagan, E. T., Ahmann, D. L., and Green, S. J.: Phase II study of recombinant leukocyte A interferon (RIFN-Alpha-A) in disseminated malignant melanoma. Cancer, 54:2844, 1984.
31. Creagan, E. T., Ahmann, D. L., Long, H. J., Frytak, S., Sherwin, S. A., and Chang, M. N.: Phase II study of recombinant interferon-gamma in patients with disseminated malignant melanoma. Cancer Treat. Rep., 71:843, 1987.
32. Creagan, E. T., Kovach, J. S., Long, H. J., and Richardson, R.L.: Phase I study of recombinant leukocyte A human interferon combined with BCNU in selected patients with advanced cancer. J. Clin. Oncol., 4:408, 1986.
33. D'Acquisto, R., Markman, M., Hakes, T., et al.: A Phase I trial of intraperitoneal recombinant gamma-interferon in advanced ovarian carcinoma. J. Clin. Oncol., 6:689, 1988.
34. DeWit, R., Boucher, C. A. B., Veenhof, K. H. N., Schattenkerk, J. K. M. E., Bakker, P. J. M., and Danner, S. A.: Clinical and virological effects of high dose recombinant interferon α in disseminated AIDS-related Kaposi's sarcoma. Lancet, 2:1214, 1988.
35. Edwards, B. S., Hawkins, M. J., and Borden, E. C.: Correlation between in vitro and systemic effects of native and recombinant interferons alpha upon human NK cell cytotoxicity. J. Biol. Response Mod., 2:409, 1983.
36. Edwards, B. S., Merritt, J. A., Fuhlbrigge, R. C., and Borden, E. C.: Low doses of interferon alpha result in more effective clinical natural killer cell activation. J. Clin. Invest., 75:1908, 1985.
37. Eggermont, A. M. M., Sugarbaker, P. H., Marquet, R. L., and Jeekel, J.: In vivo generation of lymphokine activated killer cell activity by ABPP and interleukin-2 and their antitumor effects against immunogenic and nonimmunogenic tumors in murine tumor models. Cancer Immunol. Immunother., 26:23, 1988.
38. Einhorn, S., Robert, K. H., Ostlund, L., Juliusson, G., and Biberfeld, P.: Interferon Induces Proliferation and Differentiation in Primary Chronic Lymphocytic Leukemia Cells. In The Biology of the Interferon System, 1984. Edited by H. Kirchner, and H. Schellekens. Amsterdam, Elsevier Science Publishers, 1985, p. 293.
39. Elias, L., and Sandoval, J. M.: Interferon effects upon fluorouracil metabolism by HL-60 cells. Biochem. Biophys. Res. Commun., 163:867, 1989.
40. Eriksson, B., Oberg, K., Alm, G., Karlsson, A., Lundqvist, G., Magnusson, A., Wide, L., and Wilander, E.: Treatment of malignant endocrine pancreatic tumors with human leukocyte interferon. Cancer Treat. Rep., 71:31, 1987.
41. Ernstoff, M. S., Trautman, T., Davis, C. A., Reich, S. D., Witman, P., Balser, J., Rudnick, S., and Kirkwood, J. M.: A randomized Phase I/II study of continuous versus intermittent intravenous interferon gamma in patients with metastatic melanoma. J. Clin. Oncol., 5:1804, 1987.
42. Faltynek, C. R., Princler, G. L., Rossio, J. L., Ruscetti, F. W., Maluish, A. E., Abrams, P. G., and Foon, K. A.: Relationship of the clinical response and binding of recombinant IFN α in patients with lymphoproliferative diseases. Blood, 67:1077, 1986.
43. Fellous, M., Nir, U., Wallach, D., Merlin, G., Rubinstein, M., and Revel, M.: Interferon-dependent induction of mRNA for the major histocompatibility antigens in human fibroblasts and lymphoblastoid cells. Proc. Natl. Acad. Sci. (U.S.A.), 79:3082, 1982.
44. Fisher, P. B., Prignoli, D. R., Hermo, H., Jr., Weinstein, I. B., and Pestka, S.: Effects of combined treatment with interferon and mezerein on melanogenesis and growth in human melanoma cells. J. Interferon Res., 5:11, 1985.
45. Foon, K., Maluish, A. E., Abrams, P. G., Wrightington, S., Stevenson, H. C., Alarif, A., Fer, M. F., Overton, W. R., Poole, M., Schnipper, E. F., Jaffe, E. S., and Herberman, R. B.: Recombinant leukocyte A interferon therapy for advanced hairy cell leukemia—therapeutic and immunologic results. Am. J. Med., 80:351, 1986.
46. Foon, K. A., Bottino, G. C., Abrams, P. G., Fer, M. F., Longo, D. L., Schoenberger, C. S., and Oldham, R. K.: Phase II trial of recombinant leukocyte A interferon in patients with advanced chronic lymphocytic leukemia. Am. J. Med., 78:216, 1985.
47. Foon, K. A., Sherwin, S. A., Abrams, P. B., Longo, D. L., Fer, M. F., Stevenson, H. C., Ochs, J. J., Bottino, G. C., Schoenberger, C. S., Zeffren, J., Jaffe, E. S., and Oldham, R. K.: Treatment of advanced non-Hodgkin's lymphoma with recombinant leukocyte A interferon. N. Engl. J. Med., 311:1148, 1984.
48. Freund, M., von Wussow, P., Diedrich, H., Eisert, R., Link, H., Wilke, H., Buchholz, F., LeBlanc, S., Fonatsch, C., and Deicher, H.: Recombinant human IFN alpha-2b in chronic myelogenous leukaemia: dose dependency of response and frequency of neutralizing anti-IFN antibodies. Br. J. Haematol., 72:350, 1989.
49. Gewert, D. R., Moore, G., Tilleray, V. J., and Clemens, M. J.: Inhibition of cell proliferation by interferons. 1. Effects on cell division and DNA synthesis in human lymphoblasts (Daudi) cells. Eur. J. Biochem., 139:619, 1984.
50. Goldstein, D., and Laszlo, J.: Interferon therapy in cancer: From imaginon to interferon. Cancer Res., 46:4315, 1986.
51. Goldstein, D., Sielaff, K. M., Storer, B. E., Brown, R. R., Datta, S. P., Witt, P. L., Teitelbaum, A. P., Smalley, R. V., and Borden, E. C.: Human biologic response

modification by IFN in the absence of measurable serum concentrations: a comparative trial of subcutaneous and intravenous IFN-betaser. J. Natl. Cancer Inst., 81:1061, 1989.
52. Golomb, H. M., Jacobs, A., Fefer, A., Ozer, H., Thompson, J., Portlock, C., Ratain, M., Golde, D., Vardiman, J., Burke, J. S., Brady, J., Bonnem, E., and Spiegel, R.: Alpha-2 IFN therapy of hairy-cell leukemia: A multicenter study of 64 patients. J. Clin. Oncol., 4:900, 1986.
53. Gould, M. N., Kakria, R. C., Olson, S., and Borden, E. C.: Radiosensitization of human bronchogenic carcinoma cells by interferon beta. J. Interferon Res., 4:123, 1984.
54. Gray, P. W., and Goeddel, D. V.: Structure of the human immune interferon gene. Nature, 298:859, 1982.
55. Greenway, H. T., Cornell, R. C., Tanner, D. J., Peets, E., Bordin, G. M., and Nagi, C.: Treatment of basal cell carcinoma with intralesional interferon. J. Acad. Derm., 15:437, 1986.
56. Greiner, J. W., Schlom, J., Pestka, S., Langer, J. A., Giacomini, P., Kusama, M., Ferrone, S., and Fisher, P. B.: Modulation of tumor associated antigen expression and shedding by recombinant human leukocyte and fibroblast interferons. Pharmacol. Ther., 31:209, 1987.
57. Gresser, I., Belardelli, F., Maury, C., Maunoury, M. T., and Tovey, M.G.: Injection of mice with antibody to interferon enhances the growth of transplantable murine tumors. J. Exp. Med., 158:2095, 1983.
58. Gresser, I., Maury, C., and Belardelli, F.: Anti-tumor effects of IFN in mice injected with IFN-sensitive and IFN-resistant Friend leukemia cells. VI. Adjuvant therapy after surgery in the inhibition of liver and spleen metastases. Int. J. Cancer, 39:789, 1987.
59. Gresser, I., Tovey, M. G., Maury, C., and Bandu, M. T.: Role of interferon in the pathogenesis of virus diseases in mice as demonstrated by the use of anti-interferon serum. II. Studies with herpes simplex, Moloney sarcoma, vesicular stomatitis, Newcastle disease, and influenza viruses. J. Exp. Med., 144:1316, 1976.
60. Groopman, J. E., Gottlieb, M. S., Goodman, J., Mitsuyasu, R. T., Conant, M. A., Prince, H., Fahey, J. L., Derezin, M., Weinstein, W. M., Cusaranti, C., Rothman, J., Rudnick, S. A., and Volberding, P.A.: Recombinant alpha-2 interferon therapy for Kaposi's sarcoma associated with the acquired immunodeficiency syndrome. Ann. Int. Med., 100:671, 1984.
61. Gutterman, J. U., Fine, S., and Quesada, J.: Recombinant leukocyte A IFN: pharmacokinetics, single-dose tolerance, and biologic effects in cancer patients. Ann. Int. Med., 96:549, 1982.
62. Hawkins, M. J., Borden, E. C., Merritt, J. A., Edwards, B. S., Ball, L. A., Grossbard, E., and Simon, K.J.: Comparison of the biologic effects of two recombinant human interferons alpha (rA and rD) in humans. J. Clin. Oncol., 2:221, 1984.
63. Hawkins, M. J., Krown, S. E., Borden, E. C., Krim, M., Real, F. X., Edwards, B. S., Anderson, S. A., Cunningham-Rundles, S., and Oettgen, H. F.: American Cancer Society Phase I trial of naturally produced interferon beta. Cancer Res., 44:5934, 1984.
64. Herberman, R. B., Djeu, J. Y., Ortaldo, J. R., Holden, H. T., West, W. H., and Bonnard, G. D.: Role of interferon in augmentation of natural and antibody-dependent cell-mediated cytotoxicity. Cancer Treat. Rep., 62:1893, 1978.
65. Herberman, R. B., Ortaldo, J. R., Mantovani, A., Hobbs, D. S., Kung, H. F., and Pestka, S.: Effect of human recombinant interferon on cytotoxic activity of natural killer (NK) cells and monocytes. Cell. Immunol., 67:160, 1982.
66. Horisberger, M. A., and deStaritzky, K.: A recombinant human IFN-α B/D hybrid with a broad host range. J. Gen. Virol., 68:945, 1987.
67. Huber, C., Batchelor, J. R., Fuchs, D., Hausen, A., Lang, A., Niederwieser, D., Reibnegger, G., Swetly, P., Troppmair, J., and Wachter, H.: Immune response-associated production of neopterin: release from macrophages primarily under control of interferon-gamma. J. Exp. Med., 160:310, 1984.
68. Itri, L. M., Sherman, M. I., Palleroni, A. V., Evans, L. M., Tran, L. L., Campion, M., and Chizzonite, R.: Incidence and clinical significance of neutralizing antibodies in patients receiving recombinant IFN-α_{2a}. J. Interferon Res., 9:S9, 1989.
69. Jaffe, H. S., and Herberman, R. B.: Rationale for recombinant human interferon-gamma adjuvant immunotherapy for cancer. J. Natl. Cancer Inst., 80:616, 1988.
70. Johnson, H. M., and Torres, B. A.: Peptide growth factors PDGF, EGF, and FGF regulate interferon-gamma. J. Immunol., 134:2824, 1985.
71. King, D. P., and Jones, P. P.: Induction of IA and H-2 antigens on a macrophage cell line by immune interferon. J. Immunol., 131:315, 1983.
72. Kleinerman, E. S., Kurzrock, R., Wyatt, D., Quesada, J. R., Gutterman, J. U., and Fidler, I. J.: Activation or suppression of the tumoricidal properties of monocytes from cancer patients following treatment with human recombinant gamma-interferon. Cancer Res., 46:5401, 1986.
73. Kovacs, J. A., Deyton, L., Davey, R., Falloon, J., Zunich, K., Lee, D., Metcalf, J. A., Bigley, J. W., Sawyer, L. A., Zoon, K. C., Masur, H., Fauci, A. S., and Lane, H. C.: Combined zidovudine and interferon-alpha therapy in patients with Kaposi sarcoma and the acquired immunodeficiency syndrome (AIDS). Ann. Int. Med., 111:280, 1989.
74. Krown, S. E.: Therapeutic options in renal cell carcinoma. Semin. Oncol., 12:13, 1985.
75. Krown, S. E.: Interferons and interferon inducers in cancer treatment. Semin. Oncol., 13:207, 1986.
76. Krown, S. E., Gold, J. W. M., Niedzwiecki, D., Bundow, D., Flomenberg, N., Gansbacher, B., and Brew, B. J.: Interferon alpha with zidovudine: Safety, tolerance and clinical and virological effects in patients with Kaposi sarcoma associated with the acquired immunodeficiency syndrome. Ann. Int. Med., 112:812, 1990.
77. Krown, S. E., Real, F. X., Cunningham-Rundles, S., et al.: Preliminary observations on the effect of recombinant leukocyte A interferon in homosexual men with Kaposi's sarcoma. N. Engl. J. Med., 308:1071, 1983.
78. Kurzrock, R., Talpaz, M., Kantarjian, H., Walters, R., Saks, S., Trujillo, J. M., and Gutterman, J. U.: Therapy of chronic myelogenous leukemia with recombinant IFN-γ. Blood, 70:943, 1987.
79. Kushnaryov, V. M., MacDonald, H. S., Sedmak, J. J., and Grossberg, S. E.: Murine interferon-beta receptor-mediated endocytosis and nuclear membrane binding. Proc. Natl. Acad. Sci. (U.S.A.), 82:3281, 1985.
80. Kuzmits, R., Ludwig, H., Kratzik, C., et al.: Neopterin as tumor marker: Serum and urinary neopterin concentrations in malignant diseases. J. Clin. Chem. Clin. Biochem., 24:119, 1986.
81. Lane, H. C., Kovacs, J. A., Feinberg, J., Herpin, B., Davey, V., Walker, R., Deyton, L., Metcalf, J. A., Baseler, M., Salzman, N., Manischewitz, J., Quinnan, G., Masur, H., and Fauci, A. S.: Anti-retroviral effects of interferon-α in AIDS-associated Kaposi's sarcoma. Lancet, 2:1218, 1988.
82. Larocca, A. P., Leung, S. C., Marcus, S. G., Colby, C. B., and Borden, E. C.: Evaluation of neutralizing antibodies in patients treated with recombinant IFN-βser. J. Interferon Res., 9:S51, 1989.
83. Lin, J., and Sartorelli, A. C.: Stimulation by interferon of the differentiation of human promyelocytic leukemia (HL-60) cells produced by retinoic acid and actinomycin D. J. Interferon Res., 7:379, 1987.
84. Lin, S. L., Greene, J. J., Ts'o, P. O. P., and Carter, W. A.: Sensitivity and resistance of human tumor cells to interferon and $rI_n \cdot rC_n$. Nature, 297:417, 1982.
85. Litton, G. J., Hong, R., Grossberg, S. E., Vechlekar, D., Goodavish, C. N., and Borden, E. C.: Biological and clinical effects of the oral immunomodulator 3,6-bis (2-piperidinoethoxy)acridine trihydrochloride in patients with malignancy. J. Biol. Response Mod., 9:61, 1990.
86. Lotze, M. T., Frana, L. W., Sharrow, S. O., Robb, R. J., and Rosenberg, S. A.: *In vivo* administration of purified human interleukin 2. Half-life and immunologic effects of the Jurkat cell line-derived interleukin 2. J. Immunol., 134:157, 1985.
87. Ludwig, H., Cortelezzi, A., van Camp, B. G. K., Polli, E., Scheithauer, W., Kuzmits, R., Linkesch, W., Gisslinger, H., Sinzinger, H., Fritz, E., and Flener, R.: Treatment with recombinant IFN-α-2C: Multiple myeloma and thrombocythaemia in myeloproliferative diseases. Oncology, 42:19, 1985.
88. Mahaley, M. S., Urso, M. B., Whaley, R. A., Blue, M., Williams, T. E., Guaspari, A., and Selker, R. G.: Immunobiology of primary intracranial tumors: Part 10: Therapeutic efficacy of interferon in the treatment of recurrent gliomas. J. Neurosurg., 63:719, 1985.
89. Maluish, A. E., Leavitt, R., Sherwin, S. A., Oldham, R. K., and Herberman, R. B.: Effects of recombinant interferon-alpha on immune function in cancer patients. J. Biol. Response Mod., 2:470, 1983.
90. Maluish, A. E., Urba, W. J., Longo, D. L., Overton, W. R., Coggin, D., Crisp, E. R., Williams, R., Sherwin, S. A., Gordon, K., and Steis, R. G.: The determination of an immunologically active dose of interferon-gamma in patients with melanoma. J. Clin. Oncol., 6:434, 1988.
91. Mandelli, F., Avvisati, G., Amadori, S., Boccadora, M., Gernone, A., Lauta, V. M., Marmont, F., Petrucci, M. T., Tribalto, M., Vegna, M. L., Dammacco, F., and Pileri, A.: Maintenance treatment with recombinant interferon alfa-2b in patients with multiple myeloma responding to conventional induction chemotherapy. N. Engl. J. Med., 322:1430, 1990.
92. Maniatis, T.: Mechanisms of human beta-interferon gene regulation. The Harvey Lectures, 82:71, 1988.
93. Martin, A., Nerenstone, S., Urba, W. J., Longo, D. L., Lawrence, J. B., Clark, J. W., Hawkins, M. J., Creekmore, S. P., Smith, J. W., II, and Steis, R. G.: Treatment of hairy cell leukemia with alternating cycles of pentostatin and recombinant leukocyte A interferon: Results of a Phase II study. J. Clin. Oncol., 8:721, 1990.
94. Massaro, E. R., Borden, E. C., Hawkins, M. J., Wiebe, D. A., and Shrago, E.: Effects of recombinant interferon-alpha-2 treatment upon lipid concentrations and lipoprotein composition. J. Interferon Res., 6:655, 1986.
95. Merritt, J. A., Ball, L. A., Sielaff, K. M., Meltzer, D. M., and Borden, E. C.: Modulation of 2',5'-oligoadenylate synthetase in patients treated with alpha-interferon: effects of dose, schedule, and route of administration. J. Interferon Res., 6:189, 1986.
96. Michaelvicz, R., and Revel, M.: IFNs regulate the *in vivo* differentiation of multilineage lympho-myeloid stem cells in hairy cell leukemia. Proc. Natl. Acad. Sci. (U.S.A.), 84:2307, 1987.
97. Miles, S. A., Wang, H., Cortes, E., Carden, J., Marcus, S., and Mitsuyasu, R. T.: Beta-interferon therapy in patients with poor-prognosis Kaposi sarcoma related to the acquired immunodeficiency syndrome (AIDS). Ann. Int. Med., 112:582, 1990.
98. Moertel, C. G., Rubin, J., and Kvols, L. K.: Therapy of metastatic carcinoid tumor and the malignant carcinoid syndrome with recombinant leukocyte A IFN. J. Clin. Oncol., 7:865, 1989.
99. Nagai, M., and Arai, T.: Clinical effect of interferon in malignant brain tumours. Neurosurg. Rev., 7:55, 1984.
100. Nagata, S., Mantei, N., and Weissmann, C.: The structure of the eight or more distinct chromosomal genes for human interferon-alpha. Nature, 287:401, 1980.
101. Nathan, C. F.: Secretory products of macrophage. J. Clin. Invest., 79:319, 1987.
102. Nathan, C. F., Prendergast, T. J., Wiebe, M. E., Stanley, E. R., Platzer, E., Remold, H. G., Welte, K., Rubin, B. Y., and Murray, H. W.: Activation of human macrophages comparison of other cytokines with interferon-alpha. J. Exp. Med., 160:600, 1984.
103. Nelson, B. E., and Borden, E. C.: Interferons: Biological and clinical effects. Semin. Surg. Oncol., 5:391, 1989.
104. Nolten, W. E., Goldstein, D., Lindstrom, M., McKenna, M. V., Carlson, I. H., Trump, D. L., Schiller, J. H., Borden, E. C., and Ehrlich, E. N.: Effects of cytokines on the pituitary adrenal axis in humans. J. Lab. Clin. Med., submitted, 1990.
105. Oberg, K., Alm, G., Lindstrom, H., and Lundqvist, G.: Successful treatment of therapy-resistant pancreatic cholera with human leukocyte interferon. Lancet, 1:725, 1985.
106. Oberg, K., Alm, G., Magnusson, A., Lundqvist, G., Theodorsson, E., Wide, L., and Wilander, E.: Treatment of malignant carcinoid tumors with recombinant interferon alfa-2b: development of neutralizing IFN antibodies and possible loss of antitumor activity. J. Natl. Cancer Inst., 81:531, 1989.
107. Oberg, K., Norheim, I., Lind, E., Alm, G., Lundqvist, G., Wide, L., Jonsdottir, B., Magnusson, A., and Wilander, E.: Treatment of malignant carcinoid tumors with human leukocyte interferon: Long-term results. Cancer Treat. Rep., 70:1297, 1986.
108. O'Connell, M. J., Colgan, J. P., Oken, M. M., Ritts, R. E., Jr., Kay, N. E., and Itri, L. M.: Clinical trial of recombinant leukocyte A interferons as initial therapy for favorable histology non-Hodgkin's lymphoma and chronic lymphocytic leukemia. An ECOG pilot study. J. Clin. Oncol., 4:128, 1986.
109. Oken, M. M., Kyle, R. A., Greipp, P. R., Kay, N. E., Tsiatis, A., and O'Connell, M. J.: Chemotherapy plus IFN in the treatment of multiple myeloma. Proceedings ASCO, 9:288, 1990.
110. Ostlünd, L., Einhorn, S., Robert, K. H., Juliusson, G., and Biberfeld, P.: Chronic B-lymphocytic leukemia cells proliferate and differentiate following exposure to interferon *in vitro*. Blood, 67:152, 1986.
111. Ozaki, Y., Edelstein, M. P., and Duch, D. S.: Induction of indoleamine 2,3-dioxygenase: a mechanism of the antitumor activity of IFN γ. Proc. Natl. Acad. Sci., 85:1242, 1988.
112. Ozer, H.: Biotherapy of chronic myelogenous leukemia with IFN. Semin. Oncol., 15:14, 1988.

113. Paulnock, D. M., Havlin, K. A., Storer, B. M., Spear, G. T., Sielaff, K. M., and Borden, E. C.: Induced proteins in human peripheral mononuclear cells over a range of clinically tolerable doses of interferon-gamma. J. Interferon Res., 9:457, 1989.
114. Pestka, S.: The purification and manufacture of human interferon. Sci. Am., 249:37, 1983.
115. Pestka, S., Langer, J. A., Zoon, K. C., and Samuel, C. E.: IFNs and their actions. Ann. Rev. Biochem., 56:727, 1987.
116. Pfeffer, L. M., and Tamm, I.: Comparison of the effects of α and β interferons on the proliferation and volume of human tumor cells (HeLa-S3, Daudi, P_3HR-1). J. Interferon Res., 3:395, 1983.
117. Quesada, J. R., Alexanian, R., Hawkins, M. J., Barlogie, B., Borden, E. C., and Gutterman, J.: Treatment of multiple myeloma with recombinant alpha interferon. Blood, 67:275, 1986.
118. Quesada, J. R., Hersh, E. M., Manning, J., Reuben, J., Keating, M., Schnipper, E., Itri, L., and Gutterman, J. U.: Treatment of hairy cell leukemia with recombinant alpha-interferon. Blood, 68:493, 1986.
119. Quesada, J. R., Kurzrock, R., Sherwin, S. A., and Guttermann, J. U.: Phase II studies of recombinant human interferon γ in metastatic renal cell carcinoma. J. Biol. Res. Mod., 6:20, 1987.
120. Quesada, J. R., Swanson, D. A., and Gutterman, J. U.: Phase II study of alpha interferon in metastatic renal cell carcinoma: a progress report. J. Clin. Oncol., 3:1086, 1985a.
121. Quesada, J. R., Rios, A., Swanson, D., Trown, P., and Gutterman, J. U.: Antitumor activity of recombinant derived interferon alpha in metastatic renal carcinoma. J. Clin. Oncol., 3:1522, 1985b.
122. Quesada, J. R., Talpaz, M., Rios, A., Kurzrock, R., and Gutterman, J.U.: Clinical toxicity of interferons in cancer patients: A review. J. Clin. Oncol., 4:234, 1986.
123. Rambaldi, A., Introna, M., Colotta, F., Landolfo, S., Columbo, N., Mangioni, C., and Mantovani, A.: Intraperitoneal administration of interferon β in ovarian cancer patients. Cancer, 56:294, 1985.
124. Rashidbaigi, A., Langer, J. A., Jung, V., Jones, C., Morse, H. G., Tischfield, J. A., Trill, J. J., Kung, H. F., and Pestka, S.: The gene for the human immune interferon receptor is located on chromosome 6. Proc. Natl. Acad. Sci. (U.S.A.), 83:384, 1986.
125. Ratain, M. J., Golomb, H. M., Bardawil, R. G., Vardiman, J. W., Westbrook, C. A., Kaminer, L. S., Lembersky, B. C., Bitter, M. A., and Daly, K.: Durability of responses to interferon alfa-2B in advanced hairy cell leukemia. Blood, 69:872, 1987.
126. Real, F. X., Oettgen, H. F., and Krown, S. E.: Kaposi's sarcoma and the acquired immunodeficiency syndrome: Treatment with high and low doses of recombinant leukocyte A interferon. J. Clin. Oncol., 4:544, 1986.
127. Recombinant Human Interferon Gamma (S-6810) Research Group on Renal Cell Carcinoma: Phase II study of recombinant human interferon gamma (S-6810) on renal cell carcinoma: summary of two collaborative studies. Cancer, 60:929, 1987.
128. Reid, L. M., Minato, N., Gresser, I., Holland, J., Kadish, A. R., and Bloom, B. R.: Influence of antimouse interferon serum on the growth and metastasis of tumor cells persistently infected with virus and of human prostatic tumors in athymic mice. Proc. Natl. Acad. Sci. (U.S.A.), 78:1171, 1981.
129. Reid, T. R., Race, E. R., Wolff, B. H., Friedman, R. M., Merigan, T. C., and Basham, T. Y.: Enhanced *in vivo* therapeutic response to interferon in mice with an *in vitro* interferon-resistant B-cell lymphoma. Cancer Res., 49:4163, 1989.
130. Revel, M., and Chebath, J.: IFN-activated genes. Trends in Biochemical Science, 11:166, 1986.
131. Rios, A., Mansell, P. W. A., Newell, G. R., Reuben, J. M., Hersh, E. M., and Guttermann, J. U.: Treatment of acquired immunodeficiency syndrome-related Kaposi's sarcoma with lymphoblastoid interferon. J. Clin. Oncol., 3:506, 1985.
132. Rios, A., Stringfellow, D. A., Fitzpatrick, F. A., Reele, S. B., Gutknecht, G. D., and Hersh, E. M.: Phase I study of 2-amino-5-bromo-6-phenyl-4(3H)-pyrimidinone (ABPP), an oral interferon inducer, in cancer patients. J. Biol. Response Mod., 5:330, 1986.
133. Riviere, Y., and Hovanessian, A. G.: Direct action of interferon and inducers of interferon on tumor cells in athymic nude mice. Cancer Res., 43:4596, 1983.
134. Robinson, W. A., Mughal, T. I., Thomas, M. R., Johnson, M., and Spiegel, R. J.: Treatment of metastatic melanoma with recombinant interferon alpha 2. Immunobiology, 172:275, 1986.
135. Rosenzweig, I. B., Wiebe, D. A., Borden, E. C., Storer, B., and Shrago, E. S.: Plasma lipoprotein changes in humans induced by beta interferon. Atherosclerosis, 67:261, 1987.
136. Ruzicka, F. J., Jach, M. E., and Borden, E. C.: Binding of recombinant-produced interferon beta-ser to human lymphoblastoid cells: Evidence of two binding domains. J. Biol. Chem., 262:16142, 1987.
137. Samid, D., Flessate, D. M., Greene, J. J., Chang, E. H., and Friedman, R. M.: Persisting Revertants After Interferon Treatment of Oncogene-Transformed Cells. *In* The Biology of the Interferon System 1985. Edited by W. E. Stewart, III, and H. Schellekens. Amsterdam, Elsevier Science Publishers, 1986, p. 327.
138. Sariban, E., Mitchell, T., Griffin, J., and Kufe, D. W.: Effects of interferon-γ on proto-oncogene expression during induction of human monocytic differentiation. J. Immunol., 138:1954, 1987.
139. Schiller, J. H., Bittner, G., Storer, B., and Willson, J. K. V.: Synergistic antitumor effects of tumor necrosis factor and gamma-interferon on human colon carcinoma cell lines. Cancer Res., 47:2809, 1987.
140. Schiller, J. H., Groveman, D. S., Schmid, S. M., Willson, J. K. V., Cummings, K. B., and Borden, E. C.: Synergistic antiproliferative effects of human recombinant α54- or βser interferon with γ interferon on human cell lines of various histogenesis. Cancer Res., 46:483, 1986.
141. Scott, G. M., Ward, R. J., Wright, D. J., Robinson, J. A., Onwubalili, J. K., and Gauci, C. L.: Effects of cloned IFN α2 in normal volunteers: febrile reactions and changes in circulating corticosteroids and trace metals. Antimicrob. Agents Chemother., 23:589, 1983.
142. Selby, P., Kohn, J., Raymond, J., Judson, I., and McElwain, T.: Nephrotic syndrome during treatment with IFN. Br. Med. J., 290:1180, 1985.
143. Shearer, M., and Taylor-Papadimitriou, J.: Regulation of cell growth by interferon. Cancer Metastasis Rev., 6:199, 1987.
144. Sokawa, Y., Watanabe, Y., Watanabe, Y., and Kawade, Y.: Interferon suppresses the transition of quiescent 3T3 cells to a growing state. Nature, 268:236, 1977.
145. Sreevalsan, T., Taylor-Papadimitriou, J., and Rozengurt, E.: Selective inhibition by interferon of serum-stimulated biochemical events in 3T3 cells. Biochem. Biophys. Commun., 87:679, 1979.
146. Stevenson, H. C., Dekaban, G. A., Miller, P. J., Benyajati, C., and Pearson, M. L.: Analysis of human blood monocyte activation at the level of gene expression. J. Exp. Med., 161:503, 1985.
147. Stolfi, R. L., and Martin, D. S.: Modulation of chemotherapeutic drug activity with polyribonucleotides or with interferon. J. Biol. Response Mod., 4:634, 1985.
148. Stolfi, R. L., Martin, D. S., Sawyer, R. C., and Spiegelman, S.: Modulation of 5-fluorouracil-induced toxicity in mice with interferon or with the interferon inducer, polyinosinic-polycytidylic acid. Cancer Res., 43:561, 1983.
149. Strander, H., Adamson, U., and Aparisi, T.: Adjuvant interferon treatment of human osteosarcoma. Recent Results Cancer Res., 68:40, 1978.
150. Streuli, M., Nagata, S., and Weissmann, C.: At least three human type alpha interferons: Structure of alpha 2. Science, 209:1343, 1980.
151. Sumpio, B. E., Ernstoff, M. S., and Kirkwood, J. M.: Urinary excretion of IFN, albumin and β_2-microglobulin during IFN treatment. Cancer Res., 44:3599, 1984.
152. Takikawa, O., Kuroiwa, T., Yamazaki, F., and Kido, R.: Mechanism of interferon γ action: characterization of indoleamine 2,3-dioxygenase in cultured human cells induced by interferon gamma and evaluation of the enzyme-mediated tryptophan degradation in its anticellular activity. J. Biol. Chem., 263:2041, 1988.
153. Talpaz, M., Kantarjian, H. M., McCredie, K. B., Keating, M. J., Trujillo, J., and Gutterman, J.: Clinical investigation of human alpha IFN in chronic myelogenous leukemia. Blood, 69:1280, 1987.
154. Talpaz, M., Kantarjian, H. M., McCredie, K., Trujillo, J. M., Keating, M. J., and Gutterman, J. U.: Hematologic remission and cytogenetic improvement induced by recombinant human interferon alpha (A) in chronic myelogenous leukemia. N. Engl. J. Med., 314:1065, 1986.
155. Talpaz, M., Kurzrock, R., Kantarjian, H., O'Brien, S., and Gutterman, J. U.: Recombinant IFN-α therapy of Philadelphia chromosome-negative myeloproliferative disorders with thrombocytosis. Am. J. Med., 86:554, 1989.
156. Talpaz, M., Rosenblum, M., Kurzrock, R., Reuben, J., Kantarjian, H., and Gutterman, J.: Clinical and laboratory changes induced by alpha IFN in chronic lymphocytic leukemia—A pilot study. Am. J. Hematol., 24:341, 1987.
157. Tamura, K., Makino, S., Araki, Y., Imamura, T., and Seita, M.: Recombinant IFN β and γ in the treatment of adult T-cell leukemia. Cancer, 59:1059, 1987.
158. Tan, Y. H.: Chromosome 21 and the cell growth inhibitory effect of human interferon preparations. Nature, 260:141, 1976.
159. Taniguchi, T.: Regulation of interferon-beta gene: structure and function of cis-elements and trans-acting factors. J. Interferon Res., 9:633, 1989.
160. Tokazewski-chen, S. A., Marafino, B. J., Jr., and Stebbing, N.: Effects of nephrectomy on the pharmacokinetics of various cloned human IFNs in the rat. J. Pharmacol. Exp. Ther., 227:9, 1983.
161. Torti, F. M., Shortliffe, L. D., Williams, R. D., Pitts, W. C., Kempson, R. L., Ross, J. C., Palmer, J., Meyers, F., Ferrari, M., Hannigan, J., Spiegel, R., McWhirter, K., and Freiha, F.: Alpha interferon in superficial bladder cancer: A Northern California Oncology Group study. J. Clin. Oncol., 6:476, 1988.
162. Tsuruo, T., Iida, H., Tsukagoshi, S., Oku, T., and Kishida, T.: Different susceptibilities of cultured mouse cell lines to mouse interferon. Gann, 73:42, 1982.
163. Urba, W. J., Longo, D. L., and Weiss, R. B.: Enhancement of natural killer activity in human peripheral blood by flavone acetic acid. J. Natl. Cancer Inst., 80:521, 1988.
164. Uzé, G., Lutfalla, G., and Gresser, I.: Genetic transfer of a functional human IFNα receptor into mouse cells: Cloning and expression of its DNA. Cell, 60:225, 1990.
165. Volberding, P. A., Mitsuyasu, R. T., Golando, J. P., and Spiegel, R. J.: Treatment of Kaposi's sarcoma interferon alfa-2b (Intron A). Cancer, 59:620, 1987.
166. Von Wussow, P., Jakschies, D., Freund, M., and Deicher, H.: Humoral response to recombinant IFN-α_{2b} in patients receiving recombinant IFN-α_{2b}. J. Interferon Res., 9:S25, 1989.
167. Wadler, S., Schwartz, E. L., Goldman, M., Lyver, A., Rader, M., Zimmerman, M., Itri, L., Weinberg, V., and Wiernik, P. H.: Fluorouracil and recombinant alfa-2A interferon: An active regimen against advanced colorectal carcinoma. J. Clin. Oncol., 7:1769, 1989.
168. Wagstaff, J., Scarffe, J. H., and Crowther, D.: Interferon in the treatment of multiple myeloma and the non-Hodgkin's lymphomas. Cancer Treat. Rep., 12B:39, 1985.
169. Welander, C. E.: IFN in the treatment of ovarian cancer. Semin. Oncol., 15:26, 1988.
170. Williams, R. D.: Intravesical IFN α in the treatment of superficial bladder cancer. Semin. Oncol., 15:10, 1988.
171. Wills, R. J., Dennis, S., Spiegel, H. E., Gibson, D. M., and Nadler, P. I.: IFN kinetics and adverse reactions after intravenous, intramuscular, and subcutaneous injection. Clin. Pharmacol. Ther., 35:722, 1984.
172. Yasui, H., Takai, K., Yoshida, R., and Hayaishi, O.: Interferon enhances tryptophan metabolism by inducing indoleamine 2,3-dioxygenase: its possible occurrence in cancer patients. Proc. Natl. Acad. Sci. (U.S.A.), 83:6622, 1986.
173. Young, H. A., and Ortaldo, J. R.: One-signal requirement for interferon-gamma production by human large granular lymphocytes. J. Immunol., 139:724, 1987.
174. Yung, W. K. A., Castellanos, A., Van Tassel, T., Moser, R., and Marcus, S.: A pilot study of recombinant IFN betaser in patients with recurrent gliomas. J. Neurooncol., 9:29, 1990.

Acknowledgement

Research on interferons in my laboratories is primarily supported by the National Cancer Institute, American Cancer Society, Triton Biosciences, 3M Pharmaceuticals and CIBA-GEIGY. Allison Greenwald, Kathy Edge, and Mike Recht contributed valuable assistance in manuscript completion.

Tumor Necrosis Factor

James S. Economou

History

At the turn of the century, Coley and Fehleisen attempted to induce regression of cancers by the administration of filtrates of mixtures of killed bacteria.[40] These trials were based upon the observation that a number of patients with spontaneously regressing cancers were found to have concurrent bacterial infections. Coley used killed bacteria of Streptococcus pyogenes and Serratia marcescens which came to be known as Coley's toxins. A number of patients, in fact, had dramatic regressions. The active factor in these filtrates was subsequently shown to be lipopolysaccharide (LPS). These investigations lay dormant until Old studied this phenomenon in mice.[5,40] The serum of Bacillus Calmette-Guérin (BCG) infected mice, subsequently injected with LPS, had a factor that caused the hemorrhagic necrosis of a number of experimental tumors in vivo. This activity was termed "tumor necrosis factor" (TNF).[58]

Molecular Biology

Pennica and colleagues were the first to clone human TNF in 1984.[42] TNF was purified to homogeneity from filtrates of phorbol myristate acetate stimulated HL60 cells. TNF is not glycosylated in any species, and is translated as a propeptide with a 79 amino acid leader sequence.[1] This propeptide is cleaved at approximately 8 sites during protein processing yielding a 157 amino peptide with a relative molecular mass of 17,000 daltons.[67] TNF is moderately hydrophobic and forms dimers, trimers and pentamers, a multimeric arrangement that may be required for biological activity.[1] The primary structure of TNF has been conserved in evolution and there is close homology between TNFs of several species.[1] The structure of the TNF trimer has been analyzed by X-ray crystallography at a 2.9Å level of resolution.[25] It has a topology very similar to that of viral proteins which provides for a very stable secondary structure.

In the course of cloning TNF, it was discovered that it is closely related to another cytotoxin known as lymphotoxin (LT).[34] Lymphotoxin, which has also been termed TNF beta, is tightly linked with TNF on the short arm of chromosome 6 with only about a thousand base pairs separating the 3' region of the LT gene and the 5' region of the TNF gene.[67] There is 28% amino acid homology between these two proteins and a nucleotide homology of 46%. There is particular conservation in the regions at amino acids 35–66 and 110–133. LT has an additional 18 amino acids at the N terminal region of the molecule. A polypeptide characterized by Cerami and Beutler termed "cachectin" was demonstrated in 1985 to be identical to TNF.[2]

TNF is largely produced by cells of the monocyte-macrophage lineage.[44] In fact, when stimulated with LPS, TNF may amount to approximately 1% of the total secretory product of those cells.[1] It has been shown, however, that a wide variety of other cell types produce TNF. These include T cells and B cells, natural killer (NK) cells, lymphokine activated killer (LAK) cells, astrocytes, neutrophils, and glial cells.[1,41,59,61,62] Interestingly, approximately half of the tumor cell lines tested of various tissue origins constitutively express TNF and LT mRNA.[29,39] These findings demonstrate that TNF and LT expression is a rather common phenomenon in long-term culture of tumor cell lines and raises the question whether production of these cytokines by tumor cells might be involved in certain paraneoplastic syndromes.

A potent activation signal for TNF production is LPS.[1] Depending upon the cell type, a variety of other induction signals are effective. These include phorbol esters, IL-1, IL-2, granulocyte-macrophage colony stimulating factor and anti-CD3 antibody. Interestingly, interleukin-4 down regulates TNF gene expression, as well as production of IL-1, gamma interferon and IL-6.[17,63]

TNF and LT utilize different promoters. The TNF promoter region has been the best characterized and the phorbol ester response elements are found within 95 base pairs of the transcription start site.[14] LPS response elements may be upstream in kappa B enhancer sequences.[51] TNF is profoundly regulated at the level of translation.[20,21,45] As with other inflammatory cytokines, the 3' untranslated region contains an AU rich sequence which is important in both message stability and translation rate.[53] Thus, in macrophages primed with gamma interferon a considerable amount of TNF message may accumulate in the cytoplasm, but is not translated until activitation of an appropriate signal, such as that induced by LPS.[21] This results in a translational upregulation of several orders of magnitude.

Stable TNF trimers bind to receptors on various cell types with dissociation constants ranging from 10^{-9} to 10^{-11} M.[31] There may be two different TNF receptors that differ in affinity, cell type (myeloid vs. epithelial), size and glycosylation.[47] The receptor(s) appear to bind TNF and LT with equal affinity. Several groups have cloned TNF receptors and have found them to be typical cell surface receptor proteins (signal peptide, extracellular, domains) with a significant degree of homology to the nerve growth factor receptor.[54] The mechanism of signal transduction by TNF is not known; the cytoplasmic domain has no apparent sequence homology to any known protein. A soluble form of the TNF-receptor has been described and this is potentially a protective mechanism by which cells may avoid cytotoxic action.[50]

Biological Properties
Antitumor Activity

Human and murine tumor cell lines have varying degrees of susceptibility to the cytotoxic action of TNF in vitro and in vivo.[10,60] TNF is cytotoxic or cytostatic for somewhat more than half of cancer cell lines. The concentration required to inhibit growth of nontransformed cells is several orders of magnitude higher. However, when used in vivo against experimental tumors, TNF appears to be most effective when these tumors have reached a size of approximately 5–6 mm. With the same tumor type there is little effect on smaller metastases, namely those less than 1 mm in diameter. These findings suggest that the action of TNF in vivo might be related to factors other than sensitivity of the tumor cell.

TNF has direct toxic effects on newly formed tumor vasculature which include hemorrhage, congestion and thrombosis. TNF also acts upon endothelial cells. When endothelial cells are treated with TNF they produce procoagulant activity on the cell surface which leads to fibrin formation and defective perfusion.[37,38,46] Within 24–48 hours after TNF administration, tumor vessels are packed with leukocytes, and morphological changes within the tumor are consistent with hemorrhagic necrosis.[68] This is in concert with the original observations of Old that necrosis is largely central and leaves a rim of viable tumor.[5] However, the repeated demonstration that mice bearing some experimental tumors can be either cured or sustain partial regressions when treated with recombinant TNF has generated considerable clinical interest.

Even though some cancer cells are very sensitive to TNF and others are not, treatment of insensitive cells with inhibitors of transcription or protein synthesis frequently generate sensitive targets.[40,44] These observations, in addition to providing some insight into the mechanism of the action of TNF, might be exploited in clinical applications of this cytotoxin.

The mechanism of TNF cytotoxicity is unknown, but it can occur in the absence of RNA or protein synthesis.[1] Agents that disrupt different phases of the endocytic process, such as chloroquine and colchicine, inhibit TNF killing of target cells. Microinjection of TNF into the cytoplasm causes rapid killing of cells.[55] These observations suggest that TNF may need to be internalized for certain biological effects. It has been suggested that TNF may mediate the generation of hydrogen peroxide or oxygen-free radicals. Antioxidant enzymes such as catalase, superoxide dismutase (SOD) and glutathione peroxidase protect cells from free radicals and hydrogen peroxide. Wong and Goeddel demonstrated that TNF treatment effectively and rapidly induces mRNA for MnSOD both in vitro and in vivo.[69] MnSOD is probably one of the proteins involved in protecting cells from the cytotoxic effects of TNF. In another line of investigation, Cooke and colleagues demonstrated that the E1A oncogene of the group C human adenoviruses induces the susceptibility of transformed cells to the lytic effects of TNF.[4,9] There appears to be a threshold of E1A oncogene expression required for induction of a high level of TNF susceptibility. Finally, amplified expression of the HER2/neu gene is associated with an increase in resistance to TNF, as well as resistance to macrophage-mediated cytotoxicity.[30] This oncogene is a cell surface protein closely related to the epidermal growth factor receptor. Amplification of this oncogene is associated with human breast and ovarian cancers and has been shown to correlate very closely with susceptibility to TNF.

Augmentation of Immune Responses

Several lines of evidence suggest that TNF may augment host immunity to tumors.[19,24,48] Eisenthal and Rosenberg using a mouse model, demonstrated that TNF significantly increases IL-2 induced antibody dependent cellular cytotoxicity (ADCC) activity.[15] TNF does not augment ADCC activity by itself, but significantly enhances that generated by IL-2 using both thymocytes and spleen cells as effectors. In addition, TNF appears to play a role in the generation of LAK. The addition of TNF to IL-2 driven PBL significantly enhances LAK activity.[6] Moreover, it appears that the secondary production of TNF in these IL-2 cultures plays an important role in the generation of these effector cells. The addition of IL-4 to these cultures, which inhibits the production of TNF, also inhibits the generation of LAK activity. The addition of TNF to low concentrations of IL-2 also promotes differentiation of large granular lymphocytes into LAK cells. TNF also activates neutrophils.[28,52] TNF nonspecifically increases antibody production in mice and in a variety of systems, such as listeria, appears to play an important role in antibacterial and antiviral resistance.[33] TNF induces the expression of the IL-2 receptor and promotes the proliferation of T and B cells. Thus, the use of TNF as an antitumor biological may eventually prove to act more effectively through immune effector mechanisms rather than by direct cytotoxic activity.

Macrophages play an important role in tumor immunity and several lines of evidence demonstrate that TNF has an important but not an exclusive role in macrophage-mediated cyto-toxicity.[22,43] However, neither TNF nor LT appears to mediate NK, LAK or cytotoxic T cell-mediated cytotoxicity.[23,37]

Other Biological Properties

TNF plays a major role in the pathogenesis of gram-negative shock.[36] The administration of TNF causes many of the deleterious effects of shock including fever, metabolic acidosis, diarrhea, hypotension and disseminated intravascular coagulation.[12,18] Passive immunization against TNF ameliorates many of the effects of endotoxin (LPS) administration.[3] A number of laboratories have demonstrated that moderate doses of TNF to experimental animals induces anorexia and weight loss.[64] Thus, the term "cachectin" is just as appropriate for this cytokine as tumor necrosis factor. TNF induces a number of other secondary cytokines such as IL-1 and IL-6 and these may contribute to the pathophysiological effects of this cytokine.[35]

The chronic administration of sublethal doses of TNF to rats induces a syndrome of cachexia that includes anorexia, weight loss, depletion of whole body protein and lipid stores, reduction of red blood cell mass, leukocytosis and tissue inflammation.[64] Chronic exposure to TNF during cancer or chronic disease may contribute to cachexia.

Preclinical and Clinical Trials
Preclinical Animal Trials

Since the early observations by Old, TNF has been tested in a variety of experimental systems for activity against experimental tumors. As stated earlier, some mice may be cured of experimental tumors or achieve significant regressions. TNF has been studied in animal systems in combination with other biologicals such as IL-2 and interferon gamma.[7] Rosenberg and colleagues have studied the in vivo administration of TNF in combination with high dose IL-2 in the treatment of murine experimental tumors.[32] They observed a synergistic antitumor effect of combination therapy against weakly immunogenic sarcomas growing subcutaneously and in visceral sites. Interestingly, neither of these biologicals had an effect on non-immunogenic tumors. Histologically, these tumors underwent initial necrosis and subsequent inflammatory responses. These findings suggested that IL-2 might promote the proliferation and activation of such anti-tumor effector cells in these inflammatory infiltrates. An Lyt 2 positive effector lymphocyte was felt to play an important role in TNF mediated tumor rejection. Other biologicals, such as gamma interferon, when used in combination with TNF have a synergistic antitumor effect with similar histologic findings.

TNF may be combined with IL-2 and monoclonal anti-CD3 antibody in vivo in the treatment of established murine pulmonary metastases.[70] Although the mechanism of anti-tumor activity is not firmly established, it probably permits the selective activation of cellular effectors. Moreover, this high degree of synergy permits reduced doses of IL-2 and TNF resulting in lessened toxicity.

It has been known for some time that the administration of one recombinant cytokine into patients or experimental animals generally results in the induction of secondary cytokines. This has certainly been demonstrated for TNF in which both IL-6 and IL-1 have been shown to be secondarily induced in vivo.[16] Also, the administration of IL-2 to both experimental animals and cancer patients results in the secondary production of TNF as well as gamma interferon. The secondary production of these cytokines may account for both the toxic side-effects and the antitumor activity of this type of biological therapy.

Human Clinical Trials

TNF has been administered in over a dozen phase I trials to patients with a variety of advanced cancers.[56,66] The maximum tolerated dose of TNF caused toxicity that included influenza-like syndromes, transient decrease in circulating lymphocyte and platelet counts, subclinical evidence of disseminated intravascular coagulation and the occasional occurrence of acute pulmonary toxicity.[8] In addition, TNF treatment has been associated with a capillary leak syndrome and hypotension. Metabolic alterations include a striking decrease in serum iron levels. The clinical results using TNF as a single agent have been disappointing with only an occasional minor partial response.

TNF is now being used in combination with other biologicals and chemotherapeutic agents. When administered in a phase I trial with interferon γ, there appeared to be 3-fold increase in toxicity at the same dose of TNF.[11] It was felt that interferon γ and TNF acted synergistically to induce these adverse physiological effects.

The administration of IL-2 to cancer patients results in the production of TNF.[13,23,27,57] Very high levels of TNF can be measured in the serum of some patients and these may persist in the serum even after cessation of therapy. Although

IL-2 can induce LAK activity in vivo, this has not always correlated with clinical response.[65] Blay and colleagues reported that patients with renal cell carcinoma who had a clinical response to IL-2 therapy had higher induced TNF levels than nonresponders.[4] This clinical observation suggests that the secondary induction of TNF, or perhaps other cytokines, may contribute to the antitumor effects of IL-2. Thus, the secondary production of these cytokines must be taken into consideration when designing clinical trials.

The fact that many tumor cell lines produce TNF also calls into question a clinical role for this cytokine. These TNF-producing target cells are resistant to TNF in vitro and may in part explain the refractoriness of some solid tumors.

Despite these early disappointing clinical trials, TNF may well find a useful clinical role when used in immunomodulatory doses or in combination with chemotherapy drugs or other biologicals.

References

1. Beutler, B., and Cerami, A.: Cachectin and tumour necrosis factor as two sides of the same biological coin. Nature, 320:584, 1986.
2. Beutler, B., Greenwald, D., Hulmes, J. D., Chang, M., Pan, Y.-C. E., Mathison, J., Ulevitch, R., and Cerami, A.: Identity of tumour necrosis factor and the macrophage-secreted factor cachectin. Nature, 316:552, 1985.
3. Beutler, B., Milsark, I. W., and Cerami, A. C.: Passive immunization against cachectin/tumor necrosis factor protects mice from lethal effect of endotoxin. Science, 229:869, 1985.
4. Blay, J. Y, Favrot, M. C., Negrier, S., Combaret, V., Chouaib, S., Mercatello, A., Kaemmerlen, P., Franks, C. R., and Phillip, T.: Correlation between clinical response to interleukin-2 therapy and sustained production of tumor necrosis factor. Cancer Res., 50:2371, 1990.
5. Carswell, E. A., Old, L. J., Kassel, R. L., Green, S., Fiore, N., and Williamson, B.: An endotoxin-induced serum factor that causes necrosis of tumors. Proc. Natl. Acad. Sci., 72:3666, 1975.
6. Chouaib, S., Bertoglio, J., Blay, J. Y., Marchiol-Fournigault, C., and Fradelizi, D.: Generation of lymphokine-activated killer cells: Synergy between tumor necrosis factor and interleukin-2. Proc. Natl. Acad. Sci., 85:6875, 1988.
7. Chun, M., and Hoffman, M. K.: Combination immunotherapy of cancer in a mouse model: synergism between tumor necrosis factor and other defense systems. Cancer Res., 47:115, 1987.
8. Conkling, P. R., Chua, C. C., Nadler, P., Greenberg, C. S., Doty, E., Misukonis, M. A., Haney, A. F., Bast, R. C., Jr., and Weinberg, J. B.: Clinical trials with human necrosis factor: In vivo and in vitro, effects on human mononuclear phagocyte function. Cancer Res, 48:5604, 1988.
9. Cook, J. L., May, D. L., Wilson, B. A., Holski, B., Chen, M., Shalloway, D., and Walker, T. A.: Role of tumor necrosis factor in E1A oncogene-induced susceptibility of neoplastic cells to lysis by natural killer cells and activated macrophages. J. Immunol., 142:4524, 1989.
10. Creasey, M., Doyle, L. V., Reynolds, M. T., Jung, T., Lin, L. S., and Vitt, C. R.: Biological effects of recombinant human tumor necrosis factor and its novel muteins on tumor and normal cell lines. Cancer Res., 47:145, 1987.
11. Demetri, G. D., Spriggs, D. R., Sherman, M. L., Arthur, K. A., Imamura, K., and Kufe, D. W.: A phase I trial of recombinant human tumor necrosis factor and interferon-gamma: Effects of combination cytokine administration in vivo. J. Clin. Oncol., 7:1545, 1989.
12. Dinarello, C. A., Cannon, J. G., Wolff, S. M., Bernheim, H. A., Beutler, B., Cerami, A., Figari, I. S., Palladino, M. A., Jr., and O'Connor, J. V.: Tumor necrosis factor (cachectin) is an endogenous pyrogen and induces production of interleukin-1. J. Exp. Med., 163:1433, 1986.
13. Economou, J. S., McBride, W. H., Essner, R., Rhoades, K. R., Golub, S. H., Holmes, E. C., and Morton, D. L.: Tumor necrosis factor production by interleukin-2 activates macrophages in vitro and in vivo. Immunol., 63:514, 1989.
14. Economou, J. S., Rhoades, K., Essner, R., McBride, W. H., Gasson, J. C., and Morton, D. L.: Genetic analysis of the human tumor necrosis factor/cachectin promoter region in a macrophage cell line. J. Exp. Med., 170:321, 1989.
15. Eisenthal, A., and Rosenberg, S. A.: The effect of various cytokines on the in vitro induction of antibody-dependent cellular cytotoxicity in murine cells. J. Immunol., 142:2307, 1989.
16. Elias, J. A., and Lentz, V.: IL-1 and tumor necrosis factor synergistically stimulate fibroblast IL-6 production and stabilize IL-6 messenger RNA. J. Immunol., 145:161, 1990.
17. Essner, R., Rhoades, K., McBride, W. H., Morton, D. L., and Economou, J. S.: IL-4 downregulates IL-1 and TNF gene expression in human monocytes. J. Immunol., 142:3857, 1989.
18. Fong, Y., and Lowry, S. F.: Short analytical review: Tumor necrosis factor in the pathophysiology of infection and sepsis. Clin. Immunol. Immunopath., 55:157, 1990.
19. Gordon, C., and Wofsy, D.: Effects of recombinant murine tumor necrosis factor on immune function. J. Immunol., 144:1753, 1990.
20. Han, J., Brown, T., and Beutler, B.: Endotoxin-responsive sequences control cachectin/tumor necrosis factor biosynthesis at the translational level. J. Exp. Med., 171:465, 1990.
21. Han, J., Thompson, P., and Beutler, B.: Dexamethasone and pentoxifylline inhibit endotoxin-induced cachectin/tumor necrosis factor synthesis at separate points in the signaling pathway. J. Exp. Med., 172:391, 1990.

22. Hasday, J. D., Shah, E. M., and Lieberman, A. P.: Macrophage tumor necrosis factor-α release is induced by contact with some tumors. J. Immunol., 145:371, 1990.

23. Heslop, H. E., Gottlieb, D. J., Bianchi, A. C., Meager, A., Prentice, H. G., Mehta, A. B., Hoffbrand, A. V., and Brenner, M. K.: In vivo induction of gamma interferon and tumor necrosis factor by interleukin-2 infusion following intensive chemotherapy or autologous marrow transplantation. Blood, 74:1374, 1989.

24. Hori, K., Ehrke, M. J., Mace, K., and Mihich, E.: Effect of recombinant tumor necrosis factor on tumoricidal activation of murine macrophages: Synergism between tumor necrosis factor and γ-interferon. Cancer Res., 47:5868, 1987.

25. Jones, E. Y., Stuart, D. I., and Walker, N. P. C.: Structure of tumour necrosis factor. Nature, 338:225, 1989.

26. Jongeneel, C. V., Nedospasov, S. A., Plaetinck, G., Naquet, P., and Cerottini, J. C.: Expression of the tumor necrosis factor locus is not necessary for the cytolytic activity of T lymphocytes. J. Immunol., 140:1916, 1988.

27. Kasid, A., Director, E. P., and Rosenberg, S. A.: Induction of endogenous tumor necrosis factor-α and IL-6 circulating PBMC by IL-2 administration to cancer patients. J. Immunol., 143:736, 1989.

28. Klebanoff, S. J., Vadas, M. A., Harlan, J. M., Sparks, L. H., Gamble J. R., Agosti, J. M., and Waltersdorph, A. M.: Stimulation of neutrophils by tumor necrosis factor. J. Immunol., 136:4220, 1986.

29. Kronke, M., Hensel, G., Schluter, C., Scheurich, P., Schutze, S., and Pfizenmaier, K.: Tumor necrosis factor and lymphotoxin gene expression in human tumor cell lines. Cancer Res., 48:5417, 1988.

30. Lichenstein, A., Berenson, J., Gera, J. F., Waldburger, K., Matinez-Maza, O., and Berek, J. S.: Resistance of human ovarian cancer cells to tumor necrosis factor and lymphokine-activated killer cells: Correlation with expression of HER2/neu oncogenes. Cancer Res., 50:7364, 1990.

31. Loetscher, H., Pan Y-C. E., Lahm, H. W., Gentz, R., Brockhous, M., Tabuchi, H., and Lesslauer, W.: Molecular cloning and expression of the human 55 kD tumor necrosis factor receptor. Cell, 61:351, 1990.

32. McIntosh, J. K., Mule, J. J., Krosnick, J. A., and Rosenberg, W. A.: Combination cytokine immunotherapy with tumor necrosis factor, interleukin-2 and γ-interferon and its synergistic antitumor effects in mice. Cancer Res., 49:1408, 1989.

33. Mestan, J., Digel, W., Mittnacht, S., Hillen, H., Blohm, D., Moller, A., Jacobsen, H., and Kirchner, H.: Antiviral effects of recombinant tumour necrosis factor in vitro. Nature, 323:816, 1986.

34. Muller, U., Jongeneel, C. V., Nedospasov, S. A., Lindahl, K. F., and Steinmetz, M.: Tumour necrosis factor and lymphotoxin genes map close to H-2D in the mouse major histocompatibility complex. Nature, 325:265, 1987.

35. Munker, R., Gasson, J., Ogawa, M., and Koeffler, H. P.: Recombinant human TNF induces production of granulocyte-monocyte colony-stimulating factor. Nature, 323:79, 1986.

36. Natanson, C., Eichenholz, P. W., Danner, R. L., Eichacker, P. Q., Hoffman, W. D., Kuo, G. C., Banks, S. M., MacVittie, T. J., and Parrillo, J. E.: Endotoxin and tumor necrosis factor changes in dogs simulate the cardiovascular profile of human septic shock. J. Exp. Med., 169:823, 1989.

37. Nawroth, P., Handley, D., Matsuda, G., DeWaal, R., Gerlach, H., Blohm, D., and Stern, D.: Tumor necrosis factor/cachectin-induced intra-vascular fibrin formation in meth A fibrosarcomas. J. Exp. Med., 168:637, 1988.

38. Nawroth, P. P., and Stern, D. M.: Modulation of endothelial cell hemo-static properties by tumor necrosis factor. J. Exp. Med., 163:740, 1986.

39. Naylor, M. S., Stamp, G. W. H., and Balkwill, F. R.: Investigation of cytokine gene expression in human colorectal cancer. Cancer Res., 50:4436, 1990.

40. Old, L. J.: Tumor necrosis factor (TNF). Science, 230:630, 1985.

41. Ortaldo, J. R., Ransom, J. R., Sayers, T. J., and Herberman, R. B.: Analysis of cytostatic/cytotoxic lymphokines: Relationship of natural killer cytotoxic factor to recombinant lymphotoxin, recombinant tumor necrosis factor, and leukoregulin. J. Immunol., 137:2857, 1986.

42. Pennica, D., Nedwin, G. E., Hayflick, J. S., Seeburg, P. H., Derynck, R., Palladino, M. A, Kohr, W. J., Aggarwal, B. B., and Goeddel, D. V.: Human tumour necrosis factor: Precursor structure, expression and homology to lymphotoxin. Nature, 312:724, 1984.

43. Phillip, R., and Epstein, L. B.: Tumour necrosis factor as immuno-modulator and mediator of monocyte cytotoxicity induced by itself, γ-interferon and interleukin-1. Nature 323:86, 1986.

44. Ruddle, Nancy H.: Tumor necrosis factor and related cytotoxins. Immunol. Today, 8:129, 1987.

45. Sariban, E., Imamura, K., Luebbers, R., and Kufe, D.: Transcriptional and posttranscriptional regulation of tumor necrosis factor gene expression in human monocytes. J. Clin. Invest., 81:1506, 1988.

46. Sato, N., Goto, T., Haranaka, K., Satomi, N., Narichi, H., Mano-Hirano, Y., and Sawasaki, Y.: Actions of tumor necrosis factor on culture vascular endothelial cells: Morphologic modulation, growth inhibition, and cytotoxicity. J.N.C.I., 76:1113, 1986.

47. Schall, T. J., Lewis, M., Koller, K. J., Lee, A., Rice, G. C., Wong G. H. W., Gatanaga, T., Granger, G. A., Lentz, R., Raab, H., Kohr, W. J., and Goeddel, D. V.: Molecular cloning and expression of a receptor for human tumor necrosis factor. Cell, 61:361, 1990.

48. Scheurich, P., Thomas, B., Ucer, U., and Pfizenmaier, K.: Immuno-regulatory activity of recombinant human tumor necrosis factor: TNF-α-mediated enhancement of T cell responses. J. Immunol., 138:1786, 1987.

49. Schiller, J. H., Bittner, G., Storer, B., Willson, J. K. V.: Synergistic antitumor effects of tumor necrosis factor and γ-interferon on human colon carcinoma cell lines. Cancer Res., 47:2809, 1987.

50. Seckinger, P., Zhang, J. H., Hauptmann, B., and Dayer, J. M.: Characterization of a tumor necrosis factor α (TNF-α) inhibitor: Evidence of immunological crossreactivity with the TNF receptor. Proc. Natl. Acad. Sci., 87:5188, 1990.

51. Shakhov, A. N., Collart, M. A., Vassalli, P., Nedospasov, S. A., and Jongeneel, C. V.: χBtype enhancers are involved in lipopoly-saccharide-mediated transcriptional activation of the tumor necrosis factor gene in primary macrophages. J. Exp. Med., 171:35, 1990.

52. Shau, H.: Cytostatic and tumoricidal activities of tumor necrosis factor treated neutrophils. Immunol. Letters, 17:47, 1988.

53. Shaw, G. and Kamen, R.: A conserved AU sequence from the 3′ untranslated region of GM-CSF mRNA mediates selective mRNA degradation. Cell, 46:659, 1986.

54. Smith, C. A., Davis, T., Anderson, D., Solam, L., Beckmann, M. P., Jerzy, R., Dower, S. K., Cosman, D., and Goodwin, R. G.: A receptor for tumor necrosis factor defines an unusual family of cellular and viral proteins. Science, 248:1019, 1990.

55. Smith, M. R., Munger, W. E., Kung, H. F., Takacs, L., and Durum, S. K.: Direct evidence for an intracellular role for tumor necrosis factor-α. J. Immunol., 144:162, 1990.

56. Spriggs, D. R., Sherman, M. L., Frei, E., and Kufe, D. W.: Clinical Trials With Tumor Necrosis Factor. In Tumor Necrosis Factor: Structure, Mechanism of Action, Role in Disease and Therapy. Edited by B. Bonavida, and G. Granger. Basel, Kerger, 1990, p. 233.

57. Socher, S. H., Martinez, D., Craig, J. B., Kuhn, J. G., and Oliff, A: Tumor necrosis factor not detectable in patients with clinical cancer cachexia. J.N.C.I., 80:595, 1988.

58. Staren, E. D., Essner, R. and Economou, J. S.: Overview of biological response modifiers. Semin. Surg. Oncol., 5:379, 1989.

59. Steffen, M., Ottman, O. G., and Moore, M. A. S.: Simultaneous production of tumor necrosis factor-α and lymphotoxin by normal T cells after induction with IL-2 and anti-T3. J. Immunol., 140:2621, 1988.

60. Sugarman, B. J., Aggarwal, B. B., Hass, P. E., Figari, I. S., Palladino, Jr., M. A., and Shepard, H. M.: Recombinant human tumor necrosis factor-α: Effects on proliferation of normal and transformed cells in vitro. Science, 230:943, 1985.

61. Sung, S. S. J., Jung, L. K. L., Walters, J. A., Chen, W., Wang, C. Y., and Fu, S. M.: Production of tumor necrosis factor/cachectin by human B cell lines and tonsillar B cells. J. Exp. Med., 168:1539, 1988.

62. Sung, S. S. J., Bjorndahl, J. M., Wang, C. Y., Kao, H. T., and Fu, S. M.: Production of tumor necrosis factor/cachectin by human T cell lines and peripheral blood T lymphocytes stimulated by phorbol myristate acetate and anti-CD3 antibody. J. Exp. Med., 167:937, 1988.

63. Swisher, S. G., Economou, J. S., Holmes, E. C., and Golub, S. H.: TNF-α and IFN-γ reverse IL-4 inhibition of lymphokine-activated killer cell function. Cell. Immunol., 128:450, 1990.

64. Tracey, K. J., Wei, H., Manogue, K. R., Fong, Y., Hesse, D. G., Nguyen, H. T., Kuo, G. C., Beutler, B., Cotran, R. S., Cerami, A., and Lowry, S. F.: Cachectin/tumor necrosis factor induces cachexia, anemia, and inflammation. J. Exp. Med., 167:1211, 1988.

65. Van Haelst-Pisani, C. M., Pisani, R. J., and Kovach, J. S.: Cancer Immuno-therapy: Current status of treatment with interleukin-2 and lymphokine-activated killer cells. Mayo Clin. Proc., 64:451, 1989.

66. Wanebo, H. J.: Tumor necrosis factors. Semin. Surg. Oncol., 5:402, 1989.

67. Wang, A. M., Creasey, M., Ladner, M. B., Lin, L. S., Strickler, J., Van Arsdell, J. N., Yamamoto, R., and Mark, D. F.: Molecular cloning of the complementary DNA for human tumor necrosis factor. Science, 228:149, 1985.

68. Watanabe, N., Niitsu, Y., Umeno, H., Kuriyama, H., Neda, H., Yamauchi, N., Maeda, M., and Urushizaki, I.: Toxic effect of tumor necrosis factor on tumor vasculature in mice. Cancer Res., 48:2179, 1988.

69. Wong, G. H. W., and Goeddel, D. V.: Induction of manganous superoxide dismutase by tumor necrosis factor: Possible protective mechanism. Science, 242:941, 1988.

70. Yang, S.C., Fry, K. D., Grimm, E. A., and Roth, J. A.: Successful combination immunotherapy for the generation in vivo of antitumor activity with anti-CD3, interleukin-2, and tumor necrosis factor-alpha. Arch. Surg., 125:220, 1990.

Interleukins

Edward C. Bradley
Elizabeth Grimm

Introduction

With the cloning of the IL-2 gene in 1983,[43] and the subsequent expression and clinical use of the human recombinant protein, it is now clear that it is possible to induce regression of metastatic cancer in man through the manipulation of the immune system.

This chapter deals with some of the regulatory factors of that immune system, called interleukins. These molecules have overlapping biological activities and pharmacologic functions which may prove to be more varied and complex than the limited in vitro data currently suggest.

An "interleukin" is any member of the family of soluble protein or glycoprotein products of leukocytes that regulates the responses of other leukocytes. Of disputed parentage, the term "interleukin" was widely used in the early 1970's to emphasize the role these polypeptide regulatory factors played between leukocytes, serving to coordinate the immune system, as distinct from polypeptide growth factors. While this distinction is now known to be arbitrary, since most interleukins are also growth factors and vice versa, the nomenclature has stuck and is now applied to at least 11 unique human molecules.

The interleukins are considered to be the hormones of the immune response, producing effects via autocrine and paracrine interactions. The interleukin cascade is usually initiated via antigen-specific interactions. The secreted cellular products of these interactions then function primarily at the local site of that particular immune response. The various functions of interleukins are mediated by way of interaction with specific receptors on not only leukocytes, but also other cells, including cells such as endothelial cells which are not usually thought of as being components of the immune system. These interleukins initiate, amplify, maintain, and probably terminate various differentiation, proliferation, and effector phases of the immune response. In addition to this local paracrine network of immune regulation, many interleukins exhibit potent systemic effects, via interaction with cells of the vascular endothelium, fibroblasts, keratinocytes, adipocytes, and cells of the central nervous system. Systemic effects of interleukins can be significant, especially during acute viral or allograft rejection episodes. Interleukins are pleiotropic water soluble molecules, derived from several gene families on different chromosomes. At least 11 interleukins have been described, and it is certain that more will be identified.

From an immunologic perspective, metastatic human cancers have either suppressed the immune response, are not significantly immunogenic, or both. The availability of several recombinant human interleukins has provided material in quantities sufficient to attempt short-circuiting the requirement for the antigen-specificity felt to be necessary for anti-tumor responses, thereby effecting a pharmacologic manipulation of the immune response. Many laboratory and clinical studies are under way to apply interleukins to the regulation of tumor growth through the activation of immune system components which have the potential to effect tumor destruction.

Interleukin-1

Biology

Interleukin-1 (IL-1) is a central mediator in inflammatory responses, produced primarily by activated monocytes and macrophages, which exhibits many diverse effects. Identified in 1972 as a soluble product of activated mononuclear cells required for the proliferation of thymocytes, IL-1 was originally called Lymphocyte Activating Factor. Although the major role of IL-1 in immune responses is believed to be the activation of helper T-lymphocytes by way of up-regulation of IL-2 receptors (see below), other early names for IL-1 indicate some of its diverse functions. The early names included Endogenous Pyrogen, T-Cell Replacing Factors I and II, B-Cell Activating Factor, and B-Cell Differentiation Factor. Additional functions include induction of prostaglandin release, secretion of acute phase proteins by hepatocytes, and bone resorption.[8]

Two forms of IL-1 have been characterized, designated IL-1α and IL-1β. Although each IL-1 is a glycopeptide with a molecular size of 17,000 Daltons, they are distinct gene products with individual isoelectric points (pI of IL-1α is 5.0, and of IL-1β is 7.0).[27] Biochemical data suggest that IL-1α exists primarily as a membrane bound molecule, and IL-1β as a secreted glycoprotein, although the mechanism of IL-1β secretion is currently unknown. A single class of specific receptors (80-82kD) for each IL-1 has been identified on T-cells and may be identical to the IL-1 receptors recognized to exist on fibroblasts, neutrophils, dendritic cells, endothelial cells, pre-B cells, macrophages, osteoclasts, and various bone marrow hematopoietic precursor cells. Recent evidence suggests that the IL-1 receptor complex translocates to the nucleus, but the mechanism and significance of this remains unresolved.[9]

Some tumors, including melanomas, astrocytomas, gliomas and some adult T-cell leukemic cell lines, may secrete IL-1. IL-1 may also induce differentiation in bone marrow cells, induce proliferation in pluripotent progenitors, and upregulate receptors for colony stimulating factors (CSF's) in parallel with stimulation of CSF production by lymphocytes and fibroblasts.

Preclinical Rationale for Therapeutic Trials

Because of the ability of IL-1 to induce proliferation and differentiation in bone marrow pluripotent stem cells, and because of the in vitro synergy noted between IL-1 and colony stimulating factors, IL-1 may be of clinical benefit in situations where bone marrow suppression limits the therapeutic index of irradiation or chemotherapy. In murine and primate studies in vivo, IL-1 administration accelerated recovery following chemotherapy, irradiation, or bone marrow transplantation. In these models, dose and schedule were critical in achieving a therapeutic effect without inducing significant toxicities secondary to the other, non-hematopoietic effects of IL-1. In addition to its role in proliferation, IL-1 may also alter cellular function by improving antibacterial phagocytic capabilities of leukocytes and macrophages. IL-1 has synergistic or additive capability to induce T and NK mediated tumor cytotoxicity in vitro in combination with IL-4, IL-2, TNF, or interferon gamma. IL-1 has also acted as a systemic immune adjuvant by enhancing the response in a murine model to a tumor vaccine.

Clinical Trials With IL-1

Clinical trials with recombinant IL-1 have begun in order to study systemic toxicities and effects of IL-1 as a hematopoietic stimulant. Biological activity of the molecule has been observed in man, but the most appropriate schedule and dose, as well as conclusions about clinical benefit, cannot yet be drawn.

Interleukin-2

Biology

Interleukin-2 was originally discovered in 1976 by Morgan, Ruscetti, and Gallo in human lymphocyte culture supernatants as an activity that supported the growth and proliferation of T-lymphocytes, hence the original name of T-Cell Growth Factor.[30] T-helper lymphocytes secrete IL-2, normally in response to IL-1 and antigen. Native IL-2 is a 133 amino acid glycoprotein with a molecular size of 14–16 kD by SDS-PAGE and a calculated molecular weight of 15,420 Daltons. The differential O-glycosylation is not needed for any of the biological functions known to date, but the integrity of an intrachain disulfide bond from residues 58 to 105 is required.[40]

A specific, saturable, bimolecular receptor system exists for IL-2, found primarily on T-cells, B-cells, NK cells, and their precursors. The IL-2 receptor system is composed of two molecules, a 55kD chain, known as Tac or the α-chain, and a 75kD β-chain.[44] When both receptor chains are expressed together in a noncovalent bimolecular complex, this high affinity receptor complex binds one molecule of IL-2 ($Kd = 10^{-11}M$) and transmits a signal for lymphocyte proliferation characterized by progression of the cells from G_1 through S phase of the cell cycle. Distinct, adjacent sites on the IL-2 molecule bind individually to the α-chain and to the β-chain molecules. Expression of the 55kD α-chain alone on cells has not yet been identified with any biological response, and the affinity of IL-2 interaction with this receptor com-

ponent is quite low ($Kd = 10^{-8}M$). Because of the minimal cytoplasmic portion of the 55kD receptor molecule, all investigations concur that the α-chain is incapable of transmitting signals into cells, and may act merely as an accessory molecule to "focus" low concentrations of IL-2 onto the 75kD sites.

In contrast to the ineffective role of IL-2 binding to the α-chain receptor molecule alone, the 75kD β-chain in isolation has an intermediate affinity (K_d-$10^{-9}M$) and has been shown by Tsudo to be responsible for signal transduction leading to activation of cytotoxic activity from the responding lymphocytes.[44] Activation of lymphokine-activated killing (LAK) with selectivity for tumor cells by stimulation of NK and T-lymphocytes with IL-2 is believed to occur via the β-chain. This β-chain receptor does transmit signals into the cytoplasm, and is known to be phosphorylated, possibly by way of a protein kinase C pathway.

IL-2 induces cytolytic activity in a variety of lymphocytes. IL-2 is able at relatively low concentrations to induce cytolytic activity in MHC-restricted, antigen-specific T lymphocytes (cytolytic T lymphocytes, CTL). IL-2 is also capable of activating natural killer (NK) cells which have a broader range of cellular targets. Higher concentrations of IL-2 are capable of inducing lymphokine-activated killing or LAK activity in T, large granular lymphocytes, and possibly even B-lymphocytes.[13] These LAK cells are relatively non-specific, and are capable of binding to and lysing a variety of allogeneic or autologous, transformed or non-transformed cells in vitro and in vivo.

Preclinical Rationale for Human Trials

It is well established that incubation of a variety of lymphocytes (T-, pre-T-, B-, and large granular lymphocytes) with IL-2 results in an induction of lytic activity in vitro for autologous as well as allogenic tumor cells and, to a lesser extent, non-transformed cells.[7,14] Murine splenocytes, incubated in vitro with IL-2 and then administered intraperitoneally (IP) or intravenously (IV) were curative in FBL-3 lymphoma bearing mice. IL-2 alone is also capable of inducing regression of established pulmonary metastases in a murine sarcoma model.[33] In all models studied there is a positive correlation between the tumor cytolytic activity seen and the intensity of treatment, i.e., the product of the concentration of IL-2 and the duration of exposure of target cells.

A variety of in vivo and in vitro models suggests that the degree of intrinsic immunogenicity, host immune status, and tumor burden may affect the degree of responsiveness to IL-2 therapy, and that a variety of secondary humoral and cellular factors, such as the induction of tumor necrosis factor (TNF), interferon gamma, and antibody-dependent cell-mediated cytotoxicity (ADCC) might be responsible for some of the antitumor activity seen. In spite of the complexity of the immunologic cascade triggered by IL-2 in the humoral and cellular limbs of the immune system, the reproducible observations that virtually all malignant cells can be lysed by IL-2 stimulated lymphocytes and the in vivo activity is related to the intensity of IL-2 administration have encouraged clinicians to pursue aggressive, intensive trials of IL-2 in patients with cancer.[34,36]

IL-2 Therapy in Patients

IL-2 has been primarily studied either as a single agent or in combination with the administration of cultured IL-2 stimulated autologous peripheral blood leukocytes, designated lymphokine activated killer (LAK) cells. The infusion of LAK cells has been referred to as adoptive cellular therapy. Clinical trials initially focused on renal cell carcinoma and melanoma, tumors in which a degree of intrinsic immunogenicity had been inferred because of the occurrence of occasional spontaneous remissions and a highly variable clinical course.

Because of the relatively short serum half-life (T $\frac{1}{2}$ α = 13 minutes, T $\frac{1}{2}$ β = 85 minutes) multiple dose or continuous infusion schedules were pursued.[23] Once or three-times weekly IV bolus regimens, and daily subcutaneous regimens were initially explored, and while these resulted in improvement of some immunological parameters measured ex-vivo, such as NK activity, clinical responses were rare. The greatest experience and greatest biological activity has been seen with the two most intensive schedules: q8h IV bolus daily × 5, every other week × 2, or continuous IV infusion daily × five days, every other week for two weeks.[4,32A]

LAK adoptive cellular therapy consisted of leukophoresis on the last day of the first week of the IL-2 administration, repeated up to five times. Harvested cells were then incubated in vitro for 3 or 4 days with high concentrations of IL-2 and reinfused once a day for up to 5 days during the second week of IL-2 administration.[35]

Clinical Toxicities

The multi-system toxicity seen in studies which used intensive regimens can be explained by three major groups of immunologic sequelae to the pharmacologic administration of IL-2: 1) the induction and release of secondary lymphokines, such as TNF, and interferon-gamma; 2) the activation and proliferation of lymphocytes within most organs resulting in a non-physiologic inflammation; and 3) the margination of circulating lymphocytes and vascular alterations including endothelial cell lysis and vascular leak secondary to these marginated, activated lytic cells and their factors.[7] The maximally tolerated dose of IL-2 for patients treated in an intensively monitored hospital setting is 600,000 IU/kg using the q8h bolus regimen of Rosenberg, or 18,000,000 IU/m^2 per day using the continuous infusion regimen of West. Acute toxicities, their management, and outcome, are listed in Table XVIII-5-1.[26,28,35]

IL-2 administration resulted in the induction and release of gamma interferon and TNF. Increases of these serum levels could be measured within four hours of IL-2 administration, and were temporally related to the onset of the frequently seen fever and rigors.[22] Circulating NK activity, depressed in many patients prior to therapy, often became normal, and some patients transiently developed circulating LAK cells. The induction of circulating LAK activity was associated with the dose of IL-2 and objective response to treatment.[2,3]

Acute toxicities of intensive IL-2 regimens included severe hypotension, requiring the administration of pressors such

Table XVIII-5-1.   Toxicity of IL-2

Organ System	Toxicity/Incidence	Intervention	Self-Limiting?
Cardiovascular	Hypotension/common	Dopamine	Yes
	Supraventricular arrhythmias/common	None	Yes
	Ventricular arrhythmia/rare	Lidocaine, bretyllium, cardioversion	Yes
	Myocarditis/uncommon	None	Yes
	Myocardial infarction/rare	None	Rare fatality
	Peripheral infarction/rare	None	No
	Peripheral edema/common	None	Yes
Pulmonary	Dyspnea	Oxygen	Yes
	ARDS/rare	Intubation	Rare fatality
	Pleural effusion/rare	Symptomatic	Yes
Renal	Oliguria	Low-dose dopamine, cautious fluid administration	Yes
	Pre-renal azotemia/common	None	Yes
	Anuria, acute renal failure/rare	Dialysis	Yes
Hepatic	Transaminase elevation/common	None	Yes
	Hepatic failure/rare	Supportive	Rare fatality
Hematologic	Anemia/common	Transfusion	Yes
	Thrombocytopenia/common	None	Yes
	Leukopenia	None	Yes
	Eosinophilia/common	None	Yes
Gastrointestinal	Nausea, vomiting/common	Symptomatic	Yes
	Diarrhea/common	Symptomatic	Yes
	Gastric, intestinal ulceration/common	Symptomatic	Yes
	Perforation of ulcerated site/rare	Surgical	Rare fatality
Neurologic	Confusion, altered mental status/common	Stop IL-2	Yes
	Coma/rare	Stop IL-2	Rare fatality
	Stroke	Symptomatic	Rare fatality
Other	Fever/common	Indomethacin	Yes

as dopamine in the majority of patients, as well as, fever, nausea, and vomiting. Progressive toxicities, much more prominent during the third and fourth days of each week and generally more severe during the second week of IL-2 administration, included shifts of fluid from the intravascular to extravascular sites, resulting in edema and exacerbating pleural, pericardial, and peritoneal effusions. Weight gain, oliguria, and pre-renal azotemia were common and considered to be compensatory to the decrease in intravascular volume. Other side effects were frequently seen: pulmonary interstitial edema with dyspnea and occasionally hypoxemia requiring the administration of nasal oxygen or intubation; diarrhea; generalized cutaneous erythema resulting in desquamation, particularly of the palms and soles; confusion occasionally progressing to coma; and elevation of myocardial enzymes, presumed to be secondary to myocarditis but sometimes associated with infarction. Supraventricular arrhythmias were frequent, and ventricular arrhythmias, including ventricular tachycardia, were seen but were rare. Anemia was universal, and many patients required transfusion of red blood cells during therapy. Peripheral blood lymphocyte count decreased dramatically during the first several hours of administration, presumably due to margination and sequestration during IL-2 induced activation, but gradually rose during the treatment period. Peripheral eosinophilia in some patients was profound. Infection was seen in approximately one third of patients treated. Staphylococcal bacteremias were associated with the presence of indwelling venous or arterial catheters. Centers which employed strict catheter maintenance routines and administered antibiotics prophylactically had the lowest rates of infection, but the demonstration that IL-2 impairs leukotaxis suggested that IL-2 as well as concomitant instrumentation predisposed to bacterial infection.[21] Gastric ulceration was common, and bowel perforation, often at sites of tumor involvement, was sometimes seen.

In spite of the incidence and severity of IL-2 mediated toxicities, most were reversible and did not result in prolonged hospitalization following the cessation of IL-2 administration.[25] The overall drug-related mortality in carefully selected patients treated with intensive regimens by one experienced center was less than two percent.[35]

Antitumor Activity

Anti-tumor efficacy is related to treatment intensity, and the majority of responses occurred in patients treated with intensive regimens. The overall response rate (PR + CR) in patients with renal cell carcinoma or melanoma has been between 15% and 30% in a number of centers. Complete responses, reported in approximately 5–10% of patients, have been extremely durable. Complete responses are not common in patients with bulky disease and many investigators have attempted to resect sites of bulky disease with the hope of increasing the probability of achieving a complete response. Some complete responses have lasted more than four years. The median duration of complete response has not yet been reached. The median duration of partial response is approximately one year. A number of patients with renal cell carcinoma who had partial remissions have been made surgically free of disease (surgical CR) and have

remained disease free for a prolonged period of time. It is not clear whether any benefit is gained by maintenance cycles of IL-2 following optimal response.[10,11,25,35]

Tumor response to IL-2 does not appear to be site specific, and responses have been seen in bone, hepatic, and renal sites as well as node, soft tissue, and pulmonary sites. It is not clear at this time what role, if any, LAK adoptive cellular therapy plays in the response to IL-2. While there is a trend, particularly in melanoma, for higher response rates for LAK-containing regimens the difference is slight, and one prospective randomized study failed to show a significant difference in either response rates, complete response, or duration of response between IL-2 + LAK versus IL-2 alone.[25,35] Studies comparing the regimens continue. Newer studies employing tumor infiltrating lymphocytes (TIL) as the cells administered adoptively following incubation with IL-2 are underway. Table XVIII-5-2 summarizes results of trials using intensive regimens with or without LAK adoptive cellular therapy.[25]

Combination Therapy with IL-2

IL-2 is being studied in combination with a variety of other agents which are: 1) components of the immune system, e.g. monoclonal antibodies; 2) well described immunomodulators, e.g., interferons or tumor vaccines; 3) cytotoxics used as immunomodulators, e.g. low-dose cyclophosphamide given to suppress induction of suppressor cell populations; or 4) standard agents which have activity of their own against renal cell carcinoma or melanoma, e.g. vinblastine or DTIC. Because of a well-defined response rate of renal cell carcinoma to interferon-α and the in vitro synergy of IL-2 and α-interferon, several Phase I studies have been performed with the combination.[5,17,42] The results are presented in Table XVIII-5-3.

Whether the apparent additivity of the response rates of IL-2 and IFN-α will be confirmed in Phase II studies, or whether responses will prove to be durable, remains to be seen.

Interleukin-3

Interleukin-3 (IL-3) was first described as a multilineage colony stimulating factor released from T cells in response to PHA. It is defined as a factor which causes the induction of 20α-hydroxysteroid dehydrogenase in cortisone resistant mature T lymphocytes.[19] IL-3 is larger than other lympho-

Table XVIII-5-2. Efficacy of IL-2 With or Without LAK in ECOG Grade 0 or 1 Patients with Metastatic Renal Cell Carcinoma

Number of Patients	Regimen	Response PR	CR	PR + CR (%)
90	q8h IV bolus (600,000 IU/kg)	12	4	16 (18%)
75	q8h IV bolus (600,000 IU/kg) + LAK	9	7	16 (21%)
59	Continuous infusion (18,000,000 IU/M2)	5	1	6 (10%)
48	Continuous infusion (18,000,000 IU/M2) + LAK	6	2	8 (17%)

Table XVIII-5-3. Combined IL-2 and IFN-α

Regimen	Patient Number	Response PR	CR	PR + CR (%)
IL-2, continuous infusion days 1–5 + IFN-α, days 1, 3, 5	12	3	3	6 (50%)
IL-2, continuous infusion IFN-α daily	7	3		3 (45%)
IL-2, q8h bolus, days 1–5, IFN-α, IV q8h days 1–5	14	2	1	3 (21%)

kines, with an apparent molecular weight range of 30–40kD. The variable size of IL-3 is probably a result of differences in glycosylation and post translational modification during secretion of the single peptide precursor of 166 amino acids. One form of IL-3 is the C-terminal 140 amino acids, called P-cell stimulating factor (PSF), whereas the other is the C-terminal 134 residues and is called Pan Specific Hematopoietin (PSH). A common 26 N-terminal leader sequence is cleaved during secretion of either form. The single receptor for IL-3 is of relatively high affinity ($K_d = 5 \times 10^{-11}$M), and internalizes upon IL-3 binding. This receptor has properties in common with the receptor for IL-4, IL-6 and the IL-2 p75β chain(20) which are recognized as members of a multigene family.

Only recently has the human IL-3 gene been cloned, so that most of the available information on the biologic properties of IL-3 are from murine systems.[32] As with all lymphokines, the early names indicate some of the more notable functions, which, for IL-3 include: Burst Promoting Activity, Histamine-Producing Cell Stimulating Factor, Mast Cell Growth Factor, and Multicolony Stimulating Factor. The functions of IL-3 include stimulation of mast cell proliferation, formation of neutrophils, macrophages, megakaryocytes, and mast cells from individual precursors, and inducing their colonies in soft agar. Recently, one component of the putative receptor complex for IL-3 has been cloned and expressed in murine systems but is not yet characterized in the human.[20] Although the activities of eosinophils, basophils, and monocytes have been known to be enhanced by IL-3, its ability to support multilineage colony formation early in the development of multipotent progenitors may prove to have clinical utility.[41] Because the field of colony stimulating factors is not yet consolidated, and is represented by many cytokines not considered as lymphokines, the role of IL-3 (as well as IL-1 in this regard) is quite unresolved.[47]

Preclinical Rationale for Clinical Trials

IL-3, in contrast to the hematopoietic growth factors, is active at a very early stage of hematopoietic precursor development, i.e., at the stage of the pluripotential stem cell. While IL-3 expands an early cell population, subsequent development of these cells into mature forms requires, or is augmented by, the lineage specific CSFs, such as GM-CSF. Primate models have shown that IL-3 does potentiate the in vivo production of hematopoietic precursors, but that its effect is greatly potentiated by the concurrent administration of GM-CSF, supporting the concept that IL-3 expands an early

population of cells in vivo which subsequently requires lineage-specific growth and differentiation factors to complete their development.

Clinical Trials

Trials with IL-3 have begun, designed to study whether IL-3 in patients will stimulate myelopoiesis after chemotherapy, irradiation, or bone marrow transplantation. One Phase I/II study in patients with aplastic anemia administered doses of a recombinant human IL-3 subcutaneously in doses up to 500 μg/m² daily for 15 days. Circulating platelets, reticulocytes, neutrophils, eosinophils, monocytes and lymphocytes increased in number. Side effects included mild fever, headache and cutaneous flushing. All effects in this study were transient.[12] After determining the doses and schedules that are most biologically active and safe, IL-3 will be studied in combination with GM-CSF and erythropoietin in patients undergoing intensive chemotherapy. As with all interleukins that have biological activity as growth factors, the theoretical possibility exists that certain tumors may be induced to proliferate secondary to the administration of IL-3.

Interleukin-4

Biology

Interleukin-4 (IL-4) is the product of a subset of activated T-helper cells, and was originally characterized by its ability to stimulate the proliferation of activated B-cells.[18] IL-4 has been reported to exhibit many other biological activities including induction of class II MHC molecule expression on B-cells, regulation of IgE and IgG₁ secretion, as well as the expression of specific receptors of IgE. In addition to B-cell regulation, IL-4 possesses the ability to stimulate directly as well as to inhibit various subclasses of T-cells. Additional reports indicate that IL-4 activates the mast cells that are found in connective-tissue. The various functions of IL-4 are not resolved, but its apparent ability to inhibit lymphocyte response to IL-2 while promoting antigen-specific interactions may prove applicable to tumor regulation, especially in melanoma where the tumor-specific tumor-infiltrating lymphocytes are reported to maintain tumor specificity in response to IL-4, and to lose specificity when cultured in IL-2.

Human IL-4 is expressed in a single form as evidenced by one major peak of activity on isoelectric focusing gels at a pI of 6.5–6.9. The apparent molecular weight is 12–15 kD as determined by SDS-PAGE. Similar to IL-2, the one interchain disulfide bond is required for biologic activity. Apparently, IL-4 exerts its biological activity through a single class of high affinity receptors ($K_d = 1$–2×10^{-10}M) found on both hematopoietic and nonhematopoietic lineage cells. IL-4 receptor positive cells include resting T-cells, B-cells, macrophages, myeloid progenitors, stromal cells from bone marrow, spleen, thymus, and brain, and melanoma, fibroblasts and liver. In addition to potentiating antigen-specific immune responses, potential clinical applications are suggested by the recent reports of its anti-inflammatory effects.[15]

Pre-Clinical Rationale for Clinical Trials

IL-4 is a pleiotropic B- and T-cell growth and differentiation factor. Unlike IL-2, it is species specific, and the differences between the immunologic activities of murine and human IL-4 and the absence of predictive tumor models for human IL-4 have made the pre-clinical study of recombinant human IL-4 difficult. Because of the ability of rhIL-4 to augment antigen-specific cytolytic T-cells and to induce differentiation of human B lymphocytes, including some leukemic B lymphocytes, clinical trials have been initiated to assess clinical activity in patients with solid and hematologic malignancies.

Clinical Trials with IL-4

rhIL-4 is cleared rapidly following intravenous administration, with a serum half-life of approximately 50 minutes. Serum concentrations following subcutaneous administration peak approximately two hours following administration, and are detectable for many hours. Toxicities associated with IL-4 have been positively correlated with dose, easily managed, and are reversible. Fever is common following both IV and SC administration. Malaise, headache, and nasal congestion are common and dose limiting. Anemia, thrombocytopenia, and modest elevations of hepatic transaminases, prolongation of PTT, and modest rises in creatinine have been seen. Gastric ulceration with clinically significant bleeding has occurred, possibly secondary to concomitant administration of indomethacin to inhibit fever. Hypotension and weight gain secondary to extravascular fluid retention have, unlike the case with IL-2, been prominent. Cutaneous erythema, nausea, vomiting, and diarrhea have been reported but are mild. Patients have not developed anti-IL-4 serum antibodies following IV or SC administration.

IL-4 has not shown activity in phase II trials as a single agent in patients with metastatic melanoma. Trials of IL-4 in combination with IL-2, in patients with B-cell hematologic malignancies, and in combination with TIL adoptive cellular therapy are ongoing. Some activity has been seen in Phase I studies in patients with B-cell malignancies.

Interleukin-5

Biology

Interleukin-5 is a product of activated T-lymphocytes which acts on eosinophils, B-cells, and thymocytes. In the early 1970s, it was observed that culture supernatants from parasite specific antigen-stimulated T-cell clones induced eosinophil colony formation. Subsequently, this eosinophil differentiation factor (EDF) was found to be isolated to a single peak on gel filtration, at 45 kD, which distinguished it from IL-3 and the other known colony stimulating factors. Independently, others identified a B-cell growth factor (BCGF II) produced by T-cells that were distinct from IL-4, and had physical properties identical to EDF. Today, these two distinct activities have been attributed to IL-5.[38,39,48]

Human IL-5 exists as a dimer, and exhibits a high degree of species cross reactivity. Recombinant human IL-5 encodes a 134 amino acid polypeptide, that includes a 19 residue N-terminal hydrophobic leader sequence. The core protein contains at least two glycosylation sites. Putative receptor(s) for IL-5 have been identified in murine B-cell systems, but have not as yet been found in the human. In the mouse, IL-5 has been reported to enhance IgA production, as well as to function as a killer-helper factor for induction of cytotoxic

lymphocytes. Our understanding of IL-5 is quite limited at this time. Therapeutic applications of IL-5 may include regulation of eosinophil activity and limited aspect of B- and T-lymphocyte differentiation.

Interleukin-6

Biology

Although originally reported as a fibroblast product, this 22–29 kD glycoprotein qualifies as an interleukin by virtue of its production by activated monocytes, macrophages, and T-cells.[16] IL-6's molecular size range is due to variable glycosylation, and unlike other interleukins, glycosylation may affect various activities. Human IL-6 contains multiple serine residues which have been reported to be differentially phosphorylated in different tissues. The functions of IL-6 are manifest on a variety of target cells, including T-cells, B-cells, fibroblasts, myeloid progenitors, and hepatocytes. The diverse functions associated with IL-6 include induction of plasmacytoma growth, induction of B-cell and CTL differentiation, particularly in conjunction with IL-2.

Some of the properties of IL-6 are similar to those of IL-1, such as co-stimulation of thymocyte proliferation and induction of the release of acute phase reactants from hepatocytes.[45] IL-6 can be induced in fibroblasts with poly IC, cyclohexamide, or virus, and has weak antiviral activity.

A specific saturable receptor for IL-6 has been isolated from human tonsil, with 100–1,000 receptors per resting T-cell. The apparent K_d is in the range of $1–7 \times 10^{10}$. Resting B cells do not express IL-6 receptors, but IL-6 receptors on B cells can be induced by various activating agents.

Preclinical Rationale for Use in Clinical Trials

IL-6 plays a role in vitro in the differentiation of T-lymphocytes, and, with IL-2, in augmenting cytolytic T-lymphocyte function. It induces B-lymphocytes to secrete immunoglobulins, in conjunction with other lymphokines, and potentiates the ability of IL-2 to induce LAK activity. In murine models in vivo, rhIL-6 administered as a single agent to mice bearing transplants of 34d sarcomas or adenocarcinomas significantly reduced pulmonary and hepatic metastases. While similar anti-tumor results were observed with IL-2, the therapeutic index was much greater for IL-6 supporting an immunologic rather than a direct cytotoxic mechanism for the antitumor effect. IL-6 potentiates the anti-tumor effects of TNF in murine models. These data would support clinical trials of IL-6, alone or in combination with other interleukins. Phase I trials have not yet begun.

Interleukin-7

IL-7 is a 25kD growth factor, first isolated from a murine marrow stromal cell line, and purified on the basis of its ability to stimulate growth of B-lymphocyte precursors.[31] RNA specific for IL-7 has been identified in the thymus, and costimulatory effects of IL-7 on adult T-lymphocytes suggest that it may also function in T-cell differentiation.[46] After stimulation of T-lymphocytes via an antibody to the T-cell antigen receptor, an IL-7 dependent, IL-2 independent proliferative pathway has been identified, suggesting that IL-7 may function in the absence of IL-2 to regulate T-cell proliferation.[1] The human IL-7 receptor has not yet been identified, but based on functional data, subsets of both B- and T-cells must have IL-7 receptors.

Interleukin-8

For many years, the IL-1 preparation from monocytes stimulated with various lectins was thought to be responsible for chemotaxis of polymorphonuclear neutrophils to the site of immune responses. As the ability to purify IL-1 improved, together with the advent of recombinant DNA-produced IL-1, it became clear that IL-1 was not the Monocyte-Derived Neutrophil Chemotactic Factor (MDNCF), which was identified as a distinct molecule, now known as IL-8. The cDNA sequence for IL-8 codes for a polypeptide of 99 amino acids, including a 27 amino acid signal sequence.[29] A mature protein that contains 72 amino acids is believed responsible for all the biologic activity of attracting polymorphonuclear cells. IL-8 is produced not only from monocytes, but also from fibroblasts and lymphocytes in response to either IL-1 or TNF.

A specific directional migration of PMN to very low concentrations of IL-8 (8×10^{-10}M) indicates the presence of a specific high affinity receptor.[37] Selective migration of lymphocytes at even lower IL-8 concentrations suggests a mechanism for the observed sequential PMN and then lymphocyte influx into inflammatory sites.[24] This 8kD basic heparin-binding polypeptide may have numerous clinical applications in attracting immune cells into tumors.

References

1. Armitage, R. J., Namen, A. E., Sassenfeld, H. M., and Grabstein, K. H.: Regulation of human T cell proliferation by IL-7. J. Immunol., 144:938, 1990.
2. Bradley, E. C., Doyle, M., DeGroat, S., Damle, N. K., Doyle, L. V., Rudolph, A. R., and Issel, B. F.: LAK induction in vivo in patients treated with Interleukin-2 may be necessary for tumor regression. (Abstract #1607) Proc. Am. Assoc. Cancer Res., 8:405, 1987.
3. Bradley, E. C., Konrad, M. W., and DeGroat, S.: In vivo normalization of NK activity in patients with cancer treated with Interleukin-2. (Abstract #1394) Proc. Am. Assoc. Cancer Res., 1986.
4. Bradley, E. C., Louie, A. C., Paradise, C., Carlin, D. A., Blyel, K. L., Groves, E. S., and Rudolph, A. R.: Antitumor response in patients with metastatic renal cell carcinoma is dependent upon regimen intensity. (Abstract #519) Proc. Am. Soc. Clin. Oncol., 8:133, 1989.
5. Bukowski, R. M., Murthy, S., and Sergi, J.: Phase I trial of continuous recombinant Interleukin-2 in combination with interferon-α-2a. J. Biol. Response Mod., 9:538, 1990.
6. Damle, N., Doyle, L., Bender, J., and Bradley, E. C.: Interleukin-2 activated human lymphocytes exhibit enhanced adhesion to normal vascular endothelial cells and cause their lysis. J. Immunol., 138:1779, 1987.
7. Damle, N., Doyle, L., and Bradley, E. C.: Interleukin-2 activated human killer cells are derived from phenotypically heterogenous precursors. J. Immunol., 137:2814, 1986.
8. Dinarello, C. A.: Interleukin-1 and its biologically related cytokines. Adv. Immunol., 44:153, 1989.
9. Dower, S. K., Kronheim, S. R., March, C. J., Conlon, P. J., Hopp, T. P., Gillis, S., and Urdal, D. L.: Detection and characterization of high affinity plasma membrane receptors for human Interleukin-1. J. Exp. Med., 162:501, 1985.
10. Dutcher, J. P., Creekmore, S., Weiss, G. R., Margolin, K., Markowitz, A. B., Roper, M., Parkinson, D., Ciobanu, N., Fisher, R. I., Boldt, D. H., Doroshow, J. H., Raynor, A. A., Hawkins, M., and Atkins, M.: A phase II study of Interleukin-2 and lymphokine-activated killer cell in patients with metastatic malignant melanoma. J. Clin. Oncol., 7:477, 1989.
11. Fisher, R. I., Coltman, C. A., Doroshow, J. H. , Rayner, A. A., Hawkins, M. J., Mier, J. W., Wiernik, P., McMannis, J. D., Weiss, G. R., Margolin, K. A., Gemlo, B. T., Hoth, D. F., Parkinson, D. R., and Paietta, E.: Metastatic renal cell cancer treated with IL-2 and lymphokine-activated killer cells—a phase II clinical trial. Ann. Int. Med., 108:518, 1988.
12. Ganser, A., Lindemann, A., Seipelt, E., Ottmann O. G., Eder, M., Falk, S., Herrmann, F., Kaltwasser, J. P., Meusers, P., Klausmann, M., Frisch, J., Schulz, G., Mertelsmann, R., and Hoezler, D.: Effects of recombinant human Interleukin-3 in aplastic anemia. Blood, 76:1287, 1990.
13. Grimm, E. A.: Lymphokine-Activated Killing. *In* BBA Reviews on Cancer. Edited by M. Moore. New York, Elsevier Press, 1986, p. 267.
14. Grimm, E. A., and Rosenberg, S. A.: The Human Lymphokine-Activated Killer Cell Phenomenon. *In* The Lymphokines. Edited by E. Pick. New York, Academic Press, 1984, p. 279.
15. Hart, P. H., Vitti, G. F., Burgess, D. R., Whitty, G. A., Piccoli, D. S., and Hamilton J. A.: Potential anti-inflammatory effects of Interleukin-4: Suppression of human monocyte tumor necrosis factor alpha, Interleukin-1, and prostaglandin E2. Proc. Natl. Acad. Sci. U.S.A., 86:3803, 1989.
16. Hirano, T., and Kishimoto T.: Purification to homogeneity and characterization of human B-cell differentiation factor (BCDF or BSF p-2). Proc. Natl. Acad. Sci. U.S.A., 82:5490, 1985.
17. Hirsh, M., Lipton, A., Harvey, H., Givant, E., Hopper, K. Jones, G., Zeffren, J., Levitt, D.: Phase I study of Interleukin-2 and interferon as outpatient therapy for patients with advanced malignancy. J. Clin. Oncol., 8:1657, 1990.
18. Howard, M., Farrar, J., Hilfiker, H., Johnson, B., Takatsu, K., Hamoka, T., and Paul, W. E.: Identification of T cell derived B-cell growth factor distinct from Interleukin-4. J. Exp. Med., 155:914, 1982.
19. Ihle, J. N., Pepersack, L., and Rebar, L.: Regulation of T cell differentiation: In vitro induction of 20 alpha hydroxysteroid dehydrogenase in splenic lymphocytes from athymic mice is mediated by a unique lymphokine. J. Immunol., 126:2184, 1981.
20. Itoh, N., Yonehara, S., Schreurs, J., Gorman, D. M., Maruyama, K., Ishii, A., Yahara, I., Arai, K., and Miuajima, A.: Cloning of an Interleukin-3 receptor gene: A member of a distinct receptor gene family. Science, 247:324, 1990.
21. Jablons, P., Bolton, E., Mertens, S., Rubin, M., Pizzo, P., and Lotze, M. T.: Interleukin-2 administration to cancer patients alters neutrophil FcR expression, superoxide response and chemotaxis. (Abstract #1498) Proc. Am. Assoc. Cancer Res., 30:377, 1989.
22. Konrad, M. W., DeWitt, S. K., and Bradley, E. C.: Interferon gamma induced by administration of recombinant Interleukin-2 to patients with cancer: kinetics, dose dependence, and correlation with physiological and therapeutic response. J. Immunotherapy, March, 1991.
23. Konrad, M. W., Hemstreet, G., Hersh, E. M., Mansell, P. W. A., Mertelsmann, R., Kolitz, J. E., and Bradley, E. C.: Pharmacokinetics of recombinant Interleukin-2 in humans. Cancer Res., 50:2009, 1990.
24. Larsen, C. G., Anderson, A. O., Appella, E., Oppenheim, J. J., and Matsushima, K.: The neutrophil-activating protein (NAP-1) is also chemotactic for T-lymphocytes. Science, 243:1464, 1989.
25. Louie, A. E.: Proleukin (Interleukin-2) for the treatment of metastatic renal cell carcinoma. Presented at the Biological Response Modifiers Advisory Committee Meeting of the F.D.A, July 30, 1990, Rockville, MD.
26. Louie, A., Carlin, D., Bleyl, K., Gains, K., Davis, G., Haenftling, K., Young, S., Hahn, D., Vollmer, C., Hanning, R., Rudolph, A., Paradise, C., Groves, E., and Bradley, E.: How safe is Interleukin-2. Combined results from 2,034 patients. (Abstract #706) Proc. Am. Soc. Clin. Oncol., 8:182, 1989.
27. March, C. J., Mosley, B., Larsen, A., Ceretti, D. P., Braedt, G., Proce, V., Gillis, S., Henney, C. S., Kronhein, S. R., Grabstein, K., Conlon, P. J., Hopp, T. P., and Cosman, D.: Cloning, sequence and expression of two distinct human interleukin-1 complementary DNAs. Nature, 315:641, 1985.
28. Margolin, K. A., Rayner, A. A., Hawkins, M. J., Atkins, M. B., Dutcher, J. P., Fisher, R. I., Weiss, G. R., Doroshow, J. H., Jaffe, H. S., Roper, M., Parkinson, D. R., Wiernik, P. H., Creekmore, S. P., and Boldt, D.: Interleukin-2 and lymphokine-activated killer cell therapy of solid tumors: analysis of toxicity and management guidelines. J. Clin Oncol., 7:486, 1989.
29. Matsushima, K., Morishita, K., Yoshimura, T., Lavu, S., Kobayashi, Y., Lew, W., Appella, E., Kung, H. F., Leonard, E. J., and Oppenheim, J. J.: Molecular cloning of a human monocytederived neutrophile chemotactic factor, (MDNCF) and the induction of MDCF mRNA by Interleukin-1 and tumor necrosis factor. J. Exp. Med., 167:1883, 1988.
30. Morgan, D. A., Ruscetti, F. W., and Gallo, R.: Selective in vitro growth of T-lymphocytes from normal human bone marrows. Science, 193:1007, 1976.
31. Namen, A. E., Lupton, S., Hjerrild, K., Wignall, J., Mochizuki, D. Y., Schierer, A. E., Mosley, B., March C. J., Urdal, D., Gillis, S., Cosman, D., and Goodwin, R. G.: Stimulation of B-Cell progenitors by clones murine Interleukin-7. Nature, 333:571, 1988.
32. Otsuka, T., Miyajima, A., Brown, N., Otsu, K., Abrams, J., Saeland, S., Caux, C., de Waal Malefijt, R., de Vries, J., Meyerson, P., Yokota, K., Gemmel, L., Rennick, D., Lee, F., Arai, N., Arai, K.-I., and Yokota, T.: Isolation and characterization of an expressible cDNA encoding human IL-3. Induction of IL-3 mRNA in human T cell clones. J. Immunol., 140:2288, 1988.
32A. Paciucci, P. A., Holland, J. F., Glidewell, O., and Odchimar, R.: Recombinant interleukin-2 by continuous infusion and adoptive transfer of recombinant interleukin-2 activated cells in patients with advanced cancer. J. Clin. Oncol., 17:869, 1989.
33. Papa, M. Z., Mule, J. J., Rosenberg, S. A.: Antitumor efficacy of lymphokine-activated killer cells and recombinant Interleukin-2 in vivo. Cancer Res., 46:4973, 1986.
34. Rosenberg, S. A., Lotze, M. T., Muul, L. M., Chang, A. E., Avis, F. P., Leitman, W. M., Linehan, W. M., Robertson, C. N., Lee, R. E., Rubin, J. T., Seipp, C. A., Simpson, C. G., and White, D. E.: A Progress Report on the treatment of 157 patients with advanced cancer using lymphokine-activated killer cells and IL-2 or high-dose IL-2 alone. N. Engl. J. Med., 316:889, 1987.
35. Rosenberg, S. A., Lotze, M. T., Yang, J. G., Aebersold, P. M., Linehan, W. M., Seipp, C. A., and White, D. E.: Experience with the use of high dose IL-2 in the treatment of 652 cancer patients. Ann. Surg., 210:474, 1989.
36. Rosenberg, S. A., Schwarz, S. L., and Spiess, P. J.: Combination immunotherapy for cancer: Synergistic antitumor interactions of IL-2, alpha-interferon, and tumor infiltrating lymphocytes. J. Natl. Cancer Inst., 80:1393, 1988.
37. Samanta, A. K., Oppenheim, J. J., and Matsushima, K.: Identification and characterization of specific receptors for monocyte-derived neutrophil chemotactic factor (MDNCF) on human neutrophils. J. Exp. Med., 169:1185, 1989.
38. Sanderson, C. J., O'Garra, A., Warren, D. J., and Kilaus, G. G. B.: Eosinophil differentiation factor also has B cell growth factor activity: Proposed name Interleukin-4. Proc. Natl. Acad. Sci. U.S.A., 83:437, 1986.
39. Sanderson, C. J., Warren, D. J., and Strath, M.: Identification of a lymphokine that stimulates eosinophil differentiation in vitro. J. Exp. Med., 162:60, 1985.
40. Smith, K. A.: Interleukin-2 inception, impact and implications. Science, 240:1169, 1988.
41. Sonoda, Y., Yang, Y-C., Wong, G. G., Clark, S. C., Ogawa, M.: Analysis in serum-free culture of the targets of recombinant human hemopoietic growth factors: Interleukin-3 and granulocyte/ macrophage-colony-stimulating factor are specific for early developmental stages. Proc. Natl. Acad. Sci. U.S.A., 85:4360, 1988.
42. Sznol, M., Mier, J. W., Sparano, J., Gaynor, E. R., Weiss, G. R., Margolin, K. A., Bar, M. H., Hawkins, M. J., Atkins, M. B., Dutcher, J. P., Fisher, R. I., Boldt, D. H., Doroshow, J. H., Louie, A., and Aronson, F. R.: Phase I study of high-dose Interleukin-2 in combination with interferon-α-2b. J. Biol. Response Mod., 9:529, 1990.
43. Taniguchi, T., Hatsui, H., Fujita, T., Takaoaka, C., Kashima, N., Yoshimoto, R., and Hamuro, J.: Structure and expression of a cloned cDNA for human Interleukin-2. Nature, 302:305, 1983.
44. Tsudo, M., Goldman, C. K., Bongiovanni, K. F., Chan, W. C., Winton, E. F., Yagita, M.,

Grimm, E. A., and Waldmann, T. A.: The p75 peptide is the receptor for Interleukin-2 expressed on large granular lymphocytes and is responsible for the interleukin-2 activation of these cells. Proc. Natl. Acad. Sci. U.S.A., 84:5394, 1987.

45. Van Damme, J., Van Beeumen, J., Decock, B., Van Snick, J., De Ley, M., and Billiau, A.: Separation and comparison of two monokines with lymphocyte-activating factor activity: IL-1 beta and hybridoma growth factor, (HGF). Identification of leukocyte-derived HGF as IL-6. J. Immunol., 140:1534, 1988.

46. Watson, J. D., Morrissey, P. J., Namen, A. E., Conlon, P. J., and Widmer, M. B.: Effect

of IL-7 on the growth of fetal thymocytes in culture. J. Immunol., 142:1215, 1989.

47. Weisbart, R. H., Gasson, J. C., and Golde, D. W.: Colony-stimulating factors and host defense. Ann. Intern. Med., 110:197, 1989.

48. Yokota, T., Coffman, R. L., Hagiwara H., Rennick, D. M., Takebe, Y., Yokota, K., Gemell, L., Shrader, B., Yang, G., Meyerson, P., Luh, J., Hoy, P., Pene, J., Briere, F., Spits, H., Banchereau, J., De Vries, J., Lee, F. D., Arai, N., and Arai, K-I.: Isolation and characterization of lymphokine cDNA clones encoding mouse and human IFA-enhancing factor and eosinophil colony-stimulating factor activities: Relationship to Interleukin-5. Proc. Natl. Acad. Sci. U.S.A., 84:7388, 1987.

XVIII-6

Hematopoietic Growth Factors

Janice Lynn Gabrilove

Introduction

Colony stimulating factors (CSFs) are a family of glycoproteins which regulate the self renewal, proliferation maturation, functional integrity and activation of mature blood cells which are of critical importance in general host defense, oxygen transport and hemostasis. The recent cloning of genes for several human hematopoietic growth factors has resulted in the production of recombinant forms of the proteins.[32,57,66,77,130,151–153]

The major potential clinical applications for hematopoietic growth factors reside in three general areas: 1) restoration of hematopoiesis by either preventing or accelerating recovery from iatrogenic-induced or disease related myelosuppression; 2) stimulation and production of functionally primed effector cells with anti-tumor capability and which are also able to augment general host defense; and 3) clonal extinction of malignant neoplastic disease by differentiation induction alone or by recruitment of cells into S-phase allowing them to be rendered more susceptible to killing by cycle specific agents.

The clinical ramifications, and therapeutic evaluation of hematopoietic growth factors is a rapidly moving field which holds great promise. In addition, an understanding of the mechanism and action of these factors have major basic science and clinical implications. In this chapter, we will: 1) provide an overview of how hematopoiesis is regulated; 2) review the identity and in vitro activity of the most extensively studied hematopoietic growth factors; and 3) review those clinical studies which have contributed so far to our understanding of the physiologic effects of these factors in man and their utility in the treatment of human disease.

Hematopoietic Growth Factors: Biochemical, Biological and Molecular Characterization

There is an ever increasing number of hematopoietic growth factors and interleukins which appear to be involved in the development and functional activation of blood cell elements. The molecular and biochemical characteristics, cellular sources, for many of these growth factors are summarized in Tables XVIII-6-1 and XVIII-6-2.

Granulocyte Colony Stimulating Factor (G-CSF)

Human G-CSF was first purified to homogeneity from the human bladder carcinoma cell line, 5637.[147,157A] This production of G-CSF does not appear to be a reflection of the malignant cell phenotype since the gene is identical to the gene found in normal cells.

The natural G-CSF protein has an apparent molecular weight of 19,600 daltons by SDS-PAGE. Reduction in the molecular weight to 18,000 following treatment of the native protein with neuraminidase and O-glyconase suggests that the protein contains neuraminic acid and is O-glycosylated.[158]

The gene for human G-CSF was first cloned from 5637 cells by Souza and colleagues.[130] The amino acid sequence has no significant homology to human or murine GM-CSF, IL-3, or M-CSF. A region of amino acid homology exists between G-CSF and interleukin-6 (IL-6) suggesting that there may be some similarity in the tertiary structure. Analysis of messenger RNA isolated from 5637 cells, using a G-CSF specific probe has revealed a single species of mRNA migrating at 1.65 Kd.[158] Human G-CSF has also been cloned by Nagata and colleagues from a squamous carcinoma cell line;[96] however, this clone contains nine additional bases giving rise to a protein with three additional amino acids. Furthermore, this 177 amino acid species was 100-fold less biologically active in vitro.[158] Analysis of genomic sequence has indicated that formation of this 177 amino acid species occurs as the result of splicing at an alternative splice donor site between exons two and three.[158]

The gene for G-CSF has been successfully expressed in E. coli.[130] The recombinant protein has a molecular weight of 18,000, reflecting the lack of glycosylation in the bacterially derived product. This glycosylation is not required for in vitro or in vivo biological activity.

At the myeloid progenitor cell level, G-CSF stimulates the growth of neutrophil granulocyte precursors (colony forming units, granulocyte; CFU-G),[96,114,130,147,158] and supports the survival and expansion in vitro of immature precursors of colony forming cells (Pre-CFU).[114] Originally, human G-CSF was thought to be a pluripoietin, since it appeared to support the growth of human burst forming unit erythroid (BFU-E), and uncommitted progenitors. This activity thus appeared

Table XVIII-6-1.   Summary of the Biochemical and Molecular Characteristics, Cell Sources and Targets of the CSFs

Factor cell lineage	Chromosomal location	Cell source	mRNA size (Kb)	Protein size (Kd)	Receptor mass (Kd)
GM-CSF	5q23–q32	Monocyte Fibroblast Endothelial T Lymphocyte Epithelial	1.0	14–35	50,000 130,000– 180,000
G-CSF (n)	17q11–123	Monocyte Endothelial Epithelial	2.0	18	150,000
M-CSF (CSF-1) (m)	5q23–q31	Monocyte Fibroblast Endothelial	4.0 1.8	35–45 ($\times 2$) 18–26 ($\times 2$)	160,000
IL-1 (Hemopoietin-1)	2q23–q34	Monocyte	2.3	12–19	
IL-2		T-helper cells		15.4	α55,000 β75,000
IL-3 (multi CSF) (n, m, e, b, E, M)	5q23–q31	T Lymphocyte Brain (?)	1.0	14–28	140,000
IL-4	5q23–q31	T Lymphocyte		20	
IL-5 (e)	5q31	T Lymphocyte			
IL-6 (stem cells)	7p15–p21	Monocytes Fibroblasts T Cells B Cells Endothelial	1.3	26	80,000
IL-7	?	B Lymphocytes T Lymphocytes		25	
IL-8	4q12–21	Monocytes Fibroblasts Hepatocytes Endothelial Cells		8	
IL-9 (erythroid)		T Cells	0.8	40	
Erythropoietin	7q11–q22	Kidney:? Peritubular cells Liver:? Cell Type	1.8	30.4	100,000 85,000
LIF/Hilda	22q12.1		41–58		

Abbreviations: n, neutrophil; m, monocyte; e, eosinophil; b, basophil; E, erythrocyte; M, megakaryocyte

to support mixed granulocyte, erythroid macrophage and megakaryocyte (GEMM) colonies from bone marrow.[114,130,147] However, with further depletion of accessory cells and enrichment of progenitors, G-CSF was found to no longer support the growth of erythroid or multilineage progenitors from this target cell population.[133] However, G-CSF has been shown to support the growth of megakaryocyte colonies in conjunction with interleukin-3 (IL-3).[84] G-CSF also stimulates the growth and transient clonal proliferation of enriched promyelocytes and myelocytes.[12] For cells of the mature, postmitotic compartment, G-CSF has been shown to enhance the specific binding of the chemotactic bacterial peptide formyl-methionyl-leucyl-phenylalanine (MLP),[114] to promote chemotaxis,[14] and to augment neutrophil mediated antibody dependent cellular cytotoxicity (ADCC).[113] One

important feature is that human G-CSF is not species specific in its action, and is quite active on myeloid elements of lower species.[147,158]

Granulocyte-Macrophage Colony Stimulating Factor (GM-CSF)

Human GM-CSF was first purified by Gasson and colleagues,[46] and molecularly cloned and expressed in mammalian cells by Wong and colleagues.[152] Human GM-CSF is highly and variably glycosylated, accounting for a wide range in reported molecular weights. The role of variable glycosylation with regards to cell specific production, biological activity or half life remains to be determined. Although, no

Table XVIII-6-2. Normal Hematopoietic and Nonhematopoietic Cell Types Influenced by Interleukins and Hematopoietic Growth Factors

Name	Target
IL-1α,β	T cell, B cell, neutrophils, stem cells, fibroblasts, endothelial cells, synovial cells, osteoclasts, adipocytes, hepatocytes, muscle, hypothalamus
IL-2	T cell, B cell, monocyte
IL-3	Stem cell, CFU-GEMM, CFU-GM, BFU-E, CFU-MK, basophil/mast cell, eosinophil, monocyte
IL-4	T cell, B cell, NK, LAK, monocyte/macrophage, mast cells, CFU-GM, BFU-E, CFU-MK
IL-5	Eosinophil, CFU-Eo, B cell, T cell, thymocytes
IL-6	Stem cell, CFU-GM, CFU-MK, megakaryocyte/platelet, B cell, T cell, NK, endothelial cells, hepatocytes, hypothalamus
IL-7	Pre-B cell, thymocytes, T cell
IL-8	Neutrophil, T cell, endothelium
IL-9	BFU-E, T cell, mast cells, megakaryocytes
IL-10	T_H1 helper T cells (inhibits effector function mediated by IFN-γ and IL-2); mast cells (synergy with IL-3)
KIT LIGAND	BFU-E, CFU-GEMM, HPP-CFU (synergy with IL-6, M-CSF), mast cells, primordial germ cells, melanocyte precursors
GM-CSF	CFU-GM, BFU-E, CFU-MK, neutrophil, eosinophil
G-CSF	CFU-GM, neutrophil, monocyte
M-CSF	CFU-GM, monocyte/macrophage, trophoblast
Erythropoietin	CFU-E, erythroblast
LIF/HILDA	Monocyte-macrophage, osteoblast, totipotent embryonic stem cells, hepatocytes, neurons
TGF-β	Stem cell, BFU-E, CFU-GM, monocytes, T cell, B cell, NK, fibroblast, endothelial cells, epithelium, adipocytes, muscle, osteoclasts, chondrocytes
TNF-α,β	Stem cell, CFU-GEMM, CFU-GM, BFU-E, CFU-E, CFU-MK, neutrophil, monocyte, endothelial cells, fibroblasts, adipocytes, hepatocytes, synovial cells, muscle, hypothalamus
M1P-1α	Inhibits pluripotent stem cells (HPP-CFU, CFU-s), synergistically enhances CFU-GM (with GM-CSF or M-CSF)

Abbreviations: BFU-E, erythroid burst-forming unit; CFU-E, erythroid colony-forming unit; CFU-Eo, eosinophil CFU; CFU-GEMM, granulocyte, erythroid, monocyte/macrophage CFU; CFU-GM, granulocyte, macrophage CFU; CFU-MK, megakaryocyte CFU; CFU-s, spleen CFU; HPP-CFU, high proliferative potential CFU; G-CSF, granulocyte colony stimulating factor; GM-CSF, granulocyte, macrophage CSF; M-CSF, macrophage CSF; IFN-y, interferon-y; IL, interleukin; LAK, lymphocyte activated killer (cell); LIF, leukemia inhibitory factor; NK, natural killer (cell); TGF-β, transforming growth factor-β; TNF-α,β, tumor necrosis factor-α,β.

formal comparison has been performed, both glycosylated and nonglycosylated GM-CSF are biologically active in vitro and in vivo in man.

Recombinant human GM-CSF (rhGM-CSF) supports the growth of both granulocytic and monocytic colonies in semi-solid culture;[46] however, it is also active at much earlier stages of myeloid development, as evidenced by its ability to produce colonies containing myeloid, erythroid and megakar-yocytic cells when combined with erythropoietin, a late-acting promoter of erythroid development.[41,86,128] In the presence of rhGM-CSF, mature macrophages and neutrophils demonstrate enhanced tumoricidal and phagocytic activity, intracellular killing, ADCC, superoxide production, complement-mediated (opsonized) phagocytosis, and responsiveness to chemotactic factors.[80,145] Mature eosinophils also respond to rhGM-CSF with increased ADCC activity.[80] GM-CSF is an extremely potent inducer of Mo-1, a molecule involved in granulocyte cell-to-cell adhesion and induces increased granulocyte aggregation in vitro,[5] and in vivo.[111] The clinical significance of this remains to be determined.

Macrophage Colony Stimulating Factor (M-CSF)

M-CSF is a heavily glycosylated dimer. Two forms of the glycoprotein exist, due to differential splicing of the gene.[49,66,151] The larger form encodes a 70,000 kd glycoprotein which is the major form of M-CSF in human urine, and was first cloned by Wong and colleagues.[151] A smaller form was first cloned from a human pancreatic cell line by Kawasaki and colleagues.[66] Both forms of M-CSF are biologically active. Recombinant human M-CSF (rhM-CSF) promotes the growth and maturation of monocyte and macrophage precursors. In addition, M-CSF enhances the phagocytic and tumoricidal activity of human monocyte/macrophages and induces them to secrete a variety of cytokines including tumor necrosis factor (TNF-α), interleukin-1 (IL-1) and CSFs.[49] The receptor for M-CSF is identical to the proto-oncogene c-fms.[123] Receptors for M-CSF have also been identified on tissue trophoblasts.

Erythropoietin

Erythropoietin (EPO) is a primary regulator of erythropoiesis in humans and other mammals. The cloning of the EPO gene[77] has permitted large scale production of human EPO. EPO appears to act almost exclusively on the committed erythroid progenitor and precursor cells, allowing these cells to proliferate and enter into terminal erythroid maturation, thereby expanding the production of RBCs. The EPO receptor has recently been detected only in these progenitor cells and has sequence homology with receptors for GM-CSF, IL-3, interleukin-4, interleukin-6, interleukin-7 and the beta subunit of the IL-2 receptor.[21,30] Little is known regarding the second messenger or molecular events following the binding of EPO to its receptor that leads to the proliferation and differentiation of erythroid cells.

Interleukin-1 (IL-1)

IL-1 is a mediator involved in numerous inflammatory, immunologic and hematologic responses.[32] Two forms of IL-1 have been characterized, IL-1α and IL-1β, although few differences in their respective biologic activities have been observed and both species apparently bind to the same receptor. IL-1 is a 17.5 kd protein which is produced by activated monocytes, as well as a variety of other cell types.[32,90] The major actions of IL-1 are summarized in Table XVIII-6-3. IL-1 has also been shown to stimulate the proliferation of resting stem cells in vitro and induce expression of the M-CSF, G-CSF and GM-CSF receptors.[90] In addition, IL-1 induces

Table XVIII-6-3.   Actions of IL-1 (α and β)

Endocrine Effects
  Stimulation of ACTH secretion
  Inhibition of LH + FSH induced differentiation of granulosa
    cells
  Stimulation/inhibition of insulin release
  Cytotoxic for pancreatic islet cells
Growth Effects
  Astroglial cells
  IL-2 receptor expression
Hematopoietic Effects
  Radioprotective
  Myeloprotective
  Increases procoagulant activity
  Potent stimulant of neutrophil chemotaxis

the expression of other CSFs and cytokines from monocytes, fibroblasts and endothelial cells.[90]

Interleukin-2 (IL-2)

IL-2, originally described as T-cell growth factor has been extensively studied for its role as an immunostimulant (see II, XVIII-5).

Interleukin-3 (IL-3)

Murine IL-3 was purified and characterized first by Ihle and colleagues and was subsequently shown to support the formation of multilineage colonies in vitro.[60] Gibbon and human IL-3 have recently been cloned using expression cloning techniques.[153] IL-3 is a complex glycoprotein, ranging in size from 14–28 kilodaltons. The expected size of the polypeptide is 14–15 kilodaltons.[153] The homology of murine IL-3 and human IL-3 at the amino acid level is only 29%, compared with a 93% homology between gibbon IL-3 and human IL-3.[153]

Recently, Leary and colleagues tested recombinant gibbon IL-3 on the proliferation and differentiation of an enriched population of human hematopoietic progenitors.[75] Recombinant IL-3 supported the formation of various types of single lineage, as well as multilineage colonies by CD34 [My10] positive bone marrow cells in the presence of erythropoietin. In addition, IL-3 supported the formation of blast cell colonies with high replating capability.[2,75] In these experiments, IL-3 proved to be much more effective than GM-CSF in supporting 21-day colony formation by normal human hematopoietic blasts, and the resulting colonies could be replated to yield secondary colonies with much higher efficiency than that obtained with GM-CSF-derived colonies.[2,75] These data suggest that IL-3 is probably the least restricted of the CSFs with regard to cell lineage. IL-3 acts not only at the restricted progenitor cell level, but appears to affect the functional activity of mature granulocytes and monocytes as well.[24,47A]

Interleukin-4 (IL-4)

As with most lymphokines IL-4 has been found to be multifunctional in its regulation of the immune response, acting on different cell lineages and at different stages of development and differentiation.[107,127] More recently it has been shown to have both direct and indirect effects on the reg-

ulation of hematopoiesis. The actions of IL-4 are summarized in Table XVIII-6-4.

Interleukin-5 (IL-5)

IL-5 was initially identified as a hematopoietic growth and differentiation factor with eosinophil lineage specificity. IL-5 is produced by activated T lymphocytes. In murine systems, IL-5 has also been shown to stimulate B cell proliferation.[144A] Although other lymphokines produced by T lymphocytes appear to stimulate the production of eosinophils, such as IL-2, IL-3, and GM-CSF, IL-5 appears to be the most directly and specifically involved in eosinopoiesis.[122]

Interleukin-6 (IL-6)

Human IL-6 (B cell stimulating factor 2, BSF 2) was originally identified as a factor in the culture supernatants of mitogen or antigen stimulated mononuclear cells, which induced immunoglobulin production in either Epstein Barr Virus (EBV) transformed B cells lines, or in Staphylococcus aureus Cowan 1 (SAC) stimulated normal B cells.[69,95]

The molecular cloning of the cDNA of IL-6 revealed that this factor is identical to a number of other well described regulatory molecules with a variety of biological activities (Table XVIII-6-5). These findings indicated that the actions of IL-6 were not restricted to B cells, but played an important role in various tissues and cells.[69]

IL-6 is a cytokine produced by a variety of normal cells including T and B cells, monocytes, endothelial cells, keratinocytes, astrocytes, fibroblasts, mesangial cells and bone marrow stromal cells (Table XVIII-6-5).[69] In addition, a number of cultured cell lines including monocytic leukemia cells, HTLV-1 transformed cells, T24 bladder epithelial carcinoma cell line, osteosarcoma (MG63), lung carcinoma (A549), glioblastoma (SKMG4) and astrocytoma (U373) cells also produce IL-6.[69]

A number of investigators have demonstrated the effect of IL-6 on the hematopoietic system.[69,74] Most studies have shown a synergistic effect of IL-6 with IL-3 in supporting the formation of multilineage blast colonies (both number and size) in culture. These findings have suggested either the recruitment of stem cells from G_0 or stimulation of their pro-

Table XVIII-6-4.   Actions of IL-4

1. Proliferation of human pre-B cells
2. Induces DNA synthesis in purified B cell populations
3. Increases class II antigen (Ag) expression on resting B cells
4. Induces low affinity IgE receptors
5. Increases CD23 Ag expression
6. Co-stimulant of B cell activation
7. Increases I_gE production
8. Co-stimulates growth of T cells
9. Stimulates growth of CD4, CD8, and CD3NK cells
10. Inhibits IL-2 mediated induction of LAK activity
11. Enhanced activity of Ag specific cytotoxic T cells
12. Synergizes with IL-6 and G-CSF to promote growth of high proliferative potential cells from 5FU treated mice: interacts with rhG-CSF to enhance proliferation of CFU-GM
13. Induces mRNA expression for GM-CSF, IL-3 and M-CSF from monocytes, GM-CSF, G-CSF, and M-CSF in endothelial cells

Table XVIII-6-5. Molecular Equivalents and Action of Interleukin-6 (IL-6)[1]

Molecules identical to IL-6	Major actions of IL-6
B-cell stimulatory factor 2	Induction of B cell differentiation and/or specific gene expression
Interferon Beta-2	Immunoglobulin induction in B cells
26 Kd protein	Induction of proteins in liver cells including fibrinogen,
Myeloma/plasmacytoma proteins	α-1-antichymotrypsin, α-1-acid glycoprotein, haptoglobin,
Induction of acute phase protein growth factor	C-reactive protein α-1-antitypsin and amyloid A
Hepatocyte stimulating factor	Induction of cytotoxic T-cell differentiation (with IL-2)
Macrophage granulocyte inducing factor 2	Induction of neural cell (PC12) differentiation
Cytotoxic T-cell differentiation factor	Activation of hematopoietic stem cells from G_0 to G_1
	Stimulation of cell growth
	Induction of the growth of myeloma/plasmacytoma cells
	Induction of mesangial cell growth
	Supports murine neutrophil, macrophage, eosinophil, mast cell/ megakaryocyte colonies
	Inhibition of cell growth
	Growth inhibition of myeloid leukemia cells (M1 cells)
	Growth inhibition of breast carcinoma cell lines
	Growth inhibition of human fibroblasts

[1]Adapted with permission from Kishimoto[69]

liferation.[69,74] In fact, the synergistic activity of IL-1 with IL-3 in promoting the proliferation of hematopoietic stem cells, may be secondary to the induction of IL-6 by IL-1.[74] In addition, IL-6 has demonstrated some activity in inducing differentiation of the murine myelomonocytic leukemic cells (M1) into macrophages as well as enhancing phagocytosis and the expression of Fc and C3d receptors on these same targets.[69]

Interleukin-7 (IL-7)

IL-7 was originally described as a murine stromal-cell-derived growth factor for B cell precursors. Recently, IL-7 has also been shown to be an important regulator of murine thymocytes, their fetal precursors and human peripheral blood T lymphocytes.[139]

Hematopoietic Growth Factors: In Vitro Effects on and Production by Malignant Hematopoietic Cells

Hematopoietic growth factors may not only be important physiologic regulators in maintaining hematopoiesis and augmenting host defense, but may also play a role in the pathogenesis of certain disorders. A summary of these associations is outlined in Table XVIII-6-6.

Hematopoietic growth factors, including IL-7 and IL-6, have been identified as proliferative factors for malignant lymphocytes[139] and/or plasma cells.[69] In addition, GM-CSF can synergize with IL-6 in supporting the proliferation of human myeloma cells.[69] Increased circulating levels of IL-6, as measured by bioassay, have also been reported in patients with multiple myeloma.[154] Interleukin-4 has recently been demonstrated to be the principal autocrine growth factor for and secreted by the L-428 Reed-Sternberg cell line, although other investigators have found IL-4 to inhibit clonal growth of malignant lymphoid and plasma cells.[135] In addition, Reed-Sternberg cells have recently been found to contain IL-5 mRNA which may in turn, be responsible for the eosinophillia associated with Hodgkin's disease.[122] IL-1, IL-3, GM-CSF, G-CSF, EPO, and rarely M-CSF have been reported to stim-

ulate the proliferation and/or differentiation of myeloid leukemic cells and augment the clonal growth of malignant myeloid progenitors.[49,51,58,68,73,89,97,130] Other investigators have shown that incubation of defective neutrophil granulocytes from patients with either chronic myelogenous leukemia or myelodysplastic syndrome in the presence of formyl-methionyl-leucyl phenylalanine (FMLP) can improve neutrophil function as measured by superoxide production.[157] The use of cytogenetics and premature condensation techniques or molecular analysis which takes advantage of restriction length DNA polymorphism should help clarify in future studies whether or not the normal or leukemic clone is being stimulated in these proliferation and differentiation-inducing experiments.

Several investigators have also demonstrated that leukemic cells may constitutively express transcripts and produce biologically active CSFs.[27,50,121,155,156] Alteration in the structure of both G-CSF and GM-CSF, as detected by Southern analysis, has been reported in two instances.[27] In the 5q[-] syndrome, the region of variable deletion on chromosome 5 contains the genes for IL-3, IL-5, IL-6, GM-CSF, M-CSF, and the receptor for M-CSF;[103] however, one presumably normal copy of each gene persists on the remaining intact chromosome 5. Whether or not the 5q[-] syndrome proceeding to leukemia results from a disruption, loss or mutation of a normal allelic growth factor or receptor gene, or results from the loss of a closely linked leukemia suppressor gene, remains to be determined. Recently, Furukawa and colleagues have demonstrated the expression of aberrant M-CSF genes (four copies of a rearranged M-CSF gene in addition to two copies of a structurally intact M-CSF gene) in a cell line derived from the peripheral blood of a patient with CML in blast crisis. Chromosomal analysis revealed two intact chromosome 5's and one 5q[-] fragment.

G-CSF is located in close proximity to the breakpoint on chromosome 17 involved in the 15/17 translocation in acute promyelocytic leukemia; however, no rearrangements of the gene for G-CSF have been found in this disorder.

In Vitro Effects on Non-Hematopoietic Malignant Cells. Isolated reports of receptors for G-CSF on germ cell tumor

Table XVIII-6-6.   Associations of Growth Factor Expression/Production/Detection and Disease: In Vitro and/or In Vivo

Factor	Disease State	Finding
G-CSF	Endotoxemia/Bacteremia	Increase serum levels in vivo
	AML blasts	Constitutive mRNA expression in vitro, in some cells
GM-CSF	AML blasts	Constitutive mRNA expression in vitro, in some cells
IL-1	AML blasts	Constitutive mRNA expression, in vitro, in some cells
	Diabetes	Islet cell destruction
	Rheumatoid arthritis	Increased levels in synovial fluid
IL-3	AML blasts	Constitutive mRNA expression in vitro, in some cells
IL-5	Hodgkin's disease	Reed-Sternberg cells + for message
IL-6	Lennert's T cell lymphoma	IL-6 supports in vitro growth
		Anti-IL-6 inhibits macrophage dependent growth of lymphoma
	Cardiac myxoma	Constitutive mRNA and protein by myxoma cells, in vivo
	Myeloma and plasmacytoma	In vitro constitutive production by myeloma cells and cell lines
	Castleman's disease	In vitro responsiveness related to severity of disease
	Rheumatoid arthritis	Increased levels in synovial fluid; constitutive production by T cells
	Megakaryoblastic leukemia	Constitutive expression of IL-6 receptor mRNA and IL-6 stimulated proliferation of human megakaryoblastic leukemic cells
IL-7	Acute lymphoblastic leukemia	IL-7 stimulates proliferation of ALL cells

lines,[116] for G-CSF and GM-CSF receptors on small cell carcinoma cell lines,[6] and GM-CSF receptors on sarcoma cell lines[87] have been reported. One group has reported an increase in thymidine incorporation in these same small cell carcinoma cell lines when cells are incubated with G-CSF or GM-CSF.[6] However, another group reported colony inhibition by G-CSF and GM-CSF, when these same cells were incubated with growth factor in semi-solid medium.[120]

Preclinical In Vivo Studies

In preclinical models, IL-3,[34] GM-CSF,[35,83] and G-CSF[146] have been shown to increase the number of functionally normal leukocytes in nonhuman primates. Following GM-CSF, this effect is in part due to an increase in circulating eosinophil granulocytes,[35] whereas the augmentation in white cell count following G-CSF is due predominantly to an increase in neutrophil granulocytes.[146] IL-1α has also been reported to enhance murine granulopoiesis.[132] This effect may be due either to the direct action of IL-1α or to the induction of CSFs following IL-1α administration.[132] The sequential administration of IL-3 followed by GM-CSF to nonhuman primates has been shown to augment circulating platelet counts modestly.[33]

The administration of CSFs and IL-1 in the setting of myelosuppression related to either chemotherapy or radiation treatment has also been tested in nonhuman primate and murine models.[101,144,146] Schuening and colleagues tested whether administration of rhG-CSF could reverse the otherwise lethal myelosuppressive effect of total body irradia-

tion.[124] The results demonstrated that rhG-CSF was radioprotective if given immediately following exposure to TBI. In contrast, there was no protection if 7 days elapsed before administration of the hematopoietic growth factor.[124] Although these animals were protected from lethality, profound neutropenia for a finite period did occur. Accelerated recovery or complete protection of the host from neutropenia, as well as thrombocytopenia, might be achieved with a combination of stem cell and lineage specific factors with or without the infusion of progenitors.

Administration of CSFs to Cancer Patients/ Normal Volunteers Not Receiving Myelosuppressive Treatment

Administration of both rhG-CSF and rhGM-CSF to cancer patients results in a dramatic elevation in circulating neutrophil and neutrophil-eosinophil granulocytes respectively.[28,40,56,76,92–94,112,117,131] This section will review the use of each growth factor in this setting and discuss the physiologic effects on neutrophil granulocyte production and function; other hematopoietic cell lineages; bone marrow cellularity and morphology; bone marrow and circulating progenitor cell development and growth; and pharmacokinetics.

RhG-CSF

Neutrophil Granulocytes. Morstyn and colleagues have studied different routes of administration of rhG-CSF including a twice daily intravenous infusion, subcutaneous injection as a bolus and continuous subcutaneous infusions, over five days in the absence of chemotherapy to determine the effects of rhG-CSF alone on the hematopoietic system in both previously untreated and treated patients with cancer.[92–94] The immediate effect of rhG-CSF was a decrease in circulating neutrophil counts within five minutes of intravenous administration. The magnitude of the decrease was independent of the dose over a range of 1–60 µg/kg/day. A rise in circulating neutrophils occurred after four hours which was near maximal within 24 hours.[93] Bronchud and colleagues also noted a fall in peripheral neutrophil counts within one hour followed by a rapid influx of mature neutrophils into the circulatory pool in 12 patients with small cell lung cancer treated with rhG-CSF (1–40 µg/kg/day) as continuous intravenous infusion for five days prior to receiving chemotherapy.[18] The basis of the transient fall in neutrophils has not been determined, but does not appear to be due to any selective organ sequestration.[18,108]

In all studies, a marked increase in circulating neutrophil granulocytes has been noted. A 1.8–12-fold, dose-dependent increase in absolute neutrophil count (ANC) was noted when patients were treated with a daily 30–40 minute intravenous infusion of rhG-CSF, 1–60 µg/kg/day.[40,63] The magnitude of the increase in ANC, however, was not significantly different at day 6 for the 60 µg (12-fold),[40] and 100 µg (13-fold) levels.[63] The fold-increase in circulating neutrophil counts was identical for patients who had received prior pelvic radiation therapy as compared to their previously nonirradiated cohorts. A similar dose dependent increase in circulating neutrophil counts was also noted in patients treated with either a 20 minute intravenous infusion every 12 hours, subcutaneous bolus or subcutaneous infusion for 5 days.[92–94] In the latter study, however, 2 of 3 patients who had received extensive prior chemotherapy or radiotherapy, did not exhibit a sustained increase in neutrophil counts.[92–94] A dose-dependent increase in ANC was also noted by Bronchud and colleagues in patients receiving a 1–10 µg/kg/day continuous infusion of rhG-CSF; however, a further augmentation in ANC was not noted when patients were given doses of 20 and 40 µg/kg/day.[18]

In all studies the increase in ANC was due primarily to an increase in mature segmented polymorphonuclear granulocytes, with some increase in band forms.[18,40,63,92–94,108] In patients receiving higher doses of rhG-CSF (greater than or equal to 30 µg/kg/day intravenous infusion over 30–40 minutes, or 10–40 µg/kg/day continuous intravenous infusion), the increase in ANC did not, however, appear to be due to an increase in survival of neutrophil granulocytes. In this respect, peripheral blood neutrophils obtained from patients during rhG-CSF treatment exhibited similar survival kinetics to those obtained from normal control volunteers.[18]

In all studies, morphological changes noted in neutrophil granulocytes included the appearance of toxic granulations, a decrease in nuclear lobulation, and an increase in the leukocyte alkaline phosphatase (LAP) score.[18,40,63,92–94,108] Döhle bodies, discrete round or oval areas seen in the peripheral portions of neutrophils staining sky blue with Romanowsky dyes and identified by electron microscopy to be lamellar aggregates of rough endoplasmic reticulum have also been seen.[40,63,92–94] Interestingly, Döhle bodies were first described in patients with infections, severe burns, and uncomplicated pregnancy, all situations in which, presumably, G-CSF levels are elevated.

Neutrophil Function

Neutrophil granulocytes obtained from patients treated with rhG-CSF appear to function normally in vitro and in vivo as measured by phagocytic activity (chemoluminescence)[18] migration in vitro (chemotaxis)[40,63] and in vivo as measured by employing a skin chamber technique.[138]

Other Peripheral Blood Hematopoietic Cell Lineages

Circulating eosinophil and basophil granulocytes remained unchanged following administration of rhG-CSF. Circulating monocyte counts were unchanged in patients treated with lower doses, however, a 10-fold increase in monocytes was noted following 30–100 µg of rhG-CSF/µg/day administered as a 30–40 minute intravenous infusion.[40,63] A dose-independent 2-fold increase in lymphocytes was also noted with daily intravenous administration of rhG-CSF.[40,63] No consistent effect on hemoglobin, hematocrit or platelet counts were noted in any study during the period of rhG-CSF administration.[40,63]

Bone Marrow

An increase in bone marrow myeloid to erythroid (M:E) cell ratio and cellularity was noted in all studies.[18,40,63,92–94,108] Gabrilove and colleagues noted that at the 3 µg/kg/day dose level the increased M:E ratio was due primarily to an increase in the post mitotic compartment (metamyelocytes, bands and polymorphs) whereas at the 30–60 µg/kg dose level, the increase in M:E ratio reflected an increase in the mitotic compartment, with a marked increase in the proportion of promyelocytes.[40] Similar observations were made by Morstyn and colleagues.[92–94]

Hematopoietic Progenitors

A significant increase in circulating hematopoietic progenitors was noted.[36,40] Gabrilove and colleagues reported an increase in peripheral blood day 14 CFU-GM.[40] Duhrsen and colleagues reported up to a 100-fold dose-related increase in the number of circulating progenitor cells of the granulocyte-macrophage, erythroid and megakaryocyte type.[36] In both studies, the frequency of bone marrow progenitors detected remained either unchanged or was decreased per 10^5 bone marrow cells plated.[36,40] The proportion of cycling bone marrow derived hematopoietic progenitor cells was only slightly increased by rhG-CSF treatment.[18]

Pharmacokinetics

In one study, circulating levels of rhG-CSF were assessed by a solid phase sandwich radioimmunoassay using patient serum samples collected at intervals after administration.[40] A subset of five patients receiving rhG-CSF at the 10–60 µg/kg per day dose level were studied. For a period of 40 minutes, immediately after cessation of the rhG-CSF infusion, the levels of rhG-CSF remained relatively constant and proportional to the dosage of material administered. After 40 minutes, the serum levels of rhG-CSF decayed logarithmically with time, allowing the calculation of elimination kinetics. Plasma half-lives for five patients were 3.9, 3.9, 6.3, 6.3, and 5.0 hours, respectively, for an average value of 5.1 ± 0.5 hours.[40] Furthermore, these results indicated that the elimination pathway had not reached saturation for the doses tested.[40]

In a second study, the elimination half-life was found to be dose dependent, as measured by bioassay, employing either a clonal agar differentiation assay using WEHI 3B (D+) myelomonocytic leukemia cells, or normal human or murine bone marrow progenitor cell growth. Using these assays, a dose of 0.5 and 1.5 μg/kg/day had a plasma half-life of 1.4 ± 0.3 hours, and doses of 5.0 and 30 μg/kg having a half-life of 3.7 ± 1.1 hours. These data suggest that at least one mechanism of clearance becomes saturated at a dose of 5 μg/kg.[92,94]

Following a single bolus subcutaneous injection, peak serum levels of G-CSF are reached after about 4 hours at the 10 μg/kg/day dose level with levels of detectable G-CSF being maintained for 9 hours or more.[92] When rhG-CSF was administered as a continuous subcutaneous infusion over a 5 day period at 10 μg/kg/day, a plateau serum G-CSF level was expected because the rate of infusion was constant; however, the finding that G-CSF levels fell markedly over the last 2 days of the infusion suggested that a new clearance mechanism was induced.[92] In another group of patients, a 5-day continuous subcutaneous infusion was given after an injection of melphalan.[92] In this situation, the large fall in serum G-CSF during the infusion was not seen, indicating that a high output of neutrophils from the bone marrow was required for the induced clearance seen in the first group.[92] This method of down-regulation of G-CSF may be important in returning neutrophil levels to normal after stress such as septicemia.[92] In conclusion, there appear to be at least three mechanisms for the clearance of G-CSF, but the precise nature of these mechanisms remains to be elucidated.[92]

Other Laboratory Changes

In all three studies, dose associated increases in alkaline phosphatase, presumably bone in origin, lactate dehydrogenase and leukocyte alkaline phosphatase have been observed.[3,18,40,92–94] At higher doses (>30 μg/kg/day IV) an increase in uric acid, most likely related to an increase in leukocyte turnover, has also been noted.[40,63,93] At the 100 μg dose level (IV), mild increases in SGOT and GGTP were also observed.[63] All of these values returned to normal or near baseline within 1–2 weeks after G-CSF administration. In patients administered 60–100 μg/kg/day as a short intravenous infusion, cholesterol levels demonstrated a decrease over the treatment period with variable changes in triglycerides.[63]

GM-CSF

Different rhGM-CSF preparations, both bacterial (E. coli), yeast and mammalian (CHO) cell derived, each with different specific activities, have been administered to hematologically normal and leukopenic cancer patients with success.[4,28,55,76,112,115,118,131,141]

Neutrophil Counts. A dose dependent increase in neutrophil counts has been reported in most studies.[4,28,56,76,112,115,118,141] Herrmann and colleagues, however, reported that only 4 of 15 patients had a rise above pretreatment levels in their WBC and segmented neutrophil granulocytes following IV bolus administration of 120–1500 μg/m²/day × 5 days, whereas, rhGM-CSF administered by continuous infusion resulted in a striking dose related rise in circulating neutrophil counts.[56] Similar findings were reported by Rifkin and colleagues in patients with advanced cancer treated with the same rhGM-CSF preparation.[118] Subcutaneously administered rhGM-CSF (0.3–30 μg/kg/day) for 10 days resulted in 2.2–10 fold increases in circulating neutrophil granulocytes, with an initial dose-dependent response (0.1–3 μg/kg/day) followed by a plateau in the neutrophil granulocyte response (3–15 μg/kg/day) and then a further small increment in leukocyte augmentation at the 20 μg/kg/day dose level.[76] In this study, patients who had received previous extensive chemotherapy or radiotherapy had the smallest elevations in circulating leukocytes during rhGM-CSF treatment at the 3, 10, and 15 μg/kg/day subcutaneous dose levels.[76]

Following the start of either glycosylated or non-glycosylated rhGM-CSF administration (either as a short or as a continuous intravenous infusion) an immediate, transient neutropenia, eosinopenia, and monocytopenia has been observed, which in one study appeared to be dose related[56] and not in two others.[76,112] The time of the maximum nadir was 30 minutes with a rebound in the leukocyte count to baseline or above baseline by two hours. This effect was noted even at doses which had no apparent proliferative effect and resulted in no augmentation of the circulating leukocyte count.[76,112] Radionuclide labelling studies, first reported by Devreux and colleagues showed that the leukopenia was due to sequestration within the lungs.[31] Subsequently, several groups have confirmed these initial findings.[56,108] Following subcutaneous administration of nonglycosylated rhGM-CSF, a rapid decrease in circulating leukocytes with a maximum nadir occurring by 60 minutes and lasting for up to four hours, has been observed.[76] This effect appears to be independent of the dose administered.[76]

In all studies, an apparent biphasic response to rhGM-CSF has been noted over time, with an initial plateau in WBC augmentation achieved after 3–7 days, depending upon the route of administration, followed by a second increase and plateau thereafter. Two explanations could account for the kinetics of the neutrophil response following GM-CSF administration. First, it takes seven days for cells to mature from the myeloblast to the polymorphonuclear leukocyte stage, and seven more days to see the proliferative effects of rhGM-CSF on the CFU-GM progenitor compartment reflected in the circulating counts. Alternatively, the delayed peak in the neutrophil response could be secondary to the induction of lineage specific factors such as G-CSF, M-CSF, and IL-5, which would work in concert with GM-CSF to further amplify and augment the leukocyte response. This is certainly plausible since GM-CSF has been reported to induce both G-CSF and M-CSF in vitro.[59,78] In addition, eosinophils are not noted until after seven days, perhaps suggesting that some secondary mediator plays a role. Which hypothesis is correct remains to be elucidated, but clearly it would be of interest to know if the circulating levels of G-CSF, M-CSF, or IL-5 increase during rhGM-CSF administration.

Neutrophilia following rhGM-CSF showed a left shift, and at higher doses circulating myelocytes, promyelocytes, and myeloblasts contributed to the second phase of the leukocytosis.[56,76,92]

Morphologic changes in neutrophils following rhGM-CSF have been reported to include toxic granulations,[56,76,92] and an increase in leukocyte alkaline phosphatase,[56,76] as seen with G-CSF. In addition, cytoplasmic vacuolization and hypersegmentation of polymorphonuclear granulocytes, has been reported.[56]

Neutrophil Function

Several investigators have reported preserved neutrophil function in vitro, as measured by phagocytosis and generation of superoxide.[65,111] Peters and colleagues have reported markedly impaired in vivo migration of neutrophils through a skin abrasion, in patients receiving continuous intravenous infusions of glycosylated rhGM-CSF.[108] In contrast, Toner and colleagues reported that previously treated ovarian cancer patients receiving four hour infusions of non-glycosylated rhGM-CSF at doses of 1–2 µg/kg/day did not exhibit impaired migration.[138] At higher doses of GM-CSF, however, migration was also inhibited, with the non-glycosylated growth factor.[137A] In patients suffering from or at risk for active soft tissue infection, it may be of concern that treatment with rhGM-CSF could potentially impair the ability of inflammatory cells to reach the infectious nidus.

Other Cell Lineages

A specific increase in eosinophils has been reported after five days of rhGM-CSF, administered either as an IV bolus ($\geq$ 500 µg/m^2),[56] continuous infusion (>120 µg/m^2/day)[112] or subcutaneous bolus (10–20 µg/kg/day).[76]

An increase in monocytes has also been noted following the administration of both glycosylated and non-glycosylated GM-CSF, independent of the route of administration.[4,28,56,76,112,131,141] In two studies, monocytes from patients treated with GM-CSF have been reported to exhibit enhanced tumoricidal activity in vitro;[22,150] in one other study, however, no enhanced tumoricidal activity of monocytes was observed.[71]

During subcutaneous administration of non-glycosylated rhGM-CSF, no consistent effect on hemoglobin, reticulocyte or platelet counts were noted.[76] Two other studies reported a transient decline in platelets to < 20% of pretreatment levels, but no change in hemoglobin or reticulocyte count after six or more days of glycosylated rhGM-CSF.[28,56] Lieschke and colleagues also reported the occurrence of thrombocytopenia, possibly secondary to reactivation of idiopathic thrombocytopenic purpura in a patient with a history of the disorder.[76]

Bone Marrow

Marrow biopsies obtained from patients receiving glycosylated and non-glycosylated rhGM-CSF have demonstrated an increase in myelopoiesis with an increase in myeloid to erythroid cell ratios.[4,56,76,112] In the marrow, rhGM-CSF therapy promotes a shift toward immaturity with increases, in particular, of promyelocytes and myelocytes.[56,76] Marrow eosinophilia has also been noted in patients who developed significant circulating eosinophilia.[76]

Bone Marrow and Circulating Progenitors

Socinski and colleagues were the first to report that peripheral blood day 14 CFU-GM and BFU-E increased by 18 and 8 fold per milliliter of blood, respectively, following 6 days of rhGM-CSF stimulation, whereas no significant change in bone marrow progenitors was noted.[129] Similar findings have been reported by two other groups utilizing glycosylated preparations of rhGM-CSF.[28,56]

An increase in the percentage of CFU-GM and BFU-E in S-phase has been reported in patients receiving three and six days of glycosylated GM-CSF administered as a continuous intravenous infusion.[1] An increased percentage of bone marrow myeloblasts, promyelocytes, myelocytes (but not erythroblasts) in S-phase, as measured by tritiated thymidine autoradiography, has also been reported.[1] In addition, these investigators observed an increase in the rate of cells entering cycle, from 1.3 to 3.4% per hour, and a decrease in the duration of S-phase from 14.3 to 9.1 hours, and of the cell cycle time from 86 hours to 26 hours. Finally, the proportion of S-phase bone marrow cells decreased to values lower than pretreatment levels, following discontinuation of rhGM-CSF. These findings suggest a period of relative refractoriness post-discontinuation to cell cycle active anti-neoplastic agents.[1]

Pharmacokinetics

Utilizing a radioreceptor assay, a two compartment model of rhGM-CSF elimination was reported by Herrmann and colleagues, which appeared to be independent of the administered dose.[56] In six patients, clearance of glycosylated rhGM-CSF administered over 30 minutes was found to have an alpha phase of 10 ± 3 minutes and a beta phase of 85 ± 35 minutes.[56]

More extensive pharmacokinetic analysis has been undertaken by Cebon and colleagues in patients receiving non-glycosylated GM-CSF.[25] These investigators determined the pharmacokinetics of rhGM-CSF employing both a bone marrow hematopoietic progenitor cell assay and a sensitive (0.02 ng/ml) sandwich enzyme-linked immunoabsorbent assay.[25] Utilizing the latter technique, at the lowest intravenous and subcutaneous dose levels of 0.3 µg/kg, a serum level of 14 ± 3 ng/ml and 30 pg/ml, respectively, was measured. rhGM-CSF is cleared from the blood within 120 minutes following IV administration, with two apparent phases. Following a 1 µg/kg dose of intravenously administered rhGM-CSF, peak levels of 54 ± 26 ng/ml were achieved which dropped to less than 5 ng/ml after 60 minutes and to <1 ng/ml by 120 minutes. The same dose administered subcutaneously to two patients resulted in peak levels of 0.75 ± 0.03 and 0.71 ± 0.04 ng/ml, 120 minutes after injection. At this dose level, both intravenous and subcutaneous administration were associated with at least a two-fold increase in WBC by day 10 of treatment. Higher doses of 3 and 10 µg/kg/day subcutaneously were associated with earlier initial peaks (within 15 minutes) and prolonged plateau levels of 1–3 ng/ml, which remained detectable for up to nine hours.

Overall, assuming two phases of elimination, a $T\frac{1}{2}\alpha$ of less than 5 minutes and $T\frac{1}{2}\beta$ of 50 minutes were determined following intravenous administration. In contrast, a rise in rhGM-CSF blood levels occurred within one hour, peaked by 2–4 hours and fell 2–12 hours after subcutaneous administration. The time during which rhGM-CSF remained detectable was dose dependent. At the dose level of 10 μg/kg, 0.1 ng/ml levels were detectable for 12 hours, a level is equivalent to 100 units of activity and close to that required to stimulate both progenitor cell development and granulocyte function.[25]

Laboratory Studies

An increase in serum alkaline phosphatase of 1.4-fold was noted in 7 of 16 patients receiving > 8 days of subcutaneously administered non-glycosylated GM-CSF.[76] All patients treated for 8 days at 15 and 20 μg/kg/day developed twofold or greater increases of at least two hepatic enzymes including aspartate aminotransferase. Increases in lactate dehydrogenase were also observed.[76]

Administration of CSFs to Patients Receiving Myelosuppressive Therapy

RhG-CSF

Several studies have now been completed which explore the role of rhG-CSF in either abrogating or accelerating the recovery from chemotherapy-induced neutropenia.[18,19,39,40,63,92–94] An initial study explored the efficacy of rhG-CSF in preventing chemotherapy induced myelosuppression in patients with transitional cell carcinoma of the urothelium undergoing treatment with methotrexate, doxorubicin, vinblastine and cisplatin (M-VAC).[39] RhG-CSF was administered in this study either prior to and/or during their first cycle of combination chemotherapy over a dose range of 1–60 μg/kg/day, as a short 30–40 minute intravenous infusion.[39,63] Additional patients have also been treated with a dose of 100 μg/kg/day.[63] Treatment with rhG-CSF following chemotherapy for the entire study population resulted in: 1) significantly fewer days per patient with an absolute neutrophil count of 1,000 per microliter or less; 2) fewer days of antibiotics in the setting of fever and neutropenia; and 3) a significant increase in the percentage of patients qualified to receive planned chemotherapy on day 14 of the treatment cycle. In addition, a significant decrease in the incidence and severity of mucositis was observed.[39] The protocol was subsequently amended to allow some patients to be treated during their second cycle of chemotherapy and not during their first or vice versa. These data suggest that the observations made previously are independent of the cycle in which rhG-CSF administered.[63]

In this study, patients who had received prior pelvic radiation were not protected from neutropenia and, in fact, the nadir achieved was lower when rhG-CSF was administered. However, in all cases, leukocyte counts recovered quickly, so that all such patients were eligible as scheduled for subsequent chemotherapy.[39,63]

Bronchud explored the use the rhG-CSF (1–40 μg/kg/day), administered as a continuous intravenous infusion during alternating cycles of combination chemotherapy for small cell carcinoma of the lung.[19] In this study a decrease in neutropenia, fever, and requirement for antibiotics was noted in patients during chemotherapy cycles when they received rhG-CSF as compared to when they did not.

Morstyn and colleagues initially studied the safety, biological effects and efficacy of rhG-CSF (1–60 μg/kg/day) administered either intravenously, subcutaneously or by means of a continuous subcutaneous route prior to and following high dose melphalan.[92,93] In their studies, a decrease in neutropenia was also observed when rhG-CSF was administered, independent of the route of administration, as compared to when it was not.[92,93] In addition, at doses of >30 μg/kg of rhG-CSF, the neutropenia following standard dose melphalan (25 mg/m² intravenous) was completely abrogated.[92,93] More recently, these investigators have studied the optimization of timing and duration of subcutaneously infused rhG-CSF (10 μg/kg/day) in patients receiving melphalan. The major findings were that G-CSF produced a rapid and sustained elevation in neutrophil levels even when it was begun eight days after chemotherapy. This was sufficient to abrogate leukopenia.[92,94]

One additional interesting observation was that the pharmacokinetics of rhG-CSF, administered prior to melphalan, showed a progressive fall in detectable serum levels despite a sustained rise in neutrophils. This fall was not observed when rhG-CSF was administered after melphalan, suggesting that the level of circulating neutrophil granulocytes might play a role in the half-life and clearance of the protein.[92]

RhG-CSF has been administered to patients receiving more myelosuppressive doses of chemotherapy in the setting of autologous bone marrow transplantation. Taylor and colleagues examined the ability of 60 μg/kg/day of rhG-CSF, administered as a 30 minute intravenous infusion for 28 days, to decrease the number of days required to achieve an absolute neutrophil count (ANC) 100, 500, or 1,000 cells/ul, respectively, in patients with refractory or relapsed Hodgkin's disease treated with chemotherapy and autologous bone marrow transplantation.[136] In all instances, the number of days required to achieve the desired peripheral blood count was significantly decreased as compared to historical controls.[136]

More recently, Peters and colleagues have demonstrated an accelerated recovery from neutropenia in patients treated with rhG-CSF (16–64 μg/kg/d infused continuously for 14 days) after high dose cyclophosphamide, cisplatin and carmustine followed three days later by autologous bone marrow infusion. Leukocyte counts by day 15 were 6,407 ± 1,772 cells/μl as compared to 863 ± 645 cells/μl for historical controls.[106] Granulocyte phagocytosis was found to be enhanced during rhG-CSF administration and hydrogen peroxide generation remained unchanged. In vivo migration of neutrophils to a sterile inflammatory site was preserved and comparable to patients after hematopoietic recovery who had not received growth factor. This was in contrast to the significant inhibition of neutrophil migration observed in this same patient population treated with continuous intravenous infusions of rhGM-CSF.[109]

Sheridan and colleagues studied the use of rhG-CSF after high dose chemotherapy with busulphan and autologous bone marrow transplantation (ABMT).[106] In this study, rhG-

CSF was administered as a continuous subcutaneous infusion of 20 μg/kg/day, beginning one day after ABMT, and reduced progressively when the neutrophil count exceeded 1,000 cells/μl. Of 11 patients entered, nine exceeded neutrophil counts of 500 cells/μl as early as nine days post ABMT (range 9–17) with 7 of the 9 reaching this level before day 12 as compared to 0 of 17 historical controls.[126] Similar trends in recovery for neutrophil counts to more than 1,000 cells/μl was also observed. This enhanced recovery was associated with a decrease in requirements for antibiotic use and an earlier discharge from the hospital.[126]

RhGM-CSF

Several studies exploring the role of rhGM-CSF in ameliorating myelosuppressive toxicity of chemotherapy have also been undertaken.

Antman and colleagues treated 16 patients with inoperable or metastatic sarcomas with escalating doses of rhGM-CSF before and immediately after a first cycle of mesna, doxorubacin, ifosfamide and dacarbazine chemotherapy, and compared the myelosuppressive toxicity of this to a second cycle of chemotherapy administered without concomitant growth factor. Neutropenia after cycle 1 was significantly less severe and of shorter duration than after cycle 2. The mean total leukocyte and platelet nadirs were 1.0 and 101 × 10⁹ per liter for cycle 1 as compared to 0.45 and 44 × 10⁹ per liter for cycle 2. The median intervals from day one of chemotherapy to neutrophil recovery were 15 and 19 days, respectively, and the duration of absolute neutropenia was 3.5 days as compared to 7.4 days with cycle 2.[4] Despite a decrease in the duration of neutropenia, 2 of 14 patients died of sepsis in the treatment cycle as compared to none of the 12 receiving chemotherapy alone. This raised the concern that secondary cytokines induced by the administration of rhGM-CSF, such as tumor necrosis factor (TNF), might contribute, with endotoxin, to profound septic shock in the setting of bacterial infection.[10]

Morstyn and colleagues have explored the use of rhGM-CSF to overcome the myelosuppressive toxicity of patients with small cell carcinoma of the lung receiving treatment every 28 days with carboplatin and etoposide. RhGM-CSF was administered as a 15 μg/kg/day dose subcutaneously on days 4 to 11, 4 to 18, or 4 to 25.[15,92] The results were compared to historical controls where 31 out of 82 patients developed grade IV (modified WHO classification) neutrophil toxicity.[92,93] In patients receiving rhGM-CSF, only 1 of 11 patients developed a neutrophil count of less than 500 cells/μl.[92,93]

More recently, Mertelsmann and colleagues have investigated the ability of subcutaneously administered glycosylated rhGM-CSF to abrogate hematopoietic toxicity following a variety of chemotherapy regimens for solid tumors.[85] In this study, patients underwent combination chemotherapy and, if significant neutropenia developed, a second cycle of chemotherapy was instituted with concomitant administration of hematopoietic growth factor. Results, consistent with the above, were obtained.

RhGM-CSF has also been utilized in the setting of bone marrow transplantation.[16] The first study to be reported was conducted by Peter's group in patients with either breast cancer or melanoma treated with combination chemotherapy and ABMT support.[16,109] Groups of three to four patients were treated with 2.0, 4.0, 8.0, 16.0, or 32 μg/mg/day of glycosylated (CHO cell derived) rhGM-CSF by continuous intravenous infusion beginning three hours after bone marrow infusion. Total leukocyte and granulocyte recovery was accelerated at all dose levels in these patients compared to 24 historical controls matched for age, diagnosis, and treatment. No consistent effect on platelet count recovery was noted. Less bacteremia, hepatotoxicity and nephrotoxicity occurred (perhaps related to the decrease in bacteremia) than had previously been noted for controls.[8,16,108]

Nemunaitis and colleagues administered escalating doses of glycosylated (yeast derived) rhGM-CSF, given as a two hour intravenous infusion for 14 days beginning one hour following completion of autologous or syngeneic bone marrow infusion to patients with lymphoid neoplasms in remission or in relapse.[100] In this study, rhGM-CSF was found to be biologically active at doses of 60 μg/m²/day in that 5 out of 9 patients receiving this dose recovered neutrophil counts to 500 cells/μl or more before day 14 as compared to only 1 of 6 patients receiving less than 60 μg/m², or 4 of 92 historical controls. A decrease in the number of febrile days also occurred in patients treated with 60 μg/m² or more. In addition, fewer days were required to become platelet transfusion independent in patients treated with 60 μg/m² or more of rhGM-CSF. Two patients treated with 60 μg/m² or more had received marrow treated in vitro with pan B cell antibody plus complement, both of whom recovered earlier. No enhancement of graft versus host disease was noted in the small number of patients receiving a syngeneic transplant in combination with rhGM-CSF.[100]

These studies exploring the role of rhG-CSF and rhGM-CSF in ameliorating chemotherapy-induced myelosuppression have suggested that it is possible to reduce the morbidity of chemotherapeutic regimens. From these studies, however, one cannot conclude whether a particular cytoreduction regimen, marrow purging technique or underlying disease affects the responsiveness. Larger, prospective phase III randomized trials are needed to define more precisely the possible therapeutic advantage offered by these growth factors, and to define any additional untoward effects.

By reducing morbidity and making more tolerable our present antineoplastic regimens, hematopoietic growth factors should certainly render standard cancer treatment more tolerable for patients afflicted with malignant neoplastic disease; however, an even greater question remains as to whether, by allowing one to administer dose intensified therapy, these factors will contribute to improved survival. In this regard, Bronchud and colleagues have recently explored the use of rhG-CSF to increase the intensity of treatment with doxorubicin in patients with advanced breast and ovarian cancer.[17] Treatment with escalating doses of doxorubicin was followed by an infusion of rhG-CSF 5 μg/kg/day for 11 days. In this study rhG-CSF administration resulted in a return of the absolute neutrophil count to normal or above normal levels within 12–14 days at all dose levels of doxorubicin used and allowed the administration of up to three cycles of high dose chemotherapy at 14 day intervals. An absolute neutrophil count of >2,500 cells/μl was not reached until day

19–21 after 75 μg/m² of doxorubicin without rhG-CSF. At doses of 125 μg/m² and 150 μg/m², all tumors regressed rapidly by day 12–14; however, despite the accelerated recovery from neutropenia marked epithelial toxicity was apparent and became dose limiting. In this trial, the overall response rate in patients with doxorubicin plus rhG-CSF therapy was 80% with a median time to progression of six months. Two months after treatment there was a pronounced improvement of symptoms, evidenced by the Rotterdam Symptom check list, as compared with before treatment.

Logothelis and colleagues recently reported 19 patients with progressive urothelial tumors who were treated with escalating M-VAC combination therapy plus rhGM-CSF.[79] Although a granulocyte nadir of less than 500 was still observed, 2 of 15 patients achieved complete remissions, despite prior refractoriness to lower doses of antineoplastic agents.[79]

Recently, Gianni and colleagues reported the ability of glycosylated recombinant GM-CSF to reduce the neutropenia associated with high dose cyclophosphamide in patients with non-Hodgkin's lymphoma, as well as in patients with breast cancer.[47] In this study, GM-CSF was administered at a dose of 5.5 μg/kg/day for 14 days as a continuous intravenous infusion, beginning one day after the administration of cyclophosphamide. When GM-CSF was delayed for five days following cyclophosphamide, accelerated hematopoietic recovery was not observed, suggesting that the timing of GM-CSF administration was critical.

In addition, Neidhart and colleagues demonstrated a reduction in the number of days of severe (<100 cells/μl) or moderately severe (<500 cells/μl) neutropenia, and antibiotic therapy in patients receiving rhG-CSF, 60 μg/kg/day (administered as a short intravenous infusion) while undergoing dose intensified treatment with cisplatin (150 mg/M²), etoposide (1,500 mg/M²) and cyclophopamide (5,000 mg/M²) in the absence of bone marrow transplantation.[99]

Although these studies are far from definitive, they provide an overview of the direction in which the clinical investigation of these hematopoietic growth factors is heading.

Neoplastic Disease Associated with Neutropenia

Neutropenia is also a significant problem which results directly from a number of hematopoietic disorders. Initial studies of hematopoietic growth factors in a number of hematopoietic malignancies suggest that these molecules may play an important role in the management and treatment of these disorders.

Hairy Cell Leukemia

Glaspy and colleagues conducted a study to determine whether rhG-CSF was effective in correcting severe neutropenia in patients with hairy cell leukemia.[48] RhG-CSF was administered daily, as a subcutaneous injection, beginning at a dose of 1 μg/kg/day. The dose was increased weekly for two weeks to 6 μg/kg/day and treatment continued for 5–6 weeks. Two of four patients entered had ongoing infection with conjunctivitis and periorbital skin infections; and a perirectal abscess, fever, hypotension, and urinary retention unresponsive to antibiotics and amphotericin. In 3 of 4 patients who completed the course of treatment, a significant increase

in circulating neutrophil counts was associated with an increase in myeloid bone marrow elements. In two patients with infectious complications, complete resolution of infection occurred with rhG-CSF treatment. One patient had a history of biopsy proven cutaneous leukocytoclastic vasculitis at the time of her initial presentation. An exacerbation of her dermatologic problem, consisting of acute febrile neutrophilic dermatosis (the Sweet Syndrome) occurred while receiving rhG-CSF. This most likely resulted from the increase in granulocyte reserves and neutrophil counts stimulated by rhG-CSF administration, giving rise to increased neutrophil epidermal infiltration.[48]

Myelodysplastic Syndrome (MDS)

Several hematopoietic growth factors have been tested in the treatment of (MDS) (Table XVIII-6-7). Negrin and colleagues conducted a study to determine if rhG-CSF could improve neutropenia associated with myelodysplastic syndrome (MDS).[98] Thirteen patients with MDS (two refractory anemia, eight refractory anemia with excess blasts in transformation) were treated with daily subcutaneous injections of rhG-CSF using an escalating dose, from 0.1–3.0 μg/kg/day, for 6–8 weeks. Eleven patients had significant elevations in white blood cell and absolute neutrophil counts. In five patients, a greater than two-fold increase in reticulocyte count occurred. In two of nine red cell transfusion dependent patients this led to a decrease in red cell transfusion requirements. No significant changes in platelet counts were noted during treatment.[98] Three patients subsequently received additional treatment for up to eight weeks with ANC levels remaining within the normal range. In all cases, treatment has been well tolerated. In vitro suppression of myeloid clonal self-generation was observed with the replating efficiency (PE2) decreasing to 19% of basal levels.[98] Kobayashi and colleagues also treated five MDS patients with 30 minute intravenous infusions of rhG-CSF for six days, and noted improved neutrophil counts.[72]

Several trials of rhGM-CSF have been conducted in patients with MDS.[45,137,142] The first study was conducted by Vadhan-Raj and colleagues.[142] This group of investigators explored the effect of continuously infused glycosylated rhGM-CSF given over a dose range of 30–500 μg/m², for 14 days in one patient with refractory anemia (RA), three patients with refractory anemia with excess blasts (RAEB) and four patients with refractory anemia with excess blasts in transformation (RAEBT). In this study, 5–20 fold and 5–373 fold increases in circulating WBC and ANC, respectively, were noted. Two of 4 and 2 of 8 red cell and platelet transfusion dependent patients had a significant increase in their red cell and platelet counts. No transformation to acute leukemia was noted. In patients who received more than one course of rhGM-CSF, the baseline granulocyte count improved over time with repeated cycles of treatment.[142]

Ganser and colleagues also conducted a trial of glycosylated rhGM-CSF in patients with MDS including three with RA, four with RAEB, two with RAEBT and two with chronic myelomonocytic leukemia (CMMoL).[45] RhGM-CSF was administered as an initial bolus on day 1 followed by a daily 8 hour infusion of rhGM-CSF for a total of 8–14 days. The treatment schedule included a dose escalation from 15–50

$\mu g/m^2$. Results included 1.3–18-fold increases in circulating leukocyte counts in 10 of 11 patients, an increase in monocytes and eosinophils in seven and six patients, respectively, an increase in lymphocytes affecting both T-helper and T-suppressor cells, but without evidence of activation as measured by the expression of the IL-2 receptor. Patients with greater than 14% bone marrow blasts or with pretreatment circulating blasts experienced increases in these cells. In addition, one patient with no detectable circulating blasts initially demonstrated an increase in peripheral blood blasts with treatment. No change in circulating red cell, platelet count or transfusion requirements was observed. Cytogenetic analysis revealed either increase or decrease in the number of abnormal metaphases in six patients with chromosomal abnormalities suggesting that proliferative as well as suppressive or possibly differentiating effects on marrow cells occur with rhGM-CSF treatment.[45]

Thompson and colleagues explored the use of daily subcutaneously administered non-glycosylated rhGM-CSF for ten days to seven patients with RA, eight patients with RAEB, and one patient with RAEBT.[137] Circulating granulocytes increased in a dose dependent manner. Neutrophil counts decreased to baseline after discontinuation in most patients; however, in two patients, the neutrophil count remained elevated over of at least six months of observation. Increases in monocytes and eosinophils were observed in three patients. Five of 16 patients had an increase in the percentage of bone marrow blasts, whereas four had a slight decrease, and seven remained unchanged, although the bone marrow cellularity increased.[137] Other smaller studies have suggested comparable results (Table XVIII-6-7).[3,37,55,117]

Ganser and colleagues recently conducted a Phase I/II study of rhIL-3 (250 $\mu g/M^2$–500 $\mu g/M^2$) administered subcutaneously for 15 days in nine patients with MDS (six RA and three RAEB) and concomitant severe transfusion-dependent cytopenias. Blood leukocytes increase 1.3–3.6 fold in all patients with a particular increase in eosinophil granulocytes.[44] Platelet responses were noted in two patients resulting in discontinuation of platelet transfusion requirements. Two other patients had transient thrombocytopenia with IL-3 treatment. One patient demonstrated a decrease in red cell transfusion requirements. Disease progression, as measured by an increase in circulating blasts, was noted in one patient with RAEB (see XXXVI-1).

Table XVIII-6-7. Potential Therapeutic Applications of Colony-Stimulating Factors in Hematopoietic Malignant and Nonmalignant Conditions Associated with Neutropenia

1. Angioimmunoblastic Lymphadenopathy	7. Hairy Cell Leukemia
2. Cyclic Neutropenia	8. Chronic Lymphocytic Leukemia
3. Idiopathic Neutropenia	9. Low Grade Follicular Lymphomas/ Leukemic Phase
4. Congenital Neutropenia (Kostman's Syndrome)	
5. Aplastic Anemia	10. Refractory Anemia/ Myelodysplastic Syndromes
6. AIDS	

Other Hematopoietic Growth Factors

At the present time, clinical trials of M-CSF, which has been shown to differentiate leukemic cell in vitro are underway in the treatment of MDS. Erythropoietin is also being investigated in RA, RAEB and RAEBT.

Although, these initial results utilizing growth factors appear promising for selected patients, additional studies with longer follow-up will be needed to determine efficacy, long term improvement in morbidity, and the impact upon survival and transformation to acute leukemia (see XXXVI-1).

Acute Leukemias

The use of hematopoietic growth factors in the treatment of acute myeloid leukemia (AML) has been controversial. Buchner and colleagues administered glycosylated rhGM-CSF (de-escalation in two four-day steps following neutrophil recovery after chemotherapy) to 23 patients with relapsed AML, newly diagnosed AML patients with age >65 years or ALL.[5,20] The time to achieve a neutrophil count >500 was shorter than for historical controls in 16 out of 19 patients. Platelets also appeared to recover faster in some patients. Regrowth of leukemic blasts occurred in one newly diagnosed and two secondary AML patients. Ohno and colleagues recently reported on the use of G-CSF after intensive induction therapy in relapsed or refractory AML.[20] Treatment with G-CSF accelerated neutrophil recovery significantly and decreased the incidence of documented infections in this patient population.[20] No evidence of accelerated regrowth of leukemic cells was noted.[20]

At least three studies have been initiated in Europe and the United States exploring the use of either rhGM-CSF or rhG-CSF to promote cell cycle activation and enhanced leukemic cell kill with cycle specific agents such as cytosine arabinoside. These studies, based on in vitro investigations by several groups,[13,23,134] demonstrate that, compared to cell killing with an anti-neoplastic agent alone, it is possible to augment the number of leukemic progenitors and cells of the nonprogenitor compartment killed. The clinical studies based on these observations have begun and should prove informative.[62]

Multiple Myeloma

Although neutropenia occurs, in myeloma, no study of rhG-CSF or rhGM-CSF has as yet been explored in this setting. Barlogi and colleagues have studied the use of non-glycosylated GM-CSF in a patient with refractory multiple myeloma receiving high dose melphalan.[11] Lower doses of GM-CSF (0.25 mg/M^2) appeared to hasten marrow recovery in younger aged patients or in patients who had received little prior therapy, and was associated with little toxicity. Higher doses of GM-CSF increased the incidence of side effects especially among older patients.[11]

Non-Neoplastic Disease Associated with Neutropenia

Several non-neoplastic diseases are characterized by severe neutropenia resulting in significant clinical morbidity. These are outlined in Table XVIII-6-7. We will discuss each subgroup separately.

Primary Neutropenic Disorders

Primary neutropenic disorders include cyclic neutropenia, congenital neutropenia (Kostmann's syndrome), and adult acquired idiopathic neutropenia. In addition, some of these disorders may, in fact, represent absolute or relative affinities of their respective receptors. The use of G-CSF in cyclic, congenital and idiopathic neutropenic disorders is ongoing and appears promising.

Cyclic neutropenia is a rare disorder characterized by regular and periodic disappearance of neutrophils. Usually, even at the peak of the cycle, patients are leukopenic. In addition, the typical pattern reveals that all blood counts cycle out of phase (particularly monocytes) with each other, but always with the same periodicity. Based on the preclinical observation of Lothrop and colleagues in the grey collie cyclic dog,[81] Hammond and colleagues conducted a pilot clinical trial of rhG-CSF in which patients were treated with rhG-CSF (1–10 μg/kg) intravenously or subcutaneously for several months to greater than one year.[54] Prior to therapy, the patients all had recurrent stomatitis, pharyngitis, lymphadenopathy and fever at 21 day intervals. The effects of therapy in these patients were: 1) to increase the amplitude of the neutrophil cycles; 2) shorten the cycle length from 21 to 14 days; 3) shorten the period of neutropenia to about one day; and 4) avoid a fall in count to zero during the neutropenic period. Clinically, the patients have benefitted dramatically by the abbreviated, less severe neutropenic periods.[54] With treatment, almost all of the symptoms, including the typical mouth ulcers have been eliminated.[54] In contrast, Fibbe and colleagues observed no correction of cyclic neutropenia when patients were treated with rhGM-CSF.[54]

Congenital neutropenia, or Kostmann's syndrome, is a disorder characterized by severe neutropenia with an ANC of <200 cells/μl; maturational arrest of the bone marrow myeloid precursor at the promyelocyte or myelocyte stage; early onset in infancy of severe recurrent bacterial infections; and variable monocytosis and eosinophils and plasma cells in the bone marrow. Bonilla and colleagues conducted a phase I/II trial of rhG-CSF administered intravenously and subcutaneously to patients with this disorder.[14] In the first five patients treated, an increase in circulating neutrophil counts to greater than 1,000 cells/μl has been observed with varying doses of rhG-CSF. This was associated with a decrease in infectious episodes, hospitalizations and requirements for antibiotics.[14] Similar findings have recently been reported by Welte and colleagues.[148] In this latter study, patients developed only neutrophil granulocytosis following rhG-CSF treatment. In contrast, no augmentation in neutrophil counts were seen in the same patients when rhGM-CSF was administered.[148]

Idiopathic neutropenia is characterized by progressive neutropenia associated with hypocellular bone marrows, myeloid maturation arrest, recurrent infections and oral and/or skin ulcerations. A pilot study was conducted on preclinical in vitro studies which demonstrated the efficacy of rhG-CSF in generating mature neutrophil granulocytes in bone marrow suspension cultures or neutrophil colony assays.[64] Two patients were treated with rhG-CSF, administered as a daily subcutaneous injection from 1–3 μg/kg/day. Both had

restoration of neutrophil counts to within a normal range. This in turn was associated with no further infectious episodes, and complete resolution of oral ulcerations. Both these patients have been maintained on treatment for eight months to greater than one year. No tolerance has developed and no antibody formation has been detected. Based on the three pilot studies with rhG-CSF in patients with primary neutropenic disorders, a multicenter randomized clinical trial has commenced to further explore the role of this hematopoietic growth factor in the treatment of these rare but often life-threatening diseases.

One patient with severe idiopathic agranulocytosis, was treated by Antin and colleagues with glycosylated rhGM-CSF without any apparent effect.[3] Champlin and colleagues also attempted to treat two patients with agranulocytosis with rhGM-CSF; however, treatment had to be discontinued in both patients because of dose related toxicity, before enough time had elapsed to assess, clinical response.[26]

Recently, Ganser and colleagues treated four patients with chronic neutropenia.[43] This group of patients included one patient with autoimmune neutropenia, one patient with neutropenia secondary to prior chemotherapy for Hodgkins disease, one patient with asymptomatic neutropenia of unknown cause, and one patient with congenital neutropenia with normocellular bone marrow and normal serum immunoglobulins. Patients were treated with 150 μg–1,000 μg/M² GM-CSF IV[1] or subcutaneously[3] for 12–14 consecutive days. All patients demonstrated an initial increase in leukocyte count which was associated with an increase in neutrophil and eosinophil granulocytes. All counts returned to baseline upon discontinuation of treatment. One patient with congenital neutropenia demonstrated a much smaller increment in leukocyte count.[43]

Aplastic Anemia

Five major studies have been conducted exploring the role of different glycosylated rhGM-CSF preparations in the treatment of aplastic anemia.[26,53,104,140] Antin and colleagues performed the first phase I/II study of daily glycosylated rhGM-CSF (yeast) 15–480 μg/m² administered either as a 1–4 hour intravenous infusion for 14 days.[3] Patients were allowed repeated treatments at progressively higher dose levels if no toxicity was observed. Seven red cell transfusion dependent patients with severe aplastic anemia were studied. Modest increases in granulocyte and monocyte counts, not clearly dose related, were noted in 13 of 22 and 14 of 22 courses respectively, with the median time to peak granulocyte count occurring after 4 days (range 1–21). On 5 occasions, the peak granulocyte count occurred between days 14 and 21, despite the fact that the infusion of rhGM-CSF was stopped on day 7. These findings suggest that the stimulation of early progenitors resulted in improved counts after the growth factor was no longer present. No increase in baseline counts was observed with repeated courses of rhGM-CSF in this patient population. No increases in eosinophils, immature myeloid or amelioration of red cell or platelet transfusion requirements were noted.[3]

Nissen and colleagues treated four patients with very severe aplastic anemia refractory to ATG.[104] All patients were red cell and platelet transfusion dependent and had total neutrophil counts of <50 cells/μl. Only one patient had evidence of marrow myelopoiesis. Glycosylated (CHO cell derived) rhGM-CSF was administered from 4–32 μg/kg/day either as a continuous intravenous infusion for 14 days[4] or as a subcutaneous twice daily injection.[1] In this study, only the one patient with evidence of residual marrow myelopoiesis demonstrated an increase in neutrophil counts which allowed clearance of bilateral pneumonia. No improvement in red cell or platelet transfusions was noted in any patient in this study either.[104]

Vanhan-Raj and colleagues treated eight patients with true moderate[3] to severe[5] aplastic anemia with glycosylated yeast-derived rhGM-CSF over a dose range of 60–500 μg/m[2].[140] RhGM-CSF was administered as a continuous intravenous infusion daily for two weeks. The treatment period was followed by a two week rest period and a second cycle of continuous infusion treatment. During rhGM-CSF treatment these investigators reported: 1) an increase in marrow cellularity (eight patients) and myeloid to erythroid cell ratios; and 2) an increase in circulating neutrophils (six patients), eosinophils (eight patients) and monocytes (eight patients). Despite an increase in neutrophil counts, however, four patients (three with a previous history of infectious episodes) experienced sepsis while on study. In addition, no change in red cell or platelet counts were seen.[140]

Champlin and colleagues treated 13 patients with refractory aplastic anemia with 4–64 μg/kg/day rhGM-CSF (CHO-derived) administered as a continuous intravenous infusion for 14–28 days.[26] Patients achieving complete or partial responses were subsequently treated for an additional two months. Seven patients had complete normalization of their circulating granulocyte count and three patients had an increase to >500 cells/μl. The greatest increments occurred in patients with higher pretreatment granulocyte counts. One patient had no response and in one patient, the granulocyte response was transient. All patients were monocytopenic at study entry. During treatment eight of eleven patients had normalization of monocyte counts and two achieved partial responses (>200 cells/μl). Increases in circulating eosinophils were also observed after two weeks of rhGM-CSF administration. Circulating erythrocytes, platelets, and transfusion requirements were unaffected by treatment in all but one patient who demonstrated an increase in hemoglobin from 7 to 11 and an increase in platelet count from 20,000 to 45,000 cells/μl, respectively. In addition to an augmentation of circulating blood counts, bone marrow cellularity as well as marrow and peripheral blood myeloid progenitors increased in all responding patients. In all cases, discontinuation of treatment was associated with a return to baseline peripheral blood counts and bone marrow cellularity.[26] Interestingly, in this study, the investigators noted a significant decrease in serum cholesterol in aplastic patients receiving rhGM-CSF.[102]

Recently Gluinan and colleagues conducted a trial of glycosylated (CHO derived) GM-CSF in nine pediatric patients ranging in age from 0.7–19 years (Table XVIII-6-7).[53] Seven of nine patients had received one or more courses of ATG and four patients had a history of ATG response followed by relapse. Six of eight evaluable patients had significant increases in neutrophil counts and one patient developed a trilineage response which has persisted for more than one year off study.[53]

Ganser and colleagues have studied the use of IL-3 in correcting the pancytopenia associated with aplastic anemia.[42] In a phase I/II study, 10 patients with aplastic anemia were treated with recombinant human interleukin-3 (rhIL-3) to assess the toxicity and biological effects of this multipotential hematopoietic growth factor. Doses ranging from 250–500 μg/m[2] were administered as subcutaneous bolus injections daily for 15 days. An increase in platelet counts from 1,000/μl to 31,000/μl was induced by rhIL-3 in one patient and an increase in reticulocyte counts in seven patients. The blood leukocyte counts temporarily increased in nine patients 1.1- to 2.3-fold (median, 1.7-fold), mainly due to an increase in the number of neutrophils, eosinophils, lymphocytes and monocytes. Mild side effects (headache and flushing) were observed in some patients, while low-grade fever occurred in all patients. Transient thrombocytopenia necessitating discontinuation of rhIL-3 treatment occurred in one patient.

In all of these studies, the majority of patients require continued treatment to see the desired hematologic effect. When treatment was discontinued, counts returned to baseline, and marrow cellularity decreased. This observation suggests that, in the majority of cases, normal progenitors are present but their growth is suppressed, perhaps by the inappropriate production of negative regulators, such as gamma interferon.

These studies would suggest that prospective trials are needed to determine if hematopoietic growth factors will impact favorably on the morbidity and mortality of aplastic anemia.

Acquired Immunodeficiency Syndrome (AIDS)

AIDS, while primarily due to a deficiency of T4 lymphocytes, is frequently complicated by deficits in neutrophils and monocyte number and function. CSFs may therefore be useful in AIDS by increasing the number of these host effector cells but also by enhancing their function. In addition, neutropenia is the major complication of antiviral agents, such as zidovudine (azidothymidine, AZT) presently used for either the treatment of AIDS or its complications. This toxicity, in turn limits the dose of medication which can be safely tolerated.

Three major studies have been reported which demonstrate that rhGM-CSF can augment myelopoiesis and improve neutrophil function in patients with AIDS. The first study was conducted by Groopman and colleagues who administered a continuous intravenous infusion of rhGM-CSF (0.3–4.5 μg/kg/day for 14 days) to 16 relatively well patients with AIDS and leukopenia.[52] Treatment resulted in a dramatic augmentation in circulating granulocytes and monocytes without evidence of increased viral production. Baldwin and colleagues studied the function of neutrophils produced in six of these AIDS patients treated with rhGM-CSF.[7] These investigators found that ADCC and phagocytosis improved with treatment, whereas superoxide generation was more variable.[7]

More recently, Mitsuyasu and colleagues, evaluated the toxicity, clinical, hematologic and antiviral effects of nonglycosylated rhGM-CSF administered subcutaneously daily for up to six months in 15 patients with HIV infection.[88] Cohorts of 2–4 patients were treated at doses between 0.25 and 8.0 μg/kg/day. All patients were intolerant of AZT or had severe leukopenia precluding its use. The median WBC was 2,300 (range 1,300–2,800). All patients had a three-fold increase in WBC, ANC eosinophil counts and a >2 fold increase in monocytes and lymphocytes within three weeks of treatment; however, no change in CD4:CD8 ratio, skin reactivity, hemoglobin or reticulocyte count was noted. Serum p24 antigen decreased by >50% in two patients, increased by >50% in four and remained unchanged in seven.[88]

Pluda and colleagues investigated the role of GM-CSF, first alone, and then alternating with AZT in 10 leukopenic patients with AIDS.[115] Ten patients with AIDS, five of whom could not tolerate conventional doses of AZT, were administered GM-CSF for 12 days. During this initial 12 days, an increase in WBC occurred; however, at the same time an increase in HIV p24 antigen was noted in six evaluable patients. During the subsequent treatment period of alternating AZT and GM-CSF, the serum HIV p24 antigen fell to below the post GM-CSF level. The mean T4 cell value increased in patients who had not previously received AZT, and hematologic toxicity appeared reduced. Two patients had improved tolerance of AZT.[115]

More recently, studies have been undertaken to explore the role of rhG-CSF in combination with erythropoietin and AZT in correcting neutropenia and anemia seen in association with AIDS and its treatment. The results of these studies, will certainly be of interest.

Other Hematopoietic Growth Factors

More recently, studies have been conducted exploring the use of stem cell growth factors, such as IL-1, in an attempt both to enhance stem cell proliferation, availability, and response to lineage-specific factors and to hasten the recovery of hematopoietic cells other than myeloid elements alone. To this end, a study of IL-1 has been undertaken in patients with colon cancer receiving myelosuppressive doses of 5-fluorouracil (5-FU).[29] Toxicities include fever, hypertension, hypotension, phlebitis at the site of IL-1 infusion and abdominal pain. Hematological effects of IL-1 have included leukocytosis and neutrophilic granulocytosis in all patients (peak two to eight hours). At the 0.068 μg/kg one day dose level, this granulocytosis was associated with enhanced neutrophil superoxide generation. A transient fall in platelet count within normal range three to four days after IL-1 administration was also noted, followed by a rise in platelet count four to 25 days (median 13 days) after IL-1 administration. Metabolic effects included elevated C-reactive protein and transient hypoglycemia with a mild rebound hyperglycemia. Some myeloprotective effects were noted, including more profound leukocyte and granulocyte nadirs after 5-FU alone as compared with 5-FU plus IL-1, as well as a decreased total and mean number of leukopenic and neutropenic days after 5-FU plus IL-1. At the dose levels studied so far, no favorable impact on hospitalizations for febrile neutropenia or total number of days of antibiotic treatment have been observed.[29]

Clinical investigations exploring the use of hematopoietic growth factors, such as M-CSF[8,9] and IL-4[82] to augment effector cell function have also been completed and/or underway.

Recently Bajorin and colleagues studied the ability of M-CSF to enhance antibody-dependent cellular cytotoxicity (ADCC) as well as hematopoiesis in patients with melanoma.[8,9] Biologic effects of rhM-CSF include augmentation of macrophage-mediated cytotoxicity and antibody-dependent monocyte-mediated cytotoxicity (ADMC) against human melanoma cell lines, anti-tumor activity in a mouse B-16 melanoma model, and induction of peripheral blood monocytosis in primates. In this clinical study, the safety, biologic effects and anti-tumor activity of rhM-CSF were elevated in 12 patients treated at 10, 30, 50, and 80 μg/kg/day as a continuous intravenous infusion on days 1–7 and 22–28. Increases in the percentage and absolute peripheral blood monocytes were observed at doses ≤30 μg/kg/day. At the 80 μg/kg/day level, the percentage of peripheral blood monocytes (mean ± SE) increased from 5.5 ± 0.6 pretreatment to 23.6 ± 2.7 posttreatment and monocyte counts increased from 356 ± 30/μl to 2,063 ± 359/μl. Increases in ADMC were observed in patients treated with 50 and 80 μg/kg/day. Evaluation of the effect of treatment on bone marrow progenitors is ongoing. No partial or complete responses were observed. One patient with early tumor progression had delayed regression of skin lesions; tumor biopsy revealed macrophage and CD8 + T-lymphocyte infiltration. Thrombocytopenia was mild and dose related. Changes in cholesterol and lipoproteins were dose related: at 80 μg/kg, the mean (± SE) reduction from baseline in cholesterol was 27% ± 2.9%, 32% ± 6.5 for low-density lipoprotein (LDL) and 34% ± 5.4 for high-density lipoprotein (HDL). Further dose levels are planned.

Finally, early clinical studies of IL-4 alone have been designed for further stimulation of lymphocyte-activated killer cells[82] and/or induction of other hematopoietic growth factors in vivo to augment myelopoiesis. Forty-two patients with advanced cancer have been treated in a phase I study with a daily intravenous bolus for ≥ 19 days. Effects observed include fever, chills, nausea, diarrhea, oliguria, peripheral edema and constitutional symptoms (malaise). Headache, sinus congestion, nasal fullness and gastritis have been observed in many patients. Using either a bioassay or an ELISA for IL-4, a short serum half life with an alpha distribution phase of eight minutes and a beta clearance phase of 48 minutes has been observed.

Side Effects

rhG-CSF. Treatment with rhG-CSF has been, for the most part, well tolerated. Mild to moderate medullary bone pain has been the most frequent and significant clinical side effect, observed most commonly when patients are treated with a short intravenous infusion of rhG-CSF, but also reported following subcutaneous bolus and continuous subcutaneous infusion.[1,19,40,63,92,93] The medullary bone pain is most often characterized as a pulsating deep pain or pressure localized primarily to the lower back, pelvis and/or sternum.[40] In one study, the pain was most problematic in two middle aged, moderate to severely obese post-menopausal women who received 60 and 100 μg/kg/day of rhG-CSF as a short 30–40 minute intravenous infusion.[40,63] Both of these patients experienced more diffuse bone pain, which in one patient was only relieved by indomethacin. Other occasional complaints in this setting have included chest tightness, mild headache and rarely flushing.

In one study where rhG-CSF was employed following ABMT, one patient receiving 64 μg/kg/day developed hypotension.[109] In addition, the occurrence of a maculopapular rash and an increase in serum creatinine was seen at this dose level in general patients.[108,109] Historical data for this particular ABMT setting reveals a 30% incidence of elevated creatinine in the transplant setting itself.[108,109] In two other transplant studies, the only toxicity observed was medullary bone pain.

In patients with congenital and cyclic neutropenia, splenomegaly has been reported.[14,54,148] Other unusual side effects include a flare in psoriasis in one patient with MDS,[98] the recurrence of Sweets syndrome (cutaneous neutrophilic vasculitis) in a patient with hairy cell leukemia[48] and cutaneous vasculitis in a patient with congenital neutropenic associated with an increase in ANC to >1,000 cells/μl.[148]

rhGM-CSF. A number of side effects have been reported in patients receiving both glycosylated and non-glycosylated rhGM-CSF.[4,28,56,76,92,94,112,118] Fever and bone pain are the most common side effects observed in patients treated with non-glycosylated GM-CSF. Pericarditis was determined to be dose limiting in two out of five patients treated with 20–30 μg/kg/day, whereas this side effect was not observed in 16 patients treated with lower doses.[76] In patients receiving non-glycosylated rhGM-CSF, a peculiar first dose reaction including flushing, hypotension, transient hypoxia and tachycardia has been described.[76,92] After the first dose of rhGM-CSF, subsequent doses do not elicit this response; however, if treatment is discontinued for 10 or more days and rhGM-CSF is re-introduced, the first dose again may produce this reaction.[92] Morstyn and colleagues have reported that the reaction appears to occur predominantly in patients receiving short infusions and perhaps, more commonly, in patients with pulmonary disease.[92]

The major side effects reported to be associated with glycosylated rhGM-CSF treatment include: fever, bone pain, myalgia and constitutional symptoms of weakness and fatigue.[4,16,28,56,112,118,131] The fever observed secondary to rhGM-CSF administration can be abrogated by the administration of indomethacin suggesting that it is possibly mediated by prostaglandins.[110] Short intravenous infusions of glycosylated (yeast derived), rhGM-CSF, have also been associated with dose limiting epigastric distress, nausea, and vomiting.[56,118] In two studies, at higher doses of glycosylated, (CHO cell derived) rhGM-CSF (≥ 32 μg/kg/day) used either prior to chemotherapy[4] or following ABMT,[16] generalized edema, thrombophlebitis, hypotension, and acute renal failure (one patient) have been reported. Comparable side effects with glycosylated yeast derived rhGM-CSF have not been reported;[100] however, comparable doses have not been explored in these identical settings. Treatment with both glycosylated and nonglycosylated rhGM-CSF has also, in some studies, been associated with a transient decline in platelet count.[56,76]

Other Cytokines

Side effects reported to date for IL-1 include fever, chills, phlebitis, hypotension, and abdominal pain.[29] Ganser and

colleagues reported occasional fever and hypotension in patients receiving IL-3.[42,44] M-CSF has been relatively well tolerated, with essentially no toxicity reported except for mild thrombocytopenia. Reported toxicities of IL-4 have included fever, occasional headache, episodic nasal congestion, and fluid retention in one patient.[82]

The clinical ramifications and therapeutic evaluation of hematopoietic growth factors is a rapidly moving field which holds great promise for the treatment of a variety of medical illnesses. In addition, an understanding of the mechanism and action of these factors should provide insight into the pathophysiology and manifestations of many diseases. Ultimately, combinations of hematopoietic cell factors, alone or in combination with other cytokines, low molecular weight compounds, vitamins or chemotherapeutic agents to either accelerate immune reconstitution, boost effector cell function or promote enhanced differentiation of tumor cells should prove useful in the treatment of a number of malignant, infectious and genetic disorders affecting normal hematopoiesis.

Future Directions

Hematopoietic Growth Factors in Combination

It is becoming increasingly clear that the regulation of hematopoietic cell development is very delicately controlled by an intricate network of positive and negative regulation. In order to take advantage of this complex cascade and to better affect more complete hematopoietic reconstitution, we will more than likely need to employ a combination of regulatory factors which act at different levels along the pathway of blood cell development. Considerable evidence already exists in vitro to suggest that synergism is achieved when hematopoietic growth factors which control the proliferative state of primitive hematopoietic progenitors are used in combination.[74] In addition, IL-3, an early acting factor, has been shown to synergize with GM-CSF and G-CSF to enhance the proliferation and differentiation of myeloid committed progenitors, suggesting that combinations of early acting and more lineage restricted regulatory molecules might have clinical utility in patients with iatrogenic or disease related myelosuppression.[106,119] Since individual CSFs enhance monocyte[24] and neutrophil[113] effector cell function, combinations might better augment host defense as well.

Recently, preclinical studies exploring the combination of GM-CSF and IL-3 have demonstrated that IL-3 potentiates the myeloid responsiveness of the host to subsequent administration of GM-CSF.[34] Combinations of low concentrations of IL-3 and M-CSF, which by themselves were inactive, have been shown to increase both the percentage and cycle status of macrophage colony forming cells of both high and low proliferative potential. In addition, the combination of IL-1 and G-CSF has been shown to enhance neutrophil recovery in both murine and primate non tumor-bearing and tumor-bearing models of chemotherapy-induced myelosuppression as compared to the administration of each respective growth factor alone.[91,144] These in vitro and early in vivo studies will provide the foundation for future clinical trials designed to optimize the stimulation of hematopoiesis in order to completely ablate myelosuppression.

Peripheral Blood Progenitors

The use of hematopoietic growth factors have already been shown to reduce the morbidity of myelosuppression related to the administration of chemotherapy or observed in the setting of autologous bone marrow transplantation (see XIX-1). Due to the accelerated recovery from neutropenia, dose intensification, as a strategic design to enhance the efficacy of anti-tumor regimens will be possible; however, the use of lineage specific factors alone is not likely to abrogate the myelopsuppression observed with increasing doses of cyto-toxic agents. Chemotherapy appears to do two things to the hematopoietic system: destroy the CSF responsive progen-itors; and injure the accessory cells which normally produce the appropriate regulatory stimuli. Following chemotherapy, the circulating count drops, even in the presence of coad-ministered growth factor, because the responsive progeni-tors have been temporarily injured. In the case of G-CSF, once these progenitors became available (the recovery of which may also be enhanced by the administration of this factor), they can be acted upon by the growth factor and rapidly matured and mobilized over the course of one and a half days, giving rise to the accelerated recovery in the absolute neutrophil and white blood cell count typically observed. One way to better effect recovery, therefore, would be not only to speed the recovery of the injured progenitors (which may be accomplished by coadministering an earlier acting stem cell factor), but by providing the progenitors themselves in an easily obtainable form. This can be done by collecting peripheral blood from individuals following the administration of G-CSF or GM-CSF to a chemotherapy "naive" patient, where the number of circulating progenitors has been shown to be increased up to 100-fold; or during the recovery phase of the white blood cell count, following chemotherapy plus CSF. Studies by Gianni and colleagues,[47] Peters and colleagues,[109] and Shea and colleagues,[125] have already shown that one can utilize the enhanced numbers of CSF induced progenitors to more effectively reduce myelo-suppression in the setting of high dose chemotherapy with or without autologous bone marrow transplantation. If dose intensified regimens appear promising with regard to improved response rates and possible cure for selected tumor types, the utilization of "primed" peripheral blood progenitors will likely revolutionize blood banking and become common place among our armamentarium against neoplastic disease.

References

1. Aglietta, M., Piacibello, W., Sanavio, F., Stacchine, A., Apra, F., Schena, M., Mossetti, C., Carsino, F., Cappio-Caligeris, F., and Gavosto, F.: Kinetics of human hemopoietic cells after in vivo administration of granulocyte-macrophage colony-stimulating factor. J. Clin. Invest., 83:551, 1989.
2. Andreeff, M., and Welte, K.: Hematopoietic colony stimulating factors. Sem. Onc., 16:211, 1989.
3. Antin, J. H., Smith, B. R., Holmes, W., and Rosenthal, D. S.: Phase I/II study of recombinant human granulocyte-macrophage colony-stimulating factor in aplastic anemia and myelodysplastic syndrome. Blood, 72:705, 1988.
4. Antman, K. S., Griffin, J. D., Elias, A., Socinski, M. A., Ryan, L., Cannistra, S. A., Oette, D., Whitley, M., Frei, E., and Schnipper, L. E.: Effect of recombinant human granulocyte-macrophage colony stimulating factor on chemotherapy-induced mye-losuppression. N. Engl. J. Med., 319:593, 1989.
5. Arnaout, M. A., Wang, E. A., Clark, S. C., and Sieff, C. A.: Human recombinant granulocyte-macrophage colony-stimulating factor increases cell-to-cell adhesion and surface expression of adhesion-promoting surface glycoproteins on mature gran-ulocytes. J. Clin. Invest., 78:597, 1986.
6. Baldwin, G. C., DiPersio, J., Kaufman, S. E., Quan, S. G., Golde, D. W., and Gasson, J. C.: Characterization of human GM-CSF receptors on nonhematopoietic cells. Blood, 70 Suppl. 1:519, 1987.
7. Baldwin, G. C., Gasson, J. C., Quan, S. G., Fleischmann, J., Weisbart, R., Oette, D.,
8. Mitsuyasu, R. T., and Golde, D. W.: Granulocyte-macrophage colony-stimulating factor enhances neutrophil function in acquired immunodeficiency syndrome patients. Proc. Natl. Acad. Sci., 856:2763, 1988.
8. Bajorin, D. F., Jakubowski, A., Cody, B., Chapman, P., Scheinberg, D. A., Munn, D., Cheung, N-K., Dantis, L., Templeton, M. A., Crown, J., Toner, G., Zakowski, M., Haines, C., Gabrilove, J., Oettgen, H. F., Garnick, M. B., and Houghton, A. N.: Phase I trial of recombinant macrophage colony stimulating factor (rhM-CSF) in patients (PTS) with melanoma (MEL). Blood, 74 Suppl. 1:1222, 1989.
9. Bajorin, D. F., Jakubowski, A., Cody, B., Munn, D., Cheung, N. K., Urmacher, C., Dantis, L., Templeton, M., Scheinberg, D., Chapman, P., Toner, G., Zakowski, M., Haines, C., Oettgen, H. F., Gabrilove, J. L., Garnick, M. D., and Houghton, A. N.: Recombinant macrophage colony stimulating factor (rhM-CSF): A phase I trial in patients (PTS) with melanoma (MEL). Proc. Amer. Soc. Onc., 9:708, 1990.
10. Bar, M. H., and Aronson, F. R.: Recombinant human GM-CSF in myelosuppression of chemotherapy (continued). N. Engl. J. Med., 320:939, 1988.
11. Barlogie, B., Jagamath, S., Dixon, D. O., Cheson, B., Smallwood, L., Hendrickson, A., Purvis, J. D., Bonnem, E., and Alexania, R.: High dose melphalan and granulocyte-macrophage colony stimulating factor for refractory multiple myeloma. Blood, 76:677, 1990.
12. Begley, C. G., Nicola, N. A., and Metcalf, D.: Proliferation of normal human promye-locytes and myelocytes after a single pulse stimulation by purified GM-CSF or G-CSF. Blood, 71:640, 1988.
13. Bhalla, K., Berkhofer, M., Arlin, Z., Grant, S., Latzky, J., and Graham, G.: Effect of rhGM-CSF and IL-3 on the metabolism of cytosine arabinoside in normal and leukemic human bone marrow cells. Blood, 72:348, 1988.
14. Bonilla, M. A., Gillio, A. P., Ruggeiro, M., Kernan, N. A., Brochstein, J. A., Abboud, M., Fumagalli, L., Vincent, M. E., Gabrilove, J. L., Welte, K., Souza, L. M., and O'Reilly, R.: Effects of recombinant human granulocyte colony stimulating factor on neutro-penia in patients with congenital agranulocytosis. N. Engl. J. Med., 320:1574, 1989.
15. Bonnem, E. M., and Morstyn, G.: Granulocyte-macrophage colony-stimulating factor (GM-CSF) current status and future development. Seminars Oncol., 15:46, 1988.
16. Brandt, S. J., Peters, W. P., Atwater, S. K., Kurtzberg, J., Borowitz, M. J., Jones, R. B., Shpall, E. J., Bast, Jr. R. C., Gilbert, C. J., and Oette, D. H.: Effect of recombinant human granulocyte-macrophage colony-stimulating factor on hematopoietic recon-stitution after high dose chemotherapy and autologous bone marrow transplantation. N. Engl. J. Med., 318:869, 1988.
17. Bronchud, M. H., Howell, A., Crowther, D., Hopwood, P., Souza, L., and Dexter, T. M.: The use of granulocyte colony stimulating factor to increase the intensity of treatment with doxorubicin in patients with advanced breast and ovarian cancer. Br. J. Cancer, 60:121, 1989.
18. Bronchud, M. H., Potter, M. R., Morgenstern, G., Blasco, M. J., and Scarffle, J.: In vitro and in vivo analysis of the effects of recombinant human granulocyte colony-stimulating factor in patients. Br. J. Cancer, 58:64, 1988.
19. Bronchud, M. H., Scarffe, J. H., Thatcher, N., Crowther, D., and Dexter, T. M.: Phase I/II study of recombinant human granulocyte colony stimulating factor in patients receiving intensive chemotherapy for small cell lung cancer. Br. J. Cancer, 56:809, 1987.
20. Buchner, T., Hiddemann, W., Koenigsmann, M., Zuhlsdorf, M., Wormann, B., Boeck-mann, A., Maschmeyer, G., Ludwig, W., and Schulz, G.: Chemotherapy (CT followed by recombinant human granulocyte macrophage colony stimulating factor (GM-CSF) for acute leukemias at higher age or after relapse. Proc. Amer. Soc. Clin. Onc., 8:770, 1989.
21. Bunn, H. F.: Recombinant erythropoietin therapy in cancer patients. J. Clin. Onc., 8:949, 1990.
22. Cannistra, S., Socinski, M. A., Groshek, P., Elias, A., and Antman, K.: Granulocyte-macrophage colony stimulating factor (GM-CSF) enhances monocyte tumoricidal activity. Proc. Amer. Soc. Clin. Oncol., 7:645, 1988.
23. Cannistra, S. A., Grostrek, P., and Griffin, J. D.: GM-CSF enhances the cytotoxic effects of cytosine arabinoside in acute myeloblastic leukemia and in myeloid blast crisis phase of chronic myeloid leukemia. Blood, 72:681, 1988.
24. Cannistra, S. A., Vallenga, E., Groshek, P., Rambaldi, A., and Griffin, J. D.: Human granulocyte-monocyte colony-stimulating factor and interleukin-3 stimulate monocyte cytotoxicity through a tumor necrosis factor-dependent mechanism. Blood, 71:672, 1988.
25. Cebon, J., Dempsey, P., Fox, R., Kannomakis, G., Bonnem, E., Burgess, A. W., and Morstyn, G.: Pharmacokinetics of human granulocyte-macrophage colony stimulating factor using a sensitive immunoassay. Blood, 72:1340, 1988.
26. Champlin, R. E., Nimer, S. D., Ireland, P., Oette, D. H., and Golde, D. W.: Treatment of refractory aplastic anemia with recombinant human granulocyte-macrophage col-ony-stimulating factor. Blood, 73:694, 1989.
27. Cheng, G. Y. M., Kelleher, C. A., Miyauchi, J., Wong, W. G., Clark, S. C., McCulloch, E. A., and Minden, M. D.: Structure and expression of GM-CSF and G-CSF in blast cells from patients with acute myeloblastic leukemia. Blood, 71:204, 1988.
28. Clark, J., Longo, D., Smith, J., Urba, W., Miller, R., Ruscetti, F., Hursey, J., and Steis, R.: Phase I trial of recombinant human granulocyte-macrophage colony stimulating factor (rHuGM-CSF) in cancer patients (pts). Proc. Am. Soc. Clin. Oncol., 7:614, 1988.
29. Crown, J., Gabrilove, J., Kemeny, N., Sheridan, C., Jakubowski, A., Sinha, S., Gas-paretto, C., Toner, G., Shieh, J., Meisenberg, B., Gordon, M., Botet, J., Zakowski, M., Houston, C., Dantis, L., Cheney, P., Buhles, W., Moore, M., and Kelsen, D.: Phase I-II trial of recombinant human interleukin-1B (IL-1) in patients (pts) with metastatic colorectal cancer (mcc) receiving myelosuppressive doses of 5-fluorouracil (5-FU). J. Clin. Oncol., 9:708, 1990.
30. D'Andrea A., Lodish, H., and Wong, G. C.: Expression cloning of the murine eryth-ropoietin receptor. Cell, 277:285, 1990.
31. Devreux, S., Lynch, D. C., Campos, C. D., Linch, D. C., Costa, D. C., Spittle, M. F., and Jelliffe, A. M.: Transient leucopenia induced by granulocyte-macrophage colony stimulating factor. Lancet, 1:1523, 1987.
32. Dinarello, C. A.: Biology of interleukin-1. FASEB J., 2:108, 1988.
33. Donahue, R. E., Seehra, J., Metzger, M., Lefebvre, D., Rock, B., Carbone, S., Nathan, D. C., Garnick, M., Sehgal, P. K., Laston, D., LaVallie, E., McCoy, J., Schendel, P. F., Norton, C., Turner, K., Yang, Y. C., and Clark, S. C.: Human IL-3 and GM-CSF act synergistically in stimulating hematopoiesis in primates. Science, 241:1820, 1988.
34. Donahue, R. E., Seehra, J., Norton, C., Turner, K., Metzger, M., Rock, B., Carbone,

S., Seghal, R., Yang, Y. C., and Clarks, S. C.: Stimulation of hematopoiesis in primates with human interleukin-3 and granulocyte macrophage colony stimulating factor. Blood, 70, Suppl. 1:388, 1987.
35. Donahue, R. E., Wang, E. A., Stone, D. K., Kamen, R., Wong, G. G., Sehgal, P. K., Nathan, D. G., and Clark, S. C.: Stimulation of hematopoiesis in primates by continuous infusion of recombinant human GM-CSF. Nature, 321:872, 1986.
36. Duhrsen, U., Villeval, J.-L., Boyd, J., Kannourakis, G., Morstyn, G., and Metcalf, D.: Effects of recombinant human granulocyte colony-stimulating factor on hematopoietic progenitor cells in cancer patients. Blood, 72:2074, 1988.
37. Estey, E., Kurzrock, M., Talpaz, M., Beran, M., Kantarjian, H., Keating, M., McCredie, K., Friereich, E., Deisseroth, A., and Gutterman, J.: Therapy of myelodysplastic syndromes (MDS) with GM-CSF. Proc. Am. Soc. Clin. Oncol., 8:200, 1989.
38. Fibbe, W. E., Schaafsma, M. R., Witteman, B. J. M., Falkenburg, J. H. F., Jones, T. C., and Willemze, R.: No correction of cyclic neutropenia on treatment with human recombinant GM-CSF. Blood, 72:372, 1988.
39. Gabrilove, J., Jakubowski, A., Scher, H., Sternberg, C., Wong, G., Grous, J., Yagoda, A., Fain, K., Moore, M. A. S., Clarkson, B., Oettgen, H., Alton, K., Welte, K., and Souza, L.: Granulocyte colony stimulating factor reduces neutropenia and associated morbidity of chemotherapy for transitional cell carcinoma of the urothelium. N. Engl. J. Med., 318:1414, 1988.
40. Gabrilove, J. L., Jakubowski, A., Fain, K., Grous, J., Scher, H., Sternberg, C., Yagoda, A., Clarkson, B., Bonilla, M. A., Oettgen, H. F., Alton, K., Boone, T., Altrock, B., Welte, K., and Souza, L.: A phase I study of granulocyte colony stimulating factor in patients with transitional cell carcinoma of the urothelium. J. Clin. Invest., 82:1554, 1988.
41. Gabrilove, J. L., Welte, K., Harris, P., Platzer, E., Lu, L., Levi, E., Mertelsmann, R., and Moore, M. A. S.: Pluripoietin-α: a second human hematopoietic colony stimulating factor produced by the human bladder carcinoma cell line, 5637. Proc. Natl. Acad. Sci., 83:2478, 1986.
42. Ganser, A., Lindenman, A., Seipelt, G., Ottmann, O. G., Eder, M., Falk, S., Herrmann, F., Katltwasser, J. P., Meusers, P., Klaussmann, M., Frisch, J., Schutz, G., Mertelsmann, R., and Hoelzer, D.: Effects of recombinant human interleukin-3 in aplastic anemia. Blood, 75:1287, 1990.
43. Ganser, A., Ottmann, O. G., Erdmann, H., Schulz, G., and Hoelzer, D.: The effect of recombinant human granulocyte-macrophage colony-stimulating factor on neutropenia and related morbidity in chronic severe neutropenia. Ann. Int. Med., 11:887, 1989.
44. Ganser, A., Seipelt, G., Lindemann, A., Ottman, O. G., Falk, S., Eder, M., Herrmann, F., Becher, R., Hoffken, K., Buchner, T., Klausmann, M., Frisch, J., Schulz, G., Mertelsmann, R., and Hoelzer, D.: Effects of recombinant human interleukin-3 in patients with myelodysplastic syndromes. Blood, 73:455, 1990.
45. Ganser, A., Volkers, B., Ottman, O. G., Walther, F., Becher, R., Bergmann, L., Schulz, G., and Hoelzer, D.: Recombinant human granulocyte-macrophage colony-stimulating factor in patients with myelodysplastic syndromes—a phase I/II trial. Blood, 73:31, 1989.
46. Gasson, J. C., Weisbart, R. H., Kaufman, S., Clark, S. C., Hewick, R. M., Wong, G. G., and Golde, D. W.: Purified human granulocyte macrophage colony stimulating factor: Direct action on neutrophils. Science, 226:1339, 1984.
47. Gianni, A. M., Bregni, M., Siena, S., Orazi, A., Stern, C. A., Gandola, L., and Bonadonna, G.: Recombinant human GM-CSF reduces hematologic toxicity and widens clinical applicability of high dose cyclophosphamide treatment in breast cancer and nonhodgkins lymphoma. J. Clin. Oncol., 8:768, 1990.
47A. Gillis, S.: Unpublished observation.
48. Glaspy, J. A., Baldwin, G. C., Robertson, P. A., Souza, L., Vincent, M., Ambersley, J., and Golde, D. W.: Therapy for neutropenia in hairy cell leukemia with recombinant human granulocyte colony-stimulating factor. Ann. Intern. Med., 109:789, 1988.
49. Griffin, J. D.: Clinical applications of colony stimulating factors. Oncol., 2:15, 1988.
50. Griffin, J. D., Rambaldi, A., Vallenga, E., Young, D. C., Ostapovicz, D., and Cannistra, S. A.: Secretion of interleukin-1 by acute myeloblastic leukemia cells *in vitro* induces endothelial cells to secrete colony stimulating factors. Blood, 70:1218, 1987.
51. Griffin, J. D., Young, D. C., Herrmann, D., Wiper, D., Wagner, K., and Sabbath, K. D.: Effects of recombinant human GM-CSF on proliferation of clonogenic cells in acute myeloblastic leukemia. Blood, 67:1448, 1986.
52. Groopman, J. E., Mitsuyasu, R. T., DeLeo, M. J., Oette, D. H., and Golde, D. W.: Effect of recombinant human granulocyte-macrophage colony-stimulating factor on myelopoiesis in the acquired immunodeficiency syndrome. N. Engl. J. Med., 317:593, 1987.
53. Guinan, E. C., Sieff, C. A., Oette, O. H., and Nathan, D. G.: A phase I/II trial of recombinant granulocyte-macrophage colony stimulating factor for children with aplastic anemia. Blood, 76:1077, 1990.
54. Hammond, W. P., Price, T. H., Souza, L. M., and Dale, D. C.: Treatment of cyclic neutropenia with granulocyte colony stimulating factor. N. Engl. J. Med., 320:1306, 1989.
55. Herrmann, F., Lindemann, A., Klein, H., Lubbert, M., Schultz, G., and Mertelsmann, R.: Effect of recombinant human granulocyte-macrophage colony-stimulating factor in patients with myelodysplastic syndrome with excess blasts. Leukemia, 3:335, 1989.
56. Herrmann, F., Schultz, G., Lindemann, A., Meyenburg, W., Oster, W., Krumwieh, D., and Mertelsmann, R.: Hematopoietic responses in patients with advanced malignancy treated with recombinant human granulocyte-macrophage colony stimulating factor. J. Clin. Oncol., 7:159, 1989.
57. Hirano, T., Yasukawa, K., Harada, H., Taga, T., Watanabe, Y., Matsuda, T., Kashiwamura, S., Nakajima, K., Koyama, K., Iwamatsu, A., Tsunasawa, S., Sakiyama, F., Matsui, H., Takahara, Y., Taniguchi, T., and Kishimoto, T.: Complementary DNA for a novel human interleukin (BSF-2) that induces B lymphocytes to produce immunoglobulin. Nature, 324:73, 1986.
58. Hoang, T., Nara, N., Wong, G., Clark, S., Minden, M. D., and McCulloch, E. A.: Effects of recombinant GM-CSF on the blast cells of acute myeloblastic leukemia. Blood, 68:313, 1986.
59. Horiguchi, J., Warren, M. K., and Kufe, D.: Expression of the macrophage specific CSF in human monocytes treated with granulocyte-macrophage colony stimulating factor. Blood, 69:1259, 1987.
60. Ihle, J. N., Keller, J., Henderson, L., Klein, F., and Palaszynski, E.: Procedures for the purification of interleukin-3 to homogeneity. J. Immunol., 129:2431, 1982.
61. Jacob, K., Shoemaker, C., Rudersdorf, R., Neill, S. D., Kaufman, R. J., Morfson, A., Seehra, J., Jones, S. S., Helwick, R., Fibra, F. F., Kawakita, M., Shimizu, T., and Moyake, T.: Isolation and characterization of genomie and cDNA doses of human erythropoietin. Nature, 313:806, 1985.
62. Jakubowski, A., Andreeff, M., Tafuri, A., Shieh, J. H., Sheridan, C., Sinha, S., Honge, M., Vincent, M., Alton, K., Moore, M. A. S., and Gabrilove, J. L.: *In vivo* and *in vitro* studies of rhG-CSF in acute nonlymphocytic leukemia. Blood, 74, Supp. 1:1034, 1989.
63. Jakubowski, A., and Gabrilove, J.: RhG-CSF in the treatment of bladder cancer. *In* Comparative effects of recombinant myeloid growth factors in man. Edited by W. Peters. Futura (in press), 1991.
64. Jakubowski, A., Souza, L. M., Fain, K., Clarkson, B., Moore, M. A. S., and Gabrilove, J. L.: Effects of human granulocyte colony stimulating factor in a patient with idiopathic neutropenia. N. Engl. J. Med., 320:38, 1989.
65. Kaplan, S. S., Zdziarski, V. E., Basford, R. E., Wing, E., and Shadduck, R. K.: Effect of *in vivo* recombinant human granulocyte macrophage colony stimulating factor on peripheral blood granulocyte function. Clin. Res., 36:566, 1988.
66. Kawasaki, E. S., Ladner, M. B., Wang, A. M., Van Arsdell, J., Warren, M. K., Coyne, M. Y., Schwieckart, V. L., Lee, M. T., Wilson, K. J., Boosman, A., Stanley, R. E., Ralph, P., and Mark, D. F.: Molecular cloning of a complementary DNA encoding human macrophage-specific colony-stimulating factor (CSF-1). Science, 230:281, 1950.
67. Kelleher, C., Miyauchi, J., Wong, G., Clark, S., Minden, M. D., and McCulloch, E. A.: Synergism between recombinant growth factors. GM-CSF and G-CSF, acting on the blast cells of acute myeloblastic leukemia. Blood, 69:1498, 1987.
68. Kelleher, C., Miyauchi, J., Wong, G., Clark, S., Minden, M. D., and McCulloch, E. A.: Synergism between recombinant growth factors, GM-CSF and G-CSF, acting on the blast cells of acute myeloblastic leukemia. Blood, 69:1498, 1987.
69. Kishimoto, T.: The biology of interleukin-6. Blood, 74:1, 1989.
70. Klein, B., Zhang, X. G., Jourdan, M., Content, J., Houssiau, F., Aarden, L., Piechaczyk, M., and Bataille, R.: Paracrine rather than autocrine regulation of myeloma-cell growth and differentiation by interleukin-6. Blood, 73:517, 1989.
71. Kleinerman, E. S., Knowles, R. D., Lachman, L. B., and Gutterman, J. U.: Effect of recombinant granulocyte/macrophage colony-stimulating factor on human monocyte activity *in vitro* and following intravenous administration. Cancer Res., 48:2604, 1988.
72. Kobayashi, Y., Okabe, T., Uzumaki, H., Urabe, A., and Takaku, F.: Differentiation therapy of myelodysplastic syndrome by granulocyte colony stimulating factor. Clin. Res., 36:412, 1988.
73. Lange, B., Valtieri, M., Santoli, D., Caracciolo, D., Mavilio, F., Gemperlein, I., Griffin, C., Emanuel, B., Finan, J., Nowell, P., and Rovera, G.: Growth factor requirements of childhood acute leukemia: establishment of GM-CSF dependent cell lines. Blood, 70:192, 1987.
74. Leary, A. G., Ikebuchi, K., Herai, Y., Wong, G. G., Yang, Y. C., Clark, S. C., and Ogawa, M.: Synergism between IL-6 and IL-3 in supporting proliferation of human hematopoietic stem cells: Comparison with IL-1. Blood, 71:1759, 1988.
75. Leary, A. G., Yang, Y. C., Clark, S. C., Gasson, J. C., Golde, D. W., and Ogawa, M.: Recombinant gibbon interleukin-3 supports formation of human multilineage colonies and blast cell colonies in culture: Comparison with recombinant human granulocyte-macrophage colony stimulating factor. Blood, 70:1343, 1987.
76. Lieschke, G. J., Maher, D., Cebon, J., O'Connor, M., Green, M., Sheridan, W., Boyd, A., Rallings, M., Bonnem, E., Metcalf, D., Burgess, A. W., McGran, K., Fox, R., and Morstyn, G.: Effects of bacterially synthesized recombinant human granulocyte-macrophage colony-stimulating factor in patients with advanced malignancy. Ann. Int. Med., 110:357, 1989.
77. Lin, F. K., Suggs, S., Lin, C. H., Browne, J. K., Smalling, R., Egrie, J. C., Chen, K. K., Fox, G. M., Martin, F., Slabinsky, Z., Badrawi, S. M., Lai, P. H., and Goldwasser, E.: Cloning and expression of human erythropoietin gene. Proc. Natl. Acad. Sci., 92:7580, 1985.
78. Lindemann, A., Oster, W., Riedel, D., Mertelsmann, R., and Herrmann, F.: GM-CSF induces secretion of monokines by human polymorphonuclear leukocytes. Blood, 70:223, 1987.
79. Logothelis, L., Dexeus, F., Sella, A., Amatro, R., Finn, L., and Gutterman, J.: Escalated (ESC) M-VAC (MTX 30 ug/m2, Adriamycin 60 ug/m2, Vinblastin 4 ug/m, Cisplatin 100 ug/m2) with recombinant human granulocyte macrophage stimulating factor (rhGM-CSF) for patients with advanced and chemotherapy refractory urothelium tumors: A phase I study. Proc. Amer. Soc. Clin. Oncol., 8:514, 1989.
80. Lopez, A. F., Williamson, J., Gamble, J. R., Begley, G., Harlan, J. M., Klebanoff, S. J., Waltersdorph, A., Wong, G., Clark, S. C., and Vadas, M. A.: Recombinant human granulocyte-macrophage colony-stimulating factor stimulates in vitro mature human neutrophil and eosinophil function, m-surface receptor expression and survival. J. Clin. Invest., 78:1220, 1986.
81. Lothrop, C. D., Jones, J. B., Warren, D. J., Moore, M. A. S., and Souza, L. M.: Correction of cyclic hematopoiesis with recombinant human granulocyte colony stimulating factor. Blood, 72:1324, 1988.
82. Lotze, M. T.: Cytokine therapy in patients with cancer. Presented at the fourth annual meeting of the society for biological therapy, 1989.
83. Mayer, P., Lam, C., Obenaus, H., Leihe, E., and Besemer, J.: Recombinant human GM-CSF induces leukocytosis and activates peripheral blood polymorphonuclear neutrophils in non-human primates. Blood, 70:206, 1987.
84. McNiece, I. K., McGrath, H. E., and Quesenberry, P. J.: Granulocyte colony-stimulating factor augments *in vitro* megakaryocyte colony formation by interleukin-3. Exp. Heme., 16:807, 1988.
85. Mertelsmann, R., Lindemann, L., Wieser, M., Gamm, H., Oster, W., Nuack, M., and Herrmann, R.: Prevention of chemotherapy induced neutropenia and associated morbidity in patients with advanced cancer by subcutaneous recombinant human GM-CSF (rhGM-CSF). Proc. Amer. Assoc. Cancer Res., 30:267, 1989.
86. Metcalf, D., Begley, C. G., and Johnson, G. R.: Biologic properties *in vitro* of a recombinant human granulocyte-macrophage colony stimulating factor. Blood, 67:37, 1986.
87. Mitsuyasu, R. T., and Golde, D. W.: Clinical role of GM-CSF: *In* hematopoietic growth factors. Edited by D. W. Golde. Clinics of North American (3) 411-425, 1989.
88. Mitsuyasu, R., Levine, J., Miles, S. A., DeLeo, M., Oette, D., Golde, D., and Groopman, J.: Effects of long term subcutaneous (SC) administration of recombinant granulocyte macrophage colony stimulating factor in patients with HIV-related leukopenia. Blood, 72:1297, 1988.
89. Miyauchi, J., Kelleher, C. A., Yang, Y.-C., Wong, G. C., Clark, S. C., Minden, M. D., Minkin, S., and McCulloch, E. A.: The effects of three recombinant growth factors,

IL-3, GM-CSF and G-CSF, on blast cells of acute myeloblastic leukemia maintained in short term suspension culture. Blood, 70:657, 1987.
90. Moore, M. A. S.: Growth and maturation factors in leukemia. *In* Principles of cancer biotherapy, Edited by R. K. Oldham. Raven Press, Ltd., New York, NY 2nd edition (in press), 1991.
91. Moore, M. A. S., Stolfi, R. L., and Martin, D. S.: Hematologic effects of interleukin-1β, granulocyte colony-stimulating factor in tumor-bearing mice treated with fluorouracil. Exp. Hematol., 17:805, 1989.
92. Morstyn, G., Lieschke, G. J., Cebon, J., Duhrsen, U., Villeval, J. L., and Layton, J.: Early clinical trials with colony stimulating factors. Cancer Investigation (in press):1990.
93. Morstyn, G., Souza, L. M., Keech, J., Sheridan, W., Campbell, L., Alton, N. K., Green, M., and Metcalf, D.: Effect of granulocyte colony stimulating factor on neutropenia induced by cytotoxic chemotherapy. Lancet, 1:6667, 1988.
94. Morstyn, G., Lieschke, G. J., Sheridan, W., Layton, L., Cebon, J., and Fox, R. M.: Clinical experience with recombinant granulocyte colony stimulating factor and granulocyte-macrophage colony stimulating factor. Seminars Hematol., 26:9, 1989.
95. Muraguchi, A., Kishimoto, T., Miki, Y., Kurrtani, T., Kalida, T., Yoshizaki, K., and Yamamura, Y.: T cell replacing factor (TRF). J. Immunol., 127:412, 1987.
96. Nagata, S., Tsuchinya, M., Asano, S., Kaziro, Y., Yamazaki, T., Nomura, H., and Ono, M.: Molecular cloning and expression of cDNA for human granulocyte colony stimulating factor. Nature, 319:415, 1986.
97. Nara, N., Murohashi, I., Suzuki, T., Yamashita, T., Maruyama, Y., Aoki, N., Tanikawa, S., and Onozawa, Y.: Effect of recombinant human granulocyte colony stimulating factor (G-CSF) on blast progenitors from acute myeloblastic leukemia patients. Br. J. Cancer, 56:49, 1988.
98. Negrin, R. S., Haeuber, D. H., Nagler, A., Olds, L. C., Donlon, T., Souza, L. M., and Greenberg, P. L.: Treatment of myelodysplastic syndromes with recombinant granulocyte colony stimulating factor. Ann. Intern. Med., 110:976, 1989.
99. Neidhart, J., Mangalik, A., Kohler, W., Stidley, C., Saiki, J., Duncan, P., Souza, L., and Downing, M.: Granulocyte colony-stimulating factors stimulates recovery of granulocytes in patients receiving dose-intensive chemotherapy without bone marrow transplantation. J. Clin. Oncol., 7:1685, 1989.
100. Nemunaitis, J., Singer, J. W., Buckner, D., Hill, R., Rainer, S., Donnall, T., and Appelbaum, F. R.: Use of recombinant human granulocyte-macrophage colony stimulating factor in autologous marrow transplantation. Blood, 72:834, 1988.
101. Neta, R., Dunches, S. D., and Oppenhein, J. J.: Interleukin-1 is a radioprotector. J. Immunol., 136:2483, 1986.
102. Nimer, S., Champlin, R. E., and Golde, D. W.: Serum cholesterol lowering activity of granulocyte macrophage colony stimulating factor. JAMA, 260:3297, 1988.
103. Nimer, S., and Golde, D.: The 5q- abnormality. Blood, 70:1705, 1988.
104. Nissen, C., Tichelli, A., Gratwohl, A., Speck, B., Milne, A., Gordon-Smith, E. C., and Schaedelin, J.: Failure of recombinant human granulocyte-macrophage colony-stimulating factor therapy in aplastic anemia patients with very severe neutropenia. Blood, 72:2045, 1988.
105. Ohno, R., Rononaga, M., Kobayaski, T., Kanamaru, A., Shirakawa, S., Masaoka, T., Ourone, M., Hakumei, O., Nomura, T., Sakai, Y., Hirano, M., Yokamaku, S., Nakayama, S., Yoshida, Y., Muira, A. B., Morishima, Y., Dohy, H., Niho, Y., Hamajima, N., and Takaku, F.: Effect of granulocyte colony stimulating factor after intensive induction therapy in relapsed or refractory acute leukemia. N. Engl. J. Med., 323:871, 1990.
106. Paquette, R. L., Zhou, J.-Y., Yang, Y.-C., Clark, S. C., and Koeffler, H. P.: Recombinant gibbon interleukin-3 acts synergistically with recombinant human G-CSF *in vitro*. Blood, 71:1596, 1988.
107. Peschel, C., Paul, W. E., O'Hara, J., and Green, J.: Effects of B-cell stimulatory factor-1 + interleukin-4 on hematopoietic progenitor cells. Blood, 70:254, 1987.
108. Peters, W.P.: The effect of recombinant human colony stimulating factors on hematopoietic reconstitution following autologous bone marrow transplantation. Seminars Hematol., 26:18, 1989.
109. Peters, W. P., Kurtzberg, J., Atwater, S., Borowitz, M., Gilbert, C., Rao, M., Currie, M., Shogan, J., Jones, R. B., Shpall, E. J., Stead, R., and Souza, L. M.: Comparative effects of rhG-CSF and rhG-CSF on hematopoietic reconstitution and granulocyte function following high dose chemotherapy and autologous bone marrow transplantation (ABMT). Proc. Am. Soc. Clin. Oncol., 8:691, 1989.
110. Peters, W. P., Shogan, J., Shpall, E. J., Jones, R. B., and Kim, C. S.: Recombinant human granulocyte macrophage colony stimulating factor produces fever. Lancet, 1:950, 1988.
111. Peters, W. P., Stuart, A., Affronti, M. L., Kim, C. S., and Coleman, R. E.: Neutrophil migration is defective during recombinant human granulocyte-macrophage colony stimulating factor infusion after autologous bone marrow transplantation in humans. Blood, 72:1310, 1988.
112. Phillips, N., Jacobs, S., Stoller, R., Earle, M., Przepiorka, D., and Shadduck, R. K.: Effects of recombinant human granulocyte-macrophage colony stimulating factor on myelopoiesis in patients with refractory metastatic cancer. Blood, 74:26, 1989.
113. Platzer, E., Oez, S., Welte, K., Sendler, A., Gabrilove, J. L., Mertelsmann, R., Moore, M. A. S., and Kalden, J. R.: Human pluripotent hemopoietic colony stimulating factor: Activities on human and murine cells. Immunobiology, 172:185, 1986.
114. Platzer, E., Welte, K., Gabrilove, J. V., Lu, L., Harris, P., Mertelsmann, R., and Moore, M. A. S.: Biological activities of a human pluripotent hemopoietic colony stimulating factor on normal and leukemic cells. J. Exp. Med., 162:1788, 1985.
115. Pluda, J. M., Yarchoan, R., Smith, P. D., McAtee, N., Shay, L. E., Oette, D., Meha, M., Wahl, S. M., Myers, C. E., and Broder, S.: Subcutaneous recombinant granulocyte macrophage colony stimulating factor used as a single agent and is an alternating regimen with A21d othymidine in leukopenic patients with severe human immunodeficiency virus. Blood, 76:463, 1990.
116. Rettenmier, C. N., Sacca, R., Furnan, W. L., Roussel, M. F., Holt, J. T., Nienhuis, A. W., Stanley, E. R., and Sherr, C. J.: Expression of the human c-fms proto-oncogue product (CSF-1 receptor) on peripheral blood mononuclear cells and cholocarcinoma cell lines. J. Clin. Invest., 77:1740, 1986.
117. Rifkin, R. M., Hersh, E. M., Hultquist, K. N., and Salmon, S. E.: Therapy of myelodysplastic syndrome (MDS) with subcutaneously (SC) administered recombinant human granulocyte-macrophage colony-stimulating factor. Proc. Am. Soc. Clin. Oncol., 8:178, 1989.
118. Rifkin, R., Hersh, E., and Salmon, S.: Continuous intravenous (IV) administration of recombinant human granulocyte-macrophage colony-stimulating factor (rGM-CSF) is superior to IV bolus administration: a phase I study. Proc. Am. Soc. Clin. Oncol., 7:614, 1988.
119. Robinson, B. E., McGrath, H. E., and Quesenberry, P. J.: Recombinant murine granulocyte macrophage colony-stimulating factor has megakaryocyte colony-stimulating activity and augments megakaryocyte colony stimulation by interleukin-3. J. Clin. Invest., 79:1648, 1987.
120. Ruff, M. R., Farrar, W. L., and Pert, C. B.: Interferon y and granulocyte/macrophage colony-stimulating factor inhibit growth and induce antigens characteristic of myeloid differentiation in small-cell lung cancer cell lines. Proc. Natl. Acad. Sci., 83:6613, 1986.
121. Sakai, K., Hattori, T., Matsuoka, M., Asou, N., Yamamoto, S., Sagawa, K., and Takastsuki, K.: Autocrine stimulating of interleukin-1β in acute myelogenous leukemia cells. J. Exp. Med., 166:1597, 1987.
122. Samoszuk, M., and Nansen, L.: Detection of interleukin-5 messenger RNA in Reed-Sternberg cells of hodgkin's disease with eosinophilia. Blood, 75:13, 1990.
123. Sher, C. J., Rettenmier, C. W., Sacca, R., Roussel, M. F., Look, A. T., and Stanley, R. E.: The c-fms proto-oncogene product is related to the receptor for the mononuclear phagocyte growth factor, CSF-1. Cell, 41:665, 1985.
124. Schuening, F. G., Storb, R., Goehle, S., Graham, T. C., Applebaum, F. R., Hackman, R., and Souza, L. M.: Effect of recombinant granulocyte colony stimulating factor on hematopoiesis of normal dogs and on hematopoietic recovery after otherwise lethal total body irradiation. Blood, 74:1308, 1989.
125. Shea, T. C., Mason, J. R., Storniolo, A. M., Newton, B., Breslin, M., Mullen, M., Ward, D., and Taetle, R.: Beneficial effect from sequential harvesting and reinfusing of peripheral blood stem cells (PBSC) in conjunction with rHuGM-CSF (Schering/Sandoz) and high-dose carboplatin (CBDCA). Blood, 76, Suppl. 1:651, 1990.
126. Sheridan, V., Morstyn, G., Gree, M., Boyd, A., Wolf, M., Dodds, A., McGrath, K., Maher, D., Souza, L., Alton, K., Vincent, M., and Fox, R.: Phase II study of granulocyte colony stimulating factor (G-CSF) in autologous bone marrow transplantation. Proc. Am. Soc. Clin. Oncol., 8:691, 1989.
127. Sideras, P., Nowa, T., and Honjo, T.: Structure and function of interleukin 4 and 5. Immunological Reviews, 102:189, 1988.
128. Sieff, C., Emerson, S. G., Donahue, R. E., Nathan, D. G., Wang, E. A., Wong, G. G., and Clark, S. C.: Human recombinant granulocyte-macrophage colony stimulating factor: a multi-lineage hematopoietin. Science, 230:1171, 1985.
129. Socinski, M. A., Elias, A., Schnipper, L., Cannistra, S. A., Antman, K. H., and Griffin, J. D.: Granulocyte-macrophage colony stimulating factor expands the circulating haemopoietic progenitor cell compartment in man. Lancet, 1:1194, 1988.
130. Souza, L. M., Boone, T. C., Gabrilove, J., Lai, P. H., Zsebo, K. M., Murdock, D. C., Chazin, V. R., Bruszewski, J., Lu, H., Chen, K. K., Platzer, E., Moore, M. A. S., Mertelsmann, R., and Welte, K.: Recombinant human granulocyte colony stimulating factor: effects on normal and leukemic myeloid cells. Science, 232:61, 1986.
131. Steward, W. P., Scarffe, J. H., Austen, R., Crowther, D., and Loyds, P.: Phase I study of recombinant DNA granulocyte-macrophage colony stimulating factor (rGM-CSF). Proc. Am. Soc. Clin. Oncol., 7:614, 1988.
132. Stork, J. L., Peterson, V. M., Rundus, C. H., and Robinson, W. A.: Interleukin-1 enhances murine granulopoiesis *in vivo*. Exp. Hematol., 16:163, 1987.
133. Strife, A., Labek, C., Wisniewski, D., Gulati, S., Gasson, J. C., Golde, D. W., Welte, K., Gabrilove, J. L., Clarkson, B.: Activities of four purified growth factors on highly enriched human hematopoietic progenitor cells. Blood, 69:1508, 1987.
134. Tafarri, A., Hegewisch, S., Souza, L., and Andreeff, M.: Stimulation of leukemic blast cells *in vitro* by colony stimulating factors (G-CSF, GM-CSF, and IL-3): evidence of recombinant and increased cell killing with cytosine arabanoside. Blood, 72:329, 1988.
135. Taylor C., Grogan, T. M., and Salmon, S. E.: Effects of interleukin-4 on the *in vitro* growth of human lymphoid and plasma cell neoplasms. Blood, 75:1114, 1990.
136. Taylor, K., Spitzer, G., Jagannaton, S., Dicke, K., and Souza, L. M.: Phase II study of recombinant human granulocyte colony stimulating factor (rhG-CSF) in Hodgkin's disease after high dose chemotherapy with ABMT. Blood, 72:452 1988.
137. Thompson, J. A., Lee, D. J., Kidd, P., Rubin, E., Kaufmann, J., Bonnem, E. M., and Fefer, A.: Subcutaneous granulocyte-macrophage colony stimulating factor in patients with myelodysplastic syndrome: toxicity, pharacokinetics and hematological effects. J. Clin. Oncol., 7:629, 1989.
137A. Toner, G., and Gabrilove, J. L.: Unpublished observation.
138. Toner, G. C., Jakubowski, A. A., Crown, J. P. L., Meisenberg, B., Sheridan, C., and Gabrilove, J. L.: Colony stimulating factors and neutrophil migration. Ann. Intern. Med., 110:847, 1989.
139. Touw, I., Pouwels, K., Agthoven, T. V., Gurp, R. V., Budel, L., Hoogerbrugge, H., Delwel, R., Goodwin, R., Namen, A., and Lowenberg, B.: Interleukin-7 is a growth factor of precursor B & T acute lymphoblastic leukemia. Blood, 75:2097, 1990.
140. Vadhan-Raj, S., Buescher, S., Broxmeyer, H. E., LeMaistre, A., Lepe-Zuniga, J. L., Ventura, G., Jeha, S., Herwitz, L. J., Trujillo, J. M., Gillis, S., Hittleman, W. N., and Gutterman, J. U.: Stimulation of myelopoiesis in patients with aplastic anemia by recombinant human granulocyte-macrophage colony stimulating factor. N. Engl. J. Med., 319:1628, 1988.
141. Vadhan-Raj, S., Buescher, S., LeMaistre, A., Keating, M., Walters, R., Ventura, C., Hittelman, W., Broxmeyer, H. E., and Gutterman, J. U.: Stimulation of hematopoiesis in patients with bone marrow failure and in patients with malignancy by recombinant human granulocyte-macrophage colony-stimulating factor. Blood, 72:134, 1988.
142. Vadhan-Raj, S., Keating, M., LeMaistre, A., Hittleman, W. N., McCredie, K., Trujillo, J. M., Broxmeyer, H. E., Henney, C., and Gutterman, J. U.: Effects of recombinant human granulocyte-macrophage colony-stimulating factor in patients with myelodysplastic syndromes. N. Engl. J. Med., 317:1545, 1987.
143. Vallenga, E., Young, D. C., Wagner, K., Wiper, D., Ostapovicz, D., and Griffin, J. D.: The effects of GM-CSF and G-CSF in promoting growth of cologenic cells in acute myeloblastic leukemia. Blood, 69:1771, 1987.
144. Warren, D., and Moore, M. A. S.: Interleukin-1 and granulocyte colony stimulating factor synergism: *in vivo* stimulation of stem cell recovery and hematopoietic regeneration following 5-fluorouracil treatment of mice. Proc. Natl. Acad. Sci., 84:7134, 1991.
145. Weisbart, R. H., Golde, D. W., Clark, S. C., Wong, G. G., and Gasson, J. C.: Human granulocyte-macrophage colony stimulating factor is a neutrophil activator. Nature, 314:361, 1985.
146. Welte, K., Bonilla, M. A., Gillio, A. P., Gabrilove, J., Potter, G. K., Boone, T., and

Souza, L.: *In vivo* effects of recombinant human G-CSF in therapy induced neutropenias in primates. Exp. Hematol., 15:72, 1987.

147. Welte, K., Platzer, E., Lu, L., Gabrilove, J., Mertelsmann, R., and Moore, M. A. S.: Purification and biological characterization of human pluripotent hematopoietic colony stimulating factor. Proc. Natl. Acad. Sci., 82:1526, 1985.

148. Welte, K., Zeidler, C., Reuther, A., Odenwald, E., Menzel, T., Buhrer, C., Feidert, J., Miller, W., Souza, L., and Riehm, H.: Correction of neutropenia and associated clinical symptoms with rhG-CSF in children with severe congenital neutropenia. Blood, 72:465, 1988.

149. Williams, D. E., Hangoc, G., Cooper, S., Boswell, H. S., Shadduck, R. K., Gillis, S., Waheed, A., Urdal, D., and Broxmeyer, H. E.: The effects of purified recombinant murine interleukin-3 and/or purified natural murine CSF-1 *in vivo* on the proliferation of murine high- and low-proliferative potential colony-forming cells: demonstration of *in vivo* synergism. Blood, 70:401, 1987.

150. Wing, E. J., Magee, D. M., Kaplan, S. S., and Shadduck, R. K.: Stimulation of human monocytes by recombinant granulocyte-macrophage colony stimulating factor in patients with metastatic carcinoma. Clin. Res., 36:422, 1988.

151. Wong, G. G., Temple, P. A., Leary, A. C., Witek-Giannotti, J. S., Yang, Y.-C., Ciarletta, A. B., Chung, M., Murtha, P., Kriz, R., Kaufman, R. J., Ferenz, C. R., Sibley, B. S., Turner, K. J., Hewick, R. M., Clark, S. C., Yanai, N., Yokota, H., Yamada, M., Saito, M., Motoyoshi, K., and Takaku, F.: Human CSF-1: Molecular cloning and expression of 4 kg cDNA encoding the human urinary protein. Science, 235:1504, 1987.

152. Wong, G. G., Witek, J. S., Temple, P. A., Wilkens, K. M., Leary, A. C., Luxenberg, D. P., Jones, S. S., Brown, E. L., Kay, R. M., Orr, E. C., Shoemaker, C., Golde, D.

W., Kaufman, R. J., Hewick, R. M., Wang, E. A., and Clark, S. C.: Human GM-CSF: Molecular cloning of complementary DNA and purification of the natural and recombinant proteins. Science, 228:810, 1985.

153. Yang, Y.-C., Ciarletta, A. B., Temple, P. A., Cung, M. P., Kovacic, S., Witek-Giannotti, J. S., Leary, A. C., Kritz, R., Donahue, R. E., Wong, G. G., and Clark, S. C.: Human IL-3 (multi-CSF): identification by expression cloning of a novel hematopoietic growth factor related to murine IL-3. Cell, 47:3, 1986.

154. Yee, C., Sutcliffe, S., and Minden, M. D.: Interleukin-6 (IL-6) in the plasma of lymphoma patients. Exp. Hematol., 18:377, 1990.

155. Young, D. C., and Griffin, J. D.: Autocrine secretion of GM-CSF in acute myeloblastic leukemia. Blood, 68:1178, 1986.

156. Young, D. C., Wagner, K., and Griffin, J. D.: Constitutive expression of the granulocyte-macrophage colony stimulating factor gene in acute myeloblastic leukemia. J. Clin. Invest., 79:100, 1987.

157. Yuo, A. U., Kitagawa, S., Okabe, T., Urabe, A., Komatsu, Y., Itoh, S., and Takaku, F.: Recombinant human granulocyte colony-stimulating factor repairs the abnormalities of neutrophils in patients with myelodysplastic syndromes and chronic myelogenous leukemia. Blood, 70:404, 1987.

157A. Zinzar, S. N., Svet-Moldavsky, G. J., Fogh, J., Mann, P. E., Arlin, Z., Iliescu, K., and Holland, J. F.: Elaboration of granulocyte-macrophage colony-stimulating factor by human tumor cell lines and normal urothelium. Exp. Hematol., 13:574, 1985.

158. Zsebo, K. M., Cohen, A. M., Murdock, D. C., Boone, T. C., Inque, H., Chazin, V. R., Hines, D., and Souza, L. M.: Recombinant human granulocyte colony stimulating factor: Molecular and biological characterization. Immunolobiol., 172:175, 1986.

XVIII-7

Monoclonal Serotherapy

Robert C. Bast, Jr.
Michael R. Zalutsky
Arthur E. Frankel

Introduction

Following the initial report of Kohler and Milstein,[100] monoclonal antibody technology has exerted a prompt and substantial impact on laboratory investigation. Over the last decade, availability of monoclonal reagents has permitted development of novel markers for in vitro applications, including monitoring response to treatment, detecting malignant cells histochemically, identifying subsets of patients with particularly favorable or unfavorable prognoses, and distinguishing some tumors of unknown origin. Progress in the use of monoclonal antibodies for the in vivo diagnosis and treatment of human cancer has, however, been less dramatic. Serotherapy with unmodified monoclonal antibodies has produced tumor regression in lymphomas and melanomas but has yielded more equivocal results in leukemias and gastrointestinal neoplasms.[3,206]

Obstacles to effective serotherapy include shed tumor-associated antigen, antigenic modulation, heterogeneity of antigen expression, potency of effector mechanisms, and the immune response to foreign immunoglobulin.[54,55,70,73,79] Several of these obstacles have been avoided in ex vivo applications such as the elimination of malignant cells from human bone marrow prior to autologous transplantation in patients with lymphoreticular and solid neoplasms.

In an attempt to exert greater antitumor activity in situ, monoclonal antibodies have been linked to cytotoxic drugs, radionuclides and immunotoxins. Extensive preclinical studies have been carried out and Phase I clinical trials have now been performed with each type of immunoconjugate. This chapter considers some of the possibilities and the limitations of monoclonal reagents for the treatment of cancer patients.

Therapy with Unmodified Monoclonal Antibodies

Treatment In Vivo

With rare exceptions, murine monoclonal antibodies raised against human neoplasms recognize tumor associated antigens which are also expressed by normal adult or fetal tissues. Some antigens, however, are expressed by only a small number of normal cells that may not be essential to the patient's well-being. One of the most promising reports remains that of MIller and Levy who prepared tumor specific murine monoclonal antibodies against the unique idiotopes associated with the cell surface membrane immunoglobulin present on human B-cell lymphomas.[131] The original patient treated with a specific anti-idiotypic antibody remained in complete remission for 72 months. Overall, treatment of 14 lymphoma patients with anti-idiotypic antibodies produced an objective response rate of 57%.[114] Genes encoding the cell surface membrane immunoglobulin continue to undergo point mutations resulting in loss of idiotypic determinants.[159] Use of multiple monoclonal antibodies has provided one approach to eliminating tumor cells which lack particular idiotypic determinants. Another approach has combined serotherapy with other forms of biological response modification. In a subsequent trial, 11 patients were treated with anti-idiotypic antibody and alpha interferon. Nine of the 11 patients responded objectively and one response was complete, lasting more than a year. Most of the antibodies which produced responses in vivo were of the IgG1 isotype, which is generally least efficient in fixing complement or participating in antibody dependent cell mediated cytotoxicity.

Monoclonal antibodies against differentiation antigens have been used to treat patients with acute and chronic leukemias. In the case of CD-10 positive acute lymphoblastic leukemia, anti-CD10 antibody induced prompt modulation of the common acute lymphoblastic leukemia antigen, preventing effective therapy.[163] Intravenous infusion of anti-CD5 also produced antigenic modulation and only transient, partial regression in a fraction of patients with T cell leukemia/lymphoma and chronic lymphocytic leukemia.[52] In one of the first studies of serotherapy with monoclonal reagents, a serum blocking factor was demonstrated which prevented binding of monoclonal antibody to circulating lymphosarcoma cells, consistent with the presence of shed tumor antigen.[141]

Unmodified murine monoclonal antibodies have produced regression of metastases from malignant melanoma. Intravenous administration of an IgG3 antibody that identified GD_3, a prominent ganglioside on the surface of melanoma cells, produced partial regression of soft tissue metastases in 3 of 12 patients.[87] Two additional patients experienced a mixed response. Inflammatory reactions were noted around tumor sites. Biopsies demonstrated infiltration with lymphocytes and mast cells, degranulation of the mast cells and deposition of complement components. Studies ex vivo suggest that a threshold level of GD3 expression may be required for susceptibility to host effector mechanisms.[38]

The ability of monoclonal antibodies to reach tumor cells can be limited by abnormal vascularity, elevated interstitial pressure, and relatively large distances for transport of immunoglobulins through the interstitium.[89,90] Intravenous injection of an IgG2a murine monoclonal antibody against a 250 Kd melanoma-associated chondroitin sulfate proteoglycan core protein resulted in selective localization of antibody in metastatic nodules of malignant melanoma.[171] The greater the amount of antibody administered, the greater the accumulation of murine immunoglobulin that could be demonstrated immunohistochemically in biopsied material.[171] Even after the infusion of 500 mg of antibody, however, complete saturation of antigenic sites was not achieved in all patients, consistent with limited access of antibody to tumor cells outside the vascular compartment.

Contact of antibodies with tumor cells can be enhanced by direct intratumoral injection. A human IgM monoclonal antibody reactive with the GD_2 ganglioside produced partial and complete regression of injected cutaneous melanoma nodules in 4 of 8 patients.[88] (See Plates XXXIV-1-6 and 7.) Tumor nodules that failed to respond to repeated injection had relatively lower levels of antigen than did nodules that regressed. A mononuclear infiltrate was observed at the sites of antibody injection.

Several clinical trials have utilized the 17-1A murine IgG2a antibody which reacts with human gastrointestinal carcinomas.[12,117,127,172] Responses have been reported in colorectal and pancreatic carcinoma, although evidence for tumor regression has often been equivocal and the role of antibody difficult to define. In one study, however, 6 of 22 patients (27%) experienced an objective response to prolonged treatment.[127] Injection of 17-1A has evoked a human anti-murine immunoglobulin response and some of the patient's antibodies have had anti-idiotypic specificity. Development of anti-murine immunoglobulin antibodies has generally been regarded as an undesirable consequence of injecting a foreign protein because they shorten the circulating half life of the monoclonal antibody in the circulation. Anti-idiotypic antibodies can, however, bear the internal image of the antigen and stimulate endogenous immunity in recipients.[82,83,101,133,144,210,214]

Substantial effort has been expended in the development of human monoclonal antibodies which should be less immunogenic, but their titer, specificity, isotype and affinity continue to limit the clinical utility of these reagents.[91] Immunization of patients with autologous tumor cells and Bacillus Calmette-Guérin has produced one method for expanding relevant human B cells prior to fusion.[80] One alternative approach has involved molecular engineering of murine and human immunoglobulin genes to produce chimeric antibodies with human constant and mouse variable domains.[18,134,135,136] The hypervariable complementarity-determining region (CDR) of the human heavy chain can be replaced with the CDR of a murine monoclonal immunoglobulin.[93] Although the immunogenicity of such antibodies can be substantially reduced, their injection can still evoke an anti-idiotypic response. Genetic engineering can also be utilized to produce single chain antigen binding proteins that may have more favorable pharmacokinetic properties than intact immunoglobulin or Fab fragments.[45]

To the extent that unmodified monoclonal antibodies inhibit tumor growth, several mechanisms may be important for antitumor activity including direct growth inhibition, complement dependent lysis and antibody dependent cell mediated cytotoxicity (ADCC), in addition to possible intervention in the specific immunoregulatory network of the host. Antibodies that react with the epidermal growth factor receptor (EGFR) can inhibit growth of tumor cells ex vivo in the absence of complement components or host effector cells.[123,128,165] Antibodies that block EGF binding to EGFR affect growth more readily than do antibodies that bind to other sites on the receptor. Antibodies that react with the extracellular domain of c-erbB-2 (HER-2/neu) proto-oncogene product also inhibit tumor cell growth in the absence of complement or cellular effectors.[56,218] Inhibition of ligand binding appears important for inhibition of anchorage dependent but not anchorage independent growth.[218] Recently antibodies have been described that produce apoptosis, i.e., programmed cell death, in some lymphoid cell lines and activated T cells.[48]

Murine antibodies of the IgM, IgG2a, and IgG3 isotypes can fix human complement, but often rather poorly. The rat monoclonal antibody CAMPATH 1 is an important exception to this generalization in that the antibody can mediate lysis of human cells which bear the appropriate antigen in the presence of human complement components.[205] Murine antibodies of IgG3, IgG2a and IgG2b have been reported to mediate ADCC in which large granular lymphocytes (LGL), monocytes, macrophages, or polymorphonuclear leukocytes are bound to tumor cells through Fc receptors after antibody has bound to specific antigenic determinants on the tumor cell surface. IgG3 appears to be particularly important for ADCC with LGL,[1] whereas IgG2a may interact more effectively with human monocytes.[190] In some instances it has been possible to arm mononuclear leukocytes with antibody prior to interaction with tumor targets. In vivo, ADCC may be compromised in cancer patients due to a paucity of appropriate effector cells or to the presence of circulating immune complexes which occupy or down-regulate Fc receptors. Antibodies which react against GD_3 on melanoma cells can also bind to GD_3 on the surface of T cells, enhancing their cytotoxic and proliferative responses.[84] Hybrid antibodies have been generated with one binding site for T cell associated antigens and one binding site for tumor-associated antigens.[40] Such hybrid antibodies enhance tumor cell killing by IL-2 activated T cells,[129] possibly by encouraging contact between effector cells and tumor targets.

Whatever the mechanism of tumor killing, cells which lack the relevant antigen are likely to escape elimination. Substantial heterogeneity has been observed within and between neoplasms, particularly in the case of solid tumors. When the expression of 11 distinct antigen families was studied in a panel of breast carcinomas using biotin-avidin immunoperoxidase, 16 of 18 of the tumors exhibited a distinct phenotype.[19] Similar heterogeneity was observed in epithelial ovarian carcinomas. Importantly, use of five antibodies in combination can apparently compensate for this heterogeneity.

Elimination of Malignant Cells from Bone Marrow Ex Vivo

Autologous bone marrow transplantation is likely to be most effective in those instances where tumors respond dramatically to primarily myelotoxic chemoradiotherapy and for those patients whose marrow is free of clonogenic tumor cells or can be freed from tumor by treatment ex vivo. Murine monoclonal antibodies have proven useful for the selective elimination of tumor cells while sparing clonogenic precursors. In this setting, the clinician can avoid several of the usual obstacles to serotherapy in vivo. Shed antigen can be washed from the system. Marrow can be chilled, minimizing antigenic modulation. Rabbit complement can be utilized which interacts effectively with a wide range of murine antibodies. Multiple monoclonal antibodies can be incubated with bone marrow ex vivo and immunization with foreign protein is generally not an issue. In model systems, up to 99.9% of clonogenic lymphoma cells can be eliminated from mixtures with normal human bone marrow using multiple murine monoclonal antibodies and rabbit complement[7] with or without 4-hydroperoxycyclophosphamide (4-HC).[49] Treatment with antibodies of appropriate specificity spares normal marrow precursors although 4-HC destroys mature CFU-GM.

Phase I trials in patients with acute lymphoblastic leukemia,[160,164,169] acute nonlymphocytic leukemia,[6] and neuroblastoma[96] have confirmed that reconstitution can occur in vivo after purging of malignant cells using antibody and complement or using immunomagnetic separation mediated by magnetite laden beads which are coated with an antimurine immunoglobulin. In two very similar trials, 25–30% of

children with acute lymphoblastic leukemia who had failed conventional treatment enjoyed long term disease free survival after receiving myeloblative chemoradiotherapy and an infusion of autologous bone marrow which had been treated ex vivo in the presence of rabbit complement with murine monoclonal anti-CD9 and anti-CD10 with or without anti-CD24.[160,169] Antibody and complement have also been used to purge marrow from lymphoma patients. Among 49 patients with relapsed non-Hodgkin's lymphoma, 34 remained disease-free a median of > 11 months (range > 2 to > 52 months) after receiving transplant doses of cyclophosphamide, total body irradiation (TBI) and autologous bone marrow that had been treated with anti-CD20 and rabbit complement.[196] Recent studies have permitted removal of neuroblastomas and breast cancer cells from human bone marrow using multiple monoclonal antibodies and immunomagnetic beads with or without cytotoxic drugs.[2,178]

Whether or not purging of marrow is necessary has been debated. Controlled trials have been difficult to perform. When residual lymphoma cells were detected by PCR techniques, the inability to eliminate tumor cells from marrow was the single most important prognostic indicator in predicting relapse after autologous transplantation.[77] This outcome is consistent with the usefulness of ex vivo purging of marrow at least in this setting.

Improvement of autologous bone marrow transplantation depends critically on effective removal of tumor cells from the patient as well as from the bone marrow. More effective treatment of residual disease could result from fractionated total body irradiation (TBI), use of multiple alkylating agents, treatment of disease at an earlier stage and use of adjunctive modalities such as immunotherapy. To the extent that these techniques improve control of tumor in vivo, complete elimination of tumor cells from harvested bone marrow to be reinfused will become more important. More effective purging of marrow has been achieved with several models using both immunoseparation and chemoseparation with agents such as 4-HC. Cells which evade immunoseparation are still susceptible to cytotoxic drugs. Chemoseparation appears to compensate, in part, for heterogeneity in antigenic phenotype.

Therapy with Drug-Monoclonal Antibody Conjugates

Murine monoclonal antibodies have been coupled to a variety of conventional cytotoxic agents[71,156] including antifoles, anthracyclines, vinca alkyloids, alkylating agents, and neocarzinostatin.[4,5,21,94,119,155,174,175,177,183,184,185,187,195] Prepolymerization of some drugs such as doxorubicin prior to conjugation can achieve higher ratios of drug to antibody.[212] Drugs can be bound to the amino side chains of lysine residues, provided that the most reactive residues are not found in the antibody binding site. Linkage of drugs to antibody through the carbohydrate moieties of the murine immunoglobulin has provided site-specific conjugation which generally does not impair antibody binding.[125,166]

One concern raised by some investigators is based on the observation that many cell surface antigens have $\leq 10^5$ copies per cell. Release of $\leq 3 \times 10^6$ drug molecules at the cell surface might or might not be sufficient to eliminate tumor. Another concern relates to the ability of large immunoglobulin carrier-complexes to translocate across tumor capillaries. In recent preclinical studies, however, drug-monoclonal antibody conjugates have proven substantially more effective than the free drug. Only some of these conjugates are more potent, but many are less toxic, providing an improved therapeutic index. Therapeutic advantage may relate to different rates or patterns of drug uptake when linked with monoclonal reagents. In some instances, novel linkages have been devised which would release drug at low pH or only in the presence of lysosomal proteases. Not all drug-antibody conjugates, however, must enter cells to provide effective anti-tumor therapy in nude mouse heterograft models.[189] Clinical trials have been initiated with N-acetylmelphalan or neocarzinostatin[195] conjugated to antibodies reactive with colorectal cancer and responses have been noted in 2 of 8 and 3 of 8 patients, respectively.

Other investigators have explored the use of drug-containing liposomes coated with monoclonal antibodies to deliver larger aliquots of drug.[46,124] Because of their size liposomes are likely to lodge in normal liver, spleen and lung after intravenous injection. Thus, antibody-coated liposomes may be more useful for intracavitary therapy.

Radiolabeled Monoclonal Antibodies

Monoclonal (and polyclonal) antibodies directed against human cancer-associated antigens can be exploited as carriers for the selective delivery of radionuclides to tumors. Nearly 40 years ago, Pressman and Korngold[158] demonstrated that antibody-mediated targeting of radioactivity to tumors in vivo was feasible. Subsequent work by Spar and colleagues used ^{131}I-labeled polyclonal antibodies directed against fibrinogen to show that a variety of tumors could be visualized in patients by external scanning.[186] However, because of problems with antibody specificity and limitations in imaging technology, interest in antibody imaging remained at a low level for about a decade.

The development of hybridoma methodology, in concert with parallel advances in the field of nuclear medicine instrumentation, has offered the prospect of utilizing monoclonal antibodies labeled with gamma-emitting nuclides to detect sites of tumor in a noninvasive fashion. Although radioimmunoscintigraphy will probably never have an impact in diagnostic oncology approaching initial expectations, it is clear that it is a method for defining the extent and location of disease that could well complement the anatomical information provided by other modalities such as computed tomography and magnetic resonance imaging.

Perhaps the most exciting application of radioimmunoscintigraphy is as a prelude for therapeutic approaches using antibodies labeled with β- or α-emitting nuclides. Radioimmunotherapy offers the prospect of being able to deliver curative levels of radiation to malignant cell populations while leaving normal tissues intact. The potential use of an antibody scan to select appropriate patients for labeled antibody therapy adds to the appeal of this approach.

Enthusiasm for labeled antibody imaging and therapy was heightened by multiple, separate studies performed in athymic rodent models reporting images exhibiting exquisite contrast between tumor xenograft and normal tissues,[42,150,199,203] and others demonstrating tumor regression and even cures.[39,99,105] Unfortunately, following intravenous administration of labeled antibodies into patients, most clinical series[22,31,43,63,65,78,121] report levels of radioactivity in tumors on the order of 10^{-3} percent (0.1%) injected dose per gram, uptakes which are four orders of magnitude less than those generally observed when the same antibodies are given to tumor-bearing animals.

Despite the low degree of labeled antibody uptake in tumors, successful imaging and treatment of a variety of cancers has been accomplished in some patients. However, a better understanding of the multiple factors influencing the effectiveness of labeled antibody diagnosis and therapy will be required if labeled antibodies are to make a significant impact in the clinical domain. Some of the factors which must be considered in the development of labeled antibodies for diagnostic and therapeutic applications are summarized in Table XVIII-7-1.

Radioimmunoscintigraphy

Selection of Nuclide. From an imaging perspective, the nuclide selected for use as an antibody label should decay by the emission of gamma rays with an energy of about 100–200 keV and have a half-life compatible with the pharmacokinetics of antibody localization in tumor. In addition, the absence of β emission is also desirable to minimize the radiation-absorbed dose received by the patient. The physical properties of some of the gamma-emitting nuclides that have been used for radioimmunoscintigraphy are summarized in Table XVIII-7-2. Because of its half-life, its cost, and the availability of protein radioiodination methodology, ^{131}I is the nuclide utilized most frequently for antibody imaging.[31,104] However, problems including low count rate per unit dose, scatter background, collimator penetration, and suboptimal spatial resolution make [131]I a less than ideal nuclide for both conventional planar imaging and single photon emission computed tomography (SPECT). To address these shortcomings, alternative nuclides have been evaluated. Indium-111 has been used in many clinical studies because of its acceptable imaging properties (although probably not optimal for quantitative SPECT) and the ready availability of ^{111}In-labeled antibodies from the industrial sector.

Two nuclides with ideal physical properties for antibody imaging are 6-hour half-life ^{99m}Tc and 13-hour half-life [123]I. These nuclides not only have better characteristics for conventional gamma camera imaging, but also are well-suited for SPECT, particularly when quantitative information is required. Technetium-99m is the most commonly used nuclide in nuclear medicine and would be the isotope of choice for antibody imaging if a simple method for labeling antibodies with ^{99m}Tc were available and if adequate contrast between tumor and normal tissues could be achieved in a time frame compatible with its short half-life. Iodine-123 has a longer half-life; there are methods available for radioiodinating antibodies in a stable fashion; and a scan with ^{123}I would be an ideal precursor to a therapeutic study with [131]I. Yet, the high cost and limited availability of ^{123}I are disadvantageous.

In addition to determining the quality of images, the type

Table XVIII-7-1.   Considerations for the Development of Radiolabeled Antibodies for Diagnostic Applications

Specific for a Given Antibody-Antigen System	Related to Radiolabel	Other
Antibody affinity	Stability of label in vivo	Tumor size
Antigen copies per cell	Affinity after labeling	Tumor hemodynamics
Fraction of tumor cells that are antigen-positive	Clearance of labeled catabolites	Route of antibody injection
Circulating antigen	Energy of gamma ray (imaging)	Intact antibody or fragment
	Range of beta or alpha particle (therapy)	Mouse, human or chimeric antibody
	Linear energy transfer of radiation (therapy)	

Table XVIII-7-2.   Gamma-Emitting Nuclides Utilized for Radioimmunoscintigraphy

Nuclide	Half-life	Gamma-ray Energy (keV)	Comments
^{99m}Tc	6.0 hr	140	Excellent images, routinely available, low cost
^{123}I	13.3 hr	159	Excellent images, limited supply, high cost
^{111}In	2.8 d	173, 247	Acceptable images, moderate cost
^{131}I	8.1 d	364	Poor images, widely available, beta dose to patient

of nuclide also influences the pharmacokinetics of isotope clearance following the injection of radiolabeled antibodies. Catabolism of label from radioiodinated antibodies is evidenced by uptake of activity in the thyroid and stomach and excretion of high levels of nonprotein-associated activity in the urine.[81,194] Because free iodine behaves in like fashion, and due to the structural similarity of iodotyrosine residues created on the labeled antibody to thyroid hormones, it is generally presumed that loss of label from radioiodinated antibodies occurs by dehalogenation.[58,220] With ^{111}In, retention of activity in liver and spleen is problematic making it difficult to detect hepatic metastases using ^{111}In-labeled antibodies.[137,140,161,215] The chemical form of ^{111}In in the liver is as yet unknown with multiple mechanisms for its uptake proposed including transchelation from the antibody chelate to ferroproteins as well as production of labeled immune complexes.[8,170]

In some cases, the differential catabolism of ^{131}I and ^{111}In can have a profound effect on their utility as antibody labels. Carrasquillo and colleagues have shown that T101 monoclonal antibody is effective for the detection of cutaneous T cell lymphoma when labeled with ^{111}In, but in contrast, is of minimal utility when labeled with ^{131}I.[29] This difference is probably related to the internalization of labeled T101 in T65 antigen-bearing cells. It appears likely that, with ^{131}I-labeled T101, intracellular dehalogenation causes the liberation of free iodide, whereas with ^{111}In, catabolism of label results in the production of ^{111}In-labeled ferroproteins that are retained inside the cell. Conversely, detection of malignant foci in the liver with radioiodinated antibodies is easier than with ^{111}In-labeled antibodies,[215] an observation which is related, in part, to the more rapid clearance of radioiodine-labeled catabolites from normal tissues compared to ^{111}In.

Clinical Trials. Initial radioimmunodetection studies in patients involved the use of affinity-purified, polyclonal goat antibodies directed against carcinoembryonic antigen (CEA) labeled with ^{131}I. A detection rate of 91% was reported in patients with a variety of CEA-secreting tumors.[72] This study involved the use of planar gamma camera imaging and used blood pool subtraction to increase contrast between tumor and normal tissues. However, using similar techniques, Mach and colleagues reported a sensitivity of only 39% for ^{131}I-labeled anti-CEA.[120] The discordance between the results of these studies could be related to differences in circulating CEA levels, the subjective nature of background subtraction techniques, or other variables such as those listed in Table XVIII-7-1.

External imaging studies have now been performed, primarily using mouse monoclonal antibodies labeled with either ^{111}In or ^{131}I, in patients with a variety of malignant neoplasms including melanoma,[27,30,78,197] neuroblastoma,[132] glioma,[162,221] lymphoma,[28,29] and ovarian,[76,153,208] colorectal,[34,41,57,65,122,161] and breast[53,81] carcinomas. In general, retrospective studies such as these report that, using intravenously administered radiolabeled antibodies, greater than 70% of tumors could be detected by radioimmunoscintigraphy.

Efforts to improve sensitivity and decrease false-positive detection rates have been directed at multiple facets of antibody imaging methodology. In an attempt to compensate for heterogeneity in antigen expression among tumor cells, combinations of antibodies directed against distinct cancer-associated antigens have been employed.[34] With certain antibodies, optimizing the protein dose of antibody has led to improvements in radioimmunodetection.[30,78,98] For example, Kirkwood and colleagues have reported that the percentage of known metastatic melanoma foci detected with ^{111}In-labeled anti-gp240 monoclonal antibody increased from 23% at doses less than 5 mg to 87% for doses of 20 mg.[98]

In athymic mice, monoclonal antibody F(ab')$_2$ and Fab fragments have been shown to clear from the body more rapidly than intact immunoglobulins, resulting in decreased normal tissue background.[42,199] Mach and colleagues were the first to report that the use of F(ab')$_2$ fragments improved the sensitivity of detection of colorectal cancers compared to ^{131}I-labeled intact IgG.[121,122] Since that time, the feasibility of using ^{131}I- and ^{111}In-labeled F(ab')$_2$ and Fab fragments for imaging a variety of cancers has been demonstrated.[34,86,103,150]

Because adequate contrast between tumor and normal tissue can be achieved much more rapidly with antibody fragments, nuclides with optimal imaging characteristics such as ^{123}I and ^{99m}Tc can be used despite their short half-lives. In a retrospective study of patients with colorectal cancer, Delaloye and colleagues were able to detect 82% and 89%

of tumor sites using SPECT and ^{123}I-labeled F(ab')$_2$ and Fab fragments of anti-CEA, respectively.[50] It is important to point out that, in four patients, tumor foci were imaged that were not observed by CT or ultrasound and were not suspected clinically. In a subsequent prospective study by this group using the same methodology, 10 of 21 previously unsuspected but later confirmed lesions were detected by radioimmunoscintigraphy more than one month earlier than by other diagnostic modalities, suggesting that this technique potentially could reduce the delay between diagnosis and treatment of colorectal cancer.[10]

With development of improved methods for labeling antibodies with ^{99m}Tc, clinical investigations utilizing ^{99m}Tc-labeled F(ab')$_2$ and Fab fragments have begun to appear. In a multicenter study in melanoma patients injected with antibody fragments labeled with ^{99m}Tc using a direct method, 70% of lesions were visualized, including 92 previously occult but later confirmed.[180] Using F(ab')$_2$ or Fab fragments of the 9.2.27 antibody labeled with ^{99m}Tc via a bifunctional chelating method in combination with a pre-infusion of unlabeled, nonspecific antibody, 81% of known melanoma metastases were visualized, including tumors as small as 250 mg, despite the fact that planar imaging techniques and not SPECT were utilized.[59]

As the methodology of radioimmunoscintigraphy continues to improve, the role of antibody imaging in the clinical management of cancer patients will increase and should be of particular utility in staging. Evaluation of lymph node status is critical in the staging of carcinomas of the colon, breast, prostate, ovary, and lung, as well as of melanomas and lymphomas. For this reason, immunolymphoscintigraphy has been pursued by a number of investigators.[95,106,143,201,204] With this technique, the labeled antibody is administered by a subcutaneous route in order to increase the delivery to suspected nodes and to minimize uptake by normal tissues. Although detection of more than 80% of involved nodes has been achieved,[106] there is some question as to the specificity of uptake since co-injected, nonspecific antibody has been shown to accumulate to a similar degree.[143] In addition, uptake of specific antibody in normal nodes has also been a problem[204] resulting in a high false-positive rate.

The diagnostic utility of radioimmunodetection would be enhanced if repeat studies in the same patient were possible. Unfortunately, murine monoclonal antibodies frequently elicit an immune response in the host commonly referred to as HAMA.[171,172,173] HAMA alter the pharmacokinetics of the labeled monoclonal antibody through the formation of immune complexes that are rapidly removed from the circulation and thus decrease the amount of labeled antibody available for binding to tumor. One approach to minimizing HAMA is to use antibody fragments, since they appear to be less immunogenic. Alternatively, chimeric antibodies can be generated which contain the variable region of a mouse antibody directed against the tumor and the constant regions of a human immunoglobulin.[135] Chimeric antibodies have been generated which maintain the tumor specificity of the original mouse monoclonal antibody.[191] It is encouraging to note that chimeric antibodies also appear to be less immunogenic in patients.[118]

Radioimmunotherapy

Selection of Nuclide. In developing radioimmunotherapeutic strategies, it is important to bear in mind that this type of therapy, at least initially, will probably be most useful as an adjuvant to less specific forms of treatment such as chemotherapy and teletherapy (external photon therapy). An advantage of antibody-mediated radiotherapy, in contrast to immunotoxin therapy, is the wide variation in toxicity and range of action that potentially can be achieved through the use of different nuclides that decay, producing emissions of differing qualities. Thus, it should be possible to select a nuclide with properties that are most compatible with the treatment of a tumor with a particular size, location, and radiosensitivity. Most radioimmunotherapeutic trials in patients have been performed with antibodies labeled with the β-emitter [131]I. This nuclide should continue to be of value in the future, particularly if methods of labeling shown to minimize dehalogenation and increase tumor dose in animals are of similar benefit in patients.[222]

Because beta-emitters such as ^{131}I and ^{90}Y have a range in tissue of millimeters to a few centimeters, they should be well suited to the treatment of larger tumors. In addition, their relatively long range also would facilitate the destruction of adjacent antigen-negative or poorly perfused tumor cells through radiative cross-fire. Several beta-emitting nuclides of potential utility for antibody-mediated radiotherapy are listed in Table XVIII-7-3. One advantage of these nuclides compared with ^{131}I is that their shorter half-lives might help minimize dose rate effects inherent in the use of low linear energy transfer (LET) beta radiation.

For some applications, such as the treatment of micrometastases, intra-cavitary disease, or tumors of the circulatory system, it may be preferable to use high LET radiation such as α particles or in some cases, low-energy electrons. α particles such as those emitted by [211]At (Table XVIII-7-3) have a range of tissue of only about 4–6 cell diameters. Since α particles are high LET radiation, their relative biological effectiveness is much higher than that of β particles; indeed, only 2–15 α traversals per cell are required to achieve cell killing.[20,115] In addition, since the effectiveness of α-particle irradiation is nearly oxygen independent, treatment of hypoxic regions of tumor also might be possible. When localized in the cell nucleus, low energy electrons such as those emitted by ^{125}I are also high LET radiation and might be a

Table XVIII-7-3. Nuclides of Potential Utility in Radioimmunotherapy

Nuclide	Half-life (hr)	Type of Emission	Decay Energy E_{max} (keV)
[131]I	194	β	336, 606[a]
[90]Y	64.1	β	2288
[188]Re	16.9	β	1973
[186]Re	90.6	β	934, 1072[a]
[67]Cu	61.9	β	395,[a] 484, 557
[211]At	7.2	α	5866, 7450[a]
[212]Bi	1.0	α	6051,[a] 6090
[125]I	1,450	Auger	<5

[a]Principal emission

valuable type of radiation to use with antibodies which are internalized after binding to their tumor cell targets.

Clinical Studies. The most extensive clinical experience with antibody-mediated radiotherapy is that of Order and colleagues,[107,113,147,148] who have been investigating the therapeutic efficacy of ^{131}I-labeled polyclonal antiferritin antibodies in several patient populations. In early trials, patients with hepatoma received single doses of up to 150 mCi and, with the exception of a patient who had three weeks of marrow aplasia, no toxicity was seen.[147] Radiation dosimetry calculations indicated that the absorbed doses received by the tumor, normal liver, and whole body were about 1,850, 700, and 165 cGy, respectively.[107] A more recent protocol has involved the administration of 1–4 doses of 20–30 mCi of labeled antiferritin derived from different species.[148] Measurement of tumor volume by CT was used to document complete response in 7% and partial response in 43% of patients with hepatoma. The same group has studied the therapeutic efficacy of ^{131}I-labeled antiferritin in patients with Hodgkin's disease.[52] With this relatively radiosensitive tumor, a partial remission rate of 40% was observed in patients who had not responded to chemotherapy.

A Phase I-II trial of ^{90}Y-labeled antiferritin also has been reported in patients with hepatoma.[149] The advantages of ^{90}Y are that its beta particles are more energetic than those of ^{131}I and its shorter half-life should increase radiation dose rate. Partial remissions were noted in 2 of 6 patients and some hematological toxicity was observed. When ^{90}Y-labeled antiferritin was given in multiple cycles to patients with Hodgkin's disease, complete remissions were seen in three patients.[202]

With regard to other antibodies, in patients with melanoma[11] and cutaneous T cell lymphoma,[168] responses to ^{131}I-labeled antibodies or their fragments have been transient, at best. In non-Hodgkin's lymphoma, DeNardo and colleagues have reported partial responses using multiple injections of ^{131}I-labeled Lym-1 monoclonal antibody.[51] Bernstein and colleagues have initiated a series investigating the efficacy of high doses (250–482 mCi) of ^{131}I-labeled antibody MB-1 in patients with recurrent lymphoma, and no significant non-hematological toxicity was observed.[9] Using an anti-idiotypic monoclonal antibody labeled with 10 mCi of ^{90}Y, transient partial regression of disease was reported in a patient with a B cell lymphoma.[152]

Strategies for Improving Tumor Uptake. Biopsy studies from patients who have received labeled antibodies intravenously indicate that only about 0.005% of the injected dose of radioactivity is localized per gram of tumor.[31,222] This low level of uptake is a major factor contributing to the limited efficacy of radioimmunotherapy. Multiple strategies are being investigated for improving both tumor dose and tumor–to–normal-tissue radiation-absorbed dose ratios.

Advances in monoclonal antibody labeling methodology, both in metal chelation and radiohalogenation, have resulted in more tumor uptake and lower accumulation in normal tissues. Roselli and colleagues have reported that use of an SCN-Bz-DTPA chelate for labeling antibodies with [88]Y (a long-lived analog of ^{90}Y) increased tumor uptake in an athymic mouse model more than four-fold and decreased bone uptake to a similar degree.[167] Similarly, use of an *N*-succinimidyl-3-(tri-*n*-butylstannyl)benzoate intermediate (the ATE method) for radioiodination of antibodies has been shown to increase the radiation dose to subcutaneous human glioma xenografts by more than a factor of three compared to the same antibody using a conventional method.[219,222]

Another approach for increasing tumor uptake is to attempt to manipulate tumor hemodynamics using either external beam irradiation or local hyperthermia. Although some investigators have claimed that pre-irradiation enhanced tumor uptake,[137,192] a more recent study has reported that external beam irradiation caused no statistically significant increase in tumor accumulation.[179] Interpretation of these studies is complicated by the fact that external beam irradiation can decrease tumor mass, an effect which itself can increase antibody uptake. Recently, it has been reported that local hyperthermia at 42°C could be used to increase the uptake of a radioiodinated monoclonal antibody fragment by more than two-fold in a subcutaneous glioma xenograft.[47]

Administration of the labeled antibody by a nonintravenous route is a strategy for increasing the rate and magnitude of tumor uptake while minimizing the dose to normal tissues. For example, Colcher and colleagues have shown that intraperitoneal injection of ^{131}I-labeled B72.3 increased uptake in peritoneal colorectal lesions by two- to sevenfold compared to intravenous administration.[44] Similarly, intraperitoneal administration of ^{131}I-labeled HMFG2 in patients with ovarian carcinoma increased the uptake of activity in tumor cells to levels between 4 and 7 times greater than those observed after intravenous administration.[208] However, use of the intracarotid route in patients with malignant gliomas did not result in increased uptake of labeled antibody in tumor.[223]

The therapeutic potential of antibodies administered by intracavitary routes has been investigated by several groups. Intrapleural and intrapericardial administration of ^{131}I-labeled HMFG1, HMFG2, and AUA1 antibodies to patients with malignant pleural and pericardial effusions resulted in a complete response for 10 of 13 patients.[154] The same group has extended this approach to study the efficacy of intraperitoneal delivery of ^{131}I-labeled antibodies for the treatment of epithelial ovarian carcinoma.[64] Eight patients with disease greater than 2 cm in diameter did not respond, while 9 of 16 patients with smaller volume disease experienced an objective response. In a recent study, intrathecal administration of ^{131}I-labeled antibody to patients with leptomeningeal disease resulted in objective therapeutic response in four of five patients.[99] It is important to emphasize that randomized studies using radiolabeled control antibodies will be required to determine whether these therapeutic effects are related to specific binding of the labeled antibody to the tumor.

Immunotoxins

Antibodies linked to peptide toxins provide an alternative method to increase the cytotoxic activity of monoclonal antibodies. Peptide toxins which catalytically inactivate protein synthesis are found in plants, bacteria and fungi. The plant (ricin) and bacterial (diphtheria and pseudomonas exotoxin) holotoxins consist of 60 kilodalton peptides with a 20–30 kilodalton A chain or domain covalently linked to a 30–40 kilodalton B chain or domain.[151] The B region has binding sites for normal cell surface receptors (beta-galactosyl pyranoside groups in the case of plant holotoxins although unknown for bacterial toxins).[146] After cell surface binding, the toxins are internalized into intracellular vesicles. In different compartments (endosomes for bacterial toxins and perhaps the trans-Golgi for plant toxins), the toxins translocate to the cytosol.[216] In the cytosol, the A portion of the toxins catalytically inactivate protein synthesis. The bacterial toxin A fragments ADP-ribosylate 200 elongation factor-2 molecules/minute.[130] The plant toxin A chains release adenine in an N-glycosidase reaction on adenosine 3,424 of the 28S RNA of the 60S ribosomal subunit at 100–1,000 ribosomes/minute/enzyme molecule.[62] The elongation step of protein synthesis is irreversibly stopped in each case. A single molecule of either bacterial or plant toxin can lead to cell death.[61,213]

For the synthesis of immunotoxins, the normal cell binding site of the toxin is removed and replaced with a tumor cell specific ligand. Ricin toxin can be reduced and the B chain containing the normal cell binding domain discarded.[13] Alternatively, the lectin binding sites of ricin can be blocked with oligosaccharides containing a reactive dichlorotriazine group so that normal cell binding is prevented.[102] Pseudomonas exotoxin normal cell binding site is altered by derivatizing lysine-57 with 2-iminothiolane.[92] The diphtheria toxin binding site is removed by genetic engineering to remove the 50 C-terminal amino acid residues.[138] The modified toxins are linked to monoclonal antibodies by a chemical linker. The antibody is usually derivatized with a thiolation reagent and the free thiol is then used for conjugation to toxin.[33] The toxin may have an available free thiol as in ricin toxin A chain or a thiol may be introduced when the toxin binding site is modified. Alternatively, new ligands such as interleukin-2 can be coupled to toxins such as diphtheria by an amide bond using genetic engineering. The final hybrid protein combines the extreme potency of the parent toxin with the selectivity of the attached ligand. Potent and selective immunotoxins which kill antigen bearing cells in vitro at picomolar or nanomolar concentrations have been constructed.

Pharmacology. Immunotoxins have been administered systemically to patients with refractory cancers and observations on toxicities, pharmacology, immune response and efficacy have been made (Table XVIII-7-4). The first immunotoxin trials were performed in melanoma, colorectal carcinoma, and chronic lymphocytic leukemia. Distinct pharmacologic problems appeared to reduce clinical efficacy in each case.

Spitler and colleagues administered anti-melanoma monoclonal antibody-ricin A chain conjugate as daily infusions for up to 10 days (cumulative dose up to 300 mg) to 22 patients with metastatic melanoma.[188] The immunotoxin had an IC$_{50}$ (concentration of immunotoxin inhibiting protein synthesis by 50%) of 0.35 nanomolar on melanoma cell lines. The major toxicity was a capillary leak syndrome with hypoalbuminemia, edema, and weight gain. Minor toxicities included anorexia, malaise, fatigue, fever, and decreased voltage on EKG. The half-life of the immunotoxin in the bloodstream was 30 minutes, and most patients developed antibodies to the conjugate. Spitler reported that each of five tumor samples obtained after an immunotoxin infusion showed evidence of immunotoxin localization in the tumor, but no estimate of percent saturation of tumor cells was given. One complete response was seen. The poor response rate may have been due to rapid clearance of the conjugate from the bloodstream and poor tumor capillary penetration. The immunotoxin was large (200 kilodaltons), glycosylated with mannose terminated oligosaccharides, and the ricin A chain linked by an unprotected disulfide bond.

Hertler and colleagues treated eight patients with chronic lymphocytic leukemia with one-hour infusions of anti-CD5 monoclonal antibody-ricin A chain conjugate (3, 7 or 14 mg/m^2) twice weekly for four weeks.[85] The immunotoxin had an IC$_{50}$ of greater than 10 nanomolar on fresh CLL cells. No toxicities were seen and a plasma half-life of 43 minutes was found. Though saturation of circulating leukemic cell-associated target antigen was demonstrated, no immunotoxin was detected in bone marrow or lymph node aspirates. No immune response was seen aside from a low level of human antibody to ricin A chain in one patient. No clinical responses were seen, either. While the immunotoxin had significant cytotoxicity to T leukemia cell lines, its lack of efficacy on fresh CLL cells probably contributed to the poor clinical outcome.

Byers and colleagues treated sixteen patients with metastatic colon cancer and one patient with ovarian cancer with a monoclonal antibody-ricin A chain conjugate 72 kD glycoprotein at doses of 0.02–0.2 mg/kg/day for five days by one-hour intravenous infusions.[23] The immunotoxin had an IC$_{50}$ of 0.06 nanomolar. Toxicities again included the capillary leak syndrome, as well as significant proteinuria and a reduction in electrocardiogram voltage. Transient toxic encephalopathy occurred in four patients with mental status changes and diffuse slowing or paroxysmal bursts on EEG, and normal CT scans. All patients had humoral antibody responses to both murine immunoglobulin and ricin A chain. Two partial responses were seen. As in the melanoma trial, clinical efficacy may have been limited by rapid blood clearance and poor tumor capillary permeability to the immunotoxin.

Toxicity. Subsequent clinical studies in breast cancer, ovarian cancer, T cell leukemia, cutaneous T cell lymphoma, and chronic lymphocytic leukemia were performed with either more potent immunotoxins or higher doses of previously described immunotoxins. Unexpected toxicities limited therapy and precluded significant clinical responses.

Gould and colleagues[75] and Weiner and colleagues[209] treated a total of nine patients with metastatic breast cancer with 1–8 daily infusions of 10 µg/kg/day to 100 µg/kg/day of an anti-55 kilodalton protein monoclonal antibody recombinant ricin A chain conjugate. The immunotoxin had an IC50 of 0.05 nanomolar in vitro.[11] Severe capillary leak syndrome was seen and three patients developed a profound sensory-motor peripheral neuropathy one month after therapy. Cross-reactivity of immunotoxin was documented with Schwann cells. The alpha and beta plasma half-lives of the immunotoxin were 2.2 and 9.4 hours, respectively, much longer than for native ricin A chain immunotoxins. Antibody formation was observed against both the mouse monoclonal antibody

Table XVIII-7-4. Systemic Immunotoxin Trials

Conjugate	IC50 (nM)	Total Dose (mg)	Specific Toxicity	Disease	Response Rate (CR + PR/total)	Reference
αCD5-RTA	0.1	77–112	—	GVHD	11/11	109
αCD5-RTA	0.1	55–326	—	GVHD	20/34	26
αCD5-RTA	ND	17–116	—	RA	8/16	25
αCD22-dgRTA	0.0012	9–50	—	Lymphoma	11/26	193
DAB$_{486}$IL2	1	85	—	Lymphoma	3/18	110
αCD19-bR	0.01	29	—	Lymphoma	6/22	143
αCD5-RTA	0.3	140–350	—	CTL	4/14	112
αCD5-RTA	>10	196–490	—	CLL	2/10	108
αgp72-RTA	0.06	7–70	—	Colon Cancer	2/16	23
αgp55r-RTA	0.05	5–56	Schwann	Breast CA	1/9	75,209
αproteog-RTA	0.35	≤300	—	Melanoma	1/22	188
αCD22FAb'-dgRTA	0.012	35–175	—	Lymphoma	ND	193
αTR-rRTA	0.05	0.12	—	Meninges	ND	216
αCD7-RTA	0.05	7	—	TALL	0/3	24
αTR-rRTA	0.05	4–18	CNS	Ovarian CA	0/18	16
OVB3-PE	0.0025	0.7–1.4	CNS	Ovarian CA	0/23	15
αTAC-PE	0.025	1–4	—	TALL	0/4	69
αCD5-RTA	>10	36–200	—	CLL	0/8	85

RTA = Ricin A chain; PE = pseudomonas exotoxin; CD5, CD7, CD19, and CD22 are lymphoid antigens; TR = transferrin receptor; DAB$_{486}$IL2 is a fusion protein with amino acid 1-486 of diphtheria toxin and IL2; gp72 and gp55 are epithelial antigens. Generic toxicities depended upon the toxic component. RTA yielded capillary leak syndrome with low albumin, edema, myalgias, pulmonary edema, rhabdomyolysis. PE, ricin and diphtheria toxin produced liver toxicity. dg = deglycosylated; rRTA = recombinant RTA; bR = blocked ricin; ND = not determined; RA = rheumatoid arthritis; GVHD = graft-versus-host disease; Schwann = Schwann cells in peripheral nerves; CNS = central nervous system; CTCL = cutaneous T cell lymphoma; CLL = chronic lymphocytic leukemia; TALL = T cell leukemia; Meninges = meningeal neoplasms

and recombinant ricin A chain. One partial response was seen. The severe toxicity prevented further dose escalation.

Bookman and colleagues treated 23 patients with refractory ovarian carcinoma with anti-adenocarcinoma associated antigen monoclonal antibody (OVB3)-Pseudomonas exotoxin conjugated via a non-reducible thioether bond.[15] Drug was infused intraperitoneally at doses of 5–10 μg/kg for 2–4 doses over one week (maximum total dose was 20 μg/kg). The immunotoxin had an IC50 of 0.0025 nanomolar in vitro. Abdominal pain, nausea, vomiting, malaise, fever, hepatitis, and peritoneal fibrosis occurred. A severe encephalopathy occurred in three patients, with brainstem inflammation on MRI in two patients and death in one patient. The antibody OVB3 variably reacts with an antigen in the central nervous system.[211] Intraperitoneal concentrations of immunotoxin exceeded cytotoxic levels for every patient. Host neutralizing antibody developed before day fourteen in most patients. No responses were seen. Again an apparent antibody-targeted toxicity prevented dose escalation.

Bookman, and Griffin and colleagues treated 20 patients with metastatic intraperitoneal carcinoma (i.e., ovarian, breast, mesothelioma, pancreas), utilizing anti-transferrin receptor monoclonal antibody-recombinant ricin A chain conjugate at 5–50 μg/kg daily intraperitoneally for five days.[16] The IC$_{50}$ in vitro for the OVCAR3 cell line was 0.03 nanomolar. Hypoalbuminemia, malaise, and abdominal discomfort occurred in many patients and was mild. Three patients developed transient superficial mucositis. An additional patient was treated at the 50 μg/kg dose and developed a fatal encephalopathy associated with CT scans that were negative initially but showed cerebral edema at 12 hours.[17] The antibody variably reacts with brain capillaries. Peritoneal fluid levels of immunotoxin exceeded the cytotoxic concentration by 1,000-fold at the highest doses. Serum levels of immunotoxin were undetectable except for very low levels (<100 ng/ml) in three patients at the higher dose levels. A rise of IgG and IgM antibodies against both the toxin and monoclonal antibody were observed as well as the development of neutralizing antibodies in some patients. No partial or complete responses were observed although several minor responses (decreased ascites, decreased CA125) occurred. The possible antibody targeted toxicity prevented further dose escalation.

Fitzgerald treated four patients with human T-cell leukemia (HTLV-1 positive) with anti-TAC monoclonal antibody-Pseudomonas exotoxin A conjugated with a reducible disulfide bond.[69] Daily one-hour intravenous infusions over 1–5 days with cumulative doses up to 4 mg were given. The immunotoxin had an IC$_{50}$ of 0.025 nanomolar in vitro. Significant liver toxicity was seen. The conjugate contained iminothiolate derivatized exotoxin which retained hepatocyte binding activity.[92] Neutralizing antibodies developed after one week. No lasting clinical responses were seen. The toxin-mediated toxicity prevented extension of the trial.

LeMaistre and colleagues treated 14 patients with cutaneous T cell lymphoma with anti-CD5 monoclonal antibody-ricin A chain conjugate with ten daily intravenous one hour infusions of 0.2–0.5 mg/kg/day.[111] The immunotoxin had an IC$_{50}$ of 0.3 nanomolar on cutaneous T cell lymphoma cell lines in vitro. Toxicities included the capillary leak syndrome with myalgias, dyspnea at rest, and pulmonary edema at 0.5 mg/kg/day. At lower doses a milder capillary leak occurred with hypoalbuminemia, weight gain, pedal edema, fatigue, fever, and chills. Six patients received multiple cycles of treatment and one of these patients developed urticaria on retreatment. Serum half-life was 30 minutes. All patients developed antibodies to the immunotoxin and one-half the patients showed low levels of blocking antibodies. Partial responses occurred in four patients and three of these had received more than one cycle. Patients were retreated despite the presence of antibody and responses were seen in that setting. The ricin A chain-related capillary leak syndrome limited dose escalation.

LeMaistre and colleagues treated 10 patients with chronic lymphocytic leukemia with an anti-CD5 monoclonal antibody-ricin A chain conjugate at 0.2–0.4 mg/kg/day for 14 days given as one-hour infusions.[108] Patients were retreated at 28 day intervals. Seven patients completed two cycles of treatment. Toxicities were mild at low dosages (0.33 mg/kg/day) and consisted of arthralgias, dyspnea, fever, malaise, nausea, rash and fluid retention. One patient was treated at 0.4 mg/kg/day and one patient was treated at 0.5 mg/kg/day. Both these patients had significant rhabdomyolysis and renal insufficiency. The serum half-life was approximately 40 minutes. Only two patients developed anti-immunotoxin antibodies at low levels. The two patients given 0.4–0.5 mg/kg/day doses had partial responses lasting 4 and 2+ months. The anti-CD5-ricin A chain conjugate was active in this disease when given at sufficiently high doses, but therapy was limited by the toxicity.

Thus, initial efforts to improve delivery of adequate immunotoxin to extravascular tumor deposits by raising drug potency or dose met with significant antibody and toxin-related toxicities. Antibodies with substantial normal tissue bonding (particularly to nerve or central nervous system tissue) yielded conjugates with poor therapeutic indices clinically.

Success With Accessible Target Cells. Subsequent clinical trials were made in diseases with target cells readily accessible to the bloodstream. Immunotoxins were selected with higher potency and more limited normal tissue reactivity.

Byers and colleagues treated 34 patients with acute graft–versus–host disease (GVHD) with anti-CD5 monoclonal antibody-ricin A chain conjugate.[26] A 14 day course of 0.05–0.33 mg/kg/day was given. The IC_{50} of the immunotoxin on activated donor T cells was 0.1 nanomolar.[97] Toxicities included fatigue, myalgias, hypoalbuminemia, and weight gain. Renal insufficiency occurred in six patients and was irreversible in four. Since all these patients received other potentially nephrotoxic drugs including cyclosporine, aminoglycosides, or amphotericin, the role of immunotoxin in the renal dysfunction is unclear. The blood half-life of the immunotoxin was 20–60 minutes with slower clearance at higher doses. Of 23 patients tested six developed antibodies to the monoclonal antibody and ricin A chain. No blocking antibodies or allergic reactions were seen. Of 32 evaluable patients 22 responded in at least one organ system. Twenty of these patients had durable responses. Nine patients had complete responses and seven patients had partial responses in all evaluable organ systems. Based on these excellent results with active acute GVHD, LeMaistre and colleagues used anti-CD5 monoclonal antibody-ricin A chain conjugate as prophylaxis after adult matched allogeneic bone marrow transplantation.[109] Eleven patients received 0.1 mg/kg/day from day 0, 3, 7 post transplant until day 16 post transplant.

Toxicities were mild and transient, consisting of myalgias, arthralgias, fever, proteinuria, and weight gain. Four of seven patients tested developed anti-immunotoxin antibodies at high titers (>1:1,000). Marrow engraftment was equal or better than with cyclosporine with or without methotrexate. No immunotoxin treated patient developed moderate or severe GVHD.

Byers and colleagues treated 16 rheumatoid arthritis patients with anti-CD5 monoclonal antibody-ricin A chain conjugate at 0.5–0.33 mg/kg/day over one hour for five days.[25] The abnormal target cell and its sensitivity to immunotoxin were unknown. Toxicities included hypoalbuminemia and myalgias. The β phase plasma half-life was two hours. Over one-half the patients showed significant anti-immunotoxin antibody responses. Eight out of 16 patients had a greater than 40% reduction in joint scores for over 60 days and in 3 of 8 patients the response lasted over one year.

Presumably, there is a target cell population in GVHD and rheumatoid arthritis which is sensitive to immunotoxin. Perhaps less than 90% of target cells must be killed or damaged to observe clinical benefit. Further, these cells may be circulating or be readily accessible from the bloodstream. Unfortunately, little is known of the detailed pathophysiology in vivo of these diseases.

LeMaistre and colleagues treated 18 patients with lymphoid malignant neoplasms with $DAB_{486}IL$-2.[110] This immunotoxin is a recombinant fusion protein with replacement of the diphtheria receptor binding domain with human IL-2. The IC50 on receptor positive cell lines was one nanomolar in vitro.[207] Patients received 11 doses of 0.1 mg/kg/day on days 1, 3–5, and 14–20 on a monthly basis. Some patients were treated up to six times. Dose-limiting toxicity was a transient reversible ten-fold rise in transaminases. Minor side effects included fever, dyspnea and rash. The plasma half-life was five minutes with a peak serum level of 500–900 ng/ml. Three patients pretreatment and eight patients post-treatment had anti-diphtheria toxin antibodies. No patients developed anti-IL-2 antibodies. There was one complete response, two partial responses and four minor responses lasting 3–11 months.

Stone and colleagues treated 26 patients with refractory B cell lymphoma with four infusions for one hour every other day of anti-CD22 monoclonal antibody conjugated to a deglycosylated ricin A chain.[193] Both a whole antibody linked by SMPT (a hindered disulfide) and Fab' linked by the available free thiol were used. The IC_{50} on Daudi cells of the whole antibody immunotoxin was 0.0012 nanomolar and of the Fab immunotoxin 0.012 nanomolar in vitro.[176] Doses were 8.6–50 mg for whole antibody conjugates and 35–175 mg for Fab conjugates. The beta phase half-life was 1–4 hours and serum levels reached 4 μg/ml. Toxicities included the capillary leak syndrome with weight gain, decreased serum albumin, drop in EKG voltage, fevers and myalgias. Dose-limiting toxicities included pulmonary edema, aphasia and rhabdomyolysis. The MTD was 75 mg/m² for the Fab conjugate and has not been reached for the whole antibody conjugate (>38 mg/m²). Only 1 of 26 patients developed anti-immunotoxin antibodies. Forty percent of the patients had a PR. Fifty-five percent of patients with over 50% CD22 positive tumor cells achieved a PR. There appeared to be a dose response with the whole antibody conjugate.

Nadler and colleagues treated 25 patients with refractory B leukemia or lymphoma with anti-CD19-blocked ricin conjugate (Anti-B4-bR).[142] The IC50 was 0.01 nanomolar on Daudi cells. The bolus MTD was 50 μg/kg/day for five days given over one hour, and was tolerated well. Higher doses were associated with >ten-fold transient rises in transaminases in the blood. Blood levels reached 4×10^{-9} M. One-half of the patients developed anti-ricin and anti-mouse Ig antibodies. Two partial responses and one complete response were seen in 25 patients.

The clinical responses in lymphoid malignancies may be due to more accessible target cells and the lack of a humoral immune response to the immunotoxin. Few data have been presented on tumor tissue penetration by conjugate, and this information should prove critical in the next few years in immunotoxin design both for lymphomas and other cancers.

Bone Marrow Transplantation. Many of the problems encountered in vivo have been avoided when immunotoxins have been used to treat bone marrow prior to infusion during autologous or allogeneic bone marrow transplantation. Immunotoxins have been used to purge malignant T cells from leukemic marrow. Filipovich and colleagues treated seven T-ALL patients with autologous marrow treated ex vivo with anti-CD5-ricin and anti-CD11a-ricin in the presence of 100 mM lactose.[67] One of seven patients survived disease-free for >450 days. Patient tolerance for immunotoxin treated marrow was also demonstrated by Gorin[74] and Preijers and colleagues.[157] Uckun and colleagues treated fourteen T-ALL patients with autologous marrow purged with anti-CD5-ricin plus anti-CD7-ricin and 4-hydroperoxycyclophosphamide.[198] Two of 14 patients were disease free at two years post transplant. Examination of remission marrow samples for residual leukemic progenitor cells suggested that the primary reason for recurrence of leukemia was inefficient pretransplant radiochemotherapy rather than inefficient purging of autografts.

Immunotoxins have also been used ex vivo to purge allogeneic bone marrow grafts of nonmalignant donor T cells to reduce graft–versus–host disease (GVHD). Marrow from allogeneic donors should lack contaminating tumor cells. Filipovich and colleagues treated seventeen patients with relapsed AML or ALL with HLA-MHC matched donor bone marrow which had been exposed to a mixture of three monoclonal antibody-ricin conjugates (anti-CD5, anti-CD3 and anti-CD11a) in the presence of lactose to prevent nonspecific toxicity.[68] None of the patients developed severe GVHD and only 4 of 17 experienced grade II skin GVHD. Graft rejection occurred, however, in four patients. Vallera and colleagues treated nine patients with Wiskott-Aldrich syndrome, Wolman's disease, CML, or AML with one haplotype mismatched donor marrow pretreated with the same cocktail of antibody-ricin conjugates.[200] Only one patient developed GVHD but 6 of 9 patients had marrow failure. Blythman and colleagues[14] treated 38 leukemic patients with HLA-identical marrow incubated with anti-CD5 (Fab)-ricin A chain in the presence of 20 mM ammonium chloride. Only one case of grade II GVHD occurred, but two cases of graft failure occurred. Fauser and colleagues gave HLA-identical marrow treated with anti-CD5-ricin A chain to five high risk patients and no acute GVHD or graft failure was observed.[66] While immunotoxins appear to successfully deplete T cells ex vivo without damaging stem cells, the increased graft failure which occurred limits the usefulness of this modality for GVHD prophylaxis.

Conclusions

Only two decades have passed since the earliest attempts at immunotoxin synthesis by Moolten and colleagues. We have witnessed the testing in both the laboratory and in patients of a number of immunotoxins. The potential for immunotoxins has been demonstrated in the systemic treatment of GVHD, rheumatoid arthritis, and lymphomas. Expansion of the role of immunotoxins in these diseases and in metastatic carcinomas will require a better understanding of immunotoxin pharmacology and structure-function relationships of both peptide ligands and toxins. Such a detailed analysis involves the assignment of roles to individual amino acid residues and domains in the proteins. Such unambiguous assignments are only possible if the protein is pure and changes in amino acids can be verified. A system of expression of cloned DNA sequences permits such studies. Genes have been cloned for antibody fragments, hormones, and toxins. Expression, purification and characterization in vitro and in vivo have been done for chimeras with diphtheria toxin and pseudomonas exotoxin with ligands as diverse as IL-2, CD4, alpha-MSH, anti-TAC (Fv), OVB3 (Fv), TGF-α and interleukin-6.[35,36,37,60,116,138,139,181] Hopefully, these genetically engineered molecules will be used in the next few years to define critical factors in immunotoxin design for clinical efficacy. The use of combination therapy with cytotoxic drugs,[182] small molecular weight immunotoxin enhancers,[32] cocktails of immunotoxins,[217] and the application of immunotoxins to the adjuvant setting are exciting possible future clinical avenues. The next decade may see the definition of a niche for immunotoxins in the treatment of a variety of neoplasms.

References

1. Anasetti, C., Martin, P. J., Morishita, Y., Badger, C. C., Bernstein, I. D., and Hansen, J. A.: Human large granular lymphocytes express high affinity receptors for murine monoclonal antibodies of the IgG3 subclass. J. Immunol., 138:2979, 1987.
2. Anderson, I. C., Shpall, E. J., Leslie, D. S., Nustad, K., Ugelstad, J., Peters, W. P., and Bast, R. C., Jr.: Elimination of malignant clonogenic breast cancer cells from human bone marrow. Cancer Res., 49:4659, 1989.
3. Badger, C. C., Anasetti, C., Davis, J., and Bernstein, I. D.: Treatment of malignancy with unmodified antibody. Pathol. Immunopathol. Res., 6:419, 1987.
4. Baldwin, R. W., Embleton, M. J., Gallego, J., Garnett, M., Pimm, M. V., and Price, M. R.: Monoclonal antibody drug conjugates for cancer therapy. In Monoclonal Antibodies in Cancer. Advances in Diagnosis and Treatment. Edited by J.A. Roth. New York, Futura Publishing Co., 1986, p. 215.
5. Baldwin, R. W., Embleton, M. J., Garnett, M. C., and Pimm, M. V.: Conjugates of monoclonal antibody 791T/36 with methotrexate in cancer therapy. NCI Monogr., 3:95, 1987.
6. Ball, E. D., Mills, L. E., Coughlin, C. T., Beck, J. R., and Cornwell, G. G. III: Autologous bone marrow transplantation in acute myelogenous leukemia. In vitro treatment with myeloid cell-specific monoclonal antibodies. Blood, 68:1311, 1986.
7. Bast, R. C., Jr., De Fabritiis, P., Lipton, J., Gelber, R., Maver, C., Nadler, L., Sallan, S., and Ritz, J.: Elimination of malignant clonogenic cells from human bone marrow using multiple monoclonal antibodies and complement. Cancer Res., 45:499, 1985.
8. Beatty, J. D., Beatty, B. G., O'Connor-Tressel, M., Do, T., and Paxton, R. J.: Mechanisms of tissue uptake and metabolism of radiolabeled antibody—role of antigen: antibody complex formation. Cancer Res. (Suppl.), 50:840, 1990.
9. Bernstein, I. D., Eary, J. F., Badger, C. C., Press, O. W., Appelbaum, F. R., Martin, P. J., Krohn, K. A., Nelp, W. B., Porter, B., and Fisher, D.: High dose radiolabeled antibody therapy of lymphoma. Cancer Res. (Suppl.), 50:1017, 1990.
10. Bischof-Delaloye, A., Delaloye, B., Buchegger, F., Gilgien, W., Studer, A., Curchod, S., Givel, J. C., Mosimann, F., Pettavel, J., and Mach, J. P.: Clinical value of immunoscintigraphy in colorectal carcinoma patients: A prospective study. J. Nucl. Med., 30:1646, 1989.
11. Bjorn, M. J., Ring, D., and Frankel, A.: Evaluation of monoclonal antibodies for the development of breast cancer immunotoxins. Cancer Res., 45:1214, 1985.
12. Blottiere, H. M., Maurel, C., and Douillard, J. Y.: Immune function of patients with

gastrointestinal carcinoma after treatment with multiple infusions of monoclonal antibody 17.1A. Cancer Res., 47:5238, 1987.

13. Blythman, H. E., Casellas, P., Gros, O., Gros, P., Jansen, F. K., Paolucci, F., Pau, B., and Vidal, H.: Immunotoxins: Hybrid molecules of monoclonal antibodies and a toxin subunit specifically kill tumour cells. Nature, 290:145, 1981.
14. Blythman, H., Laurent, G., Deroeg, J., Gluckman, E., Maraninchi, D., Vernant, J., Schneider, P., and Jansen, F.: Treatment of donor bone marrow with Fab T101 ricin A-chain immunotoxin for the prevention of graft-versus-host disease after allogeneic bone marrow transplantation. Second International Conference on Monoclonal Antibody Immunoconjugates for Cancer. San Diego, 1987, p. 61.
15. Bookman, M. A., FitzGerald, D., Frankel, A., Gould, B., Howell, S., Jacob, J., Longo, D., McClay, E., Reed, E., and Smith, J.: Intraperitoneal immunotoxin therapy: Two clinical studies. Antibody Immunocon. Radiopharm., 3:70, 1990a.
16. Bookman, M., Godfrey, S., Padavic, K., Griffin, T., Corda, J. P., Hamilton, T., Ozols, R. F., and Groves, E. S.: Antitransferrin receptor immunotoxin (IT) therapy: Phase-I intraperitoneal (IP) trial. Proc. Annu. Meet. Am. Soc. Clin. Oncol., 9:187, 1990b.
17. Bookman, M.: Personal communication, 1990.
18. Boulianne, G. L., Hozumi, N., and Shulman, M. J.: Production of functional chimaeric mouse/human antibody. Nature, 312:643, 1984.
19. Boyer, C. M., Borowitz, M. J., McCarty, K. S., Jr., Kinney, R. B., Everitt, L., Dawson, D. V., Ring, D., and Bast, R. C., Jr.: Heterogeneity of antigen expression in benign and malignant breast and ovarian epithelial cells. Int. J. Cancer, 43:55, 1989.
20. Brown, I.: Astatine-211: Its possible applications in cancer therapy. Int. J. Rad. Appl. Instrum. [A], 37:789, 1986.
21. Bumol, T. F., Laguzza, B. C., Baker, A. L., Todd, G. C., Pohland, R. C., and Apelgren, L. D.: Studies on 9.2.27-4-desacetyl vinblastine-3-carboxyhydrazide (9.2.27-DAVLB-hydrazide): Preclinical pharmacology and toxicology profiles for human melanoma therapy. Proc. Annu. Meet. Am. Assoc. Cancer Res., 29:A1667, 1988.
22. Buraggi, G. L., Callegaro, L., Mariani, G., Turrin, A., Cascinelli, N., Attili, A., Bombardieri, E., Terno, G., Plassio, G., and Dovis, M.: Imaging with ^{131}I-labeled monoclonal antibodies to a high-molecular-weight melanoma-associated antigen in patients with melanoma: Efficacy of whole immunoglobulin and its $F(ab')_2$ fragments. Cancer Res., 45:3378, 1985.
23. Byers, V. S., Rodvien, R., Grant, K., Durrant, L. G., Hudson, K. H., Baldwin, R. W., and Scannon, P. J.: Phase I study of monoclonal antibody-ricin A chain immunotoxin XomaZyme-791 in patients with metastatic colon cancer. Cancer Res., 49:6153, 1989.
24. Byers, V., Duerst, R., Carroll, S., Fishild, D., Kung, A., Price, M., and Baldwin, R.: Use of an anti-CD7-ricin A chain immunotoxin in the treatment of T cell acute lymphocytic leukemia. Proceedings of the Second International Symposium on Immunotoxins, Orlando, p. 11, 1990.
25. Byers, V., Strand, V., Saria, E., Ma, J., and the XOMA Rheumatoid Arthritis Treatment Group: Patients with rheumatoid arthritis treated with a pan-T lymphocyte immunotoxin: Phase II studies. Proceedings of the Second International Symposium on Immunotoxins, Orlando, p. 12, 1990.
26. Byers, V. S., Henslee, P. J., Kernan, N. A., Blazar, B. R., Gingrich, R., Phillips, G. L., LeMaistre, C. F., Gilliland, G., Antin, J. H., and Martin, P.: Use of anti-pan T-lymphocyte ricin A chain immunotoxin in steroid-resistant acute graft-versus-host disease. Blood, 75:1426, 1990.
27. Carrasquillo, J. A., Krohn, K. A., Beaumier, P., McGuffin, R. W., Brown, J. P., Hellström, K. E., Hellström, I., and Larson, S. M.: Diagnosis of and therapy for solid tumors with radiolabeled antibodies and immune fragments. Cancer Treat. Rep., 68:317, 1984.
28. Carrasquillo, J. A., Bunn, P. A., Jr., Keenan, A. M., Reynolds, J. C., Schroff, R. W., Foon, K. A., Su, M. H., Gazdar, A. F., Mulshine, J. L., and Oldham, R. K.: Radioimmunodetection of cutaneous T-cell lymphoma with ^{111}In-labeled T101 monoclonal antibody. N. Engl. J. Med., 315:673, 1986.
29. Carrasquillo, J. A., Mulshine, J. L., Bunn, P. A., Jr., Reynolds, J. C., Foon, K. A., Schroff, R. W., Perentesis, P., Steis, R. G., Keenan, A. M., Horowitz, M., and Larson, S. M.: Indium-111 Y101 monoclonal antibody is superior to iodine-131 T101 in imaging of cutaneous T-cell lymphoma. J. Nucl. Med., 28:281, 1987.
30. Carrasquillo, J. A., Abrams, P. G., Schroff, R. W., Reynolds, J. C., Woodhouse, C. S., Morgan, A. C., Keenan, A. M., Foon, K. A., Perentesis, P., Marshall, S., Horowitz, M., Szymendera, J., Englert, J., Oldham, R. K., and Larson, S. M.: Effect of antibody dose on the imaging and biodistribution of indium-111 9.2.27 anti-melanoma monoclonal antibody. J. Nucl. Med., 29:39, 1988.
31. Carrasquillo, J. A.: Radioimmunoscintigraphy with polyclonal or monoclonal antibodies. *In* Antibodies in Radiodiagnosis and Therapy. Edited by M. R. Zalutsky. Boca Raton, CRC Press Inc., 1989, p. 169.
32. Casellas, P., and Jansen, F. K.: Immunotoxin enhancers. *In* Immunotoxins. Edited by A. E. Frankel, Boston, Kluwer Academic Publishers, 1988, p. 351.
33. Chang, T. M., Dazord, A., and Neville, D. M., Jr.: Artificial hybrid protein containing a toxic protein fragment and a cell membrane receptor-binding moiety in a disulfide conjugate. II. Biochemical and biologic properties of diphtheria toxin fragment A-S-S-human placental lactogen. J. Biol. Chem., 252:1515, 1977.
34. Chatal, J. F., Saccavini, J. C., Fumoleau, P., Douillard, J. Y., Curtet, C., Kremer, M., Le Mevel, B., and Koprowski, H.: Immunoscintigraphy of colon carcinoma. J. Nucl. Med., 25:307, 1984.
35. Chaudhary, V. K., Mizukami, T., Fuerst, T. R., FitzGerald, D. J., Moss, B., Pastan, I., and Berger, E. A.: Selective killing of HIV-infected cells by recombinant human CD4-Pseudomonas exotoxin hybrid protein. Nature, 335:369, 1988.
36. Chaudhary, V. K., Queen, C., Junghans, R. P., Waldmann, T. A., FitzGerald, D. J., and Pastan, I.: A recombinant immunotoxin consisting of two antibody variable domains fused to Pseudomonas exotoxin. Nature, 339:394, 1989.
37. Chaudhary, V. K., Batra, J. K., Gallo, M. G., Willingham, M. C., FitzGerald, D. J., and Pastan, I.: A rapid method of cloning functional variable-region antibody genes in Escherichia coli as single-chain immunotoxins. Proc. Natl. Acad. Sci. USA, 87:1066, 1990.
38. Cheresh, D. A., Honsik, C. J., Staffileno, L. K., Jung, G., and Reisfeld, R. A.: Disialoganglioside GD3 on human melanoma serves as a relevant target antigen for monoclonal antibody-mediated tumor cytolysis. Proc. Natl. Acad. Sci. USA, 82:5155, 1985.
39. Cheung, N. K., Landmeier, B., Neely, J., Nelson, A. D., Abramowsky, C., Ellery, S., Adams, R. B., and Miraldi, F.: Complete tumor ablation with iodine 131-radiolabeled disialoganglioside G_{D2}-specific monoclonal antibody against human neuroblastoma xenografted in nude mice. J. Natl. Cancer Inst., 77:739, 1986.
40. Clark, M., Gilliland, L., and Waldmann, H.: Hybrid antibodies for therapy. Prog. Allergy, 45:31, 1988.
41. Cohn, K. H., Welt, S., Banner, W. P., Harrington, M., Yeh, S., Sakamoto, J., Cardon-Cardo, C., Daly, J., Kemeny, N., and Cohen, A.: Localization of radioiodinated monoclonal antibody in colorectal cancer. Initial dosimetry results. Arch. Surg., 122:1425, 1987.
42. Colcher, D., Zalutsky, M., Kaplan, W., Kufe, D., Austin, F., and Schlom, J.: Radiolocalization of human mammary tumors in athymic mice by a monoclonal antibody. Cancer Res., 43:736, 1983.
43. Colcher, D., Esteban, J. M., Carrasquillo, J. A., Sugarbaker, P., Reynolds, J. C., Bryant, G., Larson, S. M., and Schlom, J.: Quantitative analyses of selective radiolabeled monoclonal antibody localization in metastatic lesions of colorectal cancer patients. Cancer Res., 47:1185, 1987.
44. Colcher, D., Esteban, J., Carrasquillo, J. A., Sugarbaker, P., Reynolds, J. C., Bryant, G., Larson, S. M., and Schlom, J.: Complementation of intracavitary and intravenous administration of a monoclonal antibody (B72.3) in patients with carcinoma. Cancer Res., 47:4218, 1987.
45. Colcher, D., Bird, R., Roselli, M., Hardman, K. D., Johnson, S., Pope, S., Dodd, S. W., Pantoliano, M. W., Milenic, D. E., and Schlom, J.: In vivo tumor targeting of a recombinant single-chain antigen-binding protein. J. Natl. Cancer Inst., 82:1191, 1990.
46. Connor, J., Sullivan, S., and Huang, L.: Monoclonal antibody and liposomes. Pharmacol. Ther., 28:341, 1985.
47. Cope, D. A., Dewhirst, M. W., Friedman, H. S., Bigner, D. D., and Zalutsky, M. R.: Enhanced delivery of a monoclonal antibody $F(ab')_2$ fragment to subcutaneous human glioma xenografts using local hyperthermia. Cancer Res., 50:1803, 1990.
48. Debatin, K. M., Goldmann, C. K., Bamford, R., Waldmann, T. A., and Krammer, P. H.: Monoclonal-antibody-mediated apoptosis in adult T-cell leukaemia. Lancet, 335:497, 1990.
49. DeFabritiis, P., Bregni, M., Lipton, J., Reynolds, C., Nadler, L., Ritz, J., and Bast, R. C., Jr.: Antigenic heterogeneity among Burkitt's lymphoma cells surviving treatment with monoclonal antibody and complement. Leukemia Res., 10:35, 1986.
50. Delaloye, B., Bischof-Delaloye, A., Buchegger, F., von Fliedner, V., Grob, J. P., Volant, J. C., Pettavavel, J., and Mach, J. P.: Detection of colorectal carcinoma by emission-computerized tomography after injection of ^{123} I-labeled Fab or $F(ab')_2$ fragments from monoclonal anti-carcinoembryonic antigen antibodies. J. Clin. Invest., 77:301, 1986.
51. DeNardo, S. J., DeNardo, G. L., O'Grady, L. F., Levy, N. B., Mills, S. L., Macey, D. J., McGrahan, J. P., Miller, C. H., and Epstein, A. L.: Pilot studies of radioimmunotherapy of B cell lymphoma and leukemia using I-131 lym-1 monoclonal antibody. Antibody Immunocon. Radiopharm. 1:17, 1988.
52. Dillman, R. O., Shawler, D. L., Dillman, J. B., and Royston, I.: Therapy of chronic lymphocytic leukemia and cutaneous T-cell lymphoma with T101 monoclonal antibody. J. Clin. Oncol., 2:881, 1984.
53. Dillman, R. O., Beauregard, J., Ryan, K. P., Hagan, P. L., Clutter, M., Amox, D., Fincke, J. M., Bartholomew, R. M., Burnett, K. G., and Davis, G. S.: Radioimmunodetection of cancer with the use of indium-111-labeled monoclonal antibodies. NCI Monogr., 3:33, 1987.
54. Dillman, R. O.: Monoclonal antibodies for treating cancer. Ann. Int. Med., 111:592, 1989.
55. Dillman, R. O.: Human antimouse and antiglobulin responses to monoclonal antibodies. Antibody, Immunocon, Radiopharm., 3:1, 1990.
56. Drebin, J. A., Link, V. C., and Greene, M. I.: Monoclonal antibodies specific for the neu oncogene product directly mediate anti-tumor effects in vivo. Oncogene, 2:387, 1988.
57. Duda, R. B., Beatty, J. D., Sheibani, K., Williams, L. E., Paxton, R. J., Beatty, B. G., Shively, J. E., Vlahos, W. G., Werner, J. L., Kemeny, M. M.: Imaging of human colorectal adenocarcinoma with indium-labeled anticarcinoembryonic antigen monoclonal antibody. Arch. Surg., 121:1315, 1986.
58. Eary, J. F., Krohn, K. A., Kishore, R., and Nelp, W. B.: Radiochemistry of halogenated antibodies. *In* Antibodies in Radiodiagnosis and Therapy. Edited by M. R. Zalutsky. Boca Raton, CRC Press, Inc., 1989a, p. 83.
59. Eary, J. F., Schroff, R W., Abrams, P. G., Fritzberg, A. R., Morgan, A. C., Kasina, S., Reno, J. M., Srinivasan, A., Woodhouse, C. S., and Wilbur, D. S.: Successful imaging of malignant melanoma with technetium-99m-labeled monoclonal antibodies. J. Nucl. Med., 30:25, 1989.
60. Edwards, G. M., DeFeo-Jones, D., Tai, J. Y., Vuocolo, G. A., Patrick, D. R., Heimbrook, D. C., and Oliff, A.: Epidermal growth factor receptor binding is affected by structural determinants in the toxin domain of transforming growth factor-alpha-Pseudomonas exotoxin fusion proteins. Mol. Cell. Biol., 9:2860, 1989.
61. Eiklid, K., Olsnes, S., and Pihl, A.: Entry of lethal doses of abrin, ricin and modeccin into the cytosol of HeLa cells. Exp. Cell Res., 126:321, 1980.
62. Endo, Y., and Tsurugi, K.: RNA N-glycosidase activity of ricin A-chain. Mechanism of action of the toxic lectin ricin on eukaryotic ribosomes. J. Biol. Chem., 262:8128, 1987.
63. Epenetos, A. A., Snook, D., Durbin, H., Johnson, P. M., and Taylor-Papadimitriou, J.: Limitations of radiolabeled monoclonal antibodies for localization of human neoplasms. Cancer Res., 46:3183, 1986.
64. Epenetos, A. A., Munro, A. J., Stewart, S., Rampling, R., Lambert, H. E., McKenzie, C. G., Soutter, P., Rahemtulla, A., Hooker, G., and Sivolapenko, G. B.: Antibody-guided irradiation of advanced ovarian cancer with intraperitoneally administered radiolabeled monoclonal antibodies. J. Clin. Oncol., 5:1890, 1987.
65. Farrands, P. A., Perkins, A. C., Pimm, M. V., Embleton, M. J., Hardy, J. D., Baldwin, R. W., and Hardcastle, J. D.: Radioimmunodetection of human colorectal cancers by an anti-tumor monoclonal antibody. Lancet, 2:397, 1982.
66. Fauser, A. A., Langleben, A., and Shustik, C.: Ex vivo treatment of bone marrow inoculum with immunotoxin IT101 to prevent acute graft versus host disease (GVHD) in allogeneic bone marrow transplantation. J. Cell. Biochem. (Suppl.), 10D:226, 1986.
67. Filipovich, A., Ramsay, N., Hurd, D., Stong, R., Youle, R., Vallera, D., and Kersey, J.: Autologous bone marrow transplantation (BMT) for T cell leukemia and lymphoma using marrow cleaning with anti-T cell immunotoxins. Autologous BMT Meeting, University degli Studi di Parma, Parma, Italy, 1985.
68. Filipovich, A. H., Vallera, D. A., Youle, R. J., Haake, R., Blazar, B. R., Arthur, D., Neville, D. M., Jr., Ramsay, N. K., McGlave, P., and Kersey, J. H.: Graft-versus-host

disease prevention in allogeneic bone marrow transplantation from histocompatible siblings. A pilot study using immunotoxins for T cell depletion of donor bone marrow. Transplantation, 44:62, 1987.

69. FitzGerald, D.: The use of recombinant pseudomonas exotoxin in the development of conjugates directed against the interleukin-2 receptor. Third International Conference on Monoclonal Antibody Immunoconjugates for Cancer, San Diego, 1988.
70. Foon, K. A.: Biological response modifiers: The new immunotherapy. Cancer Res., 49:1621, 1989.
71. Ghose, T., and Blair, A. H.: The design of cytotoxic-agent-antibody conjugates. Crit. Rev. Ther. Drug. Carrier Syst., 3:263, 1987.
72. Goldenberg, D. M., DeLand, F., Kin, E., Bennett, S., Primus, F. J., Van Nagell, J. R., Estes, N., DeSimone, P., and Rayburn, P.: Use of radiolabeled antibodies to carcinoembyronic antigen for the detection and localization of diverse cancers by external photoscanning. N. Engl. J. Med., 298:1384, 1978.
73. Goldenberg, D. M.: Challenges to the therapy of cancer with monoclonal antibodies. J. Natl. Cancer Inst., 83:78, 1991.
74. Gorin, N. C.: Autologous bone marrow transplantation: A review of recent advances in acute leukemia. *In* Progress in Bone Marrow Transplantation. Edited by R. P. Gale, and R. Champlin. New York, Alan R. Liss, Inc., 1987, p. 723.
75. Gould, B. J., Borowitz, M. J., Groves, E. S., Carter, P. W., Anthony, D., Weiner, L. M., and Frankel, A. E.: Phase I study of an anti-breast cancer immunotoxin by continuous infusion: Report of a targeted toxic effect not predicted by animal studies. J. Natl. Cancer Inst., 81:775, 1989.
76. Granowska, M., Britton, K. E., Shepherd, J. H., Nimmon, C. C., Mather, S., Ward, B., Osborne, R. J., and Slevin, M. L.: A prospective study of ^{123}I-labeled monoclonal antibody imaging in ovarian cancer. J. Clin. Oncol., 4:730, 1986.
77. Gribben, J. G., Freedman, A. S., Neuberg, D., Roy, D. C., Blake, K. W., Woo, S. D., Grossbard, M. L., Rabinowe, S. N., Coral, F., Freeman, G. J., Ritz, J., and Nadler, L. M.: Immunologic purging of marrow assessed by PCR before autologous bone marrow transplantation for B-cell lymphoma. N. Engl. J. Med., 325:1525, 1991.
78. Halpern, S. E., Dillman, R. O., Witztum, K. F., Shega, J. F., Hagan, P. L., Burrows, W. M., Dillman, J. B., Clutter, M. L., Sobol, R. E., and Frincke, J. M.: Radioimmunodetection of melanoma utilizing In^{111}-96.5 monoclonal antibody: A preliminary report. Radiology, 155:493, 1985.
79. Harris, D. T., and Mastrangelo, M. J.: Serotherapy of cancer. Semin. Oncol., 16:180, 1989.
80. Haspel, M. V., McCabe, R. P., Pomato, N., Janesch, N. J., Knowlton, J. V., Peters, L. C., Hoover, H. C., Jr., and Hanna, M. G., Jr.: Generation of tumor cell-reactive human monoclonal antibodies using peripheral blood lymphocytes from actively immunized colorectal carcinoma patients. Cancer Res., 45:3951, 1985.
81. Hayes, D. F., Zalutsky, M. R., Kaplan, W., Noska, M., Thor, A., Colcher, D., and Kufe, D. W.: Pharmacokinetics of radiolabeled monoclonal antibody B6.2 in patients with metastatic breast cancer. Cancer Res., 46:3157, 1986.
82. Herlyn, D., Ross, A. H., and Koprowski, H.: Anti-idiotypic antibodies bear the internal image of a human tumor antigen. Science, 232:100, 1986.
83. Herlyn, D., Wettendorff, M., Schmoll, E., Iliopoulos, D., Schedel, I., Dreikhausen, U., Raab, R., Ross, A. H., Jaksche, H., Scriba, M., and Koprowski, H.: Anti-idiotype immunization of cancer patients: Modulation of the immune response. Proc. Natl. Acad. Sci. USA, 84:8055, 1987.
84. Hersey, P., MacDonald, M., Burns, C., and Cheresh, D. A.: Enhancement of cytotoxic and proliferative responses of lymphocytes from melanoma patients by incubation with monoclonal antibodies against ganglioside GD3. Cancer Immunol. Immunother., 24:144, 1987.
85. Hertler, A. A., Schlossman, D. M., Borowitz, M. J., Blythman, H. E., Casellas, P., and Frankel, A. E.: An anti-CD5 immunotoxin for chronic lymphocytic leukemia: Enhancement of cytotoxicity with human serum albumin-monensin. Int. J. Cancer, 43:215, 1989.
86. Hnatowich, D. J., Griffin, T. W., Kosciuczyk, C., Rusckowski, M., Childs, R. L., Mattis, J. A., Shealy, D., and Doherty, P. W.: Pharmacokinetics of an indium-111-labeled monoclonal antibody in cancer patients. J. Nucl. Med., 26:849, 1985.
87. Houghton, A. N., Mintzer, D., Cordon-Cardo, C., Welt, S., Fliegel, B., Vadhan, S., Carswell, E., Melamed, M. R., Oettgen, H. F., and Old, L. J.: Mouse monoclonal IgG3 antibody detecting G_{D3} ganglioside: A phase I trial in patients with malignant melanoma. Proc. Natl. Acad. Sci. USA, 82:1242, 1985.
88. Irie, R. F., and Morton, D. L.: Regression of cutaneous metastatic melanoma by intralesional injection with human monoclonal antibody to ganglioside GD2. Proc. Natl. Acad. Sci. USA, 83:8694, 1986.
89. Jain, R. K.: Transport of molecules in the tumor interstitium: A review. Cancer Res., 47:3039, 1987.
90. Jain, R. K.: Physiological barriers to delivery of monoclonal antibodies and other macromolecules in tumors. Cancer Res., 50:814, 1990.
91. James, K., and Bell, G. T.: Human monoclonal antibody production. Current status and future prospects. J. Immunol. Methods, 100:5, 1987.
92. Jinno, Y., Chaudhary, V. K., Kondo, T., Adhya, S., FitzGerald, D. J., and Pastan, I.: Mutational analysis of domain I of pseudomonas exotoxin mutations in domain I of pseudomonas which reduce cell binding and animal toxicity. J. Biol. Chem., 263:13203, 1988.
93. Jones, P. T., Dear, P. H., Foote, J., Neuberger, M. S., and Winter, G.: Replacing the complementarity-determining regions in a human antibody with those from a mouse. Nature, 321:522, 1986.
94. Kanellos, J., Pietersz, G. A., Cunningham, Z., and McKenzie, I. F. C.: Anti-tumor activity of aminopterin-monoclonal antibody conjugates; in vitro and in vivo comparison with methotrexate-monoclonal antibody conjugates. Immunol. Cell Biol., 65:483, 1987.
95. Keenan, A. M., Weinstein, J. N., Mulshine, J. L., Carrasquillo, J. A., Bunn, P. A., Jr., Reynolds, J. C., and Larson, S. M.: Immunolymphoscintigraphy in patients with lymphoma after subcutaneous injection of indium-111-labeled T101 monoclonal antibody. J. Nucl. Med., 28:42, 1987.
96. Kemshead, J. T., Heath, L., Gibson, F. M., Katz, F., Richmond, F., Treleaven, J., and Ugelstad, J.: Magnetic microspheres and monoclonal antibodies for the depletion of neuroblastoma cells from bone marrow: Experiences, improvements and observations. Br. J. Cancer, 54:771, 1986.
97. Kernan, N. A., Knowles, R. W., Burns, M. J., Broxmeyer, H. E., Lu, L., Lee, H. M., Kawahata, R. T., Scannon, P. J., and Dupont, B.: Specific inhibition of in vitro lymphocyte transformation by an anti-pan T cell (gp67) ricin A chain immunotoxin. J. Immunol., 133:137, 1984.
98. Kirkwood, J. M., Neumann, R. D., Zoghbi, S. S., Ernstoff, M. S., Cornelius, E. A., Shaw, C., Ziyadeh, T., Fine, J. A., and Unger, M. W.: Scintigraphic detection of metastatic melanoma using indium 111/DTPA conjugated anti-gp240 antibody (ZME-018). J. Clin. Oncol., 5:1247, 1987.
99. Klein, J. L., Nguyen, T. H, Laroque, P., Kopher, K. A., Williams, J. R., Wessels, B. W., Dillehay, L. E., Frincke, J., Order, S. E., and Leichner, P. K.: Yttrium-90 and iodine-131 radioimmunoglobulin therapy of an experimental human hepatoma. Cancer Res., 49:6383, 1989.
100. Kohler, G., and Milstein, C.: Continuous cultures of fused cells secreting antibody of predefined specificity. Nature, 256:495, 1975.
101. Koprowski, H., Herlyn, D., Lubeck, M., DeFreitas, E., and Sears, H. F.: Human anti-idiotype antibodies in cancer patients. Is the modulation of the immune response beneficial for the patient? Proc. Natl. Acad. Sci. USA, 81:216, 1984.
102. Lambert, J., Rao, V., Steeves, R., Keene, B., Goldmacher, V., Collinson, A., and Blattler, W.: Blocked ricin and its use in immunoconjugates: The galactose-binding sites of the cytotoxic lectin ricin can be chemically blocked by modification with reactive ligands prepared by chemical modification of N-linked oligosaccharides. Second International Symposium on Immunotoxins, Orlando, p. 46, 1990.
103. Larson, S. M., Carrasquillo, J. A., McGuffin, R. W., Krohn, K. A., Ferens, J. M., Hill, L. D., Beaumier, P. L., Reynolds, J. C., Hellstrom, K. E., and Hellstrom, I.: Use of I-131 labeled, murine Fab against a high molecular weight antigen of human melanoma: Preliminary experience. Radiology, 155:487, 1985.
104. Larson, S. M.: Clinical radioimmunodetection, 1978–1988: Overview and suggestions for standardization of clinical trials. Cancer Res. (Suppl.), 50:892, 1990.
105. Lee, Y., Bullard, D. E., Humphrey, P. A., Colapinto, E. V., Friedman, H. S., Zalutsky, M. R., Coleman, R. E., and Bigner, D. D.: Treatment of intracranial human glioma xenografts with ^{131}I-labeled anti-tenascin monoclonal antibody 81C6. Cancer Res., 48:2904, 1988.
106. Lehtovirta, P., Kairemo, K. J., Liewendahl, K., and Seppälä, M.: Immunolymphoscintigraphy and immunoscintigraphy of ovarian and fallopian tube cancer using $F(ab')_2$ fragments of monoclonal antibody OC 125. Cancer Res. (Suppl.), 50:937, 1990.
107. Leichner, P. K., Klein, J. L., Siegelman, S. S., Ettinger, D. S., and Order, S. E.: Dosimetry of ^{131}I-labeled antiferritin in hepatoma: Specific activities in the tumor and liver. Cancer Treat. Rep., 67:647, 1983.
108. LeMaistre, F., Deisseroth, A., Fogel, B., Meneghetti, C., Ma, J., Anderson, M., Saria, E., Lomen, P., and Byers, V.: Phase I trial of H65-RTA in patients with chronic lymphocytic leukemia. Blood, (In Press)a.
109. LeMaistre, F., Yau, J., Meneghetti, C., Champlin, R., Spitzer, G., Huan, S., Anderson, B., Wallerstein, R., Lomen, P., Protopsaltis, N., Jackson, L., and Deisseroth, A.: Immunoprophylaxis of graft vs. host disease with H65-RTA is associated with accelerated engraftment. Blood, (In Press)b.
110. LeMaistre, F., Rosenblum, M., Ruben, J., Parkinson, D., Meneghetti, C., Parker, K., Shaw, J., Deisseroth, A., and Woodworth, T.: Phase I study of genetically engineered DAB $_{486}$ IL-2 in IL-2 receptor expressing malignancies. Blood, (In Press)c.
111. LeMaistre, F., Meneghetti, C., Frankel, A., Rosen, S., Kornfeld, S., Saria, E., Prajesk, J., Ma, J., Fiswild, D., Scannon, P., and Byers, V.: Phase I trial of H65-RTA immunoconjugate in patients with cutaneous T cell lymphoma. Cancer Res., (In Press).
112. LeMaistre, F., Deisseroth, A., Fogel, B., Meneghetti, C., Ma, J., Anderson, M., Saria, E., Lomen, P., and Byers, V.: Phase I trial of H65-RTA in patients with chronic lymphocytic leukemia. Blood, (In Press)t.
113. Lenhard, R. E., Jr., Order, S. E., Spunberg, J. J., Asbell, S. O., and Leibel, S. A.: Isotopic immunoglobulin: A new systemic therapy for advanced Hodgkin's disease. J. Cln. Oncol., 3:1296, 1985.
114. Levy, R., and Miller, R. A.: Therapy of lymphoma directed at idiotypes. NCI Monogr., 10:61, 1990.
115. Lloyd, E. L., Gemmell, M. A., Henning, C. B., Gemmell, D. S., and Zabransky, B. J.: Cell survival following multiple-track alpha particle irradiation. Int. J. Radiat. Biol., 35:23, 1979.
116. Lorberboum-Galski, H., FitzGerald, D., Chaudhary, V., Adhya, S., and Pastan, I.: Cytotoxic activity of an interleukin 2-Pseudomonas exotoxin chimeric protein produced in Escherichia coli. Proc. Natl. Acad. Sci. USA, 85:1922, 1988.
117. LoBuglio, A. F., Saleh, M., Peterson, L., Wheeler, R., Carrano, R., Huster, W., and Khazaeli, M. B.: Phase I clinical trial of CO17-1A monoclonal antibody. Hybridoma (Suppl.), 5:117, 1986.
118. LoBuglio, A. F., Wheeler, R. H., Trang, J., Haynes, A., Rogers, K., Harvey, E. B., Sun, L., Ghrayeb, J., and Khazaeli, M. B.: Mouse/human chimeric monoclonal antibody in man: Kinetics and immune response. Proc. Natl. Acad. Sci. USA, 86:4220, 1989.
119. Luders, G., Kohnlein, W., Sorg, C., and Bruggen, J.: Selective toxicity of neocarzinostatin-monoclonal antibody conjugates to the antigen-bearing human melanoma cell line in vitro. Cancer Immunol. Immunother., 20:85, 1985.
120. Mach, J. P., Carrel, S., Forni, M., Ritschard, J., Donath, A., and Alberto, P.: Tumor localization of radiolabeled antibodies against carcinoembryonic antigen in patients with carcinoma. N. Engl. J. Med., 303:5, 1980.
121. Mach, J. P., Buchegger, F., Forni, M., Ritschard, J., Berche, C., Lumbruso, J. D., Schreyer, M., Girardet, C., Accola, R. S., and Carrel, S.: Use of radiolabeled monoclonal anti-CEA antibodies for the detection of human carcinomas by external photoscanning and tomoscintigraphy. Immunol. Today, 2:239, 1981.
122. Mach, J. P., Chatal, J. F., Lambroso, J. D., Buchegger, F., Forni, M., Ritschard, J., Berche, C., Douillard, J. Y., Carrel, S., and Herlyn, M.: Tumor localization in patients by radiolabeled monoclonal antibodies against colon carcinoma. Cancer Res., 43:5593, 1983.
123. Masui, H., Moroyama, T., and Mendelsohn, J.: Mechanism of antitumor activity in mice for anti-epidermal growth factor receptor monoclonal antibodies with different isotypes. Cancer Res., 46:5592, 1986.
124. Matthay, K. K., Heath, T. D., Badger, C. C., Bernstein, I. D., and Papahadjopoulos, D.: Antibody-directed liposomes: Comparison of various ligands for association, endocytosis, and drug delivery. Cancer Res., 46:4904, 1986.
125. McKearn, T. J., Lopes, A. D., and Radcliffe, R. D.: In vivo efficacy of site-specific anti-folate monoclonal antibody conjugates. Third International Conference on Monoclonal Antibody Immunoconjugates for Cancer, UCSD Cancer Center, San Diego, CA, 1988, p. 17.
126. Meeker, T., Lowder, J., Cleary, M. L., Stewart, S., Warnke, R., Sklar, J., and Levy,

R.: Emergence of idiotype variants during treatment of B-cell lymphoma with anti-idiotype antibodies. N. Engl. J. Med., 312:1658, 1985.
127. Mellstedt, H., Frödin, J. E., Ragnhammar, P., Masucci, G., Shetye, J., Christensson, B., Biberfeld, P., Makower, J., Pihlstedt, P., Cedermark, B., Harmenberg, U., Wahren, B., Rieger, A., Magnusson, I., Nathansson, J., and Erwald, R.: The clinical use of monoclonal antibodies MAb 17-1A, in the treatment of patients with metastatic colorectal carcinoma. Med. Oncol. Tumor Pharmacol., 6:99, 1989.
128. Mendelsohn, J.: Growth factor receptors as targets for antitumor therapy with monoclonal antibodies. Prog. Allergy, 45:147, 1988.
129. Mezzanzanica, D., Canevari, S., Menard, S., Pupa, S. M., Tagliabue, E., Lanzavecchia, A., and Colnaghi, M. I.: Human ovarian carcinoma lysis by cytotoxic T cells targeted by bispecific monoclonal antibodies: Analysis of the antibody components. Int. J. Cancer, 41:609, 1988.
130. Middlebrook, J. L., and Dorland, R. B.: Bacterial toxins: Cellular mechanism of action. Microbiol. Rev., 48:199, 1984.
131. Miller, R. A., Maloney, D. G., Warnke, R., and Levy, R.: Treatment of B-cell lymphoma with monoclonal anti-idiotype antibody. N. Engl. J. Med., 306:517, 1982.
132. Miraldi, F. D., Nelson, A. D., Kraly, C., Ellery, S., Landmeier, B., Coccia, P. F., Strandjord, S. E., and Cheung, N. K.: Diagnostic imaging of human neuroblastoma with radiolabeled antibody. Radiology, 161:413, 1986.
133. Mittelman, A., Chen, Z. J., Kageshita, T., Yang, H., Yamada, M., Baskind, P., Goldberg, N., Puccio, C., Ahmed, T., Arlin, Z., and Ferrone, S.: Active specific immunotherapy in patients with melanoma: A clinical trial with mouse antiidiotypic monoclonal antibodies elicited with syngeneic anti-high-molecular-weight-melanoma-associated antigen monoclonal antibodies. J. Clin. Invest., 86:2136, 1990.
134. Morrison, S. L., Johnson, M. J., Herzenberg, L. A., and Oi, V. T.: Chimeric human antibody molecules: Mouse antigen-binding domains with human constant region domains. Proc. Natl. Acad. Sci. USA, 81:6851, 1984.
135. Morrison, S. L.: Transfectomas provide novel chimeric antibodies. Science, 229:1202, 1985.
136. Morrison, S. L., and OI, V. T.: Genetically engineered antibody molecules. Adv. Immunol., 44:65, 1989.
137. Msirikale, J. S., Klein, J. L., Schroeder, J., and Order, S. E.: Radiation enhancement of radiolabelled antibody deposition in tumors. Int. J. Radiat. Oncol. Biol. Phys., 13:1839, 1987.
138. Murphy, J. R., Bishai, W., Borowski, M., Miyanohara, A., Boyd, J., and Nagle, S.: Genetic construction, expression and melanoma-selective cytotoxicity of a diphtheria toxin-related α-melanocyte-stimulating hormone fusion protein. Proc. Natl. Acad. Sci. USA, 83:8258, 1986.
139. Murphy, J. R., Williams, D. P., Bacha, P., Bishai, W., Waters, C., and Strom, T. B.: Cell receptor specific targeted toxins: Genetic construction and characterization of an interleukin 2 diphtheria toxin-related fusion protein. J. Recept. Res., 8:467, 1988.
140. Murray, J. L., Rosenblum, M. G., Lamki, L., Glenn, H. J., Krizan, Z., Hersh, E. M., Plager, C. E., Bartholomew, R. M., Unger, M. W., and Carlo, D. J.: Clinical parameters related to optimal tumor localization of indium-111-labeled mouse antimelanoma monoclonal antibody ZME-018. J. Nucl. Med., 28:25, 1987.
141. Nadler, L. M., Stashenko, P., Hardy, R., Kaplan, W. D., Button, L. N., Kufe, D. W., Antman, K. H., and Schlossman, S. F.: Serotherapy of a patient with a monoclonal antibody directed against a human lymphoma-associated antigen. Cancer Res., 40:3147, 1980.
142. Nadler, L., Breitmeyer, J., Coral, F., Spector, N., and Schlossman, S.: Anti-B4 blocked ricin immunotherapy for patients with B cell malignancies: Results of bolus and constant infusion phase I trials. Proceedings of the Second International Symposium on Immunotoxins, Orlando, p. 58, 1990.
143. Nelp, W. B., Eary, J. F., Jones, R. F., Hellstrom, K. E., Hellstrom, I., Beaumier, P. L., and Krohn, K. A.: Preliminary studies of monoclonal antibody lymphoscintigraphy in malignant melanoma. J. Nucl. Med., 28:34, 1987.
144. Nepom, G. T., and Hellström, K. E.: Anti-idiotypic antibodies and the induction of specific tumor immunity. Cancer Metast. Rev., 6:489, 1987.
145. Olsnes, S., Refnes, K., and Pihl, A.: Mechanism of action of the toxic lectins abrin and ricin. Nature, 249:627, 1974.
146. Olsnes, S., Saltvedt, E., and Pihl, A.: Isolation and comparison of galactose-binding lectins from *Abrus precatorius* and *Ricinus communis*. J. Biol. Chem., 249:803, 1974.
147. Order, S. E., Klein, J. L., Ettinger, D., Alderson, P., Siegelman, S., and Leichner, P.: Phase I-II study of radiolabeled antibody integrated in the treatment of primary hepatic malignancies. Int. J. Radiat. Oncol. Biol. Phys., 6:703, 1980.
148. Order, S. E., Stillwagon, G. B., Klein, J. L., Leichner, P. K., Siegelman, S. S., Fishman, E. K., Ettinger, D. S., Haulk, T., Kopher, K., and Finney, K.: Iodine 131 antiferritin, a new treatment modality in hepatoma: A Radiation Therapy Oncology Group Study. J. Clin. Oncol., 3:1573, 1985.
149. Order, S. E., Klein, J. L., Leichner, P. K., Frincke, J., Lollo, C., and Carlo, D. J.: ^{90}Yttrium antiferritin—A new therapeutic radiolabeled antibody. Int. J. Radiat. Oncol. Biol; Phys., 12:277, 1986.
150. Paik, C. H., Yokoyama, K., Reynolds, J. C., Quadri, S. M., Min, C. Y., Shin, S. Y., Maloney, P. J., Larson, S. M., and Reba, R. C.: Reduction of background activities by introduction of a diester linkage between antibody and a chelate in radioimmunodetection of tumor. J. Nucl. Med., 30:1693, 1989.
151. Pappenheimer, A. M., Jr.: Diphtheria toxin. Annu. Rev. Biochem., 46:69, 1977.
152. Parker, B. A., Vassos, A. B., Halpern, S. E., Miller, R. A., Hupf, H., Amox, D. G., Simoni, J. L., Starr, R. J., Green, M. R., and Royston, I.: Radioimmunotherapy of human B-cell lymphoma with ^{90}Y-conjugated antiidiotype monoclonal antibody. Cancer Res. (Suppl.), 50:1022, 1990.
153. Pateisky, N., Philipp, K., Skodler, W. D., Czerwenka, K., Hamilton, G., and Burchell, J.: Radioimmunodetection in patients with suspected ovarian cancer. J. Nucl. Med., 26:1369, 1985.
154. Pectasides, D., Stewart, S., Courtenay-Luck, N., Rampling, R., Munro, A. J., Krausz, T., Dhokia, B., Snook, D., Hooker, G., and Durbin, H.: Antibody-guided irradiation of malignant pleural and pericardial effusions. Br. J. Cancer, 53:727, 1986.
155. Peitersz, G. A., Smyth, M. J., Tjandra, J. J., and McKenzie, I. F.: Preclinical and clinical studies with n-acetyl melphalan (N-AcMEL) immunoconjugates and tumor necrosis factor alpha (TNF-α). Third International Conference on Monoclonal Antibody Immunoconjugates for Cancer, USCD Cancer Center, San Diego, CA, 1988, p. 20.
156. Pimm, M. V.: Drug-monoclonal antibody conjugates for cancer therapy: Potentials and limitations. Crit. Rev. Ther. Drug Carrier Syst., 5:189, 1988.
157. Preijers, F. W., De Witte, T., Wessels, J. M., De Gast, G. C., Van Leeuwen, E., Capel, P. J., and Haanen, C.: Autologous transplantation of bone marrow purged in vitro with anti-CD7-(WT1-) ricin A immunotoxin in T-cell lymphoblastic leukemia and lymphoma. Blood, 74:1152, 1989.
158. Pressman, D., and Korngold, L.: The *in vivo* localization of anti-Wagner osteogenic-sarcoma antibodies. Cancer, 6:619, 1953.
159. Raffeld, M., Neckers, L., Longo, D. L., and Cossman, J.: Spontaneous alteration of idiotype in a monoclonal B-cell lymphoma. Escape from detection by anti-idiotype. N. Engl. J. Med., 312:1653, 1985.
160. Ramsay, N., LeBien, T., Nesbit, M., McGlave, P., Weisdorf, D., Kenyon, P., Hurd, D., Goldman, A., Kim, T., and Kersey, J.: Autologous bone marrow transplantation for patients with acute lymphoblastic leukemia in second or subsequent remission: Results of bone marrow treated with monoclonal antibodies BA–1, BA–2, and BA–3 plus complement. Blood 66:508 1985.
161. Renda, A., Salvatore, M., Sava, M., Landi, R., Lastoria, S., Coppola, L., Schlom, J., Colcher, D., and Zannini, G.: Immunoscintigraphy in the follow-up of patients operated on for carcinoma of the sigmoid and rectum. Preliminary report with a new monoclonal antibody: B72.3. Dis. Colon Rectum, 30:683, 1987.
162. Richardson, R. B., Davies, A. G., Bourne, S. P., Staddon, G. E., Jones, D. H., Kemshead, J. T., and Coakham, H. B.: Radioimmunolocalization of human brain tumours: Biodistribution of radiolabelled monoclonal antibody UJ13A. Eur. J. Nucl. Med., 12:313, 1986.
163. Ritz, J., Pesando, J. M., Notis-McConarty, J., Clavell, L. A., Sallan, S. E., and Schlossman, S. F.: Use of monoclonal antibodies as diagnostic and therapeutic reagents in acute lymphoblastic leukemia. Cancer Res., 41:4771, 1981.
164. Ritz, J., Bast, R. C., Clavell, L. A., Hercend, T., Sallan, S. E., Lipton, J. M., Feeney, M., Nathan, D. G., and Schlossman, S. F.: Autologous bone-marrow transplantation in CALLA-positive acute lymphoblastic leukemia after *in vitro* treatment with J5 monoclonal antibody and complement. Lancet, 2:60, 1982.
165. Rodeck, U., Herlyn, M., Herlyn, D., Molthoff, C., Atkinson, B., Varello, M., Steplewski, Z., and Koprowski, H.: Tumor growth modulation by a monoclonal antibody to the epidermal growth factor receptor: Immunologically mediated and effector cell-independent effects. Cancer Res., 47:3692, 1987.
166. Rodwell, J. D., Alvarez, V. L., Lee, C., Lopes, A. D., Goers, J. W., King, H. D., Powsner, H. J., and McKearn, T. J.: Site-specific covalent modification of monoclonal antibodies: *In vitro* and *in vivo* evaluations. Proc. Natl. Acad. Sci. USA, 83:2632, 1986.
167. Roselli, M., Schlom, J., Gansow, O. A., Raubitschek, A., Mirzadeh, S., Brechbiel, M. W., and Colcher, D.: Comparative biodistribution of yttrium- and indium-labeled monoclonal antibody B72.3 in athymic mice bearing human colon carcinoma xenografts. J. Nucl. Med., 30:672, 1989.
168. Rosen, S. T., Zimmer, A. M., Goldman-Leikin, R., Gordon, L. I., Kazikiewicz, J. M., Kaplan, E. H., Variakojis, D., Marder, R. J., Dykewicz, M. S., and Piergies, A.: Radioimmunodetection and radioimmunotherapy of cutaneous T cell lymphomas using an ^{131}I-labeled monoclonal antibody: An Illinois Cancer Council Study. J. Clin. Oncol., 5:562, 1987.
169. Sallan, S. E., Niemeyer, C. M., Billett, A. L., Lipton, J. M., Tarbell, N. J., Gelber, R. D., Murray, C., Pittinger, T. P., Wolfe, L. C., Bast, R. C., Jr., and Ritz. J.: Autologous bone marrow transplantation for acute lymphoblastic leukemia. J. Clin. Oncol., 7:1594, 1989.
170. Sands, H., and Jones, P. L.: Methods for the study of the metabolism of radiolabeled monoclonal antibodies by liver and tumor. J. Nucl. Med., 28:390, 1987.
171. Schroff, R. W., Woodhouse, C. S., Foon, K. A., Oldham, R. K., Farrell, M. M., Klein, R. A., and Morgan, A. C., Jr.: Intratumor localization of monoclonal antibody in patients with melanoma treated with antibody to a 250,000-dalton melanoma-associated antigen. J. Natl. Cancer Inst., 74:299, 1985.
172. Sears, H. F., Herlyn, D., Steplewski, Z., and Koprowski, H.: Effects of monoclonal antibody immunotherapy on patients with gastrointestinal adenocarcinoma. J. Biol. Response Mod., 3:138, 1984.
173. Shawler, D. L., Bartholomew, R. M., Smith, L. M., and Dillman, R. O.: Human immune response to multiple injections of murine monoclonal IgG. J. Immunol., 135:1530, 1985.
174. Shawler, D. L., Johnson, D. E., Sweet, M. D., Myers, L. J., Tudor, S. D., Beidler, D. E., Koziol, J. A., and Dillman, R. O.: Preclinical trials using an immunoconjugate of T101 and methotrexate in an athymic mouse/human T-cell tumor model. J. Biol. Response Modif., 7:608, 1988.
175. Sheldon, K., Marks, A., and Baumal, R.: Sensitivity of multidrug resistant KB-C1 cells to an antibody-Dextran-Adriamycin conjugate. Anticancer Res., 9:637, 1989.
176. Shen, G. L., Li, J. L., Ghetie, M. A., Ghetie, V., May, R. D., Till, M., Brown, A. N., Relf, M., Knowles, P., and Uhr, J. W.: Evaluation of four CD22 antibodies as ricin A chain-containing immunotoxins for the in vivo therapy of human B-cell leukemias and lymphomas. Int. J. Cancer, 42:792, 1988.
177. Shouval, D., Adler, R., Wands, J. R., Hurwitz, E., Isselbacher, K. J., and Sela, M.: Doxorubicin conjugates of monoclonal antibodies to hepatoma-associated antigens. Proc. Natl. Acad. Sci. USA, 85:8276, 1988.
178. Shpall, E. J., Jones, R. B., Bast, R. C., Jr., Rosner, G. L., Vandermark, R., Ross, M., Affronti, M. L., Johnston, C., Eggleston, S., Tepperburg, M., Coniglio, D., and Peters, W. P.: 4-Hydroperoxyclophosphamide purging of breast cancer from the mononuclear cell fraction of bone marrow in patients receiving high-dose chemotherapy and autologous marrow support: A phase I trial. J. Clin. Oncol., 9:85, 1991.
179. Shrivastav, S., Schlom, J., Raubitschek, A., Molinolo, A., Simpson, J., and Hand, P. H.: Studies concerning the effect of external irradiation of localization of radiolabeled monoclonal antibody B72.3 to human colon carcinoma xenografts. Int. J. Radiat. Oncol. Biol. Phys., 16:721, 1989.
180. Siccardi, A. G.: Tumor immunoscintigraphy by means of radiolabeled monoclonal antibodies: Multicenter studies of the Italian National Research Council—Special Project "Biomedical Engineering." Cancer Res. (Suppl.), 50:899, 1990.
181. Siegall, C. B., Fitzgerald, D. J., and Pastan, I.: Cytotoxicity of IL6-PE40 and derivatives on tumor cells expressing a range of interleukin 6 receptor levels. J. Biol. Chem., 265:16318, 1990.
182. Sironi, M., Canegrati, M. A., Romano, M., Vecchi, A., and Spreafico, F.: Chemotherapy-increased antineoplastic effects of antibody-toxin conjugates. Cancer Treat. Rep., 68:643, 1984.
183. Smyth, M. J., Pietersz, G. A., and McKenzie, I. F.: The mode of action of methrotrexate-monoclonal antibody conjugates. Immunol. Cell Biol., 65:189, 1987.

184. Smyth, M. J., Pietersz, G. A., and McKenzie, I. F.: The cellular uptake and cytotoxicity of chlorambucil-monoclonal antibody conjugates. Immunol. Cell Biol., 65:315, 1987.

185. Smyth, M. J., Bogdanovski, M., McKenzie, I. F. C., and Pietersz, G. A.: Antitumor activity of idarubicin-monoclonal antibody conjugates in a disseminated thymic lymphoma model. Cancer Res., 51:310, 1991.

186. Spar, I. L., Bale, W. F., Marrack, D., Dewey, W. C., McCardle, R. J., and Harper, P. V.: 131-I labeled antibodies to human fibrinogen. Diagnostic studies and therapeutic trials. Cancer, 20:865, 1967.

187. Spearman, M. E., Goodwin, R. M., Apelgren, L. D., and Bumol, T. F.: Disposition of the monoclonal antibody-vinca alkaloid conjugate KS1/4-DAVLB (LY256787) and free r-Desacetylvinblastine in tumor-bearing nude mice. J. Pharmacol. Exper. Therapeut., 241:695, 1987.

188. Spitler, L. E., del Rio, M., Khentigan, A., Wedel, N. I., Brophy, N. A., Miller, L. L., Harkonen, W. S., Rosendorf, L. L., Lee, H. M., and Mischak, R. P.: Therapy of patients with malignant melanoma using a monoclonal antimelanoma antibody-ricin A chain immunotoxin. Cancer Res., 47:1717, 1987.

189. Starling, J., Hinson, A., and Marder, P.: Rapid internalization of antigen-immunoconjugate complexes is not required for anti-tumor activity of monoclonal antibody-drug conjugates. Third International Conference on Monoclonal Antibody Immunoconjugates for Cancer, USCD Cancer Center, San Diego, CA, 1988, p. 23.

190. Steplewski, Z., Lubeck, M. D., and Koprowski, H.: Human macrophages armed with murine immunoglobulin G2a antibodies to tumors destroy human cancer cells. Science, 221:865, 1983.

191. Steplewski, Z., Sun, L. K., Shearman, C. W., Ghrayeb, J., Daddona, P., and Koprowski, H.: Biological activity of human-mouse IgG1, IgG2, IgG3, and IgG4 chimeric monoclonal antibodies with antitumor specificity. Proc. Natl. Acad. Sci. USA, 85:4852, 1988.

192. Stickney, D. R., Gridley, D. S., Kirk, G. A., and Slater, J. M.: Enhancement of monoclonal antibody binding to melanoma with single dose radiation or hyperthermia. NCI Monogr., 3:47, 1987.

193. Stone, M., Amlot, P., Fay, J., Till, M., Ghetie, V., Collins, R., Tong, A., May, R., Newman, J., Clark, P., Thorpe, P., Uhr, J., and Vitetta, E.: Immunotoxin therapy of B cell lymphoma. Blood, (In Press).

194. Sullivan, D. C., Silva, J. S., Cox, C. E., Haagensen, D. E., Harris, C. C., Briner, W. H., and Wells, S. A.: Localization of I-131 labeled goat and primate anti-carcinoembryonic antigen (CEA) antibodies in patients with cancer. Invest. Radiol., 17:350, 1982.

195. Takahashi, T., Yamaguchi, T., Kitamura, K., Suzuyama, H., Honda, M., Yokota, T., Kotanagi, H., Takahashi, M., and Hashimoto, Y.: Clinical application of monoclonal antibody-drug conjugates for immunotargeting chemotherapy of colorectal carcinoma. Cancer, 61:881, 1988.

196. Takvorian, T., Canellos, G. P., Ritz, J., Freedman, A. S., Anderson, K. C., Mauch, P., Tarbell, N., Coral, F., Daley, H., and Yeap, B.: Prolonged disease-free survival after autologous bone marrow transplantation in patients with non-Hodgkin's lymphoma with a poor prognosis. N. Engl. J. Med., 316:1499, 1987.

197. Taylor, A., Jr., Milton, W., Eyre, H. P., Christian, P., Wu, F., Hagan, P., Alazraki, N., Datz, F. L., and Unger, M.: Radioimmunodetection of human melanoma with indium-111 labelled monoclonal antibody. J. Nucl. Med., 29:329, 1988.

198. Uckun, F. M., Kersey, J. H., Vallera, D. A., Ledbetter, J. A., Weisdorf, D., Myers, D. E., Haake, R., and Ramsay, N. K.: Autologous bone marrow transplantation in high-risk remission T-lineage acute lymphoblastic leukemia using immunotoxins plus 4-hydroperoxy-cyclophosphamide for marrow purging. Blood, 76:1723, 1990.

199. Vacca, A., Buchegger, F., Carrel, S., and Mach, J. P.: Imaging of human leukemic T-cell xenografts in nude mice by radiolabeled monoclonal antibodies and F(ab')$_2$ fragments. Cancer, 61:58, 1988.

200. Vallera, D. A.: Immunotoxins for ex vivo bone marrow purging in human bone marrow transplantation. In Immunotoxins. Edited by A. E. Frankel. Boston, Kluwer Academic Press, 1988, p. 515.

201. Vihko, P., Kontturri, M., Lukkarinen, O., Martikainen, P., Pelliniemi, L., Heikkila, J., and Vihko, R.: Immunoscintigraphic evaluation of lymph node involvement in prostatic carcinoma. Prostate, 11:51, 1987.

202. Vriesendorp, H. M., Herpst, J. M., Leichner, P. K., Klein, J. L., and Order, S. E.: Polyclonal ^{90}Yttrium labeled antiferritin for refractory Hodgkin's disease. Int. J. Radiat. Oncol. Biol. Phys., 17:815, 1989.

203. Wahl, R. L., Parker, C. W., and Philpott, G. W.: Improved radioimaging and tumor localization with monoclonal F (ab')$_2$. J. Nucl. Med., 24:316, 1983.

204. Wahl, R. L., Liebert, M., Headington, J., Wilson, B. S., Shulkin, B. L., Johnson, J. W., Mallette, S., Natale, R. B., Coon, W., and East, M.: Lymphoscintigraphy in melanoma: Initial evaluation of a low protein dose monoclonal antibody cocktail. Cancer Res. (Suppl.), 50:941, 1990.

205. Waldmann, H., Cobbold, S., Wilson, A., Clark, M., Watt, S., Hale, G., and Tighe, H.: Rat monoclonal antibodies for bone marrow transplantation—the CAMPATH series. Adv. Exp. Med. Biol., 186:869, 1985.

206. Waldmann, T. A.: Monoclonal antibodies in diagnosis and therapy. Science, 252:1657, 1991.

207. Walz, G., Zanker, B., Murphy, J. R., and Strom, T. B.: A kinetic analysis of the effects of interleukin-2 diphtheria toxin fusion protein upon activated T cells. Transplantation, 49:198, 1990.

208. Ward, B. G., Mather, S. J., Hawkins, L. R., Crowther, M. E., Shepherd, J. H., Granowska, M., Britton, K. E., and Slevin, M. L.: Localization of radioiodine conjugated to the monoclonal antibody HMFG2 in human ovarian carcinoma: Assessment of intravenous and intraperitoneal routes of administration. Cancer Res., 47:4719, 1987.

209. Weiner, L. M., O'Dwyer, J., Kitson, J., Comis, R. L., Frankel, A. E., Bauer, R. J., Konrad, M. S., and Groves, E. S.: Phase I evaluation of an anti-breast carcinoma monoclonal antibody 260F9-recombinant ricin A chain immunoconjugate. Cancer Res., 49:4062, 1989.

210. Wettendorff, M., Iliopoulos, D., Tempero, M., Kay, D., DeFreitas, E., Koprowski, H., and Herlyn, D.: Idiotypic cascades in cancer patients treated with monoclonal antibody CO17-1A. Proc. Natl. Acad. Sci., 86:3787, 1989.

211. Willingham: Personal communication, 1990.

212. Wrasidlo, W., Muller, B., Yang, H.-M., and Reisfeld, R. A.: Oligomerization of doxorubicin results in improved cytotoxicity of antibody-drug conjugates. Third International Conference on Monoclonal Antibody Immunoconjugates for Cancer, USCD Cancer Center, San Diego, CA, 1988, p. 64.

213. Yamaizumi, M., Mekada, E., Uchida, T., and Okada, Y.: One molecule of diphtheria toxin fragment A introduced into a cell can kill the cell. Cell, 15:245, 1978.

214. Yamamoto, S., Yamamoto, T., Saxton, R. E., Hoon, D. S., and Irie, R. F.: Anti-idiotype monoclonal antibody carrying the internal image of ganglioside GM3. J. Natl. Cancer Inst., 82:1757, 1990.

215. Yokoyama, K., Carrasquillo, J. A., Chang, A. E., Colcher, D., Roselli, M., Sugarbaker, P., Sindelar, W., Reynolds, J. C., Perentesis, P., Gansow, O. A.: Differences in biodistribution of indium-111- and iodine-131-labeled B72.3 monoclonal antibodies in patients with colorectal cancer. J. Nucl. Med., 30:320, 1989.

216. Youle, R. J., and Colombatti, M.: Hybridoma cells containing intracellular anti-ricin antibodies show ricin meets secretory antibody before entering the cytosol. J. Biol. Chem., 262:4676, 1987.

217. Yu, Y. H., Crews, J. R., Cooper, K., Ramakrishnan, S., Houston, L. L., Leslie, D. S., George, S. L., Lidor, Y., Boyer, C. M., Ring, D. B., and Bast, R. C., Jr.: Use of immunotoxins in combination to inhibit clonogenic growth of human breast carcinoma cells. Cancer Res., 50:3231, 1990.

218. Xu, F. J., Rodriguez, G. C., Whitaker, R., Boente, M., Berchuck, A., McKenzie, S., Houston, L., Boyer, C. M., and Bast, R. C., Jr.: Antibodies against immunochemically distinct epitopes on the extracellular domain of HER-2/neu (c-erbB-2) inhibit growth of breast and ovarian cancer cell lines. Proc. Amer. Assoc. Cancer Res., 32:260, 1991.

219. Zalutsky, M. R., and Narula, A. S.: A method for the radiohalogenation of proteins resulting in decreased thyroid uptake of radioiodine. Int. J. Rad. Appl. Instrum. [A], 38:1051, 1987.

220. Zalutsky, M. R., and Narula, A. S.: Radiohalogenation of a monoclonal antibody using an N-succinimidyl-3-(tri-n-butylstannyl) benzoate intermediate. Cancer Res., 48:1446, 1988.

221. Zalutsky, M. R., Moseley, R. P., Coakham, H. B., Coleman, R. E., and Bigner, D. D.: Pharmacokinetics and tumor localization of ^{131}I-labeled anti-tenascin monoclonal antibody 81C6 in patients with gliomas and other intracranial malignancies. Cancer Res., 49:2807, 1989.

222. Zalutsky, M. R., Noska, M. A., Colapinto, E. V., Garg, P. K., and Bigner, D. D.: Enhanced tumor localization and in vivo stability of a monoclonal antibody radioiodinated using N-succinimidyl-3-(tri-n-butylstannyl) benzoate. Cancer Res., 49:5543, 1989.

223. Zalutsky, M. R., Moseley, R. P., Benjamin, J. C., Colapinto, E. V., Fuller, G. N., Coakham, H. P., and Bigner, D. D.: Monoclonal antibody and F(ab')$_2$ fragment delivery to tumor in patients with glioma: Comparison of intracarotid and intravenous administration. Cancer Res., 50:4105, 1990.

XIX

Principles of Bone Marrow Transplantation

XIX-1

Autologous Bone Marrow Transplantation

William P. Peters

Introduction

Successful treatment of many cancers is often prevented by intrinsic tumor resistance or by tumor volume. In some cases, increasing dose intensity may overcome these constraints,[67] but this approach is limited in many cases by bone marrow or other organ tolerance. The success of allogeneic bone marrow transplantation in the treatment of relapsed acute leukemia and in certain lymphomas has demonstrated that dose intensification can, in certain circumstances, produce curative results where standard dose therapy is not curative.[218] Allogeneic marrow transplantation is, however, complicated by substantial morbidity and mortality related to graft versus host disease or complications associated with chronic immunosuppression.[219] Availability of an appropriate donor of allogeneic bone marrow has limited its application even in the setting of the leukemias and lymphomas, since only 35–40% of patients have an HLA-identical sibling. Consequently, there has been increasing interest over the past decade in the development of autologous bone marrow transplantation for leukemias, lymphomas, and for solid tumors. This is a field in rapid evolution.

Rationale and Requirements for Autologous Bone Marrow Transplantation

Requirements for successful autologous bone marrow transplantation are listed in Table XIX-1-1. The cancer being treated must be responsive to intensive cytoreductive therapy, but not be curable by conventional dose therapy. A source of cells capable of producing complete trilineage hematopoietic engraftment must also be available.[105,220] Bone

Table XIX-1-1. Requirements for Autologous Bone Marrow Transplantation

Malignancy responsive to intensive cytoreductive therapy not curable by marrow tolerable doses.
Tumor burden does not exceed therapeutic capability of cytoreductive regimen
Availability of a source of marrow progenitor cells capable of restoring hematopoiesis and free of clonogenic tumor cells

marrow has most frequently provided these cells, but other sources of hematopoietic progenitors, such as leukopheresed peripheral blood collections have also been used.[106] The requirement for freedom from malignant involvement may be critical. It is not certain, however, that the marrow needs to be completely free of limited numbers of tumor cells. Experience from the treatment of myeloma,[23] as well as the lymphomas,[17] suggest that limited marrow involvement may not preclude a successful autologous bone marrow transplant. To limit the amount of tumor cell contamination in marrow used for autologous bone marrow transplantation, strategies have been developed to remove malignant cells from the marrow, termed "purging," and have been studied in the leukemias and lymphomas, and more recently in the solid tumors.[7]

Principles

The principles which underly the use of autologous bone marrow transplantation and other methods for supportive care depend upon the disease which is being treated. Modifications of the general therapeutic strategy of dose-intensification are of necessity targeted at the particular disease. In contrast to allogeneic transplantation, in which the administration of immunosuppressive agents is required, the use of cytotoxic drugs can be directed entirely toward cytoreduction of tumor prior to autologous bone marrow transplantation.

Although there may be differences between therapeutic strategies targeted at different diseases, a number of features appear to be common between therapeutic regimens. These features are outlined in Table XIX-1-2.

Dose Intensity

The dose response relationship for many anti-tumor agents is steep both for therapeutic and for toxic effects.[67] Even for resistant tumors, in experimental systems, such relationships can be shown to be linear-log.[207] As shown in Figure XIX-1-1, cellular kill is a first-order function of dose of administered cyclophosphamide for several solid animal malignancies, even for the most resistant cell lines such as the B-16 melanoma. For more sensitive tumors, a doubling of the admin-

Table XIX-1-2.   Commonly Applied Principles in Autologous Bone Marrow Transplantation

Dose is a critical factor in treatment and even minor compromises of administered dose can result in reduction of therapeutic efficacy

Combination chemotherapy is generally required for the successful treatment of most cancers to overcome intrinsic resistance or tumor burden

Alkylating agents have properties which are particularly appropriate to use in high dose treatment settings

Alkylating agents are broadly active in many cancers

The common dose-limiting side effect is myelosuppression

At higher doses, selected alkylating agents differ in their non-myelosuppressive dose-limiting toxicities

Alkylating agents in general possess a steep dose response effect which in certain settings appears linear-log and non-saturable at clinically attainable doses

Laboratory investigations demonstrate substantial non-cross resistance among selected agents of this class

Treatment in the clinical setting of minimal disease and early stage is more likely to be associated with a valuable therapeutic outcome

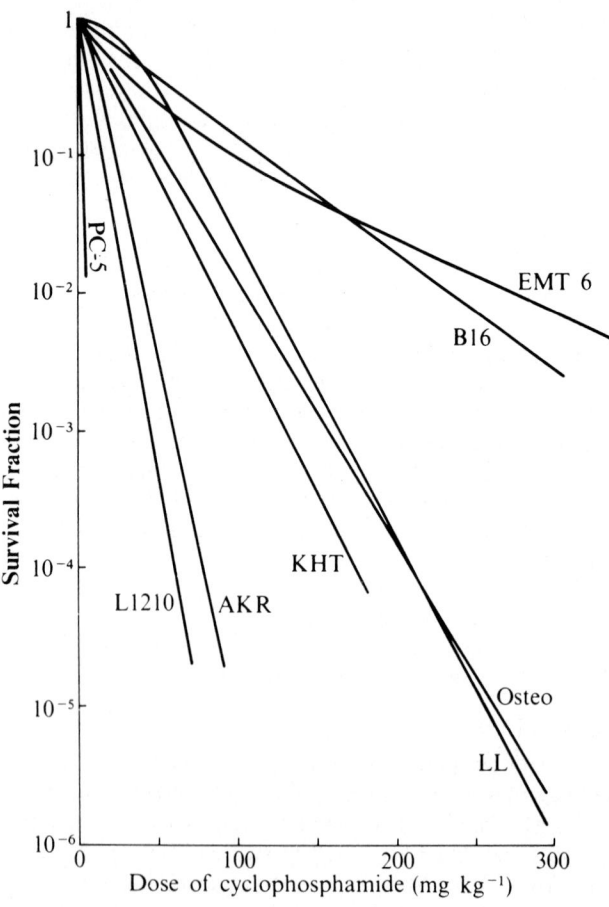

Figure XIX-1-1. First order kinetics in cell killing of several transplanted animal tumors with cyclophosphamide.

istered dose leads to a 2- to 5-fold increase in tumor cell kill in these experimental tumors. Moreover, the dose response curve does not appear to plateau. This does not apply, however, to all antineoplastic agents. While the primary limitation for many agents is toxicity in the bone marrow, other drugs are toxic for other organs at or near the myelotoxic dose. The use of high-dose chemotherapy relies on an ability to escalate dose substantially before toxicity in non-hematopoietic organs occurs (Table XIX-1-3). In autologous bone marrow transplantation, it is the difference between the response curves for tumor in normal tissues that must be exploited. In practice, this difference between the myelotoxic dose and the dose that produces unacceptable damage to other organs is usually less than 10-fold.[90]

Combination Chemotherapy

Both radiation therapy and chemotherapy have been used in autologous bone marrow transplantation. The probable occurrence of drug resistance to any single agent generally mandates the use of multiple drugs with or without radiation therapy. Agents selected should have activity against the neoplasm being teated. Many myelosuppressive agents have not, however, been tested adequately at high doses against most cancers because myelosuppression has limited the usefulness of these drugs in the absence of bone marrow support. While total body radiation has a major role in transplantation for acute leukemias and lymphomas, total body radiation is of limited value in breast cancer and other localized solid tumors where doses required for elimination of macroscopic and even microscopic disease often exceed the tolerable limits that can be administered.

Many agents are not amenable to dose escalation or do not have a linear dose response effect (see XV-3). For example, anti-metabolites such as 5-fluorouracil and methotrexate plateau in their dose response after only a small dose escalation (Figure XIX-1-2). Other agents which appear to possess a dose response effect, such as Adriamycin, while lim-

Table XIX-1-3.   Non-Hematopoietic Dose Limiting Toxicities of Various Antineoplastic Agents

Drug	Standard Tolerated Dose (mg/m²)	Maximum Tolerated Dose (mg/m²)	With Bone Marrow Support — Organ Affected by Side Effects
Doxorubicin	60–75	150	Hand-foot syndrome
Nitrogen mustard		33	CNS
Cyclophosphamide	750	7,500	Hemorrhagic myocarditis
Mitolactol (Dibromodulcitol)	300	ND	
Mitocmycin C	20	60	Venoocclusive Disease ·
Methotrexate		NA	
Melphalan	40	180–220	Enterocolitis
Carmustine	200	1,000	Pulmonary fibrosis, toxic hepatitis
Thiotepa	30	1,500	CNS syndrome
Cisplatin	120	180	Renal, neuropathy
Busulfan	2–4	1,100	Anorexia

ND, not done; NA, not achieved

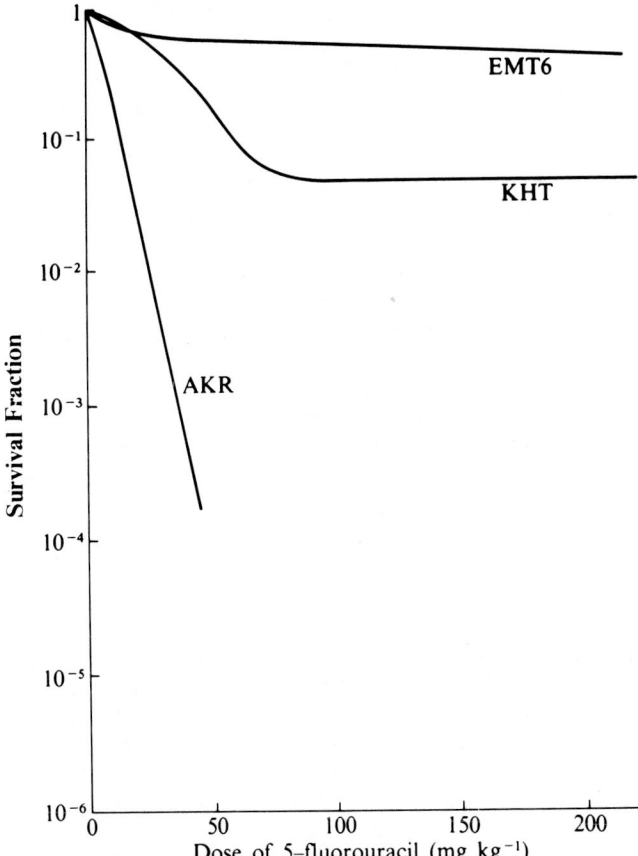

Figure XIX-1-2. Plateau in cell killing of two transplanted animal tumors using fluorouracil.

ited predominantly by myelosuppression, have non-hematopoietic toxicities which quickly limit further dose escalation.[39] Cardiotoxicity and mucosal and epithelial toxicity do not permit substantial dose escalation. It is unlikely that such compounds will play a major role in high-dose therapeutic regimens, although synergy with other active agents could be present, providing a role for these agents in high-dose programs.

Volume of Disease

Disease volume will limit the potential of intensive therapy. As tumors begin to exceed a certain volume, even high-dose therapeutic approaches may be unable to produce complete tumor regression. Consolidative radiation therapy or surgical approaches to areas of pre-treatment bulk disease may be useful.

Principles of tumor kinetic modelling should be considered in the development of therapeutic regimens using autologous bone marrow transplantation. The Golde-Coldman hypothesis suggests that spontaneous development of resistance occurs relatively early in neoplastic evolution and, hence, treatment in early stage of disease is more likely to be effective than later treatment.[73] Whether or not the dose escalation afforded by marrow protection techniques will allow sufficient increase in therapeutic effect to overcome such resistance, particularly in combination regimens, is at present uncertain for most tumors and will need to be evaluated

carefully. Norton-Simon kinetic theory would predict that the application of intensive therapy after cytoreduction would provide the most useful place in which to utilize dose intensification.[157–159] Formal testing of these hypotheses has not been evaluated at high-doses.

Procedure for Bone Marrow Transplantation

Selection of Patient

Autologous bone marrow transplantation can be utilized in older patients than can allogeneic marrow transplantation, where complications preclude use in most patients over the age of 40, due to the increasing severity of graft versus host disease. Successful autografting has been performed into the seventh decade, though such attempts in this age group are uncommon. Complicating concommitant illness and medical disability may be expected to increase the morbidity of patients treated with advanced age. Patient performance status at the start of therapy appears to be a major predictor of toxicity in autologous bone marrow transplantation.

Further evaluation of quality of life attributes need to be undertaken to evaluate the short term and long term effects of transplantation. Patients who have failed multiple therapies for their malignancy may not be good candidates for intensive therapy in that resistant tumor cells may have been selected and patient tolerance will be reduced, compromising the therapeutic efficacy of intensive therapy, and resulting in higher treatment-related toxicity.[14]

Bone Marrow Harvesting Technique and Complications

Bulk aspiration of bone marrow is generally performed under regional or general anesthesia from the posterior or anterior iliac crests.[220] The posterior and anterior iliac crests represent the most attractive areas for bulk marrow collection. Patients who have received extensive pelvic irradiation may require aspiration of marrow from the sternum, or the harvest of hematopoietic progenitor cells from the peripheral blood (see below). Approximately 1 to 3 × 10^8 nucleated cells/kg is collected, using needle aspiration from multiple sites in the iliac crests. Small aspirations (<10 cc) from multiple sites are obtained to try to minimize contamination with peripheral blood. Marrow is generally anticoagulated using heparin. After an adequate volume of marrow has been obtained, cells are usually passed through stainless steel screens to remove bone chips and to create a single cell suspension. There is disagreement about the use of screening because large cells such as megakaryocytes, other hematopoietic progenitors, or malignant cells may be removed by this technique. Nonetheless, most practitioners continue to use screens in the preparation of marrow.

Bulk marrow obtained in this way is generally concentrated by centrifugation and a buffy coat preparation obtained. The marrow is generally mixed with 10% dimethylsulfoxide or other cryoprotectants, autologous plasma, and cryopreserved at control rate in liquid nitrogen. Some authors have reported that the characteristics of the freezing process are important to marrow viability and hematopoietic reconstitution,[59,125] although others have disputed this.[86,210] Once frozen, cryopreserved marrow retains viability in liquid nitrogen for extended periods of time.[18]

Marrow harvest is associated with few complications mainly related to anesthesia. Pain in the harvest area is the most common but is generally short lived and controlled by simple analgesia. Local infection, bleeding, bone injury, nerve damage, and even air embolism has been rarely reported during marrow harvesting.[132] Efforts to perform outpatient marrow harvest procedures have been undertaken.[36]

At the time of administration, the marrow is rapidly thawed at 37°C and infused intravenously without further treatment. In some early reports, marrow was treated with enzymes followed by washing, but such processing is generally not necessary and is associated with increased febrile reactions at the time of marrow reinfusion.[66] Infused marrow stem cells circulate through the pulmonary circulation and "home" to marrow cavities. The molecular mechanism underlying this homing to marrow sites has recently been reviewed and appears to relate to the presence of unique antigens present on early marrow progenitor cells. The administration of bone marrow can be associated with hypertension and bradycardia, presumably related to the dimethylsulfoxide used as a cryoprotectant.[56] Hemolyzed red cells contaminating bulk marrow preparations produce hemoglobinuria, of which the patient should be warned; it has been associated with renal dysfunction in the early post transplant setting.[85,204] Other side effects of marrow infusion include acute anaphylaxis to infusion of autologous bone marrow apparently mediated through an IgE antibody to bovine serum albumin.[116]

Peripheral Blood Stem Cell and Progenitor Cell Collection

An alternative method for collecting cells capable of hematopoietic reconstitution involves leukopheresis to collect peripheral blood mononuclear cells. Levels of peripheral blood progenitor cells, or stem cells, increase during the recovery phase from chemotherapy, and after priming with hematopoietic colony-stimulating factors such as G-CSF or GM-CSF.[69,205] Approximately 9–10 liters of peripheral blood are processed on multiple occasions using a continuous flow centrifuge.[105] Mononuclear cells collected in this fashion are concentrated and cryopreserved as described above with marrow. Satisfactory hematopoietic reconstitution appears to correlate with the number of progenitor cells measured in the CFU-GM assay.[100] Studies in murine systems suggested that peripheral stem cells were not likely to be effective for auto-transplantation, since their capacity for cell renewal was limited when compared to that of bone marrow.[142] Transplantation experiments in dogs, however, did demonstrate that these circulating stem cells could rescue animals from supralethal radiation therapy.[45,111] The numbers of peripheral blood stem cells could be increased by exercise, ACTH, dextran or the administration of hematopoietic colony-stimulating factors.[206] Higher levels of CFU-GM have also been observed during the period of recovery from chemotherapy.[70]

During the late 1970's, Goldman and his colleagues demonstrated that circulating mononuclear cells could produce complete and sustained hematopoietic engraftment in patients with chronic myeloid leukemia after high-dose chemotherapy.[74,87] Subsequent studies have attempted to use peripheral blood progenitor cells to reconstitute patients with acute myeloid leukemia,[182] Burkitt's lymphoma,[112] Hodgkins' disease,[113] breast cancer,[107] and non-Hodgkins' lymphoma.[27,114] In these studies, rapid hematopoietic reconstitution could be consistently obtained at relatively low doses of progenitor cells measured by CFU-GM. In other studies, however, such rapid engraftment did not occur and platelet recovery was extremely slow,[44] especially in settings where the CFU-GM was low. Some patients did not attain sustained hematopoietic reconstitution.[89]

Some have claimed that peripheral blood progenitor collections have fewer contaminating malignant cells, even in patients with acute myeloid leukemia, chronic myelogenous leukemia,[115] lymphoma,[108] or solid tumors in which bone marrow contamination is evident. The level of tumor cell contamination has not been adequately measured. Recent data suggest that peripheral blood progenitor collections do contain tumor cells in neuroblastoma.[120,146,147,192]

Marrow Processing

Ex Vivo Purging. Autologous bone marrow transplantation is limited to patients in whom marrow progenitors can be obtained without contaminating clonogenic malignant cells. Many cancers involve the marrow, and in the leukemias, the primary site for disease is the marrow. A variety of methods to remove malignant cells from marrow have been utilized. Table XIX-1-4 lists various methods of ex vivo purging of bone marrow, using either direct cytotoxic activity against tumor or tumor removal methods. Randomized comparative trials establishing the efficacy of these purging methods have not yet been completed, although some trials are currently underway. Infusion of marrows contaminated with malignant cells have been suggested to result in unusual patterns of recurrence.[80]

Chemical. A variety of antineoplastic agents have been employed as a method to remove malignant cells from marrow. The most common method has involved a short-term exposure ex vivo to cytotoxic agents such as 4-hydroperoxy-cyclophosphamide (4-HC) or ASTA-Z, cyclophosphamide derivatives not requiring hepatic activation and showing antitumor activity in animal models, etoposide, cisplatin, cytosine arabinoside and others. Several considerations, including the number of malignant cells contaminating the marrow, may limit the efficacy of this approach. Some clinical trials suggest an advantage for purged versus unpurged marrows.[77] Exposure to 4-HC or other chemotherapeutic agents do not appear to exhibit major selectivity with respect to normal and leukemic clonogenic cells, nor do these agents completely inhibit the self-renewal capacity of leukemic myeloblasts in culture. In addition, the anti-leukemic and, particularly anti-solid tumor effect of 4-HC may be limited, with only modest reduction in tumor cell numbers. The use of 4-HC in acute myelocytic leukemia in second or greater complete remission has demonstrated superior long-term outcome to that expected using non-purged marrow.[189,193,239] Comparative trials of 4-HC purging technology are currently underway. The use of methods to differentially protect hematopoietic progenitors from in vitro toxic chemotherapy effects via the use of ethiofos[140] has been advocated.

Table XIX-1-4.   Methods of Ex vivo Purging of Bone Marrow

Tumoricidal Methods
  Pharmacologic
    Cyclophosphamide derivatives
      4-hydroperoxycyclophosphamide
      ASTA-Z 7557 (Mafosphamide)
    Cytosine arabinoside analogs
    Cisplatin and analogs
    Deoxynucleosides
    Deoxycoformycin
    Doxorubicin
    Verapamil
    Glucocorticoids
    Alykyl-lysophospholipids
    Etoposide
  Biophysical Agents
    Photoradiation
      Merocyanin-540 (MC-540)
      Dihematoporphyrin Ether (DHE)
    Radioisotopes
  Immunologic Methods
    Monoclonal Antibodies and Complement
    Monoclonal Antibodies and Ricin or other Toxins
    IL-2 Leukocyte Activated Killer Cells (LAK cells)
    Alpha 2b Interferon

Tumor Removal Methods
  Immunologic Methods
    Immunomagnetic beads and monoclonal antibodies
    Immunorosettes
  Physical Methods
    Counterflow Elutriation
    Centrifugation
    Immunoabsorption

The use of chemical purging has limited the use of certain hematopoietic colony stimulating factors such as GM-CSF which is then ineffective in stimulating recovery.[33] This is due to a lack of the progenitors bearing receptors capable of responding to the late acting colony stimulating factors. Other factors, such as IL-3, which act on an earlier progenitor, may be effective in this setting.[143]

Antibody. The ability of monoclonal antibodies to identify specific tumor associated antigens has been exploited in technologies to remove malignant cells. The use of anti-CALLA antibodies and complement have been used to purge leukemic cells in acute lymphocytic leukemia in childhood,[186,187] and similar technologies have been applied to lymphomas and other diseases.[8,152] Attachment of toxins such as ricin or Pseudomonas toxin to monoclonal antibodies,[22,55,59,72,145,151,179,180,194,211,212] or coupling the antibodies to immunomagnetic beads[31,50,130,178,191,199,200,231,232] produce enhanced tumor cell kill. Superior survival in children with neuroblastoma receiving marrows purged with a panel of antibodies and a magnetic separation technique has been reported.[118]

Antibody mediated purging may be limited by antigenic heterogenity of the tumor cells,[57,134] as heterogeneity in drug sensitivity among tumor clones may limit its usefulness. It is likely that combination modalities may be complementary[58,145,223–225] and lead to enhanced tumor removal.

Other. Multiple other techniques for removing malignant cells from marrow have been reported, including immuno-rosetting,[203] counter current elutriation,[103] and the use of lymphokine activated killer cells.[1,2,3,91,129,222,227] Nevertheless, despite the variety, logic, and availability of techniques, the importance and utility of removal of malignant cells has yet to be demonstrated. Some have claimed that leukemic cells do not cryopreserve as well as normal hematopoietic cells.[6]

Long-Term Culture. Recently, hematopoietic reconstitution of patients with chronic myeloid leukemia and acute myeloid leukemia has been reported using autologous marrow that had been cultured long-term in vitro. Patient preparation for marrow transplantation has been performed using busulfan and cyclophosphamide.[46,47,53] The cultured autologous transplant has been reported to result in sustained normalization of disease specific karyotypic abnormalities. Culture of CML marrow appears to yield terminally differentiated malignant cells and the outgrowth of a normal population in the in vitro setting. Expansion and collection of these cells and their subsequent re-engraftment appears to argue that two clones of cells are present in CML-affected marrow, and that reconstitution with an unaffected clone may occur.

Stem Cell Collection and Expansion. The identification of the CD34 antigen on early hematopoietic progenitors has led to attempts to isolate and expand these progenitors with subsequent use for hematopoietic reconstitution.[215] Positive selection of a stem cell may enable the elimination of most neoplastic cells and lead to sustained reconstitution. Studies in dogs,[28] primates,[29] and, more recently, in man[30] have demonstrated that sustained engraftment can be achieved with positive selection of marrow for CD34-positive/CD-33 negative hematopoietic progenitors. The importance of these observations, coupled with the recent molecular cloning of c-kit ligand[41,51,240] offers the potential for ex vivo expansion of early hematopoietic progenitors and reconstitution.[233]

Cytoreductive Therapy Administration and Supportive Care

After satisfactory collection and storage of hematopoietic progenitors, high-dose chemotherapy and/or total body irradiation is used to treat the neoplasm. Following intensive chemoradiation therapy, rapid and profound myelosuppression ensues. Hematopoietic reconstitution to a neutrophil count of $>500/mm^3$ usually requires 15–19 days, with thrombocytopenia persisting generally longer. Supportive care techniques vary from center to center, but generally include reverse isolation, transfusional therapy, and empiric and therapeutic antibacterial and antifungal therapy. Radiation of blood products is performed to eliminate the potential for graft versus host disease resulting from transfused blood products. Parenteral nutrition has frequently been utilized, since many patients, particularly those treated with total body radiation, experience severe mucositis. Studies in non-transplant patients have demonstrated the value of low bacterial content diets, and a reduced risk for systemic Aspergillus infections have been documented in patients treated in HEPA-filtered air environments.[197] Recommendations for hospital facilities and for transplant team capabilities have been developed by the American Society of Clinical Oncology and the American Society of Hematology.[12]

Specific Diseases

Acute Myelocytic Leukemia

Autologous bone marrow transplantation has been used as consolidation in patients with acute myelocytic leukemia in first, second, or subsequent remission, and studies have been performed using both purged and unpurged bone marrow. Interpretation of the available studies is complicated by differences in therapeutic regimens, differences in the interval between complete remission and autografting, and inadequate descriptions of the patient populations. Results in advanced resistant disease indicate that although complete responses occurred in more than 50% of patients, relapses were nearly universal. More recent efforts have concentrated on patients in first or second complete remission using purged or non-purged bone marrow. Most series have involved only small numbers of patients with relatively short follow-up. A recent analysis of 263 patients with acute myelocytic leukemia, autografted in first complete remission between 1982 and 1987, has been reported.[77] Leukemia-free survival at three years was 39%; among those patients whose marrow was purged with mafosphamide, who were autografted within six months of complete remission, relapse-free survival was significantly improved (Figure XIX-1-3). There is a profound influence of the time from achievement of the first complete remission to autologous bone marrow transplant upon the probability of relapse and leukemia-free survival (Figure XIX-1-4). This relationship is most likely explained by time-censoring selection bias in which patients transplanted late after complete remission is achieved, when others in the cohort have already relapsed and thus do not present for transplant, are more likely to have been cured by their chemotherapy than patients treated early in their remission. These data are consistent with earlier data of Yeager and colleagues using 4-hydroperoxycyclophosphamide[239] to purge marrow with acute myelocytic leukemia during a second complete remission. Randomized comparative data in first complete remission have not been undertaken, nor have comparative trials

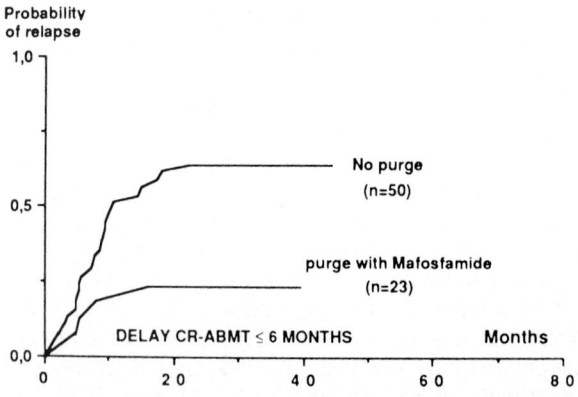

Figure XIX-1-3. Autologous bone marrow transplant in acute myeloid leukemia within six months of achieving complete remission. Patients whose marrows underwent purging with Mafosfamide had significantly fewer relapses. From Gorin et al.[77]

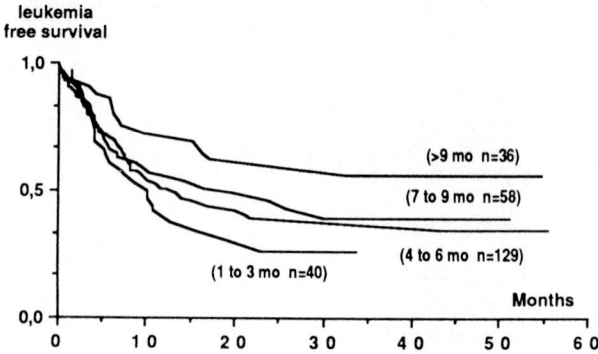

Figure XIX-1-4. Autologous bone marrow transplantation in acute myeloid leukemia appears to be more successful the later it is undertaken after attaining complete remission. This is artifactual. See text. From Gorin et al.[77]

been performed in which high-dose consolidation has not been used.

Acute Lymphocytic Leukemia

Results of autologous bone marrow transplantation in patients with acute lymphocytic lymphoblastic leukemia (ALL) have been less satisfactory. In a comparison of autografting to allografting in 91 patients with acute lymphocytic leukemia in first through fourth remission, 20% of autografted, and 27% of allografted patients became long-term disease-free survivors.[104] Although several series have demonstrated prolonged disease-free survival in some transplanted patients with high-risk ALL who have failed conventional chemotherapy, the degree of success is less than that in acute myelocytic leukemia. The major reason for treatment failure is relapse. Some authors have suggested that allograft recipients without graft versus host disease and autograft recipients have indistinguishable relapse curves, suggesting that the source of relapse in those patients is residual leukemic cells in the patient and not residual leukemic cells in the transplanted bone marrow.

Purging of ALL using monoclonal antibodies has been evaluated in several studies. A recent analysis of 47 patients comparing relapse frequency in allogeneic versus autologous bone marrow transplantation indicated that the probability of relapse was 9% for patients receiving an allogeneic bone marrow transplant, and 52% for patients receiving autologous bone marrow transplant.[32] Graft versus leukemia or tumor effect of autologous marrow may be responsible for the difference in relapse frequency. In vitro treatment with monoclonal antibodies and complement, immunotoxins, and 4-hydroperoxycyclophosphamide have been performed. The impact of purging remains less clear at present from these studies.[26,78,79] None of the data permits a conclusion that there is a benefit derived from purging bone marrow in acute lymphocytic leukemia.

Non-Hodgkins' Lymphoma

The therapeutic results of autologous bone marrow transplantation in patients with non-Hodgkins' lymphoma appears to be related to the grade and extent of disease and its resistance to previous chemotherapy. In advanced stage intermediate and high-grade lymphoma, three year progression-free survival ranges from 20–60% reflecting small study numbers and selection effects. In general results appear superior in patients with smaller volume disease, and in patients responding to induction therapy.[68,82]

Multiple conditioning regimens have been used in autologous bone marrow transplants for lymphomas, but few comparative trials between regimens have been performed. In patients with relapsed lymphoma who have a good performance status and minimal disease following conventional induction therapy, the probability of disease-free survival on an actuarial basis is 50% at 38 months (Figure XIX-1-5). This therapeutic outcome is achieved with minimal treatment-related mortality.[66] Patients in resistant relapse who have not responded to a second induction chemotherapy program fare poorly following autologous bone marrow transplantation, and few remain alive.[174] The role of purging in this setting remains controversial.

The nature of the preparative regimen may be very important with regard to both therapeutic benefit and toxicity. Dose escalations of the same drugs have resulted in frequencies of complete remission varying from 47–80%.[19] Regimens containing TBI have a higher incidence of diffuse alveolar hemorrhage than do regimens without TBI.[48,148,188]

Studies with an early combination chemotherapy regimen, BACT, used in the treatment of non-Hodgkins' lymphoma (carmustine, cytarabine, cyclophosphamide, 6-thioguanine) revealed that few patients with advanced bulky disease achieved extended disease-free survival. Canellos and his colleagues, in a survey of published reports, showed only 16 of 112 long-term disease-free survivors when ABMT was used in refractory relapse of lymphoma as opposed to 33 of 53 patients transplanted in second or subsequent remission, or in first partial remission.[43]

Hodgkins' Disease

High-dose combination chemotherapy using high-dose cyclophosphamide/BCNU/VP-16 can result in a 45% overall survival for more than six years in patients who have failed a MOPP-like regimen and Adriamycin therapy for relapsed Hodgkins' disease (Figure XIX-1-6).[95] Outcome from the autologous transplant was affected by performance status, by having received more than two chemotherapy regimens, by high tumor burden, and by the recurrence of disease within a prior radiation field. Any of these features reduced the probability of long-term survival and help to identify patients who are poor candidates for utilizing this therapeutic approach. Local radiation therapy may improve the outcome in patients with bulky disease prior to transplant.[37] Other authors have reported similar results.[4,5,37,75,83,84]

Similar treatment results have been reported from autologous bone marrow transplantation and allogeneic transplantation for Hodgkin's disease.[128] While relapses are slightly higher in autologous transplants, there is an absence of graft versus host (and graft versus lymphoma) disease. Given the difficulties often associated with allogeneic transplantation, this suggests that autologous bone marrow transplantation may represent the preferable approach for relapsed Hodgkin's patients.

Breast Cancer

Increasing interest has been focused over the past decade on the role of dose intensity in the treatment of breast cancer. Retrospective analysis and prospective clinical trials have demonstrated a dose-response relationship in terms of objective response, duration of remission, and quality of life. Responsiveness to high-dose combination chemotherapy regimens in breast cancer has been demonstrated, with most studies showing a higher complete and total response rate.[165] Most studies are small, and include heterogeneous patient populations making interpretation of data difficult.[13,14,92,93] Early studies were associated with substantial toxicity and when applied to patients who have failed a standard dose regimen for metastatic cancer, the responses are not durable.[139,166] Patients in this setting do not appear to benefit from regimens which have been tested thus far. Selection of patients at high risk for relapse and poorly responsive to standard therapies can be assisted by certain pretreatment characteristics; appropriate patients would include premenopausal women with hormone receptor neg-

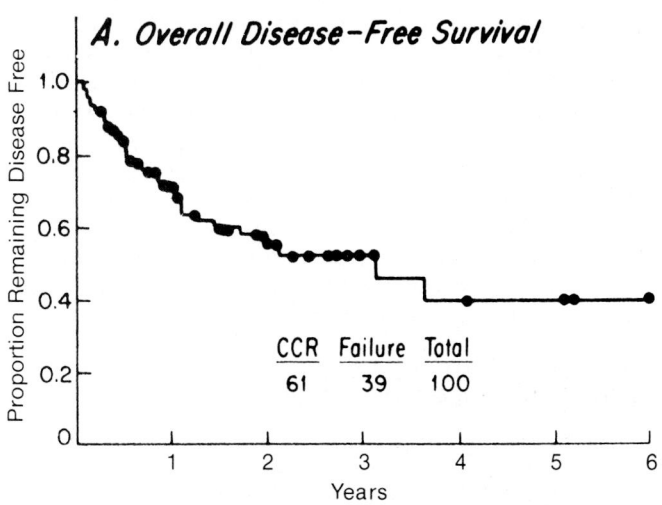

Figure XIX-1-5. Non-Hodgkin's lymphoma disease-free survival after autologous bone marrow transplant. CCR, Complete clinical remission. From Freedman et al.[66]

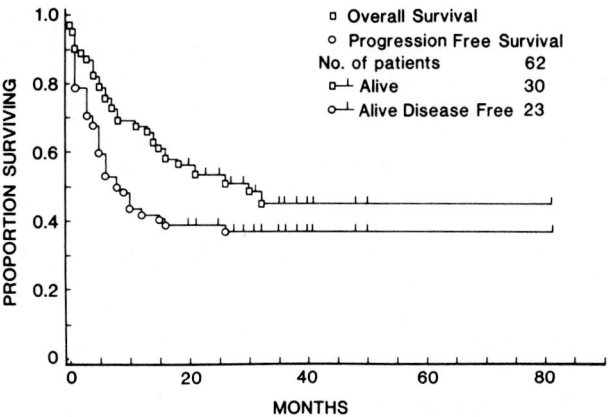

Figure XIX-1-6. Intensive chemotherapy and ABMT in relapsed Hodgkin's disease.

ative or hormone insensitive metastatic disease[141] which has not failed prior chemotherapy for metastases. More recent studies, using high dose combination alkylating agents in patients meeting these characteristics, either with no prior chemotherapy for metastases or as part of a program involving induction chemotherapy followed by high-dose consolidation, have demonstrated that between 15% and 25% of patients can achieve durable extended remissions from 3 to 6+ years.[15,60,61,167-169] Patients with limited volume disease and less prior chemotherapy respond better. Durable remissions after a single high-dose therapy and no other intervention extending beyond six years have been observed, and several studies now have found extended disease-free survival even in poor prognosis patients. High-dose consolidation with cyclophosphamide, cisplatin and carmustine with autologous bone marrow and peripheral blood progenitor cell support in the setting of high-risk primary breast cancer involving ten or more axillary lymph nodes has been studied with an apparent benefit derived from this approach compared to contemporary or historical series.[170,171] Prospective, randomized, comparative trials are in progress. While purging of bone marrow has been undertaken using chemical and monoclonal methods (see Purging above) early results do not differ from those obtained without purging techniques.

The toxicity of these treatment programs appears to be influenced by several factors, including extent of disease, performance status and the induction chemotherapy used prior to particular high-dose regimens, and the regimens themselves. Modification of treatment associated toxicity appears to be possible using hematopoietic colony stimulating factors and particularly with the use of CSF-primed peripheral blood progenitor cells. Widespread application of this technology will be dependent of the ability to achieve substantial cost-reductions given the number of potential patients for whom this technique might be relevant.

At the present time, the use of high-dose approaches should be restricted to centers possessing the expertise and facilities to safely utilize this approach and at present, only in the context of clinical trials. Very few regimens have been sufficiently tested to provide reliable information about outcome.

Small Cell Lung Cancer

Several series have examined the role of high-dose intensification in the treatment of small cell lung cancer and, in general, the results have been disappointing. Clearly, in advanced, resistant disease, high-dose consolidation appears to offer few durable remissions. Two series have reported that in patients with minimal disease treated in complete remission, approximately 15% can achieve sustained remissions in excess of two years. The technique is limited in this patient population, usually because of general poor performance, extent of disease and age of the patients presenting with this disease. A randomized trial in small-cell lung cancer showed a significant increase in disease-free survival but did not improve overall survival.[94]

Ovarian Cancer

Ovarian carcinoma has been demonstrated to display a dose-response relationship to several chemotherapy agents.

Because of the poor prognosis of patients failing initial chemotherapy for this disease, the use of high-dose chemotherapy with autologous bone marrow transplantation is attractive. Several studies have demonstrated high-response rates in ovarian cancer but the durability of these remissions has, in general, been brief.[49,54,149,156,201] While several different therapeutic regimens have been tested, long-term results and comparative effects have not been studied in detail.

Melanoma and Colon Cancer

A small series of patients have been treated with high-dose chemotherapy regimens for metastatic melanoma,[52,88,109,119,121,196,216,217,221,235] and colon cancer.[208] In general, therapeutic results in these diseases indicate that the complete response rate has not been changed substantially by the use of high-dose intensification with myelotoxic drugs, and that the application of these techniques has, as yet, not changed the ultimate outcome. Evaluation, however, has been done predominantly in the setting of advanced resistant disease, and testing in earlier settings may be valuable.

Myeloma

Most myeloma patients are usually elderly and often frail, and for these reasons have not generally been considered for high dose therapy approaches requiring bone marrow or stem cell support. However, there is an apparent steep dose response effect in refractory disease to alkylating agents with melphalan appearing preferable to cyclophosphamide in small uncontrolled observations.[24] Several large pilot studies have been reported in which high dose melphalan or thiotepa with or without total body radiation (TBI) have been used in previously treated patients.[25,76,96] Complete responses (as defined by the disappearance of monoclonal gammopathy on standard protein electrophoresis) occur in 25-50% with projected 3-4 year survival rates of 26-80% depending on response to induction therapy. Bone marrow purging of myeloma cells using anti-B cell monoclonal antibodies,[9,10,72] or 4-hydroperoxycyclophosphamide[181] has been presented but small samples and non-controlled design do not permit conclusions about efficacy. Peripheral blood cell collections have also been utilized as support after high-dose therapy.[62,183] Again, small and heterogeneous patient populations, varying treatment programs, numbers and short followup do not allow adequate assessment. In general, responses are higher, more readily achieved in patients with lower tumor burden and when secondary resistance has not yet been developed. But, there is no evidence of a plateau for disease-free survival after autologous marrow transplantation in myeloma as there appears to be after allogeneic bone marrow transplantation.[42] Further evaluation is required.

Chronic Myelogenous Leukemia

Based upon the hypothesis that there may exist normal clones within CML marrow, autologous bone marrow transplantation in patients with chronic myelocytic leukemia has been undertaken using either CML remission marrow or peripheral blood stem cell collections. Remissions of short duration were achieved, but relapse of chronic phase leukemia has been the rule. More recently, the long-term in vitro cultured bone marrow of patients with CML from which the Philadelphia chromosome has been lost has been used in these patients. Further evaluation will be required.

Gliomas

Despite in vitro evidence for a dose response effect for cytotoxic drugs in glioblastoma multiforme, the use of high-dose chemotherapy has, in general, been disappointing.[110,209] To a large extent, trials have employed single agents, most commonly BCNU or other alkylating agents, and have produced only brief remissions with significant toxicity.[71,98,153,155,190,236,238] In uncontrolled trials with this agent, no significant prolongation of survival has been achieved in either the advanced disease or in the adjuvant setting. Three studies suggested a small prolongation of survival for high-grade malignant gliomas with adjuvant high-dose BCNU and ABMT.[98,138,236] There appear to be some extended duration remissions among the patients treated in these series.[237] More recently, experience in pediatric brain tumors has suggested that a limited number of children with gliomas treated with multidrug regimens may achieve extended survival.[63]

Testicular cancer

The prognosis for patients with advanced resistant testicular cancer is poor. Recently, the use of high-dose therapy, including autologous bone marrow support, has resulted in greater than one-year disease-free survival in 40% of completely responding patients (10% of all treated) with recurrent testicular cancer.[40] Such results suggest that a fraction of these patients can be salvaged using high-dose intensification, even when there has been a failure of prior chemotherapy.[154,162]

Neuroblastoma and Ewing's Sarcoma

The prognosis for children with neuroblastoma over the age of one year is poor, with most children relapsing and dying of disease within two years. The use of phenylalanine mustard and total body irradiation in patients with neuroblastoma, with or without marrow purging, has been explored and demonstrates that about 25–35% of children with stages 3 and 4 neuroblastoma can remain continuously disease-free after this treatment.[65,117,120,175,177] Relapses after 21 months have not been observed in most series. Because of the high frequency of marrow involvement in neuroblastoma, several different approaches to purging have been applied in uncontrolled studies.[101,102,130,176,184,202,226]

Ewing's sarcoma has also attracted interest as a tumor which is potentially treatable by high-dose therapy and autologous bone marrow transplantation.[133] The low frequency of this disease has not permitted controlled trials to be undertaken.

Toxicities

Autologous bone marrow transplantation is frequently associated with both morbidity and mortality dependent upon the nature and extent of the cancer, patient performance status, prior chemotherapy, conditioning regimen and other factors. While most of the early toxicity is associated with

the conditioning regimen, complications may result from the antibiotic and antifungal regimens associated with treatment of presumed or actual infection or from other supportive care treatments such as colony stimulating factors. The timing of the toxicities associated with autologous bone marrow transplantation are usually characteristic and valuable differential diagnostic information can be derived from these considerations (Figure XIX-1-7).

Myelosuppression, Colony Stimulating Factors and Peripheral Stem Cells

The use of high-dose chemotherapy has been associated with significant periods of myelosuppression. The average time to achieve a neutrophil count greater than 500/mm³ in most studies ranges between 15 and 25 days, with thrombocytopenia lasting for a somewhat more extended period of time. In some cases, particularly in those where patients have received extensive prior chemotherapy, persistent thrombocytopenia can be a major problem, and some patients remain platelet-dependent for more than 100 days. Various explanations have been put forth for extended periods of thrombocytopenia, including reduced tolerance of megakaryocyte to cryopreservation, and removal of megakaryocytic precursors by the filtration process in which large cells are retained preferentially on the steel mesh filters used to process bone marrow.

Hematopoietic colony-stimulating factors, such as GM- and G-CSF, have been utilized more recently to accelerate hematopoietic recovery.[16,35,38,172,198] Several groups have now used CSFs as adjuncts in the bone marrow transplant setting and have reported remarkably consistent results. In each case, the use of the hemopoietin accelerated myeloid recovery after high-dose therapy with bone marrow support. Platelet reconstitution was variably improved. However, there always remained a period of absolute leukopenia which was not correctable by colony stimulating factor alone at any dose utilized. This is presumed to be related to a relative deficiency in cryopreserved marrow of the committed progenitors bearing responsive receptors for the late acting colony stimulating factors. In addition, the utilization of these compounds, either directly or indirectly, has led to a reduction of the organ system toxicity associated with high-dose chemotherapy.

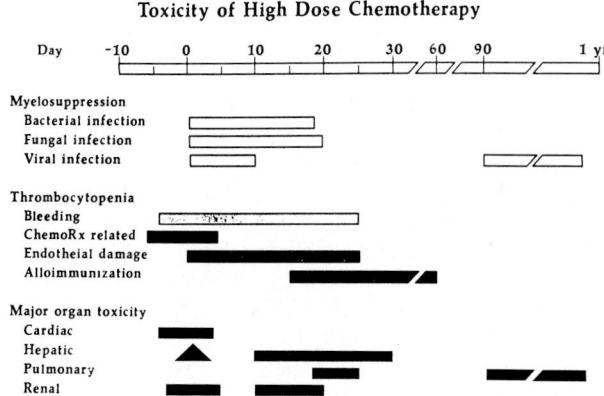

Figure XIX-1-7. Toxicities and the times they usually are most prominent after the procedure of intensive chemotherapy and ABMT.

The addition of hematopoietic progenitors derived from peripheral blood after chemotherapy, with or without colony stimulating factor priming has, in uncontrolled studies, resulted in a profound reduction of both the duration of absolute leukopenia and in the toxicity of transplantation.[69,70,173] Studies have demonstrated an accelerated rate of hematopoietic recovery after a period of absolute leukopenia, and a reduction in the infectious complications seen in these settings. Some studies have noted a reduction in the need for platelet transfusions, as well as red cell transfusions.

The major consequence of myelosuppression continues to be infectious complications. Bacterial and fungal infections are the major problems associated with autologous bone marrow transplantation although viral infections, especially reactivated viral infections of herpes simplex virus,[150] adenovirus-related hemophagocytic syndrome,[124] and transfusion associated cytomegalovirus[185,229,230,234] may all occur with autologous bone marrow transplantation.

Immune Functioning after ABMT

Immune function recovery after autologous bone marrow transplantation appears to be dependent upon the preparative regimen (busulfan), and ex vivo treatment, if any, of the graft.[11,164] In addition, there are poorly understood effects such as persistently inverted CD4/CD8 ratios,[160] and disappearance of CD4 lymphocyte circadian cycles,[135] perhaps related to differential repopulation kinetics of hematopoietic progenitors.[228]

Organ Toxicity

Organ system toxicity occurs following high-dose chemotherapy in the marrow transplant setting, generally as a direct effect of the chemotherapy and radiation therapy on organ systems. It is likely that infectious complications, as well as the need for supportive care, such as antibacterials and anti-fungals, contribute to these injuries.

During chemotherapy administration multiple complications have been described including acute fluid imbalance, syndrome of inappropriate antidiuretic hormone secretion, hemorrhagic myocarditis, nephrogenic diabetes insipidus after cyclophosphamide therapy,[64] hypertension with combination alkylating agents,[81] DIC,[85] metabolic abnormalities such as idiopathic hyperammonemia,[144] an acquired platelet secretion defect,[161] interstitial pneumonitis,[163] and late vasculitis with pulmonary hemorrhage.[195] All have been reported as complications of high-dose therapy where autologous bone marrow support has been used. In addition, failure to provide adequate bladder irrigation or to administer protective compounds such as Mesna, has been associated with the development of hemorrhagic cystitis.

Mucositis and enterocolitis are major side effects of many, though not all, regimens. TBI, etoposide, melphalan, thiotepa and regimens containing significant doses of these agents often have severe accompanying mucositis. Tissue breakdown results in a higher risk of systemic infection and often nutritional difficulties. The possibility of fungal or viral causes of mucositis and esophagitis should not be overlooked. Diarrhea in patients undergoing ABMT may result from many causes including the conditioning regimen, *C. difficile* toxin, various medications, or fungal or viral infections.

Veno-occlusive disease of the liver, reflecting endothelial damage and subsequent clot formation or fibrosis in the small hepatic venules associated with endothelial toxicity and centrolobular hemorrhage, occurs in as many as 20–40% of patients undergoing autologous bone marrow transplantation with some chemotherapy regimens. The mechanism of injury presumably reflects the deposition of activated drug metabolites into the hepatic venules after activation in the liver, with subsequent injury to endothelial cells. The syndrome is generally manifested by right upper quadrant pain, hepatomegaly, ascites, jaundice, and veno-occlusive disease. No specific therapy, but various supportive efforts have been reported. Efforts to utilize prostaglandin synthetase inhibitors or heparin to prevent the clot formation during the period of chemotherapy, diagnosis of VOD by ultrasonography,[137] or treatment by tissue plasminogen activator[21] have been studied, with success reported in non-controlled trials.

Nephrotoxicity occurring in the setting of autologous bone marrow transplantation can result from many causes, including the use of specific chemotherapeutic agents known to influence kidney function (cisplatin, nitrosoureas, phenylalanine mustard), coupled with nephrotoxic effects of antibiotics generally used during supportive care settings. Late renal dysfunction[214] probably related to radiation therapy can occur.

Pulmonary drug toxicity has been reported in the post transplant setting.[97,127] Cyclophosphamide produces a pulmonary alveolitis which has been characterized in animal systems,[34] and probably is expressed in man in a combined injury resulting from radiation therapy and cyclophosphamide as part of the preparative regimen. Pulmonary drug toxicity is commonly associated with carmustine when the acute or chronic dose exceeds 1,200 mg/m^2. The clinical syndrome is generally manifested by fever, interstitial infiltrates and dyspnea. It is characterized pathologically by type II pneumocyte proliferation, fibrosis and alveolar inflammation. Pulmonary insufficiency can be rapidly progressive and diagnostic efforts should be instituted promptly. The clinical syndrome is often confused with an infectious etiology because of the complicating fever, and delay in making a specific diagnosis can lead to rapid progression of the toxicity. While no controlled trials have been undertaken, empirical observations suggest that chemoradiation injury is worsened by exposure to high concentrations of oxygen. The use of corticosteroids in high doses is often useful in ameliorating this toxicity.[4]

The most frequent serious cardiac complication associated with autologous bone marrow transplantation is hemorrhagic myocarditis, generally due to cyclophosphamide administration alone or in combination with other drugs. The pathology suggests that the lesion is due to endothelial injury and subsequent bleeding into the myocardium. Prior radiation therapy or extensive adriamycin therapy may predispose to this injury in children. Other reported cardiac complications include non-bacterial thrombotic endocarditis and catheter associated right-sided endocarditis,[136] hypertension both during marrow infusion[213] and after chemotherapy, perhaps mediated through atrial natriuretic factor.[81]

The use of high-dose agents has resulted in a variety of central nervous system complications, including organic brain syndrome from thiotepa[235] and etoposide,[122] infectious complications,[123] and Wernicke's like encephalopathy.[131]

Cutaneous toxicity is frequently noted during autologous bone marrow transplantation from drug allergies manifested as a variety of rashes, cutaneous toxicity of chemotherapy,[126] and also a macular erythematous eruption called host versus host syndrome or autologous graft versus host disease,[99] felt to be related to a type of graft versus host disease although the mechanism is unclear.

Future Directions

Current therapeutic interventions in neoplastic diseases using high-dose therapy and autologous bone marrow transplantation do not appear to have reached their limit. Colony stimulating factors and peripheral blood progenitor cells appear to offer the potential to further increase the dose intensity of treatment programs. It appears that major improvements in toxicity are possible and thus simplification of the treatment approach should yield a more cost effective treatment. The first efforts towards reducing the hospitalization required for this approach have been undertaken.[36]

Interpretation of the outcomes in most of the diseases in which autologous bone marrow transplantation is undertaken is hampered by the lack of randomized trial designs. Primary response and outcome variables are most frequently compared to historical or contemporary results. There is little information on the relative efficacy of various high-dose regimens. However, large controlled studies are hampered by the high cost of the procedure resulting in third-party reimbursement difficulty for patients receiving high-dose procedures. Considerable controversy remains regarding the importance, if any, of purging in all disease settings and resolution of this issue will require completion of randomized comparative trials.

Retroviral vector-mediated gene transfer into pluripotent stem cells uses autologous transplantation techniques and may extend the application of this treatment approach to other non-malignant settings. The technique remains limited due to difficulties of gene packaging and expression, although early clinical trials placing new genetic material into cytotoxic T-cells have been undertaken.

References

1. Ades, E. W., Peacocke, N., and Sabio, H.: Lymphokine-activated killer cell lysis of human neuroblastoma cells: a model for purging tumor cells from bone marrow. Clin. Immunol. Immunopathol., 46:150, 1988.
2. Agah, R., Malloy, B., Kerner, M., Girgis, E., Bean, P., Twomey, P., and Mazumder, A.: Potent graft antitumor effect in natural killer-resistant disseminated tumors by transplantation of interleukin 2-activated syngeneic bone marrow in mice. Cancer Res., 49:5959, 1989.
3. Agah, R., Malloy, B., Kerner, M., and Mazumder, A.: Generation and characterization of IL-2-activated bone marrow cells as a potent graft vs tumor effector in transplantation. J. Immunol., 143:3093, 1989.
4. Ahmed, T.: Autologous marrow transplantation for Hodgkin's disease: Current techniques and prospects. Cancer Invest., 8:99, 1990.
5. Ahmed, T., Ciavarella, D., Feldman, E., Ascensao, J., Hussain, F., Engelking, C., Gingrich, S., Mittelman, A., Coleman, M., and Arlin, Z. A.: High-dose, potentially myeloablative chemotherapy and autologous bone marrow transplantation for patients with advanced Hodgkin's disease. Leukemia, 3:19, 1989.
6. Allieri, M. A., Lopez, M., Douay, et al.: Instrinsic leukemic progenitor cell sensity to cryopreservation: Incidence for autologous bone marrow transplantation. In Autologous Bone Marrow Transplantation: Proceedings of the Fourth International Symposium. Edited by K. A. Dicke, G. Spitzer, and S. Jagannath. Houston, M. D. Anderson Hospital Publishers, 1988, pp. 35–39.
7. Anderson, I. C., Shpall, E. J., Leslie, D. S., Nustad, K., Ugelstad, J., Peters, W., and Bast, R. C., Jr.: Elimination of malignant clonogenic breast cancer cells from human bone marrow. Cancer Res., 49:4659, 1989.
8. Anderson, K. C., Ritz, J., Takvorian, T., Coral, F., Daley, H., Gorgone, B. C., Freedman, A. S., Canellos, G. P., Schlossman, S. F., and Nadler, L. M.: Hematologic engraftment and immune reconstitution post transplantation with anti-B1 purged autologous bone marrow. Blood, 69:597, 1987.
9. Anderson, K., Barut, B., Takvorian, T., Freedman, A., Mauch, P., Ritz, J., and Nadler, L.: Monoclonal antibody (MoAb) purged autologous bone marrow transplantation for multiple myeloma (MM) (Abstract). Blood, 74:202a, 1989.
10. Anderson, K. C., Barut, B. A., Ritz, J., Freedman, A. S., Takvorian, T., Rabinowe, S. N., Soiffer, R., Heflin, L., Coral, F., Dear, K., Mauch, P., and Nadler, L. M.: Monoclonal Antibody-Purged Autologous Bone Marrow Transplantation Therapy for Multiple Myeloma. Blood, 77:712, 1991.
11. Anderson, K. C., Soiffer, R., DeLage, R., Takvorian, T., Freedman, A. S., Rabinowe, S. L., Nadler, L. M., Dear, K., Heflin, L., Mauch, P., and Ritz, J.: T-cell-depleted autologous bone marrow transplantation therapy: Analysis of immune deficiency and late complications. Blood, 76:235, 1990.
12. Anonymous: The American Society of Clinical Oncology and American Society of Hematology Recommended Criteria for the Performance of Bone Marrow Transplantation. J. Clin. Oncol., 8:563, 1990.
13. Anonymous: Autologous bone marrow transplantation for advanced breast cancer. Medical Letter On Drugs & Therapeutics, 33:39, 1991.
14. Antman, K., Bearman, S. I., Davidson, N., et al.: Dose intensive therapy in breast cancer: Current status. In New Strategies in Bone Marrow Transplantation. Edited by R. P. Gale, and R. E. Champlin. New York, Alan R. Liss, 1990, pp. 423–436.
15. Antman, K., Eder, A., Elias, A., Ayash, L., Wheeler, C., Schnipper, L., and Frei, E., III: High dose cyclophosphamide, thiotepa, and carboplatin intensification with autologous bone marrow support in patients with breast cancer responding to standard dose induction therapy. Proc. Am. Soc. Clin. Oncol., 9:10(33a), 1991.
16. Antman, K. H.: G-CSF and GM-CSF in clinical trials. Yale Journal of Biology & Medicine, 63:387, 1990.
17. Appelbaum, F. R., Deisseroth, A. B., Graw, R. G., Jr., Herzig, G. P., Levine, A. S., Magrath, I. T., Pizzo, P. A., Poplack, D. G., and Ziegler, J. L.: Prolonged complete remission following high-dose chemotherapy of Burkett's lymphoma in relapse. Cancer, 41:1059, 1978.
18. Areman, E. M., Sacher, R. A., and Deeg, H. J.: Cryopreservation and storage of human bone marrow: A survey of current practices. In Bone Marrow Purging and Processing. Edited by S. Gross, A. P. Gee, and D. A. Worthington-White. Alan R. Liss, Inc., New York, New York, 1990, pp. 415–433.
19. Armitage, J. O., and Bearman, P. J.: Is there an optimal conditioning regimen for patients with lymphoma undergoing autologous bone marrow transplantation and autologous bone marrow transplantation? In Autologous Bone Marrow Transplantation: Proceedings of the Fourth International Symposium. Edited by K. A. Dicke, G. Spitzer, S. Jagganath, and M. J. Evinger-Hodges. Houston, M. D. Anderson Hospital Publishers, 1988, pp. 299–303.
20. August, C. S., and Auble, B.: Autologous bone marrow transplantation for advanced neuroblastoma at the Children's Hospital of Philadelphia: An Update. In Autologous Bone Marrow Transplantation: Proceedings of the Fourth International Symposium. Houston, M. D. Anderson Hospital Press, 1989, pp. 567–573.
21. Baglin, T. P., Harper, P., and Marcus, R. E.: Veno-occlusive disease of the liver complicating ABMT successfully treated with recombinant tissue plasminogen activator (rt-PA). Bone Marrow Transplant., 5:439, 1990.
22. Barbieri, L., Dinota, A., Gobbi, M., Tazzari, P. L., Rizzi, S., Bontadini, A., Lemoli, R. M., Tura, S., and Stirpe, F.: Immunotoxins containing saporin 6 and monoclonal antibodies recognizing plasma cell-associated antigens: Effects on target cells and on normal myeloid precursors (CFU-GM). Eur. J. Haematol., 42:238, 1989.
23. Barlogie, B., Hall, R., Zander, A., Dicke, K., and Alexanian, R.: High-dose melphalan with autologous bone marrow transplantation for multiple myeloma. Blood, 67:1298, 1986.
24. Barlogie, B., Alexanian, R., Smallwood, L., Cheson, B., Dixon, D., Dicke, K., and Cabanillas, F.: Prognostic factors with high dose melphalan for refractory multiple myeloma. Blood, 72:2015, 1988.
25. Barlogie, B., and Gahrton, G.: Bone marrow transplantation in multiple myeloma. Bone Marrow Transplantation, 7:71, 1991.
26. Bast, R. C., Sallen, R. E., Reynolds, C., et al.: Autologous bone marrow transplantation with CALLA positive ALL: Update. In Proceedings of the First International Symposium of Autologous Bone Marrow Transplantation. Edited by K. A. Dicke, G. Spitzer, A. Zander, et al. Houston, University of Texas, 1985, pp. 3–6.
27. Bell, A. J., Figes, A., Oscier, D. G., and Hamblin, T. J.: Peripheral blood stem cell autografting. Lancet, I:1027, 1986.
28. Berenson, R. J., Bensinger, W. I., Kalamasz, D., Schuening, F., Deeg, H. J., Graham, T., and Storb, R.: Engraftment of dogs with Ia-positive marrow cells isolated by avidinbiotin immunoadsorption. Blood, 69:1363, 1987.
29. Berenson, R. J., Andrews, R. G., Bensinger, W. I., Kalamasz, D., Knitter, G., Buckner, C. D., and Bernstein, I. D.: Antigen CD34 + marrow cells engraft lethally irradiated baboons. J. Clin. Invest., 81:951, 1988.
30. Berenson, R. J., Bensinger, W. I., Hill, R. S., Andrews, R. G., Garcia-Lopez, J., Kalamasz, D. F., Still, B. J., Spitzer, G., Buckner, C. D., Bernstein, I. D., and Thomas, E. D.: Engraftment after infusion of CD34 + marrow cells in patients with breast cancer or neuroblastoma. Blood, 77:1717, 1991.
31. Bieva, C. J., Vander Brugghen, F. J., and Stryckmans, P. A.: Malignant leukemic cell separation by iron colloid immunomagnetic adsorption. Exp. Hematol., 17:914, 1989.
32. Blaze, D., Gaspard, M. H., Stoppa, A. M., Michel, G., Gastaut, J. A., Lepeu, G., Tubiana, N., Blanc, A. P., Rossi, J. F., Novakovitch, G., Mannoni, P., Mawas, C., Maraninchi, D., and Caccassonne, Y.: Allogeneic or autologous bone marrow transplantation for acute lymphoblastic leukemia in first complete remission. Bone Marrow Transplant. 5:7, 1990.
33. Blazer, B. R., Widmer, M. B., Kersey, J. H., Ramsay, N. K., McGlave, P. B., Urdal, D. L., Gillis, S., Henney, C., and Vallera, D. A.: Recombinant granulocyte-macrophage colony stimulating factor in human and murine bone marrow transplantation. Behring Inst. Mitt., 83:170, 1988.
34. Blumenstock, D. A., Cannon, F. D., Hales, C. A., Vlahovic, V. L., Alpern, H., and Kazemi, H.: Pulmonary function of DLA-nonidentical lung allografts in dogs treated with lethal total-body irradiation, autologous bone marrow transplantation, and methotrexate. Transplantation, 28:223, 1979.
35. Brandt, S. J., Peters, W. P., Atwater, S. K., Kurtzberg, J., Borowitz, M. J., Jones, R. B., Shpall, E. J., Gilbert, C., Bast, R. C., Jr., and Oette, D. H.: Effect of recombinant human granulocyte-macrophage colony stimulating factor on hematopoietic recon-

stitution following high-dose chemotherapy and autologous bone marrow transplantation. N. Engl. J. Med., 318:869, 1988.

36. Brandwein, J. M., Callum, J., Rubinger, M., Scott, J. G., and Keating, A.: An evaluation of outpatient bone marrow harvesting. J. Clin. Oncol., 7:648, 1989.
37. Brandwein, J., Callum, J., Sutcliffe, S. B., Scott, J. G., and Keating, A.: The evaluation of cytoreductive therapy prior to high-dose treatment with autologous bone marrow transplantation, relapsed and refractory Hodgkin's disease. Bone Marrow Transplant., 5:99, 1990.
38. Brandwein, J. M., Nayar, R., Baker, M. A., Sutton, D. M., Scott, J. G., Sutcliffe, S. B., and Heating, A.: GM-CSF therapy for delayed engraftment after autologous bone marrow transplantation. Exp. Hematol., 19:191, 1991.
39. Bronchud, M. H., Howell, A., Crowther, D., Hopwood, P., Souza, L., and Dexter, T. M.: The use of granulocyte colony-stimulating factor to increase the intensity of treatment with doxorubicin in patients with advanced breast and ovarian cancer. Br. J. Cancer, 60:121, 1989.
40. Broun, E. R., Nichols, C. R., Tricot, G., Loehrer, P. J., Williams, S. D., and Einhorn, L. H.: High dose carboplatin/VP16 plus ifosfamide with autologous bone marrow support in the treatment of refractory germ cell tumors. Bone Marrow Transplant., 7:53, 1991.
41. Broxmeyer, H. E., Cooper, S., Lu, L., Hangoc, G., Anderson, D., Cosman, D., Lyman, S. D., and Williams, D. E.: Effect of murine mast cell growth factor (c-kit proto-oncogene ligand) on colony formation by human marrow hematopoietic progenitor cells. Blood, 77:2142, 1991.
42. Buckner, C. D., Fefer, A., Bensinger, W., Storb, R., Durie, B. G., Appelbaum, F. R., Petersen, F. B., Weiden, P., Clift, R. A., Sanders, J. E., Sullivan, K. M., Witherspoon, R. P., Hill, R., Martin, P., and Thomas, E. D.: Marrow transplantation for malignant plasma cell disorders: Summary of the Seattle experience. Eur. J. Hematol. Suppl., 43:186, 1989.
43. Canellos, G. P., Nadler, L., and Takvorian, T.: Autologous bone marrow transplantation in the treatment of malignant lymphoma and Hodgkin's disease. Semin. Hematol., 25:58, 1988.
44. Castaigne, S., Calvo, F., Douay, L., Thomas, F., Benbunan, M., Gerota, J., and Degos, L.: Successful haematopoietic reconstitution using autologous peripheral blood mononuclear cells in a patient with acute promyelocytic leukemia. Br. J. Hematol., 63:209, 1986.
45. Cavins, J. A., Kasakura, S., Thomas, E. D., and Ferrebee, J. W.: Recovery of lethally irradiated dogs following infusion of autologous marrow stored at low temperature in dimethylsulfoxide. Blood, 20:730, 1962.
46. Chang, J., Morgenstern, G. R., Coutinho, L. H., Scarffe, J. H., Carr, T., Deakin, D. P., Testa, N. G., and Dexter, T. M.: The use of bone marrow cells grown in long-term culture for autologous bone marrow transplantation in acute myeloid leukaemia: An update. Bone Marrow Transplant., 4:5, 1989.
47. Chang, J., Morgenstern, G. R., Testa, N. G., and Dexter, T. M.: Marrow grown in long-term culture can be used for autologous transplantation in the treatment of acute myeloid leukaemia. Folia Haematol. (Leipz.), 116:597, 1989.
48. Chao, N. J., Duncan, S. R., Long, G. D., Horning, S. J., and Blume, K. G.: Corticosteroid therapy for diffuse alveolar hemorrhage in autologous bone marrow transplant recipients. Ann. Intern. Med., 114:145, 1991.
49. Ciobanu, N., Bunowicz, C. D., Wiernik, P. H., Strauman, T., Sheridan, C., and Bast, R. C., Jr.: CA 125 levels in patients with ovarian carcinoma undergoing autologous bone marrow transplantation. Am. J. Obstet. Gynecol., 160:354, 1989.
50. Combaret, V., Favrot, M. C., Chauvin, F., Bouffet, E., Philip, I., and Philip, T.: Immunomagnetic depletion of malignant cells from autologous bone marrow graft: From experimental models to clinical trials. Journal of Immunogenet., 16:125, 1989.
51. Copeland, N. G., Gilbert, D. J., Cho, B. C., Donovan, P. J., Jenkins, N. A., Cosman, D., Anderson, D., Lyman, S. D., and Williams, D. E.: Mast cell growth factor maps near the steel locus on mouse chromosome 10 and is deleted in a number of steel alleles. Cell, 63:175, 1990.
52. Cornbleet, M. A., McElwain, T. J., Kuman, P. J., Filshie, J., Selby, P., Carter, R. L., Hedley, D. W., Clark, M. L., and Millar, J. L.: Treatment of advanced malignant melanoma with high-dose melphalan and autologous bone marrow transplantation. Br. J. Cancer, 48:329, 1983.
53. Coutinho, L. H., Testa, N. G., Chang, J., Morgenstern, G., Harrison, C., and Dexter, T. M.: The use of cultured bone marrow cells in autologous transplantation. *In* Bone Marrow Purging and Processing. Edited by S. Gross, A. P. Gee, and D. A. Worthington-White. New York, Alan R. Liss, 1990, pp. 415–433.
54. Dauplat, J., Legros, M., Condat, P., Ferriere, J. P., Ben Ahmed, S., and Plagne, R.: High-dose melphalan and autologous bone marrow support for treatment of ovarian carcinoma with positive second-look operation. Gynecol. Oncol., 34:294, 1989.
55. Davis, B. H., and Bigelow, N. C.: Flow cytometric reticulocyte quantification using thiazole orange provides clinically useful reticulocyte maturity index. Arch. Pathol. Lab. Med., 113:684, 1989.
56. Davis, J., Rowley, S. D., and Santos, G. W.: Toxicity of autologous bone marrow graft infusion. Prog. Clin. Biol. Res., 333:531, 1990.
57. De Fabritiis, P., Bregni, M., Lipton, J., Reynolds, C., Nadler, L., Ritz, J., and Bast, R. C., Jr.: Antigenic heterogeneity among Burkitt's lymphoma cells surviving treatment with monoclonal antibody and complement. Leuk. Res., 10:35, 1986.
58. De Fabritiis, P., Bregni, M., Lipton, J., Greenberger, J., Nadler, L., Rothstein, L., Korbling, M., Ritz, J., and Bast, R. C., Jr.: Elimination of clonogenic Burkitt's lymphoma cells from human bone marrow using 4-hydroperoxycyclophosphamide in combination with monoclonal antibodies and complement. Blood, 65:1064, 1985.
59. Douay, L., Gorin, N. C., Mary, J. Y., Lemarie, E., Lopez, M., Najman, A., Stachowiak, J., Giarratana, M. C., Baillou, C., Salmon, C., and Duhamel, G.: Recovery of CFU-GM from cryopreserved marrow and in vivo evaluation after autologous bone marrow transplantation are predictive of engraftment. Exp. Hematol., 14:358–365, 1986.
60. Dunphy, F. R., Spitzer, G., Buzdar, A. U., Hortobagyi, G. N., Horwitz, L. J., Yau, J. C., Spinolo, J. A., Jagannath, S., Holmes, F., Wallerstein, R. O., Bohannan, P. O., and Dicke, K. A.: Treatment of estrogen receptor-negative or hormonally refractory breast cancer with double high-dose chemotherapy intensification and bone marrow support. J. Clin. Oncol., 8:1207, 1990.
61. Dunphy, F.R., and Spitzer, G.: Long-term complete remission of stage IV breast cancer after high-dose chemotherapy and autologous bone marrow transplantation. Am. J. Clin. Oncol., 13:364, 1990.
62. Fermand, J. P., Levy, Y., Gerota, J., Benbunan, M., Cosset, J. M., Castaigne, S., Seligmann, M., and Brouet, J. C.: Treatment of aggressive multiple myeloma by high-dose chemotherapy and total body irradiation followed by blood stem cells autologous graft. Blood, 73:20, 1989.
63. Finley, J. L., August, C., Packer, R., Zimmerman, R., Sutton, L., Fried, A., Rorke, L., Bayever, E., Kamani, N., Kramer, E., Cohen, B., Sturgill, B., Nachman, J., Strandjord, S., Turski, P., Freirdich, S., Steeves, R., and Javid, M.: High-dose multi-agent chemotherapy followed by bone marrow "rescue" for malignant astrocytomas of childhood and adolescence. J. Neurooncol., 9:239, 1990.
64. Finn, G., and Denning, D.: Transient nephrogenic diabetes insipidus following high-dose cyclophosphamide chemotherapy and autologous bone marrow transplantation. Cancer Treat. Rep., 71:220, 1987.
65. Franzone, P., Scarpati, D., Vitale, V., Corvio, R., Barra, S., Guenzi, M., Orsatti, M., and Dini, G.: Chemo-radiotherapy and autologous bone marrow transplantation in poor prognosis neuroblastoma. Radiother. Oncol., 18:102, 1990.
66. Freedman, A. S., Takvorian, T., Anderson, K. C., Mauch, P., Rabinowe, S. N., Blake, K., Yeap, B., Soiffer, R., Coral, F., Heflin, L., Ritz, J., and Nadler, L. M.: Autologous bone marrow transplantation in B-cell non-Hodgkin's lymphoma: very low treatment-related mortality in 100 patients in sensitive relapse. J. Clin. Oncol., 8:784, 1990.
67. Frei, E., III, and Canellos, G. P.: Dose, a critical factor in cancer chemotherapy. Am. J. Med., 69:585, 1986.
68. Gale, R. P., Armitage, J. O., and Dicke, K. A.: Autotransplants: Now and in the future. Bone Marrow Transplant., 7:153, 1991.
69. Gianni, A. M., Siena, S., Bregni, M., Tarella, C., Stern, A. C., Pileri, A., and Bonadonna, G.: Granulocyte-macrophage colony-stimulating factor to harvest circulating haemopoietic stem cells for autotransplantation. Lancet, II:580, 1989.
70. Gianni, A. M., Bregni, M., Siena, S., Villa, S., Sciorelli, G. A., Ravagnani, F., Pellegris, G., and Bonadonna, G.: Rapid and complete hemopoietic reconstitution following combined transplantation of autologous blood and bone marrow cells. A changing role for high dose chemo-radiotherapy? Hematol. Oncol., 7:139, 1989.
71. Giannone, L., and Wolff, S. N.: Phase II treatment of central nervous system gliomas with high-dose etoposide and autologous bone marrow transplantation. Cancer Treat. Rep., 71:759, 1987.
72. Gobbi, M., Cavo, M., Tazzari, P. L., Dinota, A., Tassi, C., Bontadini, A., Albertazzi, L., Miggiano, C., Rizzi, S., Rosti, G., Bolognesi, A., Stirpe, F., and Tura, S.: Autologous bone marrow transplantation with immunotoxin-purged marrow for advanced multiple myeloma. Eur. J. Haematol., 43:176, 1989.
73. Goldie, J. H., and Goldman, A. J.: A mathematic model for relating the drug sensitivity of tumors to the spontaneous mutation rate. Cancer Treat. Rep., 63:1727, 1979.
74. Goldman, J. M., Catovsky, D., Hows, J., Spiers, A. S. D., and Galton, D. A. G.: Cryopreserved peripheral blood cells functioning as autografts in patients with chronic granulocytic leukemia in transformation. Brit. Med. J., 11:1310, 1979.
75. Goldstone, A. H., and Gribben, J. G.: The role of autologous bone marrow transplantation in the treatment of malignant disease. Blood Rev., 1:193, 1987.
76. Gore, M. E., Selby, P. J., Viner, C., Clark, P. I., Meldrum, M., Millar, B., Bell, J., Maitland, J. A., Milan, S., Judson, I. R., Zuiable, A., Tillyer, C., Slevin, M., Malpas, J. S., and McElwain, T. J.: Intensive treatment of multiple myeloma and criteria for complete remission. Lancet, 2:879, 1989.
77. Gorin, N. C., Aegerter, P., Auvert, B., Meloni, G., Goldstone, A. H., Burnett, A., Carella, A., Korbling, M., Herve, P., Maraninchi, D., Löwenberg, R., Verdonck, L. F., de Planque, M., Hermans, J., Helbig, W., Porcellini, A., Rizzoli, V., Alesandrino, E. P., Franklin, I. M., Reiffers, J., Colleselli, P., and Goldman, J. M.: Autologous bone marrow transplantation for acute myelocytic leukemia in first remission: A European survey of the role of marrow purging. Blood, 75:1606, 1990.
78. Gorin, N. C., Herve, P., Aegerter, P., Goldstone, A., Linch, D., Maraninchi, D., Burnett, A., Helbig, W., Meloni, G., Verdonck, L. F., De Witte, T., Rizzoli, V., Carella, A., Parlier, Y., Auvert, B., and Goldman, J.: Autologous bone marrow transplantation for acute leukemia in remission. Brit. J. Haematol., 64:385, 1986.
79. Gorin, N. C., Caegerter, P., and Auvert, B.: Autologous bone marrow transplantation for acute leukemia in remission: An analysis of 1322 cases. Bone Marrow Transplant., 4:3, 1989.
80. Graeve, J.L., de Alarcon, P. A., Sato, Y., Pringle, K., and Helson, L.: Miliary pulmonary neuroblastoma. A risk of autologous bone marrow transplantation? Cancer, 62:2125, 1988.
81. Graves, S. W., Eder, J. P., Schryber, S. M., Sharma, K., Brena, A., Antman, K. H., and Peters, W. P.: Endogenous digoxin-like immunoreactive factor and digitalis-like factor associated with the hypertension of patients receiving multiple alkylating agents as part of autologous bone marrow transplantation. Clin. Sci., 77:501, 1989.
82. Gribben, J. G., Goldstone, A. H., Linch, D. C., Taghipour, G., McMillan, A. K., Souhami, R. L., Earl, H., and Richard, J. D.: Effectiveness of high-dose combination chemotherapy and autologous bone marrow transplantation for patients with non-Hodgkin's lymphomas who are still responsive to conventional-dose therapy. J. Clin. Oncol., 7:1621, 1989.
83. Gribben, J. G., Lynch, D. C., Singerl, C. R., McMillan, A. K., Jarrett, M., and Goldstone, A. H.: Successful Treatment of Refractory Hodgkin's Disease by High-Dose Combination Chemotherapy and Autologous Bone Marrow Transplantation. Blood, 73:340, 1989.
84. Gribben, J. G., Goldstone, A. H., and Linch, D. C.: Preliminary results of autologous bone marrow transplantation in the management of resistant Hodgkin's disease: Experience of the Bloomsbury Transplant Group at University College, London. Recent Results Cancer Res., 117:242, 1989.
85. Guinan, E. C., Tarbell, N. J., Niemeyer, C. M., Sallan, S. E., and Weinstein, H. J.: Intravascular hemolysis and renal insufficiency after bone marrow transplantation. Blood, 72:451, 1988.
86. Gulati, S., Shank, B., Yahalom, J., et al.: Autologous BMT for patients with poor-prognosis lymphoma and Hodgkin's disease. *In* Autologous Bone Marrow Transplantation: Proceedings of the Fourth International Symposium. Edited by K. A. Dicke, G. Spitzer, and S. Jagannath. Houston, M. D. Anderson Hospital Publishers, 1988, pp. 231-239.
87. Hanes, M. A., Goldman, J. M., Worsley, A. M., McCarthy, D. M., Wyeth, S. E., Dowding, C., Kerney, L., Th'ng, K. H., Wareham, N. H., Pollock, A., Galvin, M. C., Samson, D., Geary, C. G., Davotsky, D., and Dalton, D. A. G.: Chemotherapy and autografting for chronic granulocytic leukemia in transformation, probable prolongation of survival for some patients. Brit. J. Hematol., 58:711, 1984.
88. Hartmann, D. W., Robinson, W. A., Morton, N. J., Mangalik, A., and Glode, L. M.:

High-dose nitrogen mustard (HN2) with autologous nonfrozen bone marrow transplantation in advanced malignant melanoma. A phase I trial. Blut, 42:209, 1981.
89. Hershko, C., Ho, W. G., Gale, R. P., and Cline, M. J.: Cure of aplastic anemia in paroxysmal nocturnal haemoglobinuria by marrow transfusion from identical twins: Failure of peripheral-leukocyte transfusion to correct marrow aplasia. Lancet, I:945, 1979.
90. Herzig, G.: Autologous Marrow Transplantation in Cancer Therapy. *In* Progress in Hematology. Edited by E. B. Brown. New York, Grune & Stratton, 1981, pp. 1–23.
91. Higuchi, C. M., Thompson, J. A., Cox, T., Lindgren, C. G., Buckner, C. D., and Fefer, A.: Lymphokine-activated killer function following autologous bone marrow transplantation for refractory hematological malignancies. Cancer Res., 49:5509, 1989.
92. Hortobagyi, G. N.: The role of high-dose chemotherapy with autologous bone marrow transplantation in the treatment of breast cancer. Bone Marrow Transplant., 3:525, 1988.
93. Hortobagyi, G. N., Dunphy, F., Buzdar, A. U., and Spitzer, G.: Dose intensity studies in breast cancer—autologous bone marrow transplantation. Prog. Clin. Biol. Res., 354:195, 1990.
94. Humblet, Y., Symann, M., Bosly, A., Delaunois, L., Francis, C., Machiels, J., Beauduin, M., Doyen, C., Weynants, P., Longueville, J., and Prignot, J.: Late intensification chemotherapy with autologous bone marrow transplantation in selected small-cell carcinoma of the lung: A randomized study. J. Clin. Oncol., 5:1864, 1987.
95. Jagannath, S., Armitage, J. O., Dicke, K. A., Tucker, S. L., Valasquez, W. S., Smith, K., Vaughan, W. P., Kessinger, A., Horwitz, L. J., Hagemeister, F. B., Cabanillas, F., and Spitzer, G.: Timing of High Dose CBV and Autologous Bone Marrow Transplantation in the Management of Relapsed or Refractory Hodgkin's Disease. *In* Autologous Bone Marrow Transplantation, Proceedings of the Fourth International Symposium. Edited by K. A. Dicke, G. Spitzer, and S. Jagannath. Houston, M. D. Anderson Hospital Publishers, 1988, pp. 275–283.
96. Jagannath, S., Barlogie, B., Dicke, K., Alexarian, R., Zagars, C., Cheson, B., Lemaistre, F. C., Smallwood, L., Pruitt, K., and Dixon, D. O.: Autologous bone marrow transplantation in multiple myeloma: Identification of prognostic factors. Blood. 76:1860, 1990.
97. Jochelson, M., Tarbell, N. J., Freedman, A. S., Rabinowe, S. N., Takvorian, T., Soiffer, R., Anderson, K., Ritz, J., and Nadler, L. M.: Acute and chronic pulmonary complications following autologous bone marrow transplantation in non-Hodgkin's lymphoma. Bone Marrow Transplant., 6:329, 1990.
98. Johnson, D. B., Thompson, J. M., Corwin, J. A., Mosley, K. R., Smith, M. T., de los Reyes, R. A., Daly, M. B., Petty, A. M., Lamaster, D., Pierson, W. P., Ruxer, R. L., Jr., Leff, R. S., and Messerschmidt, G. L.: Prolongation of survival for high-grade malignant gliomas with adjuvant high-dose BCNU and autologous bone marrow transplantation. J. Clin. Oncol., 5:783, 1987.
99. Jones, R. J., Vogelsang, G. B., Hess, A. D., Farmer, E. R., Mann, R. B., Geller, R. B., Piantadosi, S., and Santos, G. W.: Induction of graft-versus-host disease after autologous bone marrow transplantation. Lancet, I:754, 1989.
100. Juttner, C. A., To, L. B., Haylock, D. N., and Dyson, P. G.: Peripheral Blood Stem Cell Selection, Collection and Autotransplantation. *In* Bone Marrow Purging and Processing. Edited by S. Gross, A. P. Gee, and D. A. Worthington-White. New York, Alan R. Liss, Inc., 1990, pp. 447–460.
101. Kemshead, J. T., and Black, J.: Developments in the biology of neuroblastoma: Implications for diagnosis and treatment. Dev. Med. Child. Neurol., 22:816, 1980.
102. Kemshead, J. T., Walsh, F., Pritchard, J., and Greaves, M.: Monoclonal antibody to ganglioside GQ discriminates between haemopoietic cells and infiltrating neuroblastoma tumour cells in bone marrow. Int. J. Cancer, 27:447, 1981.
103. Keng, P. C., Rubin, P., Constine, L. S., Frantz, C., Nakissa, N., and Gregory, P.: Characterization of the biophysical properties of human tumor and bone marrow cells as a preliminary step to the use of centrifugal elutriation in autologous bone marrow transplantation. Int. J. Radiat. Oncol. Biol. Phys., 10:1913, 1984.
104. Kersey, J. H., Weisdorf, D., Nevitt, M. E., LeBien, T. W., Woods, W. G., McLave, P. B., Kim, T., Vallera, D. A., Goldman, A. I., Bostrom, B., Perd, D., Ramsey, N.: Comparison of autologous and allogeneic bone marrow transplantation for treatment of high-risk refractory acute lymphoblastic leukemia. N. Engl. J. Med., 317:461, 1987.
105. Kessinger, A., and Armitage, J. O.: Harvesting marrow for autologous transplantation from patients with malignancies. Bone Marrow Transplant., 2:15, 1987.
106. Kessinger, A., Armitage, J. O., Smith, D. M., Landmark, J. D., Bierman, P. J., and Weisenburger, D. D.: High-dose therapy and autologous peripheral blood stem cell transplantation for patients with lymphoma. Blood, 74:1260, 1989.
107. Kessinger, A., Armitage, J. O., Landmark, J. D., and Weisenburger, D. D.: Reconstitution of human hematopoietic function with autologous cryopreserved circulating stem cells. Exp. Hematol., 114:192, 1986.
108. Kessinger, A., Bierman, P., and Armitage, J.: Refractory intermediate grade non-Hodgkin's lymphoma (NHL) treated with high dose therapy and autologous peripheral stem cell transplantation (PSCT): Response and survival. Proc. ASCO, 9:255, 1990.
109. Kessinger, A.: High-dose chemotherapy with autologous marrow transplantation for malignant melanoma. Case reports and literature review. J. Am. Acad. Dermatol., 12:337, 1985.
110. Kessinger, A.: High dose chemotherapy with autologous bone marrow rescue for high grade gliomas of the brain: A potential for improvement in therapeutic results. Neurosurgery, 15:747, 1984.
111. Korbling, M., Fliedner, T. M., Calvo, W., Ross, W. M., Northdurft, W., and Steinbach, I.: Albumin density gradient purification of canine hematopoietic stem cells (HBSC): Long-term allogeneic engraftment without graft vs. host reaction. Exp. Hematol., 7:277, 1979.
112. Korbling, M., Dorken, B., Ho, A. D., Pezzutto, A., Hunsttein, W., and Gliedner, T. M.: Autologous transplantation of blood-derived hemopoeitic stem cells after myeloablative therapy in a patient with Burkitt's lymphoma. Blood, 67:529, 1986.
113. Korbling, M., Martin, H., and Gliedner, T. M.: Autologous blood stem cell transplantation. *In* Proceedings of the Keystone Meeting on Bone Marrow Transplantation. Edited by R. P. Gale, and R. E. Champlin. New York, Alan R. Liss, 1986, pp. 1–12.
114. Korbling, M., Hess, A. D., Tutschka, P. J., Kaizer, H., Colvin, M. O., and Santos, G. W.: 4-hydroperoxycyclophosphamide: A model for eliminating residual human tumour cells and T-lymphocytes from the bone marrow graft. Br. J. Haematol., 52:89, 1982.
115. Korbling, M., Burke, P., Braine, H., Elfenbein, G., Santos, G., and Kaizer, H.: Successful engraftment of blood-derived hemopoeitic stem cells in chronic myelogenous leukemia. Exp. Hematol., 9:684, 1981.
116. Kubel, M., Helbig, W., Schwenke, H., Wotzel, M., Thierbach, V., Standke, E., and Hoffmann, F. A.: Autologous bone marrow transplantation (ABMT) using unpurged marrow as intensification for first complete remission in acute leukaemia (AL). Folia. Haematol. (Leipz.), 116:493, 1989.
117. Kushner, B. H., O'Reilly, R. J., Mandell, L. R., Gulati, S. C., LaQuaglia, M., and Cheung, N. K.: Myeloablative combination chemotherapy without total body irradiation for neuroblastoma. J. Clin. Oncol., 9:274, 1991.
118. Kvalheim, G., Fodstad, O., Pihl, A., Nustad, K., Pharo, A, Ugelstad, J., and Funderud, S.: Elimination of B-lymphoma cells from human bone marrow: Model experiments using monodisperse magnetic particles coated with primary monoclonal antibodies. Cancer Res., 47:846, 1987.
119. Lakhani, S., Selby, P., Bliss, J. M., Perren, T. J., Gore, M. E., and McElwain, T. J.: Chemotherapy for malignant melanoma: Combinations and high doses produce more responses without survival benefit. Brit. J. Cancer, 61:330, 1990.
120. Lanino, E., Melodia, A., Casalaro, A., Cornaglia-Gerraris, P.: Neuroblastoma cells circulate in peripheral blood. Ped. Hematol. Oncol., 6:193, 1989.
121. Lazarus, H. M., Herzig, R. H., Wolff, S. N., Phillips, G. L., Spitzer, T. R., Fay, J. W., and Herzig, G. P.: Treatment of metastatic malignant melanoma with intensive melphalan and autologous bone marrow transplantation. Cancer Treat. Rep., 69:473, 1985.
122. Leff, R. S., Thompson, J. M., Daly, M. B., Johnson, D. B., Harden, E. A., Mercier, R. J., and Messerschmidt, G. L.: Acute neurologic dysfunction after high-dose etoposide therapy for malignant glioma. Cancer, 62:32, 1988.
123. Leff, R. S., Martino, R. L., Pollock, W. J., and Knight, W. A., III: Pituitary abscess after autologous bone marrow transplantation. Am. J. Hematol., 31:62, 1989.
124. Levy, J., Wodell, R. A., August, C. S., and Bayever, E.: Adenovirus-related hemophagocytic syndrome after bone marrow transplantation. Bone Marrow Transplant., 6:349, 1990.
125. Leibo, S. P., Farrant, J., Mazur, P., Hanna, M. G., Jr., and Smith, L. H.: Effects of freezing on marrow stem cell suspension: Interaction of cooling and warming rates in the presence of PVP, sucrose, or glycerol. Cryobiology, 6:315, 1970.
126. Linassier, C., Colombat, P., Reisenleiter, M., Haillot, O., Chazard, M., Binet, C., Desbois, I., and Lamagnere, J. P.: Cutaneous toxicity of autologous bone marrow transplantation in nonseminomatous germ cell tumors. Cancer, 65:1143, 1990.
127. Litam, J. P., Dail, D. H., Spitzer, G., Vellekoop, L., Verma, D. S., Zander, A. R., and Dicke, K. A.: Early pulmonary toxicity after administration of high-dose BCNU. Cancer Treat. Rep., 65:39, 1981.
128. Litzow, M. R., Peterson, F. B., Appelbaum, F. R., and Buckner, C. D.: Autologous versus allogeneic bone marrow transplantation (BMT) for Hodgkin's disease. Blood, 76:550a, 1990.
129. Long, G. S., Cramer, D. V., Harnaha, J. B., and Hiserodt, J. C.: Lymphokine-activated killer (LAK) cell purging of leukemic bone marrow: Range of activity against different hematopoietic neoplasms. Bone Marrow Transplant., 6:169, 1990.
130. Lopez, M., Zucker, J. M., Urresola, R., Douay, L., Quintana, E., Kemshead, J., Gorin, N. C., and Vilcoq, J. R.: Influence of single and double immunomagnetic depletion on the hemopoietic capacity of marrow in patients with advanced neuroblastoma submitted to autologous bone marrow transplantation. Bone Marrow Transplant., 2:413, 1987.
131. Majolino, I., Caponetto, A., Scimie, R., Vasta, S., Fabbiano, F., and Caronia, F.: Wernicke-like encephalopathy after autologous bone marrow transplantation. Haematologica, 75:282, 1990.
132. Mangan, K. F., Boucek, C., Powers, D., and Shadduck, R. K.: Rapid detection of venous air embolism by mass spectrometry during bone marrow harvesting. Exp. Hematol., 13:639, 1985.
133. Marcus, R. B., Jr., Graham Pole, J. R., Springfield, D. S., Fort, J. A., Gross, S., Mendenhall, N. P., Elfenbein, G. J., Weiner, R. S., Enneking, W. F., and Million, R. R.: High-risk Ewing's sarcoma: End-intensification using autologous bone marrow transplantation. Int. J. Radiat. Oncol. Biol. Phys., 15:53, 1988.
134. Marder, R. J., Winter, J., and Epstein, A.: Heterogeneity of phenotypic expression in normal and neoplastic B-cell proliferations detected by monoclonal antibodies LN-1 and DLC-48. Am. J. Clin. Pathol., 90:149, 1988.
135. Martini, E., Gorin, N. C., Gastal, C., Doinel, C., Roquin, H., Najman, A., and Salmon, C.: Disappearance of CD4 lymphocyte circadian cycles after autologous bone marrow transplantation. Biomed. Pharmacother., 42:357, 1988.
136. Martino, P., Micozzi, A., Venditti, M., Gentile, G., Girmenia, C., Raccah, R., Santilli, S., Alessandri, N., and Mandelli, F.: Catheter-related right-sided endocarditis in bone marrow transplant recipients. Rev. Infec. Dis., 12:250, 1990.
137. Matsuishi, E., Anzai, K., Dohmen, K., Taniguchi, S., Gondo, H., Kudo, J., Shibuya, T., Ishibashi, H., Harada, M., and Niho, Y.: Sonographic diagnosis of venocclusive disease of the liver and danazol therapy for autoimmune thrombocytopenia in an autologous marrow transplant patient. Jpn. J. Clin. Oncol., 20:188, 1990.
138. Mbidde, E. K., Selby, P. J., Perren, T. J., Dearnaley, D. P., Whitton, A., Ashley, S., Workman, P., Bloom, H. J., and McElwain, T. J.: High dose BCNU chemotherapy with autologous bone marrow transplantation and full dose radiotherapy for grade IV astrocytoma. Br. J. Cancer, 58:779, 1988.
139. McGuire, W. L., Herzig, R. H., Lemaistre, C. F., and Peters, W. P.: Autologous bone marrow transplantation in breast cancer. A panel discussion. Breast Cancer Res. Treat., 11:7, 1988.
140. Meagher, R. C., Rothman, S. A., Paul, P., Koberna, P., Willmer, C., and Baucco, P. A.: Purging of small cell lung cancer cells from human bone marrow using ethiofos (WR-2721) and light-activated merocyanine 540 phototreatment. Cancer Res., 49:3637, 1989.
141. Mick, R., Begg, C. B., Antman, K. H., Korzun, A. H., and Frei, E., III: Diverse prognosis in metastatic breast cancer: Who should be offered alternative initial therapies? Breast Cancer Res. Treat., 13:33, 1989.
142. Micklem, H. S., Anderson, N., and Ross, E.: Limited potential circulating hematopoietic stem cells. Nature, 256:41, 1975.
143. Minegishi, N., Minegishi, M., Tuchiya, S., and Konno, T.: Preservation of immature hematopoietic progenitor cells responding to interleukin 3 in marrow treated with 4-hydroperoxycyclophosphamide. Tohoku J. Exp. Med., 159:113, 1989.
144. Mitchell, R. B., Wagner, J. E., Karp, J. E., Watson, A. J., Brusilow, S. W., Przepiorka, D., Storb, R., Santos, G. W., Burke, P. J., and Saral, R.: Syndrome of idiopathic hyperammonemia after high-dose chemotherapy: Review of nine cases. Am. J. Med., 85:662, 1988.

145. Montgomery, R. B., Kurtzberg, J., Rhinehardt-Clark, A., Haleen, A., Ramakrishnan, S., Olsen, G. A., Peters, W. P., Smith, C. A., Haynes, B. F., Houston, L. L., and Bast, R. C., Jr.: Elimination of malignant clonogenic T cells from human bone marrow using chemoimmunoseparation with 2'-deoxycoformycin, deoxyadenosine and an immunotoxin. Bone Marrow Transplant., 5:395, 1990.
146. Moss, T. J., Sanders, D. G., Lasky, L. C., and Bostrom, B.: Contamination of peripheral blood stem cell harvests by circulating neuroblastoma cells. Blood, 76:1879, 1990.
147. Moss, T. J., and Sanders, D. G.: Detection of neuroblastoma cells in blood. J. Clin. Oncol., 8:736, 1990.
148. Mulder, P. O., Meinesz, A. F., deVries, E. G., and Mulder, N. H.: Diffuse alveolar hemorrhage in autologous bone marrow transplant recipients [letter]. Am. J. Med., 90:278, 1991.
149. Mulder, P. O., Willemse, P. H., Aalders, J. G., deVries, E. G., Sleijfer, D. T., Sibinga, C. T., and Mulder, N. H.: High-dose chemotherapy with autologous bone marrow transplantation in patients with refractory ovarian cancer. Eur. J. Cancer Clin. Oncol., 25:645, 1989.
150. Mulder, P. O., Schroder, P., deVries, E. G., Hospers, H. G., van der Geest, S., Sleijfer, D. T., and Mulder, N. H.: Incidence and effects of herpes simplex virus infection after autologous bone marrow transplantation for solid tumours. Neth. J. Med., 34:126, 1989.
151. Myers, D. E., Uckun, F. M., Ball, E. D., and Vallera, D. A.: Immunotoxins for ex vivo marrow purging in autologous bone marrow transplantation for acute nonlymphocytic leukemia. Transplantation, 46:240, 1988.
152. Nadler, L. M., Takvorian, T., Botnick, L., Bast, R. C., Finberg, R., Hellman, S., Canellos, G. P., and Schlossman, S. F.: Anti-B1 monoclonal antibody and complement treatment in autologous bone-marrow transplantation for relapsed B-cell non-Hodgkin's lymphoma. Lancet, II:427, 1984.
153. Nakagawa, H., Murasawa, A., Taki, T., Nakajima, S., Niiyama, K., Furuta, Y., Nakamura, H., Shibata, H., and Masaoka, T.: Treatment of malignant gliomas with high-dose ACNU and autologous bone marrow transplantation [Jpn]. Gan To Kagaku Ryoho, 15:3153, 1988.
154. NIchols, C. R., Tricot, G., Williams, S. D., van Besien, K., Loehrer, P. J., Roth, B. J., Akard, L., Hoffman, R., Goulet, R., Wolff, S. N., Giannone, L., Greer, J., Einhorn, L. H., and Jansen, J.: Dose-intensive chemotherapy in refractory germ cell cancer: A phase I/II trial of high dose carboplatin and etoposide with autologous bone marrow transplantation. J. Clin. Oncol., 7:932, 1989.
155. Nomura, K., Watanabe, T., Nakamura, O., Ohira, M., Shibui, S., Takakura, K., and Miki, Y.: Intensive chemotherapy with autologous bone marrow rescue for recurrent malignant gliomas. Neurosurg. Rev., 7:13, 1984.
156. Nor'es, J. M., Dalayeun, J. F., Otmezguine, Y., Folgoas, C., and Nenna, A. D.: High-dose chemotherapy, total abdomen irradiation and autologous bone marrow infusion in ovarian cancer: An observation. Gynecol. Obstet. Ivest., 27:55, 1989.
157. Norton, L., and Simon, R.: Tumor size, sensitivity to therapy, and the design of treatment schedules. Cancer Treat. Rep., 61:1307, 1977.
158. Norton, L., and Simon, R.: The Norton-Simon hypothesis revisted. Cancer Treat. Rep., 70:163, 1986.
159. Norton, L., and Day, R.: Potential Innovation in Scheduling of Cancer Chemotherapy. *In* Important Advances in Oncology. Edited by V. T. DeVita, S. Hellman, and S. A. Rosenberg. Philadelphia, J. B. Lippincott Co., 1991, pp. 57–72.
160. Olsen, G. A., Gockerman, J. P., Bast, R. C., Jr., Borowitz, M., and Peters, W. P.: Altered immunologic reconstitution after standard-dose chemotherapy or high-dose chemotherapy with autologous bone marrow support. Transplantation, 46:57, 1988.
161. Panella, T. J., Peters, W., White, J. G., Hannun, Y. A., and Greenberg, C. S.: Platelets acquire a secretion defect after high-dose chemotherapy. Cancer, 65:1711, 1990.
162. Pcio, J. L., Droz, J. P., Ostronoff, M., et al.: High dose chemotherapy and autologous bone marrow transplantation for poor prognosis non-seminomatous germ cell tumors. *In* Autologous Bone Marrow Transplantation: Proceedings of the Fourth International Symposium. Houston, M. D. Anderson, 1989, pp. 469–476.
163. Pecego, R., Hill, R., Appelbaum, F. R., Amos, D., Buckner, C. D., Fefer, A., and Thomas, E. D.: Interstitial pneumonitis following autologous bone marrow transplantation. Transplantation, 42:515, 1986.
164. Pedrazzini, A., Freedman, A. S., Andersen, J., Heflin, L., Anderson, K., Takvorian, T., Canellos, G. P., Whitman, J., Coral, F., Ritz, J., and Nadler, L. M.: Anti-B-cell monoclonal antibody-purged autologous bone marrow transplantation for B-cell non-Hodgkin's lymphoma: Phenotypic reconstitution and B-cell function. Blood, 74:2203, 1989.
165. Peters, W. P.: Dose Intensification Using High-Dose Combination Alkylating Agents and Autologous Bone Marrow Support in the Treatment of Primary and Metastatic Breast Cancer: A Review of the Duke Bone Marrow Transplantation Program Experience. *In* High-Risk Breast Cancer. Edited by J. Ragaz, and I. M. Ariel. Berlin, Springer-Verlag, 1991, pp. 437–446.
166. Peters, W. P.: Dose intensification using combination alkylating agents and autologous bone marrow support in the treatment of primary and metastatic breast cancer: A review of the Duke Bone Marrow Transplantation Program experience. Prog. Clin. Biol. Res., 354·185, 1990.
167. Peters, W. P., Shpall, E. J., Jones, R. B., Olsen, G. A., Gockerman, J. P., Bast, R. C., and Moore, J. O.: High dose combination alkylating agents with bone marrow support as initial treatment for metastatic breast cancer. J. Clin. Oncol., 6:1368, 1988.
168. Peters, W. P., Shpall, E. J., Jones, R. B., and Ross, M.: High dose combination cyclophosphamide, cisplatin, and carmustine with bone marrow support as initial treatment for metastatic breast cancer: Three to six year follow-up. Proc. Am. Soc. Clin. Oncol., 9:10a, 1990.
169. Peters, W. P., Jones, R. B., Shpall, E. J., Gockerman, J., Kurtzberg, J., et al.: Strategies in the treatment of breast cancer with intensive chemotherapy and autologous bone marrow support. *In* Autologous Bone Marrow Transplantation: Proceedings of the Fourth International Symposium. Edited by K. A. Dicke, G. Spitzer, and S. Jagannath. Houston, M. D. Anderson Hospital Press, 1987, pp. 465–474.
170. Peters, W. P., Davis, R., Shpall, E. J., Jones, R., Ross, M., Marks, L., Norton, L., and Hurd, D.: Adjuvant chemotherapy involving high dose combination cyclophosphamide, cisplatin and carmustine, and autologous bone marrow support for stage II/III breast cancer involving ten or more lymph nodes (CALGB 8782): A preliminary report. Proc. Am. Soc. Clin. Oncol., 9:22(80a), 1990.
171. Peters, W. P.: High-Dose Chemotherapy and Autologous Bone Marrow Support for Breast Cancer. *In* Important Advances in Oncology, 1991. Edited by V. T. DeVita, S. Hellman, and S. A. Rosenberg. Philadelphia, J. B. Lippincott, 1991, pp. 135–150.
172. Peters, W. P., Kurtzberg, J., Atwater, S., Borowitz, M., Gilbert, C., Rao, M., Currie, M., Shogan, J., Jones, R. B., Shpall, E. J., and Souza, L.: Comparative effects of rHuG-CSF and rHuGM-CSF on hematopoietic reconstitution and granulocyte function following high dose chemotherapy and autologous bone marrow transplantation (ABMT). Blood, 71:130a, 1988.
173. Peters, W. P., Kurtzberg, J., Kirkpatrick, G., Atwater, S., Gilbert, C., Borowitz, M., Shpall, E., Jones, R., Ross, M., Affronti, M., Coniglio, D., Mathias, B., and Oette, D.: GM-CSF primed peripheral blood progenitor cells (PBPC) coupled with autologous bone marrow transplantation (ABMT) will eliminate absolute leukopenia following high dose chemotherapy (HDC). Blood, 74:178, 1989.
174. Philip, T., Armitage, O., Spitzer, G., Chauvin, F., Jagannath, S., Cahn, J. Y., Colombat, P., Goldstone, A. H., Gorin, N. C., Flesh, M., Laporte, J. P., Maraninchi, D., Pico, J., Bosly, A., Anderson, C., Schots, R., Biron, P., Cabanillas, F., and Dicke, K.: High Dose Therapy and Autologous Bone Marrow Transplantation after Failure of Conventional Chemotherapy in Adults with Intermediate-Grade or High-Grade Non-Hodgkin's Lymphoma. N. Engl. J. Med., 316:1493, 1987.
175. Philip, T., Bernard, J. L., Zucker, J. M., Pinkerton, R., Lutz, P., Bordigoni, P., Plouvier, E., Robert, A., Carton, R., Philippe, N., Philip, I., Chauvin, F., and Favrot, M.: High-dose chemoradiotherapy with bone marrow transplantation as consolidation treatment in neuroblastoma: An unselected group of stage IV patients over 1 year of age. J. Clin. Oncol., 5:266, 1987.
176. Philip, T., Bernard, J. L., Zucker, J. M., Souillet, G., Favrot, M., Philip, I., Bordigoni, P., Lutz, J. P., Plouvier, E., Carton, P., Robert, A., and Kemshead, J.: Purged autologous bone marrow transplantation in 25 cases of very poor prognosis neuroblastoma [letter]. Lancet, I:576, 1985.
177. Pinkerton, C. R., Hartmann, O., Dini, G., and Philip, T.: High dose chemo-radiotherapy with bone marrow rescue in stage IV neuroblastoma: EBMT Survey, 1988. *In* Autologous Bone Marrow Transplantation: Proceedings of the Fourth International Symposium. Edited by K. A. Dicke, G. Spitzer, S. Jagganath, and M. J. Evinger-Hodges. Houston, M. D. Anderson Hospital Press, 1989, pp. 543–548.
178. Pole, J. G., Gee, A., Janssen, W., Lee, C., and Gross, S.: Immunomagnetic purging of bone marrow: A model for negative cell selection. Am. J. Pediatr. Hematol. Oncol., 12:257, 1990.
179. Preijers, F. W., De Witte, T., Wessels, J. M., De Gast, G. C., Van Leeuwen, E., Capel, P. J., and Haanen, C.: Autologous transplantation of bone marrow purged in vitro with anti-CD7-(WT1-) ricin A immunotoxin in T-cell lymphoblastic leukemia and lymphoma. Blood, 74:1152, 1989.
180. Ramakrishnan, S., Uckun, F. M., and Houston, L. L.: Anti-T cell immunotoxins containing pokeweed anti-viral protein: Potential purging agents for human autologous bone marrow transplantation. J. Immunol., 135:3616, 1985.
181. Reece, D. E., Barnett, M. J., Connors, J. M., Klingemann, H. G., O'Reilly, S. E., Shepherd, J. D., and Phillips, G. L.: Intensive therapy with busulfan, cyclophosphamide and melphalan (bucy + mel) and 4-hydroperoxycyclophosphamide (4HC) purged autologous bone marrow transplantation (AUTOBMT) for multiple myeloma (MM) (Abstract). Blood, 74:754a, 1989.
182. Reiffers, J., Bernard, P., David, B., Vezon, G., Sarrat, A., Marit, G., Moulinier, J., and Broustet, A.: Successful autologous transplantation with peripheral blood hemopoietic cells in a patient with acute leukemia. Exp. Hematol., 114:312, 1986.
183. Reiffers, J., Marit, G., and Boiron, J. M.: Autologous blood stem cell transplantation in high-risk multiple myeloma. Br. J. Hematol., 72:296, 1989.
184. Reisner, Y.: Differential agglutination by soybean agglutinin of human leukemia and neuroblastoma cell lines: Potential application to autologous bone marrow transplantation. Proc. Natl. Acad. Sci. U.S.A., 80:6657, 1983.
185. Reusser, P., Fisher, L. D., Buckner, C. D., Thomas, E. D., and Meyers, J. D.: Cytomegalovirus infection after autologous bone marrow transplantation: Occurrence of cytomegalovirus disease and effect on engraftment. Blood, 75:1888, 1990.
186. Ritz, J., Sallan, S. E., Bast, R. C., Jr., Lipton, J. M., Clavell, L. A., Feeney, M., Hercend, T., Nathan, D. G., and Schlossman, S. F.: Autologous bone-marrow transplantation in CALLA-positive acute lymphoblastic leukemia after in-vitro treatment with J5 monoclonal antibody and complement. Lancet, !!:60, 1982.
187. Ritz, J., Sallan, S. E., Bast, R. C., Jr., Lipton, J. M., Nathan, D. G., and Schlossman, S. F.: *In vitro* treatment with monoclonal antibody prior to autologous bone marrow transplantation in acute lymphoblastic leukemia. Hamatol. Bluttransfus., 28:117, 1983.
188. Robbins, R. A., Linder, J., Stahl, M. G., Thompson, A. B., Haire, W., Kessinger, A., Armitage, J. O., Arneson, M., Woods, G., Vaughan, W. P., and Rennard, S. I.: Diffuse alveolar hemorrhage in autologous bone marrow transplant recipients. Am. J. Med., 87:511, 1989.
189. Rowley, S. D., Jones, R. J., Piantadosi, S., Braine, H. G., Colvin, O. M., Davis, J., Saral, R., Sharkis, S., Wingard, J., Yeager, A. M., and Santos, G. W.: Efficacy of ex vivo purging for autologous bone marrow transplantation in the treatment of acute nonlymphoblastic leukemia. Blood, 74:501, 1989.
190. Saarinen, U. M., Pihko, H., and Makipernaa, A.: High-dose thiotepa with autologous bone marrow rescue in recurrent malignant oligodendroglioma: A case report. J. Neurooncol., 9:57, 1990.
191. Saleh, R. A. Gross, S., Cassano, W., and Gee, A.: Metastatic retinoblastoma successfully treated with immunomagnetic purged autologous bone marrow transplantation. Cancer, 62:2301, 1988.
192. Sanders, D. G., Wiley, F. M., and Moss, T. J.: Serial immunocytologic analysis of blood for tumor cells in two patients with neuroblastoma. Cancer, 67:1423, 1991.
193. Santos, G. W., Yeager, A. M., and Jones, R. J.: Autologous bone marrow transplantation. Ann. Rev. Med., 40:99, 1989.
194. Schmidberger, H., King, L., Lasky, L. C., and Vallera, D. A.: Antitumor activity of L6-ricin immunotoxin against the H2981-T3 lung adenocarcinoma cell line *in vitro* and *in vivo*. Cancer Res., 50:3249, 1990.
195. Seiden, M. V., O'Donnell, W. J., Weinblatt, M., and Licht, J.: Vasculitis with recurrent pulmonary hemorrhage in a long-term survivor after autologous bone marrow transplantation. Bone Marrow Transplant., 6:345, 1990.
196. Shea, T. C., Antman, K. H., Eder, J. P., Elias, A., Peters, W. P., Schryber, S., Henner, W. D., Schoenfeld, D. A. Schnipper, L. E., and Frei, E., III: Malignant melanoma. Treatment with high-dose combination alkylating agent chemotherapy and autologous bone marrow support. Arch. Dermatol., 124:878, 1988.
197. Sherertz, R. J., Belani, A., Kramer, B. S., Elfenbein, G. J., Weiner, R. S., Sullivan, M.

L., Thomas, R. G., and Samsa, G. P.: Impact of air filtration on nosocomial Aspergillus infections. Unique risk of bone marrow transplant recipients. Am. J. Med., 83:709, 1987.

198. Sheridan, W. P., Morstyn, G., Wolf, M., Dodds, A., Lusk, J., Maher, D., Layton, J. E., Green, M. D., Souza, L., and Fox, R. M.: Granulocyte colony-stimulating factor and neutrophil recovery after high-dose chemotherapy and autologous bone marrow transplantation. Lancet, II:891, 1989.

199. Shpall, E. J., Bast, R. C., Jr., Joines, W. T., Jones, R. B., Anderson, I., Johnston, C., Eggleston, S., Tepperberg, M., Edwards, S., and Peters, W. P.: Immunomagnetic purging of breast cancer from cancer marrow for autologous transplantation. Bone Marrow Transplant., 7:145, 1991.

200. Shpall, E. J., Anderson, I. C., Bast, R. C., Jr., Joines, W. T., Jones, R. B., Ross, M., Edwards, S., Eggleston, S., Johnston, C., Tepperberg, M., et al.: Immunopharmacologic purging of breast cancer from bone marrow for autologous bone marrow transplantation. Prog. Clin. Biol. Res., 333:321, 1990.

201. Shpall, E. J., Clarke-Pearson, D., Soper, J. T., Berchuck, A., Jones, R. B., Bast, R. C., Jr., Ross, M., Lidor, Y., Vanecek, K., Tyler, T., and Peters, W. P.: High-dose alkylating agent chemotherapy with autologous bone marrow support in patients with stage III/IV epithelial ovarian cancer. Gynecol. Oncol., 38:386, 1990.

202. Sieber, F., Rao, S., Rowley, S. D., and Blum, M.: Dye-mediated photolysis of human neuroblastoma cells: Implications for autologous bone marrow transplantation. Blood, 68:32, 1986.

203. Slaper-Cortenbach, I. C., Admiraal, L. G., van Leeuwen, E. F., Kerr, J. M., von dem Borne, A. E., and Tetteroo, P. A.: Effective purging of bone marrow by a combination of immunorosette depletion and complement lysis. Exp. Hematol., 18:49, 1990.

204. Smith, D. M., Weisenburger, D. D., Bierman, P., Kessinger, A., Vaughan, W. P., and Armitage, J. O.: Acute renal failure associated with autologous bone marrow transplantation. Bone Marrow Transplant., 2:195, 1987.

205. Socinski, M. A., Cannistra, S. A., Elias, A., et al.: The in vivo effect of granulocyte-macrophage colony-stimulating factor on circulating progenitor cells in man. In Autologous Bone Marrow Transplantation: Proceedings of the Fourth International Symposium. Edited by K. A. Dicke, G. Spitzer, S. Jagannath, and M. J. Evinger-Hodges. Houston, M. D. Anderson Hospital Publishers, 1989, pp. 677–683.

206. Socinski, M. A., Cannistra, S. A., Elias, A., Antman, K. H., Schnipper, L., and Griffin, J. D.: Granulocyte-macrophage colony stimulating factor expands the circulating haemopoietic progenitor cell compartment in man. Lancet, I:1194, 1988.

207. Steel, G. G.: Growth and survival of tumor stem cells. In Growth Kinetics of Tumors. Edited by G. G. Steel. Oxford, Clarendon Press, 1977, pp. 244–267.

208. Steward, W. P., Scarffe, J. H., Dirix, L. Y., Chang, J., Radford, J. A., Bonnem, E., and Crowther, D.: Granulocyte-macrophage colony-stimulating factor (GM-CSF) after high-dose melphalan in patients with advanced colon cancer. Br. J. Cancer, 61:749, 1990.

209. Stewart, D. J.: The role of chemotherapy in the treatment of gliomas in adults. Cancer Treat. Rev., 16:129, 1989.

210. Stiff, P. J., DeRisi, M. F., Langleben, A., Gulati, S., Koester, A., Lanzotti, V., and Clarkson, B. D.: Autologous bone marrow transplantation using unfractionated cells without rate-controlled freezing in hydroxyethyl starch and dimethyl sulfoxide. Ann. N. Y. Acad. Sci., 411:378, 1983.

211. Stong, R. C., Uckun, F., Youle, R. J., Kersey, J. H., and Vallera, D. A.: Use of multiple T cell-directed intact ricin immunotoxins for autologous bone marrow transplantation. Blood, 66:627, 1985.

212. Stong, R. C., Youle, R. J., and Vallera, D. A.: Elimination of clonogenic T-leukemic cells from human bone marrow using anti-Mr 65,000 protein immunotoxins. Cancer Res., 44:3000, 1984.

213. Sugarman, J., Bashore, T. M., Ohman, E. M., Jones, R., and Peters, W. P.: Hypertension and reversible myocardial depression associated with autologous bone marrow transplantation. Am. J. Med., 88:52N, 1990.

214. Tarbell, N. J., Guinan, E. C., Niemeyer, C., Mauch, P., Sallan, S. E., and Weinstein, H. J.: Late onset of renal dysfunction in survivors of bone marrow transplantation. Int. J. Radiat. Oncol. Biol. Phys., 15:99, 1988.

215. Tarella, C., Ferrero, D., Bregni, M., Siena, S., Gallo, E., Pileri, A., and Gianni, A. M.: Peripheral blood expansion of early progenitor cells after high-dose cyclophosphamide and rhGM-CSF. Eur. J. Cancer, 27:22, 1991.

216. Tchekmedyian, N. S., Tait, N., Van Echo, D., and Aisner, J.: High-dose chemotherapy without autologous bone marrow transplantation in melanoma. J. Clin. Oncol., 4:1811, 1986.

217. Thatcher, D., Lind, M., Morgenstern, G., Carr, T., Chadwick, G., Jones, R., and Craig, P.: High-dose, double alkylating agent chemotherapy with DTIC, melphalan, and ifosfamide and marrow rescue for metastatic malignant melanoma. Cancer, 63:1296, 1989.

218. Thomas, E. D., Storb, R., Clift, R. A., Fefer, A., Johnson, L., Neiman, P. E., Lerner, K. G., Glucksberg, H., and Buckner, C. D.: Bone marrow transplantation. New Engl. J. Med., 292:832, 1975.

219. Thomas, E. D., Buckner, C. D., Clift, R. A., Fefer, A., Johnson, F. L., Neiman, P. E., Sale, G. E., Sanders, J. E., Singer, J. W., Shulman, H., Storb, R., and Weiden, P. L.: Marrow transplantation for acute nonlymphoblastic leukemia in first remission. N. Engl. J. Med., 301:597, 1979.

220. Thomas, E. D., and Storb, R.: Technique for human marrow grafting. Blood, 36:507, 1970.

221. Thomas, M. R., Robinson, W. A., Glode, L. M., Dantas, M. E., Koeppler, H., Morton, N., and Sutherland, J.: Treatment of advanced malignant melanoma with high-dose chemotherapy and autologous bone marrow transplantation. Preliminary results—Phase I study. Am. J. Clin. Oncol., 5:611, 1982.

222. Tzeng, C. H., Chuang, M. W., Wang, S. Y., Hsieh, R. K., Liu, C. J., Fan, S., and Chen, P. M.: Generation of lymphokine-activated killer (LAK) cells and possible implications in autologous bone marrow transplantation—a preliminary report. Proc. Natl. Sci. Counc. Repub. China, 14:47, 1990.

223. Uckun, F. M., Gajl-Peczalska, K., Meyers, D. E., Ramsay, N. C., Kersey, J. H., Colvin, M., and Vallera, D. A.: Marrow purging in autologous bone marrow transplantation for T-lineage acute lymphoblastic leukemia: Efficacy of ex vivo treatment with immunotoxins and 4-hydroperoxycyclophosphamide against fresh leukemic marrow progenitor cells. Blood, 69:361, 1987.

224. Uckun, F. M., Stong, R. C., Youle, R. J., and Vallera, D. A.: Combined ex vivo treatment with immunotoxins and mafosfamid: A novel immunochemotherapeutic approach for elimination of neoplastic T cells from autologous marrow grafts. J. Immunol., 134:3504, 1985.

225. Uckun, F. M., Kersey, J. H., Vallera, D. A., Ledbetter, J. A., Weisdorf, D., Myers, D. E., Haake, R., and Ramsay, N. K.: Autologous bone marrow transplantation in high-risk remission T-lineage acute lymphoblastic leukemia using immunotoxins plus 4-hydroperoxycyclophosphamide for marrow purging. Blood, 76:1723, 1990.

226. Urban, C., Slace, I., Kaulfersch, W., Greinix, H., and Hocker, P.: Treatment of stage IV neuroblastoma with high-dose melphalan and autologous bone marrow transplantation following in vitro preliminary treatment of the bone marrow with the active cyclophosphamide derivative Asta Z-7654]. Pediatr. Padol., 21:275, 1986.

227. van den Brink, M. R., Voogt, P. J., Marijt, W. A., van Luxenburg Heys, S. A., van Rood, J., and Brand, A.: Lymphokine-activated killer cells selectively kill tumor cells in bone marrow without compromising bone marrow stem cell function in vitro. Blood, 74:354, 1989.

228. Vellenga, E., Sizoo, W., Hagenbeek, A., and Lowenberg, B.: Different repopulation kinetics of erythroid (BFU-E), myeloid (CFU-GM) and T lymphocyte (TC-CFU) progenitor cells after autologous and allogeneic bone marrow transplantation. Br. J. Haematol., 65:137, 1987.

229. Verdonck, L. F., de Graan Hentzen, Y. C., Dekker, A. W., Mudde, G. C., and de Gast, G. C.: Cytomegalovirus seronegative platelets and leukocyte-poor red blood cells from random donors can prevent primary cytomegalovirus infection after bone marrow transplantation. Bone Marrow Transplant., 2:7, 1987.

230. Verdonck, L. F., and de Gast, G. C.: Is cytomegalovirus infection a major cause of T cell alterations after (autologous) bone-marrow transplantation? Lancet, I:932, 1984.

231. Vredenburgh, J. J., and Ball, E. D.: Elimination of small cell carcinoma of the lung from human bone marrow by monoclonal antibodies and immunomagnetic beads. Cancer Res., 50:7216, 1990.

232. Vredenburgh, J. J., Simpson, W., Memoli, V. A., and Ball, E. D.: Reactivity of anti-CD15 monoclonal antibody PM-81 with breast cancer and elimination of breast cancer cells from human bone marrow by PM-81 and immunomagnetic beads. Cancer Res., 51:2451, 1991.

233. Welham, M. J., Schrader, J. W.: Modulation of c-kit mRNA and protein by hemopoietic growth factors. Mol. Cell. Biol., 11:2901, 1991.

234. Wingard, J. R., Chen, D. Y., Burns, W. H., Fuller, D. J., Braine, H. G., Yeager, A. M., Kaiser, H., Burke, P. J., Graham, J. L., Santos, G. W., and Saral, R.: Cytomegalovirus infection after autologous bone marrow transplantation with comparison to infection after allogeneic bone marrow transplantation. Blood, 71:1432, 1988.

235. Wolff, S. N., Herzig, R. H., Fay, J. W., LeMaistre, C. F., Frei, E., Lahr, D., Lowder, J., Bolwell, B., Giannone, L., and Herzig, G. P.: High-dose thiotepa with autologous bone marrow transplantation for metastatic malignant melanoma: Results of phase I and II studies of the North American Bone Marrow Transplantation Group. J. Clin. Oncol., 7:245, 1989.

236. Wolff, S. N., Phillips, G. L., and Herzig, G. P.: High-dose carmustine with autologous bone marrow transplantation for the adjuvant treatment of high-grade gliomas of the central nervous system. Cancer Treat. Rep., 71:183, 1987.

237. Wolff, S. N., Phillips, G. L., Fay, J. W., Giannone, L., LeMaistre, C. F., Herzig, R. H., and Herzig, G. P.: High-Dose Chemotherapy with Autologous Marrow Transplantation for Gliomas of the Central Nervous System. In Autologous Bone Marrow Transplantation: Proceedings of the Third International Symposium. Houston, M. D. Anderson Hospital Press, 1987, pp. 557–563.

238. Yamashita, J., Kawamura, T., and Shoin, K.: High dose chemotherapy in malignant gliomas using autologous bone marrow transplantation and GM-CSF: Granulocyte-macrophage colony stimulating factors [Jpn]. No Shinkei Geka. Neurological Surgery, 18:329, 1990.

239. Yeager, A. M., Kaizer, H., Santos, G. W., Saral, R., Colvin, O. M., Stuart, R. K., Braine, H. G., Burke, P. J., Ambinder, R. F., Burns, W. H., Fuller, D. J., Davis, J. M., Karp, J. E., Stratford, W., Rowley, S. D., Sensenbrenner, L. L., Vogelsang, G. B., and Wingard, J. R.: Autologous bone marrow transplantation in patients with acute nonlymphocytic leukemia, using ex vivo marrow treatment with 4-hydroperoxycyclophosphamide. New Engl. J. Med., 315:141, 1986.

240. Zsebo, K. M., Wypych, J., McNiece, I. K., Lu, H. S., Smith, K. A., Karkare, S. B., Sachdev, R. K., Yuschenkoff, V. N., Birkett, N. C., Williams, L. R., Satyagal, V. N., Tung, W., Bosselman, R. A., Mendiaz, E. A., and Langley, K. E.: Identification, purification, and biological characterization of hematopoietic stem cell factor from buffalo rat liver—conditioned medium. Cell, 63:195, 1990.

Allogeneic Transplantation

Richard J. O'Reilly
Esperanza B. Papadopoulos

Introduction

In the 24 years since human leukocyte antigen (HLA) compatible sibling marrow grafts were first successfully applied to the curative treatment of lethal congenital immune deficiencies,[19,98] allogeneic marrow transplantation has evolved as a treatment of choice for patients with aplastic anemia,[51,219] acute leukemias relapsing early after induction of first remission,[46] chronic myelogenous leukemia,[104,233] and several lethal congenital disorders of hematopoiesis and immunity.[171] Allogeneic marrow grafts have also achieved impressive successes in the treatment of myelodysplastic syndromes,[7,165] myelofibrosis, non-Hodgkin's lymphoma,[10,166] and myeloma.[48,239] They are also being applied on a large scale for the curative treatment of the hemoglobinopathies, particularly thalassemia,[142] and are currently being explored as a method for introducing self-renewing populations of enzymatically normal progenitors of tissue macrophages for the treatment of several lethal genetic disorders of metabolism.[137]

Improvements in transplantation results over the last 10 years reflect significant advances in our understanding of the immunogenetics of histocompatibility and the cellular events contributing to graft rejection and graft vs. host disease (GvHD). There also have been advances in the development of new and more effective methods for ensuring engraftment and abrogating GvHD, and in the discovery and application of new agents for the treatment or prevention of the infectious complications to which transplant recipients are particularly susceptible. These advances will be reviewed and an attempt made to assess their impact on current clinical applications of allogeneic marrow transplants in the treatment of malignant neoplastic diseases. Subsequently, new advances will be discussed that have extended the application of marrow grafts to an increasing proportion of individuals who do not have an HLA-matched sibling donor.

Biology of Allogeneic Marrow Transplants Applied to the Treatment of Hematological Neoplasia

Genetics of Histocompatibility

Recognition of the importance of matching for the determinants of the major histocompatibility complex (MHC) in the prevention of lethal GvH reactions in rodent models[36] led to the initial successful applications of HLA-matched marrow grafts in humans.[19,98] The HLA gene complex, the major histocompatibility region in humans, is located on the short arm of chromosome 6, and is composed of a series of genes,

each possessing an extraordinary degree of allelic polymorphism (Figure XIX-2-1).[41] The HLA complex is divided into class I genes (HLA-A, -B, -C), which encode proteins expressed on the surface of all nucleated cells; class II genes (HLA-Dr, -Dq, -Dp), which encode surface proteins on a more restricted group of cell types, including early hematopoietic cells, mature macrophages and monocytes, dendritic cells, endothelial cells, B cells, and activated T cells; and class III genes, which encode other functional proteins such as the complement proteins C^2 and C^4.[41,252] The HLA genes are codominantly expressed, permitting identification of haplotypes inherited from each parent by serologic typing of HLA-A, -B, -C and -Dr determinants. Histocompatibility for determinants within the entire HLA-D region is defined by mutual unresponsiveness in mixed lymphocyte culture (MLC).[266] HLA haplotypes are usually inherited en bloc from each parent. Thus, the likelihood that any two siblings will receive the same parental haplotypes is 1:4. Because of variations in the size of families, in practice, HLA-identical siblings can be identified for 35–40% of patients.

HLA phenotypically matched or partially matched related donors can be identified for an additional 5–10% of patients in the following circumstances: the parents of the patient share one or more HLA alleles that are inherited on one of the patient's HLA haplotypes, or the patient inherits one HLA haplotype that includes HLA alleles known to be genetically linked. In the family pedigree illustrated in Figure XIX-2-2, the parents share HLA-A10, and -B35 on one haplotype. As a result, individual A could receive a single HLA allele disparate graft from her father. In this pairing, the donor possesses a unique HLA-Dr4 and the recipient an HLA-Dr7. On the other hand, patient B could receive an HLA-Dr disparate graft from either parent or from her sibling. In this case, each donor would possess a unique HLA-A and HLA-B allele that could serve as a target for graft rejection. Cells of patient B, however, would possess only the HLA-D determinant as a target for GvHD.

The family illustrated in Figure XIX-2-2 also presents a different basis for donor identification. Note that patient A inherits HLA-A3, -B7 and -Dr2 as a haplotype from her father. The HLA alleles in this haplotype are known to be in strong linkage dysequilibrium, which means that the frequency with which they are co-associated on a haplotype is far greater than would be predicted by the product of each allele's frequency in the general population. Examples of full HLA-A, -B, -D haplotypes which are detected at significantly increased frequency among individuals of Caucasian back-

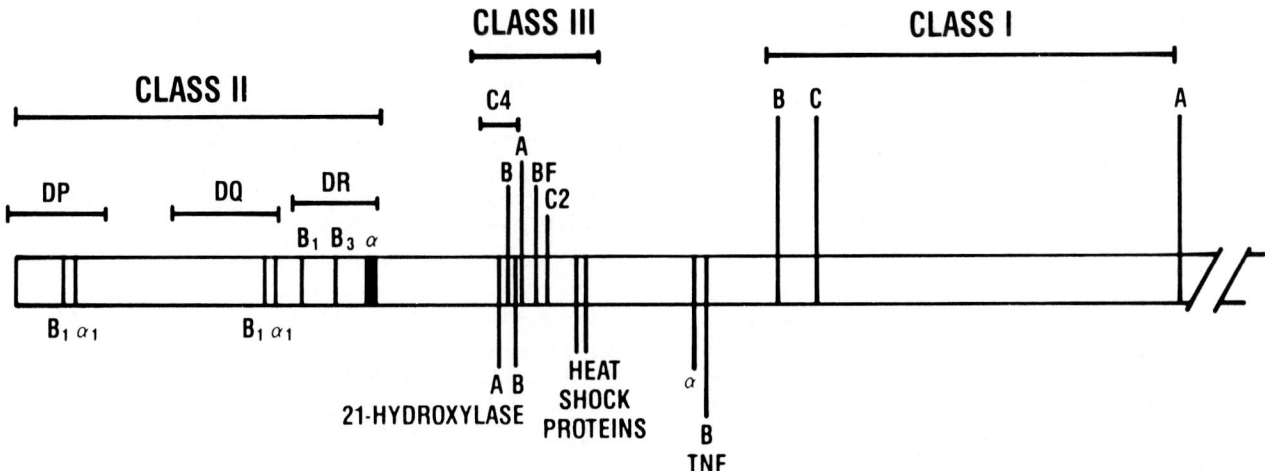

Figure XIX-2-1. A map of expressed genes of the HLA region on the short arm of chromosome 6.

ground are presented in Table XIX-2-1.[26] In the family in Figure XIX-2-2, if the father and sibling were not living, a search could be made among the offspring of maternal relatives sharing with the patient the uncommon and non-linked haplotype HLA-A10, -B35, -Dr4. In such cases, a cousin, such as individual C, could be found who derives the HLA-A3, -B7, -Dr2 haplotype from a totally different pedigree and the HLA-A10, -B35, -Dr4 from a relative of the mother.

Unrelated donors who are phenotypically matched may also be identified for a proportion of patients. Over the last six years, a National Bone Marrow Donor Registry has been established in St. Paul, Minnesota. It is connected to several donor registries and most of the major marrow transplantation centers.[153] The National Registry currently maintains a computerized bank of over 400,000 typed donors. The Anthony Nolan Foundation, a registry of over 200,000 donors based in London, is now computer-linked to this registry. Other European registries are also joining this network. Cur-

rently, these registries can probably identify serologically matched, MLC-compatible donors for up to 20–30% of patients who are of a European Caucasian background and, particularly, for patients inheriting two common HLA-A, -B, -D haplotypes.[31,208] However, the proportion of successful searches for patients who are black, oriental, or native American is very low. Furthermore, the incidence of graft rejection and severe GvHD in recipients of HLA serologically matched, MLC-compatible unrelated marrow is markedly higher than that observed in recipients of HLA-matched sibling marrow[1,30] suggesting that within the HLA region other genetic disparities may exist between unrelated HLA-matched individuals, that cannot be detected by conventional typing methods. Use of newer, more discriminatory techniques such as isoelectric focusing of class I HLA proteins[264] and analysis of DNA restriction length polymorphisms of class II HLA determinants[35] may improve selection of suitably compatible unrelated donors.[123]

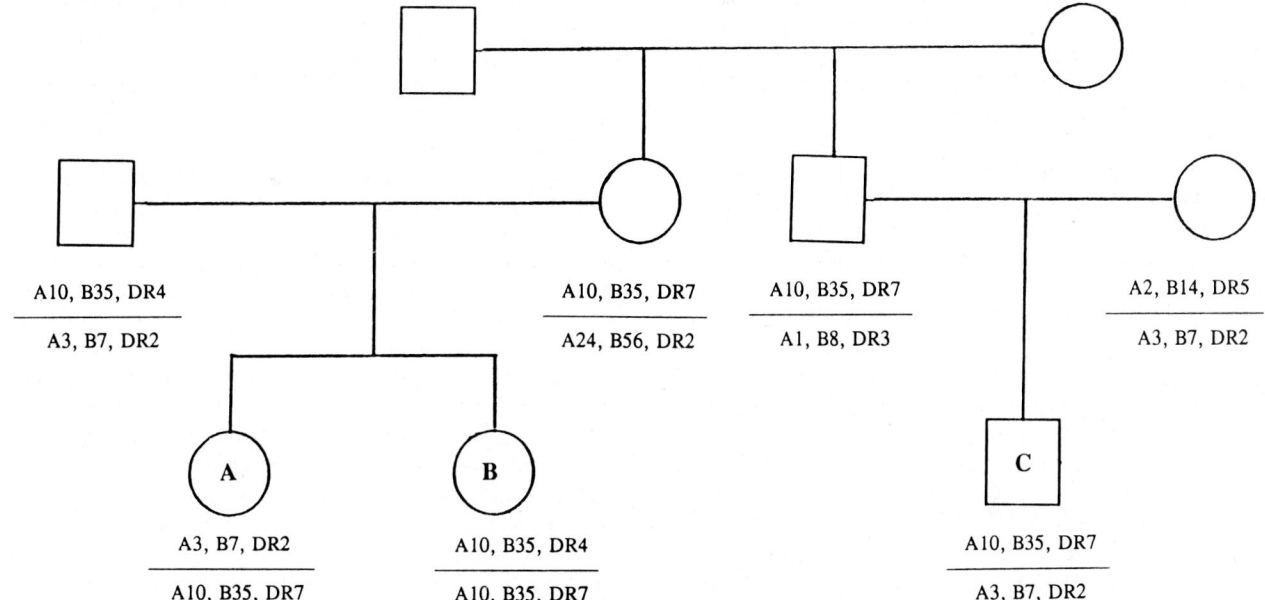

Figure XIX-2-2. An example of genetics of histocompatibility. See text.

Table XIX-2-1. Three-Locus Haplotype Frequencies (per 10,000) in Caucasians

HLA-A, B, DR (n = 1889)				
Haplotype HLA-			Haplotype frequency	Delta value
A	B	DR		
2	w62	4	86	25
2	13	7	55	2
30	13	7	83	59
2	44	7	57	−37
29	44	7	111	76
1	w57	7	101	59
2	18	w11	84	33
24	35	w11	53	23
24	35	w11	53	23
2	44	w11	61	19
3	35	1	133	72
11	35	1	79	43
2	7	2	127	−9
3	7	2	260	115
24	7	2	69	3
25	18	2	69	44
2	44	2	62	9
1	8	3	477	280
2	8	3	74	−98
3	7	4	50	−12
2	51	w11	78	18
2	w62	w11	53	10

From Bauer, et al.[26]

Preparative Cytoreduction for Allogeneic Marrow Grafts

Hematopoietic and lymphoid cells are considerably more susceptible to growth inhibition or rejection by host resistance systems than are solid organs such as the kidney or the liver. As a consequence, durable engraftment and expansion of marrow cells within an allogeneic environment can only be achieved if the host's immune system is ablated. Only patients with severe combined immune deficiency (SCID) are sufficiently compromised to permit the regular engraftment of unmanipulated HLA-matched marrow grafts. Transplants for all other conditions require intensive immunosuppressive therapy in the immediate pre-transplant period. Of the agents currently available, only total body irradiation and the alkylating agents cyclophosphamide and nitrogen mustard, administered in high doses, have been demonstrated to be sufficiently immunosuppressive to permit engraftment of foreign hematopoietic cells.[198,224,232] Total body irradiation at doses of at least 9.0–10.0 Gy induces a degree of myeloablation and immunosuppression sufficient to permit a durable engraftment of an allogeneic marrow transplant and expansion of donor progenitors in all hematopoietic lineages. Of the chemotherapeutic agents, cyclophosphamide (50 mg/kg/d × 4) is the most immunosuppressive, but it provides effective preparation only for patients with aplastic anemia.[217] For disorders that do not affect the overall cellularity of a patient's marrow, cyclophosphamide must be used in combination with a myeloablative agent such as total body irradiation, busulfan, or dimethylmyleran so that adequate space can be created for the establishment of donor hematopoietic elements within the host marrow microenvironment.[128,176]

Cytoreductive regimens developed for patients transplanted for leukemia are designed primarily to eliminate leukemia clones, but must also be sufficiently immunosuppressive and myeloablative to ensure engraftment of allogeneic hematopoietic cells. Initially, total body irradiation administered in single doses of 10 Gy was used in combination with cyclophosphamide for this purpose.[232] However, in the last 7–10 years, alternative cytoreductive regimens have been introduced that incorporate higher doses of fractionated total body irradiation[46,75] and other chemotherapeutic agents such as etoposide,[39,201] cytosine arabinoside,[58,64] or L-PAM[115] in addition to, or as substitutes for cyclophosphamide. A regimen employing high doses of busulfan and cyclophosphamide has also been developed,[240] to circumvent the use of total body irradiation. Results achieved with several of these approaches will be discussed in later sections.

The Pre-Engraftment Period

The regimens used to prepare patients for allogeneic marrow transplant regularly induce marrow aplasia and profound pancytopenia, which persist until the donor marrow graft begins to expand in the host, i.e., 2–4 weeks post-transplantation. During this interval, patients require intensive support with platelets and red cells. These and other blood products must be irradiated since they contain allogeneic lymphocytes that may induce lethal GvH reactions.[3] During this period of severe leukopenia, patients are also at high risk for local infections and sepsis caused by constituents of the microflora of the skin and gastrointestinal tract. *Pseudomonas, E. coli,* and Enterobacteriaceae derived from the mouth and intestinal tract, and skin-derived *Staphylococcus epidermitis* which frequently contaminates indwelling venous catheters, are particularly common pathogens.[256] Systemic fungal infections also contribute to morbidity and mortality. *Candida albicans* and *C. tropicalis* are particularly common.[254] However, infections with other fungal agents such as *Aspergillus, Mucor, Cryptosporidium,* and *Fusarium* are also detected at significant frequencies. Mortality due to such infections has ranged from 2–15% in reported series, despite aggressive treatment with broad-spectrum antibiotics and antifungal agents.

The incidence of serious microbial infections and their associated mortality can be significantly reduced by maintaining the patient in laminar flow isolation with skin and mucosal decontamination.[214] Less stringent measures such as oral decontamination with chlorhexidine may ameliorate mucositis, and thereby also reduce systemic infections such as candidemia.[89] Prophylactic treatment with acyclovir also reduces the incidence of herpes labialis infections, which are reactivated in a high proportion of transplant recipients after total body irradiation or cyclophosphamide therapy.[199] Recent studies indicate that the incidence of bacterial infections may also be reduced by the prophylactic administration of large doses of intravenous immune globulin.[178,222]

The cytoreductive regimens used to prepare patients for transplantation can induce acute toxicities in several other organs. For example, high doses of cyclophosphamide may induce severe or lethal cardiomyopathies, particularly in patients who have received extensive prior treatment with cardiotoxic agents such as the anthracyclines.[9,107] Cyclophosphamide may also induce severe hemorrhagic cystitis.[47,205] This complication can now be prevented, however, by the concurrent administration of mesna.[37,124]

Total body irradiation and each of the alkylating agents can induce severe enteritis, thereby further potentiating opportunities for microbial invasion. In some patients, particularly patients with antecedent hepatic dysfunction, the cytoreductive regimen may also induce significant damage to the endothelial lining of the hepatic sinusoids. The resultant edema and necrosis may induce acute and severe obstruction to the blood flow of the portal circulation resulting in the rapid onset of hepatomegaly and massive ascites, a process termed veno-occlusive disease (V.O.D.).[97,126,154] It has been estimated that up to 10% of patients transplanted for leukemia develop clinical signs and symptoms of V.O.D.[154] In milder forms, edema of the endothelial linings resolves relatively rapidly. However, in more severe forms, the obstruction leads to extensive centrilobular necrosis of the liver with severe compromise of hepatic functions, particularly the synthesis of coagulation factors and albumin. Obstruction to the portal circulation may also produce severe reductions in the central venous blood volume, thereby reducing effective perfusion of the kidneys, with resultant oliguria and prerenal azotemia. If the circulation to the kidneys is further compromised, rapid progression to renal failure is observed. The treatment of severe venoocclusive disease is largely supportive and frequently inadequate. It involves replacement of albumin and coagulation factors; careful management of parenteral fluids to maintain central venous pressure, electrolyte balance and renal output; and treatment of the respiratory and vascular complications of massive ascites and severe portal hypertension. Prophylactic therapy with heparin alone has not prevented or altered V.O.D.[28] However, thrombolysis with tissue plasminogen activator (TPA) has been used successfully in one case.[20] Prophylaxis with the vasodilator, prostaglandin E_1 has also been shown to reduce the incidence of this complication.[101]

Engraftment and Graft Failure or Rejection

Engraftment is heralded by early repopulation of myeloid and erythroid progenitors in the marrow and the emergence of neutrophils in the circulation 14–20 days post-transplant. By 28–35 days post-transplant, marrow cellularity may be normal, neutrophil counts may be stable at >1,000/μl, and platelets self-sustaining at levels of 20,000/μl or more. In a proportion of cases, despite cytogenetic evidence of engraftment of donor lymphoid and myeloid cells, recovery of white cell counts and particularly of platelet counts may be delayed for periods of 2–4 months.[42] The basis for these delayed reconstitutions is uncertain. Frequently, however, persistent cytopenias are associated with the development of GvHD or intercurrent viral infections.[27]

Graft failure, on the other hand, may be defined either as a failure to recover marrow function after transplantation or a reversion to marrow aplasia after initial hematopoietic reconstitution, which is associated with the loss of donor-type lymphoid and hematopoietic cells from the marrow and peripheral blood. Graft failures are usually detected within the first 50 days but may occur as late as 4–5 months posttransplant.

The incidence of graft failure is strongly influenced by the type of cytoreduction used to prepare the patient, the degree of HLA disparity existing between donor and recipient, and the type of transplant administered.[1,56] Among aplastic recipients of HLA-matched marrow grafts who are prepared with cyclophosphamide alone, the incidence of graft failure ranges from 10–30%, depending on the patient's prior history of transfusions.[56,215,216] In contrast, HLA-matched, unmanipulated marrow grafts are rarely rejected by leukemic patients prepared with total body irradiation and cyclophosphamide irrespective of transfusion sensitization.[74,75,232] However, HLA-disparate unmanipulated marrow grafts can be rejected after this type of cytoreduction. Indeed, the overall incidence of rejection of such grafts is 15%, and varies from 6–28% depending on the number of HLA allelic disparities unique to the donor.[1]

It is also increasingly clear that the T cells in the marrow transplant contribute to engraftment, probably by suppressing or eliminating host resistance and possibly by stimulating donor marrow cell development. In murine models of transplantation, addition of thymocytes to marrow or fetal liver hematopoietic cells potentiates their engraftment in MHC disparate irradiated hosts.[141,192] Similarly, in dogs and in man, infusions of peripheral blood leukocytes in addition to the marrow transplant can prevent rejections in heavily sensitized aplastic recipients.[212] Conversely, marrow transplants depleted of T cells so as to reduce their potential to induce GvHD have been found to be considerably more susceptible to graft failure or rejection.[113,149,174] The incidence of this complication ranges from 10–30% in leukemic recipients of T cell depleted HLA-matched marrow, despite preparation with total body irradiation and cyclophosphamide,[113,133,148] and has been reported to be as high as 40–50% in recipients of HLA non-identical T cell depleted grafts.[172]

Considerable progress has been made in identifying and characterizing the cellular mechanisms contributing to marrow graft failures. In murine models, at least two types of rejection have been identified. Lethally irradiated non-sensitized hybrid animals derived from specific genetic backgrounds are able to resist the engraftment of parental marrow cells through the inhibitory activity of natural killer cells.[130] This form of resistance does not require T cells; indeed, it is strongly expressed by athymic nude and SCID mice.[161] Presensitized mice, on the other hand, reject allogeneic marrow grafts through the activity of donor-reactive cytotoxic host T cells that survive preparative cytoreduction.[71]

Early clinical studies and experiments in canine models[213,218] documented an increased incidence of graft failure in animals that had received multiple transfusions prior to transplantation, suggesting an immunologic basis for the failures or rejections observed. Recently, direct evidence in support of this concept has been provided by a series of studies documenting the emergence of host type CD3+, CD8+, CD56− T cells exhibiting specific reactivity against donor hematopoietic cells at the time of rejection of either unmanipulated[247] or T cell depleted marrow grafts.[43,135] Unfortunately, our knowledge of the alloantigens that can stimulate rejection of a marrow graft is still rudimentary.[242] To date, only a few of these determinants have been identified. In recipients of HLA-disparate T cell depleted marrow grafts, host T cells detected in the blood at the time of rejection are CD8+Leu7− cytotoxic T cells that exhibit a striking specificity for single class I HLA alleles unique to the donor (i.e., a single HLA-A or HLA-B determinant).[135] In a small proportion of cases, CD4+ cytolytic T cells reactive against Class II HLA disparities have also been identified. Patients rejecting HLA-matched marrow grafts, on the other hand, develop CD8+ Leu7+ T cells which specifically inhibit the growth of donor colony forming hematopoietic cells (CFU$_c$, BFU$_e$) in vitro.[43] In certain cases, these T cells have been shown to be HLA-restricted and specifically reactive against the H-Y antigen expressed on cells from male donors.[109,247] Another minor alloantigen expressed on marrow cells described by Goulmy and colleagues, the HA-3 antigen, has also been implicated as a target for T cell mediated marrow graft rejections.[108]

It is uncertain whether, and to what degree, host NK cells contribute to marrow rejection in patients transplanted after treatment with regimens including cyclophosphamide. However, these cells have been implicated in the graft resistance exhibited by a proportion of patients with SCID who fail to achieve engraftment following HLA disparate T cell depleted marrow transplants administered without preparatory cytoreduction.[169]

Other processes have also been implicated in the pathogenesis of graft failure, including drug and viral induced suppression of marrow progenitors[244] and, in rare instances, an inability of the host's marrow microenvironment to support hematopoietic progenitor growth.[147]

Identification of factors potentially contributing to graft failure or rejection has spawned the development of several approaches for reversing or preventing this phenomenon which are currently in clinical trials. Intensification of preparative immunosuppressive regimens and the administration of agents such as antithymocyte globulin or T cell specific monoclonal antibodies in the early post transplant period have improved rates of engraftment in high risk groups.[45,50,117,133] Furthermore, introduction of such agents early in the course of rejection may reverse this process in a significant proportion of cases.[133] Cytokines such as GMCSF are also being explored in the treatment and prevention of graft failures.[164] In addition, preliminary evidence suggests that graft failures associated with infection due to viruses such as CMV, may be reversed when these infections are effectively treated with antiviral agents such as ganciclovir or foscarnet in combination with hyperimmune globulin preparations.[82]

Acute Graft Vs. Host Disease

Graft vs. host disease (GvHD) is a pathologic process initiated by engrafted immunocompetent donor T lymphocytes responding to alloantigens expressed on host cells, particularly cells derived from the lymphohematopoietic system.[220] These activated T lymphocytes are then thought to induce injury to host tissues either through a direct cytotoxic action, or by the activation of other cells, such as NK cells and macrophages, which are capable of non-specifically destroying host cell targets.[87] GvHD is also associated with

elevations in several cytoinhibitory cytokines such as TNF which may further contribute to the pathology observed.[180]

GvHD is most commonly manifested by a generalized maculopapular rash, hepatitis, diarrhea, and a delayed reconstitution of hematopoietic and lymphoid function.[102,246,260] Distinctive, but not pathognomonic pathologic features include infiltration of the perivascular spaces in the dermis and the dermo-epidermal junction of the skin with CD8+ cytotoxic T lymphocytes, and monocytes with secondary necrosis.[206] Similar changes are seen in the epithelium of the oropharynx, tongue, and esophagus, the bases of the intestinal crypts of the small and large bowel, and the periportal areas of the liver.[206]

Acute GvHD develops in 50–70% patients transplanted with HLA identical marrow. This process is a direct cause of death in only 5–7% of cases but contributes to the severity of viral infections such as CMV interstitial pneumonia,[159] and thereby constitutes an indirect cause of death in up to 45% of affected individuals. The minor alloantigenic disparities stimulating GvHD following HLA matched marrow grafts have not been fully defined. The incidence of severe GvH reactions complicating transplants of HLA-matched marrow has been higher in male recipients of grafts from female donors, suggesting the possibility that H-Y is an important minor alloantigen.[93,96,216] The recently described HA antigens expressed on hematopoietic and lymphoid cells are also being explored.[108] However, incompatibilities for these determinants have not, as yet, been shown to be significant predictors of GvHD in large clinical series.

GvHD of grade II–IV severity is usually treated early in its course with high doses of glucocorticosteroids.[78,131] Responses, reflected by stabilization or improvement of the skin rash and hepatic and gastrointestinal abnormalities, are usually apparent within 5–7 days of initiating this treatment. For patients with severe (Grade III–IV) or moderate (Grade II) acute GvHD which is refractory to initial steroid treatment, the prognosis has been poor. Such patients may achieve stabilization or some improvement of GvHD manifestations through the addition of antithymocyte globulin. However, 70–80% of such patients ultimately succumb to sequelae of GvHD or associated infections.[150] Unmodified T cell specific monoclonal antibodies have also failed to reverse severe acute GvHD.[189] However, promising results have recently been reported in the treatment of severe acute GvHD reactions through the use of a Ricin-A conjugated, CD5 specific T cell monoclonal antibody.[49]

Chronic Graft Vs. Host Disease

Approximately 30% of patients transplanted with HLA matched marrow develop chronic graft vs. host disease. Chronic GvHD usually develops in patients with antecedent acute GvHD, although it may develop spontaneously late after transplantation. Clinically, chronic GvHD is manifested by localized or widespread scleroderma-like changes of the skin, skin and joint contractures, xerostomia, xerophthalmia, biliary cirrhosis, malabsorption and failure to thrive.[223] The pathologic changes produced by chronic GvHD may be extensive and severely debilitating. In addition, persistent immunologic deficiencies, particularly of the humoral immune system, may be profound and render these patients highly susceptible to pyogenic infections late in the post-transplant period.[16,17] At least 20% of treated patients also develop an obliterative bronchiolitis as a manifestation of chronic GvHD, which frequently progresses to a chronic obstructive pulmonary disease with subsequent death due to respiratory failure or intercurrent pulmonary infection.[121]

Chronic GvHD is pathologically distinct from acute GvHD in that it is predominantly marked by sclerosis without a significant lymphoid infiltrate. In murine models,[175] acute GvHD is usually marked by the emergence of donor type cytotoxic T cells which are specifically lytic for host targets. In contrast, T cells cloned from animals with chronic GvHD are of a helper phenotype. They are not cytoxic against host cells; rather, they proliferate in response to either donor or host Ia+ cells and generate factors that stimulate collagen synthesis. In humans with chronic GvHD, T lymphocytes and monocytes capable of non-specific suppression of T cell transformation and B cell immunoglobulin production are regularly observed.[143,237] The T cells detected also generate cytokines stimulating fibroblast proliferation and collagen secretion. In normal individuals, such broadly reactive, and potentially autocytotoxic cells can be detected at significant frequency in the blood by limiting dilution analyses.[191] However, cells capable of specifically suppressing these cells are also present in the circulation. In patients with chronic GvHD, these specific suppressor cells are either absent or markedly reduced in number.[191] These findings, when considered in the light of studies in a murine model which mimics many features of chronic GvHD in humans, suggest that chronic GvHD may reflect ineffectively controlled immunosuppressive, and potentially autoreactive, clones of cells, possibly generated in response to populations of host-reactive donor T cells participating in acute GvHD reactions.

Treatment of chronic GvHD is still inadequate. In a series of patients treated without systemic immunosuppressive agents, only 18–23% survived over 18 months.[221] Chronic GvHD has been slowly reversed in up to 76% of patients by long-term treatment either with a combination of azathioprine and prednisone or prednisone alone.[226] Preliminary results which have been reported,[225] suggest that further improvements may be achieved with a combination of cyclosporine and prednisone.

Prevention of Graft Vs. Host Disease

Because of the high mortality associated with severe forms of acute and chronic graft vs. host disease and the limited effectiveness of its current treatment, research has been focused on the development of more effective methods for preventing this complication, or ameliorating its expression. To date, two approaches have been explored: 1) administration of immunosuppressive regimens in the immediate post-transplant period to prevent or inhibit the activation or expansion of host reactive donor T lymphocytes following engraftment of unmodified marrow, and 2) treatment of the marrow graft to remove T-cells capable of inducing graft vs. host disease.

The prophylactic administration of methotrexate in the post-transplant period has been only partially effective in abrogating GvHD in matched marrow recipients. Indeed, the frequencies of acute and chronic GvHD already cited are from series in which this agent was used for prophylaxis. While the combination of ATG and prednisone has been reported to reduce the severity of GvH, it has not improved survival.[184] In randomized trials, cyclosporine has been found to be equivalent to methotrexate in the prophylaxis of GvHD.[211] However, the prophylactic administration of a combination of methotrexate and cyclosporine reduces the incidence of severe acute GvHD, and thereby significantly improves survival.[210] Unfortunately, this combination has had little effect on either the incidence or the severity of chronic GvHD. Furthermore, this combination has not been effective in preventing severe graft vs. host reactions in HLA disparate recipients.

Other immunosuppressive agents, including thalidomide and deoxycoformycin, have achieved promising results in animal models of transplantation, but are only now being considered for clinical trials.[84,245] Prophylaxis with the T cell-specific monoclonal antibody OKT$_3$, which has been successful in preventing kidney allograft rejection, has not proved effective in preventing GvHD or altering its severity.[182] Clinical trials of prophylaxis with other T cell reactive monoclonal antibodies such as the humanized monoclonal antibody Campath 1G and XomazymeH65, a CD5 specific ricin A mouse immunotoxin, are in progress but are too early for analysis.

Alternative approaches aimed at preventing the early activation of the alloreactive donor T cells that initiate GvHD, or neutralizing the cytokines generated that potentiate GvH pathology are also being explored. In animal models and in preliminary clinical trials, antibodies to the IL-2 receptor have been shown to inhibit the expansion of alloreactive T cells, and thereby to reduce the incidence of GvHD.[2,88,118] Antibodies to tumor necrosis factor (TNF), a cytokine produced by several cells participating in GvH reactions which is strikingly elevated in the serum of patients with acute GvHD,[122] have also been found to be effective in preventing lethal GvHD in MHC incompatible mice, when administered in the early post-transplant period.[180]

While no combination of agents administered to recipients of an unmodified marrow graft has prevented the development of GvHD in HLA non-identical recipients, GvHD can be prevented in both HLA matched and HLA disparate recipients through the use of marrow grafts suitably depleted of T lymphocytes prior to infusion. The four most extensively studied techniques for T cell depletion include: lectin agglutination and E-rosette depletion, as described by Reisner and colleagues;[174,188] treatment with Campath-1, a rat monoclonal antibody which binds human complement and, therefore, can be used with the donor's own plasma as a source of complement,[113] treatment of the bone marrow with one or more T cell-specific mouse monoclonal antibodies and rabbit complement;[148,182,183] and treatment with ricin-A chain T cell immunotoxins.[90] Other techniques, which deplete T cells by treatment with monoclonal antibodies linked to magnetic beads or polystyrene membranes, or by selective elutriation, have also been developed and are being explored.[243,248]

Frame and colleagues have compared several of these techniques for their capacity to deplete clonable T cells from aliquots of the same marrow, using sensitive limiting dilution techniques.[94] These techniques may differ by 1–2 $\log_{10}$ fold in the level of T cell depletion achieved. It has recently been shown that the dose of clonable T cells in a human marrow graft is strongly correlated with the risk of developing GvHD.[134] It is therefore not surprising that in results from large series using different techniques of T cell depletion, the recorded incidences of moderate to severe acute GvHD and chronic GvHD tend to reflect the efficiency of the T cell depletion techniques used. This trend is even more striking among recipients of HLA-disparate marrow grafts. For such patients, only techniques which reduce the dose of clonable T cells to less than 1×10^5/kg have consistently prevented the development of severe acute GvHD.[173]

While several series have demonstrated that T cell depleted marrow grafts may reduce the incidence and severity of GvHD, a clear advantage of such transplants over unmodified grafts which translates into a significant improvement in long-term disease-free survival has thus far only been documented in patients with lethal congenital immune deficiencies transplanted from HLA non-identical donors.[173] Among patients transplanted for leukemia and aplastic anemia, the reductions in GvHD and GvH-associated mortality accrued by the use of T cell depleted grafts have been significantly counterbalanced by the sensitivity of such transplants to graft failure or rejection, and, in some, but not all series, by an increase in the incidence of leukemia relapse following T cell depleted transplants.[146]

Interstitial Pneumonia

Interstitial pneumonia constitutes the most common cause of death in the first three months following an HLA-matched marrow graft. Overall, 25–35% of patients transplanted for leukemia develop this process. Over 50% of cases can be ascribed to cytomegalovirus, and 10% to Pneumocytis carinii and other pathogens such as Herpes simplex, adenovirus, fungi, myobacteria or other agents.[158,163] Despite the increased use of diagnostic bronchoalveolar lavage and transbronchial or open lung biopsies, and the development of rapid, highly sensitive, immunologic and molecular techniques for detection of CMV and other viruses,[59,83] at least 40% of cases cannot be ascribed to a pathogen, and may represent processes caused by aberrant inflammatory responses induced by the combined effects of infection and/or GvHD on a lung parenchyma and supporting vasculature already damaged by radiation and chemotherapy.

Of the known pathogens, CMV has been particularly problematic. Overall, 70–90% of transplant recipients who are seropositive, or receive grafts from seropositive donors, become viremic post-transplant, usually after engraftment has been detected.[11,159] This represents 50–70% of patients transplanted. Of those who develop viremia, 30–40% develop interstitial pneumonia. In contrast, the risk of this complication among seronegative recipients of a marrow graft who receive blood cell support from seronegative donors is low.[11] These data, coupled with molecular analyses of CMV isolates, suggest that the CMV infections observed are usually due to reactivations of virus latent in the host or the donor graft.[257] Alloreactions between donor and host potentiate the risk of CMV infection and interstitial pneumonia. Thus, patients with moderate-severe GvHD have a high incidence of this

complication,[159,163,250] while recipients of syngeneic or autologous marrow grafts are at low risk.[253] Intensity of cytoreduction also increases this risk.[158,250]

In the last 3–5 years, a number of advances have been made which are reducing the incidence of interstitial pneumonias and improving the prognosis of affected patients. The introduction of cotrimoxazole prophylaxis in the pre- and post-transplant period has markedly reduced the incidence of pneumonias caused by P. carinii. For seronegative transplant recipients, the risk of developing CMV pneumonia may be drastically reduced by restricting their exposure to the virus through the exclusive use of platelets and other blood components from CMV seronegative donors for transfusion support.[144] Seroprophylaxis with CMV hyperimmune globulin is also effective in reducing the incidence of CMV pneumonia[222] in seropositive older patients. Prophylaxis with high dose acyclovir has also been reported to reduce the incidence of this complication.[160] Most importantly, although CMV pneumonia once initiated, has, in the past, been associated with a 90% mortality despite treatment with either single antiviral agents or immune globulin alone,[186] it can now be effectively treated and reversed in 50–70% of cases with a combination of the antiviral agent ganciclovir and CMV hyperimmune globulin.[81,186,200]

Late Complications of Marrow Transplants

Late complications of marrow transplantation may be divided into those resulting from the protracted period of immunodeficiency which follows a marrow graft and those resulting from the toxic and oncogenic sequelae of the cytoreductive regimens used to prepare patients for transplant.

Immunodeficiency

While the process of hematopoietic reconstitution may be largely completed within the first 40–60 days post-transplantation, redevelopment of a competent donor-derived immune system is a protracted process. T cell populations begin to redevelop within the first 2 months, but responses to mitogens and antigens may be severely depressed for at least 2–4 months post-transplant.[129,260] The risk of infections with HSV, CMV, and fungal agents falls off rapidly after the first 3–6 months post-transplant. The risk of disseminated varicella zoster virus infections, however, persists through the first year. Prior to the introduction of acyclovir, severe interstitial pneumonias and encephalitides caused by this virus were lethal in a significant proportion of cases.[140] However, treatment with intravenous acyclovir is effective and regularly leads to clearance of varicella zoster infections with low mortality.[202] Long-term prophylaxis with acyclovir may also prevent this complication.[177]

Recovery of B-cell function is more protracted, with antibody deficiency states persisting for 12–18 months.[129,143,260] In patients with chronic GvHD, severe humoral immune deficiencies may persist for 3–5 years. As a result, patients with chronic GvHD are particularly susceptible to infections, such as recurrent sinusitis, otitis media, pneumonia and sepsis, caused by the same spectrum of pyogenic bacteria that affect children with agammaglobulinemia, such as pneumococci, streptococci and Hemophilus influenzae.[18,258]

Late Cytotoxic Effects

The late effects of preparatory regimens on nonhematopoietic tissues, particularly the brain, eyes, endocrine glands and reproductive system, may be mild or severe, depending upon the type of preparatory cytoreduction used for the transplant and its dose intensity, the treatment received by the patient prior to referral for transplantation, and the age of the patient at the time of transplant. In general, patients prepared with cyclophosphamide alone sustain limited and generally transient damage to these organs, while injury induced by total body irradiation tends to be more profound and enduring. Similarly, radiation administered in a single large dose tends to be more damaging than if this dose is administered in multiple fractions.[69,195]

The most devastating of late complications resulting from damage induced by total body irradiation and chemotherapy is leukoencephalopathy.[234] This complication occurs almost exclusively in patients transplanted for leukemia who have received cranial radiation and/or extended courses of intrathecal methotrexate as treatment or prophylaxis for CNS leukemia prior to referral for transplantation. In such patients, the risk of leukoencephalopathy has been reported to be 7%.[234] This complication generally produces severe symptoms including slurred speech, confusion, ataxia, seizures, and spasticity, and may progress to coma and death. Less severe CNS toxicities may also be observed, in the form of neuropsychological dysfunctions and varying degrees of retardation.[261] However, the incidence of the latter complications has not been established. Transient neurological toxicities, including tremors, seizures and paresis, may also complicate the use of cyclosporine for prophylaxis of GvHD.[249]

Deficiencies of growth hormone and primary deficiencies of thyroid, ovarian and testicular hormones have been reported in a significant proportion of patients who have received allogeneic marrow transplants. Compensated hypothyroidism has been observed in 34–36% of patients transplanted for leukemia, and thyroid failure, requiring supplementation, in an additional 10%.[139,203] Gonadal dysfunction is a common late complication of transplantation. Among younger women prepared for transplantation with cyclophosphamide alone, deficiencies of ovarian function usually recover at a median of six months post-transplant, but, in over 35% of older women (>27 yrs.), sustained ovarian failure is observed. The incidence of this complication increases to 55% for young and 74% for older women transplanted for leukemia after preparation with total body radiation and cyclophosphamide.[193] While pregnancies and normal births have been documented among women transplanted for aplasia after cyclophosphamide alone, pregnancies have been rare in patients transplanted for leukemia. Among men transplanted after preparation with cyclophosphamide alone, Leydig cell dysfunction is uncommon. Even among leukemic male transplant recipients, deficiencies of testosterone are rare, although 76% may have compensatory elevations of FSH. However, spermatogenesis is dramatically and durably reduced or eliminated in at least 75% of patients treated with total body irradiation and up to a third of patients prepared with cyclophosphamide alone.[204]

The linear growth of children prepared for transplantation with total body irradiation is often impaired. In part, this reflects injury to the hypothalamus resulting in decreased production of growth hormone releasing factor (GHRF) and consequently abnormal growth hormone secretion.[139,195] However, total body irradiation also affects growing bone, reducing, to a variable degree, the ultimate growth potential of transplanted children. Whether and to what degree treatment with growth hormone or GHRF can partially correct short stature in these cases is now under study.

Radiation may also injure the lens of the eyes, inducing cataract formation late in the post-transplant period. In patients treated with single high doses of total body irradiation, the incidence of cataracts is 50%. This incidence is lower in patients treated with fractionated total body irradiation (10–20%).[69]

Treatment with alkylating agents such as cyclophosphamide as well as total body irradiation predisposes to secondary malignancies. To date, such neoplasms have been recorded in only a relatively small proportion of marrow transplant recipients, and predominantly among patients transplanted for leukemia.[70,259] The most common neoplasms detected are B cell lymphoproliferative disorders and immunoblastic sarcomas usually bearing EBV associated antigens or integrated EBV DNA.[259] Such lymphomas are rare following HLA-matched conventional marrow or marrow grafts depleted of T and B lymphocytes by lectin agglutination or the rat monoclonal antibody Campath-1 (<2%).[113,173,259] Although a frequency of 6.4% has been observed following transplants depleted with T cell specific mouse monoclonals,[268] the risk of B cell lymphoproliferative disease has been reported to be as high as 8–24% in patients treated with HLA-non-identical grafts depleted of T cells with T cell-specific monoclonal antibodies,[92] and in patients receiving infusions of certain T cell monoclonal antibodies for treatment of GvHD.[151] Strikingly, in several of the latter patients, the lymphomas have been of donor rather than host origin.[151] The basis for susceptibility to such B cell transformations is unclear, but may, in part, reflect an inability of such patients to generate T cells capable of regulating donor B cell expansions early in the post transplant period. Solid tumors, including basal cell carcinomas, squamous cell carcinomas of the skin, adenocarcinomas of the stomach, osteosarcomas and glioblastomas have also developed in a small proportion (1–2%) of cases followed for 1–10 years post-transplant.[259] Again, the incidence of these cancers appears to be lower than that recorded in patients given comparable or lower localized doses of radiation and chemotherapy for other neoplasms such as Hodgkin's disease. More prolonged follow-up is still needed, however, before full assessments can be made of the incidence of such tumors in transplant recipients.

HLA-Matched Marrow Transplants for Leukemia

Between 1968 and 1978, marrow transplants were almost exclusively applied to the treatment of patients with leukemia who were already refractory to chemotherapy. Overall, 13–18% of such patients achieved durable disease-free survival.[230] However, for patients transplanted when in good physical condition, the probability of extended disease-free survival was 25%. Based on these results, transplants were then applied to patients in good clinical condition, at a stage in the disease when the leukemic cell burden was low and the residual leukemic cells were likely to be still sensitive to the cytoreduction employed.[231] In 1979, the Seattle group reported a series of patients with AML transplanted in first remission of whom 63% achieved long-term disease-free survival. In this series, the risk of relapse was only 12%. This study was quickly confirmed by several transplant centers,[167] and led to the widespread exploration of HLA matched marrow grafts in the treatment of acute leukemias in first or second remission and chronic myelogenous leukemia in first chronic phase. Approximately ten years of this experience can now be evaluated. Results can also be compared with those achieved with current chemotherapy and with autologous marrow grafts at different stages in the disease course.

Marrow Transplantation for Acute Myeloid Leukemia

Transplants After First Relapse of AML

For patients with AML in second or later remission or relapse, an allogeneic HLA matched marrow graft is generally regarded as the treatment of choice. Few if any patients with AML who have failed an initial remission will survive disease-free if treated with chemotherapy alone.[54] In contrast, cytoreduction with total body irradiation or busulfan, together with cyclophosphamide, followed by an HLA-matched marrow has led to extended disease-free survival for 20–30% of adults and 30–51% of children grafted in 2° remission.[46,54,62,74] Results recently reported also indicate that similar cytoreduction followed by an autologous, drug purged marrow graft obtained during 2° remission may lead to long-term (5-year) disease-free survival in 30% of cases.[106,265] While such autologous grafts carry a higher risk of post-transplant relapse than HLA-matched marrow grafts (>50% vs. 20–25%) and a somewhat lower probability of extended disease-free survival, they are, at present, the treatment of choice for patients lacking an HLA-matched donor, and clearly superior to other chemotherapeutic approaches.

Transplants in First Remission of AML

The role of allogeneic marrow transplants in the treatment of patients with AML in first remission is considerably more controversial. Prospective clinical trials derived from six single institutions and two cooperative groups have compared HLA-matched marrow grafts and chemotherapy in the treatment of AML in 1° remission in young adults (<40 years of age).[8,57,60,65,181,267] In each of these trials, (Table XIX-2-2), the incidence of post treatment relapse was significantly lower among transplant patients (9–40%) than among patients treated with chemotherapy alone (71–90%). In each of these studies, 3–5 year disease free survival rates for patients transplanted were also superior to those achieved with chemotherapy alone. However, these differences were statistically significant in only three of the six single institution studies. Concerns regarding selection bias and the adequacy of the treatment and support administered to patients receiving chemotherapy alone have also been expressed by several investigators.[152] One issue cited is the fact that in at least two studies demonstrating significant differences, chemotherapy patients were treated at facilities different from the transplant center. However, the trend in centers in which both treatments were given at the same site was the same.[33] Randomized trials comparing results of treatment in patients assigned to transplant or chemotherapy on the basis of HLA-matched donor availability defined prior to initiation of induction chemotherapy are now in progress to resolve these issues. However, continuing improvements in chemotherapy regimens and in transplantation approaches may make these studies obsolete before they are completed (see XXXVI-2).

The role of marrow transplants in the treatment of children with AML is particularly controversial since new chemotherapeutic regimens have significantly increased the proportion of children who achieve and remain in first remission. Currently, 40–50% of children treated with such regimens who achieve a first remission are alive and in sustained remission 5 years later.[68,251] However, HLA-matched marrow grafts administered to children with AML in first remission have also achieved impressive results: 49–67% of such patients are alive and disease-free 3–5 years post-transplant.[46,196] In a recent prospective trial conducted by the CCSG, 49% of children transplanted for AML in 1° remission were alive and in sustained remission 3 years post treatment compared to 40% for patients treated with chemotherapy alone (p<.05).[86] Thus, for children with AML in first remission, HLA-matched marrow grafts appear to be superior to chemotherapy alone (see XXXIX-3).

The relative efficacy of autologous marrow grafts when compared with allogeneic marrow grafts in the treatment of patients with AML in first remission is not yet established. Several studies in which either drug-purged or untreated autologous marrow grafts, obtained in first remission, have been administered after cytoreductive regimens, including either total body irradiation or myeleran and cyclophosphamide, have been conducted in the treatment of adults. Disease-free survival rates of 45–50% have been reported.[106,157] However, these results may be skewed by the particularly good results achieved in a proportion of patients transplanted over 12 months after initial remission induction, patients who, with chemotherapy alone, are likely to have an improved prognosis. For patients transplanted within 6 months of achieving first remission, relapse rates post-transplant are 40–45%, with overall disease-free survivals ranging from 30–45% at 2–3 years.[106]

Marrow Transplantation for Acute Lymphoblastic Leukemia

Transplantation for ALL in First Remission

Current multidrug chemotherapeutic regimens combining systemic treatment and CNS prophylaxis chemotherapeutic regimens are able to induce sustained remissions or cures in 70–80% of children with ALL presenting with standard risk features.[238] Furthermore, more intensive regimens applied to children at high risk for relapse have increased their probability of sustained disease-free survival to 60–70%.[61,209] Because of these results, it has been difficult to identify pediatric patients with ALL in first remission for whom an allo-

Table XIX-2-2. Results of Prospective Trials Comparing Transplantation and Chemotherapy for the Treatment of AML in First Remission

Center	Bone Marrow Transplant		Chemotherapy		Reference
	DFS	Rate of Relapse	DFS	Rate of Relapse	
Fred Hutchinson	49%*	15%	20%	74%	Appelbaum[8]
	N = 33		N = 46		
UCLA	40%	40%*	27%	71%	Champlin[57,58]
	N = 23		N = 44		
Royal Marsden	64%	22%*	29%	68%	Powles[181]
	N = 22		N = 28		
University of Cantabria	70%*	10%*	10%	88%	Conde[65]
	N = 14		N = 25		
Memorial Sloan-Kettering Cancer Center	33%	15%*	17%	80%	Clarkson[60]
	N = 28		N = 69		
M. D. Anderson	36%*	9%*	15%	85%	Zander[267]
	N = 11		N = 27		

*Statistically significant difference

geneic transplant clearly affords an improved probability of cure. Indeed, allogeneic marrow grafts in children and adolescents with high risk features have been associated with long-term disease-free survival rates of 56–84%, which are not superior to those which can now be achieved with chemotherapy alone.[24,25,44]

The place of allogeneic marrow grafts in the treatment of adults with ALL who have achieved an initial remission is only somewhat less controversial.[53] Current chemotherapeutic regimens induce remissions in 70–85% of adults, but these remissions are sustained in only 20–43% of cases.[99,120] For patients who, at initial diagnosis, present with disease features associated with a high risk of relapse such as a high initial white cell count ($>20,000/mm^3$), older age (>60 years), central nervous system involvement, chromosomal translocations t(4:11), t(8:14) or t(9:22), null or B-cell phenotype or a failure to achieve remission within 5 weeks of initiating induction therapy, sustained remission rates range from 10–20%. However, in several series evaluating the role of HLA-matched marrow transplants applied to the treatment of high risk young adults (<40 yrs.) in first remission, such transplants have led to 3–5 year disease-free survival rates ranging from 30–71%, with relapse rates post-transplant ranging from 9–36%, depending on the type of cytoreductive regimen used[38,40,76,77,119,255] and the method of GvHD prophylaxis incorporated.[24] These promising results suggest that allogeneic marrow grafts may offer a significant advantage to the adult with ALL who presents with high risk features. Prospective trials are needed, however, to ascertain this point and also to evaluate transplantation as a general approach to the treatment of adults with both average and high risk forms of ALL who achieve a first remission (see XXXVI-5).

Transplants for ALL in Second or Greater Remission or Relapse

Results reported for series of children who have received HLA-matched marrow grafts for acute lymphoblastic leukemia when in second remission vary considerably both in the incidence of relapse post-transplant and in the proportion of patients achieving long-term disease-free survival. Trans-

plants administered after cytoreduction with variations of the Seattle regimen of single dose TB1 and cyclophosphamide have been associated with relapse rates ranging from 30–57% at 2 years, and disease-free survival rates of 33–50%.[197,263] In contrast, newer approaches incorporating higher doses of hyperfractionated total body irradiation followed by cyclophosphamide,[46] or fractionated total body irradiation administered with high dose cytosine arabinoside,[64] etoposide,[40] or altered doses of cyclophosphamide[255] have reduced the incidence of relapse post-transplant to 5–16%, and concurrently improved long-term disease-free survival to 59–64% at 5-years.

For meaningful comparisons between these transplant results and the results achievable with chemotherapy alone, it is critical to compare characteristics of the patient populations treated, particularly the duration of their first remission prior to relapse. Children with ALL who relapse early in the course of their initial chemotherapy (e.g., in the first 18 months) may be induced into a second remission with chemotherapy, but are unlikely to survive disease-free for more than 6–12 months. In contrast, chemotherapy alone may secure long-term remission or cure for up to 40% of patients with ALL who relapse after completing 18–24 months of chemotherapy (see XXXIX-2).[190] Given these statistics, it has been argued that while a transplant is indicated for children who relapse early, it may not be an appropriate option for patients relapsing after a prolonged initial remission. To address this issue, we have reanalyzed our own series from this point of view.[46] For patients whose initial remission exceeded 18 months, 77% are currently surviving disease-free at a median of 6 years post-transplant. Of those whose initial remission was less than 18 months, 46% are also disease-free at this interval. Strikingly, the incidence of relapse in the two groups is equivalent: differences in disease-free survival are based on a higher incidence of early non-leukemic mortality in transplant recipients who relapsed within the first year of their initial remission. These results strongly suggest that an allogeneic marrow graft is superior to chemotherapy for patients with ALL who relapse within 1 year of achieving their first remission. In our series, transplants may also be superior to chemotherapy when applied to patients with ALL who relapse late in their first remission. However, prospective trials comparing these two approaches are still needed to ascertain this issue.

For adults with ALL who have failed an initial remission, an HLA-matched marrow graft is the treatment of choice and the only therapy with curative potential. For adults transplanted in 2° remission, different groups have reported extended disease-free survival rates ranging from 22–43%, with relapse, post-transplant, representing the cause of failure in 26–56% of the cases.[24,75,119,255] For children and adults transplanted in later remissions or relapse, the probability of extended disease-free survival is more limited, ranging from 8–25% at 3–5 years post-grafting.[75,194,255]

Marrow Transplantation for Chronic Myelogenous Leukemia

Allogeneic bone marrow transplantation is clearly the treatment of choice in patients with chronic myelogenous leukemia (CML) who are under the age of 55 and have an HLA compatible donor. Single-agent chemotherapy applied to the treatment of CML has been only palliative, and has not been shown to significantly prolong survival.[207] Furthermore, while intensive combination chemotherapies have been used in an attempt to eradicate the Ph+ clone, suppression of Ph+ cells has been only transient. These regimens, which are associated with significant morbidity secondary to myelosuppression, have not resulted in a significant improvement in median survival.[227] Although alpha-interferon, used as first line therapy in CML, has induced hematologic remissions in as many as 70% of patients, true cytogenetic remissions have been less common, occurring in no more than 20% of patients so treated. Results reported recently, however, indicate that a number of these cytogenetic remissions may be durable in nature with some patients enjoying remissions on therapy for as long as 30 months (see XXXVI-3).[228]

Allogeneic marrow transplants, in contrast to chemotherapy alone, have induced durable eradications of Ph+ cells, and extended disease-free survival for a significant proportion of patients, dependent on the phase of disease at the time of transplant. Long-term survival rates of 55–70% have been achieved when patients are transplanted in chronic phase[103,104,155,156,241] as compared to 10 to 40% when in accelerated phase and 10% when patients receive a transplant in acute blast crisis.[55,66]

While overall survival rates as high as 70–90% at two years post-transplant have been documented for patients with CML,[229] disease-free survival rates are considerably lower. Factors shown to be associated with relapse and transplant-associated mortality have varied from one transplant group to another. However, status of disease at time of transplant is unanimously viewed as a significant predictor of subsequent relapse and survival.[72,156,233] In the three largest series reported to date,[104,155,233] patients transplanted in first chronic phase had a relapse rate of 6–30%. Those patients transplanted in accelerated phase were shown to have a 40% probability of relapse, while those patients transplanted during the blastic phase of their illness had an 80% probability of relapse. The majority of relapses occurred within the first

two years after transplant, but later relapses have been reported.

Several other factors have been examined by different transplant teams for possible association with relapse and survival. These include interval from diagnosis to transplant, influence of pretransplant splenectomy, presence of GvHD, and the use of a T cell depleted transplant. A review of the Seattle experience with allotransplants in CML demonstrated a statistically significant difference in actuarial survival between patients transplanted within the first 17 months of diagnosis as compared to those transplanted after 17 months from diagnosis, 73% vs. 54% respectively.[229] This difference, however, was not due to an increased relapse rate in the group transplanted after a longer interval from diagnosis; rather, the lower survival rate was found to be due to other complications possibly resulting from the sequelae of disease or its treatment. The International Bone Marrow Transplant Registry (IBMTR) has recently also confirmed the correlation between duration of disease prior to transplant and survival.

The influence of splenectomy prior to transplant has been reviewed by a number of investigators. There is little question that splenectomy, pre-transplant, results in more rapid engraftment and lower platelet transfusion requirements;[21,27] however, no group has documented any impact of pre-transplant splenectomy on relapse or overall survival.[233] If patients have splenomegaly at time of transplant, there is some evidence that these patients may benefit from splenectomy. A retrospective analysis of the effect of splenomegaly in patients undergoing bone marrow transplant for CML, revealed that splenomegaly significantly correlated with delayed engraftment and graft failure.[116] In that analysis, there was a higher frequency of death, secondary to graft failure, in the splenomegaly group than in the non-splenomegaly group. Additional splenic irradiation did not appear to influence the rate of engraftment in those patients with splenomegaly.

As to the effect of GvHD on relapse and survival, the IBMTR noted that the 4-year probability of survival was 74% for those patients who developed no, or mild acute GvHD compared to 35% for patients who developed moderate to severe acute GvHD.[104] Whereas acute GvHD had a negative impact on the survival rate, chronic GvHD appeared to have a favorable impact on the relapse rate. Patients who did not develop chronic GvHD exhibited a higher relapse rate than those patients who developed some degree of chronic GvHD, lending support to the theory that a graft vs. leukemia effect is associated with GvHD.

In an attempt to reduce the significant morbidity and mortality associated with GvHD, several groups have investigated the use of T cell depleted bone marrow transplants in CML.[12,104] Use of T cell depleted grafts has resulted in a significant decrease and in some cases total absence of GvHD, depending on the method of T cell depletion used. Although such an effect should result in increased survival once the morbidity and mortality of GvHD is removed, the increased incidence of graft failure and relapse post-transplant associated with the use of a T cell depleted transplant has not resulted in a significant improvement in overall disease-free survival.[104,146]

The availability of an allogeneic bone marrow transplant offers some patients with CML the chance for long-term disease-free survival. However, for a significant number of patients, i.e., those over the age of 60 and those without an HLA identical bone marrow transplant donor, the availability or efficacy of this approach is limited. The establishment of an unrelated national bone marrow registry has afforded some patients the opportunity to receive a bone marrow transplant from a phenotypically matched unrelated donor or one who is mismatched at a single HLA locus. Such transplants may result in long-term outcomes similar to those achieved with an HLA matched sibling.[29] Ultimately, better tolerated pre-transplant regimens and development of methods for securing consistent engraftment of T cell depleted marrow grafts may also extend the use of this treatment modality to older patients.

Marrow Transplants for Myelodysplastic Syndromes

The myelodysplastic syndromes are a heterogeneous series of disorders marked by peripheral cytopenias associated with normal to increased marrow cellularity and abnormal maturation of the myeloid series. In over 70% of cases, clonal cytogenetic abnormalities are observed, particularly single deletions of 5q, monosomy 7 and trisomy 8. Among these syndromes, four pathological variants, or stages, of disease have been distinguished, based on the proportion of blasts and the degree of marrow fibrosis: refractory anemia (RA), refractory anemia with excess blasts (RAEB), RAEB in leukemic transformation ($RAEB_T$) and myelofibrosis.[34] Intensive chemotherapeutic regimens have yielded only short term remissions and have been associated with significant morbidity and mortality.[127] Treatment with low dose cytosine arabinoside[111] and supportive measures, such as the use of danazol to stimulate platelets and GmCSF or GCSF to induce production of mature neutrophils,[6,63,162] may reduce the complications of peripheral cytopenias and prolong survival, but have not induced durable remissions of disease. Azacytidine has been reported to produce remissions[202A] (see XXXVI-1).

In contrast to these results, allogeneic marrow grafts administered to patients prepared with TBI or Busulfan and cyclophosphamide have led to sustained remissions of disease in 40–50% of cases.[7,14,73,112,165] Accumulated experience suggests that patients transplanted for refractory anemia enjoy somewhat better prospects for disease free survival (53–61%) than patients with RAEB (40–74%) or RAEB in transformation (14–50%). This difference reflects the extremely low incidence of disease relapse among patients transplanted for RA (0–6%), a result which has spawned exploration of preparative regimens incorporating myeloablative agents with cyclophosphamide which are associated with less extramedullary toxicity. Among patients transplanted for RAEB or $RAEB_T$, however, relapse constitutes the major cause of transplant failure.[7] Experimental protocols incorporating novel pretransplant cytoreduction regimens are being explored to reduce the incidence of this complication.

Patients with severe myelofibrosis and malignant myelosclerosis, once engrafted, may recover normal hematopoiesis and achieve complete resolution of fibrosis with sustained disease-free survival.[185,262] However, the overall success of transplants for such cases is poor due to a high rate of peritransplant mortality.[7]

Other variables which have a negative impact on the outcome of transplants for myelodysplastic syndromes include older age, and surprisingly, the absence of associated cytogenetic abnormalities.[7] While transplants in more advanced disease stages tend to be less successful, the interval between diagnosis and transplant for patients in a given stage of disease does not clearly affect outcome. Similarly, while those patients who achieve a remission with chemotherapy have a better prognosis for disease-free survival post transplant, the overall results for groups of patients who are or are not treated with chemotherapy prior to referral for transplantation are not different.[7,73]

Marrow Transplantation for Lymphoma

Current regimens employing multiple chemotherapeutic agents in dose intensive protocols induce durable curative remissions in approximately 50% of adults and over 70% of children with intermediate and high-grade lymphomas. Similarly, primary treatment of Hodgkin's disease is now curative for over 70% of cases. As a result, transplant of either allogeneic or autologous marrow, administered after myeloablative doses of total body radiation or alkylating agents together with cyclophosphamide, has largely been applied to patients who fail to attain or sustain a primary remission of disease. While experience with allogeneic marrow transplants applied to the treatment of non-Hodgkin's lymphoma is still limited,[13] it strongly indicates that disease status at time of transplant, rather than initial stage or type of lymphoma, is the most important prognostic indicator of long-term disease-free survival (DFS). For patients with chemotherapy refractory NHL, prospects for extended DFS range from 0–23%,[67,85,179] compared to 25–44% of patients grafted in a second remission and 16 of 18 (88%) patients reported who received transplants in first remission.[85,236] In large series, results of allogeneic marrow grafts have not differed in incidence of DFS or relapse post-transplant from those achieved with autologous marrow grafts if the autologous marrow was obtained during remission.[10,110] Thus, while a transplant administered after myeloablative therapy can be curative for patients with advanced NHL or Hodgkin's disease who have relapsed after chemotherapy, an allogeneic marrow graft may offer little advantage over an autologous graft except for patients whose own marrow shows histologic evidence of disease.

Marrow Transplants for Multiple Myeloma

Until recently, the treatment of multiple myeloma has been limited to combination chemotherapy alone or combined with alpha interferon.[138,145] Despite initial response rates as high as 50–60%, the median survival of patients with this disease remains at about three years.[22] Thus, attention has been focused on the use of highly intensive chemoradiotherapy regimens with hematopoietic support, either in the form of autologous marrow or peripheral blood stem cells.[4,23] Unfortunately, relapse remains a major obstacle in the use of autologous bone marrow transplantation in multiple myeloma.[5]

Recent advances in transplantation approaches and supportive care have facilitated the extension of allogeneic bone marrow transplantation to older patients. Thus, this treatment modality has now become available to selected patients with multiple myeloma, a disease characterized by a peak incidence between the ages of 50 and 70. The experience with allogeneic BMT preceded by TBI and a variety of high-dose single or multi-agent chemotherapy regimens has been limited to approximately 100 patients who comprise several separate studies reported to date.[48,95,239] At the present time, the 3-year survival for allografted patients with multiple myeloma transplanted at different stages of disease ranges between 30% and 60%.[23] Results from these studies suggest that the outcome of treatment may be dependent on the stage of disease at time of transplantation. Patients transplanted at an earlier stage and those who are not refractory to therapy prior to transplant are the ones most likely to benefit.[52,239] Complications such as GvHD and interstitial pneumonitis have a major impact on survival. In addition, whether or not a graft-vs.-myeloma effect exists, akin to the graft-vs.-leukemia effect noted in certain leukemias, is not known. These observations are consistent with the experience from the application of similar treatment regimens to other hematologic conditions.

An improvement in the outcome of allogeneic BMT in multiple myeloma will depend on initiating this form of treatment earlier in the course of the disease and better selecting those patients most likely to benefit from this approach. In addition, improved conditioning regimens and post-transplant treatment of infection and GvHD will be required if improved disease-free survival rates in this group of patients are to be achieved (see XXXVI-12).

Marrow Transplantation for Patients Lacking an HLA Identical Sibling Donor

As marrow transplantation has become recognized as a treatment of choice for many lethal congenital and acquired disorders of hematopoiesis, the need to develop effective transplantation approaches for the 60–70% of patients who lack an HLA matched sibling donor has escalated. Attention has been primarily focused on either the identification of adequately compatible alternative donors or the development of techniques whereby histoincompatible marrow can be successfully applied without risk of graft rejection or lethal graft versus host disease.

HLA-Partially Matched Related Donors

Initial attempts to identify alternative donors focused on the use of HLA haploidentical but MLC compatible related donors, since studies in murine models had suggested that marrow grafts administered to MHC Class II disparate recipients were most likely to induce lethal GvHD.[136] Early clinical experience with such transplants administered to patients with SCID indirectly supported this approach, since disparities for HLA-A and/or -B on one haplotype were tolerated without lethal GvHD.[79,132] However, in the large series of HLA partially matched transplants administered for leukemia reported by Beatty and colleagues, no single allelic disparity (e.g., HLA-A or -B or -D) was associated with a greater

severity of GvHD.[30] Indeed, marrow grafts administered to patients expressing single HLA allele disparities on one haplotype, while inducing severe GvHD in over 75% of cases, were associated with an incidence of long-term disease-free survival comparable to that achieved with HLA matched marrow grafts. Recipients exhibiting two or more HLA allelic disparities on one haplotype (e.g., HLA-A and -B, or HLA-B and -D), on the other hand, had a significantly increased risk of graft rejection (21% for two allele disparate grafts vs. 9% for one, and 7% for no allelic disparities, respectively), and severe acute and chronic graft vs. host disease. As a consequence, the proportion of patients surviving such transplants has been low (<15%).[30]

Unrelated Donors

In 1977, our group reported the first successful application of an HLA compatible marrow graft derived from an unrelated donor to the treatment of a child afflicted with SCID.[170] Thereafter, a series of case reports further documented the potential of this approach in the treatment of children with leukemia[114] and aplastic anemia.[80,105,125] The development of a statewide registry in Iowa allowed Gingrich and colleagues to administer unrelated marrow grafts to a series of 40 patients with heavily treated refractory forms of leukemia and aplastic anemia.[100] Of these patients, 6 (15%) survived disease-free for >1 year. The incidence of severe (Grade II–IV) acute GvHD was 67%; 5 of the 6 surviving patients also had chronic GvHD. However, in this series, only 6/40 were ascertained to be HLA-A, -B, -D matched with their donors. A subsequent report of the results from 4 centers which applied unrelated HLA matched marrow grafts to the treatment of 37 patients with chronic myelogenous leukemia was more encouraging: 3-year survival projections for patients transplanted in chronic phase, or in accelerated or blastic phase of CML were 55% and 22% respectively.[29] However, in series reported from individual centers, the incidence of both acute and chronic GvHD in recipients of unmodified marrow grafts from unrelated donors has been high, approximating that seen following transplants of marrow from 1–2 HLA allele disparate related donors.[32,100,101,125]

The other limitation to the use of unrelated marrow grafts is the availability of suitably matched donors. Current donor registries can provide matched donors for 20 to 30% of Caucasian individuals, particularly those who inherit common HLA haplotypes detected in Northern European Caucasian populations. However, donors of other ethnogeographic backgrounds are under-represented. Even if current registries expand to include 10^6 active donors, it will still be difficult to obtain donors for individuals whose haplotypes include HLA alleles which are rare or not genetically linked.[31,208] Thus, while unrelated donors may ultimately be found for 30% of patients, 20–30% of patients will still lack a donor. Therefore, there is a continuing need for transplantation approaches whereby consistent engraftment and functional reconstitution can be achieved in HLA disparate recipients without severe or lethal GvHD.

T Cell Depleted HLA-Non-Identical Marrow Grafts

The development of T cell depletion techniques has provided one such approach to this problem. In 1981, our group demonstrated that transplants of HLA-A, -B or HLA-A, -B, -D haplotype disparate parental marrow depleted of T cells by soybean lectin agglutination and E-rosette depletion could reconstitute hematopoietic and lymphoid function in children with leukemia[187] and severe combined immunodeficiencies (SCID)[188] without GvHD. Currently, of 33 patients with SCID transplanted with T cell depleted parental marrow in our series, 24 survive with reconstitution of immunity 1–9 years post transplant. The actuarial probability of extended disease-free survival (72%) associated with these haplotype disparate grafts does not differ significantly from that achieved with unmodified, HLA matched grafts in severe combined immune deficiency.[173] Other centers, and the European cooperative group have subsequently reported similar results.[91,92]

Transplants of T cell depleted HLA haplotype disparate marrow administered to patients for other genetic diseases or for leukemia are also associated with a low incidence of GvHD. However, the high incidence of graft rejection associated with such transplants has severely limited their effectiveness. In a recent European survey, of 23 children with genetic immune deficiencies other than SCID transplanted with T cell depleted HLA mismatched marrow after conditioning with busulfan and cyclophosphamide, 11 failed to engraft.[91] Overall, 2–4 year disease-free survival was 29% for these patients compared with a 47% disease-free survival for recipients of the HLA matched grafts. Among leukemic patients transplanted with HLA-non-identical T cell depleted marrow after cytoreduction with total body irradiation and cyclophosphamide, the incidence of graft failures or rejection has ranged from 10–50% depending on the number of disparate HLA alleles unique to the donor.[168,172] Recently, however, alternative approaches utilizing more intensive preparative cytoreduction,[45,50,235] less stringent T cell depletion,[15,50,235] and the administration of antithymocyte globulin or T cell specific immunotoxins and steroids in the early post transplant period have reduced the incidence of rejection to 0–15% without unduly increasing the risk of severe GvHD. For example, Trigg and colleagues have reported 31 children transplanted with HLA non-identical marrow depleted of T cells with CT-2 monoclonal antibody and rabbit complement after preparation with cytosine arabinoside, cyclophosphamide, and total body irradiation.[235] In this group, 13% rejected their graft; 26% developed Grade II–IV GvHD, and 54% survived 1–30 months post grafting. Similarly, Henslee and colleagues has reported a 50% extended disease-free survival rate in a series of patients transplanted for leukemia with monoclonal antibody treated, partially T cell depleted marrow after intensive cytoreduction and treatment post-transplant with a T cell specific ricin A immunotoxin.[117] In these series, results of T cell depleted transplants from related, 1–2 allele disparate donors and unrelated, HLA matched donors have yielded equivalent results. Thus, it is likely that as new approaches combining improved T cell depletion techniques and more consistently effective cyto-

reductive regimens increase the incidence and quality of engraftment, the ability to extend curative transplants to the full spectrum of patients lacking a donor will be realized.

Bibliography

1. Anasetti, C., Amos, D., Beatty, P. G., Appelbaum, F. R., Bensinger, W., Buckner, C. D., Clift, R., Doney, K., Martin, P. J., Mickelson, E., Nisperios, B., O'Quigley, J., Ramberg, R., Sanders, J. E., Stewart, P., Storb, R., Sullivan, K. M., Witherspoon, R. P., Thomas, E. D., and Hansen, J. A.: Effect of HLA compatibility of engraftment of bone marrow transplants in patients with leukemia or lymphoma. N. Engl. J. Med., 320:197, 1989.
2. Anasetti, C., Martin, P. J., Hansen, J. A., Appelbaum, F. R., Beatty, P. G., Doney, K., Harkonen, S., Jackson, A., Reichert, T., Stewart, P., Storb, R., Sullivan, K. M., Thomas, E. D., Warner, N., and Witherspoon, R. P.: A Phase I–II study evaluating the murine anti-IL-2 receptor antibody 2A3 for treatment of acute graft-versus-host disease. Transplant. Proc., 50:49, 1990.
3. Anderson, K. C., and Weinstein, H. J.: Transfusion-associated graft-versus-host disease. N. Engl. J. Med., 323:315, 1990.
4. Anderson, K. C., Barut, B. A., Ritz, J., Freedman, A. S., and Nadler, L. M.: Autologous bone marrow transplantation therapy for multiple myeloma. Eur. J. Haematol., 53 (Suppl. 51):157, 1989.
5. Anderson, M. K., Barut, B. A., Ritz, J., Freedman, A. S., Takvorian, T., Rabinowe, S. N., Soiffer, R., Heflin, L., Coral, F., Dear, K., Mauch, P., and Nadler, L. M.: Monoclonal antibody-purged autologous bone marrow transplantation therapy for multiple myeloma. Blood, 77:712, 1991.
6. Antin, J. H., Smith, B. R., Holmes, W., and Rosenthal, D. S.: Phase I/II study of recombinant human granulocyte macrophage colony-stimulating factor in aplastic anemia and myelodysplastic syndrome. Blood, 72:705, 1989.
7. Appelbaum, F. R., Barrall, J., Storb, R., Fisher, L. D., Schoch, G., Ramberg, R. E., Shulman, H., Anasetti, C., Bearman, S. I. Beatty, P., Bensinger, W. I., Buckner, C. D., Clift, R. A., Hansen, J. A., Martin, P., Petersen, F. B., Sanders, J. E., Singer, J., Stewart, P., Sullivan, K. M., Witherspoon, R. P., and Thomas, E. D.: Bone marrow transplantation for patients with myelodysplasia: Pretreatment variables and outcome. Ann. Intern. Med., 112:590, 1990.
8. Appelbaum, F. R., Dahlberg, S., Thomas, E. D., Buckner, C. D., Cheever, M. A., Clift, R. A., Crowley, J., Deeg, H. J., Fefer, A., Greenberg, P. D., Kadin, M., Smith, W., Stewart, P., Sullivan, K., Storb, R., and Weiden, P.: Bone marrow transplantation or chemotherapy after remission induction for adults with acute nonlymphoblastic leukemia: A prospective comparison. Ann. Intern. Med., 101:581, 1984.
9. Appelbaum, F. R., Strauchen, J. A., and Graw, R. G.: Acute lethal carditis caused by high-dose endoxan chemotherapy: A unique clinical and pathological entity. Lancet, 1:58, 1976.
10. Appelbaum, F. R., Sullivan, K. M., Buckner, C. D., Clift, R. A., Deeg, H. J., Fefer, A., Hill, R., Mortimer, J., Neiman, P. A., Sanders, J. E., Singer, J., Stewart, P., Storb, R., and Thomas, E. D.: Treatment of malignant lymphoma in 100 patients with chemotherapy, total body irradiation, and marrow transplantation. J. Clin. Oncol., 5:1340, 1987.
11. Apperley, J. F., and Goldman, J. M.: Cytomegalovirus: Biology, Clinical Features and Methods for Diagnosis. Bone Marrow Transplant., 3:253, 1988.
12. Apperley, J. F., Jones, L., Hale, G., Waldmann, H., Hows, J., Rombos, Y., Tsatalas, C., Marcus, R. E., Goolden, A. W. G., Gordon-Smith, E. C., Catovsky, D., Galton, D. A. G., and Goldman, J. M.: Bone marrow transplantation for patients with chronic myeloid leukaemia: T-cell depletion with Campath-1 reduces the incidence of graft-versus-host disease but may increase the risk of leukaemic relapse. Bone Marrow Transplant., 1:53, 1986.
13. Armitage, J. O.: Bone marrow transplantation in the treatment of patients with lymphoma. Blood, 73:1749, 1989.
14. Arnold, R., and Heimpel, H.: Allogeneic bone marrow transplantation for myelodysplastic syndromes (MDS). Bone Marrow Transplant., 4(Suppl. 4):101, 1989.
15. Ash, R. C., Casper, J. T., Chitambar, C. R., Hansen, R., Bunin, N., Truitt, R. L., Lawton, C., Murray, K., Hunter, H., Baxter-Lowe, L. A., Gottschall, J. L., Oldham, K., Anderson, T., Camitta, B., and Menitove, J.: Successful allogeneic transplantation on T cell depleted bone marrow from closely HLA-matched unrelated donors. N. Engl. J. Med., 332:485, 1990.
16. Atkinson, K., Norrie, S., Chan, P., Zehnwirth, B., Downs, K., and Biggs, J.: Hemopoietic progenitor cell function after HLA-identical sibling bone marrow transplantation: Influence of chronic graft-versus-host disease. Int. J. Cell Cloning, 4:203, 1986.
17. Atkinson, K., Storb, R., Prentice, R. L., Weiden, P. L., Witherspoon, R. P., Sullivan, K., Noel, D., and Thomas, E. D.: Analysis of late infections in 89 long-term survivors of bone marrow transplantation. Blood, 53:720, 1979.
18. Atkinson, K., Farewell, V., Storb, R., Tsoi, M. S., Sullivan, K. M., Witherspoon, R. P., Fefer, A., Clift, R., Goodell, B., and Thomas, E. D.: Analysis of late infections after human bone marrow transplantation. Role of non-specific suppressor cells in patients with chronic graft-versus-host disease and genotypic non-identity between marrow donor and recipient. Blood, 60:714, 1982.
19. Bach, F. H., Albertini, R. J., Joo, P., Anderson, J. L., and Bortin, M. M.: Bone marrow transplantation in a patient with the Wiskott-Aldrich Syndrome. Lancet, 2:1364, 1968.
20. Baglin, T. P., Harper, P., and Marcus, R. E.: Veno-occlusive disease of the liver complicating ABMT successfully treated with recombinant tissue plasminogen activator (rt-PA). Bone Marrow Transplant., 5:439, 1990.
21. Banaji, M., Bearman, S. I., Buckner, C. D., Clift, R. A., Bensinger, W. I., Petersen, F. B., Slichter, S. J., McGuffin, R. W., Sanders, J. E., Stewart, P. S., Hill, R. S., Deeg, H. J., Storb, R., and Thomas, E. D.: The effects of splenectomy on engraftment and platelet transfusion requirements in patients with chronic myelogenous leukemia undergoing marrow transplantation. Am. J. Hematol., 22:275, 1986.
22. Barlogie, B., Epstein, J., Selvanayagam, P., and Alexanian, R.: Plasma cell myeloma: New biological insights and advances in therapy. Blood, 73:865, 1989.
23. Barlogie, B., and Gahrton, G.: Bone marrow transplantation in multiple myeloma. Bone Marrow Transplant., 7:71, 1991.
24. Barrett, A. J., Horowitz, M. M., Gale, R. P., Biggs, J. C., Camitta, B. M., Dicke, K. A., Gluckman, E., Good, R. A., Herzig, R. H., Lee, M. B., Marmont, A. M., Masaoka, T.,

Ramsay, N. K. C., Rimm, A. A., Speck, B., Zwaan, F. E., and Bortin, M. M.: Marrow transplantation for acute lymphoblastic leukemia: Factors affecting relapse and survival. Blood, 74:862, 1989.
25. Barrett, A. J., Joshi, R., Kendra, J. R., Philips, R. H., Ashford, R., Shaw, P. J., Hugh-Jones, K., and Hobbs, J. R.: Prediction and prevention of relapse of acute lymphoblastic leukaemia after bone marrow transplantation. Br. J. Haematol., 64:179, 1986.
26. Bauer, M. P., Neugebauer, M., and Albert, E. D.: Reference tables of three-locus haplotype frequencies and delta values. *In* Caucasians, Orientals, and Negroids in Histocompatibility Testing 1984. Edited by E. D. Albert, et al: Berlin, Heidelberg, Springer-Verlag, 1984, pp. 756–760.
27. Baughan, A. S., Worsley, A. M., McCarthy, D. M., Hows, J. M., Catovsky, D., Gordon-Smith, E. C., Galton, D. A. G., and Goldman, J. M.: Haematological reconstitution and severity of graft-versus-host disease after bone marrow transplantation for chronic granulocytic leukaemia: The influence of previous splenectomy. Br. J. Haematol., 56:445, 1984.
28. Bearman, S. I., Hinds, M. S., Wolford, J. L., Petersen, F. B., Nugent, D. L., Slichter, S. J., Shulman, H. M., and McDonald, G. B.: A pilot study of continuous infusion heparin for the prevention of hepatic veno-occlusive disease after bone marrow transplantation. Bone Marrow Transplant., 5:407, 1990.
29. Beatty, P. G., Ash, R., Hows, J. M., and McGlave, P. B.: The use of unrelated bone marrow donors in the treatment of patients with chronic myelogenous leukemia: Experience of four marrow transplant centers. Bone Marrow Transplant., 4:287, 1989.
30. Beatty, P. G., Clift, R. A., Michelson, E. M., Nisperos, B., Flourney, N., Martin, P. J., Sanders, J. E., Stewart, P., Buckner, C. D., Storb, R., Thomas, E. D., and Hansen, J. A.: Marrow transplantation from related donors other than HLA-identical siblings. N. Engl. J. Med., 313:765, 1985.
31. Beatty, P. G., Dahlberg, S., Mickelson, E. M., Nisperos, B., Opelz, G., Martin, P. J., and Hansen, J. A.: Probability of finding HLA-matched unrelated marrow donors. Transplant. Proc., 45:714, 1988.
32. Beatty, P. G., Hansen, J. A., Anasetti, C., Sanders, J., Martin, P. J., Buckner, C. D., Storb, R., and Thomas, E. D.: Significance of different levels of histocompatibility in patients receiving marrow grafts from unrelated donors. Experimental Hematology, 18:509a, 1990.
33. Begg, C. B., McGlave, P. B., Bennett, J. M., Cassileth, P. A., and Oken, M. M.: A critical comparison of allogeneic bone marrow transplantation and conventional chemotherapy as treatment for acute lymphocytic leukemia. J. Clin. Oncol., 2:369, 1984.
34. Bennett, J. M., Catovsky, D., Daniel, M. T., Flandrin, G., Galton, D. A. G., Gralnick, H. R., and Sultan, C., (FAB Cooperative Group): Proposals for the classification of the myelodysplastic syndromes. B. J. Haematol., 51:189, 1982.
35. Bidwell, J. L., Bidwell, E. A., Savage, D. A., Middleton, D., Klouda, P. T., and Bradley, B. A.: A DNA-RFLP typing system that positively identifies serologically well-defined and ill-defined HLA-DR and DQ alleles including DRW 10. Transplant., 45:640, 1988.
36. Billingham, R. E.: The biology of graft-versus-host reactions. Harvey Lect., 62:21, 1966–1967.
37. Blacklock, H., Ball, L., Knight, C., Schey, S., and Prentice, G.: Experience with mesna in patients receiving allogeneic bone marrow transplants for poor prognostic leukaemia. Cancer Treat. Rev., 10(Suppl. A):45, 1983.
38. Blaise, D., Gaspard, M. H., Stoppa, A. M., Michel, G., Gastaut, J. A., Lepeu, G., Tubiana, N., Blanc, A. P., Rossi, J. F., Novakovitch, G., Mannoni, P., Mawas, C., Maraninchi, D., and Carcassone, Y.: Allogeneic or autologous bone marrow transplantation for acute lymphoblastic leukemia in first complete remission. Bone Marrow Transplant., 5:7, 1990.
39. Blume, K. G., Forman, S. J., O'Donnell, M. R., Doroshow, J. H., Krance, R. A., Nademanee, A. P., Snyder, D. S., Schmidt, G. M., Fahey, J. L., Metter, G. E., Hill, L. R., Findley, D. O., and Sniecinski, I. J.: Total body irradiation and high-dose etoposide: A new preparatory regimen for bone marrow transplantation in patients with advanced hematologic malignancies. Blood, 69:1015, 1987.
40. Blume, K. G., Forman, S. J., Snyder, D. S., Nademanee, A. P., O'Donnell, M. R., Fahey, J. L., Krance, R. A., Sniecinski, I. J., Stock, A. D., Findley, D. O., Lipsett, J. A., Schmidt, G. M., Nathwani, M. B., Hill, L. R., and Metter, G. E.: Allogeneic bone marrow transplantation for acute lymphoblastic leukemia during first complete remission. Transplant. Proc., 43:389, 1987.
41. Bodmer, W. F.: HLA 1987. *In* immunobiology of HLA, Volume II Immunogenetics and Histocompatibility. Edited by B. Dupont. New York, Springer-Verlag, 1989, pp. 1–9.
42. Bolger, G. B., Sullivan, K. M., Storb, R., Witherspoon, R. P., Weiden, P. L., Stewart, P., Sanders, J., Meyers, J. D., Martin, P. J., Doney, K. C., Deeg, H. J., Clift, R. A., Buckner, C. D., Appelbaum, F. R., and Thomas, E. D.: Second marrow infusion for poor graft function after allogeneic marrow transplantation. Bone Marrow Transplant., 1:21, 1986.
43. Bordignon, C., Keever, C. A., Small, T. N., Flomenberg, N., Dupont, B., and O'Reilly, R. J.: Graft failure after T-cell-depleted human leukocyte antigen identical marrow transplants for leukemia: In vitro analyses of host effector mechanisms. Blood, 74:2237, 1989.
44. Bordigoni, P., Vernant, J. P., Souillet, G., Gluckman, E., Marininchi, D., Milpied, N., Fischer, A., Lemoine, E. B., Jouet, J. P., and Reiffers, J.: Allogeneic bone marrow transplantation for children with acute lymphoblastic leukemia in first remission: A Cooperative Study of the Groupe d'Etude de la Greffe de Moelle Osseuse. J. Clin. Oncol., 7:747, 1989.
45. Bozdech, M. J., Sondel, P. M., Trigg, M. E., Longo, W., Kohler, P. C., Flynn, B., Billing, R., Anderson, S. A., Hank, J. A., and Hong, R.: Transplantation of HLA-haploidentical T-cell depleted marrow for leukemia: Addition of cytosine arabinoside to the pretransplant conditioning prevents rejection. Exp. Hematol., 13:1201, 1985.
46. Brochstein, J. A., Kernan, N. A., Groshen, S., Cirrincione, C., Shank, B., Emanuel, D., Laver, J., and O'Reilly, R. J.: Allogeneic bone marrow transplantation after hyperfractionated total-body irradiation and cyclophosphamide in children with acute leukemia. N. Engl. J. Med., 317:1618, 1987.
47. Brugieres, L., Hartmann, O., Travagli, J., Benhamou, E., Pico, J. L., Valteau, D., Kalifa, C., Patte, C., Flamant, F., and Lemerle, J.: Hemorrhagic cystitis following high-dose chemotherapy and bone marrow transplantation in children with malignancies: Incidence, clinical course and outcome. J. Clin. Oncol., 7:194, 1989.
48. Buckner, C. D., Fefer, A., Bensinger, W. I., Storb, R., Durie, B. G., Appelbaum, F. R., Petersen, F. B., Weiden, P., Clift, R. A., Sanders, J. E., Sullivan, K. M., Witherspoon, R. P., Hill, R., Martin, P., and Thomas, E. D.: Marrow transplantation for malignant plasma cell disorders: Summary of the Seattle experience. Eur. J. Haematol., 43(Suppl. 51):186, 1989.
49. Byers, V. S., Henslee, P. J., Kernan, N. A., Blazar, B. R., Gingrich, R., Phillips, G. L., LeMaistre, C. F., Gilliland, G., Antin, J. H., Martin, P., Tutscha, P. J., Trown, P., Ackerman, S. K., O'Reilly, R. J., and Scannon, P. J.: Use of an anti-pan T-lymphocyte Ricin A chain immunotoxin in steroid-resistant acute graft-versus-host disease. Blood, 75:1426, 1990.
50. Cahn, J. Y., Herve, P., Flesch, M., Plouvier, E., Racadot, E., Vuillier, J., Montcuquet, P., Noir, A., Rozenbaum, A., and Leconte des Floris, R.: Marrow transplantation from HLA non-identical family donors for the treatment of leukemia: A pilot study of 15 patients using additional immunosuppression and t-cell depletion. Br. J. Haematol., 69:345, 1988.
51. Camitta, B., O'Reilly, R. J., Sensenbrenner, L., Rappeport, J., Champlin, R., Doney, K., August, C., Hoffmann, R. G., Kirkpatrick, D., Stuart, R., Santos, G., Parkman, R., Gale, R. P., Storb, R., and Nathan, D.: Antithoracic duct lymphocyte globulin therapy of severe aplastic anemia. Blood, 62:883, 1983.
52. Cavo, M., Tura, S., Rosti, G., Grimaldi, M., Bandini, G., Bonelli, M. A., Calori, E., Rizzi, S., Van Lint, M. T., Bacigalupo, A., Marmnt, A., Aversa, F., Martelli, M., Polchi, P., and Lucarelli, G.: Allogeneic bone marrow transplantation for multiple myeloma. The Italian experience. Bone Marrow Transplant., 7:31, 1991.
53. Champlin, R. E., and Gale, R. P.: Acute lymphoblastic leukemia: Recent advances in biology and therapy. Blood, 73:2051, 1989.
54. Champlin, R. E., and Gale, R. P.: Acute myelogenous leukemia: Recent advances in therapy. Blood, 69:1551, 1987.
55. Champlin, R. E., Goldman, J. M., and Gale, R. P.: Bone marrow transplantation in chronic myelogenous leukemia. Semin. Hematol., 25:74, 1988.
56. Champlin, R. E., Horowitz, M. M., van Bekkum, D. W., Camitta, B. M., Elfenbein, G. E., Gale, R. P., Gluckman, E., Good, R. A., Rimm, A. A., Rozman, C., Speck, B., and Bortin, M. M.: Graft failure following bone marrow transplantation for severe aplastic anemia: Risk factors and treatment results. Blood, 73:606, 1989.
57. Champlin, R. E., Ho, W. G., Gale, R. P., Winston, D., Selch, M., Mitsuyasu, R., Lenarsky, C., Elashoff, R., Zieghelboim, J., and Feig, S. A.: Treatment of acute myelogenous leukemia: A prospective controlled trial of bone marrow transplantation versus consolidation chemotherapy. Ann. Intern. Med., 102:285, 1985.
58. Champlin, R. Jacobs, A., Gale, R. P., Ho, W., Selch, M., Lenarsky, C., and Feig, S. A.: High-dose cytarabine in consolidation chemotherapy or with bone marrow transplantation for patients with acute leukemia: Preliminary results. Semin. Oncol., XII (Suppl. 3):190, 1985.
59. Churchill, M. A., Zaia, J. A., Forman, S. J., Sheibani, K., Azumi, N., and Blume, K. G.: Quantitation of human cytomegalovirus DNA in lungs from bone marrow transplant recipients with interstitial pneumonia. J. Infect. Dis., 155:501, 1987.
60. Clarkson, B., Berman, E., Little, C., Andreeff, M., Kempin, S., Kolitz, J., Gabrilove, J., Arlin, Z., Mertelsmann, R., Cunningham, I., Castro-Malaspina, H., Gulati, S., O'Reilly, R., and Gee, T.: Update on clinical trials of chemotherapy and bone marrow transplantation in acute myelogenous leukemia in adults at Memorial Sloan-Kettering Cancer Center 1966 to 1989. Acute Myelogenous Leukemia: Progress and Controversies, Wiley-Liss, Inc., 1990, pp. 239–272.
61. Clavell, L. A., Gelber, R. D., Cohen, J. H., Hitchcock-Bryan, S., Cassady, J. R., Tarbell, N. J., Blattner, S. R., Tantravahi, R., Leavitt, P., and Sallan, S. E.: Four-agent induction and intensive asparaginase therapy for treatment of childhood acute lymphoblastic leukemia. N. Engl. J. Med., 315:657, 1986.
62. Clift, R. A., Buckner, C. D., Thomas, E. D., Kopecky, K. J., Appelbaum, F. R., Tallman, M., Storb, R., Sanders, J., Sullivan, K., Banaji, M., Beatty, P. S., Bensinger, W., Cheever, M., Deeg, J., Doney, K., Fefer, A., Greenberg, P., Hansen, J. A., Hackman, R., Hill, R., Martin, P., Meyers, J., McGuffin, R., Neiman, P., Sale, G., Shulman, H., Singer, J., Stewart, P., Weiden, P., and Witherspoon, R.: The treatment of acute nonlymphoblastic leukemia by allogeneic marrow transplantation. Bone Marrow Transplant., 2:243, 1987.
63. Clines, D. B., Cassileth, P. A., and Kiss, J.: Danazol therapy in myelodysplasia. Ann. Intern. Med., 103:58, 1985.
64. Coccia, P. F., Strandjord, S. E., Warkentin, P. I., Cheung, N. K., Gordon, E. M., Novak, L. J., Shina, D. C., and Herzig, R. H.: High-dose cytosine arabinoside and fractionated total-body irradiation: An improved preparative regimen for bone marrow transplantation of children with acute lymphoblastic leukemia in remission. Blood, 71:888, 1988.
65. Conde, E., Iriondo, A., Rayon, C., Fanjul, E., Garigo, J., Hermos, V., Coma, A., Bello, C., Carrera, D., Baro, J., and Zubizarreta, A.: Allogeneic bone marrow transplantation versus intensification chemotherapy for acute myelogenous leukaemia in first remission: A prospective controlled trial. Br. J. Haematol., 68:219, 1988.
66. Copelan, E. A., Grever, M. R., Kapoor, N., and Tutschka, P. J.: Marrow transplantation following bulsulfan and cyclophosphamide for chronic myelogenous leukaemia in accelerated or blastic phase. Br. J. Haematol., 71:487, 1989.
67. Copelan, E. A., Kapoor, N., Gibbons, B., and Tutschka, P. J.: Allogeneic marrow transplantation in non-Hodgkin's lymphoma. Bone Marrow Transplant., 5:47, 1990.
68. Creutzig, V., Ritter, J., Riehm, H., Langermann, H. J., Henze, G., Kabisch, H., Niethammer, D., Jurgens, H., Stollmann, B., Lasson, U., Kaufmann, U., Loffler, H., and Schellong, G.: Improved treatment results in childhood acute myelogenous leukemia: A Report of the German Cooperative Study AML-BFM 78. Blood, 65:298, 1985.
69. Deeg, H. J., Flournoy, N., Sullivan, K. M., Sheehan, K., Buckner, C. D., Sanders, J. E., Storb, R., Witherspoon, R. P., and Thomas, E. D.: Cataracts after total body irradiation and marrow transplantation: A sparing effect of dose fractionation. Int. J. Radiat. Oncol. Biol. Phys., 10:957, 1984.
70. Deeg, H. J., Sanders, J. E., Martin, P., Fefer, A., Neiman, P., Singer, J., Storb, R., and Thomas, E. D.: Secondary malignancies after marrow transplantation. Exp. Hematol., 12:660, 1984.
71. Dennert, G., Anderson, C. G., and Warner, J.: T killer cells play a role in allogeneic bone marrow graft rejection but not in hybrid resistance. J. Immunol., 135:3729, 1985.
72. Devergie, A., Reiffers, J., Vernant, J. P., Herve, P., Guyotat, D., Maraninchi, D., Rio, B., Michallet, M., Jouet, J. P., Milpied, N., Leblond, V., Pico, J., Attal, M., Belanger, C., Bordigoni, P., Leporrier, M., Ifrah, N., Gratecos, N., Bergerat, J. P., Legros, M., Frappaz, D., and Gluckman, E.: Long-term follow-up after bone marrow transplantation for chronic myelogenous leukemia: Factors associated with relapse. Bone Marrow Transplant., 5:379, 1990.

73. DeWitte, T., Zwaan, F.,Hermans, J., Vernant, J., Kolb, H., Vossen, J., Lonnqvist, B., Beelen, D., Ferrant, A., Gmur, J., Yin, J. L., Troussard, X., Cahn, J., Van Lint, M., and Gratwohl, A.: Allogeneic bone marrow transplantation for secondary leukaemia and myelodysplastic syndrome: A survey by the leukaemia working party of the European Bone Marrow Transplantation Group (EMBTG). Br. J. Haematol., 74:151, 1990.
74. Dinsmore, R., Kirkpatrick, D., Flomenberg, N., Gulati, S., Kapoor, N., Brochstein, J., Shank, B., Reid, A., Groshen, S., and O'Reilly, R. J.: Allogeneic bone marrow transplantation for patients with acute nonlymphocytic leukemia. Blood, 63:649, 1984.
75. Dinsmore, R., Kirkpatrick, D., Flomenberg, N., Gulati, S., Kapoor, N., Shank, B., Reid, A., Groshen, S., and O'Reilly, R. J.: Allogeneic bone marrow transplantation for patients with acute lymphoblastic leukemia. Blood, 62:381, 1983.
76. Doney, K. C., Buckner, C. D., Kopecky, K. J., Sanders, J. E., Appelbaum, F. R., Clift, R., Sullivan, K., Witherspoon, R., Storb, R., and Thomas, E. D.: Marrow transplantation for patients with acute lymphoblastic leukemia in first marrow remission. Bone Marrow Transplant., 2:355, 1987.
77. Doney, K., Fisher, L. D., Appelbaum, F. R., Buckner, C. D., Storb, R., Singer, J., Fefer, A., Anasetti, C., Beatty, P., Bensinger, W., Clift, R., Hansen, J., Hill, R., Loughran, Jr., T. P., Martin, P., Petersen, F. B., Sanders, J., Sullivan, K. M., Stewart, P., Weiden, P., Witherspoon, R., and Thomas, E. D.: Treatment of adult acute lymphoblastic leukemia with allogeneic bone marrow transplantation. Multivariate analysis of factors affecting acute graft-versus-host disease, relapse, and relapse-free survival. Bone Marrow Transplant., 7:453, 1991.
78. Doney, K. C., Weiden, P. L., Storb, R., and Thomas, E. D.: Treatment of graft-versus-host disease in human allogeneic graft recipients: A randomized trial comparing antithymocyte globulin and corticosteroids. Am. J. Hematol., 11:1, 1981.
79. Dupont, B., O'Reilly, R. J., Pollack, M. S., and Good, R. A.: Use of genotypically different donors in bone marrow transplantation. Transplant Proc., 11:219, 1979.
80. DuQuesnoy, R. J., Zeevi, A., Marrari, M., Hackbarth, S., and Camitta, B.: Bone marrow transplantation for severe aplastic anemia using a phenotypically HLA-identical, SB-compatible unrelated donor. Transplant., 35:566, 1983.
81. Emanuel, D., Cunningham, I., Jules-Elysee, K., Brochstein, J., Kernan, N. A., Laver, J., Stover, D., White, D., Fels, A., Polsky, B., Castro-Malaspina, H., Peppard, J., Bartus, P., Hammerling, U., and O'Reilly, R. J.: Cytomegalovirus pneumonia after bone marrow transplantation successfully treated with the combination of ganciclovir and high-dose intravenous immune globulin. Ann. Intern. Med., 109:777, 1988.
82. Emanuel, D., Kernan, N. H., Castro-Malaspina, H., Cunningham, I., Taylor, J., Small, T., Keever, C., Flomenberg, N., Young, J., and O'Reilly, R. J.: Cytomegalovirus-associated bone marrow failure after allogeneic bone marrow transplantation successfully treated with the combination of ganciclover and high dose CMV immune globulin. Blood, 74 (Suppl. 1):905a, 1989.
83. Emanuel, D., Peppard, J., Stover, D., Gold, J., Armstrong, F., and Hammerling, U.: Rapid immunodiagnosis of cytomegalovirus pneumonia by bronchoalveolar lavage using human and murine monoclonal antibodies. Ann. Intern. Med., 104:476, 1986.
84. Epstein, J., Bealmear, P. M., Kennedy, D. W., Herrmann, M. J., Islam, A., and Wiedlt, S. C.: Prevention of graft-versus-host disease in allogeneic bone marrow transplantation by pretreatment with 2'-deoxycoformycin. Exp. Hematol., 14:845, 1986.
85. Ernst, P., Maraninchi, D., Jacobsen, N., Kolb, H. J., Bordigoni, P., Ljungman, P., Bandini, G., Parker, A. C., Volin, L., Powles, R., Gorin, N. G., and Rio, B.: Marrow transplantation for non-Hodgkin's lymphoma: A multi-centre study from the European co-operative bone marrow transplant group. Bone Marrow Transplant., 1:81, 1986.
86. Feig, S., Nesbit, M., Buckley, J., Lampkin, B., Bernstein, I., Kim, T., Piomelli, S., Kersey, J., Coccia, P., O'Reilly, R. J., Thomas, E. D., August, C., and Hammond, D.: Superiority of allogeneic bone marrow transplantation over conventional maintenance chemotherapy in children with acute non-lymphocytic leukemia. Exp. Hematol., 15:373a, 1987.
87. Ferrara, J. L., Guillen, F. J., Dijken, P. J., Marion, A., Murphy, G. F., and Burakoff, S. J.: Evidence that large granular lymphocytes of donor origin mediate acute graft-versus-host disease. Transplant., 47:50, 1989.
88. Ferrara, J., Marion, A., McIntyre, J. F., Murphy, G. F., and Burakoff, S. J.: Amelioration of acute graft-versus-host disease due to minor histocompatibility antigens by in vitro administration of anti-interleukin-2 receptor antibody. J. Immunol., 137:1874, 1986.
89. Ferretti, G. A., Ash, R. C., Brown, A. T., Parr, M. D., Romond, E. H., and Lillich, T. T.: Control of oral mucositis and candidiasis in marrow transplantation: A prospective, double-blind trial of chlorhexidine digluconate oral rinse. Bone Marrow Transplant., 3:483, 1988.
90. Filipovitch, A. H., Vallera, D. A., Youle, R. J., Haake, R., Blazar, B. R., Arthur, D., Neville, D. M., Ramsay, N. K. C., McGlave, P., and Kersey, J. H.: Graft-versus-host disease prevention in allogeneic bone marrow transplantation from histocompatible siblings. Transplant., 44:62, 1987.
91. Fischer, A., Griscelli, C., Friedrich, W., Kubanek, B., Levinsky, R., Morgan, G., Vossen, J., Wagemaker, G., and Landais, P.: Bone marrow transplantation for immunodeficiencies and osteopetrosis: European Survey, 1968–1985. Lancet, 2:1080, 1986.
92. Fischer, A.: Bone marrow transplantation in immunodeficiency and osteopetrosis. Bone Marrow Transplant., 4(Suppl. 14):12, 1989.
93. Flowers, M. E. D., Pepe, M. S., Longton, G., Doney, K. C., Monroe, D., Witherspoon, R. P., Sullivan, K. M., and Storb, R.: Previous donor pregnancy as a risk factor for acute graft-versus-host disease in patients with aplastic anaemia treated by allogeneic marrow transplantation. Br. J. Haematol., 74:492, 1990.
94. Frame, J., Collins, N. H., Cartagena, T., Waldmann, H., O'Reilly, R. J., and Kernan, N. A.: T-cell depletion of human bone marrow: Comparison of Campath-1 plus complement, anti-t-cell Ricin A chain immunotoxin and soybean agglutinin alone or in combination with sheep erythrocytes or immunomagnetic beads. Transplant., 47:984, 1989.
95. Gahrton, G., Tura, S., Belanger, C., Cavo, M., Chapvis, B., Ferrant, A., Flesch, M., Gore, M., Gratwohl, A., Gravett, P. J., Harrouseau, J. L., Lindeberg, A., Ljungman, P., Lowenberg, B., Lucarelli, G., Michallet, M., Reiffers, J., Ringden, O., Van Lint, M. T., Vernant, J. P., Sallerfors, B., Simonsson, B., Toivanen, A., Troussard, X., Verdonck, L. F., Volin, L., and Zwaan, F. E., for the European Group for Bone Marrow Transplantation: Allogeneic bone marrow transplantation in patients with multiple myeloma. Eur. J. Haematol., 43(Suppl. 51):182, 1989.
96. Gale, R. P., Bortin, M. M., van Bekkum, D. W., Biggs, J. C., Dicke, K. A., Gluckman, E., Good, R. A., Hoffmann, R. G., Kay, H. E. M., Kersey, J. H., Marmont, A., Masaoka, T., Rimm, A. A., van Rood, J. J., and Zwaan, F. E.: Risk factors for acute graft-versus-host disease. Br. J. Haematol., 67:397, 1987.
97. Ganem, G., Girardin, M., Kuentz, M., Cordonnier, C., Marinello, G., Teboul, C., Braconnier, F., Vernant, J. P., Dhumeaux, D., and Le Bourgeois, J. P.: Veno-occlusive disease of the liver after allogeneic bone marrow transplantation in man. Int. J. Radiat. Oncol. Biol. Phys., 14:879, 1988.
98. Gatti, R. A., Meuwiissen, H. J., Allen, H. D., Hong, R., and Good, R. A.: Immunological reconstitution of sex-linked lymphopenic immunological deficiency. Lancet, 2:1366, 1968.
99. Gaynor, J., Chapmann, D., Little, C., McKenzie, S., Miller, W., Andreeff, M., Arlin, Z., Berman, E., Kempin, S., Gee, T., and Clarkson, B.: A cause-specific hazard rate analysis of prognostic factors among 199 adults with acute lymphoblastic leukemia: The Memorial Hospital Experience since 1969. J. Clin. Oncol., 6:1014, 1988.
100. Gingrich, R. D., Ginder, G. D., Goeken, D., Howe, C. W. S., Wen, B. C., Hussey, D. H., and Fyfe, M. A.: Allogeneic marrow grafting with partially mismatched, unrelated donors. Blood, 71:1375, 1988.
101. Gluckman, E., Jolivet, I., Scrobohaci, M. L., Devergie, A., Traineau, R., Bourdeau-Esperon, H., Lehn, P., Foure, P., and Drouet, L.: Use of prostaglandin E_1 for prevention of liver veno-occlusive disease in leukaemic patients treated by allogeneic bone marrow transplantation. Br. J. Haematol., 74:277, 1990.
102. Glucksberg, H., Storb, R., Fefer, A., Buckner, C. D., Neiman, P. E., Clift, R. A., Lerner, K. G., and Thomas, E. D.: Clinical manifestations of GvHD in human recipients of marrow from hla-matched sibling donors. Transplant., 18:295, 1974.
103. Goldman, J. M., Apperley, J. F., Jones, L., Marcus, R., Goolden, A. W. G., Batchelor, R., Hale, G., Waldmann, H., Reid, C. D., Hows, J., Gordon-Smith, E., Catovsky, D., and Galton, D. A. G.: Bone marrow transplantation for patients with chronic meyloid leukemia. N. Engl. J. Med., 314:202, 1986.
104. Goldman, J. M., Gale, R. P., Horowitz, M. M., Biggs, J. C., Champlin, R. E., Gluckman, E., Hoffmann, R. G., Jacobsen, S. J., Marmont, A. M., McGlave, P. B., Messner, H. A., Rimm, A. A., Rozman, C., Speck, B., Tura, S., Weiner, R. S., and Bortin, M. M.: Bone marrow transplantation for chronic myelogenous leukemia in chronic phase: Increased risk for relapse associated with t-cell depletion. Ann. Intern. Med., 108:806, 1988.
105. Gordon-Smith, E. C., Fairhead, S. M., Chipping, P. M., Hows, J., James, D. C., Dodi, A., and Batchelor, J. R.: Bone marrow transplantation for severe aplastic anemia using histocompatible unrelated volunteer donors. Br. Med. J., 2:835, 1982.
106. Gorin, N. C., Aegerter, P., and Auvert, B.: Autologous bone marrow transplantation (ABMT) for acute leukemia in remission: Fifth European Survey. Evidence in favour of marrow purging. Bone Marrow Transplant., 4(Suppl. 1):206, 1989.
107. Gottdiener, J. S., Appelbaum, F. R., Ferrans, V. J., Deisseroth, A., and Ziegler, J.: Cardiotoxicity associated with high-dose cyclophosphamide therapy. Arch. Intern. Med., 141:758, 1981.
108. Goulmy, E.: Minor histocompatibility antigens in man and their role in transplantation. *In* Transplant Reviews. Edited by J. Morris, and N. L. Tilney. NY, W. B. Saunders, 1988.
109. Goulmy, E., Termijtzlen, A., Bradley, B. A., and van Rood, J. J.: Y-antigen killing by T-cells of woman is restricted by HLA. Nature, 226:544, 1977.
110. Gribben, J., Goldstone, A. H., Ernst, P., Philip, T., Maraninchi, D., Gorin, N. C., Ricci, P., and Singer, P.: Bone marrow transplantation for non-Hodgkin's lymphoma in remission—allogeneic versus autologous. Bone Marrow Transplant., 2(Suppl. 1):204, 1987.
111. Griffin, J. D., Spriggs, D., Wisch, J. S., and Kuff, D. W.: Treatment of preleukemic syndromes with continuous intravenous infusion of low-dose cytosine arabinoside. J. Clin. Oncol., 3:982, 1985.
112. Guinan, E. C., Tarbell, N. J., Tantravahi, R., and Weinstein, H. J.: Bone marrow transplantation for children with myelodysplastic syndromes. Blood, 73:619, 1989.
113. Hale, G., Cobbold, S., and Waldmann, H.: T-cell depletion with Campath-1 in allogeneic bone marrow transplantation. Transplant., 45:753, 1988.
114. Hansen, J. A., Clift, R. A., Thomas, E. D., Buckner, C. D., Storb, R., and Giblett, E. R.: Transplantation of marrow from an unrelated donor to a patient with acute leukemia. N. Engl. J. Med., 303:565, 1980.
115. Helenglass, G., Powles, R. L., McElwain, T. J., Lakhani, A., Milan, S., Gore, M., Nandi, A., Zuiable, A., Perren, T., Foregon, G., Treleaven, J., Hamilton, C., and Millar, J.: Melphelan and total body irradiation (TBI) versus cyclophosphamide and TBI as conditioning for allogeneic matched sibling bone marrow transplants for acute myeloblastic leukemia in first remission. Bone Marrow Transplant., 3:21, 1988.
116. Helenglass, G., Treleaven, J., Parikh, P., Aboud, H., Smith, C., and Powles, R.: Delayed engraftment associated with splenomegaly in patients undergoing bone marrow transplantation for chronic myeloid leukemia. Bone Marrow Transplant., 5:247, 1990.
117. Henslee, P. J., MacDonald, J. S., and Messino, M. J.: Freedom from relapse following histoincompatible marrow transplantation in patients with high risk acute lymphoblastic leukemia. Exp. Haematol., 17:547a, 1989.
118. Herve, P., Wijdenes, J., Bergerat, J. P., Bordignon, C., Milpied, N., Cahn, J. Y., Clement, C., Beliard, R., Morel-Fourrier, B., Racadot, E., Troussard, X., Benz-Lemoine, E., Gaud, C., Legros, M., Attal, M., Kloft, M., and Peters, A.: Treatment of corticosteroid resistant acute graft-versus-host disease by in vivo administration of anti-interleukin-2 receptor monoclonal antibody (B-B10). Blood, 75:1017, 1990.
119. Herzig, R. H., Bortin, M. M., Barrett, A. J., Blume, K. G., Gluckman, E., Horowitz, M. M., Jacobsen, S. J., Marmont, A., Masaoka, T., Prentice, H. G., Ramsay, N. K. C., Rimm, A. A., Ringden, O., Speck, B., Zwaan, F. E., and Gale, R. P.: Bone marrow transplantation in high-risk acute lymphoblastic leukaemia in first and second remission. Lancet, 1:786, 1987.
120. Hoelzer, D., and Gale, R. P.: Acute lymphoblastic leukemia in adults: Recent progress, future directions. Semin. Hematol., 24:27, 1987.
121. Holland, K., Wingard, J. R., Beschorner, W. E., Saral, R., and Santos, G. W.: Bronchiolitis obliterans after bone marrow transplantation: Relationship to chronic graft-versus-host disease and serum IgG. Blood, 72:621, 1988.
122. Holler, E., Kolb, H. J., Möller, A., Kempeni, J., Liesenfeld, S., Pechumer, H., Lehmacher, W., Ruckdeschel, G., Gleixner, B., Riedner, C., Ledderose, G., Brehm, G., Mittermuller, J., and Wilmanns, W.: Increased serum levels of tumor necrosis factor α precede major complications of bone marrow transplantation. Blood, 75:1011, 1990.
123. Howell, W. M., Evans, P. R., Spellerberg, M. B., Wilson, P. J., and Smith, J. L.: A comparison of serological, cellular and DNA-RFLP methods for HLA matching in the selection of related bone marrow donors. Bone Marrow Transplant., 4:63, 1989.

124. Hows, J. M., Mehta, A., Ward, L., Woods, K., Perez, R., Gordon, M. Y., and Gordon-Smith, E. C.: Comparison of mesna with forced diuresis to prevent cyclophosphamide induced haemorrhagic cystitis in marrow transplantation: A prospective randomized study. Br. J. Cancer, 50:753, 1984.
125. Hows, J. M., Yin, J. L., Marsh, D., Swirsky, D., Jones, L., Apperley, J. F., James, D. C. O., Smithers, S., Batchelor, J. R., Goldman, J. M., and Gordon-Smith, E. C.: Histocompatible unrelated volunteer donors compared with HLA non-identical family donors in marrow transplantation for aplastic anemia and leukemia. Blood, 68:1322, 1986.
126. Jones, R. J., Lee, K. S., Beschorner, W. E., Voegl, V. G., Grochow, L. B., Braine, H. G., Vogelsang, G. B., Sensenbrenner, L. L., Santos, G. W., and Saral, R.: Veno-occlusive disease of the liver following bone marrow transplantation. Transplant., 44:778, 1987.
127. Kantarjian, H. M., Keating, M. J., Walters, R. S., Smith, T. L., Cork, A., McCredie, K. B., and Freireich, E. J.: Therapy: related leukemia and myelodysplastic syndrome: Clinical, cytogenetic and prognostic features. J. Clin. Oncol., 4:1748, 1986.
128. Kapoor, N., Kirkpatrick, D., Blaese, R. M., Oleske, J., Hilgartner, M. H., Chaganti, R. S. K., Good, R. A., and O'Reilly, R. J.: Reconstitution of normal megakaryocytopoiesis and immunologic functions in Wiscott-Aldrich Syndrome by marrow transplantation following myeloablation and immunosuppression with busulfan and cyclophosphamide. Blood, 57:692, 1981.
129. Keever, C. A., Small, T. N., Flomenberg, N., Heller, G., Pekle, K., Black, P., Kernan, N. A., and O'Reilly, R. J.: Immune reconstitution following bone marrow transplantation: Comparison of recipients of T cell depleted marrow with recipients of conventional marrow grafts. Blood, 73:1340, 1989.
130. Kiessling, R., Hochman, P. S., Haller, O., Shearer, G. M., Wigzell, H., and Cudkowicz, G.: Evidence for a similar or common mechanism for natural killer activity and resistance to hemopoietic grafts. Eur. J. Immunol., 7:655, 1977.
131. Kennedy, M. S., Deeg, H. J., Storg, R., Doney, K., Sullivan, K. M., Witherspoon, R. P., Appelbaum, F. R., Stewart, P., Sanders, J., Buckner, C. D., Martin, P., Weiden, P., and Thomas, E. D.: Treatment of acute graft-versus-host disease after allogeneic marrow transplantation: Randomized study comparing corticosteroids and cyclosporine. Am. J. Med., 78:978, 1985.
132. Kenny, A. B., and Hitzig, W. H.: Bone marrow transplantation for severe combined immunodeficiency. Eur. J. Ped., 131:155, 1979.
133. Kernan, N. A., Bordignon, C., Heller, G., Cunningham, I., Castro-Malaspina, H., Shank, B., Flomenberg, N., Burns, J., Dupont, B., Collins, N. H., and O'Reilly, R. J.: Graft failure after T-cell-depleted human leukocyte antigen identical marrow transplants for leukemia: I. Analysis of risk factors and results of secondary transplants. Blood, 74:2227, 1989.
134. Kernan, N. A., Collins, N. H., Juliano, L., Cartagena, B. S., Dupont, B., and O'Reilly, R. J.: Cloneable T-lymphocytes in T-cell depleted bone marrow transplants correlate with development of graft-versus-host disease. Blood, 68:770, 1986.
135. Kernan, N. A., Flomenberg, N., Dupont, B., and O'Reilly, R. J.: Graft rejection in recipients of T-cell depleted HLA-non-identical marrow transplants for leukemia. Transplant., 43:842, 1987.
136. Klein, J., and Park, J. M.: Graft-versus-host reaction across different regions of the H-2 complex of the mouse. J. Exp. Med., 137:1213, 1973.
137. Krivit, W., Whitley, C. B., Chang, P. N., Belani, K. G., Snover, D., Summers, C. G., and Blazar, B. R.: Lysomal storage diseases treated by bone marrow transplantation: Review of 21 Patients. *In* Bone Marrow Transplantation in Children. Edited by C. Pochedly and L. Johnson. New York, Raven Press, 1990.
138. Kyle, R. A.: Multiple myeloma. An update on diagnosis and management. Acta Oncologica, 29 Fasc. 1:1, 1990.
139. Leiper, A. D., Stanhope, R., Lau, T., Grant, D. B., Blacklock, H., Chessells, J. M., and Plowman, P. N.: The effect of total body irradiation and bone marrow transplantation during childhood and adolescence on growth and endocrine function. Br. J. Haematol., 67:419, 1987.
140. Locksley, R., Flournoy, N., Sullivan, K., and Meyers, J. D.: Infection with varicella-zoster after marrow transplantation. J. Infect. Dis., 152:1172, 1985.
141. Lowenberg, B.: Fetal Liver Transplantation. Rijswyk, Holland, Radiobiologic Institute, 1976, pp. 56–88.
142. Luccarelli, G., Galimberti, M., Polchi, P., Angelucci, E., Baronciani, D., Giardini, C., Politi, P., Durazzi, S. M. T., Muretto, P., and Albertini, F.: Bone marrow transplantation in patients with thalassemia. N. Engl. J. Med., 322:417, 1990.
143. Lum, L. G.: A Review: The kinetics of immune reconstitution after human marrow transplantation. Blood, 69:369, 1987.
144. Mackinnon, S., Burnett, A. K., Crawford, R. J., Cameron, S., Leask, B. G. S., and Somerville, R. G.: Seronegative blood products prevent primary cytomegalovirus infection after bone marrow transplantation. J. Clin. Pathol., 41:948, 1988.
145. Mandelli, F., Avvisati, G., Amadori, S., Boccadoro, M., Gernone, A., Lauta, V. M., Marmont, F., Petrucci, M. T., Tribalto, M., Vegna, M. L., Dammacco, F., and Pileri, A.: Maintenance treatment with recombinant interferon alfa-2b in patients with multiple myeloma responding to conventional induction chemotherapy. N. Engl. J. Med., 322:1430, 1990.
146. Marmont, A. M., Gale, R. P., Butturini, A., Goldman, J. M., Martelli, M. F., Prentice, H. G., Slavin, S., Storb, R., Truitt, R. L., and Van Bekkum, D. W.: T-cell depletion in allogeneic bone marrow transplantation: Progress and problems. Haematologica, 74:235, 1989.
147. Marsh, J. C. W., Harhalakis, N., Dowding, C., Laffan, M., Gordon-Smith, E. C., and Hows, J. M.: Recurrent graft failure following syngeneic bone marrow transplantation for aplastic anemia. Bone Marrow Transplant., 4:581, 1989.
148. Martin, P. J., Hansen, J. A., Buckner, C. D., Sanders, J. E., Deeg, H. J., Stewart, P., Appelbaum, F. R., Clift, R., Fefer, A., Witherspoon, R. P., Kennedy, M. S., Sullivan, K. M., Flournoy, N., Storb, R., and Thomas, E. D.: Effects of in vitro depletion of T-cells in HLA-identical allogeneic marrow grafts. Blood, 66:664, 1985.
149. Martin, P. J., Hansen, J. A., Torok-Storb, B., Durnam, D., Pzrepiorka, D., O'Quigley, J., Sanders, J., Sullivan, K. M., Witherspoon, R. P., Deeg, H. J., Appelbaum, F. R., Stewart, P., Weiden, P., Doney, K., Buckner, C. D., Clift, R., Storb, R., and Thomas, E. D.: Graft failure in patients receiving T-cell depleted HLA-identical allogeneic marrow transplants. Bone Marrow Transplant., 3:445, 1988.
150. Martin, P. J., Schoch, G., Fisher, L., Byers, V., Anasetti, C., Appelbaum, F. R., Beatty, P. G., Doney, K., McDonald, G. B., Sanders, J. E., Sullivan, K. M., Storb, R., Thomas, E. D., Witherspoon, R. P., Lomen, P., Hannigan, J., and Hansen, J. A.: A retrospective analysis of therapy for acute graft-versus-host disease: Initial treatment. Blood, 76:1464, 1990.
151. Martin, P. J., Shulman, H. M., Schubach, W. H., Hansen, J. A., Fefer, A., Miller, G., and Thomas, E. D.: Fatal Epstein-Barr-virus-associated proliferation of donor B-cells after treatment of acute graft-versus-host disease with a murine anti-T-cell antibody. Ann. Intern. Med., 101:310, 1984.
152. Mayer, R. J.: Current chemotherapeutic treatment approaches to the management of previously untreated adults with de novo acute myelogenous leukemia. Semin. Oncol., 14:385, 1987.
153. McCullough, J., Hansen, J. A., Perkins, H., Stroncek, D., and Bartsch, G.: The national marrow donor program: How it works, accomplishments to date. Oncol., 3:63, 1989.
154. McDonald, G. B., Sharma, P., Matthews, D. E., Schulman, H. M., and Thomas, E. D.: Veno-occlusive disease of the liver after bone marrow transplantation: Diagnosis, incidence, and predisposing factors. Hepatol., 4:116, 1984.
155. McGlave, P., Arthur, D., Haake, R., Hurd, D., Miller, W., Vercellotti, G., Weisdorf, D., Kim, T., Ramsay, N., and Kersey, J.: Therapy of chronic myelogenous leukemia with allogeneic bone marrow transplantation. J. Clin. Oncol., 5:1033, 1987.
156. McGlave, P. B., Arthur, D. C., Kim, T. H., Ramsay, N. K. C., Hurd, D. D., and Kersey, J.: Successful allogeneic bone marrow transplantation for patients in the accelerated phase of chronic granulocytic leukaemia. Lancet, 2:625, 1982.
157. Meloni, G., DeFabritiis, P., Carella, A. M., Mangoni, L., Porcellini, A., Marmont, A., and Mandelli, F.: Autologous bone marrow transplantation in patients with AML in first complete remission. Results of two different conditioning regimens after the same induction and consolidation therapy. Bone Marrow Transplant., 5:29, 1990.
158. Meyers, J. D., Fluornoy, N., and Thomas, E. D.: Nonbacterial pneumonia after allogeneic marrow transplantation. A review of ten year's experience. Rev. Infect. Dis., 4:1119, 1982.
159. Meyers, J. D., Fluornoy, N., and Thomas, E. D.: Risk factors for cytomegalovirus infection after human marrow transplantation. J. Infect. Dis., 153:478, 1986.
160. Meyers, J. D., Reed, E. C., Shepp, D. H., Thornquist, M., Dandlicker, P. S., Vicary, C. A., Flournoy, N., Kirk, L. E., Kersey, J. H., and Thomas E. D.: Acyclovir for prevention of cytomegalovirus infection and disease after allogeneic marrow transplantation. N. Engl. J. Med., 318:70, 1988.
161. Murphy, W. J., Kumar, V., and Bennett, M.: Rejection of bone marrow autografts by mice with severe combined immune deficiency (SCID). J. Exp. Med., 165:1212, 1987.
162. Negrin, R. S., Haeuber, D. H., Nagler, A., Kobayashi, Y., Sklar, J., Donlon, T., Vincent, M., and Greenberg, P. L.: Maintenance treatment of patients with myelodysplastic syndromes using recombinant human granulocyte colony-stimulating factor. Blood, 76:36, 1990.
163. Neiman, P. E., Reeves, W., Ray, G., Flournoy, N., Lerner, K. G., Sale, G. E., and Thomas, E. D.: A prospective analysis of interstitial pneumonia and opportunistic viral infection among recipients of allogeneic bone marrow grafts. J. Infect. Dis., 136:754, 1977.
164. Nemunaitis, J., Singer, J. W., Buckner, C. D., Durnam, D., Epstein, C., Hill, R., Storb, R., Thomas, E. D., and Appelbaum, F. R.: Use of recombinant human granulocyte-macrophage colony-stimulating factor in graft failure after bone marrow transplantation. Blood, 76:245, 1990.
165. O'Donnell, M. R., Nademanee, A. P., Snyder, D. S., Schmidt, G. M., Parker, P. M., Bierman, P. J., Fahey, J. L., Stein, A. S., Krance, R. A., Stock, A. D., Forman, S. J., and Blume, K. G.: Bone marrow transplantation for myelodysplastic and myeloproliferative syndromes. J. Clin. Oncol., 5:1822, 1987.
166. O'Leary, M., Ramsay, N. K. C., Nesbit, M. E., Hurd, D., Woods, W. G., Krivit, W., Kim, T. H., McGlave, P., and Kersey, J.: Bone marrow transplantation for non-Hodgkin's lymphoma in children and young adults. Am. J. Med., 74:497, 1983.
167. O'Reilly, R. J.: Allogeneic bone marrow transplantation: Current status and future directions. Blood, 62:941, 1983.
168. O'Reilly, R. J.: Current developments in marrow transplantation. Transplant. Proc., XIX, 1:92, 1987.
169. O'Reilly, R. J., Brochstein, J., Collins, N., Keever, C., Kapoor, N., Kirkpatrick, D., Kernan, N. A., Dupont, B., Burns, J., and Reisner, Y.: Evaluation of HLA-haplotype disparate parental marrow grafts depleted of T lymphocytes by differential agglutination with a soybean lectin and E-rosette depletion for the treatment of severe combined immunodeficiency. Vox Sang, 51(Suppl. 2):81, 1986.
170. O'Reilly, R. J., Dupont, B., Pahwa, S., Grimes, E., Smithwick, E. M., Pahwa, R., Schwartz, S., Hansen, J. A., Siegel, F. P., Sorell, M., Svejgaard, A., Jersild, C., Thomsen, M., Platz, P., L'Esperance, P., and Good, R. A.: Reconstitution in severe combined immunodeficiency by transplantation of marrow from an unrelated donor. N. Engl. J. Med., 297:1311, 1977.
171. O'Reilly, R. J., Brochstein, J., Dinsmore, R., and Kirkpatrick, D.: Marrow transplantation for congenital disorders. Semin. Hematol., 21:188, 1984.
172. O'Reilly, R. J., Collins, N. H., Kernan, N. A., Brochstein, J., Dinsmore, R., Kirkpatrick, D., Siena, S., Keeve, C., Jordon, B., Shank, B., Wolf, L., Dupont, B., and Reisner, Y.: Transplantation of marrow depleted of T-cells by soybean lectin agglutination and E-rosette depletion: Major histocompatibility complex-related graft resistance in leukemia transplant patients. Transplant Proc., 17:455, 1985.
173. O'Reilly, R. J., Keever, C. A., Small, T. A., and Brochstein, J. A.: The use of HLA-non-identical T-cell depleted marrow transplants for correction of severe combined immunodeficiency disease. Immunodeficiency Reviews, 1:273, 1989.
174. O'Reilly, R. J., Kernan, N. A., Cunningham, I., Brochstein, J., Castro-Malaspina, H., Laver, J., Flomenberg, N., Emanuel, D., Gulati, S., Keever, C., Small, T., Collins, N. H., and Bordignon, C.: Allogeneic transplants depleted of T-cells by soybean lectin agglutination and E-rosette depletion. Bone Marrow Transplant., 3(Suppl. 1):3, 1988.
175. Parkman, R.: Clonal analysis of murine graft-versus-host-disease. I. Phenotypic and functional analysis of T-lymphocyte clones. J. Immunol., 136:3543, 1986.
176. Parkman, R., Rappeport, J., Geha, R., Belli, J., Cassady, R., Levey, R., Nathan, D. G., and Rosen, F. S.: Complete correction of the Wiskott-Aldrich Syndrome by allogeneic bone marrow transplantation. N. Engl. J. Med., 298:921, 1978.
177. Perren, T. J., Powles, R. L., Easton, D., Stolle, K., and Selby, P. J.: Prevention of herpes zoster in patients by long-term oral acyclovir after allogeneic bone marrow transplantation. Am. J. Med., 85(Suppl. 2A):99, 1988.
178. Peterson, F. B., Bowden, R. A., Thornquist, M., Meyers, J. D., Buckner, C. D., Counts, G. W., Nelson, N., Newton, B. A., Sullivan, K. M., McIver, J., and Thomas, E. D.: The effect of prophylactic intravenous immune globulin on the incidence of septicemia in marrow transplant recipients. Bone Marrow Transplant., 2:141, 1987.

179. Phillips, G. L., Herzig, R. H., Lazarus, H. M., Fay, J. W., Griffith, R., and Herzig, G. P.: High-dose chemotherapy, fractionated total-body irradiation, and allogeneic marrow transplantation for malignant lymphoma. J. Clin. Oncol., 4:480, 1986.
180. Piguet, P.-F., Grau, G. E., Allet, B., and Vassali, P.: Tumor necrosis factor/cachectin is an effector of skin and gut lesions of the acute phase of graft-versus-host disease. J. Exp. Med., 166:1280, 1987.
181. Powles, R. L., Morgenstern, G., Clink, H. M., Hedley, D., Bandini, G., Lumley, H., Watson, J. G., Lawson, D., Spence, D., Barrett, A., Jameson, B., Lawler, S., Kay, H. E. M., and McElwain, T. J.: The place of bone-marrow transplantation in acute myelogenous leukaemia. Lancet, 1:1047, 1980.
182. Prentice, H. G., Janossy, G., Skeggs, D., Blacklock, H. A., Bradstock, K. F., Goldstein, G., and Hoffbrand, A. V.: Use of anti-T-cell monoclonal antibody OKT3 to prevent acute graft-versus-host disease in allogeneic bone marrow transplantation for acute leukemia. Lancet, 1:700, 1982.
183. Racadot, E., Herve, P., Beaujean, F., Vernant, J. P., Flesch, M., Plouvier, E., Andreu, G., Rio, B., Philippe, N., Souillet, G., Pico, J., Bordigoni, P., Ifrah, N., Paitre, M. L., Lutz, P., Morizet, J., and Bernard, A.: Prevention of graft-versus-host disease in HLA-matched bone marrow transplantation for malignant diseases: A multicentric study of 62 patients using 3 PAN-T monoclonal antibodies and rabbit complement. J. Clin. Oncol., 5:426, 1987.
184. Ramsay, N. K. C., Kersey, J. H., Robinson, L. L., McGlave, P. B., Woods, W. G., Krivit, W., Kim, T. H., Goldman, A. I., and Nesbit, M. E.: A randomized study of the prevention of acute graft-versus-host disease. N. Engl. J. Med., 306:392, 1982.
185. Rappeport, J., Parkman, R., Belli, J., Levey, R., Rosen, F., and Nathan, D.: Reversibility of myelofibrosis (MF) after bone marrow transplantation. Blood, 52:589a, 1978.
186. Reed, E. C., Bowden, R. A., Dandliker, P. S., Lilleby, K. E., and Meyers, J. D.: Treatment of cytomegalovirus pneumonia with ganciclovir and intravenous cytomegalovirus immunoglobulin in patients with bone marrow transplants. Ann. Intern. Med., 109:783, 1988.
187. Reisner, Y., Kapoor, N., Kirkpatrick, D., Pollack, M. S., Dupont, B., Good, R. A., and O'Reilly, R. J.: Transplantation for acute leukemia with HLA-A and B non-identical parental marrow cells fractionated with soybean agglutinin and sheep blood cells. Lancet, 2:327, 1981.
188. Reisner, Y., Kapoor, N., Kirkpatrick, D., Pollack, M. S., Cunningham-Rundles, S., Dupont, B., Hodes, M. Z., Good, R. A., and O'Reilly, R. J.: Transplantation for severe combined immunodeficiency with HLA-A, B, DR incompatible parental marrow fractionated by soybean agglutin and sheep red blood cells. Blood, 61:341, 1983.
189. Remlinger, K., Martin, P. J., Hansen, J. A., Doney, K. C., Smith, A., Deeg, H. J., Sullivan, K., Storb, R., and Thomas, E. D.: Murine monoclonal anti-T cell antibodies for treatment of steroid resistant acute graft-versus-host disease. Hum. Immunol., 9:21, 1984.
190. Rivera, G. K., Buchanan, G., Boyett, J. M., Camitta, B., Ochs, J., Kalwinsky, D., Amylon, M., Vietti, T. J., and Christ, W. M.: Intensive retreatment of childhood acute lymphoblastic leukemia in first bone marrow relapse: A pediatric oncology group study. N. Engl. J. Med., 315:273, 1986.
191. Rosenkrantz, K., Keever, C., Kirsch, J., Horvath, A., Bhimani, K., O'Reilly, R. J., Dupont, B., and Flomenberg, N.: In vitro correlates of graft-host tolerance after HLA-matched and mismatched marrow transplants: Suggestions from limiting dilution analysis. Transplant. Proc., XIX, 6(Suppl. 7):98, 1987.
192. Saltzstein, E. C., Bortin, M. M., and Rimm, A. A.: Long lived canine allogeneic radiation chimera produced with combined fetal liver and thymus cells. Proc. Soc. Exp. Biol. Med., 18:461, 1974.
193. Sanders, J. E., Buckner, C. D., Amos, D., Levy, W., Appelbaum, F. R., Doney, K., Storb, R., Sullivan, K. M., Witherspoon, R. P., and Thomas, E. D.: Ovarian function following marrow transplantation for aplastic anemia or leukemia. J. Clin. Oncol., 6:813, 1988.
194. Sanders, J. E., Fluornoy, N., Thomas, E. D., Buckner, C. D., Lum, L. G., Clift, R. A., Appelbaum, F. R., Sullivan, K. M., Stewart, P., Deeg, H. J., Doney, K., and Storb, R.: Marrow transplant experience in children with acute lymphoblastic leukemia: An analysis of factors associated with survival, relapse and graft-versus-host disease. Med. Ped. Oncol., 13:165, 1985.
195. Sanders, J. E., Pritchard, S., Mahoney, P., Amos, D., Buckner, C. D., Witherspoon, R. P., Deeg, H. J., Doney, K. C., Sullivan, K. M., Appelbaum, F. R., Storb, R., and Thomas, E. D.: Growth and development following marrow transplantation for leukemia. Blood, 68:1129, 1986.
196. Sanders, J. E., Thomas, E. D., Buckner, C. D., Flournoy, N., Stewart, P. S., Clift, R. A., Lum, L., Bensinger, W. I., Storb, R., Appelbaum, F. R., and Sullivan, K. M.: Marrow transplantation for children in first remission of acute nonlymphoblastic leukemia: An update. Blood, 66:460, 1985.
197. Sanders, J. E., Thomas, E. D., Buckner, C. D., and Doney, K.: Marrow transplantation for children with acute lymphoblastic leukemia in second remission. Blood, 70:324, 1987.
198. Santos, G. W.: Immunosuppression for clinical marrow transplantation. Semin. Hematol., 11:341, 1974.
199. Saral, R., Burns, W. H., Laskin, O. L., Santos, G. W., and Lietman, P. S.: Acyclovir prophylaxis of herpes-simplex-virus infections. A randomized double-blind, controlled trial in bone marrow transplant recipients. N. Engl. J. Med., 305:63, 1981.
200. Schmidt, G. M., Kovacs, A., Zaia, J. A., Horak, D. A., Blume, K. G., Nademanee, A. P., O'Donnell, M. R., Snyder, D. S., and Forman, S. J.: Gancyclovir/immunoglobulin combination therapy for the treatment of human cytomegalovirus-associated interstitial pneumonia in bone marrow allograft recipients. Transplant., 46:905, 1988.
201. Schmitz, N., Gassmann, W., Rister, M., Johannson, W., Suttorp, M., Brix, F., Holthuis, J. J. M., Heit, W., Hertenstein, B., Schaub, J., and Loffler, H.: Fractionated total body irradiation and high-dose VP 16-213 followed by allogeneic bone marrow transplantation in advanced leukemias. Blood, 72:1567, 1988.
202. Shepp, D. H., Dandliker, P. S., and Meyers, J. D.: Treatment of varicella-zoster virus infection in severely immunocompromised patients—a randomized comparison of acyclovir and cidarabine. N. Engl. J. Med., 314:208, 1986.
202A. Silverman, L. R., Holland, J. F., Nelson, D., Clamon, G., Powell, B. L., Bloomfield, C. D., Larson, R., Demakos, E. P., George, S. L., Davis, R. B., Liu, E., Davis, B., Schiffer, C., and McIntyre, O. R.: Trilineage response of myelodysplastic syndromes to subcutaneous azacytidine. Proc. Am. Soc. Clin. Oncol., 10:747, 1991.
203. Sklar, C. A., Tae, H. K., and Ramsay, N.: Thyroid dysfunction among long-term survivors of bone marrow transplantation. Am. J. Med., 73:688, 1982.
204. Sklar, C. A., Tae, H. K., and Ramsay, N.: Testicular function following bone marrow transplantation performed during or after puberty. Cancer, 53:1498, 1984.
205. Sladek, N. E., Smith, P. C., Bratt, P. M., Low, J. E., Powers, J. F., Borch, R. F., and Coveney, J. R.: Influence of diuretics on urinary general base catalytic activity and cyclophosphamide-induced bladder toxicity. Cancer Treat. Rep., 66:1889, 1982.
206. Slavin, R. E., and Woodruff, J. M.: The pathology of bone marrow transplantation. Path. Ann., 91:291, 1974.
207. Sokal, J. E., Baccarani, M., Russo, D., and Tura, S.: Staging and prognosis in chronic myelogenous leukemia. Semin. Hematol., 25:49, 1988.
208. Sonnenberg, F. A., Eckman, M. H., and Pauker, S. G.: Bone marrow donor registries: The relation between registry size and probability of finding complete and partial matches. Blood, 74:2569, 1989.
209. Steinherz, P. G., Gaynon, P., Miller, D. R., Reaman, G., Bleyer, A., Finklestein, J., Evans, R. G., Meyers, P., Steinherz, L., Sather, H., and Hammond, D.: Improved disease free survival of children with acute lymphoblastic leukemia at high risk for early relapse with the New York Regimen—A New Intensive Therapy Protocol: A Report from the Children's Cancer Study Group. J. Clin. Oncol., 4:744, 1986.
210. Storb, R., Deeg, H. J., Farewell, V., Doney, K., Appelbaum, F., Beatty, P., Bensinger, W., Buckner, C. D., Clift, R., Hansen, J., Hill, R., Longton, G., Lum, L., Martin, P., McGuffin, R., Sanders, J., Singer, J., Stewart, P., Sullivan, K., Witherspoon, R., and Thomas, E. D.: Marrow transplantation for severe aplastic anemia: Methotrexate alone compared with a combination of methotrexate and cyclosporine for prevention of acute graft-versus-host disease. Blood, 68:119, 1986.
211. Storb, R., Deeg, H. J., Thomas, E. D., Appelbaum, F. R., Buckner, C. D., Cheever, M. A., Clift, R. A., Doney, K. C., Flournoy, N., Kennedy, M. S., Loughran, T. P., McGuffin, R. W., Sale, G. E., Sanders, J. E., Singer, J. W., Stewart, P. S., Sullivan, K. M., and Witherspoon, R. P.: Marrow transplantation for chronic myelocytic leukemia: A controlled trial of cyclosporine versus methotrexate for prophylaxis of graft-versus-host disease. Blood, 66:698, 1985.
212. Storb, R., Doney, K. C., Thomas, E. D., Appelbaum, F., Buckner, C. D., Clift, R. A., Deeg, H. J., Goodell, B. W., Hackman, R., Hansen, J. A., Sanders, J., Sullivan, K., Weiden, P. L., and Witherspoon, R. P.: Marrow transplantation with or without donor buffy coat cells for 65 transfused aplastic anemia patients. Blood, 59:236, 1982.
213. Storb, R., Epstein, R. B., Rudolph, R. H., and Thomas, E. D.: The effect of prior transfusion on marrow grafts between histocompatible canine siblings. J. Immunol., 105:627, 1970.
214. Storb, R., Prentice, R. L., Buckner, C. D., Clift, R. A., Appelbaum, F., Deeg, H. J., Doney, K., Hansen, J. A., Mason, M., Sanders, J. E., Singer, J., and Sullivan, K. M.: Graft vs. host disease and survival in patients with aplastic anaemia treated by marrow grafts from HLA-identical siblings. N. Engl. J. Med., 308:302, 1983.
215. Storb, R., Prentice, R. L., and Thomas, E. D.: Marrow transplantation for treatment of aplastic anemia: An analysis of factors associated with graft rejection. N. Engl. J. Med., 296:61, 1977.
216. Storb, R., Prentice, R. L., and Thomas, E. D.: Treatment of aplastic anemia by marrow transplantation from HLA identical siblings. J. Clin. Invest., 59:625, 1977.
217. Storb, R., Prentice, R. L., Thomas, E. D., Appelbaum, F. R., Deeg, H. J., Doney, K., Fefer, A., Goodell, B. W., Mickelson, E., Stewart, P., Sullivan, K. M., and Witherspoon, R. P.: Factors associated with graft rejection after HLA-identical marrow transplantation for aplastic anaemia. Br. J. Haematol., 55:573, 1983.
218. Storb, R., Rudolph, R. H., Graham, T. C., and Thomas, E. D.: The influence of transfusions for unrelated donors upon marrow grafts between histocompatible canine siblings. J. Immunol., 107:409, 1971.
219. Storb, R., Thomas, E. D., Weiden, P. L., Buckner, C. D., Clift, R. A., Fefer, A., Fernando, L. P., Giblett, E. R., Goodell, B. W., Johnson, F. L., Lerner, K., Neiman, P., and Sanders, J. E.: Aplastic anemia treated by allogeneic bone marrow transplantation: A report of 49 new cases from Seattle. Blood, 48:817, 1976.
220. Streilein, W. J., and Billingham, R. E.: An analysis of graft-versus-host disease in Syrian hamsters. J. Exp. Med., 132:181, 1970.
221. Sullivan, K. M., Deeg, H. J., Sanders, J., Klosterman, A., Amos, D., Shulman, H., Sale, G., Martin, P., Witherspoon, R., Appelbaum, F., Doney, K., Stewart, P., Meyers, J., McDonald, G. B., Weiden, P., Fefer, A., Buckner, C. D., Storb, R., and Thomas, E. D.: Hyperacute graft-v-host disease in patients not given immunosuppression after allogeneic marrow transplantation. Blood, 67:1172, 1986.
222. Sullivan, K. M., Kopecky, K. J., Jocom, J., Fisher, L., Buckner, C. D., Meyers, J. D., Counts, G. W., Bowden, R. A., Petersen, F. B., Witherspoon, R. P., Budinger, M. D., Schwartz, R. S., Appelbaum, F. R., Clift, R. A., Hansen, J. A., Sanders, J. E., Thomas, E. D., and Storb, R.: Immunomodulatory and antimicrobial efficacy of intravenous immunoglobulin in bone marrow transplantation. N. Engl. J. Med., 323:705, 1990.
223. Sullivan, K. M., Shulman, H. M., Storb, R., Weiden, P. L., Witherspoon, R. P., McDonald, G. B., Schubert, M. M., Atkinson, K., and Thomas, E. D.: Chronic graft-versus-host disease in 52 patients: Adverse natural course and successful treatment with combination immunosuppression. Blood, 57:267, 1981.
224. Sullivan, K. M., Storb, R., Shulman, H. R., Shaw, C. M., Spence, A., Beckman, C., Clift, R. A., Buckner, C. D., Stewart, P., and Thomas, E. D.: Immediate and delayed neurotoxicity after mechlorethamine preparation for bone marrow transplantation. Ann. Intern. Med., 97:182, 1982.
225. Sullivan, K. M., Witherspoon, R. P., Storb, R., Deeg, H. J., Dahlberg, S., Sanders, J. E., Appelbaum F. R., Doney, K. C., Weiden, P., Anasetti, C., Loughran, T. P., Hill, R., Shields, A., Yee, G., Shulman, H., Nims, J., Strom, S., and Thomas, E. D.: Alternating day cyclosporine and prednisone for treatment of high risk chronic graft-versus-host disease. Blood, 72:555, 1988.
226. Sullivan, K. M., Witherspoon, R. P., Storb, R., Weiden, P., Flournoy, N., Dahlberg, S., Deeg, H. J., Appelbaum, F. R., McGuffin, R., McDonald, G. B., Meyers, J., Schubert, M. M., Gauvreau, J., Shulman, H. M., Sale, G. E., Anasetti, C., Loughran, T. P., Strom, S., Nims, J., and Thomas, E. D.: Prednisone and azathioprine compared with prednisone and placebo for treatment of chronic graft-versus-host disease: Prognostic influence of prolonged thrombocytopenia after allogeneic marrow transplantation. Blood, 72:546, 1988.
227. Talpaz, M., Kantarjian, H., Kurzrock, R., and Gutterman, J.: Therapy of chronic myelogenous leukemia: Chemotherapy and interferons. Semin. Hematol, 25:62, 1988.
228. Talpaz, M., Kantarjian, H., Kurzrock, R., Trugillo, J. M., and Gutterman, J. U.: Interferon-alpha produces sustained cytogenetic responses in chronic myelogenous leukemia. Ann. Intern. Med., 114:532, 1991.

229. Thomas, E. D., and Clift, R. A.: Indications for marrow transplantation in chronic myelogenous leukemia. Blood, 73:861, 1989.
230. Thomas, E. D., Buckner, C. D., Banaji, M., Clift, R. A., Fefer, A., Flournoy, N., Goodell, B. W., Hickman, R. O., Lerner, K. G., Neiman, P. E., Sale, G. E., Sanders, J. E., Singer, J., Stevens, M., Storb, R., and Weiden, P. L.: One hundred patients with acute leukemia treated by chemotherapy, total body irradiation and allogeneic marrow transplantation. Blood, 49:511, 1977.
231. Thomas, E. D., Buckner, C. D., Clift, R. A., Fefer, A., Johnson, F. L., Neiman, P. E., Sale, G. E., Sanders, J. E., Singer, J. W., Shulman, H., Storb, R., and Weiden, P. L.: Marrow transplantation for acute nonlymphoblastic leukemia in first remission. N. Engl. J. Med., 301:597, 1979.
232. Thomas, E. D., Buckner, C. D., Rudolph, R. H., Fefer, A., Storb, R., Neiman, P. E., Bryant, J. I., Chard, R. L., Clift, R. A., Epstein, R. B., Fialkow, P. J., Funk, D. D., Giblett, E., Lerner, K. G., Reynolds, F. A., and Slichter, S.: Allogeneic marrow grafting for hematologic malignancy using HLA matched donor recipient sibling pairs. Blood, 38:267, 1971.
233. Thomas, E. D., Clift, R. A., Fefer, A., Appelbau, F. R., Beatty, P., Bessinger, W. I., Buckner, C. D., Cheever, M. A., Deeg, H. J., Doney, K., Flournoy, N., Greenberg, P., Hansen, J. A., Martin, P., McGuffin, R., Ramberg, R., Sanders, J. E., Singer, J., Stewart, P., Storb, R., Sullivan, K., Weiden, P. L., and Witherspoon, R.: Marrow transplantation for the treatment of myelogenous leukemia. Ann. Intern. Med., 104:155, 1986.
234. Thompson, C. B., Sanders, J. E., Flournoy, N., Buckner, C. D., and Thomas, E. D.: The risks of central nervous system relapse and leukoencephalopathy in patients receiving marrow transplants for acute leukemia. Blood, 67:195, 1986.
235. Trigg, M. E., Gingrich, R., Goeken, N., deAlarcon, P., Klugman, M., Padley, D., Rumelhart, S., Giller, R., Wen, B. C., and Strauss, R.: Low rejection rate when using unrelated or haploidentical donors for children with leukemia undergoing marrow transplantation. Bone Marrow Transplant., 4:431, 1989.
236. Troussard, X., Leblond, V., Kuentz, M., Milpied, N., Jouet, J. P., Cordonnier, C., Leporrier, M., and Vernant, J. P.: Allogeneic bone marrow transplantation in adults with Burkitt's Lymphoma or acute lymphoblastic leukemia in first complete remission. J. Clin. Oncol., 8:809, 1990.
237. Tsoi, M. S., Storb, R., Dobbs, S., Kopecky, K. J., Santos, E., Weiden, P. L., and Thomas, E. D.: Non-specific suppressor cells in patients with chronic graft-versus-host disease after marrow grafting. J. Immunol., 123:1970, 1979.
238. Tubergen, D., Gilchest, G., Coccia, P., Nouak, L., O'Brien, R., Waskerwitz, M., Sather, H., Bleyer, A., and Hammond, D.: The role of intensified chemotherapy in intermediate risk acute lymphoblastic leukemia (ALL) of childhood. Proc. Am. Soc. Clin. Oncol., 9:216, 1990.
239. Tura, S., Cavo, J., Gobbi, M., Rosti, G., Bandini, G., Miggiano, C., Albertazzi, L., Grimaldi, M., and Visani, G.: High-dose chemoradiotherapy and allogeneic bone marrow transplantation in multiple myeloma. Eur. J. Haematol., 43(Suppl. 51):191, 1989.
240. Tutschka, P. J., Copelan, E. A., and Klein, J. P.: Bone marrow transplantation for leukemia following a new busulfan and cyclophosphamide regimen. Blood, 70:1382, 1987.
241. Tutschka, P. J., Copelan, E. A., and Kapoor, N.: Replacing total body irradiation with bulsulfan as conditioning of patients with leukemia for allogeneic marrow transplantation. Transplant. Proc., 21:2952, 1989.
242. Van Rood, J. J., de Jongh, B., Claas, F. H., Goulmy, E., Gratama, J. W., and Giphart, M. J.: New facts of HLA genetics: Are they relevant in bone marrow transplantation? Semin. Hematol., 21:65, 1984.
243. Vartdal, F., Albrechtsen, D., Ringden, O., Kvalheim, G., Lea, T., Bosnes, V., Gaudernack, G., Brinchmann, J., and Ugelstad, J.: Immunomagnetic treatment of bone marrow allografts. Bone Marrow Transplant., 2(Suppl. 2):94, 1987.
244. Verdonck, L. F., van Heugten, H., and deGast, G. C.: Delay in platelet recovery after bone marrow transplantation: Impact of cytomegalovirus infection. Blood, 66:921, 1985.
245. Vogelsang, G. B., Hess, A. D., Gorden, G., and Santos, G. W.: Treatment and prevention for acute graft-versus-host disease with thalidomide in a rat model. Transplant., 41:644, 1986.
246. Vogelsang, G. B., Hess, A. D., and Santos, G. W.: Acute graft-versus-host disease: Clinical characteristics in the cyclosporine era. Med., 67:163, 1988.
247. Voogt, P. J., Goulmy, W. E., Fibbe, W. E., Veenhof, W. F. J., Brand, A., and Falkenberg, J. H. F.: Minor histocompatibility antigen H-Y is expressed on human hematopoietic progenitor cells. J. Clin. Invest., 82:906, 1988.
248. Wagner, J. E., Santos, G. W., Noga, S. J., Rowley, S. D., Davis, J., Vogelsang, G. B.,

Farmer, E. R., Zehnbauer, B. A., Saral, R., and Donnenberg, A. D.: Bone marrow graft engineering by counterflow centrifugal elutriation: Results of a phase I-II clinical trial. Blood, 75:1370, 1990.
249. Walker, R. W., and Brochstein, J. A.: Neurologic complications of immunosuppressive agents. Neurol. Clin., 6:261, 1988.
250. Weiner, R. S., Bortin, M. B., Gale, R. P., Gluckman, E., Kay, H. E. M., Kolb, H. J., Hartz, A. J., and Rimm, A. A.: Interstitial pneumonitis after bone marrow transplantation: Assessment of risk factors. Ann. Intern. Med., 104:168, 1986.
251. Weinstein, H. J., Mayer, R. L., Rosenthal, D. S., Coral, F. S., Camitta, B. M., and Gelber, R. D.: Chemotherapy for acute myelogenous leukemia in children and adults: VAPA update. Blood, 62:315, 1983.
252. White, P.C.: Molecular genetics of the class III region of the HLA complex in immunobiology of HLA. In Volume II: Immunogenetics and Histocompatibility. Edited by B. Dupont. New York, Springer-Verlag, 1989, pp. 62–69.
253. Wingard, J. R., Chen, D. Y., Burns, W. H., Fuller, D. J., Braine, H. G., Yeager, A. M., Kaiser, H., Burke, P. J., Graham, M. L., Santos, G. W., and Saral, R.: Cytomegalovirus infection after autologous bone marrow transplantation with comparison to infection after allogeneic bone marrow transplantation. Blood, 71:1432, 1988.
254. Wingard, J. R., Merz, W. G., and Saral, R.: Candida tropicalis: A major pathogen in immunocompromised patients. Ann. Intern. Med., 91:539, 1979.
255. Wingard, J. R., Piantadosi, S., Santos, G. W., Saral, R., Vriesendorp, H. M., Yeager, A. M., Burns, W. H., Ambinder, R. F., Braine, H. G., Elfenbein, G., Jones, R. J., Kaizer, H., May, W. S., Rowley, S. D., Sensenbrenner, L. L., Stuart, R. K., Tutschka, P. J., Vogelsang, G. B., Wagner, J. E., Beschorner, W. E., Brookmeyer, R., and Farmer, E. R.: Allogeneic bone marrow transplantation for patients with high-risk acute lymphoblastic leukemia. J. Clin. Oncol., 8:820, 1990.
256. Winston, D. J., Gale, R. P., Meyers, D. V., Young, L. S., and UCLA BMT Group: Infectious complications of human bone marrow transplantation. Med., 58:1, 1979.
257. Winston, D. J., Huang, E., Miller, M. J., Lin, C. H., Ho, W. G., Gale, R. P., and Champlin, R. E.: Molecular epidemiology of cytomegalovirus infections associated with bone marrow transplantation. Ann. Intern. Med., 102:16, 1985.
258. Winston, D. J., Schiffman, G., Wang, D. C., Feig, S. A., Lin, C. H., Marso, E. L., Ho, W. G., Young, L. S., and Gale, R. P.: Pneumococcal infections after human bone marrow transplantation. Ann. Intern. Med., 91:835, 1979.
259. Witherspoon, R. P., Fisher, L. D., Schoch, G., Martin, P., Sullivan, K. M., Sanders, J., Deeg, H. J., Doney, K., Thomas, D., Storb, R., and Thomas, E. D.: Secondary cancers after bone marrow transplantation for leukemia or aplastic anemia. N. Engl. J. Med., 321:784, 1989.
260. Witherspoon, R. P., Lum, L. G., and Storb, R.: Immunologic reconstitution after human marrow grafting. Semin. Hematol., 21:2, 1984.
261. Wiznitzer, M., Packer, R. J., August, C. S., and Burkey, P. A.: Neurological complications of bone marrow transplantation in childhood. Ann. Neurol., 15:569, 1984.
262. Wolf, J. L., Spruce, W. E., Bearman, R. M., Forman, S. J., Scott, E. P., Fahey, J. L., Farbstein, M. J., Rappaport, H., and Blume, K. G.: Reversal of acute ("Malignant") myelosclerosis by allogeneic bone marrow transplantation. Blood, 59:191, 1982.
263. Woods, W. G., Nesbit, M. E., Ramsay, N. K. C., Krivit, W., Kim, T. H., Goldman, A., McGlave, P. B., and Kersey, J. H.: Intensive therapy followed by bone marrow transplantation for patients with acute lymphocytic leukemia in second or subsequent remission: Determination of prognostic factors (a report from the University of Minnesota Bone Marrow Transplantation Team). Blood, 61:1182, 1983.
264. Yang, S. Y., Morishima, Y., Collins, N. H., Alton, T., Pollack, M. S., Yunis, E. J., and Dupont, B.: Comparison of one-dimensional IEF patterns for serologically detectable HLA-A and B allotypes. Immunogenetics, 19:217, 1984.
265. Yeager, A., Kaizer, H., Santos, G. W., Saral, R., Colvin, O. M., Stuart, R. K., Braine, H. G., Burke, P. J., Ambinder, R. F., Burns, W. H., Fuller, D. J., Davis, J. M., Karp, J. E., May, W. S., and Rowley, S. D.: Autologous bone marrow transplantation in patients with acute nonlymphocytic leukemia, using ex-vivo marrow treatment with 4-hydroperoxycyclophosphamide. N. Engl. J. Med., 315:141, 1986.
266. Yunis, E. J., and Amos, D. B.: Three closely linked genetic systems relevant to transplantation. Proc. Natl. Acad. Sci., 68:3031, 1971.
267. Zander, A. R., Keating, M., Dicke, K., Dixon, D., Pierce, S., Jagannath, S., Peters, L., Horwitz, L., Cockerill, K., Spitzer, G., Vellekoop, L., Kantarjian, H., Walters, R., McCredie, K., and Freireich, E. J.: A comparison of marrow transplantation with chemotherapy for adults with acute leukemia of poor prognosis in first complete remission. J. Clin. Oncol., 6:1548, 1988.
268. Zutter, M. M., Martin, P. J., Sale, G. E., Shulman, H. M., Fisher, L., Thomas, E. D., and Durnam, D. M.: Epstein-Barr virus lymphoproliferation after bone marrow transplantation. Blood, 72:520, 1988.

XX

Principles of Psycho-Oncology

Jimmie C. Holland

Introduction

There is a far greater interest today in attaining maximum quality of life for patients at all stages of cancer; more attention is also directed toward support for families and the staff who care for cancer patients. A research effort is more actively exploring social, behavioral and psychological contributions to cancer risk, detection and survival. These aspects of cancer are components of psycho-oncology, which has emerged over the past decade as a subspecialty of oncology, with its own body of information, training and research.[29]

This new area addresses the two major psychological dimensions of cancer: the psychological response of patients to cancer at all stages of disease, and that of their families and their caretakers (psychosocial); and, the psychological, behavioral and social factors that influence risk, detection and survival (psychobiological). In order to develop these aspects of oncology, several efforts are currently being pursued: training of a group of clinicians and investigators as psycho-oncologists; developing a psychological component in the clinical training of all oncologic disciplines; encouraging research in the psychological, humanistic, ethical and spiritual aspects of patient care; incorporating concepts of quality of life in clinical care and as an outcome variable in clinical trials; and an active exploration of brain, immune and endocrine links through the new field of psychoneuroimmunology. The definition of quality of life used in oncology is the level of performance in the major domains of life function (physical, work, psychological, social and sexual) as compared to normal for that individual.

The psychological dimensions impact upon *all* aspects of oncology and the care of *all* patients. The clinical oncologic specialties (medical oncology, surgical, radiologic, gynecologic, orthopedic, urologic, pediatric and neurooncology) are all affected. Also affected by psychosocial and behavioral issues are biology, epidemiology, cancer control and prevention; bioethics, palliative and supportive care; and, clinical trials research and clinical decision making. Psychological, social and quality of life questions are being added to research studies in many of these areas which have not traditionally included such inquiry.

To address the psychological issues, most cancer centers or oncology divisions in community hospitals today have programs designed to assist patients with psychological distress and to provide support for families and staff.[38] The disciplines most often represented in these programs are nursing, social work, psychology, psychiatry and chaplaincy. Only a few centers have programs which include research and training. This chapter is an overview of present knowledge about the psychological aspects of patient care and the most significant psychiatric complications. The bibliography serves as a guide for seeking information in the separate areas, each of which has a rapidly expanding base of clinical and research information.

Historical Perspective

The stigma that cancer equals death, attached to the disease for centuries, led to the long respected dictum that doctors should not tell patients that they had cancer (Table XX-1-1). The first effective treatment for cancer was by surgery, beginning in Egypt over 500 years ago with amputations. The use of ether in 1847 and the advancement of antisepsis led to the successful surgical removal of tumors in the last half of the nineteenth century. By 1912, radiotherapy was becoming recognized as a potentially powerful additional treatment; and by 1950, chemotherapy was added. Education of the public about warning signals of cancer became important to encourage early detection. Effective cancer treatment in the first half of this century depended upon influencing patients' fatalistic attitudes. Multimodality therapy, combining surgical, radiation and chemotherapy, along with immunotherapy, began, by the 1960s, to impact significantly on the grim survival statistics, especially in children and young adults.[51]

By the late 1960s, as survival improved, the diagnosis of cancer began to be more frequently revealed to patients, particularly in the U.S. At about the same time, the concern for more humane care of patients dying of cancer increased, beginning in Europe with the hospice movement. Greater openness in revealing the diagnosis, increased concern for the dying, and enhanced concern about quality of life and the rights of patients began to direct more attention to supportive and psychological aspects of care. Evidence of the

Table XX-1-1. Key Cancer and Psycho-Oncology Events from 1850 to 1970

Year	Cancer	Behavioral/Psychosocial
1850–1900	Anesthesia (1847) Antisepsis First cancer surgery	Cancer = death; word not used
1900–1936	Surgical excision Radiation = palliative American Cancer Society started (1913)	Education about early detection
1937	National Cancer Institute founded	Enthusiasm for research Education for public
1940s	Nitrogen mustards First remission of leukemia by chemotherapy Radical surgery	Optimism about care Psychosomatic concepts Grief studied
1950s	First cure by drug alone; choriocarcinoma (1956) Combination chemotherapy	First psychologic studies of cancer patients*
1960s	Prolonged survival from combined modalities	Debate about telling diagnosis Peer support Consultation-liaison psychiatry

*Massachusetts General Hospital and Memorial Sloan-Kettering Cancer Center.

link of environmental exposures to cancer, particularly cigarette smoking, gave new impetus to examining the role of psychological and behavioral factors in cancer prevention.[32]

The stage was set by 1970 for greater interest in psychological issues; however, tools for assessment of these variables were few and early investigators were forced to develop new instruments or modify those originally developed for assessment of psychiatric patients. Investigators with knowledge of both cancer and social science research methods were few. During the 1970's and 1980's, remarkable progress was made, particularly in Europe and North America, in drawing attention to some behavioral and psychosocial issues in patient care, particularly delay, treatment compliance, and environmental exposures to tobacco.

In the early 1980's, as more clinicians and researchers began to share these interests, several national and regional groups devoted to psychosocial issues developed to provide a means of education and communication. In 1984, individuals from over 15 countries attended a meeting in New York, forming the International Psychooncology Society (IPOS). The National Cancer Institute and the American Cancer Society provided important support to encourage development of the field (Table XX-1-2). And, the psychiatric group at Memorial Sloan-Kettering Cancer Center, begun as the first psychiatric effort in a cancer hospital in 1950 by Sutherland, was reactivated in 1977 by Holland and colleagues, developing clinical and research training, publishing the first textbook of psycho-oncology, and establishing an academic chair of psychiatric oncology. This brief history underscores the relative youth of this subspecialty of oncology, as compared to the more mature fields of surgery, radiation and chemotherapy.[29] The major progress has been made in the past 20 years and most of it, since the early 1980's. The areas reviewed in this chapter reflect the rapid development of diagnostic and treatment guidelines for the clinical psychological problems (e.g., depression and anxiety) that were previously poorly defined and therefore underdiagnosed and undertreated.

Table XX-1-2. Key Psycho-Oncology Events from 1970 to 1990

Year	Behavior-Psychosocial
1972	National Cancer Program National Cancer Plan: Control and Rehabilitation (first NCI-supported psycho-oncology studies)
1975	First National Psychosocial Research Conference
1976	First Psychiatry Committee in a Cooperative Group (CALGB)
1977–1984	Psychosocial Collaborative Group (PSYCOG) (five centers)
1977–1987	Project Omega (MGH) Child studies Pain research Breast cancer studies
1977	Psychiatry Service, Memorial Sloan-Kettering Clinical Training Program Research Program Current Concepts in Psychooncology (IV) Chair of Psychiatric Oncology (1989)
1980	American Cancer Society Peer Review Committee for Psychosocial Review
1980s	Three Research Methodology Conferences

Normal Adaptation to Cancer

Reaction to Diagnosis

Learning that one has cancer, or that a close relative has it, is a catastrophic event. Information of such import is processed mentally like any news of a personal disaster, such as sudden death of a loved one. Receiving the information, despite apparent good health at the time, creates a crisis because of the meaning that individuals and society attach and have long attached to cancer: death, disability, disfigurement, dependence, and disruption of relationships to others. These easy to recall five "Ds" reflect the fears of death, of the uncertain future, and of possible physical changes

Table XX-1-3. Normal Response to Crises Encountered with Cancer

Phase	Symptoms	Time Interval
Phase I Initial response	Disbelief or denial or Despair ("I knew it all along")	Usually less than a week
Phase II Dysphoria	Anxiety, depressed mood, anorexia, insomnia, poor concentration, inability to function	Usually 1–2 weeks, but varies
Phase III Adaptation	Patient accepts validity of information and begins dealing with the options available. Finds reasons for optimism and resumes usual activities	Usually by 2 weeks, but continues over months; may or may not be successful

Modified from Massie and Holland[40]

and their impact on others. This period of crisis is an expected and normal emotional upheaval which the clinician should recognize (Table XX-1-3).[40] For most individuals, the initial period is one of disbelief and denial that the news is true. During Phase 1, they often seek to prove that it is not true ("they must have mixed up the slides"). Feeling "numb" and appearing not to understand fully the import are common reactions, however, usually lasting less than a week. Some patients, a much smaller group, experience despair instead of denial. These are individuals who always feared or expected to develop cancer. Phase II follows, characterized by a period of emotional turmoil and dysphoria in which the reality is slowly recognized. The patient often becomes anxious, depressed, has poor concentration, diminished appetite, is unable to sleep and is unable to maintain the daily routine. Thoughts of illness and death frequently recur and cannot be dispelled. This period may last one to two weeks, usually dissipating as the person begins treatment and begins to sense that all is not lost. A therapeutic alliance with the doctor encourages a return of optimism through cooperation with a treatment plan. Some patients, at times prompted by family member, seek second or multiple opinions until they find the oncologic plan that best fits their concepts.

Phase III represents the longer term adaptation, lasting weeks to months, in which the patient adjusts to the diagnosis and treatment, finds reason for compartmentalized optimism and returns to normal routines and the ways of coping that were characteristic and successful in the past. The quality of that adaptation depends upon the prior level of adjustment and emotional maturity. It is important that family, friends and staff be aware that there is no single way to cope.[57] Individuals have their own coping styles which, for better or worse, have gotten them through prior life crises. There is a strong tendency in today's society to demand that individuals with cancer have a positive attitude to "beat it." They are made to feel guilty if they do not and they are often told that absence of a positive attitude leads to faster tumor growth. While these strategies work well for some individuals, they do not for others.[26] Respect for each individual's way of coping is critically important.

This sequence of disbelief, dysphoria and adaptation may reappear with each new crisis that occurs in the course of illness. Depression becomes more prominent when the news is of progressive disease or treatment failure.

Factors in Adaptation

While the response to catastrophic news is similar at the time of diagnosis, individuals vary widely in how well or how poorly they ultimately adapt to cancer. It is, therefore, important to be able to recognize the factors which predict good or poor adjustment, thereby enabling early identification of particularly vulnerable individuals. The factors which contribute to adaptation are derived from three areas: 1) *society*-derived, which are the social attitudes and beliefs about cancer which impact upon the patient; 2) *patient*-derived, which are the personal attributes the person brings to illness; and 3) the *cancer*-derived, which represent the clinical reality of the illness to which the patient must adapt (Table XX-1-4).

Society-Derived Factors. The society-derived factors are dynamic, changing as people change their perceptions of medicine, illness and cancer. Cancer, long feared and stigmatized, is somewhat less fearsome today, as the diagnosis is more routinely given and as the public justifiably becomes more optimistic about the outcome of cancer, particularly among those in the prime of life. Coupled with society's demands for informed consent, and for knowledge of treatment options, better communication between doctor and

Table XX-1-4. Factors Which Determine Psychological Adjustment to Cancer

Society-derived
  Open discussion of diagnosis vs. unrevealed secret
  Knowledge of treatment options, prognosis, and participation as partner
  Popular beliefs (stress causes cancer)

Patient-derived
  Intrapersonal
    Patient coping ability; emotional maturity at time of cancer
    Developmental stage at time of cancer and meaning of curtailed goals (e.g., marriage, children)
  Interpersonal
    Spouse, family, friends (social support)

Cancer-derived
  Site, stage, symptoms (especially pain) and prognosis
  Treatment required (surgery, radiation, chemotherapy) and sequelae (immediate and delayed)
  Altered body structure or function; rehabilitation/restoration available
  Psychological management by the treating staff

patient has been a positive spin off. This has resulted, how-ever, in an added burden for the patient, because of the fuller knowledge of prognosis with each treatment option. Uncertainty about the future is thus far greater today. An additional burden today is the widely popularized belief that stress causes cancer. Some patients feel they themselves, by some stressful event or events that they did not manage properly, caused their cancer to develop.

Patient-Derived Factors. The patient-derived factors come from three sources which affect adaptation: developmental stage, intrapersonal, and interpersonal resources. The *developmental stage* of the person at the time cancer devel-ops, in relation to biological, personal and social life tasks and goals, determines the meaning of certain losses, such as fertility and altered appearance. Actual and potential losses have different meaning at different stages of life.

An awareness of the developmental stage of the individual,

and its expected psychological and social tasks, permits a better understanding of the meaning of cancer to an indi-vidual. Because of this insight, strategies for successful inter-vention can often be deduced. Each age has its particular life tasks which must be taken into account by the clinician. Table XX-1-5 outlines developmental stages, giving the nor-mal tasks that must be achieved at each age, the disruption which cancer produces, and the interventions which can be employed to minimize the deleterious effects of illness on development. These are particularly important in childhood and adolescence to assure maintenance of normal devel-opmental milestones. Detailed developmental tables of the life cycle have been published.[47]

The *intrapersonal resources* the person brings to the ill-ness are those that are derived by way of personality, emo-tional maturity and coping strategies.[48] A prior psychiatric disturbance usually means greater vulnerability during phys-

Table XX-1-5.   Developmental Stages and Cancer

Stage	Tasks	Disruption	Intervention
Children with Long-Term Treatment			
Childhood (Early)	Motor	Developmental	Physical/social
	Speech	Slowing	Stimulation
	Cognition	Regression	Structured play
	Family bonding	Separation anxiety	↑ Family contact
	Socialization	Withdrawal	Continuity of staff
	Confidence	↑ Fears (Pain)	Trust of staff
Childhood (Late)	Pre-pubertal	Being "different"	Maintain apperance
	Peer relations	School phobia	Minimize absences
	Intellectual and physical prowess	Death fears	Discuss illness and monitor responses
Adolescents and Young Adults with Long-Term Treatment			
Adolescence	Menarche/puberty	Alopecia/amputation "Differentness"	Maintain appearance
	Peer acceptance	↓ School/physical performance	Maintain peer contact
	↑ Independence	↑ Dependence	Support independence
	Sexual experimentation	Conflicts about self and sexuality	Counseling
	Formation of identity	Impact of illness	Counseling
Adult (Young)	Intimacy	↓ Attractiveness	Maintain appearance
	Marriage	Sterility/impotence	Sex counseling
	Parental role	↓ Family role	Homemaker Support children
	Work role	Disruption of job performance	↓ Job interruptions
Adults with Long-Term Treatment			
Middle	Changing hormonal status/menopause	Altered appearance	Maintain appearance
	Older children	Disrupted marital/family role	Counseling (patient *and* family)
	"Empty nest"	Disrupted achievements	Financial planning
	Peak of career		
Old	Aging changes	↑ Physical/emotional	Health-related
	Physical limitations	Services to maintain	Care of self
	Adjustment to increasing losses	↑ Dependence on others	Social support system
	↑ Social support needed	↑ Isolation	Promote social/familial network
	Retirement	↓ Financial security	Financial planning

Adapted from Rowland[47,48]

ical illness.[40] The patient's social environment provides the *interpersonal resources* of family, friends, and social support that materially contribute, positively or negatively. Each of these variables contributes to the strength and weakness of resources that are central to adaptation; they should be assessed in each patient. With this knowledge, an individualized plan for psychosocial support and intervention can be developed.

Much has been written on coping in general, and coping with cancer in particular. Serious illness calls on coping abilities to accomplish several goals: 1) to keep distress within manageable levels; 2) to maintain a sense of personal worth; 3) to restore or maintain relations with significant others; 4) to enhance recovery and physical function; and 5) to work out a socially acceptable post-illness status with maximal physical function.[27] Good coping strategies, taken overall, appear to be important in maintaining a sense of control, optimism, and acceptance of the facts, while seeking constructive, positive approaches to illness and treatment, and sharing information and obtaining support from others.[48] Coping ability is influenced by personality, level of illness, and other factors such as spiritual and religious beliefs. For many individuals religion supplies not only an existential view of life, death and illness, with a Supreme Being from whom help can be requested, but it also provides a supportive social community.

Prior experience with cancer is often a negative factor, especially when it relates to childhood memories of death of a parent or sibling from cancer. Chronic hypochondriasis and cancerophobia appear more common following such early experiences. Death of a relative from the same tumor adds a particularly heavy burden. Table XX-1-6 outlines the major predictors of poor coping which can readily be elicited in a standard medical history, identifying those patients who would benefit most from early intervention.[48]

Cancer-Derived Factors. The cancer-derived factors which contribute to adaptation constitute the clinical facts: stage of disease at time of diagnosis, site of the cancer, symptoms (especially pain), and prognosis; the type(s) of treatment required and their impact on function, both immediate and long-term; and, the extent of rehabilitation which is possible and the psychological management by the health care team. The wise and sensitive physician often becomes an important source of interpersonal support, offering concern and "caring" in the context of professional ministrations. The absence of such a relationship is a negative factor that must be addressed by providing added support from other members of the team, such as the nurse, social worker or mental health professional.

Psychosocial Problems

Psychosocial problems of patients are quite different, depending on stage of illness. Interventions to reduce distress must take the stage, treatment and prognosis into account in planning assistance. The relevant categories of disease in terms of management are: 1) patients receiving active treatment with cure as a goal; 2) patients receiving palliative care with control or comfort as a goal; 3) patients who have completed active treatment and who are survivors, though outcome remains uncertain; and 4) healthy individuals at known increased risk of cancer.

Adaptation to Active Treatment. In patients undergoing active treatment, the goal of psychosocial care is to support their ability to cope with the stresses of treatment, and to reduce their distress which can be viewed from the perspective of "short-term loss, long-term gain." The goal of cure encourages most individuals to tolerate the temporary side effects of chemotherapy and radiation, and to adapt to the permanent losses or organ preserving procedures that may be necessary to achieve successful antineoplastic treatment. Evidence of tumor regression is a great morale booster which encourages coping. Many clinical trials today measure these factors by assessment of quality of life which becomes an outcome variable in determining efficacy of a new agent (see quality of life assessment below). Control of anxiety, depression, delirium, nausea and vomiting, and encouraging adherence to treatment, are examples of the symptom control and support needed (see interventions below). Counseling, self-help groups, behavioral interventions and psychopharmacologic agents all represent major interventions now available to control symptoms. Most symptoms can be controlled with careful evaluation and thoughtful intervention.

Adaptation to Palliative Care. The transition from a curative approach to a palliative one is extremely difficult for the patient, family and the physician who has worked with the patient through months of vigorous treatment. This transition constitutes a crisis in treatment which carries greater anguish than that experienced at the time of the initial diagnosis. It is usually a transient period of distress, however, followed by adaptation to the new reality and a new therapeutic goal. The patient who senses the physician's commitment to continued care and maximal quality of life has an easier adjustment. Issues such as appointing a health proxy, discussion of wishes about resuscitation and life-sustaining measures are best discussed early rather than late. Decisions about where care will be given need to be discussed, as well as assessing whether the family can manage the patient at home. Patients appear to do better when care can be given at home; the grieving, surviving relative also benefits from the closeness of the last days. Increasing availability of support to help families manage at home, using nurse clinicians with expertise in pain and psychiatric management in home care programs is an encouraging sign.[15] Considerable information exists today about symptom control and comfort care in advanced stages of illness with better control of pain, anorexia, constipation, dyspnea, weakness, weight loss, and

Table XX-1-6.   Predictors of Poor Coping with Cancer*

Social isolation
Low socioeconomic status
Alcohol or drug abuse
Prior psychiatric history
Prior experience with cancer, e.g., death of a relative
Recent losses/bereavement
Inflexibility and rigidity of coping
Pessimistic philosophy of life
Absence of a belief/value system
Multiple obligations

*Adapted from Holland and Rowland[32,48]

psychological distress. There are growing numbers of controlled trials of medication, behavioral and psychological interventions for better palliation which suggest greater concern for quality of life. Many studies are being done in programs of hospice and home care which increasingly are integrated and collaborative with cancer centers.

The psychiatrist has an important consultative role in the palliative care of the patient with cancer. There are two distinct areas for which intervention is useful: for help in decisions about treatment and care; and, for assistance in control of distressing symptoms, particularly anxiety, depression and delirium associated with advanced and terminal stages of cancer.[18]

The first issue for which a consultation is requested often is to confront the reality that treatment must now be aimed at containment and comfort rather than cure. The patient, family and physician have been allied in a course of treatment with hope for cure, or at least, control of disease. The transition to containment and comfort care is difficult, with its emotional realization for all concerned that treatment goals must be altered. It is accompanied by confrontation with death and a sense of hopelessness, which may have been largely denied to this point. Some patients choose to participate in experimental programs which offer some hope and from which information may be gleaned to help other patients in the future, as in Phase I and II trials. This more aggressive approach is preferred by some patients who do not find it acceptable to give up "fighting"; by these means they can maintain hope.

A psychiatrist is helpful to the patient and staff in several areas: to help the patient and family decide where care is to be given; how aggressive they wish life sustaining efforts to be; and, how actively the family will be able to participate in care of the patient at home. The psychiatrist also has a unique opportunity to get to know the patient's family, which serves as a bridge later for acceptance of continued support during bereavement. Ideally, both patients and families are better off emotionally if terminal illness can be managed by keeping patients at home. Home care often requires active professional support to see the family through it.[15] Preexisting psychiatric disorders in the patient or family will require special, and often intensive, management during this time. A special Home Care Program has been developed at Memorial Sloan-Kettering Cancer Center for care of the patients with psychiatric difficulties complicating their care.

The second role for the psychiatrist is symptom control. This requires evaluation of mental status and mood to recognize changes indicative of delirium, anxiety, or depression. This information may not be offered by the patient to the oncologist; the psychiatrist's role may be to alert the oncologist to the problem. Pain requires control, as well as physical symptoms of nausea, vomiting, pain, hiccoughs, bowel alterations, anorexia, insomnia. Behavioral and pharmacologic approaches are useful.

Adaptation to Being a Survivor. One of the growing and increasingly vocal group of cancer patients are those who have completed active treatment and who, on returning to their lives and routine, are finding it helpful to reveal their experience and share it with others. The National Coalition of Cancer Survivors is a national advocacy group providing a voice in health policy and care and which publishes practical and sensitive "how-to" books for survivors. Delayed physical effects, risk of recurrent or second cancers, organ failure, retardation of growth, sterility, and diminished stamina are well described. For a specific example, the CNS effects of cranial radiation in children have been elucidated, with evidence of concentration deficits and altered attention span that lead to achievement problems in school. Remediation research has been slow to start, but it is beginning.[43]

Studies of young adult survivors of Hodgkin's disease, acute leukemia, and testicular cancer reveal some psychosocial characteristics which appear to apply to survivors across tumor sites (Table XX-1-7).[37] First, there is a positive effect of greater appreciation of life and often an enhanced search for the meaning of life and more worthwhile goals. Importantly, psychologically healthy individuals emerge from cancer treatment without serious psychological sequelae or serious psychiatric disorders. Subtle increased levels of anxiety are present, however, which focus on possible recurrence and death (Damocles syndrome), as well as a greater sense of vulnerability and lower self-esteem. This uncertainty is often greatest when blood tests and imaging studies are performed in periodic reassessments. Even when there is no treatment-related gonadal toxicity, there is often lower sexual desire and poorer sexual satisfaction and performance. These sexual problems likely reflect the lower self confidence in intimate relationships.[12]

Career goals suffer from difficulty in changing jobs and in pursuing career goals with the same vigor, in part based on realistic concerns about health insurance and prejudice about having had cancer. Chemotherapy results in longlasting conditioned Pavlovian responses to reminders of the treatment situation where nausea and vomiting occurred with cyclic chemotherapy. Cella and colleagues found that smells, tastes and sights which were reminders of treatment, even as long as 12 years later, resulted in a sudden sense of unexplained anxiety and nausea (rarely with vomiting) which only, on reflection, was identified by the individual as related to a reminder of prior treatment.[11] Anxiety diminishes over time, especially after five years associated with maximal risk of recurrence. It continues to be exacerbated, however, at times of periodic medical examination or appearance of minor symptoms which the person associates with possible return of cancer.

Adaptation to Increased Genetic Risk of Cancer. The explosion of information in molecular genetics has rapidly

Table XX-1-7. Psychosocial Sequelae in Cancer Survivors

Positive effect of appreciating life more
Absence of major psychiatric disorders
Presence of subtle psychological distress
  Anxiety about recurrence/illness/death (Damocles syndrome)
  Greater sense of vulnerability (less control, lower self esteem)
  Reminders (smells, sights) of chemotherapy produce anxiety
    and nausea
Marital and sexual problems (not treatment related); less sense of
  attractiveness, lower sexual desire, poorer sexual performance
Career goals altered negatively (fewer risks, less ability to change
  jobs)
Job and health insurance problems

increased identification of healthy individuals with a genetic risk of cancer. The public is now informed about the increased risk of breast, colon, ovarian and prostate cancer among first degree relatives. The psychological impact of this knowledge results in a new and increasing number of individuals who are healthy but are fearful of disease. They constitute the "worried well" who must deal with knowledge of enhanced risk despite present good health. Some perceive themselves as "walking time bombs." Some are so anxious that they find it impossible to carry out cancer detection procedures, such as regular breast self examination or mammograms, even though both become even more important in high risk individuals to assure early detection. Another cohort is comprised of individuals who have elevations of a biomarker associated with a particular tumor, such as, the prostate specific antigen (PSA), but which may be elevated by benign conditions. In the absence of clinical cancer, these individuals often experience chronically high levels of distress, and often "live by the numbers" derived from the regular monitoring. By contrast, some individuals demonstrate the "ostrich syndrome" and deny the knowledge of enhanced risk. They choose not to carry out early detection procedures, using avoidance to control their anxiety.

Another rare group are those who may now be identified to have the genetic basis for cancer proneness as the Li-Fraumeni syndrome (p53 mutation) for whom nothing is as yet available to avert development of disease. Current ethical consideration associated with identification of these individuals becomes critically important because of the potential impact upon obtaining insurance and jobs, and the psychological impact for the child and family.

Psychiatric Disorders

When patients cope with serious illness, responses of fear, worry, and sadness are expected and normal. Usually, they are transient and dissipate as a crisis passes. However, these normal emotions can become persistent, pervasive and distressing, becoming a deterrent to treatment. At that point, worry and sadness which exceed normal become identifiable as anxiety and depression. Such "symptoms" should be evaluated, and if significant, be treated. Sensitivity to this dimension of care requires ability to evaluate a psychological symptom, recognize the clusters of symptoms which represent a psychiatric disorder and be able to identify treatment options and resources.[40]

The commonest form of distress in patients with cancer is anxiety and next most common is depression; they are often seen together. Anxiety is best considered as a symptom which exists on a continuum ranging from normal fears to situational anxiety and finally, to a disabling anxiety disorder. Depression is on a continuum from sadness, which increases to reactive depression and finally to its most severe form, major depression. Prior vulnerability to depressions predicts a recurrence during physical illness.

A prevalence study of psychiatric disorders in cancer patients, uncontrolled for stage of disease, undertaken at three cancer centers, comprised of 60% inpatients and 40% outpatients, found that 53% were coping adequately, despite the stresses they were encountering. However, 47% had

levels of distress which reached diagnostic criteria for a psychiatric disorder.[19] Among the 47% of patients with a diagnosable disorder, 32% showed a mixture of reactive depression and anxiety (adjustment disorder with depressed anxious mood, in the DSM-III classification of psychiatric disorders). Six percent had major depression; 4%, organic mental disorders; 3%, personality disorder and/or alcohol abuse; and 2%, anxiety disorders. The data support the premise that the majority of psychiatric disturbances seen in cancer patients are directly related to illness. Indeed, the predominant symptoms seen in one-third of all patients were combined reactive anxiety and depression, with one or the other predominating. Farber and colleagues and Stefanek and Derogatis, studying outpatients in an oncology clinic, independently found that one-third had a significantly high level of distress.[21,54] Using a form of the SCL-90, they found that between 20–30% of patients had clinically relevant levels of distress. The percentage of distressed patients rises in hospitalized patients due to greater disability, pain, and to treatments which produce confusional states.[22] These forms of distress, from depression or anxiety, and confusional states (organic mental disorders) constitute by far the most likely psychiatric diagnoses encountered.

Anxiety Disorders. Anxiety is the most common form of psychological distress in cancer patients. It occurs from four sources: 1) situational (functional) anxiety in response to a frightening aspect of illness; 2) as a manifestation of disease; 3) as a symptom resulting from treatment; and 4) as an exacerbation of a preexisting anxiety disorder (Table XX-1-8). Situational anxiety occurs at the time of diagnosis, with anticipation of a procedure or new treatment, at transitional points in illness, after treatment is finished, and as a recurrent concern, even years later, about exacerbation of disease. Fears of recurrence appear to be present to some degree in *all* cancer survivors (Table XX-1-7). However, in some

Table XX-1-8.   Causes of Anxiety in Patients with Cancer

Situational
  Diagnosis
  Crisis
  Anticipating a frightening procedure
  Fears of recurrence

Disease-related
  Poorly controlled pain
  Abnormal metabolic states
  Hormone secreting tumors
  Paraneoplastic syndromes (remote CNS effects)

Treatment-related
  Frightening or painful procedures (MRI, scans, wound debridement)
  Anxiety-producing drugs (antiemetic neuroleptics, bronchodilators)
  Withdrawal states (opioids, benzodiazepines, alcohol)
  Conditioned (anticipatory) anxiety, nausea and vomiting with cyclic chemotherapy

Exacerbation of pre-existing anxiety disorder
  Phobias (needles, claustrophobia)
  Panic or generalized anxiety disorders
  Post-traumatic stress disorder (holocaust survivors, Vietnam veterans, recall of death of relative with cancer)

individuals the level of anxiety can be so pervasive that it interferes with ability to function and requires treatment.

Anxiety related to medical problems is seen most often as an accompaniment of poorly controlled pain; it usually disappears when pain is adequately controlled (Table XX-1-9). New unanticipated events, such as skin rash or diarrhea, can produce major anxiety as the patient wonders what else has gone wrong. Great anxiety usually attends the discovery of a new tumor or lymph node. Anxiety may also herald a change in medical status, especially in advanced cancer when complications of hypoxia, pulmonary embolus, sepsis, fever, bleeding, cardiac arrhythmia, and hypoglycemia may manifest initially with anxiety and restlessness. Hormone-secreting tumors can produce anxiety.

Among cancer treatment-related causes of anxiety the most common are: 1) anxiety related to frightening or painful procedures, especially those which occur repeatedly, such as wound debridement. About 20% of patients have trouble tolerating imaging procedures such as the MRI or CT scan due to the small, enclosed space which triggers claustrophobic fears. About 5% are unable to undergo it. Several drugs used frequently in cancer produce symptoms of anxiety: corticosteroids, neuroleptics used as antiemetics, bronchodilators, thyroxine, and stimulants. Unexplained restlessness, anxiety and agitation develop often in patients who receive large doses of metoclopramide or other neuroleptics during chemotherapy for control of nausea and vomiting as part of the extrapyramidal symptoms of akathesias and dystonias. Withdrawal states from alcohol, narcotic analgesics and sedative-hypnotics produce anxiety as a prominent symptom and must be kept in mind.

Some patients undergoing cyclic chemotherapy using an emetogenic regimen begin to develop anticipatory anxiety, nausea and vomiting by about the third cycle, a few days to hours in advance of receiving the next cycle of treatment.[3,46] This is a learned Pavlovian conditioned autonomic response to the repeated experience of nausea and vomiting. In fact, two-thirds of women receiving adjuvant chemotherapy for breast cancer develop conditioned anxiety and nausea, though not usually vomiting. The response was seen as long as 12 years later on encountering smells or tastes which reminded the person of the chemotherapy received for Hodgkin's disease.[11] Behavioral interventions and antianxiety medication are effective in controlling the symptoms. It does not develop when nausea and vomiting are controlled, as is the case with the increasingly effective antiemetic regimens.

Patients who have preexisting phobias, panic attacks, generalized anxiety or post traumatic stress disorders are at risk of exacerbation of their symptoms during cancer treatment (Table XX-1-8).[39] Phobias of needles, blood, hospitals, claustrophobia or agoraphobia are sometimes troublesome symptoms to control during treatment for cancer. Panic attacks and generalized anxiety symptoms must be controlled in order to enable the patient to tolerate anxiety-provoking medical treatment. Patients who experienced the holocaust, or who have traumatic memories of war or frightening events may experience recall of the painful memories during illness and treatment. Individuals who recall death of a relative from cancer, especially when it was the same neoplasm, have more anxiety.

The treatment of simple situational anxiety is usually handled adequately by the physician who reassures the patient, reviews frightening anticipated events, allows the person to "rehearse" them, and engenders confidence that the person can cope with the feared treatment or procedure (Table XX-1-10). The oncology nurse or social worker is often helpful in reviewing circumstances more fully and adding reassurance. For persistent or distressing anxiety, three means of treatment are available: counseling (by individual or group means, and by professional or peer counseling); behavioral, and pharmacologic means. Counseling or formal psycho-

Table XX-1-9. Anxiety Related to Common Medical Problems in Cancer*

Medical Problems	Examples
Poorly controlled pain	
Abnormal metabolic states	Hypoxia, pulmonary embolus, sepsis, fever, delirium, hypoglycemia, bleeding, coronary occlusion and heart failure, cardiac arrhythmia
Hormone-secreting tumors	Pheochromocytoma, thyroid adenoma or carcinoma, parathyroid adenoma, ACTH-producing tumors, insulinoma
Anxiety-producing drugs	Corticosteroids, neuroleptics used as antiemetics, thyroxine, bronchodilators, β-adrenergic stimulants, antihistamines, (paradoxical reactions), withdrawal states (alcohol, narcotic analgesics, sedative-hypnotics)
Side effects of treatment	Allergic skin rash to antibiotics, unexpected toxicity, e.g., diarrhea

*Adapted from Massie and Holland[39]

Table XX-1-10. Treatment of Anxiety Disorders*

Treatment Modality	Components
Supportive psychotherapy	Providing information; rehearsal of feared events; reassurance
Behavioral	Relaxation Hypnosis Systematic desensitization

Psychopharmacological	Benzodiazepines
	  Short acting (alprazolam, lorazepam, oxazepam)
	  Long acting (diazepam, clorazepate, clonazepam)
	  Beta blockers (propranolol)
	Tricyclic antidepressants (amitriptyline, doxepin, nortriptyline)
	Monoamine oxidase inhibitors (phenelzine, isocarboxazid)
	Antihistamines
	Neuroleptics (thioridazine, trifluperazine, haloperidol)
	Buspirone

Combinations of the above	

*Adapted from Massie and Holland[39]

Table XX-1-11.   Common Prescribed Benzodiazepines in Cancer Patients

Drug	Approximate Dose Equivalent	Initial Dosage PO (mg)	Half Life (Hr)	Active Metabolite
Short to Intermediate Half-Life				
Alprazolam	0.5	0.25–0.5 TID	10–15	No
Chlordiazepoxide	10.0	10–25 TID	5–30	Yes
Clonazepam	1.0	0.5 BID	18–50	No
Lorazepam*	1.0	0.5–2.0 TID	10–20	No
Oxazepam	10.0	10–15 TID	5–15	No
Temazepam**	15.0	15–30 QHS	10–15	No
Triazolam**	0.25	0.125–0.25 QHS	1.5	No
Long Half-Life				
Chlorazepate	7.5	7.5–15 BID	30–200	Yes
Diazepam	5.0	5–10	20–70	Yes

*Lorazepam can also be administered intramuscularly; other benzodiazepines are erraticaly absorbed when given intramuscularly
**Hypnotic agents

therapy, using a supportive crisis intervention model, is helpful.[41] Several behavioral interventions are effective: relaxation exercises with guided imagery and hypnosis are most frequently employed. These methods are particularly helpful to patients who wish to maintain and enhance their beleaguered sense of control over their emotions and body. Relaxation is a useful adjunct to pain control and for control of conditioned chemotherapy-related nausea and vomiting.[46]

Significant anxiety symptoms are most often treated pharmacologically by sedative-hypnotics from the benzodiazepine class of drugs, but other types of drugs are effective, such as antihistamines, beta blockers and neuroleptics in low dose (Table XX-1-10). Many patients feel it is a sign of weakness to accept medication and must be encouraged to use them during a crisis period. The benzodiazepine is chosen by the desired half-life, route of administration, metabolism and active metabolites (Table XX-1-11). Shorter half life provides better control and less likelihood of poor elimination and oversedation. Patients whose anxiety is manifested by insomnia respond to a bedtime dose of temazepam 15 mg, triazolam .25 mg, or clonazepam 1 mg. Daytime anxiety responds to lorazepam .5 mg or alprazolam .25–.50 mg TID or QID. It is important to taper these medications to prevent mild increase in anxiety or withdrawal symptoms. Buspirone is useful because it has no sedating effects and no addictive qualities. Thioridazine 10 mg QID, a neuroleptic, is useful in low dose when a benzodiazepine is contraindicated, as in older individuals.[39]

Depression. While it is expected and normal to feel sad upon learning of a diagnosis of cancer or hearing news that another crisis related to illness has occurred, some individuals experience far greater distress at a level which is abnormal and which constitutes a diagnosable depressive disorder. It is important to keep in mind that depression *does* respond to treatment and should not be left untreated because it is "based on reality." Depression is difficult to diagnose in cancer because the disease itself produces fatigue, weakness, loss of libido, of interest and of motivation and concentration.

Most depressive disorders are reactive to illness (called adjustment disorders) and are seen in about a quarter of oncology patients in the clinic; the percentage is higher in

Table XX-1-12.   Evaluation of Depression and Predisposing Factors

Evaluative Category	Findings
Family history	Depression Suicide
Personal history	Previous psychiatric illness (depression or manic episodes, alcoholism, drug abuse) Suicide attempt

Signs and symptoms	Psychological
	   Dysphoric mood (e.g., sad, depressed, anxious, crying); diurnal mood change
	   Feelings of hopelessness, helplessness
	   Loss of interest and pleasure
	   Guilt, burden on others, worthlessness
	   Poor concentration
	   Mood incongruent to disease outlook
	   Suicidal thoughts or plans
	   Delusional thoughts (psychotic symptoms rare, except in organic affective syndrome)
	Somatic, (less interpretable in more physically impaired patients)
	Insomnia
	Anorexia and weight loss
	Fatigue
	Psychomotor retardation or agitation
	Constipation
	Decreased libido

hospitalized patients.[9] The symptoms of depression are: depressed and dysphoric mood, insomnia, restlessness or psychomotor slowing and a sense of hopelessness and helplessness. Major depression is diagnosed when guilt and suicidal ideation are present. Table XX-1-12 outlines the history and symptoms that are relevant to making a diagnosis of major depression. Family history of depression, and prior personal psychiatric disorder or substance abuse should be explored. Review of symptoms should explore mental status signs and symptoms of mood, hopelessness, feeling of being a burden and suicidal ideation. While somatic symptoms are harder to interpret, insomnia, anorexia, fatigue, agitation or psychomotor retardation nevertheless are useful signs of depression when not likely related to illness; they also serve as symptoms which can be monitored for treatment effect.

Table XX-1-13 outlines the major risk factors that predict which individuals are most likely to develop significant depression during cancer. History of depression or suicide attempt, substance abuse, poor social supports or recent bereavement is important. In terms of illness, greater levels of debilitation, advanced disease and presence of another chronic illness or disability predict depression. Several medications contribute: steroids, some chemotherapeutic agents (interferon, vincristine) and medications given for other reasons. Depression appears as a part of the metabolic picture of organ failure and with some nutritional, endocrine and neurological complications of cancer.

Depression is managed first by maintaining good rapport with the patient, and assuring support from available family or friends. Supportive psychotherapeutic and behavioral interventions and psychotropic agents are important resources for treatment of depression. Behavioral interventions are effective in depression, using cognitive-behavioral methods which encourage the patient to reframe the problems more constructively; to approach each aspect intellectually with a planned response which reduces uncontrolled distressing

Table XX-1-13.   Risk Factors for Developing Depressive Symptoms in Cancer Patients

Category	Influence
Personal	History of depression (patient or family)
	History of alcoholism or substance abuse
	Prior suicide attempt
	Poor social supports
	Recent loss (bereavement)
Illness and treatment	Advanced stages of cancer
	Poorly controlled pain
	Other chronic disease/disability
	Medications
	Corticosteroids
	Prednisone, dexamethasone
	Other chemotherapeutic agents
	Vincristine, vinblastine, procarbazine, L-asparaginase, interferon, amphotericin-B
	Other medications
	Cimetidine
	Diazepam
	Indomethacin
	Levodopa
	Methyldopa
	Pentazocine
	Phenmetrazine
	Phenobarbital
	Propranolol
	Rauwolfia alkaloids
	Estrogens
	Other medical conditions
	Metabolic
	Nutritional
	Endocrine
	Neurological

emotions. This has been particularly helpful in coping with the meaning of pain, which is so frightening in cancer when it is viewed as evidence of tumor progression. Cognitive approaches also can alter distressing sensations and responses to them.[8]

Psychotropic drugs have been shown in clinical trials to be effective in control of depressive symptoms with medical illness, including cancer. Table XX-1-14 gives the most frequently used antidepressant medications in cancer patients and their starting and maintenance dose. The antidepressants commonly used are the tricyclics, second generation antidepressants, heterocyclics, monoamine oxidase inhibitors (MAOIs), psychostimulants, lithium carbonate and benzodiazepines. Tricyclics are most commonly used, started at low dose (10–25 mg at bedtime) and slowly increased by 10–25 mg increments over 4–7 day intervals. Patients are usually maintained 4–6 months on a tricyclic, chosen in part by its side effects profile. A tricyclic with sedating effects, such as amitriptyline or doxepin, is best for agitation and insomnia. Psychomotor slowing is better treated with desipramine. Nortriptyline and desipramine should be used for patients in whom minimal anticholinergic effects are desired.

Second line antidepressants are the heterocyclics. Maprotiline, amoxapine, bupropion, and trazodone are useful. In general, they have side effects similar to the tricyclics. Maprotiline can lower the seizure threshold. Fluoxetine has few side effects and has proved safe and effective in patients with depression and psychomotor retardation. Antidepressant effects may take up to 2–3 weeks to become evident with the drugs discussed above. Maximal benefit is usually obtained by four weeks.

Among the other antidepressants, psychostimulants are most widely used for promotion of well being and counteracting fatigue or advanced illness. Drowsiness associated with opioids is often diminished by dextroaphetamine, methylphenidate or pemoline, a non-controlled stimulant with no addicting potential. Alprazolam has the advantage of being effective against anxiety and depression and is useful when stronger antidepressants are contraindicated.[31]

Suicide and Cancer. Suicide is increased in incidence in patients with cancer compared to the general population, though it is not as high as often assumed.[6,7] However, it is likely that suicide by overdose at home during terminal stages of cancer is under diagnosed and under reported. Suicide is more likely to occur in advanced disease when depression, hopelessness and the presence of poorly controlled symptoms, especially pain, increase. Table XX-1-15 outlines risk factors which predict acting out suicidal thoughts. They are similar to factors predicting depression (Table XX-1-12). These factors must be assessed in evaluating a patient for suicidal risk and in evaluating strengths to be identified for support (Table XX-1-16). Evaluation of the patient with suicidal ideation should query the nature of suicidal thoughts (passive or active), past history of psychiatric problems, recent loss or bereavement, poor prior adjustment or suicidal attempt; family history of depression or suicide; present symptoms that the patient feels are poorly controlled, and the person's understanding of disease and prognosis.

It is not possible to consider suicidal thoughts and actual acts without taking into account disease stage and prog-

Table XX-1-14.   Commonly Used Antidepressants in Cancer

Drug Name	Starting Daily Dosage mg (po)	Therapeutic Daily Dosage mg (po)
Tricyclic antidepressants		
Amitriptyline	25	75–100
Doxepin	25	75–100
Imipramine	25	75–100
Desipramine	25	75–100
Nortriptyline	25	50–100
Second-generation antidepressants		
Bupropion	15	200–450
Trazodone	50	150–200
Fluoxetine	20	20–60
Heterocyclic antidepressants		
Maprotiline	25	50–75
Amoxapine	25	100–150
Monoamine oxidase inhibitors		
Isocarboxazid	10	24–40
Phenelzine	15	30–60
Tranylcypromine	10	20–40
Lithium carbonate	300	600–1200
Psychostimulants		
Dextroamphetamine	2.5 at 8 a.m. and noon	5–30
Methylphenidate	2.5 at 8 a.m. and noon	5–30
Pemoline	18.75 in a.m. and noon	37.5–150
Benzodiazepines		
Alprazolam	0.25–1.00	0.75–6.00

Table XX-1-15.   Risk Factors for Suicide in Cancer

Personal
  Prior history of suicide (personal or family)
  Prior psychiatric disorder
  Prior alcohol or drug abuse
  Depression and hopelessness
  Recent loss/bereavement
Medical
  Pain
  Delirium
  Advanced illness
  Debilitation, exhaustion, fatigue

Table XX-1-16.   Evaluation of Suicidal Risk

Establish rapport
Ask about symptoms (pain, discomfort, and adequacy of their control)
Ask about depression and suicidal thoughts at present or in the past
Ask about suicidal thoughts (Are they *passive:* "I wish I could die" or *active:* "I am thinking of ways to do it")
Asking does *not* cause suicidal thoughts; the patient is usually relieved to express them
Ask about family or friends and sense of support from others
Ask about any recent loss of close person, especially if by cancer
Ask about understanding of illness, presence of confusion, fatigue

nosis. The issues and management vary greatly with these factors. Table XX-1-17 outlines the range of issues in relation to disease stage.

To consider suicide in cancer, it is helpful to consider the issue from three perspectives: 1) suicidal thoughts in patients at all stages of disease; 2) suicidal thoughts in patients with a good prognosis; and 3) suicidal thoughts in patients with poor prognosis/poor symptom control, and patients in terminal stages.

First, almost all patients who receive a cancer diagnosis, even when the prognosis is good, carry a "secret" rarely acknowledged thought that says "I won't die in pain with advanced cancer—I'll kill myself first." This may include having a secret supply of drugs which is kept for this purpose. This usually serves as a "steam valve" with which the person is able to maintain a sense of ultimate control over the disease and an intolerable future. The thought actually serves as a protective coping device which must be recognized by

the physician and the psychiatrist as a normal and healthy means of maintaining control. For most, the time never comes to take the pills and life becomes dearer as death approaches. The intensity of suicidal thoughts is greater among patients who have seen a relative die with poor control of pain, as was more typical of earlier times, and especially if they had the same tumor. It is important that the physician listen to these fears and concerns, and even answer questions about what constitutes a lethal dose of sedative. The rapid climb of *Final Exit* by Derek Humphry of the Hemlock Society to the top of the best seller list in the U.S. shows the degree to which people fear loss of control over death and the desire to avoid meaningless life and protracted dying.[34]

However, *serious* ruminating about suicide in a patient in whom the disease is in remission, or in whom a good prognosis exists, is *not* rational. In fact, careful evaluation will very likely elicit presence of major depression, a history of sub-

Table XX-1-17. Suicide in Relation to Stage of Disease

Patients at *all* stages of cancer
  Suicidal thoughts are common and serve as a means of
    maintaining a sense of control over the disease
  Carrying out the act is viewed as for "the future when I need to
    do it"
  Some maintain a means of suicide (e.g, drugs) to assure
    ultimate control over feared intolerable symptoms

Patients in remission, with good prognosis
  Serious suicidal thoughts represent underlying psychiatric
    disorder (depression, substance abuse)
  Unlikely "rational"; treat aggressively, including hospitalization

Patients with poor prognosis and poorly controlled symptoms
  Thoughts of suicide often appear "rational"
  May request advice about physician-assisted suicide
  Need evaluation for presence of treatable depression
  Need attention to quality of life issues and comfort
  Suicidal wishes usually diminish with control of distressing
    symptoms
  Adequate symptom control by physician may hasten death
    (dual effect) but is not actual physician assisted suicide

Patients in terminal stage
  May request euthanasia by lethal injection of physician
  Request often reflects poor quality of life, hopelessness and
    depression
  Need for control of symptoms, even when hastens death
  Physicians and public need more education about available
    palliative care options
  Legalize assisted death or euthanasia in U.S.? Public and
    professional debate needed

stance abuse or recent bereavement. A study by Hietanin and Lonquist in Finland of all suicides in 1987 found that 4.3% had cancer.[28] Surprisingly, half of the cancer patients were in remission at the time of the suicide; they had greater prior psychiatric problems, particularly substance abuse, than those who suicided in advanced stages of cancer. It is important that these patients be recognized and aggressively treated for depression and suicidal risk, including psychiatric hospitalization, if necessary.

Patients with a poor prognosis, advanced disease and poorly controlled symptoms often have thoughts of suicide that are more likely to be viewed as rational. They may request help from a physician for assistance in committing suicide. Many of these patients experience reduction of the suicidal wish when their desperation is countered by good control of their symptoms and distress, especially control of pain and depression. Adequate pain control by the physician may actually also have the dual effect of hastening death, but few physicians have difficulty in carrying out such a treatment that is aimed at comfort, and when it reflects the patient's and family's wishes. Most physicians do not regard this as assisted suicide, but appropriate treatment geared to maximal comfort.

Patients who are in terminal stages and who are too weak to carry out a suicidal act are those who are most likely to request euthanasia by a lethal injection from the physician. U.S. health care, with its emphasis on tertiary care and the absence of a long preexisting relationship to patients, makes this a more difficult issue than in the Netherlands. Of the 2,000–3,000 acts of euthanasia carried out each year there,

almost all are done in patients' homes by physicians who have known them for many years and who have informed the local magistrate of the plan. Few are done in hospitals or nursing homes.

Physicians are being drawn into a public debate about the right of patients who are mentally competent to request euthanasia by a lethal injection from a physician. This is in contrast to the painstaking development of legislation to assure that patients have an opportunity to provide advance directions about life sustaining treatments by identification of a proxy to make decisions when they are no longer competent. The legislative agenda on euthanasia in several states is occurring without adequate attention to the issue of the frequency of depression in patients with advanced cancer and the fact that suicidal wishes may reflect unrecognized depression, uncontrolled pain or the sense that "my family will be better off because my care costs too much."[14] Thoughtful debate about euthanasia must weigh the rights of individuals to demand euthanasia carried out by a physician, taking into account that symptom control for many terminally ill patients is woefully inadequate, including identification and treatment of depression and hopelessness which may be at the heart of the request for euthanasia, but which remain unrecognized. Until supportive care and symptom control are more clearly acknowledged by the public and by health care policy makers, legislative efforts to legalize euthanasia may represent a slippery slope on which physicians will be required by law to make medical judgments without adequate opportunity for attention to the complex psychiatric, medical and ethical issues.

Delirium. In patients with cancer, especially with advanced stages of disease, it is prudent to consider a sudden change in mood or behavior for its possible relationship to change in neurological, vascular or metabolic status; a functional basis is far less likely. In fact, in advanced and terminal illness, 75% of hospitalized patients were found to develop a confusional state (delirium) during the period prior to death.[42] Common causes of delirium in cancer are outlined in Table XX-1-18.[22] A change in behavior in which the person becomes irritable, uncooperative, either agitated or somnolent, and misinterprets sounds or objects, is apt to represent common signs of early delirium. This picture may be followed by delusions, usually paranoid ("there are people here trying to hurt me"), frank hallucinations and difficulty in being maintained in their bed and hospital room because of mental aberrations (Table XX-1-19). It is important to have a person familiar to the patient present who can interpret what is happening, while also limiting the number of new faces and experiences. Older patients are most prone to become confused and delirium may be superimposed on dementia. Physical restraints should be used with caution to avoid falls; chemical restraint may be helpful. Low dose haloperidol in .5–1.0 mg doses 3–4 times a day often reduces confusion. Lorazepam reduces agitation in doses .5–1.0 mg TID to QID. Haloperidol and lorazepam are often given together to reduce confusion and diminish agitation. Correcting the underlying metabolic or neurologic problem is not always possible and comfort for patient and family may depend materially on being able to control these symptoms of confusion and agitation.

Table XX-1-18.   Common Causes of Delirium in Cancer Patients*

Causes	Examples
Metabolic encephalopathy due to vital organ failure	Liver, kidney, lung, thyroid, adrenal
Electrolyte imbalance	Sodium, potassium, calcium, glucose
Treatment side effects	Narcotics Anticholinergics, (narcotics, phenothiazines, antihistamines) Chemotherapeutic agents; steroids Radiation therapy
Infection	Septicemia
Hematological abnormalities	Microcytic and macrocytic anemias, coagulopathies
Nutritional	General malnutrition, thiamine, folic acid, B_{12}
Paraneoplastic syndromes	Remote effects Tumors Hormone-producing tumor

*Modified from Posner (1978); Fleishman & Lesko[22]

Table XX-1-19.   Behavioral Symptoms of Delirium in Cancer Patients*

Stage	Symptom
Early, mild	Change in sleep pattern with restlessness and transient periods of disorientation Increased irritability, anger, temper outbursts Withdrawal, refusal to talk to staff or relatives Forgetfulness, not previously present
Late, severe with behavioral changes	Refusal to cooperate with reasonable requests Angry, swearing, shouting, abusive Demanding to go home; pacing corridor Illusions (misidentifies staff, visual and sensory clues) Delusions (misinterprets events, usually paranoid, fears of being harmed) Hallucinations (visual and auditory)

*From Fleishman and Lesko[22]

Behavioral and Psychosocial Variables in Cancer Morbidity and Mortality

Many questions are raised about the role of behavioral, psychological and social variables in cancer morbidity and mortality (Table XX-1-20). There are five areas in which factors have been explored for their contribution: life style and behaviors, social environment and social support; personality and coping; affective states/life events; and psychosocial and behavioral interventions.

In terms of life style, reduced exposures to carcinogens through change in habits (e.g., smoking cessation, sunburn assistance) has the greatest potential for reducing cancer mortality. This is followed by behaviors associated with early detection of cancer (e.g., breast self examination, systematic cervical cytology and mammography). And, adherence to a

Table XX-1-20.   Primary Behaviors and Psychosocial Factors Which Impact upon Cancer Morbidity and Mortality

Life style/behaviors associated with carcinogenic exposures (tobacco, sun)
Poor socioeconomic status; poor education
Early detection and treatment compliance
Availability of social supports

treatment regimen for cancer in which compliance assures full dose of prescribed chemotherapy or radiation is critical for best outcome. Psychological issues clearly contribute to the ability to encourage behaviors that reduce exposures, assure early diagnosis and adherence.

Aspects of the social environment have increasingly been identified as contributing to cancer morbidity and mortality.[33] A study by Cella and colleagues of 2,400 patients treated by standardized protocols in the Cancer and Leukemia Group B found, after known predictors of outcome were considered, lowest education and income were correlated with shortest survival.[12] Ability to understand and comply with treatment regimens may need special attention in those with the lowest educational level. Individuals who are economically disadvantaged suffer from poor access to health care, and in addition, have such factors as nutritional deficiencies, greater presence of other medical illnesses, chronic stress of poverty and poor social supports. These are factors that have not been studied for their separate contribution to poorer survival.

Data from a meta analysis of six studies done in three different countries showed that poor or absent social ties had an impact on overall age-adjusted morbidity and mortality from a range of diseases, including cancer.[33] Similar findings found in married versus single individuals, suggest that better lifestyle, habits and earlier seeking of health care may be the factors which account for better survival. Exploration for a personality type associated with cancer, similar to the Type A personality and cardiovascular disease has not been successful.

Bereavement and depression have been most extensively studied for a role in cancer morbidity and mortality. They have also been examined for impact on immune function in physically healthy individuals. As bereavement studies have been more carefully controlled, they have failed to confirm a relationship between either cancer morbidity or mortality. Depression, likewise, has shown less likelihood of correlation with mortality. The large prospective study by Zonderman and colleagues of a nationally representative sample studied for prevalence of depression 10 years earlier found no increased cancer mortality 10 years later.[61] The fact that immune changes have accompanied depressive and grieving symptoms has been of great interest. However, questions have been raised about interpretation of psychoimmune data in terms of how clinically relevant the small changes in function which occur with emotional states may be. Chronic psychiatric disorders also have not predicted cancer mortality in several studies.

Many studies have identified the nature and frequency of distress in cancer patients. They have led to intervention studies aimed at improving coping and well being, with interests in whether they might also affect length of survival. Over 20 studies, using a range of interventions, often combining support and behavioral methods, have shown enhanced well being and improved quality of life.[41,59] A positive effect on outcome of disease and survival has been reported only by Spiegel and colleagues.[52] They found in an analysis ten years later that women with advanced breast cancer who were randomized to a weekly group psychiatric intervention for one year had survived significantly longer than those who had been assigned to the control arm.

In summary, four areas clearly show the impact of behavior and social factors on cancer morbidity and mortality: life style and behaviors; low socioeconomic and educational status; early detection and treatment compliance; and, availability of social supports (perhaps mediated through encouraging early detection and treatment compliance) (Table XX-1-20). Of great interest, but still awaiting confirmation, is whether psychosocial intervention may have a salutary effect not only on well being, but on survival as well.

Alternative Cancer Treatments

Any group of disease which has largely unknown causes, high likelihood of fatality and uncertain cure, causes great fear in the public's mind. Cancer and mental illness have historically been most feared; AIDS, for the same reasons, has been added. Diseases for which traditional medicine cannot provide a cure have always elicited an array of non-traditional treatments.[30] The history of cancer quackery is of great psychological interest since these therapies have flourished over centuries; they have only changed in type and nature. In general, the popular unconventional treatments of a particular period reflect the public's perception of cancer and medicine at that time.[10,60] Thus, balms, tonics and electrical waves were popular early in this century. They gave way to krebiozen in the 1960's, laetrile in 1970's and, most recently, to natural holistic approaches which are proposed to work by enhancing the body's defenses. The alternative therapy community tends to exist separately from mainstream medicine, assuming a polarized position. Patients are often confused as to how to relate to the two worlds.

There has been a recent effort to try to bridge this gap by preparation of a thoughtful and comprehensive report (which should be read by anyone interested in the area) of alternative therapies in the U.S., undertaken by the Office of Technological Assessment at the request of the U.S. Congress.[58] The report elucidates the present status of these therapies, outlining the four major areas of alternative therapies: psychological and behavioral approaches; nutritional; herbal; and pharmacologic/biologic. Many therapies, such as those of Gerson and of Kelly, combine several of these approaches and include a spiritual or religious context as well. The best known psychological approaches are Simonton's visualization methods to enhance immune function; Siegal's Exceptional Cancer Patients approach to improve survival by positive emotional expression. Commonweal, where Lerner combines group discussion, yoga, touch, relaxation and visualization in a week long therapeutic experience, provides these activities as complementary therapies, to be used in conjunction with traditional treatment. The fear that

patients will leave their medical treatment for an alternative appears less of a threat today.[10]

It is important to have a clear understanding of the issues, since some of the psychological and behavioral methods that are used in mainstream medicine (psychological support, visual imagery, relaxation) for enhancing quality of life and symptom control are also included in alternative therapies which promise the curing of cancer or extending survival through their use. This gray zone grows even broader in view of psychoimmune studies that show an impact of stress in healthy subjects on immune function and the study which showed greater survival among women with advanced breast cancer who received weekly psychotherapeutic group meetings.[52] It is hard for frightened individuals to view these findings only as interesting research data that warrant further study.

Many of the psychological alternative therapies suggest that the patient had a role in developing cancer, by response to stress or by personality. They also exhort the patient to be "positive," "fight," and they insist that outcome depends largely on attitude. Patients become fearful when they become depressed because being depressed "may make the cancer grow faster." These deleterious aspects of the present era, with its emphasis on psychological factors, has been examined from a sociological view.[26] Society tends to use myths to understand frightening phenomena. Often, the cancer patient is portrayed as the heroic warrior fighting the dragon, cancer. Some individuals gain strength by assuming the warrior stance and should be encouraged to maintain it. They find the cancer self-help books, visualization, and mental attitude methods helpful, and should be encouraged to use them. However, there are other patients for whom the warrior myth is distressing. They become guilty because they feel that they cannot fight hard enough. Sometimes a distraught family blames the patient for not helping enough. These individuals need to know that there are many ways of effectively coping with cancer; there is no single *right* way for all individuals. In fact, most patients do best when they rely on their own self-validated effective means of coping developed over years of trial. They can also be told that several studies have not supported longer survival in patients using unconventional therapies.[4,45]

There are several key points that have emerged from research on alternative therapies and their use that are helpful as guides. The patients who use alternative therapies today are not poorly educated individuals with advanced disease who are grasping at straws. They tend to be educated individuals, who are seeking all information at the time of diagnosis; they may be entranced by the mind-body relationship claimed by the alternative approaches. Many assume a posture of "what harm can it do." Most receive conventional therapies at the same time. Internationally, about 10–20% of patients with cancer use alternative treatments in western countries. Among them, only a small percent appear to stop conventional therapy.[10]

It is helpful to keep up with local alternative therapies in vogue, and to support patients' psychological needs in a way that they do not require seeking support from nontraditional sources. It is also important to encourage patients to discuss thoughts about alternative therapies. Angry responses from oncologists place the patient in an untenable situation which encourages lack of disclosure. A therapy that is harmful should be condemned; a therapy that is aimed at quality of life, and which is to be used as an adjunct to conventional therapy, should be condoned if it helps the patient in coping, and has no deleterious effect. However, patients should be warned that if a psychological alternative approach makes them feel distressed (e.g., guilty or depressed that they are failing) they should discontinue it. The result is sometimes experienced as blaming the victim: "You caused the cancer and now it is up to you to cure it."

Quality-of-Life Assessment

The focus of psychological studies in the last decade has increasingly been identified as "quality-of-life" research.[16,17,56] Interest in quality of life grew when the Federal Drug Administration demanded that clinical researchers after 1984 demonstrate efficacy of new anticancer agents by either improved survival or by evidence of enhanced quality of survival. Coupled with increased patient involvement in their own care and concerns about informed consent, issues of quality-of-life with one treatment versus another led to heightened interest in finding ways to measure quality of life.[20] Karnofsky and Burchenal actually described in 1949 that subjective improvement, in addition to survival, was equally important to the evaluation of patients' responses to treatment.[35] Despite that early observation, less than 5% of clinical trials had included a quality-of-life variable in 1990.[1]

There are six domains that are generally included in quality-of-life measures: physical (e.g., symptoms resulting from the disease or treatment), functional (ability to carry out daily activities), psychological, sexual, social, and work (Table XX-1-21). No "gold standard" of measurement currently exists to assess quality of life. However, there are several frequently used scales that can be employed to monitor patient adaptation and the effect of treatment. The most widely used is the Functional Living Index-Cancer (FLIC) developed by Schipper and coworkers.[23,50] A 22-item scale with physical well-being and emotional subscales, the FLIC was developed specifically for use with cancer patients. The Cancer Rehabilitation Evaluation System (CARES) is a scale that consists of 139 items concerning cancer problems across the six quality-of-life domains previously outlined.[49] A promising new quality-of-life measure has been carefully developed and tested by the European Organization for Research and Treatment of Cancer (EORTC).[1,2] The scale has a core of questions that are applicable to the quality of life of all cancer patients, and modules which query the quality of life issues related to a specific disease site (e.g., prostate, breast,

lung cancer). This is also being used by Cella in his development of Functional Assessment of Cancer Therapy (FACT) which adds an aspect of patient assessment of the discrepancy between *prior and present functions*. Aside from the Karnofsky rating scale, Spitzer and colleagues' Quality of Life Index (QL-Index) is the only observer-rated measure of quality of life that is used with some frequency.[53]

Additional scales not developed specifically for cancer, but which are widely used, are the Psychosocial Adjustment to Illness Scale (PAIS) and the Sickness Impact Profile (SIP).[5,18] The PAIS, in particular, has been used extensively with several chronic illnesses including cancer. The SIP scale is similar in format to CARES in that it lists 136 problems that can result from illness that affect quality of life.

Most quality-of-life scales presently being developed are designed to be used as self-report measures or to be completed in response to a brief structured interview.[55] Traditionally, such forms were administered at the time of clinic visits. However, use of trained telephone interviewers in cooperative group trials in the CALGB has found this approach not only more practicable, but it takes the collecting of quality of life data away from the hectic clinic setting. The method ensures consistency in terms of evaluation, promotes better compliance, and there are fewer missing data points, since questions can be clarified.[37] Findings using this type of telephone approach in which the patient has the written questions and responds to them at the interviewer's request were comparable to those attained using a face-to-face interview in a comparison study.[37,44]

Recent efforts in quality-of-life research have concentrated on the development of a unitary measure which might combine length of survival and quality of life, referred to as "quality-adjusted life years" or QALYs. "TWIST" or time without symptoms or toxicity, is another QALY method developed by Goldhirsch and coworkers.[13,24,25] In this method, the number of months in which the patient experienced symptoms (weighted as to toxicity) or was in relapse is subtracted from overall survival time, yielding a quality-adjusted life year score. In QALY research, weights, which are either empirically derived or chosen arbitrarily are assigned, to the levels of disability or symptoms in the various treatment arms. In this manner, the differences between types of symptoms upon quality of life can be mathematically taken into account.

This area of inquiry is in its infancy but it offers intriguing attempts to evaluate treatment effectiveness through the combination of physical and subjective information.[36] Information derived from quality-of-life studies will be helpful to physicians and patients in weighing the outcome of different primary treatment options.[20]

Summary

The subspecialty of psycho-oncology is a recent development within oncology, reflecting the increased interest in behavioral, psychological and social factors in cancer prevention and in the quality of life of patients with cancer at all stages. The quality of life issues are different in respect to patients under active treatment; during palliative care; for survivors; and for healthy individuals who are at known increased risk. Early identification of patients who are not

Table XX-1-21. Quality of Life Measurement: Functional Areas of Living Assessed

Physical	Symptoms of disease and treatment side effects
Functional	Ability to perform usual activities
Psychological	Mood, sense of well being
Sexual	Desire, performance
Social	Family, friends, leisure
Work	Usual level of activity

coping well with the diagnosis and treatment is important, both for compliance with treatment and for control of distress. It is important to recognize and diagnose the common psychiatric disorders, primarily anxiety and depressive symptoms, which occur in cancer patients. The modalities available to treat these symptoms that impact on the quality of life are psychotherapeutic, behavioral and pharmacologic. Referral to a mental health professional familiar with the care of patients with cancer is also important. Knowledge of alternative therapies is necessary to be able to discuss them with patients and their families. Behavioral, psychological and social factors play a role in cancer morbidity and mortality, primarily by life style and habits in cancer prevention, in the environment, poor socioeconomic conditions and poor education, behaviors which lead to early detection and compliance with therapy, and the presence of social supports which likely contribute to better health behaviors. The measurement of quality of life which assesses patients' functioning in the major domains of their lives has been a valuable addition to clinical trials research, placing emphasis on not only *quantity* of life, but its *quality* as well. This merger of medical and social science data augurs well for future research initiatives.

References

1. Aaronson, N. K.: Methodologic issues in assessing the quality of life of cancer patients. Cancer, 67:844, 1991.
2. Aaronson, N. K., Bakker, W., Stewart, A. L., van Dam, F., van Zandwijk, N., Yarnold, J. R., and Kirkpatrick, A.: Multidimensional approach to the measurement of quality of life in lung cancer clinical trials. *In* The Quality of Life of Cancer Patients. Edited by N. K. Aaronson and J. Beckmann. New York, Raven Press, 1987, p. 63.
3. Andrykowski, M. A., and Redd, W. H.: Longitudinal analysis of the development of anticipatory nausea. J. Consult. Clin. Psychol., 55:36, 1987.
4. Bagenal, F. S., Easton, D. F., Harris, E., Chilvers, C. E. D., and McElwain, T. J.: Survival of patients with breast cancer attending Bristol Cancer Help Centre. Lancet, 336:606, 1990.
5. Bergner, M., Bobbitt, R. A., Carter, W. B., and Gilson, B. S.: The Sickness Impact Profile: Development and final revision of a health status measure. Med. Care, 19:787, 1981.
6. Bolund, C.: Suicide and cancer. I. Demographical and suicidological description of suicides among cancer patients in Sweden. J. Psychosoc. Oncol., 3:17, 1985.
7. Bolund, C.: Suicide and Cancer. II. Medical and care factors in suicide by cancer patients in Sweden, 1973–1976. J. Psychosoc. Oncol., 3:31, 1986.
8. Breitbart, W., and Holland, J. C.: Psychiatric aspects of cancer pain. *In* Advances in Pain Research and Therapy: Vol. 16. Proceedings of the Second International Congress on Cancer Pain. Edited by K. M. Foley, J. J. Bonica, V. Ventafridda. New York, Raven Press, 1990, p. 73.
9. Bukberg, J., Penman, D., and Holland, J. C.: Depression in hospitalized cancer patients. Psychosom. Med., 46:199, 1984.
10. Cassileth, B. R., and Brown, H.: Unorthodox cancer medicine. CA, 38:176, 1988.
11. Cella, D. F., Pratt, A., and Holland, J. C.: Persistent anticipatory nausea, vomiting, and anxiety in cured Hodgkin's disease patients after completion of chemotherapy. Am. J. Psychiatry, 143:641, 1986.
12. Cella, D. F., Orav, E. J., Kornblith, A. B., Holland, J. C., Silberfarb, P. M., Lee, K. W., Comis, R. L., Perry, M., Cooper, R., Maurer, L. H., Hoth, D. F., Perloff, M., Bloomfield, C. D., McIntyre, O. R., Leone, L., Lesnick, G., Nissen, N., Glicksman, A., Henderson, E., Barcos, M., Crichlow, R., Faulkner, II, C. S., Eaton, W., North, W., Schein, P. S. Chu, F., King, G., and Chahinian, A. P. (for the Cancer and Leukemia Group B): Socioeconomic status and cancer survival. J. Clin. Oncol., 9:1500, 1991.
13. Coates, A., Gebski, V., Bishop, J. F., Jeal, P. N., Woods, R. L., Snyder, R., Tattersall, M. H. N., Byrne, M., Harvey, V., Gill, G., Simpson, J., Drummond, R., Browne, J., van Cooten, R., and Forbes, J. F.: Improving the quality of life during chemotherapy for advanced breast cancer: A comparison of intermittent and continuous treatment strategies. N. Engl. J. Med., 317, 1490, 1987.
14. Conwell, Y., and Caine, E. D.: Rational suicide and the right to die: Reality and myth. N. Engl. J. Med., 325:1100, 1991.
15. Coyle, N., Loscalzo, M., and Bailey, L.: Supportive home care for the advanced cancer patient and family. *In* Handbook of Psychooncology: Psychological Care of the Patient with Cancer. Edited by J. C. Holland and J. H. Rowland. New York, Oxford University Press, 1989, p. 598.
16. de Haes, J. C. J. M., and van Knippenberg, F. C. E.: The quality of life of cancer pateints: A review of the literature. Soc. Sci. Med., 20:809, 1985.
17. de Haes, J. C. J. M., van Oostrom, M. A., and Welvaart, K.: Quality of life after breast cancer surgery. J. Surg. Oncol., 28:123, 1985.
18. Derogatis, L. R., and Lopez, M.: PAIS and PAIS-SR: Administration, scoring and procedures manual. I. Baltimore, Clinical Psychometric Research, 1983.
19. Derogatis, L. R., Morrow, G. R., Fetting, D., Penman, D., Piasetsky, S., Schmale, A. M., Henrichs, M., and Carnicke, C. L. M., Jr.: The prevalence of psychiatric disorders among cancer patients. J.A.M.A., 249:751, 1983.
20. Deyo, R. A., and Patrick, D. L.: Barriers to the use of health status measures in clinical investigation, patient care, and policy research. Med. Care, 27(Suppl.):S54, 1989.
21. Farber, D. M., Wienerman, B. H., and Kuypers, J. A.: Psychosocial distress in oncology outpatients. J. Psychosoc. Oncol., 2:109, 1984.
22. Fleishman, S. B., and Lesko, L. M.: Delirium and Dementia. *In* Handbook of Psychooncology: Psychological Care of the Patient with Cancer. Edited by J. C. Holland and J. H. Rowland. New York, Oxford University Press, 1989, p. 342.
23. Ganz, P. A., Haskell, C. M., Figlin, R. A., La Soto, N., and Siau, J.: Estimating the quality of life in a clinical trial of patients with metastatic lung cancer using the Karnofsky Performance Status and the Functional Living Index-Cancer. Cancer, 61:849, 1988.
24. Gelber, R. D., and Goldhirsch, A.: A new endpoint for the assessment of adjuvant therapy in postmenopausal women with operable breast cancer. J. Clin. Oncol., 4:1772, 1986.
25. Goldhirsch, A., Gelber, R. D., Simes, R. J., Glasziou, P., and Coates, A. S.: Costs and benefits of adjuvant therapy in breast cancer: A quality-adjusted survival analysis. J. Clin. Oncol., 7:36, 1989.
26. Gray, R. E., and Doan, B. D.: Heroic self-healing and cancer: Clinical issues for the health professions. J. Palliat. Care, 6:32, 1990.
27. Hamburg, D. A., and Adams, J. E.: A perspective on coping behavior: Seeking and utilizing information in major transitions. Arch. Gen. Psychiatry, 17:277, 1967.
28. Hietanen, P., and Lonnqvist, J. : Cancer and suicide. Ann. Oncol., 2:19, 1991.
29. Holland, J. C.: Historical overview. *In* Handbook of Psychooncology: Psychological Care of the Patient with Cancer. Edited by J. C. Holland and J. H. Rowland. New York, Oxford University Press, 1989, p. 3.
30. Holland, J. C., Geary, N., and Furman, A.: Alternative cancer therapies. *In* Handbook of Psychooncology: Psychological Care of the Patient with Cancer. Edited by J. C. Holland and J. H. Rowland. New York, Oxford University Press, 1989, p. 508.
31. Holland, J. C., Morrow, G. R., Schmale, A., Derogatis, L., Stefanek, M., Berenson, S., Carpenter, P. J., Breitbart, W., and Feldstein, M., A randomized clinical trial of alprazolam versus progressive muscle relaxation in cancer patients with anxiety and depressive symptoms. J. Clin. Oncol., 9:1004, 1991.
32. Holland, J. C., and Rowland, J. H. (Eds.): Handbook of Psychooncology: Psychological Care of the Patient with Cancer. New York, Oxford University Press, 1989.
33. House, J. S., Landis, K. R., and Umberson, D.: Social relationships and health. Science, 241:540, 1988.
34. Humphry, D.: Final Exit: The Practicalities of Self-Deliverance and Assisted Suicide for the Dying. Eugene, Oregon, The Hemlock Society, 1991.
35. Karnofsky, D. A., and Burchenal, J. H.: The clinical evaluation of chemotherapeutic agents in cancer. *In* Evaluation of Chemotherapeutic Agents. Edited by C. M. McLeod. New York, Columbia University Press, 1949, p. 191.
36. Kemeny, M. M., Wellisch, D. K., and Schain, W. S.: Psychosocial outcome in a randomized surgical trial for treatment of primary breast cancer. Cancer, 62:1231, 1988.
37. Kornblith, A. B., Anderson, J., Cella, D. F., Tross, S., Zuckerman, E., Cherin, E., Henderson, E. S., Weiss, R. B., Cooper, M. R., Silver, R. T., Leone, L., Canellos, G. P., Gottlieb, A., and Holland, J. C.: Quality of life assessment of Hodgkin's Disease survivors: A model for cooperative clinical trials. Oncology, 4:93, 1990.
38. Lederberg, M. S., Massie, M. J., and Holland, J. C.: Psychiatric consultation to oncology. *In* American Psychiatric Press Review of Psychiatry: Volume 9. Edited by A. Tasman, S. M. Goldfinger, and C. A. Kaufmann. Washington, D. C., American Psychiatric Press, 1990, p. 490.
39. Massie, M. J.: Anxiety, panic, and phobias. *In* Handbook of Psychooncology: Psychological Care of the Patient with Cancer. Edited by J. C. Holland and J. H. Rowland. New York, Oxford University Press, 1989, p. 302.
40. Massie, M. J., and Holland, J. C.: Overview of Normal Reactions and Prevalence of Psychiatric Disorders. *In* Handbook of Psychooncology: Psychological Care of the Patient with Cancer. Edited by J. C. Holland and J. H., Rowland. New York, Oxford University Press, 1989, p. 273.
41. Massie, M. J., and Holland, J. C.: Psychotherapeutic Interventions. *In* Handbook of Psychooncology: Psychological Care of the Patient with Cancer. Edited by J. C. Holland and J. H. Rowland. New York, Oxford University Press, 1989, p. 455.
42. Massie, M. J., Holland, J. C., and Glass, E.: Delirium in terminally ill cancer patients. Am. J. Psychiatry, 140:8, 1983.
43. Meadows, A., and Habbie, W.: The medical consequences of cure. Cancer, 58:524, 1986.
44. Mermelstein, H., and Holland, J. C.: Psychotherapy by telephone: A therapeutic tool for cancer patients. Psychosomatics, 32:407, 1991.
45. Morgenstern, H., Gellert, G. A., Walter, S. D., Ostfeld, A. M., and Seigel, B. S.: The impact of a psychosocial support program on survival with breast cancer: The importance of selection bias in program evaluation. J. Chronic Dis., 37:273, 1984.
46. Redd, W. H., Jacobsen, P. B., Die-Trill, M., Dermatis, H., McEvoy, M., and Holland, J. C.: Cognitive/attentional distraction in the control of conditioned nausea in pediatric oncology patients receiving chemotherapy. J. Consult. Clin. Psychol., 55:391, 1987.
47. Rowland, J. H.: Developmental Stage and Adaptation: Adult Model. *In* Handbook of Psychooncology: Psychological Care of the Pateint with Cancer. Edited by J. C. Holland and J. H. Rowland. New York, Oxford University Press, 1989, p. 25.
48. Rowland, J. H.: Intrapersonal resources: Coping. *In* Handbook of Psychooncology: Psychological Care of the Patient with Cancer. Edited by J. C. Holland and J. H. Rowland. New York, Oxford University Press, 1989, p. 44.
49. Schag, C. C., and Heinrich, R. L.: CARES: Cancer Rehabilitation Evaluation System. Los Angeles, Cares Consultants, 1988.
50. Schipper, H., Clinch, J., McMurray, A., and Levitt, M.: Measuring the quality of life of cancer patients: The Functional Living Index-Cancer. Development and validation. J. Clin. Oncol., 2:472, 1984.
51. Shimkin, M.: Contrary to Nature. NIH Pub. No. 76-7291977, Washington, D.C., U.S. Department of Health and Human Services. Public Health Service, 1977.
52. Speigel, D., Kraemer, H., Bloom, J. R., and Gottheil, D.: Effect of psychosocial treatment on survival of patients with metastatic breast cancer. Lancet, 2:888, 1989.
53. Spitzer, W. O., Dobson, A. J., Hall, J., Chesterman, E., Levi, J., Shepherd, R., Battista, R. N., and Catchlove, B. R.: Measuring the quality of life of cancer patients: A concise QL-index for use by physicians. J. Chronic Dis., 34:585, 1981.
54. Stefanek, M. E., Derogatis, L. P., and Shaw, A.: Psychological distress among oncology outpatients. Psychosomatics, 28:530, 1987.
55. Stewart, A. L., Hays, R. D., and Ware, J. E.: The MOS Short-form General Health Survey: Reliability and validity in a patient population. Med. Care, 26:724, 1988.
56. Sugarbaker, P. H., Barofsky, I., Rosenberg, S. A., and Gianola, F. J.: Quality of life assessment of patients in extremity sarcoma clinical trials. Surgery, 91:17, 1982.

57. Taylor, S. E., and Aspinwall, L. G.: Psychosocial aspects of chronic illness. *In* Psychological Aspects of Serious Illness: Chronic Conditions, Fatal Diseases, and Clinical Care. Edited by P. T. Costa, Jr. and G. R. VandenBos. Washington, D.C., American Psychological Association, 1990, p.7.

58. U. S. Congress, Office of Technology Assessment. Unconventional cancer treatments (OTA-H-405). Washington, D.C., U.S. Government Printing Office, 1990.

59. Watson, M. (Ed.): Cancer Patient Care: Psychosocial Treatment Methods. Cambridge, England, Cambridge University Press, 1991.

60. Wharton, J. C.: Traditions of folk medicine in America. J.A.M.A., 257:1632, 1987.

61. Zonderman, A. B., Costa, P. T., and McCrae, R. R.: Depression as a risk for cancer morbidity and mortality in a nationally representative sample. J.A.M.A., 262:1191, 1989.

XXI

Principles of Oncology Nursing

Ellyn Rackoff Bushkin

Introduction

A textbook covering cancer medicine would be incomplete without including a description of the principles and practice of oncology nursing. Understanding the scope of oncology nursing is fundamental to the effective practice of all the oncology specialty disciplines.

Oncology nursing is a unique and dynamic nursing specialty committed to: 1) the provision of optimal care to patients diagnosed with cancer; 2) professional practice that incorporates and integrates an indepth knowledge of the pathologic, physiologic and psychosocial dynamics associated with cancer; 3) collaborative practice with all members of the health care team, especially medical oncologists; 4) providing planned patient and family education, intervention, evaluation and follow-up related to the multimodality therapies for cancer; and 5) the enhancement of practice through research, continuing education and higher education.

Oncology Nursing as a Specialty

Nurses have historically provided care to patients with cancer, but the "War on Cancer" beginning in 1971 was a catalyst for the development of oncology nursing as a separate specialty. During the 1970s, the National Cancer Institute and the American Cancer Society developed several multi-media patient education programs to provide the public with information that would change their perception of the status of cancer related issues. The recognition of cancer as a major national health problem was one of the factors that led to the formal establishment of oncology nursing. Also, in the 1970s there was a major shift in the nursing profession toward more extended and expanded roles as a means to provide comprehensive and improved patient care.

The Oncology Nursing Society (ONS) was established by a small group of nurses, many of whom worked alongside medical oncologists. Their goals were to create a means to share information; to define their evolving role; to promote the advanced practice of the oncology nurse in all care settings; and to develop relevant national and local networking as well as continuing education programs. The success of this national and international organization, with a

1034

1992 membership of over 22,000, has largely been responsible for the recognition of oncology nursing as a valued specialty. The Oncology Nursing Society and the American Nurses' Association have developed Professional Practice Standards (Table XXI-1-1) and Advanced Practice Standards (Table XXI-1-2). These standards serve as a legal definition of the highest quality of oncology nursing practice.

Oncology nurses practice in a variety of settings which include acute care hospital settings, ambulatory care clinics, private medical oncologists' offices, home care agencies and community agencies. Areas of clinical practice include surgical oncology, radiation oncology, bone marrow transplantation, gynecologic oncology, pediatric oncology, and medical oncology, which includes chemotherapy and biologic response modifiers. Oncology nurses participate in cancer screening, teach cancer detection and prevention, and provide direct patient and family care. Advanced practice of oncology nursing includes participation as principal investigators in nursing research studies, serving as patient care consultants, designing educational curricula, and holding administrative positions. Nursing care is provided to patients and families through the utilization of the *nursing process*. The nursing process includes assessment and data collection, nursing diagnosis, planning, intervention and evaluation. This process allows for an organized and systematic approach to providing nursing care.

In 1980 The Oncology Nursing Certification Corporation provided the first oncology nursing certification examination. Certification in oncology nursing promotes continuing education and communicates to the public and professionals that the oncology nurse has the specialized knowledge and expertise to care for patients with cancer. Nurses who pass the certification examination may use the OCN (oncology certified nurse) credential with their signature. Recertification is done every four years by examination. Plans are underway to develop an advanced practice certification process.

Collaborative Practice with Medical Oncologists

Physicians and nurses have always worked together. What distinguishes the collaborative practice model is the rec-

Table XXI-1-1. Professional Practice Standards

Standard I. Theory

The oncology nurse applies theoretical concepts as a basis for decisions in practice.

Standard II. Data Collection

The oncology nurse systematically and continually collects data regarding the health status of the client. The data are recorded, accessible, and communicated to appropriate members of the multidisciplinary team.

Standard III. Nursing Diagnoses

The oncology nurse analyzes assessment data to formulate nursing diagnoses.

Standard IV. Planning

The oncology nurse develops an outcome-oriented care plan that is individualized and holistic. This plan is based on nursing diagnosis and incorporates preventive, therapeutic, rehabilitative, palliative, and comforting nursing actions.

Standard V. Intervention

The oncology nurse implements the nursing care plan to achieve the identified outcomes for the client.

Standard VI. Evaluation

The oncology nurse regularly and systematically evaluates the client's responses to interventions in order to determine progress toward achievement of outcomes and to revise the data base, nursing diagnoses, and the plan of care.

Standard VII. Professional Development

The oncology nurse assumes responsibility for professional development and continuing education and contributes to the professional growth of others.

Standard X. Ethics

The oncology nurse uses the code for nurses and a Patient's Bill of Rights as guides for ethical decision making in practice.

Standard XI. Research

The oncology nurse contributes to the scientific base of nurse practice and the field of oncology through the review and application of research.

Reprinted with permission from Standards of Oncology Nursing Practice. Kansas City, KS, American Nurses Association, 1987.

Table XXI-1-2. Professional Advanced Practice Standards

Standard I. Direct Caregiver Function

The advanced practice oncology nurse who functions as a direct caregiver provides, guides, directs, and evaluates the nursing practice delivered to clients with actual or potential diagnoses of cancer.

Standard II. Coordinator Function

The advanced practice oncology nurse who functions as a coordinator uses systems theory and the change process with the interdisciplinary oncology team to determine and achieve realistic health care goals for the client, the community, and/or the health care system.

Standard III. Consultant Function

The advanced practice oncology nurse who functions as a consultant provides expert knowledge about oncology to colleagues, health professionals, allied health personnel, health care consumers, and professional/public organizations.

Standard IV. Educator Function

The advanced practice oncology nurse who functions as an educator assesses the learning needs of the client, health professionals and/or the community and then designs, implements, and evaluates educational activities.

Standard V. Researcher Function

The advanced practice oncology nurse who functions as a researcher identifies current researchable problems in oncology nursing, tests relevant theories related to oncology nursing, collaborates in research, and evaluates and implements research findings that have an impact on cancer care and cancer nursing.

Standard VI. Administrator Function

The advanced practice oncology nurse who functions as an administrator uses management theory to create an environment that provides quality care to the client and/or the community and that promotes professional nursing practice.

Standard VII. Professional Development

The advanced practice oncology nurse assumes responsibility for individual professional development and continuing education and serves as a role model and mentor to other health professionals.

Standard VIII. Ethics

The advanced practice oncology nurse applies the American Nurses' Association "Code for Nurses" and the "Patient's Bill of Rights" to ethical decision making in cancer nursing practice.

Standard IX. Legal Issues

The advanced practice oncology nurse demonstrates knowledge of the legal issues in cancer nursing practice.

Standard X. Quality Assurance

The advanced practice oncology nurse monitors and evaluates oncology nursing practice to ensure that high quality care is provided to clients and/or the community.

Standard XI. Health Care Policy

The advanced practice oncology nurse demonstrates knowledge of the political process as a mechanism to address health care policy and issues to improve health care.

Reprinted with permission from Standards of Oncology Nursing Practice. Kansas City, KS, American Nurses Association, 1987.

ognition of two professional specialists working together to provide patient and family primary care. It is a successful and professionally satisfying method of delivering patient care and conducting clinical research. Many oncology nurses first worked as data collectors and managers for cancer research studies. As the medical specialty of oncology called for increasingly more complex single and multi-modality therapy, the collaborative role of nurse and physician became the most viable way to provide uniquely comprehensive patient care.

Joint practice with physicians has given nurses the opportunity to take on the role of patient and family care coordinator. Cancer patients are provided with expert assessment, teaching, counseling, communication methods, community referrals and meticulous follow-up.

therapies, concomitant medical illnesses, and general health status.

The nurse oncologist plays a unique role in the comprehensive coordination of these therapies. This coordination of care encompasses patient assessment, documentation of data in the patient's medical record, direct patient care, and patient education throughout therapy and during follow-up intervals. In addition the nurse can serve as the patient's first line of communication. Ideally, the patient and family should be able to contact the nurse oncologist by telephone during the entire treatment program, as well as have the nurse present for all physician–patient visits. Many patients travel a long distance for cancer therapy. This has enhanced the use and value of telephone communication between patient and nurse. The importance of the telephone must be underscored for it has the potential of providing continuous patient communication; review of therapy side effects; early recognition of emergencies; and emotional support and advisement.

An overview of oncology nursing care principles entails special aspects for oncologic disciplines related to their approaches to cancer therapies. The approach to the patient is the same. The experiences that the patient will encounter in the different oncologic specialties and the impact of multidisciplinary therapy require broad understanding of these events by the nurse oncologist. Nursing care is based on The Standards of Oncology Nursing Practice[2] and incorporates assessment, planning, nursing diagnosis, intervention, and evaluation. The nurse oncologist should refer to relevant chapters of this text, as well as other sources for additional information regarding approaches to caring for patients receiving cancer therapies.

Surgery

Surgery is the oldest and most frequently used treatment for cancer. Since a definitive diagnosis of cancer requires a biopsy specimen of some kind, most patients undergo some type of biopsy as a surgical procedure early in the course of cancer treatment. In addition to diagnosis, surgery has many other applications in the management of cancer.

Surgical procedures are performed for cancer prevention, primary tumor removal, disease staging, tumor debulking, hormomal ablation, disease palliation, and reconstruction. Surgical techniques are used to insert central venous access devices for the administration of cancer therapies.

Nursing Intervention. Nursing care of the patient undergoing surgery for cancer includes fostering the patient's understanding of the specific procedure and expected outcome, preparing the patient physically and psychologically for the surgery, reducing anxiety, supporting the patient's postoperative physiological stability, relieving pain, preventing complications and promoting compliance with postoperative instructions.

The psychological impact of cancer surgery must be emphasized. The patient and his/her family may experience a wide range of emotions and reactions to the diagnosis of cancer and the need for surgery. The nurse must assess the patient's understanding of possible surgical outcomes such as change or loss of body function, limitations of mobility, and change in physical appearance as these factors may

apply to some types of cancer surgery. Based on patient assessment data care is planned to promote the patient's understanding of the surgical procedure and its outcome. The nurse prepares the patient physically for surgery, monitors the patient's return to physiological stability, monitors for surgical complications, and ensures compliance with postoperative instructions.

Patient Teaching. Patient teaching should include a discussion of the type and purpose of the surgical procedure. Such efforts should be coordinated with the surgeon so that the patient is presented with complete and consistent information and instructions. The nurse oncologist reinforces and interprets medical/surgical information to the patient and family; defines common surgical terms and discusses possible physical outcomes, such as dressing placement, loss of body function, and change in body appearance; describes postoperative devices that may be placed during the surgery such as a chest tube, nasogastric tube or central venous catheter; explains routine preoperative and postoperative procedures and schedules, and reviews deep breathing and coughing exercises.

Intervention should include early discharge planning and provision for home care if indicated. Referrals to appropriate professionals, and community support services should be considered. Other professional referrals would include clinical nurse specialists, social workers, physical and occupational therapists as indicated.

Radiation

Radiation therapy utilizes the effects of x-ray photons and gamma rays which ionize water and other compounds to damage and kill cancer cells. The radiant energy absorbed results in the release of electrons from atomic orbits, causing that atom to become ionized; and the ion can cause damage to cellular DNA and damage to the cell membrane. X-rays are generated when electrons hit a metallic target at high speed; the greater the energy (higher the speed) the higher the voltage of the x-ray emitted. Most x-rays are now delivered by linear accelerators which increase the energy of electrons by propelling them magnetically. Typical x-ray voltages of linear accelerators vary from 4 million to 20 million electron volts (MeV).

Radiation may also be delivered as atomic particles, of which only electrons have reached widespread clinical use. Electrons can also be delivered by linear accelerators. They do not have the same penetrance, but cause greater ionization when they collide with an atom. The nature of a chemical element is determined by the number of charged particles (protons) in its nucleus. The nucleus also contains uncharged particles (neutrons) that do not determine the chemical nature of the atom. Particles with the same number of protons may contain varying numbers of neutrons, thus providing several species of the same element which have different weights, called isotopes. Some of the isotopes are unstable, spontaneously decaying, with the liberation of radiant energy, and are known as radioisotopes. The half-life is a measurement of the time it takes for the unstable isotope to lose 50% of its radioactive activity. This can vary from microseconds as in a nuclear explosion to several days to thousands of years (as for radioactive carbon) depending on the element. Cobalt 60 is an unstable isotope that emits gamma rays with a mean energy equivalent to 1–2 MeV.

The amount of radiation that is delivered to tissues was measured as the radiation absorbed dose, known as the *rad*. Radiation is now denominated in grays (Gy) in honor of a British radiation scientist. It is common to think of one hundredth units, centigrays (cGy), which are equivalent to rads. Teletherapy is radiation therapy that is administered externally from a radiation machine. Radiation can also be delivered by brachytherapy, which involves implanting a radioactive isotope into or adjacent to tumors. The radioactive isotope is either sealed or unsealed. Sealed isotopes such as radium, iridium, and cesium are contained in tubes, needles, capsules, wires, or seeds. The sealed radioisotope is then placed in the affected tissue, such as needles in the tongue, a tube or capsule in the endocervical canal, or wires in the breast. These are all removable. Seeds may be placed in the depths of a dissection for carcinoma or sarcoma and remain permanently.

Unsealed isotopes are contained in solution, and enter into the metabolic pathway of the tumor to be treated, such as radioactive iodine for thyroid cancer or radioactive phosphorus for polythemia vera. The risk of spillage and contamination from isotopes in solution is high. Intracavitary colloidal suspensions of isotopes in the pleura or peritoneum are rarely used anymore.

Brachytherapy can deliver very intensive local therapy, and is usually used in a combined program with teletherapy to ensure homogeneous radiation to the entire tumor area by the implant, and to the nearby tissues that may not need the same intensity. During brachytherapy the process of afterloading refers to first placing the containers within the tissues to allow roentgenographic confirmation of proper arrangement, and to avoid personal exposure before inserting the radioactive material into the containers. Afterloading requires that the needles or tubes be placed into the treatment area and tunneled out of the skin. The procedure is done under local or general anesthesia in the operating room. The radioactive isotope or pellet or wire is later inserted into the tubes in the patient's hospital room. The patient requires a separate room during the time a gamma radiation source is in use, and staff and visitors must maintain suitable radiation precautions, particularly distance from the source. The radioactive implant may remain in place for several days. In some cases, if removal of the isotope would be difficult and the half life of the isotope is short, the implant will remain permanently.

Safety Precautions. The Nuclear Regulatory Commission has developed guidelines for occupational exposure to radiation which are of concern to all health professionals, and particularly to oncology nurses and others working in radiation oncology. Every hospital must have a radiation safety officer who is responsible for ensuring compliance with federal and state standards. Hospital personnel who care for patients receiving radiation are given special dosimetry badges to wear on their clothing which contain film that measures radiation exposure. The badges are systematically measured, and a permanent record of radiation exposure is kept for all personnel. Federal regulations stipulate the maximum permissible annual radiation exposure.

Radiation precautions must be followed when caring for a patient with a radioactive implant. Radiation safety is based on three important factors: time, distance and shielding.

Actual time spent in the patient's room is minimized and limited to a total of 30 minutes per eight hours. The amount of radiation exposure decreases by the inverse square of the distance from the source. Working twice as far from the radiation source reduces the amount of radiation to one-fourth. Thus it is important to maintain maximum physical distance from the patient whenever possible. Lead shielding provides additional protection, although lead shields and aprons have significant disadvantages. They are cumbersome to use and may actually induce a nurse to remain in the room for longer time periods. The nurse should consistently adhere to principles of time and distance while caring for the patient. Patient self care must be encouraged and all procedures and necessary precautions explained.

Nursing Care. Nursing care of the patient receiving teletherapy or brachytherapy focuses on preparing the patient physically and psychologically for the therapy; assessing the patient's understanding of the therapy and the disease; allaying anxiety related to the treatment procedure, reviewing the acute and late side effects that may be experienced; and ensuring the patient's compliance with instructions and treatment schedules.

Care for Teletherapy is planned to: 1) promote patient understanding of radiation administration procedure; 2) reassure patients that although they will be alone in a room while the radiation is administered that they will be seen and heard by the radiation technician at all times; 3) explain that during the administration they must lie still on the radiation machine table and that they will not feel the radiation administration; 4) instruct patient not to remove skin marking that designate the treatment port; 5) encourage symptom reporting; and 6) provide relief from treatment side effects.

Care for Brachytherapy is planned to: 1) promote patient understanding of radiation procedure; 2) promote patient understanding of necessary radiation precautions; 3) promote self care; 4) encourage symptom reporting, and 5) provide relief from treatment side effects. The nurse should implement measures to provide comfort by encouraging change of positions in bed; providing an alternating pressure mattress, and supporting body parts with pillows. The nurse should encourage patient communication and suggest diversionary activities such as reading, watching television, listening to music and/or relaxation exercises. The nurse should assess the patient for complaints of muscle aches and pain at the implant site and if indicated obtain a physician's order for muscle relaxants and analgesics. The nurse should explain principles of time, distance and shield to the patient, family, visitors, and other hospital staff. For receiving unsealed isotopes special precautions will be required for the disposal of body wastes and removal of linen and equipment.

Side Effects of Radiation Therapy. During radiation therapy, cells of normal tissue are subjected to the ionizing beams. Any tissue near the radiation port can be damaged. The side effects of treatment are related to the impact of radiation on normal tissue. Some side effects are acute and temporary, while other side effects develop over time and may be irreversible.

Skin. External radiation must pass through the skin to reach the tumor target. The use of megavoltage therapy has decreased the amount and severity of skin reactions because the high energy photons can penetrate without regard to the minor changes in density of the different tissues. The most common skin effect is a change in skin color within the radiation port. The skin may appear to be reddened or tanned. Reddening of skin color (erythema) is caused by dermal capillary engorgement. The erythema may cause varying degrees of itching sensations over the area. A tanning reaction is caused by increased production of pigment. Dry desquamation, which is flaking of the skin, is caused by the accumulation of dead skin cells. In cases where the basal cells of the skin are also destroyed, the dermal level is exposed which results in the leakage of serum, called moist desquamation. Skin reactions are usually temporary. In cases of severe skin reaction however, long term late effects can include scarring, changes in skin texture, and telangiectasis, dilatation of small skin venules. Necrosis, the death of skin requiring skin graft is extremely rare and suggests improper technique. Radiation recall is a delayed skin side effect in which the skin of the radiation port becomes irritated after the patient receives certain chemotherapy drugs. The skin can become erythematous and hyperpigmented. Depending on the severity of the recall reaction, vesicles and wet desquamation can develop.

Nursing Care. Patients should be informed of the possible skin side effects of radiation therapy. The nurse should observe the radiation sites for changes in color, presence of dry or moist desquamation and should assess patient symptoms. The nurse should explain the cause of the skin reactions and offer suggestions and interventions to alleviate and control these side effects.

Nursing care is planned to: 1) promote the patient's understanding of the possible skin toxicities that may result from radiation therapy and the interventions required; 2) prevent, alleviate and limit the impairment to the integrity of the skin by teaching, and demonstrating appropriate interventions; 3) promoting comfort from the skin effects of radiation therapy; and 4) patient teaching includes the following: instructing the patient to wear loosely fitting cotton clothing; gently washing the area with a mild soap and pat dry; avoiding the use of lotion, perfumes, or deodorants; avoiding pressure to the irritated area; avoiding sun exposure, swimming in salt or chlorinated water; using only water based lubricants for dry desquamation; cautioning against the application of hot and cold to irritated areas of the skin; using cool moist compresses for itching; removing water soluble emollients before treatment; using oral antihistamines and topical antipruritic lotions if prescribed by the physician; keeping moist desquamation clean, dry and exposed to air without dressings, keeping the involved area clean and *frequently* changing non-adhering, dry, dressings.

Signs and symptoms of infection to be reported promptly to caregivers: 1) elevation in body temperature; 2) severe fatigue; or 3) purulent skin drainage. Handwashing techniques must be emphasized, including keeping fingernails clean and short.

Oral hydration and good nutrition are particularly important during moist desquamation because of added losses. Hydrotherapy and/or wound debridement may be prescribed by the radiation oncologist.

Mucositis/Stomatitis. The rapidly growing cells of the mucous membrane provide a protective lining of cells in the oral cavity and genital tract. Injury to these cells can cause inflammation of the mucous membrane and underlying exposed tissues known as mucositis. In the mouth this is specifically called stomatitis and in the genital tract vulvovaginitis. Whereas mild stomatitis may be transient and easily managed, severe stomatitis can cause oral pain, infection, and can further complicate the nutritional and hydration status of the patient. Injury to the salivary glands can cause a decreased production of saliva resulting in a condition known as xerostomia or mouth dryness. Saliva is important for lubricating and cleansing the oral cavity; diluting food; and keeping an alkaline environment which limits bacterial build-up. Salivary secretions may become thick and difficult to expectorate. Teeth can be indirectly affected by radiation as a result of periodontal membrane damage and the presence of less saliva of different composition which allows for a change in the type and number of oral bacteria.

Hypogeusesthesia is the term used to describe an alteration or loss of taste sensation; this can be related to the effect of radiation on the patient's taste buds. Dysgeusia is the term used to describe the presence of unpleasant tastes, sometimes described as metallic; ageusia is the absence of taste sensation. The oral toxicities of radiation therapy can potentially undermine the hydration and nutritional status of the patient.

Nursing Care. A dental evaluation should be done first when radiation will encompass the oropharyneal region.

Stomatitis: Before the initiation of radiation therapy, the nurse should encourage oral hygiene measures after meals and before sleep. These measures include the use of a soft toothbrush and nonabrasive toothpaste, frequent oral rinsing with water, saline solution, or a nonalcohol-oral care preparation, among others an elixir of a 1:16 solution of diphenhydramine (benadryl) and water. Daily oral self examination should be taught with report of changes in oral status to the health care provider. The nurse should encourage fluid intake and discourage smoking.

If stomatitis occurs the patient should be instructed: 1) in the maintenance of nutrition with frequent liquid high caloric drinks or blenderized foods; 2) avoidance of acids such as citrus juices or vinegar; 3) avoidance of retaining food residues in the mouth; 4) the use of alkaline anesthetic mouthwashes after each and every feeding (a mixture of bicarbonate, diphenhydramine and lidocaine is helpful); and 5) realistic dialog with the physician about presciptions of analgesics, up to and including narcotic drugs for the duration of painful stomatitis. If hydration or nutrition become deficient, or pain control inadequate, the nurse oncologist must be certain these problems are appropriately addressed by the radiation oncologist.

Xerostomia: The nurse oncologist should encourage oral hygiene measures and frequent rinsing with water. Commercially available artificial saliva and lip lubricants may provide temporary relief. The patient should be instructed to avoid the use of commercial mouthwash products that contain drying agents such as alcohol. Mouth breathing should be discouraged. Encourage a fluid intake of at least 3,000 ml/day if fluid overload is not a problem. Sour hard candies can be helpful in stimulating saliva production and providing oral lubrication and creating a pleasant taste.

Thick Oral Secretions: The oncology nurse should encourage oral hygiene measures and the frequent rinsing with water or saline solution. The patient should be taught to remove thick mucus with a swab, and to use an oral gavage bag to irrigate the mouth. In severe cases oral suction equipment may be required.

Alopecia. Hair follicles are damaged or destroyed by radiation, and patients receiving radiation to the head will experience hair loss. Hair loss may be temporary or permanent depending on the amount of radiation received. Patient teaching related to alopecia is discussed below under chemotherapy. Long term, and for patients treated at high doses, delayed side effects include brain cell necrosis and infarction due to vascular injury.

Chest Radiation. Primary or metastatic lung tumors can be treated with radiation therapy. Side effects include esophagitis, pneumonitis, and as a delayed side effect, pulmonary fibrosis. The epithelium of the lungs, trachea, and esophagus can be affected by radiation resulting in inflammation, infection, and obstruction due to narrowing of these structures.

Patients receiving chest radiation may experience symptoms related to the radiation therapy concomitantly with symptoms from the disease process. Patients may require complex care based on their individual physical status. Esophagitis is an inflammation from the radiation which can result in difficulty swallowing, severe upper chest pain, and superinfection, often with candida. Esophagitis potentially compromises the patient's nutritional and hydration status.

Nursing care for the patient receiving radiation therapy to the chest and back will be planned to alleviate and limit the side effects of chest radiation through the following interventions: 1) teaching patient and family the signs and symptoms of side effects—sore throat, dyspnea, dry cough, dysphagia, hemoptysis and elevated body temperature; 2) teaching measures to conserve physical energy, and the rationale for maintaining hydration and nutrition; and 3) promoting comfort for esophagitis by suggesting a diet that includes protein and high calories for tissue repair, liquid dairy products and blenderized foods, foods served at room temperature, and avoidance of irritation from spices or mechanical trauma such as toast. For patients experiencing toxicity from chest radiation, the nurse oncologist should monitor patient status throughout therapy including the need for supplemental oxygen, the need for cough suppressant, analgesics, and nutritional supplements. Since corticosteroids, antifungal agents and other antibiotics may be indicated, the nurse oncologist must relate his or her evaluation to the radiation or medical oncologist on a timely basis.

Abdominal Radiation. Radiation can damage the rapidly growing cells of the gastrointestinal tract. When the upper abdomen receives radiation the patient may experience nausea and vomiting. This is the result of physical injury to the cells that comprise the lining of the stomach leading to irritation and inflammation. When the lower gastrointestinal tract

receives radiation, the patient may experience diarrhea and abdominal cramping. The nursing care for gastrointestinal tract side effects is similar to care for the side effects caused by chemotherapy. The principles of nursing care will be discussed below in the chemotherapy section.

Pelvic Radiation. Cancers of the cervix, endometrium, prostate, bladder, and rectum are often treated with external radiation therapy and sometimes by internal implants. Patients may experience side effects that include: diarrhea, cystitis, vaginitis, and late mucosal atrophy and sometimes stenosis. Sexual dysfunction can result from effects on the gonads, and the prostate and other male secretory glands or the vagina and female secretory glands.

Sexual Dysfunction. Radiation to the pelvis by external beam or internal implant technique can cause narrowing of the walls of the vagina, decreased vaginal secretion during sexual arousal, and inflammation and scarring of the vaginal tissues. Patients should be informed of these possible side effects and shown how to use a vaginal dilator and/or encouraged to continue sexual intercourse as a means of keeping the vaginal walls open and flexible. Artificial lubrication can be provided through the use of commercially available creams and lubricants.

Ovarian function can be totally eradicated when high levels of radiation are given to the ovaries. Radiation to the pelvis may result in premature menopause and decrease in libido. When possible, the reproductive organs are shielded from radiation. Patients must be informed of the possibility of temporary or permanent sterility. Radiation to the pelvis and gonads can result in partial and permanent sterility in males and they should be advised about the availability of sperm banks. Radiation to the prostate often diminishes potency and sexual performance. Sexual function is often altered in both sexes by fatigue and weakness during actual therapy, along with the multiple physical and psychological effects of the disease and side effects of therapy. Sexual dysfunction may persist.

Hemopoietic System. Radiation can suppress the production of blood cell precursors in the bone marrow causing anemia, leukopenia, and thrombocytopenia. Radiation to large areas of the body over bony structures such as the pelvis are most likely to produce bone marrow suppression. The patient's blood count should be monitored during the treatment course and through follow-up care. The nursing intervention required for bone marrow suppression will be discussed in Table XXI-1-5.

Chemotherapy

The use of drugs to kill cancer cells has an origin in chemical warfare. After World War I, scientists noted the bone marrow suppression effects of soldiers exposed to sulfur mustard gas. The effects of the chemical led to the hypothesis that the chemical was able to destroy rapidly growing cells. During the 1950s several drugs of the nitrogen mustard class under investigation during World War II were successfully used to shrink lymphatic tumors. Subsequently, other drugs were discovered and tested. By the 1980s chemotherapy was considered the major intervention to cure several kinds of metastatic tumors, particularly in children, and to benefit many other types of cancer. The federal government set up an organized system to evaluate new chemotherapy drugs under the National Institutes of Health at the National Cancer Institute. The National Cancer Institute is responsible for overseeing all federally sponsored clinical trials of cancer treatments, including chemotherapy.

Chemotherapy drugs are cytotoxic because they have the ability to disrupt the development and reproduction of cells. A major factor in the use of chemotherapy is the effect of the drugs on normal tissue. The multiple side effects of chemotherapy range from minor patient discomfort to life-threatening occurrences. This treatment modality has become exceedingly complex as new drugs are developed and new combinations of drugs are formulated and tested. Over 40 different chemotherapy agents are approved by the Food and Drug Administration and used to treat cancer. One or several drugs may be prescribed depending on the tumor type and stage, previous treatment course, and physical status of the patient.

Chemotherapy can be combined with the other cancer treatment modalities of radiation, surgery, or biotherapy. Chemotherapy is often used before surgery to shrink large tumors and to inhibit the microscopic spread of tumor cells. Chemotherapy is used after the surgical removal of a tumor to eliminate any microscopic spread of tumor cells. This method of chemotherapy, called adjuvant therapy, has been successfully used in the post-surgical treatment of breast, colon, lung, ovarian, testicular, and bone tumors, and in several types of childhood cancer. Chemotherapy is used in patients with clinically metastatic cancer to reduce tumor size and symptoms, and to extend useful life. The treatment goals of chemotherapy can be the cure, control, or palliation of cancer.

In order to participate in the administration, monitoring, and evaluation of chemotherapy, the nurse oncologist must understand the nature of the drugs being used. The mechanism of cell killing, the nature of the drug's interaction with the cell cycle, with target molecules and with cellular receptors all add to the nurse oncologist's appreciation of what the particular chemotherapeutic regimen is doing. These topics are covered in depth elsewhere is this text.

Combination Chemotherapy. Using more than one type of chemotherapy to treat malignant tumors is based on years of research and an increased understanding of growth, repair, and reproduction of the cancer cell. By combining drugs of different classes there is an increased chance of being effective at varying times in the cell reproduction cycle. In some instances the dosage required to kill cancer cells by a single drug would be too high to be tolerated, but combination of that drug with other active drugs would allow for the administration of lesser doses with better effects. Drugs with varying side effects can be used together. Resistance to a single drug may develop after repeated exposure, often by improved cellular repair of the injury the drug causes. Varying combinations of drugs allow independent injuries and significantly lower the chance that the cell can be resistant simultaneously to two or more agents.

Biologic Therapy

Biologic therapy is defined as treatment with chemical or biologic agents which are intended to alter the immune response of the patient to the tumor. Advances in biologic therapy are discussed in other chapters of this textbook. This approach to treatment of cancerous cells is under investigation and is predicated on the assumption that tumor characteristics can be changed (as by interferon) or that certain aspects of the immune response can be enhanced (as by levamisole or interleukin 2) as a means of recognizing and destroying or inactivating tumor cells. Biologic therapies may be primarily aimed at reconstituting normal host functions, such as granulocyte maturation and delivery.

Biologic therapy includes interferons, interleukins, vaccines, and colony stimulating factors. Biologic therapy is often used in conjunction with other forms of cancer therapies such as chemotherapy, radiotherapy and surgery.

Side Effects—Biologic Therapy. The side effects that patients experience from biologic therapy vary depending upon the type and mode of administration. Intradermal, subcutaneous, and intralesional vaccines can cause localized skin inflammation and systemic side effects of elevated body temperature, chills, diaphoresis, and fatigue. Intravenous administration of immunomodulators have a wider range of systemic side effects including fever, chills, diaphoresis, fluid retention, dyspnea, nausea, vomiting, and fatigue. Other serious disorders of organ function may be detected by chemical tests. Patients receiving investigational forms of biologic therapy are closely monitored for unknown side effects and adverse systemic reactions.

A detailed description of the current indications for chemotherapy and biotherapy can be found in several chapters of this text.

Dosage and Time Scheduling

The amount of chemotherapy and or biotherapy that is prescribed for a patient will be based on several factors including: the type of tumor to be treated; the patient's past chemotherapy and radiation therapy history; bone marrow, kidney, liver, heart, and lung function; age, weight, physical and functional status; and concomitant medical illnesses.

The dosage of most chemotherapy and or biotherapy agents is determined with relationship to the total body surface area. The patient's body surface area can be approximated in square meters (m^2) as a function of the patient's height and weight, and this can be conveniently read off a nomogram (Figure XXI-1-1). For example, if the dosage of doxorubicin is 30 mg per square meter of body surface area and the patient is 1.6 m^2, read from the nomogram based on height and weight measurements, the dose of the drug will be (30 mg/m^2 × 1.6 m^2 = 48 mg).

Treatment Schedules

Cancer therapies are administered in time intervals that allow for drug effectiveness and recovery from side effects. For example, a treatment cycle may be repeated every 21 days, or every 28 days dependent on recovery times. Other time intervals are possible. Patients are monitored at appropriate intervals throughout the cycle sometimes by phone, to determine drug side effects and toxicities. The duration of treatment prescribed will be based on tumor type, tumor response, and toxicities, along with other factors.

Continuous intravenous infusions of chemotherapy over

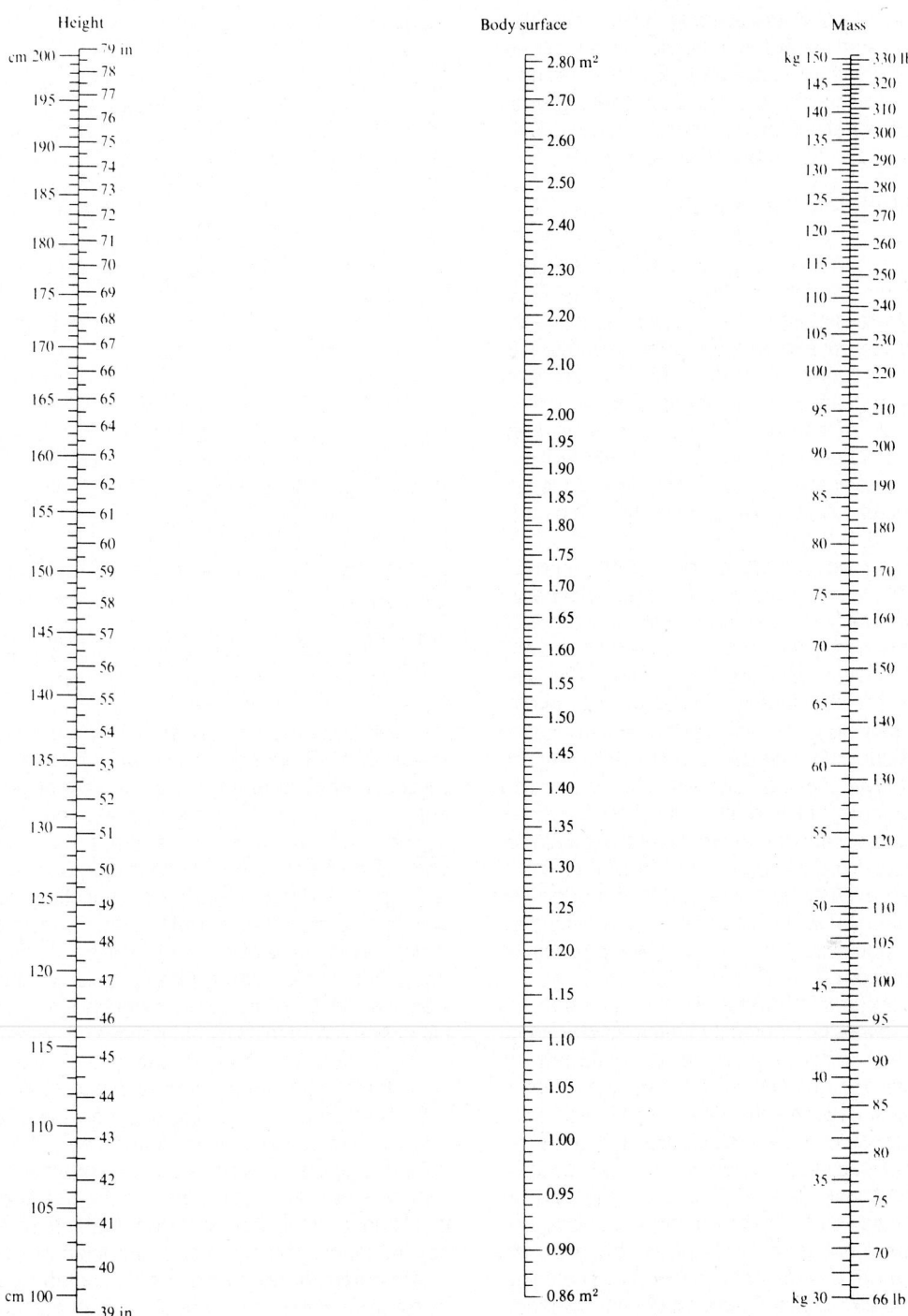

Figure XXI-1-1. Nomogram for determination of body surface from height and mass. From the formula of Du Bois and Du Bois, Arch. Inter. Med. *17*:863, 1916: $S = M^{0.725} \times H^{0.725} \times 71.84$, or $\log S = M \times 0.425 + \log H \times 0.725 + 1.8564$ (*S*: body surface i cm², *M*: mass in kg, *H*: height in cm).

several hours, days, or weeks, is based on the observations that for several neoplasms, and some drugs, constant exposure of the tumor to small amounts of drugs is effective and less toxic to normal tissues than high intermittent doses. Continuous infusions of chemotherapy may also be administered intraarterially, as into the hepatic artery.

Chemotherapy and Biologic Agent Administration

Oncology nurses have taken a primary role in the safe administration of chemotherapy and biologic response modifiers. Nurses are qualified to administer these therapies after receiving appropriate educational preparation according to the policies and procedures of the individual health care facility. Continuing education on an ongoing basis is recommended in order to maintain current knowledge and expertise related to cancer therapies, their administration, and the implications for patient care. The nurse oncologist must demonstrate meticulous patient assessment, monitoring, documentation, and evaluation skills.

Chemotherapy can be given topically, orally, intravenously, intramuscularly, subcutaneously, intraperitoneally, intrathecally, intraarterially, intravesically, and intrapleurally. Nurses are often responsible for all but the last four routes, and particularly for the administration of oral and intravenous chemotherapy. Several of the chemotherapeutic agents known as vesicants may be seriously irritating to the patient's veins and surrounding tissues. These agents, when administered through a peripheral vein must be closely monitored for tissue infiltration. Recommendations for treatment of tissue infiltration of chemotherapy vary, but the major actions that are universally accepted include: stopping the intravenous infusion; elevating the extremity; and in most cases, applying ice to the skin infiltrate. The Oncology Nursing Society has also distributed suggestions for the treatment of chemotherapy tissue infiltrations.[38]

The problem of tissue infiltration and vein damage from chemotherapy led to the development of alternative venous access devices (VAD). Venous access devices include several versions of the central venous catheter, and several versions of the implantable venous port. (see Figures XXI-1-2 and 3). Infusion pumps, both stationary and portable (see Figure XXI-1-4) can be connected to venous access devices for the continuous administration of chemotherapy.

A central venous catheter may be inserted into the subclavian vein through a trochar on a temporary basis, or on a semipermanent basis be surgically placed. The catheter tip is advanced into the superior vena cava near the right atrium. The tube is tunneled under the skin of the chest and exits with an external catheter that is anchored to the skin (see Figure XXI-1-2). The catheter has a fibrous (Velcro R) cuff to stimulate fibroblastic ingrowth to block bacterial entry alongside the tube. The external catheter can be used to obtain blood specimens, administer chemotherapy or other intravenous medications, blood and blood products, and if it has a double lumen, parenteral nutrition, which requires a specific lumen which is not subject to contamination from frequent manipulation.

Nursing Care of Central Venous Catheters. Nursing care focuses on explaining the function, and placement and

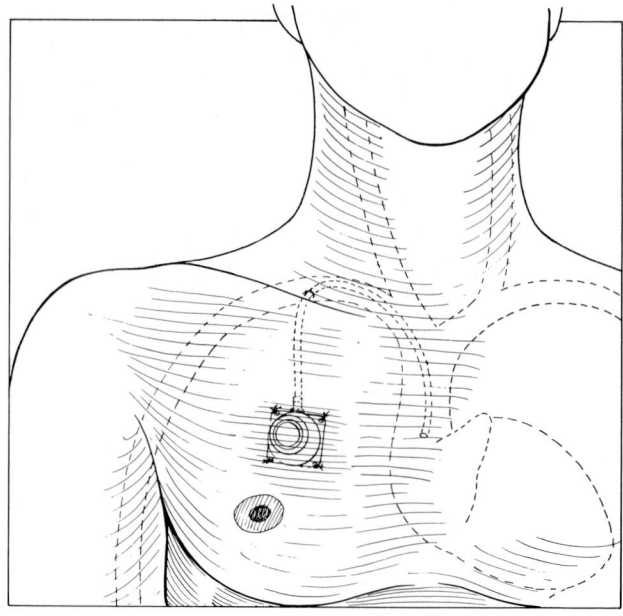

© 1990 Pharmacia Deltec Inc., St. Paul, MN

Figure XXI-1-2. Anatomical sketch of implantable central venous access system. Courtesy of Pharmacia Deltec Inc., St. Paul, MN.

teaching the care of the catheter. Care includes periodic instillation of a heparinized solution to maintain the catheter's patency, dressing changes over the entrance and exit sites, and inspection of the incision sites. Although institutional protocols of care differ, in general the patient is taught to change the dressing daily for the first two weeks, using sterile technique, and then twice weekly until healed. The catheter is anchored onto the skin with tape. Patients are instructed to observe the incision sites for swelling, erythema and drainage. Patients are further instructed how to instill a heparinized flush solution into the catheter on a precise time schedule according to institutional policy.

The nurse explains and demonstrates aseptic technique, sterile dressing changes, site inspection, and the method to flush the catheter. Occasional patients are taught to self-administer medication. In addition the nurse provides the patient and family with written instructions, encourages symptom reporting, and indicates the symptoms or findings that require immediate attention. Patients must understand how to contact the nurse and physician in an emergency.

Implanted Venous Port. An implanted venous port provides a reservoir and central venous catheter without an external catheter. A metallic chamber with a plastic resealing port is implanted under the skin. Dressing changes and frequent heparinization are not required. The port is flushed with a heparin solution by the nurse after treatment, or monthly. Patients can be taught to access the port for self administration of medications and heparinization. The risk of infection is reduced significantly by the implanted venous port. The risk of inadvertent injection of vesicant drugs into the tissue is, however, increased over exteriorized catheters, but much less than by intravenous injection.

The Ommaya reservoir is a subcutaneous port that is implanted under the scalp over a small surgical hole in the

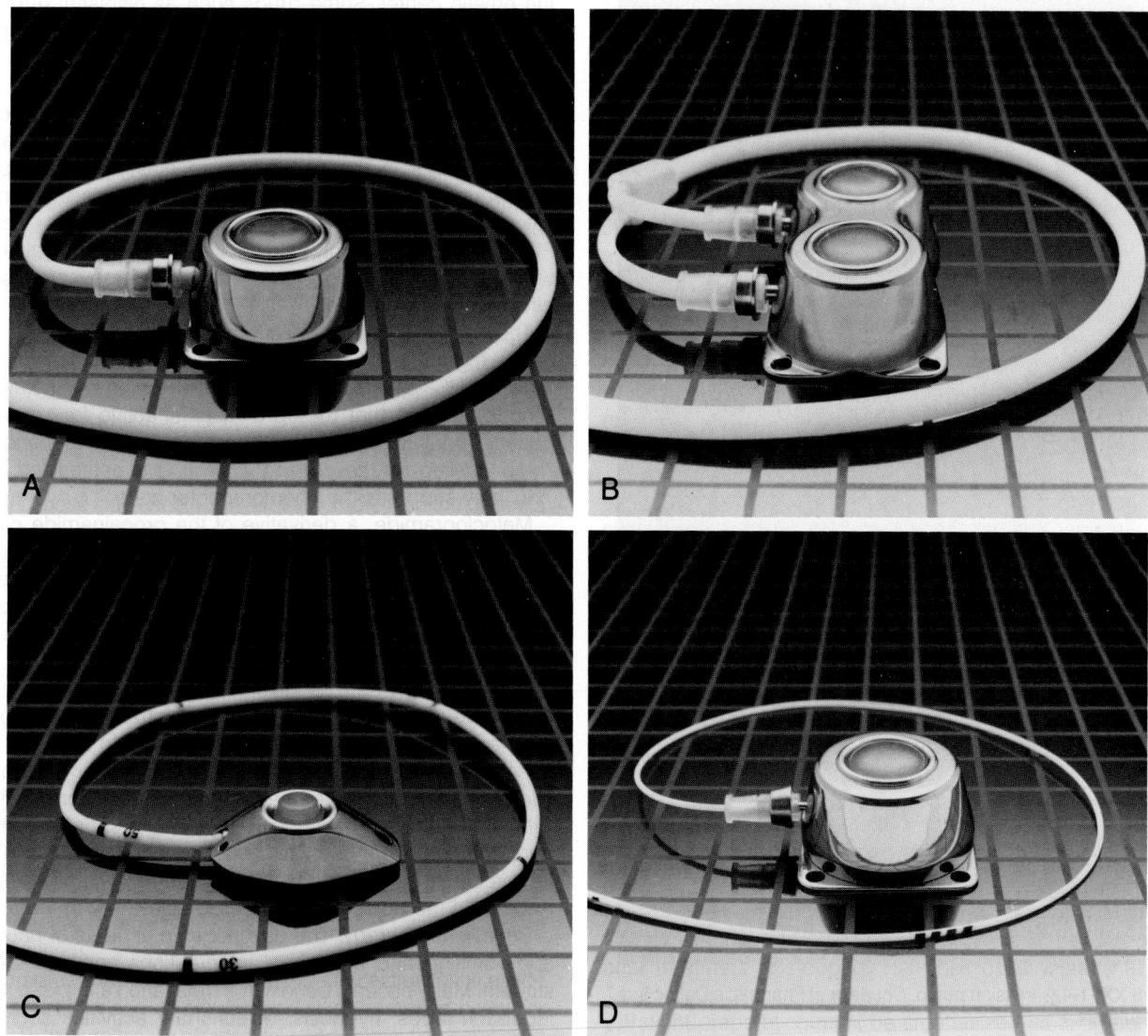

Figure XXI-1-3. Implantable access systems. A. Single lumen central venous (PORT-A-CATH^R). B. Double lumen central venous. C. Peripheral venous (P.A.S. PORT^R). D. Epidural. Courtesy of Pharmacia Deltec Inc., St. Paul, MN.

skull which allows the reservoir which is attached to a catheter to be threaded into the lateral ventricle for the administration of chemotherapy into the cerebrospinal fluid.

Catheters can also be placed intraarterially and intraperitoneally for the administration of chemotherapy. Intraarterial catheters are used when chemotherapy is to be delivered directly into an organ such as the liver. Intraperitoneal catheters are used to bathe the peritoneum with chemotherapy. Chemotherapy can also be instilled into the pleural cavity via an intrapleural catheter.

Infusion Pumps. Continuous intravenous administration of chemotherapy can be given over time intervals that span several hours to several weeks. To provide continuous infusion therapy, specialized pumps have been developed. Some of the pumps are portable and can be attached to a waist belt. The patient can be fully ambulatory and active while receiving continuous chemotherapy. The pump is filled with a solution containing the chemotherapeutic agent and attached to a central venous line. Some pumps are implanted under the skin and externally filled with chemotherapy. The pumps can be programmed to deliver small amounts of drug continuously over a given time period. More sophisticated pumps can deliver several drugs at variable rates in different time periods.

Safe Handling of Chemotherapy. The cytotoxic nature of chemotherapy agents requires that personnel who prepare and administer the drugs take precautions to protect themselves from contact with or inhalation of these agents. Protective gloves, gowns and masks are worn to guard against accidental skin contact and airborne droplets. In areas where large volumes of chemotherapy are prepared, a biologic vertical laminar air flow hood now is standard. Table XXI-1-4 describes precautions for preparation and administration and disposal of chemotherapy agents.[35]

controversial on the basis that reducing chemotherapy distribution to the scalp could theoretically create a safe area for cancer cells. Scalp hypothermia is contraindicated in cancers that are known to spread to the brain and soft tissues of the scalp. Furthermore, scalp hypothermia is relatively ineffective for high dose combination chemotherapy.

Hematologic Toxicities. The action of chemotherapy can directly affect the blood producing mechanism. Blood components (red blood cells, white blood cells and platelets) are continually being made by the rapidly growing cells of the bone marrow. The cytotoxic action of chemotherapy inhibits this production. A decrease in red blood cells (erythrocytes) causes anemia and may, if severe enough diminish oxygen transport to the tissues. White blood cells (leukocytes) are an integral component of the immune system. A decrease in the production of leukocytes reduces the system's ability to recognize and defend against foreign microorganisms, leading to increased susceptibility to infection. Platelets are blood components essential for clot formation and blood coagulation. A decrease in the number of circulating platelets causes an increased susceptibility to bleeding.

Peripheral blood counts are monitored regularly, and are always evaluated indivudually by the nurse oncologist and the medical oncologist before the beginning of a chemotherapy treatment cycle. This is a valuable double check system. Based on blood count values, therapy is sometimes modified or delayed. Hematologic toxicity from chemotherapy can result in life threatening anemia, infection and bleeding. Hematologic status can also be concomitantly compromised by invasion of the primary tumor into the bone marrow; other hematologic disorders, and malnutrition.

Renal Toxicity. Renal toxicity is a less common side effect. Impaired renal function can result from use of cisplatin, methotrexate, or mitomycin-C. With appropriate preparation, which requires meticulous nursing practice, renal toxicity can be avoided. Renal damage can result from rapid tumor destruction with liberation of large amounts of phosphates, which may precipitate as calcium phosphate.

Bladder Toxicity. Hemorrhagic cystitis is caused by mucosal irritation in the bladder. Bladder toxicity can be caused by the breakdown products of cyclophosphamide or ifosfamide which are excreted in the urine. Proper execution of the ordered hydration and neutralization with sodium methyl ethane sulfonate (MESNA) are critical areas of oncology nursing practice designed to dilute and inactivate the toxic metabolite and to eliminate its contact with the bladder mucosa by frequent voiding.

Pulmonary Toxicity. Pulmonary toxicity manifested as inflammation and fibrosis has been associated with bleomycin, methotrexate and the nitrosoureas.

Cardiotoxicity. Cardiotoxicity is a major dose limiting factor for the antitumor antibiotics doxorubicin and daunorubicin and also for idarubicin and mitoxantrone. Cardiotoxicity results from cumulative drug exposure, and can often be anticipated based on total dose, ventricular ejection fraction or echocardiography, and perceptive history of exercise and other activities. Cardiotoxic effects include arrhythmias and congestive heart failure.

Neurotoxicity. Sensory and perceptual alterations result from the effects of chemotherapy on nerve conduction fibers.

Neurotoxicity is most often associated with the vinca alkaloids (vincristine, vinblastine), and is manifested by peripheral neuropathy. The symptoms are: feeling of numbness and tingling in the hands and feet known as "paresthesias;" loss of deep tendon reflexes; generalized motor weakness; and in severe cases, atonia of the bowel and bladder. Cisplatin can cause motor and sensory neuropathy, tinnitus, and hearing loss. Procarbazine causes peripheral neuropathy and altered levels of consciousness. ifosfamide may also cause neurotoxicity in the form of somnolence.

The nurse oncologist should prepare the patient for the signs and symptoms of neurotoxicity.

Nursing Care Related to Cancer Therapies

Nursing care of the patient receiving chemotherapy, radiation therapy, and/or biologic therapy focuses on preparing the patient physically and psychologically for the therapy, assessing the patient's understanding of the therapy and the disease, allaying anxiety related to the treatment procedure, reviewing the possible side effects that may be experienced, providing information to prevent, minimize and alleviate side effects, and ensuring the patient's compliance with instructions and treatment schedules. The oncology nurse most often administers the actual chemotherapy or biotherapy and is present to monitor its acute effects.

The nurse should assess what the patient has been told about his/her disease and treatment. The nurse independently assesses the patient's general physical, psychological, and nutritional status. The oncology nurse and medical oncologist jointly review the treatment plan, expected side effects, and required patient follow-up before the therapy is administered.

Planning

Nursing care is planned in response to the particular needs which may have been identified through assessment. Care is planned to: 1) promote the patient's understanding of therapy goals, treatment time schedules, and related side effects of therapy; 2) promote physical and psychological preparation for therapy, or sometimes for multiple therapies; 3) promote physical comfort, and 4) promote compliance with instructions, treatment schedules; and symptom reporting.

Intervention

Nursing intervention involves preparing the patient and family for treatment, administering prescribed therapy, monitoring and documenting side effects of therapy, ensuring patient compliance with therapy, and teaching related to specific side effects.

The interventions in Table XXI-1-5 are presented in terms of the specific body system that may commonly be affected by the chemotherapy, radiation therapy, and or biologic therapy. Each individual patient may experience one, several or no side effects based on multiple factors. The nurse should always review the treatment plan with the physician to ensure its consistency with an approved research study or institutional protocol, or if neither, with definite therapeutic plan that has evaluation and stopping criteria. Teaching commences before therapy begins, and continues during and after treatment and may be reinforced with appropriate writ-

Table XXI-1-5. Oncology Nursing Care for Common Problems Related to Cancer Therapies

Nausea and Vomiting

Assess the patient's general appearance, skin color, and turgor. Evaluate vital signs, time, frequency, and amount of and character of emesis, serum electrolytes and chemistries for hypercalcemia, hyponatremia, uremia, dehydration. Examine abdomen, auscultate for bowel sounds (intestinal obstruction). Obtain a diet history, medication schedules, past patient measures that may have provided relief. Grade frequency and severity of emesis from 1 (minimal) to 4 (maximal)

Intervention: Involves advising the patient to eat salty foods, dry foods such as toast or crackers, take clear, cool liquids, and eat small portions of low fat foods. Patients should limit physical activity after meals and report symptoms and severity. Administer antiemetics as prescribed and suggest using antiemetics in suppository form, taking antiemetics before receiving therapy. Offer support by explaining that nausea and vomiting are expected side effects, suggesting relaxation techniques and diversionary activity, and being available for questions and follow-up.

Mucositis

Assessment: Inspect oral cavity for moisture, color, ulceration, inflammation and fungus, quality, color, and amount of saliva, condition of teeth. Ascertain patient symptoms including, pain, dysphagia, ability to open mouth, ability to eat and to take fluids, taste changes, voice changes. Grade extent and severity of mucositis from 1–4.

Intervention: Implement measures to alleviate symptoms by teaching mouth care, which includes rinsing mouth with alkaline solutions every hour (1 teaspoon of baking soda in 8 oz. of warm water), or a mouthwash containing sodium bicarbonate, diphenydramine, and lidocaine, use soft sponge or gauze instead of toothbrush, remove thick ropey saliva with gauze; irrigate mouth with sodium bicarbonate solution or diluted solution of hydrogen peroxide. Remove dentures for cleaning, keep dentures in mouth only if comfortable and not causing irritation. Suggest and evaluate effects of topical analgesics, artificial saliva, lip lubricant. Have patient avoid alcohol, smoking, commercial mouthwashes, and hot, spicy, and acidic foods and fluids. Encourge fluids, ice popsicles, a soft bland diet, using a straw to sip soups and beverages. Confer with physician regarding the need for systemic antibiotic, antifungal agents and analgesics.

Evaluation is based on the outcome of all therapeutic measures.

Diarrhea

Assessment: Frequency, character and approximate volume of bowel movements, nutrition history, height, weight, vital signs, hydration status, tissue turgor, condition of mucous membranes, serum electrolyte values. Ascertain patient's knowledge and symptoms related to diarrhea and patient initiated measures to control diarrhea.

Intervention: Implement measures to control and prevent diarrhea: Avoid irritating foods, gas forming foods, fatty foods, lactose and caffeine-containing products, smoking
Suggest: A diet low in residue, high in protein and carbohydrates, small frequent meals.
Teach perianal hygiene: Cleanse with water and mild soap after bowel movement, use sitz baths if indicated, use topical anesthetics to anal area if indicated. Administer and monitor the effects of ordered medications to control diarrhea.

Evaluate patient and family for causes of diarrhea. Evaluate dietary modifications, medication schedules, symptom reporting, and measures implemented to alleviate diarrhea.

Constipation

Assessment: History of defecation. Patient symptoms of cramping, pain, abdominal distention, hemorrhoids. Abdominal appearance, tenderness, and bowel sound patterns, usual bowel habits. Patient knowledge related to constipation. Obtain schedule of all medications. Previous medications and interventions used to treat constipation.

Intervention: Implement measures to alleviate and prevent constipation: Suggest a diet high in fiber, roughage, fluid. Drinking warm fluids to stimulate intestinal motility. Using toilet or bedside commode instead of bedpan. If patient has past history of constipation and will receive vinca alkaloid agents, suggest all the above to start with first chemotherapy dose. Avoid using enemas or suppositories without consulting physician. Administer and monitor the effects of medications prescribed to relieve constipation:
Stool softeners: dioctyl sodium sulfosuccinate, mineral oil.
Bulk producers: psyllium, hydrophilic mucilloid
Osmotic and saline laxatives: sodium, potassium, and magnesium salts.
Lactulose is especially effective for constipation caused by vinca alkaloids.
Cathartics: milk of magnesia, senna, cascara, bisacodyl.

Evaluation: Patient understanding of the causes of constipation and dietary modifications, medication schedules and symptom reporting.

Hyperpigmentation, Photosensitivity

Assessment: Inspect skin for increased pigmentation, and relationship to clothed body areas, dark veins near chemotherapy injection sites, areas of increased pigmentation in mouth and nailbeds, sunburn, rashes.

Intervention: Teach patient to avoid the rays of the direct sun, and to wear protective clothing and apply sunscreen (#15 or higher) if exposure to the sun is unavoidable. Report signs and symptoms. Follow topical medication schedules if prescribed by physician. Explain to the patient that skin reactions are expected and related to therapy, nail growth may be slowed, skin changes, vein and nail darkening are usually temporary.

Table XXI-1-5.   Oncology Nursing Care for Common Problems Related to Cancer Therapies *Continued*

Hematologic Toxicity

Leukopenia

Cancer patients are vulnerable to infection related to their disease process, malnutrition, and treatment side effects of radiation and chemotherapy. The following review of the nursing process applies to all cancer patients who are at risk for infection.

Assessment: Observe for signs and symptoms of infection. Be aware that patients with a low white blood cell count may not exhibit the normal signs of infection such as productive cough, elevated body temperature, redness of skin, edema, or pain, due to the absence of neutrophils. Monitor the white cell count, calculate the absolute neutrophil count, obtain vital signs. Inspect all body orifices including the perianal area and skin for infection. Inspect all venous access sites. Ascertain patient complaints, along with emotional status. Obtain specimens for culture if indicated, e.g., blood, urine, stool, skin, sputum, vaginal, rectal. Obtain history of medication schedule. Monitor fluid balance: intake and output, daily weight.

Intervention: Implement measures to prevent infection by protecting the patient from people with known infections, provide a separate room if possible, instruct the patient, family and visitors in good hand washing technique. Encourage fluid if not contraindicated by other medical disorders. Administer colony stimulating factor if prescribed by a physician. Suggest a low bacterial diet which excludes fresh fruits and vegetables: all foods should be cooked. Maintain skin integrity by bathing daily with antiseptic soap, include nail care. Change intravenous tubing every 24 hours. Avoid injections and skin breakdown. Monitor exit sites of central venous catheters, intravenous site or other venous access devices. Prevent respiratory infection by encouraging ambulation, coughing and deep breathing, adequate fluid intake. Prevent urinary infections by avoiding indwelling urinary catheters, adequate fluid intake, good hygienic measures after bowel movements. Prevent rectal abscess by avoiding enemas and rectal suppositories, rectal temperatures, avoiding constipation. Inspect perianal area for fissures and hemorrhoids. Have patient report any rectal pain and/or discomfort. Administer antibiotics and antifungal agents as prescribed by medical oncologist. Provide comfort measures to control fever by administering antipyretics if prescribed, providing tepid sponge bath, increased fluids. Teach the patient and family signs and symptoms of infection. Explain to the patient and family how to notify medical personnel if signs of infection appear.

Evaluation is based on the patient's knowledge related to signs and symptoms of infection. Patient understanding of interventions required to reduce the risk of infection.

Thrombocytopenia/Anemia

Assessment: Inspect patient for signs and symptoms of bleeding. Inspect skin for petechiae, ecchymosis, hematomas. Observe neurological status for changes associated with intracranial bleeding. Inspect for bleeding into joints. Inspect and test all body secretions and excreta for blood. Assessment includes monitoring of vital signs, blood pressure in reclining, sitting and standing position to assess for postural hypotension. Obtain hemoglobin, hematocrit, and platelets levels. Ascertain symptoms of fatigue, syncope, drowsiness, dyspnea, diaphoresis, chest pain, edema. Auscultate lungs for rales, pressure, abdominal girth-weight. Ascertain if patient has experienced hematemesis, melena, menometrorrhagia, hemoptysis, hematuria, epistaxis, wound bleeding. Ascertain if the patient is currently taking steroids or products which contain aspirin. Monitor all intravenous sites for bleeding.

Intervention: Implement measures to prevent and control bleeding by limiting injections and venipunctures. Use small gauge needles and apply pressure after all skin punctures. Avoid shaving with a razor blade, using a toothbrush or dental floss, straining during bowel movements, taking any medications that contain aspirin, nasotracheal, suctioning, bladder catheterization. Eliminate objects in patient's environment that may cause falls or bruising. Suggest mouth care with sponges or gauze. Increase fluid intake and stool softeners if indicated. For menstruating females: estrogen-progesterone agents can be given to stop menses if indicated. Encourage a soft diet high in fiber and protein. Limited physical activity, if indicated pad side rails, prevent falls. Use of humidifier if oxygen therapy is indicated to prevent mucosal drying. For nosebleed, place patient in high Fowler's position, apply ice packs and pressure to bridge of nose, notify physician. Administer and monitor platelet and or red blood cell transfusions if prescribed by physician. Administer antacids and ice water lavages for gastric bleeding if prescribed by physician.

Evaluation is based on patient's ability to recognize and report signs and symptoms of anemia and bleeding, as is, effectiveness of all interventions in preventing and controlling anemia and or bleeding.

Sexual Dysfunction Related to Physiological and Psychological Effects of Cancer Therapies

Assessment: Done by informing patient and partner that there may be side effects from the cancer therapies that will affect sexual functiong. Ascertain questions and concerns related to sexual function. Determine current methods of birth control.

Intervention: Inform females of possible amenorrhea, onset of early menopause with symptoms of "hot flashes," vaginal dryness, possible dyspareunia related to decreased lubrication of vaginal walls. Use water soluble lubricant or steroid cream if indicated. Explain that a decreased libido may be related to fatigue and hormonal changes. Use birth control methods if premenopausal.

Inform males of possible temporary or permanent sterility and possible impotence related to therapy, which is often temporary. Suggest sperm banking before therapy begins, if indicated. Refer patients and partners to appropriate professionals if indicated. Allow time for discussion of sexual dysfunction. Provide written information regarding contraception methods.

Evaluation: Based on the patient's understanding of possible sexual dysfunction related to therapy, and the patient's ability to identify personal strategies to assist with alterations in sexual functioning. Patient reports symptoms and concerns related to sexual dysfunction.

ten and visual learning materials. When indicated, patients and families can be referred to other professionals and community programs and agencies.

Unconventional Therapies

The very success of medical research and treatment in eradicating such diseases as polio and smallpox, has inculcated a general expectation that there must be a definitive "cure" for cancer. The search for a "miracle cure" for oncologic diseases has led patients to investigate and participate in a wide range of therapies such as diet programs, vitamin therapies, unproven and potentially unsafe biologic vaccines. Meditation and mental imaging, as primary therapy, have also been utilized by patients who are led to believe that mental conditioning can stop the growth and spread of tumor cells. Many unproven methods are costly and prevent timely treatment and restoration of health when used instead of generally accepted treatments.

Nursing Implications

Unproven methods of cancer treatment may be eagerly sought by patients and their families. Patients may request information related to alternative therapies as a means to ensure they are reviewing all treatment alternatives. The oncology nurse's primary response to such requests is to provide whatever accurate information is known related to these therapies while listening and exploring the reasons for seeking unproven methods. If unsatisfactory to the patient, the nurse should provide referrals to educational materials or other professionals who can provide additional and current information regarding the health hazards and risks of unproven cancer treatments. Among sources of information are publications of the Food and Drug Administration, the National Cancer Institute and the American Cancer Society. These agencies have literature that reviews and assesses unproven drugs, substances and treatment centers.

The nurse oncologist must be sensitive to the fact that many patients and families who seek unconventional therapy may have exhausted all conventional therapy without regression of their disease. A patient's inclination to explore unproven approaches to complex problems may be a typical life pattern, but also may be founded in desperation rather than cold reason. The nurse should remain objective and present to patients the information that will assist in their understanding the risks and implications of unproven cancer therapies. The nurse must accept the patient's right to choose whatever therapy he or she finds most desirable, even if in the nurse's judgment, it is not the correct choice. The nurse should apprise the physician of the interview. The ethical dilemma is most difficult when the patient has curable disease, but inclines toward an unproven remedy out of fear and ignorance. In such a situation support and negotiation, often most influentially by the nurse oncologist, can persuade the patient to adhere to a potentially curative regimen.

Pain Control

A major factor in advanced cancer is pain. The International Association for the Study of Pain has defined pain as "an unpleasant sensory and emotional experience associated with actual or potential tissue damage, or described in terms of such damage." The subjective nature of pain is evidenced by the unique psychological and physiological responses to pain.

Cancer pain is most often associated with tissue damage and tissue infiltration. As malignant tumors grow within a body part they stretch normal boundaries of the organ, causing severe pain. As tumors grow and occupy additional space, other organs and structures are affected. Tumor growth and tissue invasion can result in nerve compression, organ and bone invasion, obstruction of hollow organs, and stretching of capsules and tissue membranes. Primary or metastastic bone tumors cause pain related to pressure, periosteal irritation, and pathologic fractures. Pain can be experienced as an acute or chronic event. Unrelieved pain can affect a patient's lifestyle, treatment and ability to cope with his or her disease status. An indepth discussion of pain management can be found in XL-1.

Pain Management

The primary method to relieve tumor related pain is to destroy the tumor which is the cause. The surgical removal of a tumor mass or chemotherapy used to shrink a tumor mass can relieve pain. Radiation therapy can be directed to painful localized areas of tissue infiltration, particularly for bone pain. Surgical manipulation of the central nervous system can also relieve pain symptoms.

Pharmacological Agents

Analgesics, anti-inflammatory agents, and psychotropic agents are used alone or in combination for the treatment of pain. These agents control the symptom with the goal of improving the patient's comfort. Non-narcotic analgesics control pain by acting on the peripheral nervous system. Non-narcotic analgesics include aspirin, acetaminophen, and the nonsteroidal anti-inflammatory agents such as ibuprofen. Narcotics control pain by acting on the central nervous system and include codeine, morphine, hydromorphone, meperidine, and oxycodone. Non-narcotics and narcotics are often prescribed together.

Side effects from narcotics include drowsiness, constipation, nausea and vomiting, and drying of the oral mucosa. Aspirin and non-steroidal anti-inflammatory drugs can cause gastrointestinal bleeding and can interfere with platelet functioning.

Co-analgesic agents such as steroids, antipsychotic agents, muscle relaxants, and sedatives are also used to control pain related symptoms. Pharmacological agents can be given orally or parenterally, on intermittent or continuous dosing schedules. The use of oral morphine on an "around the clock schedule" has been shown to be effective in the control of severe pain. The objective of pain control is to prevent pain, not to let it periodically reappear so that it can be relieved again. Research continues in the area of self-administration and self-dose titration of parenteral and oral narcotics. The selection of pharmacological agents should be based on patient pain control history, patient preference, and patient response.

The side effects of pharmacological agents must also be considered. Narcotics can depress the function of the central nervous system. So much that enjoyable social activity becomes impossible. Counteraction with stimulants may then be of value without impairing pain relief.

Behavioral Therapies

Behavioral therapies can be used in conjunction with pharmacological therapies as a means of promoting patient participation in his/her care. Behavioral therapies, which vary in approach, are intended to decrease tension and increase muscle relaxation. These therapies can potentially assist with pain control while ameliorating nausea and vomiting related to radiation or chemotherapy. Further, general anxiety can be reduced. Diversionary activities such as exercise, hobbies, or reading assist in the redirection of pain sensations and perceptions. Relaxation therapy includes exercises, yoga, meditation, and progressive muscle relaxation. Advanced relaxation techniques can be achieved through hypnosis and guided imagery. These therapies can be learned and self-induced as a means of achieving deep relaxation. Biofeedback assists the patient with self-regulation of physiologic activities such as pulse and blood pressure, which can result in decreased tension and increased muscle relaxation.

Cutaneous Therapies

Cutaneous therapies such as skin massage, application of heat, cold, and lotions, acupuncture, and transcutaneous electronic nerve stimulation (TENS) can offer additional temporary pain relief.

Transcutaneous electronic nerve stimulation (TENS) is based on the Gate Control Theory and is accomplished through the use of a small electrical device, powered by a battery pack, that provides electrical stimulation to the skin. The large fibers of the peripheral nervous system are stimulated in an attempt to override pain stimuli and close the gate that controls pain perception.

Principles of Nursing Care Related to Pain Control

Nursing care should be planned: 1) to promote patient comfort; 2) to provide patients and their families with information related to pain control; 3) to provide information about, and assist with, behavioral and cutaneous therapies; 4) to prevent and alleviate side effects of pharmacological therapies; and 5) to promote patient compliance with therapy and required follow up.

The nurse implements measures to control and alleviate pain. Based on individual patient needs, and as prescribed by the physician, the nurse administers and monitors effects of pharmacological therapies, teaches and monitors effects of behavioral therapies, and teaches and assists with the application of cutaneous therapies.

The nurse should explain the rationale of interventions and provide time for patient and family questions. The nurse teaches the patient the names of pharmacological agents, dosage schedules, and side effects of pharmacological agents. The nurse stresses the importance of symptom reporting, interventions to alleviate nausea and vomiting, use of antiemetics, and interventions to alleviate constipation (see Table XXI-1-5). The nurse monitors effectiveness and side effects of pharmacological interventions; monitors symp-

toms, respiratory status, bowel functioning, and mental and cognitive functioning. The nurse collaborates and confers with the physician regarding effectiveness and side effects of pharmacological therapies. (Refers and consults with other professionals as indicated.) The nurse provides patient and family with written materials, ensures that the patient has a follow-up appointment, and that patient and family know how to contact medical personnel in case of an emergency.

The topic of pain control is discussed indepth elsewhere in the text, and in medical and oncology nursing literature.[4,5,8,10,12,21,31,48,52]

Nutritional Alterations Related to Cancer and Cancer Therapies

Assessment

Nursing assessment of the patient with nutritional alteration should include information covering the patient's history, treatment schedules, and current dietary intake. The patient's knowledge related to the effect of cancer and cancer treatments on nutritional status should be assessed. Nutritional status is based on observation of the patient: anthropometric measurements of subscapular skin fold thickness (SST), mid-arm muscle circumference (MAMC), and weight. Laboratory values for nutritional assessment include: hemoglobin and hematocrit, serum albumin, and blood urea nitrogen.

Assessment data should include the following: height and weight of the patient, current dietary intake, and caloric requirements. The protein, carbohydrate, fat, vitamin, mineral and fluid needs should be calculated considering the age, activity, culture, and patient food preferences. Hemoglobin, hematocrit, and serum chemistries are monitored. Triceps skin fold measurement determines external tissue mass and mid-arm muscle circumference reflects muscle. A history of cancer treatments is taken, together with side effects of cancer treatments, and patient initiated strategies to increase dietary intake. Patient assessment guidelines described in other sections of this chapter are followed.

Patients are advised to eat small, frequent meals, to avoid strong smelling foods, and increase caloric and nutrient intake. Adding wine, beer, or milk to soups and sauces helps. Combining ice cream with soda, milk shakes, or yogurt, and drinking liquid protein supplements increases intake of lean protein. Patients are taught to serve foods that are cold or at room temperature and to take advantage of "feeling well" times to prepare food to freeze for later use. Dining in an environment conducive to eating helps. Rinsing the mouth before eating, to wash away bad tastes, is useful. The patient may need help to plan meals that meet fluid and caloric needs. Keeping a food diary helps. The patient should follow interventions described for specific therapy and disease related gastrointestinal toxicities.

The nurse must consult with the physician regarding indications for enteral and parenteral nutritional supplementation, use of oral liquid supplements, and use of antiemetics, and antidiarrheals, if indicated. A patient should be referred to a dietitian if indicated. Community agencies may assist with meal preparation. It is important to provide patients with written instructions and written educational materials. Nutritional status should be monitored on a regular basis, all the while avoiding statements that may make the patient feel guilty about anorexia or weight loss.

Home Care

The diagnosis and treatment of cancer most often does not require extensive hospitalization. Many patients undergoing radiation therapy, chemotherapy, and biologic therapy may safely be treated and monitored in an ambulatory setting or at home. Advances in oncology nursing have assisted in making home therapy possible and favorable. Home care should be planned by the medical oncologist and nurse oncologist during the patient's initial assessment as well as during treatment phases. Family members and home health professionals can provide needed home care with the support and advisement of both nurse and physician. Family members may require support and teaching of basic patient care skills. When indicated, the patient should be referred to the hospital's home care department and or referred to a local home care company or visiting nurse service.

Summation

The progress of professional oncology nursing parallels the progress made in the medical and technical advances for the treatment of cancer. Nurse oncologists have earned the respect of physicians, other health care professionals, and most importantly, of patients and their families. Oncology nursing will continue to develop as a dynamic element within the health care delivery process as the number of oncology nurses increases and the level of knowledge and experience advances.

References

1. American Cancer Society: 1990 Facts and Figures. New York, The American Cancer Society, 1989.
2. American Nurses Association and the Oncology Nursing Society: Standards of Oncology Nursing Practice. Kansas City, MO, American Nurses Association, 1987.
3. Aveilanet, C.: Cancer Prevention: Cancer risk factors. Cancer Nursing, 5:295, 1982.
4. Baird, S. B., McCorkle, R., and Grant, M.: Cancer Nursing. Philadelphia, PA, W. B. Saunders, 1991.
5. Baldonado, A. A., and Stahl, D. A.: Cancer Nursing: A Holistic Multidisciplinary Approach. New York, Medical Examination Publishing Co., 1982.
6. Barckley, V.: The best of times and the worst of times: Historical reflections from an American Cancer Society National Nursing Consultant. Oncology, 12(Suppl. 1):16, 1985.
7. Borsani, G., and Carl, W.: Oral care for cancer patients. American Journal of Nursing, 83:533, 1983.
8. Carnevali, D. L., and Reiner, A. C.: The Cancer Experience: Nursing Diagnosis and Management. Philadelphia, PA, J. B. Lippincott, 1990.
9. Carpenito, L. J.: Handbook of Nursing Diagnosis. Philadelphia, PA, J. B. Lippincott Co., 1984.
10. Carrieri, V. K., Lindsay, A. M., and West, C. M.: Pathophysiological Phenomena in Nursing: Human Response to Illness. Philadelphia, W. B. Saunders Co., 1986.
11. Carter, P., Engel King, C., Rumsey, K., and Vincent, B.: Biological Response Modifier Guidelines. Recommendations for Nursing Education and Practice. Pittsburgh, PA, Oncology Nursing Society, 1989.
12. Chernecky, C. C., and Ramsey, P. W.: Critical Nursing Care of the Client with Cancer. Norwalk, Appleton-Century-Crofts, 1984.
13. Daeffler, R. J., and Petrosino, B.: Manual of Oncology Nursing Practice. Rockville, Aspen Publishing, 1990.
14. Department of Health and Human Services: Coping with Cancer. NIH Publication No. 80-2080, Bethesda, MD, 1980.
15. Department of Health and Human Services: Eating Hints, recipes and tips for better nutrition during cancer treatment. NIH Publication No. 91-2079. Bethesda, MD, National Institutes of Health, 1990.
16. Division of Cancer Prevention and Control. Screening. In Cancer Control Objectives for the Nation: 1985-2000. Edited by P. Greenwald and E. Sondik. NCI Monograph, NIH Publication 86-2880. Bethesda, MD, National Institutes of Health, 1986.
17. Dodd, M. J.: Managing Side Effects of Chemotherapy and Radiation Therapy: A Guide for Patients and Nurses. Norwalk, CT, Appleton & Lange, 1987.
18. Donovan, M. I., and Pierce, S.: Cancer Care: A Guide for Patient Education. New York, Appleton-Century-Crofts, 1981.
18A. Geigy Scientific Tables, 8TH ed., Vol. 1. Edited by C. Lentner. West Caldwell, NJ, Ciba-Geigy Corp., 1981.
19. Goodman, M., and Wickham, R.: Vascular access devices: An overview. Oncology Nursing Forum, II:16, 1984.
20. Govani, L. E., and Hayes, J. E.: Drugs and Nursing Implications, 6th Ed. Norwalk, CT, Appleton and Lange, 1988.
21. Griffiths, M. J., Murray, K. H., and Russo, P. C.: Oncology Nursing–Pathophysiology, Assessment and Intervention. New York, Macmillian, 1984.
22. Groenwald, S. L., Frogge, M. H., Goodman, M., and Yarboro, C. H.: Cancer Nursing Principles and Practice, 2nd Ed. Boston, MA, Jones and Bartlett, 1990.
23. Gullo, S. M.: Safe handling of antineoplastic drugs: Translating the recommendations into practice. Oncology Nursing Forum, 15:595, 1988.
24. Hellman, S.: Principles of Radiation Therapy. In Cancer: Principles and Practice of Oncology. 2nd ed. Edited by V. T. Devita, S. Hellman, and S. A. Rosenberg. Philadelphia, J. B. Lippincott Co., 1983.
25. Holland, J. C.: Why Patients Seek Unproven Cancer Remedies: A Psychological perspective. CA, 32:10, 1982.
26. Holland, J. C., and Rowland, J. H.: Handbook of Psychooncology: Psychological Care of the Patient with Cancer. New York, Oxford University Press, 1989.
27. Johnson, B. L., and Gross, J.: Handbook of Oncology Nursing. New York, John Wiley & Sons, 1985.
28. Johnson, J. L. B., and Blumberg, B. D.: A commentary on cancer patient education. Health Education Quarterly, 10:7, 1984.
29. Knobf, M. K., and Fischer, D. S.: Cancer chemotherapy treatment and care. 3rd ed. Boston, G. K. Hall Medical Publishers, 1989.
30. Knobf, T., Fischer, D. S., Welch-McCaffrey, D.: Cancer Chemotherapy Treatment and Care. 2nd ed. Boston, G. K. Hall Medical Publications, 1984.
31. Marino, L. B.: Cancer Nursing. St. Louis, MO, C. V. Mosby, 1981.
32. McCaffery, M., and Beebe, A.: Pain: Clinical Manual for Nursing Practice. St. Louis, C. V. Mosby Co., 1989.
33. McIntire, S. N., and Cioppa, A. N.: Cancer Nursing—A Developmental Approach. New York, John Wiley & Sons, 1984.
34. McNally, J., Stair, J., and Somerville, E.: Guidelines for Cancer Nursing Practice. Orlando, Grune & Stratton, 1985.
35. Miller, N., and Howard-Ruben, J.: Unproven methods of Cancer Management, Part 1: Backgrounds and Historical Perspectives. Oncology Nursing Forum, 10:46, 1983.
36. National Cancer Institute: Chemotherapy and You: A Guide to Self Help During Treatment. Bethesda, MD., Department of Health and Human Services. NIH Publication #88-1136, 1987.
37. Oncology Nursing Society: Antidotes for Vesicant/Irritant Drugs. Pittsburgh, PA, Oncology Nursing Press, 1989.
38. Oncology Nursing Society: Access Device Guidelines, Modules I-III. Pittsburgh, PA, Oncology Nursing Press, 1989–1990.
39. Oncology Nursing Society: Biological Response Modifier Guidelines. Pittsburgh, PA: Oncology Nursing Press, 1989.
40. Oncology Nursing Society: Cancer Chemotherapy: Guidelines and Recommendations for Nursing Education and Practice, Pittsburgh, PA, Oncology Nursing Press, 1989.
41. Oncology Nursing Society: Guidelines for Cancer Nursing Practice. Edited by J. C. McNally, J. Campbell-Stair, and E. T. Somervilee. Orlando, FL, Grune & Stratton, Inc., 1985.
42. Oncology Nursing Society: Fiscus, J. A., Hayes, N. A., Rostad, M. E., and Whedon, M. A., Safe handling of cytotoxic drugs. Independent study module. Pittsburgh, PA, The Oncology Nursing Press, p. 3, 1989.
43. Oncology Nursing Society: Committee on Clinical Practice: Standards of Advanced Practice in Oncology Nursing. Pittsburgh, PA, Oncology Nursing Press, 1990.
44. Oncology Nursing Society: Standards on Oncology Education: Patient/Family and Public. Pittsburgh, PA, Oncology Nursing Press. 1989.
45. Oncology Nursing Society and American Nurses Association Division of Medical Surgical Nursing Practice: Outcome Standards for Cancer Nursing Practice. Kansas City, MO, American Nurses Association, 1989.
46. Oppenheimer, S. B.: Cancer: A Biological and Clinical Introduction, 2nd edition, Boston, Jones and Bartlett, 1990.
47. Redman, B.: The Process of Patient Education. St. Louis, MO, C. V. Mosby Co., 1984.
48. Spross, J., and McQuire, D. B. Oncology Nursing Society Position Paper on Cancer Pain. Pittsburgh, PA, Oncology Nursing Press, 1991.
49. U. S. Department of Health and Human Services, Public Health Service, National Institutes of Health: Eating Hints, Recipes and Tips for Better Nutrition During Cancer Treatment. NIH Publication No. 81-2079, 1981.
50. U. S. Department of Health and Human Services, Public Health Services, National Institutes of Health: Radiation Therapy and You. A Guide to Self-Help During Treatment. NIH Publication No. 88-2227, 1988.
51. U. S. Department of Labor: Office of Occupational Medicine, Occupational Safety and Health Administration. Work Practice Guidelines for personnel dealing with cytotoxic (antineoplastic) drugs. Publication #8.1.1., Washington, D. C., 1986.
52. Wiernik, P. H.: Supportive Care of the Cancer Patient. New York, Futura Publishing Co., 1983.
53. Yasko, J. M.: Guidelines for Cancer Care: Symptom Management. Reston, VA, Reston Co., 1983.
54. Yasko, J. M.: Care of the Client Receiving External Radiation Therapy. Reston, VA, Reston Co., 1982.
55. Ziegfeld, C. R.: Core Curriculum for Oncology Nursing. The Oncology Nursing Society, Philadelphia, PA, W. B. Saunders Co., 1987.

XXII

Principles of
Cancer Rehabilitation Medicine

Kristjan T. Ragnarsson

Introduction

Medical advances in the diagnosis and management of cancer have markedly increased the survival rates of patients. While the treatment for some patients may now result in complete cure and no perceived physical deficits, an aggressive definitive treatment may for others result in significant physical impairment or disability. In order to ensure quick restoration of optimal function, early and continued aggressive rehabilitation interventions should be provided, i.e., physical and occupational therapy, prosthetic and orthotic devices, and assistive equipment. Application of rehabilitation techniques frequently results in a swift functional improvement and a reduction of subjective complaints even when prognosis for life is considered poor. It has always been difficult to predict with a degree of certainty the life expectancy of an individual with cancer. Modern diagnostic techniques and effective treatment of malignant neoplastic disease have invalidated old statistics and dogmas regarding life expectancy and thus made accurate prognostication even more difficult for the clinician. No cancer patient, even one with widespread metastases, should therefore be denied the benefits of aggressive treatment, including appropriate surgical intervention, chemotherapy, radiation and comprehensive rehabilitation. These interventions, when offered in an integrated and timely fashion, prolong life, protect organs and residual healthy tissue, reduce pain, maximize self-care and mobility skills, and thereby help to reduce the stigma of cancer and physical impairment while providing dignity and quality of life for the cancer patient.

Early referral for rehabilitation services and good communication between the oncologist, the surgeon, the physiatrist and the other members of the cancer rehabilitation team is essential for successful return to optimal function. Every effort should be made to coordinate the rehabilitation treatment with other types of intervention in order for them to be implemented simultaneously or in a timely manner. A comprehensive and well coordinated rehabilitation approach which concurrently deals with the physical, psychological, and social problems which are caused by the malignant neoplastic disease and the consequent disability usually yields the best results. Most important for success, however, is the patient's personal interest and ability to participate in the rehabilitation program and pursue the established functional goals supported by family and friends.

Application of Rehabilitation Concepts

A large but unknown proportion of individuals afflicted by cancer develop some form of functional impairment or disability which will interfere with self-care, mobility, and smooth transition to their former life style. These patients should be identified early and referred for rehabilitation treatment. Cancer rehabilitation can be broadly defined as the maximum restoration of physical, psychological, social, vocational, recreational and economic function within the limits imposed by the malignant neoplastic disease and its treatment. In order to make a significant and timely impact on such a wide variety of functions and needs, the efforts of a well coordinated and goal oriented multi-disciplinary cancer rehabilitation team are required (Table XXII-1-1). Due to the cancer's often uncertain prognosis, the primary goals of most cancer rehabilitation programs are focused on quick gains in mobility and self-care skills, and the provision of psycho-social support to the patient and his/her family. Flexibility in goal

Table XXII-1-1. Multidisciplinary Cancer Rehabilitation Team

Physician (physiatrist)
Rehabilitation oncology nurse
Physical therapist
Occupational therapist
Prosthetist-orthotist
Nutritionist
Speech pathologist
Social worker
Psychologist
Chaplain
Vocational counselor
Receational therapist

setting is unavoidable because of the patient's changing needs, stamina, and medical status.

Despite the potential benefits, referrals of cancer patients for rehabilitation services are often made needlessly late or not at all. This may reflect a reluctance on the part of the oncologist. Many physicians are unfamiliar with the concepts of rehabilitation treatment and its potential impact. Clinical problems amenable to rehabilitation interventions are often identified too late or not at all. Pessimistic prognostication by the oncologist and the rehabilitation specialist may hinder rehabilitation referrals as cancer patients are inappropriately compared with patients disabled by trauma, or other relatively static medical disorders. Fortunately the prognosis for most types of cancer has improved, and consequently the demand for rehabilitation services for cancer patients with disabilities has grown.

Several studies have shown that cancer rehabilitation programs result in measurable benefits when individualized, specific and realistic goals are set.[12] Comprehensive inpatient rehabilitation services may be economically provided for disabled cancer patients who are considered "cured or controlled," but precise short term rehabilitation interventions may enable even those with poor prognosis to gain the mobility and self-care skills that facilitate early hospital discharge.

The physical impairment experienced by cancer patients may result from tissue destruction caused by the cancer itself, prolonged bed rest, inactivity, or from definitive treatment, i.e, surgery, radiation, or chemotherapy. The exact nature of the impairment may vary, but in essence it is no different from impairment which is caused by trauma or noncancerous disease, and is customarily managed by the rehabilitation team. A specific rehabilitation goal must be established for each patient and an individualized program prescribed which is designed to obtain measurable early results. The main rehabilitation goals for all people with physical disabilities are: first, to develop maximum skills in the activities of daily living (ADL)(Table XXII-1-2) allowed by the disability and second, to obtain independent ambulation with or without assistive devices, i.e., wheelchairs, prostheses, orthoses, walkers, crutches, or canes. In order to reach these goals the therapist will utilize physical exercise to improve muscle strength, endurance, joint flexibility, and self-care skills, as well as apply physical modalities to decrease pain

Table XXII-1-2.   Activities of Daily Living*

Eating and drinking
Dressing and undressing
Bathing and grooming
Toileting
Managing bladder and bowel functions
Manipulating small objects
Caring for health and fitness
Moving in bed
Changing position
Walking
Climbing stairs
General wheelchair skills
Using a manual wheelchair
Using an electric wheelchair

*Rehabilitation indicators: skill indicators

and swelling. Prescription, fabrication, and fitting of prosthetic and orthotic devices and other assistive equipment, followed by training in their use, is essential for amputees and individuals with significant muscle weakness, paralysis, or unstable skeletal structures.

It is essential to provide rehabilitation interventions which also aim at the often profound psychological, sexual, social and vocational consequences of the cancer and the physical impairment in order to help the patient and his family to cope with these problems. Preferably, the anticipated psycho-social difficulties should be addressed when the initial diagnosis is made and when treatment is begun. The goal of cancer care is not just to eradicate or control the malignancy and extend the patient's life, but to maintain or re-establish a quality of life. While fatal or physically disabling consequences of cancer are quickly recognized and usually well managed by the hospital staff, the psycho-social effects of cancer, which frequently manifest after hospital discharge, may be unnoticed and therefore be untreated. As a result these may become more disabling than the physical impairment.

The rehabilitation goals of cancer patients may be broadly classified according to the different stages of the disease: 1) *Preventive rehabilitation therapy* is started early after the diagnosis of cancer is made, i.e., before or immediately after surgery, radiotherapy and or chemotherapy. At this stage no significant physical impairment exists but therapy is started in order to prevent functional loss; 2) *Restorative rehabilitation therapy* is directed at the comprehensive restoration of maximum function for patients considered "cured or controlled" but who have a residual physical impairment and disability; 3) *Supportive rehabilitation therapy* attempts to increase the self-care skills and mobility of the cancer patient with growing cancer and progressive impairment and disability for application of quick effective methods, e.g., provide appropriate assistive devices and teach simple techniques for self-care.[31] Supportive rehabilitation therapy also includes physical exercises to prevent the effects of immobilization, i.e., joint contractures, muscle atrophy, weakness, and pressure sores. These interventions sometimes may be thought of as a futile effort "to do something" in the presence of poor prognosis, but on the other hand they have few adverse effects and may lift the patient's spirit and increase his sense of well being; and 4) *Palliative rehabilitation therapy* aims to increase or maintain comfort and function of patients with terminal cancer by utilizing physical modalities, simple orthotic devices and assistive equipment in order to manage pain, joint contractures and pressure sores and to provide at least partial self-sufficiency.[31]

The Cancer Rehabilitation and Adaption Team

Organized cancer rehabilitation programs have been reported to be of significant and measurable benefits in relation to such established goals as physical function and community reintegration.[12,30] An integral part of such programs is a multi-disciplinary cancer rehabilitation and adaptation team (Table XXII-1-1) which consists of many different health professionals. The exact composition of the team may vary considerably depending on the program's philosophy and size, the type of institution and the range of disabilities encountered. The team is led by a physician who is either an oncologist or, more commonly, a physiatrist.[30] Oncology nurse, social worker, psychologist, physical and occupational therapist, vocational counselor, chaplain and nutritionist are present on most such teams.[30] Other rehabilitation professionals may contribute in an important way to the rehabilitation of cancer patients, depending on each patient's specific physical impairment, i.e., prosthetist, orthotist, speech pathologist, driver's trainer, and recreational therapist. The roles of the various team members are described hereafter.

The Physiatrist, the medical specialist that usually directs the cancer rehabilitation team, needs to be knowledgeable in oncology in addition to his expertise in the field of physical medicine and rehabilitation. The physiatrist is the team's primary link with other treating physicians. In order to establish realistic goals and prescribe an appropriate rehabilitation program, the physiatrist needs to know a) the exact cancer diagnosis with respect to organ site, histology and grade of anaplasia, b) the cancer's anatomical staging (primary site only, involvement of regional nodes or metastases), c) the patient's life expectancy, i.e., is he "cured or controlled," and if not, what is the anticipated rapidity of the cancer's progression, d) the definitive treatment plan for the cancer, i.e, the timing of surgery, chemotherapy, and/or radiation, its anticipated efficacy and potential side effects. This information the physiatrist shares with and explains to the rehabilitation team in order to develop a specific and realistic therapy plan, i.e, preventive, restorative, supportive and palliative. The physiatrist introduces the patient and the family to goals of the cancer rehabilitation team and meets regularly with the team as well as with the patient and family in order to direct and coordinate their efforts while taking into account the patient's progress and changing needs.

The Rehabilitation Oncology Nurse serves primarily as an easily accessible resource to the nursing staff that gives care to the cancer patient, as well as to the patient and the family. The nurse evaluates the patient's specific nursing needs, plans the care, helps to obtain nursing supplies, educates other nurses, the patient and his family about nursing techniques and principles of cancer treatment, facilitates patient and family self management, monitors discharge plans and assists in the discharge process. After discharge the nurse may provide advice for the care givers in the home on the management of the different and complex treatment problems that may arise.

The Physical Therapist teaches the patient to perform specific exercises to strengthen muscles, to increase stamina, and to maintain or improve joint range of motion and trunk flexibility. When indicated, training is provided in order to improve balance and coordination, as well as functional skills, i.e, transfers in and out of bed, wheelchair locomotion and ambulation with or without assistive devices. Instructions are provided to normalize gait patterns, and to safely ascend and descend stairs and curbs. Various physical modalities may be used by the therapist to reduce pain, i.e, superficial and deep heat, cold, transcutaneous electrostimulation (TENS) and massage, but the clinician needs to know that heat modalities and massage should not be applied directly over

or immediately adjacent to a site of cancer. Physical exercise perhaps is the most important therapeutic modality in rehabilitation management of physical disabilities. Muscle strengthening exercises may be either isometric, isotonic, or isokinetic. Isometric exercise does not involve joint motion, and therefore is prescribed for painful or unstable body parts, whereas isotonic exercise involves joint motion against variable resistance. Isokinetic exercise, a most effective strengthening exercise, involves use of specific devices, e.g., the Cybex apparatus, to maintain constant speed of motion independent from the force applied.[54] Passive stretching exercises are done by the therapist without the patient's direct participation in order to maintain or increase joint mobility. Task oriented exercises, e.g., ambulation or training in self care, may improve function and safety by repetition and prolonged therapy.

The Occupational Therapist focuses in particular on upper extremity exercises and training in self-care activities. The exercises are designed to improve strength, coordination, and skills in the various ADL (Table XXII-1-2). Different adaptive equipment may be provided to make the patient more proficient in self-care and activities related to work and recreation. When indicated, the therapist fabricates simple orthotic devices, e.g., hand splints for immobilization or to compensate for weak muscles. When brain dysfunction is present, a gross assessment of cognitive and visual perceptual skills is performed, and therapy is initiated to remediate for deficits in these areas. Evaluation of the home and work place is done and recommendations are offered to make these sites more accessible and conducive to complete self-sufficiency and greater productivity. Working independently, or with a recreational therapist, the occupational therapist strives to make a resumption of leisure time activities easier for the patient.

The Prosthetist/Orthotist is called upon to custom make artificial limbs (prostheses) or special braces (orthoses) for patients in need of such devices. The prosthetist/orthotist should evaluate the patient with the physiatrist and the therapist and help to select the proper components and materials for the device as well as to determine its general design and methods of fabrication based on the pathology and biomechanics involved. After delivery the physiatrist checks out the device for comfort and fit, but it is the duty of the prosthetist/orthotist to modify and service the equipment as long as it remains in use.

The Nutritionist evaluates the patient's nutritional condition, predicts the additional metabolic demands that the cancer places on the body, and recommends the optimal diet with respect to specific clinical condition, caloric intake, food ingredients of choice, optimal consistency for easy swallowing, and the individual's tastes or choice. The nutritionist judges total food intake by closely monitoring the weight and counting calories and, if nutrition is inadequate, may recommend interventions to facilitate adequate intake in the presence of poor appetite and swallowing disorders. The nutritionist should teach the patient and family general and specific dietary principles and consult with the clinical staff on the optimal parenteral nutrition when the need for that arises.

The Speech Pathologist evaluates and provides therapy

for impaired oral communication and works closely with the occupational therapist and nutritionist in the assessment and care of swallowing disorders.

The Social Worker has many important roles in the rehabilitation of the cancer patient, but, especially with respect to discharge planning, smooth transition from the hospital to the community, continuity of care, and securing appropriate follow-up services after discharge. The social worker helps the patient to secure financial resources, including health insurance coverage, social security and disability compensation, as well as to obtain authorization and payment for necessary devices and home help. Before hospital discharge, arrangements need to be made for transportation, attendant, or nursing care, home modifications and other appropriate post-hospital services. This may involve transfer to and placement at other health institutions. The social worker often acts as a liaison among the patient, the family members, and the various health care professionals.

The Rehabilitation Psychologist assesses the patient's psychological functions including intelligence, personality, i.e., ideational, emotional, behavioral, and characterological patterns, past personal history, motivation, reaction to the illness and coping skills. Following the diagnosis of cancer and development of a disability, both the patient and family members may experience reactive depression or grief, which often is expressed in diverse ways, i.e., denial, anger, anxiety, panic, fear, dependent behavior, depression and unmasking of previously controlled psychopathology. The primary role of the psychologist is to assist the patient and the family in coping, as well as to counsel and consult with the rehabilitation team members in managing the emotional reactions. The effectiveness of psycho-social intervention has been successfully demonstrated with cancer patients.[25,32]

A Chaplain is often included in the cancer rehabilitation team. The Chaplain may be able to relate to the patient and the family in a way that can help them use their faith to adjust to the illness and disability.

A Vocational Counselor should participate in the care of physically impaired cancer patients who have any potential of returning to work. An initial interview should be conducted at the hospital and vocational services continued after discharge. These services may include detailed evaluation, counselling, testing, career exploration, and educational planning. The counselor will have to proceed to the extent and at a pace which is sensitive to the patient's need and readiness to resume vocational activities, i.e., education or work. At the proper time the counselor may make visits to work or school sites and consult with employers and teachers to facilitate transition from disability to productivity as worker or student. For school age children, home tutoring may have to be arranged. Those who are unemployed may be taught skills to seek jobs successfully. The Office of Vocational Rehabilitation (OVR) exists in each state and can be a source of funding for various vocational rehabilitation services, i.e, certain aspects of rehabilitation, education, training, job placement, equipment and environmental modifications if these will enable the disabled person eventually to return to school or work. The counselor makes the initial referral to OVR and maintains a close cooperative and effective relationship with the OVR representatives.

The Recreational Therapist offers activities to meet the different needs and interests of disabled individuals both within and outside the hospital, e.g., art therapy, music therapy, attending art shows and sports events, going to theatres, restaurants, shops, etc. Family and friends may join in these recreational activities which serve to increase socialization, leisure time activities, and positive attitudes. The trips into the community may facilitate the institutional discharge for the physically disabled person and reintegration into community life.

Functional Assessment

A medical intervention should not be offered unless measurable benefits result. Unlike other fields of medicine the outcome of rehabilitation interventions cannot be measured by whether the patient lives or dies, or by disappearance of symptoms. The effectiveness of rehabilitation interventions is judged by how functionally independent the patient becomes as a result of this treatment. The terms impairment, disability, and handicap have been carefully defined by the World Health Organization in order to clarify the impact of a physical deficit on a person.[57] *Impairment* is "any loss or abnormality of psychological, physical, or anatomical structure of function," e.g., paralysis. *Disability* is "any restriction or lack (resulting from an impairment) of an ability to perform an activity in a manner within the range considered normal for a human being," e.g., paralysis resulting in an inability to walk. *Handicap* is "a disadvantage for a given individual resulting from an impairment or disability that limits or prevents the fulfillment of a role that is normal (depending on age, sex, and social and cultural factors) for that individual," e.g., paralyzed and unable to walk and thus unable to meet the requirements of the job and therefore cannot return to work.

In order to assess function accurately and to monitor changes in it, the performance in different activities of self-care, mobility, and communication, must be numerically, rated according to the patient's level of independence, i.e., completely independent, independent with devices, requires assistance (supervision, "spotting," reminding, physical help) or completely dependent. This requires collection by various means of numerous diverse data, i.e, physical examination, observation, review of records and reports from the various rehabilitation team members, as well as gathering of information directly from the patient and family. Several evaluation scales exist. Some are simple and easy to use but provide incomplete information, whereas others are detailed and time consuming as they address a whole range of quality of life factors, which include mobility, self-care, employment, income, education, family activities, living arrangements, and transportation. Computer technology has made the gathering, analysis, and plotting of data easier and has enabled clinicians to document the patient's progress numerically, both during inpatient and outpatient rehabilitation care. The functional evaluation scale which currently is gaining the widest acceptance by rehabilitation professionals is the "Functional Independence Measure" (FIM) (Table XXII-1-3), but for cancer patients the Karnofsky Performance Status Scale has been most widely used (Table XXII-1-4).[29]

Table XXII-1-3.   Functional Independence Measure (FIM)

L E V E L S	7 Complete Independence (Timely, Safely) 6 Modified Independence (Device)	NO HELPER

	Modified Dependence
	  5 Supervision
	  4 Minimal Assist (Subject = 75%+)
	  3 Moderate Assist (Subject = 50%+)
	Complete Dependence
	  2 Maximal Assist (Subject = 25%+)
	  1 Total Assist (Subject = 0%+)
		HELPER

	ADMIT	DISCHG	FOL-UP
Self Care A. Eating B. Grooming C. Bathing D. Dressing-Upper Body E. Dressing-Lower Body F. Toileting			
Sphincter Control G. Bladder Management H. Bowel Management			
Mobility Transfer: I. Bed, Chair, Wheelchair J. Toilet K. Tub, Shower			
Locomotion L. Walk/wheel Chair M. Stairs			
Communication N. Comprehension O. Expression			
Social Cognition P. Social Interaction Q. Problem Solving R. Memory			
Total FIM			

NOTE: Leave no blanks; enter 1 if patient not testable due to risk.

The Rehabilitation Process

Rehabilitation services are frequently requested too late in the care of the cancer patient. The physiatrist should be consulted as soon as it may be anticipated that the cancer will result in a physical disability. The rehabilitation interventions may thus be planned and explained to the patient before, during or immediately following definitive treatment. Physical and occupational therapy is initially provided bedside, but the patient should be mobilized out of bed as soon as possible and escorted to the rehabilitation area where facilities and equipment are conducive to better performance. Other members of the rehabilitation team become involved in the care of the disabled cancer patient as deemed appropriate by the physiatrist. If these interventions allow the patient to become self-sufficient and ambulatory, he should be discharged home directly from the acute service, when medically indicated, having received proper instructions, equipment and referrals for specific nursing interventions.

A more comprehensive and intensive rehabilitation program on an inpatient rehabilitation service is provided for physically disabled cancer patients who do not gain independence in ADL and mobility with one or two weeks of daily therapy on the acute service, whose life expectancy is greater than one year, who are medically capable of actively participating in the program for at least three hours daily, and who are motivated and mentally capable of following instructions and learning the different tasks.

The inpatient rehabilitation unit should be in a hospital with an in-house physician on call and the different medical and surgical consultation services available at all times. Here the disabled cancer patient is re-evaluated by the physiatrist who obtains a detailed medical and social history and performs a careful physical examination in order to assess the general medical and the precise musculoskeletal and neurological condition, as well as the current functional ability. The physiatrist writes the routine medical orders, e.g., for nursing care, medications, disability-specific diagnostic tests, i.e., radiological studies, urological evaluation, pulmonary function tests, electrodiagnostic studies, and blood and urine analyses. The physiatrist sets at this time the general rehabilitation goals for the patient and prescribes evaluation and interventions to be undertaken by the various members of the multi-disciplinary rehabilitation team. The physiatrist prescribes the specific exercises and training methods to be given by the physical and occupational therapist, as well as interventions by the psychologist, speech pathologist, vocational and recreational counselors, and others when they are needed.

The rehabilitation program begins promptly after transfer to the inpatient rehabilitation service. Initially the actual participation of patients on the program may be impeded by the physical deconditioning or by special evaluations and tests, but after the first few days four to six hours each day are spent in an active therapy program in addition to different ward activities, e.g., self-care training, management of bowel and bladder dysfunction, educational and recreational activities. When serious medical complications arise during the course of rehabilitation and interfere with the patient's ability to attend the rehabilitation program for at least three hours a day for more than three consecutive days, the patient should be transferred to the appropriate medical or surgical services for definitive care.

Within one week of admission an initial team conference is held where the patient's medical, functional, psychological, social, vocational, recreational status, as well as the rehabilitation potential and prognosis are presented and discussed. More specific rehabilitation goals are set, needs for equipment and personal assistance are assessed and a discharge date is predicted. Soon after this conference the physiatrist meets with the patient and the family, together or separately, to discuss these issues and answer questions regarding the patient's medical condition and rehabilitation program. Team rehabilitation conferences are held bi-weekly to discuss the progress and plans for discharge. While the patient is making continuous and measurable progress towards the set functional goals of independence in ADL and mobility, continued inpatient stay may be justified. Communication between members of the rehabilitation team, a most critical component, is facilitated through informal meetings during which specific concerns that any member of the team may have about any patient are shared and discussed. When the patient is discharged to home it is most important to ensure that needed equipment and supplies have been

Table XXII-1-4. Karnofsky Performance Status Index

General Category	Index	Specific Criteria
Able to carry on normal activity, no special care needed.	100	Normal, no complaints, no evidence of disease.
	90	Able to carry on normal activity, minor signs or symptoms of disease.
	80	Normal activity with effort, some signs or symptoms of disease.
Unable to work, able to live at home and care for most personal needs, varying amount of assistance needed.	70	Cares for self, unable to carry on normal activity or to do work.
	60	Requires occasional assistance from others, but able to care for most needs.
	50	Requires considerable assistance from others; frequent medical care.
Unable to care for self, requires institutional or hospital care or equivalent, disease may be rapidly progressing.	40	Disabled, requires special care and assistance.
	30	Severely disabled, hospitalization indicated; death not imminent.
	20	Very sick, hospitalization necessary; active supportive treatment necessary.
	10	Moribund
	0	Dead

obtained, family members or home health aides have been instructed and trained in the patient's care, follow-up by the visiting nurse service has been arranged, and referrals have been made for continued therapy and visits with various physicians, e.g., the oncologist, surgeon, physiatrist and family doctor.

Cancer of the Brain

Brain damage may result from primary tumors of the brain, metastatic disease and from treatment of the cancer, i.e., surgery, radiation or, more rarely, chemotherapy. The symptoms and disability which may result vary extensively, but in essence are similar to those that are seen in patients who have sustained traumatic brain injury or a stroke involving different parts of the brain (Table XXII-1-5). The main difference here is the potentially progressive or recurrent nature of the brain cancer and its uncertain prognosis. The greatest deficits are frequently seen immediately after surgery or during radiation and chemotherapy, after which remarkable improvement may occur. All patients with brain cancer and

Table XXII-1-5. Rehabilitation Problems Associated with Cancer of the Brain

Paralysis
Spasticity
Joint contractures
Pain
Sensory deficits
Visual field deficits
Diplopia
Aphasia
Dysarthria
Aprosodia
Dysphagia
Ataxia
Visual-perceptual deficits
Cognitive and behavioral deficits
Psycho-social-vocational problems

impaired function in mobility or ADL, should be referred for rehabilitation services. The majority can be helped with simple rehabilitation measures while others may require comprehensive inpatient rehabilitation which should be provided when longer life expectancy allows.

Most commonly the rehabilitation intervention starts after surgical resection or removal of the brain tumor. When the patient is medically stable he should be helped to sit up, get out of bed and start on active restoration program which is designed according to his general condition. The location and size of the cerebral lesion clearly determine the clinical symptoms encountered. The variability of the symptoms precludes a standard rehabilitation approach but demands an individual evaluation and treatment plan. Broadly the problems of patients with cancer of the brain are physical, psychological, social and vocational. Table XXII-1-5 shows a detailed list of problems that are most commonly found, and will be briefly discussed below.

Paralysis often in the form of hemiplegia or hemiparesis, can be a conspicuous consequence of brain cancer. While the paralysis is most profound just after the brain surgery, certain return of motor power is common and may continue for several weeks or months. As a rule, the earlier that this return is seen the greater is the recovery that can be expected. However, muscles that are still totally paralyzed four to eight weeks postoperatively generally remain so. At this point functional improvement can still occur through physical training and provision of appropriate assistive devices, e.g., orthoses or canes. While the medical condition is unstable, the patient is kept at bedrest, resting on a firm mattress with a soft surface, i.e, sheepskin, to prevent pressure sores. He should usually lie in the extended position with the affected arm abducted, externally rotated, and slightly elevated. Joint range of motion exercises should be given to the paralyzed parts and active exercises to the uninvolved parts twice a day.

Mobilization training starts when the patient is ready to be transferred out of bed. Depending on the extent of the paralysis the patient may be taught to ambulate with assistive devices or to maneuver a wheelchair. When the motor dysfunction is severe, he is first placed on a tilt table in order to decrease orthostatic hypotension and fear of the upright position, to stimulate antigravity muscles and to improve body balance. When the patient has regained some degree of body balance and lower extremity strength, he is stood up between parallel bars for balancing exercises and early ambulation training. At this stage the knee extensors on the affected side may be weak and require stabilization with a temporary knee ankle foot orthosis (KAFO) which locks the knee in extension for weight bearing. As the body balance improves and the patient has learned to lean consistently to his good side, ambulation outside of parallel bars can begin with the patient supporting himself on a broad based cane carried in the unaffected upper extremity. Usually some knee extensor strength returns, allowing the patient adequate knee support, but the ankle dorsiflexors and invertors still may be weak. Here a plastic ankle foot orthosis (AFO) may be prescribed in order to prevent foot dragging during the swing phase of gait. This orthosis is easily inserted into most shoes. It is cosmetically superior to the old metal orthoses and usually provides equal or better function. If knee extensor strength does not return, fabrication of a KAFO may be considered but the prognosis for functional ambulation with such a device is poor.

Training and elevation activities, i.e., climbing and descending stairs, ramps or curbs, is started when a good gait pattern on level ground has been achieved. Patients with severe neurological deficits may require a wheelchair either for all mobility or only at times when ambulation endurance or safety is impaired.

The major goal in the rehabilitation of the patient with cancer of the brain is independence in ADL, which may be obtained through training, prescription of proper assistive devices and possibly modification of the patients clothing and the architecture of his home.

Spasticity frequently interferes with mobility and performance of ADL. Factors which may aggravate the spasticity, e.g., skin lesions, infections, and anxiety need to be identified and treated. Thorough stretching of all joints should be performed daily. Medications, i.e, dantrolene sodium, baclofen, and diazepam, may be of certain benefit but should be used sparingly due to potential side effects. Selected nerve blocks with dilute solutions of phenol or concentrated alcohol are usually effective in reducing spasticity in the distribution of the nerve, but surgical procedures for reduction of spasticity in patients with cancer of the brain are rarely indicated.

Joint contractures, whether due to muscle imbalance, spasticity, poor nursing care, improper bed positioning or an inadequate exercise program, may change the rehabilitation prognosis significantly. A ten-degree flexion contracture of the knee, for example, will greatly increase oxygen consumption during ambulation and thus markedly reduce endurance. Knee contractures which exceed fifteen degrees will usually make functional ambulation impossible for the patient with brain cancer and hemiplegia. Development of a frozen shoulder may make independent dressing impossible. Prevention of contractures by proper joint range of motion exercises is imperative from the onset of the disability, since treatment is relatively ineffective.

Pain in different parts of the body may be experienced in patients with neurological deficits caused by cancer of the brain. Dysesthetic thalamic pain is notably refractive to treatment, although various centrally acting agents may be helpful. Pain with motion of the hemiplegic shoulder is common, perhaps due to muscle imbalance at the shoulder girdle and recurrent minor trauma to the periarticular structures. Shoulder support by an arm sling or a lap board, administration of analgetics, application of heat or cold modalities and gentle range of motion and strengthening exercises may all help to reduce the pain and improve shoulder function. Reflex sympathetic dystrophy (shoulder hand syndrome) may occur and requires similar treatment, but more effective relief may be obtained by simply administering oral steroids, i.e., prednisone 5 mg × 4 per day for 2–3 weeks.[10] Serial stellate ganglion blocks may be performed when symptoms are more persistent.

Sensory deficits of varying degrees are commonly seen in patients with brain cancer, either in the distribution of the cranial nerves or on one or both sides of the body. Cancer affecting the parietal lobes of the brain may cause severe sensory loss with little muscle weakness. This may interfere with balance and mobility since the patient who cannot feel motion is unable to control it. Although physical exercise cannot decrease the sensory loss, training with adaptive gait aids, i.e., canes, crutches or a walker, and wearing of proper shoes, may help the patient to ambulate functionally again.

Visual deficits, i.e., double vision or visual field deficits, are commonly seen as a result of cancer in the lower brain or above the tentorium respectively. While double vision may improve spontaneously, wearing of alternating or unilateral eye patches or special prism glasses may be helpful. The value of exercises for retraining the eye muscles is uncertain. Homonymous hemianopsia, i.e., blindness to the affected side of the body due to a contralateral brain tumor, rarely resolves spontaneously. While a patient with a left brain lesion usually learns easily to compensate for hemianopsia through scanning of the environment, the patient with right brain lesion may experience severe difficulties due to accompanying anosognosia, i.e., lack of awareness of the affected left side of the body and of the surroundings. However, specialized programs of cognitive remediation have been found to be effective with these patients.[26]

Aphasia may be seen in patients with cancer in the left dominant hemisphere of the brain. This is an impairment of the central language process with reduced capacity for interpretation and formulation of the symbols for communication. Although all components of language, i.e., listening, speaking, reading and writing, are usually affected, they are not affected to equal extent and thus several types of aphasia are recognized.[1,21] Expressive or nonfluent aphasia is caused by lesions in the Broca's area of the brain and are characterized by reduced language production, vocabulary and use of grammar. The patient is well aware of these difficulties and very frustrated. Less well known is receptive or fluent aphasia which is caused by lesions in the Wernicke's area of the brain. Here the patient primarily has difficulty in understanding language, both his own, and that of others. He may thus be able to speak continuously with normal speed and melody without giving any pertinent information and be unaware of his errors. Most aphasic patients however understand nonverbal sounds and enjoy listening to music and frequently some automatic speech is retained.

Different objective tests can be performed to assess the patient's language and communication skills, but many patients perform better during a conversation than on such tests, since they may be able to grasp certain key words and successfully make guesses as well as understand gesticulations, facial expressions, the tone of voice, and other situational clues. The efficiency of speech therapy is debated since most patients will have a degree of spontaneous improvement. Nonetheless, speech therapy is indicated whenever available not only for psychological support, but also to provide the necessary stimulation for the patient to utilize his maximum speech ability, to allow him to adjust to new circumstances, and to instruct the family in proper communication with the patient by such means as using short simple sentences at a normal voice volume, utilizing gestures and facial expressions while showing respect, optimism, patience and encouragement.

Dysarthria is a motor disturbance of speech which implies weakness, slowness, or incoordination of the muscles that produce speech. Understanding of written or spoken language is therefore never a problem. Articulation is usually the main problem, but disturbance of speed, rhythm, sound and intonation may also be present. Mild dysarthria accompanies many brain cancers that involve cranial nerves and cerebrum and affect the facial musculature, but it is particularly prominent in brain stem tumors. Management, which is often successful, emphasizes teaching the patient to use his remaining speech muscles more effectively or to bypass the effects of disturbed function. First the patient is guided in producing sounds, then words and finally whole sentences. If speech still remains completely unintelligible, other communication methods are introduced, i.e., writing, typing, sign language, or pictures.

Aprosodia is a little known communication disorder which is seen with lesions of the nondominant right hemisphere.[44] This condition relates to inability to express and comprehend variations in pitch, rhythm, and stress, which give emotional meaning to speech. These patients may therefore speak in a relatively flat voice and are often unable to recognize the emotional tones of speech, including the meaning of nonlanguage speech sounds, e.g., grunts, or sighs. It is important for the clinician and the family to understand this deficit and communicate with the patient strictly by words, since specific therapy does not exist. Considerable improvement usually occurs with time.

Dysphagia or impaired swallowing is frequently seen in patients with brain cancer, especially when the brain stem is involved. In its most severe form the patient may be totally unable to swallow, but in milder cases there may only be difficulty with swallowing of liquids. Aspiration with resulting pneumonia may occur, thus demanding careful evaluation of the condition and proper intervention. Serial radiographic swallowing studies should be done for proper monitoring of the condition until it is resolved or other and safer means of nutrition are established. A swallowing training program may be instituted by the speech or occupational therapist where the patient attempts to swallow food of different consistency using different techniques and positions. While a nasogastric tube can be used for several weeks while waiting for spontaneous recovery, a more persistent dysphagia warrants insertion of a gastrostomy tube for prolonged feeding.

Neuropsychological changes of different sorts may be prominently noted in cancer affecting the cerebral hemispheres. Reduced memory and judgement frequently make successful rehabilitation impossible as the patient may be unable to remember instructions. Severe agitation may need treatment with a major tranquilizer, e.g., chlorpromazine or haloperidol. Visual perceptual deficits, caused by a central disturbance in organizing visual stimuli from the environment, frequently accompany right brain damage even when visual field and acuity may be normal. These patients may experience difficulty in recognizing the three dimensions, i.e., depth and distances, the relationship of lines and objects, and vertical and horizontal lines. This may in turn affect different functions, e.g., reading, understanding maps, recognizing familiar objects, and driving vehicles safely. Similarly, these patients may be unable to recognize the emotional significance of facial expressions adding to the communication problems caused by the frequently accompanying aprosodia. There is a tendency to be impulsive and careless, to minimize or even ignore the problems in functioning, to make frequent mistakes and often to neglect their left environment (anosognosia). Patients with lesions in the left hemisphere, on the other hand, usually act and learn slowly, make few mistakes, and are aware of their deficits which frustrate them severely. In recent years neuropsychological training programs designed to help patients overcome the visual, perceptual and cognitive deficits have been reported as being successful.[27] In addition, repeated neuropsychological evaluations have been found to be sensitive indicators of recurrence.[39]

Cancer of the Spine

While primary tumors of the vertebrae, e.g., multiple myeloma, are uncommon, metastases to the spine are frequent. At autopsy more than 5% of patients with systemic cancer were found to have evidence of metastatic compression of the spinal cord.[2] This is usually an extradural anterior mass which involves bone. Intradural extramedullary tumors are usually histologically benign meningiomas or neurofibromas. Gliomas, i.e., ependymomas, astrocytomas, and medulloblastomas, are usually intramedullary, although occasionally found also in an extramedullary site. Although the histology and response to treatment is quite different for all these tumors, the neurological symptoms, signs, and rehabilitation interventions are quite similar, which permits the clinical findings and therapy for these conditions be addressed simultaneously in this chapter.

Clinical Presentation. By far the most frequent presenting symptom of a tumor of the spine is pain. The pain may be localized, diffuse, or radicular in nature. It is characteristically made worse by activity and by straining. Different from more benign back pain, the pain caused by tumors tends to be persistent, present or even worse at night, and not relieved by rest. Additional symptoms at presentation may be weakness of the legs, difficulty in walking, and urinary sphincteric problems leading to overflow symptomatology or incontinence.

Neurological deficits may develop insidiously or occur suddenly depending on the tumor's rate of growth and location, or on the occurrence of a sudden pathological fracture. Slowly progressive neurological dysfunction is often seen with tumors of the lower spine which encroach on the cauda equina, whereas tumors of the thoracic spine may cause sudden collapse of a vertebral body with direct compression of the spinal cord or of its blood supply. Although only half of all tumors of the spine are located in the thoracic region, these cause 70% of all spinal cord compressions which result in paraplegia. Such paraplegia may be neurologically complete, i.e., with total paralysis and sensory loss below the level of the lesion. More frequently, however, the neurologic lesion is incomplete, with sensation and motor function preserved to a varying degree as may be rated by the Frankel classification scale.[13,18] Impaired bladder and bowel control at first may present clinically as urinary urgency or hesitancy, but with progressive cord compression urinary retention or bowel and bladder incontinence may occur.

Treatment. Proper rehabilitation management plan and intervention depends on accurate diagnosis and staging of the tumor, exactly as does the medical and surgical management. Most patients with spinal metastases can and should be managed non-surgically with radiation, chemotherapy and orthotic stabilization of the spine, since it has been demonstrated that radiation alone provides results that are similar

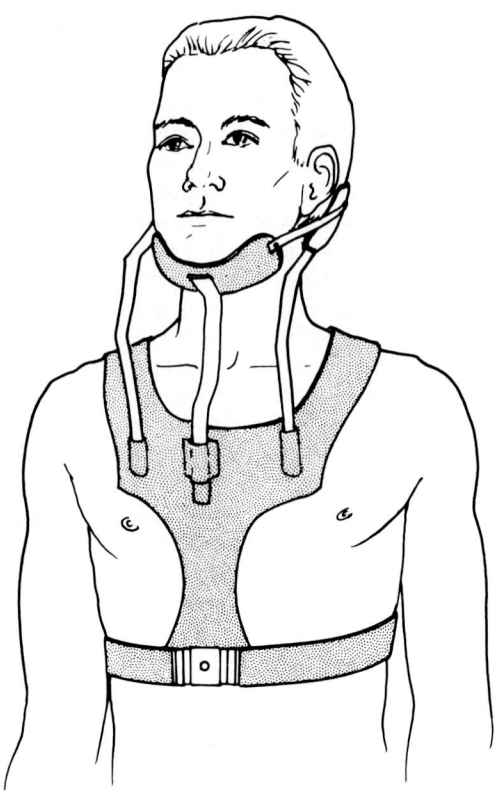

Figure XXII-1-2. Sternal-occipital-mandibular immobilizer (SOMI orthosis). (Reproduced by permission from Ragnarsson KT: Orthotics and Shoes. *In* Rehabilitation Medicine: Principles and Practice. Edited by Joel A. DeLisa, Philadelphia, J.B. Lippincott, 1988).

to those of surgery followed by radiation.[22] In general, laminectomy with decompression has been found to be of limited use compared to radiation, since the compressive lesion is usually located anteriorly to the cord and as the surgical procedure itself contributes to spinal instability. Profound neurological deficits, especially when occurring rapidly, however, may warrant surgical decompression which preferably should be done by an anterior approach followed by surgical stabilization of the spine. Surgical decompression of the spinal cord is not very effective once the patient has become completely paraplegic. Surgical stabilization may often be indicated when gross spinal instability is present. Spinal instability may be present when two of the three "columns" (anterior, middle and posterior) of the spine have been destroyed by the tumor.[16] The extent of surgical stabilization varies depending on the patient's anticipated life expectancy. Patients with short life expectancy (less than one year) benefit most from a relatively simple procedure employing methylmethacrylate, which allows immediate spinal stability and rapid mobilization of the patient, whereas patients with a more favorable prognosis may be better served with vertebrectomy, spinal instrumentation and bony fusion in conjunction with methylmethacrylate.[16]

Spinal metastases and myelomatous lesions, even when accompanied by compression fractures and minor or modest spinal instability, can be successfully managed by spinal orthotic support and radiation. Both modalities may significantly decrease pain. Lesions in the cervical spine are most

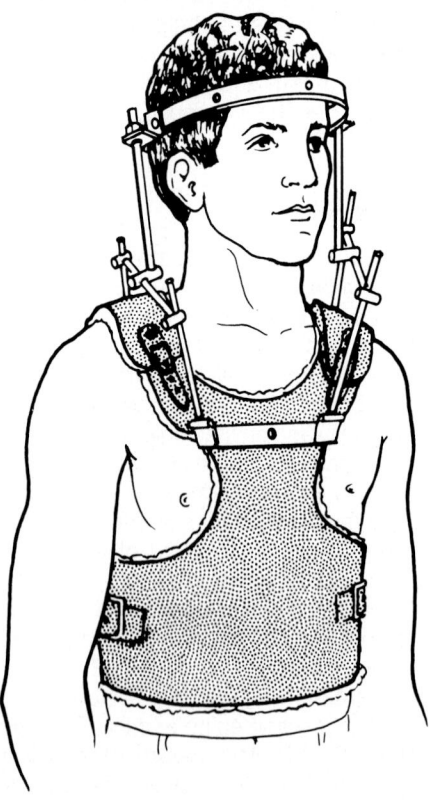

Figure XXII-1-1. Halo-orthosis. (Reproduced by permission from Ragnarsson KT: Orthotics and Shoes. *In* Rehabilitation Medicine: Principles and Practice. Edited by Joel A. DeLisa, Philadelphia, J.B. Lippincott, 1988).

rigidly immobilized by a halo brace (Figure XXII-1-1), but also may be adequately supported by SOMI brace (Sternal-occipital-mandibular-immobilizer) (Figure XXII-1-2). When such lesions are present in the upper thoracic spine, spinal orthoses may not be necessary, as this part of the spine is stabilized inherently by the rib cage. Lesions in the more mobile lower thoracic and lumbar spine are often associated with severe pain. An adjustable thoraco-lumbo sacral (TLS) orthosis (Figure XXII-1-3) with posterior stays may provide sufficient support for less severe lesions, decrease pain and allow greater mobility. The soft anterior portion of the corset, the apron, should fit snugly over the entire abdomen for optimal support. Larger lesions and post-operative conditions may require fabrication of a custom molded plastic TLS brace, a two-piece removable orthosis (Figure XXII-1-4) which firmly grabs the pelvis below and the chest above.

When neurological loss has occurred, the rehabilitation therapy must be carefully individualized, based on the extent of the neurological dysfunction, the medical/surgical condition and the patient's life expectancy. Spinal cord dysfunction with severe or complete paralysis and sensory loss and perhaps bladder and bowel dysfunction warrants a comprehensive but a relatively short term rehabilitation program involving as many members of the rehabilitation team as judged appropriate by the physiatrist. The rehabilitation programs should be designed to address each of the many clinical complications and conditions which may be seen in individuals with spinal cord dysfunction of traumatic origin (Table XXII-1-6). Early intervention should include bedside physical and occupational therapy, establishment of bowel and bladder training programs, and the application of nursing principles to prevent complications, such as pressure

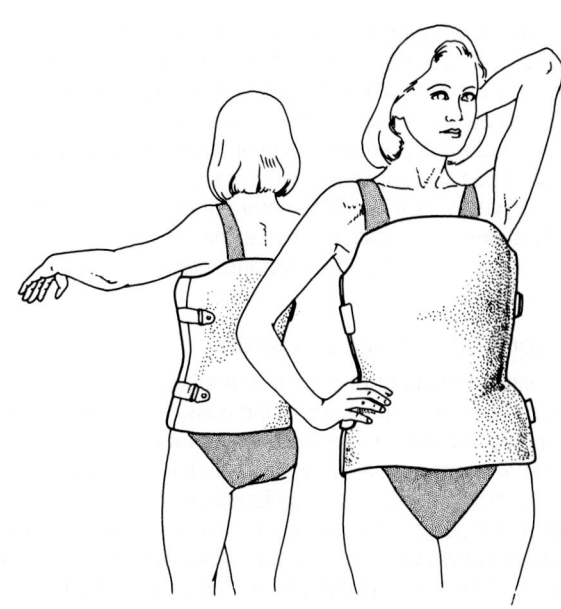

Figure XXII-1-4. Custom molded thoraco-lumbo-sacral orthosis (TLSO), a two-piece removable plastic orthosis ("body jacket"). (Reproduced by permission from Ragnarsson, KJ: Rehabilitation of patients with physical disabilities caused by tumors of the musculoskeletal system. *In* Tumors of the Musculoskeletal System. Edited by Michael M. Lewis. New York, W. B. Saunders Co., 1991.)

Table XXII-1-6. Conditions and Complications Associated with Spinal Cord Dysfunction

Loss of motor power
Loss of sensation
Pressure sores
Urinary dysfunction
Bowel dysfunction
Sexual dysfunction
Autonomic hyperreflexia
Pain
Spasticity
Joint contractures
Heterotopic ossifications
Metabolic disturbances
    a. Negative calcium balance
    b. Negative nitrogen balance
    c. Hormonal imbalance
Circulatory disturbances
    a. Orthostatic hypotension
    b. Edema
    c. Deep vein thrombophlebitis
Respiratory disturbances
Psychological problems
Social problems
Vocational problems

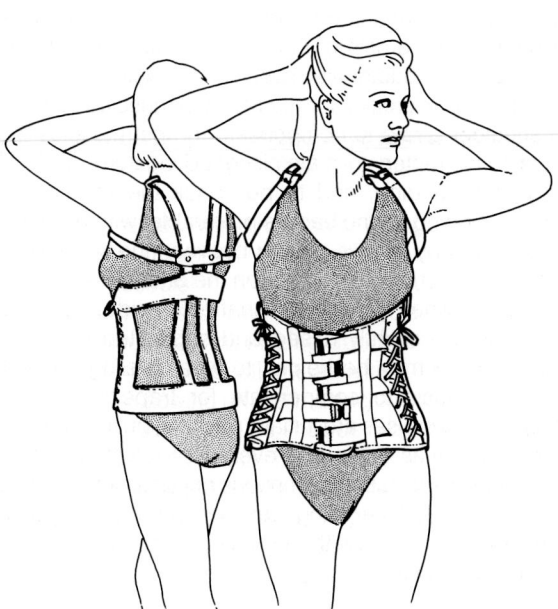

Figure XXII-1-3. Thoraco-lumbo-sacral orthosis (TLSO, Knight-Taylor brace). (Reproduced by permission from Ragnarsson, KJ: Rehabilitation of patients with physical disabilities caused by tumors of the musculoskeletal system. *In* Tumors of the Musculoskeletal System. Edited by Michael M. Lewis. New York, W. B. Saunders Co., 1991.)

sores and joint contractures which increase morbidity, worsen the functional prognosis and prolong the rehabilitation phase. Proper positioning of the patient in bed and turning at least every two hours is of paramount importance in this regard. The patient and his family are given emotional support and are educated in the medical aspects of spinal cord dysfunction and management. If prognosis is poor, i.e., less than

sure gradiated elastic sleeve should be fabricated and worn continuously. The entire limb needs to be guarded against even trivial trauma, which may be caused by constricting garments, excessive heat or exercise, in order to minimize swelling. Treatment with these physical modalities has been shown to benefit the majority of patients with post-operative lymphedema and is more effective than diuretics and surgical procedures.[59]

Cancer of the Gastrointestinal Tract

The cancer rehabilitation team is involved in the care of the patient who has cancer limited to the gastrointestinal tract when the definitive surgical treatment has resulted in an ostomy. The Enterostomal Therapist (ET nurse) plays a major role in helping the cancer patient with an ostomy, i.e., colostomy, ileostomy or urostomy, to understand the principles of ostomy care, to learn the different aspects of ostomy management, and to adjust to the altered self image.

Colostomy. The surgical treatment of cancer of the rectum usually mandates the creation of a colostomy, using the sigmoid colon. A cancer higher in the colon can frequently be resected and the bowel reconnected by anastomosis. Before undergoing a surgical procedure for cancer which will result in colostomy, the surgeon needs to discuss his plans carefully with the patient. Subsequently, the ET nurse should meet with the patient and family members to explain in simple but clear terms the nature of the colostomy, e.g., where the stoma will be located on the abdominal wall, how it will look, what coverings and collection appliances will be needed, how evacuation will occur and so on. A positive attitude on the part of the medical and nursing staff is important at this time, although the patient's fears and concerns regarding function, appearance and sexual activity need to be acknowledged and discussed. Excessive and explicit explanations, particularly regarding the details of the surgical procedure and subsequent care, should be based on a patients individual needs. Too much information that the patient is not ready to absorb may do little but increase anxiety. A visit by a person who is successfully managing his/her colostomy may be very helpful. Good pre-operative preparation reduces the patients fears and builds confidence, both of which will facilitate post-operative rehabilitation.

Post-operatively, protecting the skin and collecting the drainage should be the primary goals. This is accomplished by a properly fit appliance. Modern appliances with protective skin barriers cut to fit the exact size of the stoma will avoid post-op peristomal skin excoriation and keep the patient dry and odor free. A person with a colostomy has a choice of allowing his bowels to function normally or to irrigate as a method of attempting to control bowel movements. Often the bowel habits return to normal patterns and a well fitting appliance may be emptied or changed as needed. Proper fit of an appliance by an ET nurse allows the patient to make an informed choice as the appliances are odor proof, disposable and have protective pectin skin barriers attached to keep peristomal skin healthy and free from irritating discharge.

If the patient chooses to learn irrigation techniques this cannot always be taught in the hospital setting given current reimbursement regulations (Diagnostic Related Groups, DRG)

and pressure for early discharge. Outpatient ET services and/or Visiting Nurses often teach or continue to teach the irrigation in the home after discharge. The purpose of the irrigation is to establish a bowel routine with the goal of evacuating only after the irrigation rather than spontaneously or at inopportune moments. However, this is not always possible. Therefore the patient should always be instructed in care and use of a properly fit appliance. This may help the patient to avoid the frustrations that usually are experienced when bowel discharge continues between the irrigations. Irrigation of the colostomy may be done daily, every other day, or even every third day, and usually either in the morning or in the evening depending on the patient's preferences. Initially a full hour should be allocated for the irrigation and evacuation, although later 30 minutes may suffice to complete the task. The first irrigation is an important event that requires both sensitivity and technical skills on the part of the ET nurse. The irrigation should be done in private, preferably with the patient sitting by the toilet on a comfortable soft chair. A lubricated cone is gently inserted into the stoma and one liter of lukewarm tap water is instilled over a time period of approximately 10 minutes from an enema bag placed no higher than at the shoulder level, similar to administering an enema. The water distends the bowel, causes peristalsis and expulsion of the stools. Following evacuation the skin is cleansed with warm water and patted dry. The pouch is reapplied. A family member may want to learn instructions in colostomy care, both in order to understand the patient's plight, and to be able to assist or take over the care during periods of illness. The patient and the family are provided with information on the United Ostomy Association, its local chapters and publications as a resource for further information. After surgery, the patient is placed on a diet of clear liquids, which is followed by full fluids and later solid food. A well balanced diet and the importance of a high fiber, low fat diet is discussed. It is best to increase the diet's fiber content gradually in order to avoid gas formation and bloating by adding fruits, vegetables and whole grain food in slowly increasing amounts.

Numerous clinical problems may arise at any time after the creation of a colostomy. *Constipation* is often due to inadequate intake of fluids or dietary fiber, but may be successfully managed by increasing dietary fiber (Fiber-all) and increasing fluid intake. *Diarrhea* may be caused by different foods (spicy, greasy or fried foods, certain vegetables, fruits and juices), but small amounts of liquid stools may indicate incomplete evacuation or presence of impacted feces. *Excessive gas formation* also may result from ingestion of certain foods (baked beans, onions, greasy food), anxiety and other factors which need to be identified and treated appropriately. *Noxious odor* may be increased by different foods and liquids (cabbage, egg, onions, garlic, beer, coffee). Each person must experiment with different foods. What may adversely affect one person may not affect another. Deodorant tablets placed in the disposable colostomy pouch may help to diminish odors. *Skin excoriation and maceration* will usually respond to appropriate local care by gentle washing with soap and water and applying a properly fit appliance. *Skin infections* may be caused by fungi or bacteria. Fungal infections should be treated with nystatin powder and bacterial infections by administering topical or, occasionally, oral antibiotics. *Stomal bleeding* in small amounts is usually of little concern, but if persistent, mixed with stools or in large amounts, it will require proper diagnostic evaluation and intervention. *Sexual dysfunction* after colostomy is not common, but when impotence does occur it is primarily due to damage to the autonomic nerves in the pelvis sustained during extensive abdominal perineal resection of the cancerous bowel. Altered self image often associated with the colostomy can cause temporary dysfunction. Males may become impotent and females anorgasmic while sexual desire is not lessened.[23] Sexual counselling for both partners, good communication, and learning of new techniques for mutual satisfaction can do much to restore successful sexual activity. The colostomy patient will normally experience a reactive depression or grief, and subsequently go through the different stages of adaptation which are associated with any kind of major personal loss. The colostomy's negative influence on the patient's self-image is best counteracted by the physician and the ET nurse through making an accurate assessment of the patient's complaints and condition, planning experiences and interventions accordingly, and providing supportive counselling on an individual basis.[3]

Ileostomy. This surgical treatment for cancer is performed in some chronic cases of ulcerative colitis. The principles and techniques of stoma care are similar to those of colostomy. The stools are of a loose consistency and drain continuously from the ileostomy. It is therefore necessary that the collecting pouch be worn at all hours and that it be properly fit by an ET nurse. Small bowel content contain active digestive enzymes which can cause severe peristomal skin excoriation if leakage occurs. The collecting pouch must be emptied as needed, usually every three to six hours, by releasing the clamp from the bottom of the pouch and emptying the contents directly into the toilet. Since the fluid loss through ileostomy is greater than colostomy, fluid intake must be increased to prevent dehydration. There are no dietary restrictions except avoiding corn and peanuts, but the food should be eaten slowly and chewed well in order to avoid food blockage. Greater loss of electrolytes and certain vitamins, especially B-12, may also be experienced and require regular monitoring and supplementation. Certain coated medications and time-release capsules may pass through the gut without being digested, a fact to be considered whenever physicians prescribe medications for individuals with ileostomy. In general, the psychosocial adjustment and rehabilitation outcome for an individual with ileostomy is similar to that after any surgery requiring alteration of elimination habits that result in living with a stoma.

Cancer of the Genito-Urinary System

Invasive cancer of the bladder frequently requires radical cystectomy and a urinary diversion, i.e., creation of a new outlet for urine. More than 40 years ago Bricker developed the ileal conduit procedure by connecting the ureters to an isolated section of ileum, which is surgically closed at one end but opens at the other as a stoma on the abdominal wall, allowing free elimination of the urine. This procedure has become the traditional form of long term urinary diversion. The management principles of ileal conduit stoma care

are similar to those of colostomy and ileostomy. Since urine flows continuously from the stoma, the collecting system must be well fit and water tight in order to prevent leakage. The collecting pouch must have a drain valve for easy emptying and for connecting to a night time urine collection bag. Skin or stoma problems from the urine are not uncommon and may be caused by alkaline urine. Many physicians prescribe Vitamin C 1000 mg daily to keep urine slightly acid. The intake of 8–10 glasses of fluid daily is very important. In recent years the continent urostomy has gained considerable popularity when used with compliant patients. The Kock pouch and the Indiana pouch, with several modifications of both procedures, result in an internal reservoir.[4,8,37,45,46,51] The patient inserts a catheter into the stoma every 4–6 hours to empty the internal pouch contents. This procedure eliminates the need for external devices.

Genital Cancer. Members of the cancer rehabilitation team may occasionally be asked to provide care for the patient with cancer involving the genital organs, or when the cancer and its treatment has caused sexual dysfunction. Rehabilitation interventions for these usually involve carefully planned reconstructive surgery and psychological and sexual counselling. The form of surgical reconstruction varies quite obviously depending on the type of the cancer and the extent of the surgical resection, but also on the specific needs of the patient. The female who has undergone radical gynecological surgery with resection of the vagina may benefit from vaginal reconstruction which allows resumption of sexual intercourse.[14] The male patient, who is unable to achieve penile erection, can have a penile prosthesis implanted. The choice of prosthesis is between semi-rigid silicone rod implants and a system of inflatable cylinders implanted into the shaft of the penis with scrotal pump and fluid reservoir placed in the abdominal wall.[17,42,47] The implantation of the semi-rigid rod is a relatively simple surgical procedure followed by relatively few mechanical problems but the penis stays semi-erect permanently. The inflatable prosthesis provides a more normal appearance of the penis when flaccid and erect, but mechanical problems with the system occur quite often.

Cancer of the testes is usually treated with prompt surgical excision of one or both of the testicles followed by radiation and/or chemotherapy. Surgical implantation of a prosthetic testicle at a later date may be very gratifying for many patients concerned about their appearance and self-image.

Sexual rehabilitation obviously is not limited to those that have cancer affecting the genital organs, but rather should be available for anyone who experiences sexual dysfunction for physical or psychological reasons due to the cancer and its treatment. Different members of the rehabilitation team collaborate in providing sexual counselling for patients with different forms of cancer, both on an individual basis and by organizing courses and seminars on the physiology and anatomy of sexual function, on human sexuality and means of adjusting to sexual dysfunction. Male sexual impotence compounds the reactive depression associated with the cancer diagnosis and adds to the stigma of any physical disability. This condition is frequently met with prejudice and poor understanding, both on the part of the patient and his sexual partner. Sexual rehabilitation emphasizes that sexuality is considered to be part of the whole person and cannot be lost due to an illness or any injury. Physical disability in contrast to a physical illness does not decrease sexual drive, although it may affect sexual function both physically and psychologically. The anatomy and physiology of sexual function should be carefully explained to the disabled patients and their spouses and general guidelines for success given. Good communication and strengthening of relationships between sexual partners are emphasized. The different physical aspects of sexual performance are clarified in order to make expectations compatible with performance capability. For most cancer patients with a physical disability, impairment of mobility, sensation, continence and erection should not interfere with building a solid personal relationship, with having sensitivity to the partner's desires or being able to please and enjoy. Sexual rehabilitation is built on the concept that if sexual comfort is taught, sexual competence may result.[9] No treatment or rehabilitation of the patient with cancer can be considered complete until the clinician has adequately addressed the impact of the condition on sexual function. Sexual health cannot be separated from total health. The extra time spent considering sexual adequacy and providing guidelines for help can benefit the patient for years.

Cancer of the Limbs

Primary malignant tumors of the limbs require surgical treatment. The main surgical goal is to remove the tumor, either by an excision with wide margins through a site well clear of any malignant growth, or by a radical resection, i.e., removal of the entire bone, or the compartment afflicted by the tumor. A subsequent surgical goal is to reconstruct the resulting defect for optimal function and cosmesis. The customary and most widely accepted surgical treatment is limb amputation, although in recent years limb preservation by extended local or regional excision and reconstruction has been advocated. The survival rate and period of disease-free life after both types of surgical approaches is similar and has improved in recent years by the use of chemotherapy, radiation, or both. The return to optimal function can best be assured by a multi-disciplinary rehabilitation team approach which includes the surgeon, the medical and radiation oncologists, the physiatrist and all the members of the rehabilitation team.

Metastases to the limb bones are less common than those to the spine. While some patients may complain of localized pain, others are essentially asymptomatic until a pathological fracture occurs. Such fractures occur in approximately ten to fifteen percent of patients who have radiographic evidence of skeletal metastasis. At particular risk are women, those with advanced metastatic disease and those with a large single lytic lesion eroding the bony cortex.[5] Active rehabilitation and physical mobilization does not seem to increase the fracture risk significantly. Prophylactic surgery is generally not warranted but radiation may have some effect in reducing pain and limiting tumor growth. Where prognosis allows many months of anticipated function, prophylactic surgery for impending fracture of the femoral neck or shaft often diminishes the total disability consequent to pathologic fracture and more difficult surgical repair. Open surgical treatment of a pathological fracture with adequate internal fixation and conjunctive use of methymethacrylate may be employed successfully in order to relieve pain, increase mobility, ease nursing care and for psychological reassurance.[48] Post-operative immobilization should be brief and aggressive physical therapy should be started early in order to return the patient swiftly to previous function, as well as to minimize hospitalization.

Preoperative Rehabilitation. Rehabilitation care should start immediately after the diagnosis of primary cancer of a limb is established, regardless of whether amputation or limb sparing reconstructive surgery is planned for cancer removal, or whether chemotherapy and radiation is to be instituted pre- or post-operatively. The implications of surgery and the post-operative course should at this time be discussed with the patient and his family. Simultaneously, an appropriate physical exercise program should begin. These interventions during the emotionally stressful pre-operative days may ease the patient's adjustment and reaction to the post-operative course. Emotional support is best given by recognizing the patient's fear and anxiety and by providing in a positive way some practical information and explicit factual instructions which can be easily understood and followed. While it is important that the positive aspects of the surgical treatment be explained, i.e., that it is a swift, life-saving technique, and that modern technology and training allow significant restoration of function, it is best for the physician to resist overly optimistic predictions and to discourage unrealistic hopes until certain post-operative rehabilitation success has been ensured. On the other hand, pessimistic statements on what the patient will never be able to do are needless and usually inaccurate. A time frame is provided for post-operative rehabilitation efforts and possible return to various functional activities, taking into consideration the extent of reconstruction, level of amputation, general physical and mental status, age, athletic ability, and life style. Peer counselling by a successful rehabilitated amputee may further help the patient to anticipate post-operative events and function.

When amputation or limb sparing surgery is planned, the exact level of amputation and the surgical approach should be thoughtfully chosen, taking into account not only the location and the type of cancer, but also the probability of good wound healing and the successful fitting of a prosthesis when required. It may be helpful for the surgeon to consult with the physiatrist and prosthetist for this purpose. Pre-operatively, strengthening exercises should be started for muscles in the uninvolved extremities and the trunk, as well as for muscles to be spared in the affected limb. Specifically the patient should learn to perform isometric exercises for the quadriceps and gluteal muscles. Strengthening exercises for the unaffected limbs should focus specifically on shoulder depressors and elbow extensors which are critical for ambulation with crutches or walkers. Trunk strengthening and balancing exercises may further ensure post-operative ambulation success. Ambulation with a walker or pair of crutches, non-weight bearing on the affected limb, should be practiced pre-operatively while the patient has no fear of falling due to lack of limb support and is not impaired by incisional pain, medications, or post-operative complications. Such pre-operative therapy will not only help the patient to succeed swiftly post-operatively in ambulation and self care activities, but a quick restoration of function will ease the emotional adjustment to the disability whether it be amputation or limb sparing with an internal prosthesis.

Limb Amputation. Limb amputation for cancer at one time was discouraged as the prevailing opinion was that poor life expectancy did not justify the expense of surgery and prosthetic fitting. However, it has been shown that five year survival for patients who have undergone amputations for limb cancer (49%) compares favorably with survival of patients with amputations for limb ischemia.[53] Another study has shown that functional skills of cancer amputees are better than those who have had amputations for other reasons.[35]

Until recently amputations for cancer were done in a radical fashion and left little if any residual limb (stump), except when amputating for very distal limb tumors, since the basic clinical rule was to amputate proximally to the joint next above the tumor site. Lower limb amputations for cancer involving the knee joint or thigh thus were frequently performed by a hip disarticulation or hemipelvectomy, and upper limb amputations by shoulder disarticulation or interscapulothoracic (fore-quarter) amputations. These radical limb operations were believed to be mandatory due to the high incidence of metastases, especially metastases to the lungs. Modern diagnostic techniques now can demonstrate the presence or absence of metastases with a high degree of accuracy. According to a recent survey sarcomatous metastases apparently are not as common as was previously thought.[20] Thus, less extensive amputation techniques can now be employed, i.e., cross bone amputations with three to four inches of normal bone left as the margin. Greater residual limb length thus results and functional outcome is better for most patients. Accordingly, primary cancer in the distal femur now permits an amputation through the proximal femur, a cancer in the proximal tibia permits amputation in the mid or distal femur and cancer in the distal tibia allows a below knee amputation. Analogous amputation levels may be appropriately considered for cancer of the upper limbs.

While maximum preservation of stump length compatible with eradication of the cancer is desirable, certain amputation levels may result in stumps that are difficult to fit and therefore best avoided, i.e., the hind foot, the distal third of the leg and the femoral supracondylar region. It is critical to preserve the knee joint whenever possible in order to ensure smoothness of gait, lower energy cost and better function. Whenever possible 12–18 cm of tibia should be retained for optimal prosthetic fitting, but even a very short below knee amputation (BKA) with as little as 3 cm of tibia preserved is better than amputating above the knee. When the fibula is retained, it should be cut slightly shorter than the tibia. Disarticulation at the knee is also preferable to above knee amputation (AKA) as it provides a wide weight bearing surface, long lever arm, and proprioception. Unfortunately, this level cannot be chosen often for cancer patients due to the frequency of intra-articular spread of cancer located in the mid or proximal tibia. For prosthetic purposes, the femur should be cut at least 10 cm above the knee joint, but otherwise it is preferable to have the AKA as long as possible. A femoral stump length which measures less than 8 cm from the greater trochanter to the tip functions poorly. As a rule hip disarticulation is preferred to an amputation level above the lesser trochanter. Hip disarticulation and hemipelvec-

tomy need reconstruction with a long posterior flap in order to create a proper sitting area on the prosthesis.[15] Hemicorporectomy (translumbar amputation) has been performed on rare occasions on patients with widespread cancer of the pelvis, but without metastases elsewhere. This procedure indeed is a challenging alternative to the nonsurgical approach and has been shown to have a good rehabilitation outcome.[19] Cancers in the upper limbs unfortunately are primarily found in the proximal humerus thus requiring shoulder disarticulation or interscapulo-thoracic amputation. Here it is important to retain quality skin and maximum muscle mass for padding the shoulder, but retention of the humeral head, if possible, will result in better prosthetic fitting.

Successful prosthetic use depends to a large extent on proper surgical techniques of amputation.[7] It is not adequate only to provide a long stump, although this is important for both leverage and large total contact area for weight bearing. Optimally the stump should be firm, tapered or cylindrical in shape with all bone ends well padded. The skin must have good innervation and vascular supply, and not be adherent to bone or have sensitive scars.

Post-operative care should ensure optimal wound healing, minimize stump swelling, prevent joint contractures and improve muscle strength and function. Application of appropriate dressing and external pressure on the stump by several means is very important.[34] Stump wrapping with the customary elastic bandages needs to be done skillfully with frequent reapplications in order to maintain maximum sustained pressure and to avoid tourniquet effect. Different forms of semirigid dressings have been used, e.g., unna paste dressings, custom made elastic stump socks, plastic films and inflatable air splints, each of which has different advantages and disadvantages. Inflatable and removable air splints, recently popularized, are made of clear plastic and a zipper which allows easy inspection, as well as donning and doffing.

An elastic plaster bandage may be applied to the stump immediately after the amputation. This technique, referred to as immediate post surgical fitting, is a rigid form of dressing which can effectively reduce edema and post-operative pain. A prosthetic pylon and foot can be attached directly to the plaster in order to allow standing within two days postoperatively. Initially only minimal weight bearing is allowed, but progressive ambulation is continued and full weight bearing may be possible in three to four weeks.[6] Several disadvantages of this technique have made it difficult to implement. A removable rigid dressing provides for easier stump inspection, dressing change and adjustment for progressive stump shrinkage and may even allow attachment of a temporary adjustable prostheses.[28,58]

Post-operative Exercise Program. Physical and occupational therapy should be initiated within two days after the amputation. The preoperative exercise program is resumed for muscle strengthening and joint mobilization. Knee flexion contractures may easily develop after BKA, whereas hip flexion and abduction contractures are frequently seen with short AKA. Mobilization is started at bedside, but within a few days the patient is taken by wheelchair to the therapy area and ambulation in parallel bars or with a walker is started. The skillful amputee is subsequently provided with a pair of crutches, but when prosthetic fitting has been completed, a single cane will usually suffice. Different types of ready-made or prefabricated temporary prosthetic devices exist for the earliest ambulation efforts, but a custom fitted provisional prosthesis should be provided as soon as the surgical incision has healed. The amputee, however, may be discharged from the hospital even without a prosthesis, if he is ambulating safely with assistive gait devices and is independent in ADL. Transfer to the inpatient rehabilitation unit for more intensive therapy may be advisable at any time before these two goals are reached if the amputee is otherwise medically stable.

Prescription of an Artificial Limb. The physician needs to consider multiple factors when prescribing a limb prosthesis. The amputation level and stump condition clearly are of primary importance, but prosthetic candidacy may be affected by numerous other factors, including associated medical conditions, other physical disabilities, life expectancy, muscle strength and coordination, stamina, various psychological factors, i.e., motivation, emotional adjustment and cognition, and individual lifestyle factors, i.e., age, weight, family support, recreational interest, environment, and type of work. Extent of prosthetic usage is to some degree predictable since each symptomatic medical problem adversely affects functional prognosis. The ability of the patient to ambulate with a walker or a pair of crutches, but without a prosthesis, strongly suggests prosthetic candidacy. After carefully considering these different factors, the physiatrist may have to choose between a prosthesis which provides relatively greater safety with stability or one with greater function and mobility, between durability and low prosthetic weight, besides considering differences in cost and cosmesis. When new or advanced designs are chosen, the skill and expertise of the prosthetist are crucial factors and he must as well be easily accessible to the patient.

Most prostheses are currently fabricated from metals and plastics. The customary below knee (BK) prosthesis consists of a socket, shank and ankle-foot components, as well as a suspension system. The socket usually has a patellar tendon bearing (PTB) design and a total stump contact for maximum pressure distribution. Soft liners inside the socket add comfort by absorbing shocks. Several layers of stump socks may need to be worn to accommodate a shrinking stump. The shank is either of an endoskeletal design with an internal metal pylon or an exoskeletal structure made from laminated plastic. The solid ankle cushioned heel (SACH) foot is simple, durable, lightweight and cosmetic, and is still most commonly prescribed despite the arrival of a variety of new energy storing prosthetic feet, i.e., the Seattle and the FLEX feet designs. The prosthesis is usually attached to the residual limb by a supracondylar cuff, although several other alternatives exist. The AK amputee traditionally obtains a prosthesis with a rigid quadrilateral socket and a posterior ischial seat for additional weight bearing. The popular single axis knee joint with constant friction is simple and durable, whereas the more costly and complex polycentric or hydraulic knee units can provide better function for young physically active amputees. Stability of the knee joint during stance may be increased by posterior placement of the knee axis, but for maximum safety manual or automatic knee locks may be

added. The AK prosthesis optimally is suspended by total suction, or by partial suction and a silesian bandage or a pelvic band. An endoskeletal pylon connects the knee unit above to the prosthetic foot below. After a hip disarticulation, the amputee receives the Canadian type prostheses, which has a plastic laminated socket encircling the pelvis. This provides a resting surface for the ischial tuberosity for weight bearing. With proper molding it is suspended from the iliac crest. Similar prosthesis is worn after hemipelvectomy with the rib cage providing the weight bearing surface.

Cancer in the upper limb frequently requires shoulder disarticulation or interscapular thoracic amputation, both of which make fitting the patient with a functional body powered prosthesis difficult or impossible. Myoelectrically controlled and externally powered prostheses, however, may provide some gross function, but such prostheses are relatively expensive, heavy and require repair more often than body powered prostheses.

In recent years prosthetic techniques for all types of amputations have advanced significantly, especially with respect to evaluation methods, socket design, ankle-foot components, and cosmesis.[52]

Prosthetic Fitting and Training. Before completion of the prosthesis the amputee needs to visit the prosthetist several times to ensure optimal fit, function and comfort. When fabrication is completed, the prescribing physician checks the prosthesis for fit and comfort, socket stability, joint motions, appearance and function. The lower limb amputee receives gait training, with or without gait aids depending on motor skills, instructions in donning and doffing techniques, as well as exercises to increase muscle strength, joint range of motion, balance and posture. The upper limb amputee learns to open and close the terminal device, position the arm, manipulate objects and perform self care tasks. Initially, a prosthesis may not be worn comfortably for more 15–30 minutes at a time. The amputee thus requires frequent rest periods and short therapy sessions. After each wear the stump skin must be examined for signs of excessive pressure or poor socket fit.

At the beginning of prosthetic wear confrontational situations may develop between the amputee and the health professional, especially when the patient's expectations do not match the actual situation. New and increased demands may produce discomfort at the prosthesis-user interface and in other body parts. Disappointment with the final appearance, weight, ease of wear, level of comfort and functional limitations of the prosthesis is common. The health professional needs to understand the adjustment process and assist the amputee by paying attention to legitimate complaints, providing encouragement and making judicious adjustment of the prosthesis. Poor communication may force the amputee to obtain a new but often no better prosthesis elsewhere. Various deviations of gait occur with lower limb prosthetic use due to stump problems, inadequate prosthetic fit, psychological reactions and improper training. These need to be carefully analyzed and proper intervention offered.

Lower limb amputees ambulate at greater energy costs than non-disabled persons.[24, 55] The BK amputee expends 10–40% more oxygen than a normal person walking at the same speed and the AK amputee expends 65% more. However, in order to save energy, most amputees decrease their speed of ambulation, which is approximately 2.0–2.5 mph for BK and 1.0–1.5 mph for AK amputees compared to normal speed of 3–4 mph for non-disabled persons. The lower energy cost and greater speed of ambulation for the BK amputee clearly shows the importance of sparing the knee joint whenever possible.

Various clinical problems may occur as the result of the amputation and consequent prosthetic wear, including stump pain, skin lesions, swelling, joint contractures, and mental depression. Most amputees experience phantom sensation, which is a painless awareness of the amputated part, but more seriously, approximately 5% experience phantom pain, i.e., burning, crushing, cramping, or shooting sensations in the amputated phantom. The pain may be aggravated by stump contact and different physical activities, but the exact cause remains unknown as no detectable stump pathology or premorbid emotional problems are usually discovered. Phantom pain may be preventable or effectively managed by careful preoperative explanations of the nature of the phantom, good surgical techniques, regular examinations post-operatively, frequent manual handling and good care of the stump, as well as by effective treatment of stump infections and early provision of a functional prosthesis. Definitive treatment however is difficult, but symptoms usually improve when a relatively normal situation has been restored, e.g., ambulation with a prosthesis. Other beneficial interventions include desensitization by frequent self inspection and manipulation of the stump, by application of superficial heat or cold, deep heating with diathermy, massage, vibration, TENS, imaginary exercises of the phantom limb, active exercises of the entire body, local anesthesia of the stump and psychological interventions. Analgesic medications are relatively ineffective, but agents acting on the central nervous system may be helpful.

Actual and localized stump pain occurs frequently after amputation for various pathological reasons, such as infection, scar adhesion, muscle spasm, or poor socket fit. Skin reactions occur frequently over the stump and require meticulous care. The stump should be gently washed with soap and water and thoroughly dried each evening rather than in the morning. The prosthetic socket should be cleansed with moist soapy cloth, and stump socks should be washed immediately after removal and thoroughly dried before they are worn again. The stump should be kept dry and free of trauma to prevent maceration. Talcum powder is often used to make the skin dry and smooth but cocoa butter may be applied to lubricate the scar. During early prosthetic wear the amputee may frequently experience skin maceration, abrasions, blisters and infections of hair follicles and sweat glands, each of which requires specific treatment. Open, draining or painful skin lesions require that prosthetic wear be discontinued until healing has occurred. Gradually the skin will toughen with regular prosthetic use and skin problems become fewer in the course of time.

Reactive depression and grieving the limb loss may be anticipated but these reactions are compounded by the cancer's uncertain prognosis. Early restoration of function and psychological support provided by the entire health care team may be the best intervention, although psychiatric treatment may occasionally be indicated (see XX).

Limb Sparing Surgical Reconstruction. Local resection of cancer with limb sparing reconstruction may result in survival and disease-free period which is equal to that of amputation, and function that is superior.[49] Amputation, however, is still a primary treatment for many limb tumors since it may at times be impossible to perform a proper resection while preserving key nerves and vessels, and to reconstruct a functional limb.

Limb sparing reconstructive surgery obviously is an attractive alternative to amputation for both cosmetic and emotional reasons, but it should only be undertaken if it will restore better and longer lasting function than amputation with subsequent prosthetic fitting.[38] Depending on the location and size of the tumor, it may be a difficult procedure where muscles, bone and even joints are removed with the tumor. The bone may be replaced by transplanting a fresh frozen cadaveric bone allograft or an autologous graft, but more commonly by installing a synthetic metallic prosthetic implant.[40] An expandable and adjustable prosthesis may now be installed in growing children who formerly were felt to fare better with an amputation. Just as when amputation is planned, all patients should be carefully told preoperatively what degree of function to expect after the operation.

Rehabilitation interventions preferably should begin preoperatively when physical and/or occupational therapists should first teach the patient the exercises that will be resumed postoperatively, i.e., muscle strengthening, range of motion and ambulation exercises. Following lower limb sparing surgery the patient may begin, on the first postoperative day, exercising the uninvolved limbs, but the initiation, pace and intensity of exercises and the amount of weight bearing for the affected limb depends on the exact mode of reconstruction and the postoperative course. In general, continuous passive motion (CPM), active-assistive exercises and weight bearing as tolerated may be allowed 6–10 days postoperatively if no surgical complications occur and no specific contraindications exist. Following upper limb saving surgery, active hand and isometric shoulder muscle exercises are started on the first postoperative day, but if humeral resection was performed, active elbow and shoulder exercises should not begin for 2 or 8 weeks postoperatively depending on whether a metallic implant or allo-/autografts respectively were used. It is thus of primary importance that the rehabilitation staff know exactly which muscles, nerves and bones were resected and what the reconstruction entailed in order to plan a safe and effective rehabilitation program. Training in ADL is initiated approximately one week postoperatively. Prior to discharge, decision is made whether the patient requires a permanent orthosis or other assistive devices in order to compensate for lost function. Following discharge, most patients are referred for continued therapy and are given specific instructions for exercise and other activities at home.

Conclusion

Management of cancer appropriately focuses on prevention, early diagnosis and cure, but following effective treat-

treated if a patient were prepared for surgery by chemotherapy or radiation therapy without the surgeon's examining the tumor and the patient beforehand. In diseases where radiotherapy and chemotherapy both play a role, joint planning is mandatory.

In the absence of absolute oncologic truths, there is much room for diverse opinion. Multidisciplinary oncology implies that each discipline performs a complementary function, an estate much to be desired. The best analogy is to a symphony, each instrument playing harmoniously, rather than all on the same note, or with abandon and cacophony.

The Primary Physician

No universal blood or urine test or tests exist that can diagnose asymptomatic cancer. Isolated patients may present abnormal protein patterns or marker alterations, but such tests are not sufficiently sensitive or specific to justify them as screening tests. Until a reasonable approximation of such a desirable test is discovered, probably tumor by tumor, the most important diagnostic tool is the history. Many cancers can be found in asymptomatic status, justifying screening for cancers of the skin, oral cavity, thyroid, nodes, breast, gynecologic tract, testes, anus, prostate, and rectum. Many of these can be found by careful periodic physical examination. Some cancers are announced asymptomatically by a simple laboratory test: leukocytosis, microscopic hematuria, occult fecal blood, cervical cytology, or prostatic specific antigen. Regrettably, these diagnoses when asymptomatic are uncommon.

Most cancers are discovered when the patient exhausts other simple explanations and remedies for a new significant symptom and finally seeks medical attention. Most early symptoms of cancer are protean. The family physician has the greatest opportunity to make an early diagnosis of cancer. By attentive consideration of every minor symptom, a good doctor must sift the symptom that could be cancer from that which is not likely to be. Indeed, early symptoms that later turn out to be representations of cancer are difficult to distinguish from the vagaries of ordinary dysfunctions. It is the constellation of symptoms, their duration, and associated findings that provoke the alert physician to consider cancer in the differential diagnosis. Cough, gastritis, anorexia, hoarseness, constipation, diarrhea, weight loss, fever, fatigue, or pain which has existed unexplained for two weeks requires considering cancer in the differential diagnosis. Indeed, other more obvious possible causes may exist and lead to other diagnoses, but cancer that is not thought of is always diagnosed later than necessary. Cancer need not be characterized by symptoms that are so severe that the diagnosis becomes obvious. Cancer symptoms can be remittent. Pain at the outset is most often not constant, and when present may be poorly localized or even migratory. Systemic dysfunction early on may be so mild as not to lead to spontaneous complaint. Histories that are given are less valuable than histories that are taken.

Upon suspecting cancer, the primary physician is often able to order the appropriate tests to confirm that suspicion, and to arrange for histologic or cytologic confirmation. It is at this point that the multidisciplinary process should start.

Studies that do not establish a diagnosis of cancer could be the wrong studies. Oncologic consultation might suggest other procedures of value. The primary physician often sends a patient to a surgeon for biopsy, which when positive may be followed by resection without further consultation. We believe that after a diagnosis is suspected, or after it is proved, but before the inauguration of surgical therapy is the proper time for discussion with representatives from the many disciplines that might eventually become involved. Psychooncologic consultation and formal rehabilitation may not be necessary for every patient, but when needed, should be arranged before the definitive therapeutic program is initiated. Pathology consultation is always needed, and all oncologic specialists who will be engaged in care should avail themselves of the pathologist's interpretation; surgical, radiation and medical oncologists should see the tissue with their own eyes, as well.

The surgeon, medical oncologist, and radiation oncologist should, in many cases, have protocols for therapy of common cancers. Where possible these programs should be part of designed studies that will accumulate sufficient numbers that conclusions can be drawn. Sometimes this involves single institution (or even single practice) endeavors; whenever possible it should be part of institutional or national protocols designed to answer fundamental questions concerning the management of cancer. Where no protocol exists, agreement should be sought ahead of time that defines the procedures and sequence for this particular patient. The family physician should be a full partner in all of these decisions.

The Radiologist

Imaging specialties are essential in the discovery and staging of prospective cancer patients. Every oncologist should review relevant imaging studies with the appropriate radiologist, sonographer, or specialist in nuclear medicine. No written report compares with the surety of having personally seen the films, report in hand, or better still, with the radiologist at the viewbox. Although it is commonplace to order standard menus (a CT scan, or an MRI) considerably greater efficiency and some economy attends the oncologist who seeks advance expert consultation concerning the problem to be imaged. Special CT scans at much closer distances can provide better definition of small lesions, or special MRI views (axial, coronal, sagittal with or without gadolinium) may provide optimal visualization. Follow-up examinations using single photon emission computerized tomography (SPECT), sonographic or CT-guided needle aspiration, dynamic flow scanning and similar procedures require professional imaging input.

Oncologists can require, however, that the specialist in imaging not give an interpretation directly to the patient. Thoughtless reporting of radiologic findings to patients before they are known by the responsible oncologist causes significant difficulty in management, not only for the oncologist, but usually for the patient. Information given out of context to an individual whose personality the radiologist has not fathomed provides none of the benefits that advocates of complete disclosure maintain. The compact lies between the oncologist and the imaging specialist. The radiologist is a consultant to the oncologist, not to the patient. The responsibility for interpretation of findings to the patient, and the support that often must go with it, rests on the oncologist.

The Pathologist

The pathologist is arguably the indispensable member of every interdisciplinary team. That we are all dependent on the proper diagnosis, establishes pathology as a defining control. When a pathologist is not sure, it is not a disgrace. Other local pathologists render opinions, and the Armed Forces Institute of Pathology and several prominent universities and cancer centers are justly famed for their consultation from which pathologists, with humility but not shame, accept advice.

The ready access of the entire gastrointestinal tract to endoscopic inspection and biopsy, similar access to the external genitalia of both sexes, the accessibility of many bronchogenic carcinomas by fiberoptic bronchoscopy, and the safe intra-operative biopsies of central nervous system, pulmonary, ovarian, skeletal, and soft tissue neoplasms, mean that pre-operative or intra-operative pathologic confirmation of diagnosis should be available for nearly every tumor. Renal and testicular masses are typically removed without first establishing histologic proof, based on characteristic physical examination, sonography, other imaging techniques, and tumor associated markers. This is justified by the disadvantage of tumor spillage, and the characteristic clinical picture. For other diseases, radical surgery without pathologic basis is unnecessary and dangerous. Similarly, an inadequate surgical procedure performed because the nature of the pathologic process was not appreciated suggests insufficient or mistaken intraoperative consultation. Amputation of breast or extremity without pathologic diagnosis in advance or intraoperatively is malpractice. A surgeon may conscientiously and competently sacrifice an adjacent dispensable normal organ which appears to be involved with cancer, such as spleen, kidney, adrenal, a segment of gut, diaphragm, bladder wall or vaginal wall without histologically establishing invasion, based on surgical judgment. In other circumstances, the pathologist's imprimatur is necessary to justify cancer therapies. The same restrictions apply to radiation therapy or chemotherapy unless one stipulates and documents that the therapeutic procedure is intended "prophylactically" for subclinical disease that may exist.

The pathologist is responsible for as definitive a description of the tumor as determined effort can guarantee: its extent, its relationship to surgical margins, normal structures, and the involvement of lymph nodes, lymphatics and blood vessels. Wherever possible a specimen of fresh tissue should be maintained frozen, since increasingly, new molecular biological and biochemical techniques allow classification of tumors for receptors, oncogenes, tumor suppressor genes, and viral antigens that may some day provide prognostic information of great value. In selected circumstances, fresh tissue can be utilized for assays that predict chemotherapeutic sensitivity.

In addition to tissue preservation for more sophisticated studies if needed, pathology now allows better classification

of tumors about which some uncertainty exists concerning their type and origin. Immunopathology and cytochemistry should be able to distinguish among most anaplastic neoplasms by study with leukocyte common antigen, cytokeratin, vimentin, mucin, neuron specific enolase, and S100 protein, whether the tumor is a lymphoma, squamous carcinoma, sarcoma, adenocarcinoma, neuroectodermal tumor, or melanoma, respectively, all of which in their anaplastic state may resemble one another in hematoxylin and eosin staining. A small *fresh* sample of representative neoplasm should be placed in glutaraldehyde fixative in the operating room for eventual electron microscopy if any suggestion exists that pathologic classification might be complex. Today's research classifications may well become tomorrow's standard rubric and nomenclature. Oncologists should encourage the most discriminating description and classification of tumors.

When uncertainty exists concerning the nature of a neoplasm, additional opinions are always appropriate. Pathologic confusion is a shaky foundation on which to build therapeutic strategy.

The Surgical Oncologist

The surgical oncologist is most often likely to see a patient before other oncologic specialists. The family physician or internist most commonly seeks a diagnosis, and in circumstances where this requires biopsy, the surgeon is usually consulted. For decades, any surgeon was considered wholly competent to exercise all surgical skills, including cancer surgery. Indeed, while most surgeons may be acceptably competent, the specialty of surgical oncology is increasingly recognized by other oncologists. Surgical oncologists are surgeons with knowledge of and experience in cancer surgery that comes from additional training, limitation of the scope of general surgical practice, and familiarity with the natural history of cancers and the role of the other oncologic specialties in their diagnosis and management. Until surgical oncology becomes recognized by the proper accrediting agencies, other oncologists must exercise their judgment concerning the oncologic qualifications of their surgical confreres. Membership in the Society of Surgical Oncology, postgraduate training in a cancer institute or with a mentor known for cancer surgical expertise, limitation of surgical practice to cancer and related diseases, publications, and a personal assessment of the depth of interest and knowledge are some of the appropriate criteria.

Since a general surgeon may perform the biopsy, a surgical oncologist is rather uncommonly called upon to supersede the first surgeon on the case. Herein lies some of the problem, since the primary cancer operation is of utmost importance for determining cure. In this regard, any mass to be biopsied should be considered in the context of whether the operating surgeon will be the best choice for eventual definitive surgical therapy. Since a considerable portion of their activity deals with neoplasia, thoracic surgeons, urologic surgeons and neurosurgeons must be chosen for their general expertise, because there is not likely to be an oncologic subspecialty in the near future for those specific organ systems. On the other hand, gynecologic oncology, orthopedic oncology, otorhinolaryngologic oncology and surgical oncology are well defined, and the general gynecologist, orthopedist, otorhinolaryngologist, or surgeon is unlikely to be so well qualified as the oncologist within the specialty.

Because the implications for a proven neoplasm, potentially resectable, entail many other considerations to optimize curability, the prudent surgical oncologist surveys the potential contributions of medical oncology, radiation oncology, and other specialties before proceeding with operation.

Where appropriate and possible, patients should be entered into clinical investigative trials. There is so much that is unknown about cancer, that investigative activities should still be of prime concern to all oncologists. In institutions where investigative programs are not employed, sober consideration of joining in this effort through a community oncology program, or in alliance with some other active institution may be possible. In the absence of a structured protocol, joint assessment is appropriate to determine whether chemotherapy or radiotherapy prior to surgery may improve outcome. Most often this entails direct consultation with the medical and radiation oncologist. An opportunity for the three specialties to see the patient in the native state is of great value for subsequent planning. Confidence building makes for easy consultation over the years with colleagues that share mutual trust. The treatment of breast cancer, rectal cancer, head and neck cancer, and soft tissue sarcoma, for example, are most often best approached by multidisciplinary components from all three specialties. Whereas specific diseases may be well treated by single-modality approaches, bi-disciplinary or tri-disciplinary opinion is usually advantageous.

Surgical oncologists must also be available for surgical aspects of management later in the course of disease. End-staging laparotomy in many instances may make more sense than earlier operation, so that the medical oncologist may be certain that a complete clinical remission is pathologically confirmed rather than waiting expectantly for a lymphoma or ovarian cancer to relapse. Intestinal obstruction in the course of cancer may require operative surgical management. The surgeon may be obliged to obtain long-term or permanent venous access. A medical or radiation oncologist may discover a suspicious mass or infiltration that needs biopsy and pathologic assessment.

Palliative surgery is an area where medical and radiation oncologists often present problems to the surgeon in hopes of potential operative remedy. Debulking, diverting, and pain-relieving operations are all appropriate procedures in the proper circumstance.

Surgical oncologists also have legitimate interests in adjuvant chemotherapy and immunotherapy. For those willing to devote the time required for this undertaking, use of established drugs in adjuvant programs can be an improvement over surgical procedures alone. Indeed the National Surgical Adjuvant Breast and Bowel Project has contributed significantly to our knowledge of adjuvant therapy for these diseases (see XXXII and XXIX-10). Surgical oncologic investigators have also pioneered immunological cancer research. The rarity of surgical oncologists in practice, however, ordinarily precludes these activities for surgeons since so much of their time is ordinarily invested in pre- and post-operative care and in actual surgery. Medical oncologists must stand ready to assume primary responsibility for subsequent oncologic management. Orthopedic oncologists, otorhinolaryngologic oncologists, and neurosurgical oncologists ordinarily ally themselves with a medical oncologist with specialized interests and expertise in neoplasms of their particular discipline.

The Anesthesiologist

Few patients get to choose their anesthesiologist. Intraoperative management is consistent with that for any serious surgery. Since anesthesiologists often run the recovery room and even the intensive care units, however, their interaction with patients who may be awake can be consequential. The description of operative findings should be reserved to the surgeon. Assurance of effective pain control in the immediate post-operative period is important to avoid the exaggeration of anxiety and depression that may come with pain when first learning the significance of the operation and its findings. Patient-controlled analgesia in the immediate post-operative period, and at other times for efficient pain control, is a technique of importance to all branches of oncology, and not one that should be considered a proprietary anesthesiologic exclusive.

The Medical Oncologist

The medical oncologist usually serves the traditional role of internist in the multidisciplinary management of cancer. Whereas the surgical procedure, or even the radiotherapeutic treatment course is of short duration, the medical oncologist has continuing responsibility that may stretch over months or years of therapy, and decades of follow-up, dependent upon the neoplasm.

There is an understandable but regrettable tendency for each specialty that has interacted with a patient to schedule follow up appointments, which may entail many more visits and much greater expense than are necessary or prudent. Each therapist is entitled to see the results of the particular treatment regimen that was applied. Absence of disease in the region subjected to surgery or radiotherapy is in the purview of the treating specialist, but that is only a portion of the patient's overall health concerns. The more cogent question is the search for remediable disease in regional and distant areas, and a continuing assessment of the impact of the disease and its treatment on the patient as a whole, tasks ordinarily considered medical. A useful technique is dictation by the medical oncologist of the findings at a follow-up visit, including laboratory and radiologic results, so that the surgeon and radiologist (or other appropriate specialist) not feel excluded from knowing what is going on. The medical oncologist may superintend the medical activities of the patient that are not addressed by a family physician or internist, together with oncologic assessment that would be of importance to surgeon, radiotherapist and medical oncologist alike. In circumstances where the patient has not received adjuvant therapy by a medical oncologist, and is not undergoing treatment for metastatic disease, the involvement of a medical oncologist is discretionary on the part of the family physician or internist and other oncological specialists already engaged.

The medical oncologist should partake in the decisions of therapeutic choice, and also in the clinical staging which may determine operability. The medical oncologist should be the one to address the potential for induction or neoadjuvant chemotherapy, and the choice of regimen for postoperative chemotherapeutic or immunotherapeutic management. With few exceptions, most notable of which are the brilliant works in breast cancer done by Fisher and his colleagues and by Veronese and his colleagues (see XXXII), surgeons may be remote from recent research achievements and from the best chemotherapeutic and immunotherapeutic approaches to cancers which are appropriately treated with these therapies. A substantial portion of this treatise is devoted to activities of the medical oncologist in his diagnostic and therapeutic responsibilities.

The medical oncologist is most often the physician to reassure the patient when there is no evident cancer. Although absent tumor may only be an eclipse, the medical oncologist must keep the patient from dwelling incessantly and anxiously on imminent relapse. Indeed, the medical oncologist may need to encourage a return to normal living when the cancer is not manifest. This should never involve a lie, just a reasoned basis for hope that relapse will not occur. Osler's admonition to live life in day-tight packages is helpful.

The Radiation Oncologist

Radiation oncology is the only specialty entirely devoted to the study of cancer. The radiation oncologist must therefore be in a position to make an overall oncologic evaluation, as well as specific recommendations regarding radiotherapy.

For diseases where radiotherapy can effect curative treatment, such as localized lymphomas, cancer of the tongue and oral cavity, and cancer of the cervix, the radiation oncologist must have equal early access to the patient to set forth the possible indications for and accomplishments of radiation therapy for such tumors. Cordial interactive liaison with surgical and medical oncologists is crucial to allow this delineation of options before the patient is changed by another treatment approach.

Controversy exists over the relative debilities and late toxicities of surgery and radiotherapy. Where equal curative potential exists, there is reason to assess the disruption of anatomy and the dysfunction that might occur after surgery and radiotherapy to the same region. This produces little consensus in head and neck, early cervical, prostate and bladder cancers. The major improvement in immediate reconstructive techniques has made surgery around the oral cavity less disfiguring. Surgeons recite the dry mouth and sometimes diminished taste as late and undesirable toxicities of radiation, while radiotherapists decry the cosmetic and physiologic distortions of surgery. Similar controversy attends the dysfunction of vaginal secretions after radiation treatment for early carcinoma of the cervix, with many male gynecologic oncologists attesting the lesser implications for sexual function of total hysterectomy. In carcinomas of the bladder and prostate, the discordance is even greater,

because total cystectomy is admittedly debilitating, and American urologists question whether radiation therapy is ever equivalent, stage for stage. Thus, although radiotherapy for T1 and T2 bladder cancers is reportedly highly effective in Europe, there has been relatively little clinical investigation of this in the United States. Radical surgery for carcinoma of the prostate, until recently nearly always associated with impotence, offered sound basis for trials of radical radiotherapy. For tumors too advanced locally for surgery, radiotherapeutic consultation is usually sought. The definitive comparison of earlier stage prostatic cancer therapies has not been made.

In the area of operable oral, pharyngeal, cervical, bladder, and prostatic cancer, closer cooperation of radiation oncologist and surgeon before decisions are put into action might, if therapy is equivalent stage for stage, provide for greater organ preservation and less dysfunction. The great problem, however, is to overcome the prejudice that the results will not be the same, with each exponent nearly equally persuaded, and equally unpersuasive. Definitive clinical trials are sorely needed, but may never be done because of the evolution of the combined modality approaches.

In combined modality approaches, chemotherapy is a major component together with radiotherapy and surgery. Data abound that chemotherapy can induce major regressions when used as primary therapy for head and neck cancer and bladder cancer, as well as for breast cancer, pediatric sarcomas, and lymphomas. There is as yet no consensus about primary chemotherapy, with its major theoretical advantage of decreasing the number of cells to be killed by radiation, or to be removed by surgery. For the present, prudence supports the proposition that radiation field size and surgical boundaries can not be importantly reduced below the original extent of the tumor, where residual cells after chemotherapy may remain. One advantage of primary chemotherapy, in addition to decrease in primary tumor burden, is an early attack against undetected micrometastatic disease. Furthermore, when the tumor vasculature is intact, unimpaired by radiation angiopathy and fibrosis or surgical disruption, there is a greater chance of delivering a chemotherapeutically effective dose. Lastly, the regression of tumor seen in the primary neoplasm reinforces the confidence in using the same chemotherapeutic regimen for presumed micrometastases during the adjuvant period.

Much of the interrelation of radiation, chemotherapy and surgery is still evolving, hampered by the absence of solid data, and the paucity of attempts to compare modern multimodality regimens.

For tumors regionally beyond surgical compass, in the pharynx, parametria, pelvis, and periprostatic tissues, radiation is usually employed as primary therapy. The dismal results that often attend these advanced tumors erroneously colors the potential contributions of radiation oncology for earlier tumors, because non-participating observers ordinarily see only the failures. Substantial opportunity exists here for pilot efforts within an institution to fashion combined modality approaches for tumors which are regionally inoperable at first encounter, but which might become resectable after chemotherapy and/or radiation therapy; or which might not require surgery at all after their use. Esophageal cancer and localized pancreatic cancer appear to fit this category.

Primary brain tumors are usually best treated by primary surgery and radiotherapy, often with chemotherapy. When surgery is unfeasible, new techniques of radiosurgery, delivering precisely localized therapy from several angles, so as to spare normal brain, offer some promise.

Radiotherapy can cure localized and regionalized lymphomas of certain types. The advantages and disadvantages of combined modality therapy, or of the use of chemotherapy alone, are presented in detail for the specific diseases. There continues to be a clear indication for combined chemotherapy and radiotherapy in patients whose lymphomas are massive in size, and where confidence in tumor eradication by either modality alone is ill-founded. Radiotherapy may be a critical component in salvage regimens for relapsed leukemias and lymphomas, where maximal chemotherapy together with autologous or allogeneic marrow or stem cell transplantation is undertaken.

For palliation and pain relief, radiation therapy is indispensable to the practice of oncology. Radiotherapy can usually offer relief from the pain of tumor infiltration in bone, irrespective of tumor type. Although the extent of tumor regression (as a measure of radiosensitivity) varies, this may determine length of remission rather than initial pain relief.

The Gynecologic Oncologist

Gynecologic oncologists as a class may belong to the most integrated oncologic specialty. Gynecologic oncologists are fully qualified to diagnose and treat neoplasia of the female genital organs by surgery and chemotherapy, and to share in radiotherapeutic planning and execution to a considerable degree, particularly for brachytherapy. Highly skilled gynecologic oncologists divide on whether gastrointestinal complications of ovarian or other cancers should be handled by surgical oncologists, general surgeons, or gynecologic oncologists. Much of this depends on local custom rather than expertise at performing lysis of adhesions or enteroenterostomies. The pre-operative preparation for and execution of procedures that involve urinary tract manipulation are almost invariably conducted cooperatively with urologists.

Many medical oncologists treat gynecologic neoplasms with chemotherapy in investigational and clinical settings. This is true for adjuvant therapy as well as treatment of manifest clinical metastasis. In many academic institutions medical and gynecologic oncologists have collaborated to develop new treatment programs and to study the biology of gynecologic cancers. Local custom, the surgical obligations of gynecological oncologists and collaborative undertakings involving both specialties determine the allocation of work. A prime instance where medical oncologists should be active occurs when a gynecologist without specific oncological expertise or interest has undertaken the surgery.

The Pediatric Oncologist

Pediatric oncologists generally maintain an aloofness from adult oncologic specialties. Radiotherapists and surgeons in major centers subspecialize in pediatric neoplasia. Some gynecologists and urologists have particular interests in pediatric diseases. Orthopedic oncologists devote much of their best time to pediatric sarcomas, and thus there is no specialized subset for pediatric neoplasms. The replication in major centers of pediatric counterparts to all the medical oncologic resources, such as pediatric neurologists, radiologists, and even pathologists illustrates the specificity of pediatric oncologic information. Nearly every child in the United States can have access to programs of the Children's Cancer Study Group or the Pediatric Oncology Group. The dramatic progress in cancer therapeutics in children derives in part from the universal recognition that childhood cancer is a tragedy, and that every effort must be made to derive all possible information from every case. This allows the child to benefit from all the information that has gone before, and creates a new data base for those who will come after.

The Psycho-Oncologist

The mind is the only organ system that is affected in every patient with cancer. Nonetheless, all patients do not need formal psychiatric help. General psychiatrists often lack full understanding of the organic aspects of cancers, and the therapeutic procedures that are commonly employed; their effectiveness in dealing with these real life problems is thus diminished. Psycho-oncologists have, by dint of special education and experience, a better foundation from which to undertake supervision of those patients too difficult for oncologists of other disciplines to manage. Psycho-oncologists implement much of their influence by interaction with staff rather than patients. "Sensitivity training" has been trivialized by its use in describing lesser activities. Helping oncologists to deal sensitively and gently with their own patients is a continuing task for psycho-oncologists. Some oncologists seem to overlook the fact that a patient's cancer is usually the greatest challenge in life that he or she has ever faced. Staring into the abyss, often for the first time, requires more equanimity and fortitude than many patients can muster. Teaching doctors how to handle their own inadequacies, how to tolerate their own frustrations and failures, and how to convey a humanitarian dimension to the grim reality of their cancer therapeutics is one of psycho-oncology's best offerings. Not all the medicine comes in a bottle.

The Rehabilitation Specialist

Rehabilitation specialists provide patients the opportunity for self-reliance. Cutting the bonds of dependency can be the best of all remedies. Whether in speech, ambulation, ostomy care, physical appearance, occupational rehabilitation or sexual expression, oncologists must maintain the goal that patients should lead pain-free lives with minimal if any deficits from normal function. Early and vigorous rehabilitation efforts can make life more worth living. Oncologists could and should consult rehabilitation medicine specialists earlier and more often.

The Nurse Oncologist

The oncology nurse has become an indispensable specialist. An oncologist's nightmare is to have a complex cancer patient admitted to a general service floor. The unique medications, procedures and tests for oncology patients are themselves adequate justification for the specialty of oncology nursing. Two other attributes are critical. Oncology nurses have a greater than ordinary understanding of cancer pain, and of the psychic stresses that cancer patients may suffer. These two precious insights allow a much more aggressive advocacy for pain control, and a humanistic yet realistic support of patients and families during their crises. Oncology nurses in ambulatory settings become telephone specialists in patient management, to the great advantage and comfort of cancer patients—and to the great advantage and security of oncologists.

Nurse oncologists have become the prime movers in home care, rendering active therapy or supervision of palliative measures. As this movement gains momentum, it is probable that home hospice care will become more common and more economical. The regulatory hand of government will likely soon extend to the companies organized to provide oncology nursing at home, in an attempt to modulate the expense of the end stages of cancer.

Other Support Personnel

A few additional people are crucial in the oncologic approach to advanced cancer at home. A social worker familiar with the great stresses of cancer on every member of the family is a treasured asset. The complexities in social, economic, and service spheres can be greatly simplified by the kindly professional interest of an oncology social worker. Additional community resources such as the American Cancer Society, Cancer Care, various support groups, Meals on Wheels, companion visits, and home health care aides, often critical factors, may seem to be effortlessly mobilized by a social worker.

For those who have been guided by religious tenets and who have practiced their religion, the clergy can be extremely helpful and religious practice a strengthening act. Deathbed conversions are uncommon, however. For those who have not made religion a significant portion of their lives, visits of the clergy or allusions to afterlife provide little comfort.

The principal support throughout the cancer experience comes from a loving family. All else good may pale in comparison to the radiant affection of a spouse or other close family member. The loved one who recognizes that all the good that can be done must be done, rather than left undone, will create the palpable substance of love for the patient, without suffocation, as well as creating comforting memories for oneself, having worked well, and long, and at the end rested.

XXIV

Neoplasms of the Central Nervous System

Michael D. Prados
Charles B. Wilson

Introduction

Tumors of the central nervous system (CNS) occur in about 1–2% of the United States population, affecting more elderly adults (18 per 100,000 population per year at age 70) than adolescents and young adults (2 per 100,000 population annually) and slightly more males than females.[85,239,261] In 1989, at least 15,000 new cases of primary brain and CNS malignant neoplasms (7.3 per 100,000 population) were diagnosed in the United States and, during the same year, these tumors caused approximately 11,000 deaths.[239,261] If neoplasms metastatic to the CNS were included, these numbers would be much higher.

Despite the relatively small numbers of CNS malignant tumors overall, the morbidity and mortality they cause are significant. Among children younger than age 15 years, CNS tumors rank next to leukemia as the second leading cause of death from cancer. Among men 15–54 years old, they are the third leading cause of cancer-related mortality, and in women 15–34 years of age, they are the fourth leading cause of death.[239]

For children with primary tumors of the nervous system, the past two decades have shown an important trend toward improved survival, largely because of better therapies developed for medulloblastoma and primitive neuroectodermal tumor. During the same period, survival rates for patients with glioblastoma multiforme–the most common malignant tumor in adults–have shown only modest improvement.[239] Nonetheless, new or refined techniques in surgery, radiation therapy, and systemic chemotherapy, together with intense research efforts into molecular genetics and the immunologic aspects of the disease, give reason for optimism.

As a consequence of the therapeutic achievements made so far, a new approach to the management of malignant CNS neoplasms has developed. The truly multidisciplinary strategy includes neurosurgeons, radiation oncologists, medical and pediatric oncologists, and neurooncologists, all working in close collaboration in the care of the patient. A number of medical centers have adopted this multidisciplinary approach in treating patients who take part in clinical research trials of new drugs and therapies for CNS tumors. These trials are developed with consultation to ensure proper statistical design and interpretation, and with direct input from scientists doing basic research in the fields of immunology, molecular biology and genetics, radiobiology, biochemistry, research pharmacology, and organic chemistry. Rapid completion and statistical accuracy of the trials are assured through a referral system based on a cooperative group mechanism of patient accrual among participating centers.

There is compelling evidence that, in certain disease states, survival can be improved through this multimodality approach. In a survey of national trends in the care of patients with malignant brain tumors, for example, patients with glioblastoma multiforme who were treated in investigational protocols had an almost threefold higher 5–year survival rate (12%) than did patients who were not (4.5%).[158] Although patients increasingly are referred to centers engaged in such studies, at present less than about 10% of eligible patients are actually entered into clinical research trials each year. During this decade, while changes occur as rapidly as our technology expands, every effort must be made to maximize applications of our gains in the management of neoplastic CNS disease. There must be greater attention to attracting more patients to clinical trials and, as survival times increase, a greater emphasis on further reducing the toxicity of therapies and on issues related to the patients' quality of life.

Tumors of Glial Origin

In a review of nine registries in the United States National Cancer Institute's Surveillance, Epidemiology and End Results (SEER) Program, 1983–1985, glioblastoma multiforme was the most common malignant CNS tumor type in patients, both male and female, aged 35–64 years; among men in this age range in the San Francisco registry, for example, glioblastoma multiforme accounted for 52%, and astrocytoma for 34%, of the primary malignant CNS tumors diagnosed.[239,260] The mean age of patients with glioblastoma is 52 years; of those with astrocytoma and anaplastic astrocytoma, 48 years; and of those with oligodendroglioma, 42 years. For glioblastoma more than for other glial neoplasms, however, the incidence increases with increasing age, suggesting a different mechanism of oncogenesis.

Etiology and Epidemiology

Chromosomal abnormalities have been identified in some patients harboring gliomas; and glial neoplasms are associated with neurofibromatosis (NF), tuberous sclerosis, and, in rare cases, other genetically inherited diseases. NF types 1 and 2 are autosomal dominant diseases characterized by cutaneous neurofibromas, café au lait spots, bone abnormalities, and a variety of intracranial and/or intraspinal tumors. Reviewing 121 cases of NF1 and NF2 in children under 18 years of age, Blatt and colleagues identified 17 patients (14%) who developed brain tumors, three of whom had anaplastic astrocytomas.[28] The gene responsible for classic NF1 is located on chromosome 17. Using various DNA probes, Barker and colleagues have further identified the location of NF1 to be near the centromere of chromosome 17.[16]

Recent evidence has linked abnormalities on chromosome 22 with NF2, previously called *central NF*.[164] Patients with NF2 have bilateral eighth-nerve tumors and may have other CNS tumors, as well, including malignant glioma, meningioma, and/or schwannoma.

Abnormalities of chromosome 17 may also be involved in malignant gliomas not associated with NF. For example, a loss of constitutional heterozygosity suggesting chromosomal losses or deletions has been identified on chromosomes 1, 10, and 17 in patients who have anaplastic astrocytoma.[109] In 50% of cases in one series, which included both low-grade and high-grade astrocytomas, the loss was on the short arm of chromosome 17.[61] This area on chromosome 17 is distinct from the abnormality seen in patients with NF1, which is located on the proximal long arm.

Other chromosomal abnormalities have been described in astrocytomas, including anomalies on chromosomes 17, 10, 1, 19, 22, 7, and are likely to be found at other loci, as well. Indeed, glioblastoma tends to occur frequently in patients showing changes on chromosome 10. Fujimoto and colleagues studied 13 patients with glioblastoma, screening with polymorphic markers localized to chromosome 10.[79] In 10 of the 13 cases, loss of heterozygosity for these markers was found on chromosome 10; the smallest and most common region of loss of heterozygosity was between 10q23.3 and the middle of 10p. This finding strongly suggests that a gene or genes important in tumor development may exist on this chromosome. It seems evident that the genesis of a glial tumor can involve many genetic aberrations and a complex etiologic process involving multiple steps, including chromosomal deletions, gene amplification, chromosomal rearrangement, and overexpression of oncogenes.

There is speculation that certain gene products may be antioncogene protein products. Fearon and colleagues have described abnormalities on chromosome 17 in patients with colon cancer, as well as the related gene product designated p53.[70] They suggested that the gene may be an antioncogene, or tumor suppressor gene, that codes for the protein product. One common denominator of p53 and brain tumors is the association of Turcot syndrome both with malignant lesions of the colon and, rarely, with malignant astrocytoma and medulloblastoma. It may be that the oncogenesis of colon and brain tumors is related in part to chromosomal deletions on 17 (see I-6).[20,61]

Cavenee noted a loss of heterozygosity as measured from loci on chromosome 17p (locus D17S5) in differentiated low-grade astrocytomas, attributing the abnormality to a chromosomal loss and either duplication of the remaining homologue or mitotic recombination.[39] Similar changes were seen in anaplastic astrocytoma and glioblastoma. All patients with glioblastoma who were evaluated using probes for three loci on chromosome 10 showed a deletion at one or more of these loci, but no patient with a lower-grade astrocytoma showed similar changes on chromosome 10. These findings suggest that glioblastomas may arise from tumor cells partially deficient on both chromosomes 10 and 17 and that they may have transformed from lower-grade lesions showing changes only on 17. Genotypic analysis of this kind may be useful in predicting transformations and perhaps ultimately in therapeutic decision-making.

Also affecting the development and/or growth of astrocytomas may be genes encoding growth factors, peptides that act by binding to surface receptors on normal and neoplastic cells. Binding of the growth factor to specific receptors on cells elicits intracellular responses that modify growth and development, often signaling intracellular events such as increased protein synthesis and mitogenesis, which, when disturbed, may result in neoplastic growth. Autocrine and paracrine factors that have been identified in human gliomas include transforming growth factors alpha (TGF-α) and beta (TGF-β), bombesin, platelet-derived growth factor (PDGF), epidermal growth factor (EGF), and insulin-like growth factors I and II, as well as fibroblastic growth factor and endothelial cell growth factor. These growth factors are related to oncogenes–normal cellular genes that, when altered through mutation, amplification, or loss of control, may cause transformation. Many known oncogenes are thought to be related to the development of human brain tumors, several of which encode for either growth factors or receptors, establishing the link governing the genetic control of abnormal growth.

Neoplastic transformation is a multistep process that appears to include activation of protooncogenes and subsequent amplification or overexpression of growth factors or receptors. EGF receptor (EGF-R) is often overexpressed in glial neoplasms, and the EGF-R gene has been mapped to chromosome 7. Sang and colleagues, studying the tumorigenicity of several glioblastoma cell lines, noted the amplification and enhanced expression of the EGF-R gene in most glioblastoma cells, although there did not appear to be a good correlate with these events and tumorigenicity in nude mice.[256] Their study of protooncogene abnormalities in several neuronal and glial tumors showed extensive amplification and expression of the oncogene N-myc in neuroblastomas and retinoblastomas, and amplification of the EGF-R gene in glioblastomas. It appears, from this work, that neuronal and glial malignant changes occur from separate pathways. The exact role of EGF-R in glial oncogenesis is still undefined but conceivably the EGF-R gene acts together with one or several oncogenes to cause cellular transformation. Fujimoto and colleagues examined the accumulation and amplification of four protooncogenes—c-myc, N-myc, v-sis, and v-fos—in messenger ribonucleic acid (mRNA) in 10 primary human brain tumors.[80] V-fos amplification was seen in both glioblastoma and low-grade glioma, as well as in ependymoma and medulloblastoma. C-myc was amplified in some of the low-grade and high-grade gliomas and was strongly increased in a medulloblastoma that did not show increases in N-myc or v-sis. The amplification of two oncogenes in one tumor suggests a complicated process that may involve regulation of one oncogene by another.

PDGF, a polypeptide mitogen, is often seen in patients with glioblastoma or other gliomas. The PDGF gene has been identified in a primate retrovirus, simian sarcoma virus (SSV), as the gene involved in transformation to neoplastic growth; SSV produces glioblastoma when injected into the brain of newborn marmoset monkeys. The PDGF gene encodes for either polypeptide chain A or B which corresponds to an A-type or B-type receptor mRNA, the latter having an intracellular tyrosine kinase domain. Amino acid analysis of the B chain shows a resemblance to the protein product of the v-sis transforming gene of SSV. Human glioblastomas and other human malignant tumors express the PDGF gene and glioblastomas express both the A-type and B-type receptor mRNA. PDGF B chain and B-type receptor mRNA are also seen in proliferating endothelial cells. While the exact role of these entities in the development of glial neoplasms is not known, the possible relation of PDGF to endothelial hyperplasia suggests autocrine growth stimulation.

Inhibitory factors may also be important in tumor growth or maintenance. Human glioblastomas produce a factor that inhibits T-cell proliferation and interferes with interleukin-2 (IL-2)-dependent T-cell growth.[273] Now thought to be TGF-β, the inhibitor may prevent or modify antigen-induced immune response, in effect isolating the tumor from immune surveillance and control. TGF-β may also regulate or partially control other growth factors, including c-sis-encoded PDGF. In their study of regulation of c-sis oncogene expression in glioma cell lines, Press and colleagues found enhanced expression of the c-sis mRNA by phorbol ester, diacylglycerol, and TGF-β.[204] The TGF-β-induced c-sis expression was thought to result from an increase in transcription in the nucleus of the cell. As compared with the phorbol ester protein kinase C pathway, the signaling pathway of TGF-β has a different mechanism, probably a different protein kinase. Other oncogenes and their products found in glioblastoma include neu, n-ras, src, ros, and GLI, all of which may potentially help to explain malignant transformation and may provide clues for improving treatment.[25,63,83,123]

Tuberous sclerosis is inherited as an autosomal dominant disorder with a frequency of 1 in 30,000 population annually. Patients are born with ash-leaf unpigmented nevi and later develop adenoma sebaceum as well as other deformities. The intracranial lesions that may develop are usually benign and most often are giant cell astrocytomas.

Other than these few instances of a genetic predisposition, currently there are only sparse data to support a primary inherited genetic basis for the development of malignant glial neoplasms. Several families with a larger than expected aggregation of brain tumors are being investigated in an attempt to identify any chromosomal or DNA abnormalities present.[211]

Occupational exposure has also been investigated as a potential cause of gliomas. The tumors may be produced experimentally in rats with several chemicals, including N-nitroso compounds, aromatic hydrocarbons, triazenes, and hydrazines, or by exposure to vinyl chloride through inhalation.[160,161] Epidemiologic evidence from the National Institute for Occupational Safety and Health (NIOSH), in a study of vinyl chloride-induced angiosarcoma of the liver, has suggested that workers exposed to vinyl chloride also have an increased incidence of brain tumors, supporting its role as an oncogen; most of the 10 brain tumors noted in that study were glioblastomas, nine of which were fatal.[269] Currently there are few data to suggest that other chemical agents may be responsible for the development of malignant gliomas, and often those data are conflicting.

Virally-induced brain tumors include the Rous sarcoma virus canine gliosarcoma, the avian sarcoma virus rat glioma, and the human Jakob-Creutzfeldt (JC) virus which can produce brain tumors in monkeys.[49,107,191] Adenoviruses have been documented to produce neuroblastoma and retinoblastoma in rats and hamsters. Human brain tumors have not been shown to have a viral origin, with the possible exception of primary CNS lymphoma, which has a strong association with Epstein-Barr virus (EBV), discussed later in this chapter.

Tumors of the CNS may be a delayed consequence of radiation therapy, although rarely. Generally, these tumors develop after the patient undergoes cranial irradiation for other neoplastic diseases, such as acute leukemia, and often they are sarcomas or meningiomas.[162,206,220,242,243] Because patients with diseases such as childhood leukemia are now living longer owing to more effective therapy, usually including cranial irradiation, it is likely that more cases of secondary astrocytoma will be identified in the future. During the past few years at the University of California, San Francisco (UCSF), we have seen several cases in which malignant gliomas developed following such therapies.[44,202]

Pathology

Grading Systems for Glial Tumors. In 1926, Bailey and Cushing classified glial neoplasms using a three-tiered system: astrocytoma, astroblastoma, and spongioblastoma multiforme.[15] Since that time, many grading systems have been used. Kernohan and colleagues of the Mayo Clinic used a four-tiered system, designating the better-differentiated tumors as grades I and II, with grades III and IV corresponding to glioblastoma multiforme.[120] Ringertz introduced a three-tiered system: astrocytoma, anaplastic astrocytoma, and glioblastoma multiforme.[208] In this classification, which is used by several cooperative groups, glioblastoma multiforme is defined as an anaplastic astrocytoma that has vascular endothelial proliferation and necrosis, whereas the anaplastic astrocytomas lack necrosis and are more differentiated than the glioblastoma multiforme. The World Health Organization (WHO) classification of glial neoplasms (Table XXIV-1-1) is similar to these schemes but, in an important variation from other systems, it omits glioblastoma multiforme in the classification of astrocytomas and includes it in the group of

Table XXIV-1-1. Histological Classification of Tumors of the Central Nervous System*

I. Tumors of Neuroepithelial Tissue
  A. Astrocytic tumors
    1. Astrocytoma
      a. Fibrillary
      b. Protoplasmic
      c. Gemistocytic
    2. Pilocytic astrocytoma
    3. Subependymal giant cell astrocytoma [ventricular tumor of tuberous sclerosis]
    4. Astroblastoma
    5. Anaplastic [malignant] astrocytoma
  B. Oligodendroglial tumors
    1. Oligodendroglioma
    2. Mixed oligo-astrocytoma
    3. Anaplastic [malignant] oligodendroglioma
  C. Ependymal and choroid plexus tumors
    1. Ependymoma
      Variants:
      a. Myxopapillary ependymoma
      b. Papillary ependymoma
      c. Subependymoma
    2. Anaplastic [malignant] ependymoma
    3. Choroid plexus papilloma
    4. Anaplastic [malignant] choroid plexus papilloma
  D. Pineal cell tumors
    1. Pineocytoma [pinealocytoma]
    2. Pineoblastoma [pinealoblastoma]
  E. Neuronal tumors
    1. Gangliocytoma
    2. Ganglioglioma
    3. Ganglioneuroblastoma
    4. Anaplastic [malignant] gangliocytoma and ganglioglioma
    5. Neuroblastoma
  F. Poorly differentiated and embryonal tumors
    1. Glioblastoma
      Variants:
      a. Glioblastoma with sarcomatous component [mixed glioblastoma and sarcoma]
      b. Giant cell glioblastoma
    2. Medulloblastoma
      Variants:
      a. Desmoplastic medulloblastoma
      b. Medullomyoblastoma
    3. Medulloepithelioma
    4. Primitive polar spongioblastoma
    5. Gliomatosis cerebri
II. Tumors of Nerve Sheath Cells
  A. Neurilemmoma [schwannoma, neurinoma]
  B. Anaplastic [malignant] neurilemmoma [schwannoma, neurinoma]
  C. Neurofibroma
  D. Anaplastic [malignant] neurofibroma [neurofibrosarcoma, neurogenic sarcoma]
III. Tumors of Meningeal and Related Tissues
  A. Meningioma
    1. Meningotheliomatous [endotheliomatous, syncytial, arachnotheliomatous]
    2. Fibrous [fibroblastic]
    3. Transitional [mixed]
    4. Psammomatous

    5. Angiomatous
    6. Haemangioblastic
    7. Haemangiopericytic
    8. Papillary
    9. Anaplastic [malignant] meningioma
  B. Meningeal sarcomas
    1. Fibrosarcoma
    2. Polymorphic cell sarcoma
    3. Primary meningeal sarcomatosis
  C. Xanthomatous tumors
    1. Fibroxanthoma
    2. Xanthosarcoma [malignant fibroxanthoma]
  D. Primary melanotic tumors
    1. Melanoma
    2. Meningeal melanomatosis
  E. Others
IV. Primary Malignant Lymphomas
V. Tumors of Blood Vessel Origin
  A. Haemangioblastoma [capillary haemangioblastoma]
  B. Monstrocellular sarcoma
VI. Germ Cell Tumors
  A. Germinoma
  B. Embryonal carcinoma
  C. Choriocarcinoma
  D. Teratoma
VII. Other Malformative Tumors and Tumor-like Lesions
  A. Craniopharyngioma
  B. Rathke's cleft cyst
  C. Epidermoid cyst
  D. Dermoid cyst
  E. Colloid cyst of the third ventricle
  F. Enterogenous cyst
  G. Other cysts
  H. Lipoma
  I. Choristoma [pituicytoma, granular cell "myoblastoma"]
  J. Hypothalamic neuronal hamartoma
  K. Nasal glial heterotopia [nasal glioma]
VIII. Vascular Malformations
  A. Capillary telangiectasia
  B. Cavernous angioma
  C. Arteriovenous malformation
  D. Venous malformation
  E. Sturge-Weber disease [cerebrofacial or cerebrotrigeminal angiomatosis]
IX. Tumors of the Anterior Pituitary
  A. Pituitary adenomas
    1. Acidophil
    2. Basophil [mucoid cell]
    3. Mixed acidophil-basophil
    4. Chromophobe
  B. Pituitary adenocarcinoma
X. Local Extensions from Regional Tumors
  A. Glomus jugulare tumor [chemodectoma, paraganglioma]
  B. Chordoma
  C. Chondroma
  D. Chondrosarcoma
  E. Olfactory neuroblastoma [esthesioneuroblastoma]
  F. Adenoid cystic carcinoma [cylindroma]
  G. Others
XI. Metastatic Tumors
XII. Unclassified Tumors

From Zülch, K. J.: Histological Typing of Tumours of the Central Nervous System. *International Histological Classification of Tumours* No. 21. Geneva: World Health Organization, 1979, pp 19-24. Reproduced with permission poorly differentiated and embryonal tumors.[280] In the WHO classification, the grade III astrocytoma is considered a malignant astrocytoma, not a glioblastoma multiforme.[280] At UCSF, we use a four-tiered system: differentiated astrocytoma, moderately anaplastic astrocytoma, highly anaplastic astrocytoma, and glioblastoma multiforme (Table XXIV-1-2).

At present, no generally acknowledged grading system exists, although modified varieties of a three-grade scheme are used more often than the other systems to provide a working framework for classification and for analysis of data from clinical trials. The variations among the systems makes it extremely difficult to compile a comparative review of published clinical trials. To add to the confusion, different pathologists using the same system may disagree, one pathologist classifying a lesion as a grade II tumor while another classifies the same tumor as grade III. As judged on the basis of survival data, however, there tends to be general agreement among the various grading systems on the tumors classified as *glioblastoma multiforme* or the grade III and grade IV astrocytomas of the system devised by Kernohan and colleagues.[120] Unfortunately, the anaplastic astrocytomas other than glioblastoma multiforme are more difficult to delimit, and criteria vary considerably with respect to the proportion of mildly and moderately anaplastic astrocytomas included in a designation.

A specific description of the pathology of each tumor appears in the individual sections that follow. For this purpose, a three-tiered system is used: astrocytoma, anaplastic astrocytoma (including only highly anaplastic astrocytomas), and glioblastoma multiforme.

Proliferative Potential. Recent efforts have been directed

Table XXIV-1-2. Diagnostic Criteria for the Diagnosis of Cerebral Glioblastoma and Infiltrating Astrocytomas Used at the University of California, San Francisco*

A. Glioblastoma Multiforme
　1. At least focally highly cellular glial neoplasm and
　2. Nuclear pleomorphism and
　3. Cytoplasmic pleomorphism and
　4. Vascular endothelial proliferation
B. Highly Anaplastic Astrocytoma (infiltrating)
　1. Not a glioblastoma multiforme and
　2. At least focally moderately to highly cellular
　　and two of the following:
　3. High N/C ratio or
　4. Coarse nuclear chromatin or
　5. Much mitotic activity or
　6. Nuclear pleomorphism or
　7. Cytoplasmic pleomorphism
C. Moderately Anaplastic Astrocytoma (infiltrating)
　1. Not a highly anaplastic astrocytoma and
　2. Mild to moderate increased cellularity and
　3. Enlarged nuclei and
　4. Relatively uniform cytoplasm
D. Mildly Anaplastic Astrocytoma (infiltrating)
　1. Not a moderately anaplastic astrocytoma and
　2. Mild increase in cellularity and
　3. Nuclei enlarged, but regular and
　4. Uniform cytoplasm but not gemistocytic

*As revised at the University of California, San Francisco, 30 July 1990

toward finding markers that provide biologic correlates with tumor histopathology and are predictive of a tumor's clinical behavior. These markers include molecular probes and biologic labels introduced into tumors to permit assessment of their cellular proliferative potential. The two most commonly used markers provide a bromodeoxyuridine (BUdR) or a monoclonal antibody Ki-67 labeling index.

BUdR, a thymidine analog that incorporates into DNA during cell synthesis, is given to patients through intravenous infusion 1 hour before surgery. When tumor cells obtained during surgery are exposed to a monoclonal antibody against BUdR, the cells with the greatest proliferative potential are labeled by the marker and stain brown. Counting those cells, a labeling index can be calculated that correlates strongly, although imprecisely, with the tumor's histopathology. Cells from glioblastoma multiforme have the highest mean BUdR labeling index; those from anaplastic astrocytomas have an intermediate BUdR labeling index, and cells from lower-grade astrocytomas have a low BUdR labeling index.[102] Within tumor grades, the BUdR labeling index appears to have predictive potential, particularly in the prognosis of lower-grade lesions; in terms of statistical probabilities, low-grade astrocytomas showing a high BUdR labeling index are more likely than those with a lower labeling index to behave in a malignant fashion. For this reason, patients treated at UCSF are routinely given an intravenous bolus injection of BUdR before surgery and the tissue removed during surgery is processed to obtain the BUdR labeling index as an estimate of the malignant proliferative potential of the tumor.

The BUdR labeling technique is relatively easily performed and because of its proven accuracy in predicting a tumor's behavior, the BUdR labeling index provides important information for the planning of treatment. In assessing lower grade lesions, Hoshino and colleagues have shown the impact of the BUdR labeling index on patients' survival rates (Table XXIV-1-3).[104] Among patients with a low-grade astrocytoma, for example, the 3-year survival rate was 85% for the 60% of patients who had a labeling index of less than 1%, whereas the 40% of patients with a labeling index greater than 1% had only a 10% survival rate 3 years after surgery.

The monoclonal antibody Ki-67 index can be used in a similar fashion to the BUdR labeling index.[278] This immunohistochemical technique detects a nuclear antigen in cells in all phases of the cell cycle except the G_0 phase. The number obtained using this technique differs from the BUdR labeling index, yet it provides similar information and affords clinicians an assessment of a tumor's growth rate. Nishizaki and colleagues, assessing cell proliferation in human brain tumors using Ki-67, BUdR, and DNA content with flow cytometry, showed that both the Ki-67 labeling index and the BUdR labeling index correlated with degree of malignancy, the average Ki-67 labeling index being 1.7 times greater than the BUdR labeling index in individual tumors.[180] They also showed a direct correlation between aneuploidy and high Ki-67 and BUdR labeling indexes. All aneuploid tumors were malignant, although all malignant tumors did not show DNA aneuploidy. Assuming no sampling error, these correlations were not infallibly predictive, either in this study or in our own experience. Some tumors with a high labeling index followed a benign course and others with a relatively

Table XXIV-1-3.   BUdR Labeling Indices of 227 Neuroectodermal Tumors Treated at the University of California, San Francisco up to 1988*

Tumor type	No. of cases	Labeling index (%)		No. of cases of LI		
		Median	Range	<1%	1–5%	>5%
Medulloblastoma	13	9.8	<1.0–38.2	1	1	11
Glioblastoma multiforme	78	7.3	<1.0–30.5	0	17	61
Highly anaplastic astrocytoma	36	2.7	<1.0–21.2	5	21	10
Moderately anaplastic astrocytoma	48	<1.0	<1.0–9.3	29	16	3
Ependymoma	20	<1.0	<1.0–18.9	15	4	1
Juvenile pilocytic astrocytoma	14	<1.0	<1.0–4.3	7	7	0
Mixed glioma	12	1.7	<1.0–8.0	5	5	2
Ganglioglioma	6	<1.0	<1.0–2.4	4	2	0
Total	227	—	—	66	73	88

*Courtesy of Dr. Takao Hoshino, University of California, San Francisco, unpublished data, 1990

low labeling index have behaved aggressively. Indeed, of 78 gliomas which Jimenez and colleagues studied for DNA aneuploidy with flow cytometry, 63% were diploid and 37% aneuploid.[115] Except for two oligodendrogliomas that were aneuploid, the rest of the aneuploid lesions were astrocytomas. They found no correlation between DNA ploidy and histology or between DNA ploidy and survival. The factors that were most important in determining survival were age and vascular endothelial proliferation.

Immunopathology. Although circulating antiglioma antibodies have been shown to participate in complement-dependent and antibody-dependent reactions, further testing has proved that the antibody response is not specific, showing cross-reactivity to other tumors and to connective tissue.[26] Nonetheless, further testing in this area is warranted.

Immune cellular responses are depressed in patients with gliomas. Peripheral blood lymphocytes have reduced mitogenic activity, and recent work has suggested a possible concomitant increase in T suppressor cells.[219] The reduction in T-cell function may be a consequence of glioma-linked factors and may account for other immunologic abnormalities observed in patients with such tumors.

Many studies have evaluated the mononuclear cell infiltration observed in malignant gliomas. Rossi and colleagues evaluated 65 malignant astrocytomas for the presence of macrophages, lymphocytes, and natural killer cells.[218] Using immunoperoxidase staining with various monoclonal antibodies, they demonstrated macrophage infiltration in more than 85% of tumors; 88% contained T cells, the majority being T cytotoxic/suppressor cells. Natural killer cells were observed in 9% of tumors tested; B cells were absent in 88% of the tumors. An important finding was that human leukocyte antigen (HLA-DR) class II antigens existed not only in 100% of the tissue macrophages tested, but also in the tumor cells in 40% of these malignant astrocytomas. The detection of HLA-DR class II antigens on tumor cells is highly suggestive of a specific immune-response capability, those cells possibly serving as the antigen-presenting cell. Class II antigens are necessary for macrophage-antigen interactions to take place after antigen presentation. T cells then become activated, after which a cascade of events can take place, including the production of gamma interferon, IL-2 and subsequently natural killer cells and tumor necrosis factor. Despite this host response, tumor-related factors are known to exist

that have the ability to suppress IL-2-dependent T-cell proliferation. One of these factors is thought to be TGF-β.[273]

Host-tumor interactions are complex, yet they have potential for therapeutic immunologic interventions and suggest a possibility that the interactions might be detectable and analyzed with imaging modalities, as discussed later in this chapter. Intensive research into these events has as its goal the development of treatment strategies that are specific and nontoxic to normal tissues.

Clinical Presentation

Patients with tumors of glial origin often present with either general, nonfocal signs and symptoms or with focal manifestations related to the specific area of the brain occupied by the lesion. General signs include headache, nausea, vomiting, generalized seizures, or changes in level of consciousness. Although headache accompanies many brain tumors, few patients with headache have a brain tumor. The headaches associated with tumors may be intermittent, moderate to severe, more prominent in the early morning, and/or aggravated by maneuvers that can increase intracranial pressure, such as coughing. The pain is caused by pressure on nerve endings in the dura and blood vessels throughout the cranium. Headache associated with an increase in intracranial pressure, as occurs in most cases, is generalized and nonfocal and does not lateralize to the site of the tumor. Conversely, headaches not associated with increased intracranial pressure may truly localize a tumor: tumors in the anterior and/or middle cranial fossa may present with frontal, often supraorbital, headaches; those in the posterior fossa may present with suboccipital pain.

Seizures may be the initial manifestation of a brain tumor and eventually as many as 30% of patients with brain tumors develop seizures. Typically, seizures occur in conjunction with slower-growing, superficial tumors that involve the sensorimotor cortex. Rapidly growing tumors, such as glioblastoma multiforme, may not cause seizures as a presenting sign but may do so in time. In an adult, the new onset of seizure requires that tumor be excluded as the cause; as many as 10% of patients with generalized seizures are found to harbor a tumor. Focal seizures and partial complex seizures are more likely to reflect a tumor than is a grand-mal seizure with no focal component. Neuroimaging should be performed, and if there is a lesion, it should be subjected to histologic diagnosis. In children, seizures are due to intracranial tumors in less than 1% of cases; however, a child with seizures that are difficult to control–especially partial complex seizures–should be assessed using magnetic resonance (MR) imaging. A lesion or abnormality seen on the image may represent a neoplastic growth, often a slow-growing tumor such as a ganglioglioma. In one series of patients who were to undergo surgery for the control of seizures, 15% had a mass, and in 70% of those, the mass was a tumor.[244] At UCSF, patients with long-standing seizures often are referred for an operation to provide control and, during surgery, are found to have a tumor, a management issue discussed shortly in the section on low-grade gliomas.

Vomiting by a patient with a glial tumor may be related to a rise of intracranial pressure or, rarely, may reflect a tumor's invasion of the area postrema or vagal nucleus in the posterior fossa. Usually, the vomiting is related to increases in intracranial pressure and is accompanied by nausea. Projectile vomiting is not a usual presenting symptom, but may occur with rapid rises in intracranial pressure. Disequilibrium and even true vertigo may occur as a consequence of the increased pressure on medullary nuclei and vestibular apparatus.

Signs of intracranial glial tumors include papilledema, diplopia, cranial nerve palsies, motor and sensory abnormalities, and changes in levels of consciousness. Most patients exhibit some focal sign or symptom either at presentation or later during treatment. In following patients during treatment, the neurologic examination often provides the first clue to a change in status. Defining the etiology of a change may pose difficulties, however, requiring confirmatory neuroimaging to distinguish change caused by the tumor from change caused by edema or change as a complication of therapy. Acute changes may be related to events independent of the tumor, to irradiation and/or chemotherapy, to infections, to seizures or medications for seizure control, or to depression, hormonal imbalances such as hypothyroidism, or other medical conditions. A systematic search should be undertaken for the underlying cause of change because a change does not necessarily mean tumor progression. Acute changes caused by tumor that may be reversible with surgery include hydrocephalus due to shunt failure, hemorrhage related to tumor growth, necrosis related to irradiation, and cyst formation that may or may not be related to tumor progression.

Tumors of the frontal lobes often cause changes in mental status, including impaired intellect, reduced attention span, poor judgment, labile behavior, or dulled thought processes to the point of inability to communicate with any consistent or logical train of thought. Often, patients show losses of social inhibition alternating between vulgarity and bouts of crying. Both frontal lobes are usually affected to produce these changes, but unilateral frontal-lobe tumors may produce the same effects. Lesions that affect the premotor area may produce apraxia and mild rigidity but no loss of strength, whereas those that affect the motor cortex produce contralateral weakness. Dominant hemispheric lesions may produce motor (expressive) aphasia, often with agraphia. Patients' ability to repeat words spoken to them may be preserved, even if there is loss of volitional speech. There may be reflex changes, including abnormal grasp, suck, snout, and palmomental reflexes.

Tumors of the temporal lobes may cause abnormalities in speech, hearing, memory, and vision. Dominant temporal-lobe syndromes include auditory hallucinations, dysnomia, receptive aphasia, impairment of recent memory, and homonymous quadrantanopia. Nondominant temporal lobe findings may include spatial disorientation and problems with perception of taste, hearing, vision, and/or movement, as well as difficulty in memory retention. Seizures may accompany tumors in either temporal lobe, and often are complex partial seizures that may cause disorders of awareness and abnormal perceptions including those of the senses just described.

Lesions in the parietal lobes may cause abnormalities of sensation, including patients' inability to localize parts of their body, defects in two-point discrimination, and inability to recognize letters or numbers traced on the skin or objects placed in the hand. Neglect syndromes may occur contralateral to the side of the lesion, including lack of awareness of objects in the contralateral visual field or of movement or position of the body on the opposite side. Gerstmann's syndrome, a dominant parietal lobe disorder, includes agraphia, acalculia, finger agnosia, and right-left disorientation. Difficulty in performing complex tasks of motor function when instructed to do so may also occur. Visual field testing may reveal an inferior quadrantanopia or hemianopia.

Occipital lobe tumors cause deficits in almost all cases, including visual field defects, visual hallucinations occurring with or without seizures, and failure to recognize familiar faces or objects. Complete destruction of the occipital lobe causes contralateral homonymous hemianopia; bilateral lesions cause blindness. Visual hallucinations without seizures are strongly suggestive of an occipital lesion.

Glial tumors of the thalamus often manifest with increases in intracranial pressure, hemisensory loss or hemiparesis, and pain syndromes. Choreoathetosis may occur. Lesions of the hypothalamus produce endocrine dysfunction and visual pathway abnormalities. Patients may present with retarded growth, obesity, anorexia, and/or, in infants, the diencephalic syndrome of cachexia, euphoria, hyperkinesia, and nystagmus. Endocrine manifestations may include acromegaly, Cushing's disease, precocious puberty, infertility, loss of libido, amenorrhea, and/or galactorrhea. Diabetes insipidus and the syndrome of inappropriate antidiuretic hormone secretion may also occur. Tumors that extend into the chiasm cause visual field defects, loss of visual acuity, papilledema, and optic atrophy. Lesions in the region of the third ventricle usually manifest as a consequence of obstructive hydrocephalus, with headache, nausea, and papilledema.

Tumors of the cerebellum cause patients to show ipsilateral signs when the hemisphere is involved, including ataxia, hypotonia, nystagmus, and a tendency to fall to the affected side. They have coordination abnormalities during voluntary movement. Midline cerebellar lesions produce a wide-based unsteady gait (truncal ataxia) and nystagmus. Patients often have hydrocephalus from obstruction of the fourth ventricle and the resulting nausea, headache, and papilledema.

Lesions of the brain stem cause cranial-nerve and long-tract signs, and possibly hydrocephalus when the upper midbrain is involved or compression of the fourth ventricle occurs. Bilateral facial-nerve and abducens-nerve palsies frequently occur, as well as hemiparesis, hemiplegia, or limb and gait ataxia.

While these highlights reflect some of the more common findings associated with brain tumors, it is important to be aware that most patients who ultimately are diagnosed as having a malignant brain tumor have had signs and symptoms of their disease for weeks, months, or sometimes years before a histologic diagnosis is made. For any adult who has a new onset seizure, personality change, or new focal neurologic findings, the suspicion of a brain neoplasm should at least be considered in the differential diagnosis and the patient should be referred for neurologic evaluation.

Diagnostic Neuroimaging

Patients with signs and symptoms that suggest an intracranial mass should undergo neuroimaging studies and if they show a lesion, it should be subjected to histologic diagnosis.

Computerized Tomography. Contrast-enhanced computerized tomography (CT) scans are almost 95–97% sensitive in detecting a lesion and rarely show false-negative results. Tumors less than 1 cm in diameter can be detected with third-generation and fourth-generation CT scanners. Contrast agents must be used in order to fully characterize an abnormality; a noncontrast CT scan is not sufficient to make the diagnosis and should never be relied on to exclude a CNS lesion.

Despite the decisive superiority of contrast-enhanced CT scans to all forms of neuroimaging except magnetic resonance (MR) imaging, several limitations exist. Generally, CT is done only in the axial plane and computer reconstructions in other planes, such as coronal images, have some loss of detail. In addition, bone hardening artifacts make the evaluation of lesions in the posterior fossa difficult to interpret—this particular problem makes CT a less desirable modality for evaluating lesions in this area. Despite these limitations, contrast-enhanced CT scans are a valuable tool for both the initial evaluation and follow-up studies in many cases of malignant brain tumors.

Magnetic Resonance Imaging. MR imaging is now the neuroimaging technique most frequently used in the evaluation and follow-up review of patients with malignant brain tumors. MR imaging has several advantages over contrast-enhanced CT. The patient is not exposed to radiation. Multiple planar images are available with no loss of detail. Lesions of the spine or posterior fossa are seen in more detail than with CT, and different sequences are available to characterize the tumor. Moreover, patients are not exposed to iodinated contrast agents, obviating possible allergic reactions. The new paramagnetic agent, gadolinium (Gd) with the agent diethylenetriamine-penta-acetic acid (DPTA), permits contrast-enhanced MR images with an essentially minimal risk of allergic reactions and it shows enhancement in areas of disrupted or abnormal blood-brain barrier.

Comparison of CT and MR Imaging. In a review of the role of Gd-DPTA-enhanced MR imaging (MRI-Gd), Stack and colleagues compared such images with contrast-enhanced CT scans in patients with intracranial pathology.[245]

MR imaging sequences were obtained with T1 and T2 weighting and with T1 weighting and Gd. In all cases of high-grade gliomas, the T2-weighted (T2W) image revealed a lesion. However, the T2W sequence was not reliable in differentiating solid tumor from surrounding peritumoral edema. Even with T1-weighted (T1W) sequences done without Gd, lesions were identified, but demarcation of the tumor from surrounding normal brain was not optimally clear. When Gd was used with T1W sequences, contrast enhancement was seen in most of the tumors, distinguishing gross tumor margin from surrounding edema. Not all high-grade gliomas enhance on either CT or MRI-Gd, and the presence or absence of enhancement cannot be relied on to predict the tumor histology.

In a comparison of MRI-Gd with contrast-enhanced CT in cases of low-grade tumors, the primary advantage of MRI-Gd was the ability to view the lesions in more than one plane, even when enhancement was similar with both techniques.[245] In many cases of low-grade lesions, no enhancement is seen on either CT scans or MR images. However, there are tumors identifiable with MRI-Gd that do not show enhancement on CT scans. Some tumors are seen better on CT scans mostly because of the extent of calcification in the lesion, a feature not easily demonstrated with MR imaging, with or without Gd. In fact, CT is more desirable for following patients with calcified lesions because CT defines the anatomy more clearly.

Cases in which MR imaging may be more useful than CT include those of dural lesions. Although contrast-enhanced CT clearly defines dural-based meningiomas well, the advantage of MRI-Gd is its ability to view the lesion in multiple planes and to image the extent of dural involvement and en plaque lesions. All intracranial meningiomas enhance on MRI-Gd, making the tumor's anatomy easily identifiable for the surgeon. MRI-Gd also may reveal additional or multiple lesions not appreciated with contrast-enhanced CT scans.

In cases of metastatic disease to the brain, MRI-Gd is the technique of choice because of its sensitivity. The apparently single lesion shown on a contrast-enhanced CT scan may actually represent multiple intracranial lesions that are more accurately identified with MRI-Gd. Lesions of the brain stem, spinal cord, and leptomeninges are also more easily identified with MRI-Gd, and for brain stem tumors MRI-Gd is preferred. Tumors that involve intramedullary spinal cord often have MR signal characteristics that are different from those of a normal spinal cord, mainly because of prolonged T1 and T2 relaxation times. Tumor nodules within cysts are easily visualized with MRI-Gd, affording valuable information for the surgeon. In many cases, MRI-Gd can replace myelography, or at least complements it, after an initial myelogram is made, to the extent that lesions may be followed sequentially without the need for additional myelography.

In some cases, MRI-Gd should replace CT but, as yet, few prospective trials have evaluated both of these techniques for specific tumor types. Contrast-enhanced CT is a valuable diagnostic tool for the most common tumor type followed in our clinics—high-grade gliomas such as anaplastic astrocytoma and glioblastoma multiforme. In contrast, MRI-Gd is now preferred for lesions in the posterior fossa and is even used more frequently in evaluating supratentorial tumors. It is also preferable in defining and enumerating metastases in the brain. At UCSF, supratentorial tumors are most frequently followed using sequential contrast-enhanced CT scans, whereas lesions in the posterior fossa or spine are routinely followed with MRI-Gd.

The disadvantages of MR imaging are its cost and its inability to detect calcium or the bone changes that present with some tumors. In such cases, CT and MR imaging may be complementary, CT showing the margins of bone erosion and MR imaging, the mass within the area of bone involvement. In any case, a specific diagnosis is not possible based on the CT scan or MR image alone. The diagnosis must depend on a histopathologic analysis of surgical material.

Other Imaging Techniques. Although proton MR imaging has greatly improved our ability to detect and follow tumors in patients with malignant gliomas, it still lacks diagnostic specificity. New MR imaging techniques are being developed to investigate the biochemical basis of tumors. One such tool is phosphorus-31 MR spectroscopy (^{31}P-MRS), which is being used to evaluate such points as its applicability in assessing the response to therapy, the analysis of differences in the phosphorus spectrum between normal and abnormal brain tissue, and the correlation, if any, of this spectrum with specific tumor types. ^{31}P-MRS images are made using conventional MR imaging techniques, changing the field strengths for specific spectral imaging.

Heindel and colleagues, who studied 35 patients with ^{31}P-MRS, could monitor different phosphorus signals, including phosphomonoester (PME), phosphodiester (PDE), phosphocreatine (PCr), inorganic phosphate (Pi), and adenosine triphosphate (ATP); tissue pH could be calculated from a chemical shift of Pi and PCr.[94] Their patients with meningiomas showed markedly reduced PCr peak levels, diminished PDE levels, and occasional increases in PME, whereas those with glioblastoma multiforme had variable changes that included reduced PME and PCr. Low-grade tumors, as compared with normal brain in the same patient, often did not show changes. Hubesch and colleagues observed reductions in PCr, PME, PDE, and decreased ratios of PCr to Pi in patients with malignant glioma.[106] Measurements of tissue pH have shown inconsistent results, with a suggestion that tumors are alkaline relative to normal brain.[106]

Among other investigators using ^{31}P-MRS to study patients during treatment, Arnold and colleagues evaluated a patient before and after administration of intraarterial therapy with 1,3,bis(2-chloroethyl)-1-nitrosourea (carmustine, also BCNU).[13] As compared to the phosphorus spectrum before therapy, ^{31}P-MRS showed a decrease in PCr and PDE just after treatment and an increase in tissue pH 8 hours later. By 32 hours after treatment, the PCr and PDE had begun to increase again, with a still greater increase in tissue pH. No changes were seen on concurrent MR images or CT scans. Sagebarth and colleagues studied 12 patients with ^{31}P-MRS before and after therapy.[228] In one patient with an astrocytoma, a comparison of ^{31}P-MRS images made before and after radiation therapy showed changes in the postirradiation PME and Pi peaks. In a patient with lymphoma, ^{31}P-MRS images before radiation therapy showed high concentrations of PME and a low PCr to ATP ratio, and in the images made after irradiation, the spectrum was indistinguishable from

normal brain. The patient had improved clinically and a proton MR image also showed significant improvement. Other investigators similarly have assessed changes with therapy using ^{31}P-MRS as a potential noninvasive method for studying the biochemical characteristics of the lesion seen on proton MR imaging. One useful application of such an analysis would be to distinguish radiation-induced tissue necrosis from tumor regrowth, which at present is difficult to do using standard imaging techniques, particularly in patients treated with interstitial brachytherapy.

^{31}P-MRS is a noninvasive diagnostic and monitoring technique potentially available wherever MR imaging is used. An established means of demonstrating metabolic changes, it should become a useful tool for studying biochemical events within tumors and for following them during therapy.

Thallium-201 (^{201}Tl) single-photon emission CT (SPECT) has been used in the evaluation of many tumors, recently including primary brain tumors. There is very little uptake of thallium in normal brain and its distribution is similar to that of potassium, depending on the blood flow, blood-brain barrier permeability, and active pumping of this analog into malignant cells. It has been proposed that thallium is taken up preferentially by tumor cells, as opposed to necrotic tissue, and that the rate of uptake correlates with the tumor growth rate.[116] Mountz and colleagues calculated a tumor/cardiac ^{201}Tl uptake ratio to distinguish residual tumor from post-therapeutic changes such as necrosis in patients with brain tumors.[173] Their study suggested that an increased ratio of tumor to cardiac uptake correctly identified residual tumor, even in some cases when contrast-enhanced CT did not. The ^{201}Tl uptake ratio was also helpful in distinguishing necrosis from viable tumor in a contrast-enhancing lesion. Black and colleagues also used this method to compare ^{201}Tl uptake in brain tumor to that in noninvolved normal brain.[27] A lesion with an index greater than 1.5 was shown to be highly suggestive of a high-grade lesion.

Positron emission tomography (PET) using rubidium-82 (^{82}Rb) or fluorine-18-fluorodeoxyglucose (^{18}FDG) has shown promise in differentiating viable tumor from necrosis related to various forms of radiation therapy. Valk and colleagues followed 34 patients with high-grade malignant gliomas who had been treated with external and interstitial irradiation.[258] When a patient's CT scans and clinical history suggested either tumor recurrence or radiation necrosis, impossible to distinguish on CT scans alone, ^{82}Rb was used to define the area of blood-brain barrier breakdown and the ^{18}FDG images were used to evaluate this area. Whenever the ^{18}FDG uptake was greater in the lesion than in adjacent tissue, a diagnosis of tumor recurrence was made. As determined on the basis of the patient's clinical course and the results of subsequent surgery, the PET diagnosis was accurate in 15 of 17 patients with active regrowth of tumor and in 17 of 21 with radiation injury. Francavilla and colleagues, comparing ^{18}FDG PET scans made at early and later phases of development of the same lesion, showed changes in metabolism, the tumor's becoming hypermetabolic during malignant degeneration of a low-grade to a higher-grade glioma.[75] This work suggests that PET can be used in follow-up evaluations of patients with low-grade malignancies, to correctly diagnose malignant degeneration and thus guide subsequent management.

The hope for all of these experimental neuroimaging studies is that they may offer clinicians relatively noninvasive tools to evaluate patients, to further characterize the biochemical makeup of tumors, to help in predicting response to therapy, and to aid in quickly making a differential diagnosis, allowing for more precise treatment decisions.

Surgical Diagnosis and Resection

Despite the significant improvements in neuroimaging and its usefulness in deciding on surgical approaches, a specific diagnosis cannot be established through imaging alone.[93,212] A tissue diagnosis is necessary for prognostic reasons, and a precise tumor diagnosis is absolutely necessary to plan therapy effectively.

Surgery is undertaken in most cases with the intention of doing a biopsy for histologic diagnosis of the tumor type followed by a craniotomy and an appropriate tumor resection. Neurosurgical morbidity and mortality rates have improved to such a degree over the past several decades that a decision not to operate on an operable brain tumor is rare. At present, virtually the only reason not to operate on an otherwise healthy brain tumor patient is an MR image indicating that any diagnosis other than a diffuse brain stem lesion is extremely unlikely, that the histologic diagnosis is not necessarily of prognostic value, and that surgery has a significant risk of complications. For almost every other intracranial lesion, tissue can be obtained for histologic diagnosis either by craniotomy and biopsy or resection or by ultrasound-guided or stereotactic-guided biopsy.

From a purely oncologic point of view, surgery is still the most rapid method of tumor cell removal. Apart from diagnostic accuracy, there are several other reasons for a surgical approach to the management of malignant brain tumors. Surgery potentially increases patients' survival period, during which they may receive other therapies. Moreover, surgery reduces the tumor cell population, leaving fewer tumor cells to be eradicated with irradiation and chemotherapy. Surgery also produces partial or complete resolution of symptoms and may delay the onset of new symptoms. By changing the kinetics of tumor growth, surgery perhaps enhances the effectiveness of sequential therapies, such as irradiation and chemotherapy.

Decision-making in the neurosurgical management of a patient thought to have an intracranial neoplasm entails an understanding of the anatomy and vascularity of the tumor, its relation to adjacent structures and the neurologic function of the area, the implications of the patient's age and medical condition, and the desires of the patient and family regarding the possible outcome of treatment. Variables that affect the overall outcome must also be understood in order to plan surgery most effectively. Many slow-growing, low-grade astrocytic lesions are difficult to treat surgically, for instance, because they are diffusely infiltrative, having indistinct margins and minimal mass effect. For patients with a very large hemispheric lesion, surgery would not be used to relieve symptoms, but rather to make a diagnosis. If extensive tumor removal is virtually certain to improve overall survival, then the risk of neurologic deterioration should be discussed with the patient and weighed against the benefit of longer life.

Because the quality of patients' lives can be defined only by each patient individually, choices affecting quality of life must be decided by patients themselves if at all possible, after they are provided with the best information available concerning the risks of surgical resection in their particular case. In the case of large, diffuse hemispheric lesions, the impact of extensive tumor removal in improving survival is still debatable–a fact the patient must clearly understand. In other situations, the impact of surgery is more definable. A lesion causing severe mass effect with the potential for herniation urgently requires surgery. In a patient over 50 years of age, the most common tumor causing severe mass effect is a malignant glioma, most likely a glioblastoma multiforme. Such cases require more than simply a diagnostic biopsy–extensive tumor resection makes the diagnosis, relieves symptoms, improves survival, and affords time to discuss and implement further therapies. The benefit of initial, extensive resection to improve survival in such situations has been documented.[158] The recommended approach is to perform as nearly total a resection as is possible while preserving function. In our experience, most of the long-term survivors of malignant gliomas have had nearly total or gross-total removal of tumor.

Patients who are in poor physical health and harbor a deep-seated lesion may be treated best with stereotactic biopsy under local anesthesia to document the tumor histology before more extensive surgery is undertaken. If the histologic diagnosis is primary CNS lymphoma, for instance, then attempts at extensive tumor resection are unwarranted because they would not change the prognosis for survival. However, if the lesion is an astrocytoma, then a more definitive surgical resection is indicated.

The extent of surgical resection depends on the medical and anesthetic risks to the patient and the location and histology of the tumor. Although a tumor that is resected completely requires no further therapy, total resection is seldom an attainable goal with gliomas, the only exceptions being among such childhood tumors as hemispheric astrocytomas. For this reason, even if a lesion appears to have well-defined margins, the likelihood that some tumor cells remain after surgery is adequate reason for additional therapy to eliminate any residual tumor.

Protection of normal brain is the consideration limiting aggressive tumor removal but, within that restriction, the possibility of increasing survival has renewed surgeons' interest in pursuing extensive tumor removal, even in the knowledge that total resection is impossible and that further therapy is anticipated.[272] As opposed to a large residual tumor burden, which often has hypoxic or poorly vascularized areas that make the lesion less responsive to radiation therapy and chemotherapy, the reduced tumor burden afforded by extensive resection is more easily managed with adjuvant therapies. Particularly in young children, the negative effects of wide-field radiation therapy required to treat a large residual tumor burden is sufficient reason to aspire to total tumor removal and improvement in severe seizures refractory to medical treatment that may accompany residual and regrowing lesions.

Cortical Mapping. In light of the potential advantages of extensive resection in both children and adults, cerebral cortical mapping with neurophysiologic monitoring is an important surgical adjunct. Cortical mapping during surgery permits a more complete resection of tumor with a higher probability of retaining function and minimizing neurologic morbidity. It permits a physiologic representation to be drawn in relation to the gross anatomy of the brain, giving the surgeon a more precise knowledge of the probable effects of operating in the area of the tumor. Subcortical stimulation permits more extensive resection of lesions deep within the white matter as well.

The technique entails stimulation of excitable cortex. The cortical loci of eloquent faculties, such as language, appear to be variable and individually distinct among patients.[182] Identification of the appropriate cortical loci permits more or less extensive resection of intervening tumor while preserving eloquent function. Motor cortex can be defined with the patient under general anesthesia, but only local anesthesia can be given when localizing language functions. Nonetheless, with the patient's cooperation the process is easily managed in older children and adults.

With its other possible benefits, cortical mapping can also provide seizure control with simultaneous resection of the seizure foci, although often the focus of seizure activity is adjacent to, rather than in the area of, the tumor.[24] In some cases a better outcome is obtained by monitoring the focus of seizure activity while tumor resection is under way. Difficulties of the technique are that a longer perioperative period is often required and that patients must be awake during the mapping of eloquent brain, which is impracticable in young children. Also, patients who have complex language disturbances cannot comprehend or cooperate sufficiently to make the procedure worthwhile.

Cortical mapping with neurophysiologic monitoring requires a knowledgeable and specialized team consisting of a surgeon, anesthesiologist, neurologist, and neurophysiologist. The potential for longer survival and improved quality of life makes this technique very attractive in efforts to achieve the maximum safe resection of tumor. If properly done, it is a an extremely useful and valuable surgical tool deserving wider application.

Postoperative Imaging

Contrast enhancement on the postoperative CT or MRI-Gd image may be attributable to residual tumor volume as well as to events related to surgery, such as gliosis and revascularization. In canine models, the contrast changes attributable to surgery are not evident on CT scans until at least 1 week after surgery, suggesting that CT scans made soon after surgery demonstrate residual tumor rather than changes related to surgical resection and healing.[110] Cairncross and colleagues studied postoperative contrast enhancement in 10 patients with gliomas, noting that enhancement in the margin of resection did not occur until later than 5 days after surgery.[37] For these reasons, at UCSF, we obtain the initial postoperative CT scans or MR images within 72 hours after surgery to assess accurately the residual tumor volume and the extent of resection.

Clinical Trials

Patients entered into clinical trials are routinely followed with neuroimaging studies based on their specific diagnosis.

For patients with glioblastoma multiforme or anaplastic astrocytoma, a postoperative contrast-enhanced CT scan or MRI-Gd image should be obtained first within 72 hours after surgery, once again after the completion of radiation therapy, and then usually between each cycle of systemic chemotherapy. Sequential images or scans are analyzed for changes and, based on both the serial scans and the patient's neurologic status, the response to treatment is designated according to standardized response criteria.

In conducting clinical trials, a designation of *response* or *no response* is important to assess the impact of specific therapies. It is crucial to recognize, however, that there are no pathognomonic neurologic findings that document tumor progression with absolute certainty. Patients who have tumor progression may show no clinical signs or symptoms whatever, whereas those who show changes in clinical status may not have tumor progression but rather may exhibit complications of treatment, such as infection, cyst formation, hemorrhage, injury related to irradiation, or hydrocephalus. Only serial scans and images can be relied on to portray reliably the status or progression of tumor.

The new imaging techniques, such as MRI-Gd and PET, may make it possible to document changes related to treatment or tumor progression earlier than has been possible. In terms of managing a recurrent tumor, multiple therapies in sequence, including techniques such as interstitial brachytherapy, have increased survival rates—perhaps because the amount of tumor regrowth that must be treated is smaller as a result of earlier detection with MRI-Gd or PET.

Some tumors require surveillance more frequently than others, whether because of their estimated growth potential or because of a need to assess their response to experimental therapies independent of their growth potential. The hazards of frequent imaging are minimal, particularly with MR imaging. Cost is an important issue, however, and the clinician must weigh the information to be gained from a scan or image against the expense involved. It is difficult to place a cost factor into the formula for treatment of malignant glioma. Clearly, with more effective therapies, patients may live longer and in better health, and thus earlier intervention and closer follow-up review may actually reduce overall medical costs. In addition to the intangible benefits of improved quality of life and a sense of well-being for the patient, factors such as a patient's continued ability to work are also important to consider in assessing the cost-benefit ratio.

The discussion of individual glial tumor types that follows adds specificity to the general information about tumors of glial origin just described.

Glioblastoma Multiforme and Anaplastic Astrocytoma

These two astrocytic tumor types are treated similarly. Most series that have been reported include both tumor types, the majority being glioblastoma multiforme, but the results can be difficult to interpret because of the different classification schemes used.

Most of the grading systems for malignant astrocytomas described earlier and the UCSF system (Table XXIV-1-2) show similar survival rates within the category of *glioblastoma multiforme* or, according to Kernohan and colleagues, grade III or IV.[120,208] Nelson and colleagues reviewed a large series of patients classified according to a three-tiered system (glioblastoma multiforme, anaplastic astrocytoma, and astrocytoma) and the system of Kernohan and colleagues.[120,177] For patients with glioblastoma multiforme and those in grades III and IV, the median survival times were 8, 9, and 10 months respectively. At UCSF, the median survival time for patients with glioblastoma multiforme is 12.5–15 months overall.[152] In making a strict comparison of survival data, however, survival must take into account such very important factors as the patient's age and the extent of resection as well as the histologic variable. On that basis, patients with glioblastoma multiforme have a median survival of 10–12 months overall.

Patients with anaplastic astrocytoma, depending on the specific classification used, have widely differing reported median survival rates. The median survival at UCSF is 36 months, whereas the joint Radiation Therapy Oncology Group (RTOG)/Eastern Cooperative Oncology Group (ECOG) trial shows a median survival of 28 months.[41] Comparatively, the 2-year survival rate for these patients graded according to the UCSF (Table XXIV-1-2) and RTOG systems is close to 70%, but it is only 50% for patients classified according to the system of Kernohan and colleagues and 35% using the European Organisation for Research on Treatment of Cancer (EORTC) system.[34,35,120,208] Until an agreed upon system is adopted worldwide, there will be confusion about such data, at least within this category of tumors.

Epidemiology. Patients with glioblastoma multiforme (mean age, 54 years) are generally older than those with anaplastic astrocytoma (mean age, 45 years) and have a shorter median survival.

Pathology. For the purposes of this chapter, the diagnosis of glioblastoma multiforme requires a histologic pattern consisting of a highly cellular astrocytic tumor with nuclear and cellular pleomorphism, vascular proliferation, and mitotic figures. Necrosis frequently is present and although necrosis is requisite for a diagnosis of glioblastoma multiforme in most grading systems, it is not a requirement at UCSF. Most glioblastomas multiforme are microscopically infiltrative lesions and have a high labeling index. In contrast, anaplastic astrocytomas, which are highly cellular astrocytic neoplasms with moderate nuclear and cytoplasmic pleomorphism, may have mitotic figures and do not have necrosis. They are infiltrative with a high labeling index, although typically the labeling index is lower than that in glioblastoma multiforme.

Diagnostic Neuroimaging. The usual appearance of a glioblastoma multiforme or an anaplastic astrocytoma on MR imaging and CT is that of a single, contrast-enhancing lesion, frequently showing mass effect (Figures XXIV-1-1–XXIV-1-4). Kelly and colleagues, from multiple stereotactic biopsies, showed that the contrast-enhancing lesion on CT represents proliferative malignant cells, the central low-density region is true necrosis, and the region of low attenuation surrounding the contrast margins harbors infiltrating cells; there may also be active tumor cells within the larger area of abnormality seen on a T2W image, although the margin at which tumor cells cease to exist and only edema is present may be indistinct.[119]

Surgical Diagnosis and Treatment. Surgery for patients

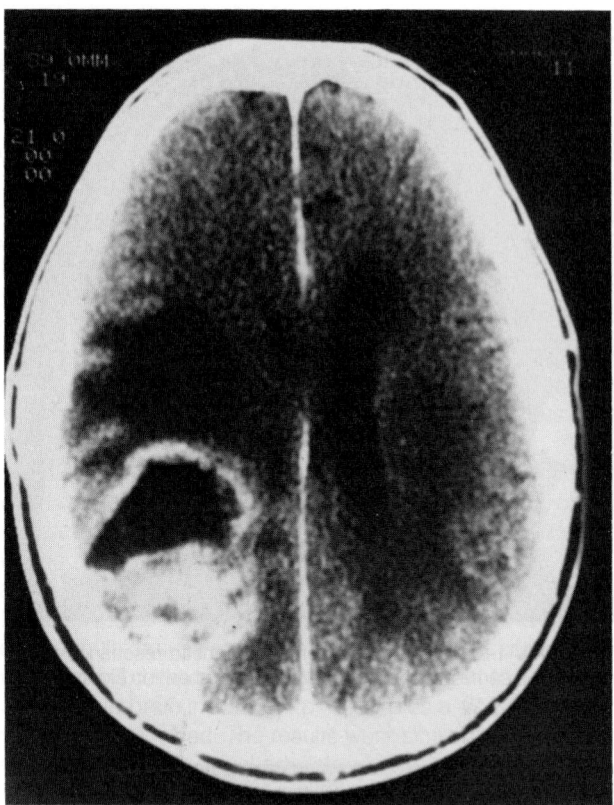

Figure XXIV-1-1.   Contrast-enhanced computed tomography (CT) scan of a primary glioblastoma multiforme.

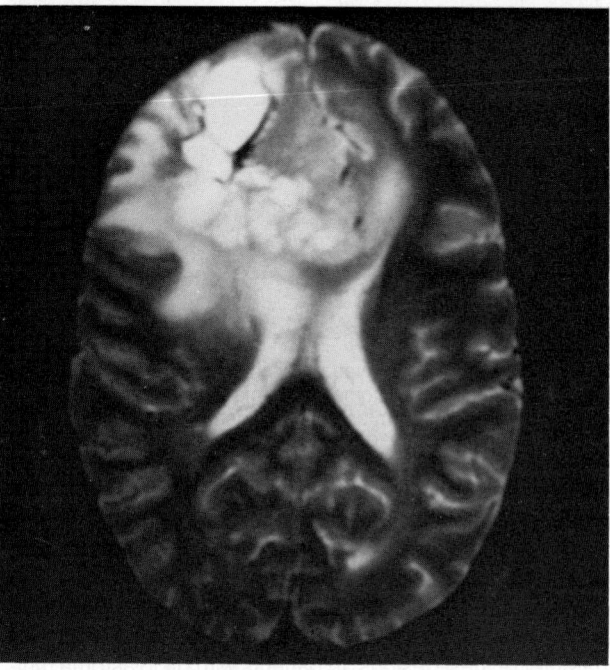

Figure XXIV-1-2.   T2-weighted axial magnetic resonance (MR) image of a glioblastoma multiforme.

tumor recurs within a 2 cm margin of the primary lesion.[44] Until local tumor control can be achieved for prolonged periods of time, there appears to be no survival advantage for the use of whole-brain irradiation.

Hyperfractionation. In standard fractionated radiation therapy, doses of 1.8–2.0 Gy are given daily until a total dose is reached. Different fractionation schemes and total delivered doses have been evaluated by the RTOG.[174,176] In hyperfractionated radiation therapy, more than one fraction of the total dose is given each day using generally smaller doses of radiation per fraction. The rationale for hyperfractionation is to reduce late effects of radiation, especially necrosis, and to prevent tumor repopulation by using more than one treatment each day.[12,62,237] Late injury effects of hyperfractionation depend more on the size of the fraction than on the intertreatment interval. Administering smaller doses minimizes the amount of sublethal radiation injury to normal brain and maximizes cellular repair. Small doses given more than once a day, usually at intervals 4–8 hours apart, produce a redistribution of proliferating tumor cells, some cells entering a radiation-sensitive stage. Nonproliferating tissue or dose-limiting tissue such as normal brain is spared this effect of redistribution or sensitization.

Douglas used a fraction scheme with 1.0 Gy doses administered three times daily, ultimately to a whole-brain radiation dose of 54 Gy with a tumor boost of another 10 Gy.[57] The survival curves for patients with glioblastoma multiforme showed better results than did those for historical controls, with a 1-year survival rate of 44%. However, in a series of trials from the BTSG, BTCG, and RTOG that evaluated hyperfractionated irradiation with or without radiation sensitizers and adjuvant chemotherapies, there was no significant difference in median survival between groups undergoing hyperfractionated irradiation to a total dose as high as 76.8 Gy and those receiving standard single-fraction radiation doses to 60 Gy.[54,86,174] Urtasun and colleagues treated patients with malignant glioma three times daily to a total dose of 61.41, 71.20, or 80.00 Gy and, when a tumor recurred, the patient received single-agent lomustine.[257] Median survivals were 45.8, 37.2, and 60.5 weeks, respectively, using this approach, again no better than historical controls.

It appears from the current data that higher doses of radiation therapy for supratentorial glioblastoma multiforme and anaplastic astrocytoma, whether in single or multiple daily fractions, do not significantly improve median survival times over those achieved with standard single-fraction 60 Gy irradiation. Newer schemes using even higher doses per fraction, termed accelerated hyperfractionation, are being investigated but the results are preliminary.

Radiation-Enhancing Agents. Because radiation is thought to be less cytocidal under hypoxic conditions, and because malignant astrocytomas are presumed to contain hypoxic tumor cells, tolerated radiation doses now used for therapy may produce poor local tumor control; increasing the radiation dose increases the risk of radiation necrosis. Studies to improve the efficacy of radiation given in the conventional dosage include investigations of hypoxic cell sensitizers. The two nitroimidazoles, misonidazole and metronidazole, given during irradiation, are electron-affinic and under conditions of hypoxia are taken up by cells and substitute for oxygen

in producing radiation-induced DNA damage.[29,176] Unfortunately, neither agent has been successful in improving survival and both have significant toxicity in clinical use. Although other imidazole compounds with potentially less toxicity are being investigated in the hope of improving efficacy, studies thus far show no hypoxic cell sensitizers that improve survival of patients with malignant glioma.

Radiation sensitizers such as the halogenated pyrimidines have been investigated in several studies. BUdR and 5-iodo-2-deoxyuridine (IUdR), two nonhypoxic cell-sensitizing agents, are given through constant infusion. They incorporate into the DNA of dividing cells in place of thymidine. Nondividing cells, such as in normal glial and neuronal tissue, do not take up these agents. Hoshino treated 107 patients with a continuous intraarterial infusion of BUdR concurrently with irradiation and found that more than 50% survived 18 months or longer.[101] The study was not repeated because of technical difficulties with the intraarterial delivery system. Greenberg and colleagues also studied intraarterial BUdR using a simplified delivery system and, as compared to historical control subjects, found a survival advantage in a small group of patients with grade III and IV malignant gliomas.[88] Preliminary data from the NCOG suggest a survival advantage with BUdR administered intravenously, as noted in patients with anaplastic astrocytoma but not in those with glioblastoma multiforme.[147] These data require confirmation by a prospective randomized trial that will open soon.

IUdR is undergoing clinical trials for use in primary and metastatic tumors. In a phase I study, continuous intravenous IUdR was delivered concurrently with hyperfractionated irradiation in a dose-escalating scheme.[122] The results suggest that IUdR is less toxic than BUdR and that the kinetics of the drug are linear at doses between 250 and 1200 mg/m², reaching steady state within 1 hour. The results of these investigations are preliminary but suggestive of increased local control rates with IUdR. The main adverse effects of these agents are myelosuppression, photosensitization, changes in the skin and nail bed, allergic reactions, and hepatic injury. However, the toxicities have been mild and generally well tolerated and further trials are planned.

High Linear Energy Transfer (LET) Irradiation. Other forms of radiation therapy less dependent on cellular oxygen include neutron and heavy-ion therapy and are called high LET irradiation. The RTOG has conducted a randomized dose-finding study of neutrons given as a boost to conventional external-beam photon therapy.[127] Patients were treated initially using whole-brain irradiation with photons to a dose of 45 Gy, then boosted with fast neutrons using six different dose levels. There was no difference between the doses in the survival obtained overall but, in patients with tumors other than glioblastoma multiforme, there was a suggestion that neutrons contributed to a poorer survival with the higher doses.

A trial with fast neutrons performed using three different schemes, and a separate study combining misonidazole with neutron therapy, both yielded negative results.[125,225] Other ions, including helium and neon ions, have been studied, and negative pi mesons have been considered because of their theoretical advantage of less resistance of hypoxic cells and more general cell cycle-specific activity. Currently, the

NCOG is conducting a trial using neon irradiation at two dose levels in patients with glioblastoma multiforme, but it is too early to report results.

Interstitial Brachytherapy. Interstitial brachytherapy, the implantation of high-activity radioactive sources or "seeds" within a tumor, has been used to treat highly anaplastic tumors and recurrent primary and metastatic tumors. Stereotactic technique and local anesthesia ensure accurate neurosurgical placement of catheters into the tumor bed, into which the radioactive seeds are afterloaded. The seeds remain in place within the tumor until the desired dose is delivered and then, in a simple maneuver done in the patient's room, the catheters and sources are removed. Patients tolerate the procedure well, the major complications being seizures during source placement and, rarely, infection. Because of its risks and the precision required for proper placement of the radioactive sources, careful selection of patients for brachytherapy is imperative. A dedicated radiation physics and oncology staff ensure the proper dosimetry.

Several radiation sources have been investigated for interstitial use, but the one most commonly used is iodine-125 (^{125}I). Gutin and colleagues have reviewed their experience at UCSF using high-activity ^{125}I interstitial brachytherapy in 45 patients with recurrent glioblastoma multiforme and 50 patients with recurrent anaplastic astrocytoma.[134] The minimum dose delivered to the tumor ranged from 50–120 Gy. The median survival was 54 weeks for patients with recurrent glioblastoma multiforme and 87 weeks for those with anaplastic astrocytoma, measured from the date of implantation. These encouraging survival data show interstitial brachytherapy to be one of the best techniques available for therapy in patients with recurrent tumors. Toxicity, however, is significant. In this series, 46% of the patients underwent reoperation for clinical deterioration caused by an increasing mass of radiation necrosis, although long-term maintenance of quality survival was achieved with an average KPS of 80.[134]

Although the results have been quite impressive, it is necessary to reduce the incidence of clinically significant necrosis with this technique. In a trial opened recently, hyperthermia is used in conjunction with brachytherapy in an attempt to increase local control, to reduce the radiation dose because heat enhances the effects of radiation therapy, and to lessen the risk of radiation necrosis. The short duration of this trial is insufficient to determine whether these goals can be achieved.

Based on the success of brachytherapy in treating patients with recurrent gliomas, several investigators have begun to evaluate this technique in patients at the time of initial diagnosis. An ongoing trial of the NCOG uses brachytherapy after conventional external-beam irradiation for the initial treatment of newly diagnosed malignant gliomas. The interstitial boost is then followed with adjuvant chemotherapy. The preliminary results suggest a survival advantage in patients with glioblastoma multiforme.[91] Among a similar pilot group of patients treated with the same strategy at UCSF, the survival data in patients with glioblastoma multiforme is encouraging, median survival being more than 80 weeks, which compares favorably with historical data for patients treated with conventional irradiation and adjuvant chemotherapy.[133]

These initial results must be confirmed in a prospective randomized trial.

Unfortunately, many patients are not candidates for brachytherapy. The tumor volume that can be implanted safely is generally less than 5 cm in any one dimension; lesions in eloquent areas of the brain are not implanted, including the corpus callosum, thalamus, and other midline deep-seated areas. The typical lesion treated is superficial, small, and in an area where necrosis produced by the procedure can be tolerated. Under these restrictions, most patients with glioblastoma multiforme, malignant astrocytoma, or even recurrent tumor are ineligible for brachytherapy, but for those who have a smaller tumor volume it is a technique that, with further investigation, could add overall to the length and quality of survival.

Radiosurgery. While more commonly used for arteriovenous malformations, radiosurgery has recently been evaluated as a possible treatment for gliomas. So far, it has been used mostly in patients with recurrent gliomas, including metastatic lesions, that have not responded to standard radiation therapy.[154] In this technique, an external beam of radiation is precisely collimated and directed to a small volume in a single large fraction. Several radiation sources have been investigated for use with radiosurgery, including heavy particles, cobalt-60 (^{60}Co), and the conventional linear accelerator. The radiation beam is directed using coordinates on a standard stereotactic head frame or using a gamma unit, a device with a sophisticated head frame that permits precise assignment of coordinates along concentric arcs to cause a convergence of the ^{60}Co source.[156] The objective of radiosurgery is to deliver a finely focused radiation beam precisely to the target. Critical evaluation in recently opened trials must address issues about dose and tumor volume and identify specific criteria for selecting tumors that would benefit from this therapy.

Multimodality Therapy. Attempts to improve the survival advantage obtained with adjuvant chemotherapy include trials of intraarterial drug delivery with the nitrosoureas and platinum compounds, and high-dose chemotherapy with autologous bone marrow transplantation (ABMT). The theoretical advantage of intraarterial therapy over intravenous infusion is in the increased uptake of drug during its first pass through the tumor capillary bed. However, while systemic toxicity may be less than with conventional chemotherapy, the local and regional toxicity is greater, substituting one toxicity for another with no obvious therapeutic advantage.

The BTCG, in a prospective randomized study comparing intraarterial with intravenous carmustine administered concurrently with radiation therapy, showed no survival advantage for patients treated through the intraarterial route but 8% of patients developed leukoencephalopathy and 16% developed unilateral blindness.[230] In a trial by Bashir and colleagues of intraarterial carmustine preceding irradiation, a high incidence of leukoencephalopathy (7%) led them to recommend that this regimen not be used in phase III studies.[18]

Mahaley and colleagues gave 40 patients cisplatin monthly as an intraarterial infusion at the time of tumor recurrence.[157] The median survival of this group was 27.5 weeks for the patients who could be evaluated. Adverse effects included renal, otologic, and neural toxicity. Newton and colleagues used cisplatin in 12 patients at the time of tumor recurrence and found that only one patient had a partial response; all the others had progressive disease or severe toxicity including seizures, weakness, coma, and visual deterioration.[179] In another recently reported trial in which 23 patients received intraarterial carboplatin monthly, 10 patients achieved either a partial response or stabilization of their disease.[73] The investigators proposed that this agent was less toxic than intraarterial cisplatin and warrants further trial.

Other nitrosoureas that have been investigated include ACNU and PCNU, and other cytotoxic agents such as teniposide are undergoing trial.[247,248,274] There is no convincing evidence that these agents improve overall survival and their toxicity is significant. Intraarterial administration of drugs should be used only in the setting of a controlled clinical trial designed to overcome toxicity and improve efficacy.

High-dose chemotherapy with ABMT has also shown only limited success. The difficulty with this approach is the end-organ toxicity of agents such as carmustine or platinum compounds, as well as the paucity of agents with activity against malignant gliomas. Carmustine has been given in large doses, resulting in pulmonary, hepatic, and infectious complications; in 11 patients treated at recurrence the median survival was 7 months.[97] Other alkylating agents investigated include thiotepa, etoposide, and busulfan. One preliminary trial, combining high-dose thiotepa and etoposide with ABMT in pediatric high-grade astrocytoma, has shown encouraging results.[71] It continues to accrue patients and the investigators plan to use this strategy in newly diagnosed patients.

Recommendation for Adjuvant Therapy. From the studies of various combinations of radiation therapy and adjuvant chemotherapy reported thus far, the standard treatment to which other therapies should be compared is still single daily fraction irradiation to a total dose of 60 Gy plus adjuvant carmustine. In patients with glioblastoma multiforme, there is no survival advantage in using whole-brain radiation therapy or other forms of chemotherapy. Adjuvant chemotherapy improves 2-year survival rates in glioblastoma patients and clearly improves median and long-term survival in patients with anaplastic astrocytoma. At least one study supports PCV chemotherapy over therapy with only carmustine in this group. In a select group of patients with glioblastoma, interstitial brachytherapy may improve survival but further trials are needed to confirm these early results.

Recurrence. The precarious character of brain tumor therapy is illustrated by astrocytomas recurring after irradiation, for which the latency period from irradiation to diagnosis may be as short as 3 years or longer than 20 years.[279] The diagnosis of tumor recurrence requires, at the minimum, an increase in tumor volume demonstrated on sequential contrast-enhanced CT scans or on MR images. While seemingly straightforward, neuroimaging studies may be difficult to interpret in the light of previous treatment, or the changes seen on the image may be only slightly worse in the case of a clinically stable patient. Changes seen on CT scans or MR images after interstitial brachytherapy are, in particular, very difficult to interpret and may represent tumor recurrence, radiation necrosis, or a combination of both. [201]Tl-

SPECT or PET studies can be helpful in differentiating these events, but neither is 100% accurate or specific.

New forms of radiation therapy, including accelerated hyperfractionation techniques and radiosurgery, have created yet another set of uncertainties similar to those attending brachytherapy. MRI-Gd is very sensitive to changes associated with radiation injury. Although the tumor volume may remain the same, the internal enhancing characteristics may vary over several images. The significance of these changes continue to be investigated—they may not represent tumor progression.

Clinical neurologic examinations are done concurrently with the neuroimaging assessment and an assessment of the patient's steroid requirements. All three factors are important in the determination of the tumor's status, but the neuroimaging study is the most important indicator of response or progression.

Once it is determined that a tumor has progressed, further treatment may include palliative care, another surgical resection, reirradiation, including brachytherapy or radiosurgery, and chemotherapy. Several factors are important in the assessment of further treatment, including the patient's age and KPS, the tumor histology, the expected outcome of additional therapies weighed against specific risks, and the needs and expectations of the patient and family. Elderly patients with poor KPS and recurrent glioblastoma multiforme have a poor prognosis and little chance of increasing their survival longer than an additional 2–3 months with further therapy. In the clinical situation of a bedridden patient with little remaining cognitive function, even maintenance of the status quo may be undesirable. Conversely, for a younger patient who is neurologically intact with a small tumor regrowth, there is a greater chance of achieving tumor control with little risk of a negative impact on quality of life. In such a case, it may be possible to achieve a median survival of greater than a year, as measured from recurrence, in selected patient groups.

Patients with recurrent malignant gliomas who are treated on research protocol studies generally live longer than those who are not, reflecting both an institutional referral bias and the benefit of further interventions that often occur in sequential treatment regimens. Patients on aggressive treatment programs are often well-motivated, young, and in relatively good neurologic condition. For these reasons, the individual characteristics of groups tested should be carefully and critically weighed in interpreting the results of trials in patients with tumor recurrence.

When tumor recurrence is diagnosed, often the first decision is whether further surgery is recommended. Several studies have addressed the impact of reoperation on quality of survival. Ammirati and colleagues reviewed 55 patients with recurrent malignant astrocytoma who underwent a second resection and reported a median survival of 36 weeks, which is similar to the reported survival of other groups.[8] In reviewing the data from 70 consecutive patients who underwent reoperation for recurrent glioblastoma multiforme and anaplastic astrocytoma, Harsh and colleagues reported a median survival of 36 weeks for patients with glioblastoma multiforme, and of 83 weeks for those with anaplastic astrocytoma measured from the date of the second operation.[92]

Age and preoperative KPS were important in predicting the quality of survival based on the KPS. Because the patients had additional therapies following their second operation, the impact of surgery must be considered in the context of multimodality treatment at recurrence. Salcman and colleagues achieved a median survival of 36 weeks in patients with recurrent glioblastoma multiforme who were treated initially with a second resection; in the group of 15 patients who survived at least 36 months from the initial diagnosis of their original tumor, each patient had undergone an average of almost three craniotomies.[224] It appears evident that a repeat surgical resection is an option with the potential for improved survival in at least some groups of patients. Appropriate selection of patients for reoperation is important, as is the use of additional therapies following surgery.

As discussed earlier, interstitial brachytherapy is an important salvage technique for the small group of patients who have a recurrent malignant glioma of sufficiently small size in an appropriate location to permit accurate and safe placement of the interstitial catheters.[134] Unfortunately most patients with recurrent tumors are not eligible for the procedure, primarily because of the size and location of their recurrence.

In patients not eligible for brachytherapy, subsequent treatment with chemotherapy is a reasonable alternative. The nitrosoureas are still the most active agents for the treatment of recurrent tumors. In patients who have never received adjuvant chemotherapy with these drugs, their use in treating recurrence often produces high response or stabilization rates. Many trials using carmustine alone or in combination with other agents show median survivals of 20–50 weeks depending on tumor histology, glioblastoma multiforme being more rapidly lethal than anaplastic astrocytoma.[136,270] Combination therapies including lomustine, such as with the PCV regimen, are also effective secondary therapies.[142]

Investigations of new agents continue in structured phase I and phase II studies, including trials with AZQ, dibromodulcitol, the biologicals such as interferons and IL-2, as well as other cytotoxic agents including cisplatin, carboplatin, etoposide, cyclophosphamide, methotrexate, thiotepa, vincristine, and recently the polyamine inhibitors α-difluoromethylornithine (DFMO) and mitoguazone, methylglyoxyl bis(guanylhydrazone) (MGBG).[124,137] Trials of drugs for recurrent tumors are often aimed at identifying new agents, or combinations of agents, that eventually may be used in phase III trials, but none can be assumed to be advantageous.

New approaches to therapy for tumor recurrence, all of which are still investigational, include intratumoral injections, intraarterial therapy, high-dose chemotherapy with ABMT, and the use of biologicals including monoclonal antibody therapy. Other avenues of treatment include methods to overcome tumor cell resistance to the nitrosoureas, whether inherent or acquired. Studies with the interferons, IL-2, and the polyamine inhibitors are assessing novel therapies for brain tumors.

Each of the interferons has been evaluated in trials of tumors at recurrence. Both α-interferon and β-interferon have shown activity; generally less activity is seen with α-interferon. Most of the trials that have been done using intrathecal, intratumoral, and systemic therapy suggest therapeutic activity. Of the 19 patients treated at recurrence with α-interferon by Mahaley and his colleagues, seven had either a response or stabilization.[159] The median survival of this group was 511 days; the patients who did not respond to the therapy survived a median of 147 days. Tumors of a smaller volume were more likely to show response than were larger lesions. Most recently β-interferon has been given intravenously in studies of both adult and childhood gliomas and high response and/or stabilization rates of up to 50% were observed when it was used at recurrence.[4,276] Unfortunately, the duration of these responses was short-lived. It is possible that these agents may be useful in combination with other agents. One ongoing trial is evaluating the use of α-interferon with carmustine as an adjuvant to surgery and irradiation. Another trial is randomizing patients to receive lomustine either alone or with α-interferon for therapy of recurrent tumor. The adverse effects of interferons include malaise, fever, weight loss, hepatotoxicity, and mild myelosuppression; one serious neurotoxic effect is an only partially reversible dementia-like state, the pathogenesis of which is uncertain.

IL-2 plus activated lymphocytes have recently been subjected to clinical trials. Merchant and colleagues treated 24 patients with intracerebral IL-2 and lymphokine-activated killer cells (LAK) at the time of recurrence.[167] During subsequent craniotomy, previously harvested cells and IL-2-activated LAK cells were injected into areas of brain up to 2 cm surrounding the surgical cavity. Subsequently, IL-2 was given through a reservoir into the tumor cavity. Among these 24 patients, the median time to tumor progression was 5 months and median survival was 9 months. Adverse effects of the therapy included increased intracranial pressure related to an increased amount of edema surrounding the tumor. Other trials have shown similar toxicity and tumor responses. Ongoing trials evaluating this approach include trials of IL-2 with LAK in combination with interferons.[166]

The polyamines influence many cellular processes and are associated with growth regulation in particular. Blockade of polyamine accumulation in cells can prevent cellular proliferation in a variety of cellular systems, including neoplastic growth. Polyamine inhibitors have been used in the treatment of brain tumors because of this property of growth inhibition and because they are relatively nontoxic. One trial investigated the use of DFMO, an irreversible inhibitor of ornithine decarboxylase, in combination with MGBG, an inhibitor of S-adenosylmethionine decarboxylase, for the treatment of recurrent gliomas.[139] The response and stabilization rate in 33 patients with recurrent anaplastic astrocytoma was 74% and the median time to tumor progression was 52 weeks. A second trial, also in patients with recurrent gliomas, combined DFMO with carmustine.[201] Of 21 patients with recurrent anaplastic astrocytomas, 57% had either a response or stabilization; the median survival was 119 weeks in this group. Both trials with the polyamine inhibitors showed little activity in patients with recurrent glioblastoma multiforme. Toxicity was mild and myelosuppression was minimal. Trials to investigate these agents are ongoing, as is laboratory research to identify other polyamine analogs and inhibitors.

Trials investigating monoclonal antibodies alone or conjugated to radiopharmaceuticals, toxins, or drugs are inconclusive as yet but show promise. Methods to overcome resistance to the nitrosoureas are also being investigated, as are trials of other mechanisms of resistance to therapy, including hypoxia-related resistance to drugs and radiation and multidrug resistance related to p-glycoprotein. Based on the potential of studies such as these, it is anticipated that research during the next decade will change the face of therapy for recurrent gliomas.

Low-Grade Astrocytoma

The low-grade astrocytomas include the lesions designated *astrocytoma* in the three-tiered systems, those in grades I and II of the classification of Kernohan and colleagues, the moderately anaplastic astrocytoma in the UCSF system (Table XXIV-1-2), as well as the mixed tumors with low-grade components of astrocytoma and oligodendroglioma.[15,120,208,280] Astrocytomas may be further classified as pilocytic, protoplasmic, or fibrillary based on their histologic appearance. The term low-grade suggests a slow biologic growth that, on one hand, would account for the appearance of a lesion in a patient with a seizure disorder that remains unchanged for many years, or, on the other hand, a lesion that may be surgically cured with total resection.

The childhood cerebellar juvenile pilocytic astrocytoma constitutes one of the most commonly occurring of these lesions and is unique and somewhat distinct from the other low-grade lesions, as it has characteristic appearances on CT scans and MR images, characteristic clinical presentations, and a characteristic response to therapy.

Etiology and Epidemiology. Low-grade astrocytomas may occur in any of many areas of the brain, including the optic nerve, cerebellum, hypothalamus, cerebral hemispheres, or brain stem. The mean age at diagnosis for patients with low-grade astrocytoma, other than juvenile pilocytic astrocytoma, is 35 years, and for those with juvenile pilocytic astrocytoma is 14 years. In children, the incidence of glial neoplasms is from 2–5 cases in each 100,000 population per year, and approximately 70% of those neoplasms are low-grade astrocytomas.[68,275] Patients with NF1 or NF2 are at increased risk for these lesions, especially for low-grade astrocytomas of the optic pathways.

Pathology. Pathologically, low-grade astrocytomas are infiltrative lesions with a population of regular, uniform cells, a slight increase in cellularity, and minimal pleomorphism. Most often, there is no clear border between the tumor and surrounding normal brain parenchyma. The astrocytes may show a fibrillary or protoplasmic morphology, or they may be mixed with abnormal oligodendrocytes or ependymal cells. Cerebellar juvenile pilocytic astrocytomas consist of spongy tissue and microcysts interlaced with bundles of neoplastic cells, and may have vascular endothelial proliferation. Lesions in the hypothalamus and optic pathways may appear identical. Biologic growth is slow, both in the infiltrative fibrillary astrocytomas and juvenile pilocytic astrocytomas.

The BUdR labeling index of infiltrative low-grade astrocytomas is usually less than 1%, consistent with its low proliferative potential, but some low-grade astrocytomas have a greater labeling index and greater biologic potential.[102] Those are often the lesions that recur quickly despite a treatment course identical to that for a similar lesion that does not regrow.

The neuroimaging studies of low-grade astrocytomas show no contrast enhancement in most cases with the exception of juvenile pilocytic astrocytoma, which uniformly shows an enhancing nodule associated with a cystic lesion. Even in lesions other than juvenile pilocytic astrocytoma, exceptions occur with respect to the presence or extent of enhancement. Some infiltrative astrocytomas enhance both with CT contrast agents and with MRI-Gd. It is not possible, therefore, to predict the histology of a lesion accurately based on enhancement, and for this reason errors are made in evaluating both the low-grade and the higher grade tumors. Tissue must be obtained in order to verify the diagnosis and, if at all possible, additional biopsy material should be submitted for proliferative studies, as with BUdR or Ki-67. MR imaging may be more sensitive than CT scanning in showing the extent of the lesion. The work of Kelly and colleagues using stereotactic biopsies, demonstrated that the area of increased signal intensity on T2W MR imaging reflects infiltrating tumor cells within otherwise normal brain tissue; this is also true of the low-density areas on CT scans, consistent with the truly infiltrative nature of these lesions.[119]

Clinical Presentation. Patients often present with seizures that may have been present for many years before the diagnosis. In most series, seizures are the most common presenting symptom, followed by headache and finally focal neurologic findings. The interval from the onset of symptoms to diagnosis may be as long as 10 years, in part because of the relative insensitivity of CT scans to detection of small low-grade lesions. Cerebellar juvenile pilocytic astrocytomas in children present with symptoms of clumsiness, ataxia, head tilt, and intermittent headaches and vomiting. Pilocytic astrocytomas of the optic nerve, chiasm, tract, and hypothalamus may present with eye movement disorders, visual field defects, and, in older children, precocious puberty. Cerebral lesions show signs and symptoms associated with the specific location of the lesion.

Diagnostic Neuroimaging. Neuroimaging studies include CT and MR imaging, MR imaging being the more sensitive technique. In general, CT scans often show a cystic or solid tumor of low density and variable amounts of contrast enhancement. Pilocytic astrocytomas reveal a cystic mass with intense contrast enhancement. Classically, the cerebellar juvenile pilocytic astrocytoma appears as a large, smooth-walled cyst with a small enhancing mural nodule.[132] In adults, the diffuse infiltrative cerebral lesions often appear solid and hypodense and may or may not enhance. Often the lesion involves an entire lobe but has indistinct margins and causes minimal mass effect. MR imaging reveals either a hypointense or isointense lesion on T1W images, with a larger area of T2 shortening very hyperintense in appearance. Gd enhancement is variably present. The MR image may show abnormalities though the CT scan appears normal, so MR images should be ordered if a tumor is suspected clinically but not seen with CT.

Treatment. The treatment of low-grade astrocytomas depends on the location of the tumor, the age of the patient, the extent of resection possible, and evaluations based on an understanding of the biology of these lesions. Childhood cerebellar juvenile pilocytic astrocytomas, for instance, are manageable in most cases with surgical resection alone.[82,252]

Only in very unusual cases do juvenile pilocytic astrocytomas recur following a gross total resection, and even the rare patient with recurrence may still enjoy a good outcome with repeat surgical interventions, with or without adjuvant radiation therapy. In contrast, infiltrative astrocytomas in adults often are not amenable to gross total surgical resection, usually require additional radiation therapy and possibly chemotherapy, and have a significantly worse prognosis with increasing age of the patient.[197]

No prospective randomized trials have established how the extent of surgery relates to survival in patients with low-grade astrocytomas. The surgical options include stereotactic biopsy, limited resections, or an attempt at total removal. The results of surgery alone suggest an excellent survival in patients with such tumors as pilocytic astrocytomas that are grossly resected, as more than 80% of patients remain alive after 10 years.[82] Most pediatric neurosurgeons attempt a gross resection of a cerebellar cystic astrocytoma because of the potential for a surgical cure. Many supratentorial juvenile pilocytic astrocytomas are deep midline lesions, however, that cannot be totally resected, in which cases the surgical approach is to remove as much tumor as can be removed safely, expecting to leave residual tumor.

Cerebral lesions are often large and in eloquent areas of the brain, creating the risk of neurologic defects if radical resection is attempted, even with cortical mapping. Leibel and colleagues in a retrospective review of cases preceding the availability of MR imaging, reported a 100% survival at 10 years following gross total resection in patients with low-grade gliomas, and no survivors following biopsy alone.[135] In a review of 194 cases, Gol reported a very short median survival (8 months) after biopsy with or without radiation therapy, and a longer survival (34 months) following subtotal resection with or without irradiation.[84] Laws and colleagues showed progressively improved survival in patients undergoing radical partial or gross total removal, as compared with those who had biopsy and/or subtotal removal.[129]

Additional therapy after surgery includes radiation therapy or chemotherapy. Laws and colleagues reviewing a large retrospective series, concluded that radiation therapy in doses over 40 Gy was beneficial in patients over the age of 40 who had undergone a subtotal resection.[130] Shaw and colleagues suggested that patients receiving more than 53 Gy did better, with a 68% 5-year survival, than those receiving a lower dose, with only 47% survival at 5 years.[232] Based on the relevant literature, Leibel suggested that postoperative irradiation increases 5-year survivals, a rate of 46% with therapy but only 19% without.[135] In contrast, Fazekas did not find a benefit to radiation in the subset of patients who underwent complete resection.[69] In reviews by Shaw and colleagues and Piepmeier, patients had similar survival times as long as radiation therapy was given, irrespective of the degree of surgery and even if only a biopsy was done.[197,232]

It would appear from these data that postoperative irradiation improves survival, but that the extent of surgical resection needed is debatable. In general, low-grade lesions that are totally removed may be followed with no further therapy as long as the patient is well-motivated and returns for frequent follow-up neuroimaging. Patients who have residual disease after surgery should probably receive postoperative irradiation to a limited field in a dose of at least 50 Gy or more.

Treatment of Young Children. In treating infants or young children, radiation therapy to the brain has been associated with intellectual deterioration, developmental delay, endocrine dysfunctions, and the long-term risk of secondary malignancy.[187] Several trials have documented the benefit of chemotherapy as primary therapy following partial surgical resection for low-grade gliomas in children, especially in the group with juvenile pilocytic astrocytoma.[188,215] Among the regimens investigated are the use of actinomycin-D with vincristine according to a protocol developed at Children's Hospital in Philadelphia,[188] and a multiagent nitrosourea-based regimen used at UCSF that includes lomustine, procarbazine, 6-thioguanine, dibromodulcitol, and vincristine.[196] The significance of these studies is that each has shown up to a 75% response or stabilization rate with chemotherapy alone, in some cases with years of disease-free survival. Ultimately, up to about one third or one half of patients require irradiation for tumor regrowth. In children under the age of 3 or 4 years, the use of chemotherapy remains a viable option for incompletely resected low-grade tumors.

Recurrence. Assessments of the proliferative potential of tumors may be helpful in decisions about the use of irradiation or chemotherapy after surgery. Hoshino and colleagues reviewing 47 patients with low-grade astrocytomas who received BUdR before surgery, reported 18 patients who had a BUdR labeling index greater than 1%.[104] Among them, 12 had tumor recurrence within 3 years after surgery, of whom nine died. In contrast, only three of the 29 patients with a BUdR labeling index less than 1% had a recurrence during the same time period. Similar analyses substantiate the impact of proliferative potential determinations in predicting biologic growth and their importance to our understanding of these low-grade lesions and their management.[103]

Recommendation. Low-grade astrocytomas that can be removed totally may be managed with surgery alone. Incompletely resected tumors may be managed with surgery and irradiation. In infants and young children, primary chemotherapy may be useful in controlling the lesion while deferring irradiation until the child is over the age of 4 or 5 years. At UCSF, our policy is to attempt as extensive a resection as is safe, using cortical mapping as needed. Patients with incompletely resected low-grade gliomas receive 54 Gy using single daily dose fractions to the tumor volume and a small margin surrounding it.

Despite the optimism associated with the treatment of lower grade lesions, many patients still die of this disease. New approaches are needed in the management of these tumors, with clinical research trials designed to answer questions concerning the optimal extent of resection, the timing and dose of radiation therapy, the use of chemotherapy, and the role, if any, of biologic or immunologic agents.

Oligodendroglioma

Etiology and Epidemiology. Constituting less than 5% of the total number of gliomas, oligodendrogliomas most often occur in young and middle-aged adults and account for only 5–6% of CNS tumors in children.[169] Oligodendrogliomas most often arise in hemispheric white matter but may be located wherever oligodendroglia cells occur in the CNS. Frequent locations are the frontal lobe (over 40%), parietal lobe (30%), and the temporal lobe (20%). They may be pure tumors or mixed, with elements of astrocytoma or ependymoma. Most often, the mixed tumors are of a low grade and the principles of treatment are those described earlier for low-grade astrocytomas. This discussion concerns only aspects of the pure oligodendrogliomas.

Pathology. Oligodendrogliomas appear as small, round cells in a monotonous pattern. The cytoplasm has distinct borders, the nuclei are dark and round, and an artifact of fixation often causes individual cells to look like fried eggs. The histologic appearance is that of a low-grade lesion with minimal anaplasia or pleomorphism. However, some oligodendrogliomas have anaplastic features with pleomorphism, in the extreme case even resembling glioblastoma multiforme. Others have intermediate features. Attempts to classify oligodendrogliomas using a grading system of A to D, from the least to the most anaplastic, have shown that survival data appear to be different only for the most anaplastic tumors.[155] It may only be important, therefore, to grade oligodendrogliomas as either highly anaplastic or not.

Clinical Presentation. Most patients with oligodendroglioma have a history of symptoms extending over many years. Seizures are common, occurring in as many as 50% of patients before diagnosis and eventually, during the course of the disease, in over 80%.[43] Other focal findings depend on the location and rate of growth of the lesion. Occasionally, a sudden onset of symptoms manifests as a consequence of hemorrhage into the tumor.

Diagnostic Neuroimaging. The CT appearance of oligodendroglioma is a hypodense or isodense lesion that may or may not enhance. Many oligodendrogliomas have calcifications scattered within the lesion, reflecting the mineralization seen histologically within blood vessel walls. There is little peritumoral edema. In some cases, the tumor appears to arise from the fourth ventricle. The MR image reflects the CT lesion, with a hypointense or isointense lesion on T1W images, a hyperintense lesion on T2W images, and areas of signal void where calcifications arise. Enhancement with Gd is variable. Spread beyond the central lesion along the leptomeninges or into the spine is unusual but may occur, especially with lesions of the fourth ventricle.

Treatment. The treatment of choice is surgery, with the goal of gross total removal if possible. The 5-year survival rate varies from 30–80% with surgery alone.[43,236] Interpreting the retrospective series, it is difficult to say with certainty that surgery alone is adequate. Lindegaard and colleagues reported an 83-month median survival for patients with grossly resected tumors and a 26-month survival with subtotal resection.[149] Earnest and colleagues, comparing results with subtotal or total removal, showed no difference in mean survival.[58] There have been no prospective, randomized trials to compare the results of surgery alone as primary therapy with those of surgery and adjuvant irradiation or chemotherapy.

Most of the reported trials of radiation therapy support its use as a treatment for oligodendrogliomas. Chin and colleagues reported a 100% 5-year survival rate in a series of 24 patients who received radiation doses from 53–70 Gy following surgery; all were alive and 79% were disease-free in that group, whereas the group who did not receive radiation had an 82% 5-year survival and only 45% were disease-free.[43]

Our experience at UCSF also supports the use of adjuvant irradiation. In a review of 32 patients, the 5-year survival rate was 85% in those who underwent irradiation but only 31% in those who did not.[236] The recently compiled 10-year survival rate in that series was 56% in patients who received radiation to a dose greater than 45 Gy, but was 18% in those receiving no radiation therapy.[266] Based on this experience, we give radiation therapy to all patients who have residual disease after surgery, using a dose of 54 Gy to a local field. Patients who have had a gross total resection and do not have highly anaplastic lesions may be observed carefully with serial CT or MR imaging; because this strategy has not been studied in controlled trials, patients are offered the option of foregoing irradiation if they are motivated and available for the frequent follow-up studies. All patients with an anaplastic lesion are treated with radiation to 60 Gy after surgery and are given adjuvant chemotherapy. The rationale for this aggressive treatment is the poor survival rates for highly anaplastic lesions (grade D), with no long-term survivors at 5 years after surgery. Patients with mixed tumors showing anaplastic elements, either in the astrocytic or oligodendroglioma components, are treated in the same fashion.

Recurrence. In patients who develop a recurrent oligodendroglioma, the recurring lesion may exhibit a more aggressive histology than did the original growth and frequently may behave like a recurrent anaplastic astrocytoma or glioblastoma multiforme. Pure anaplastic oligodendrogliomas may be very chemosensitive, particularly to nitrosourea-based combinations.[36] The polyamine inhibitors, AZQ, and thiotepa have also been active. Survival following treatment is poor, approximately 1.5–2 years from the time of recurrence.[138] If a recurrent tumor is small and in a favorable location, the treatment with first priority at UCSF is brachytherapy. Otherwise patients are treated with high-dose procarbazine, lomustine, and vincristine (PCV).

Ependymoma

Epidemiology. Ependymomas constitute about 5% of adult intracranial gliomas and up to 10% of childhood CNS tumors.[56] There is a peak incidence at age 5 years and then again at age 34 years.

Pathology. Ependymomas have cells that resemble ependymal cells and tend to occur along the surfaces of the ventricles. Alternatively, they may occur in the parenchyma adjacent to the ventricle, or anywhere along the entire length of the spinal canal and the filum terminale.[221] Over 60% of ependymomas occur below the tentorium and most of those are in the posterior fossa, predominantly in the fourth ventricle. Supratentorial tumors most commonly arise from the lateral ventricles or parenchymal areas adjacent to or separate from the ventricular wall. Tumor extension may occur along the leptomeninges, around the medulla and upper cervical cord to the conus and along nerve roots, and cells may be found in the cerebrospinal fluid (CSF).

Ependymomas are classified as either differentiated (low-grade) or anaplastic (malignant) tumors. Most are cellular tumors consisting of uniform polygonal cells in a collagenous background with well-defined cytoplasmic borders. Some groups of cells form clusters around a circumscribed central space, a configuration known as an ependymal rosette. Myxopapillary ependymomas have mucoid areas within the papillary structure and are found exclusively on the spinal cord at the cauda equina. Sometimes ependymomas are very anaplastic with features that resemble glioblastoma multiforme. Those lesions may have high mitotic activity, endothelial proliferation, and necrosis. In the WHO terminology, they are classified as anaplastic ependymomas, and in other systems as either anaplastic or malignant ependymomas.[280]

A very highly cellular, embryonal form of ependymal tumor occurring in infants and children younger than age 5 years has been termed ependymoblastoma.[170] This tumor is distinct from the other types of ependymoma just described, both biologically and pathologically. The ependymoblastoma often disseminates along the CSF pathways and requires irradiation of the craniospinal axis. Children with this tumor rarely live more than 2 to 3 years. Ependymoblastomas are most likely a form of primitive neuroectodermal tumor with ependymal differentiation and are treated in the same fashion as medulloblastoma. This variant of ependymoma should be regarded as distinct from malignant (anaplastic) ependymoma in terms of treatment.

There are conflicting data concerning the prognostic implications of anaplasia in these tumors. Ross and Rubinstein reviewed a series of 15 patients classified as having anaplastic ependymomas (excluding cases of ependymoblastoma) in an attempt to correlate pathology with survival.[217] In general, postoperative survival did not correlate with anaplastic histology. The median survival in 10 patients with malignant tumors was 8.8 years; five patients who had tumor recurrence died within 13 months to 6 years (median 2.5 years). Afra and colleagues reviewed 80 cases of supratentorial ependymoma with an overall 5-year survival of 34%.[1] They classified these lesions into a low grade, an intermediate grade, or a highly anaplastic grade similar in appearance to glioblastoma. The 5-year survival rates were 41.5%, 28.5%, and 27.2%, respectively. Ernestus and colleagues, reviewing 128 cases of intracranial ependymoma, classified the tumors into grades I to IV: grade I was called subependymoma; grade II, a typical ependymoma; grade III, a malignant ependymoma; and grade IV, identical to glioblastoma.[66] The 5-year survival rate without recurrence was 57.4% for patients with grade II, but only 24.1% for those with grade III lesions. The mean survival was 83 months for the less malignant tumors and only 18 months for the more rapidly growing ependymomas.

Clinical Presentation. Clinically, patients may present with subtle signs and symptoms for years before the diagnosis is made, or may present abruptly with obstructive hydrocephalus or an expanding ependymoma of the spinal cord. Other focal findings include visual field defects, focal seizures, headache, or nausea and vomiting.

Diagnostic Neuroimaging. The neuroimaging of ependymomas is nonspecific but some findings are useful to suggest the diagnosis, including calcification associated with a fourth ventricular tumor. Because many lesions may be confused with ependymomas, treatment should not proceed without histologic verification of the tumor and an assessment of the degree of anaplasia. The imaging studies and treatment for tumors of the spinal cord in general are covered more fully later.

Treatment. The goal of surgery for ependymoma should be removal of as much tumor as possible. Unfortunately, extensive resection is often impossible, particularly for lesions of the posterior fossa or for spinal cord ependymomas involving the cauda equina. Supratentorial lesions are more amenable to total resection and every attempt should be made to accomplish a gross removal.

In the series reported by Ernestus and colleagues, the addition of radiation therapy was particularly important in improving survival.[66] In patients with grade II tumors treated with radiation, the median survival was 185 months. The benefit of postoperative irradiation was even more striking in patients who underwent only a partial resection: the median disease-free survival was 9 months in patients undergoing surgery only, but was more than 108 months in those who received postoperative radiation therapy. Survival was only 21 months for those with grade III tumors despite irradiation.

Other trials have documented the radiosensitivity of ependymomas. The literature does not identify, however, the optimal perimeters of the radiation field for treating ependymomas in specified locations or whether the craniospinal axis should always be included in the field. The risk of spinal subarachnoid metastasis is greatest with infratentorial anaplastic ependymomas (approximately 30%) and least likely with supratentorial typical ependymomas (5–10%). There is also a risk of intraventricular and intracranial spread from a malignant supratentorial lesion. For such reasons, the extent of the irradiated field is an important issue.

Salazar and colleagues reported a local control rate of 12% using small-volume fields as compared to 78% control with whole-brain irradiation in a group of patients with low-grade ependymomas.[222] The 5-year survival rate was 12% with partial-brain and 67% with whole-brain treatment. Sheline and colleagues showed similar results but a higher intracranial recurrence rate in patients receiving partial as compared with whole-brain irradiation, although all recurrences except one were in the original site.[235] Read, however, comparing whole-brain to local-field irradiation, showed no difference in survival between the two groups.[207] Because the primary site of recurrence of low-grade ependymomas is usually within the local radiation field, whole-brain irradiation for supratentorial ependymoma is not indicated. One rational approach to low-grade ependymomas would be to treat with local irradiation, provided that accurate staging procedures to assess the extent of disease are followed, including MR imaging of the spine as well as CSF cytology for infratentorial lesions.

In the case of an anaplastic or malignant ependymoma, irradiation of the entire craniospinal axis has been suggested by many groups. Salazar and colleagues reported a 47% survival rate at 5 years when craniospinal irradiation was given, as compared with only an 8% survival for patients treated only with whole-brain irradiation.[222] Other authors have not documented increased survival rates with cranio-spinal irradiation as compared with local treatment and in most of those series, the site of tumor recurrence was most frequently in the immediate region of the original tumor.[233] For these reasons, we believe anaplastic ependymomas should be staged, including spinal MRI-Gd and CSF cytology examination, and the entire craniospinal axis should be irradiated. At UCSF, the dose directed to the tumor bed is 54 Gy, and 24 Gy is directed to the rest of the brain and spine; boosts are given to known metastatic sites of disease. Even with this schema, most recurrences occupy the primary site. An alternative to this approach may be to increase the dose of radiation to the primary site, using hyperfractionation techniques. We are now investigating the use of craniospinal hyperfractionated radiation to a dose of 72 Gy directed to the primary site and 30 Gy to the rest of the craniospinal axis. In patients with malignant tumors showing such poor-risk features as positive cytology or disseminated disease, chemotherapy is added to this protocol, the current regimen including nitrosourea therapy with cisplatin.

Chemotherapy may be useful in treating recurrent ependymoma and perhaps as an adjuvant to radiation therapy in a newly diagnosed malignant ependymoma. These tumors are sensitive to several agents, including the nitrosoureas, the platinum compounds, procarbazine, and dibromodulcitol. In a UCSF trial involving recurrent ependymomas, the median time from initiation of therapy to tumor progression was 56 weeks for patients treated with dibromodulcitol and 67 weeks for those receiving carmustine.[140] Carboplatin and cisplatin are also active agents that may be considered for use in patients who do not respond to treatment.[78,229] The role of adjuvant chemotherapy after radiation therapy in patients with primary malignant ependymomas has not been established; to date the overall survival rates have been no better than those obtained with irradiation alone.[30,72] Certain subsets of patients may prove to be helped with chemotherapy, including those who have tumors with anaplastic features and less than a complete resection. The number of patients evaluated in prospective randomized studies is too small to permit conclusions concerning the role of adjuvant chemotherapy in the treatment of ependymoma.

Brain Stem Glioma

Epidemiology. Brain stem gliomas account for 20% of childhood tumors and just short of 5% of adult tumors.[48] They are seen most frequently in children between the ages of 3 and 10 years.

Pathology. Brain stem gliomas range from well-differentiated astrocytomas, including juvenile pilocytic astrocytomas, to anaplastic astrocytomas and glioblastoma multiforme.[151] Neurosurgeons often do not biopsy a brain-stem lesion when they judge that the risks of the procedure exceed the benefit of an exact diagnosis. Even with a biopsy specimen there is a risk of sampling error and underestimation of the grade of malignancy. In most series reported, 60–80% of patients do not have a histologic diagnosis and the diagnosis of brain stem glioma is based only on clinical and radiographic findings.[3]

Clinical Presentation. The presenting neurologic findings and symptoms in patients with brain-stem glioma follow one of two patterns. In one group, the insidious onset of symptoms may precede the diagnosis by as much as a year. In another group, an abrupt onset of signs and symptoms leads quickly to an evaluation. The duration of symptoms relates to outcome, the better survival rates accruing to the patients who have symptoms for a longer period before their diagnosis, because a rapid onset of symptoms and signs tends to relate to more rapidly growing tumors. Symptoms may include nausea, headache, speech and balance abnormalities, difficulty with swallowing, and weakness or numbness of the extremities. Signs include multiple cranial nerve palsies and cerebellar and long tract signs. Signs of increased intracranial pressure may occur in association with hydrocephalus from a tumor that compresses the fourth ventricle or aqueduct. Most patients, at some point in their clinical course, manifest cranial nerve palsies of the sixth and seventh nerves.

Diagnostic Neuroimaging. Brain stem gliomas are best evaluated by MRI-Gd.[190] CT in many cases does not give the information necessary for evaluating the extent of the lesion and does not allow the spatial orientation provided by MR imaging. MR images can portray a diffuse lesion involving the pons and medulla, occasionally with extension down to the upper cervical cord or, less frequently, up into the thalamus. CT, in contrast, may miss these extensions because of a bone artifact at the base of the skull, or may not be sensitive enough to visualize the true extent of tumor. Compression of the fourth ventricle may occur, as well as involvement of the parapontine cisterns, cerebellopontine angles, or the leptomeninges. Another characteristic appearance is that of more focal brain-stem lesions, some of them with exophytic extension into the fourth ventricle, or surrounding cisterns, or extending inferiorly down to the cervicomedullary junction. Such lesions are more often found to be lower grade astrocytomas, including juvenile pilocytic astrocytoma, and have a more favorable prognosis than other brain stem gliomas. The MR imaging appearance is that of a nonenhancing tumor, most commonly isointense or hypointense on T1W images and hyperintense on T2W images. Cystic areas may be present. Dissemination along the spinal axis is possible late in the course of the illness. Staging of the spine is not suggested at the time of the primary diagnosis.

Surgical Diagnosis and Treatment. Neuroimaging of brain-stem lesions provides information sufficiently characteristic to make a diagnosis in most cases. The need for a histologic diagnosis might be questioned, especially because survival is determined more by location than by tumor grade. In the case of a diffuse, expansive pontine or pontomedullary tumor in a child who has had a rapid onset of symptoms, the outcome after therapy is at present the same, irrespective of the tumor's histologic features. A biopsy sample actually may not reflect the histologic features of the most aggressive area of the lesion. Many brain-stem lesions judged to be low-grade tumors based on a biopsy later prove to be anaplastic. In the case of a focal or exophytic lesion in the cervicomedullary junction, however, surgery may both establish the diagnosis and permit resection of some portion of the tumor. The outcome in such a case is better if the tumor is histologically verified as a low-grade lesion rather than an anaplastic glioma or a glioblastoma.

Epstein and Wisoff reviewed a series of 92 patients who underwent radical resection of a brain-stem tumor, classifying the lesions as diffuse, focal, cystic (often with a mural nodule), exophytic (dorsal or posterolateral and anterolateral), and cervicomedullary.[65] All patients had surgery with the goal of reduction of the tumor burden. All tumors that appeared as diffuse lesions on MR imaging were found to be histologically malignant. Two diffuse tumors were classified as grade II based on surgical findings, but at autopsy less than 1 month later, both proved to be disseminated glioblastomas. All tumors that appeared as focal tumors based on MR imaging and clinical findings were found to be low-grade lesions. Tumors that appeared as focal lesions on CT, or as focal lesions on MR imaging with bilateral neurologic findings, were found to behave as a diffuse lesion. It proved possible to resect totally all cystic lesions in which the mural nodule enhanced on MRI-Gd and the cyst wall did not, whereas cyst walls that enhanced indicated a more malignant potential. Cervicomedullary tumors were either low-grade astrocytomas or gangliogliomas in 80% of cases. Epstein and Wisoff concluded that surgical approaches should be guided by the appearance of the lesion on the MR image as well as the clinical findings, and that surgery affords potential benefit in some cases of a brain stem lesion.[65] There appeared to be no survival benefit from attempted resection of diffuse lesions, or even of focal pontine lesions that showed bilateral neurologic findings.

Radiation Therapy, Chemotherapy, and Other Modalities. Treatment options other than surgery for brain-stem gliomas include irradiation and chemotherapy. The overall prognosis for the diffuse malignant tumor is poor despite treatment.[2,23] Radiation therapy is the treatment of choice and adjuvant chemotherapy appears to offer no benefit. The overall 5-year survival after irradiation is 20–30% and prognosis relates to the duration of symptoms and the MR appearance of the lesion. For patients with a rapid onset of symptoms whose brain stem glioma appears as a diffuse lesion on MR imaging, the projected median survival is a year or less. Efforts to improve on these poor survival rates, including adjuvant multiagent chemotherapy, have provided no advantage.[141]

One bright spot in the treatment of brain-stem gliomas is the potential of hyperfractionated radiation therapy with treatments given twice a day. On such a schedule, higher total doses can be delivered. Treatment regimens using doses from 66–72 Gy, and currently doses of 78 Gy, have now been evaluated.[60,76,185,203] Although the results are preliminary, it appears that these hyperfractionated higher doses are tolerable in terms of the associated radiation injury, and that survival can be improved for certain groups of patients.

One trial evaluating the use of interferon in children who had failed primary radiation therapy produced some objective responders, suggesting a possible role of this biologic agent.[4] To date, nitrosourea-based regimens have not prolonged survival or achieved any beneficial response once a tumor has recurred. In a more recent study, high-dose chemotherapy with ABMT is used for recurrent tumors, with a plan to use the technique at the time of primary diagnosis as well.[71]

Spinal Cord Tumors

Etiology and Epidemiology. The most common spinal tumor is an extradural metastasis from another primary site. The most common primary spinal tumor is a spinal intradural lesion, either extramedullary or intramedullary. Primary spinal cord tumors constitute 10–15% of all primary CNS lesions.[117] The spectrum of lesions in the adult population differs from that in the pediatric age groups. In children, the most common location of the spinal lesion is intramedullary and the most frequent tumor is an astrocytoma.[205] In adults, extramedullary intradural tumors are more common and the most common are neurofibromas and meningiomas. The most frequent intramedullary tumors in adults are ependymomas and astrocytomas. In unusual cases, adult ependymomas and astrocytomas may be exophytic and extramedullary.

Clinical Presentation. Clinical symptoms of spinal cord lesions include pain, motor and sensory disturbances, and bowel, bladder, and sexual dysfunction. Extramedullary tumors grow in relation to nerve roots and produce radicular pain that frequently is worse at night and aggravated by maneuvers that increase the intracranial pressure, such as straining or coughing. Intramedullary lesions frequently do not present with pain as the initial symptom, but rather produce signs of central cord destruction, including reduced sensation to pain and extreme temperatures, long tract signs, weakness, bowel and bladder incontinence, and sexual dysfunction. Ependymomas are frequently situated at the cauda equina and produce sphincter weakness and peripheral lower-extremity weakness.

Diagnostic Neuroimaging. MR imaging is rapidly becoming the radiographic technique of choice in the evaluation of spinal cord tumors, particularly since Gd became available several years ago. The ability of MR imaging to depict the extent of the lesion and its specific location in relation to other structures, as well as its definition of cysts associated with tumors, make it preferable to other techniques. MR imaging permits an accurate prediction of the histology of the lesion in many cases; for instance, astrocytomas often show heterogeneous enhancement in an asymmetrical fashion, whereas ependymomas frequently enhance uniformly with smooth edges.[227,254,277] Tumor nodules associated with cysts are easily visualized, providing valuable information for surgical planning. Indeed, the extent of cysts above and/or below the lesion defines the level of the laminectomy and the extent of exposure needed. In order to eliminate artifacts caused by cardiac pulsations, respiration, and CSF flow, cardiac gating and other flow-compensatory mechanisms are used. For young children, sedation is often required because the acquisition of data requires that they remain motionless for a prolonged period of time.

Surgical Diagnosis and Treatment. The goal of surgery for spinal cord lesions is to remove tumor as well as to make a diagnosis. In the case of an ependymoma, meningioma, and neurofibroma, total removal is the treatment of choice. For an astrocytoma, especially a diffuse lesion occupying large areas of the spinal cord, only a biopsy and partial removal can be accomplished–although recently, some surgeons have emphasized a more aggressive approach to total removal, even with astrocytomas. Epstein, reviewing his surgical experience with 152 children with spinal cord astrocytomas, divided the lesions from a neurodiagnostic standpoint into two groups; one, holocord astrocytomas, and the second, focal astrocytomas.[64] The holocord astrocytoma was a solid lesion surrounded by a cystic component that expanded the cord caudally and rostrally and extended the entire length of the spinal cord. The focal astrocytoma usually occupied 4 to 8 segments of the cord, often causing total blockage of the spinal subarachnoid space. Surgery was directed at the solid component of the lesion with drainage of the cystic components. The tumor was removed, starting from the center of the lesion, using an ultrasonic dissector and a carbon-dioxide laser and dissecting outward until a tumor-glial interface was encountered. Physiologic monitoring was obtained by measuring evoked potentials. Postoperatively, transient increases in weakness or sensory loss were common but resolved quickly, and only one patient in this series had a significant increase in neurologic deficit. Other reports have shown that, in some cases, even a diffuse infiltrative astrocytoma of the spinal cord can be totally removed.[246] There now appears to be an increasingly widespread enthusiasm for pursuing more extensive surgical resection of intramedullary astrocytomas.

More frequently than for spinal astrocytomas, spinal ependymomas can be approached with the intention of complete surgical removal. Complete removal is potentially curative with no need for further therapy. Cooper reviewed the results obtained in 51 adults with a variety of intramedullary tumors who were treated with radical surgical resection.[49] In this series, of the 24 patients with ependymoma, only two died (one a suicide, one from a progressive tumor). In comparison, 12 of 18 patients with astrocytomas died. All patients with ependymoma who had residual tumor after surgery were treated with radiation therapy, as were all patients with an astrocytoma. The extent of surgery was considered important to outcome in the case of ependymomas, as only 1 of the 11 patients believed to have had total removal had a recurrence whereas tumor recurred in 5 of the 13 patients who had had incomplete resection. All of the patients with high-grade anaplastic astrocytomas eventually died of their tumor.

Radiation Therapy and Chemotherapy. Linstadt and colleagues reviewed the results of 42 patients with primary spinal cord tumors treated at UCSF with radiation therapy: 21 patients had ependymoma, 12 had low-grade astrocytoma, three had anaplastic astrocytoma, and six had tumors of an uncertain histology.[150] The radiation dose was in the range of 45–54.7 Gy. The projected actuarial 10-year disease-free survival for patients with localized ependymomas was 93%. Three patients had ependymoma diffusely involving the cord, one of whom died from a cerebral metastasis. The other two are alive and disease-free. The corresponding 10-year survival rate for the 12 patients with low-grade astrocytoma was 91% and no patient who had an anaplastic astrocytoma survived longer than 8 months. In both the ependymoma and low-grade astrocytoma groups, most patients who had a treatment failure had tumor regrowth in the original site of disease. One patient developed radiation myelitis following irradiation to a total dose of 50.4 Gy.

It is difficult to save a patient who has an anaplastic astro-

cytoma of the spinal cord. Most patients die of this disease despite extensive surgical resections and irradiation to the limit of cord tolerance. Other approaches to these lesions are needed. Chemotherapy only delays the inevitable. Various combinations of chemotherapy, primarily nitrosourea-based, have produced no long-term survivors and other agents, including platinum compounds, thiotepa, and cyclophosphamide, have had only limited and transient benefit. No studies of spinal anaplastic astrocytoma have evaluated hyperfractionated irradiation or radiosensitizers. These might increase the therapeutic index of radiation therapy, which is the most beneficial form of treatment. Therapeutic attempts involving high-dose chemotherapy with ABMT, just beginning in the United States, may provide further insight into the potential for treatment of these refractory tumors.

Recurrence. The recurrent spinal cord ependymoma is more amenable to therapy, including repeat surgical resections, reirradiation using hyperfractionated techniques especially for lesions of the conus, and chemotherapy with the nitrosoureas or platinum agents. When an ependymoma recurs in the spinal cord, we routinely scan the entire neuraxis to be certain of the extent of the disease, because occasionally even a histologically benign ependymoma disseminates. Using sequential therapies, it is possible to control this lesion for years.

Primary Central Nervous System Lymphoma

Primary CNS lymphoma accounts for less than 1% of all lymphomas not related to Hodgkin's disease, and for less than 1% of all primary brain tumors. Termed non-Hodgkin's lymphoma of the CNS (NHL-CNS), this rare cancer has increased in incidence during the past several decades. While the acquired immunodeficiency syndrome (AIDS) epidemic has added substantially to this increased incidence, it cannot be attributed to AIDS alone. According to Eby and colleagues, the incidence of NHL-CNS increased from 2.7 cases per 10 million to 7.5 per 10 million population during the years between 1973–1975 and 1982–1984.[59] This increase, which antedated the AIDS epidemic, comprised younger as well as older populations and men as well as women. Other than lesions caused by immunocompromise of recognized forms, the reason for the change is uncertain. Among patients with AIDS, NHL-CNS has been reported in 1.9–2.6%.[148] It is estimated that, with the increasing numbers of patients with AIDS, more than 1,800 new cases of NHL-CNS may be diagnosed in the United States in 1991.[213] This incidence would exceed that of newly diagnosed low-grade astrocytomas and approximate the numbers of newly diagnosed meningiomas.

Etiology and Epidemiology

Patients at risk for NHL-CNS include immunocompromised patients and organ-transplant recipients. In the AIDS population, there is some evidence that the Epstein-Barr virus (EBV) may be implicated in the development of this lesion. Most patients with NHL-CNS have elevated EBV antibodies. Studying NHL-CNS tissue with in situ hybridization techniques, Bashir and colleagues documented EBV sequences in four patients with immunodeficiency.[17] Four other cases of NHL-CNS not associated with immunodeficiency did not show these same sequences. In a similar review from UCSF by Baumgartner and colleagues, all cases of AIDS-related NHL-CNS studied were positive for EBV sequences.[21] Also supporting this link is the observation that, among people not in the AIDS population who have the X-linked lympho-proliferative syndrome (Duncan's syndrome), EBV-related disease is common, as is the development of NHL-CNS.[194] The association of this virus with NHL-CNS is speculative but, if proven, potential interventions with antiviral agents might be helpful in its treatment. Other syndromes associated with a high incidence of NHL-CNS include Wiskott-Aldrich syndrome and severe combined immunodeficiency syndrome (SCID). Cases of NHL-CNS have also been described in association with sarcoidosis, rheumatoid arthritis, systemic lupus erythematosus, and the vasculitic syndromes. Organ transplant patients, especially those awaiting renal or cardiac transplants, account for as many as 30% of cases of NHL-CNS.[95]

Most cases of NHL-CNS are not associated with any known risk factor, however, and patients are not immunosuppressed. The etiology of this illness is clearly multifactorial and at present is not well understood.

Pathology

The pathology of NHL-CNS resembles that of systemic NHL. The tumors are most commonly large-cell immuno-blastic lymphomas, as classified according to the International Working Formulation.[181] Small cleaved cell lymphoma and large noncleaved cell lymphoma are the next most common cell types, but others have been described as well. There may be some correlation between the tumor's histology and the prognosis for survival, longer survival being associated with the small cleaved and noncleaved cell lymphoma types.[31] However, survival depends on many factors, including the patient's age and the type of therapy, and the association of tumor type to survival may change over time.

Histologically, the lesions are often diffusely infiltrative and advance along perivascular spaces, invading blood vessel walls. There are no nodular or follicular patterns. Most NHL-CNS tumors are of B-cell origin, although rare cases of T-cell NHL-CNS have been described.[163]

Clinical Presentation

Patients with AIDS-related NHL-CNS most often present with confusion, memory loss, focal neurologic deficits, seizures, and lethargy. Most patients with AIDS have other concurrent manifestations of AIDS, including systemic infections and other CNS pathology. In 10–15% of cases, NHL-CNS is the first presentation of AIDS and any patient with NHL-CNS should be evaluated for HIV infection. The usual age range in this population is 35–40 years. The most common CNS mass lesion seen in AIDS patients is toxoplasmosis, NHL-CNS being the second most common.[214] These two illnesses may coexist in more than 10% of cases and are difficult to distinguish radiographically. Frequently, the diagnosis of NHL-CNS in patients with AIDS is made after treatment of CNS toxoplasmosis has failed.[214]

For patients with NHL-CNS who do not have AIDS, the clinical presentation differs somewhat and the patients are, on the average, older at presentation (median age, 55 years). The clinical findings include headache, focal weakness, and personality changes. There may be visual findings as well as cerebellar findings, depending on the location of the tumor. Occasionally, such patients present with clinical features of dementia or encephalitis.

Diagnostic Neuroimaging

Neuroimaging studies in the AIDS population often reveal multiple contrast-enhancing lesions, but as many as 35% may be unifocal.[241] Spinal-cord dissemination of NHL-CNS has not been described frequently in AIDS, nor has the presence of leptomeningeal disease or positive CSF cytology. Among patients with NHL-CNS who do not have AIDS, lesions are frequently multifocal, CSF is positive in as many as 10%, and involvement of the vitreous occurs in 10–20%. The appearance on MR images is that of an isointense central area on T1W images, with hyperintense regions on T2W images. The tumor often enhances on MRI-Gd. CT scans reveal a hypointense lesion that enhances with contrast. NHL-CNS has a predilection for involvement of the basal ganglia, thalami, corpus callosum, the periventricular system, and the vermis of the cerebellum. None of these findings is pathognomonic, however, and the diagnosis must be verified by biopsy.

Surgical Diagnosis and Treatment

The role of surgery is to make a diagnosis, usually by means of a stereotactic biopsy or craniotomy with sampling of the tumor. No survival advantage has been observed from attempts to totally resect the lesions.[178] In AIDS patients, because of the chance that multiple neuropathologic processes may be present, a negative biopsy evaluation for lymphoma should not exclude this diagnosis, especially if multiple lesions are present. If they are clinically suspicious, several lesions may need to be sampled.

Radiation Therapy

The treatment of choice in patients with AIDS-related NHL-CNS is radiation therapy. Whole-brain irradiation to 40 Gy over a period of 3 weeks provides good control of the tumor. Survival data from the NHL-CNS series treated at UCSF reveals a median survival of 134 days if radiation was used, but only 42 days in patients treated solely with surgery; patients with AIDS NHL-CNS frequently die of other manifestations of AIDS rather than of the lymphoma.[21] Neuroimaging after irradiation documented a complete or partial response in 70% of AIDS patients treated for NHL-CNS and stable disease in another 22%. Formenti and colleagues treated 10 patients with various doses of radiation, obtaining a median survival of 5.5 months overall.[74] Patients receiving a higher dose of radiation to 50 Gy survived for more than 12 months. The longest survivals in both series were in patients who also received chemotherapy.

For patients without AIDS, radiation therapy is also a very effective modality. High response rates are achievable using whole-brain irradiation. The RTOG currently treats patients using whole-brain irradiation to a dose of 54 Gy, obtaining a median survival of 7.5 months in patients over 60 years old and a median of 32 months in younger patients. Hochberg and Miller, treating 44 patients with 50–60 Gy to the whole brain, achieved a 79% complete-plus-partial response rate and a median survival of 21.5 months in the patients who could be evaluated.[96]

Irrespective of AIDS, a cure is rarely achieved in patients with NHL-CNS and survival is particularly poor in older patients. Systemic spread of the disease occurs in as many as 10% of patients, and a higher percentage have dissemination within the CNS.

Chemotherapy

In an attempt to improve overall survival, systemic chemotherapy has been used either adjuvantly or primarily in patients with NHL-CNS who do not have AIDS. Combination therapy using standard lymphoma regimens has proved effective in achieving objective responses with a variety of agents, including the nitrosoureas, methotrexate, doxorubicin, cyclophosphamide, vincristine, cytosine arabinoside, and procarbazine.[52,81,165,198] At UCSF, we have treated patients after surgery with a combination of irradiation and chemotherapy using the combined PCV regimen of procarbazine, lomustine (CCNU), and vincristine in the same schedule as used for malignant gliomas. Median survival has been in the range of 30 months. Other groups have used adjuvant therapies such as the CHOP regimen (consisting of cyclophosphamide, doxorubicin [hydroxydaunomycin], vincristine [Oncovin™], and prednisone), the M-BACOP regimen (consisting of methotrexate/citrovorum factor-bleomycin, doxorubicin [Adriamycin™], cyclophosphamide, vincristine, and prednisone), or single-agent high-dose methotrexate. When chemotherapy is used as the only therapy given at tumor recurrence, patients may in some cases remain in remission for years and often have a complete response. In view of these responses to chemotherapy alone, these drugs have been used before and/or after radiation therapy. Our current regimen is to administer CHOP together with high-dose methotrexate for three cycles before whole-brain irradiation to 45 Gy with a boost to 60 Gy to tumor areas. A regimen used at Memorial Sloan-Kettering Cancer Center, reported by DeAngelis and colleagues, includes high-dose systemic methotrexate as well as intrathecal methotrexate given before, and high-dose AraC given after, radiation therapy.[52] Unfortunately, there have been no randomized trials to compare the results of chemotherapy and irradiation with those obtained using radiation therapy alone. Because of the rarity of NHL-CNS and the different schedules and treatment regimens being evaluated, it is impossible to establish which may be the most effective strategy against the tumor.

In cases of AIDS-related NHL-CNS, several investigators have included chemotherapy with irradiation. Despite the fear that chemotherapy in AIDS patients may cause the underlying disease process to progress more rapidly or may produce many infectious complications, some patients have completed complicated combination chemotherapy regimens successfully. Systemic chemotherapy has been used in only a small number of cases of AIDS-related NHL-CNS. Three of the patients with the longest survival in the UCSF series just mentioned had received high-dose methotrexate, and the one with the longest survival from the series reported by Formenti and colleagues had received the BACOD reg-

imen (consisting of bleomycin, Adriamycin, Cytoxan, Oncovin, dexamethasone).[74] It may be possible to use systemic chemotherapy even in AIDS patients, if screening includes such careful selection criteria as admission only of patients who have no other manifestation of AIDS or those who have high CD4 lymphocyte counts.

Medulloblastoma and Primitive Neuroectodermal Tumors

Etiology and Epidemiology

Medulloblastoma, the most common primary malignant intracranial tumor of childhood, is not common in adults. The lesion accounts for more than 30% of all posterior fossa tumors and approximately 250 new cases are diagnosed each year in the United States. More than 80% of medulloblastomas are diagnosed in children during the first 15 years of life, the median age at diagnosis being 5 years. Medulloblastomas arise from the midline cerebellum, but histologically similar lesions may occur in the cerebral hemispheres and the pineal region.

Pathology

There is controversy about the proper nomenclature to assign to several histologically similar tumors that occur within the cerebellum, cerebrum, and pineal region—among them primitive neuroectodermal tumor and medulloblastoma.[210] For lack of a conclusive histogenesis, proposals to explain these lesions range from one speculating a single primitive cell of origin that exhibits different degrees of differentiation along astrocytic, oligodendroglial, ependymal, neuronal, melanocytic, and mesenchymal cell lines, to one at the opposite extreme describing a previously mature tumor that undergoes neoplastic "dedifferentiation" to a primitive state. Pending resolution of the debate, some pathologists and clinicians use the terms primitive neuroectodermal tumor and medulloblastoma interchangeably (PNET/MB). In fact, these tumors do have features in common and they share similar biologic properties, including the ability to disseminate throughout the nervous system and, in some cases, systemically. Until the nosology is resolved, we prefer to restrict the use of the term medulloblastoma to the characteristic lesion seen in the cerebellum, and to use the term "primitive neuroectodermal tumor" for similar lesions found elsewhere in the CNS. However, because the treatment and biology of these lesions are similar, both terms are used collectively as PNET/MB for the rest of this section.

Histologically, about one half of these tumors have recognizable cell lines combined with undifferentiated components. A relation between prognosis and the degree of cellular differentiation has been proposed, but while some reports suggest that the more undifferentiated tumors are associated with a better outcome than those with predominant differentiation along astrocytic lines, others suggest that differentiation imparts a better prognosis.[38,189] Clearly, there is no consensus concerning prognosis as it relates to histology. Cytogenic studies show frequent karyotypic abnormalities, both numerical and structural, most often involving chromosomes 1, 6, and 17.[89] Recent work suggests that the design on chromosome 17 represents a deletion resulting from a loss of heterozygosity and may play a role in the control of oncogene expression. The area on 17 is in the same region as a known tumor suppressor gene, p53. Conceivably mutations in this area may be responsible for the development of PNET/MB; however, this early work must be confirmed.

Dissemination exists in as many as 30% of patients at the time of primary diagnosis.[45,53] Disease may exist outside the primary site as nodular lesions anywhere within the neuraxis, including the spine and supratentorial fossa, and/or it may involve the CSF as indicated by positive cytology results. Occasionally, there may be disease beyond the CNS at the time of the original diagnosis, most often in the bone and/or soft tissue structures, including the lymph nodes. The prognosis is directly related to the presence and extent of disease beyond the primary tumor site.

Clinical Presentation

Most PNET/MB lesions arise from the posterior fossa in children younger than age 5 years.[184] Frequently, the tumor produces hydrocephalus and symptoms of increased intracranial pressure, including nausea, emesis, headache, diplopia, and unsteadiness. Papilledema is often found on examination. In infants less than 1 year old, increasing lethargy and enlarging head circumference are seen together with developmental delays.

Diagnostic Neuroimaging

Neuroimaging reveals a contrast-enhancing lesion in the cerebellum.[105,184] The CT appearance is that of a hypointense or isointense lesion that enhances homogeneously. MR imaging shows low signal intensity on T1W images and a high signal intensity on T2W images; Gd produces enhancement. Because of the extent of PNET/MB lesions and their relation to adjacent structures, MRI-Gd is the neuroimaging technique of choice.

Staging. Postoperative staging, assessment of the extent of disease, is required in order to treat PNET/MB properly. It should include an evaluation of the entire craniospinal axis using MRI-Gd of the brain and spinal cord, as well as a CSF sample obtained by lumbar puncture to assess the presence of malignant cells in the spinal CSF. The presence of any disease outside the primary site of the lesion adversely influences survival. In a large series reported from the Children's Cancer Study Group (CCSG) and the International Society for Pediatric Oncology (SIOP), the risk of a poor outcome is determined by the extent of disease.[5,45,53] In the CCSG trials, 58% of children without dissemination, as opposed to only 32% of those with metastatic disease, survived disease-free at 54 months.

The timing of staging is somewhat controversial. At most centers, including our own, spinal staging is done approximately 2 weeks after surgery in order to obviate misleading results caused by PNET/MB cells remaining in the CSF; it seems probable that many are nonclonogenic cells dispersed during resection. Blood within the CSF or spinal canal may produce filling defects or abnormal enhancement on myelography and MR imaging of the spine. Although such contamination should be resolved by 2 weeks postoperatively, both noncontrast and contrast MR imaging should be

done during this evaluation to maximize the likelihood of distinguishing true tumor from postoperative artifact. If the first CSF cytology shows malignant tumor cells, then another examination should be performed 1 week later. If the results are still positive, they most likely represent true dissemination. If the results of the second examination are negative, then the initial result can be considered a false-positive finding.

Other prognostic variables include the patient's age and the extent of surgical resection. Young children–those under 4 years of age–tend to have a worse outcome than older children, in some part because younger children often have disseminated disease and infants cannot be treated as aggressively with radiation therapy owing to the morbidity high-dose irradiation causes to the developing nervous system.

The size of the tumor has also been considered important, irrespective of the extent to which it is resected. According to a staging system developed by Chang and colleagues, tumors are classified according to size at the time of surgery: tumors classified as T1 or T2 lesions were less than 3 cm in diameter and did not fill the fourth ventricle completely; larger tumors, T3 or T4 lesions, filled the fourth ventricle and caused hydrocephalus (T3a lesions) or invaded the brain stem (T3b lesions) or the upper cervical cord (T4 lesions).[42] Larger lesions were considered to have a worse prognosis–but significantly so only when they were associated with dissemination, according to the CCSG and SIOP trials.[5,45,53] The impact of surgical resection on outcome, as related to tumor size, has not been fully appreciated. It would seem that even a patient with a large lesion that is totally or almost completely removed would do as well as one treated similarly who had a smaller lesion at diagnosis, assuming that there was no evidence of dissemination. In fact, the most recent study from the CCSG seems to suggest that the size of the lesion alone has no impact on survival.[67] The strongest predictors of a poor outcome are the presence of dissemination and a young age.

Surgical Diagnosis and Treatment

The goal of surgery for PNET/MB is to remove all visible tumor. Survival rates as high as 80% at 5 years after surgery have been reported following total removal, as compared to rates of 40–50% in patients having only a subtotal removal.[255] Patients undergoing biopsy only are unlikely to survive, even if they receive appropriate radiation therapy.[255] Other studies have not documented increased survival rates after total as opposed to subtotal resection, but showed significantly similar survival rates in both cases.[67] In some trials, the documented extent of resection may have been underestimated or overestimated because it was based on the operative report and not on postoperative imaging studies.[53,184] Conversely, some residual disease may not be detected with postoperative imaging, including small-volume residual tumor that may extend into the brain stem. Thus, even postoperative imaging may not show the extent of resection completely accurately. There appears to be a consensus, however, that total removal, whenever possible, is the goal of surgical therapy.

Some controversy also remains regarding hydrocephalus,

whether resection should be performed before or after a shunting procedure. The proponents of immediate surgery without shunting argue that a significant number of children do not require permanent shunting after resection and that surgery eliminates the risk of intraperitoneal spread of tumor by way of the shunt. Immediate surgery also lessens the risk of upward herniation, obviating the need for a second procedure under anesthesia. Proponents of primary shunting suggest that the subsequent surgery is easier because the brain is relaxed, resulting in less distortion of the posterior fossa, thus permitting a more complete resection. At UCSF, we favor an immediate surgical approach with the goal of total removal.

Radiation Therapy

Radiation therapy is the basis of curative treatment. Before the introduction of craniospinal axis irradiation, few patients survived for 5 years after a diagnosis of PNET/MB. Landberg and colleagues reported a 10-year survival rate of 5% for patients irradiated to the posterior fossa alone, as compared to 53% when irradiation of the craniospinal axis was used.[126] Other reports have verified the improved survival obtained with this approach and currently all patients diagnosed with PNET/MB are treated with irradiation of the craniospinal axis.[5,45,53]

The most common sites for recurrence are at the original tumor site and spinal cord metastasis. Control rates are higher and the risk of dissemination is less when a dose of 50 Gy or more is delivered to the posterior fossa. Therapy with less than 50 Gy is associated with higher local failure rates, more spinal cord metastases, and reduced survival. The question of the optimal dose to the craniospinal axis has not been completely resolved, as some uncertainty remains about the most effective dose in clinically uninvolved areas of the CNS.

Because most patients with this disease are children, concern about the delayed effects of radiation has prompted speculation about lowering the dose to the brain and spine. Late effects include hormonal abnormalities such as reduced growth hormone levels, cognitive defects such as lowered IQ score with learning disabilities, and spinal abnormalities such as reduced vertebral body height, shortened stature, and kyphoscoliosis. Standard radiation doses to the craniospinal axis have included 35–45 Gy to the brain and 30–40 Gy to the spine. Recently, several groups have reported survival outcomes similar to those in the CCSG and SIOP trials with irradiation in lowered doses to the craniospinal axis.[5,45,53] At UCSF, patients considered good-risk candidates were treated with 54 Gy to the posterior fossa and 24–30 Gy to the rest of the craniospinal axis.[144] Their survival rate at 5 years was 66%, which is comparable to survival rates from the CCSG and SIOP trials; most recurrences were in the posterior fossa.[5,45,53] Tomita and McLone also reported good survival rates when patients were treated with 25 Gy to the craniospinal axis; most of their patients had had total surgical removal of tumor.[255] Despite good local control rates, however, as many as 30–40% of patients have recurrence either within or outside of the CNS.

Chemotherapy and Multimodality Therapy

In an attempt to increase survival rates, adjuvant chemotherapy has been used with variable success in some groups of patients. In two large trials conducted by the CCSG and the SIOP, patients were randomized to receive radiation therapy either alone or with adjuvant chemotherapy.[5,67] In the CCSG trial, lomustine, vincristine, and prednisone were used; the SIOP study omitted prednisone but was otherwise similar.[5,67] A marginal benefit was suggested overall in the group receiving chemotherapy, but was significant only in patients with larger tumors and with metastatic disease (CCSG and SIOP trials), or in the case of brain stem invasion (SIOP trial only).

Overall, there is no survival advantage when chemotherapy is added to radiation therapy for patients with a newly diagnosed PNET/MB, but within certain subsets of patients there is clearly an advantage. A recent updated report of the SIOP trial revealed a 45% overall survival at 10 years, documenting patients who had a relapse after 5 years.[253] This result reaffirms the benefit of adjuvant chemotherapy in patients who have had either partial tumor removal only or brain stem involvement and disease at stage T3 or T4. In the CCSG study, patients with relatively large tumors who also had evidence of dissemination had a clear survival advantage if they received adjuvant chemotherapy.[67] Survival at 5 years in patients who had advanced tumors (T3, T4) with dissemination was 46% after irradiation and chemotherapy, but was 0% after radiation therapy alone. Conversely, in a group of 124 patients with T3 or T4 tumors without evidence of dissemination, the 5-year disease-free survival was 61% after combined therapy and 51% after irradiation alone, a statistically insignificant difference.[67] It appears from this large randomized trial that chemotherapy is primarily beneficial in the case of metastatic disease, and that the extent of surgical resection does not confer a survival advantage between patients with total removal and those with partial removal. Children younger than 4 years of age did less well, having a 5-year survival rate of only 32%. Other ongoing studies are evaluating a variety of agents, including a combination of lomustine, cisplatin, and vincristine.

Recurrence

In the CCSG trial and other studies of PNET/MB, there remains a high rate of local recurrence.[67] Attempts to improve on those rates now focus on increasing the dose of radiation using hyperfractionation techniques, a strategy that proved to be successful in the treatment of brain stem gliomas. Several ongoing studies use hyperfractionated irradiation to doses of 72 Gy to the posterior fossa as well as hyperfractionated irradiation of the craniospinal axis. These trials are just beginning to accrue patients and the results will not be fully analyzed for several years. At UCSF, good-risk patients are treated with radiation only, using hyperfractionation to 72 Gy to the posterior fossa and 30 Gy to the rest of the craniospinal axis. When poor-risk factors are found, adjuvant chemotherapy is added to this regimen.

It is difficult to save patients with PNET/MB once they have failed initial therapies; however, if they have not had chemotherapy previously, there is a role for its use. The most active agents against recurrent PNET/MB include the nitrosoureas, cyclophosphamide, melphalan, thiotepa, vincristine, procarbazine, cisplatin, and carboplatin.[77] Combination therapy with lomustine, cisplatin, and vincristine is also being evaluated;[186] others include the MOPP regimen (consisting of Mustargen, Oncovin, procarbazine, and prednisone) as used for the treatment of Hodgkin's disease,[259] PCV therapy similar to that used for malignant gliomas,[146] and a regimen called "8 in 1," in which eight drugs are delivered over a 24-hour period.[195] Unfortunately, even if the patient's initial response is good, long-term control is unlikely. In the CCSG trial described earlier, patients who were therapeutic failures of irradiation and adjuvant chemotherapy had a median survival after recurrence of only 3.9 months.[67] Patients who had undergone only irradiation could be salvaged for a median of 10.4 months. There are several options other than chemotherapy alone, such as repeat irradiation using hyperfractionation therapy combined with combination chemotherapy, and more recently the use of high-dose chemotherapy with ABMT.

We strongly recommend that patients with PNET/MB be referred to regional institutions for entry into clinical research trials, both at the time of original diagnosis and at the time of tumor recurrence.

Other Primary Tumors of the Central Nervous System

Primary Germ Cell Tumors

Etiology and Epidemiology. Primary intracranial germ cell tumors are a rare group of diverse tumors that account for less than 5% of childhood tumors and less than 1% of adult tumors. In the United States, fewer than 50 cases are diagnosed each year.[226] Most germ cell tumors occur during the second and third decades of life. For unknown reasons, their incidence is higher in Japan.[113] The most common histologic type is germinoma, believed to be the most primitive form, and the spectrum of other tumors includes embryonal carcinoma, choriocarcinoma, endodermal sinus tumor, and malignant or immature teratoma.[111] In general, these lesions are grouped together as either germinoma or nongerminoma because the former are very radiation-sensitive and the latter not. Except for the benign teratoma, all germ cell tumors are malignant neoplasms with the potential to disseminate throughout the neuraxis.

Pathology. Intracranial germ cell tumors are histologically identical to gonadal germ cell tumors, the only difference in terminology being that the term germinoma is used for the same tumor as a seminoma of the testis or dysgerminoma of the ovary. The germ cell tumor may be a mixture of several elements or may exhibit only one element. It has been suggested that germ cell tumors arise from developmental nests of primitive germ cells in midline structures, including the pineal and suprasellar regions of the brain.[114] Germinoma accounts for 65% of CNS germ cell tumors. Teratoma is the next most frequent at 18%, and choriocarcinoma is the rarest. Embryonal carcinoma and endodermal sinus tumors are intermediate in frequency. Germinomas consist of two cell populations: large round cells and a lymphocytic infiltrate. In rare cases, syncytiotrophoblasts may be present that stain positively for β-human chorionic gonadotrophin (β-HCG). Germinoma also stains positively for alkaline phosphatase. The nongerminomas, including teratomas, usually have mixtures of many cellular elements. Immunoperoxidase

staining reveals β-HCG and/or α-fetoprotein in embryonal carcinoma and choriocarcinoma, as well as in endodermal sinus tumors.[113]

Two-thirds of the germ cell tumors in the pineal region occur in male patients, whereas two thirds of suprasellar tumors affect females. Most nongerminomas arise from the pineal region, whereas germinomas may present either there or in the suprasellar region, or in both areas; 10% of germ cell tumors arise elsewhere in the brain, for example, the thalamus.

Clinical Presentation. Patients present with acute findings related to obstructive hydrocephalus and increased intracranial pressure. Other findings include abnormalities of eye movement, including upward gaze paresis, retraction nystagmus, and diminished pupillary responses. For patients with suprasellar lesions, hypothalamic and pituitary dysfunction dominate, including growth failure, precocious puberty, and diabetes insipidus. Neuroimaging studies reveal a contrast-enhancing lesion, occasionally with calcification.

Surgical Diagnosis and Treatment. Surgery is strongly recommended to determine the histology of a lesion in the pineal region. The differential diagnosis of lesions in this area includes germinoma, nongerminoma, teratoma, pineocytoma, pineoblastoma, astrocytoma, and in rare instances metastatic tumor. The therapeutic options depend on the tumor type. A negative β-HCG or α-fetoprotein finding in the CSF or serum does not exclude a nongerminoma, although the presence of these markers are indicative of these tumors.[7] A slight elevation of β-HCG may be present with germinomas as well. Modern surgical techniques make sampling or partial removal of tumors in this area safe and appropriate. In the past, because of the risks of surgery, such tumors were treated without tissue diagnosis, as if they were germinomas. If the lesion disappeared after a short course of irradiation it was believed to be a germinoma, but if it did not disappear the dilemma of its exact etiology could not be resolved. A regimen of chemotherapy for pineoblastoma, for instance, might be different from that for a mixed germ-cell tumor, as would be the decision concerning craniospinal axis irradiation.

Radiation Therapy. Radiation is directed to localized germinomas using the involved field as well as encompassing the ventricular system; 25 Gy is directed to the larger field, with a boost of an additional 20–25 Gy to the tumor bed. The field of irradiation and the dose are topics of controversy. Some authors advocate irradiation of the craniospinal axis for all patients with germinomas, especially if a biopsy has been done, because of the risk of dissemination. Wara and colleagues found that only 8.3% of 109 patients with pineal tumors developed spinal metastasis if no spinal irradiation was given.[267] The issue of craniospinal axis irradiation has not been resolved with germinomas. Jenkin and colleagues found that two of five cases of germinoma spread to the spinal subarachnoid space when spinal irradiation was not used, but no instance of spread in five patients who had spinal irradiation.[112] Currently, if CSF markers are negative and staging of the spine including cytology and MRI-Gd or myelography is negative, then wide-field irradiation including the ventricular volume is used. Germinomas are very radiation-sensitive. The survival rate for patients with biopsy-proven germinoma is as high as 70% in some series, and as high as 90% when whole-brain irradiation to at least 50 Gy was used.[251] There is some concern that the 50 Gy dose of radiation is too high and for this reason lesser doses comparable to those used for testicular seminoma (30 Gy or less) have been suggested.[112,251]

Chemotherapy. Nongerminomas are less responsive to radiation and frequently are treated initially with chemotherapy. The drugs used are similar to those used for gonadal tumors, including cisplatin, etoposide, vinblastine, bleomycin, and cyclophosphamide.[6] As many as six courses of chemotherapy with a combination of agents has been used, followed by restaging. Residual disease is then treated with radiation therapy. At UCSF a combination of cisplatin, etoposide, bleomycin and vinblastine is used, although several case reports have documented high objective response rates with cisplatin, etoposide, and bleomycin or with the two-drug combination of cisplatin and etoposide. Shorter-course therapy of only four cycles has also been used. Considering the rarity of these tumors, a consensus has not developed concerning the optimal regimen and duration of therapy. Unfortunately, the survival rate is much less with nongerminomas than with most germ cell tumors. Of 11 patients treated by Bruce and Stein, only 33% were alive at 2 years after diagnosis.[33]

In the case of disseminated germinomas, primary treatment with chemotherapy is also reasonable in order to defer or omit the use of craniospinal axis irradiation. All cases are routinely staged before treatment in order to define the therapy to be used.

Craniopharyngiomas

Etiology and Epidemiology. Craniopharyngiomas are histologically benign tumors that arise from remnants of Rathke's pouch. They are generally found in children and young adults, but exhibit a second peak incidence in late adult life. They account for as many as 4% of all brain tumors and are most often situated at the junction of the infundibular stalk and the pituitary gland. Because of their proximity to the stalk, the pituitary gland, the optic apparatus, and the third ventricle, they pose significant risks to these structures.

Pathology and Diagnosis. Most craniopharyngiomas are cystic, although some are solid or both cystic and solid. The cyst contains cholesterol-laden fluid. Calcifications are also common. These tumors may be entirely intrasellar and expand the sella turcica, may extend into the suprasellar space, or may exist primarily in the prechiasmatic cisterns and encroach on the chiasm and optic nerves, obstructing the third ventricle.[99] Patients present with hydrocephalus and/or endocrine dysfunction and visual symptoms. Neuroimaging studies reveal a cystic or mixed cystic and solid tumor, occasionally with calcifications. MR imaging is very helpful in defining the relation of the tumor to surrounding structures.

Treatment. Complete surgical removal is possible in some cases, although extensive resections involve a risk of hemorrhage, visual deterioration including loss of vision, memory deficits, diabetes insipidus, and the need for cortisol, thyroid, and/or growth hormone replacement therapy. In contrast, the risk of recurrence is greater than 50% with only a partial resection, and even after a presumed total resection, tumor may still recur in 20–25% of cases.[100] As many as 40% of these tumors cannot be removed. The dilemma concerning this "benign tumor" is therefore evident. A partial resection may avoid some neuroendocrine or visual disturbances, but frequently the tumor recurs. Extensive resection may cause deficits requiring long-term hormonal therapy, and still the tumor may recur. If possible–and if risks are thought to be minimal–an attempt at total resection should be considered for children with this disease. If postoperative neuroimaging documents total removal, radiation therapy may be deferred for years. Close follow-up review with imaging studies is required. In the case of residual disease or a less than complete removal, postoperative irradiation is recommended.

Postoperative irradiation can produce excellent long-term results. In 74 patients treated at UCSF with partial resection and postoperative irradiation, a 91% remission rate was obtained over a mean follow-up period of 4 years.[19] Of those patients with preoperative visual disturbances, 93% improved and 33% returned to normal vision. The most common radiation dose used was higher than 50 Gy. Other series have documented the benefit of irradiation after a less than complete resection. Irradiation entails some hazard, however, especially in children, and the potential for long-term negative effects on cognition, for endocrine deficits, and rarely for induced secondary tumors must be considered.[51] The treatment of recurrence after surgery alone, or surgery combined with irradiation, is difficult, mostly because of the effects of previous surgery and radiation therapy.

Cystic portions of craniopharyngiomas may become refractory to usual methods of control, including repeated cyst aspirations, multiple surgeries, and radiation therapy. Several trials have documented control with the instillation of radiation isotopes into the cyst cavity; phosphorus, gold, and yttrium isotopes have been used.[46] This technique requires careful attention to placement of the isotope, which is often done through a reservoir or using stereotactic technique. The consistency of the cyst fluid also is important because some cavities have fluid that is very thick or sludge-like, precluding adequate distribution of the isotope within the cavity. Multicystic lesions are difficult if not impossible to treat in this manner. There are other problems with this technique as well, including the risk of further radiation damage to vision when the cyst wall is very thin, allowing penetration into adjacent neural structures.

Another method of treatment for craniopharyngioma includes stereotactic radiosurgery, which permits precise localization of a radiation dose to a small field in one treatment setting.[14,46] Special units, including the focused gamma irradiation device called the gamma unit, have become available, as have specially designed linear accelerators with collimators. Although too few patients have been treated with this form of therapy to permit generalizations about results, it appears that it may prove a useful therapeutic tool. One strategy involves radiosurgery at the time of recurrence, or perhaps its use as primary therapy after partial surgical resections. The ability to localize the target precisely with radiosurgery could minimize the exposure of sensitive areas of the brain, including the pituitary gland and optic chiasm, nerves, and tracts.

Meningioma

Epidemiology. Meningiomas account for 13–17% of intracranial brain tumors. They most often occur during the fourth through the sixth decades of life with a peak occurrence in patients about 45 years of age. About 65% of all meningiomas occur in women.[90]

Pathology. Meningiomas are classified as malignant either on the basis of histologic criteria or invasiveness. Histologically malignant or anaplastic features include the presence of frequent mitotic figures (more than 1 or 2 per 10 high-powered fields), atypical mitoses, papillary structures, high cellularity, and necrosis.[108] Invasiveness is itself thought to represent malignant potential, as are the variant subtypes of hemangiopericytoma and other forms of angioblastic meningiomas. According to these criteria, the incidence of malignant meningiomas is 2–10%. There is debate over the specific features determining malignancy because some benign meningiomas have several characteristically malignant features, yet behave in a typically benign fashion. Conversely, in rare cases, meningiomas that appear benign metastasize both within the CNS and outside the cranium to the lymph nodes and lung. At UCSF, we use the criterion of invasiveness as well as the histologic criteria of increased mitoses, anaplastic features such as pleomorphism, necrosis, and a high labeling index, greater than 1%, to assign malignancy to meningiomas.

Treatment. Most meningiomas are benign tumors that are treated successfully with surgical resection alone. The goal of surgery is to remove the tumor and its dural attachment with any involved bone. Incompletely resected tumors are treated with radiation therapy.

The treatment of malignant meningiomas is as extensive a resection as possible followed by irradiation to a dose of 60 Gy using single daily fractions. We have included adjuvant chemotherapy with cyclophosphamide, Adriamycin, and vincristine with this treatment in the hope of reducing the still high recurrence rate but as yet the trial permits no conclusions about recurrence rates as compared to those in historical controls.

Options in the treatment of malignant or invasive meningioma, other than surgery and conventional radiation therapy, include the use of interstitial brachytherapy. High-activity or low-activity sources can be used to obtain good local control rates. The technique appears to confer a survival advantage. Leibel and colleagues reviewed the UCSF data obtained with brachytherapy for recurrent newly diagnosed malignant meningiomas; 13 patients were treated, two with high-activity sources and 11 with permanent low-activity radioactive iodine sources.[133] Of the patients treated with low-activity sources, eight of nine with malignant meningiomas and one of two with recurrent meningioma had stable disease ranging from 2–77 months; the two recurrences were at 8 and 22 months. One of these malignant tumors was treated with interstitial brachytherapy before the patient underwent external radiation therapy. Of the two patients treated with high-activity sources, one had recurrence after 58 months and one remains stable at 58 months. Both required reoperation for radiation necrosis, one at 12 months and one

at 35 months. None of the patients with permanent implants developed symptomatic necrosis.

Aggressive surgery may also be possible if embolism of the feeding vessels is performed before surgery to reduce the risk of bleeding during extensive resection. The most aggressive approach to these tumors would include preoperative embolization and extensive resection, followed by interstitial brachytherapy and possibly adjuvant chemotherapy. None of these approaches has been evaluated in a randomized study but because of the relative rarity of the tumor, there have been very few clinical trials in the treatment of malignant meningioma.

Recurrence. The recurrence rate for presumably completely removed meningiomas is low, generally less than 10%, but can be as high as 40–50% in patients with gross residual disease remaining postoperatively.[168] In patients who had undergone a partial resection, Wara and colleagues found recurrence in 75% of a nonirradiated group but in only 29% of the group undergoing irradiation after surgery.[268] Others do not advocate irradiation routinely for residual benign meningiomas, rather relying on a repeat surgical resection at the time of recurrence.[40,121]

Metastatic Disease to the Central Nervous System

Etiology and Epidemiology

As many as 25% of all patients with cancer develop metastasis to the brain or spinal cord, and the disease becomes clinically significant in most patients. As the population in general lives longer and as other therapies become more successful in controlling disease outside the CNS, it is likely that the incidence of CNS metastases will increase. The AIDS epidemic has produced an increasing incidence of unusual metastatic tumors, including CNS lymphoma. In the 1986 data compiled by the American Cancer Society, the number of cancer deaths from intracranial metastases was estimated at 124,000 cases, and the number of deaths from primary CNS neoplasms at 10,200 cases.[238] Clearly, metastatic tumors are an important clinical problem and a frequent cause of death.

Pathology

The most common primary sites of metastases to the CNS are the lung and breast, metastases from the lung being more frequent overall because of the larger numbers of patients with this malignancy. Other common primary sites include melanoma from any site, leukemia and lymphoma, and renal cancers. Virtually any primary cancer may spread to the CNS with involvement of brain and spinal cord parenchyma, leptomeninges, dura, and pituitary gland.[199]

Lung cancer is the most common primary source of brain parenchymal metastases, and of the various forms of lung cancer, small cell tumors are the most likely to metastasize. Metastasis to the dura, in contrast, arises more frequently from cancer of the breast or prostate, or lymphoma. Leptomeningeal disease occurs frequently as a consequence of cancer of the breast, lung, and melanoma, as well as lymphoma and leukemia. Breast cancer is the most frequent tumor to metastasize to the pituitary gland.

Clinical Presentation. The signs and symptoms of intracranial metastases are identical to those of primary brain tumors and are thus indistinguishable. Patients present with signs and symptoms related to the location of the lesion, or with more generalized signs such as personality changes, headache, generalized seizures, or weakness; dexamethasone is useful for diminishing peritumoral edema that may contribute greatly to the symptoms. An initial manifestation as a brain tumor is common for lung cancer but rare for other cancers. Every adult with symptoms of a brain tumor should have a CT scan of the lungs because plain x-ray films of the chest may not reveal small pulmonary lesions that could be the primary neoplasm. Acute findings may be the result of hemorrhage into the tumor and may be caused by hydrocephalus or by acute increases in intracranial pressure. Leptomeningeal findings include more general symptoms, such as headache and nausea, or more specific signs and symptoms related to the area most affected, such as lower cranial nerve involvement (oculomotor or facial nerve) or lower spinal-nerve invasion causing weakness, reflex changes, and bowel and bladder dysfunction. Dissemination of the tumor into the CSF (carcinomatous, lymphomatous, or leukemic meningitis) may produce hydrocephalus and may cause nuchal rigidity. Involvement of the dura may produce symptoms of pain and specific nerve-root compression. Pain over the site of the metastasis or pain radiating in a nerve-root pattern is the most common clinical finding associated with epidural spinal metastasis.

Diagnosis

Of the parenchymal lesions, approximately 50% are solitary metastases.[199] In the absence of a recognized primary tumor, the diagnosis must be verified histologically. With a known primary tumor, either before or after it is treated and in the absence of obvious systemic dissemination, we do not assume a metastatic origin but rather advocate stereotactic needle biopsy of a solitary brain tumor. In cases of a

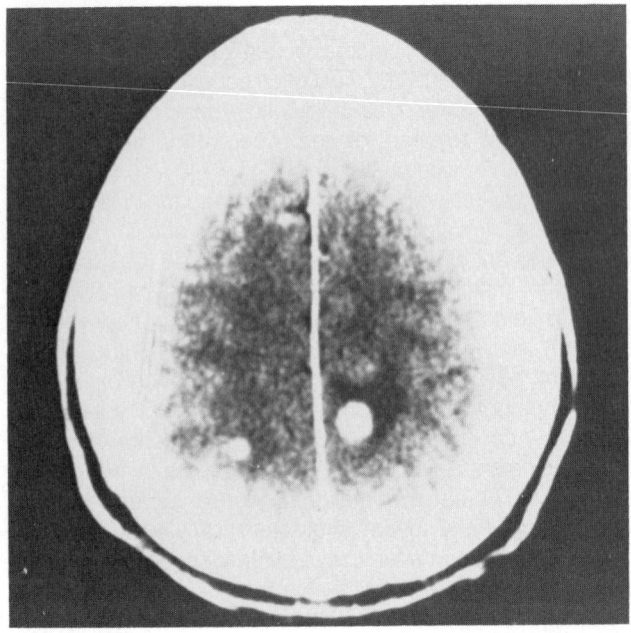

Figure XXIV-1-6. Contrast-enhanced computed tomography (CT) scan of multiple metastases from a malignant melanoma.

known systemic primary lesion, multiple lesions in the brain almost certainly are due to metastatic disease and a presumptive diagnosis of metastatic tumor to the brain would be warranted.

Radiographic findings of intracranial metastases include contrast-enhancing single or multiple lesions (Figures XXIV-1-5–XXIV-1-6). In general, metastatic brain tumors are surrounded by a large area of edema. Hemorrhage may occur, and if extensive, can obscure the tumor. Some tumors have central areas of necrosis that do not enhance, or the entire lesion may enhance uniformly with sharply demarcated borders. MRI-Gd may be more sensitive than CT because it can visualize smaller lesions and view the posterior fossa free of the bone artifacts observed with CT.[32] Areas of abnormal enhancement along the dura or leptomeninges are also better visualized with MRI-Gd.[209] If a contrast-enhanced CT scan reveals one lesion, we routinely follow CT with MRI-Gd to exclude other lesions. MR imaging of the spine, with and without Gd, is the first diagnostic test used to assess the spinal compartment.

In patients known to have a primary tumor, specific restaging may be done after a metastatic brain or spinal tumor has been documented, to assess the overall extent of tumor and to coordinate treatment strategies based on that information. At times, the site of origin of a systemic primary lesion is determined only after a CNS metastasis has been documented. Although in some cases the primary site is not determined despite extensive searches, a CNS metastasis usually is diagnosed in association with a known primary site, and usually within the first year after diagnosis of the primary lesion. Other primary tumors may not manifest a CNS recurrence for many years after the initial diagnosis, most notably in patients with breast, colon, and renal cancer. Because of the wide diversity and overall frequency of CNS spread, a

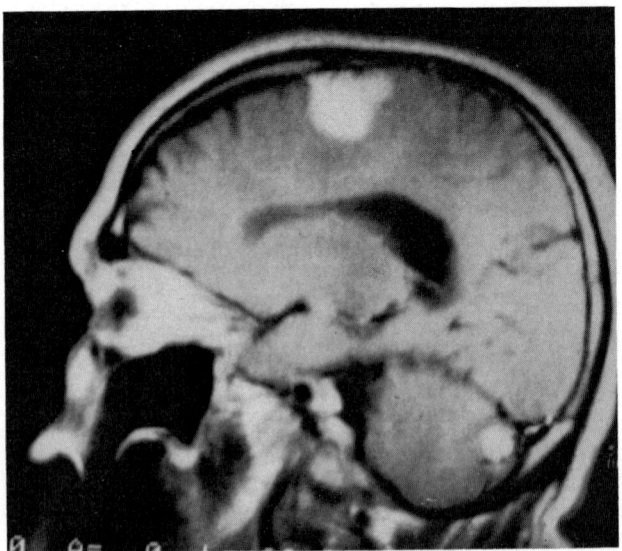

Figure XXIV-1-5. T1-weighted magnetic resonance (MR) image made with gadolinium in the sagittal plane shows multiple intracranial lesions metastatic from the kidney.

high index of suspicion is needed in evaluating predisposed patients.

Differential Diagnosis. The differential diagnosis of a space-occupying lesion or lesions in the CNS includes other primary CNS tumors, such as glioblastoma (most often found as a single enhancing tumor) or meningioma. In patients with AIDS or other causes of immunocompromise, infectious processes must be included. Clinically significant intraparenchymal hemorrhage may occur in association with chemotherapy-induced thrombocytopenia or disseminated coagulopathies, and may add confusion to the etiology of secondary bleeding. Cerebrovascular disease can cause variable enhancing lesions that may be confused with tumor, but such lesions resolve over time. The clinical setting in which the lesion exists and the patient's physical and laboratory findings should be helpful in differentiating other causes. When doubt exists regarding diagnosis and appropriate therapy, surgical biopsy or resection should be done to establish the diagnosis.

Surgery and Radiation Therapy

Brain Metastases. A decision to operate for metastatic brain tumor depends in large part on the patient's neurologic status, the extent of disease in the CNS, and most importantly the extent of systemic disease. Certainly, a decision to resect a lesion or lesions in the CNS must take into account the nature of the primary disease as well as expectations for its control. A craniotomy is seldom of benefit to a patient with melanoma that is widely disseminated both systemically and intracranially. However, a patient with controlled primary lung cancer and no other evidence of disease except a single brain metastasis is a candidate for surgical intervention. The rationale for resecting a solitary metastasis to the CNS is based partly on retrospective, uncontrolled studies comparing outcome after surgery plus irradiation with that after irradiation alone. All of those studies suggest that combined surgery and irradiation are of benefit in treating controlled primary disease and single metastases to brain. Of 125 patients treated by Sundaresen and Galicich at Memorial Sloan-Kettering Cancer Center from 1978 to 1982, for example, all had metastatic tumors resected either before or after undergoing irradiation.[249] Failure to respond to whole-brain irradiation prompted surgery in 31 cases, and 81 patients had symptomatic metastases resected and received radiation therapy postoperatively. All but six patients had single metastatic lesions; the most common primary site was the lung, followed by melanoma, kidney, and then less common primary sites such as colon, sarcoma, and breast. The median survival for the series was 12 months, 12% of the patients surviving for more than 5 years. Patients who had only CNS disease with a controlled primary site showed a distinct therapeutic advantage, their median survival being 22 months as compared to only 5 months in patients with active extracranial disease.

The period of survival after radiation therapy alone is generally shorter than that after surgery plus irradiation. In a retrospective study matching patients with lung cancer, Patchell and colleagues compared survival in those with metastatic brain tumors treated with radiation alone and those having surgery plus irradiation.[192] The median survival was

19 months in the combined treatment group but only 9 months in the group receiving radiation therapy alone. Several similar reports show survival of only 6–12 months after radiation therapy alone. Patchell and colleagues more recently reported a prospective controlled trial comparing irradiation plus surgical resection or biopsy in patients with single brain metastases.[193] The local recurrence rate was significantly greater in the group undergoing biopsy only (52%) than in the group having resection (20%), and median survival was better in the resection group (40 weeks) than in the group that had biopsy (15 weeks). They conclude that surgical resection followed by irradiation is indicated in patients with single metastatic lesions.

There is also a role for surgical resection in treating symptomatic lesions that do not respond to irradiation, for both palliation and the possibility of improved survival. Some metastatic tumors are conspicuously less responsive to irradiation and local recurrence is common. Complete removal of a single lesion, when possible, may be the best form of local control in this situation and potentially provides long-term survival.

Spinal Metastases. A decision to use surgery for spinal metastases is based largely on the status of the patient both systemically and neurologically, the extent of the lesion, and the advantages offered by other forms of treatment such as irradiation, chemotherapy, or hormonal therapy. The ideal candidate for surgical resection has a single lesion and minimal neurologic deficit. The goal of surgery is removal of the lesion, preservation of function, and maintenance of spinal integrity.[240] Extradural tumors may quickly cause irreversible deficits by compression of the spinal cord, but how long complete paralysis may exist before it becomes irreversible is not fully known. As a general guideline, complete paralysis lasting longer than 24 hours is most likely irreversible. Partial deficits may be completely reversible with rapid therapy, including high-dose corticosteroids to diminish peritumoral edema, surgery, and irradiation. If radiation therapy has not been used as primary therapy before surgery, then it should be used after surgery in most patients who have symptomatic spinal metastases.

The availability of new techniques that help achieve decompression with spinal stabilization has influenced surgeons to treat more of the patients who may benefit from surgery.[250] Nonetheless, a comparison of surgery and irradiation with regard to potential benefits still favors irradiation in most cases.[10,240,250] Appropriate indications for surgical resection include cases in which the diagnosis cannot be defined, in which spinal cord compression is progressive despite maximum radiation therapy, and, rarely, when palliation of pain is required. Ominus and colleagues achieved excellent pain relief in most of 57 patients treated surgically for spinal metastases, and 65% of those who had been bedridden before surgery recovered the ability to walk.[183] Indications for surgery further include progressive neurologic decline due to cord compression produced by a collapsed vertebral body, improvement being attributable to vertebral body resection and stabilization of the spine with methacrylate and metal or bone internal splinting.

Radiation Therapy. Radiation therapy is used in most cases of intracranial and spinal metastases. The RTOG recently reviewed their data on dose and fractionation schedules for patients with metastatic intracranial lesions.[55] No difference in outcome was observed in one series of sequential trials evaluating several regimens, including whole-brain irradiation given to a total dose of either 20 Gy within 1 week, or up to 40 Gy within 4 weeks; or in a second trial evaluating irradiation to 30 Gy within 2 weeks as compared with 50 Gy within 4 weeks. Further studies compared two other fractionation schemes: 30 Gy given in 10 fractions over 2 weeks; and 30 Gy given in six fractions over 3 weeks. Misonidazole was also evaluated in these arms in a randomized fashion and, in general, there was no significant difference in survival favoring either misonidazole or a hypofractionated scheme.

The misonidazole trials distinguished subgroups of patients destined for poor survival from those subgroups who could be expected to survive more than 200 days. Favorable factors were a patient aged 60 years or less with a single brain metastasis, a KPS of 70 or above, and primary sites that were either not identifiable or controlled. The median survival for the group in the more favorable condition was 7.4 months but it was only 2 months for patients in the less favorable group. Other studies now evaluating the role of hyperfractionated irradiation in this disease state suggest that higher doses are more effective in controlling local disease when given more often than once a day, but the final results are pending.[271]

Interstitial brachytherapy, with or without hyperthermia, and radiosurgery are also useful for brain metastases. A series reported by Prados and colleagues included several cases of long-term survival and good local control in patients treated with high-activity radioactive iodine brachytherapy.[200] Fourteen patients with metastatic tumor who either had just completed radiation therapy or had not responded to whole-brain irradiation underwent interstitial brachytherapy to boost irradiation of the immediate tumor area. Eight of the 14 were alive a median of 63 weeks later (range 52–239 weeks) and median survival of the entire group was 80 weeks. This was a select group of patients whose lesions were of a favorable size and location to permit brachytherapy. Similarly eligible patients are now being treated with a combination of interstitial brachytherapy and hyperthermia in an attempt to further improve on these results.

Radiosurgery, precisely focused irradiation of tumor, has also been used in similar groups of patients. Loeffler and colleagues treated 18 patients with stereotactic radiosurgery for recurrent or persistent brain metastases; the selection criteria included a KPS of 70 or greater and stable systemic disease.[153] All patients had previously had conventional radiation therapy. Single doses of radiation of 9–25 Gy were used. Within a median follow-up period of 9 months, all tumors had been controlled in the field and two did not respond outside the margin of the field. Although it is too early to draw conclusions, radiosurgery appears to be an attractive option in certain subsets of patients.

In cases of spinal cord compression, irradiation is effective in controlling pain and preventing disease progression–not just in patients who show only radiographic evidence of spinal metastasis but are normal on neurologic examination, but also in patients with irreversible cord compression causing paralysis and loss of bowel and bladder control. Ampil

reviewed 20 patients who had paraplegia caused by epidural cord compression, most of whom received at least 30 Gy to the tumor site; the tumors principally were metastatic from a lung or prostatic primary lesion.[10] Of this group, 78% achieved symptomatic pain relief, although none showed improvement in neurologic function and the overall median survival was only 2.5 months.

In patients with progressive neurologic decline short of complete paralysis, radiation therapy is as effective as surgery, particularly for highly radiation-sensitive tumors, including lymphomas and leukemia, oat cell tumors, breast and colon cancer, and prostatic tumors. For other tumors that are not as responsive to radiation, such as melanoma and renal cell cancers, surgical resection using new approaches may be beneficial. Radiation therapy may then be useful for small residual tumors. If the tumor can be identified by MR imaging as arising from the vertebral body, laminectomy may not be sufficient and vertebrectomy through an exterior approach may be necessary to decompress the spinal cord. Surgical resection is indicated, both for decompression and diagnosis, in cases of progressive neurologic decline when the nature of a tumor is unknown. It is also indicated for progressive neurologic decline that does not respond to radiation therapy and for pain control when other measures are ineffective.

Chemotherapy

Corticosteroids should be used routinely in the urgent treatment of epidural cord compression. Their effect is to reduce vasogenic edema secondary to tumor and to relieve pain as well as neurologic symptoms in many cases. Short courses of high-dose dexamethasone–up to 100 mg administered as a bolus and then given in divided doses on a daily basis–are given concurrently with definitive therapy, such as surgery and irradiation. Following a 3-day to 4-day course, the dose may be tapered to the lowest dose that maintains good control of symptoms. Dexamethasone is also helpful in controlling symptoms related to intracranial tumors, which frequently present with significant mass effect as a result of peritumoral edema. If the clinical situation is severe, similar doses to those used for cord compression may be used. In most cases, however, much smaller doses are required. The dose should be tapered to the lowest dose that maintains a response while more definitive therapy is given. The response to steroids is dose-dependent and may be short-lived in the case of cord compression unless definitive therapy is given.

In some cases, metastatic brain tumors may be treated with systemic chemotherapy. At UCSF, a multiagent chemotherapy regimen including lomustine, 6-thioguanine (6-TG), dibromodulcitol, procarbazine, 5-fluorouracil (5-FU) and hydroxyurea has been used for tumors that have recurred despite surgery and/or irradiation. Although the results are preliminary in this ongoing trial, this regimen controls metastatic disease in the brain and causes objective reductions in tumor size in some cases of CNS lesions metastatic from breast and lung cancer as well as melanoma.[143] Other investigators have shown objective responses in the brain using a variety of drugs. Lee and colleagues, reporting from the University of Texas M. D. Anderson Hospital, showed that among 11 evaluable patients with small cell lung cancer metastatic to the brain who received a chemotherapy regimen including doxorubicin, cyclophosphamide, etoposide, and vincristine, eight achieved at least a partial response; median survival for the group was 34 weeks.[131] Rosner and colleagues also documented objective responses in patients with metastatic breast carcinoma to brain using various combinations of cyclophosphamide, 5-FU, methotrexate, doxorubicin, and prednisone.[216] Objective responses and stable disease can be achieved with these and other drug regimens that should be considered as a therapeutic strategy against metastatic brain tumors.

Leptomeningeal Disease

The treatment of diffuse leptomeningeal disease, or neoplastic meningitis, is difficult and offers few options. Traditionally, treatment has included chemotherapy, given intrathecally or through an Ommaya reservoir, with agents such as methotrexate, cytosine arabinoside, and thiotepa. Combination therapy using two or three drugs with or without steroids has also been tried. In general, responses to treatment have been short-lived except in the case of very sensitive tumors such as leukemia, some lymphomas, and CSF spread of medulloblastoma and primitive neuroectodermal tumor. Irradiation of the craniospinal axis may be helpful, but can severely compromise the bone marrow reserve if systemic chemotherapy is given. New approaches to this disease are needed.

Benjamin and colleagues reported one patient who received intrathecal monoclonal antibody therapy conjugated to iodine-131 for carcinomatous meningitis secondary to bladder cancer.[22] The monoclonal antibody was raised against human milk fat globulin (HMFG1). The patient died within 4 days of treatment. At autopsy, the leptomeninges showed infiltration by carcinoma cells, which stained positively with HMFG1. Autoradiographic examination of the brain revealed isotope that had concentrated within the periventricular white matter and leptomeningeal layers. It appeared that labeled antibody diffused into white matter wherever contact occurred with CSF. Lashford and colleagues treated five patients who had leptomeningeal tumors with radiolabeled antibody given intrathecally, using antibodies selected for the specific tumor type from a panel of available antibodies.[128] Minimal toxicity was observed, and four of the five patients achieved an objective response varying from seven months to two years. The tumor types included pineoblastoma, lymphoma, teratoma, primitive neuroectodermal tumor, and melanoma. Moseley and colleagues found that the HMFG1 antigen could be detected in 18 of 20 cases of carcinomatous meningitis from a variety of epithelial primary tumors that included ovary, bladder, lung, breast and stomach.[172] It was also detected in two cases of neoplastic meningitis from lymphoma and medulloblastoma. Evidently this antigen could be a target for monoclonal antibody therapy for a number of tumors that invade this compartment. Moseley and colleagues also used a panel of monoclonal antibodies successfully to identify melanoma cells in cases of neoplastic meningitis. The use of specific monoclonal antibodies conjugated to radioisotopes is appealing as a therapeutic strategy for leptomeningeal disease when other therapies are not successful.[171]

Future Directions

Neurooncology is making significant progress through laboratory investigations into the molecular biology and genetics of CNS neoplasms. Clues to the etiology and pathogenesis of malignant brain tumors are being detected at a rapid pace, and, with the fundamental understanding of the nature of these tumors that this information provides, it is likely that a greater number of rationally designed, specific, nontoxic therapies may be forthcoming. For pituitary neoplasms, innovative nonsurgical approaches—particularly the synthesis of improved somatostatin analogs, modification of dopamine agonists to enhance the efficacy of long-term treatment, and maximal applications of molecular genetic techniques—offer promise of earlier diagnosis and improved treatment. For the foreseeable future, though, microsurgery affords the best prognosis for most pituitary adenomas (see XXVI-1).

Investigations into the control of growth and oncogene expression, or the lack of controlling mechanisms, afford particularly exciting avenues of research. The potential of monoclonal antibody therapies is encouraging, as are the trials of immunotherapeutic agents such as the interferons and interleukins. Radiation therapy has contributed greatly to the multidisciplinary approach to treatment, affording new fractionation schemes, interstitial brachytherapy, radiosurgery, and radiation-enhancing agents. The ability to overcome a tumor's resistance to certain drugs may additionally enhance response rates, as may revolutionary agents such as the polyamine inhibitors. Growth stimulators such as granulocyte monocyte-colony stimulating factor (GM-CSF) should permit greater dose intensity and provide additional support for high-dose chemotherapy with ABMT. Surgical techniques now permit more extensive resection with less risk than at any time in the history of neurosurgery. Perhaps the single most important ingredient in this new era of neurooncology is a willingness to abolish the pessimism of the past, replacing it with acceptance that CNS tumors should and will be treated as successfully as are tumors elsewhere in the body.

References

1. Afra, D., Müller, I., Slowik, F., Wilcke, O., Budka, H., and Turoczy, L.: Supratentorial lobar ependymomas: reports on the grading and survival periods in 80 cases, including 46 recurrences. Acta Neurochir. (Wien), 69:243, 1983.
2. Albright, A. L., Guthkelch, A. N., Packer, R. J., Price, R. A., and Rourke, L. B.: Prognostic factors in pediatric brain-stem gliomas. J. Neurosurg., 65:751, 1986.
3. Albright, A. L., Price, R. A., and Guthkelch, A. N.: Brain stem gliomas of children. A clinicopathological study. Cancer, 52:2313, 1983.
4. Allen, J., Packer, R., Bleyer, A., Zeltzer, P., Prados, M., Nirenberg, A., and Etcubanas, E.: Recombinant beta-interferon-A phase I/II dose finding trial in pediatric brain tumor patients. J. Neurooncol., Abstract, 7:S4, 1989.
5. Allen, J. C., Bloom, J., Ertel, I., Evans, A., Hammond, D., Jones, H., Levin, V., Jenkin, D., Sposto, R., and Wara, W.: Brain tumors in children: current cooperative and institutional chemotherapy trials in newly diagnosed and recurrent disease. Semin. Oncol., 13:110, 1986.
6. Allen, J. C., Bosl, G., and Walker, R.: Chemotherapy trials in recurrent primary intracranial germ cell tumors. J. Neurooncol., 3:147, 1985.
7. Allen, J. C., Nisselbaum, J., Epstein, F., Rosen, G., and Schwartz, M. K.: Alphafetoprotein and human chorionic gonadotropin determination in cerebrospinal fluid. An aid to the diagnosis and management of intracranial germ-cell tumors. J. Neurosurg., 51:368, 1979.
8. Ammirati, M., Galicich, J., Arbit, E., and Liao, Y.: Reoperation in the treatment of recurrent intracranial malignant gliomas. Neurosurgery, 21:607, 1987.
9. Ammirati, M., Vick, N., Liao, Y. L., Ciric, I., and Mikhael, M.: Effect of the extent of surgical resection on survival and quality of life in patients with supratentorial glioblastomas and anaplastic astrocytomas. Neurosurgery, 21:201, 1987.
10. Ampil, F. L.: Epidural compression from metastatic tumor with resultant paralysis. J. Neurooncol., 7:129, 1989.
11. Andreou, J., George, A. E., Wise, A., de Leon M., Kricheff, I. I., Ransohoff, J., and Foo, S. H.: CT prognostic criteria of survival after malignant glioma surgery. A.J.N.R., 4:488, 1983.

12. Arcangeli, G., Munro, R., and Morelli, B.: Multiple daily fractionation in radiotherapy: Biological rationale and preliminary clinical experience. Eur. J. Cancer, 15:1077, 1979.
13. Arnold, D. L., Shoubridge, E. A., Feindel, W., and Villemure, J. G.: Metabolic changes in cerebral gliomas within hours of treatment with intra-arterial BCNU demonstrated by phosphorus magnetic resonance spectroscopy. Can. J. Neurol. Sci., 14:570, 1987.
14. Backlund, E.: Solid Craniopharyngioma Treated by Stereotactic Radiosurgery. *In* Stereotactic Cerebral Irradiation, Inserm Symposium, No. 12. Edited by G. Szilka. New York, Elsevier/North Holland, 1979, p. 271.
15. Bailey, P., and Cushing, H.: A Classification of the Tumors of the Glioma Group on a Histogenetic Basis with a Correlated Study of Prognosis. Philadelphia, JB Lippincott, 1926.
16. Barker, D., Wright, E., Nguyen, N., Cannon, L., Fain, P., Goldgar, D., Bishop, D. T., Carey, J., Baty, J., Kivlin, J., Willard, H., Waye, J. S., Greig, G., Leinwand, L., Nakamura, Y., O'Connell, P., Leppert, M., Lalouel, J. M., White, R., and Skolnick, M.: Gene for von Recklinghausen neurofibromatosis is in the pericentromeric region of chromosome 17. Science, 236:1100, 1987.
17. Bashir, R. M., Harris, N. L., Hochberg, F. H., and Singer, R. M.: Detection of Epstein-Barr virus in CNS lymphomas by in-situ hybridization. Neurology, 39:813, 1989.
18. Bashir, R., Hochberg, F. H., Linggood, R. M., and Hottleman, K.: Pre-irradiation internal carotid artery BCNU in treatment of glioblastoma multiforme. J. Neurosurg., 68:917, 1988.
19. Baskin, D. S., and Wilson, C. B.: Surgical management of craniopharyngiomas. A review of 74 cases. J. Neurosurg., 65:22, 1986.
20. Baughman. F. A., Jr., List, C. F., Williams, J. R., Muldoon, J. P., Segarra, J. M., and Volkel, J. S.: The glioma-polyposis syndrome. N. Engl. J. Med., 281:1345, 1969.
21. Baumgartner, J. E., Rachlin, J. R., Beckstead, J. H., Meeker, T. C., Levy, R. M., Wara, W. M., and Rosenblum, M. L.: Primary central nervous system lymphomas: Natural history and response to radiation therapy in 55 patients with acquired immunodeficiency syndrome. J. Neurosurg., 73:206, 1990.
22. Benjamin, J. C., Moss, T., Moseley, R. P., Maxwell, R., and Coakham, H. B.: Cerebral distribution of immunoconjugate after treatment for neoplastic meningitis using an intrathecal radiolabeled monoclonal antibody. Neurosurgery, 25:253, 1989.
23. Berger, M. S., Edwards, M. S., LaMasters, D., Davis, R. L., and Wilson, C. B.: Pediatric brain stem tumors: Radiographic, pathological, and clinical correlations. Neurosurgery, 12:298, 1983.
24. Berger, M. S., Kincaid, J., Ojemann, G. A., and Lettich, E.: Brain mapping techniques to maximize resection, safety, and seizure control in children with brain tumors. Neurosurgery 25:786, 1989.
25. Birchmeier, C., Sharma, S., and Wigler, M.: Expression and rearrangement of the ROS1 gene in human glioblastoma cells. Proc. Natl. Acad. Sci. U.S.A., 84:9270, 1987.
26. Birkmayer, G. D., and Stass, H. P.: Humoral immune response in glioma patients: A solubilized glioma-associated membrane antigen as a tool for detecting circulating antibodies. Int. J. Cancer, 25:445, 1980.
27. Black, K. L., Hawkins, R. A., Kim, K. T., Becker, D. P., Lerner, C., and Marciano, D.: Use of thallium-201 SPECT to quantitate malignancy grade of gliomas. J. Neurosurg., 71:342, 1989.
28. Blatt, J., Jaffe, R., Deutsch, M., and Adkins, J. C.: Neurofibromatosis and childhood tumors. Cancer, 57:1225, 1986.
29. Bleehen, N. M., Wiltshire, C. R., Plowman, P. N., Watson, J. V., Gleave, J. R., Holmes, A. E., Lewin, W. S., Triep, C. S., and Hawkins, T. D.: A randomized study of misonidazole and radiotherapy for grade 3 and 4 cerebral astrocytoma. Br. J. Cancer, 43:436, 1981.
30. Bloom, H.: Intracranial tumors: Response and resistance to therapeutic endeavors, 1970-1980. Int. J. Radiat. Oncol. Biol. Phys., 8:1083, 1982.
31. Bogdahn, U., Bogdahn, S., Mertens, H. G, Dommasch, D., Wodarz, R., Wünsch, P. H., Kühl, P., and Richter, E.: Primary non-Hodgkin's lymphoma of the CNS. Acta Neurol. Scand., 73:602, 1986.
32. Brant-Zawadzki, M., Berry, I., Osaki, L., Brasch, R., Murovic, J., and Norman, D.: Gd-DPTA in clinical MR of the brain. 1. Intraaxial lesions. AJR Am. J. Roentgenol., 147:1223, 1986.
33. Bruce, J., and Stein, B.: Pineal Region Tumors. *In* Current Therapy in Neurological Surgery. Edited by D. Long. Toronto, BC Decker, 1989, p. 73.
34. Brücher, J. M., Dalesio, O., and Solbu, G.: Prospective Analysis of Grade III and IV Gliomas, with Consideration of Histologic Classification. (An EORTC Brain Tumor Group Study). *In* Brain Oncology. Edited by M. Chatel, F. Darcel, and J. Pecker. Dordrecht, Martinus Nijhoff, 1987, p. 237.
35. Burger, P. C.: Malignant astrocytic neoplasms: Classification, pathologic anatomy, and response to treatment. Semin. Oncol., 13:16, 1986.
36. Cairncross, J. G., and Macdonald, D. R.: Successful chemotherapy for recurrent malignant oligodendroglioma. Ann. Neurol., 23:360, 1988.
37. Cairncross, J. G., Pexman, J. H., Rathbone, M. P., and DelMaestro, R. F.: Postoperative contrast enhancement in patients with brain tumor. Ann. Neurol., 17:570, 1985.
38. Caputy, A. J., McCullough, D., Manz, H. J., Patterson, K., and Hammock, M. K.: A review of the factors influencing the prognosis of medulloblastoma. The importance of cell differentiation. J. Neurosurg., 66:80, 1987.
39. Cavenee, W. K.: Loss of heterozygosity in stages of malignancy. Clin. Chem., 35(Suppl. 7):B48, 1989.
40. Chan, R. C., and Thompson, G. B.: Morbidity, mortality, and quality of life following surgery for intracranial meningiomas. A retrospective study in 257 cases. J. Neurosurg., 60:52, 1984.
41. Chang, C. H., Horton, J., Schoenfeld, D., Salazer, O., Perez-Tamayo, R., Kramer, S., Weinstein, A., Nelson, J. S., and Tsukada, Y.: Comparison of postoperative radiotherapy and combined postoperative radiotherapy and chemotherapy in the multidisciplinary management of malignant gliomas. A Joint Radiation Therapy Oncology Group and Eastern Cooperative Oncology Group study. Cancer, 52:997, 1983.
42. Chang, C. H., Housepian, E. M., and Herbert, C., Jr.: An operative staging system and a megavoltage radiotherapeutic technic for cerebellar medulloblastomas. Radiology, 93:1351, 1969.
43. Chin, H. W., Hazel, J. J, Kim, T. H., and Webster, J. H.: Oligodendrogliomas. I. A clinical study of cerebral oligodendrogliomas. Cancer, 45:1458, 1980.
44. Choucair, A. K., Levin, V. A., Gutin, P. H., Davis, R. L., Silver, P., Edwards, M. S., and Wilson, C. B.: Development of multiple lesions during radiation therapy and chemotherapy in patients with gliomas. J. Neurosurg., 65:654, 1986.
45. Choux, M., Lena, G., and Hassoun, J.: Prognosis and long-term follow-up in patients with medulloblastoma. Clin. Neurosurg., 30:246, 1983.
46. Coffey, R. J., and Lunsford, D. L.: The role of stereotactic techniques in the management of craniopharyngiomas. Neurosurg. Clin. North Am., 1:161, 1990.
47. Cogen, P. H., Daneshvar, L., Metzger, A. K., and Edwards, M. S.: Deletion mapping of the medulloblastoma locus on chromosome 17p. Genomics, 8:279, 1990.
48. Cohen, M. E., and Duffner, P. K.: Brain Tumors in Children: Principles of Diagnosis and Treatment. International Review of Child Neurology series. New York, Raven Press, 1984, p. 1.
49. Cooper, P. R.: Outcome after operative treatment of intramedullary spinal cord tumors in adults: Intermediate and long-term results in 51 patients. Neurosurgery, 25:855, 1989.
50. Copeland, D. D., and Bigner, D. D.: Glial-mesenchymal tropism of in vivo avian sarcoma virus neuro-oncogenesis in rats. Acta Neuropathol. (Berl.), 41:23, 1978.
51. Danoff, B. F., Cowchock, F. S., and Kramer, S.: Childhood craniopharyngioma: Survival, local control, endocrine and neurologic function following radiotherapy. Int. J. Radiat. Oncol. Biol. Phys., 9:171, 1983.
52. DeAngelis, L. M., Yahalom, J., Heinemann, M. H., Cirrincione, C., Thaler, H. T., and Krol, G.: Primary CNS lymphoma: Combined treatment with chemotherapy and radiotherapy. Neurology, 40:80, 1990.
53. Deutsch, M.: Medulloblastoma: Staging and treatment outcome. Int. J. Radiat. Oncol. Biol. Phys., 14:1103, 1988.
54. Deutsch, M., Green, S. B., Strike, T. A., Burger, P. C., Robertson, J. T., Selker, R. G., Shapiro, W. R., Mealey, J., Jr., Ransohoff, J., Jr., Paoletti, P., Smith, K., Odom, G., Hunt, W., Young, B., Alexander, E., Walker, M., and Pistenmaa, D.: Results of a randomized trial comparing BCNU plus radiotherapy, streptozotocin plus radiotherapy, BCNU plus hyperfractionated radiotherapy, and BCNU following misonidazole plus radiotherapy in the postoperative treatment of malignant glioma. Int. J. Radiat. Oncol. Biol. Phys., 16:1389, 1989.
55. Diener-West, M., Dobbins, T. W., Phillips, T. L., and Nelson, D. F.: Identification of an optimal subgroup for treatment evaluation of patients with brain metastases using RTOG study 7916. Int. J. Radiat. Oncol. Biol. Phys., 16:669, 1989.
56. Dohrmann, G.: Ependymomas. *In* Neurosurgery, Vol. 1. Edited by R. H. Wilkins, and S. S. Rengachary. New York, McGraw Hill, 1985, p. 767.
57. Douglas, B. G.: Preliminary results using superfractionation in the treatment of glioblastoma multiforme. J. Can. Assoc. Radiol., 28:106, 1977.
58. Earnest, F., Kernohan, J., and Craig, W.: Oligodendroglioma. A review of two hundred cases. Arch. Neurol. Psychiatry, 63:964, 1950.
59. Eby, N. L., Grufferman, S., Flannelly, C. M., Schold, S. C., Jr., Vogel, F. S., and Burger, P. C.: Increasing incidence of primary brain lymphoma in the US. Cancer, 62:2461, 1988.
60. Edwards, M. S., Wara, W. M., Urtasun, R. C., Prados, M., Levin, V. A., Fulton, D., Wilson, C. B., Hannigan, J., and Silver, P.: Hyperfractionated radiation therapy for brain-stem glioma: A phase I-II trial. J. Neurosurg., 70:691, 1989.
61. el-Azouzi, M., Chung, R. Y., Farmer, G. E., Martuza, R. L., Black, P. M., Rouleau, G. A., Hettlich, C., Hedley-Whyte, E. T., Zervas, N. T., Panagopoulos, K., Nakamura, Y., Gusella, J., and Seizinger, B.: Loss of distinct regions on the short arm of chromosome 17 associated with tumorigenesis of human astrocytomas. Proc. Natl. Acad. Sci. U. S. A., 86:7186, 1989.
62. Ellis, F.: Dose, time and fractionation: a clinical hypothesis. Clin. Radiol., 20:1, 1969.
63. Engelhard, H. H., III, Butler, A. B., IV, and Bauer, K. D.: Quantification of the *c-myc* oncoprotein in human glioblastoma cells and tumor tissue. J. Neurosurg., 71:224, 1989.
64. Epstein, F.: Spinal cord astrocytomas of childhood. Prog. Exp. Tumor Res., 30:135, 1987.
65. Epstein, F., and Wisoff, J.: Surgical management of brain stem tumors of childhood and adolescence. Neurosurg. Clin. North Am., 1:111, 1990.
66. Ernestus, R. I., Wilcke, O., and Schroder, R.: Intracranial ependymomas: Prognostic aspects. Neurosurg. Rev., 12:157, 1989.
67. Evans, A. E., Jenkin, R. D. T., Sposto, R., Ortega, J. A., Wilson, C. B., Wara, W., Ertel, I. J., Kramer, S., Chang, C. H., Leiken, S. L., and Hammond, G. D.: The treatment of medulloblastoma. Results of a prospective randomized trial of radiation therapy with and without CCNU, vincristine, and prednisone. J. Neurosurg., 72:572, 1990.
68. Farwell, J. R., Dohrmann, G. J., and Flannery, J. T.: Central nervous system tumors in children. Cancer, 40:3123, 1977.
69. Fazekas, J. T.: Treatment of grades I and II brain astrocytomas. The role of radiotherapy. Int. J. Radiat. Oncol. Biol. Phys., 2:661, 1977.
70. Fearon, E. R., Hamilton, S. R., and Vogelstein, B.: Clonal analysis of human colorectal tumors. Science, 238:193, 1987.
71. Finlay, J., August, C., Packer, R., Zimmerman, R., Sutton, L., Nachman, J., Levin, A., Turski, P., Steeves, R., Longo, W., and Javid, M.: High-Dose Chemotherapy with Autologous Marrow Rescue in Children with Recurrent Brain Tumor. *In* Autologous Bone Marrow Transplantation. Proceedings of the Fourth International Symposium. Edited by K. A. Dicke, G. Spitzer, S. Jagannath, and M. J. Eringer-Hodges. Houston, The University of Texas M.D. Anderson Cancer Center, 1989, p. 449.
72. Finlay, J. L., and Goins, S. C.: Brain tumors in children. III. Advances in chemotherapy. Am. J. Pediatr. Hematol. Oncol., 9:264, 1987.
73. Follezou, J., Fauchon, F., and Chiras, J.: Intra-arterial infusion of carboplatin in the treatment of malignant gliomas: A phase II study. Neoplasma, 36:349, 1989.
74. Formenti, S. C., Gill, P. S., Lean, E., Rarick, M., Meyer, P. R., Boswell, W., Petrovich, Z., Chak, L., and Levine, A. M.: Primary central nervous system lymphoma in AIDS. Results of radiation therapy. Cancer, 63:1101, 1989.
75. Francavilla, T. L., Miletich, R. S., Di Chiro, G., Patronas, N. J., Rizzoli, H. V., and Wright, D. C.: Positron emission tomography in the detection of malignant degeneration of low-grade gliomas. Neurosurgery, 24:1, 1989.
76. Freeman, C. R., Krischer, J., Sanford, R. A., Burger, P. C., Cohen, M., and Norris, D.: Hyperfractionated radiotherapy in brain stem tumors: Results of a Pediatric Oncology Group study. Int. J. Radiat. Oncol. Biol. Phys., 15:311, 1988.
77. Friedman, H. S., Colvin, O. M., Skapek, S. X., Ludeman, S. M., Elion, G. B., Schold, S. C., Jr., Jacobsen, P. F., Muhlbaier, L. H., and Bigner, D. D.: Experimental chemotherapy of human medulloblastoma cell lines and transplantable xenografts with bifunctional alkylating agents. Cancer Res., 48:4189, 1988.

78. Friedman, H. S., and Oakes, W. J.: The chemotherapy of posterior fossa tumors in childhood. J. Neurooncol., 5:217, 1987.
79. Fujimoto, M., Fults, D. W., Thomas, G. A., Nakamura, Y., Heilbrun, M. P., White, R., Story, J. L., Naylor, S. L., Kagan-Hallet, K. S., and Sheridan, P. J.: Loss of heterozygosity on chromosome 10 in human glioblastoma multiforme. Genomics, 4:210, 1989.
80. Fujimoto, M., Sheridan, P. J., Sharp, Z. D., Weaker, F. J., Kagan-Hallet, S., and Story, J. L.: Proto-oncogene analyses in brain tumors. J. Neurosurg., 70:910, 1989.
81. Gabbai, A. A., Hochberg, F. H., Linggood, R. M., Bashir, R., and Hotleman, K.: High-dose methotrexate for non-AIDS primary central nervous system lymphoma. Report of 13 cases. J. Neurosurg., 70:190, 1989.
82. Garcia, D. M., Latifi, H. R., Simpson, J. R., and Picker, S.: Astrocytomas of the cerebellum in children. J. Neurosurg., 71(Pt. 1):661, 1989.
83. Gerosa, M. A., Talarico, D., Fognani, C., Raimondi, E., Colombatti, M., Tridente, G., De Carli, L., and Della Valle, G.: Overexpression on N-ras oncogene and epidermal growth factor receptor gene in human glioblastomas. J. Natl. Cancer Inst., 81:63, 1989.
84. Gol, A.: The relatively benign astrocytomas of the cerebrum. J. Neurosurg., 18:501, 1961.
85. Green, J. R., Waggener, J. D., and Kriegsfeld, B. A.: Classification and incidence of neoplasms of the central nervous system. Adv. Neurol., 15:51, 1976.
86. Green, S., Byar, D., and Strike, T.: Randomized comparisons of BCNU, streptozotocin, radiosensitizer, and fractionation in the postoperative treatment of malignant glioma (Study 77-02). Proc. Am. Soc. Clin. Oncol., Abstract, 3:260, 1984.
87. Green, S. B., Byar, D. P., Walker, M. D., Pistenmaa, D. A., Alexander, E., Jr., Batzdorf, U., Brooks, W. H., Hunt, W. E., Mealey, J., Jr., Odom, G. L., Paoletti, P., Ransohoff, J., Jr., Robertson, J. T., Selker, R. G., Shapiro, W. R., Smith, K. R., Jr., Wilson, C. B., and Strike, T. A.: Comparisons of carmustine, procarbazine, and high-dose methylprednisolone as additions to surgery and radiotherapy for the treatment of malignant glioma. Cancer Treat. Rep., 67:121, 1983.
88. Greenberg, H. S., Chandler, W. F., Diaz, R. F., Ensminger, W. D., Junck, L., Page, M. A., Gebarski, S. S., McKeever, P., Hood, T. W., Stetson, P. L., Litchter, A. S., and Tankanow, R.: Intra-arterial bromodeoxyuridine radiosensitization and radiation in treatment of malignant astrocytomas. J. Neurosurg., 69:500, 1988.
89. Griffin, C. A., Hawkins, A. L., Packer, R. J., Rorke, L. B., and Emanuel, B. S.: Chromosome abnormalities in pediatric brain tumors. Cancer Res., 48:175, 1988.
90. Gutherie, B. L., Ebersold, M. J., and Scheithaner, B. W.: Neoplasms of the Intracranial Meninges. *In* Neurological Surgery: A Comprehensive Reference Guide to the Diagnosis and Treatment of Neurosurgical Problems, 3rd Edition. Edited by J. R. Youmans. Philadelphia, W. B. Saunders, 1990, p. 3263.
91. Gutin, P. H.: Personal communication. 1990.
92. Harsh, G. R., IV, Levin, V. A., Gutin, P. H., Seager, M., Silver, P., and Wilson, C. B.: Reoperation for recurrent glioblastoma and anaplastic astrocytoma. Neurosurgery, 21:615, 1987.
93. Harsh, G. R., IV, and Wilson, C. B.: Neuroepithelial Tumors of the Adult Brain. In Neurological Surgery: A Comprehensive Reference Guide to the Diagnosis and Treatment of Neurosurgical Problems, 3rd Edition. Edited by J. R. Youmans. Philadelphia, W. B. Saunders, 1990, p. 3040.
94. Heindel, W., Bunke, J., Glathe, S., Steinbrich, W., and Mollevanger, L.: Combined 1H-MR imaging and localized 31P-spectroscopy of intracranial tumors in 43 patients. J. Comput. Assist. Tomogr., 12:907, 1988.
95. Helle, T. L., Britt, R. H., and Colby, T. V.: Primary lymphoma of the central nervous system. Clinicopathological study of experience at Stanford. J. Neurosurg., 60:94, 1984.
96. Hochberg, F. H., and Miller, D. C.: Primary central nervous system lymphoma. J. Neurosurg., 68:835, 1988.
97. Hochberg, F. H., Parker, L. M., Takvorian, T., Canellos, G. P., and Zervas, N. T.: High-dose BCNU with autologous bone marrow rescue for recurrent glioblastoma multiforme. J. Neurosurg., 54:455, 1981.
98. Hochberg, F. H., and Pruitt, A.: Assumptions in the radiotherapy of glioblastoma. Neurology, 30:907, 1980.
99. Hoffman, H. J.: Craniopharyngiomas. Can. J. Neurol. Sci., 12:348, 1985.
100. Hoffman, H. J.: Craniopharyngiomas. The role for resection. Neurosurg. Clin. North Am., 1:173, 1990.
101. Hoshino, T.: Radiosensitization of Brain Tumors. *In* Central Nervous System Tumors. Modern Radiotherapy and Oncology series. Edited by T. J. Deeley. London, Butterworth, 1974, p. 170.
102. Hoshino, T.: A commentary on the biology and growth kinetics of low-grade and high-grade gliomas. J. Neurosurg., 61:895, 1984.
103. Hoshino, T., Prados, M., Wilson, C. B., Cho, K. G., Lee, K. S., and Davis, R. L.: Prognostic implications of the bromodeoxyuridine labeling index of human gliomas. J. Neurosurg., 71:335, 1989.
104. Hoshino, T., Rodriquez, L. A., Cho, K. G., Lee, K. S., Wilson, C. B., Edwards, M. S., Levin, V. A., and Davis, R. L.: Prognostic implications of the proliferative potential of low-grade astrocytomas. J. Neurosurg., 69:839, 1988.
105. Hubbard, J. L., Scheithauer, B. W., Kispert, D. B., Carpenter, S. M., Wick, M. R., and Laws, E. R., Jr.: Adult cerebellar medulloblastomas: The pathological, radiographic, and clinical disease spectrum. J. Neurosurg., 70:536, 1989.
106. Hubesch, B., Sappey-Marinier, D., Roth, K., Meyerhoff, D. J., Matson, G. B., and Weiner, M. W.: ^{31}P NMR spectroscopy of normal brain and brain tumors. Radiology, 174:401, 1990.
107. Ibelgaufts, H.: DNA viruses and brain tumors. Trends Neurosci., 5:16, 1982.
108. Inoue, H., Tamura, M., Koizumi, H., Nakamura, M., Naganuma, H., and Ohye, C.: Clinical pathology of malignant meningiomas. Acta Neurochir. (Wien), 73:179, 1984.
109. James, C. D., Carlbom, E., Dumanski, J. P., Hansen, M., Nordenskjold, M., Collins, V. P., and Cavenee, W. K.: Clonal genomic alterations in glioma malignancy stages. Cancer Res., 48:5546, 1988.
110. Jeffries, B. F., Kishore, P. R., Singh, K. S., Ghatak, N. R., and Krempa, J.: Contrast enhancement in the postoperative brain. Radiology, 139:409, 1981.
111. Jellinger, K.: Primary intracranial germ cell tumours. Acta Neuropathol. (Berl.), 25:291, 1973.
112. Jenkin, R. D., Simpson, W. J., and Keen, C. W.: Pineal and suprasellar germinomas. Results of radiation treatment. J. Neurosurg., 48:99, 1978.
113. Jennings, M., Gelman, R., and Hochberg, F.: Intracranial Germ-cell Tumors: Natural History and Pathogenesis. *In* Diagnosis and Treatment of Pineal Region Tumors. Edited by E. A. Neuwelt. Baltimore, Williams & Wilkins, 1984, p. 166.
114. Jennings, M. T., Gelman, R., and Hochberg, F.: Intracranial germ-cell tumors: Natural history and pathogenesis. J. Neurosurg., 63:155, 1985.
115. Jimenez, O., Timms, A., Quirke, P., and McLaughlin, J. E.: Prognosis in malignant glioma: A retrospective study of biopsy specimens by flow cytometry. Neuropathol. Appl. Neurobiol., 15:331, 1989.
116. Kaplan, W. D., Takvorian, T., Morris, J. H., Rumbaugh C. L., Connolly, B. T., and Atkins, H. L.: Thallium-201 brain tumor imaging: A comparative study with pathologic correlation. J. Nucl. Med., 28:47, 1987.
117. Karlsson, U., and Brady, L.: Tumors of the Spinal Cord and Canal. *In* Principles and Practice of Radiation Oncology. Edited by C. A. Perez, and L. W. Brady. Philadelphia, J. B. Lippincott, 1987, p. 437.
118. Karnofsky, D. A., and Burchenal, J. H.: The clinical evaluation of chemotherapeutic agents in cancer. *In* Evaluation of Chemotherapeutic Agents. Edited by C. M. Macleod. New York, Columbia University Press, 1949, p. 122.
119. Kelly, P. J., Daumas-Duport, C., Scheithauer, B. W., Kall, B. A., and Kispert, D. B.: Stereotactic histologic correlations of computed tomography- and magnetic resonance imaging-defined abnormalities in patients with glial neoplasms. Mayo Clin. Proc., 62:450, 1987.
120. Kernohan, J., Mabon, R., Svien, H., and Adson, A.: A simplified classification of gliomas. Proc. Staff Mayo Clin., 24:71, 1949.
121. King, D. L., Chang, C. H., and Pool, J. L.: Radiotherapy in the management of meningiomas. Acta Radiol. Ther. Phys. Biol., 5:26, 1966.
122. Kinsella, T. J., Russo, A., Mitchell, J. B., Collins, J. M., Rowland, J., Wright, D., and Glatstein, E.: A phase I study of intravenous iododeoxyuridine as a clinical radiosensitizer. Int. J. Radiat. Oncol. Biol. Phys., 11:1941, 1985.
123. Kinzler, K. W., Ruppert, J. M., Bigner, S. H., and Vogelstein, B.: The GLI gene is a member of the Kruppel family of zinc finger proteins. Nature, 332:371, 1988.
124. Kornblith, P. L., and Walker, M.: Chemotherapy for malignant brain tumors J. Neurosurg., 68:1, 1988. (Erratum. J. Neurosurg., 69:645, 1988.)
125. Kurup, P. D., Pajak, T. F., Hendrickson, F. R., Nelson, J. S., Mansell, J., Cohen, L., Awschalom, M., Rosenberg, I., and Ten Haken, R. K.: Fast neutrons and misonidazole for malignant astrocytomas. Int. J. Radiat. Oncol. Biol. Phys., 2:679, 1985.
126. Landberg, T. G., Lindgren, M. L., Cavallin-Stahl, E. K., Svahn-Tapper, G. O., Sundbarg, G., Garwicz, S., Lagergren, J. A., Gunnesson, V. L., Brun, A. E., and Cronqvist, S. E.: Improvements in the radiotherapy of medulloblastoma, 1946-1975. Cancer, 45:670, 1980.
127. Laramore, G. E., Diener-West, M., Griffin, T. W., Nelson, J. S., Griem, M. L., Thomas, F. J., Hendrickson, F. R., Griffin, B. R., Myrianthopoulos, L. C., and Saxton, J.: Randomized neutron dose searching study for malignant gliomas of the brain: Results of an RTOG study. Radiation Therapy Oncology Group. Int. J. Radiat. Oncol. Biol. Phys., 14:1093, 1988.
128. Lashford, L. S., Davies, A. G., Richardson, R. B., Bourne, S. P., Bullimore, J. A., Eckert, H., Kemshead, J. T., and Coakham, H. B.: A pilot study of 131-I monoclonal antibodies in the therapy of leptomeningeal tumors. Cancer, 61:857, 1988.
129. Laws, E. R., Jr., Taylor, W. F., Bergstralh, E. J., Okazaki, H., and Clifton, M. B.: The neurosurgical management of low-grade astrocytoma. Clin. Neurosurg., 33:575, 1986.
130. Laws, E. R., Jr., Taylor, W. F., Clifton, M. B., and Okazaki, H.: Neurosurgical management of low-grade astrocytoma of the cerebral hemispheres. J. Neurosurg., 61:665, 1984.
131. Lee, J. S., Murphy, W. K., Glisson, B. S., Dhingra, H. M., Holoye, P. Y., and Hong, W. K.: Primary chemotherapy of brain metastases in small-cell lung cancer. J. Clin. Oncol., 7:916, 1989.
132. Lee, Y. Y., Van Tassel, P., Bruner, J. M., Moser, R. P., and Share, J. C.: Juvenile pilocytic astrocytomas: CT and MR characteristics. AJR Am. J. Roentgenol., 152:1263, 1989.
133. Leibel, S. A., Gutin, P. H., Sneed, P. K., Prados, M., Levin, V. A., Larson, D. A., Wara, W. M., Weaver, K. A., and Phillips, T. L.: Interstitial irradiation for the treatment of primary and metastatic brain tumors. Principles and Practice of Oncology Update Series, 3:1, 1989.
134. Leibel, S. A., Gutin, P. H., Wara, W. M., Silver, P. S., Larson, D. A., Edwards, M. S., Lamb, S. A., Ham, B., Weaver, K. A., Barnett, C., and Phillips, T. L.: Survival and quality of life after interstitial implantation of removable high-activity iodine-125 sources for the treatment of patients with recurrent malignant gliomas. Int. J. Radiat. Oncol. Biol. Phys., 17:1129, 1989.
135. Leibel, S. A., Sheline, G. E., Wara, W. M., Boldrey, E. B., and Nielsen, S. L.: The role of radiation therapy in the treatment of astrocytomas. Cancer, 35:1551, 1975.
136. Levin, V. A.: Chemotherapy of Recurrent Brain Tumors. *In* Nitrosoureas: Current Status and New Developments. Edited by A. W. Prestayko, and S. T. Crooke. New York, Academic Press, 1981, p. 159.
137. Levin, V. A.: Chemotherapy of primary brain tumors. Neurol. Clin., 3:855, 1985.
138. Levin, V. A.: Personal communication. 1990.
139. Levin, V. A., Chamberlain, M. C., Prados, M. D., Choucair, A. K., Berger, M. S., Silver, P., Seager, M., Gutin, P. H., Davis, R. L., and Wilson, C. B.: Phase I-II study of eflornithine and mitoguazone combined in the treatment of recurrent primary brain tumors. Cancer Treat. Rep., 71:459, 1987.
140. Levin, V. A., Edwards, M. S., Gutin, P. H., Vestnys, P., Fulton, D., Seager, M., and Wilson, C. B.: Phase II evaluation of dibromodulcitol in the treatment of recurrent medulloblastoma, ependymoma, and malignant astrocytoma. J. Neurosurg., 61:1063, 1984.
141. Levin, V. A., Edwards, M. S., Wara, W. M., Allen, J., Ortega, J., and Vestnys, P.: 5-Fluorouracil and 1-(2-chloroethyl)-3-cyclohexyl-1-nitrosourea (CCNU) followed by hydroxyurea, misonidazole, and irradiation for brain stem gliomas: A pilot study of the Brain Tumor Research Center and the Childrens Cancer Group. Neurosurgery, 14:679, 1984.
142. Levin, V. A., Edwards, M. S., Wright, D. C., Seager, M. L., Schimberg, T. P., Townsend, J. J., and Wilson, C. B.: Modified procarbazine, CCNU, and vincristine (PCV 3) combination chemotherapy in the treatment of malignant brain tumors. Cancer Treat. Rep., 64:237, 1980.
143. Levin, V. A., Prados, M. D., and colleagues, unpublished data, 1990.
144. Levin, V. A., Rodriguez, L. A., Edwards, M. S., Wara, W., Liu, H.-C., Fulton, D., Davis, R. L., Wilson, C. B., and Silver, P.: Treatment of medulloblastoma with procarbazine,

hydroxyurea, and reduced radiation doses to whole brain and spine. J. Neurosurg., 68:383, 1988.
145. Levin, V. A., Silver, P., Hannigan, J., Wara, W. M., Gutin, P. H., Davis, R. L., and Wilson, C. B.: Superiority of post-radiotherapy adjuvant chemotherapy with CCNU, procarbazine, and vincristine (PCV) over BCNU for anaplastic gliomas: NCOG 6G61 final report. Int. J. Radiat. Oncol. Biol. Phys., 18:321, 1990.
146. Levin, V. A., Vestnys, P. S., Edwards, M. S., Wara, W. M., Fulton, D., Barger, G., Seager, M., and Wilson, C. B: Improvement in survival produced by sequential therapies in the treatment of recurrent medulloblastoma. Cancer, 51:1364, 1983.
147. Levin, V. A., Wara, W. M., Gutin, P. H., Wilson, C. B., Phillips, T. L., Prados, M. D., Flam, M. S., and Ahn, D.: Initial analysis of NCOG 6G-82-1: Bromodeoxyuridine (BUdR) during irradiation followed by CCNU, procarbazine, and vincristine (PCV) chemotherapy for malignant gliomas (abstract). Proc. Am. Soc. Clin. Oncol., 9:91, 1990.
148. Levy, R. M., Bredesen, D. E., and Rosenblum, M. L.: Neurological manifestations of the acquired immunodeficiency syndrome (AIDS): Experience at UCSF and review of the literature. J. Neurosurg., 62:475, 1985.
149. Lindegaard, K.-F., Mork, S. J., Eide, G. E., Halvorsen, T. B., Hatlevoll, R., Solgaard, T., Dahl, O., and Ganz, J.: Statistical analysis of clinicopathological features, radiotherapy, and survival in 170 cases of oligodendroglioma. J. Neurosurg., 67:224, 1987.
150. Linstadt, D. E., Wara, W. M., Leibel, S. A., Gutin, P. H., Wilson, C. B., and Sheline, G. E.: Postoperative radiotherapy of primary spinal cord tumors. Int. J. Radiat. Oncol. Biol. Phys., 16:1397, 1989.
151. Littman, P., Jarret, P., Bilanuik, L. T., Rorke, L. B., Zimmerman, R. A., Bruce, D. A., Carabell, S. C., and Schut, L.: Pediatric brain stem gliomas. Cancer, 45:2787, 1980.
152. Liu, H., Davis, R., Vestnys, P., Resser, K., and Levin, V.: Correlation of survival and diagnosis in supratentorial malignant gliomas. J. Neurooncol., 2:268, 1984.
153. Loeffler, J. S., Kooy, H. M., Wen, P. Y., Fine, H. A., Cheng, C. W., Mannarino, E. G., Tsai, J. S., and Alexander, E., III: The treatment of recurrent brain metastases with stereotactic radiosurgery. J. Clin. Oncol., 8:576, 1990. (Comment in J. Clin. Oncol., 8:571, 1990.)
154. Loeffler, J. S., Wen, P., Fine, H., and Alexander, E.: The treatment of recurrent brain metastasis with stereotactic radiosurgery. Proc. Am. Soc. Clin. Oncol., Abstract, 9:91, 1990.
155. Ludwig, C. L., Smith, M. T., Godfrey, A. D., and Armbrustmacher, V. W.: A clinicopathological study of 323 patients with oligodendrogliomas. Ann. Neurol., 19:15, 1986.
156. Lunsford, L. D., Flickinger, J., Lindner, G., and Maitz, A.: Stereotactic radiosurgery of the brain using the first United States 201 cobalt-60 source gamma knife. Neurosurgery, 24:151, 1989.
157. Mahaley, M. S., Jr., Hipp, S. W., Dropcho, E. J., Bertsch, L., Cush, S., Tirey, T., and Gillespie, G. Y.: Intracarotid cisplatin chemotherapy for recurrent gliomas. J. Neurosurg., 70:371, 1989.
158. Mahaley, M. S., Jr., Mettlin, C., Natarajan, N., Laws, E. R., Jr., and Peace, B. B.: National survey of patterns of care for brain-tumor patients. J. Neurosurg., 71:826, 1989.
159. Mahaley, M. S., Jr., Urso, M. B., Whaley, R. A., Blue, M., Williams, T. E., Guaspari, A., and Selker, R. G.: Immunobiology of primary intracranial tumors. Part 10: Therapeutic efficacy of interferon in the treatment of recurrent gliomas. J. Neurosurg., 63:719, 1985.
160. Maltoni, C.: Occupational carcinogenesis. Predictive value of carcinogenesis bioassays. Ann. N. Y. Acad. Sci., 271:431, 1976.
161. Maltoni, C., Ciliberti, A., and Caretti, D.: Experimental contributions in identifying brain potential carcinogens in the petrochemical industry. Ann. N. Y. Acad. Sci., 381:216, 1982.
162. Malone, M., Lumley, H., and Erdohazi, M.: Astrocytoma as a second malignancy in patients with acute lymphoblastic leukemia. Cancer 57:1979, 1986.
163. Marsh, W. L., Jr., Stevenson, D. R., and Long, H. J., III: Primary leptomeningeal presentation of T-cell lymphoma. Report of a patient and review of the literature. Cancer, 51:1125, 1983.
164. Martuza, R. L., and Eldridge, R.: Neurofibromatosis 2 (bilateral acoustic neurofibromatosis). N. Engl. J. Med., 318:684, 1988.
165. McLaughlin, P., Velasquez, W. S., Redman, J. R., Yung, W. K., Hagemeister, F. B., Rodriguez, M. A., and Cabanillas, F.: Chemotherapy with dexamethasone, high-dose cytarabine, and cisplatin for parenchymal brain lymphoma. J. Natl. Cancer Inst., 80:1408, 1988.
166. Merchant, R., McVicar, D., Merchant, L., and Young, H.: Treatment of patients with recurrent glioblastoma by repeated intralesional injections of recombinant interleukin-2 alone or in combination with systemic interferon-alpha. J. Neurooncol., Abstract, 7:S19, 1989.
167. Merchant, R. E., Ellison, M. D., and Young, H. F.: Immunotherapy for malignant glioma using human recombinant interleukin-2 and activated autologous lymphocytes. A review of pre-clinical and clinical investigations. J. Neurooncol., 8:173, 1990.
168. Mirimanoff, R. O., Dosoretz, D. E., Linggood, R. M., Ojemann, R. G., and Martuza, R. L.: Meningioma: Analysis of recurrence and progression following neurosurgical resection. J. Neurosurg., 62:18, 1985.
169. Mørk, S. J., Lindegaard, K. F., Halvorsen, T. B., Lehmann, E. H., Solgaard, T., Hatlevoll, R., Harvei, S., and Ganz, J.: Oligodendroglioma: Incidence and biological behavior in a defined population. J. Neurosurg., 63:881, 1985.
170. Mørk, S. J., and Rubinstein, L. J.: Ependymoblastoma. A reappraisal of a rare embryonal tumor. Cancer, 55:1536, 1985.
171. Moseley, R. P., Davies, A. G., Bourne, S. P., Popham, C., Carrel, S., Monro, P., and Coakham, H. B.: Neoplastic meningitis in malignant melanoma: Diagnosis with monoclonal antibodies. J. Neurol. Neurosurg. Psychiatry, 52:881, 1989.
172. Moseley, R. P., Oge, K., Shafqat, S., Moseley, C. M., Sullivan, N. M., Badley, R. A., Burchell, J., Taylor-Papadimitriou, J., and Coakham, H. B.: HFMG1 antigen: A new marker for carcinomatous meningitis. Int. J. Cancer, 44:440, 1989.
173. Mountz, J. M., Stafford-Schuck, K., McKeever, P. E., Taren, J., and Beierwaltes, W. H.: Thallium-201 tumor/cardiac ratio estimation of residual astrocytoma. J. Neurosurg., 68:705, 1988.
174. Nelson, D., Curran, E., Nelson, J., Weinstein, A., Martz, K., Ahmad, K., Keller, J., Murray, K., and Hanks, G.: Hyperfractionation in malignant glioma. Report on a dose searching phase I/II protocol of the Radiation Therapy Oncology Group (RTOG). Proc. Am. Soc. Clin. Oncol., Abstract, 9:90, 1990.
175. Nelson, D. F., Nelson, J. S., Davis, D. R., Chang, C. H., Griffin, T. W., and Pajak, T. F.: Survival and prognosis of patients with astrocytoma with atypical or anaplastic features. J. Neurooncol., 3:99, 1985.
176. Nelson, D. F., Schoenfeld, D., Weinstein, A. S., Nelson, J. S., Wasserman, T., Goodman, R. L., and Carabell, S.: A randomized comparison of misonidazole sensitized radiotherapy plus BCNU and radiotherapy plus BCNU for treatment of malignant glioma after surgery: Preliminary results of an RTOG study. Int. J. Radiat. Oncol. Biol. Phys., 9:1143, 1983.
177. Nelson, J. S., Tsukada, Y., Schoenfield, D., Fulling, K., Lamarche, J., and Peress, N.: Necrosis as a prognostic criterion in malignant supratentorial, astrocytic gliomas. Cancer, 52:550, 1983.
178. Neuwelt, E. A., Frenkel, E. P., Gumerlock, M., Braziel, R., Dana, B., and Hill, S. A.: Developments in the diagnosis and treatment of primary CNS lymphoma. A prospective series. Cancer, 58:1609, 1986.
179. Newton, H. B., Page, M. A., Junck, L., and Greenberg, H. S.: Intra-arterial cisplatin for the treatment of malignant gliomas. J. Neurooncol., 7:39, 1989.
180. Nishizaki, T., Orita, T., Furutani, Y., Ikeyama, Y., Aoki, H., and Sasaki, K.: Flow-cytometric DNA analysis and immunohistochemical measurement of Ki-67 and BUdR labeling indices in human brain tumors. J. Neurosurg., 70:379, 1989.
181. Non-Hodgkin's Lymphoma Pathologic Classification Project: National Cancer Institute sponsored study of classifications of non-Hodgkin's lymphomas: Summary and description of a working formulation for clinical usage. Cancer, 49:2112, 1982.
182. Ojemann, G., Ojemann, J., Lettich, E., and Berger, M.: Cortical language localization in left, dominant hemisphere. An electrical stimulation mapping investigation in 117 patients. J. Neurosurg., 71:316, 1989.
183. Onimus, M., Schraub, S., Bertin, D., Bosset, J. F., and Guidet, M.: Surgical treatment of vertebral metastasis. Spine, 11:883, 1986.
184. Packer, R., and Finlay, J.: Medulloblastoma: Presentation, diagnosis, and management. Oncology, 2:35, 1988.
185. Packer, R. J., Littman, P. A., Sposto, R. M., D'Angio, G., Priest, J. R., Heideman, R. L., Bruce, D. A., and Nelson, D. F.: Results of a pilot study of hyperfractionated radiation therapy for children with brain stem gliomas. Int. J. Radiat. Oncol. Biol. Phys., 13:1647, 1987.
186. Packer, R. J., Siegel, K. R,, Sutton, L. N., Evans, A. E., D'Angio, G., Rorke, L. B., Bunin, G. R., and Schut, L.: Efficacy of adjuvant chemotherapy for patients with poor-risk medulloblastoma: A preliminary report. Ann. Neurol., 24:503, 1988.
187. Packer, R. J., Sposto, R., Atkins, T. E., Sutton, L. N., Bruce, D. A., Siegel, K. R., Rorke, L. B., Littman, P. A., and Schut, L.: Quality of life in children with primitive neuroectodermal tumors (medulloblastoma) of the posterior fossa. Pediatr. Neurosci., 13:169, 1987.
188. Packer, R. J., Sutton, L. N., Bilaniuk, L. T., Radcliffe, J., Rosenstock, J. G., Siegel, K. R., Bunin, G. R., Savino, P. J., Bruce, D. A., and Schut, L.: Treatment of chiasmatic/hypothalamic gliomas of childhood with chemotherapy: An update. Ann. Neurol., 23:79, 1988.
189. Packer, R. J., Sutton, L. N., Rorke, L. B., Littman, P. A., Sposto, R., Rosenstock, J. G., Bruce, D. A., and Schut, L.: Prognostic importance of cellular differentiation in medulloblastoma of childhood. J. Neurosurg., 61:296, 1984.
190. Packer, R. J., Zimmerman, R. A., Luerssen, T. G., Sutton, L. N., Bilaniuk, L. T., Bruce, D. A., and Schut, L.: Brainstem gliomas of childhood: Magnetic resonance imaging. Neurology, 35:397, 1985.
191. Palmiter, R. D., and Brinster R. L.: Transgenic mice. Cell, 41:343, 1985.
192. Patchell, R. A., Cirrincione, C., Thaler, H. T., Galicich, J. H., Kim, J. H., and Posner, J. B.: Single brain metastases: Surgery plus radiation or radiation alone. Neurology, 36:447, 1986.
193. Patchell, R. A., Tibbs, P. A., Walsh, J. W., Dempsey, R. J., Maruyama, Y., Kryscio, R. J., Markesbery, W. R., Macdonald, J. S., and Young, B.: A randomized trial of surgery in the treatment of single brain metastases to the brain. N. Engl. J. Med., 322:494, 1990. (Comment in N. Engl. J. Med., 322:544, 1990.)
194. Pattengale, P. K., Taylor, C. R., Panke, T., Tatter, D., McCormick, R. A., Rawlinson, D. G., and Davis, R. L.: Selective immunodeficiency and malignant lymphoma of the central nervous system. Possible relationship to the Epstein-Barr virus. Acta Neuropathol. (Berl.), 48:165, 1979.
195. Pendergrass, T. W., Milstein, J. M., Geyer, J. R., Mulne, A. F., Kosnik, E. J., Morris, J. D., Heideman, R. L., Ruymann, F. B., Stuntz, J. T., and Bleyer, W. A.: Eight drugs in one day chemotherapy for brain tumors: Experience in 107 children and rationale for preirradiation chemotherapy. J. Clin. Oncol., 5:1221, 1987.
196. Petronio, J., Edwards, M. S., Prados, M., Freyberger, S., Rabbitt, J., Silver, P., and Levin, V. A.: Management of chiasmal and hypothalamic gliomas of infancy and childhood with chemotherapy. J. Neurosurg., 74:701, 1991.
197. Piepmeier, J. M.: Observations on the current treatment of low-grade astrocytic tumors of the cerebral hemispheres. J. Neurosurg., 67:177, 1987.
198. Pollack, I. F., Lunsford, L. D., Flickinger, J. C., and Dameshek, H. L.: Prognostic factors in the diagnosis and treatment of primary central nervous system lymphoma. Cancer, 63:939, 1989.
199. Posner, J. B., and Chernik, N. L.: Intracranial metastases from systemic cancer. Adv. Neurol., 19:579, 1978.
200. Prados, M., Leibel, S., Barnett, C. M., and Gutin, P.: Interstitial brachytherapy for metastatic brain tumors. Cancer, 63:657, 1989.
201. Prados, M., Rodriguez, L., Chamberlain, M., Silver, P., and Levin, V.: Treatment of recurrent gliomas with 1,3-bis(2-chloroethyl)1-nitrosourea and alpha-difluoromethylornithine. Neurosurgery, 24:806, 1989.
202. Prados, M. D.: Unpublished data. 1990.
203. Prados, M. D., Wilson, C. B., and colleagues: Unpublished data. 1990.
204. Press, R. D, Misra, A., Gillaspy, G., Samols, D., and Goldthwait, D. A.: Control of the expression of c-sis mRNA in human glioblastoma cells by phorbol ester and transforming growth factor beta 1. Cancer Res., 49:2914, 1989.
205. Raffel, C., and Edwards, M. S.: Intraspinal Tumors in Children. *In* Neurological Surgery: A Comprehensive Reference Guide to the Diagnosis and Treatment of Neurosurgical Problems, 3rd Edition. Edited by J. R. Youmans. Philadelphia, W. B. Saunders, 1990, p. 3574.
206. Raffel, C., Edwards, M. S., Davis, R. L., and Ablin, A. R.: Postirradiation cerebellar glioma. Case report. J. Neurosurg., 62:300, 1985.

207. Read, G.: The treatment of ependymoma of the brain or spinal canal by radiotherapy: A report of 79 cases. Clin. Radiol., 35:163, 1984.
208. Ringertz, N.: Grading of gliomas. Acta Pathol. Microbiol. Scand., 27:51, 1950.
209. Rodesch, G., Van Bogaert, P., Mavroudakis, N., Parizel, P. M., Martin, J. J., Segebarth, C., Van Vyve, M., Baleriaux, D., and Hildebrand, J.: Neuroradiologic findings in leptomeningeal carcinomatosis: The value interest of gadolinium-enhanced MRI. Neuroradiology, 32:26, 1990.
210. Rorke, L. B.: The cerebellar medulloblastoma and its relationship to primitive neuroectodermal tumors. J. Neuropathol. Exp. Neurol., 42:1, 1983.
211. Rosenblum, M. L.: Personal Communication. 1990.
212. Rosenblum, M. L.: The Role of Surgery in Brain Tumor Management. Neurosurg. Clin. North Am., 1:1, 1990.
213. Rosenblum, M. L., Levy, R. M., and Bredesen, D. E.: Overview of AIDS and the Nervous System. In AIDS and the Nervous System. Edited by M. A. Rosenblum, R. M. Levy, and D. E. Bredesen. New York, Raven Press, 1988, p. 1.
214. Rosenblum, M. L., Levy, R. M., Bredesen, D. E., So, Y. T., Wara, W., and Ziegler, J. L.: Primary central nervous system lymphoma in patients with AIDS. Ann. Neurol., 23:S13, 1988.
215. Rosenstock, J. G., Packer, R. J., Bilaniuk, L., Bruce, D. A., Radcliffe, J. L., and Savino P.: Chiasmatic optic glioma treated with chemotherapy. A preliminary report. J. Neurosurg., 63:862, 1985.
216. Rosner, D., Nemoto, T., and Lane, W. W.: Chemotherapy induces regression of brain metastases in breast carcinoma. Cancer, 58:832, 1986.
217. Ross, G. W., and Rubinstein, L. J.: Lack of histopathological correlation of malignant ependymomas with postoperative survival. J. Neurosurg., 70:31, 1989.
218. Rossi, M. L., Hughes, J. T., Esiri, M. M., Coakham, H. B., and Brownwell, D. B.: Immunohistological study of mononuclear cell infiltrate in malignant gliomas. Acta Neuropathol. (Berl.), 74:269, 1987.
219. Roszman, T. L., Brooks, W. H., and Elliott, L. H.: Inhibition of lymphocyte responsiveness by a glial tumor cell-derived suppressive factor. J. Neurosurg., 67:874, 1987.
220. Rubinstein, A. B., Shalit, M. N., Cohen, M. L., Zandbank, U., and Reichenthal, E.: Radiation-induced cerebral meningioma: A recognizable entity. J. Neurosurg., 61:966, 1984.
221. Russell, D. S., and Rubinstein, L. J.: Pathology of Tumours of the Nervous System, 4th edition. Baltimore, Williams & Wilkins, 1977.
222. Salazar, O. M., Castro-Vita, H., VanHoutte, P., Rubin, P., and Aygun, C.: Improved survival in cases of intracranial ependymoma after radiation therapy. Late report and recommendations. J. Neurosurg., 59:652, 1983.
223. Salazar, O. M., Rubin, P., Feldstein, M. L., and Pizzutiello, R.: High dose radiation therapy in the treatment of malignant gliomas: Final report. Int. J. Radiat. Oncol. Biol. Phys., 5:1733, 1979.
224. Salcman, M., Kaplan, R. S., Ducker, T. B., Abdo, H., and Montgomery, E.: Effect of age and reoperation on survival in the combined modality treatment of malignant astrocytoma. Neurosurgery, 10:454, 1982.
225. Saroja, K. R., Mansell, J., Hendrickson, F. R., Cohen, L., and Lennox, A.: Failure of accelerated neutron therapy to control high grade astrocytomas. Int. J. Radiat. Oncol. Biol. Phys., 17:1295, 1989.
226. Schmidek, H. H.: Surgical Management of Pineal Region Tumors. In Pineal Tumors. Edited by H. H. Schmidek. New York, Masson, 1977, p. 99.
227. Scotti, G., Scialfa, G., Colombo, N., and Landoni, L.: Magnetic resonance diagnosis of intramedullary tumors of the spinal cord. Neuroradiology, 29:130, 1987.
228. Segebarth, C. M., Baleriaux, D. F., Arnold, D. L., Luyten, P. R., and den Hollander, J. A.: MR image-guided P-31 MR spectroscopy in the evaluation of brain tumor treatment. Radiology, 165:215, 1987.
229. Sexauer, C. L., Khan, A., Berger, P. C., Krischer, J. P., van Eys, J., Vats, T., and Ragab, A. H.: Cisplatin in recurrent pediatric brain tumors. A POG Phase II study. A Pediatric Oncology Group Study. Cancer, 56:1497, 1985.
230. Shapiro, W. R., and Green, S. B.: Reevaluating the efficacy of intra-arterial BCNU. J. Neurosurg., Letter, 66:313, 1987.
231. Shapiro, W. R., Green, S. B., Burger, P. C., Mahaley, M. S., Jr., Selker, R. G., VanGilder, J. C., Robertson, J. T., Ransohoff, J., Mealey, J., Jr., Strike, T. A., and Pistenmaa, D. A.: Randomized trial of three chemotherapy regimens and two radiotherapy regimens in postoperative treatment of malignant glioma. Brain Tumor Cooperative Group Trial 8001. J. Neurosurg., 71:1, 1989.
232. Shaw, E. G., Daumas-Duport, C., Scheithauer, B. W., Gilbertson, D. T., O'Fallon, J. R., Earle, J. D., Laws, E. R., Jr., and Okazaki, H.: Radiation therapy in the management of low-grade supratentorial astrocytomas. J. Neurosurg., 70:853, 1989.
233. Shaw, E. G., Evans, R. G., Scheithauer, B. W., Ilstrup, D. M., and Earle, J. D.: Postoperative radiotherapy of intracranial ependymoma in pediatric and adult patients. Int. J. Radiat. Oncol. Biol. Phys., 13:1457, 1987.
234. Sheline, G. E.: Radiation therapy of primary tumors. Semin. Oncol., 2:29, 1975.
235. Sheline, G. E. and colleagues: Unpublished data. 1990.
236. Sheline, G. E., Boldrey, E. B., Karlsberg, P., and Phillips, T. L.: Therapeutic considerations in tumors affecting the central nervous system: Oligodendrogliomas. Radiology, 82:84, 1964.
237. Sheline, G. E., Wara, W. M., and Smith, V.: Therapeutic irradiation and brain injury. Int. J. Radiat. Oncol. Biol. Phys., 6:1215, 1980.
238. Silverberg, E.: Cancer statistics. 1986. CA, 36:9, 1986.
239. Silverberg, E. and Lubera, J. A.: Cancer statistics, 1989. CA, 39:3, 1989. (Comment in CA, 39:254, 1989 and Comment in CA, 39:399, 1989.)
240. Simeone, F.: Spinal Cord Tumors in Adults. In Neurological Surgery: A Comprehensive Reference Guide to the Diagnosis and Treatment of Neurosurgical Problems, 3rd Edition. Edited by J. R. Youmans. Philadelphia, W. B. Saunders, 1990, p. 3531.
241. So, Y. T., Choucair, A., Davis, R. L., Wara, W. M., Ziegler, J. L., Sheline, G. E., and Beckstead, J. H.: Neoplasms of the Central Nervous System in Acquired Immunodeficiency Syndrome. In AIDS and the Nervous System. Edited by M. L. Rosenblum, R. L. Levy, and D. E. Bredesen. New York, Raven Press, 1988, p. 285.
242. Sogg, R. L., Donaldson, S. S., and Yorke, C. H.: Malignant astrocytoma following radiotherapy of a craniopharyngioma. Case report. J. Neurosurg., 48:622, 1978.
243. Spallone, A., Gagliardi, F. M., and Vagnozzi, R.: Intracranial meningiomas related to external cranial irradiation. Surg. Neurol., 12:153, 1979.
244. Spencer, D. D., Spencer, S. S., Matson, R. H., and Williamson, P. D.: Intracerebral masses in patients with intractable partial epilepsy. Neurology, 34:432, 1984.
245. Stack, J. P., Antoun, N. M., Jenkins, J. P., Metcalf, R., and Isherwood, I.: Gadolinium-DPTA as a contrast agent in magnetic resonance imaging of the brain. Neuroradiology, 30:145, 1988.

246. Stein, B. M.: Intramedullary spinal cord tumors. Clin. Neurosurg., 30:717, 1983.
247. Stewart, D., Grahovac, Z., Hugenholtz, H., Russell, N., Richard, M., and Benoit, B.: Combined intraarterial and systemic chemotherapy for intracerebral tumors. Neurosurgery, 21:207, 1987.
248. Stewart, D., Grahovac, Z., and Riding, M.: Intracarotid PCNU: An NCI Canada study. Proc. Am. Soc. Clin. Oncol., Abstract, 5:A136, 1986.
249. Sundaresan, N., and Galicich, J. H.: Surgical treatment of brain metastases. Clinical and computerized tomography evaluation of the results of treatment. Cancer, 55:1382, 1985.
250. Sundaresan, N., Galicich, J. H., Lane, J. M., Bains, M. S., and McCormack, P.: Treatment of neoplastic epidural cord compression by vertebral body resection and stabilization. J. Neurosurg., 63:676, 1985.
251. Sung, D. I., Harisliadis, L., and Chang, C. H.: Midline pineal tumors and suprasellar germinomas: Highly curable by irradiation. Radiology, 128:745, 1978.
252. Sutton, L.: Current management of low-grade astrocytomas of childhood. Pediatr. Neurosci., 13:98, 1987.
253. Tait, D. M., Thornton-Jones, H., Bloom, H. J., Lemerle, J., and Morris-Jones, P.: Adjuvant chemotherapy for medulloblastoma: The first multi-centre control trial of the International Society of Paediatric Oncology (SIOP I). Eur. J. Cancer, 26:464, 1990.
254. Takemoto, K., Matsumura, Y., Hashimoto, H., Inoue, Y., Fukuda, T., Shakudo, M., Nemoto, Y., Onoyama, Y., Yasui, T., Hakuba, A., Nishimura, S., and Ban, S.: MR imaging of intraspinal tumors—capability in histological differentiation and compartmentalization of extramedullary tumors. Neuroradiology, 30:303, 1988.
255. Tomita, T., and McLone, D. G.: Medulloblastoma in childhood: Results of radical resection and low-dose neuraxis radiation therapy. J. Neurosurg., 64:238, 1986.
256. U, H. S., Kelley, P. Y., Hatton, J. D., and Shew, J. Y.: Proto-oncogene abnormalities and their relationship to tumorigenicity in some human glioblastomas. J. Neurosurg., 71:83, 1989.
257. Urtasun, R., Fulton, D., Huyser-Wierenga, D., Scott-Brown, I., Shin, K., Geggie, P., and Hanson, J.: Dose intensity in radiotherapy: "Is more better" for patients with malignant gliomas? Proc. Am. Soc. Clin. Oncol., Abstract, 8:84, 1989.
258. Valk, P. E., Budinger, T. F., Levin, V. A., Silver, P., Gutin, P. H., and Doyle, W. K.: PET of malignant cerebral tumors after interstitial brachytherapy. Demonstration of metabolic activity and correlation with clinical outcome. J. Neurosurg., 69:830, 1988.
259. van Eys, J., Baram, T. Z., Cangir, A., Bruner, J. M., and Martinez-Prietro, J.: Salvage chemotherapy for recurrent primary brain tumors in children. J. Pediatr., 113:601, 1988.
260. Velema, J. P., and Percy, C. L.: Age curves of central nervous system tumor incidence in adults: Variation of shape by histologic type. J. Natl. Cancer Inst., 79:623, 1987.
261. Walker, A. E., Robins, M., and Weinfeld, F. D.: Epidemiology of brain tumors: The national survey of intracranial neoplasms. Neurology, 35:219, 1985.
262. Walker, M. D., Alexander, E., Jr., Hunt, W. E., MacCarty, C. S., Mahaley, M. S., Jr., Mealey, J., Jr., Norrell, H. A., Owens, G., Ransohoff, J., Wilson, C. B., Gehan, E. A., and Strike, T. A.: Evaluation of BCNU and/or radiotherapy in the treatment of anaplastic gliomas. A cooperative clinical trial. J. Neurosurg., 49:333, 1978.
263. Walker, M. D., Green, S. B., Byar, D. P., Alexander, E., Jr., Batzdorf, U., Brooks, W. H., Hunt, W. E., MacCarty, C. S., Mahaley, M. S., Jr., Mealey, J., Jr., Owens, G., Ransohoff, J., Jr., Robertson, J. T., Shapiro, W. R., Smith, K. R., Jr., Wilson, C. B., and Strike, T. A.: Randomized comparisons of radiotherapy and nitrosoureas for the treatment of malignant glioma after surgery. N. Engl. J. Med., 303:1323, 1980.
264. Walker, M. D., Strike, T. A., and Sheline, G. E.: An analysis of dose-effect relationship in the radiotherapy of malignant gliomas. Int. J. Radiat. Oncol. Biol. Phys., 5:1725, 1979.
265. Wallner, K. E., Galicich, J. H., Krol, G., Arbit, E., and Malkin, M. G.: Patterns of failure following treatment for glioblastoma multiforme and anaplastic astrocytoma. Int. J. Radiat. Oncol. Biol. Phys., 16:1405, 1989.
266. Wallner, K. E., Gonzales, M., and Sheline, G. E.: Treatment of oligodendrogliomas with or without postoperative irradiation. J. Neurosurg., 68:684, 1988.
267. Wara, W. M., Jenkin, R. D., Evans, A., Ertel, I., Hittle, R., Ortega, J., Wilson, C. B., and Hammond, D.: Tumors of the pineal and suprasellar region: Childrens Cancer Study Group treatment results 1960–1975: a report from the Childrens Cancer Study Group. Cancer, 43:698, 1979.
268. Wara, W. M., Sheline, G. E., Newman, H., Townsend, J. J., and Boldrey, E. B.: Radiation therapy of meningiomas. Am. J. Roentgenol. Radium Ther. Nucl. Med., 123:453, 1975.
269. Waxweiler, R. J., Alexander, V., Leffingwell, S. S., Haring, M., and Lloyd, J. W.: Mortality from brain tumor and other causes in a cohort of petrochemical workers. J. Natl. Cancer Inst., 70:75, 1983.
270. Wilson, C. B., Gutin, P., Boldrey, E. B., Crafts D., Levin, V. A., and Enot, K. J.: Single-agent chemotherapy of brain tumors. A five-year review. Arch. Neurol., 33:739, 1976.
271. Withers, H. R.: Biologic basis for altered fractionation schemes. Cancer, 55(Suppl.):2086, 1985.
272. Wood, J. R., Green, S. B., and Shapiro, W. R.: The prognostic importance of tumor size in malignant gliomas: A computed tomographic scan study by the Brain Tumor Cooperative Group. J. Clin. Oncol., 6:338, 1988.
273. Wrann, M., Bodmer, S., de Martin, R., Siepl, C., Hofer-Warbinek, R., Frei, K., Hofer, E., and Fontana, A.: T cell suppressor factor from human glioblastoma cells is a 12.5-kd protein closely related to transforming growth factor-beta. EMBO J., 6:1633, 1987.
274. Yamashita, J., Handa, H., Tokuriki, Y., Ha, Y. S., Otsuka, S.-I., Suda, K., and Taki, W.: Intra-arterial ACNU therapy for malignant brain tumors. Experimental studies and preliminary clinical results. J. Neurosurg., 59:424, 1983.
275. Young, J. L., Jr., and Miller, R. W.: Incidence of malignant tumors in U. S. children. J. Pediatr., 86:254, 1975.
276. Yung, W., Prados, M., Levin, V., Fetell, M., Bennett, J., Mahaley, S., Salcman, M., and Etcubanas, E.: Recombinant beta interferon in patients with recurrent malignant gliomas. J. Neurooncol., Abstract, 7:S32, 1989.
277. Zimmerman, R. A., and Bilaniuk, L. T.: Imaging of tumors of the spinal canal and cord. Radiol. Clin. North Am., 26:965, 1988.
278. Zuber, P., Hamou, M., and de Tribolet, N.: Identification of proliferating cells in human gliomas using the monoclonal antibody Ki-67. Neurosurgery, 22:364, 1988.
279. Zuccarello, M., Sawaya, R., and deCourten-Meyers, G.: Glioblastoma occurring after radiation therapy for meningioma: Case report and review of the literature. Neurosurgery, 19:114, 1986.
280. Zülch, K. J.: Histological Typing of Tumors of the Central Nervous System. International Histological Classification of Tumors, No. 21. Geneva, World Health Organization, 1979, p. 15.

XXV

Neoplasms of the Eye

Robert M. Ellsworth
Cynthia Boxrud

Introduction

Research in the field of ocular and orbital tumors has been highly productive in the last five years. The contributions of molecular genetics and the cloning of the retinoblastoma gene have increased our understanding of many of these neoplasms. In addition, improvements in imaging technology, specifically computed tomography (CT), ultrasonography, and magnetic resonance imaging (MRI), have expanded our ability to diagnose ocular and orbital lesions.

Cancers of the eye and orbit are similar in structure to those seen elsewhere. Their natural history and response to therapy may, however, be distinct. This chapter reviews some of these special characteristics, and describes one tumor unique to the eye: retinoblastoma.

Tumors of the Lid and Conjunctiva

Tumors of the lid are common, especially in older patients. Early diagnosis is crucial, as large tumors in the lids are difficult to excise and often require complicated postsurgical reconstruction.

Basal-Cell Carcinoma

Basal-cell carcinoma is the most common malignant tumor of the eyelid. It arises from the basal layer of the epidermis; although it grows slowly, it may spread insidiously to deeper structures and bone. Clinically, this tumor appears as a pearly-colored raised nodule, with occasional central ulceration and telangiectasias. Histologically, nests of basal cells with peripheral palisading are demonstrated. The incidence of this tumor increases in patients exposed to sunlight.

Treatment of this lesion depends on its size and location. It is preferable to attempt total excision of most basal-cell carcinomas of the eyelid, since recurrences, should they occur, are more easily managed following surgery than following radiotherapy. In addition, multiple frozen sections with careful monitoring of surgical margins have an important role in treatment.[5] If radiation must be used, a 5 mm margin around the tumor must also be irradiated, and the globe should be well-protected.

Fitzpatrick and colleagues treated 477 basal-cell and squamous-cell eyelid carcinomas in the period from 1958 to 1968.[15] Both single and fractionated exposures were used, and the doses ranged from 2,000–5,000 cGy. An overall recurrence rate of 4–8% was observed in this series (see XXXIII).

A cure rate of 90% has been reported in another large series of cases treated with either surgery or radiotherapy.[5]

Squamous-Cell Carcinoma

Squamous-cell carcinomas comprise 5% of all malignant neoplasms of the eyelid. Clinically, these tumors generally present as elevated plaques with indistinct borders, and typically affect elderly, fair-skinned individuals. They grow slowly, and when they do metastatize, the spread is usually to the regional lymph nodes. Histologically, dyskeratotic cells with keratin pearls are observed. The treatment of choice is surgery.

Squamous-cell carcinoma may involve the conjunctiva, where it is commonly located at the limbus, and it may extend to involve the corneal epithelium. This tumor can be easily confused with keratoacanthoma, a benign lesion which develops rapidly and may undergo spontaneous regression. All suspicious lesions of this type should be biopsied before treatment. Surgery is the treatment of choice, as it affords the possibility of complete excision with histologic control of the margins. However, radiation is an option, particularly in older individuals with extensive lesions (see XXXIII).[15,28]

Sebaceous Adenocarcinoma

Sebaceous adenocarcinomas arise from the meibomian glands of the tarsal plate, or from the sebaceous glands of the lashes or caruncle. They can exhibit any of a broad spectrum of clinical features, but most commonly present with a firm nodule resembling a chalazion or chronic blepharitis. Any patient who presents with a recurrent chalazion or unilateral chronic blepharitis which fails to respond to medical therapy should be biopsied to confirm the absence of this tumor.

Rao and colleagues have looked at the prognostic signs

of sebaceous-cell carcinoma.[31] A poor prognosis is associated with location in the upper lid, maximum diameter 10 mm or greater, persistence of symptoms for more than 6 months, or tumor originating in a meibomian gland. Although an occasional cure following radiotherapy has been reported in the literature, radical surgery with a wide excision offers the only real hope. As these tumors grow *en plaque*, they are sometimes difficult to excise fully. If lymph-node extension is clinically evident, lymphatic dissection should be performed promptly, at the time of lid surgery if possible. Since these tumors may be multicentric, a negative margin does not necessarily mean that complete excision has been achieved.[5]

Malignant Melanoma of the Lid and Conjunctiva

Cutaneous malignant melanoma of the eyelid, although rare (representing only about 1% of all eyelid cancer), has shown a steady increase in incidence over the last fifty years. These melanomas may arise from preexisting junctional or compound nevi, but seldom come from dermal nevi.

Melanomas of the conjunctiva may arise from acquired melanosis, preexisting nevi, or *de novo*. About 75% of cases of conjunctival melanoma have been observed to follow a condition known as primary acquired melanosis (PAM), when PAM is associated with atypia.[19,37] PAM presents as a flat, brown, "granular" lesion, often diffuse, with separate islands of pigmentation distributed over both the bulbar and palpebral conjunctiva. The areas of this pigmentation may wax and wane spontaneously, and harmlessly over a period of many years; after a mean latency of about 12 years, however, malignant changes may occur. PAM is not to be confused with benign racial melanosis, seen in deeply pigmented patients, which is a bilateral condition.

Primary acquired melanosis, when composed of epithelioid cells or exhibiting intraepithelial pagetoid extension, has between a 75% and 90% likelihood of eventuating in invasive melanoma.[19] Thickening and increased vascularity of the pigmented regions are clinical signs indicating malignant change. Whenever these signs are noted, a biopsy of the affected areas should be taken promptly.

In general, cutaneous melanoma (as seen in the lid) has a better prognosis for survival than conjunctival melanoma. The thickness of melanoma seen on histologic section has been emphasized as the most important prognostic factor: conjunctival melanomas thicker than 1.5 mm carry a grave prognosis, and those thicker than 2 mm result in 95% mortality despite any form of treatment.[37] Jakobiec and colleagues have noted that conjunctival melanomas measuring less than 0.8 mm do not tend to metastatize.[19]

Wide local excision is an acceptable treatment for early, small lesions. Larger tumors usually require more radical procedures. If invasive melanoma is discovered in the orbit or globe, exenteration is the treatment of choice, although radiotherapy can be tried in older patients or in patients with a defective fellow eye. These lesions are aggressive and tend to spread early to regional lymph nodes. Tumors arising in the lids and conjunctival fornices have a more serious prognosis than those occurring at the corneal limbus.

There is no documentation in the literature comparing the outcomes for radiotherapy and surgery in the treatment of conjunctival melanomas.

Kaposi's Sarcoma

In the past, Kaposi's sarcoma manifesting in the eyelid or conjunctiva was rarely seen in the United States, and was usually seen only in older individuals with pre-existing disease. More recently, this tumor has been observed in younger individuals suffering from acquired immunodeficiency syndrome (AIDS). Kaposi's sarcoma requires special mention because it may be the first presenting sign of AIDS.

Kaposi's sarcoma is a malignant mesenchymal tumor of the skin and mucous membranes. Clinically it presents as a deeply reddish-purple, elevated subepithelial nodule, which may affect the conjunctiva or lids. Histologically it is composed of atypical fibroblasts, well-formed capillary channels filled with blood, and vascular endothelial cells. Local radiation is an effective eradicative or palliative treatment, although recurrence elsewhere may spontaneously appear due to the underlying immunosuppressed condition of these patients.[36]

Tumors of the Orbit

Exophthalmos is the most common sign that an orbital mass exists. Marked proptosis with normal motility suggests a slow-growing, benign tumor, whereas early diplopia suggests malignancy. When a tumor grows slowly, it may fill a large volume of the orbit without causing overt symptoms. However, with rapid growth, circulatory disturbances may occur; the consequent edema of lids and conjunctiva serves as an early presentation of an orbital mass.

Signs and symptoms depend on the position and size of an orbital mass as well as its rate of growth. Tumors within the muscle cone, for example, result in eccentric proptosis and restriction of ocular movement, while vision in the affected eye remains normal.

During initial evaluation of a patient presenting with exophthalmos, it is essential to rule out masquerading conditions. These include contralateral enophthalmos, as seen in orbital fractures or metastastic schirrous carcinoma of the breast; the elongated globe of a myopic eye; asymmetry of the bony orbits; and abnormal palpebral fissures from unilateral lid retraction, a condition seen in cases of hyperthyroidism or paralysis of the vertical rectus muscles.

All patients exhibiting proptosis should receive a careful examination, with attention to ocular motility and pupillary function, and ophthalmoscopy. A careful examination of the nasal areas should be part of every workup, since neoplasms can invade the orbit from adjacent sinuses or the nasopharynx. Instruments used to measure exophthalmos are subject to error, and must be carefully calibrated; it is essential that an observer use the same instrument for serial measurements if the results are to be meaningful and statistically valid. A difference of 2 mm between the eyes is significant.

During the past decade, three emerging diagnostic techniques have revolutionized the approach to examining orbital tumors: ultrasonography, computerized tomography, and magnetic resonance imaging.

Ultrasonography, which can delineate the structures of the globe in precise detail, can give exact evidence of orbital extension of intraocular tumors such as retinoblastoma or malignant melanoma. Ultrasonography can also demonstrate pressure on the globe from extraocular tumors, and lesions involving the optic nerve. Orbital tumors have characteristic ultrasound patterns, which have been classified by Coleman in detail.[4]

Computerized tomography (CT) is perhaps the most important of the new diagnostic techniques. Thanks to its ability to resolve different soft-tissue densities within a fat-laden orbit, the precise size and location of a tumor can usually be established prior to surgery. This is of extreme importance in designing an approach to the orbit which minimizes damage to normal orbital structures, especially the optic nerve.

Magnetic resonance imaging (MRI) has recently been shown to have remarkable sensitivity in distinguishing differences in tissue composition. Its advantages are that it uses no external radiation, and it is a relatively noninvasive technique. With the use of a surface coil, an even clearer delineation of spatial relationships in the orbit can be made. As the technology improves, MRI will come to have still greater importance in the evaluation of orbital disease.

A careful review by Moss of 230 consecutive cases of unilateral exophthalmos is a great resource when approaching orbital tumors.[27] A differentiation must be made between orbital tumors in children and those in adults, since many lesions found in children are both rapid-growing and dangerous. For example, hemangioma, which is a benign lesion, is probably the most common orbital lesion in children. The presence of proptosis, however, is a most ominous sign, and the differential diagnosis in such cases must include rhabdomyosarcoma, which is a dangerous lesion but is potentially curable when diagnosed early. In adults, lesions tend to be slower-growing, and there is a greater likelihood that the condition will be relatively benign and amenable to treatment.

Table XXV-1-1 shows the frequency of the more common causes of unilateral exophthalmos.

Table XXV-1-1.   Unilateral Expanding Lesions of the Orbit (230 Consecutive Cases)

	%
1. Thyroid ophthalmopathy	16
2. Hemangioma	12
3. Malignant lymphoma	10
4. Chronic granuloma	8
5. Lacrimal gland epithelial tumors	7
6. Meningioma	5
7. Lymphangioma	4
8. Glioma of the optic nerve	3
9. Metastatic malignant tumors	3
10. Peripheral nerve tumors	3
11. Dermoid cysts	3
12. Mucocele	3
13. Rhabdomyosarcoma	3
14. Aneurysm	2
15. Angiosarcoma	2
16. Osteoma	1
17. Histiocytosis	1
18. Sarcoid	1

From Moss[21]

Thyroid-Related Orbitopathy

Thyroid-related orbitopathy (TRO), commonly known as Graves' disease, is the most common cause of unilateral and bilateral proptosis in the adult population, and therefore TRO should be included in the differential diagnosis for every orbital tumor. There is no observed relationship between the level of thyroid activity and the degree of exophthalmos. This disease is generally associated with hyperthyroidism, but it may be associated with hypothyroidism or euthyroidism.

TRO affects middle-aged females 4–5 times more often than other groups in the general population. Clinically, a broad spectrum of signs and symptoms may be observed. These range from mild lid-lag and lid retraction to severe chemosis and tremendous proptosis which may result in loss of vision. Glaucoma and nerve-bundle defects may be produced either through pressure in the nerve due to crowding at the orbital apex or intrinsic involvement of the nerve by lymphocytes and ground substance. Ocular muscle problems are due to restrictive myopathy resulting from edema, inflammation, and fibrosis.

Patients with severe thyroid ophthalmopathy present a major therapeutic challenge. There is some suggestion that rapid control of severe hyperthyroidism, either by surgery or radiotherapy using I-131, may be followed by more severe ocular signs. It is perhaps wise, therefore, to attempt to control hyperthyroidism with drugs for a period of 6 months to a year before planning more definitive therapy. This is particularly advisable for younger patients.

A diagnosis of TRO is primarily made by clinical examination. Laboratory evaluation is helpful in confirming the diagnosis. In addition to consultation with an endocrinologist, the lab workup includes measurement of titers of serum total thyroxine (T4) and serum total triiodothyronine (T3). Serum thyroid stimulating hormone (TSH) levels may be depressed in patients with hyperthyroidism. When serum T4 and T3 levels are raised even slightly above the physiological "set point," the pituitary fails to respond to exogenous thyroid releasing hormone (TRH) stimulation, and no TSH will be secreted into the systemic circulation. This serves as the basis for the TRH stimulation test, which is useful in diagnosing occult hyperthyroidism. Finally, a CT scan of the orbit shows enlarged extraocular muscles without involvement of the tendons.[18]

Many therapeutic approaches to TRO have been advocated. However, at this time, high-dose corticosteroids (100 mg prednisone equivalent per day) seem to be the most reliable modality. Satisfactory response to a combination of high-dose corticosteroids and external-beam radiotherapy at an orbital dose of 2,000 cGy has been regularly reported.

If severe proptosis threatens the function of the eye, either by optic-nerve damage, or corneal exposure and ulceration, surgical decompression should be considered. A lateral Kronlein, or an Ogura approach through the floor of the orbit with ethmoidal decompression, are used. Floor decompressions consistently result in diplopia; however, the majority of these patients had pre-existing extraocular muscle problems which contributed to this difficulty.

Hemangiomas

Hemangiomas are the most common orbital tumors in adults and infants. In a series of 28 cases, 7 occurred in infants and 21 in adults.[27,34] There is a distinct difference in the nature of these tumors between infants and adults, and treatment varies accordingly.

In infants, hemangiomas are highly cellular, angioblastic, and completely nonencapsulated. They are radiosensitive. During the first 6–12 months of life, they grow, but then normally undergo a slow spontaneous regression over a period of 6–7 years. They are commonly accompanied by hemangiomas of the skin, which have a characteristic appearance and are referred to as "strawberry nevi."

As a general rule, surgery in infants is contraindicated, and treatment consists of local or systemic corticosteroids or irradiation. Infantile capillary hemangiomas may threaten the optic nerve by compression, or cover the pupil secondary to tumor growth on the upper lid, with consequent amblyopia. In these situations, prednisone (40 mg, every other day) is given over a period of two weeks. Approximately one-half the hemangiomas treated this way show a significant response, and 50% of these maintain the improvement permanently. In the remainder, however, the tumors resume growing when the steroids are stopped. In these instances, a second course of steroids is given for 2 to 3 weeks. If the hemangiomas still fail to respond, external-beam radiotherapy can be administered to the entire orbit. The globe is completely protected, and increments of 100 to 200 cGy are given at intervals of 3 to 6 weeks until an effect is seen. In no case should the total dose exceed 800 cGy. In rare instances, excision of the tumor may be attempted. Experimental research into chemotherapeutic treatment is currently being undertaken, but no results have been published at this time.

In adults, the tumors are cavernous hemangiomas, which are not sensitive to radiation but are well-encapsulated, which makes their surgical removal effective and well-tolerated.

Lymphoid Tumors

Lymphoid tumors of the orbit encompass a broad spectrum of disease. They can range from benign reactive lymphoid hyperplasia to malignant diffuse large cell lymphoma.[66] While usually unilateral, lymphomas can involve both eyes. Malignant lymphomas may arise in the orbit; this does not necessarily imply systemic disease,[20] although about one-half of all patients presenting with apparently isolated orbital lymphoma later develop lymphoma elsewhere in the body. However, orbital lymphoma may be a manifestation of concurrent systemic lymphoma, or may be the presenting sign of lymphocytic leukemia. It has not been established whether orbital lymphoma is originally of multicentric origin or whether it spreads lymphogenously. Orbital lymphomas are rarely seen in children.

Benign reactive lymphoid hyperplasia is composed predominantly of mature lymphocytes, with some reactive germinal centers. Malignant disease is suggested by the presence of atypical and immature lymphocytes demonstrating pleomorphism and mitotic figures. Clinically, both these conditions can present as painless, progressive proptosis, accompanied by extraocular motility impairment, visual disturbances, and lacrimal-gland enlargement.

A biopsy should be performed in these cases, but this should be the limit of surgical intervention since these lesions are radiocurable. When a biopsy is taken, a fresh specimen should be reserved for immunohistopathology of cell-surface markers, in addition to the fixed specimen for light-microscopic studies. Immunopathologic identification of cell-surface markers on lymphocytes can distinguish monoclonal B- or T-cell tumors, or polyclonal proliferations. Phenotyping gives a more accurate prediction of clinical behavior, and eventually leads to greater specificity of therapy.[20]

Large cell lymphoma of the orbit is radiocurable. When large cell lymphoma involves the orbit, the radiotherapeutic treatment dose should be 4,500 cGy given over 4 weeks. Chemotherapeutic cure of systemic disease is also possible, and the possibility that disease exists outside the orbit must always be considered (see XXXVI-10).

Idiopathic Orbital Inflammation (Pseudotumor)

Traditionally there has been great confusion regarding the categorization of orbital inflammation or pseudotumor. The histologic spectrum described ranges from a granulomatous inflammation to a lymphocytic and plasmacytic infiltration which is polyclonal.

The onset is characterized by diplopia, pain on ocular motion, chemosis, proptosis, and injection. The exophthalmos observed in these cases is not severe (3 or 4 mm), as the lesions tend to grow *en plaque* along the orbital wall.

Biopsy is frequently accompanied by bleeding and aggravation of the inflammatory signs. The lesions tend to regress spontaneously; a course of radiotherapy may lead to some regression of severe proptosis. High doses of steroids have produced dramatic responses.

Lacrimal Tumors

Benign mixed tumor (BMT) is the most common epithelial tumor of the lacrimal gland. Histologically this tumor is composed of benign epithelial cells, commonly forming lumens. It is essential not to biopsy a suspected BMT, or to compromise its integrity during excision: treatment is aimed at excising the entire tumor. Incomplete removal may allow tumor cells to spill into the orbit; these cells may subsequently develop into malignant mixed tumors.[41,42]

Adenoid cystic carcinoma (cylindroma) and malignant mixed tumors are malignant tumors of the lacrimal gland. Of the two, adenoid cystic carcinoma is the more common tumor. Painful perineural infiltration often occurs in cases of adenoid cystic carcinoma. The clinical picture common to both these types of cancers is that of an insidiously enlarging mass in the upper temporal quadrant of the orbit, with absence of significant inflammation. Bone invasion occurs frequently: X-ray findings are positive in 90% of these cases. In both cases, the histopathology consists of what appear to be disarmingly benign cells. This is misleading, because these tumors are highly malignant. In a series of 24 mixed tumors, 12 eventually became malignant, and 5 required eventual exenteration.[42] Despite radical treatment, lacrimal carcinomas are frequently fatal. Although these tumors are relatively radioresistant, they can be given 5,000–6,000 cGy in association with surgery.[28]

Meningiomas

Meningiomas are thought to arise from arachnoidal villi, and most commonly originate intracranially. They produce exophthalmos with involvement of both the optic-nerve sheath and the sphenoidal ridge. Tumors of the outer ridge often present as fullness in the temporal fossa, while those of the middle ridge, on X-ray examination, show hyperostosis with direct invasion of the orbit. Those of the inner ridge involve the optic nerve early, with loss of vision, and produce late proptosis. Meningiomas of the sphenoidal ridge may be relatively inconspicuous lesions, and should always be suspected in cases with early unilateral field defects. All these tumors grow slowly over a period of years. The proper treatment is neurosurgical excision via a transfrontal approach. Arteriography and CT scanning are usually sufficient to delineate these lesions.

The behavior of meningiomas is more aggressive in pediatric patients, and the prognosis is worse.[23]

Lymphangiomas

Lymphangiomas are similar to hemangiomas. They are benign congenital vascular tumors, but, in contrast to hemangiomas, are not usually manifest at birth.[21] They grow slowly, and usually have become clinically apparent by the age of 6 or 7. Clinical onset may be abrupt, however, due to an upper-respiratory infection which causes lymphoid hyperplasia or to spontaneous hemorrhage within the tumor which causes rapid proptosis and lid ecchymosis.

Radiotherapy may control some of the lymphocytic components of the tumor, but surgery is the preferred approach. Since these tumors are not encapsulated, excision is usually incomplete. Spontaneous hemorrhage may produce rather large "chocolate cysts" within the tumor, and evacuation of these cysts may temporarily relieve the exophthalmos without causing the damage to vital orbital structures which a more invasive procedure would produce. Due to the benign nature of this lesion, radical surgery cannot be justified, particularly if the globe is functional. Due to their nature as vascular tumors, lymphangiomas are difficult to debulk and often require electrocautery. We have had superb results using a 532 nm potassium titanyl phosphate (KTP) laser (LaserScope, San Jose, CA) for these operations: the green beam produces excellent hemostasis as well as good tissue resection.

Cavernous Hemangiomas

Cavernous hemangiomas are the most common benign orbital lesions in adults. The most common presenting symptom is slowly progressive proptosis without pain. Patients may also have retinal striae and optic-nerve compression.

Histopathologically, these tumors are cavernous spaces, lined with smooth muscle, which are filled with blood. These tumors rarely undergo spontaneous regression, and surgery is therefore the treatment of choice.

Gliomas

Gliomas of the optic nerve are slow-growing pilocytic astrocytomas occurring in children and young adults. They comprise 1–5% of all intracranial tumors seen in children. Gliomas may originate in the orbital or intracanalicular por-

tion of the optic nerve, or in the optic chiasm. Loss of vision is usually early and profound. The incidence of neurofibromatosis associated with these tumors varies from 10–50%, depending upon the observer.[3] There is a female preponderance. Young children usually fare better than older ones.

The tumors enlarge the optic canal at a relatively early stage, and radiologic examinations are most valuable. Clinical examination reveals pupillary abnormalities, visual-field defects, and axial proptosis. The classic CT presentation associated with optic nerve glioma is a fusiform enlargement of the optic nerve (Fig. XXV-1-1). Plain films demonstrate enlargement of the orbit, and a J-shaped sella if the optic chiasm is involved.

When the glioma involves the optic nerve alone, removal of the entire tumor, from the apex of the orbit to the globe, is indicated. The Kronlein approach is best, but, if the optic chiasm is involved, radiotherapy with a dose of 5,000 cGy over 5 to 6 weeks is the treatment of choice. While these gliomas are radiosensitive, they are probably not fully radiocurable; however, as the growth rate is low, patients may go for many years, or even a lifetime, without experiencing catastrophic progression.

Rush and colleagues observed 85 histopathologically-proven cases of optic glioma. Of 35 cases with tumor in the optic nerve, 85% survived a mean duration of 17 years. Longevity was associated with completeness of surgical excision. Twenty-three patients with tumor in the optic chiasm survived a mean duration of 19 years, with no apparent relation to surgical method. The presence of neurofibromatosis conferred a protective benefit.[35]

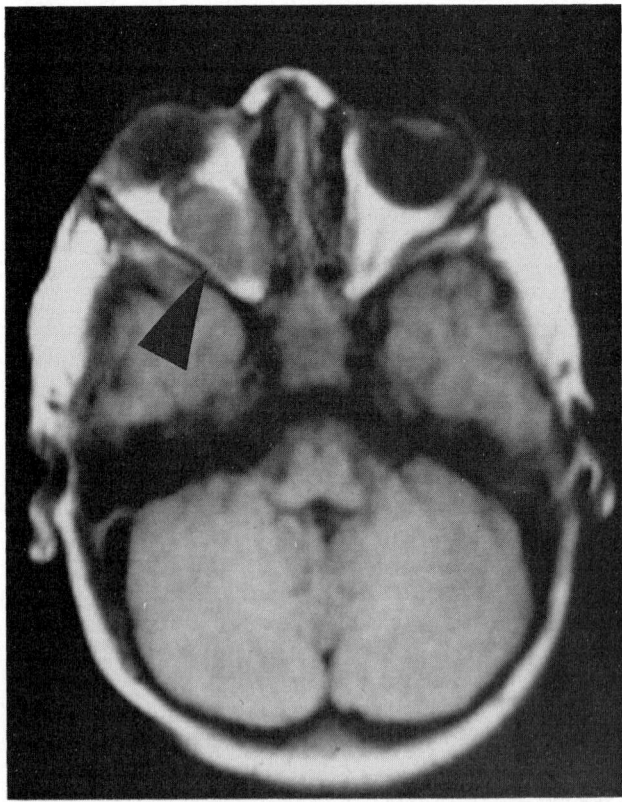

Figure XXV-1-1.   CT scan of optic glioma of right eye.

Metastatic Tumors

There is nothing clinically unique about malignant tumors which metastatize to the orbit. Such tumors are more common on the left side, due to circulatory factors, and in about 25% of cases, the condition becomes bilateral.[14]

The most striking and typical source in children is neuroblastoma from the abdomen, while in adults common sources of metastasis are carcinomas of the breast, lung, adrenals, GI tract, thyroid, and kidney. Surgical management is rarely indicated, and radiotherapy and chemotherapy are the preferred approaches. Life expectancy averages only about 8 months once orbital metastasis has become established.

Peripheral Nerve Tumors

Peripheral nerve tumors seen in the orbit include neurofibromas, neurilemmomas, and malignant schwannomas. Since the orbit is well-endowed with peripheral nerves, these tumors comprise about 4% of all orbital tumors. Neurilemmomas are focal, benign nerve-sheath tumors, encapsulated by perineurium. They can be totally removed without damage to normal perineurium. Neurofibromas, typically associated with von Recklinghausen's disease, are diffuse and often difficult to excise.

Mucoceles

Mucoceles are retention cysts, usually occurring in the frontal sinuses and pushing the globe downward and outward. Patients experience frequent episodes of orbital cellulitis.

Diagnosis can be made by observing an enlarged sinus, with thinning of its walls, on X-ray. The preferred treatment is total excision and ablation of the sinus, in the hands of an otorhinolaryngologist.

Dermoid Cysts

Dermoid cysts are among the most common orbital tumors of childhood. They are congenital ectodermal rests, which may or may not involve the underlying bone. These cysts generally occur in the first decade of life, and are most common in the anterior portion of the superior temporal orbit. Surgical removal is indicated if a pattern of growth is documented, or if the cysts present a cosmetic problem. A careful radiologic study should be made before surgery to assess possible intracranial extension.

Rhabdomyosarcoma

Rhabdomyosarcoma is the most common primary malignant orbital tumor in childhood.[21] It is both radiosensitive and radiocurable. The most common presenting sign is a mass appearing in the superior-medial orbit. Coexistent involvement of the paranasal sinuses, especially the ethmoid sinuses, must be suspected.

Rhabdomyosarcomas have traditionally been divided into three main groups. The first, embryonal rhabdomyosarcoma, comprises 74% of cases. This is composed of stellate cells with dark nuclei and a loose syncytium, resembling embryonal mesenchyme. Ribbons of eosinophilic cytoplasm and occasional cross-striations can also be seen. Alveolar rhab-

domyosarcoma, the second group, comprises 15% of all cases. This form is characterized by septa within the tumor, giving the appearance of alveoli at low magnification. Differentiated rhabdomyosarcoma, the third group, makes up the remaining 10% of cases. Cross-striations are usually seen, and some cells have ribbons of eosinophilic cytoplasm. Actin and myosin fibrils can be detected by electron microscopy when no diagnosis can be made by light microscopy; a specimen properly fixed for electron microscopy should be taken at the time of surgery.[30]

As a general rule, embryonal rhabdomyosarcomas present as masses in the superior medial wall, while alveolar rhabdomyosarcomas are located in the inferior portion of the orbit. These tumors progress rapidly over a period of days or weeks. A child may go from a barely detectable proptosis to a 10 or 12 mm difference within a week. The age for onset of tumor growth in our series of patients ranged from 5 months to 13 years, with a mean of 7 years. Rarely, the tumor has been seen at birth, and in adults. While the clinical picture is almost pathognomonic, a biopsy is essential for tissue diagnosis.

In 1959, Jones and colleagues reported a 3-year salvage rate of 47% of 44 patients treated by prompt exenteration.[21] A decade later, Cassady and colleagues suggested that localized orbital rhabdomyosarcoma might be radiocurable, basing their conclusion on the results in 17 cases.[2]

In 1977 we reanalyzed a series of 58 cases treated with radiation and chemotherapy. These cases were followed for up to 15 years, with a mean follow-up of 3 years. The observed salvage rate was 71%. As a result of this work, we have largely abandoned exenteration in treatment of orbital rhabdomyosarcoma. The current role of surgery in the treatment of rhabdomyosarcoma varies with the extent and location of tumor at diagnosis. In some cases, a debulking procedure may be desirable following chemotherapy. Most often, a biopsy for tissue diagnosis is followed by a course of radiation and chemotherapy as primary treatment.

The radiation dose used in current treatment varies from 5,000–6,000 cGy over a period of 5 weeks.[2] No effort is made to protect the eye, and ocular function is usually lost over a period of 1–2 years due to anterior segment complications (either cataract or retinal neovascularization). We feel that shielding the globe might produce shadows within the orbit, which might allow some tumor to survive.

Chemotherapy is employed for all stages of rhabdomyosarcoma, administered in accord with the Inter-group Rhabdomyosarcoma III (IRS-III) protocol (see XXXIX-8). When disease appears limited to the orbit, treatment with joint chemotherapy and radiation is superior to irradiation alone.[1]

At present, using the joint regimen of chemotherapy and radiation, our gross statstics show a salvage rate of 90%. Over the next decade, we hope that a better histologic classification and more specific chemotherapeutic methods will increase the cure rate.

The differential diagnosis of rapid progressive exophthalmos in infancy should include the following conditions: 1) *rhabdomyosarcoma*, a rapid diagnosis and treatment may be the determining factors in a satisfactory outcome; 2) *lymphangioma or hemangioma of the orbit, with hemorrhage into the tumor*, this commonly produces a rapid proptosis over a period of several days, which then stabilizes and does not progress further; 3) *metastatic neuroblastoma,* this produces a rather rapid exophthalmos, frequently with ecchymosis of the lower lid. An abdominal CT scan and careful X-ray examination of the chest and skull usually will establish the correct diagnosis before a biopsy is required; 4) *leukemia,* this may initially present with unilateral exophthalmos and an essentially normal peripheral blood picture. Examination of the bone marrow reveals the true diagnosis, as, of course, does the subsequent progressive clinical course; 5) *inflammatory disease,* principally extension of cellulitis from the adjacent sinuses. This causes apparent exophthalmos accompanied by extreme chemosis and inflammatory signs; and 6) *teratoma of the orbit,* when such a tumor breaks down, the "toxic" products liberated may produce a fairly rapid progression of exophthalmos.

The diagnosis and treatment of orbital tumors poses a challenge for the physician. Any such undertaking requires a careful history and thorough physical exam. This is particularly important, considering that lid and orbital lesions may be the only manifestations of a primary or systemic malignancy.

Imaging studies, including roentgenograms, ultrasonography, and MRI and CT scans, are used to define the size and location of the tumor, and show its relation to normal orbital structures. The importance of good tissue diagnosis cannot be overemphasized. A discussion with the pathologist prior to any surgical excision or biopsy is essential.

Management of these orbital tumors requires good surgical judgment. Not infrequently a decision must be made whether to manipulate the eye and risk damaging delicate structures in order to obtain an adequate biopsy. Often, orbital tumors are located in the apex of the orbit or along its medial wall, where many vital nerves and vessels, such as the ciliary ganglion and the nerves to the extraocular muscles, are located. These structures are difficult or impossible to visualize at the time of surgery, and great care must be taken to avoid them.

The specific etiologic diagnosis will dictate the therapeutic modality, and often the prognosis, of the patient. It is crucial for the physician to make an accurate diagnosis and implement prompt and efficient treatment.

Tumors of the Globe

Two primary tumors commonly involve the eye: retinoblastoma in infants, and uveal melanoma in adults.

Retinoblastoma

Retinoblastoma is the most common intraocular malignant neoplasm in childhood. It is a multicentric tumor which can arise in one or both retinas.[9,10,34] The tumor usually remains confined to the eye for a relatively long period of time, but may metastasize by a number of routes, and when this occurs the disease is almost invariably fatal if untreated.

The incidence worldwide varies, and in the U.S., about 300 new cases per year are seen, representing 1:20,000 live births. Between 60 and 70 of these cases are bilateral. A markedly asymmetric presentation is the rule.

As part of the new developments in molecular biology in the last decade, an important advance in our understanding of oncogenesis has been made. In 1983, Cavenee, Dryja, Phillips and colleagues presented evidence that the development of retinoblastoma tumors are related to presence of a mutant allele at a specific locus, which they termed the "retinoblastoma locus."[7,8] It is currently thought that retinoblastoma results from the absence of an "anti-cancer" gene, which restricts the uncontrolled growth of embryonic cells, rather than the presence of an oncogene which produces cancerous cells directly. This accords with Knudson's "two-hit" hypothesis, which postulated that the development of retinoblastoma required at least two separate genetic events.[25] The mechanism can best be explained by looking at hereditary retinoblastoma. Here, the germinal cells, which of course generate every retinal cell, each have one normal anti-cancer gene and one defective gene. This defective gene corresponds to the first hit in Knudson's theory; the second, normal gene can still restrict the uncontrolled growth of tumors. At a later time, if a mutagenic alteration affects the normal gene, suppressing its function as well, retinoblastoma develops following this "second hit." With the cloning of the short DNA segment containing the retinoblastoma (RB) gene,[35A] and the successful mapping of this region in the following year,[25A] it has been established that this model is substantively correct (see I-6 and III-1).

This knowledge has great implications for the management of retinoblastoma. It is currently possible to determine, via DNA analysis techniques, whether a patient has the congenital RB defect, and in the future it may be possible to assess this prenatally.

In familial retinoblastoma, the tumor is inherited as an autosomal dominant characteristic. Less than 10% of retinoblastomas present with a family history, indicating that the great majority of these tumors are spontaneous mutations. The penetrance varies with the clinical presentation. A sporadic unilateral case has only a 10–20% chance of passing the disease on to his children, but this figure is almost 50% for sporadic bilateral cases.

Clinically, the most common presentation of retinoblastoma is a white reflex, called the "cat's-eye reflex," which is seen in 56% of presenting patients. In some infants, this reflex is seen intermittently by the parents. The second most common sign is strabismus, seen in 20% of patients, which is caused when tumor infringes on the macula. Any child with abnormal ocular deviation must be evaluated immediately for the presence of tumor or retinal pathology, since retinoblastoma is such a lethal tumor. Less common presenting signs include a red, painful eye (with or without accompanying glaucoma) or orbital cellulitis.

The diagnosis is made by careful ophthalmoscopic examination of the retina, which must usually be made with the young patient under general anesthesia. Examination with a binocular indirect ophthalmoscope is invaluable. When the tumor can be clearly seen, with no overlying retinal detachment or ocular inflammation, the diagnosis is rarely in doubt. Ultrasound and CT scan can be helpful when visualization is difficult (Figure XXV-1-2). It is important to illustrate the size and location of all tumors carefully, because this is essential information for the radiotherapists. These tumors have no predilection for any particular area of the retina, but

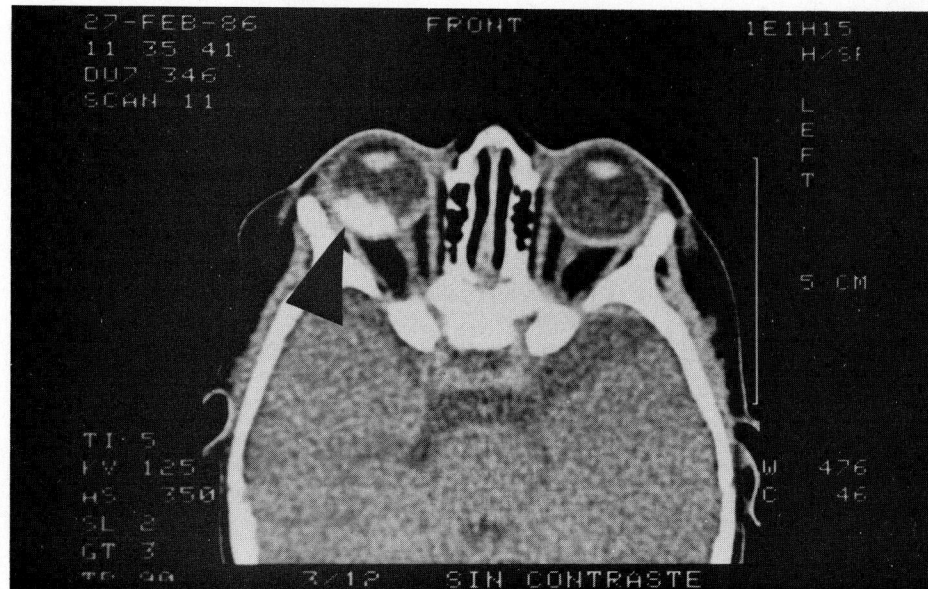

Figure XXV-1-2. CT scan showing retinoblastoma of the right eye with intra-ocular calcification (arrow).

appears to arise most commonly in the region of the ora serrata.

There are two pathognomonic clinical signs of retinoblastoma: the presence of calcium in the tumor, and seeding. Tumors which are calcified on the surface have a characteristic "cottage-cheese" appearance; calcium deeper in the tumor gives a grayish-white appearance termed "fish flesh." Seeding into the vitreous is seen most often in large tumors. These seeds are masses of tumor cells, capable of establishing new daughter tumors. They are of varying size, and float freely in the vitreous. If they come to rest on an uninvolved area of the retina where a good blood supply exists, a new tumor can readily evolve. Vitreous seeding is a poor prognostic sign for salvage of the eye.

When the tumor masses are clearly seen, there is little difficulty in the differential diagnosis. Retinoblastomas are well-circumscribed, elevated, grayish-pink tumors that are highly characteristic. Infections caused by the parasite *Toxocara canis,* and the lesions of tuberous sclerosis, may be confused with retinoblastoma in the early stages.

When there is an overlying retinal detachment or uveitis, an accurate diagnosis is far more difficult. In this situation, the most commonly confused conditions are advanced larval granulomatosis; Coats' disease, an entity defined by the presence of retinal telangiectasia which causes exudative retinal detachments; angiomatosis retinae complicated by retinal detachment; and granulomatous uveitis.

A complete diagnostic approach to retinoblastoma requires a full history and physical, as well as ophthalmoscopy under general anesthesia to assure a complete investigation of the retina. Particular attention should be made to family members of retinoblastoma patients, to look for regressed tumors. CT scans can be used to detect calcification within the tumor. Ultrasound and MRI may also be used; these can reveal gross tumor extension into the optic nerve, an orbital mass, or extension via the superior orbital fissure into the middle cranial fossa. In these advanced cases, the affected eyes are usually functionally destroyed, and often become painful;

enucleation is routinely performed, a metastatic work-up is advisable, and radiation and chemotherapy may be required.

When one eye is involved extensively and the other less so, the former is enucleated and all treatment directed toward the fellow eye. However, in patients with a family history of the disease routinely undergoing examination under anesthesia, early new tumors are occasionally found in both eyes, and in this situation there is no hesitation to treat both eyes.

Retinoblastoma is multicentric in origin. This is evidenced by the fact that 80% of involved eyes have more than one tumor. New tumors tend to arise following the initial diagnosis, especially in children aged less than 6 months. Most methods of therapy for this disease treat only the established areas of tumor, and not areas where invisibly small new tumors may be forming. For this reason, we prefer to treat all tumor-bearing eyes with an initial course of external-beam radiotherapy, with a beam energy greater than 4 MeV and a dose of 4,000 cGy over 4 weeks, to discourage all tumorigenesis. This modality is used in those cases where preservation of useful vision is possible and the tumor is not life-threatening. This level of radiation should cure the existing tumors and discourage the development of new lesions at potential, unidentifiable foci.

The children are restrained in a head case or sedated for treatment, and are treated 4 or 5 days per week for the 4-week course. An attempt is made to keep daily dose below 400 rad and weekly dose below 1,200 cGy. The entire retina is treated, up to the ora serrata, through a single 3 × 4 cm temporal portal. Care is taken to shield the lens and the anterior chamber.

The principal complication of this treatment has been obliterative vascular disease of the retina, which results in retinal and vitreous hemorrhage. This is most unusual below a dose level of 5,000 cGY, but occasionally is seen. Larger tumors, and those exhibiting seeding, are treated with a combination of radiation and chemotherapy.

The patient is examined under anesthesia 6–8 weeks following treatment, at which time the effects of the radiation are readily apparent. The retinal periphery must be examined carefully, since the radiation dose to this area might not have been completely homogeneous. If there is evidence of recurrent activity in any of the tumors, they are treated with more specific modalities. Specific measures that treat only the tumor-bearing areas of the retina include diathermy, radioactive-plaque brachytherapy, light coagulation, and cryotherapy.

Children are followed up with examination under anesthesia, at invervals of 3 to 4 months, for a period of 3 to 5 years after initial treatment. If new tumors arise, they are treated with specific measures, usually light coagulation or cryotherapy. When a tumor is large, the treatment of choice is a radioactive plaque sutured to the sclera over the tumor. A dose of 4,000 cGy to the tumor apex is required. The plaque remains on the eye until that dose is delivered, and is then removed in a second procedure. A "cure" preserving useful vision in the affected eye has been achieved in 91% of cases diagnosed early (Ellsworth-Reese Group I), and 29% of advanced cases (Group V).[12,13,34]

Retinoblastoma remains confined to the eye for a long period of time. When it does spread, it extends by way of the optic nerve into the orbit and the brain, or via the choroid into the bloodstream. At present, chemotherapy is the only effective treatment for orbital and metastatic disease. The regimen includes adriamycin, vincristine, and cytoxan. When gross involvement of the CNS has occurred, intrathecal methotrexate and radiation are used to supplement the systemic chemotherapy.

Malignant Melanoma of the Uvea

Malignant melanoma of the uvea is the most common primary intraocular tumor in adults.[34] However, metastatic spread of other cancers to the uvea, where they resemble malignant melanomas, is by far the most common cause of tumors of the globe (see below). Malignant melanoma is comparatively rare in blacks and Asians, and is rarely seen in Caucasians under the age of 20. The tumor can affect any portion of the uvea. Tumor cells tend to invade blood vessels relatively early in the course of the disease, and heterogeneous metastasis is likely by the time the initial diagnosis can be made. However, the metastatic cells may remain dormant, and not manifest for years.

An overall 5-year mortality of nearly 40% has been seen in cases of melanoma involving the choroid and ciliary body. By contrast, only a handful of deaths due to melanoma of the iris have been reported, despite the fact that iris melanomas are fairly common lesions. Little is known of the natural history of uveal melanoma without treatment. The 10- and 15-year mortality is greater than the 5-year mortality, demonstrating that delayed growth of metastases occurs.

Iris Melanoma. The clinical picture in iris melanoma varies from a dark, velvety-brown lesion involving the iris and the angle of the anterior chamber to fleshy, translucent pink, "tapioca-like" tumors, which are only lightly pigmented. A tissue diagnosis must be made, and the lesion should be totally excised at the time of biopsy. Since many of these tumors are spindle-cell melanomas with only slow growth potential, it is permissible to observe them over a period of months or years, and only perform an excisional biopsy if

they exhibit signs of growth. The presence of new blood vessels, of extension toward the chamber angle, or of distortion toward the pupil are signs of progression which indicate a biopsy should be taken. Once the tumor has invaded the chamber angle, an iridocyclectomy must be performed with a corneal or scleral graft. While this is a most satisfactory procedure in treating melanoma, it can be dangerous to the integrity of the eye. In general, an iridocyclectomy involving more than 90 degrees of the circumference of the chamber angle cannot be performed safely for mechanical reasons. For this reason, it is imperative to diagnose these tumors early, even though the low growth potential may otherwise lead to conservative management.

Choroidal Melanoma. Melanomas of the choroid are more difficult to diagnose and have a much worse prognosis than those of the iris. Again, they can grow at a relatively slow rate for a period of many months or years, and during this time they can be discovered during routine eye examinations. As the tumors grow larger, they can extend into the macular area, or produce subretinal fluid. Either of these conditions leads to a loss of vision. Such visual defects may prompt the patient to seek consultation, and therefore serve as the first presenting symptom.

The tumors can best be examined with a binocular indirect ophthalmoscope, and usually can be well visualized. If a major retinal detachment exists in the affected eye, the tumor may be difficult to see. However, the subretinal fluid behind such a detachment shifts readily, and if the patient is positioned correctly the fluid will move the detached portion of the retina away from the area of the tumor, allowing clear visualization.

When the tumor itself cannot be seen, ultrasonography may be helpful in outlining the tumor mass. A radioactive phosphorus (^{32}P) uptake test can indicate a malignant tumor, but this test does not distinguish a melanoma from a metastatic lesion.

These tumors are elevated masses, of varying size, which range in color from a dark brown to a light, almost unpigmented grayish-white. At one stage in its growth, the tumor typically assumes a mushroom shape as it penetrates the lamina vitrea and enters the vitreous. Abnormal vascular channels may be present in the dome of the tumor, and hemorrhage sometimes occurs on the surface. Crescentic hemorrhage around the edge of the tumor is unusual, but is commonly seen in some lesions which simulate melanomas. Melanomas of the choroid frequently have episodes of spontaneous necrosis within the tumor, accompanied by inflammatory signs in the eye. This may lead to a mistaken diagnosis of primary inflammatory disease.

Since enucleation historically has proven of limited value in managing this disease, it is best to observe the tumor until the diagnosis is relatively certain before considering this procedure. A delay of several weeks or months will probably not affect the long-term outcome.

A number of conditions simulate choroidal melanoma. These include metastatic tumor spread to the choroid, hematomas of the retinal pigment epithelium, hemangiomas of the choroid, melanocytomas, and macular degeneration with subretinal neovascularization.

The first of these, metastatic lesions in the uvea, are the

most common intraocular tumors. They occur most commonly from breast cancer in women and lung cancer in men. For this reason, careful examination of the chest region for a source of metastasis is in order whenever a diagnosis of uveal tumor is made. Metastatic lesions in the choroid are slightly more common in the left eye, and often occur over the posterior pole in a region supplied by the short ciliary arteries. These lesions are usually less highly elevated than true choroidal melanomas, but may be similar in color. Many are associated with extensive inferior retinal detachments.

Hematomas of the retinal pigment epithelium are elevated black masses that can look very much like melanomas. They appear suddenly, often following a bout of violent coughing, and are due to hemorrhage between the retinal pigment epithelium and the lamina vitrea. A crescentic hemorrhage is often seen along the border of a hematoma; this can vary in appearance, and eventually disappears. Careful observation over a period of several months will distinguish these lesions from melanomas.

Choroidal hemangiomas are seen in a younger age group (averaging 19 years), and may be accompanied by hemangioma of the facial region (Sturge-Weber syndrome). These tumors are generally not as highly elevated as malignant melanomas, and occur around the optic nerve head. Eventually an epichoroidal membrane develops, which may contain bone; this structure produces a relatively characteristic ophthalmoscopic picture.

Macular degeneration with subretinal neovascularization can simulate melanoma. Clinically, evidence of macular degeneration in the fellow eye is helpful in making the diagnosis.

Fluorescein patterns may appear identical in malignant melanoma, metastatic lesions, and hemangioma of the choroid. If the lesion does not fluoresce, it is not likely to be a malignant tumor, but rather a simulating lesion. While most of these merely bear watching, there are rare exceptions.

A properly performed P^{32} uptake study is almost infallible in distinguishing neoplastic from non-neoplastic tissue if it is performed, as an operative procedure, by a competent surgeon who can assure precise localization and uses proper counting equipment.

Treatment of Malignant Melanoma

In general, enucleation is the proper treatment for malignant melanoma of the choroid in younger patients. Conservatism in treating this tumor in elderly patients is reasonable, however, due to the tumor's slow growth in these cases, and radiation is an acceptable alternative.[38] If vision in the fellow eye is subnormal, and vision in the affected eye is useful, we feel every effort short of enucleation should be tried to cure the tumor.[16]

The following modalities are useful in the treatment of choroidal melanoma: diathermy, light coagulation (laser or xenon arc), cryotherapy, radiotherapy, brachytherapy (radioactive plaques), full-thickness resection of the wall of the eye, and proton-beam irradiation.

Small malignant melanomas can be cured with surface diathermy. Penetrating diathermy should not be used, as it may allow the tumor to gain access to the orbit, resulting in a fatal outcome.

Light coagulation is useful in treating lesions as large as 6 mm in diameter. The surface of these tumors is burned away repeatedly at intervals of 2 to 4 weeks, and the lesions can be obliterated completely if they do not grow too rapidly from below.

Cryotherapy has been effective in the treatment of small choroidal melanomas. However, although small lesions can be handled this way, we do not recommend it. Very little permanent effect has been seen on these tumors, although their growth rate may be impeded.

Radioactive-applicator brachytherapy appears to be a useful elective means of treating these tumors. Markings are made externally on the sclera to outline the lesion, and a radioactive plaque is chosen which overlaps this area by 1 or 2 mm around its circumference. The dose at the tumor apex is approximately 10,000 cGy. The plaque is left in place until this dose has been administered, and is then removed in a second operation.[13] Regressive changes following brachytherapy may not be seen for 4 to 6 months.

Impressive results with full eye-wall resection have been reported.[29] However, if the tumor involves the only useful eye, we feel that safer established methods are preferable, and, if the fellow eye is normal, enucleation provides a more secure prognosis.

Proton-beam irradiation is currently being researched at several sites. Seven hundred eighty consecutive patients with choroidal melanoma treated with proton-beam irradiation were evaluated in 1988. Metastasis occurred in 8%, with a median of 2.1 years between treatment and diagnosis of metastasis; this can be extrapolated to a 5-year cumulative probability of 20%. These results are comparable to those for enucleation.[17]

At present, it is common practice to observe choroidal melanomas of a diameter up to 10 mm and elevation up to 2 mm with serial photography alone, since the mortality in these cases is virtually zero. Larger melanomas, up to 15 mm in diameter and 5 mm in height, may be treated with radioactive plaques, or proton irradiation, or eye-wall resection. Any lesion greater than this should routinely be enucleated if the fellow eye is normal.

Malignant melanoma of the choroid can metastasize. The metastases can affect the orbit, subconjunctival tissue, or any distant organ, particularly the liver, and may appear after many years of apparent freedom from disease. While malignant melanoma is generally resistant to systemic chemotherapy and radiation, metastases occasionally respond dramatically better than the primary tumor. Vaccinations against malignant melanoma, and the use of specific monoclonal antibodies to aid in treatment, are under current investigation (see XXXIV).

Primary Intraocular Lymphoma (Reticulum Cell Sarcoma)

Primary intraocular lymphoma is a disease which affects adults of the middle and older ages. It can involve one or both eyes and can either occur isolated to the globe or with CNS involvement.[24] Most patients with intraocular lymphoma eventually develop CNS involvement.[2A]

Clinically, the disease most often presents with signs of uveitis unresponsive to steroids. Diagnosis is often made after vitreous biopsy. A systemic work-up is indicated including a CT scan of the head.

Management of CNS involvement generally requires brain irradiation plus intrathecal chemotherapy. However, when disease is isolated to the eye, the management is much more controversial. Radiotherapy to the ipsilateral eye and orbit is required; some oncologists institute systemic and intrathecal chemotherapy simultaneously in hopes of averting later spread. Controlled trials of therapeutic approaches have not been performed; prophylactic radiotherapy of the contralateral eye or brain, although sometimes employed, is not known to be effective.

References

1. Abramson, D. H., Ellsworth, R. M., Tretter, P., Wolff, J. A., and Kitchin, F. D.: The treatment of orbital rhabdomyosarcoma with irradiation and chemotherapy. Ophthalmology, 86:1330, 1979.
2. Cassady, J. R., Sagerman, R. H., Tretter, P., and Ellsworth, R. M.: Radiation therapy for rhabdomyosarcoma. Radiology, 91:116, 1968.
2A. Char, D. H., Ljung, B., Miller, T., and Phillips, P.: Primary Intraocular Lymphoma (ocular reticulum cell sarcoma): Diagnosis and Management. Ophthalmol., 95:626, 1988.
3. Chutorian, A. M., Schwartz, J. F., Evans, R. A., and Carter, S.: Optic glioma in children. Neurology, 14:83, 1964.
4. Coleman, D. J., Lizzi, F. L., and Jack, R. L.: Ultrasonography of the Eye and Orbit. In Ultrasonography of the Eye and Orbit. Philadelphia, Lea & Febiger, 1977.
5. Doxanos, M. T., and Green, W. R.: Sebaceous gland carcinoma. Arch. Ophthalmol., 102:245, 1984.
6. Doxanos, M. T., Green, W. R., and Ilif, C. E.: Factors in the successful surgical management of basal-cell carcinoma of the eyelids. Amer. J. Ophthalmol., 91:726, 1981.
7. Dryja, T. P., Cavenee, W., White, R., Rapaport, J. M., Petersen, R., Albert, D. M., and Bruns, G. A.: Homozygosity of chromosome 13 in retinoblastoma. N. Engl. J. Med., 310:550, 1984.
8. Dryja, T. P., Mukai, S., Peterson, R., Rapaport, J. M., Walton, D., and Yandell, D. W.: Parental origins of mutations of the retinoblastoma gene. Nature, 339:556, 1989.
9. Ellsworth, R. M.: Treatment of retinoblastoma. Am. J. Ophthalmol., 66:49, 1968.
10. Ellsworth, R. M.: The practical management of retinoblastoma. Trans. Am. Ophthalmol. Soc., 67:462, 1969.
11. Ellsworth, R. M.: Retinoblastoma. In Clinical Ophthalmology. Hagerstown, Maryland, Harper & Row, 1976.
12. Ellsworth, R. M.: Retinoblastoma. In Modern Problems in Ophthalmology. Basel, S. Karger A. G., 1977.
13. Ellsworth, R. M.: Cobalt plaques in the treatment of malignant melanoma of the choroid. In Ocular and Adnexal Tumors. Edited by F. A. Jakobiec. Birmingham, Alabama, Aesculapius Publishing Co., 1978.
14. Ferry, A. P.: The biological behavior and pathological features of carcinoma metastatic to the eye and orbit. Trans Am. Ophthalmol. Soc., 71:373, 1973.
15. Fitzpatrick, P. J., and Jamieson, D. M.: Tumors of the eyelid and their treatment by radiotherapy. Intl. J. Radiat. Oncol. Biol. Physics, 104:661, 1972.
16. Galbraith, J. E. K.: The conservative management of uveal malignancies. Aust. N. Z. J. Surg., 38:349, 1969.
17. Gragoudas, E. S., Seddon, J. M., Egan, K. M., Glynn, R. J., Goitein, M., Munzenrider, J., Verhey, L., Urie, M., and Koehler, A.: Metastasis from uveal melanoma after proton-beam irradiation. Ophthalmology, 95:992, 1988.
18. Jackson, W. B., Tolis, G., and Chertman, M.: The TRH test: Its value in the diagnosis of Graves' ophthalmopathy. Can. J. Ophthalmol., 13:10, 1978.
19. Jakobiec, F. A., and Folberg, R.: Clinicopathologic characteristics of premalignant and malignant melanocytic lesions of the conjunctiva. Ophthalmology, 96:147, 1989.
20. Jakobiec, F. A., Iwamoto, T., and Knowles, D. M.: Ocular adnexal lymphoid tumors: Correlative ultrastructural and immunological marker studies. Arch. Ophthalmol., 100:89, 1982.
21. Jones, I. S.: Lymphangiomas of the ocular adnexae: An analysis of 62 cases. Trans. Am. Ophthalmol. Soc., 57:602, 1959.
22. Jones, I. S., Reese, A. B., and Krout, J.: Orbital rhabdomyosarcoma: An analysis of 62 cases. Trans. Am. Ophthalmol. Soc., 63:223, 1965.
23. Karp, L. A., and Zimmerman, L. E.: Primary intraorbital meningiomas. Arch. Ophthalmol., 91:21, 1974.
24. Knowles, D. M, and Jakobiec, F. A.: Ocular lymphoid lesions: Clinical, pathologic, and immunologic characteristics. In Ocular and Adnexal Tumors. Edited by F. A. Jakobiec. Birmingham, Alabama, Aesculapius Publishing Co., 1978.
25. Knudson, A. G., Jr., Hethcote, H. W., and Brown, B. W.: Mutation and childhood cancer. A probabilistic model for the incidence of retinoblastoma. Proc. Natl. Acad. Sci., USA, 71:5116, 1975.
25A. McGee, T. L., Vandell, D. W., and Dryja, T. P.: Structure and partial genomic sequence of the human retinoblastoma susceptibility gene. Gene, 80:119, 1989.
26. Mohs, F. E.: Discussion paper by Robins, P., Henkind, P., and Menn, H.: Chemosurgery in the treatment of cancer of the periorbital area. Trans. Am. Acad. Ophthalmol. Otolaryngol., 75:1235, 1971.
27. Moss, H.: Expanding lesion of the orbit. Am. J. Ophthalmol., 54:761, 1962.
28. Perez, C. A., and Brady, L.: Skin cancer. In Principles and Practice of Radiation Oncology, 1987.
29. Peyman, G. A., Sonders, D. R., and May, D. R.: Local excision of malignant melanoma of the choroid. In Intraocular Tumors. New York, Appleton, Century, Crofts, 1989.
30. Polack, F. M., Kanai, A., and Hood, C. I.: Light and electron microscopic studies of orbital rhabdomyosarcoma. Am. J. Ophthalmol., 71:75, 1971.
31. Rao, N. A., Hidayat, A. A., McLean, I. W., and Zimmerman, L. E.: Sebaceous carcinoma of the ocular adnexa. Hum. Pathol., 13:113, 1982.
32. Rapaport, H.: Tumors of the hematopoietic system. In Atlas of Tumor Pathology, Section 3, Fascicle 8. Washington, D.C., AFID, 1966.
33. Reeh, M. J.: Treatment of Lid and Epibulbar Tumors. Illinois, Charles C Thomas, 1963.
34. Reese, A. B.: Tumors of the Eye. New York, Harper & Row, 1963.
35. Rush, J. A., and Younge, B. R.: Optic glioma: Long-term followup of 85 histopathologically verified cases. Ophthalmology, 89:1213, 1982.
35A. Shiang, R., Murray, J. C., Wiggs, J., and Dryja, T.: A TaqI RFLP identified at the retinoblastoma locus on chromosome 13. Nucleic Acids Res., 16:9069, 1988.
36. Shuler, J. D., Holland, G. N., Miles, S. A., Miller, B. J., and Grossman, I.: Kaposi sarcoma of the conjunctiva and eyelids associated with the acquired immunodeficiency syndrome. Arch. Ophthalmol., 107:858, 1989.
37. Silvers, D., Jakobiec, F. A., Freeman, T., Lefkowitch, J., and Elie, R.: Melanoma of the conjunctiva: A clinicopathologic study. In Ocular and Adnexal Tumors. Edited by F. A. Jakobiec. Birmingham, Alabama, Aesculapius Publishing Co., 1978.
38. Stallard, H. B.: Radiotherapy for malignant melanoma of the choroid. Br. J. Ophthalmol., 50:147, 1966.
39. Tretter, P., and Trokel, S.: Personal Communication.
40. Wolff, J. A., Pratt, C. B., and Sitarz, A. L.: Chemotherapy of metastatic retinoblastoma. In Cancer Chemotherapy Report, No. 16. Bethesda, MD, NIH, 1962.
41. Wright, J. E.: Factors affecting survival of patients with lacrimal gland tumors. Can. J. Ophthalmol., 17:3, 1982.
42. Wright, J. E., Stewart, W. B., and Krohel, G. B.: Clinical presentation and management of lacrimal gland tumors. Br. J. Ophthalmol., 63:600, 1979.

XXVI

Neoplasms of the Endocrine Glands

XXVI-1

Pituitary Neoplasms

Charles B. Wilson

Introduction

The classic histologic designation of pituitary neoplasms as chromophobic, eosinophilic, or basophilic (see Table XXIV-1-1) based on their histologic appearance as seen with light microscopy has been superceded by a system derived from the work of Landolt[46] and Kovacs and colleagues[39,40] in which adenomas are classified according to the hormone(s) they secrete (Table XXVI-1-1).[39,40,46,85] Pituitary neoplasms are generally considered either endocrine-active or endocrine-inactive. They are endocrine-active only if they secrete enough biologically active hormone to exceed normal levels in the blood and become clinically evident. Endocrine-inactive adenomas, in contrast, have secretory granules and the cellular constituents for hormone production,[46] but either they produce normal hormone in undetectably small amounts, or they secrete abnormal hormone that is not recognized by biological receptor sites or detected by radioimmunoassay, or alternatively they have lost the ability to produce hormone through degeneration or dedifferentiation. Molecular biologic studies ultimately will provide an even more informative classification of pituitary adenomas. Early evidence has shown a monoclonal origin of most adenomas, implying that somatic mutation of a single cell is likely to be the event initiating hormone hypersecretion and neoplastic transformation.[31,36] Two subsets of growth hormone (GH)-secreting adenomas have already been identified.[71,45,80] A large percentage of patients with acromegaly have somatic mutations in the α

Table XXVI-1-1. Current Morphological Classification of Pituitary Adenomas

Growth hormone cell adenoma
Prolactin cell adenoma
Mixed: growth hormone cell—prolactin cell adenoma
Corticotrophic cell adenoma
Thyrotrophic cell adenoma
Gonadotrophic cell adenoma
Undifferentiated cell adenoma
    Non-oncocytic (null cell)
    Oncocytic (oncocytoma)
Acidophilic stem cell adenoma

From Wilson, C. B.[85]

chain of the G protein (Gs) regulating the hormone-stimulatory activity of adenylyl cyclase. The adenomas with these *gsp* mutations are significantly smaller than those without mutations, and they are more sensitive to inhibitory factors such as somatostatin or dopamine—a characteristic that may prove to have therapeutic as well as diagnostic importance.

The adenoma's local growth characteristics and size, irrespective of endocrine activity, predict its nonendocrine clinical presentation.[29,84] Wilson's anatomic (radiographic and operative) scheme[84,86,87] derived from Hardy's,[26,29] classifying pituitary adenomas by the degree of sellar destruction (grade) and extrasellar extension (stage), is valuable in establishing a prognosis and helpful in designing therapy. The following generalizations provide a framework for discussion of the more prevalent pituitary neoplasms.

For patients suspected of or known to be harboring a pituitary adenoma, the diagnostic neuroimaging procedure of choice is magnetic resonance (MR) imaging. While gadolinium enhancement should be used for microadenomas (less than 10 mm in diameter),[59] its use for macroadenomas is optional. The image is preferably obtained using a 1.5 tesla MR imager with thin sections in coronal and sagittal planes.[87] Whereas adenomas that secrete growth hormone (GH), or adrenocorticotrophic hormone (ACTH), can be predicted with virtual certainty on the basis of laboratory findings alone, a confident preoperative diagnosis of a prolactin (PRL)-secreting neoplasm requires radiographic evaluation as well.

The transsphenoidal approach is the preferred surgical technique for almost all pituitary adenomas and the treatment of choice for those secreting GH (acromegaly) or ACTH (Cushing's disease or Nelson's syndrome), as well as for certain nonsecreting tumors that extend out of the sella to compress adjacent structures and produce clinical manifestations, usually impaired vision. The operative approaches to pituitary adenomas have been described.[50,86,87] The objectives of surgery are to eliminate any mass effect of the tumor, to halt endocrine hyperactivity, to retain or improve existing pituitary function,[4] to achieve these goals immediately and with minimal morbidity,[63] and to predict accurately the need for adjuvant therapy.[63] The monoclonal antibody Ki-67, which permits determinations of the frequency of proliferating cells, is a new tool for quantitative assessment of the adenoma's growth characteristics that may aid in the planning of adjuvant therapy and the estimation of prognosis.[49]

It is debated whether the initial treatment for prolactin-secreting adenomas should be medical or surgical, with bromocriptine or irradiation reserved for surgical failures. For the rare and aggressive tumors secreting thyroid-stimulating hormone, the role and timing of surgery are unclear. An endocrine-inactive tumor in an asymptomatic patient with unimpaired pituitary function should, with some exceptions, be left alone and its course observed with serial MR images. Less well defined is the most effective management for pituitary apoplexy, the symptom complex that evolves acutely or subacutely as a consequence of hemorrhage and necrosis within an adenoma. At the University of California, San Francisco (UCSF), we tend to prepare the patient quickly and proceed directly with transsphenoidal surgery. If hypopituitarism is treated with suitable replacement therapy, but no surgery, the compressive symptoms may resolve in time, but the tumor will almost certainly require treatment at a later date. Medical management does not spare the patient an operation—it merely postpones it. The only exceptions are in some cases of PRL-secreting adenomas.[87]

Prolactinomas

PRL-secreting adenomas are the most prevalent pituitary adenomas. The behavior and benign clinical manifestations of small prolactinomas distinguish them from the adenomas that produce Cushing's disease and acromegaly, two distinct metabolic entities that have severe and eventually fatal consequences independent of their effects as a mass. Unlike those lesions, prolactinomas manifest differently in men and women. Whereas large prolactinomas are slightly more prevalent in women than men, men rarely present with microadenomas.

Pathology

The level of PRL in blood, taken as an index of secretory activity, correlates directly with the size of the prolactinoma, exclusive of bulk contributed by necrosis and cysts. Necrosis is a common surgical finding in prolactinomas of all sizes. Prolactinomas, with relatively rare exceptions, grow slowly.[87]

Clinical Presentation

Prolactinomas may produce primary,[22] or secondary amenorrhea, and galactorrhea. The frequency of hyperprolactinemia in amenorrheic women is now well recognized. Equally evident is that prolactinoma is a common cause of hyperprolactinemia. Among women with prolactinomas treated at UCSF over two decades,[87] 80% had secondary amenorrhea and spontaneous or expressible galactorrhea; 10% had primary amenorrhea, one-half of whom also had galactorrhea; and 10% had oligomenorrhea with galactorrhea, secondary amenorrhea without galactorrhea, or secondary amenorrhea only. In men, a prolactinoma usually goes undetected during the initial phase of hyperprolactinemia and the diagnosis may be established only after the adenoma has become large and caused significant hypopituitarism or compressed and invaded parasellar structures; a history of lessened libido, and eventually impotence, often precedes clinical manifestations of a large mass.

Hyperprolactinemia may have extragonadal manifestations, although possibly only in patients predisposed to these disorders. A recent, rapid, often excessive, and unwanted weight gain is reported by hyperprolactinemic women with a frequency that suggests a relation. Correction of hyperprolactinemia through surgery or bromocriptine therapy is in some cases followed by impressive weight loss despite no change in dietary habits. Equally impressive is the incidence of emotional lability and its reversal after correction of hyperprolactinemia. Obesity and emotional instability may reflect multiple nonendocrine factors but hyperprolactinemia that is neither extreme nor long-standing also causes significant demineralization of bone, with its potential morbidity.[38,67]

Diagnosis

A confident preoperative diagnosis of prolactinoma requires radiographic evidence of an intrasellar tumor unless serum PRL levels exceed 200 ng/ml; even with unequivocal radiographic demonstration of a pathologic abnormality in the pituitary gland, transsphenoidal explorations have in some cases revealed either a diffusely enlarged anterior lobe (pituitary "hyperplasia") or a nonneoplastic cyst, usually in the pars intermedia.[87] Attempts to distinguish functional or nonneoplastic hyperprolactinemia from the hyperprolactinemia produced by prolactinomas on the basis of laboratory values alone have yielded conflicting conclusions. No single test or combination of tests is infallible. In men with basal PRL values over 100 ng/ml, a prolactinoma is almost always the cause of hyperprolactinemia. In women, hyperprolactinemia and basal values over 200 ng/ml almost always indicate a prolactinoma; with some exceptions, basal values of 100–200 ng/ml have nearly the same significance. Women with basal levels of 50–100 ng/ml, for which the term moderate hyperprolactinemia seems appropriate, present a quandary. Values in this range may have no recognized cause, and a confident prediction of a prolactinoma cannot be based solely on laboratory values in women whose moderate hyperprolactinemia is unrelated to medication, pregnancy, or hypothyroidism. In a few patients, moderate hyperprolactinemia is the result of a stalk section effect produced by a readily identified pathologic intrasellar or suprasellar lesion, usually an endocrine-inactive adenoma or infrequently a suprasellar tumor such as a craniopharyngioma[34] that interferes with downward blood flow through the pituitary stalk.

Treatment

Unlike long-term medical therapy for Cushing's disease and acromegaly, which is relatively ineffective, bromocriptine corrects the biochemical pathology of prolactinomas and reduces their size, at times dramatically. One view is that medical therapy should be used for all patients except the 30% or so who have unacceptable side effects from the medication. In contrast is the opinion that surgery should be the initial treatment, bromocriptine or irradiation being reserved for patients who are not cured.[9] Although some clinicians question the wisdom of treating these patients at all, the potential for adverse systemic and psychological effects from hyperprolactinemia, and the potential for invasive behavior of the tumor, provide compelling arguments for treatment, whether surgical or nonsurgical. The middle ground seems preferable. Surgery does not predictably cure these adenomas and the higher the patient's PRL level, the greater is the potential for therapeutic failure. Moreover, serious surgical complications may occur, although with an experienced surgeon the likelihood is no more than 1%. Medical management is hardly a perfect solution, however. It appears that medication must be a lifetime commitment for most if not all of the patients, a significant portion of whom have unpleasant and sometimes unacceptable side effects at effective dose levels. A few tumors are relatively resistant to bromocriptine as judged by insufficiently lowered PRL levels and, in some cases, continued tumor growth.[41] Finally, patients with macroadenomas who become pregnant may develop complications from accelerated tumor growth. Although treatment with bromocriptine usually resolves the problem, it may not.[62]

The low morbidity rates, the low incidence of recurrence, and the high likelihood of cure associated with selective transsphenoidal microsurgery support its use as the treatment of choice for patients with microprolactinomas. In patients with large, invasive tumors and extremely high PRL levels, the administration of a dopamine agonist, such as bromocriptine, either alone or in combination with surgery, pituitary irradiation, or both appears to be the appropriate mode of therapy.[83] Unless an MR image shows unquestioned invasion of the cavernous sinus, surgical cure is a reasonable expectation in any patient with a PRL level of 500 ng/ml or less.[7] The lower the PRL level, the greater the likelihood of cure. The younger the patient, the clearer are the advantages of surgery and the less desirable is medical management. Patients who cannot tolerate medication become surgical candidates, with varying expectations of cure. Irradiation sterilizes but does not inactivate prolactinomas, and is reserved for patients who are not cured with surgery and cannot tolerate medication.[10]

Recommendation

The policies currently determining recommended management at UCSF reflect our favorable experience with the microsurgical approach, the assumption that most prolactinomas grow relatively slowly, and the evidence that surgical treatment is less successful in older patients, patients with a longer duration of amenorrhea, and patients with higher PRL values and larger tumors. These recommendations apply for the cases in which the clinical presentation, laboratory data, and MR images eliminate any reasonable doubt that the patient harbors a prolactinoma.

Operative removal is recommended for most macroadenomas, virtually all of which are accompanied by PRL values greater than 100 ng/ml. For tumors smaller than 2 cm, a surgical cure is likely. For noninvasive tumors larger than 2 cm, preliminary treatment with bromocriptine should reduce tumor volume and increase the likelihood of surgical cure. Residual tumor is managed medically. Irradiation is indicated for patients who cannot tolerate bromocriptine or have tumor progression despite treatment. For macroadenomas of a size or invasiveness precluding surgical cure, an initial trial of

bromocriptine is appropriate.[82] The management of microadenomas is more controversial. At UCSF, our indications for operative removal are[86,87] a desire for pregnancy, the presence of primary amenorrhea, the patient's being male, and the patient's personal choice. For other patients, bromocriptine is prescribed, and the tumor is monitored at regular intervals with basal PRL measurements and periodic MR images; these tumors rarely expand without a concomitant rise in PRL levels. In patients electing nonoperative management initially, two subsequent developments indicate surgery: progressive elevation of PRL levels approaching 200 ng/ml in an untreated patient or a progressive elevation of PRL values in a patient taking bromocriptine; and enlargement of the tumor as determined by serial MR images.

Pregnancy. Induced pregnancy in a patient who has a prolactinoma carries a small but serious risk of complications related to rapid expansion of the tumor.[11,70] Prophylactic pituitary irradiation has been used in patients who desire pregnancy. If a tumor becomes symptomatic during pregnancy, bromocriptine can be given. We advise against pregnancy for patients known to have a prolactinoma and recommend that bromocriptine therapy be accompanied with contraception by mechanical means. As the risk of a serious complication during pregnancy seems significantly larger than the risk of transsphenoidal surgery, we advise surgical treatment when pregnancy is desired.

Growth Hormone-Secreting Pituitary Adenomas

Clinical Presentation

GH-secreting pituitary adenomas produce acromegaly and gigantism with their classic presentation marked by progressive enlargement of the hands, feet, and face. Although they progress slowly, these adenomas cause crippling cosmetic and orthopedic deformities and life-threatening metabolic effects, with 50% of untreated patients dead by the age of 50 years[21] and a death rate twice that in the general population.[88]

Diagnosis

With considerable accuracy, the diagnosis of acromegaly and gigantism can be made by history and physical examination. Evaluations of GH dynamics, including tests of glucose suppression, thyrotrophin-releasing hormone stimulation, and/or insulin-tolerance, may be performed. Patients with GH levels greater than 10 ng/ml have active disease[5] and a fasting growth hormone level in serum of less than 5 ng/ml is the benchmark normal value.[6,52,75,77–79] MR imaging is used to define the anatomical extent of the tumor.

Treatment

Although various surgical approaches have been used in the past, the treatment of choice is selective transsphenoidal removal of the adenoma. Although promising, somatostatin analogs to date do not provide a long-term alternative to operation.[61,72] Irradiation, used in the treatment of acromegaly since 1909,[25] still provides an alternative to surgery, although its efficacy is compromised by the delay in its therapeutic effect and its significant failure rate when used primarily.[3,28,35,43,64,65]

Despite the significance of clinical improvement as a measure of therapeutic success, the primary factor determining a cure is the restoration of normal GH production. Radioimmunoassays for GH and somatomedin C for the documentation of disease activity have provided quantitative information from which to assess the relative efficacy of particular forms of therapy. Based on these quantitations, transsphenoidal surgery is at present the preferable therapy in virtually every case of acromegaly. The results of transsphenoidal surgery for acromegaly at UCSF over a period of 14 years have been good,[8,63] with long-term follow-up review showing GH levels of less than 5 ng/ml in 79.4%, and less than 10 ng/ml in 92.7%, of patients operated. The rates of recurrence after an apparent surgical cure (4.3%) and complications—i.e., new anterior pituitary hypofunction in 5%, cerebrospinal fluid (CSF) leak in 2.2%, and postoperative meningitis in 1.8%—are low, with no cases of permanent diabetes insipidus or death. Because the transsphenoidal procedure is short and postoperative stress minimal, the patient's age or medical status is rarely a contraindication.[86] The surgical strategy is tailored to the size, shape, location, and consistency of the individual tumor.[28] Factors predictive of a poor prognosis are a high preoperative GH level and extrasellar extension of the tumor. For incompletely removed tumors, postoperative irradiation has a high probability (approaching 95%) of preventing future growth, but the risk of radiation-induced hypopituitarism is very high and there is a rare, but unequivocal, possibility of catastrophic complications.[63]

Mixed Adenomas

The most common mixed adenoma we encounter at UCSF contains PRL- and GH-secreting cell populations. Women with acromegaly characteristically have amenorrhea and galactorrhea whereas the men with acromegaly have either no clinical expression of hyperprolactinemia, or gynecomastia, or in rare cases gynecomastia and galactorrhea. In a few women with otherwise typical amenorrhea and galactorrhea, and no features of acromegaly, modest elevations of GH were detected unexpectedly. Transsphenoidal adenomectomy is the preferred treatment for patients with mixed adenomas.

Adrenocorticotrophic Hormone-Secreting Adenomas

Hypersecretion of ACTH by a pituitary adenoma causes Cushing's disease and Nelson's syndrome. Cushing's disease is the subset of Cushing's syndrome caused by excessive ACTH secretion by the pituitary adenoma that produces bilateral adrenal hyperplasia and hypercortisolism. Nelson's syndrome is the result of ACTH hypersecretion by a pituitary adenoma that occurs in certain patients with Cushing's syndrome following adrenalectomy and its mechanism is thought to be an absence of the negative feedback effect of cortisol on the hypothalamus which leads to chronic overstimulation of the pituitary gland by corticotrophin-releasing factor.[54]

Cushing's Disease

Cushing's disease is a serious endocrinopathy that occurs predominantly in women and has its peak incidence during the third and fourth decades of life.

Clinical Presentation. The classic features of Cushing's disease are centripetal obesity, moon facies, buffalo hump, purple abdominal striae, ecchymoses, acne, and hirsutism. Diabetes mellitus, hypertension, and osteoporosis are features that can cause significant morbidity. Weakness in the form of a proximal myopathy is often one of the most prominent findings. Mental disturbance in a patient with Cushing's disease should not be underestimated because, to the patient and family, it may be the most distressing feature of the disease.[54]

Diagnosis. The diagnosis of Cushing's disease and subsequent therapeutic decision-making are based on endocrinologic criteria. After verification of sustained hypercortisolism with loss of diurnal variation through the measurement of 17-OH corticosteroids and free cortisol in urine, the diagnosis is established by demonstrating nonsuppressibility of steroids by low-dose (1 mg) dexamethasone, less than 50% suppressibility with high-dose (8 mg) dexamethasone, and normal or slightly elevated plasma ACTH levels. Low or undetectable ACTH levels suggest Cushing's syndrome caused by an adrenal neoplasm, whereas extremely high ACTH levels suggest that the cause is an ectopic ACTH-producing tumor.[54]

Neuroimaging studies are only to provide anatomic localization after the diagnosis of Cushing's disease is established. MR imaging is the preferred neuroimaging test for localization, although it has a significant incidence of false-negative and false-positive results. If a high-quality MR image does not document an adenoma unequivocally in the case of a biochemical and clinical diagnosis, bilateral simultaneous selective venous sampling of ACTH from the cavernous sinuses is done to identify a diagnostic 2:1 ACTH gradient from cavernous sinus to peripheral venous blood.

Treatment. The decision to operate relies solely on the clinical and endocrinologic data. Transsphenoidal surgery is the initial treatment of choice.[54,55,87] Selective adenomectomy is a successful and safe treatment for Cushing's disease. The presence or absence of extrasellar extension of the adenoma is the principal determinant of the prognosis.[54] During the early postoperative period, a low-dose dexamethasone suppression test confirms a probable surgical cure. Postoperative hypoadrenalism and prolonged suppression of the pituitary-adrenal axis are noted routinely among patients who experience remission of disease after surgery. All patients are maintained on replacement hydrocortisone as long as evidence of hypoadrenalism persists.

Results in our series treated at UCSF[13,54] resemble others[15,16,27,51] in terms of the patient population and its overall results.[14–16,27,74] Remission of disease was achieved in 76% of our 216 patients and the percentage remission was significantly higher ($p < 0.001$) among patients with microadenomas than in those with macroadenomas, and also higher ($p < 0.001$) among patients with intrasellar adenomas than among those with extrasellar extension of their adenoma or perforation of the sellar floor by adenoma. Five of 6 patients in whom no grossly abnormal tissue was found during the exploration were cured by surgery. Two patients had diffuse pituitary hyperplasia. Operative mortality and morbidity were minimal. Complications occurred in 9.3% of patients, including persistent diabetes insipidus in 2.8% of patients, and visual deficits, CSF leak, and persistent sinusitis in fewer than 2% each. Adults and children do not differ in their response to transsphenoidal microsurgery[87] and transsphenoidal adenomectomy is as effective therapeutically in children as in adults. Our results, like those in other large series,[15,66] refute the notion that diffuse pituitary hyperplasia might constitute up to 25% of the cases of Cushing's disease.[44,57]

Pituitary irradiation can be used as primary or adjuvant therapy for Cushing's disease. Heavy-particle irradiation has a high cure rate and usually can be given as a single treatment with multiple ports, but it is available at only two centers in the United States and has a higher rate of complications than conventional irradiation. Because of high cure rates reported with conventional irradiation for children with Cushing's disease, some institutions use pituitary irradiation as the standard therapy for children. However, the lag period between treatment and remission of disease is typically several months. In adults, pituitary irradiation has been much less effective.

Pharmacological therapy can afford palliation for patients with Cushing's disease or Nelson's syndrome who have tumors that are resistant to surgery and radiation therapy. Various drugs[54] are used in order to reduce the secretion of ACTH by the pituitary or to block steroidogenesis by the adrenal glands. Pharmacologic agents that inhibit secretion of ACTH and corticotrophin-releasing hormone include cyproheptadine and bromocriptine; drugs that inhibit cortisol synthesis include aminoglutethimide, metyrapone, ketoconazole, and mitotane; and those that block the action of cortisol at the glucocorticoid receptor level include RU-486.[68] Except for mitotane, whose use is limited by its toxicity, the action of these drugs ceases almost immediately with discontinuation of treatment.[68] They can be used as a temporary measure, to improve a patient's condition in preparation for surgery or concurrently with pituitary irradiation, or after both surgery and irradiation have failed to produce remission (see XXVI-3).

Recommendation. Selective adenomectomy is a successful and safe treatment for Cushing's disease and is preferable to bilateral adrenalectomy, pituitary irradiation, or total hypophysectomy as the primary treatment.[54] It provides a likely selective removal of the ACTH-secreting adenoma, immediate cure of the hypercortisolism, preservation of pituitary function, and minimal morbidity. The overall percentage of remissions compares favorably with the approximately 80% obtained with primary total hypophysectomy, and adenomectomy does not entail the inevitable hypopituitarism of that procedure.[76] Because bilateral adrenalectomy is associated with a greater perioperative mortality (up to 5%), with an occasional persistence of hypercortisolism due to incomplete adrenalectomy, and frequently (8–35%) with the development of Nelson's syndrome, it should be used only as a last resort after pituitary surgery, irradiation, and pharmacological therapy have all failed.[15] Although primary irradiation of the pituitary gland can eventually produce remission in 50–80% of patients with Cushing's disease, hypercortisolism may not resolve for many months after pituitary irradiation.[2,53,69] In contrast, selective adenomectomy corrects the condition immediately.[2,15] We recommend transsphenoidal pituitary exploration as the treatment of first choice for most patients with Cushing's disease, reserving radiation therapy for patients who are either at extremely high surgical risk or harbor residual adenoma after transsphenoidal surgery. In consenting adults, if no adenoma is observed during surgical exploration, then total hypophysectomy can be performed because the result is usually a cure. For children in whom exploration shows no evidence of an adenoma, postoperative irradiation, drug therapy, or adrenalectomy is recommended.[54]

Recurrence. Because patients can develop recurrence of Cushing's disease as late as 8 years after surgery, patients in clinical remission should have periodic endocrinologic reevaluations. The anatomic reasons for the failure of initial operations include extrasellar extension and invasion of the cavernous sinus. Reoperation is a safe and effective treatment for many recurrent tumors; the majority of patients derive benefit and many are cured,[54] sometimes with the addition of chemotherapy. Medical management of recurrent tumors is effective in the long term only in patients with prolactinomas who tolerate, and whose tumors are sensitive to, bromocriptine mesylate.

Nelson's Syndrome

Nelson's syndrome occurs in 20–40% of patients who undergo bilateral adrenalectomy, once the major treatment for Cushing's disease despite its significant drawbacks. The tumors causing Nelson's syndrome are much more likely to be large and invasive than are those causing Cushing's disease[87] and while in many patients the tumor is indolent, in a significant minority it is aggressive or frankly malignant and directly causes death.[87] The intervals between adrenalectomy and transsphenoidal surgery for Nelson's syndrome range from a few months to more than two decades, reflecting the unpredictable behavior of these tumors.

Clinical Presentation. Because of the large size and invasiveness of tumors causing Nelson's syndrome, headaches and visual disturbances are more common than in association with Cushing's disease. The documentation of extremely high plasma ACTH values, often several thousand picograms per milliliter, is sufficient to make the diagnosis, which can be corroborated by MR imaging of the sella. Hyperpigmentation is the hallmark of Nelson's syndrome.[87]

Diagnosis. The diagnosis of Nelson's syndrome is straightforward. The loss of cortisol inhibition caused by adrenalectomy allows the pituitary gland to secrete very large amounts of ACTH and may promote rapid growth of the adenoma. Cutaneous melanocytes are stimulated by the high levels of ACTH to produce the characteristic hyperpigmentation of Nelson's syndrome. The development of hyperpigmentation in a patient known to have undergone adrenalectomy for Cushing's syndrome is diagnostic of Nelson's syndrome.[87]

Treatment. In cases of Nelson's syndrome, the prognosis is guarded and generally unfavorable,[55] but transsphenoidal surgery offers the best hope of controlling the disease. Craniotomy should be used only for patients in whom large parasellar or suprasellar extension or an unusually small sella turcica precludes adequate transsphenoidal access. Radiation therapy and drug therapy are important adjuvant therapies because most patients who develop the syndrome usually have large and invasive tumors with extrasellar extension by the time they come for treatment, and complete removal of the tumor is possible in fewer than 30%. Heavy-particle irradiation is more effective than conventional irradiation, but heavy-particle irradiation is suitable only for adenomas confined to the sella. Fortunately, there has been a profound reduction in the incidence of Nelson's syndrome as transsphenoidal microsurgery has replaced bilateral adrenalectomy as the primary treatment for Cushing's disease.[87]

Endocrine-Inactive Pituitary Neoplasms

Etiology and Epidemiology

Endocrine-inactive adenomas, less precisely termed nonfunctioning or nonsecreting pituitary adenomas, constitute about 25% of all clinically apparent pituitary neoplasms.[37] Although these adenomas are generally associated with the older population (mean age in both sexes, 52 years),[24] at least one study suggests that their prevalence among younger men and women may be underestimated.[60]

Pathology

Endocrine-inactive adenomas were formerly classified as *chromophobic* adenomas but this term is not useful because the agranular light microscopic appearance of the tumors is misleading—ultrastructural studies show secretory granules in "chromophobic" adenomas and sensitive radioimmunoassays show that as many as 50% of them produce a hormone.[56,84] The pituitary glycoprotein hormone alpha subunit has been demonstrated in many endocrine-inactive, undifferentiated pituitary adenomas.[30,47,48,60] It now appears likely that endocrine-inactive pituitary adenomas that are not clinically evident release small quantities of hormones, primarily gonadotrophins, and it is possible that the hormone release occurs from only a small percentage of the tumor cells.[89] Excessive secretion of gonadotrophins and/or their subunits by these adenomas is rare and may occur primarily in men. Women, however, may show an elevated ratio of alpha subunit to luteinizing hormone and follicle-stimulating hormone, which may be useful in making a diagnosis.[42] The null cell adenoma, characterized by Kovacs and colleagues appears now to be the only truly nonsecreting tumor, but it too may have an as yet unidentified secretory product.[40]

Clinical Presentation

Endocrine-inactive adenomas have an insidious clinical progression[19] and by the time patients present for a diagnosis, the tumor is usually a macroadenoma producing symptoms caused by mass effect or hypopituitarism.[37] The most frequent symptoms are headache and visual disturbances caused by the adenoma's encroachment on the visual pathway.[20,24]

Diagnosis

Both thin-section MR imaging and high-resolution computerized tomography detect the macroadenomas accurately,[73] but MR imaging is the superior technique because of the greater soft-tissue contrast it provides, permitting clear visualization of the optic chiasm, optic nerves, cavernous sinuses, and carotid arteries.[33,73] Visual evoked potential evaluations reliably assess the function of the intracranial visual pathways and can be more sensitive than conventional methods of examination.[32]

Patients suspected of having an endocrine-inactive adenoma should undergo MR imaging, assessment of pituitary hormone function, and a determination of the pituitary glycoprotein hormone alpha-subunit in serum.[37] Elevated or high-normal gonadotrophin levels suggest an underlying gonadotrophic adenoma, although pituitary adenomas secreting gonadotrophins are often diagnosed as endocrine-inactive adenomas because of the clinical findings; for example, a middle-aged woman experiencing visual disturbances.[18] Some patients have a tumor producing no hormone or a tumor with defects in hormone biosynthesis or processing that prevent detectable hormone hypersecretion. In a few patients, the endocrine-inactive pituitary adenoma interferes with the pituitary stalk and produces a moderate hyperprolactinemia (basal levels 50–100 ng/ml) as a result of a "stalk section effect."

Treatment

An endocrine-inactive tumor in an asymptomatic patient with unimpaired pituitary function should, with some exceptions, be left alone and its course followed with serial MR images.[87] For patients with symptomatic endocrine-inactive adenomas, transsphenoidal surgery with microscopic surgical technique is the preferred treatment. In some patients, transsphenoidal surgery improves pituitary function,[1,4,37,87] but even in patients with very large or giant adenomas, it permits rapid and satisfactory decompression of the optic nerves and chiasm, averts significant pituitary insufficiency in the majority of cases,[58] is well tolerated by elderly patients,[17] and is associated with low morbidity, mortality,[58] and recurrence rates.

Conventional radiation therapy is often recommended when there is evidence of residual tumor postoperatively and/or extensive extrasellar extension preoperatively,[37] but an increasing proportion of endocrine-inactive tumors is being followed, rather than referred for irradiation, after surgery because of gross total removal and potential cure.

Medical treatment of endocrine-inactive adenomas with bromocriptine, whether preoperatively or as primary therapy, is a matter of controversy. There are isolated cases in which bromocriptine is well tolerated and produces good to impressive results.[18,23] The consensus is at present, however, that with the possible exception of pituitary adenomas showing recent growth, bromocriptine is unlikely to cause growth arrest or reduce the size of endocrine-inactive pituitary adenomas.[12,81]

References

1. Adams, C. B.: The management of pituitary tumours and post-operative visual deterioration. Acta Neurochir. (Wien), 94:103, 1988.

2. Ahmed, S. R., Shalet, S. M., Beardwell, C. G., and Sutton, M. L.: Treatment of Cushing's disease with low dose radiation therapy. Br. Med. J., 289:643, 1984.
3. Aloia, J. F., Field, R. A., and Kramer, S.: Treatment of acromegaly. Arch. Intern. Med., 131:509, 1973.
4. Arafah, B. M.: Reversible hypopituitarism in patients with large nonfunctioning pituitary adenomas. J. Clin. Endocrinol. Metab., 62:1173, 1986.
5. Arosio, M., Giovanelli, M. A., Riva, E., Nava, C., Ambrosi, B., and Faglia, G.: Clinical use of pre- and postsurgical evaluation of abnormal GH responses in acromegaly. J. Neurosurg., 59:402, 1983.
6. Balagura, S., Derome, P., and Guiot, G.: Acromegaly: analysis of 132 cases treated surgically. Neurosurgery, 8:413, 1981.
7. Barrow, D. L., Mizuno, J., and Tindall, G. T.: Management of prolactinomas associated with very high serum prolactin levels. J. Neurosurg., 68:554, 1988.
8. Baskin, D. S., Boggan, J. E., and Wilson, C. B.: Transsphenoidal microsurgical removal of growth hormone-secreting pituitary adenomas. A review of 137 cases. J. Neurosurg., 56:634, 1982.
9. Baskin, D. S., and Wilson, C. B.: Bromocriptine treatment of pituitary adenomas. Neurosurgery, 8:741, 1981.
10. Belchetz, P. E., Carty, A., Clearkin, L. G., Davis, J. C., Jeffreys, R. V., and Rae, P. G.: Failure of prophylactic surgery to avert massive pituitary expansion in pregnancy. Clin. Endocrinol., 25:325, 1986.
11. Bergh, T., Nillius, S. J., and Wide, L.: Clinical course and outcome of pregnancies in amenorrhoeic women with hyperprolactinaemia and pituitary tumors. Br. Med. J., 1:875, 1978.
12. Bevan, J. S., Adams, C. B., Burke, C. W., Morton, K. E., Molyneux, A. J., Moore, R. A., and Esiri, M. M.: Factors in the outcome of transsphenoidal surgery for prolactinoma and non-functioning pituitary tumour, including pre-operative bromocriptine therapy. Clin. Endocrinol., 26:541, 1987.
13. Boggan, J. E., Tyrrell, J. B., and Wilson, C. B.: Transsphenoidal microsurgical management of Cushing's disease. Report of 100 cases. J. Neurosurg., 59:195, 1983.
14. Burch, W.: A survey of results with transsphenoidal surgery in Cushing's disease (letter). N. Engl. J. Med., 308:103, 1983.
15. Burch, W. M.: Cushing's disease. A review. Arch. Intern. Med., 145:1106, 1985.
16. Chandler, W. F., Schteingart, D. E., Lloyd, R. V., McKeever, P. E., and Ibarra-Perez, G.: Surgical treatment of Cushing's disease. J. Neurosurg., 66:204, 1987.
17. Cohen, D. L., Bevan, J. S., and Adams, C. B.: The presentation and management of pituitary tumours in the elderly. Age Ageing, 18:247, 1989.
18. Comtois, R., Bouchard, J., and Robert, F.: Hypersecretion of gonadotropins by a pituitary adenoma: pituitary dynamic studies and treatment with bromocriptine in one patient. Fertil. Steril., 52:569, 1989.
19. Dietel, P., Heberling, H. J., Lohmann, D., and Brachmann, J.: (Clinical symptoms and duration of anamnesis in patients with hypophyseal tumors.) Z. Gesamte. Inn. Med., 44:293, 1989.
20. Eitel, B.: (Ambulatory diagnosis and outpatient management of patients with hypophyseal adenomas.) Z. Gesamte. Inn. Med., 42:321, 1987.
21. Evans, H. M., Briggs, J. H., and Dixon, J. S.: The Physiology and Chemistry of Growth Hormone. *In* The Pituitary Gland, Vol. 1. Edited by G. W. Harris, and B. T. Donovan, Berkeley/Los Angeles, University of California Press, 1966, Vol. 1, p. 439.
22. Forbes, A. P., Henneman, P. H., Griswold, G. C., et al.: Syndrome characterized by galactorrhea, amenorrhea and low urinary FSH: comparison with acromegaly and normal lactation. J. Clin. Endocrinol. Metab., 14:265, 1954.
23. Garcia-Luna, P. O., Leal-Cerro, A., Pereira, J. L., Montero, C., Acosta, D., Trujillo, F., Mazuelos, C., and Astorga, R.: Rapid improvement of visual defects with parenteral depot-bromocriptine in a patient with a non-functioning pituitary adenoma. Horm. Res., 32:183, 1989.
24. Giorgis, B., Campiche, R., Burckhardt, P., and Gomez, F.: (Diagnosis, treatment and course of hypophyseal tumors.) Retrospective study of 123 cases. Schweiz. Med. Wochenschr., 116:1431, 1986.
25. Gramegna, A. G.: Un cas d'acromégalie traité par la radiothérapie. Rev. Neurol., 17:15, 1909.
26. Hardy, J.: Transsphenoidal Surgery of Hypersecreting Pituitary Tumors. *In* Diagnosis and Treatment of Pituitary Tumors. Proceedings of a conference sponsored jointly by the National Institute of Child Health and Human Development and the National Cancer Institute, January 15–17, 1973. International Congress Series, No. 303. Edited by P. O. Kohler, and G. T. Ross. Amsterdam, Excerpta Medica, 1973, pp. 179–194.
27. Hardy, J.: Microsurgery of Pituitary Disorders. *In* Functioning Pituitary Adenoma and Bromocriptine: Proceedings of the Second Workshop on Pituitary Tumors. Edited by K. Sano, K. Takakura, T. Fukushima, et al. Tokyo, Sandoz Pharmaceuticals, 1981, pp. 41–46.
28. Hardy, J., Somma, M., and Vezina, J. L.: Treatment of Acromegaly: Radiation or Surgery? *In* Current Controversies in Neurosurgery. Edited by T. P. Morley. Philadelphia, W. B. Saunders, 1976, pp. 377–391.
29. Hardy, J., and Vezina, J. L.: Transsphenoidal Neurosurgery of Intracranial Neoplasm. *In* Neoplasia in the Nervous System. Advances in Neurology series, Vol. 15. Edited by R. A. Thompson, and J. R. Green. New York, Raven Press, 1976, pp. 261–274.
30. Heitz, P. U., Landolt, A. M., Zenklusen, H. R., Kasper, M., Reubi, J. C., Oberholzer, M., and Roth, J.: Immunocytochemistry of pituitary tumors. J. Histochem. Cytochem., 35:1005, 1987.
31. Herman, V., Fagin, J., Gonsky, R., Kovacs, K., and Melmed, S.: Clonal origin of pituitary adenomas. J. Clin. Endocrinol. Metab., 71:1427, 1990.
32. Holder, G. E., and Bullock, P. R.: Visual evoked potentials in the assessment of patients with non-functioning chromophobe adenomas. J. Neurol. Neurosurg. Psychiatry, 52:31, 1989.
33. Juliani, G., Avataneo, T., Potenzoni, F., and Sorrentino, T.: (CT and MR compared in the study of hypophysis.) Radiol. Med. (Torino), 77:51, 1989.
34. Kapcala, L. P., Molitch, M. E., Post, K. D., Biller, B. J., Prager, R. J., Jackson, I. M., and Reichlin, S.: Galactorrhea, oligo/amenorrhea, and hyperprolactinemia in patients with craniopharyngiomas. J. Clin. Endocrinol. Metab., 51:798, 1980.
35. Kjellberg, R. N., Shintani, A., Frantz, A. G., and Kliman, B.: Proton-beam therapy in acromegaly. N. Engl. J. Med., 278:689, 1968.
36. Klibanski, A.: Editorial: further evidence for a somatic mutation theory in the pathogenesis of human pituitary tumors. J. Clin. Endocrinol. Metab., 71:1415A, 1990.
37. Klibanski, A.: Nonsecreting pituitary tumors. Endocrinol. Metab. Clin. North. Am., 16:793, 1987.
38. Klibanski, A., Neer, R. M., Beitinis, I. Z., Ridgeway, E. C., Zervas, N. T., and McArthur, J. W.: Decreased bone density in hyperprolactinemic women. N. Engl. J. Med., 303:1511, 1980.
39. Kovacs, K., Horvath, E., and Ezrin, C.: Pituitary adenomas. Pathol. Annu., 12 Pt 2:341, 1977.
40. Kovacs, K., Horvath, E., Ryan, N., and Ezrin, C.: Null cell adenoma of the human pituitary. Virchows Arch. (Pathol. Anat.), 387:165, 1980.
41. Kupersmith, M. J., Kleinberg, D., Warren, F. A., Budzilovitch, G., and Cooper, P.: Growth of prolactinoma despite lowering of serum prolactin by bromocriptine. Neurosurgery, 24:417, 1989.
42. Kwekkeboom, D. J., de Jong, F. H., and Lamberts, S. W.: Gonadotropin release by clinically nonfunctioning and gonadotroph pituitary adenomas in vivo and in vitro: Relation to sex and effects of thyrotropin-releasing hormone, gonadotropin-releasing hormone, and bromocriptine. J. Clin. Endocrinol. Metab., 68:1128, 1989.
43. Lamberg, B. A., Kivikangas, V., Vartianen, J., Raitta, C., and Pelkonen, R.: Conventional pituitary irradiation in acromegaly. Effect on growth hormone and TSH secretion. Acta Endocrinol. (Copenh.), 82:267, 1976.
44. Lamberts, S. W., de Lange, S. A., and Stefanko, S. Z.: Adrenocorticotropin-secreting pituitary adenomas originate from the anterior or the intermediate lobe in Cushing's disease: differences in the regulation of hormone secretion. J. Clin. Endocrinol. Metab., 54:286, 1982.
45. Landis, C. A., Harsh, G., Lyons, J., Davis, R. L., McCormick, F., and Bourne, H. R.: Clinical characteristics of acromegalic patients whose pituitary tumors contain mutant G_s protein. J. Clin. Endocrinol. Metab., 71:1416-1420, 1990.
46. Landolt, A. M.: Ultrastructure of human sella tumors. Correlations of clinical findings and morphology. Acta Neurochir. (Wien), 22(Suppl.):1, 1975.
47. Landolt, A. M. and Heitz, P. U.: Alpha-subunit-producing pituitary adenomas. Immunocytochemical and ultrastructural studies. Virchows Arch., 409(A):417, 1986.
48. Landolt, A. M., Heitz, P. U., and Zenklusen, H. R.: Production of the alpha-subunit of glycoprotein hormones by pituitary adenomas. Pathol. Res. Pract., 183:610, 1988.
49. Landolt, A. M., Shibata, T., and Kleihues, P.: Growth rate of human pituitary adenomas. J. Neurosurg., 67:803, 1987.
50. Landolt, A. M., and Wilson, C. B.: Tumors of the Sella and Parasellar Area in Adults. *In* Neurological Surgery: A Comprehensive Reference Guide to the Diagnosis and Treatment of Neurosurgical Problems, 2nd Edition. Edited by J. R. Youmans. Philadelphia, W. B. Saunders, 1982, Vol. 5, pp. 3107–3162.
51. Laws, E. R., Ebersold, M. J., Piepgras, D. G., et al: The Results of Transsphenoidal Surgery in Specific Clinical Entities. *In* Management of Pituitary Adenomas and Related Lesions with Emphasis on Transsphenoidal Microsurgery. Edited by E. R. Laws, R. V. Randall, E. B. Kern, et al. New York, Appleton-Century-Crofts, 1982, pp. 277–305.
52. Laws, E. R., Jr., Piepgras, D. G., Randall, R. V., and Abboud, C. F.: Neurosurgical management of acromegaly. Results in 82 patients treated between 1972 and 1977. J. Neurosurg., 50:454, 1979.
53. Linfoot, J. A.: Heavy Ion Therapy: Alpha Particle Therapy of Pituitary Tumors. *In* Recent Advances in the Diagnosis and Treatment of Pituitary Tumors. Edited by J. A. Linfoot. New York, Raven Press, 1979, pp. 245–267.
54. Mampalam, T. J., Tyrrell, J. B., and Wilson, C. B.: Transsphenoidal microsurgery for Cushing disease. A report of 216 cases. Ann. Intern. Med., 109:487, 1988.
55. Mampalam, T. J., and Wilson, C. B.: ACTH-Secreting Tumors, Cushing's Disease, and Nelson's Syndrome. *In* Current Therapy in Neurological Surgery–2. Edited by D. M. Long. Toronto/Philadelphia, B. C. Decker, 1989, pp. 131–135.
56. McCormick, W. F., and Halmi, N. S.: Absence of chromophobe adenomas from a large series of pituitary tumors. Arch. Pathol., 92:231, 1971.
57. McKeever, P. E., Koppleman, M. C., Metcalf, D., Quindlen, E., Kornblith, P. L., Strott, C. A., Howard, R., and Smith, B. H.: Refractory Cushing's disease caused by multinodular ACTH-cell hyperplasia. J. Neuropathol. Exp. Neurol., 41:490, 1982.
58. Mohr, G., Hardy, J., Comtois, R., and Beauregard, H.: Surgical management of giant pituitary adenomas. Can. J. Neurol. Sci., 17:62, 1990.
59. Newton, D. R., Dillon, W. P., Norman, D., Newton, T. H., and Wilson, C. B.: Gd-DTPA-enhanced MR imaging of pituitary adenomas. A.J.N.R., 10:949, 1989.
60. Oppenheim, D. S., Kana, A. R., Sangha, J. S., and Klibanski, A.: Prevalence of alpha-subunit hypersecretion in patients with pituitary tumors: clinically nonfunctioning and somatotroph adenomas. J. Clin. Endocrinol. Metab., 70:859, 1990.
61. Oppizzi, G., Petroncini, M. M., Dallabonzana, D., Cozzi, R., Verde, G., Chiodini, P. G., and Luizzi, A.: Relationship between somatomedin-C and growth hormone levels in acromegaly: Basal and dynamic evaluation. J. Clin. Endocrinol. Metab., 63:1348, 1986.
62. Richards, A. M., Bullock, M. R., Teasdale, G. M., Thomson, J. A., and Khan, M. I.: Fertility and pregnancy after operation for a prolactinoma. Br. J. Obstet. Gynaecol., 93:495, 1986.
63. Ross, D. A., and Wilson, C. B.: Results of transsphenoidal microsurgery for growth hormone-secreting pituitary adenoma in a series of 214 patients. J. Neurosurg., 68:854, 1988.
64. Roth, J., Glick, S. M., Cuatrecasas, P., and Hollander, C. S.: Acromegaly and other disorders of growth hormone secretion. Combined clinical staff conference at the National Institutes of Health. Ann. Intern. Med., 66:760, 1967.
65. Roth, J., Gorden, P., and Brace, K.: Efficacy of conventional pituitary irradiation in acromegaly. N. Engl. J. Med., 282:1385, 1970.
66. Salassa, R. M., Laws, E. R., Jr., Carpenter, P. C., and Northcutt, R. C.: Transsphenoidal removal of pituitary microadenoma in Cushing's disease. Mayo Clin. Proc., 53:24, 1978.
67. Schlechte, J., el-Khoury, G., Kathol., M., and Walkner, L.: Forearm and vertebral bone mineral in treated and untreated hyperprolactinemic amenorrhea. J. Clin. Endocrinol. Metab., 64:1021, 1987.
68. Schteingart, D. E.: Cushing's syndrome. Endocrinol. Metab. Clin. North Am., 18:311, 1989.
69. Sheline, G. E.: Conventional Radiation Therapy in the Treatment of Pituitary Tumors. *In* Clinical Management of Pituitary Disorders. Seminars in Neurological Surgery series. Edited by G. T. Tindall, and W. F. Collins. New York, Raven Press, 1979, pp. 287–314.
70. Shewchuk, A. B., Adamson, G. D., Lessard, P., and Ezrin, C.: The effect of pregnancy on suspected pituitary adenomas after conservative management of ovulation defects associated with galactorrhea. Am. J. Obstet. Gynecol., 136:659, 1980.
71. Spada, A., Arosio, M., Bochicchio, D., Bazzoni, N., Vallar, L., Bassetti, M., and Faglia, G.: Clinical, biochemical, and morphological correlates in patients bearing growth

hormone-secreting pituitary tumors with or without constitutively active adenylyl cyclase. J. Clin. Endocrinol. Metab., 71:1421, 1990.

72. Spinas, G. A., Zapf, J., Landolt, A. M., Stuckmann, G., and Froesch, E. R.: Pre-operative treatment of 5 acromegalics with a somatostatin analogue: endocrine and clinical observations. Acta Endocrinol. (Copenh.), 114:249, 1987.

73. Stein, A. L., Levenick, M. N., and Kletzky, O. A.: Computed tomography versus magnetic resonance imaging for the evaluation of suspected pituitary adenomas. Obstet. Gynecol., 73:996, 1989.

74. Tagliaferri, M., Berselli, M. E., and Loli, P.: Transsphenoidal microsurgery for Cushing's disease. Acta Endocrinol. (Copenh.), 113:5, 1986.

75. Teasdale, G.: Surgical management of pituitary adenoma. Clin. Endocrinol. Metab., 12:789, 1983.

76. Thomas, J. P., and Richards, S. H.: Long term results of radical hypophysectomy for Cushing's disease. Clin. Endocrinol. (Oxf.), 19:629, 1983.

77. Tindall, G. T., and Tindall, S. C.: Transsphenoidal Surgery for Acromegaly: Long-Term Results in 50 Patients. In Secretory Tumors of the Pituitary Gland: Progress in Endocrine Research and Therapy, Vol. 1. Edited by P. McL. Black, N. T. Zervas, E. C. Ridgway, and J. B. Martin. New York, Raven Press, 1984, pp. 175–178.

78. Tucker, H. S., Grubb, S. R., Wigand, J. P., Watlington, C. O., Blackard, W. G., and Becker, D. P.: The treatment of acromegaly by transsphenoidal surgery. Arch. Intern. Med., 140:795, 1980.

79. U, H. S., Wilson, C. B., and Tyrrell, J. B.: Transsphenoidal microhypophysectomy in acromegaly. J. Neurosurg., 47:840, 1977.

80. Vallar, L., Spada, A., and Giannattasio, G.: Altered G_s and adenylate cyclase activity in human GH-secreting pituitary adenomas. Nature, 330:566-568, 1987.

81. van Schaardenburg, D., Roelfsema, F., van Seters, A. P., and Vielvoye, G. J.: Bromocriptine therapy for non-functioning pituitary adenoma. Clin. Endocrinol. (Oxf.), 30:475, 1989.

82. Wang, C., Lam, K. S., Ma, J. T., Chan, T., Liu, M. Y., and Yeung, R. T.: Long-term treatment of hyperprolactinaemia with bromocriptine: effect of drug withdrawal. Clin. Endocrinol. (Oxf.), 27:363, 1987.

83. Weiss, M. H., Wycoff, R. R., Yadley, R., Gott, P., and Feldon, S.: Bromocriptine treatment of prolactin-secreting tumors: surgical implications. Neurosurgery, 12:640, 1983.

84. Wilson, C. B.: Neurosurgical Management of Large and Invasive Pituitary Tumors. In Clinical Management of Pituitary Disorders. Seminars in Neurological Surgery series. Edited by G. T. Tindall, and W. F. Collins. New York, Raven Press, 1979, pp. 335–342.

85. Wilson, C. B.: Surgical Management of Endocrine-Active Pituitary Adenomas. In Oncology of the Nervous System. Edited by M. D. Walker (series volume in Cancer Treatment and Research. Edited by W. L. McGuire). Boston/The Hague/Dordrecht/Lancaster, Martinus Nijhoff Publishers, 1983, pp. 117–150.

86. Wilson, C. B.: A decade of pituitary microsurgery. The Herbert Olivecrona Lecture. J. Neurosurg., 61:814, 1984.

87. Wilson, C. B.: Role of surgery in the management of pituitary tumors. Neurosurg. Clin. North Am., 1:139, 1990.

88. Wright, A. D., Hill, D. M., Lowy, C., and Fraser, T. R.: Mortality in acromegaly. Q. J. Med., 39:1, 1970.

89. Yamada, S., Asa, S. L., Kovacs, K., Muller, P., and Smyth, H. S.: Analysis of hormone secretion by clinically nonfunctioning human pituitary adenomas using the reverse hemolytic plaque assay. J. Clin. Endocrinol. Metab., 68:73, 1989.

XXVI-2

Neoplasms of the Thyroid

Blake Cady

Introduction

Thyroid cancer has always elicited concern beyond its relative incidence and death rate because of its occurrence in children and young adults and the vagaries of its clinical behavior in different age groups. In 1992 there are expected to be only 12,500 cases in the United States of which only 1,000 will die of disease. Like many endocrine gland cancers thyroid carcinoma has an extremely variable time course and biological pattern, and a variety of separate pathological forms which lead to difficulty in understanding a common theme in the disease.

Incidence

Throughout the world autopsy studies of the thyroid gland demonstrate high incidences of microscopic foci of papillary carcinoma of the thyroid or other pathological varieties ranging in size from less than a millimeter to less than a centimeter. The incidence is partly related to the number of sections taken through the thyroid gland at pathological study; whole organ sections taken at frequent intervals throughout the gland illustrate incidence of such occult cancers ranging from 6% to over 30%. In survivors of the atomic bomb explosions in Japan the incidence in the exposed population was even higher. In other countries studies have shown almost as high a rate without known exposure to atomic radiation. In the U.S. the incidence of these microscopically defined occult cancers has ranged from 6–15% in various reports. This would indicate that there are at least 15 to over 30 million cases in the U.S. of such microscopic disease. The enor-

mous gap between that figure and the 12,500 cases of cancer reported throughout the country each year provide yet another source of confusion about the biological behavior of differentiated thyroid carcinoma. It should be recognized furthermore that a significant proportion of the 12,500 cases of thyroid cancer reported in tumor registries are incidentally discovered microscopic foci of papillary carcinoma in glands that were operated on for benign conditions. Thus the actual number of clinical thyroid cancers each year in the United States is probably less than 10,000 cases.

Epidemiology and Etiology

Up to about 1950 it was a common practice in this country to give low dose radiation therapy to children for a variety of benign head and neck conditions such as enlarged tonsils or adenoids, cutaneous acne, and an enlarged thymus seen on chest X-ray in infants with respiratory symptoms. These children, when followed, were found to have an increased incidence of thyroid carcinoma in glands removed for changes in the thyroid radioactive iodine scan or clinical nodules. In those patients operated on, almost 50% had a thyroid cancer; but only about one-half of those were clinical cancers (palpable nodule) while the other half were microscopic lesions similar to those discovered on routine autopsy studies. Thus, in this group of patients who received small amounts of radiation exposure to the immature thyroid gland, an apparent increased incidence of both occult and clinical thyroid cancers did occur. Such clinical cancers associated with radiation show no apparent difference in clinical or biological behavior from other thyroid cancers in young adults and children. The practice of radiation therapy for benign conditions in childhood has entirely disappeared in the past 30 years. Radiation associated cancers due to these exposures have virtually disappeared, since the median interval from radiation to appearance of the thyroid carcinoma ranged up to 25 years.

Throughout the world there is a relationship between iodine deficiency and thyroid carcinoma incidence. Areas of relative iodine deficiency have an increased number of thyroid cancers, an increased relative proportion of follicular carcinomas and a larger number of giant and spindle cell undifferentiated carcinomas of the thyroid gland. Thus geographic regions subject to endemic goiter may well have increased incidences of thyroid carcinoma with a different pattern of pathological varieties at presentation than occur in the U.S.

Only a few carcinomas of the thyroid following radioactive iodine administration have been reported. This probably relates to the large cellular and nuclear dose of radiation therapy that occurs with radioactive iodine in contrast to the low dose of radiation given externally in treatment of benign childhood conditions. Although at extremely low doses there seems to be a linear relationship between incidence of thyroid carcinoma and radiation dose, it is known that a peak risk of induction seems to occur at about 1200 cGy above which induced carcinomas seem to occur much less often. Because of the extremely high cellular doses given when therapeutic radioactive iodine is used, i.e., Graves disease, there is little induction of clinical cancer in such patients. Also there seems to be no increased risk of thyroid cancer after diagnostic radio-active scans. Whether the use of large doses of iodine following nuclear accidents that release largely radioactive isotopes of iodine is unproven and conjectural but may be logical. The major radioisotope contamination after the Three-Mile Island accident was radioactive iodine but the doses were not high. The practicality of having iodine solutions stored in every house in a geographic area around nuclear plants, when it cannot be predicted that radioiodine isotopes will be the primary contaminant seems unnecessary, considering the low risk of eventual thyroid carcinoma and the fact that infants and children are the only ones apparently at risk for radiation induction by low dose radiation exposure. Nevertheless such a wholesale population iodine administration has been proposed.

Pathology

Thyroid carcinoma falls into two general types, differentiated and undifferentiated, and several uncommon specific types. The vast majority of thyroid carcinomas in the United States are differentiated, which consist of pure papillary, mixed papillary and follicular carcinoma (with varying proportions of each), pure follicular carcinoma (with some Hürthle cell variants) and some poorly differentiated follicular forms. Undifferentiated carcinomas generally consist of spindle and giant cell forms but small cell varieties do occur. Thyroid lymphoma is an uncommon but well recognized entity of the non-Hodgkin's type. Some small cell thyroid cancers seen in past decades, when studied by newer immunohistochemical techniques, have been shown to be thyroid lymphoma.

Some rare types such as squamous cell carcinoma and sarcoma of the thyroid do occur. Metastatic cancers to the thyroid are not uncommon, with the common primary sites being renal, lung or breast carcinomas or melanoma. A variety of other primary cancers can metastasize to the thyroid gland, however. Finally, medullary carcinoma of the thyroid is technically not a thyroid cell carcinoma but arises from the parafollicular C-cells (ultimo-branchial bodies) which migrate embryologically to lie in the anatomic thyroid gland. Medullary carcinoma occurs in both sporadic and familial forms which can be distinguished not only by family histories but by pathological features (see XXVI-4).

Differentiated Thyroid Carcinoma

Papillary and Mixed Papillary and Follicular Forms

It has been shown in studies by us[6] and by others[7] that the clinical behavior of thyroid carcinomas that have any element of papillary histologic features is similar (Figure XXVI-2-1). This is in contra-distinction to those differentiated thyroid carcinomas which are of pure follicular type (Figure XXVI-2-2). The particular clinical features of all forms of papillary carcinoma (regardless of the proportion of follicular or papillary elements) include a high incidence of multifocality

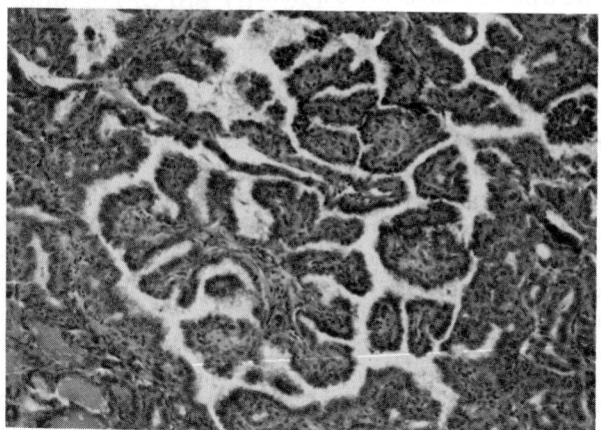

Figure XXVI-2-1. Papillary carcinoma.

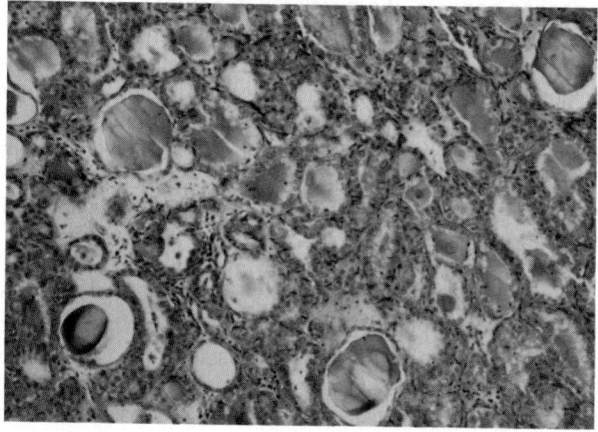

Figure XXVI-2-2. Follicular carcinoma.

Clinical Presentation

The majority of thyroid carcinomas and benign thyroid neoplasms present as a mass in the thyroid, ordinarily painless. In young patients, 25% of cases present initially as a palpable lymph node metastasis in the cervical area. Thus, marked lymphadenopathy in young adults and children should arouse suspicion of thyroid carcinoma even when a mass in the thyroid itself is not palpable. In about 10% of older patients the first manifestation is either a regional lymph node metastasis or rarely a distant metastasis. Older patients almost always have a palpable thyroid abnormality on careful inspection. While thyroid carcinoma is usually thought to present as a solitary thyroid mass, a clinically multinodular goiter with a dominant nodule or a nodule that grows rapidly on a background of an enlarged gland is a common clinical presentation of thyroid carcinoma. In the past, 75% of thyroid carcinomas occurred in women but in more recent years the proportion in men has steadily increased so that in older patients 50% of thyroid cancers are now found in men. Younger patients and children continue to display a marked female predominance of roughly 4:1. Because of the frequency of benign thyroid nodules in the population and the rarity of clinical thyroid cancers, the vast majority of thyroid nodules clinically detected will prove to be benign. Those lesions which arouse concern of cancer clinically display progressive growth, unusual hardness, fixation, accompanying hoarseness, concomitant lymph node metastases and symptoms of dysphagia or stridor. Of course, any solitary nodule, any nodule displaying the characteristics above, or any prominent nodule deserves a needle biopsy if concern about cancer is present.

Anaplastic carcinomas tend to occur in older patients, frequently with a background of a chronically enlarged thyroid presumed to be an adenomatous goiter. Lymphomas also occur in an older population and are seldom seen below the age of 40.

Diagnostic Studies

Traditionally, diagnostic studies of thyroid masses have included preliminary anatomic and functional evaluation of the thyroid gland to select patients at high risk for carcinoma. In the last decade it has become increasingly apparent that the most valuable initial diagnostic study of thyroid gland nodules or lymph node metastases in the neck is a fine needle aspiration for cytology. It has been proposed by numerous authors recently, and we strongly agree, that the most efficient, cost effective and accurate diagnostic workup of a thyroid nodule is initial fine needle aspiration. Needle aspiration cytology and biopsy of the thyroid gland can separate benign lesions from suspicious and malignant lesions with an extremely high degree of accuracy. All suspicious or malignant lesions should have an operative removal of the mass in question. Hashimoto's thyroiditis, nonspecific thyroiditis or adenomatous goiter are accurately portrayed by aspiration cytology. Interpretation of aspiration cytology as "insufficient material" should lead to a repeat needle biopsy. In the largest and most thoroughly analyzed series of needle cytologies of the thyroid, Mayo Clinic authors reported only three cases of cancer in over 400 patients initially diagnosed as benign by needle aspiration, all of whom had the nodules removed surgically. Thus the false negative rate of needle aspiration cytology was less than 1%.

Histologic and cellular details of endocrine tumors do not establish the diagnosis of carcinoma. Thus aspiration cytology of the thyroid that reveals follicular cells cannot accurately separate follicular adenomas from follicular adenocarcinomas, or even from follicular nodules in an adenomatous goiter. Extensive pathological sampling of the pseudocapsule around a follicular lesion may be required to discover capsular penetration by follicular cells which defines follicular adenocarcinoma. Fine needle aspiration of a nodule cannot be as accurate. Reports in the literature that allude to the accurate separation of follicular adenoma from follicular adenocarcinoma by needle aspiration should be viewed with great skepticism. Thus, cytology that is read as microfollicular pattern, follicular neoplasm or suspicious should all be operated upon for final definition of a follicular lesion. In contrast, most papillary carcinomas can be accurately be diagnosed as malignant by fine needle aspiration cytology because of the characteristic "Orphan Annie" (Figure XXVI-2-5) nuclei and further define or illustrate cellular features which usually are definitive in papillary carcinoma of the thyroid. Anaplastic, metastatic, and medullary carcinomas of the thyroid can also be accurately diagnosed by needle aspiration. Needle aspiration cytology of a neck node is highly accurate in diagnosing thyroid carcinoma of either papillary or follicular variants. Open biopsy of lymph nodes in the neck should never be performed without first attempting needle aspiration cytology.

The technique of fine needle aspiration of thyroid nodules is simple, uncomplicated, virtually devoid of complications and relatively easily taught and mastered. The thyroid nodule is held in the fingers of the left hand and a needle is introduced through a tiny skin wheal of anesthesia and into the thyroid nodule with the right hand. The location of the tip of the needle can be accurately surmised by the palpating fingers of the left hand. Once in place vigorous vacuum is created by a one handed syringe holder and the needle moved back and forth over a range of one centimeter or so within the palpable nodule. Before withdrawing the needle

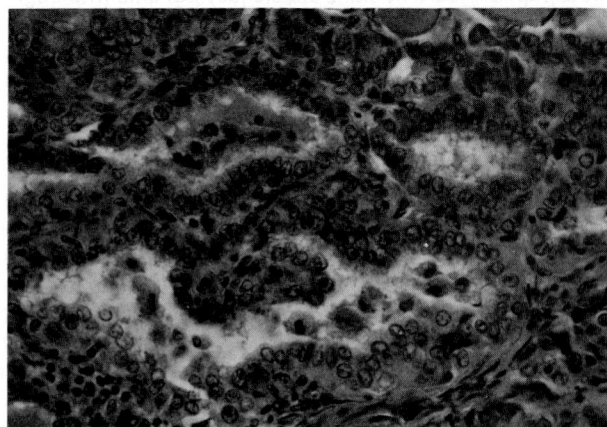

Figure XXVI-2-5. "Orphan Annie nuclei."

the syringe plunger is released eliminating the vacuum. The cellular material is then squirted onto slides, smeared as a hematology preparation and dropped promptly into fixative usually of alcoholic type as with Papanicolaou smears.

In evaluating thyroid nodules, a cytology report of insufficient material should lead to repeated aspiration, and a malignant or suspicious cytology should lead to thyroid surgery.[3] A cytology diagnosis of benign cells might then lead to further studies of anatomy or function of the thyroid gland with reassurance that the process is not cancer. Only after obtaining a fine needle aspiration cytology should other anatomic or functional studies of the thyroid gland be performed in the initial evaluation of a thyroid nodule, however. Other thyroid conditions obviously may lead to a different diagnostic sequence, but when a thyroid nodule is the clinical presentation and concern for cancer one of the primary concerns, aspiration should be the initial step. Since a thyroid cyst would be diagnosed by initial needle aspiration, ultrasound has little use. Thyroid cyst aspiration fluid should always be submitted to cytologic evaluation, however, since papillary carcinoma of the thyroid occasionally presents as a cystic lesion. Ultrasound can help diagnose a multinodular gland and may be utilized after thyroid needle aspiration.

Radioactive iodine scans and technetium scans of the thyroid gland are generally not helpful when evaluating a thyroid nodule for cancer since carcinomas and benign nodules are found to have similar frequencies of warm, cool, hot and indeterminate radionuclide uptake.

In the past it was sometimes the practice to attempt separation of suspicious and nonsuspicious nodules in the thyroid by a course of thyroid hormone for TSH suppression and evaluation of the thyroid nodule. Since some cancers respond to TSH suppression and since thyroid hormone used this way has been found to be no more effective than placebo in achieving a reduction of nodule size, this technique currently should be abandoned. Such an indirect evaluation of nodules cannot compete in any way with the direct evaluation of nodules by needle aspiration cytology in the differential diagnosis of the thyroid nodule. There still may be a role for such treatment once a needle aspiration cytology has been obtained and the nodule found not to be suspicious or requiring removal surgically.

Thyroid function tests are of no help in evaluating thyroid nodules for suspicion of carcinoma since thyroid carcinoma does not alter thyroid functional capacity. Only in the situation of extensive thyroid gland destruction from anaplastic carcinoma or lymphoma is thyroid insufficiency found as a manifestation of thyroid carcinoma.

In the presence of metastatic disease to the thyroid, other diagnostic studies are usually necessary to assess the extent of metastasis elsewhere. Magnetic resonance imaging or computerized tomographic scans of the thyroid gland itself are of little use in the ordinary differentiated thyroid carcinoma. They may provide invaluable help, however, in evaluating the unlikely possibility of resection in an anaplastic carcinoma or lymphoma or rare forms of thyroid carcinoma and should probably be reserved for such cases. All other thyroid carcinomas require exploration and resection, if at all possible, regardless of findings by imaging techniques.

Biologic Behavior of Differentiated Thyroid Carcinoma

Several recent studies have documented the critical biological features of differentiated thyroid carcinoma and have developed risk group assessments usually based on age, size, grade, presence of metastases, and extent of the primary thyroid carcinoma.[3,5,13] These prognostic scoring systems clearly illustrate that the vast majority of differentiated thyroid carcinomas fall into a low risk group with a mortality expectation of less than 2%. This low risk applies whether the cancers are papillary, mixed papillary follicular or follicular in pathological type. Follicular adenocarcinoma and papillary adenocarcinoma of the thyroid have distinctive and separable patterns of behavior but their overall prognosis is not governed by that pathological distinction as documented by numerous studies.[6,10]

In our risk group definition, low risk patients are men 40 years of age and younger, women 50 years of age and younger without distant metastases, and older patients whose carcinoma, if follicular, does not extend beyond the thyroid gland capsule, and is less than 5 cms in diameter. This "AMES" categorization (Age, Metastases, Extent and Size) corresponds closely to the "AGES" risk category (Age, Grade, Extent and Size) developed by the Mayo Clinic.[13] In our AMES prognostic scoring system, 89% of patients in the years between 1960 and 1980 were a low risk group with a death rate of only 1.8% at a median followup of 13 years.[3] The high risk AMES patients constituted 11% of the series but had a death rate of 46%. The ratio of death rates of 1:26 illustrates the power of this AMES prognostic scoring system. Thus, an easily definable clinical prognostic scoring system can enable the surgeon at the operating table to categorize easily the patient as at low risk or high risk of death from the differentiated thyroid adenocarcinoma. This assessment is critical in selecting an appropriate operative procedure, in counseling the patient, for advising on overall risk, for developing an overall therapeutic plan and for organizing a followup scheme after initial treatment.

The AMES prognostic scoring system applies to both papillary and follicular differentiated thyroid carcinomas without regard to the presence of lymph node metastases since they do not influence overall prognosis. Recent studies of the use of DNA histograms in evaluating the biological behavior and aggressiveness of thyroid carcinomas have been reported.[8] This field is still under investigation and no reliance should be placed on the use of DNA histograms at the present time. This is particularly true when realizing the accuracy reproducibility, and simplicity of the prognostic scoring groups mentioned. The DNA histograms reported are not as accurate in predicting biological outcome and aggressiveness of disease as the clinical scoring systems, and therefore, much further work needs to be done in this area. In particular, reports of differential DNA histograms in benign follicular adenoma and follicular adenocarcinomas need to be viewed with some skepticism since it is difficult even under the microscope to predict and define the technical separation of benign follicular adenoma from minor capsular invasion follicular adenocarcinoma.

Treatment of Differentiated Thyroid Carcinoma

Surgical removal is the mainstay of the treatment of differentiated thyroid carcinoma. In the last several decades the median diameter of thyroid carcinomas at presentation has fallen to 2 cms or less in almost two-thirds of cases. Therefore, bilateral thyroid operations are seldom necessary for the sake of removing the presenting mass of the differentiated thyroid carcinoma itself. The standard operation today is total thyroid lobectomy with isthmus removal. Less than a total thyroid lobectomy may be performed in certain situations such as small anterior or medially placed or isthmus thyroid carcinomas.

The major controversy today in surgery of differentiated thyroid carcinoma involves the proponents of total thyroidectomy as standard treatment for all lesions, in contrast to those authors who recommend less than a total thyroidectomy as standard surgical treatment. This controversy centers around the alleged advantages of the total removal of the thyroid gland. These advantages are stated to be: the frequent multifocality of papillary carcinoma of the thyroid, the reduced need for radioactive iodine therapy to eliminate normal residual thyroid gland when less than a total thyroidectomy is performed, the inability to use thyro-globulin as a tumor marker postoperatively when any normal thyroid tissue remains, and the conversion of longstanding unresected papillary carcinoma of the thyroid to anaplastic disease.

These four arguments for the use of total thyroidectomy are balanced by the universal reports of the higher risk of permanent hypoparathyroidism and recurrent laryngeal nerve injury when total thyroidectomy is performed in contrast to less than total thyroidectomy.[9,11] The American College of Surgeons survey of total thyroidectomy in this country indicates a risk of permanent hypoparathyroidism of 20% or more in cases reported to their registry.[9] The Mayo Clinic reports hypoparathyroidism of nearly 20% but very low rates of recurrent laryngeal nerve injury.[11] The Lahey Clinic reports, on the other hand, less than a 1% rate of hypoparathyroidism in all their cases which did not involve total thyroidectomy.[4] Individual surgeons with unusual skills at thyroid surgery have reported rates of permanent hypoparathyroidism of 1% or less with total thyroidectomy.[1] The proponents of less than total thyroidectomy point out that: 1) while papillary carcinoma is frequently multifocal, the multifocality is almost always in the form of microscopic disease which is clinically insignificant. During exploration of the thyroid at surgery the opposite thyroid lobe is palpated and if clinically apparent multifocal papillary carcinoma is detected, the opposite lobe should be removed with a bilateral thyroid operation. 2) Radioactive iodine postoperatively is seldom necessary since nearly 90% of the patients are at low risk and rarely need any radioactive iodine treatments either for diagnosis or therapy on a routine basis. 3) Thyro-globulin as a tumor marker used to follow patients seems hardly necessary when over 98% of patients in the low risk group will never die of the disease and therefore need less vigorous followup. Furthermore, high risk patients are accurately separated by clinical criteria, and when so defined, can have more extensive surgery at the time of the initial thyroid operation. In addition, almost all high risk patients who develop metastases eventually die of the disease, so early detection of metastases by tumor markers does not materially influence therapy or outcome. 4) The incidence of true conversion from papillary carcinoma to anaplastic carcinoma is extremely uncommon; in the major reported series such conversions amount to much less than 1% of cases.[17] The striking decline of the incidence of giant and spindle cell undifferentiated carcinoma of the thyroid may eventually make this estimate of risk too high.[6] Thus with few substantial gains and some major risks, it seems that advocating total thyroidectomy for all thyroid cancers is both unnecessary and potentially dangerous.

Thyroid surgery is extremely well tolerated with rare deaths after surgery and few major complications if the surgical procedure is conservative in extent. In the absence of bilateral thyroid gland dissection hypoparathyroidism does not occur and recurrent laryngeal nerve paralysis is seen in less than 1% of cases; it is usually temporary. Rarely, if a vocal cord is paralyzed preoperatively, the recurrent laryngeal nerve may be deliberately sacrificed; all functioning recurrent laryngeal nerves should be preserved if possible, however, even if it requires dissecting the nerve out of surrounding thyroid carcinoma or metastatic nodes. If the local extent of disease at initial lobectomy indicates that the patient is in the high risk group and would be a candidate for postoperative radioactive iodine (i.e., extraglandular involvement, extensive pseudocapsular involvement by follicular carcinoma, greater than 5 cm diameter, older age), the surgeon should perform either a total or subtotal contralateral lobectomy. If suspicious nodules of clinically palpable multicentric papillary carcinoma are detected in the opposite lobe, a contralateral thyroid lobectomy should be performed. By selective application of surgical removal based on risk group, only a few patients need be subjected to the increased risk of a total thyroidectomy. There is no justification for routine total thyroidectomy as a surgical approach to any benign thyroid condition.

If the primary thyroid carcinoma extends outside the thyroid gland and involves adjacent structures, these should be preserved at the initial operative approach. Thus direct involvement of the tracheal wall should be handled by sharply excising the tumor from the tracheal cartilages; the larynx or esophagus or a functioning recurrent laryngeal nerve should be preserved where such cases are in the low risk group and despite the extent of residual disease in local structures initially, as such patients seldom die of disease.[18] Sacrifice of surrounding soft tissue and strap muscles, of course, is justified whenever they are directly involved by the differentiated thyroid carcinoma. Such direct extensions of thyroid cancer into trachea, esophagus and surrounding tissues in low risk younger patients are usually treated successfully by radioactive iodine, external beam therapy and thyroid hormone suppression of thyroid stimulating hormone to provide permanent control of the disease. We have demonstrated extremely low mortality rates (11%) for such patients who technically are surgically incurable by nature of the residual gross disease at the conclusion of surgery, illustrating the unique biological behavior of differentiated thyroid carcinoma.[18]

In high risk patients with extraglandular extension of cancer, however, the prognosis is almost uniformly fatal. Extensive resections such as concomitant laryngectomy or tracheal resection is not justified initially since the outcome is seemingly not altered by such an aggressive approach, at least at the initial operative procedure. On rare occasions, when such initially unresectable disease recurs as a symptomatic or clinical problem, radical surgery such as laryngectomy may be required in unusual circumstances.

Metastatic lymph nodes in differentiated thyroid carcinoma can be resected with conservative function-preserving and tissue-sparing neck dissections. Preservation of the spinal accessory nerve should occur in every case and the internal jugular vein and sternocleidomastoid muscle can frequently be preserved also. The submandibular area need not be resected since metastases seldom occur in that area. Whether the modified dissections are "berry picking," limited resections of lymph nodes, or "functional neck dissections," a logical schema of surgical treatment of lymph node metastases is as follows: 1) lymph node metastases palpable prior to initial thyroid surgery should be treated by modified or functional neck dissection through an upward extension of the thyroid collar incision; 2) if lymph node metastases are not palpable preoperatively but are discovered at the time of the thyroid lobectomy, lymph node dissection within the confines of the collar incision and in the central compartment of the neck should be performed; and this is possible only in piecemeal fashion; 3) if obvious lymph node metastases are not palpable, preoperatively or at the time of surgery, no formal lymph node dissection need be performed.

The most frequent recurrent disease in low risk patients with papillary carcinoma of the thyroid is a cervical lymph node metastasis. Recognizing the lack of relationship of lymph node metastases to prognosis indicates that the treatment of such lymph node metastases should be conservative and is usually best accomplished by a modified neck dissection preserving all the anatomic structures previously mentioned. Radioactive iodine treatment of cervical lymph node metastases can be avoided since they are a straightforward surgical problem.

The use of radioactive iodine for therapy of distant metastatic or unresectable local differentiated thyroid carcinoma is a unique demonstration (and the first historically) of an idealized cancer treatment, since iodine is metabolized almost exclusively by thyroid tissue with minor amounts metabolized in salivary glands and gastric mucosa. Therefore radioactive iodine is a uniquely specific agent that can seek out and destroy functioning thyroid tissue wherever it occurs in the body. In actual practice, however, metastatic thyroid carcinoma is almost never as functionally efficient as normal thyroid tissue and therefore the thyroid gland must be completely removed either surgically or radiotherapeutically before metastatic disease can be induced to take up radioactive iodine. Unfortunately, only a minority of metastases from thyroid carcinoma can be induced to take up radioactive iodine, but because of its unique targeting and extremely high radiotherapeutic cellular dose, it should be attempted if diagnostic scans show appreciable uptake in the presence of distant papillary or follicular metastatic disease. Even though radioactive iodine treatment of distant metastatic disease or

local recurrence can be accomplished in the high risk patients, they seldom are cured of the cancer by radioactive iodine since the metastases tend to be heterogeneous in uptake of iodine and patients ultimately succumb to disease. In low risk patients metastases occur almost entirely in the lungs and can usually be treated effectively and in curative form by radioactive iodine. When used for pulmonary metastases, it may cause pulmonary fibrosis if doses are excessive, and this occasionally limits the ability to treat these patients.

The major controversy in the use of radioactive iodine is whether it should be used routinely as an adjuvant to surgery or in a highly selective fashion. With the definition of risk groups such as the AMES and AGES categories,[3,13] the routine use of radioactive iodine for postoperative scanning can be limited to the very selective small minority of patients at high risk (10–15% of patients). In these patients, the entire thyroid gland must be removed either surgically or by radioactive iodine (RAI) before a diagnostic scan can be utilized to detect occult metastatic disease. If metastases are discovered, RAI treatment can be attempted. External beam radiotherapy should be used for the treatment of unresectable or recurrent local neck disease if radioactive iodine cannot be utilized. External beam radiotherapy can also be used in specific metastatic sites for palliation in the absence of radioactive iodine effect.

The other adjuvant therapy currently employed universally is the suppression of thyroid stimulating hormone (TSH) by exogenous ingestion of thyroid hormone. While this has been standard practice since the first demonstration of regression of metastatic disease by TSH suppression in 1957 by Crile, patients in the low risk group with small or "occult" papillary carcinomas probably do not need such treatment. Patients with obvious clinical cancer should receive adjuvant thyroid hormone for TSH suppression but whether that actually reduces death rate is open to some question.[2]

There is no standard protocol for chemotherapeutic management of metastatic differentiated thyroid carcinoma. Adriamycin and platinum containing multiple drug programs have produced temporary palliation.

Therapy of Undifferentiated Thyroid Carcinoma

Numerous articles cite the advantages of multidisciplinary management combining radiotherapy and chemotherapy with Adriamycin containing regimens for the local and systemic treatment of anaplastic thyroid carcinoma.[14,19] Radiotherapeutic experimental techniques include hyperfractionation. Because of the small number of cases seen, it is difficult to know which program should be preferred, but Adriamycin should be a component of any multidrug protocol. It has been reported that local neck disease can be controlled without the need for surgery or tracheostomy for airway obstruction in a significant proportion of patients who formerly required tracheostomy for respiratory obstruction. Despite encouraging temporary responses to such combined treatments, few long-term survivors are reported.

Therapy of Thyroid Lymphoma

Non-Hodgkins lymphoma of the thyroid should be treated as other extranodal lymphomas. If the disease can be totally removed surgically, is of limited extent, and has not penetrated the thyroid capsule, it may be that no systemic therapy is required since cure and control rates are extremely high with or without adjuvant radiotherapy.[15] However, if the lymphoma has penetrated the thyroid capsule or is extensive in the neck or cannot be totally removed, multidrug chemotherapy programs with or without radiotherapy are essential to provide long term control.

Metastatic Disease to the Thyroid Gland

Metastases to the thyroid seldom need complicated or unusual therapy. If the metastasis is symptomatic and isolated, a resection should be considered. If it is but one component of widespread metastases, it usually need not be treated separately unless airway obstruction occurs, in which case attempt at removal or tracheostomy may be required, or local radiotherapy given.

Medullary Carcinoma of the Thyroid

Medullary carcinoma of the thyroid has unique biology and requires distinctive therapeutic planning. Since most patients that present with medullary carcinoma of the thyroid do not have a completely adequate family history available prior to surgery, total thyroidectomy should be the treatment of choice. Individual patients with medullary carcinoma of the thyroid may be the index case for a familial cluster yet to be discovered. In familial medullary thyroid carcinoma, total thyroidectomy is necessitated by both the multifocal nature of the medullary carcinoma and the C-cell hyperplasia discovered uniformly in such cases. Medullary carcinoma that presents clinically should have a *functional neck dissection* performed as part of initial surgical therapy including the central compartment of the neck. This reflects the extremely high incidence of nodal metastases in both sporadic and familial forms. However, in the familial medullary cancer that is detected by calcitonin screening without clinical signs, the incidence of lymph node metastases is extremely low. While such patients should have total thyroidectomy, lymph node resections can be more selectively applied. If the medullary carcinoma is occult or only C-cell hyperplasia exists, lymph node resection need not be performed. If the medullary carcinoma is palpable but intraglandular, it is probably wise to perform a functional neck dissection on the ipsilateral side both for prognostic and therapeutic purposes. (See XXVI-4.)

The ability to screen at risk family members of medullary thyroid carcinoma syndromes either by basal detection or stimulated calcitonin diagnostic studies permits totally curative treatment to be performed in a preclinical stage. Thus patients with multiple endocrine neoplasia (MEN) types 1, 2A or 2B, or the more restricted familial medullary thyroid cancer syndrome represent the ideal screening population where a disease precursor (C-cell hyperplasia) can be detected at totally curable preclinical stage by serum markers and curative therapy applied (total thyroidectomy). Every patient with medullary thyroid carcinoma should have extensive family screening to diagnose new familial clusters. It

should be recognized, however, that the vast majority of medullary thyroid carcinoma (+80%) appears in a sporadic form without implication of other family members.[16]

Curative treatment of metastatic medullary carcinoma is not possible and no standard therapeutic programs have been described in the literature. Radiotherapy can be utilized with some success as medullary thyroid carcinoma seems to be radiosensitive. Obviously systemic therapy could be considered with systemic manifestations of metastatic disease but there is little guidance about particular drugs or programs to be offered. Occasional surgical resection for palliation of localized symptomatic disease can be attempted.

Future Directions in Thyroid Carcinoma

It has proven impossible to mount prospective trials in differentiated thyroid carcinoma because most single institutions have insufficient cases. Attempts at multiinstitutional protocols have failed to generate research support, and thus therapeutic programs are developed by derivation from relatively small numbers of patients. The most important new research in thyroid cancer is that of identifying specific genetic markers for familial clusters of medullary carcinoma in the MEN 2 and familial cases. Such specific genetic markers will enable still more refined selection of patients for preventive surgery in these genetic varieties.

Finally, the ability clinically to separate high risk and low risk cases of thyroid cancer has been a major step forward in rationalizing therapy, but still needs to be more widely appreciated and applied in therapeutic planning.

References

1. Attie, J. N., Moskowitz, G. W., Margouleff, D., and Levy, L. M.: Feasibility of total thyroidectomy in the treatment of thyroid carcinoma: Postoperative radioactive iodine evaluation of 140 cases. Am. Jour. Surg., 138:555, 1979.
2. Cady, B., Cohn, K., Rossi, R. L., Sedgwick, C. E., Meissner, W. A., Werber, J., and Gelman, R. S.: The effect of thyroid hormone administration upon survival in patients with differentiated thyroid carcinoma. Surgery, 94:978, 1983.
3. Cady, B., and Rossi, R. L.: An expanded view of risk-group definition in differentiated thyroid carcinoma, Surgery, 104:947, 1988.
4. Cady, B., and Rossi, R. L.: Surgery of the Thyroid and Parathyroid Glands. 3rd ed. W. B. Saunders Co., Philadelphia, 1990, p. 150.
5. Cady, B., Rossi, R. L., Silverman, M. L., and Wool, M.: Further evidence of the validity of risk group definition in differentiated thyroid carcinoma. Surgery, 98:1171, 1985.
6. Cady, B., Sedgwick, C. E., Meissner, W. A., Bookwalter, J. R., Romagosa, V., and Werber, J.: Changing clinical, pathologic, therapeutic, and survival patterns in differentiated thyroid carcinoma. Ann. Surg., 184:541, 1976.
7. Cady, B., Sedgwick, C. E., Meissner, W. A., Wool, M. S., Salzman, F. A., and Werber, J.: Risk factor analysis in differentiated thyroid cancer. Cancer, 43:810, 1979.
8. Cohn, K., Backdahl, M., Forsslund, G., Auer, G., Zetterberg, A., Lundell, G., Granberg, P. O., Lowhagen, T., Willems, J. S., and Cady, B.: Biologic considerations and operative strategy in papillary thyroid carcinoma: Arguments against the routine performance of total thyroidectomy. Surgery, 96:957, 1984.
9. Foster, R. S.: Morbidity and mortality after thyroidectomy. Surg. Gyn. Ob., 146:423, 1978.
10. Franssila, K. O.: Prognosis in thyroid carcinoma. Cancer, 36:1138, 1975.
11. Grant, C., Hay, I., Gough, I. R., and Bergstralh, E. J.: Local recurrence in papillary thyroid carcinoma: Is extent of surgical resection important? Surgery, 104:954, 1988.
12. Grant, C. S., Hay, I. D., Gough, I. R., and McCarthy, P. M.: Long-term follow-up of patients with benign thyroid fine-needle aspiration cytologic diagnoses. Surgery, 106:980, 1989.
13. Hay, I., Taylor, W. F., and McConhey, W. M.: A prognostic score for predicting outcome in papillary thyroid carcinoma. Endocrinology, 119(Suppl.):T-15, 1986.
14. Kim, J. H., and Leeper, R.D.: Treatment of anaplastic giant and spindle cell carcinoma of the thyroid gland with combination Adriamycin and radiation therapy: A new approach. Cancer, 52:954, 1983.
15. Rossi, R. L., Cady, B., Meissner, W. A., Sedgwick, C. E., and Werber, J.: Prognosis of undifferentiated carcinoma and lymphoma of the thyroid. Am. J. Surg., 135:589, 1978.
16. Rossi, R. L., Cady, B., Meissner, W. A., Wool, M. S., Sedgwick, C. E., and Werber, J.: Nonfamilial medullary thyroid carcinoma. Am. J. Surg., 139:554, 1980.
17. Rossi, R. L., Cady, B., Silverman, M. L., and Wool, M. S.: Current results of conservative surgery for differentiated thyroid carcinoma. World Jour. Surg., 10:612, 1986.
18. Rossi, R. L., Cady, B., Silverman, M. L., and Wool, M.: Surgically incurable well-differentiated thyroid carcinoma. Prognostic factors and results of therapy. Arch. Surg., 123:569, 1988.
19. Werner, B., Abele, J., Alveryd, A., Bjorklund, A., Franzen, S., Granberg, P. O., Lanberg, T., Lundell, G., Lowhagen, T., Sunblad, R., et al.: Multimodality therapy in anaplastic giant cell thyroid carcinoma. World J. Surg., 8:64, 1984.

Neoplasms of the Adrenal Cortex

Mary R. Flack
George P. Chrousos

Historical Perspective

Eustachius first described the "suprarenal" glands in 1563. It was not until the nineteenth century, however, that Cuvier isolated the adrenal cortex from the medulla (1805), and Arnold defined the various histologic zones of the adrenal cortex (1866).[50] The importance of the adrenal cortex for sustaining life was suggested by Addison in 1855 and confirmed the following year in animal studies by Brown-Sequard.[1,8] In 1927, Hartman showed that purified adrenal cortical extract could be used to treat adrenal insufficiency. The active substances in these adrenal extracts would later be identified as cortisol (1949) and aldosterone (1952).[50]

Harvey Cushing first described the clinical syndrome associated with excess adrenal secretion in 1910. He attributed the syndrome to basophilic adenomas of the pituitary gland, but in 1934 Walters described this same syndrome in patients with adrenal tumors. In 1811, Rolleston noted the association of adrenal tumors with virilization, and in 1890 Thompson demonstrated decreased virilization in a woman following resection of an adrenal tumor.[50] In 1952, Rapaport reported 188 cases of malignant adrenal tumors occurring between 1930–1949 associated with excess secretion of cortisol, androgens, and estrogens.[53]

Natural History and Staging

The natural history of adrenal cancer is dismal. The survival of untreated disease is generally less than three years.[11,56,60] Macfarlane reported a mean survival of only 2.9 months in 20 patients with surgically unresectable disease.[48] Most patients have either locally invasive disease or distant metastases at the time of diagnosis.[7,11,14,56,60,63] Even with surgical treatment the prognosis is generally poor. Although there are anecdotal reports of patients living 10–15 years with adrenocortical carcinoma,[63] the mean survival of patients following tumor resection is approximately 4 years.[11,31,32,45]

The staging system for adrenal cancer (Table XXVI-3-1) depends upon tumor size, nodal involvement, invasion of adjacent organs, and distant metastases.[48,58] Stage I disease refers to a tumor less than 5 cm in diameter that is confined to the adrenal gland. Stage I adrenal cancer is rare and can be difficult to distinguish from a benign adrenal adenoma.[29,63] When it occurs and there is complete resection, the prognosis is relatively good and long-term remissions have been reported.[5,24,48,58] Given the difficulty in distinguishing adenomas from carcinomas on pathologic criteria alone, however, some tumors classified as stage I carcinoma

Table XXVI-3-1. Staging of Adrenocortical Carcinoma

Stage	T, N, M	Description
I	T1, N0, M0	Tumor less than 5 cm, confined to the adrenal gland
II	T2, N0, M0	Tumor greater than 5 cm, confined to the adrenal gland
III	T1 or T2, N1, M0	Tumor confined to the adrenal gland with involvement of local nodes or
	T3, N0, M0	Tumor extending beyond adrenal gland, but not invading adjacent organs
IV	T3 or T4, N1, M0 any T, M1	Tumor extending beyond adrenal, invading adjacent organs, with local node involvement or any tumor with metastases

Adapted from Macfarlane.[48]

may actually be adrenal adenomas, which have an excellent prognosis following resection.

Stage II disease refers to a tumor greater than 5 cm in diameter that is confined to the adrenal gland. Most patients with stage II disease will eventually have recurrent or metastatic disease, half of them within two years of tumor resection.[11] The likelihood of metastases is higher in patients with larger tumors, pathologic evidence of necrosis, vascular invasion, and increased mitotic activity. There is no single pathologic criterion, however, which accurately predicts recurrence in a given patient, except clear lymphatic or blood vessel invasion.[30,48,63] The overall five year survival for patients with stage II disease is 30–40% when all visible tumor is resected. There have been reports, however, of patients living 10–15 years after a complete resection.[1,11,15,24,58,60]

Seventy percent or more of the patients with adrenal cancer have either stage III or IV disease at the time of diagnosis.[7,11,14,56,60,63] Stage III disease refers to a tumor greater than 5 cm in diameter that is confined to the adrenal gland with involvement of adjacent nodes, or locally invasive disease without spread to adjacent organs. Despite complete resection, virtually 100% of patients with stage III disease have recurrent and/or metastatic disease within 5 years of tumor resection.[7,11,36,53,58] Tumor necrosis, vascular invasion, nuclear mitoses, pleomorphism, and involvement of the *zona reticularis* have been reported to be poor prognostic signs.[30] The overall five year survival for stage III adrenal cancer is generally less than 30%.[11,45,56,60]

Stage IV disease refers to a tumor greater than 5 cm in diameter with invasion of adjacent organs and/or distant metastases. Adrenal cancer can spread directly to adjacent organs including the kidney, mesentery, posterior abdominal wall, pancreas, diaphragm, renal vein, and inferior vena cava.[26,31,42,48] Adrenal cancer can spread via the lymphatics to regional and para aortic lymph nodes, but more commonly spreads by the hematogenous route to distant organs. The most frequent sites of metastasis are lymph nodes (25–46%), lung (47–97%), liver (53–68%), abdomen (33–43%), and bone (11–33%). Metastases have been reported in the ovary, spleen, pleura, thyroid, pharyngeal tonsils, mediastinum, myocardium, brain, spinal cord, skin, and subcutaneous tissues.[11,31,42,48,56] The survival for patients with stage IV disease is extremely poor. The 5-year survival is generally less than 15% if all the tumor cannot be resected.[11,44,48,56,60] Luton reported a mean five-year survival of 22% in their patients with metastatic disease despite medical and surgical therapy; 25% for patients under age 40, and 15% for patients over age 40.[45]

Epidemiology

Adrenal carcinoma accounts for 0.05–0.2% of all cancers with a prevalence of two per million. A bimodal age distribution has been reported with one peak occurring before age 5, and the second in the fourth to fifth decade. Adrenal cancer, however, occurs at all ages from several months to the seventh and eighth decades.[31,42,48,53,56] In large cancer registries, there is a slight male predominance,[10,17,23] while in large clinical series there is a female predominance.[31,42,53] This is most likely due to the fact that secretory tumors, which are highly represented in clinical series, occur more commonly in women, while most adrenal cancers diagnosed in men are non-secretory.[48]

There are no known causative agents for adrenocortical carcinoma. There does not appear to be any association between chronic adrenal hyperplasia and the development of adrenal cancer. The majority of adrenal cancers occur sporadically. There have been a few reports, however, of adrenocortical cancer in patients with the Li-Fraumeni hereditary multiple tumor syndrome (breast cancer, soft tissue sarcomas, gliomas).[39,40,46,47]

Diagnosis

Despite the frequent association of adrenocortical carcinoma with endocrine hypersecretion, nearly half the patients with adrenal cancer have no recognizable endocrine syndrome.[11,48,56,62] These patients present with either abdominal pain or fullness or the incidental finding of an adrenal mass on radiologic studies done for other reasons.[26,36] Rarely, patients with adrenal cancer present with anorexia, weight loss, or fever of unknown origin, all of which are poor prognostic signs.[11,26,38] Although these patients have no identifiable endocrine syndrome, there may be elevation of urine or plasma steroids in 10–20% of these patients.[14,22,45,58,60]

Over 50% of patients with adrenal cancer have an associated endocrine syndrome such as Cushing's, virilization, Cushing's plus virilization, feminization, or hyperaldosteronism. These syndromes result from the secretion of cortisol and its precursors, adrenal androgens and their precursors, or rarely estrogen and aldosterone. Adrenal cancers are inefficient in their production of steroids. This results in the secretion of large amounts of steroid precursors relative to the amount of end product (Fig. XXVI-4-1).[9,26,41] Furthermore, the amount of steroids produced is often lower than expected for the large size of these tumors.

The most common syndrome associated with adrenal cancer is Cushing's syndrome caused by the excess secretion of cortisol and its precursors. It accounts for 30–40% of patients with a clinical syndrome.[31,42,53,63] Some of the typical signs and symptoms of Cushing's (Table XXVI-3-2) may be more subtle in patients with adrenal cancer, because of the inefficient steroidogenesis by many of these neoplasms. In women, hirsutism and amenorrhea may be seen more frequently than with benign adrenal conditions due to the propensity for these tumors to secrete androgenic steroid precursors. Children rarely present with the classic clinical features of Cushing's syndrome; growth retardation and a weight gain that is inappropriate for their height are more common.[9,35,43]

Virilization is seen in 20–30% of those patients with an endocrine syndrome.[31,42,53,62] Virilization is rarely due to the secretion of testosterone itself, but is primarily associated with secretion of androgenic steroid precursors such as androstenedione, dehydroxyepiandrosterone, and 17-hydroxyprogesterone.[31,42] The signs and symptoms of excess androgen secretion in females include increased libido, excessive muscle mass, temporal balding, clitoromegaly, and heterosexual precocious puberty in girls. In males, the clinical manifestations of excess androgen secretion are obscured, except for isosexual precocious puberty in boys (Table XXVI-3-2).

The combination of Cushing's syndrome and virilization occurs in 10–30% of those patients with an endocrine syndrome.[31,42,53,62] This combined syndrome is associated with the secretion of multiple steroids and their precursors, including cortisol, androstenedione, 17-hydroxyprogesterone and dehydroepiandrosterone.[31,42] The diagnosis can only be made in women when clitoromegaly, temporal balding, or increased muscle mass are present, because amenorrhea and hirsutism can be seen in Cushing's syndrome alone.

Feminization occurs in 5–10% of men with adrenal cancer.[31,42,53,62] This presents as decreased libido, impotence, gynecomastia, and testicular atrophy. Persistent questioning and careful examination may be required to elicit these findings, but they may be the only key to an early diagnosis in males who generally have more clinically silent tumors.[48]

Pure hyperaldosteronism is rare in adrenal cancer and accounts for five percent or less of those patients with an endocrine syndrome.[3,5,7,31,42] When it does occur, it presents with hypertension, hypokalemia, and a metabolic alkalosis. Hypertension and hypokalemia, however, can occur with other syndromes in adrenal cancer due to the excess secretion of mineralocorticoid precursors, such as 11-deoxycorticosterone and corticosterone. Even more unusual presentations of adrenal cancer which have been reported include hypoglycemia, insulin resistance, and polycythemia.[10,51]

Several laboratory studies are useful in confirming excessive steroid secretion in patients with suspected adrenal cancer. Hypercortisolism is most often confirmed by measuring the urine free cortisol (UFC) in an aliquot from a 24

Table XXVI-3-2. Clinical Findings and Laboratory Studies Found in Patients With Secretory Adrenal Cancers

Endocrine Syndrome (%)	Clinical Findings	Laboratory Studies (S.I. Units)

Cushing's (30%)	Weight gain (truncal, dorsocervical and supra-clavicular). Moon facies, plethora, hypertension, striae, hirsutism, peripheral wasting and weakness, glucose intolerance, amenorrhea, acne, mental changes, osteoporosis, edema, hypokalemia[43]	Urine:
		  17-ketosteroids = 30–200 mg/d (> 100 μmol/d)
		  17-hydroxysteroids > 15 mg/g creat (> 30 μmol/d)
		  free cortisol (UFC) > 200 μg/d (> 400 nmol/d)
		  increased tetrahydro compound S
		Plasma:
		  ACTH suppressed < 11 pg/ml (< 3 pmol/L) by RIA
		  or < 5 pg/ml (< 1.2 pmol/L) by IRMA
		  DHEA-S > 3,500 ng/ml (> 10 mmol/L)

Virilization (20%)	Temporal balding, increased muscle mass, clitoromegaly, deepening of the voice in women, heterosexual precocious puberty in girls, isosexual precocious puberty in boys	Urine:
		  17-ketosteroids = 30–200 mg/24h (> 100 μmol/d)
		  increased urinary pregnenalone
		Plasma (females):
		  testosterone > 200 ng/dl (> 4 nmol/L)
		  androstenedione > 3.5 μg/L (> 12 nmol/L)

Cushing's and Virilization (30%)	Combination of the above; the finding of virilization or precocious puberty in the setting of Cushing's syndrome is highly suggestive of adrenal carcinoma	Combination of above

Feminization (15%)	Impotence, loss of libido, testicular atrophy, fatigue, inability to concentrate in men	Plasma: (males)
		  Estrone > 100 pg/ml (> 300 pmol/L)
		  Estradiol > 50 pg/ml (> 180 pmol/L)

Hyperaldosteronism (5%)	Hypertension, hypokalemia, metabolic alkalosis	Plasma: (normal salt intake) aldosterone > 30 ng/dL (> 800 pmol/L)

hour urine collection. Over 90% of patients with Cushing's syndrome have UFC values greater than 200 mcg/24 hours, while 97% of normal individuals have UFC values less than 100 mcg/24 hours. Values between 100 and 200 mcg/24 hours can be seen in patients with obesity, depression, stress, or alcoholism.[13,43] In patients with ambiguous UFC results, an overnight dexamethasone suppression test may be helpful. This test involves the oral administration of 1 mg of dexamethasone at midnight and measurement of plasma cortisol at 8 a.m. Normal individuals have cortisol values less than 5 μg/dL following dexamethasone, while patients with Cushing's syndrome generally have values greater than 5 μg/dL.[13]

Additionally, an aliquot from a 24-hour urine collection should be sent for measurement of 17-hydroxysteroids, 17-ketosteroids and creatinine. Sixty percent of patients with adrenal cancer have elevated 17-hydroxysteroid excretion and over 70% of patients have elevated 17-ketosteroid excretion. Fifty percent of patients with adrenal cancer have increased levels of both 17-hydroxy and 17-ketosteroids.[14,24,31,42,51] Extreme elevations of urinary 17-ketosteroids are often seen in patients with adrenal cancer (up to 200 mg/dL). An unusually high level of urinary ketosteroids in a patient with hypercortisolism is more suggestive of malignant adrenal disease than a benign adrenal process.[9,21,35,41,42]

There are several other tests for the differential diagnosis of Cushing's syndrome once hypercortisolism has been established. A plasma ACTH level using a reliable radioimmunoassay (usually a two-site or "sandwich" assay) can distinguish patients with ACTH-dependent Cushing's syndrome (pituitary tumors or ectopic ACTH secretion) from those with ACTH independent Cushing's syndrome (adrenal tumors or micronodular adrenal disease). Patients with pituitary disease or ectopic ACTH secretion have normal or elevated ACTH levels, while patients with primary adrenal disease, including adrenal carcinoma, have suppressed ACTH levels.[9,13,35,43] An undetectable ACTH level with the appropriate findings of a large irregular adrenal mass on computed tomography is virtually diagnostic of adrenocortical carcinoma.

The classic test for the differential diagnosis of Cushing's syndrome is the high dose dexamethasone suppression test. This test involves obtaining 24-hour urine collections for 6 consecutive days. Following 2 baseline days, dexamethasone is given orally; 0.5 mg every 6 hours for 48 hours, then 2.0 mg every 6 hours for 48 hours. Traditionally, a decline in 17-hydroxysteroid excretion to less than 50% of basal values indicates pituitary disease. Patients with adrenal cancer, however, do not have any significant decrease in their 17-hydroxysteroid excretion following high dose dexamethasone.[9,13,35,43] The high dose dexamethasone test and other tests recommended for the differential diagnosis of Cushing's syndrome, such as ovine corticotropin releasing hormone (CRH) stimulation and inferior petrosal sinus sampling, are not essential in the diagnosis of adrenal cancer, however, if the imaging studies are diagnostic and the ACTH level is suppressed.

Several other plasma and urinary steroids are elevated in patients with adrenal cancer. They include dehydroxyepiandrosterone (DHEA) and its sulfated derivative (DHEA-S), pregnenolone, 17-hydroxypregnenolone and 11-deoxycortisol in the plasma and the tetrahydro conjugate of 11-deoxycortisol (tetrahydro-compound S) in the urine (Figure XXVI-3-1).[41,42,49] While these are generally not essential in the work up of hypercortisolism, they may occasionally be a clue to the presence of adrenal malignancy in a patient with Cushing's syndrome.

The clinical diagnosis of virilization can be confirmed by

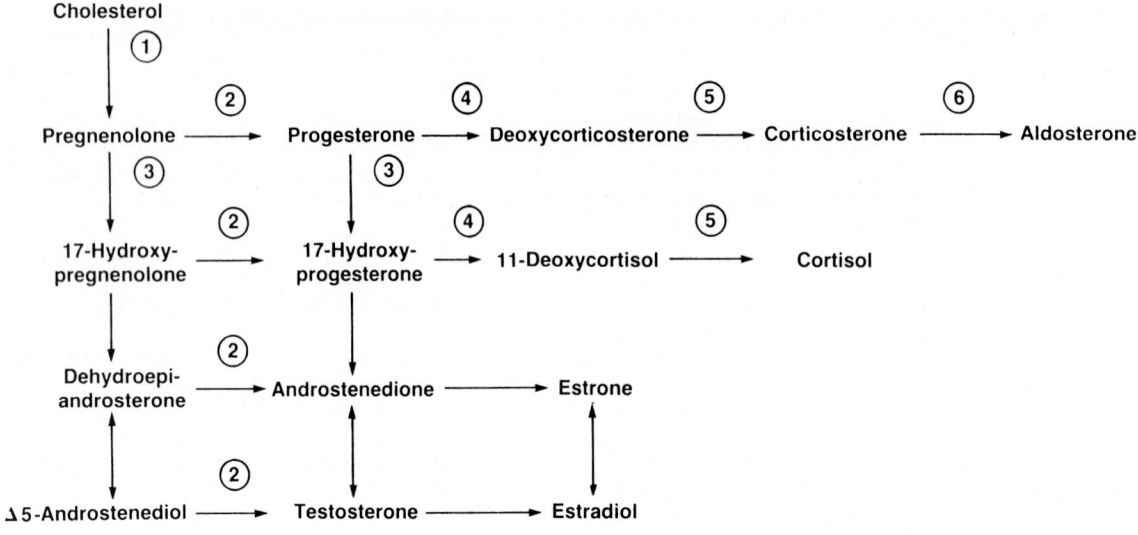

Figure XXVI-3-1. Biosynthetic pathway for the production of steroids in the adrenal cortex.

measurement of plasma androstenedione, testosterone, sex hormone binding globulin, and urinary 17-ketosteroids. Plasma levels of DHEA and DHEA-S are elevated in the majority of patients with adrenal cancer whether or not they have the clinical manifestations of virilization and/or Cushing's.[41,42,49,65] In contrast, patients with secretory adrenal adenomas have suppressed DHEA-S levels (see differential diagnosis).

The clinical diagnosis of feminization can be confirmed by measurement of elevated plasma estradiol and/or estrone. Hyperaldosteronism can be confirmed by measurement of elevated plasma and urinary aldosterone levels. Although usually not needed clinically, plasma levels of corticosterone and deoxycorticosterone are frequently elevated in patients with adrenal cancer and the clinical appearance of hyperaldosteronism.[3]

A specific diagnosis of adrenal cancer depends on the identification of an adrenal mass on computed tomography (CT) and/or magnetic resonance imaging (MRI). The finding on CT of a large unilateral adrenal mass, with irregular borders, is virtually diagnostic of adrenal cancer. If a smaller mass is present, it is more difficult to distinguish an adrenal cancer from an adrenal adenoma (see differential diagnosis). On MRI scanning, malignant adrenal lesions have an intermediate to high signal intensity on T2 weighted images, while non-functional adenomas have a low signal intensity and pheochromocytomas have an extremely high signal intensity (Figure XXV-4-2).[15,54] Iodo-cholesterol scanning shows poor adrenal uptake in adrenal cancer compared with the enhanced uptake which may be seen in adrenal hyperplasia. This study is rarely indicated, however, given the accuracy of CT and MRI.

Differential Diagnosis

"Incidentalomas"

There is a 0.5–1.0% incidence of unexpected adrenal lesions on CT or MRI scans of the upper abdomen after the age of forty. These lesions can represent benign adrenal adenomas, adrenal carcinomas, metastases from an unknown primary cancer, cysts, or rarely myelolipomas.[4,12,15] The incidental findings of these lesions has led to the diagnostic problem of distinguishing benign lesions from early adrenal cancer. With the increasing use of CT and MRI scanning, adrenal cancers as small as 3.5 cm have been identified. Resection of these small lesions will no doubt have a better prognosis, so the question of the malignant potential of these incidentally discovered lesions is important. Copeland has suggested that lesions greater than 6 cm should be considered to have high malignant potential.[12] Belldegrun and colleagues also found that most malignant lesions were greater than 6 cm in diameter, while nearly all lesions less than 6 cm were benign. However, they recommended that, due to the rare finding of small adrenal cancers, all lesions greater than 3 cm should be removed if there is no contraindication to surgery.[4]

The issue of how to proceed when an incidentaloma is discovered is controversial. The consensus of most studies[4,9,12] is that patients found to have an incidental adrenal lesion should have a preliminary screen for endocrine hypersecretion, including a complete history and physical examination and a 24-hour urine for free cortisol, 17-hydroxysteroids, 17-ketosteroids, and creatinine. If flushing or hypertension are present, urine metanephrines and catecholamines should also be included. If signs and symptoms of virilization, feminization, or hyperaldosteronism are present plasma levels of testosterone, androstenedione, DHEAS, or aldosterone should be obtained. If there is evidence of endocrine hypersecretion, the lesion should be resected.

If no endocrine hypersecretion is found, some would recommend an MRI of the adrenals.[15,54] In general, non-functioning adenomas have a low signal intensity on T2 weighted MRI; carcinomas and adrenal metastases have an intermediate to high signal intensity; while pheochromocytomas have an extremely high signal intensity. Identification of a pheochromocytoma on this study would be extremely impor-

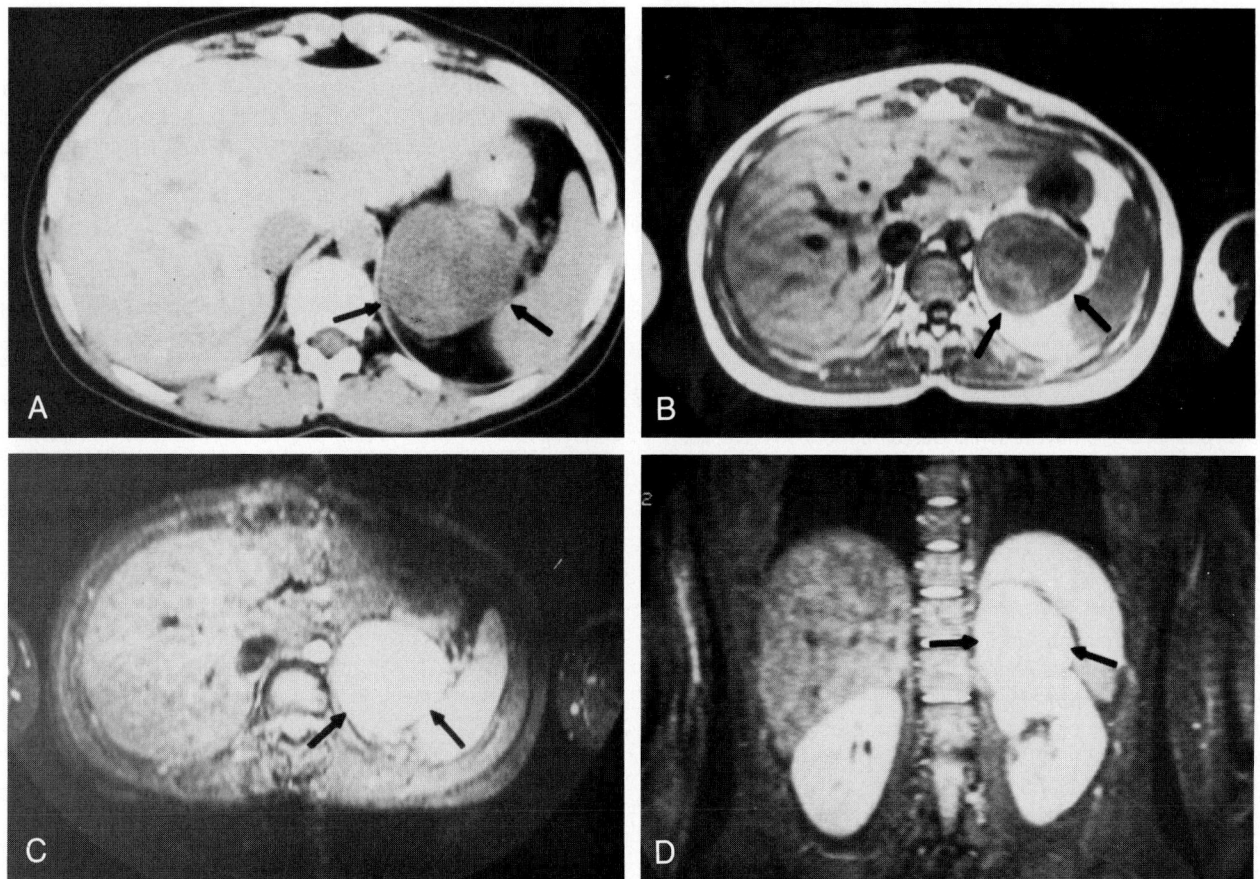

Figure XXVI-3-2. Adrenocortical carcinoma shown on **A** Computed tomography, **B** T1 weighted MRI (TR 300 ms TE 26 ms), showing signal intensity equal to liver tissue, **C** T2 weighted MRI (TR 1500 ms TI 100 ms), showing high signal intensity compared to liver, **D** T2 weighted MRI (TR 1510 ms TI 100 ms), showing the mass in relation to the upper pole of the kidney. (Courtesy of J. Doppman)

tant if manipulations such as fine needle biopsy were being considered. The absence of hypertension or the lack of elevated urine metanephrines does not rule out a pheochromocytoma in all cases. If the lesion is of intermediate to high signal intensity on T2 weighted MRI, it could still represent an adrenal metastasis from an unknown primary cancer. A reasonable effort should be made to exclude common adenocarcinomas (i.e., breast, lung, gastrointestinal tract).

If there is no endocrine syndrome or occult primary cancer found and the lesion is less than 3 cm, the patient can be reassured with perhaps one follow-up CT scan. If the lesion is 3–6 cm, there are several reasonable courses of action. If the CT appearance of the lesion is suggestive of a cyst, fine needle aspiration can be done with careful follow-up. If the patient is elderly, or there are contraindications to surgery, observation and careful follow-up are reasonable. In these cases, periodic assessment of the secretory status as well as the size of the mass should be performed, since many tumors become secretory long before they lead to a clearly recognizable endocrine syndrome. If the patient is young and there are no contraindications, surgical resection should be undertaken for lesions greater than 6 cm or lesions greater than 3–4 cm which have suspicious features such as intermediate to high signal intensity on T2 weighted MRI, irregular borders or patchy contrast uptake on CT.[4,12,15,54]

Adrenal Adenoma

In general, adrenal adenomas are highly efficient steroid secretors and tend to produce a single end-product such as cortisol, testosterone, or aldosterone, rather than multiple steroid precursors as in adrenal carcinoma.[9,26,42] A small lesion on CT scan, which avidly takes up iodocholesterol, in the setting of high levels of steroid secretion is highly suggestive of an adrenal adenoma. Following resection of an adrenal tumor, it may still be difficult to distinguish benign from malignant lesions on pathologic criteria. Hough has suggested that the presence of a diffuse growth pattern, broad fibrous bands, tumor necrosis, frequent mitoses, or vascular invasion are highly correlated with malignancy.[30] Others have emphasized the correlation between the size and weight of the lesion and the potential for malignancy.[48,55,59,63] However, there is no single criterion which distinguishes a malignant from a benign lesion in a given patient other than local invasion or metastatic disease. Thus, lesions which have a number of suspicious features on pathologic examination should be followed every three months initially for evidence of recurrence.

Therapy

Surgical resection is the only therapy which has been demonstrated to prolong survival in adrenal cancer.[11,27,48,58] Stage

I and II disease should be treated by complete resection and careful follow-up (every 3 months initially, followed by every 6–12 months). Stage III disease should be treated by resection of all visible tumor and careful follow-up. Early recognition of recurrent or metastatic disease is important since resection of isolated metastatic lesions has prolonged survival in some patients.[2] State IV disease should be treated by removal of as much tumor as possible, including resection of isolated metastases. Some centers recommend adjuvant medical treatment with mitotane following complete resection in stage III and IV disease to increase the duration between recurrences, although this has not been tested in a controlled study.[45,60]

Medical therapy is generally recommended when all the tumor cannot be removed. While partial responses have been reported with medical therapy, it is generally ineffective in prolonging overall survival in adrenal cancer. Ortho-para'DDD (mitotane) at high oral doses (up to 15 grams/day) causes remission of hypercortisolism in 50–60% of patients with adrenal cancer and Cushing's syndrome.[32] Tumor responses, however, occur much less frequently. Initially, a 20–40% partial tumor response rate was reported with mitotane treatment and there were several anecdotal reports of complete tumor responses.[6,16,32,33] More recent studies, however, involving large numbers of patients and more objective criteria for response indicate a partial response rate less than 20%.[29,45] These responses are short-lived lasting 6–10 months. Unfortunately, mitotane treatment has no effect on survival and the high doses required have considerable toxicity, including nausea, vomiting, anorexia, dizziness, lethargy, fatigue, and blood dyscrasias.

Various chemotherapeutic regimens have been used for the treatment of metastatic adrenal cancer. These have included agents such as cisplatin, etoposide, 5-fluorouracil, doxorubicin, and melphalan. In general, the response rates are less than 20% and are short-lived.[25,28,34,57,61] Radiation therapy can be used in combination with chemotherapy for palliation, particularly with bone metastases.[52]

In addition to mitotane, there are a number of other agents which can be used to treat hypercortisolism including metyrapone (250 mg QID), aminoglutethimide (250 mg QID), and ketoconazole (10 mg/kg/d). In some patients, particularly with mitotane treatment, hydrocortisone (15 mg/square meter/d) or florinef (100–400 μg/d) may be required to prevent adrenal insufficiency. Mineralocorticoid antagonists, such as spironolactone, or androgen antagonists, such as flutamide may aid in controlling the signs and symptoms of mineralocorticoid or androgen excess.[35,43]

Perspectives

One of the major problems with chemotherapy for adrenal cancer is the development of drug resistance. A surface glycoprotein (p-glycoprotein or MDR-glycoprotein) has been identified which may shuttle chemotherapeutic agents out of tumor cells. This protein is expressed in high levels in normal adrenals and in adrenal cancers.[19,20] It may contribute to the development of resistance to drugs which are transported by this glycoprotein. Agents such as verapamil and amiodarone, used in combination with chemotherapy, competitively inhibit this glycoprotein and may prolong the action of the other chemotherapeutic agents.

Experimental therapies such as Suramin, a reverse transcriptase inhibitor, and Gossypol, a plant toxin are currently being tested. Suramin has caused remissions in four of sixteen patients with adrenal cancer[37] and gossypol has caused a partial remission in one patient with adrenal cancer.[18]

References

1. Addison, T.: On the constitutional and local effects of disease of the suprarenal capsules. London, S. Highley, 1855.
2. Appelquist, P., and Kostianinen, S.: Multiple thoracotomy combined with chemotherapy in metastatic adrenal cortical carcinoma: a case report and review of the literature. J. Surg. Oncol., 24:1, 1983.
3. Arteaga, E., Biglieri, E. G., Kater, C. E., Lopez, J. M., and Schambelan, M.: Aldosterone-producing adrenocortical carcinoma. Ann. Intern. Med., 101:316, 1984.
4. Belldegrun, A., Hussain, S., Seltzer, S. E., Loughlin, K. R., Gittes, R. F., and Richie, J. P.: Incidentally discovered mass of the adrenal gland. Surg. Gynecol. Obstet., 163:203, 1986.
5. Bertagna, C., and Orth, D. N.: Clinical and laboratory findings and results of therapy in 58 patients with adrenocortical tumors admitted to a single medical center (1951 to 1978). Am. J. Med., 71:855, 1981.
6. Boven, E., Vermorken, J. B., vanSlooten, H., and Pinedo, H. M.: Complete response of metastasized adrenal cortical carcinoma with o,p'-DDD. Cancer, 53:26, 1984.
7. Brennan, M. F.: Adrenocortical Carcinoma. CA-A Cancer J. Clin., 37:348, 1987.
8. Brown-Sequard, C. E.: Recherches expérimentales sur la physiologie et la pathologie des capsules surrénales. C. R. Acad. Sci., Paris, 43:422, 1856.
9. Chrousos, G. P.: Endocrine Tumors. In Principles and Practice of Pediatric Oncology. Edited by Pizzo. Philadelphia, Lippincott, 1988, p. 733.
10. Clemmesen, J.: Statistical studies in the aetiology of malignant neoplams. Munksgaard, Copenhagen, National Anti-Cancer League, 1965.
11. Cohn, D., Gottesman, L., and Brennan, M.: Adrenocortical carcinoma. Surgery, 100:1170, 1986.
12. Copeland, P. M.: The incidentally discovered adrenal mass. Ann. Intern. Med., 98:940, 1983.
13. Crapo, L.: Cushing's syndrome: A review of diagnostic tests. Metabolism, 28:955, 1979.
14. Didolkar, M. S., Bescher, R. A., Elias, E. G., and Moore, R. H.: Natural history of adrenal cortical carcinoma: A clinicopathologic study of 42 patients. Cancer, 47:2153, 1981.
15. Doppman, J. L., Reinig, J. W., Dwyer, A. J., Frank, J. P., Norton, J., Loriaux, D. L., and Keiser, H.: Differentiation of adrenal masses by magnetic resonance imaging. Surgery, 102:1018, 1987.
16. Downing, V., Eule, J., and Huseby, R. A.: Regression of an adrenal cortical carcinoma and its neovascular bed following mitotane therapy: a case report. Cancer, 34:1882, 1974.
17. Ferber, B., Hardy, V. H., and Gerhardt, P. R.: Cancer in New York State, exclusive of New York City, 1941–1960. Albany, Bureau of Cancer Control, New York State Department of Health, 1962.
18. Flack, M. R., Wu, Y. W., Reidenberg, M. M., Pyle, R. G., Mullens, N. M., Nisula, B. C., Loriaux, D. L., and Knazek, R. A.: Treatment of adrenocortical carcinoma with gossypol. Meeting of the American Society for Cancer Research, Washington, D. C., 1990.
19. Fojo, A. T., Akiyama, S. I., Gottesman, M. M., and Pastan, I.: Reduced drug accumulation in multiple drug-resistant human KB carcinoma cell lines. Cancer Res., 45:3002, 1985.
20. Fojo, A. T., Ueda, K., Slamon, D. J., Poplack, D. G., Gottesman, M. M., and Pastan, I.: Expression of a multidrug resistance gene in human tumors and tissues. Proc. Natl. Acad. Sci., U.S.A., 1986.
21. Forbes, A. P., and Albright, F.: A comparison of the 17-ketosteroid excretion in Cushing's syndrome associated with adrenal tumor and with adrenal hyperplasia. J. Clin. Endocrinol. Metab., 11:926, 1951.
22. Fukushima, D. K., and Gallagher, T. F.: Steroid production in "nonfunctioning" adrenal cortical tumor. J. Clin. Endocrinol. Metab., 23:923, 1963.
23. Griswold, M. H., Wilder, C. S., Cutler, S. J., and Pollack, E. S.: Cancer in Connecticut, 1935–1951. Hartford, CT, Connecticut State Department of Health, 1955.
24. Hajjar, R. A., Hickey, R. C., and Samaan, N. A.: Adrenal cortical carcinoma; a study of 32 patients. Cancer, 35:549, 1975.
25. Haq, M. M., Legha, S. S., Samaan, N. A., Bodey, G. P., and Burgess, M. A.: Cytotoxic Chemotherapy in Adrenal Cortical Carcinoma. Cancer Treat. Rep., 64:909, 1980.
26. Heinbecker, P. O., and Ackerman, L. V.: Functional and nonfunctioning adrenal cortical tumors. Surg. Gynecol. Obstet., 105:21, 1957.
27. Henley, D. J., vanHeerden, J. A., Grant, C. S., Carney, J. A., and Carpenter, P. C.: Adrenal cortical carcinoma—a continuing challenge. Surgery, 94:926, 1983.
28. Hesketh, P. J., McCaffrey, R. P., Finkel, H. E., Larmon, S. S., Griffing, G. T., and Melby, J. C.: Cisplatin-based treatment of adrenocortical carcinoma. Cancer Treat. Rep., 71:222, 1987.
29. Hogan, T. F., Citrin, D. L., Johnson, M. B., Nakamura, S., Davis, T. E., and Borden, E. C.: o,p'DDD (Mitotane) therapy of adrenal cortical carcinoma. Cancer, 42:2177, 1978.
30. Hough, A. J., Hollifield, J. W., Page, D. L., and Hartmann, W. H.: Prognostic factors in adrenal cortical tumors. Am. J. Clin. Path., 72:390, 1979.
31. Hutter, A. M., and Kayhoe, D. E.: Adrenal cortical carcinoma: clinical features of 138 patients. Am. J. Med., 41:572, 1966.
32. Hutter, A. M., and Kayhoe, D. E.: Adrenal cortical carcinoma: results of treatment with o,p'DDD in 138 patients. Am. J. Med., 41:581, 1966.
33. Jarabak, J., and Rice, K.: Metastatic adrenal cortical carcinoma; prolonged regression with mitotane therapy. J.A.M.A., 246:1706, 1981.
34. Johnson, D. H., and Greco, F. A.: Treatment of metastatic adrenal cortical carcinoma with cisplatin and etoposide (VP-16). Cancer, 58:2198, 1986.

35. Kamilaris, T. C., and Chrousos, G. P.: Adrenal Diseases. In Diagnostic Endocrinology, Edited by Moore, Toronto, B. C. Decker, Inc., 1990, p. 79.
36. Kelly, W. F., Barnes, A. J., Cassar, J., White, M., Mahiter, K., Loizou, S., Welbourn, R. B., and Joplin, G. F.: Cushing's syndrome due to adrenocortical carcinoma—a comprehensive clinical and biochemical study of patients treated by surgery and chemotherapy. Acta Endocrinol., 91:303, 1979.
37. LaRocca, R. V., Stein, C. A., Danesi, R., Jamis-Dow, C. A., Weiss, G. H., and Meyers, C. E.: Suramin in adrenal cancer: modulation of steroid hormone production, cytotoxicity in vitro, and clinical antitumor effect. J. Clin. Endocrinol. Metab., 71:497, 1990.
38. Lewinsky, B. S., Grigor, K. M., Symington, T., and Neville, A. M.: The clinical and pathologic features on "non-hormonal" adrenocortical tumors. Cancer, 33:778, 1974.
39. Li, F. P., and Fraumeni, J. F.: Soft-tissue sarcomas, breast cancer, and other neoplasms; a family syndrome? Ann. Intern. Med., 71:747, 1969.
40. Li, F. P., and Fraumeni, J. F.: Prospective study of a family cancer syndrome. J.A.M.A., 247:2692, 1982.
41. Lipsett, M. B., and Wilson, H.: Adrenocortical cancer: steriod biosynthesis and metabolism evaluated by urinary metabolites. J. Clin. Endocrinol. Metab., 22:906, 1962.
42. Lipsett, M. B., Hertz, R., and Ross, G. T.: Clinical and pathophysiologic aspects of adrenocortical carcinoma. Am. J. Med., 35:374, 1963.
43. Loriaux, D. L., and Cutler, G. B.: Diseases of the adrenal glands. In Clinical Endocrinology, Edited by Kohler. Boston, John Wiley & Sons, 1986, p. 167.
44. Lubitz, J. A., Freeman, L., and Okun, R.: Mitotane use in inoperable adrenal cortical carcinoma. J.A.M.A., 223:1109, 1973.
45. Luton, J. P., Cerdas, S., Billaud, L., Thomas, G., Guilhaume, B., Bertagna, X., Laudat, M. H., Louvel, A., Chapuis, Y., Blondeau, P., Bonnin, A., and Bricaire, H.: Clinical features of adrenocortical carcinoma, prognostic factors, and the effect of mitotane therapy. N. Engl. J. Med., 322:1195, 1990.
46. Lynch, H. T., Mulcahy, G. M., Harris, R. E., Guirgis, H. A., and Lynch, J. F.: Genetic and pathologic findings in a kindred with hereditary sarcoma, breast cancer, brain tumors, leukemia, lung, laryngeal, and adrenal cortical carcinoma. Cancer, 14:2055, 1978.
47. Lynch, H. T., Katz, D. A., Bogard, P. J., and Lynch, J. F.: The sarcoma, breast cancer, lung cancer, and adrenocortical carcinoma syndrome revisited. Am. J. Dis. Child., 139:134, 1985.
48. Macfarlane, D. A.: Cancer of the Adrenal Cortex; the natural history, prognosis and treatment in a study of fifty-five cases. Ann. R. Coll. Surg. Engl., 23:155, 1958.
49. McKenna, T. J., Miller, R. B., and Liddle, G. W.: Plasma pregnenolone and 17-OH-pregnenalone in patients with adrenal tumors, ACTH excess, or Idiopathic hirsutism. J. Clin. Endocrinol. Metab., 44:231, 1977.
50. Medvei, V. C.: A History of Endocrinology. Hingham, MA, MTP Press, 1982.
51. Nader, S., Hickey, R. C., Sellin, R. V., and Samaan, N. A.: Adrenal Cortical Carcinoma; a study of 77 cases. Cancer, 52:707, 1983.
52. Percarpio, B., and Knowlton, A. H.: Radiation therapy of adrenal carcinoma. Acta Rad. Ther. Phys. Biol., 15:288, 1976.
53. Rapaport, E., Goldberg, M. B., Gordan, G. S., and Hinman, F., Jr.: Mortality in surgically treated adrenocortical tumors. Postgrad. Med., 11:325, 1952.
54. Reinig, J. W., Doppman, J. L., Dwyer, A. J., and Frank, J.: MRI of indeterminate adrenal masses. A.J.R., 147:493, 1986.
55. Richie, J. P., and Gittes, R. F.: Carcinoma of the adrenal cortex. Cancer, 45:1957, 1980.
56. Samaan, N. A., and Hickey, R. C.: Adrenal Cortical Carcinoma. Semin. Oncol., 14:292, 1987.
57. Schlumberger, M., Ostronoff, M., Bellaiche, M., Rougier, P., Droz, J. P., and Parmentier, C.: 5-Fluorouracil, doxorubicin, and cisplatin regimen in adrenal cortical carcinoma. Cancer, 61:1492, 1988.
58. Sullivan, M., Boileau, M., and Hodges, C. V.: Adrenal Cortical Carcinoma. J. Urol., 120:660, 1978.
59. Tang, C. K., and Gray, G. F.: Adrenocortical neoplasms; prognosis and morphology, Urology, 5:691, 1975.
60. Thompson, N. W., and Cheung, P. S.: Diagnosis and treatment of functioning and nonfunctioning adrenocortical neoplasms including incidentalomas. Surg. Clin. N. Amer., 67:423, 1987.
61. van Slooten, H., and van Oosterom, A. T.: CAP (cyclophosphamide, doxorubicin, and cisplatin) regimen in adrenal cortical carcinoma. Cancer Treat. Rep., 67:377, 1983.
62. van Slooten, H., Moolenaar, A. J., Van Seters, A. P., and Smeenk, D.: The treatment of adrenocortical carcinoma with o,p′DDD: Prognostic implications of serum level monitoring. 1984.
63. van Slooten, H., Schaberg, A., Smeenk, K., and Moolenaar, A. J.: Morphologic characteristics of benign and malignant adrenocortical tumors. Cancer, 55:766, 1985.

XXVI-4

Neoplasms of the Neuroendocrine System

Steven D. Averbuch
Stephen B. Baylin
A. Philippe Chahinian
Norman W. Thompson

Introduction

This chapter focuses upon three neoplasms of endocrine organs (parathyroid carcinoma, medullary thyroid carcinoma, and pheochromocytoma) and three endocrine neoplastic syndromes which are linked together by at least two major considerations. First, each of the neoplasms has histological and biochemical features which are common to all normal and neoplastic endocrine cells of the body. Histologically, these cells contain the cytoplasmic neurosecretory granules which store either small polypeptide hormones and/or biogenic amines. These secretory products reflect the specific endocrine function of the normal cells from which the neoplasms derive (Table XXVI-4-1). In terms of biochemical features, the tumors arise from the so called group of "amine precursor uptake and decarboxylation" (APUD) cells which constitute the diffuse system of neuroendocrine cells distributed throughout the body.[209,211] The "APUD" acronym denotes the capacity of these cells to synthesize and/or secrete

Table XXVI-4-1. Common Features of Amine Precursor, Uptake and Decarboxylation ("APUD") Cells

Biogenic amine synthesis
Amine precursor uptake
Amine (DOPA) decarboxylase
Small polypeptide hormone synthesis
Membrane bound neurosecretory granules

biogenic amines formed through activity of the enzyme L-dopa decarboxylase.[85]

The second feature linking these particular neoplasms and syndromes is that they can occur in individual patients as a consequence of autosomally dominant genetically transmitted disorders. Inherited genetic defects affect different groups of APUD cells and lead to neoplastic development of related cell types in diverse anatomical regions.[19] It is essential to consider these genetic disorders when approaching patients with these tumors or syndromes.

Historically, each of the three neoplasms were initially

identified as independent pathological entities. Parathyroid carcinoma was first described in 1935 by Hall and Chaffin,[100] although parathyroid adenomas and hyperplasia had been recognized as early as 1903.[10] Hazard and coworkers first recognized medullary thyroid carcinoma as a distinct entity in 1959.[105] In 1886, Frankel's postmortem discovery of bilateral adrenal tumors in a young woman following sudden death was the first report of pheochromocytoma.[78] Subsequently, complete descriptions of pheochromocytoma were made and the surgical cure of the disease was demonstrated in the 1920s.[175]

Although the first description of multiple endocrine tumors in a single individual was reported in 1903,[69] it wasn't until the 1950s that neoplasms of multiple endocrine glands in affected individuals and their families came to be recognized as three distinct syndromes, multiple endocrine neoplasia (MEN) types 1, 2a, and 2b. Wermer first described the autosomal dominant association of parathyroid adenoma or hyperplasia, pancreatic islet cell adenoma or carcinoma, and pituitary adenoma (MEN 1) in 1954;[309] Sipple first described the association of parathyroid adenoma or hyperplasia, medullary thyroid carcinoma, and familial pheochromocytoma (MEN 2a) in 1961;[265] and Williams and Pollock first described the association of medullary thyroid carcinoma, pheochromocytoma, and mucosal neuromas (MEN 2b) in 1966.[312] From these early descriptions up to the present, a number of other investigators have contributed their observations to establish these three MEN syndromes.[58,135,168,196,244,245] In addition, it is now recognized that medullary thyroid carcinoma can occur as an inherited tumor in families without other associated endocrine lesions (non-MEN familial medullary thyroid carcinoma).[72]

Based on morphological criteria, Pearse first proposed the APUD diffuse neuroendocrine system in 1968.[209] Subsequent experimental evidence has challenged the notion of a common embryologic origin of APUD cells as originally proposed by Pearse.[7,19,124,151] Thus, a neuroectodermal origin for the cells involved in the genetic medullary thyroid carcinoma syndromes separate from the endodermal origin of those in the MEN 1 syndrome is now considered likely. Nonetheless, the APUD concept as proposed by Pearse has been pivotal to exploring how single genetic defects may cause simultaneous neoplasms in the same individual and it still provides an extremely useful framework in which these closely linked neoplasms and their syndromes may be considered.

Parathyroid Carcinoma

The vast majority (>95%) of parathyroid tumors are benign, and produce signs of primary hyperparathyroidism. The emphasis in this section is on parathyroid carcinoma and the features which differentiate it from the more common benign conditions, adenomas and hyperplasia.

Epidemiology

In contrast to benign parathyroid tumors, which have an annual age-adjusted incidence of 28 per 100,000,[107] parathyroid carcinomas remain rare. Only about 200 cases have been reported.[250] Parathyroid carcinomas do not usually arise from adenoma or hyperplasia, and familial cases are exceptional.[63,250] Chronic renal failure, which leads to secondary hyperparathyroidism, has been implicated in a patient with coexisting parathyroid carcinoma, adenoma and hyperplasia.[25] Prior exposure to radiation in the neck is a well known risk factor for thyroid carcinoma and it has been reported in 9–30% of patients with hyperparathyroidism and benign parathyroid tumors, with an average latency period of 37 years.[129] A history of prior radiation has been reported in very few cases of parathyroid carcinoma, however.[250] One patient with parathyroid carcinoma had both chronic renal failure and a history of prior radiation to the neck.[121]

Natural History

Embryology and Anatomy. Embryology is the key to understanding the normal and ectopic locations of the parathyroid glands. The upper glands together with the lateral thyroid are derived from the 4th pharyngeal pouch, whereas the lower glands together with the thymus are derived from the 3rd pharyngeal pouch.[49,300] In the majority of cases, the upper parathyroid glands are found at the cricothyroid junction posteriorly (77%), less commonly behind the upper pole of the thyroid underneath its capsule (22%), and exceptionally in a retropharyngeal or retroesophageal location (1%).[300] The lower parathyroid glands are located anywhere between the lower pole of the thyroid and the thymus, 42% are found at the lower pole of the thyroid, 39% are within the thymic tongue in the lower neck, and 2% are found in the mediastinal thymus. Other ectopic locations are usually in the neck (15% juxtathyroidal, 2% in other locations)[300] and supernumerary glands have been found in 2–6% of individuals.[128] Therefore, parathyroid tumors, including carcinomas, may arise in ectopic (often mediastinal) locations or even from a fifth gland.[128,189] The average weight of the normal gland is between 40–140 mg, with a length of 3–6 mm.[49,300]

Pathological Characteristics. The normal parathyroid gland contains mainly chief cells, which are polyhedral, rich in glycogen and fat (often appearing as clear cells), and which secrete parathyroid hormone (PTH). Oxyphil cells appear later in life and increase in number with advancing age. These cells have a pyknotic nucleus and a granular eosinophilic cytoplasm packed with mitochondria.[49] They are thought to represent senescent cells, whereas the water-clear cells are thought to represent transitional cells.[259]

The distribution of parathyroid tumors in 1,200 cases of hyperparathyroidism seen at the Massachusetts General Hospital from 1932 to 1983 was as follows:[301] benign single adenoma in 83% (double adenomas <1%), hyperplasia of all 4 glands in 14% (chief cell hyperplasia in 2%, clear cell hyperplasia in 12%) and carcinoma in 2%. The majority of cases of hyperplasia occur in patients with multiple endocrine neoplasia (MEN), either type 1 or type 2a. It is often difficult to differentiate among these tumors histologically, and it is particularly difficult to ascertain their benign or malignant nature. Parathyroid carcinomas appears as grayish, hard, lobulated tumors, compared to the soft, reddish brown adenomas.[49,112,301] The carcinomas are surrounded by dense fibrotic capsules. Adherence to and invasion of surrounding structures are important signs of malignancy reported in 50% of cases.[49,112] The average size of carcinomas is 3 cm, with a mean weight of 6–12 g.[49,236] Microscopically, the carcinoma cells resemble watermelon seeds[49] and are larger and better defined than adenomatous cells. The cells are bland and uniform, however, and cellular atypia is rare, in surprising contrast to adenomas. Criteria for malignancy as described by Castleman and Roth include a trabecular pattern with thick fibrous bands, nuclear palisading, mitotic figures, and capsular and blood vessel invasion.[49] These features do not always predict for malignancy however, and even mitotic activity, "the single most valuable criterion"[49] has been challenged since it was also found in 12/17 benign adenomas and 8/10 glands containing parathyroid hyperplasia.[267] An important corollary is that when a carcinoma is suspected on clinical grounds and/or gross appearance, the surgeon should resect the tumor "en bloc" without relying on biopsy or frozen section.[250]

Biological Characteristics. Genetic studies have so far been largely limited to MEN syndromes. MEN type 1, where parathyroid hyperplasia is the rule, has been associated with loss of heterozygosity (indicating loss of a possible suppressor gene) on chromosome 11q13.[215,281] In MEN type 2 deletions are found on chromosome 1p often with a predisposing locus on chromosome 10.[215,234] Despite earlier conflicting results, it appears that parathyroid adenomas, as well as hyperplasia in MEN type 1, are monoclonal neoplasms.[9,79] A plasma factor has recently been isolated from patients with MEN 1 with a very high mitogenic activity for bovine parathyroid glands in vitro.[34] The relevance of these findings for parathyroid carcinoma has not yet been evaluated.

The use of flow cytometric DNA analysis to determine aneuploidy, S-phase fraction and proliferation index values in an attempt to distinguish parathyroid carcinoma from adenoma or hyperplasia has yielded conflicting results.[202,203] Tumor markers such as opioid peptides[32] and chromogranin A[200] have been described in benign parathyroid tumors. Production of human chorionic gonadotropin (hCG) subunits alpha and beta has been observed in parathyroid carcinoma but not in benign tumors.[276]

Clinical Features. Parathyroid carcinomas are usually slow-growing tumors with a tendency to recur locally and to metastasize late.[49] The great majority (>95%) are functional and produce a more severe picture of primary hyperparathyroidism than parathyroid adenomas or hyperplasia (Table XXVI-4-2). The major distinguishing features of malignant hyperparathyroidism are equal incidence in men and women, younger mean age by more than a decade, presence of palpable neck mass, and severe hypercalcemia, often >14 mg/dl (3.5 mmol/l). Hoarseness with recurrent nerve involvement is rare, occurring in less than 10% of patients.[112,301] Metastases are seen in 36% of patients with parathyroid carcinoma, including involvement of cervical nodes in about 20%, and distant metastases to lungs, bone, liver and other organs in 16%.[112,236,249,301] Almost all patients with malignant hyperparathyroidism are symptomatic at diagnosis, compared to only half of those with benign tumors. Symptoms are usually severe and may include a range of manifestations[8,12,46,54,106,107,144,177,208] including: 1) renal involvement with polyuria, polydipsia, urolithiasis (calcium oxalte or calcium phosphate stone), nephrocalcinosis, and decreased function; 2) bone involvement with osteitis fibrosa

Table XXVI-4-2.   Clinical Features of Primary Hyperparathyroidism Due to Parathyroid Carcinoma and Benign Tumors

	Cancer[a]	Benign[b]
Incidence	2–4%	96–98%
Female:Male	1:1	3:1
Age (years)		
Mean	45	58
Range	12–84	17–83
Palpable neck mass	42%	Rare
Serum calcium		
Mean mg/dl (mmol/l)	15 (3.75)	11–12 (2.75–3.0)
>14 mg/dl (3.5 mmol/l)	64%	<10%
Renal disease	56%	20%
Lithiasis	49%	20%
Nephrocalcinosis	23%	Rare
Decresed function	51%	14%
Bone disease	63%	6%
Osteitis fibrosa cystica	36%	4%
Renal and bone disease	39%	Rare
Gastrointestinal disease		
Peptic ulcer	11%	8%
Pancreatitis	11%	Rare
Asymptomatic	3%	47%

[a]From references 112, 236, 249, 301.
[b]From references 46, 77, 107, 144, 208.

cystica and/or osteopenia, pathologic fractures, and bone pain; 3) neuromuscular symptoms with proximal muscle weakness, easy fatigability, muscle aches, paresthesias, mental disturbances, headaches, and pruritus; 4) rheumatologic symptoms with joint pains, gout, pseudo-gout, chondrocalcinosis, and calcific tendinitis; 5) gastrointestinal symptoms with anorexia, nausea, vomiting, constipation, peptic ulcer, and pancreatitis; 6) cardiovascular manifestations with decreased Q-T interval, arrhythmias, and possibly hypertension; 7) calcifications of the cornea (band keratopathy) and other soft tissues (skin, lungs). Concomitant renal and bone involvement, exceptional in benign hyperparathyroidism, is seen in up to 39% of patients with parathyroid carcinoma.[249,301]

The existence of nonfunctioning parathyroid carcinoma has long been controversial because of the difficulties in differentiating this entity from thyroid carcinoma. Nonfunctioning tumors, occur throughout the endocrine system however, including the parathyroid. We have reported a 69 year old woman with multiple recurrences of nonfunctioning parathyroid carcinoma in the neck, a large anterior mediastinal mass and a malignant left pleural effusion.[51] A total of 11 such cases have been collected in the English literature,[186] indicating that nonfunctional cancers represent about 5% of parathyroid carcinomas. These patients have no hypercalcemia, the serum immunoreactive parathyroid hormone (iPTH) levels are within normal limits, but the biology of the tumor and its prognosis are otherwise similar to functioning carcinomas.[15,51]

Nonfunctioning parathyroid carcinomas must be distinguished from other nonfunctional parathyroid neoplasms, including oxyphil adenomas, parathyroid cysts, and metastatic carcinomas (most often from breast, lung, and renal carcinomas).[49] Electron microscopy showing lipid, glycogen and neurosecretory granules in the cytoplasm, distinguishes nonfunctional parathyroid carcinomas from thyroid carcinomas or metastatic renal cell carcinomas.[51,62] Three possible hypotheses may explain the absence of hyperparathyroidism: a lack of hormone synthesis; impairment or decrease of hormone secretion; and synthesis of an abnormal hormone. The second hypothesis seems most likely in view of the presence of secretory granules by electron microscopy, the demonstration of immunoreactivity for PTH in the tumor tissue in one case[186] and the demonstration of mRNA coding for pre-pro-PTH, the cellular precursor of PTH, in the tumor tissue of another case.[15] These investigations, in addition, further support the parathyroid origin of these nonfunctioning carcinomas.

Biochemical Features. Hypercalcemia, the hallmark of hyperparathyroidism, is usually severe in patients with parathyroid carcinoma. The serum calcium level is above 14 mg/dl (3.5 mmol/l) in about two-thirds of patients, compared to less than 10% of patients with benign hyperparathyroidism (Table XXVI-4-2). The total serum calcium, however, may be affected by several factors, principally, hypoalbuminemia and renal insufficiency.[27,54] Other laboratory features of hyperparathyroidism include hypophosphatemia, hypercalciuria (>250 mg/day in about one-quarter of patients), hyperphosphaturia, and, in some cases, hypomagnesemia, hypokalemia and hyperuricemia.[12,16,27] Increased serum chloride and decreased bicarbonate can lead to metabolic acidosis, which aggravates hypercalcemia by decreasing the binding of calcium to albumin, and by increasing the dissolution of bone mineral.[8] Urinary cyclic AMP is elevated as a result of PTH binding to renal receptors. Excessive PTH and hypophosphatemia also increase the renal production of 1,25-dihydroxyvitamin D, which is usually elevated in the serum. In cases of metabolic bone disease (without metastases), the serum alkaline phosphatase level is increased as well as the urinary excretion of hydroxyproline, and amino acid unique to collagen. Recently, elevated serum levels of osteocalcin, a major noncollagenous protein of bone, have been reported in hyperparathyroidism.[82]

Diagnostic Tests

Primary Hyperparathyroidism. The diagnosis of primary hyperparathyroidism is clinical and biochemical. Biopsy is not necessary and generally contraindicated in the majority of cases before definitive surgery for either benign or malignant parathyroid tumors.

By far the most important test to diagnose primary hyperparathyroidism is the serum level of immunoreactive (i) PTH.[8,27] Different radioimmunoassays are now available, directed either at the intact molecule, the active fragments (N-terminal), or at inactive fragments (mid-region or C-terminal region). Elevated levels of iPTH are virtually diagnostic of hyperparathyroidism and they can be very high in cases of functioning parathyroid carcinoma. Ectopic production of PTH is exceptional, and has been documented in very few cases of nonparathyroid carcinomas (see below). Two features which may be useful in differentiating parathyroid carcinoma from benign

tumors are anemia, which is more common in carcinoma (up to 80% versus less than 10%, respectively),[144,249] and elevated serum levels of hCG.

In benign hyperparathyroidism, first-time exploration of the neck by an experienced surgeon will successfully detect the tumor(s) in more than 90% of cases.[314] Imaging techniques are most useful in cases of recurrent or persistent hyperparathyroidism after initial surgery. They are also useful before initial surgery whenever a carcinoma is suspected on clinical grounds, allowing evaluation of the local extent of the tumor particularly with regard to the thyroid, trachea and esophagus, as well as possible metastases to cervical nodes and other organs.

Esophagograms with careful evaluation of the cervical esophagus can indirectly visualize parathyroid tumors.[270] Ultrasonography with high-resolution, real-time technology is an excellent non-invasive technique, although its overall results are operator dependent.[314] Retroesophageal, retrotracheal and mediastinal areas cannot usually be well assessed by this technique.[314] Computed tomography (CT) scanning can readily visualize these areas and also evaluate the extent of disease in patients with parathyroid carcinoma. Scintigraphy, formerly using radionuclides such as selenomethionine-75 or gallium-67 citrate, has been improved by computer subtraction techniques. The sequential administration of thallium 201, which concentrates both in thyroid and parathyroid, and of technetium 99m, which concentrates in the thyroid, followed by subtraction allows imaging of the parathyroid tumors.[314] This technique has high sensitivity, but its specificity can be affected by concomitant thyroid diseases, including adenomas and carcinomas. Thallium 201 can also accumulate in metastatic cancer to lymph nodes. Magnetic resonance imaging (MRI) is improving but at this time does not appear superior to CT. In a prospective comparison based on 100 patients with benign parathyroid tumors before surgery,[139] overall sensitivities were: scintigraphy, 73%, CT, 68%, MRI, 57%, sonography, 55%, with respective specificities of 94%, 92%, 87% and 95%. None of these imaging techniques had a sensitivity of more than 50% for small (<250 mg) tumors, and sensitivity was also decreased in patients who had previous surgery to the neck. For patients with parathyroid carcinoma, CT scanning appears most useful at this time since it has good sensitivity in detecting the primary tumor and allows evaluation of its local extent and metastases.

Invasive diagnostic modalities require highly skilled personnel and are currently indicated only for selected cases. Venography with venous samplings for iPTH remains one of the most sensitive techniques.[314] This method measures PTH from the venous effluents of the thyroid veins before the hormone is degraded in the peripheral blood. A unilateral gradient is in favor of a single adenoma or carcinoma, whereas a bilateral gradient usually indicates diffuse hyperplasia. Multiple venous samples are usually taken from the vertebral, thymic, and internal mammary veins in addition to the thyroid veins. It is a time-consuming but relatively safe procedure.

Angiographic studies have been obtained with a number of techniques but are rarely indicated today. The inferior thyroid artery, which originates from the thyrocervical trunk can be missed and catastrophic neurologic complications may follow inadvertent injection of contrast material into spinal branches of the thyrocervical trunk or the costocervical trunk.[277]

Sonography or CT can also guide percutaneous fine needle biopsy for diagnostic purposes. The possible risk of this biopsy is spillage of cells which, in the case of carcinoma may lead to recurrent tumors.[250] Even in cases of benign parathyroid adenomas, recurrent adenomas (parathyromatosis) have been described following spillage.

Differential Diagnosis. The major differential diagnosis of parathyroid carcinoma, besides benign parathyroid adenoma, is to rule out other causes of cancer-related hypercalcemia. In addition to the presence of lytic bone metastasis, hypercalcemia can result from humoral factors secreted by the tumor itself, "humoral hypercalcemia of malignancy" (HHM). This was hypothesized in 1941 by Fuller Albright.[1] In HHM hypophosphatemia occurs whereas most patients with hypercalcemia from bone metastasis have a normal serum phosphate level. Urinary cyclic AMP, an important marker, is increased in patients with HHM or primary hyperparathyroidism, whereas it is low in hypercalcemia related to lytic bone metastases.[39,120] Ectopic production of PTH by non-parathyroid tumors is exceptional however, and has been demonstrated only in a few cases, such as ovarian or small lung carcinomas.[197] Most often, serum levels of iPTH are low in HHM, and PTH mRNA is not expressed by these tumors.[260,278]

Great progress has been made in elucidating the syndrome of HHM. In 1987, isolation of a novel "PTH-related protein" (PTHrP) and cloning of its gene were reported.[120,278] The protein contains 141 amino-acids, compared to 84 for PTH (Table XXVI-4-3), and 8 of the 13 amino-acids of the biologically active N-terminal fragment are identical to PTH. Thereafter, the two molecules are totally different. The corresponding gene for PTHrP has been mapped to the short arm of human chromosome 12, compared to the short arm of chromosome 11 for PTH.[39,185] This similarity and proximity suggested that both genes were derived from a common ancestral gene that had duplicated and separated during evolution.[185,278] There are now at least three forms of PTHrP mRNAs known. Homology at the N-terminal region may explain

similarities in biologic activities of the two proteins, and the binding of PTHrP to PTH receptors. PTHrP increases bone resorption, increases tubular calcium reabsorption, and inhibits tubular phosphate reabsorption. Distinguishing features from primary hyperparathyroidism, however, include decreased production of 1,25 dihydroxyvitamin D, due to the limited capacity of PTHrP to stimulate 1-hydroxylase in the proximal renal tubule, and alkalosis rather than hyperchloremic acidosis (Table XXVI-4-3). In HHM serum chloride levels are usually low or normal, and bicarbonate levels are normal or high.[16] In contrast, bicarbonaturia is increased in primary hyperparathyroidism.[8,16] Hypokalemia is common in HHM (50%) and rare in primary hyperparathyroidism (17%).[16] Increased plasma levels of PTHrP have been found in about half the patients with HHM by assays using an antiserum against synthetic human PTHrP (1–34).[41] More sensitive radioimmunoassays directed at other fragments have been described.[44] The primary tumors producing PTHrP are mainly squamous carcinomas of the lung, esophagus, and head and neck although a wide range of other tumors can also cause HMM, including renal, bladder, breast, and ovarian carcinomas. This syndrome can also occur in patients with bone metastases as well.[28,217] The hypercalcemia of adult T-cell leukemias caused by HTLV-1, may also be linked to HHM, with increased PTHrP, urinary cAMP, and decreased 1,25 dihydroxyvitamin D.[39] In contrast to PTH, which is restricted to the parathyroid cells, PTHrP is found in a wide range of normal tissues, such as keratinocytes, breast tissue, milk, placenta, central nervous system, adrenals, mesothelium, and even parathyroid glands, suggesting a widespread physiologic role.[28,176] Since PTHrP is not elevated in some patients with HHM, and since some tumors producing PTHrP do not cause hypercalcemia, other factors that could act independently or synergistically with PTHrP may be implicated in HHM.[28] These may include other bone resorbing factors such as transforming growth factor alpha (TGF alpha), IL-1, and tumor necrosis factor (TNF).[185] In patients with multiple myeloma, the osteoclast activating factors produced by the malignant plasma cells are thought to be cytokines, particularly lymphotoxin or tumor necrosis factor beta.[185]

Other causes of hypercalcemia are usually easy to rule out.[27] Endocrine disorders associated with hypercalcemia include hyperthyroidism, adrenal insufficiency, pheochromocytoma, and VIPomas. The last two might coexist with hyperparathyroidism as part of MEN syndromes.[27] It has been recently suggested that pheochromocytoma may also produce HHM as described above.[275] Vitamin D excess can be seen in chronic granulomatous disorders or in some lymphomas. Medications inducing hypercalcemia include thiazide diuretics and lithium carbonate. Estrogen and antiestrogen therapy can induce hypercalcemia in patients with breast cancer and bone metastasis, perhaps based on prostaglandin secretion.[185] Vitamin A toxicity, milk-alkali syndrome and immobilization are well known causes of hypercalcemia. Familial hypocalciuric hypercalcemia can mimic primary hyperparathyroidism.[27,150] This autosomal dominant disease starts in childhood and follows a benign course with mild symptoms. In this disease, PTH levels are normal or slightly elevated and the parathyroid glands are normal or mildly hyperplastic.

Table XXVI-4-3. Biologic Characteristics and Effects of Parathyroid Hormone (PTH) and Related Peptide (PTHrP)[a]

	PTH	PTHrP
No. of Amino Acids*	84	141
Chromosome Location*	11p	12p
Serum Calcium	high	high
Urinary Calcium*	high (25%)	higher
Serum Phosphate	low	low
Urinary Phosphate	high	high
Serum pH*	acidosis	alkalosis
Nephrogenous cAMP	high	high
1,25 Dihydroxyvitamin D*	high	low
Bone Resorption	increased	increased
Bone Formation*	increased	decreased
Immunoreactive PTH*	positive	negative
Immunoreactive PTHrP*	negative	positive

[a]From references 39, 120, 185
*Denotes differentiating features

A normal serum calcium with hypophosphatemia and hyperphosphaturia should raise the possibility of oncogenic osteomalacia, a rare paraneoplastic syndrome seen in benign mesenchymal tumors and sometimes in prostate or small cell lung carcinomas and characterized by low serum levels of 1,25 dihydroxyvitamin D.[280]

Therapeutic Considerations

Surgical Management. Surgery is the primary and only curative treatment of parathyroid carcinoma, requiring expert technique and great care during the initial operation.[250] Removal of the tumor *en bloc* with all involved surrounding structures and without violating its capsule is mandatory. For Wang and Gaz all cases where the tumor capsule was violated had local tumor recurrence.[301] The surgeon must recognize the gross appearance of any enlarged gland with a thick, adherent, gray-white, fibrous capsule to suspect a carcinoma. It is equally important for the surgeon to avoid breaking into the capsule of an enlarged parathyroid tumor without these characteristic features since some carcinomas may appear to be large adenomas on gross inspection. Furthermore, even rupture of a benign tumor can result in local implementation of hyperplastic tissue that can cause a recurrence that is difficult to differentiate from carcinoma.

Simple biopsy with frozen sections should not be attempted in view of its unreliability in distinguishing benign from malignant lesions and the risk of tumor seeding.[29,250] The surgical resection should include all areas of local adherence in continuity with the tumor including the thyroid ipsilateral lobe and isthmus and involved strap muscles. If there is local invasion (rather than just adherence) of the recurrent laryngeal nerve, it should be sacrificed, since attempts to dissect it from the tumor carry the risk of local recurrence.[112] Occasionally, the trachea and/or esophagus may be involved as well. Biopsy of the lymph nodes of the tracheoesophageal groove should be performed. Lymph node metastases are uncommon during initial surgery[301] and if not present most authors do not recommend a prophylactic radical neck dissection.[250] When the gross distinction from a benign enlargement is in doubt, the other ipsilateral parathyroid should be removed to rule out the possibility of diffuse hyperplasia. Close monitoring after surgery is essential to detect hypocalcemia ("hungry bone" syndrome) which is usually temporary but may require supplements of calcium and vitamin D.[83] Recurrences are most likely to be caused by local cervical implants, pulmonary, or other distant metastases. The 5-year survival for parathyroid carcinoma is about 50% (including 30% without recurrence) and the 10-year survival varies from 13–35%.[112,236,249]

Treatment of Recurrent or Metastatic Carcinoma. Parathyroid carcinomas tend to grow slowly and metastasize late. Early recurrence, however, is an unfavorable prognostic factor and most recurrences appear within two to three years following initial surgery. Since the tumor grows slowly, and most patients die from metabolic complications of hyperparathyroidism rather than tumor burden, aggressive surgical pursuit of recurrences and metastases is indicated.[112,236] For example, repeated thoracotomies for recurrent pulmonary metastases are clearly indicated. Patients may survive many years despite repeated recurrences and

metastases.[249] Local recurrence and metastasis to cervical lymph nodes are common (30–40%). Distant metastases most commonly involve lungs (20–40%) but also other sites, including mediastinum, bone, pleura, pericardium, and pancreas.[112,249,301] Selective venous sampling for iPTH may be useful to confirm parathyroid carcinoma metastasis in some cases.

Medical Therapy for Hypercalcemia of Malignancy. The treatment of hypercalcemia in patients with parathyroid carcinoma follows the same general methods used in other forms of hypercalcemia of malignancy except that the calcium levels may be persistently elevated and more difficult to control by medical treatment, justifying attempts at palliative surgery. Serum calcium levels as high as 24 mg/dl have been reported in parathyroid carcinoma.[249]

Hydration with normal saline is the first step. Loop diuretics such as furosemide and ethacrynic acid should be added to decrease the risk of fluid overload, but only after adequate hydration is established. Plicamycin (mithramycin) is one of the most effective agents available for the treatment of hypercalcemia of malignancy,[11,27] and acts by inhibiting osteoclast function. Calcitonin inhibits osteoclastic bone resorption and also increases urinary excretion of calcium. Unfortunately its effect is limited, lasting less than 24 hours, and it loses its efficacy after repeated administration.[27]

The geminal bisphophonates are analogs of natural pyrophosphate. They bind to hydroxyapatite, inhibit bone crystal dissolution and also osteoclastic resorption.[11,225,264] Clodronate (dichloromethylene diphosphonate) has shown effectiveness in parathyroid carcinoma[251] but this agent is no longer available in the United States. The first generation bisphosphonate, etidronate (hydroxyethylidene bisphosphonate), is currently marketed in the United States. Newer compounds in this class, such as pamidronate (aminohydroxy propylidene bisphosphonate) and alendronate (aminohydroxybutylidene bisphosphonate) hold promise because of increased effectiveness by both the intravenous and oral routes. Addition of calcitonin to bisphosphonate therapy may provide a more rapid response.[222] Bisphosphonates have fewer toxic effects than plicamycin and may even be used in some patients with skeletal metastases to limit the invasion and destruction of bone and to alleviate pain in addition to controlling hypercalcemia.[11]

Gallium nitrate is an antineoplastic drug which was found to produce hypocalcemia during early clinical trials. It inhibits bone resorption and can control hypercalcemia mediated by PTH or related peptide.[302,303] At a dose of 200 mg/m^2/day for 5–7 days by continuous infusion, it was effective and shown to be superior to calcitonin or etidronate in treating hypercalcemia from various cancers.[302,304] Gallium nitrate was also effective against hypercalcemia from parathyroid carcinoma.[303] Nephrotoxicity is a potential side-effect of this agent.

The experimental agent, WR 2721 (amifostine) is an organic thiophosphate compound which is concentrated in normal tissues and much less in most neoplastic tissues.[87,225] It has been used as a protective agent against the toxicity of radiation and chemotherapy. Phase I trials revealed that WR 2721 can cause hypocalcemia, which appears related not only to inhibition of bone resorption, but also to inhibition of PTH secretion and increased urinary calcium excretion.[27,225] This agent has shown activity in the hypercalcemia of parathyroid carcinoma.[110]

Parathyroid carcinomas are resistant to radiotherapy, although radiation can occasionally be used for palliation of pain from bone metastasis.[236] There is little experience with systemic therapy. Partial and temporary remissions have been observed with hormonal therapy, including estrogens and testosterone.[51] A partial remission of 10 months duration was reported with a synthetic estrogen (phenol, 4,4'-(1,2-diethyl ethylene).[77]

Experience with chemotherapy is anecdotal. Combination chemotherapy using MACC (methotrexate, doxorubicin, cyclophosphamide and CCNU) was reported in a patient with metastatic nonfunctioning parathyroid carcinoma.[51] This combination produced objective regression of a large metastatic mediastinal mass and malignant pleural effusion for 18 months. Cisplatin given once (50 mg/m^2) at relapse produced no response. Another case of nonfunctioning carcinoma was treated with a modification of the MACC protocol (mitoxantrone substituted for doxorubicin) and had a partial response for 10+ months.[186] A combination of cyclophosphamide, 5-fluorouracil and dacarbazine produced complete regression of pulmonary metastases and a partial biochemical response of 13 months duration in a patient with a functioning parathyroid carcinoma.[42] In another patient, dacarbazine alone produced a partial response of short duration (<2 months) with marked decrease of serum calcium and iPTH.[47]

Medullary Thyroid Carcinoma (MTC)

Epidemiology

MTC is an uncommon tumor representing 5–10% of all thyroid cancers.[2] The only known etiologic factors for occurrence of this neoplasm are the autosomal dominant genetic disorders MEN 2a, MEN 2b, and familial non MEN syndromes which accounts for 20% of patients with MTC. Otherwise, MTC arises as a sporadic tumor with an equal frequency between men and women, and among different ethnic groups. The peak onset of the sporadic form of MTC is in the fifth or sixth decade of life, while this tumor appears much earlier in the MEN syndromes discussed below.[233]

Natural History

Pathological Considerations. MTC is a neoplasm of the calcitonin-secreting C-cells which are sparsely distributed in the thyroid gland.[310] In approximately 80% of patients, MTC occurs as a sporadic tumor with a unilateral origin in the thyroid. In 20% of patients, however, the neoplasm occurs in an autosomal dominant genetic syndrome, of which there are three or more that may involve other endocrine and neural lesions. In these inherited forms, MTC arises as multifocal, bilateral tumors in the thyroid.

Patients with the sporadic form of MTC present with palpable thyroid nodules and almost always have cervical lymph node involvement. MTCs are well demarcated, whitish, firm nodules which, microscopically, consist of sheets or nests of polygonal cells separated by variable amounts of fibrous

stroma (Figure XXVI-4-1). Often the tumors stain positive for amyloid. The hallmark histologic feature of MTC, however, is positive immunostaining for the peptide hormone, calcitonin, which is the major biochemical product of normal thyroid C-cells. The presence of calcitonin can help make the diagnosis of MTC when patients present with one of the several variant histological forms that have been described.[182] Immunostaining for calcitonin is also necessary for the diagnosis of the precursor lesions for MTC which occur bilaterally in the genetic forms of this tumor discussed in more detail below.

Biological Characteristics. By far the most striking biological characteristic of MTC is the occurrence of this neoplasm in a multifocal pattern in autosomal dominant genetic syndromes.[315] The molecular basis for these genetic forms of MTC is not yet understood but the known chromosomal changes and stages for development of the tumors are discussed below, in the section on inherited MTC.

The molecular basis for the loss of differentiation in the aggressive forms of MTC is not yet fully established. In contrast to many solid tumors, chromosomal changes in MTC, such as frequent allelic deletions, are not common.[148,192] Although several investigators have implicated chromosome 10,[145,171,188,261,262] the only consistent abnormalities appear to be deletions on the short arm of chromosome 1,[172] and

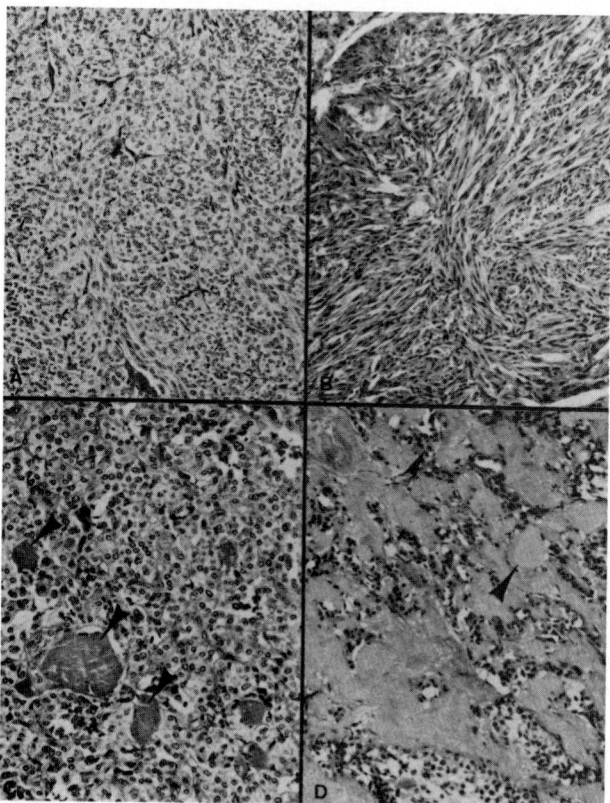

Figure XXVI-4-1. Histologic features of medullary thyroid cancer. A. Nests of polygonal cells. B. Spindle-shaped cells. C. Amyloid deposits (arrows). D. Large amount of fibrous stroma with sparse cells and amyloid nodules (arrows). (Reproduced with permission from Medelsohn et al.[181])

these could be involved with tumor progression rather than initiation.

Studies of cultured MTC cells from a patient with virulent MTC indicate that whatever chromosome regions are involved, a deficient activation of one or more cells signal transduction pathways may be a key step in progression of MTC. Activation of either the protein kinase C or protein kinase A pathways can partially differentiate cultured MTC cells as manifested by an increase in transcription of the calcitonin gene and slowing of cell growth.[191] A virtually complete differentiation response can be elicited in these same cells by insertion of a mutated Harvey *ras* oncogene.[191] In this situation, not only is there an increase in calcitonin gene expression, but the mRNA splicing for the resultant transcripts resembles the pattern of mRNA splicing in the normal thyroid C-cell. In addition, the cells acquire the typical mature neurosecretory granules of APUD cells, which are lacking in the control cultured cells. The final mediators of this response to an inserted *ras* gene are being investigated, but a coordinated increase in the protein kinase A and C pathways, plus other signal transduction input, is probably involved. A marked increase in expression of the c-*iun* oncogene,[191] which is known to participate in multiple protein kinase C mediated events, accompanies the *ras* gene induced differentiation of the MTC cells. Presumably, the increase in this transcription factor activates a series of other transcription factors which mediate maturation of the cells.

Clinical Features. The most common clinical features are a local neck mass and, less commonly, morbid signs or symptoms from distant metastases. In general, the production of secretory peptides is of no clinical significance although occasionally, apparent manifestations of MTC endocrine activity may be observed. For example, patients with MTC can develop Cushing's syndrome due to ACTH production.[180] More often, serotonin, prostaglandins, and perhaps other hormones produced by the tumor, may be implicated in the secretory diarrhea seen in up to 30% of patients with advanced MTC.[56] Although a physiologic role for calcitonin gene-related peptide (CGRP) has not been established, it is possible that, as a powerful peripheral vasodilator, CGPR, together with substance P, may play a role in the flushing observed in certain patients with advanced MTC.

Another important feature of MTC is the variable clinical behavior of this cancer. Although MTC metastasizes early, especially to cervical lymph nodes and mediastinal structures, it behaves in a relatively indolent manner in approximately 70–80% of patients.[2,233,239] Some patients, even with well documented hepatic and pulmonary metastases also take an indolent course. In another group of patients, however, MTC can behave aggressively and patients die from widespread bony and visceral metastases to lung, liver, and adrenals.[195] The overall survival rates for individuals with MTC are 80% for 5-years and 60% for 10-years (Figure XXVI-4-2A and B).[233]

The complete basis for the variable clinical behavior of MTC is not known. Inability of neoplastic C-cells to attain a fully differentiated phenotype appears to be important.[191] This deficiency in maturation is manifest as a marked decrease in the immunoreactive calcitonin and amyloid content of the tumor cells in patients with aggressive MTC.[23,191] Immuno-

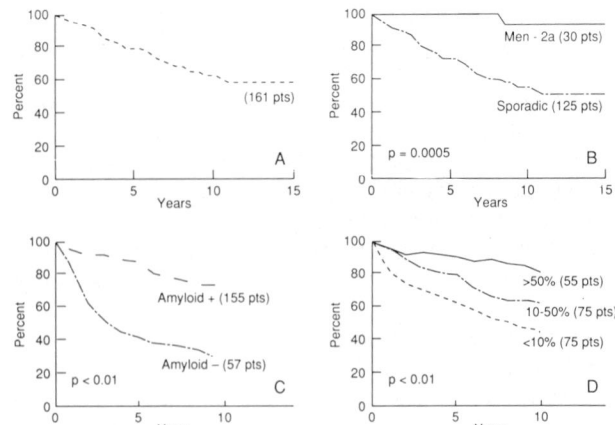

Figure XXVI-4-2. Survival of patients with medullary thyroid carcinoma (MTC). A. Adjusted survival of all patients with MTC. B. Survival of patients with sporadic MTC compared to patients with MEN 2a. C. Relative survival of patients according to amyloid positive (+) or negative (−) tumor staining characteristics. D. Relative survival of MTC patients according to percentage of tumor cells positive for calcitonin immunoreactivity. (Reproduced with permission from Saad et al.[233] and Bergholm et al.[23])

staining of such tumors reveals large areas of calcitonin negative cells which can co-exist with areas of positive staining.[156,191] This heterogeneous calcitonin staining pattern or lack of amyloid, when found in primary MTC lesions, is associated with a virulent course and poor survival at 5-years (Figures XXVI-4-2C and D).[23,156,232]

Biochemical Features. The distinguishing biochemical features of MTC relate primarily to the origin of this cancer in the calcitonin-producing C-cells of the thyroid[310] and from the general characteristics of the group of neuroendocrine cells to which these C-cells belong.

The main secretory product of the C-cells, and the biochemical marker of most clinical utility in patients with MTC, is the 32 amino acid peptide calcitonin. Calcitonins encoded by a multiexonic gene, which by alternative processing of a primary RNA transcript, generates two mRNAs. One codes for calcitonin itself and, another, for a 37 amino acid peptide called calcitonin gene-related peptide or CGRP.[4] The calcitonin mRNA predominates in normal thyroid C-cells, but, in MTC, both CGRP and calcitonin mRNAs are often found in high quantities. Both peptides may circulate at high levels in the blood of patients with MTC, but CGRP levels are much more variable and are usually lower than calcitonin levels.[170,243] During provocative diagnostic testing, as discussed below, calcitonin levels increase briskly in response to calcium and/or pentagastrin stimulation, whereas CGRP responses have been variable.[170,243]

MTC cells also express several biochemical markers that relate to the APUD features of these neuroendocrine cells, including small polypeptide hormones such as somatostatin,[226] adrenocorticotropic hormone (ACTH),[180] and gastrin-releasing peptide (GRP).[125] Like other neuroendocrine cells, MTC contains the enzyme L-dopa decarboxylase,[20] prostaglandins,[311] chromogranin A,[60] and neuron-specific enolase (NSE).[138,258] High levels of the histamine metabolizing enzyme, histaminase or diamine oxidase, are also characteristic of MTC.[20] Furthermore, these biochemical markers may occasionally be of diagnostic utility. Immunostaining of chromogranin A is positive in a very high percentage of MTC tumors, and thus may help make the diagnosis of MTC in tumors which stain poorly for calcitonin.[60,138,258]

Another biochemical marker frequently expressed by MTC is carcinoembryonic antigen (CEA). This protein is synthesized by the tumor cells at all stages of disease.[228,231] Even in the aggressive forms of MTC, where the tumor tissue becomes heterogeneous for calcitonin staining, CEA remains present. In fact, a rising blood CEA level in the face of a stable or declining calcitonin level indicates a poor prognosis in patients with MTC.[231]

Diagnostic Tests

The majority of patients with sporadic MTC present with palpable thyroid nodules which are manifested as cold nodules on ^{131}I radionuclide imaging, and as solid masses on echography. Occasionally, plain x-rays of the neck reveal a dense pattern of calcifications which is characteristic of MTC, different from the fine calcification pattern observed with papillary carcinoma. In most patients the diagnosis of MTC is made unexpectedly from examination of frozen or permanent sections of a thyroid mass removed at the time of initial surgery.

Even though virtually all patients with palpable MTC have elevated basal serum levels of calcitonin, the relative rarity of MTC makes it impractical to use this test to screen all patients who have thyroid nodules. Stimulated calcitonin secretion as described in the section on MEN 2 below, should be reserved for testing patients suspected of having MEN 2 or familial non-MEN MTC and for screening their immediate family members.[216,307] A more practical approach involves use of fine needle aspiration (FNA) biopsy to assess any patient with a suspicious thyroid nodule (Figure XXVI-4-3). The cytologic evaluation of such specimens, especially when combined with immunostaining for calcitonin, may suggest MTC and serum calcitonin immunoassays can be employed to confirm the diagnosis.

In all patients documented to have MTC, a prime consideration is the possibility that the patient may represent the index case for one of the familial forms of the disease. In the rare genetic syndrome, MEN 2b, an associated Marfan-like habitus and the presence of neuromas over the eyelids, lips and tongue should make the diagnosis obvious. For the other forms of genetic MTC, however, there are no particular physical stigmata. The possibility of familial disease then must be ruled out in virtually every patient with MTC. One extremely helpful criterion for the diagnosis of familial MTC is the presence of bilateral tumors and/or C-cell hyperplasia. Occurrence of MTC in patients younger than 40 years of age also suggests familial disease. Screening of first degree relatives with calcitonin determinations is, however, the only definitive way to exclude genetic disease. Recent studies suggest that the genetic form of MTC is found in 10–15% of cases when evaluating relatives of patients with apparently sporadic MTC.[216] The most effective approach, if possible, is first to screen the parents of a newly diagnosed MTC patient. A single negative test in the parents dramatically reduces the probability of familial disease. If the parents are not available,

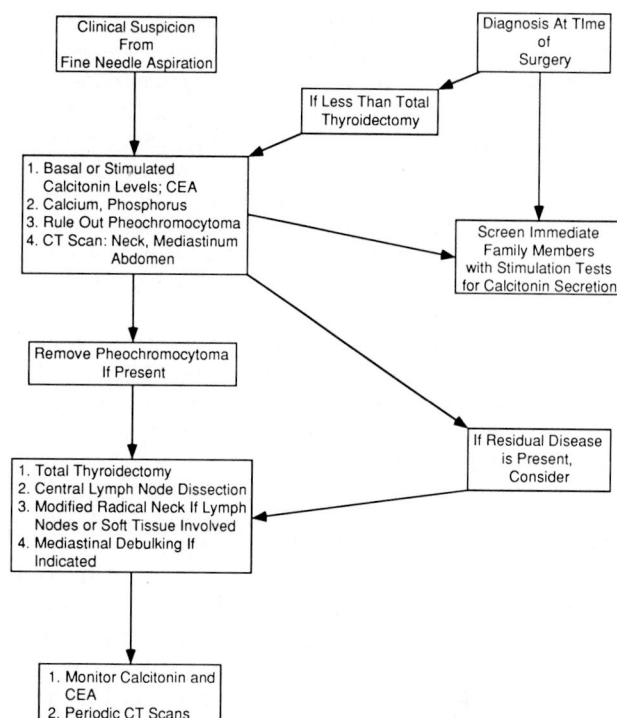

Figure XXVI-4-3. Algorithm for the diagnosis and management of medullary thyroid carcinoma.

screening of as many siblings and offspring as possible is mandatory.

Therapeutic Considerations

Surgical Management. Sporadic MCT usually presents as a solitary nodule in the upper half of the lateral lobe on either side, although in some cases, a metastatic lymph node may be detected first while the primary tumor remains occult to clinical examination. Currently, the diagnosis is frequently established before operation by FNA cytology, after which a basal serum calcitonin can be obtained to confirm the diagnosis (Figure XXVI-4-3). The calcitonin level may be of value in predicting the amount of tumor present and whether lymph nodes are likely to be involved. Urinary catecholamine levels must be obtained to rule out pheochromocytoma, even when the history is negative for MEN 2a and there are no physical findings to suggest MEN 2b, before a thyroidectomy is undertaken (Figure XXVI-4-3). If present, the pheochromocytoma should always be removed prior to the thyroidectomy.

The minimal treatment of MTC is total thyroidectomy.[102] In sporadic disease, this allows for excision of any intraglandular lymphatic spread and careful immunohistopathologic study of the contralateral lobe for possible C-cell hyperplasia. Even in some patients with metastases, given the fact that MTC is often slow growing, minimal treatment is a total thyroidectomy. Although not curative, this may prevent tumor growth which can impinge on major structures such as the trachea and esophagus. Most patients with sporadic disease have lymph node metastases when first diagnosed. A central lymph node compartment dissection, preserving the parathyroid glands and recurrent laryngeal nerves is indicated.

Dissection of the nodes includes the Delphian group, those around the upper pole of the thyroid lobe, those in the tracheo-esophageal groove along the recurrent laryngeal nerve and the anterior mediastinal lymph nodes to the level of the innominate artery. Some nodes contain metastases in nearly all patients with a palpable primary tumor within the thyroid gland at operation. If lateral lymph nodes are involved, a modified radical neck dissection should be done.[230] Occasionally, because of invasion through the lymph node capsule and involvement of contiguous structures, a formal radical dissection may be required.

In patients with MTC, discovered by calcitonin screening and no palpable tumor, central compartment lymph nodes may be tumor free. Nevertheless, even normal sized nodes should be sampled for frozen section examination to determine whether a complete and thorough central compartment dissection is required (Figure XXVI-4-3). Lateral lymph node involvement is treated by modified neck dissection, which may be bilateral, performed in one or two stages. When the lateral lymph nodes are involved with MCT, a biochemical cure as determined by calcitonin testing, is unlikely (<20%). As a result, a formal (modified) radical neck dissection has been considered by many to be futile.[230] Occasionally, this is still indicated if the procedure is required to excise all areas of gross disease because of lymph node invasion of local tissues. For this reason, when possible prior to initial surgery, or following surgery, computerized tomography or magnetic resonance image scans of the cervical, mediastinum and abdominal regions should be done to document areas of discernible metastases. When calcitonin levels remain elevated despite lack of clinically evident disease after a total thyroidectomy and central compartment dissection, controversy continues as to whether a neck dissection on one, or both sides, should be done. Tissel favors a meticulous radical neck dissection and has achieved a biochemical cure in about half of a relatively small group of patients treated this way.[288] Alternatively, others have favored regional excision of any palpable nodes or those suspected on the basis of a positive thallium scan or cervical ultrasound when the disease has been limited to the lateral neck or anterior mediastinum. One of the causes of failure after performing a radical neck dissection based entirely on an elevated calcitonin level is that clinically occult MTC already may have spread hematogenously to involve the liver, lungs, or bone. Therefore, it is reasonable to perform selective venous sampling for calcitonin to rule out disseminated disease before considering any extensive additional neck procedures.

Treatment of Recurrent or Metastatic Disease. When persistent, recurrent, or disseminated disease is present, MTC usually progresses slowly. Since effective radiation therapy or chemotherapy is not well established, it is important to consider several prognostic factors when deciding if chemotherapy is indicated. As discussed previously, tumors that have poor immunocytochemical staining for calcitonin tend to have a more aggressive course.[23,156,232] Although the serum calcitonin level correlates with the extent of disease, it does not help in identifying patients with a poorer prognosis. Rapidly rising, high serum carcinoembryonic antigen (CEA), is more predictive of a rapid disease course.[231]

Recurrent tumors may be amenable to repeated surgical resection, especially for palliation of symptoms due to local tissue invasion or due to a syndrome of hormonal excess. Radiation therapy does not have an established role in the treatment of locally advanced MTC.[239] In selected cases of patients with symptomatic bone metastases, a trial of radiation may offer transient palliative benefit.

Although most reports of chemotherapy for MTC are anecdotal, the experience provides some guidelines for therapeutic approaches. Since MTC belongs to the APUD family of neoplasms, a number of single agent and combination chemotherapy treatments that show activity in other "APUD-omas" have been used in advanced MTC.

Gottlieb and colleagues reported three partial remissions and resolution of disease related diarrhea in six patients with advanced MTC following treatment with doxorubicin.[93] Additional reports by others suggest an overall partial response rate of 30% in 46 patients with MTC treated with doxorubicin as a single agent.[118,229,256,263] The combination of streptozocin and doxorubicin was not active in a small trial of patients.[140,306] Reports of the combination of 5-fluorouracil and dacarbazine (including a complete response),[212] doxorubicin and cisplatin,[272] or of dacarbazine,[133] 5-fluorouracil,[76] or etoposide,[76,115] used as single agents suggest limited activity for these drugs.[256,313] The combination of cyclophosphamide, vincristine, and dacarbazine found to be effective in malignant pheochromocytoma[14] has been studied in three patients by us.[13,59a] Two of these patients had a partial response demonstrated by reduced serum calcitonin and/or CEA and objective regression of radiologically demonstrated masses. The other patient had stable disease for more than 17 months. Until prospective multiinstitutional studies of combination chemotherapy regimens for patients with metastatic MTC are undertaken, dacarbazine or cisplatin and doxorubicin containing regimens should be considered for individual patients with progressive, symptomatic disease.

Since biological response modifiers, such as the somatostatin analog, octreotide acetate, have been shown to reduce circulating hormones, halt progression, and occasionally reduce tumor size in various neuroendocrine tumors,[92] this agent may have a role in patients with MTC.[92,183] Long term subcutaneous injection of octreotide acetate to 21 patients with MTC reduced serum calcitonin in 11, but CEA did not change.[161,183] Flushing and diarrhea improved in some and several patients reportedly had objective tumor response. Additional clinical studies are required to determine the activity of somatostatin analogs in patients with metastatic MTC.

Pheochromocytoma

Pheochromocytoma and paraganglioma are terms describing a neoplasm of chromaffin cells found in the adrenal medulla or elsewhere within the sympathetic paraganglionic axis. The adrenal tumors are usually referred to as pheochromoctyomas, while an extra-adrenal tumor is often termed either extra-adrenal pheochromocytoma or paraganglioma, the latter usually reserved for a non-functional (i.e., non-catecholamine secreting) neoplasm. This terminology is based on historical histopathological techniques, and since these neoplasms are otherwise indistinguishable, the terminology may be confusing. Therefore, all of these neoplasms considered here will be referred to as pheochromocytomas. Additional descriptions, e.g., nonfunctional, extra-adrenal, or malignant should be included in the terminology as appropriate. Rare chromaffin neoplasms arising from special structures in the neck may be referred to as chemodectomas, glomus jugulare, or carotid body tumors.[211,255]

Epidemiology

Pheochromocytomas occur infrequently and are found in approximately 0.1–0.5% of hypertensive patients.[21,165,292] A historical autopsy series from the Mayo Clinic reported an incidence of 0.1% with one-half of the patients normotensive and three-fourths of the patients undiagnosed pre-mortem.[273] Even more recent series suggest that up to one-third of pheochromocytomas may not be diagnosed pre-mortem.[184,247] From the Mayo Clinic data, it is estimated that approximately 800 cases of pheochromocytoma are diagnosed in the U.S. each year.[21] The average annual incidence of pheochromocytoma in Sweden and Denmark is 2.1 and 1.9 cases per million population, respectively.[6,274]

Ninety percent of pheochromocytomas are sporadic neoplasms. Thus, when considering the diagnosis and management of this disease it is important also to consider the "rough rule of 10s." That is, 10% of neoplasms occur in children, 10% are associated with familial syndromes, 10% are bilateral, 10% are extra-adrenal, and 10% are malignant.[166,224,273,292] This mnemonic provides only an estimate of these presentations, and there is overlap within the pediatric, familial, and bilateral groups.[48,157] The most common familial syndromes that include pheochromocytoma as an element are the autosomal dominant multiple endocrine neoplasia (MEN) syndromes type 2a and 2b.[131,252,292] The former is characterized by parathyroid adenoma and the latter by ganglioneuromatosis and Marfanoid-like body habitus. Medullary thyroid carcinoma and pheochromocytoma are common to both syndromes. Pheochromocytomas have also been associated with von Hippel-Lindau disease, neurofibromatosis, and as a component of Carney's triad.[48,113,141,159,187] Familial pheochromocytomas typically follow a benign course, but because of their potential for causing significant morbidity or mortality, this tumor must be diagnosed and removed prior to any surgical management of thyroid or parathyroid disease.

Malignant pheochromocytoma is a rare entity among malignant diseases and its exact incidence is not known. Multiple series have estimated the frequency of malignancy among pheochromocytomas from 5–46%,[26,99,122,127,179,247,291] although the latter figure is probably inflated since it comes from a very selective referral patient population.[26] Overall, a figure of 13% of all pheochromocytomas probably represents a reliable incidence for malignant pheochromocytoma.[14] A review of SEER data for 1973–1985 suggests that the yearly age adjusted rate of malignant pheochromocytoma is .04 per 100,000 population or approximately 100 cases per year in the U.S.[14a] Extra-adrenal pheochromocytoma has been associated with a higher frequency of malignancy,[122,142,179,255,292] although this has been recently challenged.[89]

Natural History

Embryology and Anatomy. Chromaffin tissue constitutes one component of the diffuse neuroendocrine (APUD) system, thought to be derived from the embryonic neuroectodermal crest.[210,211] Although this embryologic origin of APUD tumors is now disputed,[7,19,124,151] the common genetic and clinicopathological characteristics of pheochromocytoma and APUD tumors justify their consideration as entities of a common neuroendocrine system. In the fetus and in infancy, diffuse paraganglionic chromaffin tissue is prominent but later regresses, aside from that found within the adrenal medulla.[143] Because of this, pheochromocytomas may arise from chromaffin remnants virtually anywhere, but the vast majority (90%) are found in the adrenal medulla.[141,179]

Pathological Characteristics. The typical adrenal pheochromocytoma is a sporadically occurring neoplasm, arising from either gland. When detected it is approximately 5 cm in diameter and weighs 50–100 g.[141] The adrenal mass is often pseudoencapsulated and it is highly vascularized with a beefy appearance and consistency. Larger tumors frequently contain areas of hemorrhage or empty or fluid filled cysts surrounded by connective tissue and calcifications (Figure XXVI-4-4A). The microscopic appearance of a pheochromocytoma is similar to the architecture and morphology of normal chromaffin tissue. The cells are usually round or polygonal with abundant eosinophilic or basophilic fine granular cytoplasm and are frequently arranged in cords or clusters (Fig. XXVI-4-4B).[141] Nuclear pleomorphism and hyperchromasia are common. Mitotic figures are often seen in adrenal hyperplasia and in pheochromocytoma, but they are not necessarily prominent histological features. Chromaffin cells and pheochromocytomas show a characteristic brown staining following application of chromium salts (hence, chromaffin) although this method has largely been replaced by the Grimelius argyrophile stain.[95] The demonstration of a wide array of neuroendocrine products by immunocytochemical analysis reflects the content of dense intracytoplasmic neurosecretory granules which are apparent by electron microscopic examination (Fig. XXVI-4-4C).[141] Commonly identified products include biogenic amines, neuron specific enzymes, and neuropeptides (Table XXVI-4-4).[55,86,104,131,141,155,158,166,198–200,227,240,242,296,297,305]

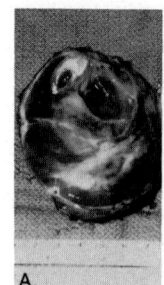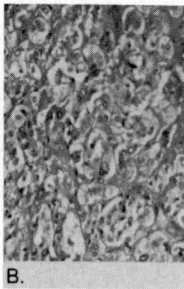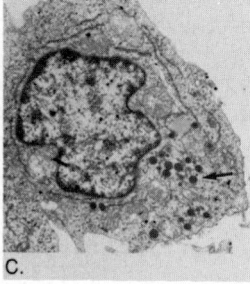

Figure XXVI-4-4. Pheochromocytoma. A. Gross appearance of a surgically removed hemisected extra-adrenal pheochromocytoma. B. Histopathological appearance of a pheochromocytoma showing typical cords of glandular cells separated by bands of stroma (hematoxylin and eosin, × 25). C. Ultrastructural appearance of a single pheochromocytoma cell showing dense neurosecretory granules (arrow) (× 6,000).

Table XXVI-4-4.   **Biological Markers in Pheochromocytoma**

	Blood	Immunocyto-chemistry	Molecular
Probe biogenic amines			
Norepinephrine	X		
Epinephrine	X		
Dopamine	X		
DOPA	X		
Serotonin	X		
Enzymes			
Neuron specific enolase	X	X	
Dopa decarboxylase		X	
Dopamine-β-hydroxylase	X	X	
Peptides			
Chromogranin A	X	X	X
Neuropeptide Y	X	X	X
Enkephalins		X	
Corticotropin releasing factor	X	X	
Somatotrophin releasing factor	X	X	
Vasoactive intestinal polypeptide (VIP)	X	X	
Somatostatin	X	X	
PTH-related peptide	X		X
Pancreatic polypeptide		X	
Calcitonin	X	X	
Calcitonin gene related peptide		X	
Substance P	X	X	
Gastrin releasing peptide		X	
Neurotensin		X	
Insulin-like growth factor II			X
Gastrin		X	
Cholecystokinin		X	

There are no pathognomonic criteria for malignancy of a pheochromocytoma other than the natural history of an individual's tumor that manifests chromaffin cell invasion or dissemination at sites where chromaffin tissue is normally not present. Malignant tumors have a predilection for spreading to bone (predominantly to spine, ribs and skull),[160] lung, liver, retroperitoneal and mediastinal lymph nodes.[14,64,255] A number of studies have attempted to identify characteristics that can discriminate malignant from benign tumors.[141,178] Among these, nuclear pleomorphism, mitotic figures, vascular invasion, cortical extension, necrosis, and immunocytochemical characteristics are not particularly useful. Some authors have shown that increased tumor size and extra-adrenal location are associated with a malignant phenotype.[178,179,292] Investigations of tumor DNA ploidy by flow cytometry have demonstrated the potential utility of this technique for defining a malignant subset.[114,136,154] Of 62 tumors studied, approximately one-third of tumors containing aneuploid, polyploid or tetraploid DNA were malignant, while all 18 that were diploid followed a benign course, a statistically significant difference.[114] However, DNA ploidy is not discriminant for malignancy since this study and others demonstrated a high prevalence of aneuploidy in benign pheochromocytomas as well.[5,206,207]

Biological Characteristics. There is sparse information regarding the molecular genetic characteristics of pheochromocytoma. Chromosomal alterations including loss of heterozygosity at specific loci may be found for those tumors associated with the familial multiple neuroendocrine syndrome MEN 2.[171,188,261,262] For sporadic pheochromocytomas and other endocrine tumors, deletions on the short arm of chromosome 1 have been reported most frequently, though the total number of samples analyzed has been relatively small.[172,290]

Clinical Features. There is no correlation between the amount of catecholamines produced and the severity of blood pressure changes.[166] Thus, patients may present anywhere in the spectrum from normotensive and asymptomatic to a severe, life-threatening hypertensive crisis causing cerebral hemorrhage, myocardial infarction, or cardiac failure.[184,241] Labile episodic or sustained hypertension each occurs in approximately one-half of patients with pheochromocytoma. Hypertensive episodes may be precipitated by physical stress, an increase in intraabdominal pressure, or by certain drugs.[131] Patients may have tachycardia or bradycardia depending on whether the tumor predominantly secretes epinephrine or norepinephrine, respectively. Characteristically, patients may also have any of several protean signs and symptoms including headaches, palpitations, anxiety, sweating, pain, nausea, constipation, and mild fasting hyperglycemia.[127,166] An important feature that distinguishes hypertension of pheochromocytoma from essential hypertension (in the absence of pharmacologic therapy) is the presence of postural hypotension.[22,166,184] Because of chronic vasoconstriction, the down regulation of peripheral alpha receptors, and the presence of vasodilatory biogenic amines or peptides, patients with pheochromocytoma are commonly hypovolemic, accounting for postural blood pressure changes.[22,131,252]

Biochemical Features. Along with other neoplasms of the diffuse neuroendocrine (APUD) system, pheochromocytomas are specialized neoplasms that can synthesize, store, and secrete biological amines and peptides. A large number of these substances have been associated with pheochromocytoma and they are often capable of producing specific clinical syndromes (Table XXVI-4-4).[55,86,104,131,166,227,240,242,296,297,305] Chromagranin A is a soluble binding protein found in the neurosecretory granule; it is the most prevalent biologic marker for pheochromocytoma.[198] This marker is not specific, however, since it is also expressed in other neuroendocrine and non-endocrine neoplasms as well.[109,199,269]

Neuropeptide Y is a peptide with potent vasoconstrictor acitivity. High neuropeptide Y immunoreactivity has been found in pheochromocytomas;[3] Grouzmann and co-workers have shown elevated plasma neuropeptide Y in patients with pheochromocytoma.[97] In their studies the highest levels of neuropeptide Y and neuron specific enolase were found in patients with malignant pheochromocytoma.[98] This finding contrasts somewhat with that of Helman and colleagues who found that neuropeptide Y RNA was highly expressed in all nine benign pheochromocytomas but only in 4 of 11 malignant pheochromocytomas.[108] Further investigations are necessary to determine the exact role for neuropeptide Y as a marker for clonal expansion of chromaffin cells[201] and whether it reliably indicates malignancy. By far, the most important secretory products of pheochromocytomas are the biogenic amines (Figure XXVI-4-5) (Table XXVI-4-4). The majority of these neoplasms secrete excess norepinephrine that results in sporadic or sustained hypertension.[165] Epinephrine is the major catecholamine secreted by normal adrenal medulla and it is frequently elevated in pheochromocytoma, especially in familial cases, but norepinephrine predominates in most tumors.[35] Dopamine, and the catecholamine precursor, dihydroxyphenylalanine (dopa) are also secreted by pheochromocytomas and there is some evidence that high circulating levels of these norepinephrine precursors are more commonly associated with a malignant phenotype.[90,220]

Diagnostic Tests

The fundamental basis for the diagnosis of pheochromocytoma is a high index of clinical suspicion with confirmation by biochemical determinations for catecholamines or catecholamine metabolites in blood or urine.[22] The most common and reliable tests are the measurements of 24-hour urinary excretion for catecholamines, metanephrines, or vanillylmandelic acid (VMA) (Figure XXVI-4-5).[35,237] Spot (2-hour)

urine specimens for metanephrines or plasma norepinephrine are preferred by some authors although these tests may be associated with a higher number of false positive or false negative outcomes.[35,214] More sophisticated catecholamine metabolite assays have been proposed to increase the specificity of urinary determinations.[65]

The clonidine suppression test, platelet catecholamine content, or leukocyte β-adrenergic receptor assays may be helpful to distinguish patients with essential hypertension from patients with pheochromocytoma that have borderline elevation of plasma or urinary catecholamines.[36,126,165,319] In more elusive cases, provocative testing with glucagon combined with baseline and post-glucagon plasma catecholamine determinations can be diagnostic for tumors with episodic catecholamine release.[96,152] This diagnostic test is associated with some risks, so that it should be conducted by experienced personnel with appropriate precautions taken.[22,96,131,152]

Anatomical localization utilizing noninvasive modern radiologic techniques is critical once the clinical and biochemical diagnoses are confirmed. Angiography, selective venogra-

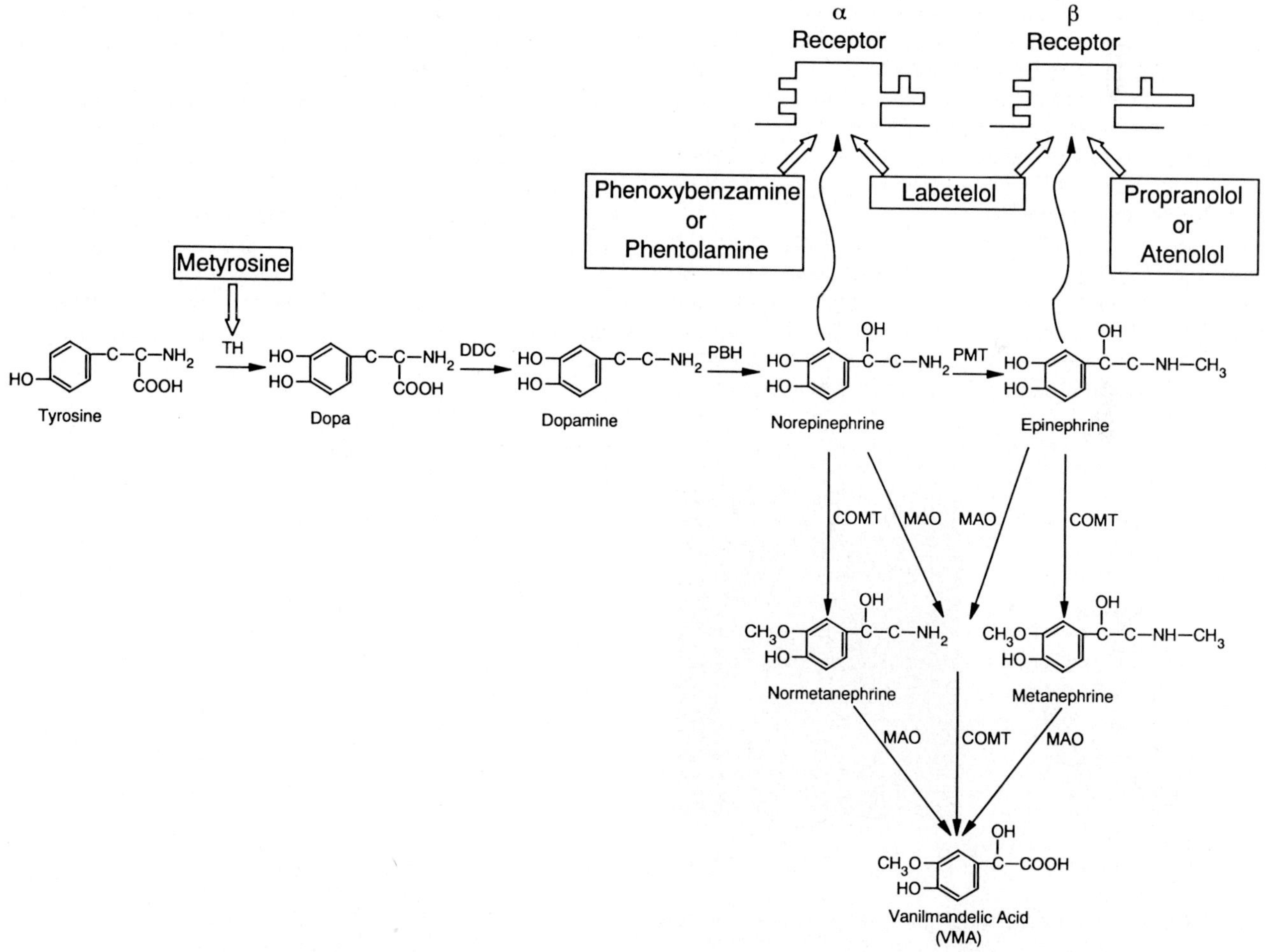

Figure XXVI-4-5. Synthetic and metabolic pathways for the catecholamines, norepinephrine and epinephrine, which are stored and secreted by chromaffin cells and pheochromocytomas. The curved arrows represent physiologic agonist-receptor interaction. The boxed arrows represent competitive antagonism at the rate-limiting step of synthesis or at receptor sites by therapeutic agents (see text). TH, tyrosine hydroxylase; DDC, dopa decarboxylase; PBH, phenylamine-β-hydroxylase; PMT, phenylethanolamine-N-methyltransferase; COMT, catechol-O-methyltransferase; MAO, monoamine oxidase.

phy, and intravenous pyelography rarely have a role in the localization of pheochromocytoma any longer. Because of its safety and high diagnostic accuracy, scintigraphic localization with radiolabelled ^{131}I-metaiodobenzylguanidine (MIBG) should be conducted in all patients with a biochemical diagnosis of pheochromocytoma. MIBG is a structural analogue of guanethidine and as such, is readily taken up by the chromaffin cell and stored in neurosecretory granules.[266] Experience reported in over 1,000 patients uniformly shows a sensitivity of approximately 90% and a specificity of nearly 100% (Figure XXVI-4-6A).[111,237,253,254] Further experience with this modality suggests that its sensitivity may be considerably less in malignant pheochromocytoma and that its specificity is limited by the fact that MIBG is readily accumulated by other neuroendocrine tumors.[111,253,298] Certain drugs (e.g., labetelol) may reduce the uptake of the MIBG into the tumor's catecholamine storage vesicles causing a false negative test.[134,253]

If nuclear scanning with MIBG suggests that tumor is confined to one or both adrenal glands, and no extra-adrenal site is detected or suspected on clinical grounds, then a chest x-ray and computed tomography (CT) of the entire abdomen with amplified views of the adrenals is all that may be required for precise localization prior to operation for tumor extirpation.[237,252,294] Occasionally, the CT characteristics of size, contrast enhancement, and consistency may provide clues regarding the probability of malignancy.[119] Because of the risk of catastrophic hemorrhage or hypertensive complications, fine needle aspiration should not be attempted for cytological diagnosis.

Although not possessing the resolution of CT, magnetic resonance imaging (MRI) may have a special role in the localization of pheochromocytomas. These tumors have a particularly intense detectable signal on T2 weighted MR images, appearing as very bright spots compared to normal tissue (Figure XXVI-4-6B).[67,223] In addition, MR image reconstruction to demonstrate coronal or sagittal views of the tumor provide important preoperative anatomic information.[74,294] The MRI is probably not necessary for routine pheochromocytomas, but it should be used for localization in the case of malignant or extra-adrenal tumors, especially in the neck, mediastinum, liver, and retroperitoneum.[246] Because of the high prevalence of bone metastases, a bone scan should be performed in patients thought to have metastatic disease, since this test has a higher sensitivity than MIBG for bone metastases.[160] If the bone scan detects lesions in the axial skeleton, a spinal MRI may be considered to rule out early spinal cord compression. In summary, each of the methods for localization of pheochromocytoma described above are complementary; they should be employed in selective combination depending on individual circumstances.[294]

Therapeutic Considerations

Medical Management. If a pheochromocytoma is suspected on clinical grounds, prompt medical therapy should be instituted even prior to biochemical confirmation (Figure XXVI-4-7). The initial therapy should include cautious volume repletion with intravenous crystalloid and pharmacological control of the blood pressure.[35,166,184,292] In severe hypertension, α-adrenergic blockade with intravenous phentolamine or vasodilation with nitroprusside may be used.[117] The mainstay of preoperative pharmacological management is α-adrenergic blockade with phenoxybenzamine in doses ranging from 10 mg twice daily up to tolerable doses that will control blood pressure, allow for restitution of normal blood volume, and block catecholamine-induced gut hypomotility (Figure XXVI-4-7).[131,237,274] The major side effect is orthostatic hypotension, and reflex supraventricular tachycardias or arrythmias may occur. The latter may be controlled with the addition of β-blocking agents such as propranolol, aten-

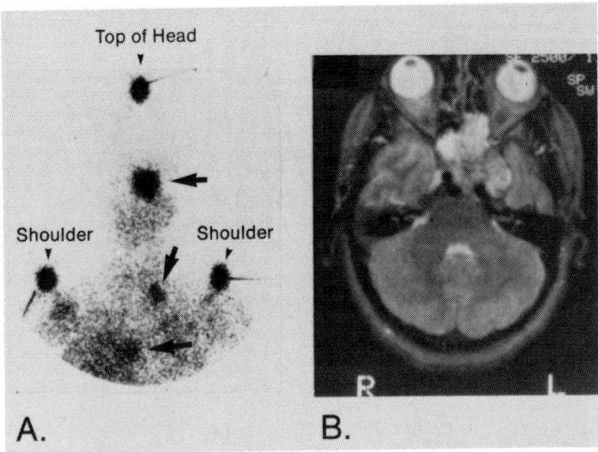

Figure XXVI-4-6. Diagnostic imaging in metastatic pheochromocytoma. A. Gamma camera image of the upper body of a patient 48 hours following injection of ^{131}I-metaiodobenzylguanidine. Areas of abnormal isotope uptake are noted at the base of the brain, the cervical region, and the mid-thoracic spine (arrows). B. T2 weighted magnetic resonance image of the same patient demonstrating a signal-intensive mass encroaching the circle of Willis, the left temporal lobe, and the left optic nerve.

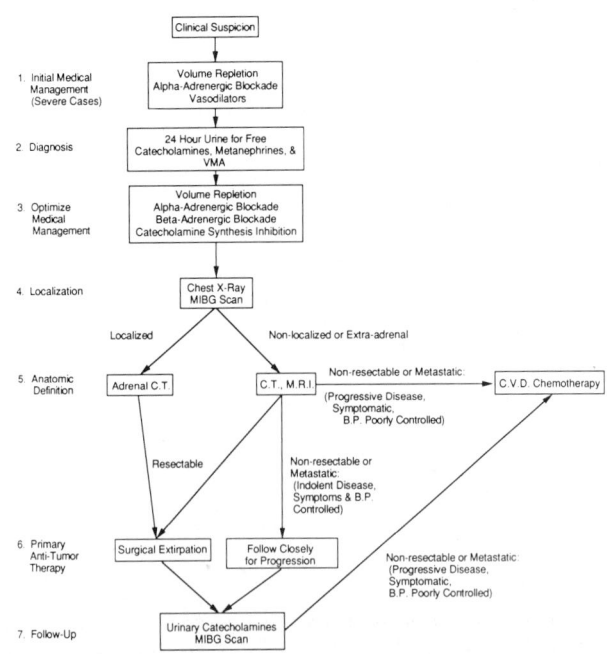

Figure XXVI-4-7. Algorithm for the diagnosis and management of pheochromocytoma.

olol, or esmolol *only after adequate α-blockade* is established since unopposed β-blockade may worsen vasoconstriction and hypertension. Additional agents may need to be added or substituted for optimal management.[22] These include the short acting α-blocker prazosin,[193] the combined α and β blocker labetolol,[190] calcium channel antagonists (nifedipine or verapamil),[197,221] and the angiotensin converting enzyme inhibitors (captopril or enalapril).[31] None of these agents has any particular advantages and some have disadvantages, so their use depends on individual circumstances and the experience of the clinician.

Metyrosine (α methyl-para-tyrosine) is a competitive inhibitor of the rate-limiting hydroxylation step of catecholamine synthesis and it is used in addition to α and β adrenergic active agents to deplete tumor catecholamines and further reduce blood pressure (Figure XXVI-4-5).[22,40] The starting dose is 250 mg four times daily and it may be titrated up to 4 g per day. The central nervous system side effects of sedation, irritability, nightmares, sleep disturbance, and hallucinations are, however, often dose-limiting.

Surgical Management of Benign or Recurrent Resectable Disease. The preoperative preparation of the patient with biochemical proof of a pheochromocytoma and appropriate localization studies are among the most important factors in reducing perioperative morbidity and mortality.[94,252] All patients, regardless of blood pressure readings, should be prepared with an alpha-blocking agent as described above for 7–14 days preoperatively. Induction of general anesthesia and manipulation of the tumor may provoke a release of massive amounts of catecholamines making prior receptor blockade important. In addition, most patients have significant reduction of intravascular fluid volume and α-blockade permits volume re-expansion. The administration of a beta-blocker may not always be necessary but clearly should be given if the patient has tachycardia, arrhythmia or a catecholamine profile showing a preponderance of epinephrine secretion. One approach is to give propranolol to most patients for 48 hours preoperatively, beginning with a dose of 10 mg four times a day. Propranolol and phenoxybenzamine may be given with a sip of water early on the morning of operation.

The operative approach is determined by the location of the tumor(s) as determined by preoperative imaging investigations. For intra-abdominal pheochromocytomas, an anterior approach is used to permit exploration of both adrenal glands and a thorough examination of the retroperitoneum for possible occult extra-adrenal pheochromocytomas.[35,94,131,184,248,292] Even when both CT and MIBG scans have localized a tumor to an adrenal gland, an anterior approach through a bucket handle or chevron upper abdominal incision is preferred in order that a thorough exploration can be performed and that the tumor may be excised with the least amount of manipulation.[50] The localized tumor is approached first. Palpation and manipulation are kept to an absolute minimum by a nearly no-touch technique. Identification and division of the central adrenal vein is done initially to minimize catecholamine release. Access to the right adrenal gland is achieved by reflecting the duodenum and pancreatic head to the left (Kocher's maneuver) and dissecting along the inferior vena cava. The left adrenal gland is approached through the lesser space after reflecting the greater omentum from the transverse colon. After removal of the adrenal containing the pheochromocytoma, the contralateral gland is carefully exposed and gently palpated. The retroperitoneum is then explored by extension of the Kocher maneuver to mobilize the right colon medially. The entire retroperitoneum, from the celiac axis to the bifurcation of the aorta, can be quickly explored for an extra-adrenal pheochromocytoma.[50] The most common location of these tumors is in the region where the left renal vein crosses the aorta. The renal hilus, and at the origin of the inferior mesenteric artery (organ of Zuckerkandl) are other possible sites that should be carefully evaluated. When extra-adrenal tumors have been localized preoperatively to other sites such as the pelvis, they are approached through incisions that allow adequate exposure for their excision. Even large malignant tumors of either adrenal gland can be removed from an upper abdominal incision rather than using a thoracoabdominal incision. In patients with large tumors some manipulation will be inevitable and blood pressure fluctuations should be expected even in those who are well prepared. For the control of hypertension intraoperatively, the rapidly acting direct vasodilating agent, sodium nitroprusside, may be used intravenously as a drip when the systolic blood pressure exceeds 160 mm Hg. The rate of infusion can be readily titrated to maintain the pressure at this level or lower. After the removal of the tumor there may be an increase in the intravascular capacity and an acute fall in blood pressure that is best managed by intravenous fluid replacement rather than vasopressor drugs.[24,50,252] Rarely, if the patient has been well prepared, an intravenous infusion of norepinephrine may be required while volume is being restored.

During operative manipulation of a pheochromocytoma, great care and gentleness are required not only to avoid episodes of severe hypertension but to avoid disruption of the tumor capsule. Malignancy cannot be determined either by the gross appearance or by histopathologic studies of the primary tumor in most cases. Some patients with proven malignant pheochromoctyoma as determined by bone, liver or lung metastases have had well encapsulated tumors without evidence of invasion or lymph node involvement. Capsular disruption by application of instruments or rough handling can result in implantation of tumor cells even when the neoplasm is considered benign.

When a pheochromocytoma is obviously malignant, as determined by preoperative studies or by the presence of metastases or local invasion found at exploration, it is not clear whether excising as much of the primary tumor and accessible metastases as is feasible will facilitate antihypertensive and chemotherapeutic drug activity postoperatively.[162,248,252,255] Although most soft tissue spread including some liver metastases are amenable to resection, the majority of patients with malignant pheochromocytomas also have bone metastases as well.[14,160]

The median time for recurrence for malignant pheochromocytoma following primary resection of disease is approximately 6 years and may be as long as 20 years.[26,160,224,247] After removal of a pheochromocytoma asymptomatic patients should have a clinical and biochemical assessment several times during the first year and then yearly follow-up with urine catecholamines.[26,35,162,184,247,252,271,291] Patients with extra-adrenal primaries or non-diploid tumors may require more frequent follow-up with urine catecholamines and perhaps an MIBG scan,[255] although the lack of discriminatory criteria for malignancy mandates lifetime follow-up of all patients following complete resection of their pheochromocytoma.[291] Pheochromocytoma during pregnancy requires special considerations.[68,103] In general, if diagnosed in the first or second trimester, surgical removal of the tumor is indicated following medical preoperative preparation. If diagnosed in the third trimester, medical management is indicated, combined with Cesarean delivery of the mature fetus.

Medical Treatment of Recurrent or Metastatic Disease. The diagnosis of malignant pheochromocytoma can be made only when the tumor is locally invasive and unresectable, recurs after primary extirpation, or is found to be metastatic. Although the natural history of the disease in each of these situations may be variable and somewhat unpredictable, advanced malignant pheochromocytoma is associated with a high morbidity and mortality.[14,99,142,153,224,248,292] These cancers also secrete catecholamines and often produce biogenic amines at a level much higher than benign neoplasms. Thus, the blood pressure elevations, cardiac effects, decreased bowel motility and other clinical complications of catecholamine excess may be severe and unrelenting. The management of these problems utilizes the same principles of pharmacologic adrenergic blockade and catecholamine synthesis inhibition as described previously.

The rarity and highly variable natural history of malignant pheochromocytoma preclude determining accurate survival estimates. Analysis of SEER data demonstrated a 5-year relative survival rate of 52% with a median survival time of 4 years.[14a] Three retrospective analyses with a long duration of patient follow-up reported a 5-year survival rate of 60%, 32%, and 44%, respectively.[99,122,224] A recent series of 22 patients treated at the National Institutes of Health and the Mount Sinai Medical Center had a 5-year survival rate of 66% with a median survival time of 74 months from the time of initial diagnosis of pheochromocytoma (Figure XXVI-4-8).[14a] All of these studies demonstrate that a significant number of patients with disseminated disease may live for long periods without specific antineoplastic therapy.[38,255] Overall, it appears that there are two distinct subsets within the population of patients with malignant pheochromocytoma: a group with aggressive disease that leads to early death (within 3 or 4 years) and a group with indolent disease that is compatible with long term survival (up to 20 or more years) (Figure XXVI-4-8).[224,292]

From the Mayo Clinic series, it appears that survival has not changed over the past several decades despite advances in diagnosis, localization, and pharmacotherapy of catecholamine excess.[224,292] Surgical debulking of malignant pheochromocytoma that cannot be completely extirpated is controversial and carries a certain operative risk without clear benefit.[162,248,252,255] The results of standard external beam radiation therapy for malignant pheochromocytoma has been limited to reports from small series of selected patients treated with a variety of techniques (Table XXVI-4-5).[64,248,257] In general, these data do not support the use of this modality except for palliation of painful bony metastases or spinal cord compression.

Targeted radiotherapy using high specific activity MIBG has been extensively investigated at the University of Michigan.[252] Because of the specificity of MIBG uptake by chromaffin tumors, this novel therapeutic approach initially generated much interest; in practice it was found that the majority of patients with malignant pheochromocytoma do not take up and retain sufficient MIBG to deliver an effective radiation dose to the tumor.[132,164,255] In their initial 63 patients screened with a tracer dose of MIBG, only 18 had sufficient uptake to permit therapeutic dosing, i.e., where between 100 to 250 mCi of MIBG will deliver 20 Gy to the tumor.[254] Out of a total of 28 patients treated by the Michigan group, eight patients had tumor and biochemical responses with most responses requiring several months and repeated dosing to become manifest.[252,253] Other investigators have reported similar results in highly selected patients (Table XXVI-4-5).[91,111,283,289,295] The cause for the insufficient uptake of MIBG for therapy by malignant chromaffin neoplasms is not fully understood, but it may be due to the fact that these neoplasms may have a less differentiated amine uptake and storage phenotype compared to benign and normal chromaffin cells.[90] Methods for accurate calculation of absorbed radiation dose are under development[137] and experimental models may provide new approaches to modulating tumor cell uptake of MIBG[30] but until such time as this and other difficulties are overcome, high dose MIBG for the treatment of pheochromocytoma has little clinical utility.

Until 1985, the data regarding standard systemic chemotherapy was limited to reports of empirically chosen single agents or combinations in small retrospective series and in anecdotal cases.[64,248] Because of its activity against gastroenteropancreatic tumors, streptozotocin was given to patients with metastatic pheochromocytoma with documented responses in some[73] but not others (Table XXVI-4-5).[101] Based on the premise that malignant pheochromocytoma and neuroblastoma are two APUD neoplasms that have many clinicopathological features in common,[90,299] a regimen highly effective in children with advanced neuroblastoma[75,132] was recently adapted for use in malignant pheochromocytoma. This regimen, a combination of cyclophosphamide, vincristine, and dacarbazine (CVD) was used in a prospective study of 14 patients with advanced, progressive and symptomatic pheochromocytoma.[14] There were 2 (14%) complete and 6 (43%) partial tumor remissions for a median duration of more than twenty-two months.

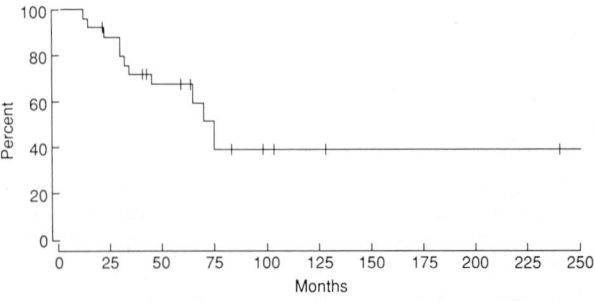

Figure XXVI-4-8. Actuarial survival of 22 patients with malignant pheochromocytoma from the time of surgical diagnosis.

Table XXVI-4-5. Treatment of Malignant Pheochromocytoma

	No. of Patients	Tumor Response	Biochem. Response	Palliation	Reference
Radiation therapy					
External beam	42	—	—	19	37, 52, 64, 91, 99, 111, 247
Targeted ^{131}I–MIBG	60	18	24	4	253, 283, 289, 295
Chemotherapy					
Streptozotocin +/− Misc. Agents	7	1	1	1	73, 101, 153, 248
Cyclophosphamide + Vincristine + Dacarbazine	23	14	17	—	13, 14, 235, 257
Cyclophosphamide +/− Misc. Agents	19	2	2	7	43, 64, 153, 248, 257
Platinum analogs +/− Doxorubicin	4	0	0	—	123, 272

Improvement in hypertension, reduction in requirement for antihypertensive medication, and improvement in overall performance status correlated well with complete and partial biochemical responses in 11 (79%) of the patients. Toxicity included moderate nausea and vomiting, myelosuppression, and mild neurotoxicity, but no unexpected adverse events. Except for some moderate degree of postural hypotension that responded promptly to volume replacement therapy, major hemodynamic side effects from chemotherapy were not observed in the patients.[14] The lack of hypertensive events in this series is probably due to the fact that patients were prepared with adequate volume repletion and pharmacologic adrenergic blockade prior to initiating chemotherapy. Since hypertensive episodes have been observed following chemotherapy,[14a,59,279] patients need to be prepared as if for surgery, and they require close monitoring during their initial chemotherapy treatment.

The CVD study is the largest prospectively studied chemotherapy series in malignant pheochromocytoma. The results have been confirmed by additional clinical experience.[13,235,257] Thus CVD should be the treatment of choice for symptomatic, disseminated pheochromocytoma. Recent experience in neuroblastoma, where CVD has been replaced by the use of new agents and more intensive regimens[219] provides a basis for possible extrapolation to pheochromocytoma in future clinical trials.

There is no information regarding the activity of interferon in malignant pheochromocytoma despite its reported activity in other neuroendocrine tumors.[204] The somatostatin analogue, octreotide acetate has been reported to produce symptomatic response in patients with endocrine syndromes caused by peptide secreting pheochromocytomas.[104]

Multiple Endocrine Neoplasia (MEN) Syndromes

There are three distinct Multiple Endocrine Neoplasia (MEN) syndromes and non-MEN familial medullary thyroid carcinoma (Table XXVI-4-6) that share two characteristics common to neuroendocrine neoplasms: 1) The tumors comprising MEN syndromes arise from APUD neuroendocrine cells, and 2) the syndromes are each inherited as an autosomal dominant trait. This second feature provides for a molecular diagnosis of affected individuals and it has led to the recent recognition of specific genetic defects that will enable a

Table XXVI-4-6. Multiple Endocrine Neoplasia Syndromes

Type	Affected Organs or Tumor	Genetic Loci
1	Pituitary Parathyroid Endocrine pancreas	11q13
2a	Parathyroid Medullary thyroid Pheochromocytoma	10
2b	Medullary thyroid Pheochromocytoma Mucosal ganglioneuromas	10
non-MEN familial medullary thyroid cancer	Medullary thyroid	10

fundamental understanding of the pathogenesis of these tumors.

Multiple Endocrine Neoplasia (MEN) Type 1

Epidemiology. Multiple endocrine neoplasia type 1 (MEN 1) syndrome is quite rare, with an estimated prevalence of between 0.02 and 0.2 per thousand and an incidence of 0.25% as determined from randomly chosen post-mortem studies.[33,66,282] However, the importance of this syndrome is related to its autosomal dominant hereditary pattern (Figure XXVI-4-9). Approximately one-third of patients with gastrinomas are associated with MEN 1 (see XXVI-5).[70,80,146,285] In contrast, insulinomas are usually sporadic and fewer than 5% are found in MEN 1 patients.[116]

Pathological Characteristics

MEN 1 is characterized by hyperplasia and/or neoplasms of the pituitary, parathyroids, and pancreatic islets. Hyperparathyroidism occurs in 90% of patients, pituitary adenomas in 40% of patients, and endocrine pancreatic tumors in 60% of patients.[66,205,238]

Although the parathyroid glands are the most frequently involved organs (95%)[282] and hyperparathyroidism is usually the first manifestation of the syndrome, its presence may not be detected until clinical disease of the pituitary or pancreas has brought the patient to medical attention. Hyperparathyroidism is often found during the second decade of life when screening immediate family members of those with proven MEN 1. In adults first suspected of the MEN 1 syndrome because of manifestations of gastrinoma, hyperparathyroidism is often diagnosed after obtaining serum calcium and

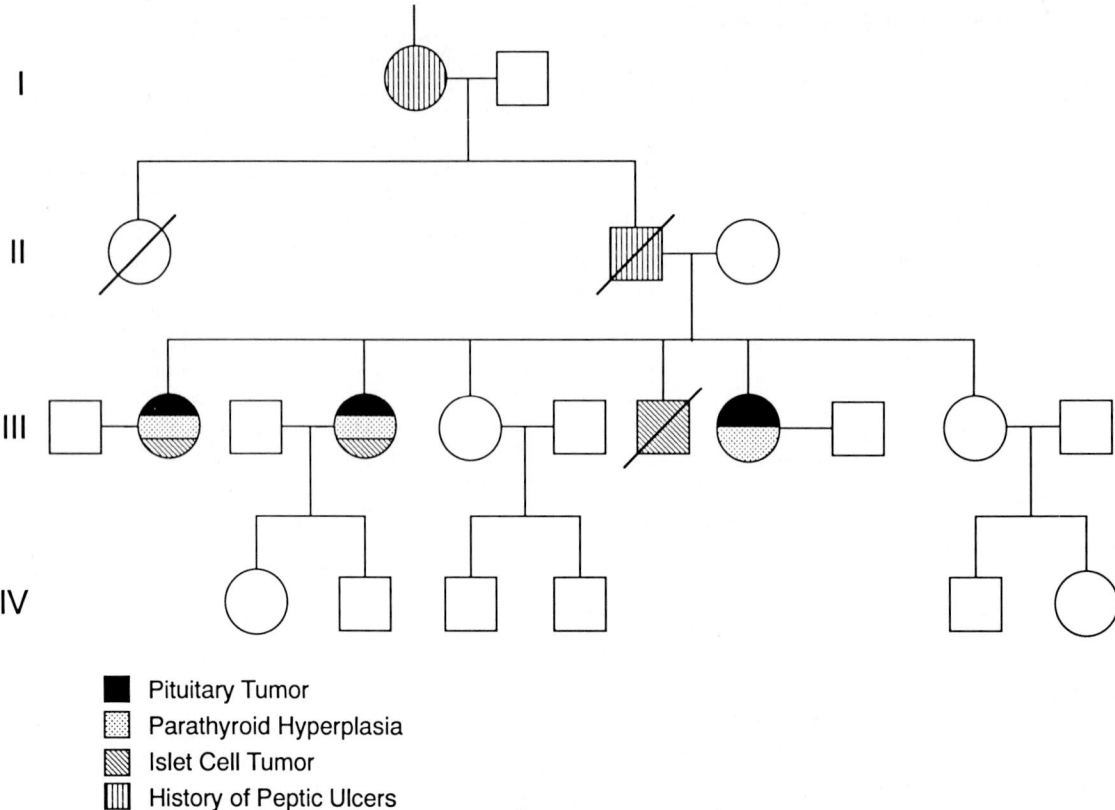

Pituitary Tumor
Parathyroid Hyperplasia
Islet Cell Tumor
History of Peptic Ulcers

Figure XXVI-4-9. Pedigree of a typical kindred with MEN type 1. (Reproduced with permission from Samaan et al.[238])

parathyroid hormone levels even though such patients may have had a decade long history of renal stones.

MEN 1 patients characteristically have nodular hyperplasia as the cause of their hyperparathyroidism. Often the individual gland involvement is variable and is best described as asymmetrical hyperplasia resulting in enlargement of only one or two glands, particularly in younger patients.

The most frequent manifestation of MEN 1 pancreatic involvement is gastrinoma, usually developing during the third or fourth decade of life. Gastrinomas in the MEN 1 syndrome are typically small, multiple adenomas of the endocrine pancreas or duodenum[213] which produce excess gastrin causing gastric hyperacidity and multiple peptic ulcerations, classically known as the Zollinger-Ellison syndrome (see XXVI-5).[318] The malignant potential of MEN 1 associated gastrinomas is probably less than sporadic tumors.[80,81,163] Insulinomas are the second most common functional tumors and may appear in the second decade. Additional tumors found are vasoactive intestinal polypeptidomas (VIPomas), glucagonomas, somatostatinomas and pancreatic polypeptidomas (PPomas) (see XXVI-5).[317] In some MEN 1 patients, tumors may develop and even metastasize to lymph nodes or liver with no clinical manifestations whatsoever. In others, more than one clinical functional syndrome may develop in the same patient either synchronously or more often metachronously.

Immunohistochemical studies of the pancreas from MEN 1 patients, have shown that most tumors that stain positively for gastrin are in the head, uncinate process, or duode-

num.[285] Many of the larger tumors in the body or tail of the pancreas in gastrinoma patients stain positively only for hormones such as pancreatic polypeptide and somatostatin. Furthermore, even though islet-cell dysplasia (nesidioblastosis, hyperplasia, microadenomas) was found in all cases, these cells failed to stain positively for either gastrin or insulin. Discrete tumors rather than diffuse islet-cell disease are usually present in patients with clinical syndromes.[194,293] The subsequent use of selective venous sampling for gastrin, insulin or other hormones in MEN 1 patients has supported this thesis.[88] It has also become apparent that gastrinomas are most likely to develop in the duodenum in MEN 1 patients.[213] These tumors may be multiple, and in some cases may be associated with pancreatic gastrinomas.

Micro- or macroadenomas of the pituitary gland are commonly detected in MEN 1 patients when biochemical and imaging studies have been performed.[33,66] The majority of patients with functional tumors secrete prolactin. Less frequently, MEN 1 patients may develop tumors secreting ACTH or growth hormone and present with Cushing's syndrome or acromegaly. In the MEN 1 patient it is especially important to establish that the Cushing's syndrome is pituitary dependent (Cushing's disease) rather than caused by an adrenal adenoma or the ectopic secretion of ACTH or corticotropin releasing factor (CRF) from islet-cell tumors or a bronchial carcinoid.

Patients with MEN 1 syndrome have an increased frequency of both functional and non-functional adrenal cortical adenomas.[18,116,173,244] Furthermore, there may be an increased frequency of adrenal cortical carcinoma in MEN 1 patients, although only five cases have been well documented.

Carcinoid tumors have been reported more frequently in MEN 1 patients than would be expected.[71] Male patients appear to have a predilection for developing carcinoid tumors within the thymus whereas bronchial carcinoids occur almost exclusively in women.

Biological Characteristics. A group of investigators from Uppsala, Sweden group mapped the MEN 1 gene locus to the long arm of chromosome 11 (11q13)[149] and several groups have now confirmed and extended the finding showing that monoclonal parathyroid and pancreatic tumor development is associated with loss of allelic heterozygosity at this site.[17,33,45,79,281] These studies have shown linkage of the MEN 1 gene with the INT-2 oncogene.[17,281]

In several patients with MEN 1, Brandi and coworkers found a circulating plasma factor that was mitogenic for parathyroid cells.[34] The significance of this factor for MEN 1 is not clear since it had no apparent mitogenic activity for pituitary or pancreatic cells.

Clinical Features. The clinical features of patients with MEN 1 depend entirely upon expression of the natural history of the individual tumor and endocrine hyperfunction. Most patients with MEN 1 pancreatic disease requiring surgical intervention present with a syndrome caused by hypersecretion of a specific hormone such as gastrin, insulin, VIP, or glucagon.[205,238] However, in some patients a tumor may be detected by imaging studies obtained after serum laboratory studies have shown an elevation of one or more hormones such as pancreatic polypeptide or somatostatin. Overall, patients with familial MEN 1 neoplasms have long survival that is sigificantly better than that for patients with sporadic endocrine pancreatic tumors.[205,238]

Diagnostic Tests. A patient presenting with hyperparathyroidism or with hypergastrinemia should be questioned carefully regarding a family history of MEN 1 syndrome.[169] Whereas biochemical tests have been the mainstay for screening of suspected kindreds, DNA linkage analysis now provides a molecularly based approach to diagnosis.[205,238] Provocative tests for gastrinoma, such as the secretin stimulated gastrin response are specific for gastrinoma in hyperparathyroid MEN 1 patients.[147] The diagnostic approach to MEN 1 patients with pancreatic disease as determined by a clinical syndrome or clearly elevated hormone level is to obtain imaging studies in an attempt to detect a primary tumor and to rule out hepatic metastases. Usually this is accomplished by abdominal CT scan and selective visceral angiography. If no hepatic metastases are found, selective venous sampling for the specific hormone(s) hypersecreted is performed. Due to their small size and multiplicity, localization procedures (see XXVI-5) for gastrinomas in MEN 1 syndrome present a special challenge. However, this procedure is particularly important since complete excision of all tumors is achievable.[184,284,293]

Therapeutic Considerations. Generally, the management of patients with MEN 1 is the same as for each sporadic tumor comprising the syndrome. Even when distant metastases are present, systemic chemotherapy is rarely indicated in this syndrome. The elements of the management of patients with MEN 1 may include: surgical removal of all four parathyroid glands, transplanting a portion of one of the glands to the forearm; subtotal pancreatoectomy, removing as many multifocal tumors as possible in patients with endocrine pancreatic tumors; and medical management of pituitary adenomas with bromocriptine for prolactinomas and octreotide for acromegaly.

The surgical treatment of the MEN 1 syndrome is dependent on the genetic expression in the individual patient. Because this may be metachronous, surgical procedures involving different endocrine organs may be required over a period of many years. Regardless of initial findings, MEN 1 patients must be followed for life for involvement of the pituitary gland, the parathyroid glands, the endocrine pancreas or duodenum, the adrenal glands, the thymus and the lungs (bronchial carcinoids). A source of persistent or recurrent disease is an overlooked supernumerary parathyroid gland which is found most commonly in the upper thymus in 6–15%. Because of this, cervical thymectomy is considered an essential component of an adequate neck exploration in the MEN 1 patient.[57] A common approach is to identify all four glands initially without impairing their blood supply. If all are enlarged, the superior glands are excised and the major portion of each inferior gland is resected leaving about 50 mg of viable parathyroid tissue based on each end artery to the gland. After several minutes of observation, the least normal appearing remnant is excised and the remaining remnant gland (50 mg) is hemoclipped to the tracheal fascia or capsule of the thyroid where it can be readily accessible in the future, if necessary. If one of the glands, even if superior, has been found to be normal sized, it is tagged with a metal clip, left in place and the other three glands are excised. Transient hypocalcemia is the desired result of these procedures and if it does not occur, it usually means a supernumerary gland has been overlooked and recurrence is likely. If properly performed, oral calcium and vitamin D therapy can usually be tapered and discontinued within weeks. If performed correctly permanent hypocalcemia should not develop. Although recurrent hypercalcemia may occur in patients after 10 years, successful surgical management is accomplished by trimming the hypertrophied remnant back to 50 mg.[53]

An alternative treatment, strongly advocated by some authors because of a recurrence rate as high as 40% after subtotal parathyroidectomy, is total parathyroidectomy, cervical thymectomy, forearm muscle autografting and cryopreservation of parathyroid tissue for possible future need.[218,308] This operation requires just as thorough cervical-mediastinal exploration as in subtotal parathyroidectomy to prevent cervical recurrence. Its advantage is that should recurrence develop from arm graft overgrowth, trimming back the implanted tissue can be performed under a local anesthesia. Its disadvantage is that all patients will require complete replacement therapy (vitamin D and oral calcium) for three months or longer, and some may be rendered permanently hypoparathyroid unless a subsequent thawed, cryopreserved transplant is successful. Both of these procedures are currently widely used in managing MEN 1 patients with hyperparathyroidism.

The surgical treatment of MEN 1 pancreatic disease is controversial.[194,293] One of the major issues centers around the fact that virtually all patients with pancreatic disease have a diffuse islet-cell dysplasia expressed as nesidioblastosis, islet-cell hyperplasia, microadenomatosis, and/or benign or malignant islet-cell tumors. As a result, it can be concluded that a cure of the pancreatic disease can only be achieved by a total pancreatectomy.[287] However, the malignant potential of MEN 1 islet cell neoplasm is relatively low and with current medical therapy, there is little justification for total pancreatectomy either because of hormone hypersecretion or potential malignancy. In contrast, there is accumulating evidence that the majority of gastrinomas are malignant and lymph node and/or hepatic metastases from them develop in most patients if followed for a long enough period. Similarly, other functional and non-functional gastroenteropancreatic neuroendocrine neoplasms may have malignant potential (See XXVI-5).

By a combination of preoperative localization and thorough exploration of both the pancreas and the duodenum, selected MEN 1 patients with hypergastrinemia can be rendered eugastrinemic, avoiding the necessity for either long term drug therapy or total gastrectomy.[194,284,293]

In patients with either insulinomas or gastrinomas, a distal pancreatectomy is performed, in most cases preserving the spleen, followed by a complete exploration of the remaining pancreatic head, uncinate process and peri-pancreatic lymph nodes.[284] Any tumor found in the head or uncinate process by palpation or intraoperative ultrasound is enucleated. In all patients with gastrinoma, a longitudinal duodenotomy is made and the mucosa from the pylorus to the third portion is evaginated into the incision and carefully palpated for small submucosal tumors, which may be as small as 1–2 mm. When present, they are locally excised as are any lymph nodes in their drainage area.[286] Using this approach, we have been able to achieve eugastrinemia in 12 patients with gastrinoma since 1978.[284] Of significance is the fact that more than one-half have had at least one peri-pancreatic lymph node involved with metastases although primary tumors were as small as 2 mm in diameter. Even though some of these patients have subsequently shown a positive response to secretin stimulation, they have not required drug therapy or gastric operations. For patients with persistent, symptomatic hypergastrinemia from unresectable or metastatic gastrinoma, medical therapy with histamine-2 blockers or proton-pump inhibitors is indicated.[174]

MEN 1 patients with hyperinsulinism usually have had more than one tumor secreting insulin. However, they are confined to the pancreas and when all are enucleated or excised (distal pancreatectomy), the syndrome is cured and recurrences appear to be rare. Octreotide acetate may be useful to palliate symptoms resulting from functional pancreatic endocrine tumors in some patients with MEN 1.[316] Positive anecdotal experience with chemotherapy in selective patients with specific endocrine syndromes has also been reported.[205,238]

In symptomatic patients or those with pituitary macroadenomas, drug therapy with bromocriptine is usually effective. However, some require transphenoidal hypophysectomy because of tumor size or failure to respond to medical therapy. Cushing's disease is best treated by transphenoidal hypophysectomy.

Surgical resection is indicated for carcinoid tumors. Unfor-tunately, the thymic carcinoids have usually been too far advanced when detected to allow for total excision and have been the cause of death in those with this tumor. Periodic mediastinal and chest CT scans should be used routinely in the follow-up of MEN 1 patients.

Multiple Endocrine Neoplasia (MEN) 2a, 2b, and Non-MEN Familial Medullary Thyroid Carcinoma

Epidemiology. The occurrence of patients with MEN 2a, 2b, or non-MEN-familial MTC syndrome is rare and the incidence is determined solely on the basis of heredity (Figure XXVI-4-10). Children of affected individuals have a 50% chance of inheriting the genetic abnormality with virtually 100% penetrance, although only 70% manifest clinical symptoms.[282] The syndromes have been described in virtually all ethnic groups throughout the world and an appreciation of the genetic inheritance patterns has provided effective screening methods to direct early treatment to reduce morbidity and mortality in affected individuals (Figure XXVI-4-3).

Pathological Characteristics. Multiple endocrine neoplasia (MEN) type 2a involves patients with virtually a 100% incidence of medullary thyroid carcinoma (MTC), a 50% incidence of clinically significant, usually bilateral pheochromocytomas and a lesser incidence of parathyroid adenomas with associated hyperparathyroidism. This syndrome always involves autosomal dominant transmission. A second syndrome, MEN 2b, occurs as an isolated congenital presentation or as a distinct autosomal dominant disease.[135] Patients with this disorder, as for MEN 2a, have 100% incidence of MTC and frequent pheochromocytomas. In addition, however, they have a characteristic physical appearance due to multiple neural defects including mucosal neuromas of the eyelids, lips and tongue.[135,312] These patients also have a marfanoid habitus with hyperflexible joints but no lens abnormalities. The neural abnormalities also include widespread ganglioneuromatosis of the gastrointestinal tract leading to abnormal gut motility. Thus, even as infants or young children, patients with MEN 2b may have diarrhea, constipation, or may present with the clinical picture of megacolon. Patients with MEN 2b seldom have hyperparathyroidism.

The third, and most recently defined form of genetic MTC, is non-MEN MTC.[72] In this autosomal dominant disease, patients have MTC but no other associated endocrine or neural tissue involvement.

The major differences in the clinical pathology of MTC and pheochromocytomas in the MEN and familial syndromes, as compared to the sporadic forms of these tumors, involve the multifocality of the lesions, the presence of hyperplastic states as precursors to frank tumors, and the different clinical behavior of the tumors in each genetic disease.

Patients diagnosed as having genetic forms of MTC may manifest bilateral C-cell hyperplasia in the thyroid as the sole lesion, or in association with frank MTC. Immunostaining of calcitonin (CT) is essential in making this diagnosis (Figure XXVI-4-3) since the hyperplasia may not be apparent on routine histologic examination. Patients diagnosed early may also have multifocal microscopic MTC diagnosed with such immunostaining. Both C-cell hyperplasia and microscopic MTC, are the only stages of this cancer consistently curable

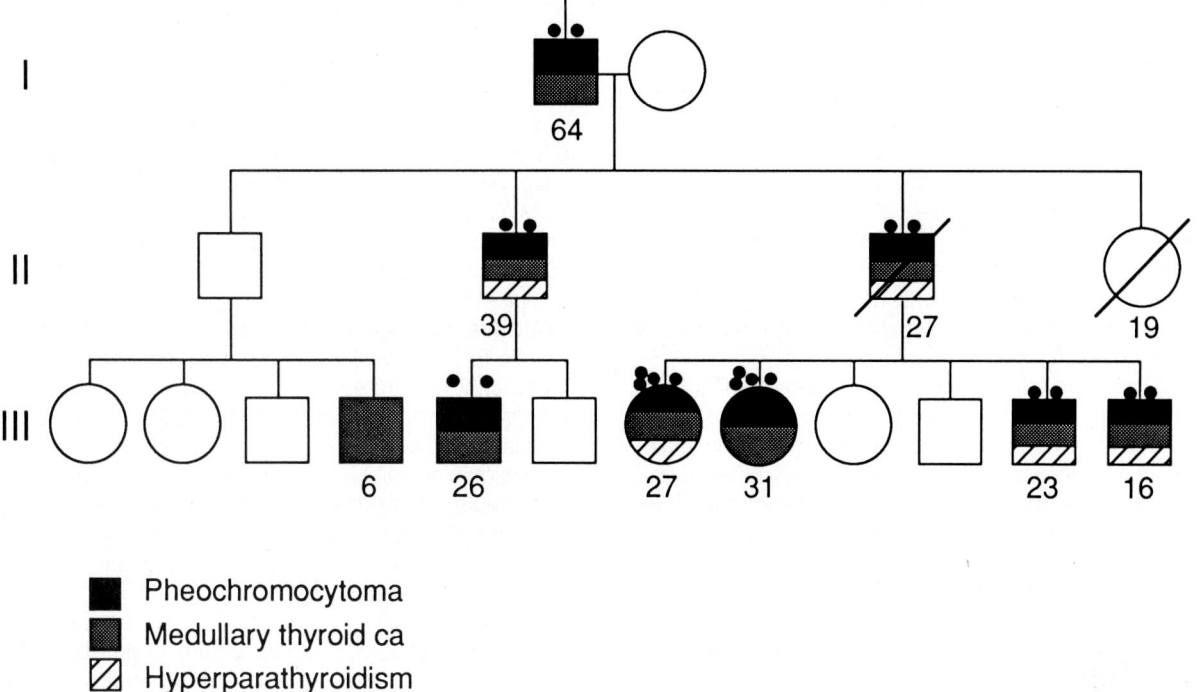

Figure XXVI-4-10. Pedigree of a typical kindred with MEN type 2a. The closed circles represent the number of pheochromocytomas found at surgery. (Courtesy of D. Pertsemlidis.)

by total thyroidectomy.[20,84] Similarly, patients with MEN 2a or 2b have a stage of adrenal hyperplasia which precedes development of pheochromocytomas. The clinical significance and management of this early condition is controversial.

Biological Characteristics. The biological properties of MTC, pheochromocytoma, and parathyroid neoplasms in the MEN syndromes are similar to those for each of the sporadic forms of these lesions described earlier. A major unanswered question remains: to identify the precise genetic events underlying the evolution of the MEN 2 and non-MEN familial MTC syndromes. At present, the gene(s) for each of these diseases has been mapped to the centromeric region of chromosome 10 (Table XXVI-4-6).[145,171,262,268] The fact that this is true for all 3 of the syndromes suggests that pleiotropic effects of a single gene abnormality may cause the different familial MTC syndromes. However, it is possible that a cluster of genes within the mapped loci control normal differentiation of the tissues involved in the syndrome under discussion and a different gene is altered for each of the genetic forms of MTC. The answer to this question must await the extensive work now ongoing to define the chromosome 10 gene(s) involved. Elucidation of such genes will also aid with the early detection of genetic MTC.

Biochemical and Clinical Features. The biochemical features of MTC, pheochromocytomas, and parathyroid neoplasms in the genetic syndromes under discussion are similar to those for the sporadic forms of each of these disorders. There are no distinguishing markers which allow the genetic forms of each neoplasm to be separated from the non-inherited types. In the case of the pheochromocytomas occurring in the MEN 2a and 2b syndromes, there is some difference in the pattern of biogenic amine synthesis in the genetic vs. the sporadic forms of this tumor. The ratio of norepinephrine to epinephrine is generally higher in the sporadic pheochromocytomas. In fact, epinephrine can actually be the dominant form in MEN 2a and 2b.[35] This probably explains the fact that patients with pheochromocytoma in the genetic setting often have less hypertension than those with the sporadic form of this adrenal tumor.

The clinical course of pheochromocytomas in MEN 2a and 2b is typically that of benign tumors with malignant pheochromocytomas having been reported only rarely.[131,252,291] The clinical behavior of MTC differs for each of the genetic syndromes under discussion. In MEN 2a, the cancer, although it metastasizes early, often behaves in a relatively indolent fashion. Thus, the survival rates for patients with this syndrome are a bit longer than that for patients with the sporadic form of MTC (Figure XXVI-4-2). Aggressive malignant behavior of MTC occurs in a small subset of patients with MEN 2a. This fact emphasizes the need to excise all tumors at the very early stages of this disease in order to prevent the consequences of widely metastatic tumor.

MTC is a particularly aggressive and lethal cancer in patients with MEN 2b.[195,244] Death from metastatic disease can occur even in young children with this disorder.[130] When the physical stigmata of MEN 2b are recognized (e.g., mucosal neuromas), even in infants, surgical intervention for MTC should be undertaken as early as is feasible.

In non-MEN familial MTC, the thyroid neoplasm behaves in its least aggressive manner.[72] The cancer generally appears in the fourth to fifth decade rather than in the 2nd decade as in MEN 2a. Although local metastases may occur frequently, the disease usually follows an indolent course and virtually never results in death of the patient.

Diagnostic Tests. Kindreds with the genetic syndromes under discussion are most frequently identified when an index patient presents with palpable MTC in the neck and/or with symptoms of pheochromocytoma. Once such a patient is under investigation, the approach is to determine if familial disease exists and to diagnose family members at risk at the very earliest stages of disease. The first step is to obtain an extensive family history. The second is to examine immediate relatives of the index patients and to perform the diagnostic tests which will detect asymptomatic disease (Figure XXVI-4-3).

Patients with the earliest subclinical stages of MTC (premalignant C-cell hyperplasia and/or microscopic carcinoma) usually do not have elevated basal serum levels of calcitonin. However, even patients with C-cell hyperplasia increase calcitonin levels abnormally in response to the secretagogues calcium and/or pentagastrin. Although several regimens for stimulating calcitonin secretion are available, the combination test devised by Wells and colleagues consisting of a 50 sec infusion of calcium gluconate (2 mg of elemental calcium/kg) followed by a 10 sec bolus of pentagastrin (Peptavalon, Ayerst, 0.5 μg/kg) seems most reliable.[307] This procedure results in less false negatives than tests performed with either of the two agents alone, is rapid, and had minimal side-effects consisting of only transient warmth, flushing and nausea. Calcitonin levels, measured at 0, 2, 3.5, and 5 minutes of the test, generally peak at the 2 or 3.5 minute points. Several commercial diagnostic laboratories, have standardized calcitonin results for this test in normal individuals. Although normal ranges vary somewhat for different calcitonin assays, in general, normal females do not have a provoked level higher than ~100 pg/ml and the limit for males is ~350 pg/ml. It is critical that the physician screening patients for MTC be thoroughly familiar with the performance of a given calcitonin assay in detecting patients with early MTC.

One important aspect of screening individuals who are at direct risk for inheriting MTC concerns the ages for initiating and stopping such testing. Both issues concern the type of genetic MTC involved. Individuals with MEN 2b can develop MTC by the age of 2 years, but usually can be identified by presence of the physical stigmata for this syndrome. For the other forms of genetic MTC, MEN 2a and familial MTC, screening can generally begin by age 3 or 4 years.

Deciding when to stop screening an individual at direct risk, who has had multiple negative tests, is a more difficult issue. Data directly related to this point are available only for MEN 2a kindreds. For this disorder, over 95% of those individuals with the gene develop a positive stimulation test for calcitonin secretion by the age of 20 to 25 years.[216] We, thus, screen kindred members at direct risk annually until this age and then biannually thereafter.

A hope for more refined diagnostic tests for inherited forms of MTC resides with the attempts to identify the gene(s) responsible for the genetic disorders in which it occurs. Polymorphic DNA probes which reside close to the gene locus on chromosome 10 have already been used in linkage studies in an attempt to identify gene carriers in known MEN 2a kindreds. For example, Sobol and colleagues were able to

provide genetic counseling to 8 out of 11 MEN 2a kindreds studied.[268] Such DNA testing is promising for early detection of gene carriers for familial MTC, but will not be maximally useful for all families with this disorder until the precise gene(s) is identified. When this is accomplished, specific probes may detect consistent DNA alterations which will allow, in individual patients, a precise diagnosis of the gene carrier state for MTC. Until this time, established standard provocative infusion tests for calcitonin secretion must be used in screening families for presence of any of the disorders involving familial MTC.

Surgical Management. The primary management for the genetic forms of MTC is, as for sporadic disease, total thyroidectomy (Figure XXVI-4-3).[230] The effectiveness of surgical treatment is dependent on the stage at which the disease is first detected and treated. The object is to use results of calcitonin stimulation tests to provide for surgery as early as possible before there are any clinical signs of disease. The stages of disease diagnosed in such a situation, C-cell hyperplasia or microscopic MTC, are the only ones usually curable by thyroidectomy.[61,307]

Patients with MEN 2 syndromes must be evaluated for possible pheochromocytomas before undergoing thyroidectomy for MCT. Operations for the adrenal disease component, if present, should always take precedence over any neck procedures to avoid potential catastrophic hypertensive crisis following anesthesia induction.

Pheochromocytomas develop in 40–50% of MEN 2 patients and arise bilaterally from medullary hyperplasia. Although the adrenal component usually develops at a later age than the thyroid disease, occasionally it may appear in childhood. Because MEN 2 tumors tend to secrete a higher proportion of epinephrine as compared to norepinephrine, hypertension may not be noted until a crisis is induced by an operation or delivery. Most commonly these patients complain of palpitations, anxiety spells, or headache early in their disease. Once the diagnosis of pheochromocytomas has been established by biochemical testing, noninvasive localization and surgical approaches are conducted as described previously for sporadic pheochromocytomas. MIBG scans may be sensitive in detecting both medullary hyperplasia and small pheochromocytomas even when CT scans have been considered normal. Since pheochromocytoma in an MEN 2 patient almost always occurs bilaterally (Figure XXVI-4-10), we advocate an anterior transabdominal approach and bilateral adrenalectomy in all MEN 2 patients. In some cases, small pheochromocytomas in the contralateral gland may be occult to palpation and apparent only after subsequent sectioning the excised adrenal gland.

Total thyroidectomy is essential in patients with the genetic forms of MTC because of the multifocal origins of the tumor in this setting. This must be extracapsular, leaving no thyroid tissue or rim of capsule. Embryologically, the C-cells are concentrated in the posterior portion of the upper two-thirds for the thyroid lobe. This is the area most frequently left by some surgeons in performing "near total" thyroidectomy. Any procedure less than a total thyroidectomy is an inadequate operation for this disease, since failure to remove all thyroid tissue inevitably leads to recurrent disease.[102,230] This point cannot be over emphasized and is particularly important in children where the disease has an excellent chance of being cured. Some have even recommended I-131 scintiscanning following total thyroidectomy and I-131 ablation of any detected thyroid remnants. In addition to thyroidectomy, central compartment lymph nodes should be excised as described previously for sporadic MTC. In MEN 2 patients diagnosed by calcitonin testing, there are usually no palpable thyroid abnormalities and perithyroidal lymph nodes are frequently free of disease. In performing both total thyroidectomy and central compartment lymph node disection, it is imperative to identify and preserve all parathyroid glands until a decision has been made about which glands should be excised. In patients with involved central compartment lymph nodes, an ipsilateral or bilateral modified neck dissection should be considered. When a modified neck dissection has not been done and the postoperative calcitonin level remains elevated, we perform selective venous sampling for calcitonin. When elevated levels are detected from one or both sides of the neck, a modified neck dissection is then recommended.

Patients with MEN 2b disease require total thyroidectomy as soon as the syndrome is recognized,[61] preferably by two years of age, because MTC develops very early in this group and is typically aggressive in biological behavior. In patients with familial MEN 2b, the characteristic physical features of typical facies, submucosal neuromas, and skeletal abnormalities are indications for thyroidectomy even without calcitonin testing. If the diagnosis has not been made until ten years or later, both central compartment and lateral node involvement require neck dissections for definitive treatment. Not infrequently, however, young adult patients have liver or bone metastases when initially diagnosed, preventing any curative operative attempts.[195]

The screening of first degree family members of those with newly discovered MTC, particularly when bilateral tumors and associated C-cell hyperplasia have been found, has led to earlier diagnosis and treatment of patients at risk during the past 15 years since calcitonin assays have been widely available (Figure XXVI-4-3). Calcitonin testing has been particularly valuable in MEN 2a family members who lack any of the characteristic features found in MEN 2b individuals. Genetic testing, when available, allows for recognition of MEN 2a family members with the trait in early infancy and eliminates the need for periodic childhood testing as currently done.

Clinical evidence of hyperparathyroidism is present in 20–30% of MEN 2a patients whereas hypercalcemia rarely occurs in MEN 2b patients. Nevertheless, one or two parathyroid glands may be abnormal in MEN 2a patients even when they are normocalcemic preoperatively. The surgical treatment of MEN 2a parathyroid disease differs from that of the MEN 1 disease in that the extent of the parathyroidectomy is tailored to the operative findings. A routine subtotal parathyroidectomy or total parathyroidecotmy and arm muscle autotransplant is not indictated. In most cases only one or two glands are enlarged. Excision of only the grossly enlarged gland(s) is sufficient treatment because recurrence, despite long term follow-up, rarely if ever occurs. Formerly, there was a high incidence of permanent hypoparathyroidism when near total or subtotal parathyroidectomy was done in this group of patients and these procedures should be avoided.[102,230]

Treatment of Recurrent or Metastatic Disease. The treatment of advanced MTC in a patient with a genetic syndrome is not distinguished from the approach used in sporadic disease. Locally recurrent disease in the neck may be amenable to further surgical management;[288] there is little evidence supporting a role for radiation therapy;[239] and in patients with progressive, symptomatic advanced disease, only anecdotal reports of combination chemotherapy have appeared.[13,212,256] We have treated a patient from the MEN 2a kindred shown in Figure XXVI-4-10. This 26 year old male with advanced MTC metastatic to lung and bones had little palliative benefit from radiation therapy to symptomatic lesions in the thoracic spine and pelvis. Following combination chemotherapy with cyclophosphamide, vincristine, and dacarbazine, the patient had a partial response with complete resolution of pulmonary metastases, improvement of bone pain and markedly reduced serum calcitonin and CEA for a duration of 14 months.[13] Although definitive supportive evidence is lacking, the anecdotal experience supports the use of dacarbazine or cisplatin containing combination chemotherapy in the treatment of patients with familial genetic forms of advanced, symptomatic MTC.

References

1. Albright, F.: Case Records of the Massachusetts General Hospital. Case 27461. N. Engl. J. Med., 225:789, 1941.
2. Alexander, H. R. and Norton, J. A.: Biology and management of medullary thyroid carcinoma of the parafollicular cells. In: Thyroid Cancer: A Lethal Endocrine Neoplasm. Moderated by J. Robbins. Ann. Intern. Med., 115:133, 1991, pp. 140-142.
3. Allen, J. M., Yeats, J. C., Causon, R., Brown, M. J., and Bloom, S. R.: Neuropeptide Y and its flanking peptide in human endocrine tumors and plasma. J. Clin. Endocrinol Metab., 64:1199, 1987.
4. Amara, S. G., Jonas, V., Rosenfeld, M. F., Ong, E. S., and Evans, R. M.: Alternative RNA processing in calcitonin gene expression generates mRNAs encoding different polypeptide products. Nature, 298:240, 1982.
5. Amberson, J. B., Vaughan, E. D., Jr., Gray, G. F., and Naus, G. J.: Flow cytometric determination of nuclear DNA content in benign adrenal pheochromocytomas. Urology, 30:1987.
6. Andersen, G. S., Toftdahl, D. B., Lund, J. O., Strandgaard, S., and Nielsen, P. E.: The incidence rate of phaeochromocytoma and Conn's syndrome in Denmark, 1977-1981. J. Hum. Hypertens., 2:187, 1988.
7. Andrew, A.: The APUD concept. Where has it led us? Brit. Med. Bull., 38:221, 1982.
8. Arnaud, C. D.: The Parathyroid Glands, Hypercalcemia and Hypocalcemia. In Cecil Textbook of Medicine. Edited by J. B. Wyngaarden, and L. H. Smith, Jr. Philadelphia, W. B. Saunders, 1988, p. 1486.
9. Arnold, A., Staunton, C. E., Kim, G.H., Gaz, R.D., and Kronenberg, H.M.: Monoclonality and abnormal parathyroid hormone genes in parathyroid adenomas. N. Engl. J. Med., 318:658, 1988.
10. Askanazy, M.: Ueber ostitis deformans ohne osteoides gowebe. Arb. Geb. Pathol. Anat. Inst. Tubingen Leipez., 4:398, 1904.
11. Attie, M.: Treatment of hypercalcemia. Endocrinol. Metab. Clin. North Am., 18:807, 1989.
12. Aurbach, G. D., Mallette, L. E., Patten, B. M., Heath, D. A., Doppman, J. L., and Bilezikian, J. P.: Hyperparathyroidism: Recent studies. Ann. Intern. Med., 79:566, 1973.
13. Averbuch, S., Wu, L., Pertsemlidis, D., and Drakes, T.: Cyclophosphamide (C), vincristine (V), and dacarbazine (D) for advanced neuroendocrine carcinomas. Proc. Am. Soc. Clin. Oncol., 9:382, 1990.
14. Averbuch, S. D., Steakley, C. S., Young, R. C., Gelmann, E. P., Goldstein, D. S., Stull, R., and Keiser, H. R.: Malignant pheochromocytoma: Effective treatment with a combination of cyclophosphamide, vincristine, and dacarbazine. Ann. Intern. Med, 109:267, 1988.
14A.Averbuch, S. D.: Unpublished observation.
15. Baba, H., Kishihara, M., Tohmon, M., Fukase, M., Kizaki, T., Okada, S., Matsuzuka, F., Kobayashi, A., Kuma, K., and Fujita, T.: Identification of parathyroid hormone messenger ribonucleic acid in an apparently nonfunctioning parathyroid carcinoma transformed from a parathyroid carcinoma with hyperparathyroidism. J. Clin. Endocrinol. Metab., 62:247, 1986.
16. Bajorunas, D. R.: Clinical manifestations of cancer-related hypercalcemia. Semin. Oncol., 17 (Suppl 5):16, 1990.
17. Bale, S. J., Bale, A. E., Stewart, K., Dachowski, L., McBride, O. W., Glaser, T., Green, J. E., Mulvihill, J. J., Brandi, M. L., Sakaguchi, K., Aurbach, G. D., and Marx, S. J.: Linkage analysis of multiple endocrine neoplasia type 1 with INT2 and other markers on chromosome 11. Genomics, 4:320, 1989.
18. Ballard, H. S., Frame, B., and Harstock, R. J.: Familial multiple endocrine adenomapeptic ulcer complex. Medicine, 43:481, 1964.
19. Baylin, S. B.: APUD cell fact and fiction. Trends Endocrin. Metab., 1:198, 1990.

20. Baylin, S. B., and Mendelsohn, G.: Medullary thyroid carcinoma: A model for the study of human tumor progression and cell heterogeneity. *In* Tumor Cell Heterogeneity, Origins and Implications. Edited by A. H. Owens Jr., D. S. Coffey, and S. B. Baylin. New York, Academic Press, 1982, p. 9.
21. Beard, C. M., Sheps, S. G., and Kurland, L. T.: Occurrence of pheochromocytoma in Rochester, Minnesota, 1950 through 1979. Mayo Clin. Proc., 58:1983.
22. Benowitz, N. L.: Pheochromocytoma. Adv. Intern. Med., 35:195, 1990.
23. Bergholm, U., Adami, H. O., Auer, G., Bergstrom, R., Backdahl, M., Grimelius, L., Hansson, G., Ljundberg, O. and Wilander, E.: Histopathologic characteristics and nuclear DNA content as prognostic factors in medullary thyroid carcinoma. A Nationwide Study in Sweden. The Swedish MTC Study Group. Cancer, 64:135, 1989.
24. Bergman, S. M., Sears, H. F., Javadpour, N., and Keiser, H. R.: Postoperative management of patients with pheochromocytoma. J. Urol., 120:109, 1978.
25. Berland, Y., Olmer, M., Lebreuil, G., and Grisoli, J.: Parathyroid carcinoma, adenoma and hyperplasia in a case of chronic renal insufficiency on dialysis. J. Clin. Nephrol., 18:154, 1982.
26. Bierewaltes, W. H., Sisson, J. C., Shapiro, B., Lloyd, R. V., Dmuchowski, C., and Rabbani, R.: Malignant potential of pheochromocytoma. Proc. Amer. Assoc. Cancer Res., 27:617, 1986.
27. Bilezikian, J. P.: Etilogies and therapy of hypercalcemia. Endocrinol. Metab. Clin. North Am., 18:389, 1989.
28. Bilezikian, J. P.: Parathyroid hormone-related peptide in sickness and in health. N. Engl. J. Med., 322:1151, 1990.
29. Black, B. K.: Carcinoma of the parathyroid. Ann. Surg., 139:355, 1954.
30. Blake, G. M., Lewington, V. J., Fleming, J. S., Zivanovic, M. A., and Ackery, D. M.: Modification by nifedipine of 131I-meta-iodobenzylguanidine kinetics in malignant phaeochromocytoma. Eur. J. Nucl. Med., 14:345, 1988.
31. Blum, R.: Enalapril in pheochromocytoma (letter). Ann. Intern. Med., 106:326, 1987.
32. Bostwick, D. G., Null, W. E., Holmes, D., Weber, E., Barchas, J. D., and Bensch, K. G.: Expression of opioid peptides in tumors. N. Engl. J. Med., 317:1439, 1987.
33. Brandi, M. L.: Multiple endocrine neoplasia type I: General features and new insights into etiology. J. Endocrinol. Invest., 14:61, 1991.
34. Brandi, M. L., Aurbach, G. D., A., Fitzpatrick, L. A., Quarto, R., Spiegel, A. M., Bliziotes, M. M., Norton, J. A., Doppman, J. L. and Marx, S. J.: Parathyroid mitogenic activity in plasma from patients with familial multiple endocrine neoplasia type 1. N. Engl. J. Med., 314:1287, 1986.
35. Bravo, E. L., and Gifford, R. W., Jr.: Pheochromocytoma: Diagnosis, localization, and management. N. Engl. J. Med., 311:1298, 1984.
36. Bravo, E. L., Tarazi, R. C., and Fouad, F. D.: Clonidine suppression test: A useful aid in the diagnosis of pheochromocytoma. N. Engl. J. Med., 305:623, 1981.
37. Brendel, A. J., Jeandot, R., Guyot, M., Lambert, B., and Drouillard, J.: Radionuclide Therapy of pheochromocytomas and neuroblastomas using iodine-131 metaiodobenzylguanidine (MIBG). Clin. Nucl. Med., 14:19, 1988.
38. Brennan, M. F., and Keiser, H. R.: Persistent and recurrent Pheochromocytoma: The Role of Surgery. World J. Surg., 6:397, 1982.
39. Broadus, A. E., Mangin, M., Ikeda, K., Insogna, K. L., Weir, E. C., Burtis, W. J., and Stewart, A. F.: Humoral hypercalcemia of cancer. Identification of a novel parathyroid hormone-like peptide. N. Engl. J. Med., 319:556, 1988.
40. Brogden, R. N., Heel, R. C., and Speight, T. M.: Alpha methyl-L-tyrosine: A review of its pharmacology and clinical use. Drugs, 21:81, 1981.
41. Budayr, A. A., Nissenson, R. A., Klein, R. F., Pun, K. K., Clark, O. H., Diep, D., Arnaud, C. D., and Strewler, G. J.: Increased serum levels of a parathyroid hormone-like protein in malignancy-associated hypercalcemia. Ann. Intern. Med., 111:807, 1989.
42. Bukowski, R. M., Sheeler, L., Cunningham, J., and Esselstyn, C.: Successful combination chemotherapy for metastatic parathyroid carcinoma. Arch. Intern. Med., 144:399, 1984.
43. Bukowski, R. M., and Vidt, D. G.: Chemotherapy trials in malignant pheochromocytoma. Report of two patients and review of the literature. J. Surg. Oncol., 27:89, 1984.
44. Burtis, W. J., Brady, T. G., Orloff, J. J., Ersbak, J. B., Warrell, R. P., Olson, B. R., Wu, T. L., Mitnick, M E., Broadus, W. E., and Stewart, A. F.: Immunochemical characterization of circulating parathyroid hormone-related protein in patients with humoral hypercalcemia of cancer. N. Engl. J. Med., 322:1106, 1990.
45. Bystrom, C., Larsson, C., Blomberg, C., Sandelin, K., Falkmer, U., Skogseid, B., Oberg, K., Werner, S., and Nordenskjold, M.: Localization of the MEN 1 gene to a small region within chromosome 11q13 by deletion mapping in tumors. Proc. Natl. Acad. Sci. USA, 87:1968, 1990.
46. Cady, B.: Hyperparathyroidism. *In* Surgery of the Thyroid and Parathyroid Glands. Edited by C. E. Sedgwick and B. Cady. Philadelphia, W. B. Saunders, 1980, p. 206.
47. Calandra, D. B., Chejfec, G., Foy, B. K., Lawrence, A. M., and Paloyan, E.: Parathyroid carcinoma: Biochemical and pathologic response to DTIC. Surgery, 96:1132, 1984.
48. Carney, J. A., Sizemore, G. W., and Sheps, S. G.: Adrenal medullary disease in multiple endocrine neoplasia, type 2: Pheochromocytoma and its precursors. Amer. J. Clin. Pathol, 66:279, 1976.
49. Castleman, B., and Roth, S. I.: Tumors of the Parathyroid Glands. *In* Atlas of Tumor Pathology. Edited by B. Castleman and S. I. Roth. Washington, D.C., Armed Forces Institute of Pathology, 1978, p. 1.
50. Caty, M. G., Coran, A. G., Geagen, M., and Thompson, N. W.: Current diagnosis and treatment of pheochromocytoma in children. Experience with 22 consecutive tumors in 14 patients. Arch. Surg., 125:978, 1990.
51. Chahinian, A. P., Holland, J. F., Nieburgs, H. E., Marinescu, A., Geller, S. A., and Kirschner, P. A.: Metastatic nonfunctioning parathyroid carcinoma: Ultrastructural evidence of secretory granules and response to chemotherapy. Am. J. Med. Sci., 282:80, 1981.
52. Charbonnel, B., Chatal, J. F., Brendel, A. J., Lanehche, B., Lumbroso, J., Marchandise, X., Mornex, R., Schlumberger, M., and Wemeau, J. L.: Le Traitement des phéochromocytomes malins par la 131-I-métaiodobenzylguanidine. Annales d'Endocrinologie, 49:344, 1988.
53. Cheung, P. S., Borgstrom, A., and Thompson, N. W.: Strategy in reoperative surgery for hyperparathyroidism. Arch. Surg., 124:676, 1989.
54. Clerkin, E. P.: Hyperparathyroidism. *In* Surgery of the Thyroid and Parathyroid Glands. Edited by B. Cady and R. L. Rossi. Philadelphia, W. B. Saunders, 1991, p. 243.
55. Conlon, M. J., McGregor, G. P., Gröndal, S., and Grimelius, L.: Synthesis of a- and β-Calcitonin Gene-Related Peptide by a Human Pheochromocytoma. Peptides, 10:327, 1989.
56. Cox, T. M., Fagan, E. A., Hillyard, C. J., Allison, D. J., and Chadwick, V. S.: Role of calcitonin in diarrhea associated with medullary carcinoma of the thyroid. Gut, 20:629, 1979.
57. Curley, I. R., Wheeler, M. H., Thompson, N. W., and Grant, C. S.: The challenge of the middle mediastinal parathyroid. World J. Surg., 12:818, 1988.
58. Cushman, P., Jr.: Familial endocrine tumors. Report of two unrelated kindreds affected with pheochromocytoma, one also with multiple thyroid carcinomas. Am. J. Med., 32:352, 1962.
59. de Asis, D. N., Ali, M. K., Soto, A., and Samaan, N. A.: Acute cardiac toxicity of antineoplastic agents as the first manifestation of pheochromocytoma. Cancer, 42:2005, 1978.
59A. de Bustros, and Baylin, S.: Personal observation.
60. Deftos, L. J., Woloszczuk, W., Krisch, I., Horvat, G., Ulrich, W., Neuhold, N., Braun, O., Reiner, A., Srikanta, S., and Krisch, K.: Medullary thyroid carcinomas express chromogranin A and a novel neuroendocrine protein recognized by monoclonal antibody HISL-19. Amer. J. Med., 85:780, 1988.
61. Delius, R. E., and Thompson, N. W.: Early total thyroidectomy in patients with multiple endocrine neoplasia IIb syndrome. Surg. Gynecol. Obstet., 169:442, 1989.
62. Dhom, G., and Hohbach, C.: Case 12. Ultrastructural Pathol., 1:141, 1980.
63. Dinnen, J. S., Greenwood, R. H., Jones J. H., Walker, D. A., and Williams, E. D.: Parathyroid carcinoma in familial hyperparathyroidism. J. Clin. Path., 30:366, 1977.
64. Drasin, H.: Treatment of malignant pheochromocytoma. West. J. Med., 128:106, 1978.
65. Duncan, M. W., Compton, P., Lazarus, L., and Smythe, G. A.: Measurement of Norepinephrine and 3,4-Dihydroxyphenylglycol in Urine and Plasma for the Diagnosis of Pheochromocytoma. N. Engl. J. Med., 319:136, 1988.
66. Eberle, F., and Grun, R.: Multiple endocrine neoplasia type I (MEN I). Ergeb. Inn. Med. Kinderheikd., 46:76, 1981.
67. Egglin, T. K., Hahn, P. F., and Stark, D. D.: MRI of the adrenal glands. Semin. Roentgenol, 23:280, 1988.
68. Ellison, G. T., Mansberger, J. A., and Mansberger, A. R., Jr.,: Malignant recurrent pheochromocytoma during pregnancy: Case report and review of the literature. Surgery, 103:484, 1988.
69. Erdheim, J.: Zur normalen und pathologischen histologie der glandula thyreoidea, parathyreoidea und hypophysis. Beitr. Pathol. Anat., 33:158, 1903.
70. Eriksson, B., Skogseid, B., Lundqvist, G., Wide, L., Wilander, E., and Oberg, K.: Medical treatment and long-term survival in a prospective study of 84 patients with endocrine pancreatic tumors. Cancer, 65:1883, 1990.
71. Farhangi, M., Taylor, J., Havey, A., and O'Dorisio, T.: Neuroendocrine (carcinoid) tumor of the lung and type 1 multiple endocrine neoplasia. South. Med. J., 80:1459, 1987.
72. Farndon, J. R., Leight, G. S., Dilley, W. G., Baylin, S. B., Smallridge, R. C., Harrison, T. S., and Wells, S. A. J.: Familial medullary thyroid carcinoma without associated endocrinopathies: A distinct clinical entity. Br. J. Surg., 73:278, 1986.
73. Feldman, J. M.: Treatment of Metastatic Pheochromocytoma With Streptozocin. Arch. Intern. Med., 143:1799, 1983.
74. Fink, I. J., Reinig, J. W., Dwyer, A. J., Doppman, J. L., LInehan, W. M., and Keiser, H. R.: MR imaging of pheochromocytomas. J. Comput. Assist. Tomogr., 9:454, 1985.
75. Finklestein, J. Z., Klemperer, M. R., Evans, A., Bernstein, I., Leikin, S., McCreadie, S., Grosfeld, J., Hittle, R., Weiner, J., Sather, H., and Hammond, D.: Multiagent chemotherapy for children with metastatic neuroblastoma. A report from Childrens Cancer Study Group. Med. Pediatr. Oncol., 6:179, 1979.
76. Fiore, J. J., Kelsen, D. P., Cheng, E., and Dukeman, M.: Phase II Trial of VP-16 in Apudomas. Proc. Amer. Assoc. Cancer Res., 15:174, 1984.
77. Flye, M. W., and Brennan, M. F.: Surgical resection of metastatic parathyroid carcinoma. Ann. Surg., 193:425, 1981.
78. Frankel, F.: Ein fall von doppelseitigem, vollig latent verlaufenen nebennierentumor und gleichzeitiger nephritis mit veranderungen am circulationsapparat und retinitis. Virchows Arch. Pathol. Anat. Physiol., 103:244, 1886.
79. Friedman, E., Sakaguchi, K., Bale, A. E., Falchetti, A., Streeten, E., Zimering, M. B., Weinstein, L. S., McBride, W. O., Nakamura, Y., Brandi, M.-L., Norton, J. A., Aurbach, G. D., Speigel, A. M., and Marx, S. J.: Clonality of parathyroid tumors in familial multiple endocrine neoplasia type 1. N. Engl. J. Med., 321:213, 1989.
80. Friesen, S. R.: The development of endocrinopathies in the prospective screening of two families with MEA-I. World J. Surg., 3:753, 1979.
81. Friesen, S. R.: Update on the diagnosis and treatment of rare neuroendocrine tumors. Surg. Clinic N. A., 67:379, 1987.
82. Fritsche, A. E.: Clinical Utility of serum osteocalcin. Cancer Invest., 8:441, 1990.
83. Fujimoto, Y., and Obara, T.: How to recognize and treat parathyroid carcinoma. Endocrinol. Metab. Clin. North Am., 67:343, 1989.
84. Gagel, R. F., Tashjian, A. H., Jr., Cummings, T., Papathanasopoulos, N., Kaplan, M. M., DeLellis, R. A., Wolfe, H. J., and Reichlin, S.: The clinical outcome of prospective screening for multiple endocrine neoplasia type 2a. N. Engl. J. Med., 318:478, 1988.
85. Gazdar, A. F., Helman, L., Israel, M. A., Russell, E. K., Linnoila, R. L., Mulshine, J., Schuller, H., and Park, J. G.: Expression of neuroendocrine cell markers L-dopa decarboxylase, chromogranin A, and dense core granules in human tumors of endocrine and non-endocrine origin. Cancer Res., 48:4078, 1988.
86. Giraud, P., Eiden, L. E., and Audigier, Y.: ACTH a-MSH and β-endorphin in human pheochromocytoma. Neuropeptides, 1:236, 1981.
87. Glover, D., Riley, L., Carmichael, K., Spar, B., Glick, J., Kligerman, M. M., Agus, Z. S., Slatopolsky, E., Attie, M., and Goldfarb, S.: Hypocalcemia and inhibition of parathyroid hormone secretion after administration of WR-2721 (A radioprotective and chemoprotective agent). N. Engl. J. Med., 309:1137, 1983.
88. Glowniak, J., Shapiro, B., Vinik, A. I., Glaser, B., Thompson, H. W., and Cho, K. J.: Percutaneous transhepatic venous sampling of gastrin: Value in sporadic and familial islet-cell tumors of G-cell. N. Engl. J. Med., 307:293, 1982.
89. Goldfarb, D. A., Novick, A. C., Bravo, E. L., Straffon, R. A., Montie, J. E., and Kay, R.: Experience with extra-adrenal pheochromocytoma. J. Urol., 142:931, 1989.
90. Goldstein, D. S., Stull, R., Eisenhofer, G., Session, J. C., Weder, A., Averbuch, S. D., and Keiser, H. R.: Plasma 3,4-dihydroxyphenylalanine (dopa) and catecholamines in neuroblastoma or pheochromocytoma. Ann. Intern. Med., 105:887, 1986.
91. Goncalves, E., Ninane, J., Wese, F., Leonet, J., Piret, L., Cornu, G., and De Meyer,

R.: Familial phaeochromocytoma: Successful treatment with ^{131}I-MIBG. Med. Ped. Oncol., 18:126, 1990.
92. Gordon, P., Comi, R. J., Maton, P. N. and Go, V. L. W.: Somatostatin and Somatostatin Analogue (SMS 201-995) in Treatment of Hormone-Secreting Tumors of the Pituitary and Gastrointestinal Tract and Non-Neoplastic Diseases of the Gut. Ann. Intern. Med. 110:35, 1989.
93. Gottlieb, J. A. and Hill, C. S., Jr.: Adriamycin (NSC-123127) Therapy in Thyroid Carcinoma. Cancer Chemother. Reports, Part 3, 6:283, 1975.
94. Gough, I. R., and Thompson, N. W.: Phaeochromocytoma. Aust. N. Z. J. Surg., 58:365, 1988.
95. Grimelius, L.: A silver nitrate stain for alpha 2 cells in human pancreatic islets. Acta Soc. Med. Upsala, 73:243, 1968.
96. Grossman, E., Goldstein, D. S., Hoffman, A., and Keiser, H. A.: Glucagon and clonidine testing in the diagnosis of pheochromocytoma. Hypertension, 17:733, 1991.
97. Grouzmann, E., Comoy, E., and Bohoun, C.: Plasma neuropeptide y concentrations in patients with neuroendocrine tumors. J. Endocrinol. Metab., 64:808, 1989.
98. Grouzmann, E., Gicquel, C., Plouin, P. F., Schlumberger, M., Comoy, E., and Bohoun, C.: Neuropeptide Y and Neuron-Specific Enolase Levels in Benign and Malignant Pheochromocytomas. Cancer, 66:1833, 1990.
99. Guo, J. Z., Gong, L. S., Chen, S. X., Luo, B. Y., and Xu, M. Y.: Malignant pheochromocytoma: Diagnosis and treatment in fifteen cases. J. Hypertens., 7:261, 1989.
100. Hall, E. M., and Chaffin, L.: Malignant tumors of the parathyroid glands. West. J. Surg. Obstet. Gynecol., 42:578, 1934.
101. Hamilton, B. P. M., Cheikh, I. E., and Rivera, L. E.: Attempted treatment of inoperable pheochromocytoma with streptozocin. Arch. Intern. Med., 137:762, 1977.
102. Harness, J. K., Fung, L., Thompson, N. W., Burney, R. E., and McLeod, M. K.: Total thyroidectomy: Complications and technique. World. J. Surg., 10:781, 1986.
103. Harper, M. A., Murnaghan, G. A., Kennedy, L., Hadden, D. R., and Atkinson, A. B.: Phaeochromocytoma in pregnancy. Five cases and a review of the literature. Br. J. Obstet. Gynae., 96:594, 1989.
104. Harrison, M., James, N., Broadley, K., Bloom, S. R., Armour, R., Wimalawansa, S., Heath, D., and Waxman, J.: Somatostatin analogue treatment for malignant hypercalcaemia. Br. Med. J., 300:1313, 1990.
105. Hazard, J. B., Hawk, W. A., and Crile, G., Jr.,: Medullary (solid) carcinoma of the thyroid—A clinicopathologic entity. J. Clin. Endocrinol. Metab., 19:152, 1959.
106. Heath, D. A.: Primary hyperparathyroidism. Clinical presentation and factors influencing clinical management. Endocrinol. Metab. Clin. North Am., 18:631, 1989.
107. Heath, H., 3rd, Hodgson, S. F., and Kennedy, M. A.: Primary hyperparathyroidism. Incidence, morbidity, and potential economic impact in a community. N. Engl. J. Med., 302:189, 1980.
108. Helman, L. J., Cohen, P. S., Averbuch, S. D., Cooper, M. J., Keiser, H. R., and Israel, M. A.: Neuropeptide Y expression distinguishes malignant from benign pheochromocytoma. J. Clin. Oncol., 7:1720, 1989.
109. Helman, L. J., Gazdar, A. F., Park, J., Cohen, P. S., Cotelingam, J. D., and Israel, M. A.: Chromogranin A Expression in Normal and Malignant Human Tissues. J. Clin. Invest., 82:686, 1988.
110. Hirschel-Scholz, S., Jung, A., Fischer, J. A., Trechsel, U., and Bonjour, J. P.: Suppression of parathyroid secretion after administration of WR-2721 in a patient with parathyroid carcinoma. Clin. Endocrinol., 23:313, 1985.
111. Hoefnagel, C. A., Voute, P. A., and deKraker, J.: Radionuclide diagnosis and Therapy of neural crest tumors using iodine-131 metaiodobenzylquanidine. J. Nucl. Med., 28:308, 1987.
112. Holmes, E. C., Morton, D. L., and Ketcham, A. S.: Parathyroid carcinoma: A collective review. Ann. Surg., 169:631, 1969.
113. Horton, W. A., Wong, V., and Eldridge, R.: Von Hippel-Lindau disease. Clinical and pathological manifestations in nine families with 50 affected members. Arch. Intern. Med., 136:769, 1976.
114. Hosaka, Y., Rainwater, L. M., Grant, C. S., Farrow, G. M., van Heerden, J. A., and Lieber, M. M.: Pheochromocytoma: Nuclear deoxyribonucleic acid patterns studied by fluorocytometry. Surgery, 100:1003, 1986.
115. Hoskin, P. J., and Harmer, C.: Chemotherapy for thyroid cancer. Radiotherapy and Oncology, 10:187, 1987.
116. Howard, T. J., and Passaro, E. J.: Gastrinoma. New medical and surgical approaches. Surg. Clinics N. A., 69:667, 1989.
117. Hull, C. J.: Phaeochromocytoma. Diagnosis, preoperative preparation and anaesthetic management. Br. J. Anaesth., 58:1453, 1986.
118. Husain, M., Alsever, R. N., Lock, J. P., George, W. F., and Katz, F. H.: Failure of Medullary Carcinoma of the Thyroid to Respond to Doxorubicin Therapy. Hormone Res., 9:22, 1978.
119. Hussain, S., Belldegrun, A., Seltzer, S. E., Richie, J. P., Gittes, R. F., and Abrams, H. L.: Differentiation of malignant from benign adrenal masses: predictive indices on computed tomography. Am. J. Roentgenol., 14:61, 1985.
120. Insogna, K. L.: Humoral hypercalcemia of malignancy. The role of parathyroid hormone-related protein. Endocrinol. Metab. Clin. North Am., 18:779, 1989.
121. Ireland, J. P., Fleming, S. J., Levison, D. A., Cattell, W. R., and Baker, L. R. I.: Parathyroid carcinoma associated with chronic renal failure and previous radiotherapy to the neck. J. Clin. Pathol., 38:1114, 1985.
122. Javadpour, N., Woltering, E., and Brennan, M. F.: Adrenal neoplasms. Curr. Prob. Surg., 17:1, 1980.
123. Jodrell, D. I., and Smith, I. E.: Carboplatin in the treatment of metastatic carcinoid tumours and paraganglioma: a phase II study. Cancer Chemother. Pharmacol., 26:62, 1990.
124. Kameda, Y., Shigemoto, H., and Ikeda, A.: Development and cytodifferentiation of C-cell complexes in dog fetal thyroids. Cell Tissue Res., 206:403, 1980.
125. Kameya, T., Bessho, T., Tsumuraya, M., Yamaguchi, K., Abe, K., Shimosato, Y., and Yanaihara, N.: Production of gastrin-releasing peptide by medullary carcinoma of the thyroid. Virchows Arch. [Pathol. Anat.], 401:99, 1983.
126. Karlberg, B. E., Hedman, L., and Lennquist, S.: The value of the clonidine suppression test in the diagnosis of pheochromocytoma. World J. Surg., 10:753, 1986.
127. Käser, H.: Clinical and diagnostic findings in patients with chromaffin tumors: Pheochromocytomas, pheochromoblastomas. Journal, 97, 1990.
128. Kastan, D. J., Kottamasu, S. R., Frame, B., and Greenwald, K.: Carcinoma in a mediastinal fifth parathyroid gland. JAMA, 257:1218, 1987.
129. Katz, A., and Braunstein, G. D.: Clinical, Biochemical, and pathologic features of radiation-associated hyperparathyroidism. Arch. Intern. Med., 143:79, 1983.
130. Kaufman, F. R., Roe, T. F., Isaacs, H., Jr., and Weitzmann, J. J.: Metastatic medullary thyroid carcinoma in young children with mucosal neuroma syndrome. Pediatrics, 70:263, 1982.
131. Keiser, H. R., Doppman, J. L., Robertson, C. N., Linehan, W. M., and Averbuch, S. D.: Diagnosis, localization, and management of pheochromocytoma. *In* Pathology of the Adrenal Glands. Edited by E. E. Lack. New York, Churchill Livingstone, 1990, p. 237.
132. Keiser, H. R., Goldstein, D. S., Wade, J. L., Douglas, F. L., and Averbuch, S. D.: Treatment of malignant pheochromocytoma with combination chemotherapy. Hypertension, 7[Suppl I]:18, 1985.
133. Kessinger, A., Foley, J. F., and Lemon, H. M.: Therapy of Malignant APUD Cell Tumors. Cancer, 51:790, 1983.
134. Khafagi, F. A., Shapiro, B., Fig, L. M., Mallette, S., and Sisson, J. C.: Labetalol reduces iodine-131 MIBG uptake by pheochromocytoma and normal tissues. J. Nucl. Med., 30:481, 1989.
135. Khairi, M. R. A., Dexter, R. N., Burzynski, N. J., and Johnston, C. C., Jr.,: Mucosal neuroma, pheochromocytoma, and medullary thyroid carcinoma. MEN type III. Medicine, 54:89, 1975.
136. Klein, F. A., Kay, S., Ratliff, J. E., White, F. K. H., and Newsome, H. H.: Flow cytometric determinations of ploidy and proliferation patterns of adrenal neoplasms: An adjunct to histological classification. J. Urol., 134:862, 1985.
137. Koral, K. F., Wang, X., Sisson, J. C., Botti, J., Meyer, L., Mallette, S., Glazer, G. M., and Adler, R. S.: Calculating radiation absorbed dose for pheochromocytoma tumors in 131-I MIBG therapy. Int. J. Rad. Oncol. Biol. Phys., 17:211, 1989.
138. Krisch, K., Krisch, I., Horvat, G., Neuhold, N., and Ulrich, W.: The value of immunohistochemistry in medullary thyroid carcinoma: A systematic study of 30 cases. Histopathology, 9:1077, 1985.
139. Krubsack, A. J., Wilson, S. D., Lawson, T. L., Kneeland, J. B., Thorsen, M. K., Collier, B. D., Hellman, R. S. and Isitman, A. T.: Prospective comparison of radionuclide, computed tomographic, sonographic, and magnetic resonance localization of parathyroid tumors. Surgery, 106:639, 1989.
140. Kvols, L. K., and Buck, M.: Chemotherapy of endocrine malignancies: A review. Sem. Oncol., 14:343, 1987.
141. Lack, E. E.: Adrenal medullary hyperplasia and pheochromocytoma. *In* Pathology of the Adrenal Glands. Edited by E. E. Lack. New York, Churchill Livingstone, 1990, p. 173.
142. Lack, E. E., Cubilla, A. L., Woodruff, J. M., and Lieberman, P. H.: Extra-adrenal paragangliomas of the retroperitoneum. Am. J. Surg. Pathol., 4:109, 1980.
143. Lack, E. E., and Kozakewich, H. P. W.: Embryology, developmental anatomy, and selected aspects of non-neoplastic pathology. *In* Pathology of the Adrenal Glands. Edited by E. E. Lack. New York, Churchill Livingstone, 1990, p. 1.
144. Lafferty, F. W.: Primary Hyperparathyroidism. Changing clinical spectrum, prevalence of hypertension and discriminant analysis of laboratory tests. Arch. Intern. Med., 141:1761, 1981.
145. Lairmore, T. C., Howe, J. R., Korte, J. A., Dilley, W. G., Aine, L., Aine, E., Wells, S. A., Jr., and Donis-Keller, H.: Familial medullary thyroid carcinoma and multiple endocrine neoplasia type 2B map to the same region of chromosome 10 as multiple endocrine neoplasia type 2A. Genomics, 9:181, 1991.
146. Lamers, C. B., Buis, J. T., and Van Tongeren, J. H.: Secretin-stimulated serum gastrin levels in hyperparathyroid patients from families with multiple endocrine adenomatosis-type I. Ann. Intern. Med., 86:719, 1977.
147. Lamers, C. B., Rotter, J. I., and Jansen, J. B.: Gastrin cell function in familial multiple endocrine neoplasia type 1. Gut, 29:1358, 1988.
148. Landsvater, R. M., Mathew, C. G., Smith, B. A., Marcus, E. M.; teMeerman, G. J., Lips, C. J., Geerdink, R. A., Nakamura, Y., Ponder, B. A., and Buys, C. H.: Development of multiple endocrine neoplasia type 2A does not involve substantial deletions of chromosome 10. Genomics, 4:246, 1989.
149. Larsson, C., Skogseid, B., Oberg, K., Nakamura, Y., and Nordenskjold, M.: Multiple endocrine neoplasia type I gene maps to chromosome 11 and is lost in insulinoma. Nature, 332:85, 1988.
150. Law, W. L., Jr., and Heath, H., III,: Familial benign hypercalcemia (hypocalciuric hypercalcemia). Clinical and pathogenetic studies in 21 families. Ann. Intern. Med., 102:511, 1985.
151. Le Douarin, N. M.: Developmental relationships between the neural crest and the polypeptide-hormone-secreting cells. *In* The Neural Crest. Edited by N. M. L. Douarin. London, Cambridge University Press, 1982, p. 91.
152. Levinson, P. D., Hamilton, B. P., Mersey, J. H., and Kowarski, A. A.: Plasma Norepinephrine and Epinephrine responses to Glucagon in Patients With Suspected Pheochromocytomas. Metabolism, 32:998, 1983.
153. Lewi, H. J. E., Reid, R., Mucci, B., Davidson, J. K., Kyle, K. F., MacPhersron, S. G., Semple, P., and Kaye, S.: Malignant pheochromocytoma. Br. J. Urol., 57:394, 1985.
154. Lewis, P. D.: A cytophotometric study of benign and malignant pheochromocytomas. Virchows Arch., 9:371, 1971.
155. Linnoila, R. I., Lack, E. E., Steinberg, S. M., and Keiser, H. R.: Decreased expression of neuropeptides in malignant paragangliomas. An immunohistochemical study. Hum. Pathol., 19:41, 1988.
156. Lippman, S. M., Mendelsohn, G., Trump, D. L., Wells, S. A., Jr., and Baylin, S. B.: The prognostic and biological significance of cellular heterogeneity in medullary thyroid carcinoma: A study of calcitonin, L-dopa decarboxylase and histaminase. J. Clin. Endocrinol. Metab., 54:233, 1982.
157. Lips, K. J. M., Veer, J. V. D. S., and Struyvenberg, A.: Bilateral occurrence of pheochromocytoma in patients with multiple endocrine neoplasia Syndrome type 2a (Sipple's syndrome). Amer. J. Med., 70:1051, 1981.
158. Lloyd, R. V., Shapiro, B., and Sisson, J. C.: An immunohistochemical study of pheochromocytomas. Arch. Pathol. Lab. Med, 108:541, 1984.
159. Loughlin, K. R., and Gittes, R. F.: Urological management of patients with von Hippel-Lindau's disease. J. Urol., 136:789, 1986.
160. Lynn, M. D., Braunstein, E. M., Wahl, R. L., Shapiro, B., Gross, M. D., and Rabbani, R.: Bone metastases in pheochromocytoma: Comparative studies of efficacy of imaging. Radiology, 160:701, 1986.
161. Mahler, C., Verhelst, J., De Longueville, M., and Harris, A.: Long-term treatment of

metastatic medullary thyroid carcinoma with the somatostatin analogue octreotide. Clin. Endocrinol., 33:261, 1990.
162. Mahoney, E. M., and Harrison, J. H.: Malignant pheochromocytoma: Clinical Course and Treatment. J. Urol., 118:225, 1977.
163. Malagelada, J. R., Edis, A. J., Adsonl, M. A., van Heerden, J. A., and Go, V. L.: Medical and surgical options in the management of patients with gastrinoma. Gastroenterol., 84:1524, 1983.
164. Mangner, T. J., Tobes, M. C., and Wieland, D. W.: Metabolism of Iodine-131 metaiodobenzylquanidine in patients with metastatic pheochromocytoma. J. Nucl. Med., 27:37, 1986.
165. Manger, W. M., and Gifford, R. W., Jr.: Pheochromocytoma. *In* Hypertension: Pathophysiology, Diagnosis, and Management, Edited by J. H. Laragh, and B. M. Brenner. New York, Raven Press, Ltd., 1990, p. 1639.
166. Manger, W. M., Gifford, R. W., and Hoffman, B. B.: Pheochromocytoma: A clinical and experimental overview. Curr. Probl. Cancer, 9:1, 1985.
167. Mannelli, M., DeFeo, M. L., Maggi, M., Geppetti, P., Baldi, E., Pupilli, C., and Serio, M.: Effect of Verapamil on Catecholamine Secretion by Human Pheochromocytoma. Hypertension, 8:813, 1986.
168. Manning, P. C., Jr., Molnar, G. D., Black, B. M., Priestley, J. T., and Woolner, L. B.: Pheochromocytoma, hyperparathyroidism, and thyroid carcinoma occurring coincidentally. N. Engl. J. Med., 268:68, 1963.
169. Marx, S. J., Sakaguchi, K., Green, J. I., Aurbach, G. D., and Brandi, M. L.: Multiple endocrine neoplasia type I: Assessment of laboratory tests to screen for the gene in a large kindred. Medicine, 65:226, 1986.
170. Mason, R. T., Shulkes, A., Zajac, J. D., Fletcher, A. E., Hardy, K. J., and Martin, T. J.: Basal and stimulated release of calcitonin gene-related peptide (CGRP) in patients with medullary thyroid carcinoma. Clin. Endocrinol., 25:675, 1986.
171. Mathew, C. G. P., Chin, K. S., Easton, D. F., Thorpe, K., Carter, C., Liou, G. I., Fong, S.-L., Bridges, C. D. B., Haak, H., Nieuwenhuijzen Kruseman, A. C., Schifter, S., Hansen, H. H., Telenius, H., Telenius-Berg, M., and Ponder, B. A. J.: A linked genetic marker for multiple endocrine neoplasia type 2A on chromosome 10. Nature, 328:527, 1987.
172. Mathew, C. G. P., Smith, B. A., Thorpe, K., Wong, Z., Royle, N. J., Jeffreys, A. J., and Ponder, B. A. J.: Deletion of genes on chromosome 1 in endocrine neoplasia. Nature, 328:524, 1987.
173. Maton, P. N., Gardner, J. D., and Jensen, R. T.: The incidence and etiology of Cushing's syndrome in patients with Zollinger-Ellison syndrome. N. Engl. J. Med., 315:1, 1986.
174. Maton, P. N., Gardner, J. D., and Jensen, R. T.: Diagnosis and management of Zollinger-Ellison Syndrome. Endocrinol. Metab. Clinics N. A., 18:519, 1989.
175. Mayo, C. H.: Paroxysmal hypertension with tumor of retroperitoneal nerve. Report of a case. J. Amer. Med. Assoc., 89:1047, 1927.
176. McAuley, P., Asa, S. L., Chiu, B., Henderson, J., Goltzman, D., and Drucker, D. J.: Parathyroid hormone-like peptide in normal and neoplastic mesothelial cells. Cancer, 66:1975, 1990.
177. McCance, D. R., Kenny, B. D., Sloan, J. M., Russell, C. J. F., and Hassen, D. R.: Parathyroid carcinoma: A review. J. Roy. Soc. Med., 80:505, 1987.
178. Medeiros, L. J., Wolf, B. C., Balogh, K., and Federman, M.: Adrenal pheochromocytoma, A clinicopathologic review of 60 cases. Hum. Pathol., 16:580, 1985.
179. Melicow, M. M.: One hundred cases of pheochromocytoma (107 tumors) at the Columbia-Presbyterian Medical Center, 1926-1976: A clinicopathological analysis. Cancer, 40:1987, 1977.
180. Melvin, K. E. W., Tashjian, A. H., Jr., Cassidy, C. E., and Givens, J. E.: Cushing's syndrome caused by ACTH- and calcitonin-secreting medullary carcinoma of the thyroid. Metabolism, 19:831, 1970.
181. Mendelsohn, G., and Baylin, S. B.: Medullary thyroid carcinoma: Diagnostic and clinical features. Lab Management, 21:21, 1983.
182. Mendelsohn, G., Bigner, S. H., Eggleston, J. C., Baylin, S. B., and Wells, S. A., Jr.,: Anaplastic variants of medullary thyroid carcinoma. A light microscopic and immunohistochemical study. Am. J. Surg. Pathol., 4:333, 1980.
183. Modigliani, E., Guliana, J. M., Maroni, M., Guillausseau, M. P., Chabrier, G., Dupont, J. L., Caron, J., Roger, P., Bentata Pessayre, M., and Jacob, C.: Effets de l'administration sous cutanée de la sandostatine (SMS 201.995) en sous cutané dans 18 cas de cancer médullaire du corps thyroïde. Annales d'Endocrinologie, 50:483, 1989.
184. Modlin, I. M., Farndon, J. R., Shepard, A., Johnston, I. D. A., Kennedy, T. L., Montgomery, D. A. D., and Welbourn, R. B.: Pheochromocytoma in 72 patients: Clinical and diagnostic features, treatment and long term results. Br. J. Surg., 66:456, 1979.
185. Mundy, G. R.: Hypercalcemia of malignancy revisited. J. Clin. Invest., 82:1, 1988.
186. Murphy, M. N., Glennon, P. G., Diocee, M. S., Wick, M. R., and Cavers, D. J.: Nonsecretory parathyroid carcinoma of the mediastinum. Light microscopic, immunocytochemical, and ultrastructural features of a case, and review of the literature. Cancer, 58:2468, 1986.
187. Nakagawara, A., Ikeda, K., and Tsuneyoshi, M.: Malignant pheochromocytoma with ganglioneuroblastomatous elements in a patient with von Recklinghausen's disease. Cancer, 55:2794, 1985.
188. Narod, S. A., Sobol, H., Nakamura, Y., Calmettes, C., Baulieu, J., Bigorgne, J., Chabrier, G., Couette, J., de Gennes, J., Duprey, J., Gardet, P., Guillausseau, P., Guilloteau, D., Houdent, C., Lefebvre, J., Modigliani, E., Parmentier, C., Pugeat, M., Siame, C., Tourniaire, J., Vandroux, J., Vinot, J., and Lenoir, G. M.: Linkage analysis of hereditary thyroid carcinoma with and without pheochromocytoma. Hum. Genet., 83:353, 1989.
189. Nathaniels, E. K., Nathaniels, A. M., and Wang, C.: Mediastinal parathyroid tumors: A clinical and pathological study of 84 Cases. Ann. Surg., 171:165, 1970.
190. Navaratnarajah, M., and White, D. C.: Labetalol and phaeochromocytoma. Br. J. Anaesth., 56:10, 1984.
191. Nelkin, B. D., de Bustros, A. C., Mabry, M., and Baylin, S. B.: The molecular biology of medullary thyroid carcinoma. JAMA, 261:3130, 1989.
192. Nelkin, B. D., Nakamura, Y., White, R. W., de Bustros, A. C., Herman, J., Wells, S. A., Jr., and Baylin, S. B.: Low incidence of loss of chromosome 10 in sporadic and hereditary human medullary thyroid carcinoma. Cancer Res., 49:4114, 1989.
193. Nicholson, J. P., Vaughn, E. D., and Pickering, T. G.: Phaeochromocytoma and prazosin. Ann. Int. Med., 99:477, 1983.
194. Norton, J. A., Doppman, J. L., Collen, M. J., Harmon, J. W., Maton, P. N., Gardner, J. D., and Jensen, R. T.: Prospective study of gastrinoma localization and resection in patients with Zollinger-Ellison syndrome. Ann. Surg., 204:468, 1986.
195. Norton, J. A., Froome, L. J., Farell, R. E., and Wells, S. A., Jr.: Multiple endocrine neoplasia type IIb: The most aggressive form of medullary thyroid cancer. Surg. Clin. North Amer., 59:109, 1979.
196. Nourok, D. S.: Familial pheochromocytoma and thyroid carcinoma. Ann. Intern. Med., 60:1028, 1964.
197. Nussbaum, S. R., Gaz, R. D,, and Arnold, A.: Hypercalcemia and ectopic secretion of parathyroid hormone by an ovarian carcinoma with rearrangement of the gene for parathyroid hormone. N. Engl. J. Med., 323:1324, 1990.
198. O'Connor, D. T., and Bernstein, K. N.: Radioimmunoassay of Chromagranin A in plasma as a measure of exocytic sympathoadrenal activity in normal subjects and patients with pheochromocytoma. N. Engl. J. Med., 311:764, 1984.
199. O'Connor, D. T., Burton, D., and Deflos, L. J.: Immunoreactive human chromogranin A in diverse polypeptide hormone producing human tumors and normal endocrine tissue. J. Clin. Endocrinol. Metab., 57:1084, 1983.
200. O'Connor, D. T., and Deftos, L. J.: Secretion of chromogranin A by peptide producing endocrine neoplasms. N. Engl. J. Med., 314:1145, 1986.
201. O'Hare, M. M. T., and Schwartz, T. W.: Expression and precursor processing of neuropeptide Y in human pheochromocytoma and neuroblastoma tumors. Cancer Res., 49:7015, 1989.
202. Obara, T., Fujimoto, Y., Hirayama, A., Kanaji, Y., Ito, Y., Kodama, T., and Ogata, T.: Flow cytometric DNA analysis of parathyroid tumors with special reference to its diagnostic and prognostic value in parathyroid carcinoma. Cancer, 65:1789, 1990.
203. Obara, T., Fujimoto, Y., Kanaji, Y., Okamoto, T., Hirayama, A., Ito, Y., and Kodama, T.: Flow cytometric DNA analysis of parathyroid tumors. Implication of aneuploidy for pathologic and biologic classification. Cancer, 66:1555, 1990.
204. Oberg, K., and Eriksson, B.: Medical treatment of neuroendocrine gut and pancreatic tumors. Acta Oncol., 28:425, 1989.
205. Oberg, K., Skogseid, B., and Eriksson, B.: Multiple endorine neoplasia type 1 (MEN-1). Clinical, biochemical and genetical investigations. Acta Oncol., 28:383, 1989.
206. Padberg, B. C., Garbe, E., Achilles, E., Dralle, H., Bressel, M., and Schröder, S.: DNA cytophotometric findings in pheochromocytoma. Henry Ford Hosp. Med. J., 37:185, 1989.
207. Padberg, C. A., Garbe, E., Achilles, E., Dralle, H., Bressel, M., and Schröder, S.: Adrenomedullary hyperplasia and phaeochromocytoma. DNA cytophotometric findings in 47 cases. Virchows Archiv. A. Pathol. Anat., 416:443, 1990.
208. Palmer, M., Ljunghall, S., Akerstrom, G., Adami, H. O., Berstrom, R., Grimelius, L., Rudberg, C., and Johansson, H.: Patients with primary hyperparathyroidism operated on over a 24 year period: Temporal trends of clinical and laboratory findings. J. Chron. Dis., 40:121, 1987.
209. Pearse, A. G. E.: Common cytochemical and ultrastructural characteristics of cells producing polypeptide hormones (the APUD) series and their relevance to thyroid and ultimobranchial C-cells and calcitonin. Proc. R. Soc. Lond. (Biol.), 170:71, 1968.
210. Pearse, A. G. E.: The Diffuse Neuroendocrine System and the APUD Concept: Related Endocrine Peptides in Brain, Intestine, Pituitary, Placenta, and Anuran Cutaneous Glands. Medical Biology, 55:115, 1977.
211. Pearse, A. G. E., and Polack, J. M.: Endocrine tumors of neural crest origin: Neurolymphomas, apudomas and the APUD concept. Med. Biol., 52:3, 1974.
212. Petursson, S. R.: Metastic medullary thyroid carcinoma: Complete response to combination chemotherapy with dacarbazine and 5-fluorouracil. Cancer, 62:1899, 1988.
213. Pipeleers-Marichal, M., Somers, G., Willems, G., Foulis, A., Imrie, C., Bishop, A. E., Polak, J. M., Hacki, W. H., Stamm, B., Heitz, P. U., and Kloppel, G.: Gastrinomas in the duodenums of patients with multiple endocrine neoplasia type 1 and Zollinger-Ellison syndrome. N. Engl. J. Med., 332:723, 1990.
214. Plouin, P. F., Dudos, J. M., and Menard, J.: Biochemical tests for diagnosis of phaeochromocytoma: Urinary versus plasma determinations. Br. Med. J., 282:1981.
215. Ponder, B.: Gene Losses in human tumours. Nature, 335:400, 1988.
216. Ponder, B. A., Ponder, M. A., Coffey, R., Pembrey, M. E., Gagel, R. F., Telenius-Berg, M., Semple, P., and Easton, D. F.: Risk estimation and screening in families of patients with medullary thyroid carcinoma. Lancet, 1:397, 1988.
217. Powell, G. J., Southby, J., Danks, J. A., Stillwell, R. G., Hayman, J. A., Henderson, M. A., Bennett, R. C., and Martin, T. M.: Localization of parathyroid hormone-related protein in breast cancer metastases: Increased incidence in bone compared with other sites. Cancer Res., 51:3059, 1991.
218. Prinz, R. A., Gamvros, O. I., and Sellu, D.: Subtotal parathyroidectomy for primary chief cell hyperplasia of the multiple endocrine neoplasia type 1 syndrome. Ann. Surg., 193:26, 1981.
219. Pritchard, J., Kiely, E., Rogers, D. W., Spitz, L., Shafford, E. A., Brereton, R., Muller, C., and Wright, V. M.: Long-term survival after advanced neuroblastoma (letter). N. Engl. J. Med., 317:1026, 1987.
220. Proye, C., Fossati, P., and Fontaine, P.: Dopamine-secreting pheochromocytoma: An unrecognized entity? Classification of pheochromocytomas according to their type of secretion. Surgery, 100:1154, 1986.
221. Proye, C., Thevenin, D., Cecat, P., Petillot, P., Carnaille, B., Verin, P., Sautier, M., and Racadot, N.: Exclusive use of calcium channel blockers in preoperative and intra-operative control of pheochromocytomas: Hemodynamics and free catecholamine assays in ten consecutive patients. Surgery, 106:1149, 1989.
222. Ralston, S. H., Alzais, A. A., Gardner, M. D., and Boyle, I. T.: A treatment of cancer associated hypercalcaemia with combined aminohydroxypropylidene diphosphonate and calcitonin. Br. Med. J., 292:1549, 1986.
223. Reinig, J. W., Doppman, J. L., Dwyer, A. J., Johnson, A. R., and Knop, R. H.: Adrenal masses differentiated by MR. Radiol., 158:81, 1986.
224. Remine, W. H., Chong, G. C., van Heerden, J. A., Sheps, S. G., and Harrison, E. G., Jr.: Current management of pheochromocytoma. Ann. Surg., 179:740, 1974.
225. Ritch, P. S.: Treatment of cancer-related hypercalcemia. Semin. Oncol., 17 (Suppl 5):26, 1990.
226. Roos, B. A., Lindall, A. W., Ells, J., Elde, R., Lambert, P. W., and Birnbaum, R. S.: Increased plasma and tumor somatostatin-like immunoreactivity in medullary thyroid carcinoma and small cell lung cancer. J. Clin. Endocrinol. Metab., 52:187, 1981.
227. Roth, K. A., Wilson, D. M., and Eberwine, J.: Acromegaly and pheochromocytoma: A multiple endocrine syndrome caused by a plurihormonal adrenal medullary tumor. J. Clin. Endocrinol. Metab., 63:1421, 1986.
228. Rougier, P., Calmettes, C., Laplanche, A., Travagli, J. P., Lefevre, M., Parmentier,

C., Milhaud, G., and Tubiana, M.: The value of calcitonin and carcinoembryonic antigen in the treatment and management of nonfamilial medullary thyroid carcinoma. Cancer, 51:855, 1983.

229. Rougier, P., Parmentier, C., Laplanche, A., Lefevre, M., Travagli, J. P., Caillou, B., Schlumberger, M., Lacour, J., and Tubiana, M.: Medullary Thyroid Carcinoma: Prognostic Factors and Treatment. Int. J. Radiat. Oncol. Biol. Phys., 9:161, 1983.

230. Russell, C. F., van Heerden, J. A., Sizemore, G. W., Edis, A. J., Taylor, W. F., ReMine, W. H., and Carney, J. A.: The surgical management of medullary thyroid carcinoma. Ann. Surg., 197:42, 1983.

231. Saad, M. F., Fritsche, H. A., and Samaan, N. A.: Diagnostic and prognostic value of carcinoembryonic antigen in medullary carcinoma of the thyroid. J. Clin. Endocrinol. Metab., 58:889, 1984.

232. Saad, M. F., Ordonez, N. G., Guido, J. J., and Samaan, N. A.: The prognostic value of calcitonin immunostaining in medullary carcinoma of the thyroid. J. Clin. Endocrinol. Metab., 59:850, 1984.

233. Saad, M. F., Ordonez, N. G., Rashid, R. K., Guido, J. J., Hill, C. S., Jr., Hickey, R. C., and Samaan, N. A.: Medullary carcinoma of the thyroid: A study of the clinical features and prognostic factors in 161 patients. Medicine, 63:319, 1984.

234. Sager, R.: Tumor suppressor genes: The puzzle and the promise. Science, 246:1406, 1989.

235. Saller, B., Jacob, K., Markl, A., Zwiebel, F. M., Engelhardt, D., and Mann, K.: Rezidivierende Hochdruckkrisen und Dyspnoe nach einseitiger Adrenalektomie wegen Phäochromozytom bei einer 44 jährigen Patientin. Internist, 31:78, 1990.

236. Samaan, N. A.: Parathyroid Carcinoma. In Cancer Medicine, 2nd Edition. Edited by J. F. Holland, and I. E. Frei. Philadelphia, Lea & Febiger, 1982, p. 1692.

237. Samaan, N. A., Hickey, R. C., and Shutts, P. E.: Diagnosis, Localization, and Management of Pheochromocytoma: Pitfalls and Follow-Up in 41 Patients. Cancer, 62:2451, 1988.

238. Samaan, N. A., Ouais, S., Ordonez, N. G., Choksi, U. A., Sellin, R. V., and Hickey, R. C.: Multiple endocrine syndrome type 1. Clinical, laboratory findings, and management in five families. Cancer, 64:741, 1989.

239. Samaan, N. A., Schultz, P. N., and Hickey, R. C.: Medullary Thyroid carcinoma: Prognosis of familial versus sporadic disease and the role of radiotherapy. J. Clin. Endocrin. Metab., 67:801, 1988.

240. Sano, T., Saito, H., Inaba, H., Hizawa, K., Saito, S., Yamanoi, A., Mizunuma, Y., Matsumura, M., Yuasa, M., and Hiraishi, K.: Immunoreactive somatostatin and vasoactive intestinal polypeptide in adrenal pheochromocytoma: An immunochemical and ultrastructural study. Cancer, 52:282, 1983.

241. Sardesai, S. H., Mourant, A. J., Sivathandon, Y., Farrow, R., and Gibbons, D. O.: Phaeochromocytoma and catecholamine induced cardiomyopathy presenting as heart failure. Br. Heart J., 63:234, 1990.

242. Sasaki, A., Yumita, S., Kimura, S., Miura, Y., and Yoshinaga, K.: Immunoreactive Corticotropin-Releasing Hormone, Growth Hormone-Releasing Hormone, Somatostatin, and Peptide Histidine Methionine Are Present in Adrenal Pheochromocytomas, but not in Extra-adrenal Pheochromacytoma. J. Clin. Endocrinol. Metab., 70:996, 1990.

243. Schifter, S.: Calcitonin gene-related peptide and calcitonin as tumour markers in MEN 2 family screening. Clin. Endocrin., 30:263, 1989.

244. Schimke, R. N.: Multiple endocrine neoplasia: How many syndromes? Amer. J. Med. Gen., 37:375, 1990.

245. Schimke, R. N., Hartmann, W. H., Prout, T. E., and Rimoin, D. L.: Syndrome of bilateral pheochromocytoma, medullary thyroid carcinoma, and multiple neuromas. N. Engl. J. Med., 279:1, 1968.

246. Schmedtje, J. F., Sax, S., Pool, J. L., Goldfarb, R. A., and Nelson, E. B.: Localization of ectopic pheochromocytomas by magnetic resonance imaging. Am. J. Med., 83:770, 1987.

247. Scott, H. W., and Halter, S. A.: Oncologic aspects of pheochromocytoma: The importance of follow-up. Surgery, 96:1061, 1984.

248. Scott, H. W., Jr., Reynolds, V., Green, N., Page, D., Oates, J. A., Robertson, D., and Roberts, S.: Clinical experience with malignant pheochromocytomas. Surg. Gynecol. Obstet., 154:801, 1982.

249. Shane, E., and Bilezikian, J. P.: Parathyroid carcinoma: A review of 62 patients. Endocr. Rev., 3:218, 1982.

250. Shane, E., and Bilezikian, J. P.: Parathyroid Carcinoma. In Textbook of Uncommon Cancer. Edited C. J. Williams, J. G. Krikorian, M. R. Green, and D. Raghavan, Chichester, John Wiley & Sons Ltd., 1988, p. 763.

251. Shane, E., Jacobs, T. P., Siris, E. S., Steinberg, S. F., Stoddart, K., Canfield, R. E, and Bilezikian, J. P.: Therapy of hypercalcemia due to parathyroid carcinoma with intravenous dichloromethylene diphosphonate. Am. J. Med., 72:939, 1982.

252. Shapiro, B., and Fig, L. M.: Management of pheochromocytoma. Endocrinol. Metab. Clin. N. A., 18:443, 1989.

253. Shapiro, B., Fig, L. M., Gross, M. D., and Khafagi, F.: Contributions of nuclear endocrinology to the diagnosis of adrenal tumors. In Recent Results in Cancer Research: Hormone-related Malignant Tumors. Edited by L. Beck, E. Grundmann, R. Ackermann and H. D. Roher. New York, Springer-Verlag, 1990, p. 113.

254. Shapiro, B., Sisson, J. C., Eyre, P., Copp, J. E., Dmuchowski, C., and Beierwaltes, W. H.: ^{131}I-MIBG—A new agent in diagnosis and treatment of pheochromocytoma. Cardiol., 72: (suppl. 1):137, 1985.

255. Shapiro, B., Sisson, J. C., Lloyd, R., Nakajo, M., Satterlee, W., and Beierwalters, W. H.: Malignant pheochromocytoma: Clinical, Biochemical and scintigraphic characterization. Clin. Endocrinol., 20:189, 1984.

256. Shimaoka, K., Schoenfeld, D. A., DeWys, W., Creech, R. H., and DeConti, R.: A randomized trial of doxorubicin versus doxorubicin plus cisplatin in patients with advanced thyroid carcinoma. Cancer, 56:2155, 1984.

257. Siddiqui, M. Z., Von Eyben, F. E., and Spanos, G.: High-votage irradiation and combination chemotherapy for malignant pheochromocytoma. Cancer, 62:686, 1988.

258. Sikri, K. L., Varndell, I. M., Hamid, Q. A., Wilson, B. S., Kameya, T., Ponder, B. A., Lloyd, R. V., Bloom, S. R., and Polack, J. M.: Medullary carcinoma of the thryoid. An immunocytochemical and histochemical study of 25 cases using eight separate markers. Cancer, 56:2481, 1985.

259. Silverman, M. L.: Pathology of Thyroid and Parathyroid Glands. In Surgery of the Thyroid and Parathyroid Glands. Edited by B. Cady and R. L. Rossi. Philadelphia, W. B. Saunders, 1991, p. 31.

260. Simpson, E. L., Mundy, G. R., D'Souza, S. M., Ibbotson, K. J., Bockman, R., and Jacobs, J. W.: Absence of parathyroid hormone messenger RNA in nonparathyroid tumors associated with hypercalcemia. N. Engl. J. Med., 309:325, 1983.

261. Simpson, N. E., and Kidd, K. K.: The mapping of the locus for multiple endocrine neoplasia type 2A by linkage with chromosome 10 markers. Horm. Metab. Res. Suppl., 21:5, 1989.

262. Simpson, N. E., Kidd, K.K., Goodfellow, P. J., McDermid, H., Myers, S., Kedd, J. R., Jackson, C. E., Duncan, A. M. V., Farrer, L. A., Brasch, K., Castiglione, C., Genel, M., Gertner, J., Greenberg, C. R., Gusella, J. F., Holden, J. J. A., and White, B. N.: Assignment of multiple endocrine neoplasia type 2A to chromosome 10 by linkage. Nature, 328:528, 1987.

263. Simpson, W. J., Palmer, J. A., Rosen, I. B., and Mustard, R. A.: Management of Medullary Carcinoma of the Thyroid. Am. J. Surg., 144:420, 1982.

264. Singer, F. R.: Role of the bisphosphonate etidronate in the therapy of cancer-related hypercalcemia. Semin. Oncol., 17 (Suppl 5):34, 1990.

265. Sipple, J. H.: The association of pheochromocytoma with carcinoma of the thyroid gland. Am. J. Med., 31:163, 1961.

266. Sisson, J. C., Frager, M. S., Valk, T. W., Gros, M. D., Swanson, D. P., Wieland, D. M., Tobes, M. C., Beierwaltes, W. H., and Thompson, N. W.: Scintigraphic localization of pheochromocytoma. N. Engl. J. Med., 305:12, 1981.

267. Snover, D. C., and Foucar, K.: Mitotic activity in benign parathyroid disease. Am. J. Clin. Pathol., 75:345, 1981.

268. Sobol, H., Narod, S. A., Nakamura, Y., Boneu, A., Calmettes, C., Chadenas, D., Charpentier, G., Chatal, J. F., Delepine, N., and Delisle, M. J.: Screening for multiple endocrine neoplasia type 2a with DNA-polymorphism analysis. N. Engl. J. Med., 321:996, 1989.

269. Sobol, R. E., Memoli, V., and Deftos, L. J.: Hormone-negative, chromogranin A-positive endocrine tumors. N. Eng. J. Med., 320:444, 1989.

270. Sofianides, T., Chang, Y.-S., Leary, J. S., and Nichols, F. X.: Localization of parathyroid adenomas by cervical esophagram. J. Clin. Endocrinol. Metab., 46:587, 1978.

271. Sparagana, M.: Late Recurrence of Benign Pheochromocytomas: The Necessity for Long Term Follow-Up. J. Surg. Oncol., 37:140, 1988.

272. Sridhar, K. S., Holland, J. F., Brown, J. C., Cohen, J. M., and Ohnuma, T.: Doxorubicin Plus Cisplatin in the Treatment of Apudomas. Cancer, 55:2634, 1985.

273. St. John Sutton, M. G., Sheps, S. G., and Lie, J. T.: Prevalence of clinically unsuspected pheochromocytoma: Review of a 50-year autopsy series. Mayo Clin. Proc., 56:354, 1981.

274. Stenstrom, G., Haljamae, H., and Tisell, L. E.: Influence of pre-operative treatment with phenoxybenzamine on the incidence of adverse cardiovascular reactions during anaesthesia and surgery for pheochromocytoma. Acta Anaesthesiol. Scand., 29:797, 1985.

275. Stewart, A. F., Hoecker, J. L., Mallette, L. E., Segre, G. V., Amatruda, T. T., Jr., and Vignery, A.: Hypercalcemia in pheochromocytoma. Evidence for a novel mechanism. Ann. Intern. Med., 102:776, 1985.

276. Stock, J. L., Weintraub, B. D., Rosen, S. W., Aurbach, G. D., Spiegel, A. M., and Marx, S. J.: Human chorionic gonadotropin subunit measurement in primary hyperparathyroidism. J. Clin. Endocrinol. Metab., 54:57, 1982.

277. Stokes, K. R.: Invasive Radiologic Evaluation of Hyperparathyroidism. In Surgery of the Thyroid and Parathyroid Glands. Edited by B. Cady and R. L. Rossi. Philadelphia, W. B. Saunders, 1991, p. 278.

278. Suva, L. J., Winslow, G. A., Wettenhall, E. H., Hammonds, R. G., Moseley, J. M., Jasgger-Diefenback, H., Rodda, C. P., Kemp, B. E., Rodriquez, H., Chen, E. Y., Hudson, P. J., Martin, T. J., and Wood, W. I.: A parathyroid hormone-related protein implicated in malignant hypercalcemia: Cloning and expression. Science, 237:893, 1987.

279. Taub, M. A., Osburne, R. C., Georges, L. P., and Sode, J.: Malignant Pheochromocytoma. Severe Clinical Exacerbation and Release of Stored Catecholamines During Lymphoma Chemotherapy. Cancer, 50:1739, 1982.

280. Taylor, H. C., Fallon, M. D., and Velasco, M. E.: Oncogenic osteomalcia and inappropriate antidiuretic hormone secretion due to oat-cell carcinoma. Ann. Intern. Med., 101:786, 1984.

281. Thakker, R. V., Bouloux, P., Wooding, C., Chotai, K., Broad, P. M., Spurr, N. K., Besser, G. M., and O'Riordan, J. L. H.: Association of parathyroid tumors in multiple endocrine neoplasia type 1 with loss of alleles on chromosome 11. N. Engl. J. Med., 321:218, 1989.

282. Thakker, R. V., and Ponder, B. A. J.: Multiple endocrine neoplasia. Bailliere's Clin. Endocrinol. Metab., 2:1031, 1988.

283. Theilade, K., Bak, M., Olsen, K., Nielsen, S. L., and Christensen, N. J.: A Case of Malignant Pheochromocytoma Treated by 131 I Metaiodobenzylguanidine. Acta Oncol., 27:296, 1988.

284. Thompson, N. W., Bondeson, A. G., Bondeson, L., and Vinik, A.: The surgical treatment of gastrinoma in MEN I syndrome patients. Surgery, 106:1081, 1989.

285. Thompson, N. W., Lloyd, R. V., Nishiyama, R. H., Vinik, A. I., Stroedel, W. E., Allo, M. D., Eckhauser, F. E., Talpos, G., and Mervak, T.: MEN I pancreas: A histological and immunohistochemical study. World J. Surg., 8:561, 1984.

286. Thompson, N. W., Vinik, A. I., and Eckhauser, F. E.: Microgastrinomas of the duodenum. A cause of failed operations for the Zollinger-Ellison syndrome. Ann. Surg., 209:396, 1989.

287. Tisell, L. E., Ahlman, H., Jansson, S., and Grimelius, L.: Total pancreatectomy in the MEN-I syndrome. Br. J. Surg., 75:154, 1986.

288. Tisell, L. E., Hansson, G., Jansson, S., and Salander, H.: Reoperation in the treatment of asymptomatic metastasizing medullary thyroid carcinoma. Surgery, 99:60, 1986.

289. Troncone, L., Rufini, V., Montemaggi, P., Danza, F. M., Lasorella, A., and Mastrangelo, R.: The diagnostic and therapeutic utility of radioiodinated metaiodobenzylguanidine (MIBG). Eur. J. Nucl. Med., 16:325, 1990.

290. Tsutsumi, M., Yokota, J., Kakizoe, T., Koiso, K., Sugimura, T., and Terada, M.: Loss of Heterozygosity on Chromosomes 1p and 11p in Sporadic Pheochromocytoma. J. Natl. Cancer Inst., 81:367, 1989.

291. van Heerden, J. A., Roland, C. F., Carney, A., Sheps, S. G., and Grant, C. S.: Long-Term Evaluation following Resection of Apparently Benign Pheochromocytoma(s)/ Paraganglioma(s). World J. Surg., 14:325, 1990.

292. van Heerden, J. A., Sheps, S. G., Hamberger, B., Sheedy, P. F., Poston, J. G., and Remine, W. H.: Pheochromocytoma. Current status and changing trends. Surgery, 91:367, 1982.

293. van Heerden, J. A., Smith, S. L., and Miller, L. J.: Management of the Zollinger-Ellison

syndrome in patients with multiple endocrine neoplasia type I. Surgery, 110:971, 1986.

294. Velchik, M. G., Alavi, A., Kressel, H. Y., and Engelman, K.: Localization of pheochromocytoma: MIBG, CT, and MRI correlation. J. Nucl. Med., 30:328, 1989.

295. Vetter, H., Fischer, M., Müller-Rensing, R., Vetter, W., and Winterberg, B.: [131I]-meta-iodobenzylguanidine in treatment of malignant phaeochromocytomas. Lancet, 2(8341):107, 1983.

296. Viale, G., Dell'Orto, P., Moro, E., Cozzaglio, L., and Coggi, G.: Vasoactive intestinal polypeptide-, somatostatin-, and calcitonin-producing adrenal pheochromocytoma associated with the watery diarrhea (WDHH) syndrome. First Case Report With Immunohistochemical Findings. Cancer, 55:1099, 1985.

297. Vinik, A. I., Shapiro, B., and Thompson, N. W.: Plasma gut hormone levels in 37 patients with pheochromocytomas. World J. Surg., 10:593, 1986.

298. Von Moll, L., McEwan, A. J., Shapiro, B., Sisson, J. C., Gross, M. D., Lloyd, R., Beals, E., Beierwaltes, W. H., and Thompson, N. W.: Iodine-131 MIBG scintigraphy of neuroendocrine tumors other than pheochromocytoma and neuroblastoma. J. Nucl. Med., 28:979, 1987.

299. Voorhess, M. L.: The catecholamines in tumor and urine from patients with neuroblastoma, ganglio-neuroblastoma and pheochromocytoma. J. Pediatr. Surg., 3:147, 1968.

300. Wang, C.: The anatomic basis of parathyroid surgery. Ann. Surg., 183:271, 1976.

301. Wang, C., and Gaz, R. D.: Natural History of Parathyroid Carcinoma. Diagnosis, treatment and results. Am. J. Surg., 149:522, 1985.

302. Warrell, R. P., Israel, R., Frisone, M., Snyder, T., Gaynor, J. J., and Bockman, R. S.: Gallium nitrate for acute treatment of cancer-related hypercalcemia. A randomized, double-blind comparison to calcitonin. Ann. Intern. Med., 108:669, 1988.

303. Warrell, R. P., Issacs, M., Alcock, N. W., and Bockman, R. S.: Gallium nitrate for treatment of refractory hypercalcemia from parathyroid carcinoma. Ann. Intern. Med., 107:683, 1987.

304. Warrell, R. P. J., Murphy, W. K., Schulman, P., O'Dwyer, P. J., and Heller, G.: A randomized double-blind study of gallium nitrate compared with etidronate for acute control of cancer-related hypercalcemia. J. Clin. Oncol., 9:1467, 1991.

305. Weinstein, R. S., and Ide, L. F.: Immunoreactive calcitonin in pheochromocytomas. Proc. Soc. Exp. Biol. Med., 165:215, 1980.

306. Weiss, R. B.: Failure of Streptozotocin in Rare Hormonally Active Malignancies. Cancer Treatment Reports, 62:847, 1978.

307. Wells, S. A., Dilley, W. G., Farndon, J. A., Leight, G. S., and Baylin, S. B.: Early diagnosis and treatment of medullary thyroid carcinoma. Arch. Intern. Med., 145:1248, 1985.

308. Wells, S. A. J., Gunnells, D. J., Gutman, R. A., Shelbourne, J. D., Schneider, A. B., and Sherwood, L. M.: The successful transplantation of frozen parathyroid in man. Surgery, 81:86, 1977.

309. Wermer, P.: Genetic aspects of adenomatosis of endocrine glands. Am. J. Med., 16:363, 1954.

310. Williams, E. D.: Histogenesis of medullary carcinoma of the thyroid. J. Clin. Pathol., 19:114, 1966.

311. Williams, E. D., Karin, S. M. M., and Sandler, M.: Prostaglandin secretion by medullary carcinoma of the thyroid. A possible cause of the associated diarrhea. Lancet, 1:22, 1968.

312. Williams, E. D., and Pollock, D. J.: Multiple mucosal neuromata with endocrine tumours: A syndrome allied to Von Recklinghausen's disease. J. Pathol. Bacteriol., 91:71, 1966.

313. Williams, S. D., Birch, R., and Einhorn, L. H.: Phase II Evaluation of Doxorubicin Plus Cisplatin in Advanced Thyroid Cancer: A Southeastern Cancer Study Group Trial. Cancer Treatment Reports, 70:405, 1986.

314. Winzelberg, G. G.: Parathyroid imaging. Ann. Intern. Med., 107:64, 1987.

315. Wolfe, H. J., Melvin, K. E W., Cervi-Skinner, S. J., Saadi, A. A., Juliar, J. F., Jackson, C. E., and Tashjian, A. H. J.: C-cell hyperplasia preceding medullary thyroid carcinoma. N. Engl. J. Med., 289:437, 1973.

316. Woltering, E. A., Mozell, E. J., O'Dorisio, T. M., Fletcher, W. S., and Howe, B.: Suppression of primary and secondary peptides with somatostatin analog in the therapy of functional endocrine tumors. Surg. Gynecol. Obstet., 167:153, 1988.

317. Wynick, D., Williams, S. J., and Bloom, S. R.: Symptomatic secondary hormone syndromes in patients with established malignant pancreatic endocrine tumors. N. Engl. J. Med., 319:605, 1988.

318. Zollinger, R. M., and Ellison, E. H.: Primary peptic ulcerations of the jejunum associated with islet cell tumor of the pancreas. Ann. Surg., 142:709, 1955.

319. Zweifler, A.J., and Julius, S.: Increased platelet catecholomine content in pheochromocytoma. A diagnostic test in patients with elevated plasma catecholamines. N. Engl. J. Med., 306:890, 1982.

XXVI-5

Neoplasms of the Gastroenteropancreatic Endocrine System

Aaron I. Vinik
Norman W. Thompson
Steven D. Averbuch

Introduction

The endocrine tumors of the gastroenteropancreatic (GEP) axis consist of cells capable of amine precursor uptake and decarboxylation and have, therefore, been named Apudomas.[252] The morphologic similarity of the Apud cells suggested a common embryologic origin, which was believed to be the neural crest but was later revised to include the neuroectoderm, or in the case of some of the endocrine cells, the dorsal placoderm. Studies by Ledouarin, Teillet, Pictet, Rall, Phelps, Andrew, and their coworkers have cast doubt on this hypothesis, and most workers agree that these tumors should be classified according to their secretory products, i.e., gastrinoma, somatostatinoma, glucagonoma, and pancreatic polypeptide (PPoma).[9,174,255] The generally held belief that the neuronal characteristics of these cells indicated an ectodermal origin during mammalian embryogenesis has largely been abandoned.

Developmental Origin of Islets During Pancreatic Embryogenesis

The developing pancreas appears as a protrusion from the dorsal surface of the embryonic gut.[256] The different islet cell types appear sequentially during development in vivo. It therefore seems reasonable to propose that coordinated growth is dependent upon specificity of growth factors.

Rosenberg and Vinik[273] have utilized a model for new islet formation (nesidioblastosis) and shown that pancreatic ductal cells are capable of differentiating upon stimulation into adult endocrine cells capable of secreting insulin in a fully regulated manner. This has led to the notion that endocrine tumors derive from a totipotential stem cell in the gut capable of differentiating into any one of a variety of cells which may be responsible for the clinical syndrome (Figure XXVI-5-1).

A great deal of interest is now being focused upon the factors responsible for initiation of growth, growth proliferation, differentiation into adult endocrine cells, and in neu-

Cell Differentiation:

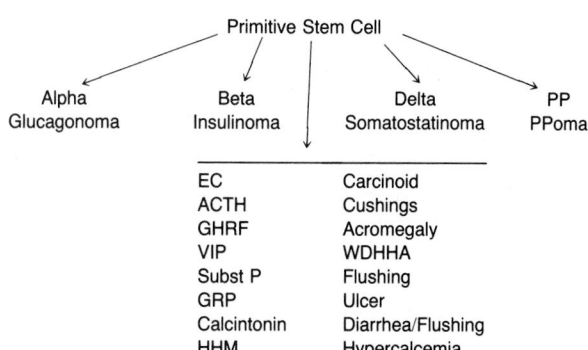

Figure XXVI-5-1. Gastroenteropancreatic tumors. ACTH, cortico-trophin; EC, enterochromaffin; GHRF, growth hormone releasing factor; GRP, gastrin releasing peptide; PP, pancreatic polypeptide; Subst P, Substance P; VIP, vasoactive intestinal peptide; WDHHA, watery diarrhea hypokalemia, hypochlorhydria, and acidosis.

Table XXVI-5-1. Characteristics of Neuroendocrine Tumors

Rare

Usually small, <1 cm

Slow growing, months to years, "Cancer in slow motion"

Usually metastasize before becoming symptomatic, often when tumor >2 cm

Expression is episodic, may be silent for years

Symptoms mimic commonplace conditions and are often misdiagnosed

Complex diagnosis, rarely made clinically, requiring sophisticated laboratory and scanning techniques

ronal systems, for growth cessation and cell maintenance. Several models of pancreatic regeneration and tumor formation have been established[40,212,261,271,272,284,304,317,319,320,362] and various growth factors implicated in the process, but none has thus far been convincing or shown to be the primary or only cause of tumor occurrence.

Growth Factors as a Cause of GEP Tumors

The coincidental findings that the multiple endocrine neoplasia, type 1 syndrome (MEN-1) (combined occurrence of tumors of the pituitary, pancreas and parathyroid glands) is associated with the loss of alleles on chromosome 11,[170,321] the same chromosome on which the insulin gene has been located;[39] and the finding of parathyroid mitogenic activity in the plasma of patients with MEN-1[188,249] suggests a genetic predisposition to tumor formation based upon elaboration of a growth factor. Cell lineage analysis data of pancreatic islets suggest that progenitor cells, which contain catecholamines, are present in pancreatic ducts and give rise to the glucagon and insulin cells of adult islets;[77] and can be stimulated to grow by plasma from patients with MEN-1. The findings that MEN-1 patients might also elaborate into their plasma, mitogenic factors for pancreatic islet-cells, led McLeod and Vinik to postulate a genetically determined circulating growth factor in the growth initiation of GEP tumors (see Table XXVI-5-1).[201]

Neuroendocrine Characteristics

A number of peptides originally isolated from gut endocrine tissues have been shown to occur in nerves. These include gastrin, cholecystokinin (CCK), vasoactive intestinal polypeptide (VIP), and substance P (SP). As a corollary, peptides which have been found primarily in nervous tissues have now been identified in gut endocrine cells and include somatostatin (SRIF), enkephalins, SP, neurotensin, and thyrotropin-releasing hormone (TRH).[25,26,315] Because many of these peptides occur both in endocrine cells and nerves, "endocrine" tumors of the gut may, in fact, be endocrine or neurocrine. Unique to the gastroenteropancreatic (GEP) axis is the ability of the endocrine cell to secrete a variety of peptides and amines. Hormonal peptides have not only been found within the same cell, e.g., motilin and serotonin in the enterochromaffin (EC) cell, but have been localized to the same secretory granule. Whether these act within the secretory granule in a paracrine manner or in some way are co-regulated is not clear. At any one point in time, several hormones and amines are co-secreted; in individual instances the symptom complex derives from one or more of the peptides and amines produced and cannot be simply ascribed to a single factor. Thus, a tumor may secrete one peptide, recur and secrete yet another; and its metastases may secrete still other peptides. In the British National Supra-Regional Survey of national health service hospitals, 58% of 353 neuroendocrine tumors had increased serum levels of two or more hormones at diagnosis. Nine percent had clinical symptoms related to different hormones. Four out of 353 developed new symptoms from secretion of a second hormone after diagnosis.[371]

Anatomic Distribution

More than 50% of neuroendocrine tumors in clinical practice are of the so-called carcinoid variety and are found incidentally at operation, after metastasis has occurred, in the small intestine, especially the appendix. The remaining fraction comprises about 50% gastrinomas, 30% insulinomas, 13% vipomas, 5–10% glucagonomas, and rarely, <5% neurotensinomas, somatostatinomas, and etopic hormone secreting tumors. Non-secretory tumors were thought to make up the bulk of pancreatic tumors, but with better immunohistochemical stains for endocrine cells, especially for neuron specific enclose (NSE), chromogranin, synaptophysin, and receptors for somatostatin,[266] there is increasing recognition that tumors masquerading as carcinomas of liver, small cell carcinoma of the lung and the like are in effect endocrine tumors (See Table XXVI-5-2). The majority of these "non-secretory" tumors actually store and secrete pancreatic polypeptide (PP) but because it has so little in the way of biologic activity the tumor remains silent.

About 60% of pancreatic endocrine tumors are concentrated in Pasarro's Triangle, an area subtended by the head of pancreas, the gastric antrum and the first portion of the duodenum.

The tumors are proliferative in nature and may take the form of hyperplasia, or neoplasia (adenoma, adenomatous hyperplasia, microadenomatosis, nesidioblastosis, or carcinoma).

Hyperplasia is relatively uncommon in benign sporadic tumors, is the rule in MEN-1 syndrome, and often is present in the area of the pancreas surrounding a benign tumor.

The tumors may be further subdivided into: *Orthoendo-*

Table XXVI-5-2.   The Clinical Syndromes

Clinical Syndrome	Tumor Type	Site	Hormone(s)
Wheezing	Carcinoid	mid foregut pancreas/foregut adrenal medulla	Serotonin, Substance P NKA, TCT, PP, CGRP, VIP
Ulcer Disease	Gastrinoma	pancreas 85% duodenum 15%	Gastrin
Hypoglycemia	Insulinoma Sarcomas Hepatoma	pancreas/uterus retro-peritoneal liver	Insulin/TNF IGF/BP
Dermatitis/Dementia Diabetes/DVT	Glucagonoma	pancreas	glucagon
Diabetes/Steatorrhea	Somatostatinoma	pancreas	Somatostatin
Cholelithiasis/neurofibromatosis	Somatostatinoma	duodenum	Somatostatin
Silent/liver Mets	PPoma	pancreas	PP
Acromegaly	GEP	pancreas	GH (GHRH)
Cushings	GEP	pancreas	ACTH/CRF
Hypercalcemia	VIPoma	pancreas	VIP
	GEP	pancreas	PTHrP
Pigmentation	GEP	pancreas	MSH

NKA = Neurokinin A	TNF = Tumor necrosis factor	GHRH = Growth hormone releasing hormone
TCT = Thyrocalcitonin	IGF = Insulin-like growth factor	ACTH = Adrenol corticotropic hormone,
PP = Pancreatic polypeptide	BP = Binding protein	corticotropin
CGRP = Calcitonin gene related peptide	GEP = Gastroenteropancreatic	CRF = Corticotropin releasing factor
VIP = Vasoactive intestinal peptide	GH = Growth hormone. somatotropin	PTHrP = Parathyroid hormone related peptide
DVT = Deep venous thrombosis		MSH = Melanocyte stimulating hormone

crine; when they secrete the normal product of the cell type, e.g., α cell glucagon. *Paraendocrine:* when they secrete a peptide or amine foreign to the organ or cell of origin. These are found in adrenal medulla, kidney, lymph nodes or in the liver. *Part of MEN-1:* when a variety of peptides or amines are secreted.

When tumors metastasize they do so to local lymph nodes, the liver, peritoneum, and rarely to bone. Metastases are notoriously highly vascular, a telltale sign of a GEP tumor auguring well for the patient. Even with extensive liver metastasis tumors can regress with treatment.

The occurrence of MEN-1 syndrome may be as frequent as one third of the cases of gastroenteropancreatic tumors, depending on the endemic area. In high risk areas measurements of ionized Ca^{2-}, prolactin and PP are important.

In the sections which follow we will focus upon the specific syndromes that are ascribed to GEP hyperfunction.

Carcinoid Tumors

Carcinoid tumors are the most commonly occurring gut endocrine tumors. The incidence of carcinoid tumors is estimated to be approximately 1.5 cases per 100,000 of the general population, i.e., about 2,500 cases/year in the United States. Nonetheless, they account for 13–34% of all tumors of the small bowel and 17–46% of all malignant tumors of the small bowel.[45] They are derived from a primitive stem cell and are generally found in the gut wall. Carcinoids may, however, occur in the pancreas, the rectum, the ovary, the lung and elsewhere. The tumors grow slowly and are often clinically silent for many years before becoming manifest, usually when metastases have occurred. They frequently metastasize to the regional lymph nodes, the liver, and less commonly to bone. The likelihood of metastases is related

to tumor size. The incidence of metastases is less than 2% with a carcinoid tumor less than 1 cm in size, but rises to 100% with tumors greater than 2 cm in diameter. These tumors may be symptomatic only episodically and their existence may go unrecognized for many years. The average time from onset of symptoms attributable to the tumor and diagnosis is a little over nine years and is usually made only when the carcinoid syndrome occurs. The carcinoid syndrome occurs, however. in less than 10% of patients with carcinoid tumors.[24] It is especially common in tumors of the ileum and jejunum, but also occurs with bronchial, ovarian and other carcinoids.[67] In this section we will discuss the incidence, natural history, clinical presentation. diagnosis, and management of carcinoid tumors.

One of the more clinically useful classifications of carcinoid tumors is according to the division of the primitive gut from which the tumor cells arise. Foregut tumors include carcinoids of bronchus, stomach, the first portion of the duodenum, and the pancreas. Midgut carcinoid tumors derive from the second portion of the duodenum, the jejunum, ileum, and right colon. Hindgut carcinoid tumors include those of the transverse colon, left colon, and rectum. This distinction assists in distinguishing a number of important biochemical and clinical differences between carcinoid tumors, since the presentation, histochemistry and secretory products are quite different (Table XXVI-5-2).

Foregut carcinoids are argentaffin negative. They have a low content of serotonin (5-hydroxytryptamine, 5HT). They often secrete the serotonin precursor 5-hydroxytryptophan (5HTP) and histamine and a multitude of polypeptide hormones. Their functional manifestations include atypical carcinoid syndrome, gastrinoma syndrome, acromegaly, Cushing's disease, and a number of other endocrine disorders. They are, furthermore, unusual in that the flush which occurs tends to be of protracted duration, is often of a purplish or violaceous hue rather than the usual pink-red color, and frequently leaves permanent telangiectasia and hypertrophy of the skin of the face and upper neck. The face assumes a leonine characteristic after repeated episodes. It is not unusual for these tumors to metastasize to bone.

Midgut carcinoids, in contrast, are argentaffin positive, have a high 5HT content, rarely secrete 5HTP and often produce a number of other vasoactive compounds such as kinins, prostaglandins, and substance P. The clinical syndrome that derives is the classic carcinoid. These tumors may produce ACTH, albeit rarely, and very infrequently metastasize to bone.

Hindgut carcinoids are argentaffin negative, rarely contain 5HT, rarely secrete 5HTP or other peptides, and are usually silent in their presentation, but may metastasize to bone.

A further point of interest is the finding that if a carcinoid tumor coexists with multiple endocrine neoplasia type I (MEN-I), more than two-thirds of the time in males the tumor is in the thymus, whereas greater than 75% of the time in females it is in the lung.

Although carcinoids are classically tumors of enterochromaffin and argentaffin cells of the digestive tract, the term "carcinoid tumor" can be expanded to cover gut tumors of paracrine- and endocrine-like cells of unknown function.[306,364] It is now established that these tumors are of neuroendocrine origin and derive from a primitive stem cell. They may differentiate into any one of a variety of adult endocrine secreting cells: B cell and insulinoma; A cell and glucagonoma; D cell and somatostatinoma; and the PP cell and PPoma, or cells capable of producing ACTH, growth hormone releasing hormone (GHRH), VIP, Substance P, gastrin releasing factor (GRF), calcitonin, and the enterochromaffin (EC) cell with its ability to co-secrete amines such as serotonin and the peptide motilin. At any one point in time, these cells may secrete one humor, whereas at other times the peptide or amine secreted may differ and yield an entirely different clinical syndrome. Indeed, metastases are known to secrete hormones that differ from the parent tumor and different metastases may secrete different hormones. Symptoms may derive from secretion of one or more of the hormones secreted.

Age Distribution

The distribution of carcinoids is gaussian in nature and the peak incidence occurs in the sixth and seventh decade but includes patients as young as 10 years of age and people in their ninth decade.

The Natural History

Carcinoid tumors are slow growing and may be present for years without overt symptoms, thus escaping attention. In the early stages, vague abdominal pain goes undiagnosed and is invariably ascribed to irritable bowel or spastic colon. Fully, one-third of patients with carcinoid tumors present with years of intermittent abdominal pain. Carcinoid tumors can present in a variety of ways. For example, duodenal tumors are known to produce gastrin and may present with the gastrinoma syndrome. Small, multiple gastric carcinoids are associated with atrophic gastritis, pernicious anemia, and chronic thyroiditis. It seems that the loss of the

inhibitory influence of gastric acid upon the G cell permits proliferation of both the G and the EC cells with the ultimate development of carcinoid tumors.[371] Patients with carcinoid tumors of the thymus most often manifest hyperparathyroidism or ectopic Cushing's syndrome. Bronchial carcinoids are associated with type I multiple endocrine neoplasia.

The major clinical manifestations of carcinoid tumors include cutaneous flushing, which occurs in 84%, GI hypermotility with diarrhea in 70%, heart disease in 37%, bronchial constriction in 17%, myopathy in 7%, and an abnormal increase in skin pigmentation in 5% of the cases.[75] When coexistence of the major symptoms of flushing and diarrhea are sought, it emerges that flushing and diarrhea occur simultaneously in 58%, diarrhea without flushing in 15%, flushing without diarrhea in 5%, and 22% of individuals have neither flushing nor diarrhea as a symptom complex.

With metastases to the liver, the correct diagnosis is generally arrived at, but with a delay of many years, however. Even then, mistaken identity is not uncommon and unless biopsy material is examined for the neuronal glycolytic enzyme neuron-specific enolase, or the secretory peptide chromogranin[49] of synaptophysin,[363] tumors may be erroneously labeled as adenocarcinomas with a negative impact upon attitudes toward management and an underestimate of survival.

Diagnosis

The diagnosis of carcinoid tumors rests upon a strong clinical suspicion in patients who present with flushing, diarrhea, wheezing, myopathy, and right heart disease, and includes appropriate biochemical and localization studies.

Biochemical Studies. The rate limiting step in carcinoid tumors for the synthesis of serotonin is the conversion of tryptophan into 5-hydroxytryptophan (5-HTP), catalyzed by the enzyme tryptophan hydroxylase. In midgut tumors, 5-HTP is rapidly converted to 5-hydroxytryptamine (5-HT) by the enzyme aromatic amino acid decarboxylase (dopadecarboxylase). 5-HT is either stored in the neurosecretory granules or may be secreted directly into the vascular compartment. Most of the secreted 5-HT is taken up by platelets and stored in their secretory granules. The rest remains free in the plasma and circulating 5-HT is then largely converted into the urinary metabolite 5-hydroxyindoleacetic acid (5-HIAA) by the enzyme monoamine oxidase (MAO) and by aldehyde dehydrogenase (AD). These enzymes are abundant in the kidney and the urine typically contains large amounts of 5-HIAA.

In patients with foregut tumors, the urine contains relatively little 5-HIAA but large amounts of 5-HTP. It is presumed that these tumors are deficient in dopa-decarboxylase which, therefore, impairs conversion of 5-HTP into 5-HT leading to 5-HTP secretion into the vascular compartment. Some 5-HTP, however, is converted to 5-HT and 5-HIAA and thus, the modest increase in these metabolites. The normal range for 5-HIAA secretion is 2–8 mg/24 hours and the quantitation of serotonin and all its metabolites usually permits the detection of 84% of patients with carcinoid tumors. No single measurement detects all cases of carcinoid syndrome, although the urine 5-HIAA appears to be the best screening procedure. Other peptides involved include substance P, neuropeptide K, pancreatic polypeptide and chromogranin A. In carcinoid tumors, neurotensin is elevated in 43%, substance P in 32%, motilin in 14%, somatostatin in 5% of cases and VIP rarely.[297] In miscellaneous illnesses, there may be elevation of the following hormones: neurotensin, substance P, and motilin in 35%, 7%, and 5% respectively. However, up to one-third of people with idiopathic flushing that do not have carcinoid syndrome have elevated levels of a number of neuropeptides.[5] Furthermore, we have examined the relationship between the products of the preprotachykinin gene, substance P and neurokinin A in healthy subjects and in patients with carcinoid tumors. Substance P was elevated 80% of the time in patients with carcinoid tumors whereas neurokinin A was raised in all patients. Why there should be a discrepancy in these two peptides which derive from a common precursor gene product remains unclear. Measurement of circulating levels enhance the ability to identify more patients with carcinoid tumors.

Localization Studies. A number of techniques have been used to identify the primary site of the tumor and to evaluate the extent of the disease and the presence of metastases. A chest X-ray or CT suffices to detect bronchial carcinoid. In contrast, carcinoids of the cecum, right colon, and hindgut carcinoids are usually demonstrable by endoscopy or barium enema examination. The greatest problems encountered are in localizing small bowel carcinoids, which may be small, and carcinoids in extra-intestinal sites. These tumors are usually not identified by upper or GI roentgenographic studies. Abdominal CT scans and ultrasound are usually not helpful because the primary tumors are below the resolution capacity of even the most sophisticated scanning apparatus. Superior mesenteric angiography may be of help, however.

Several diagnostic methods have been evaluated for the diagnosis of carcinoid tumors, including barium examinations, computed tomography, ^{131}I-metaiodobenzylguanidine (MIBG) scanning, angiography, and venous sampling with radioimmunoassay of hormones. Barium examinations are rarely diagnostic, but may demonstrate fixation, separation, thickening and angulation of the bowel loops. Computed tomography is the primary diagnostic procedure for tumor staging; it allows assessment of the extent of tumor spread to the mesentery and bowel wall as well as metastases to the lymph nodes and liver. The typical appearance of mesenteric invasion by carcinoid tumor on CT is a mesenteric mass with radiating linear densities representing thickened neurovascular bundles. Liver metastases appear as focal hypodense lesions on non-enhanced CT scanning.[114] The advantage of CT is its ability to localize precisely the tumors in relation to the adjacent structure. CT also remains the most useful roentgenographic method for evaluation of the response of metastatic carcinoid tumors to therapy. At present, the combination of computed tomography and MIBG scanning[1] are the most useful diagnostic tests for the localization of metastatic carcinoid tumors. Magnetic resonance imaging (MRI) is a very sensitive technique for the detection of liver metastases, but it appears to be less sensitive for the diagnosis of extrahepatic disease. MRI needs further evaluation before it is used as primary modality for the diagnosis and staging of carcinoid tumor.[158]

The role of angiography in the diagnosis of carcinoid tumor has been decreased by the availability of the new imaging methods. Diagnostic angiography is generally employed when non-invasive imaging studies are equivocal and surgery is contemplated. Liver metastases from carcinoid tumors vary in size and are usually vascular with abundant neovascularity, demonstrable on angiography. Percutaneous transhepatic portal and systemic venous sampling with hormone assay is not a very useful technique for the localization of carcinoid tumors.

The Scintigraphic Depiction of Carcinoids with MIBG. The first report of ^{131}I-MIBG for the imaging of a carcinoid tumor was that of Fischer and colleagues in 1984 in which hepatic metastases that were seen as photopenic areas on a ^{99m}Tc-phytate liver scan concentrated ^{131}I-MIBG.[91] Since this initial description, there have been a number of reports of successful imaging of carcinoid tumors using ^{131}I-MIBG. The number studied are far less than those reported for pheochromocytoma or neuroblastoma, but it is probably fair to say that the sensitivity is significantly lower.[124,290,291,298,357] The overall sensitivity is calculated to be 55%. Because MIBG is taken up by a wide variety of neuroendocrine tumors,[124,290,291,357] specificity depends on the certainty of the clinical and biochemical diagnosis. In the correct clinical context this is well over 95% for pheochromocytoma[189,290,291,292] and neuroblastoma,[105,179,291,331] but might well be less true for carcinoid.

In the remaining cases in whom the tumor has not been identified by the above techniques, total body venous sampling with measurement of a peptide hormone that is produced may be considered. Measurements of serotonin may be misleading but those of substance P may well direct attention to the source of overproduction of the peptide. This has proved useful in substance P producing tumors.[313]

Carcinoid Syndrome. Carcinoid syndrome occurs in less than 10% of patients with carcinoid tumors. The principal features of carcinoid syndrome include flushing, sweating, wheezing, diarrhea, abdominal pain, cardiac fibrosis and pellagra dermatosis. Diarrhea is found in 83% of cases, flushing in 49%, dyspnea in 20% and bronchospasm in 6%.[314] The relationship between diarrhea and flushing is variable. One can occur without the other and there may be no temporal relationship between the two. The specific etiologic agent(s) for each of the protean manifestations of the carcinoid tumors are not known. Serotonin,[87,204] prostaglandins,[280] 5-hydroxytryptophan,[7,244,254] substance P,[313,365] kallikrein,[178] histamine,[254] dopamine[86] and neuropeptide K,[322] are thought to be involved in the clinical manifestations of carcinoid tumors. In addition, symptoms may be related to overproduction of peptides of the proopiomelanocortin family, β endorphin and enkephalin. Pancreatic polypeptide and motilin levels are often raised,[352] may be important markers of tumor activity and may provide a means of monitoring tumor growth and response to therapy rather than contributing to specific symptomatology.

Feldman and O'Dorisio[89] examined the proportion of 43 patients with carcinoid having increased levels of serotonin and various other vasoactive peptides.[343] Serotonin, measured either as its urinary metabolite, 5-HIAA,[334] or whole blood serotonin,[64,66,360] was raised in 84% of patients with carcinoid tumors and was within normal limits in patients with other tumors and miscellaneous illnesses. Urinary 5-HIAA alone had a 73% sensitivity and 100% specificity. Seven of their patients had normal urinary 5-HIAA levels, but other elevated indices of serotonin production. Neurotensin and substance P were raised in 43% and 32% of patients and had specificity values of 60 and 85%, respectively. False positives occurred in 23% and 26% of patients with conditions other than carcinoid tumors. Motilin and somatostatin were raised in 14% and 50%, respectively.

These humors may prove useful as an aid in the localization of ostensibly occult carcinoid tumors. Whole body venous sampling with measurements of plasma serotonin erroneously localized the tumor to the neck for which a negative exploration was carried out. However, substance P levels correctly localized certain of these tumors.[313]

Diarrhea. The diarrhea syndrome which occurs with carcinoid tumors is usually of a secretory nature. Diarrhea persists with fasting or fails to disappear when feeding has been curtailed and sustenance is given by the intravenous route.

A history of improvement in the diarrhea with the administration of H_2 receptor antagonists is strongly suggestive of the gastrinoma syndrome. Hypocalcemia is frequent with VIP-secreting tumors and steatorrhea, and for all intents and purposes occurs only with the Zollinger-Ellison (ZE) syndrome. Marked metabolic acidosis with bicarbonate wasting is usually only a characteristic of VIP-secreting tumors. The villous adenoma of the rectum causing secretory diarrhea is notoriously rare and although referred to in many texts, most physicians have yet to see a case. A disturbing cause which may be very difficult to differentiate is laxative abuse and in all circumstances a KOH stool preparation to detect laxatives is mandatory. Measurement of intestinal secretion by passing a multilumen tube and quantifying electrolytes and water transport, in addition to the measurement of stool electrolytes, which should account for the total osmolarity, will help to exclude laxative abuse.

Flushing. Flushing in carcinoid syndrome is of two varieties. With midgut carcinoid, the flush is usually of a faint pink to red color and involves the face and upper trunk as far as the nipple line. The flush is initially provoked by alcohol, and food containing tyramines such as blue cheese, chocolate, red sausage, and red wine. With time the flush may occur spontaneously without provocation. It is usually ephemeral, lasting only a few minutes, may occur many times per day but does not usually leave permanent discoloration. In contrast, the flush of foregut tumors is often more intense, of protracted duration, lasting hours, purplish in hue, is frequently followed by telangiectasia and involves not only the upper trunk but also the limbs. The limbs may become acrocyanotic and the nose resembles that of rhinophyma. The skin of the face often thickens with the appearance of a leonine facies resembling that seen in leprosy and acromegaly.

Flushing cannot always be attributed to carcinoid syndrome. The differential diagnosis of flushing includes: the postmenopausal state, simultaneous ingestion of chlorpropamide and alcohol, panic attacks, medullary carcinoma of the thyroid, autonomic epilepsy, autonomic neuropathy and mastocytosis.

Flushing in carcinoid syndrome has been ascribed to pros-taglandins, kinins, and serotonin (5-HT). With the advent of sophisticated radioimmunoassay methods and region specific antisera, a number of neurohumors are now thought to be secreted by carcinoid tumors, including: serotonin,[87] dopamine,[86] histamine, and 5-HIAA,[254] kallikrein,[244] substance P,[7] neurotensin,[89] motilin,[89,313] SRIF,[89] VIP,[214] prostaglandins,[280] neuropeptide K,[322] and gastrin-releasing peptide (GRP).[89]

Feldman and colleagues have previously reported the incidence of elevated levels of plasma concentrations of neuropeptides.[89] In spite of the elevated basal concentrations of substance P and neurotensin (NT), they were able to document further increases in these neuropeptides during ethanol-induced facial flushing. We support this contention and hasten to add that neuropeptide abnormalities occur frequently in patients with all forms of flushing and may be of pathogenetic significance.[5]

Several new provocative tests have been developed for carcinoid syndrome. Ahlman recently reported the results of pentagastrin (PG) provocation in 16 patients with midgut carcinoids and hepatic metastases.[2] All patients tested had elevated urinary 5-HIAA levels and 12 had profuse diarrhea requiring medication. PG uniformly induced facial flushing and gastrointestinal symptoms in patients with liver metastases but had no effect in healthy, control patients. All patients with PG-induced GI symptoms demonstrated elevated serotonin levels in peripheral blood. Administration of a serotonin receptor antagonist had no effect on serotonin release but completely aborted GI symptoms. The authors emphasized the improved reliability of PG compared to calcium infusion, another provocative test popularized by Kaplan,[144] and pointed out that PG provocation can occasionally be falsely negative in patients with subclinical disease. Our own experience is that PG uniformly induces flushing in 11 patients with gastric carcinoid tumors associated with a rise in circulating levels of substance P in 80%.[75] Thus, substance P is one neurohumor that may be involved in the flushing of carcinoid.

Substance P (SP) has been found in tumor extracts and plasma from patients with carcinoid tumors and in one reported case was useful for tumor localization.[313] SP along with neurokinin A (NKA) and its amino-terminally extended form, neuropeptide K (NPK), comprise a group of peptides (tachykinins) with common biological properties.[58,236] Norheim measured peptide responses to pentagastrin or ingestion of food or alcohol in 16 patients with metastatic carcinoids and demonstrated two-fold or greater increases in NKA and NPK in 75% of patients and variable increases in SP in approximately 20% of patients.[131]

Conlon used region specific antisera to SP and NKA to measure circulating tachykinins during a meal-induced flush in 10 patients with metastatic carcinoid tumors.[58] Five patients had undetectable levels of NKA and SP after stimulation, suggesting that elevated tachykinin concentrations are not a constant feature of carcinoid patients. The authors also studied the effect of a somatostatin analogue administration on meal-induced tachykinin responses in three carcinoid patients. Flushing was aborted in two patients but tachykinin levels were only partially suppressed indicating that these peptides cannot be solely responsible for the carcinoid flush.

Treatment of Carcinoid

Prognosis. The general prognosis in carcinoid is excellent, compared to other visceral cancers. Based upon a world literature of some 2,837 cases, the median 5-year survival for all cases is 82%.[221] If, however, the tumor is localized, then the 5-year survival is 94%, decreasing to 64% with regional lymph node involvement and 18% with distant metastases. Davis reported a mean survival of 38 months from the first episode of flushing with 25% living for more than 6 years.[67] With regional lymph node involvement, the figure falls to about 14 months,[113] and with urinary 5-HIAA in excess of 150 mg/24 hours or inoperable tumors, the median survival is only 11 months.[221]

Surgical removal of the primary tumor is the treatment of choice for small and localized tumors and for the alleviation of any obstructive symptoms, but surgical cure of carcinoid is almost impossible in the presence of intra-abdominal and hepatic metastases. Different chemotherapeutic agents[162] and surgery or arterial embolization[192] have been used with variable success, but eventual relapse with increasing resistance to the drugs is encountered.[221] Since carcinoid is a slow growing tumor, even patients with extensive metastatic disease can enjoy a normal quality of life so long as the endocrine syndrome is quiescent. Different chemical agents such as methysergide, cyproheptadene, heparin, phenothiazines, alpha-adrenergic antagonists, corticosteroids, H_1 and H_2 anti-histamine blockers, symptomatic treatment of diarrhea with opioids, and codeine have been tried with variable results.[221] Since somatostatin has very broad inhibitory effects, somatostatin-14 has been used successfully to suppress diarrhea and flushing in patients with carcinoid tumors,[121] but its clinical use is limited by its short half-life[293] with the resulting need for continuous intravenous infusion. With the advent of the long-acting somatostatin analogue (SMS 201–995),[15] it has been used in the treatment of different neuroendocrine tumors including carcinoid.

Therapy of Carcinoid Syndrome. Various chemotherapeutic agents, including parachlorophenylalanine, cyproheptadene, methotrimeprazine, corticosteroids, aprotinin, phenoxybenzamine, and numerous antineoplastic agents have been used in Carcinoid Syndrome with variable success.[214,314] These medications either inhibit serotonin synthesis, act as systemic antagonists of serotonin, or block kallikrein release. Most recently, somatostatin 14 and its long-acting analog , octreotide, have been used successfully to control symptoms of diarrhea and flushing[121,166,306,356] in the carcinoid syndrome. We have had variable experiences with carcinoid syndrome and report below factors which determine responsiveness.

Nowadays angiography is frequently used for therapeutic purposes. Hepatic artery embolization has proved to be a relatively safe procedure for palliation of the carcinoid syndrome related to an excessive hormone production from hepatic carcinoid metastases.[50] This method is usually beneficial to the patients whose hepatic metastases have failed to respond to chemotherapy and other pharmacologic therapy (87% response rate). Gelfoam powder (particle sizes; 80–200 µm) and Ivalon particles (sizes; 149–250 µm) are the frequently used agents for devascularization of the hepatic metastases.

Evaluation of Responses to Octreotide. The responses to therapy may be divided into four groups: 1) responders were those with more than 75% improvement, i.e., a 75% drop in the frequency or intensity of a symptom, or 75% drop in the level of a biochemical marker; 2) partial responders were those with 25–75% improvement; 3) non-responders were those with less than 25% improvement; and 4) worsening was judged to occur if the clinical and/or biochemical values increased by more than 25% of their initial estimation.

Flushing. Our patients were a heterogeneous group with advanced carcinoid tumors refractory to conventional chemotherapeutic agents who were tried on the somatostatin analogue with variable clinical and biochemical responses. We have previously shown a dramatic response of flushing as a symptom during treatment with somatostatin.[306] Frolich and colleagues have also reported on the value of native somatostatin given by continuous infusion as a means of reversing the pentagastrin-induced flushing in carcinoid patients.[103] We, however, were unable to show that pentagastrin was a reliable means whereby flushing could be provoked in our patients. Kvols found that 19 of 24 patients with carcinoid tumors had a 50% reduction in flushing, three had a minor response and in two patients the octreotide failed.[167] Richter showed that 6 of 8 patients had improved symptoms.[267] Our more recent experience is that 64% of our patients presented with flushing as their major symptom. In all instances, the symptom complex improved with a clear decrease in the frequency of symptoms with doses of octreotide 1–2 µg/Kg/day. In no instance was there resistance to the drug. Tachyphylaxis did not occur and withdrawal of the drug, or substitution with distilled water, was always followed by recurrence of the symptom complex. In contrast to another study,[267] relapse of flushing did not occur with continued treatment once it was under control. However, in contrast to the reduction in a number of episodes, in certain patients the severity decreased only slightly and the duration of each episode was essentially unchanged.

The extreme example of flushing is the carcinoid crisis with a profound fall in blood pressure. It is deemed unwise to submit a patient to anesthesia or operation without premedication with a combination of adrenergic blockade, steroids, thorazine and aspirin. Kvols has presented data on one such patient, who soon after induction of anesthesia, had a fall in blood pressure which was unresponsive to intravenous fluid, calcium, neo-synephrine or epinephrine administration.[166] Within one minute of 100 µg of octreotide given intravenously, blood pressure rose and the patient made an uneventful recovery.

Thus, while it is unclear as to the mechanism of action of octreotide and the factors mediating flushing and vasodilatation, there can be no doubt that octreotide is a potent antidote to the vasoactive humors participating in the flush and hypotension. The drug may prove to be a useful adjunct in the preparation of patients for operative procedures and as a standby for the management of carcinoid crisis.

Responses of Diarrhea. Diarrhea occurred in 86% of our patients and responded variably to octreotide. Acute administration of octreotide normalized the water and electrolyte transport across the proximal intestine, as has been shown in patients with the Watery Diarrhea Hypokalemia Hypochlorhydria and Acidosis (WDHHA) syndrome.[282,356] The acute reduction in electrolyte secretion did not, however, predict the long term response of diarrhea to octreotide therapy, but this needs to be further examined in a larger number of patients. Only 58% of our patients with diarrhea had complete remission which differs from the improvement in 19 of 25 (76%) patients reported by Kvols.[167] This could be due to the fact that diarrhea in patients with carcinoid tumors has multiple etiologies, i.e., secretory, increased motility, malabsorption, partial luminal lymphatic obstruction, bacterial overgrowth, and short bowel syndrome due to surgical resection. The diarrhea may even appear to worsen with the appearance of steatorrhea and the physician is not infrequently faced with the confounding situation of not knowing to what to attribute the symptom. However, although octreotide does inhibit exocrine pancreatic secretion,[10] addition of pancreatic enzyme supplementation has not uniformly decreased octreotide-induced steatorrhea.[312] We did not find any consistent changes in frequency or consistency of bowel movements in response to pancreatic supplements in those patients with steatorrhea before treatment or the bowel habits after therapy with octreotide, a fact compatible with the notion that the steatorrhea has a complex pathogenesis and may be contributed to by alterations in bile flow, the direct effects of octreotide on nutrient absorption and intestinal motility.[128]

Effects of Octreotide on Pulmonary Function. All three of our patients with wheezing had clinical improvement and spirometric improvement was documented. Pulmonary function did not improve further after 3 months of treatment indicating an irreversible component or small airway disease secondary to long-standing smoking.[347]

Effects of Octreotide on Myopathy. One patient in our series presented with severe proximal muscle weakness with normal muscle enzymes and nerve conduction studies, but electromyographic features of a proximal myopathy. Although a neurological deficit secondary to metastatic carcinoid has been seen,[260] metabolic-induced neuromuscular disease is very rare.[18,116,370] Although our patient had a history of hypokalemia, at the time of admission his potassium was normal with no biochemical evidence of thyrotoxicosis, ectopic ACTH production or, osteomalacia. We believe that his severe myopathy was due to his carcinoid, although it might have been aggravated by severe diarrhea, weight loss and poor nutrition. Histological changes can be induced in skeletal muscle of mice by intraperitoneal injection of 5HT.[243] Three months after octreotide therapy, the patient did not have any clinical evidence of myopathy with improvement in electromyographic features.[347]

Biochemical Responses. There are conflicting reports regarding the biochemical responses of carcinoid patients to octreotide. Richter reported a significant drop in 5HT in eight patients treated with 150 μg/day of octreotide, but no changes in urinary 5-HIAA while others have found a drop in urinary 5-HIAA.[267,371] In prolonging their treatment of four of their patients to 15–30 weeks, blood serotonin remained unchanged.[312] In our patients, urinary 5-HIAA dropped in almost all patients and normalized in one-third of the patients. Four out of eight patients normalized their 24-hour 5-HIAA.

Although few of our patients had a fall in their blood sero-

tonin level, the overall post-octreotide values were not significantly lower than pre-treatment values.

There were no clinical correlations between the clinical responses and either the urinary 5-HIAA or the blood serotonin level. In contrast, for patients in whom the urinary 5-HIAA fell, there was clinical improvement in one or more of the symptoms. This may reflect the fact that there are multiple etiologic factors involved in the symptomatology of carcinoid tumors. In our patients, those who responded clinically required no more than 500 μg/day to control their symptoms, although we have examined the response to higher doses in certain instances.

Responses of Tumor Growth and Metastases to Octreotide. Due to the slow growth of carcinoid tumors, it is difficult to assess the effect of octreotide on the rate of tumor growth or regression. Shrinkage of liver metastases in patients with carcinoids[167,356] and other functioning pancreatic neuroendocrine tumors[155] has been reported. We have had variable experiences. The relationship between tumor size and growth and the biochemistry is not a simple one. In one patient the tumor clearly shrank, but ACTH levels rose to the 2,000–3,000 pg/ml range. On molecular sieve chromatography, the ACTH coeluted with native ACTH, but the patient has no clinical features of Cushing's syndrome, is gaining weight and has no diarrhea or flushing. Another patient had progression of tumor growth after 18 months of octreotide therapy, yet there was a dramatic fall in blood serotonin values and the patient is entirely asymptomatic. The opposite is also not unusual wherein there is no change in tumor size, a very well patient and hormonal levels that are unaffected by octreotide even in doses as high as 1,000 μg/day.[365]

We have follow up CT data for 14 patients. Two showed some regression of the tumor, and in one case it infarcted. Five cases showed progression and seven cases showed no changes on the CT scan followed for up to 2–5 years. It appears that cessation or reversal of growth occurs in about two-thirds of patients with carcinoid tumors treated with octreotide.

Short of an effective curative or palliative agent, octreotide can control flushing and wheezing in most and diarrhea in some patients with carcinoid tumors with improvement in their general condition. The effects of octreotide on tumor growth need to be further evaluated in relation to the slow progression and indolent nature of these tumors. Since little effective therapy is available and much may be harmful, it seems not unreasonable to offer octreotide for the control of symptoms and for palliation at this point in time. Limits of safe and effective dosage need to be established and long-term follow up is a prerequisite to defining the ultimate role of this form of peptide therapy in the carcinoid syndrome.

When, however, there is clear evidence that tumor growth is not contained by octreotide, alternative forms of treatment should be considered.[163] There are also experimental techniques which should be considered.

Internal Radiotherapy Delivered by MIBG. There is the potential to deliver therapeutic doses of radiation to those tumors in which there is intense and prolonged tumor uptake of tracer doses of MIBG. Target-to-background ratios with tracer doses that achieve diagnostic imaging may not, however, always permit the delivery of therapeutic radiation when large doses of activity are administered.[199,300-302]

MIBG therapy for carcinoid is, at the present time, to be considered highly experimental. Possible guidelines for its employment based on the experience with other neuroendocrine tumors would include:[300-302] 1) lesions not readily treatable by alternative modalities; 2) patients with life expectancies sufficient to permit beneficial effects to become apparent (e.g., greater than six months or one year);[300,301] 3) dosimetric studies for whole body and blood absorbed radiation dose using tracer doses should be undertaken to guide the size of therapeutic administrations. The bone marrow and especially the platelets appear to be the dose-limiting tissues for MIBG therapy. Typical doses to date have been in the range of 100–250 mCi per administration with cumulative doses sometimes exceeding 600 mCi;[300,302] 4) if at all possible the absorbed radiation dose to one or more representative tumors should be determined from serial scintigraphic images. From these the initial uptake and biological $T\frac{1}{2}$ of retention can be determined (the use of conjugate view technique with the inclusion of standard sources may be especially helpful).[297] Tumor volume must also be determined by CT or other modality and this, with the other parameters, can be used with Medical Internal Radiation Dose (MIRD) formulas to calculate the radiation absorbed dose[300-302,305]

Dearterialization. Several authors have described their experience with hepatic artery ligation or embolization in patients with malignant carcinoid tumors.[202,203,235] In one study, the former procedure resulted in objective tumor responses in 9 of 19 patients, stable disease in 5 of 19 patients, and progressive disease in 4 of 19 patients when they were assessed 6 and 12 months after the procedure.[235] Two patients died one and three months postoperatively from complications including liver abscesses, and the remainder of patients experienced mild abdominal pain, fever, and fatigue that was self-limiting. Hepatic artery gel foam embolization performed in eight patients resulted in three objective responses and five with stable disease. Toxicity from this procedure included fever, abdominal pain, nausea, and elevation of serum hepatic enzymes that returned to normal within 12 days. Although hepatic artery occlusion may produce subjective and objective responses in the majority of highly selected patients, the toxicity and duration of responses resulting from this therapy generally do not support its routine use.[220]

Radiation Therapy. There are no data available to support the use of radiation therapy in patients with metastatic carcinoid unless they have symptomatic bone metastases or spinal cord compression which is amenable to this modality.

Chemotherapy. In malignant carcinoid tumor, chemotherapy has not been shown to be effective for the majority, and this approach should still be considered investigational. The single agent most studied in carcinoid is 5-fluorouracil, which accounted for observed response rates of 26% and 18% in single institution and multi-institutional trials, respectively.[221,222] Melia reported a high complication rate with little benefit when 5-fluorouracil was administered by intraarterial, portal, or peripheral intravenous routes.[203] Few responses were observed following intravenous doxorubicin, 60 mg/M², every three to four weeks.[164,220,221] In spite of well established

activity in other gastroenteropancreatic cancers, streptozotocin has not demonstrated significant efficacy in patients with carcinoid.[45,221] Among other single agents, there have been anecdotal reports of objective responses to dacarbazine and dactinomycin;[150,164] however, a study in 32 patients demonstrated that dactinomycin or decarbazine had little activity against metastatic carcinoid.[338] Phase II studies in evaluable patients with carcinoid have shown rare objective responses to either cisplatin or etoposide.[149,227,338]

Initial experience with combination chemotherapy suggested that this modality may be effective against malignant carcinoid. Early non-randomized studies of combinations of cyclophosphamide plus methotrexate, streptozotocin plus 5-fluorouracil, or weekly streptozotocin plus doxorubicin reported response rates in excess of 50%; although rigid criteria for response were not always employed and complete responses were not seen.[45,149,205,221,222] Based on these observations, the Eastern Cooperative Oncology Group conducted a series of multi-institutional randomized trials of combinations that all contained streptozotocin, despite the low activity of this drug when used alone. In two studies of 170 evaluable patients, the response rates ranged from 23%–33% and there was no evidence for any difference between streptozotocin, administered every six weeks or every 10 weeks plus 5-fluorouracil versus streptozotocin plus cyclophosphamide versus single agent doxorubicin.[80,221,222] In a prospective trial, the Southwest Oncology Group reported similar response rates of brief duration following a combination of 5-fluorouracil, cyclophosphamide, and streptozotocin with or without doxorubicin.[46] Only 10% of 31 patients had objective response following streptozotocin and 5-fluorouracil in another prospective clinical trial reported by Oberg.[246]

Feldman has suggested that streptozotocin alone or in combination with 5-fluorouracil may be beneficial for patients with foregut carcinoid tumors in contrast to patients with midgut carcinoid tumors,[88] but this contrasts with the results of the Eastern Cooperative Oncology Group experience,[222] and it remains unsubstantiated. Thus, in the absence of randomized trials that contain a no treatment arm, there is no persuasive evidence that single agent or combination chemotherapy provides any significant impact on disease progression or on survival in patients with malignant carcinoid.

Biologicals. Several studies have been conducted using interferon against malignant carcinoid tumor. In the first of these, 17 of 36 (47%) patients with metastatic carcinoid tumor treated with human leukocyte interferon, 3–6 million units per day, subcutaneously, had objective hormonal responses for a median duration of 34 months.[246] Four patients had significant tumor regression and two complete responses were noted. A second study randomized 20 patients to treatment with either a combination of streptozotocin and 5-fluorouracil or human leukocyte interferon, six million units five times per week.[245] After six months, 50% of the patients treated with interferon had an objective hormonal response and no patients treated with chemotherapy responded. Finally, Oberg conducted a study in 20 patients with malignant carcinoid that suggested recombinant human interferon alpha-2b, 5×10^6 U/M² three times a week, subcutaneously for six months was as active as leukocyte interferon and that the two agents may not be cross-resistant.[246] In this study, the development of neutralizing interferon antibodies correlated with lack of response to interferon in three patients.

Additional positive outcomes using recombinant human interferon alpha-2b have been reported by several additional groups in small prospective trials.[127,300] Hanssen also gave interferon following hepatic artery embolization and they observed 5 of 7 patients with objective tumor and hormonal responses after 12 months.[127]

These encouraging results with interferon have to be interpreted with caution considering the results from another prospective study with interferon reported by Moertel and colleagues.[226] In this study, 27 previously treated patients with malignant carcinoid tumors were treated with recombinant human interferon alpha-2a, 12–24 $\times 10^6$ U/M^2 subcutaneously, three times weekly for eight weeks. Nine of 23 (39%) patients with elevated 5-HIAA had objective responses for a median of 40 weeks (range 23–127 weeks), and 4 of 20 (20%) patients had objective tumor responses for a median of seven weeks (range 4–26 weeks). The flu-like syndrome and fatigue side-effects from interferon were common in this study, requiring dose reduction in 10 patients and causing deterioration of performance status in one-half of all patients. In addition to differences in dose and in observed toxicities, the variable response rates observed among these reported studies may be related to the utilization of different recombinant interferon subtypes (alpha-2a vs. alpha-2b) and the subsequent development of neutralizing antibodies.[115] The role for the combination of recombinant human interferon alpha-2a and doxorubicin in patients with advanced pancreatic endocrine or carcinoid tumors is currently under investigation.[3]

Adjuvant Therapy. Combined modality therapy, such as the use of adjuvant chemotherapy prior to or following surgery, remains undefined for metastatic carcinoid. In the absence of well-established activity for chemotherapy in this disease, there is no rationale to support the use of adjuvant chemotherapy. In contrast, the preliminary results of the prospective experience of sequential hepatic artery occlusion and alternating combination chemotherapy at the Mayo Clinic is of some interest.[164,220,225] Following hepatic artery occlusion by surgical ligation or percutaneous embolization, twenty-one patients were treated with dacarbazine, 250 mg/M^2 daily for five days plus doxorubicin 60 mg/M^2 alternating every four to five weeks with 5-fluorouracil 400 mg/M^2 daily for five days plus streptozotocin 500 mg/M^2 daily for five days until maximum response was observed. Using this combined modality approach, Moertel reported a hormonal response rate of 86% with a median duration of response of two years.[220] The toxicity of this approach notwithstanding and pending publication of the Mayo Clinic experience or other confirmatory experience; sequential hepatic artery occlusion and combination chemotherapy may be considered for selective patients with symptomatic metastatic carcinoid refractory to somatostatin therapy.

Gastrinoma Syndrome

The gastrinoma syndrome is characterized by a severe ulcer diathesis and persistent basal gastric acid hypersecretion due to hypergastrinemia (Table XXVI-5-3).

Table XXVI-5-3. Clinical Manifestations Suggestive of Gastrinoma

Multiple upper gastrointestinal ulcers
Peptic ulcers in unusual locations (e.g., post-bulbar)
Ulcers resistant to medical therapy
Frequent and recurrent ulcers after cessation of therapy
Post-operative ulcer recurrence
Basal hyperchlorhydria
Prolonged unexplained diarrhea or steatorrhea
Symptoms of hypercalcemia, renal stones, pituitary tumors
X-ray evidence of increased gastric or duodenal folds
Family history of pituitary, pancreas, or parathyroid tumors, or kidney stones

It has been increasingly recognized that the gastrinoma syndrome can exist in multiple forms: benign sporadic; malignant metastatic; as part of the MEN-I syndrome; and as a G-cell hyperplasia syndrome apart from those rare cases in which acid hypersecretion cannot be ascribed to gastrin.[351,352] From various series, it appears that about 66% of gastrinomas are sporadic.[197] Most sporadic tumors in the pancreas are solitary and have been malignant in about 60–85% of cases. These are usually found in older subjects. Sporadic tumors generally occur in the pancreas although primary tumors may also occur in the body of the stomach, duodenum, and jejunum, and account for up to 23% of tumors found at operation.[197] Less than 40% of these are malignant. Ectopic tumors have also been identified in peripancreatic lymph nodes[95,101,197,299,308,367,374] in the splenic hilum, root of the mesentery, omentum, liver, gallbladder, and in the ovary.[21,197] Solitary tumors in these sites are less likely to be malignant, and the overall cure is higher than that reported for pancreatic tumors.[374] The likelihood of a surgeon finding the tumor in these sites, however, has been less than 50% in the past. There are still difficulties finding tumors in these locations, leading to operative failures,[308,326,367] dictating a need for improved techniques for localization.

About 33% of gastrinomas are associated with the MEN-I syndrome.[68,97,168,183,206,326] The problems attending gastrinoma in the MEN-I syndrome are quite different from those associated with the sporadic variety. If patients with hyperparathyroidism are carefully scrutinized, up to 38% are found to have gastrinomas.[98,168] Whereas 50–60% of MEN-I patients develop gastrinoma, >90% have hyperparathyroidism. Refined testing is indicated to detect the presence of gastrinoma in ulcer patients with hyperparathyroidism.[20] Tumors in the MEN-I syndrome are usually multiple, often small or undetectable, and less frequently (5–7%)[68,97,100,183] malignant. However, most cases are discovered at a younger age than in the sporadic cases and the frequency of malignancy may indeed become considerably higher. The multiplicity of the tumors and their small size may make it difficult to find the specific tumors that are secreting gastrin; and the likelihood of recurrence or persistence after excision militates against laparotomy without first identifying a specific site or sites of origin for the hypergastrinemia.

The G-cell hyperplasia syndrome has been considered by some to be a part of the gastrinoma syndrome, but in general the distinction from a tumor can be made on the basis of equivocal responses to secretin and an exaggerated response to food ingestion, directing attention to the appropriate site of gastrin overproduction.[350] There is seldom a need to pursue localization procedures.

Metastases from gastrinoma are predominantly located in the liver. The presence of gastrinoma in peripancreatic lymph glands should not be taken to indicate incurability.[169,307,308,350,367] Since it does not preclude removal of nodes and the primary tumor for possible cure. Some have advocated resection or a debulking procedure,[169,307,324,374] or even gastrectomy, which has been reported to cause regression of the primary tumor.[101,229] Nonetheless it is of vital importance to identify metastases since the tumor-related mortality can be as high as 79%.[308] High serum levels of gastrin 17 compared to gastrin 34[82,143] may be of value,[82,143] or, if available, measurement of the NH2 to COOH terminal gastrin ratio.[154,251] Elevated circulating hCG subunits strongly favor the presence of metastases.[198] In such cases, curative surgical attempts are unlikely to succeed.

Diagnosis of Gastrinoma Syndrome

The possibility of gastrinoma syndrome should be entertained in all patients with ulcer disease and in those with unexplained secretory diarrhea. Prior to development of the RIA 80% of gastrinoma patients presented with a severe ulcer diathesis, bleeding, intestinal obstruction, or perforation. Two-thirds had had at least one operation! Although this may seem extravagant, it can be calculated that one unnecessary operation costs at least 1,000 gastrin assays. Thus, if the success rate is 1:1000 it should more than compensate for the cost of the assay. Since 1970, only 20% of patients with the Zollinger-Ellison (ZE) syndrome have presented with serious ulcer complications (ulcer diabetes due to gastrinoma) and only one-third have had prior surgery.[78] Today the diagnosis of gastrinoma should be made even without ulcers, based on diarrhea or mild duodenitis.

Before carrying out an extensive work up of hypergastrinemia, however, a careful family history inquiring for features of MEN-I syndrome should be conducted. If positive or suspicious, then in most patients with MEN-I, hypercalcemia has developed before age 30. If present this indicates autosomal dominant inheritance of the MEN-I gene.[189] Measurement of serum calcium corrected for albumin will suffice since esophagogastric duodenoscopy allows the examination of gastric juice for pH and visually identifies superficial ectopic lesions missed by barium studies. A urine testing tape is useful, since in the absence of antisecretory drugs, a pH>3.0 excludes ZE syndrome.

Gastric acid secretory studies should include measurements of volume, and basal and pentagastrin-stimulated acid secretion. The diagnosis is confirmed if: 1) The volume of gastric secretion is large (>10 L/24h). 2) The basal acid output is > 15 mmol/h, or, after vagotomy or gastrectomy, >3 mmol/h. Values in the 10–15 range are borderline and <10 mmol/h excludes ZE syndrome. 3) The ratio of the basal acid output (BAO) to the maximum response to pentagastrin (MAO) is >0.6 since the gastrinoma cells are maximally stimulating acid secretion, and pentagastrin can cause no further rise. Of great importance is the need to stop H_2 blockers, K^+/H^+ ATPase inhibitors, and octreotide at least 24 hours before the study since false-negative results may occur due to iatrogenic inhibition of acid secretion.

Serum gastrin levels are usually >150 pg/ml in ZE patients, except for the small proportion who secrete a biologically active variant not recognized by the antiserum used.[154] Gastrin levels may be raised for other reasons.

On the basis of Table XXVI-5-4, it is apparent that only in conditions in which there is increased acid should ZE be considered. The most sensitive and accurate test remains the secretin stimulation test for gastrin secretion. Secretin $2\mu/kg$ is given intravenously and blood samples for gastrin drawn at 2, 5, 10, 20, and 30 minutes. A rise of >100 pg/ml is strongly suggestive of ZE. No new test has emerged with greater sensitivity or specificity. While false positives do occur they are rare and usually found in hypochlorhydric states.[352] The presence of normal hyperfunctioning antrum can usually be identified by a gastrin response to a meal greater than that to secretin.

Gastrinoma Localization

Tumor localization is needed in order to make the best treatment decisions in individual patients. The sensitivity and specificity of various localization procedures is given in Table XXVI-5-5. Selective angiography achieves visualization of the tumor in a minority of patients,[107,209,361] although it is often useful for the demonstration of hepatic metastases. CT scanning[72] and ultrasound,[72,197] even with the use of contrast, have proven to be of limited value since the density of these tumors is within the limits of the surrounding pancreatic tissue or, as occurs not infrequently, the tumors are below the resolution capacity of the technique. Furthermore, the presence of small tumors in extra-pancreatic sites and even within the body of the liver may go undetected by these means.[307,327,350,367] A technique utilizing intraoperative ultrasound of the exposed pancreas[126,275,296] has been modestly successful, suggesting that this technique may be able to eliminate some of the artifacts created by external ultrasound. Magnetic resonance imaging was greeted with some enthusiasm, but apart from enhanced capacity to visualize blood vessels, it has not generally been superior to previous techniques.[263] On occasion, a combination of techniques may be useful. Although both CT scanning and selective visceral angiography were found effective in identifying nearly all patients with metastatic disease to the liver and in some cases to retroperitoneal lymph nodes, these studies failed to identify primary tumors in more than half of the patients seen with biochemical proof of gastrinoma syndrome. Furthermore, up to 40% of patients explored with negative preoperative imaging studies had negative findings at operation.[308,374]

Table XXVI-5-4.   Causes of Hypergastrinemia

With Increased Acid	With Decreased Acid
Gastrinoma	Atrophic gastritis
G-cell hyperfunction	Pernicious anemia
Gastric outlet obstruction	Vagotomy
Short bowel syndrome	Gastric carcinoma
Retained antrum	Renal disease
Hypercalcemia	Rheumatoid arthritis
Hyperparathyroidism	Vitiligo
MEN-I	Diabetic pseudo ZE syndrome

Table XXVI-5-5.   Success of Tumor Localization in Gastrinoma

Factor	Ultrasound	Infusion	Computed Tomography	Selective Angiography		PTHVS Local	PTHVS Regional
	N*	N*	V#	N*	V#	V#	V#
Sensitivity	21	40	31	60	29	35	94
Specificity	92	100	66	100	100	89	97
Positive predictive value	80	100	83	100	100	—	94
Negative predictive value	40	50	15	60	100	89	—

PTHVS = Percutaneous transhepatic portal, pancreatic, and hepatic venous gastrin sampling
*Data from Norton[237,238]
#Data from Vinik[345,348,350]

The use of percutaneous transhepatic portal, pancreatic, and hepatic venous gastrin sampling (PTHVS) by Ingemansson in 1977[140] and Burcharth in 1979,[48] and subsequently by others,[110,250,350] suggested that this new technique was of value in those gastrinoma syndrome patients without liver metastases or these with a primary gastrinoma that was not detected by conventional imaging methods. Our initial studies were undertaken in 1978.[250,345,350] It soon became apparent that not only was a skilled angiographer imperative but also expert technique, a detailed understanding of the variable venous anatomy, a sound reliable assay method for gastrin, and thoughtful interpretation of the data in each case.[250,345,350] The technique is costly and time consuming.[154] Gradients were determined by simultaneous measurements of gastrin in peripancreatic veins and central arterial samples to avoid the misinterpretations that the rapid changes in secretory rate often associated with gastrinomas can cause. Placement of cannulae, without obstruction of the vessel, and streaming of blood in the portal vessel had to be considered. Awareness of the peculiarities of the peripancreatic venous drainage was a prerequisite to avoid erroneous localization of tumors. Furthermore, hepatic venous sampling was also considered essential to detect occult liver metastases or the rare primary gastrinoma within the liver. In our experience, it has been possible to predict the presence or absence of liver metastases, and in two patients, to identify solitary resectable primary liver gastrinomas. Our results in 46 patients with gastrin hypersecretion indicate that the technique may be uniquely valuable in sporadic or ectopic gastrinomas,[250,345,350] but false negative results have also been reported.[238] The most recent analysis of a 10-year experience supports PTHVS as a useful method to regionalize a tumor. Early results suggested that the technique was of limited value in patients with MEN-I who were much less likely to benefit from localization and excision of the tumor.[183,350] The results are based upon the demonstration of tumors in the pancreas and in ectopic sites. It is clear, however, that the surgeon would have found at least half the tumors without the aid of PTHVS. Our approach has been aggressive: if there has been a gradient (by criteria which differ from those of others), the surgeon has pursued mobilization of the head of the pancreas and duodenotomy. These procedures have not been pursued by many other surgeons because of the relatively benign course of those patients in whom no tumor is found at standard laparotomy.

With the aggressive approach, as many as 30% of patients with sporadic gastrinoma syndrome can be cured by tumor resection. Thus, in appropriate cases, an aggressive approach is distinctly advantageous in the localization and selection of operative treatment. The approach advocated by the NIH group is not to explore the head of the pancreas if localization suggests this to be the area involved and the tumor is not easily identifiable at operation.[55] Forty percent of their patients were reported to have no tumors despite positive venous gastrin gradients. It is likely, based upon the experience of others,[111,183,269,326,350] that the tumors were in the head of the pancreas, peripancreatic lymph nodes, or in the wall of the duodenum. Failure to find a tumor carries a good prognosis and none has died in an 8.5 year follow-up.[183] This must be contrasted with the 29% perioperative morbidity and mortality resulting from explorations of the head of the pancreas reported by some,[97,308,324,327,345] although one group reports 37%.[269] The ultimate answer to the vexing question of whether or not to explore the head of the pancreas will no doubt be determined by longer follow up; the approach will be dictated by the available expertise and experience of those involved.

Treatment of Gastrinoma

The treatment of the gastrinoma syndrome has undergone significant changes since the first case was described in 1955.[374] Until the development of drugs to control the excessive acid production,[70,194,196,207] the purpose of operative intervention was to excise the acid secreting stomach, which was the major cause of morbidity and mortality from massive hemorrhage or perforation. These operations were most frequently done as emergency procedures under adverse conditions and were associated with a significant increase in mortality compared to elective partial or total gastrectomies. It was soon learned that partial gastrectomy with or without vagotomy was usually ineffective and total gastrectomy became the standard operation in patients with an established diagnosis of gastrinoma.[68,197,308,374] As experience was accumulated, it became apparent that about 60% of gastrinoma syndrome patients had malignant tumors which, although relatively slow-growing, became the major contributing factor to mortality after longer follow-up.[197] Occasional cases were reported, however, in which the syndrome had been cured by tumor excision only, particularly when the primary neoplasm was in the duodenum and no metastases were found in either lymph nodes or the liver.[111,211,247,308,327] In most of these cases, a total gastrectomy was also done because the surgeon was rightfully concerned that occult metastases might be present and remain a cause of continued hypersecretion of gastrin. Most authorities now recommend a combined medical and surgical approach to the management of these tumors. If patients with MEN-I syndrome are excluded, the cure rate for excision of a gastrinoma is around 14%.[14,69,98,183,309,325,367] These studies did not, however, define the nature of the primary disease. When only extrapancreatic tumors are examined, as many as 50% may be cured by excision of the tumor,[111,197,308,367] especially those in the duodenum. Even excision of tumors in lymph nodes may result in cure.[14,111,327] For the most part, unfortunately, various reports have grouped their patients together and have not identified the subgroups defined above.

The current treatment of the MEN-I patient with gastrinoma remains controversial.[68,206,339] The total number of patients with the MEN-I syndrome and gastrinoma syndrome who have been carefully evaluated for possible palliative or curative pancreatic operations based on selective venous sampling has been so limited that a definitive statement about optimal management cannot be made at the present time. In MEN-I patients with gastrinoma syndrome, both the functional (hypergastrinemia) and malignant potential of the disease should be considered in the individual case. When there is no evidence of metastatic disease and venous sampling demonstrates an anatomically localized source of gastrin, enucleation (pancreatic head) or resection (body or tail) may offer excellent palliation, if not cure. The low incidence of malignancy in the MEN-I patients should not dictate a more cavalier approach than in sporadic cases without evidence of MEN-I.

Accurate estimates for chemotherapeutic activity in metastatic gastrinoma are difficult to ascertain since most published series have studied chemotherapy for all histological subtypes of pancreatic endocrine cancers pooled together. With respect to single agent chemotherapy, streptozotocin is probably the most active antineoplastic drug in patients with metastatic gastrinomas.[42,99,223,224] From his review, Maton has suggested that the drug appears to cause an objective response rate of 50% in patients with this disease. There is no evidence for improved outcomes when streptozotocin is used in combination with 5-fluorouracil plus or minus doxorubicin.[193,359] Inconsistencies in the reported dose and schedule of administration of streptozotocin and in the criteria used for reported objective tumor responses preclude reliable recommendations for chemotherapy with this agent in patients with metastatic gastrinoma. Among six patients with advanced gastrinoma that received dacarbazine, none had an objective response.[6,193]

Similarly, there is little experience in the use of adjuvant chemotherapy following surgical resection. In one report of four patients who underwent complete resection of locally advanced gastrinoma followed by chemotherapy with streptozotocin, doxorubicin, and 5-fluorouracil, two patients remained free of disease at 14 and 32 month follow-up evaluations.[241] The small number of patients and the relatively short follow-up period is insufficient to recommend that this approach be generally adopted, although it may be appropriate to consider for selected patients.

As discussed below for other pancreatic endocrine tumors, there appears to be a role for interferon in management,[246] although the number of reported patients with gastrinoma treated with interferon is too few to reach any firm conclusions regarding its effectiveness in this specific disease.

Insulinomas

A firmly established diagnosis of an insulin secreting lesion of the pancreas is essential to successful management. It is, therefore, of critical importance to rule out other causes of hypoglycemia associated with fasting.[85] A detailed differential diagnosis may be found in Table XXVI-5-6. Non-islet cell neoplasms associated with hypoglycemia are given in Table XXVI-5-7.

An accurate diagnosis of organic hyperinsulinism can be established with near certainty in all cases.[85] The specific causes of hyperinsulinism, given in Table XXVI-5-7, can usually be made before exploration. There are syndromes of autoimmunity which may lead to hypoglycemia which must be considered.

Antireceptor Antibodies. They usually occur in the presence of other autoimmune disease, with antireceptor antibodies mimicking the effect of insulin and reducing insulin clearance. Therefore, insulin levels may be normal or high, but C-peptide levels are low because islet cells are suppressed. Titres fall with time leading to remission, although corticosteroids have been used.

Autoimmune Hypoglycemic Disease Syndrome. This usually occurs in the presence of other autoimmune disorders (i.e., Grave's disease, rheumatoid arthritis, lupus), and generally produces reactive hypoglycemia due to prolon-

Table XXVI-5-6. Classification of Hypoglycemia

Fasting Hypoglycemia
  Hyperinsulinemia
    Islet Cell Adenoma, Carcinoma, Hyperplasia, Nesidioblastosis
  Autoimmune with Insulin Antibodies
  Counterregulatory Hormone Deficiency
    Anterior Pituitary Insufficiency—GH, ACTH
    Adrenocortical Insufficiency
    Hypothyroidism (severe)
  Large Non-Islet Tumor
  Impaired Hepatic Function
    Hepatocellular insufficiency
    Ethanol/malnutrition
    Sepsis
    Specific enzymatic defects (childhood)
  Impaired Renal Function
  Substrate Deficiency
    Fanconi syndrome (renal loss)
    Nursing
    Severe inanition
    Severe exercise
  Drug Induced
Reactive Hypoglycemia
  Alimentary
  "Pre"-diabetes
  Endocrine
  Idiopathic
Factitious
  Surreptitious Insulin Administration
  Surreptitious Sulfonylurea Administration
  Leukemoid Reaction/Polycythemia

Table XXVI-5-7. Non-islet Cell Neoplasms Associated with Hypoglycemia

Mesenchymal
  Mesothelioma
  Fibrosarcoma
  Rhabdomyosarcoma
  Leiomyosarcoma
  Hemangiopericytoma
Carcinoma
  Hepatic: hepatoma, biliary carcinoma
  Adrenocortical carcinoma
  Genitourinary: hypernephroma, Wilms', prostate
  Reproductive: cervical or breast carcinoma
Neurologic/neuroendocrine
  Pheochromocytoma
  Carcinoid
  Neurofibroma
Hematologic
  Leukemia
  Lymphoma
  Myeloma

gation of half-life of circulating insulin. Insulin levels are generally extremely elevated, often due to interference of antibodies with the particular insulin assay. Glucose tolerance testing reveals that plasma glucose is elevated early and reduced late due to the buffering effect of antibodies on the action of secreted insulin. The disease is usually self-limited, and may be precipitated in some patients by exposure to drugs containing sulfhydryl groups that react with SH groups on insulin and render it immunogenic.

The standard test used currently is a 72-hour fast while the patient is closely observed.[76,85] More than 95% of cases can be diagnosed on the basis of responses to a 72-hour fast. The normal maximal increment is 74 ± 7 μU/ml, whereas in single adenomas the rise is only 17 ± 6, in nesidioblastosis 10, and in two patients with multiple B cell adenomas and hyperplasia, 214 and 497. Serial glucose and insulin levels are obtained over the 72 hours until the patient becomes symptomatic. Because the absolute insulin level is not elevated in all patients with insulinomas, a normal level does not rule out the disease. However, a fasting insulin level greater than 24 μU/ml is found in about 50% of patients with insulinoma. This is strong evidence in favor of the diagnosis. Values of insulin greater than 7μU/ml after a more prolonged fast, in the presence of a blood glucose less than 40 mg/dl, are also highly suggestive. A refinement in the interpretation of glucose and insulin levels has been established by determining the ratio of insulin levels in μU/ml to the concomitant glucose level in mg/dl. An insulin/glucose ratio of greater than 0.3 has been found in virtually all patients proven to have an insulinoma or other islet cell disease causing organic hyperinsulinism. The accuracy of the test can be increased by calculating the amended insulin/glucose-ratio as follows:
Amended ratio = insulin (μU/ml)/glucose (mg/dl) − 30.

If the value is > 50, then organic hyperinsulinism is certain.[85] Measurements of proinsulin and C-peptide have also proven to be valuable in patients suspected of having organic hypoglycemia.[98] Normally the circulating proinsulin concentration accounts for less than 22% of the insulin immunoreactivity but is greater than 24% in more than 90% of indi-

viduals with insulinomas. Furthermore, when the proinsulin level is greater than 40%, a malignant islet cell tumor should be strongly suspected.[85,323,324] The C-peptide level is useful in ruling out factitious hypoglycemia due to self-administration of insulin. Commercial insulin preparations contain no C-peptide and low levels, combined with high insulin levels, confirms the diagnosis of self-administration of insulin. Patients who take sulfonylureas surreptitiously may have raised insulin and C-peptide values soon after ingestion, but chronic use will result in hypoglycemia without raised insulin or C-peptide levels. Only an index of suspicion and measurement of urine sulfonylureas will lead to the correct diagnosis. A variety of insulin stimulation and suppression tests were once used when precise and accurate insulin measurements were not available. Each had its limitations and all are currently considered obsolete.[85,352] The insulin response to secretin stimulation (2 u/kg IV - peak response in 1–5 min) is a valuable measure to differentiate multiple adenomas from nesidioblastosis and single adenomas.[108] Patients with single adenomas and nesidioblastosis do not respond to secretin whereas those with multiple adenomas or hyperplasia have an excessive insulin response to the administration of secretin.

Localization

Once the diagnosis of suspected hyperinsulinism is confirmed, every effort should be made to localize the source of excessive insulin production. Preoperative localization is important because approximately 30% of insulinomas are <1 cm in diameter, 10% are multiple, 10–15% are malignant, and 10% will have either islet cell hyperplasia or nesidioblastosis and no tumor at all.[76,85,111,145,175,215,310,311,350,352] Because of their small size, the techniques most commonly used to demonstrate tumors in the upper abdomen including ultrasound, computerized tomography, magnetic resonance imaging, contrast studies of the upper gastrointestinal tract, and endoscopic retrograde pancreatography are of little value. Until the past decade, the only study considered of proven value in the localization of insulinomas was selective pancreatic angiography.[76,145,268,310] Highly selective injections of contrast, subtraction procedures and magnification increase the number of insulinomas identified by this technique. In one large series, 90% of insulinomas were reported to be localized by angiography alone.[76] However, most groups report less satisfactory results.[268] In a summary of all reports in the literature, only about 60% of insulinomas have been detected by this method.[350]

Percutaneous transhepatic venous sampling (PTHVS) of insulin from pancreatic veins has been utilized, successfully localizing occult sources of hyperinsulinism.[56,139,145,147,353] We now believe that the combination of a secretin test with PTHVS provides the best means of establishing the specific cause of organic hyperinsulinism with near certainty. A skilled angiographer and careful analysis of the hormonal data in relationship to the venous anatomy in the individual case is required.

If PTHVS is not available and preoperative localization by angiography or other techniques has been negative, the surgeon may utilize intraoperative ultrasonography if a careful exploration fails to detect a tumor. Some who have utilized this technique routinely, have reported excellent results.

Ultrasonography does not identify hyperplasia or nesidio-blastosis, however, and appears to be operator dependent in its sensitivity.

Treatment of Islet B-Cell Disease with Hyperinsulinism

The treatment of pancreatic islet beta cell disease is usually surgical; in the great majority of cases it provides a complete cure. It should be performed only when the diagnosis is certain and only by a surgeon skilled in pancreatic surgery. When hypoglycemia can be controlled with diet alone, or with small, well-tolerated doses of diazoxide, and/or when the medical condition of the patient may increase the hazard of surgery sufficiently, medical management alone may be considered. Patients with diffuse hyperinsulinism for whom an operation is planned should first have a trial of treatment with diazoxide and a natriuretic benzothiadiazine. Medical treatment is required for the great majority of malignant insulinomas, since only occasionally are they cured by operation. Medical treatment for benign insulinomas is a change in meals to include "lente carbohydrate" or unrefined carbohydrate given as frequently as required to prevent hypoglycemia. Antihormonal therapy may be useful if diet is insufficient. The management of malignant insulinoma is antihormonal and anti-tumor therapy.

Medical Management of Benign Disease

Diet. The cornerstone of medical management of insulinoma and other forms of hyperinsulinism is the diet. Not uncommonly, patients may avoid symptoms of hypoglycemia for variable periods of time by spacing feedings so as to shorten the number of hours between feedings. For some the inclusion of a bedtime (11:00 p.m.) feeding is sufficient; for others a midmorning, midafternoon and/or a 3:00 a.m. snack are necessary. Even though the tumor may be stimulated occasionally to secrete insulin by the ingestion of carbohydrates, it is inadvisable to restrict the intake of carbohydrate. More slowly absorbable forms of carbohydrates (starches, bread, potatoes, and rice) are generally preferred. During hypoglycemic episodes, rapidly absorbable forms (fruit juices with added glucose or sucrose) are indicated.

In patients with severe refractory hypoglycemia the use of a continuous intravenous infusion of glucose, coupled with increased dietary intake of carbohydrate, frequently alleviates hypoglycemia long enough to institute additional therapy.

Diazoxide and Natriuretic Benzothiadiazines. Diazoxide, marketed as Proglycem®, owes its potent hyperglycemic properties to two effects.[83,84] It directly inhibits the release of insulin by B cells, through stimulation of α-adrenergic receptors, and it has an extrapancreatic hyperglycemic effect probably by inhibiting cyclic AMP phosphodiesterase, resulting in higher plasma levels of cyclic AMP and enhanced glycogenolysis. Because diazoxide induces the retention of sodium, edema is troublesome at higher dosages. The addition of a diuretic benzothiadiazine, e.g., trichlormethiazide, not only corrects or prevents edema but synergizes the hyperglycemic effect of diazoxide. At the doses needed to counteract the higher doses of diazoxide (e.g., 450–600 mg per day), natriuretic benzothiadiazines frequently induce hypokalemia. Nausea is an additional complication of higher dosages of diazoxide, and hypertrichosis may complicate long-term treatment. These compounds have been useful to elevate blood levels of glucose into the euglycemic range if operation must be delayed for weeks or months. Patients with benign insulinomas have been successfully managed for up to 16 years with diazoxide in doses of 150–450 mg/day in combination with trichlormethiazide in doses of 2–8 mg/day. If they can be tolerated, higher doses may be used in patients with malignant insulinomas.

Calcium-Channel Blockers. Calcium channel blockers theoretically are capable of inhibiting insulin secretion. Verapamil has been used successfully to alleviate the hypoglycemia caused by an insulin-secreting pancreatic tumor in a 94-year old woman.[335] Verapamil and diltiazem have been used with variable results in other patients with organic hyperinsulinism.

Propranolol. β-adrenergic receptor blocking drugs inhibit insulin secretion and may therefore be of value in treating organic hyperinsulin. Only a few reports of the use of propranolol have appeared.[36,233,287] Its use has been associated with the reduction of plasma insulin levels and with the relief of hypoglycemic attacks in patients with benign or malignant insulinoma. In a patient with a benign insulinoma, 80 mg of propranolol a day was sufficient, while a patient with malignant insulinoma in whom streptozotocin was no longer effective, 640 mg of propranolol orally per day was required.[287] Because, however, these changes can mask the adrenergic symptoms of hyperglycemia and inhibit muscle glycogenolysis, there is risk of aggravating the clinical syndrome. The drug should be used with extreme caution and careful monitoring.

Dilantin. The anticonvulsive diphenylhydantoin has been shown to inhibit the in vitro release of insulin from both the labile and storage B-cell pools. It has been used successfully to control refractory hypoglycemia as evidenced by normal overnight fasting glucose levels and absence of hypoglycemia during total fasting for up to 24 hours.[43,135] However, in only one-third or less of patients with benign insulinoma is the hyperglycemic effect of dilantin of any clinical significance. Furthermore, with the dosage required, ataxia, nystagmus, hypertrophic gums and megaloblastic anemia may be side effects. Maintenance doses of dilantin range from 300–600 mg/day. The concurrent administration of diazoxide lowers measurable blood levels of dilantin, and their concurrent use is not recommended.

Long-Acting Somatostatin Analogue. We initially reported the successful use of octreotide (Sandostatin®) in prolonging the ability to fast in a patient with a benign insulinoma,[332] and a similar experience was reported by Osei and colleagues in a patient with a malignant tumor.[248] Our more recent experience has shown a variety of responses not easily predictable by the clinical or biochemical profile. We have examined the effects of a long-acting octreotide analogue, in seven patients with endogenous hyperinsulinism, five with proven single adenomas, one with multiple adenomas, and one with organic hyperinsulinism associated with MEN-I.[310] In two patients, and possibly a third, octreotide prolonged the ability to fast without hypoglycemia with variable decreases in plasma insulin concentrations. A trial of long-term administration of octreotide in one of these patients gave only short-term relief of hypoglycemia. Octreotide did not improve or actually worsened plasma glucose levels on fasting in the other four patients. In contrast, oral administration of diazoxide to four of these patients was effective in raising plasma glucose. A child treated for nesidioblastosis did well initially but subsequently required pancreatectomy and also grew at only the 3rd percentile. It is unlikely that octreotide will be a useful addition to the therapeutic armamentarium for treatment of organic hyperinsulinism.

Glucocorticoids. The use of glucocorticoids, which increase gluconeogenesis and cause insulin resistance, can also help stabilize blood glucose at an acceptable level. Pharmacologic doses (approximately 1 mg/kg prednisone) must be used.

Glucagon. Glucagon may help raise blood glucose concentrations but may simultaneously directly stimulate the release of insulin.

Vasoactive Intestinal Peptide Tumor (VIPoma)

In 1958, Verner and Morrison first described refractory watery diarrhea and hypokalemia associated with non insulin-secreting tumors of the pancreatic islets.[341] The absence of gastric hypersecretion and even achlorhydria were documented in patients with this tumor syndrome,[230,262,341] later termed "pancreatic cholera" because the observed severe diarrhea resembled Vibrio cholera disease.[195] The acronym WDHA (watery diarrhea (100%), hypokalemia (100%), achlorhydria)[186] was proposed, although a more appropriate acronym might be WDHHA for watery diarrhea hypokalemia, hypochlorhydria, and acidosis, because of bicarbonate wasting. Several series have been reported which have confirmed the association between certain pancreatic tumors and watery diarrhea syndrome.[36,156,340]

In a review of 55 patients with the diarrhea and hypokalemia syndrome, other features were sometimes observed: alkalosis in mild cases but acidosis in severe diarrhea from bicarbonate wasting, flushing, hypercalcemia, tetany (perhaps from magnesium depletion), abnormal glucose tolerance, and dilation of the gallbladder.[340] The most prominent symptom in most patients is profuse cholera-like diarrhea, often present for three or four years prior to diagnosis, with volumes usually exceeding 6 to 8L of stool/24 hours. The stools have the appearance of dilute tea and are rich in electrolytes, with an average secretion of 300 mmol of potassium/24 hours. The diarrhea is always secretory in nature, will not disappear with fasting for 48 hours and demonstrates an increased net secretion of electrolytes in the stool. This symptom may be confused with the diarrhea found in the ZE syndrome. The distinguishing features are shown in Table XXVI-5-8.

Diarrhea which is not secretory is always due to causes other than endocrine tumors. Laxative abuse may be very difficult to exclude, however, and the measurement of stool electrolytes and osmolarity may be required. Stool electrolytes should account for the osmolarity if the condition is due to an endocrine tumor. An osmolarity that exceeds that expected from the concentration of electrolytes invariably reflects laxative abuse which must be carefully excluded.

The episodic and fulminating, secretory diarrhea associated with VIPomas results in profound hypokalemia, hypochlorhydria (rarely achlorhydria), bicarbonate wasting, and hyperchloremic metabolic acidosis. The more commonly observed hypochlorhydria is due to the direct gastric acid inhibitory effect of VIP, a biologic property shared with other members of the secretin-glucagon family: secretin, glucagon, gastric inhibitory peptide (GIP), and poly-peptide histidine and isoleucine (PPHI).[318] In the early stage of tumor growth the predominant symptoms of diarrhea are episodic and intermittent. It is generally accepted that, as the VIP tumor enlarges, the diarrhea becomes continuous and the ensuing electrolyte abnormalities life threatening.[36,156] Increased intestinal motility, as well as secretion, may contribute to the diarrhea.[305]

The clinical features of VIPomas are consistent with the known actions of VIP which include: stimulation of intestinal secretion, facial flushing, inhibition of gastric acid secretion, stimulation of glycogenolysis, and hypercalcemia.[13,34,35,112,156,265,277,340] The structural homology between VIP and secretin, glucagon, gastric inhibitory polypeptide (GIP) and peptide histidine and isoleucine (PHI)[265] may account for enhanced secretion of pancreatic juice and inhibition of gastric acid secretion. VIP has also been reported to cause gallbladder relaxation; a large distended gallbladder is often found in patients with the VIPoma syndrome. Hypercalcemia has been noted in nearly 50% of patients with the syndrome. The cause is not clear but may be related to dehydration, electrolyte disturbances secondary to diarrhea, to coincidental multiple endocrine neoplasia accompanied by hyperparathyroidism, or the secretion by the tumor of a calcitrophic peptide. Tetany has been reported in several patients and may be due to hypomagnesemia secondary to the diarrhea. Nearly 8% of patients demonstrate facial flushing. The cause of this patchy erythematous and sometimes urticarial flushing is not clear but has been attributed to VIP or prostaglandins which may be present in the tumor.

The hyperglycemia often noted in patients with the watery diarrhea syndrome is probably secondary to the profound glycogenolytic effect of high portal vein VIP on the liver.[112]

Sites of Tumors Secreting VIP. Tumors secreting vasoactive intestinal peptides usually originate usually in the pancreas or along the sympathetic chain. In a series of 62 patients, 52 patients (84%) had pancreatic tumors, and 10 patients had ganglioneuroblastomas.[177]

Of the ten patients with ganglioneuroblastomas, seven were children. There have been 18 other case reports of elevated plasma levels of VIP which have been associated with neurogenic tumors including: ganglioneuroblastoma, ganglioneuromas, neurofibroma, and pheochromocytoma.[29,53,74,138,146,160,216,328,329,373] The majority of neurogenic tumors associated with the VIPoma syndrome have been found in children. Catecholamines are frequently elevated. In patients with excess catecholamine secretion, flushing, increased sweating and hypertension may occur. Hyperglycemia and hypercalcemia have not been noted in children. Plasma levels of PP are normal and have not been detected in VIP-producing ganglioneuroblastomas. Thus, it was hoped that PP levels would distinguish pancreatic and non-pancreatic sources of VIP. However, three adults with neuro-

Table XXVI-5-8.   Differentiation of Gastrinoma and WDHHA* Syndrome

Feature	Gastrinoma	WDHHA*
Diarrhea	Acid	Alkaline (HCO_3 loss)
Gastric acid	Increased	Decreased
Gastric volume	Increased	Normal or decreased
Nasogastric suction	Diarrhea improves	Diarrhea unchanged
Motility	Increased[a]	Increased slightly[b]
Abdominal pain	Marked	Rare (initially)
Stool K+ loss	Slight	Marked
Metabolic acidosis	No (alkalosis with gastric suction)	Yes
Lesion-location	Primary pancreas (also liver, wall of stomach, and duodenum)	Primary pancreas Ganglioneuroblastoma
Mediator	Gastrin	VIP/other

*Watery diarrhea, hypokalemia, achlorhydria, and acidosis
[a]Motility enhanced secondary to gastric acid stimulation
[b]Motility may be slightly increased secondary to direct effects of either intraarterial or intraluminal VIP

genic tumors and a 64-year-old woman with a VIPoma of the lower left kidney had high serum levels of PP.[123] Excessive quantities of immunoreactive VIP and PP were found in the renal tumor tissue.

Biochemical Diagnosis and Experience. By definition, VIP levels are elevated in all patients with the VIPoma syndrome. False-positive elevations of VIP can be observed in patients with small bowel ischemia or severe low flow states caused by diarrhea and secondary dehydration not associated with VIP-producing tumors.[32,35,218] VIP is, however, not the only agent implicated in the diarrhea syndrome.

Gastrin, secretin, glucagon, enteroglucagon, gastric inhibitory polypeptide, PP, VIP, thyrocalcitonin (TCT), and prostaglandins or any one of a number of combinations have been implicated as possible etiologic agents of the diarrhea syndrome.[219] Bloom reported 1,000 patients with various forms of diarrhea.[32,33,204] Thirty-nine patients (3.9%) had greatly elevated levels of VIP; in each case, a tumor was found. In more than 50% of these patients the tumor was successfully removed, the symptoms remitted, and the plasma levels of VIP returned to normal. Twelve patients had diarrhea secondary to TCT-producing tumors of the thyroid; 13 patients had carcinoma of the lung; four patients had a villous adenoma of the rectum; and 24 patients had carcinoid tumors. All 53 of these patients had normal plasma VIP levels. Eleven additional patients had classic clinical features of the VIPoma syndrome in whom VIP levels were normal and no tumor was found; they were probably secreting an unidentified humoral substance.

Biochemical detection of VIP secreting tumors necessitates a highly sensitive and specific VIP radioimmunoassay. Range of normal VIP concentration is 0–170 pg/ml[54] similar to that (0–190 pg/ml) found by others.[34,74,276]

Information gained from a single plasma VIP level may be misleading. Between periods of watery diarrhea, the VIPoma, unlike many endocrine tumors of the gut (e.g., insulinoma or gastrinoma) may not be actively secreting VIP; thus a normal level creates a false sense of security and may delay a more vigorous search for the cause.

Treatment. In the series of 52 pancreatic cases reported by Long, most of the solitary tumors were 8 cm in diameter or greater.[177] Surgical excision of the primary pancreatic tumor relieved all symptoms in 17 patients (27%).[177] Surgical removal

of a ganglioneuroblastoma was successful in seven of 10 patients.

In patients who have diarrhea in whom no tumor is demonstrable by angiography, CT scan, ultrasound, or PTHVS, steroids have provided some symptomatic relief. A trial of inhibitors of prostaglandin synthesis, e.g., indomethacin, phenothiazines, and lithium may be warranted.[23] Octreotide has been used successfully in managing the diarrhea of VIPoma syndrome as well as diarrhea from the GEP tumors. We do not advocate blind total pancreatectomy. We have seen spontaneous remission of watery diarrhea syndrome without establishing a cause. We have also seen eventual emergence of tumors in unusual sites including the kidney and skin.

In summary, when confronted with severe chronic diarrhea, it must be established that the diarrhea is secretory in nature by fasting the patient for 48 hours and measuring stool volume. If diarrhea persists with fasting, VIP-producing tumors of the pancreas are frequently found, and plasma samples should be analyzed for VIP in these patients. If the VIP level is elevated, a VIP-secreting tumor (VIPoma) should be strongly suspected. In addition, a serum pancreatic polypeptide level should be determined simultaneously. If the tumor is located in the pancreas, this peptide will almost invariably be elevated. In children, catecholamine levels should also be obtained. If VIP levels are normal, screening for other causative agents should be performed including gastrin, substance P, SRIF, PP, TCT, serotonin, glucagon, and prostaglandins of the E series. Tumor localization should include CT scanning, celiac, superior mesenteric, and renal angiography and finally PTHVS. If a tumor is found it should be excised. In the absence of finding a tumor, symptomatic therapy is warranted, not empiric surgery. With malignant tumors, treatment with sandostatin or chemotherapy must be considered, as is discussed below.

Clinical Features of Glucagonoma Syndrome

In 1966, McGavran called attention to a syndrome that included acquired diabetes and glucagon-producing tumors.[200] It only became apparent later that these tumors were usually accompanied by a very characteristic skin rash.[316,366] The main features of the glucagonoma syndrome include a characteristic rash termed necrolytic migratory erythema (NME) (82%), painful glossitis, angular stomatitis, normochromic normocytic anemia (61%), weight loss (90%), mild diabetes mellitus (80%), hypoaminoacidemia, deep vein thrombosis (50%) and depression (50%).

The frequency of islet cell tumors has been estimated in autopsy series to be between 0 and 1.4% of all cases studied. In a very thorough study of 1366 consecutive adult autopsies, Grimelius found a tumor frequency of 0.8%.[118] All of the tumors were adenomas and all contained histochemically defined glucagon cells. None of the tumors had been suspected during life. Although these adenomas contained glucagon it is not known whether they were overproducing or even secreting glucagon. The incidence in vivo is probably 1% of all neuroendocrine tumors.

The necrolytic migratory erythomic (NME) rash of the glucagonoma syndrome has a characteristic distribution. It is usually widespread, but major sites of involvement are the perioral and perigenital regions along with the fingers, legs and feet. It may also occur in areas of cutaneous trauma. The basic process in the skin seems to be one of superficial epidermal necrosis, fragile blister formation, crusting and healing with hyperpigmentation. Skin biopsies usually show small bullae containing acantholytic epidermal cells as well as neutrophils and lymphocytes.[316] The adjacent epidermis is usually intact. The dermis contains a lymphocytic perivascular infiltrate. Different stages of the cutaneous lesions may be present simultaneously. Biopsy examination of a fresh skin lesion may be the most valuable aid in suggesting the diagnosis of the glucagonoma syndrome. Repeated biopsy samples may be necessary, however, to raise this possibility. A painful glossitis manifested by an erythematous, mildly atrophic tongue has been associated with the cutaneous lesions.

Two other features of the syndrome are noteworthy. An alarmingly high rate of thromboembolic complications occurs in patients with glucagonomas and many patients succumb to pulmonary embolism. Unexplained thromboembolic disease should alert one to the possibility of glucagonoma. Depression and other psychiatric disturbances including depression are common, but may relate in part to the chronic dermatosis.[32,151]

Several metabolic disorders are associated with cutaneous lesions closely resembling the necrolytic migratory erythemic (NME) of the glucagonoma syndrome and include acrodermatitis enteropathica, zinc deficiency induced by hyperalimentation, essential fatty acid deficiency, the dermatosis of protein calorie malnutrition of kwashiorkor, and pellagra due to niacin deficiency.[23,137,239,336] Cutaneous manifestations associated with malabsorptive states are often non-specific, affecting approximately 20% of patients with steatorrhea. Improvement in the rash associated with the glucagonoma syndrome has been reported with amino acid repletion as well as with the administration of carbohydrate. The skin rash has also been shown to improve with the administration of zinc.[136] Almost invariably the dermatosis resolves after successful removal of a glucagon-producing tumor, even if the rash has been present for several years.[228,358] In addition, in those patients who do not undergo curative

resection but are treated with chemotherapeutic agents, the dermatitis improves as glucagon levels decrease.[178,190,358]

Glucose intolerance in the glucagonoma syndrome may be related to tumor size. Fasting plasma glucagon levels tend to be higher in patients with large hepatic metastases than in persons without hepatic metastases.[228] All patients with large hepatic metastases had glucose intolerance. Massive hepatic metastases may decrease the ability of the liver to metabolize splanchnic glucagon, increasing peripheral plasma glucagon levels; but glucagon may not directly induce hyperglycemia unless metabolism of glucose by the liver is directly compromised. Another factor may be the variation in the molecular species of glucagon present in each case and its biological potency.[59]

In previously reported cases of glucagonoma in which plasma glucagon concentrations were measured by radioimmunoassay, fasting plasma glucagon concentrations were 2,100 ± 334 pg/ml. These levels are markedly higher than those reported in normal, fasting subjects (less than 150 pg/ml), or in patients with other disorders causing hyperglucagonemia including diabetes mellitus, burn injury, acute trauma, bacteremia, cirrhosis, renal failure, or Cushing's syndrome where fasting plasma glucagon concentrations are often elevated but less than 500 pg/ml.

Glucagonomas, as other islet cell neoplasms, may overproduce multiple hormones. Insulin is the most common second hormone secreted by these tumors. ACTH, pancreatic polypeptide, parathyroid hormone or substances with parathyroid hormone-like activity, gastrin, serotonin, VIP and MSH in that order of frequency.

Treatment of Glucagonomas. All reported glucagonomas with the cutaneous syndrome originated from single pancreatic tumors of considerable size (diameter 1.5–35 cm).[137,375] All tumors occurred in the tail or body of the pancreas where A cells are normally abundant deriving from the dorsal anlage of the pancreas. At the time of diagnosis, 62% of the tumors had metastases. Glucagonomas not associated with the syndrome, but characterized by morphologic and/or chemical criteria, are diagnosed in various ways. First, the tumor may appear as a malignant pancreatic tumor, discovered due to local growth, with or without metastases. Second, the tumor may be associated with an insulinoma or gastrinoma or as part of the MEN I syndrome. Glucagonoma may also occur as a single microadenoma found incidentally at autopsy in elderly patients.[151]

If the diagnosis is made while the tumor is still localized, surgical resection can be curative.[130,336,342] As in other islet cell tumors, even when malignant these tumors tend to be extremely slow growing. Effective treatment with chemotherapeutic agents is discussed below. Surgical debulking of glucagonoma tumors has also been shown to be beneficial.[228]

Somatostatinoma

Somatostatin (somatotropin release inhibiting factor–SRIF) is a tetradecapeptide that inhibits numerous endocrine and exocrine secretory functions. Almost all gut hormones studied are inhibited by SRIF, including insulin, PP, glucagon, gastrin, secretin, GIP, and motilin.[337] In addition to the inhibition of the endocrine secretions, SRIF has direct effects on a number of target organs.[61] For example, it is a potent inhibitor of basal and pentagastrin-stimulated gastric acid secretion. It also has marked effects on gastrointestinal transit time, intestinal motility, and the absorption of nutrients from the small intestine. The major effect in the small intestine appears to be a delay in the absorption of fat and reduced absorption of calcium.

The salient features of the somatostatinoma syndrome are diabetes, diarrhea/steatorrhea, gallbladder disease, hypochlorhydria, and weight loss.[104,157,172] The first cases of the somatostatinoma syndrome were reported in 1977 by Ganda and coworkers.[104] We have examined the cases reported since 1977 and describe here the features now recognized to be a part of the syndrome. For convenience, we have divided the cases into those arising from the pancreas, the intestine, and extrapancreatic tumors. It appears that the syndrome differs among tumors arising from the pancreas and the intestine or extrapancreatic sites. These will therefore be considered separately.

Clinical Features of Somatostatinoma Syndrome

Most patients were between 40 and 60 years of age. There is a 2:1 ratio of female to male patients, which contrasts with the equal sex incidence for other islet cell tumors.[60]

Plasma Somatostatin Like Immunoreactivity (SLI). The mean SLI concentration in patients with pancreatic somatostatinoma was 50 times higher than normal (range 1–250 times). Intestinal somatostatinomas, however, had only slightly elevated or normal SLI concentrations.

Diabetes Mellitus and Hypoglycemia

Seventy five percent of the patients with pancreatic tumors had diabetes mellitus. In contrast, diabetes only occurred in 11% of the patients with intestinal tumors. In all instances, the diabetes was relatively mild and could be controlled with diet and/or oral hypoglycemic agents or with small doses of insulin. It is not clear, however, whether differential inhibition of insulin and diabetogenic hormones can explain the usually mild degree of diabetes and the rarity of ketoacidosis in patients with somatostatinoma. Replacement of functional islet cell tissue by pancreatic tumor may be another reason for the development of diabetes in the majority of patients with pancreatic somatostatinoma contrasting with the low incidence in patients with intestinal tumors. These tumors are usually large and therefore, destroy substantial portions of the pancreas.

Gallbladder Disease. Fifty nine percent of the patients with pancreatic tumors and twenty seven percent of the patients with intestinal tumors had gallbladder disease. The high incidence of gallbladder disease in patients with somatostatinoma and the absence of such an association in any other islet cell tumors suggests a causal relationship between gallbladder disease and somatostatinoma. Infusion of somatostatin into normal human subjects has been shown to inhibit gallbladder emptying,[61,92] suggesting that somatostatin mediated inhibition of gallbladder emptying may be the cause for the observed high rate of gallbladder disease in patients with somatostatinoma. This thesis is supported by the observation of massively dilated gallbladders without stones or other pathology[12,253] in patients with somatostatin secreting tumors.

Diarrhea and Steatorrhea. Diarrhea consisting of 3–10 frequently foul smelling stools per day and/or steatorrhea from 20–76 g of fat per 24 hours is common with pancreatic somatastatinoma patients. This could be due to the effects of high levels of somatostatin within the pancreas, serving as a paracrine mediator to inhibit exocrine secretion, or alternatively by the somatostatinoma's causing duct obstruction. In some cases, the severity of diarrhea and steatorrhea parallels the course of the disease, worsening as the tumor advances and the metastatic disease spreads, improving after tumor resection. Somatostatin has been shown to inhibit pancreatic secretion of proteolytic enzymes, water, bicarbonate,[37] and gallbladder motility.[62] In addition, it inhibits absorption of lipids.[288] All but one patient with diarrhea and steatorrhea have had high plasma somatostatin concentrations. The rarity of diarrhea and/or steatorrhea in patients with intestinal somatostatinomas may be due to the lower SLI levels.

Hypochlorhydria. Infusion of somatostatin has been shown to inhibit gastric acid secretion in human subjects.[31] Thus, hypochlorhydria in patients with somatostatinoma in the absence of gastric mucosal abnormalities is likely to be the result of elevated somatostatin concentrations. Basal and stimulated acid secretion was inhibited in 87% of patients with pancreatic tumors tested and in only 12% of patients who had intestinal tumors.

Weight Loss. Weight loss ranging from 9–21 kg over several months occurred in one-third of patients with pancreatic tumors and one-fifth of patients with intestinal tumors. The weight loss may be related to malabsorption and diarrhea, but in small intestinal tumors, anorexia, abdominal pain and yet unexplained reasons may be relevant.

Associated Endocrine Disorders. Of great interest is the presence of cafe au lait spots, neurofibromatosis and paroxysmal hypertension in patients with intestinal tumors. Thus, approximately half of all patients have other endocrinopathies in addition to their somatostatinoma. Occurrence of multiple endocrine tumors (MEN, type 1) has been recognized in patients with islet cell tumors, and MEN 2 or 3 syndromes are present in association with pheochromocytomas and neurofibromatosis, respectively. It seems that an additional dimension of the duct associated tumors is multiple endocrine neoplasia Type 2. Secretion of different hormones by the same islet cell tumor, sometimes resulting in two distinct clinical disorders, is now being recognized with increasing frequency.[349] These possibilities should be considered during endocrine workups of patients with islet cell tumors and their relatives.

Tumor Location

Of the reported primary tumors, 60% were found in the pancreas and 40% in the duodenum or jejunum. Of the pancreatic tumors, one-half were located in the head, one-fourth in the tail, and the remaining tumors infiltrated the whole pancreas or were found in the body. Of extrapancreatic locations, approximately half originate in the duodenum, approximately half originate in the ampulla, and rarely one is found in the jejunum. Thus, about 60% of somatostatinomas originate in the upper intestinal tract, probably a consequence of the relatively large number of D cells present in this region.

Tumor Size

Somatostatinomas tend to be large, similar to glucagonomas,[22] but unlike insulinomas and gastrinomas, which are small as a rule.[142,346] Within the intestine the tumors have tended to be smaller. The symptoms associated with somatostatinomas and glucagonomas are less pronounced and probably do not develop until very high blood levels of the respective hormones have been attained. As a result, somatostatinomas and glucagonomas are likely to be diagnosed later.

Incidence of Malignancy

Eighty percent of patients with pancreatic somatostatinomas are metastatic at time of diagnosis and one-half with intestinal tumors had evidence of metastatic disease. Metastasis to the liver is most frequent and regional lymph node involvement and metastases to bone less so. Thus, in approximately 70% of the cases, metastatic disease is present at the time of diagnosis. This is similar to the high incidence of malignancy in glucagonoma[22] and in gastrinoma,[142] but it is distinctly different from the low incidence of malignant insulinoma.[346] The high prevalence of metastatic disease in somatostatinoma may also be a consequence of late diagnosis, but is apparently not dependent upon the tissue of origin.

Microscopic Appearance

On light microscopy, most tumors appear as well differentiated islet cell or carcinoid type tumors. Some show a mixed picture consisting of separate zones of differentiated and anaplastic cells. In the differentiated areas, cells are arranged in lobular or acinar patterns separated by fibrovascular stroma. Less well differentiated areas consist of sheets of cells interrupted by fibrous septa.

Diffuse positive immunoreactivity for somatostatin is usually found, in contrast to the rarity of somatostatin positive cells in gastrinomas and other tumors. There is a unique occurrence of psammoma bodies in somatostatinomas localized within the duodenum. In addition, there is abundant immunological evidence for the presence of cells containing insulin, calcitonin, gastrin and VIP, ACTH, PGE_2 and substance P. In the tumors with multiple hormones, however, SLI (somatostatin-like immunoreactivity) containing cells represent the large majority of all cells containing hormones detected by immunopathology.

Somatostatin-Containing Tumors Outside the GI Tract

Somatostatin has been found in many tissues outside the GI tract. Prominent among those are the hypothalamic and extrahypothalamic regions of the brain, the peripheral nervous system including the sympathetic adrenergic ganglia, and the C cells of the thyroid gland. Not surprisingly, therefore, high concentrations of somatostatin have been found in tumors originating from these tissues. Sano and Saito reported 7 patients with medullary carcinoma of the thyroid (MTC) who had high basal plasma SLI concentrations and high tumor SLI concentrations.[278,281] Roos reported elevated plasma SLI concentrations in 3 of 7 patients with MTC and high tissue SLI concentrations in 3 of 5 MTC tumors.[270] Some but not all of these patients exhibited the clinical somatostatinoma syndrome.

Elevated plasma SLI concentrations have also been reported in patients with small cell lung cancer.[270] One case of metastatic bronchial oat cell carcinoma caused Cushing's syndrome, diabetes, diarrhea, steatorrhea, anemia and weight loss, and had a plasma SLI concentration 20 times greater than normal.[106] We reported a patient with a bronchogenic carcinoma presenting with diabetic ketoacidosis and high levels of SLI (>5,000 pg/ml).[141] Pheochromocytomas[17,349] and catecholamine producing extra-adrenal paragangliomas[270] are other examples of endocrine tumors producing and secreting somatostatin in addition to other hormonally active substances. One-fourth of 37 patients with pheochromocytomas had elevated SLI levels.[349]

Diagnosis

In the reported series cited, somatostatinomas were often found more or less accidentally. In the majority of cases, the tumors were found either during exploratory laparotomy or during upper gastrointestinal x-ray studies, CT scans, or ultrasound or endoscopic studies performed because of various symptoms including unexplained abdominal pain, melena, hematemesis, persistent diarrhea, or in search of insulinomas or ACTH secreting tumors. Once found, the tumors were identified as somatostatinoma by demonstration of elevated tissue concentrations of SLI and/or prevalence of D cells by immunocytochemistry or by the demonstration of elevated plasma SLI concentrations. Thus, the events leading to the diagnosis of somatostatinoma usually occur in reverse order. In other islet cell tumors, the clinical symptoms and signs usually suggest the diagnosis which is then established by the demonstration of diagnostically elevated blood hormone levels following which efforts are undertaken to localize the tumors. It can be expected that the same sequence of diagnostic procedures will be followed in the future for the diagnosis of somatostatinoma mainly for two reasons: 1) the increasing familiarity of physicians with the clinical somatostatinoma syndrome. This symptom complex, while not pathognomonic, is nevertheless, sufficiently characteristic of somatostatinoma to suggest the correct diagnosis. 2) The greater availability of reliable radioimmunoassays for the determination of SLI in blood has increased the yield. Presently these assays are complicated by the need for cumbersome extraction procedures and are not readily available. However, it should be recognized that the syndrome is rare. Of 1,199 cases screened for somatostatinoma at the University of Michigan between 1982–1986, only eight had diagnostic serum levels.

The diagnosis of somatostatinoma at a time when blood SLI concentrations are normal or only marginally elevated, however, requires reliable provocative tests. Increases in plasma SLI concentrations have been reported after intravenous infusion of tolbutamide and arginine. Decreases in SLI concentrations have been observed after intravenous infusion of diazoxide. Arginine is a well established stimulant for normal D cells and thus is unlikely to differentiate between normal and supranormal somatostatin secretion. The same may be true for diazoxide, which has been shown to decrease SLI secretion from normal dog pancreas as well as in patients with somatostatinoma.[279] Tolbutamide stimulates SLI release from normal dog and rat pancreas,[37,62,279] but no change was found in circulating SLI concentrations in three normal human subjects after IV injection of 1 g of tolbutamide.[257] At present, therefore, tolbutamide appears to be a candidate for a provocative agent in the diagnosis of somatostatinoma, but its reliability will have to be established in a greater number of patients and controls. Until then, it may be necessary to measure plasma SLI concentrations during routine workups for postprandial dyspepsia and gallbladder disorders,[157] for diabetes without a family history, for unexplained steatorrhea, inasmuch as these findings can be early signs of somatostatinomas.

Treatment of Somatostatinomas

Forty percent of patients with somatostatinomas died at intervals ranging from one week to 14 months after diagnosis, while 60% of patients were alive from six months to five years after diagnosis. Thus the syndrome is associated with a high malignant potential. It is therefore important to be aggressive in management, and to attempt to remove all tumor tissue in benign cases. In patients in whom metastases have already occurred at the time of diagnosis, bulk reduction may be justified, if feasible. The optimal form of chemotherapy remains to be determined.

Pancreatic Polypeptide (PP) PPoma

Pancreatic polypeptide was discovered by serendipity. In 1972, working in separate laboratories, Chance and Jones,[54] and Kimmel, Pollack, Hazlewood, and their co-workers[152] independently purified a single major protein from a crude insulin preparation; the protein was named pancreatic polypeptide (PP).[54] In mammals 93% of the cells producing PP are located in the pancreas.

There are very dramatic effects of meal ingestion, cerebral stimulation, and hormone administration on circulating levels of PP. A biological role for PP has not been established, however.[93,109,110,117] The only physiologic effects recognized in humans are inhibition of gallbladder contraction and pancreatic enzyme secretion.[117] Thus, a tumor deriving from PP cells is predicted to be clinically silent, though this is not always the case.

Tomita reported two patients, one of whom had persistent watery diarrhea and the other of whom had high levels of circulating PP and PP-cell hyperplasia.[330] A patient with chronic duodenal ulcer and a PP tumor has been reported.[38] A tumor that invaded the bile ducts, producing biliary obstruction was a PPoma.[73] It has been suggested that the watery diarrhea syndrome, seen in gastroenteropancreatic endocrine tumors, may have its origin in PP over-production.[173] The picture is complicated by the fact that mixed tumors, PP cell hyperplasia in association with other functioning islet cell tumors, ductal hyperplasia of PP-cells, nesidioblastosis, and multiple islet tumors producing PP have also been described either alone or as part of the MEN-I syndrome.[171,258] Basal concentrations of PP in plasma may be raised above 1,000 pg/ml in 22–77% of cases of all endocrine secreting tumors, and in 29–50% of patients with the carcinoid syndrome, even if the carcinoid is located outside of the pancreas. Among 53 patients with adenocarcinomas of the pancreas, however, no instance of an elevated basal concentration of PP was found.[168,199] The diagnostic accuracy of elevated basal PP concentrations as a marker for endocrine secreting tumors can be marginally increased to around 50–60% by determining the response of PP to secretin administration.[343,344] A response of greater than 5,000 pg/min/mL (integrated response) is more than two standard deviations above that observed in healthy subjects. It appears, however, that many cases of so-called nonfunctional gastroenteropancreatic endocrine tumors are indeed PPomas, since it is our experience that 50–75% of these have raised basal PP levels, and in 67% the response to secretin is exaggerated. Thus, in the absence of factors such as chronic renal failure, which are known to cause marked elevation of PP levels, a markedly elevated PP level in an older healthy patient may occasionally be indicative of a non-functioning pancreatic endocrine tumor. Differentiation of a high basal concentration in a healthy subject from that appearing in patients with tumor has been difficult. Schwartz suggested that administration of atropine would suppress concentrations in healthy subjects and would fail to do so in patients with tumors, but this has not been subjected to extensive examination.[288]

Increased PP-cells are found in 20–67% of functioning and non-functioning tumors of the pancreas.[242] There does not appear to be a relationship between the number of cells and their function, since islet tumors containing subnormal, normal, or supernormal concentrations of PP compared with the normal pancreas may be associated with normal or high levels of circulating PP. There are now at least 21 patients in the literature with PPomas. The age ranges from 20 to 74 years with a mean of 51 years and with an equal sex incidence.

Diabetes was found in only two cases. Diarrhea, which was formerly thought to be a part of the syndrome,[173] occurred in only one-third of cases. Steatorrhea was found in 100% of patients in whom it was sought. Decreased acid secretion was only documented in 2 of 6 people studied. Fifty seven percent presented with weight loss. The PPoma syndrome is silent. These tumors are often found unsuspectedly in the course of working up patients with hepatomegaly, abdominal pain, metastases to the liver, jaundice due to obstruction of the common bile duct, or hematochezia. Upper GI bleeding may occur due to invasion of the wall of the duodenum or thrombosis of the splenic or portal vein with consequent development of varices. Not infrequently PPomas are recognized by the radiologist as highly vascular tumors with metastases to the liver. Six of the reported cases had PPomas as part of the MEN-I syndrome.

Treatment

It is our contention,[242,343,344,350,352] that not every patient with raised PP levels has a tumor. If a tumor can be identified and localized it should be removed. Raised PP levels occur as part of the MEN-I syndrome and may reflect nesidioblastosis of PP cells or multiple adenomata not amenable to resection. The frequency of malignancy of these tumors is not established and resection should be reserved for those patients with clearly identified solitary lesions.

It has been suggested that every patient who has a markedly elevated level of PP should undergo exploratory laparotomy and careful inspection of the pancreas, even if the tumor cannot be diagnosed.[102] This has not been our experience. Malignant PPomas are best treated with streptozotocin. PPomas may occur outside the pancreas, and carcinoid tumors can present a real dilemma since these may occur in the chest and elsewhere. Laparotomy is not advised. We contend that percutaneous transhepatic portal venous sampling, and if necessary total body venous sampling, should be performed to localize the source of PP overproduction. If such a locus is found, the abdominal or other exploration should be performed. In patients who have metastatic tumors and those refractory to other forms of treatment, the use of the somatostatin analogue, octreotide (Sandoz), has proved to be useful and is worthy of trial.

Neurotensinomas

Neurotensin (NT) is a 13 amino acid polypeptide first extracted from bovine brain by Carraway and Leeman.[52] It was subsequently isolated from the human gastrointestinal tract and found to have the same amino acid sequence.[125]

Neurotensin has a number of interesting pharmacologic effects which include hypotension, tachycardia and cyanosis[124,210] and stimulation of secretion from the small intestine.[8] It has also been reported to inhibit the interdigestive myoelectric complex and stimulate insulin release.[28] NT also increases venous vascular permeability[210] and raises blood glucose[51,88,232] and lowers blood pressure.[52,210]

High concentrations of neurotensin-like immunoreactivity (NTLI) are present in the ileal mucosa where it is localized to a specific "N" cell.[259] Plasma concentrations rise after food ingestion,[191] and high circulating levels[26] have been found after surgery for duodenal ulcer and jejunoileal bypass for obesity.[19] No clear physiologic role has been established for the peptide. High circulating levels have also been found in patients with VIPomas.[27,30,90,120,182,294,368]

In 1981, based upon the pharmacologic actions of neurotensin, it was predicted[344] that a syndrome of excess would emerge presenting with features consonant with the pharmacologic actions of the peptide viz: diabetes, hypotension, vasodilatation, cyanosis, and edema. In addition to these features, investigation would reveal, net secretion of fluid and electrolytes, inhibition of gastric acid secretion, infrequent interdigestive myoelectric complexes (IMMC) and prolonged T ½ of gastric emptying. The prediction that diabetes would occur was based upon the predominant stimulation of adrenomedullary secretions despite stimulation of insulin secretion.[44] The clinical features of reported cases includes diarrhea, hypotension, hypokalemia, edema, weight loss, and occasionally diabetes.[343,344]

Apart from these reported cases, Blackburn examined plasma neurotensin levels in 326 fasting patients with tumors in a variety of sites.[27] Of these patients, 180 had tumors of the pancreas including glucagonomas,[257] gastrinomas,[270] insulinomas,[157] nonsecretory tumors,[60] and VIPomas.[31] Plasma NTLI levels were raised only in six patients with VIPomas

and none of the other tumors. Twenty-one of the tumors containing VIP were removed surgically and six were found to contain NTLI. The clinical features of these six patients did not appear to differ from the remaining 15 patients.

With so few cases it is difficult to generalize on the clinical picture. Half the cases were cured by resection of tumors in the pancreas[375] or lung[372] and the remainder have responded well to streptozotocin. The syndrome appears to comprise diarrhea, diabetes, and weight loss and as such may not be readily distinguishable from the VIPoma syndrome. Neurotensinomas are probably best characterized as yet another tumor which is capable of causing the WDHHA (watery diarrhea, hypokalemia, hypochlorhydria, and acidosis) syndrome. Edema, hypotension and flushing should increase the suspicion of a neurotensinoma.

Octreotide in the Treatment of Malignant Neuroendocrine Tumors

Somatostatin, a tetradecapeptide inhibits the secretion and action of a number of peptide hormones, neurotransmitters, and exocrine secretions of the GEP axis. Its clinical use is limited because of its short half-life of 1–2 min. Development of its potent long acting octapeptide analog (Sandostatin®, Octreotide Acetate) with a half-life of >100 min was a breakthrough for clinical application.

Several aspects of treatment of gastroenteropancreatic neoplasms including: symptom reduction, hormone suppression, tumor growth and survival will be discussed below.

Symptom Control

Octreotide has a potent action in reducing symptoms in certain neuroendocrine tumors; in carcinoid, flushing is reduced in all[347] or the majority of patients.[71,167,267] The acute effects on water and electrolyte transport is a reversal from a secretory to an absorptive state. normalizing transport across the proximal intestine.[356] However, long-term responses of diarrhea differ in different reports: 9 of 14 of our patients with endocrine diarrhea responded to treatment,[347] in contrast to 19 of 25 reported by Kvols.[167] Diarrhea in VIPoma improves 95% of the time.[71] This difference might be due to involvement of different peptides causing diarrhea and different mechanisms. In five of our gastrinoma patients the presenting symptom was diarrhea which improved, as did 65% of 26 reported cases.[71] Diarrhea in 16 patients with glucagonomas also improved uniformly.[71,213] There is, however, the possibility of a rebound in symptoms and/or hormonal values during therapy. The mechanism of this is not clear, it might involve accelerated enzymatic breakdown of octreotide and/or ligand-induced changes of somatostatin receptors on the target cell preventing internalization of the hormone receptor complexes or a gradual adaptation of the target cell to the octreotide effect, as proposed by Koelz.[153]

Wheezing as one of the symptoms in carcinoid syndrome, can be reversed by octreotide and we have documented spirometric improvement in lung function.[347] In one patient who had severe proximal myopathic muscle weakness, clinical and electromyographic improvement occurred with octreotide treatment.[347] The arthropathy of carcinoid improves which may be Substance P mediated.[44] Hypoglycemia with insulinoma responds erratically due to unpredictable effects on food absorption, suppression of glucagon and insulin.[356] Of 15 patients, 50% improved, and 30% got worse.[71] The necrolytic migratory erythema of glucagonoma clears in only half of the cases (n = 16).[72]

Hormone Suppression and Biochemical Features

It has been shown that octreotide inhibits hormone secretion in some malignant GEP tumors. The most sensitive seems to be VIPoma, where lowering of VIP circulating levels parallels relief of symptoms.[282,356] Gastrin levels, however, are not equivalently lowered with octreotide. We showed that in patients with metastatic disease whose basal gastrin levels were extremely high there was no effect of lowering plasma gastrin levels. In worldwide pooled data (n = 26), 70% are reported to respond. Furthermore, ACTH overproduction heralds unresponsiveness to the drug. Glucagon levels seldom decrease.[71] The overall 5-HIAA level was significantly lower after octreotide treatment, whereas blood serotonin level did not differ significantly.[267,354] There is an overall reduction of 5-HIAA in 58% of patients.[71]

Perioperative Management

Carcinoid and other GEP tumors can be a major therapeutic problem perioperatively when vast quantities of active peptides are released into the circulation because of manipulation of tumors. Octreotide has been shown to be an effective suppressor of release and of action of peptide hormones during surgery.[332] It has been shown that profound refractory hypotension in carcinoid syndrome can be rapidly reversed by octreotide,[166] as well as gastric acid secretion and fistula drainage.[332]

Tumor Growth

Since GEP tumors grow slowly it is hard to assess the effect of treatment upon tumor growth. However, by long-term CT scan monitoring shrinkage of liver metastasis has been shown in certain patients with carcinoid and other GEP tumors.[155,167] In 85 carcinoids no change was found with <50 mg/d but Kvols[167] reported a 17% decrease in size using higher doses of 1,500 mg/d. VIPoma, glucagonoma, and gastrinoma do not generally change in size,[71] although a tumor infarction has occurred in VIPoma.[332] Tumors metastases to bone may occur despite apparent control of the primary tumor or liver metastases.[355,356]

Conclusion

The role of octreotide in the treatment of GEP tumors is still not well established. Due to the clear evidence of symptomatic relief (flushing, wheezing, diarrhea, etc) it has established a place in treatment of GEP tumors both pre- and post-operatively. Perioperative use can prevent fatal episodes of rapid extreme increases of hormones in the circulation. There is enough evidence of control of tumor growth that primary treatment of select metastatic tumors, with proper monitoring of tumor growth, is recommended (Figure XXVI-5-2).

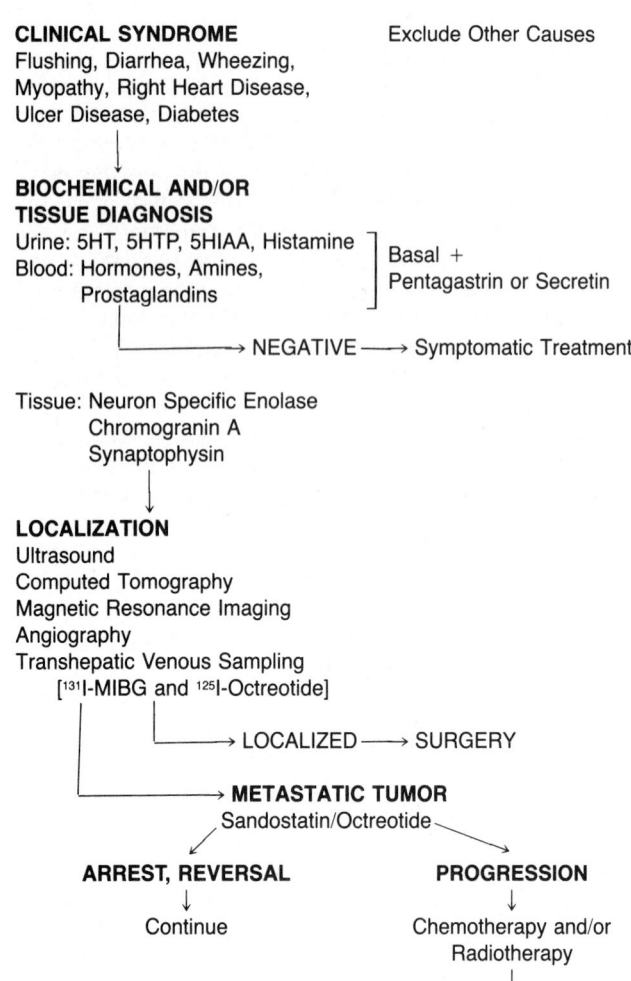

Figure XXVI-5-2. Suggested management of suspect neuroendocrine tumors.

Chemotherapy of Metastatic Islet Cell Carcinomas

Ajani performed repetitive hepatic artery embolization with polyvinyl alcohol particles in 22 patients with metastatic pancreatic endocrine tumors and they achieved partial remission of measurable hepatic tumor in 12 of 20 evaluable patients.[4] From this experience, the authors suggested this modality for prolonged palliation in selected patients. Recently, Marlink reported partial responses in all six patients with metastatic islet cell tumors following selective hepatic artery embolization;[187] however, the duration of responses was not reported.

Because of the relative rarity of gastroenteropancreatic neoplasms, chemotherapy trials have frequently combined several islet cell tumor subtypes within the same study. The experience from these studies suggests that while similar responses may be expected from chemotherapy for several of the tumor subtypes, there may be differences in responses for other types. For example, streptozotocin alone or in combination with 5-fluorouracil is extremely effective against most VIPomas[202] and moderately effective against gastrinomas and most other islet cell tumors. In contrast, streptozotocin has little activity against glucagonomas, whereas dacarbazine appears to have significant activity.[150]

Streptozotocin is a drug that is selectively cytotoxic for pancreatic islet cells. Because of this property the drug has been used to establish animal models for diabetes and islet cell hypofunction.[264] This selective cytotoxicity provided a rationale for using streptozotocin in neoplastic disorders of pancreatic endocrine cells. In several studies using intravenous and, less commonly, intraarterial administration, streptozotocin was shown to be active against several pancreatic endocrine cancers with nearly 40% tumor responses and over 50% hormonal responses reported.[42,98,223,231,285] More frequent use of this agent is limited by its significant emetogenic and renal toxicities. In the case of symptomatic hepatic metastases from glucagonoma and somatostatinoma, Friesen claims the use of intra-arterial administration of streptozotocin is effective with reduced incidence of nephrotoxicity, although this has not been confirmed.[100]

Other drugs that have single agent activity in islet cell carcinoma are chlorozotocin and doxorubicin. At a dose of 100–200 mg/M^2 chlorozotocin resulted in a 53% objective response rate in 13 previously untreated patients.[47] In 20 previously treated patients, doxorubicin, 60 mg/M^2 every three to four weeks resulted in four (20%) objective responses.[224]

Several authors have reported that dacarbazine is a highly effective agent for the treatment of pancreatic islet cell tumors, especially glucagon secreting tumors.[150] Using either 1,250 mg/M^2 in divided doses over five days or a single dose of 650 mg/M^2 Kessinger and colleagues reported two complete responses and two partial responses of elevated serum glucagon in four patients with glucagonomas.[150] Three of four additional patients with malignant islet cell carcinoma associated with glucagonoma syndrome were cited in this report

as having responded to dacarbazine alone.[150] In a recently reported prospective study of 48 evaluable patients with advanced islet cell carcinoma, Hahn reported 13 patients (27%) with objective responses (including three complete responses) following dacarbazine, 850 mg/M^2 given every four weeks.[122] Severe or lethal toxicity was experienced by 15 patients. The median survival in all patients was 19 months and the authors concluded that dacarbazine clearly had beneficial activity in patients with advanced islet cell carcinoma.[122]

None of six evaluable patients with islet cell carcinoma responded to etoposide in a phase II study.[149] No other conventional chemotherapy agents have reported activity in this disease.

In a multi-institutional study, streptozotocin combined with 5-fluorouracil was shown to be effective against malignant pancreatic endocrine tumors with an objective response rate of 63% for a duration of 17.4 months.[164,223,246] Furthermore, this combination produced a 37% complete response rate and a more prolonged median survival than streptozotocin alone. However, the combination was also associated with a high prevalence of moderately severe gastrointestinal, hematopoietic, and renal toxicity.[223] A smaller, nonrandomized series of patients receiving the same combination chemotherapy regimen produced similar results and this study also suggested that the response rate in patients with nonfunctional tumors (50%) may be less than in those with functional tumors (68%).[246] Although the regimen of streptozotocin and fluorouracil is not considered to be the most active for malignant glucagonoma, responses to the combination have been reported.[151]

In a randomized trial by the Eastern Cooperative Oncology Group, streptozotocin plus 5-fluorouracil was compared to

Table XXVI-5-9. Systemic Anticancer Therapy for Neoplasms of the Gastroenteropancreatic System

Drug	Islet Cell Neoplasm(s)	No. of Patients	Objective Biochemical or Tumor Response (%)	Reference
Single Agents				
Streptozotocin	Gastrinomas	24	50	42, 223, 224, 359
	Unspecified	125	50	42, 92, 182, 231, 334
Dacarbazine	Gastrinoma	6	0	171, 362
	Glucagonoma	10	90	172, 176, 330
	Unspecified	48	27	160
		12	50	273
Chlorozotocin	Unspecified	13	53	307
Doxorubicin	Unspecified	20	20	44
Etoposide	Unspecified	6	0	228
Interferon	Unspecified	32	73	111, 245
Octreotide acetate	VIPoma	25	75	71, 163, 246, 352
	Glucagonoma	16	55	
	Gastrinoma	36	65	
	Insulinoma	15	50	
	GRFoma	4	75	
Combination Agents				
Streptozotocin + 5-fluorouracil	Unspecified	40	63	182
		19	58	245
Streptozotocin + doxorubicin	Unspecified	31	19	231
		25	36	245
Streptozotocin + 5-fluorouracil + doxorubicin	Gastrinoma	10	40	359

Table XXVI-5-10. Systemic Anticancer Therapy for Malignant Carcinoid

Drug	No. of Patients	Objective Biochemical or Tumor Response (%)	Reference
Single Agents			
5-Fluorouracil	19	26	221, 222
Doxorubicin	33	21	150, 164, 221
Streptozotocin	23	30	45, 221
Dacarbazine	15	13	338
Dactinomycin	17	6	338
Etoposide	17	0	149
Cisplatin	15	6	227
Interferon	99	≤50	127, 245, 246, 304
	27	39	226
Octreotide acetate	85	71	71, 163, 246, 352
Combination Agents			
Streptozotocin + 5-fluorouracil	154	≤33	67, 221, 222, 246
Streptozotocin + doxorubicin	47	26	221, 222
Streptozotocin + 5-fluorouracil + doxorubicin	20	35	46

a combination of streptozotocin plus doxorubicin or to chlorozotocin.[164] Although the results have not yet been published, it is expected that this study will provide an important contribution towards further defining the optimal chemotherapeutic approach for malignant pancreatic endocrine tumors. A phase II study of the combination of streptozotocin and doxorubicin in patients with advanced miscellaneous neuroendocrine tumors (APUDomas) was conducted by Frame,[96] who reported 6 of 31 (19%) objective tumor responses for a median duration of seven months. This relatively low response rate might be improved by higher dose intensity, but this approach is untested to date.

There is no prospective investigation of adjuvant chemotherapy in patients with islet cell carcinoma.

Finally, the interferons have been reported to be active in gastroenteropancreatic endocrine neoplasms. As reviewed by Oberg and Eriksson, objective hormonal response of 73% was observed in patients with malignant pancreatic endocrine tumors treated with human leukocyte interferon, 3–6 million units per day subcutaneously.[246] Among their first 22 responders, six (27%) patients had 50% reduction in tumor mass and two patients had a complete response.[81] The median duration of response was 9.5 months; the interferon was well tolerated despite the frequent occurrence of a flu-like syndrome, weight loss, and mild myelosuppression. A summary of these studies appears in Tables XXVI-5-9 and XXVI-5-10.

Summary and Conclusions

New approaches to the diagnosis and localization of GEP tumors have been stressed, including the importance of circulating hormone levels and sophisticated immunohistochemistry, tracer scanning, and the role of peptide therapy in the management of the symptom complex, as well as the tumor. There is, however, much that remains unsolved requiring diligent research and evaluation if we are ultimately to include neuroendocrine tumors among the curable cancers.

An outline of the current approach to management of the patient suspected of harboring a GEP tumor is given in the flow diagram (Figure XXVI-5-2).

References

1. Adolph, J. M. G., Kimmig, B. N., Georgi, P., and Winkel, K.: Carcinoid tumors: CT and I-131 Meta-iodo-benzylguanidine scintigraphy. Radiology, 164:199, 1987.
2. Ahlman, H., Dahlstrom, A., Gronstad, K., Tisell, L. E., Oberg, K., Zinner, M. J., and Jaffe, B. M.: The pentagastrin test in the diagnosis of the carcinoid syndrome: Blockade of gastrointestinal symptoms by ketanserin. Ann. Surg., 201:81, 1985.
3. Ajani, J. A., Carrasco, C. H., Charnsangavej, C., Samann, N. A., Levin, B., and Wallace, S.: Islet cell tumors metastatic to the liver: Effective palliation by sequential hepatic artery embolization. Ann. Intern. Med., 108:340, 1989.
4. Ajani, J., Kavanagh, J., Patt, Y., Levin, B., Edwards, C., and Gutterman, J.: Roferon and doxorubicin combination active against advanced islet cell or carcinoid tumors. Proc. Am. Assoc. Cancer Res., 30:293, 1989.
5. Aldrich, L. B., Moattari, A. R., and Vinik, A. I.: Distinguishing features of idiopathic flushing and carcinoid syndrome. Arch. Intern. Med., 148:2614, 1988.
6. Altimari, A. F., Badrinath, K., Reisel, H. J., and Prinz, R. A.: DTIC therapy in patients with malignant intra-abdominal neuroendocrine tumors. Surgery, 102:1009, 1987.
7. Alumets, J., Hakanson, R., Ingemannson, S., and Sundler, F.: Substance P and 5-HT in granules isolated from an intestinal argentaffin carcinoid. Histochemistry, 52:217, 1977.
8. Andersson, S., Rosell, S., Hjelmquist, U., Change, D., and Folkers, K.: Inhibition of gastric and intestinal motor activity in dogs by (Gln^4)-neurotensin. Acta Physiol. Scand., 100:231, 1977.
9. Andrew, A.: An experimental investigation into the possible neural crest origin of pancreatic APUD (islet) cells. J. Embryol. Exp. Morphol., 35:577, 1976.
10. Arnold, R., and Lankisch, P. G.: Somatostatin and the gastrointestinal tract. Clin. Gastroenterol., 9:733, 1980.
11. Awrich, A. E., Peetrz, M., and Fletcher, W. S.: Dimethyltriazenoimidazole carboxamide therapy of islet cell carcinoma of the pancreas. J. Surg. Oncol., 17:321, 1981.
12. Axelrod, L., Bush, M. A., and Hirsch, H. J.: Malignant Somatostatinoma: Clinical features and metabolic studies. J. Clin. Endocrinol. Metab., 52:886, 1981.
13. Barbezat, G. O., and Grossman, M.: Intestinal secretion: Stimulation by peptides. Science, 174:422, 1971.
14. Barreras, R. F., Mack, E., Goodfriend, T., and Damm, M.: Resection of gastrinoma in the Zollinger-Ellison syndrome. Gastroenterol., 82:953, 1981.
15. Bauer, W., Briner, U., Doepfner, W., Waller, R., Huguenin, R., Marbach, P., Fletcher, T. J., and Pless, T.: SMS 201-995: A very potent and selective octapeptide analogue of somatostatin with prolonged action. Life Sci., 31:1133, 1982.
16. Bauer, R., Van de Flierdt, E., Stettmeier, H., Langhammer, H. R., and Pabst, H. W.: 1-131-MIBG therapy of carcinoid tumor of intestinal origin. (Abstract 67). Eur. J. Nucl. Med., 14:234, 1988.
17. Berelowitz, M., Szabo, M., Barowsky, H. W., Arbel, G. R., and Frohman, L. A.: Somatostatin-like immunoactivity and biological activity is present in a human pheochromocytoma. J. Clin. Endocrinol. Metab., 56:134, 1983.
18. Berry, E. M., Maunder, C., and Wilson, M.: Carcinoid myopathy and treatment with cyproheptadine (periactin). Gut, 15:34, 1974.
19. Besterman, H. S., Bloom, S. R., Sarson, D. L., Blackburn, A. M., Johnston, D. I., Patel, H. R., Stewart, J. S., Modigliani, R., Guerin, S., and Mallinson, C. N.: Gut hormone profile in coeliac disease. Lancet, 1:785, 1978.
20. Betts, J. B., O'Malley, B. P., and Rosenthal, F. D.: Hyperparathyroidism: A prerequisite for Zollinger-Ellison syndrome in MEA-1: Report of a further family and a review of the literature. Quart. J. Med., 49:69, 1980.
21. Bhagavan, B. S., Slavin, R. E., Goldberg, J., Rao, R. N.: Ectopic gastrinoma and Zollinger-Ellison syndrome. Hum. Pathol., 17:584, 1986.
22. Bhatena, S. J., Higgins, G. A., and Recant, L.: Glucagonoma and Glucagonoma Syndrome. In Glucagon. Edited by R. H. Unger and L. Orci. New York, Elsevier North Holland Inc., 1981, p. 413.

23. Binnick, A. N., Spencer, S. K., and Dennison, W. L., Jr.: Glucagonoma syndrome. Arch. Dermatol., 113:749, 1977.
24. Biorck, G., Axen, O., and Throsen, A.: Unusual cyanosis in a boy with congenital pulmonary stenosis and tricuspid insufficiency. Am. Heart J., 44:143, 1952.
25. Bissette, G., Manberg, P., Nemeroff, C. B., and Prange, A. J., Jr.: Neurotensin, a biologically active peptide. Life Sci., 23:2173, 1978.
26. Blackburn, A. M., and Bloom, S. R.: A radioimmunoassay for neurotensin in human plasma. J. Endocrinol., 83:175, 1979.
27. Blackburn, A. M., Bryant, M. G., Adrian, T. E., Bloom, S. R., Christofides, N. D., Long, R. G., Fitzpatrick, N. R., and Baron, J. H.: Pancreatic tumours produce neurotensin. J. Clin. Endocrinol. Metab., 52:820, 1981.
28. Blackburn, A. M., Fletcher, D. R., and Bloom, S. R.: Effect of neurotensin on gastric function in man. Lancet, 1:987, 1980.
29. Blair, A. W., and Ahmed, S.: Presacral vipoma in a 16-month old child. Acta Paediatr. Belg., 34:89, 1981.
30. Bloom, S. R., Lee, Y. C., Lacroute, J. M., Abbass, A., Sondag, D., Baumann, R., and Weill, J. P.: Two patients with pancreatic apudomas secreting neurotensin and VIP. Gut, 24:448, 1983.
31. Bloom, S. R., Mortimer, C. H., Thorner, M. O., Bresser, G. M., Hall, R., Comez-Pan, A., Roy, V. M., Russell, R. C., Coy, D. H., Kastin, A. J., and Schall, A. V.: Inhibition of gastrin and gastric-acid secretion by growth-hormone-release-inhibiting hormone. Lancet, 2:1106, 1974.
32. Bloom, S. R., and Polak, J. M.: Glucagonomas, VIPomas and somatostatinomas. Clin. Endocrinol. Metab., 9:285, 1980.
33. Bloom, S. R., and Polak, J. M.: Hormone Profiles. *In* Gut Hormones. Edited by S. R. Bloom and J. M. Polak. New York, Churchill Livingstone, 1981.
34. Bloom, S. R., and Polak, J. M.: VIP measurement in distinguishing Verner-Morrison syndrome and pseudo-Verner-Morrison syndrome. Clin. Endocrin., 5:223s, 1976.
35. Bloom, S. R., and Polak, J. M.: Vipomas. *In* Vasoactive Intestinal Peptides. Edited by S. I. Said. New York, Raven Press, 1982.
36. Blum, I., Doron, M., Laron, Z., Atsmon, A., and Tigva, P.: Prevention of hypoglycemic attacks by propranol suffering from insulinoma. Diabetes, 24:535, 1975.
37. Boden, G., Baile, C. A., McLaughlin, C. L., and Matschinsky, F. M.: Effects of starvation and obesity on somatostatin, insulin and glucagon release from an isolated perfused organ system. Am. J. Physiol., 241:E215, 1981.
38. Bordi, C., Togni, R., Baetens, M., Malaisse-Lagae, F., and Orci, L.: Human islet cell tumor storing pancreatic polypeptide, a light and electronic microscopic study. J. Clin. Endocrinol. Metab., 46:215, 1978.
39. Brandi, M. L., Aurbach, G. D., Fitzpatrick, L. A., Quarto, R., Spiegel, A. M., Bliziotes, M. M., Norton, J. A., Doppmann, J. L., and Marx, S. J.: Parathyroid mitogenic activity in plasma from patients with familial multiple endocrine neoplasia type 1. N. Engl. J. Med., 1986; 314:1287-1293.
40. Brockenbrough, J. S., Weir, G. C., and Bonner-Weir, S.: Discordance of exocrine and endocrine growth after 90% pancreatectomy in rats. Diabetes, 37:232, 1988.
41. Broder, L. E., and Carter, S. K.: Chemotherapy of malignant insulinomas with streptozotocin. *In* International Congress Series #314, Excerpta Medica, 1974, p. 714.
42. Broder, L. E., and Carter, S. K.: Pancreatic islet cell carcinoma: II. Results of therapy with streptozotocin in 52 patients. Ann. Intern. Med., 70(1):108, 1973.
43. Brodows, R. G., and Campbel, R. G.: Control of refractory fasting hypoglycemia in a patient with suspected insulinoma with diphenylhydantoin. J. Clin. Endocrinol. Metab., 38:159, 1974.
44. Brown, M., and Vale, W.: Effects of neurotensin and substance P on plasma insulin, gluagon and glucose levels. Endocrinology, 98:819, 1976.
45. Buchanan, K. D., Johnston, C. F., O'Hare, M. M. T., Ardill, J. E., Shaw, C., Collins, J. S., Watson, R. G., Atkinson, A. B., Hadden, P. R., and Kennedy, T. L.: Neuroendocrine tumors. A European view. Amer. J. Med., 81(Suppl 6b): 14, 1986.
46. Bukowski, R. M., Johnson, K. G., Peterson, R. F., Stephens, R. L., Rivkin, S. E., Neilan, B., and Costanzi, J. H.: A phase II trial of combination chemotherapy in patients with metastatic carcinoid tumors. Cancer, 60:2891, 1987.
47. Bukowski, R. M., McCracken, J. D., Balcerzak, S. P., and Fabian, C. J.: Phase II study of chlorozotocin in islet cell carcinoma. A Southwest Oncology Group Study. Cancer Chemother. Pharmacol., 11:48, 1983.
48. Burcharth, F., Stage, J. G., Stadil, F., Jensen, L. I., and Fischermann, K.: Localization of gastrinomas by transhepatic portal catheterization and gastrin assay. Gastroenterol., 77:444, 1979.
49. Cameron, S. J., and Doig, A.: Cerebellar tumours presenting with clinical features of phaeochromocytoma. Lancet, 1:492, 1970.
50. Carrasco, C. H., Charnsangavej, C., Ajani, J., Samaan, N. A., Richli, W., and Wallace, S.: The carcinoid syndrome: palliation by hepatic artery embolization. Am. J. Roentgenol., 147:149, 1986.
51. Carraway, R., Demers, L. M., and Leeman, S. E.: Hyperglycemic effect of neurotensin, a hypothalamic peptide. Endocrinology, 99:1452, 1976.
52. Carraway, R., and Leeman, S. E.: The isolation of a new hypotensive peptide, neurotensin, from bovine hypothalami. J. Biol. Chem., 248:6854, 1973.
53. Carson, D. J., Glasgow, J. F. T., and Ardill, J.: Watery diarrhea and elevated vasoactive intestinal polypeptide associated with a massive neurofibroma in early childhood. J. Royal Soc. Med., 73:69, 1980.
54. Chance, R. E., and Jones, W. E.: Polypeptides from bovine, ovine, human, and porcine pancreas. United States Patent Office, 842:063, 1974.
55. Cherner, J. A., Doppmann, J. L., Norton, J. A., Miller, D. L., Krudy, A. G., Raufman, J. P., Collen, M. J., Maton, P. N., Gardner, J. D., and Jensen, R. T.: Selective venous sampling for gastrin to localize gastrinomas: A prospective assessment. Ann. Int. Med., 105:841, 1986.
56. Cho, K. J., Vinik, A. I., Thompson, N. W., Shields, J. J., Porter, D. J., Brader, T. M., Cadavid, G., and Fajans, S. S.: Localization of the source of hyperinsulinism by percutaneous transhepatic portal and pancreatic vein catherterization with hormone assay. Am. J. Roentgenol., 139:237, 1982.
57. Clouse, M. E., Costello, P., Legg, M. A., Soeldner, S. J., and Cody, B.: Subselective angiography in localizing insulinomas of the pancreas. Am. J. Roentgenol., 128:741, 1977.
58. Conlon, J. M., Deacon, C. F., Richter, G., Stockman, F., and Creutzfeldt, W.: Circulating tachykinins (substance P, neurokinin A and neuropeptide K) and the carcinoid flush. Scan. J. Gastroenterol., 22:97, 1987.
59. Conlon, J. M.: The glucagon-like polypeptides—order out of chaos? Diabetologia, 18:85, 1980.
60. Crain, E. L., Jr., and Thorn, G. W.: Functioning pancreatic islet cell adenomas. Medicine, 28:427, 1949.
61. Creutzfeldt, W., and Arnold, R.: Somatostatin and the stomach: Exocrine and endocrine aspects. First International Somatostatin Symposium, Freiberg, Germany. Metabolism, 27(Suppl):1309, 1978.
62. Creutzfeldt, W., Lankisch, P. G., and Folsch, U. R.: Hemmung der Secretin und Cholezystokinin-Pankreozymin-induzierten Saft und Enzymsecretion des Pancreas und der Gallenblasen-Kontraktion beim Menschen durch Somatostatin. Dtsch. Med. Wochenschr., 100:1135, 1975.
63. Daggett, P. R., Goodburn, E. A., Kurtz, A. B., Le Quesne, L. P., Morris, D. V., Nabarro, J. D., and Raphael, M. J.: Is preoperative localization of insulinomas necessary? Lancet, 1:483, 1981.
64. Das, M. L.: A rapid sensitive method for direct estimation of serotonin in whole blood. Biochem. Med., 6:299, 1972.
65. Davies, E. R.: The radiological and scintigraphic investigation of spontaneous hypoglycaemia. Clin. Radiol., 24:177, 1973.
66. Davis, R. B.: The concentration of serotonin in normal human serum as determined by an improved method. J. Lab. Clin. Med., 54:344, 1959.
67. Davis, Z., Moertel, C. G., and Mc Lirath, D. C.: The malignant carcinoid syndrome. Surg. Gynec. Obstet. 137:637, 1973.
68. Deveney, C. W., Deveney, K. S., Stark, D., Moss, A., Stein, S., and Way, L. W.: Resection of gastrinomas. Ann. Surg., 198:546, 1983.
69. Deveney, C. W., Deveney, K. S., and Way, L. W.: The Zollinger-Ellison syndrome—23 years later. Ann. Surg., 188:384, 1978.
70. Deveney, C., Steins, S., and Way, L. W.: Cimetidine in the treatment of Zollinger-Ellison syndrome. Am. J. Surg., 146:116, 1983.
71. Dunne, M. J., Elton, R., Fletcher, T., Hofker, P., and Shui, J.: Sandostatin and Gastroenteropancreatic tumors—Therapeutic Characteristics: *In* Sandostatin in the Treatment of GEP Endocrine Tumors. Edited by T. M. O'Dorisio. Berlin, Springer Verlag, 1987, p. 93.
72. Dunnick, N. R., Doppmann, J. L., Mills, S., and McCarthy, D. M.: Computed tomographic appearance of non-beta (or non-insulin producing) pancreatic islet cell tumors. Radiology, 135:117, 1980.
73. Ebeid, A. M., Dragon, R., and Brand, D., et. al.: Clinical and pathological consideration on apudomas. (In press).
74. Ebeid, A. M., Murray, P. D., and Fisher, J. E.: Vasoactive intestinal peptide and the watery diarrhea syndrome. Ann. Surg., 187:411, 1978.
75. Eckhauser, F. E., Lloyd, R. V., Thompson, N. W., Raper, S. E., and Vinik, A. I.: Antrectomy for multicentric, argyrophil gastric carcinoids: A preliminary report. Surgery, 104:1046, 1988.
76. Edis, A. J., McIlrath, D. C., van Heerden, J. A., Fulton, R. E., Sheedy, P. F., Service, F. J., and Dale, A. J.: Insulinoma—current diagnosis and surgical management. Curr. Probl. Surg., 13:1, 1976.
77. Eisenbarth, G. S.: Expression of receptors for fetanus toxin and monoclonal antibody A^2B_2 by pancreatic islet cells. Proc. Natl. Acad. Sci., U.S.A., 77:5066, 1982.
78. Ellison, E. C., Carey, L. C., Sparks, J., O'Dorisio, T. M., Mekhjan, H. S., Fromkes, J. J., Caldwell, J. H., and Thomas, F. B.: Early surgical treatment of gastrinoma. Amer. J. Med., 82:17, 1987.
79. Elsborg, L., and Glenthoj, X.: Effect of somatostatin in necrolytic migratory erythemia in pancreatic glucagonoma (abstract). Acta Med. Scand., 218:245, 1985.
80. Engstrom, P. F., Lavin, P. T., and Folsch, E.: Streptozotocin plus fluorouracil versus doxorubicin therapy for metastatic carcinoid tumors. J. Clin. Oncol., 2:1255, 1984.
81. Eriksson, B., Oberg, K., Alm, G., et. al.: Treatment of malignant endocrine pancreatic tumors with human leukocyte interferon. Lancet, 2:1307, 1986.
82. Fabri, P. J., Johnson, J. A., and Ellison, E. C.: Prediction of progressive disease in Zollinger-Ellison syndrome—comparison of available preoperative tests. J. Surg. Research, 31:93, 1981.
83. Fajans, S. S., Floyd, J. C., Jr., Knopf, R. F., Rull, J., Guntsche, E. M., and Conn, J. W.: Benzothiadiazine suppression of insulin release from normal and abnormal islet cell tissue in man. J. Clin. Invest., 45:481, 1986.
84. Fajans, S. S., Floyd, J. C., Jr., Thiffault, C. A., Knopf, R. F., Harrison, T. S., and Conn, J. W.: Further studies on diazoxide suppression of insulin release from abnormal and normal islet tissue in man. Ann. N. Y. Acad. Sci., 150:261, 1968.
85. Fajans, S. S., and Vinik, A. I.: Diagnosis and treatment of insulinoma. *In* Diagnosis and management of endocrine-related tumors. Edited by R. J. Santen and A. Manni. Boston, Martinus Nijhoff Publishers, 1984, p. 235.
86. Feldman, J. M.: Increased dopamine production in patients with carcinoid tumors. Metabolism, 34:255, 1985.
87. Feldman, J. M.: Urinary serotonin in the diagnosis of carcinoid tumor. Clin. Chem., 32:840, 1986.
88. Feldman, J. M.: Carcinoid tumors and the carcinoid syndrome. Curr. Probl. Surg., 26:829, 1989.
89. Feldman, J. M., and O'Dorisio, T. M.: Role of neuropeptides and serotonin in the diagnosis of carcinoid tumors. Am. J. Med., 81(Suppl. 6b):41, 1986.
90. Feurle, G. E., Helmstaeder, V., Tischbirek, K., Carraway, R., Forssmann, W. G., Grube, D., and Rohe, H. D.: A multihormonal tumor of the pancreas producing neurotensin. Dig. Dis. and Sci., 26:1125, 1981.
91. Fischer, M., Kamanabroo, D., Sonderkamp, H., and Proske, T.: Scintigraphic imaging of carcinoid tumors with 1-131-metaiodobenzylguanidine. Lancet, 2:165, 1984.
92. Fisher, R. S., Rock, E., Levin, G., and Malmud, L.: Effects of somatostatin on gallbladder emptying. Gastroenterol., 92:885, 1983.
93. Floyd, J. C., Jr., Vinik, A. I., and Glaser, B., et. al.: Pancreatic polypeptide. *In* Proceedings of the 10th Congress of the International Diabetes Federation. Edited by W. Waldhusl. Amsterdam, Excerpta Medica, 1979, p. 490.
94. Folkers, K., Chang, D., Humphries, J., Carraway, R., Leeman, S. E., and Bowers, C. Y.: Synthesis and activities of neurotensin, and its acid and amide analogue: Possible natural occurrence of (Gln^4)-neurotensin. Proc. Natl. Acad. Sci., U.S.A., 73:3833, 1976.
95. Fox, P. S., Hofmann, J. W., DeCosse, J. J., and Wilson, S. D.: The influence of total gastrectomy on survival in malignant Zollinger-Ellison tumors. Ann. Surg., 180:558, 1974.
96. Frame, J., Kelsen, D., Kemeny, N., Cheng, E., Niedzwiecki, D., Heelan, R., and

Lippermann, R.: A phase II trial of streptozotocin and adriamycin in advanced APUD tumors. Amer. J. Clin. Oncol., 11:490, 1988.
97. Friesen, S. R.: The development of endocrinopathies in the prospective screening of two families with MEA-I. World J. Surg., 3:753, 1979.
98. Friesen, S. R.: Treatment of Zollinger-Ellison syndrome: A 25-year assessment. Am. J. Surg., 143:331, 1982.
99. Friesen, S. R.: Tumors of the endocrine pancreas. N. Engl. J. Med., 306:580, 1982.
100. Friesen, S. R.: Update on the diagnosis and treatment of rare neuroendocrine tumors. Surg. Clinics N. A., 67:379, 1987.
101. Friesen, S. R., Bolinger, R. E., Pearse, A. G. E., and McGuigan, J. E.: Serum gastrin levels in malignant Zollinger-Ellison syndrome after total gastrectomy and hypophysectomy. Ann. Surg., 172:504, 1970.
102. Friesen, S. R., Kimmel, J. R., and Tomita, T.: Pancreatic polypeptide as screening for pancreatic polypeptide apudomas in multiple endocrinopathies. Am. J. Surg., 139:61, 1980.
103. Frolich, J. C., Bloomgarden, Z. T., Oates, J., McGuigan, J. E., and Rabinowitz, D.: The carcinoid flush provocation by pentagastrin and inhibition by somatostatin. N. Engl. J. Med., 299:1055, 1978.
104. Ganda, P. O., Weir, G. C., Soeldner, J. S., Legg, M. A., Chick, W. L., Patel, Y. C., Ebeid, A. M., Gabbay, K. H., and Reichlin, S.: Somatostatinoma: A somatostatin-containing tumor of the endocrine pancreas. N. Engl. J. Med., 296:963, 1977.
105. Geatti, O., Shapiro, B., Sisson, J. C., Hutchinson, R. J., Mallette, S., Eyre, P., and Beierwaltes, W. H.: 1-131-metaiodobenzylguanidine (1-131-MIBG) scintigraphy for the location of neuroblastoma: Preliminary experience in 10 cases. J. Nucl. Med., 26:736, 1985.
106. Ghose, R. R., and Gupta, S. K.: Oat cell carcinoma of bronchus presenting with somatostatinoma syndrome. Thorax, 36:550, 1981.
107. Giacobazzi, P., and Passaro, E.: Preoperative angiography in the Zollinger-Ellison syndrome. Ann. Surg., 126:74, 1973.
108. Glaser, B., Shapiro, B., Fajans, S. S., and Vinik, A. I.: Effects of secretin on the normal and pathological beta cell. J. Clin. Endocrinol. Metab., 66:1138, 1988.
109. Glaser, B., Vinik, A. I., Sive, A. A., and Floyd, J. C., Jr.: Plasma human pancreatic polypeptide responses to administered secretion effects of surgical vagotomy, cholinergic blockage and chronic pancreatitis. J. Clin. Endocrinol. Metab., 50:1094, 1980.
110. Glaser, Vinik, A. I., Sive, A. A., Floyd, J. C., Jr., Fajans, S. S., and Pek, S.: Evidence for extravagal cholinergic dependence of pancreatic polypeptide responses to beef ingestion in man. (Abstract) Diabetes, 28:414, 1979.
111. Glowniak, J., Shapiro, B., Vinik, A. I., Glaser, B., Thompson, N. W., and Cho, K. J.: Percutaneous transhepatic venous sampling of gastrin: value in sporadic and familial islet-cell tumors of G-cell. N. Engl. J. Med., 307:293, 1982.
112. Go, V. L. W., and Korinik, J. K.: Effect of vasoactive intestinal polypeptide on hepatic glucose release. *In* Vasoactive Intestinal Peptide. Edited by S. I. Said. New York, Raven Press, 1982.
113. Godwin, J. D., II: Carcinoid treatment an analysis of 2,837 cases. Cancer, 36:560, 1975.
114. Gould, M., and Johnson, R. J.: Computed tomography of abdominal carcinoid tumor. Br. J. Radiol., 59:881, 1986.
115. Grander, D., Oberg, K., Lundqvist, M., Janson, E. T., Eriksson, B., and Einhorn, S.: Interferon-induced enhancement of 2′,5′-oligoadenylate synthetase in mid-gut carcinoid tumours. Lancet, 336:337, 1990.
116. Green, D., Joynt, R. J., and Van Allen, M. W.: Neuromyopathy associated with a malignant carcinoid tumor. Arch. Intern. Med., 114:494, 1964.
117. Greenberg, G. R., McCloy, R. F., Adrian, T. E., Chadwick, V. S., Baron, J. H., and Bloom, S. R.: Inhibition of pancreas and gallbladder by pancreatic polypeptide. Lancet, 2:1280, 1978.
118. Grimelius, L., and Wilander, E.: Silver stains in the study of endocrine cells of the gut and pancreas. Invest. Cell Pathol., 3:3, 1980.
119. Gunther, R. W., Klose, K. J., Beyer, R. J., Kuhn, F. P., and Klotter, H. J.: Localization of small islet cell tumors preoperative and intraoperative ultrasound, computed tomography, arteriorgraphy, digital subtraction angiography, and pancreatic venous sampling. Gastrointest. Radiol., 10:145, 1985.
120. Gutniak, M., Rosenqvist, U., Grimelius, L., Lundberg, J. M., Hokfelt, T., Rokaeus, A., Lundquist, G., Frahrenkrug, J., Sunbad, R., and Gutniak, E.: Report on a patient with watery diarrhea syndrome caused by a pancreatic tumour containing neurotensin, enkephalin and calcitonin. Acta Med. Scand., 208:95, 1980.
121. Gyr, N. E., Kayasseh, L., and Keller, U.: Somatostatin as a Therapeutic Agent. *In* Gut Hormones, 2nd Edition. Edited by S. R. Bloom and J. M. Polak. Edinburgh, Churchill Livingstone, 1981, 581.
122. Hahn, R. G., Caan, A., Kessinger, A., Foley, J. F., Doyal, Y., Petrelli, N., Tormey, D., and Smith, T.: A phase II study of DTIC in the treatment of nonresectable islet cell carcinoma: An ECOG treatment protocol. Proc. Annual Meet. Am. Soc. Clin. Oncol., 9:A417, 1990.
123. Hamilton, I., Reis, L., Bilimoria, S., and Lang, R. G.: A renal vipoma. Br. Med. J., 281(6251):1323, 1980.
124. Hammer, R. A., and Leeman, S. E.: Neurotensin: Properties and Actions. *In* Gut Hormones 2nd Edition. Edited by S. R. Bloom and J. M. Polak. Edinburgh, Churchill Livingstone, 1981, p. 290.
125. Hammer, R. A., Leeman, S. E., Carraway, R., and Williams, R.: Isolation of human intestinal neurotensin. J. Biol. Chem., 255:2476, 1980.
126. Hancke, S.: Localization of hormone-producing gastrointestinal tumors by ultrasonic scanning. Scand. J. Gastroenterol., 14(Suppl. 53):115, 1979.
127. Hanssen, L. E., Schrumpf, E., Kolbenstvedt, A. N., Tausjo, J., and Dolva, L. O.: Treatment of malignant metastatic midgut carcinoid tumours with recombinant human alfa-2b interferon with or without hepatic artery embolization. Scand. J. Gastroenterol., 24:787, 1989.
128. Hengl, G., Prager, J., and Pointner, H.: The influence of somatostatin on the absorption of triglycerides in partially gastrectomized subjects. Acta Hepato-Gastroenterologica, 26:392, 1979.
129. Heyder, N.: Localization of an insulinoma by ultrasonic endoscopy. N. Engl. J. Med., 312:860, 1985.
130. Higgins, G. A., Recant, L., and Fischman, A. B.: The glucagonoma syndrome: Surgical curable diabetes. Am. J. Surg., 137:142, 1979.
131. Hoefnagel, C. A., Marcuse, H. R., DeKraker, J., and Voute, P. A.: Detection of neuroblastoma with 1-131-meta-iodobenzylguanidine. Clin. Biol. Res., 175:389, 1985.
132. Hoefnagel, C. A., Den Hartog Jager, F. C. A., Taal, B. G., Abeling, N. G. G. M., and Engelsman, E. E.: The role of 1-131-MIBG in the diagnosis and therapy of carcinoids. Eur. J. Nucl. Med., 13:187, 1987.
133. Hoefnagel, C. A., Den Hartog Jager, F. C. A., Van Gennip, A. M., Marcuse, H. R., and Taal, B. G.: Diagnosis and treatment of a carcinoid tumor using iodine 131 metaiodobenzyl-guanidine. Clin. Nucl. Med., 11:150, 1986.
134. Hoefnagel, C. A., Voute, P. A., DeKraker, J., and Marcuse, H. R.: Radionuclide diagnosis and therapy of neural crest tumors using Iodine-131 metaiodobenzylguanidine. J. Nucl. Med., 28:308, 1987.
135. Hofeldt, F. D., Dippe, S. E., Levin, S. R., Karam, J. H., Blum, M. R., and Forsham, P. H.: Effects of diphenylhydantoin upon glucose-induced insulin secretion in three patients with insulinoma. Diabetes, 23:192, 1973.
136. Hoitsma, H. F., Cuesta, M. A., Starink, T. M., Uttendorfsky-Vander, Putten, H. J., and Vander Veen, E. A.: Zinc deficiency syndrome versus glucagonoma syndrome. Arch. Chir. Neerlandicum, 13:131, 1979.
137. Holst, J. J.: Possible entries to the diagnosis of a glucagon-producing tumour. Scand. J. Gastroent., 53(Suppl.):53, 1979.
138. Iida, Y., Nose, O., Kai, H., Okada, A., Mori, T., Lee, P. K., Kakudo, K., and Yangihara, N.: Watery diarrhea with a vasoactive intestinal peptide-producing ganglioneuroblastoma. Arch. Dis. Child., 55:929, 1980.
139. Ingemansson, S., Kuhl, C., Larsson, L., Lunderquist, A., and Lunderquist, I.: Localization of insulinomas and islet cell hyperplasia by pancreatic vein catheterization and insulin assay. Surg. Gynecol. Obstet., 146:725, 1978.
140. Ingemansson, S., Larsson, L. I., and Stadil, F.: Pancreatic vein catheterization with gastrin assay in normal patients and patients with Zollinger-Ellison Syndrome. Am. J. Surg., 134:558, 1977.
141. Jackson, J., Raju, U., Janakivamon, N., Faichney, D., Mellinger, R. C., Lloyd, R. V., and Vinik, A. I.: Metastatic pulmonary somatostatin present with diabetic ketoacidosis; clinical, biochemical and morphologic characterization. Clin. Res., 34:196A, 1986.
142. Jensen, R. T., Gardner, J. D., Raufman, J. P., Pandol, S. J., and Doppmann, J. L.: Zollinger-Ellison Syndrome: Current concepts and management. Ann. Int. Med., 98:59, 1983.
143. Johnson, J. A., Fabri, P. J., Lott, J. A.: Serum gastrins in Zollinger-Ellison syndrome—identification of localized disease. Clin. Chem., 26:867, 1980.
144. Kaplan, E. L., Jaffe, B. M., and Peskin, G. W.: A new provocative test for the diagnosis of carcinoid syndrome. Am. J. Surg., 123:173, 1972.
145. Kaplan, E., and Lee, C. H.: Recent advances in the diagnosis and treatment of insulinomas. Surg. Clin. North Am., 59:119, 1979.
146. Kaplan, S. J., Holbrook, C. T., McDaniel, H. G., Buntain, W. L., and Crist, W. M.: Vasoactive intestinal peptide secreting tumors of childhood. Am. J. Dis. Child., 134:21, 1980.
147. Katz, L. B., Aufses, A. H., Rayfield, E., and Mitty, H.: Preoperative localization and intraoperative monitoring in the management of patients with pancreatic insulinoma. Surg. Gynecol. Obstet., 163:509, 1986.
148. Kelsen, D. P., Cheng, E., and Kemeny, N.: Streptozotocin and adriamycin in the treatment of apud tumors (carcinoid, islet cell, and medullary carcinomas of the thyroid). Proc. Amer. Assoc. Cancer Res., 23:433, 1982.
149. Kelsen, D., Fiore, J., Heelan, R., Cheng, E., and Magill, G.: Phase II trial of etoposide in APUD tumors. Cancer Treat. Rep., 71:305, 1987.
150. Kessinger, A., Foley, J. F., and Lemon, H. M.: Therapy of malignant APUD cell tumors. Effectiveness of DTIC. Cancer, 51:790, 1983.
151. Khandekar, J. D., Oyer, D., Miller, H. J., and Vick, N. A.: Neurologic involvement in glucagonoma syndrome. Response to combination chemotherapy with 5-fluorouracil and streptozotocin. Cancer, 44:2014, 1979.
152. Kimmel, J., Pollack, H., and Hazelwood, R.: Isolation and characterization of chicken insulin. Endocrinology, 83:1323, 1968.
153. Koelz, A., Kraenzlin, M., Gyr, K., Meier, V., Bloom, S. R., Heitz, P., and Stalder, H.: Escape of the response to a long-acting somatostatin analogue (Sandostatin) in patients with VIPoma. Gastroenterol., 92:527, 1987.
154. Kothary, P. C., Fabri, P. J., Gower, W., O'Dorisio, T. M., Ellis, J., and Vinik, A. I.: Evaluation of NH_2-terminus gastrins in gastrinoma syndrome. J. Clin. Endocrinol. Metab., 62:970, 1986.
155. Kraenzlin, M. E., Ch'ng, K. C., Wood, S. M., Carr, D. H., and Bloom, S. R.: Long-term treatment of a VIPoma with somatostatin analogue resulting in remission of symptoms and possible shrinkage of metastases. Gastroenterol., 88:185, 1985.
156. Kraft, A. R., Tompkins, R. K., and Zollinger, R.: Recognition and management of the diarrheal syndrome caused by non-beta cell tumors of the pancreas. Am. J. Surg., 119:163, 1970.
157. Krejs, G. J., Orci, L., Conlon, M., Ravazzola, M., Davis, G. R., Raskin, P., Collins, S. M., McCarthy, D. M., Baeten, S. D., Rubenstein, A., Aldor, T. A., and Unger, R. H.: Somatostatinoma syndrome (biochemical, morphological, and clinical features). N. Engl. J. Med., 301:285, 1979.
158. Kressel, H. Y.: Strategies for magnetic resonance imaging of focal liver disease. Radiologic Clinics of North America, 26:607, 1988.
159. Krudy, A. G., Doppmann, J. L., and Jensen, R. T.: Localization of islet tumors by dynamic CT: Comparison with plain CT, arteriorgraphy, sonography and venous sampling. Am. J. Radiol., 143:585, 1984.
160. Kudo, K., Kitajima, S., Munakata, H., and Yagihashi, S.: WDHA syndrome caused by VIP-producing ganglioneuroblastoma. J. Ped. Surg., 17:426, 1982.
161. Kurose, T., Seino, Y., Ishida, H., Fujita, J., Taminato, T., Matsukura, M., and Imura, H.: Successful treatment of metastatic glucagonoma with dacarbazine. Lancet, 1:621, 1984.
162. Kvols, L. K.: Metastatic carcinoid tumors and the carcinoid syndrome. A selective review of chemotherapy and hormonal therapy. Amer. J. Med., 81(Suppl. 6b):49, 1986.
163. Kvols, L. K.: Therapy of the malignant carcinoid syndrome. Endocrinology and Metabolism Clinics of North America, 18:557, 1989.
164. Kvols, L. K., and Buck, M.: Chemotherapy of endocrine malignancies: A review. Sem. Oncol., 14:343, 1987.
165. Kvols, L. K., Buck, M., Moertel, C. G., Schutt, A. S., Rubin, J., O'Connel, M. J., and Hahn, R. G.: Treatment of metastatic islet cell carcinoma with a somatostatin analogue (SMS 201-995). Ann. Int. Med., 107:162, 1987.
166. Kvols, L. K., Martin, J. K., March, K. M., and Moertel, C. G.: Rapid reversal of carcinoid crisis with a somatostatin analogue. N. Engl. J. Med., 313:1229, 1985.

167. Kvols, L. K., Moertel, C. G., O'Connell, M. J., Schutt, A. J., Rubin, J., and Hahn, R.: Treatment of the malignant carcinoid syndrome. Evaluation of a long-acting somatostatin analogue. N. Engl. J. Med., 315:663, 1986.
168. Lamers, C. B., Buis, J. T., and Van Tongeren, J. H.: Secretin-stimulated serum gastrin levels in hyperparathyroid patients from families with multiple endocrine adenomatosis-type 1. Ann. Intern. Med., 86:719, 1977.
169. Landor, J. H.: Control of the Zollinger-Ellison syndrome by excision of primary and metastatic tumor. Am. J. Surg., 147:406, 1984.
170. Larsson, C., Skogseid, B., Oberg, K., Nakamura, Y., and Nordenskjold, M.: Multiple endocrine neoplasia type 1 gene maps to chromosome 11 and is lost in insulinoma. Nature, 332:85, 1988.
171. Larsson, L. I.: Two distinct types of islet abnormalities associated with endocrine pancreatic tumors. Virchows Arch. (Pathol. Anat.), 376:209, 1977.
172. Larsson, L. I., Hirsch, M. A., Holst, J., Ingemansson, S., Kuhl, C., Jensen, S. L., Lundquist, G., Rehfeld, J. F., and Schwartz, T. W.: Pancreatic somtatostatinoma clinical features and physiologic implications. Lancet, 1:666, 1977.
173. Larsson, L. I., Schwartz, T., Lundquist, G., Chance, R. E., Sundler, F., Rehfeld, J. F., Grimelius, L., Fahrenkrug, J., Schaffalitzky de Muckadell, O., and Moon, N.: Pancreatic polypeptide in pancreatic endocrine tumors, possible implication in watery diarrhea syndrome. Am. J. Pathol., 85:675, 1976.
174. Le Douarin, N. M., and Teillet, M. A.: The migration of neural crest cells to the wall of the digestive tract in avian embryo. J. Embryol. Exp. Morphol., 30:31, 1973.
175. Le Quesne, L. P., Nabarro, J. D. N., Kurtz, A., and Zweig, S.: The management of insulin tumors of the pancreas. Br. J. Surg., 66:373, 1979.
176. Leichter, S. B.: Clinical and metabolic aspects of glucagonoma. Medicine, 59:100, 1980.
177. Long, R. G., Byrant, M. G., Mitchell, S. J., Adrian, T. E., Polak, J. M., and Bloom, S. R.: Clinicopathological study of pancreatic and ganglioneuroblastoma tumours secreting vasoactive intestinal polypeptide (vipomas). Br. Med. J., 282:1767, 1981.
178. Lucas, K. J., and Feldman, J. M.: Flushing in the carcinoid syndrome and plasma kallikrein. Cancer, 58:2290, 1986.
179. Lumbroso, J., Guermazi, F., Hartmann, O., Coonaert, S., Rabarison, Y., Lemerle, J., and Parmentier, C.: Sensitivity and specificity of metaiodobenzylguanidine (MIBG) scintigraphy in the evaluation of neuroblastoma: analysis of 115 cases. Bull. Cancer, 75:97, 1988.
180. Lunderquist, A., and Tylen, U.: Phlebography of the pancreatic veins. Radiologe, 15:198, 1975.
181. Machina, T., Marcus, R., and Levin, S. R.: Inhibition of glucagon secretion by diphenylhydantoin in a patient with glucagonoma. West. J. Med., 132:357, 1980.
182. Maier, W., Schumacher, A., Etzrodt, H., and Arlart, I.: A neurotensinoma of the head of the pancreas: Demonstration by ultrasound and computed tomography. Europ. J. Radiol., 2:125, 1982.
183. Malagelada, J. R., Edis, A. J., Adson, M. A., Van Heerden, J. A., and Go, V. L.: Medical and surgical options in the management of patients with gastrinoma. Gastroenterol., 84:1524, 1983.
184. Manche, A., Wood, S. M., Adrian, T. E., Welbourn, K. B., and Bloom, S. R.: Pancreatic polypeptide and calcitonin secretion from a pancreatic tumor-clinical improvement after hepatic artery embolization. Postgrad. Med. J., 59:313, 1983.
185. Mandarino, L., Stenner, D., Blanchard, W., Nissen, S., Gevich, J., Ling, N., Brazeau, P., Bohlen, P., Esen, F., and Guillemer, R.: Selective effects of somatostatin-14, -25 and -28 on in vitro insulin and glucagon secretion. Nature, 291:76, 1981.
186. Marks, I. N., Bank, S., and Louw, J. H.: Islet cell tumor of the pancreas with reversible watery diarrhea and achlorhydria. Gastroenterol., 52:695, 1967.
187. Marlink, R. G., Lokich, J. J., Robins, J. R., and Clouse, M. E.: Hepatic arterial embolization for metastatic hormone-secreting tumors. Cancer, 65:2227, 1990.
188. Marx, S. J., Sakaguchi, K., Green, J., III, Aurbach, G. D., and Brandi, M. L.: Mitogenic activity on parathyroid cells in plasma from members of a large kindred with multiple endocrine neoplasia Type 1. J. Clin. Endocrinol. Metab., 67:149, 1988.
189. Marx, S. J., Vinik, A. I., Santen, R. J., Floyd, J. C., Jr., Mills, J., and Green, J., III: Multiple endocrine neoplasia type 1: Assessment of laboratory tests to screen for the gene in a large kindred. Medicine, 65:226, 1986.
190. Marynick, S. P., Fagadau, W. R., and Duncan, L. A.: Malignant glucagonoma syndrome: Response to chemotherapy. Ann. Int. Med., 93:453, 1980.
191. Mashford, M. L., Nilsson, G., Rokaeus, A., and Rossell, S.: The effect of food ingestion on circulating neurotensin-like immunoreactivity in human. Acta Physiol. Scand., 104:244, 1978.
192. Maton, P. N., Camilleri, M., Griffin, G., Hodgson, H., Allison, D. J., and Chadwick, V. S.: The role of hepatic arterial embolization in the carcinoid syndrome. Br. Med. J., Clin. Res., 287:932, 1983.
193. Maton, P. N., Gardner, J. D., and Jensen, R. T.: Diagnosis and management of Zollinger-Ellison Syndrome. Endocrinol. Metab. Clinics NA, 18:519, 1989.
194. Maton, P. N., Vinayek, R., Frucht, H., McArthur, R. A., Miller, L. S., Saced, Z. A., Gardner, J. D., and Jensen, R. T.: Long-term efficacy and safety of one prazole in patients with Zollinger-Ellison syndrome. Gastroenterol., 97:827, 1989.
195. Matsumoto, K. D., Peter, J. B., Schultze, R. G., Hakin, A. A., and Frank, P. T.: Watery diarrhea and hypokalemia associated with pancreatic islet cell adenoma. Gastroenterol., 52:965, 1967.
196. McCarthy, D. M.: Report on the U. S. experience with cimetidine in Zollinger-Ellison syndrome and other hypersecretory states. Gastroenterol., 74:453, 1978.
197. McCarthy, D. M., and Jensen, R. T.: Zollinger-Ellison syndrome: Current Issues. *In* Hormone Producing Tumors of the Gastrointestinal Tract. Edited by S. Cohen and R. Soloway. New York, Churchill Livingstone, 1985, p. 25.
198. McCarthy, D. M., Weintraub, B., and Rosen, S.: Subunits of human chorionic gonadotropin in the Zollinger-Ellison syndrome. Gastroenterol., 76:1198, 1979.
199. McEwan, A. J., Shapiro, B., Sisson, J. C., Beierwaltes, W. H., and Akery, D. M.: Radioiodo-benzylguanidine for the scintigraphic location and therapy of adrenergic tumors. Sem. Nucl. Med., 15:132, 1985.
200. McGavran, M. H., Unger, R. H., Recant, L., Polk, H. C., Kilo, C., and Levin, M. E.: A glucagon-secreting alpha-cell carcinoma of the pancreas. N. Engl. J. Med., 274:1408, 1966.
201. McLeod, M. K., Fukuuchi, A., Warnock, M., Tutera, A., and Vinik, A. I.: Mechanisms of stimulatory and inhibitory effects of somatostatin on cell proliferation in rat insulinoma (RIN m5F) cell line. Abstract, 1991.
202. Mekhjian, H. S., and O'Dorisio, T. M.: VIPoma syndrome. Sem. Oncol., 14:282, 1987.
203. Melia, W. M., Nunnerley, H. B., Johnson, P. J., and Williams, R.: Use of arterial devascularization and cytotoxic drugs in 30 patients with the carcinoid syndrome. Br. J. Cancer, 46:331, 1982.
204. Melmon, K. L., Sjoerdsma, A., Oates, J. A., and Laster, L.: Treatment of malabsorption and diarrhea of carcinoid syndrome with methysergide. Gastroenterol., 48:18, 1965.
205. Mengel, C. E., and Shaffer, R. D.: The Carcinoid Syndrome. *In* Cancer Medicine. 2nd ed. Edited by J. F. Holland and E. Frei, Philadelphia, Lea & Febiger, 1973, p. 1584.
206. Mignon, M., Ruszniewski, P., Haffar, S., Rigaud, D., Rene, E., and Bonfils, S.: Current approach to the management of tumoral process in patients with gastrinoma. World J. Surg., 10:703, 1086.
207. Mignon, M., Vallot, T., Hervoir, P., et al.: Ranirtidine Versus Cinetidine in the Management of Zollinger-Ellison Syndrome. *In* Ranitidine. Edited by A. J. Riley and P. R. Salmon. Proceedings of an International Symposium, World Congress of Enterology, Excerpta Medica, Amsterdam, p. 169, 1982.
208. Millan, V. G., Urosa, C. L., Molitch, M. E., Miller, H., and Jackson, I. M.: Localization of occult insulinoma by superselective pancreatic venous sampling for insulin assay through percutaneous transhepatic catheterization. Diabetes, 28:249, 1979.
209. Mills, S. R., Doppmann, J. L., Dunnick, N. R., and McCarthy, D. M.: Evaluation of angiography in Zollinger-Ellison syndrome. Radiology, 131:317, 1979.
210. Mitchenere, P., Adrian, T. E., Kirk, R. M., and Bloom, S. R.: Effect of gut regulatory peptides on intestinal luminal fluid in the rat. Life Sci., 29:1563, 1981.
211. Miyata, M., Nakao, K., Sakamoto, T., Tsumori, T., Hamaji, M., Himeno, S., and Kawashima, Y.: Removal of mesenteric gastrinoma: a case report. Surgery, 99:245, 1986.
212. Miyaura, C., et al.: Expression of *reg*/PSP, a pancreatic exocrine gene: Relationship to changes in islet b-cell mass. Mol. Endocrinol. (In Press), 1991.
213. Moattari, A. R., Cho, K., and Vinik, A. I.: Sandostatin in treatment of co-existing glucagonoma and pancreatic pseudocyst dissociation of responses. Surgery, 108:581, 1990.
214. Modlin, I. M.: Carcinoid syndrome. J. Clin. Gastroenterol., 2:349, 1980.
215. Modlin, I. M.: Endocrine tumors of the pancreas. Surg. Gynecol. Obstet., 149:751, 1979.
216. Modlin, I. M., and Bloom, S. R.: VIPomas and the watery diarrhea syndrome. S. Afr. Med. J., 54:53, 1978.
217. Modlin, I. M., Bloom, S. R., and Mitchell, S. J.: Experimental evidence for VIP as the cause of the watery diarrhea syndrome. Gastroenterol., 75:1051, 1978.
218. Modlin, I. M., Bloom, S. R., and Mitchell, S. J.: Plasma vasocative intestinal polypeptide (VIP) levels and intestinal ischemia. Experientia, 34:535, 1978.
219. Modlin, I. M., Mitchell, S. J., and Bloom, S. R.: The Systemic Release and Pharmacokinetics of VIP. *In* Gut Hormones. Edited by S. R. Bloom. Edinburgh, New York, Churchill Livingstone, 1978.
220. Moertel, C. G.: An odyssey in the land of small tumors. J. Clin. Oncol., 5:1502, 1987.
221. Moertel, C. G.: Treatment of the carcinoid tumor and the malignant carcinoid syndrome. J. Clin. Oncol., 1:727, 1983.
222. Moertel, C. G., and Hanley, J. A.: Combination chemotherapy trials in metastatic carcinoid tumor and the malignant carcinoid syndrome. Cancer Clin. Trials, 2:327, 1979.
223. Moertel, C. G., Hanley, J. A., and Johnson, L. A.: Streptozocin alone compared with streptoxocin plus fluorouracil in the treatment of advanced islet-cell carcinoma. N. Engl. J. Med., 303:1189, 1980.
224. Moertel, C. G., Lavin, P. T., and Hahn, R. G.: Phase II trial of doxorubicin therapy for advanced islet cell carcinoma. Cancer Treat. Rep., 66:1567, 1982.
225. Moertel, C. G., May, G. R., Martin, J. K., Rubin, J., and Schutt, A. J.: Sequential hepatic artery occlusion (HAO) and chemotherapy for metastatic carcinoid tumor and islet cell carcinoma (ICC). Proc. Am. Soc. Clin. Oncol., 4:80, 1985.
226. Moertel, C. G., Rubin, J., and Kvols, L. K.: Therapy of metastatic carcinoid tumor and the malignant carcinoid syndrome with recombinant leukocyte A interferon. J. Clin. Oncol., 7:865, 1989.
227. Moertel, C. G., Rubin, J., and O'Connell, M. J.: A phase II study of cisplatin therapy in patients with metastatic carcinoid tumor and the malignant carcinoid syndrome. Cancer Treat. Rep., 70:1459, 1986.
228. Montenegro, F., Lawrence, G. D., Macon, W., and Pass, C.: Metastatic glucagonoma. Improvement after surgical debulking. Am. J. Surg., 139:424, 1980.
229. Morowitz, D. A., and Levine, A. E.: Malignant Zollinger-Ellison syndrome: remission of primary and metastatic pancreatic tumor after gastrectomy: report of a case and review of the literature. Am. J. Gastroenterol., 81:471, 1986.
230. Murray, J. S., Paton, R. R., and Pope, C. E.: Pancreatic tumor associated with flushing and diarrhea. Report of a case. N. Engl. J. Med., 264:436, 1961.
231. Murray-Lyon, I. M., Eddleston, A. L., Williams, R., Brown, M., Hogbin, B. M., Bennett, A., Edwards, J. C., and Taylor, K. W.: Treatment of multiple hormone producing malignant islet cell tumour with streptozotocin. Lancet, 2:895, 1968.
232. Nagai, K., and Frohman, L. A.: Hyperglycemia and hyperglucagonemia following neurotensin administration. Life Sci., 19:273, 1976.
233. Neri, V., Bartorelli, A., and Faglia, G.: Effect of propranolol on the blood sugar, immunoreactive blood insulin in a patient with insulinoma. Acta Diabetol. Lat., 6:809, 1969.
234. Novin, A., Berg, M., Ericsson, M. M., Ingemannsson, S., Olsson, E., and Sundler, F.: Pancreatic polypeptide-producing tumors, report on two cases. Cancer, 53:2688, 1984.
235. Nobin, A., Mansson, B., and Lunderquist, A.: Evaluation of temporary liver dearterialization and embolization in patients with metastatic carcinoid tumour. Acta Oncol., 28:419, 1989.
236. Norheim, I., Theodorsson-Norheim, E., Brodin, E., and Oberg, K.: Tachykinins in carcinoid tumors: their use as a tumor marker and possible role in the carcinoid flush. J. Clin. Endocrinol. Metab., 63:605, 1986.
237. Norton, J. A., Doppmann, J. L., Collen, M. J., Harmon, J. W., Maton, P. N., Gardner, J. D., and Jensen, R. T.: Prospective study of gastrinoma localization and resection in patients with Zollinger-Ellison syndrome. Ann. Surg., 204:468, 1986.
238. Norton, J. A., Doppmann, J. L., Collen, M. J., et al.: Prospective study of gastrinoma localization and resection in patients with Zollinger-Ellison Syndrome. Ann. Surg. (In press).
239. Norton, J. A., Kahn, C. R., Schiebinger, R., Gorschboth, C., and Brennan, M. F.: Acid deficiency and the skin rash associated with glucagonoma. Ann. Int. Med., 91:213, 1979.

240. Norton, J. A., Sigel, B., Baker, A. R., Ettinghausen, S. E., Shawker, T. H., Krudy, A. G., Doppmann, J. L., Taylor, S. I., and Gordon, P.: Localization of an occult insulinoma by intraoperative ultrasonography. Surgery, 97:381, 1985.
241. Norton, J. A., Sugarbaker, P. H., Doppmann, J. L., Wesley, R. A., Maton, P. N., Gardner, J. D., and Jensen, R. T.: Aggressive resection of metastatic disease in selected patients with malignant gastrinoma. Ann. Surg., 203:352, 1986.
242. O'Dorisio, T. M., and Vinik, A. I.: Pancreatic polypeptide and mixed peptide-producing tumors of the gastrointestinal tract. *In* Contemporary Issues in Gastroenterology. Edited by S. Cohen and R. D. Soloway. New York, Churchill-Livingstone, 1985, p. 117.
243. O'Stern, W. K., Barnard, J. L., Jr., and Yates, R. D.: Morphologic changes in skeletal muscle induced by serotonin treatment, a light and electron microscopy study. Exp. Molec. Path., 7:145, 1967.
244. Oates, J. A., Pettinger, W. A., and Doctor, R. B.: Evidence for the release of bradykinin in the carcinoid syndrome. J. Clin. Invest., 45:173, 1966.
245. Oberg, K., and Eriksson, B.: Medical treatment of neuroendocrine gut and pancreatic tumors. Acta Oncol., 28:425, 1989.
246. Oberg, K., Alm, G., Magnusson, A., Lundqvist, G., Theodorsson, E., Wide, L., and Wilander, E.: Treatment of malignant carcinoid tumors with recombinant interferon alfa-2b: Development of neutralizing interferon antibodies and possible loss of antitumor activity. J. Natl. Cancer Inst., 81(7):531, 1989.
247. Oberhelman, H. A.: Excisional therapy for ulcerogenic tumors of the duodenum—long-term results. Archiv. Surg., 104:447, 1972.
248. Osei, K., and O'Dorisio, T. M.: Malignant insulinoma: effects of a somatostatin analogue (compound 201-995) on serum glucose, growth and gastro-entero-pancreatic hormones. Ann. Int. Med., 103:223, 1985.
249. Owerbach, D., Bell, G. I., Rutter, W. J., Brown, J. A., and Shows, T. B.: The insulin gene is activated on the short arm of chromosome 11 in humans. Diabetes, 30:267, 1981.
250. Passaro, E., Jr.: Localization of pancreatic endocrine tumors by selective portal vein catheterization and radioimmunoassay. Gastroenterol., 77:806, 1979.
251. Pauwels, S., Desmond, H., Dimaline, R., and Dockray, G. J.: Identification of progastrin in gastrinomas, antrum, and duodenum by a novel radioimmunoassay. J. Clin. Invest., 77:376, 1986.
252. Pearse, A. G. E.: Common cytochemical and ultrastructural characteristics of cells producing polypeptide hormones (the APUD series) and their relevance to thyroid and ultimobronchial C cells and calcitonin. Proc. R. Soc. Lond. (Biol.), 170:71, 1968.
253. Penman, E., Wass, J. A. U., Besser, G. M., and Rees, L. U.: Somatostatin secretion by lung and thymic tumors. Clin. Endocrinol., 13:613, 1980.
254. Pernow, B., and Waldenstrom, J.: Determination of 5-hydroxytryptamine, 5-hydroxyindoleacetic acid and histamine in 33 cases of carcinoid (argentaffinoma). Am. J. Med., 53:16, 1957.
255. Pictet, R. L., Rall, L. B., Phelps, P., and Rutter, W. J.: The neural crest and the origin of the insulin-producing and other gastrointestinal hormone-producing cells. Science, 191:191, 1967.
256. Pictet, R., and Rutter, W. J.: Development of the embryonic endocrine pancreas. *In* Handbook of Physiology, Session 7. Edited by J. Field. Baltimore, American Physiological Society, 1972, p. 25.
257. Pipeleers, D., Couturier, E., Gepts, W., Reynders, J., and Somers, G.: Five cases of somatostatinoma: Clinical heterogeneity and diagnostic usefulness of basal and tolbutamide-induced hypersomatostatinemia. J. Clin. Endocrinol. Metab., 56:1236, 1983.
258. Polak, J. M., Bloom, S. R., Adrian, T. E., Heitz, P., Bryant, M. G., and Pearse, A. G. E.: Pancreatic polypeptide in insulinomas, gastrinomas, vipomas, and glucagonomas. Lancet, 1:328, 1976.
259. Polak, J. M., Sullivan, S. N., Bloom, S. R., Buchan, A. M., Facer, P., Brown, M. R., and Pearse, A. G.: Specific localization of neurotensin to the N cell in human intestine by radioimmunoassay and immunocytochemistry. Nature, 270:183, 1977.
260. Poole, C. J. M.: Myelopathy secondary to metastatic carcinoid tumors. J. Neurol. Neurosur. Psychiatry, 47:1359, 1984.
261. Pour, P., Mohr, U., Cardesa, A., Althoff, J., and Kruger, F. W.: Pancreatic neoplasms in an animal model: Morphological, biological and comparative studies. Cancer, 36:379, 1975.
262. Priest, W. M., and Alexander, M. K.: Islet-cell tumor of the pancreas with peptic ulceration, diarrhea, and hypokalemia. Lancet, 2:1145, 1957.
263. Quint, L. E., Glaser, G. M., Francis, I. R., Vinik, A. I., and Thompson, N. W.: MR imaging and CT of pancreatic and extrapancreatic GI endocrine tumors: A comparative study. Scientific Assembly of the Radiol. Soc. of N. A., (Abstract), 1986.
264. Rakieten, N., Rakieten, M. L., and Nadkani, M. V.: Studies of the diabetogenic action of streptozotocin (NSC-37917). Cancer Chemother. Rep., 29:91, 1969.
265. Rambaud, J. C., Modiglioni, R., Matuchansky, C., Bloom, S. R., Said, S. I., Pessayre, D., and Bernier, J. J.: Pancreatic cholera: Studies on turmoral secretions and pathophysiology of diarrhea. Gastroenterol., 69:110, 1975.
266. Reubi, J. C.: Use of Receptor Autoradiography for the Visualization of Somatostatin Receptors in Human Pituitary Adenomas and Other Neuroendocrine Tumors. (Abstract No. S17), J. Endocr. Invest., 12:18, 1989.
267. Richter, G., Stockman, F., Lembeke, B., Conlon, J. M., and Creutzfeldt, W.: Short-term administration of somatostatin analogue SMS 201-995 in patients with carcinoid tumors. Scand. J. Gastroenterol., 21:193, 1986.
268. Robins, J. M., Bookstein, J. J., Oberman, H. A., and Fajans, S. S.: Selective angiography in localizing islet cell tumors of the pancreas: A further appraisal. Radiology, 106:525, 1973.
269. Roche, A., Raissonnier, A., and Gillon-Savouret, M. C.: Pancreatic venous sampling and arteriography in the localising insulinomas and gastrinomas: procedure and results in 55 cases. Radiology, 145:621, 1982.
270. Roos, B. A., Lindall, A. W., Ells, J., Elde, R., Lambert, P. N., and Birnbaum, R. S.: Increased plasma and tumor somatostatin-like immunoreactivity in medullary thyroid carcinoma and small cell lung cancer. J. Clin. Endocrinol. Metab., 52:187, 1981.
271. Rosenberg, L., Duguid, W. P., Brown, R. A., and Vinik, A. I.: Induction of neuroblastosis will reverse diabetes in the Syrian golden hamster. Diabetes, 37:334, 1988.
272. Rosenberg, L., Duguid, W. P., and Vinik, A. I.: Cell proliferation in the pancreas of the Syrian golden hamster. Dig. Dis. Sci., 32:1185, 1987.
273. Rosenberg, L., and Vinik, A. I.: Regulation of pancreatic islet growth and differentiation: Evidence for paracrine and/or autocrine growth factor(s). Clinical Research, 38:271A, 1990.
274. Rubenstein, A. H., Kuzuya, H., and Horowtiz, D. L.: Clinical significance of circulating C-peptide in diabetes mellitus and hypoglycemic disorders. Arch. Inter. Med., 137:625, 1977.
275. Rueckert, K. F., Klotter, H. J., and Kummerle, F.: Intraoperative ultrasonic localization of endocrine tumors of the pancreas. Surgery, 96:1045, 1984.
276. Said, S. I.: Vasoactive intestinal polypeptide: Elevated plasma and tissue levels in the watery diarrhea syndrome due to pancreatic and other tumors. (From the VA Hospital and Dept. of Internal Med. and Pharm., Univ. of Texas Southwestern Med. School, Dallas, Texas).
277. Said, S. I., and Mutt, V.: Isolation from porcine intestinal wall of a vasoactive octacospeptide related to secretin and to glucagon. Eur. J. Biochem., 28:129, 1972.
278. Saito, S., Saito, H., Matsumura, M., and Sano, T.: Molecular heterogeneity and biological activity of immunoreactive somatostatin in medullary carcinoma of the thyroid. J. Clin. Endocrinol. Metab., 53:1117, 1981.
279. Samols, E., Weir, G. C., Ramseur, R., Day, J. A., and Patel, Y. C.: Modulation of pancreatic somatostatin by adrenergic and cholinergic agonism and by hyper- and hypoglycemic sulfonamides. Metabolism, 24:1219, 1978.
280. Sandler, M., Karim, S. M., and Williams, E. D.: Prostaglandin in amine-peptide-secreting tumors. Lancet, 2:1053, 1968.
281. Sano, T., Kagawa, N., Hizawa, K., et. al.: Demonstration of somatostatin production in medullary carcinoma of the thyroid. Jpn. J. Clin. Oncol., 10:221, 1980.
282. Santangelo, W. C., O'Dorisio, T. M., Kim, J. G., Severino, G., and Krejs, G. J.: Pancreatic cholera syndrome-effect of a synthetic somatostatin analogue on intestinal water and ion transport. Am. Intern. Med., 103:363, 1985.
283. Santangelo, W. C., Unger, R. H., Orci, L., Pueno, M. I., Popma, J. J., and Krejs, G. J.: Somatostatin analogue-induced remission of necrolytic migratory erythema without changes in plasma glucagon concentration. Pancreas, 1:464, 1986.
284. Sarvetnick, N.: Islet cell destruction and regeneration in IFN-g transgenic mice (Abstract). J. Cell Biochem., CB019:49, 1991.
285. Schein, P. S., Kahn, R., Gorden, P., Wells, S., and DeVita, V. T.: Streptozotocin for malignant insulinomas and carcinoid tumors. Arch. Intern. Med., 132:555, 1973.
286. Schein, P. S.: Chemotherapeutic management of the hormone-secreting endocrine malignancies. Cancer, 30:1616, 1972.
287. Schusdziarra, V., Zyznar, E., Rouiller, D., Boden, G., Brown, J. C., Arimura, A., and Unger, R. H.: Splanchnic somatostatin: A hormonal regulator of nutrient homeostasis. Science, 207:530, 1980.
288. Schwartz, T. W.: Atropine suppression test for pancreatic polypeptide. Lancet, 2:43, 1978.
289. Shaklai, M., Aderka, D., Blum, I., Laron, Z., Asheror, J., Doron, M., Atsmon, A., and Pinkhas, J.: Suppression of hypoglycemia attacks and insulin release by propranolol in a patient with metastatic malignant insulinoma. Diabetes Metab., 3:155, 1977.
290. Shapiro, B.: MIBG in the diagnosis and therapy of neuroblastoma and pheo-chromocytoma. *In* Proceedings of the International Symposium on Recent Advance in Nuclear Medicine. Edited by E. Cattaruzi, E. Englaro, and O. Geatti. Surin. Biomedica, Udine, Italy, p. 11, 1987.
291. Shapiro, B.: MIBG in the management of neuroendocrine tumors. Presented at International Congress on Advances in Management of Malignancies. Ascoli Piceno, Italy. Conference Abstracts, p. 129, 1988.
292. Shapiro, B., and Sisson, J. C.: Sympatho-adrenal imaging with radioiodinated metaiodobenzylguanidine. *In* Atlas of Nuclear Medicine. Edited by D. Von Nostrand, and S. Baum. Philadelphia, J. B. Lippincott Co., 1988, p. 72.
293. Sheppard, M., Shapiro, B., Primstone, B., Kronhein, S., Berelowitz, M., and Gregory, M. J.: Metabolic clearance and plasma half disappearance time of exogenous somatostatin in man. Clinical Endocrinol. Metab., 48:50, 1979.
294. Shulkes, A., Boden, R., Cook, I., Gallagher, N., and Furness, J. B.: Characterization of a pancreatic tumor containing vasoactive intestinal peptide, neurotensin and pancreatic polypeptide. J. Clin. Endocrinol. Metab., 58:41, 1984.
295. Shulkin, B. L., Sisson, J. C., Koral, K. F., Shapiro, B., Wang, X., and Johnson, J.: Conjugate-view gamma camera method for estimating tumor uptake of Iodine-131-metaiodobenzylguanidine. J. Nucl. Med., 29:542, 1988.
296. Sigel, B., Coelho, J. C., Nyhus, L. M., Velasco, J. M., Donahue, P. E., Wood, D. K., and Spigos, D. G.: Detection of pancreatic tumors by ultrasound during surgery. Arch. Surg., 117:1058, 1982.
297. Simpson, S., Vinik, A. I., Marangos, P. J., and Lloyd, R. V.: Immunohistochemical localization of neuron-specific enolase in gastroentero-pancreatic neuroendocrine tumors. Correlation with tissue and serum levels of neuron-specific enolase. Cancer, 54:1364, 1984.
298. Sinzinger, H., Renner, F., and Granegger, S.: Unsuccessful 1-131-MIBG imaging of carcinoids and apudomas. J. Nucl. Med., 27:1221, 1986.
299. Sircus, W.: Vagotomy in Z E syndrome. Gastroenterol., 79:607, 1979.
300. Sisson, J. C., Hutchinson, R., Johnson, J., Mallette, S., Carey, J. E., Shapiro, B., and Beierwaltes, W. H.: Acute toxicity of therapeutic 1-131-MIBG relates more to whole body than to blood radiation dosimetry. J. Nucl. Med., 23:618, 1987.
301. Sisson, J. C., Shapiro, B., Beierwaltes, W. H., Glowniak, J. V., Nakajo, M., Mangner, T. J., Carey, J. E., Swanson, D. P., Copp, J. E., Satterlee, W. H., and Wieland, D. M.: Radiopharmaceutical treatment of malignant pheochromocytoma. J. Nucl. Med., 25:197, 1984.
302. Sisson, J. C., Shapiro, B., Beierwaltes, W. H., Nakajo, M., Glowniak, J., Mangner, T., Carey, J. E., Swanson, D. P., Copp, J., Satterlee, W., and Wieland, D. M.: Treatment of malignant pheochromocytoma with a new radiopharmaceutical. Trans. Assoc. Amer. Phys., 96:209, 1983.
303. Smith, F., Rosen, K., Villa-Kamoroff, L., Weir, G. C., and Bonner-Weir, S.: Enhanced IGF-I gene expression in regenerating rat pancreas is localized to capillaries and proliferating ductules. Diabetes, 39:66A, 1990.
304. Smith, D. B., Scarffe, J. H., Wagstaff, J., and Johnston, R. J.: Phase II trial of rDNA alfa 2b interferon in patients with malignant carcinoid tumor. Cancer Treat. Rep., 71:1265, 1987.
305. Snisky, C. A., Wolfe, M. M., Martin, J. L., Howe, B. A., O'Dorisio, T. M., McGuigan, J. E., and Mathias, J. R.: Myoelectric effects of vasoactive intestinal peptide of rabbit small intestine. Am. J. Physiol., 244:G46, 1983.
306. Solcia, E., Capella, C., Buffa, R., Frigerio, B., Usellini, L., and Fiocca, R.: Morphological and functional classification of endocrine cells and related growths in the gastrointestinal tract. *In* Gastrointestinal Hormones. Edited by G. B. J. Glass. New York, Raven Press, 1980, p. 1.

307. Stabile, B. E., Morrow, D. J., and Passaro, E., Jr.: The gastrinoma triangle: operative implications. Am. J. Surg., 147:25, 1984.
308. Stabile, B. E., and Passaro, E., Jr.: Benign and malignant gastrinoma. Am. J. Surg., 149:144, 1985.
309. Stage, J. G., and Stadil, F.: The clinical diagnosis of Zollinger-Ellison syndrome. Scand. J. Gastroenterol., 53:79, 1979.
310. Stefanini, P., Carboni, W., Patrassi, N., and Basoli, A.: Beta-islet cell tumors of the pancreas: Results of a study of 1,067 cases. Surgery, 75:597, 1974.
311. Stefanini, P., Carboni, W., Patrassi, N., and Benedetti-Valentini, F. J.: Surgical treatment and prognosis of insulinoma. Clin. Gastroenterol., 3:697, 1974.
312. Stockmann, F., Richter, G., Lembecke, B., Conlon, J. M., and Creutzfeldt, W.: Long-term treatment of patients with endocrine gastrointestinal tumors with the somatostatin analogue SMS 201-995. Scand. J. Gastroenterol., 21:230, 1986.
313. Strodel, W. E., Vinik, A. I., Jaffe, B. M., Eckhauser, F., and Thompson, N. W.: Substance P in localization of carcinoid tumors. J. Surg. Oncol., 27:106, 1984.
314. Strodel, W. E., Vinik, A. I., Thompson, N. W., Eckhauser, F. E., and Talpos, G. B.: Small bowel carcinoid tumors and the carcinoid syndrome. *In* Endocrine Surgery Update. Edited by N. W. Thompson and A. I. Vinik. New York, Grune & Stratton, 1983, p. 293.
315. Sundler, F., Alumets, J., and Hakanson, R.: Peptides in the gut with dual distribution in nerves and endocrine cells. *In* Gut Hormones. Edited By S. R. Bloom. Edinburg, Churchill Livingstone, 1978, p. 406.
316. Sweet, R. D.: A dermatosis specifically associated with a tumour of pancreatic alpha cells. Br. J. Dermatology, 90:301, 1974.
317. Takasawa, S., Yamamoto, K., Terazono, K., and Okamoto, H.: Novel gene activated in rat insulinoma. Diabetes, 35:1178, 1986.
318. Tatemoto, K., and Mutt, V.: Isolation of two novel candidate hormones using chemical method for finding naturally occurring polypeptide. Nature, 285:417, 1980.
319. Terazono, I., Uchiyama, Y., Ide, M., Watanabe, T., Yonekura, H., Yamamoto, H., and Okamoto, H.: Expression of *reg* protein in rat regenerating islets and its co-localization with insulin in beta cell secretory granules. Diabetologia, 33:1, 1990.
320. Terazono, K., Yamamoto, H., Takasawa, S., Shiga, K., Yonemura, Y., Tochino, Y., and Okamoto, H.: A novel gene activated in regenerating islets. J. Biol. Chem., 262:2111, 1988.
321. Thakker, R. V., Bouloux, P., Wooding, C., Chotai, K., Broad, P. M., Spurr, N. K., Besser, G. M., and O'Riordan, J. L.: Association of parathyroid tumors in multiple endocrine neoplasia type 1 with loss of alleles on chromosome 11. N. Engl. J. Med., 321:218, 1989.
322. Theodrosson-Norheim, E., Norheim, K. O., Brodin, E., Lundberg, J. M., Tatemoto, K., and Lindgren, P. G.: Neuropeptide K: A major tachykinin in plasma and tumor tissues from carcinoid patients. Biochem.-Biophys. Res. Commun., 131:77, 1985.
323. Thompson, N. W.: The surgical treatment of islet cell tumors of the pancreas. *In* Pancreatic Disease. Edited by T. L. Dent. New York, Grune & Stratton, Inc., 1981, p. 461.
324. Thompson, N. W., and Eckhauser, F. E.: Malignant islet-cell tumors of the pancreas. World J. Surg., 8:940, 1984.
325. Thompson, J. C., Lewis, B. G., Weiner, I., and Townsend, C. M., Jr.: The role of surgery in the Zollinger-Ellison syndrome. Ann. Surg., 197:594, 1983.
326. Thompson, N. W., Lloyd, R. V., Nishiyama, R. H., Vinik, A. I., Stroedel, W. E., Allo, M. D., Eckhauser, F. E., Talpos, G., and Mervak, T.: MEN I pancreas: A histological and immunohistochemical study. World J. Surg., 8:561, 1984.
327. Thompson, N. W., Vinik, A. I., Eckhauser, F. E., and Strodel, W. E.: Extrapancreatic gastrinomas. Surgery, 98:1113, 1985.
328. Tiedemann, K., Long, R. G., Pritchard, J., and Bloom, S. R.: Plasma vasoactive intestinal polypeptide and other regulatory peptides in children with neurogenic tumours. Eur. J. Pediatr., 137:147, 1981.
329. Tiedemann, K., Pritchard, J., Long, R., and Bloom, S. R.: Intractable diarrhoea in a patient with vasoactive intestinal peptide-secreting neuroblastoma. Eur. J. Pediatr., 137:217, 1981.
330. Tomita, T., Friesen, S. R., and Kimmel, J. R.: Pancreatic polypeptide cell hyperplasia with and without watery diarrhea syndrome. J. Surg. Oncol., 14:11, 1980.
331. Treuner, J., Feine, U., Niethammer, D., Muller-Schaumburg, W., Meinke, J., Elbach, E., Dopfer, R., Klingebliel, T., and Grumbach, S.: Scintigraphic imaging of neuroblastoma with I-131-MIBG. Lancet, 1:333, 1984.
332. Tsai, S. T., Eckhauser, F. E., Thompson, N. W., Stroedel, W. E., and Vinik, A. I.: Perioperative use of long-acting somatostatin analogue (SMS 201-995) in patients with endocrine tumors of the gastroenteropancreatic axis. Surgery, 100:788, 1986.
333. Tsai, S. T., Lewis, E., and Vinik, A. I.: The use of a somatostatin analogue (SMS 201-995) in the management of the flushing syndrome. Scandanavian J. Gastroenterol., 21:268, 1986.
334. Udenfriend, S., Titus, E., and Weissbach, H.: The identification of 5-hydroxy-3-indoleacetic acid in normal urine and a method for its assay. J. Biol. Chem., 216:499, 1955.
335. Ulbrecht, J. S., Schmeltz, R., Aarons, J. H., and Greene, D. A.: Insulinoma in a 94-year-old woman: Long-term therapy with verapamil. Diabetes Care, 9:196, 1986.
336. Unger, R. H., and Orci, L.: Glucagon and the A cell. Physiology and pathophysiology. N. Engl. J. Med., 304:1575, 1981.
337. Vale, W., Rivier, C., and Brown, M.: Regulatory peptides of the hypothalamus. Ann. Rev. Physiol., 39:473, 1977.
338. van Hazel, G. A., Rubin, J., and Moertel, C. G.: Treatment of metastatic carcinoid tumor with dactinomycin or decarbazine. Cancer Treat. Rep., 67:583, 1983.
339. van Heerden, J. A., Smith, S. L., and Miller, L. J.: The management of Zollinger-Ellison Syndrome in patients with multiple endocrine neoplasm Type 1. Presented at Seventh Annual Meeting, American Association of Endocrine Surgeons, April 15, 1986. Surgery (In press).
340. Verner, J. V., and Morrison, A. B.: Endocrine pancreatic islet disease with diarrhea: Report on a case due to diffuse hyperplasia of nonbeta islet tissue with a review of 54 additional cases. Arch. Intern. Med., 133:492, 1974.
341. Verner, J. V., and Morrison, A. B.: Islet cell tumor and a syndrome of refractory watery diarrhea and hypokalemia. Am. J. Med., 25:374, 1958.
342. Villar, H. V., Johnson, D. G., Lynch, P. J., Pond, G. D., and Smith, P. H.: Pattern of immunoreactive glucagon in portal, arterial and peripheral plasma before and after removal of glucagonoma. Am. J. Surg., 141:48, 1981.
343. Vinik, A. I., Achem-Karam, S., and Owyang, C.: Gastrointestinal hormones in clinical medicine. *In* Special Topics in Endocrinology and Metabolism, Volume 4. Edited by M. P. Cohen and P. P. Foa. New York, Alan R. Liss, Inc., 1983.
344. Vinik, A. I., and Glaser, B.: Pancreatic endocrine tumors. *In* Pancreatic Disease, Diagnosis and Therapy. Edited by T. L. Dent. New York, Grune & Stratton, 1981, 25:427.
345. Vinik, A. I., Glowniak, J., Glaser, B., Shapiro, B., Funakoshi, A., Cho, K. J., Thompson, N. W., and Fajans, S. S.: Localization of gastroenteropancreatic (GEP) tumors. *In* Surgery 2, Endocrine Surgery. Edited by I. D. A. Johnston and N. W. Thompson. London, Butterworth's International Medical Reviews, London, 1983, 6:76.
346. Vinik, A. I., Levitt, N. S., Pimstone, B. L., and Wagner, L.: Peripheral plasma somatostatin-like immunoreactive responses to insulin hypoglycemia and mixed meal in healthy subjects in non-insulin-dependent maturity-onset diabetes. J. Clin. Endocrin. Metab., 52:330, 1980.
347. Vinik, A. I., and Moattari, A. R.: Use of somatostatin analogue in the management of carcinoid syndrome. Dig. Dis. and Sci., 34(3):14s, 1989.
348. Vinik, A. I., Moattari, A. R., Cho, K., and Thompson, N. W.: Transhepatic portal vein catherization for localization of sporadic and MEN gastrinomas: a 10 year experience. Surgery, 107:246, 1990.
349. Vinik, A. I., Shapiro, B., and Thompson, N. W.: Plasma gut hormone levels in 37 patients with pheochromocytomas. World J. Surg., 10:593, 1985.
350. Vinik, A. I., Strodel, W. E., Cho, K. J., Eckhausaer, F. E., and Thompson, N. W.: Localization of hormonally active gastrointestinal tumors. *In* Endocrine Surgery Update. Edited by N. W. Thomson and A. I. Vinik. New York, Grune & Stratton, 1983.
351. Vinik, A. I., Stroedel, W. M., Lloyd, R. V., and Thompson, N. W.: Unusual gastroenteropancreatic tumors and their hormones. *In* Endrocrine Surgery Update. Edited by N. W. Thompson and A. I. Vinik. New York, Grune & Stratton, 1983, p. 293.
352. Vinik, A. I., Strodel, W. E., and O'Dorisio, T. M.: Endocrine tumors of the gastroenteropancreatic axis. *In* Diagnosis and Management of Endocrine-Related Tumors. Edited by R. J. Santen and A. Manni. Boston, Martinus Nijhoff Publishers, 1984, p. 305.
353. Vinik, A. I., and Thompson, N. W.: Controversies in the management of Zollinger Ellison syndrome. Ann. Int. Med., 105:956, 1986.
354. Vinik, A. I., Thompson, N. W., Eckhauser, F., and Moattari, A. R.: Clinical features of carcinoid syndrome and the use of somatostatin analogue in its management. Acta Oncol., 28:389, 1989.
355. Vinik, A. I., Tsai, S. T., Moattari, A. R., and Cheung, P.: Somatostatin analogue (SMS 201-995) in patients with gastrinomas. Surgery, 104:834, 1988.
356. Vinik, A. I., Tsai, S., Moattari, A. R., Cheung, P., Eckhauser, F., and Cho, K.: Somatostatin analogue (SMS 20-1995) in the management of gastroenteropancreatic tumors and diarrhea syndromes. Amer. J. Med., 81:23, 1986.
357. von Moll, L., McEwan, A. J., Shapiro, B., Sisson, J. C., Gross, M. D., Lloyd, R., Beals, F., Beierwaltes, W. H., Thompson, N. W., and Lloyd, R.: Iodine-131-MIBG scintigraphy of neuroendocrine tumors other than pheochromocytoma and neuroblastoma. J. Nucl. Med., 28:979, 1987.
358. von Schenck, H., Thorell, J. I., Berg, J., Bojs, G., Dymling, J. F., Hallengren, B., Liungberg, O., and Tibblin, S.: Metabolic studies and glucagon gel filtration pattern before and after surgery in a case of glucagonoma syndrome. Acta Med. Scand., 205:155-162, 1979.
359. von Schrenck, T., Howard, J. M., Doppmann, J. L., Norton, J. A., Maton, P. N., Smith, F. P., Vinayek, R., Frucht, H., Wank, S. A., and Gardner, J. D.: Prospective study of chemotherapy in patients with metastatic gastrinoma. Gastroenterol., 94:1326, 1988.
360. Walker, T. P.: The determination of serotonin (5-hydroxytryptamine) in human blood. J. Lab. Clin. Med., 55:824, 1959.
361. Wank, S. A., Doppmann, J. L., Miller, D. L., Maton, P. N., Vinayek, R., Slaff, J. I., Norton, J. A., Gardner, J. D., and Jensen, R. T.: Prospective study of the ability of computed axial tomography to localize gastrinomas in patients with Zollinger Ellison syndrome. Gastroenterol., 92:905, 1987.
362. Watanabe, T., Yonekura, H., Terazono, K., Yamamoto, H., and Okamoto, H.: Complete nucleotide sequence of human *reg* gene and its expression in normal and tumoral tissues. J. Biol. Chem., 265:7432, 1990.
363. Weidenmann, B., Franke, W. W., Kuhn, C., Moll, R., and Gould, V. E.: Synaptophysin: a marker protein for neuroendocrine cells and neoplasms. Proc. Natl. Acad. Sci. USA, 83:3500, 1986.
364. Weil, C.: Gastroenteropancreatic endocrine tumors. Klin. Wochenschr., 63:433, 1985.
365. Wilander, E., Grimelius, L., Portela-Gomes, G., Lundquist, G., Skoog, V., and Westerwark, P.: Substance P and enteroglucagon-like immunoreactivity in argentaffin and argyrophil mid-gut carcinoid tumors. Scand. J. Gastroenterol., 53:19, 1979.
366. Wilkinson, D. S.: Necrolytic migratory erythema with carcinoma of the pancreas. Trans. St. Johns Hosp. Dermatol. Soc., 59:244, 1973.
367. Wolfe, M. M., Alexander, R. W., and McGuigan, J. E.: Extrapancreatic, extraintestinal gastrinoma. N. Engl. J. Med., 306:1533, 1982.
368. Wood, J. R., Wood, S. M., Lee, Y. C., and Bloom, S. R.: Neurotensin-secreting carcinoma of the bronchus. Postgraduate Med. J., 59:46, 1983.
369. Wood, S. M., Kraenzlin, M. E., Adrian, T. E., and Bloom, S. R.: Treatment of patients with pancreatic endocrine tumors using a new long-acting somatostatin analogue: symptomatic and peptide responses. Gut, 26:438, 1985.
370. Wroe, S. J., Ardon, M., and Bouden, A. R.: Myasthenia gravis associated with a hormone producing malignant carcinoid tumor. J. Neurol. Neurosurg. Psychiatry, 48:719, 1985.
371. Wynick, D., Williams, S. J., and Bloom, R. S.: Symptomatic secondary hormone syndromes in patients with established malignant pancreatic endocrine tumors. N. Engl. J. Med., 319:605, 1988.
372. Yallow, R. S., and Berson, S. A.: Immunoassay of endogenous plasma insulin in man. J. Clin. Invest., 39:1157, 1960.
373. Yamaguchi, K., Abe, K., Adachi, I., Tanaka, M., Ueda, M., Oka, Y., Miyakaw, S., Kameya, T., and Yangihara, N.: Clinical and hormonal aspects of the watery diarrhea-hypokalemia-achlorhydria (WGHA) syndrome due to vasoactive intestinal polypeptide (VIP)-producing tumor. Endocrinol. Japan, 27:79, 1980.
374. Zollinger, R. M.: Gastrinoma: factors influencing prognosis. Surgery, 97:49, 1985.
375. Zollinger, R. M., and Ellison, E. H.: Primary peptic ulcerations of the jejunum associated with islet cell tumors of the pancreas. Ann. Surg., 39:231, 1955.

(Studies of A. I. Vinik, reported here, were supported by a grant from the NIH #1-RO1CA54641-01)

patients (in the U.S., 43,000 annual diagnoses of HNSCC versus 168,000 diagnoses of lung, and 111,000 diagnoses of colon cancers) that requires grouping many different types in each HNSCC therapy trial.[64]

New strategies for the management of this devastating group of UADT cancers are badly needed. A team concept is required. Already the role of each treatment modality is becoming more clearly defined. New combined-modality approaches (e.g., sequential and synchronous chemoradiotherapy) and advances in organ preservation and chemoprevention are beginning to offer realistic hopes for improvements in HNSCC patients' survival rates and quality of life. HNSCC research, both clinical and basic, is becoming a model for research into other epithelial cancers. This chapter reviews both the current status of and future investigative directions for the epidemiology, biology, chemoprevention, diagnosis and therapy of head and neck cancer.

Etiology and Epidemiology

Overview

The complex process of head and neck carcinogenesis involves dynamic interactions among many factors.[23,67,88,160,343,402,458,583] Approximately 90% of head and neck cancers occur after exposure to known UADT carcinogens. Chief among HNSCC-related carcinogens are tobacco-like substances, such as betel leaf. Alcohol use is closely linked to tobacco in this regard and is part of a group of agents that can potentiate tobacco-related carcinogenesis. Important etiologic factors besides tobacco and alcohol are viruses, genetic predisposition, occupation, radiation exposure, and diet.

Incidence of HNSCC increases with age, and HNSCC patients typically are older than 50.[100,174] Several retrospective series report a worse prognosis in younger patients (30 years or younger). Other data suggest, however, that the natural history of HNSCC is the same in stage-matched patients regardless of age.[42,111,433,602,636] Confounding factors in younger patients include genetic susceptibility and immunologic profile.[573]

Complicating the issues of HNSCC etiology and epidemiology are carcinomas of the salivary gland and nasopharynx. Both cancers are distinct from head and neck cancers at other sites and therefore, will be considered separately after a general discussion of etiologic factors in head and neck cancer.

Tobacco and Alcohol Exposure

Tobacco is a weak carcinogen that initiates a linear dose-response carcinogenic effect in which duration is more important than intensity of exposure.[417,790] The major carcinogenic activity of cigarette smoke resides in the particulate (tar) fraction, which contains a complex mixture of interacting cancer initiators, promoters and co-carcinogens. The pooling of saliva containing these carcinogens in gravity-dependent regions may account for the frequent location of oral SCC along the lateral and ventral surfaces of the tongue and in the floor of the mouth.[483] In heavy smokers, approximately 15 years must pass before risk is approximately back to the level of people who never smoked.[88,417,790]

Tobacco is smoked and chewed in daunting quantities. Estimated 1986 world figures for smoking and smokeless tobacco use are one billion and 600 million people, respectively.[417,420] Smoking rates are rising by 2% per year in developing countries, offsetting a 1.5% annual decrease in developed nations. Smokeless tobacco use is a growing international problem in many parts of the world, including Asia and Africa.[660] Although overall U.S. rates have not changed in 30 years, dramatic increases in smokeless tobacco use have occurred among younger people, which may account for the excess of oral cancer mortality rates in this group.[100,148,166,174,630,660,775]

Striking variations in head and neck cancer sites and incidences occur among different regions, cultures and demographic groups, mainly because of differing patterns of tobacco use.[58,67,166,174,660] SCC of the oral cavity and hypopharynx accounts for only 3% of all cancers in the United States, where smokers outnumber chewers, but for 50% of all cancers in Bombay, where "pan" (betel leaf, lime, catechu and areca nut) is commonly chewed.[67,660] SCC of the hard palate is endemic in other parts of Asia where reverse chutta (homemade cigar) smoking—burning end held in the mouth—is common. Oral cancer incidence is highest in Southeast Asia, lip cancer in Newfoundland, and nasopharyngeal cancer in southern China. The male-to-female ratios of HNSCC incidence run the gamut from 12:1 in France to 1:1 in Bangalore, India. In the U.S. this ratio has changed from about 4:1 40 years ago to about 2:1 today. U.S. head-and-neck cancer rates have changed over time as tobacco-use habits have shifted. Among American women and nonwhite men, HNSCC incidence and mortality rates have increased over the last 50 years—trends most striking for oral cancer (seven-fold increase in women).[150,174] Increased U.S. tobacco use among women, adolescents, and children augurs increasing national death rates from head and neck cancer in the next several decades.[148]

Although primary, tobacco is not the only factor in the complex causality equation for these cancers. Alcohol is an important *promoter* of carcinogenesis and is a contributive factor in at least 75% of UADT cancers.[58] It has only a modest independent effect, however.[655] Studies attempting to correlate types of alcoholic beverages with specific cancer risks have been conflicting. Most investigators believe that ethanol itself is the important factor.[360] The major clinical significance of alcohol consumption is that it potentiates the carcinogenic effect of tobacco at every level of tobacco use, and the causative effect is most striking at the highest levels of exposure to both. The magnitude of the effect is midway between additive and multiplicative.

Smoking marijuana appears to confer even greater risk for HNSCC (but not for lung cancer) than does cigarette smoking.[89,186] Marijuana smoke has 4-times higher tar burdens and 50% higher concentrations of benzpyrene and aromatic hydrocarbons than are present in tobacco smoke.

Viruses

Viral agents have been implicated in the pathogenesis of oral, laryngeal, and nasopharyngeal carcinoma (NPC).[69,219,316,369]

Seroepidemiologic studies in oral SCC suggest that herpes simplex virus type 1 (HSV-1) may act as a mutagen in the development of this cancer. These studies have shown that patients with oral SCC have increased levels of HSV-1 IgA and IgM antibodies that are of prognostic significance.[609,611] Recent laboratory work, however, has raised questions about the importance of HSV-1 in oral carcinogenesis, since HSV-1 gene products appear in oral SCC tissue only in isolated cases.[610] If not critical by itself, HSV-1 still may be a cofactor with other viral or chemical agents in causing oral carcinogenesis.

More recently, an association between head and neck cancer and human papilloma viruses (HPVs) has been hotly pursued.[70,164,369,431,599,674] HPVs are a family of at least 65 viral subtypes that have been best studied in cervical carcinogenesis and recently linked to other epithelial cancers.[369] Early studies suggested that the HPV-to-verrucous carcinoma relationship is stronger than that between HPV and other types of oral SCC, but they have not been confirmed. Immunohistochemical analysis of HPV capsid antigen and in situ hybridization studies of HPV DNA suggested the association of HPVs (numbers 6, 11, 16, and 18) with oral carcinogenesis.[164,431,674] These uncontrolled small studies generated conflicting results, however, and suggested marked overlap between viral expressions in oral SCC and in normal oral mucosa. Laryngeal papillomatosis is associated with HPVs 6 and 11, whereas laryngeal SCC is associated with HPVs 16 and 18.[369] HPV DNA is not limited to lesion sites, but is present also in clinically and histologically normal UADT epithelium. New work using polymerase chain reaction (PCR) probes in controlled studies, coupled with standard epidemiologic data, should provide major insights into the role of HPVs in head-and-neck carcinogenesis.

Genetic Links

Levels of aryl hydrocarbon hydroxylase—the enzyme that activates polycyclic aromatic hydrocarbons (major carcinogens in cigarette smoke)—are greater in laryngeal cancer patients than in controls. An association between the development of HNSCC in patients and specific human leukocyte antigens has also been reported. Recent data from several groups suggest that HNSCC patients have increased sensitivity to clastogen-induced chromosome damage when compared with case controls. A multiplicative risk of HNSCC has been reported when analyzing mutagen-induced chromosome damage and carcinogenic exposure.[654] Along with environmental factors, genetic factors may become useful components of quantitative risk-assessment models.[417,576]

Occupation

Although occupational exposures play a minor role overall in the development of HNSCC, they are major risk factors for adenocarcinoma of the sinonasal region.[33,88] The most important exposures occur in the environments of nickel refining, woodworking and leather working. Asbestos exposure has been associated with certain UADT cancers, most notably in the larynx.[95]

Radiation

Apparently, there is no strong association between exposure to ionizing radiation and the development of squamous carcinoma of the head and neck. Other than in lip cancer, which like skin cancer is associated with ultraviolet-B exposure, only two associations are known to exist between radiation and UADT cancers—paranasal sinus cancers related to radium dial painting and thyroid cancers related to radiotherapy.[273] Therapeutic irradiation of HNSCC does not appear to induce second primary tumors in the aerodigestive tract.[419]

Diet

Considerable epidemiologic evidence suggests that vitamin A and β-carotene play a protective role in epithelial neoplasia.[98,275,425,460,521] Deficiencies of carotenoids appear to be a risk factor for squamous UADT and lung cancers. It is not known, however, which of the more than 500 carotenoids are protective, or what protective role other micronutrients in carotenoid-rich foods may play.[425,456] Several groups specifically studied the association between dietary vitamin A and/or β-carotene and risk for oral cancer. Winn and colleagues found that the risk of oral SCC in women is inversely related to the consumption of fresh fruits and vegetables.[776] Diets are complex and difficult to assess and validate; in particular, there are often inaccuracies in translating foods into constituent nutrients. Further studies are needed to define sharply the relationship between dietary-intake and serum levels of the various carotenoid components. Even in positive studies, it is impossible to determine which of the vast array of compounds is most beneficial; and controlling for other dietary variables and confounding risk factors has remained a difficult methodologic problem. Smoking has been associated with reduced dietary intake and serum levels of carotenoids.[253]

Despite their many problems, prospective and retrospective nutritional (serum and dietary) epidemiologic studies, along with basic science research, have provided important clues to the development and prevention of specific cancers. Several large-scale clinical chemoprevention trials of β-carotene and/or retinol in epithelial neoplasia have been designed on the basis of data from these studies.[47,147,275,279,309,425]

Salivary Gland and Nasopharyngeal Carcinoma

As stated in the overview above, nasopharyngeal and salivary carcinomas, each accounting for 0.2% of all U.S. cancers, are distinct from those in other head and neck sites.[174] Neither has been strongly linked etiologically to tobacco and neither demonstrates the multiple-primary or second-primary patterns of the other head and neck cancer sites.[307] Salivary gland cancer incidence has been stable for the past 25 years in the U.S. These tumors are similar to nonmelanoma skin cancers and lip cancer in their epidemiologic association with ultraviolet-B and ionizing radiation exposure.[40,528,617,656]

Nasopharyngeal carcinoma (NPC) presents in a younger population than other head and neck cancer sites. Its incidence increases with age, and plateaus at 50–60 years. In all races, NPC is 2–3-fold more common in males. NPC is 20 times more common in the Far East than in North America, although within the latter it has an increased frequency among Alaskan natives. This carcinoma's pattern shows incidences decreasing in a gradient from southern to northern regions of China (30–50 per 100,000 person-years down to 2 or 3 per 100,000). Among Chinese in Hong Kong and Singapore, this is the most common cancer in people 15–34 years old.[101,217,251] Immigrant studies indicate that incidence differences seemingly associated with ethnicity are really largely associated with environment. Americans with Chinese ancestry have an incidence halfway between those of native Chinese and American whites. These are but a few of the wide variations in NPC incidences produced by geographic, ethnic and cultural differences.[101,217,251,307]

Two major, independent risk factors for NPC are salted fish as a diet standard and the Epstein-Barr virus (EBV).[793] Seven studies have used case-control methodology to look at whether eating salted fish correlates with NPC incidence.[500] These studies were variously performed in high- and low-risk areas of China. All seven identified salted fish as an independent risk factor (attributable risk of 50%).

Even stronger than that of salted fish is the epidemiologic link between EBV and NPC.[127,217,218,251] Regardless of histopathologic subtype (WHO I–III), geographic or ethnic setting, sporadic or endemic pattern, premalignant or malignant status, NPC is an EBV-associated malignancy. Type II and III NPC cells have EBV nuclear antigen (EBNA), DNA and transmissible virus.[99,127] The association between EBV and well-differentiated (WHO type I) NPC was recognized only recently with the detection of EBV genome in type I lesions by recombinant DNA technology.[538] NPC may be the best example of a virus-related epithelial carcinoma and has served as a model for the study of virus-induced carcinogenesis anywhere in the body. The fundamental and early role of EBV in the pathogenesis of NPC is suggested by the recent finding of EBV DNA in premalignant nasopharyngeal lesions. The 20% transformation rate of these lesions, however, indicates the importance of other factors in nasopharyngeal tumorigenesis.

Several serologic associations exist between EBV and types II and III NPC.[99,555,796] Elevated IgG response to EBV capsid antigen (EBVCA) is most sensitive, seen in nearly 100% of types II and III NPC, but least NPC-specific. The IgA EBVCA serologic measure is more specific but less sensitive. The most specific but least sensitive of current serologic tests is IgA response in a *diffuse* pattern to EBV early antigen (EBVEA)—positive in 40–60% of NPC patients and in fewer than 2% of other HNSCC patients and controls.[251,796] These data illustrate that IgA response to both EBVCA and EBVEA is useful for recognizing occult disease in treated patients and for screening high-risk groups.

Etiologic and Epidemiologic Goals

The ultimate goals of epidemiology and etiology are disease prevention and early detection. Studying incidence patterns and risk factors facilitates research and intervention strategies designed ultimately to reduce cancer mortality. Cancers of the head and neck are a devastating group of diseases for which many etiologic factors are known. The strong relationship of NPC with EBV has important diagnostic and therapeutic implications,[218] and offers the unique opportunity to develop effective screening for early detection with viral markers in high-risk areas and vaccines for disease prevention.[209] Significant efforts should be made toward eliminating or at least diminishing the effects of the major known causes of head and neck cancer.[222] For example,

given the double-barreled multiplicative effect of tobacco and alcohol, substantially reducing the use of either could dramatically reduce rates of HNSCC.[417] Unfortunately, both smoking and drinking have proved so far to be highly resistant to primary-prevention (use-reduction) approaches. Some success has been achieved in getting patients to quit smoking after treatment of primary HNSCC: fear of recurrent disease disposes them to heed their physicians' advice. Effective tobacco- and alcohol-cessation programs are prerequisite to the control and prevention of HNSCC.

Biology

Carcinogenesis (Field Cancerization). Slaughter's classic 1953 report[628] on oral cancer proposed that UADT carcinogenesis is a process of "field cancerization"—the repeated exposure of a region's entire tissue area to carcinogenic insult (e.g., tobacco and alcohol), which exposure increases the tissue's risk for developing multiple independent premalignant and malignant foci.[418,419,670] This concept (also called field carcinogenesis or condemned-mucosa syndrome) may explain the clinical occurrence of multiple primary and second primary tumors in HNSCC. The data indicate that second primaries, whether synchronous or metachronous, generally are of squamous histology, develop at a constant rate (2–5% of treated patients per year), are not treatment related, and occur in the aerodigestive field at risk ("carcinogen playground"), i.e., the head and neck, the upper two-thirds of the esophagus, and the lung.[130,175,418,419,724] These characteristics of second primaries support the field cancerization hypothesis.

Despite intensive study, much of the complex fundamental biology of HNSCC remains poorly understood. Like other epithelial neoplasms, UADT carcinogenesis appears to evolve through a complex multistep process involving certain biomolecular changes preceding premalignant lesions preceding invasive cancer.[640] An excellent system for studying these steps is the 7,12-dimethylbenz(a)anthracene (DMBA)-induced hamster cheek pouch model.[612,614] Typical of HNSCCs, oral cancer in this model develops in an orderly histologic sequence that mimics, in fast-forward, the human situation: hyperplasia (at 4 weeks), dysplasia (8 weeks), and SCC (16 weeks).

On the basis of animal studies, epithelial carcinogenesis has been divided into three phases: initiation, promotion, and progression. Although human neoplasia does not fit neatly into this tripartite framework, the framework serves as a useful model for understanding pharmacologic interventions. Pharmacologic interventions at each phase have attendant advantages and disadvantages.[47] Chemoprevention's greatest potential is in the promotion and progression phases of carcinogenesis.

Occurring within the three-phase model described above, multiple subtle steps of UADT carcinogenesis involve: genetic alterations; dysregulated epithelial differentiation; abnormal proliferation; and altered regulatory effects. Although the earliest genetic changes precede relatively simultaneous occurrences of altered differentiation and proliferation, continuing genetic changes accompany the latter changes as carcinogenesis progresses. One important focus of combined clinical and basic research is to establish specific probes and markers of these carcinogenic steps. These probes would help identify individuals at highest risk of UADT cancer and would act as intermediate-endpoint markers for early evaluations of the efficacy of chemopreventive agents.[423]

Genetic Alterations. Degree of genetic damage reflects degrees of carcinogen exposure and inherent tissue sensitivity. Genomic changes accumulate presumably in the entire carcinogen-exposed tissue; however, clonal malignant foci develop only in specific sites where tumorigenesis is possible. Nonspecific (random) genomic alterations indicted by micronuclei, sister-chromatid exchanges and aneuploidy can occur in normal, premalignant and malignant aerodigestive tract tissue.[49,187,254,556,560] Although the fundamental genetic events associated with UADT cancers have not yet been established, several non-random chromosomal alterations (e.g., alterations in chromosomes 1, 3, 5, 7, 8, 9, 10, 11, and 13) have been detected in HNSCC (fresh tissue and cell-line studies).[49,411,768] Short-term cultures of oral premalignant cells may reveal early non-random cytogenetic changes.[331,563]

Carcinogenesis is thought to be regulated fundamentally by the cellular balance between oncogenes and tumor-suppressor genes. This dynamic relationship has been demonstrated in colon cancer[731] and is under intensive study in HNSCC.[420] Aberrant expressions (amplifications or mutations) of specific families of cellular oncogenes—such as *myc, ras, neu, bcl, int* and *hst*—are associated with ADT carcinogenesis.[43,220,238,244,405,568,641] Up to one-third of cases of primary HNSCC demonstrate amplification of either the *int*-2 or *hst*-1 gene (both members of the fibroblast growth-factor gene family) on chromosome 11q13.[43,635,707] Little is known, however, about when these events take place during the multistep process or what role their gene products play in regulating growth and differentiation. The families of *ras*, *neu* and n-*myc* oncogenes are amplified in the more advanced stages of oral SCC, and activated oncogenes of these families in vitro alter response to differentiation agents and promote uncontrolled cellular growth, aneuploidy and tumorigenicity.[220,238,641]

Differentiation Alterations. Dysregulation of differentiation is another hallmark of multistep carcinogenesis.[658] Human oral and esophageal epithelium is stratified squamous in type. Oral mucosa is noncornified except for the mucosa on the gingiva and dorsal surface of the tongue, which undergo keratinization. Cytokeratins, a family of at least 19 intermediate-sized filaments that range from 40–68 kDa are expressed in different complex patterns that correlate with distinct types of epithelial differentiation.[128,495]

Major alterations in keratin expression occur during carcinogenesis.[128] For example, K1 (68 kDa) is absent in normal oral tissue but often is expressed in noncornified UADT epithelium subjected to experimental vitamin A deficiency and cigarette-smoke exposure, and in animal and human oral premalignant and well-differentiated malignant lesions.[420] The expression of K19 (40 kDa) is increased in basal and suprabasal layers of lesions with moderate to severe dysplasia, but is lost if the tissue proceeds to terminal squamous differentiation. In HNSCC, K19 is weekly expressed in well-differentiated lesions and strongly expressed in poorly differentiated lesions.[122,331] K13 expression patterns are completely opposite to those of K19—strongly expressed in normal tissue and weak expression or absent in severe dysplasia and poorly differentiated HNSCC.[420] The spatial distribution of involucrin, transglutaminase I and other differentiation antigens is also altered in dysplasia and carcinoma.[90,128,151,420]

Proliferation Alterations. The third major phase of multistep carcinogenesis is dysregulated proliferation. The transition from normal epithelium to hyperplasia and dysplasia is associated with an increased growth fraction and cells proliferating beyond the basal layer. Older histologic assays have correlated this process with increased frequencies of mitotic figures; more recently, DNA flow cytometry and monoclonal-antibody probes to nuclear antigens (e.g., Ki-67 and proliferating-cell nuclear antigen, PCNA) have revealed some strong positive correlations in ADT epithelium between abnormal suprabasal proliferation and later carcinogenic stages (severe dysplasia).[122,423]

Altered Regulatory Effects. Epithelial carcinogenesis is associated also with the abnormal expression of cellular factors that regulate growth and development. The importance of these factors is inferred from their differential expression in normal and malignant tissues. For example, high expression of epidermal growth factor-receptor (EGF-R) is found in a significant fraction of experimental and human SCCs of the UADT.[195,786] EGF-R gene activation occurs early in experimental oral carcinogenesis, and foci of cells expressing EGF-R can be found in human premalignant lesions. Similarly, high expression of transforming-growth factor-α (TGF-α) has been associated with malignant transformation of a variety of tumors (including oral cancers), and is frequently accompanied by elevated levels of EGF-R in SCC.[699] The relationship between high TGF-α and high EGF-R suggests that an autocrine loop mechanism drives the dysregulation of proliferation.

Immunology

A variety of immunologic abnormalities occur in HNSCC, but precise cause-and-effect relationships between abnormalities and cancer remain unclear.[370,512] Two immunologic responses are cell-mediated (macrophage, natural-killer [NK] and T-cell) immunity and humoral (antibody-mediated) immunity. Both of these have important implications for HNSCC prognosis and therapy.

Cell-mediated immunity apparently is involved in tumor control.[567,572] Defective cell-mediated immunity as determined by NK activity, skin tests, and other measures correlates with advanced disease, early recurrence and poor survival.[512] Large variations in tumor-infiltrating lymphocyte (TIL) levels in HNSCC have been reported. TILs in HNSCC are primarily CD3+ T cells (NK cells are rare), and 30–50% of TILs express HLA-DR-activation antigens. The prognostic significance of tumor-infiltrating cell subsets is unclear.[311,782]

Most recent work in HNSCC immunology has focused on humoral immune status. A large body of growing evidence suggests that humoral immunity plays a negative role in HNSCC.[512,669] Increased serum levels of IgA, IgM, and immune complexes are associated with advanced disease and poor prognosis in HNSCC.[492] Increased IgA can block many aspects of the host cell-mediated immune response, including cytotoxic effects of sensitized lymphocytes, NK cells and macrophages, and IgG-mediated antibody-dependent cell-mediated cytotoxicity (ADCC). In contrast, increased IgE is associated with a good prognosis in HNSCC. The ratio of IgA to IgE, therefore, may be more predictive of prognosis than either IgA or IgE is individually. Posttreatment patterns of IgA and immune complexes differ—immune complex levels more accurately reflect tumor burden.[512]

Although multiple and prominent immunologic deficits occur in HNSCC, immunologic therapeutic approaches (IFN-α, IL-2, plasmapheresis) have yielded only modest response rates and short response durations (see Immunobiologic Therapy below).

Biologic Goals

The basic genetic and phenotypic alterations associated with UADT carcinogenesis and field cancerization are under intensive study. Although this work has already identified several nonrandom chromosomal alterations, activated oncogenes, and deleted tumor-supressor genes in HNSCC, no consistent patterns have emerged. The recent development of antibody probes for key gene products and molecular probes for gene transcripts should allow future study to identify the timing and sequence of gene alterations during multistep UADT carcinogenesis. This work will allow improved understanding of carcinogenesis, identification of intermediate endpoint biomarkers (see Chemoprevention below), and development of new chemopreventive and therapeutic approaches.

The mechanisms of HNSCC invasion and metastasis are not well established. Recent studies have identified specific membrane proteins and binding sites required for SCC invasion and metastasis (in animal models) and associated with early recurrence (in clinical studies).[90] This work opens novel therapeutic possibilities for the use of directed monoclonal antibodies/inhibitors to block key binding sites and thus prevent tumor invasion and metastasis.

Profound and complex immunologic alterations characterize HNSCC patients. These changes include increased humoral and depressed cellular immunity likely of intrinsic (genetic) and extrinsic (malnutrition, alcohol) etiology. Regardless of the precise mechanistic details, the characterization of these defects provides avenues for the development of new therapeutic approaches. For example, the immunosuppressive effect of immune complexes has led to early trials of plasmapheresis alone and integrated into systemic therapy regimens. The depressed cellular immunity has led to the use of biologic-response modifiers such as IL-2 and interferons. Although current immunologic therapy approaches have produced only modest activity, treatment strategies should improve and become more focused as our basic understanding of immune defects in HNSCC and of immune therapy in general improves.

Chemoprevention Approaches

Overview

The control and management of HNSCC are hindered tremendously by poor overall survival rates and the high risk of second primary tumors in early-stage cases. Compound-

ing these issues are severe disfigurements and debilities resulting from definitive local therapy of head and neck tumors. Although tobacco and alcohol cessation are of primary importance, cessation approaches have not succeeded in significantly reducing exposure to these carcinogens. Consequently, chemoprevention very recently has come to the forefront of head and neck cancer research efforts.

In the mid-1970s Michael Sporn of the NCI coined the term "chemoprevention"—the pharmacologic inhibition of carcinogenesis or its reversal in premalignant stages.[657,658] Current HNSCC chemopreventive study focuses strongly on retinoids and carotenoids in oral premalignancy (leukoplakia) and in adjuvant prevention of second primary tumors. The term "retinoid" was coined in 1976 also by Dr. Sporn.[659] Ultimately this study hopes to find effective agents or dietary manipulations with *little* or *no* toxicity for use in largely healthy subjects at risk.[47,63,472] Another major focus of this work is on potential biologic markers of intermediate endpoints.[423]

Because chemoprevention is far less familiar than are etiology or standard treatment strategies in HNSCC, we will discuss this new approach at length. This section begins with a general discussion of preclinical drug investigation before narrowing down to the investigative foci mentioned in the preceding paragraph.

Preclinical Study

UADT models have enabled the identification of several promising chemopreventive agents against oral carcinogenesis, including retinoic acid, β-carotene, vitamin E, selenium and inhibitors of prostaglandin and protease synthesis.[420,589,614,704] Retinoic acid is highly effective in both the buccal and lingual SCC models; β-carotene's experimental chemopreventive activity is only in the buccal model.[272,615,616]

Vast data from epidemiologic, in vitro and animal studies strongly support the role of retinoids (a class of more than 2,500 natural derivatives and synthetic analogs of vitamin A) in the prevention of epithelial carcinogenesis.[62,158,271,420,565,658,659,780] Retinoids are potent modulators of epithelial-cell differentiation in a number of normal, premalignant and malignant cell systems.[331,420,422] Retinoids suppress the promotion and progression phases of carcinogenesis in a variety of human and animal epithelial tissues, including the skin, trachea, lungs, and oral mucosa.[420,422,614] Recent investigation suggests that retinoids modulate carcinogenesis primarily by directly regulating gene expression. This activity may be mediated by nuclear retinoic acid receptors (RARs), which have strong sequence homology in the DNA-binding zinc finger region to the steroid and thyroid hormone-receptor family.[55,212,331]

Epidemiologic data reviewed above suggest that carotenoids—especially β-carotene (a dimer that is metabolized into two retinol molecules)—have potential as dietary inhibitors of carcinogenesis.[425,427,456,521] Like that of retinoids, the mechanism of carotenoid action is unclear but may relate to carotenoids' antioxidant (free-radical-scavenger) or immunomodulatory properties.[80,456] Other data suggest that β-carotene's anticarcinogenic potential relates to its metabolic conversion to retinol and retinoic acid.[55,420]

Clinical Trials

Oral Premalignancy. A Model System of Human Epithelial Carcinogenesis. Most clinical chemoprevention study in HNSCC to date has been of the retinoid 13-*cis*-retinoic acid (13cRA), endogenous in human serum at low levels, and the natural carotenoid (β-carotene) used at pharmacologic doses in oral premalignant lesions, or leukoplakias.[418] Leukoplakia is a clinical descriptive term which includes any white patch or plaque on the oral mucosa that cannot be removed by scraping, reversed by elimination of obvious local irritants (e.g., dentures) or classified clinically or histologically as any other specific disease.[614,620] Oral premalignancy's broader definition also includes normal-appearing mucosa at risk of malignant transformation—via field carcinogenesis (see above).

Leukoplakia is classified as a premalignant lesion in part because of its epidemiologic, geographic, and etiologic similarities to oral SCC,[65] frequent occurrence adjacent to oral SCC in over 30% (range 10–100%) of cancers,[66,193] and the relationship between its malignant transformation rates and the presence and degree of dysplasia (see below). Red (erythroplasia) or speckled sites within lesions are highly associated with dysplastic epithelium and, therefore, are useful indicators of logical biopsy sites. Standard management is close follow-up or surgical excision. Resectability often is limited by the extent and location of the lesion(s). Furthermore, local therapy does not prevent multifocal development of de novo lesions. A significant number of leukoplakia patients would benefit from effective chemoprevention.

Histologic assessment is critically important since even pure white lesions can be associated with severe dysplasia or even frankly invasive SCC. Hyperplastic lesions are associated with low (<5%) transformation and high (>30%) spontaneous regression rates, whereas dysplastic lesions (only 10–15% of all leukoplakias) are associated with 10-fold higher transformation and 10-fold lower spontaneous regression rates.[622] These features underscore two issues critical to oral chemoprevention trials: first, all clinical premalignant lesions must be evaluated histologically; and second, to establish drug efficacy, randomized trials must be stratified by histology to control for lesions' variable natural histories. In clinical trials, the term oral premalignancy refers to the clinical spectrum of lesions defined above, with further classification and stratification based on histologic differences.

These many characteristics of oral leukoplakia—tobacco-related; precursor of SCC; easily monitored; availability of preclinical models—make it an ideal human system for the study of chemopreventive agents with potential for applicability to other tobacco-related epithelial neoplastic disorders. Oral premalignancy chemoprevention studies already have contributed to the design of a retinoid trial that achieved the significant suppression of second primary tumors in patients with HNSCC.[323,324]

The first clinical studies of vitamin A in oral premalignancy were conducted in the 1950s (Table XXVII-1-1). These early studies indicated vitamin A's activity and led to important observations regarding patterns of response, relapse and toxicity that are still relevant today. They used extremely high doses of topical and systemic vitamin A. Despite early promising results and insights, however, further work in this area was suspended for 20 years.

Stich and colleagues were the first to resume vitamin A clinical study, conducting a series of vitamin A and β-carotene trials in Asian betel nut chewers.[666–668] Their initial work in these high-risk groups indicated that vitamin A and/or β-carotene effectively suppressed the expression of micronuclei (a genotoxic marker). However, canthaxanthine (a synthetic carotenoid not converted to retinol) was ineffective, suggesting that the protective effect was from retinoid (converted from β-carotene) rather than from carotenoid activity. In one trial, this group treated leukoplakia patients for 6 months with β-carotene, β-carotene plus vitamin A, or placebo. Lesion resolution in 15% of the β-carotene group was countered by the development of new lesions in 15%.[667] The resolution and new lesion rates for the β-carotene plus vitamin A group were 28% and 8%, respectively. Four other β-carotene trials have been reported with conflicting results (Table XXVII-1-1) including a 71% response with 30 mg/d × 3 months[247] vs. less than 30% with more dose-intensive regimens (90–120

Table XXVII-1-1. Chemoprevention Trials with Vitamin A and β-Carotene in Oral Leukoplakia

Investigators	Dose and Schedule	N	Clinical Response
Wulf[789]	Vitamin A (100,000 IU/day × 3 mo)	20	90%
Silverman[a 621,623]	Vitamin A (75–900,000 IU/day × 6–39 wks)	503[b]	57%
Stich[668]	β-Carotene (180 mg/wk × 10 wks)	23	0%
Stich[667]	Placebo	33	3%[c]
	β-Carotene (180 mg/wk × 6 mo)	27	15%[c,d]
	β-Carotene (180 mg/wk × 6 mo) plus vitamin A (100,000 IU/wk × 6 mo)	51	28%[c,d]
Stich[666]	Vitamin A (200,000 IU/wk × 6 mo)	21	57%[c]
Garewal[247]	β-Carotene (30 mg/day × 3 mo)	24	71%
Toma[700]	β-Carotene (90 mg/day × 6 mo)	24	27%
Malaker[441]	β-Carotene (120 mg/day × 3 mo)	18	22%

[a] Topical only

[b] Total from this report and literature review

[c] Only complete resolution reported

[d] The rates of lesion resolution and *new* lesion development during therapy were identical (15%) in the β-carotene arm; the respective rates in the β-carotene plus vitamin A arm were 28% (resolution) and 8% (new lesion)

poor prognosis.[361,392] Mitotic rate and labelling index have also been used to reflect proliferative activity, but large scale studies in head and neck cancers have been lacking.

Features reflecting aggressive disease include lymphatic invasion, perineural invasion, lymph node metastases and penetration of tumor through the capsule of involved lymph nodes (extracapsular spread). The presence of regional lymph node metastases is the single most important determinant of prognosis in head and neck cancer and is associated with a 50% decrease in survival rates compared to patients without regional metastases.

More recently, the histologic pattern of invasion of these cancers has been systematically studied. Tumors which invade with thin, finger-like projections or single disassociated cells behave more aggressively regardless of differentiation grade and tend to be associated with vascular and neural invasion.[351] The presence of extracapsular spread of tumor in the neck has been directly associated with high rates of distant metastases. These various histologic features play an important role in therapeutic decision making.

Diagnosis

The identification and appropriate management of pre-malignant mucosal lesions in the head and neck is an important aspect of patient management that has a major impact on overall survival rates. Since stage (extent) of disease at the time of diagnosis is the most important prognostic factor in the treatment of HNSCC, identification and early treatment of small cancers correlates with excellent survival statistics. Most early premalignant changes or in situ carcinomas of the oral mucosa occur as red (erythroplasia) or white (leukoplakia) patches that should be readily apparent on visual examination.[454] In areas less easily visualized directly such as the larynx and hypopharynx, early lesions cause symptoms such as chronic hoarseness, chronic sore throat, referred otalgia, or dysphagia. These symptoms demand visualization of the involved structures by direct or indirect laryngoscopy.

Appropriate management of leukoplakia and erythroplasia lesions includes a high index of suspicion, particularly when they occur in high risk populations. Management varies with location, extent and histology. The diffuse field effect and multifocal nature of the epithelial carcinogenic process supports the need for effective systemic chemoprevention (see Chemoprevention Approaches above). White lesions can be confused with mucositis, histoplasmosis, candidiasis, lichen planus or local tissue irritation from mechanical, thermal or chemical trauma. Lesions that persist despite removal of local irritating factors that are associated with ulceration, vertical growth, induration, recent change in size or pain should undergo biopsy. Topical supravital staining of suspicious lesions with toluidine blue can be helpful in identifying areas of biopsy and in screening high risk populations.[455,620]

Dysphagia, odynophagia, otalgia (referred), hoarseness, mucosal irregularities and ulceration, pain, weight loss and the presence of an unexplained neck mass are the common presenting complaints of HNSCC.[343] The predominant symptoms vary with site: chronic dysphagia or odynophagia (6

weeks or more) demands thorough visualization of the oropharynx, hypopharynx, and esophagus; chronic hoarseness demands visualization of the larynx; chronic, unilateral serous otitis media is a result of cancer of the nasopharynx until proven otherwise; and unilateral nasal polyps, nasal obstruction or epistaxis are common presenting signs of nasal cavity or paranasal sinus neoplasm. A firm or hard unilateral neck mass represents cancer until proven otherwise. Over 80% of the time, such a mass represents neoplasm and 80% of these neoplasms are due to metastatic spread from an UADT primary.

In patients presenting with a suspicious neck mass, complete head and neck examination usually reveals the primary malignant tumor.[343] If not, a thorough search for occult primary cancers both above and below the clavicles is warranted. Technological advances in fiberoptic, and flexible and rigid endoscopes now provide excellent upper airway visualization that previously required special skills in indirect mirror examination. Endoscopic evaluation should include the nasopharynx, oropharynx, hypopharynx, larynx, and esophagus. This endoscopic evaluation should be preceded by a barium swallow and chest radiographs. Most commonly, occult primaries responsible for neck metastases occur in the nasopharynx, tongue base, tonsil or hypopharynx. In the absence of an identifiable mass, random biopsies of these sites are indicated during endoscopic evaluation. Metastasis to a solitary left supraclavicular lymph node (Virchow's node) is occasionally seen with intra-abdominal cancer. Only after a thorough search for a primary tumor has been completed should a neck mass undergo open surgical excision or biopsy.[343] At time of excision or open biopsy of a neck mass, the surgeon and patient should be prepared for definitive neck dissection should the mass prove to be metastatic squamous carcinoma. The recent introduction of fine needle aspiration of neck masses has gained wide acceptance in the early evaluation of such masses and frequently supplements the diagnostic work up.[218,343] The dangers of inadvertent aspiration of unsuspected vascular lesions and false negative results are inherently obvious. Further, accuracy of the cytologic interpretation of the aspirate is directly dependent on the skill and experience of the pathologist. Three-dimensional imaging with computerized tomography (CT) and magnetic resonance imaging (MRI) are frequently used to supplement the clinical evaluation and staging of the primary tumor and regional lymph nodes.

Table XXVII-1-4. Clinical Tumor Stage and Groupings for Head and Neck Cancer

Stage 0	Tis	N0	M0
Stage 1	T1	N0	M0
Stage 2	T2	N0	M0
Stage 3	T3	N0	M0
	T1	N1	M0
	T2	N1	M0
	T3	N1	M0
Stage 4	T4	Any N	M0
	Any T	N2,3	M0
	Any T	Any N	M1

Staging

Staging criteria for cancers arising in the upper aerodigestive tract, paranasal sinuses and salivary glands have been developed by the American Joint Committee on Cancer (AJCC) and undergo regular re-evaluation and modification. The stage groupings utilized for head and neck cancer are based on T (primary tumor), N (regional node), and M (distant metastases) designations. The criteria have been developed based on anatomic site and extent of cancer and allow classification of patients into groups with differing prognosis. Because of variations in the growth and behavior of head and neck cancers according to site of origin, differences exist in the staging criteria for each anatomic site and region in the head and neck. Despite the variations in primary tumor staging parameters, the characteristics used for staging regional nodes and distant metastases are uniform for all sites (Tables XXVII-1-4 and XXVII-1-5).

Careful documentation of tumor extent and accurate staging classification is also important for the comparison of the results of different treatment regimens. Accurate evaluation of the results of a given treatment or the efficacy of new treatment strategies requires comparisons to patient groups with tumors of similar extent and behavior. Re-staging after treatment, or for recurrent cancers, must be clearly designated and separate from primary staging of previously untreated cancers. Post-surgical, or pathologic staging, is gaining increasing importance in the primary treatment of head and neck cancers because of the increasing use of post-operative radiation therapy and/or adjuvant chemotherapy for patients with specific tumor characteristics such as histologically proven lymph node metastases, close surgical margins, or extracapsular spread into the soft tissues of the neck.[357,358]

Treatment

General Principles

After an histologic diagnosis has been established and tumor extent determined, the selection of appropriate treatment for a specific cancer is dependent on a complex array of variables including tumor site, respective morbidity of various treatments, patient performance and nutritional status, concomitant health problems, social and logistical factors, therapy anticipated for potential recurrences or second primaries and patient preference. These variables are each considered with respect to the established effectiveness of various treatment regimens available (Table XXVII-1-6).

Several generalizations are useful in therapeutic decision making, but variations on these themes are numerous. Surgical resection and radiation therapy are the mainstays of treatment for most head and neck cancers. For small primary cancers without regional metastases (Stage I or II), wide surgical excision alone or curative radiation therapy alone are used. Functional and cosmetic results are usually better following radiotherapy. Local tumor control rates are generally better with primary surgical resection, but local recurrences after primary radiation therapy can often be successfully treated with subsequent salvage surgery resulting in similar overall survival rates. Surgical complication rates are generally increased following radiation. Salvage of surgical recurrences by radiation therapy is less effective than surgical salvage of radiation failures.

For more extensive primary tumors or regional metastases (Stage III or IV), planned combinations of pre- or post-operative radiation and complete surgical excision are generally used.[255] For selected patients with advanced cancers of specific sites such as the larynx, treatment approaches with radiation alone, and surgery held in reserve for salvage of recurrences have been utilized in attempts to preserve structure and function. Although these organ preserving techniques are successful in many patients, they are generally associated with lower overall survival rates.[154,169,372,396,510,527]

The overall management goals in treating patients with head and neck cancer are to achieve the highest cure rates at the lowest cost in terms of functional and cosmetic morbidity. These goals include early diagnosis, effective rehabilitation and appropriate palliation when cancers are incurable. The achievement of these goals requires the close interaction and cooperation of a multidisciplinary team of practitioners representing surgery, radiation, chemotherapy,

---

Table XXVII-1-5. Clinical Tumor Staging Characteristics for Regional Lymph Nodes and Distant Metastases

Regional Lymph Nodes (N)

Nx	Regional lymph nodes cannot be assessed
N0	No regional lymph node metastases
N1	Metastasis in a single ipsilateral lymph node, 3 cm or less in greatest dimension
N2a	Metastasis in a single ipsilateral lymph node, more than 3 cm, but not more than 6 cm in greatest dimension
N2b	Metastasis in multiple ipsilateral lymph nodes, none greater than 6 cm in greatest dimension
N2c	Metastasis in bilateral or contralateral lymph nodes, none greater than 6 cm in greatest dimension
N3	Metastasis in a lymph node greater than 6 cm in greatest dimension

Distant Metastasis (M)

Mx	Presence of distant metastasis cannot be assessed
M0	No distant metastasis
M1	Distant metastasis

Table XXVII-1-6. Therapeutic Approaches in Head and Neck Cancer

Established
  Definitive surgery (S)
  Definitive radiation therapy (RT)
  Surgery and planned preoperative or postoperative RT
  Definitive RT with surgery reserved for salvage of recurrence
  Palliative radiation therapy
  Palliative chemotherapy

Investigational
  Induction chemotherapy and S or RT
  Induction chemotherapy with curative RT (organ preservation)
  Concomitant chemoradiotherapy
  S or RT and adjuvant chemotherapy
  RT and adjunctive hyperthermia or radio-sensitizers
  Altered fractionation RT
  Immunobiologic therapy
  Chemoprevention

prosthedontics, dentistry, social services, dietetics, physical medicine, pathology, nursing, and sometimes psychiatry.

Effective rehabilitation is an important part of the overall treatment of head and neck cancers. Modern advances in surgical reconstruction, microvascular free tissue transfer and prosthedontics have significantly improved functional performance.[26] Rehabilitation concerns must be addressed at initial treatment planning and carefully integrated with the various treatment modalities used. (See XXII.) Pre-treatment dental evaluations, and speech and swallowing assessments are routine. Needed dental care and/or extractions should be planned prior to chemotherapy, or radiation, to reduce dental associated sepsis, mucositis and osteoradionecrosis. The overall impact of treatment and rehabilitation decisions on a patient's quality of life are important issues that may require utilization of specialized social or psychiatric support systems for the patient and family. Finally, the prolonged nature of treatment for advanced disease, which may extend over many months, requires consideration of the social and financial impact of treatment decisions on the patient, his family and employer.

Biopsies of primary tumors should not be excisional unless the biopsy procedure is sufficient for definitive treatment and the surgeon performing the excision is responsible for providing curative treatment. Oncologic principles of surgical resection must not be compromised by ill-conceived reconstructive efforts or attempts at modifying the necessary resection in order to minimize functional or cosmetic morbidity. Head and neck cancers are serious threats to life and it achieves no worthwhile purpose to secure some temporary preservation of function at the cost of high morbidity and death from recurrent cancer. Positive surgical margins after tumor resection, or gross residual cancer, portends inevitable treatment failure. Appropriate management must also include utilization of precise modern techniques of conservative surgical resection (e.g., Moh's technique of serial pathology-guided partial excisions until achieving clean margins, partial laryngectomy, functional neck dissection), that in selected patients have cure rates similar to more radical techniques.[404]

Radiotherapy

General. Radiation therapy is an effective modality in treating local/regional disease. For early lesions, it gives results comparable to those achieved by surgery. For certain tumor sites such as the larynx, it is preferred over surgery in the treatment of early tumors because it maintains organ function. When lesions are intermediate in size, it is used adjuvantly (following surgical excision) to improve local/regional control.

Vikram and colleagues found that the rates of local/regional tumor recurrence were markedly higher if there was a greater than 6 week delay between surgery and postoperative radiotherapy.[728] For very advanced, inoperable lesions, and for lesions arising in certain sites such as the nasopharynx radiation therapy may be the only modality that offers a potential for cure. Recently, its therapeutic effectiveness has been enhanced by the concomitant use of chemotherapy.

Ionizing radiation (high-energy photons, electrons, neutrons, charged particles) interacts with matter in subtle ways.[292]

Tumors can vary dramatically in their ability to repair the DNA damage inflicted by radiation. Hyperthermia and concomitant chemotherapy are methods of reducing this repair ability. HNSCCs are generally characterized as moderately radioresponsive, meaning that fairly large dosages of radiation are required to achieve high probabilities of tumor control. Fortunately, the required dosages are within the tolerance of the various critical structures of the head and neck.

The effectiveness of a given quantity of radiation depends on the manner in which it is given.[292] Many different radiation treatment schedules are in use, and under investigation, in controlled clinical trials. Over the last 20 years in the U.S., however, a regimen of 180–200 cGy once a day for 5 days a week has become standard for most head and neck cancer patients. This schema evolved empirically to allow the regeneration of normal tissues during the course of radiotherapy. Radiation kills the stem cells in the basal layer, and then several weeks later the cells in the superficial layers are not replaced when they are lost through normal physiological processes. This denudes the epithelium, giving rise to the mucositis reaction that can greatly inhibit a patient's ability to swallow liquids and solids. Patients must be monitored closely during radiotherapy to ensure that this problem is minimized. It is important to note that this reaction does not occur immediately but develops after several weeks of treatment. A similar process takes place in skin layers exposed to therapeutic radiation, giving rise to a sunburn-like desquamation. Certain chemotherapeutic agents (5-Fluorouracil, actinomycin D, doxorubicin, and mitomycin C) can potentiate these reactions.

Although mucositis can delay the delivery and increase the overall treatment time, the major limiting factors for final dose determination are the long term effects of radiation on normal tissues. The late effects of head and neck irradiation can include thickening or fibrosis of the subcutaneous tissues, or fibrosis in the temporomandibular joint (which can cause trismus). In contrast to acute reactions, the magnitude of the late effects is determined more by the total dose given than by the daily fraction size. Salivary gland function and taste perception are altered by radiation.[488–490] The loss of saliva is significant after about 1,000 cGy is given to the glands; this decreased salivary output may persist for years. Taste loss is significant after 4,000–4,500 cGy to the oral cavity.

The decrease in saliva and changes in its chemical composition cause alterations in the microorganisms inhabiting the mouth, which in turn can cause a marked increase in the number of caries. Aggressive dental prophylaxis can reduce this problem, and workup by a dentist with expertise in these problems is mandatory *before* radiotherapy is initiated. The incidence of osteoradionecrosis can be considerably reduced if the necessary repairs and/or extractions are done pre-treatment rather than waiting until problems occur in a heavily irradiated field.[39,493] A delay of 2–3 weeks is required between extractions and the initiation of radiotherapy to allow adequate healing.

Technological Advances. Advances in radiotherapy have been tied to advances in technology. Modern radiotherapy departments use linear accelerators rather than ^{60}Co units, producing sharper field edges and higher dose rates. Megavoltage electron beams are used to treat the posterior neck nodes to tumoricidal dosages without risk of spinal cord damage. Custom blocking techniques reduce the radiation dosage to normal tissues and thus reduce treatment related morbidity. Computed tomography and magnetic resonance imaging are used to localize tumors for radiation therapy treatment planning. Figure XXVII-1-4 shows a reconstructed computed tomography scan with a large tumor of the maxillary, ethmoid, and frontal sinuses outlined on anterior and lateral projections. Information from such scans is input into treatment-planning computers to design individualized optimal treatment plans. Figure XXVII-1-5 shows the isodose distribution from a treatment plan for the tumor shown in Figure XXVII-1-4. Two levels are shown. Note how the radiation dose distribution lies deeper in the region of the maxillary and ethmoid sinuses but is "pulled" anteriorly at a level through the frontal sinus, thus sparing the frontal lobe. Noncoplanar field configurations, often using vertex presentations are now fairly standard techniques in many radiotherapy centers. Treatment field arrangements are verified immediately using a fluoroscopic simulator. With such techniques, there should be many fewer marginal misses than in the past.

Curative Radiotherapy. HNSCCs respond to radiation injury through a loss of reproductive capability, resulting in a clonogenic cell death. This cell-killing ability is essentially an exponential function of the radiation dosage (within the context of a given radiation fractionation schema), and so the dosage required for a given level of tumor control is approximately proportional to the number of clonogenic cells in the tumor.[292] Subclinical microscopic disease requires a dosage of

approximately 5,000 cGy, a 1 cm³ tumor requires approximately 6,500 cGy, and large (T_3 or T_4) tumors require dosages in the range of 7,000–7,500 cGy to maximize the chances of achieving tumor control.[224,400] Patients with head and neck tumors are generally treated with shrinking field techniques, wherein the various regions at risk receive dosages commensurate with the tumor mass they are thought to contain. A typical head and neck treatment regimen involves at least three separate alterations in radiation field geometry. Dosages greater than 7,500 cGy may be achieved using interstitial radioactive implants, which allow the delivery of ultrahigh dosages to small volumes with the dose levels to critical normal tissues kept within safe limits. Table XXVII-1-7 shows representative local control rates and survival data for patients with SCCs of common head and neck sites treated with definitive radiotherapy.[400] While the local/regional control rates are excellent for the small lesions, there is obviously room for improvement regarding the larger lesions.[281]

The choice between radiotherapy and surgery as definitive primary treatment is dependent on the interplay among many factors.[475] For early lesions of the larynx and the tip of the tongue, the two modalities yield equivalent local/regional control and survival. However, the functional result is better with radiotherapy, and so it is the treatment of choice. For early lesions of the lip or skin cancers of the nose or eyelid, the ultimate cosmetic result is better with radiotherapy. For sites such as the nasopharynx that are surgically unapproachable, radiotherapy is the only tenable form of definitive treatment. For early lesions of the tonsil and tongue (base and lateral aspect), the results are equivalent to surgery and informed patient choice should guide the treatment decision.

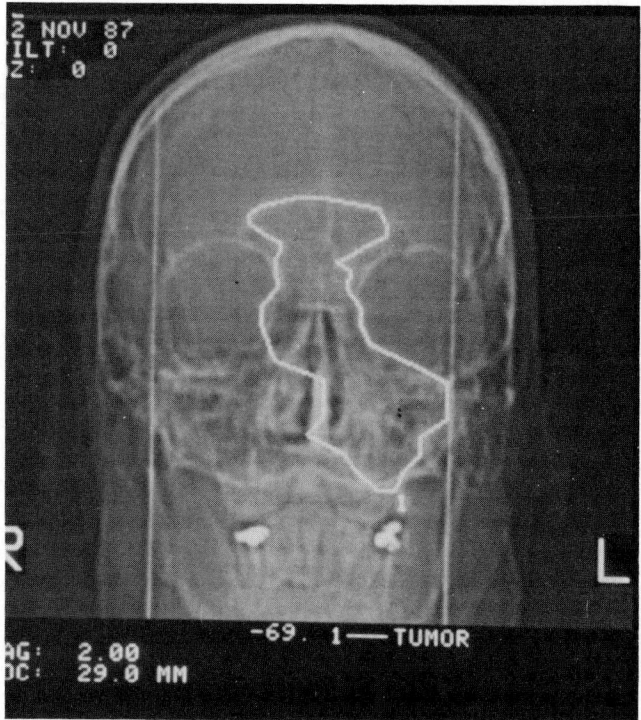
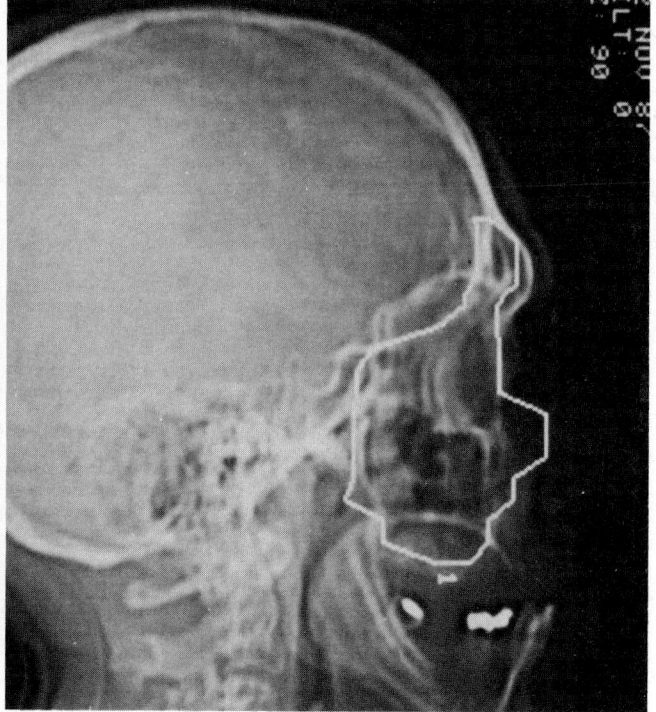

Figure XXVII-1-4. A large tumor of the maxillary, ethmoid and frontal sinuses outlined on a CT scan reconstruction showing the patient in anterior and lateral views. This information is used to design radiation therapy treatment fields.

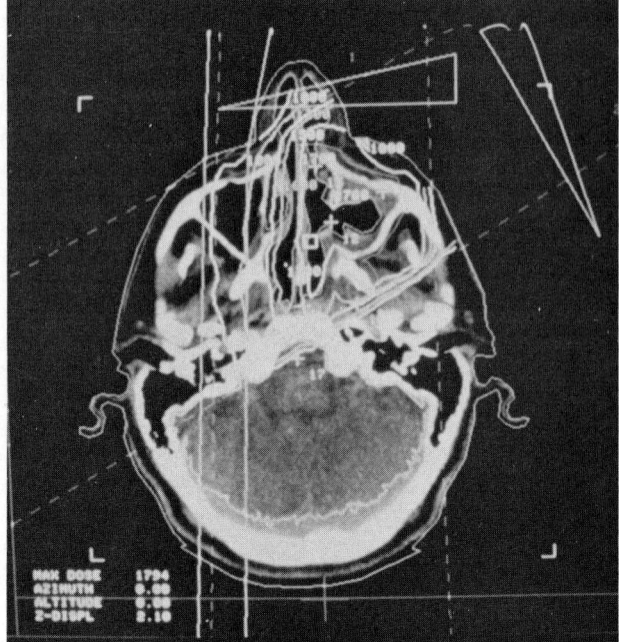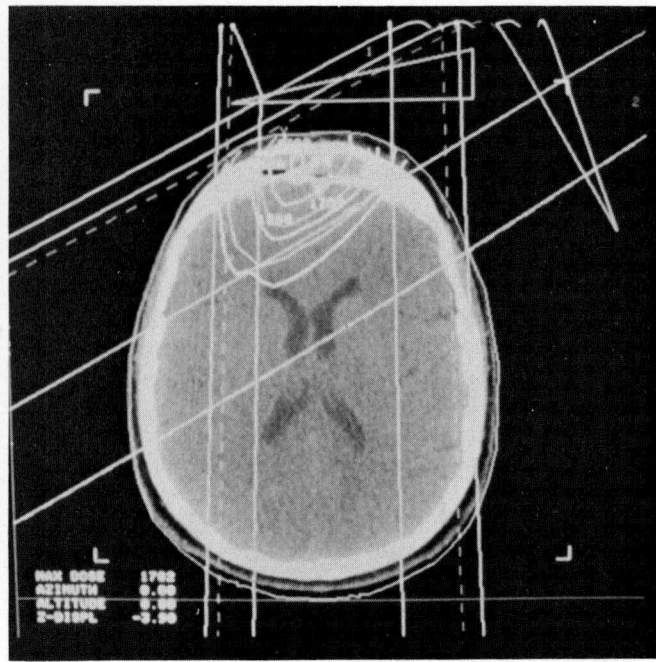

Figure XXVII-1-5. Radiation isodose distributions overlying transverse CT scan images at two different levels for the tumor shown in Figure XXVII-1-4. Note how the radiation isodoses extend posteriorly to cover the tumor in the maxillary and ethmoid sinus regions but are pulled anteriorly at the superior level thus sparing the normal brain tissue at this level while adequately treating the frontal sinuses.

Radiotherapy is also given following diagnosis of SCC metastatic to the cervical lymph nodes from an unknown primary site. The treatment fields encompass the probable sites of tumor origin: nasopharynx, tonsillar fossa, base of tongue, and hypopharynx; patient survival at 2–3 years ranges from 30–60%.[290]

Accelerated and Hyperfractionated Radiotherapy. An area of current clinical interest in radiotherapy is the use of non-standard fractionation patterns in radiotherapy in an attempt to improve the therapeutic response ratio. Late radiation effects limit the total amount of radiation that can be safely given in the standard treatment schema. The slowly proliferating normal tissues are the dose limiting structures for these late effects. Such tissues tend to have large shoulders on their cell survival curves which indicates an increased ability to repair sublethal radiation damage compared to that of rapidly proliferating normal tissues.[292] Hence, a logical approach would be to give smaller radiation treatment fractions so as not to exceed the shoulder on the late effects tissue cell survival curves and then to go to a higher total dose. The assumption is implicitly made that the tumor will behave like the rapidly proliferating normal tissues in that it will not have a large shoulder on its radiation cell survival curve and hence a therapeutic gain will result. To avoid inordinately prolonging the overall treatment time and hence allowing tumor repopulation kinetics to become the dominant effect, multiple daily fractions must be given.[292,695] A sufficient time interval (generally ≥ 6 hours) must be allowed between treatments to allow for adequate repair of sublethal and potentially-lethal damage.

Hyperfractionation refers to giving multiple daily doses such that the overall treatment time is about the same as for a course of conventionally-fractionated once a day radio-

therapy. The RTOG has been systematically exploring this approach using twice daily treatments of 120 cGy. Initially, a randomized trial was performed that randomized this treatment to a total dose of 6,000 cGy vs. conventional fractionation.[442] A total of 210 patients was entered onto this study. There was no difference in either local/regional control or survival, but the acute effects were well tolerated. This is important since the daily dose rate determines the acute effects, and on radiobiological grounds it should be possible to use a total dose considerably above 6,000 cGy. Currently the RTOG is conducting a phase II randomized trial to determine the maximum total hyperfractionated dose that can safely be given to the head and neck region. A preliminary report on this work suggests improved local control at 2 years with increasing radiation dose on the three lower dose arms: 25% for 6,720 cGy, 37% for 7,200 cGy, and 42% for 7,680 cGy (P = .08).[135] No survival differences were noted. The incidence of grade 4 necrosis was 10.0% on the 6,720 cGy arm, 5.1% on the 7,200 cGy arm, and 13.9% on the 7,680 cGy arm. Data on the 8,160 cGy arm are not yet available. The EORTC has investigated 3 daily fractions of 160 cGY each for 10 days, a 3-week break in treatment, followed by a boost of 6,720 cGy with or without misonidazole (a hypoxic cell radiosensitizer), compared to a third arm of standard fraction radiotherapy alone in a total of 523 patients. No significant differences in local or regional control or survival have been reported among the three arms.[713] Early mucosal reactions were more severe on the hyperfractionation arms but late effects were equivalent. The EORTC has also conducted a phase III trial comparing twice daily treatment of 115 cGy to a total dose of 8,050 cGy vs. 200 cGy once a day to a total dose of 7,000 cGy in 254 patients. The 3-year

Table XXVII-1-7. Representative Local Control Rates and Survival for Patients with Squamous Cell Carcinoma of Common Head and Neck Sites Treated with Definitive Radiotherapy

Stage by Site	Local Control (%)	Survival* (%)
Oral cavity		
Oral tongue		
T1	80–90	75–80
T2	60–85	40–60
T3	30–50	20–30
T4	25–45	10–15
Floor of mouth		
T1	75–85	70–85
T2	60–80	50–60
T3	30–50	15–40
T4	5–30	5–20
Oropharynx		
Base of tongue		
T1	80–95	65–85
T2	60–75	40–55
T3	40–65	15–20
T4	30–50	5–20
Tonsil/tonsillar fossa		
T1	75–95	65–85
T2	60–80	55–60
T3	35–70	20–40
T4	20–30	10–15
Soft palate		
T1	90–100	90–95
T2	75–85	65–75
T3	60–70	30–40
T4	25–35	10–15
Nasopharynx		
T1	70–85	60–75
T2	50–60	50–65
T3	20–45	25–50
T4	15–35	5–30
Hypopharynx		
Pyriform sinus		
T1	60–70	30–50
T2	40–50	20–45
T3	30–40	15–25
T4	10–25	5–20
Larynx		
Supraglottic		
T1	80–90	65–90
T2	60–80	50–65
T3	35–70	35–55
T4	30–60	15–40
Glottis		
T1	85–95	80–95
T2	65–75	60–85
T3	20–35	35–60
T4	15–30	10–30

*Adapted from Laramore.[400] Local control is for radiation alone. Survival data include surgical salvage for radiation failures. Overlap in the two sets of figures is due to data coming from different patient series, which are a heterogeneous mix of nodal stages, Karnofsky scores, tumor differentiation.

local/regional control rate was 59% on the hyperfractionation arm vs. 43% on the standard arm.[328]

Accelerated fractionation refers to giving multiple daily doses of such a size that the overall treatment time is shortened relative to that of conventional radiotherapy. The fraction size and the total dose given are generally slightly less than that of conventional radiotherapy. C.C. Wang has developed a twice daily schema utilizing 160 cGy fractions.[749,751] The total daily dose is thus 320 cGy, which is too high for the rapidly proliferating normal tissues (e.g., mucosa) to tolerate without a planned interruption in treatment to allow for recovery and repopulation. No randomized trial has been carried out to evaluate it, but an historical comparison indicates a possible benefit to its use. Other accelerated fractionation schemes have been utilized in various pilot studies but no randomized trials have taken place.[276,467,476,498] Because of the acute toxicity with these regimens, a controlled trial is warranted before acceptance into standard practice.

Combined Surgery and Radiotherapy

Very few well-designed randomized trials have compared surgery alone to combined therapy in any disease site. When treatment is surgery or radiotherapy alone, local/regional control rates for stage I and II lesions are in the range of 75–90% (depending on disease site). The local/regional control rates with single-modality therapy are much less satisfactory in stage III and IV lesions, for which the standard medial practice of today employs both modalities.

Radiotherapy can be given either preoperatively or postoperatively. The aims of preoperative radiotherapy are to sterilize microscopic disease outside the resection field and to shrink the tumor bulk, thus making the surgery easier to perform. Theoretically, preoperative radiotherapy should also reduce the risk of the dissemination of viable tumor cells at surgery. A dosage of 5,000 cGy over 5–5½ weeks is usually given.[226] There appear to be no significant problems with delayed wound healing at this dosage.

When radiotherapy is postoperative, the surgical resection bed has a disrupted blood supply and conventional wisdom says that higher dosages of radiation are needed because of the increased likelihood of hypoxic tumor cells, which are less radiosensitive. Generally, one delivers 5,500–6,000 cGy in 180 to 200 cGy fractions in a postoperative setting. Higher dosages are used if the surgical margins are compromised and there is a high likelihood of the presence of macroscopic residual disease. Postoperative radiotherapy has the advantage of being given to only those patients thought to be at a significant risk for local/regional tumor recurrence based on a thorough review of the pathologic data. It has the further advantage of not delaying the surgical procedure, which for patients with operable disease is the most important treatment modality.

Preoperative and postoperative radiotherapy were compared in a randomized clinical trial by the RTOG. A total of 277 patients with tumors of the oral cavity, oropharynx, supraglottic larynx, or hypopharynx were entered into the study.[396] Patients in the preoperative arm received 5,000 cGy followed by surgery in 4–6 weeks, whereas patients in the postoperative arm received 6,000 cGy starting 2–4 weeks after the surgical resection. At higher percentage of patients in the postoperative arm completed the combined course of therapy within protocol guidelines (74% vs. 56%). The 4-year competing-risk local/regional tumor control was 65% in the postoperative arm vs. 48% in the preoperative arm (P = 0.04). For the subgroup of 194 patients who completed overall treatment within protocol guidelines, the local/regional control rates were 74% in the postoperative arm and 56% in the preoperative arm. There were no significant differences between the two study arms in complication or survival rates.

In general, there is little role for debulking surgery in head and neck tumors. When gross tumor is left behind, high-dosage radiation delivered as in definitive radiotherapy is required. This means that 6,500–7,500 cGy must be given in 6½ to 8 weeks, which is generally more difficult to tolerate after a radical surgical procedure.

Chemotherapy—General. Chemotherapeutic strategies for HNSCC are reviewed in detail in Chemotherapy Approaches below. Systemic approaches to salivary gland tumors, nasopharyngeal carcinoma, advanced skin cancer, esthesioneuroblastoma and other non-squamous cancers are distinct from head and neck cancers at other sites and therefore are discussed separately below.

Natural History and Treatment by Site

Oral Cavity

Both tumor growth and treatment significantly compromise speech and deglutition, particularly for those patients in whom cancer involves the tongue, floor of mouth, or mandible. Furthermore, the diversity of potential sites of cancer development in the oral cavity and variations of lymphatic drainage and rates of node metastases lend added complexity to treatment planning.[714,740] Despite the fact that this region is readily amenable to visual examination and bimanual palpation, more than 50% of patients are diagnosed in advanced stages. The current T staging of oral cavity primaries are listed in Table XXVII-1-8.

Lip. SCCs of the lip are the most common oral cavity cancer. Over 90% occur on the lower lip, usually on the exposed vermilion border, midway between the midline and the oral commissure. Upper lip cancers most commonly are basal cell carcinomas.[448] Well differentiated and verrucous cancers rarely metastasize. Poorly differentiated and spindle cell varieties tend to grow aggressively, metastasize commonly and infiltrate neural pathways.[579]

The treatment of lip cancers must consider adequate removal of tissue to encompass the disease yet provide the patient with a lip that functions in speech, chewing, and oral competence, and provides adequate cosmesis.[24,752] These goals are achieved equally well with either primary radiation or surgery when the tumors are less than 2 cm in size or are very superficial. Larger lesions are best treated with surgical resection and reconstruction[354] where there is greater accuracy in evaluating the extent of tumor and nerve or cervical lymphatic involvement. Frequently, adjacent precancerous changes are present which can be treated with Moh's surgery, or vermilionectomy of the remainder of the lip, to prevent recurrences or development of second primary tumors.[464,774] For large lesions, primary reconstruction with local and regional flaps avoids defects which result from tissue loss with radiotherapy, provides for future reconstructive and treatment options and eliminates the risk of osteoradionecrosis of the mandible. Lesions demonstrating extensive infiltration, bone involvement or lymphatic metastases are increasingly managed with combined surgery and postoperative radiation.

Radiation therapy techniques for management of lip cancers includes external irradiation, interstitial implants (usually radium needles or iridium-192), or combinations of both. Local tumor control rates with irradiation exceed 80%[359,438,525] with determinant survival at 5 years, including surgical salvage, in excess of 95%. Similar tumor control and survival rates are reported with primary surgical excision.[25] Confirmed regional metastases decrease the survival rates to 36–55%.[146,359] Five-year survival rates for patients with carcinomas of the upper lip are lower than for lower lip lesions and range from 40–60%.[482,585] Involvement of both lips or the lateral commissure is uncommon. The prognosis for commissure lesions is not as good as for cancers of other areas of the lip. Cross and colleagues report 5-year survival rate of 34% for patients with oral commissure carcinoma (Table XXVII-1-9).[146]

Tongue. Tongue cancers account for 25% of oral cavity SCC and most commonly arise in the oral portion or anterior two-thirds of the tongue on the lateral edge or ventral surface. Infiltration of the underlying tongue musculature occurs early. The intrinsic tongue muscles are loosely arranged, interdigitating and endowed with a rich vascular and lymphatic supply which may explain the early high rate of regional metastases.

Most patients present with T2 lesions. Prognosis is directly

Table XXVII-1-8. Primary Tumor Staging Characteristics for Oral Cavity Carcinoma

Tx	Primary tumor cannot be assessed
T0	No evidence of primary tumor
Tis	Carcinoma in situ
T1	Tumor 2 cm or less in greatest dimension
T2	Tumor more than 2 cm, but less than 4 cm in greatest dimension
T3	Tumor more than 4 cm in greatest dimension
T4	(lip) Tumor invades adjacent structures, e.g., through cortical bone, tongue, skin of neck
T4	(oral cavity) Tumor invades adjacent structures, e.g., cortical bone, deep tissues (extrinsic muscle of tongue, maxillary sinus, skin)

Table XXVII-1-9. Five-Year Survival Rates for Patients with Carcinoma of the Lip

Investigator	Number of Patients	5-Year Survival (%)	
		Determinant	Absolute
Burkell[78]	534	89	80
Gladstone[260]	519	82	65
Schreiner[585]	636	74	59
Wookey[788]	1,128	85	58
Molnar[482]	2,066	86	76
Cross[146]	563	58	50
Jorgensen[359]	869	97	84
MacKay and Sellers[438]	3,166	89	65

related to the degree of infiltration and presence of regional metastases. The biologic aggressiveness of small (<4 cm) tongue cancers is noteworthy and is reflected in higher rates of occult regional metastases than similarly staged lesions arising from other oral sites (Table XXVII-1-10). Occult node metastases are present in 30–40% of early lesions.[162,184,214,648] Approximately 40% of patients have clinical evidence of node metastases at diagnosis.[647] Primary echelon node drainage is to the upper deep cervical lymphatics. Involvement of mid and lower neck nodes (Level III & IV) is not uncommon. Bilateral nodal involvement may be present with cancers of the tip of the tongue or those involving the midline of the tongue. Local-regional recurrence in patients with tongue cancer accounts for 60–70% of cancer deaths.[84,720,743] Distant metastases account for 15% of deaths and second primaries for 20–40%.

The management of carcinomas of the tongue has been significantly influenced by a better appreciation of the aggressiveness of small, deeply infiltrative lesions, the high rate of occult lymph node metastases and an interest in improving treatment without compromising oral function. Although surgical excision has been the mainstay of treatment, combined surgery and adjuvant radiation therapy to include the primary site and regional nodes is commonly used for most advanced (Stage III and IV) cancers and is being used increasingly for small Stage II cancers. For Stage I cancers, surgical excision is effective and expeditious with good preservation of function. For Stage II lesions that are infiltrative, hemiglossectomy achieves excellent tumor control rates and can be combined with selective dissection of neck nodes to provide accurate staging information and determination of the need for adjuvant radiation. Hemiglossectomy results in significant functional morbidity in terms of articulation and deglutition. Because of this, radiation therapy alone has been used in some cases. For radiation to be as effective as surgery in controlling these cancers, interstitial brachytherapy combined with external radiation is essential. Radiation doses of 80–85 Gy are generally given via external megavoltage radiation or in combination with brachytherapy. Interstitial treatment requires precise placement and spacing of implants. Accurate dosimetry is enhanced by using afterloading techniques in which the radioactive source is inserted into previously placed hollow tubes. Tracheostomy at time of implant should be considered because of the potential development of tongue edema after implantation. Occult or apparent neck disease is usually treated using external radiation or radiation combined with

neck dissection.[162] Extension of cancer to the floor of mouth or mandible may necessitate partial mandibulectomy or segmental mandibular resection. Modern reconstructive techniques with vascularized composite bone and soft tissue free flaps, titanium metal prostheses, pedicled myocutaneous regional flaps and free bone grafts have improved the function and cosmetic results of major mandibular resections. In most cases, if the neck must be surgically entered to accomplish adequate resection of the primary tumor, a neck dissection is performed simultaneously. When tumors grossly involve bone, radiation therapy is less effective in these poorly vascularized osseous tissues and requires high doses that are associated with osteoradionecrosis. After local failure of interstitial implants complication rates for salvage surgical resections are extremely high and are associated with significant morbidity from fistulization, radionecrosis and failure of primary reconstructive efforts. In many cases, construction of control fistulas and delayed reconstruction with well-vascularized flaps is advantageous. Although the surgical salvage of radiation failures is often successful in early lesions, success drops to less than 50% in advanced lesions.

For more advanced primary lesions (Stage III & IV), external radiation *and* surgery are generally used. Radiation has been administered either as planned pre-operative or postoperative therapy. Although no prospective controlled trials have proven the superiority of combined therapy over surgery alone, many studies indicate improved local/regional control rates.[227,407,408,724,729] These improvements have generally been offset, in part, by an increased frequency of distant metastases and second primaries. Surgical management generally consists of partial glossectomy and neck dissection frequently combined with mandibulectomy. Where tumors extend to the midline or involve the tongue base, subtotal or total glossectomy may be necessary. Modern reconstructive techniques have improved the functional results of these aggressive resections. Provisions for temporary tracheostomy and prolonged enteral nutrition should be made. Total glossectomy or sacrifice of both hypoglossal nerves frequently necessitates permanent feeding gastrostomy or jejunostomy. Current experience indicates that total glossectomy can be accomplished without the need for laryngectomy.[51]

Tumor resection is more difficult after pre-operative radiation therapy unless precise tattooing of intended resection margins is accomplished prior to therapy. Likewise, the rates of surgical complications, fistulization, exposed bone and radionecrosis are increased with preoperative radiation.

Table XXVII-1-10. Occult Lymph Node Metastases for Oral Cavity Carcinoma by Level*

Level (# positive/total)	Tongue (18/58) %	Floor of Mouth (15/57) %	Gingiva (20/52) %	Retromolar Trigone (7/16) %	Buccal (5/9) %
I	14	16	27	19	44
II	19	12	21	12	11
III	16	7	6	6	0
IV	3	2	4	6	0
V	0	0	2	0	0

*Modified from Shah et al.[594]

Because of this, most centers have adopted a policy of post-operative radiation. With postoperative radiation, higher doses can be delivered, the extent of disease is precisely defined, the histologic status of the lymph nodes is known, and high risk areas of close margins or residual cancer can be treated to high dose. Both ipsilateral and contralateral necks are irradiated with dosage determined by disease extent. Post-operative radiation should begin within 4–6 weeks of resection. Interstitial implants are not used. Close surgical margins require high doses (70 Gy) because of the difficulty in eradicating even small amounts of tumor in the tongue after glossectomy.[30] Curative radiation alone with surgical salvage has been shown to be inferior to combined therapy in control of local/regional disease, and in the complication rate, even though survival rates are similar with these approaches.[395,396] Even with combined therapy, estimated 2-year disease-free and overall survival rates for advanced disease are only 51% and 53%, respectively.[783] Five-year survival rates range from 50–70% for Stages I and II to 15–30% for Stages III and IV (Table XXVII-1-11).[84]

The management of the neck is of particular interest in patients with tongue cancer because of the high rate of occult node metastases. For lesions T2 or greater in size, rates of occult metastases exceed 40% and some form of neck treatment is generally indicated. When the primary tumor can be adequately excised via transoral technique, irradiation of both necks may be substituted for elective neck dissections, particularly if adjuvant radiation for control of the primary tumor is anticipated. When radiation alone is selected for treatment of primary tumors with neck node metastases, this treatment is often combined with therapeutic neck dissection.[162]

Floor of Mouth. Floor of mouth cancers occur with a frequency similar to tongue cancer. Early spread to adjacent areas (gingiva and periosteum of the mandible) is common. The periosteum is a natural barrier to spread. Fixation of the tongue is a sign of deep invasion. Tumor may extend to or through the mylohyoid muscle which serves as a natural barrier to direct spread below the hyoid bone. Lymph node metastases at presentation are seen in approximately 40% of patients and an additional 20% have occult lymphatic metastases.[184] The occult metastatic rate increases with the T stage of the primary: T2 tumors have a 40%, and T3 tumors a 70% occult metastases rate.

First echelon nodes of lymphatic drainage include the submandibular and deep cervical jugulodigastric nodes (Level I and II). Submental node involvement is unusual. Evaluation for early mandibular involvement is facilitated by palpation since fixation to the mandible indicates periosteal involve-

ment and direct bone invasion is present in 50–60% of such tumors.

Small cancers (T1, T2) are treated effectively by wide resection or radiation therapy. Little morbidity results from surgical resection of superficial lesions. Lateral floor of mouth tumors can often be resected transorally and the resection defect closed with advancement of adjacent mucosa or with skin grafts. Early cancers involving the mandible are best treated surgically because bone involvement compromises radiation efficacy.

Radiation therapy for small floor of mouth cancers usually involves combinations of external radiation and brachytherapy. Decision-making concerning primary therapy involves consideration of the expected functional result, management of the neck nodes and risk of osteoradionecrosis. Radiotherapy for moderate size (T2) anterior floor of mouth lesions and small or deeply invasive cancers offers the advantage of treating bilateral first echelon lymph nodes. Rates of occult nodal metastases range from 30–40%. Resection of cancers which extend to involve the tongue cause greater functional impairment and radiation therapy achieves a better functional result and equally good local control rates. Regional lymphatics are electively irradiated.

More advanced floor of mouth cancers (T3, T4) are generally treated with resection combined with postoperative radiation of the primary and regional nodes. These resections require a transcervical approach and are combined with neck dissection and mandibular resections as needed. Large surgical defects are reconstructed with skin grafts, local flaps, or myocutaneous pedicled regional flaps. Mandibular reconstruction for segmental defects is performed primarily with free or pedicled bone grafts or alloplastic materials.

Doses of radiation therapy for local/regional tumor control are based on actual tumor volume rather than T stage.[466] Interstitial doses of 65–75 Gy are recommended for early lesions (1–3 cm) if brachytherapy alone is used, or external beam radiation of 50 Gy combined with 25–30 Gy of interstitial radiation. Post-operative doses are given by external radiation only at doses of 65 Gy over 6–7 weeks, or preoperative doses of 50 Gy over 6 weeks. No significant differences in overall survival rates have been shown comparing pre-operative to postoperative radiation regimens.[396]

Treatment results are influenced by the size of the primary tumor, presence of lymph node metastases, degree of mandibular involvement and adequacy of resection. Five-year survival rates for localized Stage I and II carcinomas of the floor of mouth range from 60–80% (Table XXVII-1-12). Cancers that cross the midline, involve the tongue, or involve

Table XXVII-1-11.   Overall Five-Year Survival Rates (%) for Patients with Squamous Carcinoma of the Tongue

Investigator	N	Stage I	Stage II	Stage III	Stage IV
Callery[84]	252	75	60	40	20
Decroix[162]	602	59	45	25	13
Wallner[743]	424	68	50	33	20
Ildstad[338]	122	48	48	18	26
O'Brien[504]	97	73*	62*	—	—
Average	(N = 1,497)	65	53	29	20

*Disease-free survival

Table XXVII-1-12. Overall Five-Year Survival Rates (%) in Patients with Squamous Carcinoma of the Floor of Mouth

Investigator	N	Stage I	Stage II	Stage III	Stage IV
Harrold[296]	634	69	49	25	7
Panje[510]	103	57	60	43	19
Trible[703]	56	100	65	37	11
Nason[496]	198	69	64	46	26
Shaha[601]	320	88	80	66	32
Fu[241]	153	83	71	43	10
Average	(N = 1,464)	78	65	43	18

the mandible are associated with 50–60% 5-year survival rates.[510] Survival rates for more advanced lesions (Stage III and IV) are less than 50%. Lymph node metastases decrease survival rates to approximately 25%. The major advantage in combined treatment (radiation and surgery) in these patients is improved control of ipsilateral and contralateral neck disease. Because rates of occult nodal disease are high in advanced primary lesions, elective treatment of the neck with radiation or bilateral neck dissection is indicated. Recurrence in the untreated, clinically negative neck is the most frequent site of failure in patients treated only with surgery.[601] The debate over performing elective neck dissection versus irradiation remains unresolved. If adequate primary tumor margins are uncertain or if multiple histologically positive lymph node metastases are detected, postoperative radiation to the ipsilateral and contralateral neck is administered. The development of second primary cancers is a major cause of morbidity and death. Fu and colleagues reported 55 of 153 (36%) of patients developed second primaries of whom 30 died from their second cancer.[241] Distant metastases occur in 10–15% of patients.[241,601]

Gingiva and Buccal Mucosa. Gingival cancers occur most commonly (80%) in the lower gingiva posterior to the bicuspid teeth.[83] For both sites, trismus is an ominous sign. Clinical staging criteria are similar to other oral sites. Overall, regional metastases occur in 30% of gingival cancers[81] and approximately 50% of buccal cancers.[57] Occult metastases occur in 10–20% of patients. Exophytic tumors tend to be papillary or verrucous in appearance and can be confused with benign hyperkeratosis.

Small, superficial gingival cancers can be effectively treated with surgical resection or radiation therapy with excellent preservation of function. Generally, the amount of bone resected for small lesions is minimal and resection can be accomplished transorally. Even larger lesions requiring partial maxillectomy or alveolectomy can be resected without external incision. External beam irradiation is not as effective in local tumor control once gross bone involvement has occurred. The intermediate (T2 or larger) lesions are best handled surgically; the risk of osteoradionecrosis is thereby avoided. For large lesions (T3 and T4) segmental mandibulectomy or maxillectomy is required and adjuvant radiation is frequently recommended. Elective neck dissection is not indicated unless the en bloc resection of a large primary tumor requires neck exposure. For patients in whom no neck dissection is performed, elective neck irradiation should be considered. Clinically positive neck nodes warrant neck dissection combined with resection of the primary tumor.

Buccal carcinomas of early stage (I or II) can be treated equally well with surgery or radiation. Radiation therapy offers the advantage of including the draining lymphatics in the treatment fields, but also risks post-treatment fibrosis and trismus. Large primary tumors or tumors with regional metastases are managed surgically with the need for adjuvant radiation determined by the adequacy of resection and risk of suspected residual disease. Neck dissection is preferred in all cases of clinically positive lymph nodes.

Overall survival rates for gingival and buccal cancers depend on tumor size, bone involvement and node metastases. Five-year survival rates for lower gingival lesions do not differ from upper gingiva and range from 78% for Stage I to 15% for Stage IV disease.[436] Surgical results are clearly superior to radiation when bone involvement is present. Survival rates (5-year) for Stage I and II buccal carcinomas range from 65–75%. Determinant survival for Stage III and IV disease varies from 20% to 30%.[57] For both gingival and buccal mucosal cancers, overall survival rates have improved over recent years when surgical management has replaced radiation therapy as primary treatment.

Retromolar Trigone. Cancers arising of the retromolar trigone (the narrow band of mucosa that lies behind the mandibular molar teeth and covers the ascending ramus) are rarely confined to that gingiva, but involve adjacent buccal mucosa, anterior tonsillar pillar, floor of mouth or posterior gingiva. Thus, retromolar trigone cancers that involve the anterior tonsillar pillar behave more like oropharyngeal cancers than oral cavity primaries. The risk of clinically positive and occult lymph node metastases is higher than with other gingival cancers. The frequent involvement of periosteum mandates partial (rim or marginal) mandibulectomy as part of surgical management even for small lesions. Primary radiation therapy is reserved for superficial lesions that cover a large surface area, such as extension to soft palate or buccal mucosa. Moderately advanced or deeply invasive lesions are best treated with surgical resection (mandibulectomy and neck dissection) followed by radiation therapy, unless the functional or cosmetic result would be unacceptable to the patient.

Oropharynx

The clinical staging of oropharyngeal cancers is dependent primarily on tumor size and is similar to the staging of oral cavity cancers (Table XXVII-1-13). Tumors may arise from any site in the oropharynx, but most commonly arise from the tonsillar area and palatine arch. The most common presenting symptom is chronic sore throat (often unilateral) and referred otalgia. Change in voice, dysphagia, and tris-

Table XXVII-1-13. Primary Tumor Staging Characteristics for Cancer of the Oropharynx

Tx	Primary tumor cannot be assessed
T0	No evidence of primary tumor
Tis	Carcinoma in situ
T1	Tumor <2 cm in greatest dimension
T2	Tumor >2 cm, but not more than 4 cm in greatest dimension
T3	Tumor >4 cm in greatest dimension
T4	Tumor invades adjacent structures, e.g., through cortical bone, soft tissue of neck, deep muscle of tongue

mus are late signs. Regional lymphatic metastases occur frequently and are related to the depth of tumor invasion and tumor size. Upper cervical nodes are generally invaded first, but clinical involvement of lower nodes can occur with skipping of upper first-echelon nodes. Bilateral lymphatic metastases can occur, particularly with cancers of the soft palate, tongue base and midline pharyngeal wall.

Tonsil

These cancers tend to be superficial, better differentiated and earlier stage than other oropharyngeal tumors. The treatment of early tonsillar neoplasms (Stage I, II) is usually radiation therapy alone. Transoral wide local excision of small, superficial lesions is effective. Deeply invasive cancers require extensive resections of pharyngeal wall or mandible.[544]

Radiation for early cancers offers the advantage of treating upper echelon lymph nodes. Treatment is usually unilateral unless extension to tongue base or midline soft palate is present which warrants treatment of contralateral lymphatics. Ipsilateral treatment portals allow sparing the contralateral mucosa and salivary glands. Because much of the tumor may be hidden from external beam photons by the mandible, deeper dose-calculation with electron beam therapy is used which can be combined with a small interstitial implant if invasion of adjacent tongue is present. Early cancers of the tonsillar pillar are less effectively treated with radiation alone than are cancers confined to the tonsillar fossa.[481]

Radical radiotherapy to lymph nodes controls approximately 90% of limited nodal disease (N_1) if the primary tumor is controlled , but nodal failure increases to greater than 20% if failure occurs at the primary tumor site. Overall 5-year survival rates for patients with advanced primary tumors or regional metastases are generally less than 25% with single modality therapy.[105,248,481,694] Combinations of surgery and radiation therapy offer improved rates of local and regional tumor control which, in some studies, has translated into improved survival.[154,481,618] Similar tumor control and survival rates have been reported for Stage III (T_3N_0) patients without nodal metastases who are treated with radiation alone or combined surgery and radiation or surgery alone (Table XXVII-1-14).[16,518] In general, preoperative or postoperative radiation for advanced (Stage III, IV) cancers of the tonsillar fossa is recommended, combined with radical resection to include the tonsillar fossa, adjacent mandible and regional lymphatics (composite neck resection). Postoperative rather than preoperative radiation is currently preferred because it allows more accurate assessment of surgical margins, local extent of disease and degree of lymphatic involvement, and is associated with lower rates of surgical complications.

Tongue Base

Base of the tongue cancer poses a more difficult therapeutic problem than tonsillar carcinomas. Five-year survival rates are lower, metastases more common, early diagnosis less common, and treatment morbidity is greater. Because of the functional difficulties from wide local excision, even of small tongue base cancers, most early (T_1, T_2) tumors are treated with definitive radiation. Three-quarters of patients are first seen with Stage III or IV disease primarily because of the early development of regional metastases, even with T_1 or T_2 tumors. Understaging of the primary tumor is frequent because these cancers tend to be diffusely infiltrative beyond their clinical appearance. This may account for similarities in local tumor control rates for both "early" and advanced lesions. The poor outcome is largely due to late diagnosis.

The staging of tongue base carcinomas is principally dependent on primary tumor size and extent of regional metastases. Lymph node involvement is present in approximately 60% of patients with small (T_1, T_2) primaries[759] and is the major determinant of prognosis. Overall 5-year survival rates range from 11 to 45%.[32,756] Five-year survival rates decrease from greater than 60% for N_0 patients to less than 30% for N_+ patients.[32,34,759]

The results of radiation therapy alone as definitive treatment for small primary tumors (T_1, T_2) are better for exophytic than for deeply invasive tumors.[759] Radiation alone is generally reserved for those patients without clinical node metastases, but can be combined with salvage neck dissection for patients with clinically positive nodes that persist after completion of radiation. Local recurrence is more frequent after radiation alone in most series,[32,558,759] and salvage of local failure with subsequent surgery is poor. In selected patients, interstitial radiation therapy has been used to treat residual palpable disease after external beam radiation in anticipation of better local control. The use of brachytherapy is associated with high rates of soft tissue necrosis and osteoradionecrosis, however.[246,315] The results of supplemental interstitial therapy appear to be highly dose and technique dependent with the best results reported with extensive percutaneous lateral cervical loop implants to include treatment of the lateral oropharyngeal wall and pharyngoepiglottic fold.[267] The acute morbidity of implantation techniques is severe and results in massive tongue edema necessitating tracheostomy in all patients. The role of radiation therapy alone seems best reserved for small, exophytic primary tumors without node metastases.

Surgical management of small primary tongue base tumors (T_1) achieves results similar to radiation alone. In most cases, primary tumors are moderately advanced and require transcervical resection via mandibulotomy or lateral pharyngotomy approaches, combined with elective or therapeutic neck dissection. Local tumor control rates are superior to radiation alone,[32,759] but regional control is poor if clinically positive nodes are present. Elective neck dissection can serve an important role as a staging procedure to determine if metastases are present, thereby providing rationale for adjuvant radiation therapy. To date, no prospective randomized trial

Table XXVII-1-14. Three-Year and Five-Year Survival Rates (%) in Patients with Squamous Carcinoma of the Tonsil

Investigator	N	Stage I	Stage II	Stage III	Stage IV	Duration
Perez[518]	218	76	40	42	25	3-year
Spiro[646]	117	89	83	58	49	3-year
Dasmahapatra[154]	174	83	72	23	15	5-year
Amornarn[16]	185	100	73	52	21	5-year
Mizono[481]	171	92	77	56	29	5-year determinant
Givens[259]	104	93	57	27	17	5-year determinant

data are available to demonstrate improved survival comparing surgery alone to combined surgery with either pre- or postoperative radiation for patients with tongue base cancer. Survival rates do not differ substantially by stage of disease for patients with tongue base cancers except for those with Stage IV disease (Table XXVII-1-15).

Soft Palate and Pharyngeal Wall

These cancers are less common than other oropharyngeal neoplasms. Most soft palate cancers occur on the anterior surface of the palate and tend to be superficial. Regional metastases are uncommon, although lateral extension to the tonsillar area results in increased rates of lymph node involvement and lesions close to the midline result in bilateral or contralateral neck metastases in 15% of patients. Occult node metastases are estimated to occur in 16% of patients.[416] Posterior wall lesions tend to be superficial with less tumor bulk than similarly staged lesions elsewhere in the oropharynx. Tumor extension to the tongue base decreases survival and increases the rate of metastases which are often bilateral. Advanced lesions with deep invasion have ready access to the prevertebral space, infratemporal fossa and skull base and can be associated with extensive submucosal spread with clinical "skip" areas.

Radiation alone as curative treatment is preferred in most cases even for T_3 or T_4 primary tumors.[225] Resection of all but the smallest soft palate lesions is associated with significant functional disability. The rates of occult regional metastases are difficult to determine because elective irradiation of bilateral nodal groups is included as part of primary treatment. Clinically positive lymph nodes at presentation occur in 30% of patients. Small primary tumor with positive nodes can be effectively treated with definitive radiation to the primary tumor and radiation combined with neck dissection for the nodes. Extensive pharyngeal wall cancers or palate cancers with extension to the tonsil and those cases with advanced regional metastases are usually treated with combined surgical resection and postoperative radiation. Overall 5-year survival rates for soft palate and faucial pillar

cancers are 60–70% and range from 80–90% for T_1 or T_2 lesions to 30–60% for Stage III and IV lesions.[759] Local/regional recurrence is the most frequent cause of failure.[761]

Hypopharynx

SCC of the hypopharynx represents one of the most lethal sites. Lymph node metastases are clinically evident at time of diagnosis in 70–80% of patients[35,200,474] and are indicative of advanced disease. Bilateral and contralateral lymph node metastases occur in 10–20% of cases particularly if tumors cross the midline of the hypopharynx. Primary tumor extension beyond the hypopharynx is common.[91,527] Hypopharyngeal cancers are characterized by a propensity to spread submucosally to involve the oropharynx or esophagus. Ulcerated, deep infiltration and "skip areas" are common. This leads to difficulties in adequately assessing the margins of the tumor and contributes to poor local tumor control even with the addition of adjuvant radiation.[194] The majority (>75%) of hypopharyngeal cancers arise in the pyriform sinus while 20% occur in the posterior pharyngeal wall. Postcricoid cancers are rare (<5%). Posterior pharyngeal wall cancers tend to grow superficially and only involve the prevertebral fascia in advanced lesions. Pyriform cancers spread early to other contiguous structures such as the larynx, postcricoid area, thyroid gland and thyroid and cricoid cartilages. Most pyriform sinus cancers arise in the apex of the sinus. The postcricoid mucosa is contiguous with the apex of the pyriform and tumor can spread circumferentially to involve the entire lower hypopharynx. Because of the locale of hypopharyngeal cancers and their growth patterns and proximity to the larynx, surgical management generally entails partial or total pharyngectomy combined with laryngectomy.[577]

The staging of hypopharyngeal cancer is based primarily on the subsite of the pharynx involved, presence of vocal cord fixation and extent of lymph node metastases (Table XXVII-1-16). Distant metastases at the time of diagnosis are rare. Staging evaluation is critical for treatment planning and must include endoscopic evaluation to determine precisely the tumor margins, extent of invasion of adjacent structures

Table XXVII-1-15. Overall Survival Rates (%) in Patients with Squamous Carcinoma of the Tongue Base According to T Class and Tumor Stage

Investigator	N	T class				Stage				Rate
		T1	T2	T3	T4	I	II	III	IV	
Thawley[696]	101	57	72	30	22	50	44	45	28	5-year
Weber[759]	173	100	58	38	20	100	72	50	30	5-year
Barrs[32]	119	63	56	31	—	68	55	55	11	3-year

Table XXVII-1-16. Primary Tumor Staging Characteristics for Carcinoma of the Hypopharynx

Tx	Primary tumor cannot be assessed
T0	No evidence of primary tumor
Tis	Carcinoma in situ
T1	Tumor limited to one subsite of the hypopharynx
T2	Tumor invades more than one subsite of the hypopharynx or adjacent site, without fixation of hemilarynx
T3	Tumor invades more than one subsite of the hypopharynx or adjacent site, with fixation of hemilarynx
T4	Tumor invades adjacent structures, e.g., cartilage or soft tissue of neck

and presence of second primary tumors or "skip areas." Determination of the precise site of origin and inferior extent of a tumor can be difficult with large tumors or with those obstructing the esophageal inlet.

Because of the necessity of removing the larynx as part of the surgical treatment of most hypopharyngeal cancers, radiation therapy alone as treatment has been extensively investigated.[478] Retrospective analyses have consistently demonstrated that survival rates are lower and local/regional failure rates higher with radiation alone compared to surgery or surgery and radiotherapy.[91,192,194,200,527,543] However, for small (T_1) cancers of the hypopharynx, and in particular, for superficial posterior pharyngeal wall lesions, radiation therapy alone has been used effectively, with surgery reserved for salvage.[540,652] Radiation therapy offers the advantage of treating bilateral occult lymph node disease including retropharyngeal nodes that are frequently involved when cancer arises from the posterior pharyngeal wall.[29] Small cancers of the hypopharynx can be treated equally effectively with surgical resection, often with sparing of the larynx for posterior wall lesions or with supraglottic laryngectomy for superficial cancers of the medial or lateral pyriform when the apex mucosa is tumor-free. Most patients, however, present with advanced primary tumors (T_2–T_4) and positive lymph nodes. In such patients local control rates with radiation alone decrease to 50% and salvage surgery is rarely successful. Thus, surgical management has become the mainstay of treatment for most hypopharyngeal cancers. Resections may entail partial pharyngectomy, pharyngolaryngectomy or total pharyngectomy combined with neck dissection. Tumors arising in the lower laryngopharynx or postcricoid mucosa often spread to involve the esophagus. Distal submucosal spread in the esophagus can be extensive and require partial or total esophagectomy. Reconstruction with transposition of the stomach (gastric pull-up) or jejunal free graft is currently recommended.[294,312,578] Tumor recurrences after adequate surgery most commonly occur in the neck, particularly the contralateral neck.[91] Treatment approaches with combined preoperative or postoperative radiation have improved control of lymph node disease, but survival rates have not improved substantially over surgery alone because of increased rates of distant metastases. Postoperative radiation is currently preferred to preoperative radiation because of lower local recurrence rates, fewer complications and less difficulty in accurately assessing tumor margins.[194] The clear superiority of combined surgery and radiation over surgery alone has not been established.[91,194,715,792] Although several studies demonstrate improved survival with combined therapy[192,200] direct comparisons to surgery alone are difficult because of differences in patient selection factors, tumor extent and degree of lymph node involvement. Well-designed, randomized trials to compare surgery alone to combined therapy have not been performed.

The presence of lymph node metastases, extracapsular lymph node involvement and direct extension of the primary tumor into the soft tissues of the neck are major negative prognostic factors. Overall 5-year survival rates range from 10–30% for posterior pharyngeal wall cancers,[76,152,540,652,745] and to 20–40% for pyriform sinus cancers (Table XXVII-1-17).[35,192,200,527,543,715] Local/regional recurrence develops in >80% of patients at 2 years, and accounts for the greatest number of deaths from disease.[350,715] Distant metastases are rarely evident at the time of presentation. Development of distant metastases may appear many years after primary therapy and seem to correlate with extent of regional lymph node involvement.[200] Rates of distant metastases range from 20–30%[200,715] but make up only 13% of deaths.[192]

Larynx

Because of the prominent role the larynx plays in speech communication, swallowing, respiration and protection of the lower airway, the treatment of cancer of larynx presents formidable functional consequences in addition to the intrinsic threat to life posed by these cancers. Unique to this particular site of head and neck cancer, quality of life issues have been incorporated into treatment decision making more extensively than for other cancer sites.[462] Cancer of the larynx is generally diagnosed at an earlier stage of development than other head and neck sites primarily due to early manifestation of symptoms. As a result, cure rates are generally higher than for other sites.

The 3 laryngeal subdivisions (see Anatomy above) form the basis for classifying cancers arising at the different sites within the larynx and have clinical importance in the embryologic development, vascular and lymphatic anatomy and the patterns of tumor growth within the larynx, and in the frequency of metastases. The characteristics used in clinical staging of primary tumors arising in each of these major subdivisions differ (Table XXVII-1-18).

Considerable attention has been devoted to anatomic studies of the vascular and lymphatic compartments of the larynx.[237,382,536,764] These studies have formed the basis for defining natural anatomic barriers to cancer spread within the larynx and have contributed to the development of precise surgical techniques for partial laryngeal resections for small cancers.

The true vocal cords present an effective apparent boundary between supraglottic and subglottic lymphatic spread within the larynx. This separation breaks down with tumors involving the anterior or posterior commissures and with deep invasive tumors that extend vertically across the true and false vocal cords (transglottic cancers). Normally the internal perichondrium of the thyroid cartilage also presents an effective barrier to cancer spread. However, cancer involvement of the anterior commissure or transglottic extension is associated with invasion of the thyroid cartilage in 40–60% of cases.[381]

Table XXVII-1-17. Overall Five-Year Survival Rates (%) in Patients with Squamous Carcinoma of the Hypopharynx

Investigator	(n)	Stage I	Stage II	Stage III	Stage IV	Overall
Dubois[192]	(457)	60	47	23	8	16
Bataini[35]	(384)	36	33	24	10	19
Razack[543]	(120)	77	63	25	5	28
Carpenter[91]	(162)	100	66	51	0	47
Pingree[527]	(1,208)		35*		23*	25

*Stages I and II combined; III and IV combined

Table XXVII-1-18. Primary Tumor Staging Characteristics for Carcinoma of the Larynx

Supraglottis
T1 Tumor limited to one subsite, normal vocal cord mobility
T2 Tumor invades more than one subsite, normal vocal cord mobility
T3 Tumor limited to larynx with vocal cord fixation and/or invades postcricoid area, medial wall of pyriform sinus or pre-epiglottic tissues
T4 Tumor invades thyroid cartilage and/or extends to tissues beyong larynx, e.g., oropharynx, soft tissue of neck

Glottis
T1 Tumor limited to vocal cord(s) with normal mobility
T2 Tumor extends to supraglottis and/or subglottis and/or impaired vocal cord mobility
T3 Tumor limited to larynx with vocal cord fixation
T4 Tumor invades thyroid cartilage and/or extends to tissues beyond the larynx

Subglottis
T1 Tumor limited to the subglottis
T2 Tumor extends to vocal cord(s) with normal or impaired mobility
T3 Tumor limited to larynx with vocal cord fixation
T4 Tumor invades cricoid or thyroid cartilage and/or extends to tissues beyong the larynx

Early diagnosis is critical for achieving high survival rates and larynx preservation.[168] Most cancers that are diagnosed at an early stage of development arise in the glottic larynx. This is because minimal changes in the mass of the vibrating vocal cord due to tumor growth result in changes in its vibrating characteristics which are evident as dysphonia or hoarseness. Supraglottic cancers are usually more advanced than glottic cancers at the time of diagnosis. Cancers arising in the supraglottic larynx do not generally produce early symptoms of hoarseness. Rather, the earliest symptoms of a supraglottic cancer are usually sore throat, dysphagia, referred otalgia or development of a neck mass representing regional metastasis. Airway obstruction may be an early symptom with subglottic cancers.

Modern clinical evaluation of laryngeal cancers includes indirect mirror-assisted or fiberoptic laryngoscopy, direct laryngoscopy, computerized tomography and more recently MRI scanning of the larynx and neck. These radiologic assessments are of value in assessing direct extension to the pre-epiglottic and paraglottic spaces of the larynx, detecting cartilage invasion and evaluating the soft tissues and lymph nodes of the neck. These studies have replaced conventional tomography and contrast laryngograms. Precise evaluation of tumor extent demands direct laryngoscopy

under anesthesia. With large obstructive tumors, this may necessitate prior tracheostomy. In some patients with large obstructive lesions, debulking the tumor mass at the time of direct laryngoscopy can obviate the need for tracheostomy and thereby reduce the risk of tumor seeding of the tracheostomy site. Even with precise clinical evaluation, inaccurate estimation of tumor extent (usually underestimation) occurs in 30–40% of cases.[526] Most often this involves failure to identify invasion of the laryngeal cartilage framework.

Supraglottic primary tumors account for 25–50% of all laryngeal cancers.[170] A knowledge of the laryngeal compartments aids in understanding the spread, and staging of supraglottic and glottic cancers. The staging of supraglottic cancers is based on the subsite or region of the supraglottis involved by cancer. Subsites include the false vocal cords, arytenoids, lingual and laryngeal surfaces of the epiglottis and aryepiglottic folds. The epiglottis itself is also subdivided into the region extending above the plane of the hyoid and that below the hyoid. Suprahyoid epiglottic tumors tend to have a better prognosis than infrahyoid cancers with the exception of these invading the aryepiglottic fold (marginal area) to involve the pyriform sinus. Early cancers (T_1 and T_2) involve one or more subsites, but have normal vocal cord motion. Those cancers that cause fixation of the vocal cord or involve the postcricoid region, medial wall of the pyriform sinus or pre-epiglottic space are staged T_3. Those that extend beyond the larynx or invade thyroid cartilage are staged T_4.

Glottic carcinomas are also staged according to subsites involved. Cancers limited to the true vocal cords are T_1 (T_{1a}: one vocal cord involved, T_{1b}: both vocal cords involved) and those with extension to the false cord above or supraglottis below are staged T_2. Vocal cord fixation are classified T_3 while those with cartilage involvement or extension outside the larynx are T_4.

Subglottic cancers which are limited to the subglottic region (T_1) or to subglottis and true vocal cords (T_2) are early cancers. Fixation of the vocal cord (T_3) and cartilage invasion or extension outside the larynx (T_4) are associated with worse prognosis. The nodal classification for staging is the same as for other HNSCC sites.

Curative radiotherapy is the treatment of choice for early stage laryngeal lesions. It is for the moderately-advanced lesions that one must consider the trade-offs between definitive radiotherapy, with surgery held in reserve for salvage vs. a combined surgical-radiotherapeutic approach. The patient must be brought into the decision making process when the various treatment options are being formulated since he/she may well decide to lose a few percentage points in terms of survival probability in return for a higher probability of voice preservation if the chosen treatment is successful.

The design of the radiation portals must be tailored to the individual patient but some general comments can be made. In general, supraglottic tumors have access to a richer lymphatic drainage than tumors of the glottic larynx and so radiation fields tend to be larger in order to treat the larger volume at risk for metastatic disease.[446] Typically one treats the primary tumor volume and regions at risk for subclinical metastatic disease to 5,000 cGy and then reduces the field size to areas of gross disease, and delivers an additional 2,000–2,400 cGy. The spinal cord is shielded at 4,500 cGy and megavoltage electron beams used to treat the posterior cervical nodes to higher doses as required. Because of the V-shape of the anterior neck, wedge compensating filters are often required in order to ensure uniform radiation dose distributions. If the anterior supraclavicular fossa is at risk for micrometastatic disease, it is treated to 5,000 cGy using an anterior field suitably matched to the upper neck fields. Early stage ($T_{1-2} N_0$) glottic lesions are generally treated with relatively small fields localized to the primary tumor. Tumors of the subglottic larynx can spread to the upper paratracheal nodes as well as to the nodes in the cervical chain, and radiation fields for this disease must, therefore, include the upper mediastinum.[228]

The treatment of more advanced laryngeal cancers (T_3, T_4) generally includes both radiation therapy and surgery, although controversy exists on the role of primary radiation therapy with surgery salvage, and the emerging role of chemotherapy and altered fractionation radiation to avoid laryngopharyngectomy in selected patients with advanced laryngeal and hypopharyngeal cancers. Much of the controversy surrounds quality of life issues as they relate to preservation of the larynx.[462,726]

Many surgical procedures for laryngeal carcinoma involve the creation of a tracheal stoma. This area is sometimes at significant risk for tumor recurrence. Once a stomal recurrence has developed, the prognosis is very grave regardless of whether it is treated with surgery or radiotherapy. Sisson and colleagues report on a series of 28 patients with stomal recurrences treated with one or more surgical resections.[626] The 5-year survival was only 17%. Schneider and colleagues report on patients with tracheal recurrences treated with radiotherapy—good palliation of local pain and/or bleeding was achieved, but the 2-year survival was only 6%.[581] Given the poor results with salvage therapy, it is clearly better to prevent stomal recurrence in the first place. If risk factors for stomal recurrence are present (Table XXVII-1-21), then the tracheal stoma should be irradiated as part of the initial management.

Supraglottic. Important factors in selecting therapy for supraglottic cancers are tumor location and pre-epiglottic extension. Tumors limited to the suprahyoid epiglottis are amenable to radiation with fields that encompass neck regions at risk for lymphatic metastases. Tumors involving the aryepiglottic folds, pyriform sinuses or infrahyoid epiglottis tend to be more aggressive, deeply infiltrative and frequently involve the pre-epiglottic space. Radiation alone is less effective than surgery, resulting in more frequent local recurrences that require surgical salvage. Often these recurrences are difficult to detect early enough to allow salvage by laryngeal conservation surgery and therefore require salvage total laryngectomy. Persistent post-radiation edema of the supraglottic larynx is not uncommon and contributes to difficulty in detecting recurrence which occurs in 40–50%.[243,746,753]

Pre-epiglottic extension of cancer carries a poor prognosis. However, these situations can be managed effectively with horizontal supraglottic laryngectomy which allows preservation of the voice. Indeed, even advanced tumors with extension of cancer to the valleculae and tongue base can often be treated by supraglottic laryngectomy with results equal to total laryngectomy. Very superficial tumors of the suprahyoid epiglottis can also be treated with simple epiglottectomy. Because supraglottic laryngectomy is associated with variable degrees of postoperative aspiration, adequate pulmonary status is a prerequisite for this surgery, as is intact mobility of the true vocal cords.

In every patient undergoing supraglottic laryngectomy, preoperative permission must be obtained for total laryngectomy in case the surgical findings dictate that more extensive surgery is needed to extirpate the cancer. Approximately 20% of patients require prolonged tracheostomy, and this is usually related to edema secondary to postoperative radiation. The rates of persistent swallowing difficulties are low, however, and the need for completion laryngectomy for persistent aspiration ranges only from 0–5%.[61,406,437]

The frequency of neck node metastases is high with T_2 or greater tumors. Treatment of the clinically negative neck may be accomplished with surgery or radiation. Surgical approaches should include removal of primary nodal groups at risk (Levels II, III, IV) for occult disease and complete neck dissection for histologically confirmed nodal metastases. The discovery of occult nodal metastases is associated with a high frequency of contralateral neck metastases and warrants consideration of postoperative radiation or contralateral selective neck dissection. Treatment of both necks is especially important with midline primary tumors. Most authors advocate elective (for N_0) modified radical or selective dissection of nodal groups.[60,77,173,398] Others argue that neck dissection can be delayed until clinically evident metastases occur.[494,596] For T_1 and T_2 lesions, most authors demonstrate overall cure rates of 68–73%[77,115,383] with determinate 3-year survival rates of 80–85%[60,171,412] when elective neck dissection is included. Most recurrences occur in the neck and this argues for prophylactic neck treatment.

Radiation is also effective for early lesions. Local control rates for patients with supraglottic tumors treated with radiation alone range from 68–94% and survival rates from 50–89%. The latter set of survival figures are comparable to those for planned surgery and adjuvant radiotherapy which range from 46–90%. While the figures are comparable for T_1 and T_2 lesions, there is a trend favoring the combined approach for larger lesions. Nonrandomized series from different institutions are not strictly comparable since unstated patient selection factors are generally involved. For example, the excellent local control results by Goepfert and colleagues for T_3 and T_4 lesions are for a selected set of tumors that were exophytic in nature.[263] Survival rates tend to run lower than local control rates for supraglottic tumors because of

Table XXVII-1-19. Overall Five-Year Survival Rates (%) for Patients with Squamous Carcinoma of the Supraglottic Larynx

Investigator	N	Stage I	Stage II	Stage III	Stage IV
Flynn[229]	234	93	49	50	33
Fu[240]	173	64	80	35	10
Shah and Tollefsen[598]	290	83	72	42	0*
Coates[115]	212	69	73	51	—
DeSanto[170] **	236	80	65	62	52
Goepfert[263]	241	100	68	59	32

*3 patients
**Determinant survival, 2–13 yr. follow-up

deaths from second primaries and other intercurrent diseases. Cure rates range from 73–75%[298,719,747] and increases to 80–85% with the addition of surgical salvage.[341,465,643] Most recurrences are local and preservation of voice is successful in 65–70% of patients when salvage surgery is included.[643]

The treatment of more advanced supraglottic cancers (T_3, T_4) remains controversial. In cases with clinically evident regional metastases, combined surgery and postoperative radiation are usually recommended since this treatment approach is associated with better local control rates[633] and better control rates for neck disease in both the ipsilateral and contralateral neck.[240] Approximately 50% of patients have clinically palpable lymph nodes at the time of diagnosis and 20–25% have bilateral nodal involvement. In the clinically negative neck, elective neck dissection shows cancer metastases in 15–30% of patients. Failure to control disease in the neck is a major cause of mortality in advanced supraglottic cancers. In most reports, radiation alone for control of supraglottic cancers with N_2 or N_3 nodes is clearly inferior to combined therapy. Although the issue of optimal initial management for the patient with N_0 disease has not been settled, an individualized approach has been recommended in which bilateral selective node dissections are performed and postoperative radiation reserved for patients with proven regional metastases.[406,637]

Overall 5-year survival rates for supraglottic cancers range from 40–50% (Table XXVII-1-19).[447,643] Local failures occur in approximately 10% of patients and regional failures in 15–20%. Rates of distant metastases range from 11–18%[256,435,447,643] with rates approaching 30% in patients with Stage IV disease.[643] Second primaries (20–25% of failures) are a major cause of death.[447,643] Intercurrent illness accounts for up to 20% of deaths.[447,712]

Glottic. The treatment of glottic cancer is greatly influenced by the secondary goal of voice preservation. Mobility of the vocal cords is a critical factor in selecting treatment. For small cancers (T_1, T_2) with mobile vocal cords, radiation therapy alone for cure achieves excellent local control rates (T_1, 85–95%, T_2, 65–75%) and overall survival rates similar to surgical resection.[302,366] Voice quality, although often impaired by radiation, is generally better than that following surgical resection.[367,497] Local control rates are 10–15% better with primary surgery, but local recurrences after definitive radiation can often be salvaged by subsequent surgery and this combined approach results in overall survival figures comparable to primary surgery. Tumor involvement of the anterior commissure or arytenoids is associated with higher

local recurrence rates with radiation alone, and such patients are often selected for primary surgery. As with supraglottic cancers, careful clinical tumor staging is necessary since underestimation of tumor extent is common.[526] The "irradiate and watch" treatment strategy is predicated on close follow-up in order to detect recurrences when they are still salvageable by surgery. Delay in diagnosis of recurrent glottic cancers after radiation is more frequent than with supraglottic cancers[172] and often requires total laryngectomy for cure. Thus, unreliable patients, or patients who are difficult to examine, may be more suitable for primary surgical treatment.

Survival figures in radiotherapy series are comparable to local control figures reflecting the effectiveness of surgical salvage and the fact that few patients with early stage glottic cancer die of their disease. Five-year survival rates for T_1 lesions range from 80–95% with either primary surgery or radiation (Table XXVII-1-20). Rates for T_2 lesions are generally in the range of 70–80%, but these rates are decreased 10–15% (local control rates drop 20–25%) when the mobility of the vocal cords is impaired,[301] or transglottic spread is present.[479] Lesions with impairment due to invasion of muscle behave more like T_3 cancers and have a poorer response to radiation alone.[300,363,377,711,712] Transglottic cancers and those with subglottic extension have higher rates of regional metastases and often require total laryngectomy for cure. In selected patients with these more advanced lesions or impaired vocal cord mobility, extended hemilaryngectomy, or more extensive subtotal laryngectomy with resection of a major portion of the cricoid cartilage, can achieve excellent cure rates.[50,514] Voice quality is diminished with these extensive procedures, and chronic aspiration or permanent tracheostomy is often a result. Although further study is required, hemilaryngectomy with postoperative radiation therapy has been advocated for some patients with close or involved surgical margins.[264]

The management of advanced glottic cancers (Stage III, IV) generally consists of total laryngectomy with or without postoperative radiation therapy. Local control rates with radiotherapy alone for T_3 and T_4 lesions run between 20–35% with survival rates running between 36–57% for T_3 lesions and 10% or less for T_4 lesions. In patients without regional metastases, local tumor control rates with surgery alone are excellent. Significant increases in local control with the addition of radiation therapy have not been clearly demonstrated. However, in patients with regional metastases, overall prognosis is poor and recurrence in the neck is a major problem. Better regional tumor control rates are achieved with the

Table XXVII-1-20. Overall Five-Year Survival Rates (%) for Patients with Squamous Carcinoma of the Glottic Larynx

Investigator	N	Stage I	Stage II	Stage III	Stage IV
Maipang[440]	143	93	83	—	—
Kelly[377] †	148	82	79	—	—
Hendrickson[308] ‡	525	82	68	61	37*
Kaplan[363]	283	96	88	65	57*
Yuen[794]	192	—	—	80	63
Skolnick[627]	264	82	70	53	20

*<10 patients
†3-year rates
‡4-year disease-free rates

Table XXVII-1-21. Risk Factors for Tracheal Stomal Recurrence

Extensive primary lesion (T_3 or T_4)
Subglottic tumor extension
Preliminary emergency tracheostomy for airway obstruction
Inadequate tumor margins on the pathologic specimen
Tumor involvement of the paratracheal lymphatics
Large, fixed nodes or multiple involved cervical nodes
Perineural or venous invasion by tumor

addition of adjuvant radiation therapy, and this justifies its use in these advanced cases.[263] Because rates of occult regional metastases approach 30% in patients with advanced glottic (T_3, T_4) cancers, elective modified or selective node dissections for staging purposes are frequently performed. Demonstration of histologically positive nodal metastases has been used as an indication for postoperative radiation. Surgery alone is curative in 50–80% of patients without nodal metastases,[169,363,410,719,794] and decreases to less than 40% if metastases are present.[145,479,627]

Considerable controversy surrounds the use of definitive radiation with surgical salvage in patients with advanced (T_3N_0, T_4N_0) but localized glottic cancers.[169,299] A very large, long-term British study has demonstrated that salvage laryngectomy was possible in <50% of patients who suffered tumor recurrence after definitive radiation.[772] The radiation alone concept, however, presumes equal overall survivorship compared to primary laryngectomy with associated low complication rates. Overall survival rates range from 50–55%[145,299,372] with larynx preservation in 60–70% of these patients.[145,299,479] High complication rates, however, have been reported with late surgical salvage of radiation failures.[145] The overall patterns are confusing and based entirely on retrospective series. The resolution of this controversy in management will require carefully designed prospective studies that include assessments of not only survival, but voice and quality of life issues and complication rates.

A subset of laryngeal cancers that warrant special consideration are those which involve both the glottic and supraglottic regions (transglottic). These cancers are usually advanced and are associated with a high incidence (30–50%) of regional metastases,[459,479] extralaryngeal spread and vocal cord fixation. Although clinical understaging is common, occasionally these cancers are quite superficial and amenable to conservation surgical techniques. Most patients, however, require total laryngectomy. In a careful review of 152 cases of transglottic carcinomas, Mittal reported a 55%

cure rate with combined therapy compared to a 5-year survival of 8% with radiation alone.[479]

Subglottic. Primary subglottic carcinomas account for <5% of laryngeal cancers. The limited data support the use of primary radiotherapy for early stage (T_1, T_2) lesions. They usually are advanced at diagnosis, however, with regional metastases in 20% of patients.[600] Many reported series contain glottic primaries with subglottic extension. Surgical treatment generally requires total laryngectomy combined with resection of adjacent soft tissues (thyroid gland, strap muscles, paratracheal lymph nodes). Five-year survival rates of 36% for radiation therapy and 42% for surgery[719] have been reported. Cure rates as high as 70% have been reported in a small number of patients treated with combined therapy.[600] The addition of adjuvant radiation offers the advantage of improved regional control rates and treatment of paratracheal and upper mediastinal lymph nodes. Histologically positive lymph nodes can be found in 65% of cases. The risk of stomal recurrence increases substantially with cancers that involve the subglottic larynx, particularly if prior tracheostomy was necessary for impending airway obstruction.[376] Early aggressive treatment (often within 24 hours) has been recommended for patients requiring tracheostomy for subglottic extension of laryngeal cancers.[155]

Patterns of failure for glottic carcinoma differ somewhat from other laryngeal sites. Local failures are uncommon with primary surgical therapy and account for less than 10% of recurrences. However, after primary radiation therapy for local glottic primaries, recurrences account for 10–50% of failures.[372,772] Regional nodal recurrences occur in 15–30% of patients with advanced disease who are treated with surgery alone.[794] This contrasts to supraglottic cancers where regional recurrences are the major site of failure.

It has previously been thought that distant metastases from laryngeal cancers were uncommon, accounting for less than 10% of failures. Distant spread is approximately four times more common with supraglottic than with glottic cancers.[537] Rates of distant metastasis associated with glottic cancer have, however, increased with the use of combined therapy and have been reported in approximately 20% of patients with advanced disease.[372] Rates appear directly related to extent of nodal disease with reported rates as high as 40–50% of failures attributed to distant metastases in patients with N_2 or N_3 disease.

Carcinoma In Situ. A special issue relates to the treatment of carcinoma in situ of the vocal cords.[141,258] This disease often can be managed with vocal cord stripping, but if enough serial sections are examined, foci of invasive carcinoma are often found. Pene and Fletcher report on a series of 79 patients with carcinoma in situ and 7 patients with leukoplakia/atypical hyperplasia that were treated with radiotherapy.[515] Patients were staged as either T_1 or T_2 using the same criteria as for invasive tumors. Local control rates were the same as for invasive lesions—89% for T_1 and 74% for T_2. However, only 2/12 failures were on the initially involved cord suggesting that most were not true recurrences but rather new disease developing in dysplastic epithelium. Furthermore, it took about 5 years for 80% of the failures to develop which further suggests a second process. Most of the failures after primary radiotherapy tend to be invasive while failures after vocal cord stripping tend to be equally-divided between carcinoma in situ and invasive disease.

Very superficial cancers limited to the free edge of the vocal cord or carcinoma in situ can be effectively treated by limited excision by conventional means, or with laser excision, with excellent voice preservation.[507,769] More extensive disease requires cordectomy or vertical hemilaryngectomy.[502] Numerous methods have been devised for reconstructing the vocal cords after conservation surgery, but voice results are generally inferior to radiation alone and associated problems with glottic insufficiency, prolonged tracheostomy and aspiration are more common.

Paranasal Sinus and Nasal Cavity

Paranasal sinus and nasal cavity tumors represent 0.2% of all human cancers. Roughly two-thirds occur in the maxillary sinus and one-third in the ethmoid sinus. Frontal and sphenoid sinus cancers are rare—0.3% of sinus tumors. These cancers are associated epidemiologically with occupational exposures (wood working, nickel refining), inhaling noxious fumes (dioxane, nitrosamine), and tobacco (see Epidemiology above). Although 80% of paranasal sinus cancers are squamous cell, a variety of other cell types exist.[36]

These tumors notoriously present at a late stage—over 80% have bony involvement at diagnosis by radiographic or clinical examination. This fact relates to their vague and often ignored symptoms—sinusitis is the most common. The natural history is characterized by local invasion into adjacent structures—base of skull and orbit. While nodal and distant metastases are staged according to the AJC criteria for the HNSCC, a staging system for primary tumors exists only for the maxillary sinus.

The complex anatomy of the paranasal sinuses and nasal cavity and their proximity to the orbit and skull base pose major problems in staging and treatment planning. The maxillary sinus can be visualized as a pyramidal chamber, which is bordered inferiorly by the alveolar ridge and palate, medially by the nasal cavity, and laterally by the cheek. This tumor can invade superiorly to the orbit; inferiorly into the alveolar ridge impinging on the superior alveolar nerve and posteriorly involving the trunk of the maxillary branch of the trigeminal nerve.

The ethmoid sinus is a complex of air cells between the medial walls of the orbits. The sphenoid sinus is a deep midline structure. Lateral wall invasion commonly results in an abducens paralysis, but can also cause facial paresthesias and numbness in divisions one and two of the trigeminal

nerve and ocular palsies. Invasion superiorly into the orbit often involves the optic nerve.

The treatment of tumors of the paranasal and nasal cavity has traditionally been linked to advances in surgical excision along with muscle preservation or reconstitution for effective prosthesis. Early reports indicated poor results with 5-year survivors of 20–40%. Surgical approaches have become more aggressive over the last two decades producing variable success and complication rates. Traditional surgical therapy of paranasal/nasal sinus tumors consists of a medial maxillectomy for low grade lesions. The area of the premaxilla can be preserved if there is no tumor invasion into the anterior maxillary sinus wall or into the hard palate. The total maxillectomy involves transection of the malar bone from the zygomatic process of the frontal bone and the transection of the zygomatic arch and hard palate. This is followed by skin grafting. Recent work suggests that transcranial resection produces comparable short-term results with a low complication rate.[54]

Single modality therapy is effective in early stage disease. Radiation of the cervical or retropharyngeal lymph nodes is limited to the presence of positive nodes or high risk lesions. Results of pre- versus postsurgical radiation are mixed. Wang found a 58% 3-year disease-free survival with pre-operative radiation vs. a 36% 3-year disease-free survival with postoperative radiotherapy.[747] However, Jesse found no difference between the two groups.[353] A recent series suggests that in patients with resectable tumors, survival rates are better in patients treated with surgery and postoperative radiotherapy.[339] Radiotherapy data are mixed with 5-year survivals ranging from 0–50%.

In maxillary sinus tumors without bone invasion surgery or radiation are equally effective. Once bone invasion has occurred, however, combination radiation and surgery is the suggested therapy. An exception is seen in a study which achieved a 3-year disease-free survival of 40%, and a 5-year disease-free survival of 35%, in a group of 20 patients of whom 18 had T_4 lesions, using megavoltage beams, meticulous technique and effective doses.[2,14]

SCC of the nasal vestibule, a distinct type of skin cancer, is related more to tobacco usage than to sunlight exposure and presents a difficult management problem. Nasal vestibule cancers have a distinctly more aggressive natural history with a worse prognosis than skin cancers of other sites and therefore require more immediate evaluation and treatment.[262] Unexpected deep extension may occur in the nasal vestibule itself, upper lip, and other midface regions.[509] Radiation is now the favored approach for patients without regional node disease because recurrence rates and survival data appear equivalent to those seen with surgery, the cosmetic outcome is much better than with surgery, and the morbidity is low.[102] Furthermore, many of the radiation failures can be salvaged surgically. In patients without clinical neck node involvement, either surgery or radiotherapy yields 10–20% recurrence overall and only a 3% recurrence rate after primary single-modality therapy of lesions smaller than 2 cm.[785] Large lesions, or those infiltrating the upper lip, may be treated with external beam radiation combined with radioactive implants or paired wedged beam radiation. Regional neck node involvement is uncommon (6%) at presentation and confers a poor prognosis with a high (>50%) recurrence rate despite aggressive local therapy (surgery and radiotherapy).

Salivary Gland

Anatomy. Tumors can arise not only in the major glands but also in the small foci of salivary gland tissue scattered throughout the upper respiratory and digestive tract. The most common sites of minor salivary gland tumors are the palate, base of tongue, and buccal mucosa.[203,285,653] The majority of salivary gland tumors arise in the parotid glands, and about 80% of these are benign. Tumors arising in the submandibular, submaxillary, or minor salivary glands are much more likely to be malignant.

The largest salivary glands are the parotids, which lie anterior to the external auditory canals. The facial nerve passes through the parotid and divides it into superficial and deep lobes. About 80% of the parotid gland lies in the superficial lobe and 20% lies in the deep lobe. The internal carotid artery, the internal jugular vein, the cervical sympathetic chain, and cranial nerves IX, X, XI, and XII are in close proximity to the deep lobe of the parotid. This nodal group then drains into the nodes at the angle of the mandible, the subdigastric nodes, or the upper portion of the posterior cervical chain. Depending on histology, these nodes are frequently involved. Certain histologies such as adenoid cystic carcinoma tend to invade major nerve sheaths—the facial nerve and the auricular-temporal branch of cranial nerve V.

The second largest glands are the submaxillary glands, located in the submaxillary triangle of the neck, which lies just anterior, and inferior to, the angle of the mandible. Certain tumors of the submandibular glands may invade along nerve sheaths or perineural lymphatics to spread to the mandible or the base of the skull. The sublingual glands are the smallest of the major salivary glands and are located deep to the floor of the mouth.

Histopathology. Benign lesions account for about 80% of tumors arising in the parotid glands, 50% in the submandibular glands, and 25% in minor salivary glands. A list of such tumors is given in Table XXVII-1-22.

The basic histologic classification of malignant salivary tumors was developed by Foote and Frazell (Table XXVII-1-23).[231] Mucoepidermoid carcinomas constitute about 26%, 21%, and 10%, respectively, of malignant salivary gland tumors of the palatal, parotid, and sublingual glands.[461] They are the most common malignant tumor of the parotid.[355] Well-differentiated tumors are characterized by a slow growth rate, a low recurrence rate after complete surgical excision

Table XXVII-1-22. Benign Tumors of the Salivary Glands

Adenomas
Pleomorphic adenoma
Monomorphic adenoma
Warthin's tumor (adenolymphoma)
Sebaceous lymphadenoma
Oncocytoma
Myoepithelioma
Vascular tumors
Hemangiomas
Lymphangiomas

Table XXVII-1-23. Malignant Tumors of the Salivary Glands

Mucoepidermoid carcinoma
Low grade
High grade
Acinic cell carcinoma
Adenoid cystic carcinoma
Adenocarcinoma
Malignant mixed tumor (carcinoma ex-pleomorphic adenoma)
Squamous cell carcinoma

(about 15%), and rare metastatic spread. High-grade tumors are more aggressive; the local recurrence rate after surgery approaches 60%.[461] About 50% of patients with high-grade mucoepidermoid carcinoma present with regional metastasis, and 30% develop distant metastasis.[649]

Acinic cell carcinomas are usually well differentiated and account for about 13% of the cancers arising in the parotid glands. Lymph node metastasis occurs in about 16% of cases.[461] Local recurrences and distant metastases many years after treatment are common.[36,650]

Adenoid cystic carcinomas (cylindromas) account for approximately 12% of parotid gland cancers and approximately 58% of malignant neoplasms arising in the submandibular or minor salivary glands.[124,204,461,651] An outstanding feature of this neoplasm is its propensity to invade major nerves and to spread along the perineural sheath. This must be taken into account in designing treatment. Although these tumors often follow an indolent course, as many as 40% of patients ultimately develop regional and/or distant metastasis.[399,730]

Adenocarcinomas account for about 12% of parotid gland cancers, where the majority of them are high grade, and they are common tumors of the minor salivary glands. About 36% of patients either present with or subsequently develop regional lymph node.[649] Distant metastases (bone, lungs) are common.

Carcinomas ex-pleomorphic adenoma, arise from pre-existing benign pleomorphic adenomas. The risk of malignant transformation increases with time—1.6% for adenomas of less than 5 years' duration and 9.4% for adenomas present for more than 15 years.[53] True malignant mixed tumors are very rare, constituting about 2–5% of all malignant salivary gland tumors and is an aggressive tumor: the neck nodes become involved in about 25% of patients.

Primary SCC of the salivary gland is rare, accounting for less than 3% of all parotid neoplasms. However, given the rich lymphatic network that permeates the parotids, SCCs of the skin of the forehead, temple, or ear may metastasize to this region. Such primary sites must be excluded before the diagnosis of primary SCC of the parotid can be made. About 50% of patients with primary SCC of the parotid ultimately develop positive regional nodes.

The presentation of malignant salivary gland tumors is variable, depending on site and histology. Facial nerve paralysis is uncommon and generally indicates a malignant lesion. Tumors of the deep lobe of the parotid may produce dysphagia, earache, or trismus. When the parapharyngeal space is invaded, there may be cranial nerve IX, X, XI, or XII involvement. The usual presentation of a submandibular gland tumor is painless swelling below the mandible.

Staging. Recently, the AJCC and the UICC have agreed to changes in the staging system for salivary gland tumors to bring the two schema into agreement. T-stage criteria are reproduced in Table XXVII-1-24, along with stage groupings. The N- and M-stage criteria are the same as for the more common HNSCCs.

Treatment. The treatment of benign salivary gland tumors is primarily surgical. However, there is a role for postoperative radiation in high-risk situations. If the mass is incompletely resected, particularly after a first recurrence, postoperative radiation is effective in preventing subsequent recurrences.[157,755] These tumors must be followed for extended periods because of the late recurrence and spontaneous transformation.[36]

Surgery is the primary form of treatment for patients with resectable salivary gland cancer. Early-stage (T_1/T_2), low-grade mucoepidermoid cancers are generally treated with local excision. Such tumors arising in the parotid are treated with a total parotidectomy with preservation of the facial nerve. Early-stage, high-grade tumors of all other histologies are treated with surgical resection plus dissection of the regional lymph nodes. Such tumors arising in the parotid require a total parotidectomy, but usually the facial nerve can be spared. Patients with clinically positive neck nodes should have radical neck dissection on the involved side. For many years, salivary gland tumors were thought to be resistant to conventional photon irradiation, but now it is recognized that this treatment can be highly effective when given in a postoperative setting to eradicate subclinical disease. Postoperative radiotherapy is indicated[684] when: 1) tumor is high grade (any histology, excepting low-grade mucoepidermoid carcinoma) or is metastatic SCC, regardless of the surgical margins; 2) the surgical margins are close or microscopically positive (which includes most tumors involving the deep lobe

of the parotid gland), regardless of the grade; 3) resection has been performed for *recurrent disease,* regardless of the histology or margin status; 4) tumor has invaded skin, bone, nerve, or extraparotid tissue; 5) regional nodes are confirmed as positive on neck dissection; and 6) there is gross residual or unresectable disease.

In the past, patients with T_3 or T_4 parotid disease required radical parotidectomy with sacrifice of the facial nerve. Now, nerve-sparing surgery may be used followed by radiotherapy. Dosages given to the primary resection site are in the range of 5,500–6,500 cGy depending on the postsurgical tumor status. In the case of low-grade mucoepidermoid carcinomas, it is generally not necessary to treat the neck nodes in the N_0 neck. For other histologies, the neck nodal drainage is generally treated to dosages in the range of 5,000 cGy. In the case of adenoid cystic carcinomas, the radiation fields must include the courses of the adjacent cranial nerves because perineural spread is common.

The results of treatment depend on both histology and site. In a series from M. D. Anderson Cancer Center, 5-year survivals were: 100% for 11 patients with acinic cell carcinoma, 95% for 20 patients with adenoid cystic carcinoma, 90% for 10 patients with low-grade mucoepidermoid carcinoma, 82% for 20 patients with high-grade mucoepidermoid carcinoma, 70% for 30 patients with adenocarcinoma, and 59% for 16 patients with malignant mixed tumor. In a retrospective review of 407 patients treated at Princess Margaret Hospital, primary parotid disease was controlled by surgery alone in 24% cases, and by surgery and radiotherapy in 74% of cases.[223] In a surgical series of submandibular tumors,[125] 8 of 17 patients with adenoid cystic histology were free of disease after five years compared with only 3 of 17 with mucoepidermoid histology. Minor salivary gland tumors arising in the paranasal sinuses often present in advanced stage. Goepfert and colleagues found a 2-year local control rate of 47% (9/19) in patients treated with surgery alone compared with 76% (26/34) in patients treated with surgery and postoperative radiotherapy.[265]

For patients with large, inoperable salivary gland cancers, fast-neutron radiotherapy is an alternative. A randomized clinical trial was performed comparing neutron irradiation and photon irradiation in patients with large, inoperable lesions.[282] After only 32 patients had been entered, the trial was closed early for ethical reasons. The tumor clearance rate at the primary site was 85% for the neutron group vs. 33% for the photon group ($P = 0.01$); the clearance rate in the neck for patients with clinically positive nodes was 86% for neutrons, vs. 25% for photons. Actuarial projections showed the 2-year survival at 62% for the neutron group, compared with 25% for the photon group ($P = 0.10$). Review of the non-randomized trials showed the local/regional control rate to be 67% (194/289) with definitive neutron radiation, and 24% (61/254) with definitive photon irradiation.[281] Fast-neutron radiation is particularly of interest in situations that would require sacrifice of the facial nerve were surgery used instead. Its role in the high-risk, postoperative setting is currently under investigation.

Control of local/regional disease is only a part of the problem. Table XXVII-1-25 shows the incidence of distant metastasis from a series of parotid tumors as a function of histol-

Table XXVII-1-24. Staging of Salivary Gland Primary Tumors According AJCC, 1988

T Stage

Tx	Primary tumor cannot be assessed
T0	No evidence of primary tumor
T1	Tumor less than or equal to 2 cm in greatest diameter
T2	Greatest diameter of tumor more than 2 cm but less than 4 cm
T3	Greatest diameter of tumor more than 4 cm but less than 6 cm
T4	Tumor more than 6 cm in greatest diameter

Subdivisions

The above categories are subdivided into (a) no local extension or (b) local extension. Local extension is defined as clinical or macroscopic evidence of tumor invading the skin, soft tissues of the neck, bone, or nerve.

Stage Grouping

Stage I	T1a	N0	M0	
	T2a	N0	M0	
Stage II	T1b	N0	M0	
	T2b	N0	M0	
	T3a	N0	M0	
Stage III	T3b	N0	M0	
	T4a	N0	M0	
	any T	N1	M0	(excluding T4b)

Table XXVII-1-25.   Distant Metastasis Rates in Parotid Carcinomas by Histology

Histologic Type	No. with Metastases/ Total (%)
Mucoepidermoid	14/183 (8%)
Acinic cell	2/14 (14%)
Adenoid cystic	22/53 (42%)
Malignant mixed tumor	3/14 (21%)
Adenocarcinoma	25/91 (27%)
Squamous cell	2/13 (15%)

From Johns and Kaplan[356]

ogy.[356] This ranges from a low of 8% for mucoepidermoid tumors to a high of 42% for adenoid cystic tumors.

Although early-stage low-grade tumors have high cure rates with surgery-radiotherapy, standard local therapy is not so successful in locally or regionally advanced, metastatic or high-grade disease. Therefore, a moderate amount of phase II chemotherapeutic study has been conducted in search of effective systemic therapy for these difficult cases.[545]

Whereas adenoid cystic carcinoma is a slow-growing neoplasm, the mucoepidermoid subtype appears to grow faster and more closely resemble HNSCC in its biologic and clinical behavior. The single-agent response patterns reflect these differences. Paralleling results in HNSCC, methotrexate has yielded a 36% response rate in mucoepidermoid cancer. In salivary gland cancers of other histologies, however, methotrexate has produced only a 6% response rate. In contrast to methotrexate, doxorubicin is relatively inactive in mucoepidermoid carcinoma and HNSCC but active in other salivary gland histologic subtypes.[718] These suggestions must be interpreted with great caution, since they are based in large part on retrospective data and very small patient numbers. Furthermore, response rates do not correlate well with survival—with the more chemo-resistant but slow-growing adenoid cystic subtype having the longest survival.

Several single-agent studies have been conducted in salivary gland cancers. Promising results have been achieved with cisplatin, methotrexate, doxorubicin and 5-fluorouracil. Tannock and colleagues conducted a single-institution review of results with non-cisplatin single agents in adenoid cystic cancer.[681] Although achieving one of the lowest response rates (29%), compared with other single-agent or combination trials, it also revealed the longest median survival rate (nearly two years). More recently, regimens including cisplatin have been tested. Cisplatin alone or in combination has been evaluated in over 130 patients and has yielded response rates in the range of 17–100%. Studies have evaluated single-agent cisplatin, mainly in adenoid cystic carcinomas, and yielded conflicting results (Table XXVII-1-26). The combination of cyclophosphamide, doxorubicin, and cisplatin (CAP) is the most extensively studied regimen. A recent study with a dose-intensive cisplatin-based regimen combining all four drugs active in this disease produced high toxicity without an improvement in response or survival over single-agent cisplatin or other combinations.[180] Hormonal therapy (based on supportive preclinical work) appears to have limited activity.[178,605]

Nasopharyngeal Carcinoma

In the U.S., nasopharyngeal carcinoma (NPC) accounts for 2% of all HNSCCs (see Epidemiology above). Its unusual epidemiologic and natural history features include a remarkable tendency toward early regional and distant dissemination.[101,217] NPC also is extremely sensitive to radiotherapy and cytotoxic chemotherapy.

Natural History. In the adult the nasopharynx is a chamber that is approximately cuboidal in shape and 4 cm on an edge. Anteriorly it is bounded by the choana of the nasal cavity, superiorly it is bounded by the base of the skull, inferiorly it is bounded by the soft palate, and its posterior wall is the mucosa that overlies the superior constrictor muscles of the pharynx and the C1 and C2 vertebral bodies. The lateral walls contain the Eustachian tube orifices. The epithelium of the superior lateral walls contains pseudostratified columnar cells and occasional goblet cells while the inferior lateral and posterior walls are stratified squamous in nature. The region is richly endowed with lymphatics which drain to the retropharyngeal and deep cervical nodes.

Malignant neoplasms of the nasopharynx are primarily epithelial with the presence of keratin associated with a poorer prognosis. The World Health Organization (WHO) recognizes three histopathologic types of NPC: type 1, differentiated SCC (of varying degrees); type 2, nonkeratinizing carcinoma; and type 3, undifferentiated or lymphoepithelial carcinoma.[519] Mixed patterns are common. About 75% of nasopharyngeal carcinomas are type 1 or 2 (or predominantly one or both of these types). The term lymphoepithelial carcinoma (type 3) is used when numerous infiltrating lymphocytes are seen.

About one-third of patients present with a neck mass without other complaints and about 70–75% of patients have enlarged neck nodes at presentation. Other common complaints are epistaxis, nasal stuffiness, headache, or hearing loss (generally unilateral). The tumor can spread laterally and superiorly to cause bony destruction of the base of the skull. Frequently there are cranial nerve findings with the 6th nerve being most commonly involved.[101] There are two principal cranial nerve syndromes associated with NPC: the retroparotidian syndrome involving the 9th, 10th, 11th, and 12th cranial nerves and the petro-sphenoidal syndrome involving the 3rd, 4th, 5th, and 6th cranial nerves (and occasionally the 2nd cranial nerve via extension through the foramen lacerum into the middle cranial fossa). Evaluation of the nasopharynx should consist of direct visualization with either a mirror or a fiberoptic scope. A CT and/or MRI scan is important in evaluating base of skull involvement and the possible presence of occult involved lymph nodes.

Staging. The staging for nodal disease is the same as for other head and neck cancers. The staging for the primary site is based upon regions of tumor involvement rather than size of the lesion as follows: Tis, carcinoma in situ; T_1, tumor confined to one site of the nasopharynx or no tumor visible (positive biopsy only); T_2, tumor involving two sites of the nasopharynx; T_3, tumor extends into nasal cavity or oropharynx; and T_4, tumor invades base of skull and/or cranial nerve involvement.

Treatment. Standard treatment for NPC is radiotherapy

Table XXVII-1-26.   Phase II Chemotherapy Results in Salivary Gland Cancers*

Author	No. of Patients	Histology	Agent(s)	Objective Response Rate (%)	Median Survival (mo)**
Tannock[681]	17	AC	Mult	29	21
Alberts[6]	5	Mult	CDP	100	8
Schramm[584]	10	AC	P	70	7–18
Posner[532]	13	Mult	CD	38	8
	3	Mucd	PBM	66	6
Suen[672]	14	AC	P	64	—
Sessions[593]	14	AC	P	50	—
Creagan[137]	34	Mult	P-based	38	15
Eisenberger[196]	4	Mult	CDP	100	11 +
Dreyfuss[190]	13	Mult	CDP	46	—
Triozzi[705]	21	AC	COF	25	—
Venook[717]	17	Mult	PDF	35	15
Licitra[415]	23	Mult	P	17	—
Dimery[180]	16	Mult	FACP	50	18

Abbreviations: AC, adenoid cystic carcinoma; Mucd, mucoepidermoid carcinoma; Mult, multiple; D, doxorubicin; B, bleomycin; C, cyclophosphamide; F, 5-fluorouracil; M, methotrexate; O, vincristine; P, cisplatin; V, vinblastine; —, no data
*Excluding isolated case reports
**From diagnosis

for early and locally advanced disease. Surgical resection even for early-stage disease is technically difficult because of the anatomic location of the primary tumor and the frequent bilateral cervical and retropharyngeal node involvement. The role of the surgeon is limited to obtaining tissue for diagnosis and occasionally to resecting residual adenopathy after definitive radiotherapy. Fortunately these tumors tend to be fairly radiosensitive and even large lymph nodes often respond to moderate doses of radiotherapy.[401] Prior to initiating therapy a dental consultation is advised since it is necessary to irradiate the parotid glands bilaterally and the resulting xerostomia predisposes to serious oral problems.

The initial radiation fields encompass the adjacent base of the skull as well as the nasopharynx itself. The fields are bilaterally directed and include the retropharyngeal drainage, the anterior and posterior cervical chains. A dose of 4,500 cGy is given using megavoltage photons and then the fields are reduced to spare the spinal cord and an additional 500 cGy given. Megavoltage electrons are used to bring the posterior cervical nodes to this same dose. Then the fields are reduced in size and an additional 2,000–2,200 cGy given to the nasopharyngeal primary. Regions of positive cervical adenopathy are also boosted with megavoltage photons and/or electrons to total doses of 6,500–7,500 cGy depending on the original size of the node and its response to the first phase of therapy.[280] In selected patients, the boost dose to the nasopharynx itself can be given with an intracavitary implant.[750] Critical normal structures in the treatment region include the cervical cord, the brain stem, optic nerves, and orbital contents. Proper shielding and limiting the delivered dose to these structures is necessary to avoid untoward complications. An anterior supraclavicular field is generally matched to the initial large lateral fields and approximately 5,000 cGy given to treat submicroscopic disease in this area.

Treatment results are related to both stage and histopathology but many series do not adequately document outcome as a function of these variables. Huang combines the above listed T_1, T_2 and T_3 stages into his T_1/T_2 categories.[334] For a clinically negative neck he reports a 5-year survival of 65%. For groups corresponding to T_4N_0–N_2 and T_4N_3 he finds respective 5-year survivals of 41.3% and 23%. Vikram and colleagues note a 5-year local/regional control rate for early T-stage N_0 patients of 65%.[727] Scanlon and colleagues show a clear worsening of prognosis with increasing cervical adenopathy with 5-year survivals of 67%, 24%, and 14% when the patient has no clinical adenopathy, unilateral adenopathy, or bilateral adenopathy.[570] It is important to note that these series were treated prior to routine CT/MRI scanning which would have the tendency to increase the clinical stage of the neck disease.

A clear correlation exists between the degree of cervical adenopathy and the subsequent development of distant metastases with patients with bilateral adenopathy having a 5-year actuarial risk of approximately 80% of developing distant metastases. Common sites of distant metastases are the lung, bone, and liver. In selected cases, a failure at the primary site alone can be salvaged using a combination of external beam radiotherapy and an intracavitary implant.[748] However, the morbidity associated with this may be substantial.

Although effective in early stages, standard radiotherapy (despite achieving high complete response rates) produces 5-year survivals in stage III disease of only 10%–45% and in stage IV disease of 0–30%.[322,520] Despite major differences between NPC and other HNSCCs, many chemotherapy studies have included NPC patients, which confounds study results. Chemotherapeutic strategies in NPC now treat this disease as a distinct entity. With the exception of parts of China, the problem of small patient numbers is obviously even greater in NPC trials then in many other HNSCC trials.

Early U.S. reports of chemotherapy in NPC were single-institution retrospective surveys of recurrent or metastastic NPC patients treated over a many year period with a variety of agents. Active single agents include cisplatin, bleomycin, methotrexate, 5-fluorouracil, doxorubicin, and vinca alkaloids. (Interferon data are reviewed in Immunobiologic Therapy below.) Retrospective surveys from the early 1980s reported 40–70% response rates (<20% CR) with a variety of cisplatin- and non-cisplatin-based *combination* regimens in recurrent disease. More recent series with intensive cisplatin-based regimens in recurrent disease have reported higher and more durable complete response rates.[22]

The use of combined-modality treatments (sequential chemotherapy and radiotherapy) is under active study in advanced NPC.[322] Neoadjuvant series have reported 60–80% response rates (10–30% complete) with cisplatin- and non-cisplatin-based regimens. Results of a large series from Taiwan treating 1,206 patients with a variety of chemotherapeutic agents given with split-course radiotherapy suggested that the combined-modality approach was more effective than radiotherapy alone in historical controls.[335]

At least seven small, single-arm sequential-therapy studies have been reported, all but one with cisplatin-based regimens.[21,322,380,638,680] Tannock and colleagues reported the largest series of 49 consecutive patients treated with methotrexate, cisplatin and 3-day continuous infusion bleomycin followed by radiotherapy.[680] The overall response rate was high, but complete response was low—22% (8/36) in patients with measurable nodal disease. After radiotherapy, the complete response rate jumped to 82%. This group compared their results with 140 stage-matched historical controls and reported no differences in disease-free or overall survival. Furthermore, there was no apparent reduction in distant metastases in the chemotherapy group. This study was not confirmed by three similar series[110,182,520]—complete response rates were equivalent in the combined-modality and radiotherapy groups; however, the disease-free and median survivals of the combined-modality group were higher.

The need for effective adjuvant therapy in NPC is indicated by the high recurrence rate despite high initial complete response rates with primary therapy. The only randomized adjuvant trial in adult NPC reported no differences between the adjuvant arm and non-adjuvant arm in respect to patterns of failure, disease-free survival and overall survival (See Primary Chemotherapy below). Three problems with this trial were the inclusion of radiotherapy partial responders in the "adjuvant" arm, the long delay between radiotherapy and chemotherapy (>65 days in 20% of patients) and the use of a non-cisplatin regimen that is not well studied in any HNSCC site.[561]

Advanced Skin Cancer

Although the skin of the head and neck accounts for less than 10% of the body's surface area, 70–80% of cutaneous malignancies occur in this region. As a result of greater sun exposure in occupational and recreational activities, and the depleted ozone layer (with increased UV-B exposure), the incidence of skin cancer seems to be increasing, and the initial age at presentation decreasing.[760] About 3,000 yearly deaths in the U.S. are attributable to non-melanoma cutaneous malignancies; morbidity occurs in a many-fold greater number of people, however, in terms of medical costs, cosmetic deformity and loss of function. Treatment is protracted because of the recurrent nature of the disease, need for repeated reconstructive efforts and propensity of second primary skin cancers to occur. Most early lesions are successfully controlled on the first attempt with conservative local therapy. But advanced skin cancer of the head and neck is not controlled easily, and its frequently devastating physical consequences can have tremendous influence on patients' psychological well-being.

No standard systemic therapy exists for unresectable, recurrent or metastatic skin SCC. Although data are limited, cytotoxics, retinoids and α-interferon do have activity,[317,424,426,539,677,760] and should be considered in the multimodality approach for advanced, recurrent disease.

Melanoma of the head and neck region is considered in Section XXXIV.

Sarcomas

Sarcomas arising from bone or extraskeletal soft tissues of the head and neck are rare. The most commonly encountered include osteogenic sarcoma, malignant fibrous histiocytoma, rhabdomyosarcoma, fibrosarcoma, synovial sarcoma, angiosarcoma and chrondrosarcoma. Complete excision is the mainstay of treatment with radiation or chemotherapy playing a less well defined role in most head and neck sarcomas with the exception of rhabdomyosarcoma.[457]

Osteogenic sarcoma is the most common malignant neoplasm of bone, although it is rare in the oral and facial bones. Less than 10% of all osteogenic sarcomas occur in the skull, with most of them in the mandible or maxilla. Among American children, osteogenic sarcoma is the most frequent primary malignant tumor of the jaw. Craniofacial osteogenic sarcomas tend to have a better prognosis than those arising in long bones, with best survival seen in tumors of the maxilla. Overall 5 year survival is <35%.[249]

Approximately 10% of *chondrosarcomas* occur in head and neck sites.[79] The most common sites include the jaws, paranasal sinuses, and larynx. Chondrosarcomas of the larynx deserve special note because they tend to be low grade, well differentiated sarcomas with low metastatic capability. Successful management usually consists of complete surgical excision often with voice conservation techniques. This is in contrast to chondrosarcomas arising from skull base or maxilla where complete excisions are less likely, ultimate tumor control rates less and where adjuvant radiation may contribute to local control of disease.[453] Survival rates for chondrosarcoma are directly related to resectability, site and tumor grade. Five-year survival rate for low grade, completely resected tumors range from 70–90% and overall survival rates range from 0–50% for unresectable or high grade tumors.[79,213]

Rhabdomyosarcoma is the most common soft tissue sarcoma in children and in the head and neck presents most frequently in the orbit, sometimes by invasion from the adjacent nasal cavity or sinus. Other sites of involvement include the nasopharynx, ear, paranasal sinuses and soft tissues of the oral cavity and neck. Histologically, the embryonal variety is the most common. Of prognostic importance in rhabdomyosarcomas of the head and neck is the site of origin. Orbital sites have the most favorable and parameningeal sites the least favorable prognosis. Five-year survival rates for these sites of childhood rhabdomyosarcoma are 89%,

55%, and 47%, respectively.[457] The parameningeal group consists of sites at high risk for meningeal spread of tumor and includes the infratemporal fossa, ear, nasopharynx, nasal cavity, and paranasal sinuses. Prior to the mid 1960s, surgical excision was the mainstay of therapy with survival rates <20% and with more than 80% of patients developing metastatic disease within 1 year of diagnosis.[673] The addition of chemotherapy and radiation has achieved 5-year survival rates of 83% for localized, completely resected disease and 70% for grossly resected disease with microscopic residual and 52% for patients with gross residual disease.[475]

Malignant fibrous histiocytoma is the most common soft tissue sarcoma in adults, however, only 3–10% occur in the head and neck.[31] The paranasal sinuses are the most common head and neck site of origin followed by craniofacial bones, larynx, soft tissues of the neck and oral cavity. Those tumors arising in the sinonasal tract or facial bones tend to be very aggressive with high rates of local recurrence and distant metastases (25–30%). Regional node metastases are rare. Two-year survival rates range from 30–40%.[31]

Lymphomas can arise in any structure in the head and neck region, and they must enter into the differential diagnosis of every neoplasm (see XXXVI-9 and XXXVI-10).

Small Cell Undifferentiated Cancer

A variety of small cell neoplasms occur in the head and neck which pose particular diagnostic problems for the pathologist. They probably derive from cells of embryonic neuroectodermal or neuroendocrine origin. In general, these tumors tend to behave aggressively. Some are unique to the head and neck such as esthesioneuroblastoma, but others such as neuroendocrine carcinoma, carcinoids, and Merkel cell carcinoma have counterparts that occur at sites outside the head and neck. Differentiation of distinct entities frequently requires electron microscopy, special stains (PAS, Grimelius) or immuno-histochemical stains for keratin, neuron-specific enolase and polypeptide hormones such as calcitonin, somatostatin or ACTH. Some tumors may have a mixed histologic appearance with evidence of squamous or glandular differentiation.

Esthesioneuroblastoma

Esthesioneuroblastoma (olfactory neuroblastoma) is an uncommon tumor (3% of nasal tumors) arising from the olfactory epithelium of the superior nasal cavity and cribriform plate.[202,595,706] A bimodal age distribution exists and the etiology is not known. Intracranial spread through the natural foramina of the cribriform plate occurs commonly. The type and extent of primary therapy depends on tumor size and location. Generally, early stage disease is treated with a single modality approach such as complete surgical excision, usually with craniofacial resection techniques that encompass the entire cribriform plate and ethmoid complex. Adjuvant radiation is used for extensive tumors or for tumors where microscopic residual disease is suspected.

Despite aggressive local therapy this tumor has a high propensity for multiple local recurrences. The distant metastasis rate is 10–20%. Overall survival correlates with stage with a 3-year survival of 50% in stage C (Kadish system) after surgery and radiotherapy. Chemotherapy has been increasingly integrated into the management of stage C disease and in recurrent/metastatic disease. Although the data are limited, drug response patterns are similar to lung and other small cell cancers—cyclophosphamide, vinca alkaloids, doxorubicin, cisplatin, and epipodophyllotoxins appear active.[268] The most frequently reported regimen, cyclophosphamide/vincristine (with or without doxorubicin), produces overall response rates of 50–70%. A retrospective series recently reported significantly improved survival with multimodality therapy (including primary chemotherapy) over local therapy alone for stage C disease.[642] No improvement in DFS was noted, however, despite multiagent chemotherapy and craniofacial resection. In an attempt to increase DFS, high-dose chemotherapy and autologous bone marrow transplant was investigated.[664] The series included eight heavily pretreated patients, 5 with esthesioneuroblastoma and 3 with sinonasal undifferentiated carcinoma. Prolonged DFS (17+ to 60 months) was reported in 4 patients.

Neuroendocrine Carcinoma

The most common sites of origin for neuroendocrine carcinoma in the head and neck are the larynx and paranasal sinuses, although similar cancers have been reported in the trachea and parotid gland.[37,767] Although biochemical evidence of hormone production is common, paraneoplastic syndromes are rare. Prognosis is directly related to site of origin and degree of histologic differentiation. Five-year survival rates of 70% for paranasal sinus sites has been reported compared to <20% for laryngeal neuroendocrine tumors.[37] Biologic behavior also varies according to histologic spectrum from low grade, well-differentiated "carcinoid type" tumors to intermediate grade or moderately differentiated neuroendocrine carcinoma to highly aggressive undifferentiated carcinomas. A particularly virulent entity of undifferentiated carcinoma has been recently described in the sinonasal tract.[413] Management of low grade tumors consists of conservative resection often combined with radiation. Because of the rapid occurrence of distant metastases with high grade or undifferentiated tumors, chemotherapy combined with radiation therapy or surgery is under study.

Merkel Cell Carcinoma

Merkel cell carcinomas arise from Merkel cells located in the basal layer of the epidermis and occur most commonly as a primary neuroendocrine carcinoma of the skin. Merkel cells are tactile cells of neuroectodermal origin and histologically show ultrastructural neurosecretory granules and immunohistochemical staining for neuron-specific enolase. The skin of the head and neck is a common site of origin. These tumors generally occur in elderly patients. Although previously viewed as fairly indolent cancers of the skin, more recent reports indicate the true biologic aggressiveness of these cancers with an 80% rate of regional metastases and 50% rate of distant dissemination.[266] Overall 5-year survival rates are <20%. Wide local excision and regional node dissection is effective in controlling localized disease. Adjuvant radiation is indicated for large tumors, tumors with close surgical margins or lymphatic invasion. Because of the propensity for distant metastases and evidence that these cancers are quite sensitive to chemotherapy,[252,791] this modality may be explored.

Chemotherapy Approaches in HNSCC

Overview

Chemotherapy is investigational in primary (advanced untreated) HNSCC.[8,46,92,104,106,109,320,342,632,644,663,679,685,777] Data from the many different single- and combined-agent trials do not indicate that chemotherapy currently is able to improve survival prospects over those of local therapy of surgery and/or irradiation alone. Chemotherapy does play a role in the palliation of recurrent disease and recently has proven effective in primary-therapy trials of organ-preservation.

Research into breast, lung, prostate and colon cancers benefits from large, relatively homogeneous study groups.[64] HNSCC research, on the other hand, suffers from great disease heterogeneity and low incidence in the United States, factors contributing to confusion and conflicting reports regarding chemotherapy outcome (response and survival) and underscoring the importance of large multicenter randomized chemotherapy trials. A large-scale study of laryngeal cancer by the Veterans Affairs is contributing important data on organ preservation (see Primary Chemotherapy below) and demonstrating the importance of multicenter studies of specific HNSCC sites.[710] Single-arm trials should be limited to feasibility testing of new drugs and innovative study designs.

Prognostic Factors. Prognostic factors for chemotherapy response generally accepted as standard include performance status, nutritional status, degree of tumor differentiation, tumor burden (size of primary tumor, resectability and extent of regional nodal metastases), disease stage and primary cancer site.[108,120,143,392,632,783] In head and neck cancer, however, correlative results are conflicting, and it is difficult in most cases to say which of these standard factors have significant effects on response. One clear exception relates to site: undifferentiated nasopharyngeal cancer is the most responsive and adenoid cystic salivary gland cancer the least responsive to chemotherapy.

Recent work looking for additional prognostic factors in HNSCC has focused on immunologic studies and tumor DNA content.[342,512] Clq-binding macromolecules and circulating immune complexes are the best studied immunologic factors; both appear to be inversely correlated with response of previously untreated patients to cisplatin-based chemotherapy.[574,575] DNA content studies report a direct correlation between aneuploidy and complete response rate to cisplatin-based regimens.[208] However promising such studies of biologic factors are, further data are required.

Chemotherapy Response. Comparing the results of HNSCC chemotherapy trials can be difficult because of inconsistent standards for response determination.[632] Confusion regarding tumor measurements can arise because of superinfection from ulcerative lesions or, in studies in recurrent disease, from scarring after local therapy. Timing of response determination also varies. Clinical response determinations 4–6 weeks after therapy often describe persistent nonmalignant abnormalities (e.g., fibrosis, edema) that resolve after longer follow-up. This is a problem with bulky tumors

treated with chemoradiotherapy. These responses may be variably reported as complete or partial.

All investigators agree that a *complete* response to chemotherapy is of overwhelming importance to a patient's survival outlook. The current direction of response reporting in primary HNSCC trials is to differentiate between responses at primary sites and those at regional sites. Pathologic documentation of primary-site clinical complete response is critical, and the number and depth of biopsies must be rigorously defined. There is disagreement, however, over the comparative importance of histologic and clinical complete responses.[7,215,503] Much of the discrepancy in this area of research may relate to lack of thoroughness in clinical staging and lack of uniform specifications for the number and depth of postchemotherapy biopsies. Although critical in screening for new drug activity, partial responses do not increase survival in primary or recurrent disease.

Toxicities. Chemotherapy-related toxicities frequently encountered in HNSCC are reviewed briefly in the following discussions of each agent. They are classic toxicities seen with the use of these agents in other cancers.[94] Toxicities that are not well established or that are unique to drugs not currently in common use are not mentioned here but only in the applicable discussion of each drug.

The most frequent and dose-limiting toxicities with current chemotherapeutic approaches in HNSCC fall into three areas: myelosuppression, mucositis, and the legendary toxicities associated with cisplatin. Myelosuppression is a well-known and long-standing side effect of chemotherapy. Its mitigation is being pursued in an encouraging new line of work with hematopoietic growth factors (see XVIII-6). Mucositis is becoming the limiting acute toxicity in the chemotherapy of HNSCC. Two of the most promising new approaches for controlling advanced HNSCC—concomitant chemoradiotherapy and chemical/pharmacologic modulation of 5-fluorouracil—are severely limited by this toxic effect. How to best mitigate mucositis is not clear.

Several promising strategies to limit therapy-induced mucositis in HNSCC are under study.[245,277,287,477,524,645] In a randomized study, sucralfate rinses decreased mucositis associated with cisplatin and 5-fluorouracil.[524] Antimicrobial mouthwashes containing amphotericin B, polymyxin B, and tobramycin have been reported to limit the radiation-induced oral mucositis by selectively decreasing colonization of the oral cavity by fungi and aerobic gram-negative bacteria.[645] A novel approach for reducing drug-induced mucositis is the use of *circadian* infusion schedules of anticancer therapy.[287] Two other approaches which have yielded promising results include the use of G-CSF and cryotherapy.

Cisplatin toxicities (renal, otologic, neurologic, and gastrointestinal) may be solved largely by substituting carboplatin, a platinum analogue.[87,742] Nevertheless, cisplatin will remain a leading agent against HNSCC when management is hampered by myelosuppression. Recent availability of specific $5HT_3$ (serotonin) receptor antagonists (e.g., ondansetron) will greatly enhance the control of the major acute problem of cisplatin-induced nausea and vomiting. Cisplatin's relative lack of mucositis also will contribute to its continued utility because of the association of this toxic effect with some of the newer strategies, especially concomitant chemoradiotherapy.

Preclinical data and suggestive results of single-arm clinical trials have pointed to other ways to control cisplatin toxicity. One such new strategy is the use of a heterogeneous group of agents called "chemoprotectors"—a group including thiol-containing compounds (e.g., sodium diethyldithiocarbamate, sodium thiosulfate, WR-2721) and probenecid. However, none of these toxicity-reduction strategies has yet proved itself in randomized clinical trials.[45,511]

Preclinical Screening. Preclinical drug screening for active new agents and combinations is of highest priority. Many groups are developing panels of HNSCC cell lines for this research, and these lines are as heterogeneous as the disease itself. The establishment of panels of site-specific HNSCC cell lines may be important for future chemosensitivity studies. However, different cell lines from the same HNSCC may have different chemosensitivity patterns.[393]

In addition to drug screening, the in vitro work has allowed the study of chemical modulation of active drugs. This work has shown that leucovorin, hydroxyurea, α-interferon and methotrexate potentiate 5-fluorouracil cytoxicity. In vitro interactions between chemotherapy (e.g., hydroxyurea, 5-fluorouracil) and irradiation and between chemotherapy (cisplatin-5-fluorouracil) and hyperthermia have also led to clinical trials. In vivo (xenograft) work has identified promising new drugs such as 2',2'-difluorodeoxycytidine.[68,716]

Chemotherapy of Recurrent HNSCC

The majority of patients included in the following discussion has recurrent disease and constitutes the principal study group; a minority has metastatic or advanced unresectable disease. We refer to this patient group generically as "recurrent," although many studies discussed under this rubric include the minority cases also.

The exclusive arena for testing new chemotherapeutic single agents and the principal arena for trials of new combinations of agents in HNSCC is in recurrent disease. So far, chemotherapy has had no impact on overall survival in recurrent HNSCC. The purely clinical, noninvestigational goal of chemotherapy in recurrent disease has been to achieve palliation, unlike the goal of primary chemotherapy trials, which is to cure locally advanced, untreated cancer. The overall prognosis in recurrent HNSCC is dismal (6–10 months median survival).

Lumped diagnostically under HNSCC is a diverse group of cancers with markedly variable natural histories (fully discussed in the "Biology" section above) and, therefore, markedly variable responses to chemotherapy. Important diversities also occur in HNSCC relapse patterns: at the primary site, in regional nodes and at distant sites after definitive local therapy. These and many other diversities make it extremely difficult to interpret results of chemotherapy trials in cancers of this region.

Many chemotherapy studies encompass all guises of recurrent HNSCC. That gamut runs from minimal, resectable disease seen locally after radiation therapy to bulky regional and distant disease occurring after surgery, radiotherapy and even after primary and/or salvage chemotherapy. Often these last salvage patients are excluded from further che-

motherapy trials because of extremely poor risk. Other poor-risk patients, for example, those with unresectable disease resistant to neoadjuvant chemotherapy or with short disease-free intervals or persistent disease after primary therapy, are included in many trials. Although patients with advanced *resectable* disease should be included in trials of primary therapy,[108,779] the varying definition of resectable among different head and neck surgeons can place these patients in "recurrent" trials.

Many of the factors mentioned above can confound results. In some trials, confounding factors suppress response; in others, they may enhance response, such as trial populations with significantly larger percentages of advanced primary disease since drug responsiveness is generally better in untreated disease. We have tried to note in the following discussions of trials all confounding factors of which we are aware.

Single Agent Trials. Four drugs have major activity in recurrent HNSCC: methotrexate, cisplatin, bleomycin, and 5-fluorouracil. Response rates of different trials with the same agent have varied markedly due to HNSCC's great heterogeneity and because of differences in trial designs. Pooling results with these drugs as single agents shows response rates in the range of 15–35% and remission durations of 3–5 months (Table XXVII-1-27). Cyclophosphamide and hydroxyurea also have reported activity, although experience is less.

Methotrexate, according to many oncologists, is the standard palliative therapy for recurrent or metastatic HNSCC.[320,409] Standard dose and schedule for palliation is 40 mg/m²/week IV or IM,[86] with dose escalations until achieving mild toxicity or any tumor response. This methotrexate dose and schedule is relatively nontoxic, inexpensive and convenient—features critical to palliative therapy.

Preclinical work and early single-arm HNSCC clinical studies suggested a dose-response effect with high-dose methotrexate plus delayed leucovorin. However, five randomized trials of standard-dose methotrexate versus high-dose (up to 100-fold increases) methotrexate plus delayed leucovorin failed to confirm the single-arm results. Pooled response rates for the two arms (high- vs. low-dose) from all of the five randomized studies are nearly identical (Table XXVII-1-28).

The issue of high-dose methotrexate recently has been revived, however. A randomized, placebo-controlled trial of standard-dose methotrexate with leucovorin or without it, revealed that even delayed leucovorin (given 24 hours after high-dose methotrexate) not only suppressed toxicity but

Table XXVII-1-27. Single-Agent Activity in Recurrent Head and Neck Cancer*

Agent	N	Response (%)
Methotrexate	998	31
Bleomycin	347	21
Cisplatin	288	28
Carboplatin	115	26
5-Fluorouracil	118	15
Cyclophosphamide	86	36
Hydroxyurea	38	32

*See text

Table XXVII-1-28.   Randomized Trials of Weekly Standard-Dose vs. High-Dose Methotrexate in HNSCC

| Author | Standard Dose | | High-Dose | | |
	Dose[a]	Response (%)	Dose[a]	Respnse (%)	Leucovorin (mg)
Levitt[414]	80–240	7/16 (44)	240–1,080	15/25 (60)	40/m² IV then 25/m² every 6 hr × 4 at 36 hr
Vogler[733]	60	12/44 (27) 19/61 (31)[b]	500	11/49 (22)	5 every 6 hr × 6 at 36 hr
Woods[787]	50	7/27 (26)[c] 6/23 (26)	500–5000	10/22 (46) 7/27 (26)	15 every 6 hr × 2 at 24 hr
DeConti[161]	40–60	21/81 (26)	120[d] (2 wks)	19/90 (21)	25 every 6 hr × 8 at 42 hr
Taylor[689]	40	4/18 (22)	1,500	6/19 (32)	25 × 2 then 10 every 6 hr at 30 hr
Total	40–240	76/270 (28)	120–5,000	68/232 (29)	

[a]mg/m² per week
[b]Standard dose used in two different schedules; both were compared to a single high-dose regimen
[c]Three dose levels tested; middle dose (500 mg) was used at high dose vs. 50 mg, and as standard dose vs. 5,000 mg
[d]240 mg/m² per 2 week

also antitumor activity as well.[73] This study indicates the need for further work in optimizing methotrexate/leucovorin doses and schedules.

Cisplatin is perhaps the most important chemotherapeutic drug for HNSCC.[92,777,778] Most studies have given cisplatin in an intermittent standard-dose bolus schedule (80–120 mg/m² every 3–4 weeks). Altered drug schedules designed to enhance therapeutic index in HNSCC have been tested. A small randomized comparison of schedules showed no difference in activity between bolus cisplatin at 120 mg/m²/day and the less-toxic schedule of 20 mg/m²/day for 5 days.[566] Cisplatin given as a continuous infusion has pharmacokinetic advantages and equivalent activity in HNSCC to that of the same dose given in boluses.[234,344]

The dose-response relationship between cisplatin and HNSCC has been studied by several groups but remains unproved. Single-arm studies of regional and high-dose (150–200 mg/m²) systemic cisplatin have produced single-agent response rates of over 70% and definite objective responses in patients failing standard-dose cisplatin.[236,305,485] The only randomized HNSCC trial, however, tested a lower "high-dose" regimen and failed to confirm cisplatin's dose-response effect.[722] This trial, which directly compared 120 mg/m² to 60 mg/m² via intravenous bolus, was stopped early because of very similar response rates between the two arms (16.1% and 17.8%, respectively) and identical median survivals (34 weeks).

Bleomycin has been studied extensively as a single agent and in combinations in HNSCC. Its spectrum of toxicity is distinctive. Dose-intensity is directly associated with mucositis; and total cumulative dosage is directly associated with skin toxicity and with the most feared side effect, pulmonary fibrosis. Bleomycin's lack of myelosuppression, even with prolonged continuous infusion, promotes its use in combinations. Continuous infusion regimens produce less pulmonary toxicity but are not clearly more active clinically than intermittent-bolus schedules in HNSCC.[516,531,619]

5-Fluorouracil is less active than methotrexate, cisplatin or bleomycin in HNSCC (Table XXVII-1-27). It has been given in varying doses as an intravenous bolus daily (for 5 days), weekly or every 3 or 4 weeks. The dose-limiting toxicity of

bolus administration is myelosuppression; *prolonged* administration is limited by mucositis, diarrhea and cutaneous erythema. Schedule dependency of 5-fluorouracil treatment has received little study in HNSCC.[682] Continuous-infusion regimens were designed initially to reduce myelosuppression and seemed to have enhanced activity.[9] Recent studies suggest an association between continuous-infusion 5-fluorouracil and cardiac ischemia.[547]

Despite 5-fluorouracil's modest single-agent activity in HNSCC, preclinical studies indicating its synergistic interaction with cisplatin and enhanced cytotoxicity with chemical modulators (e.g., leucovorin stabilization of the thymidylate synthetase ternary complex) have translated into major clinical advances in this area (see Promising New Combinations below). Therefore, 5-fluorouracil is now one of the most promising antineoplastics in HNSCC research.

Other active agents (producing response rates of 15–30%) which are not widely utilized in HNSCC include cyclophosphamide and hydroxyurea.[403] These agents (or their analogs) used in combination with other agents or modalities are under investigation and may play a greater role in the future.

Randomized trials have compared different single agents in recurrent HNSCC. Two phase III studies have directly compared cisplatin and methotrexate (randomized, two-arm design). In the first of these studies, Hong and colleagues gave cisplatin at 50 mg/m² on days 1 and 8 every month versus methotrexate at 40–60 mg/m² per week.[325] Each arm produced similar response rates, 28.6% and 23.5%, respectively. These data were confirmed by the second phase III trial.[283]

New drug development in HNSCC is following five major avenues: high-dose therapy; altered schedules (e.g., continuous infusion); chemical/pharmacologic modulation of activity and/or toxicity of currently active drugs (primarily 5-fluorouracil); structurally and mechanistically new drugs; and new analogues of known active drugs with increased therapeutic indices. The first four avenues of study are discussed elsewhere in this section. Work along the last approach, analogue development, is discussed here.

The methotrexate analogues trimetrexate, piritrexim and

edatrexate all appear to be active in HNSCC (response rates of 20–30%), and may have pharmacologic advantages and less renal toxicity.[94,557,582,708] In preclinical studies, some lack of cross-resistance between these analogues and methotrexate has been observed. The dose-limiting toxicity of piritrexim is myelosuppression and mucositis is the major problem with edatrexate.

Driven by the major activity and legendary toxicities of cisplatin, analogue development has moved faster with this drug than with other drugs. Carboplatin is a second-generation platinum complex with activity equivalent to and toxicity less than cisplatin.[87,742] Bolus carboplatin has pharmacokinetic and toxicity profiles similar to those of continuous-infusion cisplatin and has significantly less renal, otologic, neurologic and gastrointestinal (nausea/vomiting) toxicity than bolus cisplatin. Reversible myelosuppression (primarily thrombocytopenia) is the dose-limiting toxicity for carboplatin.

Single-agent studies of carboplatin given monthly in bolus (400 mg/m^2), or fractionated (80 mg/m^2/day for 5 days) schedules produced objective response rates of 20–30% in recurrent and metastatic HNSCC.[138,159,197,199,329] These single-arm data were confirmed in a cooperative group randomized phase II trial of two second-generation platinum complexes—carboplatin (response rate 24%) and iproplatin (response 12%).[10] In contrast to the proven activity of carboplatin, this and other trials of iproplatin in recurrent HNSCC have been uniformly disappointing[1] with overall response rates of less than 10% and major toxicity (myelosuppression, nausea/vomiting).

An intriguing concept currently under study in a number of solid tumors is combined use of carboplatin and cisplatin. In part, this is a dose-response inquiry aimed at allowing higher doses of platinum by varying the types and thereby lowering the intensities of platinum toxicities. Two recent single-arm studies in advanced and recurrent disease, however, did not show increased response (17% in one, 33% in the other).[183,535]

Bleomycin and 5-fluorouracil analogues, used systemically, in HNSCC have shown no therapeutic advantages over the parent compounds.[9,499]

Several currently available agents deserve further study in HNSCC including ifosfamide[387,723] and etoposide (VP-16-213).[116,144,284]

General classes of drugs with limited single-agent activity include the anthracyclines, vinca alkaloids, mitomycin (and analogues), and nitrosoureas.[257] The major role for anthracyclines in head and neck cancer appears to be in the therapy of non-squamous cancers (salivary gland cancer, small cell carcinoma, sarcoma, and esthesioneuroblastoma). Following is a partial list of drugs that are inactive in recurrent HNSCC or do not appear to have advantages over parent compounds in single-agent trials: PCNU, bisantrene, hexamethylmelamine, mitoguazone, m-AMSA, aclacinomycin, doxorubicin, epirubicin, mitoxantrone, tallysomycin S$_{10}$b, vindesine, dibromodulcitol, triazinate, gallium nitrate, 6-thioguanine, triazofurin, homoharringtonine, porfiromycin, mitozolomide, and lomustine.[8,320]

Multiagent Trials. Nearly all possible combinations and combination doses/schedules of methotrexate, cisplatin, bleomycin and 5-fluorouracil and other agents listed in Table XXVII-1-27 have been tried in numerous single-arm studies in recurrent HNSCC.[18] Results have covered a wide range of response rates, including generally low complete response rates, in heterogeneous subsets of patients. In the late 1970s, work focused on cisplatin-bleomycin combinations, which appeared from single-arm studies to be more active than non-cisplatin combinations.[320,777,779] The highest complete response rate to a high-dose cisplatin-bleomycin combination strategy in recurrent disease was 24%.[291]

The cisplatin/5-fluorouracil regimen in HNSCC was an important advance launched by preclinical studies indicating synergy between these drugs and by concern over bleomycin's pulmonary toxicity. Pioneering clinical work by the Wayne State group in the early 1980s yielded major objective response rates of 78% (27% complete responses) in recurrent disease.[388] Lower response rates have been reported by other centers, however, including disappointing phase II response rates of 11%, with an every-28-day schedule; 25% using the identical regimen (drugs, doses, schedules and cycle number) in patients with recurrent (chemotherapy-naive) disease; and less than 10% in patients failing prior chemotherapy.[8,104,153,468] Enthusiasm for this combination in recurrent disease is further diminished by the negative long-term results[735] and recent results of randomized trials comparing cisplatin-5-fluorouracil with other combinations and even single agents (Tables XXVII-1-29 and XXVII-1-30). Several phase II and III trials (over 200 reported patients) of the less-toxic carboplatin/5-fluorouracil regimen report response rates equivalent to cisplatin/5-fluorouracil.[199,310,450]

Based on preclinical synergy and activity in other human tumors, the cisplatin-etoposide and cisplatin-cytarabine combinations have been studied in HNSCC. Cisplatin-etoposide produced equivalent activity and toxicity to single-agent cisplatin in a phase III trial.[444] Despite 4 negative phase II trials,[44,136,445,534] cisplatin-cytarabine produced significantly higher response rates compared to cisplatin/5-fluorouracil in a small randomized trial.[270]

Randomized Studies. Only two of the 11 trials comparing multiagent to single-agent (methotrexate in 7 trials and cisplatin in 5) therapies produced significant differences in response, and the overall single-agent and multiagent median survivals are identical at 5.5 months (Table XXVII-1-29).

Jacobs and colleagues recently reported a 3-arm comparative trial of cisplatin and 5-fluorouracil as single agents and in combination.[346] Although no major survival differences occurred, the response rate was highest in the cisplatin/infusional 5-fluorouracil combination (Table XXVII-1-29).

Recently, the Southwest Oncology Group (SWOG) reported an interim analysis of its 3-arm randomized phase III study comparing cisplatin/5-fluorouracil, carboplatin (300 mg/m^2)/5-fluorouracil and single-agent methotrexate in recurrent HNSCC.[235] The response rate and toxicity of cisplatin/5-fluorouracil were significantly greater than they were in the methotrexate arm. The carboplatin/5-fluorouracil arm did not differ significantly from the 2 other arms in response or toxicity. Median survival was poor and not significantly different among the three groups. Interpretation of these results is clouded by atypical toxicity patterns. Moderate to severe

Table XXVII-1-29.   Randomized Trials of Chemotherapy in Recurrent Head and Neck Cancer: Single Agents Versus Multiple Agents

Author	Agents	No. Patients	% Response (Complete)	Median Survival (mo)
Davis[156]	P v PBM	30 v 27	13(3) v 11(0)	4.2 v 5.2[a]
DeConti[161]	M/MI v MICA	81/80 v 76	26(–) 24(–) v 18(–)	5.0/4.4 v 3.2
Drelichman[189]	M v POB	24 v 27	33(8) v 41(11)	5.5 v 3.2
Jacobs[348]	P v PM	40 v 39	18(8) v 33(15)	6.2 v 6.9
Vogl[362,732]	M v PBM	83 v 80	35(8) v 48(16)[b]	5.6 v 5.6
Morton[486] [c]	P/B v PB	31/22 v 38	13(3)/14(0) v 24(5)	3.7/2.8 v 3.8
Williams[773]	M v PVB	98 v 92	16(0) v 24(1)	7.3 v 6.8
Jacobs[346]	P/F v PF	83/83 v 79	17(4)/13(2) v 32(6)[d]	5.0/6.1 v 5.5
Eisenberger[198]	M v CpM	20 v 20	25(5) v 25(0)	6 v 6
Forastiere[235]	M v CpF/PF	88/87 v 87	11(1) v 18(2)/30(5)[e]	5.6 v 5.2/6.6
Liverpool[85,429]	P/M v PF/PM	50/50 v 50/50	29(2)/12(0) v 24(6);22(0)	2.7/8.7 v 5.3/6.7[f]
Total (Median Response—*Single Agent* v Multiagent)			16(3) v 24(5)	5.5 v 5.5

Abbreviations: P, cisplatin; Cp, carboplatin; F, 5-fluorouracil; M, methotrexate; B, bleomycin; C, cyclophosphamide; O, vincristine; V, vinblastine; A, cytarabine; I, leucovorin; —, not available; v, versus. Italic = single agents

[a] Median partial response duration

[b] Initial report significant (P = .04, 1-sided T-test); final report (P = .07, 1-sided T-test)

[c] Four-arm study with a no treatment (supportive care) control arm. Single arm cisplatin associated with a significantly increased median survival v control arm

[d] PF v P, P = .035; PF v F, P = .005

[e] Response rate significant PF v M, P = .02

[f] Taken from interim report, not available in final report.

Table XXVII-1-30.   Randomized Trials of Cisplatin/5-Fluorouracil vs Other Agent(s)

Author	No.	Agents	% Response (Complete)	Survival
Neoadjuvant				
Clark[107]	56	PF v PBMI (2 cycles)	77(19) v 70(19)	P = NS
Gonzales[270]	36	PF v PA (3 cycles)	83(16) v 89(35)[a]	P = NS
Recurrent				
Kish[386]	40	PF v PF (bolus)	72(22) v 20(10)[b]	P = NS
Clavel[113]	382	PV v PBMO	31(2) v 34(10)	P = NS
Jacobs[346]	104	PF v P/F	32(6) v 17(4)/13(2)[c]	P = NS
Forastiere[235]	262	PF v CpF/M	30(5) v 18(2)/11(1)	P = NS
Amrein[17]	55	PF v PFBMI	46(0) v 63(7)	P = NS
Liverpool[429]	200	PF v P/M/PM	24(6) v 29(2)/12(0)/22(0)	P = NS

Abbreviations: P, cisplatin; Cp, carboplatin; F, 5-Fluorouracil; B, bleomycin; M, methotrexate; A, cytarabine; O, vincristine; I, leucovorin; NS, not statistically significant (P > 0.05)

[a] Significant difference complete response (P < .05)

[b] Significant difference (P < .01)

[c] PF v P, P = .035; PF v F, P = .005

myelosuppression (leukopenia) was significantly more frequent in the cisplatin arm, suggesting suboptimal dosing of carboplatin.

Carboplatin's reduced renal toxicity led to a recent study of this agent combined with methotrexate versus methotrexate alone.[198] In the combination arm, renal toxicity was not excessive, but significant myelosuppression led to frequent carboplatin dose reductions in most combined-treatment patients, which underscores the difficulty in combining carboplatin with other myelosuppressive drugs. The two study arms showed identical response rates and median survivals.

Five studies compared single-agent cisplatin to cisplatin combinations. Despite promising single-arm studies, cisplatin combinations have not performed better than cisplatin alone in phase III trials (Table XXVII-1-29). Multiagent survival rates are equivalent to single-agent cisplatin.[429,486]

Two phase III trials compared cisplatin-based combinations to similar regimens without cisplatin.[2,112] These trials reported significant increases in response rates with the cisplatin regimen but no survival differences.

A randomized trial designed to test the schedule dependency of 5-fluorouracil in the cisplatin-5-fluorouracil combination compared cisplatin (100 mg/m^2) bolus plus 5-fluorouracil given by continuous infusion (1,000 mg/m^2/day × 4 days) to the same bolus dose of cisplatin plus 5-fluorouracil as a bolus (600 mg/m^2 day 1 and day 8).[386] The continuous-infusion regimen produced a higher response rate of 72% (22% complete) compared to the bolus-group response rate of 20% (10% complete) (P < 0.01). Despite the lower total dose, the bolus arm was associated with greater toxicity (myelosuppression). The interpretation of this study is clouded by the bolus-5-fluorouracil arm's unusual day 1 and 8 schedule, and more than 4-fold lower total dose of 5-fluorouracil. Furthermore, single-arm trials of different schedules (e.g., cisplatin and 5-fluourouracil given as daily intravenous bolus for 5 days)[378,471] or different sequences,[379] produced response rates comparable to those, in similar risk patients, of the standard regimen of cisplatin plus continuous-infusion 5-fluorouracil.

Single-arm clinical trials of methotrexate pretreatment and 5-fluorouracil in advanced and recurrent HNSCC yielded mixed results: response rates ranging from 16–94%.[529,554] However, three randomized studies differing somewhat in design and results, clearly indicate that the methotrexate/5-fluorouracil sequence—predicted by preclinical studies to be active—does not produce a response or survival advantage over simultaneous administration or the reverse sequence (Table XXVII-1-31).[72,74,75,114]

Conclusions. All these data for recurrent, unresectable, and metastatic disease fail to show that multiagent therapy is more effective than single-agent therapy. Although combination chemotherapy for recurrent or metastatic HNSCC may produce higher response rates than single agents, none of the 11 randomized combination trials (including those comparing cisplatin/5-fluorouracil) produced improved survival over single-agent treatment (Tables XXVII-1-29 and XXVII-1-30).

Single-agent and combination chemotherapy can provide effective palliation for these patients. Because of its documented activity, acceptable toxicity, convenience of administration and low cost, methotrexate remains the single-agent standard of comparison, but other agents are active. Indeed, cisplatin is at least comparable to methotrexate in response and survival rates, albeit with increased toxicity. Single-agent carboplatin is active against HNSCC, but has not been compared adequately to cisplatin in this setting.[87] Nevertheless, carboplatin may be preferred as palliation for selected patients due to its favorable toxicity profile.

The current standard chemotherapy options for recurrent HNSCC are all palliative. The development of new, more-active drugs and combinations must assume highest priority. The combination of cisplatin and infusion 5-fluorouracil has generally been the combination of choice for palliation in patients able (according to performance status) to tolerate the increased toxicity associated with combination therapy. (See below for cisplatin-leucovorin-fluorouracil combination.) The results of large phase II trials with long follow-up[735] and of recent phase III trials (Table XXVII-1-30), however, indicate no advantage over other combinations (in response or survival) or over less-toxic single-agent therapy (in survival). Choice of regimen depends on the important balance between efficacy and toxicity (quality of life), which must be considered on a case-by-case basis.

Regional Cytotoxic Therapy

Preclinical data support regional therapy in HNSCC, as do the predominantly local-regional tumor spread and a relatively selective access to tumor blood supply.[27,121,179,432,487,491,592,632,683,770] High total-body clearance and low regional exchange rates are the major pharmacokinetic factors that allow optimization of regional drug delivery. Total-body clearance for drugs active in HNSCC is highest for floxuridine (FUDR) and lowest for methotrexate, with cisplatin at the low end.[592] Single arm clinical and pharmacokinetic studies of regional therapy in HNSCC have reported low regional exchange rates, increased intratumoral drug levels, enhanced toxicity in the infused area (mucositis, alopecia), reduced systemic toxicity and modest increases in response rates (complete and partial) without apparent survival benefit over the systemic route (see XV-4).

Although cisplatin is not ideal for regional therapy from a pharmacokinetic perspective, it is very active and achieves an estimated fourfold greater intratumoral drug concentration when given intraarterially (i.e., regionally) rather than intravenously. A recent dose-intensive trial of regional cisplatin (100 mg/m²/week) in 25 patients with unresectable HNSCC produced an overall response rate of 80% overall,[485] exceeding the 30% average single-agent response rate achieved with systemic therapy (Table XXVII-1-27). The complete response rate was 32% at the primary site and 50% at regional sites.

Perhaps the most promising combination is cisplatin and floxuridine (FUDR)—the latter has the most favorable regional pharmacokinetic profile of any drug active in HNSCC.[233] A recent phase II study of 15 heavily pretreated HNSCC patients (12 with prior chemotherapy) reported a 47% response rate (complete in less than 10%) with minimal toxicity. The exceptional response rate with this combination in prior chemotherapy failure suggests potential in primary therapy.

The future of regional drug therapy in HNSCC is uncertain.

Table XXVII-1-31. Randomized Trials of Sequential Methotrexate-5-Fluorouracil

Author	No.	Chemotherapy	% Response (Complete)	Median Survival (mo.)
Browman[72,75]	79	M-F[a] v MF[b]	38 (5) v 62(12)	19 v 18
Coates[114]	70	M-F[a] v F-M	51(11) v 40(6)[c]	13.3 v 13.0
			65(12) v 39(4)[d]	13.3 v not reached
Browman[74] [e]	113	M-F[f] v MF[b]	47 (5) v 45(10)	34 v 33

[a] 1-hour sequential methotrexate-5-fluorouracil
[b] Simultaneous
[c] All patients (advanced plus recurrent)
[d] Advanced untreated only
[e] Mostly advanced (11% recurrent). Toxicity (mucositis) increased in sequential arm (p < .05)
[f] 18-hour sequential methotrexate-5-fluorouracil

Table XXVII-1-32.   Randomized Trials of Single Agent Induction Chemotherapy for Head and Neck Cancer

Author	N	Induction Schedule	% Response (Complete)	% Disease-Free Survival (yr)[a]		% Survival (yr)[a]	
				Control	Chemotherapy	Control	Chemotherapy
Von Essen[741]	98 (bm)	M	53 (—)	23 (2–14 mo)	15	—	—
Richard[549] [b]	39 (oc,op)	M (ia)	—	—	—	4 (5)	4
Knowlton[389]	96	M/MI	27 (—)	—	—	10.4 (5)	9
Lustig[434]	75	M	14 (—)	—	—	10 (3)	20
Fazekas[216,395]	638	M	—	—	—	3–16 (5)	9–22 (5)[c]
Arcangeli[20]	142 (oc,op,ma)	M (ia)	>33 (—)	—	—	25 (5)	43 (5)[d]
Taylor[688] [e]	82	ML (PD)	34 (6)	20 (6)	43	39 (6)	37
Rentschler[546] [e]	60	M	73 (4)	57 (5)	47	20 (6)	23

Abbreviations: p, primary site; ia, intra-arterial; bm, buccal mucosa cancer; oc, oral cavity; op, oropharynx; ma, maxillary antrum; M, methotrexate; L, leucovorin; P, cisplatin; D, doxorubicin.

[a] published values or estimated from published data/survival curves
[b] significantly favored methotrexate in response and 9-month survival rate
[c] rates by primary site (overall rates not reported)
[d] $p < .05$; most significant in oral cavity and early stage disease
[e] trials include induction *plus* adjuvant therapy

Enthusiasm is waning for this area of investigation. Despite theoretical advantages, numerous positive single-arm studies and improved methodology, intraarterial therapy has not produced clearly better results than intravenous therapy.[770] Also, local complication rates of intraarterial therapy potentially are more severe. Apparent increases in primary-site complete response rates are negated by high failure rates in the neck (regional nodes) and distant sites. Intraarterial approaches associated with high local control rates may, however, have a role in organ preservation. Intraarterial therapy has been used in sinus tumors to avoid craniofacial resection. Further advances await clarification of the pharmacologic advantage of regional therapy, study of new regional approaches (e.g., chemoembolization), development of more effective systemic therapy to prevent distant relapse, effective concomitant regional chemoradiotherapy and ultimately phase III comparison of regional and systemic chemotherapy.

Immunobiologic Therapy

Immunotherapeutic approaches to head and neck cancer have been disappointing. Early clinical trials adding non-specific immunoadjuvants to chemotherapy were negative. Despite limited encouraging results,[691] most of the nine phase III adjuvant trials with bacillus Calmette-Guérin (BCG), thymosin, *Cornyebacterium parvum,* and levamisole were negative.[15,38,149,506,675,691,744]

Cytokines. Cytokines have received limited study in HNSCC. A promising early report of low-dose interferon-α (responses in 7 of 12 recurrent disease patients, 58%) has not been confirmed. Several studies using recombinant IFN-α have reported response rates in the 10% range.[221,463,480,512]

Two factors led to the study of interferons in NPC: 1) these patients have increased antibody-dependent cytotoxicity and a selective deficit in anti-EBV T-cell activity, and 2) interferons have anti-viral activity against EBV and are immunomodulators. Several small series of type I interferons have produced a response rate of 16% (25 treated patients).[126,127]

Despite the wealth of supportive preclinical single-agent and combined agent data,[552] clinical results with IFN-gamma have been uniformly poor—the agent has been inactive in both phase I and II trials in HNSCC and NPC.[177]

Several human HNSCC cell lines express high-affinity interleukin-2 (IL-2) receptors and are growth-inhibited by IL-2 in vitro and in vivo.[512] It has been shown also in HNSCC that tumor-infiltrating lymphocytes can be increased 30,000-fold by IL-2.[311] Systemic IL-2, given alone or with IFN-α, however, has produced objective responses of short duration.[512] Significant toxicity and modest activity have limited this line of work.

Differentiation Agents. Although preclinical studies have identified several promising agents, only the retinoids have been studied clinically, in HNSCC.[420] Two HNSCC trials, one recently reported randomized phase II trial, of over 30 heavily pretreated patients, produced a 15% response to 13-*cis*-retinoic acid.[421,422] Studies have been conducted in Japan of the 5-fluorouracil-vitamin A-radiotherapy regimen (which reportedly has in vitro synergy) in hundreds of HNSCC patients.[678] The Japanese results are encouraging, but it is difficult to draw firm conclusions because the trials were not controlled.

Plasma-Exchange Approaches. Plasmapheresis in HNSCC is based on the adverse role of humoral immunity in this disease. Increased levels of IgA and immune complexes, which may suppress cell-mediated immunity, are poor prognostic signs in these patients (see Biology above). Plasmapheresis can achieve a decrease in the serum levels of IgA and immune complexes, a rise in serum IgE, and partial restoration of some in vitro lymphocyte function; this treatment has been associated with objective tumor regression in HNSCC.[371,512,590] These data are very preliminary. Plasmapheresis followed by cytotoxic or biologic therapy is a provocative new strategy that is entering clinical study.

Goals. Study is now focusing on the best ways to combine cytokines, differentiation agents, cytotoxic agents and irradiation. There is no question that several biologic agents (e.g., IFN-α, IL-2, 13-*cis*-retinoic acid) used systemically have produced objective tumor regression in HNSCC patients. Overall, however, response rates have been low and remissions incomplete and of short duration. Preclinical mechanistic data provide a basis for clinical dosing and scheduling decisions, although major differences and complex dose-response relationships occur in man. Based on preclinical data, type I interferons are under phase I/II clinical study as radiosensitizers.[96,318] Small series of regional cytokine therapy (IFN-α and IL-2) and of adoptive cellular therapy have reported objective responses in advanced HNSCC.[337,340,591]

The integration of biologic agents into cytotoxic regimens as primary therapy is more complex. Early results suggest that IFN-α may enhance both the activity *and* toxicity of 5-fluorouracil.[94] It is not yet clear if the therapeutic index of the IFN-α/5-fluorouracil regimen is greater than that of high-dose single-agent 5-fluorouracil. The possible contribution of additional anti-tumor activity by IFN-α immune modulation in vivo is under study. In recurrent HNSCC, adding IFN-α[613] or IL-2[181] to the cisplatin/5-fluorouracil regimen was associated with significant toxicity and relatively low response rates (30% and 35%). A new area of highly specific immunologic therapy in HNSCC is the use of monoclonal antibodies;[797] clinical work in this area is just beginning.

As a rule, immunobiologic therapy is more effective when tumor volume is low, well differentiated, or only partially transformed (premalignant). Carefully controlled trials monitoring clinical response and markers of biologic activity will be required to clearly define the roles of these agents—alone and in combination—as primary, adjuvant and chemopreventive therapy.

Primary Chemotherapy

Although chemotherapy has not improved the short survival of patients with recurrent or metastatic HNSCC, promising results are beginning to emerge from the intense study of chemotherapy as an adjunct to standard *primary* treatment (surgery and/or radiotherapy) of advanced local disease. The role of primary chemotherapy is not yet established, however, and its use is restricted to the setting of clinical trials. A patient's prognosis and treatment depend on the primary tumor site and TNM stage. Primary chemotherapy is not called for in early-stage ($T_{1-2}N_{0-1}M_0$) disease, usually cured through standard treatment. After cure, early-stage patients require chemoprevention, however, because of their high risk of second primary tumors.[419]

Chemotherapy can play a role in the primary treatment of more than 60% of all HNSCC patients, or those who are diagnosed with advanced or extensive ($T_{3-4}N_{2-3}M_0$) local-regional disease. This is because advanced HNSCC is both a local-regional and systemic phenomenon. Although optimal surgery or radiotherapy has improved local or regional control, it has not improved survival, mainly because of metastatic disease. Two years after standard treatment, clinical evaluations indicate that less than 40% of these patients will be disease free: local invasion and regional lymph node metastases are diagnosed in 60% and distant metastases in 15–25%.[588] The rate of distant metastases is actually far greater. Autopsy series show that occult distant metastases are present in up to 50% of HNSCC fatalities.[91,165,274,330,394,504,537,586,795]

Severe morbidities after surgery, high mortality rates, and the poor outcome of chemotherapy for recurrent tumors led to clinical investigations of many therapeutic variations of primary chemotherapy, either alone or added to combined-modality approaches. These approaches fall into three main categories: 1) neoadjuvant, primary or induction, chemotherapy (*before* standard surgery and/or radiotherapy); 2) maintenance, or true adjuvant, chemotherapy (*following* definitive standard primary therapy); and 3) concomitant chemotherapy (in combination with radiotherapy usually in unresectable HNSCC). The principal goals of primary chemotherapy in HNSCC are to enhance local-regional control (relapse prevention, organ preservation and primary curative treatment), decrease distant metastases and improve overall survival.

Many reports have used the terminology of primary chemotherapy loosely. Some authors refer to adjuvant chemotherapy as any and all primary chemotherapy.[104,342,632,663] They intend this phrase merely to distinguish from treatment of recurrent disease. In this section, however, we distinguish between neoadjuvant, adjuvant and curative primary chemotherapy. We use the term "adjuvant chemotherapy" only to refer to prevention of relapse after standard therapy. "Neoadjuvant chemotherapy" refers specifically to tumor reduction prior to definitive therapy. And "curative chemotherapy" applies to treatments (limited so far to chemotherapy given concomitantly with radiotherapy) intended to achieve definitive control of local, regional and micrometastatic disease.

Although many phase II studies of chemotherapy in HNSCC have been conducted, the great heterogeneity of head and neck disease and patient populations mandates controlled trials to establish the role of chemotherapy. Innovative single-arm phase I–II trials are important, however, for testing promising new agents and combinations before phase III study.

The following discussion focuses primarily on results from randomized phase III chemotherapy trials in primary HNSCC. These trials are categorized as neoadjuvant, concomitant, adjuvant and neoadjuvant (or concomitant) plus adjuvant therapy. Unlike trials in more common solid tumors (e.g., breast and colon), HNSCC randomized trials have been critically flawed by their small sizes.[109,632,663] None has been large enough to detect a probable degree of survival improvement of 5–10%; the median difference that could be detected with confidence was 25%. Of course, randomized trials are not needed to detect such a dramatic improvement. HNSCC's comparative scarcity and tremendous heterogeneity account for this problem of small trial populations and create the need for multicenter cooperative studies in HNSCC.

Neoadjuvant. Neoadjuvant (induction) therapy, is defined as the use of chemotherapy before definitive (curative) therapy, which generally is surgery and/or radiotherapy. The sequence of chemotherapy followed by definitive radiotherapy frequently is referred to as *sequential* chemoradiotherapy. This approach specifically excludes or limits the extent of surgery except in treatment failures and is growing in importance as an "organ preservation" approach for locally advanced resectable disease.[322] The neoadjuvant concept recently has been expanded to include very novel studies of neoadjuvant chemotherapy followed by a primary curative component of concomitant chemoradiotherapy.[13]

The use of chemotherapy as induction treatment prior to local therapy for advanced HNSCC has been evaluated for over 15 years.[104,109,119,201,319,320,322,326,342,384,632,777,779] The strong rationale for this approach comes from mathematical models of cell kinetics and acquired drug resistance and from preclinical in vivo data.[109,571] The principal objectives of induction are as follows: to promote regression and so enhance subsequent local-regional therapy; to identify patients with responding lesions that might be controlled by more conservative local treatment (organ preservation) rather than by extensive surgical procedures; to identify responding tumors that may benefit from adjuvant chemotherapy following surgery or radiotherapy;[106,210] and to provide early treatment for micrometastatic disease.[109]

Early nonrandomized neoadjuvant trials based their selections of agents on trials in recurrent disease. Single-agent early trials achieved response rates of 30–40%.[104,319–321,326,517,606,777] Gradually, neoadjuvant studies expanded to include multiagent therapy.[320] The first major advance of chemotherapy in this area came in the late 1970s when Randolph and colleagues reported a 71% objective response rate (20% complete responses) in 21 HNSCC patients receiving cisplatin and continuous-infusion bleomycin.[541,779] Single-arm studies that followed and confirmed Randolph's initial report achieved overall response rates in advanced untreated HNSCC ranging from 37% to 87%, including complete response rates generally less than 20%.[104,109,291,319–321,326,517,606] The addition of other drugs to cisplatin/bleomycin to create three- and four-drug regimens produced significant increases in toxicity without improving response or survival rates.[104,777,779]

The next major advance occurred in the early 1980s when Wayne State investigators reported a neoadjuvant trial of cisplatin-infusional 5-fluorouracil, which produced a response rate of 88% (complete, 54%). The unprecedented complete response rate of greater than 50% was perhaps the most important finding because of the significant impact complete responses have on survival. Wayne State data suggested that 5-fluorouracil was better given for 5 days than for 4 and, most important, that three cycles were significantly more active than were two; their complete response rates doubled between the second and third cycles.[8,559,758] Subsequent studies used a variety of doses and schedules of cisplatin and 5-fluorouracil, and confirmed the activity of this combination, although generally at lower objective (mean, 77%; range, 38–100%) and complete (mean, 34%; range, 13–54%) response rates.[8,9,104,109,632] The RTOG used the Wayne State regimen and corroborated its activity by achieving a 38% complete response rate.

More recently, many uncontrolled trials have attempted to further enhance the activity of cisplatin/5-fluorouracil. They have given high-dose cisplatin with fixed-dose 5-fluorouracil; high-dose 5-fluorouracil with fixed-dose cisplatin; cisplatin intraarterially rather than intravenously; increased numbers of courses beyond three; other cytotoxic drugs such as bleomycin, methotrexate, cyclophosphamide, mitoguazone or vinca alkaloids; and dose-intensive multicourse alternating regimens.[8,9,104,109,207,277,385,709] These trials have produced increased toxicity and no consistent improvements in response or survival. Phase II and Phase III trials of carboplatin/5-fluorouracil yielded response rates of 70–80% (complete in

30–40%)—results comparable to cisplatin/5-fluorouracil.[199,450]

Non-cisplatin combinations are under development because of cisplatin's relatively high toxicity. Alternative foundations used most commonly are 5-fluorouracil, cyclophosphamide, bleomycin, and methotrexate, with or without vinca alkaloids. Response rates have ranged from 11% to 69%. One of the best studied of these regimens is Price and Hill's schedule A developed over 10 years ago, a complex combination of vincristine, bleomycin, methotrexate/leucovorin, 5-fluorouracil, hydrocortisone, and doxorubicin based on stem-cell kinetics and cell-cycle specificity.[313,314] Doxorubicin was later excluded.

Randomized trials of neoadjuvant therapy vs. standard local therapy have been conducted with single-agent and multiagent regimens (Tables XXVII-1-33 and XXVII-1-34). Eight of these trials using single-agent neoadjuvant treatment have been reported. All used methotrexate (standard- or high-dose with leucovorin). The only trial reporting significantly improved survival used methotrexate intraarterially in SCC of the oral cavity, oropharynx and maxillary antrum.[20]

Fourteen randomized multiagent neoadjuvant (9 with cisplatin-based regimens) trials with local therapy control groups have been reported to date. Although none have shown that neoadjuvant therapy significantly improves survival, these trials' many design limitations make it impossible to draw definitive conclusions. These limitations include suboptimal patient numbers, relatively inactive induction regimens, variations in local-regional therapies (surgery alone, surgery and radiotherapy, radiotherapy alone) and heterogeneous study populations with multiple primary sites, and resectable and unresectable cases (Table XXVII-1-33). None of the neoadjuvant regimens produced a CR rate of over 50% (median 10%; range, 0–46%). Ten of the 14 randomized studies had such small study numbers that they could not detect significant survival differences below 25%. Only four randomized trials evaluated enough patients (more than 75 patients per study arm) to reveal smaller differences.

Organ preservation is second to improving survival as a goal of primary chemotherapy. Those patients fortunate enough to survive their cancer often face a lifetime of significant morbidity because of cosmetic and functional debilities from surgical resection. Despite marked advances in reconstructive surgery and rehabilitation, patients who have undergone laryngectomy, glossectomy, or composite resection still have major debility. Unfortunately, the importance of organ and function preservation often is ignored. Many opt to receive the less effective therapy of radiation alone to avoid curative surgery.[462] They risk shorter survival rather than face increased survival with severe surgical morbidity. An active area of HNSCC research involves chemoradiotherapy (sequential or concomitant) to facilitate organ-preserving approaches for advanced disease.[322] This research is designed to preserve anatomical structures without compromising survival. In such studies, extensive surgery is reserved to salvage patients who fail to respond to initial therapy or who recur.

Laryngeal preservation is the most advanced application of organ-preservation chemotherapy. In advanced laryngeal SCC (T_3 or T_4, or nodal metastasis), total laryngectomy

Table XXVII-1-33.   Randomized Trials of Neoadjuvant (Induction) Multiagent Chemotherapy for Head and Neck Cancer

Author	N	Induction Therapy Regimen (No. Cycles)	% Response (Complete)	Local Therapy	% Disease-Free Survival (yr)[a] Control	Chemotherapy	% Survival (yr)[a] Control	Chemotherapy
Petrovich[522]	23	MLO (2) (ia)	25 (0)	R	—	—	9 (2)	17
Richard[548]	225 (oc,op)	OB (12d)	—	S ± R	—	—	— (3)[b]	—
Shetty[607]	42 (tb)	OBMFMc (2)	—	R	50 (0.54)	50 (0.58)	—	—
Stolwijk[665]	68	VBMCF (2)	21 (0)	S ± R	—	—	77 (1)	58
Kun[397,702] c	83	CMBF (2)	67 (5)	R ± S	64 (2)	59	43 (2)	31
Szpirglas[676] d	114	DOBP (3)	53 (11)	R	3 (3+)	5	5 (3+)	11
Toohill[289,701]	60	PF (3)	85 (19)	R + S	70 (2)	70	70 (2)	56
Schuller[587] e	158	PMBO (3)	70 (18)	S + R	23 (5)	23	28 (5)	28
Martin[451]	107 (oc,op)	PFBML (3)	48 (6)	S + R; R	42 (2)	49[f]	—	—
Carugati[93] g	120	PB+/−M (1)	44–59 (—)	—	25 (5)	33	18 (5)	38
Jaulerry[352]	100	PBVdMc (2)	50 (10)−p	R	38 (2)	44	45 (2)	34
VACSP[327,710] d	332 (lc)	PF (2)	85 (31)	R	—	—	56 (3)	53
Martin[449]	75	PF (3)	68 (46)	S + R; R	61 (1)	73	—	—
Paccagnella[508]	221	PF (4)	70 (29)	S + R	58	62	—	—
Martin[450]	218 (op)	CpF (3)	81 (34)	S + R; R	21 (2)	22	60 (2)	65

Abbreviations: P, cisplatin; Cp, carboplatin; F, 5-flourouracil; M, methotrexate; L, leukovorin; B, bleomycin; O, vincristine; Vd, Videsine; Mc, mitomycin-C; R, radiotherapy; S, surgery; p, primary site; oc, oral cavity; op, oropharynx; tb, tongue base; lc, laryngeal cancer; ia, intra-arterial

[a] Published values or estimated from published data/survival curves
[b] Reduction in local-regional recurrence (P < .05) in chemotherapy arm
[c] Freedom from local-regional recurrence (53 v 35%, P = .06)
[d] Reduced distant metastasis rate in chemotherapy arm (P < .05)
[e] Low-dose cisplatin (50 mg/m²/cycle; distant metastases lower (49% v 28%, P = .07) in chemotherapy arm
[f] Disease-free survival favored control arm at 1 year (70 v 54%, P = .01)
[g] 3-arm study—2 chemotherapy arms combined for analysis

Table XXVII-1-34.   The Veterans Affairs Cooperative Studies Program Trial in Laryngeal Cancer: Patterns of Failure

Failure Site/Type	Surgery + Radiotherapy	Chemotherapy + Radiotherapy
Local recurrence	4	20
Regional recurrence	9	14
Distant metastasis	29	18
Second primary tumor	10	3
Total	52 (31%)	55 (33%)

From VACSP[327,710]

improves survival at the price of impaired speech, and up-front irradiation preserves the voice at the price of a decreased chance of survival. Survival remains low with strategies to combine radiotherapy and surgery because of high incidences of local-regional and distant recurrence.

Loss of natural speech, of course, is the chief forfeit of surgery for laryngeal cancer. Laryngectomy also can result in the need of a neck stoma (for breathing), an inability to smell or sneeze, a diminished sense of taste, and problems with swallowing. Cosmetic and psychological consequences can be great.

Although preservation of the voice long has been an important goal of the treatment of these patients, interest in the issue has heightened over recent years. A trend of decreasing use of radical surgery so as to preserve normal function and improve quality of life is developing in a variety of other solid tumor settings, as well. Two examples are limb preservation in osteosarcoma and breast preservation in breast cancer.

Based on promising pilot data[206,322,345,368] in 1985, the Veterans Affairs Cooperative Studies Program (VACSP) initiated a multi-institutional randomized prospective trial that attempted laryngeal preservation in previously untreated patients with locally advanced resectable laryngeal cancer (Figure XXVII-1-6). Patterns of treatment failure differed (Table XXVII-1-34). At a median follow-up of 43 months, an increased local-regional recurrence rate and a decreased distant metastasis rate occurred in the sequential chemoradiotherapy group in comparison to the surgery-radiotherapy group. The findings also indicated that delay of definitive local therapy in chemotherapy nonresponders was not detrimental. Chemotherapy responders and nonresponders in the experimental arm had about the same rate of survival. Estimated 3-year survival rates were similar (53% and 56%) in the two study arms, and laryngeal preservation was achieved in 66% of the chemotherapy recipients. Sequential chemoradiotherapy was least effective in advanced regional disease (N_2,N_3)—over 50% of this patient subgroup required salvage laryngectomy.[710]

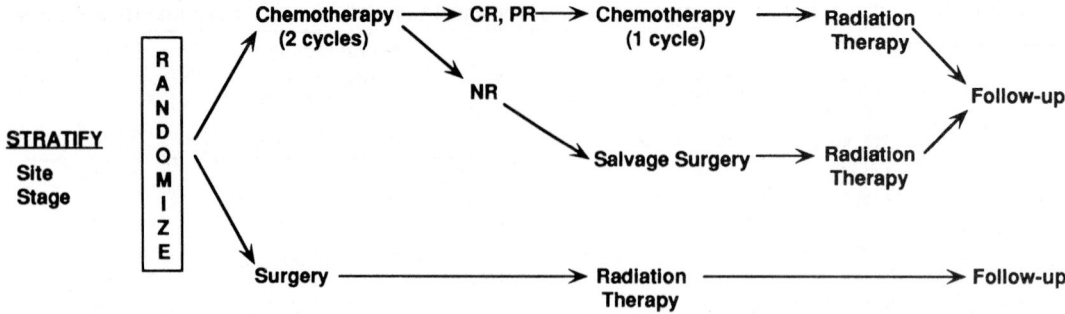

Figure XXVII-1-6.   Veterans Affair Laryngeal Cancer Study Group trial schema: induction chemotherapy plus radiation compared with surgery plus radiation in patients with advanced laryngeal cancer (see text).

These early results from the large VACSP trial indicate that sequential induction chemotherapy and definitive radiotherapy can be an effective strategy for achieving laryngeal preservation in a high percentage of patients without compromising overall survival. The trial's success argues strongly for adoption of this new treatment strategy in order to spare patients the functional, psychological and cosmetic deformities resulting from laryngectomy.

Future trials aimed at laryngeal preservation will need to establish chemotherapy regimens that achieve higher complete response rates, investigate innovative fractionated-radiation schemes and assess concomitant chemoradiation programs—approaches detailed elsewhere in this chapter. Expansion of this work to other HNSCC sites and to locally advanced regional and unresectable disease is in progress with promising early Phase III results.[167,322,368,450]

Promising new combinations are being tried to overcome the major disappointment of neoadjuvant chemotherapeutic approaches—i.e., despite achieving high response rates of 70–90% (20–50% complete) in advanced untreated patients, neoadjuvant chemotherapy has had no clear impact on patterns of failure (notably systemic recurrence) or survival.[326,517,587,663,679,685,697] Data suggest that neoadjuvant regimens capable of significantly improving survival must be able to produce reproducible complete response rates of over 50%.[109,685] So far, complete response rates in phase II trials have appeared to be inflated and always drop in phase III trials. Although developed most often in recurrent disease, promising new dose-intensive regimens are designed for later integration into primary chemotherapy. The following discussion includes trials of new combinations in both the recurrent-disease and neoadjuvant settings.

Preclinical data suggested a promising new line of work to potentiate 5-fluorouracil cytotoxicity—perhaps the most exciting and innovative chemotherapeutic area in HNSCC. Laboratory studies indicate that 5-fluorouracil resistance can be overcome by adding reduced folates (e.g., leucovorin) before 5-fluorouracil exposure due to enhanced stability of the active ternary complex with thymidylate synthetase. Although still in development, combining leucovorin with cisplatin and 5-fluorouracil (PFL regimen) already has produced the highest complete response rates reported in locally advanced HNSCC. This application of leucovorin must be distinguished from leucovorin rescue (reducing toxicity) in combination with high-dose methotrexate. Leucovorin significantly increases the toxicity of 5-fluorouracil while enhancing its activity.

Vokes and colleagues were among the first to test this concept clinically in HNSCC.[734,737] Using a variation of the PFL regimen in untreated advanced disease, investigators from the Dana-Farber Cancer Institute gave high-dose leucovorin (500 mg/m²/day for 6 days), cisplatin (25 mg/m²/day for 5 days), and 5-fluorouracil (800 mg/m²/day for 5 days) all by continuous infusion, starting the 5-fluorouracil 24 hours after the cisplatin and leucovorin.[191] Preclinical data suggested that prior exposure to cisplatin and leucovorin enhanced the cytotoxicity of 5-fluorouracil. The striking finding in this phase II study was an apparent shift in the degree of response. The 80% objective response rate is in line with cisplatin/5-fluorouracil and other cisplatin-based regimens; however, the overall clinical complete response rate was 66%, the highest complete response rate reported to date with any chemotherapy regimen in advanced HNSCC. The clinical complete response rate at the primary site was 77%, and 74% of these patients had a pathologic complete response. The clinical complete response in the regional (neck) nodes was 67% (83% in N_2 and 46% in N_3 disease). Toxicities were notable, including moderate-to-severe mucositis in 94% of patients, nausea and vomiting in 37% and diarrhea in 17%, necessitating dose reductions after the first cycle in 31% of patients. Rash developed in 26% and significant myelosuppression was uncommon (<10%). As with the cisplatin/5-fluorouracil regimen, three cycles were critical in PFL administration—the complete response rate jumped from 26% to 66% with the third cycle.

All the PFL data reveal an extremely promising portrait that remains to be established. The activity and toxicity are similar to those reported in a recent high-dose 5-fluorouracil study.[277] No randomized, controlled study of this regimen has been reported. Comparative studies of this regimen versus cisplatin or cisplatin/5-fluorouracil are needed.

Concomitant Chemoradiotherapy. This is the most promising primary chemotherapy approach to prolong survival of patients with locally advanced resectable and unresectable disease. It is the only systemic approach consistently shown to improve local-regional control and survival in randomized trials (*significant* improvements in disease-free survival in 11 trials and overall survival in six). Schedules of concomitant chemoradiotherapy can be *synchronous*, both modalities administered close together, or *alternating*, both administered in a non-overlapping fashion. Both of these schedules offer distinct therapeutic advantages over regimens of strictly sequential treatment.

Radiotherapy and chemotherapy given concomitantly is a dose-intensive approach that exploits the independent complementary activity of radiotherapy locally and chemotherapy distantly (spacial cooperation) and the potentially enhanced local activity (within the radiotherapy field).[239,738] Chemoradiotherapy approaches must attempt to incorporate full doses of both modalities. Suboptimal doses and/or schedules of either (e.g., low-dose cisplatin or split-course radiotherapy) will compromise dose-intensity and, ultimately, survival. Dose intensities possible with concomitant chemoradiotherapy are higher in 2–3 months than those allowed by sequential chemoradiotherapy given over twice the period of time. Even if no direct drug-radiation synergy occurs, concomitant therapy should produce additive effects and avoid critical delays of either therapy. Unfortunately, the concomitant approach incurs severe toxicity (primarily mucositis), which is difficult to balance effectively with desired activity.[687]

Concomitant single-agent chemoradiotherapy has been under investigation in head and neck cancer for the last three decades. Numerous phase II trials have reported encouraging but inconclusive results. All cytotoxic drugs with major activity in this disease have been studied.[239,687,738] Frequently, these have been administered in low doses during full course conventional radiotherapy. We will focus on the major findings from the phase III trials (Table XXVII-1-35).

Bleomycin, an active single agent and radiosensitizer, has been included in numerous single-arm trials. Eight randomized studies of this drug alone with concomitant radiotherapy have been published. Of the four trials with relatively large study cohorts (exceeding 100 patients)—two reported significant long-term survival improvements in the concomitant arm.[242,604] A key feature of one positive trial was the use of very-low-dose bleomycin, suggesting that the subtherapeutic dose of bleomycin enhanced radiosensitivity of the tumor.[242]

5-Fluorouracil, a radioenhancer in vitro[82] and active also in head and neck cancer, has been tested in 2 randomized trials. Both trials were positive (significant improvements in disease-free survival in 2, overall survival in 1). University of Wisconsin investigators reported the largest trial in patients with unresectable SCC of the oral cavity, oropharynx, and base of tongue.[19,269,430] The concomitant arm included radiotherapy with 5-fluorouracil administered by intravenous bolus 10 mg/kg/d for the first three days then 5 mg/kg/d three times during each treatment week. In this study, both local control and survival rates were significantly improved in the concomitant arm. The survival difference was greatest in the oral cavity subgroup.

Methotrexate, a drug that produces severe mucositis at full doses (especially combined with radiotherapy), has been evaluated in 2 randomized trials. The largest concomitant trial[286] gave only two doses (100 mg/m^2 on days 0 and 14 with leucovorin rescue in selected patients with elevated methotrexate serum levels) along with nonstandard radiotherapy (40–55 Gy radiotherapy in 15–16 fractions over 3 weeks). At a median follow-up of 32 months, relapse-free (p < .016) and overall survivals (p = .075) were better in the methotrexate arm. The improvements in local control

(p = 0.002) and survival (p = 0.009) were most striking in the oropharyngeal subset. The need for salvage surgery also was reduced in the methotrexate arm. Furthermore, toxicity was equivalent in the two treatment arms.

Hydroxyurea is a ribonucleotide reductase inhibitor with S phase-specific cytotoxicity[94,738] and single-agent activity in HNSCC (Table XXVII-1-27). Stefani and colleagues conducted the largest randomized placebo-controlled trial of concomitant hydroxyurea and radiotherapy and found no increase in response or survival with this combination. Toxicity and distant metastases were increased in the concomitant arm.

Mitomycin C, a bioreductive alkylating agent, is differentially metabolized, selectively toxic to hypoxic (radiotherapy-resistant) cells and produces little mucositis, which provides a favorable toxicity profile for chemoradiotherapy studies.[373] Weissberg and colleagues reported the only randomized comparison in HNSCC of radiotherapy alone versus radiotherapy plus mitomycin.[763] Mitomycin was given at a dose of 15 mg/m^2 on the fifth day of radiotherapy, and in some cases on a second occasion six weeks later. Despite limited single-agent activity in HNSCC, at a median follow-up exceeding five years, the actuarial disease-free (P = .07) and local-regional-disease-free (87% vs. 66%, P = .02) survivals were higher in patients treated with mitomycin.

Cisplatin is ideal for concomitant chemoradiotherapy in HNSCC. It has established single-agent activity and synergistic interaction in vitro and non-overlapping toxicities (no mucositis) in vivo with radiotherapy.[134,176] Cisplatin has recently received extensive clinical evaluation in concomitance with radiotherapy. Despite high complete local control rates from phase II trials (Table XXVII-1-36), study follow-ups are short and the impact on disease-free and overall survival is unclear. Only one phase III study of this approach has been completed.[304] This randomized study compared cisplatin (20 mg/m^2 weekly) during radiation to conventional radiotherapy in patients with inoperable HNSCC. Preliminary results indicate that concomitant therapy increased overall response but not complete response, disease-free or overall survival rates. Concomitant therapy's complete response rate of only 34% in this phase III trial stands in marked contrast to the 84% complete response rate achieved with the same dose and schedule in a pilot trial.[303]

The *optimal* dose, schedule and sequence of cisplatin with radiotherapy has undergone extensive evaluation.[134,188] Preclinical (in vitro and in vivo) and clinical chemoradiotherapy data suggest that cisplatin used predominantly as a cytotoxic agent (large and infrequent doses) is more active than cisplatin used predominantly as a radiosensitizer (small and frequent weekly or daily doses). The clinical data are more difficult to sort out—based on comparisons of dose and schedule from many uncontrolled single-institution trials of heterogeneous and small patient groups and multiple variables (doses, schedules and routes of cisplatin administration; differing schedules, fractionation programs and total doses of radiotherapy) (Table XXVII-1-36). The many dose-schedule clinical trials of cisplatin with irradiation suggest that cisplatin at 100 mg/m^2 on days 1, 22, and 43 of radiation treatment is most promising, mostly based on a large cooperative-group phase II trial with long-term follow-up.[443] Fifty-

Table XXVII-1-35.   Phase III Studies of Concomitant Single Agent Chemotherapy (CT) and Radiotherapy (RT) in Head and Neck Cancer

Drug Author	N	% Complete Response Rate		% Disease-Free Survival (yr)[a]		% Survival (yr)[a]	
		RT	RT + CT	RT	RT + CT	RT	RT + CT
Bleomycin							
Scandolaro[569]	30	43	50			50(2)	50
Kapstad[364,365]	29	14[b]	27[b]	64(2+)	87	—	—
Shanta[604]	157 (oc)	19	79*	17(5)	72*	24(5)	66*
Morita[484]	45 (t)	61 (or)	64	65(2)	73	—	—
Shetty[607]	38 (tb)	—	—	50(0.54)	50(0.29)	—	—
Vermund[721]	222	58	63	58(5)	53	42(5)	38
Fu[242]	104	45	67	26(5)	64*	14(5)	28
Eschwege[211]	199	69	65	—	—	22(6)	24
Parvinen[513]	46	35	38	—	—	38(5)	35
5-Fluorouracil							
Shigematsu[608]	63 (ia;ci;ma)	—	—	18(2)	40*	61(2)	68
Lo[19,269,430]	136 (oc,op,tb)	32	44	18(2)	49*	13(5)	32*,d
Methotrexate							
Condit[123]	40	60	45	—	—	—	—[e]
Gupta[286]	313	—	—	48(5)	60*	27(5)	42[f]
Hydroxyurea							
Richards[550,551]	40	20	65*	—	—	35(5)	50
Stefani[661]	126	47	42	31(2)	22	51(2)	29
Hussey[336]	40	56	67	38(2)	38	27(2)	30
Mitomycin C							
Weissberg[763]	117	—	—	49(5)	75[g]	40(5)	48
Cisplatin							
Haselow[304]	319	30	34[h]	—	—	—	—

Abbreviations: RT, radiotherapy; CT, chemotherapy; —, not available; ci, continuous infusion; ia, intra-arterial; oc, oral cavity; t, tongue; ma, maxillary antrum; op, oropharynx; tb, tongue base; or, overall response rate

* P < 0.05
[a] Published or estimated from data/survival curves
[b] Histologic CR
[c] Histologic CR increased in RT + CT (P < .05)
[d] Even greater significance in tonsil and intraoral
[e] Only 25 completed therapy and no survival data reported
[f] Overall survival (P = 0.075)—oropharyngeal (P < .002)
[g] P < .07
[h] Overall response greater in CT + RT (P < .05)

eight percent of the patients received adequate radiotherapy (>64.5 Gy) and the full 3 cycles of cisplatin. The complete response rate was 71% and the 3-year absolute survival was 43%—results superior to those in historical controls (radiotherapy only). Acute and chronic toxicities were acceptable.

The activity of intermittent standard or high-dose cisplatin regimens is further supported by evidence that it can salvage patients that fail to respond to induction therapy with cisplatin and infusion 5-fluorouracil.[205] Some recent single-arm work suggests that local control rates may be further improved with regional or higher-dose cisplatin and hyperfractionated or accelerated radiotherapy schedules. Randomized trials in HNSCC of this cisplatin dose and schedule are currently in progress.[118]

As a relatively new agent, carboplatin has not yet received adequate clinical evaluation in concomitance with radiotherapy.[134] Preliminary data limited to 3 phase I/II trials with differing doses and schedules of carboplatin and of radiotherapy in unresectable disease have produced complete responses in the range of 50–70%. These carboplatin trials included patients with more advanced primary and nodal stage disease[624] than many concomitant cisplatin trials.[443] Further study to establish optimal doses and schedules is needed.

The same RTOG concomitant cisplatin-radiotherapy regimen[443] has been tested in 27 locally advanced NPC patients (26 stage IV). The complete response rate was 89%; disease-free and overall survival rates were higher, and distant metastasis rates lower than those of historical controls (radiotherapy alone) from the RTOG data base.[11]

Pure radiosensitizer trials (i.e., drugs without independent activity in HNSCC) have been generally negative.[28,713] Misonidazole, the best-studied agent in this class, has achieved no improvement in survival in several randomized trials in a total of over 1,000 HNSCC patients.[713] A recent double-blind, randomized Italian study of lonidamine with or without hyperfractionated radiotherapy reported improvements in complete response, response duration and local control.[439] The estimated 2-year disease-free survival was 51% in the lonidamine arm vs. 25% without the drug.

Concomitant multi-agent chemoradiotherapy began as a result of positive studies with concomitant single-agent che-

Table XXVII-1-36. Synchronous Single-Agent Platinum Chemo-Radiotherapy Trials

Author	Dose (mg/m²) and Schedule	Radiotherapy	N	Response (Complete %)
Cisplatin				
Haselow[303]	10–30 (weekly)	Conventional	32	27 (84)
Bloom[56]	20 (5 d every 3 wk)	Conventional	34	18 (53)
Miller[473]	80 (d 1,23,43)	Conventional	22	10 (45)
Slotman[629]	20 (d 1–4, 21–24)	Conventioal	18	13 (72)
Snyderman[634]	15 (d 1–5, 21–25)	Conventional	29	9 (31)
Crispino[140] b	20 (weekly)	Conventional	19	10 (53)
Tobias[698]	10c × 6 weeks	Conventional	16	9 (56)
Chang[97]	20 (d 1–4) × 3 cycles	Conventional	22	18 (82)
Choi[103]	5–7 CI (2–3 wk) × 2 courses	Conventional/ Hyperfraction	23	16 (70)
Cognetti[118]	100 (d 1,21,43)	Conventional	30d	13d(44)
Wheeler[771]	40 (5 d every 4–5 wk) × 3 cycles	Conventional	18	17 (94)
Gasparini[250]	80 (d 1,21,42)	Conventional	18	11 (61)
Al-Sarraf[11]	100 (d 1,21,42)	Conventional	27 (npc)	24 (89)
Fontanesi[230]	100 (d 1,22,42)	Hyperfraction	20	16 (80)
Harrison[295]	100 (d 1 22)	Conventional/ Hyperfraction	22	14 (64)
Haselow[304]	20 (weekly)	Conventional	159	54 (34)
Marcial[443]	100 (d 1,21,42)	Conventional	124	88 (71)
Shankar[603]	100 (d 1,28,56)	Accelerated	19	14 (68)
Carboplatin				
Sinibaldi[624]	60–100 weekly	Conventional	29	15 (52)
Schnabel[580]	70 (d 1–5, 29–33)	Conventional	54	36 (67)
Volling[738]	20–60 (4 d wk 1,2,5; 2 d/wk 6)	Accelerated	23	13 (57)
Total			500	346 (69%)

Abbreviations: d, day; wk, week; CI, continuous infusion; npc, nasopharyngeal carcinoma

a From randomized trial

b Split-course radiotherapy

c Total dose per day

d Percentage accurate; numbers estimated from abstract

motherapy and radiotherapy. The primary goal of these combined-agent trials was to reduce distant failures, which seem to be resistant to single-agent chemoradiotherapy therapy; the secondary goal is to further enhance already excellent local control rates with concomitant approaches. Due to acute toxicity (mucositis), many trials used split-course radiotherapy—a period (or cycle) or concurrent chemoradiotherapy is followed by a planned interruption in all therapy to allow time for normal tissue recovery. Much of this work has been done in phase I/II feasibility trials designed to sort out issues of maximized dose-intensity and minimized normal tissue toxicity. A popular variant of, or hybrid between, synchronous and sequential combined-agent-chemoradiotherapy is the *alternating* approach.[505,725] Its rationale comes in part from preclinical in vivo work (murine model) indicating that the approach reduces normal-tissue toxicity and therefore represents a compromise between synchronous and sequential chemoradiotherapy.

A distinct advantage of single-agent over combined-agent concomitant trials is the simplicity of study design and more effective (continuous, uninterrupted) conventional or hyperfractionated radiotherapy. The split-course radiotherapy necessary with combined agents is inferior to uninterrupted radiotherapy. The rationale for pursuing combined-agent trials is based on the assumption that combined agents are better than single agents—an assumption that has not been proven in HNSCC. Survival rates with single-agent cisplatin are equivalent to any combination chemotherapy. Combined modality approaches requiring reduced dose intensities of cisplatin may produce results inferior to cisplatin alone at high doses.

Cisplatin-based concomitant multiagent regimens have been studied in several recent phase II trials. An increasing trend toward employing combinations of cisplatin and 5-fluorouracil with conventional or hyperfractionated split-course radiotherapy has been reported.[3,132,133,375,469,686,687,690] Preclinical studies have demonstrated synergistic interactions between any two of these three treatments. Doses and schedules of cisplatin, 5-fluorouracil, and radiotherapy have varied considerably. The modulation of 5-fluorouracil by leucovorin and hydroxyurea as part of concomitant chemoradiotherapy regimens is under study.[297,736,765,766]

Taylor and colleagues administered a regimen of concomitant cisplatin (60 mg/m²) and 5-fluorouracil (800 mg/m² × 5 days) with conventionally fractionated (total 70 Gy) radiation given every other week for 7 cycles.[687,690] Results from 53 unresectable patients indicate a high rate of clinical complete (55%) and partial (43%) responses, and a median failure-free survival of 51 months (range 12–83). The overall median survival was 37 months. Further, survival of patients with a partial response to therapy was remarkably high and not significantly different from that of patients achieving a complete response.

However promising they may be, studies of concomitant cisplatin, 5-fluorouracil (with or without modulators of 5-fluorouracil) and radiotherapy must be interpreted with caution in light of their radical designs and markedly increased normal-tissue toxicity. One study of alternating cisplatin/5-fluorouracil and hyperfractionated radiotherapy was terminated early because of excessive toxicity.[132] Moreover, potential therapeutic gains with the concomitant regimen may be compromised by a significant decrease in the dose intensity of radiotherapy. Despite these potential drawbacks, the preliminary experience with concomitant cisplatin, 5-fluorouracil and radiotherapy is promising and deserves future comparisons to conventional and hyperfractionated radiotherapy. These innovative concomitant approaches await confirmation of efficacy in randomized trials.

Randomized trials have compared concomitant chemoradiotherapy with either radiotherapy alone (five trials) or sequential (neoadjuvant) chemoradiotherapy (five trials).[4,5,48,117,118,133,374,375,469,470,639,686,697] Although the work is still ongoing, preliminary data favor the concomitant approach. In the trials of concomitant treatment versus radiotherapy alone,[48,374,375,469,697] early results in unresectable disease suggest improved complete response,[469] disease-free survival,[48,697] and survival.[48] Five randomized studies are designed to compare concomitant chemoradiotherapy to neoadjuvant, or sequential, chemoradiotherapy.[5,118,133,470,639,686] Concomitant therapy produced significantly increased disease-free survival in 3 trials[4,5,133,470,639] and overall survival in 1.[133]

Adjuvant. Adjuvant (maintenance) chemotherapy to eradicate micrometastases following local therapy (adjuvant therapy in the strict sense) has not been studied extensively in HNSCC. The principal objectives of adjuvant trials have been to control subclinical persistent disease after surgery or radiotherapy and to decrease the rates of local-regional and distant relapse. The ideal study design would include: enrollment of (high-risk) patients with resectable advanced disease; *early* administration after local therapy to avoid drug resistance; and an effective regimen. Although no study has met all these criteria, promising leads for future studies have emerged.

Six randomized studies have evaluated the impact of adjuvant multiagent chemotherapy with no clear survival impact: significant differences occurred in two trials (Table XXVII-1-37), one small positive trial[52] and one large negative trial of delayed adjuvant therapy.[185]

Neoadjuvant (or Concomitant) Plus Adjuvant Chemotherapy. This is perhaps the most important primary-therapy study design (Table XXVII-1-38). The largest of these is an NCI-sponsored multi-institutional trial, begun in 1978, called the Head and Neck Contracts Program.[306,347] Over 400 patients with resectable stage III or IV disease were randomized to: 1) induction chemotherapy (one cycle of cisplatin and bleomycin) followed by standard therapy (surgery *and* radiotherapy in all study arms); or 2) induction chemotherapy followed by standard therapy followed by six cycles of adjuvant monthly cisplatin (80 mg/m²) by 24-hour continuous infusion; or 3) standard therapy only. At a median follow-up of more than 5 years, the disease-free and overall survivals were not significantly different among the three arms. This study has been criticized because of its one cycle of induction chemotherapy, considered suboptimal (3% complete response, 34% objective response), and a striking noncompliance rate in the adjuvant-therapy arm (47% never received any maintenance therapy). Subset analyses of this study suggested improved disease-free and/or overall survival in 3 subgroups: oral cavity, T_{1-2} primary lesions, and N_{1-2} regional disease.[347]

An important aspect of the planned design of one study, the administration of adjuvant therapy to only those who responded to the chemotherapy, reported a definite disease-free survival improvement in the adjuvant arm.[210] These promising results are not definitive in light of the extremely small sample sizes, but they do justify future large-scale study of this strategy.

Table XXVII-1-37. Randomized Trials of Adjuvant Chemotherapy for Head and Neck Cancer

Author	N	Adjuvant Chemotherapy	% Disease-Free Survival (yr)[a]		% Survival (yr)[a]	
			Control	Chemotherapy	Control	Chemotherapy
Szpirglas[675]	95 (at,fom)	M1B (3-arm)	47 (2)	52	58 (4)	58
Bitter[52]	33 (oc)	MBO	24 (3)	68[b]	29 (3)	65[b]
Huang[332,333]	126	MBVL	58 (—)	72[c]	—	—
Rossi[561]	229 (npc)	ODC	56 (4)	58	67 (4)	59
Domenge[185]	287 (ecs)	PBM	— (3)	—	— (3)[d]	—
Intergroup[12e]	448	PF	—[f]	—	—[f]	—

Abbreviations: at, anterior tongue; fom, floor of mouth; oc, oral cavity; npc, nasopharyngeal carcinoma; ecs, extracapsular spread; LF, 5-Flourouracil; M, methotrexate; B, bleomycin; O, vincristine; V, vinblastine; L, lomustine; D, doxorubicin; C, cyclophosphamide; P, cisplatin; I, leucovorin; —, not available.

[a] published values or estimated from published data/survival curves

[b] statistically significant

[c] significant ony for patients receiving more than 2 cycles

[d] statistically significant favoring control

[e] significant reduction in incidence of distant metastasis in chemotherapy arm (P = 0.05)

[f] no significant differences in median disease-free or overall survival rates

Table XXVII-1-38. **Randomized Trials of Induction Plus Adjuvant Chemotherapy for Head and Neck Cancer**

Author	N	Induction (Schedule)	% Response (Complete)	Local Therapy	Adjuvant (Cycles)	% Disease-Free Survival (yr)[a]		% Survival (yr)[a]	
						Control	Chemotherapy	Control	Chemotherapy
Tejada[692]	82	PM (—)	66 (4)	S ± R	PM (—)	576[b]	530[b]		
Stell[625,662]	86	BOFML CMp (2 cycles)	—	R	BOFML/CMp (12 cycles)	—	—	18 (8)	16
Taylor[688]	82	M (d 1,5,9)	40 (6)	S ± R	M (1 yr) or PD (4 cycles)	37 (3)	50	41 (3)	41
Kun[397,702]	83	BCMF (2 cycles)	67 (5)	S + R; R	BCMF[c] (2 cycles)	64 (2)	59[d]	43 (2)	31
Ervin[210]	114	PBML (2 cycles)	78 (26)	S + R; R	PBM (3 cycles)	61 (2)	84[e]	—	—
HNCP[306]	462 (see text)	PB (1 cycle)	37 (3)	S + R	P (6 cycles)	55 (5)	49-I 64-Ad	35 (5)	37-I 45-Ad
Rentschler[546]	60	M (4 doses)	73 (5)—p 60 (7)—r	S + R	M (12 weekly)	59 (3)	66	55 (3)	55

Abbreviations: M, methotrexate; P, cisplatin; d, doxorubicin; C, cyclophosphamide; F, fluorouracil; O, vicristine (oncovin); V, vinblastine; Mp, 6-mercaptopurine; L, leucovorin; Vds, vindesine; MMC, mitomycin-C; A, cytosine arabinoside (ara-C), S, surgery; R, radiotherapy; I, induction only; Ad, adjuvant; p, primary site; r, regional disease
[a] Published values or estimated from published data/survival curves
[b] Mean disease-free survival in days
[c] Adjuvant therapy stopped early in trial because of non-compliance
[d] Local-regional free survival significantly different P < .02
[e] Only 46 patients randomized to the adjuvant trial—benefit greatest for partial responders (P = 0.14 overall)

Summary and Future Directions. Advanced local disease is the focus of primary chemotherapy investigation in HNSCC. Advanced local HNSCC is not controlled adequately by standard surgery and/or radiotherapy alone: two-year disease-free survival after standard therapy is less than 40%. Preclinical work strongly supports the early integration of chemotherapy into the primary management of advanced HNSCC.[94,571]

Primary chemotherapy in HNSCC falls into three main treatment categories: 1) *neoadjuvant chemotherapy,* designed to reduce tumor burden prior to definitive local control; 2) *concomitant chemoradiotherapy,* designed to be a third definitive treatment (in addition to surgery and radiotherapy) for controlling advanced local HNSCC; and 3) *adjuvant chemotherapy,* designed to maintain, or prevent recurrence in, patients after definitive local control.

Major goals of the first treatment category, neoadjuvant chemotherapy, are to prolong disease-free and overall survivals and to improve quality of life for surviving patients by providing effective organ-preservation approaches for the control of advanced HNSCC. Data from the numerous phase I and II neoadjuvant studies reveal many positive features of this approach—multiagent response rates of 70–90% (complete in 20–50%) with 30–70% of clinical complete responders having complete pathologic tumor regression in biopsies or surgical specimens. Initial tumor stage or extent—whether defined by overall stage, T stage, N stage or resectability—is predictive of response to chemotherapy and survival. Response to chemotherapy is predictive of response to radiotherapy. Further, chemotherapy responders have a better prognosis than do nonresponders,[119,517,644] but whether this is a benefit of chemotherapy or a result of unknown factors in the responding subset of patients is not clear.[679,685]

Local-regional control is adequate with surgery or radiotherapy alone in selected patients who respond completely to induction. Induction chemotherapy does not significantly increase the toxicity of subsequent radiotherapy, surgery or chemotherapy.[533] Major concerns with the neoadjuvant approach are the possibilities of delaying and compromising definitive local therapy and the risk that responding patients may refuse definitive local therapy. Furthermore, neoadjuvant chemotherapy definitely prolongs the treatment course, is expensive and compromises later palliative chemotherapy in recurring patients. Of the nearly 30 phase III trials incorporating neoadjuvant chemotherapy, only one (using single-agent regional chemotherapy), reported significantly improved survival over that of patients receiving standard local therapy.[20] These trials were flawed in many aspects, including study size, heterogeneous patient populations/disease sites/local therapies and ineffective chemotherapy (median CR rate 10% in multiagent trials).

One randomized neoadjuvant trial, the VACSP did have a large sample size, a relatively homogeneous patient population (advanced operable laryngeal cancer patients) and a relatively effective regimen of chemotherapy (cisplatin and infusion 5-fluorouracil at full doses). Although this trial produced a respectable complete response rate it did not increase survival. Still, neoadjuvant chemotherapy could not be evaluated as an independent variable because the local-regional treatments in the two study arms were not identical. Even so, this study achieved the positive results of laryngeal preservation in over 60% of patients and a significant decrease in distant relapse rate in the neoadjuvant arm.

Phase I and II trials must continue to translate the preclinical study data into trials of new, more active regimens. Regimens deserving further study include combined cisplatin/5-fluorouracil/leucovorin and other combinations with agents such as IFN-α and hydroxyurea that enhance 5-fluorouracil cytotoxicity. Neoadjuvant trials also should investigate the issue of optimal numbers of chemotherapy cycles on response (clinical/histologic) and on survival.[109] Future work should study the integration of biologic response modifiers, differentiation agents, other cytotoxic drugs (e.g., ifosfamide) and irradiation into primary therapy.

The second major category of primary chemotherapy is that of regimens designed to achieve definitive local and distant control. So far, concomitant chemoradiotherapy is the only approach in this category that has shown potential by increasing survival in randomized testing. This survival benefit has appeared in trials in both resectable and unresectable HNSCC. Although early trials have used suboptimal intensities, concomitant chemoradiotherapy is designed ultimately to maximize dose intensities of both treatment modalities. All the positive single-agent concomitant trials used suboptimal doses of active drugs (e.g., bleomycin and methotrexate) and full doses of relatively inactive drugs (e.g., mitomycin C). This indicates that chemotherapy enhances radiotherapy. Recent data from numerous phase II trials now support the promise of concomitant cisplatin/radiotherapy. The lack of overlapping toxicities allows optimal administration of both modalities. Randomized trials are required, however.

Concomitant multiagent chemoradiotherapy (which includes synchronous therapy with split-course radiotherapy and alternating chemoradiotherapy) greatly increases acute toxicity and so requires creative study designs to make this approach feasible. The major problem with multiagent regimens is the need to lower radiotherapy's dose intensity, which compromises local control rates. "Aggressive" multiagent chemoradiotherapy programs paradoxically may ultimately be of decreased rather than increased dose intensity. Nevertheless, early results from all ten randomized trials are encouraging, with survival favoring the experimental (concomitant) arm. Five trials had no standard local therapy only arms. These studies have been criticized for comparing only two experimental arms. Although faulty, this study design has a silver lining—it has provided the best support for concomitant chemoradiotherapy.[5,133,470,639] Before accepting concomitant chemoradiotherapy as standard, the results of these and other planned randomized trials (especially those with standard-therapy arms) will need to mature with more patients, longer follow-ups and careful assessments of toxicity and quality of life.

Concomitant therapy does not appear to significantly increase surgical complications[692] and clearly it has altered the natural history of locally advanced unresectable HNSCC. It has produced lower local-regional failure rates, which suggests that a direct chemotherapy-radiotherapy interaction occurs at primary sites. The lack of impact on distant relapse rates, however, suggests that concomitant chemoradiotherapy should be followed by adjuvant therapy, and support for this approach comes from randomized trials.[242,501,663]

No survival benefit is evident in trials of adjuvant chemotherapy, the third major treatment category. The adjuvant approach in HNSCC has not been adequately tested, however. Regimens, cycle number and timing may not have been

optimal, study size and stratification (by site and stage, for example) have not been adequate to allow for this disease's heterogeneity, post-operative delays in initiating adjuvant therapy have compromised results, and toxicity and noncompliance rates have been uniformly high. In the HNCP study, nearly 50% of the patients randomized to adjuvant therapy did not receive any chemotherapy after surgery, and only 8% of all the patients in the adjuvant arm completed the full six cycles.[306] Still, this series produced a significant reduction in distant relapse rate, notwithstanding the inclusion of all the many untreated patients in the analysis of this effect. This result underscores the potential value of adjuvant chemotherapy.

The collective data suggest that adjuvant chemotherapy may be useful in the management of selected head and neck cancer patients: those with disease in specific primary sites (e.g., the oral cavity), those with small-volume disease, and those with response who retain a high risk of relapse (Tables XXVII-1-37 and XXVII-1-38). The data indicate further that trials should incorporate active regimens of chemotherapy in the immediate postoperative period, either before or concomitant with radiotherapy. It also seems evident that large-scale studies designed to detect modest but clinically important survival differences will be required to test the role of adjuvant chemotherapy in HNSCC.

Timing of therapy may be crucial. A novel strategy to circumvent the toxicity of adjuvant chemotherapy given after radiotherapy is adjuvant chemotherapy sandwiched between standard local therapies.[104,109] This interposition of chemotherapy between surgery and radiotherapy is a carefully conceived strategy.[12,349] Initiating chemotherapy *after* surgery means that tumor margins are not obscured by prior chemotherapy responses (nor in this protocol are they obscured by responses to prior radiotherapy). It eliminates the problem of patients who refuse surgery because they have responded to chemotherapy, and it allows chemotherapy to attempt its effect in an already debulked tumor. Drug delivery before radiotherapy is through an intact vascular supply. Furthermore, this approach avoids the expected toxicity of postirradiation chemotherapy.

Ultimately, the optimum control of advanced HNSCC certainly will require primary chemotherapy in all three of its strategic roles, i.e., as neoadjuvant, primary curative and adjuvant therapy. Meta-analysis, or analysis of pooled data from all randomized trials, reveals that primary chemotherapy has produced a significant reduction in local-regional failure.[663] This effect is most pronounced with concomitant chemoradiotherapy.[20,286,430]

Unfortunately, the greatest hope for primary chemotherapy—that it would eradicate systemic disease—has not been fulfilled. This is so even though elegant mathematical and preclinical models support the early use of chemotherapy to eradicate micrometastases and, thus, prevent distant relapse. Heterogeneous cancer cell populations and relatively low growth fractions may be the major hurdles to developing effective chemotherapy for this disease. Significant decreases[12,109,306,327,676,710] and increases[15,661,663,679,721] in distant relapse rates have been reported from the more than 50 phase III trials incorporating primary chemotherapy (Tables XXVII-1-32, -33, -35, -37 and -38). All types of analyses, including meta-analysis of the 50+ trials, indicate that neither single-agent nor multiagent regimens have consistently diminished distant relapse rates.

Although overall results show no improvement, three recent trials were well-designed, large-scale, cooperative group trials that achieved significantly reduced distant relapse rates.[12,306,327,710] Through their large patient bases, these trials were able to show statistically significant, small improvements and therefore suggest that currently available platinum-based chemotherapy may have clinically important, albeit modest, activity in micrometastatic disease. Future work should build on these findings and must continue to search for more effective programs in the systemic control of advanced HNSCC.

References

1. Abele, R., Clavel, M., Rossi, A., Bruntsch, U., and Pinedo, H. M.: Iproplatin (CHIP, JM-9) in advanced squamous cell carcinoma of the head and neck: A phase II study of the EORTC early clinical trials group. (Abstract #575) Proc. Am. Soc. Clin. Oncol., 5:147, 1986.
2. Abele, R., Honegger, H. P., Grossenbacher, R., Mermillod, B., Kaplan, E., Gervasi, A., Wolfensbeager, M., Lehmann, W., and Cavalli, F.: A randomized study of methotrexate, bleomycin, hydroxyurea with versus without ciplatin in patients with previously untreated and recurrent squamous cell carcinoma of the head and neck. Eur. J. Cancer Clin. Oncol., 23:47, 1987.
3. Adelstein, D. J., Sharan, V. M., Earle, A. S., Shah, A. C., Vlastou, C., Haria, C. D., Carter, S. G., Damm, C., and Hines, J. D.: Simultaneous radiotherapy and chemotherapy with 5-fluorouracil and cisplatin for locally confined squamous cell head and neck cancer. N.C.I. Monogr., 6:347, 1988.
4. Adelstein, D. J., Sharan, V. M., Earle, A. S., Shah, A. C., Vlastou, C., Haria, C. D., Damm, C., Carter, S. G., and Hines, J. D.: A prospective randomized trial of simultaneous (SIM) vs. sequential (SEQ) chemoradiotherapy (CRT) for squamous cell head and neck cancer (SCHNC). (Abstract #648) Proc. Am. Soc. Clin. Oncol., 8:167, 1989.
5. Adelstein, D. J., Sharan, V. M., Earle, A. S., Shah, A. C., Vlastou, C., Haria, C. D., Damm, D., Carter, S. G., and Hines, J. D.: Simultaneous versus sequential combined technique therapy for squamous cell head and neck cancer. Cancer, 65:1685, 1990.
6. Alberts, D. S., Manning, M. R., Coulthard, S. W., Koopmann, C. F., Jr., and Herman, T. S.: Adriamycin/cis-platinum/cyclophosphamide combination chemotherapy for advanced carcinoma of the parotid gland. Cancer, 47:645, 1981.
7. Al-Kourainy, K., Kish, J., Ensley, J., Tapazoglou, E., Jacobs, J., Weaver, A., Crissman, J., Cunnings, G., and Al-Sarraf, M.: Achievement of superior survival for histologically negative versus histologically positive clinically complete responders to cisplatin combination in patients with locally advanced head and neck cancer. Cancer, 59:233, 1987.
8. Al-Sarraf, M.: Chemotherapeutic management of head and neck cancer. Cancer and Metastasis Rev., 6:181, 1987.
9. Al-Sarraf, M.: Clinical trials with fluorinated pyrimidines in patients with head and neck cancer. Invest. New Drugs, 7:71, 1989.
10. Al-Sarraf, M., Metch, B., Kish, J., Ensley, J., Rinehart, J. J., Schuller, D. E., and Coltman, C. A., Jr.: Platinum analogs in recurrent and advanced head and neck cancer: A Southwest Oncology Group and Wayne State University Study. Cancer Treat. Rep., 71:723, 1987.
11. Al-Sarraf, M., Pajak, T. F., Cooper, J. S., Mohiuddin, M., Herskovic, A., and Ager, P. J.: Chemo-radiotherapy in patients with locally advanced nasopharyngeal carinoma: a radiation therapy oncology group study. J. Clin. Oncol., 8:1342, 1990.
12. Al-Sarraf, M., Scott, C. B., Ahmad, R., Schwade, J. G., Schuller, D., Laramore, G. E., and Jacobs, J.: Phase III study comparing sequential chemotherapy (CT) and radiotherapy (RT) to RT for Resected and Negative Margins Squamous Cell Carcinoma of the Head & Neck: Intergroup study #0034. Proc. Am. Soc. Clin. Oncol., 11:1992.
13. Al-Sarraf, M., Tapazoglou, F., Ensley, J. F., Ahmad, K., Jacobs, J. R., Suchowski, C., and Kish, J. A.: Significant loco-regional control of advanced head and neck cancer (HN-CA) with concurrent cisplatin and radiotherapy (RT) after initial response to induction chemotherapy (CT). (Abstract #670) Proc. Am. Soc. Clin. Oncol., 9:173, 1990.
14. Amendola, B. E., Eisert, D., Hazra T. A., and King, E. R.: Carcinoma of the maxillary antrum: Surgery or radiation therapy? Int. J. Radiat. Oncol. Biol. Phys., 7:743, 1981.
15. Amiel, J. L., Sancho-Garnier, H., Vandenbrouck, C., Eschwege, F., Droz, J. P., Schwaab, G., Wibault, P., Stromboni, M., and Rey, A.: First results of a randomized trial on immunotherapy of head and neck tumors. Recent Results. Cancer Res., 68:318, 1978.
16. Amornarn, R., Prempre, T., Jaiwatana, J., and Wixwnberg, M. J.: Radiation management of carcinoma of the tonsillar region. Cancer, 54:1293, 1984.
17. Amrein, P. C.: Cisplatin and 5-fluorouracil vs. the same plus bleomycin and methotrexate in recurrent squamous cell carcinoma of the head and neck (SCC H+N). (Abstract #676) Proc. Am. Soc. Clin. Oncol., 9:175, 1990.
18. Amrein, P. C., Fingert, H., and Weitzman, S. A.: Cisplatin-vincristine-bleomycin therapy in squamous cell carcinoma of the head and neck. J. Clin. Oncol., 1:421, 1983.
19. Ansfield, F. J., Ramirez, G., Davis, H. L., Jr., Korbitz, B. C., Vermund, H., and Gollin, F. F.: Treatment of advanced cancer of the head and neck. Cancer, 25:78, 1970.
20. Arcangeli, G., Nervi, C., Righini, R., Creton, G., Mirri, M. A., and Guerra, A.: Combined radiation and drugs: the effect of intra-arterial chemotherapy followed by radiotherapy in head and neck cancer. Radiother. Oncol., 1:101, 1983.
21. Atichartakarn, V., Kraiphibul, P., Clongsusuek, P., Pochanugool, L., Kulapaditharom, B., and Ratantharathorn, V.: Nasopharyngeal carcinoma: Result of treatment with cis-diamminedichloroplatinum II, 5 fluorouracil, and radiation therapy. Int. J. Radiat. Oncol. Biol. Phys., 14:461, 1988.
22. Bachouchi, M., Cvitkovic, E., Azli, N., Gasmi, J., Cortes-Funes, H., Boussen, H., Rahal, M., Kalifa, C., Schwaab, G., and Eschwege, F.: High complete response in advanced nasopharyngeal carcinoma with bleomycin, epirubicin, and cisplatin before radiotherapy. J. Natl. Cancer Inst., 82:616, 1990.
23. Baden, E.: Prevention of cancer of the oral cavity and pharynx. CA, 37:49, 1987.
24. Bailey, B. J.: Management of carcinoma of the lip. Laryngoscope, 87:250, 1977.
25. Baker, S. R., and Krause, C. J.: Carcinoma of the lip. Laryngoscope, 90:19, 1980.
26. Baker, S. R., and Sullivan M. J.: Osteocutaneous free scapular flap for one-stage mandibular reconstruction. Arch. Otolaryngol., 114:267, 1988.
27. Baker, S. R., and Wheeler, R. H.: Intraarterial chemotherapy for head and neck cancer, Part I: Theoretical considerations and drug delivery systems. Head Neck Surg., 6:664, 1983.
28. Bakowski, M. T., MacDonald, E., Mould, R. F., Cawte, P., Sloggem, J., Barrett, A., Dalley, V., Newton, K. A., Westbury, G., James, S. E., and Hellman, K.: Double blind controlled clinical trial of radiation plus razoxane (ICRF 159) versus radiation plus placebo in the treatment of head and neck cancer. Int. J. Radiat. Oncol. Biol. Phys., 4:115, 1978.
29. Ballantyne, A. J.: Methods of repair after surgery for cancer of the pharyngeal wall, postcricoid area and cervical esophagus. Am. J. Surg., 122:482, 1971.
30. Bamberg, M., Schulz, U., and Scherer, E.: Postoperative split course radiotherapy of squamous cell carcinoma of the oral tongue. Int. J. Radiat. Oncol. Biol. Phys., 5:515, 1979.
31. Barnes, L., and Kanbour, A.: Malignant fibrous histiocytoma of the head and neck. Arch. Otolaryngol. Head Neck Surg., 114:1149, 1988.
32. Barrs, D. M., DeSanto, L. W., and O'Fallon, W. M.: Squamous cell carcinoma at the tonsil and tongue-base regions. Arch. Otolaryngol., 105:479, 1979.
33. Barton, R. T., and Hogetveit, A. C.: Nickel-related cancers of the respiratory tract. Cancer, 45:3061, 1980.
34. Bataini, P., Bernier, J., Jaulerry, C., Brunin, F., and Pontvert, D.: Impact of cervical disease and its definitive radiotherapeutic management on survival: Experience in 2013 patients with squamous cell carcinoma of the oropharynx and pharyngolarynx. Laryngoscope, 100:716, 1990.
35. Bataini, P., Brugere, J., Bernier, J., Jaulerry, C. H., Picot, C., and Ghossein, N. A.: Results of radical radiotherapeutic treatment of carcinoma of the pyriform sinus: Experience of the Institute Curie. Int. J. Rad. Oncol. Biol. Phys., 8:1277, 1982.
36. Batsakis, J. G.: Tumors of the head and neck. *In* Clinical and Pathological Considerations. Edited by Batsakis, J. G. Baltimore, Williams & Wilkins, 1974.
37. Baugh, R. F., Wolf, G. T., and McClatchey, K. D.: Small cell carcinoma of the head and neck. Head Neck Surg., 8:343, 1986.
38. Beatty, J. D., Terz, J. J., Brown, P. W., Lawrence, W., Jr., Schuller, G. B., and Kaplan, A. M.: Adjuvant intralesional and systemic Corynebacterium parvum immunotherapy for surgically treated head and neck cancer. Surg. Forum, 29:155, 1978.
39. Bedwinek, J. M., Shukovsky, L. J., Fletcher, G. H., and Daly, T. E.: Osteonecrosis in patients treated with definitive radiotherapy for squamous cell carcinomas of the oral cavity and naso- and oropharynx. Radiology, 119:665, 1976.
40. Belsky, J. L., Tachikawa, C., Cihak, R. W., and Yamamoto, T.: Salivary gland tumors in the atomic bomb survivors. Hiroshima-Nagasaki, 1957 to 1970. JAMA, 219:864, 1972.
41. Bendich, A.: The safety of beta-carotene. Nutr. Cancer, 11:207, 1988.
42. Benninger, M. S., Roberts, J. K., Levine, H. L., Wood, B. G., and Tucker, H. M.: Squamous cell carcinoma of the head and neck in patients 40 years of age and younger. Laryngoscope, 98:531, 1988.
43. Berenson, J. R., Yang, J., Koga, H., Slamon, D., and Mickel, R. A.: Bcl-1 and Int-2 coamplification in squamous cell carcinomas of the head and neck and lung. (Abstract #1749) Proc. Am. Asoc. Cancer Res., 30:440, 1989.
44. Bernstein, J. I., Jacobs, C., Meyers, F., Rich-Goffinet, L., and Tanakal, L.: A phase II study of cisplatin and cytosine arabinoside for recurrent squamous cell carcinoma of the head and neck. Am. J. Clin. Oncol., 9:58, 1986.
45. Berry, M., Jacobs, C., Sikic, B., Halsey, J., and Borch, R. F.: Modification of cisplatin toxicity with diethyldithiocarbamate. J. Clin. Oncol., 8:1585, 1990.
46. Bertino, J. R., Boston, B., and Capizzi, R. L.: The role of chemotherapy in the management of cancer of the head and neck: a review. Cancer, 36:752, 1975.
47. Bertram, J. S., Kolonel, L. N., and Meyskens, F. L., Jr.: Rationale and strategies for chemoprevention of cancer in humans. Cancer Res., 47:3012, 1987.
48. Bezwoda, W. R., de Moor, N. G., and Deman, D. P.: Treatment of advanced head and neck cancer by means of radiation therapy plus chemotherapy: a randomized trial. Med. Pediatr. Oncol., 6:353, 1979.
49. Bijman, J. T., Wagener, D., van Rennes, H., Wessels, J. M., and van den Brock, P.: Flow cytometric evaluation of cell dispersion from human head and neck tumors. Cytometry, 6:334, 1985.
50. Biller, H. F., and Lawson, W.: Partial laryngectomy for vocal cord cancer with marked limitations or fixation of the vocal cord. Laryngoscope, 96:61, 1986.
51. Biller, H. F., Lawson, W., and Baek, S. M.: Total glossectomy. A technique of reconstruction eliminating laryngectomy. Arch. Otolaryngol., 109:69, 1983.
52. Bitter, K.: Postoperative chemotherapy versus postoperative cobalt 60 radiation in patients with advanced oral carcinoma: Report on a randomized study (abst). Head Neck Surg., 3:264, 1981.
53. Bjorkland, A., and Eneroth, C. M.: Management of parotid gland neoplasms. Am. J. Otolaryngol., 1:155, 1980.
54. Blacklock, J. B., Weber, R. S., Lee, Y. Y., and Goepfert, H.: Transcranial resection of tumors of the paranasal sinuses and nasal cavity. J. Neurosurg., 71:10, 1989.
55. Blomhoff, R., Green, M. H., Berg, T., and Norum, K. R.: Transport and storage of vitamin A. Science, 250:399, 1990.
56. Bloom, E. J., Green, M. D., Cooper, J. S., Cohen, N., and Muggia, F. M.: Concomitant use of cis-platinum (CDDP) chemotherapy and radiation therapy (RT) in the treatment of advanced head and neck cancer. (Abstract #C-533) Proc. Am. Soc. Clin. Oncol., 4:137, 1985.
57. Bloom, N. D., and Spiro, R. H.: Carcinoma of the cheek mucosa: a retrospective analysis. Am. J. Surg., 140:556, 1980.
58. Blot, W. J., McLaughlin, J. K., Winn, D. M., Austin, D. F., Grumbers, R. S., Preston-Martin, S., Bernstein, L., Schoenberg, J. B., Stemhagen, A., and Fraumeni, J. F., Jr.:

Smoking and drinking in relation to oral and pharyngeal cancer. Cancer Res., 48:3282, 1988.
59. Bluhm, R., Branch, R., Johnson, P., and Stein, R.: Aplastic anemia associated with canthaxanthin ingested for 'tanning' purposes. JAMA, 264:1141, 1990.
60. Bocca, E.: Supraglottic cancer. Laryngoscope, 85:1318, 1975.
61. Bocca, E., Pignataro, O., and Oldini, C.: Supraglottic laryngectomy: 30 years of experience. Ann. Otol. Rhinol. Laryngol., 92:14, 1983.
62. Bollag, W.: Vitamin A and retinoids: from nutrition to pharmacotherapy in dermatology and oncology. Lancet, 1:860, 1983.
63. Boone, C. W., Kelloff, G. J., and Malone, W. E.: Identification of candidate cancer chemopreventive agents and their evaluation in animal models and human clinical trials: a review. Cancer Res., 50:2, 1990.
64. Boring, C. C., Squires, T. S., and Tong, T.: Cancer statistics, 1992. CA, 42:19, 1992.
65. Bouquot, J. E., Kurland, L. T., and Weiland, L. H.: Carcinoma in situ of the upper aerodigestive tract. Incidence, time trends, and follow-up in Rochester, Minnesota, 1935–1984. Cancer, 61:1691, 1988.
66. Bouquot, J. E., Weiland, L. H., and Kurland, L. T.: Leukoplakia and carcinoma in situ synchronously associated with invasive oral/oropharyngeal carcinoma in Rochester, Minn., 1935–1984. Oral Surg. Oral Med. Oral Pathol., 65:199, 1988.
67. Boyle, P., Macfarlane, G. J., McGinn, R., Zheng, T., La Vecchia, C., Maisonneuve, P., and Scully, C.: International epidemiology of head and neck cancer. *In* Multiple Primary Tumors in the Head and Neck. By de Vries, N., and Gluckman, J. L., 1990, pp. 80–138.
68. Braakhuis, B. J. M., van Dongen, G. A. M. S., Vermorken, J. B., and Snow, G. B.: Preclinical in vivo activity of 2′,2′-difluorodeoxycytidine (Gemcitabine) against human head and neck cancer. Cancer Res., 51:211, 1991.
69. Bradford, C. R., Hoffman, H. T., Wolf, G. T., Carey, T. E., Baker, S. R., and McClatchey, K. D.: Squamous carcinoma of the head and neck in organ transplant recipient: possible role of oncologic viruses. Laryngoscope, 100:190, 1990.
70. Brandsma, J. L., and Abramson, A. L.: Association of papillomavirus with cancer of the head and neck. Arch. Otolaryngol. Head Neck Surg., 115:621, 1989.
71. Broders, A. C.: The microscopic grading of cancer. Surg. Clinic N. Am., 21:947, 1941.
72. Browman, G. P., Archibald, S. D., Young, J. E., Hrynink, W. M., Russell, R., Kiehl, K., and Levine, M. N.: Prospective randomized trial of one-hour sequential versus simultaneous methotrexate plus 5-fluorouracil in advanced and recurrent squamous cell head and neck cancer. J. Clin. Oncol., 1:787, 1983.
73. Browman, G. P., Goodyear, M. D., Levine, M. N., Russell, R., Archibald, S. D., and Young, J. E.: Modulation of the antitumor effect of methotrexate by low-dose leucovorin in squamous cell head and neck cancer: a randomized placebo-controlled clinical trial. J. Clin. Oncol., 8:203, 1990.
74. Browman, G. P., Levine, M. N., Goodyear, M. D., Russell, R., Archibald, S. D., Jackson, B. S., Young, J. E., Basrur, V., and Johanson, C.: Methotrexate/fluorouracil scheduling influences normal tissue toxicity but not antitumor effects in patients with squamous cell head and neck cancer: Results from a randomized trial. J. Clin. Oncol., 6:963, 1988.
75. Browman, G. P., Levine, M. N., Russell, R., Young, J. E., and Archibald, S. D.: Survival results from a phase III study of simultaneous versus 1-hour sequential methotrexate-5-fluorouracil chemotherapy in head and neck cancer. Head Neck Surg., 8:146, 1986.
76. Bryce, D.: The conventional surgical management of carcinoma of the hypopharynx. J. Laryngol. Otol., 85:1221, 1971.
77. Bryce, D. P.: The management of laryngeal cancer. J. Otolaryngol., 8:105, 1979.
78. Burkell, C. C.: Cancer of lip. Can. Med. Assoc. J., 62:28, 1950.
79. Burkey, B. B., Hoffman, H. T., Baker, S. R., Thornton, A. F., and McClatchey, K. D.: Chondrosarcoma of the head and neck. Laryngoscope, 100:1301, 1990.
80. Burton, G. W., and Ingold, K. U.: Beta-carotene: an unusual type of lipid antioxidant. Science, 224:569, 1984.
81. Byers, R. M., Newman, R., Russell, N., and Yue, A.: Results of treatment of squamous carcinoma of the lower gum. Cancer, 47:236, 1981.
82. Byfield, J. E., Calabro-Jones, P., Klisak, I., and Kulhanian, F.: Pharmacologic requirements for obtaining sensitization of human tumor cells in vitro to combined 5-fluorouracil or ftorafur and x-rays. Int. J. Radiat. Oncol. Biol. Phys., 8:1923, 1982.
83. Cady, B., and Catlin, D.: Epidermoid carcinoma of the gum. Cancer, 23:551, 1969.
84. Callery, C. D., Spiro, R. H., and Strong, E. W.: Changing trends in the management of squamous carcinoma of the tongue. Am. J. Surg., 148:449, 1984.
85. Campbell, J. B., Dorman, E. B., McCormick, M., Miles, J., Morton, K. P., Rugman, F., Stell, P. M., Stoney, P. J., Vaughn, E. D., and Wilson, J. A.: A randomized phase III trial of cisplatinum, methotrexate, cisplatinum + methotrexate, and cisplatinum + 5-fluoro-uracil in end-stage head and neck cancer. Acta Otolaryngol., (Stockh.) 103:519, 1987.
86. Campbell, M. A., Perrier, D. G., Dorr, R. T., Alberts, D. S., and Finley, P. R.: Methotrexate bioavailability and pharmokinetics. Cancer Treat., 69:833, 1985.
87. Canetta, R., Bragman, K., Smaldone, L., and Rozencweig, M. I.: Carboplatin: current status and future prospects. Cancer Treat. Rev., 15(Suppl. B):17, 1988.
88. Cann, C. I., Fried, M. P., and Rothman, K. J.: Epidemiology of squamous cell cancer of the head and neck. Otolaryngol. Clin. North Am., 18:367, 1985.
89. Caplan, G. A., and Brigham, B. A.: Marijuana smoking and carcinoma of the tongue. Is there an association? Cancer, 66:1005, 1990.
90. Carey, T. E., Wolf, G. T., Hsu, S., Poore, J., Peterson, K., and McClatchey, K. D.: Expression of A9 antigen and loss of blood group antigens as determinants of survival in patients with head and neck squamous carcinoma. Otolaryngol. Head Neck Surg., 91:221, 1987.
91. Carpenter, R. J., DeSanto, L. W., Devine, K. D., and Taylor, W. F.: Cancer of the hypopharynx: Analysis of treatment and results in 162 patients. Arch. Otolaryngol., 102:716, 1976.
92. Carter, S. K., and Livingston, R. B.: The chemotherapy of head and neck cancer. *In* Principles of Cancer Treatment. Carter, S. K., Glatstein, E., and Livingston, R. B., (eds.). New York, McGraw-Hill, 1982.
93. Carugati, A., Pradier, R., and de la Torre, A.: Combination chemotherapy (CT) pre radical treatment of head and neck squamous cell carcinoma (SCC). (Abstract #589) Proc. Amer. Soc. Clin. Oncol., 7:152, 1988.
94. Chabner, B. A., and Collins, J. M.: Cancer Chemotherapy: Principles and Practice. J. B. Lippincott Company, Philadelphia, 1990.
95. Chan, C. K., and Gee, J. B. L.: Asbestos exposure and laryngeal cancers: An analysis of the epidemiologic evidence. J. Occup. Med., 30:23, 1988.
96. Chang, A. Y., and Keng, P. C.: Potentiation of radiation cytotoxicity by recombinant interferons, a phenomenon associated with increased blockage at the G_2-M phase of the cell cycle. Cancer Res., 47:4338, 1987.
97. Chang, H., Leone, L., Tefft, M., and Nigri, P. T.: Simultaneous cis-platinum and radiotherapy as an induction therapy for advanced head and neck squamous cell carcinoma. (Abstract #579) Proc. Am. Soc. Clin. Oncol., 8:150, 1988.
98. Chaudhy, N. A., Jafarey, N. A., and Ibrahim, K.: Plasma vitamin A and carotene levels in relation to the clinical stages of carcinoma of the oral cavity and oropharynx. JPMA, 30:221, 1980.
99. Chen, J. Y., Chen, C. J., Liu, M. Y., Cho, S. M., Hsu, M. M., Lynn, T. C., Shieh, T., Tu, S. M., Beasley, R. P., and Hwang, L. Y.: Antibody to Epstein-Barr virus specific DNase as a marker for field survey of patients with nasopharyngeal carcinoma in Taiwan. J. Med. Virol., 27:269, 1989.
100. Chen, K., Katz, R. V., and Krutchkoff, D. J.: Intraoral squamous cell carcinoma: Epidemiologic patterns in Connecticut from 1935 to 1985. Cancer, 66:1288, 1990.
101. Chiang, T. C., and Griem, M. L.: Nasopharyngeal cancer. Surg. Clin. N. Amer., 53:121, 1973.
102. Chobe, R., McNeese, M., Weber, R., and Fletcher, G. H.: Radiation therapy for carcinoma of the nasal vestibule. Otolaryngol. Head Neck Surg., 98:67, 1988.
103. Choi, K., Aziz, H., Stark, R., Sohn, C., Rosenthal, J., Braverman, A., Khil, S., Isaacson, S., Marti, J., and Rotman, M.: Concomitant radiation and infusion cis-platinum in advanced cancers of the head and neck: influence of radiation fractionation. (Abstract #607) Proc. Am. Soc. Clin. Oncol., 8:157, 1988.
104. Choksi, A. J., Dimery, I. W., and Hong, W. K.: Adjuvant chemotherapy of head and neck cancer: the past, the present, and the future. Semin. Oncol., 15(Suppl. 3):45, 1988.
105. Chung, T. S., and Stefani, S.: Distant metastases of carcinoma of tonsillar region: a study of 475 patients. J. Surg. Oncol., 14:5, 1980.
106. Clark, J. R., Fallon, B. G., Dreyfuss, A. I., Norris, C. M., Jr., Anderson, J. W., Ervin, T. J., Anderson, R. F., Chaffey, J. T., Miller, D., and Frei, E., III: Chemotherapeutic strategies in the multidisciplinary treatment of head and neck cancer. Semin. Oncol., 15(Suppl. 3):35, 1988.
107. Clark, J., Fallon, B., Norris, C., Miller, D., Fabian, R., Weichselbaum, R., Anderson, R., Chaffey, J., Ervin, T., and Frei, E.: A randomized trial of two induction regimens for advanced squamous cell carcinoma of the head and neck (SCCHN): Preliminary results. (Abstract #515) Proc. Am. Soc. Clin. Oncol., 5:132, 1986.
108. Clark, J. Fallon, B., Weichselbaum, R., Miller, D., Norris, C., Frei, E., and Ervin, T.: The influence of resectability on response to induction chemotherapy and survival in advanced squamous cell carcinoma of the head and neck (SCCHN). (Abstract #C-542) Proc. Am. Soc. Clin. Oncol., 4:139, 1985.
109. Clark, J. R., and Frei, E., III: Chemotherapy for head and neck cancer: progress and controversy in the management of patients with MO disease. Semin. Oncol., 16(Suppl. 6):44, 1989.
110. Clark, J. R., Norris, C. M., Jr., Dreyfuss, A. I., Fallon, B. G., Balogh, K., Anderson, R. F., Jr., Chaffey, J. T., Anderson, J. W., and Miller, D.: Nasopharyngeal carcinoma: The Dana-Farber Cancer Institute experience with 24 patients treated with induction chemotherapy and radiotherapy. Ann. Otol. Rhinol. Laryngol., 96:608, 1987.
111. Clark, R. M., Rosen, I. B., and Laperriere, N. J.: Malignant tumors of the head and neck in a young population. Am. J. Surg., 144:459, 1982.
112. Clavel, M., Cognetti, F., Dodion, P., Wildiers, J., Rosso, R., Rossi, A., Gignoux, B., Van Rymenart, M., Cortez-Funes, H., and Dalesio, O.: Combination chemotherapy with methotrexate, bleomycin, and vincristine with or without cisplatin in advanced squamous cell carcinoma of the head and neck. Cancer, 60:1173, 1987.
113. Clavel, M., Vermorken, J., Cognetti, F., De Mulder, P., Schornagel, J., Verweij, J., Kirkpatrick, A., and Dalesio, O.: Chemotherapy in recurrent and/or metastatic head and neck squamous cell carcinoma (SCCHN). Prognostic factors from 589 patients (pts) treated in three protocols. (Abstract #692) Proc. Am. Soc. Clin. Oncol., 9:179, 1990.
114. Coates, A. S., Tattersall, M. H., Swanson, C., Hedley, D., Fox, R. M., and Raghavan, D.: Combination therapy with methotrexate and 5-fluorouracil: a prospective randomized clinical trial of order of administration. J. Clin. Oncol., 2:756, 1984.
115. Coates, H. L., DeSanto, L. W., Devine, K. D., and Elveback, L. R.: Carcinoma of the supraglottic larynx. A review of 221 cases. Arch. Otolaryngol., 102:686, 1976.
116. Cobleigh, M. A., Hill, J. H., Lad, T.E., Shevrin, D. E., and Applebaum, E. L.: Phase II study of etoposide in previously untreated squamous cell carcinoma of the head and neck. Cancer Treat. Rep., 71:321, 1987.
117. Cognetti, F., Carlini, P., and Pinnaro, P.: Prospective randomized trial of neoadjuvant cisplatin and 5-FU followed by radiotherapy versus concurrent cisplatin and radiotherapy in locally advanced head and neck squamous cell cancer: Preliminary results (abstr). Proceedings Second Inter. Conf. Head and Neck Cancer, Boston, MA, July 31–August 5, 1988.
118. Cognetti, F., Carlini, P., Pinnaro, P., Ruggeri, E. M., Perrino, A., Del Vecchio, M. R., Ambesi Impiombato, F., and Calabresi, F.: Preliminary results of a randomized trial of sequential versus simultaneous chemo and radiotherapy (CT-xRT) in patient (pts) with locally advanced unresectable squamous cell carcinoma of the head and neck (SCCHN). (Abstract #661) Proc. Am. Soc. Clin. Oncol., 8:170, 1989.
119. Cognetti, F., Pinnaro, P., Carlini, P., and Ruggeri, E. M.: Neoadjuvant chemotherapy in previously untreated patients with advanced head and neck squamous cell cancer. Cancer, 62:251, 1988.
120. Cognetti, F., Pinnaro, P., Ruggeri, E. M., Carlini, P., Perrino, A., Impiobato, F. A., Calabresi, F., Chilelli, M. G., and Giannarelli, D.: Prognostic factors for chemotherapy response and survival using combination chemotherapy as initial treatment of advanced head and neck squamous cell cancer. J. Clin. Oncol., 7:829, 1989.
121. Collins, J. M.: Pharmacologic rationale for regional drug delivery. J. Clin. Oncol., 2:498, 1984.
122. Coltrera, M. D., Zarbo, R. J., Gown, A. M., et al.: Comparison of two putative markers of premalignant change in the oral cavity: suprabasal expression of CK-19 and proliferating cell nuclear antigen (PCNA). Third International Head and Neck Oncology Research Conference, Las Vegas, Nevada, 1990.
123. Condit, P. T.: Treatment of carcinoma with radiation therapy and methotrexate. Mo. Med., 65:832, 1968.
124. Conley, J., and Dingman, D. K.: Adenoid cystic carcinoma in the head and neck (cylindroma). Arch. Otolaryngol., 100:81, 1974.

125. Conley, J., Myers, E., and Cole, R.: Analysis of 115 patients with tumors of the submandibular gland. Ann. Otol. Rhinol. Laryngol., 81:323, 1972.
126. Connors, J. M., Andiman, W. A., Howarth, C. B., Liu, E., Merigam, T. C., Savage, M. E., and Jacobs, C.: Treatment of nasopharyngeal carcinoma with human leukocyte interferon. J. Clin. Oncol., 3:813, 1985.
127. Connors, J. M., and Jacobs, C.: Nasopharyngeal carcinoma: Relationship to Epstein-Barr virus and treatment with interferon. *In* Cancers of the Head and Neck. Edited by Jacobs, C. Boston, Martinus Nijhoff Publishers, 1987, pp. 167–175.
128. Conti, C. J.: Markers of keratinocyte differentiation in preneoplastic and neoplastic lesions. *In* Immunocytochemistry in Tumor Diagnosis. Edited by Russo, J. Proceedings of the Workshop on Immunocytochemistry in Tumor Diagnosis. Detroit, Michigan. Boston, Martinus Nijhoff Publishers, 1984, pp. 59–71.
129. Cooke, L. D., Cooke, T. G., Bootz, F., Forster, G., Helliwell, T. R., Spiller, D., and Stell, P. M.: Ploidy as a prognostic indicator in end stage squamous cell carcinoma of the head and neck region treated with cisplatinum. Br. J. Cancer, 61:759, 1990.
130. Cooper, J. S., Pajak, T. F., Rubin, P., Tupchong, L., Brady, L. W., Leibel, S. A., Laramore, G. E., Marcial, V. A., Davis, L. W., Cox, J. D., et al: Second malignancies in patients who have head and neck cancers: Incidence, effect on survival and implications for chemoprevention based on the RTOG experience. Int. J. Radiat. Oncol. Biol. Phys., 17:449, 1989.
131. Cordero, A. A., Allevato, M. A. J., Barclay, C. A., et al.: Treatment of lichen planus and leukoplakia with the oral retinoid RO 10-9359. *In* Retinoids, Advances in Basic Research and Therapy. Edited by Orfanos, C. E., et al. Berlin, Springer-Verlag Publishers, 1981, pp. 273–278.
132. Corvo, R., Merlano, M., Looney, W. B., Benasso, M., Bacigalupo, A., and Margarino, G.: Integration of chemotherapy in an MFD-radiotherapy plan for advanced inoperable squamous cell carcinoma of the head and neck. Head Neck, 12:60, 1990.
133. Corvo, R., Merlano, M., Scarpati, D., Grimaldi, A., Benasso, M., Franzone, P., Santelli, A., Scasso, F., Rosso, R., and Vitale, V.: Sequential or alternate chemo-radiotherapy in the treatment of advanced head and neck tumors. Results of a randomized study. Radiol. Med., 75:653, 1988.
134. Coughlin, C. T., and Richmond, R. C.: Biologic and clinical developments of cisplatin combined with radiation: concepts, utility, projections for new trials, and the emergence of carboplatin. Semin. Oncol., 16:31, 1989.
135. Cox, J. D., Pajak, T. F., Marcial, V. A., Hanks, G. E., Mohiuddin, M., Fu, K. K., Byhard, R. W., and Rubin, P.: Dose response for local control with hyperfractionated radiation therapy in advanced carcinomas of the upper aerodigestive tracts: preliminary report of Radiation Therapy Oncology Group protocol 83-13. Int. J. Radiat. Oncol. Biol. Phys., 18:515, 1990.
136. Craig, J. B., Powell, B. L., Jackson, D. V., Atkins, J. N., Smith, L. R., White, D. R., Richards, F., and Capizzi, R. L.: Phase II trial of high-dose cytarabine and cisplatin in locoregional previously untreated squamous carcinoma of the head and neck. A Piedmont Oncology Association Study. Cancer Treat. Rep., 71:151, 1987.
137. Creagan, E. T., Woods, J. E., Schutt, A. J., and O'Fallon, J. R.: Cyclophosphamide, adriamycin and cis-diamminedichloroplatinum (II) in the treatment of advanced nonsquamous cell head and neck cancer. Cancer, 52:2007, 1983.
138. Creekmore, S. P., Micetich, K. C., Vogelzang, N., Canzoneri, C., Choudhurg, A., and Fisher, R. I.: Low toxicity and significant tumor responses in phase II trials of carboplatin (CBDCA) in head & neck, non-small cell lung, urothelial, and ovarian cancers. (Abstract #C-562) Proc. Am. Soc. Clin. Oncol., 4:144, 1985.
139. Crile, G.: Excision of cancer of the head and neck. JAMA, 258:1780, 1906.
140. Crispino, O., Tancini, O., Barni, S., Colombo, A., Paolorossi, F., Frigerio, F., Lissoni, P., Buratti, C., and Ferri, L.: Simultaneous cisplatinum (CDDP) and radiotherapy in patients with locally advanced head and neck cancer. (Abstract #482) Proc. Am. Soc. Clin. Oncol., 6:123, 1987.
141. Crissman, J. D.: Laryngeal keratosis and subsequent carcinoma. Head Neck Surg., 1:386, 1979.
142. Crissman, J. D., Liu, W. Y., Gluckman, J. L., and Cummings, G.: Prognostic value of histopathologic parameters in squamous cell carcinoma of the oropharynx. Cancer, 54:2995, 1984.
143. Crissman, J. D., Pajak, T. F., Zarbo, R. J., Marcial, V. A., and Al-Sarraf, M.: Improved response and survival to combined cisplatin and radiation in non-keratinizing squamous cell carcinomas of the head and neck. An RTOG Study of 114 advanced stage tumors. Cancer, 59:1391, 1987.
144. Crivellari, D., Veronesi, A., Magri, M. D., Tirelli, U., Comoretto, R., Barzan, L., Caruso, G., Carbone, A., and Grigoletto, E.: Phase II trial of oral VP 16-213 (etoposide) in patients with advanced head and neck cancer. Tumori, 71:499, 1985.
145. Croll, G. A., Gerritsen, G. J., Tiwari, R. M., and Snow, G. B.: Primary radiotherapy with surgery in reserve for advanced laryngeal carcinoma: Results and complications. Eur. J. Surg. Oncol., 15:350, 1989.
146. Cross, J. E.: Carcinoma of the lip: A review of 563 case records of carcinoma of the lip at the Pondville Hospital. Surg. Gynec. Obstet., 87:153, 1948.
147. Cullen, J. W.: The National Cancer Institute's intervention trials. Cancer, 62:1851, 1988.
148. Cullen, J. W., Blot, W., Henning Field, J., Boyd, G., Mecklenberg, R., and Massey, M. M.: The Health Consequences of Using Smokeless Tobacco. Summary of the Advisory Committee's Report to the Surgeon General. Public Health Rep., 101:355, 1986.
149. Cunningham, T. J., Antemann, R., Paonessa, D., Sponzo, R. W., and Steiner, D.: Adjuvant immuno-and/or chemotherapy with neuraminidase-treated autogenous tumor vaccine and Bacillus Calmette-Guerin for head and neck cancers. Ann. N. Y. Acad. Sci., 277:339, 1976.
150. Current trends: Deaths from oral cavity and pharyngeal cancer—United States, 1987. JAMA, 264:678, 1990.
151. Dabelsteen, E., Vedtofte, P., Hakomori, S., and Young, W. W., Jr.: Accumulation of a blood group antigen precursor in oral premalignant lesions. Cancer Res., 43:1451, 1983.
152. Dalley, V. M.: Cancer of the laryngopharynx. J. Laryngol. Otol., 20:1859, 1968.
153. Dasmahapatra, K. S., Citrin, P., Hill, G. J., Yee, R., Mohit-Tabatabai, M. A., and Rush, B. F., Jr.: A prospective evaluation of 5-fluorouracil plus cisplatin in advanced squamous cell cancer of the head and neck. J. Clin. Oncol., 3:1486, 1985.
154. Dasmahapatra, K. S., Mohit-Tabatabai, M. A., Rush, B. F., Jr., Hill, G. J., Feuerman, M., and Ohanian, M.: Cancer of the tonsil: Improved survival with combination therapy. Cancer, 57:451, 1986.
155. Davis, R. K., and Shapshay, S. M.: Peristomal recurrence: Pathophysiology, prevention and treatment. Otolaryngol. Clin. North Am., 13:499, 1980.
156. Davis, S., and Kessler, W.: Randomized comparison of cis-diamminedichloroplatinum versus cis-diamminedichloroplatinum, methotrexate, and bleomycin in recurrent squamous cell carcinoma of the head and neck. Cancer Chemother. Pharmacol., 3:57, 1979.
157. Dawson, A. K., and Orr, J. A.: Long term results of local excision and radiotherapy in pleomorphic adenoma of the parotid. Int. J. Radiat. Oncol. Biol. Phys., 11:451, 1985.
158. Dawson, M. I., and Okamura, W. H.: Chemistry and Biology of Synthetic Retinoids. Boca Raton, Florida, CRC Press, 1990.
159. de Andres Basauri, L., Lopez Pousa, A., Alba, E., and Sanpedro, F.: Carboplatin, an active drug in advanced head and neck cancer. Cancer Treat. Rep., 70:1173, 1986.
160. Decker, J., and Goldstein, J. C.: Risk factors in head and neck cancer. N. Engl. J. Med., 306:1151, 1982.
161. DeConti, R. C., and Schoenfeld, D.: A randomized prospective comparison of intermittent methotrexate, methotrexate with leucovorin, and a methotrexate combination in head and neck cancer. Cancer, 48:1061, 1981.
162. Decroix, Y., and Ghossein, N. A.: Experience of the Curie Institute in treatment of cancer of the mobile tongue I: Treatment policies and results. Cancer, 47:496, 1981.
163. De Luca, L. M., Shores, R. L., Spangler, E. F., and Wenk, M. L.: Inhibition of initiator-promoter-induced skin tumorigenesis in female SENCAR mice fed a vitamin A-deficient diet and reappearance of tumors in mice fed a diet adequate in retinoid or beta-carotene. Cancer Res., 49:5400, 1989.
164. De Villiers, E. M., Weidauer, H., Otto, H., and zur Hausen, M.: Papillomavirus DNA in human tongue carcinomas. Int. J. Cancer, 36:575, 1985.
165. Dennington, M. L., Carter, D. R., and Meyers, A. D.: Distant metastases in head and neck epidermoid carcinoma. Laryngoscope, 90:196, 1980.
166. Depue, R. H.: Rising mortality from cancer of the tongue in young white males (Letter). N. Engl. J. Med., 315:647, 1986.
167. Demard, F., Chauvel, P., Santini, J., Vallicioni, J., Thyss, A., and Schneider, M.: Response to chemotherapy as justification for modification of the therapeutic strategy for pharyngolaryngeal carcinomas. Head Neck Surg., 12:225, 1990.
168. DeSanto, L. W.: The options in early laryngeal carcinoma. N. Engl. J. Med., 306:910, 1982.
169. DeSanto, L. W.: T3 glottic cancer: options and consequences of the options. Laryngoscope, 94:1311, 1984.
170. DeSanto, L. W.: Cancer of the supraglottic larynx: A review of 260 patients. Otolaryngol. Head Neck Surg., 93:705, 1985.
171. DeSanto, L. W.: Early supraglottic cancer. Ann. Otol. Rhinol. Laryngol., 99:593, 1990.
172. DeSanto, L. W., Lillie, J. C., and Devine, K. D.: Surgical salvage after radiation for laryngeal cancer. Laryngoscope, 87:649, 1976.
173. DeSanto, L. W., Lillie, J. C., and Devine, K. D.: Cancer of the larynx: Supraglottic cancer. Surg. Clin. North Am., 57:505, 1077.
174. Devesa, S. S., Silverman, D. T., Young, J. L., Jr., Pollack, E. S., Brown, J. W., Percy, C. L., Myers, M. H., McKay, F. W., and Fraumeni, J. F., Jr.: Cancer incidence and mortality trends among whites in the United States, 1947–84. J. Natl. Cancer Inst., 79:701, 1987.
175. DeVries, N., and Snow, G. B.: Prevention of second primary cancers in head and neck cancer patients: new perpectives. Am. J. Otolaryngol., 9:151, 1988.
176. Dewit, L.: Combined treatment of radiation and cisdiamminedichloroplatinum (II): A review of experimental and clinical data. Int. J. Radiat. Oncol. Biol. Phys., 13:403, 1987.
177. Dimery, I. W., Jacobs, C., Tseng, A., Jr., Saks, S., Pearson, G., Hons, W. K., and Gutterman, J. U.: Recombinant interferon-gamma in the treatment of recurrent nasopharyngeal carcinoma. J. Biol. Response Mod., 8:221, 1989.
178. Dimery, I. W., Jones, L. A., Verjan, R. P., Raymond, A. K., Goepfert, H., and Hong, W. K.: Estrogen receptors in normal salivary gland and salivary gland carcinoma. Arch. Otolaryngol. Head Neck Surg., 113:1082, 1987.
179. Dimery, I., Lee, Y. Y., VanTassel, P., Goepfert, H., Byers, R., Guillamondegui, O., McCarthy, K., and Hong, W. K.: Combined intra-arterial (I.A.) and systemic chemotherapy (CT) for paranasal sinus carcinoma (PNSC). Proc. Am. Soc. Clin. Oncol., 7:150, 1988.
180. Dimery, I. W., Legha, S. S., Shirinian, M., and Hong, W. K.: Fluorouracil, doxorubicin, cyclophosphamide, and cisplatin combination chemotherapy in advanced or recurrent salivary gland carcinoma. J. Clin. Oncol., 8:1056, 1990.
181. Dimery, I. W., Martin, T., Bradley, E., Kramer, A., and Hong, W.: Phase I trial of interleukin-2 (rIL-2) plus cisplatin (CDDP) and 5-fluorouracil (5-FU) in recurrent or advanced squamous cell carcinoma of the head and neck. Proc. Amer. Soc. Clin. Oncol., 8:170, 1989.
182. Dimery, I. W., Peters, L. J., Goepfert, H., Neely Atkinson, E., McCarthy, K., Byers, R., Weber, R. S., and Hong, W. K.: Survival in Stage IV Nasopharyngeal Carcinoma after Combination Chemotherapy and Radiotherapy. Edited by Salmon, S. E. Philadelphia, W. B. Saunders Company, 1990, pp. 82–100.
183. Dimery, I. W., Brooks, B. J., Winn, R., Martin, T., Shirinian, M., and Hong, W. K.: Phase II trial of carboplatin plus cisplatin in recurrent and advanced squamous cell carcinoma of the head and neck. J. Clin. Oncol., 9:1939, 1991.
184. DiTroia, J. F.: Nodal metastases and prognosis in carcinoma of the oral cavity. Otolaryngol. Clin. North Am. 5:333, 1972.
185. Domenge, C., Marandas, P., Vignond, J., et al.: Postsurgical adjuvant chemotherapy in extracapsular spread invaded lymph node of epidermoid carcinoma of the head and neck: A randomized multicentric trial. Proceedings of the 2nd International Conference on Head and Neck Cancer: Combined Therapy. (Abstract #108) Boston, July 31–August 5, 1988, p. 74.
186. Donald, P. J.: Marijuana smoking—possible cause of head and neck carcinoma in young patients. Otolaryngol. Head Neck Surg., 94:517, 1986.
187. Doseva, D., Christov, K., Kristeva, K.: DNA content in reactive hyperphasia, precancerosis, and carcinomas of the oral cavity. Acta Histochem., 75:113, 1984.
188. Douple, E. B.: Platinum-radiation interactions, N.C.I. Monogr., 6:315, 1988.
189. Drelichman, A., Cunnings, G., and Al-Sarraf, M.: A randomized trial of cis-platinum, oncovin and bleomycin (COB) versus methotrexate in patients with advanced squamous cell carcinoma of the head and neck. Cancer, 52:399, 1983.
190. Dreyfuss, A. I., Clark, J. R., Fallon, B. G., Posner, M. R., Norris, C. M., Jr., and Miller,

D.: Cyclophosphamide, doxorubicin, and cisplatin combination chemotherapy for advanced carcinomas of salivary gland origin. Cancer, 60:2869, 1987.
191. Dreyfuss, A. I., Clark, J. R., Wright, J. E., Norris, C. M., Jr., Busse, P. M., Lucarini, J. W., Fallon, B. G., Casey, D., Andersen, J. W., and Klein, R.: Continuous infusion high-dose leucovorin with 5-fluorouracil and cisplatin for untreated stage IV carcinoma of the head and neck. Ann. Intern. Med., 112:167, 1990.
192. Dubois, J. B., Guerrier, B., DiRuggiero, J. M., and Pourquier, H.: Cancer of the pyriform sinus: Treatment by radiation therapy alone and with surgery. Radiol., 160:831, 1986.
193. Einhorn, J., and Wersall, J.: Incidence of oral carcinoma in patients with leukoplakia of the oral mucosa. Cancer, 20:2189, 1967.
194. Eisbach, K. J., and Krause, C. J.: Carcinoma of the pyriform sinus: a comparison of treatment modalities. Laryngoscope, 87:1904, 1977.
195. Eisbruch, A., Blick, M., Lee, J. S., Sacks, P. G., and Gutterman, J.: Analysis of the epidermal growth factor receptor gene in fresh human head and neck tumors. Cancer Res., 47:3603, 1987.
196. Eisenberger, M. A.: Supporting evidence for an active treatment program for advanced salivary gland carcinomas. Cancer Treat. Rep., 69:319, 1985.
197. Eisenberger, M., Hornedo, J., Silva, H., Donehower, R., Spaulding, M., and Van Echo, D.: Carboplatin (NSC-241-240): an active platinum analog for the treatment of squamous-cell carcinoma of the head and neck. J. Clin. Oncol., 4:1506, 1986.
198. Eisenberger, M., Krasnow, S., Ellenberg, S., Silva, H., Abrams, J., Sinibaldi, V., Van Echo, D., and Aisner, J.: A comparison of carboplatin plus methotrexate verus methotrexate alone in patients with recurrent and metastatic head and neck cancer. J. Clin. Oncol., 7:1341, 1989.
199. Eisenberger, M., Van Echo, D., and Aisner, J.: Carboplatin: The experience in head and neck cancer. Semin. Oncol., 16(Suppl. 5):34, 1989.
200. El Badawi, S. A., Goepfert, H., Fletcher, G. H., Herson, J., and Oswald, M. J.: Squamous cell carcinoma of the pyriform sinus. Laryngoscope, 92:357, 1982.
201. Elias, E. G., Chretien, P. B., Monnard, E., Kahn, T., Bouchelle, W. H., Wiernik, P. H., Lipson, S. D., Mande, K. R., and Zentai, T.: Chemotherapy prior to local therapy in advanced squamous cell carcinoma of the head and neck: preliminary assessment of an intensive drug regimen. Cancer, 43:1025, 1979.
202. Elkon, D., Hightower, S. I., Lim, M. L., Cantrell, R. W., and Constable, W. C.: Esthesioneuroblastoma. Cancer, 44:1087, 1979.
203. Eneroth, C. M.: Salivary gland tumors in the parotid gland, submandibular gland and the palate region. Cancer, 27:1418, 1971.
204. Eneroth, C. M., and Hamberger, C. A.: Principles of treatment of different types of parotid tumors. Laryngoscope, 84:1732, 1974.
205. Ensley, J. F., Ahmed, K., and Kish, J. A.: Salvage of patients with advanced squamous cell cancers of the head and neck (SCCHN) following induction chemotherapy failure using radiation and concurrent cisplatinum (CACP). *In* Adjuvant Therapy of Cancer IV. Edited by Salmon, S. 1990, pp. 92–100.
206. Ensley, J. F., Jacobs, J. R., Weaver, A., Kinzie, J., Crissman, J., Kish, J. A., Cummings, G., and Al Sarraf, M.: Correlation between response to cisplatinum-combination chemotherapy and subsequent radiotherapy in previously untreated patients with advanced squamous cell cancers of the head and neck. Cancer, 54:811, 1984.
207. Ensley, J., Kish, J., Tapazoglou, E., Jacobs, J., Weaver, A., Atkinson, D., Ahmed, K., Mathog, R., and Al Sarraf, M.: An intensive, five course, alternating combination chemotherapy induction regimen used in patients with advanced, unresectable head and neck cancer. J. Clin. Oncol., 6:1147, 1988.
208. Ensley, J. F., Maciorowski, Z., Pietraszkiewicz, H., deBaud, F., Sakr, W., Kish, J., Al Sarraf, M., and Tapazoglou, E.: Clinical applications of cellular DNA content parameters determined by flow cytometry in squamous cell cancers of the head and neck. *In* Adjuvant Therapy of Cancer VI. Edited by Salmon, S. 1990, pp. 101–108.
209. Epstein, M. A.: Vaccination against Epstein-Barr virus: Current progress and future strategies. Lancet, 1:1425, 1986.
210. Ervin, T. J., Clark, J. R., Weichselbaum, R. R., Fallon, B. G., Miller, D., Fabian, R. L., Posner, M. R., Norris, C. M., Jr., Tuttle, S. A., and Schoenfeld, D. A.: An analysis of induction and adjuvant chemotherapy in the multidisciplinary treatment of squamous-cell carcinoma of the head and neck. J. Clin. Oncol., 5:10, 1987.
211. Eschwege, F., Sancho-Garnier, H., Gerard, J. P., Madelain, M., DeSaulty, A., Jortay, A., and Cachin, Y.: Ten-year results of randomized trial comparing radiotherapy and concomitant bleomycin to radiotherapy alone in epidermoid carcinomas of the oropharynx: Experience of the European Organization for Research and Treatment of Cancer. N.C.I. Monographs, 6:275, 1988.
212. Evans, R. M.: The steroid and thyroid hormone receptor superfamily. Science, 240:889, 1988.
213. Evans, H. L., Ayala, A. G., and Romsdahl, M. M.: Prognostic factors in chondrosarcoma of bone. A clincopathologic analysis with emphasis on histologic grading. Cancer, 40:818, 1977.
214. Fakih, A. R., Rao, R. S., Borges, A. M., and Patel, A. R.: Elective versus therapeutic neck dissection in early carcinoma of the oral tongue. Am. J. Surg., 158:309, 1989.
215. Fallon, B. G., Clark, J. R., Norris, C. M., Jr., Balogh, K., Domanowski, G., Andersen, J., Dreyfuss, A. I., Anderson, R. F., Chaffey, J. T., Miller, D., and Frei, E., III: Induction chemotherapy for advanced cell carcinoma of the head and neck: An analysis of clinical and histopathologic correlates after a complete response to chemotherapy. *In* Head and Neck Oncology Research. Edited by G. T. Wolf and T. E. Carey. Amsterdam and Berkeley, Kugler and Ghedini, 1987, pp. 281–286.
216. Fazekas, J. T., Sommer, C., and Kramer, S.: Adjuvant intravenous methotrexate or definitive radiotherapy alone for advanced squamous cancers of the oral cavity, oropharynx, supraglottic larynx or hypopharynx. Int. J. Radiat. Oncol. Biol. Phys., 6:533, 1980.
217. Fedder, M., and Gonzalez, M. F.: Nasopharyngeal carcinoma: Brief review. Am. J. Med., 79:365, 1985.
218. Feinmesser, R., Miyazaki, I., Cheung, R., Freeman, J. L., Noyek, A. M., and Dosch, H. M.: Diagnosis of nasopharyngeal carcinoma by DNA amplification of tissue obtained by fine-needle aspiration. N. Engl. J. Med., 326:17, 1992.
219. Fey, S. J., and Larsen, P. M.: DNA viruses and human cancer. Cancer Letters, 41:1, 1988.
220. Field, J. K., Spandidos, D. A., Stell, P. M., Vaughan, E. D., Evan, G. I., and Moore, J. P.: Elevated expression of the c-myc oncoprotein correlates with poor prognosis in head and neck squamous cell carcinoma. Oncogene., 4:1463, 1989.
221. Fierro, R., Johnson, J., Myers, E., Colao, D., Pelch, K., Rust, D., Wagner, R., Whiteside, J., and Vlock, D.: Phase II trial of non-recombinant interferon alpha (INF) in recurrent squamous cell carcinoma of the head and neck. (Abstract #605), (SCCHN) Proc. Am. Soc. Clin. Oncol., 7:156, 1988.
222. Fiore, M. C., Pierce, J. P., Remington, P. L., and Fiore, B. J.: Cigarette smoking: The clinician's role in cessation, prevention, and public health. Dis.-Mon., 36:181, 1990.
223. Fitzpatrick, P. J., and Therialut, C.: Malignant salivary gland tumors. Int. J. Radiat. Oncol. Biol. Phys., 12:1743, 1986.
224. Fletcher, G. H.: Clinical dose-response curves of human malignant epithelial tumors. Br. J. Radiol., 46:1, 1973.
225. Fletcher, G. H.: Squamous cell carcinomas of the oropharynx. Int. J. Radiol. Oncol. Biol. Phys., 5:2073, 1979.
226. Fletcher, G. H.: Lucy Wortham James Lecture: Subclinical disease. Cancer, 53:1274, 1984.
227. Fletcher, G. H., and Jesse, R. H.: The contribution of supervoltage roentgen therapy to the integration of radiation and surgery in head and neck squamous cell carcinoma. Cancer, 15:566, 1962.
228. Fletcher, G. H., Lindberg, R. D., Hamberger, A., and Horiot, J. C.: Reasons for irradiation failure in squamous cell carcinoma of the larynx. Laryngoscope, 85:987, 1975.
229. Flynn, M. B., Jesse, R. H., and Lindberg, R. D.: Surgery and irradiation in the treatment of squamous cell cancer of the supraglottic larynx. Am. J. Surg., 124:477, 1972.
230. Fontanesi, J., Kun, L. E., Beckford, N., Babin, R., Kavanagh, K., Lester, E., Pao, W. J., Tai, D., and Eddy, T.: Hyperfractionated irradiation and concomitant cisplatin for advanced squamous cell carcinoma head and neck: Early experience. Third International Head and Neck Oncology Research Conference, Las Vegas, Nevada, 1990.
231. Foote, F. W., Jr., and Frazell, E. L.: Tumors of the major salivary glands. Cancer, 6:1065, 1953.
232. Foote, R. L., Buskirk, S. J., Stanley, R. J., Grambsh, P. M., Olsen, K. D., De Santo, L. W., Earle, J. D., and Weiland, L. H.: Patterns of failure after total laryngectomy for glottic carcinoma. Cancer, 64:143, 1989.
233. Forastiere, A. A., Baker, S. R., Wheeler, R., and Medvec, B.R.: Intra-arterial cisplatin and FUDR in advanced malignancies confined to the head and neck. J. Clin. Oncol., 5:1601, 1987.
234. Forastiere, A. A., Belliveau, J. F., Goren, M. P., Vogel, W. C., Posner, M. R., and O'Leary, G. P., Jr.: Pharmacokinetic and toxicity evaluation of five-day continuous infusion versus intermittent bolus cis-diamminedichloroplatinum(II) in head and neck cancer patients. Cancer Res., 48:3869, 1988.
235. Forastiere, A., Metch, B., Keppen, M., Schuller, D., Ensley, J., and Coltman, C., Jr.: Randomized comparison of cisplatin (CDDP) + 5-fluorouracil (5-FU) vs. carboplatin (CBP) + 5-FU vs. methotrexate (MTX) in advanced squamous cell carcinoma of the head and neck. (Abstract #421) Proc. Am. Soc. Clin. Oncol., 8:168, 1989, (and personal communication).
236. Forastiere, A. A., Takasugi, B. J., Baker, S. R., Wolf, G. T., and Kudla-Hatch, V.: High-dose cisplatin in advanced head and neck cancer. Cancer Chemother. Pharmacol., 19:155, 1987.
237. Freeland, A. P., Van Nostrand, A. W., and Jahn, A. F.: Metastasis to the larynx. J. Otolaryngol., 8:448, 1979.
238. Friedman, W. H., Rosenblum, B. N., Loewenstein, P., Thornton, H., Katsantonis, G., and Green, M.: Oncogenes: their presence and significance in squamous cell cancer of the head and neck. Laryngoscope, 95:313, 1985.
239. Fu, K. K.: Biological basis for the interaction of chemotherapeutic agents and radiation therapy. Cancer, 55:2123, 1985.
240. Fu, K. K., Eisenberg, L., Dedo, H. H., and Phillips, T. L.: Results of integrated management of supraglottic carcinoma. Cancer, 40:2874, 1977.
241. Fu, K. K., Lichter, A., and Galante, M.: Carcinoma of the floor of mouth: an analysis of treatment results and the sites and causes and failures. Int. J. Radiol. Oncol. Biol. Phys., 1:829, 1976.
242. Fu, K. K., Phillips, T. L., Silverberg, I. J., Jacobs, C., Goffinet, D. R., Chun, C., Friedman, M. A., Kohler, M., McWhirter, K., and Carter, S. K.: Combined radiotherapy and chemotherapy with bleomycin and methotrexate for advanced inoperable head and neck cancer: update of a Northern California Oncology Group randomized trial. J. Clin. Oncol., 5:1410, 1987.
243. Fu, K. K., Woodhouse, R. J., Quivey, J. M., Phillips, T. L., and Dedo, H. H.: The significance of laryngeal edema following radiotherapy of carcinoma of the vocal cord. Cancer, 49:655, 1982.
244. Gallick, G. E., Sacks, P. G., Maxwell, S. A., Steck, P. A., and Gutterman, J. U.: Head and neck squamous cell carcinoma cell lines as a model system for the study of oncogene expression during tumor progression and metastasis. Prog. Clin. Biol. Res., 212:97, 1986.
245. Garbrilove, J. L., Jakubowski, A., Scher, H., Sternberg, C., Wong, G., Grovs, J., Yagoda, A., Fain, K., Moore, M. A., and Clarkson, B.: Effect of granulocyte colony-stimulating factor on neutropenia and associated morbidity due to chemotherapy for transitional-cell carcinoma of the urothelium. N. Engl. J. Med., 318:1414, 1988.
246. Gardner, K. E., Parsons, J. T., Mendenhall, W. M., Million, R. R., and Cassisi, N. J.: Time dose relationships for local tumor control and complications following irradiation of squamous cell carcinoma of the base of tongue. Int. J. Radiol. Oncol. Biol. Phys., 13:507, 1987.
247. Garewal, H. S., Meyskens, F. L., Killen, D., Reeves, D., Kiersch, T. A., Elletson, H., Strosberg, A., King, D., and Steinbronn, K.: Response of oral leukoplakia to beta-carotene. J. Clin. Oncol., 8:1715, 1990.
248. Garrett, P. G., Beale, F. A., Cummins, B. J., Harwood, A. R., Keane, T. J., Payne, D. G., and Rider, W. D.: Cancer of the tonsil: Results of radical radiation therapy with surgery in reserve. Am. J. Surg., 146:432, 1983.
249. Garrington, G. E., Scotfield, H. H., Coryn, J., and Hooker, S. P.: Osteosarcoma of the jaws. Analysis of 56 cases. Cancer, 20:377, 1967.
250. Gasparini, G., Recher, G., Favretto, S., Visona, A., Bevilacqua, P., and Del Fior, S.: Simultaneous cis-platinum (CDDP) and radiotherapy (RT) in inoperable or advanced squamous cell carcinoma of the head and neck (H&N). (Abstract #663) Proc. Am. Soc. Clin. Oncol., 8:170, 1989.
251. Gastpar, H., Wilmes, E., and Wolf, H.: Epidemiologic, etiologic and immunologic aspects of nasopharyngeal carcinoma (NPC). J. Med., 12:257, 1981.
252. George, T. K., Sant Agnese, A. D., and Bennett, J. M.: Chemotherapy for metastatic merkel cell carcinoma. Cancer, 56:1034, 1985.
253. Gerster, H.: Beta-carotene and smoking. J. Nutr. Growth Cancer, 4:45, 1987.
254. Ghosh, R., Sharma, J. K., and Ghosh, P. K.: Sister chromatid exchanges in the

lymphocytes of patients with oral leukoplakia. Cancer Genet. Cytogenet., 36:177, 1988.

255. Ghossein, N. A., and Bataini, J. P.: The role of radiotherapy in the treatment of neck metastases from head and neck cancer. *In* Head and Neck Cancer. Edited by G. T. Wolf. Boston, Martinus Nijhoff, 1984, pp. 169–199.
256. Ghossein, N. A., Bataini, J. P., Ennuyen, A., Stacey, P., and Krishnaswamy, V.: Local control and site of failure in radially irradiated supraglottic laryngeal cancer. Radiology, 112:187, 1974.
257. Giaccone, G.,Bagatella, M., Donadio, M., and Calciati, A.: Phase II study of divided-dose vinblastine in advanced cancer patients. Tumori, 75:248, 1989.
258. Gillis, T. M., Incze, J., Strong, M. S., Vaughan, C. W., and Simpson, G. T.: Natural history and management of keratosis, atypia carcinoma-in situ, and microinvasive cancer of the larynx. Am. J. Surg., 146:512, 1983.
259. Givens, C. D., Johns, M. E., and Cantrell, R. W.: Carcinoma of the tonsil: Analysis of 162 cases. Arch. Otolaryngol., 107:730, 1981.
260. Gladstone, W. S., and Kerr, H. O.: Epidermiod carcinoma of the lower lip: Results of radiation therapy of the local lesions. Am. J. Roentgen., 79:101, 1958.
261. Glick, J. H., Marcial, V., Richter, M., and Velez-Garcia, E.: The adjuvant treatment of inoperable Stage III and IV epidermoid carcinoma of the head and neck with platinum and bleomycin infusions prior to definitive radiotherapy: an RTOG pilot study. Cancer, 46:1919, 1980.
262. Goepfert, H., Guillamondegui, O. M., Jesse, R. H., and Lindberg, R. D.: Squamous cell carcinoma of nasal vestibule. Arch. Otolaryngol. Head Neck Surg., 100:8, 1974.
263. Goepfert, H., Jesse, R. H., Fletcher, G. H., and Hamberger, A.: Optimal treatment for technically resectable squamous cell carcinoma of the supraglottic larynx. Laryngoscope, 85:14, 1975.
264. Goepfert, H., Lindberg, R. D., and Jesse, R. H.: Combined laryngeal conservation surgery and irradiation: Can we expand on the indications for conservative therapy? Otolaryngol. Head Neck Surg., 89:974, 1981.
265. Goepfert, H., Luna, M., Lindberg, R., and White, A.: Malignant salivary gland tumors of the paranasal sinuses and nasal cavity. Arch. Otolaryngol., 109:662, 1983.
266. Goepfert, H., Remmler, D., Silva, E., and Wheeler, B.: Merkel cell carcinoma (endocrine carcinoma of the skin) of the head and neck. Arch. Otolaryngol., 110:707, 1984.
267. Goffinet, D. R., Fee, W. E., Wells, J., Austin-Seymour, M., Clarke, D., Mariscal, J. M., and Goode, R. L.: 192 Ir pharyngoepiglottic fold interstitial implants: the key to successful treatment of base of tongue carcinoma by radiation therapy. Cancer, 55:941, 1985.
268. Goldsweig, H. G., and Sundaresan, N.: Chemotherapy of recurrent esthesioneuroblastoma. Am. J. Clin. Oncol.. 13:139, 1990.
269. Gollin, F. F., Ansfield, F. J., Brandenburg, J. H., Ramirez, G., and Vermund, H.: Combined therapy in advanced head and neck cancer: a randomized study. Am. J. Roentgenol. Radium. Ther. Nucl. Med., 114:83, 1972.
270. Gonzalez, M. F., Valdivieso, J. G., Sartiano, G. P., Hollman, J. M., and Worster, C. F.: Comparative study with two platinum containing combinations in locally advanced head and neck squamous cell carcinoma (HNSCC). (Abstract #572) Proc. Am. Soc. Clin. Oncol., 5:146, 1986.
271. Goodman, D. S.: Vitamin A and retinoids in health and disease. N. Engl. J. Med., 310:1023, 1984.
272. Goodwin, W. J., Bordash, G. D., Huijing, F., and Altman, N.: Inhibition of hamster tongue carcinogenesis by selenium and retinoic acid. Ann. Otol. Rhinol. Laryngol., 95:162, 1986.
273. Goolden, A. W. G.: Radiation Cancer. A review with special reference to radiation tumours in the pharynx, larynx, and thyroid. Br. J. Radiol., 30:626, 1957.
274. Gowan, G. F., and deSuto-Nagy, G.: The incidence and sites of distant metastases in head and neck carcinoma. Surg. Gynecol. Obstet., 116:603, 1953.
275. Graham, S.: Epidemiology of retinoids and cancer. J. Nat. Cancer. Inst., 73:1423, 1984.
276. Gray, A. J.: Treatment of advanced head and neck cancer with accelerated fractionation. Int. J. Radiat. Oncol. Biol. Phys., 12:9, 1986.
277. Greenberg, B., Ahmann, F., Garewal, H., Koopmann, C., Coulthard, S., Berzes, M., Alberts, D., Shimm, D., and Slymen, D.: Neoadjuvant therapy for advanced head and neck cancer with allopurinol-modulated high dose 5-fluorouracil and cisplatin. A Phase I–II study. Cancer, 59:1860, 1987.
278. Greenberg, E. R., Baron, J. A., Stukel, T. A., Stevens, M. M., Mandel, J. S., Spencer, S. K., Elias, P. M., Lowe, N., Nierenberg, D. W., and Bayrd, G.: A clinical trial of beta carotene to prevent basal-cell and squamous-cell cancers of the skin. N. Engl. J. Med., 323:789, 1990.
279. Greenwald, P., Sondik, E., and Lynch, B. S.: Diet and chemoprevention in NCI's research strategy to achieve national cancer control objectives. Annu. Rev. Public Health, 7:267, 1986.
280. Griem, M. L., and Chiang, D. T. C.: Nasopharynx. *In* Radiation Therapy of Head and Neck Cancer. Edited by G. E. Laramore. Berlin, Springer-Verlag, 1989.
281. Griffin, T. W., Pajak, T. F., Gillespie, B. W., Davis, L. W., Brady, L. W., Rubin, P., and Marcial, V. A.: Predicting the response of head and neck cancers to radiation therapy with a multivariate modelling system: an analysis of the RTOG head and neck registry. Int. J. Radiat. Oncol. Biol. Phys., 10:481, 1984.
282. Griffin, T. W., Pajak, T. F., Laramore, G. E., Duncan, W., Richter, M. P., Hendrickson, F. R., and Maor, M. H.: Neutron vs photon irradiation of inoperable salivary gland tumors: results of an RTOG-MRC Cooperative Randomized Study. Int. J. Radiat. Oncol. Biol. Phys., 15:1085, 1988.
283. Grose, W. E., Lehane, D. E., Dixon, D. O., Fletcher, W. S., and Stuckey, W. J.: Comparison of methotrexate and cisplatin for patients with advanced squamous cell carcinoma of the head and neck region: A Southwest Oncology Group study. Cancer Treat. Rep., 69:577, 1985.
284. Grunberg, S. M., Felman, I. E., Gala, K. V., Johnson, K. B., and Owens, J. C.: Phase II study of etoposide (VP-16) in the treatment of advanced head and neck cancer. Am. J. Clin. Oncol., 8:393, 1985.
285. Guillamondegui, O. M., Byers, R. M., and Tapley, N. du V.: Malignant tumors of the salivary gland. *In* Textbook of Radiotherapy 3rd edition. Edited by G. H. Fletcher. Philadelphia, Lea & Febiger, 1980.
286. Gupta, N. K., Pointon, R. C., and Wilkinson, P. M.: A randomized clinical trial to contrast radiotherapy with radiotherapy and methotrexate given synchronously in head and neck cancer. Clin. Radiol., 38:575, 1987.
287. Guthrie, T. H., Brubaker, L. H., Porubsky, E. S., Isaacs, J. H., Erwin, S. A., and Roberts, W. H.: Circadian cisplatin (C), bleomycin (B) and 5-fluorouracil (F) in advanced squamous cell carcinoma of the head and neck (SCCH). (Abstract #689) Proc. Am. Soc. Clin. Oncol., 9:178, 1990.
288. Guthrie, T. H., Jr., Porubsky, E. S., Luxenberg, M. N., Shah, K. J., Wurtz, K. L., and Watson, P. R.: Cisplatin-based chemotherapy in advanced basal and squamous cell carcinoma of the skin: Results in 28 patients including 13 patients receiving multimodality therapy. J. Clin. Oncol., 8:342, 1990.
289. Haas, C., Anderson, T., Byhardt, R., Cox, J., Duncavage, J., Grossman, T., Haas, J., Libnoch, J., Malin, T., Ritch, P., and Toohill, R.: Randomized neo-adjuvant study of 5-fluorouracil (FU) and cis-platinum (DDP) for patients (PTS) with advanced resectable head and neck squamous carcinoma (ARHSC). (Abstract #735) Proc. Am. Assoc. Cancer Res., 27:185, 1986.
290. Haas, J. S., and Cox, J. D.: Cervical nodal metastasis from an unknown primary carcinoma. *In* Radiation Therapy of Head and Neck Cancer. Edited by G. E. Laramore. Berlin, Springer-Verlag, 1988.
291. Haines, I., Bosl, G., Pfister, D., Spiro, R., Gerold, F., Sessions, R., Shah, J., Strong, E., Vikram, B., and Harrison, L.: Very-high-dose cisplatin with bleomycin infusion as initial treatment of advanced head and neck cancer. J. Clin. Oncol., 5:1594, 1987.
292. Hall, E. J.: Radiobiology for the Radiologist, 3rd ed. Hagerstown, MD, Harper & Row, 1988.
293. Han, J., Jiao, L., Lu, Y., Sun, Z., Gu, Q. M., and Scanlon, K. J.: Evaluation of N-4-(Hydroxycarbophenyl) retinamide as a cancer prevention agent and as a cancer chemotherapeutic agent. In Vivo, 4:153, 1990.
294. Harrison, D. F. N.: Surgical management of hypopharyngeal cancer. Arch. Otolaryngol. Head Neck Surg., 105:149, 1979.
295. Harrison, L., Bosl, G., Fass, D., Armstrong, J., Pfister, D. G., Motzer, R., Weisen, S., Teeple, C., Sessions, R., Shah, J., Spiro, R., and Strong, E.: A new chemo-radiation program for advanced, unresectable head and neck cancer. Third International Head and Neck Oncology Research Conference, Las Vegas, Nevada. 1990.
296. Harrold, C. C.: Management of cancer of the floor of mouth. Am. J. Surg., 122:487, 1971.
297. Hartenstein, R., Wendt, T. G., and Kastenbauer, E. R.: 5-Fluorouracil/folinic acid/cisplatin-combination and accelerated split-course radiotherapy in advanced head and neck cancer. Adv. Exp. Med. Biol., 244:275, 1988.
298. Harwood, A. R., Beale, F. A., Cummings, B. J., Keane, T. J., Payne, D. G., Rider, W. D., Rawlinson, E., and Elhakim, T.: Supraglottic laryngeal carcinoma: an analysis of dose-time-volume factors in 410 patients. Int. J. Radiat. Oncol. Biol. Phys., 9:311, 1983.
299. Harwood, A. R., Bryce, D. P., and Rider WD: Management of T3 glottic cancer. Arch. Otolaryngol., 106:697, 1980.
300. Harwood, A. R., and DeBoer, G.: Prognostic factors in T2 glottic cancer. Cancer, 45:991, 1980.
301. Harwood, A. R., Hawkins, N. V., Keane, T., Cummings, B., Beale, F. A., Rider, W. D., and Bryce, D. P.: Radiotherapy in early glottic cancer. Laryngol., 90:465, 1980.
302. Harwood, A. R., Hawkins, N. V., Rider, W. D., and Bryce, D. P.: Radiation therapy of early glottic cancer I. Int. J. Radiat. Oncol. Biol. Phys., 5:473, 1979.
303. Haselow, R. E., Adams, G. S., and Oken, M. M.: Simultaneous cis-platinum (DDP) and radiation therapy (RT) for locally advanced unresectable head and neck cancer. (Abstract #C-780) Proc. Am. Soc. Clin. Oncol., 2:160, 1983.
304. Haselow, R. E., Warshaw, M. G., and Oken, M. M.: Radiation alone versus radiation with weekly low dose cis-platinum in unresectable cancer of the head and neck. *In* Head and Neck Cancer, Volume II. Edited by W. E. Fee, Jr., H. Goepfert, M. E. Johns, E. W. Strong, and P. H. Ward, Jr. Philadelphia, B. C. Decker, 1990, pp. 279–281.
305. Havlin, K. A., Kuhn, J. G., Myers, J. W., Ozols, R. F., Mattox, D. E., Clark, G. M., and von Hoff, D. D.: High-dose cisplatin for locally advanced or metastatic head and neck cancer: A phase II pilot study. Cancer, 63:423, 1989.
306. Head and Neck Contracts Program: Adjuvant chemotherapy for advanced head and neck squamous carcinoma. Final report of the Head and Neck Contracts Program. Cancer, 60:301, 1987.
307. Henderson, B. E., Louie, E., SooHoo Jing, J., Buell, P., and Gardner, M. B.: Risk factors associated with nasopharyngeal carcinoma. N. Engl. J. Med., 295:1101, 1977.
308. Hendrickson, F. R.: Radiation therapy treatment of larynx cancers. Cancer, 55:2058, 1985.
309. Hennekens, C. H.: Micronutrients and cancer prevention. N. Eng. J. Med., 315:1288, 1986.
310. Henriquez, I., Martin Algarra, S., Bilbao, I., and Calvo, F. A.: Continuous intra-arterial (ia) infusion of carboplatin (CBDCA) and 5-fluorouracil (5FU) in unresectable locally advanced (stage III–IV) head and neck cancer. (Abstract #684) Proc. Am. Soc. Clin. Oncol., 8:176, 1989.
311. Heo, D. S., Whiteside, T. L., Johnson, J. T., Chen, K. N., Barnes, E. L., and Herberman, R. B.: Long term interleukin 2 dependent growth and cytotoxic activity of tumor-infiltrating lymphocytes from human squamous cell carcinomas of the head and neck. Cancer Res., 47:6353, 1987.
312. Hester, T. R., McConnel, F. M., Nahal, F., Juriewicz, M. J., and Brown, R. G.: Reconstruction of the cervical esophagus, hypopharynx and oral cavity using free jejunal transfer. Am. J. Surg., 140:487, 1980.
313. Hill, B. T., and Price, L. A.: Long term survival advantage in patients with advanced oropharyngeal squamous cell carcinoma receiving two courses of initial schedule a non-cisplatin containing combination chemotherapy before definitive local therapy. (Abstract #685) Proc. Am. Soc. Clin. Oncol., 9:177, 1990.
314. Hill, B. T., Price, L. A., and MacRae, K.: Importance of primary site in assessing chemotherapy response and 7-year survival data in advanced squamous-cell carcinomas of the head and neck treated with initial combination chemotherapy without cisplatin. J. Clin. Oncol., 4:1340, 1986.
315. Hintz, B. L., Kagan, R., Wollin, M., Rao, A. R., Ryoo, M. C., Nussbaum, H., and Rowland, J.: Treatment selection for base of tongue carcinoma. J. Surg. Oncol., 41:165, 1989.
316. Hollingshead, A. C., Lee, O., Chretien, P. B., Tarpley, J. L., Rawls, W. E., and Adam, E.: Antibodies to herpesvirus nonvirion antigens in squamous carcinomas. Science, 182:713, 1973.
317. Holoye, P. Y., Byers, R. M., Gard, D. A., Goepfert, H., Guillamondegui, O. M., and Jesse, R. H.: Combination chemotherapy of head and neck cancer. Cancer, 42:1661, 1978.
318. Holsti, L. R., Mattson, K., Niiranen, A., Standertskiold-Nordenstam, C. G., Stenman,

S., Sovijarvi, A., and Cantell, K.: Enhancement of radiation effects by alpha interferon in the treatment of small cell carcinoma of the lung. Int. J. Radiat. Oncol. Biol. Phys., 13:1161, 1987.

319. Hong, W. K., Bhutani, R., Shapshay, S. M., and Strong, M. S.: Induction chemotherapy in advanced previously untreated squamous cell head and neck cancer with cisplatin and bleomycin. *In* Cisplatin: Current Status and New Developments. Prestayki, A. W., Crooke, S. T., and Carter, S. K. (eds.). New York, Academic Press, 1980, pp. 431–444.

320. Hong, W. K., and Bromer, R.: Chemotherapy in head and neck cancer. Current concepts. N. Engl. J. Med., 308:75, 1983.

321. Hong, W. K., Bromer, R. H., Amato, D. A., Shapshay, S., Vincent, M., Vaughan, C., Willett, B., Katz, A., Welch, J., Fofonoff, S., and Strong, M. S.: Patterns of relapse in locally advanced head and neck cancer patients who achieved complete remission after combined modality therapy. Cancer, 56:1242, 1985.

322. Hong, W. K., Choksi, A., and Dimery, I. W.: Sequential induction chemotherapy and radiotherapy for advanced head and neck cancer: Potential impact of treatment in advanced laryngeal and nasopharyngeal carcinomas. Head and Neck Cancer, 282–285, 1990.

323. Hong, W. K., Endicott, J., Itri, L. M., Doos, W., Batsakis, J. G., Bell, R., Fofonoff, S., Byers, R., Atkinson, E. N., and Vaughan, C.: 13-cis-retinoic acid in the treatment of oral leukoplakia. N. Engl. J. Med., 315:1501, 1986.

324. Hong, W. K., Lippman, S. M., Itri, L. M., Karp, D. D., Lee, J. S., Byers, R. M., Schantz, S. P., Kramer, A. M., Lotan, R., Peters, L. J., Dimery, I. W., Brown, B. W., and Goepfert, H.: Prevention of second primary tumors with isotretinoin in squamous cell carcinoma of the head and neck. N. Engl. J. Med., 323:795, 1990.

325. Hong, W. K., Schaefer, S., Issell, B., Cummings, C., Luedke, D., Bromer, R., Fofonoff, S., D'Aoust, J., Shapshay, S., Welch, J., Levin, E., Vincent, M., Vaughan, C., and Strong, S.: A prospective randomized trial of methotrexate versus cisplatin in the treatment of recurrent squamous cell carcinoma of the head and neck. Cancer, 52:206, 1983.

326. Hong, W. K., Shapshay, S. M., Bhutani, R., Craft, M. L., Ucmakli, A., Yamaguchi, K. T., Vaughan, C. W., and Strong, M. S.: Induction chemotherapy in advanced squamous head and neck carcinoma with high-dose cis-platinum and bleomycin infusion. Cancer, 44:19, 1979.

327. Hong, W. K., Wolf, G. T., Fisher, S., Spaulding, M., Endicott, J., Laramore, G., Hillman, R., McClatchey, K., and Fye, C.: Laryngeal preservation with induction chemotherapy (CT) and radiotherapy (XRT) in the treatment for advanced laryngeal cancer: interim survival data of VA Laryngeal Cancer Study Group #286. (Abstract #650) Proc. Am. Soc. Clin. Oncol., 8:167, 1989.

328. Horiot, J. C., van den Bogaert, W., Ang, K. K., van der Schueren, E., Bartelink, H., Gonzales, D., de Pauw, M., and van Glabbeke, M.: European Organization for Research on Treatment of Cancer trials using radiotherapy with multiple fractions per day: A 1978–1987 survey. Front. Radiat. Ther. Oncol., 22:149, 1988.

329. Hornedo-Muguiro, J., So, M., Spaulding, M. B., Van Echo, D. A., Donehouser, R., Ettinger, D., and Aisner, J.: Phase II trial of carboplatin (CBDCA) in aerodigestive malignancies. (Abstract #C-530) Proc. Am. Soc. Clin. Oncol., 4:136, 1985.

330. Hoye, R. C., Herrold, K. M., and Smith, R.: A clincopathological study of epidermoid carcinoma of the head and neck. Cancer, 15:741, 1962.

331. Hu, L., Crowe, D. L., Rheinwald, J. G., Chambon, P., and Gudas, L. J.: Abnormal expression of retinoic acid receptors and keratin 19 by human oral and epidermal squamous cell carcinoma cell lines. Cancer Res., 51:3972, 1991.

332. Huang, A. T., Cole, T. B., Fishburn, R., and Jelovsek, S. B.: Adjuvant chemotherapy after surgery and radiation for stage III and IV head and neck cancer. Ann. Surg., 200:195, 1984.

333. Huang, A. T., Fisher, S. R., and Cole, T. B.: A study of postoperative and/or postradiation adjuvant chemotherapy (abstr). Proceedings of the 2nd International Head and Neck Oncology Research Conference, Arlington, VA, Sept. 10–13, 1987.

334. Huang, S. C.: Nasopharyngeal cancer: A review of 1605 patients treated radically with cobalt 60. Int. J. Radiat. Oncol. Biol. Phys., 6:401, 1980.

335. Huang, S. C., Lui, L. T., and Lynn, T. C.: Nasopharyngeal cancer: study III. A review of 1206 patients treated with combined modalities. Int. J. Radiat. Oncol. Biol. Phys., 11:1789, 1985.

336. Hussey, D. H., and Abrams, J. P.: Combined therapy in advanced head and neck cancer: hydroxyurea and radiotherapy. Prog. Clin. Cancer, 6:79, 1975.

337. Ikic, D., Padovan, I., Brodarec, I., Knezevic, M., and Soos, E.: Application of human leucocyte interferon in patients with tumours of the head and neck. Lancet, 1:1025, 1981.

338. Ildstad, S. T., Bigelow, M. E., and Remensnyder, J. P.: Squamous cell carcinoma of the tongue: A comparison of the anterior two thirds of the tongue with its base. Am. J. Surg., 146:456, 1983.

339. Isaacs, J. H., Mooney, S., Mendenhall, W. M., and Parsons, J. T.: Cancer of the maxillary sinus treated with surgery and/or radiation therapy. The American Surgeon, 56:327, 1990.

340. Ishikawa, T., Ikawa, T., Eura, M., Fukiage, T., and Masuyama, K.: Adoptive immunotherapy for head and neck cancer with killer cells induced by stimulation with autologous or allogeneic tumour cells and recombinant interleukin-2. Acta Otolaryngol. (Stockh.), 107:346, 1989.

341. Issa, P. Y.: Cancer of the supraglottic larynx treated by radiotherapy exclusively. Int. J. Radiat. Oncol. Biol. Phys., 15:843, 1985.

342. Jacobs, C.: Adjuvant chemotherapy for head and neck cancer. J. Clin. Oncol., 7:823, 1989.

343. Jacobs, C.: The internist in the management of head and neck cancer. Ann. Intern. Med., 113:771, 1990.

344. Jacobs, C., Bertino, J. R., Goffinet, D. R., Fu, W. E., and Good, R. L.: 24-hour infusion of cis-platinum in head and neck cancers. Cancer, 42:2135, 1978.

345. Jacobs, C., Goffinet, D. R., Goffinet, L., Kohler, M., and Fee, W. E.: Chemotherapy as a substitute for surgery in the treatment advanced resectable head and neck cancer: A report from the Northern California Oncology Group. Cancer, 60:1178, 1987.

346. Jacobs, C., Lyman, G., Velez-Garcia, E., Sridhar, K. S., Knight, W., Hochster, H., Goodnough, L. T., Mortimer, J. E., Einhorn, L. H., Schacter, L., Cherng, N., Dalton, T., Burroughs, J., and Rozencweig, M.: A phase III randomized study comparing cisplatin and fluorouracil as single agents and in combination for advanced squamous cell carcinoma of the head and neck. J. Clin. Oncol., 10:257, 1992.

347. Jacobs, C., and Makuch, R.: Efficacy of adjuvant chemotherapy for patients with resectable head and neck cancer: A subset analysis of the Head and Neck Contracts Program. J. Clin. Oncol., 8:838, 1990.

348. Jacobs, C., Meyers, F., Hendrickson, C., Kohler, M., and Carter, S.: A randomized phase III study of cisplatin with or without methotrexate for recurrent squamous cell carcinoma of the head and neck. A Northern California Oncology Group study. Cancer, 52:1563, 1983.

349. Jacobs, J. R., Pajak, T. F., Al-Sarraf, M., Kinzie, J., Stetz, J., Davis, L. W., Leibel, S., and Laramore, G. E.: Chemotherapy following surgery for head and neck cancer. A Radiation Therapy Oncology Group Study. Am. J. Clin. Oncol., 12:185, 1989.

350. Jacobs, J. R., Sessions, D. G., and Ogura, J. H.: Recurrent carcinoma of the larynx and the hypopharynx. Otolaryngol. Head Neck Surg., 88:425, 1980.

351. Jakobsson, P. A., Eneroth, D. M., Killander, D., Moberger, G., and Martensson, B.: Histologic classification and grading of malignancy in carcinoma of the larynx. Acta Radiol. Ther. Phys. Biol., 12:1, 1973.

352. Jaulerry, C., Mosseri, V., Brunin, F., Rodriguez, J., Pontuert, D., Brugere, J., Jouve, M., Pouillart, P., and Bataini, P.: Induction chemotherapy in advanced head and neck cancer. Final results of a randomized trial. Int. J. Radiat. Oncol. Biol. Phys., 15(Suppl. 1):137, 1989.

353. Jesse, R. H.: Radiation in the treatment of squamous carcinoma of paranasal sinus. Am. J. Surg., 110:552, 1965.

354. Jesse, R. H.: Extensive cancer of the lip. Surgical therapy. Arch. Surg., 94:509, 1967.

355. Johns, M. E., and Goldsmith, M. M.: Incidence, diagnosis, and classification of salivary gland tumors. Oncology, 3:47, 1989.

356. Johns, M. E., and Kaplan, M. J.: Malignant neoplasms. *In* Otolaryngology Head and Neck Surgery, Vol. II. Edited by C. W. Cummings, J. M. Fredreickson, L.A. Harker, C. J. Krause, and D. E. Schuller, St. Louis, Mosby, 1986, p. 1049.

357. Johnson, J. T., Myers, E. N., Bedetti, C. D., Barnes, E. L., Schramm, V. L., Jr., and Thearle, P. B.: Cervical lymph node metastases. Incidence and implications of extracapsular carcinoma. Arch. Otolaryngol., 111:534, 1985.

358. Johnson, J. T., Myers, E. N., Schramm, V. L., Jr., Mayernik, D. G., Nolan, T. A., Sigler, B. A., and Wagner, R. L.: Adjuvant chemotherapy for high-risk squamous cell carcinoma of the head and neck. J. Clin. Oncol., 5:456, 1987.

359. Jorgensen, K., Elbrond, O., and Anderson, A. P.: Carcinoma of the lip. A series of 869 cases. Acta Radiol. Ther. Phys. Biol., 12:177, 1973.

360. Kabat, G. C., and Wynder, E. L.: Type of alcoholic beverage and oral cancer. Int. J. Cancer, 43:190, 1989.

361. Kalnins, I. K., Leonard, A. G., Sako, K., Razack, M. S., and Shedd, D. P.: Correlation between prognosis and degree of lymph node involvement in carcinoma of the oral cavity. Am. J. Surg., 134:540, 1977.

362. Kaplan, B. H., Schoenfeld, D., and Vogl, S. E.: Treatment of recurrent (REC) or metastatic (MET) squamous cancer of the head and neck (SCH&N) with methotrexate (M), M plus Corynebacterium parvum (CP) or M plus bleomycin (B) plus diamminedichloroplatinum (D): A prospective randomized trial of the Eastern Cooperative Oncology Group. (Abstract #C-780) Proc. Am. Assoc. Cancer Res., 22:532, 1981.

363. Kaplan, M. J., Johns, M. E., Clark, D. A., and Cantrell, R. W.: Glottic carcinoma: The role of surgery and irradiation. Cancer, 53:2641, 1984.

364. Kapstad, B., Bang, G., Rennaes, S., and Dahler, A.: Combined preoperative treatment with cobalt and bleomycin in patients with head and neck carcinoma a controlled clinical study. Int. J. Radiat. Oncol. Biol. Phys., 4:85, 1978.

365. Kapstad, B.: Cobalt and bleomycin against carcinomas of head and neck. A controlled clinical study. Acta Otolaryngol. (Suppl.), 360:171, 1979.

366. Karim, A. B. M. F., Snow, G. B., Hasman, A., Chang, S. C., Kelhotz, A., and Hoekstra, F.: Dose response in radiotherapy for glottic carcinoma. Cancer, 41:1728, 1978.

367. Karim, A. B., Snow, G. B., Siek, H. T., and Njo, K. H.: The quality of voice in patient irradiated for laryngeal carcinoma. Cancer, 51:47, 1983.

368. Karp, D., Vaughan, C., Carter, R., Willett, B., Heeren, T., Calarese, P., Zeitels, S., Strong, M. S., and Hong, W.: Voice preservation using induction chemotherapy (CT) plus radiation therapy (RT) as an alternative to laryngectomy in advanced head and neck cancer: long term follow up. Am. J. Clin. Oncol., 14:273, 1991.

369. Kashima, H. K.: Epidemiology and carcinogens in head and neck cancer. *In* Head and Neck Cancer. Edited by W. E. Fee, H. Goepfert, M. E. Johns, E. W. Strong, and P. H. Ward. Philadelphia, B. C. Decker, 1990, pp. 39–43.

370. Katz, A. E.: Immunobiologic staging of patients with carcinoma of the head and neck. Laryngoscope, 93:445, 1983.

371. Katz, D. E., Seder, R. H., and Keggins, J. J.: Plasmapheresis in Patients with Advanced Carcinoma of the Head and Neck. *In* Head and Neck Oncology Research. Edited by G. T. Wolf and T. E. Carey. Amsterdam, Kugler and Ghedini, 1988, pp. 151–157.

372. Kazem, I., and van den Broek, P.: Planned preoperative radiation therapy vs definitive radiotherapy for advanced laryngeal carcinoma. Laryngoscope, 94:1355, 1984.

373. Keane, T. J., Harwood, A. R., Beale, F. A., Cummings, B. J., Payne, D. G., Elhakim, T., and Rawlingson, E.: A pilot study of mitomycin-C/5-fluorouracil infusion combined with split course radiation therapy for carcinomas of the larynx and hypopharynx. J. Otolaryngol., 15:286, 1986.

374. Keane, T. J., Harwood, A. R., and Danjoux, C.: Results of a randomized trial of radiation compared to radiation and chemotherapy for advanced laryngeal and hypopharyngeal squamous carcinoma. (Abstract #55). Proc. 2nd Int. Conf. on Head Neck Cancer, Boston, MA, July, 31–August, 5, 1988.

375. Keegan, P., Pillsbury, H. C., Weissler, M., Rosenman, J., Varia, M., and Tepper, J.: Hyperfractionated radiotherapy with or without simultaneous cisplatin and fluorouracil (5-FU) in the treatment of advanced head and neck cancer. (Abstract #667) Proc. Am. Soc. Clin. Oncol., 9:172, 1990.

376. Keim, W. F., Shapiro, M. J., and Rosin, H. D.: Study of post laryngectomy stomal recurrence. Arch. Otolaryngol., 81:183, 1965.

377. Kelly, M. D., Hahn, S. S., Spaulding, C. A., Kersh, C. R., Constable, W. C., and Cantrell, R. W.: Definitive radiotherapy in the management of stage I and II carcinomas of the glottis. Laryngoscope, 98:235, 1989.

378. Kerpel-Fronius, S., Mechl, Z., Csetenyi, J., Nagykalnai, T., Gyergyay, F., Jassem, J., Vuletic, L., Kolaric, K., and Eckhardt, S.: Pharmacokinetic and response rate of 5-fluorouracil (5-FU) given in daily 4 H infusion combined with cisplatin (CDDP) in head and neck cancer (H&N CA): Phase I–II. A South-East European Oncology Group (SEEOG) study. (Abstract #581) Proc. Amer. Soc. Clin. Oncol., 8:150, 1988.

379. Khojasteh, A., Reynolds, R., Ruble, K., Garcia, A., Coleman, J., and Gohel, M.: A phase III, comparison of sequence-dependent schedules of cisplatin (DDP) and 5-

fluorouracil (5FU) in carcinoma of head and neck (H&N Ca). An up date report. (Abstract #611) Proc. Amer. Soc. Clin. Oncol., 8:158, 1988.
380. Khoury, G. G., and Paterson, I. C.: Nasopharyngeal carcinoma: A review of cases treated by radiotherapy and chemotherapy. Clin. Radiol., 38:17, 1987.
381. Kirchner, J. A.: Two hundred laryngeal cancers: patterns of growth and spread as seen in serial sections. Laryngoscope, 87:474, 1977.
382. Kirchner, J. A., Cornog, J. L., and Holmes, R. E.: Transglottic cancer. Its growth and spread within the larynx. Arch. Otolaryngol., 99:247, 1974.
383. Kirchner, J. A., and Som, M. L.: Clinical and histologic observation on supraglottic cancer. Am. Otol. Rtinol. Laryngol., 80:638, 1971.
384. Kirkwood, J. M., Miller, D., Weichselbaum, R., and Pitman, S.: Predefinitive and postdefinitive chemotherapy for locally advanced squamous cell carcinoma of the head and neck. Laryngoscope, 89:573, 1979.
385. Kish, J. A., Ensley, J. F., Jacobs, J. R., Binns, P., and Al Sarraf, M.: Evaluation of high-dose cisplatin and 5-FU infusion as initial therapy in advanced head and neck cancer. Am. J. Clin. Oncol., 11:553, 1988.
386. Kish, J. A., Ensley, J. F., Jacobs, J., Weaver, A., Cummings, G., and Al Sarraf, M.: A randomzed trial of cisplatin (CACP) + 5-fluorouracil (5-FU) infusion and CACP + 5-FU bolus for recurrent and advanced squamous cell carcinoma of the head and neck. Cancer, 56:2740, 1985.
387. Kish, J. A., Tapazoglou, E., Ensley, J., and Al-Sarraf, M.: Activity of ifosfamide (NSC-109724) in recurrent head and neck cancer patients. (Abstract #1130) Proc. Am. Assoc. Cancer. Res., 31:190, 1990.
388. Kish, J. A., Weaver, A., Jacobs, J., Cummings, G., and Al Sarraf, M.: Cisplatin and 5-fluorouracil infusion in patients with recurrent and disseminated epidermoid cancer of the head and neck. Cancer, 53:1819, 1984.
389. Knowlton, A. H., Percarpio, B., Bobrow, S., and Fischer, J. J.: Methotrexate and radiation therapy in the treatment of advanced head and neck tumors. Radiology, 116:709, 1975.
390. Koch, H. F.: Biochemical treatment of precancerous oral lesions: the effectiveness of various analogues of retinoic acid. J. Maxillofac, Surg., 6:59, 1978.
391. Koch, H. F.: Effect of retinoids on precancerous lesions of oral mucosa. *In* Retinoids, Advances in Basic Research and Therapy. Edited by C. E. Orfanos, et al. Berlin, Springer-Verlag, 1981, pp. 307–12.
392. Kokal, W. A., Gardive, R. L., Sheibani, K., Zak, I. W., Beatty, J. D., Riihimaki, D. U., Wagman, L. D., and Terz, J. J.: Tumor DNA content as a prognostic indication in squamous cell carcinoma of the head and neck region. Am. J. Surg., 156:276, 1988.
393. Komiyara, S., Matsui, K., Kudoh, S., Nogae, I., Kuratoma, Y., Saburi, Y., Asoh, K., Kohno, K., and Kuwano, M.: Establishment of tumor cell lines from a patient with head and neck cancer and their different sensitivities to anti-cancer agents. Cancer, 63:675, 1989.
394. Kotwall, C., Sako, K., Razack, M. S., Rao, U., Bakamjian, V., and Shedd, D. P.: Metastatic patterns in squamous cell cancer of the head and neck. Am. J. Surg., 154:439, 1987.
395. Kramer, S.: Methotrexate and radiation therapy in the treatment of advanced squamous cell carcinoma of the oral cavity, oropharynx, supraglottic larynx, and hypopharynx: (Preliminary report of a controlled clinical trial of the Radiation Therapy Oncology Group). Can. J. Otolaryngol., 4:213, 1975.
396. Kramer, S., Gleber, R. D., Snow, J. B., Marcial, V. A., Lowry, L. D., Davis, L. W., and Chandler, R.: Combined radiation therapy and surgery in the management of advanced head and neck cancer: final report of the study 73-03 of the Radiation Therapy Oncology Group. Head Neck Surg., 10:19, 1987.
397. Kun, L. E., Toohill, R. J., Holoye, P. Y., Duncavage, J. A., Byhardt, R. W., Ritch, P. S., Grossman, T. W., Hoffmann, R. G., Cox, J. D., and Malin, T.: A randomized study of adjuvant chemotherapy for cancer of the upper aerodigestive tract. Int. J. Radiat. Oncol. Biol. Phys., 12:173, 1986.
398. Laccourreye, H., Brasnu, D. F., and Beutter, P.: Carcinoma of the laryngeal margin. Head Neck Surg., 5:500, 1983.
399. Lampe, I., and Zatzkin, H.: Pulmonary metastases of pseudoadenomatous basal cell carcinoma (mucous and salivary gland tumor). Radiology, 53:379, 1949.
400. Laramore, G. E.: Radiation Therapy of Head and Neck Cancer. Berlin, Springer-Verlag, 1988.
401. Laramore, G. E., Clubb, B., Quick, C., Amer, M. H., Ali, M., Greer, W., Mahboubi, E., El-Senoussi, M., Schultz, H., and El-Akkad, S. M.: Nasopharyngeal carcinoma in Saudi Arabia: a retrospective study of 166 cases treated with curative intent. Int. J. Radiat. Oncol. Biol. Phys., 15:1119, 1988.
402. Larsson, L. G., Sandstrom, A., and Westling, P.: Relationship of Plummer-Vinson disease to cancer of the upper alimentary tract in Sweden. Cancer Res., 35:3308, 1975.
403. Lee, G., Pitman, S. W., and Bertino, J. R.: Weekly hydroxyurea in squamous head and neck cancer. (Abstract #C-572) Proc. Am. Soc. Clin. Oncol., 4:147, 1985.
404. Lee, J. G., and Krause, C. J.: Radical neck dissection: Elective, therapeutic and secondary. Arch. Otolaryngol., 101:656, 1975.
405. Lee, J. S., Kim, J. S., Blick, M., Hong, W. K., and Lotan, R.: Effects of retinoic acid on oncogene expression in a human head and neck squamous carcinoma cell line. *In* Head and Neck Oncology Research. Edited by G. T. Wolf and T. E. Carey, Berkeley, CA, Kugler & Ghedini, 1987, pp. 43–48.
406. Lee, N. K., Goepfert, H., and Wendt, C. D.: Supraglottic laryngectomy for intermediate-stage cancer: UT MD Anderson Cancer Center experience with combined therapy. Laryngoscope, 100:831, 1990.
407. Leipzig, B., Cummings, C. W., Chung, C. T., Johnson, J. T., and Sagerman, R. H.: Carcinoma of the anterior tongue. Ann. Otol. Rhinol. Laryngol., 91:94, 1982.
408. Leonard, J. R., Litton, W. B., Latourette, H. B., and McCube, B. F.: Combined radiation and surgical therapy: tongue, tonsil and floor of mouth. Ann. Otol. Rhinol. Laryngol., 77:514, 1968.
409. Leone, L. A., Albala, M. M., and Rege, V. B.: Treatment of carcinoma of the head and neck with intravenous methotrexate. Cancer, 21:828, 1968.
410. Leroux, R. J.: A statistical study of 620 laryngeal carcinomas of the glottic region personally operated upon more than 5 years ago. Laryngoscope, 85:1440, 1985.
411. Lester, E. P., and Tharapel, S. A.: Chromosome abnormalities in squamous carcinoma cell lines of head and neck origin. Third International Head and Neck Oncology Research Conference, Las Vegas, Nevada, 1990.
412. Levendag, P., Sessions, R., Vikran, B., Strong, E. W., Shah, J. P., Spiro, R., and Gerold, F.: The problem of neck relapse in early stage supraglottic larynx cancer. Cancer, 63:345, 1989.
413. Levine, P. A., Frierson, H. F., Stewart, F. M., Mills, S. E., Fechner, R. E., and Cantrell, R. W.: A distinctive and highly aggressive neoplasm. Laryngoscope, 97:905, 1987.
414. Levitt, M., Mosher, M. B., DeConti, R. C., Farber, L. R., Skeel, R. T., Marsh, J. C., Mitchell, M. S., Papac, R. J., Thomas, E. D., and Bertino, J. R.: Improved therapeutic index of methotrexate with "leucovorin rescue." Cancer Res., 33:1729, 1973.
415. Licitra, L., Marchini, S., Spinazze, S., De Braud, F., Rossi, A., Salvatori, P., and Bonadonna, G.: Phase II study with cisplatin (DDP) for advanced carcinoma of salivary gland origin. (Abstract #584) Proc. Amer. Soc. Clin. Oncol., 8:151, 1988.
416. Lindberg, R. D., Barkley, H. T., Jesse, R. H., and Fletcher, G. H.: Evolution of the clinically negative neck in patients with squamous cell carcinoma of the faucial arch. Am. J. Roentgenol., 111:60, 1971.
417. Lippman, S. M., Bassford, T. L., Meyskens, F. L.: A quantitatively scored cancer-risk assessment tool: Its development and use. J. Cancer Education, 7:15, 1992.
418. Lippman, S. M., and Hong, W. K.: Retinoid Chemoprevention of Upper Aerodigestive Tract Carcinogenesis. *In* Important Advances In Oncology. DeVita, V. T., Hellman, S., and Rosenberg, S. A. (eds.). Philadelphia, Lippincott, 1992, pp. 91–107.
419. Lippman, S. M., and Hong, W. K.: Second malignant tumors in head and neck squamous cell carcinoma: the overshadowing threat for patients with early-stage disease (Editorial). Int. J. Radiat. Oncol. Biol. Phys., 17:691, 1989.
420. Lippman, S. M., and Hong, W. K.: Differentiation Therapy for Head and Neck Cancer. *In* Multimodality Therapy for Head and Neck Cancer. Edited by G. Snow, and J. R. Clark. Verlag Press, 1992.
421. Lippman, S. M., Kessler, J. F., Al-Sarraf, M., Alberts, D. S., Itri, L. M., Mattox, D., Von Hoff, D. D., Loescher, L., and Meyskens. F. L.: Treatment of advanced squamous cell carcinoma of the head and neck with isotretinoin: A phase II randomized trial. Invest. New Drugs, 6:51, 1988.
422. Lippman, S. M., Kessler, J. F., and Meyskens, F. L., Jr.: Retinoids as preventive and therapeutic anticancer agents. Cancer Treat. Rep., 71:391, 493, 1987.
423. Lippman, S. M., Lee, J. S., Lotan, R., Hittelman, W., Wargovich, M. J., and Hong, W. K.: Biomarkers as intermediate endpoints in chemoprevention trials. J. Natl. Cancer Inst., 82:555, 1990.
424. Lippman, S. M., and Meyskens, F. L.: Treatment of advanced squamous cell carcinoma of the skin with isotretinoin. Ann. Intern. Med., 107:499, 1987.
425. Lippman, S. M., and Meyskens, F. L.: Retinoids for the Prevention of Cancer. *In* Nutrition and Cancer Prevention: The Role of Micronutrients. Edited by T. E. Moon, and M. Micozzi. New York, Marcel Dekker, Inc, 1989, pp. 243–272.
426. Lippman, S. M., Parkinson, D. R., Itri, L. M., Weber, R. S., Schantz, S. P., Ota, D. M., Schusterman, M. A., Krakoff, I. H., Gutterman, J. U., and Hong, W. K.: 13-*cis*-retinoic acid and interferon α-2a: Effective combination therapy for advanced squamous cell carcinoma of the skin. J. Natl. Cancer Inst., 84:235, 1992.
427. Lippman, S. M., and Spitz, M. R.: Intervention in the premalignant process. Cancer Bull., 43:473, 1991.
428. Lippman, S. M., Toth, B. B., Batsakis, J. G., Lee, J. S., Weber, R. S., Craddock, C., Martin, J. W., Hays, G., Lotan, R., and Hong, W. K.: Phase-III Trial to Maintain Remission of Oral Premalignancy: Low-dose 13-cis retinoic acid (13cRA) versus beta-carotene. Proc. Am. Soc. Clin. Oncol., 11: 1992
429. Liverpool Head and Neck Oncology Group. A phase II randomized trial of cisplatinum, methotrexate, cisplatinum + methotrexate and cisplatinum + 5-FU in end stage squamous cell carcinoma of the head and neck. Liverpool Head and Neck Oncology Group. Br. J. Cancer, 61:311, 1990.
430. Lo, T. C., Wiley, A. L., Jr., Ansfield, F. J., Brandenburg, J. H., Davis, M. L., Jr., Gollin, F. F., Johnson, R. O., Ramirez, G., and Vermund, H.: Combined radiation therapy and 5-fluorouracil for advanced squamous cell carcinoma of the oral cavity and oropharynx: A randomized study. Am. J. Roentgenol., 126:229, 1976.
431. Loning, T., Ikenberg, H., Becker, J., Gissman, L., Hoepfer, I., and zur Hausen, M.: Analysis of oral papillomas, leukoplakias, and invasive carcinomas of human papillomavirus type related DNA. J. Invest. Dermatol., 84:417, 1985.
432. LoRusso, P., Tapazoglou, E., Kish, J. A., Ensley, J. F., Cummings, G., Kelly, J., and Al-Sarraf, M.: Chemotherapy for paranasal sinus carcinoma. A 10-year experience at Wayne State University. Cancer, 62:1, 1988.
433. Lund, V. J., and Howard, D. J.: Head and neck cancer in the young: A prognostic conundrum? J. Laryngology and Otology, 104:544, 1990.
434. Lustig, R. A., DeMare, P. A., and Kramer, S.: Adjuvant methotrexate in the radiotherapeutic management of advanced tumors of the head and neck. Cancer, 37:2703, 1976.
435. Lutz, C. K., Johnson, J. T., Wagner, R. L., and Myer, E. N.: Supraglottic carcinoma: Patterns of recurrence. Ann. Otol. Rhinol. Laryngol., 99:12, 1990.
436. MacComb, W. S., and Fletcher, G. H.: Cancer of the Head and Neck. Baltimore, Williams & Wilkins, 1967.
437. Maceri, D. R., Laupe, H. B., Makielski, K. H., Passamani, P. P., and Krause, C. J.: Conservation laryngeal surgery. A critical analysis. Arch. Otolaryngol., 111:361, 1985.
438. Mackay, E. N., and Sellers, A. H.: A statistical review of carcinoma of the lip. Can. Med. Assoc. J., 90:670, 1964.
439. Magno, L., Terraneo, F., Scandolaro, L., Bertoni, F., De Gregorio, M., and Ciottoli, G. B.: Lonidamine (L) and radiotherapy in head and neck cancer: A preliminary report. (Abstract #494) Proc. Am. Soc. Clin. Oncol., 6:126, 1987.
440. Mainpang, T., Razack, M. S., Sako, K., and Chen, T. Y.: Surgical salvage for recurrent "early" glottic cancers. J. Surg. Oncol., 40:32, 1989.
441. Malaker, K., Anderson, B., Beecroft, W., and Hodson, D.: Management of oral mucosal dysplasia with β-carotene and retinoic acid: a pilot cross-over study. Cancer Detect. Prev., 15:335, 1991.
442. Marcial, V. A., Pajak, T. F., Chang, C., Tupchong, L., and Stetz, J.: Hyperfractionated photon radiation therapy in the treatment of advanced squamous cell carcinoma of the oral cavity, pharynx, larynx, and sinuses, using radiation therapy as the only planned modality: (preliminary report) by the Radiation Therapy Oncology Group (RTOG). Int. J. Radiat. Oncol. Biol. Phys., 13:41, 1987.
443. Marcial, V. A., Pajak, T. F., Mohiuddin, M., Cooper, J. S., Al Sarraf, M., Mowry, P. A., Curran, W., Crissman, J., Rodriguez, M., and Velez-Garcia, E.: Concomitant cisplatin chemotherapy and radiotherapy in advanced mucosal squamous cell carcinoma of the head and neck. Cancer, 66:1861, 1990.
444. Marechal, F., Nasca, S., Morel, M., Jezekova, D., Coninx, P., Legros, M., Nguyen, T. D., and Cattan, A.: A phase III of cisplatinum versus cisplatinum-etoposide for

previously untreated squamous cell carcinoma of the head and neck. Anticancer Res., 7:455, 1987.
445. Margolin, K., Doroshow, J., Leong, L., Akman, S., Carr, B. I., Odujinrin, O., and Flanagin, B.: Combination chemotherapy with cytosine arabinoside (Ara-C) and cis-diamminedichloroplatinum (CDDP) for squamous cancers of the upper aerodigestive tract. Am. J. Clin. Oncol., 12(6):494, 1989.
446. Marks, J. E., Breaux, S., Smith, P. G., Thawley, S. E., Spector, G. G., and Sessions, D. G.: The need for elective irradiation of occult lymphatic metastases from cancer of the larynx and piriform sinus. Head Neck Surg., 8:3, 1985.
447. Marks, J. E., Freeman, R. B., Lee, F., and Ogua, J. H.: Carcinoma of the supraglottic larynx. AJR Am. J. Roentgenol., 132:255, 1979.
448. Martin, H., MacComb, W. S., and Blady, J. V.: Cancer of the lip. Ann. Surg., 114:226, 1941.
449. Martin, M., Hazan, A., Vergnes, L., Peytral, C., Lelievre, G., Senechaut, J. P., Mazeron, J. P., and Peynegre, R.: Randomized study of 5 fluorouracil (5.F.U.) and cis platinum (D.D.P) as neoadjuvant therapy in head and neck cancer. A preliminary report. (Abstract #680) Proc. Am. Soc. Clin. Oncol., 8:175, 1989.
450. Martin, M., Lelievre, G., Gehanno, P., Depondt, J., Guerrier, B., Peytral, C., Hazan, A., Dubreuil, P., Margotton, A., and Pellae-Cosser, B.: Induction carboplatin (CBDCA) and 5 Fluorouracil (5FU) Treatment Versus No Chemotherapy Before Locoregional Treatment for Oro and Pharyngolaryngeal Cancers: Preliminary results of a randomized study. Proc. Am. Soc. Clin. Oncol., 11: 1992.
451. Martin, M., Mazeron, J. J., Brun, B., Vergnes, L., Lelievre, G., Feuillade, F., Juvanon, J. M., Haddad, E., Delacour, I. S., Peynegre, R., and Pierquin, B.: Neo-adjuvant polychemotherapy of head and neck cancer: Results of a randomized study. (Abstract #590) Proc. Am. Soc. Clin. Oncol., 7:152, 1988.
452. Martin, S. A., Marks, J. E., Lee, J. Y., Bauer, W. C., and Ogura, J. H.: Carcinoma of the pyriform sinus: Predictors of TNM relapse and survival. Cancer, 46:1974, 1980.
453. Marwood, A. R., Krajbich, J. I., and Fornasier, V. L.: Radiotherapy of chondrosarcoma of bone. Cancer, 45:2769, 1980.
454. Mashberg, A. L.: Erythroplasia vs leukoplakia in the diagnosis of early asymptomatic oral squamous carcinoma. N. Engl. J. Med., 297:109, 1977.
455. Mashberg, A., and Samit, A. M.: Early detection, diagnosis and management of oral and oropharyngeal cancer. CA, 39:67, 1989.
456. Mathews-Roth, M. M.: Beta-Carotene, Canthaxanthin, and Phytoene. *In* Nutrition and Cancer Prevention: The Role of Micronutrients. T. E. Moon, and M. Micozzi. New York, Marcel Dekker, Inc. 1989, pp. 272–290.
457. Mauer, H. M., Beltangady, M., Gehan, E. A., Christ, W., Hammond, D., Hays, D. M., Heyn, R., Lawrence, W., Newton, W., and Ortega, J.: The intergroup rhabdomyosarcoma study—I: A final report. Cancer, 61:209, 1985.
458. McCoy, G. D., Hecht, S. S., and Wynder, E. L.: The roles of tobacco, alcohol, and diet in the etiology of upper alimentary and respiratory tract cancers. Prev. Med., 9:622, 1980.
459. McGovern, M. H., Bauer, W. C., and Ogura, J. H.: The incidence of cervical lymph node metastases from epidermoid carcinoma of the larynx and their relationship to certain characteristics of the primary tumor. Cancer, 14:55, 1961.
460. McLaughlin, J. K., Gridley, G., Block, G., Winn, D. M., Preston-Martin, S., Schoenberg, J. B., Greenberg, R. S., Stemhagen, A., Austin, D. F., and Ershow, A. G.: Dietary factors in oral and pharyngeal cancer. J. Natl. Cancer Inst., 80:1237, 1988.
461. McNeese, M. D., and Fletcher, G. H.: Tumors of the Major and Minor Salivary glands. *In* Radiation Therapy of Head and Neck Cancer. Edited by G. E. Laramore. Berlin, Springer-Verlag, 1988.
462. McNeil, B. J., Weichselbaum, R., and Parker, S. G.: Speech and survival: tradeoffs between quality and quantity of life in laryngeal cancer. N. Engl. J. Med., 305:982, 1981.
463. Medenica, R. N., and Slack, N.: Clinical results of leukocyte interferon-induced tumor regression in resistant human metastatic cancer resistent to chemotherapy and/or radiotherapy-pulse therapy schedule. Cancer Drug Deliv., 2:53, 1985.
464. Mehregan, D. A., and Roenigk, R. K.: Management of superficial squamous cell carcinoma of the lip with Mohs micrographic surgery. Cancer, 66:463, 1990.
465. Mendenhall, W. M., Parsons, J. T., Stringer, S. P., Cassisi, N. J., and Million, R. R.: Carcinoma of the supraglottic larynx: a basis for comparing the results of radiotherapy and surgery. Head Neck, 12:204, 1990.
466. Mendenhall, W. M., VanCise, W. S., Bova, F. J., and Million, R. R.: Analysis of time-dose factors in squamous cell carcinoma of the oral tongue and floor of mouth treated with radiation therapy alone. Int. J. Radiol. Oncol. Biol. Phys., 7:1005, 1981.
467. Meoz, R. T., Fletcher, G. H., Peters, L. J., Barkley, H. T., and Thames, H. D.: Twice daily fractionation schemes for advanced head and neck cancer. Int. J. Radiat. Oncol. Biol. Phys., 10:831, 1984.
468. Merlano, M., Conte, P. F., Tatarek, R., Scarsi, P., Barbieri, A., Benedetti, G., and Rosso, R.: Ineffectiveness of 5-fluorouracil and cisplatin as a second line chemotherapy in head and neck cancer. Tumori, 70:267, 1984.
469. Merlano, M., Corvo, R., Brema, F., Benasso, M., Bacigalupo, A., Toma, S., Rubagotti, A., Pronzato, P., and Rosso, R.: Alternating chemotherapy (CDDP + 5FU) and radiotherapy in advanced squamous cell carcinoma of the head and neck (SCC-HN). A randomized trial. (Abstract #682) Proc. Am. Soc. Clin. Oncol., 8:175, 1989.
470. Merlano, M., Rosso, R., Sertoli, M. R., Bonelli, L., Margarino, G., Grimaldi, A., Benasso, M., Gardin, G., Corvo, R., and Scarpati, D.: Sequential versus alternating chemotherapy and radiotherapy in stage III–IV squamous cell carcinoma of the head and neck: A phase III study. J. Clin. Oncol., 6:627, 1988.
471. Merlano, M., Tatarek, R., Grimaldi, A., Margarino, G., and Rosso, R.: Phase I–II trial with cisplatin and 5-FU in recurrent head and neck cancer: an effective outpatient schedule. Cancer Treat. Rep., 69:961, 1985.
472. Meyskens, F. L., Jr.: Coming of Age—the chemoprevention of cancer. N. Engl. J. Med., 323:825, 1990.
473. Miller, B., Yu, A., Tefft, M., and Leone, L.: Improved response rate in patients with advanced unresectable cancer of the head and neck. (Abstract #C-552) Proc. Am. Soc. Clin. Oncol., 4:142, 1985.
474. Million, R. R., and Cassisi, N. J.: Radical irradiation for carcinoma of the pyriform sinus. Laryngoscope, 91:439, 1981.
475. Million, R. R., Cassisi, N. J., and Wittes, R. E.: Cancer in the head and neck. *In* Cancer—Principles and Practice of Oncology. Edited by V. T. Devita, S. Hellman, and S. A. Rosenberg. Philadelphia, Lippincott, 1982. pp. 301–395.
476. Million, R. R., Parsons, J. T., and Cassisi, N. J.: Twice a day irradiation technique for squamous cell carcinoma of the head and neck. Cancer, 55:2096, 1985.
477. Mills, E. E.: The modifying effect of beta-carotene on radiation and chemotherapy induced oral mucositis. Br. J. Cancer, 57:416, 1988.
478. Mirimanoff, R. O., Wang, C. C., and Doppke, K. P.: Combined surgery and post-operative radiotherapy for advanced laryngeal and hypopharyngeal tumors. Int. J. Radiat. Oncol. Biol. Phys., 11:499, 1985.
479. Mittal, B., Marks, J. E., and Ogura, J. H.: Transglottic carcinoma. Cancer, 53:151, 1984.
480. Miyake, H., Horiuchi, M., Togawa, K., Kawamoto, K., Kaneko, T., Iruyama, Y., Hondo, Y., Baba, S., Matsunaga, T., and Ishikawa, T.: Recombinant interferon alpha 2 (sch 30500) in patients with head and neck cancer. Gan To Kagaku Ryoho, 12:1651, 1985.
481. Mizono, G. S., Diaz, R. F., Fu, K. K., and Boles, R.: Carcinoma of the tonsillar region. Laryngoscope, 96:240, 1986.
482. Molnar, L., Ronay, P., and Tapolcsanyi, L.: Carcinoma of the lip: Analysis of the material of 25 years. Oncology, 29:101, 1974.
483. Moore, C., and Catlin, D.: Anatomic origins and locations of oral cancer. Am. J. Surg., 114:510, 1967.
484. Morita, K.: Clinical significance of radiation therapy combined with chemotherapy. Strahlentherapie, 156:228, 1980.
485. Mortimer, J. E., Taylor, M. E., Schulman, S., Cummings, C., Weymuller, E., Jr., and Laramore, G.: Feasibility and efficacy of weekly intraarterial cisplatin in locally advanced (stage III and IV) head and neck cancers. J. Clin. Oncol., 6:969, 1988.
486. Morton, R. P., Rugman, F., Dorman, E. B., Stoney, P. J., Wilson, J. A., McCormick, M., Veevers, A., and Stell, P. M.: Cisplatinum and bleomycin in the treatment of advanced or recurrent squamous cell carcinoma of the head and neck: A randomized factorial phase III controlled trial. Sonderb.-Strahlenther. Oncol., 81:141, 1987.
487. Moseley, H. S., Thomas, L. R., Everts, E. C., Stevens, K. R., and Ireland, K. M.: Advanced squamous cell carcinoma of the maxillary sinus: Results of combined regional infusion chemotherapy, radiation therapy and surgery. Am. J. Surg., 141:522, 1981.
488. Mossman, K. L.: Quantitative radiation dose response relationships for normal tissues in man. II. Response of the salivary glands during radiotherapy. Radiat. Res., 95:392, 1983.
489. Mossman, K. L., Chencharick, J. D., Scheer, A. C., Walker, W. P., Ornitz, R. D., Rogers, C. C., and Hendin, R. I.: Radiation induced changes in gustatory function: Comparison of effects of neutron and photon irradiation. Int. J. Radiat. Oncol. Biol. Phys., 5:521, 1979.
490. Mossman, K. L., Shatzman, A. R., and Chencharick, J. D.: Effects of radiotherapy on human parotid saliva. Radiat. Res., 88:403, 1981.
491. Muggia, F. M., and Wolf, G. T.: Intra-arterial chemotherapy of head and neck cancer: Worth another look? Cancer Clin. Trials, 3:375, 1980.
492. Mukhopadhyaya, R., Rao, R. S., Fakih, A. R., and Gangal, S. G.: Detection of circulating immune complexes in patients with squamous cell carcinoma of the oral cavity. J. Clin. Lab Immunol., 21:189, 1986.
493. Murray, C. G., Herson, J., Daly, T. E., and Zimmerman, S. O.: Radiation necrosis of the mandible a 10 year study. Part I factors influencing the onset of necrosis. Int. J. Radiat. Oncol. Phys., 6:543, 1980.
494. Nadol, J. B., Jr.: Treatment of carcinoma of the epiglottis. Ann. Otol. Rhinol. Laryngol., 90:442, 1981.
495. Nagle, R. B., Moll, R., Weidauer, H., Nemetschek, H., and Franke, W. W.: Different patterns of cytokeratin expression in the normal epithelia of the upper respiratory tract. Differentiation, 30:130, 1985.
496. Nason, R. W., Sako, K., Beecroft, W. A., Razack, M. S., Bakamjian, V. Y., and Shedd, D. P.: Surgical management of squamous cell carcinoma of the floor of mouth. Am. J. Surg., 158:292, 1989.
497. Nass, J. M., Brady, L. W., Glassburn, J. R., Prasasvinichai, S., and Schatanoff, D.: Radiation therapy of glottic carcinoma. Int. J. Radiat. Oncol. Biol. Phys., 1:867, 1976.
498. Nguyen, T. D., Demange, L., Froissart, D., Panis, X., and Liorette, M.: Rapid hyper-fractionated radiotherapy. Clinical results in 178 advanced squamous cell carcinomas of the head and neck. Cancer, 56:16, 1985.
499. Nicaise, C., Hong, W. K., Dimery, W., Usakewicz, J., Rozencweig, M., and Krakoff, I.: Phase II study of tallysomycin $S_{10}b$ in patients with advanced head and neck cancer. Invest. New Drugs, 8:325, 1990.
500. Ning, J. P., Yu, M. C., Wang, Q. S., and Henderson, B. E.: Comsumption of salted fish and other risk factors for nasopharyngeal carcinoma (NPC) in Tianjin, a low-risk region for NPC in the People's Republic of China. J. Natl. Cancer Inst., 82:291, 1990.
501. Nissenbaum, M., Browde, S., Bezwoda, W. R., de Moor, N. G., and Derman, D. P.: Treatment of advanced head and neck cancer: Multiple daily dose fractionated radiation therapy and sequential multimodal treatment approach. Med. and Pediatr. Oncol., 12:204, 1984.
502. Norris, C. M.: Laryngectomy and neck dissection. Otolaryngol. Clin. North Am., 69:667, 1969.
503. Norris, C. M., Jr., Clark, J. R., Frei, E., Ervin, T. J., Fallon, B., Tuttle, S. A., Fabian, R. L., and Miller, P.: Pathology of surgery after induction chemotherapy: an analysis of resectability and locoregional control. Laryngoscope, 96:292, 1986.
504. O'Brien, P. H., Carlson, R., and Steubber, E. A.: Distant metastases in head and neck epidermoid carcinoma. Laryngoscope, 90:196, 1980.
505. O'Connor, D., Clifford, P., Edwards, W. G., Dallen, V. M., Durden-Smith, J., Hollis, B. A., and Calman, F. M.: Long-term results of VBM and radiotherapy in advanced head and neck cancer. Int. J. Radiat. Oncol. Biol. Phys., 8:1525, 1982.
506. Olivari, A. J., Glait, H. M., Guardo, A., Califano, L., and Pradier, R.: Levamisole in squamous cell carcinoma of the head and neck. Cancer Treat. Rep., 63:983, 1979.
507. Ossoff, R. H., Shapshay, S. M., and Sisson, G. A.: Endoscopic management of selected early vocal cord carcinoma. Ann. Otol. Rhinol. Laryngol., 94:560, 1985.
508. Paccagnella, A., Cavaniglia, G., Zorat, P. L., Pappagallo, G. L., Orlando, A., Balli, M., Bononi, A., Puccetti, C., Fila, G., Vinante, O., Sala, O., Calzavara, F., and Fiorentino, M. V.: Chemotherapy (CT) before loco-regional treatment (LRT) in stage III + IV head and neck cancer: intermediate results of an ongoing randomized phase III trial. A GSTTC study. (Abstract #669) Proc. Amer. Soc. Clin. Oncol., 9:173, 1990.
509. Panje, W. R., and Ceilley, R. I.: The influence of embryology of the mid-face on the spread of epithelial malignancies. Laryngoscope, 89:1914, 1979.
510. Panje, W. R., Smith, B., and McCabe, B. F.: Epidermoid carcinomas of the floor of

mouth. Surgical therapy vs combined therapy vs radiation therapy. Otolaryngol. Head Neck Surg., 88:714, 1980.
511. Paredes, J., Hong, W. K., Felder, T., Dimery, I. W., Choksi, A. J., Newman, R. A., Castellanos, A. M., Robbins, K. T., McCarthy, K., and Atkinson, N.: Prospective randomized trial of high-dose cisplatin and 5-FU infusion with or without sodium diethyldithiocarbamate (DDT) in recurrent and/or metastatic squamous cell carcinoma of the head and neck. J. Clin. Oncol., 6:955, 1988.
512. Parkinson, D. R., and Schantz, S.: The immunobiological therapy of head and neck cancer. *In* Multimodality Therapy for Head and Neck Cancer. Edited by G. Snow, and J. R. Clark. Verlag Press. In press, 1992.
513. Parvinen, L. M., Parvinen, M., Nordman, E., and Kortekangas, A. E.: Combined bleomycin treatment and radiation therapy in squamous cell carcinoma of the head and neck region. Acta Radiol. Oncol., 24:487, 1985.
514. Pearson, B. W., Woods, R. D., II, and Hartman, D. E.: Extended hemilaryngectomy of T3 glottic carcinoma with preservation of speech and swallowing. Laryngoscope, 90:1950, 1980.
515. Pene, F., and Fletcher, G. H.: Results in irradiation of the in situ carcinomas of the vocal cord. Cancer, 37:2586, 1976.
516. Peng, Y.-M., Alberts, D. S., Chen, H.-S., Mason, N., and Moon, T. E.: Antitumor activity and plasma kinetics of bleomycin by continuous and intermittent administration. Br. J. Cancer, 41:644, 1980.
517. Pennacchio, J. L., Hong, W. K., Shapshay, S., Gillis, T., Vaughan, C., Bhutani, P., Ucmakli, A., Katz, A. E., Bromer, R., Willet, B., and Strong, S. M.: Combination of cis-platin and bleomycin prior to surgery and/or radiotherapy compared with radiotherapy alone for the treatment of advanced squamous cell carcinoma of the head and neck. Cancer, 50:2795, 1982.
518. Perez, C. A., Purdy, J. A., Breaux, S. R., Ogura, J. H., and von Essen, S.: Carcinoma of the tonsillar fossa. Cancer, 50:2314, 1982.
519. Peters, L. J., Batsakis, J. G., Goepfert, H., and Hong, W. K.: The diagnosis and management of nasopharyngeal cancer in caucasians. *In* Textbook of Uncommon Cancer. Edited by C. J. Williams, J. G. Krikorian, M. R. Green, and D. Raghaven. Chichester, England, John Wiley and Sons, 1988, pp. 975–1006.
520. Peters, L. J., Harrison, M. L., Dimery, I. W., Fields, R., Goepfert, M., and Oswald, M. J.: Acute and late toxicity associated with sequential bleomycin-containing chemotherapy regimens and radiation therapy in the treatment of carcinoma of the nasopharynx. Int. J. Radiat. Oncol. Biol. Phys., 14:623, 1988.
521. Peto, R., Doll, R., Buckley, J. D., and Sporn, M. B.: Can dietary beta-carotene materially reduce human cancer rates? Nature, 290:201, 1981.
522. Petrovich, Z., Block, J., Kuisk, H., Mackintosh, R., Casciato, D., Jose, L., and Berton, R.: A randomized comparison of radiotherapy with radiotherapy-chemotherapy combination in stage IV carcinoma of the head and neck. Cancer, 47:2259, 1986.
523. Petrovich, Z., Kuisk, H., Jose, L., Barton, R., and Rice, D.: Advanced carcinoma of the tonsil. Treatment results. Acta Radiol. Oncol., 19:425, 1980.
524. Pfeiffer, P., Madsen, E. L., Hansen, O., and May, O.: Effect of prophylactic sucralfate suspension on stomatitis induced by cancer chemotherapy. A randomized, double-blind cross-over study. Acta Oncol., 29:171, 1990.
525. Pigneux, J., Richaud, P. M., and Lagarde, C.: The place of interstitial therapy using 192 Indium in the management of carcinoma of the lip. Cancer, 43:1073, 1979.
526. Pillsbury, H. R., and Kirchner, J. A.: Clinical vs histopathologic staging in laryngeal cancer. Arch. Otolaryngol., 105:157, 1979.
527. Pingree, T. F., Davis, R. K., Reichman, O., and Derrick, L.: Treatment of hypopharyngeal carcinoma: A 10 year review of 1362 cases. Laryngoscope, 97:901, 1987.
528. Pinkston, J. A., Wakabuyashi, T., Yamamoto, T., Asano, M., Harada, Y., Kumagami, H., and Takeuchi, M.: Cancer of the head and neck in atomic bomb survivors: Hiroshima and Nagasaki, 1957–1976. Cancer, 48:2172, 1981.
529. Pitman, S. W., Kowal, C. D., and Bertino, J. R.: Methotrexate and 5-fluorouracil in sequence in squamous head and neck cancer. Semin. Oncol., 10 (Suppl. 2):15, 1983.
530. Pomp, J., Levendag, P. C., and van Putten, L.: Reirradiation of recurrent tumors in the head and neck. Am. J. Clin. Oncol., 11:543, 1988.
531. Popkin, J. D., Hong, W. K., Bromer, R. H., Moffer, S. M., Doos, W. G., Willett, B. L., Katz, A. E., Vaughn, C. W., and Strong, M. S.: Induction bleomycin infusion in head and neck cancer. Am. J. Clin. Oncol. (CCT). 7:199, 1984.
532. Posner, M. R., Ervin, T. J., Weichselbaum, R. R., Fabian, R. L., and Miller, D.: Chemotherapy of advanced salivary gland neoplasms. Cancer, 50:2261, 1982.
533. Posner, M. R., Weichselbaum, R. R., Fitzgerald, T. J., Clark, J. R., Rose, C., Fabian, R. L., Norris, C. M., Jr., Miller, D., Tuttle, S. A., and Ervin, T. J.: Treatment complications after sequential combination chemotherapy and radiotherapy with or without surgery in previously untreated squamous cell carcinoma of the head and neck. Int. J. Radiat. Oncol. Biol. Phys., 11:1887, 1985.
534. Powell, B. L., Craig, J. B., Muss, H. B., Zekan, P. J., Cooper, M. R., Schnell, F. M., Hampton, J. W., White, D. R., Smith, L. R., and Capizzi, R. L.: Phade II trial of high-dose cytosine arabinoside and cisplatin in recurrent squamous carcinoma of the head and neck. Am. J. Clin. Oncol., 11:550, 1988.
535. Powell, B. L., Stanley, V., Brockschmidt, J., White, D., Muss, H., Livesay, L., McNeill, J., Schifeling, D., Jackson, D., Baker, A., Caldwell, D., O'Rourke, M., Paschal, B., Brodkin, R., and Pavy, M.: Combination carboplatin (CBDCA) and cisplatin (CDDP) for advanced squamous carcinoma of the head and neck (SCHN). (Abstract #693) Proc. Am. Soc. Clin. Oncol., 9:179, 1990.
536. Pressman, J. J., Dowdy, A., and Libby, M.: Further studies upon the submucosal compartments and lymphatics of the larynx by the injection of dye and radioisotopes. Ann. Otol. Rhinol. Laryngol., 65:963, 1956.
537. Probert, J. C., Thompson, R. W., and Bagshaw, M. A.: Patterns of spread of distant metastases in head and neck cancer. Cancer, 33:127, 1974.
538. Raab-Traub, N., Flynn, K., Pearson, G., Huang, A., Levine, P., Lanier, A., and Pagano, J.: The differentiated form of nasopharyngeal carcinoma contains Epstein-Barr virus DNA. Int. J. Cancer, 39:25, 1987.
539. Rahal, M., Sadek, H., Azli, M., Cvitkovic, E., Djemma, A., Wendling, J. L., Filali, T., Avril, M. F., and Armand, J. P.: Advanced loco-regional skin carcinoma. Primary chemotherapy with cisplatin (CDDP), bleomycin (BLM) and 5-JP: fluorouracil (5 FU). (Abstract #1142) Proc. Am. Soc. Clin. Oncol., 8:293, 1989.
540. Raine, C. H., Stell, P. M., and Dalby, J.: Squamous cell carcinoma of the posterior wall of the hypopharynx. J. Laryngol. Otol., 96:997, 1982.
541. Randolph, V. L., Vallejo, A., Spiro, R. H., Shah, J., Strong, E. W., Huvos, A. G., and Wittes, R. E.: Combination therapy of advanced head and neck cancer: induction of remissions with diamminedichloroplatinum (II) bleomycin and radiation therapy. Cancer, 41:460, 1978.
542. Raque, C. J., Biondo, R. V., Keeran, M. G., Honeycutt, W. M., and Jansen, G. T.: Snuff dippers keratosis (snuff-induced leukoplakia). South. Med. J., 68:565, 1975.
543. Razack, M. S., Sako, K., Marchetta, F. C., Calamel, P., Bakamjian, V., and Shedd, D. P.: Carcinoma of the hypopharynx: Success and failure. Am. J. Surg., 134:489, 1977.
544. Remmier, D., Medina, J. E., Byers, R. M., Meoz, R., and Pfalzgraf, K.: Treatment of choice for squamous carcinoma of the tonsillar fossa. Head Neck Surg., 7:206, 1985.
545. Rentschler, R., Burgess, M. A., and Byers, R.: Chemotherapy of malignant major salivary gland neoplasms: A 25-year review of M. D. Anderson Hospital experience. Cancer, 40:619, 1977.
546. Rentschler, R. E., Wilbur, D. W., Petti, G. H., Chonkich, G. D., Hilliard, D. A., Camacho, E. S., and Thorpe, R. B.: Adjuvant methotrexate escalated to toxicity for resectable stage III and IV squamous head and neck carcinomas—A prospective, randomized study. J. Clin. Oncol., 5:278, 1987.
547. Rezkalla, S., Ensley, J., Turi, Z., Kloner, R. A., Kish, J., Tapazoglou, E., Bhasin, S., Revels, S., Olivienstein, A., Wynne, J., and Al-Sarraf, M.: 5-fluorouracil (5FU) cardiotoxicity: A controlled, prospective investigation of ischemic changes during 5-FU infusions. (Abstract #580) Proc. Am. Soc. Clin. Oncol., 8:150, 1988.
548. Richard, J., Molinari, R., Sancho-Garnier, H., et al.: A randomized trial comparing surgery preceded or not by intra-arterial chemotherapy in squamous cell carcinomas of the head and neck. Proceedings of the International Conference on Head and Neck Cancer, Baltimore, Md., 1984, p. 113.
549. Richard, J. M., Sancho, H., Lepintre, Y., Rodary, J., and Pierquin, B.: Intra-arterial methotrexate chemotherapy and telecobalt therapy in cancer of the oral cavity and oropharynx. Cancer, 34:491, 1974.
550. Richards, G. J., Jr., and Chambers, R. G.: Hydroxyurea: A radiosensitizer in the treatment of neoplasms of the head and neck. Am. J. Roentgenol. Radium. Ther. Nucl. Med., 105:555, 1969.
551. Richards, G. J., Jr., and Chambers, R. G.: Hydroxyurea in the treatment of neoplasms of the head and neck: A resurvey. Am. J. Surg., 126:513, 1973.
552. Richtsmeier, W. J.: Interferon gamma induced oncolysis: An effect of head and neck squamous carcinoma cultures. Arch. Otolaryngol. Head Neck Surg., 114:432, 1988.
553. Riley, R. W., Fee, W. E., Jr., Goffinet, D., Cox, R., and Goode, R. L.: Squamous cell carcinoma of the base of the tongue. Otolaryngol. Head Neck Surg., 91:143, 1983.
554. Ringborg, U., Ewert, G., Kinnman, J., Lundgvist, P. G., and Strander, H.: Sequential methotrexate-5-fluorouracil treatment of squamous cell carcinoma of the head and neck. Cancer, 52:971, 1983.
555. Ringborg, U., Henle, W., Henle, G., Ingimarson, S., Klein, G., Silfversward, C., and Strander, H.: Epstein-Barr virus—specific serodiagnostic tests in carcinomas of the head and neck. Cancer, 52:1237, 1983.
556. Roa, R. A., Carey, T. E., Passamani, P. P., Greenwood, J. H., Hsu, S., Ridings, E. O., Schwartz, D. R., Wolf, G. T., and Hudson, J. L.: DNA content of human squamous cell carcinoma cell lines. Analysis by flow entometry and chromosome enumeration. Arch. Otolaryngol., 111:565, 1985.
557. Robert, F.: Trimetrexate as a single agent in patients with advanced head and neck cancer. Semin. Oncol., 15(Suppl. 2):22, 1988.
558. Rollo, J., Rozenbom, C. V., Thawley, S., Korba, A., Ogura, J., Perez, C. A., Powers, W. E., and Bauer, W. C.: Squamous carcinoma of the base of the tongue: A clinicopathologic study of 81 cases. Cancer, 47:333, 1981.
559. Rooney, M., Kish, J., Jacobs, J., Kinzie, J., Weaver, A., Crissman, J., and Al Sarraf, M.: Improved complete response rate and survival in advanced head and neck cancer after three-course induction therapy with 120-hour 5-FU infusion and cisplatin. Cancer, 55:1123, 1985.
560. Rosin, M. P., Dunn, B. P., and Stich, H. F.: Use of intermediate endpoints in quantitating the response of precancerous lesions to chemopreventive agents. Can. J. Physiol. Pharmacol., 65:483, 1987.
561. Rossi, A., Molinari, R., Boracchi, P., Del Vecchio, M., Marubini, E., Nava, M., Morandi, L., Zucali, R., Pilotti, S., and Grandi, C.: Adjuvant chemotherapy with vincristine, cyclophosphamide, and doxorubicin after radiotherapy in local-regional nasopharyngeal cancer: Results of a 4-year multicenter randomized study. J. Clin. Oncol., 6:1401, 1988.
562. Ryssel, H. J., Brunner, K. W., and Bollag, W.: Die perorale Anwendung von Vitamin-A-Saure bei Leukoplakien, Hyperkeratosen and Plattenepithelkarzinomen: Ergebnisse und Vertaglichkeit. Schweiz Med. Wschr., 101:1027, 1971.
563. Sacks, P. G., Hong, W. K., and Hittelman, W. N.: In vitro studies of the premalignant process: initial culture of oral premalignant lesions. Cancer Bull., 43:485, 1991.
564. Sacks, P., Oke, V., and Mehta, K.: Antiproliferative effects of free and liposome-encapsulated retinoic acid in squamous carcinoma model: Monolayer and multicellular tumor spheroids. J. Cancer Res. Clin. Oncol., 1992, (in press).
565. Saffiotti, U., Montesano, R., Sellakumar, A. R., and Borg, S. A.: Experimental cancer of the lung. Inhibition by vitamin A of the induction of tracheobroncial squamous metaplasia and squamous cell tumours. Cancer, 20:857, 1967.
566. Sako, K., Razack, M. S., and Kalnins, I.: Chemotherapy for advanced and recurrent squamous cell carcinoma of the head and neck with high and low dose cis-diamminedichloroplatinum. Am. J. Surg., 136:529, 1978.
567. Saranath, D., Mukhopadhyaya, R., Rao, R. S., Fakih, A. R., Naik, S. L., and Gangal, S. G.: Cell-mediated immune status in patients with squamous cell carcinoma of the oral cavity. Cancer, 56:1062, 1985.
568. Saranath, D., Panchal, R. G., Nair, R., Mehta, A. R., Sanghavi, V., Sumegi, J., Klein, G., and Deo, M. G.: Oncogene amplification in squamous cell carcinoma of the oral cavity. Jpn. J. Cancer Res., 80:430, 1989.
569. Scandolaro, L., and Bertoni, F.: Tolleranza cutanea e mucosa e risposte cliniche a breve termine nella associazione tra radioterapia e bleomycina per tumori del distretto cervico-cefalico. Acta Otorhinol. Ital., 2:213, 1982.
570. Scanlon, P. W., Rhodes, R. E., Woolner, L. B., Devine, K. D., and McBean, J. B.: Cancer of the nasopharynx. One hundred forty-two patients treated in the 11-year period 1950–1960. Amer. J. Roentgen., 99:313, 1967.
571. Schabel, F. M., Jr.: Concepts for treatment of micrometastases developed in murine systems. Amer. J. Roentgenol., 126:500, 1976.
572. Schantz, S. P., and Guillamondegui, O. M.: Developing perspectives in head and neck tumor immunology. Prob. Gen. Surg., 5:99, 1988.

573. Schantz, S. P., Hsu, T. C., Ainslie, N., and Moser, R. P.: Young adults with head and neck cancer express increased susceptibility to mutagen-induced chromosome damage. JAMA, 262:3313, 1989.
574. Schantz, S. P., Savage, H. E., Brown, B. W., Reuben, J. M., Hong, W. K., and Rossen, R. D.: Association of levels of Clq binding macromolecules with induction chemotherapy response in head and neck cancer patients. Cancer Res., 48:5868, 1988.
575. Schantz, S. P., Savage, H. E., Race, T., Liu, F. J., Brown, B. W., Rossen, R. D., and Hong, W. K.: Immunologic determinants of head and neck cancer response to induction chemotherapy. J. Clin. Oncol., 7:857, 1989.
576. Schantz, S. P., Spitz, M. R., and Hsu, T. C.: Mutagen sensitivity in patients with head and neck cancers: A biologic marker for risk of multiple primary malignancies. J. Natl. Cancer Inst., 82:1773, 1990.
577. Schechter, G. L., and Kalafsky, J. T.: Cancer of the hypopharynx and cervical esophagus: management concepts. Oncology, 2:17,34, 1988.
578. Schechter, G. L., Baker, J. W., El-Mahdi, A. M., and Bumata, J. T.: Combined treatment of advanced cancer of the laryngopharynx and cervical esophagus. Laryngoscope, 92:11, 1982.
579. Schmidseder, R., and Dick, H.: Spread of epidermoid carcinoma of the lip along the inferior alveolar nerve. Oral. Surg. Oral. Med. Oral. Pathol., 43:517, 1977.
580. Schnabel, T., Zamboglou, N., Pape, H., Achterrath, W., Lenaz, L., Schmitt, G., and Preusser, P.: Phase II trial with carboplatin and simultaneous radiation in previously untreated advanced squamous cell carcinoma of the head and neck (SCCHN). (Abstract #680) Proc. Am. Soc. Clin. Oncol., 9:176, 1990.
581. Schneider, J. J., Lindberg, R. D., and Jesse, R. H.: Prevention of tracheal stoma recurrences after total laryngectomy by postoperative irradiation. J. Surg. Oncol., 7:187, 1975.
582. Schornagel, J., Cappelaere, P., Verwey, J., Cognetti, F., de Mulder, P., Clavel, M., Vemorklen, J., and Snow, G.: A randomized phase II study of 10-ethyl-10-deazaaminopterin (10-EdAM) and methotrexate (MTX) in advanced head and neck squamous cell carcinoma (AHNC), and EORTC study. (Abstract #679) Proc. Am. Soc. Clin. Oncol., 8:174, 1989.
583. Schottenfeld, D.: Epidemiology, etiology, and pathogenesis of head and neck cancer. *In* Head and Neck Cancer. Edited by P. B. Chretien, M. E. John, and D. P. Shedd. New York, B. C. Decker, Inc., 1985, pp. 6–18.
584. Schramm, V. L., Jr., Srodes, C., and Myers, E. N.: Cisplatin therapy for adenoid cystic carcinoma. Arch. Otolaryngol., 107:739, 1981.
585. Schreiner, B. F., and Christy, C. J.: Results of irradiation treatment of cancer of the lip: Analysis of 636 cases from 1926–1936. Radiol., 39:293, 1942.
586. Schuller, D. E., McGuirt, W. F., and Krause, C. J.: Symposium: Adjuvant cancer therapy of head and neck tumors. Increased survival with surgery alone vs. combined therapy. Laryngoscope, 89:1735, 1979.
587. Schuller, D. E., Metch, B., Stein, D. W., Mattox, D., and McCracken, J. D.: Preoperative chemotherapy in advanced resectable head and neck cancer: final report of the Southwest Oncology Group. Laryngoscope, 98:1205, 1988.
588. Schuller, D. E., Stein, D. W., and Metch, B.: Analysis of treatment failure patterns. A Southwest Oncology Group Study. Arch. Otolaryngol. Head Neck Surg., 115:834, 1989.
589. Schwartz, J., Shklar, G., Reid, S., and Trickler, D.: Prevention of experimental oral cancer by extracts of Spirulina-Dunaliella algae. Nutr. Cancer, 11:127, 1988.
590. Seder, R. H., Vaughan, C. W., Oh, S. K., Keegins, J. J., Hayes, J. A., Blanchard, G. C., Vincent, M. E., and Katz, A. E.: Tumor repression and temporary restoration of immune response after plasmapheresis in patients with recurrent oral cancer. Cancer, 60:318, 1987.
591. Selvaggi, K. J., Vlock, D. R., Johnson, J. T., Snyderman, C. H., Rubin, J., Kirkwood, J., Haselow, R., Letessier, E., Whiteside, T., and Prescott, K.: Phase Ib trial of peritumoral and intranodal injections of IL-2 in patients with advanced squamous cell carcinoma of the head and neck (SCCHN)—preliminary results. (Abstract #691) Proc. Am. Soc. Clin. Oncol., 9:178, 1990.
592. Sessions, R. B., Lehane, D. E., Bryan, R. N., and Horowitz, B. L.: Intra-arterial cisplatin in the treatment of aerodigestive squamous carcinoma and nasopharyngeal carcinoma. *In* Head and Neck Cancer. Edited by P. B. Chretian, M. E. Johns, D. P. Shedd, E. W. Strong, and P. H. Ward. Philadelphia, B. C. Decker, Inc., 1985, pp. 451–455.
593. Sessions, R. B., Lehane, D. E., Smith, R. J., Bryan, R. N., and Suen, J. Y.: Intra-arterial cisplatin treatment of adenoid cystic carcinoma. Arch. Otolaryngol., 108:221, 1982.
594. Shah, J. P., Caudela, F. C., and Poddar, A. K.: The patterns of cervical lymph node metastases from squamous carcinoma of the oral cavity. Cancer, 66:109, 1990.
595. Shah, J. P., and Feghali, J.: Esthesioneuroblastoma. Am. J. Surg., 142:456, 1981.
596. Shah, J. P., and Jollefsen, H. R.: Epidermoid carcinoma of the supraglottic larynx. Role of neck dissection in initial surgical treatment. Am. J. Surg., 128:494, 1974.
597. Shah, J. P., Strong, E. W., DeCosse, J. J., Itri, L., and Sellers, P.: Effect of retinoids on oral leukoplakia. Am. J. Surg., 146:466, 1983.
598. Shah, J. P., and Tolletsen, H. R.: Epidermoid carcinoma of the supraglottic larynx. Role of neck dissection in initial surgical treatment. Am. J. Surg., 128:494, 1974.
599. Shah, K. V.: Papillomavirus infections of the respiratory tract, the conjunctiva, and the oral cavity. *In* Papillomaviruses and Human Cancer. Edited by Herbert Pfister. 1990, pp. 73–261.
600. Shaha, A. R., and Shah, J. P.: Carcinoma of the subglottic larynx. Am. J. Surg., 144:456, 1982.
601. Shaha, A., Spiro, R., Shah, J., and Strong, E. W.: Squamous carcinomas of the floor of mouth. Am. J. Surg., 148:455, 1984.
602. Sham, J. S., Poon, Y. F., Wei, W. I., and Choy, D.: Nasopharyngeal carcinoma in young patients. Cancer, 65:2606, 1990.
603. Shankar, P. G., Taylor, S. A., and Gemer, L. S.: Accelerated fractionation radiation therapy and concurrent cis-platin chemotherapy for advanced head and neck cancer. (Abstract #696) Proc. Am. Soc. Clin. Oncol., 9:180, 1990.
604. Shanta, V., and Krishnamurthi, S.: Combined bleomycin and radiotherapy in oral cancer. Clin. Radiol., 31:617, 1980.
605. Shapira, A., Virolainen, E., Jameson, J. J., Ossakow, S. J., and Carey, T. E.: Growth inhibition of laryngeal UM-SCC cell lines by tamoxifen: Comparison with effects on the MCF-7 breast cancer cell line. Arch. Otolaryngol. Head Neck Surg., 112:1151, 1986.
606. Shapshay, S. M., Hong, W. K., Incze, J. S., Sismanis, A., Bhutani, R., Vaughn, C. W., and Strong, M. S.: Prognostic indicators in induction cis-platinum bleomycin chemotherapy for advanced head and neck cancer. Am. J. Surg., 140:543, 1980.
607. Shetty, P., Mehta, A., Shinde, S., Mazumdar, A., and Hingorani, C.: Controlled study in squamous cell carcinoma of base of tongue using conventional radiation, radiation with single drug and radiation with multiple drug chemotherapy. (Abstract #C-595) Proc. Am. Soc. Clin. Oncol., 4:152, 1985.
608. Shigematsu, Y., Sakai, S., and Fuchihata, H.: Recent trials in the treatment of maxillary sinus carcinoma with special reference to the chemical potentiation of radiation therapy. Acta Otolaryng., 71:63, 1971.
609. Shillitoe, E. J., Greenspan, D., Greenspan, J. S., and Silverman, S., Jr.: Five-year survival of patients with oral cancer and its association with antibody to herpes simplex virus. Cancer, 58:2256, 1986.
610. Shillitoe, E. J., Hwang, C. B., Silverman, S., Jr., and Greenspan, J. S.: Examination of oral cancer tissue for the presence of the proteins ICP4, ICP5, ICP6, ICP8, and gB of herpes simplex virus type 1. J. Natl. Cancer Inst., 76:371, 1986.
611. Shillitoe, E. J., and Silverman, S., Jr.: Oral cancer and herpes simplex virus: a review. Oral Surg. Oral Med. Oral Pathol., 48:216, 1979.
612. Shin, D. M., Gimenez, I. B., Lee, J. S., Nishioka, K., Wargovich, M. J., Thacher, S., Lotan, R., Slaga, T. J., and Hong, W. K.: Expression of epidermal growth factor receptor, polyamine levels, ornithine decarboxylase activity, micronuclei, and transglutaminase I in a 7,12-dimethylbenz(a)anthracene-induced hamster buccal pouch carcinogenesis model. Cancer Res., 50:2505, 1990.
613. Shirinian, M., Choksi, A. J., Dimery, I., Heyne, K., Lippman, S., Guillory, C., and Hong, W. K.: Phase I/II study of cisplatin (P) + 5-fluorouracil (F) + α-interferon (IFN) for recurrent squamous cell carcinoma of the head and neck (SCCHN). Proc. Am. Soc. Clin. Oncol., 11: 1992.
614. Shklar, G.: Oral leukoplakia. N. Engl. J. Med., 315:1544, 1986.
615. Shklar, G., Marefat, P., Konhauser, A., Trickler, D. P., and Wallace, K. D.: Retinoid inhibition of lingual carcinogenesis. Oral Surg. Oral Med. Oral Pathol., 49:325, 1980.
616. Shklar, G., Schwartz, J., Grau, D., Trickler, D. P., and Wallace, K. D.: Inhibition of hamster buccal pouch carcinogenesis by 13-cis-retinoic acid. Oral Surg. Oral Med. Oral Pathol., 50:45, 1980.
617. Shore-Friedman, E., Abrahams, C., Recant, W., and Schneider, A. B.: Neurilemonas and salivary gland tumors of the head and neck following childhood irradiation. Cancer, 51:2159, 1983.
618. Shresbury, D., Adams, G. L., Duvall, A. J., III, Maisel, R. H., and Haselow, R. E.: Carcinoma of the tonsillar region: a comparison of radiation therapy with combined preoperative radiation and surgery. Otolaryngol. Head Neck Surg., 89:979, 1981.
619. Sikic, B. T., Collins, J. M., Mimnaugh, E. G., and Gram, T. E.: Improved therapeutic index of bleomycin when administered by continuous infusion in mice. Cancer Treat. Rep., 62:2011, 1978.
620. Silverman, S.: Early diagnosis of oral cancer. Cancer, 62:1796, 1988.
621. Silverman, S., Eisenberg, E., and Renstrup, G.: A study of the effects of high doses of vitamin A on oral leukoplakia (hyperkeratosis), including toxicity, liver function and skeletal metabolism. J. Oral Therap. and Pharm., 2:9, 1965.
622. Silverman, S., Jr., Gorsky, M., and Lozada, F.: Oral leukoplakia and malignant transformation: A follow-up study of 257 patients. Cancer, 53:563, 1984.
623. Silverman, S., Renstrup, G., and Pindborg, J. J.: Studies in oral leukoplakias. III. Effects of vitamin A comparing clinical, histopathologic, cytologic and hematologic responses. Acta Odont. Scandinav., 21:271, 1963.
624. Sinibaldi, V., Eisenberger, M., and Jacobs, M.: Treatment of advanced unresectable stage IV squamous cell carcinoma of the head and neck (SCCHN) with combined carboplatin (CBDCA) and radiotherapy (RT). (Abstract #659) Proc. Am. Soc. Clin. Oncol., 8:169, 1989.
625. Siodlak, M. Z., Dalby, J. E., Bradley, P. J., Campbell, J. B., Strickland, P., Fraser, J. G., Willatt, D. J., Flood, L. M., and Stell, P. M.: Induction VBM plus radiotherapy, versus radiotherapy alone for advanced head and neck cancer: Long-term results. Clin. Otolaryngol., 14:17, 1989.
626. Sisson, G. A., Bytell, D. E., Edison, B. D., and Yeh, S.: Transsternal radical neck dissection for control of stomal recurrences—end results. Laryngoscope, 85:1504, 1975.
627. Skolnick, E. M., Yee, K. F., Wheatley, M. A., and Martin, L. O.: Carcinoma of the laryngeal glottis therapy and end results. Laryngoscope, 85:1453, 1975.
628. Slaughter, D. P., Southwick, H. W., and Smejkal, W.: "Field cancerization" in oral stratification squamous epithelium: Clinical implications of mutocentric origin. Cancer, 6:963, 1953.
629. Slotman, G. J., Cummings, F. J., Glicksman, A. R., Doolittle, C. L., and Leone, L. A.: Preoperative simultaneously-administered cis-platinum plus radiation therapy for advanced squamous cell carcinoma of the head and neck. Head Neck Surg., 8:159, 1986.
630. Smokeless tobacco use in the United States. N.C.I. Monogr., 8:1, 1989.
631. Snow, G. B., Annyas, A. A., van Slooten, E. A., Bartelink, H., and Hart, A. A.: Prognostic factors of neck node metastases. Clin. Otolaryngol., 7:185, 1982.
632. Snow, G. B., Vermorken, J. B., and Pinedo, H. M.: Adjuvant chemotherapy: the EORTC Trials. *In* Head and Neck Oncology. Edited by H. J. G. Bloom, et al. New York, Raven Press, 1986, pp. 83–92.
633. Snow, J. B., Gelber, R. D., Kramer, S., Davis, L. W., Marcial, V. A., and Lowry, L. D.: Comparison of preoperative and postoperative radiation therapy for patients with carcinoma of the head and neck. Interim Report. Act. Otolaryngol., 91:611, 1981.
634. Snyderman, N. L., Wetmore, S. J., and Suen, J. Y.: Cisplatin sensitization to radiotherapy in stage IV squamous cell carcinoma of the head and neck. A follow-up report. Arch. Otolaryngol. Head Neck Surg., 112:1147, 1986.
635. Somers, K. D., Cartwright, S. L., and Schechter, G. L.: Coamplification of INT-2 and HST-1 genes in squamous cell carcinoma of the head and neck. Third International Head and Neck Oncology Research Conference, Las Vegas, Nevada, 1990.
636. Son, Y. H., and Kapp, D. S.: Oral cavity and oropharyngeal cancer in a younger population: Review of literature and experience at Yale. Cancer, 55:441, 1985.
637. Soo, K. C., Shah, J. P., Gopinath, K. S., Gerold, F. P., Jaques, D. P., and Strong, E. W.: Analysis of prognostic variables and results after supraglottic partial laryngectomy. Am. J. Surg., 156:301, 1988.
638. Souhami, L., and Rabinowits, M.: Combined treatment in carcinoma of the nasopharynx. Laryngoscope, 98:881, 1988.
639. South East Cooperative Oncology Group: A randomized trial of combined multidrug chemotherapy and radiotherapy in advanced squamous cell carcinoma of the head and neck. Eur. J. Surg. Oncol., 12:289, 1986.
640. Sozzi, G., Miozzo, M., Tagliabue, E., Calderone, C., Lombardi, L., Pilotti, S., Pastorino,

U., Pierotti, M. A., and Porta, G. D.: Cytogenetic abnormalities and overexpression of receptors for growth factors in normal bronchial epithelium and tumor samples in lung cancer patients. Cancer Res., 51:400, 1991.
641. Spandidos, P. A., Lamothe, A., and Field, J. K.: Multiple transcriptional activation of cellular oncogenes in human head and neck solid tumors. Anticancer Res., 5:221, 1985.
642. Spaulding, C. A., Kranyak, M. S., Constable, W. C., and Stewart, F. M.: Esthesioneuroblastoma: a comparison of two treatment eras. Int. J. Rad. Oncol. Biol. Phys., 15:581, 1988.
643. Spaulding, C. A., Krochak, R. J., Hahn, S. S., and Constable, W. C.: Radiotherapeutic management of cancer of the supraglottis. Cancer, 57:1292, 1986.
644. Spaulding, M. B., Lore, J. M., and Sundquist, N.: Long-term follow-up of chemotherapy in advanced head and neck cancer. Arch. Otolaryngol. Head Neck Surg., 115:68, 1989.
645. Spijkervet, F., Vermey, A., Panders, A. V., Saene, H., and Mehta, D.: Prevention of irradiation mucositis in head-neck cancer patients. (Abstract #673) Proc. Am. Soc. Clin. Oncol., 9:174, 1990.
646. Spiro, J. D., and Spiro, R. H.: Carcinoma of the tonsillar fossa: an update. Arch. Otolaryngol. Head Neck Surg., 115:1186, 1989.
647. Spiro, R. H.: Squamous cancer of the tongue. Cancer, 35:252, 1985.
648. Spiro, R. H., Alfonso, A. E., Farr, H. W., and Strong, E. W.: Cervical node metastases from epidermoid carcinoma of the oral cavity and oropharynx. A critical assessment of current staging. Am. J. Surg., 128:562, 1974.
649. Spiro, R. H., Huvos, A. G., and Strong, E. W.: Cancer of the parotid gland: a clinicopathologic study of 288 primary cases. Am. J. Surg., 130:452, 1975.
650. Spiro, R. H., Huvos, A. G., and Strong, E. W.: Acinic cell carcinoma of salivary origin: a clinicopathologic study of 67 cases. Cancer, 41:924, 1978.
651. Spiro, R. H., Huvos, A. G., and Strong, E. W.: Adenoid cystic carcinoma: factors influencing survival. Am. J. Surg., 138:579, 1979.
652. Spiro, R. H., Kelly, J., Vega, A. L., Harrison, L. B., and Strong, E. W.: Squamous carcinoma of the posterior pharyngeal wall. Am. J. Surg., 160:420, 1990.
653. Spiro, R. H., Koss, L. G., Hajdu, S. I., and Strong, E. W.: Tumors of minor salivary gland origin a clinicopathologic study of 492 cases. Cancer, 31:117, 1973.
654. Spitz, M. R., Fueger, J. J., Beddingfield, N. A., Annegers, J. F., Hsu, T. C., Newell, G. R., and Schantz, S. P.: Chromosome sensitivity to bleomycin-induced mutagenesis: an independent risk factor for upper aerodigestive tract cancers. Cancer Res., 49:4626, 1989.
655. Spitz, M. R., Fueger, J. J., Geopfert, H., Hong, W. K., and Newell, G. R.: Squamous cell carcinoma of the upper aerodigestive tract: A case comparison analysis. Cancer, 61:203, 1988.
656. Spitz, M. R., Sider, J. G., Newell, G. R., and Batsakis, J. G.: Incidence of salivary gland cancer in the United States relative to ultraviolet radiation exposure. Head Neck Surg., 10:305, 1988.
657. Sporn, M. B.: Approaches to prevention of epithelial cancer during the preneoplastic period. Cancer Res., 36:2699, 1976.
658. Sporn, M. B.: Carcinogenesis and cancer: Different perspectives on the same disease. Cancer Res., 51:6215, 1991.
659. Sporn, M. B., Dunlop, N. M., Newton, D. L., and Smith, J. M.: Prevention of chemical carcinogenesis by vitamin A and its synthetic analogs (retinoids). Fed. Proc., 35:1332, 1976.
660. Squier, C. A.: Smokeless tobacco and oral cancer: A cause for concern? CA, 34:242, 1984.
661. Stefani, A., and Chung, T. S.: Hydroxyurea and radiotherapy in head and neck cancer—long term results of a double blind randomised prospective study. Radiat. Oncol. Biol. Phys., 6:1398, 1980.
662. Stell, P. M., Dalby, J. E., Strickland, P., Fraser, J. G., Bradley, P. J., and Flood, L. M.: Sequential chemotherapy and radiotherapy in advanced head and neck cancer. Clin. Radiol., 34:463, 1983.
663. Stell, P. M., and Rawson, N. S.: Adjuvant chemotherapy in head and neck cancer. Br. J. Cancer, 61:779, 1990.
664. Stewart, F. M., Lazarus, H. M., Levine, P. A., Stewart, K. A., Tabbara, I. A., and Spaulding, C. A.: High-dose chemotherapy and autologous marrow transplantation for esthesioneuroblastoma and sinonasal undifferentiated carcinoma. Am. J. Clin. Oncol., 12:217, 1989.
665. Stolwijk, C., Wagener, D. J., van den Broek Levendaj, P. C., Kazem, I., Bruaset, I., and DeMulder, P. H.: Randomized adjuvant chemotherapy trial for advanced head and neck cancer. Neo-Neth. J. Med., 28:347, 1985.
666. Stich, H. F., Hornby, A. P., Mathew, B., Sankaranarayanan, R., and Nair, M. K.: Response of oral leukoplakias to the administration of vitamin A. Cancer Lett., 40:93, 1988.
667. Stich, H. F., Rosin, M. P., Hornby, A. P., Mathew, B., Sankaranarayanan, R., and Nair, M. K.: Remission of oral leukoplakias and micronuclei in tobacco/betel quid chewers treated with beta-carotene and with beta-carotene plus vitamin A. Int. J. Cancer, 42:195, 1988.
668. Stich, H. F., Hornby, A. P., and Dunn, B. P.: A pilot beta-carotene intervention trial with Inuits using smokeless tobacco. Int. J. Cancer, 36:321, 1985.
669. Strome, M., Clark, J., Fried, M., Rodliff, S., and Blazar, B. A.: Prognostic Implications of Defining Natural Killer Cell Function and T-cell Sub-sets in Patients with Squamous Cell Carcinoma. *In* Head and Neck. Edited by W. Fee, W. Goepfert, M. E. Johns, E. W., Strong, and P. H. Ward. Philadelphia, B. C. Decker, 1990, pp. 89–93.
670. Strong, M. S., Incze, J., and Vaughan, C. W.: Field cancerization in the aerodigestive tract—Its etiology, manifestation, and significance. J. Otolaryngol., 13:1, 1984.
671. Stuttgen, G.: Oral vitamin A acid therapy. Acta Derm. Venereol. Suppl., 74:174, 1975.
672. Suen, J. Y., and Johns, M. E.: Chemotherapy for salivary gland cancer. Laryngoscope, 92:235, 1982.
673. Sutow, W. W., Sullivan, M. P., Reid, H. L., Taylor, M. G., and Griffith, K. M.: Prognosis in childhood rhabdomyosarcoma. Cancer, 25:1238, 1970.
674. Syrjanen, S. M., Syrjanen, K. J., and Happonen, R. P.: Human papillomavirus (HPV) DNA sequences in oral precancerous lesions and squamous cell carcinoma demonstrated by in situ hybridization. J. Oral. Pathol., 17:273, 1988.
675. Szpirglas, H., Chastang, C., and Bertrand, J. C.: Adjuvant treatment of tongue and floor of the mouth cancers. Recent Results Cancer Res., 68:309, 1978.
676. Szpirglas, H., Nizri, D., Marneur, M., et al.: Neo-adjuvant chemotherapy. A randomized trial before radiotherapy in oral and oro-pharyngeal carcinomas: end results. Head and Neck Oncology Research. Proceedings of the 2nd Internation. Arlington VA, pp. 261–264, Sept. 10–12, 1987.
677. Taguchi, T.: Clinical studies of recombinant interferon alfa-2a (Roferon-A) in cancer patients. Cancer, 57:1705, 1986.
678. Takaku, F.: Clinical trials and cancer risk in Japan. J. Natl. Cancer Inst., 73:1483, 1984.
679. Tannock, I. F., and Browman, G.: Lack of evidence for a role of chemotherapy in the routine management of locally advanced head and neck cancer. J. Clin. Oncol., 4:1121, 1986.
680. Tannock, I., Payne, D., Cummings, B., Hewitt, K., and Panzarella, T.: Sequential chemotherapy and radiation for nasopharyngeal cancer: Absence of long-term benefit despite a high rate of tumor response to chemotherapy. J. Clin. Oncol., 5:629, 1987.
681. Tannock, I. F., and Sutherland, D. J.: Chemotherapy for adenocystic carcinoma. Cancer, 46:452, 1980.
682. Tapazoglou, E., Kish, J., Ensley, J., and Al-Sarraf, M.: The activity of a single-agent 5-fluorouracil infusion in advanced and recurrent head and neck. Cancer, 57:1105, 1986.
683. Tapazoglou, E., Lorusso, P., Kish, J., Ensley, J., and Al-Sarraf, M.: The management of paranasal sinus cancer. Second International Head and Neck Oncology Research Conference: 357–364, 1987.
684. Tapley, N.–du V.: Irradiation treatment of malignant tumors of the salivary glands. Ear Nose Throat J., 56:110, 1977.
685. Taylor, S. G., IV: Why has so much chemotherapy done so little in head and neck cancer? (Editorial) J. Clin. Oncol., 5:1, 1987.
686. Taylor, S., Murthy, A., Showel, J., Griem, K., Hartsell, W., Kiel, K., Kies, M., Mittal, B., Pelzer, H., Vokes, E., Vannetzel, J. M., Coupez, D. J., Colin, P., and Dray, M.: Analysis of sequential v. simultaneous chemotherapy and radiation in unresectable head and neck cancer: ICC and PCP studies. Proc. Am. Soc. Clin. Oncol., 11: 1992.
687. Taylor, S. G., IV: Combined Chemotherapy and Radiation for Unresectable Head and Neck Cancer. *In* Carcinomas of the Head and Neck: Evaluation and Management. Edited by C. Jacobs. Boston, MA, Kluwer Academic Publishers, 1990, pp. 195–208.
688. Taylor, S. G., IV, Applebaum, E., Showel, J. L., Norusis, M., Holinger, L. D., Hutchinson, J. L., Jr., Murthy, A. K., and Caldarelli, D. D.: A randomized trial of adjuvant chemotherapy in head and neck cancer. J. Clin. Oncol., 3:672, 1985.
689. Taylor, S. G., IV, McGuire, W. P., Hauck, W. W., Showel, J. L., and Lad, T. E.: A randomized comparison of high-dose infusion methotrexate versus standard-dose weekly therapy in head and neck squamous cancer. J. Clin. Oncol., 2:1006, 1984.
690. Taylor, S. G., IV, Murthy, A. K., Caldarelli, D. D., Showel, J. L., Kiel, K., Griem, K. L., Mittal, B. B., Kies, M., Hutchinson, J. C., Jr., and Molinger, L. D.: Combined simultaneous cisplatin/fluorouracil chemotherapy and split course radiation in head and neck cancer. J. Clin. Oncol., 7:846, 1989.
691. Taylor, S. G., Sisson, G. A., Bytell, D. E., and Raynor, W. J.: A randomized trial of adjuvant BCG immunotherapy in head and neck cancer. Arch. Otolaryngol., 109:544, 1983.
692. Tejada, F., and Chandler, J. R.: Combined therapy for stage III and IV head and neck cancer (H&N). (Abstract C-774) Proc. Am. Soc. Clin. Oncol., 1:199, 1982.
693. Tepperman, B. S., and Fitzpatrick, P. J.: Second respiratory and upper digestive tract cancers after oral cancer. Lancet, 2:547, 1981.
694. Terz, J. J., and Farr, H. W.: Carcinoma of the tonsillar fossa. Surg. Gynecol. Obstet., 125:581, 1967.
695. Thames, H. D., Peters, L. J., Withers, H. R., and Fletcher, G. H.: Accelerated fractionation vs hyperfractionation: rationales for several treatments per day. Int. J. Radiat. Oncol. Biol. Phys., 9:127, 1983.
696. Thawley, S. E., Simpson, J. R., Marks, J. E., Perez, C. A., and Ogura, J. H.: Preoperative irradiation and surgery for carcinoma of the base of the tongue. Ann. Otol. Rhinol. Laryngol., 92:485, 1983.
697. Tobias, J. S.: Has chemotherapy proved itself in head and neck cancer? Br. J. Cancer, 61:649, 1990.
698. Tobias, J. S., Smith, B. J., Blackman, G., and Finn, G.: Concurrent daily cisplatin and radiotherapy in locally advanced squamous carcinoma of the head and neck and bronchus. Radiother. Oncol., 9:263, 1987.
699. Todd, R., Donoff, B. R., Gertz, R., Chang, A. L., Chow, P., Matossian, K., McBride, J., Chiang, T., Gallager, G. T., and Wong, D. T.: TGF-alpha and EGF-receptor mRNAS in human oral cancer. Carcinogenesis, 10:1553, 1989.
700. Toma, S., Albanese, E., DeLorenzi, M., Nicolo, G., Mangiante, P., Galli, A., and Cancedda, R.: Beta-carotene in the treatment of oral leukoplakia. (Abstract #695) Proc. Am. Soc. Clin. Oncol., 9:179, 1990.
701. Toohill, R. J., Anderson, T., Byhardt, R. W., Cox, J. D., Duncavage, J. A., Grossman, T. W., Haas, C. D., Haas, J. S., Hartz, A. J., and Libroch, J. A.: Cisplatin and fluorouracil as neoadjuvant therapy in head and neck cancer. A preliminary report. Arch. Otolaryngol. Head Neck Surg., 113:758, 1987.
702. Toohill, R. J., Duncavage, J. A., Malin, T. C., Wilson, J. F., Haas, J. S., Anderson, T., Ritch, P. S., Libnoch, J., Grossmam, T. W., Teplin, R. W., Byhardt, R. W., Cox, J. D., Holoye, P. Y., Haas, C. D., and Hoffmann, R. G.: The effects of delay in standard treatment due to induction chemotherapy in two randomized prospective studies. Laryngoscope, 97:407, 1987.
703. Trible, W. M.: Cancer of the oral cavity: Five year end results in 237 patients. Ann. Otol. Rhinol. Laryngol., 78:716, 1969.
704. Trickler, D., and Shklar, G.: Prevention by vitamin E of experimental oral carcinogenesis. J. Natl. Cancer Inst., 78:165, 1987.
705. Triozzi, P. L., Brantley, A., Fisher, S., Cole, T. B., Crocker, I., and Huang, A. T.: 5-Fluorouracil, cyclophosphamide, and vincristine for adenoid cystic carcinoma of the head and neck. Cancer, 59:887, 1987.
706. Trojanowski, J. Q., Lee, V., Pillsbury, N., and Lee. S.: Neuronal origin of human esthesioneuroblastoma demonstrated with antineurofilament monocional antibodies. N. Engl. J. Med., 307:159, 1982.
707. Tsuda, T., Tahara, E., Kajiyama, G., Sakamoto, M., Tejada, M., and Sugimura, T.: High incidence of coamplification of hst-1 and int-2 genes in human esophageal carcinomas. Cancer Res., 49:5505, 1989.
708. Uen, W., Huang, A. T., Mennel, R., Jones, S. E., Spaulding, M. B., Killion, K., Havlin, K., Keegan, P., and Clendeninn, N. J.: A phase II study of piritrexim in patients with advanced squamous head and neck cancer. Cancer, 69:1008, 1992.
709. Urba, S., Forastiere, A. A., Wolf, G. T., Sullivan, M., Thronton, A., and Husted, S.:

Induction chemotherapy (CT) with intensive continuous infusion high dose cisplatin (CDDP), 5-fluorouracil (5FU) and mitoguazone (MGBG) for advanced head and neck cancer (H&N CA). (Abstract #663) Proc. Am. Soc. Clin. Oncol., 9:171, 1990.
710. VA Laryngeal Cancer Study Group: Induction chemotherapy plus radiation compared with surgery plus radiation in patients with advanced laryngeal cancer. N. Engl. J. Med., 324:1685, 1991.
711. Van den Bogaert, W., Ostyn, F., and Van der Schueren, E.: The significance of extension and impaired mobility in cancer of the vocal cord. Int. J. Radiat. Oncol. Biol. Phys., 9:181, 1983.
712. Van den Bogaert, W., Ostyn, F., and Van der Schueren, E.: The differential clinical presentation, behaviour and prognosis of carcinomas originating in the epilarynx and the lower supraglottic. Radiother. Oncol., 1:117, 1983.
713. Van den Bogaert, W., Van der Schueren, E., Horiot, J. C., Chaplin, G., Devilhena, M., Rapso, S., Leonor, J., Schraub, S., Chenal, C., Barthelme, E., Daban, A., Eschwege, F., Gonzales, D., Leer, J. W., Hamers, H., Svoboda, V., Rigon, A., Arcangeli, G., Sack, H., de Pauw, M., and van Glabbeke, M.: Early results of the EORTC randomized clinical trial on multiple fractions per day (MFD) and misonidazole in advanced head and neck cancer. Int. J. Radiat. Oncol. Biol. Phys., 12:587, 1986.
714. Van den Brouck, C., Sancho-Garnier, H., Chassagne, D., Saravane, D., Chachin, Y., and Micheau, C.: Elective versus therapeutic radical neck dissection in epidermoid carcinoma of the oral cavity: Results of a randomized clinical trial. Cancer, 46:386, 1980.
715. Van den Brouck, C., Eschwege, F., De La Rochefordiere, A., Sicot, H., Mamelle, G., Le Ridant, A. M., Bosq, J., and Domenge, C.: Squamous cell carcinoma of the pyriform sinus: Retrospective study of 351 cases treated at the Institute Gustave-Roussy. Head Neck Surg., 10:4, 1987.
716. van Dongen, G., Braakhuis, B. J., Bagnay, M., Leyva, A., and Snow, G. B.: Activity of differentiation-inducing agents and conventional drugs in head and neck cancer xenografts. Acta Otolaryngol. (Stockh.), 105:488, 1988.
717. Venook, A. P., Tseng, A., Jr., Meyers, F. J., Silverberg, I., Boles, R., Fu, K. K., and Jacobs, C. D.: Cisplatin, doxorubicin, and 5 fluorouracil chemotherapy for salivary gland malignancies: a pilot study of the Northern California Oncology Group. J. Clin. Oncol., 5:951, 1987.
718. Vermeer, R. J., and Pinedo, H. M.: Partial remission of advanced adenoid cystic carcinoma obtained with adriamycin: A case report with a review of the literature. Cancer, 43:1604, 1979.
719. Vermund, H.: Role of radiotherapy in cancer of the larynx as related to the TNM system of staging. Cancer, 25:485, 1970.
720. Vermund, H., Brennhovd, I., Kaalhus, O., and Poppe, E.: Incidence and control of occult neck node metastases from squamous cell carcinoma of the anterior two-thirds of the tongue. Int. J. Radiol. Oncol. Biol. Phys., 10:2025, 1984.
721. Vermund, H., Kaalhus, O., Winther, F., Trausj, J., Thorud, E., and Marang, R.: Bleomycin and radiation therapy in squamous cell carcinoma of the upper aero-digestive tract: A phase III clinical trial. Int. J. Radiat. Oncol. Biol. Phys., 11:1877, 1985.
722. Veronesi, A., Zagonel, V., Trielli, U., Galligioni, E., Tumolo, S., Barzan, L., Lorenzini, M., Comoretto, R., and Grigoletto, E.: High-dose versus low-dose cisplatin in advanced head and neck squamous carcinoma: a randomized study. J. Clin. Oncol., 3:1105, 1985.
723. Verweij, J., Alexieva-Figusch, J., de Boer, M. F., Reichquelt, B., and Stoter, G.: Ifosfamide in advanced head and neck cancer. A phase II study of the Rotterdam Cooperative Head and Neck Cancer Study Group. Eur. J. Cancer Clin. Oncol., 24:795, 1988.
724. Vikram, B.: Changing patterns of failure in advanced head and neck cancer. Arch. Otolaryngol., 110:564, 1984.
725. Vikram, B.: Cisplatin-based chemotherapy rapidly alternating with accelerated radiation therapy for carcinomas of the hypopharynx and upper esophagus. Third International Head and Neck Oncology Research Conference, Las Vegas, Nevada, 1990.
726. Vikram, B., Bosl, G. J., Pfister, D., Assad, W., Strong, E. W., Spiro, R. H., Sessions, R. B., Gerold, F. P., and Shah, J. P.: New strategies for avoiding total laryngectomy in patients with head and neck cancer. N.C.I. Monogr., 6:361, 1988.
727. Vikram, B., Mishra, U. B., Strong, E. W., and Manolatos, S.: Patterns of failure in carcinoma of the nasopharynx I: failure at the primary site. Int. J. Radiat. Oncol. Biol. Phys., 11:1455, 1985.
728. Vikram, B., Strong, E. W., Shah, J., and Spiro, R. H.: Elective postoperative irradiation in stages III and IV epidermoid carcinoma of the head and neck. Am. J. Surg., 140:580, 1980.
729. Vikram, B., Strong, E. W., Shah, J. P., and Spiro, R.: Failure at the primary site following multimodality treatment in advanced head and neck cancer. Head Neck Surg., 6:720, 1984.
730. Vikram, B., Strong, E. W., Shah, J. P., and Spiro, R. H.: Radiation therapy in adenoid-cystic carcinoma. Int. J. Radiat. Oncol. Biol. Phys., 10:221, 1984.
731. Vogelstein, B., Fearon, E. R., Hamilton, S. R., Kern, S. E., Preisinger, A. C., Leppert, M., Nakamura, Y., White, R., Smith, A. M., and Bos, J. L.: Genetic alterations during colorectal-tumor development. N. Engl. J. Med., 319:525, 1988.
732. Vogl, S. E., Schoenfeld, D. A., Kaplan, B. H., Lerner, H. J., Engstrom, P. F., and Horton, J.: A randomized prospective comparison of methotrexate with a combination of methotrexate, bleomycin, and cisplatin in head and neck cancer. Cancer, 56:432, 1985.
733. Vogler, W. R., Jacobs, J., Moffitt, S., et al: Methotrexate therapy with or without citrovorum factor in carcinoma of the head and neck, breast, and colon. Cancer Clin. Trials, 2:227, 1979.
734. Vokes, E. E., Choi, K. E., Schilsky, R. L., Moran, W. J., Guarnieri, C. M., and Panje, W. R.: Cisplatin, fluorouracil, and high-dose leucovorin for recurrent or metastatic head and neck cancer. J. Clin. Oncol., 6:618, 1988.
735. Vokes, E. E., Mick, R., Lester, E. P., Panje, W. R., and Weichselbaum, R. R.: Cisplatin and fluorouracil chemotherapy does not yield long-term benefit in locally advanced head and neck cancer: Results from a single institution. J. Clin. Oncol., 9:1376, 1991.
736. Vokes, E. E., Panje, W. R., Schilsky, R. L., Mick, R., Awan, A. M., Moran, W. J., Goldman, M. D., Tybor, A. G., and Weichselbaum, R. R.: Hydroxyurea, fluorouracil, and concomitant radiotherapy in poor-prognosis of head and neck cancer: A phase I–II study. J. Clin. Oncol., 7:761, 1989.
737. Vokes, E. E., Schilsky, R. L., Weichselbaum, R. R., Kozloff, M. F., and Parje, W. R.: Induction chemotherapy with cisplatin, fluorouracil, and high-dose leucovorin for locally advanced head and neck cancer: A clinical and pharmacologic analysis. J. Clin. Oncol., 8:241, 1990.
738. Vokes, E. E., and Weichselbaum, R. R.: Concomitant chemoradiotherapy: Rationale and clinical experience in patients with solid tumors. J. Clin. Oncol., 8:911, 1990.
739. Volling, P., Mueller, R. P., Staar, S., Schroeder, M., Achterrath, W., and Lenaz, L.: Pilot study with carboplatin (CBDCA) and simultaneous accelerated radiation (RT) in advanced squamous cell carcinoma of the head and neck (SCCHN). (Abstract #681) Proc. Am. Soc. Clin. Oncol., 9:176, 1990.
740. Volterrani, F., Chiesa, F., and Molinari, R.: Argument in favor of precautional treatment of cervical nodes in clinically no oral cancer. Tumori, 68:241, 1982.
741. von Essen, C. P., Joseph, L. B., Simon, G. T., Singh, A. D., and Singh, S. P.: Sequential chemotherapy and radiation therapy of buccal mucosa carcinoma in South India. Methods and preliminary results. Am. J. Roentgenol. Radium Ther. Nucl. Med., 102:530, 1968.
742. Von Hoff, D. D.: Whither carboplatin—a replacement for or an alternative to cisplatin? J. Clin. Oncol., 5:169, 1987.
743. Wallner, P. E., Hanks, G. E., Kramer, S., and McLean, C. J.: Patterns of care study: Analysis of outcome survey data—anterior two thirds of tongue and floor of mouth. Am. J. Clin. Oncol., 9:50, 1986.
744. Wanebo, H. J., Hilal, E. Y., Strong, E. W., Pinsky, C. M., Mike, V., and Oettgen, H. F.: Adjuvant trial of levamisole in patients with squamous cancer of the head and neck: a preliminary report. Recent Results Cancer Res., 68:324, 1978.
745. Wang, C. C.: Radiotherapeutic management of carcinoma of the posterior pharyngeal wall. Cancer, 27:894, 1971.
746. Wang, C. C.: Megavoltage radiation therapy for supraglottic carcinoma: results of treatment. Radiology, 109:183, 1973.
747. Wang, C. C.: Radiation therapy for head and neck neoplasms: Indications, techniques and results. Boston, John Wright P. S. G., 1983.
748. Wang, C. C.: Re-irradiation of recurrent nasopharyngeal carcinoma—treatment techniques and results. Int. J. Radiat. Oncol. Biol. Phys., 13:952, 1987.
749. Wang, C. C.: Local control of oropharyngeal carcinoma after two accelerated hyperfractionation radiation therapy schemes. Int. J. Radiat. Oncol. Biol. Phys., 14:1143, 1988.
750. Wang, C. C., Busse, J., and Gitterman, M.: A simple afterloading application for intracavitary irradiation of the nasopharynx. Radiology, 115:737, 1975.
751. Wang, C. C., Suit, H. D., and Blitzer, P. H.: Twice a day radiation therapy for supraglottic carcinoma. Int. J. Radiat. Oncol. Biol. Phys., 12:3, 1986.
752. Ward, G. E., and Hendrick, J. W.: Results of treatment of carcinoma of the lip. Surg., 27:321, 1950.
753. Ward, P. H., Calcaterra, T. C., and Kagan, A. R.: The regimen of postradiation edema and recurrent or residual carcinoma of the larynx. Laryngoscope, 85:522, 1975.
754. Warren, S., and Gates, O.: Multiple primary malignant tumors: A survey of the literature and statistical study. Am. J. Cancer, 51:1358, 1932.
755. Watson, T. A.: Irradiation in the management of tumors of the head and neck. Am. J. Surg., 110:542, 1965.
756. Wawro, N. W., Babcock, A., and Ellison, L.: Cancer of the tongue: Experience at the Hartford Hospital from 1931–1963. Am. J. Surg., 119:455, 1970.
757. Weaver, A., Fleming, S., Ensley, J., Kish, J. A., Jacobs, J., Kinzie, J., Crissman, J., and Al Sarraf, M.: Superior clinical response and survival rates with initial bolus of cisplatin and 120 hour infusion of 5-fluorouracil before definitive therapy for locally advanced head and neck cancer. Am. J. Surg., 148:525, 1984.
758. Weaver, A., Flemming, S., Kish, J., Vandenberg, M., Jacob, J., and Crissman, J.: Cis-platinum and 5-fluorouracil as induction therapy for advanced head and neck cancer. Am. J. Surg., 144:445, 1982.
759. Weber, R. S., Gidley, P., Morrison, W. H., Peters, L. J., Hankins, P., Wolf, P., and Guillamondegui, O.: Treatment selection for carcinoma of the base of the tongue. Am. J. Surg., 160:415, 1990.
760. Weber, R. S., Lippman, S. M., and McNeese, M. D.: Advanced basal and squamous cell carcinoma of the head and neck. *In* Carcinomas of the Head and Neck. Edited by C. Jacobs. Norwell, MA, Kluwer Academic Publishers, 1990, pp. 61–81.
761. Weber, R. S., Peters, L. J., Wolf, P. S., and Guillamondegui, O.: Squamous cell carcinoma of the soft palate, uvula and anterior faucial pillar. Otolaryngol. Head Neck Surg., 99:16, 1988.
762. Weinstein, I. B.: Cancer prevention: Recent progress and future opportunities. Cancer Res., 51:5080, 1991.
763. Weissberg, J. B., Son, Y. H., Papac, R. J., Sasaki, C., Fischer, D. B., Lawrence, R., Rockwell, S., Sartorelli, A. C., and Fischer, J. J.: Randomized clinical trial of mitomycin C as an adjunct to radiotherapy in head and neck cancer. Int. J. Radiat. Oncol. Biol. Phys., 17:3, 1989.
764. Welsh, L. W., Welsh, J. J., and Rizzo, T. A., Jr.: Laryngol spaces and lymphatics: current anatomic concepts. Ann. Otol. Rhinol. Laryngol. Suppl., 105:19, 1983.
765. Wendt, T. G., Hartenstein, R. C., and Wustrow, T. P.: 4-years-update of simultaneous chemo-radiotherapy with 5-FU/folinic acid (FA)/cisplatin (DDP) and accelerated radiation in inoperable head and neck cancer (HNC). (Abstract #658) Proc. Am. Soc. Clin. Oncol., 8:169, 1989.
766. Wendt, T. G., Hartenstein, R. C., Wustrow, T. P., and Lissner, J.: Cisplatin, fluorouracil with leucovorin calcium enhancement, and synchronous accelerated radiotherapy in the management of locally advanced head and neck cancer: A phase II study. J. Clin. Oncol., 7:471, 1989.
767. Wenig, B. M., Hyam, V. J., and Heffner, D. K.: Moderately differentiated neuroendocrine carcinoma of the larynx. Cancer, 62:2658, 1988.
768. Wennerberg, J., Heim, S., Jin, Y., et al: Rearrangements involving chromosome bands 1p22 and 11q13 in squamous cell carcinomas of the head and neck. Third International Head and Neck Oncology Research Conference, Las Vegas, Nevada, 1990.
769. Wetmore, S. J., Key, M. J., and Suen, J. Y.: Laser therapy for T1 glottic carcinoma of the larynx. Arch. Otolaryngol. Head Neck Surg., 112:853, 1986.
770. Wheeler, R. H., Baker, S. R., and Medvec, B. R.: Single-agent and combination-drug regional chemotherapy for head and neck cancer using an implantable infusion pump. Cancer, 54:1504, 1984.
771. Wheeler, R., Salter, M., Stephens, S., Hardy, I., Peters, G., Urist, M., and Maddox, W.: Simultaneous therapy with high-dose cisplatin and radiation for unresectable squamous cell cancer of the head and neck: a phase I–II study. N.C.I. Monogr., 6:339, 1988.
772. Wiernik, G., Bates, T. D., Bleehen, M. N., Brindle, J. M., Bullimore, J., Fowler, J. F.,

Haybittle, J. L., Howard, N., Laing, A. H., and Lindup, R.: Final report of the general clinical result of the British Institute of Radiology fractionation study of the 3F wk versus 5F wk in radiotherapy of carcinoma of the laryngo-pharynx. Br. J. Radiol., 63:169, 1990.

773. Williams, S. D., Velez-Garcia, E., Essessee, I., Ratkin, G., Birch, R., and Einhorn, L. H.: Chemotherapy for head and neck cancer: Comparison of cisplatin + vinblastine + bleomycin versus methotrexate. Cancer, 57:18, 1986.

774. Wilson, J. S., and Walker, E. P.: Reconstruction of the lower lip. Head Neck Surg., 4:29, 1981.

775. Winn, D. M., Blot, W. J., Shy, C. M., Pickle, L. W., Toledo, A., and Fraumeni, J. F., Jr.: Snuff dipping and oral cancer among women in the southern United States. N. Engl. J. Med., 304:745, 1981.

776. Winn, D. M., Ziegler, R. G., Pickle, L. W., Gridley, G., Blot, W. J., and Hoover, R. N.: Diet in the etiology of oral and pharyngeal cancer among women from the southern United States. Cancer Res., 44:1216, 1984.

777. Wittes, R. E.: Chemotherapy of head and neck cancer. Otolaryngol. Clin. North Am., 13:515, 1980.

778. Wittes, R. E., Cvitkovic, E., Shah, J., Gerold, F. P., and Strong, W. E.: Cis-dichloro-diammineplatinum (II) in the treatment of epidermoid carcinoma of the head and neck. Cancer Treat. Rep., 61:359, 1977.

779. Wittes, R., Heller, K., Randolph, V., Howard, J., Vallejo, A., Farr, H., Harrold, C., Gerold, F., Shah, J., Shapiro, R., and Strong, E.: cis-Dichlorodiammineplatinum(II)-based chemotherapy as initial treatment of advanced head and neck cancer. Cancer Treat. Rep., 63:1533, 1979.

780. Wolbach, S. B., and Howe, P. R.: Tissue changes following deprivation of fat soluble A vitamin. J. Exp. Med., 42:753, 1925.

781. Wolf, G. T., Carey, T. E., Schmaltz, S. P., McClatchey, K. D., Poore, J., Glaser, L., Hayashida, D. J., and Hsu, S.: Altered antigen expression predicts outcome in squamous cell carcinoma of the head and neck. J. Natl. Cancer Inst., 82:1566, 1990.

782. Wolf, G. T., Hudson, J. L., Peterson, K. A., Miller, H. L., and McClatchey, D.: Lymphocyte subpopulation infiltrating squamous carcinomas of the head and neck: correlations with extent of tumor and prognosis. Otolaryngol. Head Neck Surg., 95:142, 1986.

783. Wolf, G. T., Makuch, R. W., and Baker, S. R.: Predictive factors for tumor response to pre-operative chemotherapy in patients with squamous carcinoma. The Head and Neck Contracts Group. Cancer, 54:2869, 1984.

784. Wolf, G. T., Truelson, J. M., Beals, T., and Fisher, S.: Nuclear area and adjusted DNA index: A new correlate of prognosis in squamous carcinoma of the larynx. Proc. Am. Assoc. Cancer Res., 31:189, 1990.

785. Wong, C. S., and Cummings, B. J.: The place of radiation therapy in the treatment of squamous cell carcinoma of nasal vestibule: A review. Acta Oncol., 27:203, 1988.

786. Wong, D. T.: Amplification of the c-erb B1 oncogene in chemically-induced oral carcinomas. Carcinogenesis, 8:1963, 1987.

787. Woods, R. L., Fox, R. M., and Tattersall, M. H.: Methotrexate treatment of squamous-cell head and neck cancers: dose-response evaluation. Br. Med. J. (Clin. Res.), 282:600, 1981.

788. Wookey, H., Ash, C., Welsh, W. K., and Mustard, R. A.: The treatment of oral cancer by a combination of radiotherapy and surgery. Ann. Surg., 134:529, 1951.

789. Wulf, K.: Zur vitamin A behandlung der leukoplakien. Arch. Klin. exp. Derm., 206–495, 1957.

790. Wynder, E. L., and Hoffman, D.: Tobacco. In Cancer Epidemiology and Prevention. Edited by D. Schottenfeld, and J. F. Fraumeni, Jr. Philadelphia, W. B. Saunders, 1982, pp. 277–292.

791. Wynne, C. J., and Kearsley, J. H.: Merkel cell tumor: A chemosensitive skin cancer. Cancer, 62:28, 1988.

792. Yates, A., and Crumley, R. L.: Surgical treatment of pyriform sinus cancer: A retrospective study. Laryngoscope, 94:1586, 1984.

793. Yu, M. C.: Diet and nasopharyngeal carcinoma. Prog. Clin. Biol. Res., 346:93, 1990.

794. Yuen, A., Medina, J. E., Goepfert, H., and Fletcher, G.: Management of stage T3 and T4 glottic carcinoma. Am. J. Surg., 148:467, 1984.

795. Zbaeren, P., and Lehmann, W.: Frequency and sites of distant metastases in head and neck squamous cell carcinoma. Arch. Otolaryngol. Head Neck Surg., 113:762, 1987.

796. Zeng, Y.: Seroepidemiological studies on nasopharyngeal carcinoma in China. Adv. Cancer Res., 44:121, 1985.

797. Zenner, H. P.: Selective killing of laryngeal carcinoma cells by a monoclonal immuno-toxin. Ann. Otol. Rhinol. Laryngol., 95:115, 1986.

XXVII-2

Odontogenic Tumors

George T. Gallagher
Gerald Shklar

Introduction

Odontogenic tumors comprise an unusual group of lesions of the jaws, derived from primordial tooth-forming tissues, and presenting in a large number of histologic patterns. Some of these lesions, particularly the odontomas, are now interpreted as developmental malformations or hamartomatous lesions, rather than true neoplasms. Other lesions, such as ameloblastoma, are accepted as true neoplasms and must be diagnosed and treated as such. The true odontogenic tumors are essentially benign lesions, but infiltrate the adjacent bone between the spicules of the medulla. This form of bony infiltration, common to all benign tumors of bone, such as giant cell tumors, is not the true invasiveness of malignant tumors, but represents a clinical problem, in that the tumor can recur after surgical therapy if the bony margins still contain some of the tumor infiltration.

In general terms, odontogenic tumors tend to be more common in younger patients, but can occur at any age.[29] They originate in the jaws and usually are found in the tooth-bearing sites. The odontomas are often associated with impacted or missing teeth. Since the odontomas represent maldevelopment of a tooth bud, that tooth will not develop. The common sites for odontogenic tumors are the mandibular molar region and the maxillary cuspid region. The odontogenic tumors are slowly growing and asymptomatic. Pain is not a feature of benign tumors of the jaws, but is a common symptom of malignant tumors of the jaws. The odontogenic tumors are expansile lesions and may expand the bony cortex, but will not invade or perforate it. Radiographically, the odontomas will present as mixed radiolucent and radiopaque lesions. Among true neoplasms, the radiographic appearance may vary from entirely radiolucent to mixed.

The odontomas usually occur in cyst-like cavities with a connective tissue lining. They can be removed surgically by simple enucleation and will not recur since they are not true neoplasms and do not infiltrate the contiguous bone. The neoplasms, such as ameloblastoma, are to be regarded as benign tumors and treated by conservative surgical removal. Simple enucleation rarely offers a permanent cure for ameloblastoma since recurrence of the tumor will eventually occur from the infiltrative foci at the tumor margin. A block resection is favored, leaving the cortical lower border of the mandible intact. These benign tumors are relatively unaffected by radiation, and the risks of radiation in stimulating the development of a malignant tumor or of radiation necrosis is unwarranted for a benign tumor.

Over the years, very extensive and complicated classifications have been used for the odontogenic tumors and related lesions. A simple classification will suffice, based upon the derivation of the lesions and the degree of cellular differentiation involved (Table XXVII-2-1).

Other lesions, which probably are different from odontogenic lesions, but which are frequently included in this general topic are: *Periapical Cemental Dysplasia* and *Gigantiform Cementoma; Peripheral Odontogenic Fibroma* and *Odontogenic Epithelial Hamartoma* of gingiva; *Craniopharyngioma; Adamantinoma* of long bones; *Teratoma*.

Odontogenic lesions share two major characteristics: 1) They arise from tissue with the potential for differentiation into tooth or periodontal ligament structures. 2) They are found predominantly to arise at tooth-bearing sites. Variable, but distinctive features of odontogenic lesions include: 3) Formation of tooth-related extracellular substance, some of which may calcify and be visible on radiographs. 4) Epithelial-mesenchymal interactions ("induction").

Odontogenic lesions vary widely in their degree of differentiation, and there is a rough correlation between the degree of differentiation and the biologic behavior associated with any given lesion. True malignant transformation of benign odontogenic lesions, or the development of malignancy, *de novo,* from odontogenic tissues have both been reported, but such occurrences are extremely rare. In general, the less-differentiated odontogenic lesions (the immature ones) are more likely to have indistinct radiographic borders, invasive growth patterns, and relatively aggressive clinical behavior, while the mature or well-differentiated entities are more likely to produce recognizable extracellular product, to be well-circumscribed, and to be self-limiting in terms of growth.

Although odontogenic lesions may be discovered at any age, certain lesions are typically found in patients of particular age groups, and at certain sites; knowledge of these patterns, plus careful radiographic interpretation, enables the astute clinician to make an accurate clinical diagnosis of odontogenic lesions fairly frequently.

Clinical, Radiographic, Histologic Features

Epithelial Odontogenic Lesions

Enamel Pearl is a developmental defect whereby enamel is deposited on the root surface of a tooth separate from the coronal enamel. Such defects are most commonly found in the furcation region of maxillary molars. On the radiograph, enamel pearls appear as rounded, well-circumscribed densities associated with tooth roots.

These nodules are of little clinical significance, except that they may be complicating factors in periodontal disease, and they may contain cores of dentin and projections of dental pulp which could complicate their removal.

Squamous Odontogenic Tumor (S.O.T.). A well-differentiated odontogenic tumor composed of islands or sheets of squamous epithelium that lack recognizable features of enamel organ differentiation.[16,28] The typical clinical presentation is of a slowly-growing, well-circumscribed radiolucent lesion in a young adult, that is associated with the cervical portion of a tooth root. No site is really typical, but maxillary anterior and mandibular posterior regions have been most frequently affected. Multifocal lesions have been reported more frequently than in the case of other odontogenic tumors. This is an uncommon lesion, so it should not be high on the differential diagnostic list when considering radiolucent jaw lesions; if the clinical situation fits, however, and at exploration one discovers that a solid fleshy lesion is associated with a vital tooth root, then the S.O.T. becomes more likely.

Microscopically, the lesion consists of bland nests of squamous cells. No palisading or polarization of peripheral cells should be demonstrable.

Aggressive behavior or recurrences seem to be rare in S.O.T., but care must be taken to differentiate the lesion histologically from acanthomatous ameloblastoma, odontogenic carcinoma, and central mucoepidermoid carcinoma, all of which are more serious.

Nests of squamous epithelium may be found in the walls of odontogenic cysts, or in small gingival nodules, that resemble the S.O.T. microscopically; these may be called Odontogenic Epithelial Hamartomas if they seem to lack the characteristics of a true tumor.

Adenomatoid Odontogenic Tumor (A.O.T.). A well-circumscribed odontogenic tumor composed of sheets and nests of spindle-shaped epithelial cells resembling somewhat the stellate reticulum of the enamel organ, along with palisaded, polarized ameloblast-like cells which frequently produce extracellular product.[1,8,15] The typical clinical presentation is that of a well-circumscribed radiolucency (sometimes with small foci of calcification) associated with an unerupted tooth in the anterior maxilla of a young female patient. In general, affected patients are likely to be in the second and third decade of life, females are more frequently affected

Table XXVII-2-1. Classification of Odontogenic Tumors

	Epithelial	Mixed	Mesenchymal
Immature	Ameloblastoma	Ameloblastic fibroma	Myxoma
Intermediate	Calcifying odontogenic cyst (Gorlin lesion) Calcifying epithelial odontogenic tumor	Ameloblastic fibro-odontoma	Cementoblastoma (True cementoma)
Mature	Adenomatoid odontogenic tumor	Odontoma	Odontogenic fibroma (central ossifying/ cementifying fibroma)
	Squamous odontogenic tumor Enamel pearl?		

than males, the maxilla is more frequently affected than the mandible, the anterior regions are more frequently affected than the posterior, and most A.O.T.'s are associated with unerupted tooth crowns (that is, they are in a dentigerous relationship to a tooth). No other odontogenic lesion has this clinical pattern.

A.O.T. is not common, but many may have been misdiagnosed in the past; true incidence is difficult to know. A.O.T. should be considered in the differential diagnosis of a radiolucent lesion about the crown of an impacted maxillary canine, especially.

Microscopically the main cell type consists of basophilic spindle-shaped epithelial cells in sheets and whorls. Focally, one finds columnar cells in duct-like array or forming rosettes, and frequent deposits of eosinophilic, hyaline material ("membrana preformativa") are seen. Dystrophic calcifications are not uncommon, and these are usually found within the epithelium. Pleomorphism and mitotic activity are not expected.

A.O.T. is differentiated from ameloblastoma microscopically by the absence of polarized or palisaded cells at the periphery of the epithelial aggregates, and by the production of extracellular product and calcifications. A.O.T. is distinguished from C.E.O.T. (see below) by the predominantly spindle-cell morphology it exhibits, and its failure to produce amyloid.

Clinical behavior is generally that of a slow-growing, expansile lesion that seldom, if ever, would be expected to recur after conservative removal.

Calcifying Epithelial Odontogenic Tumor (C.E.O.T.). A moderately differentiated odontogenic tumor composed of somewhat pleomorphic and polyhedral epithelial cells in sheets and nests, along with extracellular material which has the characteristics of amyloid. Calcifications are quite commonly found, associated both with the epithelial cells and with the amyloid material. This lesion is also sometimes called Pindborg Tumor, after the pathologist who first described it as distinct from ameloblastoma.[11,19,27,31] The typical clinical presentation is similar in most respects to that of ameloblastoma, in that there is a predominance of cases in adults, in the mandible, and in the posterior region. The lesion exhibits radiolucency, sometimes with small focal opacities, and may not be associated with a tooth (Figure XXVII-2-1).

The histologic appearance is quite characteristic; the growth pattern is usually that of a solid lesion with amorphous amphiphilic extracellular material mixed with islands or sheets of polyhedral epithelial cells, some of which may undergo degeneration. The nuclei of the cells may be large and basophilic, but mitotic activity is absent. Special stains for amyloid are positive when applied to the extracellular material. Calcifications are frequently spherical and lamellar (Figure XXVII-2-2).

No ameloblastic differentiation is noted in the epithelial islands, and the cohesive nature of the epithelial cell nests, along with the absence of mitotic activity militate against a malignant interpretation.

This lesion, while uncommon, should be considered in the differential diagnosis of posterior jaw radiolucencies in the adult, especially if there are foci of radiopacity within the lesion. The clinical course is usually that of slow growth and

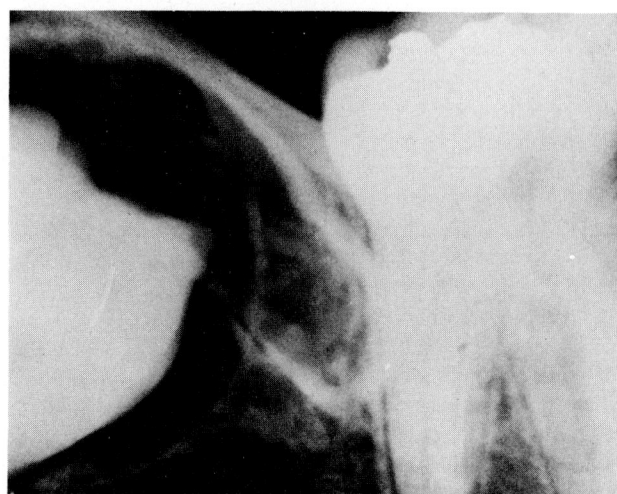

Figure XXVII-2-1. Calcifying epithelial odontogenic tumor with impacted third molar tooth.

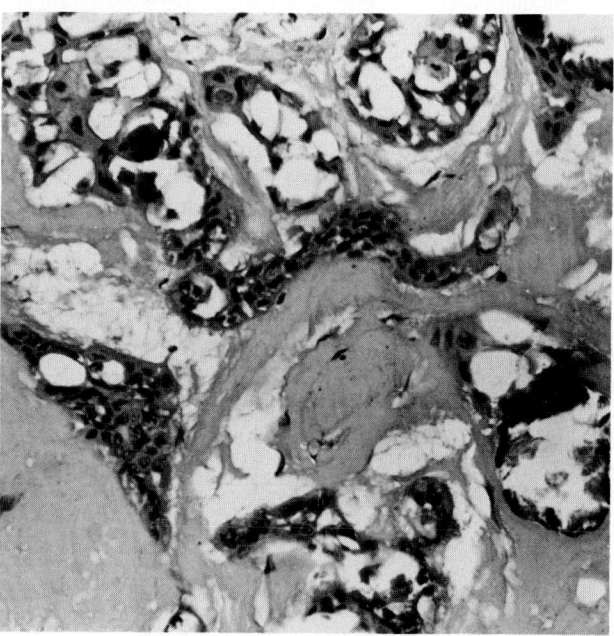

Figure XXVII-2-2. Microscopic appearance of calcifying epithelial odontogenic tumor showing clusters of epithelial cells, calcifications, and amyloid material.

uncommon recurrence, but radiographic evidence of poorly circumscribed borders should suggest the need for removal of bone to insure tumor-free margins.

Calcifying Odontogenic Cyst (C.O.C.). This term is applied to a heterogeneous group of lesions which have in common the histologic finding of ghost-cell keratinization.[22] Many lesions histologically designated as C.O.C. (or Gorlin cyst) are probably best viewed as simple odontogenic cysts which happen to contain ghost cells, as nothing about that alteration *per se* seems to predispose to altered biologic behavior. Often the lesions demonstrate radiopaque foci, and this usually designates a moderately well-differentiated odontogenic lesion. Many C.O.C.'s are associated with either impacted teeth or odontomas.

Histologically, ghost cells are squamous epithelial cells which lose their nuclei as they keratinize, leaving empty space in the cytoplasm where the nuclei had been. Frequently, foci of keratinizing cells escape into the connective tissue, whereupon a foreign-body reaction with inflammation and giant cells supervenes. Calcium may deposit in the foci of keratinization, but no tooth-related matrix is generally produced. In one rare variant form, designated the Type II ghost cell lesion, a tumor-like proliferation of epithelium with ghost cells is noted, along with production (perhaps by mesenchyme) of an osteoid or dentin-like extracellular substance.

The clinical course of most ghost-cell lesions is similar to that of a dentigerous cyst, with relatively easy removal and a low frequency of recurrence. A few of the rare variants may behave more aggressively.

Ameloblastoma. This immature benign odontogenic lesion replicates the histologic appearance of the early enamel organ, with palisaded, polarized ameloblast-like cells at the border between epithelium and connective tissue, and stellate reticulum-like cells centrally.[24,35,37] No extracellular product is produced.

The typical clinical presentation is that of a slowly growing, radiolucent, destructive lesion in the mandibular molar-ramus region of a young adult (over 50% are first discovered between the ages of 20 and 40 years).[2,18,24] The radiolucency usually has well-circumscribed borders. Early lesions usually appear unilocular,[30] (Figure XXVII-2-3) while established ones are generally multilocular (Figures XXVII-2-4 and XXVII-2-5). Calcifications within the lesion are never found. Approximately 20% of ameloblastomas appear in the dentigerous relationship to unerupted teeth, and these usually are noted before the age of 30. Some ameloblastoma-like lesions may arise from cyst lining[23,32] and proliferate entirely *within* the cyst lumen; if there is no invasive component, such lesions are termed, unicystic ameloblastoma, and probably behave as cysts, with little potential for recurrence. "Mural" ameloblastomas are those which arise in cyst linings and proliferate

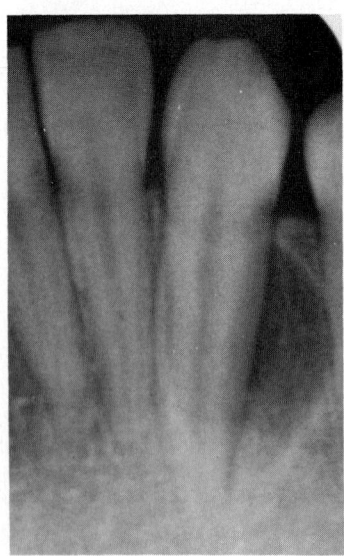

Figure XXVII-2-3.   Unilocular ameloblastoma between mandibular cuspid and bicuspid teeth.

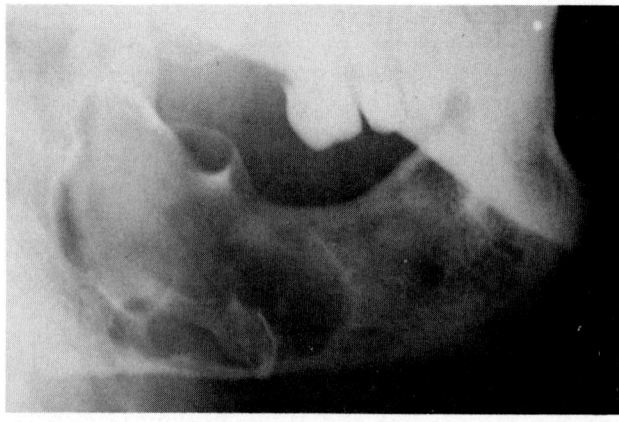

Figure XXVII-2-4.   Large cystic ameloblastoma in posterior mandible.

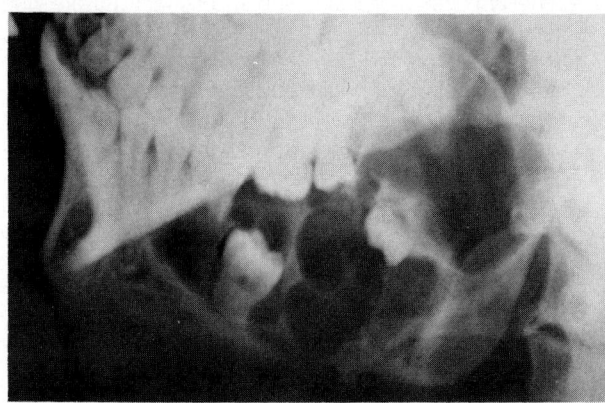

Figure XXVII-2-5.   Large multilocular ameloblastoma of mandible with two impacted teeth. The entire body and ramus of the mandible are involved.

away from the cyst lumen, invading bone; these lesions behave as conventional ameloblastomas, with a high recurrence potential.

Microscopically, in ameloblastoma one sees proliferating epithelial islands and strands, a mature collagenous stroma, and an invasive pattern of growth (Figure XXVII-2-6). The identification of mature collagen fibers in the stroma is very important for distinguishing the ameloblastoma from ameloblastic fibroma, a mixed odontogenic tumor. The tumor cells exhibit both palisading (alignment of the cell nuclei at one level in the cells) and polarization (migration of the nuclei to one end of the cell). Of great importance, also, is the nature of the polarization; in ameloblasts, secretion of matrix occurs toward connective tissue, with the nuclei polarized *away* from connective tissue, an orientation which is almost unique to this cell type. Little or no inductive effect occurs in ameloblastoma, so we see no mesenchymal differentiation, and no matrix production by the tumor cells. (In *normal* tooth formation we do not speak of "ameloblast" until actual enamel matrix formation is initiated; columnar cells with palisaded, polarized nuclei which are not yet producing matrix are most properly called "preameloblasts.")

Histologic patterns of ameloblastoma have led to classification of subgroups such as acanthomatous ameloblastoma[3]

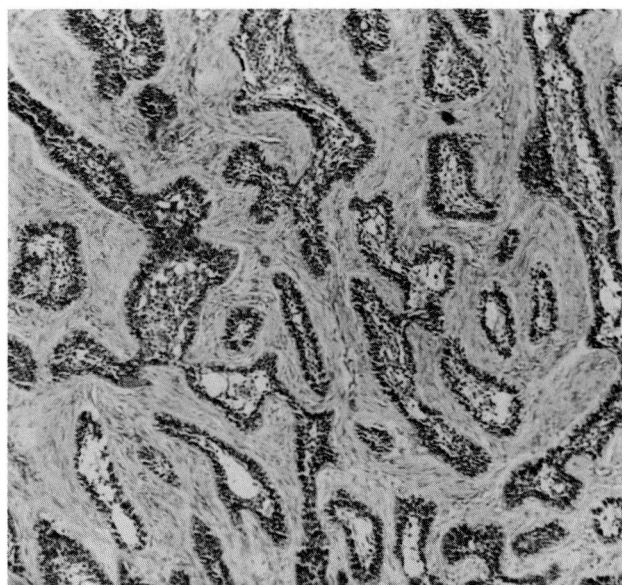

Figure XXVII-2-6. Microscopic appearance of ameloblastoma showing cords and nests of ameloblastic cells with a central stellate reticulum. The ameloblastic structures are surrounded by a fibrous connective tissue matrix.

with development of keratin-like substance within the epithelial islands or plexiform ameloblastoma,[13] with an extensive network of strands with a loose inner reticulum. These histologic variants do not appear to relate to different clinical behavior of the lesions.

The stellate reticulum within the nests and cords of columnar epithelium tends to undergo degeneration, forming microscopic cysts, (Figure XXVII-2-7).[20] The microcysts then expand to form large cystic spaces within the tumor and give the ameloblastoma its multicystic gross and radiologic appearance (Figure XXVII-2-8). No calcifications are found in ameloblastomas, not even dystrophic calcification.

Ameloblastoma is a slowly growing lesion (mitoses are hardly ever seen), but, unlike its better-differentiated epithelial relatives, it displays a marked propensity for invasive growth, spreading between trabeculae of medullary bone for a moderate distance beyond its apparent radiographic or surgical margins. Seldom, however, does the tumor penetrate the cortical plate of bone, although expansion of bony cortex is sometimes seen in longstanding lesions.

The clinical behavior of the tumor relates mainly to the difficulty at surgery of establishing tumor-free margins; recurrence is predictable unless 1–2 cm of clinically uninvolved bone is resected in addition to that which is obviously infiltrated by tumor. Curettage is inadequate treatment; recommended approaches involve en bloc excision, usually with preservation of the inferior border of the mandible. Maxillary lesions, although less frequently encountered,[5,36] are more dangerous than mandibular ones, due to the tendency for the lesion to spread more extensively in the more porous maxillary bone and the possibility of the involvement of the cranial base. Patients who have been treated for ameloblastoma should be followed carefully with radiographs, in order to recognize recurrence early.

Craniopharyngioma is a tumor which occurs within the

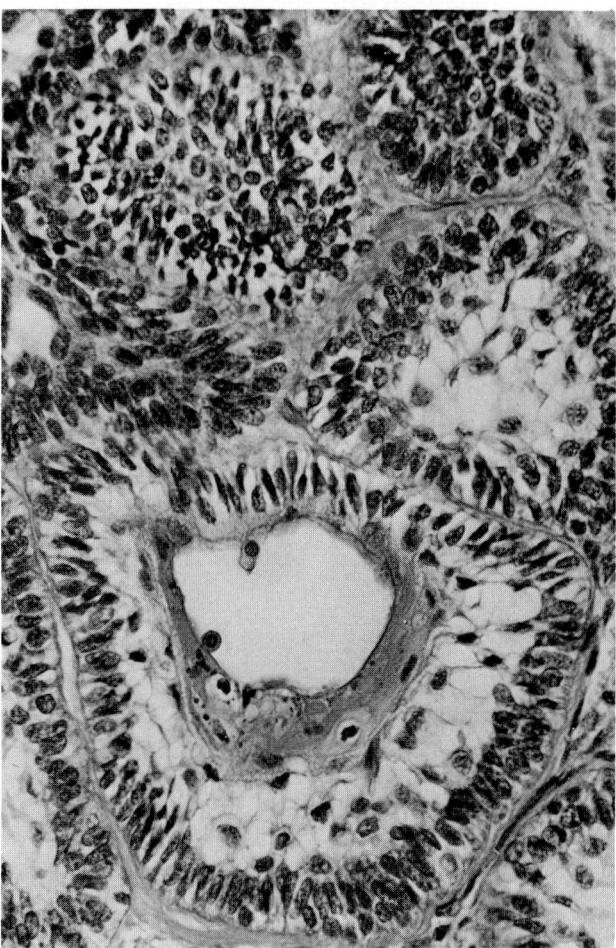

Figure XXVII-2-7. High power view showing crystic degeneration of stellate reticulum. The ameloblastic cells are columnar.

skull, in the region around the pituitary gland, and which is said to arise from remnants of the stomadeal ectoderm that invaginates to form Rathke's pouch. Fusion of Rathke's pouch with a process of the forebrain produces the anterior and posterior pituitary in the adult. Although epithelial remnants of the craniopharyngeal duct are said to be quite common, craniopharyngioma develops infrequently, accounting for fewer than 5% of all C.N.S. tumors (see XXIV).[6]

Clinical features of craniopharyngioma relate to destruction of the pituitary (diabetes insipidus) or compression of nearby cranial nerves; radiographically a suprasellar mass, often with calcifications (75% of cases) is the usual finding. Although the most common presenting age is in the second and third decades, any age may be affected.

Microscopic findings are quite variable; lesions in children seem to be rather invasive, with epithelium in islands or sheets, often showing ghost cell keratinization, calcification, and foreign-body reactions similar to that which is seen in the C.O.C. (see above). Adult lesions may be more squamous in their morphology, without calcifications or necrosis. The resemblance of those lesions to ameloblastoma, although frequently cited, is usually not great.

Prognosis in craniopharyngioma must be guarded, since complete excision is difficult and damage to vital structures

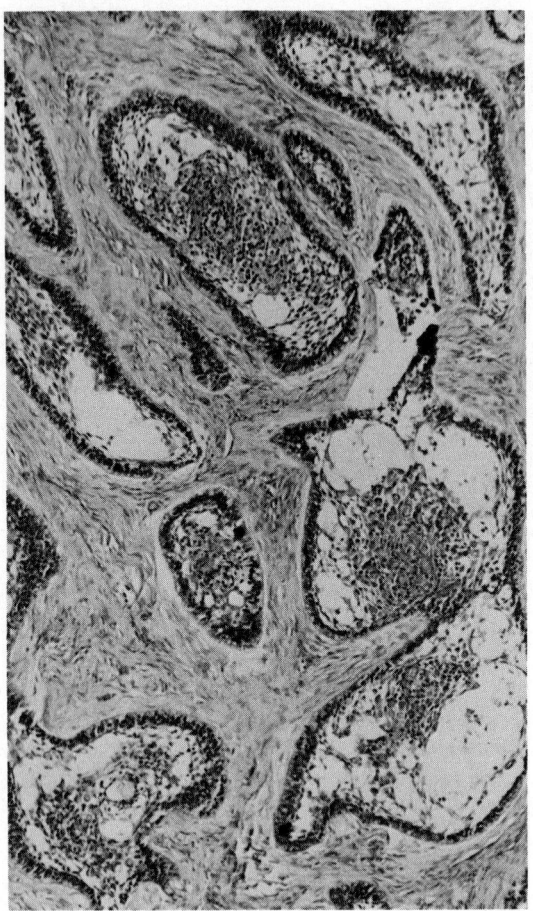

Figure XXVII-2-8. Cystic development within the islands of an ameloblastoma.

is a risk. Subtotal removal followed by radiation results in outcomes at least as favorable as treatment by total removal alone[38] and superior to surgery alone.[39]

Adamantinoma is a tumor of long bones with a striking predilection for occurrence in the tibial diaphysis (79% of reported cases).[26] Its name implies a relationship to enamel organ, given originally because odontogenic lesions are the only other primary tumors in which epithelial elements are seen to arise within bone. Although recent studies show that the cells in adamantinoma are probably, in fact, epithelial (the cells have desmosomes and produce keratin), there is no good explanation of the origin of the lesion. No enamel organ differentiation is found in these lesions, nor is toothy product produced.

The clinical course is quite variable, with some lesions behaving quite aggressively and sometimes metastasizing. Histologic features cannot be used to predict clinical behavior.

Mixed Odontogenic Lesions

Odontoma. This is a term applied to odontogenic proliferations in which enamel, dentin and pulp are present within the lesion; this represents terminally differentiated odontogenic tissue. Although toothy tissues are present, the structures formed are arranged either as collections of small,

morphologically atypical teeth ("compound" odontoma), or as a disorderly mass of dental tissues which lack recognizable tooth form altogether ("complex" odontoma).

The typical clinical presentation of odontoma is that of a well-circumscribed radiopacity, usually located either in the anterior maxilla (compound type) or posterior mandible (complex type), which may be associated with an unerupted tooth, but which is otherwise asymptomatic. An important finding is the presence of toothy structures, or a radiodensity indicative of the presence of enamel (Figure XXVII-2-9). Generally, a radiolucent rim is noted between the opaque area and the surrounding bone. The common presenting age is during the 2nd decade, but since the growth of the lesion is self-limiting, it may persist and be discovered during later life. In occasional cases, a dentigerous cyst may develop in association with an odontoma, and this would appear as a larger surrounding radiolucency.

Microscopically, one sees mixtures of odontogenic epithelium and mesenchyme, with recognizable enamel matrix, dentin, pulp and periodontal ligament. Two major subgroups of odontomas are recognized. In a *compound composite odontoma,* all dental tissues are present and are arranged in the form of numerous miniature teeth. In a *complex composite odontoma* the dental tissues are arranged in a hap-

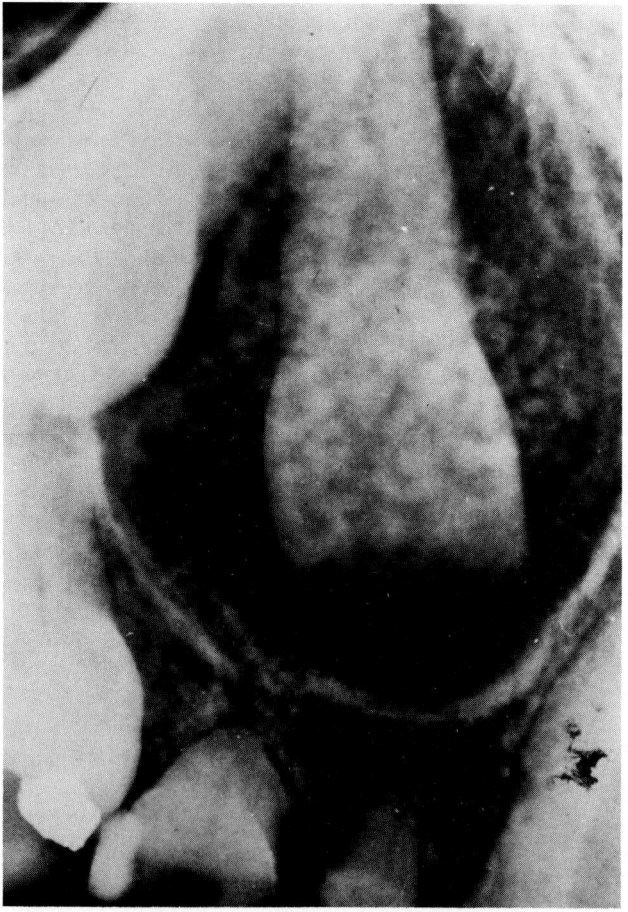

Figure XXVII-2-9. Radiograph of complex composite odontoma with impacted maxillary central incisor tooth. The calcified materials within the odontoma appear as opaque granules.

hazard pattern and do not resemble tooth-like structures (Figure XXVII-2-10). No proliferations of immature odontogenic tissues should be found in the uncomplicated odontoma; rare cases of ghost-cell lesion or ameloblastoma in association with odontomas have been reported, but these lesions' behavior is usually dominated by the epithelial proliferation and may be more aggressive.

The clinical behavior of odontomas is more in keeping with the view that they are developmental disorders of the odontogenic apparatus rather than true neoplasms. They are usually surgically removed so that normal alignment of teeth is not jeopardized by pressure of the odontoma. The surgical procedure is usually quite straightforward. Complications are rare, and recurrences are not expected.

Ameloblastic Fibro-odontoma. The name applied to an odontogenic lesion which exhibits mixed epithelial-mesenchymal proliferation and both mature and immature areas.[33] There has been a controversy as to whether, with the passage of time, such lesions would become completely mature odontomas. At present, the prevailing opinion is that at least some ameloblastic fibro-odontomas would never be expected to progress to maturity.

The usual clinical presentation of ameloblastic fibro-odontoma is somewhat similar to that described in connection with an odontoma developing in a dentigerous cyst; there is an expansile lesion which is mostly radiolucent and well-circumscribed, but which contains foci of radiopacity that may resemble teeth. Teenagers and young adults are most commonly affected.

The microscopic appearance is that of a combination of ameloblastic fibroma and odontoma, frequently with fairly well-formed teeth. Since tooth-like structures are frequently removed from soft tissues before histologic processing, the

diagnosis might be missed on the basis of the soft-tissue specimen alone.

Clinical behavior of this lesion seems to be similar to that of the ameloblastic fibroma. There are reported instances in which lesions have behaved rather aggressively following multiple attempted excisions and recurrences.

Ameloblastic Fibroma. An immature mixed odontogenic neoplasm within which is commonly observed a very slight inductive effect, but in which no extracellular matrix is elaborated.[33,40] The usual clinical presentation is that of a radiolucent, expansile lesion in the posterior mandible of a young person. The radiographic appearance is indistinguishable from ameloblastoma (no calcified foci are present), but the lesion occurs usually in children or teenagers rather than in adults. A dentigerous relationship to an unerupted tooth seems to be relatively uncommon, but the lesion may present as if it were a primordial cyst (a radiolucency replacing a tooth).

Microscopically, the lesion exhibits proliferating odontogenic epithelium which may resemble dental lamina (cords of cuboidal cells) or enamel organ (like ameloblastoma). In addition, there is invariably a substantial amount of immature mesenchymal tissue, consisting of spindle shaped or stellate fibroblastic cells which are widely separated by myxoid-appearing extracellular material. No mature collagen fibers are seen. The mesenchymal tissue resembles dental papilla, and a hyalinized basement membrane-like product is frequently observed at the interface between mesenchyme and epithelium ("inductive" effect). No calcified material is present. Mitotic activity should be absent.

The expected clinical course is that of a slowly growing noninvasive lesion; although the ameloblastic fibroma may become quite large, and produce substantial clinical deformity, it is usually easily excised. Recurrence may occur if tumor is left behind, however, and there are reports of lesions which seemed to have evolved into mesenchymal malignancies when subjected to multiple incomplete surgical attempts. Hypercellularity and mitotic activity among the mesenchymal components are worrisome pathologic findings in this regard. Probably a valid approach to the ameloblastic fibroma involves an initial attempt at conservative removal by curettage; those lesions which recur should probably be treated at the second attempt by a more aggressive, *en bloc* type excision. Radiation treatment would seem to be contraindicated, as in most benign conditions.

Mesenchymal Odontogenic Lesions

Odontogenic Fibroma. This name is applied to lesions of the jaws which behave as though they are neoplastic, and which show a propensity for production of extracellular mesenchymal matrix substances that are associated with periodontal ligament.

The clinical presentation is of an expansile central lesion which begins as a radiolucency,[12] but which develops progressive diffuse radioopacity with the passage of time. The molar region of the mandible is the most common site, and the lesion usually appears spherical, displacing the cortical plate of bone as it expands, but without penetration or periosteal reactive bone formation. No connection with tooth roots is generally observed, nor is there pain. A radiolucent

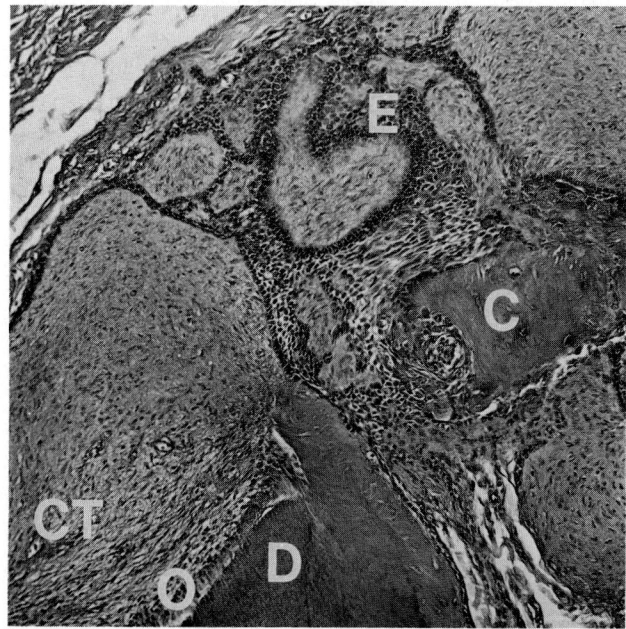

Figure XXVII-2-10. Microscopic features of complex composite odontoma showing cementum (C), dentin (D), ameloblastic epithelium (E), and connective tissue (CT) resembling dental pulp and differentiating into odontoblasts (O).

rim separates the lesion from surrounding bone. Young adults are most commonly affected.[9]

Microscopically, the lesion consists of mature fibroblastic elements, with varying amounts of collagen, osteoid or cementum in a manner reminiscent of periodontal ligament (Figure XXVII-2-11). "Cementifying fibroma" or "cemento-ossifying fibroma" are names which have been applied to these lesions, according to the amount and types of product observed, but distinctions of this sort have little, if any, clinical relevance. Just as epithelial nests may be observed in periodontal ligament, some odontogenic fibromas possess epithelial elements; these are most frequently sparsely distributed, rudimentary epithelial nests, without apparent inductive influence.

The expected clinical behavior is that of a slow-growing benign neoplasm. Excision is usually relatively easy and recurrence is uncommon. Lesions which present as described here seem to have little malignant potential.

Peripheral Odontogenic Fibroma. A lesion of gingival soft tissue which may resemble the central lesion histologically, but which usually behaves as a self-limiting reactive nodule. The presence of odontogenic epithelial nests and/or calcified product has led to the suggestion that these might be neoplasms of odontogenic tissues, but in the absence of unlimited growth potential, this hypothesis is hard to support. Epithelial nests are common in gingiva (dental lamina rests of Serres), and gingival fibroblasts seem to readily express potential for calcified matrix production; although the occasional true neoplasm of gingival mesenchyme probably does occur, the vast majority of gingival "fibromas" are unlikely to be neoplastic.

Cementoblastoma. A distinctive odontogenic lesion which is always attached to the root of a tooth, and which exhibits robust cementum production. The usual clinical presentation

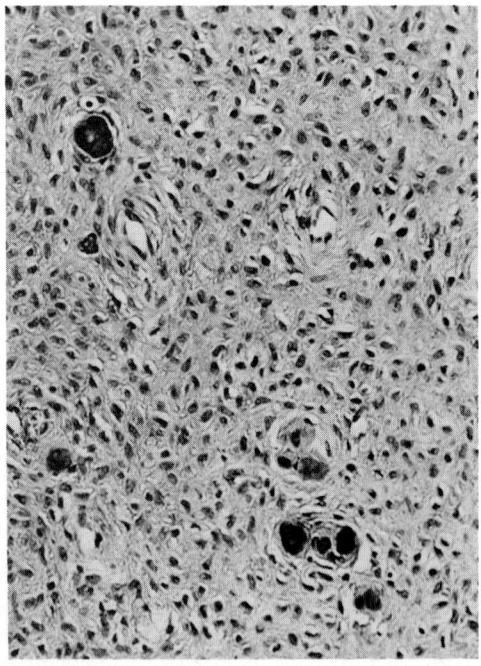

Figure XXVII-2-11. Microscopic appearance of odontogenic fibroma with some cementum forming.

is associated with pain and tenderness in a mandibular posterior tooth of a teenager or young adult. Radiographically there is a radiolucency with localized disruption of the periodontal ligament space and lamina dura, usually involving a single root. The tooth possesses a vital pulp (confusion with periapical cyst or granuloma may occur if the tooth happens to be carious, but the cemental lesion, *per se,* is not associated with pulpal pathosis). As the lesion enlarges, radioopacity develops, first in the central portions, and, in the well developed lesion, the opacity is connected to the cementum of the root, with a peripheral radiolucent rim.

The microscopic appearance may be somewhat alarming, with large numbers of hyperchromatic, basophilic cells depositing cementum matrix, which may resemble osteoid in some cases. Actual cellular atypia is absent, and if the clinical information is available the microscopic interpretation is not too difficult. Mitotic activity is not prominent.

The clinical course is of unlimited expansile growth; if the tooth is extracted without curettage of the lesion, the cementoblastoma continues to grow. In times past, the affected tooth was always sacrificed; recently there have been reports of attempts to treat the lesion via apicoectomy, with salvage of the tooth and later endodontic therapy. Malignant transformation is not reported.

Osteoblastoma and Osteoid Osteoma. These are lesions of bone with a histologic resemblance to one another, and to cementoblastoma. They are not associated with the roots of teeth, and they occur in bone generally, not being confined to occurrence within the jaws. These lesions are best considered as benign tumors of bone, and so will not be further treated here (see XXXV-1).

Cementoma. A term used with respect to a cemental lesion which is probably not neoplastic, but which is of great clinical importance. Cementoblastoma is sometimes called "true cementoma" to distinguish it from this other condition, which would be better termed *periapical cemental dysplasia.* The clinical presentation of periapical cemental dysplasia is that of asymptomatic periapical radiolucencies involving, usually, mandibular anterior teeth. The patients are frequently young adult black females. The teeth possess vital pulps. The lesion(s) may be single or multiple, and the lesion evolves radiographically in a predictable fashion: the radiolucencies may be observed to enlarge to a certain size, after which the lesions stop growing and begin to opacify. Finally, the lesions opacify completely, and seem to become confluent with the tooth and the surrounding bone (Figure XXVII-2-12). If there is no clinical intervention, no adverse sequelae result.

The microscopic appearance varies depending upon the stage at which biopsy is performed, but the lesion is indistinguishable from fibro-osseous lesions or odontogenic fibroma.

The importance of the lesion lies in the fact that needless extraction or endodontic therapy may be carried out if the lesion is not recognized by the clinician. Periodic follow-up is the only management required.

Gigantiform Cementoma. Another lesion with a marked predilection for black females, and this is characterized by diffuse patchy radioopacities throughout the jaws. There is a histologic resemblance to other osteoid or cementum forming jaw lesions, but the true nature of the condition is still

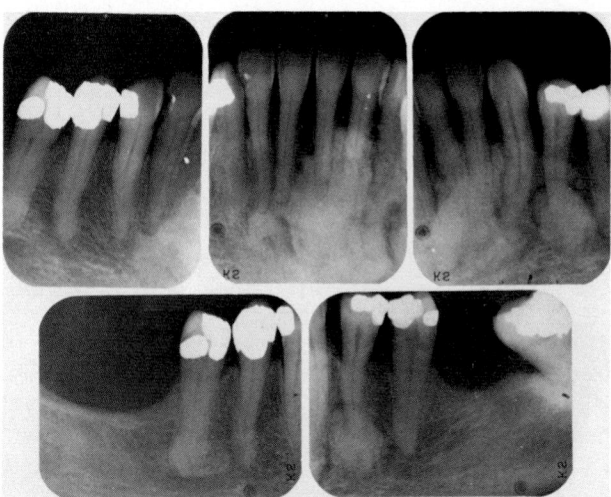

Figure XXVII-2-12. Multiple cementomas of the mandible at the apices of the teeth (periapical cemental dysplasia).

unknown. It seems unlikely to be a neoplastic disorder, but rather to represent a florid development of periapical cemental dysplasia. The relationship of the lesion to infection or other inflammatory influences has been postulated, but is unproven. Management is conservative, but the condition may be associated with pain, and the clinical problems may become complex. As with periapical cemental dysplasia, the diagnosis is usually made on clinical and radiographic grounds, and biopsy should be *avoided* whenever possible.

Myxoma. Myxoma refers to a proliferation of fibroblastic elements which do not produce mature extracellular product. Although soft-tissue myxomatous tumors have been reported throughout the body, myxomas of bone seem to occur only in the jaws, and are presumed, therefore, to arise from odontogenic tissues. The usual clinical presentation is that of an expansile, ill-defined radiolucency of the jaw in a young adult. Symptoms are variable, and growth is usually slow.

Myxoma is relatively invasive, and at surgery a gelatinous consistency may be noted. The microscopic appearance is that of bony replacement by a myxoid mass, without mature collagen formation. No giant cells, adipocytes or neurogenic elements should be noted. Mitoses should not be found. The tissue somewhat resembles dental papilla.

The clinical course is unpredictable, since complete excision by conservative approaches is often very difficult. Persistent destructive growth is frequently encountered, and wide margins may be required for definitive treatment. Although mitotic activity, hypercellularity, and more rapid growth may characterize some lesions, metastatic spread seems distinctly uncommon.

Malignant Odontogenic Tumors

The odontogenic tumors and tumor-like lesions are to be considered benign and managed as such. Malignant odontogenic tumors have been described but are *exceedingly* rare. They are either an ameloblastic sarcoma,[7,21] in which an ameloblastoma-like component is seen within a fibrosarcoma, or a carcinoma[34] arising from ameloblastic cells, either within an ameloblastoma, or de novo from ameloblastic cells

within the mandible. As in all malignant tumors, they are characterized microscopically by hypercellularity, pleomorphism, and abnormal and increased mitotic activity. Pain and paresthesia are clinical features of all malignant tumors of the jaws. The prognosis and management of ameloblastic sarcoma is similar to fibrosarcoma of the jaws. The carcinomas arising in the jaws are undifferentiated and aggressive with a poor prognosis.

Management

The treatment of odontogenic tumors is surgical, conservative, and based on proper microscopic and clinical evaluation.[14] The odontomas are well-circumscribed, non-infiltrative, and usually surrounded with a connective tissue membrane. They can be enucleated and the healing is uneventful. The ameloblastoma is an infiltrative tumor of bone and simple enucleation will not remove finger-like projections of tumor into medullary bone at the margins of the lesion. This explains the recurrence of ameloblastoma following incomplete surgical removal. A block-resection is favored, leaving the lower border of the mandible intact. The cortex is rarely infiltrated. The block-resection may involve the sacrifice of adjacent teeth.

Radiation therapy is not indicated for odontogenic tumors, although some recent reports have reconsidered the question, using current techniques.[4] The ameloblastoma is relatively resistent to radiation and the risks of radiation are unwarranted for the management of a benign lesion where access is relatively easy and total surgical removal can be effected without significant complications.

References

1. Abrams, A. M., Melrose, R. J., and Howell, F. J.: Adenoameloblastoma: A clinical pathological study of ten new cases. Cancer, 22:175, 1968.
2. Adekeye, E. O.: Ameloblastoma of the jaws: A survey of 109 Nigerian patients. J. Oral Surg., 38:36, 1980.
3. Anneroth, G., Heindahl, A., and Wersall, J.: Acanthomatous ameloblastoma. Int. J. Oral Surg., 9:231, 1980.
4. Atkinson, C. H., Harwood, A. R., and Cummings, B. J.: Ameloblastoma of the jaw: A reappraisal of the role of megavoltage irradiation. Cancer, 53:869, 1984.
5. Batsakis, J. G., and McClatchey, K. D.: Ameloblastoma of the maxilla and peripheral ameloblastoma. Ann. Otol. Rhinol. Laryngol., 92:532, 1983.
6. Bernstein, M., and Buchino, J.: The histologic similarity between craniopharyngioma and odontogenic lesions: A reappraisal. Oral Surg., 56:501, 1983.
7. Cataldo, E., Nathanson, N., and Shklar, G.: Ameloblastic sarcoma of the mandible. Oral Surg., 16:953, 1963.
8. Courtney, R. M., and Kerr, D. A.: The odontogenic adenomatoid tumor. Oral Surg., 39:424, 1975.
9. Dahl, E., Wolfson, S., and Haugen, J.: Central odontogenic fibroma. J. Oral Surg., 39:120, 1981.
10. Eversole, L. R., Tomich, C. E., and Cherrick, H. M.: Histogenesis of odontogenic tumors. Oral Surg., 32:569, 1971.
11. Franklin, C. D., and Pindborg, J. J.: The calcifying epithelial odontogenic tumor. Oral Surg., 42:753, 1976.
12. Gardner, D. G.: The central odontogenic fibroma: An attempt at clarification. Oral Surg., 50:425, 1980.
13. Gardner, D. G., and Corio, R. L.: Plexiform unicystic ameloblastoma: A variant of ameloblastoma with a low-recurrence rate after enucleation. Cancer, 53:1730, 1984.
14. Gardner, D. G., and Pecak, A. M. J.: The treatment of ameloblastoma based on pathologic and anatomic principles. Cancer, 46:2514, 1980.
15. Giansanti, J. S., Someren, A., and Waldron, C. A.: Odontogenic adenomatoid tumor (adenoameloblastoma). Oral Surg., 30:69, 1970.
16. Goldblatt, L. I., Brannon, R. B., and Ellis, G. L.: Squamous odontogenic tumor: Report of five cases and review of the literature. Oral Surg., 54:187, 1982.
17. Gorlin, R. J., Chaudhry, A. P., and Pindborg, J. J.: Odontogenic tumors, classification, histopathology and clinical behavior in man and domestic animals. Cancer, 14:73, 1961.
18. Kahn, M. A.: Ameloblastoma in young persons: A clinicopathologic analysis and etiologic investigation. Oral Surg., 67:706, 1989.
19. Krolls, S. O., and Pindborg, J. J.: Calcifying epithelial odontogenic tumor. A survey of 23 cases and discussion of histomorphologic variations. Arch. Pathol., 98:206, 1974.
20. Leider, A., Eversole, L., and Barkin, M.: Cystic ameloblastoma. Oral Surg., 60:624, 1985.
21. Leider, A. S., Nelson, J. F., and Trodahl, J. N.: Ameloblastic fibrosarcoma of the jaws. Oral Surg., 33:559, 1972.

22. McGowan, R. H., and Browne, R. M.: The calcifying odontogenic cyst: a problem of preoperative diagnosis. Br. J. Oral Surg., 20:203, 1982.
23. McMillan, M. D., and Smillie, A. C.: Ameloblastomas associated with dentigerous cysts. Oral Surg., 51:489, 1981.
24. Mehlisch, D. R., Dahlin, D. C., and Masson, J. K.: Ameloblastoma: A clinicopathologic report. J. Oral Surg., 30:9, 1972.
25. Minderjahn, A.: Incidence and clinical differentiation of odontogenic tumors. J. Maxillofac. Surg., 7:142, 1979.
26. Perez-Atayde, A., Kozakewich, H., and Vawter, G.: Adamantinoma of the tibia. Cancer, 55:1015, 1985.
27. Pindborg, J. J., Kramer, I. R. H., and Torloni, H.: Histologic typing of odontogenic tumors, jaw cysts, and allied lesions. International Histological Classification of Tumors, No. 5, Geneva, World Health Organization, 1971.
28. Pullon, P. A., Shafer, W. G., Elzay, R. P., Kerr, D. A., and Corio, R. L.: Squamous odontogenic tumor: Report of six cases of a previously undescribed lesion. Oral Surg., 40:616, 1975.
29. Regezi, J. A., Kerr, D. A., and Courtney, R. M.: Odontogenic tumors: an analysis of 706 cases. J. Oral Surg., 36:771, 1978.
30. Robinson, L., and Martinez, M. G.: Unicystic ameloblastoma. A prognostically distinct entity. Cancer, 40:2278, 1977.
31. Sadeghi, E. M., and Hopper, T. L.: Calcifying epithelial odontogenic tumor. J. Oral Surg., 40:225, 1982.
32. Shteyer, A., Lustmann, J., and Lewin-Epstein, J.: The mural ameloblastoma: Review of literature. J. Oral Surg., 36:866, 1978.
33. Slootweg, P. J.: An analysis of the interrelationship of the mixed odontogenic tumor—ameloblastic fibroma, ameloblastic fibro-odontoma, and the odontomas. Oral Surg., 51:266, 1981.
34. Slootweg, P. J., and Muller, H.: Malignant ameloblastoma or ameloblastic carcinoma. Oral Surg., 57:168, 1984.
35. Small, I. A., and Waldron, C. A.: Ameloblastomas of the jaws. Oral Surg., 8:281, 1955.
36. Tsaknis, P. J., and Nelson, J. F.: The maxillary ameloblastoma: An analysis of 24 cases. J. Oral Surg., 38:336, 1980.
37. Waldron, C., and El-Mofty, S.: A histopathologic study of 116 ameloblastomas with special reference to the desmoplastic variant. Oral Surg., 63:441, 1987.
38. Weiss, M., Sutton, L., Marcial, V., Fowble, B., Packer, R., Zimmerman, R., Shut, L., Bruce, D., and D'Angio, G.: The role of radiation therapy in the management of childhood craniopharyngioma. Int. J. Radiat. Oncol. Biology Phys., 17:1313, 1989.
39. Wen, B. C., Hussey, D. H., Staples, J., Hitchon, P. W., Jani, S. K., Vigliotti, A. P., and Doornbos, J. F.: A comparison of the roles of surgery and radiation therapy in the management of craniopharyngiomas. Int. J. Radiat. Oncol. Biol. Phys., 16:17, 1989.
40. Zallen, R. D., Preskar, M. H., and McClary, S. A.: Ameloblastic fibroma. J. Oral Surg., 40:513, 1982.

Index

Page numbers followed by the letter "t" refer to tables; page numbers in *italic* refer to illustrations.